Casarett and Doull's
TOXICOLOGY

The Basic Science of Poisons

> What is there that is not poison?
>
> All things are poison and nothing (is)
>
> without poison. Solely the dose
>
> determines that a thing is not a poison.
>
> *Paracelsus (1493–1541)*

Casarett and Doull's
TOXICOLOGY

The Basic Science of Poisons

Eighth Edition

editor

Curtis D. Klaassen, PhD
University Distinguished Professor
Division of Gastroenterology
Department of Internal Medicine
College of Medicine
University of Kansas
Kansas City, Kansas

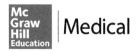 **Medical**

New York Chicago San Francisco Lisbon London Madrid Mexico City
Milan New Delhi San Juan Seoul Singapore Sydney Toronto

ett and Doull's Toxicology
e Basic Science of Poisons, Eighth Edition

4 5 6 7 8 9 QVS/QVS 21 20 19 18 17

Set ISBN 978-0-07-176923-5
Set MHID 0-07-176923-4

Book ISBN 978-0-07-176925-9
Book MHID 0-07-176925-0

DVD ISBN 978-0-07-176924-2
DVD MHID 0-07-176924-2

This book was set in Times by Thomson Digital.
The editors were James F. Shanahan and Christie Naglieri.
The production supervisor was Sherri Souffrance.
Project management was provided by Charu Bansal, Thomson Digital.
The designer was Janice Bielawa; the cover designer was LaShae V. Ortiz.
Quad/Graphics was printer and binder.

Library of Congress Cataloging-in-Publication Data

Casarett and Doull's toxicology : the basic science of poisons / editor, Curtis D. Klaassen. — 8th ed.
    p. ; cm.
  Toxicology
  Includes bibliographical references and index.
  ISBN 978-0-07-176923-5 (hard cover : alk. paper) — ISBN 0-07-176923-4
  I. Klaassen, Curtis D. II. Casarett, Louis J. III. Doull, John, 1923- IV. Title: Toxicology.
  [DNLM: 1. Poisoning—physiopathology. 2. Poisons. 3. Toxicology—methods. QV 600]
  615.9—dc23

                                                                    2012024293

McGraw-Hill Education books are available at special quantity discounts to use as premiums and sales promotions, or for use in corporate training programs. To contact a representative please e-mail us at bulksales@mcgraw-hill.com.

Dedication

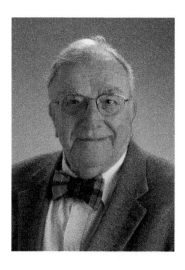

This edition of *Casarett & Doull's Toxicology the Basic Science of Poisons* is dedicated to John Doull, M.D., Ph.D., the co-founder and co-editor of the first editions of this textbook, for his many contributions to the discipline of toxicology. Dr. Doull was born in Baker, Montana, on September 13, 1922, recently celebrating his 90th birthday. He obtained a B.A. with a chemistry major from Montana State College in 1944. John spent 2 years in the Navy during WWII, before attending graduate school at the University of Chicago, an outstanding center of toxicology research and education. There he was mentored by two prominent researchers in the history of toxicology, E. M. K. Geiling and Kenneth DuBois. John received his Ph.D. in 1950 and M.D. in 1953, followed by an appointment as Assistant Professor and then Associate Professor at the University of Chicago.

After 2 decades in Chicago, John became Professor of Pharmacology and Toxicology at the University of Kansas Medical School in Kansas City, Kansas, in 1967. Dr. Doull initiated the toxicology research and education programs in the Department of Pharmacology and Toxicology. Within his first year at KU Medical School, John and his colleague, Dan Azarnoff, M.D., obtained an NIH Center grant, which provided faculty salaries, scientific equipment and supplies, as well as research space for the toxicology program. During the next 4 decades, John saw the toxicology program flourish with the receipt of a NIEHS Toxicology Training grant, a NIH COBRE grant, the hiring of more than 20 faculty, and the training of more than 200 graduate and postdoctoral students in toxicology.

Dr. Doull was also active in toxicology at the national level. He has been a charter member of the Society of Toxicology since its establishment in 1961. He served on numerous SOT committees including president of the Society from 1986 to 1987. John was also a member of 20 committees of the National Academy of Science, and was chair of 7 of those committees. In addition, he served on 10 committees for the Environmental Protection Agency, as well as committees for the National Toxicology Program, and the Food and Drug Administration. For the National Institute of Health, John was a member of the Toxicology Study Section (1965–70) and NIEHS Council (1975–80), the National Institute of Occupational Health and Safety, Chairman of the TLV Committee of the American Conference of Governmental Industrial Hygienists (1989–97), the Toxicology Forum, and others too numerous to list.

In addition to these numerous contributions to the discipline of toxicology, it is probably the co-founding of this textbook that has had and will have the greatest impact in elevating the discipline of toxicology. This textbook helps to define the discipline of toxicology and has been used in educating toxicologists for almost 40 years.

Contents

Contributors

S. Satheesh Anand, PhD, DABT
Senior Research Toxicologist
Haskell Global Centers for Health and Environmental Sciences
Newark, Delaware
Chapter 24

Michael Aschner, PhD
Professor
Department of Pediatrics
Vanderbilt University Medical Center
Nashville, Tennessee
Chapter 16

Thomas M. Badger, PhD
Distinguished Faculty Scholar
Professor
Departments of Pediatrics and Physiology/Biophysics
University of Arkansas for Medical Sciences
Director
Arkansas Children's Nutrition Center
Little Rock, Arkansas
Chapter 27

John C. Bloom, VMD, PhD
President
Bloom Consulting Services, LLC
Special Government Employee
FDA
Adjunct Professor of Pathology
Schools of Veterinary Medicine
University of Pennsylvania and Purdue University
Indianapolis, Indiana
Chapter 11

Windy A. Boyd, PhD
Biologist
Biomolecular Screening Branch
National Toxicology Program Division
National Institute of Environmental Health Sciences, NIH
Research Triangle Park, North Carolina
Chapter 23

William K. Boyes, PhD
Neurotoxicology Branch
Toxicity Assessment Division
National Health and Environmental Effects Research Laboratory
Office of Research and Development
US Environmental Protection Agency
Research Triangle Park, North Carolina
Chapter 17

John T. Brandt, MD
Eli Lilly & Co. (retired)
Indianapolis, Indiana
Chapter 11

James V. Bruckner, PhD
Professor of Pharmacology & Toxicology
Department of Pharmaceutical & Biomedical Sciences
College of Pharmacy
University of Georgia
Athens, Georgia
Chapter 24

David B. Buckley, PhD
Chief Scientific Officer
XenoTech, LLC
Lenexa, Kansas
Chapter 6

George A. Burdock, PhD, DABT, FACN
President
Burdock Group Consultants
Orlando, Florida
Chapter 31

Louis R. Cantilena Jr., MD, PhD
Professor, Medicine and Pharmacology
Department of Medicine
Uniformed Services University
Bethesda, Maryland
Chapter 33

Daniel L. Costa, PhD
Office of Research and Development
National Program Director for Air, Climate, and Energy
     Research Program
US Environmental Protection Agency
Research Triangle Park, North Carolina
Chapter 29

Lucio G. Costa, PhD
Professor
Department of Environmental and Occupational Health Sciences
School of Public Health
University of Washington
Seattle, Washington
Chapter 22

Maciej Czerwinski, PhD
Principal Scientist
XenoTech, LLC
Lenexa, Kansas
Chapter 6

Richard T. Di Giulio, PhD
Professor
Nicholas School of the Environmental
Duke University
Durham, North Carolina
Chapter 30

David L. Eaton, PhD
Professor
Department of Environmental and Occupational Health Sciences
Associate Vice Provost for Research
University of Washington
Seattle, Washington
Chapter 2

Elaine M. Faustman, PhD
Professor
Institute for Risk Analysis and Risk Communication
Department of Environmental and Occupational Health Sciences
School of Public Health
University of Washington
Seattle, Washington
Chapter 4

Jodi A. Flaws, PhD
Professor
Department of Comparative Biosciences
University of Illinois
Urbana, Illinois
Chapter 21

Paul M.D. Foster, PhD
Chief
Toxicology Branch
Division of the National Toxicology Program
National Institute of Environmental Health Sciences
Research Triangle Park, North Carolina
Chapter 20

Donald A. Fox, PhD
Professor of Vision Sciences
Biology and Biochemistry, Pharmacology, and Health and
     Human Performance
University of Houston
Houston, Texas
Chapter 17

Jonathan H. Freedman, PhD
Laboratory of Toxicology and Pharmacology
National Institute of Environmental Health Sciences
Research Triangle Park, North Carolina
Chapter 23

Michael A. Gallo, PhD
Environmental and Occupational Health Sciences Institute
Rutgers-The State University of New Jersey
UMDNJ-Robert Wood Johnson Medical School
Piscataway, New Jersey
Chapter 1

Steven G. Gilbert, PhD
Director
Institute of Neurotoxicology & Neurological Disorders
Seattle, Washington
Chapter 2

Bruce A. Goldberger, PhD
Professor and Director of Toxicology
Departments of Pathology and Psychiatry
University of Florida College of Medicine
Gainesville, Florida
Chapter 32

Terry Gordon, PhD
Professor
Department of Environmental Medicine
NYU School of Medicine
Tuxedo, New York
Chapter 29

L. Earl Gray Jr., PhD
Reproductive Toxicology Branch
United States Environmental Protection Agency
Adjunct Professor
North Carolina State University
Raleigh, North Carolina
Chapter 20

Zoltán Gregus, MD, PhD, DSc, DABT
Professor
Department of Pharmacology and Therapeutics
Toxicology Section
University of Pecs
Medical School
Pecs, Hungary
Chapter 3

David G. Hoel, PhD
Principal Scientist
Exponent, Inc
Alexandria, Virginia
Distinguished University Professor
Department of Medicine
Medical University of South Carolina
Charleston, South Carolina
Chapter 25

George R. Hoffmann, PhD
Professor
Department of Biology
College of the Holy Cross
Worcester, Massachusetts
Chapter 9

Michael P. Holsapple, PhD, ATS
Senior Research Leader
Systems Toxicology
Health and Life Sciences Global Business
Battelle Memorial Institute
Columbus, Ohio
Chapter 12

Patricia B. Hoyer, PhD
Professor
Department of Physiology
College of Medicine
The University of Arizona
Tucson, Arizona
Chapter 21

Robert H. Hurt, PhD
Professor
School of Engineering
Director
Institute for Molecular and Nanoscale Innovation
Brown University
Providence, Rhode Island
Chapter 28

Hartmut Jaeschke, PhD, ATS
Professor and Chair
Department of Pharmacology, Toxicology & Therapeutics
University of Kansas Medical Center
Kansas City, Kansas
Chapter 13

Norbert E. Kaminski, PhD
Professor
Department of Pharmacotherapy and Toxicology
Director
Center for Integrative Toxicology
Michigan State University
East Lansing, Michigan
Chapter 12

Agnes B. Kane, MD, PhD
Professor
Department of Pathology and Laboratory Medicine
Brown University
Providence, Rhode Island
Chapter 28

Y. James Kang, DVM, PhD, FATS
Professor and Distinguished University Scholar
Department of Pharmacology and Toxicology
University of Louisville School of Medicine
Louisville, Kentucky
Chapter 18

Barbara L.F. Kaplan, PhD
Assistant Professor
Center for Integrative Toxicology
Department of Pharmacology and Toxicology and Neuroscience
    Program
Michigan State University
East Lansing, Michigan
Chapter 12

Faraz Kazmi, BS
Senior Scientist
XenoTech, LLC
Lenexa, Kansas
Chapter 6

Rebecca D. Klaper, PhD
School of Freshwater Sciences
University of Wisconsin-Milwaukee
Milwaukee, Wisconsin
Chapter 28

James E. Klaunig, PhD, ATS, IATP
Professor
Environmental Health
Indiana University
Bloomington, Indiana
Chapter 8

Frank N. Kotsonis, PhD
Retired Corporate Vice President
Worldwide Regulatory Sciences
Monsanto Corporation
Skokie, Illinois
Chapter 31

Lois D. Lehman-McKeeman, PhD
Distinguished Research Fellow
Discovery Toxicology
Bristol-Myers Squibb Company
Princeton, New Jersey
Chapter 5

George D. Leikauf, PhD
Professor
Department of Environmental and Occupational Health
Graduate School of Public Health
University of Pittsburgh
Pittsburgh, Pennsylvania
Chapter 15

Gary E. Marchant, PhD, JD
Regents Professor and Faculty Director
Center for Law, Science & Innovation
Sandra Day O'Connor College of Law
Arizona State University
Tempe, Arizona
Chapter 35

Theodora M. Mauro, MD
Professor and Vice-Chair
Dermatology Department
University of California, San Francisco
Service Chief
Dermatology
San Francisco Veterans Medical Center
San Francisco, California
Chapter 19

Virginia C. Moser, PhD, DABT, FATS
Toxicologist
Toxicity Assessment Division
National Health and Environmental Effects Research Laboratory
US Environmental Protection Agency
Research Triangle Park, North Carolina
Chapter 16

Michael C. Newman, MS, PhD
A. Marshall Acuff Jr. Professor
Virginia Institute of Marine Science
College of William & Mary
Gloucester Point, Virginia
Chapter 30

Gunter Oberdörster, DVM, PhD
Professor
Department of Environmental Medicine
University of Rochester
School of Medicine & Dentistry
Rochester, New York
Chapter 28

Brian W. Ogilvie, BA
Principal Scientist
XenoTech, LLC
Lenexa, Kansas
Chapter 6

Gilbert S. Omenn, MD, PhD
Professor of Internal Medicine, Human Genetics and Public
    Health
Director
Center for Computational Medicine and Bioinformatics
University of Michigan Department of Computational Medicine
    and Bioinforamatics
Ann Arbor, Michigan
Chapter 4

Oliver Parkinson, PhD
XPD Consulting, LLC
Shawnee, Kansas
Chapter 6

Andrew Parkinson, PhD
CEO
XPD Consulting, LLC
Shawnee, Kansas
Chapter 6

Martin A. Philbert, PhD
Professor of Toxicology and Dean
School of Public Health
University of Michigan
Ann Arbor, Michigan
Chapter 16

R. Julian Preston, MA, PhD
Associate Director for Health
National Health and Environmental Effects Research Laboratory
US Environmental Protection Agency
Research Triangle Park, North Carolina
Chapter 9

Robert H. Rice, PhD
Professor
Department of Environmental Toxicology
University of California
Davis, California
Chapter 19

Rudy J. Richardson, ScD, DABT
Toxicology Program
University of Michigan School of Public Health
Neurology Department
University of Michigan School of Medicine
Ann Arbor, Michigan
Chapter 16

John M. Rogers, PhD
Toxicity Assessment Division
National Health and Environmental Effects Research Laboratory
Office of Research and Development
United States Environmental Protection Agency
Research Triangle Park, North Carolina
Chapter 10

Martin J. Ronis, BA, MA, Nat Sci Cantab, PhD
Professor
Department of Pharmacology & Toxicology
College of Medicine
University of Arkansas for Medical Sciences
Associate Director for Basic Research
Arkansas Children's Nutrition Center
Arkansas Children's Hospital Research Institute
Little Rock, Arkansas
Chapter 27

Andrew E. Schade, MD, PhD
Senior Director
Clinical Diagnostics Laboratory
Diagnostics Research and Development
Eli Lilly and Co.
Indianapolis, Indiana
Chapter 11

Rick G. Schnellmann, PhD
Professor and Chair
Department of Pharmaceutical and Biomedical Sciences
Medical University of South Carolina
Charleston, South Carolina
Chapter 14

Kartik Shankar, PhD, DABT
Arkansas Children's Nutrition Center
Department of Pediatrics
University of Arkansas for Medical Sciences
Little Rock, Arkansas
Chapter 27

Danny D. Shen, PhD
Professor
Departments of Pharmaceuticals and Pharmacy
School of Pharmacy
University of Washington
Seattle, Washington
Chapter 7

Courtney E.W. Sulentic, PhD
Associate Professor
Department of Pharmacology & Toxicology
Boonshoft School of Medicine
Wright State University
Dayton, Ohio
Chapter 12

Peter S. Thorne, MS, PhD
Professor and Head
Department of Occupational and Environmental Health
College of Public Health
The University of Iowa
Iowa City, Iowa
Chapter 34

Erik J. Tokar, PhD
Biologist
Inorganic Toxicology Group
Division of the National Toxicology Program
National Toxicology Program
National Institute of Environmental Health Sciences
Research Triangle Park, North Carolina
Chapter 23

Michael P. Waalkes, PhD
Chief
National Toxicology Group
Division of the National Toxicology Program
National Toxicology Program
National Institute of Environmental Health Sciences
Research Triangle Park, North Carolina
Chapter 23

D. Alan Warren, MPh, PhD
Program Director
Environmental Health Science
University of South Carolina Beaufort
Beaufort, South Carolina
Chapter 24

John B. Watkins, III, PhD
Associate Dean and Director
Medical Sciences Program
Indiana University School of Medicine
Bloomington, Indiana
Chapter 26

Diana G. Wilkins, MS, PhD
Director
Center for Human Toxicology
Research Associate Professor
Department of Pharmacology and Toxicology
University of Utah
Salt Lake City, Utah
Chapter 32

Preface

The eighth edition of *Casarett and Doull's Toxicology: The Basic Science of Poisons*, as the previous seven, is meant to serve primarily as a text for, or an adjunct to, graduate courses in toxicology. Because the seven previous editions have been widely used in courses in environmental health and related areas, an attempt has been made to maintain those characteristics that make it useful to scientists from other disciplines. This edition will again provide information on the many facets of toxicology, especially the principles, concepts, and modes of thoughts that are the foundation of the discipline. Mechanisms of toxicity are emphasized. Research toxicologists will find this book an excellent reference source to find updated material in areas of their special or peripheral interests.

The design of the eighth edition has been changed markedly, in that for the first time the figures and tables are presented in full color to allow for clearer interpretation of the basic concepts throughout the text. The rainbow of colors used in this edition makes this edition much more "user-friendly." Each book will come with a DVD with image bank features of all illustrations and tables from the text in a presentation-ready format. The book will also be available in a variety of eBook formats for all popular devices such as iPad and Kindle.

The overall framework of the eighth edition is similar to that of the seventh edition. The seven units are "General Principles of Toxicology" (Unit I), "Disposition of Toxicants" (Unit II), "Non-Organ-Directed Toxicity" (carcinogenicity, mutagenicity, and teratogenicity) (Unit III), "Target Organ Toxicity" (Unit IV), "Toxic Agents" (Unit V), "Environmental Toxicology" (Unit VI), and "Applications of Toxicology" (Unit VII).

This edition reflects the marked progress made in toxicology during the last few years. For example, the importance of apoptosis, cytokines, growth factors, oncogenes, cell cycling, receptors, gene regulation, transcription factors, signaling pathways, transgenic animals, "knock-out" animals, "humanized" mice, polymorphisms, microarray technology, genomics, proteonomics, epigenetics, etc, in understanding the mechanisms of toxicity is included in this edition. More information on environmental hormones is included. Two new chapters have been added to this edition, namely the "Toxic Effects of Calories" and the "Toxic Effects of Nanoparticles." References in this edition include not only traditional journal and review articles, but internet sites too. (Readers who would like a Power-Point version of the figures and tables can obtain the same from the publisher.)

The editor is grateful to his colleagues in academia, industry, and government who have made useful suggestions for improving this edition, both as a book and as a reference source. The editor is especially thankful to all the contributors, whose combined expertise has made possible a volume of this breadth. I especially recognize John Doull, the original editor of this book, for his continued support.

Preface to the First Edition

This volume has been designed primarily as a textbook for, or adjunct to, courses in toxicology. However, it should also be of interest to those not directly involved in toxicologic education. For example, the research scientist in toxicology will find sections containing current reports on the status of circumscribed areas of special interest. Those concerned with community health, agriculture, food technology, pharmacy, veterinary medicine, and related disciplines will discover the contents to be most useful as a source of concepts and modes of thought that are applicable to other types of investigative and applied sciences. For those further removed from the field of toxicology or for those who have not entered a specific field of endeavor, this book attempts to present a selectively representative view of the many facets of the subject.

Toxicology: The Basic Science of Poisons has been organized to facilitate its use by these different types of users. The first section (Unit I) describes the elements of method and approach that identify toxicology. It includes those principles most frequently invoked in a full understanding of toxicologic events, such as dose–response, and is primarily mechanistically oriented. Mechanisms are also stressed in the subsequent sections of the book, particularly when these are well identified and extend across classic forms of chemicals and systems. However, the major focus in the second section (Unit II) is on the systemic site of action of toxins. The intent therein is to provide answers to two questions: What kinds of injury are produced in specific organs or systems by toxic agents? What are the agents that produce these effects?

A more conventional approach to toxicology has been utilized in the third section (Unit III), in which the toxic agents are grouped by chemical or use characteristics. In the final section (Unit IV) an attempt has been made to illustrate the ramifications of toxicology into all areas of the health sciences and even beyond. This unit is intended to provide perspective for the nontoxicologist in the application of the results of toxicologic studies and a better understanding of the activities of those engaged in the various aspects of the discipline of toxicology.

It will be obvious to the reader that the contents of this book represent a compromise between the basic, fundamental, mechanistic approach to toxicology and the desire to give a view of the broad horizons presented by the subject. While it is certain that the editors' selectivity might have been more severe, it is equally certain that it could have been less so, and we hope that the balance struck will prove to be appropriate for both toxicologic training and the scientific interest of our colleague.

L.J.C.
J.D.

Although the philosophy and design of this book evolved over a long period of friendship and mutual respect between the editors, the effort needed to convert ideas into reality was undertaken primarily by Louis J. Casarett. Thus, his death at a time when completion of the manuscript was in sight was particularly tragic. With the help and encouragement of his wife, Margaret G. Casarett, and the other contributors, we have finished Lou's task. This volume is a fitting embodiment of Louis J. Casarett's dedication to toxicology and to toxicologic education.

J.D.

Dose and Dose-Rate matter

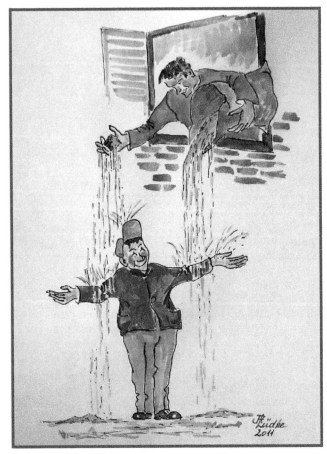

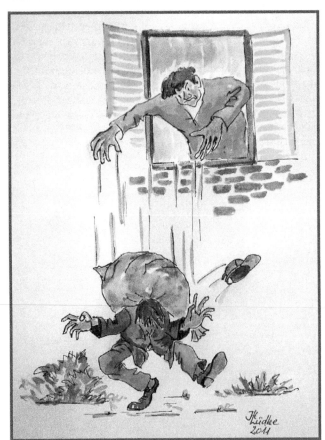

General Principles
of Toxicology

Unit

chapter 1

History and Scope of Toxicology

Michael A. Gallo

Toxicology has been defined as the study of the adverse effects of xenobiotics and thus is a borrowing science that has evolved from ancient poisoners. Modern toxicology goes beyond the study of the adverse effects of exogenous agents to the study of molecular biology, using toxicants as tools. Historically, toxicology formed the basis of therapeutics and experimental medicine. Toxicology in this century (1900 to the present) continues to develop and expand by assimilating knowledge and techniques from most branches of biology, chemistry, mathematics, and physics. A recent addition to the field of toxicology (1975 to the present) is the application of the discipline to safety evaluation and risk assessment.

The contributions and activities of toxicologists are diverse and widespread. In the biomedical area, toxicologists are concerned with mechanisms of action and exposure to chemical agents as a cause of acute and chronic illness. Toxicologists contribute to physiology and pharmacology by using toxic agents to understand physiological phenomena. They are involved in the recognition, identification, and quantification of hazards resulting from occupational exposure to chemicals and the public health aspects of chemicals in air, water, other parts of the environment, foods, and drugs. Traditionally, toxicologists have been intimately involved in the discovery and development of new drugs and pesticides. Toxicologists also participate in the development of standards and regulations designed to protect human health and the environment from the adverse effects of chemicals. Environmental toxicologists (a relatively new subset of the discipline) have expanded toxicology to study the effects of chemicals in flora and fauna. Molecular toxicologists are studying the mechanisms by which toxicants modulate cell growth and differentiation and cells respond to toxicants at the level of the gene. In all branches of toxicology, scientists explore the mechanisms by which chemicals produce adverse effects in biological systems. Clinical toxicologists develop antidotes and treatment regimes to ameliorate poisonings and xenobiotic injury. Toxicologists carry out some or all of these activities as members of academic, industrial, and governmental organizations. In doing so, they share methodologies for obtaining data about the toxicity of materials and the responsibility for using this information to make reasonable predictions regarding the hazards of the material to people

and the environment. These different but complementary activities characterize the discipline of toxicology.

Toxicology, like medicine, is both a science and an art. The science of toxicology is defined as the observational and data-gathering phase, whereas the art of toxicology consists of the utilization of the data to predict outcomes of exposure in human and animal populations. In most cases, these phases are linked because the facts generated by the science of toxicology are used to develop extrapolations and hypotheses to explain the adverse effects of chemical agents in situations where there is little or no information. For example, the observation that the administration of 2,3,7,8-tetrachlorodibenzo-*p*-dioxin (TCDD) to female Sprague–Dawley rats induces hepatocellular carcinoma is a fact. However, the conclusion that it will also do so in humans is a prediction or hypothesis. It is important to distinguish facts from predictions. When we fail to distinguish the science from the art, we confuse facts with predictions and argue that they have equal validity, which they clearly do not. In toxicology, as in all sciences, theories have a higher level of certainty than do hypotheses, which in turn are more certain than speculations, opinions, conjectures, and guesses. An insight into modern toxicology and the roles, points of view, and activities of toxicologists can be obtained by examining the historical evolution of the discipline.

HISTORY OF TOXICOLOGY

Antiquity

Toxicology dates back to the earliest humans, who used animal venoms and plant extracts for hunting, warfare, and assassination. Elucidating the mechanisms of the toxicity of venoms continues today in the field of toxinology. The knowledge of these poisons must have predated recorded history. It is safe to assume that prehistoric humans categorized some plants as harmful and others as safe. The same is probably true for the classification of snakes and other animals. The Ebers Papyrus (circa 1500 BC) contains information pertaining to many recognized poisons, including hemlock (the state poison of the Greeks), aconite (a Chinese arrow poison), opium (used as both a poison and an antidote), and metals such as arsenic lead, copper, and antimony. There is also an indication that plants containing substances similar to digitalis and belladonna alkaloids were known. Hippocrates (circa 400 BC) added a number of poisons and clinical toxicology principles pertaining to bioavailability in therapy and overdosage, while the *Book of Job* (circa 400 BC) speaks of poison arrows (Job 6:4). In the literature of ancient Greece, there are several references to poisons and their use. Some interpretations of Homer have Odysseus obtaining poisons for his arrows (Homer, circa 600 BC). Theophrastus (370–286 BC), a student of Aristotle, included numerous references to poisonous plants in *De Historia Plantarum*. Dioscorides, a Greek physician in the court of the Roman emperor Nero, made the first attempt at a classification of poisons, which was accompanied by descriptions and drawings. His classification into plant, animal, and mineral poisons not only remained a standard for 16 centuries but also is still a convenient classification (Gunther, 1934). Dioscorides also dabbled in therapy, recognizing the use of emetics in poisoning and the use of caustic agents and cupping glasses in snakebite. Poisoning with plant and animal toxins was quite common. Perhaps the best known recipient of poison used as a state method of execution was Socrates (470–399 BC), whose cup of hemlock extract was apparently estimated to be the proper dose. Expeditious suicide on a voluntary basis also made use of toxicological knowledge. Demosthenes (385–322 BC), who took poison hidden in his pen, was one of many examples. The mode of suicide calling for one to fall on his sword, although manly and noble, carried little appeal and less significance for the women of the day. Cleopatra's (69–30 BC) knowledge of natural primitive toxicology permitted her to use the more genteel method of falling on her asp.

The Romans too made considerable use of poisons in politics. One legend tells of King Mithridates VI of Pontus, whose numerous acute toxicity experiments on unfortunate criminals led to his eventual claim that he had discovered an antidote for every venomous reptile and poisonous substance (Guthrie, 1946). Mithridates was so fearful of poisons that he regularly ingested a mixture of 36 ingredients (Galen reports 54) as protection against assassination. On the occasion of his imminent capture by enemies, his attempts to kill himself with poison failed because of his successful antidote concoction, and he was forced to use a sword held by a servant. From this tale comes the term "mithridatic," referring to an antidotal or protective mixture. The term "theriac" also has become synonymous with "antidote," although the word comes from the poetic treatise *Theriaca* by Nicander of Colophon (204–135 BC), which dealt with poisonous animals; his poem *Alexipharmaca* was about antidotes.

Poisonings in Rome reached epidemic proportions during the 4th century BC (Livy). It was during this period that a conspiracy of women to remove men from whose death they might profit was uncovered. Similar large-scale poisoning continued until Sulla issued the *Lex Cornelia* (circa 82 BC). This appears to be the first law against poisoning, and it later became a regulatory statute directed at careless dispensers of drugs. Nero (AD 37–68) used poisons to do away with his stepbrother Brittanicus and employed his slaves as food tasters to differentiate edible mushrooms from their more poisonous kin.

Middle Ages

Come bitter pilot, now at once run on
The dashing rocks thy seasick weary bark!
Here's to my love! O true apothecary!
Thy drugs are quick. Thus with a kiss I die.

Romeo and Juliet, act 5, scene 3

Before the Renaissance, the writings of Maimonides (Moses ben Maimon, AD 1135–1204) included a treatise on the treatment of poisonings from insects, snakes, and mad dogs (*Poisons and their Antidotes*, 1198). Maimonides, like Hippocrates before him, wrote on the subject of bioavailability, noting that milk, butter, and cream could delay intestinal absorption. Maimonides also refuted many of the popular remedies of the day and stated his doubts about others. It is rumored that alchemists of this period (circa AD 1200), in search of the universal antidote, learned to distill fermented products and made a 60% ethanol beverage that had many interesting powers.

In the early Renaissance, the Italians, with characteristic pragmatism, brought the art of poisoning to its zenith. The poisoner became an integral part of the political scene. The records of the city councils of Florence, particularly those of the infamous Council of Ten of Venice, contain ample testimony about the political use of poisons. Victims were named, prices set, and contracts recorded; when the deed was accomplished, payment was made.

An infamous figure of the time was a lady named Toffana who peddled specially prepared arsenic-containing cosmetics (*Agua Toffana*). Accompanying the product were appropriate instructions for its use. Toffana was succeeded by an imitator with organizational genius, Hieronyma Spara, who provided a new fillip by directing her activities toward specific marital and monetary objectives. A local club was formed of young wealthy married women, which soon became a club of eligible young wealthy widows, reminiscent of the matronly conspiracy of Rome centuries earlier. Incidentally, arsenic-containing cosmetics were reported to be responsible for deaths well into the 20th century (Kallet and Schlink, 1933).

Among the prominent families engaged in poisoning, the Borgias were the most notorious. However, many deaths that were attributed to poisoning are now recognized as having resulted from infectious diseases such as malaria. It appears true, however, that Alexander VI, his son Cesare, and Lucrezia Borgia were quite active. The deft application of poisons to men of stature in the Catholic Church swelled the holdings of the papacy, which was their prime heir.

In this period Catherine de Medici exported her skills from Italy to France, where the prime targets of women were their husbands. However, unlike poisoners of an earlier period, the circle represented by Catherine and epitomized by the notorious Marchioness de Brinvillers depended on developing direct evidence to arrive at the most effective compounds for their purposes. Under the guise of delivering provender to the sick and the poor, Catherine tested toxic concoctions, carefully noting the rapidity of the toxic response (onset of action), the effectiveness of the compound (potency), the degree of response of the parts of the body (specificity, site of action), and the complaints of the victim (clinical signs and symptoms).

The culmination of the practice in France is represented by the commercialization of the service by Catherine Deshayes, a midwife sorceress who earned the title "La Voisin." Her business was dissolved by her execution in 1680. Her trial was 1 of the most famous of those held by the Chambre Ardente, a special judicial commission established by Louis XIV to try such cases without regard to age, sex, or national origin. La Voisin was convicted of many poisonings, with over 2000 infants among her victims.

Age of Enlightenment

All substances are poisons; there is none which is not a poison. The right dose differentiates poison from a remedy.

Paracelsus

A significant figure in the history of science and medicine in the late Middle Ages was the renaissance man Philippus Aureolus Theophrastus Bombastus von Hohenheim-Paracelsus (1493–1541). Between the time of Aristotle and the age of Paracelsus, there was little substantial change in the biomedical sciences. In the 16th century, the revolt against the authority of the Catholic Church was accompanied by a parallel attack on the godlike authority exercised by the followers of Hippocrates and Galen. Paracelsus personally and professionally embodied the qualities that forced numerous changes in this period. He and his age were pivotal, standing between the philosophy and magic of classical antiquity and the philosophy and science willed to us by figures of the 17th and 18th centuries. Clearly, one can identify in Paracelsus's approach, point of view, and breadth of interest numerous similarities to the discipline that is now called toxicology.

Paracelsus, a physician–alchemist and the son of a physician, formulated many revolutionary views that remain an integral part of the structure of toxicology, pharmacology, and therapeutics today (Pagel, 1958). He promoted a focus on the "toxicon," the primary toxic agent, as a chemical entity, as opposed to the Grecian concept of the mixture or blend. A view initiated by Paracelsus that became a lasting contribution held as corollaries that (1) experimentation is essential in the examination of responses to chemicals, (2) one should make a distinction between the therapeutic and toxic properties of chemicals, (3) these properties are sometimes but not always indistinguishable except by dose, and (4) one can ascertain a degree of specificity of chemicals and their therapeutic or toxic effects. These principles led Paracelsus to introduce mercury as the drug of choice for the treatment of syphilis, a practice that survived 300 years but led to his famous trial. This viewpoint presaged the "magic bullet" (arsphenamine) of Paul Ehrlich and the introduction of the therapeutic index. Further, in a very real sense, this was the first sound articulation of the dose–response relation, a bulwark of toxicology (Pachter, 1961).

The tradition of the poisoners spread throughout Europe, and their deeds played a major role in the distribution of political power throughout the Middle Ages. Pharmacology as it is known today had its beginnings during the Middle Ages and early Renaissance. Concurrently, the study of the toxicity and the dose–response relationship of therapeutic agents were commencing.

The occupational hazards associated with metalworking were recognized during the 15th century. Early publications by Ellenbog (circa 1480) warned of the toxicity of the mercury and lead exposures involved in goldsmithing. Agricola published a short treatise on mining diseases in 1556. However, the major work on the subject, *On the Miners: Sickness and Other Diseases of Miners* (1567), was published by Paracelsus. This treatise addressed the etiology of miners' disease, along with treatment and prevention strategies. Occupational toxicology was further advanced by the work of Bernardino Ramazzini. His classic, published in 1700 and entitled *Discourse on the Diseases of Workers*, set the standard for occupational medicine well into the 19th century. Ramazzini's work broadened the field by discussing occupations ranging from miners to midwives and including printers, weavers, and potters.

The developments of the industrial revolution stimulated a rise in many occupational diseases. The recognition, in 1775, of the renowned 18th-century English surgeon Percival Pott (1714–1788) of the role of soot in scrotal cancer among chimney sweeps was the first reported example of polyaromatic hydrocarbon (PAH) carcinogenicity, a problem the mechanism of which still intrigues toxicologists today. These findings led to improved medical practices, particularly in prevention of occupationally related diseases. It should be noted that Paracelsus and Ramazzini also pointed out the toxicity of smoke and soot.

The 19th century dawned in a climate of industrial and political revolution. Organic chemistry was in its infancy in 1800, but by 1825 phosgene ($COCl_2$) and mustard gas (bis[β-chloroethyl]sulfide) had been synthesized. These 2 agents, along with chlorine gas, were used by the German forces in World War I as chemical warfare agents. They were stockpiled throughout World War II, and used by Iraq in the Iran–Iraq War in the 1980s (*Marine Corps History*). By 1880 over 10,000 organic compounds had been synthesized including chloroform, carbon tetrachloride, diethyl ether, and carbonic acid, and petroleum and coal gasification by-products were used in trade. Determination of the toxicological potential of these newly created chemicals became the underpinning of the science of toxicology as it is practiced today. However, there was little interest during the mid-19th century in hampering industrial development. Hence, the impact of industrial toxicology discoveries was not felt until the passage of worker's insurance laws, first in Germany (1883), then in England (1897), and later in the United States (1910). Experimental toxicology accompanied the growth of organic chemistry and developed rapidly during the 19th century. Magendie (1783–1885), Orfila (1787–1853), and Bernard (1813–1878) carried out truly seminal research in experimental toxicology and medicine, and laid the groundwork for pharmacology, drug safety toxicology, and experimental therapeutics as well as occupational toxicology.

Orfila, a Spanish physician in the French court, was the first toxicologist to use autopsy material and chemical analysis systematically as legal proof of poisoning. His introduction of this detailed type of analysis survives as the underpinning of forensic toxicology (Orfila, 1818). Orfila published the first major work devoted expressly to the toxicity of natural agents (1814–1815). Magendie, a physician and experimental physiologist, studied the mechanisms of action of emetine, strychnine, and "arrow poisons" (Olmsted, 1944). His research into the absorption and distribution of these compounds in the body (the precursor to ADME studies today) remains a classic in toxicology and pharmacology. One of Magendie's more famous students, Claude Bernard, continued the study of arrow poisons (Bernard, 1850) but also added works on the mechanism of action of carbon monoxide. Bernard's treatise, *Introduction to the Study of Experimental Medicine* (translated by Greene and Schuman in 1949), is a classic in the development of toxicology.

Many German scientists contributed greatly to the growth of toxicology in the late 19th and early 20th centuries. Among the giants of the field are Oswald Schmiedeberg (1838–1921) and Louis Lewin (1850–1929). Schmiedeberg made many contributions to the science of toxicology, not the least of which was the training of approximately 120 students who later populated the most important laboratories of pharmacology and toxicology throughout the world. Schmiedeberg's research focused on the synthesis of hippuric acid in the liver and the detoxification mechanisms of the liver in several animal species (Schmiedeberg and Koppe, 1869). Lewin, who was educated originally in medicine and the natural sciences, trained in toxicology under Liebreich at the Pharmacological Institute of Berlin (1881). His contributions on the chronic toxicity of narcotics and other alkaloids remain a classic. Lewin also published much of the early work on the toxicity of methanol, glycerol, acrolein, and chloroform (Lewin, 1920, 1929).

20TH CENTURY TOXICOLOGY: THE AWAKENING OF UNDERSTANDING

The doubter is a true man of science; he doubts only himself and his interpretations, but he believes in science.

Claude Bernard

The latter part of the 19th century saw the introduction of "patent medicines" in many parts of the world.

Toxicology evolved rapidly during the 20th century. The early controversies focusing on patent medicines and sale of consumer products of questionable safety (Kallett and Schlink) were followed by the rapid advances in analytical chemistry methods that fostered the advancement of forensic toxicology specifically at the New York City Medical Examiner's Office. However, the exponential growth of the discipline can be traced to the World War II era with its marked increase in the production of drugs, pesticides, munitions, synthetic fibers, and industrial chemicals. The history of many sciences represents an orderly transition based on theory, hypothesis testing, and synthesis of new ideas. Toxicology, as a gathering and an applied science, has, by contrast, developed in fits and starts. It calls on almost all the basic sciences to test its hypotheses. This fact, coupled with the health and occupational regulations that have driven toxicology research since 1900, has made toxicology exceptional in the history of science. The differentiation of toxicology as an art and a science, though arbitrary, permits the presentation of historical highlights along 2 major lines.

Modern toxicology can be viewed as a continuation of the development of the biological and physical sciences in the late 19th and 20th centuries (Table 1-1). During the second half of the 19th century, the world witnessed an explosion in science that produced the beginning of the modern era of medicine, synthetic chemistry, physics, and biology. Toxicology has drawn its strength and diversity from its proclivity to borrowing. With the advent of anesthetics and disinfectants and the advancement of experimental pharmacology in the late 1850s, toxicology as it is currently understood got its start. The introduction of ether, chloroform, and carbonic acid led to several iatrogenic deaths. These unfortunate outcomes spurred research into the causes of the deaths and early experiments on the physiological mechanisms by which these compounds caused both beneficial and adverse effects. By the late 19th century the use of organic chemicals was becoming more widespread, and benzene, toluene, and the xylenes, as well as the chlorinated solvents related to chloroform, went into large-scale commercial production. During this period, the use of patent medicines, consisting primarily of "medicinal herbs," nonsugar sweeteners, and alcohol, was prevalent, and there were several incidents of poisonings from these medicaments. In 1902 Congress approved $5000 to fund the "Poison Squad," professional tasters under the direction of Harvey Washington Wiley that harkened back to the food tasters used by royalty to avoid intentional poisoning from their foods. The case of "Doctor" Munyan versus Harvey Wiley, MD (1844–1930), a classic battle between the federal government and the most infamous purveyor of patent medicines, over mislabeling, false advertisement, lack of efficacy, and serious toxicity led to further Congressional action. The adverse reactions to patent medicines and mislabeled foods coupled with the response to Upton Sinclair's exposé of the Chicago meat-packing industry in *The Jungle* (*1905*) culminated in the passage of the Wiley Bill (*The Pure Foods Act of 1906*).

Table 1-1

Selection of Developments in Toxicology

Development of early advances in analytical methods
  Marsh: development of method for arsenic analysis
  Reinsh: combined method for separation and analysis of As and Hg
  Fresenius and von Babo: development of screening method for general poisons
  Stas-Otto: detection and identification of phosphorus

Early mechanistic studies
  F. Magendie: study of "arrow poisons," mechanism of action of emetine and strychnine
  C. Bernard (1850): carbon monoxide combination with hemoglobin, study of mechanism of action of strychnine, site of action of curare
  R. Bohm (ca. 1890): active anthelmintics from fern, action of croton oil catharsis, poisonous mushrooms

Introduction of new toxicants and antidotes
  R. A. Peters, L. A. Stocken, and R. H. S. Thompson: development of British anti-Lewisite (BAL) as a relatively specific antidote for arsenic, toxicity of monofluorocarbon compounds
  K. K. Chen: introduction of modern antidotes (nitrite and thiosulfate) for cyanide toxicity
  C. Voegtlin *et al.* (1923): mechanism of action of As and other metals on the SH groups
  P. Müller: introduction and study of dichlorodiphenyltrichloroethane (DDT) and related insecticide compounds
  G. Schrader: introduction and study of organophosphorus compounds
  R. N. Chopra: indigenous drugs of India

Miscellaneous toxicological studies
  R. T. Williams: study of detoxication mechanisms and species variation
  A. Rothstein: effects of uranium ion on cell membrane transport
  R. A. Kehoe: investigation of acute and chronic effects of lead
  A. Vorwald: studies of chronic respiratory disease (beryllium)
  H. Hardy: community and industrial poisoning (beryllium)
  A. Hamilton: introduction of modern industrial toxicology
  H. C. Hodge: toxicology of uranium, fluorides; standards of toxicity
  A. Hoffman: introduction of lysergic acid and derivatives; psychotomimetics
  R. A. Peters: biochemical lesions, lethal synthesis
  A. E. Garrod: inborn errors of metabolism
  T. T. Litchfield and F. Wilcoxon: simplified dose–response evaluation
  C. J. Bliss: method of probits, calculation of dosage–mortality curves

This was the first of many US pure food and drug laws (see Hutt and Hutt, 1984, for regulatory history of foods). The Wiley Bill as it was known was widely supported in Congress at its passage. However, the support did not last. The Bill required prior toxicity testing, the establishment of a government analytical laboratory, and the removal of toxic compounds, particularly ethanol, herbal mixtures, and coloring agents. It also prohibited false advertising. After enactment of the Bill, individual federal leaders including Congressmen and judges, as well as "Dr" Munyan (who claimed his remedies were effective and had cured thousands), campaigned against its enforcement. Parts of the Bill were overturned by Justice Oliver Wendell Holmes and the US Supreme Court in 1911 stating that "hype is not false advertising." In part because of the opposition to the Bill, Wiley left the government to direct the fledgling Consumer Union in 1912. Today, a century later, similar battles are being fought over dietary supplements and food additives.

A working hypothesis about the development of toxicology is that the discipline expands in response to legislation, which itself is a response to a real or perceived tragedy. The Wiley Bill was the first such reaction in the area of food and drugs, and the workers' compensation laws cited above were a response to occupational toxicities. In addition, the National Safety Council was established in 1911, and the Division of Industrial Hygiene was established by the US Public Health Service in 1914. A corollary to this hypothesis might be that the founding of scientific journals and/or societies is sparked by the development of a new field. The *Journal of Industrial Hygiene* began in 1918. The major chemical manufacturers in the United States (Dow, Union Carbide, and Du Pont) established internal toxicology research laboratories to help guide decisions on worker health and product safety.

During the 1890s and early 1900s, European scientists Becquerel, Roentgen, and the Curies reported the discovery of radioactivity and x-rays. This opened up for exploration a very large area in physics, biology, and medicine. Interestingly, many of these early researchers died of radiation poisoning. Radiation exposure became widespread in consumer usage. Radium-containing rocks were touted as health cures, and the Radiothor and radium dial watches were widespread. The adverse effects were virtually unknown and radiation would not actively affect the science of toxicology until the World War II era.

However, another discovery, that of vitamins, or "vital amines," led to the use of the first large-scale bioassays (multiple animal studies) to determine whether these new synthetic chemicals were beneficial or harmful to laboratory animals, and by extension to humans. The initial work in this area took place at around the time of World War I in several laboratories, including the laboratory of Philip B. Hawk in Philadelphia. Hawk and a young associate, Bernard L. Oser, were responsible for the development and verification of many early toxicological assays that are still used in a slightly amended form. The results from these animal studies formed the underpinnings of risk assessment. Oser's contributions to food and regulatory toxicology were extraordinary. These early bioassays were made possible by a major advance in toxicology: the availability of developed and refined strains of inbred laboratory rodents (Donaldson, 1912) and the rapid development of analytical chemistry.

The 1920s saw many events that began to mold the fledgling field of toxicology. The discovery by Paul Ehrlich (1854–1915) of arsenicals for the treatment of syphilis (arsenicals had been used in agriculture since the mid-19th century) resulted in acute and chronic toxicity. Arsenic remains a major toxicant in many developing nations. Prohibition of alcoholic beverages in the United States opened the door for early studies of neurotoxicology, with the discovery that triorthocresyl phosphate (TOCP), methanol, and lead (all found in bootleg liquor) are neurotoxicants. TOCP, which was a recent gasoline additive, caused a syndrome that became known as "ginger-jake" walk, a spastic gait resulting from drinking ginger beer adulterated with TOCP. Methanol, used as a cheap ethanol substitute, blinded and killed many unsuspecting people (see *Poisoners Handbook*, 2011). Mueller's discovery of dichlorodiphenyltrichloroethane (DDT) and several other organohalides, such as hexachlorobenzene and hexachlorocyclohexane, during the late 1920s resulted in widespread use of these insecticidal agents. Toxicity testing of the new organohalide compounds was in its infancy. Understanding of the modes of action and persistence of these compounds would have to wait 40 years.

Other scientists were hard at work attempting to elucidate the structures and activity of the estrogens and androgens. Work on the steroid hormones led to the use of several assays for the determination of the biological activity of organ extracts and synthetic compounds. Allen and Doisy published the first uterotrophic assay (1928) that accelerated the study of estrogenic chemicals. Modifications of this assay are used today in studying endocrine disruption by xenobiotics. Efforts to synthesize estrogen-active chemicals were spearheaded by E. C. Dodds and his co-workers, one of whom was Leon Golberg, a young organic chemist and a future leader in toxicology. Dodds's work on the bioactivity of the estrogenic compounds resulted in the synthesis of diethylstilbestrol (DES), hexestrol, other stilbenes, and bisphenol A (BPA) and the discovery of the strong estrogenic activity of substituted stilbenes. Golberg's intimate involvement in this work stimulated his interest in biology, leading to degrees in biochemistry and medicine and a career in toxicology in which he oversaw the creation of the laboratories of the British Industrial Biological Research Association (BIBRA) and the Chemical Industry Institute of Toxicology (CIIT). Interestingly, the initial observations that led to the discovery of DES were the findings of feminization of animals treated with the experimental carcinogen 7,12-dimethylbenz[a]anthracene (DMBA).

Occupational illnesses became more pronounced after the 1920s, and occupational toxicology developed into a field of its own. The seminal works of Alice Hamilton (1869–1970) (Exploring the Dangerous Trades) and Ethel Browning (Toxicity of Industrial Solvents, 1937) are critical readings.

The 1930s saw the world preparing for World War II and a major effort by the pharmaceutical and chemical industry in Europe and the United States to manufacture the first mass-produced antibiotics. One of the first journals expressly dedicated to experimental toxicology, *Archiv für Toxikologie*, began publication in Europe in 1930, the same year that Herbert Hoover signed the act that established the National Institutes of Health (NIH) in the United States.

The discovery of sulfanilamide was heralded as a major event in combating bacterial diseases. However, for a drug to be effective, there must be a reasonable delivery system, and sulfanilamide is highly insoluble in an aqueous medium. Therefore, it was originally prepared in ethanol (elixir). However, it was soon discovered that the drug was more soluble in *di*ethylene glycol. The drug was sold in glycol solutions but was labeled as an elixir, and several patients (mostly children) died of acute kidney failure resulting from the metabolism of the glycol to oxalic acid and glycolic acid, with the acids and the active drug crystallizing in the kidney tubules. This tragic event led to the passage of the Copeland Bill in 1938, the second major bill involving the formation of the US Food and Drug Administration (FDA). The sulfanilamide disaster played a critical role in the further development of toxicology, resulting in work by Eugene Maximillian Geiling in the Pharmacology Department of the University of Chicago that elucidated the mechanism of toxicity of both sulfanilamide and diethylene glycol. Studies of the glycols were simultaneously carried out at the US FDA by a group led by Arnold Lehman. The scientists associated with Lehman and Geiling were to become the leaders of toxicology (especially the Society of Toxicology) over the next 40 years. With few exceptions, toxicology in the United States owes its heritage to Geiling's innovativeness and ability to stimulate and direct young scientists, and Lehman's vision of the use of experimental toxicology in public health decision making. Because of Geiling's reputation, the US government turned to this group for help in the war effort. There were 3 main areas in which the Chicago group took part during World War II: the toxicology and pharmacology of organophosphate (OP) chemicals, antimalarial drugs, and radionuclides. Each of these areas produced teams of toxicologists who became academic, governmental, and industrial leaders in the field.

It was also during this time that DDT and the phenoxy herbicides were developed for increased food production and, in the case of DDT, control of insect-borne diseases. These efforts between 1940 and 1946 led to an explosion in toxicology. Thus, in line with the hypothesis advanced above, the crisis of World War II caused the next major leap in the development of toxicology.

If one traces the history of the toxicology of metals over the past 45 years, the role of the Chicago and Rochester groups is quite visible. This story commences with the use of uranium for the "bomb" and continues today with research on the role of metals in their interactions with DNA, RNA, and growth factors. Indeed, the Manhattan Project created a fertile environment that resulted in the initiation of quantitative biology, radiotracer technology, and inhalation toxicology. These innovations have revolutionized modern biology, chemistry, therapeutics, and toxicology.

Inhalation toxicology began at the University of Rochester under the direction of Stafford Warren, who headed the Department of Radiology. He developed a program with colleagues such as Harold Hodge (pharmacologist), Herb Stokinger (chemist), Sid Laskin (inhalation toxicologist), and Lou and George Casarett (toxicologists). These young scientists were to go on to become giants in the field. The other sites for the study of radionuclides were Chicago for the "internal" effects of radioactivity and Oak Ridge, Tennessee, for the effects of "external" radiation. The work of the scientists on these teams gave the scientific community data that contributed to the early understanding of macromolecular binding of xenobiotics, cellular mutational events, methods for inhalation toxicology and therapy, and toxicological properties of trace metals, along with a better appreciation of the complexities of the dose–response curve.

Another seminal event in toxicology that occurred during the World War II era was the discovery by Lange and Schrader in 1938 of OP cholinesterase inhibitors including sarin, tabun (chemical warfare agents), and less potent OP insecticides. This class of chemicals was destined to become a driving force in the study of neurophysiology and toxicology for several decades. Again, the scientists in Chicago played major roles in elucidating the mechanisms of action of this new class of compounds. Geiling's group, Kenneth DuBois in particular, was the leader in this area of toxicology and pharmacology. DuBois's colleagues, particularly Sheldon Murphy, continued to be in the forefront of this special area. The importance of the early research on the OPs has taken on special meaning in the years since 1960, when these nonbioaccumulating insecticides were destined to replace DDT and other organochlorine insecticides. Today, a third generation of insecticides has replaced much of the OP use.

Early in the 20th century, it was demonstrated experimentally that quinine has a marked effect on the malaria parasite (it had been known for centuries that cinchona bark extract is efficacious for "Jesuit fever" [malaria]). This discovery led to the development of quinine derivatives for the treatment of the disease and the formulation of the early principles of chemotherapy. The Pharmacology Department of the University of Chicago was charged with the development of antimalarials for the war effort. The original protocols called for testing of efficacy and toxicity in rodents and perhaps dogs and then the testing of efficacy in human volunteers. One of the investigators charged with generating the data needed to move a candidate drug from animals to humans was Fredrick Coulston. This young parasitologist and his colleagues, working in Chicago, were to evaluate potential drugs in animal models and then establish human clinical trials. It was during these experiments that the use of nonhuman primates came into vogue for toxicology testing. It had been noted by Russian scientists that some antimalarial compounds caused retinopathies in humans but did not apparently have the same adverse effect in rodents and dogs. This finding led the Chicago team to add 1 more step in the development process: toxicity testing in rhesus monkeys just before efficacy studies in people. This resulted in the prevention of blindness in untold numbers of volunteers and perhaps some of the troops in the field. It also led to the school of thought that nonhuman primates may be one of the better models for humans and the establishment of primate colonies for the study of toxicity. Coulston pioneered this area of toxicology and remained committed to it.

Another area not traditionally thought of as toxicology but one that evolved during the 1940s as an exciting and innovative field is experimental pathology. This branch of experimental biology developed from bioassays of estrogens and early experiments in chemical- and radiation-induced carcinogenesis. It is from these early studies that hypotheses on tumor promotion and cancer progression have evolved.

Toxicologists today owe a great deal to the researchers of chemical carcinogenesis of the 1940s. Much of today's work can be traced to Elizabeth and James Miller at Wisconsin. This husband and wife team started under the mentorship of Professor Rusch, the director of the newly formed McArdle Laboratory for Cancer Research, and Professor Baumann. The seminal research of the Millers led to the discovery of the role of reactive intermediates in carcinogenicity and that of mixed-function oxidases in the endoplasmic reticulum. These findings, which initiated the great works on the cytochrome P450 family of proteins, were aided by 2 other major discoveries for which toxicologists (and all other biological scientists) are deeply indebted: paper chromatography in 1944 and the use of radiolabeled dibenzanthracene in 1948. Other major events of note in drug metabolism included the work of Bernard Brodie on the metabolism of methyl orange in 1947. This piece of seminal research led to the examination of blood and urine for chemical and drug metabolites. It became the tool with which one could study the relationship between blood levels and biological action. The classic treatise of R. T. Williams, *Detoxication Mechanisms*, was published in 1947. This text described the many pathways and possible mechanisms of detoxication and opened the field to several new areas of study.

The decade after World War II was not as boisterous as the period from 1935 to 1945. The first major US pesticide act was signed into law in 1947. The significance of the initial Federal Insecticide, Fungicide, and Rodenticide Act was that for the first time in US history a substance that was neither a drug nor a food had to be shown to be safe and efficacious. This decade, which coincided with the Eisenhower years, saw the dispersion of the groups from Chicago, Rochester, and Oak Ridge and the establishment of new centers of research. Adrian Albert's classic *Selective Toxicity* was published in 1951. This treatise, which has appeared in several editions, presented a concise documentation of the principles of the site-specific action of chemicals.

THE SECOND HALF OF THE 19TH CENTURY

You too can be a toxicologist in two easy lessons, each of ten years.
Arnold Lehman (circa 1955)

The mid-1950s witnessed the strengthening of the US FDA's commitment to toxicology under the guidance of Arnold Lehman. Lehman's tutelage and influence are still felt today. The adage "You too can be a toxicologist" is as important a summation of toxicology as the often-quoted statement of Paracelsus: "The dose makes the poison." The period from 1955 to 1958 produced 2 major events that would have a long-lasting impact on toxicology as a science and a professional discipline. Lehman, Fitzhugh, and their co-workers formalized the experimental program for the appraisal of food, drug, and cosmetic safety in 1955, updated by the US FDA in 1982, and the Gordon Research Conferences established a conference on toxicology and safety evaluation, with Bernard L. Oser as its initial chairman. These 2 events led to close relationships among toxicologists from several groups and brought toxicology into a new phase. At about the same time, the US Congress passed and the president of the United States signed the additives amendments to the Food, Drug, and Cosmetic Act. The Delaney Clause (1958) of these amendments stated broadly that any chemical found to be carcinogenic in laboratory animals or humans could not be added to the US food supply. The impact of this legislation cannot be overstated. Delaney became a battle cry for many groups and resulted in the inclusion at a new level of biostatisticians and mathematical modelers in the field of toxicology. It fostered the expansion of quantitative methods in toxicology and led to innumerable arguments about the "1-hit" theory of carcinogenesis. Regardless of one's view of Delaney, it has served as an excellent starting point for understanding the complexity of the biological phenomenon of carcinogenicity and the development of risk assessment models. One must remember that at the time of Delaney, the analytical detection level for most chemicals was 20 to 100 ppm (today, parts per quadrillion). Interestingly, the Delaney Clause has been invoked only on a few occasions, and it has been stated that Congress added little to the food and drug law with this clause (Hutt and Hutt, 1984).

Shortly after the Delaney amendment and after 3 successful Gordon Conferences, the first American journal dedicated to toxicology was launched by Coulston, Lehman, and Hayes. *Toxicology and Applied Pharmacology* has been a flagship journal of toxicology ever since. The founding of the Society of Toxicology (1961) followed shortly afterward, and this journal became its official publication of the SOT through the 20th century. The society's founding members were Fredrick Coulston, William Deichmann, Kenneth DuBois, Victor Drill, Harry Hayes, Harold Hodge, Paul Larson, Arnold Lehman, and C. Boyd Shaffer. These researchers

deserve a great deal of credit for the growth of toxicology. DuBois and Geiling published their *Textbook of Toxicology* in 1959.

In 1975, Louis Casarett and John Doull followed this short text with what has become the most widely accepted general toxicology text—*Toxicology: The Basic Science of Poisons*. This volume is the eighth addition of the classic text.

The 1960s were a tumultuous time for society, and toxicology was swept up in the tide, starting with the tragic thalidomide incident, in which several thousand children were born with serious birth defects. Dr Frances O. Kelsey, a protégé of E. M. K. Geiling, was instrumental in keeping this notorious teratogen off the US market. Interestingly, as the mechanism of thalidomide became known later in the 20th century, the drug and its derivatives were developed for several life-threatening diseases. The publication of Carson's *Silent Spring* (1962) energized the field of environmental toxicology that developed at a feverish pitch. Attempts to understand the effects of chemicals on the embryo and fetus and on the environment as a whole gained momentum. New legislation was passed, and new journals were founded. The education of toxicologists spread from the deep traditions of Chicago and Rochester to Harvard, Miami, Albany, Iowa, Jefferson, and beyond. Geiling's fledglings spread as Schmiedeberg's had a half century before. Many new fields were influencing and being assimilated into the broad scope of toxicology, including environmental sciences, aquatic and avian biology, cell biology, analytical chemistry, and genetics.

During the 1960s the analytical tools used in toxicology were developed to a level of sophistication that allowed the detection of chemicals in tissues and other substrates at part per billion concentrations (see *The Vanishing Zero*, 1972). Today parts per quadrillion and less are detected. Pioneering work in the development of point mutation assays that were replicable, quick, and inexpensive led to a better understanding of the genetic mechanisms of carcinogenicity (Ames, 1983). The combined work of Ames and the Millers (Elizabeth C. and James A.) at McArdle Laboratory allowed the toxicology community to make major contributions to the understanding of the carcinogenic process.

The low levels of detection of chemicals and the ability to detect point mutations rapidly created several problems and opportunities for toxicologists and risk assessors that stemmed from interpretation of the Delaney amendment. Cellular and molecular toxicology developed as a subdiscipline, and risk assessment became a major product of toxicological investigations.

The establishment of the National Center for Toxicologic Research (NCTR), the expansion of the role of the US FDA, and the establishment of the US Environmental Protection Agency (EPA) and the National Institute of Environmental Health Sciences (NIEHS) were considered clear messages that the government had taken a strong interest in toxicology. Several new journals appeared during the 1960s, and new legislation was written quickly after *Silent Spring* and the thalidomide disaster.

Elwood Jensen and his colleagues discovered the high-affinity estradiol-binding protein (the estrogen receptor) in the mid-1960s. The end of the 1960s witnessed the "discovery" of TCDD as a contaminant in the herbicide Agent Orange (the original discovery of TCDD toxicity was reported in 1957). The research on the toxicity of this compound has produced some very good and some very poor research in the field of toxicology. The discovery of a high-affinity cellular binding protein, using techniques established by Jensen, was designated the "Ah" receptor (see Poland and Knutsen, 1982, for a review) at the McArdle Laboratory. Works on the genetics of the receptor at NIH (Nebert and Gonzalez, 1987) revolutionized the field of toxicology. The importance of TCDD to toxicology lies in the fact that it forced researchers, regulators, and the legal community to look at the role of mechanisms of toxic action in a different fashion.

At least one other event precipitated a great deal of legislation during the 1970s: Love Canal. The "discovery" of Love Canal led to major concerns regarding hazardous wastes, chemical dump sites, and disclosure of information about those sites. Soon after Love Canal, the EPA listed several equally contaminated sites in the United States. The agency was given the responsibility to develop risk assessment methodology to determine health risks from exposure to effluents and to attempt to remediate these sites. These combined efforts led to broad-based support for research into the mechanisms of action of individual chemicals and complex mixtures. Love Canal and similar issues created the legislative environment that led to the Toxic Substances Control Act and eventually to the Superfund Bill. These omnibus bills were created to cover the toxicology of chemicals from initial synthesis to disposal (cradle to grave).

The expansion of legislation, journals, and new societies involved with toxicology was exponential during the 1970s and 1980s and shows no signs of slowing down. Currently, in the United States there are dozens of professional, governmental, and other scientific organizations with thousands of members and over 120 journals dedicated to toxicology and related disciplines.

In addition, toxicology continues to expand in stature and in the number of programs worldwide. The International Congress of Toxicology is made up of toxicology societies from Europe, South America, Asia, Africa, and Australia and brings together the broadest representation of toxicologists.

The original Gordon Conference series that celebrated its 50th anniversary in 2007 has evolved to *Cellular & Molecular Mechanisms of Toxicity*, and several other conferences related to special areas of toxicology are now in existence. The Society of Toxicology formed specialty sections and regional chapters to accommodate the over 6000 scientists involved in toxicology today. The SOT celebrated its 50th anniversary in March 2011. Texts and reference books for toxicology students and scientists abound. Toxicology has evolved from a borrowing science to a seminal discipline seeding the growth and development of several related fields of science and science policy.

The history of toxicology has been interesting and varied but never dull. Perhaps as a science that has grown and prospered by borrowing from many disciplines, it has suffered from the absence of a single goal, but its diversification has allowed for the interspersion of ideas and concepts from higher education, industry, and government. As an example of this diversification, one now finds toxicology graduate programs in medical schools, schools of public health, and schools of pharmacy as well as programs in environmental science and engineering and undergraduate programs in toxicology at several institutions. Surprisingly, courses in toxicology are now being offered in several liberal arts undergraduate schools as part of their biology and chemistry curricula. This has resulted in an exciting, innovative, and diversified field that is serving science and the community at large.

THE 21ST CENTURY

Genetics loads the gun but the environment pulls the trigger.

Judith Stein

The sequencing of the human genome and several other genomes has markedly affected all biological sciences. Toxicology is no exception. Today new animal models, especially zebrafish, *C. elegans*, and *D. melanogaster* (all of which have orthologs of human genes), are widely used in toxicology. The understanding of epigenetics is opening novel approaches to the fetal origin of adult diseases including cancers, diabetes, and neurodegenerative diseases and disorders. These are discussed in subsequent chapters.

Few disciplines can point to both basic sciences and direct applications at the same time. Toxicology—the study of the adverse effects of xenobiotics—may be unique in this regard. The mechanisms of action of the xenobiotics studied by toxicologists, in the tradition of Claude Bernard, continue to be the tools of modern biology.

REFERENCES

Albert A. *Selective Toxicity*. London: Methuen; 1951.

Ames BN. Dietary carcinogens and anticarcinogens. *Science*. 1983;221:1249–1264.

Bernard C. Action du curare et de la nicotine sur le systeme nerveux et sur le systme musculaire. *C R Soc Biol*. 1850;2:195.

Bernard C. *Introduction to the Study of Experimental Medicine*. Greene HC, Schuman H, trans. New York: Dover; 1949.

Carson R. *Silent Spring*. Boston: Houghton Mifflin; 1962.

Donaldson HH. The history and zoological position of the albino rat. *Natl Acad Sci*. 1912;15:365–369.

DuBois K, Geiling EMK. *Textbook of Toxicology*. New York: Oxford University Press; 1959.

Gunther RT. *The Greek Herbal of Dioscorides*. New York: Oxford University Press; 1934.

Guthrie DA. *A History of Medicine*. Philadelphia: Lippincott; 1946.

Hutt PB, Hutt PB II. A history of government regulation of adulteration and misbranding of food. *Food Drug Cosmet J*. 1984;39:2–73.

Kallet A, Schlink FJ. *100,000,000 Guinea Pigs: Dangers in Everyday Foods, Drugs and Cosmetics*. New York: Vanguard; 1933.

Lewin L. *Die Gifte in der Weltgeschichte: Toxikologische, allgemeinverstandliche Untersuchungen der historischen Quellen*. Berlin: Springer; 1920.

Lewin L. *Gifte und Vergiftungen*. Berlin: Stilke; 1929.

Nebert D, Gonzalez FJ. P450 genes: structure, evolution and regulation. *Annu Rev Biochem*. 1987;56:945–993.

Olmsted JMD. *François Magendie: Pioneer in Experimental Physiology and Scientific Medicine in XIX Century France*. New York: Schuman; 1944.

Orfila MJB. *Traite des Poisons Tires des Regnes Mineral, Vegetal et Animal, ou, Toxicologie Generale Consideree sous les Rapports de la Physiologie, de la Pathologie, de la Medecine Legale*. Paris: Crochard; 1814–1815.

Orfila MJB. *Secours a Donner aux Personnes Empoisonees et Asphyxiees*. Paris: Feugeroy; 1818.

Pachter HM. *Paracelsus: Magic into Science*. New York: Collier; 1961.

Pagel W. *Paracelsus: An Introduction to Philosophical Medicine in the Era of the Renaissance*. New York: Karger; 1958.

Paracelsus (Theophrastus ex Hohenheim Eremita). *Von der Besucht*. Dillingen; 1567.

Poland A, Knutson JC. 2,3,7,8-Tetrachlorodibenzo-*p*-dioxin and related halogenated aromatic hydrocarbons, examination of the mechanism of toxicity. *Annu Rev Pharmacol Toxicol*. 1982;22:517–554.

Schmiedeberg O, Koppe R. *Das Muscarin das giftige Alkaloid des Fliegenpilzes*. Leipzig: Vogel; 1869.

US FDA. *Toxicologic Principles for the Safety Assessment of Direct Food Additives and Color Additives Used in Food*. Washington, DC: US Food and Drug Administration, Bureau of Foods; 1982.

Voegtlin C, Dyer HA, Leonard CS. On the mechanism of the action of arsenic upon protoplasm. *Public Health Rep*. 1923;38:1882–1912.

Williams RT. *Detoxication Mechanisms*. 2nd ed. New York: Wiley; 1959.

SUPPLEMENTAL READING

Adams F, trans. *The Genuine Works of Hippocrates*. Baltimore: Williams & Wilkins; 1939.

Beeson BB. Orfila—pioneer toxicologist. *Ann Med Hist*. 1930;2:68–70.

Bernard C. Analyse physiologique des proprietes des systemes musculaire et nerveux au moyen du curare. *C R Acad Sci (Paris)*. 1856;43:325–329.

Bryan CP. *The Papyrus Ebers*. London: Geoffrey Bales; 1930.

Clendening L. *Source Book of Medical History*. New York: Dover; 1942.

Gaddum JH. *Pharmacology*. 5th ed. New York: Oxford University Press; 1959.

Garrison FH. *An Introduction to the History of Medicine*. 4th ed. Philadelphia: Saunders; 1929.

Hamilton A. *Exploring the Dangerous Trades*. Boston: Little, Brown; 1943 [reprinted by Northeastern University Press, Boston, 1985].

Hays HW. *Society of Toxicology History, 1961–1986*. Washington, DC: Society of Toxicology; 1986.

Holmstedt B, Liljestrand G. *Readings in Pharmacology*. New York: Raven Press; 1981.

chapter 2

Principles of Toxicology

David L. Eaton and Steven G. Gilbert

INTRODUCTION TO TOXICOLOGY

Toxicology is the study of the adverse effects of chemical or physical agents on living organisms. A *toxicologist* is trained to examine and communicate the nature of those effects on human, animal, and environmental health. Toxicological research examines the cellular, biochemical, and molecular mechanisms of action as well as functional effects such as neurobehavioral and immunological, and assesses the probability of their occurrence. Fundamental to this process is characterizing the relation of exposure (or dose) to the response. *Risk assessment* is the quantitative estimate of the potential effects on human health and environmental significance of various types of chemical exposures (eg, pesticide residues in food, contaminants in drinking water). The variety of potential adverse effects and the diversity of chemicals in the environment make toxicology a broad science, which often demands specialization in one area of toxicology. Our society's dependence on chemicals and the need to assess potential hazards have made toxicologists an increasingly important part of the decision-making processes.

Different Areas of Toxicology

The professional activities of toxicologists fall into 3 main categories: descriptive, mechanistic, and regulatory (Fig. 2-1). Although each has distinctive characteristics, each contributes to the other, and all are vitally important to chemical risk assessment (see Chap. 4).

A *mechanistic toxicologist* is concerned with identifying and understanding the cellular, biochemical, and molecular mechanisms by which chemicals exert toxic effects on living organisms (see Chap. 3 for a detailed discussion of mechanisms of toxicity). The results of mechanistic studies are very important in many areas of applied toxicology. In risk assessment, mechanistic data may be very useful in demonstrating that an adverse outcome (eg, cancer, birth defects) observed in laboratory animals is directly relevant to humans. For example, the relative toxic potential of organophosphorus (OP) insecticides in humans, rodents, and insects can be accurately predicted on the basis of an understanding of common mechanisms (inhibition of acetylcholinesterase) and differences in biotransformation for these insecticides among the different species. Similarly, mechanistic data may be very useful in identifying

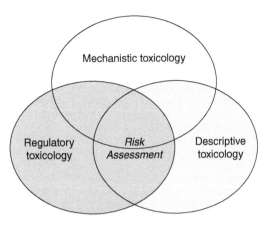

Figure 2-1. *Graphical representation of the interconnections between different areas of toxicology.*

adverse responses in experimental animals that may not be relevant to humans. For example, the propensity of the widely used artificial sweetener saccharin to cause bladder cancer in rats may not be relevant to humans at normal dietary intake rates. This is because mechanistic studies have demonstrated that bladder cancer is induced only under conditions where saccharin is at such a high concentration in the urine that it forms a crystalline precipitate (Cohen, 1998). Dose–response studies suggest that such high concentrations would not be achieved in the human bladder even after extensive dietary consumption.

Mechanistic data are also useful in the design and production of safer alternative chemicals and in rational therapy for chemical poisoning and treatment of disease. For example, the drug thalidomide was originally marketed in Europe and Australia as a sedative agent for pregnant women. However, it was banned for clinical use in 1962 because of devastating birth defects that occurred if the drug was ingested during a critical period in pregnancy. But mechanistic studies over the past several decades have demonstrated that this drug may have a unique molecular mechanism of action that interferes with the expression of certain genes responsible for blood vessel formation (angiogenesis). With an understanding of this mechanism, thalidomide has been "rediscovered" as a valuable therapeutic agent that may be highly effective in the treatment of certain infectious diseases (eg, leprosy) and multiple myeloma. This provides an interesting example of how a highly toxic drug with selectivity toward a specific population (pregnant women) can be used relatively safely with proper precautions. Following its approval for therapeutic use in 1998, a program was established that required all clinicians, pharmacists, and patients who receive thalidomide to enroll in a specific program (System for Thalidomide Education and Prescribing Safety [STEPS]). The population at risk for the potential teratogenic effects of thalidomide (all women of childbearing age) was required to use 2 forms of birth control, and also have a negative pregnancy test within 24 hours of beginning therapy, and periodically thereafter. Among the patients registered with the STEPS program, 6000 were females of childbearing age. Remarkably, after 6 years of use, only 1 patient actually received thalidomide during her pregnancy. She initially tested negative at the beginning of therapy; on a subsequent test she was identified as positive, and the drug was stopped. The pregnancy ended up as a miscarriage (Uhl *et al.*, 2006). Thus, a clear understanding of mechanism of action led to the development of strict prescribing guidelines and patient monitoring, thereby allowing a potentially dangerous drug to be used safely and effectively to treat disease in tens of thousands of patients who would otherwise not have benefited from the therapeutic actions of the drug (Lary *et al.*, 1999).

In addition to aiding directly in the identification, treatment, and prevention of chemical toxicity, an understanding of the mechanisms of toxic action contributes to the knowledge of basic physiology, pharmacology, cell biology, and biochemistry. The advent of new technologies in molecular biology and genomics now provides mechanistic toxicologists with the tools to explore exactly how humans may differ from laboratory animals in their response to toxic substances. These same tools are also being utilized to identify individuals who are genetically susceptible to factors in the environment or respond differently to a chemical exposure. For example, a small percentage of the population genetically lacks the ability to detoxify the chemotherapeutic drug, 6-mercaptopurine, used in the treatment of some forms of leukemia. Young children with leukemia who are homozygous for this genetic trait (about 1 in 300) may experience serious toxic effects from a standard therapeutic dose of this drug (Weinshilboum *et al.*, 1999). Numerous genetic tests for polymorphisms in drug-metabolizing enzymes and transporters are now available that can identify genetically susceptible individuals in advance of pharmacological treatment (Eichelbaum *et al.*, 2006).

The development of new approaches to identifying associations between diseases or adverse outcomes and common genetic variants (polymorphisms) has changed from a focus on individual candidate genes to "genome-wide association studies" (GWAS). GWAS are based on a rapid scan of hundreds of thousands of specific genetic variants (markers called "tag SNP") across the genome of persons affected by a particular disorder or adverse-response phenotype and persons who are not affected, with robust statistical tests to identify associations between a specific genetic marker and the phenotype (eg, disease state or adverse drug response). These tools have resulted in the discovery of many "gene–environment interactions," including associations between adverse drug responses and particular genetic polymorphisms (Wang *et al.*, 2011). Moving from the single, "candidate gene" approach to genome-wide studies has led to the development of the relatively new fields of pharmacogenomics and toxicogenomics. These areas provide an exciting opportunity for mechanistic toxicologists to identify and protect genetically susceptible individuals from harmful environmental exposures, and to customize drug therapies that enhance efficacy and minimize toxicity, based on an individual's genetic makeup.

A *descriptive toxicologist* is concerned directly with toxicity testing, which provides information for safety evaluation and regulatory requirements. The appropriate toxicity tests (as described later in this chapter and other chapters) in cell culture systems or experimental animals are designed to yield information to evaluate risks posed to humans and the environment from exposure to specific chemicals. The concern may be limited to effects on humans, as in the case of drugs and food additives. Toxicologists in the chemical industry, however, must be concerned not only with the risk posed by a company's chemicals (insecticides, herbicides, solvents, etc) to humans but also with potential effects on fish, birds, and plants, as well as other factors that might disturb the balance of the ecosystem. Descriptive toxicology is of course not divorced from mechanistic studies, as such studies provide important clues to a chemical's mechanism of action, and thus contribute to the development of mechanistic toxicology through hypothesis generation. Such studies are also a key component of risk assessments that are used by regulatory toxicologists. The development of so-called omics technologies (genomics, transcriptomics, proteomics, metabonomics/metabolomics, etc) forms the basis of the subdiscipline of toxicogenomics. The application of these technologies to toxicity testing is in many ways "descriptive" in nature, yet affords great mechanistic insights into how chemicals produce their toxic effects. This exciting area of toxicology is discussed in more detail later in the chapter.

A *regulatory toxicologist* has the responsibility for deciding, on the basis of data provided by descriptive and mechanistic toxicologists, whether a drug or other chemical poses a sufficiently low risk (or, in the case of drugs, a favorable risk/benefit profile) to be marketed for a stated purpose or subsequent human or environmental exposure resulting from its use. The Food and Drug Administration (FDA) is responsible for allowing drugs, cosmetics, and food additives to be sold in the market according to the Federal Food, Drug and Cosmetic Act (FFDCA). The US Environmental Protection Agency (EPA) is responsible for regulating most other chemicals according to a variety of different legislative acts, including the Federal Insecticide, Fungicide and Rodenticide Act (FIFRA), the Toxic Substances Control Act (TSCA), the Resource Conservation and Recovery Act (RCRA), the Safe Drinking Water Act, and the Clean Air Act. In 1996, the US Congress passed the Food Quality Protection Act (FQPA) that fundamentally changed the pesticide and food safety laws to consider stricter safety standards particularly for infants and children, who were recognized as more susceptible to health effects of pesticides. The EPA is also responsible for enforcing the Comprehensive Environmental Response, Compensation and Liability Act (CERCLA, later revised as the Superfund Amendments Reauthorization Act [SARA]), more commonly called the Superfund Act. This regulation provides direction and financial support for the cleanup of waste sites that contain toxic chemicals that may present a risk to human health or the environment. The Occupational Safety and Health Administration (OSHA) of the Department of Labor was established to ensure that safe and healthful conditions exist in the workplace. The National Institute for Occupational Safety and Health (NIOSH) as part of the Centers for Disease Control and Prevention (CDC) in the Department of Health and Human Services (DHHS) is responsible for conducting research and making recommendations for the prevention of work-related injury and illness. The Consumer Product Safety Commission (CPSC) is responsible for protecting consumers from hazardous household substances, whereas the Department of Transportation (DOT) ensures that materials shipped in interstate commerce are labeled and packaged in a manner consistent with the degree of hazard they present. The Nuclear Regulatory Commission (NRC), established in 1974, regulates the civilian use of nuclear material to protect public health and safety, and the environment. Regulatory toxicologists are also involved in the establishment of standards for the amount of chemicals permitted in ambient air, industrial atmospheres, and drinking water, often integrating scientific information from basic descriptive and mechanistic toxicology studies with the principles and approaches used for risk assessment (see Chap. 4).

In addition to the above categories, there are other specialized areas of toxicology such as forensic, clinical, and environmental toxicology. *Forensic toxicology* is a hybrid of analytic chemistry and fundamental toxicological principles. It is concerned primarily with the medicolegal aspects of the harmful effects of chemicals on humans and animals. The expertise of forensic toxicologists is invoked primarily to aid in establishing the cause of death and determining its circumstances in a post-mortem investigation (see Chap. 31). *Clinical toxicology* designates an area of professional emphasis in the realm of medical science that is concerned with disease caused by or uniquely associated with toxic substances (see Chap. 32). Generally, clinical toxicologists are physicians who receive specialized training in emergency medicine and poison management. Efforts are directed at treating patients poisoned with drugs or other chemicals and at the development of new techniques to treat those intoxications. Public information about treatment and prevention is often provided through the national network of poison control centers. *Environmental toxicology* focuses on the impacts of chemical pollutants in the environment on biological organisms. Although toxicologists concerned with the effects of environmental pollutants on human health fit into this definition, it is most commonly associated with studies on the impacts of chemicals on nonhuman organisms such as fish, birds, terrestrial animals, and plants. *Ecotoxicology* is a specialized area within environmental toxicology that focuses more specifically on the impacts of toxic substances on population dynamics in an ecosystem. The transport, fate, and interactions of chemicals in the environment constitute a critical component of both environmental toxicology and ecotoxicology.

Toxicology and Society

Information from the toxicological sciences, gained by experience or research, has a growing influence on our personal lives as well as on human and environmental health across the globe. Knowledge about the toxicological effects of a compound affects consumer products, drugs, manufacturing processes, waste cleanup, regulatory action, civil disputes, and broad policy decisions. The expanding influence of toxicology on societal issues is accompanied by the responsibility to be increasingly sensitive to the ethical, legal, and social implications of toxicological research and testing.

The convergence of multiple elements has highlighted the evolving ethical dynamics of toxicology. First, experience and new discoveries in the biological sciences have emphasized our interconnectedness with nature and the need for well-articulated visions of human, animal, and environmental health. One vision is that we have "condition(s) that ensure that all living things have the best opportunity to reach and maintain their full genetic potential" (Gilbert, 2005a). Second, we have experience with the health consequences of exposure to such things as lead, asbestos, and tobacco, along with the detailed mechanistic research to understand the long-term risks to individuals and society. This has precipitated many regulatory and legal actions and public policy decisions, not to mention costly and time-consuming lawsuits. Third, we have an increasingly well-defined framework for discussing our social and ethical responsibilities. There is growing recognition that ethics play a crucial role in public health decision making that involves conflicts between individual, corporate, and social justice goals (Callahan and Jennings, 2002; Kass, 2001; Lee, 2002). Fourth is the appreciation that all research involving humans or animals must be conducted in a responsible and ethical manner. Fifth is managing both the uncertainty and biological variability inherent in the biological sciences. Decision making often includes making judgments with limited or uncertain information, which often includes an overlay of individual values and ethics. Finally, individuals involved in toxicological research must be aware of and accountable to their own individual biases and possible conflicts of interest and adhere to the highest ethical standards of the profession (Maurissen *et al.*, 2005; Coble *et al.*, 2009; Gilbert and Eaton, 2009).

Ethical reasoning and philosophy has a long and deep history, but more pragmatic bioethical reasoning can be traced to Leopold, who is arguably America's first bioethicist: "A thing is right when it tends to preserve the integrity, stability, and beauty of the biotic community. It is wrong when it tends otherwise" (Leopold, 1949). The essence of toxicology is to understand the effects of chemicals on the biotic community. This broader definition of an ethic became more focused with examples such as the mercury poisoning in Minamata Bay, Japan, thalidomide, and the effects of pesticides as brought to public awareness by Carson's *Silent Spring* (Carson, 1962). In the United States, these events supported the public and political will to establish the EPA and strengthen the FDA and other regulations designed to protect human and environmental health. The knowledge that some segments of our society were deferentially at risk from chemical exposures evolved into an appreciation of environmental justice (Corburn, 2002; EPA, 2005; Lee, 2002; Morello-Frosch *et al.*, 2002). The EPA defines environmental justice as "the fair treatment and meaningful involvement of all people regardless of race, color, national origin, or income with respect to the development, implementation, and enforcement of environmental laws, regulations, and policies…" (EPA, 2005). Environmental justice is now an important component of numerous community-based programs of interest, and is relevant to the field of toxicology (Nweke, 2011). There is growing recognition of the direct financial and indirect costs to individuals and society from environmental exposures that are not equally distributed across society (Landrigan *et al.*, 2002).

On a parallel track, biomedical ethics developed out of the lessons of World War II and related abuses of human subjects. The 4 principle of biomedical ethics—respect for autonomy, beneficence (do good), nonmaleficence (do no harm), and justice (be fair)—became well established as a basis for decision making in health care settings (Beauchamp and Childress, 1994). These principles formed the basis of rules and regulations regarding the conduct of human research. The demands of ethics and science made it clear that the highest standards of care produced the best results in both human and animal research. Rules and regulations regarding the housing and conduct of animal studies evolved similarly. Professional toxicology societies now require their members to adhere to the highest ethical standards when conducting research with humans or animals. A further refinement and expansion of biomedical ethical principles is the development of community-based participatory research that takes into consideration community needs to ensure the best results and benefit to the community (Arcury *et al.*, 2001; Gilbert, 2006; O'Fallon and Dearry, 2002).

A glance at the daily newspaper confirms the number of current, sometimes controversial issues that are relevant to the field of toxicology. Decisions and action are often demanded or required even when there is a certain level of uncertainty in the toxicological data. The classic example of this challenge is establishing causation of the health effects of tobacco products. In part to address issues related to the health effects of tobacco products, Hill, a distinguished epidemiologist, defined a set of guidelines for evaluating "causation"—for example, whether a causal connection between a particular "exposure" and a particular outcome, condition, or disease can be scientifically established (Hill, 1965). These criteria are briefly summarized as follows:

1. Strength of association (relationship between independent and dependent variables)
2. Consistency of findings (replication of results by different studies)
3. Biological gradient (strength of the dose–response relationship)
4. Temporal sequence ("cause" before effect)
5. Biological or theoretical plausibility (mechanism of action)
6. Coherence with established knowledge (no competing hypotheses)
7. Specificity of association (cause is tightly linked to an outcome)

Although the guidelines provided by Hill were originally designed for interpretation of epidemiological data, they are equally applicable to establishing causation in toxicology, which often relies on a mix of both epidemiological and toxicological data.

Quantitative risk assessment was developed in part to address issues of uncertainty related to potential harm. The risk assessment process summarizes data for risk managers and other decision makers, who must take into consideration to some degree the qualitative elements of ethical, social, and political issues. Whereas risk management clearly has an ethical and values-based aspect, risk assessment is not immune from the influence of one's values, bias, or perspective. Ultimately action is required and as Hill (1965) noted: "All scientific work is incomplete—whether it be observational or experimental. All scientific work is liable to be upset or modified by advancing knowledge. That does not confer upon us a freedom to ignore the knowledge we already have or postpone the action that it appears to demand at a given time." These so-called Bradford Hill criteria were developed largely as a "weight-of-evidence" approach for interpreting a body of epidemiology data, yet are relevant as well to toxicology. Guzelian *et al.* (2005) provided a more detailed, evidence-based approach for determining causation in toxicology, primarily for application in the legal arena.

Although the scientific data may be the same, there are substantial differences in how toxicological data are used in a regulatory framework to protect public health versus establishing individual causation in the courtroom (Eaton, 2003). The approach to regulatory decision making is in part directed by policy. For example, the experience with thalidomide and other drugs motivated the US Congress to give the FDA broad power to ensure the efficacy and safety of new medicines or medical procedures. In this situation the pharmaceutical company or proponents of an activity must invest in the appropriate animal and human studies to demonstrate safety of the product. In general, a relatively precautionary approach has historically been taken with regard to drugs and medical devices. The approach to industrial chemicals is defined by the Toxic Substance Control Act and does not stipulate such a rigorous approach when introducing a new chemical into commerce.

Building on the work of Hill and others particularly from Europe, the Precautionary Principle was defined at the Wingspread Conference, in 1998: "When an activity raises threats of harm to human health or the environment, precautionary measures should be taken even if some cause and effect relationships are not fully established scientifically" (Gilbert, 2005b; Myers and Raffensperger, 2006; Raffensperger and Tickner, 1999). The precautionary principle incorporates elements of science and ethical philosophy into a single statement, acknowledging that ethics and values are part of the decision-making process. Although the conceptual value of the precautionary principle to public health protection is obvious, its actual implementation in toxicological risk assessment is not straightforward, and remains a point of considerable debate (Marchant, 2003; Goldstein, 2006; Peterson, 2006). The challenge remains to develop a regulatory environment that is responsive to issues of public health and the stewardship of societal resources (Simon, 2011).

With the increased relevance of toxicological data and evaluation in issues fundamental to society, there has been increased awareness of the possibility of conflicts of interest influencing the decision-making process (Maurissen *et al.*, 2005). The disclosure of conflicts of interest as well as the development of appropriate guidelines continues to be a challenge (NAS, 2003; Goozner, 2004; Krimsky and Rothenberg, 2001). These issues go to the core of one's individual values and integrity in the interpretation and communication of research results. Many professional societies, including the Society of Toxicology (http://www.toxicology.org/ai/asot/ethics.asp), have developed codes of ethics for their members. Conflict of interest has also been addressed by most publishers of toxicology journals (Krimsky and Sweet, 2009).

Table 2-1

Approximate Acute LD$_{50}$s of Some Representative Chemical Agents

AGENT	LD$_{50}$ (mg/kg)*
Ethyl alcohol	10,000
Sodium chloride	4000
Ferrous sulfate	1500
Morphine sulfate	900
Phenobarbital sodium	150
Picrotoxin	5
Strychnine sulfate	2
Nicotine	1
D-Tubocurarine	0.5
Hemicholinium-3	0.2
Tetrodotoxin	0.10
Dioxin (TCDD)	0.001
Botulinum toxin	0.00001

*LD$_{50}$ is the dosage (mg/kg body weight) causing death in 50% of exposed animals.

As the field of toxicology has matured and its influence on societal issues has increased, so has the need for the profession to make a commitment to examine the ethical, legal, and social implications of research and practice of toxicology.

General Characteristics of the Toxic Response

One could define a poison as any agent capable of producing a deleterious response in a biological system, seriously injuring function or producing death. This is not, however, a useful working definition for the very simple reason that virtually every known chemical has the potential to produce injury or death if it is present in a sufficient amount. Paracelsus (1493–1541), a Swiss/German/Austrian physician, scientist, and philosopher, phrased this well when he noted, "What is there that is not poison? All things are poison and nothing [is] without poison. Solely the dose determines that a thing is not a poison."

Among chemicals there is a wide spectrum of doses needed to produce deleterious effects, serious injury, or death. This is demonstrated in Table 2-1, which shows the dosage of chemicals needed to produce death in 50% of treated animals (lethal dose 50 [LD$_{50}$]). Some chemicals produce death in microgram doses and are commonly thought of as being extremely poisonous. Other chemicals may be relatively harmless after doses in excess of several grams. It should be noted, however, that measures of acute lethality such as LD$_{50}$ do not accurately reflect the full spectrum of toxicity, or hazard, associated with exposure to a chemical. For example, some chemicals with low acute toxicity may have carcinogenic, teratogenic, or neurobehavioral effects at doses that produce no evidence of acute toxicity. In addition, there is growing recognition that genetic factors can account for individual susceptibility to a range of responses. Finally, it should be recognized that, for a given chemical, multiple different effects can occur in a given organism, each with its own "dose–response relationship." In some circumstances, effects that occur at low doses may not be evident at higher doses because other adverse responses overwhelm or mask more subtle effects that may occur at low doses. Although some have argued that such low-dose effects, not seen at higher doses, make the classical interpretation of the "dose–response" relationship no longer relevant, such low-dose effects also follow their own "dose–response" relationship, but with a "saturation" of the effect occurring at higher doses that induces other molecular, biochemical, and cellular effects that tend to obscure the effects seen at lower doses. The effects of exogenous chemicals that bind to and activate or inhibit endogenous hormone receptors (so-called endocrine disruptors—see Chap. 21) may often have "low-dose" effects that are quite different from those seen at much higher doses.

CLASSIFICATION OF TOXIC AGENTS

Toxic agents are classified in a variety of ways, depending on the interests and needs of the classifier. In this textbook, for example, toxic agents are discussed in terms of their target organs (liver, kidney, hematopoietic system, etc), use (pesticide, solvent, food additive, etc), source (animal and plant toxins), and effects (cancer, mutation, liver injury, etc). The term *toxin* generally refers to toxic substances that are produced by biological systems such as plants, animals, fungi, or bacteria. The term *toxicant* is used in speaking of toxic substances that are produced by or are a by-product of anthropogenic (human-made) activities. Thus, zearalenone, produced by a mold, is a toxin, whereas "dioxin" (2,3,7,8-tetrachlorodibenzo-*p*-dioxin [TCDD]), produced during the production and/or combustion of certain chlorinated organic chemicals, is a toxicant. Some toxicants can be produced by both natural and anthropogenic activities. For example, polyaromatic hydrocarbons are produced by the combustion of organic matter, which may occur both through natural processes (eg, forest fires) and through anthropogenic activities (eg, combustion of coal for energy production; cigarette smoking). Arsenic, a toxic metalloid, may occur as a natural contaminant of groundwater or may contaminate groundwater secondary to industrial activities. Generally, such toxic substances are referred to as toxicants, rather than toxins, because, although they are naturally produced, they are not produced by biological systems. Distinguishing a "toxin" from a "toxicant" is not always easy. For example, many pesticides, such as the pyrethroids, are synthetic analogs of natural products, such that one would call the pyrethrum found in the chrysanthemum flower a "toxin," but the synthetic (and slightly altered in structure) form produced for use in pesticide formulations would be a "toxicant." Thus, although technically incorrect, many physicians and others involved in the diagnosis and treatment of poisonings often use the term "toxin" to refer to any toxic substance, regardless of origin.

Toxic agents may also be classified in terms of their physical state (gas, dust, liquid, size, eg, nanotoxicology), their chemical stability or reactivity (explosive, flammable, oxidizer), general chemical structure (aromatic amine, halogenated hydrocarbon, etc), or poisoning potential (extremely toxic, very toxic, slightly toxic, etc). Classification of toxic agents on the basis of their biochemical mechanisms of action (eg, alkylating agent, cholinesterase inhibitor, endocrine disruptor) is usually more informative than classification by general terms such as irritants and corrosives. But more general classifications such as air pollutants, occupation-related agents, and acute and chronic poisons can provide a useful focus on a specific problem. It is evident from this discussion that no single classification is applicable to the entire spectrum of toxic agents and that a combination of classification systems or a classification based on other factors is generally needed to provide the best characterization of a toxic substance. Nevertheless, classification systems that take into consideration both the chemical and the biological properties of an agent and the exposure characteristics are most likely to be useful for regulatory or control purposes and for toxicology in general.

SPECTRUM OF UNDESIRED EFFECTS

The spectrum of undesired effects of chemicals is often broad. Some effects are deleterious and others are not. In therapeutics, for example, each drug produces a number of effects, but usually only one effect is associated with the primary objective of the therapy; all the other effects are referred to as *undesirable* or *side effects* of that drug for that therapeutic indication. However, some of these side effects may be desired for another therapeutic indication. For example, the "first-generation" antihistamine diphenhydramine (Benadryl) is effective in reducing histamine responses associated with allergies, but it readily enters the brain and causes mild central nervous system (CNS) depression (drowsiness, delayed reaction time). With the advent of selective histamine receptor antagonists that do not cross the blood–brain barrier and thus do not have this CNS-depressant side effect, diphenhydramine is used less commonly today as an antihistamine. However, it is widely used as an "over-the-counter" sleep remedy, often in combination with analgesics (eg, Tylenol PM, Excedrin PM), taking advantage of the CNS-depressant effects. Some side effects of drugs are never desirable and are always deleterious to the well-being of humans. These are referred to as the *adverse, deleterious,* or *toxic* effects of the drug.

Allergic Reactions

Chemical allergy is an immunologically mediated adverse reaction to a chemical resulting from previous sensitization to that chemical or to a structurally similar one. The term *hypersensitivity* is most often used to describe this allergic state, but *allergic reaction* and *sensitization reaction* are also used to describe this situation when preexposure of the chemical is required to produce the toxic effect (see Chap. 12). Once sensitization has occurred, allergic reactions may result from exposure to relatively very low doses of chemicals; therefore, population-based dose–response curves for allergic reactions have seldom been obtained. Because of this omission, some people assumed that allergic reactions are not dose-related. Thus, they do not consider the allergic reaction to be a true toxic response. However, for a given allergic individual, allergic reactions are dose-related. For example, it is well known that the allergic response to pollen in sensitized individuals is related to the concentration of pollen in the air. In addition, because the allergic response is an undesirable, adverse, deleterious effect, it obviously is also a toxic response. Sensitization reactions are sometimes very severe and may be fatal.

Most chemicals and their metabolic products are not sufficiently large to be recognized by the immune system as a foreign substance and thus must first combine with an endogenous protein to form an antigen (or immunogen). A molecule that must combine with an endogenous protein to elicit an allergic reaction is called a *hapten*. The hapten–protein complex (antigen) is then capable of eliciting the formation of antibodies, and usually at least one or two weeks is required for the synthesis of significant amounts of antibodies. Subsequent exposure to the chemical results in an antigen–antibody interaction, which provokes the typical manifestations of allergy. The manifestations of allergy are numerous.

They may involve various organ systems and range in severity from minor skin disturbance to fatal anaphylactic shock. The pattern of allergic response differs in various species. In humans, involvement of the skin (eg, dermatitis, urticaria, and itching) and involvement of the eyes (eg, conjunctivitis) are most common, whereas in guinea pigs, bronchiolar constriction leading to asphyxia is the most common. However, chemically induced asthma (characterized by bronchiolar constriction) certainly does occur in some humans, and the incidence of allergic asthma has increased substantially in recent years. Hypersensitivity reactions are discussed in more detail in Chap. 12.

Idiosyncratic Reactions

Chemical idiosyncrasy refers to a genetically determined abnormal reactivity to a chemical (Goldstein *et al.*, 1974; Levine, 1978; Uetrecht, 2007). The response observed is usually qualitatively similar to that observed in all individuals but may take the form of extreme sensitivity to low doses or extreme insensitivity to high doses of the chemical. However, while some people use the term *idiosyncratic* as a catchall to refer to all reactions that occur with low frequency, it should not be used in that manner (Goldstein *et al.*, 1974). A classic example of an idiosyncratic reaction is provided by patients who exhibit prolonged muscular relaxation and apnea (inability to breathe) lasting several hours after a standard dose of succinylcholine. Succinylcholine usually produces skeletal muscle relaxation of only short duration because of its very rapid metabolic degradation by an enzyme that is present normally in the bloodstream called plasma butyrylcholinesterase (also referred to as pseudocholinesterase). Patients exhibiting this idiosyncratic reaction have a genetic polymorphism in the gene for the enzyme butyrylcholinesterase, which results in a protein that is less active in breaking down succinylcholine. Family pedigree and molecular genetic analyses have demonstrated that the presence of low plasma butyrylcholinesterase activity is due to the presence of one or more single-nucleotide polymorphisms (SNPs) in this gene (Bartels *et al.*, 1992). Similarly, there is a group of people who are abnormally sensitive to nitrites and certain other chemicals that have in common the ability to oxidize the iron in hemoglobin to produce *methemoglobin,* which is incapable of carrying oxygen to the tissues. The unusual phenotype is inherited as an autosomal recessive trait and is characterized by a deficiency in NADH-cytochrome b_5 reductase activity. The genetic basis for this idiosyncratic response has been identified as a single nucleotide change in codon 127, which results in replacement of serine with proline (Kobayashi *et al.*, 1990). The consequence of this genetic deficiency is that these individuals may suffer from a serious lack of oxygen delivery to tissues after exposure to doses of methemoglobin-producing chemicals that would be harmless to individuals with normal NADH-cytochrome b_5 reductase activity.

It is now recognized that many of the so-called idiosyncratic adverse drug reactions and many drug–drug interactions are due to specific genetic polymorphisms in drug-metabolizing enzymes, transporters, or receptors. As discussed previously, the growing field of pharmacogenomics and toxicogenomics has helped to identify the molecular basis for many previously described idiosyncratic responses to drugs and other toxic substances (Wang *et al.*, 2011). However, not all "idiosyncratic" responses to toxic substances are easily described by a single genetic polymorphism in a drug-metabolizing enzyme. It is generally thought that most, but not all, idiosyncratic drug responses are due to a combination of individual differences in the ability to: (1) form a reactive intermediate (usually through oxidation to an electrophilic intermediate), (2) detoxify that reactive intermediate (usually through hydrolysis or conjugation), and/or (3) exhibit differences in immune response to adducted proteins (Uetrecht, 2007). The role of the immune system in mediating rare drug-induced toxic reactions in the liver, skin, and other organ systems is widely recognized, and specific genetic variants in certain parts of the genome that code for the major histocompatibility complexes (MHCs) give rise to specific immune responses to proteins that have been damaged by reactive intermediates of certain drugs. Thus, it is only the individuals who genetically form sufficient amounts of a reactive drug metabolite, *and* who then have an immune response to the modified protein, who have an adverse response to the drug (Uetrecht, 2007).

For example, troglitazone, introduced into the marketplace in 1997 as an effective treatment for type II diabetes, was subsequently withdrawn from the market because of a relatively rare (1 adverse response per 30,000 patients) but often fatal hepatotoxic response. Subsequent studies of tissues from patients who had developed hepatotoxic responses at the normal therapeutic doses revealed that individuals who lacked functional genes for 2 forms of glutathione *S*-transferase (GSTM1 and GSTT1) were more than 3 times as likely to develop troglitazone-induced hepatotoxicity than individuals with 1 or more functional GSTM1 or T1 genes (Ikeda, 2011). However, this does not explain the rarity of the adverse response, since there were many individuals who lacked GSTM1 and T1 genes who took troglitazone with no evident hepatotoxicity. Further studies have suggested that the idiosyncratic hepatotoxicity from troglitazone also has an immune system component, and genetic differences in specific human lymphocyte antigen (HLA) loci might contribute to idiosyncratic drug-induced hepatotoxicity (Ikeda, 2011).

Immediate versus Delayed Toxicity

Immediate toxic effects can be defined as those that occur or develop rapidly after a single administration of a substance, whereas delayed toxic effects are those that occur after the lapse of some time. Carcinogenic effects of chemicals usually have a long latency period, often 20 to 30 years after the initial exposure, before tumors are observed in humans. For example, daughters of mothers who took diethylstilbestrol (DES) during pregnancy have a greatly increased risk of developing vaginal cancer, in young adulthood, approximately 20 to 30 years after their in utero exposure to DES (Hatch *et al.*, 1998). Also, delayed neurotoxicity is observed after exposure to some OP insecticides that act by covalent modification of an enzyme referred to as *neuropathy target esterase* (NTE), a neuronal protein with serine esterase activity (Glynn *et al.*, 1999). Binding of certain OP chemicals to this protein initiates degeneration of long axons in the peripheral and CNS. The most notorious of the compounds that produce this type of neurotoxic effect is triorthocresylphosphate (TOCP). The effect is not observed until at least several days after exposure to the toxic compound. In contrast, most substances produce immediate toxic effects but do not produce delayed effects.

Reversible versus Irreversible Toxic Effects

Some toxic effects of chemicals are reversible, and others are irreversible. If a chemical produces pathological injury to a tissue, the ability of that tissue to regenerate largely determines whether the effect is reversible or irreversible. Thus, for a tissue such as liver, which has a high ability to regenerate, most injuries are reversible, whereas injury to the CNS is largely irreversible because differentiated cells of the CNS cannot divide and be replaced (although recovery from chemically induced damage to the CNS can occur,

primarily through the "plasticity" of the brain that allows developed neurons to learn new functions; see Chap. 16). Carcinogenic and teratogenic effects of chemicals, once they occur, are usually considered irreversible toxic effects.

Local versus Systemic Toxicity

Another distinction between types of effects is made on the basis of the general site of action. Local effects are those that occur at the site of first contact between the biological system and the toxicant. Such effects are produced by the ingestion of caustic substances or the inhalation of irritant materials. For example, chlorine gas reacts with lung tissue at the site of contact, causing damage and swelling of the tissue, with possibly fatal consequences, even though very little of the chemical is absorbed into the bloodstream. The alternative to local effects is systemic effects. Systemic effects require absorption and distribution of a toxicant from its entry point to a distant site at which deleterious effects are produced. Most substances except highly reactive materials produce systemic effects. For some materials, both effects can be demonstrated. For example, tetraethyl lead produces effects on skin at the site of absorption and then is transported systemically to produce its typical effects on the CNS and other organs. If the local effect is marked, there may also be indirect systemic effects. For example, kidney damage after a severe acid burn is an indirect systemic effect because the toxicant does not reach the kidney.

Most chemicals that produce systemic toxicity do not cause a similar degree of toxicity in all organs; instead, they usually elicit their major toxicity in only 1 or 2 organs. These sites are referred to as the *target organs* of toxicity of a particular chemical. The target organ of toxicity is often not the site of the highest concentration of the chemical. For example, lead is concentrated in bone, but its toxicity is due to its effects in soft tissues, particularly the brain. DDT is concentrated in adipose tissue but produces no known toxic effects in that tissue.

The target organ of toxicity most frequently involved in systemic toxicity is the CNS (brain and spinal cord). Even with many compounds having a prominent effect elsewhere, damage to the CNS can be demonstrated by the use of appropriate and sensitive methods. Next in order of frequency of involvement in systemic toxicity are the circulatory system; the blood and hematopoietic system; visceral organs such as the liver, kidney, and lung; and the skin. Muscle and bone are least often the target tissues for systemic effects. With substances that have a predominantly local effect, the frequency with which tissues react depends largely on the portal of entry (skin, gastrointestinal tract, or respiratory tract).

Interaction of Chemicals

Because of the large number of different chemicals an individual may come in contact with at any given time (workplace, drugs, diet, hobbies, etc), it is necessary, in assessing the spectrum of responses, to consider how different chemicals may interact with each other. Interactions can occur in a variety of ways. Chemical interactions are known to occur by a number of mechanisms, such as alterations in absorption, protein binding, and the biotransformation and excretion of 1 or both of the interacting toxicants. In addition to these modes of interaction, the response of the organism to combinations of toxicants may be increased or decreased because of toxicological responses at the site of action.

The effects of 2 chemicals given simultaneously produce a response that may simply be additive of their individual responses or may be greater or less than that expected by addition of their individual responses. The study of these interactions often leads to a better understanding of the mechanism of toxicity of the chemicals involved. A number of terms have been used to describe pharmacological and toxicological interactions. An *additive* effect occurs when the combined effect of 2 chemicals is equal to the sum of the effects of each agent given alone (eg, 2 + 3 = 5). The effect most commonly observed when 2 chemicals are given together is an additive effect. For example, when 2 OP insecticides are given together, the cholinesterase inhibition is usually additive. A *synergistic* effect occurs when the combined effects of 2 chemicals are much greater than the sum of the effects of each agent given alone (eg, 2 + 2 = 20). For example, both carbon tetrachloride and ethanol are hepatotoxic compounds, but together they produce much more liver injury than the mathematical sum of their individual effects on liver at a given dose would suggest. *Potentiation* occurs when 1 substance does not have a toxic effect on a certain organ or system but when added to another chemical makes that chemical much more toxic (eg, 0 + 2 = 10). Isopropanol, for example, is not hepatotoxic, but when it is administered in addition to carbon tetrachloride, the hepatotoxicity of carbon tetrachloride is much greater than when it is given alone. *Antagonism* occurs when 2 chemicals administered together interfere with each other's actions or 1 interferes with the action of the other (eg, 4 + 6 = 8; 4 + (−4) = 0; 4 + 0 = 1). Antagonistic effects of chemicals are often very desirable in toxicology and are the basis of many antidotes. There are 4 major types of antagonism: functional, chemical, dispositional, and receptor. *Functional antagonism* occurs when 2 chemicals counterbalance each other by producing opposite effects on the same physiological function. For example, advantage is taken of this principle in that the blood pressure can markedly fall during severe barbiturate intoxication, which can be effectively antagonized by the intravenous administration of a vasopressor agent such as norepinephrine or metaraminol. Similarly, many chemicals, when given at toxic dose (TD) levels, produce convulsions, and the convulsions often can be controlled by giving anticonvulsants such as the benzodiazepines (eg, diazepam). *Chemical antagonism or inactivation* is simply a chemical reaction between 2 compounds that produces a less toxic product. For example, 2,3-dimercaptosuccinic acid (DMSA; Succimer) chelates with metal ions such as arsenic, mercury, and lead and decreases their toxicity. The use of antitoxins in the treatment of various animal toxins is also an example of chemical antagonism. The use of the strongly basic low-molecular-weight protein protamine sulfate to form a stable complex with heparin, which abolishes its anticoagulant activity, is another example. *Dispositional antagonism* occurs when the disposition—that is, the absorption, distribution, biotransformation, or excretion of a chemical—is altered so that the concentration and/or duration of the chemical at the target organ are diminished. Thus, the prevention of absorption of a toxicant by ipecac or charcoal and the increased excretion of a chemical by administration of an osmotic diuretic or alteration of the pH of the urine are examples of dispositional antagonism. If the parent compound is responsible for the toxicity of the chemical (such as the anticoagulant warfarin) and its metabolic breakdown products are less toxic than the parent compound, increasing the compound's biotransformation (metabolism) by administering a drug that increases the activity of the metabolizing enzymes (eg, a "microsomal enzyme inducer" such as phenobarbital) will decrease its toxicity. However, if the chemical's toxicity is largely due to a metabolic product (as in the case of the organophosphate insecticide parathion), inhibiting its biotransformation by an inhibitor of microsomal enzyme activity (SKF-525A or piperonyl butoxide) will decrease its toxicity. *Receptor antagonism* occurs when 2 chemicals that bind to the same receptor produce less of an effect when given together than the addition of their separate effects

(eg, 4 + 6 = 8) or when 1 chemical antagonizes the effect of the second chemical (eg, 0 + 4 = 1). Receptor antagonists are often termed *blockers*. This concept is used to advantage in the clinical treatment of poisoning. For example, the receptor antagonist naloxone is used to treat the respiratory depressive effects of morphine and other morphine-like narcotics by competitive binding to the same receptor. Another example of receptor antagonism is the use of the antiestrogen drug tamoxifen to lower breast cancer risk among women at high risk for this estrogen-related cancer. Tamoxifen competitively blocks estradiol from binding to its receptor. Treatment of organophosphate insecticide poisoning with atropine is an example not of the antidote competing with the poison for the receptor (cholinesterase) but of blocking the receptor (cholinergic receptor) for the excess acetylcholine that accumulates by poisoning of the cholinesterase by the organophosphate (see Chap. 22).

Tolerance

Tolerance is a state of decreased responsiveness to a toxic effect of a chemical resulting from prior exposure to that chemical or to a structurally related chemical. Two major mechanisms are responsible for tolerance: 1 is due to a decreased amount of toxicant reaching the site where the toxic effect is produced (*dispositional tolerance*) and the other is due to a reduced responsiveness of a tissue to the chemical. Comparatively less is known about the cellular mechanisms responsible for altering the responsiveness of a tissue to a toxic chemical than is known about dispositional tolerance. Two chemicals known to produce dispositional tolerance are carbon tetrachloride and cadmium. The barbiturate, phenobarbital, produces tolerance to itself by increasing the expression of enzymes in the liver that are responsible for its biotransformation to pharmacologically inactive products, a process known as "biotransformation enzyme induction." The mechanism of cadmium tolerance is explained by induction of metallothionein, a metal-binding protein. Subsequent binding of cadmium to metallothionein rather than to critical cellular macromolecules decreases its toxicity.

CHARACTERISTICS OF EXPOSURE

Toxic effects in a biological system are not produced by a chemical agent unless that agent or its metabolic breakdown (biotransformation) products reach appropriate sites in the body at a concentration and for a length of time sufficient to produce a toxic manifestation. Many chemicals are of relatively low toxicity in the "native" form but, when acted on by enzymes in the body, are converted to intermediate forms that interfere with normal cellular biochemistry and physiology. Thus, whether a toxic response occurs is dependent on the chemical and physical properties of the agent, the exposure situation, how the agent is metabolized by the system, the concentration of the active form at the particular target site(s), and the overall susceptibility of the biological system or subject. Thus, to characterize fully the potential hazard of a specific chemical agent, we need to know not only what type of effect it produces and the dose required to produce that effect but also information about the agent, the exposure, and its disposition by the subject. Two major factors that influence toxicity as it relates to the exposure situation for a specific chemical are the route of exposure and the duration and frequency of exposure.

Route and Site of Exposure

The major routes (pathways) by which toxic agents gain access to the body are through the gastrointestinal tract (ingestion), the lungs (inhalation), or the skin (topical, percutaneous, or dermal). Toxic agents generally produce the greatest effect and the most rapid response when given directly into the bloodstream (the intravenous route). An approximate descending order of effectiveness for the other routes would be inhalation, intraperitoneal, subcutaneous, intramuscular, intradermal, oral, and dermal. The "vehicle" (the material in which the chemical is dissolved) and other formulation factors can markedly alter absorption after ingestion, inhalation, or topical exposure. In addition, the route of administration can influence the toxicity of agents. For example, an agent that acts on the CNS, but is efficiently detoxified in the liver, would be expected to be less toxic when given orally than when given via inhalation, because the oral route requires that nearly all of the dose pass through the liver before reaching the systemic circulation and then the CNS.

Occupational exposure to toxic agents most frequently results from breathing contaminated air (inhalation) and/or direct and prolonged contact of the skin with the substance (dermal exposure), whereas accidental and suicidal poisoning occurs most frequently by oral ingestion. Comparison of the toxic dose (TD) of a toxic substance by different routes of exposure often provides useful information about its extent of absorption. In instances when the TD after oral or dermal administration is similar to the TD after intravenous administration, the assumption is that the toxic agent is absorbed readily and rapidly. Conversely, in cases where the TD by the dermal route is several orders of magnitude higher than the oral TD, it is likely that the skin provides an effective barrier to absorption of the agent. Toxic effects by any route of exposure can also be influenced by the concentration of the agent in its vehicle, the total volume of the vehicle and the properties of the vehicle to which the biological system is exposed, and the rate at which exposure occurs. Studies in which the concentration of a chemical in the blood is determined at various times after exposure are often needed to clarify the role of these and other factors in the toxicity of a compound. For more details on the absorption of toxicants, see Chap. 5.

Duration and Frequency of Exposure

Toxicologists usually divide the exposure of experimental animals to chemicals into 4 categories: acute, subacute, subchronic, and chronic. Acute exposure is defined as exposure to a chemical for less than 24 hours, and examples of exposure routes are intraperitoneal, intravenous, and subcutaneous injection; oral intubation; and dermal application. Whereas acute exposure usually refers to a single administration, repeated exposures may be given within a 24-hour period for some slightly toxic or practically nontoxic chemicals. Acute exposure by inhalation refers to continuous exposure for less than 24 hours, most frequently for 4 hours. Repeated exposure is divided into 3 categories: subacute, subchronic, and chronic. *Subacute exposure* refers to repeated exposure to a chemical for 1 month or less, *subchronic* for 1 to 3 months, and *chronic* for more than 3 months, although usually this refers to studies with at least 1 year of repeated dosing. These 3 categories of repeated exposure can be by any route, but most often they occur by the oral route, with the chemical added directly to the diet.

In human exposure situations, the frequency and duration of exposure are usually not as clearly defined as in controlled animal studies, but many of the same terms are used to describe general exposure situations. Thus, workplace or environmental exposures may be described as *acute* (occurring from a single incident or episode), *subchronic* (occurring repeatedly over several weeks or months), or *chronic* (occurring repeatedly for many months or years).

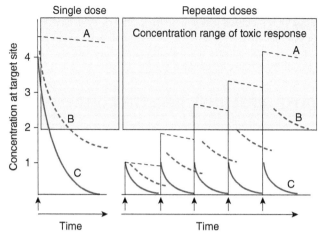

Figure 2-2. *Diagrammatic view of the relationship between dose and concentration at the target site under different conditions of dose frequency and elimination rate.* (Line A) A chemical with very slow elimination (eg, half-life of 1 year). (Line B) A chemical with a rate of elimination equal to frequency of dosing (eg, 1 day). (Line C) Rate of elimination faster than the dosing frequency (eg, 5 hours). Blue shaded area is representative of the concentration of chemical at the target site necessary to elicit a toxic response.

For many chemicals, the toxic effects that follow a single exposure are quite different from those produced by repeated exposure. For example, the primary acute toxic manifestation of benzene is CNS depression, but repeated exposures can result in bone marrow toxicity and an increased risk for leukemia. Acute exposure to chemicals that are rapidly absorbed is likely to produce immediate toxic effects but also can produce delayed toxicity that may or may not be similar to the toxic effects of chronic exposure. Conversely, chronic exposure to a toxic chemical may produce some immediate (acute) effects after each administration in addition to the long-term, low-level, or chronic effects of the toxic substance. In characterizing the toxicity of a specific chemical, it is evident that information is needed not only for the single-dose (acute) and long-term (chronic) effects but also for exposures of intermediate duration. The other time-related factor that is important in the temporal characterization of repeated exposures is the frequency of exposure. The relationship between elimination rate and frequency of exposure is shown in Fig. 2-2. A chemical that produces severe effects with a single dose may have no effect if the same total dose is given in several intervals. For the chemical depicted by line B in Fig. 2-2, in which the half-life for elimination (time necessary for 50% of the chemical to be removed from the bloodstream) is approximately equal to the dosing frequency, a theoretical toxic concentration (shown conceptually as 2 concentration units in Fig. 2-2) is not reached until the fourth dose, whereas that concentration is reached with only 2 doses for chemical A, which has an elimination rate much slower than the dosing interval (time between each repeated dose). Conversely, for chemical C, where the elimination rate is much shorter than the dosing interval, a toxic concentration at the site of toxic effect will never be reached regardless of how many doses are administered. Of course, it is possible that residual cell or tissue damage occurs with each dose even though the chemical itself is not accumulating. The important consideration, then, is whether the interval between doses is sufficient to allow for complete repair of tissue damage. It is evident that with any type of repeated exposure, the production of a toxic effect not only is influenced by the frequency of exposure but may also, in fact, be totally dependent on the frequency rather than the duration of exposure. Chronic toxic effects may occur, therefore, if the chemical accumulates in the biological system (rate of absorption exceeds the rate of biotransformation and/or excretion), if it produces irreversible toxic effects, or if there is insufficient time for the system to recover from the toxic damage within the exposure frequency interval. For additional discussion of these relationships, see Chaps. 5 and 7.

DOSE–RESPONSE RELATIONSHIP

The characteristics of exposure and the spectrum of toxic effects come together in a correlative relationship customarily referred to as the *dose–response relationship.* Whatever response is selected for measurement, the relationship between the degree of response of the biological system and the amount of toxicant administered assumes a form that occurs so consistently as to be considered the most fundamental and pervasive concept in toxicology.

From a practical perspective, there are 2 types of dose–response relationships: (1) the individual dose–response relationship, which describes the response of an *individual* organism to varying doses of a chemical, often referred to as a "graded" response because the measured effect is continuous over a range of doses, and (2) a quantal dose–response relationship, which characterizes the distribution of individual responses to different doses in a *population* of individual organisms. It is also important to recognize that a given chemical may have multiple different molecular, biochemical, and cellular effects, each with its own "dose–response" relationship. Thus, the nature of a toxic response might very well be different at low doses than at higher doses. In the case of population-level "dose–response" characterization, the observed response is an integration of multiple individual "dose–response relationships" occurring in different cell types, and at different molecular sites within those cells. Subtle effects that occur at low doses may be masked or overwhelmed by more evident responses occurring at higher doses.

Individual, or Graded, Dose–Response Relationships

Individual dose–response relationships are characterized by a dose-related increase in the severity of the response. The dose relatedness of the response often results from an alteration of a specific biochemical process. For example, Fig. 2-3 shows the dose–response relationship between different dietary doses of the organophosphate insecticide chlorpyrifos and the extent of inhibition of 2 different enzymes in the brain and liver: acetylcholinesterase and carboxylesterase. In the brain, the degree of inhibition of both enzymes is clearly dose-related and spans a wide range, although the amount of inhibition per unit dose is different for the 2 enzymes. From the shapes of these 2 dose–response curves it is evident that, in the brain, cholinesterase is more easily inhibited than carboxylesterase. The toxicological response that results is directly related to the degree of cholinesterase enzyme inhibition in the brain. Thus, clinical signs and symptoms for chlorpyrifos would follow a dose–response relationship similar to that for brain cholinesterase. However, as noted above, for many chemicals, more than 1 effect may result because of multiple different target sites in different tissues. Thus, the observed response to varying doses of a chemical in the whole organism is often complicated by the fact that most toxic substances have multiple sites or mechanisms of toxicity, each with its own "dose–response" relationship and subsequent adverse effect. Note that when these dose–response data are plotted using the base 10 log of the dose on the abscissa (Fig. 2.3B), a better "fit" of the data to a straight line usually occurs. This is typical of many graded as well as quantal dose–response relationships.

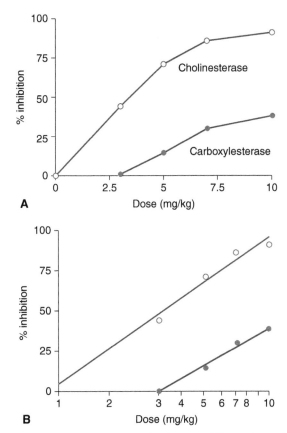

Figure 2-3. *Dose–response relationship between different doses of the organophosphate insecticide chlorpyrifos and esterase enzyme inhibition in the brain.* Open circles and blue lines represent acetylcholinesterase activity and closed circles represent carboxylesterase activity in the brains of pregnant female Long–Evans rats given 5 daily doses of chlorpyrifos. (**A**) Dose–response curve plotted on an arithmetic scale. (**B**) Same data plotted on a semi-log scale. (Data from Lassiter *et al.*, 1999, with permission.)

Quantal Dose–Response Relationships

In contrast to the "graded" or continuous-scale dose–response relationship that occurs in individuals, the dose–response relationships in a *population* are by definition quantal—or "all or none"—in nature, that is, at any given dose, an individual in the population is classified as either a "responder" or a "nonresponder." Although these distinctions of "quantal population" and "graded individual" dose–response relationships are useful, the 2 types of responses are conceptually identical. The ordinate in both cases is simply labeled *the response,* which may be the degree of response in an individual or system or the fraction of a population responding, and the abscissa is the range in administered doses.

A widely used statistical approach for estimating the response of a population to a toxic exposure is the "effective dose" (ED). Generally, the midpoint, or 50%, response level is used, giving rise to the "ED_{50}" value. However, any response level, such as an ED_{01}, ED_{10}, or ED_{30}, could be chosen. A graphical representation of an approximate ED_{50} is shown in Fig. 2-4. Note that these data are "quantal." Where death is the end point, the ED_{50} would be referred to as the LD_{50}. Historically, determination of the LD_{50} was often the first experiment performed with a new chemical. Today, it is widely recognized that the LD_{50} is of marginal value as a measure of hazard, although it does provide a useful "ball park" indication of the relative hazard of a compound to cause serious, life-threatening poisoning from a single exposure. Although death is an obvious quantal end point to measure, it should be noted that any

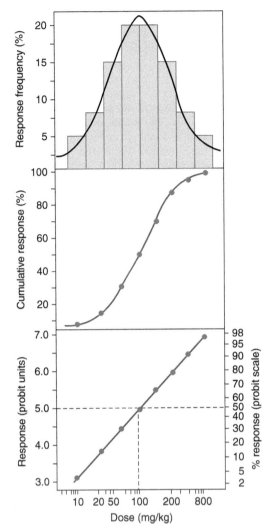

Figure 2-4. *Diagram of quantal dose–response relationship.* The abscissa is a log dosage of the chemical. In the top panel the ordinate is response frequency, in the middle panel the ordinate is percent response, and in the bottom panel the response is in probit units (see text).

differences in susceptibility to chemicals among individuals; this is known as biological variation. Animals responding at the left end of the curve are referred to as *hypersusceptible*, and those at the right end of the curve are called *resistant*. If the numbers of individuals responding at each consecutive dose are added together, a cumulative, quantal dose–response relationship is obtained. When a sufficiently large number of doses is used with a large number of animals per dose, a sigmoid dose–response curve is observed, as depicted in the middle panel of Fig. 2-4. With the lowest dose (6 mg/kg), 1% of the animals respond. A normally distributed sigmoid curve such as this one approaches a response of 0% as the dose is decreased and approaches 100% as the dose is increased, but—theoretically—it never passes through 0% and 100%. However, the minimally ED of any chemical that evokes a stated all-or-none response is called the *threshold dose* even though it cannot be determined experimentally.

For a normally distributed population response, the sigmoid curve has a relatively linear portion between 16% and 84%. These values represent the limits of 1 standard deviation (SD) of the mean (and the median) in a population with truly normal or Gaussian distribution. However, it is usually not practical to describe the dose–response curve from this type of plot because one does not usually have large enough sample sizes to define the sigmoid curve adequately. In a normally distributed population, the mean ±1 SD represents 68.3% of the population, the mean ±2 SD represents 95.5% of the population, and the mean ±3 SD equals 99.7% of the population. Because quantal dose–response phenomena are usually normally distributed, one can convert the percent response to units of deviation from the mean or normal equivalent deviations (NEDs). Thus, the NED for a 50% response is 0; an NED of +1 is equated with an 84.1% response. Traditionally, units of NED are converted by the addition of 5 to the value to avoid negative numbers; these converted units are called *probit units* (Bliss, 1957). The probit (from the contraction of *prob*ability un*it*), then, is an NED plus 5. In this transformation, a 50% response becomes a probit of 5, a +1 deviation becomes a probit of 6, and a −1 deviation is a probit of 4.

The data given in the top 2 panels of Fig. 2-4 are replotted in the bottom panel with the response plotted in probit units. The data in the middle panel (which was in the form of a sigmoid curve) and the top panel (a bell-shaped curve) form a straight line when transformed into probit units. In essence, what is accomplished in a probit transformation is an adjustment of quantal data to an assumed normal population distribution, resulting in a straight line. The ED_{50} is obtained by drawing a horizontal line from the probit unit 5, which is the 50% response point, to the dose–effect line. At the point of intersection, a vertical line is drawn, and this line intersects the abscissa at the ED_{50} point. It is evident from the line that information with respect to the ED for 90% or for 10% of the population also may be derived by a similar procedure. Mathematically, it can be demonstrated that the range of values encompassed by the confidence limits is narrowest at the midpoint of the line (ED_{50}) and widest at both extremes (ED_{10} and ED_{90}) of the dose–response curve (dotted lines in Fig. 2-5). In addition to the ED_{50}, the slope of the dose–response curve can also be obtained. Fig. 2-5 demonstrates the dose–response curves for the response of 2 compounds. Compound A exhibits a "flat" dose–response curve, showing that a large change in dosage is required before a significant change in response will be observed. However, compound B exhibits a "steep" dose–response curve, where a relatively small change in dosage will cause a large change in response. It is evident that the ED_{50} for both compounds is the same (8 mg/kg). However, the slopes of the dose–response curves are quite different. At one half of ED_{50} of the compounds (4 mg/kg), less than 1% of the animals exposed to compound B would respond but 20% of the animals given compound A would respond.

quantal response could be used. For example, the LD_{50} of lead or DDT is not a relevant end point when characterizing hazards of the agents to children or wildlife, respectively. Even continuous variables can be converted to quantal responses if desired. For example, an antihypertensive drug that lowers blood pressure might be evaluated in a population by assigning a "responder" as an individual whose blood pressure was lowered by 10 mm Hg or more. Note that, in this example, an individual who responded to a change in blood pressure of 50 mm Hg would classified the same as an individual with a change in only 10 mm Hg, yet an individual with a change in 8 mm Hg would be classified as a "nonresponder." The top panel of Fig. 2-4 shows that quantal dose responses typically exhibit a normal or Gaussian distribution. The frequency histogram in this panel also shows the relationship between dose and effect. The bars represent the percentage of animals that responded at each dose minus the percentage that responded at the immediately lower dose. One can clearly see that only a few animals responded to the lowest dose and the highest dose. Larger numbers of animals responded to doses intermediate between these 2 extremes, and the maximum frequency of response occurred in the middle portion of the dose range. Thus, we have a bell-shaped curve known as a *normal frequency distribution*. The reason for this normal distribution is that there are

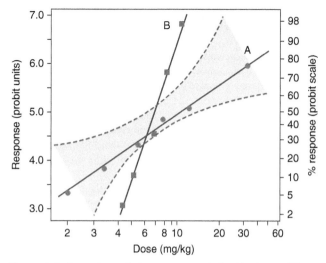

Figure 2-5. *Comparison of dose–response relationship for 2 different chemicals, plotted on a log dose-probit scale.* Note that the slope of the dose–response is steeper for chemical B than for chemical A. Dotted lines represent the confidence limits for chemical A.

In Figs. 2-4 and 2-5 the dosage has been given on a log basis. Although the use of the log of the dosage is empiric, log dosage plots for normally distributed quantal data provide a more nearly linear representation of the data. It must be remembered, however, that this is not universally the case. Some radiation effects, for example, give a better probit fit when the dose is expressed arithmetically rather than logarithmically. There are other situations in which other functions (eg, exponentials) of dosage provide a better fit to the data than does the log function. It is also conventional to express the dosage in milligrams per kilogram. It might be argued that expression of dosage on a mole-per-kilogram basis would be better, particularly for making comparisons among a series of compounds. Although such an argument has considerable merit, dosage is usually expressed in milligrams per kilogram.

One might also view dosage on the basis of body weight as being less appropriate than other bases, such as surface area. The term *allometry* refers to the field of study that examines the relationships between body weight and other biological and physical parameters such as rate of basal metabolism (caloric consumption), heart rate, blood flow, etc. Allometric studies revealed that the relationship between body weight and various other physiological parameters can be closely estimated by the following formula: $Y = aW^b$, where Y is the biological parameter of interest and a and b are constants that relate Y to body weight (Rodricks *et al.*, 2008). In general, organ sizes between species seem to scale best when b is equal to 1, whereas metabolically derived parameters scale better when b is 0.67 to 0.75. The relationship between body surface area and body weight across most mammalian species is closely described by the formula SA = 10.5 × (body weight [grams])$^{0.67}$ (Harkness and Wagner, 1995). Empirical comparisons of toxicity data across species confirm that this relationship is appropriate for toxicological scaling. For example, Travis and White (1988) analyzed a number of toxicity testing data sets for 27 different chemotherapeutic drugs for which toxicity data were available in mouse, rat, hamster, dog, monkey, and human. They found that the exponent of body weight that gave the best correlation with toxicity was 0.73, with 95% confidence bounds of 0.69 to 0.77 (Rodricks *et al.*, 2008). Table 2-2 illustrates the differences in comparative doses when scaling is done by body weight (mg/kg) versus an allometric approach that uses an exponent of either 0.67 or 0.75. Thus, if a scaling factor of (BW)$^{2/3}$ is used, a mouse would need to receive a dose 13 times greater than that required for humans for an equivalent toxic response, whereas the dose would be 7 times greater if a scaling factor of (BW)$^{3/4}$ was used. However, not all toxic responses will necessarily scale across species in the same way. For example, acute lethality seemed to correlate better across species when body weight, rather than body surface area, was used (Rhomberg and Wolff, 1998). The selection of the most appropriate scaling factor should also take into account pharmacokinetic differences, including physiologically based pharmacokinetic modeling (PBPK). When toxicity is attributable to the formation of a toxic metabolite, or when xenobiotic biotransformation is saturated at high doses, a scaling factor of 1 may be more appropriate than 0.75 (Kirman *et al.*, 2003).

Shape of the Dose–Response Curve

Essential Nutrients The shape of the dose–response relationship has many important implications in toxicity assessment. For example, for substances that are required for normal physiological

Table 2-2					
Allometric Scaling of Dose Across Different Species					
			FOLD DIFFERENCE, RELATIVE TO HUMANS, NORMALIZED BY BODY WEIGHT		
SPECIES	WEIGHT (kg)	SURFACE AREA (cm^2)*	mg/kg	(BW)$^{2/3}$	(BW)$^{3/4}$
Mouse	0.30	103	1	13.0	7.0
Rat	0.2	365	1	6.9	4.3
Guinea pig	0.4	582	1	5.5	3.6
Rabbit	1.5	1410	1	3.5	2.6
Cat	2	1710	1	3.2	2.4
Monkey	4	2720	1	2.6	2.0
Dog	12	5680	1	1.8	1.5
Human	70	18,500	1	1.0	1.0

*Surface area of animals is closely approximated by the following formula: SA = 10.5 × (body weight [grams])$^{2/3}$.

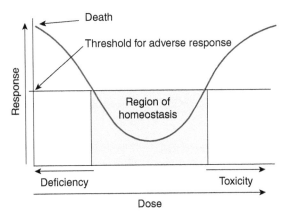

Figure 2-6. *Individual dose–response relationship for an essential substance such as a vitamin or trace element.* It is generally recognized that, for most types of toxic responses, a threshold exists such that at doses below the threshold, no toxicity is evident. For essential substances, doses below the minimum daily requirement, as well as those above the threshold for safety, may be associated with toxic effects. The blue shaded region represents the "region of homeostasis"—the dose range that results in neither deficiency nor toxicity.

function and survival (eg, vitamins and essential trace elements such as chromium, cobalt, and selenium), the "graded" dose–response relationship in an individual over the entire dose range is actually U-shaped (Fig. 2-6). That is, at very low doses, there is a high level of adverse effect, which decreases with an increasing dose. This region of the dose–response relationship for essential nutrients is commonly referred to as a *deficiency*. As the dose is increased to a point where the deficiency no longer exists, no adverse response is detected and the organism is in a state of homeostasis. However, as the dose is increased to abnormally high levels, an adverse response (usually qualitatively different from that observed at deficient doses) appears and increases in magnitude with increasing dose, just as with other toxic substances. Thus, it is recognized that high doses of vitamin A can cause liver toxicity and birth defects, high doses of selenium can affect the brain, and high doses of estrogens may increase the risk of breast cancer, even though low doses of all these substances are essential for life.

Hormesis There is considerable evidence to suggest that some nonnutritional toxic substances may also impart beneficial or stimulatory effects at low doses but that, at higher doses, they produce adverse effects. This concept of "hormesis" was first described for radiation effects but may also pertain to most chemical responses (Calabrese and Blaine, 2005). Thus, in plotting dose versus response over a wide range of doses, the effects of hormesis may also result in a "U-shaped" dose–response curve. In its original development, the concept of hormesis pertained to the ability of substances to stimulate biological systems at low doses but to inhibit them at high doses. The application of the concept of hormesis to whole-animal toxicological dose–response relationships may also be relevant but requires that the "response" on the ordinate be variant with dose. For example, chronic alcohol consumption is well recognized to increase the risk of esophageal cancer, liver cancer, and cirrhosis of the liver at relatively high doses, and this response is dose-related (curve A, Fig. 2-7). However, there is also substantial clinical and epidemiological evidence that low to moderate consumption of alcohol reduces the incidence of coronary heart disease and stroke (curve B, Fig. 2-7) (Hanna *et al.*, 1997). Thus, when all responses are plotted on the ordinate, a "U-shaped" dose–response curve is obtained (curve C, Fig. 2-7). U-shaped dose–response relationships

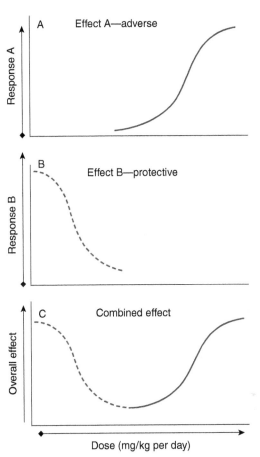

Figure 2-7. *Hypothetical dose–response relationship depicting characteristics of hormesis.* Hormetic effects of a substance are hypothesized to occur when relatively low doses result in the stimulation of a beneficial or protective response (**B**), such as induction of enzymatic pathways that protect against oxidative stress. Although low doses provide a potential beneficial effect, a threshold is exceeded as the dose increases and the net effects will be detrimental (**A**), resulting in a typical dose-related increase in toxicity. The complete dose–response curve (**C**) is conceptually similar to the individual dose–response relationship for essential nutrients shown in Fig. 2-6.

have obvious implications for the process of low-dose extrapolation in risk assessment.

Threshold Another important aspect of the dose–response relationship at low doses is the concept of the threshold. It has long been recognized that acute toxicological responses are associated with thresholds, that is, there is some dose below which the probability of an individual responding is zero. Obviously, the identification of a threshold depends on the particular response that is measured, the sensitivity of the measurement, and the number of subjects studied. For the individual dose–response relationship, thresholds for most toxic effects certainly exist, although interindividual variability in response and qualitative changes in response pattern with dose make it difficult to establish a true "no effects" threshold for any chemical. The biological basis of thresholds for acute responses is well established and frequently can be demonstrated on the basis of mechanistic information (Aldridge, 1986). The traditional approaches to establishing acceptable levels of exposure to chemicals are inherently different for threshold versus nonthreshold responses. The existence of thresholds for chronic responses is less well defined, especially in the area of chemical carcinogenesis. It is, of course, impossible to scientifically prove the absence of a threshold, as one can never prove a negative.

Nevertheless, for the identification of "safe" levels of exposure to a substance, the absence or presence of a threshold is important for practical reasons (see Chap. 4). A classic example of the difficulty of establishing thresholds experimentally is provided by the "ED_{01}" study, where over 24,000 mice and 81 different treatment groups were used to determine the shape of the dose–response relationship for the prototypical carcinogen 2-acetylaminofluorene (2-AAF). The study was designed to identify a statistically significant response of 1% (0.01 probability). The mice were exposed to 2-AAF at 1 of 7 different doses in the dose range of 30 to 150 ppm (plus 0 dose control) (Littlefield *et al.*, 1979). Eight "sacrifice intervals" were used to determine how quickly tumors developed. Both types of tumors demonstrated increasing incidence with increasing dose, but the shapes of the 2 curves are dramatically different. For liver tumors, no clear threshold was evident, whereas for bladder tumors, an apparent threshold was evident. However, the apparent threshold, or "no observable adverse effect level" (NOAEL), for bladder cancer was lower at 33 months (45 ppm) than at 24 months (75 ppm). Of course, the ability to detect a low incidence of tumors depends on the number of animals used in the study. Thus, although a threshold (a dose below which no response occurs) appears evident for bladder tumors, one cannot say for certain that tumors would not occur if more animals had been included in the lower-dose groups. A different animal model that relies on relatively brief exposure of rainbow trout embryos to carcinogens has allowed an even more statistically stringent analysis of the shape of the dose–response curve at low doses for mutagenic carcinogens. Using this model with 2 different genotoxic carcinogens, dibenzo[*d,e,f,p*]chrysene (DBC, also referred to as dibenzo[*a,l*]pyrene) and aflatoxin B_1 (AFB_1), estimates of the shape of the dose–response curve down to a response level of 1 additional tumor in 5000 animals could be obtained, because very large numbers of animals could be exposed. In both studies, over 40,000 trout were exposed to different doses ranging over a factor of 200 (AFB_1, lowest dose 0.5 ppb, highest dose 110 ppb) to 500 (DBC, lowest dose 0.45 ppm, highest dose 225 ppm), with over 8000 animals in the control and low-dose groups (Williams, 2012). Both of these chemicals are potent mutagens, so it was assumed that both the rate of DNA adduct formation and the tumor incidence would be linear throughout the dose range. However, for DBC, there was a clear deviation from linearity at the lower doses, such that the extrapolated dose–response curve crossed the *y*-axis at 1 cancer in a million exposed animals at a dose 500- to 1500-fold (depending on the statistical model) higher than would have been predicted from the linear extrapolation below the 10% response range (ED_{10}) (Bailey *et al.*, 2009) (Fig. 2-8). Remarkably, although the tumor response exhibited a clear "threshold," the formation of DBC–DNA adducts was quite linear through the lowest dose used. In contrast, in a similarly designed study using the potent carcinogen, AFB_1, both tumor response and AFB–DNA adduct formation appear approximately linear down through the lowest dose; the liver tumor response to AFB_1 remained linear to the lowest dose, although the slope was about 1.5 and the predicted dose resulting in 1 cancer in a million exposed animals was about 10-fold higher than that predicted from the extrapolated LED_{10} line, although the lowest doses tested yielded tumor incidence that was close (within a factor of 2) to the background tumor rate (Fig. 2-9) (Williams *et al.*, 2009a; Williams, 2012).

(See Chap. 4 for more discussion on statistical issues related to extrapolation of dose–response curves and the determination of NOAELs.)

In evaluating the shape of the dose–response relationship in populations, it is realistic to consider inflections in the shape of the dose–response curve rather than absolute thresholds. That is, the

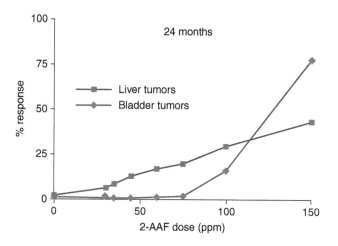

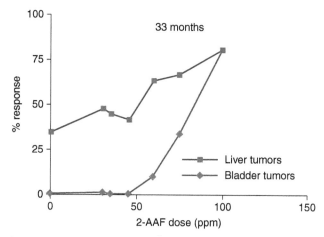

Figure 2-8. *Dose–response relationship for carcinogens—rodents and 2-AAF.*

slope of the dose–response relationship at high doses may be substantially different from the slope at low doses, usually because of dispositional differences in the chemical. Saturation of biotransformation pathways, protein-binding sites or receptors, and depletion of intracellular cofactors represent some reasons why sharp inflections in the dose–response relationship may occur. For example, the widely used analgesic acetaminophen has a very low rate of liver toxicity at normal therapeutic doses. Even though a toxic metabolite (*N*-acetyl-*p*-benzoquinone imine [NAPQI]) is produced in the liver

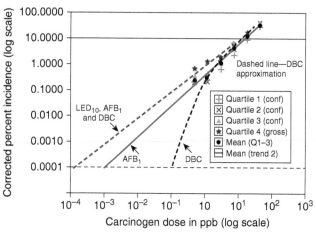

Figure 2-9. *Dose–response relationship for carcinogens—fish and aflatoxin B1.* (Reproduced with permission from Williams, 2012.)

at therapeutic doses, it is rapidly detoxified through conjugation with the intracellular antioxidant glutathione. However, at very high doses, the level of intracellular glutathione in the liver is depleted and NAPQI accumulates, causing serious and potentially fatal liver toxicity. This effect is analogous to the rapid change in pH of a buffered solution that occurs when the buffer capacity is exceeded. Some toxic responses, most notably the development of cancer after the administration of genotoxic carcinogens, are often considered to be linear at low doses and thus do not exhibit a threshold. In such circumstances, there is no dose with "zero" risk, although the risk decreases proportionately with a decrease in the dose. The existence or lack of existence of a threshold dose for carcinogens has many regulatory implications and is a point of considerable controversy and research in the field of quantitative risk assessment for chemical carcinogens (see Chap. 4).

Nonmonotonic Dose–Response Curves For chemicals that exert their primary toxic effects via modification of hormonal responses (endocrine disruptors), it is possible that effects occur at relatively low doses that are not seen at higher doses, thereby seemingly defying the traditional concept of "dose–response".

The characterization of so-called nonmonotonic dose–response (NMDR) curves is an important refinement in our understanding of dose–response relationships in toxicology (Fig. 2-10). Indeed, some chemicals, such as the plastics monomer bisphenol A (BPA), exhibit relatively little evident toxicity at high doses in traditional acute toxicity testing procedures, yet may have important biological effects when exposure occurs during sensitive periods of development, even at doses well below those shown to cause evident toxicity. For example, human pituitary cells cultured in the presence of BPA elicited significant responses at concentrations of 0.001 and

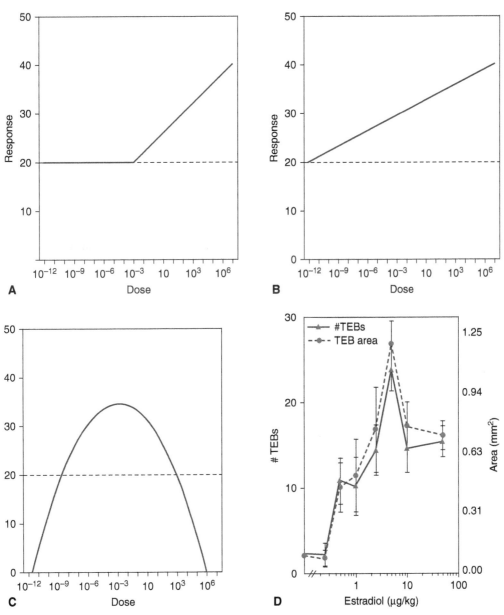

Figure 2-10. *Hypothetical dose–response curves for the (A) threshold responses, (B) nonthreshold linear response, and (C and D) nonmonotonic dose–response (NMDR).* Curves A and B reflect traditional dose–response relationships. However, in the NMDR curve (C), an increase in dose does not necessarily correspond to an increase in response, such that, in this example, doses from 10^{-12} to 10^{-3} dose units result in an increase in response, and doses from 10^{-3} to 10^6 dose units result in a decrease in response. Curve D represents the NMDR curves observed in mammary gland morphological parameters after administration of estradiol to ovariectomized females. The *left y-axis* is the number of terminal end buds (TEBs), and the *right y-axis* is total area of all TEBs; the TEB is an estrogen-dependent structure. (Based on Vandenberg *et al.*, 2009.)

0.01 nM, but not at 1 and 10 nM, yet the response was seen at 100 nM (Vandenberg *et al.*, 2009). Several other studies have found that BPA and other endocrine-active xenobiotics can elicit NMDR relationships for a variety of other specific receptors and/or cell signaling pathways (reviewed in Vandenberg *et al.*, 2009).

Specific cellular/molecular mechanisms that might explain NMDR curves include: (1) upregulation of some receptors at low concentrations, with downregulation of the same receptors at higher levels, and/or (2) integration of 2 or more monotonic dose–response curves that occur through different molecular/cellular pathways with common end points but opposite effects (Vandenberg *et al.*, 2009). Since endocrine-active xenobiotics may act as weak agonists for specific hormone receptors, it is reasonable that low doses could have different effects than high doses if, as partial agonists, they competitively inhibit endogenous ligands at higher concentrations, but have either no or positive agonist effects at low concentrations. Another explanation for NMDR curves is that we simply do not understand all the varied and interconnected molecular pathways that work in concert to produce an observable response at the organismal level. Indeed, BPA has been shown to have multiple different effects on a myriad of putative molecular pathways involved in hormone function, so it perhaps is not surprising to see NMDR functions over dose ranges of many orders of magnitude (Vandenberg *et al.*, 2009).

Assumptions in Deriving the Dose–Response Relationship

A number of assumptions must be considered before dose–response relationships can be used appropriately. The first is that the response is due to the chemical administered. To describe the relationship between a toxic material and an observed effect or response, one must know with reasonable certainty that the relationship is indeed a causal one. For some data, it is not always apparent that the response is a result of chemical exposure. For example, an epidemiological study might result in the discovery of an "association" between a response (eg, disease) and 1 or more variables. Frequently, the data are presented similarly to the presentation of "dose response" in pharmacology and toxicology. Use of the dose response in this context is suspect unless other convincing evidence supports a causal connection between the estimated dose and the measured end point (response). Unfortunately, in nearly all retrospective and case–control studies and even in many prospective studies, the dose, duration, frequency, and routes of exposure are seldom quantified, and other potential etiologic factors are frequently present. In its most strict usage, then, the dose–response relationship is based on the knowledge that the effect is a result of a known toxic agent or agents.

A second assumption seems simple and obvious: the magnitude of the response is in fact related to the dose. Perhaps because of its apparent simplicity, this assumption is often a source of misunderstanding. It is really a composite of 3 other assumptions that recur frequently:

1. There is a molecular target site (or sites) with which the chemical interacts to initiate the response.
2. The production of a response and the degree of response are related to the concentration of the chemical at the target site.
3. The concentration at the site is, in turn, related to the dose administered.

The third assumption in using the dose–response relationship is that there exist both a quantifiable method of measuring and a precise means of expressing the toxicity. For any given dose–response

relationship, a great variety of criteria or end points of toxicity could be used. The ideal criterion would be one closely associated with the molecular events resulting from exposure to the toxicant. It follows from this that a given chemical may have a family of dose–response relationships, 1 for each toxic end point. For example, a chemical that produces cancer through genotoxic effects, liver damage through inhibition of a specific enzyme, and CNS effects via a different mechanism, may have 3 distinct dose–response relationships, 1 for each end point. Early in the assessment of toxicity, little mechanistic information is usually available; thus, establishing a dose–response relationship based on the molecular mechanism of action is usually impossible. Indeed, it might not be approachable even for well-known toxicants. In the absence of a mechanistic, molecular ideal criterion of toxicity, one looks to a measure of toxicity that is unequivocal and clearly relevant to the toxic effect. Such measures are often referred to as "effects-related biomarkers." For example, with a new compound chemically related to the class of organophosphate insecticides, one might approach the measurement of toxicity by measuring the inhibition of cholinesterase in blood. In this way, one would be measuring, in a readily accessible system and using a technique that is convenient and reasonably precise, a prominent effect of the chemical and one that is usually pertinent to the mechanism by which toxicity is produced.

The selection of a toxic end point for measurement is not always so straightforward. Even the example cited above may be misleading, as an organophosphate may produce a decrease in blood cholinesterase, but this change may not be directly related to its toxicity. As additional data are gathered to suggest a mechanism of toxicity for any substance, other measures of toxicity may be selected. Although many end points are quantitative and precise, they are often indirect measures of toxicity. Changes in enzyme levels in blood can be indicative of tissue damage. For example, alanine aminotransferase (ALT) and aspartate aminotransferase (AST) are used to detect liver damage. Use of these enzymes in serum is yet another example of an effects-related biomarker because the change in enzyme activity in the blood is directly related to damage to liver cells. Much of clinical diagnostic medicine relies on effects-related biomarkers, but to be useful the relationship between the biomarker and the disease must be carefully established. Patterns of isozymes and their alteration may provide insight into the organ or system that is the site of toxic effects. As discussed later in this chapter, the new tools of toxicogenomics provide an unprecedented opportunity to discover new "effects-related biomarkers" in toxicology.

Many direct measures of effects are also not necessarily related to the mechanism by which a substance produces harm to an organism but have the advantage of permitting a causal relation to be drawn between the chemical and its action. For example, measurement of the alteration of the tone of smooth or skeletal muscle for substances acting on muscles represents a fundamental approach to toxicological assessment. Similarly, measures of heart rate, blood pressure, and electrical activity of heart muscle, nerve, and brain are examples of the use of physiological functions as indices of toxicity. Measurement can also take the form of a still higher level of integration, such as the degree of motor activity or behavioral change.

The measurements used as examples in the preceding discussion all assume prior information about the toxicant, such as its target organ or site of action or a fundamental effect. However, such information is usually available only after toxicological screening and testing based on other measures of toxicity. With a new substance, the customary starting point is a single-dose acute toxicity test designed to provide preliminary identification of target organ toxicity. Studies specifically designed with lethality as an end point are no longer recommended by the United States or international agencies. Data from acute studies provide essential information for choosing doses for repeated dosing studies as well as choosing specific toxicological end points for further study. Key elements of the study design must be a careful, disciplined, detailed observation of the intact animal extending from the time of administration of the toxicant to any clinical signs of distress, which may include detailed behavioral observations or physiological measures. It is recommended that these observations be taken over a 14-day period. From properly conducted observations, immensely informative data can be gathered by a trained toxicologist. Second, an acute toxicity study ordinarily is supported by histological examination of major tissues and organs for abnormalities. From these observations, one can usually obtain more specific information about the events leading to the various end points, the target organs involved, and often a suggestion about the possible mechanism of toxicity at a relatively fundamental level.

Evaluating the Dose–Response Relationship

Comparison of Dose Responses Fig. 2-11 illustrates a hypothetical quantal dose–response curve for a desirable effect of a chemical (effective dose, ED) such as anesthesia, a toxic effect (toxic dose, ED) such as liver injury, and the lethal dose (LD). As depicted in Fig. 2-11, a parallelism is apparent between the ED curve and the curve depicting mortality (LD). It is tempting to view the parallel dose–response curves as indicative of identity of mechanism—that is, to conclude that the lethality is a simple extension of the therapeutic effect. Whereas this conclusion may ultimately prove to be correct in any particular case, it is not warranted solely on the basis of the 2 parallel lines. The same admonition applies to any pair of parallel "effect" curves or any other pair of toxicity or lethality curves.

Therapeutic Index The hypothetical curves in Fig. 2-11 illustrate 2 other interrelated points: the importance of the selection of the toxic criterion and the interpretation of comparative effect. The concept of the "therapeutic index" (TI), which was introduced by Paul Ehrlich in 1913, can be used to illustrate this relationship. Although the TI is directed toward a comparison of the therapeutically ED to the TD of a chemical, it is equally applicable to considerations of comparative toxicity. The TI in its broadest sense is defined as the ratio of the dose required to produce a toxic effect to

the dose needed to elicit the desired therapeutic response. Similarly, an index of comparative toxicity is obtained by the ratio of doses of 2 different materials to produce an identical response or the ratio of doses of the same material necessary to yield different toxic effects.

The most commonly used index of effect, whether beneficial or toxic, is the median effect dose (ED_{50}). The TI of a drug is an approximate statement about the relative safety of a drug expressed as the ratio of the adverse end point or TD (historically the LD) to the therapeutic dose:

$$TI = \frac{TD_{50}}{ED_{50}}.$$

From Fig. 2-11 one can approximate a TI by using these median doses. The larger the ratio, the greater is the relative safety. The ED_{50} is approximately 20, and the TD_{50} is about 60; thus, the TI is 3, a number indicating that reasonable care in exposure to the drug is necessary to avoid toxicity. However, the use of the median effective and median toxic doses is not without disadvantages, because median doses tell nothing about the slopes of the dose–response curves for therapeutic and toxic effects.

Margins of Safety and Exposure One way to overcome this deficiency is to use the ED_{99} for the desired effect and the TD_1 for the undesired effect. These parameters are used in the calculation of the margin of safety (MOS):

$$MOS = \frac{TD_1}{ED_{99}}.$$

The quantitative comparisons described above have been used mainly after a single administration of chemicals. However, for chemicals for which there is no beneficial or effective dose and exposures are likely to occur repeatedly, the ratio of TD_1 to ED_{99} has little relevance. Thus, for nondrug chemicals, the term *MOS* has found use in risk assessment procedures as an indicator of the magnitude of the difference between an estimated "exposed dose" to a human population and the NOAEL or other benchmark dose determined in experimental animals.

A measure of the degree of accumulation of a chemical and/or its toxic effects can also be estimated from quantal toxicity data. The *chronicity index* of a chemical is a unitless value obtained by dividing its 1-dose TD_{50} by its 90-dose (90-day) TD_{50}, with both expressed in milligrams per kilogram per day. Theoretically, if no cumulative effect occurs over the doses, the chronicity index will be 1. If a compound were absolutely cumulative, the chronicity index would be 90.

Historically, statistical procedures similar to those used to calculate the LD_{50} can also be used to determine the lethal time 50 (LT_{50}), or the time required for half the animals to die (Litchfield, 1949). The LT_{50} value for a chemical indicates the time course of the toxic effects but does not indicate whether 1 chemical is more toxic than another.

Frequently, dose–response curves from repeated-dose experimental animal studies (subacute, subchronic, or chronic) are used to estimate the NOAEL, or some other "benchmark" measure of minimal toxic response, such as the dose estimated to produce toxic effects in 10% of the population (TD_{10}) (see also Chap. 4). These estimates of minimal TD, derived from quantal dose–response curves, can be used in risk assessment to derive a "margin of exposure" (MOE) index. This index compares the estimated daily exposure, in milligrams per kilogram per day, that might occur under a given set of circumstances with some estimated value from the quantal dose–response relationship (eg, NOAEL or TD_{10}). Like the

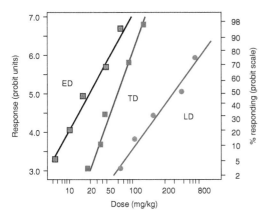

Figure 2-11. *Comparison of effective dose (ED), toxic dose (TD), and lethal dose (LD).* The plot is of log dosage versus percentage of population responding in probit units.

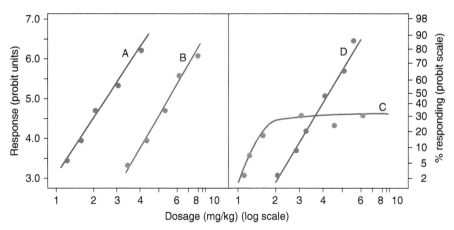

Figure 2-12. *Schematic representation of the difference in the dose–response curves for 4 chemicals (**A-D**), illustrating the difference between potency and efficacy (see text).*

MOS, the MOE is often expressed as a ratio of these 2 values. Thus, for example, if an estimate of human exposure to a pesticide residue yielded a value of 0.001 mg/kg per day, and a TD_{10} of 1 mg/kg per day was determined for that same pesticide, the MOE would be 1000. This value indicates that the estimate of daily exposure under the described set of conditions is 1/1000 the estimated daily dose that would cause evident toxicity in 10% of exposed animals. (See Chap. 4 for a more complete discussion of benchmark doses, NOAELs, and MOE.)

Potency versus Efficacy To compare the toxic effects of 2 or more chemicals, the dose response to the toxic effects of each chemical must be established. One can then compare the potency and maximal efficacy of the 2 chemicals to produce a toxic effect. These 2 important terms can be explained by reference to Fig. 2-12, which depicts dose–response curves to 4 different chemicals for the frequency of a particular toxic effect, such as the production of tumors. Chemical A is said to be more potent than chemical B because of their relative positions along the dosage axis. Potency thus refers to the range of doses over which a chemical produces increasing responses. Thus, A is more potent than B and C is more potent than D. Maximal efficacy reflects the limit of the dose–response relationship on the response axis to a certain chemical. Chemicals A and B have equal maximal efficacy, whereas the maximal efficacy of C is less than that of D.

VARIATION IN TOXIC RESPONSES

Selective Toxicity

Selective toxicity means that a chemical produces injury to 1 kind of living matter without harming another form of life even though the 2 may exist in intimate contact (Albert, 1973). The living matter that is injured is termed the *uneconomic form* (or undesirable), and the matter protected is called the *economic form* (or desirable). They may be related to each other as parasite and host or may be 2 tissues in 1 organism. This biological diversity interferes with the ability of ecotoxicologists to predict the toxic effects of a chemical in 1 species (humans) from experiments performed in another species (laboratory animals). However, by taking advantage of the biological diversity, it is possible to develop chemicals that are lethal for an undesired species and harmless for other species. In agriculture, for example, there are fungi, insects, and even competitive plants that injure the crop, and thus selective pesticides are needed. Similarly, animal husbandry and human medicine require

chemicals, such as antibiotics, that are selectively toxic to the undesirable form but do not produce damage to the desirable form.

Drugs and other chemicals used for selective toxic purposes are selective for 1 of 2 reasons. Either (1) the chemical is equally toxic to both economic and uneconomic cells but is accumulated mainly by uneconomic cells or (2) it reacts fairly specifically with a cytological or a biochemical feature that is absent from or does not play an important role in the economic form (Albert, 1973). Selectivity resulting from differences in distribution usually is caused by differences in the absorption, biotransformation, or excretion of the toxicant. The selective toxicity of an insecticide spray may be partly due to a larger surface area per unit weight that causes the insect to absorb a proportionally larger dose than does the mammal being sprayed. The effectiveness of radioactive iodine in the treatment of hyperthyroidism (as well as its thyroid carcinogenicity) is due to the selective ability of the thyroid gland to accumulate iodine. A major reason why chemicals are toxic to one, but not to another, type of tissue is that there are differences in accumulation of the ultimate toxic compound in various tissues. This, in turn, may be due to differences in the ability of various tissues to transport or biotransform the chemical into the ultimate toxic product.

Selective toxicity caused by differences in comparative cytology is exemplified by a comparison of plant and animal cells. Plants differ from animals in many ways—for example, absence of a nervous system, an efficient circulatory system, and muscles as well as the presence of a photosynthetic mechanism and cell walls. The fact that bacteria contain cell walls and humans do not has been utilized in developing selective toxic chemotherapeutic agents, such as penicillin and cephalosporins, that kill bacteria but are relatively nontoxic to mammalian cells.

Selective toxicity can also be a result of a difference in biochemistry in the 2 types of cells. For example, bacteria do not absorb folic acid but synthesize it from *p*-aminobenzoic acid, glutamic acid, and pteridine, whereas mammals cannot synthesize folic acid but have to absorb it from the diet. Thus, sulfonamide drugs are selectively toxic to bacteria because the sulfonamides, which resemble *p*-aminobenzoic acid in both charge and dimensions, antagonize the incorporation of *p*-aminobenzoic acid into the folic acid molecule—a reaction that humans do not carry out.

Species Differences

Although a basic tenet of toxicology is that "experimental results in animals, when properly qualified, are applicable to humans," it is important to recognize that both quantitative and qualitative differences in response to toxic substances may occur among different species. As discussed above, there are many reasons for selective toxicity among different species. Even among phylogenetically similar species (eg, rats, mice, guinea pigs, and hamsters), large differences in response may occur. For example, the LD_{50} for the highly toxic dioxin, TCDD, differs by more than 1000-fold between guinea pigs and hamsters. Not only the lethal dose for TCDD but also the particular target organs affected vary widely among species. Species differences in response to carcinogenic chemicals represent an important issue in regulatory risk assessment. As discussed in Chap. 4, extrapolation of laboratory animal data to infer human cancer risk is currently a key component of regulatory decision making. The validity of this approach of course depends on the relevance of the experimental animal model to humans. Large differences in carcinogenic response between experimental animal species are not unusual. For example, mice are highly resistant to the hepatocarcinogenic effects of the fungal toxin AFB_1. Dietary doses as high as 10,000 ppb failed to produce liver cancer in mice, whereas in rats dietary doses as low as 15 ppb produced a significant increase in liver tumors (Wogan et al., 1974). The mechanistic basis for this dramatic difference in response appears to be entirely related to species differences in the expression of a particular form of glutathione S-transferase (mGSTA3-3) that has unusually high catalytic activity toward the carcinogenic epoxide of aflatoxin (Eaton and Gallagher, 1994). Mice express this enzyme constitutively, whereas rats normally express a closely related form with much less detoxifying activity toward aflatoxin epoxide. Interestingly, rats do possess the gene for a form of glutathione S-transferase with high catalytic activity toward aflatoxin epoxide (rGSTA5-5) that is inducible by certain dietary antioxidants and drugs. Thus, dietary treatment can dramatically change the sensitivity of a species to a carcinogen.

Other examples in which large species differences in response to carcinogens have been observed include the development of renal tumors from 2,3,5-trimethylpentane and D-limonene in male rats (Lehman-McKeeman and Caudill, 1992), the production of liver tumors from "peroxisomal proliferators" such as the antilipidemic drug clofibrate and the common solvent trichloroethylene (Roberts, 1999), and the induction of nasal carcinomas in rats after inhalation exposure to formaldehyde (Monticello and Morgan, 1997).

Identifying the mechanistic basis for species differences in response to chemicals is an important part of toxicology because only through a thorough understanding of these differences can the relevance of animal data to human response be verified.

Individual Differences in Response

Even within a species, large interindividual differences in response to a chemical can occur because of subtle genetic differences. Hereditary differences in a single gene that occur in more than 1% of the population are referred to as *genetic polymorphism* and may be responsible for idiosyncratic reactions to chemicals, as discussed earlier in this chapter. However, genetic polymorphism may have other important but less dramatic effects than those described for acute idiosyncratic responses (such as that occurring in pseudocholinesterase-deficient individuals after succinylcholine exposure). For example, it is recognized that approximately 50% of the Caucasian population has a gene deletion for the enzyme glutathione S-transferase M1. This enzyme has no apparent significant physiological function, and thus homozygotes for the gene deletion (eg, those who lack both copies of the normal gene) are functionally and physiologically normal. However, epidemiological studies have indicated that smokers who are homozygous for the null

allele may be at slightly increased risk of developing lung cancer compared with smokers who have 1 or both copies of the normal gene (Mohr et al., 2003). Chap. 6 provides additional examples of genetic differences in biotransformation enzymes that may be important determinants of variability in individual susceptibility to chemical exposures.

Genetic polymorphism in physiologically important genes may also be responsible for interindividual differences in toxic responses. For example, studies in transgenic mice have shown that mice possessing 1 copy of a mutated *p53* gene (a so-called tumor suppressor gene; see Chap. 8) are much more susceptible to some chemical carcinogens than are mice with 2 normal copies of the gene (Tennant et al., 1999). In humans, there is evidence that possessing 1 mutated copy of a tumor suppressor gene greatly increases the risk of developing certain cancers. For example, retinoblastoma is a largely inherited form of cancer that arises because of the presence of 2 copies of a defective tumor suppressor gene (the Rb gene) (Wiman, 1993). Individuals with 1 mutated copy of the Rb gene and 1 normal copy are not destined to acquire the disease (as are those with 2 copies of the mutated gene), although their chance of acquiring it is much greater than that of persons with 2 normal Rb genes. This is the case because both copies of the gene must be nonfunctional for the disease to develop. With 1 mutated copy present genetically, the probability of acquiring a mutation of the second gene (potentially from exposure to environmental mutagens) is much greater than the probability of acquiring independent mutations in both copies of the gene as would be necessary in people with 2 normal Rb alleles. (See Chap. 8 for additional discussion of tumor suppressor genes.)

As our understanding of the human genome increases, more "susceptibility" genes will be discovered, and it is likely that the etiology of many chronic diseases will be shown to be related to a combination of genetics and environment. Simple blood tests may ultimately be developed that allow an individual to learn whether he or she may be particularly susceptible to specific drugs or environmental pollutants. Although the public health significance of this type of information could be immense, the disclosure of such information raises many important ethical and legal issues that must be addressed before wide use of such tests.

The study of "gene–environment" interactions, or "ecogenetics" (Costa and Eaton, 2006), is a rapidly developing field of substantial relevance to toxicology. It is likely that the majority of chronic diseases develop as a result of the complex interplay between multiple genes and the myriad of environmental factors, including diet, lifestyle, and occupational and/or environmental exposures to toxic substances. The growing field of epigenetics, discussed in more detail later in this chapter, is likely to have an equally great impact on the science of toxicology, as it is likely that many xenobiotics will be found to exert many of their chronic adverse effects through subtle effects on gene expression.

DESCRIPTIVE ANIMAL TOXICITY TESTS

Two main principles underlie all descriptive animal toxicity testing. The first is that the effects produced by a compound in laboratory animals, when properly qualified, are applicable to humans. This premise applies to all of experimental biology and medicine. Most, if not all, known chemical carcinogens in humans are carcinogenic in some species, but not necessarily in all species of laboratory animals. It has become increasingly evident that the converse—that all chemicals identified as carcinogenic in laboratory animals are also carcinogenic in humans—is not true (Dybing and Sanner, 1999; Grisham, 1997; Hengstler et al., 1999). However, for regulatory and risk assessment purposes, positive carcinogenicity tests in animals are usually interpreted as indicative of potential human carcinogenicity. If a clear understanding of the mechanism of action of the carcinogen indicates that a positive response in animals is not relevant to humans, a positive animal bioassay may be considered irrelevant for human risk assessment (see Chap. 4). This species variation in carcinogenic response appears to be due in many instances to differences in biotransformation of the procarcinogen to the ultimate carcinogen (see Chap. 6).

The second principle is that exposure of experimental animals to chemicals in high doses is a necessary and valid method of discovering possible hazards in humans. This principle is based on the quantal dose–response concept that the incidence of an effect in a population is greater as the dose or exposure increases. Practical considerations in the design of experimental model systems require that the number of animals used in toxicology experiments always be small compared with the size of human populations at risk. Obtaining statistically valid results from such small groups of animals requires the use of relatively large doses so that the effect will occur frequently enough to be detected. However, the use of high doses can create problems in interpretation if the response(s) obtained at high doses does not occur at low doses. Thus, for example, it has been shown that bladder tumors observed in rats fed very high doses of saccharin will not occur at the much lower doses of saccharin encountered in the human diet. At the high concentrations fed to rats, saccharin forms an insoluble precipitate in the bladder that subsequently results in chronic irritation of bladder epithelium, enhanced cell proliferation, and ultimately bladder tumors (Cohen, 1998, 1999). In vitro studies have shown that precipitation of saccharin in human urine will not occur at the concentrations

that could be obtained from even extraordinary consumption of this artificial sweetener. As noted above and shown in Fig. 2-8, even for mutagenic chemicals that form DNA adducts, the response at high doses, as seen for DBC, may not be linear at low doses, although for another DNA-reactive carcinogen, AFB_1, the high-dose data were reflective of low-dose response in an approximately linear fashion. Examples such as these illustrate the importance of considering the molecular, biochemical, and cellular mechanisms responsible for toxicological responses when extrapolating from high to low dose and across species.

Toxicity tests are not designed to demonstrate that a chemical is safe but to characterize the toxic effects a chemical can produce. Although there are no set toxicology tests that have to be performed on every chemical intended for commerce, a tiered approach typical of many hazard assessment programs is illustrated in Fig. 2-13. Depending on the eventual use of the chemical, the toxic effects produced by structural analogs of the chemical, as well as the toxic effects produced by the chemical itself, contribute to the determination of the toxicology tests that should be performed. The FDA, EPA, and Organization for Economic Cooperation and Development (OECD) have written good laboratory practice (GLP) standards and other guidance that stipulate that procedure must be defined and accountability documented. These guidelines are expected to be followed when toxicity tests are conducted in support of the introduction of a chemical to the market.

The following sections provide an overview of basic toxicity testing procedures in use today. For a detailed description of these tests, the reader is referred to several authoritative texts on this subject (Barile, 2010; Hayes, 2008; Jacobson-Kram and Keller, 2006; Eaton and Gallagher, 2010).

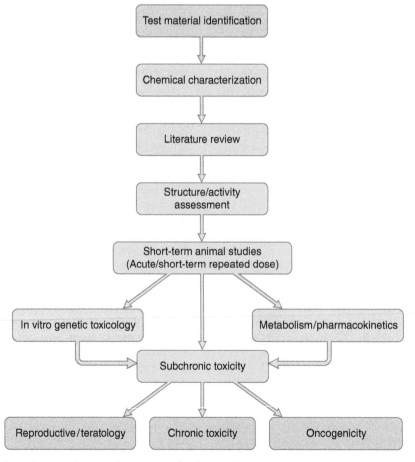

Figure 2-13. *Typical tiered testing scheme for the toxicological evaluation of new chemicals.* (From Wilson *et al.* 2008, Fig. 19-1, p. 918.)

Table 2-3

International Conference on Harmonization (ICH) Codification of "Safety" Protocols

Carcinogenicity studies

S1A	Need for Carcinogenicity Studies of Pharmaceuticals
S1B	Testing for Carcinogenicity of Pharmaceuticals
S1C(R1)	Dose Selection for Carcinogenicity Studies of Pharmaceuticals & Limit Dose

Genotoxicity studies

S2A	Guidance on Specific Aspects of Regulatory Genotoxicity Tests for Pharmaceuticals
S2B	Genotoxicity: A Standard Battery for Genotoxicity Testing of Pharmaceuticals

Toxicokinetics and pharmacokinetics

S3A	Note for Guidance on Toxicokinetics: The Assessment of Systemic Exposure in Toxicity Studies
S3B	Pharmacokinetics: Guidance for Repeated Dose Tissue Distribution Studies

Toxicity testing

	Single Dose Toxicity Tests
S4	Duration of Chronic Toxicity Testing in Animals (Rodent and Non Rodent Toxicity Testing)

Reproductive toxicology

S5(R2)	Detection of Toxicity to Reproduction for Medicinal Products & Toxicity to Male Fertility

Biotechnological products

S6	Preclinical Safety Evaluation of Biotechnology-Derived Pharmaceuticals

Pharmacology studies

S7A	Safety Pharmacology Studies for Human Pharmaceuticals
S7B	The Non-Clinical Evaluation of the Potential for Delayed Ventricular Repolarization (QT Interval Prolongation) by Human Pharmaceuticals

Immunotoxicology studies

S8	Immunotoxicity Studies for Human Pharmaceuticals

Joint safety/efficacy (multidisciplinary) topic

M3(R1)	Non-Clinical Safety Studies for the Conduct of Human Clinical Trials for Pharmaceuticals

Titles and abbreviations adopted in November 2005. Data from http://www.ich.org/fileadmin/Public_Web_Site/ICH_Products/Guidelines/Guidelines_Index.pdf.

Although different countries have often had different testing requirements for toxicity testing/product safety evaluation, efforts to "harmonize" such testing protocols have resulted in more standardized approaches. The International Conference on Harmonization (ICH) of Technical Requirements for Registration of Pharmaceuticals for Human Use includes regulatory authorities from Europe, Japan, and the United States (primarily the FDA), as well as experts from the pharmaceutical industry in the 3 regions, who worked together to develop internationally recognized scientific and technical approaches to pharmaceutical product registration. ICH has adopted guidelines for most areas of toxicity testing (Table 2-3). In addition to safety assessment (ICH guidelines designated with an "S"), ICH has also established guidelines on quality (Q), efficacy (E), and multidisciplinary (M) topics. (See http://www.ich.org/products/guidelines.html for a description of current ICH guidelines and reviews by Pugsley *et al.* (2008, 2011) for a detailed discussion of in vitro and in vivo approaches to safety pharmacology that has been informed by the ICH regulatory guidance document for preclinical safety testing of drugs.)

Typically, a tiered approach is used, with subsequent tests dependent on results of initial studies. A general framework for how new chemicals are evaluated for toxicity is shown in Fig 2-13. Early studies require careful chemical evaluation of the compound or mixture to assess purity, stability, solubility, and other physicochemical factors that could impact the ability of the test compound to be delivered effectively to animals. Once this information is obtained, the chemical structure of the test compound is compared with similar chemicals for which toxicological information is already available. Structure–activity relationships may be derived from a review of existing toxicological literature, and can provide additional guidance on design of acute and repeated-dose experiments, and what specialized tests need to be completed. Once such basic information has been compiled and evaluated, the test compound is then administered to animals in acute and repeated-dose studies.

Because of increased societal pressure to reduce or eliminate the use of animals in toxicity testing, while also ensuring that new chemicals do not represent unreasonable risks to human health or the environment, regulatory agencies have been encouraging new approaches to descriptive toxicity tests that do not rely on laboratory animals. For example, the European Union (EU) promulgated an important regulatory initiative for the Registration, Evaluation, Authorisation and Restriction of Chemicals (REACH). The implementation of REACH "will have significant impact on applied toxicology and exposure assessment by stimulating innovation in sampling and analysis, toxicology testing, exposure modeling, alternative toxicity testing, and risk assessment practices"

(Williams *et al.*, 2009b). Alternative, in vitro approaches to toxicity assessment are likely to transform the way that product safety evaluation is done in the future, although the standard approaches to hazard evaluation described in this section are likely to continue as the mainstay of toxicity evaluation for the next decade, irrespective of the fact that some areas, such as acute toxicity testing and eye irritation, are likely to be largely replaced by in vitro tests in the next decade (Ukelis *et al.*, 2008).

The development of new "omics" technologies (discussed later in this section) may have profound implications for toxicity testing in the future (NAS/NRC, 2007). The recognition that many of the existing chemicals in commercial use today, as well as new chemicals being introduced into commerce, have little toxicological information about them has prompted calls for new "high-throughput" approaches to toxicity testing that will allow at least basic hazard characterization for the thousands of untested chemicals currently in the marketplace, as well as the many new chemicals that are introduced each year. A report from the National Academy of Sciences/National Research Council in 2007 called for a "paradigm shift" in how toxicity testing is done (NAS/NRC, 2007). A key component of this new vision on toxicity testing is the use of an extensive battery of in vitro tests to evaluate "pathways" of toxicity (NAS/NRC, 2010). The hope is that new technologies in genomics, transcriptomics, proteomics, metabolomics, and bioinformatics (discussed later in this chapter) can be combined with automated high-throughput technologies to create a tiered structure for toxicity testing. The approach to using biochemical and molecular pathway-based analyses, rather than apical end points (eg, target organ damage, mutagenesis, carcinogenesis, reproductive and developmental effects), to identify potentially problematic chemicals early in their development is particularly attractive from a time frame and economic perspective (NAS/NRC, 2010). However, it is also recognized that validation of such tests is critically important to the reliable use of such screening technologies, and that the traditional in vivo studies described in the following section will continue to serve an important role in hazard evaluations for years to come, especially as a means of validating new high-throughput screening approaches.

Acute Toxicity Testing

Generally, the first toxicity test performed on a new chemical is acute toxicity, determined from the administration of a single exposure. The objectives of acute toxicity testing are to: (1) provide an estimate of the intrinsic toxicity of the substance, often times expressed as an approximate LD (eg, LD_{50}), (2) provide information on target organs and other clinical manifestations of toxicity, (3) identify species differences and susceptible species, (4) establish the reversibility of the toxic response, and (5) provide information that will assist in the design and dose selection for longer-term (subchronic, chronic) studies. It should be noted that the ICH recommended in 1991 (D'Arcy and Harron, 1992) the elimination of LD_{50} determinations for pharmaceuticals, although other regulatory requirements, for example, pesticide registration, may still require determinations of LD_{50}s.

The LD_{50} and other acute toxic effects are determined after 1 or more routes of administration (1 route being oral or the intended route of exposure) in 1 or more species. The species most often used are the mouse and rat. Studies are performed in both adult male and female animals. Food is often withheld the night before dosing. The number of animals that die in a 14-day period after a single dosage is tabulated. In addition to mortality and weight, daily examination of test animals should be conducted for signs

of intoxication, lethargy, behavioral modifications, morbidity, food consumption, and so on.

Determination of the LD_{50} has become a public issue because of increasing concern for the welfare and protection of laboratory animals. The LD_{50} is not a biological constant. Many factors influence toxicity and thus may alter the estimation of the LD_{50} in any particular study. Factors such as animal strain, age, and weight, type of feed, caging, pretrial fasting time, method of administration, volume and type of suspension medium, and duration of observation have all been shown to influence adverse responses to toxic substances. These and other factors have been discussed in detail in earlier editions of this textbook (Doull, 1980). Because of this inherent variability in LD_{50} estimates, it is now recognized that for most purposes it is only necessary to characterize the LD_{50} within an order of magnitude range such as 5 to 50 mg/kg, 50 to 500 mg/kg, and so on.

There are several traditional approaches to determining the LD_{50} and its 95% confidence limit as well as the slope of the probit line. The reader is referred to the classic works of Litchfield and Wilcoxon (1949), Bliss (1957), and Finney (1971) for a description of the mechanics of these procedures. Other statistical techniques that require fewer animals, such as the "moving averages" method of Thompson and Weill (Weil, 1952), are available but do not provide confidence limits for the LD_{50} and the slope of the probit line. Finney (1985) has succinctly summarized the advantages and deficiencies of many of the traditional methods. For most circumstances, an adequate estimate of the LD_{50} and an approximation of the 95% confidence intervals can be obtained with as few as 6 to 9 animals, using the "up-and-down" method as modified by Bruce (1985). When this method was compared with traditional methods that typically utilize 40 to 50 animals, excellent agreement was obtained for all 10 compounds tested (Bruce, 1987). In mice and rats the LD_{50} is usually determined as described above, but in the larger species only an approximation of the LD_{50} is obtained by increasing the dose in the same animal until serious toxic effects are evident.

Alternative in vitro approaches to estimating the LD_{50} have been proposed. For example, the *Registry of Cytotoxicity* (RC), originally published in German in 1998 (Halle, 2003), was developed by linear regression analysis of the mean IC_{50} values determined in mammalian cells in culture and the LD_{50} values reported in the literature from various laboratory species. Using this approach, the authors predicted (within a reasonable dose range) the acute oral LD_{50} for 252 of 347 xenobiotics, and the intravenous LD_{50} for rats and/or mice for 117 of 150 xenobiotics (Halle, 2003). Of course, such in vitro approaches do not fully account for dispositional effects that could result in large species differences in acute toxicity, but do provide a rapid first approximation of acute toxicity without the use of experimental animals.

If there is a reasonable likelihood of substantial exposure to the material by dermal or inhalation exposure, acute dermal and acute inhalation studies are performed. When animals are exposed acutely to chemicals in the air they breathe or the water they (fish) live in, the dose the animals receive is usually not known. For these situations, the lethal concentration 50 (LC_{50}) is usually determined, that is, the concentration of chemical in the air or water that causes death to 50% of the animals. In reporting an LC_{50}, it is imperative that the time of exposure be indicated. The acute dermal toxicity test is usually performed in rabbits. The site of application is shaved. The test substance is kept in contact with the skin for 24 hours by wrapping the skin with an impervious plastic material. At the end of the exposure period, the wrapping is removed and the skin is wiped to remove any test substance still remaining. Animals are observed at various intervals for 14 days, and the LD_{50} is calculated. If no toxicity is evident at 2 g/kg, further acute dermal toxicity testing is usually not performed. Acute inhalation studies are performed that are similar to other acute toxicity studies except that the route of exposure is inhalation. Most often, the length of exposure is 4 hours.

By themselves LD_{50} and LC_{50} values are of limited significance given the growing sophistication of target organ toxicity end points and mechanistic analysis. The most meaningful scientific information derived from acute toxicity tests comes from clinical observations and post-mortem examination of animals rather than from the specific LD_{50} value.

Skin and Eye Irritations

The ability of a chemical to irritate the skin and eye after an acute exposure is usually determined in rabbits. For the dermal irritation test (Draize test), rabbits are prepared by removal of fur on a section of the back by electric clippers. The chemical is applied to the skin (0.5 mL of liquid or 0.5 g of solid) under 4 covered gauze patches (1 in square; 1 intact and 2 abraded skin sites on each animal) and usually kept in contact for 4 hours. The nature of the covering patches depends on whether occlusive, semiocclusive, or nonocclusive tests are desired. For occlusive testing, the test material is covered with an impervious plastic sheet; for semiocclusive tests, a gauze dressing may be used. Occasionally, studies may require that the material be applied to abraded skin. The degree of skin irritation is scored for erythema (redness), eschar (scab), and edema (swelling) formation, and corrosive action. These dermal irritation observations are repeated at various intervals after the covered patch has been removed. To determine the degree of ocular irritation, the chemical is instilled into 1 eye (0.1 mL of liquid or 100 mg of solid) of each test rabbit. The contralateral eye is used as the control. The eyes of the rabbits are then examined at various times after application.

Controversy over this test has led to the development of alternative in vitro models for evaluating cutaneous and ocular toxicity of substances. The various in vitro methods that have been evaluated for this purpose include epidermal keratinocyte and corneal epithelial cell culture models. Several commercially available "reconstructed human epidermis" models have been developed explicitly for the purposes of in vitro skin irritation and corrosion tests (Netzlaff et al., 2005).

Sensitization

Information about the potential of a chemical to sensitize skin is needed in addition to irritation testing for all materials that may repeatedly come into contact with the skin. Numerous procedures have been developed to determine the potential of substances to induce a sensitization reaction in humans (delayed hypersensitivity reaction), including the Draize test, the open epicutaneous test, the Buehler test, Freund's complete adjuvant test, the optimization test, the split adjuvant test, and the guinea pig maximization test (Hayes et al., 2008; Rush et al., 1995). Although they differ in regard to route and frequency of duration, they all utilize the guinea pig as the preferred test species. In general, the test chemical is administered to the shaved skin topically, intradermally, or both and may include the use of adjuvant to enhance the sensitivity of the assay. Multiple administrations of the test substance are generally given over a period of 2 to 4 weeks. Depending on the specific protocol, the treated area may be occluded. Approximately 2 to 3 weeks after the last treatment, the animals are challenged with a nonirritating concentration of the test substance and the development of erythema is evaluated.

Subacute toxicity tests are performed to obtain information on the toxicity of a chemical after repeated administration and as an aid to establish doses for subchronic studies. A typical protocol is to give 3 to 4 different dosages of the chemicals to the animals by mixing it in their feed. For rats, 10 animals per sex per dose are often used; for dogs, 3 dosages and 3 to 4 animals per sex are used. Clinical chemistry and histopathology are performed after either 14 or 28 days of exposure, as described in the section "Subchronic."

Subchronic

The toxicity of a chemical after subchronic exposure is then determined. Subchronic exposure can last for different periods of time, but 90 days is the most common test duration. The principal goals of the subchronic study are to establish a NOAEL and to further identify and characterize the specific organ or organs affected by the test compound after repeated administration. One may also obtain a "lowest observed adverse effect level" (LOAEL) as well as the NOAEL for the species tested. The numbers obtained for NOAEL and LOAEL will depend on how closely the dosages are spaced and the number of animals examined. Determinations of NOAELs and LOAELs have numerous regulatory implications. For example, the EPA utilizes the NOAEL to calculate the *reference dose* (RfD), which may be used to establish regulatory values for "acceptable" pollutant levels (Barnes and Dourson, 1988) (see Chap. 4). An alternative to the NOAEL approach referred to as the *benchmark dose* uses all the experimental data to fit 1 or more dose–response curves (Crump, 1984). These curves are then used to estimate a benchmark dose that is defined as "the statistical lower bound on a dose corresponding to a specified level of risk" (Allen et al., 1994a). Although subchronic studies are frequently the primary or sole source of experimental data to determine both the NOAEL and the benchmark dose, these concepts can be applied to other types of toxicity testing protocols, such as that for chronic toxicity or developmental toxicity (Allen et al., 1994a,b; Faustman et al., 1994) (see also Chap. 4 for a complete discussion of the derivation and use of NOAELs, RfDs, and benchmark doses). If chronic studies have been completed, these data are generally used for NOAEL and LOAEL estimates in preference to data from subchronic studies.

A subchronic study is usually conducted in 2 species (usually rat and dog for FDA, and mouse for EPA) by the route of intended exposure (usually oral). At least 3 doses are employed (a high dose that produces toxicity but does not cause more than 10% fatalities, a low dose that produces no apparent toxic effects, and an intermediate dose) with 10 to 20 rodents and 4 to 6 dogs of each sex per dose. Each animal should be uniquely identified with permanent markings such as ear tags, tattoos, or electronically coded microchip implants. Only healthy animals should be used, and each animal should be housed individually in an adequately controlled environment. When the test compound is administered in the diet over a prolonged period of time (subchronic and chronic studies), the concentration in the diet should be adjusted periodically (weekly for the first 12–14 weeks) to maintain a constant intake of material based on food consumption and rate of change in body weight (Wilson et al., 2008). Animals should be observed once or twice daily for signs of toxicity, including changes in body weight, diet consumption, changes in fur color or texture, respiratory or cardiovascular distress, motor and behavioral abnormalities, and palpable masses. All premature deaths should be recorded and necropsied as soon as possible. Severely moribund animals should be terminated immediately to preserve tissues and reduce unnecessary suffering.

At the end of the 90-day study, all the remaining animals should be terminated and blood and tissues should be collected for further analysis. The gross and microscopic condition of the organs and tissues (about 15–20) and the weight of the major organs (about 12) are recorded and evaluated. Hematology and blood chemistry measurements are usually done before, in the middle of, and at the termination of exposure. Hematology measurements usually include hemoglobin concentration, hematocrit, erythrocyte counts, total and differential leukocyte counts, platelet count, clotting time, and prothrombin time. Clinical chemistry determinations commonly made include glucose, calcium, potassium, urea nitrogen, ALT, serum AST, gamma-glutamyltranspeptidase (GGT), sorbitol dehydrogenase, lactic dehydrogenase, alkaline phosphatase, creatinine, bilirubin, triglycerides, cholesterol, albumin, globulin, and total protein. Urinalysis is usually performed in the middle of and at the termination of the testing period and often includes determination of specific gravity or osmolarity, pH, proteins, glucose, ketones, bilirubin, and urobilinogen as well as microscopic examination of formed elements. If humans are likely to have significant exposure to the chemical by dermal contact or inhalation, subchronic dermal and/or inhalation experiments may also be required. Subchronic toxicity studies not only characterize the dose–response relationship of a test substance after repeated administration but also provide data for a more reasonable prediction of appropriate doses for chronic exposure studies.

For chemicals that are to be registered as drugs, acute and subchronic studies (and potentially additional special tests if a chemical has unusual toxic effects or therapeutic purposes) must be completed before the company can file an Investigational New Drug (IND) application with the FDA. If the application is approved, clinical trials can commence. At the same time phase I, phase II, and phase III clinical trials are performed, chronic exposure of the animals to the test compound can be carried out in laboratory animals, along with additional specialized tests.

Chronic

Long-term or chronic exposure studies are performed similarly to subchronic studies except that the period of exposure is longer than 3 months. In rodents, chronic exposures are usually for 6 months to 2 years. Chronic studies in nonrodent species are usually for 1 year but may be longer. The length of exposure is somewhat dependent on the intended period of exposure in humans. For example, for pharmaceuticals, the ICH S4 guidance calls for studies of 6 months in duration in rodents, and 9 months in nonrodents. However, if the chemical is a food additive with the potential for lifetime exposure in humans, a chronic study up to 2 years in duration is likely to be required.

Dose selection is critical in these studies to ensure that premature mortality from chronic toxicity does not limit the number of animals that survive to a normal life expectancy. Most regulatory guidelines require that the highest dose administered be the estimated maximum tolerable dose (MTD, also commonly referred to as the "minimally toxic dose"). This is generally derived from subchronic studies, but additional longer studies (eg, 6 months) may be necessary if delayed effects or extensive cumulative toxicity are indicated in the 90-day subchronic study. The MTD has had various definitions (Haseman, 1985). It has been defined by some regulatory agencies as the dose that suppresses body weight gain slightly (ie, 10%) in a 90-day subchronic study (Reno, 1997). However, regulatory agencies may also consider the use of parameters other than weight gain, such as physiological and pharmacokinetic considerations and urinary metabolite profiles, as indicators

of an appropriate MTD (Reno, 1997). Generally, 1 or 2 additional doses, usually fractions of the MTD (eg, one-half and one-quarter MTD), and a control group are tested.

Chronic toxicity tests may include a consideration of the carcinogenic potential of chemicals so that a separate lifetime feeding study that addresses carcinogenicity does not have to be performed. However, specific chronic studies designed to assess the carcinogenic potential of a substance may be required (see below).

Developmental and Reproductive Toxicity

The effects of chemicals on reproduction and development also need to be determined. *Developmental toxicology* is the study of adverse effects on the developing organism occurring anytime during the life span of the organism that may result from exposure to chemical or physical agents before conception (either parent), during prenatal development, or postnatally until the time of puberty. *Teratology* is the study of defects induced during development between conception and birth (see Chap. 10). *Reproductive toxicology* is the study of the occurrence of adverse effects on the male or female reproductive system that may result from exposure to chemical or physical agents (see Chap. 20).

Several types of animal tests are utilized to examine the potential of an agent to alter development and reproduction. (For a detailed description of reproductive and developmental toxicity testing procedures, see Christian [2008].) General fertility and reproductive performance (segment I) tests are usually performed in rats with 2 or 3 doses (20 rats per sex per dose) of the test chemical (neither produces maternal toxicity). Males are given the chemical 60 days and females 14 days before mating. The animals are given the chemical throughout gestation and lactation. Typical observations made include the percentage of females that become pregnant, the number of stillborn and live offspring, and the weight, growth, survival, and general condition of the offspring during the first 3 weeks of life.

The potential of chemicals to disrupt normal embryonic and/or fetal development (teratogenic effects) is also determined in laboratory animals. Current guidelines for these segment II studies call for the use of 2 species, including 1 nonrodent species (usually rabbits). Teratogens are most effective when administered during the first trimester, the period of organogenesis. Thus, the animals (usually 12 rabbits and 24 rats or mice per group) are usually exposed to 1 of 3 dosages during organogenesis (days 7-17 in rodents and 7-19 in rabbits), and the fetuses are removed by cesarean section a day before the estimated time of delivery (gestational days 29 for rabbit, 20 for rat, and 18 for mouse). The uterus is excised and weighed and then examined for the number of live, dead, and resorbed fetuses. Live fetuses are weighed; half of each litter is examined for skeletal abnormalities and the remaining half for soft tissue anomalies.

The perinatal and postnatal toxicities of chemicals also are often examined (segment III). This test is performed by administering the test compound to rats from the 15th day of gestation throughout delivery and lactation and determining its effect on the birth weight, survival, and growth of the offspring during the first 3 weeks of life.

In some instances a multigenerational study may be chosen, often in place of segment III studies, to determine the effects of chemicals on the reproductive system. At least 3 dosage levels are given to groups of 25 female and 25 male rats shortly after weaning (30–40 days of age). These rats are referred to as the F_0 generation. Dosing continues throughout breeding (about 140 days of age), gestation, and lactation. The offspring (F_1 generation) have thus been exposed to the chemical in utero, via lactation, and in the feed thereafter. When the F_1 generation is about 140 days old, about 25 females and 25 males are bred to produce the F_2 generation, and administration of the chemical is continued. The F_2 generation is thus also exposed to the chemical in utero and via lactation. The F_1 and F_2 litters are examined as soon as possible after delivery. The percentage of F_0 and F_1 females that get pregnant, the number of pregnancies that go to full term, the litter size, the number of still-born, and the number of live births are recorded. Viability counts and pup weights are recorded at birth and at 4, 7, 14, and 21 days of age. The fertility index (percentage of mating resulting in pregnancy), gestation index (percentage of pregnancies resulting in live litters), viability index (percentage of animals that survive 4 days or longer), and lactation index (percentage of animals alive at 4 days that survived the 21-day lactation period) are then calculated. Gross necropsy and histopathology are performed on some of the parents (F_0 and F_1), with the greatest attention being paid to the reproductive organs, and gross necropsy is performed on all weanlings.

The International Conference on Harmonization (ICH) guidelines provide for flexible guidelines that address 6 "ICH stages" of development: premating and conception (stage A), conception to implantation (stage B), implantation to closure of the hard palate (stage C), closure of the hard palate to end of pregnancy (stage D), birth and weaning (stage E), and weaning to sexual maturity (stage F). All of these stages are covered in the segment I to segment III studies described above (Christian, 2008).

Numerous short-term tests for teratogenicity have been developed (Faustman, 1988). These tests utilize whole-embryo culture, organ culture, and primary and established cell cultures to examine developmental processes and estimate the potential teratogenic risks of chemicals. Many of these in utero test systems are under evaluation for use in screening new chemicals for teratogenic effects. These systems vary in their ability to identify specific teratogenic events and alterations in cell growth and differentiation. In general, the available assays cannot identify functional or behavioral teratogens (Faustman, 1988).

Mutagenicity

Mutagenesis is the ability of chemicals to cause changes in the genetic material in the nucleus of cells in ways that allow the changes to be transmitted during cell division. Mutations can occur in either of 2 cell types, with substantially different consequences. Germinal mutations damage DNA in sperm and ova, which can undergo meiotic division and therefore have the potential for transmission of the mutations to future generations. If mutations are present at the time of fertilization in either the egg or the sperm, the resulting combination of genetic material may not be viable, and the death may occur in the early stages of embryonic cell division. Alternatively, the mutation in the genetic material may not affect early embryogenesis but may result in the death of the fetus at a later developmental period, resulting in abortion. Congenital abnormalities may also result from mutations. Somatic mutations refer to mutations in all other cell types and are not heritable but may result in cell death or transmission of a genetic defect to other cells in the same tissue through mitotic division. Because the initiating event of chemical carcinogenesis is thought to be a mutagenic one, mutagenic tests are often used to screen for potential carcinogens.

Numerous in vivo and in vitro procedures have been devised to test chemicals for their ability to cause mutations. Some genetic alterations are visible with the light microscope. In this case, cytogenetic analysis of bone marrow smears is used after the animals have been exposed to the test agent. Because some mutations are

incompatible with normal development, the mutagenic potential of a chemical can also be evaluated by the dominant lethal test. This test is usually performed in rodents. The male is exposed to a single dose of the test compound and then is mated with 2 untreated females weekly for 8 weeks. The females are killed before term, and the number of live embryos and the number of corpora lutea are determined.

The test for mutagens that has received the widest attention is the *Salmonella*/microsome test developed by Ames *et al.* (1975). This test uses several mutant strains of *Salmonella typhimurium* that lack the enzyme phosphoribosyl ATP synthetase, which is required for histidine synthesis. These strains are unable to grow in a histidine-deficient medium unless a reverse or back mutation to the wild type has occurred. Other mutations in these bacteria have been introduced to enhance the sensitivity of the strains to mutagenesis. The 2 most significant additional mutations enhance penetration of substances into the bacteria and decrease the ability of the bacteria to repair DNA damage. Because many chemicals are not mutagenic or carcinogenic unless they are biotransformed to a toxic product by enzymes in the endoplasmic reticulum (microsomes), rat liver microsomes are usually added to the medium containing the mutant strain and the test chemical. The number of reverse mutations is then quantified by the number of bacterial colonies that grow in a histidine-deficient medium.

Strains of yeast have recently been developed that detect genetic alterations arising during cell division after exposure to nongenotoxic carcinogens as well as mutations that arise directly from genotoxic carcinogens. This test identifies deletions of genetic material that occur during recombination events in cell division that may result from oxidative damage to DNA, direct mutagenic effects, alterations in fidelity of DNA repair, and/or changes in cell cycle regulation (Galli and Schiestl, 1999). Mutagenicity is discussed in detail in Chap. 9.

With the advent of techniques that readily allow manipulation of the mouse genome, transgenic animals have been developed that allow for in vivo assessment of mutagenicity of compounds. For example, 2 commercially available mouse strains, the "MutaMouse" and "Big Blue," contain the *lac* operon of *E. coli* that has been inserted into genomic DNA using a lambda phage to DNA to produce a recoverable shuttle vector. Stable, homozygous strains of these transgenic animals (both mice and rats have been engineered) can be exposed to potential mutagenic agents. Following in vivo exposure, the target *lac* genes can be recovered from virtually any cell type or organ and analyzed for mutations (Brusick *et al.*, 2008).

Oncogenicity Bioassays

Oncogenicity studies are both time consuming and expensive, and are usually only done when there is reason to suspect that a chemical may be carcinogenic, or when there may be wide spread, long-term exposures to humans (eg, widely used food additives, drinking water contaminants, or pharmaceuticals that are likely to be administered repeatedly for long periods of time). Chemicals that test positive in several mutagenicity assays are likely to be carcinogenic, and thus are frequent candidates for oncogenicity bioassay assessment. In the United States, the National Toxicology Program (NTP) has the primary responsibility for evaluating non-drug chemicals for carcinogenic potential. For pharmaceuticals, the FDA may require the manufacturer to conduct oncogenicity studies as part of the preclinical assessment, depending on the intended use of the drug, and the results of mutagenicity assays and other toxicological data.

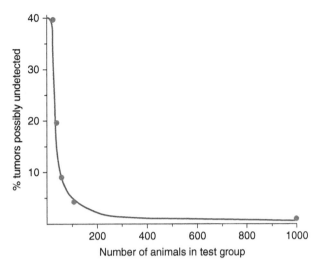

Figure 2-14. *Statistical limitations in the power of experimental animal studies to detect tumorigenic effects.*

Studies to evaluate the oncogenic (carcinogenic) potential of chemicals are usually performed in rats and mice and extend over the average lifetime of the species (18 months to 2 years for mice, 2–2.5 years for rats). To ensure that 30 rats per dose survive the 2-year study, 60 rats per group per sex are often started in the study. Both gross and microscopic pathological examinations are made not only on animals that survive the chronic exposure but also on those that die prematurely. The use of the MTD in carcinogenicity has been the subject of controversy. The premise that high doses are necessary for testing the carcinogenic potential of chemicals is derived from the statistical and experimental design limitations of chronic bioassays. Consider that a 0.5% increase in cancer incidence in the United States would result in over 1 million additional cancer deaths each year—clearly an unacceptably high risk. However, identifying with statistical confidence a 0.5% incidence of cancer in a group of experimental animals would require a minimum of 1000 test animals, and this assumes that no tumors were present in the absence of exposure (zero background incidence).

Fig. 2-14 shows the statistical relationship between minimum detectable tumor incidence and the number of test animals per group. This curve shows that in a chronic bioassay with 50 animals per test group, a tumor incidence of about 8% could exist even though no animals in the test group had tumors. This example assumes that there are no tumors in the control group. These statistical considerations illustrate why animals are tested at doses higher than those that occur in human exposure. Because it is impractical to use the large number of animals that would be required to test the potential carcinogenicity of a chemical at the doses usually encountered by people, the alternative is to assume that there is a relationship between the administered dose and the tumorigenic response and give animals doses of the chemical that are high enough to produce a measurable tumor response in a reasonable size test group, such as 40 to 50 animals per dose. The limitations of this approach are discussed in Chap. 4. For nonmutagenic pharmaceutical agents, ICH S1C provides the following guidance on dose selection for oncogenicity studies: "The doses selected for rodent bioassays for non-genotoxic pharmaceuticals should provide an exposure to the agent that (1) allow an adequate margin of safety over the human therapeutic exposure, (2) are tolerated without significant chronic physiological dysfunction and are compatible with good survival, (3) are guided by a comprehensive set of animal and human data that focus broadly on the properties of the agent and the suitability of the animal (4) and permit data interpretation in the context of clinical use."

Another approach for establishing maximum doses for use in chronic animal toxicity testing of drugs is often used for substances for which basic human pharmacokinetic data are available (eg, new pharmaceutical agents that have completed phase I clinical trials). For chronic animal studies performed on drugs where single-dose human pharmacokinetic data are available, a daily dose that would provide an area under the curve (AUC) in laboratory animals equivalent to 25 times the AUC in humans given the highest (single) daily dose to be used therapeutically may be used, rather than the MTD. Based on a series of assumptions regarding allometric scaling between rodents and humans (Table 2-2), the ICH noted that it may not be necessary to exceed a dose of 1500 mg/kg per day where there is no evidence of genotoxicity, and where the maximum recommended human dose does not exceed 500 mg per day.

Most regulatory guidelines require that both benign and malignant tumors be reported in oncogenicity bioassays. Statistical increases above the control incidence of tumors (either all tumors or specific tumor types) in the treatment groups are considered indicative of carcinogenic potential of the chemical unless there are qualifying factors that suggest otherwise (lack of a dose response, unusually low incidence of tumors in the control group compared with "historic" controls, etc; Huff, 1999). Thus, the conclusion as to whether a given chronic bioassay is positive or negative for carcinogenic potential of the test substance requires careful consideration of background tumor incidence. Properly designed chronic oncogenicity studies require that a concurrent control group matched for variables such as age, diet, and housing conditions be used. For some tumor types, the "background" incidence of tumors is surprisingly high. Fig. 2-15 shows the background tumor incidence for

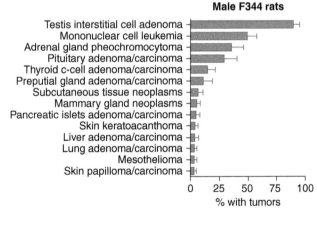

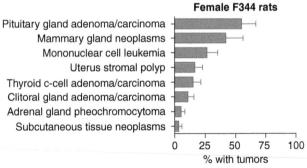

Figure 2-15. *Most frequently occurring tumors in untreated control rats from recent NTP 2-year rodent carcinogenicity studies.* The values shown represent the mean ± SD of the percentage of animals developing the specified tumor type at the end of the 2-year study. The values were obtained from 27 different studies involving a combined total of between 1319 and 1353 animals per tumor type.

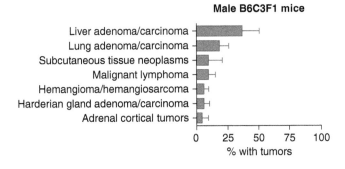

Male B6C3F1 mice

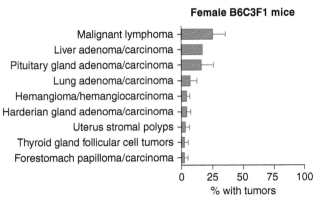

Female B6C3F1 mice

Figure 2-16. *Most frequently occurring tumors in untreated control mice from recent NTP 2-year rodent carcinogenicity studies.* The values shown represent the mean ± SD of the percentage of animals developing the specified tumor type at the end of the 2-year study. The values were obtained from 30 different studies involving a total of between 1447 and 1474 animals per tumor type.

various tumors in male and female F344 rats used in 27 NTP 2-year rodent carcinogenicity studies. The data shown represent the percent of animals in control (nonexposed) groups that developed the specified tumor type by the end of the 2-year study. These studies involved more than 1300 rats of each sex. Fig. 2-16 shows similar data for control (nonexposed) male and female B6C3F1 mice from 30 recent NTP 2-year carcinogenicity studies and includes data from over 1400 mice of each sex. There are several key points that can be derived from these summary data:

1. Tumors, both benign and malignant, are not uncommon events in animals even in the absence of exposure to any known carcinogen.
2. There are numerous different tumor types that develop "spontaneously" in both sexes of both rats and mice, but at different rates.
3. Background tumors that are common in 1 species may be uncommon in another (eg, testicular interstitial cell adenomas are very common in male rats but rare in male mice; liver adenomas/carcinomas are about 10 times more prevalent in male mice than in male rats).
4. Even within the same species and strain, large gender differences in background tumor incidence are sometimes observed (eg, adrenal gland pheochromocytomas are about 7 times more prevalent in male F344 rats than in female F344 rats; lung and liver tumors are twice as prevalent in male B6C3F1 mice as in female B6C3F1 mice).
5. Even when the general protocols, diets, environment, strain and source of animals, and other variables are relatively constant, background tumor incidence can vary widely, as shown by the relatively large SDs for some tumor types in the NTP

bioassay program. For example, the range in liver adenoma/carcinoma incidence in 30 different groups of unexposed (control) male B6C3F1 mice went from a low of 10% to a high of 68%. Pituitary gland adenomas/carcinomas ranged from 12% to 60% and 30% to 76% in unexposed male and female F344 rats, respectively, and from 0% to 36% in unexposed female B6C3F1 mice.

Taken together, these data demonstrate the importance of including concurrent control animals in such studies. In addition, comparisons of the concurrent control results to "historic" controls accumulated over years of study may be important in identifying potentially spurious "false-positive" results. The relatively high variability in background tumor incidence among groups of healthy, highly inbred strains of animals maintained on nutritionally balanced and consistent diets in rather sterile environments highlights the dilemma in interpreting the significance of both positive and negative results in regard to the human population, which is genetically diverse, has tremendous variability in diet, nutritional status, and overall health, and lives in an environment full of potentially carcinogenic substances, both natural and human-made.

Finally, it should be noted that both inbred and outbred strains have distinct background tumor patterns and the NTP and most other testing programs select strains based on the particular needs of the agent under study. For example, the NTP used the Wistar rat for chemicals that may have the testis as a target organ, based on acute, subchronic, or other bioassay results. Similarly, the NTP used the Sprague–Dawley strain of rat in studies of estrogenic agents such as genistein because its mammary tumors are responsive to estrogenic stimulation, as are humans'.

Neurotoxicity Assessment

Neurotoxicity or a neurotoxic effect is defined as an adverse change in the chemistry, structure, or function of the nervous system following exposure to a chemical or physical agent. The structure, function, and development of the nervous system and its vulnerability to chemicals are examined in Chap. 16. When evaluating the potential neurological effects of a compound, effects may be on the central or peripheral nervous system or related to exposure that occurred during development or as an adult. The developing nervous system is particularly sensitive to chemical exposures (see Chap. 10).

In vitro systems often using cell culture techniques are a rapidly developing area of neurotoxicity assessment. Specific cell lines are available to examine effects on neuron or glial cells such as proliferation, migration, apoptosis, synaptogenesis, and other end points. In vitro assays have a number of potential advantages including minimizing the use of animal, lower costs, and adaptable to high-throughput screening. It is also possible to use an in vitro model to examine the interaction of chemicals, such as food additives, on neuronal cells (Lau *et al.*, 2006). The principles and challenges of in vitro neurotoxicity testing are well described (Claudio, 1992; Tiffany-Castiglioni, 2004).

Procedures for the neurobehavioral evaluation of animals were initially developed as part of the scientific investigation of behavioral motivation. Some of these procedures were then used to evaluate the neuropharmacological properties of new drugs. Now animals are commonly used to evaluate the neurotoxic properties of chemicals. A wide range of adult and developmental animal tests are used to access neurobehavioral function. In addition, neuropathological assessment is an important part of the neurotoxicity evaluation and best practices have been developed for developmental neurotoxicity (DNT) (Bolon et al., 2006). Irwin developed a basic screen for behavioral function in mice (Irwin, 1968), which was subsequently refined to the functional observational battery (FOB) (Moser, 2000). The FOB can also be used in the evaluation of drug safety (Redfern et al., 2005).

The US EPA established a protocol for the evaluation of DNT in laboratory animals (US EPA 870.6300 and OECD 426) (EPA, 1998; OECD, 2004). These protocols include tests of neurobehavioral function, such as auditory startle, learning and memory function, changes in motor activity, and neuropathological examination and morphometric analysis. Methods and procedures for DNT evaluation are well established (Claudio et al., 2000; Cory-Slechta et al., 2001; Dorman et al., 2001; Garman et al., 2001; Mileson and Ferenc, 2001). Recent studies examine the neurotoxicity of multiple chemical exposures in animals (Moser et al., 2006). Methods are also available to examine cognitive measures on weanling rodents in DNT studies (Ehman and Moser, 2006). Nonhuman primates have been invaluable in evaluating the effects of neurotoxicants and the risk assessment process (Burbacher and Grant, 2000). Sophisticated assessment of operant behavior, and learning and memory assessment of rodents, has been used to evaluate the effects of lead (Cory-Slechta, 1995, 1996, 2003). Monkeys can also be used to evaluate the low-level effects of neurotoxicants such as mercury on vision, auditory function, and vibration sensitivity (Burbacher et al., 2005; Rice and Gilbert, 1982, 1992, 1995). There is remarkable concordance between human and animal neurotoxicity assessment, for example, in lead, mercury, and PCBs (Rice, 1995).

Human testing for the neurological effects of occupational exposures to chemicals (Anger, 2003; Farahat et al., 2003; Kamel et al., 2003; McCauley et al., 2006), and even the neurotoxic effects of war (Binder et al., 1999, 2001), is advancing rapidly. These methods have also been applied to Hispanic workers (Rohlman et al., 2001b) and populations with limited education or literacy (Rohlman et al., 2003). The WHO has also recommended a test battery for humans (Anger et al., 2000). There are also neurobehavioral test batteries for assessing children (Rohlman et al., 2001a). Evaluation of the childhood neurological effects of lead (Lanphear et al., 2005; Needleman and Bellinger, 1991) and mercury (Myers et al., 2000) has added enormously to our understanding of the health effects of these chemicals and to the methodology of human neurobehavioral testing.

In summary, the neurotoxicological evaluation is an important aspect of developing risk assessments for environmental chemicals and drugs.

Immunotoxicity Assessment

Under normal conditions, the immune system is responsible for host defense against pathogenic infections and certain cancers. However, environmental exposures can alter immune system development and/or function and lead to hypersensitivity, autoimmunity, or immunosuppression, the outcome of which may be expressed as a pathology in most any organ or tissue (see Chap. 12). Our understanding of the biological processes underlying immune system dysfunction remains incomplete. However, advances in molecular biology (including use of transgenic/knockout mice), analytic methods (including gene expression arrays and multiparameter flow cytometry), animal models (including adoptive transfers in immunocompromised mice and host resistance to viral, bacterial, or tumor cell challenge), and other methods are greatly advancing our knowledge.

From a toxicologist's perspective, evaluation of immune system toxicity represents special challenges. Development of hypersensitivity can take various forms, depending on the mechanism underlying the associated immune response, and standard assumptions regarding dose–response relationships may not necessarily apply. For example, a single or incidental exposure to beryllium has been associated with chronic beryllium disease in some individuals. We are only just beginning to understand the biological basis underlying such individual susceptibility. In the case of chronic beryllium disease, a genetic polymorphism in a gene involved in antigen recognition may be associated with increased susceptibility (see Bartell et al., 2000). Although our ability to predict immunogenicity remains poor, research efforts are continuing to identify aspects of the chemical and the individual that confer immunogenicity and underlie hypersensitivity. For example, the increasing incidence of allergic asthma among preschool-age children in the United States since the 1980s may be associated with exposure to allergens (eg, dust mites, molds, and animal dander), genetic factors, and other factors in the in utero and postnatal environment (see Donovan and Finn, 1999; Armstrong et al., 2005).

Immunosuppression is another form of immune system toxicity, which can result in a failure to respond to pathogenic infection, a prolonged infection period, or expression of a latent infection or cancer. Various chemicals have been associated with immunosuppression. Broad-spectrum and targeted immunosuppressive chemicals are designed and used therapeutically to reduce organ transplant rejection or suppress inflammation. However, a large number of chemicals have been associated with immunosuppression, including organochlorine pesticides, diethylstilbesterol, lead, and halogenated aromatic hydrocarbons (including TCDD), and exposures that occur during critical stages may present special risk to development (Holladay, 2005).

Autoimmunity is a specific immune system disorder in which components of the immune system attack normal (self) tissues. Cases of autoimmunity have been reported for a wide range of chemicals including therapeutic drugs, metals, pesticides, and solvents. As with other forms of immune system toxicity, autoimmunity can present in most any tissue.

Finally, new forms of immunotoxicity are appearing based on novel forms of clinical therapy and immunomodulation. These include the variously classified "tumor lysis syndromes" and "cytokine storms" that arise from massive cytokine dysregulation. A recent example involved 6 healthy volunteers who had enrolled in a phase 1 clinical trial in the United Kingdom who developed a severe cytokine response to an anti-CD28 monoclonal antibody leading to systemic organ failures (Bhogal and Combes, 2006). Such cases are stark reminders of the challenges we face in understanding how the immune system is regulated, developing reliable test systems for identifying such risks prior to human use, and developing safe means for testing these agents in humans.

As described in Chap. 12, current practice for evaluating potential toxic effects of xenobiotic exposures on the immune system involves a tiered approach to immunotoxicity screening (Luster et al., 2003). This tiered approach is generally accepted worldwide in the registration of novel chemical and therapeutic products. Most recently, final guidance to the pharmaceutical industry was published in April 2006 by the ICH of Technical Requirements for Registration of Pharmaceuticals for Human Use (Table 2-3). This guidance, which applies to the nonclinical (animal) testing of human pharmaceuticals, is the accepted standard in the United States, EU, and Japan, and demonstrates the continued commitment by these regulatory bodies to understand the potential risks posed by novel therapeutics.

Tiered testing relies on the concept that standard toxicity studies can provide good evidence for immunotoxicity when considered with known biological properties of the chemical, including structural similarities to known immunomodulators, disposition, and other clinical information, such as increased occurrence of infections or tumors. Evaluation of hematological changes, including differential effects on white blood cells and immunoglobulin changes, and alterations in lymphoid organ weights or histology, can provide strong evidence of potential effects to the immune system. Should such evaluations indicate a potential effect on immune system function, more detailed evaluations may be considered, including the evaluation of functional effects (eg, T-cell-dependent antibody response or natural killer cell activity), flow cytometric immunophenotyping, or host resistance studies. Thus, as with other areas of toxicology, the evaluation of immune system toxicity requires the toxicologist to be vigilant in observing early indications from a variety of sources in developing a weight-of-evidence assessment regarding potential injury/dysfunction.

Other Descriptive Toxicity Tests

Most of the tests described above will be included in a "standard" toxicity testing protocol because they are required by the various regulatory agencies. Additional tests may be required or included in the protocol to provide information relating a special route of exposure, such as inhalation. Inhalation toxicity tests in animals usually are carried out in a dynamic (flowing) chamber rather than in static chambers to avoid particulate settling and exhaled gas complications. Such studies usually require special dispersing and analytic methodologies, depending on whether the agent to be tested is a gas, vapor, or aerosol; additional information on methods, concepts, and problems associated with inhalation toxicology is provided in Chaps. 15 and 28. The duration of exposure for inhalation toxicity tests can be acute, subchronic, or chronic, but acute studies are more common with inhalation toxicology. Other special types of animal toxicity tests include toxicokinetics (absorption, distribution, biotransformation, and excretion), the development of appropriate antidotes and treatment regimens for poisoning, and the development of analytic techniques to detect residues of chemicals in tissues and other biological materials.

TOXICOGENOMICS

In the past decade, numerous new genome-based technologies have become available that allow for the large-scale analysis of biological responses to external stimuli. Traditional scientific approaches to elucidate the biochemical and molecular effects of toxic substances focused largely on examining biochemical pathways that were logically connected to observed responses identified through gross pathology, histology, blood chemistry, or behavioral observations. Such "hypothesis-driven" research into understanding mechanism of action remains a mainstay of current scientific investigations in toxicology. However, technologies now available allow one to examine the entire "universe" of biological responses to a toxic substance (Fig. 2-17). These new "hypothesis-generating" technologies include genomics (characterization of much or all of the genome of an organism), transcriptomics (characterization of most or all of the messenger RNAs [mRNAs], or transcriptome, expressed in a given cell/tissue), proteomics (characterization of most or all of the proteins expressed in a given cell/tissue), and metabonomics (characterization of most or all of the small molecules in a cell or tissue, including substrates, products, and cofactors of enzyme reactions). Other "omics" approaches (eg, "lipidomics,"

"nutrigenomics") are being devised to look broadly at the biological response of an organism to change. The integration of all of these levels of molecular function (genomics, transcriptomics, proteomics, metabonomics, etc) to the understanding of how a living organism functions at the cellular level is sometimes referred to as "systems biology" (Weston and Hood, 2004). Because each level of analysis generates a very large quantity of data, the collection, organization, evaluation, and statistical analysis is in itself an enormous undertaking. The field of "bioinformatics" has been developed to address the many computational and statistical challenges of "omics" data. In the field of toxicology, the term "toxicogenomics" is used to define the area of research that "combines transcript, protein and metabolite profiling with conventional toxicology to investigate the interaction between genes and environmental stress in disease causation" (Waters and Fostel, 2004). A conceptual model for how the various new "omics" technologies can be incorporated into toxicological evaluation is shown in Fig. 2-17.

Genomics

The genome of an organism represents the full complement of genes that are determined at fertilization by the combination of the parental DNA. Thus, each cell of an organism has the same genome, characterized by the nucleotide sequences inherited from its parents. The human genome consists of approximately 3 billion base pairs of deoxyribonucleotides. Within the human genome, there is, on average, about 0.1% variability in DNA sequence between any 2 individuals, and it is these differences that contribute to the uniqueness of each person. Most of this variability exists as "SNPs," although larger segments of DNA may be variable between individuals, including the duplication or loss of entire genes. The identification of particular genetic variants, such as the GSTM1 polymorphism, which might contribute to interindividual differences in susceptibility to chemicals or other environmental factors discussed previously, represents a relatively new and growing area of study that aims to understand the complex interactions between the human genome and the environment (Costa and Eaton, 2006).

Although the genome provides the blueprint for biological function, in order for the genomic information to be utilized in a cell, it must be expressed. Expression of the genome occurs when the coding sequence of DNA is converted to mRNA. For any given cell, transcription of the genomic information contained in that cell is only partial. It is the differential expression of genes in a given cell that is largely responsible for the diverse function of the thousands of different cells, tissues, and organs that constitute an individual organism. Thus, understanding which genes are expressed in a given tissue, at what level, and how toxicants perturb the "transcriptome" is of great relevance to toxicology. In addition to coding for mRNAs that provide the blueprint for protein synthesis, genomic DNA also generates small interfering RNAs (siRNA, microRNAs) that are biologically active and can participate in the regulation of gene expression.

Epigenetics/Epigenomics

The expanding research into the relatively new field of epigenomics will have important implications for public health and toxicology. The concept of epigenetics, meaning something acting "above or in addition" to genes, was proposed many decades ago, although the application to the full genome (epigenomics) rather than to single or a few genes (epigenetics) is new. Conrad Hal Waddington first postulated in the 1930s that it was not just the genes that shaped development but also the environment that shapes the genes

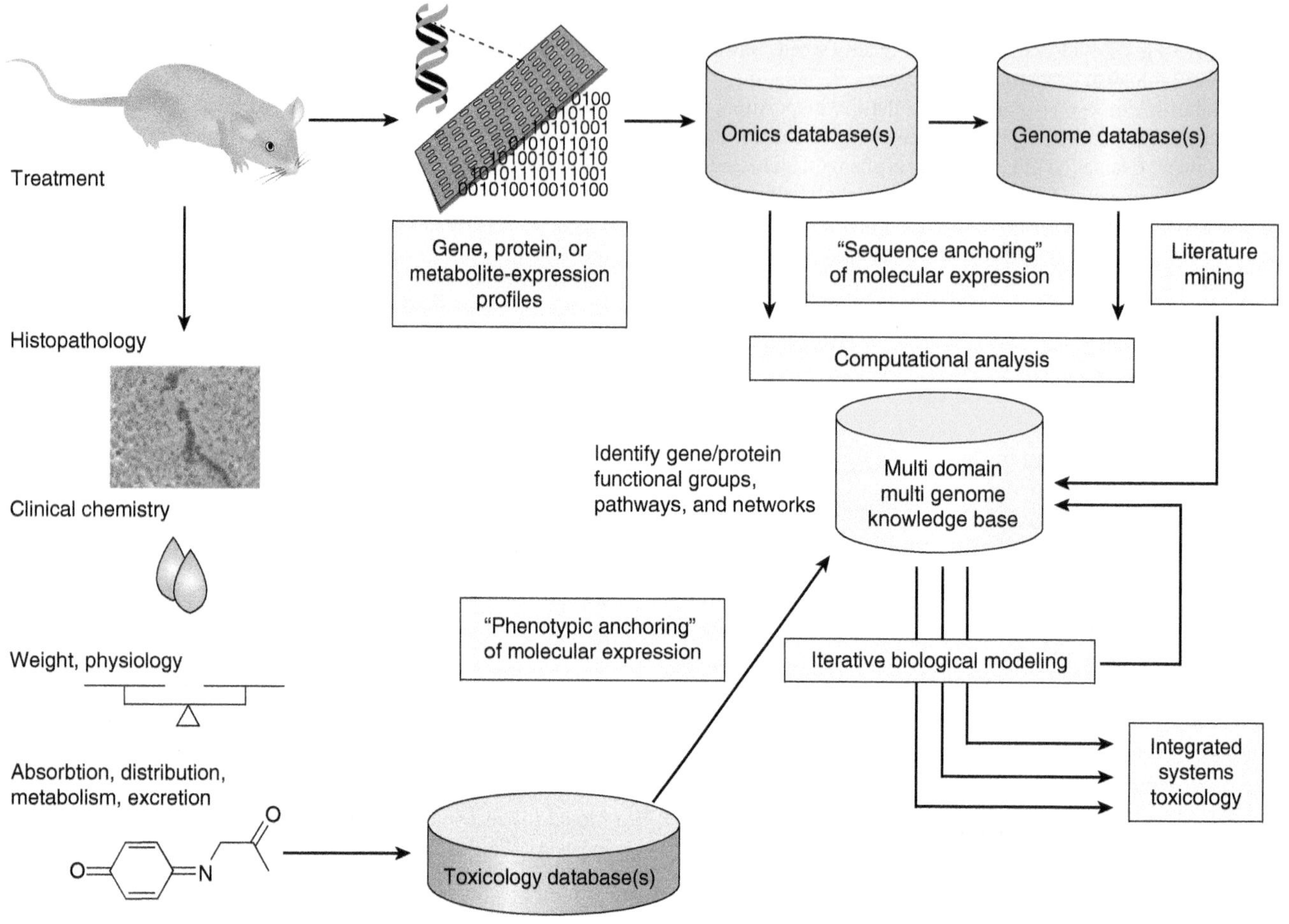

Figure 2-17. *Conceptual approach for incorporating "omics" technologies and resulting large databases into toxicological evaluation.* Data from experiments that evaluate the effects of a chemical on global patterns of gene expression (transcriptomics), protein content (proteomics), and small molecules/metabolites (metabonomics/metabolomics), combined with genomic information from both the test species (eg, rats, mice) and the target species of interest (eg, humans), are analyzed by computational tools (bioinformatics) for unique or potentially predictive patterns of toxicity. Essential to the use of omics data for predictive toxicology/safety assessment is the ability to reliably tie observed omics patterns to traditional measures of toxicity, such as histopathology and clinical chemistry (phenotypic anchoring). (From Waters and Fostel, 2004, with permission.)

(Holliday, 2006). Understanding a possible mechanism had to wait for a far deeper understanding of DNA and its role in development. Epigenetics has been defined in various ways, with perhaps the strictest definition being "a mitotically or meiotically heritable change in gene expression that occurs independently of an alteration in DNA sequence" (Youngson and Whitelaw, 2008). Typically gene expression is silenced or suppressed, or in some instances activated, by DNA methylation or histone deacetylation—changes that do not alter the nucleotide sequence of the silenced genes (Fig. 2-18). Epigenetic changes can potentially be transgenerational, as suggested in some animal models, which has important implications for toxicological assessment (Rosenfeld, 2010; Skinner, 2011). Given the growing recognition of epigenetics as a means by which environmental factors can alter biological responses, genomic analyses in toxicology may also include techniques to identify toxicant-induced changes in DNA methylation patterns (Watson and Goodman, 2002; LeBaron et al., 2010).

Although classical approaches to toxicology have thoroughly documented the potential for a variety of environmental toxicants, such as thalidomide, alcohol, lead, mercury, and PCBs, to cause adverse effects on the developing organism, more subtle epigenetic changes, which are not associated with either cytotoxicity or mutations, can also result from environmental exposures and

thus may have important toxicological implications. Epigenetic changes have been demonstrated to occur from exposure to a variety of environmental hazards, including tobacco smoke, metals, alcohol, phthalates, and BPA (Cheng et al., 2012; Perera and Herbstman, 2011; Bernal and Jirtle, 2010; Baccarelli and Bollati, 2009). Furthermore, epigenetic changes can occur through nutrition, methyl content of diet, intake of folic acid and vitamins, or even social and maternal behavior toward the offspring (Cummings et al., 2010). Epigenetic changes have been causally implicated in cancer, neurodevelopment disorders, autoimmune diseases, diabetes and metabolic disorders, asthma, behavioral disorders, and endocrine disorders (Godfrey et al., 2011; Nystrom and Mutanen, 2009; Zhang and Ho, 2011; Attig et al., 2010). There is also concern chemicals in the environment may induce epigenetic changes in wildlife that could be an important consideration in ecotoxicology (Vandegehuchte and Janssen, 2011; Head et al., 2012). Thus, epigenetic changes induced by xenobiotics, dietary factors, and maternal behavior have important implications for safety assessment and risk assessment for xenobiotics (LeBaron et al., 2010; Goodman et al., 2010; Szyf, 2007).

Thus, it is now evident that methylation of DNA is an important determinant of gene expression in cells and tissues, and exogenous chemicals can interfere with transcriptional function

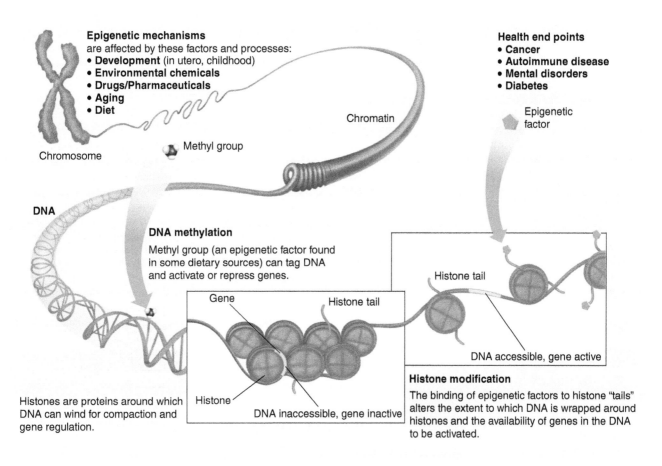

Epigenetic mechanisms
are affected by these factors and processes:
• **Development** (in utero, childhood)
• **Environmental chemicals**
• **Drugs/Pharmaceuticals**
• **Aging**
• **Diet**

Chromosome

Methyl group

Chromatin

DNA

DNA methylation
Methyl group (an epigenetic factor found in some dietary sources) can tag DNA and activate or repress genes.

Gene

Histone tail

Histones are proteins around which DNA can wind for compaction and gene regulation.

Histone

DNA inaccessible, gene inactive

Health end points
• **Cancer**
• **Autoimmune disease**
• **Mental disorders**
• **Diabetes**

Epigenetic factor

Histone tail

DNA accessible, gene active

Histone modification
The binding of epigenetic factors to histone "tails" alters the extent to which DNA is wrapped around histones and the availability of genes in the DNA to be activated.

Figure 2-18. *Process and consequence of epigenetic regulation of gene expression* (National Institute of Health).

via alternating DNA methylation (Watson and Goodman, 2002). Importantly, although such epigenetic changes do not result in the alteration of the genomic sequence, they theoretically can result in heritable phenotypic changes; although proof of multigenerational epigenetic changes from environmental exposures has yet to be demonstrated in humans (Baccarelli and Bollati, 2009), several animal models have demonstrated transgenerational epigenetic changes (Skinner, 2011). Thus, genomic analyses in toxicology may also include techniques to identify toxicant-induced changes in DNA methylation patterns to access epigenetic changes and the potential consequences (Watson and Goodman, 2002; Szyf, 2007).

Transcriptomics

Among the first changes that a cell will exhibit following exposure to a toxic substance is a change in gene expression. The transcriptome (all of the mature mRNA species present in a cell at a given point in time) is dynamic, and represents the steady state between the rate of synthesis (transcription) and degradation of mRNAs in a cell. Toxicologists have utilized the so-called Northern blot analysis to assess the level of expression of individual genes in cells or tissues for decades. The "reverse transcriptase polymerase chain reaction" (RT-PCR) allows one to quantitatively measure the relative number of mRNA species in a sample for specific genes. Using general primers, it is also possible to amplify the entire transcriptome quantitatively to make many complete copies of the transcriptome in a test tube. Thus, large amounts of material for analysis can be obtained from a relatively small number of cells. Finally,

using microarray technologies, where tens of thousands of unique oligonucleotides (or cDNAs) are anchored on a solid matrix, toxicologists can now quantitatively assess the expression of thousands of unique mRNAs in a single sample, thus capturing an "expression profile" of the entire transcriptome in 1 analysis.

There is great promise that gene expression profiles may be used to provide signatures of specific types of toxic responses, such as a cellular response to DNA damage or oxidative stress. There is also hope that such signature changes in gene expression could be used to facilitate more accurate cross-species extrapolation, allowing comparison of, for example, toxicant-induced changes in gene expression in rat hepatocytes with that of human hepatocytes under identical experimental conditions. However, 1 of the major challenges in toxicogenomics is the recognition that transcriptional regulation is highly dynamic, and that gene expression profiles can change dramatically with both dose and time. Because microarray experiments are relatively expensive and highly data intensive, it becomes both costly and challenging to conduct and analyze experiments with extensive dose and time course data (although costs are declining). Although changes in gene expression often contribute to, or are reflective of, phenotypic changes that occur in response to a toxic substance, the transcriptome is still somewhat far removed from the ultimate biochemical functions that dictate the actual biological function of the cell. Because the functional expression of a gene generally requires the translation of the mRNA to a protein, there is also great interest in looking at the "proteome"—the entire complement of *proteins* that are present in a cell or tissue at a given point in time.

Proteomics

Analysis of the proteome of a cell or tissue is much more difficult than analysis of the transcriptome, primarily because it is not yet possible to "amplify" the number of copies of proteins in a cell. Furthermore, unambiguous identification of specific proteins is much more difficult than that for individual mRNAs. Identification of specific proteins is generally done using a combination of separation techniques (eg, 2D gel electrophoresis, high-performance liquid chromatography), followed by tandem mass spectrometry for identification (Aebersold and Mann, 2003). Because of size limitations for accurate mass spectrometry, protein mixtures are usually digested to smaller peptide fragments. The mixture of peptide fragments is resolved into individual components, and the identity of the specific peptides is determined based on high-resolution mass analysis and sequential degradation (sequential loss of single amino acids) of the peptides by various means (Aebersold and Mann, 2003). The large and complex set of peptide mass fragments is then analyzed by computers and compared with a large database of mass fragments of known peptides/proteins. Because as few as 5 amino acid sequences may provide unique identification of a specific protein, the presence and relative abundance of specific proteins in a sample can then be reconstructed through bioinformatic analyses. As with transcriptomics, it is hoped that changes in protein expression can be used as specific biomarkers for particular types of toxic responses. Of course, such conceptual approaches have been used for years, for example, use of serum transaminase proteins as indicators of liver damage, or the presence of prostate-specific antigen (PSA) in serum as a potential biomarker of early stage prostate hyperplasia or cancer. The potential power of proteomics lies in the ability to identify unique patterns of protein expression, or identification of unique proteins or peptides, that are predictive of early toxic response or later development of disease.

Metabonomics/Metabolomics

These 2 terms are often used interchangeably to describe the analysis of the "universe" of small molecules that serve as substrates, products, and cofactors of the milieu of enzymatic reactions and other metabolic processes that define living cells, and thus the organism. Metabonomics has been defined as "the comprehensive and simultaneous systematic profiling of metabolite levels and their systematic and temporal change through such effects on diet, lifestyle, environment, genetic and pharmaceuticals, both beneficial and adverse, in whole organisms" (Lindon et al., 2003, 2006). The term "metabolomics" has been used principally in studies in plants and in vitro or single-cell systems (Fiehn, 2002). Regardless of the specific term used (metabonomics will be used here), the concept of quantitatively analyzing toxicant-induced changes in the "metabolic profile" (the "metabonome") of a cell, tissue, or body fluid in some ways represents the "Holy Grail" of toxicogenomics, because the changes in these small molecules must represent a biologically relevant integration of all of the molecular, biochemical, and cellular perturbations that lead to the development of toxicity (Fig. 2-17). In other words, changes in the metabonome should reflect the biologically relevant changes in gene transcription, translation, protein function, and other cellular processes, including temporal and adaptive responses, while ignoring biologically irrelevant changes in these factors. Although conceptually superior to either transcriptomics or proteomics for predictive toxicology, metabonomics lags significantly in technological development of readily accessible tools for thorough analysis of the metabonome.

Two approaches for identifying and measuring hundreds, or even thousands, of small molecules in biological samples have emerged—nuclear magnetic resonance (NMR) and mass spectrometry (Lindon et al., 2003, 2006). Both have their advantages and limitations, and it is likely that the most successful approaches to applying metabonomics to toxicological problems will utilize both techniques (Pan and Raftery, 2007).

Bioinformatics

One feature in common among all of the various "omics" technologies is the ability to generate very large volumes of data (literally millions of data points from a single experiment). Both the data management and statistical evaluation of toxicogenomics studies represent an enormous challenge. The emerging field of bioinformatics has developed to address these challenges. Numerous commercial platforms for conducting microarray analysis of the transcriptome are available, and sophisticated software is available for both data management and analysis. One of the major challenges in statistical analysis of large data sets is the large number of "false positives" that will result from multiple comparisons. In a typical gene array experiment, it is not uncommon for an investigator to make >20,000 different comparisons. At the typical "95%" statistical confidence limit, one would expect more than 1000 of the noted differences to occur just by chance alone. Thus, more rigorous statistical methods have been developed to reduce the so-called false discovery rate in such experiments (Storey et al., 2005; Gao, 2006).

Challenges in Using "Omics" Technologies for Predictive Toxicology and Risk Assessment

A conceptual framework for incorporating these new technologies into toxicology, sometimes referred to as "systems toxicology," is shown in Fig. 2-18. Several key components of such an approach include: (1) large databases of treatment-specific information, such as results of transcriptomic, proteomic, and metabonomic analyses from target tissues and/or body fluids derived from toxicant-treated animals, (2) genomic databases that describe the DNA sequence information from the species of interest, (3) computational tools that extract information from these and other databases and the published literature to identify critical pathways and networks that are altered by the toxicant treatment, and (4) comparison with traditional toxicological end points to ensure that the observed "omics responses" are closely aligned with the toxicant-related pathophysiology in the animal (histopathology, clinical chemistry, etc)—a process called "phenotypic anchoring" (Waters and Fostel, 2004).

Toxicogenomics tools are becoming indispensable for research aimed at identifying the mechanisms and mode of action of toxic substances. However, the incorporation of such approaches into routine toxicity assessment presents numerous challenges. Numerous working group reports and publications have addressed the challenges of incorporating toxicogenomics data into predictive toxicology and risk assessment (Bammler et al., 2005; Maggioli et al., 2006; Boverhof and Zacharewski, 2006).

One of the major challenges to incorporating toxicogenomic data into risk assessment is related to the highly dynamic processes that preceded an observed toxic response. Traditional measure of toxicity, such as histopathological changes in a tissue, tends to be stable or even irreversible, whereas the myriad of molecular, biochemical, and cellular changes that give rise to the toxic response(s) are highly dynamic, frequently changing by the hour. Thus, the profiles of mRNAs, proteins, and/or metabolites captured at a single point in time may be dramatically different, depending on the specific point in time the sample was collected. Many of the observed changes may be the result of direct effects of the toxicant on specific targets, whereas others will be compensatory or feedback mechanisms invoked in response to the initial damage. Nevertheless, patterns of change in transcript, protein, and/or metabolite profiles are likely to provide informative "signatures" of toxic response that will be of great value in predictive toxicology. Such approaches may be particularly useful in pharmaceutical development, where toxicogenomic profiles may help to accelerate preclinical evaluation of drug candidates by identifying "class prediction" profiles indicative of certain types of desirable (pharmacological efficacy) as well as adverse (eg, DNA damage, oxidative stress) responses.

Finally, it is likely that the introduction of omics technologies to toxicity testing will eventually contribute to the reduction, refinement, and replacement (the "3Rs") of animals in toxicity testing and product safety evaluations (Kroeger, 2006).

REFERENCES

Aebersold R, Mann M. Mass spectrometry-based proteomics. *Nature.* 2003;422:198–207.

Albert A. *Selective Toxicity.* London: Chapman and Hall; 1973.

Aldridge WN. The biological basis and measurement of thresholds. *Annu Rev Pharmacol Toxicol.* 1986;26:39–58.

Allen BC, Kavlock RJ, Kimmel CA, et al. Dose–response assessment for developmental toxicity: II. Comparison of generic benchmark dose estimates with no observed adverse effect levels. *Fundam Appl Toxicol.* 1994a;23:487–495.

Allen BC, Kavlock RJ, Kimmel CA, et al. Dose–response assessment for developmental toxicity: III. Statistical models. *Fundam Appl Toxicol.* 1994b;23:496–509.

Ames BN, McCann J, Yamasaki E. Methods for detecting carcinogens and mutagens with the *Salmonella*/mammalian-microsome mutagenicity test. *Mutat Res.* 1975;31:347–364.

Anger WK. Neurobehavioural tests and systems to assess neurotoxic exposures in the workplace and community. *Occup Environ Med.* 2003;60:531–538, 474.

Anger WK, Liang YX, Nell V, et al. Lessons learned—15 years of the WHO-NCTB: a review. *Neurotoxicology.* 2000;21(5):837–846.

Arcury TA, Quandt SA, Dearry A. Farmworker pesticide exposure and community-based participatory research: rationale and practical applications. *Environ Health Perspect.* 2001;109(suppl 3):429–434.

Armstrong JM, Loer-Martin D, Leibnitz R. Developmental immunotoxicant exposure and exacerbated postnatal immune responses: asthma. In: Holladay SD, ed. *Developmental Immunotoxicology.* Boca Raton: CRC Press; 2005:229–281.

Attig L, Gabory A, Junien C. Nutritional developmental epigenomics: immediate and long-lasting effects. *Proc Nutr Soc.* 2010;69:221–231.

Baccarelli A, Bollati V. Epigenetics and environmental chemicals. *Curr Opin Pediatr.* 2009;21:243–251.

Bailey GS, Reddy AP, Pereira CB, et al. Non-linear cancer response at ultra-low dose: a 40,800-animal ED001 tumor and biomarker study. *Chem Res Toxicol.* 2009;22:1264–1276.

Bammler T, Beyer RP, Bhattacharya S, et al. Standardizing global gene expression analysis between laboratories and across platforms. *Nat Methods.* 2005;2:351–356.

Barile FA. Clinical Toxicology: Principles and Mechanisms, 2nd ed. New York, *Informa Healthcare.* 2010.

Barnes DG, Dourson M. Reference dose (RfD): description and use in health risk assessments. *Regul Toxicol Pharmacol.* 1988;8:471–486.

Bartell SM, Takaro TK, Ponce RA, et al. Risk assessment and screening strategies for beryllium exposure. *Technology.* 2000;7:241–249.

Bartels CF, James K, La Du BN. DNA mutations associated with the human butyrylcholinesterase J-variant. *Am J Hum Genet.* 1992;50: 1104–1114.

Beauchamp TL, Childress JF. *Principles of Biomedical Ethics.* 4th ed. New York: Oxford University Press; 1994.

Bernal AJ, Jirtle RL. Epigenomic disruption: the effects of early developmental exposures. *Birth Defects Res A Clin Mol Teratol.* 2010;88(10):938–944.

Bhogal N, Combes R. TGN1412: time to change the paradigm for the testing of new pharmaceuticals. *Altern Lab Anim.* 2006;34:225–239.

Binder LM, Storzbach D, Anger WK, et al. Subjective cognitive complaints, affective distress, and objective cognitive performance in Persian Gulf War veterans. *Arch Clin Neuropsychol.* 1999;14:531–536.

Binder LM, Storzbach D, Campbell KA, et al. Neurobehavioral deficits associated with chronic fatigue syndrome in veterans with Gulf War unexplained illnesses. *J Int Neuropsychol Soc.* 2001;7: 835–839.

Bliss CL. Some principles of bioassay. *Am Sci.* 1957;45:449–466.

Bolon B, Garman R, Jensen K, Krinke G, Stuart B. A "best practices" approach to neuropathologic assessment in developmental neurotoxicity testing—for today. *Toxicol Pathol.* 2006;34(3):296–313.

Boverhof DR, Zacharewski TR. Toxicogenomics in risk assessment: applications and needs. *Toxicol Sci.* 2006;89:352–360.

Bruce RD. An up-and-down procedure for acute toxicity testing. *Fundam Appl Toxicol.* 1985;5:151–157.

Bruce RD. A confirmatory study of the up-and-down method for acute oral toxicity testing. *Fundam Appl Toxicol.* 1987;8:97–100.

Brusick DJ, Fields WR, Myhr BC, Doolittle DJ. Genetic toxicology. In: Hayes AW, ed. *Principles and Methods of Toxicology.* 5th ed. New York: Informa Healthcare; 2008:1179–1222:chap 23.

Burbacher TM, Grant KS. Methods for studying nonhuman primates in neurobehavioral toxicology and teratology. *Neurotoxicol Teratol.* 2000;22:475–486.

Burbacher TM, Grant KS, Mayfield DB, et al. Prenatal methylmercury exposure affects spatial vision in adult monkeys. *Toxicol Appl Pharmacol.* 2005;208:21–28.

Calabrese EJ, Blain R. The occurrence of hormetic dose responses in the toxicological literature, the hormesis database: an overview. *Toxicol Appl Pharmacol.* 2005;202:289–301.

Callahan D, Jennings B. Ethics and public health: forging a strong relationship. *Am J Public Health.* 2002;92:169–176.

Carson R. *Silent Spring.* Boston: Houghton Mifflin; 2002, c 1962.

Cheng TF, Choudhuri S, Muldoon-Jacobs K. Epigenetic targets of some toxicologically relevant metals: a review of the literature. *J Appl Toxicol.* 2012;32(9):643–653.

Christian MS. Test methods for assessing female reproductive and developmental toxicology. In: Hayes AW, ed. *Principles and Methods of Toxicology.* 5th ed. New York: Informa Healthcare; 2008:1641–1712: chap 34.

Claudio L. An analysis of the U.S. Environmental Protection Agency neurotoxicity testing guidelines. *Regul Toxicol Pharmacol.* 1992;16(2): 202–212.

Claudio L, Kwa WC, Russell AL, Wallinga D. Testing methods for developmental neurotoxicity of environmental chemicals. *Toxicol Appl Pharmacol.* 2000;164(1):1–14.

Coble Y, Coussens C, Quinn K. *Environmental Health Sciences Decision Making: Risk Management, Evidence, and Ethics: Workshop Summary.* Washington, DC: National Academies Press; 2009.

Cohen SM. Cell proliferation and carcinogenesis. *Drug Metab Rev.* 1998;30:339–357.

Cohen SM. Calcium phosphate–containing urinary precipitate in rat urinary bladder carcinogenesis. *IARC Sci Publ.* 1999;147:175–189.

Corburn J. Environmental justice, local knowledge, and risk: the discourse of a community-based cumulative exposure assessment. *Environ Manage.* 2002;29:451–466.

Cory-Slechta DA. Relationships between lead-induced learning impairments and changes in dopaminergic, cholinergic, and glutamatergic neurotransmitter system functions. *Annu Rev Pharmacol Toxicol.* 1995;35: 391–415.

Cory-Slechta DA. Legacy of lead exposure: consequences for the central nervous system. *Otolaryngol Head Neck Surg.* 1996;114: 224–226.

Cory-Slechta DA. Lead-induced impairments in complex cognitive function: offerings from experimental studies. *Child Neuropsychol.* 2003;9:54–75.

Cory-Slechta DA, Crofton KM, Foran JA, et al. Methods to identify and characterize developmental neurotoxicity for human health risk assessment. I: behavioral effects. *Environ Health Perspect.* 2001;109(suppl 1): 79–91.

Costa LG, Eaton DL. *Gene–Environment Interactions: Fundamentals of Ecogenetics.* New York: Wiley Press; 2006:557 pp.

Crump KS. An improved procedure for low-dose carcinogenic risk assessment from animal data. *J Environ Pathol Toxicol Oncol.* 1984;5:339–348.

Cummings JA, Clemens LG, Nunez AA. Mother counts: how effects of environmental contaminants on maternal care could affect the offspring and future generations. *Front Neuroendocrinol.* 2010;31:440–451.

D'Arcy PF, Harron DWG, eds. *Proceedings of the First International Conference on Harmonisation.* Belfast: Queen's University of Belfast; 1992.

Donovan CE, Finn PW. Immune mechanisms of childhood asthma. *Thorax.* 1999;54:938–946.

Dorman DC, Allen SL, Byczkowski JZ, et al. Methods to identify and characterize developmental neurotoxicity for human health risk assessment. III: pharmacokinetic and pharmacodynamic considerations. *Environ Health Perspect.* 2001;109(suppl 1):101–111.

Doull J. Factors influencing toxicity. In: Doull J, Klaassen CD, Amdur MO, eds. *Casarett and Doull's Toxicology: The Basic Science of Poisons.* 2nd ed. New York: Macmillan; 1980:70–83.

Dybing E, Sanner T. Species differences in chemical carcinogenesis of the thyroid gland, kidney and urinary bladder. *IARC Sci Publ.* 1999;147:15–32.

Eaton DL. Scientific judgment and toxic torts: a primer in toxicology for judges and lawyers. *J Law Policy.* 2003;12:5–42.

Eaton DL, Gallagher EP. Introduction to principles of toxicology. In: McQueen C, ed. *Comprehensive Toxicology: Volume 1, General Principles.* 2nd ed. New York: Elsevier; 2010:1–46.

Ehman KD, Moser VC. Evaluation of cognitive function in weanling rats: a review of methods suitable for chemical screening. *Neurotoxicol Teratol.* 2006;28(1):144–161.

Eichelbaum M, Ingelman-Sundberg M, Evans WE. Pharmacogenomics and individualized drug therapy. *Annu Rev Med.* 2006;57:119–137.

EPA. *Health Effects Test Guidelines.* OPPTS 870.6300. Developmental Neurotoxicity Toxicity Study. Washington, DC: U.S. Environmental Protection Agency; 1998.

EPA. *Environmental Justice.* Washington, DC: Environmental Protection Agency; 2005. Available at: http://www.epa.gov/compliance/environmentaljustice/.

Farahat TM, Abdelrasoul GM, Amr MM, et al. Neurobehavioural effects among workers occupationally exposed to organophosphorous pesticides. *Occup Environ Med.* 2003;60:279–286.

Faustman EM. Short-term tests for teratogens. *Mutat Res.* 1988;205:355–384.

Faustman EM, Allen BC, Kavlock RJ, et al. Dose–response assessment for developmental toxicity: I. Characterization of database and determination of no observed adverse effect levels. *Fundam Appl Toxicol.* 1994;23:478–486.

Fiehn O. Metabolomics—the link between genotypes and phenotypes. *Plant Mol Biol.* 2002;48:155–171.

Finney DJ. *Probit Analysis.* Cambridge: Cambridge University Press; 1971.

Finney DJ. The median lethal dose and its estimation. *Arch Toxicol.* 1985;56:215–218.

Galli A, Schiestl RH. Cell division transforms mutagenic lesions into deletion-recombinagenic lesions in yeast cells. *Mutat Res.* 1999;429:13–26.

Gao X. Construction of null statistics in permutation-based multiple testing for multi-factorial microarray experiments. *Bioinformatics.* 2006;22:1486–1494.

Garman RH, Fix AS, Jortner BS, et al. Methods to identify and characterize developmental neurotoxicity for human health risk assessment. II: neuropathology. *Environ Health Perspect.* 2001;109(suppl 1):93–100.

Gilbert G. Ethical, legal, and social issues: our children's future. *Neurotoxicology.* 2005a;26:521–530.

Gilbert SG. Public health and the precautionary principle. *Northwest Public Health.* 2005b;(spring/summer):4.

Gilbert SG. Supplementing the traditional institutional review board with an environmental health and community review board. *Environ Health Perspect.* 2006;114:1626–1629.

Gilbert SG, Eaton DL. Ethical, legal, social, and professional issues in toxicology. In: Ballantyne B, Marrs TC, Syversen T, eds. *General and Applied Toxicology.* 3rd ed. West Sussex, UK: Wiley; 2009:chap 116.

Glynn P, Read DJ, Lush MJ, et al. Molecular cloning of neuropathy target esterase (NTE). *Chem Biol Interact.* 1999;119(120):513–517.

Godfrey KM, Sheppard A, Gluckman PD, et al. Epigenetic gene promoter methylation at birth is associated with child's later adiposity. *Diabetes.* 2011;60:1528–1534.

Goldstein A, Aronow L, Kalman SM. *Principles of Drug Action.* New York: Wiley; 1974.

Goldstein BD. The precautionary principle: is it a threat to toxicological science? *Int J Toxicol.* 2006;25:3–7.

Goodman JI, Augustine KA, Cunnningham ML, et al. What do we need to know prior to thinking about incorporating an epigenetic evaluation into safety assessments? *Toxicol Sci.* 2010;116:375–381.

Goozner M. *Unrevealed: Non-Disclosure of Conflicts of Interest in Four Leading Medical and Scientific Journals.* Washington, DC: Center for Science in the Public Interest; 2004.

Grisham JW. Interspecies comparison of liver carcinogenesis: implications for cancer risk assessment. *Carcinogenesis.* 1997;18:59–81.

Guzelian PS, Victoroff MS, Halmes NC, et al. Evidence-based toxicology: a comprehensive framework for causation. *Hum Exp Toxicol.* 2005;24:161–201.

Halle W. The Registry of Cytotoxicity: toxicity testing in cell cultures to predict acute toxicity (LD50) and to reduce testing in animals. *Altern Lab Anim.* 2003;31(2):89–198.

Hanna EZ, Chou SP, Grant BF. The relationship between drinking and heart disease morbidity in the United States: results from the National Health Interview Survey. *Alcohol Clin Exp Res.* 1997;21:111–118.

Harkness JE, Wagner JE. *The Biology and Medicine of Rabbits and Rodents.* 4th ed. New York: Williams and Wilkins; 1995.

Haseman JK. Issues in carcinogenicity testing: dose selection. *Fundam Appl Toxicol.* 1985;5:66–78.

Hatch EE, Palmer JR, Titus-Ernstoff L, et al. Cancer risk in women exposed to diethylstilbestrol in utero. *JAMA.* 1998;280:630–634.

Hayes AW, ed. *Principles and Methods of Toxicology.* 5th ed. New York: Informa Healthcare; 2008.

Hayes BB, Patrick E, Maibach HJ. Dermatotoxicology. In: Hayes AW, ed. *Principles and Methods of Toxicology.* New York: Informa Healthcare; 2008:1359–1406:chap 27.

Head JA, Dolinoy DC, Basu N. Epigenetics for ecotoxicologists. *Environ Toxicol Chem.* 2012;31(2):221–227.

Hengstler JG, Van der Burg B, Steinberg P, et al. Interspecies differences in cancer susceptibility and toxicity. *Drug Metab Rev.* 1999;31: 917–970.

Hill AB. The environment and disease: association or causation? *Proc R Soc Med.* 1965;58:295–300.

Holladay SD, ed. *Developmental Immunotoxicology.* Boca Raton: CRC Press; 2005:364.

Holliday R. Epigenetics: a historical overview. *Epigenetics.* 2006;1:76–80.

Huff JE. Value, validity, and historical development of carcinogenesis studies for predicting and confirming carcinogenic risk to humans. In: Kitchin KT, ed. *Carcinogenicity Testing: Predicting & Interpreting Chemical Effects.* New York: Marcel Dekker; 1999:21–123.

Ikeda T. Drug-induced idiosyncratic hepatotoxicity: prevention strategy developed after the troglitazone case. *Drug Metab Pharmacokinet.* 2011;26(1):60–70.

Irwin S. Comprehensive observational assessment: Ia. A systematic, quantitative procedure for assessing the behavioral and physiologic state of the mouse. *Psychopharmacologia.* 1968;13(3):222–257.

Jacobson-Kram D, Keller KA. *Toxicology Testing Handbook: Principles, Applications and Data Interpretation.* 2nd ed. New York: Informa Healthcare; 2006.

Kamel F, Rowland AS, Park LP, et al. Neurobehavioral performance and work experience in Florida farmworkers. *Environ Health Perspect.* 2003;111:1765–1772.

Kass NE. An ethics framework for public health. *Am J Public Health.* 2001;91:1776–1782.

Kirman CR, Sweeney LM, Meek ME, Gargas ML. Assessing the dose-dependency of allometric scaling performance using physiologically based pharmacokinetic modeling. *Regul Toxicol Pharmacol.* 2003; 38(3):345–367.

Kobayashi Y, Fukumaki Y, Yubisui T, et al. Serine–proline replacement at residue 127 of NADH-cytochrome b5 reductase causes hereditary methemoglobinemia, generalized type. *Blood.* 1990;75:1408–1413.

Krimsky S, Rothenberg LS. Conflict of interest policies in science and medical journals: editorial practices and author disclosures. *Sci Eng Ethics.* 2001;7:205–218.

Krimsky S, Sweet E. An analysis of toxicology and medical journal conflict-of-interest polices. *Account Res.* 2009;16:235–253.

Kroeger M. How omics technologies can contribute to the "3R" principles by introducing new strategies in animal testing. *Trends Biotechnol.* 2006;24:343–346.

Landrigan PJ, Schechter CB, Lipton JM, et al. Environmental pollutants and disease in American children: estimates of morbidity, mortality, and costs for lead poisoning, asthma, cancer, and developmental disabilities. *Environ Health Perspect.* 2002;110:721–728.

Lanphear BP, Hornung R, Khoury J, et al. Low-level environmental lead exposure and children's intellectual function: an international pooled analysis. *Environ Health Perspect.* 2005;113:894–899.

Lary JM, Daniel KL, Erickson JD, et al. The return of thalidomide: can birth defects be prevented? *Drug Saf.* 1999;21:161–169.

Lassiter TL, Barone S Jr, Moser VC, Padilla S. Gestational exposure to chlorpyrifos: dose–response profiles for cholinesterase and carboxylesterase activity. *Toxicol Sci.* 1999;52:92–100.

Lau K, McLean WG, Williams DP, Howard CV. Synergistic interactions between commonly used food additives in a developmental neurotoxicity test. *Toxicol Sci.* 2006;90:178–187.

LeBaron MJ, Rasoulpour RJ, Klapacz J, et al. Epigenetics and chemical safety assessment. *Mutat Res.* 2010;705(2):83–95.

Lee C. Environmental justice: building a unified vision of health and the environment. *Environ Health Perspect.* 2002;110(suppl 2):141–144.

Lehman-McKeeman LD, Caudill D. Biochemical basis for mouse resistance to hyaline droplet nephropathy: lack of relevance of the alpha 2u-globulin protein superfamily in this male rat-specific syndrome. *Toxicol Appl Pharmacol.* 1992;112:214–221.

Leopold A. *A Sand County Almanac: With Essays on Conservation.* Oxford: Oxford University Press; 1949 [reprinted, 2001].

Levine RR. *Pharmacology: Drug Actions and Reactions.* Boston: Little, Brown, and Company; 1978.

Lindon JC, Holmes E, Nicholson JK. Metabonomics techniques and applications to pharmaceutical research & development. *Pharm Res.* 2006;23:1075–1088.

Lindon JC, Nicholson JK, Holmes E, et al. Contemporary issues in toxicology the role of metabonomics in toxicology and its evaluation by the COMET project. *Toxicol Appl Pharmacol.* 2003;187:137–146.

Litchfield J, Wilcoxon F. Simplified method of evaluating dose–effect experiments. *J Pharmacol Exp Ther.* 1949;96:99–113.

Litchfield JT. A method for rapid graphic solution of time-percent effective curve. *J Pharmacol Exp Ther.* 1949;97:399–408.

Littlefield NA, Farmer JH, Gaylor DW, et al. Effects of dose and time in a long-term, low-dose carcinogenicity study. In: Staffa JA, Mehlman MA, eds. *Innovations in Cancer Risk Assessment (ED01 Study).* Park Forest South, IL: Pathotox Publishers; 1979.

Luster MI, Dean JH, Germolec DR. Consensus workshop on methods to evaluate developmental immunotoxicity. *Environ Health Perspect.* 2003;111:579–583.

Maggioli J, Hoover A, Weng L. Toxicogenomic analysis methods for predictive toxicology. *J Pharmacol Toxicol Methods.* 2006;53:31–37.

Marchant G. From general policy to legal rule: aspirations and limitations of the precautionary principle. *Environ Health Perspect.* 2003;111:1799–1803.

Maurissen JP, Gilbert SG, Sander M, et al. Workshop proceedings: managing conflict of interest in science. A little consensus and a lot of controversy. *Toxicol Sci.* 2005;87:11–14.

McCauley LA, Anger WK, Keifer M, et al. Studying health outcomes in farmworker populations exposed to pesticides. *Environ Health Perspect.* 2006;114:953–960.

Mileson BE, Ferenc SA. Methods to identify and characterize developmental neurotoxicity for human health risk assessment: overview. *Environ Health Perspect.* 2001;109(suppl 1):77–78.

Mohr LC, Rodgers JK, Silvestri GA. Glutathione S-transferase M1 polymorphism and the risk of lung cancer. *Anticancer Res.* 2003;23:2111–2124.

Monticello TM, Morgan KT. Chemically-induced nasal carcinogenesis and epithelial cell proliferation: a brief review. *Mutat Res.* 1997;380:33–41.

Morello-Frosch R, Pastor M Jr, Porras C, Sadd J. Environmental justice and regional inequality in southern California: implications for future research. *Environ Health Perspect.* 2002;110(suppl 2):149–154.

Moser VC. The functional observational battery in adult and developing rats. *Neurotoxicology.* 2000;21(6):989–996.

Moser VC, Simmons JE, Gennings C. Neurotoxicological interactions of a five-pesticide mixture in preweanling rats. *Toxicol Sci.* 2006;92:235–245.

Myers GJ, Davidson PW, Cox C, et al. Twenty-seven years studying the human neurotoxicity of methylmercury exposure. *Environ Res.* 2000;83:275–285.

Myers NJ, Raffensperger C, eds. *Precautionary Tools for Reshaping Environmental Policy.* Cambridge: MIT Press; 2006.

NAS. *Policy on Committee Composition and Balance and Conflicts of Interest for Committees Used in the Development of Reports.* Washington, DC: National Academies Press; 2003.

NAS/NRC. *Toxicity Testing in the 21st Century: A Vision and a Strategy.* Washington, DC: National Academy Press; 2007.

NAS/NRC. *Toxicity-Pathway-Based Risk Assessment: Preparing for Paradigm Change: A Symposium Summary.* Washington, DC: National Academies Press; 2010.

Needleman HL, Bellinger D. The health effects of low level exposure to lead. *Annu Rev Public Health.* 1991;12:111–140.

Netzlaff F, Lehr CM, Wertz PW, Schaefer UF. The human epidermis models EpiSkin, SkinEthic and EpiDerm: an evaluation of morphology and their suitability for testing phototoxicity, irritancy, corrosivity, and substance transport. *Eur J Pharm Biopharm.* 2005;60(2):167–178.

Nweke OC. A framework for integrating environmental justice in regulatory analysis. *Int J Environ Res Public Health.* 2011;8(6):2366–2385.

Nystrom M, Mutanen M. Diet and epigenetics in colon cancer. *World J Gastroenterol.* 2009;15:257–263.

OECD. *Draft Guidance Document on Reproductive Toxicity Testing and Assessment, Series on Testing and Assessment No. 43.* Paris, France: Environment Directorate, Organisation for Economic Cooperation and Development; 2004.

O'Fallon LR, Dearry A. Community-based participatory research as a tool to advance environmental health sciences. *Environ Health Perspect.* 2002;110(suppl 2):155–159.

Pan Z, Raftery D. Comparing and combining NMR spectroscopy and mass spectrometry in metabolomics. *Anal Bioanal Chem.* 2007;387(2): 525–527.

Perera F, Herbstman J. Prenatal environmental exposures, epigenetics, and disease. *Reprod Toxicol.* 2011;31:363–373.

Peterson M. The precautionary principle is incoherent. *Risk Anal.* 2006;26:595–601.

Pugsley MK, Authier S, Curtis MJ. Principles of safety pharmacology. *Br J Pharmacol.* 2008;154(7):1382–1399.

Pugsley MK, Towart R, Authier S, Gallacher DJ, Curtis MJ. Innovation in safety pharmacology testing. *J Pharmacol Toxicol Methods.* 2011; 64(1):1–6.

Raffensperger C, Tickner J, eds. *Protecting Public Health & the Environment: Implementing the Precautionary Principle.* Washington, DC: Island Press; 1999.

Redfern WS, Strang I, Storey S, et al. Spectrum of effects detected in the rat functional observational battery following oral administration of non-CNS targeted compounds. *J Pharmacol Toxicol Methods.* 2005;52:77–82.

Reno FE. Carcinogenicity studies. In: Sipes IG, McQueen CA, Gandolfi AJ, eds. *Comprehensive Toxicology.* Williams PD, Hottendorf GH, eds. *Toxicological Testing and Evaluation.* Vol. 2. New York: Pergamon Press; 1997:121–131.

Rhomberg LR, Wolff SK. Empirical scaling of single oral lethal doses across mammalian species based on a large database. *Risk Anal.* 1998;18:741–753.

Rice DC. Neurotoxicity of lead, methylmercury, and PCBs in relation to the Great Lakes. *Environ Health Perspect.* 1995;103(suppl 9):71–87.

Rice DC, Gilbert SG. Early chronic low-level methylmercury poisoning in monkeys impairs spatial vision. *Science.* 1982;216(4547):759–761.

Rice DC, Gilbert SG. Exposure to methyl mercury from birth to adulthood impairs high-frequency hearing in monkeys. *Toxicol Appl Pharmacol.* 1992;115:6–10.

Rice DC, Gilbert SG. Effects of developmental methylmercury exposure or lifetime lead exposure on vibration sensitivity function in monkeys. *Toxicol Appl Pharmacol.* 1995;134:161–169.

Roberts RA. Peroxisome proliferators: mechanisms of adverse effects in rodents and molecular basis for species differences. *Arch Toxicol.* 1999;73:413–418.

Rodricks JV, Gaylor DW, Turnbull D. Quantitative extrapolations in toxicology. In: Hayes AW, ed. *Principles and Methods in Toxicology.* 5th ed. New York: Informa Healthcare; 2008:453–474:chap 9.

Rohlman DS, Anger WK, Tamulinas A, et al. Development of a neurobehavioral battery for children exposed to neurotoxic chemicals. *Neurotoxicology.* 2001a;22:657–665.

Rohlman DS, Bailey SR, Anger WK, McCauley L. Assessment of neurobehavioral function with computerized tests in a population of Hispanic adolescents working in agriculture. *Environ Res.* 2001b;85:14–24.

Rohlman DS, Gimenes LS, Eckerman DA, et al. Development of the Behavioral Assessment and Research System (BARS) to detect and characterize neurotoxicity in humans. *Neurotoxicology.* 2003;24:523–531.

Rosenfeld CS. Animal models to study environmental epigenetics. *Biol Reprod.* 2010;82:473–488.

Rush RE, Bonnette KL, Douds DA, et al. Dermal irritation and sensitization. In: Derelanko MJ, Hollinger MA, eds. *CRC Handbook of Toxicology.* New York: CRC Press; 1995:105–162.

Simon T. Just who is at risk? The ethics of environmental regulation. *Hum Exp Toxicol.* 2011;30:795–819.

Skinner MK. Role of epigenetics in developmental biology and transgenerational inheritance. *Birth Defects Res C Embryo Today.* 2011;93:51–55.

Storey JD, Xiao W, Leek JT, et al. Significance analysis of time course microarray experiments. *Proc Natl Acad Sci U S A.* 2005;102:12837–12842.

Szyf M. The dynamic epigenome and its implications in toxicology. *Toxicol Sci.* 2007;100(1):7–23.

Tennant RW, Stasiewicz S, Mennear J, et al. Genetically altered mouse models for identifying carcinogens. *IARC Sci Publ.* 1999;146:123–150.

Tiffany-Castiglioni E, ed. *In Vitro Neurotoxicology: Principles and Challenges (Methods in Pharmacology and Toxicology).* Totowa, NJ: Humana Press; 2004.

Travis CC, White RK. Interspecific scaling of toxicity data. *Risk Anal.* 1988;8:119–125.

Uetrecht J. Idiosyncratic drug reactions: current understanding. *Annu Rev Pharmacol Toxicol.* 2007;47:513–539.

Uhl K, Cox E, Rogan R, et al. Thalidomide use in the US: experience with pregnancy testing in the S.T.E.P.S. programme. *Drug Saf.* 2006;29:321–329.

Ukelis U, Kramer PJ, Olejniczak K, Mueller SO. Replacement of in vivo acute oral toxicity studies by in vitro cytotoxicity methods: opportunities, limits and regulatory status. *Regul Toxicol Pharmacol.* 2008;51(1):108–118.

Vandegehuchte MB, Janssen CR. Epigenetics and its implications for ecotoxicology. *Ecotoxicology.* 2011;20:607–624.

Vandenberg LN, Maffini MV, Sonnenschein C, Rubin BS, Soto AM. Bisphenol-A and the great divide: a review of controversies in the field of endocrine disruption. *Endocr Rev.* 2009;30(1):75–95.

Wang L, McLeod HL, Weinshilboum RM. Genomics and drug response. *N Engl J Med.* 2011;364(12):1144–1153.

Waters MD, Fostel JM. Toxicogenomics and systems toxicology: aims and prospects. *Nat Rev Genet.* 2004;5:936–948.

Watson RE, Goodman JI. Epigenetics and DNA methylation come of age in toxicology. *Toxicol Sci.* 2002;67:11–16.

Weil C. Tables for convenient calculation of median-effective dose (LD50 or ED50) and instruction in their use. *Biometrics.* 1952;8:249–263.

Weinshilboum RM, Otterness DM, Szumlanski CL. Methylation pharmacogenetics: catechol *O*-methyltransferase, thiopurine methyltransferase, and histamine *N*-methyltransferase. *Annu Rev Pharmacol Toxicol.* 1999;39:19–52.

Weston AD, Hood L. Systems biology, proteomics, and the future of health care: toward predictive, preventive, and personalized medicine. *J Proteome Res.* 2004;3:179–196.

Williams DE. The rainbow trout liver cancer model: response to environmental chemicals and studies on promotion and chemoprevention. *Comp Biochem Physiol C Toxicol Pharmacol.* 2012;155(1):121–127.

Williams DE, Orner G, Willard KD, et al. Rainbow trout (*Oncorhynchus mykiss*) and ultra-low dose cancer studies. *Comp Biochem Physiol C Toxicol Pharmacol.* 2009a;149(2):175–181.

Williams ES, Panko J, Paustenbach DJ. The European Union's REACH regulation: a review of its history and requirements. *Crit Rev Toxicol.* 2009b;39(7):553–575.

Wilson NH, Hardisty JF, Hayes JR. Short-term, subchronic and chronic toxicology studies. In: Hayes AW, ed. *Principles and Methods of Toxicology.* New York: Informa Healthcare; 2008;1223–1264:chap 24.

Wiman KG. The retinoblastoma gene: role in cell cycle control and cell differentiation. *FASEB J.* 1993;7:841–845.

Wogan GN, Paglialunga S, Newberne PM. Carcinogenic effects of low dietary levels of aflatoxin B1 in rats. *Food Cosmet Toxicol.* 1974;12:681–685.

Youngson NA, Whitelaw E. Transgenerational epigenetic effects. *Annu Rev Genomics Hum Genet.* 2008;9:233–257.

Zhang X, Ho SM. Epigenetics meets endocrinology. *J Mol Endocrinol.* 2011;46:R11–R32.

chapter 3

Mechanisms of Toxicity

Zoltán Gregus

Depending primarily on the degree and route of exposure, chemicals may adversely affect the function and/or structure of living organisms. The qualitative and quantitative characterization of these harmful or toxic effects is essential for an evaluation of the potential hazard posed by a particular chemical. It is also valuable to understand the mechanisms responsible for the manifestation of toxicity—that is, how a toxicant enters an organism, how it interacts with target molecules, and how the organism deals with the insult.

An understanding of the mechanisms of toxicity is of both practical and theoretical importance. Such information provides a rational basis for interpreting descriptive toxicity data, estimating the probability that a chemical will cause harmful effects, establishing procedures to prevent or antagonize the toxic effects, designing drugs and industrial chemicals that are less hazardous, and developing pesticides that are more selectively toxic for their target organisms. Elucidation of the mechanisms of chemical toxicity has led to a better understanding of fundamental physiologic and biochemical processes ranging from neurotransmission (eg, curare-type arrow poisons) through deoxyribonucleic acid (DNA)

repair (eg, alkylating agents) to transcription, translation, and signal transduction pathways (eg, chemicals acting through transcription factors [TFs], such as the aryl hydrocarbon receptor [AhR]). Pathologic conditions such as cancer and Parkinson disease are better understood because of studies on the mechanism of toxicity of chemical carcinogens and 1,2,3,6-tetrahydro-1-methyl-4-phenylpyridine (MPTP), respectively. Continued research on mechanisms of toxicity will undoubtedly continue to provide such insights.

This chapter reviews the cellular mechanisms that contribute to the manifestation of toxicities. Although such mechanisms are also dealt with elsewhere in this volume, they are discussed in detail in this chapter in an integrated and comprehensive manner. We provide an overview of the mechanisms of chemical toxicity by relating a series of events that begins with exposure, involves a multitude of interactions between the invading toxicant and the organism, and culminates in a toxic effect. This chapter focuses on mechanisms that have been identified definitively or tentatively in humans or animals.

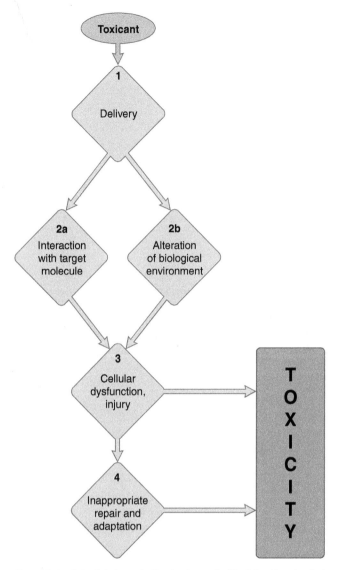

Figure 3-1. *Potential stages in the development of toxicity after chemical exposure.*

As a result of the huge number of potential toxicants and the multitude of biological structures and processes that can be impaired, there are a tremendous number of possible toxic effects. Correspondingly, there are various pathways that may lead to toxicity (Fig. 3-1). A common course is when a toxicant delivered to its target reacts with it, and the resultant cellular dysfunction manifests itself in toxicity. An example of this route to toxicity is that taken by the puffer fish poison, tetrodotoxin. After ingestion, this poison reaches the voltage-gated Na$^+$ channels of neurons (step 1). Interaction of tetrodotoxin with this target (step 2a) results in blockade of Na$^+$ channels, inhibition of the activity of motor neurons (step 3), and ultimately skeletal muscle paralysis. No repair mechanisms can prevent the onset of such toxicity.

Sometimes a xenobiotic does not react with a specific target molecule but rather adversely influences the biological (micro) environment, causing molecular, organellar, cellular, or organ dysfunction leading to deleterious effects. For example, 2,4-dinitrophenol, after entering the mitochondrial matrix space (step 1), collapses the outwardly directed proton gradient across the inner membrane by its mere presence there (step 2b), causing mitochondrial dysfunction (step 3), which is manifest in toxic

effects such as hyperthermia and seizures. Chemicals that precipitate in renal tubules and block urine formation represent another example for such a course (step 2b).

The most complex path to toxicity involves more steps (Fig. 3-1). First, the toxicant is delivered to its target or targets (step 1), after which the ultimate toxicant interacts with endogenous target molecules (step 2a), triggering perturbations in cell function and/or structure (step 3), which initiate repair mechanisms at the molecular, cellular, and/or tissue levels as well as adaptive mechanisms to diminish delivery, boost repair capacity, and/or compensate for dysfunction (step 4). When the perturbations induced by the toxicant exceed repair and adaptive capacity or when repair and adaptation becomes malfunctional, toxicity occurs. Tissue necrosis, cancer, and fibrosis are examples of chemically induced toxicities whose development follow this 4-step course.

STEP 1—DELIVERY: FROM THE SITE OF EXPOSURE TO THE TARGET

Theoretically, the intensity of a toxic effect depends primarily on the concentration and persistence of the ultimate toxicant at its site of action. The ultimate toxicant is the chemical species that reacts with the endogenous target molecule (eg, receptor, enzyme, DNA, microfilamental protein, lipid) or critically alters the biological (micro) environment, initiating structural and/or functional alterations that result in toxicity. Often the ultimate toxicant is the original chemical to which the organism is exposed (parent compound). In other cases, the ultimate toxicant is a metabolite of the parent compound or a reactive oxygen or nitrogen species (ROS or RNS) generated during the biotransformation of the toxicant. Occasionally, the ultimate toxicant is an unchanged or altered endogenous molecule (Table 3-1).

The concentration of the ultimate toxicant at the target molecule depends on the relative effectiveness of the processes that increase or decrease its concentration at the target site (Fig. 3-2). The accumulation of the ultimate toxicant at its target is facilitated by its absorption, distribution to the site of action, reabsorption, and toxication (metabolic activation). Conversely, presystemic elimination, distribution away from the site of action, excretion, and detoxication oppose these processes and work against the accumulation of the ultimate toxicant at the target molecule.

Absorption versus Presystemic Elimination

Absorption Absorption is the transfer of a chemical from the site of exposure, usually an external or internal body surface (eg, skin, mucosa of the alimentary and respiratory tracts), into the systemic circulation. Whereas transporters may contribute to the gastrointestinal (GI) absorption of some chemicals (eg, salicylate and valproate by monocarboxylate transporters, some β-lactam antibiotics and ACE inhibitor drugs by peptide transporters (PEPT), Fe^{2+}, Cd^{2+}, as well as some other divalent metal ions by the divalent metal ion transporter, and arsenate by phosphate transporters), the vast majority of toxicants traverse epithelial barriers and reach the blood capillaries by diffusing through cells. The rate of absorption is related to the concentration of the chemical at the absorbing surface, which depends on the rate of exposure and the dissolution of the chemical. It is also related to the area of the exposed site, the characteristics of the epithelial layer through which absorption takes place (eg, the thickness of the stratum corneum in the skin), the intensity of the subepithelial microcirculation, and the physicochemical properties of the toxicant. Lipid solubility is usually the most important

Table 3-1

Types of Ultimate Toxicants and Their Sources

Parent xenobiotics as ultimate toxicants

Pb ions
Tetrodotoxin
TCDD
Methylisocyanate
HCN
CO

Xenobiotic metabolites as ultimate toxicants

Amygdalin	→	HCN
Arsenate	→	Arsenite
Fluoroacetate	→	Fluorocitrate
Ethylene glycol	→	Oxalic acid
Hexane	→	2,5-Hexanedione
Acetaminophen	→	N-Acetyl-p-benzoquinoneimine
CCl_4	→	$CCl_3OO^\bullet$
Benzo[a]pyrene (BP)	→	BP-7,8-diol-9,10-epoxide
Benzo[a]pyrene (BP)	→	BP-radical cation

Reactive oxygen or nitrogen species as ultimate toxicants

Hydrogen peroxide		
Diquat, doxorubicin, nitrofurantion ⎫	→	Hydroxyl radical (HO$^\bullet$)
Cr(V), Fe(II), Mn(II), Ni(II) ⎭		
Paraquat → $O_2^{\cdot} + NO^\bullet$	→	Peroxynitrite (ONOO$^-$)

Endogenous compounds as ultimate toxicants

Sulfonamides → albumin-bound bilirubin	→	Bilirubin
$CCl_3OO^\bullet$ → unsaturated fatty acids	→	Lipid peroxyl radicals
$CCl_3OO^\bullet$ → unsaturated fatty acids	→	Lipid alkoxyl radicals
$CCl_3OO^\bullet$ → unsaturated fatty acids	→	4-Hydroxynon-2-enal
HO$^\bullet$ → proteins	→	Protein carbonyls

property influencing absorption. In general, lipid-soluble chemicals are absorbed more readily than are water-soluble substances.

Presystemic Elimination During transfer from the site of exposure to the systemic circulation, toxicants may be eliminated. This is not unusual for chemicals absorbed from the GI tract because they must first pass through the GI mucosal cells, liver, and lung before being distributed to the rest of the body by the systemic circulation. The GI mucosa and the liver may eliminate a significant fraction of a toxicant during its passage through these tissues, decreasing its systemic availability. For example, ethanol is oxidized by alcohol dehydrogenase in the gastric mucosa (Lim *et al.*, 1993), cyclosporine is returned from the enterocyte into the intestinal lumen by multidrug resistance protein (MDR1, also known as P-glycoprotein, an ATP-dependent xenobiotic transporter) and is also hydroxylated by cytochrome P450 (CYP3A4) in these cells (Lin *et al.*, 1999), morphine is glucuronidated in intestinal mucosa and liver, and manganese is taken up from the portal blood into liver and excreted into bile. Such processes may prevent a considerable quantity of chemicals from reaching the systemic blood. Thus, presystemic or first-pass elimination reduces the toxic effects of chemicals that reach their target sites by way of the systemic circulation. In contrast, the processes involved in presystemic elimination may contribute to injury of the digestive mucosa, liver, and lungs by chemicals such as ethanol, iron salts, α-amanitin, and paraquat because these processes promote their delivery to those sites.

Distribution To and Away from the Target

Toxicants exit the blood during the distribution phase, enter the extracellular space, and may penetrate into cells. Chemicals dissolved in plasma water may diffuse through the capillary endothelium via aqueous intercellular spaces and transcellular pores called fenestrae and/or across the cell membrane. Lipid-soluble compounds move readily into cells by diffusion. In contrast, highly ionized and hydrophilic xenobiotics (eg, tubocurarine and aminoglycosides) are largely restricted to the extracellular space unless specialized membrane carrier systems are available to transport them.

During distribution, toxicants reach their site or sites of action, usually a macromolecule on either the surface or the interior of a particular type of cell. Chemicals also may be distributed to the site or sites of toxication, usually an intracellular enzyme, where the ultimate toxicant is formed. Some mechanisms facilitate, whereas others delay, the distribution of toxicants to their targets.

Mechanisms Facilitating Distribution to a Target Distribution of toxicants to specific target sites may be enhanced by (1) the porosity of the capillary endothelium, (2) specialized membrane transport, (3) accumulation in cell organelles, and (4) reversible intracellular binding.

Porosity of the Capillary Endothelium Endothelial cells in the hepatic sinusoids and in the renal peritubular capillaries have larger

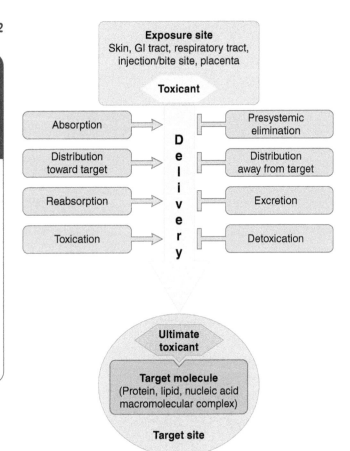

Figure 3-2. *The process of toxicant delivery is the first step in the development of toxicity.*

fenestrae (50–150 nm in diameter) that permit passage of even protein-bound xenobiotics. This favors the accumulation of chemicals in the liver and kidneys.

Specialized Transport Across the Plasma Membrane Specialized ion channels and membrane transporters can contribute to the delivery of toxicants to intracellular targets. For example, aquaglyceroporin channels may mediate influx of arsenite, which is present at physiologic pH as uncharged $As(OH)_3$, voltage-gated Ca^{2+} channels permit the entry of cations such as lead or barium ions into excitable cells, and Na^+,K^+-ATPase promotes intracellular accumulation of thallous ion. By mimicking Na^+, Li^+ may enter excitable cells through voltage-gated Na^+ channels and, from the tubular fluid, into the principal cells of the renal collecting duct via the epithelial Na^+ channels. Paraquat enters into pneumocytes via hitherto unspecified transporters and an MPTP metabolite (MPP^+) is taken up into extrapyramidal dopaminergic neurons by the dopamine transporter. Organic cation transporters (OCT) mediate the uptake of small-molecular-weight organic cations (eg, metformin, cimetidine, and cisplatin) from blood into liver cells (by OCT1) and into renal proximal tubular cells (by OCT2). The hepatocellular uptake of α-amanitin is mediated by the Na-dependent bile acid transporter (NTCP). Specific organic anion-transporting polypeptide (OATP) transporters mediate the hepatic uptake and hepatotoxicity of microcystin, a cyclic heptapeptide toxin produced by blue-green algae. In mice, Oatp1b2 (the rodent ortholog of OATP1B1/1B3) is essential, as Oatp1b2-null mice are resistant to microcystin-induced liver injury (Lu *et al.*, 2008). Organic anion transporters such as human OAT1 and OAT3 mediate renal tubular uptake of ochratoxin and mercuric ion (the latter as the

dicysteine conjugate Cys-Hg-Cys), whereas both OAT1 and amino acid transporters can carry methylmercury as its cysteine conjugate CH_3-Hg-Cys, and an MPTP metabolite (MPP^+) enters into extrapyramidal dopaminergic neurons by means of the dopamine transporter. Endocytosis of some toxicant–protein complexes, such as Cd-metallothionein (MT) or hydrocarbons bound to the male rat–specific α_{2u}-globulin, by renal proximal tubular cells can also occur. Particles, such as asbestos and manufactured nanomaterial, may also enter cells by endocytosis, depending on their size and shape. Lipoprotein receptor–mediated endocytosis contributes to entry of lipoprotein-bound toxicants into cells equipped with such transporters. Membrane recycling can internalize cationic aminoglycosides associated with anionic phospholipids in the brush border membrane of renal tubular cells (Laurent *et al.*, 1990). This process may also contribute to cellular uptake of heavy metal ions. Such uptake mechanisms facilitate the entry of toxicants into specific cells, rendering those cells targets. Thus, carrier-mediated uptake of paraquat by pneumocytes and internalization of aminoglycosides by renal proximal tubular cells expose those cells to toxic concentrations of those chemicals.

Accumulation in Cell Organelles Amphipathic xenobiotics with a protonable amine group and lipophilic character accumulate in lysosomes as well as mitochondria and cause adverse effects there. Lysosomal accumulation occurs by pH trapping, that is, diffusion of the amine (eg, amiodarone, amitriptyline, fluoxetine) in unprotonated form into the acidic interior of the organelle, where the amine is protonated, preventing its efflux. The entrapped amine inhibits lysosomal phospholipases, impairing degradation of lysosomal phospholipids and causing phospholipidosis. Mitochondrial accumulation takes place electrophoretically. The amine is protonated in the intermembrane space (to where the mitochondria eject protons). The cation thus formed will then be sucked into the matrix space by the strong negative potential there (–220 mV), where it may impair β-oxidation and oxidative phosphorylation. By such mechanisms, the valued antiarrhytmic drug amiodarone is entrapped in the hepatic lysosomes and mitochondria, causing phospholipidosis (Kodavanti and Mehendale, 1990) and microvesicular steatosis with other liver lesions (Fromenty and Pessayre, 1997), respectively. The cationic metabolite of MPTP (MPP^+) also electrophoretically accumulates in the mitochondria of dopaminergic neurons, causing mitochondrial dysfunction and cell death, whereas highly lipophilic local anesthetics (eg, tetracaine, bupivacaine), when overdosed or inadvertently injected into a blood vessel, accumulate in cardiac mitochondria, compromising mitochondrial energy production and causing cardiac failure. Human equilibrative nucleoside transporter 1 (ENT1) in the mitochondrial inner membrane appears responsible for targeting fialuridine (an already withdrawn thymidine nucleoside analogue antiviral drug) into human mitochondria, where it inhibits mitochondrial DNA synthesis, thereby inducing hepatotoxicity. The fact that ENT1 is not localized in rodent mitochondria may account for the dramatic difference in mitochondrial toxicity of fialuridine between humans and rodents (Lee *et al.*, 2006).

Reversible Intracellular Binding Binding to the pigment melanin, an intracellular polyanionic aromatic polymer, is a mechanism by which chemicals, such as organic and inorganic cations and polycyclic aromatic hydrocarbons, can accumulate in melanin-containing cells in retina, substantia nigra, and skin (Larsson, 1993). The release of melanin-bound toxicants is thought to contribute to the retinal toxicity associated with chlorpromazine and chloroquine, injury to substantia nigra neurons by MPTP and manganese, and the induction of melanoma by polycyclic aromatics.

Keratins are the major structural proteins in the epidermis and its appendages (nail and hair), constituting up to 85% of fully differentiated keratinocytes (skin cells). As keratins are abundant in cysteine residues, they can sequester thiol-reactive metal ions and metalloid compounds, whose nail and hair contents are indicative of exposure. Release of keratin-bound arsenic in keratinocytes may adversely affect these cells, leading to dermal lesions common in arsenicism.

Mechanisms Opposing Distribution to a Target Distribution of toxicants to specific sites may be hindered by several processes. The processes include (1) binding to plasma proteins, (2) specialized barriers, (3) distribution to storage sites such as adipose tissue, (4) association with intracellular binding proteins, and (5) export from cells.

Binding to Plasma Proteins As long as xenobiotics such as DDT (an insecticide) and TCDD (often called dioxin, an environmental pollutant) are bound to high-molecular-weight proteins or lipoproteins in plasma, they cannot leave the capillaries by diffusion. Even if they exit the bloodstream through fenestrae, they have difficulty permeating cell membranes. Dissociation from proteins is required for most xenobiotics to leave the blood and enter cells. Therefore, strong binding to plasma proteins delays and prolongs the effects and elimination of toxicants.

Specialized Barriers Brain capillaries have very low aqueous porosity because their endothelial cells lack fenestrae and are joined by extremely tight junctions. This blood–brain barrier prevents the access of hydrophilic chemicals to the brain except for those that can be actively transported. In the choroid plexus, where the capillaries are fenestrated, the choroidal epithelial cells are sealed together by tight junctions, forming the blood–cerebrospinal fluid barrier. Water-soluble toxicants also have restricted access to reproductive cells, which are separated from capillaries by other cells. The oocyte in the ovary is surrounded by multiple layers of granulosa cells, and the spermatogenic cells are supported by Sertoli cells that are tightly joined in the seminiferous tubules to form the blood–testis barrier (see Chap. 20). Transfer of hydrophilic toxicants across the placenta is also restricted. However, none of these barriers are effective against lipophilic substances.

Distribution to Storage Sites Some chemicals accumulate in tissues (ie, storage sites) where they do not exert significant effects. For example, highly lipophilic substances such as chlorinated hydrocarbon insecticides concentrate in adipocytes, whereas lead is deposited in bone by substituting for Ca^{2+} in hydroxyapatite. Such storage decreases the availability of these toxicants for their target sites and acts as a temporary protective mechanism. However, insecticides may return to the circulation and be distributed to their target site, the nervous tissue, when there is a rapid lipid loss as a result of fasting. This contributes to the lethality of pesticide-exposed birds during migration or during the winter months, when food is restricted. The possibility that lead is mobilized from the bone during pregnancy is of concern.

Association with Intracellular Binding Proteins Binding to nontarget intracellular sites also reduces the concentration of toxicants at the target site, at least temporarily. MT, a cysteine-rich cytoplasmic protein, serves such a function in acute cadmium intoxication (Klaassen *et al.*, 1999).

Export from Cells Intracellular toxicants may be transported back into the extracellular space. This occurs in brain capillary endothelial cells. In their luminal membrane, these cells contain ATP-dependent membrane transporters (ATP-binding cassette [ABC] transporters) such as the MDR1, or P-glycoprotein, which extrudes chemicals and contributes to the blood–brain barrier (Schinkel, 1999). Compared with normal mice, mice with disrupted *mdr1a* gene exhibit 100-fold higher brain levels of and sensitivity to ivermectin, a neurotoxic pesticide and human antihelmintic drug that is one of many P-glycoprotein substrates (Schinkel, 1999). The ooctye is also equipped with P-glycoprotein that provides protection against chemicals that are substrates for this efflux pump (Elbling *et al.*, 1993). Hematopoietic stem cells (and perhaps other stem cells) are also protected by ABC transporters, such as MDR1, MRP1, and breast cancer resistance protein (BCRP), of which the latter confers these cells resistance to mitoxantrone. ABC transporters that export drugs were first identified in tumor cells that often overexpress them, thereby making these cells resistant to antitumor drugs these transporters pump out (see Chap. 5).

Excretion versus Reabsorption

Excretion Excretion is the removal of xenobiotics from the blood and their return to the external environment. It is a physical mechanism, whereas biotransformation is a chemical mechanism for eliminating the toxicant.

For nonvolatile chemicals, the major excretory structures in the body are the renal glomeruli, which hydrostatically filter small molecules (<60 kDa) through their pores, and the proximal renal tubular cells and hepatocytes, which actively transport chemicals from the blood into the renal tubules and bile canaliculi, respectively. These cells are readily exposed to blood-borne chemicals through the large endothelial fenestrae; they have transporters of the solute carrier (SLC) family (eg, OAT, OCT, and OATP type) that mediate the basolateral uptake of particular chemicals and transporters of the ABC carrier family (eg, MRP and MDR type) that mediate the luminal export of certain chemicals (see Chap. 5). Renal transporters have a preferential affinity for smaller (<300 Da), and hepatic transporters for larger (>400 Da) amphiphilic molecules. A less common "excretory" mechanism consists of diffusion and partition into the excreta on the basis of their lipid content (see below) or acidity. For example, morphine is transferred into milk and amphetamine is transferred into gastric juice by nonionic diffusion. This is facilitated by pH trapping of those organic bases in those fluids, which are acidic relative to plasma (see Chap. 5).

The route and speed of excretion depend largely on the physicochemical properties of the toxicant. The major excretory organs—kidney and liver—can efficiently remove only highly hydrophilic, usually ionized chemicals such as organic acids and bases. The reasons for this are as follows: (1) in the renal glomeruli, only compounds dissolved in plasma water can be filtered; (2) transporters in hepatocytes and renal proximal tubular cells are specialized for secretion of highly hydrophilic organic acids and bases; (3) only hydrophilic chemicals are freely soluble in the aqueous urine and bile; and (4) lipid-soluble compounds are readily reabsorbed by transcellular diffusion.

There are no efficient elimination mechanisms for nonvolatile, highly lipophilic chemicals such as polyhalogenated biphenyls and chlorinated hydrocarbon insecticides. If they are resistant to biotransformation, such chemicals are eliminated very slowly and tend to accumulate in the body on repeated exposure. Three rather inefficient processes are available for the elimination of such chemicals: (1) excretion by the mammary gland after the chemical is dissolved in milk lipids; (2) excretion in bile in association with biliary micelles and/or phospholipid vesicles; and (3) intestinal excretion, an incompletely understood transport from blood into the intestinal lumen. Volatile, nonreactive toxicants such as gases and volatile liquids diffuse from pulmonary capillaries into the alveoli and are exhaled.

Reabsorption Toxicants delivered into the renal tubules may diffuse back across the tubular cells into the peritubular capillaries. This process is facilitated by tubular fluid reabsorption, which increases the intratubular concentration as well as the residence time of the chemical by slowing urine flow. Reabsorption by diffusion is dependent on the lipid solubility of the chemical. For organic acids and bases, diffusion is inversely related to the extent of ionization, because the nonionized molecule is more lipid-soluble. The ionization of weak organic acids, such as salicylic acid and phenobarbital, and bases, such as amphetamine, procainamide, and quinidine, is strongly pH-dependent in the physiologic range. Therefore, their reabsorption is influenced significantly by the pH of the tubular fluid. Acidification of urine favors the excretion of weak organic bases, whereas alkalinization favors the elimination of weak organic acids. Some organic compounds may be reabsorbed from the renal tubules by transporters. For example, PEPT can move peptidomimetic drugs, such as some β-lactam antibiotics and angiotensin-converting enzyme inhibitors, across the brush border membrane. Carriers for the physiologic oxyanions mediate the reabsorption of some toxic metal oxyanions in the kidney. Thus, chromate and molybdate are reabsorbed by the sulfate transporter, whereas arsenate is reabsorbed by the phosphate transporter.

Toxicants delivered to the GI tract by biliary, gastric, and intestinal excretion and secretion by salivary glands and the exocrine pancreas may be reabsorbed by diffusion across the intestinal mucosa. Because compounds secreted into bile are usually organic acids, their reabsorption is possible only if they are sufficiently lipophilic or are converted to more lipid-soluble forms in the intestinal lumen. For example, glucuronides of toxicants such as diethylstilbestrol (DES) and glucuronides of the hydroxylated metabolites of polycyclic aromatic hydrocarbons, chlordecone, and halogenated biphenyls are hydrolyzed by the β-glucuronidase of intestinal microorganisms, and the released aglycones are reabsorbed (Gregus and Klaassen, 1986). Glutathione conjugates of hexachlorobutadiene and trichloroethylene are hydrolyzed by intestinal and pancreatic peptidases, yielding the cysteine conjugates, which are reabsorbed and serve as precursors of some nephrotoxic metabolites (Anders, 2004).

Toxication versus Detoxication

Toxication A number of xenobiotics (eg, strong acids and bases, nicotine, aminoglycosides, ethylene oxide, methylisocyanate, heavy metal ions, HCN, CO) are directly toxic, whereas the toxicity of others is due primarily to metabolites. Biotransformation to harmful products is called *toxication or metabolic activation*. With some xenobiotics, toxication confers physicochemical properties that adversely alter the microenvironment of biological processes or structures. For example, oxalic acid formed from ethylene glycol may cause acidosis and hypocalcaemia as well as obstruction of renal tubules by precipitation as calcium oxalate. Occasionally, chemicals acquire structural features and reactivity by biotransformation that allows for a more efficient interaction with specific receptors or enzymes. For example, the organophosphate insecticide parathion is biotransformed to paraoxon, an active cholinesterase inhibitor; the rodenticide fluoroacetate is converted in the citric acid cycle to fluorocitrate, a false substrate that inhibits aconitase; as a result of its CYP2E1-catalyzed oxidation, the general anesthetic methoxyflurane releases fluoride ion that inhibits several enzymes (including enolase in the glycolytic pathway) and that

contributes to renal injury after prolonged anesthesia; some cephalosporin antibiotics (eg, cephoperazone) may cause hemorrhage because they undergo biotransformation with release of 1-methyltetrazole-5-thiol that inhibits vitamin K epoxide reductase and thus impairs activation of clotting factors; and fialuridine, an antiviral drug withdrawn from development because it produced lethal hepatotoxicity in patients involved in the clinical trial, is phosphorylated to the triphosphate, which inhibits DNA polymerase-γ and thus impairs synthesis of mitochondrial DNA (Lewis *et al.*, 1996). Most often, however, toxication renders xenobiotics and occasionally other molecules in the body, such as oxygen and nitric oxide (•NO), indiscriminately reactive toward endogenous molecules with susceptible functional groups. This increased reactivity may be due to conversion into (1) electrophiles, (2) free radicals, (3) nucleophiles, or (4) redox-active reactants.

Formation of Electrophiles Electrophiles are molecules containing an electron-deficient atom with a partial or full positive charge that allows it to react by sharing electron pairs with electron-rich atoms in nucleophiles. The formation of electrophiles is involved in the toxication of numerous chemicals (Table 3-2) (see Chap. 6). Such reactants are often produced by insertion of an oxygen atom, which withdraws electrons from the atom it is attached to, making that electrophilic. This is the case when aldehydes, ketones, epoxides, arene oxides, sulfoxides, nitroso compounds, phosphonates, and acyl halides are formed (Table 3-2). In other instances, conjugated double bonds are formed, which become polarized by the electron-withdrawing effect of an oxygen, making one of the double-bonded carbons electron-deficient (ie, electrophilic). This occurs when α,β-unsaturated aldehydes and ketones as well as quinones, quinoneimines, and quinone methides are produced (Table 3-2). Formation of many of these electrophilic metabolites is catalyzed by cytochrome P450s (Leung *et al.*, 2012).

Cationic electrophiles may be produced as a result of heterolytic bond cleavage. For example, methyl-substituted aromatics, such as 7,12-dimethylbenzanthracene, and aromatic amines (amides), such as 2-acetylaminofluorene, are hydroxylated to form benzylic alcohols and *N*-hydroxy arylamines (amides), respectively (Miller and Surh, 1994). These metabolites are then esterified, typically by sulfotransferases. Heterolytic cleavage of the C–O or N–O bonds of these esters results in a hydrosulfate anion and the concomitant formation of a benzylic carbonium ion or arylnitrenium ion, respectively (see Chap. 6). The antiestrogen tamoxifen undergoes similar activation by hydroxylation and sulfation to form a carbocationic metabolite (Kim *et al.*, 2004). After being C-hydroxylated by CYP2E1, the hepatocarcinogen dimethylnitrosamine undergoes spontaneous decomposition, finally a heterolytic cleavage of the C–N bond to form methyl carbonium cation ($^+CH_3$) (see Chap. 6). In a similar process, the tobacco-specific nicotine-derived nitrosamine ketone (NNK), the most potent carcinogen in tobacco, may generate either methyl carbonium cation or piridyloxobutyl carbonium cation, depending on the site of C-hydroxylation that initiates its decomposition. Formally, spontaneous heterolytic cleavage of the C–Cl bond results in formation of reactive episulfonium ion from the vesicant chemical warfare agent sulfur mustard (2,2′-bis-chloroethylsulfide). An episulfonium ion metabolite is also the ultimate toxicant produced from the fumigant 1,2-dibromoethane following its conjugation with glutathione to form *S*-(2-bromoethyl) glutathione conjugate, a so-called half-sulfur mustard (Anders, 2004). The oxidation of mercury (Hg^0) to Hg^{2+} by catalase and reduction of CrO_4^{2-} into DNA-reactive Cr^{3+} by ascorbate (Quievryn *et al.*, 2002) are examples for formation of electrophilic toxicants from inorganic chemicals. Reduction of arsenate (containing As^V)

Table 3-2

Toxication by Formation of Electrophilic Metabolites

ELECTROPHILIC METABOLITE	PARENT TOXICANT	ENZYMES CATALYZING TOXICATION	TOXIC EFFECT
Nonionic electrophiles			
Aldehydes, ketones			
Acetaldehyde	Ethanol	ADH	Hepatic fibrosis (?)
Zomepirac glucuronide	Zomepirac	GT → isomerization	Immune reaction (?)
2,5-Hexanedione	Hexane	CYP	Axonopathy
α,β-Unsaturated aldehydes, ketones			
Acrolein	Allyl alcohol	ADH	Hepatic necrosis
Acrolein	Allyl amine	MAO	Vascular injury
Acrolein	Cyclophosphamide	CYP → sp. cl.	Hemorrhagic cystitis
Muconic aldehyde	Benzene	Multiple	Bone marrow injury
Atropaldehyde (2-phenylacrolein)	Felbamate	Esterase → ADH → sp. cl.	Bone marrow and liver injury
4-Hydroxynon-2-enal	Fatty acids	Lipid peroxidation	Cellular injury (?)
Quinones, quinoneimines			
DES-4,4′-quinone	DES	Peroxidases	Carcinogenesis (?)
N-Acetyl-p-benzoquinoneimine	Acetaminophen	CYP, peroxidases	Hepatic necrosis
Epoxides, arene oxides			
Aflatoxin B₁ 8,9-epoxide	Aflatoxin B₁	CYP	Carcinogenesis
2-Chlorooxirane	Vinyl chloride	CYP	Carcinogenesis
Bromobenzene 3,4-oxide	Bromobenzene	CYP	Hepatic necrosis
Benzo[a]pyrene 7,8-diol 9,10-oxide	Benzo[a]pyrene	CYP	Carcinogenesis
Sulfoxides			
Thioacetamide S-oxide	Thioacetamide	FMO	Hepatic necrosis
Nitroso compounds			
Nitroso-sulfamethoxazole	Sulfamethoxazole	CYP	Immune reaction
Phosphonates			
Paraoxon	Parathion	CYP	ChE inhibition
Acyl halides			
Phosgene	Chloroform	CYP	Hepatic necrosis
Trifluoroacetyl chloride	Halothane	CYP	Immune hepatitis
Thionoacyl halides			
2,3,4,4-Tetrachlorothiobut-3-enoic acid chloride	HCBD	GST → GGT → DP → CCβL	Renal tubular necrosis
Thioketenes			
Chloro-1,2,2-trichlorovinyl-thioketene	HCBD	GST → GGT → DP → CCβL	Renal tubular necrosis
Cationic electrophiles			
Carbonium ions			
Benzylic carbocation	7,12-DMBA	CYP → ST	Carcinogenesis
Carbonium cation	DENA	CYP → sp. ra.	Carcinogenesis
Nitrenium ions			
Arylnitrenium ion	AAF, DMAB, HAPP	CYP → ST	Carcinogenesis
Sulfonium ions			
Episulfonium ion	1,2-dibromoethane	GST	Carcinogenesis
Metal ions			
Mercury(II) ion	Elemental Hg	Catalase	Brain injury
Diaquo-diamino platinate(II)	Cisplatinum	sp. ra.	Renal tubular necrosis

KEY: AAF, 2-acetylaminofluorene; ADH, alcohol dehydrogenase; CCβL, cysteine conjugate β-lyase; ChE, cholinesterase; CYP, cytochrome P450; DENA, diethylnitrosamine; DMAB, N,N-dimethyl-4-aminoazobenzene; 7,12-DMBA, 7,12-dimethylbenzanthracene; DES, diethylstilbestrol; DP, dipeptidase; FMO, flavin-containing monooxygenase; GT, UDP-glucuronosyltransferase; GGT, gamma-glutamyltransferase; GST, glutathione S-transferase; HAPP, heterocyclic arylamine pyrolysis products; HCBD, hexachlorobutadiene; ST, sulfotransferase; sp. cl., spontaneous cleavage; sp. ra., spontaneous rearrangement.

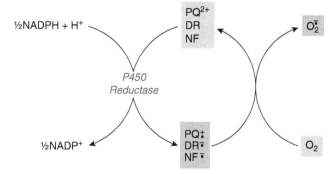

Figure 3-3. *Production of superoxide anion radical ($O_2^{\bullet-}$) by paraquat (PQ^{2+}), doxorubicin (DR), and nitrofurantoin (NF).* Note that formation of $O_2^{\bullet-}$ is not the final step in the toxication of these xenobiotics, because $O_2^{\bullet-}$ can yield the much more reactive hydroxyl radical, as depicted in Fig. 3-4.

to arsenite (containing As^{III}) by glutathione is greatly accelerated via incorporation of arsenate into arsenate esters or anhydrides. These arsenylated metabolites (eg, ribose-1-arsenate, glucose-1-arsenate, ADP-arsenate) can be formed by phosphorolytic enzymes (eg, purine nucleoside phosphorylase and glycogen phosphorylase) and by ATP synthase, which accept arsenate instead of phosphate as their substrate. This is how such enzymes promote reduction of arsenate into the more toxic thiol-reactive arsenite (Gregus *et al.*, 2009; Németi *et al.*, 2010).

Formation of Free Radicals A free radical is a molecule or molecular fragment that contains one or more unpaired electrons in its outer orbital. Radicals are formed by (1) accepting an electron, (2) losing an electron, or (3) homolytic fission of a covalent bond.

1. Xenobiotics such as paraquat, doxorubicin, and nitrofurantoin can accept an electron from reductases to give rise to radicals (Fig. 3-3). These radicals typically transfer the extra electron to molecular oxygen, forming a superoxide anion radical ($O_2^{\bullet-}$) and regenerating the parent xenobiotic, which is ready to gain a new electron (Kappus, 1986). Through this "redox cycling,"

one electron acceptor xenobiotic molecule can generate many $O_2^{\bullet-}$ molecules. There are also endogenous sources of $O_2^{\bullet-}$. This radical is generated in large quantities by NADPH oxidase (Nox) in activated macrophages and granulocytes during "respiratory burst," and in smaller quantities by many other cells, such as endothelial cells and vascular smooth muscle cells, which also express Nox in the plasma membrane (Bokoch and Knaus, 2003). Growth factor receptor stimulation in these non-phagocytotic cells is coupled to Nox activation. $O_2^{\bullet-}$ is also produced by the mitochondrial electron transport chain, especially by complexes I and III. The significance of $O_2^{\bullet-}$ stems to a large extent from the fact that $O_2^{\bullet-}$ is a starting compound in two toxication pathways (Fig. 3-4); one leads to formation of hydrogen peroxide (HOOH) and then hydroxyl radical (HO$^{\bullet}$), whereas the other produces peroxynitrite (ONOO$^-$) and ultimately nitrogen dioxide ($^{\bullet}$NO$_2$), and carbonate anion radical (CO$_2^{\bullet-}$).

2. Nucleophilic xenobiotics such as phenols, hydroquinones, aminophenols, aromatic amines (eg, benzidine), hydrazines, phenothiazines (eg, chlorpromazine; see Fig. 3-6), and thiols are prone to lose an electron and form free radicals in a reaction catalyzed by peroxidases (Aust *et al.*, 1993). Some of these chemicals, such as catechols and hydroquinones, may undergo two sequential one-electron oxidations, producing first semiquinone radicals and then quinones. Quinones are not only reactive electrophiles (Table 3-2) but also electron acceptors with the capacity to initiate redox cycling or oxidation of thiols and NAD(P)H. Polycyclic aromatic hydrocarbons with sufficiently low ionization potential, such as benzo[*a*]pyrene and 7,12-dimethylbenzanthracene, can be converted via one-electron oxidation by peroxidases or cytochrome P450 to radical cations, which may be the ultimate toxicants for these carcinogens (Cavalieri and Rogan, 1992). Like peroxidases, oxyhemoglobin (Hb-FeII-O$_2$) can catalyze the oxidation of aminophenols to semiquinone radicals and quinoneimines. This is another example of toxication, because these products, in turn, oxidize ferrohemoglobin (Hb-FeII) to methemoglobin (Hb-FeIII), which cannot carry oxygen.

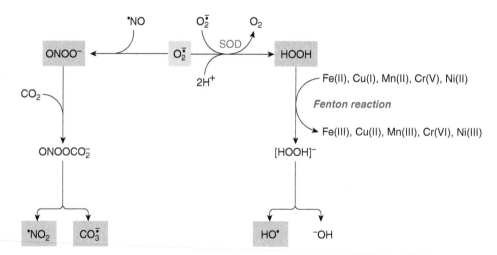

Figure 3-4. *Two pathways for toxication of superoxide anion radical $O_2^{\bullet-}$ via nonradical products (ONOO$^-$ and HOOH) to radical products ($^{\bullet}NO_2$, $CO_3^{\bullet-}$, and HO$^{\bullet}$).* In one pathway, conversion of $O_2^{\bullet-}$ to HOOH is spontaneous or is catalyzed by SOD. Homolytic cleavage of HOOH to hydroxyl radical and hydroxyl ion is called the Fenton reaction and is catalyzed by the transition metal ions shown. Hydroxyl radical formation is the ultimate toxication for xenobiotics that form $O_2^{\bullet-}$ (see Fig. 3-3) or for HOOH, the transition metal ions listed, and some chemicals that form complexes with these transition metal ions. In the other pathway, $O_2^{\bullet-}$ reacts avidly with nitric oxide ($^{\bullet}$NO), the product of $^{\bullet}$NO synthase (NOS), forming peroxynitrite (ONOO$^-$). Spontaneous reaction of ONOO$^-$ with carbon dioxide (CO$_2$) yields nitrosoperoxy carbonate that is homolytically cleaved to nitrogen dioxide ($^{\bullet}$NO$_2$) and carbonate anion radical (CO$_2^{\bullet-}$). All 3 radical products indicated in this figure are oxidants, whereas $^{\bullet}$NO$_2$ is also a nitrating agent (see Fig. 3-8).

3. Free radicals are also formed by homolytic bond fission, which can be induced by electron transfer to the molecule (reductive fission). This mechanism is involved in the conversion of CCl_4 to the trichloromethyl free radical ($Cl_3C^\bullet$) by an electron transfer from cytochrome P450 or the mitochondrial electron transport chain (reductive dehalogenation) (Recknagel *et al.*, 1989). The $Cl_3C^\bullet$ reacts with O_2 to form the even more reactive trichloromethylperoxy radical ($Cl_3COO^\bullet$) (Hippeli and Elstner, 1999).

The hydroxyl radical ($HO^\bullet$), a free radical of paramount toxicological significance, is also generated by homolytic fission. Such a process yields large amounts of $HO^\bullet$ from water on ionizing radiation. Reductive homolytic fission of HOOH to the harmful $HO^\bullet$ and the harmless HO^- (hydroxide anion) is called the Fenton reaction (Fig. 3-4). This is catalyzed by transition metal ions, typically Fe(II), Cu(I), Cr(V), Ni(II), or Mn(II), and is a major toxication mechanism for HOOH and its precursor $O_2^{\bullet-}$, as well as for transition metals. Moreover, the toxicity of chemicals, such as nitrilotriacetic acid, bleomycin, and orellanin (Hippeli and Elstner, 1999), which chelate transition metal ions is also based on Fenton chemistry, because chelation increases the catalytic efficiency of some transition metal ions. Complexation with some endogenous oligopeptides also increases the catalytic efficiency of weakly Fenton-active metal ions, such as Ni(II). The pulmonary toxicity of inhaled mineral particles such as asbestos and silica is caused, at least in part, by the formation of $HO^\bullet$ triggered by Fe ions on the particle surface (Vallyathan *et al.*, 1998; Castranova, 2004). HOOH is a direct or indirect by-product of several enzymatic reactions, including monoamine oxidase, acyl-coenzyme A oxidase, xanthine oxidase (Harrison, 2002), aldehyde oxidase, and CYP2E1 (Caro and Cederbaum, 2004). It is produced in large quantities by spontaneous or superoxide dismutase (SOD)–catalyzed dismutation of $O_2^{\bullet-}$.

Homolytic cleavage is also involved in free radical generation from $ONOO^-$ (Squadrito and Pryor, 1998) (Fig. 3-4). The facile reaction of $ONOO^-$ with the ubiquitous CO_2 yields nitrosoperoxycarbonate ($ONOOCO_2^-$), which can spontaneously homolyze into 2 radicals, the oxidant and nitrating agent nitrogen dioxide ($^\bullet NO_2$) and the oxidant carbonate anion radical ($CO_2^{\bullet-}$). Thus, formation of $ONOO^-$ and the latter radicals represents a toxication mechanism for $O_2^{\bullet-}$ and $^\bullet NO$. As $^\bullet NO$ is the product of nitric oxide synthase (NOS), this mechanism is especially relevant in and around cells that express NOS constitutively (ie, neurons and endothelial cells) as well as in and around cells that express the inducible form of NOS in response to cytokines. Inside the cell, a predominant site for formation of $ONOO^-$ as well as its products $CO_3^{\bullet-}$ and $^\bullet NO_2$ is the mitochondria, wherein the lipophilic $^\bullet NO$ can readily diffuse and where the electron transport chain and the citric acid cycle produce $O_2^{\bullet-}$ and CO_2, respectively (Denicola and Radi, 2005).

Formation of Nucleophiles The formation of nucleophiles is a relatively uncommon mechanism for activating toxicants. Examples include the formation of cyanide from amygdalin, which is catalyzed by bacterial β-glucosidase in the intestine; from acrylonitrile after epoxidation and subsequent glutathione conjugation; and from sodium nitroprusside by thiol-induced decomposition. Carbon monoxide is a toxic metabolite of dihalomethanes that undergo oxidative dehalogenation. Hydrogen selenide, a strong nucleophile and reductant, is formed from selenite by reaction with glutathione or other thiols.

Formation of Redox-Active Reactants There are specific mechanisms for the creation of redox-active reactants other than those already mentioned. Examples include the formation of the methemoglobin-producing nitrite from nitrate by bacterial

reduction in the intestine or from esters of nitrous or nitric acids in reaction with glutathione. Dapsone hydroxylamine and 5-hydroxyprimaquine, hydroxylated metabolites of the respective drugs, produce methemoglobin by cooxidation (Fletcher *et al.*, 1988). Reductants such as ascorbic acid and reductases such as NADPH-dependent flavoenzymes reduce Cr(VI) to Cr(V) (Shi and Dalal, 1990). Xenobiotic radicals formed in redox cycling (eg, those depicted in Fig. 3-3) as well as $O_2^{\bullet-}$ can reduce Fe(III) bound to ferritin and consequently release it as Fe(II). Cr(V) and Fe(II) thus formed catalyze $HO^\bullet$ formation (Fig. 3-4).

In summary, the most reactive metabolites are electron-deficient molecules and molecular fragments such as electrophiles and neutral or cationic free radicals. Although some nucleophiles are reactive (eg, HCN, CO), many (eg, hydroquinones) are activated by conversion to electrophiles. Similarly, free radicals with an extra electron (eg, those shown in Fig. 3-3) cause damage by giving rise to the neutral $HO^\bullet$ radical after the formation and subsequent homolytic cleavage of HOOH.

Detoxication Biotransformation that eliminates an ultimate toxicant or prevents its formation is called detoxication. In some cases, detoxication may compete with toxication for a chemical. Detoxication can take several pathways, depending on the chemical nature of the toxic substance.

Detoxication of Toxicants with No Functional Groups In general, chemicals without functional groups, such as benzene and toluene, are detoxicated in 2 phases. Initially, a functional group such as hydroxyl or carboxyl is introduced into the molecule, most often by cytochrome P450 enzymes. Subsequently, an endogenous acid, such as glucuronic acid, sulfuric acid, or an amino acid, is added to the functional group by a transferase. With some exceptions, the final products are inactive, highly hydrophilic organic acids that are readily excreted. Carbonyl reduction, catalyzed by at least 5 enzymes (eg, 11-β-hydroxysteroid dehydrogenase-1, carbonyl reductase, and 3 members of aldo-keto reductase superfamily), initiates detoxication of the potent carcinogen NNK (4-(methylnitrosamino)-1-(3-pyridyl)-1-butanone). The formed nicotine-derived nitrosamine alcohol is then readily glucuronidated at its hydroxyl moiety and is excreted into urine (Maser, 2004).

Detoxication of Nucleophiles Nucleophiles are generally detoxicated by conjugation at the nucleophilic functional group. Hydroxylated compounds are conjugated by sulfation, glucuronidation, or rarely by methylation, whereas thiols are methylated or glucuronidated and amines and hydrazines are acetylated. These reactions prevent peroxidase-catalyzed conversion of the nucleophiles to free radicals and biotransformation of phenols, aminophenols, catechols, and hydroquinones to electrophilic quinones and quinoneimines. An alternative mechanism for the elimination of thiols, amines, and hydrazines is oxidation by flavin-containing monooxygenases (Krueger and Williams, 2005). Some alcohols, such as ethanol, are detoxicated by oxidation to carboxylic acids by alcohol and aldehyde dehydrogenases. A specific detoxication mechanism is the biotransformation of cyanide to thiocyanate by rhodanese or mercaptopyruvate sulfurtransferase.

Detoxication of Electrophiles A general mechanism for the detoxication of electrophilic toxicants is conjugation with the thiol nucleophile glutathione (Ketterer, 1988). This reaction may occur spontaneously or can be facilitated by glutathione *S*-transferases. Metal ions—such as Ag^+, Cd^{2+}, Hg^{2+}, and CH_3Hg^+ ions—readily react with and are detoxicated by glutathione. Specific mechanisms for the detoxication of electrophilic chemicals include epoxide hydrolase-catalyzed biotransformation of epoxides and arene oxides to diols and dihydrodiols, respectively, and carboxyles-terase-catalyzed hydrolysis of organophosphate ester pesticides. Others are two-electron reduction of quinones to hydroquinones by NAD(P)H:quinone oxidoreductase (NQO1) and NRH:quinone oxidoreductase (NQO2), reduction of α,β-unsaturated aldehydes (eg, the lipid peroxidation product 4-oxonon-2-enal) to alcohols or to their saturated derivative by carbonyl reductase (Maser, 2006), or oxidation of α,β-unsaturated aldehydes to acids by aldehyde dehydrogenases. Complex formation of thiol-reactive metal ions by MT and the redox-active ferrous iron by ferritin are special types of detoxications. Covalent binding of electrophiles to proteins can also be regarded as detoxication provided that the protein has no critical function and does not become a neoantigen or otherwise harmful. Carboxylesterases, for example, inactivate organophosphates not only by hydrolysis but also by covalent binding.

Detoxication of Free Radicals Because $O_2^{\bullet-}$ can be converted into much more reactive compounds (Fig. 3-4), its elimination is an important detoxication mechanism. This is carried out by SOD, high-capacity enzymes located in the cytosol (Cu, Zn-SOD) and the mitochondria (Mn-SOD), which convert $O_2^{\bullet-}$ to HOOH (Fig. 3-5). Subsequently, HOOH is reduced to water by catalase in the peroxisomes (also in the mitochondria in cardiac muscle), by the selenocysteine-containing glutathione peroxidases in the cytosol and mitochondria, and by peroxiredoxins in the cytosol, mitochondria, and endoplasmic reticulum (EPR) (Fig. 3-5) (Rhee *et al.*, 2005).

No enzyme eliminates HO•. Whereas some relatively stable radicals, such as peroxyl radicals (see Fig. 3-9), can readily abstract a hydrogen atom from glutathione, α-tocopherol (vitamin E), or ascorbic acid (vitamin C), thus becoming nonradicals, these antioxidants are generally ineffective in detoxifying HO• (Sies, 1993). This is due to its extreme reactivity and thus short half-life (10^{-9} seconds), which provides little time for the HO• to reach and react with antioxidants. Therefore, the only effective protection against HO• is to prevent its formation by elimination of its precursor, HOOH, via conversion to water (Fig. 3-5).

ONOO⁻ (which is not a free radical oxidant) is significantly more stable than HO• (half-life of about 1 second). Nevertheless, the small biological antioxidant molecules (glutathione, uric acid, ascorbic acid, α-tocopherol) are relatively inefficient in intercepting it, because ONOO⁻ rapidly reacts with CO_2 (Squadrito and Pryor, 1998) to form reactive free radicals (Fig. 3-4). More efficient are the selenocysteine-containing glutathione peroxidase and peroxiredoxins, which can reduce ONOO⁻ to nitrite (ONO⁻) the same way they reduce HOOH to water (Fig. 3-5). Selenoprotein P, which contains 10 selenocysteine residues and coats the surface of endothelial cells, also reduces ONOO⁻ and may serve as a protectant against this oxidant in blood. In addition, ONOO⁻ reacts with oxyhemoglobin, heme-containing peroxidases, and albumin, all of which

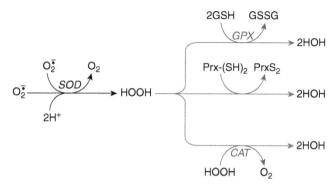

Figure 3-5. *Detoxication of superoxide anion radical ($O_2^{\bullet-}$) by superoxide dismutase (SOD), and of HOOH by glutathione peroxidase (GPX), peroxiredoxin (Prx-(SH)₂), and catalase (CAT).* When GPX reduces HOOH, it forms glutathione disulfide (GSSG) as a by-product, which is reduced back to GSH by glutathione reductase using NADPH. When Prx-(SH)₂ reduces HOOH, its catalytic thiol group (-R-S-H) becomes first oxidized into a sulfenic acid group (-R-S-OH), which in turn reacts with another SH group of Prx, forming HOH and Prx disulfide (PrxS₂). The latter can be reduced back into Prx-(SH)₂ by the thioredoxin–thioredoxin reductase–NADPH system, as shown in Fig. 3-22. When HOOH is produced in large excess, the sulfenic acid group (-R-S-OH) in Prx may react with a second molecule of HOOH, causing its overoxidation into a sulfinic acid group (-R-S(O)-OH). This can be reduced back into -R-S-OH group by the ATP-dependent sulfiredoxins, thus reactivating Prx-(SH)₂ (Lowther and Haynes, 2011). Further oxidation into a sulfonic acid form (-R-S(O)-(OH)₂) is irreversible and results in the loss of the peroxidase function of Prx; however, in this form Prx functions as a molecular chaperone (see later). Thus, out of the 3 enzymes eliminating HOOH, the capacity of Prx becomes limited at moderate overload of HOOH, whereas catalase activity is not capacity-limited even at high HOOH overload (Neumann *et al.*, 2009).

could be important sinks for ONOO⁻. Furthermore, elimination of the 2 ONOO⁻ precursors—that is, •NO by reaction with oxyhemoglobin (to yield methemoglobin and nitrate) and $O_2^{\bullet-}$ by SODs (see above)—is a significant mechanism in preventing ONOO⁻ buildup (Squadrito and Pryor, 1998).

Peroxidase-generated free radicals are eliminated by electron transfer from glutathione. This results in the oxidation of glutathione, which is reversed by NADPH-dependent glutathione reductase (Fig. 3-6). Thus, glutathione plays an important role in the detoxication of both electrophiles and free radicals.

Detoxication of Protein Toxins Presumably, extracellular and intracellular proteases are involved in the inactivation of toxic polypeptides. Several toxins found in venoms, such as α- and β-bungarotoxin, erabutoxin, and phospholipase, contain intramolecular disulfide bonds that are required for their activity. These proteins are inactivated by thioredoxin, an endogenous dithiol protein that reduces the essential disulfide bond (Lozano *et al.*, 1994).

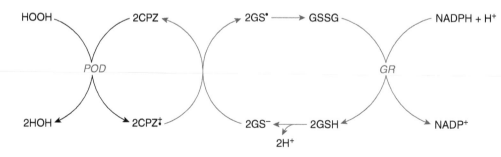

Figure 3-6. *Detoxication of peroxidase (POD)–generated free radicals such as chlorpromazine free radical (CPZ•⁺) by glutathione (GSH).* The by-products are glutathione thiyl radical (GS•) and glutathione disulfide (GSSG), from which GSH is regenerated by glutathione reductase (GR).

When Detoxication Fails Detoxication may be insufficient for several reasons:

1. Toxicants may overwhelm detoxication processes, leading to saturation of the detoxication enzymes, consumption of the cosubstrates, or depletion of cellular antioxidants such as glutathione, ascorbic acid, and α-tocopherol. This results in the accumulation of the ultimate toxicant.

2. Occasionally, a reactive toxicant inactivates a detoxicating enzyme. For example, $ONOO^-$ incapacitates Mn-SOD, which normally would counteract $ONOO^-$ formation (Murphy, 1999) (see Fig. 3-4).

3. Some conjugation reactions can be reversed. For example, 2-naphthylamine, a bladder carcinogen, is *N*-hydroxylated and glucuronidated in liver, with the glucuronide excreted into urine. While in the bladder, the glucuronide is hydrolyzed, and the released arylhydroxylamine is converted by protonation and dehydration to the reactive electrophilic arylnitrenium ion (Bock and Lilienblum, 1994). Isocyanates and isothiocyanates form labile glutathione conjugates from which they can be released. Thus, methylisocyanate readily forms a glutathione conjugate in the lung after inhalation. From there, the conjugate is distributed to other tissues, where the reactive electrophilic parent compound may be regenerated (Baillie and Kassahun, 1994). Such conjugates are considered transport forms of toxicants.

4. Sometimes detoxication generates potentially harmful by-products, such as the glutathione thiyl radical and glutathione disulfide, which are produced during the detoxication of free radicals (Fig. 3-6). Glutathione disulfide can form mixed disulfides with protein thiols, whereas the thiyl radical ($GS^{•}$), after reacting with thiolate (GS^-), forms glutathione disulfide radical anion ($GSSG_2^{•}$), which can reduce O_2 to $O_2^{•}$. Conjugation with glutathione may lead to HCN generation in the course of acrylonitrile biotransformation, the first step of which is epoxidation of acrylonitrile ($H_2C=CH-CN$). Whereas glutathione conjugation detoxifies this epoxide if it takes place at the carbon adjacent to the nitrile group (-CN), it causes release of this group as HCN if glutathione conjugates with the epoxide at the carbon not linked to the nitrile moiety.

STEP 2—REACTION OF THE ULTIMATE TOXICANT WITH THE TARGET MOLECULE

Toxicity is typically mediated by a reaction of the ultimate toxicant with a target molecule (step 2a in Fig. 3-1). Subsequently, a series of secondary biochemical events occur, leading to dysfunction or injury that is manifest at various levels of biological organization, such as at the target molecule itself, cell organelles, cells, tissues and organs, and even the whole organism. Because interaction of the ultimate toxicant with the target molecule triggers the toxic effect, consideration is given to (1) the attributes of target molecules, (2) the types of reactions between ultimate toxicants and target molecules, and (3) the effects of toxicants on the target molecules (Fig. 3-7). Finally, consideration is given to toxicities that are initiated not by reaction of the ultimate toxicant with target molecules, but rather by alteration of the biological (micro)environment (step 2b in Fig. 3-1) in which critical endogenous molecules, cell organelles, cells, and organs function.

Attributes of Target Molecules

Practically all endogenous compounds are potential targets for toxicants. The identification and characteristics of the target molecules

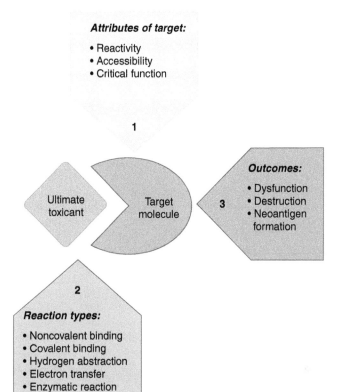

Figure 3-7. *Reaction of the ultimate toxicant with the target molecule: the second step in the development of toxicity.*

involved in toxicity constitute a major research priority, but a comprehensive inventory of potential target molecules is impossible. Nevertheless, the most prevalent and toxicologically relevant targets are macromolecules such as nucleic acids (especially DNA) and proteins. Among the small molecules, membrane lipids are frequently involved, whereas cofactors such as coenzyme A and pyridoxal rarely are involved.

To be a target, an endogenous molecule must possess the appropriate reactivity and/or steric configuration to allow the ultimate toxicant to enter into covalent or noncovalent reactions. For these reactions to occur, the target molecule must be accessible to a sufficiently high concentration of the ultimate toxicant. Thus, endogenous molecules that are exposed to reactive chemicals or are adjacent to sites where reactive metabolites are formed are frequently targets. Technical advances in the field of proteonomics make it increasingly possible to identify potential protein targets of reactive chemicals as chemical–protein adducts. A compendium of proteins adducted by reactive toxicant metabolites has been established at the University of Kansas (http://tpdb.med-chem.ku.edu/tpdb.html). The first target for reactive metabolites is often the enzyme that catalyzes their production or the adjacent intracellular structures. For example, thyroperoxidase, the enzyme involved in thyroid hormone synthesis, converts some nucleophilic xenobiotics (such as methimazole, amitrole, and resorcinol) into reactive free radicals that inactivate thyroperoxidase (Engler *et al.*, 1982). This is the basis for the antithyroid as well as the thyroid tumor–inducing effect of these chemicals. Carbon tetrachloride, which is activated by cytochrome P450, destroys this enzyme as well as the neighboring microsomal membranes (Osawa *et al.*, 1995). Several mitochondrial enzymes are convenient targets for nephrotoxic cysteine conjugates such as dichlorovinyl cysteine, because these conjugates are converted to electrophiles by mitochondrial enzymes with cysteine conjugate β-lyase activity (eg, aspartate aminotransferase and branched chain amino acid aminotransferase) that can readily channel their reactive products to neighboring enzymes such as α-ketoglutarate dehydrogenase (Anders, 2004). Reactive metabolites that are unable to find appropriate endogenous reaction partners in close proximity to their site of formation may diffuse until they encounter such reactants. For example, hard electrophiles such as the arylnitrenium ion metabolite of *N*-methyl-4-aminoazobenzene react readily with hard nucleophilic atoms in nucleic acids, and thus target DNA in the nucleus, even though the electrophiles are produced in the cytoplasm. Vinyl chloride epoxide, formed in the hepatocytes from vinyl chloride, reaches its DNA targets in the neighboring endothelial cells (which are more sensitive to this genotoxin than the liver cells), initiating hepatic hemangiosarcoma.

Not all targets for chemicals contribute to the harmful effects. Thus, while carbon monoxide causes toxicity by binding to ferrohemoglobin, it also associates with the iron in cytochrome P450 with little or no consequence. Covalent binding of toxicants to various intracellular proteins, including enzymes and structural proteins, has been demonstrated, yet it is often uncertain which protein(s) is/are involved in binding that is toxicologically relevant (Cohen *et al.*, 1997; Pumford and Halmes, 1997; Rombach and Hanzlik, 1999). Arylation of some hepatic mitochondrial proteins by acetaminophen (4′-hydroxyacetanilide) is thought to be causally related to the liver injury induced by this drug because the nonhepatotoxic regioisomer of acetaminophen (3′-hydroxyacetanilide) does not readily bind covalently to these proteins (Cohen *et al.*, 1997; Jaeschke and Bajt, 2006). In contrast, arylation of a number of hepatic cytoplasmic proteins by acetaminophen is likely to be inconsequential because the nonhepatotoxic regioisomer of this drug also arylates those proteins (Nelson and Pearson, 1990). Covalent binding to proteins without adverse consequences may even represent a form of detoxication by sparing toxicologically relevant targets. This principle is best exemplified by covalent binding of organophosphate insecticides to plasma cholinesterase, which is a significant protective mechanism, as it counteracts phosphorylation of acetylcholinesterase, the target molecule. Thus, to conclusively identify a target molecule as being responsible for toxicity, it should be demonstrated that the ultimate toxicant (1) reacts with the target and adversely affects its function, (2) reaches an effective concentration at the target site, and (3) alters the target in a way that is mechanistically related to the observed toxicity.

Types of Reactions

The ultimate toxicant may bind to the target molecules noncovalently or covalently and may alter it by hydrogen abstraction, electron transfer, or enzymatically.

Noncovalent Binding This type of binding can be due to apolar interactions or the formation of hydrogen and ionic bonds and is typically involved in the interaction of toxicants with targets such as membrane receptors, intracellular receptors, ion channels, and some enzymes. For example, such interactions are responsible for the binding of strychnine to the glycine receptor on motor neurons in the spinal cord, TCDD to the AhR, saxitoxin to sodium channels, phorbol esters to protein kinase C (PKC), and warfarin to vitamin K 2,3-epoxide reductase. Such forces also are responsible for the intercalation of chemicals such as acridine yellow and doxorubicin into the double helix of DNA. These chemicals are toxic because the steric arrangement of their atoms allows them to combine with complementary sites on the endogenous molecule more or less as a key fits into a lock. Noncovalent binding usually is reversible because of the comparatively low bonding energy.

Covalent Binding Being practically irreversible, covalent binding is of great toxicological importance because it permanently alters endogenous molecules (Boelsterli, 1993). Covalent adduct formation is common with electrophilic toxicants such as nonionic and cationic electrophiles and radical cations. These toxicants react with nucleophilic atoms that are abundant in biological macromolecules, such as proteins and nucleic acids. Electrophilic atoms exhibit some selectivity toward nucleophilic atoms, depending on their charge-to-radius ratio. In general, soft electrophiles prefer to react with soft nucleophiles (low charge-to-radius ratio in both), whereas hard electrophiles react more readily with hard nucleophiles (high charge-to-radius ratio in both). Examples are presented in Table 3-3. Metal ions such as silver and mercury are also classified as soft electrophiles. These prefer to react covalently with soft nucleophiles (especially thiol groups). Conversely, hard electrophiles such as lithium, calcium, and barium react preferentially as cations with hard nucleophiles (eg, carboxylate and phosphate anions). Metals falling between these 2 extremes, such as chromium, zinc, and lead, exhibit universal reactivity with nucleophiles. The reactivity of an electrophile determines which endogenous nucleophiles can react with it and become a target.

Table 3-3

Examples of Soft and Hard Electrophiles and Nucleophiles

ELECTROPHILES		NUCLEOPHILES
Carbon in polarized double bonds (eg, quinones, α,β-unsaturated ketones)	*Soft*	Sulfur in thiols (eg, cysteinyl residues in proteins and glutathione)
Carbon in epoxides, strained-ring lactones, aryl halides		Sulfur in methionine
Aryl carbonium ions		Nitrogen in primary and secondary amino groups of proteins (eg, lysine ε-amino group)
Benzylic carbonium ions, nitrenium ions		Nitrogen in amino groups in purine bases in nucleic acids
Alkyl carbonium ions		Oxygen of purines and pyrimidines in nucleic acids
	Hard	Phosphate oxygen in nucleic acids

SOURCE: Based on Coles (1984).

A covalent reaction of special biological significance can take place between HOOH (a soft electrophile) and protein thiol groups, preferentially those with low pK_a value, that is, with a propensity of being in the strongly nucleophilic thiolate anion form (Prot-S⁻) at physiologic pH. This reaction produces protein sulfenic acid (Prot-S-OH):

$$\text{Prot-SH} + \text{HOOH} \rightarrow \text{Prot-S-OH} + \text{HOH.}$$

The S atom in a sulfenic acid is electrophilic as it is made electron-deficient by the electron-withdrawing effect of O. Therefore, a protein–sulfenic acid can react with another thiol group of the same or a different protein or of glutathione (GSH), resulting in, respectively, formation of an intramolecular disulfide, intermolecular disulfide, or a mixed disulfide of the protein and glutathione (ie, glutathionylation of the protein):

$$\text{Prot}_1\text{-S-OH} + \text{Prot}_2\text{-SH} \rightarrow \text{Prot}_1\text{-S-S-Prot}_2 + \text{HOH;}$$

$$\text{Prot-S-OH} + \text{GSH} \rightarrow \text{Prot-S-SG} + \text{HOH.}$$

Not only HOOH but also hydroperoxides (eg, lipid hydroperoxides, LOOH; see Fig. 3-9) may enter into such reactions, producing protein–sulfenic acids, protein–disulfides, and glutathionylated proteins, which can be considered as posttranslational modifications with a role in redox signaling (Forman *et al.*, 2004).

Neutral free radicals such as HO•, •NO₂, and Cl₃C• can also bind covalently to biomolecules. The addition of Cl₃C• to double-bonded carbons in lipids or to lipid radicals yields lipids containing chloromethylated fatty acids. The addition of hydroxyl radicals to DNA bases results in the formation of numerous products, including 8-hydroxypurines, 5-hydroxymethylpyrimidines, and thymine and cytosine glycols (Breen and Murphy, 1995).

Nucleophilic toxicants are in principle reactive toward electrophilic endogenous compounds. Such reactions occur infrequently because electrophiles are rare among biomolecules. Examples include the covalent reactions of amines and hydrazides with the aldehyde pyridoxal, a cosubstrate for several enzymes, including glutamate decarboxylase. Carbon monoxide, cyanide, hydrogen sulfide, and azide form coordinate covalent bonds with iron in various heme proteins. Other nucleophiles react with hemoglobin in an electron transfer reaction (see below).

Hydrogen Abstraction Neutral free radicals, such as those generated in reactions depicted in Fig. 3-4, can readily abstract H atoms from endogenous compounds, converting those compounds into radicals. Abstraction of hydrogen from thiols (R-SH) creates thiyl radicals (R-S•), which on radical recombination with HO• form sulfenic acids (R-S-OH) that are precursors of disulfides (R-S-S-R) (see above). Radicals can remove hydrogen from CH₂ groups of free amino acids or from amino acid residues in proteins and convert them to carbonyls. These carbonyls react covalently with amines, forming cross-links with DNA or other proteins. Hydrogen abstraction from deoxyribose in DNA yields the C-4′ radical, the first step to DNA cleavage (Breen and Murphy, 1995). Abstraction of hydrogen from fatty acids produces lipid radicals and initiates lipid peroxidation. As depicted in Fig. 3-8, nitration of tyrosine residues in proteins purportedly involves H abstraction followed by radical recombination, that is, covalent binding between the resultant tyrosyl radical and •NO₂ (Squadrito and Pryor, 1998).

Electron Transfer Chemicals can oxidize Fe(II) in hemoglobin to Fe(III), producing methemoglobinemia. Nitrite can oxidize hemoglobin, whereas *N*-hydroxyl arylamines (such as dapsone hydroxylamine), phenolic compounds (such as 5-hydroxy

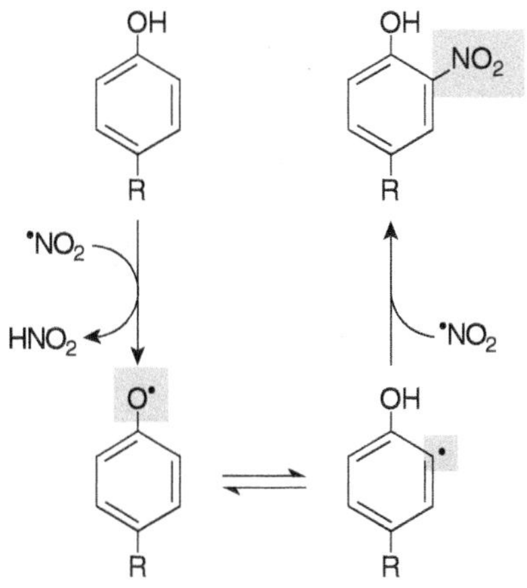

Figure 3-8. *Formation of 3-nitrotyrosine residues in proteins by reaction with nitrogen dioxide (•NO₂).* •NO₂ is an oxidizing and nitrating species generated from ONOO⁻ (Fig. 3-4). In addition, •NO₂ is a contaminant in cigarette smoke, exhaust of gas engines and stoves, as well as the causative agent of "silo-filler's disease."

primaquine), and hydrazines (such as phenylhydrazine) are cooxidized with oxyhemoglobin, forming methemoglobin and HOOH (Coleman and Jacobus, 1993).

Enzymatic Reactions A few toxins act enzymatically on specific target proteins. For example, the plant toxins ricin and abrin are *N*-glycosidases; they hydrolyze a specific glycosidic bond in ribosomal RNA, blocking protein synthesis. Botulinum toxin acts as a Zn-protease; it hydrolyzes the fusion proteins that assist in exocytosis of the neurotransmitter acetylcholine in cholinergic neurons, most importantly motor neurons, causing paralysis. The lethal factor component of anthrax toxin is also a Zn-protease, which inactivates mitogen-activated protein kinase kinase (MAPKK), inducing cell death. Other bacterial toxins catalyze the transfer of ADP-ribose from NAD⁺ to specific proteins. Through such a mechanism, diphtheria toxin blocks the function of elongation factor 2 in protein synthesis and cholera toxin activates a G protein. Snake venoms contain hydrolytic enzymes that destroy biomolecules.

In summary, most ultimate toxicants act on endogenous molecules on the basis of their chemical reactivity. Those with more than one type of reactivity may react by different mechanisms with various target molecules. For example, quinones may act as electron acceptors and initiate thiol oxidation or free radical reactions that lead to lipid peroxidation, but they may also act as soft electrophiles and bind covalently to protein thiols. The lead ion acts as a soft electrophile when it forms coordinate covalent bonds with critical thiol groups in δ-aminolevulinic acid dehydratase, its major target enzyme in heme synthesis (Goering, 1993). However, it behaves like a hard electrophile or an ion when it binds to PKC or blocks calcium channels, substituting for the natural ligand Ca²⁺ at those target sites.

Effects of Toxicants on Target Molecules

Reaction of the ultimate toxicant with endogenous molecules may cause dysfunction or destruction; in the case of proteins, it may render them foreign (ie, an antigen) to the immune system.

Dysfunction of Target Molecules Some toxicants activate protein target molecules, mimicking endogenous ligands. For example, morphine activates opioid receptors, clofibrate is an agonist on the peroxisome proliferator–activated receptor, and phorbol esters and lead ions stimulate PKC.

More commonly, chemicals inhibit the function of target molecules. Several xenobiotics—such as atropine, curare, and strychnine—block neurotransmitter receptors by attaching to the ligand-binding sites, whereas others interfere with the function of ion channels. Tetrodotoxin and saxitoxin, for example, inhibit opening of the voltage-activated sodium channels in the neuronal membrane, whereas DDT and the pyrethroid insecticides inhibit their closure. Some toxicants block ion transporters, others inhibit mitochondrial electron transport complexes, and many inhibit enzymes. Chemicals that bind to tubulin (eg, vinblastine, colchicine, paclitaxel, trivalent arsenic) or actin (eg, cytochalasin B, phalloidin) impair the assembly (polymerization) and/or disassembly (depolymerization) of these cytoskeletal proteins.

Protein function is impaired when conformation or structure is altered by interaction with the toxicant. Many proteins possess critical moieties, especially thiol groups, which are essential for catalytic activity or assembly to macromolecular complexes. Proteins that are sensitive to covalent and/or oxidative modification of their thiol groups include the enzymes glyceraldehyde 3-phosphate dehydrogenase (see Table 3-6) and pyruvate dehydrogenase (see Fig. 3-16), the Ca^{2+} pumps (see Fig. 3-17, Table 3-7), the DNA repair enzyme O^6-methylguanine-DNA-methyltransferase, the DNA-methylating enzyme C^5-cytosine-DNA-methyltransferase, ubiquitin-activating and -conjugating enzymes (E1 and E2), peroxiredoxins, protein tyrosine phosphatases (PTP, eg, cdc25), the lipid phosphatase PTEN (phosphatase and tensin homologue; see Fig. 3-12) (Rhee *et al.*, 2005), caspases (see Fig. 3-19), the TF AP-1, and the electrophile sensor protein Keap1 (see Fig. 3-27), just to name a few. These and many other proteins are inactivated by thiol-reactive chemicals, causing impaired maintenance of the cell's energy and metabolic homeostasis.

Binding of thiol-reactive chemicals to specific proteins may also initiate a signal. For example, thiol-reactive and oxidant chemicals, such as acrolein, methyl isocyanate, the lacrimator chloroacetophenone, and corrosive gases (eg, phosgene, chloropicrin, and chlorine), react with cysteine thiol groups of the TRPA1 receptor (a cation channel) in the membrane of sensory neurons. Excitation of these neurons located in the cornea and the mucous membranes of the eye and the respiratory tract elicits irritation, pain, lacrimation, bronchial secretion, sneezing, coughing, and bronchospasm (Bessac and Jordt, 2010). If moderate, these responses are alerting and protective, but are incapacitating and detrimental when exaggerated at high exposure. Keap1 may be regarded as an intracellular sensor of similar chemicals, as covalent and/or oxidative modification of thiol groups in Keap1 triggers the adaptive electrophile stress response, which is cytoprotective (see Fig. 3-27; Klaassen and Reisman, 2010). Conversion of the catalytic thiol group (-SH) in PTP and the lipid phosphatase PTEN to sulfenic acid group (-S-OH) on reaction with HOOH or lipid hydroperoxides (see reaction scheme above) inactivates these enzymes. PTPs keep protein kinase–mediated signal transduction pathways under control and PTEN controls the phosphatidilinositol-3-kinase (PI3K)–Akt pathway, both activated by growth factors (see Fig. 3-12). Therefore, inactivation of PTPs and PTEN permits these signalings to surge, thereby initiating, for example, a proliferative response. However, this concept may be an oversimplification because similar inactivation of cdc25 (another PTP) may compromise mitosis, as cdc25 normally dephosphorylates and activates cyclins 1 and 2, which are positive regulators of cell division (see Fig. 3-25). Formation of protein sulfenic acids by the oxidative stress product HOOH is thus considered as an initiating event of redox signaling (Forman *et al.*, 2004). Redox signaling is controlled by the production of HOOH (eg, by Nox activated on growth factor receptor stimulation) and its

enzymatic elimination. At low level, HOOH is removed effectively by peroxiredoxins (Fig. 3-5); however, these enzymes are incapacitated by overoxidation of their catalytic thiol groups at high HOOH levels (see Fig. 3-5). This modification can be reversed by sulfiredoxins (Lowther and Haynes, 2011). Furthermore, protein sulfenic acid formation is readily reversed by reaction of the sulfenic acid with a thiol (eg, glutathione), resulting in a protein disulfide (eg, protein-S-SG; see the scheme above), which in turn is reduced by thioredoxin or glutaredoxin as shown in Fig. 3-22, thereby regenerating PTPs and PTEN in their active thiol form. Therefore, peroxiredoxins, sulfiredoxins, thioredoxin, thioredoxin reductase, glutaredoxin, glutathione, and NADPH are all important negative regulators of oxidative signaling (Neumann *et al.*, 2009). Protein tyrosine nitration (see Fig. 3-8) may also alter protein function or may interfere with signaling pathways that involve tyrosine kinases and phosphatases.

Toxicants may interfere with the template function of DNA. The covalent binding of chemicals to DNA causes nucleotide mispairing during replication. For example, covalent binding of aflatoxin 8,9-oxide to N-7 of guanine results in pairing of the adduct-bearing guanine with adenine rather than cytosine, leading to the formation of an incorrect codon and the insertion of an incorrect amino acid into the protein. Such events are involved in the aflatoxin-induced mutation of the Ras proto-oncogene and the p53 tumor suppressor gene (Eaton and Gallagher, 1994). 8-Hydroxyguanine (8-OH-Gua) and 8-hydroxyadenine are mutagenic bases produced by HO$^\bullet$ that can cause mispairing with themselves as well as with neighboring pyrimidines, producing multiple amino acid substitutions (Breen and Murphy, 1995). Cr(III) produced from chromate (Cr(VI)) via reduction by ascorbate, alone or complexed to ascorbate, forms a coordinate covalent bond with phosphate in DNA, thereby inducing a mutation (Quievryn *et al.*, 2002). Chemicals such as doxorubicin, which intercalate between stacked bases in the double-helical DNA, push adjacent base pairs apart, causing an even greater error in the template function of DNA by shifting the reading frame.

Destruction of Target Molecules In addition to adduct formation, toxicants alter the primary structure of endogenous molecules by means of cross-linking and fragmentation. Bifunctional electrophiles, such as 2,5-hexanedione, carbon disulfide, acrolein, 4-oxonon-2-enal, 4-hydroxynon-2-enal, and nitrogen mustard alkylating agents, cross-link cytoskeletal proteins, DNA, or DNA with proteins. HOOH and hydroxyl radicals can also induce cross-linking by converting proteins into either reactive electrophiles (eg, protein sulfenic acids and protein carbonyls, respectively), which react with a nucleophilic group (eg, thiol, amine) in another macromolecule. Radicals (eg, those shown in Fig. 3-4) may induce cross-linking of macromolecules by converting them into radicals, which react with each other by radical recombination. Cross-linking imposes both structural and functional constraints on the linked molecules.

Some target molecules are susceptible to spontaneous degradation after chemical attack. Free radicals such as $Cl_3COO^\bullet$ and HO$^\bullet$ can initiate peroxidative degradation of lipids by hydrogen abstraction from fatty acids (Recknagel *et al.*, 1989). The lipid radical (L$^\bullet$) formed is converted successively to lipid peroxyl radical (LOO$^\bullet$) by oxygen fixation, lipid hydroperoxide (LOOH) by hydrogen abstraction, and lipid alkoxyl radical (LO$^\bullet$) by the Fe^{2+}-catalyzed Fenton reaction. Subsequent fragmentation gives rise to hydrocarbons such as ethane and reactive aldehydes such as 4-hydroxynon-2-enal and malondialdehyde (Fig. 3-9). Thus, lipid peroxidation not only destroys lipids in cellular membranes but also generates endogenous toxicants, both free radicals (eg, LOO$^\bullet$, LO$^\bullet$) and electrophiles (eg, 4-oxonon-2-enal, 4-hydroxynon-2-enal). These substances can

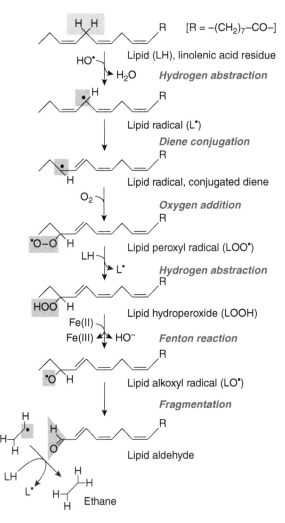

Figure 3-9. *Lipid peroxidation initiated by the hydroxyl radical (HO•).* Many of the products, such as the radicals and the α,β-unsaturated aldehydes, are reactive, whereas others, such as ethane, are nonreactive but are indicators of lipid peroxidation.

readily react with adjacent molecules, such as membrane proteins, or diffuse to more distant molecules such as DNA. F_2-isoprostanes are stable peroxidation products of arachidonic acid; these are not only sensitive markers of lipid peroxidation but also potent pulmonary and renal vasoconstrictors (Basu, 2004).

Apart from hydrolytic degradation by toxins and radiolysis, toxicant-induced fragmentation of proteins is not well documented. There are, however, examples for destruction of the prosthetic group in enzymes. For instance, cytochrome P450 converts allyl isopropyl acetamide into a reactive metabolite, which alkylates the heme moiety of the enzyme. This leads to loss of the altered heme and to porphyria (De Matteis, 1987). Arsine (AsH$_3$) acutely induces heme release from oxyhemoglobin, which may underlie its hemolytic effect. Aconitase is attacked by ONOO⁻ at its [4Fe-4S]$^{2+}$ cluster, in which one of the Fe atoms is genuinely labile (as is complexed to inorganic sulfur and not to enzyme-bound cysteines like the others). As a result of the oxidant action of ONOO⁻, the labile Fe is lost, inactivating the enzyme (Castro *et al.*, 1994) and compromising the citric acid cycle where aconitase functions.

Several forms of DNA fragmentation are caused by toxicants. For instance, attack of DNA bases by HO• can result in the formation of imidazole ring–opened purines or imidazole ring–contracted pyrimidines, which block DNA replication. Formation of a bulky adduct at guanine *N*-7 destabilizes the *N*-glycosylic bond, inducing depurination. Depurination results in apurinic sites that are mutagenic. Single-strand breaks (SSB) typically are caused by hydroxyl radicals via abstraction of H from desoxyribose in DNA yielding the C-4′ radical, followed by O$_2^{•-}$ addition, Criegee rearrangement, and cleavage of the phosphodiester bond (Breen and Murphy, 1995). Multiple hydroxyl radical attacks on a short length of DNA, which occur after ionizing radiation, cause double-strand breaks (DSB) that are typically lethal to the affected cell.

Neoantigen Formation Whereas the covalent binding of xenobiotics or their metabolites is often inconsequential with respect to the function of the immune system, in some individuals these altered proteins, which carry the xenobiotic adduct as a hapten, evoke an immune response. Some chemicals (eg, dinitrochlorobenzene, penicillin, and nickel ion) are sufficiently reactive to bind to proteins spontaneously. Others may obtain reactivity by autooxidation to quinones (eg, urushiols, the allergens in poison ivy) or by enzymatic biotransformation (Park *et al.*, 2005). For example, CYP2E1 biotransforms halothane to an electrophile, trifluoroacetyl chloride, which binds as a hapten to microsomal and cell surface proteins in the liver, inducing a hepatitis-like immune reaction in sensitive patients.

Haptenized proteins released from cells may evoke antibody-mediated (humoral) and/or T-cell-mediated (cellular) immune response. In the humoral response, B cells play the leading role: they bind the complete antigen through their B-cell receptors and associate with T-helper cells (CD4⁺). Antigen binding (as signal #1) and cell surface costimulatory molecules on T-helper cells (as signal #2) induce differentiation of B cells into plasma B cells that manufacture and secrete antibody. By binding to the antigen, the antibody assists in destruction of the antigen by phagocytosis; however, harmful consequences may also result. For example, when penicillin-bound proteins as antigens react with IgE-type antibodies on the surface of mast cells, the reaction triggers release of mast cell mediators (eg, histamine, leukotrienes), which in turn may cause bronchoconstriction (asthma), vasodilatation, and plasma exudation (wheal, anaphylactic shock).

In cellular immune response, T cells are the main mediators. In the sensitization phase, T-helper cells become activated by two signals coming from antigen-presenting cells, such as macrophages in internal tissues and dendritic cells in tissues that are in contact with external environment (ie, skin and mucosal lining of the respiratory and GI tract). The APC phagocytoses the haptenized protein and migrates to lymph nodes where most T cells are located. Meanwhile, the APC processes the antigen into appropriate peptides, externalizes, and transfers the processed antigen to the major histocompatibility complex (MHC) on its surface. On reaching the lymph node, the APC presents the MHC-bound peptide to the T-cell receptor (TCR) of T-helper cells (signal #1). In addition, cell surface coactivator molecules (eg, CD80 and CD86) on APC bind to their counterparts (eg, CD28) on T cells (signal #2). Without signal #2 (which verifies that the antigen detected is foreign) the T cell becomes functionally inert (anergic). On receiving both signals, the helper T cell becomes specific to one particular antigen, expresses the T-cell growth factor IL-2 and its receptor, proliferates, differentiates, and is released into the circulation. On reexposure to the allergen, the elicitation phase commences. Antigen-specific T cells enter the exposure site (eg, the skin) and using IL-2 and other cytokines, they can activate cytotoxic T cells (CD8⁺) and induce expression of adhesion molecules at the site of allergen contact. Whereas this response is protective against virus-infected cells and tumor cells, it causes inflammation and cell injury in cells containing xenobiotic neoantigens. This model describes the response to contact allergens, such as nickel and urushiols, and is the basis of detecting contact allergens in mice with the local lymph node assay.

Besides the above-described classical mechanism of neoantigen-initiated APC-mediated T-cell activation, xenobiotics may cause T-cell activation by more direct ways. For example, Ni ions may not only form coordinate covalent bonds with proteins, making them neoantigens, but also apparently cross-link MHC of APC with the TCR of T cells, activating the latter. Moreover, some drugs (eg, sulfamethoxazole), which can be biotransformed into adduct forming metabolites (eg, nitroso-sulfamethoxazole) that triggers T-cell activation by the classical mechanism, purportedly may also stimulate the TCR of T cells directly, without involvement of APC.

Regarding contact allergens, a new concept has emerged: to elicit allergic contact dermatitis chemicals should not only initiate formation of antigen-specific T cells (as described above) but also evoke a less specific inflammatory reaction (referred to as innate immune signal). For example, nickel alone cannot give a positive response in the local lymph node assay in mice; however, it can when coadministered with lipopolysaccharide (LPS), a bacterial cell wall component. LPS acts through Toll-like receptor 4 (TLR4) on resident skin cells (macrophages, dendritic cells, fibroblasts) to trigger inflammatory gene expression via signaling pathways that involves NF-κB. However, nickel alone can evoke contact dermatitis in sensitive humans, apparently because it activates the human TLR4 that, unlike the mouse receptor, contains 2 nonconserved histidine residues (Schmidt and Goebeler, 2011). The need for an innate immune signal may account for the observation that contact allergy may be facilitated by an injury evoking inflammatory response, such as toxic cell injury by an irritant chemical or microbial infection.

Drug-induced lupus and possibly many cases of drug-induced agranulocytosis are thought to be mediated by immune reactions triggered by drug–protein adducts. The causative chemicals are typically nucleophiles, such as aromatic amines (eg, aminopyrine, clozapine, procainamide, and sulfonamides), hydrazines (eg, hydralazine and isoniazid), and thiols (eg, propylthiouracil, methimazole, and captopril). These substances can be oxidized by myeloperoxidase of granulocytes and monocytes (the precursors of APC) or by the ROS/RNS such cells produce (HO•, ONOO−, hypochlorous acid [HOCl], see Fig. 3-26) to reactive metabolites that bind to the surface proteins of these cells, making them antigens (Uetrecht, 1992). The reactive metabolites may also activate monocytes and thus promote the immune reaction. Activation of CD4+ T cells by inhibition of promoter methylation of specific genes by procainamide and hydralazine as a possible lupus-inducing mechanism is discussed in the section "Dysregulation of Transcription."

Toxicity Not Initiated by Reaction with Target Molecules

Some xenobiotics not only interact with a specific endogenous target molecule to induce toxicity but also, instead, alter the biological microenvironment (see step 2b in Fig. 3-1). Included here are (1) chemicals that alter H+ ion concentrations in the aqueous biophase, such as (a) acids and substances biotransformed to acids, such as methanol and ethylene glycol, (b) protonophoric uncouplers such as 2,4-dinitrophenol and pentachlorophenol, which dissociate their phenolic protons in the mitochondrial matrix, thus dissipating the proton gradient that drives ATP synthesis, and (c) cationic amphiphilic drugs (eg, chloroquine and amiodarone)

that diffuse into lysosomes and accumulate there after being protonated at their amino groups; (2) solvents and detergents that physicochemically alter the lipid phase of cell membranes and destroy transmembrane solute gradients that are essential to cell functions; and (3) other xenobiotics that cause harm merely by occupying a site or space. For example, some chemicals (eg, the ethylene glycol-derived Ca-oxalate, methotrexate, and acyclovir) form water-insoluble precipitates in renal tubules. The poorly water-soluble complex produced in renal tubules from melamine and its derivative cyanuric acid caused the renal injury observed in cats and dogs fed adulterated pet food (Dobson *et al.*, 2008) and is probably also responsible for a similar disorder that occurred in children fed melamine-contaminated infant formula. By occupying bilirubin binding sites on albumin, compounds such as the sulfonamides induce bilirubin toxicity (kernicterus) in neonates. Carbon dioxide displaces oxygen in the pulmonary alveolar space and causes asphyxiation.

STEP 3—CELLULAR DYSFUNCTION AND RESULTANT TOXICITIES

The reaction of toxicants with a target molecule may result in impaired cellular function as the third step in the development of toxicity (Fig. 3-1). Each cell in a multicellular organism carries out defined programs. Certain programs determine the destiny of cells—that is, whether they undergo division, differentiation (ie, express proteins for specialized functions), or apoptosis. Other programs control the ongoing (momentary) activity of differentiated cells, determining whether they secrete more or less of a substance, whether they contract or relax, and whether they transport and metabolize nutrients at higher or lower rates. For regulation of these cellular programs, cells possess signaling networks (such as those shown in Figs. 3-12 and 3-15) that can be activated and inactivated by external signaling molecules. To execute the programs, cells are equipped with synthetic, metabolic, kinetic, transport, and energy-producing systems as well as structural elements, organized into macromolecular complexes, cell membranes, and organelles, by which they maintain their own integrity (internal functions) and support the maintenance of other cells (external functions).

As outlined in Fig. 3-10, the nature of the primary cellular dysfunction caused by toxicants, but not necessarily the ultimate outcome, depends on the role of the target molecule affected. If the target molecule is involved in cellular regulation (signaling), dysregulation of gene expression and/or dysregulation of momentary cellular function occur primarily. However, if the target molecule is involved predominantly in the cell's internal maintenance, the resultant dysfunction can ultimately compromise the survival of the cell. The reaction of a toxicant with targets serving external functions can influence the operation of other cells and integrated organ systems. The following discussion deals with these consequences.

Toxicant-Induced Cellular Dysregulation

Cells are regulated by signaling molecules that activate specific cellular receptors linked to signal transducing networks that transmit the signals to the regulatory regions of genes and/or to functional proteins. Receptor activation may ultimately lead to (1) altered gene expression that increases or decreases the quantity of specific proteins and/or (2) a chemical modification of specific proteins, typically by phosphorylation, which activates or inhibits proteins. Programs controlling the destiny of cells primarily affect gene

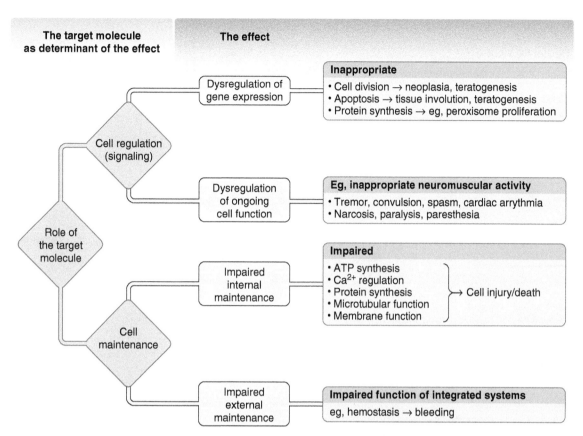

Figure 3-10. *The third step in the development of toxicity: alteration of the regulatory or maintenance function of the cell.*

expression, whereas those regulating the ongoing activities primarily influence the activity of functional proteins; however, one signal often evokes both responses because of branching and interconnection of signaling networks.

Dysregulation of Gene Expression Gene expression is the process by which information from a gene is used in the synthesis of a functional gene product. The genetic information may be transcribed from DNA into messenger RNA (mRNA), which in turn is translated into a protein product. The nonprotein-coding genes may be transcribed into other RNAs, among them the recently discovered small silencing RNA or microRNA (miRNA), which can repress translation of mRNA into proteins, thereby regulating protein synthesis posttranscriptionally (Fig. 3-11). Chemicals may dysregulate the expression of genes encoding mRNA, miRNA, or both, in either way causing altered synthesis of specific proteins. Dysregulation of gene expression may occur at elements that are directly responsible for transcription, at components of the intracellular signal transduction pathway, and at the synthesis, storage, or release of the extracellular signaling molecules. Dysregulation of gene expression initiated by chemicals at these 3 levels is discussed below.

Dysregulation of Transcription Transcription of genetic information from DNA to mRNA and miRNA is controlled largely by interplay between TFs and the regulatory or promoter region of genes coding for mRNA and miRNA (Fig. 3-11). By binding to distinctive nucleotide sequences in this region, ligand- and signal-activated TFs facilitate or impede the formation of the preinitiation complex, thereby promoting or repressing transcription of the adjacent gene. Xenobiotics may interact with the TFs (or other components of the preinitiation complex) and/or may alter the promoter region of the gene.

Dysregulation of Transcription by Chemicals Acting Through Ligand-Activated Transcription Factors Several endogenous compounds, such as hormones (eg, steroids, thyroid hormones) and vitamins (retinoids and vitamin D), influence gene expression by binding to and activating TFs or intracellular receptors (Table 3-4). Xenobiotics may mimic the natural ligands. For example, fibric acid–type lipid-lowering drugs, phthalate esters, and compound Wy-14,643 substitute for polyunsaturated fatty acids as ligands for the peroxisome proliferator–activated receptor (PPARα) (Poellinger *et al.*, 1992), and xenoestrogens (eg, DES, DDT, methoxychlor) substitute estradiol, an endogenous ligand for estrogen receptors (ER).

Acting through ligand-activated TFs, natural or xenobiotic ligands when administered at extreme doses or at critical periods during ontogenesis may cause toxicity by inappropriately influencing the fate of cells and inducing cell death or mitosis (Table 3-4). Glucocorticoids such as dexamethasone induce apoptosis of lymphoid cells. Whereas desirable in the treatment of lymphoid malignancies, this is an unwanted response in many other conditions. TCDD, a ligand of the AhR, produces thymic atrophy by causing apoptosis of thymocytes. Estrogens exert mitogenic effects in cells that express the ER, such as those found in female reproductive organs, mammary gland, and liver. ER-mediated proliferation appears to be responsible, at least in part, for formation of tumors in these organs during prolonged estrogen exposure (Green, 1992), as well as for induction of the rare vaginal adenocarcinoma in late puberty after transplacental exposure to the synthetic estrogen DES. Stimulation of these receptors during a critical prenatal period of differentiation reprograms the estrogen target tissue (ie, Mullerian duct), resulting in benign and malignant abnormalities in the reproductive tract later in life (Newbold, 2004). Mice exposed neonatally to DES served

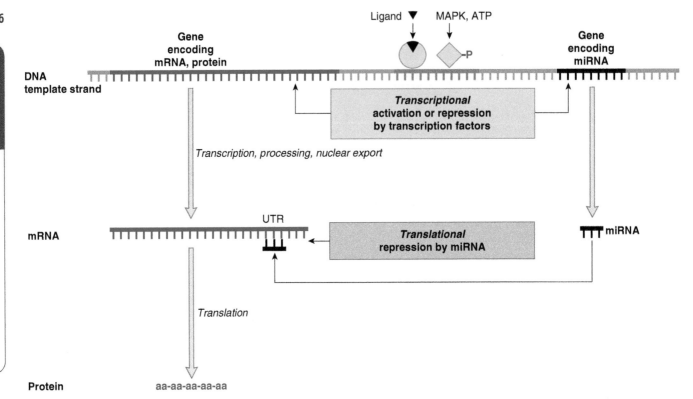

Figure 3-11. *Basic steps of gene expression—transcription factors regulate transcription, whereas microRNAs regulate (repress) translation.* In the process of gene expression, information from a gene is used in the synthesis of a functional gene product. This simplified figure depicts how the synthesis of two important functional gene products, that is, proteins and microRNAs (miRNA, also called small silencing RNA), are interrelated. As described in the text, these normally controlled processes may be dysregulated by endobiotics and xenobiotics as well as during pathologic processes, such as carcinogenesis.

Genetic information in a protein-coding gene (red in the DNA strand) is transcribed into a precursor messenger RNA (mRNA), which is processed into the mature mRNA by capping at the 5′ end, splicing (ie, removing noncoding introns) and polyadenylation at the 3′ end (not shown). After export from the nucleus, the mRNA associates with the ribosome and serves as a template to determine the amino acid (aa) sequence of the protein being synthesized (translation).

DNA sequences between protein-coding genes (ie, intergenic regions) may code for miRNAs. These are small noncoding RNA molecules (21–25 nucleotides in length) that may control the translation of more than 60% of mRNAs into proteins. The gene for miRNA (black in the DNA strand) codes for an initial transcript, termed pri-miRNA, which may be several kilobases long (not shown; Wahid *et al.*, 2010). The pri-miRNA is then cut shorter in the nucleus by an RNase (Drosha), assisted by its partner protein DiGeorge syndrome critical region in gene 8 (DGCR8), to become pre-miRNA (60–70 nucleotides in length). After export into the cytoplasm, the pre-miRNA is further truncated by another RNase (Dicer) and its partner TRBP to form the mature miRNA. Finally, miRNA associates with an Argonaute protein, thus forming microRNA-induced silencing complex (miRISC). The miRNA guides miRISC to specifically recognize mRNAs, called target mRNAs. The miRNA binds with base pairing to the untranslated region (UTR) of the target mRNA and miRISC downregulates its translation into protein by translational repression and/or mRNA cleavage. Because miRNAs bind to their target mRNAs by partial complementarity over a short sequence, one miRNA may have several hundreds of mRNA targets; therefore, a single miRNA can silence the expression of many proteins. Often a single pri-miRNA is processed into a cluster of miRNAs; therefore, their expression pattern is usually similar. A well-known example is the miR17-92 cluster comprising 7 miRNAs that are often overexpressed in cancer.

Ligand- and signal-activated transcription factors (represented by the round and the rectangular symbols, respectively) can bind to the promoter regions (green in the DNA strand) of the protein-coding genes and the miRNA-coding genes and upregulate or downregulate their transcription, thereby directly influencing the expression of mRNA and/or miRNA and ultimately affecting the synthesis of specific proteins. Transcription factors and miRNAs thus regulate diverse cellular pathways. It is important to note that miRNAs, as a rule, repress the translation of proteins. Therefore, upregulation of miRNA transcription results in downregulation of protein translation from the target mRNAs, whereas downregulation of miRNA causes derepression of protein translation from the target mRNAs, thereby increasing the synthesis of specific proteins.

to model DES-induced late carcinogenesis in the reproductive tract. Compared with the wild-type animals, mice overexpressing estrogen receptor-α (ERα) were exceedingly sensitive to DES-induced uterine adenocarcinoma, whereas ERα-knockout mice were resistant, indicating the role of ERα in tumorigenesis. It has been speculated that environmental xenoestrogens such as DDT, polychlorinated biphenyls, bisphenol A, and atrazine contribute to an increased incidence of breast cancer. Zearalenone, a mycoestrogen feed contaminant, causes vulval prolapse in swine, an example of an ER-mediated proliferative lesion. The mitogenic and hepatic tumor-promoting effects of peroxisome proliferators in rodents are also receptor-mediated, because they are not observed in PPARα-null mice (Peters *et al.*, 1998). Humans do not respond with hepatocellular and peroxisomal proliferation to

fibrates and express PPARα at low levels and often in nonfunctional forms. Humanized mice (ie, PPARα-null mice transfected with human PPARα) also fail to respond with hepatocellular and peroxisomal proliferation to fibrates, indicating that the human receptor cannot signal for proliferation (Gonzalez and Yu, 2006). In addition, pathways downstream of the receptor are also inappropriate to produce such a response in humans, because transfection of rat PPARα into human hepatocytes failed to make the peroxisomes inducible by PPARα ligands in the human cells. Chemicals that act on ligand-activated TFs, such as glucocorticoids, TCDD, and retinoids, induce fetal malformations that may be regarded as inappropriate gene expression. Candidate target genes are the homeobox genes that determine the body plan during early ontogenesis.

Table 3-4

Toxicants Acting on Ligand-Activated Transcription Factors

LIGAND-ACTIVATED TRANSCRIPTION FACTOR	ENDOGENOUS LIGAND	EXOGENOUS LIGAND	EFFECT
Estrogen receptor (ER)	Estradiol	Ethynylestradiol Diethylstilbestrol DDT, methoxychlor Zearalenone	Mammary and hepatic carcinogenesis Porcine vulval prolapse
Glucocorticoid receptor (GR)	Cortisol	Dexamethasone	Apoptosis of lymphocytes Teratogenesis (cleft palate)
Retinoic acid receptor (RAR, RXR)	All-*trans*-retinoic acid	13-*cis*-Retinoic acid	Teratogenesis (craniofacial, cardiac, thymic malformations)
Aryl hydrocarbon receptor (AhR)	Unknown	TCDD PCBs PAHs	Thymic atrophy Wasting syndrome Teratogenesis (cleft palate) Hepatocarcinogenesis in rats Enzyme induction (eg, CYP1A1)
Peroxisome proliferator–activated receptor (PPARα)	Fatty acids	Fibrate esters (eg, clofibrate) Phthalate esters (eg, DEHP)	Hepatocarcinogenesis in mice Peroxisome proliferation Enzyme induction (eg, CYP4A1, acyl-CoA oxidase)
Constitutive androstane receptor (CAR)	3α,5α-Androstenol 3α,5α-Androstanol (inhibitors)	TCPOBOP, phenobarbital[*] DDT, PCP, chlorpromazine	Enzyme induction (eg, CYP2B, CYP3A) Hepatocarcinogenesis in mice
Pregnane X receptor (PXR)	Pregnenolone Progesterone	PCN, dexamethasone Spironolactone, cyproterone Rifampicin, zearalenone Litocholic acid	Enzyme induction (eg, CYP3A) Transporter induction (eg, Oatp1a4, Mdr1, Mrp1, Mrp2, Mrp3)

TCPOBOP, 1,2-bis[2-(3,5-dichloropyridyloxy)]benzene.
[*]*Phenobarbital indirectly activates CAR, not as a ligand.*

In addition to altering the fate of specific cells, compounds that act on ligand-activated TFs can also evoke changes in the metabolism of endobiotics and xenobiotics by inducing overexpression of relevant enzymes. For example, the PPARα-ligand fibrates induce lipoprotein lipase and enzymes involved in fatty acid oxidation. Unlike the hepatic proliferative effects of PPARα agonists, these effects occur not only in rodents but also in humans, and form the basis of the use of fibrates as lipid-lowering drugs. TCDD, phenobarbital, and pregnenolone 16α-carbonitrile (PCN) activate AhR, the constitutive androstane receptor (CAR), and the pregnane X receptor (PXR), respectively (Table 3-4), thereby exerting their well-known cytochrome P450-inducing effects. However, rodent, rabbit, and human PXRs and CARs exhibit low degree of sequence conservation in their ligand-binding domains. This accounts for marked species differences in the induction potential of their ligands, such as PCN, rifampicin, and TCPOBOP (Gonzalez and Yu, 2006). Genes of several xenobiotic-metabolizing enzymes may be activated by these chemicals. For example, TCDD increases the expression of cytochrome P450 1A1, UDP-glucuronosyltransferase-1, and several subunits of mouse and rat glutathione *S*-transferase in an AhR-dependent manner. In AhR-null mice, TCDD induces neither these enzymes nor the adverse effects listed in Table 3-4 (Gonzalez and Fernandez-Salguero, 1998). CYP1A1 becomes also strongly expressed in the epithelial cells of the dioxin-induced cystic lesions in the human skin and thus CYP1A1 induction (which is detectable immunohistochemically in these structures) may serve as a biomarker of human dioxin exposure (Saurat *et al.*, 2012). Chloracne, as this multiple dermal lesion has been called inappropriately, is now identified as hamartoma. Dioxin-induced hamartomas appear in the epidermis and are characterized by (1) nonmalignant proliferation of columnar epithelial cells enclosing cysts with inflammatory signs and (2) involution of sebaceous glands. Whole genome microarray analysis of TCDD-induced hamartomas revealed severe dysregulation of gene expression, with marked overexpression of some genes, such as those coding for CYP1A1, inflammatory proteins, and gremlin 2 (a cytokine that inhibits bone morphogenic protein, a transforming growth factor-β [TGF-β]–like growth factor), and repression of many others, such as those encoding several sebaceous lipid synthesis enzymes and solute carriers (Saurat *et al.*, 2012). Mechanistic interpretation of many of these TCDD-induced alterations in gene expression and their role in development of dioxin-induced dermal hamartomas is still uncertain.

The above-mentioned alterations in cell fate and function caused by endobiotics and xenobiotics that act on ligand-activated TFs may in part be mediated by transcriptional upregulation or downregulation of protein-coding genes, that is, genes that are transcribed into mRNA, which in turn is translated into protein (Fig. 3-11). For example, the drug-metabolizing enzymes are induced by TCDD (see above) because the promoter regions of their genes contain a dioxin (or xenobiotic) response element (DRE or

XRE). The TCDD-activated AhR complexed with its nuclear translocator protein Arnt (also called HIF-1β) binds to this sequence and promotes the transcription of these genes and secondarily the synthesis of enzyme proteins. The cyclooxygenase-2 (COX-2) gene, whose product is involved in the synthesis of inflammatory prostaglandins, also contains DRE/XRE permitting its transactivation by TCDD-activated AhR. Similarly, the ligand-activated PPARα, after dimerizing with RXR, upregulates the transcription of genes encoding enzymes involved in fatty acid transport and β-oxidation by interacting with the peroxisome proliferator response element (PPRE) located in the promoter of these genes.

As discovered recently, the effects of endobiotics and xenobiotics that act on ligand-activated TFs may also be mediated by transcriptional upregulation or downregulation of genes coding for miRNAs. Because miRNAs repress the translation of target mRNAs into proteins, upregulation of miRNA transcription results in increased repression of protein translation, whereas downregulation of miRNA causes derepression of protein translation from the target mRNAs, and in turn increases the synthesis of specific proteins (Fig. 3-11). The mechanism of hepatocellular proliferation in mice exposed to the peroxisome proliferator Wy-14,643 involves transcriptional downregulation by the Wy-14,643-activated mouse PPARα of the gene coding for let-7c, a miRNA (Gonzalez and Shah, 2008). Let-7c is known to target c-Myc mRNA and represses its translation into c-Myc protein. Therefore, declining levels of let-7c in response to Wy-14,643 result in derepression of c-Myc mRNA and a consequential surge in c-Myc protein synthesis. As c-Myc is a TF signaling for mitosis (see Figs. 3-12 and 3-32), its increased abundance in the liver induces hepatocellular proliferation. Interestingly, the proliferative action of c-Myc also involves miRNA gene regulation: c-Myc upregulates miR-17-92, a cluster of miRNAs, which in turn repress the translation of p21, a cyclin-dependent kinase inhibitor with antimitotic action (see Fig. 3-32), and Bim, a proapoptotic protein (see Fig. 3-15), thereby permitting mitosis and opposing apoptosis. In contrast to normal mice, PPARα-humanized mice (expressing the human PPARα) exhibit neither downregulation of let-7c gene expression nor hepatocellular proliferation on Wy-14,643 treatment, supporting a causative relationship between these events. The mode of action of some other ligand-activated TFs also involves downregulation of miRNA gene transcription with subsequent derepression of the target mRNAs, causing their increased translation into specific proteins. For example, dexamethasone downregulates the expression of the miRNA cluster miR-17-92, which results in elevated levels of Bim, a proapoptotic member of the Bcl family of proteins (see Fig. 3-15). In addition, glucocorticoids can also upregulate the transcription of the Bim gene. Overexpression of the Bim protein, at both transcriptional and translational levels, may be the principal mechanism of glucocorticoid-induced apoptosis in lymphoid cells (Molitoris et al., 2011). Glucocorticoids also cause skeletal muscle wasting, partly because they stimulate the production of myostatin by the muscle. Acting on the muscle in a paracrine manner, this TGF-β-like signaling protein negatively regulates muscle mass (see Fig. 3-30). Glucocorticoids decrease the expression of miR-27a and b (which normally repress the translation of myostatin mRNA, as this mRNA contains a recognition sequence for miR-27a and b in its 3'-untranslated region), thereby increasing the synthesis of myostatin protein. Whereas TCDD, acting through the AhR and the XRE in the COX-2 gene promoter, can transcriptionally upregulate COX-2 expression as mentioned above, studies on mice indicate that TCDD can induce COX-2 protein also by downregulating of miR-101a gene, because one of the targets for miR-101a is the mRNA that translates into the COX-2 enzyme (Yoshioka et al., 2011). It appears

that COX-2 induction plays a role in TCDD-induced liver injury in mice. Furthermore, the expression of drug-metabolizing enzymes is regulated not only by TFs (see above and in Table 3-4) but also by miRNAs. For example, the translation of CYP3A4 (which forms the genotoxic metabolites of aflatoxin B_1 and benzo[a]pyrene) and CYP2E1 (which contributes to toxification of acetaminophen, carbon tetrachloride, and dimethylnitrosamine) is repressed by miR-27b and miR-378, respectively (Yokoi and Nakajima, 2011). The complexity of protein expression regulation is underlined by the recent recognition that while TFs can control the expression of miRNAs at their transcription, miRNAs can control the expression of TFs at their translation (Yokoi and Nakajima, 2011).

Finally, ligand-activated TFs do not act only by regulating gene expression through binding to their cognate response element but also by interacting with other proteins, including other nuclear receptors or their associates. Such interactions underlie, for example, the antiestrogenic effect of TCDD and dioxin-like chemicals, which involves at least two mechanisms. First, the TCDD-ligated AhR can associate with the ER, facilitating its nuclear export and proteasomal degradation. In addition, dimerization of the TCDD-ligated AhR with its partner Arnt reduces the availability of this protein for ER that employs Arnt as a transcriptional coactivator (Denison et al., 2011).

Dysregulation of Transcription by Chemicals Altering the Regulatory Region of Genes Xenobiotics may dysregulate transcription by also altering the regulatory gene regions through direct chemical interaction or by changing their methylation pattern. It has been hypothesized that thalidomide (or its hydrolysis product) exerts teratogenic effect in the embryo by intercalating to GGGCGG sequences (also called GC boxes) that are binding sites for Sp1 and Egr-1 TFs (Stephens et al., 2000). Thalidomide would thus impair insulin-like growth factor-1 (IGF-1) and fibroblast growth factor-2 (FGF2) signaling pathways necessary for angiogenesis and limb formation, because both pathways encompass multiple proteins whose genes contain GC boxes in the regulatory region but lack TATA and CCAAT boxes (eg, specific integrins, FGF2, IGF-1, and IGF-1 receptor substrate-1). Another chemical feature of thalidomide that may account for impaired Sp1-mediated transcriptional activation is that the hydrolysis product of this drug is a glutamine analogue and thus mimics the glutamine-rich activation domain of Sp1 protein.

As described in more detail in the section "Carcinogenesis," methylation of cytosines in CpG islands located in the promoter of genes is a major epigenetic mechanism, which together with coupled histone modifications (eg, acetylation, methylation) influences the transcriptional activity of the adjacent gene. Increased promoter methylation (hypermethylation) silences genes, whereas decreased methylation (hypomethylation) permits their activation. Importantly, when DNA replication occurs, the methylation pattern is copied from the parent strand to the daughter strand by DNA methyltransferase-1 (DNMT1), making the pattern heritable. Nevertheless, promoter methylation is subject to environmental influences, which can thus cause heritable changes in gene regulation. Altered promoter methylation has been implicated in chemically induced systemic lupus erythemathosus (SLE), in developmental deficiencies manifested postnatally or even in subsequent generations, and in cancer. The antiarrhythmic drug procainamide and the antihypertensive hydralazine often induce SLE, an autoimmune inflammatory disease. Both drugs inhibit DNA methylation and induce global DNA hypomethylation in CD4+ T lymphocytes with concomitant overexpression of proteins important in inflammation, such as CD11a (an integrin subunit), CD70 (a B-cell costimulatory molecule), and perforin (a cell-killing molecule) (Ballestar et al., 2006). Idiopathic lupus also involves global DNA hypomethylation in T cells with overexpression of these proinflammatory proteins. Therefore, promoter hypomethylation and overexpression of critical genes that convert T cells into aggressive inflammatory cells appears fundamental in the pathogenesis of both idiopathic and drug-induced SLE.

DNA methylation is an important process also in genomic imprinting that takes place during formation of germ cells. The vast majority of genes in both germ cells (ie, the sperm and the egg) similarly undergo or avoid epigenetic alterations (eg, methylation and related histone modifications); therefore, the offspring carries equally expressed 2 copies (ie, maternal and paternal alleles) of most genes. However, a relatively few (100–200) genes (called the imprinted genes) are epigenetically altered (generally methylated and thus typically silenced) only in the male or female germ cells; therefore, either the paternal or the maternal gene copy is expressed in the offspring, whereas the other allele is not expressed. For example, the insulin-like growth factor-2 gene, which encodes an autocrine growth factor important in fetal growth, is expressed only from the paternal allele. Because the genomically imprinted genes have only a single active copy, they are especially susceptible for epigenetic dysregulation. Dysregulation of imprinting can range from loss of imprinting, which results in biallelic expression and double amounts of the gene product, to silencing of both alleles. Although prenatal exposure to chemicals, such as TCDD and ethanol, influences genomic imprinting (Wu *et al.*, 2004; Stouder *et al.*, 2011), mechanistic interpretation of the role of such epigenetic alterations in chemically induced embryonic, early postnatal, or transgenerational defects in somatic or germ cell development is still uncertain due to the complexity of gene regulation.

The genome is especially susceptible to epigenetic alterations during early development, as in the preimplantation mammalian embryo, the genome (except for the imprinted genes) undergoes extensive demethylation, and appropriate patterns of cytosine methylation are reestablished after implantation. Developing mammalian germ cells are also subject to such changes: primordial germ cells undergo genomic demethylation while they migrate into the early gonad, and then they undergo remethylation during sex determination in the gonad, for example, testis development. During this period (embryonic 11–15 days in the rat), the androgen receptor and ER-β are expressed in the developing testis, and ligands of these nuclear receptors can influence the methylation process. Indeed, transient exposure of gestating female rats during the period of gonadal sex determination to vinclozolin (an agricultural fungicide with antiandrogenic activity) or methoxychlor (a DDT-type insecticide with estrogenic activity) decreased the spermatogenic capacity (with reduced sperm number and viability) in the adult male offspring and increased the incidence of male infertility (Anway *et al.*, 2005). Importantly, these effects were transferred through the male germ line to nearly all males of the subsequent 3 generations. These adverse transgenerational effects on reproduction correlate with altered DNA methylation patterns in the germ line. Thus, endocrine disruptors have the potential to epigenetically reprogram the germ line and promote transgenerational disease state, although the relevance of these findings under human exposure conditions is still uncertain.

Transcription is also severely dysregulated in cancer cells by altered promoter methylation (ie, global DNA hypomethylation and tumor suppressor gene hypermethylation). DNA methylation, including its biochemistry, its influence on histone modifications (acetylation and methylation), and its role in chemical carcinogenesis, is discussed in this chapter in the section "Epigenetic Mechanisms in Carcinogenesis: Inappropriate Activation or Responsiveness of the Regulatory Region of Critical Genes."

Dysregulation of Signal Transduction Extracellular signaling molecules (such as growth factors, cytokines, hormones, neurotransmitters, and some secreted proteins) engage cell surface receptors and intracellular signal transducing networks and ultimately activate TFs. Fig. 3-12 depicts a simplified scheme for some of these networks and identifies some signal-activated TFs that are turned on by these systems and that in turn control the transcriptional activity of genes that determine the fate of cells by influencing mitosis and/or apoptosis. Among these TFs are c-Fos and c-Jun proteins, which bind in dimeric combinations (called AP-1) to the tetradecanoylphorbol acetate (TPA) response element (TRE), for example, in the promoter of the cyclin D gene whose product promotes the cell division cycle (see Figs. 3-25 and 3-32). Other signal-activated TFs that upregulate the transcription of cyclin D gene by binding to their cognate nucleotide sequences include c-Myc, E2F, NF-κB, CREB, and STAT. Mitogenic signaling molecules thus induce cell proliferation. In contrast, TGF-β activates SMADs and induces the expression of cyclin-dependent kinase inhibitor proteins (eg, p15, p21, and p57), which mediate its antimitotic effect (Johnson and Walker, 1999) (see Fig. 3-32), as well as the proapoptotic protein Bim (see Fig. 3-19), which conveys its apoptotic action.

In addition to the proliferatory signaling pathways illustrated in Fig. 3-12, Figs. 3-13 and 3-14 depict 2 other pathways, the activation of which can also promote cell division. These are set in motion by secreted glycoproteins, the Wnt and Hedgehog (Hh) ligands, which act on specific cell surface receptors, ultimately activating the transcriptional coactivator β-catenin and the TF Gli, respectively, which in turn can also activate the transcription of cyclin D gene, among many others. The Wnt–β-catenin and Hh–Gli systems are especially important in certain proliferative processes, such as embryogenesis, development of adult stem cells as well as progenitor cells, tissue regeneration after injury, and oncogenesis.

The signal from the cell surface receptors to the TFs is relayed mainly by successive protein–protein interactions and protein phosphorylations at specific serine, threonine, or tyrosine hydroxyl groups. Cell surface growth factor receptors (item 4 in Fig. 3-12) are in fact phosphorylating enzymes (ie, receptor protein tyrosine kinases). Their ligands induce them to phosphorylate themselves, which, in turn, enable these receptors to bind adapter proteins. Through these, the growth factor receptors can initiate proliferative signaling via two important pathways: (1) by activating Ras, they set in motion the mitogen-activated protein kinase (MAPK) cascade (Qi and Elion, 2005), and (2) by activating PI3K, they start the PI3K–Akt pathway. A crucial step in the latter is the PI3K-catalyzed phosphorylation of a plasma membrane lipid to generate phosphatidylinositol-3,4,5-triphosphate (PIP_3) that recruits protein kinase Akt to the membrane for activation. Because Akt (also called protein kinase B) has numerous substrates, the PI3K–Akt pathway branches (Morgensztern and McLeod, 2005). Fig. 3-12 shows the branch that leads to activation of the TF NF-κB, a prolife pathway. In addition, Akt may also indirectly activate the mammalian target of rapamycin (mTOR), a ubiquitous protein kinase, whose phosphorylated products promote the trophic state of cells by boosting protein synthesis and restraining autophagy (see Fig. 3-29). Furthermore, Akt catalyzes the inactivating phosphorylation of two important signaling proteins. One is glycogen synthase kinase 3 (GSK), a ubiquitous multifunctional constitutively active protein kinase, whose inactivation by Akt (or by some other Ser/Thr kinases) causes numerous effects ranging from promotion of glycogen synthesis from UDP-glucose to suppression of apoptosis (see later), and whose incapacitation by Wnt and Hh signaling permits β-catenin and Gli, respectively, to escape degradation and act as transcription activators (see Figs. 3-13 and 3-14). The other is the FoxO family of TFs, whose inactivation by Akt-catalyzed phosphorylation prevents protein degradation in the skeletal muscle and promotes proliferation, thereby countering muscle atrophy (see Fig. 3-30).

The intracellular signal transducer proteins are typically but not always activated by phosphorylation, which is catalyzed by protein kinases, and are usually inactivated by dephosphorylation, which is carried out by protein phosphatases. Interestingly, growth factor receptors can amplify their signals by inducing formation of HOOH. As discussed earlier, by attacking protein thiolate groups and converting them into sulfenic acid groups, HOOH reversibly inactivates PTP and PTEN, a lipid phosphatase that eliminates PIP_3 (see Fig. 3-12; Rhee et al., 2005). The source of HOOH is $O_2^{\cdot-}$ produced by the enzyme complex Nox, which is activated by growth factor receptors via the $PI3K \rightarrow PIP_3 \rightarrow$ Rac (a G-protein that associates with Nox) pathway. Even if once thought to be restricted to phagocytes, Nox occurs in the plasma membrane of many other cells, such as endothelial cells and vascular smooth muscle cells (Bokoch and Knaus, 2003). Although Nox in these cells is much less efficient to produce $O_2^{\cdot-}$ than Nox in phagocytes, the nonphagocytotic Nox releases $O_2^{\cdot-}$ into the cytoplasm, whereas the phagocytotic Nox delivers it to the external face of the plasma membrane (El-Benna et al., 2005).

Chemicals may cause aberrant signal transduction in a number of ways, most often by altering protein phosphorylation, occasionally by interfering with the GTPase activity of G proteins (eg, Ras), by disrupting normal protein–protein interactions or by establishing abnormal ones, or by altering the synthesis or degradation of signaling proteins. Such interventions may ultimately influence cell cycle progression.

Chemically Altered Signal Transduction with Proliferative Effect Xenobiotics that facilitate phosphorylation of signal transducers often promote mitosis and tumor formation. Such are the phorbol esters and fumonisin B that activate PKC. These chemicals functionally mimic diacylglycerol (DAG), one of the physiologic activators of PKC (Fig. 3-12). The other physiologic PKC activator Ca^{2+} is mimicked by Pb^{2+}, whose effect on $PKC\alpha$ is concentration-dependent: stimulatory at picomolar concentration, when Pb^{2+} occupies only high-affinity binding sites on PKC, and inhibitory at micromolar concentration, where the low-affinity sites are also occupied (Sun et al., 1999). Lead salts do induce marked hepatocellular proliferation in rats. The activated PKC promotes mitogenic signaling at least in two ways: (1) by phosphorylating Raf, the first protein kinase in the MAPK pathway (Fig. 3-12), and (2) by phosphorylating a protein phosphatase that dephosphorylates the TF c-Jun at specific sites (Thr 231, Ser 234, and Ser 249), thereby permitting its binding to DNA. Protein kinases may also be activated by interacting proteins that had been altered by a xenobiotic. For example, the TCDD-liganded AhR binds to MAPK. This so-called nongenomic effect of TCDD may contribute to overexpression of cyclins and cyclin-dependent kinases in guinea pig liver (Ma and Babish, 1999).

Hyperphosphorylation of proteins may result not only from increased phosphorylation by kinases but also from decreased dephosphorylation by phosphatases. Inhibition of phosphatases, including the lipid phosphatase PTEN (see Fig. 3-12), appears to be the underlying mechanism of the mitogenic effect of various chemicals, oxidative stress, and ultraviolet (UV) irradiation (Herrlich et al., 1999). PTP and dual-specificity phosphatases (ie, enzymes that remove phosphate from phosphorylated tyrosine as well as serine and threonine residues) as well as PTEN contain a catalytically active cysteine, and are susceptible to inactivation by

HOOH via sulfenic acid formation and by covalent reaction with other SH-reactive chemicals (Forman et al., 2004; Rhee et al., 2005). Indeed, xenobiotics such as the SH-reactive iodoacetamide, the organometal compound tributyltin, arsenite, as well as HOOH cause phosphorylation of the epidermal growth factor (EGF) receptor (item 4 in Fig. 3-12) by interfering with the PTP that would dephosphorylate and thus "silence" this receptor (Herrlich et al., 1999; Chen et al., 1998). Arsenite-induced oxidative stress (Lynn et al., 2000; Smith et al., 2001) may in fact result from activation of growth factor receptors. These signal via the $PI3K \rightarrow PIP_3 \rightarrow$ Rac pathway to the neighboring Nox, which also resides in the plasma membrane. Overproduction of $O_2^{\cdot-}$ by the activated Nox in endothelial cells and vascular smooth muscle cells might contribute to the vasculotoxic effects of arsenic. Arsenite may also inactivate the dual-specificity phosphatase that dephosphorylates and "silences" certain MAPKs (c-jun N-terminal kinase [JNK], p38), whereas methylmethane sulfonate (MMS) appears to inhibit a protein phosphatase that inactivates Src, a protein tyrosine kinase (Herrlich et al., 1999). The thiol-oxidizing agent diamide (which increases phosphorylation of MAPKs) and phenolic antioxidants (which form phenoxyl radicals and increase c-Fos and c-Jun expression) (Dalton et al., 1999) may also act by incapacitating PTP. Protein phosphatase 2A (PP2A) is the major soluble Ser/Thr phosphatase in cells and is likely responsible, at least in part, for reversing the growth factor–induced stimulation of MAPK, thereby keeping the extent and duration of MAPK activation under control (Goldberg, 1999). PP2A also removes an activating phosphate from a mitosis-triggering protein kinase ($p34^{cdc2}$). Several natural toxins are extremely potent inhibitors of PP2A, including the blue-green algae poison microcystin-LR and the dinoflagellate-derived okadaic acid (Toivola and Eriksson, 1999), which are tumor promoters in experimental animals subjected to prolonged low-dose exposure. It is to be noted, however, that acute high-dose exposure to microcystin induces severe liver injury, whereas such exposure to okadaic acid is the underlying cause of the diarrhetic shellfish poisoning. In these conditions, hyperphosphorylation of proteins other than those involved in proliferative signaling (eg, hepatocellular microfilaments in microcystin poisoning) may be primarily responsible for the pathogenesis.

Apart from phosphatases, there are also inhibitory binding proteins that can keep signaling under control. Such is IκB, which binds to NF-κB, preventing its transfer into the nucleus and its function as a TF. On phosphorylation by its designated IκB kinase (IKK), IκB is degraded by the proteasome and NF-κB is set free. IKK can be phosphorylated (activated) by other protein kinases, such as Raf (a member of the MAPK cascade) and Akt (a member of the PI3K–Akt pathway) (Fig. 3-12). NF-κB is an important contributor to proliferative and prolife signaling, because via the above pathways, growth factor receptor stimulation can cause IκB phosphorylation and thus the release of NF-κB, and because the released NF-κB transactivates genes whose products accelerate the cell division cycle (eg, cyclin D1 and c-Myc) and inhibit apoptosis (eg, antiapoptotic Bcl proteins and the caspase inhibitor of apoptosis proteins [IAP]) (Karin, 2006). NF-κB activation, via the Akt-mediated IKK phosphorylation, is involved in the proliferative (and possibly carcinogenic) effect of arsenite, nicotine, and the NNK. In addition, because NF-κB also targets the genes of several cytokines (eg, TNF, IL-1β), chemokines (eg, monocyte chemotactic protein-1 [MCP-1], cytokine-induced neutrophil chemoattractant [CINC]-1), cell adhesion molecules (eg, ICAM-1, E- and P-selectins), enzymes producing inflammatory lipid mediators (eg, PLA2, COX-2), and acute-phase proteins (eg, C-reactive protein, α1-acid glycoprotein), and because such cytokines acting on their receptors (items 2 and 3 in Fig. 3-12) activate

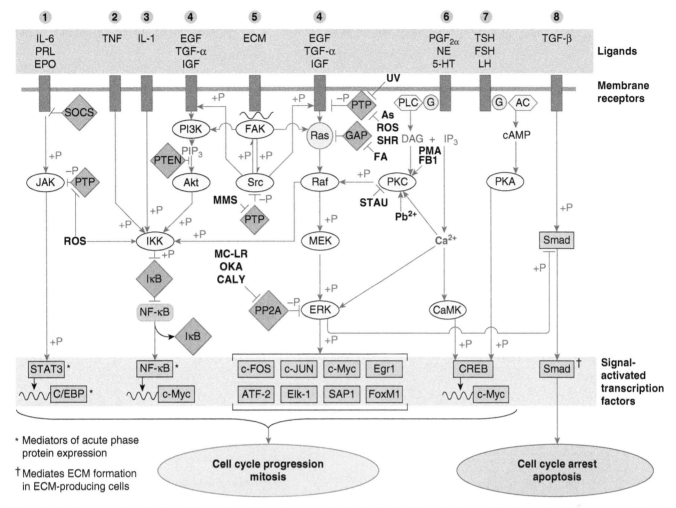

Figure 3-12. *Some signal transduction pathways from cell membrane receptors to signal-activated nuclear transcription factors that influence transcription of genes involved in cell-cycle regulation.* The symbols of cell membrane receptors are numbered 1 to 8 and some of their activating ligands are indicated. Circles represent G proteins, oval symbols protein kinases, rectangles transcription factors, wavy lines genes, and diamond symbols inhibitory proteins, such as protein phosphatases (PTP, PP2A) and the lipid phosphatase PTEN, the GTPase-activating protein GAP, and inhibitory binding proteins, such as IκB and suppressor of cytokine signaling (SOCS). Arrowheads indicate stimulation or formation of second messengers (eg, DAG, IP_3, PIP_3, cAMP, Ca^{2+}), whereas blunt arrows indicate inhibition. Phosphorylation and dephosphorylation are indicated by +P and −P, respectively. Abbreviations for interfering chemicals are printed in black (As, arsenite; CALY, calyculin A; FA, fatty acids; FB1, fumonisin B; MC-LR, microcystin-LR; OKA, okadaic acid; MMS, methylmethane sulfonate; PMA, phorbol miristate acetate; ROS, reactive oxygen species; SHR, SH-reactive chemicals, such as iodoacetamide; STAU, staurosporin).

Two important proliferative signaling can be evoked by growth factors, such as EGF, acting on their tyrosine kinase receptors (#4), which are duplicated in the figure for clarity. These receptors use adaptor proteins (Shc, Grb2, and SOS; not shown) to activate Ras by converting it from inactive GDP-bound form to active GTP-bound state, which in turn activates the MAP-kinase phosphorylation cascade built up from specific forms of MAPKKK, MAPKK, and MAPK proteins (here Raf, MEK, and ERK, respectively). The phosphorylated MAPK (eg, ERK) moves into the nucleus and phosphorylates transcription factors (eg, c-Fos), thereby enabling them to bind to cognate sequences in the promoter regions of genes (eg, cyclin genes) to facilitate transcription. The same growth factor receptors (#4) can signal through the phosphatidilinositol-3-kinase (PI3K)–Akt–IκB-kinase (IKK)–IκB–NF-κB pathway (see the text for more details). There are numerous interconnections between the signal transduction pathways. For example, the G-protein-coupled receptor (#6) can relay signal into the MAPK pathway via phospholipase C (PLC)–catalyzed formation of second messengers that activate protein kinase C (PKC), whereas signals from TNF and IL-1 receptors (#2 and 3) are channeled into the PI3K–Akt–NF-κB pathway by phosphorylating IKK. (Note that TNF may also signal for apoptosis when its receptor recruits an adaptor molecule FADD; see Fig. 3-19.) The integrin receptor (#5), whose ligands are constituents of the extracellular matrix (ECM), can also engage the growth factor receptors and Ras as well as PI3K via focal adhesion kinase (FAK) and the tyrosine kinase Src. The cell cycle acceleration induced by these and other signal transduction pathways is further enhanced by the ERK-catalyzed inhibitory phosphorylation of Smad that blocks the cell-cycle arrest signal from the TGF-β receptor (#8). Activation of protein kinases (PKC, CaMK, MAPK) by Ca^{2+} can also trigger mitogenic signaling. Several xenobiotics that are indicated in the figure may dysregulate the signaling network. Some may induce cell proliferation by either activating mitogenic protein kinases (eg, PKC) or inhibiting inactivating proteins, such as protein phosphatases (PTP, PP2A), GAP, or IκB. Others, for example, inhibitors of PKC, oppose mitosis and facilitate apoptosis.

This scheme is oversimplified and tentative in several details. Virtually all components of the signaling network (eg, G proteins, PKCs, MAPKs) are present in multiple, functionally different forms whose distribution may be cell-specific. The pathways depicted are not equally relevant for all cells. In addition, these pathways regulating gene expression not only determine the fate of cells but also control certain aspects of the ongoing cellular activity. For example, NF-κB induces synthesis of acute-phase proteins.

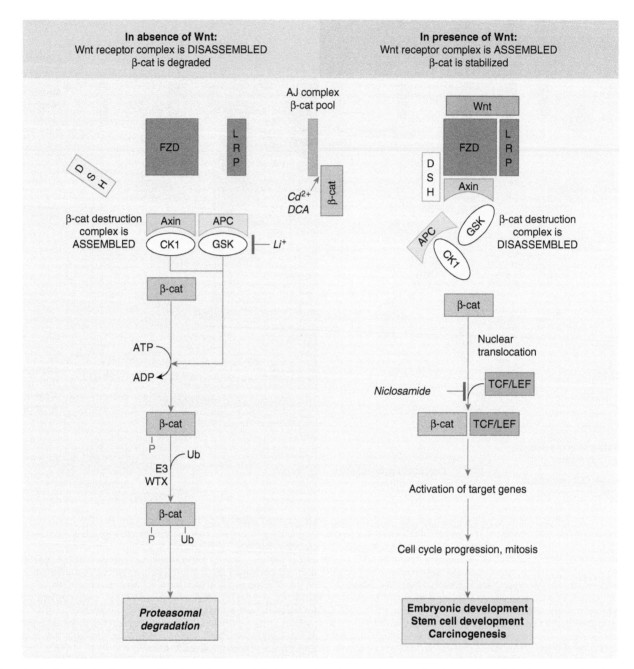

Figure 3-13. *The Wnt signaling—a proliferative pathway especially important in embryogenesis, stem cell and progenitor cell development, and carcinogenesis.* Wnt ligands are a secreted proteins covalently modified by palmitoylation and glycosylation. They act in autocrine, paracrine, or endocrine manner through their cell surface receptor frizzled (FZD) and coreceptor lipoprotein receptor–related protein (LRP).

In the absence of Wnt (as in the left side of the figure) intracellular proteins, including Axin, adenomatous polyposis coli (APC), casein kinase 1 (CK1), and glycogen synthase kinase 3 (GSK), form the so-called β-catenin (β-cat) destruction complex. The kinase members of this complex phosphorylate β-cat, thereby targeting it for ubiquitination by an E3 ubiquitin ligase (which is facilitated by WTX) and subsequent proteasomal degradation.

On binding of Wnt to FZD and LRP (as in the right side of the figure) the Wnt receptor complex assembles, and with recruitment of Axin into this complex, the β-cat destruction complex becomes disassembled. Consequently, β-cat escapes phosphorylation, ubiquitination, and degradation. Therefore, β-cat accumulates in the cell, translocates into the nucleus, and is recruited to its target genes by TCF/LEF family of transcription factors. Wnt signaling thus upregulates the transcription of numerous genes, including cyclin-D1, c-Myc, ABCB1 (P-glycoprotein), and S100A4 (a Ca²⁺-binding protein involved in cell cycle progression, cell motility, and metastasis development). Interestingly, β-cat is not only a transcriptional coactivator but also a structural protein that associates with E-cadherin at adherens junctions (AJ), thus participating in cell–cell adhesion. The disruption of E-cadherin–β-cat complexes causes an increase in β-cat-mediated transcription of Wnt-responsive genes. In contrast, stabilization of the E-cadherin–β-cat complex brings about reduced β-cat-mediated Wnt signaling.

Chemicals that influence Wnt signaling may interfere with embryonic development, cell proliferation, and carcinogenesis. Inhibition of GSK activity (eg, by Li⁺ ion) can lead to stabilization of β-cat and activation of β-cat-dependent gene transcription. Cd²⁺ disrupts the E-cadherin/β-cat complex of epithelial AJ, and the resultant β-cat-mediated proliferation of renal tubular cells could contribute to cadmium-induced nephrocarcinogenesis (Thévenod and Chakraborty, 2010). By a similar mechanism, deoxycholic acid (DCA) increases the proliferation and invasiveness of colon cancer cells. Inactivating mutations of APC and WTX, negative regulators of Wnt signaling, typically occur in colon cancer and Wilms tumor, respectively. The antihelminthic drug niclosamide inhibits formation of the β-cat-TCF/LEF complex at the promoter of S100A4 gene and thus counters colon cancer metastasis. DSH, disheveled; LEF, lymphoid enhancer-binding factor; TCF, T-cell factor; WTX, Wilms tumor suppressor.

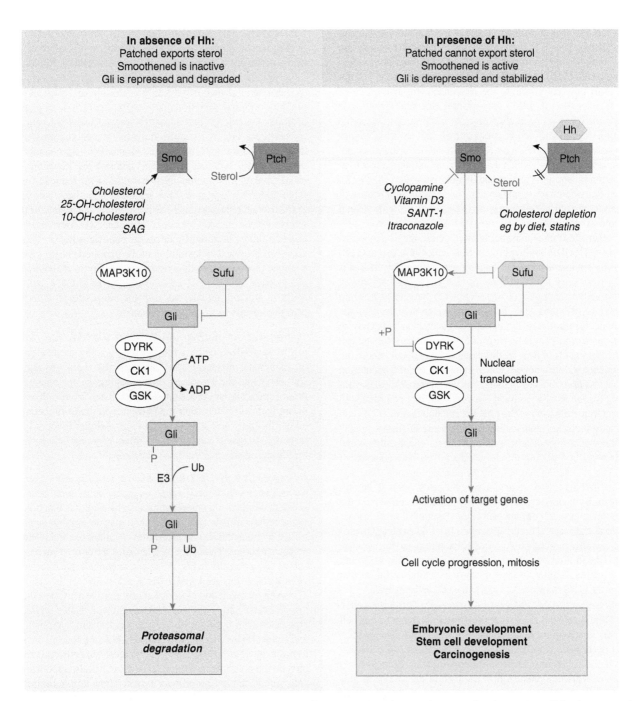

Figure 3-14. *The hedgehog (Hh) signaling—a proliferative pathway especially important in embryogenesis, stem cell and progenitor cell development, and carcinogenesis.* Hh ligands are secreted proteins covalently modified by palmitate and cholesterol. They act in autocrine, paracrine, or endocrine manner through their membrane receptor Patched (Ptch), which is the key inhibitor of Hh signaling in the unligated form (Katoh and Katoh, 2008).

In the absence of Hh (as in the left side of the figure) Ptch impedes the Hh pathway by inhibiting the activity of Smoothened (Smo), a positive regulator of signaling. According to the model presented in the figure, Ptch is a sterol pump that exports sterols (cholesterol or an oxysterol), thereby removing these activator molecules from Smo and making Smo idle. The repression of Smo by Ptch incapacitates the downstream Hh effectors, the glioma-associated family of transcription factors (Gli). This occurs partly because Gli is suppressed by Sufu (suppressor of fused) and partly because protein kinases, such as the dual-specificity tyrosine-(Y)-phosphorylation regulated kinase (DYRK), casein kinase 1 (CK1), and glycogen synthase kinase 3 (GSK), phosphorylate Gli, thereby marking Gli for ubiquitination by a ubiquitin ligase (E3) and subsequent degradation by the proteasome.

Binding of Hh to Ptch (as in the right side of the figure) abrogates its sterol-exporting activity; therefore, the sterol can activate Smo. In a manner incompletely understood, the active Smo suppresses Sufu, thereby permitting Gli activation, and activates mitogen-activated protein kinase kinase kinase 10 (MAP3K10), which in turn phosphorylates and inhibits DYRK, thereby preventing phosphorylation, ubiquitination, and proteasomal degradation of Gli. Thereafter the active Gli accumulates in the cell, translocates into the nucleus, and binds to its target genes. Hh signaling thus upregulates the transcription of numerous genes, including those that encode Ptch and Gli (a positive feedback loop), cyclin-D1 and -D2 (for cell cycle acceleration), several transcription factors such as those of the Forkhead box protein family (for cell fate determination), receptor ligands such as Jagged 2 (a ligand protein that activates Notch and related receptors), and ligand-binding proteins such as the Secreted frizzled-related protein 1 (SFRP1) that binds Wnt protein, thus preventing Wnt signaling (Fig. 3-13).

Chemicals that activate or inhibit Smo (shown in the left and right sides of the figure, respectively) may interfere with embryonic development. For example, the plant alkaloid cyclopamine inhibits Smo and causes cyclopia, a birth defect, in lambs. Smo inhibitors are potentially anticarcinogenic, whereas Smo activators may promote carcinogenesis by increased Hh signaling. Inactivating mutation of Ptch, the main inhibitor of Hh signaling, typically occurs in basal cell carcinoma of the skin that may be induced by UV and ionizing radiation, as well as arsenic exposure (Tang *et al.*, 2007). SAG, Smoothened Agonist; SANT-1, Smoothened Antagonist 1.

NF-κB, this TF plays a leading role also in inflammatory and acute-phase reactions, as well as in cancer caused by chronic inflammation (Karin, 2006; Waddick and Uckun, 1999). Conversely, inactivation of a subtype of NF-κB protein (RelA/p65) by binding to the TCDD-ligated AhR may contribute to the immunosuppressive effect of TCDD (Denison *et al.*, 2011). The proliferative Wnt signaling is also restrained by a set of binding proteins and protein kinases, the so-called β-catenin destruction complex that includes axin, adenomatous polyposis coli (APC), casein kinase 1 (CK1), and glycogen synthase kinase 3 (GSK), which destroy the transcriptional coactivator β-catenin by phosphorylation and ubiquitination (see Fig. 3-13). Impaired function of this complex (eg, by inactivating mutation of APC) can lead to unleashing the transcriptional coactivator β-catenin and in turn to colon cancer.

Another site from which aberrant mitogenic signals may originate is the GTP/GDP-binding protein Ras, which is active in GTP-bound form but inactive in GDP-bound form. The activity of Ras is normally terminated via stimulation of its own GTPase activity by a GTPase-activating protein (GAP) (Fig. 3-12) that returns Ras into its inactive GDP-bound state. Fatty acids, which may accumulate, for example, in response to phospholipase A activation and exposure to peroxisome proliferators (Rose *et al.*, 1999), inhibit GAP and can delay the turning off of Ras. As discussed in more detail later in the chapter, genotoxic carcinogens may mutate Ras, and if the mutation leads to a loss of its GTPase activity, this would result in permanent signaling for the MAPK pathway—a condition that contributes to malignant transformation of the affected cell population.

Finally, increased mobilization of a mitogenic TF from a "silent" intracellular pool may also be a mechanism for chemically altered signal transduction with proliferative effect. This may underlie, at least in part, the nephrocarcinogenicity of cadmium and the colon tumor–promoting action of secondary bile acids, such as deoxycholic acid. By disrupting the E-cadherin/β-catenin complex in the adherens junctions (AJ) of renal and colonic epithelial cells, respectively, these chemicals mobilize β-catenin from AJ (where this protein serves a structural function) into the cytoplasm and the nucleus. There β-catenin functions as a TF of Wnt signaling (Fig. 3-13) and activates the transcription of several genes, including cyclin D1 that promotes the G1/S transition of cells in the cell division cycle.

Chemically Altered Signal Transduction with Antiproliferative Effect Turning off the increased proliferative signaling after cell injury may compromise replacement of injured cells. This prediction has been made from a study on cultured Hepa 1–6 cells that exhibited the following, seemingly consequential alterations on exposure to acetaminophen (follow the path in Fig. 3-12): inhibition of Raf → diminished degradation of IκB → diminished binding of NF-κB to DNA → diminished expression of c-Myc mRNA (Boulares *et al.*, 1999). Downregulation of a normal mitogenic signal is a step away from survival and toward apoptosis. Indeed, inhibitors of PKC (staurosporin), PI3K (wortmannin), and IκB degradation (gliotoxin) (Waddick and Uckun, 1999) are apoptosis inducers. TGF-β and glucocorticoids increase IκB synthesis and, in turn, decrease NF-κB activation and c-Myc expression (Waddick and Uckun, 1999). These mechanisms may contribute to the apoptotic effect of TGF-β and glucocorticoids, the latter in lymphoid cells.

Offsetting the Hh–Gli pathway (Fig. 3-14), a key mitogenic signaling pathway controlling embryonic development, is the mechanism of the teratogenic action of cyclopamine (ie, cyclopia). This severe cephalic malformation was observed in the offspring of sheep grazing in a field where *Veratrum californicum* grew. This plant contains the steroidal alkaloid cyclopamine, which is an inhibitor of Smoothened, a positive regulator of Hh signaling (Chen *et al.*, 2002).

Dysregulation of Extracellular Signal Production Hormones of the anterior pituitary exert mitogenic effects on endocrine glands in the periphery by acting on cell surface receptors. Pituitary hormone production is under negative feedback control by hormones of the peripheral glands. Perturbation of this circuit adversely affects pituitary hormone secretion and, in turn, the peripheral gland. For example, xenobiotics that inhibit thyroid hormone production (eg, the herbicide amitrole and the fungicide metabolite ethylenethiourea) or enhance thyroid hormone elimination (eg, phenobarbital) reduce thyroid hormone levels and increase the secretion of thyroid-stimulating hormone (TSH) because of the reduced feedback inhibition. The increased TSH secretion stimulates cell division in the thyroid gland, which is responsible for the goiters or thyroid tumors caused by such toxicants (see Chap. 21). Decreased secretion of pituitary hormone produces the opposite adverse effect, with apoptosis followed by involution of the peripheral target gland. For example, estrogens produce testicular atrophy in males by means of feedback inhibition of gonadotropin secretion. The low sperm count in workers intoxicated with the xenoestrogen chlordecone probably results from such a mechanism.

Dysregulation of Ongoing Cellular Activity Ongoing control of specialized cells is exerted by signaling molecules acting on membrane receptors that transduce the signal by regulating Ca^{2+} entry into the cytoplasm or stimulating the enzymatic formation of intracellular second messengers. The Ca^{2+} or other second messengers ultimately alter the phosphorylation of functional proteins, changing their activity and, in turn, cellular functions almost instantly. Toxicants can adversely affect ongoing cellular activity by disrupting any step in signal coupling.

Dysregulation of Electrically Excitable Cells Many xenobiotics influence cellular activity in excitable cells, such as neurons, skeletal, cardiac, and smooth muscle cells. Cellular functions such as the release of neurotransmitters and muscle contraction are controlled by transmitters and modulators synthesized and released by adjacent neurons. The major mechanisms that control such cells are shown schematically in Fig. 3-15, and chemicals that interfere with these mechanisms are listed in Table 3-5.

Altered regulation of neural and/or muscle activity is the basic mechanism of action of many drugs and is responsible for toxicities associated with drug overdosage, pesticides, and microbial, plant, and animal toxins (Herken and Hucho, 1992). As neurons are signal-transducing cells, the influence of chemicals on neurons is seen not only on the neuron affected by the toxicant but also on downstream cells influenced by the primary target. Thus, tetrodotoxin, which blocks voltage-gated Na^+ channels (item 7 in Fig. 3-15) in motor neurons, causes skeletal muscle paralysis. In contrast, cyclodiene insecticides, which block GABA receptors (item 3 in Fig. 3-15) in the central nervous system, induce neuronal excitation and convulsions (Narahashi, 1991).

Perturbation of ongoing cellular activity by chemicals may be due to an alteration in (1) the concentration of neurotransmitters, (2) receptor function, (3) intracellular signal transduction, or (4) the signal-terminating processes.

Alteration in Neurotransmitter Levels Chemicals may alter synaptic levels of neurotransmitters by interfering with their synthesis, storage, release, or removal from the vicinity of the receptor. The convulsive effect of hydrazine and hydrazides (eg, isoniazid) is due to their ability to decrease the synthesis of the inhibitory neurotransmitter GABA (Gale, 1992). Reserpine causes its several adverse effects by inhibiting the neuronal storage of norepinephrine, 5-hydroxytryptamine, and dopamine, thereby depleting these

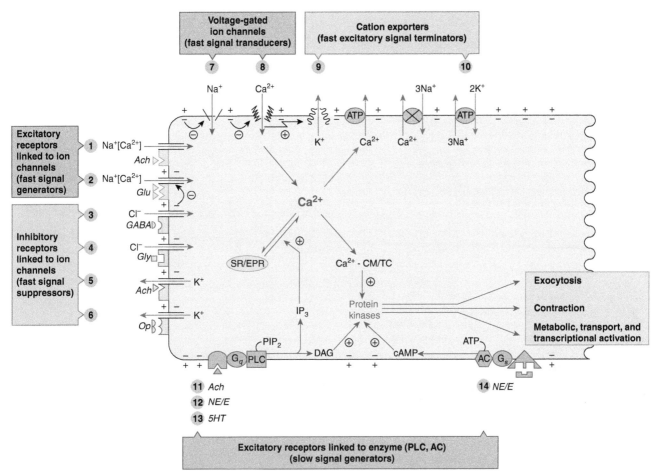

Figure 3-15. *Signaling mechanisms for neurotransmitters.* This simplified scheme depicts major cellular signaling mechanisms that are operational in many neurons and muscle and exocrine cells. Chemicals acting on the numbered elements are listed in Table 3-5. Fast signaling is initiated by the opening of ligand-gated Na^+/Ca^{2+} channels (1, 2). The resultant cation influx decreases the inside negative potential (ie, evokes depolarization) and thus triggers the opening of the voltage-gated Na^+ and Ca^{2+} channels (7, 8). As a second messenger, the influxed Ca^{2+} activates intracellular Ca^{2+}-binding proteins such as calmodulin (CM) and troponin C (TC), which, in turn, enhance the phosphorylation of specific proteins, causing activation of specific cellular functions. The signal is terminated by channels and transporters (eg, 9, 10) that remove cations from the cells and thus reestablish the inside negative resting potential (ie, cause repolarization) and restore the resting Ca^{2+} level. Fast signaling can be suppressed by opening the ligand-activated Cl^- or K^+ channels (3–6), which increases the inside negativity (ie, induces hyperpolarization) and thus counteracts opening of the voltage-gated Na^+ and Ca^{2+} channels (7, 8). Signal transduction from other receptors (11–13) that are coupled to G_q proteins involves generation of the second messenger inositol 1,4,5-trisphosphate (IP_3) and diacylglycerol (DAG) by phospholipase C (PLC), whereas signaling from receptor 14 that is coupled to G_s protein involves production of cyclic AMP (cAMP) by adenylyl cyclase (AC). These second messengers in turn influence cellular activities by mobilizing Ca^{2+} from the sarcoplasmic or endoplasmic reticulum (SR and EPR), as IP_3 does, or by activating protein kinases, as cAMP and DAG do, which activate PKA and PKC, respectively. For clarity, this figure does not depict that inhibitory receptors 5 and 6 are G_i protein–coupled and that besides opening K^+ channels, they also inhibit AC. Ach, acetylcholine; Glu, glutamate; GABA, γ-aminobutyric acid; Gly, glycine; Op, opioid peptides; NE, norepinephrine; E, epinephrine; 5HT, 5-hydroxytryptamine; G, G protein; PIP_2, phosphatidylinositol 4,5-bisphosphate. Encircled positive and negative signs indicate activation and inhibition, respectively.

transmitters. Skeletal muscle paralysis caused by botulinum toxin is due to inhibition of acetylcholine release from motor neurons and the lacking stimulation of the acetylcholine receptors at the neuromuscular junction (receptor 1 in Fig. 3-15). In contrast, inhibition of acetylcholinesterase by organophosphate or carbamate insecticides or chemical warfare agents (eg, soman) prevents the hydrolysis of acetylcholine, resulting in massive stimulation of cholinergic receptors (receptors 1, 5, and 11 in Fig. 3-15) and a cholinergic crisis (Table 3-5). Inhibition of the neuronal reuptake of norepinephrine by cocaine or tricyclic antidepressants is responsible for overexcitation of $α_1$-adrenergic receptors on vascular smooth muscles, resulting in nasal mucosal ulceration and myocardial infarction in heavy cocaine abusers, whereas overstimulation of $β_1$-adrenergic receptors contributes to life-threatening arrhythmias. Similar cardiac complications may result from amphetamine abuse, because amphetamine enhances the release of norepinephrine from adrenergic neurons and competitively inhibits neuronal reuptake of

this transmitter. A hypertensive crisis can occur with the combined use of tricyclic antidepressants and monoamine oxidase inhibitors, drugs that block different mechanisms of norepinephrine elimination (Hardman *et al.*, 1995). Concomitant use of drugs that increase the level of serotonin (5-HT) by enhancing its neuronal release and decreasing its neuronal reuptake (eg, fluoxetine) or its biotransformation (eg, monoamine oxidase inhibitors) induce the serotonin syndrome with cognitive and behavioral changes, autonomic dysfunction, and neuromuscular abnormalities. It is thought that cytotoxic antineoplastic drugs (eg, cisplatin) and radiation cause nausea and emesis, a disturbing reaction to chemotherapy and radiotherapy, by inducing release of 5-HT from enterochromaffin cells of the intestinal mucosa, which stimulates the 5-HT$_3$ receptors (5-HT-gated cation channel, functionally similar to item 1 in Fig. 3-15) on the adjacent vagal afferent neurons, thereby evoking the vomiting reflex (Endo *et al.*, 2000). Intestinal release of 5-HT and stimulation of vagal afferent neurons are also involved in the

Table 3-5

Agents Acting on Signaling Systems for Neurotransmitters and Causing Dysregulation of the Momentary Activity of Electrically Excitable Cells such as Neurons and Muscle Cells

RECEPTOR/CHANNEL/PUMP		AGONIST/ACTIVATOR		ANTAGONIST/INHIBITOR	
NAME	LOCATION	AGENT	EFFECT	AGENT	EFFECT
1. Acetyl-choline nicotinic receptor	Skeletal muscle	Nicotine Anatoxin-a Cytisine *Ind*: ChE inhibitors	Muscle fibrillation, and then paralysis	Tubocurarine, lophotoxin α-Bungarotoxin α-Cobrotoxin α-Conotoxin Erabutoxin b *Ind*: botulinum toxin	Muscle paralysis
	Neurons	See above	Neuronal activation	Pb^{2+}, general anesthetics	Neuronal inhibition
2. Glutamate receptor	CNS neurons	*N*-Methyl-D-aspartate Kainate, domoate Quinolinate Quisqualate *Ind*: hypoxia, HCN → glutamate release	Neuronal activation → convulsion, neuronal injury ("excitotoxicity")	Phencyclidine Ketamine General anesthetics	Neuronal inhibition → anesthesia Protection against "excitotoxicity"
3. GABA$_A$ receptor	CNS neurons	Muscimol, Avermectins, Sedatives (barbiturates, benzodiazepines), General anesthetics (halothane), Alcohols (ethanol)	Neuronal inhibition → sedation, general anesthesia, coma, depression of vital centers	Bicuculline Picrotoxin Pentylenetetrazole Cyclodiene insecticides Lindane, TCAD *Ind*: isoniazid	Neuronal activation → tremor, convulsion
4. Glycine receptor	CNS neurons, motor neurons	Avermectins (?), General anesthetics	Inhibition of motor neurons → paralysis	Strychnine *Ind*: tetanus toxin	Disinhibition of motor neurons → tetanic convulsion
5. Acetylcholine M$_2$ muscarinic receptor	Cardiac muscle	*Ind*: ChE inhibitors	Decreased heart rate and contractility	Belladonna alkaloids (eg, atropine), atropine-like drugs (eg, TCAD)	Increased heart rate
6. Opioid receptor	CNS neurons, visceral neurons	Morphine and congeners (eg, heroin, meperidine) *Ind*: clonidine	Neuronal inhibition → analgesia, central respiratory depression, constipation, urine retention	Naloxone	Antidotal effects in opiate intoxication
7. Voltage-gated Na$^+$ channel	Neurons, muscle cells, etc	Aconitine, veratridine Grayanotoxin Batrachotoxin Scorpion toxins Ciguatoxin DDT, pyrethroids	Neuronal activation → convulsion	Tetrodotoxin, saxitoxin μ-Conotoxin Local anesthetics Phenytoin Quinidine	Neuronal inhibition → paralysis, anesthesia Anticonvulsive action
8. Voltage-gated Ca^{2+} channel	Neurons, muscle cell, etc	Maitotoxin (?) Atrotoxin (?) Latrotoxin (?)	Neuronal/muscular activation, cell injury	ω-Conotoxin Pb^{2+}	Neuronal inhibition → paralysis
9. Voltage/Ca^{2+}-activated K$^+$ channel	Neurons, smooth and skeletal muscle, cardiac muscle	Pb^{2+}	Neuronal/muscular inhibition	Ba^{2+}, apamin (bee venom), dendrotoxin, 20-HETE, hERG inhibitors (eg, cisapride, terfenadine)	Neuronal/muscular activation → convulsion/spasm vasoconstriction, PMV tachycardia (torsade de pointes)

(continued)

Table 3-5

(Continued)

RECEPTOR/CHANNEL/PUMP		AGONIST/ACTIVATOR		ANTAGONIST/INHIBITOR	
NAME	LOCATION	AGENT	EFFECT	AGENT	EFFECT
10. Na⁺,K⁺-ATPase	Universal			Digitalis glycosides Oleandrin Chlordecone	Increased cardiac contractility, excitability Increased neuronal excitability → tremor
11. Acetylcholine M₃ muscarinic receptor	Smooth muscle, glands	*Ind*: ChE inhibitors	Smooth muscle spasm, salivation, lacrimation	Belladonna alkaloids (eg, atropine), atropine-like drugs (eg, TCAD)	Smooth muscle relaxation → intestinal paralysis, decreased salivation, decreased perspiration
Acetylcholine M₁ muscarinic receptor	CNS neurons	Oxotremorine *Ind*: ChE inhibitors	Neuronal activation → convulsion	See above	
12. Adrenergic α₁ receptor	Vascular smooth muscle	(Nor)epinephrine *Ind*: cocaine, tyramine, amphetamine, TCAD	Vasoconstriction → ischemia, hypertension	Prazosin	Antidotal effects in intoxication with α₁-receptor agonists
13. 5-HT₂ receptor	Smooth muscle	Ergot alkaloids (ergotamine, ergonovine)	Vasoconstriction → ischemia, hypertension	Ketanserine	Antidotal effects in ergot intoxication
14. Adrenergic β₁ receptor	Cardiac muscle	(Nor)epinephrine *Ind*: cocaine, tyramine, amphetamine, TCAD	Increased cardiac contractility and excitability	Atenolol, metoprolol	Antidotal effects in intoxication with β₁-receptor agonists

CNS, central nervous system; ChE, cholinesterase; Ind, indirectly acting (ie, by altering neurotransmitter level); 20-HETE, 20-hydroxy-5,8,11, 14-eicosatetraenoic acid; PMV, polymorphic ventricular; TCAD, tricyclic antidepressant.

*Numbering of the signaling elements in this table corresponds to the numbering of their symbols in Fig. 3-12. This tabulation is simplified and incomplete. Virtually all receptors and channels listed occur in multiple forms with different sensitivity to the agents. The reader should consult the pertinent literature for more detailed information.

emetic effect of ipecac syrup and its alkaloids (cephaelin and emetine). The α_2-adrenergic receptor agonist clonidine induces release in the brain of β-endorphin, an endogenous peptide that stimulates opioid receptors (item 6 in Fig. 3-15). This explains why clonidine intoxication mimics several symptoms of morphine poisoning, including depressed respiration and pinpoint pupils.

Toxicant–Neurotransmitter Receptor Interactions Some chemicals interact directly with neurotransmitter receptors, including (1) agonists that associate with the ligand-binding site on the receptor and mimic the natural ligand, (2) antagonists that occupy the ligand-binding site but cannot activate the receptor, (3) activators, and (4) inhibitors that bind to a site on the receptor that is not directly involved in ligand binding. In the absence of other actions, agonists and activators mimic, whereas antagonists and inhibitors block, the physiologic responses characteristic of endogenous ligands. For example, muscimol, a mushroom poison, is an agonist at the inhibitory $GABA_A$ receptor (item 3 in Fig. 3-15), whereas barbiturates, benzodiazepines, general anesthetics, and alcohols are activators (Narahashi, 1991). Thus, all these chemicals cause inhibition of central nervous system activity, resulting in sedation, general anesthesia, coma, and ultimately blockade of the medullary

respiratory center, depending on the dose administered. There are also similarities in the responses evoked by agonist/activators on excitatory receptors and those elicited by antagonists/inhibitors on inhibitory sites. Thus, glutamate receptor agonists and muscarinic receptor agonists cause neuronal hyperactivity in the brain and ultimately convulsions, as do inhibitors of $GABA_A$ receptor. It is also apparent that chemicals acting as agonists/activators on inhibitory receptors and those acting as antagonists/inhibitors on excitatory receptors may exert similar effects. Moreover, general anesthetic solvents induce general anesthesia not only by activating the inhibitory ligand-gated chloride-ion channels (ie, $GABA_A$ and glycine receptors; see items 3 and 4, respectively, in Fig. 3-15) but also by inhibiting the excitatory ligand-gated cation channels (ie, neuronal nicotinic acetylcholine receptor and glutamate receptors; see items 1 and 2, respectively, in Fig. 3-15) (Franks and Lieb, 1998; Perouansky et al., 1998). Because there are multiple types of receptors for each neurotransmitter, these receptors may be affected differentially by toxicants. For example, the neuronal nicotinic acetylcholine receptor is extremely sensitive to inhibition by lead ions, whereas the muscular nicotinic receptor subtype is not (Oortgiesen et al., 1993). Other chemicals that produce neurotransmitter receptor–mediated toxicity are listed in Table 3-5.

Some sensory neurons have membrane receptors that are stimulated by noxious chemicals and operate as ligand-gated cation channels. Such are the transient receptor potential (TRP) channels, whose opening cause influx of Na^+ and Ca^{2+} that depolarize and activate the neuron. The TRPV1 receptor is excited by capsaicin, the pungent ingredient of red peppers, and mediates the burning sensation of the tongue and reflex stimulation of the lacrimal gland associated with exposure to pepper spray (also called OC tear gas). The TRPA1 receptor, however, is activated by thiol-reactive and oxidant chemicals, such as the lacrimator compounds in tear gas (eg, chloroacetophenone, chlorobenzalmalonitrile, and dibenzoxazepine), acrolein, methyl isocyanate, corrosive gases (eg, phosgene, chloropicrin, and chlorine) and other irritants. These chemicals evoke sensations (irritation and pain), secretory and respiratory reflexes (lacrimation, bronchial secretion, sneezing, coughing, and bronchospasm), and neurogenic inflammation through the TRPA1 receptor (Bessac and Jordt, 2010).

Toxicant–Signal Transducer Interactions Many chemicals alter neuronal and/or muscle activity by acting on signal transduction processes. Voltage-gated Na^+ channels (item 7 in Fig. 3-15), which transduce and amplify excitatory signals generated by ligand-gated cation channels (receptors 1 and 2 in Fig. 3-15), are activated by a number of toxins derived from plants and animals (Table 3-5) as well as by synthetic chemicals such as DDT, resulting in overexcitation (Narahashi, 1992). In contrast, chemicals that block voltage-gated Na^+ channels (such as tetrodotoxin and saxitoxin) cause paralysis. The Na^+ channels are also important in signal transduction in sensory neurons; therefore, Na^+-channel activators evoke sensations and reflexes, whereas Na^+-channel inhibitors induce anesthesia. This explains the reflex bradycardia and burning sensation in the mouth that follow the ingestion of monkshood, which contains the Na^+-channel activator aconitine, as well as the use of Na^+-channel inhibitors such as procaine and lidocaine for local anesthesia.

Toxicant–Signal Terminator Interactions The cellular signal generated by cation influx is terminated by removal of the cations through channels or by transporters (Fig. 3-15). Inhibition of cation efflux may prolong excitation, as occurs with the blockade of Ca^{2+}-activated K^+ channels (item 9 in Fig. 3-15) by Ba^{2+}, which is accompanied by potentially lethal neuroexcitatory and spasmogenic effects. The arachidonic acid metabolite 20-hydroxy-5,8,11,14-eicosatetraenoic acid (20-HETE) also blocks Ca^{2+}-activated K^+ channels, causing vasoconstriction. Induction by cyclosporine of 20-HETE production in renal proximal tubular cells and the resultant decrease in renal cortical blood flow may underlie the nephrotoxic effect of cyclosporine (Seki et al., 2005). Blockade of specific voltage-gated K^+ channels (called hERG channels; item 9 in Fig. 3-15) in the heart delays cardiac repolarization (as indicated by prolonged QT time in ECG) and may evoke polymorphic ventricular tachycardia (termed torsade de pointes), which may cause sudden death if degenerates into ventricular fibrillation (Sanguinetti and Mitcheson, 2005). Several drugs with such an effect (eg, astemizole, cisapride, grepafloxacin, terfenadine) have been withdrawn from clinical use. Glycosides from digitalis and other plants inhibit Na^+,K^+-ATPase (item 10 in Fig. 3-15) and thus increase the intracellular Na^+ concentration, which, in turn, decreases Ca^{2+} export by Ca^{2+}/Na^+ exchange (Fig. 3-15). The resultant rise in the intracellular concentration of Ca^{2+} enhances the contractility and excitability of cardiac muscle. Inhibition of brain Na^+,K^+-ATPase by chlordecone may be responsible for the tremor observed in chlordecone-exposed workers (Desaiah, 1982). Lithium salts, although used therapeutically, have the potential to produce hyperreflexia, tremor, convulsions, diarrhea, and cardiac arrhythmias (Hardman et al., 1995).

Lithium also markedly potentiates cholinergic-mediated seizures. Besides inhibition of Li^+-sensitive enzymes (eg, inositol monophosphatase, bisphosphate 3′-nucleotidase, and GSK), another possible reason for these toxic effects is inefficient repolarization of neurons and muscle cells in the presence of Li^+. Whereas Li^+ readily enters these cells through Na^+ channels, contributing to the signal-induced depolarization, it is not a substrate for the Na^+,K^+ pump. Therefore, the cells fail to repolarize properly if a fraction of intracellular Na^+ is replaced by Li^+.

Failure of the Na^+,K^+ pump is also believed to contribute to the neuronal damage resulting from hypoxia, hypoglycemia, and cyanide intoxication. Inasmuch as 70% of the ATP produced in neurons is used to drive the Na^+,K^+ pump, cessation of ATP synthesis causes a cell to become or remain depolarized. The depolarization-induced release of neurotransmitters such as glutamate from such neurons is thought to be responsible for the hypoxic seizures and further amplification of neuronal injury by the neurotoxic actions of glutamate (Patel et al., 1993).

Dysregulation of the Activity of Other Cells While many signaling mechanisms also operate in nonexcitable cells, disturbance of these processes is usually less consequential. For example, rat liver cells possess α_1-adrenergic receptors (item 12 in Fig. 3-15) whose activation evokes metabolic changes, such as increased glycogenolysis and glutathione export, through elevation of intracellular Ca^{2+}, which may have toxicological significance.

Many exocrine secretory cells are controlled by muscarinic acetylcholine receptors (item 11 in Fig. 3-15). Salivation, lacrimation, and bronchial hypersecretion after organophosphate insecticide poisoning are due to stimulation of these receptors. In contrast, blockade of these receptors contributes to the hyperthermia characteristic of atropine poisoning. Kupffer cells, resident macrophages in the liver, secrete inflammatory mediators (see Fig. 3-26) that can harm neighboring cells. Because Kupffer cells possess glycine receptors, that is, glycine-gated Cl^- channels (item 4 in Fig. 3-15), the secretory function of these macrophages (eg, secretion of inflammatory mediators) can be blocked by administration of glycine, which induces hyperpolarization via influx of Cl^-. Such intervention alleviates ethanol-induced liver injury (Yin et al., 1998).

The discovery that some sulfonamides produce hypoglycemia in experimental animals led to the development of oral hypoglycemic agents for diabetic patients. These drugs inhibit K^+ channels in pancreatic β cells, inducing sequential depolarization, Ca^{2+} influx through voltage-gated Ca^{2+} channels, and exocytosis of insulin (Hardman et al., 1995). The antihypertensive diazoxide acts in the opposite fashion on K^+ channels and impairs insulin secretion. Whereas this effect is generally undesirable, it is exploited in the treatment of inoperable insulin-secreting pancreatic tumors.

Toxic Alteration of Cellular Maintenance

Numerous toxicants interfere with cellular maintenance functions. In a multicellular organism, cells must maintain their own structural and functional integrity as well as provide supportive functions for other cells. Execution of these functions may be disrupted by chemicals, resulting in a toxic response.

Impairment of Internal Cellular Maintenance: Mechanisms of Toxic Cell Death For survival, all cells must synthesize endogenous molecules; assemble macromolecular complexes, membranes, and cell organelles; maintain the intracellular environment; and produce energy for operation. Chemicals that disrupt these functions, especially the energy-producing function of mitochondria and protein synthesis controlling function of the genome, jeopardize survival and may cause toxic cell death.

There are three critical biochemical disorders that chemicals inflicting cell death may initiate, namely, ATP depletion, sustained rise in intracellular Ca^{2+}, and overproduction of ROS and RNS. In the following discussion, these events and the chemicals that may cause them are individually characterized. Then it is pointed out how their concerted action may induce a bioenergetic catastrophe, culminating in necrosis. Finally, there follows a discussion of the circumstances under which the cell can avoid this disordered decay and how it can execute death by activating catabolic processes that bring about an ordered disassembly and removal of the cell, called apoptosis.

Primary Metabolic Disorders Jeopardizing Cell Survival: ATP Depletion, Ca²⁺ Accumulation, ROS/RNS Generation

Depletion of ATP ATP plays a central role in cellular maintenance both as a chemical for biosynthesis and as the major source of energy. It is utilized in numerous biosynthetic reactions, activating endogenous compounds by phosphorylation and adenylation, and is incorporated into cofactors as well as nucleic acids. It is required for muscle contraction and polymerization of the cytoskeleton, fueling cellular motility, cell division, vesicular transport, and the maintenance of cell morphology. ATP drives ion transporters, such as the Na^+,K^+-ATPase in the plasma membrane, the Ca^{2+}-ATPase in the plasma and the ER membranes, and H^+-ATPase in the membrane of lysosomes and neurotransmitter-containing vesicles. These pumps maintain conditions essential for various cell functions. For example, the Na^+ concentration gradient across the plasma membrane generated by the Na^+,K^+ pump drives Na^+–glucose and Na^+–amino acid cotransporters as well as the Na^+/Ca^{2+} antiporter, facilitating the entry of these nutrients and the removal of Ca^{2+}.

Chemical energy is released by hydrolysis of ATP to ADP or AMP. The ADP is rephosphorylated in the mitochondria by ATP synthase (Fig. 3-16). Coupled to oxidation of hydrogen to water, this process is termed *oxidative phosphorylation*. In addition to ATP synthase, oxidative phosphorylation requires the (1) delivery of hydrogen in the form of NADH to the initial electron transport complex; (2) delivery of oxygen to the terminal electron transport complex; (3) delivery of ADP and inorganic phosphate to ATP synthase; (4) flux of electrons along the electron transport chain to O_2, accompanied by ejection of protons from the matrix space across the inner membrane; and (5) return of protons across the inner membrane into the matrix space down an electrochemical gradient to drive ATP synthase (Fig. 3-16).

Several chemicals impede these processes, interfering with mitochondrial ATP synthesis (Commandeur and Vermeulen, 1990; Wallace and Starkov, 2000; Wallace, 2008). These chemicals are divided into 5 groups (Table 3-6). Substances in class A interfere with the delivery of hydrogen to the electron transport chain. For example, fluoroacetate inhibits the citric acid cycle and the production of reduced cofactors. Class B chemicals such as rotenone and cyanide inhibit the transfer of electrons along the electron transport chain to oxygen. Class C agents interfere with oxygen delivery to the terminal electron transporter, cytochrome oxidase. All chemicals that cause hypoxia ultimately act at this site. Chemicals in class D inhibit the activity of ATP synthase, the key enzyme for oxidative phosphorylation. At this site, the synthesis of ATP may be inhibited in one of four ways: (1) direct inhibition of ATP synthase, (2) interference with ADP delivery, (3) interference with inorganic phosphate delivery, and (4) deprivation of ATP synthase from its driving force, the controlled influx of protons into the matrix space. Protonophoric chemicals (uncouplers) such as 2,4-dinitrophenol and pentachlorophenol import protons into the mitochondrial matrix, dissipating the proton gradient that drives the controlled influx of protons into the matrix, which, in turn, drives ATP synthase. Finally, chemicals causing mitochondrial DNA injury, and thereby impairing synthesis of specific proteins encoded by the mitochondrial genome (eg, subunits of complex I and ATP synthase), are listed in group E. These include the dideoxynucleoside antiviral drugs used against AIDS, such as zidovudine. Table 3-6 lists other chemicals that impair ATP synthesis.

ATP synthase is also present at sites in addition to the mitochondria, such as the outer segment disk of the retinal rods as well as the plasma membrane of certain cells and the concentric membranes that form the myelin sheath around the axon of neurons. Unlike its mitochondrial counterpart, the ATP synthase in plasma and myelin

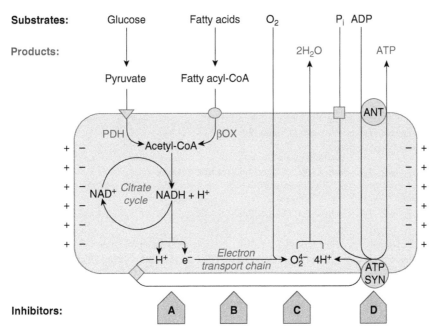

Figure 3-16. *ATP synthesis (oxidative phosphorylation) in mitochondria.* Arrows with letters A to D point to the ultimate sites of action of 4 categories of agents that interfere with oxidative phosphorylation (Table 3-6). For simplicity, this scheme does not indicate the outer mitochondrial membrane and that protons are extruded from the matrix space along the electron transport chain at 3 sites. βOX, beta-oxidation of fatty acids; e⁻, electron; P_i, inorganic phosphate; ANT, adenine nucleotide translocator; ATP SYN, ATP synthase (F_oF_1-ATPase).

Table 3-6

Agents Impairing Mitochondrial ATP Synthesis[*]

A. Inhibitors of hydrogen delivery to the electron transport chain acting on/as

1. Glycolysis (critical in neurons): hypoglycemia; iodoacetate, koningic acid, and NO^+ at GAPDH
2. Gluconeogenesis (critical in renal tubular cells): coenzyme A depletors (see below)
3. Fatty acid oxidation (critical in cardiac muscle): hypoglycin, 4-pentenoic acid, 4-ene-valproic acid
4. Pyruvate dehydrogenase: arsenite, DCVC, p-benzoquinone
5. Citrate cycle
   (a) Aconitase: fluoroacetate, $ONOO^-$
   (b) Isocitrate dehydrogenase: DCVC
   (c) Succinate dehydrogenase: malonate, DCVC, PCBD-Cys, 2-bromohydroquinone, 3-nitropropionic acid, cis-crotonalide fungicides
6. Depletors of TPP (inhibit TPP-dependent PDH and α-KGDH): ethanol (when chronically consumed)
7. Depletors of coenzyme A (CoA)
   (a) Thiol-reactive electrophiles: 4-(dimethylamino)phenol, p-benzoquinone
   (b) Drugs enzymatically conjugated with CoA: salicylic acid (the metabolite of aspirin), valproic acid
8. Depletors of NADH
   (a) See group A.V.1. in Table 3-7
   (b) Activators of poly(ADP-ribose) polymerase: agents causing DNA damage (eg, MNNG, hydrogen peroxide, $ONOO^-$)

B. Inhibitors of electron transport acting on/as

1. Inhibitors of electron transport complexes
   (a) NADH–coenzyme Q reductase (complex I): rotenone, amytal, MPP^+, paraquat
   (b) Coenzyme Q–cytochrome c reductase (complex III): antimycin-A, myxothiazole
   (c) Cytochrome oxidase (complex IV): cyanide, hydrogen sulfide, azide, formate, $^\bullet NO$, phosphine (PH_3)
   (d) Multisite inhibitors: dinitroaniline and diphenylether herbicides, $ONOO^-$
2. Electron acceptors: CCl_4, doxorubicin, menadione, MPP^+

C. Inhibitors of oxygen delivery to the electron transport chain

1. Chemicals causing respiratory paralysis: CNS depressants (eg, opioids), convulsants
2. Chemicals impairing pulmonary gas exchange: CO_2, "deep pulmonary irritants" (eg, NO_2, phosgene, perfluoroisobutene)
3. Chemicals inhibiting oxygenation of Hb: carbon monoxide, methemoglobin-forming chemicals
4. Chemicals causing ischemia: ergot alkaloids, cocaine

D. Inhibitors of ADP phosphorylation acting on/as

1. ATP synthase: oligomycin, cyhexatin, DDT, chlordecone
2. Adenine nucleotide translocator: atractyloside, DDT, free fatty acids, lysophospholipids
3. Phosphate transporter: N-ethylmaleimide, mersalyl, p-benzoquinone
4. Chemicals dissipating the mitochondrial membrane potential (uncouplers)
   (a) Cationophores: pentachlorophenol, dinitrophenol-, benzonitrile-, thiadiazole herbicides, salicylate, CCCP, cationic amphiphilic drugs (bupivacaine, perhexiline), valinomycin, gramicidin, calcimycin (A23187)
   (b) Chemicals permeabilizing the mitochondrial inner membrane: PCBD-Cys, chlordecone
5. Multisite inhibitor drugs: phenformin, propofol, salicylic acid (when overdosed)

E. Chemicals causing mitochondrial DNA damage and/or impaired transcription of key mitochondrial proteins

1. Antiviral drugs: zidovudine, zalcitabine, didanosine, fialuridine
2. Antibiotics: chloramphenicol (when overdosed), linezolid
3. Ethanol (when chronically consumed)

CCCP, carbonyl cyanide m-chlorophenylhydrazone; DCVC, dichlorovinyl-cysteine; GAPDH, glyceraldehyde 3-phosphate dehydrogenase; α-KGDH, α-ketoglutarate dehydrogenase; MNNG, N-methyl-N′-nitro-N-nitrosoguanidine; MPP^+, 1-methyl-4-phenylpyridinium; PCBD-Cys, pentachlorobutadienylcysteine; PDH, pyruvate dehydrogenase; TPP, thyamine pyrophosphate.

[*]The ultimate sites of action of these agents are indicated in Fig. 3-13.

membranes forms ATP on the external membrane face and is called ecto-ATP synthase. It is hypothesized that ATP produced by the myelinic ATP synthase (supported by the colocalized respiratory chain complexes and O_2 well dissolved in the myelin lipids) is delivered into the axon through gap junctions that traverse the myelin membranes and the axolemma (Morelli *et al.*, 2011). Myelinic ATP supply to axons, in which mitochondria are sparse, may explain why demyelinated axons die and why the white matter (composed of myelinated axons) is sensitive to hypoxia. Oxidative phosphorylation of ADP in isolated myelin vesicles (which are devoid of mitochondria) is sensitive to chemicals listed in Table 3-6 as mitochondrial

electron transport chain inhibitors (eg, antimycin and cyanide), ATP synthase inhibitors (eg, oligomycin), and uncouplers (eg, CCCP and valinomycin). If the trophic role of myelin in axonal maintenance under in vivo conditions becomes validated, it will be necessary to evaluate whether the ATP-synthesizing machinery of myelin is a relevant target for known neurotoxicants, such as lead, methyl mercury, hexachlorophene, and the methanol-derived formic acid.

Impairment of oxidative phosphorylation is detrimental to cells because failure of ADP rephosphorylation results in the accumulation of ADP and its breakdown products as well as depletion of ATP. Accordingly, hepatocytes exposed to KCN and iodoacetate exhibit a rapid rise in cytosolic H^+ and Mg^{2+} as a result of the hydrolysis of adenosine diphosphates and triphosphates (existing as Mg salts) and the release of phosphoric acid and Mg^{2+} (Herman *et al.*, 1990). The increased conversion of pyruvate to lactate also may contribute to the acidosis. The lack of ATP compromises the operation of ATP-requiring ion pumps, leading to the loss of ionic and volume-regulatory controls (Buja *et al.*, 1993). Shortly after intracellular acidosis and hypermagnesemia, liver cells exposed to KCN and iodoacetate exhibit a rise in intracellular Na^+, probably as a result of the failing Na^+ pump, after which plasma membrane blebs appear. The intracellular phosphoric acidosis is beneficial for the cells presumably because the released phosphoric acid forms insoluble calcium phosphate, preventing the rise of cytosolic Ca^{2+}, with its deleterious consequences (see below). In addition, a low pH also directly decreases the activity of phospholipases and inhibits mitochondrial permeability transition (MPT; see later). Terminally, the intracellular pH rises, increasing phospholipase activity, and this contributes to irreversible membrane damage (ie, rupture of the blebs) not only by degrading phospholipids but also by generating endogenous detergents such as lysophospholipids and free fatty acids. The lack of ATP aggravates this condition because the reacylation of lysophospholipids with fatty acids is impaired.

Sustained Rise of Intracellular Ca^{2+} Intracellular Ca^{2+} levels are highly regulated (Fig. 3-17). The 10,000-fold difference between extracellular and cytosolic Ca^{2+} concentration is maintained by the impermeability of the plasma membrane to Ca^{2+} and by transport mechanisms that remove Ca^{2+} from the cytoplasm (Richter and Kass, 1991). Ca^{2+} is actively pumped from the cytosol across the plasma membrane and is sequestered in the ER and mitochondria (Fig. 3-17). Because mitochondria are equipped with a low-affinity

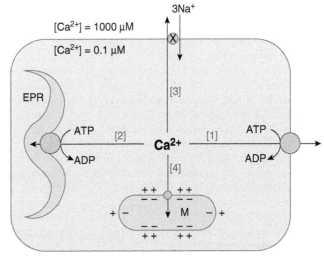

Figure 3-17. *Four mechanisms for the elimination of Ca^{2+} from the cytoplasm: Ca^{2+}-ATPase-mediated pumping into (1) the extracellular space as well as (2) the endoplasmic reticulum (EPR) and ion-gradient-driven transport into (3) the extracellular space (by the Ca^{2+}/Na^+ exchanger) as well as (4) the mitochondria (M; by the Ca^{2+} uniporter). Some chemicals that inhibit these mechanisms are listed in Table 3-7, group B.*

Ca^{2+} transporter, they play a significant role in Ca^{2+} sequestration only when the cytoplasmic levels rise into the micromolar range. Under such conditions, a large amount of Ca^{2+} accumulates in the mitochondria, where it is deposited as calcium phosphate.

Toxicants induce elevation of cytoplasmic Ca^{2+} levels by promoting Ca^{2+} influx into or inhibiting Ca^{2+} efflux from the cytoplasm (Table 3-7). Opening of the ligand- or voltage-gated Ca^{2+} channels

---

Table 3-7

Agents Causing Sustained Elevation of Cytosolic Ca^{2+}

A. Chemicals inducing Ca^{2+} influx into the cytoplasm
  I. Via ligand-gated channels in neurons
   1. Glutamate receptor agonists ("excitotoxins"): glutamate, kainate, domoate
   2. TRPV1 receptor (capsaicin receptor) agonists: capsaicin, resiniferatoxin
   3. TRPA1 receptor agonists: SH-reactive electrophiles, such as lacrimators (eg, chlorobenzalmalonitrile), acrolein, methyl isocyanate, phosgene, chloropicrin
  II. Via voltage-gated channels: maitotoxin (?), $HO^•$
  III. Via "newly formed pores": maitotoxin, amphotericin B, chlordecone, methylmercury, alkyltins
  IV. Across disrupted cell membrane
   1. Detergents: exogenous detergents, lysophospholipids, free fatty acids
   2. Hydrolytic enzymes: phospholipases in snake venoms, endogenous phospholipase A_2
   3. Lipid peroxidants: carbon tetrachloride
   4. Cytoskeletal toxins (by inducing membrane blebbing): cytochalasins, phalloidin
  V. From mitochondria
   1. Oxidants of intramitochondrial NADH: alloxan, *t*-BHP, NAPBQI, divicine, fatty acid hydroperoxides, menadione, MPP$^+$
   2. Others: phenylarsine oxide, gliotoxin, $^•NO$, $ONOO^-$
  VI. From the endoplasmic reticulum
   1. IP_3 receptor activators: γ-HCH (lindane), IP_3 formed during "excitotoxicity"
   2. Ryanodine receptor activators: δ-HCH

B. Chemicals inhibiting Ca^{2+} export from the cytoplasm (inhibitors of Ca^{2+}-ATPase in cell membrane and/or endoplasmic reticulum)
  I. Covalent binders: acetaminophen, bromobenzene, CCl_4, chloroform, DCE
  II. Thiol oxidants: cystamine (mixed disulfide formation), diamide, *t*-BHP, $O_2^{\overline{•}}$, and HOOH generators (eg, menadione, diquat)
  III. Others: vanadate, Cd^{2+}, thapsigargin (specific SERCA inhibitor)
  IV. Chemicals impairing mitochondrial ATP synthesis (see Table 3-6)

KEY: DCE, 1,1-dichloroethylene; t-BHP, t-butyl hydroperoxide; HCH, hexachlorocyclohexane; MPP$^+$, 1-methyl-4-phenylpyridinium; NAPBQI, N-acetyl-p-benzoquinoneimine; SERCA, sarco/endoplasmic reticulum calcium ATPase.

or damage to the plasma membrane causes Ca^{2+} to move down its concentration gradient from extracellular fluid to the cytoplasm. Toxicants also may increase cytosolic Ca^{2+} by inducing its leakage from the mitochondria or the EPR. They also may diminish Ca^{2+} efflux through inhibition of Ca^{2+} transporters or depletion of their driving forces. Several chemicals that can cause a sustained rise in cytoplasmic Ca^{2+} levels are listed in Table 3-7.

Sustained elevation of intracellular Ca^{2+} is harmful because it can result in (1) depletion of energy reserves, (2) dysfunction of microfilaments, (3) activation of hydrolytic enzymes, and (4) generation of ROS and RNS. There are at least 3 mechanisms by which sustained elevations in intracellular Ca^{2+} unfavorably influence the cellular energy balance. First, high cytoplasmic Ca^{2+} concentrations cause increased mitochondrial Ca^{2+} uptake by the Ca^{2+} "uniporter," which, like ATP synthase, utilizes the inside negative mitochondrial membrane potential ($\Delta\Psi m$) as the driving force. Consequently, mitochondrial Ca^{2+} uptake dissipates $\Delta\Psi m$ and inhibits the synthesis of ATP. Moreover, chemicals that oxidize mitochondrial NADH activate a transporter that extrudes Ca^{2+} from the matrix space (Richter and Kass, 1991). The ensuing continuous Ca^{2+} uptake and export ("Ca^{2+} cycling") by the mitochondria further compromise oxidative phosphorylation. Second, Ca^{2+} may also impair ATP synthesis by causing oxidative injury to the inner membrane by mechanisms described later. Third, a sustained rise in cytoplasmic Ca^{2+} not only impairs ATP synthesis but also increases ATP consumption by the Ca^{2+}-ATPases working to eliminate the excess Ca^{2+}.

A second mechanism by which an uncontrolled rise in cytoplasmic Ca^{2+} causes cell injury is microfilamental dissociation (Nicotera *et al.*, 1992; Leist and Nicotera, 1997). The cell-wide network of actin filaments maintains cellular morphology by attachment of the filaments to actin-binding proteins in the plasma membrane. An increase of cytoplasmic Ca^{2+} causes dissociation of actin filaments from α-actinin and fodrin, proteins involved in anchoring the filaments to the plasma membrane. This represents a mechanism leading to plasma membrane blebbing, a condition that predisposes the membrane to rupture.

A third event whereby high Ca^{2+} concentrations are deleterious to cells is activation of hydrolytic enzymes that degrade proteins, phospholipids, and nucleic acids (Nicotera *et al.*, 1992; Leist and Nicotera, 1997). Many integral membrane proteins are targets for Ca^{2+}-activated neutral proteases, or calpains (Liu *et al.*, 2004). Calpain-mediated hydrolysis of actin-binding proteins may also cause membrane blebbing. Indiscriminate activation of phospholipases by Ca^{2+} causes membrane breakdown directly and by the generation of detergents. Activation of a Ca^{2+}-Mg^{2+}-dependent endonuclease causes fragmentation of chromatin. Elevated levels of Ca^{2+} can lock topoisomerase II in a form that cleaves but does not religate DNA. In summary, intracellular hypercalcemia activates several processes that interfere with the ability of cells to maintain their structural and functional integrity. The relative importance of these processes in vivo requires further definition.

Overproduction of ROS and RNS There are a number of xenobiotics that can directly generate ROS and RNS, such as the redox cyclers (Fig. 3-3) and the transition metals (Fig. 3-4). In addition, overproduction of ROS and RNS can be secondary to the intracellular hypercalcemia, as Ca^{2+} activates enzymes that generate ROS and/or RNS in the following ways:

1. Activation of the dehydrogenases in the citric acid cycle by Ca^{2+} accelerates the hydrogen output from the citrate cycle and, in turn, the flux of electrons along the electron transport chain (see Fig. 3-16). This, together with the suppressed

ATP-synthase activity (owing to the Ca^{2+}-induced uncoupling), increases the formation of $O_2^{\bullet-}$ by the mitochondrial electron transport chain.

2. Ca^{2+}-activated proteases proteolytically convert xanthine dehydrogenase into xanthine oxidase, whose by-products are $O_2^{\bullet-}$ and HOOH (Harrison, 2002).

3. Neurons and endothelial cells constitutively express NOS that is activated by Ca^{2+}. Given the extremely high reactivity of $\bullet$NO with $O_2^{\bullet-}$, coproduction of these radicals will inevitably lead to formation of $ONOO^-$, a highly reactive oxidant (Murphy, 1999) (Fig. 3-4). Moreover, $ONOO^-$ can increase its own formation by incapacitating the highly sensitive Mn-SOD, which would eliminate $O_2^{\bullet-}$, a precursor of $ONOO^-$.

Interplay between the Primary Metabolic Disorders Spells Cellular Disaster The primary derailments in cellular biochemistry discussed above do not remain isolated but interact and amplify each other in a number of ways (Fig. 3-18):

1. Depletion of cellular ATP reserves deprives the endoplasmic and plasma membrane Ca^{2+} pumps of fuel, causing elevation of Ca^{2+} in the cytoplasm. With the influx of Ca^{2+} into the mitochondria, $\Delta\Psi m$ declines, hindering ATP synthase.

2. As stated above, intracellular hypercalcemia facilitates formation of ROS and RNS, which oxidatively inactivate the thiol-dependent Ca^{2+} pump, which, in turn, aggravates the hypercalcemia.

3. The ROS and RNS can also drain the ATP reserves. $\bullet$NO is a reversible inhibitor of cytochrome oxidase; NO^+ (nitrosonium cation, a product of $\bullet$NO) S-nitrosylates and thus inactivates glyceraldehyde 3-phosphate dehydrogenase, impairing glycolysis, whereas $ONOO^-$ irreversibly inactivates respiratory chain complexes I, II, III, and aconitase (by reacting with their Fe-S center) (Murphy, 1999). Therefore, $\bullet$NO and $ONOO^-$ inhibit cellular ATP synthesis.

4. Furthermore, $ONOO^-$ can induce DNA SSB, which activates poly(ADP-ribose) polymerase (PARP) (Szabó, 1996). As part of the repair strategy, activated PARP transfers multiple ADP-ribose moieties from NAD^+ to nuclear proteins and PARP itself (D'Amours *et al.*, 1999). Consumption of NAD^+ severely compromises ATP synthesis (see Fig. 3-16), whereas

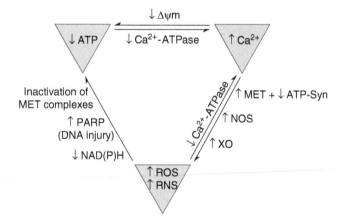

Figure 3-18. *Interrelationship between the primary metabolic disorders (ATP depletion, intracellular hypercalcemia, and overproduction of ROS/RNS) that ultimately cause necrosis or apoptosis. See text for details. ATP-Syn, ATP synthase; MET, mitochondrial electron transport; NOS, nitric oxide synthase; PARP, poly(ADP-ribose) polymerase; ROS, reactive oxygen species; RNS, reactive nitrogen species; XO, xanthine oxidase; $\Delta\Psi m$, mitochondrial membrane potential.*

resynthesis of NAD+ consumes ATP. Hence, a major consequence of DNA damage by ONOO− is a cellular energy deficit (Murphy, 1999).

The chain of events and their contribution to the worsening metabolic conditions are somewhat cell- and toxicant-specific. For example, cyanide toxicity in neurons is associated with depolarization and glutamate release (Patel *et al.*, 1993), followed by Ca^{2+} influx through voltage-gated as well as glutamate-gated channels (see items 8 and 2, respectively, in Fig. 3-15). As they express Ca^{2+}-activated NOS, neurons are also prone to generate "nitrosative stress," which affects not only themselves but also perhaps more significantly the neighboring astrocytes (Szabó, 1996). In contrast, in cyanide- and iodoacetate-poisoned liver cells, the increase in cytoplasmic Ca^{2+} is not an early event (Herman *et al.*, 1990). A nitrosative stress critically contributes to propagation of acetaminophen-induced hepatocellular injury, in which the initiating event is covalent binding of *N*-acetyl-*p*-benzoquinoneimine (NAPBQI) to mitochondrial proteins (Jaeschke and Bajt, 2006). This purportedly causes a surge in mitochondrial ($O_2^{\bullet}$) generation, followed by in situ formation of ONOO−. Owing to depletion of the protective glutathione by NAPBQI, ONOO− readily nitrates mitochondrial proteins. Concomitantly, covalent binding incapacitates the plasma membrane Ca^{2+} pump and the resultant hypercalcemia further deteriorates mitochondrial function and ATP production. It appears that in this and many other cytotoxicities the interplay of ATP depletion, intracellular hypercalcemia, and overproduction of ROS and RNS, involving multiple vicious cycles (Fig. 3-18), can progressively aggravate the biochemical disorder until it becomes a disaster.

Mitochondrial Permeability Transition and the Worst Outcome: Necrosis Mitochondrial Ca^{2+} uptake, decreased $\Delta\Psi m$, generation of ROS and RNS, depletion of ATP, and consequences of the primary metabolic disorders (eg, accumulation of inorganic phosphate, free fatty acids, and lysophosphatides) are all considered as causative factors of an abrupt increase in the mitochondrial inner-membrane permeability, termed MPT. This is thought to be caused by misfolded proteins from the inner and outer membranes, which aggregate and open a proteinaceous pore ("megachannel") that spans both mitochondrial membranes (Kroemer *et al.*, 1998; Kim *et al.*, 2003; Rodriguez-Enriquez *et al.*, 2004). As this pore is permeable to solutes of size <1500 Da, its opening permits free influx of protons into the matrix space, causing rapid and complete dissipation of $\Delta\Psi m$ and cessation of ATP synthesis as well as osmotic influx of water, resulting in mitochondrial swelling. Ca^{2+} that accumulates in the matrix space effluxes through the pore, flooding the cytoplasm. Such mitochondria not only are incapable of synthesizing ATP but also even waste the remaining resources because depolarization of the inner membrane forces the ATP synthase to operate in the reverse mode, as an ATPase, hydrolyzing ATP. Then even glycolysis may become compromised by the insufficient ATP supply to the ATP-requiring glycolytic enzymes (hexokinase, phosphofructokinase). A complete bioenergetic catastrophe ensues in the cell if the metabolic disorders evoked by the toxic chemical (such as ones listed in Tables 3-6 and 3-7) are so extensive that most or all mitochondria in the cell undergo MPT, causing depletion of cellular ATP (see Fig. 3-20). Degradative processes already outlined (eg, oxidative and hydrolytic degradation of macromolecules and membranes as well as disintegration of intracellular solute and volume homeostasis) will go to completion, causing a complete failure in maintenance of cellular structure and functions and culminating in cell lysis or necrosis.

An Alternative Outcome of MPT: Apoptosis Chemicals that adversely affect cellular energy metabolism, Ca^{2+} homeostasis, and redox state and then ultimately cause necrosis may also induce apoptosis, another form of cell demise. Whereas the necrotic cell swells and lyses, the apoptotic cell shrinks; its nuclear and cytoplasmic materials condense, and then it breaks into membrane-bound fragments (apoptotic bodies) that are phagocytosed (Wyllie, 1997).

As discussed above, the multiple metabolic defects that a cell suffers in its way to necrosis are causal yet rather random in sequence. In contrast, the routes to apoptosis are ordered, involving cascade-like activation of catabolic processes that finally disassemble the cell. A scheme of the apoptotic pathways is presented in Fig. 3-19. Pathways initiated by EPR stress will be dealt with in the section "Mechanisms of Adaptation."

It appears that most if not all chemical-induced cell deaths will involve the mitochondria, and the resulting mitochondrial dysfunction (such as Ca^{2+} accumulation, dissipation of $\Delta\Psi m$, and overproduction of ROS/RNS) may ultimately trigger either necrosis or apoptosis, and that MPT can be a crucial event in both. A related event is release into the cytoplasm of cytochrome *c* (cyt *c*), a small positively charged heme protein that normally resides in the mitochondrial intermembrane space attached electrostatically to cardiolipin, a specific inner membrane phospholipid with excess negative charge. Peroxidation of cardiolipin by HOOH, a process catalyzed by cyt *c*, results in detachment of cyt *c* from the lipid, which may be a critical first step of cyt *c* release into the cytoplasm (Orrenius *et al.*, 2011).

The significance of cyt *c* release is two-fold (Cai *et al.*, 1998): (1) as cyt *c* is the penultimate link in the mitochondrial electron transport chain, its loss will block ATP synthesis, increase formation of $O_2^{\bullet}$ (instead of O_2^{4-} as shown in Fig. 3-16), and potentially thrust the cell toward necrosis. (2) Simultaneously, the unleashed cyt *c* (and some other proteins set free from the mitochondria) represents a signal or an initial link in the chain of events directing the cell to the apoptotic path (Cain, 2003) (Fig. 3-19). Cyt *c* together with dATP/ATP induces the cytoplasmic adapter protein apoptotic protease activating factor (Apaf-1) to oligomerize and bind the latent procaspase-9 (forming a complex called apoptosome), facilitating its conversion to active caspase-9.

Caspases are cysteine proteases (ie, they possess a catalytically active cysteine) that cleave proteins after specific aspartate residues. They reside mostly in the cytoplasm in inactive forms, as procaspases, which are activated by either dimerization (initiators) or proteolytic cleavage (effectors) (Boatright and Salvesen, 2003). Perhaps in order to guarantee that inadvertent activation of caspases should not occur, IAPs, such as XIAP and cIAP, reside in the cytoplasm and physically capture caspases that might have become activated (Cain, 2003). Therefore, cyt *c* alone probably could not induce sufficiently strong caspase activation if it were not for proteins that physically remove the IAPs from the caspases just being activated. These proteins, named Smac and Omi (or Diablo and HtrA2, respectively), are not only the helpers of cyt *c* but also residents of the mitochondrial intermembrane space, from where they are jointly mobilized to promote the caspase cascade. Some caspases on the "top" of the cascade (eg, 8 and 9) cleave and activate procaspases. Thereby these initiator caspases carry the activation wave to the so-called effector caspases (eg, 3, 6, and 7), which cleave specific cellular proteins, activating or inactivating them. It is the hydrolysis of these specific proteins that accounts directly or indirectly for the morphological and biochemical alterations in apoptotic cells. For example, proteolytic inactivation of PARP prevents futile DNA repair and wasting of ATP; caspase-mediated cleavage of Beclin 1 aborts autophagy, hydrolysis of the inhibitor of

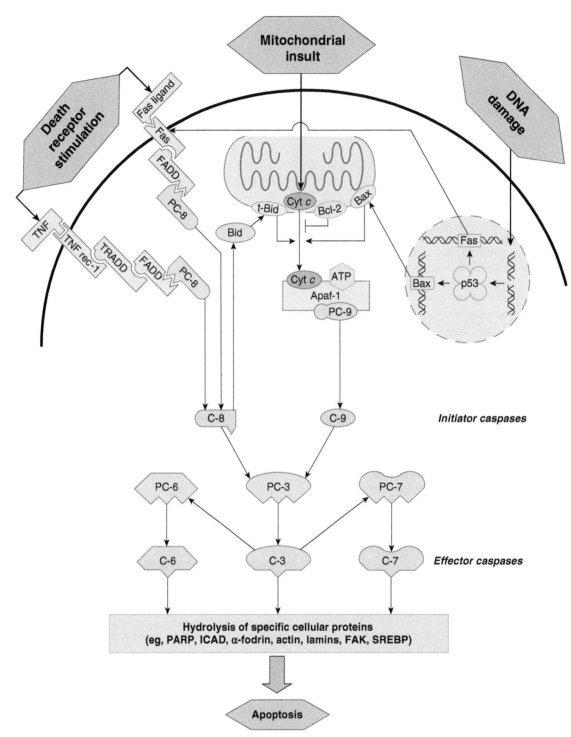

Figure 3-19. *Apoptotic pathways initiated by mitochondrial insult, nuclear DNA insult, and death receptor stimulation.* The figure is a simplified scheme of 3 pathways to apoptosis. (1) Mitochondrial insult (see text) ultimately opens the permeability transition pore spanning both mitochondrial membranes and/or causes release of cytochrome *c* (Cyt *c*) and other proapoptotic and antiapoptotic proteins (not shown) from the mitochondria. Cyt *c* release is facilitated by Bax or truncated Bid (tBid) proteins and opposed by Bcl-2 protein. (2) DNA insult, especially double-strand breaks, activates p53 protein that increases the expression of Bax (which mediates Cyt *c* release) and the membrane receptor protein Fas. (3) Fas ligand, tumor necrosis factor (TNF), or TNF-related apoptosis-inducing ligand (TRAIL, not shown) binds to and activates their respective receptor, Fas, TNF receptor-1 (TNFR1), and TRAIL receptors (not shown). The ligand-bound death receptors and the released Cyt *c* interact with specific adapter proteins (ie, FADD, TRADD, and Apaf-1) through which specific initiator procaspases (PC, eg, PC-8 and PC-9) become active caspases (C). The latter in turn cleave and activate other proteins, for example, Bid and the main effector procaspase PC-3. The active effector caspase-3 activates other effector procaspases (PC-6, PC-7). Finally, C-3, C-6, and C-7 cleave specific cellular proteins, leading to morphological and biochemical features of apoptosis. These pathways are not equally relevant in all types of cells and other apoptotic pathways, such as those triggered by TGF-β as an extracellular signaling molecule (which upregulates the proapoptotic Bim protein) and ceramide as an intracellular signaling molecule, also exist. Note that through TNFR1 TNF may signal not only for apoptosis (via TNFR1–TRADD–FADD association, as shown above) but also for cell survival (via TNFR1–TRADD–TRAF2 association). The survival pathways thus triggered are the NF-κB and the MAPK (specifically Jun kinase) pathways (see Fig. 3-12). FAK, focal adhesion kinase; ICAD, inhibitor of caspase-activated DNase; PARP, poly(ADP-ribose) polymerase; SREBP, sterol regulatory element–binding protein.

caspase-activated DNase (ICAD) permits caspase-activated DNase (CAD) to translocate to the nucleus and cleave internucleosomal DNA; cleavage of structural proteins (α-fodrin, actin, lamins) aids in disassembly of the cell; incapacitation of focal adhesion kinase (see Fig. 3-12) permits detachment of the cell from the extracellular matrix (ECM); and hydrolytic activation of sterol regulatory element–binding proteins may contribute to accumulation of sterols and externalization of phosphatidylserine in the plasma membrane that identify the apoptotic cell to phagocytes (and the latter also enables experimental detection of apoptotic cells with fluorescently labeled annexin-V that binds to phosphatidylserine residues on the cell surface). Besides caspases, DNA fragmentation can be induced by apoptosis-inducing factor (AIF) and endonuclease G that are also released from the mitochondrial intermembrane space and may contribute to DNA fragmentation during apoptosis and acetaminophen-induced caspase-independent hepatocellular necrosis (Jaeschke and Bajt, 2006). Prerequisite for the release of AIF is its hydrolysis by the Ca^{2+}-activated protease calpain localized to the intermembrane space. Oxidative modification of AIF by mitochondrial ROS increases its affinity to calpain (Orrenius et al., 2011).

The decisive mitochondrial event of cell death, that is, release of cyt c and other proapoptotic proteins (eg, Smac, Omi, AIF), is controlled by the Bcl-2 family of proteins, which includes members that facilitate (eg, Bax, Bak, Bad, Bid, Bim, BNIP3, Puma, Noxa) and those that inhibit (eg, Bcl-2, Bcl-XL) these processes. The death-promoting members can oligomerize and form pores in the mitochondrial outer membrane (MOM). By doing so, they may facilitate release of cyt c and other intermembrane proapoptotic proteins via MPT induced by toxic insult of the mitochondria; however, mitochondrial outer membrane permeabilization (MOMP) alone by Bax and its congeners is sufficient to evoke egress of cyt c from the mitochondria. MOMP induced by Bax, Bak, and/or Bid is responsible for cyt c release in apoptosis initiated at extramitochondrial targets, including death receptors and the nuclear DNA (see below). The death suppressor Bcl-2 and Bcl-XL can dimerize with the death-inducing counterparts and neutralize them. Thus, the relative amount of these antagonistic proteins functions as a regulatory switch between cell survival and death (Reed et al., 1998).

The proapoptotic Bax and Bid proteins, which can induce MOMP, represent links whereby death programs initiated extramitochondrially, for example, by DNA damage in the nucleus or by stimulation of the so-called death receptors (Fas receptor and TNF receptor-1 [TNR1]) at the cell surface, can engage the mitochondria into the apoptotic process (Green, 1998) (Fig. 3-19). DNA damage evoked by ionizing and UV radiations, alkylating chemicals, and topoisomerase II inhibitors, such as doxorubicin (Adriamycin), induces stabilization and activation of p53 protein that can promote apoptosis at dual cellular locations and by dual mechanisms. In the nucleus, p53 acts as a TF, which increases expression of proapoptotic members of the Bcl-family of proteins, such as Bax, Puma, and Noxa (Liu and Chen, 2006) (see also Fig. 3-33). Cytoplasmic p53 participates in protein–protein interactions. In such a manner, p53 abrogates the function of antiapoptotic proteins (eg, Bcl-X_L) and activates the MOMP-forming function of proapoptotic Bax and Bak (Green and Kroemer, 2009). As discussed further on, DNA damage is potentially mutagenic and carcinogenic; therefore, apoptosis of cells with damaged DNA is an important self-defense of the body against oncogenesis. Furthermore, the antitumor drugs targeting the nuclear DNA exert their desirable toxic effects against tumor cells (and also their undesirable cytotoxic effects against rapidly dividing normal cells such as hematopoietic cells and small intestinal mucosal cells) by inducing apoptosis primarily via a p53-dependent mechanism.

Stimulation of the Fas receptor (also known as CD95 or Apo-1), TNR1, or TNF-related apoptosis-inducing ligand (TRAIL) receptors (DR4 and DR5, not shown) by their ligands induces receptor oligomerization and recruitment of adapter proteins. The thus formed death-inducing protein complex (DISC) activates caspase-8, an initiator caspase that sets the caspase cascade in motion (Fig. 3-19). In addition, death receptor activation can also engage the mitochondria into the apoptosis program via caspase-8-mediated cleavage of Bid to its active form. The Fas system is involved in cell-mediated cytotoxicity, as cytotoxic T lymphocytes express the Fas ligand that activates the Fas receptor in the membrane of potential target cells, such as those of the liver, heart, and lung. Cholestatic liver injury involves apoptosis induced by the retained hydrophobic bile acids mediated partly through their mitochondrial effect (ie, MPT) and through the death receptors (Higuchi and Gores, 2003). By activating PKC, toxic bile acids promote trafficking of Fas receptor and TRAIL receptor-2 (also known as DR5) from the Golgi complex into the plasma membrane of liver cells, where the increased receptor density induces spontaneous (ie, ligand-independent) receptor oligomerization and caspase activation. Increased expression of soluble FasL and Fas receptor is thought to play a causative role in the apoptosis of pulmonary alveolar epithelial cells underlying acute lung injury (or acute respiratory distress syndrome) (Martin et al., 2005), a potentially lethal outcome of various pathologies and heroin intoxication. The Fas system also mediates germ cell apoptosis in the testes of rodents exposed to mono-(2-ethylhexyl)phthalate or 2,5-hexanedione, the ultimate toxicant formed from hexane. These chemicals damage the microtubules in the Sertoli cells that normally nurse the germ cells. Unable to support the germ cells, Sertoli cells overexpress the Fas ligand to limit the number of germ cells (which upregulate their Fas receptor) by deleting them via apoptosis (Cohen et al., 1997; Lee et al., 1997).

Thus, apoptosis can be executed via multiple pathways, most involving caspase activation. The route preferred will depend, among others, on the initial insult (Fig. 3-19) as well as on the type and state of the cell. For example, T lymphocytes lacking the Bax gene can still undergo p53-dependent death in response to ionizing radiation, probably by increasing Fas expression (Fig. 3-19), whereas Bax-null fibroblasts cannot. AIF appears to play a critical role in neuronal cell death (Orrenius et al., 2011), whereas TRAIL is an important death inducer in various tumor cells. In contrast, keratinocytes and endothelial cells are resistant to death ligand-mediated apoptosis, as they strongly express cFLIP, an inhibitor of caspase-8.

What Determines the Form of Cell Death? For reasons discussed later, it is not inconsequential for the surrounding tissue whether a cell dies by apoptosis or necrosis. Therefore, considerable research has focused on what determines the form of cell death. Interestingly, there are some common features in the process of apoptosis and necrosis. Both forms of cell death caused by cytotoxic agents may involve similar metabolic disturbances and MPT (Kim et al., 2003; Kroemer et al., 1998; Qian et al., 1999), and blockers of the latter (eg, cyclosporin A, Bcl-2 overexpression) prevent both apoptosis and necrosis in different settings. Furthermore, many xenobiotics—such as the hepatotoxicant 1,1-dichloroethylene, thioacetamide, and cadmium as well as the nephrotoxicant ochratoxin—can cause both apoptosis and necrosis (Corcoran et al., 1994). However, toxicants tend to induce apoptosis at low exposure levels or early after exposure at high levels, whereas they cause necrosis later at high exposure levels. This indicates that the severity of the insult determines the mode of cell death. Based on experimental evidence, it appears that a larger toxic insult causes necrotic cell death rather than apoptosis because it incapacitates the cell to undergo apoptosis. This incapacitation may result from three causatively related cellular events, that is, increasing number of mitochondria undergoing MPT, depletion of ATP, and failed activation of caspases or their inactivation.

Lemasters and coworkers (Kim *et al.*, 2003; Rodriguez-Enriquez *et al.*, 2004) used confocal microscopy to visualize mitochondria in cells exposed to an apoptogenic stimulus and found that MPT does not occur uniformly in all mitochondria. They proposed a model in which the number of mitochondria undergoing MPT (which probably depends on the degree of chemical exposure) determines the fate of the cell. According to this model, when only a few mitochondria develop MPT, they are removed by selective autophagy (mitophagy; see the section "Cellular Repair") and the cell survives. When more mitochondria suffer MPT, the autophagic mechanism becomes overwhelmed, and the released proapoptotic factors (eg, cyt *c*, Smac, and Omi) initiate caspase activation (Fig. 3-19). By hydrolyzing Beclin 1, a component of the autophagic mechanism, caspase-8 aborts mitophagy (Li *et al.*, 2011), and by hydrolyzing other cellular proteins (see above) and DNA, caspases and AIF, respectively, promote apoptosis. When eventually MPT involves virtually all mitochondria, cytolysis occurs. Fig. 3-20 illustrates an expanded version of this model.

For reasons discussed above, ATP is bound to become severely depleted in cells in which most mitochondria suffer MPT. The degree of ATP depletion may decide the fate of the cell. In experimental models as distinct as Ca^{2+}-exposed hepatocytes, Fas-stimulated T lymphocytes, and HOOH-exposed endothelial cells,

necrosis occurs instead of apoptosis when cells are depleted of ATP, whereas apoptosis takes place rather than necrosis when ATP depletion is alleviated by providing substrates for ATP generation (Leist *et al.*, 1997; Kim *et al.*, 2003; Lelli *et al.*, 1998). Lack of ATP can prevent execution of the apoptotic program, because apoptosis involves ATP-requiring steps, such as activation of procaspase-9 in the apoptosome complex (Fig. 3-19).

Failure of caspase activation can also result from direct action of reactive toxicants on these enzymes. The active site of caspases is composed of a pentapeptide (QACXG) with a reactive cysteine in it. At high concentrations, soft electrophiles, disulfides (eg, glutathione disulfide), and oxidants (eg, ROS), can react with this cysteine, causing caspase inactivation and ablation of the apoptotic program, with necrosis rather than apoptosis as the final outcome. Such a scenario has been demonstrated for cell death evoked by tributyltin, pyrrolidine dithiocarbamate, and arsenic trioxide (Orrenius, 2004) and might also underlie the acetaminophen-induced hepatocellular necrosis, which involves cyt *c* release with no caspase activation or apoptosis (Jaeschke and Bajt, 2006).

Induction of Cell Death by Unknown Mechanisms In addition to chemicals that ultimately injure mitochondria by disrupting oxidative phosphorylation and/or intracellular Ca^{2+} homeostasis, there are toxicants that cause cell death by affecting other functions or structures primarily. Included here are (1) chemicals that directly damage the plasma membrane, such as lipid solvents, detergents, and venom-derived hydrolytic enzymes; (2) xenobiotics that damage the lysosomal membrane, evoking release of lysosomal hydrolases and Fe^{2+}, such as aminoglycoside antibiotics and hydrocarbons binding to α_{2u}-globulin that injure renal tubular cells; (3) toxins that destroy the cytoskeleton, such as the microfilament toxins (eg, phalloidin and cytochalasins) and the microtubule toxins (eg, colchicine and 2,5-hexanedione); (4) the protein phosphatase inhibitor and hepatotoxicant microcystin, which causes hyperphosphorylation of microfilaments and other cellular proteins (Toivola and Eriksson, 1999); (5) toxins that disrupt protein synthesis, such as α-amanitin and ricin; and (6) cholesterol-lowering drugs (statins) that inhibit HMG-coenzyme A reductase, the rate-limiting enzyme in the mevalonate pathway, and rarely cause myotoxicity.

The events leading to cell death after exposure to these chemicals are generally unknown. It is likely that cell death caused by these chemicals is ultimately mediated by impairment of oxidative phosphorylation, sustained elevation of intracellular Ca^{2+}, and/or overproduction of ROS/RNS, and that it takes the form of necrosis if these processes are abrupt, but apoptosis if they are protracted. For example, direct injury of the plasma membrane would lead rapidly to increased intracellular Ca^{2+} levels. Neurofilamental toxins that block axonal transport cause energy depletion in the distal axonal segment. HMG-coenzyme A reductase inhibitors not only diminish the synthesis of cholesterol but may also compromise formation of other products of the mevalonate pathway. Such are the mitochondrial electron-transporting molecule ubiquinone (also called coenzyme Q) and isopentenyl pyrophosphate, which is utilized for isopentenylation of selenocysteinyl-tRNA, an obligatory step for synthesis of selenoproteins, including the antioxidant glutathione peroxidase (see Fig. 3-5) and thioredoxin reductase (see Fig. 3-22). These alterations may contribute to statin-induced myopathy and rhabdomyolysis.

Impairment of External Cellular Maintenance Toxicants may also interfere with cells that are specialized to provide support to other cells, tissues, or the whole organism. Chemicals acting on the liver illustrate this type of toxicity. Hepatocytes produce and

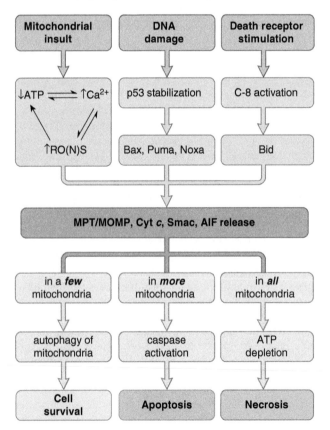

Figure 3-20. *"Decision plan" on the fate of injured cell.* See the text for details. MOMP, mitochondrial outer membrane permeabilization; MPT, mitochondrial permeability transition; Puma, p53-upregulated modulator of apoptosis; RO(N)S, reactive oxygen or nitrogen species.

release into the circulation a number of proteins and nutrients. They remove cholesterol and bilirubin from the circulation, converting them into bile acids and bilirubin glucuronides, respectively, for subsequent excretion into bile. Interruption of these processes may be harmful to the organism, the liver, or both. For example, inhibition of hepatic synthesis of coagulation factors by coumarins does not harm the liver, but may cause death by hemorrhage (Hardman *et al.*, 1995). This is the mechanism of the rodenticidal action of warfarin. In the fasting state, inhibitors of hepatic gluconeogenesis, such as hypoglycin (the ackee fruit-derived causative agent of Jamaican vomiting sickness; methylene cyclopropyl alanine), may be lethal by limiting the supply of glucose to the brain. Similarly, Reye syndrome, which is viewed as a hepatic mitochondrial injury caused by a combination of a viral disease (which may induce hepatic NOS) and intake of salicylate (which provokes MPT) (Fromenty and Pessayre, 1997; Kim *et al.*, 2003), causes not only hepatocellular injury but also severe metabolic disturbances (hypoglycemia, hyperammonemia) that affect other organs as well. Chemical interference with the β-oxidation of fatty acids or the synthesis, assembly, and secretion of lipoproteins overloads the hepatocytes with lipids, causing hepatic dysfunction (Fromenty and Pessayre, 1997). α-Naphthylisothiocyanate (ANIT) causes separation of the intercellular tight junctions that seal bile canaliculi (Krell *et al.*, 1987), impairing biliary secretion and leading to the retention of bile acids and bilirubin; this adversely affects the liver as well as the entire organism.

STEP 4—INAPPROPRIATE REPAIR AND ADAPTATION

The fourth step in the development of toxicity is inappropriate repair and adaptation (Fig. 3-1). As noted previously, many toxicants alter macromolecules, which eventually cause damage at higher levels of the biological hierarchy in the organism. Progression of toxic lesions can be intercepted by repair mechanisms operating at molecular, cellular, and tissue levels (Fig. 3-21). Another strategy whereby the organism can resist the noxious chemical is by increasing its own readiness to cope with it and with its harmful effects. This phenomenon is called adaptation. Because the capacity of the organism to repair itself and adapt to the toxic exposure and effects is so important in determining the outcome of chemical exposure, the mechanisms of repair and adaptation will be discussed below.

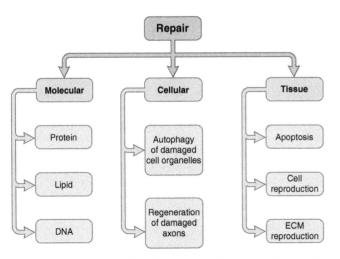

Figure 3-21. *Repair mechanisms.* Dysfunction of these mechanisms results in dysrepair, the fourth step in the development of numerous toxic injuries. ECM, extracellular matrix.

Mechanisms of Repair

Molecular Repair Damaged molecules may be repaired in different ways. Some chemical alterations, such as oxidation of protein thiols and methylation of DNA, are simply reversed. Hydrolytic removal of the molecule's damaged unit or units and insertion of a newly synthesized unit or units often occur with chemically altered DNA and peroxidized lipids. In some instances, the damaged molecule is totally degraded and resynthesized. This process is time-consuming but unavoidable in cases such as the regeneration of cholinesterase after organophosphate intoxication.

Repair of Proteins Thiol groups are essential for the function of numerous proteins, such as receptors, enzymes, cytoskeletal proteins, and TFs. Oxidation of protein thiols (Prot-SHs) to protein disulfides (Prot-SS, $Prot_1$-SS-$Prot_2$), protein–glutathione mixed disulfides (Prot-SSG), and protein sulfenic acids (Prot-SOH) can be reversed by reduction (Watson *et al.*, 2004; Gravina and Mieyal, 1993) (Fig. 3-22). The endogenous reductants are thioredoxins and glutaredoxins, small, ubiquitous proteins with two redox-active cysteines in their active centers (Holmgren *et al.*, 2005). These proteins as well as thioredoxin reductase have two isoenzymes; those labeled 1 are located in the cytosol, whereas those labeled 2 are mitochondrial. Because the catalytic thiol groups in these proteins become oxidized, they are reduced by NADPH, which is generated by $NADP^+$-dependent isocitrate dehydrogenase localized in various cell compartments (cytosol, mitochondria, peroxisomes), as well as by the cytosolic glucose-6-phosphate dehydrogenase and 6-phosphogluconate dehydrogenase in the pentose phosphate pathway. ROS may oxidize methionines in proteins into sulfoxides (protein-Met-S=O), forming both the S and R epimers, which can be reduced by methionine sulfoxide reductase (Msr) A and B enzymes, respectively (Moskovitz, 2005). Msr enzymes can reverse this modification at the expense of oxidation of their catalytic cysteine to sulfenic acid (Msr-Cys-S-OH). This then reacts with a neighboring thiol (in MsrA), forming an intramolecular disulfide, or with glutathione (in some other Msr proteins), forming a protein–glutathione disulfide. Finally the disulfide enzyme is reduced by thioredoxin or glutaredoxin, respectively, with subsequent steps depicted in Fig. 3-22. Reduction of methionine sulfoxides in lens proteins (eg, α-crystallin) is especially critical for maintenance of the transparency of the eye lens. MsrA knockout mice develop cataract on repeated exposure to hyperbaric oxygen (Kantorow *et al.*, 2010). Repair of oxidized hemoglobin (methemoglobin) occurs by means of electron transfer from cytochrome b_5, which is then regenerated by a NADH-dependent cytochrome b_5 reductase (also called methemoglobin reductase).

Soluble intracellular proteins such as cytosolic enzymes are typically folded into a globular form with their hydrophobic amino acid residues hidden inside, whereas the hydrophilic residues are located externally together with a hydrophobic cleft that constitutes the ligand (substrate) binding site. Physical or chemical insults may evoke an unduly large opening of this cleft that may lead to unfolding of the protein (denaturation) and its aggregation. Molecular chaperones such as the heat-shock proteins (Hsp, eg, Hsp90, Hsp70, and Hsp40) can prevent protein unfolding by "clamping down" onto the exposed hydrophobic region of their client protein, using the energy of ATP hydrolysis to execute their conformational change that entails this maneuver. According to a recent model (Pratt *et al.*, 2010), Hsp90 plays the leading role in stabilizing the cleft and impeding further unfolding, which would eventually lead to degradation of the protein by the ubiquitin–proteasome system (UPS) as described below. Indeed, the benzoquinone ansamycin Hsp90

Thioredoxin pathway

Glutaredoxin pathway

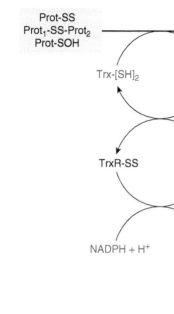

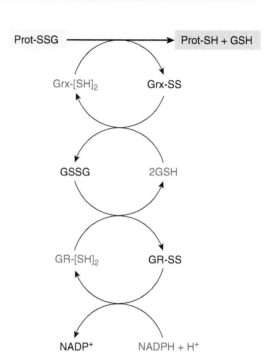

Figure 3-22. *Repair of proteins oxidized at their thiol groups.* Protein disulfides (Prot-SS, Prot$_1$-SS-Prot$_2$) and protein sulfenic acids (Prot-SOH) are reduced by thioredoxin (Trx-[SH]$_2$) or thioredoxin-like proteins. Protein–glutathione mixed disulfides (Prot-SSG) are reduced by glutaredoxin (Grx-[SH]$_2$), which is also called thioltransferase. The figure also indicates how Trx-[SH]$_2$ and Grx-[SH]$_2$ are regenerated from their disulfides (Trx-SS and Grx-SS, respectively). In the mitochondria, Trx-SS also can be reduced by the dithiol dihydrolipoic acid, a component of the pyruvate- and α-ketoglutarate dehydrogenase complexes. GSH, glutathione; GSSG, glutathione disulfide; GR-[SH]$_2$ and GR-SS, glutathione reductase (dithiol and disulfide forms, respectively); TrxR-[SH]$_2$ and Trx-SS, thioredoxin reductase (dithiol and disulfide forms, respectively).

inhibitors (eg, geldanamycin and herbimycin) promote degradation of Hsp90 client proteins by the UPS.

When unfolding progresses beyond a limit, Hsp90 dissociates. This may occur in response to chemical-induced protein damage, such as that inflicted by mechanism-based enzyme inactivators that are converted into reactive metabolites that bind covalently to the catalytic site of the enzyme. Dissociation of Hsp90 from the unfolding protein allows Hsp70 and its co-chaperone Hsp40 to recruit the Hsp70-dependent E3 ubiquitin ligases (eg, CHIP and Parkin) that in turn direct ubiquitin-charged E2 enzymes to the Hsp70-bound client protein to tag it with a polyubiquitin chain as the final step in a process presented in Fig. 3-23 (Bedford *et al.*, 2011). The protein tagged with a Lys48-linked polyubiquitin chain is then recognized and degraded in the proteasomes. The 26S proteasome is large barrel-shaped multiprotein complex that binds the ubiquitinated protein, deubiquitinates and unfolds it using ATP, and finally hydrolyzes the protein with its threonine-containing protease active sites into small peptides. The UPS controls the cellular level of numerous regulatory proteins (eg, p53, IκB, Nrf2, β-catenin, cyclins) and also has a prominent role in eliminating oxidized or otherwise damaged and unfolded intracellular proteins (Poppek and Grune, 2006). NOS exposed to its mechanism-based inactivator guanabenz that causes loss of tetrahydrobiopterin from the substrate-binding cleft will suffer this fate (Pratt *et al.*, 2010). CYP2E1, in which the heme becomes cross-linked to the protein as a consequence of reductive dechlorination of CCl$_4$ to the trichloromethyl free radical by this enzyme, is also eliminated by proteasomal degradation.

Oligomerization and aggregation of damaged and unfolded proteins preclude the proteasome from degrading them; such substrates can even trap proteasomes, rendering them nonfunctional.

After ubiquitination, protein aggregates can be eliminated by autophagy, a process described in more detail in the section "Cellular Repair." Ubiquitin on the modified proteins is recognized and bound by autophagic adaptor proteins, such as p62 or Nbr1, which interact with LC3 to deliver them to autophagosomes, newly formed vesicles that encapsulate their protein cargo. After fusing of autophagosomes with lysosomes, the damaged protein is hydrolyzed by proteases. Lysosomal proteases degrade, for example, the immunogenic trifluoroacetylated proteins that are formed in the liver during halothane anesthesia (Cohen *et al.*, 1997). Erythrocytes have ATP-independent, nonlysosomal proteolytic enzymes that rapidly and selectively degrade proteins denatured by HO• (Davies, 1987). Red blood cells containing protein aggregates (Heinz body) after exposure to methemoglobin-forming chemicals are removed via phagocytosis by macrophages in the spleen.

Repair of Lipids Phospholipids containing fatty acid hydroperoxides are preferentially hydrolyzed by phospholipase A2, with the peroxidized fatty acids replaced by normal fatty acids (van Kuijk *et al.*, 1987). Peroxidized lipids (eg, fatty acid hydroperoxides and phospholipid-associated hydroperoxides) may be reduced by the glutathione peroxidase–glutathione–glutathione reductase system (see Fig. 3-24) or by the peroxiredoxin–thioredoxin–thioredoxin reductase system (shown in part in Fig. 3-22). Again, NADPH is needed to "repair" the reductants that are oxidized in the process.

Repair of DNA Despite its high reactivity with electrophiles and free radicals, nuclear DNA is remarkably stable, in part because it is packaged in chromatin and because several repair mechanisms are available to correct alterations. The mitochondrial DNA, however,

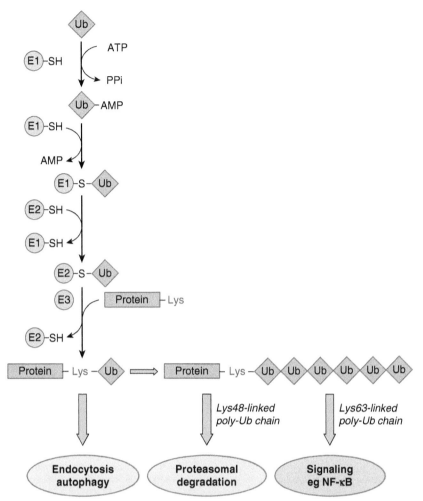

Figure 3-23. *The process of ubiquitination and its possible outcomes.* Ubiquitin (Ub) is a small (8.6 kDa) ubiquitous protein that when covalently linked to a target protein (as a monomer or as a polymer of Ub units) alters its fate and/or function. Ubiquitination is a posttranslational protein modification that takes place in an enzymatic cascade composed of 3 types of proteins—the E1 Ub-activating enzyme, the E2 Ub-conjugating enzyme, and the E3 Ub ligase. Humans possess 8 E1, over 30 E2, and hundreds of E3 enzymes. E1 first activates Ub in an ATP-consuming reaction by adenylating the terminal carboxyl group of Ub, thus forming Ub-AMP, and then it transfers Ub from Ub-AMP to its catalytic SH group, forming a high-energy thioester bond between E1 and Ub. In the subsequent transthiolation reaction, Ub is transferred from E1 to the catalytic SH group of E2. Thereafter, E3 binds both the target protein and the Ub-charged E2 and catalyzes the transfer of Ub from E2 to the target protein, forming an isopeptide bond between the terminal carboxyl group of Ub and the ε-amino group of a lysine in the substrate. Most E3 ligases, including the so-called RING finger domain-containing E3 ligases (which constitute 1 of the largest enzyme groups in the cell), ubiquitinate proteins this way. However, the HECT domain-containing E3 ligases, which possess an active site cysteine, take Ub from E2 in a transthiolation reaction, and then they (rather than E2) transfer Ub to the target protein. As Ub contains 7 lysine residues, it can also be ubiquitinated. Multiple rounds of ubiquitination generate polyubiquitin chains. In general, monoubiquitination triggers endocytosis or autophagy of the protein. Substrates that are tagged with Lys48-linked Ub chains are recognized and degraded by the 26S proteasome into small peptides, with the Ubs released for reuse. Proteins polyubiquitinated with Lys63-linked Ub chains are generally not degraded but are essential components of signaling pathways, functioning as scaffolds to assemble signaling complexes. For example, the activation of transcription factor NF-κB on signaling (see Fig. 3-12) involves assembly of a signaling complex by means of Lys63-linked Ub chains. Ubiquitination can be reversed by deubiquitinating enzymes, which are Ub-specific proteases (cysteine proteases or zinc metalloproteases). These may rescue a substrate from degradation by removing a degradative Ub signal or may change or remove a nondegradative Ub signal. Instead of Ub, proteins may also be modified by covalent attachment of Ub-like proteins, such as NEDD8, SUMO, and ISG15, using the enzymatic machinery described above.

lacks histones and efficient repair mechanisms and therefore is more prone to damage. Different types of damages are corrected by specialized mechanisms, each employing a different set of repair proteins (Christmann *et al.*, 2003).

Direct Repair Certain covalent DNA modifications are directly reversed by enzymes such as DNA photolyase, which cleaves adjacent pyrimidines dimerized by UV light. Inasmuch as this chromophore-equipped enzyme uses the energy of visible light to correct damage, its function is restricted to light-exposed cells.

Minor adducts, such as methyl groups, attached to DNA bases by alkylating agents (eg, MMS) may be removed by special enzymes (Christmann *et al.*, 2003). Such groups attached to the O^6 position of guanine are cleaved off by O^6-methyguanine-DNA-methyltransferase (MGMT). While repairing the DNA, this alkyltransferase sacrifices itself, transferring the adduct onto one of its cysteine residues. This results in its inactivation, ubiquitination, and proteasomal degradation. Thus, like glutathione, which is depleted during detoxication of electrophiles, MGMT is consumed during the repair of DNA. Methyl groups attached to N^1 of adenine and guanine, and N^3 of thymine and cytosine are removed by oxidative demethylation catalyzed by DNA dioxygenases (ABH2 and ABH3). These peculiar O_2, Fe^{2+}, ascorbate, and 2-oxoglutarate-dependent

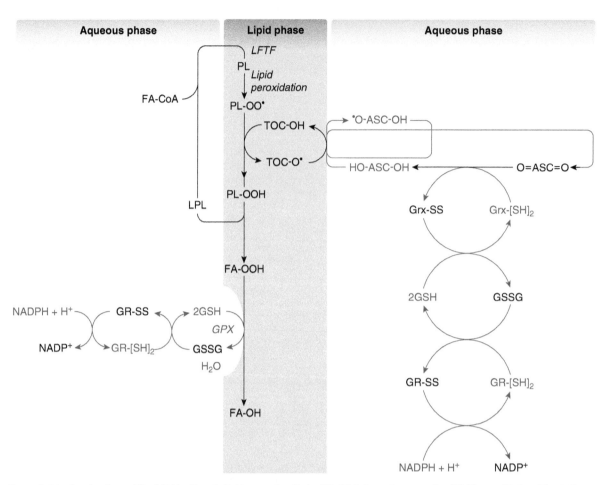

Aqueous phase   **Lipid phase**   **Aqueous phase**

Figure 3-24. *Repair of peroxidized lipids.* Phospholipid peroxyl radicals (PL-OO•) formed as a result of lipid peroxidation (Fig. 3-9) may abstract hydrogen from α-tocopherol (TOC-OH) and yield phospholipid hydroperoxide (PL-OOH). From the latter, the fatty acid carrying the hydroperoxide group is eliminated via hydrolysis catalyzed by phospholipase (PLase), yielding a fatty acid hydroperoxide (FA-OOH) and a lysophospholipid (LPL). The former is reduced to a hydroxy fatty acid (FA-OH) by glutathione peroxidase (GPX), utilizing glutathione (GSH), or peroxiredoxins (not shown), whereas the latter is reacylated to phospholipid (PL) by lysophosphatide fatty acyl-coenzyme A transferase (LFTF), utilizing long-chain fatty acid–coenzyme A (FA-CoA). The figure also indicates regeneration of TOC-OH by ascorbic acid (HO-ASC-OH), regeneration of ascorbic acid from dehydroascorbic acid (O=ASC=O) by glutaredoxin (Grx-[SH]$_2$), and reduction of the oxidized glutaredoxin (Grx-SS) by GSH. Oxidized glutathione (GSSG) is reduced by glutathione reductase (GR-[SH]$_2$), which is regenerated from its oxidized form (GR-SS) by NADPH, the ultimate reductant. NADPH is produced by NADP⁺-dependent isocitrate dehydrogenases and during metabolism of glucose via the pentose phosphate shunt. TOC-O•, tocopheroxyl radical; •O-ASC-OH, ascorbyl radical.

enzymes oxygenate the methyl group adduct, which in turn leaves as formaldehyde, whereas 2-oxoglutarate is oxidatively decarboxylated to succinate.

Excision Repair Base excision and nucleotide excision are two mechanisms for removing damaged bases from DNA (see Chaps. 8 and 9). Lesions that do not cause major distortion of the helix typically are removed by base excision, in which the altered base is recognized by a relatively substrate-specific DNA glycosylase that hydrolyzes the *N*-glycosidic bond, releasing the modified base and creating an apurinic or apyrimidinic (AP) site in the DNA. For example, 8-OH-Gua, a major mutagenic product of oxidative stress, is removed from the DNA by a specific 8-OH-Gua DNA glycosylase. The AP site is recognized by the AP endonuclease, which hydrolyzes the phosphodiester bond adjacent to the abasic site. After its removal, the abasic sugar is replaced with the correct nucleotide by a DNA polymerase and is sealed in place by a DNA ligase. Interestingly, AP endonuclease is a bifunctional protein and is also called redox factor-1 (Ref-1). In concert with thioredoxin and thioredoxin reductase, it maintains TFs with sensitive thiol groups in their DNA-binding domain (Fos, Jun, NF-κB) in an active reduced state (Hansen *et al.*, 2006).

Bulky lesions such as adducts produced by aflatoxins or aminofluorene derivatives and dimers caused by UV radiation are removed by nucleotide excision repair system, which consists of approximately 30 proteins (Christmann *et al.*, 2003). Lesions in the nontranscribed strands or the nontranscribed regions of the genome are corrected by the global genomic repair system. This involves proteins that recognize the distorted double helix at the lesion, unwind the DNA, and excise a number of intact nucleotides on both sides of the lesion together with the one containing the adduct. The excised section of the strand is restored by insertion of nucleotides into the gap by DNA polymerase and ligase, using the complementary strand as a template. Lesions in the transcribed DNA strand blocking the RNA polymerase in the actively transcribed genes are removed by another variation of nucleotide excision repair, the transcription-coupled repair system. This involves assembly of repair proteins to remove the stalled RNA polymerase before excision of the damage and filling the gap. Resynthesis of the removed section of the strand is designated "unscheduled DNA synthesis" and can be detected by the appearance of altered deoxynucleosides in urine. Excision repair has a remarkably low error rate of less than one mistake in 10⁹ bases repaired.

PARP appears to be an important contributor to excision repair. On base damage or SSB, PARP binds to the injured DNA and becomes activated. The active PARP cleaves NAD^+ to use the ADP-ribose moiety of this cofactor for attaching long chains of polymeric ADP-ribose to nuclear proteins, such as histones. Because one ADP-ribose unit contains two negative charges, the poly(ADP-ribosyl)ated proteins accrue negativity and the resultant electrorepulsive force between the negatively charged proteins and DNA causes decondensation of the chromatin structure. It is hypothesized that PARP-mediated opening of the tightly packed chromatin allows the repair enzymes to access the broken DNA and fix it. Thereafter, poly(ADP-ribose) glycohydrolase gains access to the nucleus from its perinuclear localization and reverses the PARP-mediated modification of nuclear proteins (D'Amours et al., 1999). Other features of PARP that are relevant in toxicity—such as destruction of PARP by caspases during apoptosis as well as the significance of NAD^+ (and consequently ATP) wasting by PARP in necrosis—have been discussed earlier in this chapter.

Nonhomologous End Joining This process repairs DSB that may be formed when two SSB occur in close proximity, or when DNA with SSB undergoes replication. This repair system directly ligates the broken ends without the need for a homologous template. DSBs are recognized by the Ku protein (a heterodimer of Ku70 and Ku80) that binds to the DNA end. Ku then binds and activates DNA-dependent protein kinase catalytic subunit (DNA-PKcs), leading to recruitment and activation of end-processing enzymes, DNA polymerases, and DNA ligase. Although the nonhomologous end joining is error-prone, it can operate in any phase of the cell cycle and is the mechanism for DSB repair in nondividing terminally differentiated cells (eg, neurons). By contrast, the other and more faithful mechanism for DSB repair, homologous recombination, can function only after replication (in S and G2 phases), when sister chromatid sequences are available for use as templates (see below), and thus is not an option in nondividing cells.

Recombinational (or Postreplication) Repair Homologous recombination can be used to fix postreplication gaps and DSBs (Li and Heyer, 2008). The former defect may result when excision of a bulky adduct or an intrastrand pyrimidine dimer fails to occur before DNA replication begins. At replication, such a lesion prevents DNA polymerase from polymerizing a daughter strand along a sizable stretch of the parent strand that carries the damage. Then the replication results in two homologous ("sister") yet dissimilar DNA duplexes; one has a large postreplication gap in its daughter strand and an intact duplex synthesized at the opposite leg of the replication fork. This intact sister duplex is utilized to complete the postreplication gap in the damaged sister duplex. This is accomplished by recombination ("crossover") of the appropriate strands of the two homologous duplexes. After separation, the sister duplex that originally contained the gap carries in its daughter strand a section originating from the parent strand of the intact sister, which in turn carries in its parent strand a section originating from the daughter strand of the damaged sister. This strand recombination explains the phenomenon of "sister chromatid exchange," which is indicative of DNA damage corrected by recombinational repair. After completing the postreplication gap by recombination, the damage still present in the parent strand may be removed by nucleotide excision.

In addition to eliminating postreplication gaps, homologous recombination can also repair DSB in a complex process employing numerous proteins. These include, for example, the MRN complex (the trimer of Mre11, Rad50, and Nbs1 proteins, which binds to the DSB and is involved in end processing by generation of single-stranded DNA), Rad51, Rad54, and the breast cancer susceptibility proteins BRCA1 and BRCA2 (which assist the single-stranded DNA in invading the undamaged template in an ATP-dependent process), as well as polymerases, nucleases, helicases, and other components, which mediate DNA ligation and substrate resolution. A combination of excision and recombinational repairs occurs in restoration of DNA with interstrand cross-links caused by bifunctional electrophiles, such as nitrogen mustard-type drugs and cisplatin.

Cellular Repair Autophagic removal of damaged cell organelles may be viewed as a universal mechanism of cellular repair, whereas clearance and regeneration of damaged axons is a mechanism specific for nerve cells.

Autophagy of Damaged Cell Organelles Cells suffering mild injury may repair themselves by removing and degrading damaged components, such as organelles and protein aggregates, in a process called autophagy, meaning eating of self (Rabinowitz and White, 2010). While autophagy serves the purpose of cell restitution in all cells, it is particularly important in terminally differentiated cells, such as neurons and myocytes, where cell renewal by cell replication is not possible. In addition, autophagy of normal cell constituents is an ultimate means of nutrient generation (see the section "Adaptation to Energy Depletion—The Energy Stress Response").

In autophagy, a so-called isolation membrane (or phagophore) emerges possibly from the EPR, which engulfs the cytoplasmic material and then encapsulates it in a double-membrane vesicle (called autophagosome). This vesicle moves along microtubules, driven by dynein motors, to the lysosome and on fusing with the lysosome generates an autolysosome. The cargo as well as the inner membrane of the original autophagosome is then degraded by lysosomal hydrolytic enzymes, such as proteases, lipases, nucleases, and glycosidases (which work optimally at the acidic pH in the lysosomes) to amino acids, lipids, nucleosides, and carbohydrates. These breakdown products are then released by lysosomal permeases and transporters into the cytosol, where they may be further metabolized or used for synthesis of new macromolecules.

Autophagic removal of damaged cell organelles is a method of their quality control, disposal and recycling. This is well exemplified by deletion of depolarized mitochondria through selective autophagy or mitophagy in cells exposed to mitochondrial poisons, such as the protonophoric uncoupler CCCP, valinomycin, and paraquat (see Table 3-6). Several proteins mediate this process (Mehrpour et al., 2010; Youle and Narendra, 2011), including (1) Pink1 (a protein kinase) localized in the MOM that accumulates there on dissipation of the mitochondrial membrane potential, (2) the cytosolic Parkin (an E3 ubiquitin ligase) that is recruited to the mitochondria by Pink1 and that then polyubiquitinates itself and other proteins, among them (3) the MOM protein mitofusins (Mfn1, Mfn2) and voltage-dependent anion channel (VDAC), (4) p62 (an autophagic adaptor protein) that binds to both ubiquitinated proteins and to (5) the cytosolic LC3 (microtubule-associated protein light chain 3), which, after cleavage to LC3-I, becomes conjugated with phosphatidylethanolamine by (6) a ubiquitin-like conjugation system that requires Atg7 (E1-like), Atg3 (E2-like), and the Atg12-Atg5:Atg16L complex (E3-like), (7) the phosphatidylinositol 3-kinase vesicular protein sorting 34 (Vps34), which is activated by interacting with (8) Beclin 1 (Bcl-2-interacting protein-1). The lipidated LC-3 (called LC3-II) can integrate into the membrane of autophagosome and can recruit the ubiquitin-tagged mitochondria into this structure. The latter protein (which later decomposes in the lysosome) is a marker for autophagosomes.

Removal of damaged mitochondria by autophagy is important not only for maintaining a functional mitochondrial pool but also for limiting oxidative cell damage and preventing apoptosis because injured mitochondria may be sources of ROS and apoptotic factors, such as cyt c, Smac, and AIF (see Fig. 3-20). Indeed, overexpression of Parkin suppresses cell death (Tanaka, 2010). In contrast, loss-of-function mutations in the genes encoding Pink1 and Parkin cause early onset monogenic forms of Parkinson disease probably through defective mitophagy of damaged mitochondria in the dopaminergic nigrostriatal neurons (Youle and Narendra, 2011). Autophagy also contributes to structural restitution of liver cells. For example, left-over peroxisomes after exposure to peroxisome proliferators (eg, fibrate esters) and lipid droplets in hepatic steatosis are also cleared by autophagy.

Regeneration of Damaged Axons Peripheral neurons with axonal damage can regenerate their axons with the assistance of macrophages and Schwann cells. Macrophages remove debris by phagocytosis and produce cytokines and growth factors, which activate Schwann cells to proliferate and transdifferentiate from myelinating operation mode into a growth-supporting mode. Distal to the injury, Schwann cells play an indispensable role in promoting axonal regeneration by increasing their synthesis of cell adhesion molecules (eg, N-CAM), by elaborating ECM proteins for base membrane construction, and by producing an array of neurotrophic factors (eg, brain-derived neurotrophic factor, glial cell line–derived neurotrophic factor, and nerve growth factor) and their receptors (Boyd and Gordon, 2003). While comigrating with the regrowing axon, Schwann cells physically guide as well as chemically lure the axon to reinnervate the target cell.

In the mammalian central nervous system, axonal regrowth is prevented partly by the nonpermissive external environment. At the site of injury, the oligodendrocytes produce growth inhibitory myelin-associated proteins (eg, Nogo, NI 35, myelin-associated glycoprotein, oligodendrocyte myelin glycoprotein, ephrin, and semaphorin), which act through specific receptors, whereas the astrocytes produce chondroitin sulfate proteoglycans and fibrotic scar (whose components include laminin, fibronectin, and collagen IV) (Johnson, 1993) that hinder axonal regrowth. Signaling by TGF-β through Smad2 TF (see pathway #8 in Fig. 3-12) plays a leading role in overexpression of these extrinsic growth inhibitory factors. In addition, CNS neurons lose their intrinsic growth capacity postnatally, which occurs simultaneously with increased expression of some neuronal growth inhibitory Krüppel-like TFs, such as KLF4. For these reasons, damage to central neurons is irreversible but is compensated for in part by the large number of reserve nerve cells that can take over the functions of lost neurons. For example, in Parkinson disease, symptoms are not observed until there is at least an 80% loss of nigrostriatal neurons.

Tissue Repair In tissues with cells capable of multiplying, damage is reversed by deletion of the injured cells and regeneration of the tissue by proliferation. The damaged cells are eliminated by apoptosis or necrosis.

Apoptosis: An Active Deletion of Damaged Cells Apoptosis initiated by cell injury can serve as tissue repair for two reasons: first, because it may intercept the process leading to necrosis, as discussed earlier (see Fig. 3-20). Necrosis is a more harmful sequel than apoptosis for the tissue in which the injured cell resides. A cell destined for apoptosis shrinks; its nuclear and cytoplasmic materials condense, and then it breaks into membrane-bound fragments (apoptotic bodies) that are phagocytosed (Bursch *et al.*, 1992). During necrosis, cells and intracellular organelles swell and disintegrate with membrane lysis. Whereas apoptosis is orderly, necrosis

is a disorderly process that ends with cell debris in the extracellular environment. The constituents of the necrotic cells attract aggressive inflammatory cells, and the ensuing inflammation amplifies cell injury (see further on). With apoptosis, dead cells are removed without inflammation. Second, apoptosis may intercept the process leading to neoplasia by eliminating the cells with potentially mutagenic DNA damage. This function of apoptosis is discussed in more detail in the final section of this chapter.

It must be emphasized, however, that apoptosis of damaged cells may serve tissue restoration only for tissues that are made up of constantly renewing cells (eg, the bone marrow, the respiratory and GI epithelium, and the epidermis of the skin), or of conditionally dividing cells (eg, hepatic and renal parenchymal cells), because in these tissues the apoptotic cells are readily replaced. The role of apoptosis as a tissue repair strategy is markedly lessened in organs containing nonreplicating and nonreplaceable cells, such as the neurons, cardiac muscle cells, and female germ cells, because deletion of such cells, if extensive, can cause a deficit in the organ's function. Apoptosis may also be harmful when it occurs at a critical location. For example, in the pulmonary alveolar epithelium, an extremely tight barrier, apoptosis could cause flooding of the alveolar space with interstitial fluid, a potentially lethal outcome.

Proliferation: Regeneration of Tissue Tissues are composed of various cells and the ECM. Tissue elements are anchored to each other by transmembrane proteins. Cadherins allow adjacent cells to adhere to one another, whereas connexins associate into tubular structures and connect neighboring cells internally (gap junctions). Integrins link cells to the ECM. Therefore, repair of injured tissues involves not only regeneration of lost cells and the ECM but also reintegration of the newly formed elements. In parenchymal organs such as liver, kidney, and lung, various types of cells are involved in the process of tissue restoration. Nonparenchymal cells of mesenchymal origin residing in the tissue, such as resident macrophages and endothelial cells, and those migrating to the site of injury, such as blood monocytes, produce factors that stimulate parenchymal cells to divide and stimulate some specialized cells (eg, the stellate cells in the liver) to synthesize ECM molecules.

Replacement of Lost Cells by Mitosis Soon after injury, cells adjacent to the damaged area enter the cell division cycle (Fig. 3-25). Enhanced DNA synthesis is detected experimentally as an increase in the labeling index (which is the proportion of cells that incorporate administered ^{3}H-thymidine or bromodeoxyuridine into their nuclear DNA during the S phase of the cycle), or by increased expression of proliferating cell nuclear antigen (PCNA, a trimeric protein that functions as a sliding clamp to hold DNA polymerase-δ to the template DNA strand during DNA replication). Also, mitotic cells can be observed microscopically. As early as 2 to 4 hours after administration of a low dose of carbon tetrachloride to rats, the mitotic index in the liver increases dramatically, indicating that cells already in the G_2 phase progress rapidly to the M phase. The mitotic activity of the hepatocytes culminates at 36 to 48 hours, after a full transit through the cycle, indicating that quiescent cells residing in G_0 enter and progress to mitosis (M). Peak mitosis of nonparenchymal cells occurs later, after activation and replication of parenchymal cells. In severe toxic liver injury, when hepatocyte replication is impaired (eg, in rats dosed with galactosamine or acetylaminofluorene, and in humans intoxicated with acetaminophen), restoration of the liver may depend on stem cell–derived cells, called oval cells, which are located in the terminal bile ductules. These cells proliferate and differentiate into both hepatocytes and biliary epithelial cells (Fausto *et al.*, 2006; Vessey and Hall, 2001). As oval cells produce α-fetoprotein, the increase in serum

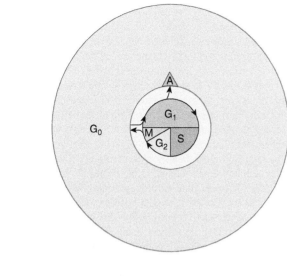

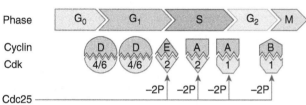

Figure 3-25. *The cell division cycle and the participating cyclins and cyclin-dependent protein kinases.* Areas representing phases of the cycle are meant to be proportional to the number of cells in each phase. Normally, most cells are in G_0 phase, a differentiated and quiescent state. After receiving signals to divide, they progress into the G_1 phase of the cell division cycle. G_0/G_1 transition involves activation of immediate early genes so that cells acquire replicative competence. Now increasingly responsive to growth factors, these cells progress to the phase of DNA synthesis (S). If this progression is blocked (eg, by the accumulated p53 protein), the cells may undergo apoptosis (A). After DNA replication, the cells prepare further for mitosis in the G_2 phase. Mitosis (M) is the shortest phase of the cell cycle (approximately 40 minutes out of the 40-hour-long cycle of hepatocytes) and most likely requires the largest energy expenditure per unit of time. The daughter cells produced may differentiate and enter into the pool of quiescent cells (G_0), substituting for those which had been lost. During the cycle, the levels of various cyclins temporarily surge by synthesis and degradation (see figure). These proteins bind to and activate specific cyclin-dependent protein kinases (Cdk, see figure), which, in turn, phosphorylate and thus activate enzymes and other proteins required for DNA replication and cell division (Johnson and Walker, 1999) (see Fig. 3-32). In addition to cyclines, phosphorylation also regulates the activity of Cdks: phosphorylation by Wee1 protein kinase (not shown) inactivates Cdk1 and Cdk2, whereas dephosphorylation by cdc25 phosphatases activates them. After tissue necrosis, the number of cells entering the cell division cycle markedly increases at areas adjacent to the injury. The proportion of cells that are in S phase in a given period is reflected by the labeling index, whereas the percentage of cells undergoing mitosis is the mitotic index (see text).

α-fetoprotein levels indicates an improved outcome of acetaminophen-induced injury. Hepatic sinusoidal endothelial cells originate from bone marrow progenitors and when they are chemically injured (eg, by monocrotaline) bone marrow–derived precursor cells move into the sinusoids and contribute to their replacement, as demonstrated in a rat model of hepatic sinusoidal obstruction syndrome (Harb *et al.*, 2009). Accordingly, bone marrow infusion ameliorates, and myelosuppression aggravates, such liver injury. In an ozone-exposed lung, the nonciliated Clara cells and type II pneumocytes undergo mitosis and terminal differentiation to replace, respectively, the damaged ciliated bronchial epithelial cells and

type I pneumocytes (Mustafa, 1990). In some tissues, such as intestinal mucosa and bone marrow, stem cells first divide to provide self-renewal and then differentiate to replace more mature cells lost through injury.

Sequential changes in gene expression occur in cells that are destined to divide. In rats subjected to partial hepatectomy to study regeneration of the liver, oligonucleotide microarray analysis revealed that more than 150 genes are involved in the early gene response with upregulation or downregulation (Su *et al.*, 2002). The overexpressed genes include those that code for TFs important in proliferative signaling, such as c-*fos*, c-*jun*, *Egr1*, and c-*myc* (see Fig. 3-12), the genes of the antiapoptotic protein Bcl-X$_L$ (see Fig. 3-19), and that of mdm2 that constrains p53, a proapoptotic and cell cycle inhibitory TF (see Fig. 3-32). Interestingly, some genes whose products decelerate the cell cycle also become temporarily overexpressed (eg, the cyclin-dependent kinase inhibitor p21 and gadd45; see Fig. 3-32), suggesting that this duality keeps tissue regeneration precisely regulated. Nevertheless, the genetic expression is apparently reprogrammed so that DNA synthesis and mitosis gain priority over specialized cellular activities. For example, as a result of dedifferentiation, regenerating hepatocytes underexpress cytochrome P450, *N*-acetyltransferase-2, as well as PPARα, and hepatic stellate cells cease to accumulate fat and vitamin A.

It has been speculated that the regenerative process is initiated by the release of chemical mediators from damaged cells. The nonparenchymal cells, such as resident macrophages and endothelial cells, are receptive to these chemical signals and produce a host of secondary signaling molecules, cytokines, and growth factors that promote and propagate the regenerative process (Fig. 3-26). In rodents subjected to partial hepatectomy, the initial or priming phase of liver regeneration is controlled by the cytokines TNF and IL-6, whose hepatic mRNA and serum levels increase. TNF originates from the Kupffer cells. This cytokine acts on these macrophages in an autocrine manner, activating its receptor (item 2 in Fig. 3-12) and the coupled signal transducing network. This in turn causes activation of NF-κB, which increases IL-6 expression. The secreted IL-6 then acts on the hepatocytes and through its receptor (item 1 in Fig. 3-12) activates Janus kinase (JAK) and induces TFs (eg, Stat3, C/EBPβ), which activate several target genes. This cytokine network promotes transition of the quiescent liver cells (G_0) into cell cycle (G_1) and makes them receptive to growth factors ("priming"). Growth factors, especially the hepatocyte growth factor (HGF), transforming growth factor-α (TGF-α), and heparin-binding epidermal growth factor–like growth factor (HB-EGF), initiate the progression of the "primed" cells in the cycle toward mitosis (Costa *et al.*, 2003; Fausto *et al.*, 2006). Despite its name, neither the formation nor the action of HGF is restricted to the liver. It is produced by resident macrophages and endothelial cells of various organs—including liver, lung, and kidney—and in a paracrine manner activates receptors on neighboring parenchymal cells (Fig. 3-26). In rats intoxicated with carbon tetrachloride, the synthesis of HGF in hepatic and renal nonparenchymal cells increases markedly (Noji *et al.*, 1990) and HGF levels in blood rise rapidly (Lindroos *et al.*, 1991). The communication between parenchymal and nonparenchymal cells during tissue repair is mutual. For example, TGF-α, a potent mitogen produced by regenerating hepatocytes, acts both as an autocrine and a paracrine mediator on liver cells as well as on adjacent nonparenchymal cells (Fig. 3-26). By activating their receptors (item 4 in Fig. 3-12), these growth factors initiate signaling through the MAPK pathway and the PI3K–Akt pathway (Fig. 3-12), thereby mediating activation of TFs (c-Jun, c-Fos, c-Myc, FoxM1B, NF-κB, Stat3). These, among others, induce cyclins and the protein phosphatase cdc25, two groups of short-lived regulatory proteins. Then cyclins activate

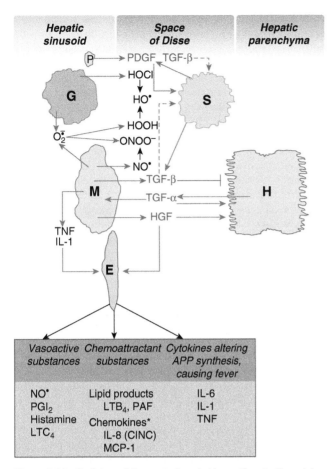

Figure 3-26. *Mediators of tissue repair and side reactions to tissue injury in liver: (1) growth factors promoting replacement of cells and the extracellular matrix; (2) mediators of inflammation, acute-phase protein (APP) synthesis, and fever; and (3) cytotoxic mediators of inflammatory cells.* HGF, hepatocyte growth factor; PDGF, platelet-derived growth factor; TGF-α, transforming growth factor-alpha; TGF-β, transforming growth factor-beta; NO•, nitric oxide; PGI$_2$, prostacyclin; LTC$_4$, leukotriene C$_4$; IL, interleukin; LTB$_4$, leukotriene B$_4$; PAF, platelet-activating factor; CINC (the rat homologue of IL-8), cytokine-induced neutrophil chemoattractant; MCP-1, monocyte chemotactic protein; TNF, tumor necrosis factor. Cells presented are E, endothelial cells; G, granulocyte; H, hepatocyte; M, macrophage (Kupffer cell); S, stellate cell (also called perisinusoidal, Ito, or fat-storing cell). *Rather than the endothelial cells, other stromal cells are the main sources of chemokines (eg, stellate cells for MCP-1). Solid arrows represent effects of growth factors on cell division, whereas the dashed arrow shows the effect on extracellular matrix formation. When directed to a cell, pointed and blunted arrows indicate stimulation and inhibition, respectively. See text for further details.

Cdks by associating with them (Fig. 3-25), whereas cdc25 activates Cdk1 and Cdk2 by dephosphorylating their 2 amino acid residues (Thr14 and Tyr15). The activated Cdks accelerate the cell cycle mainly by phosphorylation of pRb. This in turn releases the TF E2F, which induces enzymes and regulatory proteins needed for cell cycle progression (Fig. 3-32). The growth factor signaling also activates mTOR that upregulates mRNA translation, thereby meeting the demand for increased protein synthesis (see Fig. 3-29). Similar signaling appears to mediate regeneration of the *S*-(1,2-dichlorovinyl)-L-cysteine-injured kidney that exhibits increased expression of the cytokine IL-6, the growth factors TGF-α and HB-EGF, the growth factor receptors EGFR (also receptor for TGF-α) and IGF-1R, and the MAP kinase isoform Erk1 (Vaidya *et al.*, 2003).

Although the cytokine- and growth factor–controlled mitotic cell replacement is likely an essential part in the repair

of most tissues built up of cells with proliferative capacity, there are also tissue-specific features of tissue repair. For example in the liver, bile acids also stimulate hepatocyte proliferation through their nuclear receptor, FXR (Huang *et al.*, 2006). In mice subjected to partial hepatectomy, liver regrowth is hastened by bile acid feeding, but is markedly delayed when FXR is deleted or recirculation of bile acids from the intestine to the liver is prevented. Epithelia composed of a single cell layer form important barriers; therefore, replacement of mortally injured epithelial cells, which become detached from the basement membrane, is an urgent need. This can be achieved more rapidly by cell migration than by mitotic cell replacement. For example, in the damaged mucosa of the GI tract, cells of the residual epithelium rapidly migrate to the site of injury as well as elongate and become thin to reestablish the continuity of the surface even before this could be achieved by cell replication. Cell movement involves orderly dissociation of cadherin-mediated cell–cell contacts (involving β-catenin phosphorylation) and integrin-mediated cell–ECM contacts at focal adhesions (involving FAK phosphorylation), assembly of actin stress fibers, and formation of lamellopodia (cell projection filled with F-actin meshwork). Mucosal repair is dictated not only by growth factors and cytokines operative in tissue repair elsewhere but also by trefoil factors (TFFs). TFFs are small (7–12 kDa) protease-resistant proteins that are abundantly secreted from specific mucosal cells (eg, intestinal goblet cells) and are associated with the mucous layer of the GI tract (Taupin and Podolsky, 2003). TFF expression is rapidly upregulated at the margins of mucosal injury by cytokine and growth factor signaling. Whereas growth factors (eg, HGF and EGF) exert both motogenic (motility-increasing) and mitogenic effects on enterocytes, TFFs are potent motogens, but are not mitogens. Although TFFs do not act alone, they are the only peptides shown to be essential for restitution of the injured intestinal mucosa. Normal mice exposed to dextran sodium sulfate in the drinking water develop diffuse colonic mucosal injury, some exhibiting bloody diarrhea. In contrast, the majority of TFF3-null mice develop frank bloody diarrhea and die in response to dextran sodium sulfate. The immediate target molecule (eg, receptor) for TFFs remains unknown. Migration of the surviving cells also precedes mitotic cell replacement in the tubular epithelium of the injured kidney. It appears that ECM components, such as collagen IV, beneath the tubular epithelial cells aid in the restitution of the injured epithelium and reestablishment of its polarity (Nony and Schnellmann, 2003).

Replacement of the Extracellular Matrix The ECM is composed of proteins, glycosaminoglycans, and the glycoprotein and proteoglycan glycoconjugates (Gressner, 1992). In liver, these molecules are synthesized by stellate or fat-storing cells located in the space of Disse, between the hepatic sinusoid and the hepatocytes (Fig. 3-26). The stellate cells become activated during liver regeneration, undergoing mitosis and major phenotypic changes. The latter changes include not only increased synthesis and secretion of ECM constituents but also expression of α-smooth muscle actin as well as the myogenic TF MyoD and loss of fat, vitamin A, and PPARγ content. Thus, resting stellate cells become transdifferentiated into myofibroblast-like contractile and secretory cells. Activation of stellate cells is mediated chiefly by 2 growth factors—platelet-derived growth factor (PDGF) and TGF-β (Fig. 3-26). Both may be released from platelets (which accumulate and degranulate at sites of injury) and later from the activated stellate cells themselves. The main sources of TGF-β, however, are the neighboring tissue macrophages residing in the hepatic sinusoids (Gressner, 1992). A dramatic increase in TGF-β mRNA levels in Kupffer cells is observed with in situ hybridization after carbon tetrachloride–induced hepatic necrosis. Proliferation of stellate cells is induced by the potent mitogen PDGF. Through its receptor (like item 4 in Fig. 3-12), PDGF activates the PI3K–Akt pathway, which not only signals for proliferation but also inactivates the FoxO1 TF, which would halt the cell cycle in G1 phase by increasing the expression of p27, a cyclin-dependent kinase inhibitor. TGF-β acts on the stellate cells to induce their transdifferentiation and to stimulate the synthesis of ECM components, including collagens, fibronectin, tenascin, and proteoglycans. TGF-β acts through its Ser/Thr kinase receptor (item 8 in Fig. 3-12), which phosphorylates the TFs Smad2 and 3 (Flanders, 2004). TGF-β also plays a central role in ECM formation in other tissues. In kidney and lung, for example, TGF-β targets the mesangial cells and the septal fibroblasts, respectively. Remodeling of the ECM is aided by matrix metalloproteinases, which hydrolyze specific components of the matrix, as well as by tissue inhibitors of matrix metalloproteinases. The former group of these proteins originates from various types of nonparenchymal cells, including inflammatory cells; however, their inhibitors are mainly produced by stellate cells (Arthur *et al.*, 1999).

The way in which tissue regeneration is terminated after repair is unclear, but the gradual dominance of TGF-β, which is a potent antimitogen and apoptogen, over mitogens is a contributing factor in the termination of cell proliferation. ECM production may be halted by an intracellular negative feedback mechanism in the ECM-producing cells, that is, by induction of Smad7 (an inhibitory Smad), which competitively inhibits phosphorylation of the receptor-activated Smads (Smad2 and 3). In addition, extracellular products of the proliferative response, such as the proteoglycan decorin and the positive acute-phase protein α_2-macroglobulin, can bind and inactivate TGF-β; thereby they may contribute to its silencing (Gressner, 1992).

Side Reactions to Tissue Injury In addition to mediators that aid in the replacement of lost cells and the ECM, resident macrophages and endothelial cells activated by cell injury also produce other mediators that induce ancillary reactions with uncertain benefit or harm to tissues (Fig. 3-26). Such reactions include inflammation, altered production of acute-phase proteins, and generalized reactions such as fever.

Inflammation—Leukocyte Invasion Alteration of the microcirculation and accumulation of inflammatory cells are the hallmarks of inflammation. These processes are largely initiated by resident macrophages secreting cytokines, such as TNF and interleukin-1 (IL-1), in response to tissue damage (Baumann and Gauldie, 1994) (Fig. 3-26). These cytokines, in turn, stimulate neighboring stromal cells, such as the endothelial cells and fibroblasts, to release mediators that induce dilation of the local microvasculature and cause permeabilization of capillaries. Activated endothelial cells also facilitate the egress of circulating leukocytes into the injured tissue by releasing chemoattractants and expressing cell adhesion molecules, which are cell surface glycoproteins (Jaeschke, 1997). One group of cell adhesion molecules, called selectins, located on the membrane of endothelial cells, interact with their ligands on the surface of leukocytes, thereby slowing down the flow of these cells and causing them to "roll" on the capillary surface. Subsequently a stronger interaction (adhesion) is established between the endothelial cells and leukocytes with participation of intercellular adhesion molecules (eg, ICAM-1) expressed on the endothelial cell membrane and integrins expressed on the membrane of leukocytes. This interaction is also essential for the subsequent transendothelial migration of leukocytes. This is facilitated by gradients of chemoattractants that induce expression of leukocyte integrins. Chemoattractants originate from various

stromal cells and include chemotactic cytokines (or chemokines), such as the MCP-1 and IL-8 (whose rat homologue is the CINC-1), as well as lipid-derived compounds, such as platelet-activating factor (PAF) and leukotriene B$_4$ (LTB$_4$). Ultimately all types of cells in the vicinity of injury express ICAM-1, thus promoting leukocyte invasion; the invading leukocytes also synthesize mediators, thus propagating the inflammatory response. Production of most inflammatory mediators is induced by signaling, turned on by TNF and IL-1, which results in activation of TFs, notably NF-κB and C/EBP (Poli, 1998) (see Fig. 3-12). Genes of many of the proteins mentioned above (eg, selectins, ICAM-1, MCP-1, IL-8) and below (eg, inducible NOS, acute-phase proteins) as well as the genes of TNF and IL-1 themselves contain binding sites for the NF-κB (Lee and Burckart, 1998).

Inflammation—ROS and RNS Production Macrophages, as well as leukocytes, recruited to the site of injury undergo a respiratory burst, discharging free radicals and enzymes (Weiss and LoBuglio, 1982) (Fig. 3-26). Free radicals are produced in the inflamed tissue in three ways, each of which involves a specific enzyme: Nox, NOS, or myeloperoxidase.

Nox is an electron-transporting protein complex composed of two transmembrane proteins (one of them the FAD- and heme-containing catalytic subunit) and 4 cytoplasmic proteins (including the G-protein Rac) (El-Benna *et al.*, 2005). In resting cells Nox is dormant; however, in activated cells the cytoplasmic subunits become extensively phosphorylated and move to the membrane to assemble the Nox complex. Constituents of microorganisms, such as the bacterial LPS (the active endotoxin component of gram-negative bacteria), acting through the cell surface Toll-like receptors (TLR), and PKC activators, such as phorbol miristate acetate (PMA), may evoke Nox activation. Unlike in nonphagocytic cells, in macrophages and granulocytes activation causes a sudden and rapid electron transfer from NADPH through the FAD and heme in Nox to the molecular oxygen, releasing the thus formed superoxide anion radical ($O_2^{\bullet-}$) in a burst ("respiratory burst") at the external membrane surface into the phagocytic vacuole:

$$NADPH + 2O_2 \rightarrow NADP^+ + H^+ + 2O_2^{\bullet-}.$$

The $O_2^{\bullet-}$ can give rise to the hydroxyl radical (HO$^\bullet$) in two sequential steps: the first is spontaneous or is catalyzed by SOD, and the second, the Fenton reaction, is catalyzed by transition metal ions (see also Fig. 3-4):

$$2O_2^{\bullet-} + 2H^+ \rightarrow O_2 + HOOH;$$
$$HOOH + Fe^{2+} \rightarrow Fe^{3+} + HO^- + HO^\bullet.$$

Macrophages, but not granulocytes, generate another cytotoxic free radical, nitric oxide ($^\bullet$NO). This radical is produced from arginine by NOS (Wang *et al.*, 1993), which is inducible in macrophages by bacterial endotoxin and the cytokines IL-1 and TNF:

$$\text{L-Arginine} + O_2 \rightarrow \text{L-citrulline} + {^\bullet}NO.$$

Subsequently, $O_2^{\bullet-}$ and $^\bullet$NO, both of which are products of activated macrophages, can react with each other, yielding peroxynitrite anion; on reaction with carbon dioxide, this decays into two radicals, nitrogen dioxide and carbonate anion radical (Fig. 3-4):

$$O_2^{\bullet-} + {^\bullet}NO \rightarrow ONOO^-;$$
$$ONOO^- + CO_2 \rightarrow ONOOCO_2^-;$$
$$ONOOCO_2^- \rightarrow {^\bullet}NO_2 + CO_3^{\bullet-}.$$

Granulocytes, but not macrophages, discharge the lysosomal enzyme myeloperoxidase into engulfed extracellular spaces, the phagocytic vacuoles (Wang *et al.*, 1993). Myeloperoxidase catalyzes the formation of HOCl, a powerful oxidizing agent, from HOOH and chloride ion:

$$HOOH + H^+ + Cl^- \rightarrow HOH + HOCl.$$

Like HOOH, HOCl can form $HO^\bullet$ as a result of electron transfer from Fe^{2+} or from $O_2^{\bullet-}$ to HOCl:

$$HOCl + O_2^{\bullet-} \rightarrow O_2 + Cl^- + HO^\bullet.$$

All these reactive chemicals, as well as the discharged lysosomal proteases, are destructive products of inflammatory cells. Although these chemicals exert antimicrobial activity at the site of microbial invasion, at the site of toxic injury they can damage the adjacent healthy tissues and thus contribute to propagation of tissue injury (see the section "Tissue Necrosis"). Moreover, in some chemically induced injuries, inflammation plays the leading role. For example, ANIT, a cholestatic chemical, causes neutrophil-dependent hepatocellular damage. ANIT apparently acts on bile duct epithelial cells, causing them to release chemoattractants for neutrophil cells, which on invading the liver, injure hepatocytes (Hill *et al.*, 1999). Kupffer cell activation, TNF release, and subsequent inflammation are also prominent and causative events in galactosamine-induced liver injury in rats (Stachlewitz *et al.*, 1999).

Whereas it is well recognized that chemical-inflicted tissue injury can induce inflammation as a side reaction of tissue repair, it is becoming clear that inflammation (even if harmless alone) can precipitate an overt tissue injury on chemical exposure that is noninjurious alone. For example, a small harmless quantity of the macrophage activator LPS converts the nontoxic doses of monocrotaline, aflatoxin B$_1$, and allyl alcohol into markedly hepatotoxic doses (Roth *et al.*, 2003). Moreover, in rats pretreated with LPS, unlike in untreated animals, chlorpromazine, ranitidine, and trovafloxacin caused liver injury. These drugs (and many others) when given to patients can induce rare, unexpected, and not obviously dose-related liver injury. Therefore, it is hypothesized that such idiosyncratic drug reactions develop when some endotoxin exposure decreases the threshold for drug toxicity by priming the Kupffer cells that produce ROS and inflammatory mediators discussed above. Manifest or subclinical infection, GI disturbance, or alcohol consumption (which greatly increases the intestinal permeability for endotoxin) may be the source of endotoxin. It is not surprising that most idiosyncratic drug reactions affect the liver, because this organ contains 80% to 90% of the body's fixed macrophages (ie, Kupffer cells), because the liver is the first organ to be exposed to LPS translocating from the intestinal lumen, and because the Kupffer cells not only are activated by LPS but also remove it from the circulation, thereby protecting other organs from its inflammatory effects (Roth *et al.*, 2003). However, the causative relationship between inflammation and idiosyncrasy needs further substantiation.

Altered Protein Synthesis: Acute-Phase Proteins Cytokines released from macrophages and endothelial cells of injured tissues also alter protein synthesis, predominantly in the liver (Baumann and Gauldie, 1994) (Fig. 3-21). Mainly IL-6 but also IL-1 and TNF act on cell surface receptors and increase or decrease the transcriptional activity of genes encoding certain proteins called positive and negative acute-phase proteins, respectively, utilizing primarily the TFs NF-κB, C/EBP, and STAT (Poli, 1998; see Fig. 3-15). Many of the hepatic acute-phase proteins, such as C-reactive protein and hepcidin, are secreted into the circulation, and their elevated levels in serum are diagnostic of tissue injury, inflammation, or neoplasm. Increased sedimentation of red blood cells, which is also indicative of these conditions, is due to enrichment of blood plasma with positive acute-phase proteins such as fibrinogen.

Apart from their diagnostic value, positive acute-phase proteins may play roles in minimizing tissue injury and facilitating repair. For example, many of them, such as α$_2$-macroglobulin and α$_1$-antiprotease, inhibit lysosomal proteases released from the injured cells and recruited leukocytes. Haptoglobin binds hemoglobin in blood, MT complexes metals in the cells, heme oxygenase oxidizes heme to biliverdin, and opsonins facilitate phagocytosis. Thus, these positive acute-phase proteins may be involved in the clearance of substances released on tissue injury. Induction of hepcidin, which triggers degradation of the iron exit channel ferroportin (see the section "Mechanisms of Adaptation") and thus decreases the duodenal Fe^{2+} absorption and Fe^{2+} export from macrophages, may be protective by limiting iron availability in the circulation for pathogens and by minimizing the Fe^{2+}-catalyzed Fenton reaction (Fig. 3-4), the source of reactive hydroxyl radicals that may cause tissue injury.

Negative acute-phase proteins include some plasma proteins, such as albumin, transthyretin, and transferrin, as well as hepatic enzymes (eg, several forms of cytochrome P450 and glutathione *S*-transferase), ligand-activated TFs (eg, PPARα and the bile acid receptor FXR), and transporters, such as bile acid transporters at the sinusoidal and canalicular membrane of hepatocytes (NTCP and bile salt export pump [BSEP], respectively) and the bile canalicular export pump Mrp2. Because the latter enzymes and transporters play important roles in the toxication, detoxication, and excretion of endobiotics and xenobiotics, the disposition and toxicity of bile acids and toxicants may be altered markedly during the acute phase of tissue injury.

Although the acute-phase response is phylogenetically preserved, some of the acute-phase proteins are somewhat species-specific. For example, during the acute phase of tissue injury or inflammation, C-reactive protein and serum amyloid A levels dramatically increase in humans but not in rats, whereas the concentrations of α$_1$-acid glycoprotein and α$_2$-macroglobulin increase markedly in rats but only moderately in humans.

Generalized Reactions Cytokines released from activated macrophages and endothelial cells at the site of injury also may evoke neurohumoral responses. Thus, IL-1, TNF, and IL-6 alter the temperature set point of the hypothalamus, triggering fever. IL-1 possibly also mediates other generalized reactions to tissue injury, such as hypophagia, sleep, and "sickness behavior" (Rothwell, 1991). In addition, IL-1 and IL-6 act on the pituitary to induce the release of ACTH, which in turn stimulates the secretion of cortisol from the adrenals. This represents a negative feedback loop because corticosteroids inhibit cytokine gene expression.

Mechanisms of Adaptation

Adaptation may be defined as a harm-induced capability of the organism for increased tolerance to the harm itself. It involves responses acting to preserve or regain the biological homeostasis in the face of increased harm. Theoretically, adaptation to toxicity may result from biological changes causing (1) diminished delivery of the causative chemical(s) to the target, (2) decreased size or susceptibility of the target, (3) increased capacity of the organism to repair itself, and (4) strengthened mechanisms to compensate the toxicant-inflicted dysfunction. Mechanistically, adaptation involves sensing the noxious chemical and/or the initial damage or dysfunction, and a response that typically occurs through altered gene expression. Such mechanisms will be briefly overviewed below.

Adaptation by Decreasing Delivery to the Target The
first step in the development of toxicity is delivery of the ultimate

toxicant (a xenobiotic, its metabolite or xenobiotic-generated ROS and RNS) to the target (Fig. 3-2). Certain chemicals induce adaptive changes that lessen their delivery by diminishing the absorption, increasing their sequestration by intracellular binding proteins, enhancing their detoxication, or promoting their cellular export.

Repression of Iron Absorption Adaptive mechanisms triggered by iron itself adjust the intestinal absorption of this essential yet potentially harmful metal ion, a catalyst of hydroxyl radical formation by the Fenton reaction (Fig. 3-4), to its demand. Fe^{2+} is taken up from the intestinal lumen into the enterocyte by the proton-coupled divalent metal transporter 1 (DMT1) localized in the luminal membrane and is exported across the basolateral membrane of these cells through the ferroportin iron channel. High iron intake diminishes the expression of both DMT1 and ferroportin in the enterocytes, whereas low intake has the opposite effect.

The expression of DMT1 is regulated at the translational level by the intracellular iron-regulatory proteins (IRP) that contain a [4Fe-4S] cluster. Iron supply influences the Fe content of this cluster and in turn affects the capacity of IRP to bind to mRNAs containing iron response element (IRE) in their untranslated regions and to alter translation. In iron deficiency, loss of Fe from the [4Fe-4S] cluster allows the thus formed IRP1 apoprotein to bind to and protect DMT1 mRNA from enzymatic degradation. On becoming more abundant, DMT1 mRNA translates into more DMT1 protein. Conversely, iron overload saturates IRP1 with Fe, making it incapable of binding to and stabilizing the DMT1 mRNA. The consequential loss of DMT1 mRNA and its translation into less DMT1 protein then limits Fe^{2+} absorption. This physiologically important adaptive mechanism may have toxicological corollary. Since DMT1 also mediates the transport of Cd^{2+}, DMT1 overexpression in iron deficiency increases intestinal absorption of this highly toxic metal ion (Park *et al.*, 2002).

Ferroportin allows exit of iron not only from enterocytes but also from macrophages (which obtain iron from phagocytosed senescent or damaged erythrocytes) and hepatocytes (which store iron). The abundance of ferroportin in the plasma membrane of these cells is regulated directly by hepcidin, a peptide hormone secreted by the hepatocytes of the liver (Ganz, 2011). By binding to ferroportin, hepcidin triggers the internalization and lysosomal hydrolysis of ferroportin. Hepatic production of hepcidin is sensitive to iron supply. Iron deficiency decreases hepcidin secretion, precluding ferroportin degradation and thus increasing the abundance of this iron exporter in the basolateral membrane of enterocytes. This (together with the upregulated DMT1 in the apical membrane of these cells) permits increased iron absorption from the duodenum. In contrast, iron overload increases the secretion of hepcidin, which in turn induces degradation of ferroportin, thereby preventing iron export from the enterocytes. Thus, decreased synthesis of DMT1 (see above) and degradation of ferroportin act in concert to shut down iron absorption from the intestine and protect against iron excess from the diet, from lysed red blood cells, or from ferritin. The toxicological significance of this mechanism is exemplified by findings with diquat, a redox cycling hepatotoxic herbicide that (like paraquat, see Fig. 3-3) can accept an electron, forming diquat monocation radical ($DQ^{\bullet+}$), which in turn transfers the electron to O_2, producing superoxide anion radical ($O_2^{\bullet-}$). Soon after diquat injection to rats, hepatic free iron increased dramatically (purportedly because both $DQ^{\bullet+}$ and $O_2^{\bullet-}$ had reductively released Fe^{2+} from ferritin) followed by a rise in hepatic hepcidin mRNA first, and later by a decrease in plasma iron (Higuchi *et al.*, 2011), a seemingly appropriate protective response.

Inappropriately elevated hepcidin, however, may cause iron deficiency. For example, one might speculate that elevated plasma levels of prohepcidin observed in chronic lead intoxication contribute to lead-induced anemia.

Hepcidin production by hepatocytes is transcriptionally regulated by Smad4 and STAT3 TFs through their cognate response elements in the hepcidin gene (Ganz, 2011). Two pathways converge on Smad4: one signals the amount of intracellular iron, whereas the other signals the quantity of plasma iron. Increase in intracellular iron in the liver cells is detected by unidentified sensors that induce secretion of bone morphogenetic protein (BMP6, a TGF-β-like signaling molecule) acting in an autocrine or paracrine manner on its cell surface BMP receptor that activates Smad4 by phosphorylation (like TGF-β does in pathway 8 shown in Fig. 3-12). Increase in plasma iron is detected by the transferrin receptor (TFR) of hepatocytes when activated by transferrin saturated with iron. Then TFR relays the signal through adapter proteins to the BMP receptor, which thus becomes increasingly sensitive to its ligand, BMP6. The pathway descending to STAT3 is initiated by IL-6 (see Fig. 3-12, item 1), a cytokine that triggers the acute-phase response, explaining why hepcidin is also a positive acute-phase protein (see above). In summary, the pathways initiated by transferrin and BMP receptors upregulate the hepatic production of hepcidin that reduces iron absorption in response to iron overload, whereas the pathway triggered by IL-6 has a similar effect in response to inflammation, tissue injury, or cancer, conditions with increased IL-6 production. The latter disorders may cause anemia by this mechanism.

Induction of Ferritin and Metallothionein Adaptive cellular accumulation of the binding proteins ferritin and MT is protective against their respective ligands, iron and cadmium ions. Interestingly, upregulation of ferritin by iron overload, like downregulation of DMT1, is also translationally mediated by IRP1. However, the apoIRP1 (which is formed in iron deficiency) acts oppositely on ferritin mRNA and blocks its translation. Iron overload relieves this blockade, as it yields IPR1 with the [4Fe-4S] cluster, which does not bind to the IRE in ferritin mRNA, thus causing a surge in ferritin translation. Ferritin is protective as it removes Fe^{2+} from the Fenton reaction (Fig. 3-4) and incorporates it as Fe^{3+} through its ferroxidase activity.

MT is greatly induced by cadmium and elevated levels of MT protect the liver by restricting distribution of this toxic metal ion to sensitive intracellular targets (Klaassen *et al.*, 1999). Induction of MT by Cd^{2+} is likely indirect, mediated by Zn (displaced from intracellular binding sites), which activates the metal-responsive transcription factor 1 (MTF-1) that in turn augments transcription of the MT gene by binding to the metal-responsive elements in its promoter (Lichtlen and Schaffner, 2001).

Induction of Detoxication—The Electrophile Stress Response, Part 1 Adaptive increases in detoxication (ie, elimination of xenobiotics, their reactive metabolites, harmful endobiotics, or ROS and RNS by biotransformation) and cellular export have a major role in limiting toxicity. Such adaptation is typically induced by compounds with thiol reactivity (ie, soft electrophiles, oxidants, and those generating oxidative stress), which are sensed by the cytosolic Keap1–Nrf2 protein complex. The response is initiated by the TF Nrf2, which activates genes with electrophile response element (EpRE) in their regulatory region (Fig. 3-27; Dinkova-Kostova *et al.*, 2005). Normally Nrf2 is retained in the cytoplasm by Keap1, a cysteine-rich homodimeric protein. Keap1 keeps Nrf2 inactive and at low intracellular levels by anchoring it to the cytoskeleton and also by linking it to cullin 3, a component in certain E3 ubiquitin ligase complexes, thereby initiating ubiquitination of

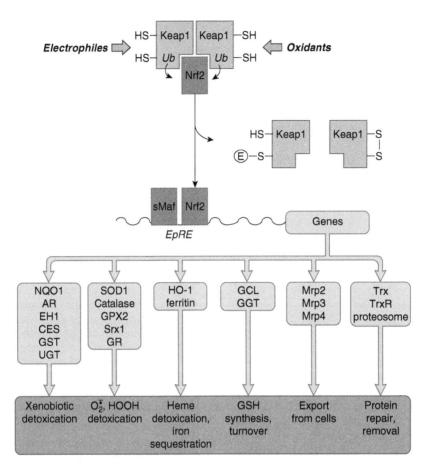

Figure 3-27. *Signaling by Keap1/Nrf2 mediates the electrophile stress response.* Normally NF-E2-related factor 2 (Nrf2) is kept inactive and at a low intracellular level by interacting with Keap1 that promotes its proteasomal degradation by ubiquitination. Electrophiles covalently bind to, whereas oxidants oxidize the reactive thiol groups of Keap1, causing Keap1 to release Nrf2. Alternatively, Nrf2 release may follow its phosphorylation by protein kinases. After being released from Keap1, the active Nrf2 accumulates in the cell, translocates into the nucleus, and forms a heterodimer with small Maf proteins to activate genes that contain electrophile response element (EpRE) in their promoter region. These include enzymes, binding proteins, and transporters functioning in detoxication and elimination of xenobiotics, ROS, and endogenous reactive chemicals, as well as some proteins that can repair or eliminate oxidized proteins. Induction of such proteins represents an electrophile stress response that provides protection against a wide range of toxicants. Nrf1, a transcription factor structurally related to Nrf2, also interacts with Keap1 and Maf proteins as well as EpRE and its role is partially overlapping with that of Nrf2. *Abbreviations*: AR, aldose reductase; CES carboxylesterase; EH1, microsomal epoxide hydrolase; GCL, glutamate–cysteine ligase; GGT, gamma-glutamyl transpeptidase; GPX2, glutathione peroxidase 2; GR, glutathione reductase; GST, glutathione *S*-transferase; HO-1, heme oxygenase 1; NQO1, NAD(P)H:quinone oxidoreductase; Mrp2, Mrp3, and Mrp4, multidrug resistance protein 2, 3, and 4; SOD1, superoxide dismutase 1; Srx1, sulfiredoxin 1; UGT, UDP-glucuronosyltransferase; Trx, thioredoxin; TrxR, thioredoxin reductase.

Nrf2 for subsequent proteasomal degradation. On disruption of the Keap1–Nrf2 complex, the active Nrf2 escapes rapid degradation and accumulates in the cell. Electrophiles, such as quinones (eg, t-butylquinone), quinoneimines (eg, NAPBQI derived from acetaminophen), quinone methides (eg, metabolite of butylated hydroxytoluene), α,β-unsaturated aldehydes and ketones (eg, the lipid peroxidation products 4-oxonon-2-enal, 4-hydroxynon-2-enal, and 15-A$_{2t}$-isoprostane), isothiocyanates (eg, ANIT), thiol-reactive metal ions (eg, Cd^{2+}), and trivalent arsenicals, as well as direct and indirect oxidants (eg, HOOH, diquat, quinones) may attack Keap1 at its reactive cysteine thiol groups by binding to them covalently or oxidizing them, thereby forcing Keap1 to release Nrf2. After being released from Keap1, Nrf2 translocates into the nucleus, forms a heterodimer with small Maf proteins, and activates genes through binding to EpREs.

There are many genes with EpRE motifs that encode proteins known to be important in detoxication and export (Fig. 3-27). These include genes that code for (1) enzymes that detoxify xenobiotics (eg, NQO1, NQO2, AR, EH-1, CES1e1, CES2a6, GST, and UGT), (2) enzymes that eliminate $O_2^{\bullet-}$ (ie, SOD1) and HOOH (eg, GPX2, catalase, and Srx1; the latter reduces the overoxidized peroxiredoxins that in turn can reduce not only HOOH [see Fig. 3-5] but also lipid hydroperoxides and peroxinitrite), (3) proteins that detoxify heme (HO-1) and Fe^{2+} (ferritin), (4) enzymes involved in the synthesis of GSH and its regeneration from GSSG (eg, GCL and the NADPH-forming G6PDH), and (5) transporters that pump xenobiotics and their metabolites out of cells (eg, Mrp2, 3, and 4. Other Nrf2-induced proteins of known toxicological relevance will be mentioned later.

As demonstrated in Fig. 3-28 through the example of t-butyl-hydroquinone (tBHQ), these Nrf2-mediated adaptive changes facilitate elimination and detoxication of electrophilic chemicals, as well as ROS that may be generated by them, and assist in repairing or removing damaged proteins (to be discussed later); therefore, Nrf2 conveys protection against a wide range of toxicants. Indeed, Nrf2 knockout mice are more sensitive to the hepatotoxicity of acetaminophen, pentachlorophenol, and carbon tetrachloride, the pulmonary toxicity of butylated hydroxytoluene, hyperoxia, or cigarette smoke,

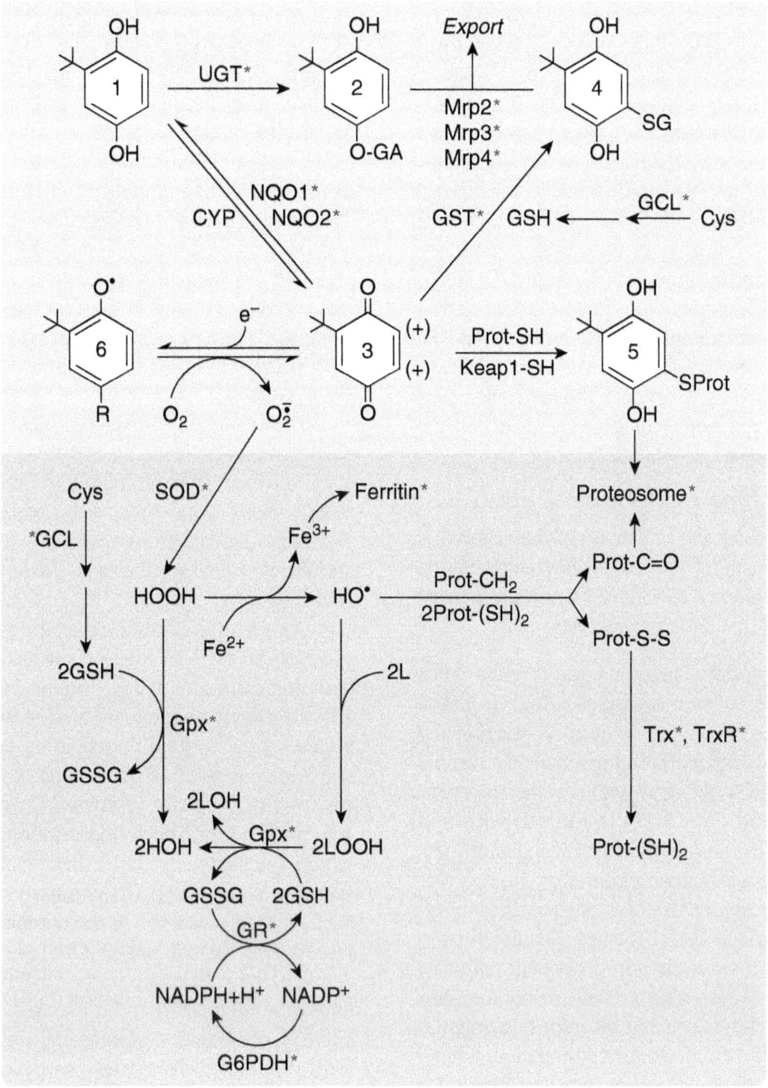

Figure 3-28. *Adaptive changes in response to the t-butylhydroquinone (tBHQ)–induced electrophile stress that influence the metabolic fate and some effects of tBHQ and of superoxide anion radical generated in the course of tBHQ biotransformation.* This figure illustrates the numerous proteins (ie, enzymes, exporters, repair proteins) that, when induced in response to the *t*BHQ-induced electrophile stress, facilitate the detoxication and export of *t*BHQ and/or its metabolites, the detoxication of ROS formed during the biotransformation of *t*BHQ, and repair or removal of proteins damaged by the reactive metabolites. Proteins induced by Nrf2 as a result of adaptation to the electrophile stress are marked with an asterisk.

*t*BHQ (1) can be detoxified by UDP-glucuronosyltransferase to form *t*BHQ glucuronide (2) and toxified by cytochrome P450–catalyzed dehydrogenation to *t*-butylquinone (*t*BQ; 3), which contains electrophilic carbon atoms (+), and is believed to be the actual inducer of electrophile stress response. *t*BQ can undergo 3 biotransformations. First, it can be detoxified by conjugation with glutathione (GSH) to form *t*BHQ-SG (4), which, together with *t*BHQ-glucuronide, is exported from the cell by Mrp2, 3, and 4. Second, *t*BQ can covalently bind to SH groups in proteins (5), including Keap1. Third, by accepting an electron (e), *t*BQ can form *t*-butylsemiquinone radical (6), which can pass the electron to molecular oxygen to form superoxide anion radical ($O_2^{\bullet-}$), completing a redox cycle. In a process catalyzed by superoxide dismutase (SOD), $O_2^{\bullet-}$ can form HOOH, which is detoxified by GSH-peroxidase (GPX), using GSH (whose synthesis is rate-limited by GCL), or toxified by Fe^{2+}-catalyzed Fenton reaction to form hydroxyl radical (HO$^\bullet$). HO$^\bullet$ can react with proteins to form oxidized proteins (Prot-C=O, Prot-S-S), which can be degraded in the proteasome, or Prot-S-S can also be repaired through reduction by the thioredoxin (Trx)–thioredoxin reductase (TrxR) system. HO$^\bullet$ can also react with lipid (L) and form lipid hydroperoxide (LOOH), which can be reduced to lipid alcohol (LOH) by GPX at the expense of GSH. This results in formation of glutathione disulfide (GSSG), which can be reduced back to GSH by glutathione reductase (GR) at the expense of NADPH generated by glucose-6-phosphate dehydrogenase (G6PDH). Virtually all of these processes become more effective after the electrophile stress response.

the neurotoxicity of 3-nitropropionic acid, and the carcinogenicity of benzo[*a*]pyrene (Klaassen and Reisman, 2010). Conversely, liver-specific deletion of Keap1 constitutively activates Nrf2 in hepatocytes, causing them to overexpress many detoxifying enzymes and become resistant to acetaminophen-induced hepatotoxicity.

Nrf2 can be activated by treatment with several chemicals of low toxicity that are thiol-reactive as soft electrophiles or oxidants.

These include *t*BHQ, butylated hydroxyanisole (BHA), sulforaphane (a compound in broccoli with an electrophilic isothiocyanate group), curcumin (a compound in turmeric containing 2 α,β-unsaturated ketone groups), resveratrol (a hydroquinone-type compound in red grapes that may undergo oxidation to a quinone and redox cycling, like shown for *t*BHQ in Fig. 3-28), derivatives of oleanolic acid, such as 2-cyano-3,12-dioxooleana-1,9(11)-dien-28-oic acid (CDDO, which contains 2 electrophilic enone groups), and oltipraz (a dithiolenethione compound whose metabolites can form mixed disulfides with thiols, probably also with those on Keap1). These chemicals induce Nrf2 target genes (Fig. 3-27) and protect from toxicant-induced tissue injury and cancer. For example, treatment with oleanolic acid or CDDO ameliorates acetaminophen-induced hepatotoxicity and aflatoxin-induced hepatocarcinogenesis (Klaassen and Reisman, 2010). The superpotent Nrf2 agonist CDDO is now tested clinically for use in chronic kidney diseases. Of these chemopreventive agents, some (eg, tBHQ, BHA, and resveratrol) are antioxidants; hence the inappropriate names "antioxidant response" and "antioxidant response element" (ARE) for the Nrf2-mediated adaptive alterations and the cognate DNA-binding site for Nrf2, respectively. It became apparent only later that the electrophilic quinone metabolites of these chemicals are the inducers and not the antioxidants.

Adaptation by Decreasing the Target Density or Responsiveness

Decreasing the density and sensitivity of the xenobiotic target is an adaptation mechanism for several cell surface receptors. Such alterations underlie the tolerance induced by opioids, abused drugs of considerable clinical toxicological interests.

Induction of Opioid Tolerance The main target of opioids (eg, morphine, heroine, methadone) is the μ-opioid receptor. Stimulation of this G_i protein–coupled inhibitory receptor by an agonist results in adenyl cyclase inhibition (causing decline in cyclic AMP levels and PKA activity) and K^+ channel opening (causing hyperpolarization) (Fig. 3-15) in neurons with opioid receptors, such as those in the midbrain periaqueductal gray. Even brief stimulation induces adaptive alterations: the receptor is desensitized by G-protein receptor kinase–mediated phosphorylation and β-arrestin binding, and then becomes uncoupled from the G protein and internalized via a clathrin-dependent pathway. Whereas some receptors are recycled to the cell membrane, others are degraded in the lysosomes, causing receptor downregulation (Bailey and Connor, 2005). On prolonged stimulation, adenyl cyclase signaling undergoes a compensatory increase. Tolerance to opioids, though far from being clarified mechanistically, may result from downregulation of the receptors and upregulation of adenyl cyclase signaling. These changes would require increasing doses of agonist to produce an effect (ie, inhibition of adenyl cyclase signaling) as intensive as after its first application. These adaptive changes could also explain the withdrawal reaction, that is, appearance of clinical symptoms (dysphoria, excitement, pain sensation), contrasting with the pharmacologic effects of opioids (euphoria, sedation, analgesia), on abrupt termination of drug treatment, because withdrawal of the opioid would disinhibit the reinforced signaling it had inhibited. Nevertheless, mechanistic relationships between tolerance and the withdrawal reaction remain controversial (Bailey and Connor, 2005). An important clinical feature of opioid tolerance is that the tolerance to the respiratory depressive effect is short-lived and sensitivity returns after some abstinence. Therefore, abusers often kill themselves with a dose tolerated earlier.

Adaptation by Increasing Repair

There are several repair mechanisms that can be induced after toxicant exposure. Some of these may aid in repairing damaged molecules, proteins, and DNA, others in regenerating the injured tissue.

Induction of Enzymes Repairing Oxidized Proteins—The Electrophile Stress Response, Part 2 After sublethal exposure to chemicals, such as tBHQ, 4-hydroxynon-2-enal, and Cd^{2+}, not only enzymes functioning in xenobiotic detoxication but also some of those mediating protein repair become overexpressed as part of the above-described electrophile response. The induced proteins include thioredoxin 1 (Trx1) and thioredoxin reductase 1 (TR1), which can reduce oxidized proteins (protein disulfides, -sulfenic acids, and -methionine sulfoxides) (Fig. 3-22), and several subunits of the proteasome complex, which hydrolyzes damaged proteins. These repair proteins are transcribed from genes containing EpRE, and their transcription is controlled by Nrf2 (Fig. 3-27). As Trx1 and TR1 are reduction partners for ribonucleotide reductase, they support this enzyme in forming deoxyribonucleotides for DNA synthesis. Thus, induction of Trx1 and TR1 also assists DNA repair.

Induction of Chaperones Repairing Misfolded Proteins—The Heat-Shock Response The cellular abundance of many molecular chaperones, which can disaggregate and refold denatured proteins, also increases after physical and chemical stresses (eg, heat, ionizing radiation, oxidants, electrophile reactants, and metal ions). Two adaptive reactions involving overexpression of chaperones are known; they are the heat-shock response and the EPR stress response.

Although first observed as a result of hyperthermia, the heat-shock response is an adaptive mechanism also triggered by various pathologic conditions (eg, trauma, tissue ischemia) and by virtually all reactive chemicals and/or their metabolites (eg, electrophiles, oxidants, lipid peroxidation products, metal ions, arsenite) that denature proteins. Thus, it takes place simultaneously with the electrophile response discussed above. This reaction, however, is governed by heat-shock transcription factors (HSF), mainly HSF1, which transactivate genes that encode Hsp through heat-shock response elements (HSE) within the promoter region. HSF1, like Nrf2, normally resides in the cytoplasm, where it associates with Hsp90, Hsp70, and Hsp40. On heat- or chemical-induced protein damage, these Hsps are purportedly sequestered by damaged proteins, allowing HSF1 to be released. HSF1 then migrates into the nucleus, trimerizes, undergoes phosphorylation, and stimulates the transcription of Hsp genes. As described in the section "Repair of Proteins," the chaperones Hsp90 and Hsp70, together with co-chaperone proteins, are especially important in maintaining the integrity of hundreds of proteins (Pratt *et al.*, 2010). The client proteins include not only those carrying out housekeeping functions but also those involved in signaling and apoptosis. Therefore, induction of Hsps has pleiotropic effects besides increased protection from cytotoxicity. However, when the proteotoxic stress induces excessive protein unfolding, Hsp70 and Hsp40 recruit the ubiquitin system (Fig. 3-23) to tag the aberrant proteins for proteasomal degradation (Bedford *et al.*, 2011).

Induction of Chaperones Repairing Misfolded Proteins—The Endoplasmic Reticulum Stress and the Unfolded Protein Response All proteins that are destined for export or insertion into cellular membranes pass through the EPR. In this Ca^{2+}-rich oxidative environment, they may be subjected to N-glycosylation at asparagine residues by oligosaccharyltransferase, formation of disulfide bonds by protein disulfide isomerases, and folding assisted by EPR-resident chaperones, such as the glucose-regulated proteins Grp78 (also called binding immunoglobulin protein [BiP]) and Grp94 as well as the Ca^{2+}-binding proteins calreticulin and calnexin. Damage of proteins being processed in the EPR by reactive metabolites produced in situ by CYP enzymes (eg, the quinoneimine metabolite of acetaminophen, $Cl_3C^•$ and $Cl_3COO^•$ radicals formed from CCl_4, and ROS generated by CYP2E1 during oxidation of ethanol) and/or depletion of Ca^{2+} in the EPR lumen (eg, by inactivation of the EPR Ca^{2+}-ATPase by reactive metabolites) causes accumulation of unfolded or misfolded proteins, a condition known as EPR stress (Cribb *et al.*, 2005; Nagy *et al.*, 2007; Malhi and Kaufman, 2011). Protein folding disorder can also be experimentally induced by some natural compounds that disturb the homeostasis of EPR at specific steps, such as thapsigargin (which blocks SERCA-mediated Ca^{2+} uptake into EPR; see Table 3-7), tunicamycin (which inhibits *N*-glycosylation of proteins), castanospermine (which interferes with maturation of nascent glycoproteins by deglucosylation), and brefeldin A (which inhibits transport of proteins from EPR to Golgi).

When the load of unfolded or misfolded proteins in the EPR exceeds the capacity of EPR-resident chaperones, these proteins trigger a complex adaptive response, called unfolded protein response (UPR). This may constrain exacerbation of the disorder (1) by attenuation of mRNA translation to decrease the functional load on the EPR, (2) by increased transcription of EPR chaperones to boost the folding capacity, (3) by initiating the translocation of aberrant proteins via translocon peptide channels from the EPR into the cytosol for proteasomal degradation, and (4) by eliminating the affected cell via apoptosis, if the EPR stress is sustained or massive. The eukaryotic translation initiation factor 2α (eIF2α) and TFs X-box binding protein 1 (XBP1), ATF6, ATF4, and C/EBP homologous protein (CHOP) (or Gadd153) are the major executioners of this adaptive response.

Three transmembrane EPR proteins sense the overload of the EPR lumen with misfolded proteins and transduce this signal to initiate the UPR. These are (1) PERK, (2) inositol-requiring enzyme 1α (IRE1α), a protein with kinase and endoribonuclease (RNase) activities, and (3) the precursor form ATF6 (activating TF 6). Normally, these sensor proteins are turned off by being associated at their luminal domain with the EPR-resident soluble chaperone BiP (or Grp78). However, when EPR stress occurs, the unfolded proteins that accumulate in the lumen of the EPR sequester BiP away from these sensors, thereby turning them on to signal for the UPR. PERK stripped off BiP is activated by dimerization and trans-autophosphorylation. With its kinase activity thus raised, PERK catalyzes the phosphorylation of the eIF2α, with the phosphorylated eIF2α causing a global translation attenuation and decreased synthesis of most (but not all) proteins. The second EPR stress sensor IRE1α also undergoes dimerization and trans-autophosphorylation on dissociation from BiP. These changes boost the RNase activity of IRE1α, enabling it to cleave and process a mRNA into one that translates into XBP1, an active TF, another executioner of UPR. The third sensor ATF6 resides as a 90 kDa precursor protein in the EPR with its Golgi localization sequences masked by BiP. On dissociation from BiP, ATF6 translocates to the Golgi, undergoes a so-called regulated intramembrane proteolysis (by site-1 and site-2 proteases), yielding a 50 kDa fragment, the active TF ATF6. XBP1 and ATF6 bind alone or as heterodimers to cognate DNA sequences, such as EPR response element (ERSE) and unfolded protein response element (UPRE), and activate the transcription of genes coding for chaperone proteins that promote protein folding (eg, Grp78, Grp94, Mdg1/Erdj4, Herp) and for proteins that assist in degradation of misfolded proteins (eg, EPR degradation-enhancing α-mannosidase-like protein [EDEM]).

On excessive EPR stress, the three activated sensors, that is, PERK, ATF6, and IRE1α, may act in concert to initiate apoptosis (Malhi and Kaufman, 2011). While PERK-catalyzed phosphorylation of eIF2α decreases the synthesis of most proteins (as stated above), it increases the synthesis of some, including that of ATF4. This TF (as well as ATF6) promotes the expression of CHOP, yet another TF. CHOP in turn can transcriptionally induce the expression of the proapoptotic Bim protein and the cell surface death receptor TRAIL-2, while inhibiting the expression of the antiapoptotic Bcl-2 protein (see Fig. 3-19). The activated IRE1α may initiate cell death via recruiting the adaptor protein TNF receptor-associated factor-2 (TRAF2), with subsequent activation of apoptosis signal-regulating kinase 1 (ASK1) and JNK. By phosphorylation, JNK can activate the proapoptotic Bim and inactivate the antiapoptotic Bcl-2 proteins (Malhi and Kaufman, 2011). The IRE1α–TRAF2 complex may also recruit and activate procaspase 12. Alternatively, Ca^{2+} released from the EPR can activate calpains, which cleave the EPR-associated procaspase 12 into active caspase 12. The latter then engages the caspase cascade (see Fig. 3-19) by activating effector caspases therein to sacrifice the cell by apoptosis. Several toxicants have been shown to induce EPR stress in experimental animals and in isolated cells by demonstrating expression of some elements of the UPR on toxicant exposure (Cribb *et al.*, 2005; Nagy *et al.*, 2007; Malhi and Kaufman, 2011).

Induction of Enzymes Repairing DNA—The DNA Damage Response (DDR) DDR is initiated by detection of the DNA damage. Double-stranded DNA breaks are recognized by the MRN complex (the trimer of Mre11, Rad50, and Nbs1 proteins) or the Ku protein (the dimer of Ku70 and Ku80; see the section "Repair of DNA") that bind and activate protein kinases ataxia telangiectasia mutated (ATM) and DNA-PKcs, respectively. A third kinase, ataxia telangiectasia and Rad3-related (ATR), is activated in response to persistent single-stranded DNA coated with replication protein A (RPA), an intermediate during nucleotide excision or recombination DNA repair processes. Directly or through checkpoint kinases (Chk1, Chk2), these kinases phosphorylate p53 (Christmann *et al.*, 2003; McGowan and Russell, 2004), a protein that can play the role of a TF regulating gene expression and the role of an associate protein affecting the function of its interacting protein partner. Normally, p53 is kept inactive and at low levels by its binding protein mdm2 (see Fig. 3-33), which ubiquitinates p53, facilitating its proteasomal degradation. On phosphorylation, p53 escapes from mdm2, allowing its activation and stabilization. Indeed, the levels of p53 protein in cells increase dramatically in response to DNA damage caused by UV or gamma irradiation or genotoxic chemicals. p53 then facilitates DNA repair by a number of mechanisms. For example, mainly by transcriptionally upregulating the cyclin-dependent kinase inhibitor protein p21, p53 arrests cells in G1 phase of the cell cycle (see Fig. 3-33), allowing more time for DNA repair. As a TF, p53 also increases expression of proteins directly involved in DNA repair (Harms *et al.*, 2004). Such proteins include (a) growth arrest and DNA damage inducible (gadd45), which interacts with histones and facilitates access of proteins (eg, topoisomerase) to DNA, (b) XPE and XPC, members of the xeroderma pigmentosum group of proteins important in UV-induced DNA damage recognition before nucleotide excision repair, (c) MSH2 operating in mismatch repair, (d) PCNA that holds DNA polymerase-δ to DNA during DNA replication as well as reparative DNA synthesis in the excision and the recombination repair processes, and (e) a form of ribonucleotide reductase that provides deoxyribonucleotides for sealing DNA gaps. As a partner protein, p53 supports the function of several proteins of the nucleotide excision machinery (eg, TFIH, XPB, XPD). (Other roles p53 plays in apoptosis and in carcinogenesis as a tumor suppressor protein are illustrated in Figs. 3-19 and 3-33 and discussed elsewhere in this chapter.) The DNA-damage-activated protein kinases (ATM, ATR, and DNA-PK) also phosphorylate histone H2AX adjacent to the damage, which then becomes ubiquitinated. These markings in turn recruit repair proteins (including BRCA1) and induce chromatin relaxation for better access of repair enzymes to the lesion. The DDR-initiating kinases have numerous other protein substrates, including other kinases; therefore, DDR may extend to diverse cellular functions. It is important to realize that while both the complex DDR and distinct DNA repair mechanisms (eg, direct repair by MGMT) protect normal cells that suffered DNA damage from transformation into cancer cells (a process to be discussed below), these mechanisms, if remain operative in cancer cells, can protect them from mortal DNA damage inflicted by radiotherapy or chemotherapy, and thereby DDR and DNA repair can contribute to resistance of tumor cells to anticancer treatments.

Adaptive Increase in Tissue Repair—A Proliferative Response
Many toxicants potentially injurious to cells, for example, electrophiles, oxidants, and those inducing oxidative stress, can initiate mitogenic signaling as a prelude to tissue repair via cell replacement. It appears that the need for mitogenesis is sensed by PTP (eg, PTP1B) and the lipid phosphatase PTEN, which contains reactive cysteine thiols at their active site (Rhee *et al.*, 2005). These phosphatases serve as brakes on the growth factor receptor–initiated mitogenic signaling, as PTPs dephosphorylate (and inactivate) the receptors themselves (eg, EGFR, PDGFR, IGFR) as well as some protein kinases (eg, Src and JAK), whereas PTEN dephosphorylates PIP_3, an important second messenger in the PI3K–Akt–IKK–NF-κB pathway (Fig. 3-12). Electrophiles covalently bind to essential cysteine-SH groups in these phosphatases. HOOH can oxidize the critical -SH group in PTEN to an intramolecular disulfide, whereas it oxidizes the -SH group of PTP1B, through sulfenic acid (-S-OH), to a 5-membered cyclic sulfenyl amide species in which the sulfur atom is covalently linked to the nitrogen of the neighboring serine (Rhee *et al.*, 2005). Inactivation of PTPs and PTEN, which decrease the proliferative signal transduction, amplifies intracellular signaling for mitosis and survival.

It has been known for some time that oxidative stress, if not severe, activates the TF NF-κB (Dalton *et al.*, 1999). For example, silica, which can produce ROS on its surface, activates NF-κB as well as PI3K when added to various cells (Castranova, 2004). In light of new information discussed above, NF-κB activation is now attributed to the fact that this TF is situated downstream of growth factor receptors (which are negatively controlled by the ROS-sensitive PTP) and PIP_3 (which is eliminated by ROS-sensitive PTEN) (Fig. 3-12). Furthermore, NF-κB is at the focal point of proliferative and prolife signaling, as it transactivates genes producing cell cycle accelerators (eg, cyclin D1 and c-Myc) and apoptosis inhibitors (eg, antiapoptotic Bcl proteins and the caspase IAPs) (Karin, 2006). In addition, NF-κB also transactivates the genes of ferritin, GST, SOD1, HO-1, a proteasome subunit, and gadd45, facilitating detoxication and molecular repair. All these roles of NF-κB explain its involvement in tolerance to chemically induced tissue injury, resistance against cholestatic liver injury caused by bile acids, adaptation to ionizing radiation, as well as the phenomenon termed preconditioning. This is a tolerance to ischemic tissue injury (eg, myocardial infarction), a tolerance induced by temporarily enhanced ROS formation evoked by hyperoxia or brief periods of ischemia–reperfusion.

In addition to signaling for cell replacement in damaged tissue—in which NF-κB plays a leading role—the growing cells need to boost protein synthesis. This is done under the control of the protein kinase mTOR. As shown in Fig. 3-29, mTOR activation results from signaling through both pathways coupled to growth factor receptors, that is, the MAPK pathway leading to phosphorylation of the MAPK isoform Erk and the PI3K pathway leading to phosphorylation of Akt (see Fig. 3-12). Importantly,

these pathways are subject to activation in response to oxidant or electrophile exposure as they are controlled by PTPs and PTEN (Fig. 3-12). Erk and Akt protein kinases activate mTOR through a complex mechanism (Fig. 3-29), and mTOR in turn phosphorylates and regulates effectors of protein synthesis, such as the translation repressor protein 4EBP1 and the protein kinase S6K, which modifies ribosomes increasing their translational efficiency (Shaw and Cantley, 2006). As described in the sections "Adaptation to Hypoxia—The Hypoxia Response" and "Adaptation to Energy Depletion—The Energy Stress Response," mTOR signaling is switched off in the cell to save energy as a measure to adapt to the energy shortage caused by hypoxia or toxic impairment of ATP synthesis.

Adaptation by Compensating Dysfunction Dysfunctions caused by toxicants or drug overdose manifested at the level of organism (eg, hypoxia), organ system (eg, hypotension and hypertension), or organ (eg, renal tubular dysfunction) may evoke compensatory mechanisms.

Adaptation to Hypoxia—The Hypoxia Response When O_2 delivery is impaired and hypoxia persists for more than a few minutes, a response involving gene expression alteration is initiated. This reaction is mainly orchestrated by hypoxia-inducible factor-1α (HIF-1α), a ubiquitous TF whose activity and cellular abundance is greatly increased in response to hypoxia (Maxwell and Salnikow, 2004; Pouyssegur *et al.*, 2006). HIF-1α is maintained at very low intracellular levels because of continuous hydroxylation of its 2 proline residues by HIF-prolyl hydroxylases. This permits a ubiquitin ligase subunit (called von Hippel Lindau protein [VHL]) to capture HIF-1α and initiate its destruction by proteasomal degradation. Indeed, HIF-1α is one of the shortest lived proteins with a half-life of less than 5 minutes. In addition, HIF-1α is kept transcriptionally inactive by hydroxylation at one of its asparagine residues by HIF-asparagine hydroxylases, which prevents interaction of HIF-1α with transcriptional coactivators, such as p300 and CREB-binding protein (CBP). These two types of HIF hydroxylases are O_2 sensors: they use O_2 as a substrate to carry out proline/asparagine hydroxylations with concomitant oxidative decarboxylation of 2-oxoglutarate to succinate, with the K_M of O_2 being close to the ambient O_2 concentration. As the O_2 concentration falls, decreases in the hydroxylation rate of HIF-1α as well as its VHL-mediated ubiquitination and proteasomal degradation occur, and this increases its abundance and transcriptional activity. HIF hydroxylases belong to the Fe^{2+} and ascorbate-dependent dioxygenases (the largest group of nonheme oxidases); therefore, not only hypoxia but also Fe^{2+} deficiency impairs their activity. The latter feature explains why iron chelators (eg, deferoxamine) or Fe^{2+}-mimicking metal ions (eg, Co^{2+} and Ni^{2+}) also induce and activate HIF-1α (Maxwell and Salnikow, 2004). When induced after hypoxic conditions, HIF-1α dimerizes with HIF-1β (also called Arnt, which, coincidentally, is the dimerization partner for the Ah receptor as well). The HIF complex transactivates a vast array of genes with hypoxia response element (HRE) in their promoter. Many of the gene products assist in acclimatization to hypoxia (Pouyssegur *et al.*, 2006). These include (1) erythropoietin (EPO) that is produced largely in kidney and activates erythropoiesis in bone marrow, (2) proteins involved in iron homeostasis (eg, transferrin, TFR, ceruloplasmin, and heme oxygenase) that may increase availability of iron for erythropoiesis, (3) vascular endothelial growth factor (VEGF) and angiopoietin-2 that stimulate blood vessel growth (ie, angiogenesis), (4) proteins facilitating anaerobic ATP synthesis from glucose (ie, glycolysis), such as the glucose transporter GLUT1 and

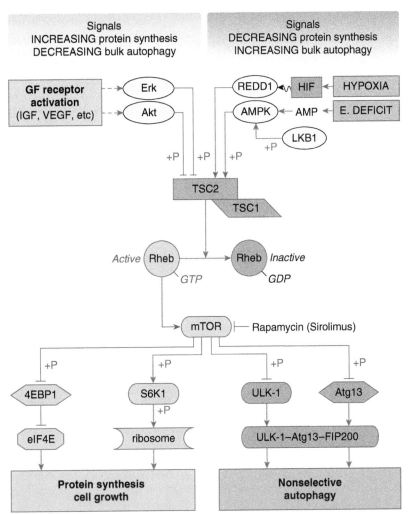

Figure 3-29. *Modulation of protein synthesis and autophagy by signaling through the mTOR kinase pathway as a means for cellular adaptation— increased signaling via mTOR promotes protein synthesis at translational level and suppresses autophagy, thereby permitting cell growth and proliferation, whereas attenuated signaling via mTOR permits energy saving (by halting protein synthesis) and a desperate attempt for energy generation (by starting autophagy) when hypoxia, nutrient shortage, or toxic injury causes energy deficit.* Growth factor receptors signaling via either the MAPK pathway (leading to phosphorylation of Erk) or the PI3K pathway (leading to phosphorylation of Akt) (see Fig. 3-12) activate the serine/threonine kinase, mammalian target of rapamycin (mTOR; rapamycin is also called sirolimus) by an indirect mechanism. The protein kinases Erk and Akt catalyze inactivating phosphorylation of TSC2, a member of TSC1/2 complex. TSC2 is a GTPase-activating protein whose substrate is Rheb, a small G protein (Ras homologue), which is active in the GTP-bound form and inactive in the GDP-bound form. With its GTPase activating capacity blocked by Erk or Akt, TSC2 cannot convert Rheb-GTP into inactive Rheb-GDP, and thus Rheb-GTP activates mTOR. In turn, mTOR phosphorylates 2 substrates that are necessary to initiate translation of mRNA into proteins, that is: (1) eukaryotic initiation factor 4E-binding protein-1 (4EBP1), which thus releases the translational initiation factor eIF4E, and (2) ribosomal protein S6 kinase-1 (S6K1), which phosphorylates ribosomal protein S6, thereby increasing translational efficiency of mRNAs that encode ribosomal proteins ("ribosomal biogenesis"). Simultaneously, mTOR phosphorylates and inactivates unc-51-like kinase-1 (ULK-1) and Atg13, thereby preventing nonselective or bulk autophagy that is dependent on formation of the stable complex of ULK-1, Atg13, and focal adhesion kinase family-interacting protein of 200 kDa (FIP200).

Protein synthesis for cell growth and proliferation is halted, whereas bulk autophagy is facilitated in times of energy deficit resulting from hypoxia, nutrient shortage, or toxic impairment of ATP production. Then AMP levels increase and AMP binds to the AMP-activated protein kinase (AMPK), facilitating its phosphorylation by protein kinase LKB1. Activated AMPK phosphorylates TSC2 (at a site different from that targeted by Akt and Erk), thereby increasing the GTPase-activating capacity of TSC2. This in turn switches Rheb off, making mTOR inactive. This suspends mRNA translation and starts autophagy. Hypoxia can initiate this process in a more specific way as well, that is, via stabilization of the hypoxia-inducible factor (HIF). This transcription factor induces the synthesis of REDD1 (by a mechanism that is not completely understood), which activates TSC2. See text for further details on cellular responses to hypoxia and energy deficit.

some glycolytic enzymes, (5) proteins that correct acidosis caused by glycolytic overproduction of lactate (eg, a monocarboxylate transporter and a Na$^+$/H$^+$ exchanger for export of lactate and H$^+$, respectively), (6) the REDD1 signal transducer protein that initiates a complex signaling pathway that leads to suspension of the ATP-consuming protein synthesis via inactivation of the protein kinase mTOR (Fig. 3-29), and (7) many other proteins, such as

those that promote ECM remodeling (eg, matrix metalloproteinase-2) and cell migration (perhaps to facilitate access of the cells to the blood vessel), as well as BNIP3, a proapoptotic MOM protein that is also involved in autophagy of mitochondria in reticulocytes (perhaps to induce apoptosis of cells subjected to extreme hypoxia and to facilitate the terminal differentiation of red blood cells). Experiments on mice kept in low O$_2$ environment (hypoxic preconditioning) demonstrated that HIF-1α became stabilized in the retina of these animals, hypoxia-responsive genes (EPO, VEGF) were induced, and the retina became resistant to light toxicity (Grimm et al., 2005). Adaptation to hypoxia also occurs, for example, in response to high-altitude hypoxia, chronic cardiorespiratory dysfunction, and ischemic preconditioning, along with other adaptive responses discussed above. The hypoxia response is also expected to develop as a result of toxicities causing hypoxia acutely or subacutely (eg, respiratory muscle weakness after organophosphate intoxication, diquat-induced pulmonary injury) or as a delayed sequel (eg, respiratory surface restriction in hard metal disease).

Adaptation to Energy Depletion—The Energy Stress Response
Cells try to maintain their adenosine nucleotide pool in triphosphorylated, energized state, which is in the form of ATP. When the rephosphorylation rate of AMP and ADP to ATP does not keep up with the rate of ATP use, because, for example, oxidative phosphorylation is impaired or ATP use for muscle contraction or ion pumping is excessive, the ratio of AMP to ATP increases. A cellular mechanism has evolved to sense this menacing energy deficit and, in order to compensate, boosts ATP production and curtails ATP consumption (Hardie et al., 2006). The sensor is a ubiquitous heterotrimeric intracellular protein complex called AMP-activated protein kinase (AMPK). AMP strongly activates AMPK allosterically, and also by making it susceptible for phosphorylation by protein kinase LKB1 (or by the calmodulin-dependent protein kinase kinase [CaMKK] in neurons). The phosphorylated, and thus activated AMPK, targets 2 sets of proteins. One set includes those whose activation facilitates ATP production from catabolism of glucose and fatty acids as well as by promoting the biogenesis of mitochondria. For example, AMPK activation increases (a) glucose uptake (via recruiting to the cell membrane or activating glucose transporters GLUT4 and GLUT1), (b) glycolysis (via phosphorylation and activation of 6-phosphofructo-2-kinase [PFK-2] whose product, fructose-2,6-bisphosphate, is a glycolytic activator), and (c) fatty acid oxidation in mitochondria (via phosphorylation and inactivation of acetyl-CoA-carboxylase, whose product, malonyl-CoA, is an allosteric inhibitor of carnitine palmitoyltransferase-1 [CPT-1], which mediates uptake of long-chain fatty acid CoA esters into mitochondria). Another set of proteins, which are inactivated by AMPK (directly or indirectly), includes those that are involved in biosynthetic ATP-consuming reactions. Thus, AMPK inhibits (a) glycogen synthesis via phosphorylation and inactivation of glycogen synthase, (b) lipid synthesis by phosphorylating and inactivating acetyl-CoA-carboxylase, whose product, malonyl-CoA, is an essential substrate for fatty acid synthesis, (c) cholesterol synthesis by phosphorylating and inactivating HMG-CoA reductase, (d) glucose synthesis via inactivating phosphorylation of a transcriptional coactivator, TORC2, which then decreases expression of key gluconeogenetic enzymes, such as phosphoenolpyruvate carboxykinase (PEPCK) and glucose-6-phosphatase, and (e) protein synthesis, and thus cell growth, by inhibiting the protein kinase mTOR (Fig. 3-29). AMPK-mediated modulation of cellular energy supply and consumption involves mainly kinase reactions rather than new protein synthesis. Therefore, this adaptation is a rapid process. It can be a response to any harmful condition that compromises oxidative phosphorylation, such as hypoxia, hypoglycemia (especially in neurons), and chemically induced mitochondrial toxicity. For example, cells exposed to arsenite exhibit rapid increases in the AMP/ATP ratio and AMPK activity, with concomitant declines in HMG-CoA reductase activity as well as fatty acid and cholesterol synthesis (Corton et al., 1994).

Apart from the above-described rapid AMPK-dependent reprogramming of the cell's intermediary metabolism from energy-consuming operation to the energy-producing mode, there is an ultimate means for the cell to generate fuel for ATP production in case of nutrient shortage. This slower process involves consumption of the cell's own constituents (lipid droplets, glycogen particles, proteins, and organelles) by nonselective or bulk autophagy (Rabinowitz and White, 2010) involving their lysosomal hydrolysis in order to gain fuel (amino acids, fatty acids, nucleosides, and carbohydrates). An essential actor in this form of autophagy is a protein complex of unc-51-like kinase-1 (ULK-1), autophagy-related protein 13 (Atg13), and focal adhesion kinase family-interacting protein of 200 kDa (FIP200), which is an initiator of autophagosome formation (Fig. 3-29). When nutrients are abundant, the ULK-1–Atg13–FIP200 complex associates with mTOR complex 1 (mTORC1), with both ULK-1 and mTOR kinase being bound by Raptor, a scaffolding protein in mTORC1. Then mTOR phosphorylates and inactivates ULK-1 and Atg13, thus inhibiting autophagy. In nutrient shortage, signaling pathways, such as those activated by AMP and hypoxia (see Fig. 3-29), inactivate mTOR kinase, thereby forcing mTORC1 to release the complex of ULK-1–Atg13–FIP200, which in turn initiates autophagosome nucleation (Hosokawa et al., 2009).

In summary, mTOR kinase is a key regulator of the cell's energy homeostasis, permitting or limiting cell growth according to availability of resources, the use of which can also be controlled by mTOR through switching autophagy on and off. In the presence of abundant nutrients and growth factors, mTOR is activated, thereby promoting cell growth and metabolic activity while suppressing nonselective autophagy. In nutrient deprivation or stress (eg, energetic failure, hypoxia), signaling pathways inactivate mTOR kinase activity. This both suppresses cell growth to reduce energy demand and induces autophagy to enable stress adaptation and survival (Fig. 3-29).

After surveying the major cellular adaptation mechanisms to toxicants, it is easy to recognize that one noxious effect may initiate several adaptive responses. For example, cells exposed to a hypoxic environment can rapidly respond with both AMPK-mediated program of energy stabilization and HIF-1α-directed adaptation to oxygen shortage. Theoretically, an electrophile toxicant that can bind covalently to cellular macromolecules and can also generate oxidative stress, such as a redox cycling quinone, would be expected to induce a number of adaptive processes, including the electrophile response, the heat-shock response, the EPR stress response, the DDR, and the proliferative response, and if it compromises ATP synthesis as well, it even induces the energy stress response.

Adaptation by Neurohumoral Mechanisms There are numerous adaptive responses to dysfunctions of organs or organ systems that are mediated by humoral or neuronal signals between cells located in the same or different organs. For example, the rapid hyperventilation evoked by acute hypoxia or HCN inhalation is mediated by a neural reflex initiated by glomus cells in the carotid body. These chemosensitive cells generate a Ca^{2+} signal via the above-described AMP sensor, AMPK, which becomes activated by hypoxia or CN$^-$ through impairment of oxidative phosphorylation in these cells, causing rise in the AMP/ATP ratio (Evans et al., 2005). Besides CN$^-$, mitochondrial electron transport inhibitors (eg, rotenone, antimycin A, myxothiazole), uncouplers (eg, 2,4-dinitrophenol), or ATP-synthase inhibitors (eg, oligomycin) (see Table 3-6 and Fig. 3-16) as well as AMPK activators mimic the response to hypoxia in these cells. There are numerous other neurohumoral adaptive mechanisms in the body, such as the sympathetic reflex as well as activation of the renin–angiotensin–aldosterone system in response to hypotension, and the feedback systems between endocrine glands and the hypothalamus–hypophysis, which correct abnormal hormone levels. For information on these and other mechanisms, the reader is referred to textbooks of physiology.

When Repair and Adaptation Fail

When Repair Fails Although repair mechanisms operate at molecular, cellular, and tissue levels, for various reasons they often fail to provide protection against injury. First, the fidelity of the repair mechanisms is not absolute (eg, the nonhomologous end joining that restores DNA DSB), making it possible for some lesions to be overlooked or erroneously fixed. However, repair fails most typically when the damage overwhelms the repair mechanisms, as when protein thiols are oxidized faster than they can be reduced. In other instances, the capacity of repair may become exhausted when necessary enzymes or cofactors are consumed. For example, alkylation of DNA may lead to consumption of MGMT (a selfsacrificing enzyme), lipid peroxidation can deplete α-tocopherol, and overproduction of oxidized or otherwise damaged proteins can exhaust the pool of ubiquitin. Sometimes the toxicant-induced injury adversely affects the repair process itself. For example, ethanol generates ROS via CYP2E1 that impairs the proteasomal removal of damaged proteins. Autophagic removal of cell constituents may be compromised by lysosomotropic drugs (lipophilic amines) that increase the pH in these organelles, thus decreasing the activity of lysosomal hydrolases. This may underlie the mechanism of chloroquine-induced myopathy in rats. Thiol-reactive chemicals may inactivate ubiquitin-activating enzymes (E1), ubiquitin-conjugating enzymes (E2), and the HECT domain-containing ubiquitin ligases (E3), each of which contains a catalytically active cysteine, as well as the lysosomal cysteine proteases (eg, cathepsins B, H, and L), thereby compromising the clearance of damaged proteins by both the UPS and autophagy. Indeed, diminished proteolysis occurs in hepatocytes exposed to toxic concentrations of acetaminophen. These repair mechanisms are especially important in neurons, as genetic deletion of proteins mediating UPS and autophagy causes accumulation of intraneuronal inclusions, neuronal loss, or neurodegeneration. In fact, human neurodegenerative diseases can be directly attributed to some dysfunction of the UPS and/or autophagy (Bedford et al., 2011). The finding that individual overexpression of some E2 and E3 enzymes confers resistance to methylmercury toxicity in yeast (Hwang et al., 2006) lends some support to the speculation that impairment of the UPS and/or autophagy might contribute to the neurotoxicity of methylmercury. After exposure to necrogenic chemicals, mitosis of surviving cells may be blocked and restoration of the tissue becomes impossible (Mehendale, 2005). Finally, some types of toxic injuries cannot be repaired effectively, as occurs when xenobiotics are covalently bound to proteins or when protein carbonyls are formed. Thus, toxicity is manifested when repair of the initial injury fails because the repair mechanisms become overwhelmed, exhausted, or impaired or are genuinely inefficient.

It is also possible that repair contributes to toxicity. This may occur in a passive manner, for example, if excessive amounts of NAD$^+$ are cleaved by PARP when this enzyme assists in repairing broken DNA strands, or when too much NAD(P)H is consumed for the repair of oxidized proteins and endogenous reductants. Either event can compromise oxidative phosphorylation, which is also dependent on the supply of reduced cofactors (see Fig. 3-16), thus causing or aggravating ATP depletion that contributes to cell injury.

Excision repair of DNA and reacylation of lipids also contribute to cellular deenergization and injury by consuming significant amounts of ATP. However, repair also may play an active role in toxicity. This is observed after chronic tissue injury, when the repair process goes astray and leads to uncontrolled proliferation instead of tissue remodeling. Such proliferation of cells may yield neoplasia, whereas overproduction of ECM results in fibrosis. A specific case is when the cellular repair processes that normally degrade damaged proteins, such as the UPS and the autophagy pathway, become inappropriately stimulated by adverse signaling, causing degradation of ordinary intracellular proteins. This occurs in muscle wasting induced by glucocorticoids, such as cortisol and dexamethasone. This condition appears to be secondary to suppression of the growth-promoting IGF-1–PI3K–Akt signaling that leaves FoxO TFs unchecked, which in turn increase the expression of muscle-specific ubiquitin ligases (MAFbx, also called atrogin-1, and MuRF1) as well as several components of the autophagy–lysosome pathway (Fig. 3-30).

When Adaptation Fails Although adaptation mechanisms, such as the Nrf2-mediated electrophile response and the NF-κB-induced proliferative reaction, boost the capacity of the organism to withstand toxicant exposure and damage, excessive exposure can overwhelm these protective responses. Moreover, toxicants may impair the adaptive process. For example, moderate oxidative stress activates NF-κB, AP-1, and Nrf2 to initiate adaptive protection. However, extensive oxidant exposure aborts this program because it leads to oxidation of thiol groups in the DNA-binding domain of these TFs (Hansen et al., 2006). Similarly, Hg^{2+} can incapacitate NF-κB, thus inhibiting the prolife program activated by this TF. This promotes Hg^{2+}-induced renal tubular cell injury (Dieguez-Acuna et al., 2004).

Some adaptive mechanisms may be harmful under extreme conditions. For example, acute tubular injury, which impairs tubular reabsorption and causes polyuria, triggers a tubuloglomerular feedback mechanism that reduces glomerular blood flow and filtration. Ultimately, this may precipitate anuric renal failure. It is possible that an adaptive mechanism that is beneficial in the short term may become harmful when forced to operate for a prolonged period of time. Bulk autophagy likely contributes to lethal wasting syndrome induced by TCDD in experimental animals. Chronic inflammation, tissue injury, or cancer may lead to iron deficiency and anemia because IL-6 (the acute-phase-triggering cytokine overproduced in these conditions) upregulates hepcidin secretion from the liver, which in turn reduces intestinal iron absorption. As discussed earlier, NF-κB activation is indispensable for repair via proliferation of the acutely injured tissue. However, NF-κB also targets cytokine genes, and the cytokines (eg, TNF, IL-1β) in turn activate NF-κB through their receptors (see Fig. 3-12). This vicious cycle may lead to chronic inflammation and cancer when repetitive tissue injury maintains NF-κB signaling (Karin, 2006). This occurs after occupational exposure to silica (Castranova, 2004). Sustained activation of HIF-1α in tumors facilitates invasiveness, in part by increasing VEGF expression and angiogenesis. In the kidney, HIF-1α may be involved in fibrogenesis, as it targets critical genes, such as tissue inhibitor of metalloproteinase-1 (TIMP-1).

Toxicity Resulting from Inappropriate Repair and Adaptation

Like repair, dysrepair occurs at the molecular, cellular, and tissue levels. Some toxicities involve dysrepair at an isolated level. For example, hypoxemia develops after exposure to methemoglobin-forming chemicals if the amount of methemoglobin produced overwhelms

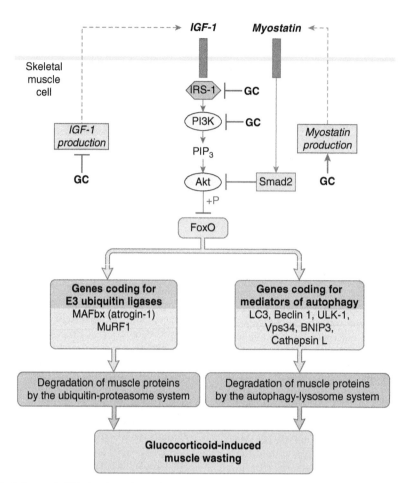

Figure 3-30. *A model of glucocorticoid-induced muscle wasting: by attenuating the IGF-1–PI3K–Akt growth signaling pathway, glucocorticoids disinhibit FoxO transcription factors that upregulate the degradation of muscle proteins by both the ubiquitin–proteasome system and the autophagy–lysosome pathway.* The trophic condition of the skeletal muscle is positively regulated by IGF-1, a muscle anabolic growth factor. IGF-1 acts in autocrine and paracrine manner on its tyrosine kinase receptor to trigger signaling through insulin receptor substrate 1 (IRS-1), phosphatidylinositol 3-kinase (PI3K), and the lipid mediator phosphatidylinositol (3,4,5)-trisphosphate (PIP$_3$), causing activation of the serine/threonine protein kinase Akt (see also Fig. 3-12). As shown in Fig. 3-29, Akt activation leads to activation of mTOR, which boosts protein translation and halts bulk autophagy. In addition, the active Akt also phosphorylates and inactivates Forkhead box O transcription factors (eg, FoxO1 and FoxO3), thereby preventing them from translocating into the nucleus and activating the expression of genes whose products would mediate degradation of muscle proteins. These mechanisms collectively contribute to muscle hypertrophy.

Glucocorticoids (GC) induce muscle atrophy mainly by suppressing the IGF-1–PI3K–Akt signaling pathway in the skeletal muscle. Under this condition the phosphorylation of FoxO by Akt ceases, and then the nonphosphorylated FoxO translocates into the nucleus and activates the transcription of its target genes. Among these are the genes coding for muscle-specific E3 ubiquitin ligases, that is, muscle atrophy F-box (MAFbx, also called atrogin-1) and muscle ring finger 1 (MuRF1). By ubiquitinating their substrates, which include structural proteins (eg, myosin heavy chain) and regulatory proteins (eg, the transcription factor MyoD and the translation initiation factor eIF3f), these ubiquitin ligases promote their proteasomal degradation. FoxO also turns on the other degradative machinery, the autophagy–lysosome system (Mehrpour *et al.*, 2010), by increasing the expression of a number of its components, such as LC3, Beclin 1, ULK-1, Vps34, BNIP3, and cathepsin L (see more details in the sections "Cellular Repair" and "Adaptation to Energy Depletion—The Energy Stress Response").

GC suppress the IGF-1–PI3K–Akt signaling by multiple mechanisms. They decrease production of IGF-1 by the muscle, downregulate the expression of IRS-1, and inhibit PI3K activity (apparently by direct interaction of the activated GC receptor with the regulatory subunit of PI3K). In addition, GC upregulate the expression of myostatin in the muscle probably by downregulating the expression of miRNA-27a and b, which target myostatin mRNA (see elsewhere). Myostatin is a TGF-β family member protein, which is a negative regulator of muscle mass. It acts by both endocrine and paracrine fashion on its receptor (similar to item 8 in Fig. 3-12) and activates Smad2, which inhibits Akt (Glass, 2010). Other mechanisms may also contribute to GC-induced muscle wasting (Hasselgren *et al.*, 2010).

the capacity of methemoglobin reductase. Because this repair enzyme is deficient at early ages, neonates are especially sensitive to chemicals that cause methemoglobinemia. Formation of cataracts purportedly involves inefficiency or impairment of lenticular repair enzymes, such as the endopeptidases and exopeptidases, which normally reduce oxidized crystalline and hydrolyze damaged proteins to their constituent amino acids. Dysrepair also is thought to contribute to the formation of Heinz bodies, which are protein aggregates formed in oxidatively stressed and aged red blood cells. Defective proteolytic degradation of the immunogenic

trifluoroacetylated proteins may make halothane-anesthetized patients victims of halothane hepatitis.

Several types of toxicity involve failed and/or derailed repairs at different levels before they become apparent. This is true for the most severe toxic injuries, such as tissue necrosis, fibrosis, and chemical carcinogenesis.

Tissue Necrosis As discussed above, several mechanisms may lead to cell death. Most or all involve molecular damage that is potentially reversible by repair mechanisms. If repair mechanisms operate effectively, they may prevent cell injury or at least retard its progression. For example, prooxidant toxicants cause no lipid fragmentation in microsomal membranes until α-tocopherol is depleted in those membranes. Membrane damage ensues when this endogenous antioxidant, which can repair lipids containing peroxyl radical groups (Fig. 3-24), becomes unavailable (Scheschonka et al., 1990). This suggests that cell injury progresses toward cell necrosis if molecular repair mechanisms are inefficient or the molecular damage is not readily reversible.

Progression of cell injury to tissue necrosis can be intercepted by 2 repair mechanisms working in concert: apoptosis and cell proliferation. As discussed above, injured cells can initiate apoptosis, which counteracts the progression of the toxic injury. Apoptosis does this by preventing necrosis of injured cells and the consequent inflammatory response, which may cause injury by releasing cytotoxic mediators. Indeed, the activation of Kupffer cells, the source of such mediators in the liver, by the administration of bacterial LPS (endotoxin) greatly aggravates the hepatotoxicity of galactosamine. In contrast, when the Kupffer cells are selectively eliminated by pretreatment of rats with gadolinium chloride, the necrotic effect of carbon tetrachloride is markedly alleviated (Edwards et al., 1993). Blockade of Kupffer cell function with glycine (via the inhibitory glycine receptor; see item 4 in Fig. 3-15) also protects the liver from alcohol-induced injury (Yin et al., 1998).

Another important repair process that can halt the propagation of toxic injury is proliferation of cells adjacent to the injured cells. This response is initiated soon after cellular injury. A surge in mitosis in the liver of rats administered a low (non-necrogenic) dose of carbon tetrachloride is detectable within a few hours. This early cell division is thought to be instrumental in the rapid and complete restoration of the injured tissue and the prevention of necrosis. This hypothesis is corroborated by the finding that in rats pretreated with chlordecone, which blocks the early cell proliferation in response to carbon tetrachloride, a normally nonnecrogenic dose of carbon tetrachloride causes hepatic necrosis (Mehendale, 2005). The sensitivity of a tissue to injury and the capacity of the tissue for repair are apparently two independent variables, both influencing the final outcome of the effect of injurious chemical—that is, whether tissue restitution ensues with survival or tissue necrosis occurs with death. For example, variations in tissue repair capacity among species and strains of animals appear to be responsible for certain variations in the lethality of hepatotoxicants (Soni and Mehendale, 1998).

It appears that the efficiency of repair is an important determinant of the dose–response relationship for toxicants that cause tissue necrosis. Following chemically induced liver or kidney injury, the intensity of tissue repair increases up to a threshold dose, restraining injury, whereupon it is inhibited, allowing unrestrained progression of injury (Mehendale, 2005). Impaired signaling to mitosis (see Fig. 3-12), caused by high tissue concentrations of toxicants (eg, acetaminophen in the liver or S-(1,2-dichlorovinyl)-L-cysteine in the kidney) and their reactive metabolites may account for lagging tissue repair (Boulares et al., 1999; Vaidya et al., 2003), but maintenance of DNA and protein synthesis, mitotic machinery, and energy supply may also be impaired at high-dose chemical exposures. That is, tissue necrosis is caused by a certain dose of a toxicant not only because that dose ensures sufficient concentration of the ultimate toxicant at the target site to initiate injury but also because that quantity of toxicant causes a degree of damage sufficient to compromise repair, allowing for progression of the injury. Experimental observations with hepatotoxicants indicate that apoptosis and cell proliferation are operative with latent tissue injury caused by low (non-necrogenic) doses of toxicants, but

are inhibited with severe injury induced by high (necrogenic) doses. For example, 1,1-dichloroethylene, carbon tetrachloride, and thioacetamide all induce apoptosis in the liver at low doses, but cause hepatic necrosis after high-dose exposure (Corcoran et al., 1994). Similarly, there is an early mitotic response in the liver to low-dose carbon tetrachloride, but this response is absent after administration of the solvent at necrogenic doses (Mehendale, 2005). This suggests that tissue necrosis occurs because the injury overwhelms and disables the repair mechanisms, including (1) repair of damaged molecules, (2) elimination of damaged cells by apoptosis, and (3) replacement of lost cells by cell division.

As in tissues and organs several types of cells are integrated and support the function of each other, toxic injury to different cell types may exacerbate the tissue damage and promote its progression to tissue necrosis. This principle is exemplified by the acetaminophen-induced hemorrhagic hepatic necrosis. Even before causing manifest injury to the parenchymal liver cells, acetaminophen overdose in mice has a deleterious effect on the sinusoidal endothelial cells (McCuskey, 2008). These cells swell and lose normal function (eg, endocytosis); their fenestrae coalesce into gaps that permit red blood cells to penetrate into the space of Disse. The subsequent collapse of sinusoids reduces blood flow, thus impairing oxygen and nutrient supply of hepatocytes that also endure direct damage by the reactive metabolite of acetaminophen.

Fibrosis Fibrosis is a pathologic condition characterized by excessive deposition of an ECM of abnormal composition. Hepatic fibrosis, or cirrhosis, results from chronic consumption of ethanol or high-dose retinol (vitamin A), treatment with methotrexate, and intoxication with hepatic necrogens such as carbon tetrachloride and iron. Pulmonary fibrosis is induced by drugs such as bleomycin and amiodarone and prolonged inhalation of oxygen or mineral particles. Doxorubicin may cause cardiac fibrosis, whereas drugs acting as agonists on 5-HT_{2B} receptors of human valvular interstitial cells, such as bromocriptine, ergotamine, methysergide, and fenfluramine after long-term use as well as 5-HT itself when overproduced in carcinoid syndrome, induce proliferative valve disease with fibrosis. Exposure to high doses of ionizing radiation induces fibrosis in many organs. Most of these agents generate free radicals and cause chronic cell injury.

Fibrosis is a specific manifestation of dysrepair of the chronically injured tissue. As discussed above, cellular injury initiates a surge in cellular proliferation and ECM production, which normally ceases when the injured tissue is remodeled. If increased production of ECM is not halted, fibrosis develops.

The cells that manufacture the ECM during tissue repair (eg, stellate cells and myofibroblasts in liver, mesangial cells in the kidney, fibroblast-like cells in lungs and skin) are the ones that overproduce the matrix in fibrosis. These cells are controlled and phenotypically altered ("activated") by cytokines and growth factors secreted by nonparenchymal cells, including themselves (see Fig. 3-26). TGF-β appears to be the major mediator of fibrogenesis, although other factors are also involved. These include growth factors, such as connective tissue growth factor (CTGF, a TGF-β-induced growth factor) and PDGF, vasoactive peptides, such as endothelin-1 and angiotensin-II, and the adipocyte-derived hormone leptin (Lotersztajn et al., 2005). The evidence is compelling to indicate that TGF-β, acting through its receptor (item 8 in Fig. 3-12), and receptor-activated TFs (Smad2 and 3), is a highly relevant causative factor of fibrosis. For example, subcutaneous injection of TGF-β induces local fibrosis, whereas overexpression of TGF-β in transgenic mice produces hepatic fibrosis. Smad3-null mice are relatively resistant to radiation-induced cutaneous fibrosis, bleomycin-induced pulmonary fibrosis, and CCl_4-induced hepatic fibrosis. TGF-β antagonists, such as anti-TGF-β immunoglobulin and decorin, as well as Smad3 antagonists, such as halofuginone and overexpressed Smad7 protein (which is antagonistic to Smad2 and 3), ameliorate chemically induced fibrogenesis (Flanders, 2004). In several types of experimental fibrosis and in patients with active liver cirrhosis, overexpression of TGF-β in affected tissues has been demonstrated. Specific factors may also be involved in the pathomechanism of chemically induced fibrosis. For example, in alcoholic liver cirrhosis stellate cells may be activated directly by acetaldehyde (formed by alcohol dehydrogenase), by ROS (generated by the ethanol-induced CYP2E1), and by bacterial endotoxin (LPS), which is increasingly absorbed from the gut, the permeability of which is enhanced by chronic alcohol exposure. LPS can stimulate stellate cells both directly and indirectly through Kupffer cells (see Fig. 3-26) because both cells express TLR through which LPS acts.

The increased expression of TGF-β is a common response mediating regeneration of the ECM after an acute injury. However, whereas TGF-β production ceases when repair is complete, this does not occur when tissue injury leads to fibrosis. Failure to halt TGF-β overproduction could be caused by continuous injury or a defect in the regulation of TGF-β. Indeed, after acute CCl_4-induced liver injury, hepatic stellate cells exhibit a TGF-β-mediated induction of Smad7 (which purportedly terminates the fibrotic signal by inhibiting activation of Smad2 and Smad3 by TGF-β receptor); however, after chronic injury, Smad7 induction fails to occur (Flanders, 2004).

The fibrotic action of TGF-β is due to increased production and decreased degradation of ECM components. TGF-β stimulates the synthesis of individual ECM components (eg, collagens) by specific target cells via the Smad pathway (see Fig. 3-12) and also by down-regulation of the transcription of miR-29 miRNA family members, which inhibit the translation of collagen. Downregulation of miR-29 family members occurs in murine hepatic stellate cells exposed to TGF-β, in the stellate cells of mice with hepatic fibrosis induced by CCl_4 or bile duct ligation, and in the liver of patients with advanced liver cirrhosis (Roderburg *et al.*, 2011). TGF-β inhibits ECM degradation by disproportionately increasing the expression of inhibitor proteins that antagonize ECM-degrading enzymes, such as TIMP-1 and plasminogen activator inhibitor-1 (PAI-1), compared with the expression of ECM-degrading metalloproteinases (Arthur *et al.*, 1999; Flanders, 2004). Interestingly, TGF-β induces transcription of its own gene in target cells (Flanders, 2004), suggesting that the TGF-β produced by these cells can amplify in an autocrine manner the production of the ECM. This positive feedback (autoinduction) may facilitate fibrogenesis.

Fibrosis involves not only excessive accumulation of the ECM but also changes in its composition. The basement membrane components, such as collagen IV and laminin, as well as the fibrillar-type collagens (collagen I and III), which confer rigidity to tissues, increase disproportionately during fibrogenesis (Gressner, 1992).

Fibrosis is detrimental in a number of ways:

1. The scar compresses and may ultimately obliterate the parenchymal cells and blood vessels.
2. Deposition of basement membrane components between the capillary endothelial cells and the parenchymal cells presents a diffusional barrier that contributes to malnutrition of the tissue cells.
3. An increased amount of ECM and its rigidity unfavorably affect the elasticity and flexibility of the whole tissue,

compromising the mechanical function of organs such as the heart and lungs.

4. Furthermore, the altered extracellular environment is sensed by integrins. Through these transmembrane proteins and the coupled intracellular signal transducing networks (see Fig. 3-12), fibrosis may modulate several aspects of cell behavior, including polarity, motility, and gene expression (Raghow, 1994).

Carcinogenesis Chemical carcinogenesis involves malfunctions in various repair and adaptive mechanisms. At the molecular level, a crucial feature of carcinogenesis is altered expression of critical proteins, that is, proto-oncogenic proteins and tumor suppressor proteins. This may result (1) from mutation of critical genes due to insufficient adaptive response to DNA damage and missed DNA repair or (2) from inappropriate transcriptional control at the regulatory regions of critical genes that gives rise to overexpression or underexpression of their products. (Note that the genes that we designate here as "critical" include those that are transcribed into mRNAs that in turn translate into proto-oncogenic or tumor suppressor proteins, as well as those that are transcribed into miRNAs that in turn regulate the translation of proto-oncogenic or tumor suppressor proteins. These proteins will be defined below.) At the cellular level, the fundamental feature of tumorigenesis is proliferation of cells, which may result (1) from failure to execute apoptosis and/or (2) from failure to restrain cell division.

As to be described in more detail later, carcinogenesis entails gene expression alterations initiated by two fundamentally distinct types of mechanisms that often work simultaneously and in concert, that is, genetic and epigenetic mechanisms. Genetic mechanisms bring about a *qualitative* change in gene expression, that is, expression of an altered gene product, a mutant protein, or miRNA, with gain or loss in activity. In contrast, epigenetic mechanisms cause *quantitative* change in gene expression resulting in more or less gene product. Whereas genetic mechanisms alter the coding sequences of critical genes, epigenetic mechanisms eventually influence the regulatory (promoter) region of genes. Thus, chemical and physical insults may induce neoplastic transformation of cells by affecting critical genes through genotoxic and nongenotoxic (ie, epigenetic) mechanisms. However, either mechanism ultimately induces cancer by causing cellular failures in executing apoptosis and/or restraining cell division, thereby giving rise to an uncontrollably proliferating cell population.

Genotoxic Mechanisms of Carcinogenesis: Chemical Damage and Disrepair in the Coding Region of Critical Genes Leading to Mutation Chemicals that react with DNA may cause damage such as adduct formation, oxidative alteration, and strand breakage. In most cases, these lesions are repaired or the injured cells are eliminated. If neither event occurs, a lesion in the parental DNA strand may induce a heritable alteration, or mutation, in the daughter strand during replication. The mutation may remain silent if it does not alter the protein encoded by the mutant gene or if the mutation causes an amino acid substitution that does not affect the function of the protein. Alternatively, the genetic alteration may be incompatible with cell survival. The most unfortunate scenario for the organism occurs when the altered genes express mutant proteins that reprogram cells for multiplication and escaping apoptosis (ie, immortalization). When such cells undergo mitosis, their descendants also have a similar propensity for proliferation. Moreover, because enhanced DNA replication and cell division increases the likelihood of mutations (for reasons discussed below), these cells eventually acquire additional mutations that may further augment their growth advantage over their normal

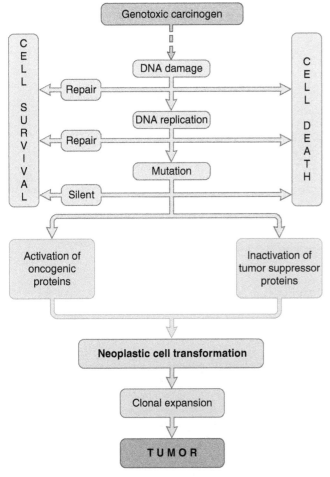

Figure 3-31. *The process of carcinogenesis initiated by genotoxic carcinogens.* The figure indicates that activating mutation of proto-oncogenes that encode permanently active oncoproteins and inactivating mutation of tumor suppressor genes that encode permanently inactive tumor suppressor proteins can cooperate in neoplastic transformation of cells. It is important to realize that overexpression of normal proto-oncogenes (eg, by hypomethylation of their promoter) and underexpression (silencing) of normal tumor suppressor genes (eg, by hypermethylation of their promoter) may also contribute to such transformation (see text for explanation).

counterparts. The final outcome of this process is a nodule, followed by a tumor consisting of rapidly proliferating transformed cells (Fig. 3-31).

The critical role of DNA repair in preventing carcinogenesis is attested by the human heritable disease xeroderma pigmentosum. Affected individuals lack excision repair proteins of the XP series and exhibit a greatly increased incidence of sunlight-induced skin cancers. Cells from these patients are also hypersensitive to DNA-reactive chemicals, including aflatoxin B_1, aromatic amines, polycyclic hydrocarbons, and 4-nitroquinoline-1-oxide (Lehmann and Dean, 1990). Also, mice with ablated PARP gene are extremely sensitive to γ-rays and N-methyl-N-nitrosourea and show genomic instability, as indicated by sister chromatid exchanges and chromatid breaks following genotoxic insult (D'Amours et al., 1999).

A small set of cellular genes is the target for genetic alterations that initiate neoplastic transformations. Included are proto-oncogenes and tumor suppressor genes (Barrett, 1992).

Mutation of Proto-Oncogenes Proto-oncogenes are highly conserved genes encoding proteins that stimulate the progression of cells through the cell cycle, or oppose apoptosis (Smith et al., 1993). The products of proto-oncogenes that accelerate the

cell division cycle include (1) growth factors; (2) growth factor receptors; (3) intracellular signal transducers such as G proteins, protein kinases, cyclins, and cyclin-dependent protein kinases; and (4) nuclear TFs (see Figs. 3-12 and 3-32). A notable proto-oncogene product that inhibits apoptosis is Bcl-2 (see Fig. 3-19).

Fig. 3-32 depicts several proto-oncogene products that are closely involved in initiating the cell division cycle. The legend of that figure outlines some important details on the function of these proteins and their interaction with tumor suppressor proteins (to be discussed below). Transient increases in the production or activity of proto-oncogene proteins are required for regulated growth, as during embryogenesis, tissue regeneration, and stimulation of cells by growth factors or hormones. In contrast, permanent activation and/or overexpression of these proteins favor neoplastic transformation. One mechanism whereby genotoxic carcinogens induce neoplastic cell transformation is by producing an activating mutation of a proto-oncogene. Such a mutation is so named because the altered gene (then called an oncogene) encodes a permanently active protein that forces the cell into the division cycle.

An example of mutational activation of an oncogene protein is that of the Ras proteins. Ras proteins are G-proteins with GTP/GDP-binding capacity as well as GTPase activity (Anderson et al., 1992). They are localized on the inner surface of the plasma membrane and function as crucial mediators in the signaling pathways initiated by growth factors (see Figs. 3-12 and 3-32). Ras is located downstream from growth factor receptors and nonreceptor protein tyrosine kinases and upstream from mitogen-activated protein kinase (MAPK) cascade whose activation finally upregulates the expression of cyclin D and initiates the mitotic cycle (Fig. 3-32). In this pathway, Ras serves as a molecular switch, being active in the GTP-bound form and inactive in the GDP-bound form. Some mutations of the Ras gene (eg, a point mutation in codon 12) dramatically lower the GTPase activity of the protein. This in turn locks Ras in the permanently active GTP-bound form. Continual rather than signal-dependent activation of Ras can lead eventually to uncontrolled cell division and transformation. Indeed, microinjection of Ras-neutralizing monoclonal antibodies into cells blocks the mitogenic action of growth factors as well as cell transformation by several oncogenes. Ionizing radiation and carcinogenic chemicals (eg, N-methyl-N-nitrosourea, polycyclic aromatic hydrocarbons, benzidine, aflatoxin B_1) induce mutations of Ras proto-oncogenes that lead to constitutive activation of Ras proteins (Anderson et al., 1992). Most of these chemicals induce point mutations by transversion of G_{35} to T in codon 12.

Another example for activating mutation of a proto-oncogene is B-Raf mutation, although Ras and Raf mutations are mutually exclusive (Shaw and Cantley, 2006). Raf proteins are protein kinases, lying just downstream from Ras and being the first signal transducers in the MAP kinase pathway (see Fig. 3-12). After recruitment by Ras to the cell membrane, Raf is activated by the growth factor receptor (see item 4 in Fig. 3-12) through phosphorylation in its activating segment. B-Raf mutations occur in mouse liver tumors induced by diethylnitrosamine (Jaworski et al., 2005) in 66% of malignant melanomas and a wide range of human cancers. All mutations are within the activation segment of B-Raf, with a single amino acid substitution (V599E) accounting for the majority. The mutant B-Raf protein has elevated kinase activity probably because substitution of the nonpolar valine with the negatively charged glutamate mimics an activating phosphorylation. Thus, the constitutively active B-Raf continually sends Ras-independent proliferative signal down the MAPK pathway. Indeed, transfection of the mutant B-Raf gene into cells induced neoplastic transformation even in the absence of Ras proteins (Davies

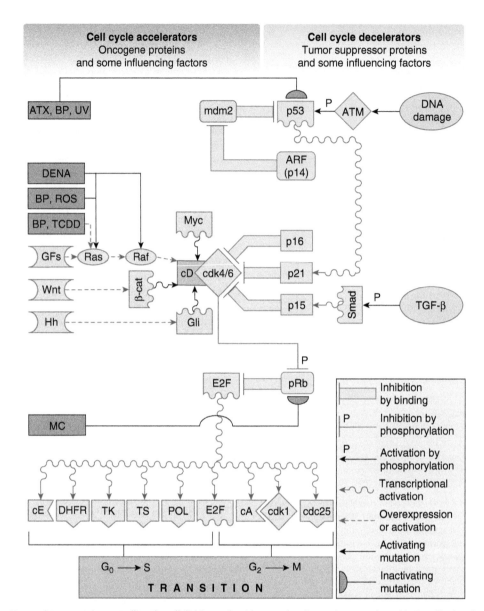

Figure 3-32. *Key regulatory proteins controlling the cell division cycle with some signaling pathways and xenobiotics affecting them.* Proteins on the left, represented by brown symbols, accelerate the cell cycle and are oncogenic if permanently active or expressed at high level. In contrast, proteins on the right, represented by blue symbols, decelerate or arrest the cell cycle and thus suppress oncogenesis, unless they are inactivated (eg, by mutation).

Accumulation of cyclin D (cD) is a crucial event in initiating the cell division cycle. cD activates cyclin-dependent protein kinases 4 and 6 (cdk4/6), which in turn phosphorylate the retinoblastoma protein (pRb) causing dissociation of pRb from transcription factor E2F (Johnson and Walker, 1999). Then the unleashed E2F is able to bind to and transactivate genes whose products are essential for DNA synthesis, such as dihydrofolate reductase (DHFR), thymidine kinase (TK), thymidylate synthetase (TS), and DNA polymerase (POL), or are regulatory proteins, such as cyclin E (cE), cyclin A (cA), and cyclin-dependent protein kinase 1 (cdk1), which promote further progression of the cell cycle. Expression of cD is increased, for example, by growth factors signaling through Ras proteins and the MAPK pathway (see Fig. 3-12) as well as by Wnt and Hedgehog (Hh) ligands that ultimately signal through B-cat and Gli transcription factors, respectively (see Figs. 3-13 and 3-14). Some carcinogens, for example, benzpyrene (BP) and reactive oxygen species (ROS), and diethylnitrosamine (DENA) may cause mutation of the *Ras* or *Raf* gene that results in permanently active mutant Ras or Rab protein, but BP as well as TCDD may also induce simple overexpression of normal Ras protein.

Cell cycle progression is counteracted, for example, by pRb (which inhibits the function of E2F), by cyclin-dependent protein kinase inhibitors (such as p15, p16, and p21), by p53 (which transactivates the *p21* gene), and by ARF (also called p14 that binds to mdm2, thereby neutralizing the antagonistic effect of mdm2 on p53). Signals evoked by DNA damage and TGF-β will ultimately result in accumulation of p53 and p15 proteins, respectively, and deceleration of the cell cycle. In contrast, mutations that disable the tumor suppressor proteins facilitate cell cycle progression and neoplastic conversion and are common in human tumors. Aflatoxin B$_1$ (ATX), BP, and UV light cause such mutations of the *p53* gene (Bennett *et al.*, 1999), whereas *pRb* mutations occur invariably in methylcholanthrene (MC)–induced transplacental lung tumors in mice (Miller, 1999).

et al., 2002). Another proto-oncogene product that often undergoes activating mutation in breast and colon tumors is p110-α, the catalytic subunit of PI3K (Shaw and Cantley, 2006). This can cause permanent proliferative signaling via the GF receptor–PI3K–Akt pathway (see Fig. 3-12).

Whereas constitutive activation of oncogene proteins, as a result of point mutation, is a common initiator of chemical carcinogenesis, permanent overexpression of such proteins also can contribute to neoplastic cell transformation. Overexpression of proto-oncogene proteins may result from amplification of the proto-oncogene, that is, the formation of more than one copy (Anderson et al., 1992). Such an event may be initiated by DNA strand breaks, and therefore often observed after exposure to ionizing radiation; however, proto-oncogene amplification also occurs in spontaneous human cancer. An example for a proto-oncogene protein that is overexpressed in response to gene damage is the antiapoptotic Bcl-2 protein (see Fig. 3-19). The aberrantly increased expression of Bcl-2 is caused by a chromosomal translocation and is responsible for B-cell lymphoma, a spontaneous human malignancy (see later). Overexpression of proto-oncogene proteins as a result of nongenotoxic, epigenetic mechanisms will be discussed later.

Mutation of Tumor Suppressor Genes Tumor suppressor genes encode proteins that inhibit the progression of cells in the division cycle, or promote DNA repair or apoptosis on DNA damage. Fig. 3-32 depicts such proteins, which include, for example, cyclin-dependent protein kinase inhibitors (eg, p15, p16, and p21), TFs (eg, p53 and Smad) that activate genes encoding cyclin-dependent protein kinase inhibitors, proteins (eg, pRb) that block TFs involved in DNA synthesis and cell division, and proteins (eg, ARF) that block inhibitors of tumor suppressor proteins. Other notable tumor suppressor gene products include, for example, the protein kinases (eg, ATM, ATR) that sense the DNA damage and signal for the p53-controlled response shown in Fig. 3-33, proteins involved in DNA repair, such as O^6-methyguanine-DNA methyltransferase (which removes alkyl groups adducted to guanine) as well as BRCA1 and BRCA2 proteins (which contribute to recombinational DNA repair), proapoptotic proteins (eg, Bax, Puma, Noxa, and Bim) induced after DNA damage (Fig. 3-33), the suppressor of cytokine signaling (Socs) protein (Fig. 3-12), the phosphatase PTEN (which dephosphorylates the membrane lipid PIP_3, an essential intermediate in the PI3K–Akt pathway) that turns off the PI3K–Akt pathway-mediated proliferative signaling (Fig. 3-12), and the tuberous sclerosis complex-2 (TSC2) that prevents activation of mTOR (Fig. 3-29). Uncontrolled proliferation can occur when the mutant tumor suppressor gene encodes a protein that cannot suppress cell division. Inactivating mutations of specific tumor suppressor genes in germ cells are responsible for the inherited predisposition to cancer, as in familial retinoblastoma (pRb; see Fig. 3-32), Wilms tumor (WT1, WTX, and β-catenin; see Fig. 3-13), familial polyposis (Smad4; see Figs. 3-12 and 3-32), and Li–Fraumeni syndrome (p53; see Figs. 3-19, 3-32, and 3-33). Mutations of tumor suppressor genes in somatic cells contribute to nonhereditary cancers. The genes of p16, PTEN, and pRb are frequently mutated in human cancer. The best known tumor suppressor gene involved in both spontaneous and chemically induced carcinogenesis is p53.

The p53 tumor suppressor gene encodes a 53 kDa protein with multiple functions (Fig. 3-33). Acting as a transcriptional modulator, the p53 protein (1) activates protein-coding genes whose products arrest the cell cycle (eg, p21 and gadd45), repair damaged DNA (eg, XPE, MSH2), or promote apoptosis (eg, Bax, Puma, and Fas receptor); (2) activates miRNA-coding genes whose products (eg,

miR-34a) repress the translation of mitogenic TFs and cell cycle accelerator proteins (eg, Myc, E2F3, cyclin D, and CDK4/6); and (3) represses protein-coding genes that encode cell cycle accelerators (eg, cyclin B1, Cdk1), or antiapoptotic proteins (eg, Bcl-2 and IGF-1 receptor) (Bennett et al., 1999; Liu and Chen, 2006). DNA damage activates protein kinases (ATM, ATR, Chk1, Chk2) to phosphorylate and stabilize the p53 protein, causing its accumulation (Fig. 3-33). The accumulated p53 may induce cell cycle arrest and apoptosis of the affected cells. Thus, p53 eliminates cancer-prone cells from the replicative pool, counteracting neoplastic transformation; therefore, it is commonly designated as guardian of the genome.

Indeed, cells that have no p53 are a million times more likely to permit DNA amplification than are cells with a normal level of this suppressor gene. Furthermore, mice with the p53 gene deleted develop cancer by 6 to 9 months of age, attesting to the crucial role of the p53 tumor suppressor gene in preventing carcinogenesis.

Mutations in the p53 gene are found in 50% of human tumors and in a variety of induced cancers. The majority are "missense mutations" that change an amino acid and result in a faulty or altered protein (Bennett et al., 1999). The faulty p53 protein forms a complex with endogenous wild-type p53 protein and inactivates it. Thus, the mutant p53 not only is unable to function as a tumor suppressor protein but also prevents tumor suppression by the wild-type p53.

Carcinogens may cause characteristic mutations in the p53 tumor suppressor gene. An example is the point mutation in codon 249 from AGG to AGT, which changes amino acid 249 in the p53 protein from arginine to serine. This mutation predominates in hepatocellular carcinomas in individuals living where food is contaminated with aflatoxin B_1 (Bennett et al., 1999). Because in human hepatocytes the CYP-activated metabolites of aflatoxin B_1 induce the transversion of G to T in codon 249 of the p53 tumor suppressor gene (Aguilar et al., 1993), it appears likely that this mutation in primary human liver cancer is indeed caused by this mycotoxin. Although the incriminated mutation probably contributes to the hepatocarcinogenicity of aflatoxin B_1 in humans, it is not involved in aflatoxin B_1–induced hepatocarcinogenesis in rats, as the transformed liver cells from the toxin-exposed rats do not show this mutation.

Another example for inactivating mutation of a tumor suppressor gene of environmental origin is that of Patched, which often occurs in basal cell carcinoma of the skin that may be induced by UV and ionizing radiation, as well as arsenic exposure (Tang et al., 2007). Normal Patched, the membrane receptor of the Hh ligand, suppresses the mitogenic Hh pathway in absence of Hh ligand, which would inhibit Patched (Fig. 3-14). Mutant Patched loses its power to restrain this signaling network, which thus promotes cell division even in absence of its inhibitor ligand.

In addition to aberrations in critical protein-coding genes, damage in genes coding for miRNA (which repress the translation of critical proteins; see Fig. 3-11) may also contribute to carcinogenesis. For example, amplification of miR-21 (which is oncogenic by repressing the translation of PTEN; see Fig. 3-12) and deletion of miR-15 and miR-16 (which is tumor suppressive by repressing the translation of cdc25A; see Fig. 3-25) occur in spontaneous human malignancies. Therefore, miRNA gene damage may also underlie the mechanism of chemical carcinogenesis. The role of altered miRNA expression as an epigenetic mechanism of chemical carcinogenesis will be discussed below.

Epigenetic Mechanisms in Carcinogenesis: Inappropriate Activation or Responsiveness of the Regulatory Region of Critical Genes Whereas some chemicals cause cancer by reacting with DNA and inducing a mutation, others do not damage DNA,

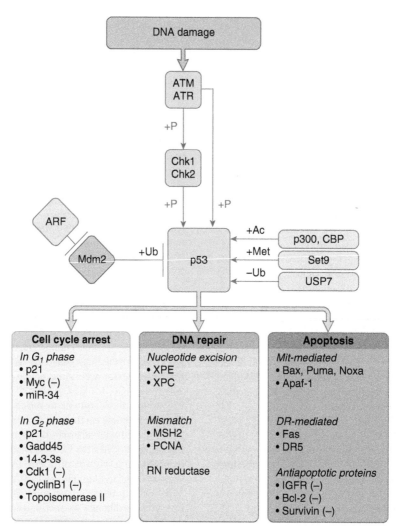

Figure 3-33. *The guardian of the genome: p53 tumor suppressor protein—its role and regulation.* When activated on DNA damage, the p53 protein may mediate cell cycle arrest, DNA repair, and apoptosis. When inducing these effects, p53 acts chiefly as a transcription factor that can activate the transcription of most target genes, while repressing some of others, such as those marked with (–) in the figure (Liu and Chen, 2006). For example, p53 transactivates *p21* and *gadd45* genes (whose products are inhibitors of cyclin–cyclin-dependent protein kinase complexes) and arrest the cell cycle in G_1 and G_2 phases, respectively, but p53 represses the *Cdk1* and *cyclin B1* genes (whose products are indispensable for the cells to transit from G_2 phase to M) (see Fig. 3-25). p53 also induces the expression of miR-34 (a microRNA), which in turn represses the translation of cyclin D, CDK4/6, and E2F, important cell cycle accelerator proteins (see Fig. 3-32) (Chen *et al.*, 2010). p53 also transactivates the genes of some DNA repair proteins and proapoptotic proteins (eg, bax and fas; see Fig. 3-19) and represses the genes of antiapoptotic proteins (eg, Bcl-2 and IGF-1 receptor), whereby it promotes apoptosis. These (and other) p53-induced proapoptotic mechanisms may be cell-specific, that is, all are not necessarily occurring in the same cell at the same time.

The intracellular level and activity of p53 depends primarily on the presence of mdm2 protein, which inactivates p53 by ubiquitinating it; monoubiquitination causes export of p53 from the nucleus, whereas polyubiquitination promotes its proteasomal degradation. The influence of mdm2 on p53 may be disrupted by overexpression of the ARF (or p14) protein (which binds to mdm2 and removes it from p53) or by posttranslational modification of p53 through phosphorylation by protein kinases (see below), acetylation by acetyltransferases (eg, p300 and CBP), methylation by methyltransferases (eg, Set9) and deubiquitination by ubiquitin-specific-processing protease 7 (USP7, also called HAUSP) (Liu and Chen, 2006). These mechanisms release p53 from mdm2 and stabilize the p53 protein, thereby greatly increasing its abundance and activity. Phosphorylation of p53 is induced by DNA damage. This is sensed by kinases, such as ataxia telangiectasia mutated (ATM) and ataxia telangiectasia related (ATR), which directly or through checkpoint kinases (Chk1, Chk2) phosphorylate p53 to induce cell cycle arrest, DNA repair, or apoptosis (McGowan and Russell, 2004).

It is important to emphasize that there is also a p53-independent mechanism to arrest the cells suffering DNA damage before mitosis. Like induction of p53, this is also initiated by the activated Chk1, which phosphorylates and inactivates cdc25A, a protein phosphatase, which normally would dephosphorylate Cdk1 and activate the Cdk1–cyclin B complex (see Fig. 3-25). Thus, when cdc25A is inactivated, Cdk1 stalls and mitosis is delayed. Interestingly, p53 assists in keeping Cdk1, this mitosis-driving molecular motor, off track as it induces 14-3-3σ, a cytoplasmic binding protein, which associates with both cdc25A and the Cdk1–cyclin B complex and sequesters them in the cytoplasm.

By arresting division of cells with potentially mutagenic DNA damage, facilitating the DNA repair or eliminating such cells, p53 protein counteracts neoplastic development. *p53*-null mice, like *ARF*-null mice, develop tumors with high incidence. Mutational inactivation of the p53 protein is thought to contribute to the carcinogenic effect of aflatoxin B$_1$, sunlight, and cigarette smoke in humans. Overexpression of mdm2 can lead to constitutive inhibition of p53 and thereby promotes oncogenesis even if the *p53* gene is unaltered. See the text for more details.

yet induce cancer after prolonged exposure (Barrett, 1992). These chemicals are designated *nongenotoxic* (or epigenetic) *carcinogens* and include (1) xenobiotic mitogens, that is, chemicals that promote proliferative signaling, such as the PKC activator phorbol esters and fumonisin B$_1$, as well as the protein phosphatase inhibitor okadaic acid (see Fig. 3-12); (2) endogenous mitogens, such as growth factors (eg, TGF-α) and hormones with mitogenic action on specific cells, for example, estrogens on mammary gland or liver cells, TSH on the follicular cells of the thyroid gland, and luteinizing hormone on Leydig cells in testes; (3) toxicants that, when given chronically, cause sustained cell injury (such as chloroform and D-limonene); (4) xenobiotics that are nongenotoxic carcinogens in rodents but not in humans, such as phenobarbital, DDT, TCDD, and peroxisome proliferators (eg, fibrates, WI-14643, dihalogenated and trihalogenated acetic acids); and (5) ethionine and diethanolamine, which interfere with formation of the endogenous methyl donor *S*-adenosyl methionine (Poirier, 1994). Because several of the listed chemicals promote the development of tumors after neoplastic transformation has been initiated by a genotoxic carcinogen, they are referred to as *tumor promoters*. Despite the initial belief that promoters are unable to induce tumors by themselves, studies suggest that they can do so after prolonged exposure.

It appears that nongenotoxic chemicals, like the genotoxic ones, eventually also influence the expression of proto-oncogenes and/or tumor suppressor genes, but in a different manner. When continuously present, nongenotoxic carcinogens can permanently induce the synthesis of normal proto-oncogene proteins and/or repress the synthesis of normal tumor suppressor proteins, rather than inducing the synthesis of permanently active mutant proto-oncogene proteins or permanently inactive mutant tumor suppressor proteins, as the mutagenic genotoxic carcinogens do.

Carcinogens may alter the synthesis of proto-oncogene proteins and tumor suppressor proteins at transcriptional and/or translational levels. Chemicals may modify transcription of the genes into mRNAs for proto-oncogene and tumor suppressor proteins by perturbing the signal transduction to the promoter region of these genes and/or by altering the signal receptivity of this gene region by DNA methylation and histone modifications. Translation of proto-oncogene proteins and tumor suppressor proteins from their mRNA may be controlled by specific miRNAs, which repress this process (Fig. 3-11). Carcinogen-induced perturbations in signaling and promoter alterations may not only influence transcription of protein-coding genes but also affect the transcription of miRNA-coding genes. The resultant changes in the abundance in miRNAs in turn alter, in a reciprocal (inverse) manner, the synthesis of proto-oncogene proteins and tumor suppressor proteins, provided the miRNA in question targets the mRNA of such a protein. The forthcoming discussion deals with the importance of signaling, DNA as well as histone modifications, and miRNA expression in carcinogenesis.

Role of Signaling in Carcinogenesis An important target of nongenotoxic carcinogens is the promoter region of critical genes where they can act via two distinct modes. First, they may alter the abundance and/or activity of TFs, typically by influencing upstream signaling elements ranging from extracellular signaling molecules (eg, TSH) to intracellular transducer proteins (eg, PKC). Obviously both xenobiotic and endogenous mitogens mentioned above can thus activate proliferative pathways (see Fig. 3-12) that descend to TFs (eg, Myc) that act on the promoter of proto-oncogenes coding for mRNAs of proto-oncogene proteins (eg, cyclins), and, as to be discussed below, on the promoter of genes coding for oncogenic miRNAs (eg, miR-17-92). It is easy to recognize that

even nongenotoxic carcinogens of the cytotoxic type act in this manner. As described under tissue repair, cell injury evokes the release of mitogenic growth factors such as HGF and TGF-α from tissue macrophages and endothelial cells. Thus, cells in chronically injured tissues are exposed continuously to endogenous mitogens. Although these growth factors are instrumental in tissue repair after acute cell injury, their continuous presence is potentially harmful because they may ultimately transform the affected cells into neoplastic cells. Indeed, transgenic mice that overexpress TGF-α develop hepatomegaly at a young age and tumors by 12 months (Fausto *et al.*, 2006). Mitogenic cytokines secreted by Kupffer cells are apparently involved in hepatocyte proliferation and, possibly, tumor formation induced by peroxisome proliferators in rats (Rose *et al.*, 1999) and in the formation of the endothelial cell–derived hepatic hemangiosarcoma in mice exposed to 2-butoxyethanol (Corthals *et al.*, 2006).

Role of DNA Methylation and Histone Modification in Carcinogenesis As a second mode of action, nongenotoxic carcinogens may alter expression of critical genes by modifying the responsiveness of the promoter region of these genes to TFs. Promoter responsiveness is typically controlled by DNA methylation. This takes place at C$_5$ of specific cytosine residues located in CpG islands (ie, clusters of CpG dinucleotides) in the promoter and is catalyzed by DNA cytosine methyltransferases (eg, DNMT1, DNMT3a, and DNMT3b) using *S*-adenosyl methionine as the methyl donor. It is well known that promoter methylation decreases the transcriptional activity of genes. For example, tissue-specific genes (eg, the genes of GI TFFs) are hypermethylated in tissues where they are not expressed, but are typically hypomethylated in tissues where they are expressed.

Promoter methylation can silence genes because it weakens binding of TFs to the promoter and because it triggers secondary alterations in histone proteins that reduce the accessibility of the promoter for TFs (Esteller, 2005). The latter mechanism involves modification of the protruding amino-terminal tails of core histone proteins by deacetylation and methylation of lysine residues. This makes the histone more compact, thereby diminishing access of TFs and other proteins involved in transcription initiation to the gene promoter. Histone deacetylases that remove the acetyl group from histone tails may be recruited by DNMTs directly, or through proteins that recognize and bind to the methylated CpG dinucleotides (eg, MeCP1, MeCP2, MBD2, MBD3). Some of these methyl-CpG-binding domain-containing proteins (eg, MBD2, MBD3) also have histone deacetylase activity. Finally, both DNMTs and MBDs can recruit histone methyltransferases to methylate histone tail lysines.

While methylation of CpG dinucleotides codes for gene silencing via histone deacetylation and methylation ("histone code"), hypomethylated genes are alert. In fact, CpG islands in the 5′-end region (promoter, untranslated region, exon 1) of genes are relatively hypomethylated in normal tissues, except for tissue- or germ-line-specific genes, and genomically imprinted genes (see earlier). Thus, if the appropriate TFs are available for a particular gene, and if the CpG island remains hypomethylated, the histones acetylated and hypomethylated, then the gene will be transcribed (Esteller, 2005). Histones are acetylated by histone acetyltransferases, such as p300 and CBP, which also acetylate other proteins, including p53 (see Fig. 3-33), and are also transcriptional coactivators.

It is well documented that the normal methylation pattern of DNA is disrupted in cancer cells. Such cells are characterized by global (average) hypomethylation, that is, decreased content of genomic 5′-methylcytosine. Paradoxically, DNA hypomethylation occurs in the face of hypermethylation of the CpG islands in the promoter region tumor suppressor genes, which are normally demethylated (Esteller, 2005). The frequently hypermethylated tumor suppressor genes in human cancers are, for example, the Cdk inhibitor p15 and p16, the mdm2-binding protein ARF, pRb that tethers E2F (see Fig. 3-30), the DNA repair enzyme MGMT, and the lipid phosphatase PTEN (see Fig. 3-12). Importantly, both global hypomethylation and tumor suppressor gene hypermethylation intensify with increased malignancy of the tumor. Relevance of hypermethylation-induced silencing of tumor suppressor genes in carcinogenesis is supported by the finding that inhibitors of DNMTs (such as 5-aza-2′-deoxycytidine) can stop the growth of cancer cells and induce their differentiation by demethylating the dormant tumor suppressor genes, thereby restoring their expression (Esteller, 2005). The consequence of global hypomethylation of DNA is less clear. Nevertheless, hypomethylation of proto-oncogenes and increased expression of their products is a plausible mechanism (Goodman and Watson, 2002), although others have also been proposed (eg, chromosomal instability, reactivation of transposable DNA elements, and loss of genomic imprinting). On comparing mouse strains, it has been suggested that their sensitivity to chemical carcinogens may be related inversely to their capacity to maintain normal patterns of DNA methylation. It is worth noting that DNA methylation is more stable in human cells than in rodent cells (Goodman and Watson, 2002).

It appears that some of the nongenotoxic carcinogens alter DNA methylation. Inhibition of DNA methylation is a plausible mechanism that underlies tumorigenesis induced by ethionine, which depletes S-adenosyl-methionine (the methyl donor for DNMTs), and diethanolamine, which inhibits cellular uptake of choline, a dietary methyl group source for methylation of homocysteine to methionine. On prolonged administration, virtually all nongenotoxic rodent liver carcinogens listed above decrease DNA methylation. In addition to global DNA hypomethylation, promoter hypomethylation of the following proto-oncogenes have been observed in mouse or rat liver: Ras or Raf, following phenobarbital treatment, c-Jun, c-Myc, and IGF-2, after treatment with dichloroacetic acid, dibromoacetic acid, or trichloroacetic acid, and c-Myc after WY-14643 dosing. Long-term arsenic exposure of mice also induces hypomethylation of hepatic DNA globally and in the promoter of ERα, a hormone-activated TF. This is associated with an increase of cyclin D, a potentially ERα-linked gene (Chen et al., 2004). In contrast, in human keratinocytes TCDD induces promoter hypermethylation in the tumor suppressor genes p16 and p53 as well as immortalization of these cells (Ray and Swanson, 2004). Although the mechanisms that initiate altered promoter methylation are currently unknown, it is possible that that altered promoter methylation plays a role in tumor promotion by these nongenotoxic carcinogens.

Role of MicroRNAs in Carcinogenesis As miRNAs almost always repress the translation of proteins from their mRNAs (Fig. 3-11), a miRNA plays an oncogenic role if it represses the translation of tumor suppressor proteins, that is, proteins that counter cell division, repair DNA, or promote apoptosis. For example, the miR-17-92 cluster is considered oncogenic, because its members promote mitosis by repressing the translation of PTEN (an inhibitor of the mitogenic PI3K–Akt signaling; see Fig. 3-12) and p21 (a cyclin-dependent kinase inhibitor; see Fig. 3-32) and because they inhibit apoptosis by repressing the translation of the proapoptotic protein Bim. Other examples for oncogenic miRNAs include miR-29b (which also targets the mRNAs of p21 and Bim), as well as miR-221/222, the targets of which include mRNAs translating into tumor suppressor proteins, such as PTEN, p27, p57, FOXO3 (see Fig. 3-30), TIMP3 (metalloproteinase inhibitor 3), and Bim

(Chen et al., 2010; Garofalo and Croce, 2011). Overexpression of such oncogenic miRNAs promotes neoplastic cell transformation, whereas their underexpression opposes it.

Conversely, a miRNA has tumor suppressive role if it represses the translation of proto-oncogene proteins, that is, proteins that facilitate cell division or oppose apoptosis. For example, the let-7 family of miRNAs is regarded tumor suppressive as they silence the translation of Ras and Myc proteins, components of proliferative signaling (see Fig. 3-12). Furthermore, miR-15a and miR-16-1 repress the translation of protein phosphatase cdc25, which dephosphorylates and thus activates CDK1 and 2 that drives the cell cycle (see Fig. 3-25), and of Bcl-2, which inhibits apoptosis (see Fig. 3-19). Another tumor suppressor miRNA is miR-34, whose targets include the mRNAs that translates into the mitogenic TFs Myc and E2F3, as well as the cell cycle accelerator proteins cyclin D and CDK4/6 (see Figs. 3-25 and 3-32) (Chen, 2010; Garofalo and Croce, 2011). Upregulation of such tumor suppressive miRNAs counters neoplastic cell transformation, whereas their downregulation stimulates it.

Expression of miRNAs, like that of mRNAs coding for proteins, can be regulated at the promoter region of their genes by TFs as well as DNA methylation and histone modification. For example, Myc activates the transcription of the oncogenic miR-17-92, whereas p53 activates the transcription of the tumor suppressive miR-34. Therefore, the latter event is part of the adaptive DNA damage stress response discussed earlier and depicted in Fig. 3-33. Indeed, genotoxic carcinogens such as N-ethyl-N-nitrosourea and tamoxifen (which forms a DNA-reactive metabolite in rats, but not in humans) as well as ionizing radiation typically induce overexpression of mi-34.

The role of miRNAs in tumorigenesis induced by nongenotoxic carcinogens is well exemplified by the rodent hepatocarcinogenesis induced by the PPARα-activator WY-14643. This process involves transcriptional downregulation of the gene coding for let-7c and consequential derepression of the translation of c-Myc mRNA into c-Myc protein. Due to its increased abundance, this TF (see Figs. 3-12 and 3-32) increasingly activates the gene coding for cyclin D, a mitogenic protein, as well as the gene coding for miR-17-92, an oncogenic miRNA. miR-17-92 in turn represses the translation of proteins that counter mitosis (eg, PTEN and p21) and promote apoptosis (eg, Bim), thus forcing hepatocytes to proliferate (Gonzalez and Shah, 2008).

Cooperation of Genotoxic and Epigenetic Mechanisms in Carcinogenesis Genotoxic and epigenetic mechanisms most likely complement and amplify each other in chemical carcinogenesis. One chemical may exert both genotoxic and epigenetic effects. For example, estrogens produce mutagenic free radicals via redox cycling of their quinone and hydroquinone metabolites and induce receptor-mediated proliferative effect (Newbold, 2004). Well-known genotoxic carcinogens can also cause epigenetic alterations. For example, 2-acetylaminofluorene does not only form DNA adducts but also induces DNA methylation in the promoter of Rassf1a and p16 genes as well as histone methylation around the promoter of Rassf1a, p16, Socs1, Cdh1, and Cx26 genes, thereby silencing all these genes that encode tumor suppressor proteins (Pogribny et al., 2011). The p16, ARF, and MGMT tumor suppressor genes are also hypermethylated in aflatoxin B_1–induced mouse lung tumor and in 7,12-dimethylbenzanthracene-induced skin tumor. The antiestrogen tamoxifen, a hepatocarcinogen in rats (but not in humans), exerts genotoxic effect and induces global hypomethylation of DNA and histones in rat liver (Tryndyak et al., 2006). Thus, epigenetic alterations evoked by genotoxic carcinogens may drive the process of carcinogenesis after the initiating genotoxic event (Pogribny *et al.*, 2011). Conversely, global DNA hypomethylation and tumor suppressor gene hypermethylation may increase the occurrence of mutations in cells exposed to non-genotoxic carcinogens. In this sense, epigenetic mechanisms may also initiate carcinogenesis (Goodman and Watson, 2002).

Failure to Execute Apoptosis Promotes Mutation and Clonal Growth As discussed earlier, in cells suffering DNA damage, the stabilized p53 protein may induce cell death by apoptosis (Fig. 3-33). Apoptosis thus eliminates cells with DNA damage, preventing mutations to initiate carcinogenesis. Initiated preneoplastic cells have much higher apoptotic activity than do normal cells (Bursch *et al.*, 1992) and this can counteract their clonal expansion. In fact, facilitation of apoptosis can induce tumor regression. This occurs when hormone-dependent tumors are deprived of the hormone that promotes growth and suppresses apoptosis. This is the rationale for the use of tamoxifen, an antiestrogen, and gonadotropin-releasing hormone analogues to combat hormone-dependent tumors of the mammary gland and the prostate gland, respectively (Bursch *et al.*, 1992).

Thus, inhibition of apoptosis is detrimental because it facilitates both mutations and clonal expansion of preneoplastic cells. Indeed, apoptosis inhibition plays a role in the pathogenesis of human B-cell lymphomas, in which a chromosomal translocation results in aberrantly increased expression of Bcl-2 protein, which overrides programmed cell death after binding to and inactivating the proapoptotic Bax protein (see Fig. 3-19). Increased levels of Bcl-2 are also detected in other types of cancer, and a high Bcl-2/Bax ratio in a tumor is a marker for poor prognosis (Jäättelä, 1999). Other antiapoptotic proteins, such as Hsp27, Hsp70, and Hsp90 (Sreedhar and Csermely, 2004) and IAP family members, may also contribute to progression of neoplasia. Survivin, a member of the IAP family, is expressed in all cancer cells but not in adult differentiated cells (Jäättelä, 1999).

Inhibition of apoptosis is one mechanism by which the rodent tumor promoter phenobarbital promotes clonal expansion of preneoplastic cells. This has been demonstrated in rats given a single dose of *N*-nitrosomorpholine followed by daily treatments with phenobarbital for 12 months to initiate and promote, respectively, neoplastic transformation in liver (Schulte-Hermann *et al.*, 1990). From 6 months onward, phenobarbital did not increase DNA synthesis and cell division in the preneoplastic foci, yet it accelerated foci enlargement. The foci grow because phenobarbital lowers apoptotic activity, allowing the high cell replicative activity to manifest itself. The peroxisome proliferator nafenopin, a nongenotoxic hepatocarcinogen, also suppresses apoptosis in primary rat hepatocyte cultures (Bayly *et al.*, 1994). Based on a recent study with WY-14643, another peroxisome proliferator (Gonzalez and Shah, 2008), it may be suggested that miR-17-92 upregulation and consequential suppression of Bim translation accounts for apoptosis inhibition.

Failure to Restrain Cell Division Promotes Mutation, Proto-Oncogene Expression, and Clonal Growth Enhanced mitotic activity, whether it is induced by oncogenes inside the cell or by external factors such as xenobiotic or endogenous mitogens, promotes carcinogenesis for a number of reasons:

1. First, the enhanced mitotic activity increases the probability of mutations. This is due in part to activation of the cell division cycle, which invokes a substantial shortening of the G_1 phase, allowing less time for the repair of injured DNA before replication, thus increasing the chance that the damage will yield a mutation. Although repair still may be feasible after replication, postreplication repair is error-prone. In addition, activation of the cell division cycle increases the proportion of cells that replicate their DNA at any given time. During replication, DNA becomes unpacked and its amount doubles, greatly increasing the effective target size for DNA-reactive mutagenic chemicals, including ROS.

2. Enhanced mitotic activity may compromise DNA methylation, which occurs in the early postreplication period and is carried out by DNMTs that copy the methylation pattern of the parental DNA strand to the daughter strand (maintenance methylation). Limitation of DNMTs by shortened G_2 phase or by presence of other transacting factors might impair methylation and may contribute to overexpression of proto-oncogens, starting a vicious cycle.

3. During cell division, the cell-to-cell communication through gap junctions (constructed from connexins) and AJ (constructed from cadherins) is temporarily disrupted. Several tumor promoters, such as phenobarbital, phorbol esters, and peroxisome proliferators, decrease gap junctional intercellular communication. It has been hypothesized that this contributes to neoplastic transformation. Increased susceptibility of connexin-knockout mice to spontaneous and chemically induced liver tumors supports this hypothesis (Chipman *et al.*, 2003). Lack of the AJ contributes to the invasiveness of tumor cells (see below).

4. Another mechanism by which proliferation promotes the carcinogenic process is through clonal expansion of the initiated cells to form nodules (foci) and tumors.

In summary, transformation of normal cells with controlled proliferative activity to malignant cells with uncontrolled proliferative activity is driven by 3 major forces: (1) accumulation of genetic damage in the form of mutant proto-oncogenes (which encode permanently activated cell cycle accelerator and/or antiapoptotic proteins) and mutant tumor suppressor genes (which encode permanently inactivated cell cycle decelerator and/or proapoptotic proteins); (2) increased transcription and/or translation of normal proto-oncogenes (causing expression of more cell cycle accelerator and/or antiapoptotic proteins); and (3) silencing of normal tumor suppressor genes at transcriptional and/or translational level (causing expression of less cell cycle decelerator and/or proapoptotic proteins). Uncontrolled proliferation results from offset of the balance between mitosis and apoptosis (Fig. 3-34).

Genotoxic carcinogens appear to induce cancer primarily by inducing activating mutations in proto-oncogenes or inactivating mutations in tumor suppressor genes, and secondarily by causing inappropriate expression rate of these critical genes. In contrast, nongenotoxic carcinogens cause cancer primarily by transcriptional or translational upregulation of the synthesis of proto-oncogene proteins or downregulation of the synthesis of tumor suppressor proteins. Secondarily, however, nongenotoxic carcinogens may also increase mutation of critical genes, which is initiated by genotoxic agents or spontaneous DNA damage. In human cells, spontaneous DNA damage may give rise to mutation at a frequency of 1 out of 10^8 to 10^{10} base pairs (Barrett, 1992). Genotoxic carcinogens increase this frequency 10- to 1000-fold. Nongenotoxic carcinogens also increase the rate of spontaneous mutations through a mitogenic effect (see above) and increase the number of cells with DNA damage and mutations by facilitating their division and inhibiting their apoptosis. Both enhanced mitotic activity and decreased apoptotic activity expand the population of transformed cells.

According to an emerging theory, cancers may form by genotoxic and/or epigenetic mechanisms in pluripotent stem cell

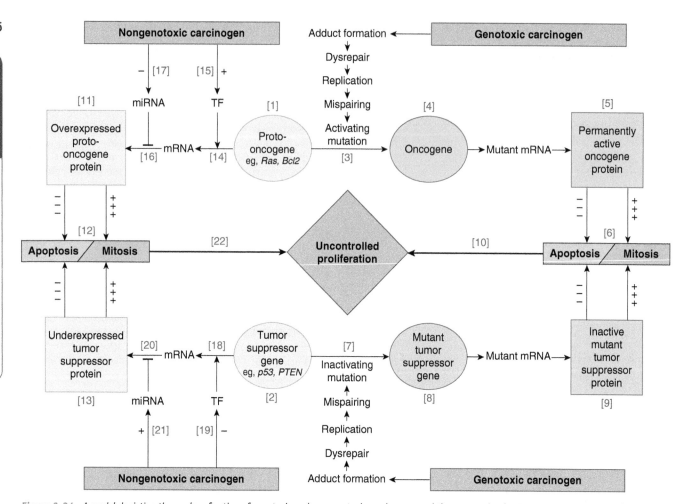

Figure 3-34. *A model depicting the modes of action of genotoxic and nongenotoxic carcinogens and the cooperation between proto-oncogenes and tumor suppressor genes in transformation of normal cells with controlled proliferation into neoplastic cells with uncontrolled proliferation.* When produced in appropriate quantities, the normal proteins encoded by proto-oncogenes [1] and tumor suppressor genes [2] reciprocally influence mitosis and apoptosis and thus ensure controlled cell proliferation. However, the balance between the effects of these 2 types of proteins on the fate of cells is offset by carcinogens via genotoxic and nongenotoxic mechanisms resulting in uncontrolled proliferation.

A genotoxic (or DNA-reactive) carcinogen may induce cell proliferation in 2 ways. In the first way, it inflicts DNA damage (eg, by forming DNA adducts) that ultimately brings about an activating mutation [3] in a proto-oncogene [1] and the mutant proto-oncogene (then called an oncogene) [4] in turn encodes a constitutively (ie, permanently) active oncogene protein [5] that continuously signals for mitosis or against apoptosis [6], depending on its function. In the second way, the DNA-reactive chemical produces DNA damage that eventually yields an inactivating mutation [7] in a tumor suppressor gene [2], with the mutant gene [8] encoding an inactive tumor suppressor protein [9] that cannot restrain mitosis or evoke apoptosis (eg, in response to DNA damage). In both instances, the rate of mitosis will exceed the rate of apoptosis [6] and uncontrolled proliferation of the affected cells will ensue [10]. Such a scenario may underlie the carcinogenicity of aflatoxin B$_1$, which induces mutation sometimes in the *Ras* proto-oncogene and often in the *p53* tumor suppressor gene (see text for details).

Nongenotoxic (epigenetic) carcinogens may also induce cell proliferation by 2 modes of action: first, by causing the overexpression of normal proto-oncogenes [1], yielding increased quantity of their protein products [11], which in turn excessively stimulate mitosis or inhibit apoptosis [12]. The second mode involves the underexpression of normal tumor suppressor genes [2], yielding diminished quantity of their protein products [13], which thus fail to restrain mitosis or promote apoptosis appropriately [12]. Nongenotoxic carcinogens may induce the synthesis of proto-oncogene proteins [11] at transcriptional and/or translational levels. They may facilitate the transcription of a proto-oncogene [1] into its mRNA [14] either by increasing the abundance of active transcription factors (TFs) at the promoter region of the gene or by facilitating the accessibility of TFs to the promoter (eg, by hypomethylation of this region) [15]. Nongenotoxic carcinogens may promote the translation of the mRNA into proto-oncogene protein [16] by decreasing the expression of microRNA (miRNA) [17] that normally represses the translation of this protein [16]. (Such miRNAs have tumor suppressor roles.) Nongenotoxic (also called epigenetic) carcinogens also may reduce the synthesis of tumor suppressor proteins [13] at transcriptional and/or translational levels. They may diminish the transcription of a tumor suppressor gene [2] into its mRNA [18] either by decreasing the abundance of active TFs at the promoter region of the gene or by impeding the accessibility of TFs to the promoter (eg, by hypermethylation of this region) [19]. Nongenotoxic carcinogens may downregulate the translation of the mRNA into a tumor suppressor protein [20] by increasing the expression of a miRNA [21] that normally represses the translation of this protein [20]. (Such miRNAs have oncogenic roles.) Eventually, overexpression of proto-oncogene proteins and/or underexpression of tumor suppressor proteins produce mitosis rate that exceeds the rate of apoptosis [12], thereby leading to uncontrolled proliferation of the affected cells [22]. Examples for nongenotoxic carcinogens acting by these mechanisms are given in the text.

In effect, the modes of action of these 2 types of chemical carcinogens are more complex: genotoxic carcinogens may also exert epigenetic effects and nongenotoxic carcinogens may increase the frequency of spontaneous mutations as well as the division and survival of cells carrying mutations (see the text for details).

populations. Such cells are characterized by quiescence, self-renewal, and conditional immortality, thus would potentially supply a lifelong, latent neoplastic population after carcinogen attack. Stem cells may be an especially likely target for transplacental carcinogens, such as DES or arsenic (Tokar *et al.*, 2011), because they are abundant during fetal development and have the longevity to carry the molecular lesion to the adult period of life.

Finally, further changes in gene expression may occur in these proliferating cells making them capable of invading the tissue and forming metastasis. These alterations confer the cells capacity for increased mobility by (1) their transdifferentiation into a mobile fibroblastoid phenotype (called epithelial-to-mesenchymal transition [EMT]), (2) disruption of the AJ that anchor cells to their neighbor (by downregulation of E-cadherin expression), and (3) degradation of the surrounding ECM (by upregulation of matrix metalloproteinases). Signaling systems that orchestrate EMT include those triggered by TGF-β (Fig. 3-12), the Wnt ligand (see Fig. 3-13), and the Hh ligand (see Fig. 3-14) (Katoh and Katoh, 2008).

CONCLUSIONS

This overview systematically surveys the mechanisms of the potential events that follow toxicant exposure and contribute to toxicity.

This approach is also useful in the search for mechanisms responsible for (1) selective toxicity, that is, differences in the sensitivity to toxicants of various organisms, such as different species and strains of animals, organs, and cells, and (2) alteration of toxicity by exogenous factors such as chemicals and food and physiologic or pathologic conditions such as aging and disease. To identify the mechanisms that underlie selective toxicity or alterations in toxicity, all steps where variations might occur must be considered systematically. Selective or altered toxicity may be due to different or altered (1) exposure; (2) delivery, thus resulting in a different concentration of the ultimate toxicant at the target site; (3) target molecules; (4) biochemical processes triggered by the reaction of the chemical with the target molecules; (5) repair at the molecular, cellular, or tissue level; or (6) altered gene expression-based stress responses as well as circulatory and thermoregulatory reflexes by which the affected organism can adapt to some of the toxic effects.

In this chapter, a simplified scheme has been used to give an overview of the development of toxicity (Fig. 3-1). In reality, the route to toxicity can be considerably more diverse and complicated. For example, one chemical may yield several ultimate toxicants, one ultimate toxicant may react with several types of target molecules, and reaction with one type of target molecule may have a number of consequences. Thus, the toxicity of one chemical may involve several mechanisms that can interact with and influence each other in an intricate manner.

This chapter has emphasized the significance of the chemistry of a toxicant in governing its delivery to and reaction with the target molecule as well as the importance of the biochemistry, molecular and cell biology, immunology, and physiology of the affected organism in its response to the action of the toxicant. An organism has mechanisms that (1) counteract the delivery of toxicants, such as detoxication; (2) reverse the toxic injury, such as repair mechanisms; and (3) offset some dysfunctions, such as adaptive responses. Thus, toxicity is not an inevitable consequence of toxicant exposure because it may be prevented, reversed, or compensated for by such mechanisms. Toxicity develops if the toxicant exhausts or impairs the protective mechanisms and/or overrides the adaptability of biological systems.

REFERENCES

Aguilar F, Hussain SP, Cerutti P. Aflatoxin B1 induces the transversion of G → T in codon 249 of the p53 tumor suppressor gene in human hepatocytes. *Proc Natl Acad Sci U S A.* 1993;90:8586–8590.

Anders MW. Glutathione-dependent bioactivation of haloalkanes and haloalkenes. *Drug Metab Rev.* 2004;36:583–594.

Anderson MW, Reynolds SH, You M, Maronpot RM. Role of protooncogene activation in carcinogenesis. *Environ Health Perspect.* 1992;98:13–24.

Anway MD, Cupp AS, Uzumcu M, Skinner MK. Epigenetic transgenerational actions of endocrine disruptors and male fertility. *Science.* 2005;308:1466–1469.

Arthur MJP, Iredale JP, Mann DA. Tissue inhibitors of metalloproteinases: role in liver fibrosis and alcoholic liver disease. *Alcohol Clin Exp Res.* 1999;23:940–943.

Aust SD, Chignell CF, Bray TM, et al. Free radicals in toxicology. *Toxicol Appl Pharmacol.* 1993;120:168–178.

Bailey CP, Connor M. Opioids: cellular mechanisms of tolerance and physical dependence. *Curr Opin Pharmacol.* 2005;5:60–68.

Baillie TA, Kassahun K. Reversibility in glutathione-conjugate formation. *Adv Pharmacol.* 1994;27:163–181.

Ballestar E, Esteller M, Richardson BC. The epigenetic face of systemic lupus erythematosus. *J Immunol.* 2006;176:7143–7147.

Barrett JC. Mechanisms of action of known human carcinogens. In: Vainio H, Magee PN, McGregor DB, McMichael AJ, eds. *Mechanisms of Carcinogenesis in Risk Identification.* Lyons, France: International Agency for Research on Cancer; 1992:115–134.

Basu S. Isoprostanes: novel bioactive products of lipid peroxidation. *Free Radic Res.* 2004;38:105–122.

Baumann H, Gauldie J. The acute phase response. *Immunol Today.* 1994;15:74–80.

Bayly AC, Roberts RA, Dive C. Suppression of liver cell apoptosis in vitro by the nongenotoxic hepatocarcinogen and peroxisome proliferator nafenopin. *J Cell Biol.* 1994;125:197–203.

Bedford L, Lowe J, Dick LR, Mayer RJ, Brownell JE. Ubiquitin-like protein conjugation and the ubiquitin–proteasome system as drug targets. *Nat Rev Drug Discov.* 2011;10:29–46.

Bennett WP, Hussain SP, Vahakangas KH, et al. Molecular epidemiology of human cancer risk: gene–environment interactions and *p53* mutation spectrum in human lung cancer. *J Pathol.* 1999;187:8–18.

Bessac BF, Jordt SE. Sensory detection and responses to toxic gases: mechanisms, health effects, and countermeasures. *Proc Am Thorac Soc.* 2010;7:269–277.

Boatright KM, Salvesen GS. Mechanisms of caspase activation. *Curr Opin Cell Biol.* 2003;15:725–731.

Bock KW, Lilienblum W. Roles of uridine diphosphate glucuronosyltransferases in chemical carcinogenesis. In: Kauffman FC, ed. *Conjugation–Deconjugation Reactions in Drug Metabolism and Toxicity.* Berlin: Springer-Verlag; 1994:391–428.

Boelsterli UA. Specific targets of covalent drug–protein interactions in hepatocytes and their toxicological significance in drug-induced liver injury. *Drug Metab Rev.* 1993;25:395–451.

Bokoch GM, Knaus UG. NADPH oxidases: not just for leukocytes anymore! *Trends Biochem Sci.* 2003;28:502–508.

Boulares HA, Giardina C, Navarro CL, et al. Modulation of serum growth factor signal transduction in Hepa 1–6 cells by acetaminophen: an inhibition of c-*myc* expression, NF-κB activation, and Raf-1 kinase activity. *Toxicol Sci.* 1999;48:264–274.

Boyd JG, Gordon T. Neurotrophic factors and their receptors in axonal regeneration and functional recovery after peripheral nerve injury. *Mol Neurobiol.* 2003;27:277–324.

Breen AP, Murphy JA. Reactions of oxyl radicals with DNA. *Free Radic Biol Med.* 1995;18:1033–1077.

Buja LM, Eigenbrodt ML, Eigenbrodt EH. Apoptosis and necrosis: basic types and mechanisms of cell death. *Arch Pathol Lab Med.* 1993;117:1208–1214.

Bursch W, Oberhammer F, Schulte-Hermann R. Cell death by apoptosis and its protective role against disease. *Trends Pharmacol Sci.* 1992;13:245–251.

Cai J, Yang J, Jones DP. Mitochondrial control of apoptosis: the role of cytochrome c. *Biochim Biophys Acta*. 1998;1366:139–149.

Cain K. Chemical-induced apoptosis: formation of the Apaf-1 apoptosome. *Drug Metab Rev*. 2003;35:337–363.

Caro AA, Cederbaum AI. Oxidative stress, toxicology, and pharmacology of CYP2E1. *Annu Rev Pharmacol Toxicol*. 2004;44:27–42.

Castranova V. Signaling pathways controlling the production of inflammatory mediators in response to crystalline silica exposure: role of reactive oxygen/nitrogen species. *Free Radic Biol Med*. 2004;37: 916–925.

Castro L, Rodriguez M, Radi R. Aconitase is readily inactivated by peroxynitrite, but not by its precursor, nitric oxide. *J Biol Chem*. 1994;269: 29409–29415.

Cavalieri EL, Rogan EG. The approach to understanding aromatic hydrocarbon carcinogenesis: the central role of radical cations in metabolic activation. *Pharmacol Ther*. 1992;55:183–199.

Chen D, Farwell MA, Zhang B. MicroRNA as a new player in the cell cycle. *J Cell Physiol*. 2010;225:296–301.

Chen H, Li S, Liu J, et al. Chronic inorganic arsenic exposure induces hepatic global and individual gene hypomethylation: implications for arsenic hepatocarcinogenesis. *Carcinogenesis*. 2004;25:1779–1786.

Chen JK, Taipale J, Cooper MK, Beachy PA. Inhibition of Hedgehog signaling by direct binding of cyclopamine to Smoothened. *Genes Dev*. 2002;16: 2743–2748.

Chen T. The role of microRNA in chemical carcinogenesis. *J Environ Sci Health C Environ Carcinog Ecotoxicol Rev*. 2010;28:89–124.

Chen W, Martindale L, Holbrook NJ, Liu Y. Tumor promoter arsenite activates extracellular signal-regulated kinase through a signaling pathway mediated by epidermal growth factor receptor and Shc. *Mol Cell Biol*. 1998;18:5178–5188.

Chipman JK, Mally A, Edwards GO. Disruption of gap junctions in toxicity and carcinogenicity. *Toxicol Sci*. 2003;71:146–153.

Christmann M, Tomicic MJ, Roos W, Kaina B. Mechanism of human DNA repair: an update. *Toxicology*. 2003;193:3–34.

Cohen SD, Pumford NR, Khairallah EA, et al. Contemporary issues in toxicology: selective protein covalent binding and target organ toxicity. *Toxicol Appl Pharmacol*. 1997;143:1–2.

Coleman MD, Jacobus DP. Reduction of dapsone hydroxylamine to dapsone during methaemoglobin formation in human erythrocytes in vitro. *Biochem Pharmacol*. 1993;45:1027–1033.

Coles B. Effects of modifying structure on electrophilic reactions with biological nucleophiles. *Drug Metab Rev*. 1984;15:1307–1334.

Commandeur JNM, Vermeulen NPE. Molecular and biochemical mechanisms of chemically induced nephrotoxicity: a review. *Chem Res Toxicol*. 1990;3:171–194.

Corcoran GB, Fix L, Jones DP, et al. Apoptosis: molecular control point in toxicity. *Toxicol Appl Pharmacol*. 1994;128:169–181.

Corthals SM, Kamendulis LM, Klaunig JE. Mechanisms of 2-butoxyethanol-induced hemangiosarcomas. *Toxicol Sci*. 2006;92:378–386.

Corton JM, Gillespie JG, Hardie DG. Role of the AMP-activated protein kinase in the cellular stress response. *Curr Biol*. 1994;4:315–324.

Costa RH, Kalinichenko VV, Holterman AX, Wang X. Transcription factors in liver development, differentiation, and regeneration. *Hepatology*. 2003;38:1331–1347.

Cribb AE, Peyrou M, Muruganandan S, Schneider L. The endoplasmic reticulum in xenobiotic toxicity. *Drug Metab Rev*. 2005;37: 405–442.

Dalton TP, Shertzer HG, Puga A. Regulation of gene expression by reactive oxygen. *Annu Rev Pharmacol Toxicol*. 1999;39:67–101.

D'Amours D, Desnoyers S, D'Silva I, Poirier GG. Poly(ADP-ribosyl)ation reactions in the regulation of nuclear functions. *Biochem J*. 1999;342:249–268.

Davies H, Bignell GR, Cox C, et al. Mutations of the BRAF gene in human cancer. *Nature*. 2002;417:949–954.

Davies KJ. Protein damage and degradation by oxygen radicals: I. General aspects. *J Biol Chem*. 1987;262:9895–9901.

De Matteis F. Drugs as suicide substrates of cytochrome P450. In: De Matteis F, Lock EA, eds. *Selectivity and Molecular Mechanisms of Toxicity*. Houndmills, England: Macmillan; 1987:183–210.

Denicola A, Radi R. Peroxynitrite and drug-dependent toxicity. *Toxicology*. 2005;208:273–288.

Denison MS, Soshilov AA, He G, Degroot DE, Zhao B. Exactly the same but different: promiscuity and diversity in the molecular mechanisms of action of the aryl hydrocarbon (dioxin) receptor. *Toxicol Sci*. 2011;124:1–22.

Desaiah D. Biochemical mechanisms of chlordecone neurotoxicity: a review. *Neurotoxicology*. 1982;3:103–110.

Dieguez-Acuna FJ, Polk WW, Ellis ME, et al. Nuclear factor κB activity determines the sensitivity of kidney epithelial cells to apoptosis: implications for mercury-induced renal failure. *Toxicol Sci*. 2004;82: 114–123.

Dinkova-Kostova AT, Holtzclaw WD, Kensler TW. The role of Keap1 in cellular protective responses. *Chem Res Toxicol*. 2005;18:1779–1791.

Dobson RL, Motlagh S, Quijano M, et al. Identification and characterization of toxicity of contaminants in pet food leading to an outbreak of renal toxicity in cats and dogs. *Toxicol Sci*. 2008;106:251–262.

Eaton DL, Gallagher EP. Mechanisms of aflatoxin carcinogenesis. *Annu Rev Pharmacol Toxicol*. 1994;34:135–172.

Edwards MJ, Keller BJ, Kauffman FC, Thurman RG. The involvement of Kupffer cells in carbon tetrachloride toxicity. *Toxicol Appl Pharmacol*. 1993;119:275–279.

El-Benna J, Dang PM, Gougerot-Pocidalo MA, Elbim C. Phagocyte NADPH oxidase: a multicomponent enzyme essential for host defenses. *Arch Immunol Ther Exp*. 2005;53:199–206.

Elbling L, Berger W, Rehberger A, et al. P-glycoprotein regulates chemosensitivity in early developmental stages of the mouse. *FASEB J*. 1993; 7:1499–1506.

Endo T, Minami M, Hirafuji M, et al. Neurochemistry and neuropharmacology of emesis—the role of serotonin. *Toxicology*. 2000;153: 189–201.

Engler H, Taurog A, Nakashima T. Mechanism of inactivation of thyroid peroxidase by thioureylene drugs. *Biochem Pharmacol*. 1982;31: 3801–3806.

Esteller M. Aberrant DNA methylation as a cancer-inducing mechanism. *Annu Rev Pharmacol Toxicol*. 2005;45:629–656.

Evans AM, Mustard KJ, Wyatt CN, et al. Does AMP-activated protein kinase couple inhibition of mitochondrial oxidative phosphorylation by hypoxia to calcium signaling in O_2-sensing cells? *J Biol Chem*. 2005;280:41504–41511.

Fausto N, Campbell JS, Riehle KJ. Liver regeneration. *Hepatology*. 2006;43:S45–S53.

Flanders KC. Smad3 as a mediator of the fibrotic response. *Int J Exp Pathol*. 2004;85:47–64.

Fletcher KA, Barton PF, Kelly JA. Studies on the mechanisms of oxidation in the erythrocyte by metabolites of primaquine. *Biochem Pharmacol*. 1988;37:2683–2690.

Forman HJ, Fukuto JM, Torres M. Redox signaling: thiol chemistry defines which reactive oxygen and nitrogen species can act as second messengers. *Am J Physiol Cell Physiol*. 2004;287:C246–C256.

Franks NP, Lieb WR. Which molecular targets are most relevant to general anaesthesia? *Toxicol Lett*. 1998;100–101:1–8.

Fromenty B, Pessayre D. Impaired mitochondrial function in microvesicular steatosis. Effects of drugs, ethanol, hormones and cytokines. *J Hepatol*. 1997;26:43–53.

Gale K. Role of GABA in the genesis of chemoconvulsant seizures. *Toxicol Lett*. 1992;64–65:417–428.

Ganz T. Hepcidin and iron regulation, 10 years later. *Blood*. 2011;117: 4425–4433.

Garofalo M, Croce CM. MicroRNAs: master regulators as potential therapeutics in cancer. *Annu Rev Pharmacol Toxicol*. 2011;51:25–43.

Glass DJ. Signaling pathways perturbing muscle mass. *Curr Opin Clin Nutr Metab Care*. 2010;13:225–229.

Goering PL. Lead–protein interactions as a basis for lead toxicity. *Neurotoxicology*. 1993;14:45–60.

Goldberg Y. Protein phosphatase 2A: who shall regulate the regulator? *Biochem Pharmacol*. 1999;4:321–328.

Gonzalez FJ, Fernandez-Salguero P. The aryl hydrocarbon receptor. Studies using the AhR-null mice. *Drug Metab Dispos*. 1998;26:1194–1198.

Gonzalez FJ, Shah YM. PPARalpha: mechanism of species differences and hepatocarcinogenesis of peroxisome proliferators. *Toxicology.* 2008; 246:2–8.

Gonzalez FJ, Yu AM. Cytochrome P450 and xenobiotic receptor humanized mice. *Annu Rev Pharmacol Toxicol.* 2006;46:41–64.

Goodman JI, Watson RE. Altered DNA methylation: a secondary mechanism involved in carcinogenesis. *Annu Rev Pharmacol Toxicol.* 2002;42:501–525.

Gravina SA, Mieyal JJ. Thioltransferase is a specific glutathionyl mixed disulfide oxidoreductase. *Biochemistry.* 1993;32:3368–3376.

Green DR. Apoptotic pathways: the roads to ruin. *Cell.* 1998;94:695–698.

Green DR, Kroemer G. Cytoplasmic functions of the tumour suppressor p53. *Nature.* 2009;458:1127–1130.

Green S. Nuclear receptors and chemical carcinogenesis. *Trends Pharmacol Sci.* 1992;13:251–255.

Gregus Z, Klaassen CD. Enterohepatic circulation of toxicants. In: Rozman K, Hanninien O, eds. *Gastrointestinal Toxicology.* Amsterdam: Elsevier/ North Holland; 1986:57–118.

Gregus Z, Roos G, Geerlings P, Németi B. Mechanism of thiol-supported arsenate reduction mediated by phosphorolytic-arsenolytic enzymes. II. Enzymatic formation of arsenylated products susceptible for reduction to arsenite by thiols. *Toxicol Sci.* 2009;110:282–292.

Gressner AM. Hepatic fibrogenesis: the puzzle of interacting cells, fibrogenic cytokines, regulatory loops, and extracellular matrix molecules. *Z Gastroenterol.* 1992;30(suppl 1):5–16.

Grimm C, Hermann DM, Bogdanova A, et al. Neuroprotection by hypoxic preconditioning: HIF-1 and erythropoietin protect from retinal degeneration. *Semin Cell Dev Biol.* 2005;16:531–538.

Hansen JM, Go Y-M, Jones DP. Nuclear and mitochondrial compartmentation of oxidative stress and redox signaling. *Annu Rev Pharmacol Toxicol.* 2006;46:215–234.

Harb R, Xie G, Lutzko C, et al. Bone marrow progenitor cells repair rat hepatic sinusoidal endothelial cells after liver injury. *Gastroenterology.* 2009;137:704–712.

Hardie DG, Hawley SA, Scott JW. AMP-activated protein kinase—development of the energy sensor concept. *J Physiol.* 2006;574:7–15.

Hardman JG, Gilman AG, Limbird LL, eds. *Goodman & Gilman's The Pharmacological Basis of Therapeutics.* 9th ed. New York: McGraw-Hill; 1995.

Harms K, Nozell S, Chen X. The common and distinct target genes of the p53 family transcription factors. *Cell Mol Life Sci.* 2004;61:822–842.

Harrison R. Structure and function of xanthine oxidoreductase: where are we now? *Free Radic Biol Med.* 2002;33:774–797.

Hasselgren PO, Alamdari N, Aversa Z, et al. Corticosteroids and muscle wasting: role of transcription factors, nuclear cofactors, and hyperacetylation. *Curr Opin Clin Nutr Metab Care.* 2010;13:423–428.

Herken H, Hucho F, eds. *Selective Neurotoxicity.* Berlin: Springer-Verlag; 1992.

Herman B, Gores GJ, Nieminen AL, et al. Calcium and pH in anoxic and toxic injury. *Crit Rev Toxicol.* 1990;21:127–148.

Herrlich P, Rahmsdorf HJ, Bender K. Signal transduction induced by adverse agents: "activation by inhibition." The UV response 1997. In: Puga A, Wallace KB, eds. *Molecular Biology of the Toxic Response.* Philadelphia: Taylor & Francis; 1999:479–492.

Higuchi H, Gores GJ. Bile acid regulation of hepatic physiology: IV. Bile acids and death receptors. *Am J Physiol.* 2003;284:G734–G738.

Higuchi M, Yoshikawa Y, Orino K, Watanabe K. Effect of diquat-induced oxidative stress on iron metabolism in male Fischer-344 rats. *Biometals.* 2011;24:1123–1131.

Hill DA, Jean PA, Roth RA. Bile duct epithelial cells exposed to alpha-naphthylisothiocyanate produce a factor that causes neutrophil-dependent hepatocellular injury in vitro. *Toxicol Sci.* 1999;47:118–125.

Hippeli S, Elstner EF. Transition metal ion-catalyzed oxygen activation during pathogenic processes. *FEBS Lett.* 1999;443:1–7.

Holmgren A, Johansson C, Berndt C, Lonn ME, Hudemann C, Lillig CH. Thiol redox control via the thioredoxin and glutaredoxin systems. *Biochem Soc Trans.* 2005;33:1375–1377.

Hosokawa N, Hara T, Kaizuka T, et al. Nutrient-dependent mTORC1 association with the ULK-1-Atg13–FIP200 complex required for autophagy. *Mol Biol Cell.* 2009;20:1981–1991.

Huang W, Ma K, Zhang J, et al. Nuclear receptor-dependent bile acid signaling is required for normal liver regeneration. *Science.* 2006;312: 233–236.

Hwang GW, Ishida Y, Naganuma A. Identification of F-box proteins that are involved in resistance to methylmercury in *Saccharomyces cerevisiae. FEBS Lett.* 2006;580:6813–6818.

Jäättelä M. Escaping cell death: survival proteins in cancer. *Exp Cell Res.* 1999;248:30–43.

Jaeschke H. Cellular adhesion molecules: regulation and functional significance in the pathogenesis of liver diseases. *Am J Physiol.* 1997;273:G602–G611.

Jaeschke H, Bajt ML. Intracellular signaling mechanisms of acetaminophen-induced liver cell death. *Toxicol Sci.* 2006;89:31–41.

Jaiswal AK. Nrf2 signaling in coordinated activation of antioxidant gene expression. *Free Radic Biol Med.* 2004;36:1199–1207.

Jaworski M, Buchmann A, Bauer P, Riess O, Schwarz M. B-raf and H-ras mutations in chemically induced mouse liver tumors. *Oncogene.* 2005;24:1290–1295.

Johnson AR. Contact inhibition in the failure of mammalian CNS axonal regeneration. *Bioessays.* 1993;15:807–813.

Johnson DG, Walker CL. Cyclins and cell cycle checkpoints. *Annu Rev Pharmacol Toxicol.* 1999;39:295–312.

Kantorow M, Lee W, Chauss D. Focus on molecules: methionine sulfoxide reductase A. *Exp Eye Res.* 2012;100:110–111.

Kappus H. Overview of enzyme systems involved in bio-reduction of drugs and in redox cycling. *Biochem Pharmacol.* 1986;35:1–6.

Karin M. Nuclear factor-κB in cancer development and progression. *Nature.* 2006;441:431–436.

Katoh Y, Katoh M. Hedgehog signaling, epithelial-to-mesenchymal transition and miRNA (review). *Int J Mol Med.* 2008;22:271–275.

Ketterer B. Protective role of glutathione and glutathione transferases in mutagenesis and carcinogenesis. *Mutat Res.* 1988;202:343–361.

Kim JS, He L, Lemasters JJ. Mitochondrial permeability transition: a common pathway to necrosis and apoptosis. *Biochem Biophys Res Commun.* 2003;304:463–470.

Kim SY, Suzuki N, Laxmi YR, Shibutani S. Genotoxic mechanism of tamoxifen in developing endometrial cancer. *Drug Metab Rev.* 2004;36:199–218.

Klaassen CD, Liu J, Choudhuri S. Metallothionein: an intracellular protein to protect against cadmium toxicity. *Annu Rev Pharmacol Toxicol.* 1999;39:267–294.

Klaassen CD, Reisman SA. Nrf2 the rescue: effects of the antioxidative/electrophilic response on the liver. *Toxicol Appl Pharmacol.* 2010;244:57–65.

Kodavanti UP, Mehendale HM. Cationic amphiphilic drugs and phospholipid storage disorder. *Pharmacol Rev.* 1990;42:327–353.

Krell H, Metz J, Jaeschke H, et al. Drug-induced intrahepatic cholestasis: characterization of different pathomechanisms. *Arch Toxicol.* 1987;60:124–130.

Kroemer G, Dallaporta B, Resche-Rigon M. The mitochondrial death/ life regulator in apoptosis and necrosis. *Annu Rev Physiol.* 1998;60: 619–642.

Krueger SK, Williams DE. Mammalian flavin-containing monooxygenases: structure/function, genetic polymorphisms and role in drug metabolism. *Pharmacol Ther.* 2005;106:357–387.

Larsson BS. Interaction between chemicals and melanin. *Pigment Cell Res.* 1993;6:127–133.

Laurent G, Kishore BK, Tulkens PM. Aminoglycoside-induced renal phospholipidosis and nephrotoxicity. *Biochem Pharmacol.* 1990;40: 2383–2392.

Lee EW, Lai Y, Zhang H, Unadkat JD. Identification of the mitochondrial targeting signal of the human equilibrative nucleoside transporter 1 (hENT1): implications for interspecies differences in mitochondrial toxicity of fialuridine. *J Biol Chem.* 2006;281:16700–16706.

Lee J, Richburg JH, Younkin SC, Boekelheide K. The Fas system is a key regulator of germ cell apoptosis in the testis. *Endocrinology.* 1997;138:2081–2088.

Lee JI, Burckart GJ. Nuclear factor kappa B: important transcription factor and therapeutic target. *J Clin Pharmacol.* 1998;38:981–993.

Lehmann AR, Dean SW. Cancer-prone human disorders with defects in DNA repair. In: Cooper CS, Grover PL, eds. *Chemical Carcinogenesis and Mutagenesis II*. Berlin: Springer-Verlag; 1990:71–101.

Leist M, Nicotera P. Calcium and neuronal death. *Rev Physiol Biochem Pharmacol*. 1997;132:79–125.

Leist M, Single B, Castoldi AF, et al. Intracellular adenosine triphosphate (ATP) concentration: a switch in the decision between apoptosis and necrosis. *J Exp Med*. 1997;185:1481–1486.

Lelli JL, Becks LL, Dabrowska MI, Hinshaw DB. ATP converts necrosis to apoptosis in oxidant-injured endothelial cells. *Free Radic Biol Med*. 1998;25:694–702.

Leung L, Kalgutkar AS, Obach RS. Metabolic activation in drug-induced liver injury. *Drug Metab Rev*. 2012;44:18–33.

Lewis W, Levine ES, Griniuviene B, et al. Fialuridine and its metabolites inhibit DNA polymerase γ at sites of multiple adjacent analog incorporation, decrease mtDNA abundance, and cause mitochondrial structural defects in cultured hepatoblasts. *Proc Natl Acad Sci U S A*. 1996;93:3592–3597.

Li H, Wang P, Sun Q, et al. Following cytochrome c release, autophagy is inhibited during chemotherapy-induced apoptosis by caspase 8-mediated cleavage of Beclin 1. *Cancer Res*. 2011;71:3625–3634.

Li X, Heyer WD. Homologous recombination in DNA repair and DNA damage tolerance. *Cell Res*. 2008;18:99–113.

Lichten P, Schaffner W. The "metal transcription factor" MTF-1: biological facts and medical applications. *Swiss Med Wkly*. 2001;131:647–652.

Lim RT Jr, Gentry RT, Ito D, et al. First-pass metabolism of ethanol is predominantly gastric. *Alcohol Clin Exp Res*. 1993;17:1337–1344.

Lin JH, Chiba M, Baillie TA. Is the role of the small intestine in first-pass metabolism overemphasized? *Pharmacol Rev*. 1999;51:135–137.

Lindroos PM, Zarnegar R, Michalopoulos GK. Hepatocyte growth factor (hepatopoietin A) rapidly increases in plasma before DNA synthesis and liver regeneration stimulated by partial hepatectomy and carbon tetrachloride administration. *Hepatology*. 1991;13:743–750.

Liu G, Chen X. Regulation of the p53 transcriptional activity. *J Cell Biochem*. 2006;97:448–458.

Liu X, Van Vleet T, Schnellmann RG. The role of calpain in oncotic cell death. *Annu Rev Pharmacol Toxicol*. 2004;44:349–370.

Lotersztajn S, Julien B, Teixeira-Clerc F, et al. Hepatic fibrosis: molecular mechanisms and drug targets. *Annu Rev Pharmacol Toxicol*. 2005;45:605–628.

Lowther WT, Haynes AC. Reduction of cysteine sulfinic acid in eukaryotic, typical 2-Cys peroxiredoxins by sulfiredoxin. *Antioxid Redox Signal*. 2011;15:99–109.

Lozano RM, Yee BC, Buchanan BB. Thioredoxin-linked reductive inactivation of venom neurotoxins. *Arch Biochem Biophys*. 1994;309:356–362.

Lu H, Choudhuri S, Ogura K, et al. Characterization of organic anion transporting polypeptide 1b2-null mice: essential role in hepatic uptake/toxicity of phalloidin and microcystin-LR. *Toxicol Sci*. 2008;103:35–45.

Lynn S, Gurr JR, Lai HT, Jan KY. NADH oxidase activation is involved in arsenite-induced oxidative DNA damage in human vascular smooth muscle cells. *Circ Res*. 2000;86:514–519.

Ma X, Babish JG. Activation of signal transduction pathways by dioxins. "Activation by inhibition." The UV response 1997. In: Puga A, Wallace KB, eds. *Molecular Biology of the Toxic Response*. Philadelphia: Taylor & Francis; 1999:493–516.

Malhi H, Kaufman RJ. Endoplasmic reticulum stress in liver disease. *J Hepatol*. 2011;54:795–809.

Martin TR, Hagimoto N, Nakamura M, Matute-Bello G. Apoptosis and epithelial injury in the lungs. *Proc Am Thorac Soc*. 2005;2:214–220.

Maser E. Significance of reductases in the detoxification of the tobacco-specific carcinogen NNK. *Trends Pharmacol Sci*. 2004;25:235–237.

Maser E. Neuroprotective role for carbonyl reductase? *Biochem Biophys Res Commun*. 2006;340:1019–1022.

Maxwell P, Salnikow K. HIF-1, an oxygen and metal responsive transcription factor. *Cancer Biol Ther*. 2004;3:29–35.

McCuskey RS. The hepatic microvascular system in health and its response to toxicants. *Anat Rec (Hoboken)*. 2008;291:661–671.

McGowan CH, Russell P. The DNA damage response: sensing and signaling. *Curr Opin Cell Biol*. 2004;16:629–633.

Mehendale HM. Tissue repair: an important determinant of final outcome of toxicant-induced injury. *Toxicol Pathol*. 2005;33:41–51.

Mehrpour M, Esclatine A, Beau I, Codogno P. Overview of macroautophagy regulation in mammalian cells. *Cell Res*. 2010;20:748–762.

Miller JA, Surh Y-J. Sulfonation in chemical carcinogenesis. In: Kauffman FC, ed. *Conjugation–Deconjugation Reactions in Drug Metabolism and Toxicity*. Berlin: Springer-Verlag; 1994:429–457.

Miller MS. Tumor suppressor genes in rodent lung carcinogenesis. Mutation of p53 does not appear to be an early lesion in lung tumor pathogenesis. *Toxicol Appl Pharmacol*. 1999;156:70–77.

Molitoris JK, McColl KS, Distelhorst CW. Glucocorticoid-mediated repression of the oncogenic microRNA cluster miR-17~92 contributes to the induction of Bim and initiation of apoptosis. *Mol Endocrinol*. 2011;25:409–420.

Morelli A, Ravera S, Panfoli I. Hypothesis of an energetic function for myelin. *Cell Biochem Biophys*. 2011;61:179–187.

Morgensztern D, McLeod HL. PI3K/Akt/mTOR pathway as target for cancer therapy. *Anticancer Drugs*. 2005;16:797–803.

Moskovitz J. Methionine sulfoxide reductases: ubiquitous enzymes involved in antioxidant defense, protein regulation, and prevention of aging-associated diseases. *Biochim Biophys Acta*. 2005;1703:213–219.

Murphy MP. Nitric oxide and cell death. *Biochim Biophys Acta*. 1999;1411:401–414.

Mustafa MG. Biochemical basis of ozone toxicity. *Free Radic Biol Med*. 1990;9:245–265.

Nagy G, Kardon T, Wunderlich L, et al. Acetaminophen induces ER dependent signaling in mouse liver. *Arch Biochem Biophys*. 2007;459:273–279.

Narahashi T. Transmitter-activated ion channels as the target of chemical agents. In: Kito S, Segawa T, Olsen R, eds. *Neuroreceptor Mechanisms in the Brain*. New York: Plenum Press; 1991:61–73.

Narahashi T. Nerve membrane Na⁺ channels as targets of insecticides. *Trends Pharmacol Sci*. 1992;13:236–241.

Nelson SD, Pearson PG. Covalent and noncovalent interactions in acute lethal cell injury caused by chemicals. *Annu Rev Pharmacol Toxicol*. 1990;30:169–195.

Németi B, Regonesi ME, Tortora P, Gregus Z. Polynucleotide phosphorylase and mitochondrial ATP synthase mediate reduction of arsenate to the more toxic arsenite by forming arsenylated analogues of ADP and ATP. *Toxicol Sci*. 2010;117:270–281.

Neumann CA, Cao J, Manevich Y. Peroxiredoxin 1 and its role in cell signaling. *Cell Cycle*. 2009;8:4072–4078.

Newbold RR. Lessons learned from perinatal exposure to diethylstilbestrol. *Toxicol Appl Pharmacol*. 2004;199:142–150.

Nicotera P, Bellomo G, Orrenius S. Calcium-mediated mechanisms in chemically induced cell death. *Annu Rev Pharmacol Toxicol*. 1992;32:449–470.

Noji S, Tashiro K, Koyama E, et al. Expression of hepatocyte growth factor gene in endothelial and Kupffer cells of damaged rat livers, as revealed by in situ hybridization. *Biochem Biophys Res Commun*. 1990;173:42–47.

Nony PA, Schnellmann RG. Mechanisms of renal cell repair and regeneration after acute renal failure. *J Pharmacol Exp Ther*. 2003;304:905–912.

Oortgiesen M, Leinders T, van Kleef RG, Vijverberg HP. Differential neurotoxicological effects of lead on voltage-dependent and receptor-operated ion channels. *Neurotoxicology*. 1993;14:87–96.

Orrenius S. Mitochondrial regulation of apoptotic cell death. *Toxicol Lett*. 2004;149:19–23.

Orrenius S, Nicotera P, Zhivotovsky B. Cell death mechanisms and their implications in toxicology. *Toxicol Sci*. 2011;119:3–19.

Osawa Y, Davila JC, Nakatsuka M, et al. Inhibition of P450 cytochromes by reactive intermediates. *Drug Metab Rev*. 1995;27:61–72.

Park BK, Kitteringham NR, Maggs JL, Pirmohamed M, Williams DP. The role of metabolic activation in drug-induced hepatotoxicity. *Annu Rev Pharmacol Toxicol*. 2005;45:177–202.

Park JD, Cherrington NJ, Klaassen CD. Intestinal absorption of cadmium is associated with divalent metal transporter 1 in rats. *Toxicol Sci*. 2002;68:288–294.

Patel MN, Yim GK, Isom GE. N-Methyl-D-aspartate receptors mediate cyanide-induced cytotoxicity in hippocampal cultures. *Neurotoxicology.* 1993;14:35–40.

Perouansky M, Kirson ED, Yaari Y. Mechanism of action of volatile anesthetics: effects of halothane on glutamate receptors in vitro. *Toxicol Lett.* 1998;100–101:65–69.

Peters JM, Aoyama T, Cattley RC, et al. Role of peroxisome proliferator-activated receptor α in altered cell cycle regulation in mouse liver. *Carcinogenesis.* 1998;19:1989–1994.

Poellinger L, Göttlicher M, Gustafsson JA. The dioxin and peroxisome proliferator-activated receptors: nuclear receptors in search of endogenous ligands. *Trends Pharmacol Sci.* 1992;13:241–245.

Pogribny IP, Muskhelishvili L, Tryndyak VP, Beland FA. The role of epigenetic events in genotoxic hepatocarcinogenesis induced by 2-acetylaminofluorene. *Mutat Res.* 2011;722:106–113.

Poirier LA. Methyl group deficiency in hepatocarcinogenesis. *Drug Metab Rev.* 1994;26:185–199.

Poli V. The role of C/EBP isoforms in the control of inflammatory and native immunity functions. *J Biol Chem.* 1998;273:29279–29282.

Poppek D, Grune T. Proteasomal defense of oxidative protein modifications. *Antioxid Redox Signal.* 2006;8:173–184.

Pouyssegur J, Dayan F, Mazure NM. Hypoxia signaling in cancer and approaches to enforce tumor regression. *Nature.* 2006;441:437–443.

Pratt WB, Morishima Y, Peng HM, Osawa Y. Proposal for a role of the Hsp90/Hsp70-based chaperone machinery in making triage decisions when proteins undergo oxidative and toxic damage. *Exp Biol Med (Maywood).* 2010;235:278–289.

Pumford NR, Halmes NC. Protein targets of xenobiotic reactive intermediates. *Annu Rev Pharmacol Toxicol.* 1997;37:91–117.

Qi M, Elion EA. MAP kinase pathways. *J Cell Sci.* 2005;118:3569–3572.

Qian T, Herman B, Lemasters JJ. The mitochondrial permeability transition mediates both necrotic and apoptotic death of hepatocytes exposed to Br-A23187. *Toxicol Appl Pharmacol.* 1999;154:117–125.

Quievryn G, Messer J, Zhitkovich A. Carcinogenic chromium(VI) induces cross-linking of vitamin C to DNA in vitro and in human lung A549 cells. *Biochemistry.* 2002;41:3156–3167.

Rabinowitz JD, White E. Autophagy and metabolism. *Science.* 2010;330:1344–1348.

Raghow R. The role of extracellular matrix in postinflammatory wound healing and fibrosis. *FASEB J.* 1994;8:823–831.

Ray SS, Swanson HI. Dioxin-induced immortalization of normal human keratinocytes and silencing of p53 and p16INK4a. *J Biol Chem.* 2004;279:27187–27193.

Recknagel RO, Glende EA Jr, Dolak JA, Waller RL. Mechanisms of carbon tetrachloride toxicity. *Pharmacol Ther.* 1989;43:139–154.

Reed JC, Jurgensmeier JM, Matsuyama S. Bcl-2 family proteins and mitochondria. *Biochim Biophys Acta.* 1998;1366:127–137.

Rhee SG, Kang SW, Jeong W. Intracellular messenger function of hydrogen peroxide and its regulation by peroxiredoxins. *Curr Opin Cell Biol.* 2005;17:183–189.

Richter C, Kass GE. Oxidative stress in mitochondria: its relationship to cellular Ca^{2+} homeostasis, cell death, proliferation, and differentiation. *Chem Biol Interact.* 1991;77:1–23.

Roderburg C, Urban GW, Bettermann K, et al. Micro-RNA profiling reveals a role for miR-29 in human and murine liver fibrosis. *Hepatology.* 2011;53:209–218.

Rodriguez-Enriquez S, He L, Lemasters JJ. Role of mitochondrial permeability transition pores in mitochondrial autophagy. *Int J Biochem Cell Biol.* 2004;36:2463–2472.

Rombach EM, Hanzlik RP. Detection of adducts of bromobenzene 3,4-oxide with rat liver microsomal protein sulfhydryl groups using specific antibodies. *Chem Res Toxicol.* 1999;12:159–163.

Rose ML, Rusyn I, Bojes HK, et al. Role of Kupffer cells in peroxisome proliferator-induced hepatocyte proliferation. *Drug Metab Rev.* 1999;31:87–116.

Roth RA, Luyendyk JP, Maddox JF, Ganey PE. Inflammation and drug idiosyncrasy—is there a connection? *J Pharmacol Exp Ther.* 2003;307:1–8.

Rothwell NJ. Functions and mechanisms of interleukin 1 in the brain. *Trends Pharmacol Sci.* 1991;12:430–436.

Sanguinetti MC, Mitcheson JS. Predicting drug–hERG channel interactions that cause acquired long QT syndrome. *Trends Pharmacol Sci.* 2005;26:119–124.

Saurat JH, Kaya G, Saxer-Sekulic N, et al. The cutaneous lesions of dioxin exposure: lessons from the poisoning of Victor Yushchenko. *Toxicol Sci.* 2012;125:310–317.

Scheschonka A, Murphy ME, Sies H. Temporal relationships between the loss of vitamin E, protein sulfhydryls and lipid peroxidation in microsomes challenged with different prooxidants. *Chem Biol Interact.* 1990;74:233–252.

Schinkel AH. P-glycoprotein, a gatekeeper in the blood–brain barrier. *Adv Drug Deliv Rev.* 1999;36:179–194.

Schmidt M, Goebeler M. Nickel allergies: paying the Toll for innate immunity. *J Mol Med.* 2011;89:961–970.

Schulte-Hermann R, Timmermann-Trosiener I, Barthel G, Bursch W. DNA synthesis, apoptosis, and phenotypic expression as determinants of growth of altered foci in rat liver during phenobarbital promotion. *Cancer Res.* 1990;50:5127–5135.

Seki T, Ishimoto T, Sakurai T, et al. Increased excretion of urinary 20-HETE in rats with cyclosporine-induced nephrotoxicity. *J Pharmacol Sci.* 2005;97:132–137.

Shaw RJ, Cantley LC. Ras, PI(3)K and mTOR signalling controls tumour cell growth. *Nature.* 2006;441:424–430.

Shi X, Dalal NS. NADPH-dependent flavoenzymes catalyze one electron reduction of metal ions and molecular oxygen and generate hydroxyl radicals. *FEBS Lett.* 1990;276:189–191.

Sies H. Strategies of antioxidant defense. *Eur J Biochem.* 1993;215:213–219.

Smith KR, Klei LR, Barchowsky A. Arsenite stimulates plasma membrane NADPH oxidase in vascular endothelial cells. *Am J Physiol.* 2001;280:L442–L449.

Smith MR, Matthews NT, Jones KA, Kung HE. Biological actions of oncogenes. *Pharmacol Ther.* 1993;58:211–236.

Soni MG, Mehendale HM. Role of tissue repair in toxicologic interactions among hepatotoxic organics. *Environ Health Perspect.* 1998;106:1307–1317.

Squadrito GL, Pryor WA. Oxidative chemistry of nitric oxide: the roles of superoxide, peroxynitrite, and carbon dioxide. *Free Radic Biol Med.* 1998;25:392–403.

Sreedhar AS, Csermely P. Heat-shock proteins in the regulation of apoptosis: new strategies in tumor therapy: a comprehensive review. *Pharmacol Ther.* 2004;101:227–257.

Stachlewitz RF, Seabra V, Bradford B, et al. Glycine and uridine prevent D-galactosamine hepatoxicity in the rat: role of the Kupffer cells. *Hepatology.* 1999;29:737–745.

Stephens TD, Bunde CJ, Fillmore BJ. Mechanism of action in thalidomide teratogenesis. *Biochem Pharmacol.* 2000;59:1489–1499.

Stouder C, Somm E, Paoloni-Giacobino A. Prenatal exposure to ethanol: a specific effect on the H19 gene in sperm. *Reprod Toxicol.* 2011;31:507–512.

Su AI, Guidotti LG, Pezacki JP, et al. Gene expression during the priming phase of liver regeneration after partial hepatectomy in mice. *Proc Natl Acad Sci U S A.* 2002;99:11181–11186.

Sun X, Tian X, Tomsig JL, Suszkiw JB. Analysis of differential effects of Pb^{2+} on protein kinase C isozymes. *Toxicol Appl Pharmacol.* 1999;156:40–45.

Szabó C. DNA strand breakage and activation of poly-ADP ribosyltransferase: a cytotoxic pathway triggered by peroxynitrite. *Free Radic Biol Med.* 1996;21:855–869.

Tanaka A. Parkin-mediated selective mitochondrial autophagy, mitophagy: Parkin purges damaged organelles from the vital mitochondrial network. *FEBS Lett.* 2010;584:1386–1392.

Tang JY, So PL, Epstein EH Jr. Novel Hedgehog pathway targets against basal cell carcinoma. *Toxicol Appl Pharmacol.* 2007;224:257–264.

Taupin D, Podolsky DK. Trefoil factors: initiators of mucosal healing. *Nat Rev Mol Cell Biol.* 2003;4:721–732.

Thévenod F, Chakraborty PK. The role of Wnt/beta-catenin signaling in renal carcinogenesis: lessons from cadmium toxicity studies. *Curr Mol Med.* 2010;10:387–404.

Toivola DM, Eriksson JE. Toxins affecting cell signalling and alteration of cytoskeletal structure. *Toxicol In Vitro.* 1999;13:521–530.

Tokar EJ, Ou W, Waalkes MP. Arsenic, stem cells, and the developmental basis of adult cancer. *Toxicol Sci.* 2011;120:S192–S203.

Tryndyak VP, Muskhelishvili L, Kovalchuk O, et al. Effect of long-term tamoxifen exposure on genotoxic and epigenetic changes in rat liver: implications for tamoxifen-induced hepatocarcinogenesis. *Carcinogenesis.* 2006;27:1713–1720.

Uetrecht JP. The role of leukocyte-generated reactive metabolites in the pathogenesis of idiosyncratic drug reactions. *Drug Metab Rev.* 1992;24:299–366.

Vaidya VS, Shankar K, Lock EA, et al. Molecular mechanisms of renal tissue repair in survival from acute renal tubule necrosis: role of ERK1/2 pathway. *Toxicol Pathol.* 2003;31:604–618.

Vallyathan V, Shi X, Castranova V. Reactive oxygen species: their relation to pneumoconiosis and carcinogenesis. *Environ Health Perspect.* 1998;106:1151–1155.

van Kuijk FJGM, Sevanian A, Handelman GJ, Dratz EA. A new role for phospholipase A2: protection of membranes from lipid peroxidation damage. *TIBS.* 1987;12:31–34.

Vessey CJ, Hall PM. Hepatic stem cells: a review. *Pathology.* 2001;33:130–141.

Waddick KG, Uckun FM. Innovative treatment programs against cancer: II. Nuclear factor-κ B (NF-κB) as a molecular target. *Biochem Pharmacol.* 1999;57:9–17.

Wahid F, Shehzad A, Khan T, Kim YY. MicroRNAs: synthesis, mechanism, function, and recent clinical trials. *Biochim Biophys Acta.* 2010;1803:1231–1243.

Wallace KB. Mitochondrial off targets of drug therapy. *Trends Pharmacol Sci.* 2008;29:361–366.

Wallace KB, Starkov AA. Mitochondrial targets of drug toxicity. *Annu Rev Pharmacol Toxicol.* 2000;40:353–388.

Wang JF, Komarov P, de Groot H. Luminol chemiluminescence in rat macrophages and granulocytes: the role of NO, and HOCl. *Arch Biochem Biophys.* 1993;304:189–196.

Watson WH, Yang X, Choi YE, Jones DP, Kehrer JP. Thioredoxin and its role in toxicology. *Toxicol Sci.* 2004;78:3–14.

Weiss SJ, LoBuglio AF. Phagocyte-generated oxygen metabolites and cellular injury. *Lab Invest.* 1982;47:5–18.

Wu Q, Ohsako S, Ishimura R, Suzuki JS, Tohyama C. Exposure of mouse preimplantation embryos to 2,3,7,8-tetrachlorodibenzo-*p*-dioxin (TCDD) alters the methylation status of imprinted genes H19 and Igf2. *Biol Reprod.* 2004;70:1790–1797.

Wyllie AH. Apoptosis: an overview. *Br Med Bull.* 1997;53:451–465.

Yin M, Ikejima K, Arteel GE, et al. Glycine accelerates recovery from alcohol-induced liver injury. *J Pharmacol Exp Ther.* 1998;286:1014–1019.

Yokoi T, Nakajima M. Toxicological implications of modulation of gene expression by microRNAs. *Toxicol Sci.* 2011;123:1–14.

Yoshioka W, Higashiyama W, Tohyama C. Involvement of microRNAs in dioxin-induced liver damage in the mouse. *Toxicol Sci.* 2011;122:457–465.

Youle RJ, Narendra DP. Mechanisms of mitophagy. *Nat Rev Mol Cell Biol.* 2011;12:9–14.

chapter 4

Risk Assessment

Elaine M. Faustman and Gilbert S. Omenn

INTRODUCTION AND HISTORICAL CONTEXT

In the 1970s Congress established a basic plan for environmental laws that authorized regulatory actions to protect public health and the environment. These science-based actions provided the foundation for environmental and human health risk assessment. Toxicological research and toxicity testing constitute the scientific core of risk assessment, which is used for evaluating potential adverse health impacts from chemical exposures. However, such considerations for risk evaluation were not new, since for decades the American Conference of Governmental Industrial Hygienists (ACGIH) set threshold limit values for occupational exposures and the US Food and Drug Administration (FDA) established acceptable daily intakes (ADIs) for pesticide residues and food additives. In 1958, the US Congress instructed the FDA in the Delaney Clause to prohibit the addition of all substances found to cause cancer in animals or humans to the food supply. Pragmatically, this policy allowed food sources that had nondetectable levels of these additives to be declared "safe." As advances in analytical chemistry revealed that "nondetects" were not equivalent to "not present," regulatory agencies were forced to develop "tolerance levels" and "acceptable risk levels." Risk assessment methodologies blossomed in the 1970s with the rising need to address these issues and statues and to provide a common framework for considering human and ecological health effects (Albert, 1994).

Risk assessment was defined as a specific activity in 1983 in the National Research Council (NRC) publication *Risk Assessment in the Federal Government: Managing the Process (Red Book)*. This book detailed steps for hazard identification, dose–response assessment, exposure analysis, and characterization of risks (NRC, 1983). These 4 basic framework steps now form the foundation framework for risk assessment and risk management approaches for many contexts such as children's health and ecological health and they provide a consistent context for risk assessment frameworks across agencies nationally and worldwide. Risk assessment frameworks have been used by the Health and Safety Executive Risk Assessment Policy Unit of the United Kingdom (Great Britain and Health and Safety Executive, 1999) and by the World Health Organization (NRC, 2009; WHO, 2010) and all of these build from these common components. Fig. 4-1 illustrates a framework with bidirectional arrows demonstrating an ideal situation where mechanistic research feeds directly into risk assessments and critical data uncertainty drives research. The common elements of the basic risk assessment framework are shown in red highlight. Initially, attention in risk assessment was focused on cancer risks; in subsequent years, noncancer end points were examined with similar methods and risk assessments were performed across life stages and for ecosystems. Continuing advances in toxicology, epidemiology, exposure assessment, biologically based modeling of adverse responses, and modeling of variability and uncertainty, as well as the rapidly growing area of genomics, have contributed to improvements in risk assessment. Risk assessment links with the public policy objectives from risk management often require extrapolations that go far beyond the observation of actual effects. Extrapolating data to address risks continues to generate controversy.

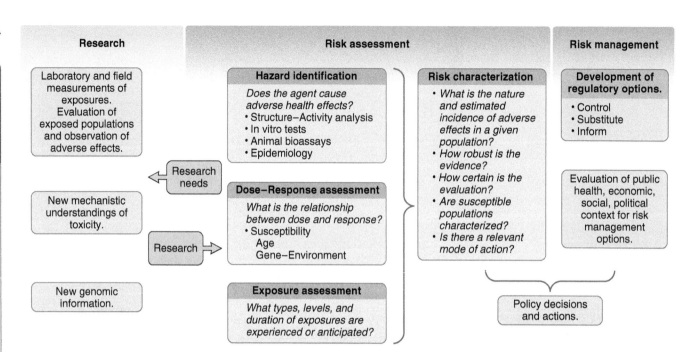

Figure 4-1. *Risk assessment/risk management framework.* This framework shows, under the red highlight, the 4 key steps of risk assessment: hazard identification, dose–response assessment, exposure assessment, and risk characterization. It shows an interactive, 2-way process where research needs from the risk assessment process drive new research, and new research findings modify risk assessment outcomes. (Adapted from Calkins *et al.* (1980), NRC Committee on Risk Assessment Methodology (1993), NRC (1994), Faustman and Omenn (1996), Risk Commission (1997), and Gargas *et al.* (1999); reprinted with permission from the National Academic Press, National Academy of Sciences.)

The National Academy of Sciences (NAS) 1994 report entitled *Science and Judgment in Risk Assessment* captured in its title the combination of qualitative and quantitative approaches essential for effective assessment of risks (NRC, 1994). The report discussed in detail the challenges and provided approaches for incorporating new scientific findings into the risk assessment process. It also highlighted ways to deal with uncertainty when insufficient scientific information was available. To address these challenges, the Presidential/Congressional Commission on Risk Assessment and Risk Management (Risk Commission, 1997) formulated a comprehensive framework that (1) placed each environmental problem or issue into public health and/or ecological context and (2) proactively called for engaging relevant stakeholders, often affected or potentially affected community groups, from the very beginning of the 6-stage process shown in Fig. 4-2. This report emphasized that particular exposures and potential health effects must be evaluated across sources and exposure pathways and in light of multiple end points, not just one chemical, in one environmental medium (air, water, soil, food, products), for one health effect at a time. The single-chemical, single-exposure approach had been the general approach up to this time. The importance of defining the risk problem based on this initial input is critical to risk assessment. Problem formulation and scoping has now been defined as Phase 1 for risk-based decision making and has been outlined by the US Environmental Protection Agency (EPA) (US EPA, 2011b) and reinforced by Science and Decisions, the *Silver Book* (NRC, 2009).

DEFINITIONS

Risk assessment is the systematic scientific evaluation of potential adverse health effects resulting from human exposures to hazardous agents or situations (NRC, 1983, 1994; Omenn, 2000). Risk is defined as the probability of an adverse outcome based

on the exposure and potency of the hazardous agent(s). Although historically there have been differences in how the term hazard has been used, international risk harmonization activities have allowed for current consensus on hazard as reference to intrinsic

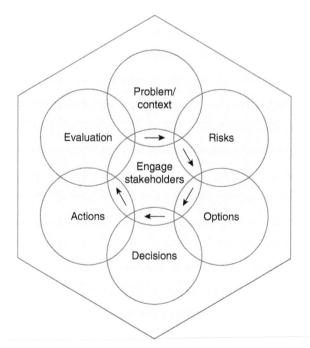

Figure 4-2. *Risk management framework for environmental health from the US Commission on Risk Assessment and Risk Management.* The framework comprises 6 stages: (1) formulating the problem in a broad public health context; (2) analyzing the risks; (3) defining the options; (4) making risk reduction decisions; (5) implementing those actions; and (6) evaluating the effectiveness of the actions taken. Interactions with stakeholders are critical and thus have been put at the center of the framework (Charnley and Omenn, 1997; Risk Commission, 1997).

Table 4-1

Objectives of Risk Assessment

1. Protect human and ecological health
   Toxic substances
2. Balance risks and benefits
   Drugs
   Pesticides
3. Set target levels of risk
   Food contaminants
   Water pollutants
4. Set priorities for program activities
   Regulatory agencies
   Manufacturers
   Environmental/consumer organizations
5. Estimate residual risks and extent of risk reduction after steps are taken to reduce risks

toxic properties, whereas exposure becomes an essential consideration along with hazard for risk. Risk assessment requires an integration of both qualitative and quantitative scientific information. For example, qualitative information about the overall evidence and nature of the end points and hazards is integrated with quantitative assessment of the exposures, host susceptibility factors, and the magnitude of the hazard. A description of the uncertainties and variability in the estimates is a significant part of risk characterization and an essential component of risk assessment. Analogous approaches are applied to ecological risks, as demonstrated by EPA's ecological risk assessment guidelines (US EPA, 2011b). The objectives of risk assessment are outlined in Table 4-1.

The phrase "characterization of risk" reflects the combination of qualitative and quantitative analysis. Increasingly, the use of the term "hazard characterization" versus "hazard identification" has been seen in both the US EPA (2012a) and WHO (1999) documents. This shift recognizes the difficulties in evaluating only hazard information without dose–response information. Unfortunately, many users equate risk assessment with quantitative risk assessment, generating a number for an overly precise risk estimate, while ignoring crucial information about the uncertainties of the risk assessment, mode of action (MOA), and type of effect across species or context.

Risk management refers to the process by which policy actions are chosen to control hazards identified in the risk assessment stage of the framework (Fig. 4-2). Risk managers consider scientific evidence and risk estimates—along with statutory, engineering, economic, social, and political factors—in evaluating alternative options and choosing among those options (Risk Commission, 1997).

Risk communication is the challenging process of making risk assessment and risk management information comprehensible to the public, community groups, lawyers, local elected officials, judges, business people, labor, environmentalists, etc (Morgan, 1993; Sandman, 1993; Fischhoff et al., 1996; NRC, 1996). Such communication requires an understanding of level of risk response needed, how and which individuals and organizations should be informed, and what the audience hears versus what was intended as the risk communication message. Involving stakeholders in the initial problem formulation, as well as in the translation of the bottom line has become an essential part of risk management. Part of this analytical–deliberative process is the crucial, too-often neglected or delayed need for considering the fears, perceptions, priorities, and proposed remedies of these stakeholders (Risk Commission, 1997; Drew et al., 2003, 2006; Judd et al., 2005; Kramer et al., 2006; Cullen et al., 2008). Underestimating potential public and media attitudes toward local polluters, other responsible parties, and relevant government agencies may lead to what has been labeled "the outrage factor" (Sandman, 1993), greatly influencing the communication process and the choices for risk management. Sometimes the decision makers and stakeholders simply want to know the "bottom line": whether a substance or a situation is "safe" or not. Others will be keenly interested in knowing how and why the risk estimates are uncertain and may be well prepared to challenge underlying assumptions about context and methodology. Stakeholders can also be part of a risk management solution (Judd et al., 2005; Drew et al., 2006). Perception of risk is further discussed at the end of this chapter.

DECISION MAKING

Risk management decisions are reached under diverse statutes in the United States. Table 4-2 lists examples of major environmental statutes and the year of initial enactment. Some statutes specify reliance on risk alone, whereas others require a balancing of risks and benefits of the product or activity. Risk assessments provide a valuable framework for priority setting within regulatory and health agencies, in the chemical development process within companies, and in resource allocation by environmental organizations. Similar approaches for risk assessment have been developed in many other countries and through such international organizations as the International Programme on Chemical Safety (IPCS) within the WHO. Currently within the IPCS, there are significant efforts toward a global harmonization of risk assessment methodology (WHO, 2006). The *WHO Human Health Risk Assessment Toolkit: Chemical Hazards* is an example (WHO, 2010). Their goals include use of a common risk assessment framework and development of confidence and acceptance of different risk assessment approaches through a common understanding and agreement on basic principles of testing and evaluation.

A major challenge for risk assessment, risk communication, and risk management is to work across disciplines to demonstrate the biological plausibility and clinical significance of the conclusions from epidemiologic studies, animal bioassays, short-term in vitro and in vivo tests, and structure–activity studies of chemicals thought to have potential adverse effects. Biomarkers of exposure, effect, or individual susceptibility can link the presence of a chemical in various environmental compartments to specific sites of potential action in target organs and to host health impacts (NRC, 1989a,b, 1992a,b; Adami et al., 2011). Mechanistic investigations of the actions of specific chemicals can help us penetrate the "black box" approach of simply counting tumors, for example, in exposed animals in routine bioassays. Greater appreciation of the mechanisms and extent of individual variation in susceptibility to adverse health impacts among humans can improve protection of susceptible populations and better relate findings in animals to the characterization of risk for humans. Identifying individual behavioral and social risk factors can be critically important both to the characterization of risk and to the reduction of risk.

HAZARD IDENTIFICATION

Assessing Toxicity of Chemicals—Introduction

In order to assess the toxicity of chemicals, information from four types of studies is used: structure–activity relationships (SAR), in vitro or short-term studies, in vivo animal bioassays, and

Table 4-2

Examples of Major Toxic Chemical Laws in the United States by Responsible Agency and Year of Initial Enactment

EPA	Air pollutants	Clean Air Act, 1970
	Water pollutants	Federal Water Pollution Control Act, 1948
	Drinking water	Safe Drinking Water Act, 1974
	Pesticides	Fungicides, Insecticides & Rodenticides Act (FIFRA), 1947
		Food Quality Protection Act (FQPA), 1996
	Ocean dumping	Marine Protection, Research and Sanctuaries Act (MPRSA) or
		Ocean Dumping Act, 1972
	Toxic chemicals	Toxic Substances Control Act (TSCA), 1976
	Hazardous wastes	Resource Conservation and Recovery Act (RCRA), 1976
	Abandoned hazardous wastes	Superfund (CERCLA), 1980
CEQ	Environmental impacts	National Environmental Policy Act (NEPA), 1969
OSHA	Workplace	Occupational Safety and Health (OSH) Act, 1970
FDA	Foods, drugs, and cosmetics	Food and Drugs Act, 1906
		Food, Drugs and Cosmetics Act (FDC), 1938
		FDA Modernization Act, 1997
CPSC	Dangerous consumer products	Consumer Product Safety Act (CPSA), 1972
DOT	Transport of hazardous materials	Hazardous Materials Transportation Act (HMTA), 1975

EPA, Environmental Protection Agency; CEQ, Council for Environmental Quality (now Office of Environmental Policy); OSHA, Occupational Safety and Health Administration; FDA, Food and Drug Administration; CPSC, Consumer Product Safety Commission; DOT, Department of Transportation.

information from human epidemiologic studies. In many cases, toxicity information for chemicals is limited. For example, in 1998, the EPA evaluated high production volume (HPV) chemicals (those produced in excess of one million lb per year) to ascertain the availability of chemical hazard data. Their study found that for 43% of these HPV chemicals, there were no publicly available studies for any of the basic toxicity end points (US EPA, 1998a). In response, EPA established a voluntary program called the HPV Challenge Program (US EPA, 2011c). Industry participants in this program committed to filling the data gaps for HPV chemicals. Since its inception, there have been over 2200 chemicals sponsored for additional testing. International efforts such as the Organization for Economic Cooperation and Development's screening information data set (OECD/SIDS) program are also addressing data needs related to HPV, highlighted by the publication of their *Manual for Investigation of HPV Chemicals* (OECD, 2011).

Data requirements for specific chemicals can vary greatly by compound type and applicable regulatory statutes. Introduced in 2003 and approved in 2006, the European Union released a regulatory framework for Registration, Evaluation and Authorisation of Chemicals (REACH) (REACH, 2011). Under the REACH framework, since 2007, all stakeholders submit dossiers that include physical, chemical, and toxicological data as well as risk assessment studies for all chemicals in use in Europe. Such chemical safety assessments are submitted prior to approval in approaches similar to premanufacturing notices (PMNs) in the United States for the US EPA (US EPA, 2011d). Table 4-3 shows requirements and costs for one example class of agents, pesticides (Stevens, 1997; US EPA, 1998b; EPA, 2000), in the United States (40 CFR 158.340). It also illustrates current international efforts to align these testing guidelines by listing examples of the harmonized 870 test guidelines (US EPA, 2010a). The emphasis in REACH is on non–in vivo animal tests. Also, REACH has brought about new international labeling laws for hazard identification.

Assessing Toxicity of Chemicals—Approaches

Structure–Activity Relationships Given the cost of two to four million dollars and the three to five years required for testing a single chemical in a lifetime rodent carcinogenicity bioassay, initial decisions on whether to continue development of a chemical, to submit PMN, or to require additional testing may be based largely on results from SARs and limited short-term assays.

A chemical's structure, solubility, stability, pH sensitivity, electrophilicity, volatility, and chemical reactivity can be important information for hazard identification. Historically, certain key molecular structures have provided regulators with some of the most readily available information on the basis of which to assess hazard potential. For example, 8 of the first 14 occupational carcinogens were regulated together by the Occupational Safety and Health Administration (OSHA) as belonging to the aromatic amine chemical class. The EPA Office of Toxic Substances relies on SARs to meet deadlines to respond to PMN for new chemical manufacture under the Toxic Substances Control Act (TSCA). Structural alerts such as N-nitroso or aromatic amine groups, amino azo dye structures, or phenanthrene nuclei are clues to prioritize chemicals for additional evaluation as potential carcinogens. SAR information for specific noncancer health end points can be challenging. The database of known developmental toxicants limits SARs to a few chemical classes, including chemicals with structures related to those of valproic acid, retinoic acid, phthalate esters, and glycol ethers (NRC, 2000). More recently, omic technologies have been used to supplement SAR relationship databases, as seen with the creation of the National Cancer Institute's (NCI) gene expression database (http://dtp.nci.nih.gov/) and the US EPA Computational Toxicity Program Screening Database (ToxCast™) (US EPA ACToR, 2011).

SARs have been used for assessment of complex mixtures of structurally related compounds. A prominent application has been the assessment of risks associated with 2,3,7,8-tetrachlorodibenzo-*p*-dioxin (TCDD), related chlorinated and brominated

Table 4-3

Example EPA/FIFRA Requirements for Hazard Evaluation of Pesticides

GUIDELINE NO.	REVISED 870 GUIDELINE	TYPE OF TOXICITY STUDY	TEST SYSTEM	OBJECTIVE	APPROXIMATE COST/STUDY* (US$)
81-1	1100	Acute oral	Rats	Define toxic dose by ingestion	2700
81-2	1200	Acute dermal	Rabbits	Define toxic dose by absorption through skin	2000
81-3	1300	Acute inhalation	Rats	Define toxic dose by inhalation	6800
81-4	2400	Ocular	Rabbits	Assess eye irritation/injury	2000
81-5	2500	Skin irritation	Rabbits	Assess skin irritation/injury	130
81-6	2600	Sensitization	Guinea pigs	Assess allergic potential	4000
81-7	6100–6855	Neurotoxicity†,‡	Hens/rats	Assess nervous system injury	34,000‡
84-2	5100–5915	Mutagenicity§	In vivo/in vitro	Determine genotoxic potential; screen for carcinogenicity	6800
82-1	3050–3465	Range-finding§ Subacute (28- to 90-day*)	Rats Mice	Determine effects following repeated doses; set dose level	95,000 95,000
			Dogs Rabbits	For longer studies	136,000 101,000
			Rats Mice	Identify target organs; set dose Levels for chronic studies	258,000 258,000
83-5	4200–4300	Carcinogenicity/ chronic toxicity	Rats	Determine potential to induce tumors; define dose–response relationships (lifetime)	1,900,000
83-2			Mice		1,087,000
83-1			Dogs	Determine long-term toxic effects (1 year)	543,000
83-3	3550–3800	Reproduction and teratogenicity	Rats	Determine potential to cause fetal abnormalities and effects on development, fertility, pregnancy, and development of offspring over at least 2 generations	686,000
83-4			Rabbits		
85-1	7485	Toxicokineties	Rats, mice	Determine and quantitate the metabolic fate of a pesticide	135,000

*Indicates per assay cost using Consumer Price Index (CPI) conversion factors to determine 2010 value (oregonstate.edu/cla/polisci/sahr/sahr). Estimates were provided using guideline 81 series.

†Required for organophosphate insecticides only.

‡Additional neurotoxicity tests 81-7, 81-8, 82-6, 82-7, and 83-6 have been added to requirements for certain materials and can include tests such as functional observational battery, motor activity, developmental landmarks, and learning and memory assessments (Sette, 1991). Costs listed for this type of study are only those for the initial study, not additional testing.

§Range-finding studies are not required, but provide justification for setting dose levels in required studies. EPA-required studies can include reverse mutation assays in Salmonella, forward mutation assays in mammalian cells—for example, Chinese hamster ovary cells and mouse lymphoma L5178Y (the locus cells)—and in vivo cytogenetics (Dearfield, 1990).

SOURCE: Adapted from Stevens (1997), and updated with newly revised EPA 870 guideline information (US EPA, 2010a). For details on changes in the health effects test guidelines reflective of the harmonization of the toxicology guidelines between the Office of Pollution Prevention and Toxics (OPPT) and the Office of Pesticide Programs (OPP), within the EPA and with the Organization for Economic Cooperation and Development (OECD) guidelines, see EPA (US EPA, 2010a, 2011a) (http://www.epa.gov/OPPTS_Harmonized/870_Health_Effects_Test_Guidelines).

dibenzo-p-dioxins, dibenzofurans, and planar biphenyls, and chemicals generally present as mixtures in the environment. Toxicity equivalence factors (TEFs) are used to evaluate health risks associated with closely related chemicals. For the TCDD class, this is based on a common mechanism of aryl hydrocarbon (Ah) receptor induction (US EPA, 1994a). The estimated toxicity of environmental mixtures containing these chemicals is calculated as the sum of the product of the concentration of each chemical multiplied by its TEF value. The World Health Organization has organized efforts to reach international consensus on the TEFs used for polychlorinated biphenyls (PCBs), polychlorinated dibenzo-p-dioxins (PCDDs), and polychlorinated dibenzofurans (PCDFs) for both humans and wildlife, and has updated its values and published the supporting database (Van den Berg et al., 1998, 2006; Haws et al.,

2006). Under the auspices of WHO, the dioxin-like PCB congeners have been assigned TEFs reflecting their toxicity relative to TCDD, which itself has been assigned a TEF of 1.0.

Computerized SAR methods have, in general, given disappointing results in the National Toxicology Program (NTP) rodent carcinogenicity prediction challenges (Ashby and Tennant, 1994; Omenn et al., 1995; Benigni and Zito, 2004). More successes are those of pharmaceutical companies using combinatorial chemistry and 3-dimensional (3D) molecular modeling approaches to design ligands (new drugs) that can sterically fit into the "receptors of interest." However, for environmental pollutants where selective binding to specific receptors is rare, these applications of SAR have had limited success within risk assessment. A renewed interest in quantitative SAR (QSAR) approaches has resulted from the need to evaluate nano-engineered materials where the tremendous number of unique new products has highlighted the necessity of using QSAR approaches to handle the avalanche of novel untested materials (Maynard et al., 2006; Liu et al., 2011).

Efforts within REACH have also emphasized the potential for use of SAR as similar chemicals are collectively evaluated using a concept of "read-across." Substances whose physicochemical, toxicological, and ecotoxicological properties are similar can be grouped as a "category" of substances when they have a common functional group, common precursor or breakdown product, or a common pattern of potency.

In Vitro and Short-Term Tests The next level of biological information obtained within the hazard identification process includes assessment of the test chemical in in vitro or short-term tests, ranging from bacterial mutation assays performed entirely in vitro to more elaborate short-term tests, such as skin painting studies in mice or altered rat liver foci assays conducted in vivo. For example, EPA mutagenicity guidelines call for assessment of reverse mutations using the Ames *Salmonella typhimurium* assay; forward mutations using mammalian cells, mouse lymphoma L5178Y, Chinese hamster ovary, or Chinese hamster lung fibroblasts; and in vivo cytogenetics assessment (bone marrow metaphase analysis or micronucleus tests) (US EPA, 2005). Chap. 8 discusses uses of these assays for identifying chemical carcinogens and Chap. 9 describes in detail various assays of genetic and mutagenic end points. Other assays evaluate specific health end points such as developmental toxicity (Faustman, 1988; Whittaker and Faustman, 1994; Brown et al., 1995; Lewandowski et al., 2000; NRC, 2000; Spielmann et al., 2006), reproductive toxicity (Gray, 1988; Harris et al., 1992; Shelby et al., 1993; Yu et al., 2009), neurotoxicity (Atterwill et al., 1992; Costa, 2000), and immunotoxicity (ICCVAM, 1999, 2011a) (Chap. 12). Less information is available on the extrapolation of these test results for noncancer risk assessment than for the mutagenicity or carcinogenicity end points; however, mechanistic information obtained in these systems has been applied to risk assessment (Abbott et al., 1992; US EPA, 1994b; Leroux et al., 1996; NRC, 2000).

Overall, progress in developing and validating new in vitro assays has been slow and frustrating. The Interagency Coordinating Committee on the Validation of Alternative Methods (ICCVAM) of NTP reinvigorated the validation process in the United States as a result of Public Law 103-43 and coordinates cross-agency issues relating to development, validation, acceptance, and national/international harmonization of toxicological test methods for use in risk assessments. The committee has put forth recommendations for over 40 alternative safety testing methods using various short-term/in vitro assays, such as the cell-free corrosivity test, and for the mouse local lymph node assay for assessing chemical potential to elicit allergic reactions (ICCVAM, 1999, 2011a; NIEHS, 1999a,b). In 2006 the committee released a document that extensively reviews in vitro acute toxicity methods (National Toxicology Program Center for the Evaluation of Alternative Toxicological Methods (US) and Interagency Coordinating Committee on the Validation of Alternative Methods (US), 2006). The European Centre on the Validation of Alternative Methods (ECVAM) has been very active given the visibility of animal rights issues in the European Union, and this Center was originally formed to "support the development, validation, and acceptance of methods that could reduce, refine, or replace [3 Rs] the use of laboratory animals" (http://ecvam.jrc. cec.eu.int/index.htm). Early successes of ECVAM are described in Hartung et al. (2003). However, a recent report for the Center for Alternatives for Animal Testing highlights the slow progress on full replacement of animal testing, especially for repeated dose toxicity testing, carcinogenicity, or reproductive toxicity testing (Adler et al., 2011; Hartung et al., 2011). It does highlight numerous successes for evaluating sensitization and toxicokinetics (TK). International efforts to reduce the number of animals required for chemical safety testing have been established between ICCVAM, Korea, Japan, Canada, and ECVAM (http://iccvam.niehs.nih.gov/docs/about_docs/ICATM-MOC-Mar11.pdf).

The validation and application of short-term assays is particularly important to risk assessment because such assays can be designed to provide information about mechanisms of effects, and, moreover, they are fast and inexpensive compared with lifetime bioassays (McGregor et al., 1999). Validation of in vitro assays, like other kinds of tests, requires determination of their sensitivity (eg, ability to identify true carcinogens), specificity (eg, ability to recognize noncarcinogens as noncarcinogens), and predictive value for the toxic end point under evaluation. The societal costs of relying on such tests, with false positives (noncarcinogens classified as carcinogens) and false negatives (true carcinogens not detected), are the subject of a value-of-information model for testing in risk assessment and risk management (Lave and Omenn, 1986; Omenn and Lampen, 1988).

Efforts to improve our ability to utilize short-term tests for carcinogenicity prediction include increased attention to improving the mechanistic basis of short-term testing. Examples of this approach include the development and application of several knockout transgenic mouse models as shorter-term in vivo assays to identify carcinogens (Nebert and Duffy, 1997; Tennant et al., 1999). Specific assays for evaluating mechanisms such as the function of the estrogen receptor are an example where in vitro test methods are used to predict endocrine disruptor actions (ICCVAM, 2011b, 2012). The primary use of short-term tests in the United States continues to be for mechanistic evaluations with the hope of informing chemical-specific information or overall MOA. In that context, results from short-term assays have impacted risk assessments. For example, evidence of nonmutagenicity in both in vitro and in vivo short-term assays plays an essential role, allowing regulators to consider nonlinear cancer risk assessment paradigms for nongenotoxic carcinogens (US EPA, 1999a). Mechanistic information from short-term in vitro assays can also be used to extend the range of biological observations available for dose–response assessment. In addition, for developmental toxicity assessment, assay methods that acknowledge the highly conserved nature of developmental pathways across species have accelerated the use of a broader range of model organisms and assay approaches for noncancer risk assessments (NRC, 2000). *Toxicity Testing in the 21st Century* and *Toxicity Pathway-Based Risk Assessment* emphasized such approaches for using model organisms and tiered toxicity strategies for Risk Assessment (NRC, 2007a; NRC, 2010).

Animal Bioassays Animal bioassays are a key component of the hazard identification process. A basic premise of risk assessment is that chemicals that cause tumors in animals can cause tumors in humans. All human carcinogens that have been adequately tested in animals produce positive results in at least one animal model. Thus, "although this association cannot establish that all chemicals and mixtures that cause cancer in experimental animals also cause cancer in humans, nevertheless, in the absence of adequate data on humans, it is biologically plausible and prudent to regard chemicals and mixtures for which there is sufficient evidence of carcinogenicity in experimental animals as if they presented a carcinogenic risk to humans" (IARC, 2000)—a reflection of the "precautionary principle." The US EPA cancer guidelines (US EPA, 2005) also assume relevance of animal bioassays unless lack of relevance for human assessment is specifically determined. In general, the most appropriate rodent bioassays are those that test exposure and biological pathways of most relevance to predicted or known human exposure pathways. Bioassays for reproductive and developmental toxicity and other noncancer end points have a similar rationale. The National Toxicology Program (NTP) serves as a resource for conducting, designing, and evaluating bioassays for cancer as well as noncancer evaluation. The NTP Office of Human Health Assessment and Translation serves as a resource to the public and regulatory agencies regarding the interpretation and assessment of adverse effects of chemicals (National Toxicology Program, 2011b). The WHO International Agency for Research on Cancer (IARC) has evaluated over 900 agents "of which more than 400 have been identified as carcinogenic, probably carcinogenic or possibly carcinogenic to humans" (WHO, 2011b).

Consistent features in the design of standard cancer bioassays include testing in two species and both sexes, with 50 animals per dose group and near-lifetime exposure. Important choices include the strains of rats and mice, the number of doses, and dose levels (typically 90%, 50%, and 10%–25% of the maximally tolerated dose [MTD]), and details of the required histopathology (number of organs to be examined, choice of interim sacrifice pathology, etc). The NTP Web site lists details on study designs and protocols (National Toxicology Program, 2011a). Positive evidence of chemical carcinogenicity can include increases in number of tumors at a particular organ site, induction of rare tumors, earlier induction (shorter latency) of commonly observed tumors, and/or increases in the total number of observed tumors. Recently, NTP has added an in utero exposure period to the start of their cancer bioassays to more directly evaluate the significance of early life exposures for cancer incidence.

The cancer bioassay, originally designed for hazard identification, is frequently used to evaluate dose–response. The relatively limited number of evaluated doses and the use of high doses have caused issues for low-dose extrapolations and have limited the use of cancer bioassays as a "gold standard" for prediction of human carcinogenicity risk (McClain, 1994; Cohen, 1995; Risk Commission, 1997; Rodericks et al., 1997; Capen et al., 1999; Rice et al., 1999). Tumors may be increased only at the highest dose tested, which is usually at or near a dose that causes systemic toxicity (Ames and Gold, 1990). Second, even without toxicity, the high dose may trigger different events than do low-dose exposures and high doses can saturate important metabolism and elimination pathways.

Rats and mice give concordant positive or negative results in approximately 70% of bioassays, so it is unlikely that rodent/human concordance would be higher (Lave et al., 1988). Haseman and Lockhart (1993) concluded that most target sites in cancer bioassays showed a strong correlation (65%) between males and females—especially for forestomach, liver, and thyroid tumors—so

they suggested, for efficiency, that bioassays could rely on a combination of male rats and female mice. Even when concordant, positive results are observed, there can still be large differences in potency, as observed in aflatoxin-induced tumors in rats and mice. In this example, an almost 100,000-fold difference in susceptibility to aflatoxin B_1 (AFB$_1$)–induced liver tumors is seen between the sensitive rat and trout species and the more resistant mouse strains. Genetic differences in the expression of cytochrome P450 and glutathione S-transferases explain most of these species differences and suggest that humans may be as sensitive to AFB$_1$-induced liver tumors as rats (Eaton and Gallagher, 1994; Eaton et al., 1995, 2001). These species differences have been supported by research results (Groopman and Kensler, 1999; Kensler et al., 2011) and have been extended within epidemiologic studies to demonstrate the interaction of hepatitis C infection with AFB$_1$ exposure to fully explain elevated human liver cancer risks.

Lifetime bioassays have been enhanced with the collection of additional mechanistic data and with the assessment of multiple noncancer end points. It is feasible and desirable to integrate such information together with data from mechanistically oriented short-term tests and biomarker and genetic studies in epidemiology (Perera and Weinstein, 2000). In the example of AFB$_1$-induced liver tumors, AFB$_1$–DNA adducts have proved to be an extremely useful biomarker. A highly linear relationship was observed between liver tumor incidence (in rats, mice, and trout) and AFB$_1$–DNA adduct formation over a dose range of 5 orders of magnitude (Eaton and Gallagher, 1994). Such approaches may allow for an extension of biologically observable phenomena to doses lower than those leading to frank tumor development and help to address the issues of extrapolation over multiple orders of magnitude to predict response at environmentally relevant doses.

Table 4-4 presents some mechanistic details about rodent tumor responses that are no longer thought to be predictive of cancer risk for humans. This table lists examples of both qualitative and quantitative considerations useful for determining relevance of rodent tumor responses for human risk evaluations. An example of qualitative considerations is the male rat kidney tumors observed following exposure to chemicals that bind to α_{2u}-globulin (eg, unleaded gasoline, 1,4-dichlorobenzene, D-limonene). The α_{2u}-globulin is a male-rat-specific low-molecular-weight protein not found in female rats, humans, or other species, including mice and monkeys (McClain, 1994; Neumann and Olin, 1995; Oberdorster, 1995; Omenn et al., 1995; Risk Commission, 1997; Rodericks et al., 1997).

Table 4-4 also illustrates quantitative considerations important for determining human relevance of animal bioassay information. For example, doses of compounds so high as to exceed solubility in the urinary tract outflow lead to tumors of the urinary bladder in male rats following crystal precipitation and local irritation leading to hyperplasia. Such precipitates are known to occur following saccharin or nitriloacetic acid exposure (Cohen et al., 2000). The decision to exclude saccharin from the NTP list of suspected human carcinogens reaffirms the nonrelevance of such high-dose responses for likely human exposure considerations (Neumann and Olin, 1995; National Toxicology Program, 2005). A gross overloading of the particle clearance mechanism of rat lungs via directly administered particles, as was seen in titanium dioxide (TDO) exposures, resulted in EPA's delisting TDO as a reportable toxicant for the Clean Air Act Toxic Release Inventory (US EPA, 1988; Oberdorster, 1995).

Other rodent responses not likely to be predictive for humans include localized forestomach tumors after gavage. Ethyl acrylate, which produces such tumors, was delisted on the basis of extensive

Table 4-4

Examples of Mechanistic Considerations for Carcinogens: Explanation for Special Cases of Rodent Bioassay Data Lacking Relevance for Human Risk Evaluation

SYSTEM	TARGET ORGAN	MECHANISM FOR SUSCEPITBLE SPECIES	SPECIES DIFFERENCES	ILLUSTRATIVE CHEMICAL AGENTS
Urinary tract	Renal tumors in male rats	Chemicals bind to α_{2U}-globulin, accumulation in target kidney cells, increased necrosis, increased regenerative hyperplasia, renal tubular calcification neoplasia	α_{2U}-Globulin male-rat-specific low-molecular-weight protein not found in female rats, humans, mice, monkeys	Unleaded gasoline, 1,4-dichlorobenzene, D-limonene, isophorone, dimethyl-methylphosphonate, perchloroethylene, pentachloroethane, hexachloroethane
	Bladder	Reactive hyperplasia from cytotoxic precipitated chemicals	Rodent exposure levels exceed solubility, not relevant for human exposure	Saccharin, melamine, nitrilotriacetic acid, fosetyl-A2
Gastric	Forestomach	Direct oral gavage, local cytotoxicity, hyperplasia	Rodent gavage treatment, exposure conditions not relevant for human exposure	BHA, propionic acid, ethyl acrylate
Endocrine	Thyroid gland tumors	Alteration in thyroid homeostasis, decreased thyroid hormone production, sustained increase in thyroid-stimulating hormone (TSH), thyroid tumors	Lack of thyroid-binding protein in rodents versus humans, decreased $t_{1/2}$ for T_4, increased TSH levels in rodents	Ethylene bisdithiocarbamate, fungicides, amitrol, goitrogens, sulfamethazine
Respiratory	Rat lung	Overwhelming clearance mechanisms	High-dose effects seen with rodent models	Various particles, titanium dioxide

SOURCE: McClain (1994), Neumann and Olin (1995), Oberdorster (1995), Omenn et al. (1995), Risk Commission (1997), and Rodericks et al. (1997)

mechanistic studies (National Toxicology Program, 2005). In general, for risk assessment, it is desirable to use the same route of administration as the likely exposure pathway in humans to avoid such extrapolation issues. Despite the example of forestomach tumors, tumors in unusual sites—such as the pituitary gland, the eighth cranial nerve, or the Zymbal gland—should not be immediately dismissed as irrelevant, since organ-to-organ correlation is often lacking (NRC, 1994). The EPA cancer guidelines provide a good list of considerations for evaluating relevance in the sections on evaluating weight of evidence (US EPA, 2005).

In an attempt to improve the prediction of cancer risk to humans, transgenic mouse models have been developed as possible alternative to the standard 2-year cancer bioassay. Transgenic models use knockout or transgenic mice that incorporate or eliminate a gene that has been linked to human cancer. NTP evaluated some of these models and found the p53-deficient (p53+/− heterozygous) and Tg.AC (v-Ha-ras transgene) models to be particularly useful in identifying carcinogens and mechanisms of action (Bucher, 1998; Chhabra et al., 2003). The use of transgenic models has the power to improve the characterization of key cellular and MOA of toxicological responses (Mendoza et al., 2002; Gribble et al., 2005). However, these studies have been used primarily for mechanistic characterization than for hazard identification. Transgenic models have been shown to reduce cost and time as compared with the standard 2-year assay but they have also been shown to be somewhat limited in their sensitivity (Cohen, 2001). As stated in the current EPA cancer guidelines, transgenic models should not be used to replace the standard 2-year assay, but can be

used in conjunction with other types of data to assist in the interpretation of additional toxicological and mechanistic evidence (US EPA, 2005). A series of genetically defined (fully sequenced genomes, 20 × coverage) mice referred to as the Collaborative Cross have been established to investigate genetic and environmental influences on toxicological response in mice (Chesler et al., 2008) and these strains should improve our understanding of mammalian genes that predispose to cancer (Koturbash et al., 2011).

Use of Epidemiologic Data in Risk Assessment The most convincing lines of evidence for human risk are well-conducted epidemiologic studies in which a positive association between exposure and disease has been observed (NRC, 1983). Environmental and occupational epidemiologic studies are frequently opportunistic. Studies begin with known or presumed exposures, comparing exposed with nonexposed individuals, or with known cases, compared with persons lacking the particular diagnosis.

Table 4-5 shows examples of epidemiologic study designs and provides clues on types of outcomes and exposures evaluated. Although convincing, there are important limitations inherent in epidemiologic studies. Robust exposure estimates are often difficult to obtain as they are frequently done retrospectively (eg, through retrospective job history records). Also, since many important health effects have long latency before clinical manifestations appear, reconsideration of relevant populations can be challenging. Another challenge for interpretation is that there are often exposures to multiple chemicals, especially when a lifetime exposure period is

Table 4-5

Example of 3 Types of Epidemiologic Study Designs

METHODOLOGICAL ATTRIBUTES	TYPE OF STUDY		
	COHORT	CASE–CONTROL	CROSS-SECTIONAL
Initial classification	Exposure–nonexposure	Disease–nondisease	Either one
Time sequence	Prospective	Retrospective	Present time
Sample composition	Nondiseased individuals	Cases and controls	Survivors
Comparison	Proportion of exposed with disease	Proportion of cases with exposure	Either one
Rates	Incidence	Fractional (%)	Prevalence
Risk index	Relative risk–attributable risk	Relative odds	Prevalence
Advantages	Lack of bias in exposure; yields incidence and risk rates	Inexpensive, small number of subjects, rapid results, suitable for rare diseases, no attrition	Quick results
Disadvantages	Large number of subjects required, long follow-up, attrition, change in time of criteria and methods, costly, inadequate for rare diseases	Incomplete information, biased recall, problem in selecting control and matching, yields only relative risk—cannot establish causation, population of survivors	Cannot establish causation (antecedent consequence), population of survivors, inadequate for rare diseases

SOURCE: Gamble and Battigelli (1978, 1991).

considered. There is frequently a trade-off between detailed information on relatively few persons and very limited information on large numbers of persons. Contributions from lifestyle factors, such as smoking and diet, are important to assess as they can have a significant impact on cancer development. Human epidemiologic studies can provide both very useful information for hazard assessment and quantitative information for data characterization. Good illustrations of epidemiologic studies and their interpretation for toxicological evaluation are available (Gill *et al.*, 2011 and Regalado *et al.*, 2006).

Three types of epidemiologic study designs—cross-sectional studies, cohort studies, and case–control studies—are detailed in Table 4-5. Cross-sectional studies survey groups of humans to identify risk factors (exposure) and disease but are not useful for establishing cause and effect. Cohort studies can evaluate individuals selected on the basis of their exposure to a chemical under study. Thus, based on exposure status, these individuals are monitored for development of disease. These prospective studies monitor over time individuals who initially are disease-free to determine the rates at which they develop disease. In case–control studies, subjects are selected on the basis of disease status: disease cases and matched cases of disease-free individuals. Exposure histories of the 2 groups are compared to determine key consistent features in their exposure histories. All case–control studies are retrospective studies.

In risk assessment, epidemiologic findings are judged by the following criteria: strength of association, consistency of observations (reproducibility in time and space), specificity (uniqueness in quality or quantity of response), appropriateness of temporal relationship (did the exposure precede responses?), dose–responsiveness, biological plausibility and coherence, verification, and analogy (biological extrapolation) (Hill, 1965; Faustman *et al.*, 1997; World Health Organization and International Programme on

Chemical Safety, 1999; Adami *et al.*, 2011). These same criteria have been used for evaluating MOAs where integrated considerations of both human and animal studies are done.

Epidemiologic study designs should also be evaluated for their power of detection, appropriateness of outcomes, verification of exposure assessments, completeness of assessing confounding factors, and general applicability of the outcomes to other populations at risk. Power of detection is calculated using study size, variability, accepted detection limits for end points under study, and a specified significance level (Healey, 1987; EGRET, 1994; Dean *et al.*, 1995). Meta-analysis is used with epidemiologic studies to combine results from different studies using weighting of results to account for sample size across studies. The importance of human studies for risk assessment is shown in evaluations with arsenic and dioxin (US EPA, 2010b).

Advance from the human genome project have increase sophistication of molecular biomarkers and have improved the mechanistic bases for epidemiologic hypotheses. This has allowed epidemiologists to get within the "black box" of statistical associations and forward our understanding of biological plausibility and clinical relevance. "Molecular epidemiology," the integration of molecular biology into traditional epidemiologic research, is an important focus of human studies where improved molecular biomarkers of exposure, effect, and susceptibility have allowed investigators to more effectively link molecular events in the causal disease pathway. Epidemiologists can now include the contribution of potential genetic factors with environmental risk factors for the determination of the etiology, distribution, and prevention of disease. Highlighting the potential power of genetic information to epidemiologic studies, the Human Genome Epidemiology (HuGE) Network was launched in 1998, providing a literature database of published, population-based epidemiologic studies of human genes (Khoury, 1999).

With the advance of genomics, the range of biomarkers has grown dramatically and includes identification of single-nucleotide polymorphisms (SNPs), genomic profiling, transcriptome analysis, and proteomic analysis (Simon and Wang, 2006). Implications of these improvements for risk assessment are tremendous, as they provide an improved biological basis for extrapolation across the diversity of human populations and allow for improved cross-species comparisons with rodent bioassay information because of evolutionarily conserved response pathways (NRC, 2000). In addition, genomics allows for "systems-based" understanding of disease and response, moving risk assessment away from a linear, single-event-based concept and improving the biological plausibility of epidemiologic associations (Toscano and Oehlke, 2005; NRC, 2010).

Integrating Qualitative Aspects of Risk Assessment

Qualitative assessment of hazard information should include a consideration of the consistency and concordance of findings, including a determination of the consistency of the toxicological findings across species and target organs, an evaluation of consistency across duplicate experimental conditions, and a determination of the adequacy of the experiments to consistently detect the adverse end points of interest.

Qualitative assessment of animal or human evidence is done by many agencies, including the EPA and IARC. Similar evidence classifications have been used for both the animal and human evidence categories by both agencies. These evidence classifications have included levels of "sufficient, limited, inadequate, and no evidence" (US EPA, 1994b, 2005) or "evidence suggesting lack of carcinogenicity" (IARC, 2000). For both agencies, these classifications are used for an overall weight-of-evidence approach for carcinogenicity classification.

Weight of evidence is an integrative step used by the EPA to "characterize the extent to which the available data support the hypothesis that an agent causes cancer in humans" (US EPA, 2005). It is the process of "weighing" all of the evidence to reach a conclusion about carcinogenicity. With this method, the likelihood of human carcinogenic effect is evaluated within an evaluation of the conditions under which such effects may be expressed. Weight of evidence can consider both the quality and quantity of data as well as any underlying assumptions. The evidence includes data from all of the hazard assessment and characterization studies such as SAR data, in vivo and/or in vitro studies, and epidemiologic data. Using this type of information and weight-of-evidence approach, the EPA includes hazard descriptors to define carcinogenic potential and to provide a measure of clarity and consistency in the characterization narrative: "carcinogenic to humans," "likely to be carcinogenic to humans," "suggestive evidence of carcinogenic potential," "inadequate information to assess carcinogenic potential," and "not likely to be carcinogenic to humans." In this section, approaches for evaluating cancer end points are discussed for carcinogens. Similar weight-of-evidence approaches have been proposed for reproductive risk assessment (refer to sufficient and insufficient evidence categories in EPA's guidelines for reproductive risk [US EPA, 1996a] and considerations by NTP).

The Institute for Evaluating Health Risks defined an "evaluation process" by which reproductive and developmental toxicity data can be consistently evaluated and integrated to ascertain their relevance for human health risk assessment (Moore et al., 1995; Faustman et al., 2011). This evaluation process has served as the basis for US EPA's guidelines for developmental toxicity

risk assessment (US EPA, 1991) and for NTP's *Office of Health Assessment and Translation (Formerly CERHR)* (National Toxicology Program, 2011b). Application of such carefully deliberated approaches for assessing noncancer end points has helped avoid the tendency to list chemicals as yes or no (positive or negative) without human relevancy information.

Mode of Action The EPA has emphasized in their revised cancer guidelines the importance of using "weight of evidence" to arrive at insights to possible "MOA" (US EPA, 2005). MOA information describes key events and processes leading to molecular and functional effects that would in general explain the overall process of cancer development. In many cases these could be plausible hypothesized MOAs for specific toxicity end points, but the detailed mechanistic nuances of the pathway might not yet be fully known. EPA is using such MOA information to suggest non-default approaches for cancer risk assessments and for evaluating toxicity of compounds with common MOAs in cumulative risk assessments (US EPA, 1996a, 1998a).

Within the EPA's carcinogenic risk assessment guidelines, the MOA framework considers evidence from animal studies, relevance to humans, and life stage or population susceptibility (US EPA, 2005). Chemical-specific adjustment factors for interspecies differences and human variability have been proposed and build upon guidance developed by the WHO's International Programme on Chemical Safety Harmonization Project (WHO, 2000). Critical to the MOA development is the use of "criteria of causality" considerations, which build upon Hill criteria used in epidemiology (Hill, 1965; Faustman et al., 1996; US EPA, 1999a; Klaunig et al., 2003), and consider dose–response relationships and temporal associations, as well as the biological plausibility, coherence, strength, consistency, and specificity of the postulated MOA.

DOSE–RESPONSE ASSESSMENT

Integrating Quantitative Aspects of Risk Assessment

Quantitative considerations in risk assessment include dose–response assessment, exposure assessment, variation in susceptibility, and characterization of uncertainty. For dose–response assessment, varying approaches have been proposed for threshold versus nonthreshold end points. Traditionally, in the United States, threshold approaches have been applied for assessment of noncancer end points, and nonthreshold approaches have been used for cancer end points. As we have learned more about nongenotoxic mechanisms of carcinogenicity, these processes have been evaluated using threshold approaches. Each approach and its inherent assumptions are discussed below, as are efforts to include more detailed mechanistic considerations to harmonize these approaches (Bogdanffy et al., 2001).

In general, human exposure data for prediction of human response to environmental chemicals are quite limited; thus, animal bioassay data have primarily served as the basis for most quantitative risk assessments and have required extrapolation for human health risk prediction. The risk assessor, however, is normally interested in low environmental exposures when considering human risk, exposures that are well below the experimentally observable range of responses in most animal assays. Thus, methods for extrapolating from high dose to low dose as well as extrapolating from animal risk to human risk are required and comprise a major emphasis of dose–response assessment.

The fundamental basis of the quantitative relationships between exposure to a chemical and the incidence of an adverse response is the dose–response assessment. Analysis of dose–response relationships must start with the determination of the critical effects to be quantitatively evaluated. It is usual practice to choose the most robust data sets with adverse effects occurring at the lowest levels of exposure from studies using the most relevant exposure routes. The "critical" adverse effect is defined as the significant adverse biological effect that occurs at the lowest exposure level (Barnes and Dourson, 1988). EPA has issued toxicity-specific guidelines that are useful in identifying such critical effects (for developmental toxicity [US EPA, 1991], reproductive toxicity [US EPA, 1996a], neurotoxicity [US EPA, 1998c], and cancer [US EPA, 1994b, 1996a, 1999a, 2005]). IPCS has compiled a document cited as the *Principles for Modeling Dose–Responses for the Risk Assessment of Chemicals* (International Programme on Chemical Safety, 2006). It outlines key concepts and considerations for dose–response evaluations within the context of a risk assessment.

Threshold Approaches Approaches for characterizing threshold dose–response relationships include identification of "no observed adverse effect level" (NOAEL) or "lowest observed adverse effect levels" (LOAELs). On the dose–response curve illustrated in Fig. 4-3, the doses tested in the bioassay are given as F, G, H, and I. The statistical significance of points G, H, and I is indicated using an asterisk (*). The NOAEL (F) is identified as the highest nonstatistically significant dose tested; in this example the NOAEL occurs at approximately 2 mg/kg body weight. Point G is the LOAEL (~2.3 mg/kg body weight), as it is the lowest dose tested with a statistically significant effect. Lines A to D represent possible extrapolations below the point of departure (POD), which is represented on this figure as a square (■) and is labeled as point E. The POD is used to specify the estimated dose near the

lower end of the observed dose range, below which extrapolation to lower exposures is necessary (US EPA, 2005). In Fig. 4-3, the POD occurs at 10% effective dose or ED_{10}. The type of extrapolation below the POD is depending on the type of data available. The importance of choosing an appropriate POD and extrapolation type is discussed further in the following sections of this chapter. From these modeled approaches, model D shows a model where the threshold (T) represents the dose below which no additional increase in response is observed.

In general, most animal bioassays are constructed with sufficient numbers of test animals to detect biological responses at the 10% response range; however, this is also dependent on end point and the background rate of the end point in control animals. The risk assessor should always understand the biological significance of the responses being evaluated in order to put statistical observations in context. Significance thus usually refers to both biological and statistical criteria (Faustman *et al.*, 1994) and is dependent on the number of dose levels tested, the number of animals tested at each dose, and background incidence of the adverse response in the nonexposed control groups. The NOAEL should not be perceived as risk-free, as several reports have shown that the response of NOAELs for continuous end points averages 5% risk, and NOAELs based on quantal end points can be associated with risk of greater than 10% (Allen *et al.*, 1994a; Faustman *et al.*, 1994).

As described in Chap. 2, approaches for characterizing dose–response relationships include identification of effect levels such as LD_{50} (dose producing 50% lethality), LC_{50} (concentration producing 50% lethality), ED_{10} (dose producing 10% response), as well as NOAELs. NOAELs have traditionally served as the basis for risk assessment calculations, such as reference doses (RfDs) or ADI values. RfDs or concentrations (RfCs) are estimates of daily exposure (oral or inhalation, respectively) to an chemical that is assumed to be without adverse health impact in humans. The ADIs are used by WHO for pesticides and food additives to define "the daily intake of chemical, which during an entire lifetime appears to be without appreciable risk on the basis of all known facts at that time" (WHO, 1962; Dourson *et al.*, 1985). RfDs (first introduced in Chap. 2) and ADI values typically are calculated from NOAEL values by dividing by uncertainty factor (UF) and/or modifying factor (MF) (Dourson and Stara, 1983; Dourson and DeRosa, 1991; US EPA, 1991):

$$RfD = \frac{NOAEL}{UF \times MF},$$

$$ADI = \frac{NOAEL}{UF \times MF}.$$

Tolerable daily intakes (TDI) can be used to describe intakes for chemicals that are not "acceptable" but are "tolerable" as they are below levels thought to cause adverse health effects. These are calculated in a manner similar to ADI. Historically, dividing by the UFs allows for interspecies (animal-to-human) and intraspecies (human-to-human) variability with default values of 10 each. An additional UF is used to account for experimental inadequacies—for example, to extrapolate from short-exposure-duration studies to a situation more relevant for chronic study or to account for inadequate numbers of animals or other experimental limitations. If only a LOAEL value is available, then an additional 10-fold factor is commonly used to arrive at a value more comparable to a NOAEL. For developmental toxicity end points, it has been demonstrated that the application of the 10-fold factor for LOAEL-to-NOAEL

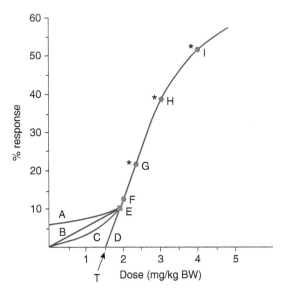

Figure 4-3. *Dose–response curve.* This figure is designed to illustrate a typical dose–response curve with points F to I indicating the biologically determined responses. Statistical significance of these responses is indicated with the symbol "*." Point E (■) represents a dose near the lower end of the observed dose–response range, below which extrapolation to lower doses can occur for cancer risk estimates (US EPA, 2005). Point F is the highest nonstatistically significant response point; hence, it is the "no observed adverse effect level" (NOAEL) for this example. Point G is the "lowest observed adverse response level" (LOAEL). Curves A to D show some options for extrapolating the dose–response relationship below the range of biologically observed data points and POD.

conversion is too large (Allen *et al.*, 1994a). Traditionally, a safety factor of 100 would be used for RfD calculations to extrapolate from a well-conducted animal bioassay (10-fold factor for animal-to-human variability) and to account for human variability in response (10-fold factor for human-to-human variability).

MFs are values that can be used to adjust the UFs if data on mechanisms, pharmacokinetics, or relevance of the animal response to human risk are available. For example, if there is kinetic information suggesting there is very similar metabolism for a particular compound in rats and humans, producing the same active target metabolite, then—rather than using a 10-fold UF to divide the NOAEL from the animal toxicity study to obtain a human relevant RfD—a factor of 3 for that UF might be used. Of particular interest is the addition of an extra 10-fold factor through the Food Quality Protection Act (FQPA) to ensure protection of infants and children (US EPA, 1996b). Under this law an additional UF is added to ensure protection of children's health and it is currently being used for determining allowable pesticide chemical residues. This factor is designed to take into account potential prenatal and postnatal toxicity and to overcome the incompleteness of toxicity and exposure data (FQPA, PL 104-170). Illustrative discussions on how such a legislatively mandated UF might be applied are available for chlorpyrifos (Schardein and Scialli, 1999; US EPA, 2000a). In this case, this uncertainty factor was reduced due to the availability of specific animal experiments assessing developmental toxicity at sensitive life stages (Zhao *et al.*, 2006; US EPA, 2011e).

To reduce uncertainty in calculating RfDs and ADIs, there has been a transition from the use of traditional 10-fold UFs to the use of data-derived and chemical-specific adjustment factors. Such efforts have included reviewing the human pharmacologic literature from published clinical trials (Silverman *et al.*, 1999) and developing human variability databases for a large range of exposures and clinical conditions (Renwick, 1991, 1999; Johnson *et al.*, 1997). Toward this goal, Renwick has separated the intraspecies and interspecies UFs into 2 components: toxicokinetics (TK) and toxicodynamic (TD) aspects (Renwick, 1991, 1999; Johnson *et al.*, 1997). Fig. 4-4 shows these distinctions. A key advantage of this approach is that it provides a structure for incorporating scientific information on specific aspects of the overall toxicological process into the RfD calculations; thus, relevant data can replace a portion of the overall "uncertainty" surrounding these extrapolations. Current WHO guidance uses a 4.0- and 2.5-fold factor for the TK and TD interspecies components, respectively (WHO, 2005), and interindividual TK and TD factors of 3.16 (Renwick and Lazarus, 1998).

The recent NAS publications (*Silver Book*) have emphasized the need to consider population variability and context in risk assessment. In examples described in this NRC report, high background incidence of cancers or other adverse health outcomes in the population should be considered before setting "acceptable" levels of additional risks (NRC, 2009).

NOAEL values have also been utilized for risk assessment by evaluating a "margin of exposure" (MOE), where the ratio of the NOAEL determined in animals and expressed as mg/kg per day is compared with the level to which a human may be exposed. For example, consider the case where human exposures to a specific chemical are calculated to be solely via drinking water, and the total daily intake of the compound is 0.04 mg/kg per day. If the NOAEL for neurotoxicity is 100 mg/kg per day, then the MOE would be 2500 for the oral exposure route for neurotoxicity. Such a large value is reassuring to public health officials. Low values of MOE indicate that the human levels of exposure are close to levels for the NOAEL in animals. There is usually no factor included in this calculation for differences in human or animal susceptibility or animal-to-human extrapolation; thus, MOE values of less than 100 have been used by regulatory agencies as flags for requiring further evaluation.

The NOAEL approach has been criticized on several points, including that (1) the NOAEL must, by definition, be one of the experimental doses tested and (2) once this is identified, the rest of the dose–response curve is ignored. Because of these limitations, an alternative to the NOAEL approach, the benchmark dose (BMD) method, was proposed (Crump, 1980). In this approach, the dose–response is modeled and the lower confidence bound for a dose at a specified response level (benchmark response [BMR]) is calculated. The BMR is usually specified at 1%, 5%, or 10%. Fig. 4-5 shows the BMD using a 10% BMR (BMD_{10}) and a 95% lower confidence bound on dose ($BMDL_{10}$). The BMD_x (with x representing the percent BMR) is used as an alternative to the NOAEL value for RfD calculations. Thus, the RfD would be:

$$RfD = \frac{BMD_x \text{ or } MBDL_x}{UF \times MF}.$$

EPA has developed software for the application of BMD methods and a technical guidance document to provide guidelines for application of BMDs for both cancer and noncancer end points (EPA, 2000). It recently released an updated version (2.2) of its BMD software (http://www.epa.gov/ncea/bmds/index.html). The 2009 WHO

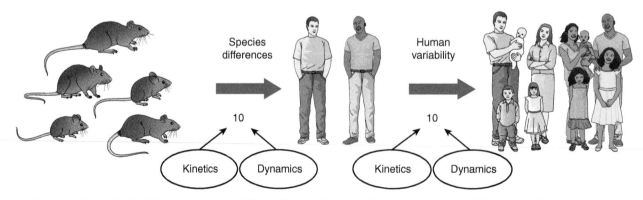

Figure 4-4. *Toxicokinetic (TK) and toxicodynamic (TD) considerations inherent in interspecies and interindividual extrapolations. TK refers to the processes of absorption, distribution, elimination, and metabolism of a toxicant. TD refers to the actions and interactions of the toxicant within the organism and describes processes at organ, tissue, cellular, and molecular levels. This figure shows how uncertainty in extrapolation both across and within species can be considered as being due to 2 key factors: a kinetic component and a dynamic component. Challenges remain for extrapolating information on human variation to specific populations (NRC, 2009). Refer to the text for detailed explanations.*

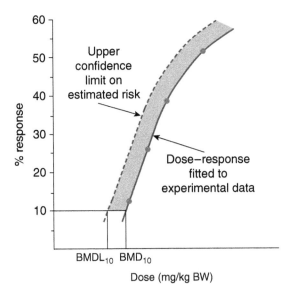

Figure 4-5. *Illustration of benchmark dose (BMD) approach.* This figure shows the $BMDL_{10}$ and BMD_{10}, the lower confidence limit and dose (ED_{10}) associated with a 10% incidence of adverse response, respectively (Kavlock *et al.*, 1995; US EPA, 2005). For reference, points are labeled as described in the legend for Fig. 4-3.

guidelines for dose–response modeling for risk assessment also discuss BMD approaches (International Programme on Chemical Safety, 2006). Both the EPA and WHO guidelines distinguish NOAEL versus BMD-based approaches. Harmonization of approaches available for assessments is discussed in the WHO documents.

The BMD approach has been applied to study noncancer end points, including developmental (Allen *et al.*, 1994a) and reproductive toxicity (Auton, 1994). The most extensive studies with developmental toxicity have shown that BMD_{05} values were similar to a statistically derived NOAEL for a wide range of developmental toxicity end points and that results from using generalized dose–response models were similar to biologically based dose–response (BBDR) models designed specifically to represent unique features of developmental toxicity testing (Faustman *et al.*, 1999).

Advantages of the BMD approach include (1) the ability to take into account the dose–response curve; (2) the inclusion of a measure of variability (confidence limit); and (3) the use of a consistent BMR level for RfD calculations across studies. Limitations in the animal bioassays in regard to minimal test doses for evaluation, shallow dose responses, and use of study designs with widely spaced test doses will limit the utility of these assays for any type of quantitative assessments, whether NOAEL- or BMD-based approaches.

Nonthreshold Approaches As Fig. 4-3 shows, numerous dose–response curves can be proposed in the low-dose region of the dose–response curve if a threshold assumption is not made. Because the risk assessor generally needs to extrapolate beyond the region of the dose–response curve for which experimentally observed data are available, the choice of models to generate curves in this region has received lots of attention. For nonthreshold responses, methods for dose–response assessments have models for extrapolation to de minimus (10^{-4} to 10^{-6}) risk levels at very low doses, far below the biologically observed response range and far below the effect levels evaluated for threshold responses.

EPA cancer guidelines define the dose–response methods as requiring two steps: (1) defining the "POD" or the lowest dose associated with adverse effects within the range of the experimental data and (2) the extrapolation from the POD to low environmentally

relevant exposure levels based on experimental data. The extrapolation can be done with a linear model or a nonlinear model with this choice dependent on the amount and type of experimental data available. Risk estimates using the linear model (biological response increases proportionally with level of exposure) are generally higher than those using nonlinear models. For example, in 2003, the EPA released a Dioxin Reassessment and used the BMD dose–response method. The reassessment used a POD based on a 1% response with a linear extrapolation model based on the position that the scientific data were inadequate to rule out the EPA's standard default linear assumption. The EPA Dioxin Reassessment was evaluated in a National Academies Report in 2006 (National Academy of Science, 2006) and this review discussed remaining extrapolation issues. In EPA's recent draft of dioxin risk assessment (US EPA, 2010b) revised TCDD cancer risk assessment is presented using the upper bound on the regression slope for estimating cancer mortality risk from the epidemiology evaluation by Cheng *et al.* (2006). The top 5% of exposure estimates from this epidemiologic study were excluded as the dose-related changes in cancer mortality plateaued at high doses. EPA lagged exposures by 15 years and adjusted cancer risk based on cumulative TCDD fat concentrations. Their analysis included an estimate of TCDD cancer risks above the TCDD background levels found in the NIOSH worker cohort analyzed by Chang *et al.* Below the POD, the EPA assumed a default linear slope value. (For more information, please go to US EPA as this draft document is undergoing final comments and discussion.) This document represents one of the most recent interpretations of cancer risk assessment by EPA for data-rich compounds with multiple cancer risk estimates for animal and human studies as well as how extensive mechanistic and kinetic information is considered. This draft report provides insight into recent interpretations of US EPA cancer guidelines (US EPA, 2005).

Statistical or Probability Distribution Models Two general types of dose–response models exist for extrapolation: statistical (or probability distribution models) and mechanistic models (Krewski and Van Ryzin, 1981). The distribution models are based on the assumption that each individual has a tolerance level for a test chemical and that this response level is a variable following a specific probability distribution function. These responses can be modeled using a cumulative dose–response function. Chap. 2 discusses the common normal distribution pattern (see Fig. 2-3). A log probit model estimates the probability of response at a specified dose (d); thus, $P(d) = \phi[a + \beta \log d]$, where ϕ is the cumulative function for a standard normal distribution of the log tolerances with standard deviations σ and mean μ, a equals μ/σ, and β equals the slope of the probit line ($-1/\sigma$). The probit curve at low doses usually assumes an S shape. Chap. 2 discusses determination of the LD_{50} value from such a curve. However, extrapolation of the experimental data from 50% response levels to a "safe," "acceptable," or "de minimus" level of exposure—for example, one in a million risk above background—illustrates the huge gap between scientific observations and highly protective risk limits (sometimes called virtually safe doses [VSDs] or those corresponding to a 95% upper confidence limit on adverse response rates).

The log-logistic model was derived from chemical kinetic theory. The probability of response at dose d is defined as $P(d) = [1 \exp(a + \beta \log d)]^{-1}$. Like the probit model, this model defines sigmoidal curves that are symmetrical around the 50% response level; however, the log-logistic curves approach the 0% and 100% response levels with a shallow curve shape. The logit and probit curves are indistinguishable in fitting the data in the region of the response curve where experimentally derived data are present (Brown, 1984; Hartung, 1987; Allen *et al.*, 1994b).

Models Derived from Mechanistic Assumptions This modeling approach designs a mathematical equation to describe dose–response relationships that are consistent with postulated biological mechanisms of response. These models are based on the idea that a response (toxic effect) in a particular biological unit (animal, human, pup, etc) is the result of the random occurrence of one or more biological events (stochastic events).

Radiation research has spawned a series of such "hit models" for cancer modeling, where a hit is defined as a critical cellular event that must occur before a toxic effect is produced. The simplest mechanistic model is the one-hit (one-stage) linear model in which only one hit or critical cellular interaction is required for a cell to be altered. For example, based on somatic mutation theory, a single mutational change would be sufficient for a cell to become cancerous through a transformational event and dose-independent clonal expansion. The probability statement for these models is $P(d) = 1 - \exp^{(-\lambda d)}$, where λd equals the number of hits occurring during a time period. Using this approach, a single molecule of a genotoxic carcinogen would have a minute but finite chance of causing a mutational event.

As theories of cancer have grown in complexity, so too have these hit-based mechanistic models. Multihit models have been developed that can describe hypothesized single-target multihit events, as well as multi-target, multi-hit events in carcinogenesis. The probability statements for these models are $P(d) = \int^{\lambda d} x^{k-1} \exp(-x)/\Gamma(k) dx$, where $\Gamma(k)$ denotes the gamma function with k being the critical number of hits for the adverse response. The Weibull model has a dose–response function with characteristics similar to those of the multihit models, where the response equation is $P(d) = 1 - \exp[-\lambda d^k]$. Here again, k is the critical number of hits for the toxic cellular response.

Armitage and Doll (1957) developed a multistage model for carcinogenesis that was based on these equations and on the hypothesis that a series of ordered stages was required before a cell could undergo mutation, initiation, transformation, and progression to form a tumor. This relationship was generalized by Crump (1984) by maximizing the likelihood function over polynomials, so that the probability statement is:

$$P(d) = 1 - \exp[-(\lambda_0 + \lambda_1 d^1 + \lambda_2 d^2 + \cdots + \lambda_k d^k)].$$

If the true value of λ_1 is replaced with λ_1^* (the upper confidence limit of λ_1), then a linearized-multistage model can be derived where the expression is dominated by $\lambda_1^* d$ at low doses. The slope on this confidence interval, q_1^*, has been used by EPA for quantitative cancer assessment. To obtain an upper 95% confidence interval on risk, the q_1^* value (risk/Δ dose in mg/kg per day) is multiplied by the amount of exposure (mg/kg per day). Thus, the upper bound estimate on risk (R) is calculated as:

$$R = q_1^* \text{ [risk (mg/kg per day)}^{-1}] \times \text{exposure (mg/kg per day)}.$$

This relationship has been used to calculate a "VSD," which represents the lower 95% confidence limit on a dose that gives an "acceptable level" of risk (eg, upper confidence limit for 10^{-6} excess risk). The Integrated Risk Information System (IRIS) (US EPA, 2011e) developed by EPA gives q^* values for many environmental carcinogens (US EPA, 2000b). Because both the q_1^* and VSD values are calculated using 95% confidence intervals, the values are believed to represent conservative, protective estimates.

The EPA has utilized the LMS model to calculate "unit risk estimates" in which the upper confidence limit on increased individual lifetime risk of cancer for a 70-kg human breathing 1 µg/m³ of contaminated air or drinking 2 L per day of water containing 1 ppm (1 mg/L) is estimated over a 70-year life span. The example given in Fig. 4-6 shows the calculation of incremental lifetime cancer risk (ILCR) of skin cancer using soil exposure and q^* values for inorganic arsenic. If a POD-based approach is used for low-dose extrapolation, the model would be used to extrapolate from the POD or upper confidence limit and these slopes would be considered for the q^* values.

Toxicological Enhancements of the Models Three exemplary areas of research that have improved the models used in risk extrapolation are time to tumor information, physiologically based TK modeling, and BBDR modeling (Albert, 1994). Chap. 7 discusses in detail improvements in our estimation of exposure and offers approaches on how to model "target internal effective dose" in risk assessment rather than just using single-value "external exposure doses." In this chapter we discuss the BBDR modeling.

BBDR modeling aims to make the generalized mechanistic models discussed in the previous section more clearly reflect specific biological processes. Measured rates are incorporated into the mechanistic equations to replace default or computer-generated values. For example, the Moolgavkar–Venson–Knudson (MVK) model is based on a two-stage model for carcinogenesis, where two mutations are required for carcinogenesis and birth and death rates of cells are modeled through clonal expansion and tumor formation. This model has been applied effectively to human epidemiologic data on retinoblastoma. In animal studies, kidney and liver tumors in the 2-acetylaminofluorene (2-AAF) "mega mouse" study, rat lung tumors following radiation exposure, rat liver tumors following N-nitrosomorpholine exposure, respiratory tract tumors following benzo[a]pyrene exposure, and mouse liver tumors following chlordane exposure have been modeled (Cohen and Ellwein, 1990; Moolgavkar and Luebeck, 1990).

There have been concerted research efforts to improve our mechanistic understanding of response at lower and lower exposures. Two excellent examples of the use of biomarkers to supplement our exploration of these dose–response relationships are seen in Bailey *et al.* (2009) and Vlaanderen *et al.* (2011). Hormetic responses are U-shaped dose–response relationships where small doses of a chemical can be beneficial but high doses are toxic. These are discussed in Chap. 2. These responses pose challenges to risk assessors. In general, science-based mechanistic conditions of low-dose response are always critical. See approaches used by the Institute of Medicine for vitamins and essential elements as these compounds consistently exhibit hormesis (Institute of Medicine (US), 2008).

Development of BBDR models for end points other than cancer is limited; however, several approaches have been explored in developmental toxicity, utilizing MOA information on cell cycle kinetics, enzyme activity, and cytotoxicity as critical end points (Faustman *et al.*, 1989, 2005a; Shuey *et al.*, 1994; Leroux *et al.*, 1996; Gohlke *et al.*, 2002, 2004, 2005, 2007; Daston *et al.*, 2004). Approaches have been proposed that link pregnancy-specific TK models with temporally sensitive TD models for developmental impacts (Faustman *et al.*, 1999; Faustman and Omenn, 2006). Unfortunately, there is a lack of specific, quantitative biological information on both kinetics and dynamics for most toxicants and end points (NRC, 2000; Faustman *et al.*, 2005a).

EXPOSURE ASSESSMENT

The primary objectives of exposure assessment are to determine source, type, magnitude, and duration of contact with the chemical(s) of interest. This is a critical element of the risk assessment process, as hazard does not occur in the absence of exposure. However, it is

A. Ingestion of arsenic from soil—point estimation method

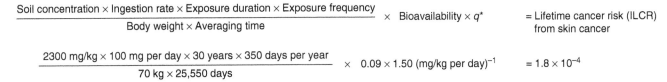

$$\frac{\text{Soil concentration} \times \text{Ingestion rate} \times \text{Exposure duration} \times \text{Exposure frequency}}{\text{Body weight} \times \text{Averaging time}} \times \text{Bioavailability} \times q^* = \text{Lifetime cancer risk (ILCR) from skin cancer}$$

$$\frac{2300 \text{ mg/kg} \times 100 \text{ mg per day} \times 30 \text{ years} \times 350 \text{ days per year}}{70 \text{ kg} \times 25{,}550 \text{ days}} \times 0.09 \times 1.50 \text{ (mg/kg per day)}^{-1} = 1.8 \times 10^{-4}$$

B. Ingestion of arsenic from soil—probabilistic methods

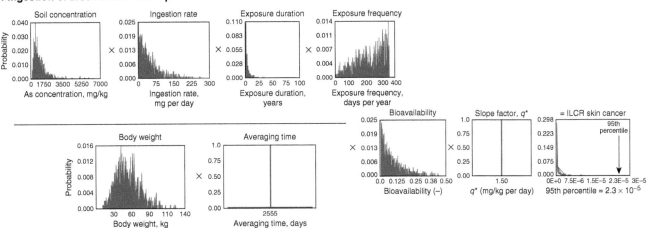

Figure 4-6. *Example of risk calculations for incremental lifetime cancer risk (ILCR) of skin cancer due to ingestion of arsenic in soil.* (**A**) Point exposure estimation method for calculation of ILCR. Point estimates for arsenic exposure input parameters are used in this example to calculate the ILCR. This exposure estimate is multiplied by the bioavailability of arsenic in soil to calculate the absorbed dose. Multiplication of the dose by the slope factor (q^*) yields the lifetime risk. (**B**) Probabilistic exposure methods for calculating the ILCR from arsenic ingestion. In this example, the soil concentration, ingestion rate, exposure duration and frequency, body weight, and bioavailability are modeled as distributions. Note that q^* and averaging time (years) are given as single-point estimations. This method yields a distribution of ILCR, with a 95th percentile upper confidence interval of 2.3×10^{-5}. Data from Calabrese *et al.* (1989), US EPA (1989, 1992, 1999a), Davis *et al.* (1990), Israeli and Nelson (1992), Brorby and Finley (1993), and Agency for Toxic Substances and Disease Registry (2007).

also frequently identified as the key area of uncertainty in the overall risk determination. Here, the primary focus is on uses of exposure information in quantitative risk assessment.

The primary goal of exposure calculations is not only to determine the type and amount of total exposure but also to find out specifically who may be exposed and how large a dose may be reaching target tissues. A key step in making an exposure assessment is determining what exposure pathways are relevant for the risk scenario under development. Fig. 4-7 shows an example exposure diagram used to illustrate possible exposure pathways from a hazardous chemical release. The subsequent steps entail quantitation of each pathway identified as a relevant exposure and then summarizing these pathway-specific exposures for calculation of overall exposure. Such calculations can include an estimation of total exposures for a specified population as well as calculation of exposure for highly exposed individuals. The EPA has published numerous documents that provide detailed definitions and guidelines for determining such exposures (US EPA, 1992, 2008, 2011a), with the recognition that special considerations need to be adopted when assessing childhood exposures (US EPA, 2008).

Conceptually, calculations are designed to represent "a plausible estimate" of exposure of individuals in the upper 90-95th percentile of the exposure distribution. Upper bound estimations would be "bounding calculations" designed to represent exposures at levels that exceed the exposures experienced by all individuals in the exposure distribution and are calculated by assuming upper limits for all exposure variables. A calculation for individuals exposed at concentrations near the middle of the exposure distribution is a central estimate. Fig. 4-7 gives example risk calculations using two types of exposure estimation procedures (US EPA, 1989, 1992, 2011a). Part A shows an example point estimation method for the calculation of arsenic (As) exposure via a soil ingestion route. In this hypothetical scenario, As exposure is calculated using point estimates for the upper 95th percent confidence limit of the arithmetic mean for each value in the lifetime average daily dose (LADD) equation. The LADD is calculated as follows:

$$\text{LADD} = \frac{\text{concentration of the toxicant in soil} \times \text{contact rate} \times \text{exposure duration}}{\text{bodyweight} \times \text{lifetime}}.$$

In this scenario, the average time (AT) is lifetime (25,550 days) and the contact or ingestion rate (CR) is equal to 100 mg soil per day. The exposure frequency and duration (EDF) is equal to the exposure frequency (daily exposure = 365 days per year) times the exposure duration (30 years). To obtain the ILCR, the LADD must be multiplied by the bioavailability to obtain an absorbed dose and q^* where the upper 95% CLM slope (q^*) is 1.5 × change in risk per mg/kg body weight per day in this example.

Many exposures are now estimated using probability distributions for exposures rather than single-point estimates for the factors within the LADD equation (Finley *et al.*, 1994; Cullen and Frey, 1999). Such approaches can provide a reality check and can be useful for generating more realistic exposure profiles reflective of population exposures. Good sources for US exposures can be obtained from the EPA *Exposure Factors Handbook* (US EPA, 2011a). Fig. 4-7B shows how this is done using an example arsenic risk scenario with soil As concentration, ingestion rate, exposure duration, frequency, body weight, and bioavailability modeled as

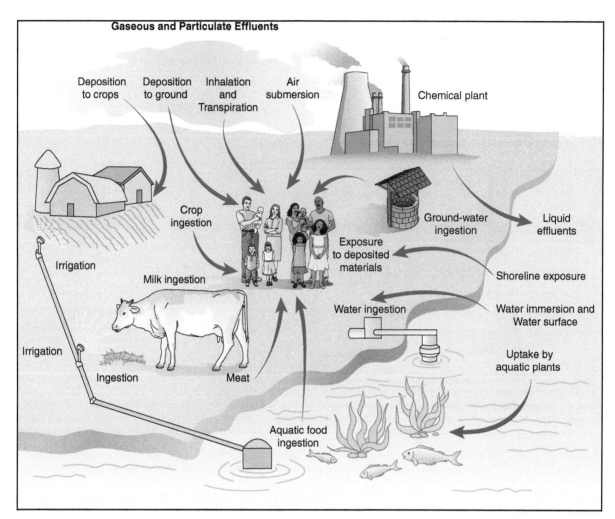

Figure 4-7. *Exposure pathway schematic.* Within the risk assessment process, a critical early step is the identification of the exposure pathway(s). To fully characterize exposure, the site- and chemical-specific exposure pathways must be identified. This hypothetical exposure pathway schematic illustrated the various ways in which contaminants can move from the source through media to points of exposure. (Adapted from Sexton *et al.* (1992); reproduced with permission from Taylor & Francis Group, LLC, http://www.taylorandfrancis.com.)

distributed variables. Using Monte Carlo simulation techniques, an overall ILCR distribution can be generated and a 95th percentile for population risk obtained.

The FQPA of 1996 has highlighted the need for considerations of potential special risks for children and the need to evaluate child-specific exposures as well as cumulative exposures and risks (US EPA, 1996b). In 2006, the EPA released a supplemental document with child-specific exposure factors to address the special considerations necessary when evaluating childhood exposures (US EPA, 2008). Table 4-6 shows example exposure factors for drinking water intake for children and adults. The EPA *Child-Specific Exposure Factors Handbook*, which is online, provides useful information about such exposure distributions. The FQPA also identified the need to evaluate total exposures by determining aggregate exposure measures for all exposures to a single substance. Cross-media exposure analyses, such as those conducted for lead and mercury, are good examples of the value of looking at such total exposures in evaluating human risks, and complex models are available for some compounds (see EPA's integrated exposure uptake biokinetic [IEUBK] model for lead in children; US EPA, 2010c). Cumulative exposures and cumulative risk refer to the total exposure and risks from a group of compounds. In FQPA chemicals with similar modes of toxicity are evaluated using cumulative exposure and risk estimates. For example, EPA is identifying and categorizing pesticides

that act by a common MOA, and cumulative exposures to classes of organophosphates with similar MOAs (cholinesterase inhibition) have been used as examples of classes of pesticides for which cumulative exposure and cumulative risk estimates are needed (US EPA, 1996c; ILSI, 1999; Ryan, 2010). WHO has recently published a framework for combined exposures (Meek *et al.*, 2011).

Additional considerations for exposure assessments include how time and duration of exposure are evaluated in risk assessments. In general, estimates for cancer risk use average exposure over a lifetime (see LADD example above). In a few cases, short-term exposure limits (STELs) are required (eg, ethylene oxide) and characterization of brief but high levels of exposure is significant. In these cases exposures are not averaged over the lifetime and the effects of high, short-term doses are estimated. With developmental toxicity, a single exposure can be sufficient to produce an adverse developmental effect if exposures occur during a window of developmental susceptibility; thus, daily doses are used, rather than lifetime weighted averages (US EPA, 1991; Weller *et al.*, 1999).

RISK CHARACTERIZATION

Risk characterization is a summary of the risk assessment components and serves to outline the key findings and inform the risk manager in public health decisions. It is an analysis and integration

Table 4-6

Example Exposure Factor Handbook Information: Drinking Water Intake for Children

AGE GROUP	MEAN	INTAKE (mL PER DAY), 95TH PERCENTILE	MEAN	INTAKE (mL/kg PER DAY), 95TH PERCENTILE
Newborn (<1 month)	184	839	52	232
Infants (1 to <3 months)	227	896	48	205
Infants (3 to <6 months)	362	1056	52	159
Infants (6 to <12 months)	360	1055	41	126
Child (1 to <2 years)	271	837	23	71
Child (2 to <3 years)	317	877	23	60
Child (3 to <6 years)	380	1078	22	61
Child (6 to <11 years)	447	1235	16	43
Child (11 to <16 years)	606	1727	12	34
Child (16 to <18 years)	731	1983	11	31
Adult (18 to <21 years)	826	2540	12	35

SOURCE: Ershow and Cantor (1989) and US EPA (2008, 2011a).

of the conclusions from the hazard assessment, the dose–response, and the exposure assessment. EPA outlines the science policy and elements for completing a risk characterization in their *Risk Characterization Handbook* (US EPA, 2000c). As shown in Fig. 4-1, risk characterization considers the nature, estimated incidence, and reversibility of adverse effects in a given population; how robust the evidence is; how certain the evaluation is; if susceptible populations are characterized; and if there is a relevant mode of action.

For many years there has been an information sharing process aimed at harmonization of chemical testing regimes and clinical trials methodologies, so that data might be accepted in multiple countries. Efforts by WHO and IPCS have included the Harmonization of Approaches to the Assessment of Risk from Exposure to Chemicals Project (WHO, 2011a). This project has the goal of globally harmonizing but not standardizing the approaches to risk assessment by increasing understanding and developing basic principles and guidance on specific chemical risk assessment issues. The WHO has worked to harmonize dose–response methodologies (DRM) and released a report providing descriptive guidance for risk assessors in using DRM in hazard characterization (International Programme on Chemical Safety, 2006). Examples of other reports include those on terminology (International Programme on Chemical Safety, 2004) and exposure assessment (World Health Organization, 2006) and *Uncertainty and Data Quality in Exposure Assessment* (International Programme on Chemical Safety, 2008).

Uncertainty analysis is an essential component in our final risk characterization and includes factors such as variability and lack of knowledge (NRC, 1994). Variability refers to true differences such as is reflected in temporal, spatial, or interindividual differences. It usually cannot be reduced with further study. Lack of knowledge can also be discussed as a source of uncertainty and these factors may be reduced with further study. For example, if only a few environmental samples are taken from a contaminated site for analysis, then uncertainty can be reduced by taking further samples. Formal methods for dealing with uncertainty analysis are described in several references including IPCS (2008) and Bogen *et al.* (2009). Using probabilistic-based approaches (PRA) for exposure assessment and assuming distributional versus

dichotomous data for exposure factors is one way of addressing uncertainty that is commonly applied.

Variation in Susceptibility

Risk assessment methodologies incorporating human variability have been slow to develop. Generally, assay results utilize means and standard deviations to measure variation, or even standard errors of the mean. This ignores variability in response due to specific differences in age, sex, health status, and genetics. Default factors of 10× are overutilized to describe cross- and between-species differences and TK and dynamic data are rare. Nevertheless, EPA and OSHA are expected under the Clean Air Act and the Occupational Safety and Health Act to promulgate standards that protect the most susceptible subgroups or individuals in the population (Omenn *et al.*, 1990; Cullen and Frey, 1999; Faustman and Omenn, 2006; Kramer *et al.*, 2006; Cullen *et al.*, 2008). Sensitive or susceptible populations have been defined and interpreted for the Clean Air Act and in this context "particularly sensitive citizens, such as bronchial asthmatics and emphysematics", are to be protected by the standards. This illustrates not only the importance but also the challenge to risk assessors to ensure protection for human populations.

Ecogenetics has been defined as the study of critical genetic determinants that define susceptibility to environmentally influenced adverse health effects (Costa and Eaton, 2006). Ecogenetic variation can affect biotransformation systems that activate and detoxify chemicals or alter the response in target tissues. With the completion of the Human Genome Project in April 2003, the identification of human polymorphisms has greatly expanded our potential for understanding how genetic variability can impact biological response and susceptibility. There have been numerous activities initiated with the goal of understanding the linkage between genes and the environment. The following databases and initiatives are designed to identify polymorphisms, including single-nucleotide polymorphisms (SNP), insertions, deletions, amplifications, and alternative splicing. These include the International HapMap Project (HapMap, 2009), the DNA Polymorphism Discovery Resource (National Human Genome Research Institute, 2010), the National Center for Biotechnology Information (NCBI) SNP databases (NCBI, 2011a,b), and the NIH

GAIN program (National Human Genome Research Institute, 2010). Using the information from such databases, researchers hope to identify genetic similarities and differences in human beings with the goal of identifying genes that affect health, disease, and individual responses to medications and environmental factors (Omen, 2012). Recent observations now demonstrate that not only genetics is significant, but also epigenetics (Sartor et al., 2012). SNP arrays are now available that can identify and characterize approximately 1×10^6 SNPs in the human population. Arrays also exist that evaluate SNPs in pathways significant for drug metabolism enzymes and transporters. These are in FDA-approved pathways and have been used for evaluation of appropriate drug therapies. However, they are just starting to be used for environmental risk assessment (Guerrette et al., 2011). Next-generation sequencing, where coverage of the genome can be extended to 40×, has revealed rare copy number variants that can be linked to disease and provide another level of understanding concerning human variation (Sudmant et al., 2010). It should be noted that this genetic information on individuals can raise ethical, social, and legal concerns regarding protections of individuals and their rights (Hsieh, 2004). Recent legislation that protects individuals from discrimination on the basis of genetic variation helps to ensure protection and not exclusion for all workers (Human Genome Program, 2008; United States Act, 2008).

One of the key challenges for toxicologists doing risk assessments will be the interpretation and linking of observations from highly sensitive molecular and genome-based methods with the overall process of toxicity (Eisen et al., 1998; Limbird and Taylor, 1998; Andersen and Barton, 1999; NRC, 2000). The basic need for linkage of observations was highlighted in early biomarker work. NRC reports on biomarkers (NRC, 1989a,b, 1992a,b) drew distinctions for biomarkers of effect, exposure, and susceptibility across a continuum of exposure, effect, and disease/toxicity. Biomarkers of early effects, such as frank clinical pathology, arise as a function of exposure, response, and time. Early, subtle, and possibly reversible effects can generally be distinguished from irreversible disease states. Chemical-specific biomarkers have the potential to provide critical information, but there is an inherent complexity in pulling the information together. If biomarkers are considered a reflection of exposure or disease state, then considerations have to be made regarding the interactions between genes and the environment and the difference between a population-based assessment and individual assessment (Groopman and Kensler, 1999).

Nowhere is the challenge for interpretation of early and highly sensitive response biomarkers clearer than in the complicated data from gene expression arrays (toxicogenomics). Our continued ability to monitor changes in response in thousands of genes has proven challenging for toxicologists. Emphasis on toxicity-based risk assessment methods and analysis has been strongly encouraged by several significant NAS reports (NRC, 2000, 2007a,b; NRC, 2010) as well as development and application of pathway-based methods (Yu et al., 2006). Toxicogenomics projects have confirmed the repeatability and cross-platform concordance of microarray data (Bammler et al., 2005; Guo et al., 2006; Nature Biotechnology Editorial, 2006; Patterson et al., 2006) and standards for data interpretation (minimum information about a microarray experiment [MIAME]) accepted (Brazma et al., 2001).

Microarray analysis for risk assessment requires sophisticated analyses beyond basic cluster analysis (Eisen et al., 1998) to arrive at a functional interpretation and linkage to conventional toxicological (apical) end points. Because of the vast number of measured responses with gene expression arrays, pattern analysis techniques are being used through pathway mapping platforms such as MAPPFinder and GenMAPP (Moggs et al., 2004; Currie et al.,

2005). The Gene Ontology Consortium has developed a controlled vocabulary (ontology) for sharing biological information across species. Database users can then annotate their gene products with gene ontology (GO) terms, establishing a consistent description and definition across databases and studies, and this facilitates risk assessment. Through the power of GO terms, analysis methods are being developed to allow for a quantitative time- and dose-dependent interpretation of genomic response using systems-based approaches to integrate responses at the biological and cellular level (Yu et al., 2006). A very good approach to integrated analysis of multiple omics datasets is Conceptgen (Sartor et al., 2010).

Both the EPA and FDA have formally recognized the power of genomic information as well as its potential limitations. Both agencies have issued interim policies guiding how to include genomic information into risk assessments and they have agreed to use genomic information in conjunction with (but not in isolation of) standard risk assessment data (FDA, 2011; US EPA, 2011f). Extensive research efforts by the US EPA Computational Toxicology program will facilitate future risk assessment uses (US EPA, 2012b).

INFORMATION RESOURCES

There are numerous information resources available for risk assessment and a few are listed below to provide the reader with examples but not a comprehensive list of risk assessment resources and databases. Such resources include the Toxicology Data Network (http://toxnet.nlm.nih.gov/) from the US National Library of Medicine, the US NTP (National Toxicology Program, 2011a) including the *Report on Carcinogens* and the *Office of Health Assessment and Translation*, the WHO IPCS (WHO, 2011a), and the IARC (WHO, 2011b). The WHO Toolkit for Risk Assessment is especially user friendly for new risk assessors (WHO, 2010). WHO, through its IPCS, produces useful risk documents entitled *Concise International Chemical Assessment Documents* that cover a variety of chemical substances (WHO, 2011c). The Codex Alimentarius Commission created by FAO and WHO produces guidelines and reports relevant for food safety and standards (FAO and WHO, 2011). The IRIS is US EPA's human health assessment program that evaluates health risks for over 500 chemical substances (US EPA, 2011e). IRIS lists specific risk values used by the US EPA. It is anticipated that additional databases will be available from REACH.

There is a need for a note of caution for users of these risk-relevant databases as with most databases there is a need to consider multiple contributions to differences between recommended values. These differences can be due to variations in how and when new scientific information is incorporated in the evaluations. Also, different regulatory drivers for national values or issues related to legal priorities or delays in implementing draft to final recommended values can occur. Such factors have contributed to differences in arsenic and dioxin risk estimates in the United States.

Recently, new toxicogenomic databases that identify and, in some cases, provide characterization of chemicals have become available. The NCBI (2011a,b) provides access to an enormous set of biomedical and genomic information. Its portfolio of comprehensive data and tools can be valuable for risk assessment and the aim to integrate with toxicologically relevant end points and disease is laudable. It has Chemicals and Bioassays, Data and Software, DNA and RNA, Protein Domains and Structures, Genes and Expression, genetic information databases linked with decision outcomes, Genomes and Gene Maps, and Cross-Species Homology. Resources covering databases and tools help in the study of SARs. A publicly available functional genomics data repository (Gene Expression Omnibus [GEO] database) supports MIAME-compliant data submission, and allows for easily accessible microarray- and sequence-based data, which are searchable for specific profiles of interest based on gene annotation or precomputed profile characteristics. Also variations such as data on genomic variation, interaction of genotypes and phenotypes, and the single-nucleotide polymorphisms (dbSNP) can be obtained through the NCBI. ACToR (http://actor.epa.gov/actor/faces/ACToRHome.jsp), EPA's online database on chemical toxicity data and potential chemical risks to human health and the environment, is another useful resource for risk assessments. It allows users to search and query data including Toxicity Reference Database (ToxRefDB) (30 years and $2 billion worth of animal toxicity studies), ToxCastDB (data from screening 1000 chemicals in over 500 high-throughput assays), ExpoCastDB, and DSSTox (provides high-quality chemical structures and annotations). The ToxRefDB captures thousands of in vivo animal toxicity studies on hundreds of chemicals. Another curated Comparative Toxicogenomics Database (CTD, http://ctd.mdibl.org/) includes data describing cross-species chemical–gene/protein interactions and chemical– and gene–disease relationships to illuminate molecular mechanisms underlying variable susceptibility and environmentally influenced diseases. These data provide insight into complex chemical–gene and protein interaction networks. These databases can be especially useful for hazard identification and mechanistic information; few emphasize exposure information.

RISK PERCEPTION AND COMPARATIVE ANALYSES OF RISK

It is well known that individuals respond differently to information about hazardous situations and products (Fischhoff, 1981; Fischhoff et al., 1993, 1996; Sandman, 1993; NRC, 1996; Risk Commission, 1997; Institute of Medicine, 1999; Slovic, 2010). Understanding these behavioral responses at the individual, community, and population levels is critical in stimulating constructive risk communication and evaluating potential risk management options for risk assessment issues. In a classic study, students, League of Women Voters members, active club members, and scientific experts were asked to rank 30 activities or agents in order of their annual contribution to deaths (Slovic et al., 1979, 2005). Club members ranked pesticides, spray cans, and nuclear power as safer than did other laypersons. Students ranked contraceptives and food preservatives as riskier and mountain climbing as safer than did others. Experts ranked electric power, surgery, swimming, and x-rays as more risky, but nuclear power and police work as less risky than did laypersons. From studies like these, we now know that there are cultural and gender differences in perception of risks. There are also group differences in perceptions of risk from chemicals among toxicologists, correlated with their employment in industry, academia, or government (Neal et al., 1994). Recent risk perception research has emphasized the importance of knowing the balance between analytical thinking and "affect." Our immediate emotional reaction can shape our initial risk perceptions ("affect"), while our thoughtful, deliberate "analytical" thinking also impacts our risk understanding but the latter is a slower response. Understanding this balance can help us explain why there is a complex relationship between perceived risk and benefits (Slovic, 2010).

Psychological factors such as dread, perceived uncontrollability, and involuntary exposure interact with factors that represent the extent to which a hazard is familiar, observable, and "essential" for daily living (Lowrance, 1976; Morgan, 1993). Fig. 4-8 presents a grid on the parameters controllable/uncontrollable and observable/not observable for a large number of risky activities;

for each of the two-paired main factors, highly correlated factors are described in the boxes.

Public demand for government regulations often focuses on involuntary exposures (especially in the food supply, drinking water, and air) and unfamiliar hazards, such as radioactive waste, electromagnetic fields, asbestos insulation, and genetically modified crops and foods. The public can respond negatively when they perceive that information about hazards or new technologies has been withheld or under-rated. This can explain some of the very strong responses to genetically modified foods, HIV-contaminated blood transfusions in the 1980s, or hazardous chemical and radioactive wastes. Loss of trust is exemplified by Japanese reactions following the Fukushima Daiichi nuclear reactor meltdown (March 2011), where initial perceived benefits of nuclear power were transformed to distrust during follow-up actions and responses to the earthquake and tsunami.

Perceptions of risk led to the addition of an extra safety factor (default value 10) for children in the FQPA of 1996. Engineering-based "as low as reasonably achievable" (ALARA) approaches also reflect the general "precautionary principle," which is strongly favored by those who, justifiably, believe we are far from knowing all risks given frequently limited toxicity testing data (Roe et al., 1997).

EMERGING CONCEPTS

In order for risk assessment to inform environmental risk management, there is a need to ensure that the initial "problem formulation" of the risk question(s) is succinctly framed to answer questions in the real world. Environmental health is very dynamic and many divergent emerging environmental challenges such as climate change, energy shortages, and engineered nanoparticles will require an expansion of our context well beyond single-chemical, single-exposure scenarios. In order to accomplish this goal, several factors need to be considered. These factors include defining not only health but also well-being and sustainability and will require a context of global and international scale.

Well-being is increasingly being used to describe human health and the goal of sustainable environmental risk management. The WHO has championed the use of well-being rather than health to describe the Millennium Development Goals (WHO, 2011d). Well-being goes beyond "disease-free" existence to freedom from want (including food and water security) and fear (personal safety) and sustainable futures. Concepts such as food security (abundance and quality of foods), water security (plentiful supplies and high quality of water), and sustainability form internationally recognized environmental and developmental goals. Sustainability embraces the risk management concept that "development that meets the needs of the present, without compromising the ability of future generations" to thrive and hence well-being is one of the goals of environmental actions and decisions. Recognition that environmental problems are global is essential to our understanding of how we manage risks and how we address sustainability (Leiserowitz et al., 2006; Gohlke et al., 2008; Kite-Powell et al., 2008). Ocean health and air pollution are excellent examples of the need for understanding the global context where pollutants do not honor country and national borders. World Trade Organization (WTO) agreements have also placed risk assessment approaches in the forefront as tools for managers working to meet the global goals for sustainable trade and economic health. At the most basic level new risk assessments are being done with a new global emphasis (Carruth and Goldstein, 2004; US EPA Office of Research and Development, 2011). Recent reorganization of EPA along management lines of sustainability now provides an integrative framework for working toward sustainability goals. As a response for this broader framing of health impacts, the EPA

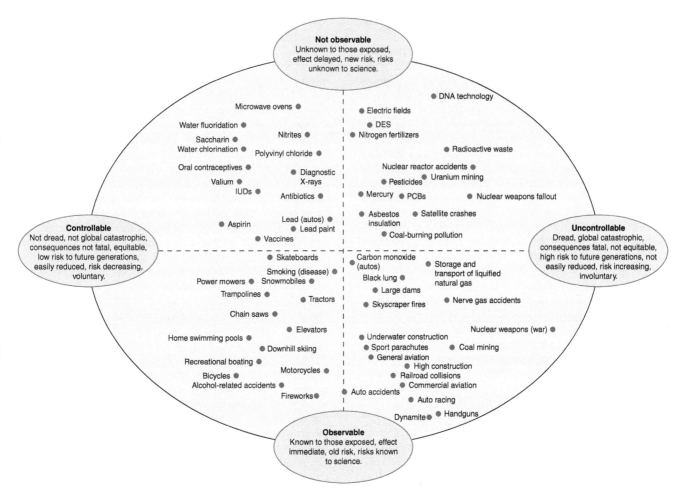

Figure 4-8. *Perceptions of risk illustrated using a "risk space" axis diagram.* Risk space has axes that correspond roughly to a hazard's perceived "dreadedness" and to the degree to which it is familiar or observable. Risks in the upper right quadrant of this space are most likely to provoke calls for government regulation.

Office of Research and Development realigned their research within a new structure of Chemical Safety for Sustainability; Sustainable and Healthy Communities; Safe and Sustainable Water Resources; and Air, Climate and Energy. Risk assessment is viewed as one of the critical approaches for integrating these goals and toxicology is one of the tools used within that approach (Teichman and US EPA, 2011).

PUBLIC HEALTH RISK MANAGEMENT

Associated with concepts of well-being and sustainability is a public health orientation to risk assessment and risk management. Public health as a discipline is very compatible with toxicology, where toxicological tests are performed to identify and characterize potential health risks and to prevent the unsafe use of such agents. Public health also has an emphasis on approaches for identifying, characterizing, and preventing risks.

Within public health risk management, there are three stages of prevention: *primary*, whose goal is prevention and risk or hazard avoidance; *secondary*, whose goal is mitigation or preparedness including risk or vulnerability reduction and risk transfer; and *tertiary*, where prompt response or recovery is an approach for decreasing residual risk or risk reduction (Frumkin, 2010). Fig. 4-9 shows an overview of risk assessment and management for public health where concepts of capacity assessment, vulnerability, and impact assessment are included. In this context, vulnerability assessment would include consideration of exposure and susceptibility as

part of the vulnerability assessment. Hazard analysis refers to both hazard identification and probability-based frequency of anticipated events. Capacity assessment has been used for identifying strengths and resiliency of a system to impact. Recent disasters such as Hurricane Katrina, the Gulf Oil Spill, and the Fukushima Daiichi nuclear reactor meltdown all point to the need for environmental risk assessment to be considered as a part of an even larger context in order to understand critical infrastructure for determining human and environmental risks. Life-cycle analysis, green chemistry, and built environment all require such a broad context for evaluation (Keim, 2002; NRC, 2009). Fig. 4-4 also suggests that understanding population variability and vulnerability in a context of "built environment" is important. The "built environment" encompasses all man-made resources and infrastructure, including buildings, spaces, and transportation systems, which support human activity and have a strong influence on public health (Perdue *et al.*, 2003). These types of frameworks can allow for easier consideration of public health concepts for sustainability, environmental disaster response, and life-cycle systems analysis than many of our traditional frameworks for environmental chemical risk assessment, which can be done in relative isolation.

SUMMARY

The NRC and Risk Commission frameworks for risk assessment and risk management provide a consistent framework-based approach for evaluating risks and taking action to reduce

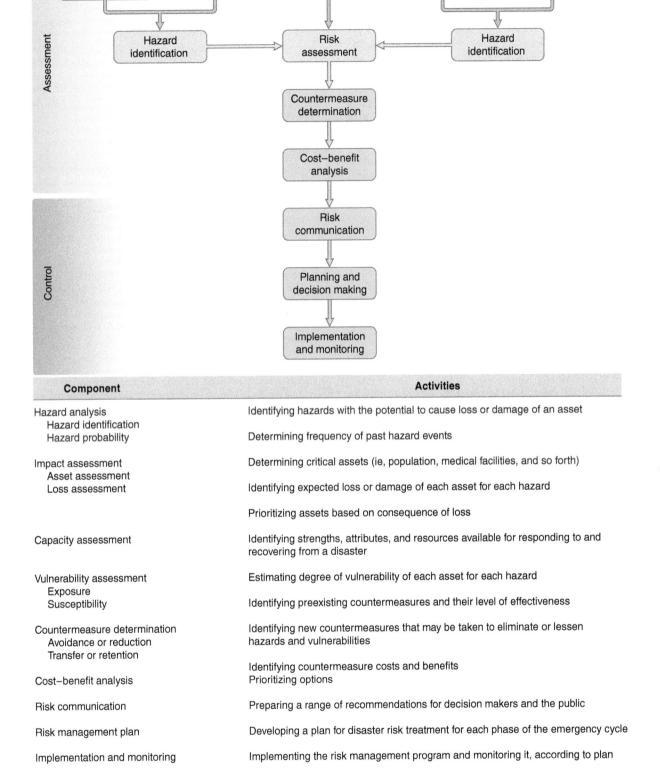

Component	Activities
Hazard analysis Hazard identification	Identifying hazards with the potential to cause loss or damage of an asset
Hazard probability	Determining frequency of past hazard events
Impact assessment Asset assessment	Determining critical assets (ie, population, medical facilities, and so forth)
Loss assessment	Identifying expected loss or damage of each asset for each hazard
	Prioritizing assets based on consequence of loss
Capacity assessment	Identifying strengths, attributes, and resources available for responding to and recovering from a disaster
Vulnerability assessment Exposure	Estimating degree of vulnerability of each asset for each hazard
Susceptibility	Identifying preexisting countermeasures and their level of effectiveness

Countermeasure determination
  Avoidance or reduction
  Transfer or retention
	Identifying new countermeasures that may be taken to eliminate or lessen hazards and vulnerabilities

Cost–benefit analysis	Identifying countermeasure costs and benefits Prioritizing options
Risk communication	Preparing a range of recommendations for decision makers and the public
Risk management plan	Developing a plan for disaster risk treatment for each phase of the emergency cycle
Implementation and monitoring	Implementing the risk management program and monitoring it, according to plan

Figure 4-9. *Overview and process for environmental risk management.* This scheme shows a broad context for thinking about risk management that includes considerations of vulnerabilities and impact analysis frequently discussed in environmental engineering and public health. (Adapted from Frumkin *et al.* (2010); reproduced with permission from John Wiley & Sons, Inc.)

risks. The objectives of risk assessments vary with the issues, risk management needs, and statutory requirements. Hence, setting the context and problem formation for risk evaluation is essential (NRC, 2009). The frameworks are sufficiently flexible to address various objectives and to accommodate new knowledge while also providing guidance for priority setting in industry, environmental organizations, and government regulatory and public health agencies. Risk assessment analyzes the science and, if incomplete, identifies uncertainty and provides approaches for moving forward with decisions (NRC, 2009). Toxicology, epidemiology, exposure assessment, and clinical observations can be linked with biomarkers, cross-species investigations of mechanisms of effects, and systematic approaches to risk assessment, risk communication, and risk management. Advances in toxicology are certain to improve the quality of risk assessments for a broad array of health end points as scientific findings substitute data for assumptions and help to describe and model uncertainty more credibly.

REFERENCES

Abbott BD, Harris MW, Birnbaum LS. Comparisons of the effects of TCDD and hydrocortisone on growth factor expression provide insight into their interaction in the embryonic mouse palate. *Teratology.* 1992;45: 35–53.

Adami HO, Berry SC, Breckenridge CB, et al. Toxicology and epidemiology: improving the science with a framework for combining toxicological and epidemiological evidence to establish causal inference. *Toxicol Sci.* 2011;122:223–234.

Adler S, Basketter D, Creton S, et al. Alternative (non-animal) methods for cosmetics testing: current status and future prospects—2010. *Arch Toxicol.* 2011;85:367–485.

Agency for Toxic Substances and Disease Registry. *Toxicological Profile for Arsenic.* Atlanta, GA: Department of Health and Human Services; 2007.

Albert RE. Carcinogen risk assessment in the US Environmental Protection Agency. *Crit Rev Toxicol.* 1994;24:75–85.

Allen BC, Kavlock RJ, Kimmel CA, Faustman EM. Dose response assessments for developmental toxicity: II. Comparison of generic benchmark dose estimates with no observed adverse effect levels. *Fundam Appl Toxicol.* 1994a;23:487–495.

Allen BC, Kavlock RJ, Kimmel CA, Faustman EM. Dose-response assessment for developmental toxicity. 3. Statistical-models. *Fundam Appl Toxicol.* 1994b;23(4):496–509.

Ames BN, Gold LS. Too many rodent carcinogens: mitogenesis increases mutagenesis. *Science.* 1990;247:970–971.

Andersen ME, Barton HA. Biological regulation of receptor–hormone complex C in relation to dose–response assessments of endocrine-active compounds. *Toxicol Sci.* 1999;48:38–50.

Armitage P, Doll R. A two-stage theory of carcinogenesis in relation to the age distribution of human cancer. *Br J Cancer.* 1957;11:161–169.

Ashby J, Tennant RW. Prediction of rodent carcinogenicity of 44 chemicals: results. *Mutagenesis.* 1994;9:7–15.

Atterwill CK, Johnston H, Thomas SM. Models for the in vitro assessment of neurotoxicity in the nervous system in relation to xenobiotic and neurotrophic factor-mediated events. *Neurotoxicology.* 1992;13:39–54.

Auton TR. Calculation of benchmark doses from teratology data. *Regul Toxicol Pharmacol.* 1994;19:152–167.

Bailey GS, Reddy AP, Pereira CB, et al. Nonlinear cancer response at ultralow dose: a 40800-animal ED(001) tumor and biomarker study. *Chem Res Toxicol.* 2009;22:1264–1276.

Bammler T, Beyer RP, Bhattacharya S, et al. Standardizing global gene expression analysis between laboratories and across platforms. *Nat Methods.* 2005;2:351–356.

Barnes DG, Dourson MJ. Reference dose (Rfd): description and use in health risk assessment. *Regul Toxicol Pharmacol.* 1988;8:471–486.

Benigni R, Zito R. The second National Toxicology Program comparative exercise on the prediction of rodent carcinogenicity: definitive results. *Mutat Res.* 2004;566:49–63.

Bogdanffy MS, Daston G, Faustman EM, et al. Harmonization of cancer and noncancer risk assessment: proceedings of a consensus-building workshop. *Toxicol Sci.* 2001;61:18–31.

Bogen KT, Cullen AC, Frey HC, Price PS. Probabilistic exposure analysis for chemical risk characterization. *Toxicol Sci.* 2009;109:4–17.

Brazma A, Hingamp P, Quackenbush J, et al. Minimum information about a microarray experiment (MIAME)—toward standards for microarray data. *Nat Genet.* 2001;29:365–371.

Brorby G, Finley G. Standard probability density functions for routine use in environmental health risk assessment. In: Society for Risk Analysis annual meeting; 1993; Savannah, GA.

Brown CC. High-to-low-dose extrapolation in animals. In: Rodricks JV, Tardiff RG, eds. *Assessment and Management of Chemical Risks.* Washington, DC: American Chemical Society; 1984:57–79.

Brown NA, Spielmann H, Bechter R. Screening chemicals for reproductive toxicity: the current alternatives: the report and recommendations of an ECVAM/ETS workshop. *Altern Lab Anim.* 1995;23:868–882.

Bucher JR. Update on National Toxicology Program (NTP) assays with genetically altered or "transgenic" mice. *Environ Health Perspect.* 1998;106:619–621.

Calabrese EJ, Pastides H, Barnes R. How much soil do young children ingest: an epidemiologic study. In: Kostecki PT, Calabrese EJ, eds. *Petroleum Contaminated Soils.* Chelsea, MI: Lewis Publishers; 1989:363–397.

Calkins DR, Dixon RI, Gerber CR. Identification, characterization, and control of potential human carcinogens: a framework for federal decision-making. *J Natl Cancer Inst.* 1980;61:167–175.

Capen CC, Dybing E, Rice JM, Wilbourn JD, eds. *Species Differences in Thyroid, Kidney and Urinary Bladder Carcinogenesis.* IARC Scientific Publications No. 147. International Agency for Research on Cancer and World Health Organization; 1999.

Carruth RS, Goldstein BD. The asbestos case: a comment on the appointment and use of nonpartisan experts in World Trade Organization dispute resolution involving health risk. *Risk Anal.* 2004;24:471–481.

Charnley G, Omenn GS. A summary of the findings and recommendations of the commission on risk assessment and risk management (and accompanying papers prepared for the commission). *Hum Ecol Risk Assess.* 1997;3:701–711.

Cheng H, Aylward L, Beall C, et al. TCDD exposure-response analysis and risk assessment. *Risk Anal.* 2006;26(4):1059–1071.

Chesler EJ, Miller DR, Branstetter LR, et al. The Collaborative Cross at Oak Ridge National Laboratory: developing a powerful resource for systems genetics. *Mamm Genome.* 2008;19:382–389.

Chhabra RS, Bucher JR, Wolfe M, Portier C. Toxicity characterization of environmental chemicals by the US National Toxicology Program: an overview. *Int J Hyg Environ Health.* 2003;206:437–445.

Cohen SM. Human relevance of animal carcinogenicity studies. *Regul Toxicol Pharmacol.* 1995;21:75–80 [discussion 81–86].

Cohen SM. Alternative models for carcinogenicity testing: weight of evidence evaluations across models. *Toxicol Pathol.* 2001;29(suppl):183–190.

Cohen SM, Arnold LL, Cano M, Ito M, Garland EM, Shaw RA. Calcium phosphate-containing precipitate and the carcinogenicity of sodium salts in rats. *Carcinogenesis.* 2000;21:783–792.

Cohen SM, Ellwein LB. Proliferative and genotoxic cellular effects in 2-acetylaminofluorene bladder and liver carcinogenesis: biological modeling of the EDO1 study. *Toxicol Appl Pharmacol.* 1990;104:79–93.

Costa L, Eaton D. Introduction. In: Costa L, Eaton D, eds. *Gene–Environment Interactions: Fundamentals of Ecogenetics.* Hoboken, NJ: John Wiley and Sons Inc; 2006.

Costa LG. Biochemical and molecular neurotoxicology. In: Maines MD, Costa LG, Reed DJ, eds. *Current Protocols in Toxicology.* New York: Wiley; 2000.

Crump KS. An improved procedure for low-dose carcinogenic risk assessment from animal data. *J Environ Pathol Toxicol.* 1980;5:339–348.

Crump KS. A new method for determining allowable daily intakes. *Fundam Appl Toxicol.* 1984;4:854–871.

Cullen AC, Corrales MA, Kramer CB, Faustman EM. The application of genetic information for regulatory standard setting under the Clean Air Act: a decision-analytic approach. *Risk Anal.* 2008;28:877–890.

Cullen AC, Frey HC. *Probabilistic Techniques in Exposure Assessment: A Handbook for Dealing with Variability and Uncertainty in Models and Inputs.* New York: Plenum Press; 1999.

Currie RA, Bombail V, Oliver JD, et al. Gene ontology mapping as an unbiased method for identifying molecular pathways and processes affected by toxicant exposure: application to acute effects caused by the rodent non-genotoxic carcinogen diethylhexylphthalate. *Toxicol Sci.* 2005;86:453–469.

Daston G, Faustman EM, Ginsberg G, et al. A framework for assessing risks to children from exposure to environmental agents. *Environ Health Perspect.* 2004;112:238–256.

Davis S, Waller P, Buschborn R. Quantitative estimates of soil ingestion in normal children between the ages of 2 and 7 years: population-based estimates using aluminum, silicon, and titanium as soil tracer elements. *Arch Environ Health.* 1990;45:112–122.

Dean AG, Dean JA, Coulombier D. *Epi Info, Version 6: A Word Processing, Database, and Statistics Program for Public Health on IBM-Compatible Microcomputers.* Atlanta, GA: Centers for Disease Control and Prevention (CDC); 1995.

Dearfield KL. *Pesticide Assessment Guidelines. Subdivision F, Hazard Evaluation: Humans and Domestic Animals.* Series 83-3. 1990.

Dourson MJ, Hertzberg RC, Hartung R, Blackburn K. Novel methods for the estimation of acceptable daily intake. *Toxicol Ind Health.* 1985;1:23–41.

Dourson ML, DeRosa CT. The use of uncertainty factors in establishing safe levels of exposure. In: Krewski D, Franklin C, eds. *Statistics in Toxicology.* New York: Gordon & Breach; 1991:613–627.

Dourson ML, Stara JF. Regulatory history and experimental support of uncertainty (safety factors). *Regul Toxicol Pharmacol.* 1983;3:224–238.

Drew CH, Grace DA, Silbernagel SM, et al. Nuclear waste transportation: case studies of identifying stakeholder risk information needs. *Environ Health Perspect.* 2003;111:263–272.

Drew CH, Kern M, Martin T, Blozek ML, Power M, Faustman EM. The Hanford Openness Workshops: fostering open and transparent long-term decision making at the department of energy. In: Leschine TM, ed. *Long-Term Management of Contaminated Sites (Research in Social Problems and Public Policy, Volume 13).* Emerald Group Publishing Limited; 2006;13–48.

Eaton DL, Bammler TK, Kelly EJ. Interindividual differences in response to chemoprotection against aflatoxin-induced hepatocarcinogenesis: implications for human biotransformation enzyme polymorphisms. *Adv Exp Med Biol.* 2001;500:559–576.

Eaton DL, Gallagher EP. Mechanisms of aflatoxin carcinogenesis. *Annu Rev Pharmacol Toxicol.* 1994;34:135–172.

Eaton DL, Gallagher EP, Bammler TK, Kunze KL. Role of cytochrome P4501a2 in chemical carcinogenesis—implications for human variability in expression and enzyme-activity. *Pharmacogenetics.* 1995;5:259–274.

EGRET. *Statistics and Epidemiology Research Corporation (SERC).* Seattle: Statistics and Epidemiology Research Corporation; 1994.

Eisen MB, Spellman PT, Brown PO, Botstein D. Cluster analysis and display of genome-wide expression patterns. *Proc Natl Acad Sci U S A.* 1998;95:14863–14868.

EPA. *Benchmark Dose Technical Guidance Document. External Review Draft.* Washington, DC: Risk Assessment Forum; 2000.

Ershow AG, Cantor KP. Federation of American Societies for Experimental Biology. Life Sciences Research Office, and National Cancer Institute (US). Division of Cancer Etiology. Epidemiology and Biostatistics Program. *Total Water and Tapwater Intake in the United States: Population-based Estimates of Quantities and Sources.* Bethesda, MD: Life Sciences Research Office Federation of American Societies for Experimental Biology; 1989.

FAO, WHO. *Codex Alimentarius Commission—International Food Standards.* 2011. Available at: http://www.codexalimentarius.org/.

Faustman E, Omenn G. Risk assessment and the impact of ecogenetics. In: Costa L, Eaton D, eds. *Gene–Environment Interactions: Fundamentals of Ecogenetics.* Hoboken, NJ: Wiley and Sons; 2006.

Faustman EM. Short-term test for teratogens. *Mutat Res.* 1988;205:355–384.

Faustman EM, Allen BC, Kavlock RJ, Kimmel CA. Dose–response assessment for developmental toxicity: I. Characterization of data base and determination of no observed adverse effect levels. *Fundam Appl Toxicol.* 1994;23:478–486.

Faustman EM, Gohlke J, Judd NL, Lewandowski TA, Bartell SA, Griffith WC. Modeling developmental processes in animals: applications in neurodevelopmental toxicology. *Environ Toxicol Pharmacol.* 2005a;19:615–624.

Faustman EM, Gohlke JM, Ponce RA, et al. Experimental approaches to evaluate mechanisms of developmental toxicity. In: Hood R, ed. *Developmental and Reproductive Toxicology: A Practical Approach.* 3rd ed. Boca Raton: CRC Press, Inc.; 2011.

Faustman EM, Lewandowski TA, Ponce RA, Bartell SM. Biologically based dose–response models for developmental toxicants: lessons from methylmercury. *Inhal Toxicol.* 1999;11:101–114.

Faustman EM, Omenn GS. Risk assessment. In: Klaassen CD, ed. *Casarett and Doull's Toxicology.* 5th ed. New York: McGraw-Hill; 1996:75–88.

Faustman EM, Ponce RA, Seeley MR, Whittaker SG. Experimental approaches to evaluate mechanisms of developmental toxicity. In: Hood R, ed. *Handbook of Developmental Toxicology.* Boca Raton, FL: CRC Press; 1996:13–41.

Faustman EM, Ponce RA, Seeley MR, Whittaker SG. Experimental approaches to evaluate mechanisms of developmental toxicity. In: Hood R, ed. *Handbook of Developmental Toxicology.* Boca Raton: CRC Press, Inc, 1997;13–41.

Faustman EM, Wellington DG, Smith WP, Kimmel CS. Characterization of a developmental toxicity dose response model. *Environ Health Perspect.* 1989;79:229–241.

FDA US. *Critical Path Initiative. Science & Research.* Silver Spring, MD: US Food and Drug Administration; 2011. Available at: http://www.fda.gov/ScienceResearch/SpecialTopics/CriticalPathInitiative/default.htm.

Finley G, Proctor D, Scott P. Recommended distributions for exposure factors frequently used in health risk assessment. *Risk Anal.* 1994;14:533–553.

Fischhoff B. Cost–benefit analysis: an uncertain guide to public policy. *Am N Y Acad Sci.* 1981;363:173–188.

Fischhoff B, Bostrom A, Quandrel MJ. Risk perception and communication. *Annu Rev Public Health.* 1993;14:183–203.

Fischhoff B, Bostrom A, Quandrel MJ. Risk perception and communication. In: Detels R, Holland W, McEwen J, Omenn GS, eds. *Oxford Textbook of Public Health.* New York: Oxford University Press; 1996:987–1002.

Frumkin H. Nature contact: a health benefit? In: Frumkin H, ed. *Environmental Health: From Global to Local.* 2nd ed. San Francisco, CA: Jossey-Bass; 2010.

Gamble JF, Battigelli MC. Epidemiology. In: Clayton GD, Clayton FE, eds. *Patty's Industrial Hygiene and Toxicology.* New York: Wiley; 1978;113–127.

Gamble JF, Battigelli MC. Occupational epidemiology: some guideposts. In: Clayton GD Clayton FE, eds. *Patty's Industrial Hygiene and Toxicology.* New York: Wiley; 1991.

Gargas ML, Finley BL, Paustenback DJ, Long TF. Environmental health risk assessment: theory and practice. In: Ballantyne B, Marrs T, Syversen T, eds. *General and Applied Toxicology.* New York: Grove's Dictionaries; 1999:1749–1809.

Gill EA, Curl CL, Adar SD, et al. Air pollution and cardiovascular disease in the Multi-Ethnic Study of Atherosclerosis. *Prog Cardiovasc Dis.* 2011;53(5):353–360.

Gohlke JM, Griffith WC, Bartell SM, Lewandowski TA, Faustman EM. A computational model for neocortical neuronogenesis predicts ethanol-induced neocortical neuron number deficits. *Dev Neurosci.* 2002;24:467–477.

Gohlke JM, Griffith WC, Faustman EM. The role of cell death during neocortical neurogenesis and synaptogenesis: implications from a computational model for the rat and mouse. *Brain Res Dev Brain Res.* 2004;151:43–54.

Gohlke JM, Griffith WC, Faustman EM. A systems-based computational model for dose–response comparisons of two mode of action hypotheses for ethanol-induced neurodevelopmental toxicity. *Toxicol Sci.* 2005;86:470–484.

Gohlke JM, Griffith WC, Faustman EM. Computational models of neocortical neuronogenesis and programmed cell death in the developing mouse, monkey, and human. *Cereb Cortex.* 2007;17:2433–2442.

Gohlke JM, Hrynkow SH, Portier CJ. Health, economy, and environment: sustainable energy choices for a nation. *Environ Health Perspect.* 2008;116:A236–A237.

Gray TJB. Application of in vitro systems in male reproductive toxicology. In: Lamb JC IV, Foster PMD, eds. *Physiology and Toxicology of Male Reproduction.* San Diego, CA: Academic Press; 1988: 250–253.

Great Britain, Health and Safety Executive. *Reducing Risks, Protecting People: Health & Safety Executive.* Suffolk, UK: HSE Books; 1999.

Gribble EJ, Hong SW, Faustman EM. The magnitude of methylmercury-induced cytotoxicity and cell cycle arrest is p53-dependent. *Birth Defects Res A Clin Mol Teratol.* 2005;73:29–38.

Groopman JD, Kensler TW. The light at the end of the tunnel for chemical-specific biomarkers: daylight or headlight? *Carcinogenesis.* 1999;20:1–11.

Guerrette Z, Moreira EG, Griffith WC, et al. Cytochrome P450 3A5 genotype is correlated with acetylcholinesterase inhibition levels after exposure to organophosphate pesticides. Abstract 2111. *The Toxicologist CD—An Official Journal of the Society of Toxicology.* Volume 120, March 2011.

Guo L, Lobenhofer EK, Wang C, et al. Rat toxicogenomic study reveals analytical consistency across microarray platforms. *Nat Biotechnol.* 2006;24:1162–1169.

HapMap. *International HapMap Project.* 2009. Available at: http://snp.cshl.org/index.html.en.

Harris MW, Chapin RE, Lockhart AC. Assessment of a short-term reproductive and developmental toxicity screen. *Fundam Appl Toxicol.* 1992;19:186–196.

Hartung R. Dose–response relationships. In: Tardiff RG, Rodricks JV, eds. *Toxic Substances and Human Risk: Principles of Data Interpretation.* New York: Plenum Press; 1987:29–46.

Hartung T, Blaauboer BJ, Bosgra S, et al. An expert consortium review of the EC-commissioned report "alternative (non-animal) methods for cosmetics testing: current status and future prospects—2010". *ALTEX.* 2011;28:183–209.

Hartung T, Bremer S, Casati S, et al. ECVAM's response to the changing political environment for alternatives: consequences of the European Union chemicals and cosmetics policies. *Altern Lab Anim.* 2003;31:473–481.

Haseman JK, Lockhart AM. Correlations between chemically related site-specific carcinogenic effects in long-term studies in rats and mice. *Environ Health Perspect.* 1993;101:50–54.

Haws LC, Su SH, Harris M, et al. Development of a refined database of mammalian relative potency estimates for dioxin-like compounds. *Toxicol Sci.* 2006;89:4–30.

Healey GF. Power calculations in toxicology. *Altern Lab Anim.* 1987;15:132–139.

Hill AB. The environment and disease: association or causation. *Proc R Soc Med.* 1965;58:295–300.

Hsieh A. A nation's genes for a cure to cancer: evolving ethical, social and legal issues regarding population genetic databases. *Columbia J Law Soc Probl.* 2004;37:359–411.

Human Genome Program. *Breaking News: GINA Becomes Law May 2008.* Genetics Privacy and Legislation. 2008. Available at: http://www.ornl.gov/sci/techresources/Human_Genome/elsi/legislat.shtml. Accessed 2011.

IARC. *IARC Monographs on the Evaluation of Carcinogenic Risks to Humans.* Lyon, France: World Health Organization; 2000.

ICCVAM. *The Murine Local Lymph Node Assay: A Test Method for Assessing the Allergic Contact Dermatitis Potential of Chemicals/Compounds: The Results of an Independent Peer Review Evaluation.* Research Triangle Park, NC: National Institute of Environmental Health Sciences; 1999. NIH publication no. 99-4494.

ICCVAM. *ICCVAM Test Method Evaluation Report on using the LLNA for Testing Pesticide Formulations, Metals, Substances in Aqueous Solutions, and Other Products.* Research Triangle Park, NC: National Institute of Environmental Health Sciences; 2011a. NIH publication no. 10-7512.

ICCVAM. *Independent Scientific Peer Review Panel Report Evaluation of the LUMI-CELL®ER (BG1Luc ER TA) Test Method.* Research Triangle Park, NC: National Institute of Environmental Health Sciences, National Institutes of Health; 2011b.

ICCVAM. *Validation of the BG1Luc Estrogen Receptor Transcriptional Activation Test Method.* 2012. Available at: http://iccvam.niehs.nih.gov/methods/endocrine/end_eval.htm.

ILSI. *A Framework for Cumulative Risk Assessment.* Washington, DC: International Life Science Institute; 1999.

Institute of Medicine. *Toward Environmental Justice. Research, Education, and Health Policy Needs.* Washington, DC: National Academy Press; 1999.

Institute of Medicine (U.S.). *Development of DRIs 1994–2004 Lessons Learned and New Challenges: Workshop Summary.* Washington, DC: National Academies Press; 2008.

International Program on Chemical Safety. World Health Organization, United Nations Environment Programme, International Labour Organisation, and Inter-Organization Programme for the Sound Management of Chemicals. *IPCS Risk Assessment Terminology.* Harmonization Project Document. Geneva: World Health Organization; 2004.

International Programme on Chemical Safety. Dose–response modelling: principles for modeling dose–response for the risk assessment of chemicals. In: *Environmental Health Criteria Series, No. 234.* Geneva: World Health Organization; 2006.

International Programme on Chemical Safety. *Uncertainty and Data Quality in Exposure Assessment.* Geneva: World Health Organization; 2008.

Israeli M, Nelson CB. Distribution and expected time of residence for United States households. *Risk Anal.* 1992;12:65–72.

Johnson DE, Wolfgang GHI, Gledin MA, Braeckman RA. Toxicokinetics and toxicodynamics. In: Sipes I, McQueen C, Gandolfi A, eds. *Comprehensive Toxicology.* Oxford, UK: Pergamon, Elsevier Sciences; 1997:169–181.

Judd NL, Drew CH, Acharya C, et al. Framing scientific analyses for risk management of environmental hazards by communities: case studies with seafood safety issues. *Environ Health Perspect.* 2005;113:1502–1508.

Kavlock RJ, Allen BC, Faustman EM, Kimmel CA. Dose response assessments for developmental toxicity: IV. Benchmark doses for fetal weight changes. *Fundam Appl Toxicol.* 1995;26:211–222.

Keim M. Intentional chemical disasters. In: Hogan D, Burstein J, eds. *Disaster Medicine.* Philadelphia: Lippincott Williams & Wilkins; 2002:340–348.

Kensler TW, Roebuck BD, Wogan GN, Groopman JD. Aflatoxin: a 50-year odyssey of mechanistic and translational toxicology. *Toxicol Sci.* 2011;120(suppl 1):S28–S48.

Khoury MJ. Human genome epidemiology: translating advances in human genetics into population-based data for medicine and public health. *Genet Med.* 1999;1:71–73.

Kite-Powell HL, Fleming LE, Backer LC, et al. Linking the oceans to public health: current efforts and future directions. *Environ Health.* 2008;7:S6.

Klaunig JE, Babich M, Baetcke K, et al. PPARα agonist-induced rodent tumors: modes of action and human relevance. *Crit Rev Toxicol.* 2003;33:655–780.

Koturbash I, Scherhag A, Sorrentino J, et al. Epigenetic mechanisms of mouse interstrain variability in genotoxicity of the environmental toxicant 1,3-butadiene. *Toxicol Sci.* 2011;122:448–456.

Kramer CB, Cullen AC, Faustman EM. Policy implications of genetic information on regulation under the Clean Air Act: the case of particulate matter and asthmatics. *Environ Health Perspect.* 2006;114:313–319.

Krewski D, Van Ryzin J. Dose response models for quantal response toxicity data. In: Csorgo M, Dawson D, Rao J, Seleh A, eds. *Statistics and Related Topics.* Amsterdam: North-Holland; 1981:201–229.

Lave LB, Ennever F, Rosenkranz HS, Omenn GS. Information value of the rodent bioassay. *Nature.* 1988;336:631–633.

Lave LB, Omenn GS. Cost-effectiveness of short-term tests for carcinogenicity. *Nature.* 1986;334:29–34.

Leiserowitz AA, Kates RW, Parris TM. Sustainability values, attitudes, and behaviors: a review of multinational and global trends. *Annu Rev Environ Resour.* 2006;31:413–444.

Leroux BG, Leisenring WM, Moolgavkar SH, Faustman EM. A biologically based dose–response model for development. *Risk Anal.* 1996;16:449–458.

Lewandowski TA, Ponce RA, Whittaker SG, Faustman EM. In vitro models for evaluating developmental toxicity. In: Gad S, ed. *Vitro Toxicology.* New York: Taylor & Francis; 2000:139–187.

Limbird LE, Taylor P. Endocrine disruptors signal the need for receptor models and mechanisms to inform policy. *Cell.* 1998;93:157–163.

Liu R, Rallo R, George S, et al. Classification NanoSAR development for cytotoxicity of metal oxide nanoparticles. *Small.* 2011;7:1118–1126.

Lowrance WW. *Of Acceptable Risk: Science and the Determination of Safety.* Los Altos, CA: William Kaufmann; 1976.

Maynard AD, Aitken RJ, Butz T, et al. Safe handling of nanotechnology. *Nature.* 2006;444:267–269.

McClain RM. Mechanistic considerations in the regulation and classification of chemical carcinogens. In: Kotsonis F, Mackey M, Hjelle J, eds. *Nutritional Toxicology.* New York, Raven Press; 1994:278–304.

McGregor DB, Rice JM, Venitt S. *The Use of Short- and Medium-Term Tests for Carcinogens and Data on Genetic Effects in Carcinogenic Hazard Evaluation.* Lyon, France: IARC; 1999.

Meek ME, Boobis AR, Crofton KM, Heinemeyer G, Van Raaij M, Vickers C. Risk assessment of combined exposure to multiple chemicals: a WHO/IPCS framework. *Regul Toxicol Pharmacol.* 2011;60(2): S1–S14.

Mendoza MA, Ponce RA, Ou YC, Faustman EM. p21(WAF1/CIP1) inhibits cell cycle progression but not G2/M-phase transition following methylmercury exposure. *Toxicol Appl Pharmacol.* 2002;178:117–125.

Moggs JG, Tinwell H, Spurway T, et al. Phenotypic anchoring of gene expression changes during estrogen-induced uterine growth. *Environ Health Perspect.* 2004;112:1589–1606.

Moolgavkar SH, Luebeck G. Two-event model for carcinogenesis: biological, mathematical, and statistical considerations. *Risk Anal.* 1990;10:323–341.

Moore JA, Daston GP, Faustman EM. An evaluative process for assessing human reproductive and developmental toxicity of agents. *Reprod Toxicol.* 1995;9:61–95.

Morgan GM. Risk analysis and management. *Sci Am.* 1993;269:32–41.

National Academy of Science. *Health Risks from Dioxin and Related Compounds: Evaluation of the EPA Reassessment.* Washington, DC: National Academies Press; 2006.

National Human Genome Research Institute. *A DNA Polymorphism Discovery Resource.* 2010. Available at: http://www.genome.gov/10001552.

National Toxicology Program. *11th Report on Carcinogens.* 2005. Available at:http://ntp.niehs.nih.gov/index.cfm?objectid=32BA9724-F9721F9726-9975E-9727FCE50709CB50704C50932.

National Toxicology Program Center for the Evaluation of Alternative Toxicological Methods (U.S.), Interagency Coordinating Committee on the Validation of Alternative Methods (U.S.). *ICCVAM Test Method Evaluation Report In Vitro Cytotoxicity Test Methods for Estimating Starting Doses for Acute Oral Systemic Toxicity.* Bethesda, MD: National Institutes of Health; 2006. NIH publication no. 07-4519.

Nature Biotechnology Editorial. Making the most of microarrays. *Nat Biotechnol.* 2006;24:1039–1039.

NCBI. *dbSNP Short Genetic Variations.* 2011a. Available at: http://www.ncbi.nlm.nih.gov/SNP/.

NCBI. *National Center for Biotechnology Information.* 2011b. Available at: http://www.ncbi.nlm.nih.gov/.

Neal N, Malmfors T, Slovic P. Intuitive toxicology: expert and lay judgments of chemical risks. *Toxicol Pathol.* 1994;22:198–201.

Nebert DW, Duffy JJ. How knockout mouse lines will be used to study the role of drug-metabolizing enzymes and their receptors during reproduction, development, and environmental toxicity, cancer and oxidative stress. *Biochem Pharmacol.* 1997;53:249–254.

Neumann DA, Olin SS. Urinary bladder carcinogenesis: a working group approach to risk assessment. *Food Chem Toxicol.* 1995;33:701–704.

NIEHS. *Corrositex: An In Vitro Test Method for Assessing Dermal Corrosivity Potential of Chemicals.* Washington, DC: ICCVAM; 1999a: 33109–33111.

NIEHS. *The Murine Local Lymph Node Assay: A Test Method for Assessing the Allergic Contact Dermatitis Potential of Chemicals/Compounds.* Washington, DC: ICCVAM; 1999b:14006–14007.

NRC. *Risk Assessment in the Federal Government: Managing the Process.* Washington, DC: National Academy Press; 1983.

NRC. *Biological Markers in Pulmonary Toxicology.* Washington, DC: National Academy Press; 1989a.

NRC. *Biological Markers in Reproductive Toxicology.* Washington, DC: National Academy Press; 1989b.

NRC. *Biological Markers in Immunotoxicology.* Washington, DC: National Academy Press; 1992a.

NRC. *Environmental Neurotoxicology.* Washington, DC: National Academy Press; 1992b.

NRC. *Science and Judgement in Risk Assessment.* Washington, DC: National Academy Press; 1994.

NRC. *Understanding Risk: Informing Decisions in a Democratic Society.* Stern PC, Fineberg HV, eds. Washington, DC: National Academy Press; 1996.

NRC. *Scientific Frontiers in Developmental Toxicology and Risk Assessment.* Washington, DC: National Research Council; 2000.

NRC. *Toxicity Testing in the 21st Century: A Vision and a Strategy.* Washington, DC: National Academies Press; 2007a.

NRC. *Applications of Toxicogenomic Technologies to Predictive Toxicology and Risk.* Washington, DC: National Academies Press; 2007b.

NRC. *Science and Decisions: Advancing Risk Assessment.* Washington, DC: National Academies Press; 2009.

NRC. *Toxicity Pathway-Based Risk Assessment Preparing for Paradigm Change, A Symposium Summary.* Washington, DC: National Academies Press; 2010.

NRC Committee on Risk Assessment Methodology. *Issues in Risk Assessment: Use of Maximum Tolerated Dose in Animal Bioassays for Carcinogenicity.* Washington, DC: National Academy Press; 1993.

NTP. *National Toxicology Program.* 2011a. Available at: http://ntp.niehs.nih.gov/.

NTP. *Office of Health Assessment and Translation (Formerly CERHR).* National Toxicology Program; 2011b. Available at: http://ntp.niehs.nih.gov/?objectid=497C419D-E834-6B35-8AF15D389859AF07.

Oberdorster G. Lung particle overload: implications for occupational exposure to particles. *Regul Toxicol Pharmacol.* 1995;12:123–135.

OECD. *Organisation for Economic Co-Operation and Development.* 2011. Available at: www.oecd.org.

Omenn GS. The genomic era: a crucial role for the public health sciences. *Environ Health Perspect.* 2000;108:A204–A205.

Omenn GS. Gene-environment interactions: eco-genetics and toxicogenomics. In: Ginsburg GS, Willard HF, eds. *Genomic and Personalized Medicine.* 2nd ed. Elsevier; 2012.

Omenn GS, Lampen A. Scientific and cost-effectiveness criteria in selecting batteries of short-term tests. *Mutat Res.* 1988;205:41–49.

Omenn GS, Omiecinski CJ, Eaton DE. Eco-genetics of chemical carcinogens. In: Cantor C, Caskey C, Hood L, eds. *Biotechnology and Human Genetic Predisposition to Disease.* New York: Wiley-Liss; 1990:81–93.

Omenn GS, Stuebbe S, Lave LB. Predictions of rodent carcinogenicity testing results: interpretation in light of the Lave–Omenn value-of-information model. *Mol Carcinogen.* 1995;14:37–45.

Patterson TA, Lobenhofer EK, Fulmer-Smentek SB, et al. Performance comparison of one-color and two-color platforms within the MicroArray Quality Control (MAQC) project. *Nat Biotechnol.* 2006;24: 1140–1150.

Perdue WC, Stone LA, Gostin LO. The built environment and its relationship to the public's health: the legal framework. *Am J Public Health.* 2003;93:1390–1394.

Perera FP, Weinstein IB. Molecular epidemiology: recent advances and future directions. *Carcinogenesis.* 2000;21:517–524.

REACH. *Registration, Evaluation, Authorisation and Restriction of Chemicals.* 2011. Available at: http://ec.europa.eu/enterprise/sectors/chemicals/reach/index_en.htm.

Regalado J, Perez-Padilla R, Sansores R, et al. The effect of biomass burning on respiratory symptoms and lung function in rural Mexican women. *Am J Respir Crit Care Med.* 2006;174(8):901–905.

Renwick AG. Safety factors and the establishment of acceptable daily intakes. *Food Addit Contam.* 1991;8:135–150.

Renwick AG. Toxicokinetics. In: Ballantyne B, Marrs T, Syversen T, eds. *General and Applied Toxicology.* New York: Grove's Dictionaries; 1999:67–95.

Renwick AG, Lazarus NR. Human variability and noncancer risk assessment—an analysis of the default uncertainty factor. *Regul Toxicol Pharmacol.* 1998;27:3–20.

Rice JM, Baan RA, Blettner M. Rodent tumors of urinary bladder, renal cortex, and thyroid gland. IARC monographs: evaluations of carcinogenic risk to humans. *Toxicol Sci.* 1999;49:166–171.

Risk Commission. *The Presidential/Congressional Commission on Risk Assessment and Risk Management.* Washington, DC: Government Printing Office; 1997.

Rodericks JV, Rudenko I, Starr TB, Turnbull D. Risk assessment. In: Sipes I, McQueen C, Gandolfi A, eds. *Comprehensive Toxicology.* Oxford, UK: Pergamon Elsevier Sciences; 1997.

Roe D, Pease W, Florini K, Silbergeld E. *Toxic Ignorance: The Continuing Absence of Basic Health Testing for Top-Selling Chemicals in the United States.* Washington, DC: Environmental Defense Fund Inc; 1997.

Ryan PB. Exposure assessment, industrial hygiene, and environmental management. In: Frumkin H, ed. *Environmental Health: From Global to Local.* 2nd ed. San Francisco, CA: Jossey-Bass; 2010.

Sandman PM. *Responding to Community Outrage: Strategies for Effective Risk Communication.* Fairfax, VA: American Industrial Hygiene Association; 1993.

Sartor MA, Dolinoy DC, Rozek LS, Omenn GS. Bioinformatics for high-throughput toxico-epigenomics studies. In: Sahu SC, ed. *Toxicology and Epigenetics.* New York: John Wiley and Sons; 2012.

Sartor MA, Mahavisno V, Keshamouni VG, et al. ConceptGen: a gene set enrichment and gene set relation mapping tool. *Bioinformatics.* 2010;26:456–463.

Schardein JL, Scialli AR. The legislation of toxicologic safety factors: the Food Quality Protection Act with chlorpyrifos as a test case. *Reprod Toxicol Rev.* 1999;13:1–14.

Sette WF. *Pesticide Assessment Guidelines, Subdivision D, Hazard evaluation, Human and Domestic Animals, Addendum 10.* Neurotoxicity Series 81, 82 and 83 PB91-154617. Washington, DC: National Technical Information Services; 1991.

Sexton K, Selevan SG, Wagener DK, Lybarger JA. Estimating human exposures to environmental pollutants: availability and utility of existing databases. *Arch Environ Health.* 1992;47:398–407.

Shelby MD, Bishop JB, Mason JM, Tindall KR. Fertility, reproduction and genetic disease: studies on the mutagenic effects of environmental agents on mammalian germ cells. *Environ Health Perspect.* 1993;200:283–291.

Shuey DL, Lau C, Logsdon TR. Biologically based dose–response modeling in developmental toxicology: biochemical and cellular sequelae of 5-fluorouracil exposure in the developing rat. *Toxicol Appl Pharmacol.* 1994;126:129–144.

Silverman KC, Naumann BD, Holder DJ. Establishing data-derived adjustment factors from published pharmaceutical clinical trial data. *Hum Ecol Risk Assess.* 1999;5:1059–1089.

Simon R, Wang SJ. Use of genomic signatures in therapeutics development in oncology and other diseases. *Pharmacogenomics J.* 2006;6:166–173.

Slovic P. *The Feeling of Risk: New Perspectives on Risk Perception.* London, Washington, DC: Earthscan, in association with the International Institute for Environment and Development; 2010. The Earthscan Risk in Society Series.

Slovic P, Baruch F, Lichtenstein S. Rating the risks. *Environment.* 1979;21:1–20, 36–39.

Slovic P, Peters E, Finucane ML, MacGregor DG. Affect, risk, and decision making. *Health Psychol.* 2005;24:S35–S40.

Spielmann H, Seiler A, Bremer S, et al. The practical application of three validated in vitro embryotoxicity tests—the report and recommendations of an ECVAM/ZEBET workshop (ECVAM workshop 57). *Altern Lab Anim.* 2006;34:527–538.

Stevens JT. Risk assessment of pesticides. In: Williams P, Hottendorf G, eds. *Comprehensive Toxicology.* Oxford, UK; Pergamon Elsevier Sciences; 1997:17–26.

Sudmant PH, Kitzman JO, Antonacci F, et al. Diversity of human copy number variation and multicopy genes. *Science.* 2010;330:641–646.

Teichman K; U.S. EPA. *Presentation to the Science Advisory Board and Board of Scientific Counselors (Overview).* June 2011. Available at: http://my.brainshark.com/Dr-Kevin-Teichman-SAB-BOSC-Presentation-720933584.

Tennant RW, Stasiewicz S, Mennear J. Genetically altered mouse models for identifying carcinogens. In: McGregor DB, Rice JM, Venitt S, eds. *The Use of Short- and Medium-Term Tests for Carcinogens and Data on Genetic Effects in Carcinogenic Hazard Evaluation.* Vol. 146. Lyon, France: IARC Scientific Publications; 1999:123–150.

Toscano WA, Oehlke KP. Systems biology: new approaches to old environmental health problems. *Int J Environ Res Public Health.* 2005;2:4–9.

United States Act. *The Genetic Information Nondiscrimination Act of 2008 (GINA).* Public Law 110-233; May 21, 2008.

US EPA. Proposed guidelines for assessing female reproductive risk. *Fed Reg.* 1988;53:24834–24847.

US EPA. *Risk Assessment Guidance for Superfund. Vol. 1. Human Health Evaluation Manual, Part A.* Washington, DC: Office of Policy Analysis and Office of Emergency and Remedial Response; 1989.

US EPA. Guidelines for developmental toxicity risk assessment. *Fed Reg.* 1991;56:63798–63826.

US EPA. Guidelines for exposure assessment. *Fed Reg.* 1992;57:22888–22938.

US EPA. *Health Assessment Document for 2,3,7,8-Tetrachlorodibenzo-p-Dioxin (TCDD) and Related Compounds.* Washington, DC: Office of Research and Development; 1994a.

US EPA. *Guidelines for Carcinogen Risk Assessment (Draft Revisions).* Washington, DC: Office of Health and Environmental Assessment; 1994b.

US EPA. Guidelines for reproductive toxicity risk assessment. *Fed Reg.* 1996a;61:56278–56322.

US EPA. *Food Quality Protection Act (FQPA).* Washington, DC: Office of Pesticide Programs; 1996b.

US EPA. *Food Quality Protection Act (FQPA) of 1996.* 1996c. Available at: http://epa.gov/pesticides/regulating/laws/fqpa/index.htm.

US EPA. *Chemical Hazard Availability Study.* Washington, DC: Office of Pollution Prevention and Toxics; 1998a.

US EPA. Guidance for identifying pesticides that have a common mechanism of toxicity: notice of availability and solicitation of public comments. *Fed Reg.* 1998b;63:42031–42032.

US EPA. *Guidelines for Neurotoxicity Risk Assessment.* EPA Technical Report. Risk Assessment Forum. Washington, DC: United States Environmental Protection Agency; 1998c.

US EPA. *Guidelines for Carcinogen Risk Assessment, Draft.* NCEA-F-0644. Washington, DC: EPA; 1999a.

US EPA. *Chlorpyrifos: re-evaluation report of the FQPA Safety Factor Committee.* HED Doc. No. 014077. Washington, DC: US Environmental Protection Agency; 2000a.

US EPA. *Integrated Risk Information System.* 2000b. Available at: http://www.epa.gov/iris/index.html.

US EPA. *Risk Characterization Handbook.* Washington, DC: U.S. Environmental Protection Agency Science Policy Council; 2000c.

US EPA. *Guidelines for Carcinogen Risk Assessment (Cancer Guidelines), Federal Register Notice.* 2005.

US EPA. *Child-Specific Exposure Factors Handbook (Final Report).* Washington, DC: Office of Research and Development and the National Center for Environmental Assessment; 2008. EPA/600/R-06/096F.

US EPA. *The Office of Chemical Safety and Pollution Prevention (OCSPP) Harmonized Test Guidelines: Series 870—Health Effects Test Guidelines. 870 Series Final Guidelines.* 2010a. Available at: http://www.epa.gov/ocspp/pubs/frs/publications/Test_Guidelines/series870.htm.

US EPA. *EPA's Reanalysis of Key Issues Related to Dioxin Toxicity and Response to NAS Comments Draft.* 2010b. NAS comments are published by the National Research Council of the National Academies and available from the National Technical Information Service, Springfield, VA, and online at http://www.epa.gov/ncea.

US EPA. Integrated exposure uptake biokinetic model for lead in children, Windows® version (IEUBKwin v1.1 build 11). Washington, D.C.: U.S. Environmental Protection Agency; 2010c. Available from the National Technical Information Service: http://www.epa.gov/superfund/lead/products.htm.

US EPA. *Exposure Factors Handbook: 2011 Edition. Final Report: EPA*. Washington, DC: Office of Health and Environmental Assessment; 2011a.

US EPA. *Ecological Risk Assessments. Pesticides: Environmental Effects*. 2011b. Available at: http://www.epa.gov/pesticides/ecosystem/ecorisk.htm.

US EPA. *High Production Volume (HPV) Challenge*. 2011c. Available at: http://www.epa.gov/hpv/.

US EPA. *PMN Forms and Information. New Chemicals*. 2011d. Available at: http://www.epa.gov/oppt/newchems/pubs/pmnforms.htm.

US EPA. *Integrated Risk Information System (IRIS)*. 2011e. Available at: http://www.epa.gov/IRIS/.

US EPA. *Interim Genomics Policy*. Office of the Science Advisor (OSA); 2011f. Available at: http://www.epa.gov/spc/genomics.htm.

US EPA. Integrated Risk Information System (IRIS): Glossary of IRIS Terms. 2012a. Available at: http://www.epa.gov/iris/help_gloss.htm.

US EPA. Computational Toxicology Research. 2012b. Available at: http://www.epa.gov/ncct/.

US EPA ACToR. *ACToR*. United States Environmental Protection Agency; 2011. Available at: http://actor.epa.gov/actor/faces/ACToRHome.jsp.

US EPA Office of Research and Development. Presentations for the Science Advisory Board and Board of Scientific Counselors. In: Preparation for the June 29–30, 2011 Joint Meeting; 2011. Available at: http://yosemite.epa.gov/sab/sabproduct.nsf/F53952681221F76F852578AF007EE972/$File/SABBOSC+Presentations.pdf.

Van den Berg M, Birnbaum L, Bosveld ATC. Toxic equivalency factors (TEFs) for PCBs, PCDDs, PCDFs for humans and wildlife. *Environ Health Perspect*. 1998;106:775–792.

Van den Berg M, Birnbaum LS, Denison M, et al. The 2005 World Health Organization reevaluation of human and mammalian toxic equivalency factors for dioxins and dioxin-like compounds. *Toxicol Sci*. 2006;93:223–241.

Vlaanderen J, Portengen L, Rappaport SM, Glass DC, Kromhout H, Vermeulen R. The impact of saturable metabolism on exposure–response relations in 2 studies of benzene-induced leukemia. *Am J Epidemiol*. 2011;174:621–629.

Weller E, Long N, Smith A. Dose–rate effects of ethylene oxide exposure on developmental toxicity. *Toxicol Sci*. 1999;50:259–270.

Whittaker SG, Faustman EM. *In Vitro Assays for Developmental Toxicity*. New York: Raven Press; 1994.

WHO. *Principles in Governing Consumer Safety in Relation to Pesticide Residues: Report of a Meeting of a W.H.O. Expert Committee on Pesticide Residues Held Jointly with the F.A.O. Panel of Experts on the Use of Pesticides in Agriculture*. World Health Organization Technical Report Series, No. 240. 1962.

WHO. *Joint IPCS/OECD Project on the Harmonization of Chemical Hazard/Risk Assessment Terminology (Harmonization Project)*. 2000.

WHO. *Chemical-Specific Adjustment Factors for Interspecies Differences and Human Variability: Guidance Document for Use of Data in Dose/Concentration–Response Assessment*. 2005.

WHO. *IPCS Harmonization Project. Programmes and Projects*. 2011a. Available at: http://www.who.int/ipcs/methods/harmonization/en/.

WHO. *The International Agency for Research on Cancer (IARC)*. 2011b. Available at: http://www.iarc.fr/.

WHO. *Concise International Chemical Assessment Documents*. International Programme on Chemical Safety (IPCS); 2011c. Available at: http://www.who.int/ipcs/publications/cicad/en/.

WHO. *Millennium Development Goals (MDGs). Health Topics*. 2011d. Available at: http://www.who.int/topics/millennium_development_goals/en/.

WHO, International Programme on Chemical Safety, Inter-Organization Programme for the Sound Management of Chemicals. *WHO Human Health Risk Assessment Toolkit: Chemical Hazards*. IPCS Harmonization Project Document No. 8. Geneva: World Health Organization; 2010.

World Health Organization. *Principles of Characterizing and Applying Human Exposure Models*. IPCS Harmonization Project Document No. 3. Geneva: World Health Organization; 2006.

World Health Organization, International Programme on Chemical Safety. *Principles for the Assessment of Risks to Human Health from Exposure to Chemicals. Environmental Health Criteria*. Geneva: WHO; 1999.

Yu X, Griffith WC, Hanspers K, et al. A system based approach to interpret dose and time-dependent microarray data: quantitative integration of GO ontology analysis for risk assessment. *Toxicol Sci*. 2006;92:560–577.

Yu XZ, Hong S, Moreira EG, Faustman EM. Improving in vitro Sertoli cell/gonocyte co-culture model for assessing male reproductive toxicity: lessons learned from comparisons of cytotoxicity versus genomic responses to phthalates. *Toxicol Appl Pharmacol*. 2009;239:325–336.

Zhao Q, Dourson M, Gadagbui B. A review of the reference dose for chlorpyrifos. *Regul Toxicol Pharmacol*. 2006;44:111–124.

Unit II

Disposition of Toxicants

Absorption, Distribution, and Excretion of Toxicants

Lois D. Lehman-McKeeman

INTRODUCTION

The disposition of a chemical or xenobiotic is defined as the composite actions of its absorption, distribution, biotransformation, and elimination. This chapter will focus on the contribution of absorption, distribution, and elimination to xenobiotic toxicity, whereas Chap. 6 is dedicated to biotransformation. The quantitative characterization of xenobiotic disposition is termed pharmacokinetics or toxicokinetics and is reviewed in Chap. 7.

The various factors and organs involved in affecting disposition of a toxicant are depicted in Fig. 5-1. The diagram is a pictoral overview of the processes of absorption, distribution, and excretion, and its complexity is intended to illustrate that, although they will be discussed separately, the processes that determine disposition are likely to occur simultaneously. Moreover, the disposition of any compound is a fundamental factor that contributes to its potential for toxicity. Specifically, the toxicity of a substance is directly dependent on the dose, where "dose" is defined as the amount that ultimately reaches the site or sites of action (tissue, cell, or molecular target). Therefore, the disposition of a chemical determines its concentration at the site of action such that the concerted actions of absorption, distribution, and elimination also determine the potential for adverse events to occur.

The skin, lungs, and alimentary canal are the main barriers that separate higher organisms from an environment containing a large number of chemicals (Fig. 5-1). Toxicants must cross one or several of these incomplete barriers to exert deleterious effects, and only chemicals that are caustic and corrosive (acids, bases, salts, oxidizers), which act directly at the point of contact, are exceptions to this generalization. A chemical absorbed into the bloodstream or lymphatics through any of the major barriers is distributed, at least to some extent, throughout the body, including the site where it produces damage. This site is called the target organ or target tissue. A chemical may have one or several target organs, and, in turn, several chemicals may have the same target organ or organs. However, target organ concentration is not the only factor that can influence the susceptibility of organs to toxicants, and the organ or tissue with the highest concentration of a toxicant is not necessarily the site where toxicity is observed. A classic example of this distinction is dichlorodiphenyltrichloroethane (DDT), a chlorinated hydrocarbon insecticide that achieves high concentrations in fat depots but is not toxic to that tissue.

Poor absorption of a toxicant resulting from a low amount absorbed or from a low rate of absorption will limit or prevent toxicity because a chemical may never attain a sufficiently high concentration at a potential site of action to cause toxicity. Similarly, a chemical that is well absorbed but rapidly biotransformed or eliminated from an organism is less likely to be toxic because rapid excretion prevents it from reaching a sufficiently high concentration at a potential site of action to cause toxicity. These are examples of how the disposition of toxicants contributes to the fundamental concept that the "dose makes the poison."

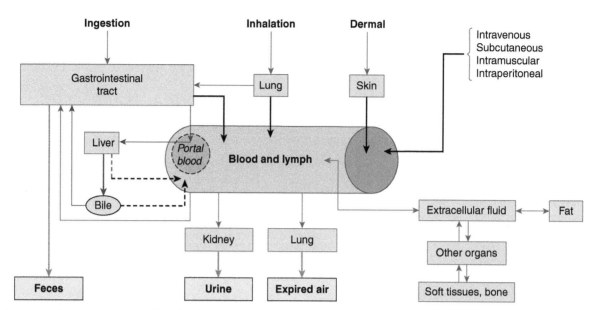

Figure 5-1. *Summary of the disposition of toxicants as determined by absorption, distribution, and excretion in the body.* Black lines represent major pathways of absorption into the body, blue designates distribution, and green lines identify pathways of final excretion (elimination) from the body, with the exception of enterohepatic circulation, which is designated in red.

The processes comprising xenobiotic disposition are interrelated and influence each other. The integrated relationship of these processes is illustrated in Fig. 5-1. In this chapter, the qualitative aspects of absorption, distribution, and excretion are presented with emphasis on the functional features and molecular determinants of these processes. As all these processes involve passage across biological membranes, we begin with a discussion of this important and ubiquitous barrier.

CELL MEMBRANES

Toxicants usually pass through a number of cells, such as the stratified epithelium of the skin, the thin cell layers of the lungs or the gastrointestinal (GI) tract, capillary endothelium, and ultimately the cells of the target organ. The plasma membranes surrounding all these cells are remarkably similar. The basic unit of the cell membrane is a lipid bilayer composed primarily of phospholipids, glycolipids, and cholesterol. The phospholipids, primarily phosphatidylcholine and phosphatidylethanolamine are most abundant. Phospholipids are amphiphilic, consisting of a hydrophilic polar head and a hydrophobic lipid tail. In membranes, the polar head groups are oriented toward the outer and inner surfaces of the membrane, whereas the hydrophobic tails are oriented inward and face each other to form a continuous hydrophobic inner space. The thickness of the cell membrane is about 7 to 9 nm. Numerous proteins are inserted or embedded in the bilayer, and some transmembrane proteins traverse the entire lipid bilayer, functioning as important biological receptors or allowing the formation of aqueous pores, ion channels, and transporters (Fig. 5-2). The fatty acids of the membrane do not have a rigid crystalline structure but are semifluid at physiological temperatures. Overall, hydrophobic interactions are the major driving force in the formation of membrane lipid bilayers, and the fluid character of membranes is determined largely by the structure and relative abundance of unsaturated fatty acids. The more unsaturated fatty acids the membranes contain, the more fluid-like they are, facilitating more rapid active or passive transport.

The membrane barrier is differentially permeable and regulates what enters into or exits from cells. Toxicants cross membranes either by passive processes in which the cell expends no energy or by mechanisms in which the cell provides energy to translocate the toxicant across its membrane.

Passive Transport

Simple Diffusion Most toxicants cross membranes by simple diffusion, following the principles of Fick's law, which establishes that chemicals move from regions of higher concentration to regions of lower concentration without any energy expenditure. Small hydrophilic molecules (up to about 600 Da) permeate membranes through aqueous pores (Benz *et al.*, 1980), in a process termed paracellular diffusion, whereas hydrophobic molecules diffuse across the lipid domain of membranes (transcellular diffusion). The smaller a hydrophilic molecule is, the more readily it traverses membranes by simple diffusion through aqueous pores. Consequently, a small, water-soluble compound such as ethanol is rapidly absorbed into the blood from the GI tract and is distributed just as rapidly throughout the body by simple diffusion from blood into all tissues.

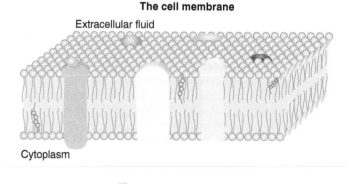

Figure 5-2. *Schematic model of a biological membrane.*

Table 5-1

Octanol/Water Partition Coefficients (P) of Different Molecules Expressed as log P

COMPOUND	LOG P
Paraquat	Charged molecule
Cephalosporin C	–4.72
Glycine	–3.21
Glutathione	–3.05
Cysteine	–2.35
Glucose	–2.21
Ethylene glycol	–1.37
Lead acetate	–0.63
p-Aminohippuric acid	–0.25
Dimercaprol	0.18
Scopolamine	0.30
Aspirin (acetyl salicylic acid)	1.02
Colchicine	1.19
Atropine	1.32
Benzoic acid	1.88
Benzene	2.14
Salicylic acid	2.19
Methyl salicylate	2.34
2,4-D	2.73
Warfarin	2.89
Digitoxin	3.05
Parathion	3.47
DDT	6.76
TCDD	7.05

2,4-D, 2,4-dichlorophenoxyacetic acid; DDT, dichlorodiphenyltrichloroethane; TCDD, 2,3,7,8-tetrachlorodibenzo-p-dioxin.

For larger organic molecules with differing degrees of lipid solubility, the rate of transport across membranes correlates with lipophilicity. Lipid solubility is generally determined by the octanol/water partition coefficient, *P*, which is defined as the ratio of the concentration of neutral compound in organic and aqueous phases under equilibrium conditions. It is usually expressed in logarithmic form as log P, and numerous examples are listed in Table 5-1. The log P is an extremely informative physicochemical parameter relative to assessing potential membrane permeability, with positive values associated with high lipid solubility. In contrast, charged molecules such as paraquat do not have a measurable log P. As illustrated by the compounds in Table 5-1, amino acids such as glycine are highly water soluble and have a negative log P, whereas the environmental contaminants DDT and 2,3,7,8-tetrachlorodibenzo-p-dioxin (TCDD) are very lipid soluble and have a high, positive log P. There are a variety of experimental methods for empirical determination of log P, along with computational tools that can be used to predict log P for any chemical (Mannhold *et al.*, 2009).

Many chemicals are weak organic acids or bases, which in solution are ionized according to Arrhenius' theory. The ionized form usually has low lipid solubility and thus does not permeate readily through the lipid domain of a membrane. There may be some transport of organic anions and cations (depending on their molecular weight) through the aqueous pores, but this is a slow and inefficient process. In contrast, the nonionized form of weak organic acids and bases is lipid soluble to some extent, resulting in diffusion across the lipid domain of a membrane. The rate of movement of the nonionized form is proportional to its lipid solubility such that the extent to which a compound is nonionized determines its diffusion.

The molar ratio of ionized to nonionized molecules of a weak organic acid or base in solution depends on the ionization constant, which is defined as the pH at which a weak organic acid or base is 50% ionized (denoted as pK_a or pK_b for acids and bases, respectively). Like pH, pK_a and pK_b are defined as the negative logarithm of the ionization constant of a weak organic acid or base. An organic acid with a low pK_a is relatively a strong acid, and one with a high pK_a is a weak acid. The opposite is true for bases. The numerical value of pK_a does not indicate whether a chemical is an organic acid or a base. Knowledge of the chemical structure is required to distinguish between organic acids and bases.

The Henderson–Hasselbalch equation describes the derivation of pH as a function of the pK_a in a biological system. Two equivalent forms of this equation are

$$pH = pK_a + \log \frac{[\text{ionized}]}{[\text{nonionized}]}$$

$$pH = pK_a - \log \frac{[\text{nonionized}]}{[\text{ionized}]}$$

Rearranging these equations enables determination of the extent to which a weak acid or base is ionized or nonionized at any pH as follows:

$$\text{For acids: } pK_a - pH = \log \frac{[\text{nonionized}]}{[\text{ionized}]}$$

$$\text{For bases: } pK_a - pH = \log \frac{[\text{nonionized}]}{[\text{ionized}]}$$

The effect of pH on the degree of ionization of an organic acid (benzoic acid) and an organic base (aniline) is illustrated in Fig. 5-3. According to the Brönsted–Lowry acid–base theory, an acid is a proton (H⁺) donor and a base is a proton acceptor. Thus, the ionized and nonionized forms of an organic acid represent an acid–base pair, with the nonionized moiety being the acid and the ionized moiety being the base. At a low pH, a weak organic acid such as benzoic acid is largely nonionized. At pH 4, exactly 50% of benzoic acid is ionized and 50% is nonionized because this is the pK_a of the compound. As the pH increases, more and more protons are neutralized by hydroxyl groups, and benzoic acid continues to dissociate until almost all of it is in the ionized form. For an organic base such as aniline, the inverse is true. At a low pH, when protons are abundant, almost all of aniline is ionized. This form of aniline is an acid because it can donate protons. As the pH increases, ions from aniline continue to dissociate until almost all the aniline is in the nonionized form, which is the aniline base. As transmembrane passage is largely restricted to the nonionized form, benzoic acid is more readily translocated through a membrane from an acidic environment, whereas more aniline is transferred from an alkaline environment.

Filtration When water flows in bulk across a porous membrane, any solute small enough to pass through the pores flows with it. Passage through these channels is called filtration, as it involves

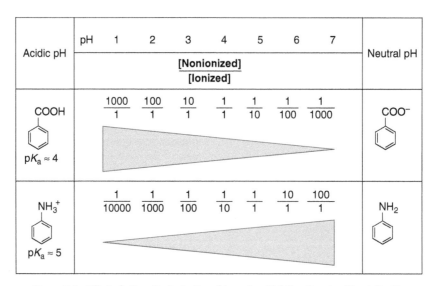

Acidic pH	pH	1	2	3	4	5	6	7	Neutral pH
				[Nonionized]					
				[Ionized]					
COOH pK$_a \approx$ 4		$\frac{1000}{1}$	$\frac{100}{1}$	$\frac{10}{1}$	$\frac{1}{1}$	$\frac{1}{10}$	$\frac{1}{100}$	$\frac{1}{1000}$	COO$^-$
NH$_3^+$ pK$_a \approx$ 5		$\frac{1}{10000}$	$\frac{1}{1000}$	$\frac{1}{100}$	$\frac{1}{10}$	$\frac{1}{1}$	$\frac{10}{1}$	$\frac{100}{1}$	NH$_2$

Figure 5-3. *Effect of pH on the ionization of benzoic acid (pK$_a$ = 4) and aniline (pK$_a$ = 5).*

bulk flow of water caused by hydrostatic or osmotic force. One of the main differences between various membranes is the size of these channels. In renal glomeruli, a primary site of filtration, these pores are relatively large (about 70 nm) allowing molecules smaller than albumin (approximately 60 kDa) to pass through. In contrast, there are no aqueous pores at cellular tight junctions, and channels in most cells are much smaller (3–6 Å), thereby only permitting substantial passage of molecules with molecular weights of no more than a few hundred daltons (Schanker, 1962; Lin, 2006).

Special Transport

There are numerous compounds whose movement across membranes cannot be explained by simple diffusion or filtration. Some compounds are too large to pass through aqueous pores or too insoluble in lipids to diffuse across the lipid domains of membranes. Nevertheless, they are often transported very rapidly across membranes, even against concentration gradients. To explain these phenomena, specialized transport systems have been identified. These systems are responsible for the transport (both influx and efflux) across cell membranes of many nutrients, such as sugars and amino and nucleic acids, along with numerous foreign compounds. Based on the sequencing of the human genome, there are at least 500 genes whose putative function involves membrane transport (Venter *et al.*, 2001). However, not all of these genes contribute to the disposition of toxicants. Throughout this chapter, membrane-associated transporters known to contribute to the disposition and subsequent effects of xenobiotics will be emphasized. Importantly, the role of xenobiotic transporters in chemical disposition is an expanding research field, and new information regarding their function, molecular regulation, and genetic polymorphisms continues to inform and modify traditional concepts in toxicology.

Active Transport
Active transport is characterized by (1) movement of chemicals against electrochemical or concentration gradients, (2) saturability at high substrate concentrations, (3) selectivity for certain structural features of chemicals, (4) competitive inhibition by chemical cogeners or compounds that are carried by the same transporter, and (5) requirement for expenditure of energy, so that metabolic inhibitors block the transport process.

Substances actively transported across cell membranes presumably form a complex with a membrane-bound macromolecular carrier on one side of the membrane. The complex subsequently traverses to the other side of the membrane, where the substance is released. Afterward, the carrier returns to the original surface to repeat the transport cycle.

Facilitated Diffusion
Facilitated diffusion applies to carrier-mediated transport that exhibits the properties of active transport except that the substrate is not moved against an electrochemical or concentration gradient, and the transport process does not require the input of energy; that is, metabolic poisons do not interfere with this transport. The transport of glucose from the GI tract across the basolateral membrane of the intestinal epithelium, from plasma into red blood cells, and from blood into the central nervous system (CNS) occurs by facilitated diffusion.

Xenobiotic Transporters
Significant advances in identifying and understanding the carrier-mediated transport systems for xenobiotics have been made in the recent years. In total, it is estimated that at least 5% of all human genes are transporter related, indicative of the importance of the transport function in normal biological and toxicological outcomes (Hediger *et al.*, 2004). Transporters mediate the influx (uptake) or efflux of xenobiotics and can be divided into 2 categories, determined by whether they mediate active or facilitated transfer of compounds. The first active, energy-dependent xenobiotic transporter identified was a phosphoglycoprotein overexpressed in tumor cells that showed resistance to anticancer drugs. The gene conferred multidrug resistance (MDR) to the cells, and was also called P-glycoprotein (P-gp or MDR1; gene name *MDR1*). This transporter functions as an efflux pump, which in cancerous cells, exudes cytotoxic drugs out of the tumor cells, and thus contributes to their resistance (Ambudkar *et al.*, 1999). MDR1 was the first member of a large superfamily of transport proteins known as ATP-binding cassette (ABC) transporters, with 7 subfamilies of ABC transporters now identified (Box 5-1). These are classified as subfamilies A to G with 49 genes in humans (Ueda, 2011). Many of these transporters play key roles in the homeostasis of numerous endogenous substrates. For example, ABCA1 is a major regulator of cholesterol in cells, mediating its efflux from liver, and ABCB4 specifically transports phospholipid substrates. In this chapter, transporters that play important roles in xenobiotic disposition and toxicity are described, with emphasis on the human genes and proteins. For example, in humans, the major

form of MDR1 involved in xenobiotic transport is a single protein (ABCB1; MDR1), whereas in rodents there are 2 drug-transporting MDR1 homologs identified as Mdr1a and Mdr1b.

The second important ABC transport subfamily is the ABCC subfamily, which is also known as the multiresistant drug protein (MRP) family (see Box 5-1). ABCC1 (MRP1) was also originally isolated from multidrug resistant cells. Members of this family excrete chemicals from cells, with MRP2 and MRP3 particularly important in the efflux of xenobiotic metabolites, especially those conjugated with UDP-glucuronic acid or glutathione. The breast cancer resistance protein (BCRP) is a member of the ABCG subfamily (ABCG2) and was originally isolated from a breast cancer cell line. It is expressed in a variety of normal tissues and contributes to the disposition of the efflux transport of numerous endogenous and xenobiotic sulfate conjugates. It is also highly expressed in numerous stem cells, particularly the side population of human

bone marrow and other organs where is it purported to provide protection from xenobiotics (Ni et al., 2010).

ABC transporters exhibit the characteristics of active transport outlined above, and most notably, they require expenditure of energy to function. For most ABC transporters, the binding and hydrolysis of ATP provides the energy required to move their substrates across membranes. The typical structure of most ABC transporters consists of two types of structural domains including hydrophobic membrane spanning domain (MSD) and the hydrophilic, intracellular nucleotide binding domain (NBD) where ATP binds and is hydrolyzed (Fig. 5-4). The typical structural organization of the ABC transporter, as exemplified by MDR1, is a tandem repeat of two domains (1 MSD followed by 1 NBD). The two repeated halves are joined by a polypeptide linker sequence. MRPs are distinguished from MDR1 in that they comprise 5 domains, with an extra MSD that comprises 5 transmembrane segments and

---

Box 5-1

Human ABC Transporters: Gene Family Overview and Major Transporters Involved in Xenobiotic Disposition

ABC SUBFAMILY	GENES IN FAMILY	GENE SYMBOLS
A	12	ABCA1-10, 12, 13
B	11	ABCB1-11
C	13	ABCC1-13*
D	4	ABCD1-4
E	1	ABCE1
F	3	ABCF1-3
G	5	ABCG1, 2, 4, 5, 8

*ABCC13 is reported to be a pseudogene.

Bolded subfamily designations are those with a major role in xenobiotic disposition.

GENE SYMBOL	COMMON NAME	GENERAL FUNCTION
ABCB1	Multidrug resistant protein/P-glycoprotein (MDR)	Efflux from gut, brain, placenta; biliary excretion
ABCB11	Bile salt export pump (BSEP)	Bile salt transport
ABCC1	Multidrug resistance–associated protein 1 (MRP1)	Multidrug resistance in many tissues; export pump
ABCC2	Multidrug resistance–associated protein 2 (MRP2)	Organic anion efflux, glucuronide and glutathione conjugates, biliary excretion
ABCC3	Multidrug resistance–associated protein 3 (MRP3)	Organic anion efflux, glucuronide and glutathione conjugates
ABCC4	Multidrug resistance–associated protein 4 (MRP4)	Nucleoside transport and organic anion efflux
ABCC5	Multidrug resistance–associated protein 5 (MRP5)	Mainly nucleoside transport
ABCC6	Multidrug resistance–associated protein 6 (MRP6)	Some glutathione conjugates
ABCC10	Multidrug resistance–associated protein 7 (MRP7)*	Organic anions, vinca alkaloids
ABCC11	Multidrug resistance–associated protein 8 (MRP8)*	Cyclic nucleotides and organic anions
ABCC12	Multidrug resistance–associated protein 9 (MRP9)*	Not defined
ABCG2	Breast cancer resistance protein (BCRP)	Organic anion efflux, many sulfate conjugates, biliary excretion

*There is little functional information available for MRP7, MRP8, and MRP9. A single nucleotide polymorphism in MRP8 is known to determine wet or dry earwax.

SOURCE: Compiled from Kruh et al. (2007), Klaassen and Aleksunes (2010), and Ueda et al. (2011).

Box 5-2

Major Members of the Human Solute Carrier Transporter Families Involved in Xenobiotic Disposition

TRANSPORTER	GENE FAMILY	HUMAN PROTEINS	GENE NAME	FUNCTION
Organic anion transporting polypeptide (OATP)	SLCO	OATP1A2	SLCO1A2	Transport of organic anions, cations, and neutral compounds
		OATP1B1	SLCO1B1	
		OATP1B3	SLCO1B3	
		OATP1C1	SLCO1C1	
		OATP2A1	SLCO2A1	
		OATP2B1	SLCO2B1	
		OATP3A1	SLCO3A1	
		OATP4A1	SLCO4A1	
		OATP4C1	SLCO4C1	
		OATP5A1	SLCO5A1	
		OATP6A1	SLCO6A1	
Organic cation transporter (OCT)	SLC22	OCT1	SLC22A1	Transport of organic cations
		OCT2	SLC22A2	
		OCT3	SLC22A3	
Organic cation/carnitine transporter (OCTN)	SLC22	OCTN1	SLC22A4	Organic cations; OCTN2 specific for carnitine
		OCTN2	SLC22A5	
Organic anion transporter (OAT)	SLC22	OAT1	SLC22A6	Transport of organic anions
		OAT2	SLC22A7	
		OAT3	SLC22A8	
		OAT4	SLC22A11	
		OAT5	SLC22A10	
Peptide transporter (PEPT)	SLC15	PEPT1	SLC15A1	Transport of di- and tripeptides, some xenobiotics
		PEPT2	SLC15A2	
Multidrug and toxin extrusion transporter (MATE)	SLC47	MATE1	SLC47A1	Efflux of organic cations; MATE2K localized to kidney
		MATE2K	SLC47A2	

Gene and protein members of the solute carrier families are compiled from Mizuno et al. (2003), Hagenbuch and Meier (2004), Sahi (2005), Lin (2006), Hagenbuch and Guo (2008), Kusuhara and Sugiyama (2009), and Klaassen and Aleksunes (2010).

the barrier function of numerous tissues sites including the blood–brain barrier (BBB), the blood–testis barrier, and the maternal–fetal barrier or placenta. Hence, they play a central role in the disposition and toxicity of xenobiotics. Their function in absorption, distribution, and excretion will be discussed throughout the remaining sections of this chapter.

The second major family of xenobiotic transporters is the solute carriers (SLCs), which function predominantly as facilitative transporters. There are 43 SLC gene families identified, and many of the nearly 300 genes comprising the 43 distinct SLC families play important roles in the disposition of endogenous compounds, including glucose, neurotransmitters, nucleotides, essential metals, and peptides. Additionally, there are several families that are vital to xenobiotic disposition, regulating the movement of many diverse organic anions and cations across cell membranes (Hediger et al., 2004; Klaassen and Aleksunes, 2010).

The major human solute carriers involved in xenobiotic disposition are summarized in Box 5-2. The organic-anion transporting peptides (OATPs, SLCO family) are important membrane transport proteins that mediate the sodium-independent transport of a wide range of compounds, including organic acids, bases, and neutral compounds. Although they are largely regarded as influx pumps, solutes can move bidirectionally, and these proteins appear to be especially important in the hepatic uptake of xenobiotics. In human liver, OATP1B1, OATP1B3, OATP1A2, and OATP2B1 have

an extracytosolic amino terminus, whereas BCRP is a "half-transporter" with a single MSD of 6 transmembrane segments preceded by a single NBD. Recent evidence suggests that BCRP forms a homodimer or a homotetramer to function as an efflux pump (Leslie et al., 2005; Ni et al., 2010). These differences in structure account for differences in molecular weight (approximately 170, 190, and 70 kDa for MDR1, MRP1, and BCRP, respectively), but there is considerable overlap in many of the xenobiotics that are transported by these proteins.

Members of the ABC transport family are expressed constitutively in many cells, and collectively they play important roles in absorption from the GI tract and elimination into bile or into urine for a wide range of xenobiotics. They are also critical to maintaining

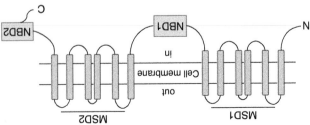

Figure 5-4. Diagrammatic representation of the structure of MRD1, illustrating the membrane spanning domain and ATP-binding domains (NBD).

been identified, whereas the major Oatps in rat liver are Oatp1a1, Oatp1a4, and Oatp1b2. For OATPs, the mechanism of transport is anion exchange such that the cellular influx of an organic compound is thought to be coupled to the efflux of bicarbonate, glutathione, or glutathione conjugates.

The organic-anion transporter (OAT; SLC22) family is particularly important in the renal uptake of anions, and human proteins (OAT1-5) have been identified in the kidney, whereas Oat1 and Oat3 are the major transporters identified in rodent kidneys. The organic-cation transporter (OCT; also SLC22) family is important in both the renal and hepatic uptake of xenobiotics. In this family, OCT1 is expressed in human liver, whereas only OCT2 has been detected in human kidney. In rats, Oct1 is found in liver, whereas both Oct1 and Oct2 are expressed in rat kidney. Novel organic-cation transporters (OCTNs; also SLC22) have also been identified which transport exogenous cations along with important endogenous compounds such as carnitine. OAT's transport substrates against an electrochemical gradient in exchange for intracellular dicarboxylates, such as α-ketoglutarate, whereas the driving force for OCT-mediated transport is the electrochemical gradient of the transported cation, typical of facilitated diffusion (described above). Peptide transporters (PEPT1 and PEPT2; SLC15) are responsible for the transport of di- and tri-peptides as well as drugs and toxicants such as the β-lactam antibiotics. Finally, the multidrug and toxin extrusion transporters (MATEs; SLC47) are a unique gene family of solute carriers expressed predominantly in liver and kidney that function specifically as cation efflux pumps.

Additional Transport Processes Other forms of specialized transport have been proposed, but their overall importance is not as well established as that of active transport and facilitated diffusion. Phagocytosis and pinocytosis are proposed mechanisms for cell membranes flowing around and engulfing particles. This type of transfer has been shown to be important for the removal of particulate matter from the alveoli by phagocytes and from blood by the reticuloendothelial system of the liver and spleen.

ABSORPTION

The process by which toxicants cross body membranes to enter the bloodstream is referred to as absorption. There are no specific systems or pathways for the sole purpose of absorbing toxicants. Xenobiotics penetrate membranes during absorption by the same processes as do biologically essential substances such as oxygen, foodstuffs, and other nutrients. The main sites of absorption are the GI tract, lungs, and skin. However, absorption may also occur from other sites, such as the subcutis, peritoneum, or muscle, if a chemical is administered by special routes. Experimentalists and medical professionals often distinguish between parenteral and enteral administration of drugs and other xenobiotics. Enteral administration includes all routes pertaining to the alimentary canal (sublingual, oral, and rectal), whereas parenteral administration involves all other routes (intravenous, intraperitoneal, intramuscular, subcutaneous, etc.).

Absorption of Toxicants by the Gastrointestinal Tract

The GI tract is one of the most important sites where toxicants are absorbed. Many environmental toxicants enter the food chain and are absorbed together with food from the GI tract. This site of absorption is also particularly relevant to toxicologists because accidental ingestion is the most common route of unintentional exposure to a toxicant (especially for children) and intentional overdoses most frequently occur via the oral route.

The GI tract may be viewed as a tube traversing the body. Although it is within the body, its contents remain outside of the body. Therefore, unless a noxious agent has direct caustic or irritating properties, toxicants remaining in the GI tract may damage the cells that make up the organ, but usually do not produce systemic injury until they are absorbed.

Absorption of toxicants can take place along the entire GI tract, even in the mouth and the rectum. Therefore, although the majority of drugs are given orally, drugs such as nitroglycerin are administered sublingually whereas others are administered as rectal suppositories. If a toxicant is an organic acid or base, it tends to be absorbed by simple diffusion in the part of the GI tract where it exists in its most lipid-soluble (nonionized) form. Because gastric juice is acidic (pH about 2) and the intestinal contents are nearly neutral, the lipid solubility of weak organic acids or bases can differ markedly in these 2 areas of the GI tract. The Henderson–Hasselbalch equations (discussed above) determine the fraction of a toxicant that is in the nonionized (lipid-soluble) form and estimate the rate of absorption from the stomach or intestine. As illustrated in Fig. 5-3, a weak organic acid such as benzoic acid is present mainly in the nonionized (lipid-soluble) form in the stomach and predominantly in the ionized form in the intestine. Therefore, weak organic acids are absorbed more readily from the stomach than from the intestine. In contrast, organic bases (except very weak organic bases) are likely to be ionized and not lipid soluble in the stomach, but are more likely to be in the nonionized form in the intestine, suggesting that the absorption of such compounds occurs predominantly in the intestine rather than in the stomach. However, the Henderson–Hasselbalch calculations are not an absolute determination of absorption because other factors—including the mass action law, surface area, and blood flow rate—have to be taken into consideration in examining the absorption of weak organic acids or bases. For example, only 1% of benzoic acid is present in the lipid-soluble form in the neutral pH of the intestine. Therefore, one might conclude that the intestine has little capacity to absorb this organic acid. However, absorption is a dynamic process. The blood keeps removing benzoic acid from the lamina propria of the intestine, and according to the mass action law, the equilibrium will always be maintained at 1% in the nonionized form, providing continuous availability of benzoic acid for absorption. Moreover, absorption by simple diffusion is also proportional to the surface area. The small intestine has a very large surface because the villi and micro-villi increase the surface area approximately 600-fold, such that the overall capacity of the intestine for absorption of benzoic acid is quite large. Similar considerations are also valid for the absorption of all weak organic acids from the intestine.

The mammalian GI tract has numerous specialized transport systems (carrier-mediated) for the absorption of nutrients and electrolytes (Table 5-2). The absorption of some of these substances is complex and depends on several additional factors. For example, iron absorption is determined by the need for iron and takes place in 2 steps: iron first enters the mucosal cells of the GI tract and then moves into the blood. The first step is relatively rapid, whereas the second is slow. Consequently, iron accumulates within the mucosal cells as a protein–iron complex termed ferritin. When the concentration of iron in blood drops below normal values, some iron is liberated from the mucosal stores of ferritin and transported into the blood. As a consequence, the absorption of more iron from the intestine is triggered to replenish these stores. Calcium is also absorbed by a 2-step process: absorption into the lumen followed by exudation into the interstitial fluid. The first step is faster than the

Numerous xenobiotic transporters are expressed in the GI tract where they function to increase or decrease absorption of xenobiotics (Fig. 5-5). Several proteins in the SLC families are expressed in the intestine where they are predominantly localized on the apical brush-border membranes of the enterocytes and increase uptake from the lumen into the enterocytes. In humans, OATP1A2 and OATP2B1 are the most abundant and important members of this family that are expressed in the intestine, although OATP3A1 and OATP4A1 have also been identified. In contrast, in rodents Oatp1a5 is the predominant uptake transporter. OCT1 and OCT2 are also present in the intestine, with OCTN2 specifically involved in the uptake of carnitine. The peptide transporter, PEPT1 is highly expressed in the GI tract and mediates the transport of peptide-like drugs such as antibiotics, particularly those containing a β-lactam structure. The OCTs, particularly OCT1 and OCT2, also contribute to xenobiotic uptake into enterocytes, but are expressed on the baso-lateral membrane (Klaassen and Aleksunes, 2010; Tamai, 2012). The primary active efflux transporters such as MDR1, MRP2, and BCRP are also expressed on enterocyte brush-border membranes where they function to excrete their substrates into the lumen, thereby decreasing the net absorption of xenobiotics. MRP3 is also found in the intestine, but is localized to the basolateral membrane. The expression of the intestinal transporters varies across the GI tract. For example, MDR1 expression increases from the duodenum

second, and therefore intracellular calcium rises in mucosal cells during absorption. Vitamin D is required for both steps of calcium transport.

Some xenobiotics are absorbed by the same specialized transport systems for nutrients, thereby leading to potential competition or interaction. For example, 5-fluorouracil is absorbed by the pyrimidine transport system (Yuasa et al., 1996), thallium utilizes the system that normally absorbs iron (Leopold et al., 1969), lead can be absorbed by the calcium transporter (Fullmer, 1992), and cobalt and manganese compete for the iron transport system (Flanagan et al., 1980).

to colon, whereas MRP2 and most of the uptake transporters are expressed most highly in the duodenum and decrease to in the terminal ileum and colon. BCRP is found throughout the small intestine and colon.

The efflux transporters are particularly relevant to the disposition of toxicants, as there will be a net reduction in the absorption of chemicals that are substrates for these transporters, and this is a desirable outcome for toxic chemicals. For example, the dietary

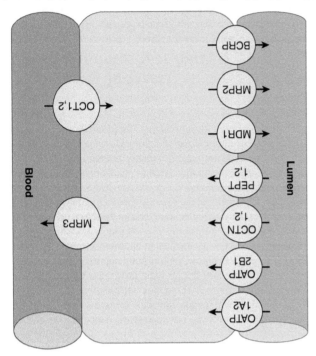

Figure 5-5. *Schematic model showing the important xenobiotic transport systems present in the human gastrointestinal tract.*

Table 5-2
Distribution of Specialized Transport Systems in the Small Intestine of Man and Animals

SUBSTRATES	UPPER	MIDDLE	LOWER	COLON
Sugar (glucose, galactose, etc)	++	+++	++	0
Neutral amino acids	++	+++	++	0
Basic amino acids	++	+	++	?
Gamma globulin (newborn animals)	+	++	+++	?
Pyrimidines (thymine and uracil)	+	+	?	?
Triglycerides	++	++	+	?
Fatty acid absorption and conversion to triglyceride	+++	++	+	0
Bile salts	0	+	+++	
Vitamin B_{12}	0	+	+++	0
Na^+	+++	++	+++	+++
H^+ (and/or HCO_3^- secretion)	0	+	++	++
Ca^{2+}	+++	++	+	?
Fe^{2+}	+++	++	+	?
Cl^-	+++	++	+	0

SOURCE: Data from Wilson (1962).

of chemicals, an extremely lipid-soluble chemical is unlikely to dissolve in the aqueous fluids within the GI tract, which limits its absorption from the GI tract. Similarly, if the toxicant is a solid and is relatively insoluble in GI fluids, it will also have limited contact with the GI mucosa and its rate of absorption will be low (Lipinski et al., 2001).

In addition to the characteristics of the compounds themselves, there are numerous additional factors relating to the GI tract itself that influence the absorption of xenobiotics. These factors include pH, the presence of food, digestive enzymes, bile acids, and bacterial microflora in the GI tract, along with the motility and permeability of the GI tract. Chemical resistance or lack of resistance to alteration by the acidic pH of the stomach, enzymes of the stomach or intestine, or the intestinal microflora are extremely important. A toxicant may be hydrolyzed by stomach acid, biotransformed by enzymes in the GI tract or modified by the resident microflora to new compounds with a toxicity different from that of the parent compound. For example, snake venoms, which are proteinaceous moieties, are much less toxic by the oral route relative to intravenous exposure because they are degraded by digestive enzymes of the GI tract.

Intestinal microflora can also influence absorption and toxicity of compounds. For example, a variety of nitroaromatic compounds are reduced by intestinal bacteria to potentially toxic and carcinogenic aromatic amines. Nitroreduction of 2,6-dinitrotoluene to the mutagenic 2,6-diaminotoluene in the GI tract produces long-term adverse effects, including mutagenicity and carcinogenicity, which are not observed in germ-free animals (Rickert et al., 1984). Similarly, the nitroaromatic perfume, musk xylene, can inhibit the activity of cytochrome P450 enzymes in the liver only after it is reduced to an amine derivative by resident microflora in the GI tract and subsequently absorbed (Lehman-McKeeman et al., 1997). It has also been shown that ingestion of well water with a high nitrate content produces methemoglobinemia much more frequently in infants than in adults. In this case, bacteria in the GI tract convert nitrate to nitrite, increasing the likelihood of methemoglobinemia (Mensinga et al., 2003). Infants are more susceptible to methemoglobinemia because the higher pH of the neonatal GI tract is permissive for the growth of bacteria (such as *Escherichia coli*) that convert nitrate to nitrite. One example wherein intestinal microflora reduce the potential toxicity is that of the mycotoxin, deoxynivalenol, which is found in numerous grains and foodstuffs. Strict anaerobes detoxify this compound leading to the absorption of a less toxic reductive metabolite (Awad et al., 2010). The contribution of bacteria in the GI tract to other aspects of xenobiotic disposition, particularly enterohepatic circulation, is discussed in greater detail later in this chapter.

Agents such as the chelator, ethylenediaminetetraacetic acid (EDTA), increase absorption of some toxicants by increasing intestinal permeability. An increase in permeability is thought to result from the chelation of calcium that is involved in the formation and maintenance of tight intercellular junctions (Ballard et al., 1995) such that binding of calcium reduces the integrity of the cell junctions, allowing more paracellular absorption. Furthermore, simple diffusion is proportional not only to the surface area and the permeability but also to the residency time within various segments of the GI tract. Therefore, the rate of absorption of a toxicant remaining for longer periods in the intestine increases, whereas that with a shorter residency time decreases. Experiments have shown that the oral toxicity of some chemicals is increased by diluting the dose (Borowitz et al., 1971). This phenomenon may be explained by more rapid stomach emptying induced by increased dosage volume, which in turn leads to greater absorption in the duodenum because of the larger surface area there. Furthermore, some agents

carcinogen, 2-amino-1-methyl-6-phenylimidazo (4,5-b)pyridine (PhIP), a heterocyclic amine produced during the cooking of meat, is a substrate for MRP2. Studies comparing the disposition of PhIP in wild-type and Mrp2-deficient rats showed that MRP is very important in limiting the oral absorption of this harmful compound (Dietrich et al., 2001). However, although limiting absorption of toxicants and carcinogens is beneficial, these transporters can also function to limit the oral absorption of drugs. For example, the immunosuppressive drug cyclosporine and the chemotherapeutic anticancer drugs paclitaxel (taxol), colchicine, and vincristine are not readily absorbed from the GI tract because they are good substrates for MDR1.

The number of toxicants actively absorbed by the GI tract is low; most enter the body by simple diffusion. Although lipid-soluble substances are absorbed more rapidly and extensively than are water-soluble substances, the latter may also be absorbed to some degree. After oral ingestion, about 10% of lead, 4% of manganese, 1.5% of cadmium, and 1% of chromium salts are absorbed. If a compound is very toxic, even small amounts of absorbed material produce serious systemic effects. An organic compound that would not be expected to be absorbed on the basis of the pH-partition hypothesis is the fully ionized quaternary ammonium compound pralidoxime chloride (2-PAM; molecular weight 137), yet it is absorbed almost entirely from the GI tract. The mechanism by which some lipid-insoluble compounds are absorbed is not entirely clear. It appears that organic ions of low molecular weight (<200) can be transported across the mucosal barrier by paracellular transport, that is, passive penetration through aqueous pores at the tight junctions or by active transport as discussed above. Particles and particulate matter can also be absorbed by the GI epithelium. In this case, particle size is a major determinant of absorption, whereas factors such as the lipid solubility or ionization characteristics are less important. For particles, size is inversely related to absorption such that absorption increases with decreasing particle diameter (Florence et al., 1995). This explains why metallic mercury is relatively nontoxic when ingested orally and why powdered arsenic was found to be significantly more toxic than its coarse granular form (Schwarze, 1923). Large particles (greater than about 20 μm in diameter) enter intestinal cells by pinocytosis, a process that is much more prominent in newborns than in adults, after which they are carried through the intestinal epithelium in intact vesicles and discharged into the interstices of the lamina propria. Absorption into gut-associated lymphoid tissue (such as Peyer's patches) and the mesenteric lymph supply also plays a key role in systemic absorption of particles (Jani et al., 1990; Florence et al., 1995).

There is increasing interest in particles of very small diameter that may be used in a variety of chemical and biological processes. Nanoparticles or nanomaterials are typically less than 100 nm in size, and numerous issues have been raised regarding the toxic potential of these entities (Chap. 28). Although the absorption of large particles is typically limited, absorption of nanoparticles by the GI tract in rats is as high as 30% for particles that are less than 50 nm in diameter (Jani et al., 1990). Additionally, surface characteristics of nanoparticles contributes to their absorption, with hydrophobic, nonionized particles being more extensively absorbed than those modified to possess an ionized surface as is the case with larger particles, the gut-associated lymphoid tissue appears to be the predominant absorption pathway for nanoparticles from the GI tract (Stern and McNeil, 2008). Overall, the absorption of a toxicant from the GI tract depends on its physical properties, including lipid solubility and its dissolution rate. Although it is often generalized that an increase in lipid solubility increases the absorption used as laxatives alter absorption of xenobiotics by increasing intestinal motility, whereas agents used as antidiarrheals may increase absorption by slowing intestinal motility.

The amount of a chemical that enters the systemic circulation after oral administration depends on several factors. The amount absorbed into the cells of the GI tract is important, and transporters can influence this amount by affecting the uptake or efflux from the cells. Further, before a chemical enters the systemic circulation, it can be biotransformed by the cells in the GI tract or extracted by the liver and excreted into bile with or without prior biotransformation. This phenomenon of the removal of chemicals before entrance into the systemic circulation is referred to as presystemic elimination or first-pass effect. The lung can also contribute to the biotransformation or elimination of chemicals before their entrance into the systemic circulation, although its role is less well defined than that of the intestine and the liver. Chemicals that have a high first-pass effect will appear to have a lower absorption because they are eliminated as quickly as they are absorbed. For toxicants, a high first-pass effect will serve to limit exposure and typically minimizes toxic potential.

A number of other factors have been shown to alter absorption. For example, although lead and many other heavy metal ions are not absorbed readily from the GI tract. EDTA and other chelators increase the lipid solubility and thus the absorption of complexed ions. Thus, it is important not to administer a chelator orally when excess metal is still present in the GI tract after oral ingestion. Furthermore, metal ions can affect absorption of other ions. For example, cadmium decreases the absorption of zinc and copper, calcium decreases cadmium absorption, and magnesium decreases absorption of fluoride (Pfeiffer, 1977). Consumption of grapefruit juice can also influence GI absorption through the actions of naringin, a flavonoid that inhibits the function of several transporters including MDR1 and OATP1A2 (Bailey, 2010). By reducing MDR1-dependent efflux, grapefruit juice increases GI absorption of numerous pharmaceutical agents (such as calcium-channel blockers and cholesterol-lowering agents), and, in some cases, this effect leads to toxic or adverse reactions resulting from increased exposure to the drugs. Alternatively, inhibition of OATPs reduces absorption and could limit toxicity.

Species differences in absorption across the GI tract are widely recognized. As one example, absorption of nadolol after intraperitoneal and oral dosing was compared across species by calculating the exposure as plasma area-under-the-curve (AUC) and was found to be essentially complete in dogs, substantially less in humans, and limited in rats. Urinary and fecal excretion of nadolol support the bioavailability data, as the low oral absorption of nadolol in rats is consistent with the large amount of drug recovered in feces (Table 5-3). However, excretory data further indicate that in addition to the nonabsorbed portion of this compound, biliary and possibly nonbiliary sources also contribute to the fecal excretion of this compound. Similar comparisons across species provide further evidence for species differences in the absorption of numerous compounds, indicating that nadolol is not an exceptional case (Calabrese, 1984). The factors that contribute to species differences in absorption are not fully understood. Anatomical considerations are likely to contribute to species differences in intestinal absorption, and substantial functional differences exist between species. Because most xenobiotics are transported across the GI mucosa by passive diffusion, and because this transport is surface area- and site-dependent, it is likely that these factors will also contribute to species differences. Furthermore, species differences in the pH along the GI tract exist (Table 5-4), varying by as much as 2 pH units. The magnitude of this diversity can translate into differences up to 2 orders of magnitude in the concentration of the nonionized versus ionized moiety of a weak

Table 5-3

Absorption and Excretion of Radioactivity in Rats, Dogs, and Humans After Nadolol Dosages*

SPECIES	DOSE (mg/kg)	ROUTE	PERCENT OF DOSE EXCRETED FECES	PERCENT OF DOSE EXCRETED URINE	PERCENT OF DOSE ABSORBED
Rat	20	ip	62	31	(100)
	20	po	11	84	18
Dog	25	ip	75	12	(100)
	25	po	76	28	102
Human	2	ip	73	23	(100)
	2	po	25	77	34

*po and ip denote oral and intraperitoneal administration, respectively.

SOURCE: Data from Dreyfuss et al. (1978).

organic acid or base available for absorption. In addition, the GI absorption is often higher in dogs compared to other species because paracellular absorption is thought to occur to a greater extent in dogs. Another factor that may result in species-dependent absorption of xenobiotics is the presence and function of the GI microflora. Bacteria in the GI tract are highly abundant, with strict anaerobes (oxygen intolerant) being the most prevalent. More than 400 species of bacteria have been found in the GI tract. In general, the intestinal microflora in animals is remarkably similar, although qualitative and quantitative differences have been reported (Rowland et al., 1985). For example, rabbit and humans are distinguished from other species in that the number of microbes found in the upper regions of the GI tract is relatively low (Table 5-5). The more acidic pH of the stomach in rabbits and humans contributes to the lower number of microbes found in this region. Importantly, bacterial metabolism is a prerequisite for absorption of some xenobiotics, and species differences in absorption may result from differences in the type and number of microbes in the GI tract.

Absorption of Toxicants by the Lungs

Toxic responses to chemicals can occur from absorption following inhalation exposure. Relevant examples include carbon monoxide poisoning and silicosis, an important occupational disease. These toxicities result from absorption or deposition of airborne poisons in the lungs.

Table 5-4

pH of the Gastrointestinal Contents of Various Species*

SPECIES	STOMACH	JEJUNUM	CECUM	COLON	FECES
			pH		
Monkey	2.8	6.0	5.0	5.1	5.5
Dog	3.4	6.6	6.4	6.5	6.2
Rat	3.8	6.8	6.8	6.6	6.9
Rabbit	1.9	7.5	6.6	7.2	7.2

*SOURCE: Data from Smith (1965).

Table 5-5

Number of Microbes and Their Distribution Along the Gastrointestinal Tract of Various Species*

SPECIES	STOMACH	JEJUNUM	COLON	FECES
Monkey	23	24	41	38
Dog	19	20	40	43
Rat	18	23	37	38
Rabbit	4	5	13	13
Man	2	4	10	—

Expressed as log_{10} of viable counts.
SOURCE: Modified from Smith (1965) and Rowland et al. (1985).

A major group of toxicants that are absorbed by the lungs are gases (eg, carbon monoxide, nitrogen dioxide, and sulfur dioxide), vapors of volatile or volatilizable liquids (eg, benzene and carbon tetrachloride), and aerosols. Because the absorption of inhaled gases and vapor differs from that of aerosols, aerosols are discussed separately below. However, the absorption of gases and vapors is governed by the same principles, and therefore the word gas is used to represent both in this section.

Gases and Vapors A vapor is the gas form of substance that can also exist as a liquid or solid at atmospheric pressure and normal temperature. Most organic solvents evaporate and produce vapors, and some solids can also sublimate into a gaseous form. Vapor pressure is that exerted by a vapor above its own liquid in a closed system, such that liquids that have a high vapor pressure have a higher tendency to evaporate. A toxicant with a high vapor pressure at room temperature is considered to be volatile. Examples of the vapor pressure of several toxicants are presented in Table 5-6.

The absorption of inhaled gases takes place mainly in the lungs. However, when inhaled, gases first pass through the nose, filtering through delicately scrolled, simple epithelial-lined turbinates, which serve to increase the surface area of exposure. Because the mucosa of the nose is covered by a film of fluid, gas molecules can be retained by the nose and do not reach the lungs if they are very water soluble or react with cell surface components. Therefore, the nose acts as a "scrubber" for water-soluble

Table 5-6

Vapor Pressures of Common Solvents or Toxicants

SUBSTANCE	VAPOR PRESSURE (SI UNITS; kPa)	VAPOR PRESSURE (mm Hg)
Ethylene glycol	0.5	3.75
Water	2.3	17.5
Ethanol	5.83	43.7
Chloroform	30	225
Acetaldehyde	98.7	740
Formaldehyde	435.7	3268

SI units are the International System of units for pressure with the Pascal (Pa) as the standard unit. All values obtained at 20°C.

and highly reactive gases, partially protecting the lungs from potentially injurious insults. Although these actions may serve to reduce systemic exposure or to protect the lungs, they also increase the risk that the nose could be adversely affected. Such is the case with formaldehyde (Kerns et al., 1983) and vinyl acetate (Bogdanffy et al., 1999), which cause tumors of the nasal turbinates in rats.

Absorption of gases in the lungs differs from intestinal and percutaneous absorption of compounds in that the dissociation of acids and bases and the lipid solubility of molecules are less important factors in pulmonary absorption because diffusion through cell membranes is not rate-limiting in the pulmonary absorption of gases. There are at least 3 reasons for this. First, ionized molecules are of very low volatility, so that they do not achieve significant concentrations in normal ambient air. Second, type I pneumocytes (epithelial cells lining the alveoli; Chap. 15) are very thin and the capillaries are in close contact with the pneumocytes, so that the distance for a chemical to diffuse is very short. Third, chemicals absorbed by the lungs are removed rapidly by the blood, and blood moves very quickly through the extensive capillary network in the lungs.

When a gas is inhaled into the lungs, gas molecules diffuse from the alveolar space into the blood and then dissolve. Except for some gases with a special affinity for certain body components (eg, the binding of carbon monoxide to hemoglobin), the uptake of a gas by a tissue usually involves the simple physical process of dissolving. The end result is that gas molecules partition between two media, namely air and blood during the absorptive phase and blood and other tissues during the distributive phase. As the inspired gas remains in contact with blood in the alveoli, more molecules dissolve in blood until gas molecules in blood are in equilibrium with gas molecules in the alveolar space. At this equilibrium, the ratio of the concentration of chemical in the blood and chemical in the gas phase is constant. This solubility ratio is called the blood-to-gas partition coefficient, and it is unique for each gas. Note that although the ratio is constant, the concentrations achieved vary in accordance with Henry's law, which dictates that the amount of gas dissolved in a liquid is proportional to the partial vapor pressure of the gas in the gas phase at any given concentration before or at saturation. Thus, the higher the inhaled concentration of a gas (ie, the higher the partial pressure), the higher the gas concentration in blood, but the blood:gas ratio does not change unless saturation has occurred. When equilibrium is reached, the rate of transfer of gas molecules from the alveolar space to blood equals the rate of removal by blood from the alveolar space. For example, chloroform has a relatively high blood-to-gas partition coefficient (approximately 20), whereas ethylene has a low coefficient (0.14). By comparison, a smaller percentage of the total ethylene in the lungs is removed into the blood during each circulation because the low blood-to-gas partition coefficient dictates that blood is quickly saturated with this gas. Therefore, an increase in the respiratory rate or minute volume does not change the transfer of such a gas to blood. In contrast, an increase in the rate of blood flow increases the rate of uptake of a compound with a low solubility ratio because of more rapid removal from the site of equilibrium, that is, the alveolar membranes. It has been calculated that the time to equilibrate between the blood and the gas phase for a relatively insoluble gas is about 10 to 20 minutes.

A gas with a high blood-to-gas partition coefficient, such as chloroform, is readily transferred to blood during each respiratory cycle so that little if any remains in the alveoli just before the next inhalation. The more soluble a toxic chemical is in blood, the more of it will be dissolved in blood by the time equilibrium is reached. Consequently, the time required to equilibrate with blood is much longer for a gas with a high blood-to-gas partition coefficient than for a gas with a low ratio. This has been calculated to take a minimum of one hour for compounds with a high solubility ratio, although it may take even longer if the gas also has high tissue affinity (ie, high fat solubility). With highly soluble gases, the principal factor limiting the rate of absorption is respiration. Because the blood is already removing virtually all gases with a high solubility ratio from the lungs, increasing the blood flow rate does not substantially increase the rate of absorption. However, the rate can be accelerated greatly by increasing the rate of respiration.

The blood carries the dissolved gas molecules to the rest of the body. In each tissue, the gas molecules are transferred from the blood to the tissue until equilibrium is reached at a tissue concentration dictated by the tissue-to-blood partition coefficient. After releasing part of the gas to tissues, blood returns to the lungs to take up more of the gas. The process continues until a gas reaches equilibrium between blood and each tissue according to the tissue-to-blood partition coefficients characteristic of each tissue. This equilibrium is referred to as steady state, and at this time, no net absorption of gas takes place as long as the exposure concentration remains constant.

AEROSOLS AND PARTICLES

Absorption of aerosol and particles is distinguished from gases and vapors by the factors that determine absorption from the inhalation route of exposure. The absorption of gases and vapors by inhalation is determined by the partitioning of the compound between the blood and the gas phase along with its solubility and tissue reactivity. In contrast, the important characteristics that affect absorption after exposure to aerosols are the aerosol size and water solubility of any chemical present in the aerosol.

The site of deposition of aerosols and particulates depends largely on the size of the particles. This relationship is discussed in detail in Chap. 15. In general, the smaller the particle, the further into the respiratory tree the particle will deposit (Fig. 5-6). Particles ranging from 5 μm or larger, described as "course particles" usually are deposited in the nasopharyngeal region. Those deposited on the unciliated anterior or rostral portion of the nose tend to remain at the site of deposition until they are removed by nose wiping, blowing, or sneezing. The mucous blanket of the ciliated nasal surface propels insoluble particles by the movement of the cilia. These particles and particles inhaled through the mouth are swallowed within minutes. Soluble particles may dissolve in the mucus and be carried to the pharynx or may be absorbed through the nasal epithelium into the blood.

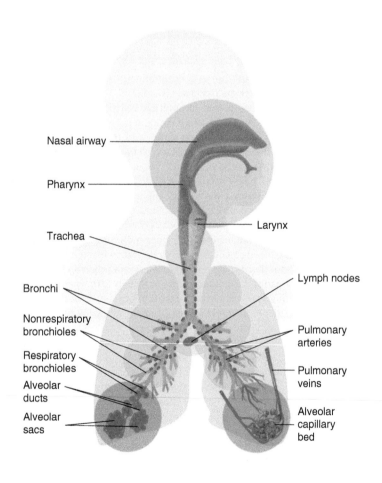

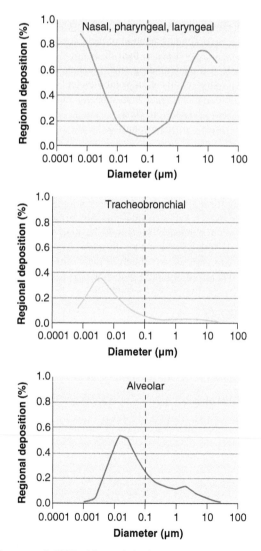

Figure 5-6. *Representation of particle distribution in the lungs relative to size.* (Oberdorster *et al.*, 2005, with permission.)

Particulate matter with diameters of approximately 2.5 μm, referred to as "fine particles" are deposited mainly in the tracheobronchiolar regions of the lungs, from which they may be cleared by retrograde movement of the mucus layer in the ciliated portions of the respiratory tract (also known as the mucociliary escalator). The rate of cilia-propelled movement of mucus varies in different parts of the respiratory tract, although in general it is a rapid and efficient transport mechanism. Toxicants or viral infections that damage cilia may impair the efficiency of this process. Measurements have shown transport rates between 0.1 and 1 mm/min, resulting in removal half-lives between 30 and 300 minutes. Coughing and sneezing greatly increase the movement of mucus and particulate matter toward the mouth. Particles eventually may be swallowed and absorbed from the GI tract or expectorated.

Particles 1 μm and smaller penetrate to the alveolar sacs of the lungs. Ultrafine- or nanoparticles, particularly those that are approximately 10 to 20 nm in size, have the greatest likelihood of depositing in the alveolar region. These extremely small particles may be absorbed into blood or cleared through the lymphatics after being scavenged by alveolar macrophages (Oberdorster et al., 2005).

In addition to being a major determinant of lung deposition, as particle size decreases, the number of particles in a unit of space increases along with the total surface area of the particles. This relationship, illustrated in Table 5-7, indicates that nanoparticles have the propensity to deliver high amounts of particulates to the lung. However, it appears that the surface properties of nanoparticles may be more important determinants of toxic potential than their size or surface area. The contribution of nanoparticles to toxic responses, with special emphasis on their disposition (and factors that influence disposition including size, composition, surface structure, surface group modification, solubility, and aggregation) are major areas of toxicological and human health effects research (Nel et al., 2006; Stern and McNeil, 2008).

The mechanisms responsible for the removal or absorption of particulate matter from the alveoli are less clear than those responsible for the removal of particles deposited in the tracheobronchial tree. Removal appears to occur by three major mechanisms. First, particles may be removed from the alveoli by a physical process. As described earlier, it is thought that particles deposited on the fluid layer of the alveoli are aspirated onto the mucociliary escalator of the tracheobronchial region. From there, they are transported to the mouth and may be swallowed. The origin of the thin fluid layer in the alveoli is probably a transudation of lymph and secretions of lipids and other components by the alveolar epithelium. The alveolar fluid flows by an unknown mechanism to the terminal

bronchioles. This flow seems to depend on lymph flow, capillary action, the respiratory motion of the alveolar walls, the cohesive nature of the respiratory tract's fluid blanket, the propelling power of the ciliated bronchioles, and the surface tension within the fluid layer. Second, particles from the alveoli may be removed by phagocytosis. The principal cells responsible for engulfing alveolar debris are the resident alveolar macrophages. These phagocytic cells are found in large numbers in normal lungs and contain many phagocytized particles of both exogenous and endogenous origin. They apparently migrate to the distal end of the mucociliary escalator and are cleared and eventually swallowed. Third, removal may occur via the lymphatics. The endothelial cells lining lymphatic capillaries are permeable to very large molecules and particles (molecular weight >1000 kDa), although the rate of penetration is low when molecular weight exceeds 10 kDa. Nevertheless, the lymphatic system plays a prominent role in collecting high-molecular-weight proteins leaked from cells or blood capillaries and particulate matter from the interstitium and the alveolar spaces. Particulate matter may remain in lymphatic tissue for long periods, and this explains the phenomenon of "dust store of the lungs."

In general, the overall removal of particles from the alveoli is relatively inefficient. The rate of clearance by the lungs can be predicted by a compound's solubility in lung fluids. The lower the solubility, the lower the removal rate. Thus, it appears that removal of particles that enter the alveoli is largely due to dissolution and vascular transport. Some particles may remain in the alveoli indefinitely. This may occur when long-lived alveolar macrophages phagocytose indigestible dust particles and secrete cytokines that stimulate the development of a local network of type I and III collagen fibers to form an alveolar dust plaque or nodule.

Absorption of Toxicants Through the Skin

Skin is the largest body organ and provides a relatively good barrier for separating organisms from their environment. Overall, human skin comes into contact with many toxic chemicals, but exposure is usually limited by its relatively impermeable nature. However, some chemicals can be absorbed by the skin in sufficient quantities to produce systemic effects. For example, there are several insecticides for which fatal exposures have occurred in agricultural workers after absorption through intact skin (see Chap. 19). In addition, there are numerous chemicals that increase tumor development in other organs after dermal application.

The skin comprises 2 major layers, the epidermis and dermis (Fig. 5-7). The epidermis is the outermost layer and contains keratinocytes that are metabolically competent and able to divide. Proliferating keratinocytes in the stratum germinativum displace maturing keratinocyte layers upward until they reach the outermost layer, the stratum corneum. The stratum corneum contains densely packed keratinized cells that have lost their nuclei and are biologically inactive. The stratum corneum is replaced approximately every 3 to 4 weeks in adult humans. This complex process involves dehydration and polymerization of intracellular matrix forming keratin-filled dried cell layers. During the process, the cell walls apparently double in thickness and transform into a dry, keratinous semisolid state with much lower permeability for diffusion of toxicants. The stratum corneum is unique anatomically and represents the single most important barrier to preventing fluid loss from the body while also serving as the major barrier to prevent the absorption of xenobiotics into the body.

The dermis is situated beneath the epidermis and consists primarily of fibroblasts. This region also contains the vascular network that provides the dermis and epidermis with blood supply and

Table 5-7

Particle Number and Surface Area for 10 μg/m³ Airborne Particles

PARTICLE DIAMETER (μm)	PARTICLES/mL AIR	PARTICLE SURFACE AREA (μm²/mL AIR)
5	0.15	12
2	2	30
0.5	153	120
0.02	2,400,000	3016
0.05	153,000,000	12,000

SOURCE: Modified from Oberdorster et al. (2005) and Nel et al. (2006).

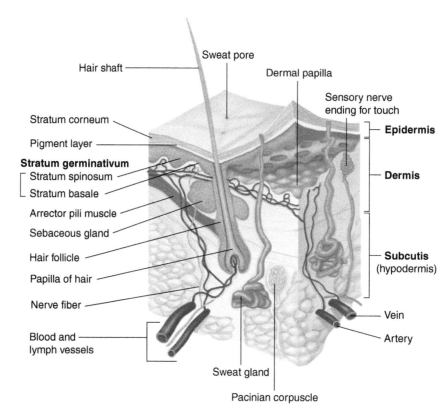

Figure 5-7. *Diagram of a cross section of human skin illustrating the various layers, cellular composition, and blood supply.* (www.dentalarticles.com/visual/d/skin-layers.php)

serves to carry absorbed compounds into the body. Although the major anatomical area that controls absorption across the skin is the stratum corneum, compounds may also be absorbed through dermal appendages, including sweat and sebaceous glands and hair follicles found in the dermis. Sweat glands and hair follicles are scattered in varying densities on skin. These appendages account for no more than 1% of the total cross-sectional area of the total skin surface, and, in general, passage through these areas is much more rapid than passage through the stratum corneum. Ultimately, to be absorbed a chemical must pass the barrier of the stratum corneum and then traverse the other six layers of the skin (Dugard, 1983; Poet and McDougal, 2002).

In contrast to the complexity of the GI tract, the skin is a simpler penetration barrier for chemicals because passage through the stratum corneum is the rate-determining step. All toxicants move across the stratum corneum by passive diffusion. In general, lipophilic (fat-soluble) compounds are absorbed more readily across the stratum corneum, whereas the penetration of hydrophilic (water-soluble) compounds is more limited. Nonpolar toxicants diffuse through the skin in a manner that is proportional to their lipid solubility and inversely related to molecular weight. However, although lipophilic compounds may pass more readily through the stratum corneum, their passage through the dermis may become rate-limiting. Hydrophilic compounds are more likely to penetrate the skin through appendages such as hair follicles.

Human stratum corneum is significantly different in structure and chemistry in various regions of the body, and these differences affect the permeability of the skin to chemicals. Skin from the palmar and plantar regions is much different from skin from other areas of the body in that the stratum corneum of the palms and soles is adapted for weight bearing and friction and there are no hair follicles present. The stratum corneum of the rest of the body surface is adapted for flexibility and fine sensory discrimination. The

permeability of the skin also depends on both the diffusivity and the thickness of the stratum corneum. Although the stratum corneum is much thicker on the palms and soles (400–600 μm in callous areas) than on the arms, back, legs, and abdomen (8–15 μm), it has much higher diffusivity per unit thickness. In contrast, the skin of the scrotum is characterized by a thin stratum corneum and a high diffusivity. Consequently, as illustrated by the comparative absorption of malathion across different human skin sites (Table 5-8), toxicants are likely to readily cross scrotal skin, whereas absorption across forehead skin is less extensive, and penetration across the palm is lowest because of the thickness of the stratum corneum and the lack of dermal appendages.

The second phase of percutaneous absorption consists of diffusion of the toxicant through the lower layers of the epidermis (stratum germinativum, spinosum, and granulosum) and the dermis. Despite possessing tight intercellular junctions, these cell layers are

Table 5-8

Absorption of Malathion Across Different Human Skin Regions

ANATOMICAL REGION	ABSORPTION (%)	STRATUM CORNEUM THICKNESS (μm)	HAIR FOLLICLES/ cm^2
Scrotum	101.6	5	60
Forehead	23.2	13	770
Hand (back)	12.5	49	18
Palm	5.8	400	—

SOURCE: Adapted from Poet and McDougal (2002).

far inferior to the stratum corneum as diffusion barriers. In contrast to the stratum corneum, they contain a porous, nonselective, aqueous diffusion medium. Toxicants pass through this area by diffusion and enter the systemic circulation through the numerous venous and lymphatic capillaries in the dermis. The rate of diffusion depends on blood flow, interstitial fluid movement, and perhaps other factors, including interactions with dermal constituents.

There are several factors that can influence the absorption of toxicants through the skin, including (1) the integrity of the stratum corneum, (2) the hydration state of the stratum corneum, (3) temperature, (4) solvents as carriers, and (5) molecular size. Because the stratum corneum plays a critical role in determining cutaneous permeability, removal of this layer causes a dramatic increase in permeability of the epidermis for a variety of large or small molecules, both lipid-soluble and water-soluble (Poet and McDougal, 2002). Caustic agents, such as acids and alkalis, that damage the stratum corneum increase its permeability. The most frequently encountered penetration-enhancing damage to the skin results from burns and various skin diseases. Water also plays an extremely important role in skin permeability. Under normal conditions, the stratum corneum is partially hydrated, containing about 7% water by weight. This amount of water increases the permeability of the stratum corneum approximately 10-fold over the permeability that exists when it is completely dry. On contact with water, the stratum corneum can increase its weight of tightly bound water up to 5-fold, which increases permeability an additional 2- to 3-fold. In many studies, the site of application will be covered with plastic wrap (occlusive application), originally described by Draize *et al.* (1944), to hydrate the stratum corneum and enhance the absorption of some toxicants. Similarly, an increase in temperature will increase dermal penetration by increasing dermal blood flow. This is particularly important for occupational exposures to chemicals such as insecticides in which agricultural workers are likely to be working strenuously at relatively high temperatures. Such environmental conditions increase dermal penetration and may increase the risk of systemic toxicity.

Solvents used to dissolve compounds of interest can also influence dermal penetration. In general, lower absorption will be observed if a toxicant is highly soluble in the vehicle, whereas low solubility of the toxicant in the vehicle will tend to increase dermal penetration. In addition, solvents such as dimethyl sulfoxide (DMSO) facilitate the penetration of toxicants through the skin by increasing the permeability of the stratum corneum. Although the mechanism by which DMSO enhances skin permeability is not fully understood, it has been suggested that it (1) removes much of the lipid matrix of the stratum corneum, making holes on artificial shunts in the penetration barrier; (2) alters keratin configuration to change protein structure; and (3) functions as a swelling agent (Williams and Berry, 2004).

With respect to molecular size, it is generally recognized that compounds above 400 Da exhibit poor dermal penetration. As such, nanoparticles may exhibit higher dermal absorption and systemic exposures in light of their small size. However, although nanoparticles appear to penetrate the skin as a function of their size, their overall absorption is relatively low. For nanomaterials, hair follicles can contribute to dermal penetration, and as a general rule, particles that are approximately 300 to 600 nm penetrate deeply in to hair follicles, where the extensive capillary network around the follicles facilitates uptake (Lademann *et al.*, 2011). Based on these features, nanoparticle formulations may facilitate absorption from the skin. In contrast, nanosized particles of titanium dioxide and zinc oxide, which are widely used in sunscreens, do not appear to penetrate beyond the stratum corneum, a feature that is consistent with their skin protective effects (Newman *et al.*, 2009).

Dermal absorption has been studied in most laboratory animals including rats, mice, rabbits, guinea pigs, primates, and pig, and dermal absorption varies widely across these species. As a general rule, dermal absorption across rodent skin is greater than human skin, whereas the cutaneous permeability characteristics of guinea pigs, pigs, and monkeys are more similar to those observed in humans (Wester and Maibach, 1993). Species differences in percutaneous absorption account for the differential toxicity of insecticides in insects and humans. For example, the LD_{50} of injected DDT is approximately equal in insects and mammals, but DDT is much less toxic to mammals than to insects when it is applied to the skin. This appears to be due to the fact that DDT is poorly absorbed through the skin of mammals but passes readily through the chitinous exoskeleton of insects. Furthermore, insects have a much greater body surface area relative to weight than mammals.

Species differences in dermal absorption of xenobiotics result from several anatomic, physiological, and biochemical factors (Dugard, 1983; Poet and McDougal, 2002). First, the composition and thickness of the stratum corneum along with the nature of the dermal appendages are highly variable across species. The stratum corneum is much thicker in humans than in most laboratory animals, making human skin typically less permeable than animal skin. However, the thinner stratum corneum in animals is often compensated for by a relatively thick hair cover, diminishing direct contact of the skin with a xenobiotic. Sweat and pilosebaceous ducts also vary across species. For example, eccrine sweat glands are located in the pads of the extremities of all mammals. However, the general body surface of humans contains 100 to 600/m^2 of coiled tubular sweat glands, whereas rodents, rabbits, cats, and dogs have none. The number of pilosebaceous ducts in humans and pigs is similar (about 40/cm^2), but rodents may have up to 100 times more. Another important potential rate-limiting step in the dermal absorption of chemicals is the cutaneous blood flow. In humans, the skin plays an important thermoregulatory function as opposed to furred animals. Consequently, there is a much more extensive vasculature in humans than in most mammals (Calabrese, 1984). Biotransformation reactions in skin can also facilitate absorption, and the presence of metabolizing enzymes is highly variable across species. Xenobiotic transporters, including members of the ABCC family and the SLCO and SLC families have been identified in skin with expression predominantly in keratinocytes. Differences in levels or patterns of expression of these transporters may also contribute to species differences in dermal absorption of toxicants (Kao *et al.*, 1985; Baron *et al.*, 2001).

Overall, commonly used laboratory animals are typically not good models of human absorption of toxicants. An example of the species differences and lack of concordance with human data for dermal absorption of the herbicide 2,4-dichlorophenoxyacetic acid (2,4-D) is illustrated in Table 5-9. As illustrated by these data, absorption through rat skin was higher than in other species. In general, absorption through primate or pig skin is considered to most closely predict human dermal absorption (Wester and Maibach, 1993). Additionally, in vitro methods using human skin may provide reasonable alternatives to the use of laboratory animals for evaluating dermal absorption of toxicants (Bronaugh *et al.*, 1982).

Absorption of Toxicants After Special Routes of Administration

Toxicants usually enter the bloodstream after absorption through the skin, lungs, or GI tract. However, in studying the effects of chemicals in laboratory animals, other routes of administration may also be used. The most common routes are (1) intravenous,

Table 5-9

Comparison of Dermal Absorption of 2,4-D Across Species

SPECIES	WASH TIME (HOUR)	COLLECTION TIME (HOUR)	% ABSORBED
Rat	24	336	20
Rabbit	24	336	12
Monkey	24	336	6
Human	4	120	3.7

NOTE: Data from Ross et al. (2005) and represent application of the dimethylamine salt of 2,4-dichlorophenoxyacetic acid (2,4-D). In all cases, the dose applied was 4 µg/cm². For rats, rabbits, and monkeys, the application site was washed after 24 hours, whereas human skin was washed after 4 hours. The collection time denotes the interval over which data were collected to determine absorption.

(2) intraperitoneal, (3) subcutaneous, and (4) intramuscular. The intravenous route introduces the toxicant directly into the bloodstream, eliminating the process of absorption. Intraperitoneal injection results in rapid absorption of xenobiotics because of the rich peritoneal and mesenteric blood supply and the relatively large surface area of the peritoneal cavity. In addition, this route of administration circumvents the delay and variability of gastric emptying. Intraperitoneally administered compounds are absorbed primarily through the portal circulation and therefore pass through the liver before reaching other organs. Subcutaneous and intramuscular injections usually result in slower absorption rates, but toxicants enter directly into the general circulation. The rate of absorption by these two routes can be altered by changing the blood flow to the injection site. For example, epinephrine causes vasoconstriction and will decrease the rate of absorption if it is coinjected intramuscularly with a toxicant. The formulation of a xenobiotic may also affect the rate of absorption, as toxicants are typically absorbed more slowly from suspensions than from solutions.

The toxicity of a chemical may or may not depend on the route of administration. If a toxicant is injected intraperitoneally, most of the chemical enters the liver via the portal circulation before reaching the general circulation. Therefore, with intraperitoneal administration, a compound may be completely extracted and biotransformed by the liver with subsequent excretion into bile without gaining access to the systemic circulation. Propranolol (Shand and Rangno, 1972) and lidocaine (Boyes *et al.*, 1970) are classical examples of drugs with efficient extraction during the first pass through the liver. A chemical with a high first-pass effect that is toxic in an organ other than the liver and GI tract is likely to be less toxic when administered

intraperitoneally than when administered by other routes (intravenously, intramuscularly, or subcutaneously) because the intraperitoneal route favors extraction in the liver to reduce what is available systemically. In contrast, compounds with no appreciable biotransformation in the liver are likely to show similar toxicity independent of the route of administration if the rates of absorption are equal. Therefore, preliminary information on the contribution of biotransformation and excretion of xenobiotics to toxic outcome can be derived by comparing toxic responses after administration by different routes.

DISTRIBUTION

After gaining entry into the bloodstream, regardless of route of exposure, a toxicant distributes to tissues throughout the body. The rate of distribution to organs or tissues is determined primarily by blood flow and the rate of diffusion out of the capillary bed into the cells of a particular organ or tissue, and usually occurs rapidly. The final distribution depends largely on the affinity of a xenobiotic for various tissues. In general, the initial phase of distribution is dominated by blood flow, whereas the eventual distribution is determined largely by affinity. The penetration of toxicants into cells occurs by passive diffusion or special transport processes, as discussed previously. Small water-soluble molecules and ions apparently diffuse through aqueous channels or pores in the cell membrane. Lipid-soluble molecules readily permeate the membrane itself. Very polar molecules and ions of even moderate size (molecular weight of 50 or more) cannot enter cells easily except by special transport mechanisms because they are surrounded by a hydration shell, making their actual size much larger.

Volume of Distribution

A key concept in understanding the disposition of a toxicant is its volume of distribution (Vd), a primary determinant of the concentration of a toxicant in blood that is used to quantify distribution throughout the body. It is defined as the volume in which the amount of drug would need to be uniformly dissolved in order to produce the observed blood concentration. Total body water is derived from that which is either extracellular or intracellular and represents three distinct compartments: plasma water and interstitial water comprise the extracellular compartment and are distinguished from intracellular water (Box 5-3). If a chemical distributes only to the plasma compartment (no tissue distribution), it has a high plasma concentration and hence, a low Vd. In contrast, if a chemical distributes throughout the body (total body water), the effective plasma concentration is low and hence, a high Vd. However, the distribution of toxicants is complex and under most circumstances cannot be simply equated with distribution into one of the water compartments of the body. Binding to and/

Box 5-3

Estimates of the Size of the Major Compartments That Contribute to Volume of Distribution

COMPARTMENT	PERCENTAGE OF TOTAL	LITER IN 70-kg HUMAN	PLASMA CONCENTRATION AFTER 1 g OF CHEMICAL (mg/L)
Plasma water	4.5	3	333
Total extracellular water	20	14	71
Total body water	55	38	26
Tissue binding	—	—	0–25

or dissolution in various storage sites of the body, such as fat, liver, and bone, are usually more important factors in determining the distribution of chemicals.

Some toxicants do not readily cross cell membranes and therefore have restricted distribution, whereas other toxicants rapidly pass through cell membranes and are distributed throughout the body. Some toxicants selectively accumulate in certain parts of the body as a result of protein binding, active transport, or high solubility in fat. The target organ for toxicity may be the site of accumulation, but this is not always the case. If a toxicant accumulates at a site other than the target organ or tissue, the accumulation is likely to be protective because plasma levels and consequently its concentration at the site of action is reduced. In this case, it is assumed that the chemical in the storage depot is toxicologically inactive. However, a chemical in a storage depot is also in equilibrium with the free fraction of the toxicant in plasma, so that it is released into the circulation as the unbound fraction of toxicant is eliminated. Examples illustrating a wide range of Vd are noted in Table 5-10, and the factors that contribute to the Vd are discussed below.

Storage of Toxicants in Tissues

Because only the free fraction of a chemical is in equilibrium throughout the body, binding to or dissolving in certain body constituents greatly alters the distribution of a xenobiotic. Some xenobiotics attain their highest concentrations at the site of toxic action, such as carbon monoxide, which has a very high affinity for hemoglobin, and paraquat, which accumulates in the lungs. Other chemicals concentrate at sites other than the target organ. For example, lead is stored in bone, but manifestations of lead poisoning appear in soft tissues. The compartment where a toxicant is concentrated is described as a storage depot. Toxicants in these depots are always in equilibrium with the free fraction in plasma, so that as a chemical is biotransformed or excreted from the body, more is released

Table 5-10

Examples of Factors that Contribute to Volume of Distribution (Vd)

COMPOUND	Vd (L/kg)	FACTORS INFLUENCING DISTRIBUTION
Warfarin	0.1	High plasma protein binding with little distribution into tissues
Ethanol	0.5	Distribution in total body water
Propranolol	4.3	Distributed to peripheral tissues
Tamoxifen	50	Extensive distribution to peripheral tissues and high protein binding
Chloroquine	100	High tissue uptake and trapping in lysosomes

from the storage site. As a result, the biological half-life of stored compounds can be very long.

Plasma Proteins as Storage Depot Binding to plasma proteins is the major site of protein binding, and several different plasma proteins bind xenobiotics and some endogenous constituents of the body. As depicted in Fig. 5-8, albumin is the major protein in plasma and it binds many different compounds. α_1-Acid glycoprotein, although present at a much lower concentration than albumin, is also an important protein in plasma, and compounds with basic characteristics tend to bind to it. Transferrin, a β-globulin, is important for the transport of iron in the body. The other major metal-binding protein in plasma is ceruloplasmin, which carries copper. The α- and β-lipoproteins are very important in the transport of

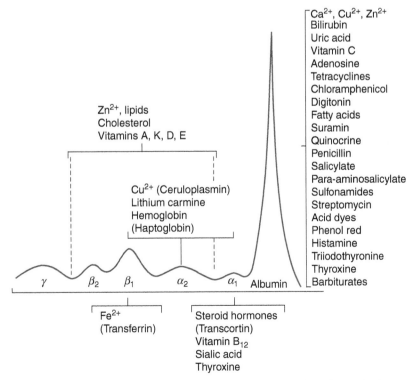

Figure 5-8. *Schematic representation of the electrophoretic separation of plasma proteins and xenobiotics that interact with these proteins.*

lipid-soluble compounds such as vitamins, cholesterol, and steroid hormones as well as xenobiotics. Plasma γ-globulins are antibodies that function specifically in immunological reactions. Overall, plasma proteins bind acidic compounds such as phenylbutazone, basic compounds such as imipramine, and neutral compounds such as digitoxin.

Albumin, present in the plasma at a concentration of 500 to 600 μM, is the most abundant protein in plasma and serves as both a depot and multivalent transport protein for many endogenous and exogenous compounds. Protein–ligand interactions occur primarily as a result of hydrophobic forces, hydrogen bonding, and Van der Waals forces. Because of their high molecular weight, plasma proteins and the toxicants bound to them cannot cross capillary walls. Consequently, the fraction of a toxicant bound to plasma proteins is not immediately available for distribution into the extravascular space or filtration by the kidneys. However, the interaction of a chemical with plasma proteins is a reversible process, and as unbound chemical diffuses out of capillaries, bound chemical dissociates from the protein until the free fraction reaches equilibrium between the vascular space and the extravascular space. In turn, diffusion in the extravascular space to sites more distant from the capillaries continues, and the resulting concentration gradient provides the thermodynamic force for continued dissociation of the bound fraction in plasma. Active transport processes are not limited by the binding of chemicals to plasma proteins.

The binding of toxicants to plasma proteins is usually determined by equilibrium dialysis or ultrafiltration. The total amount in plasma is determined prior to these separation methods, and the fraction that passes through a dialysis membrane or appears in the ultrafiltrate is the unbound (or free) fraction. The bound fraction is determined as the difference between the total and unbound fractions. The extent of plasma protein binding varies considerably among xenobiotics. Some, such as antipyrine, are not bound; others, such as secobarbital, are bound to about 50%; and some, such as warfarin, are 99% bound. For warfarin, the high protein binding is the single most important determinant of its Vd, which is limited to the plasma compartment (Table 5-10).

The binding of chemicals to plasma proteins is an important concept in toxicology for two reasons. Toxicity is typically manifested by the amount of a xenobiotic that is unbound. Therefore, a compound with a high degree of plasma protein binding may not show toxicity when compared to one that is less extensively bound to plasma proteins. Ironically, a high degree of protein binding also tends to increase the risk of adverse effects resulting from interactions with other highly bound compounds. In particular, severe toxic reactions can occur if a toxicant with a high degree of protein binding is displaced from plasma proteins by another chemical, increasing the free fraction of the toxicant in plasma. This interaction increases the equilibrium concentration of the toxicant in a target organ, thereby increasing the potential for toxicity. For example, if a compound is 99.9% bound to plasma protein (0.1% free), then an interaction that decreases protein binding to 99.5%, which may seem to be a minor change, is effectively a 5-fold increase in the free plasma concentration (0.5% free). Most research on the adverse interactions associated with binding of xenobiotics to plasma proteins has been conducted with drugs. For example, if a strongly bound sulfonamide is given concurrently with an antidiabetic drug, the sulfonamide may displace the antidiabetic drug and induce a hypoglycemic coma. Similarly, interactions resulting from displacement of warfarin can lead to inappropriate blood clotting and possible deleterious effects. Xenobiotics can also compete with and displace endogenous compounds that are bound to plasma

Table 5-11

Plasma Protein Binding and Half-life of Clofibric Acid in the Mouse, Rat, and Man

SPECIES	PLASMA PROTEIN BINDING (%)	HALF-LIFE (HR)
Human	97	21
Rat	75	6
Mouse	45	2

SOURCE: Data from Cayen (1980).

proteins. The importance of this phenomenon was demonstrated in a notable clinical trial comparing the efficacy of tetracycline with that of a penicillin–sulfonamide mixture in the management of bacterial infections in premature infants (Silverman et al., 1956). The penicillin–sulfonamide mixture led to much higher mortality than did the tetracycline because the sulfonamide displaced a considerable amount of bilirubin from albumin. Free bilirubin then diffused into the brain of the newborns (because the BBB is not fully developed), causing a severe form of brain damage termed kernicterus. In addition to drugs, some chemicals, such as the insecticide dieldrin, also bind avidly to plasma proteins (99%). Therefore, it is to be expected that chemical–chemical interactions that alter plasma protein binding occur with many different xenobiotics.

Plasma protein binding can also give rise to species differences in the disposition of xenobiotics. For example, plasma protein binding of clofibric acid is considerably different between mice, rats, and humans and correlates with the half-lives of this compound in these species (Table 5-11). Because clofibric acid is primarily eliminated in all three species by renal glomerular filtration without tubular reabsorption, differences in the free fraction of this compound in plasma across the species contribute to the observed species differences in drug half-life. Additional factors that influence plasma protein binding across species include differences in the concentration of albumin, in binding affinity, and/or in competitive binding of endogenous substances.

Liver and Kidney as Storage Depots The liver and kidney have a high capacity for binding many chemicals. These two organs probably concentrate more toxicants than do all the other organs combined, and, in most cases, active transport or binding to tissue components are likely to be involved.

Hepatic uptake of lead illustrates how rapidly liver binds foreign compounds: just 30 minutes after a single dose, the concentration of lead in liver is 50 times higher than the concentration in plasma (Klaassen and Shoeman, 1974). In addition, some proteins serve to sequester xenobiotics in the liver or kidney. For example, metallothionein (MT), a specialized metal-binding protein, sequesters both essential and toxic metals including zinc and cadmium (Cd) with high affinities in the kidney and liver. In liver, Cd bound to MT serves to concentrate and sequester the heavy metal while preventing its excretion into bile. In kidney, however, the Cd–MT complex is very toxic and is mechanistically involved in the chronic toxicity of Cd (Klaassen and Liu, 1997). Another protein that sequesters certain toxicants in the kidney is α2u-globulin. This protein, which is synthesized in large quantities only in male rats, binds to a diverse array of xenobiotics including metabolites of D-limonene (a major constituent of orange juice) and 2,4,4-trimethylpentane (found in unleaded gasoline). The chemical-α2u-globulin complex is taken up by the kidney, where it accumulates within the lysosomal compartment and damages the proximal tubule cells. Ultimately, the accumulation of this complex in the kidney is responsible for male-rat specific nephrotoxicity and carcinogenicity (Lehman-McKeeman, 2010).

As noted in Table 5-10, chloroquine has a very high Vd, which is determined largely by extensive storage in peripheral tissues. This compound is an example of a wide range of chemicals referred to as cationic amphiphiles. At physiological pH, chloroquine is non-ionized, but once in cells, it is taken up into the acidic milieu of the lysosome where it becomes highly ionized (as per Henderson–Hasselbalch equations) and is subsequently trapped in this compartment. A variety of xenobiotics share these attributes, which ultimately lead to lysosomal dysfunction and the accumulation of phospholipids, referred to as phospholipidosis (Hanumegowda *et al.*, 2010).

Fat as Storage Depot There are many organic compounds that are highly stable and lipophilic, leading to their accumulation in the environment. The lipophilic nature of these compounds also permits rapid penetration of cell membranes and uptake by tissues, and it is not surprising that highly lipophilic toxicants are distributed and concentrated in body fat where they are retained for a very long time. The environmental accumulation and potential toxicological significance of long-term storage of numerous compounds including the pesticides aldrin, chlordane, DDT, dieldrin, endrin, heptachlor, mirex, and toxaphene, along with polychlorinated and polybrominated biphenyls, polybrominated flame retardants, dioxins, and furans is a major issue in toxicology. There is extensive research efforts designed to assess the potential for these compounds to produce carcinogenic, developmental, and endocrine effects, which is directly related to their accumulation and storage in body fat (Jandacek and Tso, 2001).

Toxicants appear to accumulate in fat by dissolution in neutral fats, which constitute about 50% and 20% of the body weight of obese individuals and lean athletic individuals, respectively. Thus, toxicants with a high lipid/water partition coefficient may be stored in body fat, and higher amounts are likely to be retained in obese individuals. Storage lowers the concentration of the toxicant in the target organ such that toxicity is likely to be less severe in an obese person than in a lean individual. However, of more practical toxicological concern is the possibility that a sudden increase in the concentration of a chemical in blood and the target organ of toxicity may occur if rapid mobilization from fat occurs. Several studies have shown that signs of intoxication can be produced by short-term starvation of experimental animals that were previously exposed to persistent organochlorine insecticides.

There have been numerous attempts to alter storage of lipophilic toxins in adipose tissues in animal models and humans. Changes in body fat composition appear to be the most effective in reducing body burdens, and interventions designed to reduce the absorption of these compounds from the GI tract appear to be somewhat helpful in reducing storage depots of persistent organic pollutants in fat (Jandacek and Tso, 2001).

Bone as Storage Depot Compounds such as fluoride, lead, and strontium may be incorporated and stored in the bone matrix. For example, 90% of the lead in the body is eventually found in the skeleton. Skeletal uptake of xenobiotics is essentially a surface chemistry phenomenon, with exchange taking place between the bone surface and the fluid in contact with it. The fluid is the extracellular fluid, and the surface is that of the hydroxyapatite crystals of bone mineral. Many of those crystals are very small, resulting in a large surface area relative to the mass of the bone. The extracellular fluid brings the toxicant into contact with the hydration shell

of the hydroxyapatite, allowing diffusion through it and penetration of the crystal surface. As a result of similarities in size and charge, F⁻ may readily displace OH⁻, whereas lead or strontium may substitute for calcium in the hydroxyapatite lattice matrix through an exchange–adsorption reaction.

Foreign compounds deposited in bone are not sequestered irreversibly by that tissue. Toxicants can be released from the bone by ionic exchange at the crystal surface and dissolution of bone crystals through osteoclastic activity. An increase in osteolytic activity such as that seen after parathyroid hormone administration leads to enhanced mobilization of hydroxyapatite lattice, which can be reflected in an increased plasma concentration of toxicants. Ultimately, deposition and storage of toxicants in bone may or may not be detrimental. Lead is not toxic to bone, but the chronic effects of fluoride deposition (skeletal fluorosis) and radioactive strontium (osteosarcoma and other neoplasms) are well documented.

Blood–Brain Barrier

Access to the brain is restricted by the presence of two barriers: the BBB and the blood–cerebral spinal fluid barrier (BCSFB). Although neither represents an absolute barrier to the passage of toxic chemicals into the CNS, many toxicants do not enter the brain in appreciable quantities because of these barriers.

The BBB is formed primarily by the endothelial cells of blood capillaries in the brain (Fig. 5-9). Each endothelial cell forms a tight junction with adjacent cells, essentially forming a tight seal between the cells and preventing diffusion of polar compounds through paracellular pathways. Diffusion of more lipophilic compounds through endothelial cell membranes is counteracted by xenobiotic efflux transporters present in the endothelial cells. Glial cells, particularly astrocytes, contribute to the BBB by secreting chemical factors that modulate endothelial cell permeability, and astrocytes and perivascular microglial cells extend processes that support the integrity of the BBB. For small- to medium-sized water-soluble molecules, the tighter junctions of the capillary endothelium and the lipid membranes of the glial cell processes represent the major barrier. Although the absorption of lipid-soluble compounds is favored in the brain, such compounds must traverse the membranes of the endothelial cells, not be substrates for xenobiotic transporters, and then traverse the glial cell processes to enter the brain.

Although the BBB is a physical structure that limits distribution to the brain, active transport processes also play a pivotal role in determining the concentration of xenobiotics in the brain. Numerous ATP-dependent transporters have been identified as part of the BBB, comprising various members of the ABC and SLC families (Fig. 5-9) (Kusuhara and Sugiyama, 2005; Deeken and Loscher, 2007; Miller, 2010). Efflux transporters, including MDR1, BCRP, MRP1, 2, 4, and 5 are located on the apical (blood side)

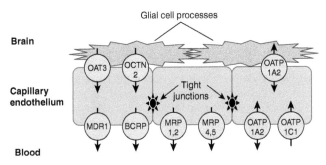

Figure 5-9. *Schematic model showing the xenobiotic transporting systems that contribute to the human blood–brain barrier.*

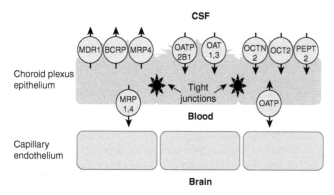

Figure 5-10. *Schematic model showing the xenobiotic transporting systems that contribute to the human blood–cerebral spinal fluid barrier.*

plasma membrane and function to move xenobiotics absorbed into the capillary endothelial cells out into the blood, thereby limiting distribution into the brain. Uptake transporters, including OATP1A2 and OATP1C1 are found on both the basolateral and apical side of the endothelium, and can drive a concentrative efflux if coupled energetically to the electrical potential difference across the endothelial cell membrane. OATP1C1 is suggested to specifically transport thyroid hormone into the brain. Finally, uptake transporters on the apical membranes include OAT3 and CTN2. In combination, these transporters can efficiently efflux a wide range of anionic, cationic, uncharged, and numerous drug conjugates from the brain.

The BCSFB is found between the circulating blood and the circulating cerebral spinal fluid in the brain (Fig. 5-10). It comprises elements of the choroid plexus, the arachnoid membrane, and certain periventricular locations (including the area postrema). The choroid plexus has highly permeable endothelial cells on the blood side but is lined by epithelial cells on the CSF side that form the barrier. Xenobiotic transporters also contribute to removing compounds that may enter the endothelial cells. Blood flow through the choroid plexus is about 10 times higher than in the brain, a feature that provides the high turnover of biological fluids necessary to support the dynamic changes in nutrients required for neuronal function. Furthermore, the protein concentration in CSF is much lower than that in other body fluids. The low protein content of the CSF also limits the movement of water-insoluble compounds by paracellular transport, which is possible in a largely aqueous medium only when such compounds are bound to proteins. In general, toxicants achieve concentrations in the CSF that are no higher than the concentration of the unbound toxicant in the plasma. The BCSFB is more of an anatomical entity than a true barrier, but it does provide some protection against the distribution of toxicants to the CNS, thereby affording some protection against toxicity.

Xenobiotic transporters are also expressed in the epithelial cells of the choroid plexus, but within the BSCFB, MDR1 and Mrp1 are thought to play the most important roles (Fig. 5-10). In this barrier, MDR1 is expressed on the luminal side, with efflux from the choroidal epithelial cells into the CSF. In contrast, MRP1 is expressed on the basolateral side of the choroidal epithelium, catalyzing the transport of xenobiotics out of the cells and into the vascular compartment, and it has been suggested that MDR1 and MRP1 may play an important function to coordinate the absorption and secretion of toxicants into the CNS at the BSCFB (Deeken and Loscher, 2007). Members of the OATP, OAT, OCT, and PEPT families are also expressed in the choroid plexus (Klaassen and Aleksunes, 2010). The function of these proteins is not well

characterized, but studies in rodents suggest that Oatps, particularly Oatp1a4, play an important role in regulating xenobiotic concentrations in the CSF.

The importance of transport processes to the maintenance of the BBB has been demonstrated in genetically modified mouse models. Compounds that are substrates for MDR1 achieve much higher brain levels in P-gp null (Mdr1a$^{-/-}$/Mdr1b$^{-/-}$) mice relative to wild-type mice, and are likely to show increased toxicity as well. Seminal studies demonstrated that MDR1 null mice were far more sensitive to the insecticide, ivermectin, and the anticancer agent, vinblastine. The brain uptake of these compounds was increased 26- and 80-fold, respectively, and the sensitivity to neurotoxicity or lethality was increased up to 100-fold (Schinkel *et al.*, 1994; Lankas *et al.*, 1997). Expression of Mrp1 in the choroid plexus has been shown to modulate the concentrations of toxicants in the cerebral spinal fluid, but no studies have yet shown a correlation to neurotoxic potential relative to Mrp1 function.

In addition to their role in regulating distribution of xenobiotics into the CNS, transporter function is also implicated in neurological diseases. MDR1 and BCRP contribute to the efflux of β-amyloid from the brain. This protein is known to accumulate in Alzheimer's disease, and there is evidence that MDR1 levels are decreased in Alzheimer's patients, with a concomitant increase in BCRP expression. There is also ongoing work to determine the potential for MDR1 to remove toxicants from the brain in a manner that may ultimately be protective against the development of Parkinson's disease (Miller, 2010). These observations require more research, with particular emphasis on how altered transporter function or expression may be affected by toxicant exposures that could contribute to human diseases.

The effectiveness of the BBB varies from one area of the brain to another. For example, the cortex, the lateral nuclei of the hypothalamus, the area postrema, the pineal body, and the posterior lobe of the hypophysis are more permeable than are other areas of the brain. It is not clear whether this is due to the increased blood supply to those areas, or because the BSCFB represents a more permeable barrier, or both. In general, the entrance of toxicants into the brain follows the same principle that applies to transfer across other cells in the body. Only the free fraction of a toxicant (ie, not bound to plasma proteins) equilibrates rapidly with the brain. Lipid solubility plays an important role in determining the rate of entry of a compound into the CNS, as does the degree of ionization, as discussed earlier. Lipid solubility enhances the rate of penetration of toxicants into the CNS, whereas ionization greatly diminishes it. 2-PAM, a quaternary nitrogen derivative, does not readily penetrate the brain and is ineffective in reversing the inhibition of brain cholinesterase caused by organophosphate insecticides. Some very lipophilic compounds may enter the brain but are so efficiently removed by xenobiotic transporters that they do not reach appreciable concentrations. This is particularly true for agents such as cyclosporin. TCDD, which is highly lipophilic, is also not readily distributed into the brain, but it is not known whether transporters influence its distribution to the brain. It is likely that strong binding to plasma proteins or lipoproteins, as well as the composition of the brain (mainly phospholipids), limits the entry of very lipophilic compounds into the brain. Some xenobiotics, although very few, may enter the brain by carrier-mediated processes. For example, methylmercury combines with cysteine, forming a sulfhydryl complex that is similar to methionine, which can be utilized as the large neutral amino acid carrier of the capillary endothelial cells for uptake into the brain (Clarkson, 1987).

The BBB is not fully developed at birth, and this is one reason why some chemicals are more toxic in newborns than adults. The

Table 5-12

Features of the Placental Barrier Based on Separation of Fetal and Maternal Blood

TYPE	SPECIES	MATERNAL TISSUE ENDOTHELIUM	CONNECTIVE TISSUE	EPITHELIUM
Epitheliochorial	Pig, horse, donkey	+	+	+
Synepitheliochorial	Cow, sheep, goat	+	+	−
Endotheliochorial	Cat, dog, elephant	+	−	−
Hemochorial	Human, monkey	−	−	−
Hemoendothelial	Rat, rabbit, guinea pig	−	−	−

Fetal layers that separate maternal and fetal blood also include the endothelial, connective tissue, and epithelial components in all types of placentas.
In the hemoendothelial type, only the fetal epithelium is present.
SOURCE: Modified from Morris et al. (1994), Enders and Carter (2004).

example of kernicterus resulting from increased brain levels of bilirubin in infants was noted earlier. In addition, morphine is 3 to 10 times more toxic to newborn than to adult rats because of the higher permeability of the brain of a newborn to morphine. Similarly, lead produces encephalomyelopathy in newborn rats but not in adults, apparently because of differences in the stages of development of the BBB.

Passage of Toxicants Across the Placenta

The term placental barrier has been associated with the concept that the main function of the placenta is to protect the fetus against the passage of noxious substances from the mother. However, the placenta is a multifunctional organ that also provides nutrition for the conceptus, exchanges maternal and fetal blood gases, disposes of fetal excretory material, and maintains pregnancy through complex hormonal regulation. Placental structure and function show more species differences than any other mammalian organ. Anatomically, the placental barrier consists of several cell layers interposed between the fetal and maternal circulations, but the number of cell layers varies across species and with the stage of gestation. The maximum number of cell layers in placentas is 6 (3 maternal and 3 fetal layers), and when all 6 layers are present, the placenta is termed epitheliochorial (Table 5-12). Those in which the maternal epithelium is absent are referred to as syndesmochorial. When only the endothelial layer of the maternal tissue remains, the tissue is termed endotheliochorial; when even the endothelium is gone (as in humans), the chorionic villi bathe in the maternal blood, and the tissue is called hemochorial. In some species, the maternal layers are absent along with the fetal endothelial and connective tissue, and these are called hemoendothelial. Within the same species, the placenta may also change its histological classification during gestation. For example, at the beginning of gestation, the placenta of a rabbit has 6 major layers (epitheliochorial), and at the end it has only one (hemoendothelial). Overall, there are marked species differences in placental structure. The animal models that are most similar to the organization of the human placenta based on its hemochorial histological organization are rodents and primates, but the decidual nature of the rodent placenta still differs markedly from that of humans (Myllynen et al., 2005; Leiser and Kauffman, 1994).

Most of the vital nutrients necessary for the development of the fetus are transported by active transport systems. For example, vitamins, amino acids, essential sugars, and ions such as calcium and iron are transported from mother to fetus against

a concentration gradient (Ganapathy et al., 2000). In contrast, most toxic chemicals pass the placenta by simple diffusion. The only exceptions are a few antimetabolites that are structurally similar to endogenous purines and pyrimidines, which are the physiological substrates for active transport from the maternal to the fetal circulation. The placenta also has biotransformation capabilities that may prevent some toxic substances from reaching the fetus (Syme et al., 2004; Prouillac and Lecoeur, 2010). Among the substances that cross the placenta by passive diffusion, more lipid-soluble substances rapidly attain a maternal–fetal equilibrium. Under steady-state conditions, concentrations of a toxic compound in the plasma of the mother and fetus are usually the same.

Many foreign substances can cross the placenta, and the same factors that dictate the passage of xenobiotics across biological membranes are important determinants of the placental transfer. These include previously discussed attributes including degree of ionization, lipophilicity, protein binding, and molecular weight along with blood flow and the concentration gradient across the barrier. In addition to chemicals, viruses (eg, rubella virus), cellular pathogens (eg, syphilis spirochetes), and globulin antibodies can traverse the placenta. In this regard, the placental barrier is not as precise an anatomical unit like the BBB. The human placenta includes the syncytiotrophoblast and cytotrophoblast layers. The apical membrane of the syncytiotrophoblast, which forms a continuous epithelial layer, is bathed in maternal blood and the basolateral surface is in contact with the discontinuous cytotrophoblast layer, the stromal tissue, or the fetal vasculature. To reach the fetus, toxins must traverse the apical and basolateral membranes of the syncytiotrophoblast as well as the endothelium of the fetal capillaries. Xenobiotic transporters are differentially expressed in these various cells and contribute to the barrier function that restricts distribution of toxicants to the fetus. The transporters are also critical to the movement of nutrients from the maternal circulation to the fetus along with the transfer of toxicants or waste products from the fetus back to the maternal circulation. Of the various cells in the placenta, the syncytiotrophoblasts appear to have the most extensive cohort of xenobiotics transporters (Fig. 5-11). In particular, BCRP is highly expressed in these cells. In fact, BCRP expression is highest in the human placenta relative to any other organ. BCRP, MDR1, and several MRPs are also expressed on the apical border of the syncytiotrophoblast where they play important roles in protecting the fetus from toxicants while regulating the movement of essential nutrients. Several uptake transporters are also expressed on the apical membrane, including OCTNs and OATPs. In contrast,

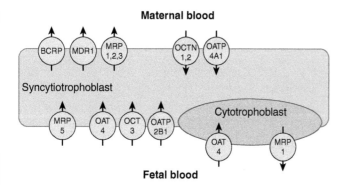

Figure 5-11. *Schematic model showing the transport systems that contribute to the barrier function of the human placenta.*

the efflux transporter, MRP5 is expressed on the basolateral side of the synctiotrophoblast along with uptake transporters including OAT4, OCT3, and OATP2B1. Expression of transporters in other cells of the placenta is less characterized, but it appears that the cytotrophoblasts express MRP1 and OAT4 (Prouillac and Lecoeur, 2010; Klaassen and Aleksunes, 2010).

There are several examples illustrating that placental transporters protect the developing fetus from toxicant exposure and possible abnormal development. For example, the fetal concentration of the antibiotic nitrofurantoin is increased 5-fold in Bcrp-null mice, demonstrating that it prevents fetal exposure to this drug (Zhang *et al.*, 2007). Furthermore, homozygous offspring of female MDR1 null mice (Mdr1a$^{-/-}$/Mdr1b$^{-/-}$) develop cleft palate when treated with a photoisomer of avermectin, whereas heterozygous littermates showed intermediate susceptibility and wild-type mice were resistant to this adverse effect (Lankas *et al.*, 1998). Finally, it has been shown that some anticonvulsants, including known developmental toxicants such as valproic acid and phenytoin (see Chap. 10), inhibit OCTN2 function in human placental membrane vesicles (Wu *et al.*, 2004). This transporter is critical for the uptake of carnitine, leading to the hypothesis that inhibition of carnitine uptake by valproic acid (or other drugs) with subsequent fetal deficiency of carnitine may be involved in the adverse developmental effects associated with a variety of anticonvulsant drugs.

Despite the presence of biotransformation systems and xenobiotic transporters designed to nourish and protect the fetus, the transfer of xenobiotics across the placenta can still occur. One important consequence of placental transfer is that of transplacental carcinogenesis. In this case exposing the mother during gestation increases the likelihood of tumor development in the offspring later in life (see Chap. 8). The most well-known transplacental carcinogen in humans is diethylstilbestrol (Newbold and McLachlan, 1996), but other compounds such as the antiviral drug zidovudine (Diwan *et al.*, 1999) and inorganic arsenic (Waalkes *et al.*, 2003; Tokar *et al.*, 2011) induce tumors in mice when exposed to these chemicals only during gestation.

Redistribution of Toxicants

The most critical factors that affect the distribution of xenobiotics are the organ blood flow and its affinity for a xenobiotic. The initial phase of distribution is determined primarily by blood flow to the various parts of the body. Therefore, a well-perfused organ such as the liver may attain high initial concentrations of a xenobiotic. However, chemicals may have a high affinity for a binding site (eg, intracellular protein or bone matrix) or to a cellular constituent (eg, fat), and with time, will redistribute to these high affinity sites. For example, although 50% of a dose of lead

is found in the liver two hours after administration, one month later, 90% of the lead remaining in the body is associated with the crystal lattice of bone. Similarly, persistent organic pollutants do not distribute rapidly to fat, but accumulate selectively in adipose tissue over time.

EXCRETION

Toxicants are eliminated from the body by several routes. The kidney is perhaps the most important organ for the excretion of xenobiotics because more chemicals are eliminated from the body by this route than by any other (see Chap. 14). Biotransformation to more water-soluble products is usually a prerequisite to the excretion of xenobiotics through urine (see Chap. 6). The second important route of elimination of many xenobiotics is through feces, and the third, primarily for gases, is through the lungs. Biliary excretion of xenobiotics and/or their metabolites is most often the major source of fecal excretion, but a number of other sources can be significant for some compounds. All body secretions appear to have the ability to excrete chemicals; toxicants have been found in sweat, saliva, tears, and milk.

Urinary Excretion

The kidney is a very efficient organ for the elimination of toxicants from the body. The functional unit of the kidney is the nephron, comprising the glomerulus, a capillary tuft that initiates the process of filtration of the blood, and tubular elements within the renal cortex and medulla that function to produce and concentrate urine. Toxic compounds are excreted in urine by the same mechanisms the kidney uses to remove the end products of intermediary metabolism from the body, including glomerular filtration, tubular excretion by passive diffusion, and active tubular secretion. In general, the excretion of small molecular weight (<350 Da), water-soluble compounds is favored in urine.

The kidney receives about 25% of the cardiac output, about 20% of which is filtered at the glomeruli. The glomerular capillaries have large pores (approximately 70 nm), which filter compounds up to a molecular weight of about 60 kDa (smaller than albumin). Thus, the degree of plasma protein binding affects the rate of glomerular filtration because protein–xenobiotic complexes, particularly those bound to albumin, will not be filtered. Glomerular filtration rates vary considerably across species, ranging from a high of approximately 10 mL/min/kg in mice to about 1.8 mL/min/kg in humans. This difference appears to be determined by the relative number of nephrons per kilogram of body weight, with mice being the highest (Lin, 1995; Walton *et al.*, 2004).

A toxicant filtered at the glomerulus may remain in the tubular lumen and be excreted in urine. Depending on the physicochemical properties of a compound, it may be reabsorbed across the tubular cells of the nephron back into the bloodstream. The principles governing the reabsorption of toxicants across the kidney tubules are the same as those discussed earlier in this chapter for passive diffusion across cell membranes. Thus, toxicants with a high lipid/water partition coefficient are reabsorbed efficiently, whereas polar compounds and ions are excreted in urine. The pH of urine may vary but it is usually slightly acidic (approximately 6–6.5). Just as the Henderson–Hasselbach calculations determine the absorption of nonionized compounds from the GI tract, they also determine urinary excretion. In this case, urinary excretion of the ionized moiety is favored, such that bases are excreted to a greater extent at lower pH whereas excretion of acids predominates at higher urinary pH. A practical application of this knowledge is illustrated by the treatment of phenobarbital poisoning with sodium bicarbonate. The percentage of ionization is increased markedly within physiologically attainable pH ranges for a weak organic acid such as phenobarbital (pK_a = 7.2) such that alkalinization of urine increases the fraction of drug in the ionized state, thereby increasing the urinary excretion of phenobarbital. Similarly, excretion of salicylate can be accelerated by administering sodium bicarbonate. In a similar manner, urinary acidification can be used to increase the excretion of a weak base such as phencyclidine (PCP) in drug abusers.

Toxic agents can also be excreted from plasma into urine by passive diffusion through the tubule. This process is probably of minor significance because filtration is much faster than excretion by passive diffusion through the tubules, providing a favorable concentration gradient for reabsorption rather than excretion. Exceptions to this generalization may be some organic acids ($pK_a \approx$ 3–5) and bases ($pK_a \approx$ 7–9) that would be largely ionized and thus trapped at the pH of urine (pH $\approx$ 6). For renal excretion of such compounds, the flow of urine is likely to be important for the maintenance of a concentration gradient, favoring excretion. Thus, diuretics can hasten the elimination of weak organic acids and bases because they increase urine flow.

Xenobiotics can also be excreted into urine by active secretion. This process involves the uptake of toxicants from the blood into the cells of the renal proximal tubule, with subsequent efflux from the cell into the tubular fluid from which urine is formed. Fig. 5-12 illustrates the various families of transporters expressed in the human kidney that are directly involved in xenobiotic disposition. There are numerous other transporters such as specific glucose transporters or nucleotide transporters that play a role predominantly in the flux of endogenous substances, which are not presented here. Transporters may be expressed on the apical cell membrane where efflux pumps contribute to tubular secretion and influx pumps are important for reabsorption. Transporters localized to the basolateral membranes serve to transport xenobiotics to and from the systemic circulation or the renal tubular cells and also contribute to reabsorptive and excretory processes. Renal functional activity, as may be altered by toxicant exposure, can also be evaluated by determining the renal clearance of transporter substrates such as the widely used organic anion, p-aminohippurate (PAH).

Transporters expressed on the basolateral side of the renal tubules in humans that contribute mainly to excretion include OATs,

OCTs, and OATP4C1. The OAT family is a major contributor to urinary excretion as these proteins mediate the renal uptake of organic acids such as PAH and the renal exchange of dicarboxylates. In humans, OAT1, 2, 3 are expressed on the basolateral membrane, whereas OAT4 is localized to the brush-border membrane. In contrast, in rodents, Oat1 and 3 are localized to the basolateral membranes. Although the OATs play an important role in the physiological exchange of metabolites in the kidney, they can also contribute to the development of renal toxicity. In particular, the clinical use of antiviral drugs cidofovir and adefovir is limited by nephrotoxicity that is mediated by the accumulation of these drugs in the proximal tubule by OAT1 (Ho et al., 2000). Additionally, OAT1 mediates the uptake of methylmercury and ochratoxin A, and as such, may play a role in the nephrotoxicity associated with these toxicants (Rizwan and Burckhardt, 2007).

The OCT family is responsible for the renal uptake of some cations, particularly those of low molecular weight. Substrates for OCTs include endogenous compounds such as choline, tetraethylammonium (TEA), and certain cationic drugs including cisplatin, cimetidine, metformin, and acyclovir. OCT2 is highly expressed in human kidney, whereas Oct1 and 2 are expressed on the basolateral membranes of the rodent kidney (Shitara et al., 2005). The antineoplastic drug, cisplatin, is a substrate and inhibitor of OCT2, and the dose-limiting nephrotoxicity associated with this drug may be directly related to uptake-mediated concentration of drug in the proximal tubule epithelium (Zolk and Fromm, 2011).

A second cation transporter is OCTN, and 2 isoforms, OCTN1 and OCTN2 are localized to the brush-border membranes in human and rodent kidney. Substrates include cations such as TEA, and OCTN2 is particularly important in the renal reabsorption of carnitine, which is an essential cofactor for fatty acid β-oxidation.

In kidney, peptide transporters, localized to the brush-border membrane of the proximal tubule are important for the reuptake of di- and tripeptides. Two transporters, PEPT1 and PEPT2 have been identified in the human and rodent kidney, with PEPT1 localized in the upper region of the proximal tubule (pars convoluta) and PEPT2 expressed in the lower region (pars recta) of the convoluted tubule.

MDR1, MRP2, and MRP4 are also found on the luminal brush border of the proximal tubule, where they contribute to the efflux of xenobiotics out of the cells and into the tubular fluid, thereby enhancing excretion. In general, these efflux transporters work in

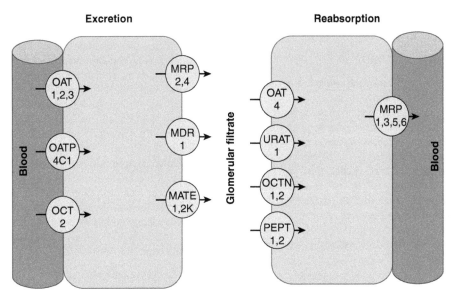

Figure 5-12. *Schematic model showing the transport systems in the human proximal tubule of the kidney.*

concert with uptake transporters to accomplish the urinary excretion of xenobiotics. For example, following OAT-mediated uptake of adefovir (described above), MRP4 transports the potentially toxic drug out of the cell and into the tubular fluid. Similarly, MATE1 and MATE2K are expressed on the apical membrane of renal tubular cells and contribute to the functional coordination of the urinary excretion of cationic compounds. For example, there is a recognized interplay between OCT2-mediated uptake of organic cations, such as metformin, followed by the secretion into the tubular fluid by MATE1 and MATE2K. This is particularly important in the case of metformin because the drug does not undergo extensive hepatic metabolism and is eliminated from the body almost exclusively by urinary excretion (Zolk and Fromm, 2011).

Mrp1 is also expressed in the rodent kidney, but it is primarily found in the epithelial cells of the loop of Henle and the collecting ducts, whereas in humans, MRP1 has been detected in the glomerulus. In Mrp1($^{-/-}$) null mice, the anticancer drug VP-16 causes polyuria indicative of damage to the collecting duct, suggesting that Mrp1 is likely to be involved in the clearance of the compound from the kidney (Wihnholds et al., 1998).

Finally, in humans, BCRP does not appear to be expressed in appreciable levels in the kidney, whereas it is expressed at high levels in the apical brush border of rat and mouse kidney. This transporter appears to play an important role in the efflux of certain sulfate conjugates of xenobiotics. The contribution of this species difference in renal BCRP expression with respect to toxic responses remains to be fully evaluated.

As in all active transport systems, there is competition for renal secretion of xenobiotics. This fact was taken advantage of during World War II, when penicillin was in short supply. Penicillin is actively secreted by the organic acid systems (OATs) of the kidney. To lengthen its half-life and duration of action, another acid was sought to compete with penicillin for renal secretion, and probenecid was successfully introduced for this purpose. Uric acid is also secreted actively by renal tubules, and a unique member of the OAT family, the urate transporter (URAT1; SLC22A12) is expressed only in the kidney where it functions specifically as a mechanism for reabsorption of urate. Various uricosuric agents, including probenecid and phenylbutazone inhibit URAT1 to facilitate the excretion of uric acid from the body.

Because many functions of the kidney are incompletely developed at birth, some xenobiotics are eliminated more slowly in newborns than in adults, and therefore may be more toxic to newborns. For example, the clearance of penicillin by premature infants is only about 20% of that observed in older children. In contrast, some compounds, such as cephaloridine, are nephrotoxic in adult animals but not in newborns. The reduced toxicity results directly from the lack of active uptake of cephaloridine by the kidneys in newborns, such that the chemical is not concentrated in the tubules.

The renal proximal tubule reabsorbs small plasma proteins that are filtered at the glomerulus. This largely occurs by pinocytosis at the brush-border membrane of the proximal tubule epithelium. If a toxicant binds to those small proteins, it can be carried into the proximal tubule cells and exert toxicity. As discussed previously, cadmium bound to MT is readily taken up by the kidney and is the major cause of Cd-induced nephrotoxicity (Klaassen and Liu, 1997). Similarly, chemicals such as limonene and 2,4,4-trimethyl pentane bind to the male-rat-specific protein, α_{2u}-globulin, and are taken up by the proximal tubule to produce hyaline droplet nephropathy and eventually renal tumors in male rats (Lehman-McKeeman, 2010).

Species differences in regard to the urinary excretion of weak organic acids and bases are observed frequently, as the pH of urine

Table 5-13

Urinary and Biliary Excretion of Griseofulvin and/or Metabolites in Rats and Rabbits

	RATS[*]		RABBITS[*]	
	URINE	BILE	URINE	BILE
Total	12	77	78	11
Phase I metabolites	ND[†]	23	70	3
Phase II metabolites	ND	54	8	8

[*]Expressed as percent of dose.
[†]ND, not determined.
SOURCE: Data from Symchowicz et al. (1967), with permission.

varies widely among species. Differences in renal clearance also can occur for compounds filtered at the glomeruli because of differences in plasma protein binding. Similarly, differences in xenobiotic transporter expression, regulation, and function can contribute to differences in the renal excretion of toxicants.

Additional factors affecting the excretion of xenobiotics are exemplified by the disposition of griseofulvin in rats and rabbits (Table 5-13). Rabbits metabolize griseofulvin to 6-demethylgriseofulvin (a phase-I metabolite), a low-molecular-weight species that is predominantly excreted in urine. In contrast, rats metabolize griseofulvin to many conjugates (phase-II metabolites) that are higher-molecular-weight species (>350) that are preferentially excreted in bile. In this example, species differences in biotransformation ultimately determine the route of excretion of griseofulvin.

Fecal Excretion

Fecal excretion, the second major pathway for the elimination of xenobiotics, is a complex process that is not as well understood as urinary excretion. Excretion of toxicants via the feces can result from direct elimination of nonabsorbed compounds in the GI tract, from delivery to the GI tract via the bile and from secretion into intestinal luminal contents from the enterocytes.

Nonabsorbed Ingesta In addition to undigested material, varying proportions of nutrients and xenobiotics that are present in food or are ingested voluntarily (drugs) pass through the alimentary canal unabsorbed, contributing to fecal excretion. The physicochemical properties of xenobiotics and the biological characteristics that facilitate absorption were discussed earlier in this chapter. Although most chemicals are lipophilic to some extent and thereby available for absorption, it is rare for 100% of a compound to be absorbed. However, some macromolecules and some high-molecular-weight compounds that are essentially completely ionized are not absorbed at all. For example, the absorption of polymers or quaternary ammonium bases is quite limited in the intestine. Consequently, most of a dose of orally administered sucrose polyester, cholestyramine, or paraquat can be found in feces. The nonabsorbed portion of xenobiotics contributes to the fecal excretion of most chemicals to some extent. One other factor contributing to fecal excretion is intestinal secretion, which likely occurs by passive diffusion out of enterocytes or via exfoliation of intestinal cells during the normal turnover of this epithelium.

Biliary Excretion The biliary route of elimination is a significant source contributing to the fecal excretion of xenobiotics and is even more important for the excretion of metabolites. The liver plays an important role in removing toxic chemicals from blood after absorption from the GI tract because blood from the GI tract passes via the portal circulation through the liver before reaching the general circulation. A compound can be extracted by the liver, thereby preventing its distribution to other parts of the body. The liver is also the main site for biotransformation of toxicants, and metabolites may be excreted directly into bile. In this manner, the liver can remove xenobiotics and their metabolites before entering the general circulation. Furthermore, xenobiotics and/or their metabolites excreted into bile enter the intestine and may be excreted with feces. However, if the physicochemical properties favor reabsorption, an enterohepatic circulation may ensue (discussed below).

Toxic chemicals bound to plasma proteins are fully available for active biliary excretion. The factors that determine whether a chemical will be excreted into bile or into urine are not fully understood. However, as a general rule, low-molecular-weight compounds (<325) are poorly excreted into bile, whereas compounds or their conjugates with molecular weights exceeding about 325 can be excreted in appreciable quantities. Glutathione and glucuronide conjugates have a high predilection for excretion into bile, but there are marked species differences in the biliary excretion of foreign compounds with consequences for the biological half-life of a compound and its toxicity. Table 5-14 provides examples of species differences in biliary excretion, and demonstrates that species variation in biliary excretion is also compound specific. It is therefore difficult to categorize species into "good" or "poor" biliary excretors, but, in general, rats and mice tend to be better biliary excretors than are other species (Klaassen and Watkins, 1984).

Foreign compounds excreted into bile are often divided into 3 classes on the basis of the ratio of their concentration in bile versus that in plasma. Class A substances have a ratio of nearly 1 and include sodium, potassium, glucose, mercury, thallium, cesium, and cobalt. Class B substances have a ratio of bile to plasma greater than 1 (usually between 10 and 1000). Class B substances include bile acids, bilirubin, lead, arsenic, manganese, and many other xenobiotics. Class C substances have a ratio below 1 (eg, inulin, albumin, zinc, iron, gold, and chromium). Compounds rapidly excreted into bile are usually class B substances. However, a compound does not have to be highly concentrated in bile for biliary excretion to be of quantitative importance. For example, mercury is not concentrated in bile, yet bile is the main route of excretion for this slowly eliminated substance.

Biliary excretion is regulated predominantly by xenobiotic transporters present on the canalicular membrane, which include MRP2, BCRP, MDR1, MATE1, and BSEP (Fig. 5-13). MRP2 is extremely important in biliary excretion because it is largely

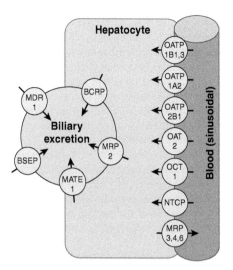

Figure 5-13. *Schematic model showing the xenobiotic transporting systems present in the human liver.*

responsible for the transport of organic anions including glucuronide and glutathione conjugates of many xenobiotics. BCRP has particular affinity for sulfated conjugates of toxicants, whereas MDR1 primarily transports a variety of substrates into bile. MATE1 is specifically involved in biliary excretion of organic cations, and BSEP is critical for the secretion of bile salts and the regulation of bile flow.

The important contribution of MRP2 to biliary excretion of toxicants was established in part by the characterization of 2 naturally occurring mutant strains of rat, the Groningen/Yellow transport deficient (TR⁻) and the Eisai hyperbilirubinemic rat (EHBR), both of which lack functional Mrp2 protein. These rats are phenotypically similar to humans suffering from Dubin–Johnson syndrome, a rare inherited disorder associated with mutations in MRP2 and characterized by chronic conjugated hyperbilirubinemia. The mutant rats also present with conjugated hyperbilirubinemia, show reduced biliary excretion of glutathione, and are defective in the normal biliary excretion of glucuronide and glutathione conjugates of many xenobiotics. An Mrp2⁻/⁻ null mouse has been developed, and like its mutant rat counterparts, shows marked reductions in bile flow, biliary glutathione concentrations, and reduced ability to eliminate xenobiotics. For example, plasma levels of the food-derived carcinogen, PhIp, increased 1.9-fold in Mrp2⁻/⁻ null mice compared to wild-type controls, demonstrating that functional Mrp2 plays a role in reducing exposure to toxic chemicals (Vlaming *et al.*, 2006). Finally, species differences in Mrp2 function may contribute to the qualitative differences

Table 5-14

Biliary Excretion of Xenobiotic Conjugates Across Species

(MOLECULAR WEIGHT)	INDOCYANINE GREEN, (775)	PHENOLPHTHALEIN GLUCURONIDE, (495)	SULFADIMETHYOXINE n-GLUCURONIDE, (487)	STILBESTROL GLUCURONIDE, (445)
		% EXCRETED IN BILE		
Rat	82	54	43	95
Dog	97	81	43	65
Rabbit	97	13	10	32
Guinea pig	Not done	6	12	20

SOURCE: Data modified from Lin (1995).

observed across species in biliary excretion. In a direct comparison of the transport of 2,4-dinitrophenyl-S-glutathione (DNP-SG) across canalicular membrane vesicles from various species, clearance ranged from a high rate of 64.2 μL/min/mg protein in rats to a low of 3.8 μL/min/mg protein in humans, with intermediate values for other species including mouse, guinea pig, rabbit, and dog (Ishizuka *et al.*, 1999). Such differences in transporter function and expression are likely to contribute to species differences in biliary excretion illustrated in Table 5-14.

Although the highest levels of BCRP are found in the placenta, the transporter is expressed on the bile canalicular membrane of hepatocytes where it preferentially transports sulfate conjugates of xenobiotics. Known substrates for BCRP include estrone 3-sulfate and 4-methylembelliferone sulfate and methotrexate. MDR1 is important in the biliary elimination of compounds such as doxorubicin and vinblastine.

As described earlier, MATE1 and MATE2K are involved in the urinary excretion of organic cations such as metformin. MATE1, but not MATE2K, is also expressed on the bile canaliculus, where it also functions to transport organic cations into bile. In the case of metformin, a drug that works to inhibit gluconeogenesis in the liver, biliary excretion reduces hepatic drug concentrations, and thereby limits pharmacological activity.

The biliary excretion of xenobiotics mediated by MRP2, BCRP, and MDR1 usually results in increased excretion of toxicants out of hepatocytes and into bile. In doing so, these transporters increase excretion of xenobiotics and generally limit the likelihood of toxicity in the liver. However, adverse reactions can occur if the function of these transporters is inhibited, as evidenced by the examples illustrated above for the genetic mutant or knockout models. Furthermore, although BSEP does not appear to play a major role in the excretion of xenobiotics, some compounds can inhibit the function of this transporter, thereby decreasing the biliary excretion of bile acids and leading to cholestasis (defined as a decrease in bile flow with increased serum bilirubin) and cholestatic liver injury (Arrese and Ananthanarayanan, 2004). For example, inhibition of BSEP by the pharmaceutical agent, troglitazone, and to a much greater extent, troglitazone sulfate, competitively inhibits BSEP function, leading to intrahepatic cholestasis, which may contribute to the hepatotoxicity of troglitazone. Furthermore, inhibition of BSEP contributes to the cholestasis observed with steroids such as estradiol. Collectively, the ability of a chemical to interfere with the normal function of BSEP may be involved in hepatotoxicity (Morgan *et al.*, 2010).

Although the transporters located on the canalicular membrane are directly responsible for biliary excretion of xenobiotics, other xenobiotic transporters localized to the sinusoidal membranes are also important in determining hepatic concentrations of toxicants and thereby contribute to hepatic disposition and biliary elimination. Transporters present on sinusoidal membranes include the ABC transport family members, MRP3, MRP4, and MRP6, along with OATPs, OATs, and OCT. The Na$^+$/taurocholate cotransporting polypeptide is also found on the sinusoidal membrane where it functions specifically in the uptake of bile acids into the liver.

MRP3 transports many of the same organic anions that are substrates for MRP2 from the liver into the blood circulation. It has recently been shown to be important in the excretion of acetaminophen- and morphine glucuronide conjugates from liver into blood (Borst *et al.*, 2006). In humans, it is upregulated during cholestasis and in patients with Dubin–Johnson syndrome, and in a similar manner, it is increased in TR$^-$ and EHBR rats. The increase in MRP3 is recognized as a compensatory response that

helps to protect hepatocytes from toxic chemicals for cells deficient in MRP2. MRP4 is specifically involved in the cellular efflux of purine analogs, nucleoside antiviral drugs, and cyclic nucleotides, including cAMP and cGMP. It has also been shown to be a carrier for some xenobiotics including conjugated and unconjugated compounds (Borst *et al.*, 2006). A major role for MRP6 in xenobiotic disposition has not been established, but mutations in human MRP6 are associated with pseudoxanthoma elasticum, a hereditary disease affecting the elasticity of connective tissues (Bergen *et al.*, 2007).

Transporters present on the sinusoidal membranes of hepatocytes also contribute to hepatic uptake and efflux, and thereby contribute to hepatobiliary clearance of xenobiotics. In humans, OATP1B1 and 1B3 contribute to the uptake of many organic anions. Several plant toxins including phalloidin (from mushrooms) and mycrocystin-LR (from blue–green algae) are transported by the OATP1B proteins, and Oatp1b2-null mice are resistant to hepatotoxicity induced by both of these toxins (Lu *et al.*, 2008). The Oatps exhibit broad substrate specificity and play an important role in the hepatic uptake of numerous drugs and xenobiotics along with a variety of hormones, including thyroxin, and hormone conjugates. OAT2 is expressed in liver and transports small organic anions such as indomethacin and salicylate along with prostaglandins (Anzai *et al.*, 2006). OCT1 is also expressed in human and rodent liver, and contributes to the uptake of organic cations. This includes numerous endogenous compounds such as choline and dopamine as well as cationic xenobiotics such as metformin. Oct1 null mice are generally resistant to lactic acidosis than is caused by metformin (Wang *et al.*, 2003), suggesting a role for this uptake transporter (along with the biliary transporters highlighted above) in the elimination and toxic potential of this compound. In concert, the OATPs, OAT, and OCT family of transporters are important in the uptake of toxicants into the liver, a step that will also influence the contribution of hepatic metabolism, efflux into the bile, or efflux back into the circulation.

An important concept relating to biliary excretion is the phenomenon of enterohepatic circulation. After a compound is excreted into bile, it enters the intestine where it can be reabsorbed or eliminated with feces (illustrated in Fig. 5-1). Many organic compounds are conjugated with UDP-glucuronic acid, sulfate, or glutathione (see Chap. 6) before excretion into bile, and these polar metabolites are not sufficiently lipid soluble to be reabsorbed. However, enzymes found in the intestinal microflora may hydrolyze glucuronide and sulfate conjugates, liberating a more lipophilic moiety and increasing the likelihood of reabsorption. Reabsorption of the liberated xenobiotic completes a cycle in which the compound can return to the liver, where it can again be metabolized and excreted back into bile. Repeated enterohepatic cycling can lead to very long half-lives of xenobiotics in the body. Therefore, it is often desirable to interrupt this cycle to hasten the elimination of a toxicant from the body (Genius, 2011). This principle has been utilized in the treatment of dimethylmercury poisoning; ingestion of a polythiol resin binds the mercury and thus prevents its reabsorption (Magos and Clarkson, 1976).

An increase in hepatic excretory function also has been observed after pretreatment with some drugs (Klaassen and Watkins, 1984). For example, it has been demonstrated that phenobarbital increases plasma disappearance of bromosulfophthalein (BSP) by enhancing its biliary excretion. The increase in bile flow caused by phenobarbital is an important factor in increasing the biliary excretion of BSP. However, other factors, including induction of phase-II enzymes (see Chap. 6) and xenobiotic transporters may also enhance biliary elimination. Induction of metabolizing enzymes and transporters work in concert to increase the clearance of a toxicant from the plasma. In particular, induction of these processes increases the capacity for a xenobiotic to be (1) taken up into the liver; (2) metabolized to conjugates that are likely to be excreted into bile; and (3) excreted into bile and removed from the general circulation. However, not all microsomal enzyme inducers increase bile flow and excretion, as agents such as 3-methylcholanthrene and benzo[a]pyrene are relatively ineffective in this regard.

The toxicity of some compounds can also be directly related to their biliary excretion. For example, the intestinal toxicity of several xenobiotics and drugs is increased by their excretion into bile. This is the case for nonsteroidal anti-inflammatory drugs that cause intestinal ulcerations that can be abolished by bile-duct ligation (Duggan *et al.*, 1975). More recently, irinotecan, an anticancer drug, was found to induce severe GI toxicity (severe diarrhea) in humans and rats. The mechanism for the effect of this drug involved metabolism to an active metabolite that was a good substrate for MRP2. The excretion into bile mediated by MRP2 results in high concentrations of the toxic metabolite in the intestinal lumen and toxicity ensues. The toxicity of irinotecan can be modulated by inhibiting MRP2 function (Chu *et al.*, 1997).

Many xenobiotic transporters are not expressed early in development, and the hepatic excretory system is not fully developed in newborns. As a result, there are numerous examples of compounds that are more toxic to newborns than to adults (Klaassen and Slitt, 2005). For example, ouabain is about 40 times more toxic in newborn than in adult rats. This is due to an almost complete inability of the newborn rat liver to remove ouabain from plasma. The development of hepatic excretory function can be promoted in newborns by administering microsomal enzyme inducers.

Finally, the plasma clearance or biliary excretion of organic acids, such as BSP or indocyanine green (ICG), has been used to evaluate liver function. In particular, ICG is a valuable diagnostic agent in clinical practice. It is injected intravenously after which its disappearance from plasma is easily monitored. A change in plasma clearance of ICG does not distinguish between changes in hepatic blood flow or cellular function, but is highly suggestive of reduced hepatic function, including reduced biliary excretion, consistent with liver dysfunction or injury (Sakka, 2007).

Exhalation

Substances that exist predominantly in the gas phase at body temperature are eliminated mainly by the lungs. Because volatile liquids are in equilibrium with their gas phase in the alveoli, they may also be excreted via the lungs. The amount of a liquid eliminated via the lungs is proportional to its vapor pressure. A practical application of this principle is seen in the breath analyzer test for determining the amount of ethanol in the body. Highly volatile liquids such as diethyl ether and certain volatile anesthetics (nitrous oxide) are excreted almost exclusively by the lungs.

No specialized transport systems have been described for the excretion of toxic substances by the lungs. Some xenobiotic transporters, including MRP1 and MDR1, have been identified in the lung, but overall, compounds excreted via exhalation in the lung are most likely to be eliminated by simple diffusion. Elimination of gases is roughly inversely proportional to the rate of their absorption. Therefore, gases with low solubility in blood, such as ethylene, are rapidly excreted, whereas chloroform, which has a much higher solubility in blood, is eliminated very slowly by the

lungs. Trace concentrations of highly lipid-soluble anesthetic gases such as halothane and methoxyflurane may be present in expired air for as long as 2 to 3 weeks after a few hours of anesthesia. Undoubtedly, this prolonged retention is due to deposition in and slow mobilization from adipose tissue of these very lipid-soluble agents. The rate of elimination of a gas with low solubility in blood is perfusion-limited, whereas that of a gas with high solubility in blood is ventilation-limited.

Other Routes of Elimination

Cerebrospinal Fluid A specialized route of removal of toxic agents from a specific organ is represented by the cerebrospinal fluid (CSF). All compounds can leave the CNS with the bulk flow of CSF through the arachnoid villi. In addition, lipid-soluble toxicants also can exit at the site of the BBB. As discussed earlier, toxicants also can be removed from the CSF by active transport, using the transport systems present in the BCSFB.

Milk The secretion of toxic compounds into milk is extremely important because (1) a toxic material may be passed with milk from the mother to the nursing offspring and (2) compounds can be passed from cows to people via dairy products. Toxic agents are excreted into milk by simple diffusion. Because milk has an acidic pH (about 6.5), basic compounds may be concentrated in milk, whereas acidic compounds may attain lower concentrations in milk than in plasma (Findlay, 1983; Wilson, 1983). More important, about 3% to 4% of milk consists of lipids, and the lipid content of colostrum after parturition is even higher. Lipid-soluble xenobiotics diffuse along with fats from plasma into the mammary glands and are excreted with milk during lactation. Many of the same compounds that can accumulate in fat such as aldrin, chlordane, DDT, and polychlorinated and polybrominated biphenyls, dibenzo-*p*-dioxins, and furans (Van den Berg *et al.*, 1987; Li *et al.*, 1995) have been found in human breast milk, and milk can be a major route of their excretion. More recently, other persistent compounds such as nitromusk perfume ingredients have been identified in milk, but it is unclear as to whether the presence of these compounds is directly responsible for possible adverse effects (Leibl *et al.*, 2000). Species differences in the excretion of xenobiotics with milk are to be expected, as the proportion of milk fat derived from the circulation versus that synthesized de novo in the mammary gland differs widely among species. Metals chemically similar to calcium, such as lead, and chelating agents that form complexes with calcium also can be excreted into milk to a considerable extent.

BCRP is expressed in the alveolar epithelial cells of mammary glands and actively secretes a variety of compounds into milk. Endogenous compounds such as vitamin B_{12} (riboflavin) are actively transported into breast milk by BCRP, as well as numerous toxicants including heterocyclic amines and aflataxon. The contribution of BCRP to toxicants in the mammary gland and breast milk is paradoxical in that secretion into the milk is likely to be protective to the mother, while simultaneously increasing the potential for exposure in suckling infants or dairy consumers to a variety of toxic chemicals (Van Herwaarden and Schinkel, 2006; Vlaming *et al.*, 2009).

Sweat and Saliva The excretion of toxic agents in sweat and saliva is quantitatively of minor importance. Again, excretion depends on the diffusion of the nonionized, lipid-soluble form of an agent. Toxic compounds excreted into sweat may produce dermatitis. Substances excreted in saliva enter the mouth, where they are usually swallowed to become available for GI absorption.

COMPUTATIONAL AND EXPERIMENTAL APPROACHES TO ASSESS XENOBIOTIC DISPOSITION

In general, the empiric determination of xenobiotic absorption, distribution, and elimination in experiments involving laboratory animals or studies in human subjects is the most reliable means by which disposition can be studied. However, such studies may require the development of sophisticated analytical methods, the use of radioactive compounds and in the case of human studies, controlled laboratory conditions and constant monitoring. As such, these types of studies are not always practical or feasible, and a variety of computational models, nonanimal tools or in vitro cellular systems have been developed to predict dispositional attributes of drugs and toxicants. A brief overview of several of the most widely used tools is presented here, but it is noted that this is a dynamic and rapidly changing field. In general, these models are particularly useful in studying absorption and excretion, particularly biliary excretion. Tissue distribution, with particular emphasis on target organ dosimetry can also be assessed with pharmacokinetic models (Chap. 7).

Absorption A variety of models are used to estimate log P because the lipid solubility is an important, general feature of any toxicant (Mannhold *et al.*, 2009). Additionally, based on the general principles outlined earlier, computational tools to estimate permeability have been developed. One such model predicts poor absorption as a function of the calculated log P (Clog P), the molecular weight and the presence of hydrogen bond donors and acceptors. The concept, based on these 4 elements is referred to as the "rule of 5" because the determinants are based on multiples of 5 and include (1) molecular weight greater than 500; (2) Clog P greater than 5; (3) more than 5 H-bond donors; and (4) 10 H-bond acceptors (Lipinski *et al.*, 2001).

The human colon adenocarcinoma cell line, Caco-2, is widely used to evaluate xenobiotic permeability. These cells form a confluent epithelial monolayer with well-defined tight junctions and typical microvilli on the apical surface. A variety of xenobiotic transporters are expressed on Caco-2 cells. The uptake transporters, OATP2B1, PEPT1, and OCTN2 are expressed on the apical membrane along with efflux transporters, MDR1, MRP2, and BCRP. On the basolateral membrane, efflux transporters MRP3, 4, and 6 have been identified (Sun *et al.*, 2008).

Caco-2 cells are specifically used to estimate the fraction of xenobiotic that will be absorbed in the GI tract. Movement across the apical (A) and basolateral (B) membranes is also used to determine whether a xenobiotic is substrate or inhibitor of xenobiotic transporters. Transport in the A→B direction is indicative of absorption, whereas movement in the B→A direction suggests that carrier-mediated efflux is favored.

Another model used to predict absorption are artificial membranes such as that exemplified by the parallel artificial membrane permeability assay (PAMPA). As an artificial membrane, this system lacks transporters or paracellular pathways and is most useful for assessing the non-energy-dependent diffusion of toxicants.

Dermal exposure can be evaluated in a variety of in vitro systems, either with skin biopsy samples or with models developed to represent human skin. Mathematical models, with emphasis on the lipid matrix as the principal pathway of permeation, have also been developed and used with increasing frequency. Such methods emphasize log P and molecular size in model development (Lian *et al.*, 2008).

Hepatobiliary Excretion The development of sandwich-cultured hepatocytes has become a valuable tool for studying how xenobiotics move in and out of the liver, with emphasis on transport function, including transporter regulation and species differences in transporter function that may contribute to organ toxicity. Briefly, when hepatocytes are cultured between 2 layers of gelled collagen (hence the sandwich configuration), they retain molecular and biochemical characteristics more consistent with their properties in the whole organ than monolayer cultures of cells. These features include the formation of canalicular networks necessary for biliary excretion. This system has been optimized to assess toxicant accumulation, estimate biliary excretion, and investigate the interplay between metabolism and transport, and has proven to be useful in vitro system to aid in the evaluation of hepatobiliary disposition (Swift *et al.*, 2010).

Xenobiotic transporter function can also be evaluated with membrane vesicles isolated from specific organs or with expressed cell systems. The development of a variety of transporter-deficient models, particularly in mice, have also proven to be very useful for assessing transporter activity and contribution to toxicity as have been described throughout this chapter (Klaassen and Lu, 2008).

CONCLUSION

Humans are in continuous contact with toxic chemicals. Toxicants are in the food we eat, the water we drink, and the air we breathe. Depending on their physical and chemical properties, toxic chemicals may be absorbed by the GI tract, the lungs, and/or the skin. Fortunately, the body has the ability to biotransform and excrete these compounds into urine, feces, and air. However, when the rate of absorption exceeds the rate of elimination, toxic compounds may accumulate and reach a critical concentration at a certain target site, and toxicity may ensue. Whether a chemical elicits toxicity depends not only on its inherent potency and site specificity but also on whether, and if so how, it is absorbed, distributed, and eliminated. Therefore, knowledge of the disposition of chemicals is of great importance in judging the toxicity of xenobiotics. For example, for a potent CNS suppressant that displays a strong hepatic first-pass effect, oral exposure is of less concern than is exposure by inhalation. Also, 2 equipotent gases, with the absorption of one being perfusion rate-limited and that of the other being ventilation rate-limited, will exhibit completely different toxicity profiles at a distant site because of differences in the concentrations attained in the target organ.

Many chemicals have very low inherent toxicity but can be metabolically activated into toxic metabolites, and toxicity may be determined by the rate of formation of toxic metabolites. Alternatively, a very potent toxicant may be detoxified rapidly by biotransformation. The fundamental and overarching concept is that adverse effects are related to the unbound concentration of the "toxic chemical" at the site of action (in the target organ), whether a chemical is administered or generated by biotransformation in the target tissue or at a distant site. Accordingly, the toxic response exerted by chemicals is critically influenced by the rates of absorption, distribution, biotransformation, and excretion.

REFERENCES

Ambudkar SV, Dey S, Hrycyna CA, Ramachandra M, Pastan I, Gottesman MM. Biochemical, cellular and pharmacological aspects of the multidrug transporter. *Annu Rev Pharmacol Toxicol.* 1999;39:361–398.

Anzai N, Kanai Y, Endou H. Organic anion transporter family: current knowledge. *J Pharmacol Sci.* 2006;100:411–426.

Arrese M, Ananthanarayanan M. The bile salt export pump: molecular properties, function and regulation. *Pflugers Arch.* 2004;449:123–131.

Awad Wa, Ghareeb K, Bohm J, Zentek J. Decontamination and detoxification strategies for the Fusarium mycotoxin deoxynivalenol in animal feed and the effectives of microbial biodegradation. *Food Add Contam.* 2010;27:510–520.

Bailey DG. Fruit juice inhibition of uptake transport: a new type of food-drug interaction. *Br J Clin Pharmacol.* 2010;70:645–655.

Ballard ST, Hunter JH, Taylor AE. Regulation of tight-junction permeability during nutrient absorption across the intestinal epithelium. *Annu Rev Nutr.* 1995;15:35–55.

Baron JM, Holler D, Schiffer R, et al. Expression of multiple cytochrome P450 enzymes and multidrug resistance-associated transport proteins in human skin keratinocytes. *J Invest Dermatol.* 2001;116:541–548.

Benz R, Janko K, Länger P. Pore formation by the matrix protein (porin) to *Escherichia coli* in planar bilayer membranes. *Ann NY Acad Sci.* 1980;358:13–24.

Bergen AA, Plomp AS, Hu X, deJong PT, Gorgels TG. ABCC6 and pseudo-xanthoma elasticum. *Pflugers Arch.* 2007;453:685–691.

Bogdanffy MS, Manning LA, Sarangapani R. High-affinity nasal extraction of vinyl acetate vapor is carboxylesterase dependent. *Inhal Toxicol.* 1999;11:927–941.

Borowitz JL, Moore PF, Him GKW, Miya TS. Mechanism of enhanced drug effects produced by dilution of the oral dose. *Toxicol Appl Pharmacol.* 1971;19:164–168.

Borst P, Zelcer N, van de Wetering K. MRP2 and 3 in health and disease. *Cancer Lett.* 2006;234:51–61.

Boyes RN, Adams HJ, Duce BR. Oral absorption and disposition kinetics of lidocaine hydrochloride in dogs. *J Pharmacol Exp Ther.* 1970; 174:1–8.

Bronaugh RL, Stewart RF, Congdon ER, Giles AL Jr. Methods for in vitro percutaneous absorption studies. I. Comparison with in vivo results. *Toxicol Appl Pharmacol.* 1982;62:474–480.

Calabrese EJ. Gastrointestinal and dermal absorption: interspecies differences. *Drug Metab Rev.* 1984;15:1013–1032.

Cayen MN. Metabolic disposition of antihyperlipidemic agents in man and laboratory animals. *Drug Metab Rev.* 1980;11:291–323.

Chu XY, Kato Y, Niinuma K, Sudo KI, Hakusui H, Sugiyama Y. Multi-specific organic anion transporter (cMOAT) is responsible for the biliary excretion of the camptothecin derivative irinotecan, CPT-11 and its metabolites in rats. *J Pharmacol Exp Ther.* 1997;281:304–314.

Clarkson TW. Metal toxicity in the central nervous system. *Environ Health Perspect.* 1987;75:59–64.

Deeken JG, Loscher W. The blood-brain barrier and cancer: transporters, treatment and trojan horses. *Clin Cancer Res.* 2007;13:1663–1674.

Dietrich CG, Rudi de Waart D, Ottenhoff R, Schoots IG, Oude Elferink RPJ. Increased bioavailability of the food-derived carcinoge 2-amino-1-methyl-6-phenylimidazo[4,5]pyridine in MRP2-deficient rats. *Mol Pharmacol.* 2001;59:974–980.

Diwan BA, Riggs CW, Logsdon D, et al. Multiorgan transplacental and neonatal carcinogenicity of 3′-axido-3′-deoxythymidine in mice. *Toxicol Appl Pharmacol.* 1999;161:82–99.

Draize JH, Woodard G, Calvery HO. Methods for the study of irritation and toxicity of substances applied topically to the skin and mucous membranes. *J Pharmacol Exp Ther.* 1944;82:377–390.

Dreyfuss J, Shaw JM, Ross JJ. Absorption of the adrenergic-blocking agent, nadol, by mice, rats, hamsters, rabbits, dogs, monkeys and man: unusual species differences. *Xenobiotica.* 1978;8:503–510.

Dugard PH. Skin permeability theory in relation to measurements of percutaneous absorption in toxicology. In: Marzulli FN, Maibach HI, eds. *Dermatotoxicology.* 2nd ed. Washington/New York/London: Hemisphere; 1983:91–116.

Duggan DE, Hooke KF, Noll RM, Kwan KC. Enterohepatic circulation of indomethacin and its role in intestinal irritation. *Biochem Pharmacol.* 1975;24:1749–1754.

Enders AC, Carter AM. What can comparative studies of placental structure tell us?—A review. *Placenta.* 2004;25(suppl A): S3-S9.

Findlay JWA. The distribution of some commonly used drugs in human breast milk. *Drug Metab Rev.* 1983;14:653–686.

Flanagan PR, Haist J, Valberg LS. Comparative effects of iron deficiency induced by bleeding and low-iron diet on the intestinal absorptive interactions of iron, cobalt, manganese, zinc, lead and calcium. *J Nutr.* 1980;110:1754–1763.

Florence AT, Hillery AM, Hussain N, Jani PU. Factors affecting the oral up-take and translocation of polystyrene nanoparticles: histological and analytical evidence. *J Drug Target.* 1995;3:65–70.

Fullmer CS. Intestinal interactions of lead and calcium. *Neurotoxicology.* 1992;13:799–807.

Ganapathy V, Prasad PD, Ganapathy ME, Leibach FH. Placental transporters relevant to drug disposition across the maternal-fetal interface. *J Pharmacol Exp Ther.* 2000;294:413–420.

Genius SJ. Elimination of persistent toxicants from the human body. *Human Exp Toxicol.* 2011;30:3–18.

Hagenbuch B, Guo C. Xenobiotic transporters of the human organic anion transporting polypeptides (OATP) family. *Xenobiotica.* 2008;38:778–801.

Hagenbuch B, Meier PJ. Organic anion transporting polypeptides of the OATP/SLC21 family: phylogenetic classification as OATP/SLCO superfamily, new nomenclature and molecular/functional properties. *Pflugers Arch.* 2004;447:653–665.

Hanumegowda UM, Wenke G, Regueiro-Ren A, Yordanova R, Corradi JP, Adams, SP. Phospholipidosis as a function of basicity, lipophilicity and volume of distribution of compounds. *Chem Res Toxicol.* 2010;23:749–755.

Hediger MA, Romero MF, Peng J-B, Rolfs A, Takanaga H, Bruford EA. The ABCs of solute carriers: physiological, pathological and therapeutic implications of human membrane transport proteins. *Pflugers Arch.* 2004;447:465–468.

Ho ES, Lin DC, Mendel DB, Cihlar T. Cytotoxicity of antiviral nucleotides adefovir and cidofovir induced by the expression of the human renal organic anion transporter I. *J Am Soc Nephrol.* 2000;11:383–393.

Ishizuka H, Donno K, Shiina T, et al. Species differences in the transport activity for organic anions across the bile canalicular membrane. *J Pharmacol Exp Ther.* 1999;290:1324–1330.

Jandacek RJ, Tso P. Factors affecting the storage and excretion of toxic lipophilic xenobiotics. *Lipids.* 2001;36:1289–1305.

Jani P, Halbert GW, Langridge J, Florence AT. Nanoparticle uptake by the rat gastrointestinal mucosa: quantitation and particle size dependency. *J Pharm Pharmacol.* 1990;42:821–826.

Kao J, Patterson FU, Hall J. Skin penetration and metabolism of topically applied chemicals in six mammalian species, including man: an in vitro study with benzo(a)pyrene and testosterone. *Toxicol Appl Pharmacol.* 1985;81:502–516.

Kerns WD, Pavkov KL, Donofrio DJ, Gralla EJ, Swenberg JA. Carcinogenicity of formaldehyde in rats and mice after long-term inhalation exposure. *Cancer Res.* 1983;43:4382–4392.

Klaassen CD, Aleksunes LM. Xenobiotic, bile acid and cholesterol transporters: function and regulation. *Pharmacol Rev.* 2010;62:1–96.

Klaassen CD, Liu J. Role of metallothionein in cadmium-induced hepatotoxicity and nephrotoxicity. *Drug Metab Rev.* 1997;29:79–102.

Klaassen CD, Lu H. Xenobiotic transporters: ascribing function from gene knockout and mutation studies. *Toxicol Sci.* 2008;101:186–196.

Klaassen CD, Shoeman DW. Biliary excretion of lead in rats, rabbits and dogs. *Toxicol Appl Pharmacol.* 1974;29:434–446.

Klaassen CD, Slitt AL. Regulation of hepatic transporters by xenobiotic receptors. *Curr Drug Metab.* 2005;6:309–328.

Klaassen CD, Watkins JB. Mechanisms of bile formation, hepatic uptake, and biliary excretion. *Pharmacol Rev.* 1984;36:1–67.

Kruh GD, Guo U, Hopper-Borge E, Belinsky MG, Chen Z-S. ABCC10, ABCC11 and ABCC12. *Pflugers Arch-Eur J Physiol.* 2007;453:675–684.

Kusuhara H, Sugiyama Y. Active efflux across the blood-brain barrier: role of the solute carrier family. *NeuroRx.* 2005;2:73–85.

Kusuhara H, Sugiyama Y. In vitro-invio extrapolation of transporter-mediated clearance in the liver and kidney. *Drug Metab Pharmacokinet.* 2009;24:37–52.

Lademann J, Richter H, Schanzer S, et al. Penetration and storage of particles in human skin: perspectives and safety aspects. *Eur J Pharm Biopharm.* 2011;77:465–468.

Lankas GR, Cartwright ME, Umbenhauer D. P-glycoprotein deficiency in a subpopulation of CF-1 mice enhances avermectin-induced neurotoxicity. *Toxicol Appl Pharmacol.* 1997;143:357–365.

Lankas GR, Wise LD, Cartwright ME, et al. Placental p-glycoprotein deficiency enhances susceptibility to chemically induced birth defects in mice. *Reprod Toxicol.* 1998;12:457–463.

Lehman-McKeeman LD. α2u-Globulin nephropathy. In: Schnellman RG, ed. *Comprehensive Toxicology.* 2nd ed. New York: Elsevier; 2010:507–521.

Lehman-McKeeman LD, Johnson DR, Caudill D. Induction and inhibition of mouse cytochrome P450 2B enzymes by musk xylene. *Toxicol Appl Pharmacol.* 1997;142:169–177.

Leibl B, Mayer R, Ommer S, Sonnichsen C, Koletzko B. Transition of nitro musks and polycyclic musks into human milk. *Adv Exp Med Biol.* 2000;478:289–305.

Leiser P, Kaufmann R. Placental structure: in a comparative aspect. *Exp Clin Endocrinol.* 1994;102:122–134.

Leopold G, Furukawa E, Forth W, Rummel W. Comparative studies of absorption of heavy metals in vivo and in vitro. *Arch Pharmacol Exp Pathol.* 1969;263:275–276.

Leslie EM, Deeley RG, Cole SPC. Multidurg resistance proteins: role of P-glycoprotein, MRP1, MRP2, and BCRP (ABCG2) in tissue defense. *Toxicol Appl Pharmacol.* 2005;204:216–237.

Li X, Weber LWD, Rozman KK. Toxicokinetics of 2,3,7,8-tetrachlorodiben zo-p-dioxin (TCDD) in female Sprague-Dawley rats including placental and lactational transfer to fetuses and neonates. *Fundam Appl Toxicol.* 1995;27:70–76.

Lian G, Chen L, Han L. An evaluation of mathematical models for predicting skin permeability. *J Pharm Sci.* 2008;97:585–598.

Lin JH. Species similarities and differences in pharmacokinetics. *Drug Metab Dispos.* 1995;23:1008–1021.

Lin JH. Tissue distribution and pharmacodynamics: a complicated relationship. *Curr Drug Metab.* 2006;7:39–65.

Lipinski CA, Lombardo F, Dominy BW, Feeney PJ. Experimental and computational approaches to estimate solubility and permeability in drug discovery and development settings. *Adv Drug Deliv Rev.* 2001;46:3–26.

Lu H, Choudhuri S, Ogura K, et al. Characterization of organic anion transporting polypeptide 1b2-null mice: essential role in hepatic uptake/toxicity o phalloidin and microcystin-LR. *Toxicol Sci.* 2008;103:35–45.

Magos L, Clarkson TW. The effect of oral doses of a polythiol resin on the excretion of methylmercury in mice treated with cystein, d-penicillamine or phenobarbitone. *Chem Biol Interact.* 1976;14:325–335.

Mannhold R, Poda GI, Ostermann C, Tetko IV. Calculation of molecular lipophilicity: state-of-the-art and comparison of Log P methods on more than 96,000 compounds. *J Pharm Sci.* 2009;98:861–893.

Mensinga TT, Speijers GJ, Meulenbelt J. Health implications of exposure to environmental nitrogenous compounds. *Toxicol Rev.* 2003;22:41–51.

Miller DS. Regulation of P-glycoprotein and other ABC drug transporters at the blood-brain barrier. *Trends Pharm Sci.* 2010;31:246–254.

Mizuno N, Niwa T, Yotsumoto Y, Sugiyama Y. Impact of drug transporter studies on drug discovery and development. *Pharmacol Rev.* 2003;55:425–461.

Morgan RE, Trauner M, van Staden CJ, et al. Interference with bile salt export pump function is a susceptibility factor for human liver injury in drug development. *Toxicol Sci.* 2010;118:485–500.

Morris FH Jr, Boyd DH, Mahendran D. Placental transport. In: Knobel E, Neill JD, eds. *The Physiology of Reproduction.* New York, NY: Raven Press; 1994:813–861.

Myllynen P, Pasanen M, Pelkonen O. Human placenta: a human organ for developmental toxicology research and biomonitoring. *Placenta.* 2005;26:361–371.

Nel A, Xia T, Madler L, Li N. Toxic potential of materials at the nanolevel. *Science.* 2006;311:622–627.

Newbold RR, McLachlan JA. Transplacental hormonal carcinogenesis: diethylstilbestrol as an example. *Prog Clin Biol Res.* 1996;394:131–147.

Newman MD, Stotland M, Ellis JI. The safety of nanosized particles in titanium dioxide and zinc oxide-based suncreens. *J Am Acad Dermatol.* 2009;61:685–692.

Ni Z, Bikadi Z, Rosenberg MF, Mao Q. Structure and function of the human breast cancer resistance protein (BCRP/ABCG2). *Curr Drug Metab.* 2010;11:603–617.

Oberdorster G, Oberdorster E, Oberdorster J. Nanotoxicology: an emerging discipline evolving from studies of ultrafine particles. *Environ Health Perspect.* 2005;113:823–839.

Pfeiffer CJ. Gastroenterologic response to environmental agents—absorption and interactions. In: Lee DHK, ed. *Handbook of Physiology. Section 9: Reactions to Environmental Agents.* Bethesda, MD: American Physiological Society; 1977:349–374.

Poet TS, McDougal JN. Skin absorption and human risk assessment. *Chem Biol Interact.* 2002;140:19–34.

Prouillac C, Lecoeur S. The role of the placenta in fetal exposure to xenobiotics: importance of membrane transporters and human models for transport studies. *Drug Metab Dispos.* 2010;38:1623–1635.

Rickert DE, Butterworth BE, Popp JA. Dinitrotoluene: acute toxicity, oncogenicity, genotoxicity and metabolism. *CRC Crit Rev Toxicol.* 1984;13:217–234.

Rizwan AN, Burckhardt G. Organic anion transporters of the SLC22 family: biopharmaceutical, physiological and pathological roles. *Pharm Res.* 2007;24:9181–2004.

Ross JH, Driver JH, Harris SA, Maibach HI. Dermal absorption of 2,4-D: a review of species differences. *Regul Toxicol Pharmacol.* 2005;41:82–91.

Rowland IR, Mallet AK, Wise A. The effect of diet on mammalian gut flora and its metabolic activities. *CRC Crit Rev Toxicol.* 1985;16:31–103.

Sahi J. Use of in vitro transporter assays to understand hepatic and renal disposition of new drug candidates. *Expert Opin Drug Metab Toxicol.* 2005;1:409–427.

Sakka SG. Assessing liver function. *Curr Opin Crit Care.* 2007;13:207–214.

Schanker LS. Passage of drugs across body membranes. *Pharmacol Rev.* 1962;74:501–530.

Schinkel A, Smith JJM, van Tellingen O, et al. Disruption of the mouse mdr1a p-glycoprotein gene leads to a deficiency in the blood–brain barrier and to increased sensitivity to drugs. *Cell.* 1994;47:491–502.

Schwartze EW. The so-called habituation to arsenic: variation in the toxicity of arsenious oxide. *J Pharmacol Exp Ther.* 1923;20:181–203.

Shand DG, Rangno RE. The deposition of propranolol: I. Elimination during oral absorption in man. *Pharmacology.* 1972;7:159–168.

Shitara Y, Sato H, Sugiyama Y. Evaluation of drug–drug interaction in the hepatobiliary and renal transport of drugs. *Annu Rev Pharmacol Toxicol.* 2005;45:689–723.

Silverman WA, Andersen DH, Blanc WA, Crozier DN. A difference in mortality rate and incidence of kernicterus among premature infants allotted to two prophylactic antibacterial regimens. *Pediatrics.* 1956;18:614–625.

Smith HW. Observations on the flora of the alimentary tract of animals and factors affecting its composition. *J Pathol Bacteriol.* 1965;89:95–107.

Stern ST, McNeil SE. Nanotechnology safety concerns revisited. *Toxicol Sci.* 2008;101:4–21.

Sun H, Chow ECY, Liu S, Du Y, Pang KS. The Caco-2 cell monolayer: usefulness and limitations. *Expert Opin Drug Metab Toxicol.* 2008;4:395–411.

Swift B, Pfeifer ND, Brouwer KLR. Sandwich-cultured hepatocytes: an in vitro model to evaluate hepatobiliary transporter-based drug interactions and hepatotoxicity. *Drug Metab Rev.* 2010;42:446–471.

Symchowicz S, Staub MS, Wong KKA. Comparative study of griseofulvin-^{14}C metabolism in the rat and rabbit. *Biochem Pharmacol.* 1967;16:2405–2411.

Syme MR, Paxton JW, Keelan JA. Drug transfer and metabolism by the human placenta. *Clin Pharmacokinet.* 2004;43:487–514.

Tamai I. Oral drug delivery using intestinal OATP transporters. *Adv Drug Deliv Rev.* 2012;64:508–514.

Tokar EJ, Qu W, Waalkes MP. Arsenic, stem cells and the developmental basis of adult cancer. *Toxicol Sci.* 2011;120(suppl 1):S192–S203.

Ueda K. ABC proteins protect the human body and maintain optimal health. *Biosci Biotechnol Biochem.* 2011;75:401–409.

Van den Berg M, Heeremans C, Veerhoven E, Olie K. Transfer of polychlorinated dibenzo-p-dioxins and dibenzofurans to fetal and neonatal rats. *Fundam Appl Toxicol.* 1987;9:635–644.

Van Herwaarden AE, Schinkel AH. The function of breast cancer resistance protein in epithelial barriers, stem cells and milk secretion of drugs and xenotoxins. *Trends Pharmacol Sci.* 2006;27:10–16.

Venter JC, Adams MD, Myers EW, et al. The sequence of the human genome. *Science.* 2001;291:1304–1351.

Vlaming ML, Lagas JS, Schinkel AH. Physiological and pharmacological roles of ABCG2 (BCRP): recent findings in Abcg2 knockout mice. *Adv Drug Deliv Rev.* 2009;61:14–25.

Vlaming MLH, Morhmann K, Wagenaar E, et al. Carcinogen and anticancer drug transport by Mrp2 in vivo: Studies using Mrp2 (Abcc2) knockout mice. *J Pharmacol Exp Ther.* 2006;318:319–327.

Wang DS, Kusuhara H, Kato Y, Jonker JW, Schinkel AH, Sugiyama Y. Involvement of organic cation transporter 1 in the lactic acidosis caused by metformin. *Mol Pharmacol.* 2003;63:844–848.

Waalkes MP, Ward JM, Liu J, Diwan BA. Transplacental carcinogenesis of inorganic arsenic in drinking water: induction of hepatic, ovarian, pulmonary and adrenal tumors in mice. *Toxicol Appl Pharmacol.* 2003;186:7–17.

Walton K, Dorne JLCM, Renwick AG. Species-specific uncertainty factors for compounds eliminated principally by renal excretion in humans. *Food Chem Toxicol.* 2004;42:261–274.

Wester RC, Maibach HI. Animal models for percutaneous absorption. In: Wang RGM, Knaak JB, Maibach HI, eds. *Health Risk Assessment—Dermal and Inhalation Exposure and Absorption of Toxicants.* Boca Raton: CRC Press; 1993:89–103.

Wihnholds J, Scheffer GL, van der Valk M, et al. Multidrug resistance protien 1 protects the oropharyngeal mucosal layer and the testicular tubules against drug-induced damage. *J Exp Med.* 1998;188:797–808.

Williams AC, Berry BW. Penetration enhancers. *Adv Drug Deliv Rev.* 2004;56:603–618.

Wilson JT. Determinants and consequences of drug excretion in breast milk. *Drug Metab Rev.* 1983;14:619–652.

Wilson TH. *Mechanisms of Absorption.* Philadelphia: WB Saunders; 1962:40–68.

Wu SP, Shyu MK, Liou HH, Gau CS, Lin CJ. Interaction between anticonvulsants and human placental carnitine transporter. *Epilepsia.* 2004;45:204–210.

Yuasa H, Matsuhisa E, Watanabe J. Intestinal brush border transport mechanism of 5-fluorocuracil in rats. *Biol Pharm Bull.* 1996;19:94–99.

Zhang Y, Wang H, Unadkat JD, Mao Q. Breast cancer resistance protein limits fetal distribution of nitrofurantoin in the pregnant mouse. *Drug Metab Dispos.* 2007;35:2154–2158.

Zolk O, Fromm MF. Transporter-mediated drug uptake and efflux: important determinants of adverse drug reactions. *Clin Pharmacol Ther.* 2011;89:798–805.

chapter 6

Biotransformation of Xenobiotics

Andrew Parkinson, Brian W. Ogilvie, David B. Buckley,
Faraz Kazmi, Maciej Czerwinski, and Oliver Parkinson

INTRODUCTION

In 2003, my father (and Oliver's grandfather), Edward William Parkinson, died of Lou Gehrig disease, otherwise known as amyotrophic lateral sclerosis (ALS) in America and as motor neuron disease (MND) in Britain. He died beeping. The beeping came from a portable, electronic syringe that periodically injected my father with glycopyrrolate, an anticholinergic drug that blocks the production of saliva that many ALS patients have difficulty swallowing. Glycopyrrolate is a quaternary ammonium salt; hence, it is positively charged at physiological pH. As such, glycopyrrolate does not readily cross lipid bilayers, which is why it is injected intravenously or intramuscularly; it has few CNS effects (it does not readily cross the blood–brain barrier), and a relatively small volume of distribution at steady state (V_{ss} = 0.42 L/kg). Unchanged glycopyrrolate is rapidly eliminated in urine. The mean elimination half-life increases from 19 minutes in patients with normal kidney function to 47 minutes in patients with severe kidney impairment, indicating that renal disease impairs the elimination of glycopyrrolate. Although it is excreted in urine largely as unchanged drug, glycopyrrolate reinforces a number of principles about xenobiotic biotransformation, the most important of which is: xenobiotic biotransformation is the process—actually a series of enzyme-catalyzed processes—that alters the physiochemical properties of foreign chemicals (xenobiotics) from those that favor

absorption across biological membranes (namely, lipophilicity) to those favoring elimination in urine or bile (namely, hydrophilicity). Without xenobiotic biotransformation, the numerous foreign chemicals to which we are exposed (which includes both man-made and natural chemicals such as drugs, industrial chemicals, pesticides, pollutants, pyrolysis products in cooked food, alkaloids, secondary plant metabolites, and toxins produced by molds, plants, etc) either unintentionally or, in the case of drugs, intentionally would—if they are sufficiently lipophilic to be absorbed from the gastrointestinal tract and other sites of exposure—eventually accumulate to toxic levels. Furthermore, absent xenobiotic biotransformation, many of the drugs in use today would have an unacceptably long duration of action. In contrast, drugs that are not lipophilic, such as glycopyrrolate, are not absorbed from the gastrointestinal tract unless their uptake is mediated by a transporter protein (hence, they are not orally active), and if they are administered parenterally, they are not obligated to undergo biotransformation (because they are already hydrophilic) to facilitate their elimination from the body.

The enzymes that catalyze xenobiotic biotransformation are often called drug-metabolizing enzymes. The acronym ADME stands for *a*bsorption, *d*istribution, *m*etabolism, and *e*limination. This acronym is widely used in the pharmaceutical industry to describe the 4 main processes governing drug disposition. The acronym is sometimes extended to include drug transport (AMDET) or drug toxicity (ADME-Tox). This chapter describes some fundamental principles of xenobiotic biotransformation, and describes the major enzyme systems involved in the biotransformation (or metabolism) of drugs and other xenobiotics. The examples given are biased toward drugs and human enzyme systems for 2 reasons. First, many of the fundamental principles of xenobiotic biotransformation stem from such studies. This is especially true of drugs with a narrow therapeutic index (where the toxic dose is not much greater than the therapeutic dose), which have revealed a large number of genetic and environmental factors that affect xenobiotic biotransformation and, hence, drug toxicity. Second, adverse drug events (ADEs) are one of the leading causes of death in the United States. Lazarou *et al.* (1998) estimated that in 1994 over 2 million hospitalized patients had serious ADEs (also known as adverse drug reactions or ADRs) and 106,000 had fatal outcomes, placing ADEs only behind heart disease, cancer, stroke, and pulmonary disease as a leading cause of death. Of the 548 new chemical entities approved by the Food and Drug Administration (FDA) between 1974 and 1999, ~10% (56 drugs) required black box warnings or were withdrawn from the market because of ADEs that included hepatotoxicity, cardiotoxicity (several as a result of drug–drug interactions), myelotoxicity, immunotoxicity, and warnings to pregnant women (Lasser *et al.*, 2002; Thomas, 2002). Between 1998 and 2005 the number of serious ADEs reported voluntarily to the FDA through the Adverse Events Reporting System (AERS), known as MedWatch reports, increased 2.6-fold (from 34,966 in 1998 to 89,842 in 2005) and the number of ADE-related fatalities increased 2.7-fold (from 5519 in 1998 to 15,107 in 2005) (Moore *et al.*, 2007). These increases in ADE incidence were 4 times greater than the increase in the total number of outpatient prescriptions written during the same period. In many cases, xenobiotic biotransformation is central to understanding these ADEs.

PRINCIPLES OF XENOBIOTIC BIOTRANSFORMATION

It is difficult to make categorical statements about xenobiotic biotransformation because there is an exception to every rule. Nevertheless, the following points, which might be considered principles or rules, apply in the majority of cases:

Point 1   Xenobiotic biotransformation or drug metabolism is the process of converting lipophilic (fat-soluble) chemicals, which are readily absorbed from the gastrointestinal tract and other sites, into hydrophilic (water-soluble) chemicals, which are readily excreted in urine or bile. There are exceptions even to this most basic rule. For example, acetylation and methylation are biotransformation reactions that can actually decrease the water solubility of certain xenobiotics. As a general rule, xenobiotics with a log $D_{7.4} > 0$ require biotransformation to facilitate their elimination (Williams *et al.*, 2003b).

Point 2   The biotransformation of xenobiotics is catalyzed by various enzyme systems that can be divided into 4 categories based on the reaction they catalyze:

1. Hydrolysis (eg, carboxylesterase)
2. Reduction (eg, carbonyl reductase)
3. Oxidation (eg, cytochrome P450 [CYP])
4. Conjugation (eg, UDP-glucuronosyltransferase [UGT])

The mammalian enzymes involved in the hydrolysis, reduction, oxidation, and conjugation of xenobiotics are listed in Table 6-1, together with their principal subcellular location. The conjugation reactions include glucuronidation, sulfonation (often

called sulfation), acetylation, methylation, conjugation with glutathione (GSH; mercapturic acid synthesis), and conjugation with amino acids (such as glycine, taurine, and glutamine). Examples of the major chemical groups that undergo biotransformation together with the enzymes that commonly mediate their biotransformation are given in Table 6-2 (Williams *et al.*, 2003b; Testa and Krämer, 2008, 2010).

Xenobiotic biotransformation is generally catalyzed by enzymes, but there are exceptions. For example, hydrolysis of certain carboxylic and phosphoric acid esters, reduction of sulfoxides to sulfides (eg, rabeprazole), isomerization involving enol–keto tautomerization (eg, thalidomide), and the conjugation of certain xenobiotics with GSH can occur nonenzymatically at an appreciable rate. Certain reactions are catalyzed by gastric acid, such as the hydrolysis of esters and the conversion of indole-3-carbinol to a dimer that is a potent agonist of the aryl hydrocarbon receptor (AhR) and, consequently, an inducer of various enzymes including certain CYP enzymes (CYP1A1, 1A2, 1B1, and 2S1) (Grose and Bjeldanes, 1992).

Point 3   In general, individual xenobiotic-biotransforming enzymes are located in a single organelle. In Table 6-1, some enzymes are listed with 2 or more subcellular locations. However, in such cases, the enzyme name generally refers to 2 or more enzymes, each with its own distinct subcellular location. For example, the epoxide hydrolase located in microsomes is the same enzyme located in the plasma membrane but is a different enzyme from the epoxide hydrolase located in cytosol (ie, they are distinct gene products). From a practical perspective, it is noteworthy that during the homogenization of tissue and the preparation of subcellular fractions, a certain degree of cross-contamination of organelles occurs. For example, microsomes contain detectable levels of monoamine oxidase (MAO) and other outer mitochondrial enzymes, such as the mitochondrial amidoxime-reducing component (mARC) due to their contamination with the outer mitochondrial membrane. On the other hand, some xenobiotic-biotransforming enzymes are present in 2 or more subcellular locations. Some CYP enzymes, such as CYP2E1, are present in microsomes and the inner mitochondrial membrane, which has implications for the site of xenobiotic toxicity, as discussed in the section "CYP2E1."

Point 4   In general, xenobiotic biotransformation is accomplished by a limited number of enzymes with broad substrate specificities. In humans, for example, 2 CYP enzymes—namely, CYP2D6 and CYP3A4—metabolize over half the orally effective drugs in current use (Gonzalez *et al.*, 2011). The broad and sometimes overlapping substrate specificities of xenobiotic-biotransforming enzymes preclude the possibility of naming the individual enzymes after the reactions they catalyze (which is how most other enzymes are named). Many of the enzymes involved in xenobiotic biotransformation are arranged in families and subfamilies and named according to nomenclature systems based on the primary amino acid sequence of the individual enzymes. CYP2D6, for example, is in CYP family 2, subfamily D, and gene number 6. Some enzymes are given the same name across all mammalian species, whereas others are named in a species-specific manner. For example, some CYP enzymes, such as CYP1A1, CYP1A2, and CYP1B1, are so named in all mammalian species, whereas CYP enzymes in the CYP2, CYP3, and CYP4 families (with certain exceptions such as CYP2E1) are named in a species-specific manner. The convention of using italic and regular letters to distinguish between the gene and gene products (mRNA and protein), respectively, and the convention of using lower case letters to designate mouse genes and gene products will not be followed in this chapter.

Table 6-1

General Pathways of Xenobiotic Biotransformation and Their Major Subcellular Location

REACTION	ENZYME OR SPECIFIC REACTION	LOCALIZATION
Hydrolysis	Carboxylesterase	Microsomes, cytosol, lysosomes, blood
	Butyrylcholinesterase	Plasma and most tissues
	Acetylcholinesterase	Erythrocytes and most tissues
	Paraoxonases	Plasma, microsomes, inner mitochondrial membrane
	Alkaline phosphatase	Plasma membrane
	Peptidase	Blood, lysosomes
	β-Glucuronidase	Microsomes, lysosomes, microflora
	Epoxide hydrolase	Microsomes, plasma membrane, cytosol
Reduction	Azo- and nitro-reduction	Microflora
	Carbonyl (aldo-keto) reduction	Cytosol, microsomes, blood
	Disulfide reduction	Cytosol
	Sulfoxide reduction	Cytosol
	Quinone reduction	Cytosol, microsomes
	Dihydropyrimidine dehydrogenase	Cytosol
	Reductive dehalogenation	Microsomes
	Dehydroxylation (mARC*)	Mitochondria
	Dehydroxylation (aldehyde oxidase)	Cytosol
Oxidation	Alcohol dehydrogenase	Cytosol
	Aldehyde dehydrogenase	Mitochondria, cytosol
	Aldehyde oxidase	Cytosol
	Xanthine oxidoreductase	Cytosol
	Class I amine oxidases	
	MAO-A and B	Outer mitochondrial membrane, platelets
	PAO	Cytosol, peroxisomes, plasma
	SMOX	Cytosol, nucleus
	Class II amine oxidases (CuAOs)	
	SSAOs (eg, AOC3)	Cytosolic and membrane-associated forms
	DAOs	Microsomes and extracellular matrix
	LOX	Extracellular matrix
	Peroxidases	Microsomes, lysosomes, saliva
	Flavin monooxygenases	Microsomes
	Cytochrome P450	Microsomes, mitochondria
Conjugation	UDP-glucuronosyltransferase	Microsomes
	Acyl-CoA synthetase	Mitochondria
	Sulfotransferase	Cytosol
	Glutathione transferase	Cytosol, microsomes, mitochondria
	Amino acid transferase	Mitochondria, microsomes
	N-Acetyltransferase	Mitochondria, cytosol
	Methyltransferase	Cytosol, microsomes, blood

*mARC: mitochondrial amidoxime-reducing component.

The structure (ie, amino acid sequence) of a given xenobiotic-biotransforming enzyme may differ among individuals, which can give rise to differences in rates of drug metabolism. In general, a variant form of a xenobiotic-biotransforming enzyme (known as an *allelic variant* or *allelozyme*) has diminished enzymatic activity or level of expression compared with that of the wild-type enzyme, although this is not always the case (see the sections "Alcohol Dehydrogenase," "Aldehyde Oxidase," "Cholinesterases (AChE and BChE)," "Carboxylesterases," "Epoxide Hydrolase," "Flavin Monooxygenases," "Glutathione Conjugation," "Paraoxonases (Lactonases)," "Sulfonation," "CYP1A1, 1A2, and 1B1," "CYP1A1, 1A2, and 1B1," "CYP2C8," "CYP2C19," and "CYP3A5"). The impact of amino acid substitution(s) on the catalytic activity of a xenobiotic-biotransforming enzyme may be substrate-dependent, such that an allelic variant may interact normally with some substrates (and inhibitors) but interact atypically with others.

The broad substrate specificity of xenobiotic-biotransforming enzymes makes them catalytically versatile but slow compared with most other enzymes (with the exception of hydrolytic reactions). The sequential oxidation, conjugation, and transport of a xenobiotic tend to proceed quicker at each subsequent step, which prevents the accumulation of intracellular metabolites. Were it not for the low catalytic turnover of CYP (one molecule of which may take several seconds or minutes to oxidize a single drug molecule), it would not be possible to achieve the once-a-day dosing characteristic of a large number of drugs.

Table 6-2

Common Chemical Groups and Enzymes Possibly Involved in Their Metabolism

CHEMICAL GROUP	ENZYME(S)	REACTION(S)	CHEMICAL GROUP	ENZYME(S)	REACTION(S)
Alkane R—CH₂—R	CYP	Hydroxylation, dehydrogenation	Aldehyde (R—C(=O)—H)	CYP, ALDH Aldehyde oxidase	Oxidative deformylation, oxidation to carboxylic acid
Alkene (R₂C=CR₂)	CYP, GST	Epoxidation, glutathionylation	Aliphatic amide (R—C(=O)—NH—R)	Amidase (esterase)	Hydrolysis
Alkyne R—C≡C—R	CYP	Oxidation to ketocarbenes and carboxylic acid	Aniline (phenyl—NH₂)	CYP, NAT, UGT, peroxidase, SULT	N-Hydroxylation, N-acetylation, N-glucuronidation, N-oxidation, N-sulfonation
Aliphatic alcohol R—CH₂—OH	CYP, ADH, catalase, UGT, SULT	Oxidation, glucuronidation, and sulfonation	Aromatic azaheterocycles (quinoline)	UGT, CYP, aldehyde oxidase	N-Glucuronidation, hydroxylation, N-oxidation, ring cleavage, oxidation
Aliphatic amine R—NH₂	CYP, FMO, MAO, UGT, SULT, MT, NAT, peroxidase	N-Dealkylation, N-oxidation, deamination, N-glucuronidation, N-carbamoylglucuronidation, N-sulfonation, N-methylation, N-acetylation	Carbamate R—NH—C(=O)—O—R	CYP, esterase	Oxidative cleavage, hydrolysis
Amidine HN=CR—NH₂	CYP	N-Oxidation	Ester R—CH₂—O—C(=O)—R	CYP, esterase	Oxidative cleavage, hydrolysis
Arene (phenyl—R)	CYP	Hydroxylation and epoxidation	Ether R—CH₂—O—CH₂—R	CYP	O-Dealkylation
Carboxylic acid R—COOH	UGT, amino acid transferases, acyl-CoA synthetase	Gluconidation, amino acylation, coenzyme A thioesterification	Ketone R—CH₂—C(=O)—R	CYP, FMO, SDR, AKR	Baeyer–Villiger oxidation, reduction
Epoxide	Epoxide hydrolase, GST	Hydrolysis, glutathionylation	Phenol (phenyl—OH)	CYP, UGT, SULT, MT	Ipso-substitution, glucuronidation, sulfonation, methylation
Lactone	Lactonase (paraoxonase)	Hydrolysis (ring opening)	Thioether R—CH₂—S—CH₂—R	CYP, FMO	S-Dealkylation, S-oxidation

ADH, alcohol dehydrogenase; ALDH, aldehyde dehydrogenase; AKR, aldo-keto reductases; FMO, flavin monooxygenase; GST, glutathione S-transferase; MT, methyltransferase; SDR, short-chain dehydrogenases/reductases; SULT, sulfotransferase; UGT, UDP-glucuronosyltransferase. Data from Williams et al. (2003b).

Point 5 Hydrolysis, reduction, and oxidation expose or introduce a functional group (such as –OH, –NH$_2$, –SH, or –COOH) that can be converted to a water-soluble conjugate (see Table 6-2). For subsequent conjugation, the functional group introduced or exposed by hydrolysis, reduction, or oxidation must be nucleophilic (in the case of glucuronidation, sulfonation, methylation, acetylation, and conjugation with glycine or taurine) or electrophilic (in the case of glutathionylation).

The first 3 reactions (hydrolysis, reduction, and oxidation) are often called Phase 1 reactions, and the conjugation reactions are often called Phase 2 reactions. The classification of xenobiotic-biotransforming enzymes into Phase 1 and Phase 2 (and the extension of this system to classify xenobiotic transporters as Phase 3) has been criticized by Josephy *et al.* (2005), as being both misleading and contrary to the original principles of Williams (1959), the drug metabolism pioneer who coined the phrases to distinguish reactions that resulted in either a decrease or increase in xenobiotic toxicity (Phase 1) from reactions that resulted in only a decrease in toxicity (Phase 2). Notwithstanding the arguments against the Phase 1–Phase 2 classification, which were summarized in the previous version of this chapter (Parkinson and Ogilvie, 2008), the terms are widely used today not as R. T. William's originally intended but to distinguish biotransformation reactions involving oxidation, reduction, or hydrolysis (Phase 1) from those involving conjugation (Phase 2). The original idea that Phase 2 metabolism results in only detoxication is incorrect. Indeed, on a case-by-case basis, all xenobiotic-metabolizing enzymes are capable of increasing the toxicity of one or more xenobiotics, including the conjugating enzymes that R. T. Williams classified as Phase 2 (detoxifying) enzymes. For example, conjugation of carboxylic acid–containing drugs with glucuronic acid or coenzyme A (CoA) to form acyl glucuronides and acyl-CoA thioesters, respectively, is thought to be responsible for the hepatotoxicity observed with numerous nonsteroidal anti-inflammatory drugs (NSAIDs). In fact, in the United States, NSAIDs and other carboxylic acid–containing drugs represent the largest category of drugs whose clinical development was halted or whose regulatory approval was subsequently withdrawn because of liver toxicity in humans (Fung *et al.*, 2001). Although Phase 1 biotransformation often precedes Phase 2 metabolism, some drugs, such as acetaminophen (Tylenol), are conjugated directly (by glucuronidation and sulfonation), whereas other drugs, such as gemfibrozil and diclofenac, undergo Phase 1 metabolism (by CYP [CYP2C8]) *after* Phase 2 metabolism (glucuronidation) (Ogilvie *et al.*, 2006).

Point 6 Oxidation, reduction, hydrolysis, methylation, and acetylation generally cause a modest increase in the water solubility of a xenobiotic, whereas glucuronidation, sulfonation, glutathionylation, and amino acid conjugation generally cause a marked increase in hydrophilicity. The impact of biotransformation on the physiochemical properties and disposition of xenobiotics and their metabolites can be appreciated from modern approaches to drug development. For a drug to be absorbed by passive diffusion in the gut (so that it can be orally effective and distribute throughout the body) it must generally have a log P of 0 to 5 and a calculated total polar surface area (TPSA) less than 100 Å^2 (Smith and Dalvie, 2012). Water-soluble drugs (those with a negative log P) might be orally active if their absorption is mediated by an intestinal drug transporter. Extremely lipophilic drugs (log $P > 5$) tend to be too insoluble or they dissolve too slowly to be well absorbed from the intestine unless the dose is particularly low. Drugs must undergo desolvation (ie, they must dissociate from water molecules) to penetrate the lipid bilayer of cells. Drugs begin to lose their lipoidal permeability when their TPSA increases above ~75 Å^2 and lose it

entirely at a TPSA of around 150 Å^2. When drugs meet the aforementioned criteria (log $P = 0$–5, TPSA < 100 Å^2), their metabolites formed by oxidation, reduction, hydrolysis, methylation, or acetylation also tend to meet these same criteria; hence, the metabolites formed by these reactions, like the parent drug, readily diffuse across biological membranes down a concentration gradient (unless their diffusion into tissues such as the brain is restricted by efflux transporters). Metabolites formed by conjugation reactions (other than methylation and acetylation) contain a negatively charged glucuronide, sulfate, or amino acid (glycine or taurine) moiety (or a zwitterionic GSH moiety) and consequently have a much lower log P and a much greater TPSA than the parent drug, so much so that they cannot readily diffuse passively across biological membranes. The elimination of such conjugates from the liver (where they are largely formed) requires active transport across the canalicular (apical) membrane so they can be eliminated in bile or across the sinusoidal (basolateral) membrane, which enables their transport into blood (where they are generally highly bound to albumin given their anionic nature [negative charge]) and then to the kidney for elimination in urine (by either glomerular filtration or possibly active transport [tubular secretion]). Drug conjugates are actively transported into bile primarily by MRP2 (ABCC2) on the canalicular membrane and actively transported into blood primarily by MRP1 (ABCC1; in the case of GSH conjugates) and MRP3 (ABCC3; in the case of glucuronide and sulfate conjugates) on the sinusoidal membrane, although on a case-by-case basis other transporters may be involved (Borst *et al.*, 2006).

Point 7 Not all biotransformation reactions are catalyzed by the mammalian enzymes listed in Table 6-1. Some biotransformation reactions are catalyzed by enzymes in the gut microflora (largely anaerobic bacteria in the colon), whereas the biotransformation of still other xenobiotics is catalyzed by enzymes that participate in intermediary (endobiotic) metabolism. This principle is illustrated in Fig. 6-1 for 3 xenobiotics that are all converted to benzoic acid and then hippuric acid. The conversion of toluene to hippuric acid is catalyzed by some of the xenobiotic-biotransforming enzymes listed in Table 6-1: microsomal CYP converts toluene to benzoic acid in 3 oxidative steps (R-CH$_3$ → R-CH$_2$OH → RCHO → RCOOH), which introduces a functional group (namely, –COOH) that is conjugated with glycine to produce hippuric acid, which is excreted in urine. Cinnamic acid is also converted to benzoic acid but, in this case, the reaction is catalyzed by the mitochondrial enzymes involved in the β-oxidation of fatty acids. Quinic acid is also converted to benzoic acid, but this reductive, multistep reaction is catalyzed by gut microflora. Incidentally, the conversion of benzoic acid to hippuric acid is of historical interest because it is generally recognized as the first xenobiotic biotransformation reaction to be discovered (in dogs by Woehler in 1828, and in humans by Ure in 1841).

Some drugs are intentionally designed to be biotransformed by endobiotic-metabolizing enzymes. For example, the anti-HIV drug zidovudine (AZT) is converted to a triphosphate nucleoside by enzymes in the salvage pathway (nucleoside kinase, nucleoside monophosphate kinase [NMK], and nucleoside diphosphate kinase [NDK]). HIV reverse transcriptase inhibitors, such as zidovudine, are administered as nonphosphorylated analogs to facilitate their absorption and cellular uptake. Conversely, some drugs are administered as a phosphorylated prodrug (eg, fosamprenavir) to promote their water solubility and rate of dissolution. The luminal surface of the small intestine contains high levels of alkaline phosphatase, which hydrolyzes prodrugs such as fosamprenavir and thereby releases the active drug at the surface of the enterocyte, where it is readily absorbed. Generally speaking, kinase and

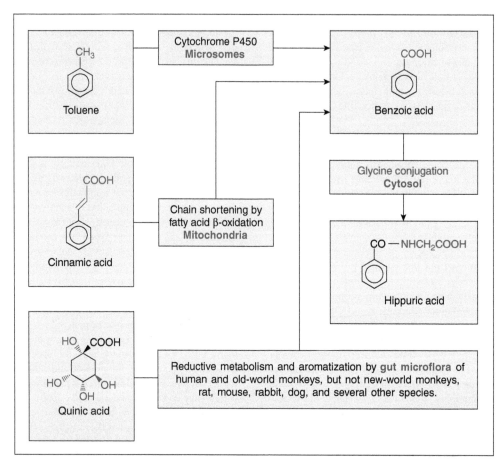

Figure 6-1. *Examples of xenobiotic biotransformation by different enzyme systems: a xenobiotic-biotransforming enzyme (cytochrome P450), an endobiotic-metabolizing enzyme, and gut microflora.*

alkaline phosphatase are not usually considered to be xenobiotic-biotransforming enzymes.

Point 8 Just as some xenobiotics are biotransformed by the so-called endobiotic-metabolizing enzymes (Point 7), certain endobiotics are biotransformed by the so-called xenobiotic-metabolizing enzymes. For example, the same CYP enzymes implicated in xenobiotic biotransformation also contribute to the hepatic catabolism of steroid hormones, and the same UGTs that conjugate xenobiotics also glucuronidate bilirubin, thyroid hormones, and steroid hormones. Interestingly, the CYP and UGT enzymes that play a major role in steroid metabolism (namely, CYP3A4 and UGT1A1) display positive homotropic cooperativity (ie, the enzymes have Hill coefficients >1) such that the rate of metabolism of steroid hormones by these enzymes is slow at low substrate concentrations but increases dramatically as the concentration of steroid hormone increases. Benzoic acid, a xenobiotic, is conjugated with glycine (as shown in Fig. 6-1), and so are bile acids (endobiotics). Certain leukotrienes are GSH conjugates. Conjugates of endogenous substrates, such as the glucuronide and sulfate conjugates of steroid and THs, tend to be transported out of the hepatocyte by MRP2, the same canalicular transporter that transports drug conjugates into bile. From the few examples in Points 7 and 8, it is apparent that, on a case-by-case basis, there is often no clear-cut distinction between endobiotic- and xenobiotic-biotransforming enzymes.

The human genome project has helped to establish that what were once thought to be 2 distinct enzymes, one involved in the metabolism of endobiotics and one involved in the metabolism of xenobiotics, are in fact one and the same enzyme. For example, the microsomal enzyme known as 11β-hydroxysteroid dehydrogenase is identical to the xenobiotic-metabolizing enzyme known as microsomal carbonyl reductase (gene symbol HSD11B1; aka SDR26C1). Likewise, hepoxilin A₃ hydrolase was thought to represent a fifth class of epoxide hydrolases, but was subsequently identified as the same enzyme as soluble epoxide hydrolase (sEH) (Cronin *et al.*, 2011).

Point 9 Several xenobiotic-biotransforming enzymes are inducible, meaning their expression can be increased (upregulated) usually in response to exposure to high concentrations of xenobiotics. Induction is mediated by ligand-activated receptors (so-called xenosensors) that are activated by xenobiotics (ligands) to DNA-binding proteins that upregulate the transcription of various genes encoding xenobiotic-biotransforming enzymes, especially CYP enzymes, which are usually induced to the greatest extent (in terms of fold increase). The major xenosensors are aryl hydrocarbon receptor (AhR), which induces CYP1 enzymes, the constitutive androstane receptor (CAR), which induces CYP2B, 2C, and 3A enzymes, the pregnane X receptor (PXR), which also induces CYP2B, 2C, and 3A enzymes, and the peroxisome proliferator–activated receptor-α (PPARα), which induces CYP4 enzymes. CAR and PXR are closely related nuclear receptors, and they tend to be activated by the same ligands and bind to the same DNA-response elements (ie, the same discrete regions of DNA that control gene expression), for which reason there is said to be considerable *cross-talk* between these 2 xenosensors. Certain xenosensors are activated by endogenous ligands (eg, bilirubin, bile acids, and fatty acids activate CAR, PXR, and PPARα, respectively), and certain nuclear receptors, such as the vitamin D receptor (VDR), can mimic PXR and induce CYP3A4, which inactivates the active metabolite of vitamin D. These examples illustrate how xenosensors are not just involved in xenobiotic disposition but also play a role in endobiotic homeostasis. Two proteins called Kelch-like ECH-related protein (KEAP)-1 and nuclear factor E2 p45-related factor-2 (Nrf2) function as xenosensors inasmuch as they induce enzymes in response to oxidative stress, which is often associated with xenobiotic biotransformation. Binding of the transcription factor Nrf2 to the region of DNA known as the antioxidant response element (also known as the electrophilic response element [EpRE]) induces enzymes that detoxify electrophiles and metabolites that generate reactive oxygen species (ROS), including glutathione transferase (GST; GSTA1), microsomal epoxide hydrolase (mEH), aldo-keto reductase (AKRs; AKR7A, also known as aflatoxin aldehyde reductase), NAD(P)H-quinone oxidoreductase (NQO1, also known as DT-diaphorase), microsomal heme oxygenase, and glutamate–cysteine ligase (GCL), which catalyzes the rate-limiting step in GSH synthesis. Induction of GCL increases the rate of GSH synthesis under conditions of oxidative stress and a decrease in GSH concentration (Lee and Johnson, 2004).

Induction is a reversible, adaptive response to xenobiotic exposure. The induced enzymes (and transporters) usually accelerate the elimination of the xenobiotic that triggered the induction process, in which case the xenobiotic is said to be an autoinducer (one that induces its own metabolism). However, xenobiotics often induce enzymes that are not capable of metabolizing them, in which case the induction is said to be gratuitous. Induction is a pleiotropic response: activation of AhR, CAR, PXR, PPARα, and Nrf2 all results in alterations in the expression of numerous genes.

Suppression (downregulation) of drug-metabolizing enzymes is often association with inflammatory diseases (such as arthritis), cancer, infectious diseases (both bacterial and viral), vaccination, and treatment with certain proinflammatory biologics (therapeutic proteins). These disease processes activate nuclear factor kappa-B (NF-κB) (and other nuclear receptors), which suppresses the expression and induction of CYP and other xenobiotic-metabolizing enzymes because activated NF-κB suppresses all 4 xenosensors (AhR, CAR, PXR, and PPARα), as well as several other nuclear receptors. By reversing the disease process—such as lessening the inflammation associated with rheumatoid arthritis—some biologics (large drug molecules such as monoclonal antibodies and other types of therapeutic proteins) can reverse the suppression of drug-metabolizing enzymes and restore their activity to normal (predisease) levels (Morgan, 2009; Huang et al., 2010).

Point 10 The ability of certain xenobiotic-biotransforming enzymes to metabolize hormones and other endobiotics (Point 8) and the ability of certain xenobiotics to induce xenobiotic-biotransforming enzymes (Point 9) have implications for understanding an important mechanism by which certain xenobiotics can alter homeostasis or cause toxicity. Persistent exposure to xenobiotics that are enzyme inducers (especially CAR and PPARα activators) can increase the rate of steroid hormone oxidation by CYP and increase the rate of thyroid hormone glucuronidation and sulfonation that, in rodents, can lead to the development of Leydig cell tumors (due to elevated levels of LH and FSH) and thyroid follicular tumors (due to elevated levels of thyroid-stimulating hormone [TSH]), respectively (Grasso et al., 1991). Persistent exposure to enzyme inducers can also cause liver tumors, although the mechanism is not fully understood. Activation of certain xenosensors (CAR or PPARα) is critical to liver tumor development in mice, although upregulation of xenobiotic-biotransforming enzymes is less important than other xenosensor-dependent events, such as, in the case of the CAR activator phenobarbital, altered DNA methylation of numerous genes, upregulation of GADD45B (an antiapoptotic factor) and MDM2

(a negative regulator of the tumor suppressor p53), and the down-regulation of gap junctional proteins (connexin 32), which diminishes cell–cell communication (Omiecinski et al., 2011b).

Phenobarbital, Wy-14643, methapyrilene, and Ponceau S are representatives of 4 classes of nongenotoxic rodent tumorigens (epigenetic tumor promoters) that cause hepatocellular hyperplasia and hypertrophy in association with proliferation of the endoplasmic reticulum, peroxisomes, mitochondria, and lysosomes, respectively (Grasso et al., 1991). In the first 2 cases, the hepatocellular changes depend on activation of CAR (in the case of phenobarbital) and PPARα (in the case of Wy-14643). Prolonged activation of these receptors in rodents results in the development of liver and/or thyroid tumors. However, this is thought to be a rodent-specific phenomenon because, in the case of phenobarbital and other enzyme-inducing antiepileptic drugs (EIAEDs), there is compelling epidemiological evidence that these chemicals do not cause liver tumors in humans even after >30 years of treatment (Parkinson et al., 2006).

The major UGT responsible for conjugating bilirubin is UGT1A1, which is inducible by CAR activators such as phenobarbital and scoparone (6,7-dimethylesculetin). At one time, the management of neonatal jaundice included treatment with phenobarbital to induce bilirubin conjugation, but this practice has been discontinued. However, the Chinese herbal Yin Zhi Huang (active ingredient scoparone) is still used to treat neonatal jaundice. Bilirubin is also a CAR agonist, and high levels of bilirubin induce UGT1A1 and bilirubin/bilirubin glucuronide transporters (MRP2 [ABCC2] and MRP3 [ABCC3]) to increase the rate of bilirubin elimination when bilirubin levels are elevated (eg, during hemolytic anemia).

Although prolonged activation of PXR in rats is associated with thyroid tumor promotion due to induction of triiodothyronine (T3) glucuronidation (Richardson and Klaassen, 2010), this effect is thought not to occur in humans. However, prolonged activation of PXR by rifampin in humans (which induces hepatic and intestinal CYP3A4) is associated with osteomalacia caused by an enhanced rate of conversion of the active metabolite of vitamin D to inactive metabolites by CYP3A4 (Xu et al., 2006; Zhou et al., 2006a).

Point 11 Xenobiotic biotransformation can alter the biological properties of a xenobiotic. It can make the xenobiotic less toxic (detoxication), but in some cases it can make it more toxic (activation). The oxidation of ethanol (alcohol) to acetaldehyde is an example of xenobiotic activation, and the subsequent oxidation of acetaldehyde to acetic acid is an example of detoxication. The biotransformation of drugs can result in (1) a loss of pharmacological activity (eg, the conversion of acetaminophen to acetaminophen glucuronide and the conversion of morphine to morphine-3-glucuronide), (2) no change in pharmacological activity (eg, the conversion of fluoxetine to its *N*-demethylated metabolite norfluoxetine), or (3) an increase in pharmacological activity (eg, the conversion of codeine to morphine, as well as the conversion of morphine to morphine-6-glucuronide). When the parent drug is pharmacologically active, diminished metabolism (due to a genetic deficiency or enzyme inhibition) can result in an exaggerated pharmacological response (Type A toxicity), such as the prolonged or increased hypotension caused by debrisoquine, alprenolol, bufuralol, metropolol, propranolol, and timolol in individuals lacking CYP2D6 (Turner et al., 2001; Ingelman-Sundberg, 2005). When a metabolite is the pharmacologically active component, diminished formation (due to a genetic deficiency or enzyme inhibition) can result in little or no pharmacological response (Type F toxicity), such as the diminished effects of codeine and tamoxifen in individuals lacking CYP2D6 and the diminished effects of clopidogrel in individuals lacking CYP2C19 (discussed in the sections "CYP2D6" and "CYP2C19").

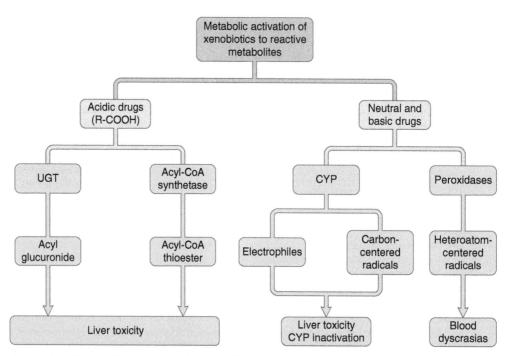

Figure 6-2. *Some major pathways of metabolic activation of xenobiotics to reactive metabolites that cause toxicity.*

Point 12 In many cases, the toxicity of a xenobiotic is due to the parent compound (the compound that was absorbed), in which case xenobiotic biotransformation serves as a detoxication mechanism. This principle is underscored by the clinical observation that the incidence of ADEs is often higher in individuals with a poor metabolizer (PM) phenotype (discussed later in Point 24). However, xenobiotic-biotransforming enzymes can convert certain xenobiotics to reactive metabolites (eg, electrophiles and radicals), and this activation process plays an important role in chemical toxicity and chemical mutagenicity/carcinogenicity; the former often involves the covalent binding of reactive metabolites to critical cellular nucleophiles such as proteins, whereas the latter involves covalent binding to one or more purine or pyrimidine bases in DNA. Formation of reactive metabolites can also lead to irreversible CYP inhibition (a process known as metabolism-dependent inhibition [MDI] or time-dependent inhibition [TDI]), which is an important cause of drug–drug interactions. As illustrated in Fig. 6-2, carboxylic acid–containing drugs (especially the acetic and propionic acid–containing NSAIDs that cause liver toxicity) can be converted to reactive acyl glucuronides and/or acyl-CoA thioesters, whereas many neutral and basic drugs are converted by CYP to electrophilic metabolites or carbon-centered radicals that may cause liver toxicity (or damage to the cells harboring the activating CYP). Several nitrogen- and sulfur-containing drugs can be activated by peroxidases to heteroatom-centered radicals that can cause blood dyscrasias such as agranulocytosis/neutroprenia, aplastic anemia, and thrombocytopenia (Tang and Lu, 2010; Walsh and Miwa, 2011). In Fig. 6-2, the scheme depicting the formation and toxicity of reactive metabolites is an oversimplification. Furthermore, some drugs can be converted to 2 or more reactive metabolites. Tienilic acid, for example, contains a carboxylic acid group, which is converted to a reactive acyl glucuronide and acyl-CoA thioester, and a furan (a neutral group), which is converted by CYP to an epoxide and other reactive metabolites (such as an enedial).

CYP is particularly effective at converting proximate carcinogens to ultimate carcinogens by converting the former to electrophilic metabolites that bind to and mutate DNA, thereby leading to mutations and tumor initiation. The Ames bacterial mutagenicity

assay, which is representative of several mutagenicity tests, is performed in the absence and presence of CYP (ie, liver microsomes) to evaluate the mutagenic potential of both the parent compound and any electrophilic metabolites, respectively. Polycyclic aromatic hydrocarbons (PAHs; combustion pollutants and components of tobacco smoke), aromatic amines (industrial chemicals), aflatoxin (a mycotoxin), cooked food pyrolysis products, and tobacco-specific nitrosamines are all examples of proximate carcinogens that require metabolic activation to form electrophilic, DNA-binding metabolites (ultimate carcinogens).

Certain anticancer drugs require activation by xenobiotic-metabolizing enzymes in order to exert their antineoplastic effects. For example, cyclophosphamide is activated by CYP (CYP2B6 and CYP3A4), and canfosfamide is activated by GST, namely, GSTP1-1, which is often overexpressed in tumors thereby conferring resistance against certain anticancer drugs (see the section "Glutathione Conjugation") (Gonzalez and Tukey, 2006).

Liver microsomes are widely used in 3 in vitro systems to investigate the potential of drugs or drug candidates to be converted to reactive metabolites. First, liver microsomes from Aroclor 1254–treated (induced) rats are used in the Ames bacterial mutagenicity assay. A limitation of this assay is that it is well suited to identify reactive metabolites formed by CYP but not by other xenobiotic-biotransforming enzymes, examples of which are given in the section "Conjugation." This limitation has been addressed through genetic engineering of *Salmonella typhimurium* so that test bacteria express one or more human xenobiotic-metabolizing enzymes (Iwata *et al.*, 1998; Glatt and Meinl, 2004b). Second, human and rat liver microsomes are widely used to assess the formation of reactive metabolites that bind covalently to microsomal protein or GSH (or a related nucleophile such as *N*-acetylcysteine [NAC]). This system does a poor job of distinguishing hepatotoxic drugs from nonhepatotoxic drugs (Obach *et al.*, 2008), but the distinction is improved when covalent binding is assessed in human hepatocytes and dose is taken into account (Bauman *et al.*, 2009; Nakayama *et al.*, 2009). Third, human liver microsomes are widely used to evaluate a drug candidate's potential to cause irreversible inhibition of the major drug-metabolizing CYP enzymes.

False-negative results can occasionally occur when metabolism by a non-CYP enzyme is instrumental to CYP inactivation, such as the need to glucuronidate gemfibrozil in order to inactivate CYP2C8. In such cases of so-called system-dependent inhibition the use of human hepatocytes offers advantages over human liver microsomes (Parkinson *et al.*, 2010).

Structural alerts (functional groups) for the bioactivation of xenobiotics to reactive metabolites that cause toxicity and/or CYP inactivation include the following (which is not an exhaustive list): (1) acetic and propionic acids (activated by UGT and/or acyl-CoA synthetase), (2) nitro aromatics (activated by reductases and/or CYP), and (3) a large number of functional groups that are activated by CYP and, in some cases, peroxidases: acetylenes, activated aromatics, 3-alkly indoles, anilines, cyclopropylamines, formamides, furans, hydrazines, pyrroles, sulfonylureas, thiazolidinones, thioamides, thiophenes, and thioureas (Walsh and Miwa, 2011).

Point 13 The toxicity and potential carcinogenicity of electrophilic metabolites produced by CYP and other xenobiotic-biotransforming enzymes is reduced and often altogether eliminated by their conjugation with GSH, which is often described as a non-critical cellular nucleophile. Conjugation with GSH can occur both enzymatically (by GST) and nonenzymatically. In the majority of cases, conjugation with GSH represents a detoxication reaction, one that protects critical cellular nucleophiles, such as protein and DNA, from covalent modification. However, there are cases (eg, methyl-bromide and dibromoethane) where conjugation with GSH actually produces a DNA-reactive (mutagenic) metabolite. Activation of haloalkanes and dihaloalkanes (which are used industrially as fumigants) is usually catalyzed by the Theta class of GSTs (Josephy, 2010). Depletion of GSH or genetic deficiency of a particular GST can predispose to certain drug toxicities. For example, the genetic loss of glutathione transferase-Mu (GSTM1) predisposes to the hepatotoxic effects of carbamazepine and valproic acid (Saruwatari *et al.*, 2010), whereas the combined loss of GSTM1 and glutathione transferase-Theta (GSTT1) is a risk factor for troglitazone hepatotoxicity (Ikeda, 2011).

Point 14 The biotransformation of some xenobiotics results in the production of ROS, which can cause cell toxicity (including DNA damage) through oxidative stress and lipid peroxidation. GSH, GSTs, and glutathione peroxidases (GPXs) all limit the toxic effects of ROS just as they limit the toxicity of reactive metabolites formed directly from xenobiotics. Oxidative stress and the formation of electrophilic metabolites reduce GSH levels and thus result in the concurrent oxidation of KEAP-1, which then releases Nrf2, which in turn upregulates the expression of enzymes that detoxify electrophilic metabolites (eg, epoxides) and those metabolites that generate ROS (eg, quinones) (see Point 9). Certain xenobiotics and ischemic reperfusion injury cause an accumulation of unfolded proteins in the endoplasmic reticulum (where proteins are folded and posttranslationally modified), which gives rise to the unfolded protein response (UPR; also known as endoplasmic reticulum stress [ER stress]), which activates Nrf2 and Bax-inhibitor-1 (BI-1). The heme oxygenase induced by Nrf2 as well as BI-1 (which complexes with NADPH-cytochrome P450 reductase) protects cells from oxidative stress by inhibiting the production of ROS by CYP2E1 and other CYP enzymes (discussed in the section "CYP2E1").

Point 15 The balance between activation and detoxication by xenobiotic-biotransforming enzymes is often a key determinant of chemical toxicity, and is often the basis for organ or species differences in toxicity. For example, aflatoxin is converted by liver microsomal CYP to a reactive epoxide that is thought to be responsible for the hepatotoxic and hepatocarcinogenic effect of this mycotoxin. The fact that this reaction occurs in the liver explains why aflatoxin causes liver toxicity and liver tumors. On this basis, mice would be expected to be more sensitive than rats to the hepatotoxic effects of aflatoxin because mice catalyze the epoxidation of aflatoxin faster than rats. However, through GSH conjugation, mice also detoxify aflatoxin epoxide faster than rats. Consequently, despite their slower rate of activation, rats are more susceptible than mice to the toxic effects of aflatoxin. Coumarin is hepatotoxic to rats, but not to humans. This species difference is attributable to differences in the metabolites formed by CYP. Rats convert coumarin to a reactive epoxide that rearranges to a reactive aldehyde, whereas humans convert coumarin to the relatively non-toxic metabolite 7-hydroxycoumarin (umbelliferone).

Point 16 Exposure to xenobiotics (especially drugs) is largely through oral ingestion, and the small intestine and liver are highly developed to limit systemic exposure to orally ingested xenobiotics, a process known as *first-pass elimination (or presystemic elimination)*. The enterocytes at the tips of the small intestinal villi express the efflux transporters P-glycoprotein (ABCB1 or MDR1) and BCRP (ABCG2), which serves to limit xenobiotic absorption. The enterocytes express high levels of certain CYP and UGT enzymes, which biotransform a wide variety of xenobiotics. The liver expresses a number of uptake transporters that actively remove xenobiotics from the blood. They also express a number of efflux transporters that actively discharge xenobiotics or their metabolites (especially conjugates) into the bile canaliculus for biliary excretion, or that actively discharge xenobiotic metabolites (especially conjugates) across the sinusoidal membrane back into the blood for urinary excretion. The liver expresses the largest number and, with few exceptions, the highest concentrations of xenobiotic-biotransforming enzymes.

Although the liver contains higher concentrations of most xenobiotic-biotransforming enzymes, and because the number of hepatocytes in the liver exceeds the number of enterocytes in the small intestine, it might be assumed that, compared with the liver, the small intestine would make only a small contribution to first-pass metabolism, but this is not the case in part because in the small intestine xenobiotics are recycled by P-glycoprotein (ABCB1) and BCRP (ABCG2) on the lumenal surface of enterocytes, which delays absorption and increases the opportunity for xenobiotic biotransformation by intestinal enzymes such as CYP (especially CYP3A4), UGT, and sulfotransferase (SULT) (Benet, 2009). Furanocoumarins in grapefruit juice inhibit intestinal but not hepatic CYP3A4 and yet grapefruit juice increases systemic exposure to felodipine and other drugs that undergo first-pass metabolism by CYP3A4 (Paine *et al.*, 2006). The impact of the CYP3A4 inhibitor ketoconazole on the disposition of the CYP3A4 substrate midazolam depends on whether midazolam is given orally or intravenously. When midazolam is given intravenously, such that its clearance is dependent only on hepatic metabolism, ketoconazole causes a 3- to 5-fold increase in the area-under-the-plasma-concentration-time curve (AUC). However, when midazolam is given orally, ketoconazole causes a 10- to 15-fold increase in AUC, the difference reflecting the significant role of intestinal metabolism to the presystemic clearance of midazolam. In rats, administration of the general CYP inhibitor 1-aminobenzotriazole (ABT) by the intravenous route (which inhibits only hepatic CYP enzymes) and the oral route (which inhibits both intestinal and hepatic CYP enzymes) can be used to assess the relative role of the intestine and liver to the first-pass metabolism of a drug or other xenobiotic (Strelevitz *et al.*, 2006).

The small intestine and liver are exposed to high concentrations of xenobiotics, and they possess high levels of the enzymes that potentially convert xenobiotics to reactive or toxic metabolites.

It is perhaps not surprising, therefore, that both tissues possess protective mechanisms to minimize the risk of xenobiotic toxicity and carcinogenicity. As already mentioned, both tissues have enzymes and transporters that facilitate the elimination of xenobiotics and their metabolites. In both tissues, several of the xenobiotic-biotransforming enzymes and transporters are inducible, enabling the liver and the small intestine to respond to high levels of xenobiotics by enhancing the rate of xenobiotic biotransformation and elimination. In the small intestine, the enterocytes at the villus tips undergo extensive turnover, such that the mature cells that are exposed to high levels of xenobiotics and/or reactive metabolites are quickly lost (exfoliated) and replaced in a matter of days. In liver, high levels of GSH (5-10 mM), a large proportion of diploid (binucleated) cells, and a high regenerative capacity all protect the liver from xenobiotic toxicity or help the liver to repair chemical-mediated toxicity. In addition, severely damaged hepatocytes can undergo apoptosis (cell-programmed death) to eliminate precancerous cells (ie, cells with extensive DNA damage).

Point 17 Some of the same mechanisms that protect the small intestine and liver from xenobiotic toxicity also protect certain organs such as the brain and reproductive organs. Xenobiotics that enter the systemic circulation are often excluded from the brain by the blood–brain barrier, which poses a physical barrier to xenobiotic transport (in the form of tight junctions) and a biochemical barrier notably in the form of the efflux transporters *P*-glycoprotein (ABCB1) and BCRP (ABCG2). Germ cells in the testis are protected in part by a blood–testis barrier, by high levels of GSH (and GST and GPX), and by high cell turnover (as in the case of enterocytes). The ovum, with virtually no cell turnover, possesses high levels of GSH (8 mM or more), which protects it from DNA-reactive electrophiles and from the oxidative stress that accompanies both xenobiotic exposure and fertilization. Efflux transporters and GSTs are often overexpressed in tumor cells as a result of chromosomal rearrangements that place the genes encoding these proteins under the control of a strong promoter. The overexpression of a transporter and/or GST can confer resistance to certain cancer chemotherapeutic agents (many of which are intended to be converted to reactive metabolites that damage DNA and kill tumor cells).

Point 18 In view of the important role of CYP in the metabolic activation of proximate carcinogens to ultimate carcinogens, it may seem paradoxical to list CYP induction among the defense mechanisms that protect organisms from the carcinogenic effects of xenobiotics. Activation by CYP is definitely required for certain xenobiotics to exert their carcinogenic effects, and induction of CYP is associated with an increase in the toxicity of certain xenobiotics. However, contrary to expectation, treatment of rodents with a CYP inducer prior to treatment with a known proximate carcinogen (such as aflatoxin, various nitrosamines, or PAHs) is generally associated with a decrease, not an increase, in tumor incidence (Parkinson and Hurwitz, 1991). The route of exposure to the carcinogen can affect the impact of enzyme induction; it protects against orally administered drugs but may increase the tumorigenicity of carcinogens applied directly to their site of action (Nebert *et al.*, 2004), and prolonged treatment of rodents with an enzyme inducer *after* application of the initiating carcinogen can lead to an increase in tumor incidence because many enzyme inducers act as tumor promoters (see Point 10). Nevertheless, for the most part, enzyme induction provides protection against chemical toxicity and carcinogenesis (Nebert and Dalton, 2006; Shimada, 2006; Ma and Lu, 2007).

Point 19 Although the small intestine and liver contain the highest concentrations, xenobiotic-biotransforming enzymes are nevertheless widely distributed throughout the body. In terms of specific content (ie, the amount of enzyme on a per-milligram-protein basis), some of the highest concentrations of xenobiotic-metabolizing enzymes are to be found in nasal epithelium, a portal of entry for many volatile xenobiotics. The presence of high levels of xenobiotic-biotransforming enzymes in nasal epithelium is of interest because numerous xenobiotics cause nasal cytotoxicity and cancer in rodents (reviewed in Jeffrey *et al.*, 2006). Xenobiotic-biotransforming enzymes in the lung, eye, and skin can be especially important for the metabolism of drugs delivered by inhalation, eye drop, or topical application, respectively. The kidney expresses several xenobiotic-biotransforming enzymes, in addition to numerous transporters that actively secrete xenobiotics (especially acidic metabolites) into urine. The kidney also metabolizes GSH conjugates formed in the liver and converts them to mercapturic acids (*N*-acetylcysteine conjugates).

Point 20 Species differences in xenobiotic-biotransforming enzymes are often the basis for species differences in both the qualitative and quantitative aspects of xenobiotic biotransformation and toxicity. As mentioned in Point 15, species difference in coumarin metabolism and toxicity (activation by epoxidation in rats, detoxication by aromatic hydroxylation in humans) reflects a species difference in hepatic microsomal CYP, whereas species differences in GST activity account for the difference between rats and mice in terms of their susceptibility to aflatoxin-induced liver toxicity. Species differences in the fetal expression of xenobiotic-biotransforming enzymes have raised questions about the suitability of laboratory animals to assess the risk of human teratogenicity because human fetal liver expresses CYP3A7, an enzyme capable of activating aflatoxin to reactive metabolites, whereas no such enzyme is expressed in the fetus of rodents (Li *et al.*, 1997; Pang *et al.*, 2012). Biotransformation, inhibition, and induction can occur in a species-specific manner. For example, furafylline and omeprazole are inhibitors and inducers of human CYP1A2, respectively, but they do not inhibit or induce CYP1A2 in rodents. Such species differences are the impetus for the development of chimeric mice (in which the mouse hepatocytes are replaced with human hepatocytes) (Strom *et al.*, 2010) and so-called humanized mice, which involves substituting the murine genes that encode xenobiotic-metabolizing enzymes (and the receptors that regulate their expression) with their human counterparts (Gonzalez, 2003; Gonzalez and Yu, 2006).

In some species, entire pathways of xenobiotic biotransformation are low or absent from a particular species. For example, cats and dogs are considered poor glucuronidators and poor acetylators of xenobiotics, respectively. Because of their inability to glucuronidate drugs, cats are sensitive to acetaminophen hepatotoxicity (Baillie and Rettie, 2011). Dogs are poor acid secretors, which disfavors the gastric absorption of acidic drugs. Interestingly, although dogs can conjugate acidic drugs, they are poor metabolizers of acidic drugs in terms of oxidative biotransformation by CYP enzymes (Baillie and Rettie, 2011). Metabolism by gut microflora can occur in a species-dependent manner. For example, as shown in Fig. 6-1, quinic acid is converted to benzoic acid in humans and old-world monkeys but not in new-world monkeys, mice, rats, and most other laboratory animals (Adamson *et al.*, 1970).

Point 21 In sexually mature rats and, to a lesser extent, mice there are marked gender differences in the expression of certain xenobiotic-biotransforming enzymes (both oxidative and conjugating enzymes) (Waxman and Holloway, 2009). In other species, including humans, gender differences either do not exist or generally represent less than a 2-fold difference, whereas the differences in rodents can be an order of magnitude or greater (Parkinson *et al.*, 2004; Soldin *et al.*, 2011). Against a large background of interindividual variation in each gender, it is often difficult to discern gender differences in xenobiotic biotransformation in humans, although, in general, women appear to have lower CYP1A2 and higher CYP3A4 activity than men (Parkinson *et al.*, 2004). It is particularly interesting that, compared with men, women appear to have a higher incidence of idiosyncratic drug toxicity (Walgren *et al.*, 2005), which has been the cause of a number of drug withdrawals and black box warnings (see Point 22).

Point 22 Idiosyncratic drug reactions (IDRs) are rare adverse events (generally <0.1%) that do not involve an exaggerated pharmacological response, do not occur in most patients at any dose, and typically do not occur immediately after exposure but do so after weeks or months of repeated administration (Walgren *et al.*, 2005). IDRs are also known as Type B or hypersensitivity reactions and they can be divided into allergic and nonallergic IDRs. The former tend to develop relatively quickly (in days or weeks) and, after the drug is discontinued, patients respond robustly when rechallenged with the same or a closely related drug, whereas the latter tend to develop relatively slowly (with symptoms sometimes appearing after 6 months or more of drug treatment) and patients may or may not respond to rechallenge with the drug. Evidence for an immune component (ie, an acquired immune response) to allergic IDRs is often circumstantial or lacking, as is the evidence for the lack of an immune component to nonallergic IDRs, which possibly involve an innate immune response. Hepatotoxicity is a prevalent IDR. Drugs that were withdrawn from the US market or carry a black box warning for idiosyncratic hepatotoxicity are listed in Table 6-3. The drugs are structurally diverse and fall into numerous therapeutic classes.

Several factors predispose to IDRs including gender (women are more prone than men), age (the elderly are more prone), ethnicity, viral infection (a particularly strong predisposing factor), and other disease states (such as diabetes and obesity), possibly alcohol consumption, comedications that cause pharmacokinetic drug–drug interactions, genetic polymorphisms in xenobiotic-biotransforming enzymes and transporters (discussed in Point 23), and genetic polymorphisms that affect immune function especially allelic variants of human leukocyte antigens (HLA haplotypes), part of the major histocompatibility complex (MHC) (Alfirevic and Pirmohamed, 2010; Chalasani and Björnsson, 2010).

The best understood IDR is the skin hypersensitivity reaction to the anti-HIV drug abacavir, which is determined in a highly predictable manner by an individual's HLA subtype (Alfirevic and Pirmohamed, 2010). Abacavir binds to the antigen-presenting groove of MHC I molecule in patients carrying the B*5701 allele (in patients of all ethnic groups). In vitro studies have demonstrated that treatment of antigen-presenting cells positive for B*5701, but not for the related alleles B*5702 or B*5801, with abacavir can stimulate a CD8+ T-cell response. Topical exposure to abacavir (patch test) reveals activated CD8+ T cells in skin biopsies. Genetic testing for B*5701 is highly predictive; abacavir hypersensitivity is almost never seen in individuals without the B*5701 allele and it is seen in about half of B*5701-positive carriers. Genetic testing for B*5701 prior to abacavir treatment is required by the FDA and is cost effective (the cost of treating the severe skin lesions that occur in 5%–9% of abacavir-treated patients outweighs the costs of genetic testing). The strongest association (odds ratio >1000) between HLA alleles (HAL B*1502) and IDR is seen with carbamazepine-induced skin lesions (Stevens–Johnson syndrome [SJR] and toxic epidermal necrolysis [TEN]) in Han Chinese, Thai, Malay, and Indian populations. However, B*1502 is neither predictive of SJS/TEN in Japanese or Caucasian populations (in whom HLA-A*3101 is a moderate risk factor) (McCormack *et al.*, 2011) nor predictive

of other carbamazepine-induced IDRs such as maculopapular exanthema or drug reaction with systemic symptoms (DRESS) in Asian populations (Alfirevic and Pirmohamed, 2010).

Hypersensitivity to abacavir is unusual for 2 reasons. First, an individual's HLA haplotype (the expression of B*5701) is the dominant determining factor. Second, the parent drug, which binds to the antigen-binding grove of B*5701, rather than a (reactive) metabolite, appears to be the precipitating factor, although it is possible that a metabolite formed in peripheral blood mononuclear cells (PBMCs) may contribute to or be responsible for the IDR. In other IDRs, especially drug-induced liver injury (DILI), there is evidence that a reactive metabolite triggers the idiosyncratic response by forming a protein adduct (hapten) that triggers an acquired immune response (activation of killer T cells and/or antibody-producing B lymphocytes). There is strong evidence including the production of antibodies against drug-modified proteins that the idiosyncratic DILI caused by halothane and tienilic acid are due to the formation of reactive metabolites, which is why, during the process of drug development, considerable attention is devoted to avoiding drug candidates that are converted to reactive metabolites that bind covalently to protein (see Point 12) (Obach *et al.*, 2008; Bauman *et al.*, 2009; Nakayama *et al.*, 2009; Tang and Lu, 2010; Ikeda, 2011; Park *et al.*, 2011; Walsh and Miwa, 2011). However, formation of reactive metabolites (which occurs in all individuals) is insufficient to account for the rarity of idiosyncratic DILI. For many drugs that cause idiosyncratic DILI, HLA haplotype is a factor but not to the extent seen with abacavir (Alfirevic and Pirmohamed, 2010).

In several cases, the drugs that cause idiosyncratic liver injury (those listed in Table 6-3) have closely related structures that do not cause idiosyncratic DILI. For example, rosiglitazone and pioglitazone contain the same thiazolidinedione ring that in troglitazone is converted to a reactive metabolite, and yet only troglitazone has been withdrawn from the market because of idiosyncratic hepatotoxicity. This difference may be due to the much larger daily dose of troglitazone (300 mg) compared with rosiglitazone (4-8 mg) and pioglitazone (15-45 mg). Uetrecht (2001) has proposed the general rule that drugs administered at a daily dose of 10 mg or less do not cause idiosyncratic toxicity, and this rule is consistent with the dosing information shown in Table 6-3. Both dose (more than 50 mg/day) and extent of hepatic metabolism (greater than 50%) are now recognized as risk factors for idiosyncratic drug-induced liver injury (Lammert *et al.*, 2008 and 2010; Chalasani and Björnsson, 2010). Other examples of closely related drugs where one does and one does not cause hepatotoxicity include tolcapone/entacapone, ticlopidine/clopidogrel, amineptine/tianeptine, tamoxifen/toremifene, ibufenac/ibuprofen, ebrotidine/famotidine, and niperotidine/ranitidine (Walgren *et al.*, 2005). Labetalol has 2 chiral centers and is a racemic mixture of 4 enantiomers, one of which is dilevalol. Although labetrol carries a black box warning for hepatotoxicity, dilevalol was not approved by the FDA because it caused a high incidence of liver toxicity during clinical trials. In some cases the difference is thought to be due to differences in dose (which is invariably higher for the drug partner that causes hepatotoxicity), but in other cases the basis for the difference is not known. Furthermore, more than 20 drugs (many of which do not cause idiosyncratic toxicity) bind covalently to their pharmacological target, including aspirin, omeprazole (and other proton pump inhibitors), clopidogrel, and neratinib (Singh *et al.*, 2011).

Just as the acquired immune system can be activated by drugs that cause Type B toxicity (idiosyncratic toxicity) so the innate immune system can be activated by drugs that cause Type C (off-target) toxicity. For example, acetaminophen (Tylenol), which is a

Table 6-3

Drugs That Have Been Withdrawn or Carry a Black Box Warning for Idiosyncratic Hepatotoxicity[*]

DRUG NAME	TYPICAL DOSE	INDICATION	REACTIVE METABOLITE AND EVIDENCE OF METABOLISM-DEPENDENT ENZYME INHIBITION	INDUCTION,[†] IMMUNOLOGICAL AND OTHER MECHANISTIC ASPECTS
Drugs withdrawn				
Benoxaprofen	300-600 mg	NSAID	Acyl glucuronide	Inducer (rat AhR and PPARα agonist)
Bromfenac	25-50 mg	NSAID	Acyl glucuronide	
Iproniazid	25-150 mg	Depression	Multiple. MDI of MAO-B	Anti-MAO-B and antimitochondria
Nefazodone	200 mg	Depression	Quinoneimine. MDI of CYP3A4	
Tienilic acid	250-500 mg	Diuretic	Thiophene epoxide, sulfoxide. MDI of CYP2C9	Anti-LKM$_2$ (anti-CYP2C9)
Troglitazone	400 mg	Diabetes	Quinone methide, sulfenic acid, α-ketoisocyanate	Inducer (CAR/PXR agonist)
Black box warnings				
Acitretin	25-50 mg	Psoriasis	No. Acitretin, a retinoid, is esterified to etretinate	Etretinate was withdrawn in 2002
Bosentan	125-250 mg	PAH	No	Inhibits BSEP. Inducer (PXR agonist)
Dacarbazine	140-315 mg	Melanoma, lymphoma	Methyl diazohydroxide and methyl cation (CH_3^+)	Hepatotoxic to laboratory animals
Dantrolene	300-400 mg	Muscle relaxant	Nitro-reduction intermediates bind to GSH	Inducer (AhR agonist)
Felbamate	1200 mg	Epilepsy	2-Phenylpropenal (atropaldehyde)	Inducer (PXR agonist)
Flutamide	750 mg	Prostate cancer	Nitro-reduced, nitrogen radicals, and *ortho*-quinoneimines bind to protein and GSH[‡]	Inhibits mitochondrial respiration
Gemtuzumab	9 mg/m²	AML	Reductive activation to a diradical	Designed to intercalate and bind DNA
Isoniazid	300 mg	Tuberculosis	Multiple. MDI of CYP1A1, 2A6, 2C19, and 3A4	Radicals formed by myeloperoxidase
Ketoconazole	200 mg	Fungal infections	Dialdehyde	Autoinhibitor (inhibits CYP3A4)
Naltrexone	50 mg	Alcoholism, addiction	No	
Nevirapine	200-400 mg	AIDS	Quinonemethide. MDI of CYP3A4[§]	Inducer (PXR agonist)
Pemoline	37.5-112.5 mg	Hyperactivity	No	
Tolcapone	300 mg	Parkinsonism	Nitro-reduction and then quinoneimine formation	Uncouples mitochondrial respiration
Trovafloxacin	100-500 mg	Antibiotic	No, but it has a lipophilic difluorinated side chain present in a toxic fluoroquinolone—now withdrawn	Eosinophilia suggests an immune-mediated hepatitis
Valproic acid (VPA)	1000-4200 mg	Epilepsy	CoA thioesterification and epoxidation of 4-ene-VPA	Disrupts mitochondrial β-oxidation

AhR, aryl hydrocarbon receptor; AIDS, acquired immunodeficiency syndrome; AML, acute myeloid leukemia; anti-LKM$_2$, autoantibodies against liver and kidney microsomes (anti-LKM$_1$ contains antibodies against CYP2D6, whereas anti-LKM$_2$ contains antibodies against CYP2C9); BSEP, bile salt export pump (a bile canalicular transporter); CYP, cytochrome P450; GSH, glutathione; MAO, monoamine oxidase; MDI, metabolism-dependent inhibitor (aka suicide inactivator); NSAID, nonsteroidal anti-inflammatory drug; PAH, pulmonary arterial hypertension; PPARα, peroxisome proliferator–activated receptor-alpha; PXR, pregnane X receptor; VPA, valproic acid.

[*]*Data adapted from Walgren et al. (2005).*

[†]*The receptor agonist assignment is based on the CYP-induced enzyme (CYP1A for AhR; CYP2B, CYP2C, and/or CYP3A for CAR/PXR; CYP4A for PPARα).*

[‡]*Wen et al. (2008).*

[§]*Chen et al. (2008).*

leading cause of acute liver failure in humans (Kaplowitz, 2005), is activated to a reactive metabolite (*N*-acetylbenzo-p-quinoneimine) that binds covalently to mitochondrial proteins, which leads to cell death. The cell damage (necrosis) caused by acetaminophen causes the release of cellular constituents such as fragmented DNA (and other molecules that make up the so-called danger-associated molecular pattern [DAMP]) that bind to Toll-like receptors and other receptors that activate macrophages, which in turn recruit neutrophils and monocytes to the site of injury (Jaeschke *et al.*, 2012). Whether activation of the innate immune system in this way is detrimental (by leading to a second round of hepatocellular damage) or beneficial (by limiting damage and promoting tissue repair)

Table 6-4

The Relationship Between Genotype and Phenotype for the Polymorphically Expressed Enzyme CYP2D6 with Active (wt), Partially Active (*x), and Inactive (*y) Alleles

GENOTYPE	ALLELES	CONVENTIONAL	ACTIVITY SCORE*	ACTIVITY SCORE PHENOTYPE†
Duplication of active alleles ($n = 2$ or more)	(wt/wt)n	UM‡	$2 \times n$	UM
Two fully active wild-type (wt) alleles	wt/wt	EM	$1 + 1 = 2$	High EM
One fully active + 1 partially active allele	wt/*x	EM	$1 + 0.5 = 1.5$	Medium EM
One fully active + 1 inactive allele	wt/*y	EM	$1 + 0 = 1$	Low EM
Two partially active alleles	*x/*x	EM or IM	$0.5 + 0.5 = 1$	Low EM
One partially active + 1 inactive allele	*x/*y	IM	$0.5 + 0 = 0.5$	IM
Two inactive alleles	*y/*y	PM	$0 + 0 = 0$	PM

Data adapted from Gaedigk et al. (2008) and Zineh et al. (2004).

In the case of CYP2D6, various activity scores have been assigned as follows:
  Activity score = 1.0 for each *1 (wt), *2, *35, and *41 [2988G].
  Activity score = 0.75 for each *9, *29, *45, and *46.
  Activity score = 0.5 for each *10, *17, and *41 [2988A].
  Activity score = 0 for each *3, *4, *5, *6, *7, *8, *11, *12, *15, *36, *40, and *42.

†*Activity scores are classified as follows:*
  UM activity score ≥2.0 (eg, [*1/*1]n, where n is 2 or more gene duplications).
  High EM activity score = 1.75 to 2.0 (eg, *1/*1).
  Medium EM activity score = 1.5 (eg, *1/*17 or *9/*9).
  Low EM activity score = 1.0 to 1.25 (eg, *1/*4, *17/*17, or *9/*17).
  IM activity score = 0.5 to 0.75 (eg, *4/*9 or *4/*17).
  PM activity score = 0 (eg, *4/*4).

‡*The phenotypes are ultrarapid metabolizer (UM), extensive metabolizer (EM), intermediate metabolizer (IM), and poor metabolizer (PM), based on the particular combination of alleles that are fully active (wt), partially active (*x), or inactive (*y).*

is controversial. However, it is noteworthy that, in the case of Type C toxicity, the innate immune system is activated by cellular components released from damaged cells (DAMP) and not by the drug or its metabolites (although in the example given it is recognized that the reactive metabolite of acetaminophen plays a critical role in causing the cell damage that subsequently activates the innate immune system). This contrasts with the direct role of the drug and/or its metabolites (including reactive metabolites) in Type B toxicity. In the case of idiosyncratic toxicity, the drug/metabolite plays a key role in activating the acquired immune system.

Point 23 The same dose of drug (or any other xenobiotic) administered to humans often results in large interindividual differences in exposure to the parent compound (typically measured as the plasma AUC). This variation can reflect genetically determined differences in the activity of xenobiotic-biotransforming enzymes or transporters (genetic polymorphisms) or environmental factors, such as drug–drug interactions.

The study of the causes, prevalence, and impact of heritable differences in xenobiotic-biotransforming enzymes is known as *pharmacogenetics*. It is the basis for the concept of individualized medicine, whereby the dosage of drugs with a narrow therapeutic index (such as anticancer drugs) is adjusted in accordance with an individual's genotype (ie, drug-metabolizing potential).

Genetic variation in a xenobiotic-metabolizing enzyme produces 4 discernible phenotypes: poor metabolizers (PMs), intermediate metabolizers (IMs), extensive metabolizers (EMs), and ultrarapid metabolizers (UMs), which arise from the expression of no functional alleles (−/−) for PMs, one nonfunctional allele and one partially functional allele or two partially active alleles (−/* or */*) for IMs, one or two functional alleles (+/−, +/*, or +/+) for

EMs, and gene duplication ([+/+]n) for UMs. This traditional classification scheme has been revised on the basis of an activity score, which assigns to each allelic variant a functional activity value from one (for the wild-type or *1 allele) to zero (for any completely nonfunctional allele), as shown in Table 6-4 (Zineh *et al.*, 2004).

For those enzymes that are polymorphically expressed, such as CYP2D6, the incidence of the PM (and UM) genotype can vary widely from one ethnic group to the next. For example, the CYP2D6 PM genotype is common among Caucasians but not Asians, whereas the converse is true of the CYP2C19 PM genotype.

When the clearance of a drug is largely determined by a polymorphically expressed enzyme, such as CYP2D6, exposure to the parent drug follows the rank order: PMs > IMs > EMs > UMs. Exposure to metabolites (especially the maximum concentration, C_{max}) follows the opposite rank order. The difference in exposure between PMs and EMs (ie, the fold increase in C_{max} or AUC associated with the PM phenotype vs the EM phenotype) depends on fractional metabolism (fm), a measure of how much of the drug's clearance is determined by CYP2D6 (or whatever enzyme is responsible for metabolizing the drug in question). The fold increase in AUC (AUC_{PM}/AUC_{EM}) is equal to $1/(1 - fm)$; hence, the impact of the polymorphism increases dramatically as fm approaches unity. If CYP2D6 accounted for half of a drug's clearance (fm = 0.5), exposure to that drug would increase 2-fold in CYP2D6 PMs. However, if CYP2D6 accounted for 90% of a drug's clearance (fm = 0.9), then exposure to that drug would increase 10-fold in CYP2D6 PMs. This is why PMs are often at increased risk of ADEs either due to an exaggerated pharmacological response to the drug or due to its toxic side effects. An exception is omeprazole and other proton pump inhibitors, which actually provide improved control over gastroesophageal reflux disease (GERD) in CYP2C19 PMs compared with EMs (Furuta *et al.*, 2005).

There are a minority of cases where the UMs, not the PMs, are at increased risk, especially in cases where the polymorphic enzyme catalyzes the formation of a pharmacologically active or toxic metabolite. For example, CYP2D6 converts the prodrug codeine to the active metabolite morphine, and there are reports of morphine intoxication in CYP2D6 UMs, one case being the death of a baby being breastfed by a CYP2D6 UM mother who was prescribed codeine (Gasche *et al.*, 2004; Koren *et al.*, 2006).

Many cases have now been described where the PM phenotype requires dosage adjustment to prevent off-target (Type C) toxicity or an exaggerated pharmacological response (Type A toxicity). For example, CYP2D6 PMs are at increased risk for perhexiline hepatotoxicity and at increased risk for an exaggerated pharmacological response to debrisoquine and sparteine, 3 drugs that were not approved in the United States because of the high incidence of adverse events in the PMs. On the other hand, when drugs are converted to active metabolites by CYP2D6, PMs derive inadequate therapeutic effect (Type F toxicity). For example, CYP2D6 converts codeine to morphine; hence, codeine is a less effective analgesic in PMs. Similarly, CYP2D6 converts the breast cancer drug tamoxifen to endoxifen (which is 30- to 100-fold more potent than tamoxifen in suppressing estrogen-dependent cell proliferation); hence, CYP2D6 PMs are at increased risk for breast cancer recurrence following tamoxifen adjuvant therapy (Goetz *et al.*, 2005). Other examples of genetic polymorphisms that affect drug disposition in humans include CYP2C8 (repaglinide, paclitaxel), CYP2C9 (warfarin), CYP2C19 (clopidogrel, omeprazole, lansoprazole, and pantoprazole), CYP3A5 (tacrolimus), UGT1A1 (irinotecan), UGT2B7 (morphine), thiopurine methyltransferase (TPMT) (6-mercaptopurine), *N*-acetyltransferase 2 (NAT2) (isoniazid), catechol-*O*-methyltransferase (COMT) (levodopa), dihydropyrimidine dehydrogenase (DPD) (5-fluorouracil), and the efflux transporter P-glycoprotein (digoxin) (Robert *et al.*, 2005; Relling and Giacomini, 2006). Details of these genetic polymorphisms are given later in the chapter. Many of the drugs identified in parentheses have a narrow therapeutic index. Some victim drugs have a high therapeutic index; hence, they are therapeutically effective in PMs to UMs and cause roughly the same incidence of adverse effects regardless of genotype. However, in the case of victim drugs with a narrow therapeutic index, dosage must be increased in UMs to achieve a therapeutic effect and/or it must be decreased in PMs to prevent ADEs.

Genetic polymorphisms in xenobiotic-biotransforming enzymes have an impact on the incidence of certain environmental diseases. For example, ethnic differences in the incidence of polymorphisms in alcohol dehydrogenase (ADH) and aldehyde dehydrogenase (ALDH) impact the incidence of alcoholism (Li, 2000). Genetic polymorphisms in CYP2A6 impact the incidence of cigarette-smoking-induced lung cancer. Individuals lacking CYP2A6 are PMs of nicotine (so they tend to smoke less than CYP2A6 EMs) and are poor activators of tobacco-specific mutagens (so they form fewer DNA-reactive metabolites than do CYP2A6 EMs) (Kamataki *et al.*, 2005).

Genetic polymorphisms can be the underlying cause of a disease. For example, the severe and mild hyperbilirubinemia associated with Crigler–Najjar syndrome and Gilbert syndrome, respectively, reflect a complete and partial loss of the UGT responsible for conjugating bilirubin, namely, UGT1A1. The hyperbilirubinemic Gunn rat is the rodent equivalent of Crigler–Najjar

syndrome. Genetic polymorphisms in CYP1B1 are associated with primary congenital glaucoma.

Genetic polymorphisms have been described in laboratory animals. For example, laboratory-bred rabbits have about 50:50 chance of being a poor or rapid acetylator of certain drugs (such as isoniazid) because NAT2 is polymorphically expressed in rabbits. CYP1A2 is polymorphically expressed in dogs.

Point 24 Environmental factors can introduce as much variation in drug metabolism as can genetic factors, and this is especially true of drug–drug interactions. To take CYP3A4 as an example, PMs can be created pharmacologically with inhibitors (such as ketoconazole and erythromycin), whereas UMs can be created pharmacologically with inducers (such as rifampin and the herbal agent St. John's wort). Whereas the impact of genetic polymorphisms on drug disposition and safety is often identified during clinical trials, the impact of drug–drug interactions may not be identified until after the drug has been approved and is under postmarketing surveillance.

Drugs (and other xenobiotics) can be viewed from a *victim* and *perpetrator* perspective. A drug whose clearance is largely determined by a single route of elimination, such as metabolism by a single CYP enzyme, is considered a victim drug (also known as a sensitive or object drug). Such drugs have a high victim potential because a diminution or loss of that elimination pathway, either due to a genetic deficiency in the relevant CYP enzyme or due to its inhibition by another, concomitantly administered drug, will result in a large decrease in victim drug clearance and a correspondingly large increase in exposure (the magnitude of which will depend on f_m, as indicated in Point 23). Perpetrators are those drugs (or other environmental factors) that inhibit or induce the enzyme that is otherwise responsible for clearing a victim drug. In other words, perpetrators are drugs that cause drug–drug interactions. Perpetrators are also known as precipitants. Genetic polymorphisms that result in the partial or complete loss of enzymatic activity can also be viewed as perpetrators inasmuch they cause a decrease in the clearance of—and an increase in exposure to—victim drugs. A combination of 2 perpetrators (such as 2 drugs that inhibit different enzymes or an inhibitory drug plus a genetic polymorphism) can have a dramatic effect on the disposition of a victim drug if they impair *parallel* pathways of clearance, a phenomenon called *maximum exposure* (Collins *et al.*, 2006). This is illustrated by voriconazole, whose metabolic clearance is determined by CYP2C19 and CYP3A4 (which represent 2 parallel pathways of clearance). Based on plasma AUC, CYP2C19 PMs (individuals lacking CYP2C19) are exposed to roughly twice as much voriconazole compared with CYP2C19 EMs. Loss of CYP3A4 (and only CYP3A4) by administering ritonavir to CYP2C19 EMs also causes about a doubling in systemic exposure to voriconazole. However, when ritonavir is administered to CYP2C19 PMs (such that *both* CYP2C19 and CYP3A4 are inactive), exposure to voriconazole increases more than 25-fold. This example illustrates how 2 drugs (ritonavir and voriconazole) can interact dramatically in some individuals (CYP2C19 PMs) but not others (CYP2C19 EMs). Conversely, a perpetrator drug that inhibited only CYP2C19 would cause such inhibition only in CYP2C19 EMs (the PMs having no enzyme to inhibit). Many other examples of perpetrator–perpetrator–victim interactions (maximum exposure) are reviewed in Ogilvie and Parkinson (in press).

Terfenadine (Seldane), cisapride (Propulsid), astemizole (Hismanal), and cerivastatin (Baycol) are all victim drugs, so much so that they have all been withdrawn from the market (Fung *et al.*, 2001). The first 3 are all victim drugs because they are extensively metabolized by CYP3A4. Inhibition of CYP3A4 by various antimycotic drugs, such as ketoconazole, and antibiotic drugs, such as erythromycin, decreases the clearance of terfenadine, cisapride, and astemizole and increases their plasma concentrations to levels that, in some individuals, cause ventricular arrhythmias (QT prolongation) that can result in fatal heart attacks. Cerivastatin is extensively metabolized by CYP2C8. Its metabolism is inhibited by gemfibrozil (actually by gemfibrozil glucuronide), and the combination of cerivastatin (Baycol) and gemfibrozil (Lopid) is associated with a high incidence of fatal, cerivastatin-induced rhabdomyolysis (Ogilvie *et al.*, 2006).

Mibefradil (Posicor) is the only drug withdrawn from the US market largely because of its perpetrator potential. This calcium channel blocker not only causes extensive inhibition of CYP3A4 but also causes prolonged inhibition of the enzyme by virtue of being a metabolism-dependent inhibitor of CYP3A4. By inactivating CYP3A4 in an irreversible manner—such that restoration of normal CYP3A4 activity requires the synthesis of new enzyme—mibefradil inhibits CYP3A4 long after treatment with the drug is discontinued.

The in vitro technique of reaction phenotyping (also known as enzyme mapping) is the process of identifying which enzyme or enzymes are largely responsible for metabolizing a drug candidate (Williams *et al.*, 2003b; Ogilvie *et al.*, 2008). Reaction phenotyping allows an assessment of the victim potential of a drug candidate or other xenobiotic. Drug candidates can also be evaluated in vitro for their potential to inhibit or induce CYP enzymes, which allows an assessment of their perpetrator potential (Tucker *et al.*, 2001; Bjornsson *et al.*, 2003; http://www.fda.gov/Drugs/DevelopmentApprovalProcess/DevelopmentResources/DrugInteractionsLabeling/ucm080499.htm; Huang *et al.*, 2008; EMA, 2012; FDA, 2012.

Herbal remedies can also interact with drugs. For example, St. John's wort contains hyperforin, which is a potent PXR agonist and, as such, is an inducer of CYP3A4 (along with several other xenobiotic-metabolizing enzymes) and *P*-glycoprotein (ABCB1). To prevent a loss of therapeutic efficacy, the use of St. John's wort is not recommended for patients on antirejection drugs (such as cyclosporine and tacrolimus), anti-HIV drugs (such as indinavir and nevirapine), anticoagulants (such as warfarin and phenprocoumon), or oral contraceptive steroids (Pal and Mitra, 2006). Food can affect drug disposition in a number of ways. It can affect absorption, which is why some drugs are taken with meals and others are taken between meals. Large quantities of cruciferous vegetables (eg, broccoli and Brussels sprouts) can induce hepatic CYP1A2 (Conney, 1982), whereas grapefruit juice can inhibit intestinal CYP3A4 (Paine *et al.*, 2006).

Point 25 Although drug–drug interactions can cause an increase in the incidence of adverse events or, in the case of induction, a loss of therapeutic efficacy, not all drug–drug interactions are undesirable. For example, some anti-HIV drugs, such as ritonavir, inhibit CYP3A4 and thereby improve the pharmacokinetic profile of other anti-HIV drugs, such as saquinavir and lopinavir. Tumors often overexpress various transporters and GSTs, which limit the effectiveness of several anticancer drugs. Drugs that inhibit transporters and GST are being developed to enhance the efficacy of anticancer drugs.

Point 26 Although the amount of functional enzyme determines whether an individual is a PM, IM, EM, or UM, disease states and cofactor levels can impact the rate of xenobiotic metabolism. Not surprisingly, severe liver disease decreases the rate of metabolism of a large number of drugs whose clearance is determined by hepatic metabolism, as can kidney disease that decreases the hepatic

expression of CYP2D6 (Rostami-Hodjegan *et al.*, 1999). For certain xenobiotic-metabolizing enzymes, particularly the conjugating enzymes, cofactor availability can impact the rate of xenobiotic biotransformation. The liver usually has sufficient NADPH to saturate reactions catalyzed by CYP, but it does not have sufficient levels of UDP-glucuronic acid (UDPGA) or 3′-phosphoadenosine-5′-phosphosulfate (PAPS) to saturate the enzymes responsible for glucuronidating or sulfonating xenobiotics. Consequently, alterations in the levels of these cofactors can impact the rate or extent of glucuronidation and sulfonation. For example, fasting lowers hepatic levels of these cofactors, and fasting decreases the extent to which acetaminophen is conjugated. Consequently, fasting increases the extent to which acetaminophen is metabolized to a toxic metabolite by CYP (including CYP2E1, which is induced by fasting), for which reason fasting is suspected of being one of the risk factors for acetaminophen hepatotoxicity (Whitcomb and Block, 1994).

Point 27 Stereochemical aspects can play an important role in the interaction between a xenobiotic and its biotransforming enzyme (from both a substrate and an inhibitor perspective), and xenobiotic-biotransforming enzymes can play a key role in converting one stereoisomer to another, a process known as *mutarotation* or *inversion of configuration.*

A xenobiotic that contains a chiral center can exist in 2 mirror-image forms called stereoisomers or enantiomers. The biotransformation of some chiral xenobiotics occurs stereoselectively, meaning that one enantiomer (stereoisomer) is biotransformed faster than its antipode. For example, the antiepileptic drug Mesantoin®, which is a racemic mixture of *R*- and *S*-mephenytoin, is biotransformed stereoselectively in humans, such that the *S*-enantiomer is rapidly hydroxylated (by CYP2C19) and eliminated faster than the *R*-enantiomer. The ability of some chiral xenobiotics to inhibit xenobiotic-biotransforming enzymes can also occur stereoselectively. For example, quinidine is a potent inhibitor of CYP2D6, whereas quinine, its antipode, has relatively little inhibitory effect on this enzyme. In some cases, achiral molecules (or achiral centers) are converted to a mixture of enantiomeric metabolites, and this conversion may proceed stereoselectively such that one enantiomer is formed preferentially over its antipode. Inversion of configuration is the process whereby one enantiomer is converted to its antipode via an achiral intermediate. This interconversion can occur nonenzymatically, as in the case of thalidomide, or it can be catalyzed by a xenobiotic-metabolizing enzyme, as in the case of lisofylline, or by an endobiotic-metabolizing enzyme, as in the case of simvastatin (Fig. 6-3).

In the case of thalidomide, inversion of configuration (as shown in Fig. 6-3) occurs spontaneously, although the process is facilitated by albumin (Eriksson *et al.*, 1998). In the mid-to-late 1950s, mainly in Europe, thalidomide was prescribed to pregnant women in the first trimester to treat morning sickness. Unfortunately, whereas (*R*)-thalidomide is an effective sedative, the (*S*)-enantiomer is a teratogen that produces phocomelia (limb shortening) and other congenital defects in the offspring largely as a result of its ability to inhibit angiogenesis (vasculogenesis). The teratogenic effect of thalidomide cannot be circumvented by administering only the (*R*)-enantiomer because spontaneous or albumin-facilitated racemization quickly produces the teratogenic (*S*)-enantiomer. Thalidomide blocks the release of tumor necrosis factor-α (TNFα) and it has been approved for the treatment of erythema nodosum leprosum (an acute inflammatory reaction associated with lepromatous leprosy), and is useful in the treatment of several other inflammatory conditions and immune-mediated diseases. Because of its ability to inhibit angiogenesis (the process that supplies tumors with

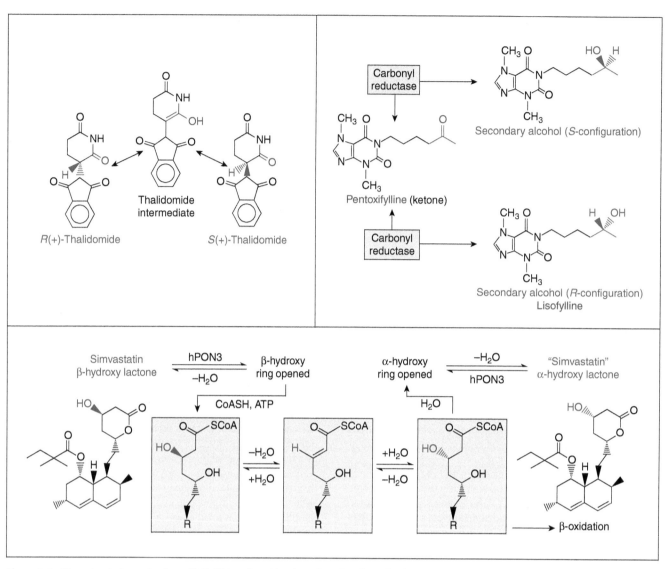

Figure 6-3. *Stereochemical aspects of xenobiotic biotransformation: inversion of configuration by nonenzymatic means (thalidomide), by carbonyl reductase (lisofylline), and by hydrolysis and condensation (lactonization) of a lactone ring (simvastatin).*

new blood vessels), thalidomide is also under investigation as an anticancer drug. It is ironic that a drug with antivascular side effects that was originally prescribed as a sedative is now in clinical trials for vascular diseases with sedation as a side effect (Franks *et al.*, 2004).

Ketones can be reduced by carbonyl reductases to a mixture of enantiomeric secondary alcohols, and this can occur with a high degree of stereoselectivity. For example, pentoxifylline is reduced by carbonyl reductases in blood and liver to a mixture of secondary alcohols with the major metabolite having an *S*-configuration, as shown in Fig. 6-3. Interestingly, the minor metabolite, a secondary alcohol with the *R*-configuration, has pharmacological properties distinct from those of its *S*-antipode and its ketone precursor, pentoxifylline. This minor metabolite is known as lisofylline, which is under clinical investigation for the treatment of various diseases. Through the action of carbonyl reductase, lisofylline is oxidized to pentoxifylline and then reduced to its antipode (ie, *R*-alcohol → ketone → *S*-alcohol), the net result being an inversion of configuration (Lillibridge *et al.*, 1996). The same type of interconversion explains why the administration of pure *R*-albuterol to human volunteers results in the formation of *S*-albuterol, just

as the administration of pure *S*-albuterol leads to the formation of *R*-albuterol (Boulton and Fawcett, 1997).

In the case of simvastatin (which contains a β-hydroxylactone), the interconversion of 2 secondary alcohols (β-hydroxylactone ↔ α-hydroxy-lactone) involves hydrolysis of the lactone ring (by paraoxonase 3 [PON3] in humans) followed by formation of an acyl-CoA thioester with CoA, the first step in the β-oxidation of fatty acids, followed by dehydration to an achiral intermediate. Reversal of the steps by a combination of hydrolysis and lactonization (condensation) restores the lactone ring with the hydroxyl group in the original β-configuration or in the opposing α-configuration. In humans, both the initial hydrolysis of the lactone ring and the final lactonization (condensation) reaction are catalyzed by PON3 (Draganov and La Du, 2004). Conversion to an acyl-CoA thioester also plays a role in the chiral inversion of ketoprofen. In this case, only the *R*-enantiomer is converted to an acyl-CoA thioester, which isomerizes and undergoes hydrolysis to the *S*-enantiomer. Although both *R*- and *S*-ketoprofen are converted to acyl glucuronides, the former is hydrolyzed twice as quickly as the latter, which further contributes to the accumulation of the *S*-enantiomer (Regan *et al.*, 2010).

Point 28 Mass spectrometry is widely used to characterize the structure of metabolites, and many instruments now come equipped with software to assist in this process, based on the fact that certain xenobiotic reactions are associated with discrete changes in mass (Holčapek et al., 2008). For example, the loss of 2 atomic mass units (amu) signifies dehydrogenation, whereas the loss of 14 amu usually signifies demethylation ($-CH_2$). Several reactions result in an increase in mass, including reduction (+2 amu = 2H), methylation (+14 amu = CH_2), oxidation (+16 amu = O), hydration (+18 amu = H_2O), acetylation (+42 amu = C_2H_2O), glucosidation (+162 = $C_6H_{10}O_5$), sulfonation (+80 amu = SO_3), glucuronidation (+176 amu = $C_6H_8O_6$), carbamoyl glucuronidation (+220 amu = $C_7H_8O_8$), and conjugation with GSH (+305 amu = $C_{10}H_{15}N_3O_6S$), glycine (+57 amu = C_2H_3NO), taurine (+107 amu = $C_2H_5NO_2S$), and glutamine (+107 amu = $C_5H_7NO_3$) (Holčapek et al., 2008). Conjugation of acidic drugs with CoA (to form acyl-CoA thioesters) increases mass by 749 amu, but these conjugates are not transported out of cells and, hence, are not detected in blood, bile, or urine.

Occasionally, routine changes in mass can arise from unexpected reactions. For example, ziprasidone is converted to 2 metabolites, each of which involves an increase of 16 amu, which normally indicates addition of oxygen (eg, hydroxylation, sulfoxidation, N-oxygenation). One of the metabolites is indeed formed by addition of oxygen to ziprasidone (sulfoxidation), as shown in Fig. 6-4 (Beedham et al., 2003). However, the other metabolite is formed by a combination of reduction (+2 amu) and methylation (+14). Therefore, nominal changes in mass can sometimes leave in doubt the biotransformation event that led to metabolite formation, which accounts for the popularity of accurate mass spectrometry, a technique that can distinguish, in the case of ziprasidone, for example, oxidation from a combination of reduction and methylation.

Mass spectrometry can typically provide information on which region of a molecule has undergone biotransformation, but in some cases it cannot distinguish between several closely related possibilities. For example, based on mass spectrometry alone, it might be possible to ascertain that a certain phenyl group has been hydroxylated. However, analysis by nuclear magnetic resonance (NMR) may be required to ascertain whether the hydroxylation occurred at the ortho, meta, or para position.

Point 29 As mentioned in Point 19, xenobiotic-biotransforming enzymes are widely distributed throughout the body. The advent of high-throughput assays based on quantitative real-time reverse-transcription polymerase chain reaction (QPCR) has facilitated comprehensive measurements of the levels of mRNA encoding numerous xenobiotic-biotransforming enzymes, transporters, and xenosensors in a wide range of human tissues (Nishimura et al., 2003, 2004; Furukawa et al., 2004; Nishimura and Naito, 2005, 2006). These data are very informative as far as mRNA expression is concerned, but it can be difficult to draw conclusions about the activity of a given enzyme in a given tissue based on mRNA levels alone. For instance, based on mRNA levels in human liver, the levels of the major xenobiotic-biotransforming CYP enzymes follow the rank order: CYP2E1 > 2A6 > 2C8 > 2C18 ≈ 1A2 ≈ 4A11 ≈ 2C9 ≈ 3A4 (Nishimura et al., 2003). This contrasts substantially from the levels of CYP protein (as determined by LC–MS/MS), which follow the rank order: CYP2C9 > 3A4 ≈ 2E1 ≈ 2A6 > 2C8 > 1A2 > 2D6 > 2B6 ≈ 2C19 > 3A5 ≈ 3A43 ≈ 3A7 (Kawakami et al., 2011; Ohtsuki et al., 2012). In the case of CYP2E1, hepatic mRNA levels are more than 17 times higher than the levels of CYP3A4 mRNA, but CYP2E1 protein levels in microsomes are comparable to those of CYP3A4. This discrepancy is due to the fact that, under normal conditions, most of the mRNA encoding CYP2E1 is sequestered in the cytoplasm and is not available for translation (Gonzalez, 2007). The mRNA for FMO2 is present at very high levels in human lung, but is not translated into functional enzyme due to the presence of a truncation mutation in Caucasians and Asians. However, about 33% of sub-Saharan Africans, 26% of African Americans, 7% of Puerto Ricans, and 2% of Mexicans have one normal allele and express a functional protein (Cashman and Zhang, 2006; Veeramah et al., 2008). Human CYP2A7 and CYP4B1 are full-length genes that encode enzymes incapable of incorporating heme and are therefore nonfunctional.

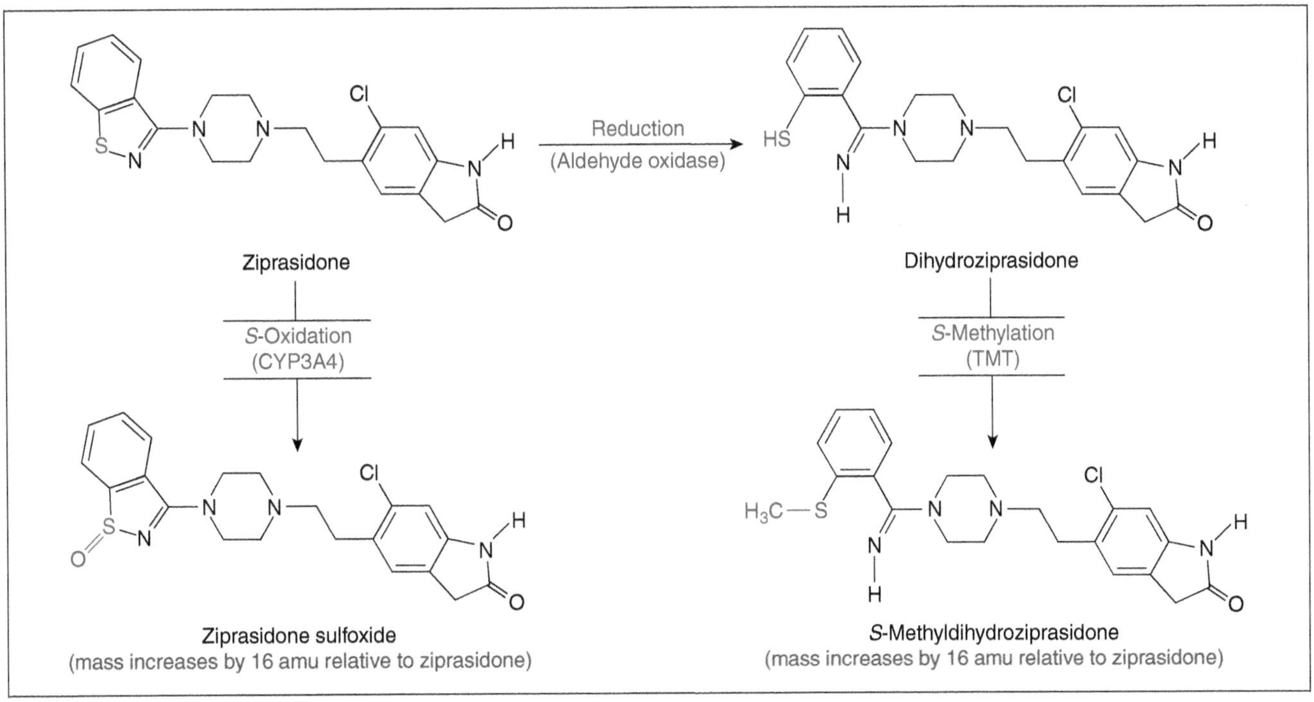

Figure 6-4. Conversion of ziprasidone to 2 different metabolites, both involving a mass increase of 16 amu (relative to ziprasidone).

Mass spectrophotometric techniques for the quantitative analysis of proteins have been applied to drug-metabolizing enzymes and transporters (Kawakami *et al.*, 2011; Sakamoto *et al.*, 2011; Ohtsuki *et al.*, 2012). The levels of CYP and UGT enzymes in human liver microsomes have been determined by LC–MS/MS and are described in the sections "Cytochrome P450" and "Glucuronidation and Formation of Acyl-CoA Thioesters."

HYDROLYSIS, REDUCTION, AND OXIDATION

Hydrolysis

Mammals contain a variety of enzymes that hydrolyze xenobiotics containing such functional groups as a carboxylic acid ester (delapril and procaine), amide (procainamide), thioester (spironolactone), carbamate (irinotecan), phosphoric acid ester (paraoxon),

acid anhydride (diisopropylfluorophosphate [DFP]), lactone (lovastatin), and thiolactone (erdosteine), most of which are shown in Figs. 6-5 and 6-6. The major hydrolytic enzymes are the carboxylesterases, cholinesterases, and paraoxonases (for which lactonase is a more encompassing name), but they are by no means the only hydrolytic enzymes involved in xenobiotic biotransformation. The first 2 classes of hydrolytic enzymes, the carboxylesterases and cholinesterases, are known as serine esterases because their catalytic site contains a nucleophilic serine residue that participates in the hydrolysis of various xenobiotic and endobiotic substrates and the stoichiometric (one-to-one) binding of organophosphorus (OP) compounds and other cholinergic neurotoxins.

Approximately 100 human gene products encode serine hydrolases that are classified as esterases, amidases, thioesterases, lipases, peptidases, or proteases (Evans and Cravatt, 2006; Ross and Crow, 2007; Testa and Krämer, 2008, 2010). The active-site serine residue of carboxylesterases, cholinesterases, and other

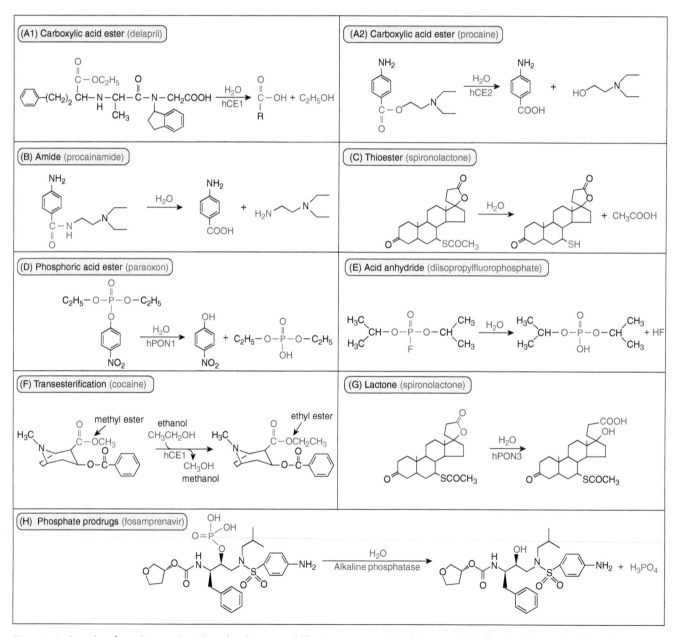

Figure 6-5. *Examples of reactions catalyzed by carboxylesterases, cholinesterases, organophosphatases, and alkaline phosphatase.* CES1 and CES2 (human carboxylesterases 1 and 2); PON1 and PON3 (human paraoxonase 1 and 3).

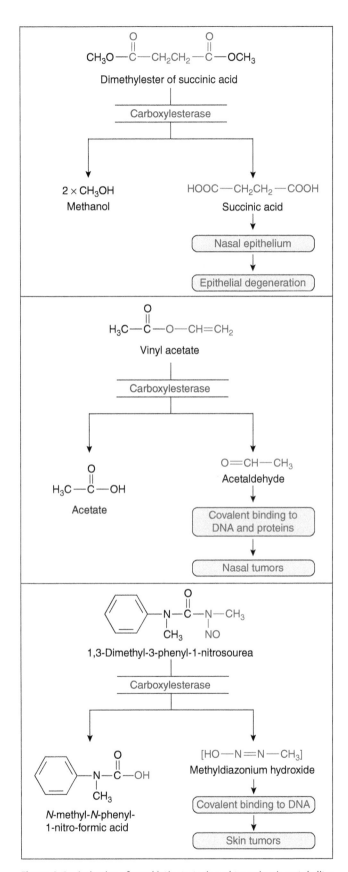

Figure 6-6. *Activation of xenobiotics to toxic and tumorigenic metabolites by carboxylesterases.*

serine hydrolases becomes phosphorylated (or phosphonylated) by OP compounds, such as those used as insecticides, herbicides, fungicides, nematicides, and plant growth regulators. Binding of OP compounds to carboxylesterases, cholinesterases, and other targets, some of which have been identified as receptors and enzymes involved in the hydrolysis of endobiotics (reviewed in Casida and Quistad, 2005), plays a key role in limiting the binding of OP compounds to acetylcholinesterase (AChE). Phosphorylation of AChE, which hydrolyzes acetylcholine and thereby terminates its neurotransmitter activity, is the principal mechanism of OP toxicity in mammals, insects, and nematodes, with 70% to 90% inhibition usually proving lethal. Reversal of this phosphorylation event with pyridinium oximes such as pralidoxime (2-PAM) and obidoxime (toxogonin) is one of the strategies to treat OP poisoning (Casida and Quistad, 2005).

Albumin, lipases, peptidases, proteases, ALDHs, and carbonic anhydrases have all been shown to have hydrolytic (esteratic) activity toward various xenobiotics. CYP can catalyze the cleavage of certain xenobiotics containing a carboxylic acid ester, phosphoric acid ester, or carbamate (see the section "Cytochrome P450" for examples).

In the presence of an alcohol, carboxylesterases and certain other hydrolytic enzymes can catalyze the transesterification of xenobiotics, which accounts for the conversion of cocaine (a methyl ester) to ethylcocaine (the corresponding ethyl ester) (Fig. 6-5). The same transesterification occurs with clopidogrel, which is converted from a methyl to an ethyl ester (Tang *et al.*, 2006). Transesterification occurs when ethanol, not water, cleaves the catalytic transition state, that is, the esteratic bond between the active serine residue on the enzyme and the carbonyl group on the xenobiotic:

$$\text{Enzyme–O–CO-R} + CH_3CH_2OH$$
$$\rightarrow \text{enzyme–OH} + CH_3CH_2\text{–O–CO-R.}$$

In humans, the hydrolysis of xenobiotics (including many prodrugs) is largely catalyzed by microsomal carboxylesterases in liver (CES1 and CES2) and intestine (CES2), and by cholinesterases, paraoxonases, and albumin in blood (some of these enzymes are present in plasma; others are bound to erythrocytes in a species-dependent manner) (Li *et al.*, 2005). Compared with many other mammalian species humans are unusual because they lack a plasma carboxylesterase (Li *et al.*, 2005). However, human erythrocytes contain esterase D, a carboxylesterase used as a genetic marker for retinoblastoma (Wu *et al.*, 2009). On a case-by-case basis, specific enzymes other than those mentioned above can be involved in xenobiotic hydrolysis. For example, the valine ester prodrugs of acyclovir (valacyclovir) and gangciclovir (valgangciclovir) are hydrolyzed by valacyclovirase (gene code BPHL), a serine- and α/β-fold-hydrolase that hydrolyzes other antiviral and anticancer nucleoside drugs such as zidovudine, floxuridine, and gemcitabine (Lai *et al.*, 2008).

In general, esters are hydrolyzed more rapidly than amides, which can impact the duration and site of action of drugs. For example, procaine, a carboxylic acid ester, is rapidly hydrolyzed, which is why this drug is used mainly as a local anesthetic. In contrast, procainamide, the amide analog of procaine, is hydrolyzed much more slowly; hence, this drug reaches the systematic circulation, where it is useful in the treatment of cardiac arrhythmia. In general, enzymatic hydrolysis of amides occurs more slowly than esters, although electronic factors can influence the rate of hydrolysis. The presence of electron-withdrawing substituents weakens an amide bond, making it more susceptible to enzymatic hydrolysis.

The hydrolysis of xenobiotics by carboxylesterases and other hydrolytic enzymes is not always a detoxication process. Fig. 6-5 shows some examples in which carboxylesterases convert xenobiotics to toxic and tumorigenic metabolites.

In 1953, Aldridge classified hydrolytic enzymes on the basis of their interaction with OP compounds, classifying those that hydrolyze OP compounds as A-esterases, those that are inhibited by OP compounds as B-esterases, and those that do not interact with OP compounds as C-esterases. Although the terms are still used, the classification system of Aldridge can be somewhat confusing because it divides the paraoxonases into the A- and C-esterase classes: the human paraoxonase PON1 hydrolyzes OP compounds and so can be classified as an A-esterase, whereas PON2 and PON3 can be classified as C-esterases because they neither hydrolyze OP compounds nor, in most cases, are inhibited by them. Furthermore, carboxylesterases and cholinesterases, 2 distinct classes of hydrolytic enzymes, are both B-esterases according to Aldridge because both are inhibited by OP compounds.

Carboxylesterases Carboxylesterases are predominantly microsomal enzymes (~60 kDa glycoproteins) that are present in liver, intestine, and a wide variety of tissues, including plasma in rats and mice but not humans. The 2 major human carboxylesterases involved in xenobiotic hydrolysis are CES1 and CES2, which differ in their tissue distribution and substrate specificity. Both enzymes are expressed in liver microsomes (although CES1 predominates) but only CES2 is expressed in intestinal microsomes (Nishimura and Naito, 2006; Ross and Crow, 2007). CES1 prefers to hydrolyze xenobiotics with a small alcoholic leaving group, whereas CES2 prefers to hydrolyze xenobiotics with a large alcoholic leaving group. In other words, methyl and ethyl esters tend to be hydrolyzed by CES1. This is illustrated in Fig. 6-5 for the hydrolysis of delapril by CES1 (which releases ethanol, a small alcohol) and the hydrolysis of procaine by CES2 (which releases a large alcohol). In the case of cocaine (the structure of which is shown in Fig. 6-5), the ethyl ester is hydrolyzed by CES1 (to release a small alcohol), whereas the benzoic ester is hydrolyzed by CES2 (to release a large alcohol). CES1 also catalyzes the transesterification of the methyl ester of cocaine, as shown in Fig. 6-5. CES1 is more active than CES2 at catalyzing the hydrolysis of oseltamivir, benazepril, cilazepril, quinapril, temocapril, imidapril, meperidine, delapril, and clopidogrel, whereas CES2 is more active than CES1 at hydrolyzing aspirin, heroin, cocaine benzoyl ester, 6-acetylmorphine, oxybutynin, and the anticancer drug irinotecan (also known as CPT-11) (Satoh and Hosokawa, 2006; Shi *et al.*, 2006; Tang *et al.*, 2006). Individual pyrethroids such as *trans*-permethrin represent an example of xenobiotics that are hydrolyzed by both CES1 and CES2 (Ross and Crow, 2007).

In addition to hydrolyzing xenobiotics, carboxylesterases hydrolyze numerous endogenous compounds, such as long- and short-chain acyl-glycerols (both monoacylglycerols and diacylglycerols), long-chain acyl-carnitine, long-chain acyl-CoA thioesters (eg, palmitoyl-CoA), retinyl ester, platelet-activating factor, and other esterified lipids. Carboxylesterases can also catalyze the synthesis of fatty acid ethyl esters, which represents a nonoxidative pathway of ethanol metabolism in adipose and certain other tissues. In the case of platelet-activating factor, carboxylesterases catalyze both the deacetylation of PAF and its subsequent esterification with fatty acids to form phosphatidylcholine (Satoh and Hosokawa, 1998).

In addition to CES1 and CES2, human liver microsomes contain another serine hydrolase known as AADAC, which stands for arylacetamide deacetylase. This enzyme catalyzes the hydrolysis of the phenacetin (a discontinued drug), 2-acetylaminofluorene (2-AAF; a carcinogen), and flutamide (an antiandrogen drug) (Watanabe *et al.*, 2010). AADAC deacetylates phenacetin and 2-aminofluorene (2-AF) to aromatic amines that can be *N*-hydroxylated by CYP and then conjugated to form reactive metabolites. Examples of this type of metabolic activation are given later in the sections "Azo- and Nitro-Reduction" and "Conjugation").

CES1 (the major liver form, which is also expressed in lung and other tissues) and CES2 (the major intestinal form, which is also expressed in kidney and brain) represent 2 of the 5 families of human carboxylesterases (Satoh and Hosokawa, 2006; Holmes *et al.*, 2010). The other enzymes are CES3 (expressed in brain, liver, and colon), CES4A (previously called CES6 or CES8, which is expressed in brain, lung, and kidney), and CES5A (previously called CES7, which is expressed in brain, lung, and testis). A larger number of carboxylesterases have been identified in rats and mice (Holmes *et al.*, 2010). Human CES1 is encoded by 2 genes (CSE1A1 and CES1A2) that differ only in the amino acid sequence of the encoded signal recognition peptide (SRP) that directs the enzyme to the endoplasmic reticulum (Satoh and Hosokawa, 2006).

Genetic polymorphisms that affect carboxylesterase activity or expression levels underscore the importance of CES1 and CES2 in drug metabolism. Genetic polymorphisms of CES1 affect the disposition of methylphenidate (Ritalin, a methyl ester) and the antiviral prodrug oseltamivir (an ethyl ester) (Zhu and Markowitz, 2009). A phenotype for CES1 that might be classified as high EM has been described. It arises from a single-nucleotide polymorphism (SNP) in the promoter region of CES1A2 (but not CES1A1) that increases the expression of CES1 and thereby increases the rate of hydrolysis of imidapril to its active metabolite imidaprilat, an angiotensin-converting enzyme (ACE) inhibitor, which increases its antihypertensive effect (Geshi *et al.*, 2005). Genetic polymorphisms of CES2 affect the disposition of the anticancer drug irinotecan (CPT-11, a carbamate), which is converted by CES2 to the active metabolite SN-38, a topoisomerase inhibitor (Kubo *et al.*, 2005). However, genetic polymorphisms of UGT1A have a greater impact on the disposition and toxicity of irinotecan, as detailed in the section "Glucuronidation and Formation of Acyl-CoA Thioesters."

Certain carboxylesterases also have a physiological function in anchoring other proteins to the endoplasmic reticulum. For example, the lysosomal enzyme β-glucuronidase is also present in the endoplasmic reticulum, where it is anchored in the lumen by egasyn, a microsomal carboxylesterase designated Ces1e in mouse and rat (Holmes *et al.*, 2010). Egasyn binds to β-glucuronidase at its active-site serine residue, which effectively abolishes the carboxylesterase activity of egasyn, although there is no corresponding loss of β-glucuronidase activity. Binding of OP compounds to egasyn causes the release of β-glucuronidase into plasma, which serves as the basis for a test for OP exposure (Fujikawa *et al.*, 2005). The retention of β-glucuronidase in the lumen of the ER is thought to be physiologically significant. Glucuronidation by microsomal UGTs is a major pathway in the clearance of many of the endogenous aglycones (such as bilirubin) and xenobiotics (such as drugs). However, hydrolysis of glucuronides by β-glucuronidase complexed with egasyn in the lumen of the ER appears to be an important mechanism for recycling endogenous compounds, such as steroid hormones (Dwivedi *et al.*, 1987). The acute-phase response protein, C-reactive protein, is similarly anchored in the endoplasmic reticulum by egasyn.

The mechanism of catalysis by carboxylesterases is analogous to the mechanism of catalysis by serine proteases. In the case of carboxylesterases, it involves charge relay among a catalytic triad comprising an acidic amino acid residue (glutamate [Glu_{335}]),

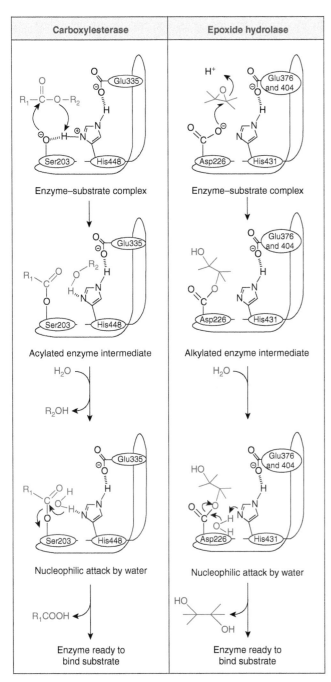

Carboxylesterase	Epoxide hydrolase

Enzyme–substrate complex · Enzyme–substrate complex

Acylated enzyme intermediate · Alkylated enzyme intermediate

Nucleophilic attack by water · Nucleophilic attack by water

Enzyme ready to bind substrate · Enzyme ready to bind substrate

Figure 6-7. *Catalytic cycle of microsomal carboxylesterase (left) and microsomal epoxide hydrolase (right), 2 α/β-hydrolase fold enzymes.*

a basic residue (histidine [His$_{448}$]), and a nucleophilic residue (serine [Ser$_{203}$]) (Yan *et al.*, 1994; Satoh and Hosokawa, 1998). (These amino acid residues, numbered for a rat carboxylesterase, differ slightly in other species, but the overall location and function of these residues are the same in all mammalian carboxylesterases.) The mechanism of catalysis of carboxylesterases is shown in Fig. 6-7, and is discussed in more detail in the section "Epoxide Hydrolases." OP compounds bind to the nucleophilic OH-group on the active-site serine residue to form a phosphorus–oxygen bond, which is not readily cleaved by water. Therefore, OP compounds bind stoichiometrically to carboxylesterases and inhibit their enzymatic activity, for which reason they are also classified as B-esterases (Aldridge, 1953). Surprisingly, the stoichiometric binding of OP compounds to carboxylesterases and cholinesterases is

an important determinant of OP toxicity, as outlined in the section "Cholinesterases (AChE and BChE)."

As mentioned previously in this section, a plasma carboxylesterase, namely, Ces1c (previously known as Es1), is present in mouse plasma but not human plasma and accounts, at least in part, for the relative resistance of mice to the OP nerve agent soman. Duysen *et al.* (2011) demonstrated that plasma carboxylesterase knockout mice are considerably more susceptible to soman toxicity than wild-type mice.

Given the lack of plasma carboxylesterase in humans, the hydrolysis of xenobiotics in human blood is catalyzed by cholinesterases and paraoxonases (with a significant contribution from albumin on a case-by-case basis), as described in the following sections.

Cholinesterases (AChE and BChE) Humans have 2 cholinesterases, namely, acetylcholinesterase (AChE; gene name ACHE) and butyrylcholinesterase (BChE, also known as pseudocholinesterase; gene name BCHE), which are related enzymes (about 54% identical). They are present in most tissues. The levels of BChE are higher than those of AChE except in brain and muscle, tissues where AChE terminates the action of the neurotransmitter acetylcholine. In human plasma, the levels of BChE are 100- to 1000-fold greater than those of AChE, although the latter enzyme is present in erythrocytes (Li *et al.*, 2005). As the names imply, AChE and BChE have high activity toward acetylcholine and butyrylcholine, respectively. AChE is highly selective for acetylcholine and plays little or no significant role in the hydrolysis of xenobiotics, whereas BChE hydrolyzes numerous drugs (and other xenobiotics) including aspirin, bambuterol, chlorpropaine, cocaine, flestolol, heroin, irinotecan, isosorbide diaspirinate, methylprednisolone acetate, mivacurium, moxisylyte, *n*-octanoyl ghrelin, procaine, succinylcholine (suxamethonium), and tetracaine (Li *et al.*, 2005). Eserine (physostigmine) is an inhibitor of both enzymes, whereas BW284C51 is a selective inhibitor of AChE, and iso-OMPA, bambuterol, tolserine, and bis-norcymserine are selective inhibitors of BChE (Liederer and Borchardt, 2006; Masson and Lockridge, 2010). Drugs that selectively inhibit brain AChE and BChE activity, such as rivastigmine (Exelon®), have been used to treat Alzheimer disease. Other drugs that inhibit AChE and are used to treat Alzheimer disease include tacrine (Cognex®), gelantamine (Reminyl®), and donepezil (Aricept®).

Both enzymes exist in 6 different forms with differing solubility: monomer (G1), dimer (G2), tetramer (G4), tailed tetramers (A4), double tetramers (A8), and triple tetramers (A12). G1, G2, and G4 contain 1, 2, and 4 subunits, each with a catalytic site. These various forms can each exist in 3 states: soluble (hydrophilic), immobilized (asymmetric), and amphiphilic globular (membrane-bound through attachment to the phospholipid bilayer) (Nigg and Knaak, 2000). All forms are expressed in muscle. In the case of AChE, the major form in brain is the tetramer G4 (anchored with a 20-kDa side chain containing fatty acids), but the major form in erythrocytes is the dimer G2 (anchored with a glycolipid-phosphatidylinositol side chain). In the case of BChE, the major form in plasma is the tetramer G4 (a glycoprotein with Mr 342 kDa). In both AChE and BChE, the esteratic site (containing the active-site serine residue) is adjacent to an anionic (negatively charged) site that interacts with the positively charged nitrogen on acetylcholine and butyrylcholine.

Genetic variants of AChE that eliminate its activity have not been described, which is not surprising given the key role that AChE plays in terminating neurotransmission by acetylcholine, although AChE knockout mice (AChE$^{-/-}$) are born alive and, despite developmental abnormalities, survive up to 21 days (Xie *et al.*, 2000).

Based on measurements of erythrocyte AChE activity, familial reductions of 30% have been reported, and a reduction of 50% has been linked to paroxysmal nocturnal hemoglobinuria (Nigg and Knaak, 2000).

More than 70 genetic variants of BChE have been described following the discovery of poor metabolizers (PMs) of succinylcholine (suxamethonium) and, later, mivacurium. Succinylcholine and mivacurium are muscle relaxants whose duration of action is determined by plasma BChE. Succinylcholine (1.5-2.0 mg/kg) is a rapidly acting muscle relaxant (the onset of paralysis takes 30-60 seconds) with a short duration of action (8-15 minutes) making it well suited for intubating patients. In some individuals, succinylcholine causes prolonged (60-120 minutes) paralysis (muscular relaxation and apnea), which led to the discovery of 2 BChE genetic polymorphisms (now known as BCHE*A and BCHE*K) (Cerf *et al.*, 2002). The so-called A variant of BChE (Asp$_{70}$Gly) has markedly reduced enzymatic activity (less than 10% of the wild-type enzyme) but is relatively rare; about 1 in 300 Caucasians are homozygous for the A variant. The K variant (Ala$_{539}$Thr) is considerably more common (with one in 63 individuals being homozygous) but the K variant still retains approximately two thirds of its enzymatic activity. Consequently, the A variant causes a greater impairment of succinylcholine (and mivacurium) metabolism than does the K variant (La Du, 1992; Lockridge, 1992; Levano *et al.*, 2008). Although the A variant has markedly diminished activity toward succinylcholine (due to a ~100-fold decrease in affinity [K_m]), it nevertheless has appreciable activity toward other substrates, such as acetylcholine and benzoylcholine. Wild-type BChE and the A variant are equally sensitive to the inhibitory effect of OP compounds, but the allelic variant is relatively resistant to the inhibitory effect of dibucaine, a local anesthetic, which forms the basis of a diagnostic test for its presence (frequently called a test for atypical pseudocholinesterase). The percent inhibition of hydrolysis of benzoylcholine by dibucaine (with both the substrate and inhibitor at 10 μM) is called the dibucaine number; it is 80% or more with wild-type BChE and about 40% with the A variant in most but not all cases (Cerf *et al.*, 2002). The discovery of the A variant of BChE (the so-called atypical pseudocholinesterase) is of historical interest because it ushered in the new field of pharmacogenetics, a field pioneered by Dr Werner Kalow, after whom the K variant of BChE is named.

Carboxylesterases and cholinesterases in the blood and tissues play an important role in limiting the amount of cholinergic neurotoxins that reach AChE in the brain, marked inhibition (70%–90%) of which is lethal to mammals, insects, and nematodes. The cholinergic neurotoxins that are bound covalently to—or are hydrolyzed by—these enzymes include OP nerve agents (such as soman and sarin), OP pesticides (such as parathion, malathion, and chlorpyros, which are converted to oxons by CYP), carbamate pesticides (such as aldicarb, carbaryl, carbofuran), the naturally occurring OP compound anatoxin-a(S) from blue-green algae, physostigmine (eserine) from the Calabar bean, huperzine A from the club moss *Huperzia serrata*, solandine from green potatoes, and cocaine from the *Erythroxylum coca* plant. The covalent interaction between OP compounds and brain AChE is analogous to their binding to the active-site serine residue in all serine esterases (B-esterases). As previously mentioned, certain OP compounds are hydrolyzed by A-esterases (the paraoxonase PON1) but bind stoichiometrically and, for the most part, irreversibly to B-esterases (carboxylesterases and cholinesterases). Surprisingly, stoichiometric binding of OP compounds to carboxylesterase and cholinesterase (and perhaps to numerous other enzymes and receptors that have structural features common to serine esterases) plays an important role in limiting

the toxicity of OP compounds. Numerous studies have shown an inverse relationship between serine esterase activity and susceptibility to the toxic effect of OP compounds. Factors that decrease serine esterase activity potentiate the toxic effects of OP compounds, whereas factors that increase serine esterase activity have a protective effect. For example, the susceptibility of animals to the toxicity of parathion, malathion, and diisopropylfluorophosphate (DFP) is inversely related to the level of plasma esterase activity (which reflects BChE activity and, in some species, carboxylesterase activity). Differences in the susceptibility of several mammalian species to OP toxicity can be abolished by pretreatment with selective serine esterase inhibitors such as cresylbenzodioxaphosphorin oxide, the active metabolite of tri-*ortho*-tolylphosphate (which is also known as tri-*ortho*-cresylphosphate [TOCP]). Knockout mice that lack plasma carboxylesterase (Ces1c, previously known as Es1) or AChE are more susceptible to the toxic effects of OP compounds, as are PON1 knockout mice in some but not all cases (discussed in the section "Paraoxonases (Lactonases)") (Xie *et al.*, 2000; Duysen *et al.*, 2011). Somewhat surprisingly, BChE knockout mice are not more sensitive to OP toxicity than wild-type mice (Duysen *et al.*, 2007), but this may not reflect the situation in humans because mouse plasma contains a carboxylesterase, whereas humans do not (see the section "Carboxylesterases"). In humans, BChE plays an important role in preventing OP compounds from reaching AChE in the brain. Carboxylesterases, cholinesterases, and paraoxonases are not the only enzymes involved in the detoxication of OP pesticides. Certain OP compounds are detoxified by CYP, flavin monooxygenases, and GSTs. However, paraoxonases, enzymes that catalyze the hydrolysis of certain OP compounds, appear to play a limited role in determining susceptibility to OP toxicity, as outlined in the following section.

Once bound to the active site of cholinesterase or carboxylesterase, OP compounds can undergo dealkylation reactions that further retard their release from the active-site serine residue of these enzymes. This process is called "aging." In many cases the phosphorylated or phosphonylated enzyme can be reactivated by displacement of the OP adduct with nucleophilic compounds such as fluoride, hydroxamates, and oximes. The pyridinium oximes pralidoxime (2-PAM) and obidoxime (toxogonin) are used therapeutically as antidotes to OP poisoning. More potent oximes (HI-6 and MMB-4) are under development (Masson and Lockridge, 2010). Cocaine is hydrolyzed by CES1 and CES2 in liver and intestine, and by BChE in plasma. Genetic polymorphisms that reduce BChE activity toward succinylcholine (such as the A variant described earlier in this section) also reduce its activity toward cocaine (again by decreasing K_m), which exacerbates cocaine toxicity (Masson and Lockridge, 2010). Despite its important role in cocaine toxicity, BChE hydrolyzes cocaine slowly. Masson and Lockridge (2010) reviewed efforts based on molecular dynamics simulation to improve the hydrolytic function of BChE through site-directed mutagenesis. A BChE variant with 4 mutations hydrolyzes cocaine with a catalytic efficiency 1500- to 5000-fold greater than that of the wild-type enzyme, whereas a variant with 5 mutations is 6500 times more active. The latter man-made variant is of therapeutic interest for the treatment of cocaine overdose. Other variants of BChE are being developed with improved hydrolysis of OP compounds for the treatment of OP poisoning and protection against OP nerve agents.

Paraoxonases (Lactonases) Paraoxonases catalyze the hydrolysis of a broad range of organophosphates, organophosphinites, aromatic carboxylic acid esters (such as phenylacetate), cyclic carbonates, lactones, and oxidized phospholipids. They are calcium-dependent enzymes containing a critical sulfhydryl (−SH) group; as such they are inhibited by EDTA, metal ions (Cu and Ba), and various mercurials such as phenylmercuric acetate (PMA), *para*-chloromercuribenzoate (PCMB), and the PCMB hydrolysis product, *para*-hydroxymercuribenzoate. (*Note*: Calcium must be added to measure paraoxonase activity in plasma prepared from EDTA-anticoagulated blood.) Based on the observation that A-esterases are inhibited by PCMB but not OP compounds, Augustinsson (1966) postulated that, in the case of paraoxonases, OP compounds bind to a nucleophilic SH-group on an active-site cysteine residue and form a phosphorus–sulfur bond, which is readily cleaved by water. A strong argument against this postulate is the fact that there is no loss of enzymatic activity when the only potential active-site cysteine residue in human paraoxonase (Cys_{283}) is substituted with serine or alanine (Sorenson *et al.*, 1995). However, substitution with serine or alanine renders paraoxonase resistant to inhibition by PCMB, placing Cys_{283} near but not in the active site of paraoxonase. Paraoxonase requires Ca^{2+}, for both stability and catalytic activity, which raises the possibility that the hydrolysis of OP compounds by paraoxonase involves metal-catalyzed hydrolysis, analogous to that proposed for calcium-dependent phospholipase A2 or zinc-dependent phosphotriesterase activity (Sorenson *et al.*, 1995). A structurally modified but catalytically active form of recombinant PON1 has been crystallized and shown by x-ray analysis to contain 2 calcium ions in a 6-fold β-propeller protein similar to that found in squid diisopropylfluorophosphatase (DFPase), a paraoxonase-like enzyme (Otto *et al.*, 2009).

Humans express 3 paraoxonases designated PON1, PON2, and PON3. PON1 is present in liver microsomes and plasma, where it is associated exclusively with high-density lipoprotein (HDL). PON2 is not present in plasma but it is expressed in the inner mitochondrial membrane of vascular cells and many tissues (Devarajan *et al.*, 2011). PON3 is expressed in liver and kidney microsomes and plasma. Only PON1 has appreciable arylesterase activity and the ability to hydrolyze the toxic oxon metabolites of OP insecticides such as parathion (paraoxon), diazinon (diazoxon), and chlorpyrifos (chlorpyrifos oxon) (Gupta and DuBois, 1998; Draganov and La Du, 2004). However, all 3 enzymes can catalyze the hydrolysis of various lactones, for which reason the name "lactonase" is more encompassing. A lactone derived from arachidonic acid (5-hydroxy-cicosate traeomic acid-1,5-lactone) is one of the few substrates hydrolyzed by all 3 paraoxonases (Gupta *et al.*, 2009). Lactone hydrolysis of the statins lovastatin and simvastatin is catalyzed only by PON3. Reports of the same reaction being catalyzed by PON1 appear to be attributable to trace contamination with PON3 (Draganov and La Du, 2004). However, both PON1 and PON3 hydrolyze the lactone form of atorvastatin, which reverses the lactonization of atorvastatin, a reaction that involves formation of an acyl glucuronide of atorvastatin by UGT1A3 (Riedmaier *et al.*, 2011). PON1 hydrolyzes thiolactones such as homocysteine thiolactone (an endobiotic substrate) and a thiolactone metabolite of clopidogrel (discussed later in the section "CYP2C19"), whereas PON3 hydrolyzes the lactone spironolactone (a diuretic drug) (Gupta *et al.*, 2009). PON1 is the major plasma enzyme responsible for hydrolyzing the prodrug olmesartan medoxomil to its active metabolite (Ishizuka *et al.*, 2012) and is one of the plasma enzymes responsible for hydrolyzing the structurally related prodrugs prulifloxacin and ceftobiprole medocaril to their active metabolites (Eichenbaum *et al.*, 2012).

PON2, located on the inner mitochondrial membrane, appears to play no significant role in xenobiotic biotransformation, although it can hydrolyze the lactone dihydrocoumarin. In the inner mitochondrial membrane, PON2 is bound to coenzyme Q_{10}

and complexed with respiratory complex III where it protects the mitochondrion from oxidative damage from superoxide anion and its derivative ROS (hydrogen peroxide, peroxynitrite, and hydroxy radicals) (Devarajan *et al.*, 2011).

PON1 has 2 prominent polymorphisms in the coding region, namely, $Q_{192}R$ ($Glu_{192}Arg$) and $L_{55}M$ ($Leu_{55}Met$), and several polymorphisms in the promoter region. Polymorphisms in the promoter region and the $L_{55}M$ polymorphism in the coding region do not affect PON1 activity but they do affect expression levels (Gupta *et al.*, 2009; Furlong *et al.*, 2010). The commonest genetic polymorphism, $Q_{192}R$, affects PON1 activity in a substrate-dependent manner. The glutamine (Q_{192}) and arginine (R_{192}) allelozymes have the same hydrolytic activity toward *para*-nitrophenylacetate (a measure of arylesterase activity) and diazoxon (the oxon of diazinon) but R_{192} is more active toward paraoxon (the oxon of parathion), chlorpyrifos oxon, the prodrugs olmesartan medoxomil and prulifloxacin, and the lactone pilocarpine, whereas Q_{192} is more active toward soman, sarin, the thiolactone metabolite of clopidogrel (Bouman *et al.*, 2011; discussed later in the section "CYP2C19"), and lipid peroxides, the significance of which is discussed later in this section (Gupta *et al.*, 2009; Furlong *et al.*, 2010; Eichenbaum *et al.*, 2012; Ishizuka *et al.*, 2012).

There is evidence to suggest that PON1 protects against atherosclerosis by hydrolyzing specific derivatives of oxidized cholesterol and/or phospholipids in atherosclerotic lesions and in oxidized low-density lipoprotein (LDL). For example, mice lacking PON1 (knockout mice or PON1 null mice) are predisposed to atherogenesis, whereas mice overexpressing PON1 are protected (Draganov and La Du, 2004; Gupta *et al.*, 2009). Some studies show that individuals who are homozygous for the R_{192} allele are at increased risk of atherosclerosis and ischemic stroke compared with individuals who are homozygous for the Q_{192} allele, suggesting that the absence of the latter enzyme, the PON1 allelozyme with high activity toward lipid peroxides and offering more protection against LDL oxidation, is a risk factor for cardiovascular disease (Gupta *et al.*, 2009; Dahabreh *et al.*, 2010). However, the association is controversial. A complicating factor is that the R_{192} allelozyme is expressed at higher levels than the Q_{192} enzyme, which may partially offset its lower ability to hydrolyze lipid peroxides. Bayrak *et al.* (2011) proposed that, in terms of assessing the risk of atherosclerosis, an assessment of both plasma PON1 activity and genotype is more reliable than genotype alone. This seems appropriate in view of the finding that several environmental factors affect PON1 levels, which are upregulated by hypolipidemic drugs (fenofibrate and statins) and cardioprotective dietary components such as polyphenols (such as resveratrol), oleic acid, and olive oil, and downregulated by diabetes and a high-fat (proatherogenic) diet (Gupta *et al.*, 2009).

It seems reasonable to assume that PON1 would play an important role in determining the susceptibility of humans to OP toxicity based on 3 considerations: first, PON1 hydrolyzes OP compounds (rather than simply bind them stoichiometrically like BChE). Second, the concentration of PON1/3 in human plasma is 10 times greater than that of BChE (50 mg/mL *vs* 5 mg/mL) (Li *et al.*, 2005). Third, human plasma does not contain carboxylesterase (Li *et al.*, 2005). PON1/3 may protect against OP toxicity in some but not all cases. PON1 knockout mice are no more susceptible than wild-type mice to the toxic effects of paraoxon (the active metabolite of parathion), and administration of human PON1 (either the R_{192} or the Q_{192} allelozyme) to PON1 knockout mice does not confer protection against paraoxon. However, administration of either the R_{192} or Q_{192} human allelozymes to PON1 knockout mice does protect against diazoxon toxicity, and administration of the R_{192} allelozyme (but not the Q_{192} allelozyme) protects against chlorpyrifos oxon (Cole *et al.*, 2010). The allelozyme-dependent pattern of protection corresponds with the rate of hydrolysis of these OP oxons by R_{192} and Q_{192} (high and equal for diazoxon, high but greater with R_{192} for chlorpyrifos oxon, and low but greater with R_{192} for paraoxon). Although the concentration of BChE in human plasma is only one tenth that of PON1/3 (~50 nM *vs* 500 nM), its apparent second-order rate constant with OP compounds is very high (10^7 to 10^9 M^{-1} min^{-1}) compared with the catalytic efficiency of PON1 ($10^5 M^{-1} min^{-1}$) (Masson and Lockridge, 2010).

Diisopropylfluorophosphatase (DFPase), a squid enzyme that catalyzes the release of fluoride from DFP (Fig. 6-5), is a hydrolytic enzyme related to the paraoxonases. It hydrolyzes the nerve gas agents sarin and soman (Liederer and Borchardt, 2006). Human paraoxonases do not hydrolyze DFP but are inhibited by this OP compound.

Prodrugs and Alkaline Phosphatase

Many prodrugs are designed to be hydrolyzed by hydrolytic enzymes (Liederer and Borchardt, 2006). Some prodrugs, such as propranolol ester, are hydrolyzed by both carboxylesterases and cholinesterases (both AChE and BChE), whereas others are preferentially or specifically hydrolyzed by carboxylesterases (capecitabine, irinotecan), BChE (bambuterol, methylprednisolone acetate), hPON1 (prulifloxacin, olmesartan medoxomil), or PON3 (lovastatin, simvastatin). On a case-by-case basis, specific enzymes other than those mentioned above can be involved in xenobiotic hydrolysis. For example, the valine ester prodrugs of acyclovir (valacyclovir) and gangciclovir (valgangciclovir) are hydrolyzed by valacyclovirase (gene code BPHL), a serine- and α/β-fold-hydrolase that hydrolyzes other antiviral and anticancer nucleoside drugs such as zidovudine, floxuridine, and gemcitabine (Lai *et al.*, 2008). Some prodrugs are hydrolyzed with a high degree of stereoselectivity. For example, in the case of prodrugs of ibuprofen and flurbiprofen, the *R*-enantiomer is hydrolyzed about 50 times faster than the *S*-enantiomer. The acyl glucuronides of ibuprofen and other NSAIDs are also hydrolyzed stereoselectively (see the section "Glucuronidation and Formation of Acyl-CoA Thioesters").

Some prodrugs, such as fosphenytoin (Cerebyx®) and fosamprenavir (Lexiva®), are designed to be hydrolyzed by alkaline phosphatase, high concentrations of which are present on the luminal surface of the enterocytes lining the wall of the small intestine. Hydrolysis of these prodrugs by alkaline phosphatase releases the active drug at the surface of the enterocytes, where it can be readily absorbed. Soluble epoxide hydrolase (sEH) is a bifunctional enzyme; its C-terminus contains an epoxide hydrolase domain, whereas its N-terminus contains a phosphatase domain, as described in the section "Epoxide Hydrolases." Although it may play a role in the hydrolysis of endogenous phosphates, such as polyisoprenyl phosphates and lysophosphatidic acids (Oguro and Imaoka, 2012), sEH is an intracellular enzyme and, as such, can play no significant role in the hydrolysis of phosphate/phosphonate prodrugs.

As a result of their ability to hydrolyze prodrugs, hydrolytic enzymes may have clinical applications in the treatment of certain cancers. They might be used, for example, to activate prodrugs in vivo and thereby generate potent anticancer agents in highly selected target sites (eg, at the surface of tumor cells, or inside the tumor cells themselves). For example, carboxylesterases might be targeted to tumor sites with hybrid monoclonal antibodies (ie, bifunctional antibodies that recognize the carboxylesterase and the tumor cell), or the cDNA encoding a carboxylesterase might be targeted to the tumor cells via a viral vector. In the case of irinotecan, this therapeutic strategy would release the anticancer drug SN-38 in the vicinity of the tumor cells, which would reduce the systemic levels and side effects of this otherwise highly toxic drug (Senter *et al.*, 1996). Some prodrugs, such as capecitabine, are activated by hydrolytic enzymes in the tumors themselves.

Peptidases

With the advent of recombinant DNA technology, numerous human peptides have been mass-produced for use as therapeutic agents, and several recombinant peptide hormones, growth factors, cytokines, soluble receptors, and humanized monoclonal antibodies currently are used clinically. To avoid acid precipitation and proteolytic degradation in the gastrointestinal tract, peptides are administered parenterally. Nevertheless, peptides are hydrolyzed in the blood and tissues by a variety of peptidases, including aminopeptidases and carboxypeptidases, which hydrolyze amino acids at the N- and C-terminus, respectively, and endopeptidases, which cleave peptides at specific internal sites (trypsin, for example, cleaves peptides on the C-terminal side of arginine or lysine residues) (Humphrey and Ringrose, 1986; Testa and Krämer, 2008, 2010). Peptidases cleave the amide linkage between adjacent amino acids; hence, they function as amidases. As in the case of carboxylesterases, the active site of peptidases contains either a serine or cysteine residue, which initiates a nucleophilic attack on the carbonyl moiety of the amide bond. As previously noted, the mechanism of catalysis by serine proteases, such as chymotrypsin, is similar to that by serine esterases (B-esterases).

β-Glucuronidase

β-Glucuronidase is present in liver lysosomes and microsomes (where it is bound to the lumen of the endoplasmic reticulum by egasyn [Ces1e], as mentioned in the section "Carboxylesterases") and in gut microflora. The enzyme hydrolyzes xenobiotic glucuronides (in which the glucuronide is in the β-configuration). When a drug is glucuronidated directly and excreted in bile, hydrolysis by β-glucuronidase in the gut can release the aglycone (the parent drug) and result in a second phase of drug absorption, a process called enterohepatic circulation. In the case of the anticancer drug irinotecan, which is hydrolyzed to SN-11 (the pharmacologically active and toxic metabolite) and then glucuronidated, hydrolysis of SN-11-glucuronide by microflora β-glucuronidase is undesirable because it releases SN-11 in the colon and causes dose-limiting diarrhea. To reduce the risk of such an adverse event, an inhibitor of gut β-glucuronidase has been developed, which is described in more detail in the section "Glucuronidation and Formation of Acyl-CoA Thioesters."

Epoxide Hydrolases

Epoxide hydrolases catalyze the *trans*-addition of water to alkene epoxides and arene oxides (oxiranes), which can form during the CYP-dependent oxidation of aliphatic alkenes and aromatic hydrocarbons, respectively. As shown in Fig. 6-8, the products of this hydrolysis are vicinal diols with a *trans*-configuration (ie, *trans*-1,2-dihydrodiols), a notable exception being the conversion of leukotriene A_4 (LTA_4) to leukotriene B_4 (LTB_4), in which case the 2 hydroxyl groups that result from epoxide hydrolysis appear on nonadjacent carbon atoms. Epoxide hydrolases play an important role in detoxifying electrophilic epoxides that might otherwise bind to proteins and nucleic acids and cause cellular toxicity and genetic mutations. In the case of PAHs, however, microsomal epoxide hydrolase plays a critical role in forming diol epoxides, the ultimate carcinogenic metabolites of benzo[*a*]pyrene (B[*a*]P), 7,12-dimethylbenz[*a*]anthracene (DMBA), and many other PAHs (discussed later in this section).

There are 4 distinct forms of epoxide hydrolase in mammals: microsomal epoxide hydrolase (mEH; gene name EPHX1), soluble epoxide hydrolase (sEH; gene name EPHX2), cholesterol-5,6-epoxide hydrolase (ChEH; gene yet to be characterized), and leukotriene A_4 hydrolase (LTA_4 hydrolase; gene name LTA4H) (Fretland

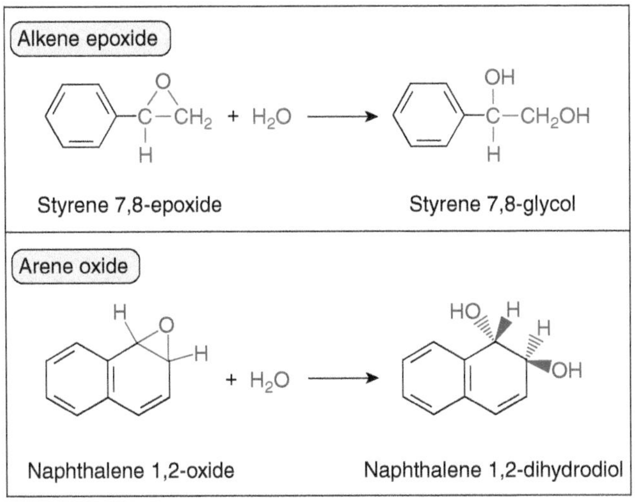

Figure 6-8. *Examples of the hydrolyation of an alkene epoxide (top) and an arene oxide (bottom) by epoxide hydrolase.*

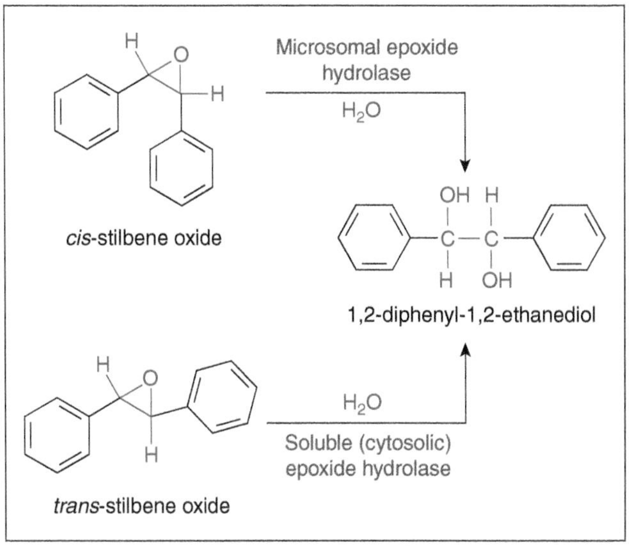

Figure 6-9. *Stereoselective hydrolyation of stilbene oxide by microsomal and soluble epoxide hydrolase.*

and Omiecinski, 2000; Morisseau and Hammock, 2005). Hepoxilin A_3 hydrolase was thought to represent a fifth class of epoxide hydrolase but it was subsequently identified as being the same enzyme as sEH (Cronin *et al.*, 2011). As their names imply, cholesterol-5,6-epoxide hydrolase (ChEH) and LTA_4 hydrolase hydrolyze endogenous epoxides specifically, and have virtually no capacity to detoxify xenobiotic oxides. LTA_4 hydrolase is distinct from the other epoxide hydrolases because it is a bifunctional zinc metalloenzyme that has both epoxide hydrolase and peptidase activity, and because the 2 hydroxyl groups introduced during the conversion of LTA_4 to LTB_4 are 8 carbon atoms apart. sEH is a bifunctional enzyme; its C-terminus contains an epoxide hydrolase domain, whereas its N-terminus contains a phosphatase domain. The latter domain is structurally related to members of haloacid dehalogenase (HAD) superfamily, which includes dehalogenases, phosphonatases, phosphomutases, phosphatases, and ATPases. The phosphatase domain of sEH is thought to play a role in the hydrolysis of endogenous phosphates, such as polyisoprenyl phosphates (which regulate cholesterol levels) and lysophosphatidic acids (Imig and Hammock, 2009; Oguro and Imaoka, 2012).

mEH hydrolyzes a wide variety of xenobiotics with an alkene epoxide or arene oxide. sEH hydrolyzes some xenobiotic epoxides and oxides, such as *trans*-stilbene oxide, but it also plays an important role in the hydrolysis of endogenous fatty acid epoxides, such as the epoxyeicosatrienoic acids (EETs) that are formed by epoxidation of arachidonic acid by CYP (particularly CYP2J2 and CYP2C9) and the leukotoxins that are formed by the epoxidation of linoleic acid by leukocytes (Fretland and Omiecinski, 2000; Morisseau and Hammock, 2005; Imig and Hammock, 2009). EETs are endothelin-derived hyperpolarizing factors (EDHFs) (ie, vasodilators) that possess anti-inflammatory properties and protect tissues from ischemic injury. Hydrolysis of EETs by sEH terminates their vasodilatory and anti-inflammatory effects. Accordingly, sEH is a potential therapeutic target for the treatment of various cardiovascular diseases such as hypertension and atherosclerosis (Imig and Hammock, 2009; Wang *et al.*, 2010c). Several disubstituted ureas (including the anticancer drug sorafenib) have been identified as competitive inhibitors of sEH that are both potent (K_i values in the nanomolar range) and specific (they do not inhibit the phosphatase domain of sEH and they do not potently inhibit mEH). In addition to their vasodilatory and anti-inflammatory effects, EETs promote endothelial cell proliferation and migration; hence, they are angiogenic (ie, they stimulate blood vessel supply). A potential side effect of sEH inhibitors, therefore, may be potentiation of EET-mediated angiogenic resulting in accelerated tumorigenesis (Imig and Hammock, 2009; Wang *et al.*, 2010c).

Although the levels vary from one tissue to the next, mEH has been found in the microsomal fraction (and in some cases the plasma membrane) of virtually all tissues, including the liver, testis, ovary, lung, kidney, skin, intestine, colon, spleen, thymus, brain, and heart. sEH is also widely distributed in tissues; high levels of sEH are present in the cytosol (and in some cases the lysosomes) of liver, kidney, brain, and vasculature and lower levels are present in lung, spleen, and testis. In general, mEH prefers monosubstituted epoxides and disubstituted epoxides with a *cis* configuration, such as *cis*-stilbene oxide, whereas sEH prefers tetrasubstituted and trisubstituted epoxides and disubstituted epoxides with a *gem* configuration (both substituents on the same carbon atom) or the *trans* configuration, such as *trans*-stilbene oxide, as shown in Fig. 6-9. In rodents, both sEH and mEH are inducible enzymes; sEH is under the control of PPARα, so it is induced following treatment of rats and mice with peroxisome proliferators, whereas mEH is under the control of Nrf2, so it is induced in response to oxidative stress or exposure to electrophiles and GSH depletors (see the section "Quinone Reduction—NQO1 and NQO2"). Treatment of mice with the CAR agonist phenobarbital induces mEH about 2- to 3-fold, whereas treatment with Nrf2 activators such as butylated hydroxytoluene (BHT), butylated hydroxyanisole (BHA), and ethoxyquin induces mEH by an order of magnitude or more. mEH is one of several proteins (so-called preneoplastic antigens) that are overexpressed in chemically induced foci and nodules that eventually develop into liver tumors.

Many epoxides and oxides are intermediary metabolites formed during the CYP-dependent oxidation of unsaturated aliphatic and aromatic xenobiotics. These electrophilic metabolites might otherwise bind to proteins and nucleic acids and cause cellular toxicity and genetic mutations. In general, sEH and mEH are found in the same tissues and cell types that contain CYP. For example, the distribution of epoxide hydrolase parallels that of CYP in liver, lung, and testis. In other words, both enzymes are located in the centrilobular region of the liver (zone 3), in Clara and type II cells in the lung, and in Leydig cells in the testis. The colocalization of epoxide hydrolase and CYP presumably ensures the rapid detoxication of alkene epoxides and arene oxides generated during the oxidative metabolism of xenobiotics.

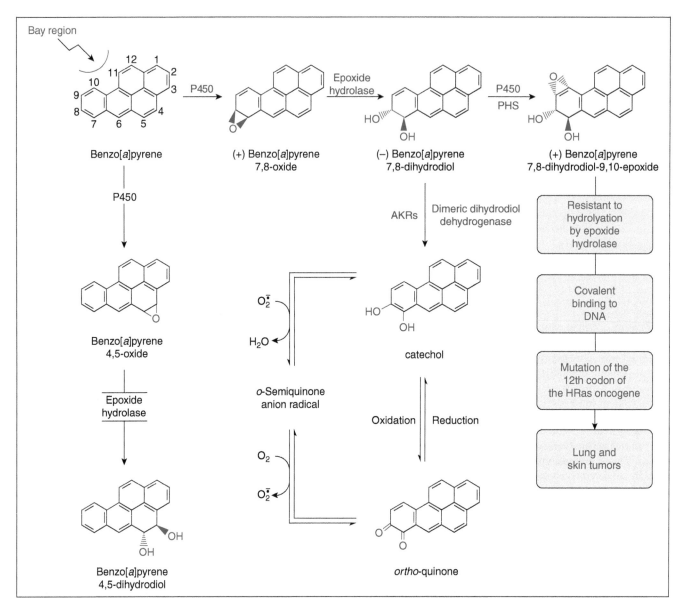

Figure 6-10. *Role of epoxide hydrolase in the inactivation of benzo[a]pyrene 4,5-oxide and in the conversion of benzo[a]pyrene to its tumorigenic bay-region diol epoxide.* Also shown is the role of dimeric dihydrodiol dehydrogenase, and the aldo-keto reductase (AKR) superfamily, in the formation of reactive catechol and *ortho*-quinone metabolites of benzo[a]pyrene.

Electrophilic epoxides and arene oxides are constantly produced during the CYP-dependent oxidation of unsaturated aliphatic and aromatic xenobiotics, and are potentially reactive to cellular macromolecules such as DNA and protein. Epoxide hydrolase can rapidly convert these potentially toxic metabolites to the corresponding dihydrodiols, which are less reactive and easier to excrete. Thus, epoxide hydrolases are widely considered as a group of detoxication enzymes. In some cases, however, further oxidation of a dihydrodiol can lead to the formation of diol epoxide derivatives that are no longer substrates for epoxide hydrolase because the oxirane ring is protected by bulky substituents that sterically hinder interaction with the enzyme. This point proved to be extremely important in elucidating the mechanism by which PAHs cause tumors in laboratory animals (Conney, 1982). Tumorigenic PAHs, such as B[a]P, are converted by CYP (particularly by CYP1B1 and CYP1A1) to a variety of arene oxides that bind covalently to DNA, making them highly mutagenic to bacteria. One of the major arene oxides formed from B[a]P, namely, the 4,5-oxide, is highly mutagenic to bacteria but weakly mutagenic to mammalian cells. This discrepancy reflects the

rapid inactivation of B[a]P 4,5-oxide by epoxide hydrolase in mammalian cells. However, one of the arene oxides formed from B[a]P, namely, B[a]P 7,8-dihydrodiol-9,10-oxide, is not a substrate for epoxide hydrolase and is highly mutagenic to mammalian cells and considerably more potent than B[a]P as a lung tumorigen in mice.

B[a]P 7,8-dihydrodiol-9,10-oxide is known as a bay-region diol epoxide, and analogous bay-region diol epoxides are now recognized as tumorigenic metabolites of numerous PAHs. A feature common to all bay-region epoxides is their resistance to hydrolyation by mEH, which results from steric hindrance from the nearby dihydrodiol group. As shown in Fig. 6-10, B[a]P 7,8-dihydrodiol-9,10-oxide is formed in 3 steps: B[a]P is converted to the 7,8-oxide, which is converted to the 7,8-dihydrodiol, which is converted to the corresponding 9,10-epoxide (which can exist in 4 diastereomeric forms). The first and third steps are epoxidation reactions catalyzed by CYP (especially CYP1B1 and CYP1A1) or prostaglandin H synthase, but the second step is catalyzed by mEH. Consequently, even though mEH plays a major role in detoxifying several B[a]P, such as the 4,5-oxide, it nevertheless plays a role in converting B[a]P to its ultimate tumorigenic metabolite, B[*a*]P 7,8-dihydrodiol-9,10-oxide. Diol epoxides are also the carcinogenic metabolites of DMBA and many other PAHs (Shimada, 2006).

The importance of mEH in the conversion of PAHs to their ultimate carcinogenic metabolites, namely, diol epoxides, is illustrated by the observation that mEH knockout mice (mEH-null mice) are completely resistant to the tumorigenic effects of DMBA (Shimada, 2006). Genetic polymorphisms of human mEH also impact cigarette-smoking-induced cancer of the lung and upper aerodigestive tract (UADT) in a manner consistent with the protective effect conferred by a lack of mEH in DMBA-treated mice (Li *et al.*, 2011b). More than 110 SNPs have been identified in the human EPHX1 gene, 2 of which have been studied in detail: One of them ($Tyr_{113}His$) decreases mEH activity (by about 40%) and the other ($His_{139}Arg$) increases mEH activity (by about 25%). The low-activity mEH (observed in individuals who are homozygous or heterozygous for the His_{133} allelozyme) protects from tobacco-induced cancer of the lung and UADT, whereas the high-activity variant (observed in individuals who are homozygous or heterozygous for the Arg_{139} allelozyme) predisposes to these cancers (Li *et al.*, 2011b).

Not all epoxides are highly reactive and toxic to the cells that produce them. Some drugs actually contain an epoxide, such as scopolamine, tiotropium, and troleandomycin. Vitamin K epoxide is also a nontoxic epoxide, which is formed and consumed during the vitamin K–dependent γ-carboxylation of prothrombin and other clotting factors in the liver. Vitamin K epoxide is not hydrated by mEH but is reduced by vitamin K epoxide reductase. This enzyme is inhibited by warfarin and related coumarin anticoagulants, which interrupts the synthesis of several clotting factors. The major metabolite of carbamazepine is an epoxide, which is so stable that carbamazepine 10,11-epoxide is a major circulating metabolite in patients treated with this antiepileptic drug. (Carbamazepine is converted to a second epoxide, which is less stable and more cytotoxic, as shown in the section "Cytochrome P450.") Circulating levels of carbamazepine 10,11-epoxide are elevated in individuals expressing the low-activity variant of mEH (the His_{133} allelozyme) but, with one possible exception, this genetic polymorphism is not associated with an increase in the adverse effects of this or other anticonvulsant drugs (Daly, 1999). The exception is a case report of a man who had a defect in mEH expression and suffered acute and severe phenytoin toxicity (Morisseau and Hammock, 2005). Certain drugs, such as valpromide (the amide analog of valproic acid) and progabide (a γ-aminobutyric acid [GABA] agonist), cause clinically significant inhibition of mEH and may impair epoxide hydrolase activity more than genetic polymorphisms. These 2 drugs potentiate the neurotoxicity of carbamazepine by inhibiting mEH, leading to increased plasma levels of carbamazepine 10,11-epoxide and presumably its more toxic 2,3-epoxide (Kroetz *et al.*, 1993). mEH can be inhibited in vitro by certain epoxides, such as 1,1,1-trichloropropene oxide and cyclohexene oxide, and stimulated by several alcohols, ketones, and imidazoles.

The microsomal and soluble forms of epoxide hydrolase show no evident sequence identity and, accordingly, are immunochemically distinct proteins (Beetham *et al.*, 1995). Nevertheless, mEH and sEH catalyze reactions by the same mechanism, and similar amino acids are involved in catalysis, namely, a nucleophilic acid (Asp_{226} in mEH and Asp_{334} in sEH), a basic histidine (His_{431} in mEH and His_{523} in sEH), an orienting acid (Glu_{404} in mEH and Asp_{495} in sEH), and polarizing tyrosine residues (Tyr_{299} and Tyr_{374} in mEH and Tyr_{382} and Tyr_{465} in mEH) (Morisseau and Hammock, 2005). The mechanism of catalysis by epoxide hydrolase is similar to that of carboxylesterase, in that the catalytic site comprises 3 amino acid residues that form a catalytic triad, as shown in Fig. 6-7. The attack of the nucleophile Asp_{226} on the carbon of the oxirane ring initiates enzymatic activity, leading to the formation of an α-hydroxyester-enzyme intermediate, with the negative charge developing on the oxygen atom stabilized by a putative oxyanion hole. The His_{431} residue (which is activated by Glu_{376} and Glu_{404}) activates a water molecule by abstracting a proton (H^+). The activated (nucleophilic) water then attacks the Cγ atom of Asp_{226}, resulting in the hydrolysis of the ester bond in the acyl–enzyme intermediate, which restores the active enzyme and results in formation of a vicinal diol with a *trans*-configuration (Armstrong, 1999). The second step, namely, cleavage of the ester bond in the acyl–enzyme intermediate, resembles the cleavage of the ester or amide bond in substrates for serine esterases and proteases.

Although both epoxide hydrolase and carboxylesterase have a catalytic triad comprising a nucleophilic, basic, and acidic amino acid residue, there are striking differences in their catalytic machinery, which account for the fact that carboxylesterases primarily hydrolyze esters and amides, whereas epoxide hydrolases primarily hydrolyze epoxides and oxides. In the triad, both enzymes have histidine as the base and either glutamate or aspartate as the acid, but they differ in the type of amino acids for the nucleophile. Even during catalysis, there is a major difference. In carboxylesterases, the same carbonyl carbon atom of the substrate is attacked initially by the nucleophile Ser_{203} to form an α-hydroxyester-enzyme ester that is subsequently attacked by the activated water to release the alcohol product. In contrast, 2 different atoms in epoxide hydrolase are targets of nucleophilic attacks. First the less hindered carbon atom of the oxirane ring is attacked by the nucleophile Asp_{226} to form a covalently bound ester, and next this ester is hydrolyzed by an activated water molecule that attacks the Cγ atom of the Asp_{226} residue, as illustrated in Fig. 6-7. Therefore, in carboxylesterase, the oxygen introduced to the product is derived from the activated water molecule. In contrast, in epoxide hydrolase, the oxygen introduced to the product is derived from the nucleophile Asp_{226} (Fig. 6-7).

Carboxylesterases and epoxide hydrolases exhibit no primary sequence identity, but they share surprising similarities in the topology of the structure and sequential arrangement of the catalytic triad. Both are members of the α/β-hydrolase fold enzymes, a superfamily of proteins that includes lipases, esterases, and haloalkane dehydrogenases (Beetham *et al.*, 1995). Functionally, proteins in this superfamily all catalyze hydrolytic reactions; structurally, they all contain a similar core segment that is composed of 8 β-sheets connected by α-helices. They all have a catalytic triad and the arrangement of the amino acid residues in the triad (ie, the order of the nucleophile, the acid, and the base in the primary sequence) is the mirror image of the arrangement in other hydrolytic enzymes such as trypsin. All 3 active-site residues are located on loops that are the best conserved structural features in the fold, which likely provides catalysis with certain flexibility to hydrolyze numerous structurally distinct substrates.

Reduction

Certain metals (eg, pentavalent arsenic) and xenobiotics containing an aldehyde, ketone, alkene, disulfide, sulfoxide, quinone, *N*-oxide, hydroxamic acid, amidoxime, isoxazole, isothiazole, azo, or nitro group are often reduced in vivo, although it is sometimes difficult to ascertain whether the reaction proceeds enzymatically or nonenzymatically by interaction with reducing agents (such as the reduced forms of glutathione, FAD, FMN, and NAD[P]). Some of these functional groups can be either reduced or oxidized.

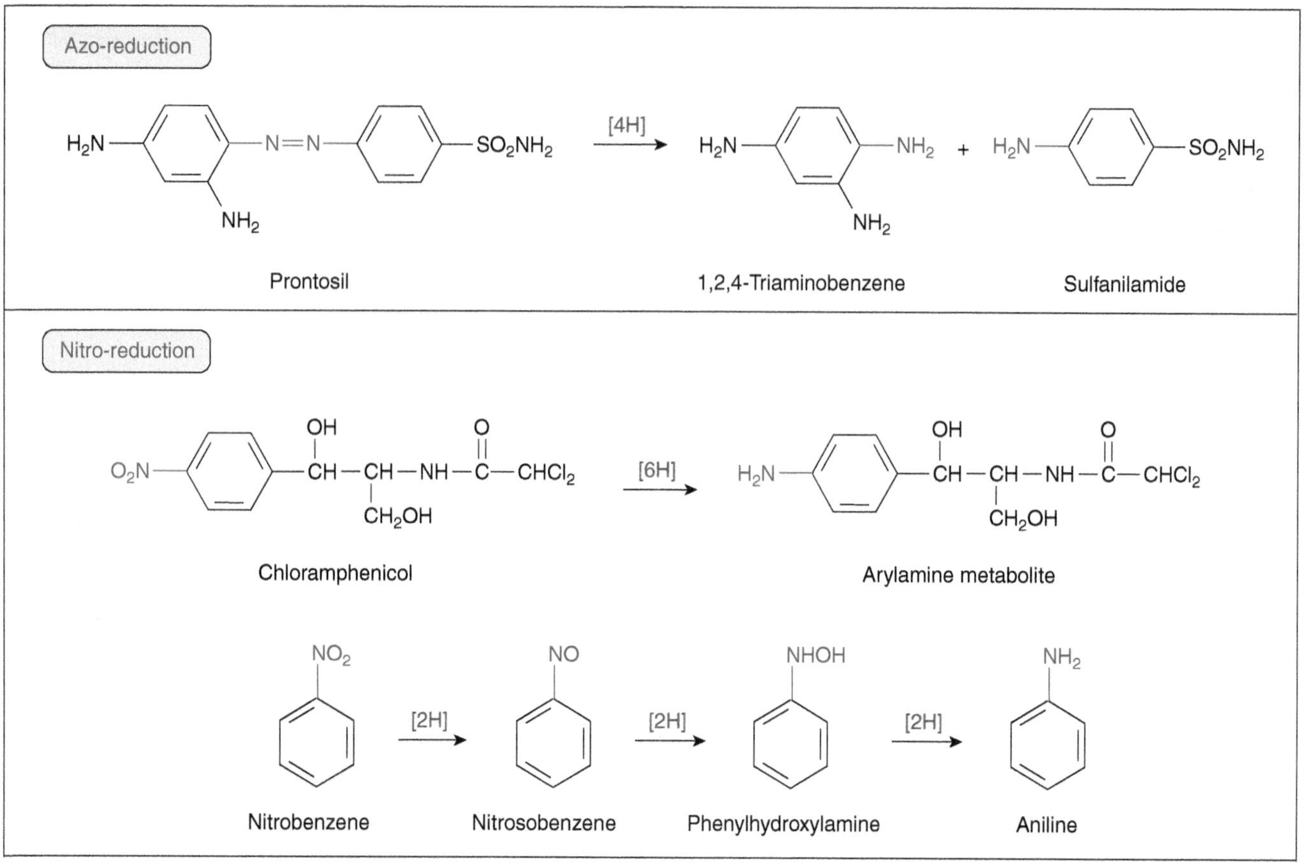

Figure 6-11. *Examples of drugs that undergo azo-reduction (prontosil) and nitro-reduction (chloramphenicol and nitrobenzene).*

For example, aldehydes (R-CHO) can be reduced to an alcohol (R-CH₂OH) or oxidized to a carboxylic acid (R-COOH), whereas sulfoxides (R₁-SO-R₂) can be reduced to a sulfide (R₁-S-R₂) or oxidized to a sulfone (R₁-SO₂-R₂). Likewise, some enzymes, such as alcohol dehydrogenase (ADH), aldehyde oxidase (AO), and CYP, can catalyze both reductive and oxidative reactions depending on the substrate or conditions (eg, aerobic vs anaerobic). In the case of halogenated hydrocarbons, such as halothane, dehalogenation can proceed by an oxidative or reductive pathway, both of which are catalyzed by the same enzyme (namely, CYP). In some cases, such as azo-reduction, nitro-reduction, and the reduction of certain alkenes, the reaction is largely catalyzed by intestinal microflora.

Azo- and Nitro-Reduction Prontosil and chloramphenicol are examples of drugs that undergo azo- and nitro-reduction, respectively, as shown in Fig. 6-11. Reduction of prontosil is of historical interest. Treatment of streptococcal and pneumococcal infections with prontosil marked the beginning of specific antibacterial chemotherapy. Subsequently, it was discovered that the active drug was not prontosil but its metabolite, sulfanilamide (*para*-aminobenzene sulfonamide), a product of azo-reduction. During azo-reduction, the nitrogen–nitrogen double bond is sequentially reduced and cleaved to produce two primary amines, a reaction requiring four reducing equivalents. Nitro-reduction requires six reducing equivalents, which are consumed in three sequential reactions, as shown in Fig. 6-11 for the conversion of nitrobenzene to aniline.

Azo- and nitro-reduction reactions are generally catalyzed by intestinal microflora. However, under certain conditions, such as low oxygen tension, the reactions can be catalyzed by liver microsomal CYP and NAD(P)H-quinone oxidoreductase (NQO1, a cytosolic flavoprotein that is also known as DT-diaphorase) and,

in the case of nitroaromatics, by cytosolic AO. The anaerobic environment of the lower gastrointestinal tract is well suited for azo- and nitro-reduction, which is why intestinal microflora contributes significantly to these reactions. The reduction of quinic acid to benzoic acid is another example of a reductive reaction catalyzed by gut microflora, as shown in Fig. 6-1.

Nitro-reduction by intestinal microflora is thought to play an important role in the toxicity of several nitroaromatic compounds including 2,6-dinitrotoluene, which is hepatotumorigenic to male rats. The role of nitro-reduction in the metabolic activation of 2,6-dinitrotoluene is shown in Fig. 6-12 (Long and Rickert, 1982; Mirsalis and Butterworth, 1982). The biotransformation of 2,6-dinitrotoluene begins in the liver, where it is oxidized by CYP and conjugated with glucuronic acid. This glucuronide is excreted in bile and undergoes biotransformation by intestinal microflora. One or both of the nitro groups are reduced to amines by nitroreductase, and the glucuronide is hydrolyzed by β-glucuronidase. The reduced/deconjugated metabolites are absorbed and transported to the liver, where the newly formed amine group is N-hydroxylated by CYP and conjugated with acetate or sulfonate. These conjugates form good leaving groups, which renders the nitrogen highly susceptible to nucleophilic attack from proteins and DNA; this ostensibly leads to mutations and the formation of liver tumors. Compared with females, male rates are more susceptible to hepatotumorigenicity of 2,6-dinitrotoluene due to their higher rate of bile secretion and therefore their higher rate of biliary excretion of 2,6-dinitrobenzylalcohol glucuronide. The complexity of the metabolic scheme shown in Fig. 6-12 underscores an important principle, namely, that the activation of some chemical tumorigens to DNA-reactive metabolites involves several different biotransforming enzymes and may take place in more than one

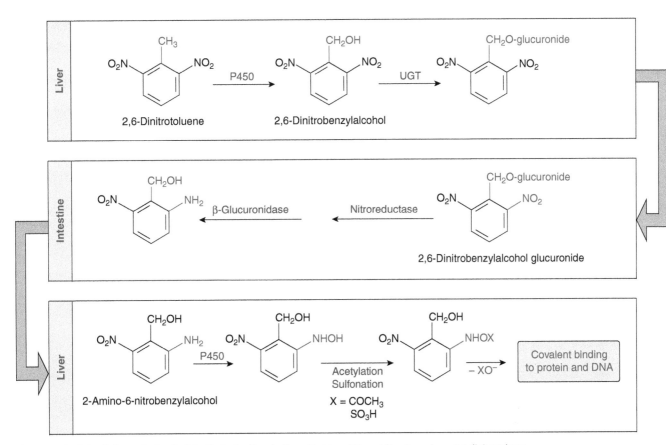

Figure 6-12. *Role of nitro-reduction by intestinal microflora in the activation of the rat liver tumorigen, 2,6-dinitrotoluene.*

tissue. Consequently, the ability of 2,6-dinitrotoluene to bind to DNA and cause mutations is not revealed in most of the short-term assays for assessing the genotoxic potential of chemical agents. These in vitro assays for genotoxicity do not make allowance for biotransformation by intestinal microflora or, in some cases, the conjugating enzymes.

Nitro-reduction by intestinal microflora also plays an important role in the biotransformation of musk xylene (1,3,5-trinitro-2-*t*butyl-4,6-dimethylbenzene). Reduction of one or both of the nitro groups is required for musk xylene to induce (as well as markedly inhibit) liver microsomal CYP (namely, CYP2B) in rodents (Lehman-McKeemanm *et al.*, 1999).

Carbonyl Reduction—AKRs and SDRs A variety of xenobiotics contain a carbonyl function (R-CHO and R_1-CO-R_2) that undergoes reduction in vivo. The reduction of aldehydes to primary alcohols and of ketones to secondary alcohols is generally catalyzed in mammals by NAD(P)H-dependent reductases belonging to one of several superfamilies, the aldo keto reductases (AKRs), the short-chain dehydrogenases/reductases (SDRs), the medium-chain dehydrogenases/reductases (MDRs), ALDHs, and NAD(P)H-quinone oxido reductases (NQO) as shown in Table 6-5 (Jez and Penning, 2001; Oppermann *et al.*, 2001; Matsunaga *et al.*, 2006; Malatkova *et al.*, 2010; Skarydova and Wsol, 2011). The AKRs are members of a superfamily of cytosolic enzymes that reduce both xenobiotic and endobiotic compounds, as their alternative names imply (Table 6-5). Dimeric dihydrodiol dehydrogenase and various members of the AKR superfamily, functioning as dihydrodiol dehydrogenases, can oxidize the *trans*-dihydrodiols of various polycyclic aromatic hydrocarbon oxiranes (formed by epoxide hydrolase) to the corresponding *ortho*-quinones, as shown previously in Fig. 6-10. The role of AKR as an oxidizing enzyme is

discussed in the section "Dimeric Dihydrodiol Dehydrogenase." As mentioned earlier (see Point 9 in the section "Introduction"), one of the AKRs, namely, AKR7A (also known as aflatoxin aldehyde reductase), is one of the many enzymes induced following activation of Nrf2 by oxidative stress, exposure to electrophiles, or depletion of GSH. Humans contain at least 71 SDR members, three of which, namely, cytosolic carbonyl reductases (CBR1 and CBR3) and a microsomal carbonyl reductase (HSD11B1), play a role in the reduction of a wide variety of carbonyl-containing xenobiotics (other species express more than two carbonyl reductases) (see http://www.sdr-enzymes.org). Erythrocytes also contain carbonyl reductase, which contributes significantly to the reduction of haloperidol, as shown in Fig. 6-13. From the alternative names given in Table 6-5, it is apparent that the both cytosolic and microsomal carbonyl reductases have been studied for their role in endobiotic metabolism, namely, the reduction of prostaglandin derivatives and 11β-hydroxysteroids, respectively (Kavanagh *et al.*, 2008).

In certain cases, the reduction of aldehydes to alcohols can be catalyzed by ADH, as shown in Fig. 6-13 for the conversion of the sedative–hypnotic, chloral hydrate, to trichloroethanol. As shown in Table 6-5, ADHs belong to the medium chain dehydrognases/reductases (MDRs). They typically convert alcohols to aldehydes, for which reason they are discussed later in the section "Alcohol Dehydrogenase." In the case of chloral hydrate, the reverse reaction is favored by the presence of the trichloromethyl group, which is a strong electron-withdrawing group.

The SDR carbonyl reductases are monomeric, NADPH-dependent enzymes present in erythrocytes and both the cytosolic and microsomal fractions of the liver, kidney, brain, and many other tissues. The major circulating metabolite of the antipsychotic drug, haloperidol, is a secondary alcohol formed by carbonyl reductases in the blood and liver, as shown in Fig. 6-13. Other xenobiotics

Table 6-5

Human Aldo-Keto Reductases (AKRs), Short-Chain Dehydrogenases/Reductases (SDRs), Medium-Chain Dehydrogenases/Reductases (MDRs), and Quinone Reductases (NQOs)

ENZYME SUPERFAMILY	EXAMPLE ENZYMES	ALTERNATIVE NAMES	SUBCELLULAR LOCALIZATION
Aldo-keto reductase (AKR), 15 enzymes	AKR1A1	Aldehyde reductase	Cytosol
	AKR1B1	Aldose reductase	Cytosol
	AKR1B10	Small intestine reductase (small intestine and liver)	Cytosol
	AKR1B15	Putative aldo-keto reductase family 1 member B15	Membrane-associated
	AKR1C1	20α-Hydroxysteroid dehydrogenase, dihydrodiol dehydrogenase (DD1)	Cytosol
	AKR1C2	3α-Hydroxysteroid dehydrogenase, dihydrodiol dehydrogenase (DD2), bile acid binding protein	Cytosol
	AKR1C3	3α-Hydroxysteroid dehydrogenase, 17β-hydroxysteroid dehydrogenase type V, dihydrodiol dehydrogenase (DD3)	Cytosol
	AKR1C4	3α-Hydroxysteroid dehydrogenase, chlordecone reductase, dihydrodiol dehydrogenase (DD4)	Cytosol
	AKR1D1	Δ^4-3-Ketosteroid-5β-reductase	Cytosol
	AKR1E2	AKRDC1; AKR1CL2; LoopADR	Unknown
	AKR6A3, 6A5, 6A9	Shaker-channel subunit Kvb1, Kvb2, Kvb3 (KCNAB1-3)	Cytosol
	AKR7A2	Aflatoxin B$_1$ aldehyde reductase 2	Golgi
	AKR7A3	Aflatoxin B$_1$ aldehyde reductase 3	Cytosol
Short-chain dehydrogenase/reductases (SDR), 73 enzymes	Cytosolic carbonyl reductases (gene symbols CBR1 and 3)	Xenobiotic ketone reductase with pH 6.0 activity; prostaglandin 9-ketoreductase; human placental NADP-linked 15-hydroprostaglandin dehydrogenase, SDR21C1 and C2	Cytosol
	Microsomal carbonyl reductase (gene symbol HSD11B1)	11β-Hydroxysteroid dehydrogenase; 11β-HSD1; 11β-reductase, 11-oxidoreductase, SDR26C1	Microsomes
Medium-chain dehydrogenase/reductases (MDR), 7 ADH enzymes	ADH1A	Class I ADH; ADH1, α, β, γ; hADH1, 2, 3	Cytosol
	ADH1B	Class I ADH; ADH2, β, γ; ADHII; hADH4	Cytosol
	ADH1C	Class I ADH; ADH3, γ	Cytosol
	ADH4	Class II ADH; π, hADH7	Cytosol
	ADH5	Class III ADH; χ, ADH3	Cytosol
	ADH6	Class V ADH	Cytosol
	ADH7	Class IV ADH; μ (σ)	Cytosol
NQO, 2 enzymes	NQO1	DT diaphorase, menadione reductase	Cytosol
	NQO2	N-Ribosyldihydronicotinamide dehydrogenase	Cytosol

NQO, NAD(P)H-quinone oxidoreductase. Members of the aldo-keto reductase superfamily can be found at http://www.med.upenn.edu/akr/members.shtml. Information on human SDR membranes can be found at http://www.sdr-enzymes.org/resources.htm.

that are reduced by carbonyl reductases include pentoxifylline (see Fig. 6-3), acetohexamide, daunorubicin, doxorubicin, loxoprofen, menadione, 4-nitroacetophenone, timiperone, and *R*-warfarin (Rosemond and Walsh, 2004). As shown in Fig. 6-3, the reduction of ketones to secondary alcohols by carbonyl reductases may proceed with a high degree of stereoselectivity, as in the case of pentoxifylline (Lillibridge *et al.*, 1996).

Liver cytosol contains at least two carbonyl reductases (CBR1 and CBR3) and microsomes contain at least one other form of carbonyl reductase (HSD11B1), and these can differ in the degree to which they stereoselectively reduce ketones to secondary alcohols. For example, keto-reduction of pentoxifylline produces two enantiomeric secondary alcohols: one with the *R*-configuration (which is known as lisofylline) and one with the *S*-configuration, as shown in Fig. 6-3. Reduction of pentoxifylline

by cytosolic carbonyl reductases results in the stereospecific formation of the optical antipode of lisofylline, whereas the same reaction catalyzed by microsomal carbonyl reductase produces both lisofylline and its optical antipode in a ratio of about 1 to 5 (Lillibridge *et al.*, 1996).

The well-known microsomal carbonyl reductase is 11β-hydroxysteroid dehydrogenase (gene symbol HSD11B1, aka SDR26C1) (Skarydova and Wsol, 2011). However, there are several other microsomal carbonyl-reducing enzymes, such as the six human retinol dehydrogenases (eg, RDHs) and the six human 17β-hydroxysteroid dehydrogenases. Although these enzymes have not been well characterized for their ability to reduce carbonyl-containing xenobiotics, there is indirect evidence from the ratio of enantiomers of metabolites that multiple microsomal enzymes may play a role in the metabolism of some

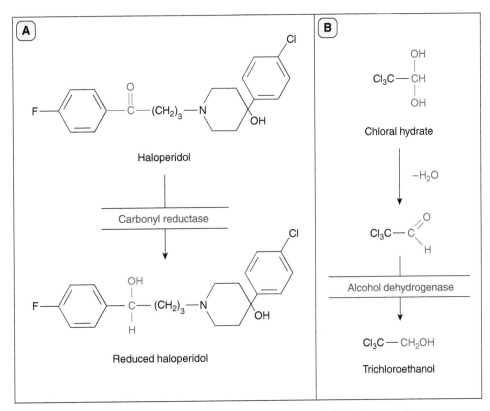

Figure 6-13. *Reduction of xenobiotics by carbonyl reductase (A) and alcohol dehydrogenase (B).*

xenobiotics such as 7α-methyl-19-nortestotsterone (Skarydova and Wsol, 2011). There are at least two monomeric cytosolic carbonyl reductases (gene symbols CBR1 [aka SDR21C1] and CBR3 [aka SDR21C2]) that have broad, and somewhat overlapping, substrate specificities toward many endobiotics and xenobiotics such as menadione, isatin, 4-(methylnitrosamino)-1-(3-pyridyl)-1-butanone (NNK), daunorubicin, and doxorubicin (Malatkova *et al.*, 2010). A human tetrameric mitochondrial carbonyl reductase, namely, CBR4 (aka SDR45C1), has also been identified with activity toward 9,10-phenanthrenequinone and 1,4-benzoquinone, and therefore acts as a mitochondrial quinone reductase (Malatkova *et al.*, 2010).

In rat liver cytosol, the reduction of quinones is primarily catalyzed by NQO1 and NQO2 (see the section "Quinone Reduction—NQO1 and NQO2"), whereas in human liver cytosol, quinone reduction is catalyzed by both NQO and carbonyl reductases.

Various members of the AKR superfamily have been implicated in the reduction of such carbonyl-containing xenobiotics as the tobacco-specific nitrosamine NNK, acetohexamide, daunorubicin, naloxone, naltrexone, befunolol, ethacrynic acid, ketoprofen, ketotifen, haloperidol, loxoprofen, metyrapone, oxo-nortryptyline, and numerous aromatic and aliphatic aldehydes (Rosemond and Walsh, 2004). Putative AKR1A, 1B, 1C1 to 4, or 1D1-selective inhibitors, statil, flufenamic acid, phenolphthalein, and finasteride, respectively, can aid in the evaluation of which reductive enzyme(s) is(are) involved in the formation of specific metabolites. Many of the xenobiotics reduced by AKRs are also reduced by SDRs, and in most cases the relative contribution of individual carbonyl-reducing enzymes is not known. Genetic polymorphisms of human AKR1C3, AKR1C4, AKR7A2, and cytosolic carbonyl reductase (CBR1) have been associated with decreased metabolism of carbonyl-containing xenobiotics such as doxorubicine and daunorubicine in vitro (Gonzalez-Covarrubias *et al.*, 2007; Bains *et al.*, 2010).

Allelic variants of human cytosolic AKR1C2 with reduced enzymatic activity toward the androgen 5α-dihydrotestosterone (DHT) have also been identified (Takahashi *et al.*, 2009). There appear to be no reports of clinically significant drug–drug interactions involving the inhibition or induction of AKRs or SDRs (Rosemond and Walsh, 2004).

Disulfide Reduction Some disulfides are reduced and cleaved to their sulfhydryl components, as shown in Fig. 6-14 for the alcohol deterrent, disulfiram (Antabuse). As shown in Fig. 6-14, disulfide reduction by glutathione is a 3-step process, the last of which is catalyzed by glutathione reductase. The first steps can be catalyzed by glutathione transferase, or they can occur nonenzymatically.

Sulfoxide and N-Oxide Reduction Thioredoxin-dependent enzymes in liver and kidney cytosol have been reported to reduce sulfoxides, which themselves may be formed by CYP or flavin monooxygenases (Anders *et al.*, 1981). Recycling through these counteracting enzyme systems, a process known as retro-reduction or futile cycling (Hinrichs *et al.*, 2011), may prolong the half-life of certain xenobiotics. As shown in Fig. 6-15 sulindac is a sulfoxide that undergoes reduction to a sulfide, which is excreted in bile and reabsorbed from the intestine (Ratnayake *et al.*, 1981). This enterohepatic cycling prolongs the duration of action of the drug such that this NSAID need only be taken twice daily. In human liver, glutaredoxin (GLRX) and thioredoxin may also be involved in reducing the mixed disulfide formed between xenobiotics and glutathione, as is the case in the formation of the pharmacologically active metabolite of the P2Y$_{12}$ inhibitor prasugrel (Hagihara *et al.*, 2011).

Sulfoxide reduction may also occur nonenzymatically at an appreciable rate, as in the case of the proton pump inhibitor rabeprazole (Miura *et al.*, 2006). Diethyldithiocarbamate methyl ester, a metabolite of disulfiram, is oxidized to a sulfine, which is reduced

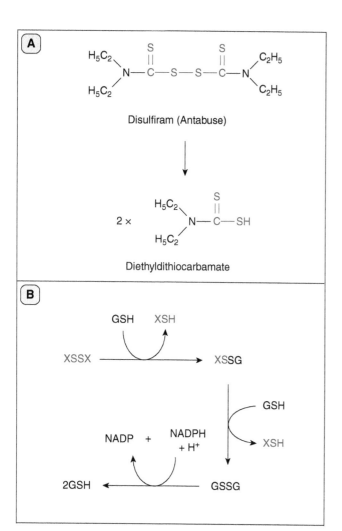

Figure 6-14. *Biotransformation of disulfiram by disulfide reduction* (**A**) *and the general mechanism of glutathione-dependent disulfide reduction of xenobiotics* (**B**). GSH, glutathione; XSSX, xenobiotic disulfide; GSSG, reduced glutathione. The last reaction in "B" is catalyzed by glutathione reductase.

to the parent methyl ester by glutathione. In the latter reaction, two molecules of gluathione are oxidized with reduction of the sulfine oxygen to water (Madan *et al.*, 1994) as shown below:

$$R_1R_2C=S^+\text{--}O^- + 2GSH \rightarrow R_1R_2C=S + GSSG + H_2O.$$

Just as sulfoxide reduction can reverse the effect of sulfoxidation, so the reduction of *N*-oxides can reverse the *N*-oxygenation of amines, which is catalyzed by flavin monooxygenases and CYP. Under reduced oxygen tension, reduction of the *N*-oxides of imipramine, tiaramide, indicine, and *N,N*-dimethylaniline can be catalyzed by mitochondrial and/or microsomal enzymes in the presence of NADH or NADPH (Sugiura and Kato, 1977). The NADPH-dependent reduction of *N*-oxides in liver microsomes appears to be catalyzed by CYP (Sugiura *et al.*, 1976), although in some cases NADPH-cytochrome P450 reductase may play an important role.

As a class, *N*-oxides are not inherently toxic compounds. However, certain aromatic and aliphatic *N*-oxides have been exploited as bioreductive drugs (also known as DNA-affinic drugs) for the treatment of certain cancers and infectious diseases (Wardman *et al.*, 1995). In these cases, *N*-oxides have been used as prodrugs that are converted to cytotoxic or DNA-binding drugs under hypoxic conditions. The fact that *N*-oxides of certain drugs

are converted to toxic metabolites under hypoxic conditions is the basis for their selective toxicity to certain solid tumors (namely, those that are hypoxic and, hence, resistant to radiotherapy) and anaerobic bacteria. For example, tirapazamine (SR 4233) is a benzotriazine di-*N*-oxide that is preferentially toxic to hypoxic cells, such as those present in solid tumors, apparently due to its rapid activation by one-electron reduction of the *N*-oxide to an oxidizing nitroxide radical, as shown in Fig. 6-15 (Walton *et al.*, 1992). This reaction is catalyzed by CYP and NADPH-cytochrome P450 reductase (Saunders *et al.*, 2000). Two-electron reduction of the di-*N*-oxide, SR 4233, produces a mono-*N*-oxide, SR 4317, which undergoes a second *N*-oxide reduction to SR 4330. Like SR 4233, the antibacterial agent, quindoxin, is a di-*N*-oxide whose cytotoxicity is dependent on reductive activation, which is favored by anaerobic conditions. AQ4N is a di-*N*-oxide prodrug that is converted by *N*-oxide reduction to the potent topoisomerase II inhibitor 4QA (1,4-bis{[2-(dimethylamino)ethyl]amino}-5,8-dihydroxy-anthracene-9,10-dione) (Nishida *et al.*, 2010). The reductive reaction is catalyzed by CYP2S1 and CYP2W1, two hypoxia-inducible CYP enzymes expressed in many solid tumors. The induction of CYP2S1 and CYP2W1 in hypoxic tumor cells provides a basis for their application in the selective bioreductive activation of antineoplastic drugs (Nishida *et al.*, 2010).

Bioreductive alkylating agents, which include such drugs as mitomycins, anthracyclins, and aziridinylbenzoquinones, represent another class of anticancer agents that require activation by reduction. However, for this class of agents, bioactivation also involves a two-electron reduction reaction, which is largely catalyzed by NQO, which is described in the next section.

Quinone Reduction—NQO1 and NQO2 Quinones can be reduced to hydroquinones by two closely related, cytosolic flavoproteins, namely, NQO1 and NQO2. The former enzyme, NAD(P)H-quinone oxidoreductase-1, is also known as DT-diaphorase. The latter enzyme, NAD(P)H-quinone oxidoreductase-2, is also known as NRH-quinone oxidoreductase because it prefers the unusual electron donor dihydronicotinamide riboside (NRH) over NAD(P)H. Although they are closely related enzymes (both contain two 27-kDa subunits each with an FAD prosthetic group), NQO1 and NQO2 have different substrate specificities, and they can be distinguished on the basis of their differential inhibition by dicoumarol and quercetin (which are selective inhibitors of NQO1 and NQO2, respectively). NQO2 may have a physiological role in the metabolism of vitamin K hydroquinone (Chen *et al.*, 2000).

An example of the type of reaction catalyzed by NQO is shown in Fig. 6-16. Formation of the hydroquinone involves a two-electron reduction of the quinone with stoichiometric oxidation of NAD[P]H *without* oxygen consumption. (The two-electron reduction of certain quinones can also be catalyzed by carbonyl reductase, especially in humans.) In contrast, NADPH-cytochrome P450 reductase, a microsomal flavoprotein, catalyzes the one-electron reduction of quinones to semiquinone radicals that, in addition to being reactive metabolites themselves, cause oxidative stress by reacting with oxygen to form reactive oxygen species, which leads to nonstoichiometric oxidation of NADPH and oxygen consumption, as shown in Fig. 6-16. The two-electron reduction of quinones is a nontoxic reaction—one that is not associated with semiquinone formation and oxidative stress—provided the resultant hydroquinone is sufficiently stable to undergo glucuronidation or sulfonation. However, there are quinone-containing xenobiotics that, despite undergoing two-electron reduction by NQO, produce semiquinone free radicals, oxidative stress, DNA damage, and cytotoxicity. Many of these xenobiotics are being developed as anticancer drugs because

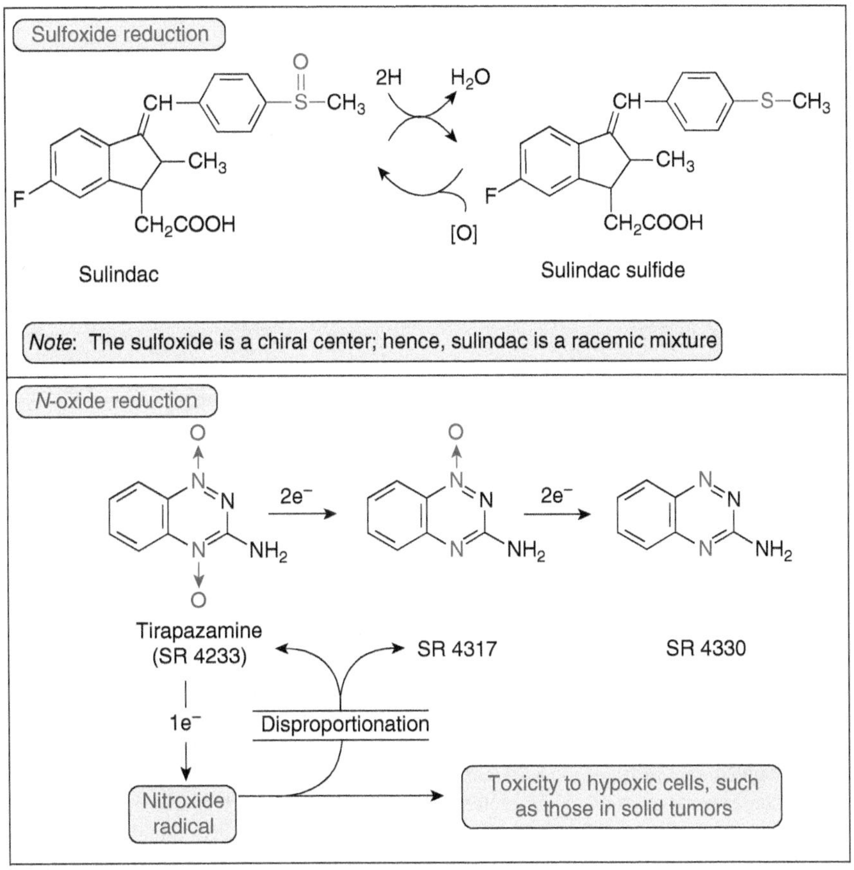

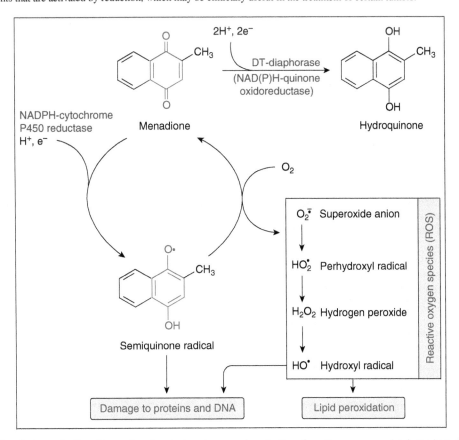

Figure 6-15. *Examples of sulfoxide and N-oxide reduction.* Note that tirapazamine (3-amino-1,2,4-benzotriazine-1,4-dioxide) is a representative of a class of agents that are activated by reduction, which may be clinically useful in the treatment of certain tumors.

Figure 6-16. *Two-electron reduction of menadione to a hydroquinone, and production of reactive oxygen species during its 1-electron reduction to a semiquinone radical.*

NQO1 is often overexpressed in tumor cells. The impact of the null allele NQO1*2 (discussed below in this section) on the sensitivity and resistance to antitumor quinones remains to be established (Siegel *et al.*, 2011). The properties of the hydroquinone determine whether, during the metabolism of quinone-containing xenobiotics, NQO functions as a protective antioxidant or a pro-oxidant activator leading to the formation of reactive oxygen species and reactive semiquinone free radicals. The latter are thought to form not from the one-electron reduction of the quinone but from the two-electron reduction of the quinone (Q) to the hydroquinone (QH_2), which then undergoes one-electron oxidation or perhaps disproportionation to form the reactive semiquinone (QH):

$$QH_2 + Q \leftrightarrow 2QH.$$

Drugs or drug candidates that are activated by NQO to anticancer agents include the aziridinylbenzoquinone diaziquone, the anthraquinone mitoxantrone, the indolquinones mitomycin C and EO9 (an analog of mitomycin C that is more rapidly reduced by NQO1), and the anthracycline antibiotics daunorubicin and doxorubicin (Gutierrez, 2000). These so-called bioreductive alkylating agents are reduced by NQO1 to generate semiquinone free radicals and other reactive intermediates that undergo nucleophilic additions with DNA, resulting in single-strand DNA breaks. The reason such drugs are preferentially toxic to tumor cells is that tumor cells, especially those in solid tumors, are hypoxic, and hypoxia induces the synthesis of NQO1 (by a mechanism that involves the activator protein 1 [AP-1] and NF-κB response elements in the 5′-promoter region of the NQO1 gene). Therefore, tumor cells often express high levels of NQO1, which predisposes them to the toxic effects of quinone-reductive anticancer drugs such as mitomycin C. Interestingly, mitomycin C also upregulates the expression of NQO1, which may enable this anticancer drug to stimulate its own metabolic activation in tumor cells (Yao *et al.*, 1997). Some cancer chemotherapeutic agents, such as the *N*-oxide SR 4233 (tirapazamine), are inactivated, not activated, by NQO, as shown in Fig. 6-15.

NQO can activate certain nitroaromatic compounds ($R-NO_2$) to the corresponding hydroxylamine (R-NHOH), which can be activated by acetylation or sulfonation (by pathways analogous to those shown in Fig. 6-12). Dinitropyrenes and the nitroaromatic compound CB 1954 are activated by NQO. The latter compound was under consideration as an anticancer agent. However, although it is activated by reduction by rat NQO, the nitroaromatic compound CB 1954 is not activated by human NQO.

Oxidative stress is an important component to the mechanism of toxicity of several xenobiotics that either contain a quinone or can be biotransformed to a quinone (Anders, 1985). The production of superoxide anion radicals and oxidative stress are responsible, at least in part, for the cardiotoxic effects of doxorubicin (adriamycin) and daunorubicin (daunomycin), the pulmonary toxicity of paraquat and nitrofurantoin, and the neurotoxic effects of 6-hydroxydopamine. Oxidative stress also plays an important role in the destruction of pancreatic β cells by alloxan and dialuric acid. Tissues, low in superoxide dismutase activity, such as the heart, are especially susceptible to the oxidative stress associated with the redox cycling of quinones. This accounts, at least in part, for the cardiotoxic effects of adriamycin and related anticancer agents, although other susceptibility factors have been proposed (Mordente *et al.*, 2001).

As already mentioned in this section, it is now apparent that the structure of the hydroquinones produced by NQO determines whether the two-electron reduction of quinones results in xenobiotic detoxication or activation. Hydroquinones formed by two-electron reduction of unsubstituted or methyl-substituted 1,4-naphthoquinones (such as menadione) or the corresponding quinone epoxides are relatively stable to autoxidation, whereas the methoxyl, glutathionyl, and hydroxyl derivatives of these compounds undergo autoxidation with production of semiquinones and reactive oxygen species. The ability of glutathionyl derivatives to undergo redox cycling indicates that conjugation with glutathione does not prevent quinones from serving as substrates for NQO. The glutathione conjugates of quinones can also be reduced to hydroquinones by carbonyl reductases, which actually have a binding site for glutathione. In human carbonyl reductase, this binding site is Cys_{227}, which is involved in binding both substrate and glutathione (Tinguely and Wermuth, 1999). Although oxidative stress is an important mechanism by which quinones cause cellular damage (through the intermediacy of semiquinone radicals and the generation of reactive oxygen species), it should be noted that quinones are Michael acceptors, and cellular damage can occur through direct alkylation of critical cellular proteins and/or DNA (Bolton *et al.*, 2000).

NQO1 is inducible up to 10-fold by two classes of inducers, which have been categorized as *bifunctional* and *monofunctional* inducers (Prochaska and Talalay, 1988). The bifunctional inducers include compounds such as β-naphthoflavone, benzo[*a*]pyrene, 3-methylcholanthrene, and 2,3,7,8-tetrachlorodibenzo-*p*-dioxin (TCDD or dioxin), which are AhR agonists that induce both oxidative enzymes (such as the CYP enzyme CYP1A1) and conjugating enzymes (such as GST and UGT). The monofunctional inducers are Nrf2 activators that tend to induce conjugating and other non-CYP enzymes (although in mice, monofunctional inducers can induce CYP2C55 and 2U1, as well as AO). The AhR agonists (the so-called bifunctional inducers) signal through the xenobiotic-response element (XRE), whereas Nrf2 activators (the so-called monofunctional inducers) signal through the antioxidant response element (ARE), which is also known as the electrophilic response element (EpRE). (Response elements are short sequences of DNA, often located in the 5′-promoter region of a gene, that bind the transcription factors that control gene expression.) The monofunctional inducers can be subdivided into two chemical classes: those that activate Nrf2 by causing oxidative stress through redox cycling (eg, the quinone, menadione, and the phenolic antioxidants *tert*-butylhydroquinone and 3,5-di-*tert*-butylcatechol) and those that activate Nrf2 by causing oxidative stress by depleting glutathione (eg, fumarates, maleates, acrylates, isothiocyanates, and other Michael acceptors that react with glutathione).

NQO1 is under the control of both AhR and Nrf2. The flavonoid β-naphthoflavone and the PAH B[*a*]P induce NQO1 (and other enzymes) by both mechanisms; the parent compound activates AhR, whereas electrophilic and/or redox active metabolites activate Nrf2. The situation with B[*a*]P is quite intriguing. This PAH binds directly to AhR, which binds to XRE and induces the synthesis of CYP1A1 and CYP1B1, which in turn convert B[*a*]P to electrophilic metabolites (such as arene oxides and diol epoxides) and redox active metabolites (such as catechols), as shown in Fig. 6-10. These electrophilic and redox active metabolites activate Nrf2 and induce various enzymes that protect against oxidative stress. However, the catechol metabolites of B[*a*]P are further converted by AKRs and/or dimeric dihydrodiol dehydrogenase to *ortho*-quinones (Fig. 6-10), and are thereby converted back into planar, hydrophobic compounds that are highly effective ligands for the AhR (Burczynski and Penning, 2000). This may be toxicologically important, because the AhR may translocate *ortho*-quinone metabolites of B[*a*]P into the nucleus, where they might damage DNA (Bolton *et al.*, 2000).

Sulforaphane and various isothiocyanates are Nrf2 activators that are present in broccoli and are thought to be responsible for the anticarcinogenic effects of this cruciferous vegetable (Zhang *et al.*, 1992). These Nrf2 activators induce GST (GSTA1), mEH, AKR (AKR7A, also known as aflatoxin aldehyde reductase), NQO1 (also known as DT-diaphorase), glutamate cysteine ligase, as well as genes involved in apoptosis. One isothiocyanate in particular, phenethyl isothiocyanate, has been found to activate Nrf2 and activate numerous genes in addition to those encoding xenobiotic-biotransforming enzymes and oxidant defense systems. Microarray studies carried out in wild-type and Nrf2 knockout mice treated with phenethyl isothiocyanate showed that the most highly inducible genes include the very low-density lipoprotein (VLDL) receptor, G-protein signaling modulator 2, early growth response 1, pancreatic lipase-related protein 2, histocompatibility 2 (K region), general transcription factor IIB, myoglobin, potassium voltage-gated channel Q2, and SLC39A10 (Hu *et al.*, 2006). As with other xenosensors, activation of Nrf2 results in a pleiotypic response in which a large number of genes are activated (or repressed). As mentioned above (this section), hypoxia and the anticancer agent mitomycin C are also inducers of NQO1, which has implications for cancer chemotherapy.

NQO1 and NQO2 are polymorphically expressed enzymes, and several lines of evidence suggest that NQO1 and/or NQO2 plays a key role in protecting bone marrow from the hematotoxic effects of benzene or other environmental factors (Iskander and Jaiswal, 2005). In humans, a high percentage of individuals with myeloid and other types of leukemia are homozygous or heterozygous for a null mutant allele of NQO1. This polymorphism, NQO1*2, is a SNP ($C_{609}T$) that changes Pro_{187} to Ser_{187}, which destabilizes the protein and targets it for rapid degradation by the ubiquitin proteasomal pathway; this polymorphism is also associated with increased risk of colorectal and esophageal cancers (Ross, 2005; Chen *et al.*, 2012). Mice lacking NQO1 or NQO2 (knockout or null mice) have no developmental abnormalities but have increased granulocytes in the blood and myelogenous hyperplasia of the bone marrow (due to decreased apoptosis). Mice lacking NQO1 are substantially more susceptible than wild-type mice to benzene-induced hematotoxicity (Iskander and Jaiswal, 2005; Ross, 2005). The hematotoxicity of benzene is thought to involve its conversion to hydroquinone in the liver and its subsequent oxidation to benzoquinone by myeloperoxidase in the bone marrow (discussed later in the section "Peroxidase-Dependent Cooxidation"). NQO would be expected to play a role in detoxifying benzoquinone, as predicted, loss of NQO potentiates benzene hematotoxicity. However, loss of NQO also impairs apoptosis, which also represents a plausible explanation for the association between loss of NQO and increased susceptibility to benzene hematotoxicity. The latter mechanism (ie, impaired apoptosis) likely accounts for the observation that NQO1 and NQO2 null mice are more susceptible than wild-type mice to skin carcinogenesis by B[*a*]P and DMBA, an effect attributable to the diol epoxides, not the quinone metabolites, of these PAHs (Iskander and Jaiswal, 2005).

Dihydropyrimidine Dehydrogenase In 1993, 15 Japanese patients died as a result of an interaction between two oral medications: sorivudine (a new antiviral drug for herpes zoster) and tegafur (a prodrug that is converted in the liver to the anticancer agent, 5-fluorouracil). The deaths occurred within 40 days of the Japanese

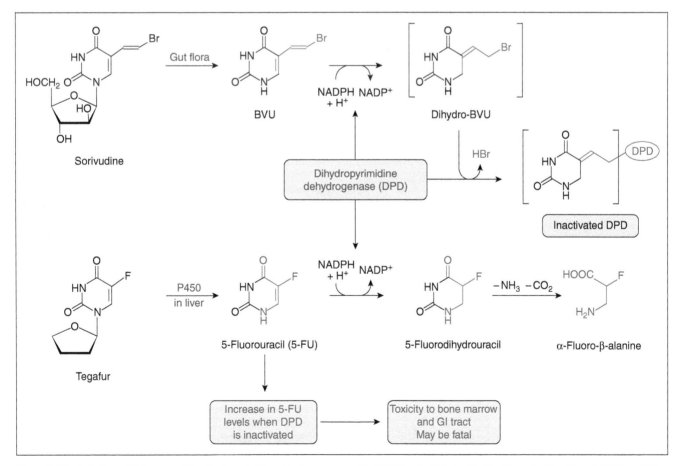

Figure 6-17. *Reduction of 5-fluorouracil by dihydropyrimidine dehydrogenase and its inhibition (suicide inactivation) by sorivudine. Note*: Inhibition of dihydropyrimidine dehydrogenase is the mechanism of fatal interactions between sorivudine and the 5-fluorouracil prodrug, tegafur.

government's approval of sorivudine for clinical use. The mechanism of the lethal interaction between sorivudine and tegafur is illustrated in Fig. 6-17, and involves inhibition of dihydropyrimidine dehydrogenase (DPD), an NADPH-requiring, homodimeric protein (Mr ~210 kDa) containing FMN/FAD and an iron–sulfur cluster in each subunit. The enzyme is located mainly in liver cytosol, where it catalyzes the reduction of 5-fluorouracil and related pyrimidines. Sorivudine is converted in part by gut flora to (E)-5-(2-bromovinyl) uracil (BVU), which lacks antiviral activity but which is converted by DPD to a metabolite that binds covalently to the enzyme. The irreversible inactivation (aka suicidal inactivation) of DPD by sorivudine causes a marked inhibition of 5-fluorouracil metabolism, which increases blood levels of 5-fluorouracil to toxic and, in some cases, lethal levels (Ogura et al., 1998; Kanamitsu et al., 2000).

Several genetic polymorphisms that result in a partial or complete loss of DPD activity, affecting ~8% of the population, have been described (van Kuilenburg et al., 2004; Robert et al., 2005). Severe 5-fluorouracil toxicity has also been documented in individuals who are heterozygous for loss-of-function allelic variants of DPD, and 5-fluorouracil lethality has been documented in rare individuals who are completely deficient in DPD (1 individual in about 10,000). 5-Fluorouracil is one of the most frequently prescribed anticancer drugs, for which reason assessing an individual's DPD genotype (by analyzing DNA for allelic variants) or phenotyping (by measuring DPD activity in peripheral blood mononuclear cells) is advocated prior to 5-fluorouracil or capecitabine (a 5-flurouracil prodrug) therapy so that the dosage of these anticancer drugs can be adjusted on an individual basis.

Dehalogenation There are three major mechanisms for removing halogens (F, Cl, Br, and I) from aliphatic xenobiotics (Anders, 1985). The first, known as *reductive dehalogenation*, involves replacement of a halogen with hydrogen, as shown below:

$$X-\underset{\underset{X}{|}}{\overset{\overset{X}{|}}{C}}-\underset{\underset{H}{|}}{\overset{\overset{X}{|}}{C}}-X \quad \xrightarrow[-HX]{+2H} \quad X-\underset{\underset{X}{|}}{\overset{\overset{X}{|}}{C}}-\underset{\underset{H}{|}}{\overset{\overset{X}{|}}{C}}-H$$

Pentahaloethane   Tetrahaloethane

In the second mechanism, known as *oxidative dehalogenation*, a halogen and hydrogen on the same carbon atom are replaced with oxygen. Depending on the structure of the haloalkane, oxidative dehalogenation leads to the formation of an acylhalide or aldehyde, as shown below:

$$X-\underset{\underset{X}{|}}{\overset{\overset{X}{|}}{C}}-\underset{\underset{H}{|}}{\overset{\overset{X}{|}}{C}}-X \quad \xrightarrow[-HX]{+[O]} \quad X-\underset{\underset{X}{|}}{\overset{\overset{X}{|}}{C}}-\overset{\overset{X}{|}}{C}=O$$

Pentahaloethane   Tetrahaloacetylhalide

$$X-\underset{\underset{X}{|}}{\overset{\overset{X}{|}}{C}}-\underset{\underset{H}{|}}{\overset{\overset{X}{|}}{C}}-H \quad \xrightarrow[-HX]{+[O]} \quad X-\underset{\underset{X}{|}}{\overset{\overset{H}{|}}{C}}-\overset{\overset{H}{|}}{C}=O$$

Tetrahaloethane   Trihaloacetaldehyde

A third mechanism of dehalogenation involves the elimination of two halogens on adjacent carbon atoms to form a carbon-carbon double bond, as shown below:

$$X-\underset{\underset{X}{|}}{\overset{\overset{X}{|}}{C}}-\underset{\underset{H}{|}}{\overset{\overset{X}{|}}{C}}-X \quad \xrightarrow[-2HX]{+2H} \quad \underset{X}{\overset{X}{}}C=C\underset{H}{\overset{X}{}}$$

Pentahaloethane   Trihaloethylene

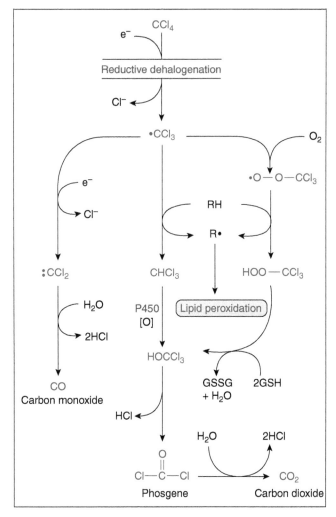

Figure 6-18. *Reductive dehalogenation of carbon tetrachloride to a trichloromethyl free radical that initiates lipid peroxidation.* RH, unsaturated lipid; R•, lipid dienyl radical; GSH, reduced glutathione; GSSG, oxidized glutathione.

A variation on this third mechanism is *dehydrohalogenation*, in which a halogen and hydrogen on adjacent carbon atoms are eliminated to form a carbon–carbon double bond.

Both reductive and oxidative dehalogenations are catalyzed by CYP. (The ability of CYP to catalyze both reductive and oxidative reactions is explained later in the section "Cytochrome P450.") Dehalogenation reactions leading to double bond formation are catalyzed by CYP and GST. These reactions play an important role in the biotransformation and metabolic activation of several halogenated alkanes, as the following examples illustrate.

The hepatotoxicity of carbon tetrachloride (CCl_4) and several related halogenated alkanes is dependent on their biotransformation by reductive dehalogenation (Plaa, 2000). The first step in reductive dehalogenation is a one-electron reduction catalyzed by CYP, which produces a potentially toxic, carbon-centered radical and inorganic halide. In the case of CCl_4, reductive dechlorination produces a trichloromethyl radical (•CCl_3), which initiates lipid peroxidation and produces a variety of other metabolites, as shown in Fig. 6-18.

Halothane can also be converted by reductive dehalogenation to a carbon-centered radical, as shown in Fig. 6-19. The mechanism is identical to that described for carbon tetrachloride, although in the case of halothane the radical is generated through loss of

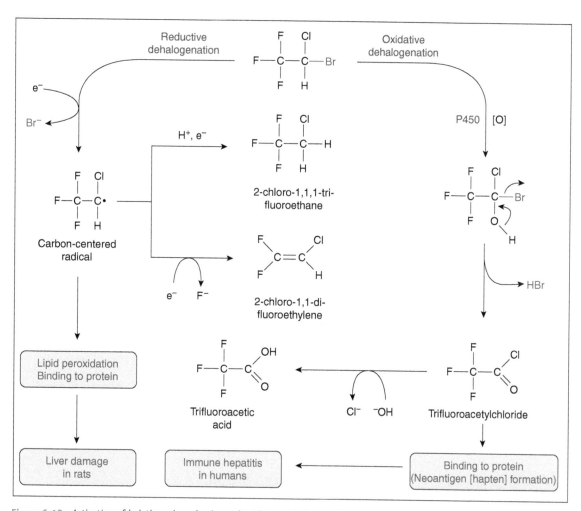

Figure 6-19. *Activation of halothane by reductive and oxidative dehalogenation and their role in liver toxicity in rats and humans.*

bromine, which is a better leaving group than chlorine. Fig. 6-19 also shows that halothane can undergo oxidative dehalogenation, which involves oxygen insertion at the C–H bond to generate an unstable halohydrin ($CF_3COHClBr$) that decomposes to a reactive acylhalide (CF_3COCl), which can bind to cellular proteins (particularly to amine groups) or further decompose to trifluoroacetic acid (CF_3COOH).

Both the oxidative and reductive pathways of halothane metabolism generate reactive intermediates capable of binding to proteins and other cellular macromolecules. The relative importance of these two pathways to halothane-induced hepatotoxicity is species dependent. In rats, halothane-induced hepatotoxicity is promoted by those conditions favoring the reductive dehalogenation of halothane, such as moderate hypoxia (10%–14% oxygen) plus treatment with the CYP inducers, phenobarbital, and pregnenolone-16α-carbonitrile (PCN). In contrast to the situation in rats, halothane-induced hepatotoxicity in guinea pigs is largely the result of oxidative dehalogenation of halothane (Lunam *et al.*, 1989). In guinea pigs, halothane hepatotoxicity is not enhanced by moderate hypoxia and is diminished by the use of deuterated halothane, which impedes the oxidative dehalogenation of halothane because the CYP-dependent insertion of oxygen into a carbon–deuterium bond is energetically less favorable (and therefore slower) than inserting oxygen into a carbon–hydrogen bond.

Halothane hepatitis in humans is a rare but severe form of liver necrosis associated with repeated exposure to this volatile anesthetic. In humans, as in guinea pigs, halothane hepatotoxicity

results from the oxidative dehalogenation of halothane, as shown in Fig. 6-19. Serum samples from patients suffering from halothane hepatitis contain antibodies directed against neoantigens formed by the trifluoroacetylation of proteins. These antibodies have been used to identify which specific proteins in the endoplasmic reticulum are targets for trifluoroacetylation during the oxidative dehalogenation of halothane (Pohl *et al.*, 1989).

The concept that halothane is activated by CYP to trifluoroacetylhalide, which binds covalently to proteins and elicits an immune response, has been extended to other volatile anesthetics, such as enflurane, methoxyflurane, and isoflurane. In other words, these halogenated aliphatic hydrocarbons, like halothane, may be converted to acylhalides that form immunogens by binding covalently to proteins. In addition to accounting for rare instances of enflurane hepatitis, this mechanism of hepatotoxicity can also account for reports of a *cross-sensitization* between enflurane and halothane, in which enflurane causes liver damage in patients previously exposed to halothane.

One of the metabolites generated from the reductive dehalogenation of halothane is 2-chloro-1,1-difluoroethylene (Fig. 6-19). The formation of this metabolite involves the loss of two halogens from adjacent carbon atoms with formation of a carbon–carbon double bond. This type of dehalogenation reaction can also be catalyzed by GSTs. GSH initiates the reaction with a nucleophilic attack either on the electrophilic carbon to which the halogen is attached (mechanism A) or on the halogen itself (mechanism B), as shown in Fig. 6-20 for the dehalogenation of 1,2-dihaloethane to ethylene.

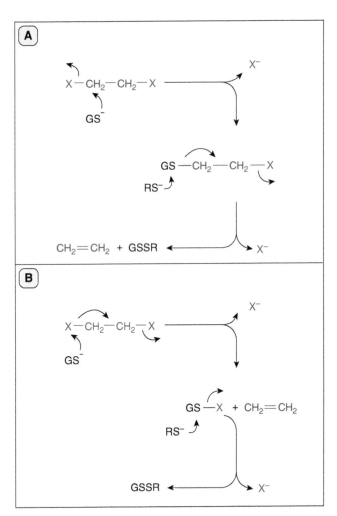

Figure 6-20. *Glutathione-dependent dehalogenation of 1,2-dihaloethane to ethylene.* (**A**) Nucleophilic attack on carbon and (**B**) nucleophilic attack on halide.

The insecticide DDT is detoxified by dehydrochlorination to DDE by a lyase (ie, DDT-dehydrochlorinase), as shown in Fig. 6-21. The activity of this GSH-dependent reaction correlates well with resistance to DDT in houseflies.

Dehydroxylation—mARC, Cytochrome b_5, b_5 Reductase, and Aldehyde Oxidase Mitochondrial amidoxime reducing component (mARC) is a molybdenum-containing enzyme that, in the presence of NADH, cytochrome b_5, and NADH-cytochrome b_5 reductase, can catalyze the N-dehydroxylation of various amidoximes and related N-hydroxy compounds, as shown in Fig. 6-22 (Havemeyer *et al.*, 2010). Reactions catalyzed by mARC/cytochrome b_5/NADH-cytochrome b_5 reductase include the N-dehydroxylation of amidoximes formed during the activation of the antiparasitic prodrug pafuramidine (DB-289), the N-dehydroxylation of N-hydroxysulfonamides, and the N-dehydroxylation of N-hydroxy-valdecoxib

to its active principal, a cyclooxygenase-2 (COX-2) inhibitor (Saulter *et al.*, 2005; Havemeyer *et al.*, 2010). The mARC complex can also N-dehydroxylate the aryl hydroxylamine metabolites of carcinogenic arylamines such as 4-aminobiphenyl and 2-amino-1-methyl-6-phenyl-imidazol[4,5-*b*]pyridine (PhIP), N-hydroxy metabolites that are formed by CYP1A1, 1A2, 1B1, lactoperoxidase, and myeloperoxidase (see the sections "Cytochrome P450" and "Peroxidase-Dependent Cooxidation") (Kurian *et al.*, 2006). Because these carcinogenic aryl hydroxylamines can be further activated by glucuronidation, sulfonation, or acetylation in various tissues (see the sections "Glucuronidation and Formation of Acyl-CoA Thioesters," "Sulfonation," and "Acetylation"), reduction by mARC/cytochrome b_5/NADH-cytochrome b_5 reductase represents a competing detoxication pathway. Gut microflora can also catalyze dehydroxylation reactions as shown in Fig. 6-1 for quinic acid. Gut microflora can also reduce N- and S-oxides formed by FAD-containing monooxygenase (FMO) and/or CYP, as described for trimethylamine (TMA) N-oxide in the section "Flavin Monooxygenases."

Aldehyde Oxidase—Reductive Reactions Aldeyde oxidase (AO) is a cytosolic molybdoenzyme that catalyzes the oxidation of some xenobiotics and the reduction of others. The types of oxidative and reductive reactions catalyzed by AO are shown in Fig. 6-23. In contrast to the large number of drugs that are known to be (or suspected of being) oxidized by AO in vivo, only a few drugs are known to be (or suspected of being) reduced by AO in vivo, including nitrofurazone, zonisamide, and ziprasidone. The reductive metabolism of ziprasidone by AO is shown in Fig. 6-4. The features of AO and the oxidative reactions it catalyzes are discussed later in the section "Aldehyde Oxidase."

Oxidation

Alcohol, Aldehyde, Ketone Oxidation–Reduction Systems Alcohols, aldehydes, and ketones are oxidized by a number of enzymes, including alcohol dehydrogenase, aldehyde dehydrogenase, AKRs (such as those with dihydrodiol dehydrogenase activity), the molybdenum-containing enzymes (namely, AO and xanthine dehydrogenase [XD]/xanthine oxidase [XO]), and CYP. For example, simple alcohols (such as methanol and ethanol) are oxidized to aldehydes (namely, formaldehyde and acetaldehyde) by ADH. These aldehydes are further oxidized to carboxylic acids (formic acid and acetic acid) by ALDH, as shown in Fig. 6-24. Many of the aforementioned enzymes can also catalyze the reduction of xenobiotics, as discussed in the section "Reduction."

Alcohol Dehydrogenase ADHs belong to the MDRs, as shown in Table 6-5. ADHs are zinc-containing, cytosolic enzymes present in several tissues including liver (which has the highest levels), kidney, lung, and gastric mucosa (Agarwal, 1992; Ramchandani, 2004). These enzymes oxidize several types of alcohols including hydroxysteroids, retinol, ethanol, lipid peroxidation products, and other simple and complex (eg, ring-containing) alcohols. Human ADHs are dimeric proteins consisting of two ~40-kDa subunits designated α, β, γ, π, χ, σ (also previously known as μ), or ADH6

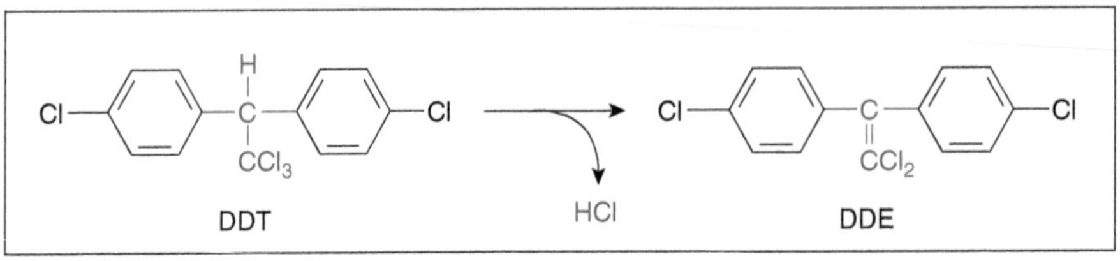

Figure 6-21. *Dehydrochlorination of the pesticide DDT to DDE, a glutathione-dependent reaction.*

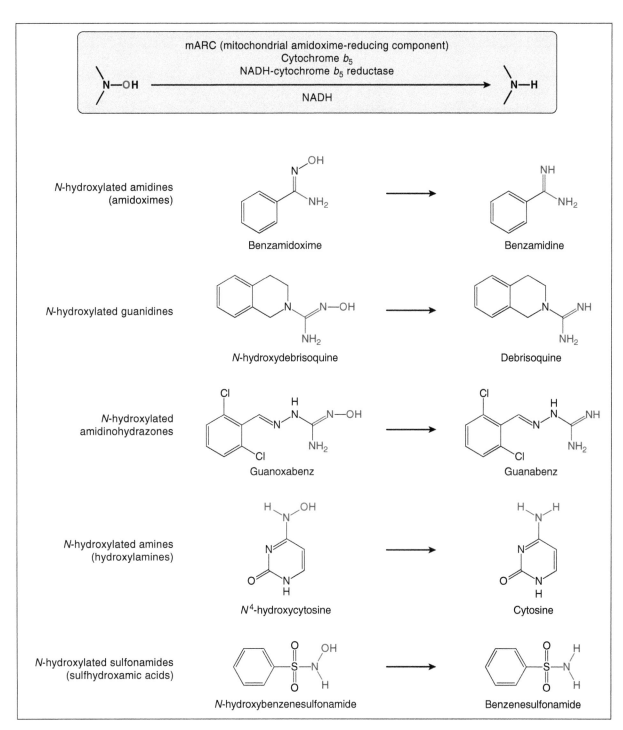

Figure 6-22. *Dehydroxylation reactions catalyzed by the molybdoenzyme mitochondrial amidoxime-reducing component (mARC), cytochrome b₅, and NADH-cytochrome b₅ reductase.* *Note*: Aldehyde oxidase can also catalyze dehydroxylation reactions as shown in Fig. 6-23.

(the latter having no subunit designation). As shown in Table 6-5, there are 7 human ADHs, and these are categorized into 5 classes (I-V) based on patterns of tissue-specific expression, catalytic properties, and amino acid sequence. Class I comprises 3 hepatically expressed genes: ADH1A, ADH1B, and ADH1C, which were formerly known as ADH1, -2, and -3, respectively. The class I isozymes consist of homodimeric and heterodimeric forms of the 3 subunits (eg, αα, αβ, ββ, βγ, γγ, etc). Class II contains ADH4, which is composed of 2 pi subunits (ππ). Class III contains ADH5, which is composed of 2 chi subunits (χχ). Class IV contains ADH7, which is composed of 2 sigma subunits (σσ). Class V contains ADH6 (for which there is no subunit designation) (Brennan

et al., 2004; Ramchandani, 2004). Therefore, there are over 20 human ADH isozymes and these differ in their substrate specificity and catalytic efficiency toward ethanol (Ramchandani, 2004). The human ADH genes have similar sequences (ie, 60%–70% identical coding regions), and all have 9 exons and 8 introns with the exception of ADH6, which lacks the last exon (Han et al., 2005). In addition, several hundred genetic variants have been described across the human ADH cluster which lies on chromosome 4q (Li et al., 2008). Alcohols can be oxidized to aldehydes by non-ADH enzymes in microsomes and peroxisomes, although these are quantitatively less important than ADH for ethanol oxidation (Lieber, 2004). The microsomal ethanol oxidizing system (formerly known

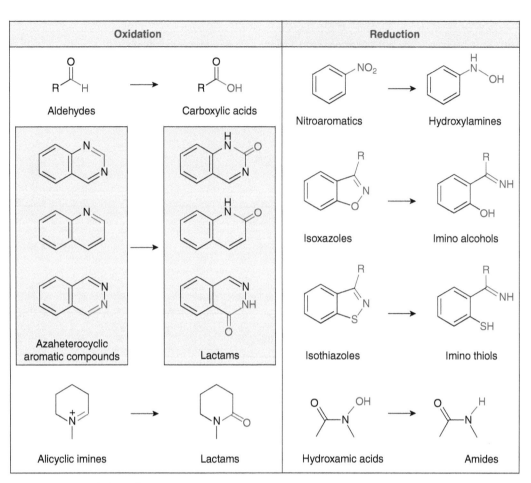

Figure 6-23. *Examples of oxidation and reduction catalyzed by aldehyde oxidase.*

as MEOS) is the CYP enzyme, CYP2E1. The corresponding peroxisomal enzyme is catalase. The oxidation of ethanol to acetaldehyde by these 3 enzyme systems is shown in Fig. 6-25.

Class I (ADH1A, 1B, 1C) The class I ADH isozymes (ADH1A or α-ADH, ADH1B or β-ADH, and ADH1C or γ-ADH) are responsible for the oxidation of ethanol and other small, aliphatic alcohols, and they are strongly inhibited by pyrazole and its 4-alkyl derivatives (eg, 4-methylpyrazole). High levels of class I ADH isozymes are expressed in liver and adrenals, with lower levels in kidney, lung, blood vessels (in the case of ADH1B), gastric mucosa (in the case of ADH1C), and other tissues, but not brain. It is noteworthy that the liver expresses a very large amount of ADHs (approximately 3% of all soluble protein) and also expresses the widest variety of isozymes (Ramchandani, 2004).

The class I ADH isozymes differ in their capacity to oxidize ethanol. Polymorphisms have been well described for the class I ADH isozymes. Even the allelozymes, which differ in a single amino acid, differ markedly in their affinity (K_m) and/or capacity

(V_{max}) for oxidizing ethanol to acetaldehyde. There are at least 3 allelic variants of ADH1B (ie, *1, *2, and *3), with a single amino acid change at position 48. The homodimer, $\beta_2\beta_2$, and heterodimers containing at least 1 β_2 subunit (ie, the ADH1B*2 allelozymes) are especially active in oxidizing ethanol at physiological pH. ADH1B*2 (formerly known as ADH2*2) is known as *atypical* ADH, and is responsible for the unusually rapid conversion of ethanol to acetaldehyde in up to 90% of the Pacific Rim Asian population (eg, Japanese, Chinese, Korean), whereas only ~10% of Caucasians express this allele. The ADH1B*3 is relatively common in individuals of African descent. The latter 2 alleles have greater activity toward ethanol than the ADH1B1*1 allele (Kimura and Higuchi, 2011). These population differences in ADH1B allelozyme expression contribute to ethnic differences in alcohol consumption and toxicity, as discussed in the section "Aldehyde Dehydrogenase."

Unlike the allelic variants of ADH1B, the allelic variants of ADH1C do not differ markedly in their ability to oxidize ethanol.

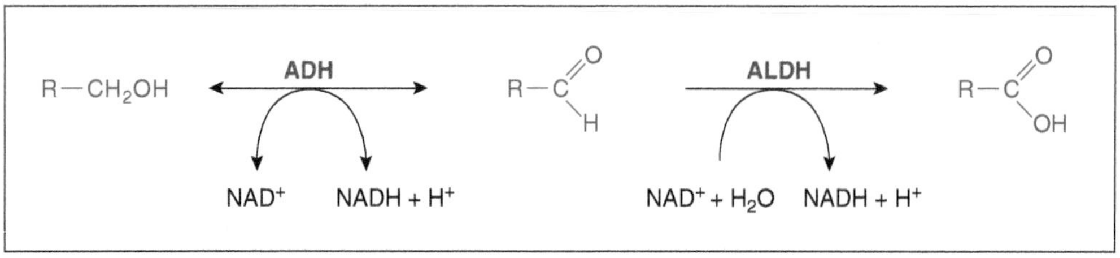

Figure 6-24. *Oxidation of alcohols to aldehydes and carboxylic acids by alcohol dehydrogenase (ADH) and aldehyde dehydrogenase (ALDH).*

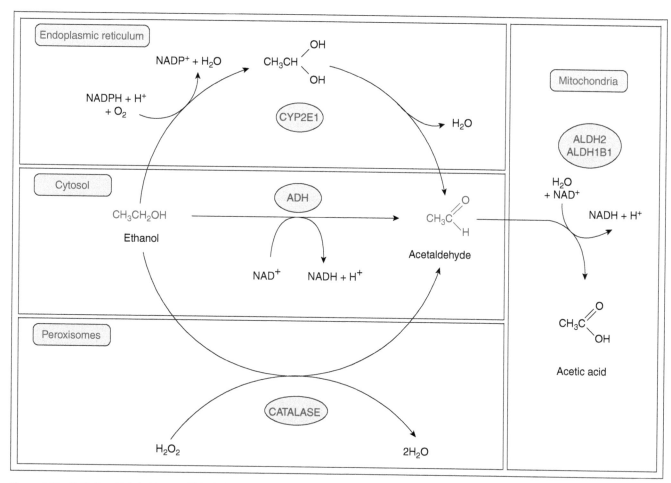

Figure 6-25. *Oxidation of alcohol to acetaldehyde by alcohol dehydrogenase (ADH), cytochrome P450 (CYP2E1), and catalase. Note*: The oxidation of alcohol to acetic acid involves multiple organelles.

However, as in the case of the ADH1B allelozymes, the expression of the ADH1C allelozymes also varies from one ethnic group to the next. The 2 allelozymes of ADH1C, namely, ADH1C*1 (γ_1-ADH) and ADH1C*2 (γ_2-ADH), are, respectively, expressed ~50:50 in Caucasians and 90:10 in Pacific Rim Asians, with the *2 allele having somewhat higher activity toward ethanol than the *1 allele (Li, 2000; Kimura and Higuchi, 2011). An additional SNP in ADH1C has been found in up to 20% of some Native American populations (Ramchandani, 2004).

Class II (ADH4) The class II enzyme ADH4 (π-ADH) is mainly expressed in liver (and to some extent in other gastrointestinal tissues), where it preferentially oxidizes larger alcohols (Ramchandani, 2004). ADH4 differs from the ADH1 isozymes in that it is less sensitive to pyrazole inhibition, but may play some role in ethanol oxidation, especially at high concentrations (Lockley *et al.*, 2005; Edenberg, 2007; Kimura and Higuchi, 2011). Some studies support a role for polymorphisms of ADH4 in the susceptibility to alcoholism (Kimura and Higuchi, 2011).

Class III (ADH5) The class III enzyme ADH5 (a homodimer of the χ-subunit) preferentially oxidizes long-chain alcohols (pentanol and larger), omega-hydroxy-fatty acids, and other alcohols (such as cinnamyl alcohol). Like ADH4, ADH5 is less sensitive to pyrazole inhibition than ADH1 enzymes. However, in contrast to ADH4, which is largely confined to the liver, ADH5 is ubiquitous, being present in virtually all tissues (including brain), where it catalyzes the rate-limiting step in detoxifying formaldehyde through oxidation of *S*-hydroxymethylglutathione

(which is formed spontaneously from formaldehyde and GSH) to *S*-formylglutathione. In fact, ADH5 and the GSH-dependent formaldehyde dehydrogenase (also referred to in literature as FDH, ADH3, or *S*-nitrosoglutathione reductase [GSNOR]) are identical enzymes (Koivusalo *et al.*, 1989; Edenberg, 2007; Just *et al.*, 2011). This enzyme appears to be the ancestral form of ADH from which all other vertebrate ADHs have evolved, and so far functional polymorphisms have not been identified in ADH5 (Just *et al.*, 2011).

Class IV (ADH7) The class IV enzyme ADH7 (σ-ADH; also referred to as the μ subunit) is a low-affinity (high K_m), high-capacity (high V_{max}) enzyme, and is the most active of the medium-chain ADHs in oxidizing retinol (a member of the vitamin A family). It is the major ADH expressed in human stomach and other areas of the UADT (eg, stomach, esophagus, pharynx, gingiva, mouth, and tongue), as well as the eyes (Han *et al.*, 2005). In contrast to the other ADHs, ADH7 is not expressed in adult human liver (Ramchandani, 2004). Among the human ADH forms, ADH7 has the highest activity toward ethanol (Han *et al.*, 2005). Inasmuch as ADH7 is expressed in the upper gastrointestinal tract, where chronic alcohol consumption leads to cancer development, there is considerable interest in the role of ADH7 in the preabsorptive conversion of ethanol to acetaldehyde (a suspected upper GI tract carcinogen or cocarcinogen) and in its role in the metabolism of retinol (a vitamin required for epithelial cell growth and differentiation), which might be inhibited by alcohol consumption (Seitz and Oneta, 1998). The role for a protective effect of high-activity polymorphisms against alcoholism remains to be fully elucidated, with some studies showing a positive association (Han *et al.*, 2005), and others no association (Duell *et al.*, 2011). However, the A92G SNP (rs1573496; C → G) in ADH7 has been found to confer a reduced risk of squamous cell carcinoma of the head and neck in Caucasians (Wei *et al.*, 2010).

Compared with hepatic ADH, gastric ADH has a lower affinity (higher K_m) but higher capacity (larger V_{max}) for oxidizing ethanol, the former being dominated by the class I ADH isozymes and the latter by the class IV enzyme ADH7. Although ethanol is largely biotransformed by hepatic ADH1, gastric ADH7 nevertheless can limit the systemic bioavailability of alcohol. This first-pass elimination of alcohol by gastric ADH7 can be significant depending on the manner in which the alcohol is consumed; large doses over a short time produce high ethanol concentrations in the stomach, which compensate for the low affinity (high K_m) of gastric ADH7. Young women have lower gastric ADH7 activity than do men, and gastric ADH7 activity tends to be lower in alcoholics (Frezza *et al.*, 1990). Some alcoholic women have no detectable gastric ADH7, and blood levels of ethanol after oral consumption of alcohol are the same as those that are obtained after intravenous administration. Gastric ADH7 activity decreases during fasting, which is one reason alcohol is more intoxicating when consumed on an empty stomach. Several commonly used drugs (eg, cimetidine, ranitidine, aspirin) are noncompetitive inhibitors of gastric ADH7. Under certain circumstances these drugs increase the systemic availability of alcohol, although the effect is too small to have serious medical, social, or legal consequences (Levitt, 1993). About 30% of Asians appear to be genetically deficient in ADH7, the main gastric ADH. In addition to biotransforming ethanol and retinol, ADH7 also detoxifies the dietary carcinogen, nitrobenzaldehyde. It has been suggested that a lack of ADH7 in some Japanese subjects may impair their ability to detoxify nitrobenzaldehyde and may possibly be linked to the high rate of gastric cancer observed in the Japanese population (Seitz and Oneta, 1998).

Class V (ADH6) The mRNA for class V ADH (namely, ADH6, for which there is no subunit designation) (Brennan *et al.*, 2004; Ramchandani, 2004) has been found in fetal and adult liver (Edenberg, 2007). However, the protein has not yet been isolated from human tissue, so little is known about its in vivo function. ADH6 has been expressed in vitro and metabolizes ethanol with a K_m of approximately 28 mM and has higher affinity for benzyl alcohol (K_m 0.12 mM) and propanol (K_m 3.2 mM) (Zhi *et al.*, 2000).

Aldehyde Dehydrogenase ALDHs oxidize 4 major types of aldehydes: (1) saturated alkanals (eg, formaldehyde, acetaldehyde), (2) unsaturated alkenals (eg, acrolein), (3) aromatic aldehydes (eg, benzaldehyde), and (4) dicarbonyls (eg, glyoxal, malondialdehyde) to their corresponding carboxylic acids, generally with NAD$^+$ as the cofactor. However, it should be noted that ALDH1L1 prefers NADP$^+$ over NAD$^+$, and ALDH3B1 can use either cofactor in a substrate-dependent manner. In addition, ALDH6A1 requires acetyl- or propionyl-CoA (Marchitti *et al.*, 2007, 2008). Most of the enzymes also have esterase activity (Yoshida *et al.*, 1998; Marchitti *et al.*, 2008). Several ALDH enzymes are involved in the oxidation of xenobiotic aldehydes, such as those formed from ethanol, allyl alcohol, carbon tetrachloride, cyclophosphamide, and ifosfamide (Marchitti *et al.*, 2007). Formaldehyde dehydrogenase, which specifically oxidizes formaldehyde that is complexed with GSH, is not a member of the ALDH family but is a class III ADH (ADH5) (Koivusalo *et al.*, 1989; Edenberg, 2007; Just *et al.*, 2011). At least 19 ALDH genes have been identified in humans, and a correspondingly large number of ALDH genes appear to be present in other

mammalian species (Sládek, 2003; Vasiliou *et al.*, 2004; Marchitti *et al.*, 2007, 2008). The name, tissue distribution, subcellular location, and major substrate for the human ALDHs are summarized in Table 6-6. The ALDHs differ in their primary amino acid sequences. They may also differ in the quaternary structure. For example, ALDH3A1 is a dimer of two 85-kDa subunits, whereas ALDH1A1 and ALDH2 are homotetramers of 54-kDa subunits (Goedde and Agarwal, 1992; Marchitti *et al.*, 2008).

As shown in Fig. 6-25, ALDH2 is a mitochondrial enzyme that, by virtue of its high affinity, is primarily responsible for oxidizing simple aldehydes, such as acetaldehyde (K_m for acetaldehyde <1 μM) and, by acting as a nitrate reductase, ALDH2 is the principal enzyme necessary for the activation of nitroglycerin (Marchitti *et al.*, 2008). In fact, the genetic polymorphism ALDH2*2 is associated with decreased nitroglycerin efficacy in certain Chinese populations (Marchitti *et al.*, 2008). Several genetic polymorphisms in human ALDH2 have been described, including the well-described ALDH2*2 point mutation (Glu$_{487}$ → Lys$_{487}$), which results in a loss of activity due to a greatly diminished affinity for NAD$^+$ (Marchitti *et al.*, 2008). The mutant ALDH2*2 allele is dominant, such that heterotetrameric ALDH2 proteins containing even a single ALDH2*2 subunit are inactive (Marchitti *et al.*, 2008). A high percentage (40%–50%) of individuals of Asian descent are deficient in ALDH2 activity due to the presence of the ALDH2*2 allele. This same population also has a high incidence of the atypical form of ADH1B (ie, ADH1B*2), which means that they rapidly convert ethanol to acetaldehyde but only slowly convert acetaldehyde to acetic acid. (They also have a relatively high prevalence of a deficiency of ADH7 activity, which impairs gastric metabolism of ethanol.) As a result, many Asian subjects experience a flushing syndrome after consuming alcohol due to a rapid buildup of acetaldehyde, which triggers the dilation of facial blood vessels through the release of catecholamines. Some Native American populations also experience a flushing syndrome after consuming alcohol, possibly because they express ADH1B*2 (Ramchandani, 2004) or a different allelic variant of ALDH2 and/or because acetaldehyde oxidation in blood erythrocytes is impaired in these individuals, possibly due to the expression of a variant form of ALDH1A1. Both the functional genetic variants of ADH that rapidly convert ethanol to acetaldehyde (ie, ADH1B*2) and the genetic variants of ALDH that slowly detoxify acetaldehyde (ie, ALDH2*2) protect against heavy drinking and alcoholism. Inhibition of ALDH by disulfiram (Antabuse) causes an accumulation of acetaldehyde in alcoholics. The nauseating effect of acetaldehyde serves to deter continued ethanol consumption (Goedde and Agarwal, 1992). However, it is important to note that a predisposition toward alcoholism is not simply determined by factors that affect the pharmacokinetics of ethanol and its metabolites. Studies in humans and rodents implicate 5-HT1B, 2A, 3A, and 3B receptors, dopamine-related genes, GABA receptors, cholinergic muscarinic receptor 2, the endogenous opioid system, tryptophan hydroxylase, and neuropeptide Y as candidate targets of genetic susceptibility in the pharmacodynamic actions of ethanol (Li, 2000; Kimura and Higuchi, 2011). MAO may also be a risk factor for alcoholism, as discussed later (see the section "Amine Oxidases").

Genetic deficiencies in other ALDHs impair the metabolism of other aldehydes, which is the underlying basis of certain diseases. For example, polymorphisms in certain ALDH genes may alter the risk for, or cause, the following: spina bifida (ALDH1A2), Sjögren–Larsson syndrome (ALDH3A2), paranoid schizophrenia (ALDH3B1), type II hyperprolinemia (ALDH4A1), γ-hydroxybutyric aciduria (ALDH5A1), methylmalonic aciduria (ALDH6A1), pyroxidine-dependent seizures

Table 6-6

Properties of the Human Aldehyde Dehydrogenases (ALDHs)

ALDH	ALTERNATIVE NAMES	FORM	TISSUE	SUBCELLULAR LOCALIZATION	MAJOR SUBSTRATE
1A1	ALDH1, ALDH11, RALDH1	Homotetramer	Liver, kidney, lung, stomach, testis, lens, retina, CNS, etc	Cytosol	Retinal
1A2	RALDH2	Homotetramer	Intestine, testis, lung, liver, kidney, retina, CNS, etc	Cytosol	Retinal, nitroglycerin
1A3	ALDH6, RALDH3	Homodimer	Prostate, salivary gland, stomach, kidney, breast, CNS, etc	Cytosol	Retinal, aliphatic aldehydes
1B1	ALDH5	Homotetramer	Muscle, liver, kidney, lung, testis, muscle, heart, CNS, etc	Mitochondria	Acetaldehyde, aliphatic aldehydes
1L1	FDH	Homotetramer	Liver, kidney, pancreas, lung, prostate, heart, muscle, testis, ovary, CNS, etc	Cytosol, mitochondria	10-Formyltetrahydrofolate, propanal, and acetaldehyde
1L2	mtFDH	Homotetramer	Spleen, cervix, uterus, corpus callosum	Mitochondria	10-Formyltetrahydrofolate
2	ALDM, ALDHI	Homotetramer	Liver, kidney, lung, heart, stomach, muscle, CNS, etc	Mitochondria	Acetaldehyde
3A1	ALDH3	Homodimer	Cornea, esophagus, trachea, stomach, lung, bladder, etc	Cytosol, nucleus	Aromatic and medium-chain aliphatic aldehydes
3A2	ALDH10, FALDH	Homodimer	Adrenals, kidney, liver, lung, intestine, pancreas, stomach, heart, muscle, CNS, etc	Microsomes, peroxisomes	Fatty and aromatic aldehydes
3B1	ALDH4, ALDH7	Unknown	Kidney, lung, liver, cerebral astrocytes, testis, macrophages, pancreas, spleen	Cytosol (membrane-bound in some tissues)	Medium- and long-chain aliphatic and aromatic aldehydes
3B2	ALDH8	Unknown	Parotid, adrenals, prostate, lung, kidney, liver, CNS	Microsomes	Unknown[*]
4A1	ALDH4, P5CDH	Homodimer	Liver, muscle, kidney, CNS	Mitochondria	Glutamate γ-semialdehyde, short- and medium-chain aliphatic aldehydes
5A1	SSDH, SSADH	Homotetramer	Liver, kidney, muscle, heart, CNS	Mitochondria	Succinate semialdehyde
6A1	MMSDH	Homotetramer	Kidney, liver, heart, muscle, CNS	Mitochondria	Malonate semialdehyde
7A1	ATQ1, EPD	Homotetramer	Cochlea, eye, ovary, heart, kidney, liver, CNS, etc	Cytosol, nucleus, mitochondria	α-Aminoadipic semialdehyde
8A1	ALDH12	Unknown	Liver, kidney, CNS, breast, testis, prostate, etc	Cytosol	9-cis-Retinal
9A1	ALDH4, ALDH7, ALDH9, γABHD	Homotetramer	Liver, kidney, muscle, CNS	Cytosol	γ-Aminobutyraldehyde
16A1	MGC10204	Unknown	CNS, uterus, placenta, bone marrow, heart, kidney, lung	Cytosol	Unknown
18A1	GSAS, Δ¹-P5CS[†]	Unknown	Pancreas, ovary, testis, kidney, heart, colon, muscle, CNS, etc	Mitochondria	Glutamic γ-semialdehyde

γABHD, 4-aminobutyraldehyde; FALDH, fatty aldehyde dehydrogenase; SSDH, succinic dehydrogenase; MMSDH, methylmalonate semialdehyde dehydrogenase. Data from Strickland et al. (2011), Marchitti et al. (2007, 2008, 2010), Sládek (2003), and Vasiliou et al. (2004).

[*]ALDH3B2 contains an in-frame stop codon, suggesting the possibility that it is a pseudogene, although transcripts have been found in various tissues.

[†]Δ¹-Pyrroline-5-carboxylate synthase, P5CS.

(ALDH7A1), nonalcoholic steatohepatits (NASH) (ALDH9A1), and hyperammonemia and/or hypoprolinemia (ALDH18A1) (Marchitti et al., 2008).

The toxicological consequences of an inherited (ie, genetic) or acquired (eg, drug-induced) deficiency of ALDH illustrate that aldehydes are more cytotoxic than the corresponding alcohol. This is especially true of allyl alcohol (CH_2=CHCH$_2$OH), which is converted by ADH to the highly hepatotoxic aldehyde, acrolein (CH_2=CHCHO) (Marchitti et al., 2007, 2008).

The oxidation of ethanol by ADH and ALDH leads to the formation of acetic acid, which is rapidly oxidized to carbon dioxide and water. However, in certain cases, alcohols are converted to toxic carboxylic acids, as in the case of methanol and ethylene glycol, which are converted via aldehyde intermediates to formic acid and oxalic acid, respectively. Formic and oxalic acids are considerably more toxic than acetic acid. For this reason, methanol and ethylene glycol poisonings are commonly treated with ethanol, which competitively inhibits the oxidation of methanol and ethylene glycol by ADH and ALDH. The potent inhibitor of ADH, 4-methylpyrazole (fomepizole) (Lockley et al., 2005), is also used to treat methanol and ethylene glycol poisonings.

The reduction of aldehydes and ketones to primary and secondary alcohols by carbonyl reductases has already been discussed (see the section "Carbonyl Reduction—AKRs and SDRs"). In contrast to ADH and ALDH, carbonyl reductases typically use NADPH as the source of reducing equivalents. Aldehydes, especially aromatic aldehydes, can also be oxidized by AO and xanthine oxidoreductase (XOR), which are discussed in the section "Molybdenum Hydroxylases (Molybdoenzymes)."

Dimeric Dihydrodiol Dehydrogenase As mentioned in the section "Carbonyl Reduction—AKRs and SDRs," several members of the AKR superfamily are dihydrodiol dehydrogenases that oxidize the trans-dihydrodiols of various PAHs to the corresponding ortho-quinones, as shown in Fig. 6-10 (Penning, 1997; Burczynski and Penning, 2000). There is also a dihydrodiol dehydrogenase (gene symbol DHDH; completely unrelated to AKRs or SDRs) that encodes a dimeric enzyme that oxidizes trans-dihydrodiols of aromatic hydrocarbons to the corresponding catechols in a NADP$^+$-dependent manner (Carbone et al., 2008). The overall reaction catalyzed by dimeric dihydrodiol dehydrogenase is a 2-electron oxidation of one of the hydroxyl groups of a trans-dihydrodiol to an intermediate ketol, which rapidly enolizes to the catechol (Carbone et al., 2008). It also activates naphthalene trans-dihydrodiol to 1,2-dihydroxynaphthalene, which rapidly auto-oxidizes to 1,2-naphthoquinone, a cytotoxic ortho-quinone that may be responsible for naphthalene-induced cataracts (Carbone et al., 2008). Dimeric dihydrodiol dehydrogenase is not active toward hydroxysteroids, but it does oxidize several endogenous sugars, including D-glucose and D-xylose, and may therefore play a role in the metabolism of dietary sugars with subsequent generation of NADPH. Dimeric dihydrodiol dehydrogenase can also catalyze reductions in the presence of NADPH, such as the carbonyl reduction of methylglyoxal and 3-deoxyglucosone, nitrobenzaldehydes, and camphoroquine (Carbone et al., 2008). Dimeric dihydrodiol dehydrogenase can be inhibited by L-ascorbic and isoascorbic acids and also by 4-hydroxyphenylketones and 2,6-dihydroxyanthraquinone, and is inactivated by magnesium chloride and some phosphate salts (Carbone et al., 2008). This enzyme was first characterized in rabbit liver, where it oxidizes benzene dihydrodiol to the genotoxic and immunotoxic catechol. It has also been isolated from pig, dog, and cynomolgus monkey (Macaca fascicularis). The purified enzyme is composed of identical subunits with molecular weights of 32 to 36 kDa, and amino acid sequence in humans indicates that each subunit is composed of 335 amino acids (Carbone et al., 2008). Dimeric dihydrodiol dehydrogenase is ubiquitously expressed in dogs and pigs, but only in the kidney of monkey, lens and intestine of rabbit, and apparently only the intestine of humans (Carbone et al., 2008).

It should be noted that PAHs can be oxidized by CYP to an arene oxide, an electrophilic and potentially toxic metabolite that is detoxified by its conversion to a trans-dihydrodiol by epoxide hydrolase. By oxidizing the trans-dihydrodiol to an ortho-quinone, AKRs generate yet another potentially toxic metabolite. These roles of AKRs (which can act as monomeric dihydrodiol dehydrogenases) in the metabolism of PAHs are well known but the activity of dimeric dihydrodiol dehydrogenase toward the trans-dihydrodiols of PAHs has not yet been reported (Carbone et al., 2008). In terms of their ability to cause oxidative stress and cellular toxicity, ortho-quinones can be considered equivalent to para-quinones, which were discussed earlier in the section "Quinone Reduction—NQO1 and NQO2."

Molybdenum Hydroxylases (Molybdoenzymes) There are 5 human molybdenum-containing enzymes (molybdoenzymes), namely, AO (gene symbol AOX1), XOR (also known as XO or XD, gene symbol XDH), sulfite oxidase (gene symbol SUOX), and the more recently discovered "mitochondrial amidoxime-reducing component" (mARC-1 and -2; gene symbols MOSC1 and MOSC2) (Havemeyer et al., 2011). AO and XOR are the 2 major molybdoenzymes that participate in the biotransformation of xenobiotics. The human mARC (consisting of mARC-1 and -2) is involved in the activation of amidoxime prodrugs and detoxication of some N-hydroxylated xenobiotics, as described in the section "Dehydroxylation—mARC, Cytochrome b_5, b_5 Reductase, and Aldehyde Oxidase." Sulfite oxidase will not be described in detail here except that, as its name implies, the enzyme oxidizes sulfite, an irritating air pollutant, to sulfate, which is relatively innocuous, and is also required to metabolize the sulfur-containing amino acids cysteine and methionine in foods.

Genetic polymorphisms can affect all molybdoenzymes or individual enzymes. Homozygosity for nonfunctional forms of some of the genes involved in the synthesis of the active molybdenum cofactor (MoCo), namely, MOCS1, MOCS2, MOCOS, or GPHN, results in a complete lack of activity of all molybdoenzymes, and is clinically indistinguishable from isolated SUOX deficiency (Reiss and Hahnewald, 2010), a rare condition that gives rise to progressive neurological damage and death in early childhood (Reiss and Johnson, 2003; Feng et al., 2007). Isolated XOR deficiency results in the classical type I xanthinuria, which can lead to xanthine stones (calculi) because of the inability to oxidize xanthine and hypoxanthine to uric acid, but it is not life-threatening (Reiss and Hahnewald, 2010). Although no isolated forms of AO deficiency have been described, type II xanthinuria results from a combined deficiency of XOR and AO as evidenced by the inability to oxidize both xanthine and hypoxanthine as well as allopurinol to oxypurinol. Certain polymorphisms in AO do appear to cause a decrease or complete loss of activity toward certain substrates, as discussed in the section "Aldehyde Oxidase" (Hartmann et al., 2012). Not surprisingly, given its recent discovery, isolated mARC deficiency has not yet been described.

XOR and AO comprise the human members of the "XO family" of molybdoenzymes. Both enzymes are only active as homodimers, each with an ~145-kDa monomer consisting of an N-terminal region that binds 2 nonidentical iron–sulfur clusters of the [2Fe–2S] type, followed by an FAD-binding region and C-terminal domains that bind the molybdenum center (Wahl *et al.*, 2010). In XOR, however, an additional NAD⁺ binding site is present. In XOR and AO, the molybdenum is ligated to an oxo ligand, a hydroxyl group, 2 dithiolene sulfurs, and a sulfido group (as shown in the upper left panel of Fig. 6-27). The molybdenum–sulfur bond is inserted through a posttranslational reaction catalyzed by MoCo sulfurase (gene symbol *MOCOS*), which substitutes one of the oxo groups of the MoCo with a sulfo double bond and is essential for the activity of these enzymes (Garattini *et al.*, 2008). In contrast, in sulfite oxidase (the only fully accepted human member of the "sulfite oxidase family" of molybdoenzymes), the molybdenum is coordinated by the 2 sulfurs on the pterin, 2 oxo ligands, and a protein-derived cysteinyl sulfur (Wahl *et al.*, 2010). Sulfite oxidase does not require posttranslational sulfuration of the MoCo to become active. The two 35 kDa human mARC enzymes may represent a separate family of molybdoenzymes in that they do not contain an FAD domain and may bind molybdenum in a manner different than either the XO or sulfite oxidase families. However, there is some evidence to suggest that the mARCs are in fact members of the human sulfite oxidase family of molybdoenzymes (Havemeyer *et al.*, 2011). In addition, the mARCs share significant sequence similarity with the C-terminal domain of MOCOS and appear to require cytochrome b_5, cytochrome b_5 reductase, and NADH for catalytic activity (Wahl *et al.*, 2010). Furthermore, whereas XOR, AO, and SUOX are localized in the cytosol, the 2 mARC proteins appear to be localized to the outer mitochondrial membrane (Havemeyer *et al.*, 2011).

The catalytic cycle for XOR and AO involves an interaction between the molybdenum center with a reducing substrate, which results in the reduction of the MoCo, after which reducing equivalents are transferred intramolecularly to the flavin cofactors (which act as electron sinks), with reoxidation occurring via the flavin moiety by molecular oxygen (in the case of AO and the XO form of XOR) or NAD⁺ (in the case of the XD form of XOR). Electrons are transferred from the MoCo to the flavin cofactor through the intermediacy of the iron–sulfur centers. During substrate oxidation, AO and XOR are reduced and then reoxidized by molecular oxygen; hence, they function as true oxidases. The oxygen incorporated into the xenobiotic is derived from water rather than oxygen, which distinguishes these oxidases from oxygenases. The main functional difference between AO and XOR is the ability of the latter to use both NAD⁺ (in its XD form) *and* molecular oxygen (in its XO form), as the final acceptors of the reducing equivalents (Garattini and Terao, 2011). Reduction of oxygen by the XO form of XOR leads to the formation of hydrogen peroxide or superoxide anion (in a substrate-dependent manner) as follows:

$$RH + H_2O + O_2 \rightarrow ROH + H_2O_2;$$
$$RH + H_2O + 2O_2 \rightarrow ROH + 2O_2^- + 2H^+.$$

Additional details of the catalytic cycle are described in the section "Xanthine Oxidoreductase." XOR and AO catalyze the oxidation of carbon atoms with a low electron density such as the electron-deficient sp^2-hybridized carbon atom, double bonded to nitrogen in aromatic azaheterocycles (R_1-CH=N-R_2) or oxygen in various aldehydes (R_1-CH=O). In aromatic azaheterocycles (such as purines, pyrimidines, pteridines, quinolines, iminium ions, and diazanaphthalenes), oxidation by AO (and in most cases by XOR) occurs at the carbon with the lowest electron density, which is typically the α-carbon (next to the nitrogen) but in some cases the γ-carbon (2 carbons removed) (Strolin-Benedetti, 2011). This contrasts with oxidation by CYP, which generally catalyzes the oxidation of carbon atoms with a high electron density. For this reason, xenobiotics that are good substrates for molybdoenzymes

(nucleophilic oxidizing enzymes) tend to be poor substrates for CYP (an electrophilic oxidizing enzyme), and vice versa (Pryde *et al.*, 2010). AO and, to a lesser extent, XOR hydroxylate the carbonyl carbon in certain aldehydes and convert them to carboxylic acids (R-CHO → R-COOH). Both molybdoenzymes hydroxylate the α-carbon in aromatic azaheterocycles (R_1-CH=N-R_2) to form α-hydroxyimines (R_1-COH=N-R_2) that rapidly tautomerize to the corresponding lactam (R_1-CO–NH-R_2) (α-aminoketone). Certain aromatic aldehydes, such as tamoxifen aldehyde and benzaldehyde, are good substrates for AO and XOR, whereas aliphatic aldehydes tend to be poor substrates. Consequently, AO and XOR contribute negligibly to the metabolism of acetaldehyde under normal conditions. Some reactions catalyzed by AO and XOR are shown in Fig. 6-26. It should be noted that although AO and XOR tend to oxidize similar substrates, there are some differences in substrate specificity (eg, vanillin is rapidly oxidized by AO, but there is little contribution of XOR) (Strolin-Benedetti, 2011). An interesting difference between XOR and AO is their regioselective oxidation of the purine prodrug 6-deoxyacyclovir, which is oxidized by XOR in the 6-membered ring to form the active drug acyclovir (discussed below) but is oxidized by AO in the 5-membered ring to form the pharmacologically inactive metabolite 6-deoxy-8-hydroxyacyclovir (Testa and Krämer, 2008, 2010). In the case of nonaromatic azaheterocycles the preferred substrate is the protonated form (−CH=NH⁺−) because this form lowers the electron density at the α-carbon. For this same reason, *N*-alkylation of aromatic azaheterocycles to form a quaternary (positively charged) nitrogen next to the α-carbon improves oxidation by AO (more so than by XOR), as in the case of *N*-methylnicotinamide. Under certain conditions, both enzymes can also catalyze the reduction of xenobiotics (Testa and Krämer, 2008, 2010). Examples of reductive reactions catalyzed by AO are shown in Fig. 6-23.

Xanthine Oxidoreductase XD and XO are 2 forms of the same cytosolic enzyme (XOR, gene symbol XDH) that differ in the electron acceptor used in the final step of catalysis. In the case of XD, the final electron acceptor is NAD⁺ (dehydrogenase activity), whereas in the case of XO the final electron acceptor is oxygen (oxidase activity). Although both XOR and AO are expressed in many tissues, the highest XOR expression in humans is found in the proximal intestine, liver, and lactating mammary glands (Strolin-Benedetti, 2011). XD is converted reversibly to XO by oxidation of sulfhydryl groups or irreversibly by proteolytic cleavage (Testa and Krämer, 2008, 2010). In humans, XOR is encoded by a single gene (ie, XDH). Under normal physiological conditions, XD is the predominant form of the enzyme found in vivo. However, during tissue processing, the dehydrogenase form tends to be converted to the oxidase form; hence, most in vitro studies are conducted with XO or a combination of XO and XD. The induction (upregulation) of XD and/or the conversion of XD to XO in vivo is thought to play an important role in ischemia–reperfusion injury, lipopolysaccharide (LPS)–mediated tissue injury, and alcohol-induced hepatotoxicity (Pacher *et al.*, 2006). During ischemia, XO levels increase because hypoxia induces XOR gene transcription, and because XD is converted to XO. During reperfusion, XO contributes to oxidative stress and lipid peroxidation because the oxidase activity of XO involves the reduction of molecular oxygen, which can lead to the formation of ROS of the type shown in Fig. 6-16. Similarly, treatment with LPS, a bacterial endotoxin that triggers an acute inflammatory response, increases XO activity both by inducing XOR transcription and by converting XD to XO. The associated increase in oxidative stress has been implicated in LPS-induced cytotoxicity. Ethanol facilitates the conversion of XD to XO, and the conversion

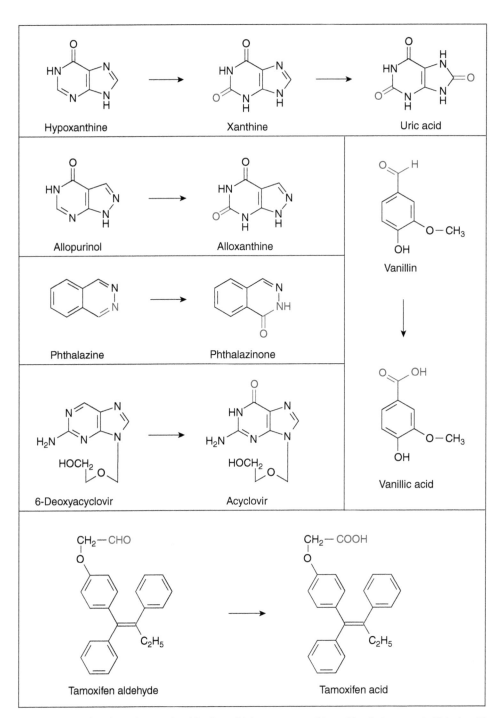

Figure 6-26. *Examples of reactions catalyzed by the molybdoenzymes, xanthine oxidoreductaase, and aldehyde oxidase.*

of ethanol to acetaldehyde provides a substrate and, hence, a source of electrons for the reduction of oxygen. Hereafter, the 2 forms of the enzyme will be referred to as XOR.

Typical reactions catalyzed by XOR are shown in Fig. 6-26. XOR contributes significantly to the first-pass elimination of several purine derivatives (eg, 6-mercaptopurine and 2,6-dithiopurine), and limits the therapeutic effects of these cancer chemotherapeutic agents. In contrast, certain prodrugs are activated by XOR. For example, the antiviral prodrugs 6-deoxyacyclovir and 2′-fluoroarabino-dideoxypurine, which are relatively well absorbed after oral dosing, are oxidized by XOR to their respective active forms, acyclovir and 2′-fluoroarabino-dideoxyinosine, which are otherwise poorly absorbed (see Fig. 6-26). Furthermore,

XOR has been implicated in the bioactivation of mitomycin C and related antineoplastic drugs, although this bioactivation reaction is thought to be largely catalyzed by NQO1 (DT-diaphorase), as discussed previously in the section "Quinone Reduction— NQO1 and NQO2." Other xenobiotic substrates of XOR include 6-thioxanthine, methotrexate, and the benzylic aldehyde metabolite of tolbutamide (Chladek *et al.*, 1997; Testa and Krämer, 2008, 2010; Kudo *et al.*, 2010).

XOR catalyzes an important physiological reaction, namely, the sequential oxidation of hypoxanthine to xanthine and uric acid, as shown in Fig. 6-26 (Rajagopalan, 1980). By competing with hypoxanthine and xanthine for oxidation by XOR, allopurinol inhibits the formation of uric acid, making allopurinol a useful

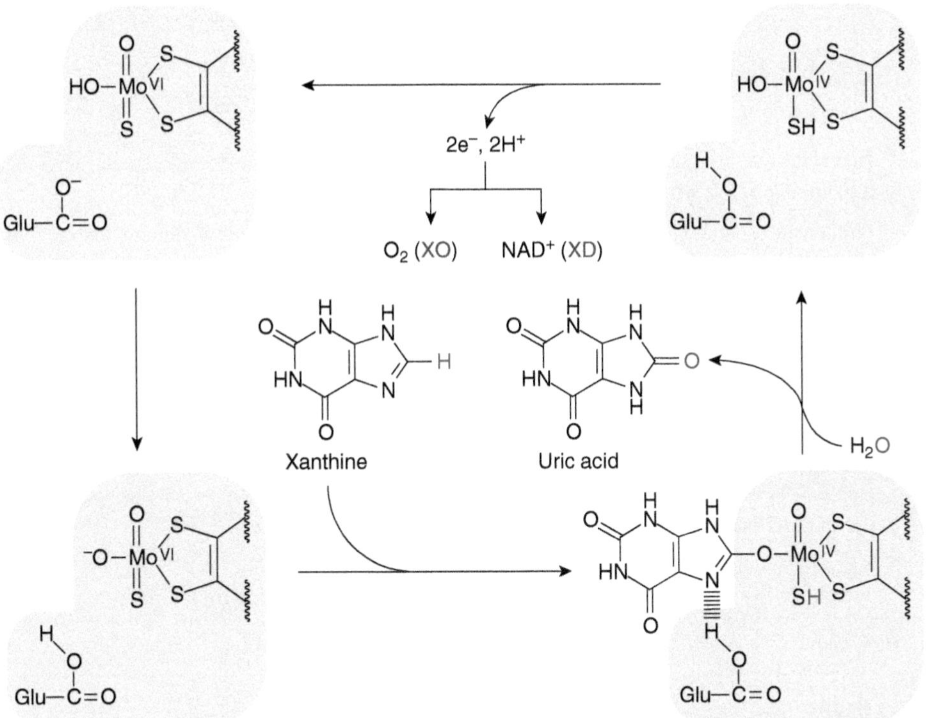

Figure 6-27. *Catalytic cycle of the molybdoenzyme xanthine oxidoreductase.* Xanthine oxidoreductase is a molybdoenzyme with xanthine dehydrogenase (XD) and xanthine oxidase (XO) activities. During the final step of the catalytic cycle, the enzyme is reoxidized by transferring electrons to NAD$^+$ (in the case of XD) or oxygen (in the case of XO). The same mechanism of catalysis likely applies to aldehyde oxidase, although there is no dehydrogenase form of this molybdoenzyme.

drug in the treatment of gout (a complication of hyperuricemia). Allopurinol can also be used to evaluate the contribution of XOR to xenobiotic biotransformation in vivo. Like allopurinol, hydroxylated coumarin derivatives, such as umbelliferone (7-hydroxycoumarin) and esculetin (7,8-dihydroxycoumarin), are potent inhibitors of XOR. Allopurinol and other XOR inhibitors are being evaluated for the treatment of various types of ischemia–reperfusion and vascular injury that appear to be mediated, at least in part, by XOR (Pacher *et al.*, 2006).

Monomethylated xanthines are preferentially oxidized to the corresponding uric acid derivatives by XOR. In contrast, dimethylated and trimethylated xanthines, such as theophylline (1,3-dimethylxanthine) and caffeine (1,3,7-trimethylxanthine), are oxidized to the corresponding uric acid derivatives primarily by CYP. Through 2 sequential *N*-demethylation reactions, CYP converts caffeine to 1-methylxanthine, which is converted by XOR to 1-methyluric acid. The urinary ratio of 1-methylxanthine to 1-methyluric acid provides an in vivo marker of XOR activity.

The mechanism of catalysis by molybdoenzymes depicted in Fig. 6-27 is based on studies of XOR by Okamoto *et al.* (2004), Amano *et al.* (2007), and Alfaro and Jones (2008). The molybdopterin active center of the enzyme consists of molybdenum (Mo) bound to the following groups: pterin cofactor, thioxo (=S), oxo (=O), and hydroxyl (–OH). For simplicity, this cofactor will be written as S=Mo–OH. The hydroxyl group (S=Mo–OH) is activated by a nearby glutamic acid residue in the enzyme to S=Mo–O$^-$, which initiates a concerted nucleophilic attack on the substrate at the electron-deficient carbon atom double bonded to the nitrogen (H–CR$_1$=N-R$_2$) with hydride transfer from the α-carbon to the thioxo group to form the intermediate (HS–Mo–O–CR$_1$=N-R$_2$). The oxygen bound to the α-carbon in the substrate (eg, xanthine) is replaced by oxygen from water to complete formation of product (eg, uric acid). The resting enzyme is restored by the removal of 2 reducing equivalents, which

may be transferred to NAD$^+$ (in the case of XD) or oxygen (in the case of XO), as shown in Fig. 6-27. In the XO mode, XOR (and AO, which exists only in the XO mode) can transfer both reducing equivalents to a single molecule of oxygen to produce hydrogen peroxide or it can transfer the 2 electrons to 2 molecules of oxygen to produce superoxide anion. In addition to the concerted mechanism described above, a stepwise mechanism involving a tetrahedral intermediate is also possible (Alfaro and Jones, 2008).

Aldehyde Oxidase The term AO is something of a misnomer, in that this enzyme does not solely act on aldehyde-containing substrates (see Table 6-7). AO is the second of 2 molybdoenzymes that play an important role in xenobiotic biotransformation, the other being XOR (discussed in the preceding section). Whereas XOR exists in 2 forms, a dehydrogenase form (XD) that relays electrons to NAD$^+$ and an oxidase form (XO) that relays electrons to molecular oxygen, AO exists only in the oxidase form because it lacks an NAD$^+$ binding site (Garattini and Terao, 2011). Another significant difference between these 2 molybdoenzymes is that high levels of XOR appear to be widely distributed throughout the body, whereas high levels of AO (or at least its mRNA) are found in the liver and adrenal gland, with somewhat less expression in the small and large intestines, ovary, prostate, proximal-, distal-, and collecting tubules of the kidney, the epithelia of trachea and bronchium, and the alveolar cells of the lung, with only detectable levels of transcript in the endocrine tissues, esophagus, pancreas, brain, and few other tissues, at least in humans (Pryde *et al.*, 2010; Garattini and Terao, 2011). The human AOX1 gene is complex with 35 exons, and exists as an active homodimer. There is also considerable interindividual variability in the levels of AO in humans, which may be due to genetic (as discussed further below) as well as environmental factors such as age, disease state (eg, cancer, inflammatory conditions leading to altered levels

Table 6-7

Substrates Associated with Oxidation by Aldehyde Oxidase

SUBSTRATE GROUPS	EXAMPLE SUBSTRATES
Aldehydes	Acetaldehyde, benzaldehyde, citalopram aldehyde, phenylacetaldehyde, pyridoxal, retinal, tamoxifen aldehyde, tolbutamide aldehyde, vanillin
Aromatic azaheterocycles	Phthalazines, cinchona alkaloids, quinazolines, carbazeran, chloroquinazolinone, famciclovir, 6-mercaptopurine, N-methyl-nicotinamide, N-methyl-phthalazinium, phenanthridine, 3-descladinosyl-11,12-dideoxy-6-omethyl-3-oxo-12,11-(oxycarbonyl-(1-(1R-([1,8]naphthyridin-4-yl)-ethyl)azetidin-3-yl)imino)erythromycin A, 2,4-diaminopteridine, N-{trans-4-[2-(6-cyano-3,4-dihydroisoquinolin-2(1H)-yl)ethyl]cyclohexyl}quinoline-4-carboxamide (SB-277011), methotrexate, 6-thioxanthine, zebularine, 5-fluoro-pyrimidinone, 5-ethinylpyrimidinone, caffeine, 6-deoxyacyclovir, 8-hydroxy-6-deoxyacyclovir, allopurinol, pyrazinamide, N-[(20-dimethylamino) ethyl]acridine-4-carboxamide (DACA), 2-[4-(7-chloro-2-quinoxalinyloxyphenoxy]-propionic acid (XK-469), dibenzo[b,f]-1,4-oxazepine, briminodine, 3-tert-butyl-7-(5-methylisoxazol-3-yl)-2-(1-methyl-1H-1,2,4-triazol-5-ylmethoxy)-pyrazolo[1,5-d][1,2,4]triazine (MRK-016), 6-(2,4-difluoro-phenoxy)-2-((R)-2-hydroxy-1-methyl-ethylamino)-8-((S)-2-hydroxy-propyl)-8H-pyrido[2,3-d]pyrimidin-7-one (RO1), zaleplon
Iminium ions	Nicotine iminium ion, N-methyl-nicotinamide iminium ion, iminium ion of 3-methyl-5-[(2S)-1-methyl-2-pyrrolidinyl]isoxazole (ABT-418), prolintane iminium ion, azapetine iminium ion

Data from Pryde et al. (2010) and Hartmann et al. (2012).

of various cytokines), smoking, and drug use (Pryde *et al.*, 2010). Apart from these differences, many of the features of XOR apply to AO, including subcellular location (cytosol), enzyme structure and cofactor composition, typical mechanism of catalysis, preference for oxidizing sp^2-hybridized carbon atoms adjacent to the nitrogen atoms in nitrogen heterocycles, and its preference for oxidizing aromatic aldehydes over aliphatic aldehydes. Other AO substrate types include nitro- or nitroso-containing compounds as well as aldehyde or iminium ion intermediates formed by CYP, ADHs, or MAOs (Pryde *et al.*, 2010). Furthermore, AO also transfers electrons to molecular oxygen, which can generate ROS (eg, superoxide anion, which dismutates to hydrogen peroxide) and lead to oxidative stress and lipid peroxidation (Garattini and Terao, 2011). However, in contrast to XOR, the physiological functions of AO remain largely unknown, although endogenous compounds such as indole-3-acetate, retinaldehyde, retinoic acid, nicotinamide, and pyridoxal are substrates for AO (Garattini and Terao, 2011).

Many SNPs in the human AOX1 gene have been described in the NCBI dbSNP database (http://www.ncbi.nlm.nih.gov/projects/SNP). In a population of 180 Italian individuals, relatively frequent nonsense, synonymous, or missense SNPs in AO have been described, with a total of 51 SNPs identified, with 10 individuals being homozygous for a SNP (Hartmann *et al.*, 2012). Two of the SNPs resulted in a fast metabolizer phenotype (FMs; $N_{1135}S$, frequency = 2.9%, and $H_{1297}R$, frequency = 5.3%) and 1 in a PM phenotype (ie, $R_{921}H$, frequency = 0.3%). In addition, a relatively frequent nonsense mutation in exon 5 (Y_{126}stop, frequency = 0.026) was identified that results in a very short and nonfunctional 126-amino acid protein, but no subjects were homozygous for this loss-of-function mutation. An important point about these polymorphisms described so far is that the effects appear to be somewhat substrate-dependent based on the functional characterization of purified, heterologously expressed variants described above with the AO substrates benzaldehyde, phthalazine, phenanthridine, and chloroquinazolinone (Hartmann *et al.*, 2012).

Substrates for AO do not appear to correlate with any specific area of "chemical space" based on physicochemical properties, which have a wide variety of lipophilicity, polar surface area, polarity, and structure, in contrast to P450 substrates, for which

there is a high correlation between higher log *P* and P450-mediated metabolism as measured by microsomal stability in the presence of NADPH (see Table 6-7 for example substrates) (Pryde *et al.*, 2010). Therefore, although it has been assumed that, in general, xenobiotics that are good substrates for AO are poor substrates for CYP, and vice versa (Rettie and Fisher, 1999), there is some overlap, and structural motifs alone may be a better predictor of AO substrates (Pryde *et al.*, 2010). Naphthalene (with no nitrogen atoms) is oxidized by CYP, but not by AO, whereas the opposite is true of pteridine (1,3,5,8-tetraazanaphthalene), which contains 4 nitrogen atoms. The intermediate structure, quinazolone (1,3-diazanaphthalene), is a substrate for both enzymes. This complementarity in substrate specificity reflects the opposing preference of the 2 enzymes for oxidizing carbon atoms; CYP prefers to oxidize carbon atoms with high electron density, whereas AO (and XOR) prefers to oxidize carbon atoms with low electron density. Because of their opposing mechanisms of action (electrophilic for CYP, nucleophilic for AO), the common practice in drug development of adding a fluorine atom to block a site of oxidation by CYP (to improve metabolic stability) can potentially increase the rate of metabolism by AO. In nearly all cases, oxidation of aromatic heterocycles by AO occurs at the α-carbon but occasionally, depending on ring structure, the γ-carbon (or even the β-carbon) has the lowest electron density and is the site of oxidation. Examples of γ-carbon (or β-carbon) oxidation by AO include N-methylnicotinamide, quinolone, cinnoline, and N-[(2'-dimethylamino)ethyl]acridine-4-carboxamide (DACA) (Schofield *et al.*, 2000; Testa and Krämer, 2008, 2010). In terms of its role in drug metabolism, it is reasonable to conclude that human AO does play—and will continue to play—a significant role in the oxidation of a wide range of structurally diverse nitrogen heterocyclic substrates (Pryde *et al.*, 2010).

As shown in Figs. 6-23 and 6-26, AO can oxidize a number of substituted pyrroles, pyridines, pyrimidines, purines, pteridines, and iminium ions (see Table 6-7 for additional examples) by the mechanism described for XOR in the previous section (Alfaro and Jones, 2008). AO can oxidize aldehydes to their corresponding carboxylic acids, but the enzyme shows a marked preference for aromatic aldehydes (eg, benzaldehyde, tamoxifen aldehyde). Consequently, AO contributes negligibly to the oxidation of aliphatic aldehydes, such as acetaldehyde. Rodrigues (1994) found that, in a bank of human liver samples, AO activity toward N^1-methylnicotinamide varied more than 40-fold, whereas activity toward 6-methylpurine varied less than 3-fold. Although this suggests human liver cytosol contains 2 or more forms of AO, subsequent Southern blot analysis has provided evidence for only a single copy of the AO gene in humans (Terao *et al.*, 1998), although genomic analysis of chromosome 2q has revealed the presence of 2 nearby pseudogenes (Garattini and Terao, 2011). Species differences in the number of functional AOX genes are discussed further below.

The substrate specificity of AO differs among mammalian species, often leading to erroneous conclusions about the potential metabolic stability of certain drugs in humans, as detailed below. AO activity among animal species can vary depending on the particular substrate, but in general it is high in monkeys and humans, low in rats, and essentially absent in dogs (because the latter only express AOX3L1 and AOX4) (Garattini and Terao, 2011). These differences have been ascribed to the size of the active site (Pryde *et al.*, 2010). However, large differences in activity have also been found among individual strains of rats and mice (eg, high activity in Sea:SD rats and low in WKA/Sea rats; large differences between Sprague–Dawley and Wistar as well as between C129/C57 and CB57B1/6J mice) (Pryde *et al.*, 2010). Gender differences between rats and mice due to hormonal regulation further complicate attempts to extrapolate stability of AO substrates from toxicologically relevant species to humans (eg, 2- to 4-fold higher activity in male mice than in female) (Pryde *et al.*, 2010). Finally, whereas humans encode only a single functional AO (namely, AOX1; the others being transcribed pseudogenes, ie, AOX3P and 3L1P), mice and rats possess 4 functional AOX genes (namely, AOX1, 3, 4, and 3L1) (Garattini and Terao, 2011). Rhesus monkeys possess 2 functional AO (AOX3 and AOX3L1). In the mouse and monkey, AOX3L1 is expressed only in nasal mucosa (Garattini and Terao, 2011). A further complication is the observation of species differences in the relative roles of AO and XOR in xenobiotic biotransformation. For example, the 6-oxidation of antiviral deoxyguanine prodrugs is catalyzed exclusively in rats by XOR, but by AO in humans (Rettie and Fisher, 1999). Similarly, only human AO catalyzes the oxidation of 6-deoxypenciclovir to penciclovir (Strolin-Benedetti, 2011).

AO in human liver has proven to be rather unstable, which complicates an in vitro assessment of species differences in AO activity in frozen stocks of human liver cytosol (Rodrigues, 1994; Rettie and Fisher, 1999; Garattini and Terao, 2011). In addition, few human cell lines express functional AO (eg, HepG2 cells express the AOX1 transcript, but lack the functional enzyme) (Garattini and Terao, 2011). Fresh or cryopreserved human hepatocytes are therefore most likely to have relevant levels of AO activity.

AO is the second of 2 enzymes involved in the formation of cotinine, a major metabolite of nicotine excreted in the urine of cigarette smokers. The initial step in this reaction is the formation of a double bond (C=N) in the pyrrole ring, which produces nicotine $\Delta^{1',5'}$-iminium ion. Like nicotine, several other drugs are oxidized either sequentially or concomitantly by CYP and AO, including quinidine, azapetine, cyclophosphamide, carbazeran, and prolintane. Other drugs that are oxidized by AO include bromonidine, citalopram, proprionaldehyde, O^6-benzylguanine, 6-mercaptopurine, metyrapone, quinine, pyrazinamide, methotrexate, vanillin, isovanillin, zaleplon, and famciclovir (an antiviral prodrug that is converted by AO to penciclovir) (for additional examples, see Table 6-7). Several pyrimidine derivatives are oxidized by AO, including 5-ethyl-2(1*H*)-pyrimidone, which is converted by AO to 5-ethinyluracil. Like sorivudine, 5-ethinyluracil is a metabolism-dependent (suicide) inactivator of DPD (see Fig. 6-17).

Raloxifene is an extraordinarily potent inhibitor of human AO (K_i values as low as 0.9 nM), whereas it is at least 3 orders of magnitude less potent in other species (Obach, 2004; Pryde *et al.*, 2010). Perphenazine and menadione are also potent inhibitors of AO (IC_{50} ~0.03 and ~0.2 µM) and are often used together with allopurinol to discriminate between AO- and XOR-catalyzed reactions. The ability of proadifen to inhibit AO is noteworthy because this methadone analog, commonly known as SKF 525A, is widely used as a CYP inhibitor. Hydralazine is an irreversible (time-dependent) inhibitor of AO. Nitroso-imidacloprid has been characterized as a mechanism-based inhibitor of rabbit AO with a K_i value of 1.3 mM and k_{inact} of 0.35/min (Dick *et al.*, 2007). Several other inhibitors of AO have also been described, but raloxifene is probably the most useful for in vitro studies to evaluate the contribution of AO to the metabolism of a substrate (Pryde *et al.*, 2010). For instance, if a substrate that undergoes oxidative metabolism is found (1) to have higher in vitro turnover in human hepatocytes than in human liver microsomes, (2) is oxidized in human liver S9 or cytosol in the absence of NADPH, and (3) contains a structure amenable to oxidation by aldehyde oxidase, then raloxifene can be used to confirm involvement of aldehyde oxidase in the metabolism of the substrate (Pryde *et al.*, 2010).

Under certain conditions, AO and XOR can also catalyze the reduction of xenobiotics, including azo-reduction (eg, 4-dimethylaminoazobenzene), nitro-reduction (eg, 1-nitropyrene, imidacloprid and other nitroguanidines, nitromethylenes), *N*-oxide reduction (eg, *S*-(−)-nicotine-1′-*N*-oxide, imipramine *N*-oxide, and cyclobenzaprine *N*-oxide), nitrosamine reduction (eg, *N*-nitrosodiphenylamine), hydroxamic acid reduction (eg, *N*-hydroxy-2-acetylaminofluorene [NOH-AAF]), sulfoxide reduction (eg, sulindac; see Fig. 6-15, fenthion sulfoxide), quinone reduction (eg, diethylstilbestrol quinone), epoxide reduction (eg, B[*a*]P, 4,5-oxide), and heterocycle reduction (eg, ziprasidone and zonisamide) (Testa and Krämer, 2008, 2010; Pryde *et al.*, 2010). Oximes (C=NOH) can also be reduced by AO to the corresponding ketimines (C=NH), which may react nonenzymatically with water to produce the corresponding ketone or aldehyde (C=O) and ammonia (Testa and Krämer, 2008, 2010). The reduction of ziprasidone by AO is shown in Fig. 6-4, and examples of other reductive reactions catalyzed by AO are shown in Fig. 6-23. Xenobiotic reduction by AO in vitro requires anaerobic conditions or the presence of a reducing substrate, such as N^1-methylnicotinamide, 2-hydroxypyrimidine, or benzaldehyde. These "cosubstrates" reduce the enzyme, which in turn catalyzes azo-reduction, nitroreduction, etc, by relaying electrons to xenobiotics (rather than molecular oxygen). These unusual requirements make it difficult to assess the degree to which AO functions as a reductive enzyme in vivo.

Amine Oxidases Human amine oxidases can be divided into 2 classes: (I) the familiar FAD-containing mitochondrial MAOs, MAO-A and -B (gene symbols MAOA and MAOB), as well as polyamine oxidase (PAO; gene symbol PAOX) and spermine oxidase (gene symbol SMOX); and (II) the copper-containing amine oxidases (CuAOs) that contain a tightly bound Cu^{II} and a quinone residue (typically 2,4,5-trihydroxyphenylalanine quinone [TPQ]) as the redox cofactor (Largeron, 2011). The latter class of human amine oxidases belongs to the larger class of so-called quinoproteins class, which are present in plants, animals, fungi, yeast, and bacteria. In humans the CuAOs include (1) the intracellular lysyl oxidase (gene symbol LOX), (2) diamine oxidase (DAO; also known as AOC1 [from "amine-oxidase, copper-containing] and DAO [gene symbol ABP1, from "amiloride binding protein"]), and (3) the 2 known so-called semicarbazide-sensitive copper-containing amine oxidases (or SSAOs), which are located in plasma and the plasma membranes of various tissues (gene symbols AOC2 for the retina-specific amine oxidase and AOC3 for the gene encoding what is probably the originally identified SSAO, which is the same as vascular adhesion protein [VAP1]) (Largeron, 2011).

Class I amine oxidases differ markedly from class II amine oxidases in their substrate specificity, but there is some overlap. For instance, dopamine and tyramine are good substrates for MAOs, SSAOs, and DAO, whereas benzylamine is a good substrate for both MAOs and the CuAOs (Largeron, 2011). Features of some of these enzymes will be discussed below, with examples of reactions catalyzed by MAO, DAO, and PAO shown in Fig. 6-28.

Class I Amine Oxidases: MAO-A and B, PAO, and SMOX MAO (gene symbols MAOA and MAOB), spermine oxidase (gene symbol SMOX), and PAO (gene symbol PAOX) are involved in the oxidative deamination of primary, secondary, and tertiary amines (Benedetti, 2001; Agostinelli *et al.*, 2004; Edmondson *et al.*, 2004). Substrates for these enzymes include several naturally occurring amines, such as the monoamine serotonin (5-hydroxytryptamine), and monoacetylated derivatives of the polyamines spermine and spermidine. A number of xenobiotics are substrates for these enzymes, particularly MAOs. Oxidative deamination of a primary amine produces ammonia and an aldehyde, whereas oxidative deamination of a secondary amine produces a primary amine and an aldehyde. (The products of the former reaction—that is, an aldehyde and ammonia—are those produced during the reductive biotransformation of certain oximes by AO, as described in the section "Aldehyde Oxidase.") The aldehydes formed by MAO are usually oxidized further by other enzymes to the corresponding carboxylic acids, although in some cases they are reduced to alcohols.

MAO is located throughout the brain, and is present at high levels in the liver, kidney, intestine, heart, blood platelets, and blood vessels (but absent from erythrocytes) in the outer membrane of mitochondria (although some activity has been found in other cellular compartments, possibly because human liver microsomes prepared from frozen tissue are contaminated with the outer mitochondrial membrane) (Pearce *et al.*, 1996a; Testa and Krämer, 2008, 2010). Although MAOs are expressed in most tissues, there are some that express predominantly one form over the other. For example, MAO-A is the predominant form in human placenta, whereas MAO-B is the predominant form in human platelets, lymphocytes, and chromaffin cells (Strolin Benedetti *et al.*, 2007). MAO substrates include milacemide (Fig. 6-28), a dealkylated metabolite of propranolol (Fig. 6-28), primaquine, haloperidol, citalopram, sertraline, doxylamine, 1-methyl-4-phenyl-1,2,5,6-tetrahydropyridine (MPTP), β-phenylethylamine, tyramine, catecholamines (eg, dopamine, norepinephrine, epinephrine), tryptophan derivatives (tryptamine, serotonin), and tryptophan analogs known as triptans, which include the antimigraine drugs almotriptan, sumatriptan, zolmitriptan, and rizatriptan (Strolin Benedetti *et al.*, 2007; Testa and Krämer, 2008, 2010). In the case of the triptans, when a nitrogen exists in either a pyrrolidine or a piperidine ring, MAOs are not involved in their metabolism. Also, as a general rule, the introduction of a methyl group in the α-position relative to the nitrogen atom in what would otherwise be an MAO substrate renders it resistant to oxidative deamination by MAO (Strolin Benedetti *et al.*, 2007).

MAO-A preferentially oxidizes serotonin (5-hydroxytryptamine), norepinephrine, and the dealkylated metabolite of propranolol, and is preferentially inhibited by clorgyline, whereas MAO-B preferentially oxidizes β-phenylethylamine, benzylamine, and

citalopram, and is preferentially inhibited by L-deprenyl (selegiline) (Strolin Benedetti *et al.*, 2007). Species differences in the substrate specificity of MAO have been documented. For example, dopamine is oxidized by MAO-B in humans, but by MAO-A in rats, and by both enzymes in several other mammalian species. The distribution of MAO in the brain shows little species variation, with the highest concentration of MAO-A in the locus coeruleus, and the highest concentration of MAO-B in the raphe nuclei. MAO-A is expressed predominantly in catecholaminergic neurons, whereas MAO-B is expressed largely in serotonergic and histaminergic neurons and glial cells. The distribution of MAO throughout the brain does not always parallel that of its substrates. For example, serotonin is preferentially oxidized by MAO-A, but MAO-A is not found in serotonergic neurons.

The mechanism of catalysis by MAO is illustrated as follows:

$$RCH_2NH_2 + FAD \rightarrow RCH=NH + FADH_2;$$
$$RCH=NH + H_2O \rightarrow RCHO + NH_3;$$
$$FADH_2 + O_2 \rightarrow FAD + H_2O_2.$$

The substrate is oxidized by the enzyme, which itself is reduced (FAD $\rightarrow$ FADH$_2$). The oxygen incorporated into the substrate is derived from water, not molecular oxygen; hence, the enzyme functions as a true oxidase. The catalytic cycle is completed by reoxidation of the reduced enzyme (FADH$_2$ $\rightarrow$ FAD) by oxygen, which generates hydrogen peroxide (which may be a cause of oxidative stress). The initial step in the catalytic cycle is abstraction of hydrogen from the α-carbon adjacent to the nitrogen atom; hence, the oxidative deamination of xenobiotics by MAO is generally blocked by substitution of the α-carbon. For example, amphetamine and other phenylethylamine derivatives carrying a methyl group on the α-carbon atom are not oxidized well by MAO. (Amphetamines can undergo oxidative deamination, but the reaction is catalyzed by CYP.) The abstraction of hydrogen from the α-carbon adjacent to the nitrogen atom can occur stereospecifically; therefore, only one enantiomer of an α-substituted compound may be oxidized by MAO. For example, whereas MAO-B catalyzes the oxidative deamination of both *R*- and *S*-β-phenylethylamine, only the *R*-enantiomer is a substrate for MAO-A. The oxidative deamination of the dealkylated metabolite of propranolol is catalyzed stereoselectively by MAO-A, although in this case the preferred substrate is the *S*-enantiomer (which has the same absolute configuration as the *R*-enantiomer of β-phenylethylamine) (Benedetti and Dostert, 1994).

Clorgyline and L-deprenyl (selegiline) are metabolism-dependent inhibitors (ie, mechanism-based or suicide inactivators) of MAO-A and MAO-B, respectively. Both enzymes are irreversibly inhibited by phenelzine, a hydrazine that can be oxidized either by abstraction of hydrogen from the α-carbon atom, which leads to oxidative deamination with formation of benzaldehyde and benzoic acid, or by abstraction of hydrogen from the terminal nitrogen atom, which leads to formation of phenylethyldiazene and covalent modification of the enzyme, as shown in Fig. 6-28.

MAO has received considerable attention for its role in the activation of MPTP to a neurotoxin that causes symptoms characteristic of Parkinson disease in humans and monkeys but not rodents (Gerlach *et al.*, 1991). In 1983, Parkinsonism was observed in young individuals who, in attempting to synthesize and use a narcotic drug related to meperidine (Demerol®), instead synthesized and self-administered MPTP, which causes selective destruction of dopaminergic neurons in the substantia nigra. MPTP crosses the blood–brain barrier, where it is oxidized by MAO in the astrocytes (a type of glial cell) to 1-methyl-4-phenyl-2,3-dihydropyridine

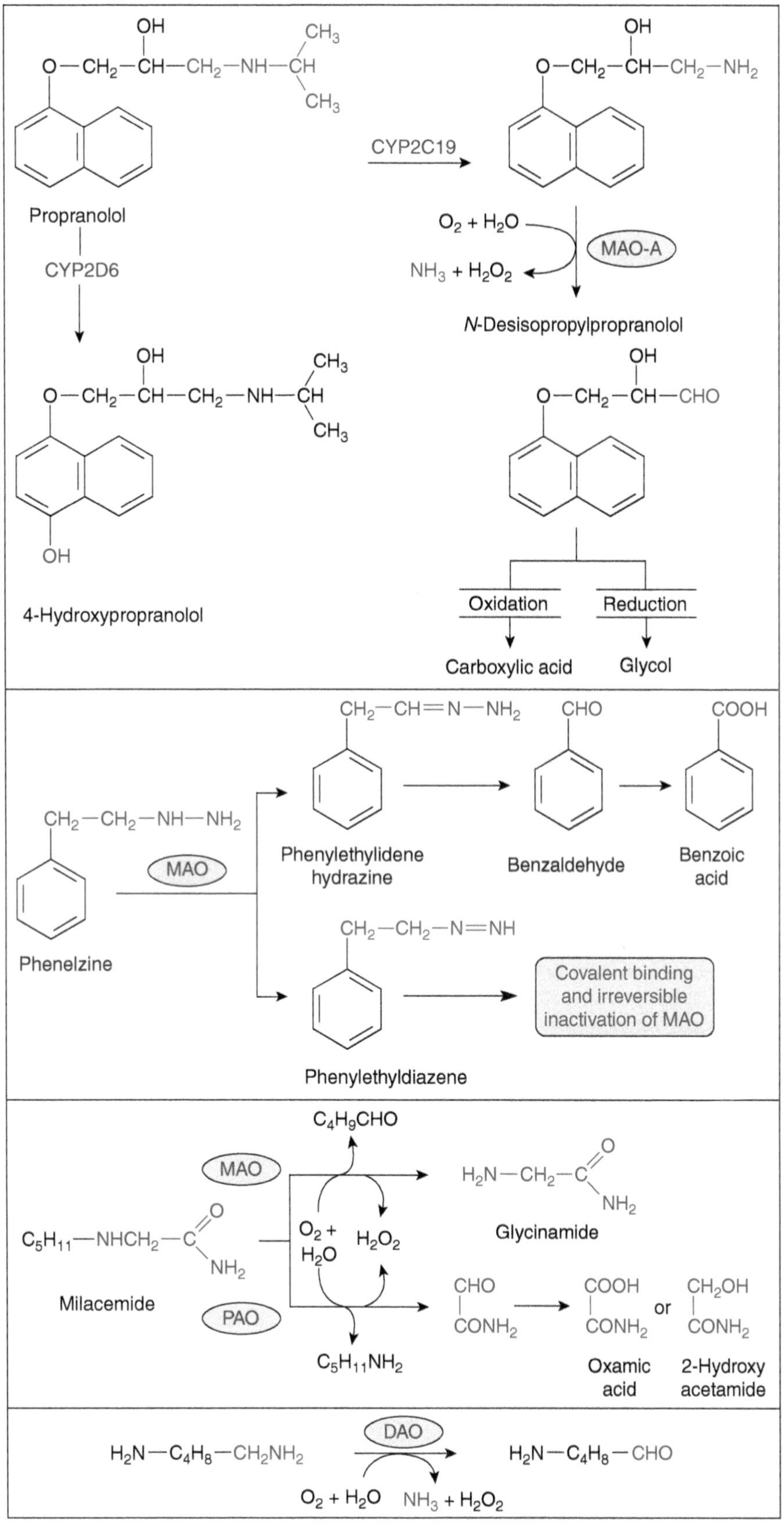

Figure 6-28. *Examples of reactions catalyzed by selected amine oxidases.* Note that phenelzine is a metabolism-dependent (mechanism-based) inhibitor of MAO-A and MAO-B.

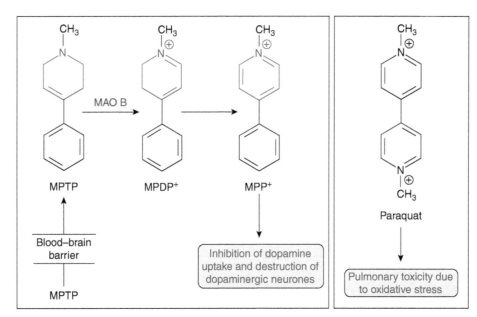

Figure 6-29. *Activation of 1-methyl-4-phenyl-1,2,5,6-tetrahydropyridine (MPTP) to the neurotoxic metabolite, 1-methyl-4-phenylpyridine (MPP+), by monoamine oxidase B.* The toxic pyridinium metabolite, MPP+, is structurally similar to the herbicide paraquat MPDP+, 1-methyl-4-phenyl-2,3-dihydropyridine.

(MPDP+), which in turn autoxidizes to the neurotoxic metabolite, 1-methyl-4-phenylpyridine (MPP+), as shown in Fig. 6-29. Because it is transported by the dopamine transporter, MPP+ concentrates in dopaminergic neurons, where it impairs mitochondrial respiration. The neurotoxic effects of MPTP can be blocked with pargyline (an inhibitor of both MAO-A and MAO-B) and by L-deprenyl (a selective inhibitor of MAO-B) but not by clorgyline (a selective inhibitor of MAO-A). This suggests that the activation of MPTP to its neurotoxic metabolite is catalyzed predominantly by MAO-B. This interpretation is consistent with the finding that MAO-B knockout mice (ie, transgenic mice that lack MAO-B) do not sustain damage to the dopaminergic terminals of nigrostriatal neurons after MPTP treatment (Shih *et al.*, 1999; Quinn *et al.*, 2007).

Both genetic and environmental factors appear to play important roles in the etiology of Parkinson disease. Apart from MPTP, Parkinsongenic neurotoxins to which humans are exposed have not been identified unequivocally; hence, the environmental factors that cause Parkinson disease remain to be identified. It is interesting that the bipyridyl herbicide, paraquat, is similar in structure to the toxic metabolite of MPTP, as shown in Fig. 6-29. Some epidemiological studies have shown a positive correlation between herbicide exposure and the incidence of Parkinsonism in some but not all rural communities. Haloperidol can also be converted to a potentially neurotoxic pyridinium metabolite (Subramanyam *et al.*, 1991).

MAO-B may be among the genetic factors that affect susceptibility to Parkinson disease. MAO-B activity in the human brain increases with aging, perhaps due to a proliferation of glial cells. It has been proposed that increased oxidation of dopamine by MAO-B in the elderly may lead to a loss of dopaminergic neurons in the substantia nigra, which underlies Parkinson disease. Such damage may be caused by the oxidative stress associated with the oxidative deamination of dopamine by MAO-B. In support of this proposal, patients with Parkinson disease have elevated MAO-B activity in the substantia nigra, and the MAO-B inhibitors L-deprenyl (selegiline), lazabemide, and rasagiline provide some symptomatic relief and can delay the progression of symptoms and need for levodopa (Sano *et al.*, 1997; Löhle and Reichmann, 2011). Furthermore, there are allelic variants of MAO-B, some of

which (such as alleles 1, A, B4, and G) appear to be associated with an increased risk of developing Parkinson disease, especially in women (Shih *et al.*, 1999; Kang *et al.*, 2006). No such association has been found between Parkinson disease and MAO-A gene polymorphisms (Williams-Gray *et al.*, 2009). Cigarette smoking, which carries a number of health risks, nevertheless provides some protection against Parkinson disease (Gorell *et al.*, 1999; Gu *et al.*, 2010). Although the mechanism of protection remains to be determined, it is interesting to note that cigarette smokers are known to have decreased levels of MAO-B (and MAO-A) (Shih *et al.*, 1999), the degree of which is proportional to cigarette usage (ie, it is dose related) (Whitfield *et al.*, 2000).

MAO-A knockout mice have elevated brain levels of serotonin and a distinct behavioral syndrome, including enhanced aggression in adult males. The enhanced aggressive behavior exhibited by MAO-A knockout mice is consistent with the abnormal aggressive behavior in individuals who lack MAO-A activity due to a point mutation in the MAO-A gene (Shih *et al.*, 1999). Other polymorphisms in the MAO-A gene appear to be risk factors for alcoholism among Euro-Americans and Han Chinese (Shih *et al.*, 1999). MAO-B may also be a factor in alcoholism inasmuch as alcoholics (especially male Type 2 alcoholics) tend to have lower MAO activity in platelets, which only contain MAO-B. However, MAO-B activity is not lower in alcoholics when cigarette smoking status is taken into account, which suggests that MAO-B activity tends to be lower in alcoholics because smoking and alcohol dependence are strongly associated with each other (Whitfield *et al.*, 2000).

Although not present in mitochondria, the PAO, PAOX (approved name: "polyamine oxidase [exo-N4-amino]"), and SMOX (approved name: "spermine oxidase") resemble MAO in their cofactor requirement and basic mechanism of action. These enzymes use oxygen as an electron acceptor, which results in the production of hydrogen peroxide. However, spermine and spermidine are first acetylated by spermidine/spermine N^1-acetyltransferases (gene symbols SAT1 and 2), and subsequently oxidized by PAOX, which produces not only hydrogen peroxide but also 3-acetamidopropanal (Hakkinen *et al.*, 2010). SMOX has very different substrate specificity, preferring nonacetylated polyamines (but not spermidine). The polyamines, spermine, spermidine, and the diamine precursor, putrescine (discussed below), are ubiquitous in mammalian cells. The intracellular levels of these amines are strictly controlled by several enzymes (including PAOX and SMOX) as well as various transporters (Hakkinen et al., 2010). Dysregulation of polyamine metabolism is associated with cancer and other diseases. Because of differences in polyamine regulation in various parasites, several xenobiotic polyamine synthesis inhibitors or substrates have been investigated as antiparasitic, chemopreventive, or chemotherapeutic drugs, including N-alkylated polyamine analogs such as diethylnorspermine, as well as some N-benzyl-substituted polyamines (Hakkinen et al., 2010).

The MAO inhibitor pargyline also inhibits PAOX. The anticonvulsant milacemide is one of the few xenobiotic substrates for PAOX (the structure of which is unrelated to polyamines), although it is also a substrate for MAO (Fig. 6-28) (Strolin Benedetti et al., 1992). By converting milacemide to glycine (via glycinamide), MAO plays an important role in the anticonvulsant therapy with milacemide (Benedetti and Dostert, 1994).

Class II Amine Oxidases (CuAOs): SSAOs, DAO, and LOX The term SSAO is confusing because the term has been previously used to refer only to amine oxidases that are active only toward primary amines, although this has not been proven, and several publications that mention SSAOs actually describe DAO. There are at least 3 types of SSAOs (Largeron, 2011). The first (which probably includes the original SSAO) has the recommended name PrAOs, for "primary amine oxidases," and includes gene symbols AOC2 and AOC3, the latter of which is probably the originally identified SSAO. The second SSAO is DAO (represented by AOC1; gene symbol ABP1, for "amiloride-binding protein"). A third type of SSAO is lysyl oxidase (LOX) (Largeron, 2011). All of these enzymes are CuAOs. In general, the SSAOs (ie, PrAOs) do oxidize primary monoamines and have little or no activity toward diamines. DAO (ABP1) oxidizes both diamines such as histamine and some primary amines. Neither DAO nor SSAOs have activity toward secondary and tertiary amines (Largeron, 2011). These PrAOs can be either soluble or membrane associated and are expressed in the liver, lung, lymph nodes, small intestine, and blood plasma (Testa and Krämer, 2008, 2010). The PrAO/SSAO known as AOC3 is a 180 kDa dimeric endothelial transmembrane glycoprotein that mediates leukocyte extravasation, for which reason it is widely known as the "vascular adhesion protein 1" [VAP1] (Kaitaniemi et al., 2009).

SSAOs/PrAOs catalyze fundamentally the same reaction catalyzed by MAO (Kaitaniemi et al., 2009):

$$RCH_2NH_2 + H_2O + O_2 \rightarrow RCHO + H_2O_2 + NH_3.$$

The endogenous roles of the CuAOs include regulating levels of endogenous and exogenous levels of primary monoamines and polyamines by catalyzing their oxidative deamination (eg, methylamine, putrescine, and cadaverine [and specific lysine residues of extracellular matrix proteins in the case of LOX]), which produces an aldehyde, hydrogen peroxide, and ammonia (Yraola et al., 2009; Largeron, 2011). Because all of the latter species are potentially cytotoxic, these metabolic pathways can activate endobiotics and xenobiotics. The activity of plasma CuAOs is generally increased in various disease states, including Alzheimer disease, congestive heart failure, cirrhosis, Type 1 and 2 diabetes, atherosclerosis, and other inflammatory conditions, which leads to the overproduction of toxic species, especially aldehydes and hydrogen peroxide, and may further contribute to the disease process (Largeron, 2011).

Although CuAOs do not play a large role in xenobiotic oxidation, there is some evidence for the involvement of SSAOs

in the oxidative deamination of a few xenobiotics, including allylamine, primaquine, mescaline, amlodipine, and amifostine (Testa and Krämer, 2008, 2010; Largeron, 2011). The calcium channel blocker amlodipine is first oxidized (mainly by CYP3A4) to dehydroamlodipine, with subsequent deamination to an aldehyde (consistent with the action of an SSAO) and finally oxidation to the corresponding carboxylic acid by an ALDH and/or AO (Largeron, 2011). Amifostine is a thiophosphate prodrug used as a cytoprotective adjuvant used in cancer chemotherapy and radiotherapy; it is rapidly converted to 2-[3-aminopropylamino] ethanethiol by alkaline phosphatase followed by oxidative deamination catalyzed by one or more CuAOs to an aldehyde that spontaneously decomposes to acrolein and cysteamine (Largeron, 2011). Benzylamine (and several analogs) may be used in vitro as a substrate for SSAOs (Yraola et al., 2009). MAO-B can also catalyze the deamination of benzylamine, but MAO-B acts by removal of the *pro-R* H-atom, whereas SSAOs act by removal of the *pro-S* H-atom (Testa and Krämer, 2008, 2010). There also appear to be some substrate selectivity between the individual SSAOs, AOC2 and 3, in that the preferred in vitro substrates of AOC2 (highly expressed in the retina) include 2-phenylethylamine, tryptamine, and tyramine, rather than the benzylamines and methylamine, which appear to be the preferred substrates for AOC3 (Kaitaniemi et al., 2009).

DAO is a cytosolic, copper-containing, pyridoxal phosphate-dependent enzyme that is highly expressed in lung, liver, kidney, intestine, and placenta, among other tissues, for which 2 crystal structures have been described (McGrath et al., 2010). It is located in the extracellular space (secreted form) or in the endoplasmic reticulum (Testa and Krämer, 2008, 2010). Its preferred substrates include histamine and simple alkyl diamines with a 4- or 5-carbon chain length such as putresine (1,4-diaminobutane) and cadaverine (1,5-diaminopentane) (McGrath et al., 2010). Diamines with carbon chains longer than 9 are not substrates for DAO, although they can be oxidized by MAO. DAO or a similar enzyme is present in cardiovascular tissue and appears to be responsible for the cardiotoxic effects of allylamine, which is converted by oxidative deamination to acrolein. Although histamine is a substrate for DAO (which catalyzes oxidative deamination of the primary amine to imidazole acetaldehyde by the secreted DAO) (McGrath et al., 2010), there is little DAO in brain (nor is there a receptor-mediated uptake system for histamine, in contrast to other neurotransmitters). For this reason, the major pathway of histamine metabolism in the brain is by methylation (see the section "Methylation").

Aromatization The conversion of MPTP to MPP$^+$ (Fig. 6-29) is an example of a xenobiotic whose oxidation involves the introduction of multiple double bonds to achieve some semblance of aromaticity (in this case, formation of a pyridinium ion). Aromatization of xenobiotics is an unusual reaction, but some examples have been documented. A mitochondrial enzyme in guinea pig and rabbit liver can oxidize several cyclohexane derivatives to the corresponding aromatic hydrocarbon, as shown in Fig. 6-30 for the aromatization of cyclohexane carboxylic acid (hexahydrobenzoic acid) to benzoic acid. Mitochondria from rat liver are less active, and those from cat, mouse, dog, monkey, and human are inactive (Mitoma et al., 1958). The reaction requires magnesium, CoA, oxygen, and ATP. The first step is the formation of hexahydrobenzoyl-CoA, which is then dehydrogenated to the aromatic product. Glycine stimulates the reaction, probably by removing benzoic acid through conjugation to form hippuric acid. The conversion of androgens to estrogens involves aromatization of the A-ring of the steroid nucleus. This reaction is catalyzed by CYP19A1, one of the CYP enzymes involved in steroidogenesis. The major substrate of CYP19A1 is

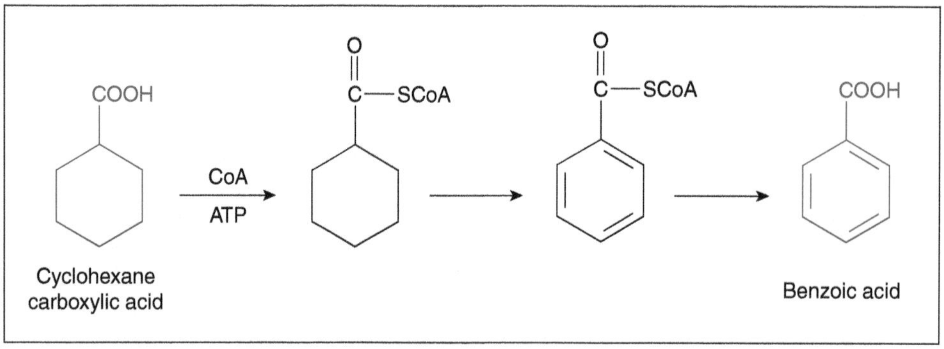

Figure 6-30. *Aromatization of cyclohexane carboxylic acid, a reaction catalyzed by rabbit and guinea pig liver mitochondria.*

androstenedione, which is converted to estrone by 3 successive oxidation steps (Kuhl and Wiegratz, 2007). Gut microflora can catalyze aromatization reactions, as shown in Fig. 6-1 for the conversion of quinic acid to benzoic acid.

Evidence for the apparent aromatization of a few xenobiotics by other P450 enzyme has also been described. For instance, 19-nortestosterone derivatives can be converted to aromatic metabolites, namely, ethinylestradiol (from norethisterone and norethynodrel) and 7α-methylethinylestradiol (from tibolone) (Kuhl and Wiegratz, 2007). Formation of these A-ring aromatized steroids occurs in the liver, which does not express the steroidogenic enzyme CYP19A1 (aromatase). In addition, indoline (and some derivatives) is aromatized to indole in human liver microsomes, and mainly by recombinant human CYP3A4 (as well as CYP1A2, 2B6, 2C19, 2D6, and 2E1) by a dehydrogenation pathway (Sun et al., 2007). The aromatization mechanism involves two one-electron oxidations, which is different from that catalyzed by CYP19A1, which catalyzes 2 sequential carbon oxidations followed by cleavage of a carbon–carbon bond (Sun et al., 2007). The indoline-containing diuretic, indapamide, is also dehydrogenated to the aromatic indole by CYP3A4 (Sun et al., 2009). This type of dehydrogenation can lead to P450 inactivation, as exemplified by the mechanism-based inhibition of CYP3A4 by the 3-alkylindole-containing TNFα inhibitor, SPD-304, which forms an electrophilic 3-methylenindolenine (Sun and Yost, 2008).

Peroxidase-Dependent Cooxidation The oxidative biotransformation of xenobiotics generally requires the reduced pyridine nucleotide cofactors, NADPH and NADH, although oxidation by AO and MAO is a notable exception. Another exception is xenobiotic biotransformation by peroxidases, which are heme-containing enzymes that couple the reduction of hydrogen peroxide (or a lipid hydroperoxide) to the one-electron oxidation of other substrates (O'Brien, 2000; Tafazoli and O'Brien, 2005). Several different peroxidases catalyze the biotransformation of xenobiotics (in addition to performing important physiological functions), and these enzymes occur in a variety of tissues and cell types. Peroxidases do not play an important role in the first-pass metabolism or clearance of drugs and most other xenobiotics because their contribution is usually negligible compared with CYP and other oxidative enzymes. However, peroxidases do play an important role in xenobiotic toxicity, especially the activation of drugs associated with idiosyncratic hepatotoxicity, blood dyscrasias (eg, agranulocytosis, neutropenia, aplastic anemia, and thrombocytopenia), and skin rashes, and the activation of xenobiotics (including the activation of proximate carcinogens to ultimate carcinogens) in skin, bladder, bone marrow, and various other extrahepatic tissues. As shown in Fig. 6-2, peroxidases form reactive intermediates by converting nitrogen- and sulfur-containing xenobiotics to heteroatom-centered radicals (Tang and Lu, 2010; Walsh and Miwa, 2011).

In humans, the family of peroxidases includes myeloperoxidase (gene symbol MPO), eosinophil peroxidase (EPO; gene symbol EPX), lactoperoxidase (gene symbol LPO), thyroid peroxidase (gene symbol TPO), catalase, 2 forms of prostaglandin H synthase (also known as PHS1 and 2 or cyclooxygenase-1 [COX-1] and COX-2; gene symbols PTGS1 and 2), as well as the selenium-containing glutathione peroxidases (gene symbols GPX1-8). Some basic features of these peroxidases are summarized in Table 6-8.

Table 6-8

Characteristics of Some Human Peroxidases

PEROXIDASES	CELLULAR LOCATION	SUBCELLULAR LOCATION	HOMOLOGY WITH MPO
Myeloperoxidase (MPO)	Neutrophils, leukocytes	Lysosomes (human milk)	100%
Eosinophil peroxidase (EPO)	Eosinophils	Lysosomes	70%
Lactoperoxidase (LPO)	Mammary duct epithelial cells	Saliva, tears (bovine milk)	61%
Thyroid peroxidase (TPO)	Thyroid follicular cells	Microsomes, Golgi	47%

Prostaglandin-H synthase
  PHS1 (COX-1)[*]
  PHS2 (COX-2)[*]
	
	Numerous extrahepatic tissues
	Inflammatory cells
		
		Microsomes
		Microsomes	

Data from O'Brien (2000).

[*]*There are 2 forms of prostaglandin H synthase, PHS1 and PHS2; they are the peroxidase component of the bifunctional enzymes known as COX-1 and COX-2 (gene symbols PTGS1 and PTGS2), respectively.*

These peroxidases all have physiological functions: MPO, EPO, and LPO are lysosomal enzymes present in neutrophils, eosinophils, and secretory cells of exocrine glands, respectively. During infection, MPO and EPO are released into phagocytic vacuoles (granules) and into the plasma, whereas LPO is released into saliva and tears, where they kill microorganisms and thereby provide protection against infectious agents such as bacteria and parasites. (Peroxidases are also present in milk: LPO is the predominant peroxidase in cow's milk, whereas MPO is the predominant peroxidase in human milk.) The hydrogen peroxide required by MPO and EPO is produced by a membrane-bound NADPH oxidase that is activated by the presence of infectious agents. Unlike MPO, EPO, and LPO, which are soluble enzymes, TPO is a membrane-bound peroxidase located on the apical membrane of thyroid follicular cells; it catalyzes the iodination of tyrosine residues and the oxidative coupling of di-iodinated and monoiodinated tyrosine residues in thyroglobulin to form T3- and thyroxine (T4)–bound thyroglobulin, from which thyroid hormones are released. An NAD(P)H-oxidase known as p138 TOX (gene symbol DUOX2), which is also localized on the apical plasma membrane, produces the hydrogen peroxide required by TPO to synthesize thyroid hormones. PHS1 and PHS2 are the peroxidase component of COX-1 and COX-2; they are enzymes that convert arachidonic acid (and closely related fatty acids) to a variety of eicosanoids (prostaglandins, leukotrienes, thromboxane, and prostacyclin). In contrast to the other peroxidases, PHS1 and PHS2 do not require a source of hydrogen peroxide (although they can use it); hence, their activity is not dependent on an H_2O_2-generating NAD(P)H-oxidase. Catalase is also a peroxidase. This peroxisomal enzyme catalyzes the disproportionation of hydrogen peroxide to water and oxygen ($2H_2O_2 \rightarrow 2H_2O + O_2$). At low concentrations of hydrogen peroxide, catalase can catalyze the oxidation of ethanol (see Fig. 6-25) and various other small molecules. GPXs are a family of selenium-containing enzymes that also detoxify hydrogen peroxide (and lipid hydroperoxides) by reducing it to water, which is associated with the formation of oxidized GSH as follows:

$$2GSH + HOOH \rightarrow GS\text{-}SG + 2H_2O.$$

In mammalian peroxidases (in contrast to plant peroxidases), the heme prosthetic group is covalently attached to the enzyme. Iron is bound to 4 pyrrole nitrogen atoms with the nitrogen on the imidazole ring of histidine serving as the usual fifth ligand. The sixth coordination position is vacant so that peroxidases can interact with hydrogen peroxide (or other hydroperoxides), just as the sixth coordinate position of hemoglobin and myoglobin (both of which have low peroxidase activity) is available to bind molecular oxygen (Tafazoli and O'Brien, 2005). The oxidation of a xenobiotic ($X \rightarrow XO$ or $2XH \rightarrow 2X^\bullet + H_2O$) by peroxidase involves the conversion of hydrogen peroxide to water or the conversion of a hydroperoxide to the corresponding alcohol ($ROOH \rightarrow ROH$), during which the peroxidase (Fe^{III}) is converted to spectrophotometrically distinct states known as compound I and compound II, shown as follows for the conversion of a xenobiotic phenol (XOH) to the corresponding phenoxyl radical ($XO^\bullet$) (Tafazoli and O'Brien, 2005):

$$\text{Peroxidase} + ROOH \rightarrow \text{compound I} + ROH;$$
$$\text{Compound I} + XOH \rightarrow \text{compound II} + XO^\bullet + H^+;$$
$$\text{Compound II} + XOH \rightarrow \text{peroxidase} + XO^\bullet + H_2O.$$

In this example, the hydroperoxide is converted to the corresponding alcohol ($ROOH \rightarrow ROH$), and the peroxyl oxygen atom is reduced to water (H_2O) by the one-electron oxidation of 2 molecules of xenobiotic (XOH) to produce 2 xenobiotic radicals ($XO^\bullet$). In some cases, the oxygen from the hydroperoxide is incorporated into the xenobiotic itself ($XH \rightarrow XOH$). Examples of each reaction are given later in this section. The conversion of ROOH to ROH involves the release of an oxygen atom that coordinates with the heme iron (initially in the ferric or Fe^{III} state). This iron-bound oxygen formally contains only 6 (instead of 8) valence electrons, making it a powerful oxidizing species. One electron is removed from the iron to produce $Fe^{IV}=O$, and a second electron is removed from the tetrapyrrole ring to produce a π-porphyrin cation radical ($Por^{\bullet+}$), which corresponds to compound I ($Fe^{IV}=O\text{-}Por^{\bullet+}$). The transfer of an electron from a xenobiotic ($XOH \rightarrow XO^\bullet + H^+$) to the porphyrin cation radical produces compound II ($Fe^{IV}=O\text{-}Por$). In some cases, such as PHS, the electron donated to the initial Fe=O complex comes directly or indirectly from an amino acid rather than the tetrapyrrole ring, and this accounts in part for some of the differences among the various peroxidases (such as the ability of TPO to catalyze the iodination of tyrosine residues and the subsequent formation of thyroid hormones).

Although peroxidases are renowned for catalyzing one-electron oxidation reactions, they can catalyze the 2-electron oxidation of iodide (I^-) to hypoiodous acid (HOI) and iodine which, in the case of TPO, is important for the synthesis of thyroid hormones:

$$\text{Peroxidase compound I(O)} + I^- + H^+ \rightarrow HOI;$$
$$\text{Peroxidase compound I(O)} + 2 \times I^- + H^+ \rightarrow I_2 \text{ (iodine)} + OH^-.$$

MPO, EPO, and LPO can all oxidize the pseudohalide thiocyanate (SCN^-) faster than iodide, which in turn is oxidized faster than bromide, which is oxidized much faster than chloride. In fact, MPO is the only peroxidase with appreciable ability to oxidize chloride to hypochlorous acid (HOCl). There is an inverse relationship between the rate of conversion of halides to hypohalous acids and their physiological plasma concentrations: chloride = 100 to 140 mM, bromide = 20 to 100 μM, and iodide = 0.1 to 0.5 μM. Consequently, the relatively low rate of chloride oxidation is offset by the high levels of chloride such that about half (20%–70%) of the hydrogen peroxide produced by activated neutrophils is converted to HOCl, which reacts with GSH, proteins, thiols, amines, unsaturated fatty acids, and cholesterol, all of which disrupt cell membranes and lead to cell lysis and death (of both infectious organisms and host cells). Formation of HOCl by MPO is important not only from a physiological perspective but also from a drug metabolism and toxicity perspective, as discussed later in this section. The preferred "halide" substrate for MPO is thiocyanate, which is present in plasma at concentrations ranging from 20 to 120 μM, which is sufficiently high that oxidation of thiocyanate consumes the other half of the hydrogen peroxide produced by activated neutrophils. Whereas MPO oxidizes chloride to HOCl, which is cytotoxic, it oxidizes thiocyanate to thiocyanogen (SCN_2), which rapidly hydrolyzes to hypothiocyanic acid (HOSCN). HOSCN is much less reactive and cytotoxic than HOCl, such that the oxidation of thiocyanate by peroxidases is a mechanism to remove hydrogen peroxide without forming HOCl. This represents an important mechanism of hydrogen peroxide detoxication in saliva, which contains low levels of catalase but high levels (1-5 mM) of thiocyanate, and in the stomach, where the levels of thiocyanate in parietal cells are 3 times greater than plasma levels, which allows gastric peroxidase to inactivate hydrogen peroxide that otherwise stimulates gastric acid secretion by stimulating histamine release from mast cells. Inactivation of gastric peroxidase by aspirin, dexamethasone, indomethacin, or methimazole can result in gastric ulceration due to impaired detoxication of hydrogen peroxide and impaired synthesis of cytoprotective prostaglandins (O'Brien, 2000).

MPO and EPO can be distinguished by (1) their cellular distribution (neutrophils/leukocytes vs eosinophils); (2) their ability to oxidize halides (MPO is better than EPO at converting chloride to HOCl, whereas EPO is better than MPO at converting bromide to hypobromous acid), and (3) their sensitivity to inhibitors (MPO is more sensitive to the inhibitory effect of cyanide over azide, whereas the opposite is true of EPO).

The level of EPO (or a related peroxidase) in uterine epithelial cells is regulated by estrogen; uterine peroxidase activity is inducible several hundred-fold by estrogenic steroids, including the synthetic estrogens diethylstilbestrol and tamoxifen. The level of TPO in thyroid follicular cells is regulated by TSH. The enzyme is inactivated by a variety of ethylenethiourea drugs, such as propylthiouracil and methimazole (which is used as an antithyroid drug in patients with Graves disease), as well as a number of naturally occurring flavonoid/resorcinol compounds that also have antithyroid effects. By inactivating TPO and impairing thyroid hormone synthesis, these chemicals trigger a large and prolonged increase in TSH that in rodents (but apparently not in humans) can result in thyroid follicular cell tumor formation.

MPO is an abundant enzyme in granulocytes, where it accounts for 5% of the dry weight. It can be used as a diagnostic marker to differentiate myeloid leukemia from lymphoid leukemia. MPO is one of the peroxidases implicated in the formation of reactive metabolites of drugs that cause idiosyncratic agranulocytosis (or other blood dyscrasias), including clozapine, aminopyrine, vesnarinone, propylthiouracil, dapsone, remoxipride, sulfonamides, procainamide, amodiaquine, and ticlopidine (Liu and Uetrecht, 2000; O'Brien, 2000; Tafazoli and O'Brien, 2005; Testa and Krämer, 2008, 2010). The nitro-reduced metabolite of tolcapone can be converted to a reactive *ortho*-quinoneimine by MPO and potentially lead to hepatotoxicity (Testa and Krämer, 2008, 2010). Many of these drugs are aromatic amines, and both MPO and PHS have also been implicated in the activation of several carcinogenic aromatic amines, such as benzidine, methylaminoazobenzene, and aminofluorene. Furthermore, inactivating polymorphisms in MPO (such as MPO-463A) appear to afford protection against both the activation of aromatic amines and PAH in tobacco smoke and the tumor-promoting effects of hydrogen peroxide formed by tobacco smoke–activated neutrophils (O'Brien, 2000).

In the presence of hydrogen peroxide and chloride (which are converted to HOCl by MPO), activated neutrophils and monocytes (including Kupffer cells) oxidize the aforementioned drugs to reactive intermediates (such as nitrogen-centered radicals, hydroxylamines, *N*-chloramines, and, in the case of aromatic amines with a hydroxyl group in the *para*-position, quinoneimines or the corresponding semiquinoneimine radicals). In the case of ticlopidine, MPO converts the thiophene ring of this antiplatelet drug to a thiophene-*S*-chloride, a reactive metabolite that rearranges to 2-chloroticlopidine (minor) and dehydro-ticlopidine (major), or reacts with GSH, as shown in Fig. 6-31. When catalyzed by activated neutrophils, ticlopidine oxidation is inhibited by low concentrations of azide and catalase. When catalyzed by purified myeloperoxidase, ticlopidine oxidation requires hydrogen peroxide and chloride, although all components of this purified system can be replaced with HOCl. It is not known whether drugs that cause agranulocytosis are activated in the bone marrow by neutrophils or their precursors that contain myeloperoxidase, or are activated in neutrophils in the general circulation. In the latter case, agranulocytosis would presumably involve an immune response triggered by neoantigens formed in neutrophils by the covalent modification of cellular component by one or more of the reactive metabolites formed by MPO. MPO is also present in Kupffer cells, which release the enzyme in the liver upon activation by hydrogen peroxide. It is possible to increase the toxicity of hydralazine (which is associated with the development of hepatitis and centrilobular necrosis) toward cultured hepatocytes by the inclusion of a hydrogen peroxide–generating system (Tafazoli and O'Brien, 2008).

MPO has also been implicated in the formation of pro-oxidant phenoxyl radicals of etoposide, a topoisomerase inhibitor that can cause myelogenous leukemia, and both MPO and PHS have been implicated in the formation of phenoxyl radicals of benzene, an industrial solvent linked to bone marrow suppression and leukemia. MPO and PHS cannot oxidize benzene itself. Liver CYP converts benzene to phenol, which in turn is oxidized to hydroquinone, which can be converted to DNA-reactive metabolites by MPO in bone marrow leukocytes and by PHS in bone marrow. The myelosuppressive effect of benzene can be blocked by the PHS inhibitor, indomethacin, which suggests an important role for PHS-dependent activation in the myelotoxicity of benzene. The formation of phenol and hydroquinone in the liver is also important for myelosuppression by benzene. However, such bone marrow suppression cannot be achieved simply by administering phenol or hydroquinone to mice, although it can be achieved by coadministering hydroquinone with phenol. Phenol stimulates the MPO- and PHS-dependent activation of hydroquinone. Therefore, bone marrow suppression by benzene involves the CYP-dependent oxidation of benzene to phenol and hydroquinone in the liver, followed by the phenol-enhanced, MPO- and PHS-catalyzed peroxidative oxidation of hydroquinone to reactive intermediates that bind to protein and DNA in the bone marrow (Fig. 6-32). It is noteworthy that the CYP enzyme responsible for hydroxylating benzene has been identified as CYP2E1 (see the section "Cytochrome P450"). Although CYP2E1 was first identified in liver, this same enzyme has been identified in bone marrow where it can presumably convert benzene to phenol and possibly hydroquinone. The importance of CYP2E1 in the metabolic activation of benzene was confirmed by the demonstration that CYP2E1 knockout mice are relatively resistant to the myelosuppressive effects of benzene (Gonzalez, 2003; Gonzalez and Yu, 2006). MPO has also been shown to convert phenol to diols. Benzene-diols are good substrates of EPO, LPO, and MPO and their oxidation by peroxidases leads to oxidative stress (Testa and Krämer, 2008, 2010).

Prostaglandin H synthase (formally known as prostaglandin-endoperoxide synthase 1 and 2, and also widely known as cyclooxygenase 1 and 2; gene symbols PTGS1 and 2 and collectively referred to below as "PHS") is one of the most extensively studied peroxidases involved in xenobiotic biotransformation. As shown in Fig. 6-33, PHS is a dual-function enzyme composed of a *cyclooxygenase*, which converts arachidonic acid to PGG_2, a 15-hydroperoxide-endoperoxide (which involves the addition of 2 molecules of oxygen to each molecule of arachidonic acid), and a *peroxidase* that converts the 15-hydroperoxide to the corresponding 15-alcohol PGH_2, which can be accompanied by the oxidation of xenobiotics (a "cosubstrate") and formation of ROS (Ramkissoon and Wells, 2011). PHS1 is localized in the endoplasmic reticulum and nuclear envelope and is constitutively expressed in a wide variety of tissues that synthesize and release eicosanoids (prostaglandins, leukotrienes, thromboxane, prostacyclin), which generally bind to G-coupled cell surface receptors and regulate cellular function, largely in a paracrine (local) fashion (Ramkissoon and Wells, 2011). In contrast, PHS2 is expressed in cells that respond to inflammatory cytokines, mitogens, tumor promoters, and AhR agonists (ie, agents such as TNFα, LPS, phorbol esters, TPA, TCDD) such as the macula densa of the kidney, the vas deferens, and certain regions of the brain (Ramkissoon and Wells, 2011). PGH2 produces prostaglandins that activate receptors on the

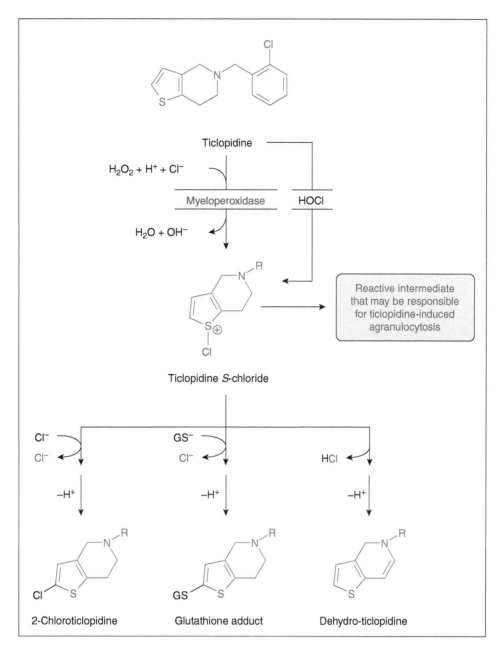

Figure 6-31. *Activation of ticlopidine to a reactive thiophene-S-chloride by myeloperoxidase.*

nuclear membrane, and high levels of the enzyme are expressed in colorectal and other tumors, which appear to be important for tumor promotion and angiogenesis (the process of stimulating the blood vessel supply). Both enzymes play an important role in the activation of xenobiotics to toxic or tumorigenic metabolites, particularly in extrahepatic tissues that contain low levels of CYP. PHS2 (COX-2) also plays an important role in the subsequent response of tissues to cell damage and tumor initiation, and is a possible target for the treatment or prevention of certain types of cancer. Increasing evidence suggests that inhibition of COX-2 by NSAIDs may be part of the mechanism whereby these drugs protect against colon and other gastrointestinal cancers (Dubé *et al.*, 2007; Wu *et al.*, 2010). PHS has been evaluated for its contribution to the activation of phenytoin and other antiepileptic drugs, B[*a*]P, thalidomide, methamphetamine, and 3,4-methylenedioxymethamphetamine (Ramkissoon and Wells, 2011).

In certain cases, the oxidation of xenobiotics by peroxidases involves direct transfer of the peroxide oxygen to the xenobiotic, as shown in Fig. 6-33 for the conversion of substrate X to product XO. An example of this type of reaction is the PHS-catalyzed epoxidation of B[*a*]P 7,8-dihydrodiol to the corresponding 9,10-epoxide (see Fig. 6-10). Although PHS can catalyze the final step (ie, 9,10-epoxidation) in the formation of this tumorigenic metabolite of B[*a*]P, it cannot catalyze the initial step (ie, 7,8-epoxidation), which is catalyzed by CYP. Several lines of evidence suggest that both PHS1 and PHS2 play an important role in PAH-induced skin carcinogenesis. First, both PHS1 knockout and PHS2 knockout mice are resistant to PAH-induced skin cancer. (It is noteworthy that PHS1 knockout mice appear normal despite having only 1% of the prostaglandin levels of wild-type mice, whereas only 60% of PHS2 knockout mice survive until weaning, and the 40% that survive past weaning usually die within a year of kidney disease.) Both resveratrol (an inhibitor of PHS1 and CYP1A1) and SC-58125 (an inhibitor of PHS2) block PAH-induced skin cancer in mice.

PHS can also catalyze the 8,9-epoxidation of aflatoxin B$_1$, which is one of the most potent hepatotumorigens known.

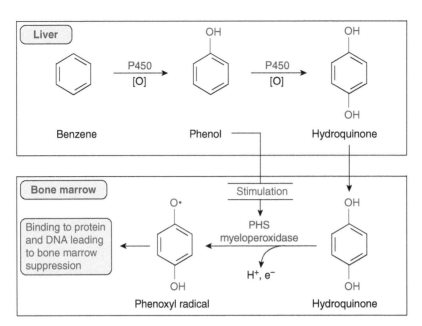

Figure 6-32. *Role of cytochrome P450 and peroxidases in the activation of benzene to myelotoxic metabolites.*

Epoxidation by CYP is thought to be primarily responsible for the hepatotumorigenic effects of aflatoxin B₁. However, aflatoxin B₁ also causes neoplasia of rat renal papilla. This tissue has very low levels of CYP, but contains relatively high levels of PHS, which is suspected, therefore, of mediating the nephrotumorigenic effects of aflatoxin (Fig. 6-34).

The direct transfer of the peroxide oxygen from a hydroperoxide to a xenobiotic is neither the only mechanism of xenobiotic oxidation by peroxidases nor the most common. Xenobiotics that can serve as electron donors, such as amines and phenols, can be oxidized to free radicals during the reduction of a hydroperoxide. In this case, the hydroperoxide is still converted to the corresponding alcohol, but the peroxide oxygen is reduced to water instead of being incorporated into the xenobiotic. For each molecule of hydroperoxide reduced (which is a 2-electron process), 2 molecules of xenobiotic can be oxidized (each by a one-electron process). Important classes of compounds that undergo one-electron oxidation reactions by peroxidase include aromatic amines, phenols, hydroquinones, and polycyclic hydrocarbons. Many of the metabolites produced are reactive electrophiles. For example, PAHs, phenols, and hydroquinones are oxidized to electrophilic quinones. Acetaminophen is similarly converted to a quinoneimine, namely, *N*-acetyl-benzoquinoneimine, a cytotoxic electrophile that binds to cellular proteins, as shown in Fig. 6-35. The formation of this toxic metabolite by CYP causes centrilobular necrosis of the liver. However, acetaminophen can also damage the kidney medulla, which contains low levels of CYP but relatively high levels of PHS; hence, PHS may play a significant role in the nephrotoxicity of acetaminophen. The 2-electron oxidation of acetaminophen to *N*-acetyl-benzoquinoneimine by PHS likely involves the formation of a one-electron oxidation product, namely, *N*-acetyl-benzosemiquinoneimine radical. Formation of this semiquinoneimine radical by PHS likely contributes to the nephrotoxicity of acetaminophen and related compounds, such as phenacetin and 4-aminophenol. Metabolites of the NSAID diclofenac (namely, 4′-hydroxydiclofenac and 5-hydroxydiclofenac) can also be converted to benzoquinoneimines by peroxidases (Testa and Krämer, 2008, 2010).

Like the kidney medulla, urinary bladder epithelium also contains low levels of CYP but relatively high levels of PHS. Just as

PHS in kidney medulla can ostensibly activate aflatoxin and acetaminophen to nephrotoxic metabolites, so PHS in urinary bladder epithelium can potentially activate certain aromatic amines, such as benzidine, 4-aminobiphenyl, and 2-aminonaphthalene, to DNA-reactive metabolites that cause bladder cancer in certain species, including humans and dogs. PHS can convert aromatic amines to reactive radicals, which can undergo nitrogen–nitrogen or nitrogen–carbon coupling reactions, or they can undergo a second one-electron oxidation to reactive diimines. Binding of these reactive metabolites to DNA is presumed to be one of the underlying mechanisms by which several aromatic amines cause bladder cancer in humans and dogs. In some cases the one-electron oxidation of an amine leads to *N*-dealkylation. For example, PHS catalyzes the *N*-demethylation of aminopyrine, although in vivo this reaction is mainly catalyzed by CYP. In contrast to CYP, PHS does not appear to catalyze the *N*-hydroxylation of carcinogenic aromatic amines (an important step in their metabolic activation), although MPO and LPO have been shown to catalyze this reaction. In liver, activation of aromatic amines by *N*-hydroxylation is catalyzed predominantly by CYP1A2, whereas this same reaction in the bladder epithelium appears to be catalyzed by another enzyme, possibly a CYP enzyme other than CYP1A2, such as CYP2A13, CYP4B1, or CYP2S1 (Nakajima *et al.*, 2006), or a peroxidase other than PHS.

Many of the aromatic amines known or suspected of causing bladder cancer in humans have been shown to cause bladder tumors in dogs. In rats, however, aromatic amines cause liver tumors by a process that is thought to involve *N*-hydroxylation by CYP, followed by conjugation with acetate or sulfonate, as shown in Fig. 6-12. This species difference has complicated an assessment of the role of PHS in aromatic amine–induced bladder cancer, because such experiments must be carried out in dogs. However, another class of compounds, the 5-nitrofurans, such as *N*-[4-(5-nitro-2-furyl)-2-thiazole]formamide (FANFT) and its deformylated analog 2-amino-4-(5-nitro-2-furyl)thiazole (ANFT), are substrates for PHS and are potent bladder tumorigens in rats. The tumorigenicity of FANFT is thought to involve deformylation to ANFT, which is oxidized to DNA-reactive metabolites by PHS. The ability of FANFT to cause bladder tumors in rats is blocked by the COX inhibitor, aspirin, which suggests that PHS plays an important role in the metabolic

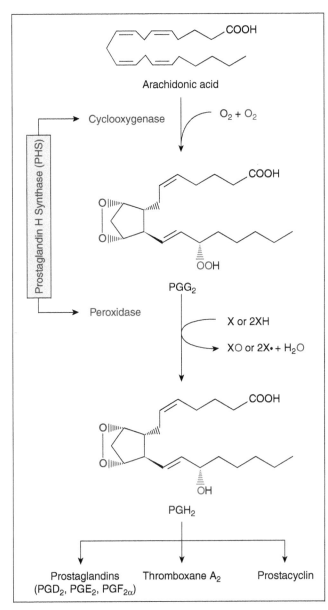

Figure 6-33. *Cooxidation of xenobiotics (X) during the conversion of arachidonic acid to PGH₂ by prostaglandin H synthase.*

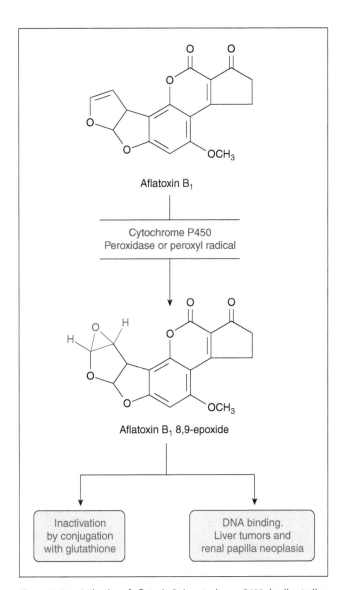

Figure 6-34. *Activation of aflatoxin B₁ by cytochrome P450, leading to liver tumor formation, and by peroxidases, leading to renal papilla neoplasia.*

activation and tumorigenicity of this nitrofuran. Unexpectedly, combined treatment of rats with FANFT and aspirin causes forestomach tumors, which are not observed when either compound is administered alone.

Increased expression of PHS2 (COX-2) has been documented in a number of tumors, including human colorectal, gastric, esophageal, pulmonary, and pancreatic carcinomas (Gupta and DuBois, 1998; Molina *et al.*, 1999; Dubé *et al.*, 2007; Wu *et al.*, 2010). Aspirin and other NSAIDs block the formation of colon cancer in experimental animals, and there is epidemiological evidence that long-term use of certain NSAIDs (aspirin and sulindac), but not acetaminophen (which does not inhibit COX-2), decreases the incidence of colorectal polyps and cancer in humans, and also decreases the number of deaths from esophageal, gastric, and rectal cancers. The incidence of intestinal neoplasms in Apc^Δ716 knockout mice is dramatically suppressed by crossing these transgenic animals with PHS2 (COX-2) knockout mice (Oshima *et al.*, 1996). From these few examples it is apparent that PHS2 may play at least 2 distinct roles in tumor formation; it may convert certain xenobiotics to

DNA-reactive metabolites (and thereby *initiate* tumor formation), and it may *promote* subsequent tumor growth, perhaps through formation of growth-promoting eicosanoids, such as PGE2, which can activate EGFR, ERKs, etc (Wu *et al.*, 2010).

Many phenolic compounds can serve as reducing substrates for PHS peroxidase. The phenoxyl radicals produced by one-electron oxidation reactions can undergo a variety of reactions, including binding to critical nucleophiles, such as protein and DNA, reduction by antioxidants such as GSH, and self-coupling. The reactions of phenoxyl radicals are analogous to those of the nitrogen-centered free radicals produced during the one-electron oxidation of aromatic amines by PHS.

It was previously mentioned in this section that phenol can enhance the peroxidative metabolism of hydroquinone, which is an important component to benzene myelotoxicity. An analogous interaction has been described between the phenolic antioxidants, BHT, and BHA. In mice, the pulmonary toxicity of BHT, which is a relatively poor substrate for PHS, is enhanced by BHA, which is a relatively good substrate for PHS. The mechanism by which BHA enhances the pulmonary toxicity of BHT involves the peroxidase-dependent conversion of BHA to a phenoxyl radical that interacts with BHT, converting it to a phenoxyl radical (by one-electron

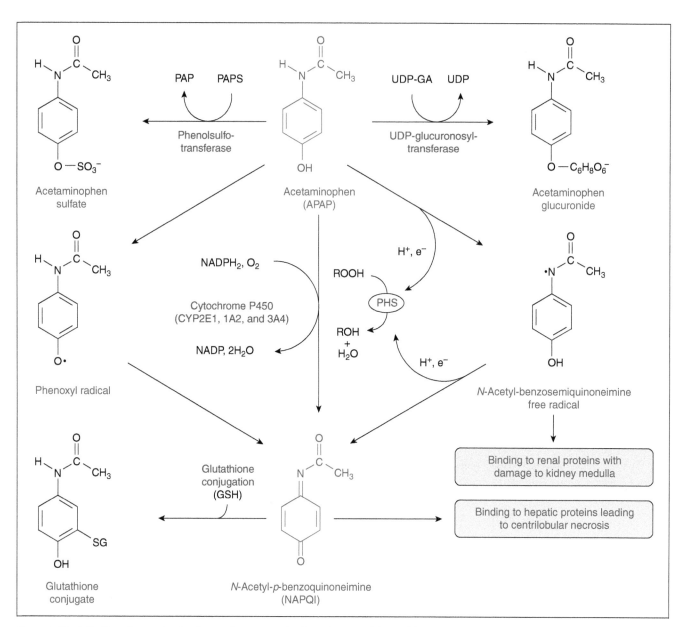

Figure 6-35. *Activation of acetaminophen by cytochrome P450, leading to hepatotoxicity, and by prostaglandin H synthase (PHS), leading to nephrotoxicity.* Conjugation with sulfonate, glucuronic acid, or glutathione represents detoxication reactions.

oxidation) or a quinone methide (by 2-electron oxidation), as shown in Fig. 6-36. Formation of the toxic quinone methide of BHT can also be catalyzed by CYP, which is largely responsible for activating BHT in the absence of BHA. A similar outcome occurs with quercetin, which is oxidized to a quinonemethide in the presence of peroxidases (Testa and Krämer, 2008, 2010).

Several reducing substrates, such as phenylbutazone, retinoic acid, 3-methylindole, sulfite, and bisulfite, are oxidized by PHS to carbon- or sulfur-centered free radicals that can trap oxygen to form a peroxyl radical, as shown in Fig. 6-37 for phenylbutazone. The peroxyl radical can oxidize xenobiotics in a peroxidative manner. For example, the peroxyl radical of phenylbutazone can convert B[*a*]P 7,8-dihydrodiol to the corresponding 9,10-epoxide.

PHS is unique among peroxidases because it can both generate hydroperoxides and catalyze peroxidase-dependent reactions, as shown in Fig. 6-33. Xenobiotic biotransformation by PHS is controlled by the availability of arachidonic acid. The biotransformation of xenobiotics by other peroxidases is controlled by the availability of hydroperoxide substrates. Hydrogen peroxide is a

normal product of cellular respiration, and lipid peroxides can form during lipid peroxidation. The level of these peroxides and their availability for peroxidase reactions depends on the efficiency of hydroperoxide scavenging by GPX and catalase.

Flavin Monooxygenases Liver, kidney, intestine, brain, and lung (among other tissues) contain one or more FAD-containing monooxygenases (FMO) that oxidize soft nucleophilic nitrogen, sulfur, selenium, phosphorus, and rarely—iodine, carbon, and boron—atoms of xenobiotics (Ziegler, 1993; Lawton *et al.*, 1994; Cashman, 1995, 1999, 2008; Rettie and Fisher, 1999; Cashman and Zhang, 2006; Mitchell, 2008; Testa and Krämer, 2008, 2010). Among these types of substrates, the best tend to be those with lone pairs of electrons available to form a polar, coordinate covalent (dative) bond (eg, hydroxylamines and piperidines) (Cashman, 2008; Testa and Krämer, 2008, 2010). The mammalian FMO gene family comprises 5 enzymes (designated FMO1-FMO5) that contain 532 to 558 amino acid residues each and are 48% to 60% identical in amino acid sequence within a species, whereas orthologous

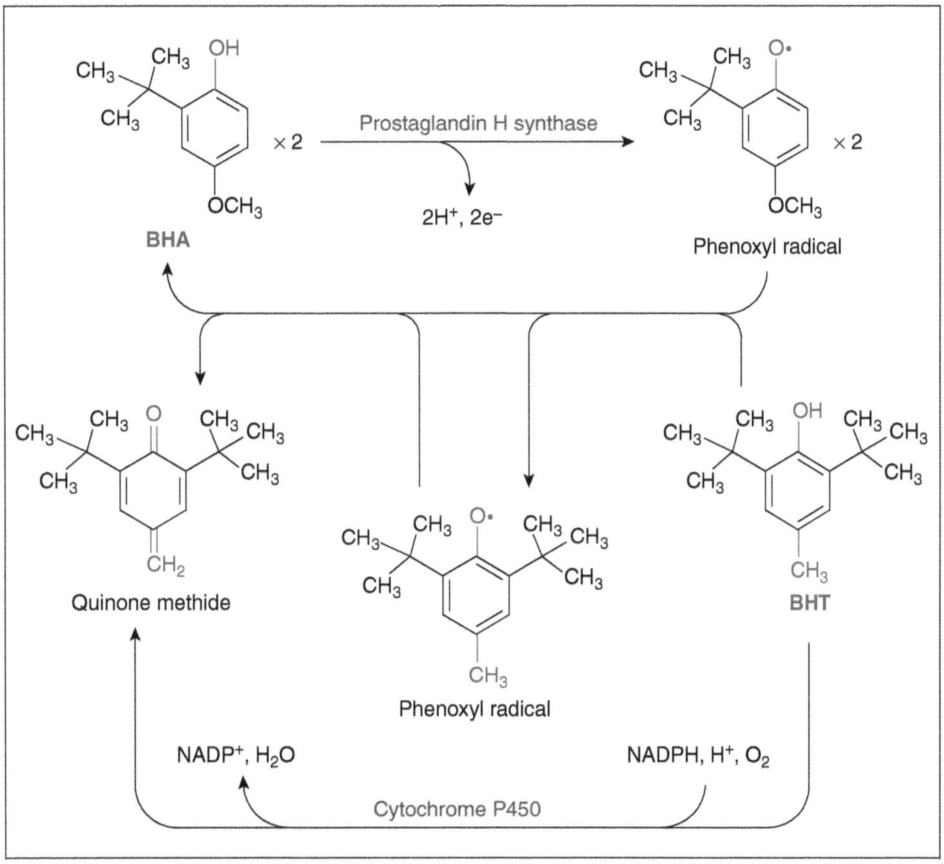

Figure 6-36. *Metabolite interaction between the phenolic antioxidants, butylated hydroxytoluene (BHT), and butylated hydroxyanisole (BHA).* Note that activation of BHT to a toxic quinone methide can be catalyzed by cytochrome P450 or, in the presence of BHA, by prostaglandin H synthase (PHS).

forms are 82% to 86% identical across species (Hines *et al.*, 2002). The human enzymes range in apparent molecular weight from 52 to 64 kDa (Testa and Krämer, 2008, 2010). Up to 6 human FMO pseudogenes have also been observed, including one that shares 71% sequence identity with FMO3, namely, FMO6, for which 9 distinct transcripts were identified in liver, but not kidney. All of these variant FMO6 transcripts arise by alternative splicing and lead to truncated, and therefore nonfunctional, enzymes. The possibility remains that rare SNPs in the FMO6 pseudogene could lead to normal expression of FMO6 in some individuals, but this has not yet been documented (Hines *et al.*, 2002). Each FMO enzyme contains a highly conserved glycine-rich region (residues 4-32) that binds 1 mol of FAD (noncovalently) near the active site, which is adjacent to a second highly conserved glycine-rich region (residues 186-213) that binds NADPH (or NADH). Other structural motifs have been reviewed in detail by Ziegler (2002).

Like CYP, the FMOs are microsomal enzymes that require O_2 and NADPH (or NADH in some cases) (Lai *et al.*, 2011), and many of the reactions catalyzed by FMO also can be catalyzed by CYP. However, whereas CYP catalyzes 2 sequential one-electron oxidations, FMO catalyzes a single 2-electron oxidation (Cashman, 2008). In contrast to CYP enzymes, FMOs are not readily induced or inhibited, such that metabolism of a drug by FMO tends to decrease its victim potential (ie, its potential to be the object of drug–drug interactions) (Cashman, 2008). However, basal expression levels appear to vary as much as 20-fold between individuals, with the differences appearing to be caused by mutations in the promoter regions of at least FMO1 and 3 (Testa and Krämer, 2008, 2010). Consequently, the disposition of a drug primarily metabolized by

FMO would likely show considerable interindividual variation and, for reasons outlined later in this section, infants and young children would likely be PMs.

Several in vitro techniques have been developed to distinguish reactions catalyzed by FMO from those catalyzed by CYP. In general, and in contrast to CYP, FMO is heat labile and can be inactivated in the absence of NADPH by warming microsomes to 50°C for one minute (Ogilvie *et al.*, 2008). However, even the often-used procedure of preincubating human liver microsomes at 37°C prior to addition of NADPH can cause significant inactivation of FMO, possibly leading to an underestimation of the role of FMO in the metabolism of xenobiotics (Cashman, 2008). By comparison, CYP can be inactivated with nonionic detergent, such as 1% Emulgen 911, which has a minimal effect on FMO activity. The pH optimum for FMO-catalyzed reactions (pH 8-10) tends to be higher than that for most (but not all) CYP reactions (pH 7-8). Based on the latter approach, a higher rate of formation of *N*-oxides from tertiary amines in microsomal incubations at pH 10 relative to pH 7.4 provides strong evidence for the role of FMO in *N*-oxide formation (Cashman, 2008). Antibodies raised against purified CYP enzymes can be used not only to establish the role of CYP in a microsomal reaction but also to identify which particular CYP enzyme catalyzes the reaction. In contrast, antibodies raised against purified FMO do not inhibit the enzyme. The use of chemical inhibitors to ascertain the relative contribution of FMO and CYP to microsomal reactions is often complicated by a lack of specificity. For example, both cimetidine and SKF 525A, which are well-recognized CYP inhibitors, are substrates for FMO. Conversely, the FMO inhibitor methimazole is known to cause direct inhibition of CYP2B6 and

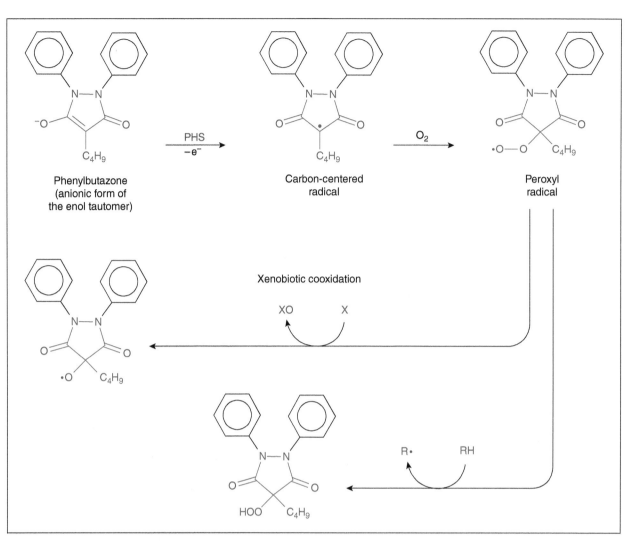

Figure 6-37. *Oxidation of phenylbutazone by prostaglandin H synthase (PHS) to a carbon-centered radical and peroxyl radical.* Note that the peroxyl radical can oxidize xenobiotics (X) in a peroxidative manner.

CYP2C9, and MDI of CYP3A4 (Parkinson *et al.*, 2011). Excellent FMO substrates, such as the strong nucleophile mercaptoimidazole, can potentially be used as competitive inhibitors of FMO-mediated *N*-oxidation of tertiary amines (Cashman, 2008). Zwitterions, positively multiple charged compounds, and diamines such as cadaverine are generally not FMO substrates (Krueger *et al.*, 2006). The situation is further complicated by the observation that the various forms of FMO differ in their thermal stability and sensitivity to detergents and other chemical modulators (examples of which are described later in this section).

FMO catalyzes the oxidation of nucleophilic tertiary amines to *N*-oxides, secondary amines to hydroxylamines and nitrones, and primary amines to hydroxylamines and oximes. Amphetamine, benzydamine, chlorpromazine, clozapine, guanethidine, imipramine, methamphetamine, olanzapine, and tamoxifen are examples of nitrogen-containing drugs that are *N*-oxygenated by FMO (and by CYP in most cases). Only sp[3]-hybridized electron-rich (nucleophilic) nitrogen atoms—those with pK_a values 5 to 10—are substrates for *N*-oxygenation by FMO, hence the preference of FMO for tertiary and cyclic amines. Therefore, in general, FMO *N*-oxygenates tertiary aliphatic amines and aliphatic cyclic amines (CYP can also) but FMO does not usually *N*-oxygenate aromatic amines (pyridines and anilines such as clozapine) (Testa and Krämer, 2008, 2010). Heteroaromatics (with an sp[2]-hybridized

nitrogen) and amides (which have low basicity [low pK_a]) are not *N*-oxygenated by FMO but they may be *N*-oxygenated by CYP. Thus, CYP can *N*-oxygenate both tertiary/cyclic amines and pyridines. In the case of anilines (arylamines), however, CYP (as will peroxidases, but rarely FMO) will *N*-hydroxylate them (Testa and Krämer, 2008, 2010). The *N*-oxygenation of primary and secondary aliphatic amines by FMO is more complex. For instance, the aliphatic *secondary* amine, methamphetamine (R-NH–CH$_3$), is *N*-oxygenated by FMO3 first to a hydroxylamine (R-NOH–CH$_3$) and then to a dihydroxylated intermediate (R-N$^+$(OH)$_2$–CH$_3$) that loses water to form a nitrone (R-N$^+$O–CH$_3$). The resulting nitrone can spontaneously hydrolyze to a ketone (phenylacetone in this case), such that this overall reaction represents an alternative deamination pathway (Testa and Krämer, 2008, 2010). In the case of the aliphatic *primary* amine, amphetamine (R-CH$_2$–NH$_2$), FMO again catalyzes 2 sequential *N*-hydroxylation reactions but in this case the *N*-dihydroxylated metabolite R-CH$_2$–N(OH)$_2$ loses water to form an oxime (R-CH=NOH). Primary aliphatic amines tend to be poor substrates for CYP; in fact, primary alkylamines, such as the *N*-demethylated metabolite of fluoxetine, are metabolically stable and potent inhibitors of CYP (discussed later in the section "Inhibition of Cytochrome P450").

FMO also oxygenates several sulfur-containing xenobiotics (such as thiols, thioethers, thiones, and thiocarbamates) and phosphines to *S*- and *P*-oxides, respectively. Cimetidine and sulindac sulfide are examples of sulfur-containing drugs that are converted to sulfoxides by FMO. As in the case of *N*-oxygenation, *S*-oxygenation requires a soft nucleophilic heteroatom, such as that found in thioethers. Both FMO and CYP can convert thioethers to sulfoxides (R_1-S-R_2 → R_1-SO-R_2) but only CYP can convert sulfoxides to sulfones (R_1-SO-R_2 → R_1-SO$_2$-R_2). Electron-withdrawing groups next to the sulfur (as in the case of sulfoxides and many heteroaromatics) decrease the nucleophilicity of the sulfur atom and decrease or abolish its oxygenation by FMO, whereas electronic-donating groups have the opposite effect, which is why thioamides are excellent substrates for *S*-oxygenation by FMO. Fig. 6-15 shows how sulindac, a sulfoxide, is reduced to sulindac sulfide, only to be oxidized by FMO back to the parent drug in what is often called a futile cycle as discussed further below in this section. Hydrazines, iodides, selenides, and boron-containing compounds are also substrates for FMO. Examples of FMO-catalyzed reactions are shown in Fig. 6-38A and B. One of the more unusual reactions catalyzed by FMO1 is the oxidative defluorination of 4-fluoro-*N*-methylaniline to 4-hydroxy-*N*-methylaniline (ie, 4-*N*-methylaminophenol) through the intermediacy of a reactive quinoneimine (Driscoll *et al.*, 2010). In the case of 4-fluoro-*N*-methylaniline, this oxidative defluorination reaction is facilitated by delocalization of the lone pair of electrons on the aniline nitrogen.

In general, the metabolites produced by FMO are the products of a chemical reaction between a xenobiotic and a peracid or peroxide, which is consistent with the mechanism of catalysis of FMO (discussed later in this section). The reactions catalyzed by FMO are generally detoxication reactions, although there are exceptions to this rule, which are described below (this section). Inasmuch as FMO attacks nucleophilic heteroatoms, it might be assumed that substrates for FMO could be predicted from their pK_a values (ie, from a measure of their basicity). Although there is some truth to this—for example, xenobiotics containing an sp^3-hybridized nitrogen atom with a pK_a of 5 to 10 are generally good substrates for FMO—predictions of substrate specificity based on pK_a values alone are not very reliable presumably because steric effects influence access of substrates to the FMO active site, which is consistent with the reported lack of rabbit FMO2 activity toward imipramine and chlorpromazine (Rettie and Fisher, 1999; Krueger *et al.*, 2006).

The mechanism of catalysis by FMO is depicted in Fig. 6-39. After the FAD moiety is reduced to FADH$_2$ by NADPH, the oxidized cofactor, NADP$^+$, remains bound to the enzyme. FADH$_2$ then binds oxygen to produce a peroxide (ie, the C(4a)-hydroperoxyflavin of FAD). The FAD-hydroperoxide is relatively stable, probably because the active site of FMO comprises non-nucleophilic, lipophilic amino acid residues, and this is thought to be the enzyme's resting state (ie, the FAD-hydroperoxide is the form in which FMO exists prior to substrate binding). During the oxygenation of xenobiotics (depicted as X → XO in Fig. 6-39), the nucleophilic heteroatom (N or S) attacks the terminal oxygen of the C(4a)-hydroperoxyflavin resulting in oxygen transfer to the xenobiotic (to form an *N*-oxide or sulfoxide) and formation of C(4a)-hydroxyflavin. From the latter step, it is understandable why the metabolites produced by FMO are generally the products of a chemical reaction between a xenobiotic and a peroxide or per-acid. The final step in the catalytic cycle involves dehydration of C(4a)-hydroxyflavin (which restores FAD to the ground state) and release of NADP$^+$. This final step is important because it is rate-limiting, and it occurs after substrate oxygenation. Consequently, this step determines the upper limit of the rate of substrate oxidation. Therefore, all good substrates for FMO are converted to products at roughly the same maximum rate (ie, V_{max} is determined

by the final step in the catalytic cycle). Binding of NADP$^+$ to FMO during catalysis is important because it prevents the reduction of oxygen to H$_2$O$_2$. In the absence of bound NADP$^+$, FMO would function as an NADPH-oxidase that would consume NADPH and cause oxidative stress through excessive production of H$_2$O$_2$. In some cases the reactive C(4a)-hydroperoxyflavin can function as an "enzymatic peroxide" to catalyze a Baeyer–Villiger oxidation, which involves the insertion of an oxygen atom into a carbon–carbon bond next to a carbonyl group (eg, aldehyde or ketone), to form an ester (eg, oxidation of salicylaldehyde by pig FMO1) (Lai *et al.*, 2011). However, this reaction has not been described in humans with the notable exception of FMO5 (and only FMO5), which mediates the Baeyer–Villiger lactonization of ER-879819, the ketone metabolite of the poly(ADP-ribose) polymerase inhibitor, E7016 (Lai *et al.*, 2011).

The oxygenation of substrates by FMO does not lead to inactivation of the enzyme, even though some of the products are strong electrophiles capable of binding covalently to critical and non-critical nucleophiles such as protein and GSH, respectively. The products of the oxygenation reactions catalyzed by FMO and/or the oxygenation of the same substrates by CYP can inactivate CYP. For example, the FMO-dependent *S*-oxygenation of spironolactone thiol (which is formed by the deacetylation of spironolactone by carboxylesterases, as shown in Fig. 6-5) leads to the formation of an electrophilic sulfenic acid (R-SH → R-SOH) that can undergo redox cycling, or be further converted to the reactive sulfinic acid (R-SO$_2$H) or sulfanyl radical (HS$^•$) that inactivates CYP and binds covalently to other proteins (Decker *et al.*, 1991; Krueger *et al.*, 2006; Testa and Krämer, 2008, 2010).

In humans, FMO plays a role in the biotransformation of several drugs (eg, albendazole, amphetamine, benzydamine, chlorpheniramine, cimetidine, clindamycin, clozapine, codeine, dasatinib, deprenyl, ethionamide, fenbendazole, guanethidine, itopride, methimazole, olanzapine, olopatadine, pargyline, ranitidine, sulindac sulfide, tamoxifen, tazarotene, thiacetazone, thioridazine, tozasertib, vandetanib, voriconazole, xanomeline, zimeldine, hydrazines such as procarbazine, and various dimethylaminoalkyl phenothiazine derivatives such as chlorpromazine and imipramine) and other xenobiotics (eg, aldicarb, cocaine, diallyl disulfide, *N,N*-dimethylaniline, disulfoton, fenthion, methyl-*p*-tolyl sulfide, methamphetamine, nicotine, phorate, thioacetamide, thiobenzamide, and tyramine), and in the activation of 3,3′-iminodipropionitrile to the neurotoxic *N*-hydroxy-3,3′-iminodipropionitrile (Ballard *et al.*, 2007; Testa and Krämer, 2008, 2010; Wang *et al.*, 2008; Francois *et al.*, 2009; Weil *et al.*, 2010; Strolin-Benedetti, 2011). As discussed later in this section, FMO also plays a role in the metabolism of some endogenous substrates such as TMA, cysteamine, cysteine conjugates, methionine, and lipoic acid (6,8-dithiooctanoic acid).

The major flavin monooxygenase in human liver microsomes, FMO3, is predominantly if not solely responsible for converting (*S*)-nicotine to (*S*)-nicotine *N*-1′-oxide (which is one of the reactions shown in Fig. 6-38A). The reaction proceeds stereospecifically; only the *trans* isomer is produced by FMO3, and this is the only isomer of (*S*)-nicotine *N*-1′-oxide excreted in the urine of cigarette smokers or individuals wearing a nicotine patch (Cashman and Zhang, 2006). Therefore, the urinary excretion of *trans*-(*S*)-nicotine *N*-1′-oxide can be used as an in vivo probe of FMO3 activity in humans. However, common polymorphisms in FMO1 (eg, FMO1*6) have been shown to be associated with nicotine dependence in European patients (Hinrichs *et al.*, 2011). Furthermore, recombinant human FMO1 catalyzes the *N*-oxidation of (*S*)-nicotine approximately 4-fold more efficiently than recombinant human FMO3, and does so nonstereospecifically (ie, 55:45 *cis:trans* ratio of (*S*)-nicotine

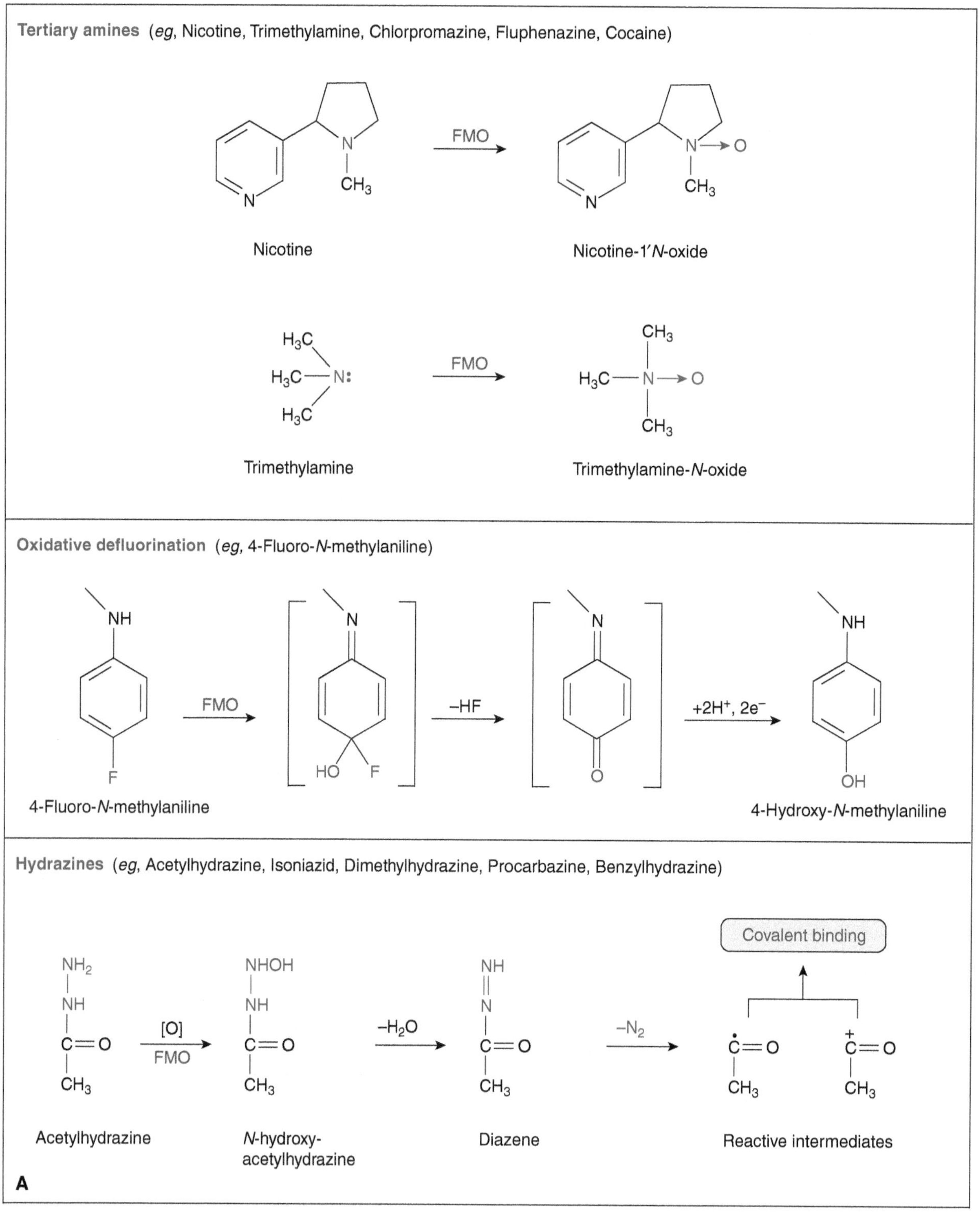

Figure 6-38. *Examples of reactions catalyzed by flavin monooxygenases (FMO).* (**A**) Nitrogen-containing xenobiotics.

N-1′-oxide, similar to the situation with pig, rat, and rabbit FMO1), whereas FMO3 forms predominantly the *trans*-(*S*)-nicotine *N*-1′-oxide (as described above) (Hinrichs *et al.*, 2011). FMO1 is extrahepatic, with high expression levels in the kidney, and some expression in the intestine and brain. If FMO1 contributes significantly to the metabolism of nicotine in the brains of smokers, it is possible that the *N*-oxide formed by FMO1 could be reduced back to nicotine in the brain by AO, a process known as retro-reduction or futile cycling (Hinrichs *et al.*, 2011).

FMO3 is also the principal enzyme involved in the *S*-oxygenation of cimetidine, an H$_2$-antagonist that was once widely used in the treatment of gastric ulcers and other acid-related disorders (this reaction is shown in Fig. 6-38B). Cimetidine is stereoselectively sulfoxidated by FMO3 to an 84:16 mixture of (+) and (−) enantiomers, which closely matches the 75:25 enantiomeric composition of cimetidine *S*-oxide in human urine. Therefore, the urinary excretion of cimetidine *S*-oxide, like that of (*S*)-nicotine *N*-1′-oxide, is an in vivo indicator of FMO3 activity in humans.

DISPOSITION OF TOXICANTS

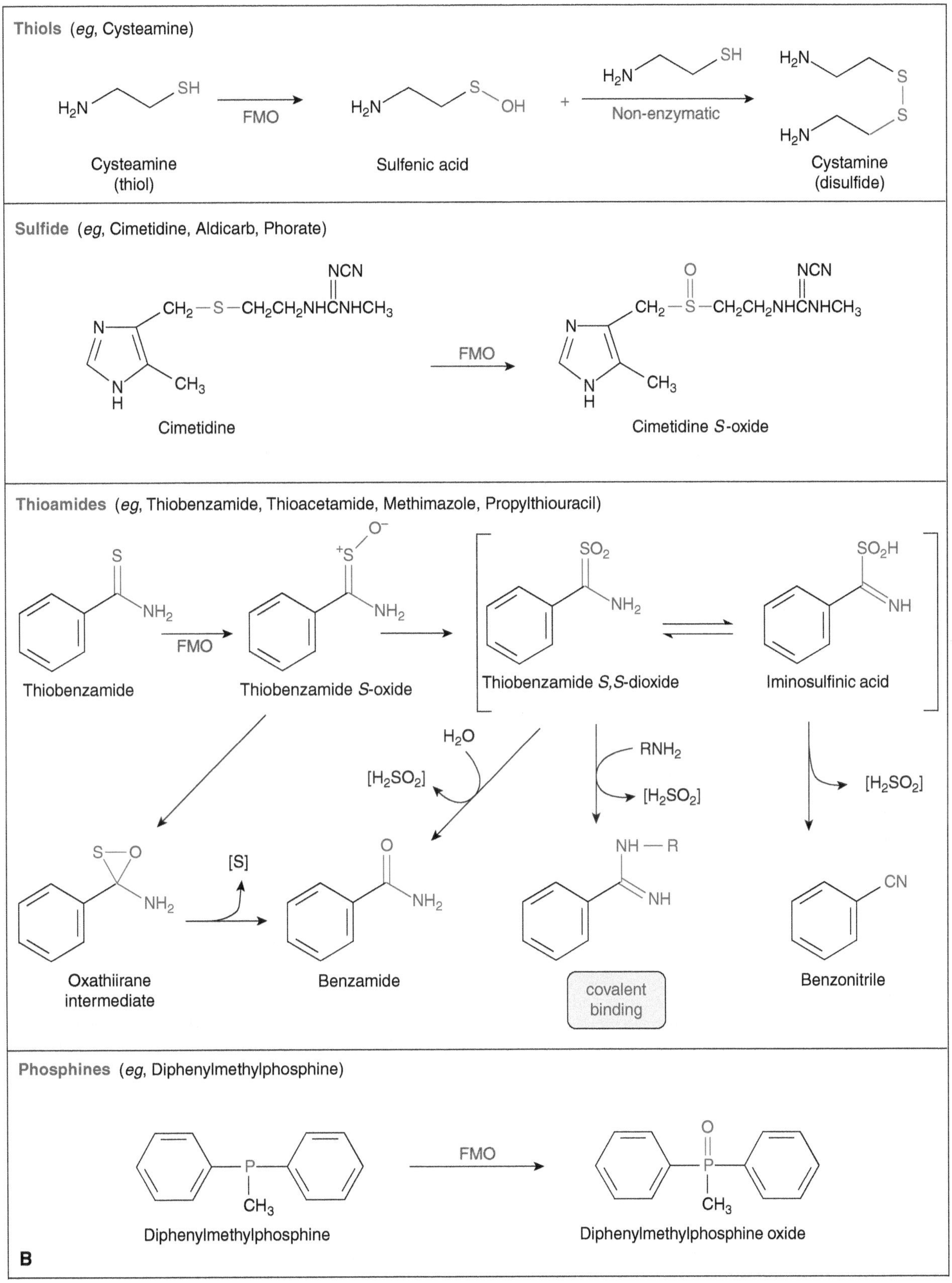

Figure 6-38. (*Continued*) (**B**) Sulfur- and phosphorus-containing xenobiotics.

Sulindac is a sulfoxide that exists in 2 stereochemical forms (as do most sulfoxides), and a racemic mixture of *R*- and *S*-sulindac is used therapeutically as a NSAID. As shown in Fig. 6-15, the sulfoxide group in sulindac is reduced to the corresponding sulfide (which is achiral), which is then oxidized back to sulindac by

retro-reduction (futile cycling). In human liver, the sulfoxidation of sulindac sulfide is catalyzed by FMO3 with little or no contribution from CYP. At low substrate concentrations (30 μM), FMO3 converts sulindac sulfide to *R*- and *S*-sulindac in an 87:13 ratio (Hamman *et al.*, 2000). Consequently, although sulindac is administered as

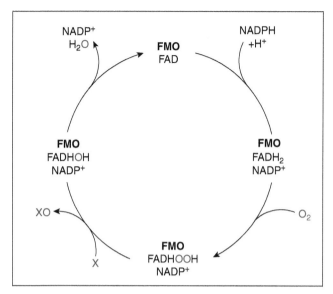

Figure 6-39. *Catalytic cycle of flavin monooxygenase (FMO).* X and XO are the xenobiotic substrate and oxygenated product, respectively. The C(4a)-hydroperoxyflavin and C(4a)-hydroxyflavin of FAD are depicted as FADHOOH and FADHOH, respectively.

a racemic mixture (ie, a 1:1 mixture of *R*- and *S*-enantiomers), the reduction of this drug to the corresponding sulfide and its preferential sulfoxidation by FMO3 to *R*-sulindac results in stereoselective enrichment of *R*-sulindac in plasma and urine.

This retro-reduction of sulfide *S*-oxides or amine *N*-oxides formed by FMO (or CYP) back to the parent may occur more often than is currently recognized, but it can be observed in vitro when the levels of an *N*- or *S*-oxide metabolite increase rapidly at first but then quickly reach a plateau as a balance between oxidation and reduction is reached (Cashman, 2008). There are at least 7 systems that can catalyze the retro-reduction of FMO metabolites: (1) AO, (2) quinone reductase, (3) hemoglobin itself or other heme-containing proteins such as CYP (which may or may not be enzymatically catalyzed), (4) XOR, (5) NADPH-cytochrome P450 reductase, (6) the mARC with NADH-cytochrome b_5/cytochrome b_5, and (7) gut microflora (Cashman, 2008; Testa and Krämer, 2008, 2010). For instance, amitriptyline *N*-oxide, imipramine *N*-oxide, cyclobenzaprine *N*-oxide, and brucine *N*-oxide are reduced back to the parent tertiary amine by quinone reductase, heme, and/or gut microflora (Cashman, 2008; Testa and Krämer, 2008, 2010). Nicotine *N*-oxide is retro-reduced to nicotine by AO (Cashman, 2008). Recombinant human CYP1A1, 2A6, 2D6, and 3A4 can also retro-reduce tamoxifen *N*-oxide to the tertiary amine (Cashman, 2008). The retro-reduction of TMA *N*-oxide to TMA by gut microflora is discussed later in this section (Cashman, 2008; Testa and Krämer, 2008, 2010).

In the case of sulindac sulfide, stereoselective sulfoxidation occurs not only with human FMO3 (the major drug-metabolizing FMO in human liver) but also with porcine FMO1 (the major form expressed in pig liver) and rabbit FMO2 (the major form expressed in rabbit lung) (Hamman *et al.*, 2000). However, this conformity is the exception, rather than the rule. For example, in contrast to the stereoselective oxygenation of (*S*)-nicotine and cimetidine by human FMO3 (see above), FMO1 (which is the major FMO expressed in pig, rat, and rabbit liver) converts (*S*)-nicotine to a 1:1 mixture of *cis*- and *trans*-(*S*)-nicotine *N*-1′-oxide, and similarly converts cimetidine to a 1:1 mixture of (+) and (−) cimetidine *S*-oxide, respectively. Therefore, statements concerning the role of FMO in

the disposition of xenobiotics in humans may not apply to other species, or vice versa.

Several sulfur-containing xenobiotics are oxygenated by FMO to electrophilic reactive intermediates. Such xenobiotics include various thiols, thioamides, 2-mercaptoimidazoles, thiocarbamates, and thiocarbamides. The electrophilic metabolites of these xenobiotics do not inactivate FMO, but they can covalently modify and inactivate neighboring proteins, including CYP. Some of these same xenobiotics are substrates for CYP, and their oxygenation to electrophilic metabolites leads to inactivation of CYP, a process known variously as MDI, mechanism-based inhibition, and suicide inactivation. 2-Mercaptoimidazoles undergo sequential *S*-oxygenation reactions by FMO, first to sulfenic acids and then to sulfinic acids (R-SH → R-SOH → R-SO$_2$H). These electrophilic metabolites, such as the sulfenic acid metabolite produced from spironolactone thiol (see above), bind to critical nucleophiles (such as proteins) or interact with GSH to form disulfides. The thiocarbamate functionality present in numerous agricultural chemicals is converted by FMO to *S*-oxides (sulfoxides), which can be further oxygenated to sulfones. These reactions involve *S*-oxygenation adjacent to a ketone, which produces strong electrophilic acylating agents, which may be responsible for the toxicity of many thiocarbamate herbicides and fungicides. The hepatotoxicity of thiobenzamide is dependent on *S*-oxidation by FMO and/or CYP. As shown in Fig. 6-38B, the *S*-oxidation of thiobenzamide produces an *S*-oxide, which can rearrange to an oxathiirane (a 3-membered ring of carbon, sulfur, and oxygen) on photolysis or thermolysis. However, such oxathiiranes are readily reduced back to the *S*-oxide. In vivo, the *S*,*S*-dioxide is more likely to form, which readily tautomerizes to iminosulfinic acid, binds covalently to protein (which leads to hepatocellular necrosis), or rearranges to benzamide, a reaction known as *oxidative group transfer*. In general, thiols with a negative charge on the S-atom (eg, dithioacids) tend to be good substrates of FMOs, whereas less nucleophilic S-atoms tend to be oxidized by CYP (Testa and Krämer, 2008, 2010).

Endogenous FMO substrates include cysteamine, which is oxidized to the disulfide, cystamine, and TMA, which is converted to TMA *N*-oxide (Fig. 6-38). By converting cysteamine to cystamine, FMO may serve to produce a low-molecular weight disulfide exchange agent, which may participate in the formation of disulfide bridges during peptide synthesis or the renaturation of proteins. By converting TMA to TMA *N*-oxide, FMO3 (but neither FMO1 nor 5) converts a malodorous and volatile dietary product derived from the reduction of dietary TMA *N*-oxide by gut bacteria (eg, from choline, lecithin, carnitine, and especially fish, which contain large amounts of TMA *N*-oxide) to an inoffensive metabolite. TMA smells of rotting fish (because bacteria in dead fish rapidly convert the high levels of TMA *N*-oxide to TMA), and people who are genetically deficient in FMO3 suffer from trimethylaminuria or *fish odor syndrome*, which is caused by the excretion of TMA in urine, sweat, and breath (Ayesh and Smith, 1992; Phillips and Shephard, 2008). Although the lack of functional FMO3 (and hence trimethylaminuria) occurs only rarely (eg, ~1% of British Caucasians), it is now known to be caused by one of at least 30 mutations that decrease or abolish FMO3 activity (Cashman *et al.*, 2000; Cashman and Zhang, 2006; Phillips and Shephard, 2008). As might be expected, trimethylaminuria is associated with an impairment of nicotine *N*-oxidation and other pathways of drug biotransformation that are primarily catalyzed by FMO3 (Rettie and Fisher, 1999). For instance, benzydamine *N*-oxygenation and oxidation of sulindac sulfide has been correlated with FMO3 genotype in trimethylaminurics (Cashman and Zhang, 2006; Testa and Krämer, 2008, 2010; Francois *et al.*,

Table 6-9

Putative Tissue Levels of Flavin Monooxygenase (FMO) Enzymes Present in Animals and Humans

	FMO1	FMO2	FMO3	FMO4	FMO5
Liver					
Mouse	Low	None	High	Unknown	Low
Rat	High	Unknown	Low	Unknown	Low
Rabbit	High	None	Low	Unknown	Low
Human*	Trace	Low	Very high	High	Very high
Kidney					
Mouse	High	Unknown	High	Unknown	Low
Rat	High	Unknown	High	High	Low
Rabbit	Low	Low	Trace	High	Low
Human*	High	High	Low	Medium	Medium
Lung					
Mouse	Unknown	High	Trace	None	Low
Rat	Unknown	Unknown	Unknown	None	Low
Rabbit	Unknown	Very high	Unknown	None	None
Human*	Low	Variable†	Medium	Low	Medium
Small intestine					
Human*	Low	Low	Trace	Trace	High

Data from Cashman and Zhang (2006) and Zhang and Cashman (2006).

Human tissue levels are based on FMO mRNA levels.

†*FMO2 mRNA levels in human lung are high, but this mRNA is not translated into functional enzyme due to the presence of a truncation mutation in Caucasians and Asians. Approximately 33% of sub-Saharan Africans, 26% of African Americans, 7% of Puerto Ricans, and 2% of Mexicans have 1 normal allele and express a functional protein (Veeramah et al., 2008).*

2009). Some polymorphisms decrease while others increase the activity of FMO3 toward certain substrates, while others affect the promoter region and alter the amount of enzyme expressed (Phillips and Shephard, 2008).

Humans and other mammals express 5 different flavin monooxygenases (FMO1, FMO2, FMO3, FMO4, and FMO5) in a species- and tissue-specific manner, as shown in Table 6-9, based on mRNA levels, which may not reflect protein levels (adapted from Cashman, 1995; Cashman and Zhang, 2006; Zhang and Cashman, 2006). The major hepatic FMOs expressed in humans are FMO3 and FMO5, whereas FMO1 is the major FMO expressed in rat, rabbit, and pig liver. In humans FMO1 is expressed in fetal liver and is very rapidly downregulated after birth (although not in kidney) while hepatic FMO3 is gradually upregulated over months to years, in contrast to other mammals (Shephard *et al.*, 2007; Phillips and Shephard, 2008; Testa and Krämer, 2008, 2010). This delay between the hepatic silencing of FMO1 and expression of FMO3 means that most infants probably have very little drug-metabolizing FMO present in the liver for several months (Shimizu *et al.*, 2011). In addition, given the fact that apparently only FMO3 catalyzes the *N*-oxidation of TMA produced from gut bacteria, this begs the question of why all infants do *not* have *fish odor syndrome*. In a cohort of 6 patients with genetically confirmed trimethylaminuria, the average age of presentation was 6 (±3.6) years (Chalmers *et al.*, 2006). As a genetic deficiency of FMO3, trimethylaminuria is obviously present from birth. However, the phenotype only becomes apparent when an affected child is weaned, and foods with high amounts of choline (eg, eggs, liver, etc) or TMA *N*-oxide (eg, seafood) are introduced (Chalmers *et al.*, 2006). Diagnostic delay also presumably leads to the higher than expected average age of presentation. Transient trimethylaminuria can however occur in neonates and infants

if their diet sporadically contains higher than usual levels of choline, etc (Testa and Krämer, 2008, 2010).

Previously, FMO3 has been considered to be the dominant FMO in human liver, and although FMO5 expression is higher, it has activity toward fewer xenobiotic substrates, and likely plays only a minor role in xenobiotic metabolism, with the exception of E7016, the poly(ADP-ribose) polymerase inhibitor noted above (Cashman and Zhang, 2006; Lai *et al.*, 2011). FMO5 is also the most highly expressed FMO in the small intestine, in terms of mRNA. In humans, high levels of FMO1 are expressed in the kidney, and low levels of FMO2 are expressed in the lungs of Caucasians and Asians.

Lung microsomes from most mammals, particularly rabbit, mouse, monkey, and other nonhuman primates, contain high levels of functional FMO2, and of the FMO transcripts detected in human lung, the FMO2 transcript is found at the highest levels by far (Zhang and Cashman, 2006). The uncharacteristically low level of active FMO2 in human lung is caused by a mutation (a C → T transition at codon 472 in exon 9) in the major human FMO2*2A allele found in essentially all Caucasian and Asian populations, which results in a premature stop codon and the synthesis of a nonfunctional, truncated protein (one lacking the last 64 amino acid residues from the C-terminus) (Dolphin *et al.*, 1998; Veeramah *et al.*, 2008; Francois *et al.*, 2009). In contrast, 26% of African Americans, 7% of Puerto Ricans, and 2% of Mexicans have one normal allele and express a functional protein (Cashman and Zhang, 2006). In sub-Saharan Africa, approximately 33% of individuals possess at least one functional FMO2*1 allele, and in some subpopulations the incidence approaches 50% (Veeramah *et al.*, 2008). In pulmonary microsomes from individuals who express one or more functional FMO2 alleles, the protein level is equal to or greater than that of CYP enzymes. Functional FMO2 has high activity toward thioureas and thioamides, which implies that individuals who express a functional FMO2 may be more susceptible to the toxic effects of sulfenic or sulfinic acids formed from *S*-oxygenation of phenylthiourea, α-naphthylthiourea, and ethylenethiourea, whereas Caucasians and Asians may be more susceptible to thioether-containing organophosphate pesticides such as phorate and disulfoton, for which the parent compounds are more toxic than products of the FMO2-catalyzed reaction (Cashman and Zhang, 2006; Veeramah *et al.*, 2008). FMO2 has also been shown to catalyze *S*-oxygenation of the second-line antitubercular drugs ethionamide and thiacetazone, leading to the formation of reactive metabolites such as the sulfenic and sulfinic acids, carbodiimide derivatives, and *S*-oxides (Francois *et al.*, 2009). Because these second-line antitubercular agents are prodrugs that must be converted by the mycobacteria in FMO-like reactions to the reactive products, it is possible that administration to individuals with at least one FMO2*1 allele could decrease their efficacy and increase pulmonary toxicity.

FMO4 is expressed at low levels in the brain of several mammalian species, where it might terminate the action of several centrally active drugs and other xenobiotics. It is unstable, however, which makes its characterization somewhat difficult (Cashman and Zhang, 2006).

The various forms of FMO are distinct gene products with different physical properties and substrate specificities. For example, FMO2 *N*-oxygenates *n*-octylamine, whereas such long aliphatic primary amines are not substrates for FMO1, although they stimulate its activity toward other substrates (in some cases causing a change in stereospecificity). Conversely, short-chain tertiary amines, such as chlorpromazine, orphenadrine, and imipramine, are substrates for FMO1 but not FMO2. FMO2 exhibits no activity toward phenothiazine derivatives with only a 3-carbon side chain or 1,3-diphenylthiourea (Krueger *et al.*, 2006). FMO3 is highly selective in the *N*-oxygenation of TMA, whereas FMO5 is selective for the *N*-oxygenation of short-chain aliphatic primary amines such as *N*-octylamine, but has little activity toward other typical FMO substrates, with the exception of E7016, the poly(ADP-ribose) polymerase inhibitor noted previously (Krueger *et al.*, 2006; Lai *et al.*, 2011). The substrate specificity of FMO4 also is somewhat restricted. Certain substrates are oxygenated stereospecifically by one FMO enzyme but not another. For example, FMO2 and FMO3 convert (*S*)-nicotine exclusively to *trans*-(*S*)-nicotine *N*-1′-oxide, whereas the *N*-oxides of (*S*)-nicotine produced by FMO1 are a 1:1 mixture of *cis* and *trans* isomers. FMO2 is heat stable under conditions that completely inactivate FMO1, and FMO2 is resistant to anionic detergents that inactivate FMO1. Low concentrations of bile acids, such as cholate, stimulate FMO activity in rat and mouse liver microsomes but inhibit FMO activity in rabbit and pig liver.

The FMO enzymes expressed in liver microsomes are not under the same regulatory control as CYP enzymes. In rats, the expression of FMO1 is suppressed rather than induced by treatment with phenobarbital or 3-methylcholanthrene (although some studies point to a modest [~3-fold] induction of rat FMO1 by 3-methylcholanthrene). Indole-3-carbinol, which induces the same CYP enzymes as 3-methylcholanthrene, causes a marked decrease in FMO activity in rat liver and intestine. A similar decrease in FMO3 activity occurs in human volunteers following the consumption of large amounts of Brussels sprouts, which contain high levels of indole-3-carbinol and related indoles. The decrease in FMO3 activity may result from direct inhibition of FMO3 by indole-3-carbinol and its derivatives rather than from an actual decrease in enzyme levels (Cashman, 1999). Increased levels of nitric oxide (NO), as occurs during acute inflammation (eg, sepsis or endotoxemia), which activates nitric oxide synthase-2 (NOS-2), can inhibit FMO (as well as CYP) (Mitchell, 2008). However, the AhR agonist, TCDD, was found to induce FMO2 and FMO3 mRNA levels in mice by 30- and 80-fold, respectively (Tijet *et al.*, 2006).

The levels of FMO3 and, to a lesser extent, the levels of FMO1 in mouse liver microsomes are sexually differentiated (female > male) due to suppression of expression by testosterone. The opposite is true of FMO1 levels in rat liver microsomes, the expression of which is positively regulated by testosterone and negatively regulated by estradiol. In pregnant rabbits, lung FMO2 is positively regulated by progesterone and/or corticosteroids.

Species differences in the relative expression of FMO and CYP appear to determine differences in the toxicity of the pyrrolizidine alkaloids, senecionine, retrorsine, and monocrotaline. These compounds are detoxified by FMO, which catalyzes the formation of tertiary amine *N*-oxides, but are activated by CYP, which oxidizes these alkaloids to pyrroles that generate toxic electrophiles through the loss of substituents on the pyrrolizidine nucleus (details of which appear in the section "Cytochrome P450"). Rats have a high pyrrole-forming CYP activity and a low *N*-oxide-forming FMO activity, whereas the opposite is true of guinea pigs. This likely explains why pyrrolizidine alkaloids are highly toxic to rats but not to guinea pigs. Many of the reactions catalyzed by FMO are also catalyzed by CYP, but differences in the oxidation of pyrrolizidine alkaloids by FMO and CYP illustrate that this is not always the case. Species differences in the levels of FMO can also complicate the findings of preclinical toxicology and metabolism studies because most toxicologically useful small animal species express FMO1 as the dominant hepatic FMO in contrast to human, in which FMO3 is the dominant form (Cashman, 2008). However, one animal model that may be more similar to the human hepatic expression of FMO is the female mouse, which has relatively high levels of FMO3 and 5 (Cashman, 2008).

Cytochrome P450 Of all the xenobiotic-biotransforming enzymes, the CYP enzyme system ranks first in terms of catalytic versatility and the sheer number of xenobiotics it detoxifies or activates to reactive intermediates. The highest levels of CYP enzymes involved in xenobiotic biotransformation are found in liver endoplasmic reticulum (microsomes), but CYP enzymes are present in virtually all tissues. Some of the so-called microsomal CYP enzymes are also located on the inner membrane of mitochondria, the importance of which is discussed in the section "CYP2E1." CYP enzymes play a very important role in determining the intensity and duration of action of drugs, and they also play a key role in the detoxication of xenobiotics. CYP enzymes in liver and extrahepatic tissues play important roles in the activation of xenobiotics to toxic and/or tumorigenic metabolites. The catalytic versatility of CYP enzymes is apparent from Table 6-2, which shows some of the many chemical groups that can be metabolized by CYP.

Microsomal and mitochondrial CYP enzymes play key roles in the biosynthesis or catabolism of steroid hormones, bile acids, fat-soluble vitamins such as vitamins A and D, fatty acids, and eicosanoids such as prostaglandins, thromboxane, prostacyclin, and leukotrienes, which underscores the catalytic versatility of CYP.

The human CYP superfamily contains 55 functional genes and 60 pseudogenes (Zhou *et al.*, 2009a; Guengerich *et al.*, 2010; http://drnelson.uthsc.edu/CytochromeP450.html). Many sources place the number of functional genes at 57; however, the 2 additional genes, namely, CYP2A7 (originally named IIA4) and CYP4B1, encode enzymes incapable of incorporating heme, rendering them catalytically inactive (note, however, that functional CYP4B1 is expressed in other mammalian species) (Yamano *et al.*, 1990; Ding *et al.*,

Table 6-10

Classification of the 55 Functional Human CYP Enzymes

XENOBIOTICS		FATTY ACIDS/ EICOSANOIDS	STEROIDOGENIC	BILE ACIDS	VITAMIN D	RETINOIC ACID	UNKNOWN
CYP1A1	CYP2F1	CYP2U1	CYP11A1	CYP7A1	CYP2R1	CYP26A1	CYP4A22
CYP1A2	CYP2J2*,†	CYP4A11	CYP11B1	CYP7B1	CYP24A1	CYP26B1	CYP4X1
CYP1B1	CYP2S1	CYP4F2‡,§	CYP11B2	CYP8B1	CYP26C1**		CYP20A1
CYP2A6	CYP2W1	CYP4F3§	CYP17A1	CYP27A1†	CYP27B1		CYP27C1
CYP2A13	CYP3A4†,††	CYP4F8	CYP19A1	CYP39A1			
CYP2B6	CYP3A5	CYP4F11	CYP21A2	CYP46A1			
CYP2C8*	CYP3A7	CYP4F12§		CYP51A1‡‡			
CYP2C9*	CYP3A43	CYP4F22					
CYP2C18		CYP4V2					
CYP2C19		CYP4Z1					
CYP2D6		CYP5A1§§					
CYP2E1		CYP8A1***					

Note: CYP2A7 and 4B1 are full-length genes that probably encode inactive enzymes due to lack of heme incorporation.

Also involved in fatty acid and eicosanoid metabolism.

†*Also involved in vitamin D metabolism.*

‡*Also involved in vitamin E and vitamin K metabolism.*

§*Also involved in xenobiotic metabolism.*

**Also involved in retinoic acid metabolism.*

††*Also involved in bile acid synthesis.*

‡‡*Also involved in cholesterol biosynthesis.*

§§*Thromboxane A synthase (TBXAS1).*

***Prostaglandin I₂ (prostacyclin) synthase (PTGIS).*

1995; Baer and Rettie, 2006). As shown in Table 6-10, the 55 human CYP enzymes can be broadly categorized on the basis of their role in (1) xenobiotic biotransformation, (2) fatty acid/eicosanoid hydroxylation/epoxidation, (3) steroidogenesis, (4) bile acid synthesis, vitamin D activation/inactivation, (5) retinoic acid metabolism, and (6) unknown function (a diminishing group of so-called orphan enzymes). In several cases, there is no clear functional distinction in terms of endobiotic and xenobiotic metabolism because, as noted in Table 6-10, there are many examples of CYP enzymes playing an important role in the metabolism of both an endobiotic and a drug or other xenobiotic. CYP2J2 and, in animals, CYP4B1 are examples of enzymes that ride the xenobiotic–endobiotic fence. In terms of endobiotic metabolism, CYP enzymes play a role in both catabolism and anabolism (several different CYP enzymes play a role in steroid hormone and bile acid synthesis). For example, CYP enzymes both activate vitamin D_3 to $1\alpha,25$-dihydroxyvitamin D_3 ($1,25\text{-}(OH)_2\text{-}D_3$) (CYP2R1, CYP2J2, CYP3A4, CYP27A1, and CYP27B1) and inactivate the active metabolite (CYP24A1 and CYP3A4). Arachidonic acid is epoxidated by CYP2C8, CYP2C9, and especially CYP2J2 to vasodilatory epoxyeicosatrienoic acids (EETs) but is converted by ω-hydroxylation to the vasoconstrictor 20-hydroxyeicosatetraenoic acid (20-HETE) by various CYP4A and CYP4F enzymes. The major xenobiotic-biotransforming CYP enzymes in human liver microsomes belong to families 1, 2, and 3, which are shown in Table 6-11 along with their homologs in the nonclinical species widely used in drug safety testing.

All CYP enzymes are heme-containing proteins. In some cases, such as many members of the CYP4 family, the heme moiety is covalently attached to the protein but in most other cases it

is attached noncovalently (Ortiz de Montellano, 2008). The heme iron in CYP is usually in the ferric (Fe^{III}) state. When reduced to the ferrous (Fe^{II}) state, CYP can bind ligands such as O_2 and carbon monoxide (CO). The complex between ferrous CYP and CO absorbs light maximally at 450 nm, from which CYP derives its name (*Pigment 450*). The absorbance maximum of the CO complex differs slightly among different CYP enzymes and ranges from 447 to 452 nm. All other hemoproteins that bind CO absorb light maximally at ~420 nm. The unusual absorbance maximum of CYP is due to an unusual fifth ligand to the heme (a cysteine thiolate). The amino acid sequence around the cysteine residue that forms the thiolate bond with the heme moiety is highly conserved in all CYP enzymes. When this thiolate bond is disrupted, CYP is converted to a catalytically inactive form called cytochrome P420. By competing with oxygen, CO inhibits CYP. The inhibitory effect of CO can be reversed by irradiation with light at 450 nm, which photodissociates the CYP–CO complex. These properties of CYP are of historical importance (Omura, 2011). The observation that treatment of rats with certain chemicals, such as 3-methylcholanthrene, causes a shift in the peak absorbance of CYP (from 450 to 448 nm) provided some of the earliest evidence for the existence of multiple forms of CYP in liver microsomes. The conversion of CYP to cytochrome P420 by detergents and phospholipases helped to establish the hemoprotein nature of CYP. The inhibition of CYP by CO and the reversal of this inhibition by photodissociation of the CYP–CO complex established CYP as the microsomal and mitochondrial enzyme involved in drug biotransformation and steroid biosynthesis (Omura, 2011).

The basic reaction catalyzed by CYP enzymes is monooxygenation in which one atom of oxygen is incorporated into a substrate,

Table 6-11

Homologs of the Major Xenobiotic-Metabolizing CYP Enzymes in Liver Microsomes from Humans and Nonclinical Species

SUBFAMILY	HUMAN	MONKEY	DOG	RAT	MOUSE
CYP1A	1A2 (1A1, IB1)	1A2 (1A1, IB1)	1A2 (1A1, IB1)	1A2 (1A1, IB1)	1A2 (1A1, IB1)
CYP2A	2A6, 2A13	2A23, 2A24	2A13, 2A25	2A1, 2A2, 2A3	2A4, 2A5, 2A12, 2A22
CYP2B	2B6	2B6, 2B17	2B11	2B1, 2B2, 2B3	2B9, 2B10
CYP2C	2C8, 2C9, 2C18, 2C19	2C20, 2C43, 2C76	2C21, 2C41	2C6, 2C7, 2C11, 2C12, 2C13, 2C22, 2C23, 2C24, 2C46, 2C77, 2C79, 2C80, 2C81	2C29, 2C37, 2C38, 2C39, 2C40, 2C44, 2C50, 2C54, 2C55, 2C65, 2C66, 2C67, 2C68, 2C69, 2C70
CYP2D	2D6	2D17, 2D19, 2D29, 2D30	2D15	2D1, 2D2, 2D3, 2D4, 2D5, 2D18	2D9, 2D10, 2D11, 2D12, 2D13, 2D22, 2D26, 2D34, 2D40
CYP2E	2E1	2E1	2E1	2E1	2E1
CYP2J	2J2	2J2	2J2	2J3, 2J4, 2J10, 2J13, 2J16	2J5, 2J6, 2J7, 2J8, 2J9, 2J11, 2J12, 2J13
CYP3A	3A4, 3A5, 3A7, 3A43	3A8	3A12, 3A26	3A1/23, 3A2, 3A9, 3A18, 3A23, 3A62, 3A73	3A11, 3A13, 3A16, 3A25, 3A41, 3A44, 3A57, 3A59

Note: CYP1A1 and CYP1B1 are extrahepatic enzymes, although CYP1A1 is an AhR-inducible hepatic enzyme. Data from Baillie and Rettie (2011) and Nelson (2009).

designated RH, and the other is reduced to water with reducing equivalents derived from NADPH, as follows:

$$\text{Substrate (RH)} + O_2 + NADPH + H^+ \rightarrow$$
$$\text{Product (ROH)} + H_2O + NADP^+$$

Although CYP functions as a monooxygenase, the products are not limited to alcohols and phenols due to rearrangement reactions (Guengerich, 1991, 2001b, 2007; Isin and Guengerich, 2007). During catalysis, CYP binds directly to the substrate and molecular oxygen, but it does not interact directly with NADPH or NADH. The mechanism by which CYP receives electrons from NAD(P)H depends on the subcellular localization of CYP. In the endoplasmic reticulum, which is where most of the CYP enzymes involved in xenobiotic biotransformation are localized, electrons are relayed from NADPH to CYP via a flavoprotein called NADPH-cytochrome P450 reductase (also known as an oxidoreductase; gene symbol POR). Within this flavoprotein, electrons are transferred from NADPH to CYP via FMN and FAD. In mitochondria, which house many of the CYP enzymes involved in steroid hormone biosynthesis and vitamin D metabolism, electrons are transferred from NAD(P)H to CYP via 2 proteins: an iron–sulfur protein called ferredoxin (gene symbol FDX1) and an FMN-containing flavoprotein called ferredoxin reductase (gene symbol FDXR). These proteins are also known as adrenodoxin and adrenodoxin reductase. In bacteria such as *Pseudomonas putida*, which express P450cam (CYP101A1), electron flow is similar to that in mitochondria (NADH → flavoprotein → putidaredoxin → P450).

There are some notable exceptions to the general rule that CYP requires a second enzyme (ie, a flavoprotein) for catalytic activity. One exception applies to 2 CYP enzymes involved in the conversion of arachidonic acid to eicosanoids, namely, thromboxane A synthase (CYP5A1, gene symbol TBXAS1) and prostaglandin I_2 synthase, which is also known as prostacyclin synthase (CYP8A1, gene symbol PTGIS). These 2 CYP enzymes convert the endoperoxide,

PGH_2, to thromboxane (TXA_2) and prostacyclin (PGI_2) in platelets and the endothelial lining of blood vessels, respectively. In both cases, CYP functions as an isomerase and catalyzes a rearrangement of the oxygen atoms introduced into arachidonic acid by cyclooxygenase (see Fig. 6-33). The plant CYP, allene oxide synthase (CYP74A1), and certain invertebrate CYP enzymes also catalyze the rearrangement of oxidized chemicals (Guengerich, 2001b).

The second exception is represented by CYP102 (P450BM3) from the bacterium *Bacillus megaterium*, which produces a CYP enzyme linked directly to a flavoprotein to form a single, self-sufficient fusion protein. Some bacterial CYP enzymes are thermophilic (such as CYP119, CYP174A1, and CYP231A2), which has attracted attention for their potential industrial applications (Nishida and Ortiz de Montellano, 2005). The thermophilic P450 enzyme from *Sulfolobus acidocaldarius*, namely, CYP119, was used to confirm (and settle a long-standing debate) that the final step in the catalytic cycle of CYP is formation of compound I ($por^{\bullet+}Fe^{IV}=O$), as in the case of peroxidases, which is discussed later in this section (Rittle and Green, 2010). Most mammalian CYP enzymes are not synthesized as a single enzyme containing both the hemoprotein and flavoprotein moieties, but this arrangement is found in the nitric oxide (NO) synthases. In addition to its atypical structure, the P450 enzyme expressed in *B. megaterium*, CYP102, is unusual for another reason: it is inducible by phenobarbital, which provided insight into the mechanism of CYP induction.

Phospholipids and cytochrome b_5 also play an important role in CYP reactions (McLaughlin *et al.*, 2010). CYP and NADPH-cytochrome P450 reductase are embedded in the phospholipid bilayer of the endoplasmic reticulum, which facilitates their interaction. With the notable exception of CYP2W1 (discussed later in this section), CYP and NADPH-cytochrome P450 reductase face the cytoplasmic side of the endoplasmic reticulum. When the C-terminal region that anchors NADPH-cytochrome P450 reductase in the membrane is cleaved with trypsin, the truncated flavoprotein can no longer support CYP reactions, although it is still capable of reducing cytochrome c and other soluble electron acceptors. The ability of phospholipids to facilitate the interaction between NADPH-cytochrome P450 reductase and CYP does not appear to depend on the nature of the polar head group (serine, choline, inositol, ethanolamine), although certain CYP enzymes (those in the CYP3A subfamily) have a requirement for phospholipids containing unsaturated fatty acids. In vitro experiments established that cytochrome b_5 can stimulate various CYP reactions by either increasing V_{max} or decreasing K_m, which was initially interpreted as evidence that cytochrome b_5 can donate the second of 2 electrons required by CYP. However, the same stimulation occurs with heme-depleted cytochrome b_5 (Yamazaki *et al.*, 1996, 2001). The stimulatory effect of cytochrome b_5 is now attributed to its effect on CYP conformation and/or its ability to facilitate the interaction between CYP and NADPH-cytochrome P450 reductase. Experiments in conditional knockout mice establish that cytochrome b_5 has an important stimulatory effect on CYP in vivo (McLaughlin *et al.*, 2010). Liver microsomes contain numerous forms of CYP but contain a single form of NADPH-cytochrome P450 reductase (POR) and cytochrome b_5 (CYB5A).

For each molecule of NADPH-cytochrome P450 reductase in rat liver microsomes, there are 5 to 10 molecules of cytochrome b_5 and 10 to 20 molecules of CYP. In human liver microsomes the ratio of CYP to NADPH-cytochrome P450 reductase is slightly lower (closer to 5:1). NADPH-cytochrome P450 reductase will reduce electron acceptors other than CYP, which enables this enzyme to be measured based on its ability to reduce cytochrome c (which is why NADPH-cytochrome P450 reductase is often called NADPH-cytochrome c reductase). NADPH-cytochrome P450 reductase can transfer electrons much faster than CYP can use them, which more than likely accounts for the low ratio of NADPH-cytochrome P450 reductase to CYP in liver microsomes. Low levels of NADPH-cytochrome P450 reductase may also be a safeguard to protect cells from the often deleterious one-electron reduction reactions catalyzed by this flavoprotein (see Fig. 6-16). NADPH-cytochrome P450 reductase also supports heme oxygenase, a Nrf2-inducible enzyme, the significance of which is discussed in the section "CYP2E1."

Whereas microsomal cytochrome b_5 is encoded by CYB5A, CYB5B encodes the cytochrome b_5 found in the outer mitochondrial membrane where it supports the molybdoenzyme mARC in the dehydroxylation of certain amidoximes and related compounds (see the section "Dehydroxylation—mARC, Cytochrome b_5, b_5 Reductase, and Aldehyde Oxidase" and Fig. 6-22).

The catalytic cycle of CYP involves 8 steps (A → H), as shown in Fig. 6-40 for the oxidation of a substrate (RH) to its hydroxylated metabolite (ROH) (Dawson, 1988; Guengerich, 2007; Rittle and Green, 2010; Johnston *et al.*, 2011; Hrycay and Bandiera, 2012). In this scheme, iron is shown bound to its fifth ligand, a heme thiolate provided by a highly conserved cysteine (Cys) residue. The first steps of the cycle (A → G) involve the activation of oxygen to compound I, and the final steps involve substrate oxidation by compound I (G → H) followed by release of the metabolite (ROH) to restore the enzyme to its resting (ferric) state (H → A). Following the binding of substrate (RH) to CYP (A → B), the heme iron is reduced from the ferric (Fe^{III}) to the ferrous (Fe^{II}) state by the introduction of a single electron from NADPH-cytochrome P450 reductase (B → C). In many cases the reduction of CYP is facilitated by substrate binding because binding of the substrate in the vicinity of the heme moiety converts the heme ferric iron from a low-spin to a high-spin state, although some enzymes, such as CYP1A2 and CYP2E1, are naturally in the high-spin state and can be reduced in the absence of substrate. It is at stage C, when the iron is in

the ferrous state, that CYP can bind oxygen and CO. It is at this stage of the cycle that, under reduced oxygen tension, CYP can reduce certain substrates (see "Other Reactions" at the bottom of the catalytic cycle shown in Fig. 6-40). In the third step (C → D) oxygen binds to the ferrous iron, which transfers an electron to oxygen to form ferrisuperoxo anion (ie, ferric-bound superoxide anion), designated $Cys–Fe^{III}O_2^-$. At this stage the cycle can be interrupted (uncoupled) to release superoxide anion and restore the enzyme to its resting (ferric) state (see "Other Reactions" in Fig. 6-40). In the fourth step (D → E), a second electron is introduced from NADPH-cytochrome P450 reductase, which is delocalized over the thiolate bond, to form the supernucleophilic ferriperoxo intermediate $^-Cys–Fe^{III}O_2^-$. Uncoupling of the cycle at this stage releases hydrogen peroxide and restores the enzyme to its resting (ferric) state (see "Other Reactions" in Fig. 6-40). In the fifth step (E → F), addition of a proton (H^+) converts the supernucleophilic ferriperoxo intermediate to its corresponding hydroperoxide, the ferrihydroperoxy intermediate $^-Cys–Fe^{III}OOH$. In the sixth step (F → G), addition of a second proton and release of water converts the ferrihydroperoxy intermediate to compound I, an iron^{IV}-oxo porphyrin radical cation species (an oxidizing species previously described in the section "Peroxidase-Dependent Cooxidation"). The formation of compound I (por$^{•+}Fe^{IV}$=O) by protonation of the ferrihydroperoxy intermediate involves the heterolytic cleavage of oxygen with the 2-electron oxygen atom going to water, a reaction facilitated by the strong electron-donating effects of the heme thiolate anion. Heterolytic (2-electron) cleavage of oxygen to produce compound I places the iron in the perferryl (Fe^V) oxidation state, which is a considerably stronger oxidant than that formed by homolytic cleavage of oxygen, which produces the less reactive Por Fe^{IV}–OH with iron in oxidation state IV. (*Note*: It is somewhat confusing that compound I is written as por$^{•+}Fe^{IV}$=O because, without taking the porphyrin ring into account, the formula gives the erroneous impression that the iron is in the Fe^{IV} [ferryl] state, whereas it is actually in the Fe^V [perferryl] state.) In the seventh step (G → H), the highly electrophilic oxygen from compound I is transferred to the substrate (RH) to produce metabolite (ROH). In the final step (H → A), the metabolite is released, which restores the enzyme to its initial resting (ferric) state.

Compound I is the electrophilic oxo species responsible for the vast majority of CYP-catalyzed reactions (Hrycay and Bandiera, 2012). It can be formed as described above with NADPH and oxygen, or it can be formed by oxygen transfer from various organic hydroperoxides and peracids (X-OOH, such as cumene hydroperoxide, *tert*-butylhydroperoxide, and *meta*-chloroperbenzoic acid) in a one-step reaction called the "peroxide shunt," as shown in "Other Reactions" in Fig. 6-40. Formation of CYP compound I from peroxy compounds (P450 + X-OOH → P450 compound I + X-OH) is identical to the formation of compound I in peroxidases (see the section "Peroxidase-Dependent Cooxidation"). However, by virtue of its unusual fifth ligand (the heme thiolate from cysteine) and, perhaps more importantly, its active site topology, CYP can catalyze a far greater array of oxidative reactions (or catalyze them much faster) than those typically seen with peroxidases (even chloroperoxidase, which is unusual among peroxidases for containing a Cys thiolate as the fifth ligand to the heme like that in CYP). CYP reactions supported by organic peroxides and peracids are not affected by CO, an inhibitor of reactions supported by NADPH/O_2.

Although P450 compound I generated by the peroxide shunt is as catalytically versatile as that generated by NADPH/O_2, differences in the ratio of metabolites formed from a single substrate, differences in the relative rates of oxidation of 2 or more substrates, and differences in kinetic isotope effects (the influence of deuterium

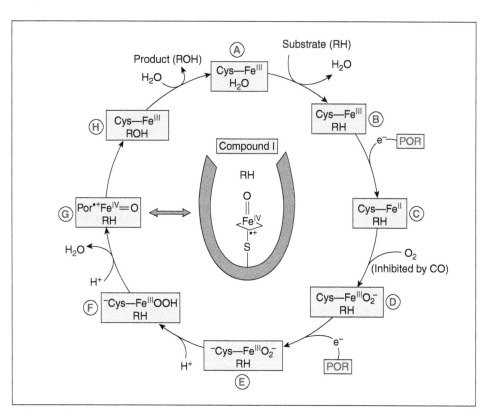

Other reactions

One-electron reduction	C (Cys—Fe^{II} RH)	$\longrightarrow$	A (Cys—Fe^{III} + RH$^{\bullet}$)
Superoxide anion production	D (Cys—Fe^{III}O$_2^-$ RH)	$\longrightarrow$	B (Cys—Fe^{III} RH) + O$_2^{\bar{\bullet}}$
Hydrogen peroxide production	E ($^-$Cys—Fe^{III}O$_2^-$ RH) + 2H$^+$	$\longrightarrow$	B (Cys—Fe^{III} RH) + H$_2$O$_2$
Hydrogen peroxide shunt	B (Cys—Fe^{III} RH) + H$_2$O$_2$	$\longrightarrow$	F ($^-$Cys—Fe^{III}OOH RH) + H$^+$
Peroxide shunt to form Compound I	B (Cys—Fe^{III} RH) + XOOH	$\longrightarrow$	G (Por$^{\bullet+}$Fe^{IV}=O RH) + XOH

Figure 6-40. *Catalytic cycle of cytochrome P450.* Cytochrome P450 is represented as Cys-Fe^{III}, where Cys represents the fifth ligand (a cysteine thiolate) to the ferric heme iron. RH and ROH represent the substrate and product (hydroxylated metabolite), respectively. The intermediates in the catalytic cycle are as follows: A, ferric resting state; B, substrate bound; C, ferrous intermediate; D, ferrisuperoxo anion intermediate; E, ferriperoxo intermediate with an electron delocalized over the Cys thiolate bond; F, ferrihydroperoxy intermediate (with a negative charge on the Cys thiolate bond); G, compound I, an iron^{IV}-oxo porphyrin cation, which is responsible for most substrate oxidation reactions; H, enzyme in its resting state prior to the release of product formed by hydrogen abstraction followed by oxygen rebound (see text for details). Fe^{II}, Fe^{III}, Fe^{IV}, and Fe^{V} refer to iron in the ferrous, ferric, ferryl, and perferryl state, respectively. It should be noted that although it is written as por$^{\bullet+}$Fe^{IV}=O, compound I is in the highly oxidized perferryl (Fe^{V}) state when the oxidation state of the porphyrin ring is also taken into account.

substitution at the site of oxidation) have led to the "multiple oxidants" hypothesis. The concept is supported by the finding that site-directed mutagenesis of a highly conserved threonine residue in bacterial and mammalian CYP enzymes can differentially affect reaction rates. For example, site-directed mutagenesis (Thr268Ala) of the bacterial enzyme CYP102A1 (P450BM3) increases the rate of sulfoxidation relative to *N*-demethylation of a single substrate, namely, dimethyl-(4-methylsulfanylphenyl)amine, whereas another mutation (Phe87Ala) has the opposite effect. Although the concept that CYP forms 2 or more oxidizing species is well accepted, the basis for the multiplicity is a source of considerable debate (Chandrasena *et al.*, 2004; Jin *et al.*, 2004; Newcomb and Chandrasena, 2005; Sheng *et al.*, 2009; Hrycay and Bandiera, 2012). The 2 major competing theories are the 2-state and the 2-oxidant hypotheses, both of which have supporting evidence. The 2-state

hypothesis posits that compound I is the only oxidizing species but it exists in 2 states, a low-spin state (that favors *N*-demethylation) and a high-spin state (that favors sulfoxidation) (Newcomb and Chandrasena, 2005; Hrycay and Bandiera, 2012). The 2-oxidant hypothesis posits that compound I is the major electrophilic oxidizing species but that its precursor, the ferrihydroperoxo intermediate ($^-$Cys–Fe^{III}OOH), can function as a relatively strong nucleophilic but weak electrophilic oxidizing species (Chandrasena *et al.*, 2004; Jin *et al.*, 2004; Sheng *et al.*, 2009). This is supported by the observation that hydrogen peroxide (which does not form compound I but instead forms the preceding ferrihydroperoxo intermediate or its equivalent, namely, ferric iron–bound hydrogen peroxide) can support certain reactions that are not supported by organic hydroperoxides and peracids. The 2 mechanisms of generating multiple oxidizing species are not mutually exclusive and both may be needed to explain all the catalytic properties of CYP. There are also competing theories concerning the mechanism of substrate oxidation by P450 compound I (Hrycay and Bandiera, 2012). Hereafter, the mechanism of carbon hydroxylation is discussed in terms of just one possibility, namely, hydrogen atom transfer (HAT) from the site of substrate hydroxylation by compound I to form a carbon radical followed by oxygen rebound in a nonconcerted, stepwise manner even though experiments with so-called ultrarapid radical clocks support a nonradical mechanism (Newcomb and Chandrasena, 2005; Hrycay and Bandiera, 2012). In reactions involving heteroatoms (N and S) the initial step involves (among other possibilities) single electron transfer (SET) leading to *S*- and *N*-oxygenation or HAT leading to *S*- and *N*-dealkylation, as discussed later in this section (Li *et al.*, 2009a; Roberts and Jones, 2010).

CYP catalyzes several types of oxidation reactions, including:

1. Hydroxylation of an aliphatic or aromatic carbon
2. Epoxidation of a double bond
3. Heteroatom (S-, N-, and I-) oxygenation and *N*-hydroxylation
4. Heteroatom (*O*-, *S*-, and *N*-) dealkylation
5. Oxidative group transfer
6. Cleavage of esters and carbamates
7. Dehydrogenation

In the first 3 cases, oxygen from P450 compound I is incorporated into the substrate, which otherwise remains intact. In the fourth case, oxygenation of the substrate is followed by a rearrangement reaction leading to cleavage of an amine (*N*-dealkylation) or an ether (*O*- and *S*-dealkylation). Oxygen from P450 compound I is incorporated into the alkyl-leaving group, producing an aldehyde or ketone. In the fifth case, oxygenation of the substrate is followed by a rearrangement reaction leading to loss of a heteroatom (oxidative group transfer). The sixth case, the cleavage of esters and carbamates, resembles heteroatom dealkylation in that the functional group is cleaved with incorporation of oxygen from P450 compound I into the leaving group, producing an aldehyde. In the seventh case, 2 hydrogens are abstracted from the substrate with the formation of a double bond (C=C, C=O, or C=N), with the reduction of oxygen from P450 compound I to water. It should be noted that this long list of reactions does not encompass all the reactions catalyzed by CYP (Guengerich, 2001b, 2007). CYP can catalyze reductive reactions (such as azo-reduction, nitro-reduction, *N*-oxide reduction, sulfoxide reduction, and reductive dehalogenation), ring expansion or ring formation, dearylation, dearomatization, isomerization (such as the conversion of PGH$_2$ to thromboxane and prostacyclin), and oxidative dehalogenation (as described previously for FMO; see Fig. 6-38). During the synthesis of steroid hormones, CYP catalyzes the cleavage of carbon–carbon bonds, which occurs during the conversion of cholesterol to pregnenolone by cholesterol side-chain cleavage enzyme (CYP11A1, which is also known as P450$_{scc}$) and the aromatization of a substituted cyclohexane, which occurs during the conversion of androgens to estrogens by aromatase (CYP19A1, also known as CYP19 and P450$_{arom}$).

Examples of aliphatic and aromatic hydroxylation reactions catalyzed by CYP are shown in Figs. 6-41 and 6-42, respectively. The hydroxylation of aromatic hydrocarbons may proceed via an oxirane intermediate (ie, an arene oxide) that isomerizes to the corresponding phenol. Alternatively, aromatic hydroxylation can proceed by a mechanism known as direct insertion. The *ortho*- and *para*-hydroxylation of chlorobenzene proceed via 2,3- and 3,4-epoxidation, whereas *meta*-hydroxylation proceeds by direct insertion, as shown in Fig. 6-43. When aromatic hydroxylation involves direct insertion, hydrogen abstraction (ie, cleavage of the

C–H bond) is the rate-limiting step, so that substitution of hydrogen with deuterium or tritium considerably slows the hydroxylation reaction. This *isotope effect* is less marked when aromatic hydroxylation proceeds via an arene oxide intermediate. Arene oxides are electrophilic and, therefore, potentially toxic metabolites that are detoxified by such enzymes as epoxide hydrolase (see Figs. 6-8 to 6-10) and GST (see the section "Glutathione Conjugation"). Depending on the ring substituents, the rearrangement of arene oxides to the corresponding phenol can lead to an intramolecular migration of a substituent (such as hydrogen or a halogen) from one carbon to the next. This intramolecular migration occurs at the site of oxidation and is known as the NIH shift, so named for its discovery at the National Institutes of Health.

Aliphatic hydroxylation involves insertion of oxygen into a C–H bond. The initial step involves HAT to form a carbon radical followed by oxygen rebound, shown as follows:

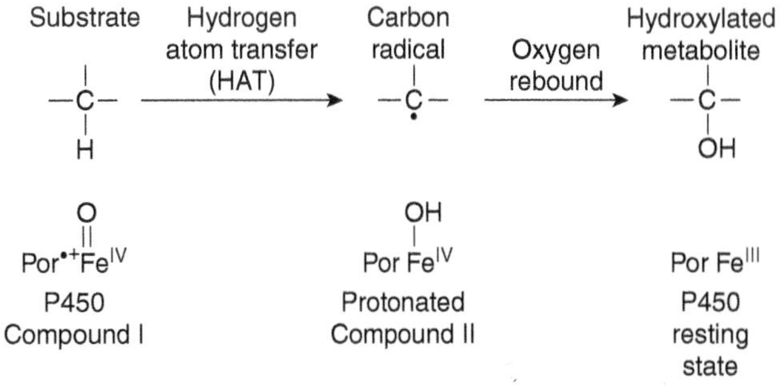

In the case of simple, straight-chain hydrocarbons, such as *n*-hexane, aliphatic hydroxylation occurs at both the terminal methyl groups and the internal methylene groups. In the case of fatty acids (both saturated and unsaturated) and their derivatives (ie, retinoic acid and eicosanoids such as prostaglandins and leukotrienes), aliphatic hydroxylation occurs at the ω-carbon (terminal methyl group) and the ω-1 carbon (penultimate carbon), as shown for lauric acid in Fig. 6-41. For thermodynamic reasons, most CYP enzymes preferentially catalyze the ω-1 hydroxylation of fatty acids and their derivatives, but one group of CYP enzymes (those encoded by the CYP4 gene family) preferentially catalyzes the less energetically favorable ω-hydroxylation of fatty acids, which can be further oxidized to dicarboxylic acids and undergo chain shortening by β-oxidation (Baer and Rettie, 2006; Johnston *et al.*, 2011).

Like CYP, the molybdoenzymes AO and XO can also catalyze the carbon oxidation of xenobiotics as outlined in the section "Molybdenum Hydroxylases (Molybdoenzymes)." As an electrophilic oxidizing enzyme, CYP generally prefers to catalyze the oxidation of carbon atoms with a high electron density, whereas the nucleophilic oxidizing enzymes AO and XO preferentially catalyze the oxidation of carbon atoms with a low electron density (such as the sp^2 carbon atom double bonded to a nitrogen atom in various nitrogen heterocycles). For this reason, xenobiotics that are good substrates for CYP enzymes tend to be poor substrates for AO, and vice versa (Pryde *et al.*, 2010).

Xenobiotics containing a carbon–carbon double bond (ie, alkenes) can be epoxidated (ie, converted to an oxirane) in an analogous manner to the oxidation of aromatic compounds to arene oxides. Just as arene oxides can isomerize to phenols, so aliphatic epoxides can isomerize to the corresponding ene-ol, the formation of which may involve an intramolecular migration (NIH shift) of a substituent at the site of oxidation (examples of intramolecular shifts accompanying epoxidation are given in the section "Activation of Xenobiotics by Cytochrome P450"). Like arene oxides, aliphatic epoxides are also potentially toxic metabolites that are inactivated

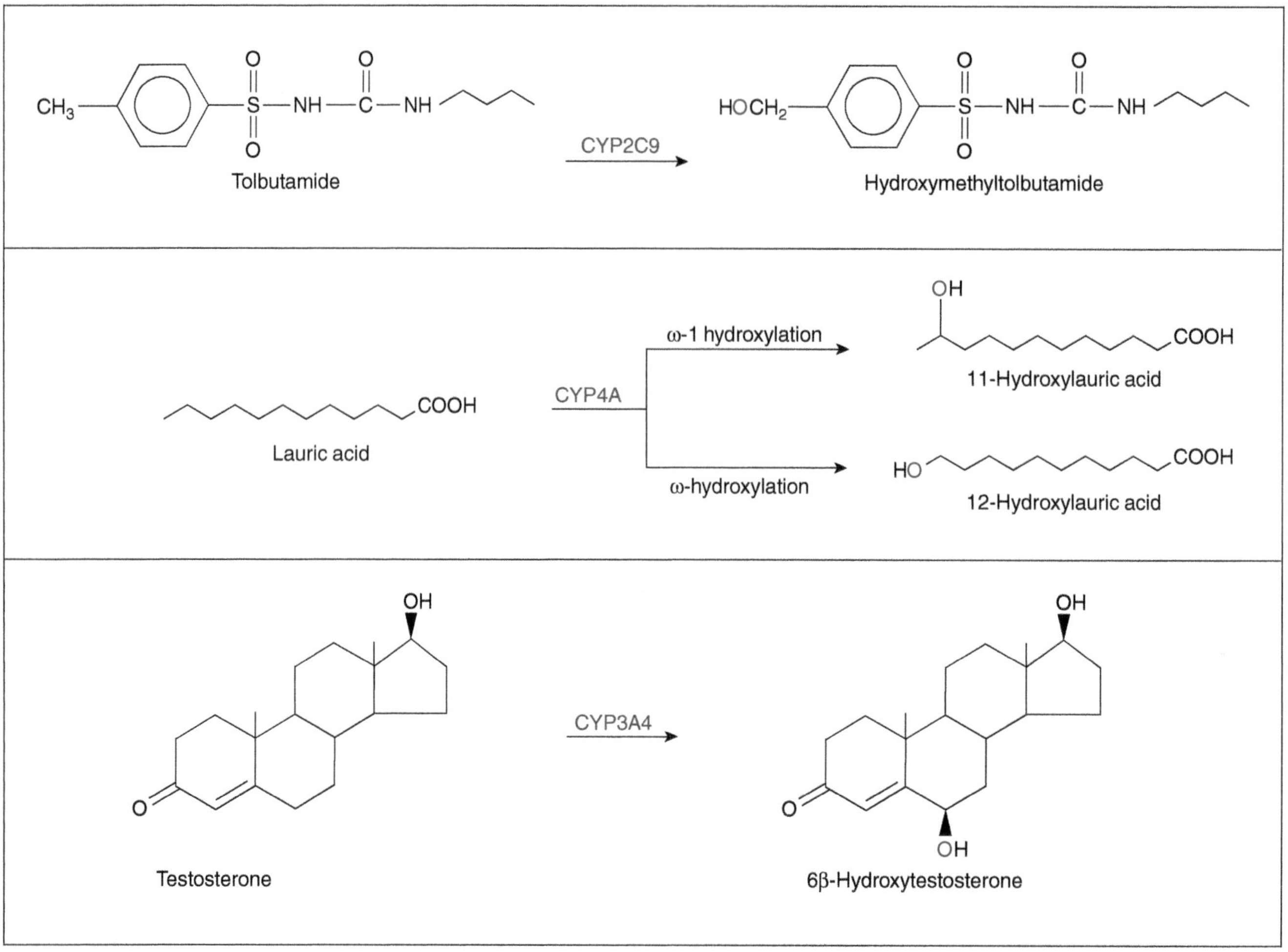

Figure 6-41. *Examples of reactions catalyzed by cytochrome P450: hydroxylation of aliphatic carbon.*

by other xenobiotic-metabolizing enzymes such as epoxide hydrolase and GST. Alkynes can be epoxidated by CYP to ketocarbenes (which can be further oxidized to carboxylic acids). The conversion of an alkyne to a ketocarbene via epoxidation or other possible oxidation intermediates is shown in the following scheme:

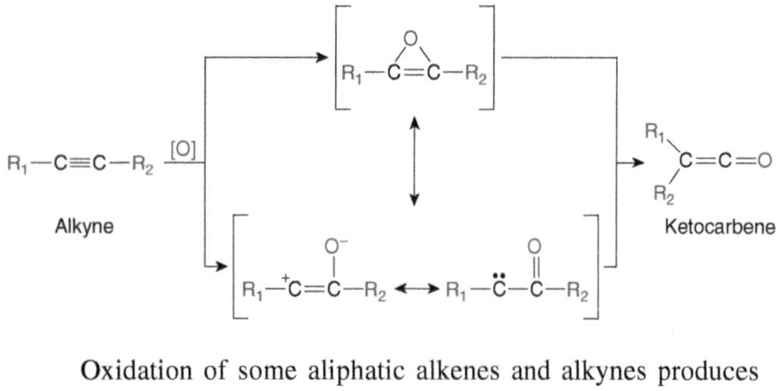

Oxidation of some aliphatic alkenes and alkynes produces metabolites that are sufficiently reactive to bind covalently to the heme moiety of CYP, a process known as suicide inactivation or MDI (discussed later in the section "Inhibition of Cytochrome P450"). As previously discussed in the section "Epoxide Hydrolases," not all epoxides are highly reactive electrophiles. Although the 3,4-epoxidation of coumarin produces a hepatotoxic metabolite, the 10,11-epoxidation of carbamazepine produces a stable, relatively nontoxic metabolite (Fig. 6-43). EETs are endogenous epoxides with vasodilatory, anti-inflammatory, and angiogenic properties (Imig and Hammock, 2009; Wang *et al.*, 2010c). They are formed

by CYP2C8, CYP2C9, and CYP2J2 (discussed later in this section) and inactivated by sEH (see the section "Epoxide Hydrolases").

In the presence of NADPH and O_2, liver microsomes catalyze the oxygenation of several sulfur-containing xenobiotics, including chlorpromazine, cimetidine, lansoprazole, pantoprazole, and omeprazole. Sulfur-containing xenobiotics can potentially undergo 2 consecutive sulfoxidation reactions: one that converts the sulfide (S) to the sulfoxide (SO), which occurs during the sulfoxidation of chlorpromazine and cimetidine, and one that converts the sulfoxide (SO) to the sulfone (SO_2), which occurs during the sulfoxidation of omeprazole and lansoprazole, as shown in Fig. 6-44. Albendazole is converted first to a sulfoxide and then to a sulfone. Both CYP and FMO can sulfoxidate sulfides to sulfoxides (S → SO) but only CYP can covert sulfoxides to sulfones (SO → SO_2) (see the section "Flavin Monooxygenases") (Testa and Krämer, 2008, 2010). Accordingly, the sulfoxidation of the proton pump inhibitors omeprazole, lansoprazole, and pantoprazole to sulfones is catalyzed by CYP (CYP3A4) and not by FMO. Examples of sulfoxidation reactions catalyzed by FMO and/or CYP are shown in Figs. 6-38B and 6-44. In the presence of NADPH and O_2, liver microsomes catalyze the oxygenation of several nitrogen-containing xenobiotics, including chlorpromazine, doxylamine, oflaxacin, morphine, nicotine, MPTP, methapyrilene, methaqualone, metronidazole, pargyline, pyridine, senecionine, strychnine, TMA, trimipramine, and verapamil, all of which are converted to stable *N*-oxides. Whereas *S*-oxygenation might be catalyzed by both CYP and FMO, *N*-oxygenation is more likely to be catalyzed by just one of these enzymes. FMO

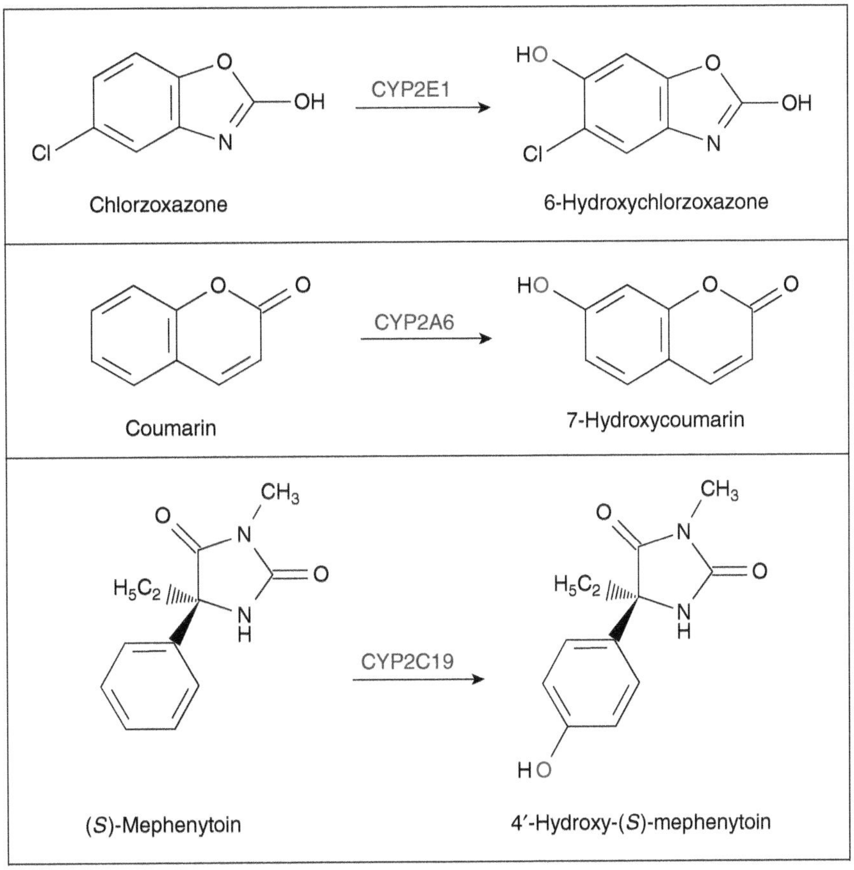

Figure 6-42. *Examples of reactions catalyzed by cytochrome P450: hydroxylation of aromatic carbon.*

prefers to *N*-oxygenate aliphatic amines (particularly tertiary and cyclic amines) with a highly nucleophilic/basic nitrogen atom (pK_a 5–10) but, in contrast to CYP, FMO cannot *N*-oxygenate aromatic amines, for which reason the *N*-oxygenation of pyridines and (iso) quinolones is usually catalyzed only by CYP, as is the case for pyridine-containing xenobiotics such as the tobacco-specific nitrosamine NNK and the antihistamine temelastine, and the isoquinoline-containing muscle relaxant 6,7-dimethoxy-4-(4′-chlorobenzyl) isoquinoline. Methods to distinguish the role of CYP versus FMO in microsomal *N*- and *S*-oxygenation reactions are described in the section "Flavin Monooxygenases."

Although direct oxygen transfer is possible (Li *et al.*, 2009a), the initial step in heteroatom oxygenation by CYP could involve SET from the heteroatom (*N*, *S*, or *I*) to P450 compound I, shown as follows for sulfoxidation:

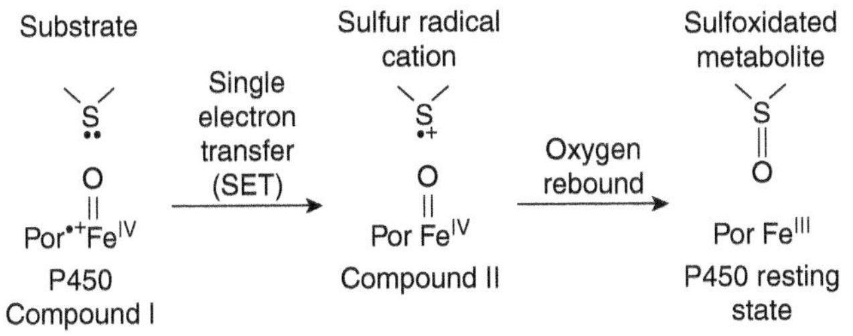

SET from *N*, *O*, or *S* to P450 compound I may also be the initial step in heteroatom dealkylation, but in this case abstraction of the electron from the heteroatom is quickly followed by abstraction of a proton (H⁺) from the α-carbon atom (the carbon atom attached to the heteroatom) to form a carbon radical. Oxygen rebound leads

to hydroxylation of the α-carbon, which then rearranges to form the corresponding aldehyde or ketone with cleavage of the α-carbon from the heteroatom, as shown in the following scheme for the *N*-dealkylation of an *N*-alkylamine:

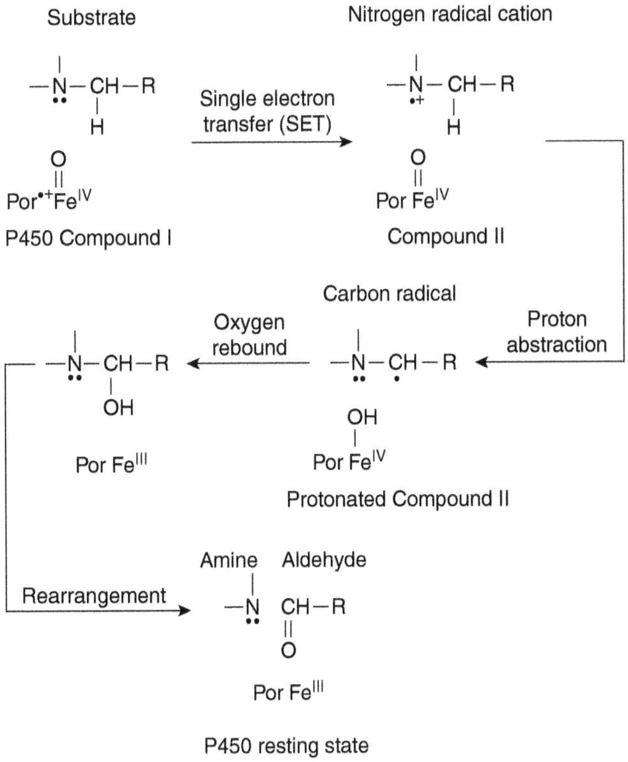

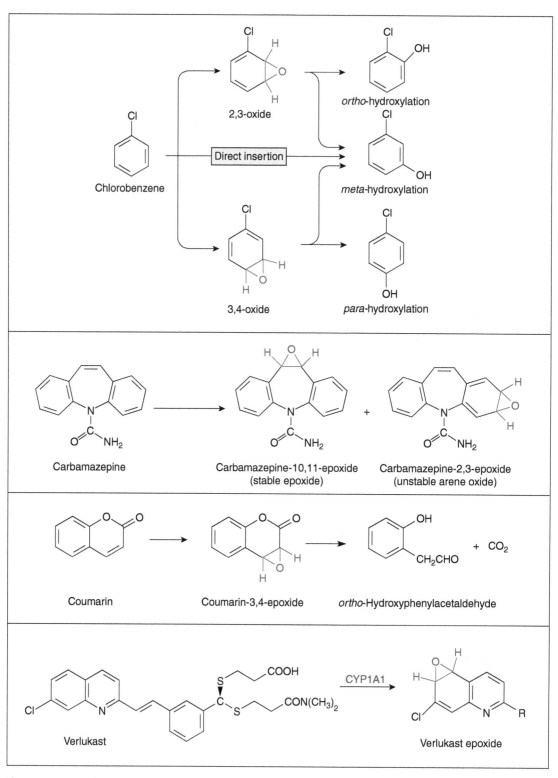

Figure 6-43. *Examples of reactions catalyzed by cytochrome P450: epoxidation.*

Alternatively, it seems more likely that the initial step in heteroatom dealkylation may be HAT from the α-carbon atom to compound I to produce a carbon radical that undergoes oxygen rebound and rearrangement as shown in the following scheme (Li et al., 2009a; Roberts and Jones, 2010):

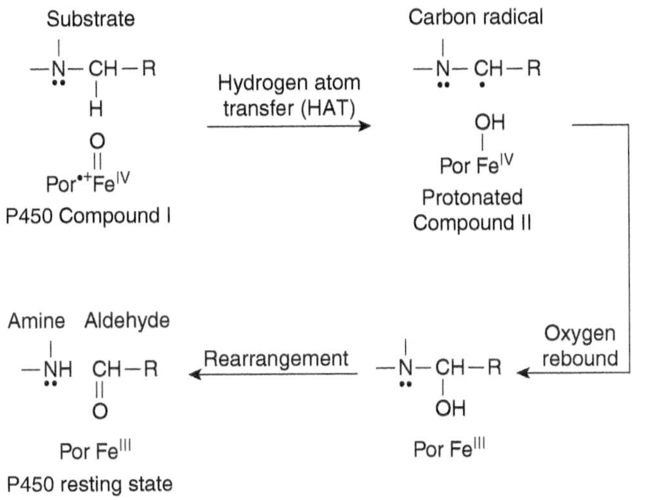

In general, CYP catalyzes the N-dealkylation, not the N-oxygenation, of amines. N-Oxygenation by CYP can occur if the nitrogen is next to an electron-donating group (making the nitrogen electron rich) or if α-protons are either absent (eg, aromatic amines) or inaccessible (eg, quinidine). In the case of aromatic amines (anilines; aryl-NH$_2$), N-oxidation by CYP usually results in the formation of hydroxylamines (aryl-NHOH). Some hydroxylamines are further oxidized to the corresponding nitroso metabolite, as observed with sulfamethoxazole (aryl-NH$_2$ → aryl-NOH → aryl-NO). Primary aromatic amides (aryl-CONH$_2$) are not substrates for N-oxidation, but secondary aromatic amides (aryl-NHCOR) are often N-hydroxylated by CYP (often by CYP1A2) to produce N-hydroxyamines (also known as hydroxamic acids). N-Hydroxylamines and hydroxyamides are of toxicological interest because under acidic conditions they can dissociate to form reactive nitrenium ions. Phenacetin, an aromatic amide (aryl-NH–CO–CH$_3$), causes kidney toxicity because it is converted by N-hydroxylation to a hydroxamic acid (aryl-NOH–CO–CH$_3$) that in the low pH of urine undergoes acid-catalyzed conversion to a reactive nitrenium ion (aryl-NOH–CO–CH$_3$ + H$^+$ → aryl-N$^+$–CO–CH$_3$ + H$_2$O) (Testa and Krämer, 2008, 2010). N-Hydroxylation of aromatic amines with subsequent O-acetylation or O-sulfonation is 1 mechanism by which tumorigenic aromatic amines, such as 2-AAF and 4-aminobiphenyl, are converted to electrophilic reactive intermediates that bind covalently to DNA (discussed later in the sections "Glucuronidation and Formation of Acyl-CoA Thioesters" and "Acetylation").

Numerous xenobiotics are N-, O-, or S-dealkylated by CYP (but not by FMO), and some examples of these heteroatom dealkylation reactions are shown in Fig. 6-45. The dealkylation of xenobiotics containing an N-, O-, or S-methyl group results in the formation of formaldehyde, which can easily be measured by a simple colorimetric assay to monitor the demethylation of substrates in vitro. The expiration of ^{13}C- or ^{14}C-labeled carbon dioxide following the demethylation of drugs containing a ^{13}C- or ^{14}C-labeled methyl group has been used to probe CYP activity in vivo (Watkins, 1994). The activity of the human CYP enzymes involved in the N-demethylation of aminopyrine, erythromycin, and caffeine can be assessed by this technique. Although caffeine has 3 N-methyl groups, all of which can be removed by CYP, the major pathway in humans involves N$_3$-demethylation of caffeine to paraxanthine (see Fig. 6-45). Fig. 6-45 also presents an example of a xenobiotic (octamethylcyclotetrasiloxane, a component of cosmetics and deodorants) that undergoes silicone demethylation by CYP (Varaprath et al., 1999).

Whereas the metabolism of N-methyl amines by CYP generally results in N-demethylation, with the hydroxylation of the methyl group leading to the release of formaldehyde, the metabolism of N-methyl amides and carbamates by CYP can result in the formation of a stable methyl-hydroxylated metabolite, one that does not release formaldehyde (which would otherwise complete an N-demethylation reaction) possibly because of the hydroxymethyl metabolite formation of a 6-membered configuration that is stabilized by hydrogen bonding, illustrated as follows:

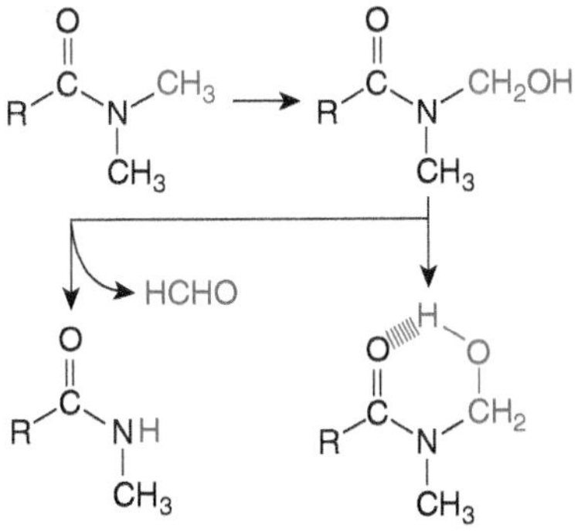

Zolpidem and camazepam are amide- and carbamate-containing drugs, respectively, that undergo such N-methyl-hydroxylation reactions.

Seto and Guengerich have shown that the N-demethylation and N-deethylation of N-ethyl-N-methylaniline not only proceed at different rates (with N-demethylation proceeding up to 20 times faster than N-deethylation) but also proceed by different mechanisms (Seto and Guengerich, 1993; Guengerich, 2001a). The initial step in the N-deethylation reaction involves HAT from the α-carbon atom (ie, the carbon atom attached to the nitrogen), whereas the initial step in the N-demethylation reaction involves a much faster reaction, namely, a SET from the nitrogen atom, which is transferred to P450 compound I. Although the N-demethylation of N,N-substituted amines proceeds by the relatively rapid process of SET, the N-demethylation of N,N-substituted amides, where the adjacent carbonyl causes electrons to be withdrawn from the nitrogen atom, proceeds by the relatively slow process of HAT, for which reason the latter reactions, in contrast to the former, show a large intrinsic isotope effect when the hydrogen atoms are replaced with deuterium (because it requires more energy to break a C–D bond than a C–H bond).

In addition to N-dealkylation, some primary amines can also undergo oxidative deamination by CYP, which is an example of oxidative group transfer. The mechanism of oxidative deamination is similar to that of N-dealkylation: the α-carbon adjacent to the primary amine is hydroxylated, which produces an unstable intermediate that rearranges to eliminate ammonia with the formation of an aldehyde or ketone. The conversion of amphetamine to phenylacetone is an example of CYP-catalyzed oxidative deamination, as shown in Fig. 6-46. However, primary aliphatic amines tend to be poor substrates for CYP; in fact, primary alkylamines, such as the N-demethylated metabolite of fluoxetine, are metabolically stable and potent inhibitors of CYP inhibitors (discussed later in the section "Inhibition of Cytochrome P450"). Oxidative deamination is also catalyzed by MAO and FMO (Testa and Krämer, 2008, 2010).

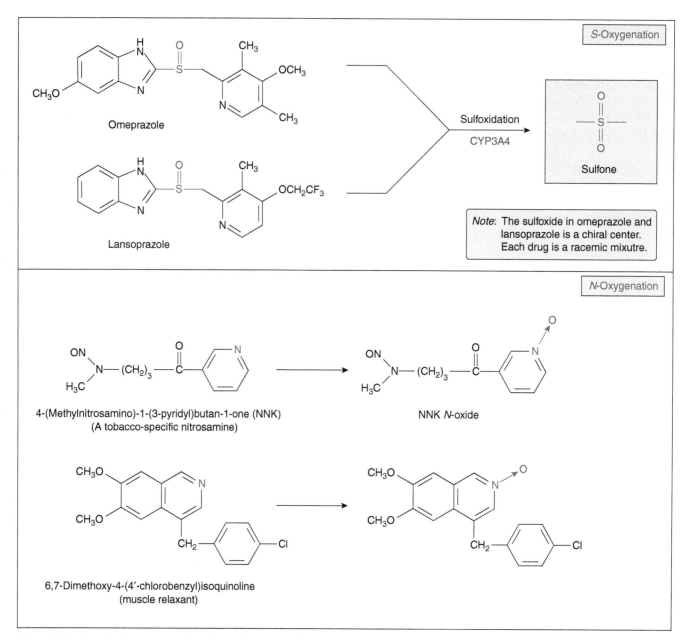

Figure 6-44. *Examples of reactions catalyzed by cytochrome P450: heteroatom oxygenation.*

In the example given above, however, the substrate, amphetamine, contains an α-methyl group that renders it a poor substrate for MAO (as described in the section "Amine Oxidases").

In addition to oxidative deamination, CYP catalyzes 2 other types of oxidative group transfer, namely, oxidative desulfuration and oxidative dehalogenation. In all cases the heteroatom (*N*, *S*, or halogen) is replaced with oxygen. As shown in Fig. 6-47, oxidative desulfuration converts parathion, which has little insecticidal activity, to paraoxon, which is a potent insecticide. The same reaction converts thiopental to pentobarbital. Diethyldithiocarbamate methyl ester, a metabolite of disulfiram, also undergoes oxidative desulfuration. The initial reaction involves *S*-oxidation by CYP or FMO to a sulfine ($R_1R_2C=S \rightarrow R_1R_2C=S^+-O^-$). In the presence of GSH and GST, this sulfine either is converted back to the parent compound ($R_1R_2C=S^+-O^- + 2GSH \rightarrow R_1R_2C=S + H_2O$) or undergoes desulfuration ($R_1R_2C=S + 2GSH \rightarrow R_1R_2C=O + GSSG + H_2S$) (Madan *et al.*, 1994). CYP catalyzes both reductive and oxidative dehalogenation reactions (Guengerich, 1991). During oxidative dehalogenation,

a halogen and hydrogen from the same carbon atom are replaced with oxygen ($R_1R_2CHX \rightarrow R_1R_2CO$) to produce an aldehyde or acylhalide, as shown in Fig. 6-19 for the conversion of halothane ($CF_3CHClBr$) to trifluoroacetylchloride (CF_3COCl). Oxidative dehalogenation does not involve a direct attack on the carbon–halogen bond, but it involves the formation of an unstable halohydrin by oxidation of the carbon atom bearing the halogen substituent. The carbon–halogen bond is broken during the rearrangement of the unstable halohydrin. When the carbon atom contains a single halogen, the resulting product is an aldehyde, which can be further oxidized to a carboxylic acid or reduced to a primary alcohol. When the carbon atom contains 2 halogens, the dihalohydrin intermediate rearranges to an acylhalide, which can be converted to the corresponding carboxylic acid (see Fig. 6-19). Aldehydes and, in particular, acylhalides are reactive compounds that can bind covalently to protein and other critical cellular molecules. The immune hepatitis caused by repeated exposure of humans to halothane and related volatile anesthetics is dependent on oxidative dehalogenation by

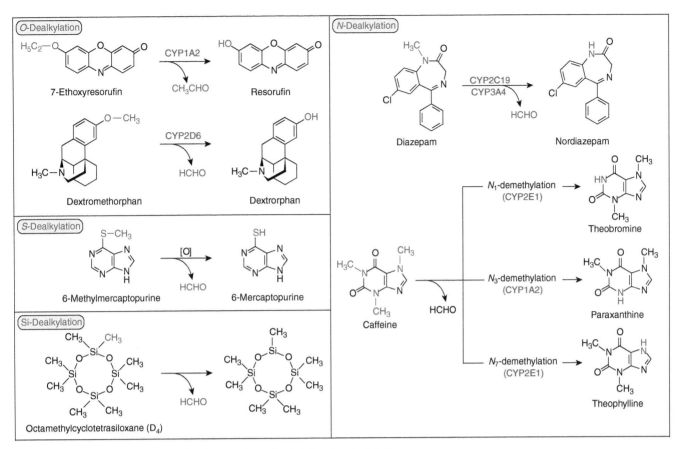

Figure 6-45. *Examples of reactions catalyzed by cytochrome P450: heteroatom dealkylation.*

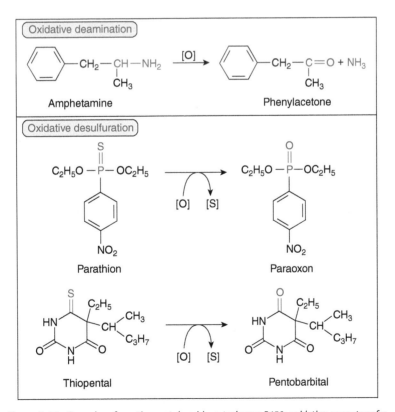

Figure 6-46. *Examples of reactions catalyzed by cytochrome P450: oxidative group transfer.*

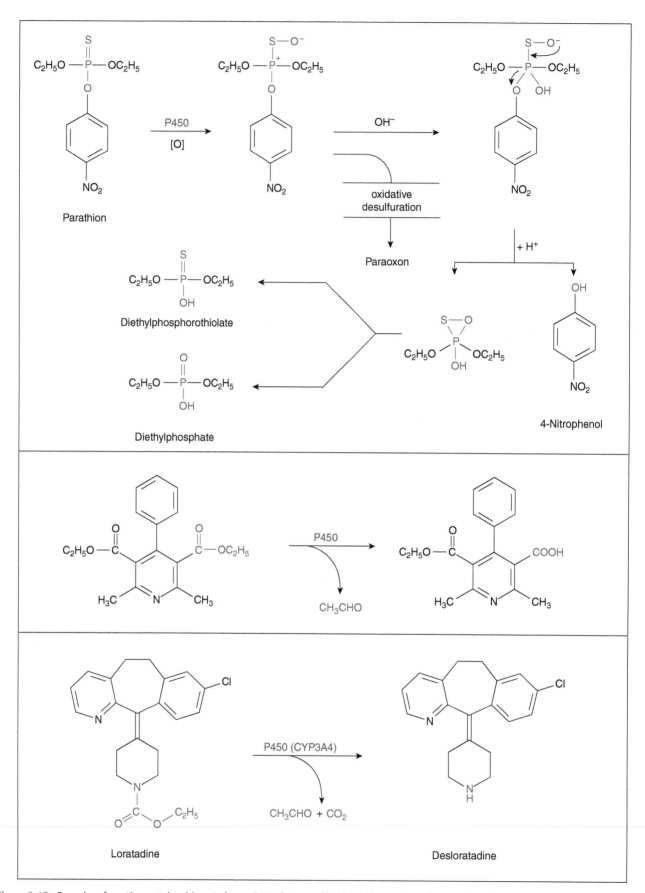

Figure 6-47. *Examples of reactions catalyzed by cytochrome P450 that resemble hydrolytic reactions: cleavage of a thiophosphate (parathion), a carboxylic acid ester (2,6-dimethyl-4-phenyl-3,5-pyridinecarboxylic acid diethyl ester), and a carbamate (loratadine).*

CYP, with neoantigens produced by the trifluoroacetylation of proteins, as shown in Fig. 6-19. Another example of oxidative dehalogenation by CYP is provided by studies of dasatinib metabolism by Li *et al.* (2009b), who, in order to prevent the formation of a reactive quinoneimine metabolite that bound to GSH, used fluoro and chloro substitution in an attempt to block *para*-hydroxylation of the substituted aniline in dasatinib, which is a metabolism-dependent inhibitor of CYP3A4. The halogen substitutions did not block the formation of GSH adducts of the *para*-hydroxylated metabolite. The mechanism of oxidative dehalogenation of the substituted aniline in dasatinib (followed by glutathionylation) was presumed to arise from an epoxide intermediate that underwent dehalogenation during its conjugation with GSH. Another example of oxidative defluorination is shown in Fig. 6-38 for the oxidative defluorination of 4-fluoro-*N*-methylaniline by FMO (Driscoll *et al.*, 2010).

CYP can catalyze the reductive dehalogenation of halogenated alkanes (see Figs. 6-18 and 6-19) and the reduction of certain azo- and nitro-containing xenobiotics, although these latter reactions are largely catalyzed by gut microflora (see Figs. 6-11 and 6-12). The ability of CYP to reduce xenobiotics can be understood from the catalytic cycle shown in Fig. 6-40. Binding of a substrate to CYP is followed by a one-electron reduction by NADPH-cytochrome P450 reductase. Under aerobic conditions, reduction of the heme iron to the ferrous state permits binding of oxygen. Anaerobic conditions, in contrast, interrupt the cycle at this point, which allows CYP to reduce those substrates capable of accepting an electron. Therefore, CYP can catalyze reduction reactions, such as azo-reduction, nitro-reduction, *N*-oxide reduction, sulfoxide reduction, and reductive dehalogenation, particularly under conditions of low oxygen tension. In effect, the substrate rather than molecular oxygen accepts electrons and is reduced. In fact, oxygen acts as an inhibitor of these reactions because it competes with the substrate for the reducing equivalents. The toxicity of many halogenated alkanes is dependent on their biotransformation by reductive dehalogenation. The first step in reductive dehalogenation is a one-electron reduction catalyzed by CYP, which produces a potentially toxic, carbon-centered radical and inorganic halide. The conversion of CCl_4 to a trichloromethyl radical and other toxic metabolites is shown in Fig. 6-18. The activation of the prodrug AQ4N (ie, 1,4-bis{[2-(dimethylamino-*N*-oxide)ethyl]amino}-5,8-dihydroxyanthracene-9,10-dione) by *N*-oxide reduction to form 4QA (ie, 1,4-bis{[2-(dimethylamino)ethyl]amino}-5,8-dihydroxyanthracene-9,10-dione), a potent topoisomerase II inhibitor, by the hypoxia-inducible enzymes CYP2S1 and CYP2W1 represents a potentially new cancer chemotherapy, as discussed later in this section.

The oxidative desulfuration of parathion (see Fig. 6-46) involves the production of an intermediate that rearranges to paraoxon (as shown in Fig. 6-47). This same intermediate can decompose to 4-nitrophenol and diethylphosphorothioic acid, which are the same products formed by the hydrolysis of parathion (Fig. 6-47). In addition to facilitating the hydrolysis of phosphoric acid esters, CYP also catalyzes the cleavage of certain carboxylic acid esters and carbamates, as shown in Fig. 6-47. Carboxylic acid esters typically are cleaved by carboxylesterases and cholinesterases (see the section "Hydrolysis"), which results in the formation of an acid and an alcohol ($R_1COOCH_2R_2 + H_2O \rightarrow R_1COOH + R_2CH_2OH$). In contrast, CYP converts carboxylic acid esters to an acid plus aldehyde ($R_1COOCH_2R_2 + [O] \rightarrow R_1COOH + R_2CHO$), as shown in Fig. 6-47. The deacylation of loratadine, a carbamate, is the major route of biotransformation of this nonsedating antihistamine. The reaction is catalyzed predominantly by CYP (namely, CYP3A4 with a minor contribution from CYP2D6), with little contribution from carboxylesterases (Yumibe *et al.*, 1996).

CYP can also catalyze the dehydrogenation of a number of compounds, including acetaminophen, nifedipine, and related dihydropyridine calcium channel blockers, sparteine, nicotine, and testosterone, as shown in Fig. 6-48. Dehydrogenation by CYP converts acetaminophen to its hepatotoxic metabolite, *N*-acetylbenzo-*p*-quinoneimine (NAPQI), as shown in Fig. 6-35. The formation of a double bond during the conversion of digitoxin (dt_3) to 15′-dehydro-dt_3 leads to cleavage of the terminal sugar residue to produce digitoxigenin bisdigitoxoside (dt_2) (Fig. 6-48), which can similarly be converted to 9′-dehydro-dt_2, which undergoes digitoxosyl cleavage to digitoxigenin monodigitoxoside (dt_1). In contrast to digitoxin, the latter metabolite is an excellent substrate for glucuronidation. In rats, the CYP enzymes responsible for converting digitoxin to dt_1 (namely, the CYP3A enzymes) and the UGT responsible for glucuronidating dt_1 are inducible by dexamethasone, PCN, and spironolactone, all of which protect rats from the toxic effects of digitoxin. The dehydrogenation of nicotine produces nicotine $\Delta^{1',5'}$-iminium ion, which is oxidized by cytosolic AO to cotinine, a major metabolite of nicotine excreted in the urine of cigarette smokers (see Fig. 6-48). Although nicotine can be *N*-oxygenated by FMO, dehydrogenation by CYP2A6 is responsible for 80% of the clearance of nicotine from cigarette smoking (Hukkanen *et al.*, 2005).

Testosterone is dehydrogenated by CYP to 2 metabolites: 6-dehydrotestosterone, which involves formation of a carbon–carbon double bond, and androstenedione, which involves formation of a carbon–oxygen double bond, as shown in Fig. 6-48. The conversion of testosterone to androstenedione is one of several cases where CYP converts a primary or secondary alcohol to an aldehyde or ketone, respectively. The reaction can proceed by formation of a *gem*-diol (2 hydroxyl groups on the same carbon atom), with subsequent dehydration to a keto group, as shown in Fig. 6-25 for the conversion of ethanol to acetaldehyde. However, *gem*-diols are not obligatory intermediates in the oxidation of alcohols by CYP, and in fact the conversion of testosterone to androstenedione by CYP2B1 (the major phenobarbital-inducible CYP enzyme in rats) does not involve the intermediacy of a *gem*-diol but proceeds by direct dehydrogenation (Fig. 6-48). In contrast, a *gem*-diol is involved in the formation of androstenedione from *epi*-testosterone (which is identical to testosterone except the hydroxyl group at C_{17} is in the α-configuration, not the β-configuration) (Wood *et al.*, 1988). The fact that formation of androstenedione from *epi*-testosterone involves formation of a *gem*-diol, whereas its formation from testosterone does not, makes it difficult to generalize the mechanism by which CYP converts alcohols to aldehydes and ketones.

Liver microsomes from all mammalian species contain numerous CYP enzymes (Table 6-11), each with the potential to catalyze the various types of reactions shown in Figs. 6-41 to 6-48. In other words, all of the CYP enzymes expressed in liver microsomes have the potential to catalyze xenobiotic hydroxylation, epoxidation, dealkylation, oxygenation, dehydrogenation, and so forth. The broad and often overlapping substrate specificity of liver microsomal CYP enzymes precludes the possibility of naming these enzymes for the reactions they catalyze, which are now categorized into families and subfamilies and named individually on the basis of their amino acid sequence. As shown in Tables 6-10 and 6-11, the CYP enzymes involved in xenobiotic biotransformation belong mainly to the CYP1, 2, and 3 gene families, although on a case-by-case basis CYP enzymes in other gene families play a key role in xenobiotic biotransformation. The CYP enzymes involved in endobiotic metabolism generally have the same name in all mammalian species. Some of the xenobiotic-biotransforming CYP enzymes have the same name in all mammalian species, whereas others are named in a species-specific manner. For example, all mammalian

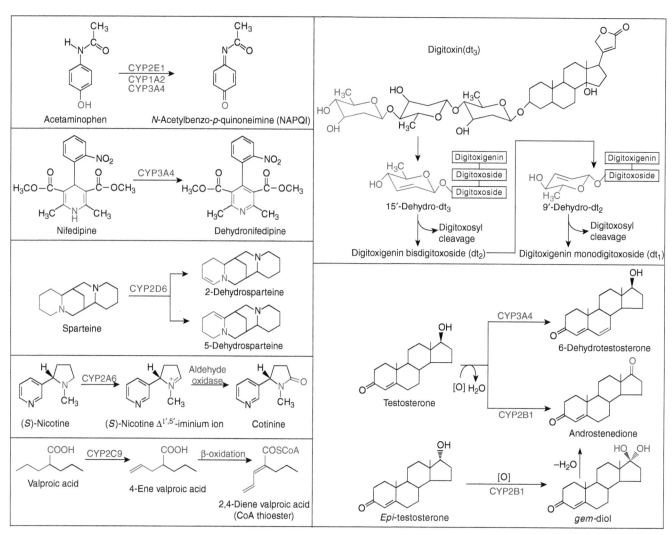

Figure 6-48. *Examples of reactions catalyzed by cytochrome P450: dehydrogenation.*

species contain 2 CYP enzymes belonging to the CYP1A subfamily, and in all cases these are known as CYP1A1 and CYP1A2 because the function and regulation of these enzymes are highly conserved among mammalian species. The same is true of CYP1B1, 2E1, 2R1, 2S1, 2U1, and 2W1, all of which are highly conserved homologs that can be given the same name across mammalian species. In most other cases, functional or evolutionary relationships are not immediately apparent; hence, the CYP enzymes are named in a species-specific manner, and the names are assigned in chronological order regardless of the species of origin. For example, human liver microsomes express CYP2D6, but this is the only functional member of the CYP2D subfamily found in human liver. CYP2D7 and 2D8 are human pseudogenes. The other members of this subfamily (ie, CYP2D1-CYP2D5 and CYP2D9 onward) are the names given to CYP2D enzymes in other species.

Without exception, the levels and activity of each CYP enzyme have been shown to vary from one individual to the next, due to environmental and/or genetic factors. Decreased CYP enzymatic activity can result from (1) a genetic mutation that either blocks the synthesis of a CYP enzyme or leads to the synthesis of a catalytically compromised, inactive, or unstable enzyme, which gives rise to the PM and IM genotypes; (2) exposure to an environmental factor (such as an infectious disease or an inflammatory process) that suppresses CYP enzyme expression, or (3) exposure to a xenobiotic that inhibits or inactivates a preexisting CYP enzyme. By inhibiting

CYP, one drug can impair the biotransformation of another, which may lead to an exaggerated pharmacological or toxicological response to the second drug. In this regard, inhibition of CYP by a drug (and suppression of CYP by infection, vaccination, or inflammation) essentially mimics the effects of a genetic deficiency in CYP enzyme expression (ie, these environmental factors mimic the IM or PM genotype depending on the degree to which they decrease CYP activity). Genetic deficiencies in CYP expression, CYP inhibition, and, to a lesser extent, CYP suppression all contribute significantly to interindividual variability in drug metabolism and toxicity, and inhibition of CYP activity is a major cause of drug–drug interactions. Examples of the impact of these genetic and environmental factors on drug metabolism and toxicity are given later in this section in the overviews of individual CYP enzymes and in the section "Inhibition of Cytochrome P450."

Increased CYP enzymatic activity can result from (1) gene duplication leading to overexpression of a CYP enzyme, which gives rise to the UM genotype; (2) gene mutations in the coding or promoter region that increase expression, activity, or stability of CYP; (3) exposure to drugs and other xenobiotics that induce the synthesis or retard the degradation of CYP; or (4) exposure to drugs and other xenobiotics that stimulate the activity of a preexisting enzyme (a process known as homotropic or heterotropic activation depending on whether the drug stimulates its own metabolism or the metabolism of other drugs, respectively). Activation of CYP has been documented in vitro and in some in situ situations, such as the pronounced (up to 25-fold) activation of *R*-warfarin 10-hydroxylation by quinidine in rabbit liver microsomes and perfused rabbit liver (Chen *et al.*, 2004a). However, in general, activation does not appear to be a major cause of drug–drug interactions. Although duplication of functional CYP2D6 genes has been documented (and shown to be relevant to drug metabolism and safety [see the section "CYP2D6"]), induction of CYP by xenobiotics is the most common mechanism by which CYP enzyme activity is increased to a pharmacologically relevant extent. By inducing CYP, one drug can stimulate the metabolism of a second drug and thereby decrease or ameliorate its therapeutic effect. Enzyme induction is a particular concern when it compromises the therapeutic effectiveness of drugs that have a narrow therapeutic index and are being used to treat a life-threatening illness, such as anti-HIV drugs, antirejection drugs (such as cyclosporine and tacrolimus), and oral anticoagulants (such as warfarin), or when it is used with drugs that exhibit a quantal (all-or-nothing) dose–response relationship, such as oral contraceptive steroids (which either block or do not block ovulation and thereby provide or do not provide protection against pregnancy).

The environmental factors known to affect P450 levels include medications (eg, prescription drugs as well as herbal remedies), foods (eg, cruciferous vegetables, charcoal-broiled beef), social habits (eg, alcohol consumption, cigarette smoking), and disease status (diabetes, infection, inflammation, vaccination, liver and kidney disease, and both hyperthyroidism and hypothyroidism). When environmental factors influence CYP enzyme levels, considerable variation may be observed during repeated measures of xenobiotic biotransformation (eg, drug metabolism) in the same individual. Such variation is not observed when alterations in CYP activity are determined genetically.

Due to their broad substrate specificity, it is possible that 2 or more CYP enzymes can contribute to the metabolism of a single compound. Three human CYP enzymes, CYP1A2, CYP2E1, and CYP3A4, can convert the commonly used analgesic, acetaminophen, to its hepatotoxic metabolite, NAPQI (Figs. 6-34 and 6-48). It is also possible for a single CYP enzyme to catalyze 2 or more metabolic pathways for the same drug. For example, CYP2D6 catalyzes both the *O*-demethylation and 5-hydroxylation (aromatic ring hydroxylation) of methoxyphenamine, and CYP3A4 catalyzes the 3-hydroxylation and *N*-oxygenation of quinidine, the 1′- and 4-hydroxylation of midazolam, the *tert*-butyl-hydroxylation and *N*-dealkylation of terfenadine, and several pathways of testosterone oxidation, including 1β-, 2β-, 6β-, and 15β-hydroxylation and dehydrogenation to 6-dehydrotestosterone (Figs. 6-41 and 6-48).

The pharmacological or toxic effects of certain drugs are exaggerated in a significant percentage of the population due to a heritable deficiency in a CYP enzyme (Meyer, 1994; Tucker, 1994; Zhou *et al.*, 2009b). The observation that individuals who are genetically deficient in a particular CYP enzyme are PMs of one or more drugs illustrates a very important principle, namely, that the rate of elimination of drugs can be largely determined by a single CYP enzyme. This observation seems to contradict the fact that CYP enzymes have broad and overlapping substrate specificities. The resolution to this apparent paradox lies in the fact that although more than one human CYP enzyme can catalyze the biotransformation of a xenobiotic, they may do so with markedly different affinities. Consequently, xenobiotic biotransformation in vivo, where only low substrate concentrations are usually achieved, is often determined by the CYP enzyme with the highest affinity (lowest apparent K_m) for the xenobiotic. For example, the 5-hydroxylation of lansoprazole, which represents the key route of elimination of this proton pump inhibitor, is catalyzed by both

CYP2C19 and CYP3A4. However, these reactions are catalyzed by CYP3A4 with such low affinity that the 5-hydroxylation (and hence the clearance) of lansoprazole in vivo is largely determined by CYP2C19 (Pearce *et al.*, 1996b). When several CYP enzymes catalyze the same reaction, their relative contribution to xenobiotic biotransformation is determined by the kinetic parameter, V_{max}/K_m, which is a measure of in vitro intrinsic clearance at low substrate concentrations (<10% of K_m).

A drug whose clearance is largely determined by a single CYP enzyme (or any single route of elimination) is said to have high *victim* or *object* potential, meaning its rate of clearance will be decreased by genetic polymorphisms and inhibitory drugs that result in a loss of that particular CYP activity and increased by drugs and other xenobiotics that induce that particular CYP enzyme. For example, a drug that is largely cleared by CYP2D6 will be slowly metabolized in CYP2D6 PMs and rapidly metabolized in CYP2D6 UMs, whereas a drug whose clearance is largely determined by CYP3A4 will be slowly metabolized in the presence of ketoconazole (and other CYP3A4 inhibitors) and rapidly metabolized in the presence of rifampin or St. John's wort (and other CYP3A4 inducers). The extent to which genetic polymorphisms and CYP inhibitors/inducers impact the disposition of a drug (or any other xenobiotic) is determined by fm, the fraction of clearance attributable to the affected enzyme. This principle applies to all xenobiotic-biotransforming enzymes and is explained in detail in Point 24 in the section "Introduction." Point 24 also covers the principle of drug–drug interactions in terms of perpetrator–victim interactions (in which the disposition of one drug, the victim, is impacted by a single perpetrator such as an inhibitory drug or a genetic polymorphism) and perpetrator–perpetrator–victim interactions, otherwise known as "maximum exposure," which involves the dramatic (synergistic) impact of 2 perpetrators blocking 2 parallel pathways of clearance of the victim drug (Collins *et al.*, 2006; Ogilvie and Parkinson, in press).

Accordingly, for drugs under development, considerable attention is paid to identifying which CYP enzyme or enzymes are involved in eliminating the drug, a process known as *reaction phenotyping* or *enzyme mapping*. Four in vitro approaches have been developed for reaction phenotyping (Ogilvie *et al.*, 2008). Each has its advantages and disadvantages, and a combination of approaches is usually required to identify which human CYP enzyme is responsible for metabolizing a xenobiotic. The 4 approaches to reaction phenotyping are as follows:

1. Correlation analysis, which involves measuring the rate of xenobiotic metabolism by several samples of human liver microsomes and correlating reaction rates with the variation in the level or activity of the individual CYP enzymes in the same microsomal samples. This approach is successful because the levels of the CYP enzymes in human liver microsomes vary enormously from sample to sample as shown in Table 6-12.

2. Chemical inhibition, which involves an evaluation of the effects of known CYP enzyme inhibitors on the metabolism of a xenobiotic by human liver microsomes. Chemical inhibitors of CYP, which are discussed later, must be used cautiously because most of them can inhibit more than one CYP enzyme. Some chemical inhibitors are metabolism-dependent inhibitors that require biotransformation to a metabolite that inactivates or noncompetitively inhibits CYP.

3. Antibody inhibition, which involves an evaluation of the effects of inhibitory antibodies against selected CYP enzymes on the biotransformation of a xenobiotic by human liver microsomes. Due to the ability of antibodies to inhibit selectively

Table 6-12

Specific Content of Individual Cytochrome P450 (CYP) Enzymes in Human Liver Microsomes (HLM)

| ENZYME | POOLED HLM* | INDIVIDUAL HLM (N = 17)[†] | | |
		MEAN	RANGE (MINIMUM–MAXIMUM)	FOLD VARIATION (MAXIMUM/MINIMUM)
CYP1A2	17.7	25.1	3.26–65.5	20.1
CYP2A6	49.2	56.2	5.45–168	30.8
CYP2B6	6.86	6.72	4.05–14.9	3.7
CYP2C8	29.3	30.0	5.66–83.5	14.8
CYP2C9	80.2	76.3	40.2–115	2.9
CYP2C19	3.64	5.31	2.08–22.2	10.7
CYP2D6	11.5	17.2	6.16–36.4	5.9
CYP2E1	51.3	66.1	36.3–147	4.0
CYP3A4	64.0	60.4	6.22–270	43.4
CYP3A5	3.54	3.86	2.48–17.1	6.9
CYP3A7	ND	2.40	BLQ–9.39	NA
CYP3A43	1.30	4.10	BLQ–6.42	NA
CYP4A11	ND	21.8	9.29–46.5	5.0
P450 OR	ND	71.6	41.7–99.0	2.4

ND, not determined; BLQ, below limit of quantitation; NA, not applicable; P450 OR, NADPH-cytochrome P450 reductase.
Data from Kawakami et al. (2011).
[†]*Data from Ohtsuki et al. (2012).*

and noncompetitively, this method alone can potentially establish which human CYP enzyme is responsible for biotransforming a xenobiotic. Unfortunately, the utility of this method is limited by the availability of specific inhibitory antibodies.

4. Biotransformation by purified or recombinant (cDNA-expressed) human CYP enzymes, which can establish whether a particular CYP enzyme can or cannot biotransform a xenobiotic, but it does not address whether that CYP enzyme contributes substantially to reactions catalyzed by human liver microsomes. The information obtained with purified or recombinant human CYP enzymes can be improved by taking into account large differences in the extent to which the individual CYP enzymes are expressed in human liver microsomes. The specific content of the major xenobiotic-biotransforming enzymes in human liver microsomes has been determined by mass spectrometry and the values are summarized in Table 6-12. The extrapolation of metabolic rates obtained with recombinant enzymes to those expected to occur in liver microsomes can be based on specific content, relative activity factors (RAF), or a combination of both called intersystem extrapolation factor (ISEF) (Proctor *et al.*, 2004; Ogilvie *et al.*, 2008).

Some CYP enzymes, such as CYP1A1 and CYP1B1, are expressed at such low levels in human liver microsomes that they do not contribute significantly to the hepatic biotransformation of xenobiotics that are excellent substrates for these enzymes. Other CYP enzymes are expressed in some but not all livers, as discussed later under each individual enzyme subheading. It should be

emphasized that reaction phenotyping in vitro is not always carried out with pharmacologically or toxicologically relevant substrate concentrations. As a result, the CYP enzyme that appears responsible for biotransforming the drug in vitro may not be the CYP enzyme responsible for biotransforming the drug in vivo (Ogilvie *et al.*, 2008). This may be particularly true of CYP3A4, which metabolizes several drugs with high capacity but low affinity.

Reaction phenotyping (often in conjunction with clinical observation) has been used to characterize the substrate specificity of many of the CYP enzymes expressed in human liver microsomes, as discussed later under each individual enzyme subheading.

Examples of reactions catalyzed by individual human CYP enzymes are shown in Figs. 6-41 to 6-48, and lists of substrates, inhibitors, and inducers for each CYP enzyme are given in Table 6-13. The examples listed in Table 6-13 are largely based on examples cited by the US FDA (http://www.fda.gov/Drugs/DevelopmentApprovalProcess/DevelopmentResources/DrugInteractionsLabeling/ucm080499.htm), which has provided, where possible, the following lists to guide the conduct of in vitro and in vivo pharmacokinetic drug–drug interaction studies: (1) preferred and acceptable CYP substrates and chemical inhibitors for reaction phenotyping in vitro; (2) sensitive probe substrates to monitor CYP activity in vivo (a sensitive substrate is one whose clearance is largely [>80%] determined by a single CYP enzyme such that loss of that CYP enzyme causes a 5-fold or higher increase in exposure); (3) drugs that are strong or weak inhibitors of CYP enzymes in vivo; (4) preferred and acceptable inhibitors and inducers for use as positive controls for CYP inhibition and induction studies in vitro; and (5) drugs that are effective

Table 6-13

Examples of Clinically Relevant Substrates, Inhibitors, and Inducers of the Major Human Liver Microsomal P450 Enzymes Involved in Xenobiotic Biotransformation

	CYP1A2	CYP2A6	CYP2B6	CYP2C8	CYP2C9	CYP2C19	CYP2E1
Substrates	Alosetron*	Coumarin[†]	Bupropion*[†]	Amodiaquine[‡]	Celecoxib*	Clobazam*	Aniline[‡]
	Caffeine*[‡§]	Nicotine[†]	Efavirenz*[†§]	Cerivastatin	Diclofenac[†]	Esomeprazole	Acetaminophen
	Duloxetine*	Efavirenz	Propofol[†]	Montelukast	Fluoxetine[†]	Fluoxetine[‡]	Chlorzoxazone[†]
	7-Ethoxyresorufin[†]		S-Mephenytoin[‡]	Paclitaxel[†,**]	Flurbiprofen[‡]	S-Mephenytoin*[‡,**]	Lauric acid[‡]
	Melatonin*		Cyclophosphamide	Rosiglitazone[‡§]	Phenytoin[**]	Lansoprazole*[§]	4-Nitrophenol[‡]
	Phenacetin[†]		Ketamine	Repaglinide*[§]	Tolbutamide[†§]	Moclobemide	
	Ramelteon*		Meperidine		S-Warfarin[†§,**]	Omeprazole*[‡§]	
	Tacrine*[‡]		Nevirapine			Pantoprazole[§]	
	Tizanidine*,[**]						
	Theophylline[‡§,**]						
Inhibitors	Acyclovir[††]	Methoxsalen[†]	Clopidogrel[†,††]	Fluvoxamine[††]	Amiodarone[§‡‡]	Allicin[††]	Clomethiazole[‡]
	Allopurinol[††]	Pilocarpine[‡]	3-Isopropenyl-3-methyl diamantane[‡]	Gemfibrozil glucuronide[‡,§,§§§]	Capecitabine[††]	Armodafinil[††]	Diallyldisulfide[‡]
	Caffeine[††]	Tranylcypromine[†]	2-Isopropenyl-2-methyladamantane[‡]	Ketoconazole[††]	Cotrimoxazole[††]	Carbamazepine[††]	Diethyldithiocarbamate[‡]
	Cimetidine[††]	Tryptamine[‡]	Phencyclidine[‡]	Montelukast[†]	Etravirine[††]	Cimetidine[††]	Disulfiram[§]
	Ciprofloxacin[§§]		Prasugrel[††]	Pioglitazone[‡]	Fluconazole[‡,§,‡‡]	Esomeprazole[‡‡]	
	Daidzein[††]		Sertraline[‡]	Quercetin[†]	Fluoxetine[††]	Etravirine[††]	
	Disulfiram[††]		Thio-TEPA[‡]	Rosiglitazone[‡]	Fluvastatin[††]	Felbamate[††]	
	Echinacea[††]		Ticlopidine[‡,††]	Rosuvastatin	Fluvoxamine[‡,††]	Fluconazole[§§]	
	Enoxacin[§§]		Phenylethylpiperidine	Trimethoprim[††]	Metronidazole[††]	Fluoxetine[‡‡]	
	Famotidine[††]				Miconazole[‡‡]	Fluvoxamine[§,§§]	
	Fluvoxamine[§,§§]				Oxandrolone[‡‡]	Human growth hormone (rhGH)[††]	
	Furafylline[†]				Sulfaphenazole[†]	Ketoconazole[††]	
	Methoxsalen[‡‡]				Sulfinpyrazone[††]	Moclobemide[§,‡‡]	
	Mexiletine[‡‡]				Tienilic acid	Nootkatone[†]	
	α-Naphthoflavone[‡]				Tigecycline[††]	Omeprazole[§,‡‡]	
	Norfloxacin[††]				Voriconazole[††]	Oral contraceptives[††]	
	Oral contraceptives[‡‡]				Zafirlukast[‡]	Ticlopidine[‡‡,§§]	
	Propafenone[‡‡]					Voriconazole[‡‡]	
	Propranolol[‡‡]						
	Phenylpropanolamine[‡‡]						
	Terbinafine[††]						
	Thiabendazole[‡‡]						
	Ticlopidine[††]						
	Vemurafenib[‡‡]						
	Verapamil[‡‡]						
	Zileuton[‡]						

(continued)

Table 6-13 (Continued)

	CYP1A2	CYP2A6	CYP2B6	CYP2C8	CYP2C9	CYP2C19	CYP2E1
Inducers	3-Methylcholanthrene[†]	Dexamethasone[†]	Efavirenz[***]	Phenobarbital[‡]	Aprepitant[†††]	Artemisinin[†††]	Ethanol[§]
	β-Naphthoflavone[†]	Pyrazole[‡]	Nevirapine[†††]	Rifampin[†,§,***]	Bosentan[†††]	Phenobarbital	Isoniazid
	Omeprazole[†,†††]		Phenobarbital[†]		Carbamazepine[***]	Rifampin[†,§,***]	
	Lansoprazole[‡]		Phenytoin[‡]		Phenobarbital[†††]		
	Montelukast[***]		Rifampin[***]		Rifampin[***]		
	Moricizine[†††]				St. John's wort[†††]		
	Phenobarbital[†††]						
	Phenytoin[***]						
	TCDD						

Substrates

CYP2D6

Atomoxetine[*,§]	Methylphenidate
Amitriptyline	Mexiletine
Aripiprazole	Morphine
Brofaromine	Nebivolol[*]
(±)-Bufuralol[†]	Nortriptyline
(S)-Chlorpheniramine	Ondansetron
Chlorpromazine	Paroxetine
Clomipramine	Perhexilene
Codeine	Perphenazine[*]
Debrisoquine[‡]	Pimozide[**]
Desipramine[*,§]	Propafenone
Dextromethorphan[*,†,§]	(+)-Propranolol[*]
Dolasetron	Sparteine
Duloxetine	Tamoxifen
Fentanyl	Thioridazine[**]
Haloperidol (reduced)	Timolol
Imipramine	Tolterodine[*]
Loperamide	Tramadol
(R)-Metoprolol[*]	(R)-Venlafaxine[*]

CYP3A4

Alfentanil[*,**]	Cyclosporine[**]	Etoricoxib	Methylprednisolone	Saquinavir[*]
Alfuzosin	Darifenacin[*]	Felodipine[*,§]	Mexazolam	Sildenafil[*,§]
Alprazolam	Darunavir[*]	Fentanyl[*]	Midazolam[*,†,§]	Sibutramine
Amlodipine	Dasatinib[*]	Fluticasone[*]	Mifepristone	Simvastatin[*,§]
Amprenavir	Depsipeptide	Gallopamil	Mosapride	Sirolimus[*,**]
Aprepitant[*]	Dexamethasone	Gefitinib	Nicardipine	Sunitinib
Artemether	Dextromethorphan[‡]	Gepirone	Nifedipine[‡]	Tacrolimus[**]
Astemizole[**]	Diergotamine[**]	Gestodene	Nimodipine	Tadalafil
Atazanavir	α-Dihydroergocriptine	Granisetron	Nisoldipine[*]	Telithromycin
Atorvastatin	Dihydroergotamine[**]	Halofantrine	Nitrendipine	Terfenadine[‡,***]
Azithromycin	Disopyramide	Imatinib	Norethindrone	Testosterone[†]
Barnidipine	Docetaxel	Indinavir[*]	Oxatomide	Tiagabine
Bexarotene	Domperidone	Isradipine	Oxybutynin	Ticagrelor[*]
Bortezomib	Dronedarone[*]	Itraconazole	Perospirone	Tipranavir[*]
Brotizolam	Dutasteride	Karenitecin	Pimozide[**]	Tirilazad
Budesonide[*]	Ebastine	Ketamine	Pranidipine	Tofisopam
Buspirone[*,§]	Eletriptan[*,§]	Laquinimod	Praziquantel	Tolvaptan[*]
Capravirine	Eplerenone[**]	Levomethadyl	Quetiapine[*]	Triazolam[*,‡,§]
Carbamazepine	Ergotamine[**]	Lonafarnib	Quinidine[**]	Trimetrexate
Cibenzoline	Erlotinib	Loperamide	Quinine	Vardenafil[*]
Cilastazol	Erythromycin[‡]	Lopinavir[*]	Reboxetine	Vinblastine
Cisapride[**]	Eplerenone	Lovastatin[*,§]	Rifabutin	Vincristine
Clarithromycin	Ethosuximide	Lumefantrine	Ritonavir	Vinorelbine
Clindamycin	Etoperidone	Lurasidone[*]	Rosuvastatin	Ziprasidone
Clopidogrel	Everolimus[*]	Maraviroc[*]	Ruboxistaurin	Zonisamide
Conivaptan[*]	Ethinyl estradiol	Medroxyprogesterone	Salmetrol	

Inhibitors	Amiodarone†† Buproprion§§ Celecoxib‡‡ Chlorpheniramine Cimetidine†† Cinacalet‡‡ Clobazam†† Clomipramine Desvenlafaxine†† Diltiazem‡‡ Diphenhydramine†† Duloxetine‡‡ Echinacea†† Escitalopram†† Febuxostat†† Fluoxetine§,§§ Gefitinib†† Haloperidol	Hydralazine†† Hydroxychloroquine†† Imatinib†† Methadone†† Mibefradil Oral contraceptives†† Paroxetine§,§§ Pazopanib†† Propafenone†† Quinidine†,§§ Ranitidine†† Ritonavir§,§§ Sertraline†† Telithromycin†† Terbinafine‡‡ Verapamil†† Vemurafenib††	Alprazolam†† Amiodarone†† Amlodipine†† Amprenavir†† Aprepitant‡‡ Atazanavir§,‡‡ Atorvastatin†† Azamulin‡ Bicalutamide†† Bosentan Boceprevir§§ Cilostazol††	Cimetidine†† Ciprofloxacin‡‡ Clarithromycin§,§§ Conivaptan§§ Crizotinib‡‡ Cyclosporine†† Darunavir‡‡ Diltiazem‡‡ Erythromycin‡‡ Felbamate Fluconazole‡‡ Fluoxetine††	Fluvoxamine†† Fosamprenavir‡‡ Gestodene Ginkgo†† Goldenseal†† Grapefruit Juice‡‡,§§ Imatinib‡‡ Indinavir§,§§ Isoniazid†† Itraconazole†,§,§§ Ketoconazole†,§,§§ Lapatinib‡‡	Lopinavir§§ Mibefradil§§ Nefazodone§,§§ Nelfinavir§,§§ Nilotinib†† Oral contraceptives†† Pazopanib‡‡ Posaconazole§§ Ranitidine†† Ranolazine†† Ritonavir§,‡‡,§§ Roxithromycin	Saquinavir§,§§ St. John's wort Telaprevir§§ Telithromycin§,§§ Ticagrelor†† Tipranavir‡ Troleandomycin‡ Verapamil‡‡‡ Voriconazole§§ Zileuton§§
Inducers	NA		Amprenavir††† Aprepitant††† Armodafinil††† Avasimibe‡‡‡ Bosentan*** Carbamazepine§,‡‡‡ Clobazam Echinacea††† Clotrimazole Cyproterone acetate	Dexamethasone‡ Echinacea††† Efavirenz*** Etravirine*** Etoposide Guggulsterone Hyperforin Lovastatin Modafinil***	Mifepristone Nafcillin*** Nelfinavir Nifedipine Omeprazole Paclitaxel‡ PCBs Phenobarbital‡ Phenytoin‡,‡‡‡	Pioglitazone††† Prednisone††† Rifabutin Rifampin†,§,‡‡‡ Rifapentine‡ Ritonavir Rufinamide††† St. John's wort‡‡‡ Simvastatin	Spironolactone Sulfinpyrazole Topotecan Troglitazone‡ Troleandomycin Vemurafenib††† Vitamin E Vitamin K_2 Yin Zhi Huang

Note: All FDA classifications are based on information available as of February 21, 2012 at the following URL: http://www.fda.gov/Drugs/DevelopmentApprovalProcess/DevelopmentResources/DrugInteractionsLabeling/ucm093664.htm.

*Classified by the FDA as a "sensitive substrate" (ie, drugs whose plasma AUC values have been shown to increase by ≥5-fold when coadministered with a known CYP inhibitor).

†FDA-preferred in vitro substrate, inhibitor, or inducer.

‡FDA-acceptable in vitro substrate, inhibitor, or inducer.

§FDA-provided examples of in vivo substrates, inhibitors, or inducers for oral administration. Substrates in this category have plasma AUCs that are increased by at least 2-fold (5-fold for CYP3A4 substrates) when coadministered with inhibitors of the enzyme. Inhibitors in this category increase the AUC of substrates for that enzyme by at least 2-fold (5-fold for CYP3A4). Inducers in this category decrease the plasma AUC of substrates for that enzyme by at least 30%.

**Classified by the FDA as a "substrate with narrow therapeutic range" (ie, drugs whose exposure-response indicates that increases in their exposure levels by concomitant use of CYP inhibitors may lead to serious safety concerns such as torsades de pointes).

††Classified by the FDA as a "weak inhibitor" (ie, caused a ≥1.25-fold but <2-fold increase in plasma AUC or 20%–50% decrease in the clearance of sensitive CYP substrates when the inhibitor was given at the highest approved dose and the shortest dosing interval in clinical evaluations).

‡‡Classified by the FDA as a "moderate inhibitor" (ie, caused a ≥2-fold but <5-fold increase in plasma AUC or 50%–80% decrease in the clearance of sensitive CYP substrates when the inhibitor was given at the highest approved dose and the shortest dosing interval in clinical evaluations).

§§Classified by the FDA as a "strong inhibitor" (ie, caused a ≥5-fold increase in plasma AUC or ≥80% decrease in the clearance of CYP substrates in clinical evaluations).

***Classified by the FDA as a "moderate inducer" (ie, caused a ≥50%–80% decrease in AUC of CYP substrates in clinical evaluations).

†††Classified by the FDA as a "weak inducer" (ie, caused a ≥20%–50% decrease in AUC of CYP substrates in clinical evaluations).

‡‡‡Classified by the FDA as a "strong inducer" (ie, caused a ≥80% decrease in AUC of CYP substrates in clinical evaluations).

inducers of CYP enzymes in vivo (FDA; http://www.fda.gov/Drugs/DevelopmentApprovalProcess/DevelopmentResources/DrugInteractionsLabeling/ucm080499.htm).

The global features of the major xenobiotic-biotransforming human CYP enzymes are as follows:

1. Two CYP enzymes, namely, CYP2D6 and CYP3A4, metabolize the majority of orally effective drugs, but they often metabolize different drugs and they do not metabolize all drugs; consequently, there are many drugs whose clearance is largely determined by CYP enzymes other than CYP2D6 or CYP3A4. Interindividual variation in CYP2D6, which is largely confined to the liver, is largely determined by genetic factors, whereas interindividual variation in CYP3A4, which is expressed in liver and small intestine, is largely determined by environmental factors (such as inhibitory and inducing drugs).

2. The induction of CYP3A4 is often associated with induction of CYP2A6, 2B6, 2C8, 2C9, and 2C19. CYP1A2 and CYP2E1 are also inducible enzymes, but they are induced by different mechanisms and xenobiotics. Consequently, CYP1A2, 2E1, and 3A4 represent 3 distinct classes of inducible human CYP enzymes. CYP induction is invariably associated with the upregulation of other xenobiotic-biotransforming enzymes, as discussed later in the section "Induction of Cytochrome P450—Xenosensors." CYP2D6 is considered a noninducible enzyme, although its levels increase during pregnancy and decrease following renal impairment (Rostami-Hodjegan *et al.*, 1999; Sit *et al.*, 2010).

3. Genetic polymorphisms have been identified for all of the human CYP enzymes involved in drug metabolism. Zhou *et al.* (2009a) estimated that each human CYP gene contains an average of ~15 nonsynonymous SNPs, many of which are associated with altered drug metabolism or susceptibility to disease (a selection of which will be discussed later under each individual enzyme subheading). The incidence of CYP polymorphisms varies greatly among different ethnic groups. In the case of CYP2D6, genetic polymorphisms are common among Caucasian and impact the metabolism, safety, and efficacy of many drugs, as summarized in Point 23 in the section "Introduction." Based on CYP2D6 genotype, individuals can be categorized as PMs, IMs, EMs, and UMs (and the EMs can be subdivided into low, medium, and high EMs), as shown in Table 6-4. There is a vast literature describing SNPs and other genetic polymorphisms affecting the human CYP enzymes involved in xenobiotic biotransformation, too large—and often too confusing—to be summarized here (reviewed in Zhou *et al.*, 2009a). (Information on CYP genetic polymorphisms can be found at http://www.cypalleles.ki.se.) Genetic polymorphisms in the coding region can increase or decrease CYP activity, sometimes in a substrate-dependent manner, making generalizations difficult. They can also alter the stability of CYP enzymes without altering their enzymatic activity. Genetic polymorphisms in the promoter region can impair transcription (and thereby decrease CYP levels) or increase CYP levels by increasing its constitutive expression or inducibility by activated xenosensors. In many cases neither the impact of a particular SNP is known nor is it known in many cases whether the SNP is in linkage disequilibrium with another genetic polymorphism. Studies on a genetic polymorphism in CYP2C8—the *3 allele—illustrate the complexity of this field of research. The *3 allele of CYP2C8 is in partial linkage disequilibrium with the *2 allele of CYP2C9 (ie, individuals with one allelic variant will likely have the second too). Furthermore, based on in vitro studies CYP2C*3 was considered a *loss-of-function* allele, but in vivo studies with 3 different CYP2C8 substrates established that the CYP2C8*3 allele is a *gain-of-function* allele. These findings sound a word of caution about interpreting the impact of genetic polymorphisms on drug disposition, adverse effects, efficacy, and disease processes. That said, there are many cases of CYP genetic polymorphisms having a reproducible, clinically relevant impact on drug disposition, examples of which are given below under each individual enzyme subheading.

There are also many reports of CYP polymorphisms predisposing individuals to diseases or conferring protection against them. This literature is often confusing. For example, in the case of CYP2J2 (which converts arachidonic acid to EETs that are thought to be cardioprotective), a genetic polymorphism in the promoter region that causes a decrease in CYP2J2 expression was examined in 4 separate studies for its effects on coronary artery disease (CAD) (reviewed in Zordoky and El-Kadi, 2010). The CYP2J2 polymorphism was associated with an increased risk of CAD in one study (in Germans) and a decreased risk in another study (in African Americans) and had no discernible effect in 2 other studies (in Swedes and a Caucasian population). Four other studies on the impact of the same genetic polymorphism of CYP2J2 (ie, lower expression) on hypertension gave similar results: 1 showed increased risk (in Russians), one showed decreased risk (in Caucasians [but only in males]), and 2 showed no association. Given the incongruity of these studies, the impact of genetic polymorphisms on disease will not be discussed below with the notable exception of the impact of CYP1A and CYP2A6 polymorphisms on cigarette-smoking-induced cancer of the lung and upper aerodigestive tract (UADT).

The salient features of each of the major xenobiotic-biotransforming CYP enzymes, with emphasis on the CYP enzymes in human liver microsomes, are summarized in the following subsections.

CYP1A1, 1A2, and 1B1 All mammalian species examined possess 3 members of the CYP1 family, namely, CYP1A1, CYP1A2, and CYP1B1. They have attracted considerable attention because they are highly inducible by AhR agonists such as TCDD and PAHs and because they play a major role in the activation/detoxication of carcinogenic/mutagenic compounds such as PAHs, aflatoxin B_1, various aromatic amines/amides, and PhIP and 2-amino-3-methylimidazol[4,5f]quinoline (IQ), 2 representatives of the many heterocyclic amines (products of amino acid pyrolysis) known as cooked food mutagens. A possible d'Artagnan to these 3 musketeers is CYP2S1, which resembles CYP1A1 and CYP1B1 in being an AhR-inducible, extrahepatic enzyme capable of metabolizing PAHs, but it will be discussed later in the section "CYP2R1, 2S1, 2U1, and 2W1." High levels of CYP1A2 are expressed in liver (see Table 6-12) but not in extrahepatic tissues. In contrast, liver contains low or undetectable levels of CYP1A1 and CYP1B1 but these enzymes are expressed in a great number of extrahepatic tissues (Shimada, 2006). Only CYP1A2 contributes significantly to the in vivo clearance of drugs (extensively reviewed by Zhou *et al.*, 2010b).

The ability of CYP1 enzymes to activate a wide variety of compounds to mutagenic metabolites underscores the widespread practice of using liver microsomes from Aroclor 1254–induced rats in the Ames bacterial mutagenicity assay (because these microsomes have high levels of CYP1A1 and CYP1A2, among many other induced CYP enzymes). This and many other in vitro studies, including heterologous expression of CYP1 enzymes in mammalian cells, have established that CYP1A1 and CYP1B1 are adept at oxidizing PAHs such as B[a]P and DMBA to DNA-reactive diol epoxides, as illustrated in Fig. 6-10. (A second pathway of DMBA activation is shown later in the section "Sulfonation.") Similar in vitro studies have clearly established that CYP1A2 is highly effective in catalyzing the initial step (N-hydroxylation) in the activation of numerous carcinogenic aromatic amines (4-aminobiphenyl, 2-aminonaphthalene, 2-AF), aromatic amides (2-acetylaminofluorine), and heterocyclic amines (PhIP, IQ, etc) to mutagenic metabolites (these activation pathways will be discussed in the sections "Glucuronidation and Formation of Acyl-CoA Thioesters" for 2-aminonaphthalene, "Sulfonation" for 2-AAF, and "Acetylation" for 2-aminofluorence and 2-AAF). In the case of PAHs, it was noted that these carcinogens are also AhR agonists; hence, it was long assumed that PAHs can induce CYP1 enzymes and thereby induce their own activation to carcinogenic metabolites. Consequently, it came as a huge surprise when experiments with knockout mice indicated that these in vitro findings did not translate in a predictable manner to the in vivo situation (reviewed in Nebert and Dalton, 2006; Shimada, 2006; Ma and Lu, 2007).

Compared with their wild-type littermates, CYP1A1, CYP1A2, and CYP1B1 knockout mice would be expected to be less susceptible and possibly resistant to the tumorigenic effects of PAHs such as B[a]P and DMBA, and to aromatic amines such as 4-aminobiphenyl and cooked food mutagens. However, contrary to expectation, deletion of CYP1A1 *potentiated* the toxicity of oral B[a]P, which caused increased spleen and thymus weight, leukocytopenia, and extreme hypercellularity in the bone marrow (and death within 30 days) in CYP1A1 knockout mice but not in wild-type mice. CYP1A1 knockout mice also had *higher* levels of B[a]P–DNA adducts in extrahepatic tissues. However, both wild-type mice and CYP1A1 knockout mice were susceptible to B[a]P toxicity when the PAH was administered by intraperitoneal injection instead of the oral route of administration. These findings strongly suggest that induction of CYP1A1 in the intestine and liver and metabolism of PAHs in these presystemic organs provide protection against orally administered PAHs (Nebert and Dalton, 2006; Shimada, 2006; Ma and Lu, 2007).

Contrary to expectation, deletion of CYP1A2 similarly potentiates the toxicity and liver tumorigenicity of aromatic/heterocyclic amines. Deletion of CYP1A2 (CYP1A2 null mice) increased the toxicity of 4-aminobiphenyl (methemoglobinemia), adduct formation in liver and bladder (2 targets of arylamine carcinogenicity in rodents), and the incidence of hepatocellular tumors and preneoplastic foci. Deletion of CYP1A2 likewise increased adduct and tumor formation by the cooked food mutagens (heterocyclic amines) known as PhIP and IQ. These results strongly suggest that the role of CYP1A2 in aromatic/heterocyclic amine/amide metabolism is protective, and that enzymes other than CYP1A2 (such as peroxidases, extrahepatic CYP enzymes, and/or UGTs) play an important role in their activation (or, alternatively, it is the parent compound that causes tumor formation) (Nebert and Dalton, 2006; Shimada, 2006; Ma and Lu, 2007).

In contrast to the unexpected results observed with CYP1A1 and CYP1A2 knockout mice, gene deletion of CYP1B1 does in fact have the anticipated protective effect against PAH tumorigenicity. CYP1B1 mice are completely protected against DMBA tumor formation (Nebert and Dalton, 2006; Shimada, 2006; Ma and Lu, 2007). Similar protection against DMBA and/or B[a]P has been achieved with CYP1B1 inhibitors such as 1-ethinylpyrene (an irreversible inhibitor of both CYP1B1 and CYP1A1) and the specific (or more selective) CYP1B1 inhibitor 1,4-phenylenebis(methylene)-selonocyanate (p-XSC). These results suggest CYP1B1 plays a

key role in activating PAHs to diol epoxides that cause skin and mammary tumors in experimental animals. Of particular interest is the finding that, although both CYP1A1 and CYP1B1 convert PAHs to DNA-reactive diol epoxides, the latter enzyme does so with higher affinity (Nebert and Dalton, 2006; Shimada, 2006; Ma and Lu, 2007).

The studies in knockout mice establish that induction of CYP1A1 protects against *oral* PAH toxicity (through first-pass [presystemic] elimination) but does not protect against parenterally administered PAH toxicity. In humans, the most prevalent exposure to parenterally administered PAHs is through cigarette smoking. Not surprisingly, therefore, a large number of studies have examined the impact of genetic polymorphisms in CYP1A1 and, to a lesser extent, in CYP1B1 on the incidence of lung and UADT cancers in cigarette smokers and, in some cases, nonsmokers (Chen *et al.*, 2010, 2011b; Zhan *et al.*, 2011). Allelic variants that increase CYP1A1 and CYP1B1 have been investigated for their potential to predispose to environmental tobacco smoke (ETS)–induced lung, UADT, and other cancers. In the case of CYP1A1, the focus has been on 2 mutually linked polymorphisms, namely, *2A and *2B; the former is point mutation in the 3′-flanking region and is commonly called the *MspI* polymorphism. By itself *MspI* has no effect on CYP1A1 activity or expression. However, *MspI* (*2A) is linked to *2B, a point mutation in exon 7 that leads to an Ile$_{462}$Val substitution, which is near the heme-binding site. The latter polymorphism is associated with increased activity or inducibility of CYP1A1 (Crofts *et al.*, 1994). In the case of CYP1B1, the focus of attention has been on the *3 allele caused by a Leu$_{432}$Val substitution that increases CYP1B1 activity (Li *et al.*, 2000). Studies of the impact of these gain-of-function polymorphisms of CYP1A1 and CYP1B1 on the incidence of lung and other cancers are numerous and the outcomes varied. Within a study, an association between gain-of-function alleles and cancer incidence is often found in a subgroup based on ethnicity or gender, and in some studies the association (increased risk) is observed in both smokers and nonsmokers. In the case of CYP1A1, 2 meta-analysis studies, one based on 18,397 subjects (Zhan *et al.*, 2011) and the other based on 30,368 subjects (Chen *et al.*, 2011b), concluded that the overall risk of cigarette smoking lung cancer posed by the gain-of-function polymorphism in CYP1A1 was low (odds ratio ~1.2) but that slightly higher risks could be discerned in subgroups based on ethnicity. In the case of CYP1B1, a meta-analysis based on 6501 subjects similarly concluded that the overall risk of cigarette smoking lung cancer posed by the gain-of-function polymorphism in CYP1B1 was low (odds ratio 1.46) but variable among different ethnic groups (Chen *et al.*, 2010). The authors concluded that the gain-of-function polymorphism in CYP1B1, which had a larger odds ratio than that of CYP1A1, was a low-penetrant risk for developing lung cancer.

The early studies of CYP1A1 induction were based on measurement of aryl hydrocarbon hydroxylase (AHH) activity, which took advantage of the conversion of B[a]P to the fluorescent metabolite 3-hydroxy-B[a]P (Conney, 1982). This assay was supplanted when it was discovered that CYP1A1 and CYP1A2 catalyze 7-ethoxyresorufin O-dealkylation (EROD) to form the highly fluorescent metabolite resorufin, which is one of the reactions shown in Fig. 6-45 (Burke and Mayer, 1974). These studies are of historical interest because they provided some of the earliest evidence for the existence of multiple forms of CYP, one of which (namely, CYP1A1) was highly inducible by 3-methylcholanthrene. Why was 3-methylcholanthrene studied for its effects on AHH activity? It was studied because of the observation reported in 1952 that treating rats with a low dose of one carcinogen, namely, 3-methylcholanthrene, could delay or entirely prevent liver tumor formation by a second carcinogen, namely, 3′-methyl-4-dimethylaminoazobenzene (reviewed by Ma and Lu, 2007). Therefore, the more recent studies in knockout mice reinforced (arguably rediscovered) the protective effect of CYP1 induction. The possibility that CYP1A induction is associated with adverse effects stemmed in part from the discovery that TCDD (or dioxin), an industrial and environmental chemical that is highly toxic to certain species, is an extraordinarily potent inducer of CYP1A enzymes in rodents, and that strain differences in TCDD toxicity in mice correlate with CYP inducibility (Poland and Glover, 1974). As outlined in the section "Induction of Cytochrome P450—Xenosensors," TCDD is the most potent AhR agonist known, and it is this xenosensor, not the induction of CYP1A enzymes per se, that mediates the toxicity of TCDD, which is abrogated in AhR knockout mice. However, the impact of CYP1 gene deletion on the teratogenic effects of TCDD is interesting. Gene deletion of CYP1A1 or CYP1B1 has no effect on TCDD teratogenicity. However, gene deletion of CYP1A2 in dams predisposes to TCDD teratogenicity by exposing the embryos to higher levels of TCDD. The loss of CYP1A2 does result in decreased metabolism of TCDD, which is essentially metabolically stable, but is likely due to loss of hepatic binding of TCDD to CYP1A2 (Dragin et al., 2006).

CYP1B1 is expressed in the eye, and genetic polymorphisms that decrease CYP1B1 function are associated with primary congenital glaucoma. CYP1B1 knockout mice also have structural eye defects, which suggest that CYP1B1 has an important physiological role in eye development. In addition to metabolizing PAHs, CYP1B1 also catalyzes the 4-hydroxylation of 17β-estradiol, which produces a catechol that can potentially oxidize to a toxic *ortho*-quinone. Methylation of 4-hydroxyestradiol acts as a detoxication pathway in some tissues, as discussed in the section "Methylation." In addition to being under the transcriptional control of AhR, the expression of human CYP1B1 is controlled posttranscriptionally by the microRNA known as miR-27b, a small noncoding RNA that blocks the synthesis of CYP1B1 by binding to near-perfect matching sequences in the 3′ untranslated region of CYP1B1. The level of miR-27b is decreased and the level of CYP1B1 is correspondingly increased (overexpressed) in breast cancerous cells (and other cancerous tissues) (Tsuchiya et al., 2006). The overexpression of CYP1B1 in malignant cells (coupled with its ability to activate xenobiotics to reactive metabolites) is being exploited to activate a prodrug to a cytotoxic metabolite as a possible cancer treatment. A related approach is the development of CYP1B1 DNA vaccine, which has been shown in clinical trials to kill CYP1B1-expressing cancer cells (Maecker et al., 2003).

Of the 3 CYP1 enzymes, only CYP1A2 contributes significantly to the in vivo clearance of drugs (extensively reviewed by Gunes and Dahl, 2008; Zhou et al., 2010b). Drugs and other xenobiotics that are substrates, inhibitors, or inducers of human CYP1A2 are shown in Table 6-13. CYP1A2 catalyzes the O-dealkylation of phenacetin and the 4-hydroxylation of acetanilide, both of which produce acetaminophen, which can be converted by CYP1A2 and other CYP enzymes to a toxic NAPQI (Fig. 6-35). As shown in Fig. 6-45, CYP1A2 catalyzes the N_3-demethylation of caffeine to paraxanthine. By measuring rates of formation of paraxanthine in blood, urine, or saliva or by measuring the exhalation of isotopically labeled CO_2 from [13]C- or ^{14}C-labeled caffeine, the N_3-demethylation of caffeine can be used as an in vivo probe of CYP1A2 activity, which varies enormously from 1 individual to the next.

As in the case of CYP1A1 and CYP1B1, the function and regulation of CYP1A2 is reasonably conserved across mammalian species, but there are some notable differences. For example, furafylline is a metabolism-dependent inhibitor of human but not rodent CYP1A2 (Racha et al., 1998) and omeprazole and other

proton pump inhibitors are inducers of human but not rodent CYP1A2 (Diaz et al., 1990).

Although the levels of CYP1A2 vary enormously from 1 individual to the next, genetic defects in CYP1A2 (ie, CYP1A2 PMs) are extremely rare. Several clinical studies have reported gender differences in CYP1A2, with most—but not all—studies reporting slightly higher CYP1A2 in males compared with females (with wide variation in both genders). Rasmussen et al. (2002) reported that, based on a clinical study of caffeine metabolism in 378 individuals, males have higher CYP1A2 activity than females. Although oral contraceptive treatment reduces CYP1A2 activity, the gender difference reported by Rasmussen et al. was significant even when women on oral contraceptive steroids were excluded from the analysis. Rasmussen et al. (2002) also demonstrated a strong correlation in CYP1A2 activity between identical (monozygous) twins and concluded that, despite the large number of environmental factors that can potentially influence CYP1A2 expression (such as cigarette smoking and treatment with proton pump inhibitors, which induce CYP1A2, and oral contraceptive therapy, which suppresses CYP1A2), genetic factors account for 70% to 75% of the observed variation in CYP1A2 activity. Some but not all studies suggest an association between genetic polymorphisms that impair CYP1A2 function and elevated levels of clozapine. Decreased levels of clozapine are observed in cigarette smokers (Gunes and Dahl, 2008). In conjunction with caffeine consumption, a genetic polymorphism that decreases CYP1A2 expression and impairs caffeine metabolism is associated with a small increase in the risk of hypertension and nonfatal myocardial infarction (Zordoky and El-Kadi, 2010).

CYP2A6, CYP2A7, and 2A13 Enzymes belonging to the *CYP2A* gene family show marked species differences in catalytic function. For example, 2 of the 3 CYP2A enzymes expressed in rat liver, namely, CYP2A1 and CYP2A2, primarily catalyze the 7α- and 15α-hydroxylation of testosterone, respectively. In contrast, the CYP2A enzyme expressed in human liver, namely, CYP2A6, catalyzes the 7-hydroxylation of coumarin, as shown in Fig. 6-42. Just as rat CYP2A1 and CYP2A2 have little or no capacity to 7-hydroxylate coumarin, human CYP2A6 has little or no capacity to hydroxylate testosterone. Mouse liver microsomes contain 4 CYP2A enzymes, one of which catalyzes the 7α-hydroxylation of testosterone (CYP2A12), one of which catalyzes the 15α-hydroxylation of testosterone (CYP2A4), and one of which catalyzes the 7-hydroxylation of coumarin (CYP2A5). Functionally, CYP2A5 can be converted to CYP2A4 by a single amino acid substitution ($Phe_{209}Leu$). In other words, this single amino substitution converts CYP2A5 from a coumarin 7-hydroxylating enzyme to a testosterone 15α-hydroxylating enzyme (Lindberg and Negishi, 1989). Differences in CYP2A function have important implications for the adverse effects of coumarin, which is hepatotoxic to rats but not humans. Whereas coumarin is detoxified in humans by conversion to 7-hydroxycoumarin, which is subsequently conjugated with glucuronic acid and excreted, a major pathway of coumarin biotransformation in rats involves formation of the hepatotoxic metabolite, coumarin 3,4-epoxide, as shown in Fig. 6-43. In addition to catalyzing the 7-hydroxylation of coumarin, CYP2A6 converts 1,3-butadiene to butadiene monoxide and nicotine to nicotine $\Delta^{1',5'}$-iminium ion, which is further oxidized by AO to cotinine, as shown in Fig. 6-48.

Humans possess 2 functional CYP2A genes, namely, CYP2A6 and 2A13, and one nonfunctional CYP2A gene, namely, CYP2A7. CYP2A7 (originally named IIA4) is a full-length gene that encodes an enzyme incapable of incorporating heme, rendering it catalytically inactive (Yamano et al., 1990; Ding et al., 1995). CYP2A6 is expressed in the liver but few extrahepatic tissues (with the notable exception of mammary gland), whereas CYP2A13 is expressed mainly in the lung (bronchus and trachea) and bladder, with lower levels in reproductive organs such as testis, ovary, uterus, and mammary gland. Hepatic CYP2A6 plays a major role in the metabolism of coumarin and nicotine, and plays a role in the metabolism of tegafur, fadrozole, methoxyflurane, and valproic acid. 8-Methoxypsoralen, a structural analog of coumarin, is a potent, metabolism-dependent inhibitor of CYP2A6 (and CYP2A13), whereas the aromatase inhibitor letrozole is a potent competitive inhibitor (Jeong et al., 2009). Other inhibitors of CYP2A6 are listed in Table 6-13. CYP2A13 does not appear to contribute to drug clearance, but it may play an important role in the activation of xenobiotics to toxic and carcinogenic metabolites in lung and bladder. Both CYP2A6 and CYP2A13 activate nitrosamines to DNA-reactive (mutagenic) metabolites, especially those nitrosamines with bulky alkyl substituents such as NNK, N'-nitrosonorcotinine, and related nitrosamines found in tobacco smoke. (CYP2E1 also activates nitrosamines, but it preferentially activates nitrosamines with small alkyl substituents such as N-nitrosodimethylamine.)

The identification of 3 Japanese individuals who were PMs of SM-12502, an antiplatelet drug whose clearance is largely determined by CYP2A6, led to the identification of a genetic polymorphism that, in homozygous individuals, leads to the complete loss of CYP2A6 (CYP2A6*4/*4). The incidence of the CYP2A6 PM genotype is high in Asians (up to 15%) and relatively low in Caucasians (0%–4.2%) and black Africans and African Americans (0.9%–1.9%) (Liu et al., 2011). Individuals who are genetically deficient in CYP2A6 have a considerably lower risk of cigarette-smoking-induced lung cancer presumably because these individuals have a reduced capacity for activating tobacco-smoke nitrosamines to carcinogenic metabolites (Kamataki et al., 2005). In support of this interpretation, the CYP2A inhibitor 8-methoxypsoralen protects mice from NNK-induced lung adenomas. CYP2A6 PMs are not only PMs of nitrosamines but also PMs of nicotine. Therefore, decreased cigarette consumption may also contribute to the lowered risk of lung cancer in CYP2A6 PMs. CYP2A6 is detectable in human lung, but the levels are considerably less than those of CYP2A13, which can activate the same carcinogens as CYP2A6. Therefore, it is not immediately obvious why a genetic deficiency in CYP2A6 protects against lung cancer. A similar situation occurs with CYP2D6 inasmuch as individuals lacking this hepatic enzyme (ie, CYP2D6 PMs) also have a slightly decreased risk of cigarette-smoking-induced lung cancer (Rostami-Hodjegan et al., 1998).

It seems somewhat paradoxical but just as CYP2A6 PMs have a decreased risk of lung cancer, so they have an increased risk of nasopharyngeal cancer, which is rare in Caucasians (Western countries) but endemic in Southern China and Southeast Asia. It has been postulated that, in the absence of CYP2A6, higher levels of nitrosamines and other carcinogens reach the nasal epithelium where they can be activated to carcinogenic metabolites by CYP2E1 and CYP2A13, both of which are expressed in nasal epithelium (Tiwawech et al., 2006).

Like CYP2A6, CYP2A13 can activate several carcinogens including many of the nitrosamines (eg, NNK) and aromatic amines (eg, 4-aminobiphenyl) that are present in cigarette smoke, and the mycotoxin aflatoxin B_1. CYP2A13 is suspected of playing a role in the activation of carcinogens in tobacco smoke because it is localized in the 2 sites where cigarette smoking causes cancer, namely, the lung bronchus and bladder (Nakajima et al., 2006).

In view of high prevalence of the CYP2A6 PM genotype in Chinese populations, it is noteworthy that the estimated 300 million cigarette smokers in China consume approximately one third of the world's cigarettes. Although CYP2A6 PMs smoke fewer cigarettes than CYP2A6 EMs, the protective effect of this loss-of-function polymorphism does not prevent an estimated 1 million smokers dying annually from tobacco-related diseases each year in China, a number that is predicted to rise to 2.2 million by 2020 (Liu et al., 2011).

CYP2B6 CYP2B6 is expressed in human liver and, to a lesser extent, in kidney, intestine, and lung. It plays a significant role in the metabolism of the antidepressant bupropion, the antiretrovirals efavirenz and nevirapine, the anesthetics propofol and ketamine, the antineoplastics cyclophosphamide, ifosfamide, and tamoxifen, the antimalarial artemisinin, the synthetic opioids methadone and pethidine (Demerol), the anti-Parkinsonian selegiline, and the endocrine disrupter methoxychlor (Wang and Tompkins, 2008). The activation of cyclophosphamide by CYP2B6 (and CYP3A4) is shown in Fig. 6-50. CYP2B6 also catalyzes the N-demethylation of S-mephenytoin but not the 4'-hydroxylation, which is catalyzed by CYP2C19. Some but not all of these substrates can be used in vitro or in vivo to assess CYP2B6 activity, as shown in Table 6-13. Several drugs have been shown to inhibit CYP2B6 (Table 6-13), and many of them do so in a metabolism-dependent manner, such as clopidogrel, ticlopidine, and thio-TEPA, all of which inactivate other CYP enzymes. 2-Phenyl-2-(1-piperidinyl) propane (PPP) is a potentially selective inactivator of CYP2B6 for in vitro studies (Walsky et al., 2006; Walsky and Obach, 2007). CYP2B6 is an inducible enzyme; it is generally coinduced with CYP3A4 and several CYP2C enzymes by xenobiotics that activate CAR and/or PXR, such as rifampin, the EIAEDs such as phenobarbital, phenytoin, carbamazepine, clotrimazole, and felbamate, and the herbal preparation of St. John's wort, which is the topic of a subsequent section (see the section "Induction of Cytochrome P450—Xenosensors").

There is considerable interindividual variation in CYP2B6 activity, partly due to environmental factors (such as treatment with enzyme inducers) and partly due to genetic factors. Several SNPs that, to varying degrees, impair CYP2B6 expression and/or activity have been identified. The CYP2B6*6 allele ($Gln_{172}His$, $Lys_{262}Arg$) is common in Asians (15%–40%), Caucasians (20%–30%), and African Americans (over 50%), which is associated with a marked decrease in CYP2B6 activity. One functional consequence of the CYP2B6*6 polymorphism is impaired clearance of efavirenz, leading to increased plasma levels and adverse effects (Wang and Tompkins, 2008). CYP2B6*6 is also associated with impaired cyclophosphamide metabolism and S-mephenytoin N-demethylation. Another loss-of-function allele, namely, CYP2B6*5 ($Arg_{487}Cys$), is common in Caucasians (14%–25%) and curiously results in a decrease in CYP2B6 expression and activity but only in females (Wang and Tompkins, 2008).

CYP2C Enzymes Humans express 4 CYP2C enzymes, namely, CYP2C8, CYP2C9, 2C18, and 2C19. With the exception of CYP2C18, these CYP2C enzymes play a significant role in drug metabolism, and their inhibition or induction is the basis of a number of clinically important drug interactions. In the case of CYP2C9 and 2C19, genetic polymorphisms give rise to a relatively common IM or even PM phenotype, which also impacts the metabolism and safety or efficacy of certain drugs. As a general rule, CYP2C8 metabolizes large, acidic drugs, including several glucuronide conjugates, whereas CYP2C9 metabolizes (or is inhibited by) smaller acid- or sulfonamide-containing drugs, and CYP2C19 metabolizes neutral or weakly basic drugs often with a high degree of stereoselectivity (ie, it preferentially metabolizes one enantiomer over the other). All 4 enzymes appear to be inducible by CAR/PXR agonists such as phenobarbital, rifampin, and St. John's wort (hyperforin); hence, they tend to be coinduced together with CYP2B6 and

CYP3A4. Substrates, inhibitors, and inducers of CYP2C8, 2C9, and 2C19 are listed in Table 6-13.

CYP2C8, CYP2C9, and CYP2C19 are abundant enzymes in human liver (see Table 6-12) but low levels of CYP2C8 and 2C9 are also expressed in a wide range of tissue and in vascular endothelium where, together with CYP2J2, they epoxidate arachidonic acid to vasoactive EETs (see the sections "CYP2J2" and "Epoxide Hydrolases") (Chen and Goldstein, 2009; Zordoky and El-Kadi, 2010). CYP2C8 and CYP2C9 can also hydroxylate *all-trans*-retinoic acid and 9-*cis*- and 13-*cis*-retinoic acid (Marill *et al.*, 2000, 2002).

CYP2C8 and CYP2C9 show a marked preference for metabolizing large and small acidic drugs, respectively, and these substrates are ionized (negatively charged) at physiological pH and highly bound to albumin in plasma. In many cases substrates for CYP2C8, which metabolizes large acidic drugs, are also substrates for one or more of the organic anion polypeptide transporters (OATPs) in the intestine and liver. Accordingly, drug interactions with CYP2C8 may also involve drug interactions at the level of OATP especially if transporter-mediated uptake into liver becomes a rate-limiting step in clearance.

As shown in Table 6-11, rats and mice express a large number of CYP2C enzymes (13 and 15, respectively). The expression of CYP2C11 in adult male but not adult female rats (together with male-predominant expression of CYP3A2, which also has a broad substrate specificity) is a key factor underlying many gender differences in xenobiotic and steroid metabolism in mature rats (Waxman and Holloway, 2009).

CYP2C8 CYP2C8 has been implicated in the metabolism of over 60 drugs including the thiazolidinediones rosiglitazone, pioglitazone, and troglitazone (withdrawn), amiodarone, amodiaquine, carbamazepine, cerivastatin (withdrawn), chloroquine, cilostazol, *R*-ibuprofen, lovastatin, morphine, paclitaxel (Taxol®), repaglinide, rosuvastatin, simvastatin, tazarotene (a retinoid derivative), torsemide, verapamil, and zopiclone (Lai *et al.*, 2009). However, with the exception of the antidiabetic drug, repaglinide, all of the above drugs are metabolized to a significant extent by enzymes other than CYP2C8, and in the case of repaglinide its disposition is influenced by the transporter OATP1B1 (SLCO1B1). Repaglinide is classified by the FDA as a sensitive CYP2C8 substrate with the qualification that it is only suitable as an in vivo probe for drug–drug interaction studies if the investigational drug being evaluated as a CYP2C8 inhibitor does not inhibit OATP1B1. In the presence of the CYP2C8/OATP1B1 inhibitor gemfibrozil, exposure to repaglinide (based on plasma AUC) increases about 8-fold (from 5.5- to 15-fold) but gemfibrozil causes only a ~2.3-fold increase in the plasma AUC of rosiglitazone, another potential in vivo probe of CYP2C8.

Substrates for CYP2C8 tend to be large and acidic as evidenced by the observation that CYP2C8 metabolizes several glucuronides (Nishihara *et al.*, 2012, and references therein). For example, whereas 17β-estradiol and diclofenac are metabolized by CYP2C9, the glucuronide metabolites of these compounds (namely, estradiol-17β-glucuronide and diclofenac acyl glucuronide) are metabolized by CYP2C8 (at the same site as that metabolized by CYP2C9, which is distal to the glucuronide moiety). The importance of CYP2C8-dependent metabolism of glucuronides is discussed in the section "Glucuronidation and Formation of Acyl-CoA Thioesters." The ability of CYP2C8 to metabolize glucuronide conjugates plays an important role in the mechanism by which the hypolipidemic drug gemfibrozil inhibits the metabolism, and thereby increases the toxicity (a sometimes fatal muscle disorder known as rhabdomyolysis) of cerivastatin (Baycol), a member of the statin class of cholesterol synthesis inhibitors that was withdrawn from the market (Ogilvie *et al.*, 2006; Baer *et al.*, 2009). Gemfibrozil glucuronide, but not gemfibrozil itself, is an irreversible metabolism-dependent inhibitor of CYP2C8 (Ogilvie *et al.*, 2006). During the benzylic hydroxylation of gemfibrozil, CYP2C8 forms a benzylic radical (as shown previously in the scheme for the mechanism of carbon hydroxylation [this section]) that evades oxygen rebound and alkylates the heme moiety (at the α-meso position), which inactivates the enzyme (Baer *et al.*, 2009). The sometimes fatal interaction between gemfibrozil (the perpetrator drug) and cerivastatin (the victim drug) was a significant factor in the decision to withdraw cerivastatin from the US, European, and Japanese markets.

A large number of genetic polymorphisms have been identified in the CYP2C8 gene, one of which is particularly noteworthy, namely, the *3 allele, which is common in Caucasians (~12%) but rare in Asians, black Africans, and African Americans (Daily and Aquilante, 2009). CYP2C8*3 is a double mutation (Arg$_{139}$Lys and Lys$_{399}$Arg). It is of particular interest for 2 reasons. First, the *3 allele of CYP2C8 is in partial linkage disequilibrium with the *2 allele of CYP2C9, meaning individuals often carry both allelic variants, which complicates the clinical assessment of either one of these genetic polymorphisms on drug metabolism or diseases processes. Second, CYP2C8*3 is of particular interest because of the disconnect between in vitro and in vivo findings. In vitro studies identified the CYP2C8*3 as a *loss-of-function* allelic variant. However, clinical studies established that *3 is a *gain-of-function* allelozyme that is associated with increased clearance of repaglinide, rosiglitazone, and pioglitazone, but not paclitaxel (Daily and Aquilante, 2009). Both the linkage between the *3 allele for CYP2C8 and the *2 allele for CYP2C9 and the discrepancy between in vitro and in vivo findings on CYP2C8*3 sound a word of caution about interpreting the impact of genetic polymorphisms on drug disposition, adverse effects, efficacy, and disease processes.

CYP2C9 CYP2C9 plays a role in the metabolism of over 100 drugs including NSAIDs (eg, diclofenac, celecoxib, ibuprofen, flurbiprofen, naproxen, piroxicam, mefenamic acid, and suprofen), oral hypoglycemics (eg, glyburide, glipizide, glimepiride, tolbutamide), oral anticoagulants (eg, *S*-warfarin, *S*-acenocoumarol, and phenprocoumon), diuretics and uricosurics (eg, sulfinpyrazone sulfide, torsemide, tienilic acid [ticrynafen]), angiotensin II blockers (eg, candesartan, irbesartan, losartan), anticonvulsants (eg, phenytoin), and many others (Zhou *et al.*, 2009b). It also metabolizes Δ^9-tetrahydrocannabinol. Substrates and inhibitors of CYP2C9 tend to be carboxylic acid–, tetrazole-, or sulfonamide-containing compounds, but there are exceptions to this general rule. In fact, the most potent CYP2C9 inhibitors known, namely, benzbromarone and 2-methyl-3-(3′,5′-diiodo-4′-hydroxybenzoyl)benzofluran, are neither acid- nor sulfonamide-containing compounds but they resemble these agents in that they are phenolic anions (negatively charged) at physiological pH (Rettie and Jones, 2005).

CYP2C9 is a polymorphically expressed enzyme. Of the more than 30 variants identified, 2 particular loss-of-function alleles, the *2 and *3 variants, are recognized for their clinically significant impact on drug disposition and safety (Zhou *et al.*, 2009b; Van Booven *et al.*, 2010). CYP2C9*2 (Arg$_{144}$Cys) is prevalent in Caucasians (10%–15%) but not in Asians or African Americans, as is the case with the *3 allele of CYP2C8. These 2 alleles (on different enzymes) are in partial linkage disequilibrium as noted above in the preceding section. CYP2C9*3 (Ile$_{359}$Leu) is widespread across all ethnic groups, being highest in Caucasians (5%–16%) followed by African Americans (~10%) and Asians (1%–5%)

(Van Booven et al., 2010). CYP2C9*2 and *3 have moderately and markedly decreased catalytic activity, respectively. Individuals who are homozygous for the *3 allele are considered CYP2C9 PMs. They are PMs of S-warfarin, tolbutamide, and phenytoin. These 3 drugs have a low therapeutic index, and their dose must be reduced in CYP2C9 PMs to prevent adverse drugs events. Dosage adjustment is also required when these drugs are combined with a CYP2C9 inhibitor or inducer, examples of which are given in Table 6-13. In the case of the anticoagulant warfarin, CYP2C9 genotype is 1 of 3 important genetic factors that affect dosing requirements, the second being the therapeutic target of warfarin vitamin K epoxide reductase complex 1 (VKORC1) (McDonald et al., 2009; Lurie et al., 2010). A third genetic factor is a genetic polymorphism in CYP4F2 (Val$_{433}$Met) that impairs the metabolism of vitamin K$_1$. Individuals with this CYP4F2 polymorphism require a higher warfarin dose to compete with the increased levels of the vitamin K$_1$ in the liver (McDonald et al., 2009; Lurie et al., 2010).

Tienilic acid, suprofen, and silybin are all metabolism-dependent inhibitors of CYP2C9. Tienilic acid is of interest because it was withdrawn from the market due to its hepatotoxicity (see Table 6-3). CYP2C9 converts tienilic acid to an electrophilic thiophene sulfoxide that can react either with water to give 5-hydroxytienilic acid or with a nucleophilic amino acid in CYP2C9 to form a covalent adduct, which inactivates the enzyme (Lecoeur et al., 1994). Antibodies directed against the adduct between CYP2C9 and tienilic acid are thought to be responsible for the immunoallergic hepatitis that develops in about 1 out of every 10,000 patients treated with this uricosuric diuretic drug. As shown in Table 6-3, these autoantibodies against CYP2C9 are known as anti-LKM$_2$ because they are directed against liver and kidney microsomes. The subscript number 2 distinguishes these antibodies against CYP2C9 from those against CYP2D6, which are known as anti-LKM$_1$. It should be noted that tienilic acid can also be activated to a reactive acyl glucuronide, as outlined in the section "Glucuronidation and Formation of Acyl-CoA Thioesters."

CYP2C18 In contrast to the other 3 CYP2C enzymes expressed in human liver, CYP2C18 plays little or no role in drug metabolism. CYP2C18 is the most abundant CYP2C enzyme in skin and lung, and it is also expressed in brain, uterus, mammary gland, kidney, and duodenum. CYP2C18 is more than an order of magnitude more active than either CYP2C9 or CYP2C19 at catalyzing the *para*-hydroxylation of phenytoin to HPPH, and CYP2C18 can further hydroxylate HPPH to a catechol (Kinobe et al., 2005). Autoxidation of this catechol to an *ortho*-quinone is thought to be responsible, at least in part, for rare incidences of hypersensitivity reactions to phenytoin. Therefore, although hepatic CYP2C9 and CYP2C19 are largely responsible for determining the systemic clearance of phenytoin, it is possible that CYP2C18 is responsible for activating phenytoin by the catechol/quinone pathway in the skin, the tissue where the first signs of hypersensitivity to phenytoin are observed.

CYP2C19 CYP2C19 is a polymorphically expressed enzyme that metabolizes several drugs with a high degree of stereospecificity such that, in the case of drugs administered as a racemic mixture, it metabolizes one enantiomer faster than the other, as in the case of mephenytoin (Mesantoin®), which is of historical interest with respect to CYP2C19. A genetic polymorphism for the metabolism of S-mephenytoin was first described in 1984 (reviewed in Wilkinson et al., 1989). The deficiency affects the 4′-hydroxylation (aromatic ring hydroxylation) of this anticonvulsant drug (see Fig. 6-42). The other major pathway of S-mephenytoin metabolism, namely, N-demethylation to S-nirvanol, is not affected. (This pathway was subsequently shown to be catalyzed by CYP2B6.) Consequently,

PMs excrete little or no 4′-hydroxymephenytoin in their urine, but they do excrete increased amounts of the N-demethylated metabolite, S-nirvanol (S-phenylethylhydantoin). The enzyme responsible for this genetic polymorphism is CYP2C19, and it is highly stereoselective for the S-enantiomer of mephenytoin (de Morais et al., 1994). In contrast to the S-enantiomer, the R-enantiomer is not converted to 4′-hydroxymephenytoin, but it is N-demethylated to R-nirvanol (R-phenylethylhydantoin). Individuals who are genetically deficient in CYP2C19 are at increased risk of adverse events from Mesantoin® (a racemic mixture of the S- and R-enantiomers of mephenytoin). An exaggerated central response has been observed in CYP2C19 PMs administered Mesantoin® at doses that were without effect in CYP2C19 EMs.

CYP2C19 plays an important role in the metabolism of the proton pump inhibitors omeprazole, lansoprazole, pantoprazole, and rabeprazole, representative structures of which are shown in Fig. 6-44. The sulfoxide group in proton pump inhibitors is a chiral center, and CYP2C19 preferentially metabolizes one enantiomer over the other: it preferentially hydroxylates the R-enantiomer in the case of omeprazole, and it preferentially hydroxylates the S-enantiomer in the case of lansoprazole. These reactions are equivalent inasmuch as these 2 proton pump inhibitors are hydroxylated on opposite ends of the molecule (on the pyridine ring in the case of omeprazole and on the benzimidazole ring in the case of lansoprazole), meaning the sulfoxide in each case binds to the active site of CYP2C19 in the same orientation (Kim et al., 2003). CYP2C19 PMs are poor metabolizers of omeprazole and lansoprazole. However, CYP2C19 PMs are not at increased risk for ADEs but actually derive greater therapeutic benefit (better control of GERD) from standard doses of proton pump inhibitors (Furuta et al., 2005). Esomeprazole, the S-enantiomer of omeprazole, was approved for the treatment of GERD and related gastric acid disorders. Compared with the R-enantiomer, esomeprazole is not rapidly metabolized by CYP2C19, and its improved pharmacokinetic behavior provides CYP2C19 EMs with the same therapeutic benefit as CYP2C19 PMs administered omeprazole. This is due in part to the ability of esomeprazole to function as a metabolism-dependent inhibitor of CYP2C19 and inhibit its own metabolism in CYP2C19 EMs (Ogilvie et al., 2011). Other substrates, inhibitors, and inducers of CYP2C19 are listed in Table 6-13.

Two genetic polymorphisms, the *2 and *3 alleles (and their variants *2A, *2B, and *2C, and *3A and *3B), are responsible for the majority of CYP2C9 PMs (Zhou et al., 2009a). Both the *2 and *3 are null alleles; hence, individuals homozygous for either allele (*2/*2 and *3/*3) and heterozygotes (*2/*3) are devoid of functional CYP2C19. The incidence of the CYP2C19 PM genotype varies considerably from one ethnic group to the next: it ranges from 13% to 23% in Japanese, Chinese, Korean, Vietnamese, and Indian populations, but the incidence is considerably lower in black African and African Americans (3%–5%), and in Caucasians (1%–7% depending on geographical location) (Zhou et al., 2009a). A high incidence of CYP2C19 PMs is found in Australian aboriginals (~26%) and in South Pacific Polynesian populations (~14%). In the Polynesian island of Vanuatu, 79% of the population has been identified as CYP2C19 PMs. When administered standard drug doses, CYP2C19 PMs have elevated plasma levels of proton pump inhibitors (omeprazole, lansoprazole, pantoprazole, and, to a lesser extent, rabeprazole), diazepam, escitalopram, sertraline, and voriconazole, not to mention the S-enantiomer of mephenytoin in individuals administered Mesantoin, which was the original observation that led to the discovery the CYP2C19 PM genotype. No CYP2C19 UMs individuals with functional CYP2C19 gene duplications have been identified; however, CYP2C19*17 (Ile$_{331}$Val) has

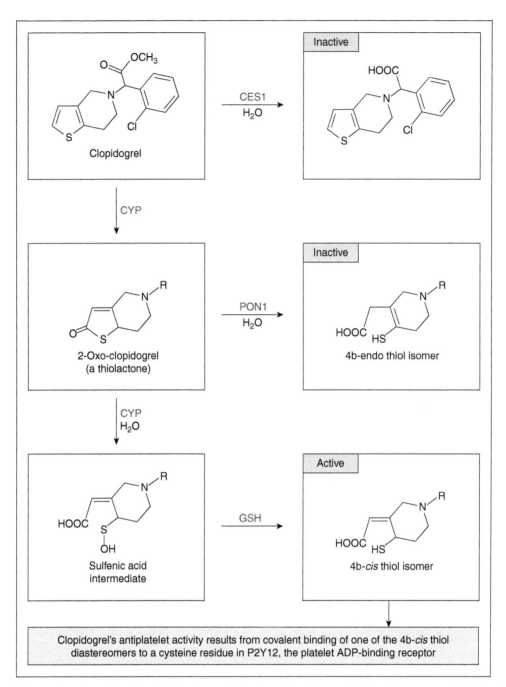

Figure 6-49. *Biotransformation of clopidogrel to inactive metabolites by carboxylesterase (CES1) and paraoxonase (PON1) and its active, antiplatelet metabolite by cytochrome P450 (especially CYP2C19).*

been identified as a gain-of-function allele with allele frequencies of about 20% in Caucasians and black Africans but only ~2% in Asian populations (Li-Wan-Po *et al.*, 2010). Based on the magnitude of the increase in clearance of drugs such as escitalopram, CYP2C19 activity in individuals who are homozygous for this gain-of-function allele (*17/*17) can be considered high-activity EMs rather than UMs (Li-Wan-Po *et al.*, 2010). CYP2C19 is regulated by CAR/PXR; hence, its activity in IMs and EMs can be increased by enzyme-inducing drugs (see Table 6-13).

CYP2C19 has attracted considerable attention for its role in converting the antiplatelet drug clopidogrel to its pharmacologically active metabolite. This activation process is shown in Fig. 6-49. It is unusual for several reasons. First, the therapeutically active component is a reactive metabolite that binds covalently to the ADP-binding

receptor ($P2Y_{12}$) on platelets. Second, the oxidative pathway leading to formation of this active metabolite is in competition with 2 hydrolytic pathways, one that hydrolyzes clopidogrel, which is catalyzed by CES1 (a carboxylesterase), and another that hydrolyzes the first oxidative metabolite (a thiolactone), which is catalyzed by PON1 (a paraoxonase). Third, the active metabolite formed by CYP and the inactive metabolite formed from the intermediary thiolactone by PON1 are isomers, as shown in Fig. 6-49 (based on studies by Dansette *et al.*, 2011). Fourth, clopidogrel provides an example of Type F toxicity whereby PMs (individuals who fail to produce the active metabolite) derive diminished therapeutic benefit and, in the case of clopidogrel, are at increased risk of thrombosis and CAD, whereas high-activity EMs who produce too much of the active metabolite (and hence too much platelet inhibition) are at increased risk from bleeding and hemorrhage. Much of the pharmacogenomic data strongly implicate CYP2C19 as the most important enzyme for clopidogrel activation, based on poor response to clopidogrel in carriers of the loss-of-function CYP2C19 alleles (ie, the *2 and *3 alleles), and also increased bleeding in carriers of the gain-of-function CYP2C19*17 allele (Sibbing *et al.*, 2010; Scott *et al.*, 2011). A dominant role for PON1 in clopidogrel activation has been proposed (Bouman *et al.*, 2011). This rather compelling (but controversial) proposal was explained by Dansette *et al.* (2011) by showing that the ring-opened thiol produced by PON1 (with the double bond in the α/β position relative to the thiol) is an inactive isomer of the true active metabolite produced by CYP2C19 (with the double bond in the β/γ position relative to the thiol), as shown in Fig. 6-49.

Because of its tendency to cause gastric bleeding as an adverse event, clopidogrel was often prescribed together with a proton pump inhibitor (to raise gastric pH and lessen the severity of gastric bleeding). It was established that omeprazole and its *S*-enantiomer esomeprazole, but not pantoprazole or lansoprazole, compromise the antiplatelet effect of clopidogrel. It was subsequently established that omeprazole (and its *S*-enantiomer esomeprazole), but not pantoprazole or lansoprazole, is a metabolism-dependent inhibitor of CYP2C19 (Ogilvie *et al.*, 2011). This drug–drug interaction and the pharmacogenomic data strongly implicate CYP2C19 as the major enzyme responsible for converting clopidogrel to its pharmacologically active metabolite.

CYP2D6 In the late 1950s, clinical trials in the United States established that sparteine was as potent as oxytocin for inducing labor at term. However, the duration and intensity of action of sparteine was dramatically increased in ~7% of all patients tested. The exaggerated response to sparteine included prolonged (tetanic) uterine contraction and abnormally rapid labor. In some cases, sparteine caused the death of the fetus. The drug was not recommended for clinical use because these adverse effects were unpredictable and occurred at doses that were well tolerated by other patients. The antihypertensive drug, debrisoquine, was subsequently found to cause a marked and prolonged hypotension in 5% to 10% of patients, and a genetic polymorphism for the metabolism of debrisoquine and sparteine was discovered in 1977–1979. PMs lack CYP2D6, which catalyzes the 4-hydroxylation of debrisoquine and the dehydrogenation (Δ^2- and Δ^5-oxidation) of sparteine (see Fig. 6-48).

Genetic polymorphisms of CYP2D6 have been so extensively studied that it is possible not only to categorize individuals into 4 phenotypes, namely, PMs, IMs, EMs, and UMs but also to subdivide the EMs into 3 categories, namely, High-Activity EM, medium-activity EM, and Low-Activity EM, as summarized in Table 6-4. More than 100 allelic variants of CYP2D6 have been identified (Zhou *et al.*, 2009a; http://www.cypalleles.ki.se/cyp2d6.htm). Many of the allelic variants that result in a partial or complete loss of CYP2D6 activity are listed in the legend to Table 6-4. The incidence of the CYP2D6 PM genotype varies considerably from one ethnic group to the next: it is 5% to 7% in Caucasians, 2% to 4% in black Africans and African Americans, and 1% to 2% in Asian (Thai, Chinese, and Japanese) populations. Similarly, the incidence of the CYP2D6 gene duplication, which gives rise to the CYP2D6 UM genotype, varies among ethnic groups: it is up to 29% in Ethiopians, 20% in Saudi Arabians, 5% to 10% in Southern European Caucasians, but only 1% to 2% of Northern European Caucasians, 5% to 10% of Turkish subjects, and 2% or less in black African, African-American, and Asian subjects.

CYP2D6 plays a major role in drug metabolism, second only to CYP3A4 in terms of the sheer number of drugs it metabolizes (Zhou, 2009a,b; Zhou *et al.*, 2009a). CYP2D6 prefers to metabolize lipophilic amines, which is the fundamental structure of most cardiovascular and CNS drugs. Accordingly, CYP2D6 metabolizes various tricyclic antidepressants, nontricyclic antidepressants, SSRIs, neuroleptics, β-blockers, antiarrhymthics, antiemetics, opioids, and antihistamines, examples of which are given in Table 6-13. CYP2D6 plays an important role in tamoxifen metabolism (discussed later in this section). CYP2D6 also metabolizes several drugs of abuse including methamphetamine ("meth" or "ice"), methylenedioxymethamphetamine (NMDA or "ecstasy"), *N*-ethyl-3,4-methylenedioxyamphetamine (MDE or "eve"), and 3,4-methylenedioxyamphetamine (MDA or "the love drug"). Those drugs of abuse containing a methylenedioxy (benzodioxole) moiety are also metabolism-dependent inhibitors of CYPD6 (Van *et al.*, 2006). CYP2D6 also metabolizes the neurotoxin MPTP (see Fig. 6-29 and the section "Amine Oxidases"). Individuals lacking CYP2D6 have an exaggerated response to some but not all the drugs mentioned above or shown in Table 6-13. Large increases (>5-fold) in systemic exposure are observed in CYP2D6 PMs with atomoxetine, desipramine, dextromethorphan, metropolol, perphenazine, and respiridone, some of which are useful in vivo probes of CYP2D6 activity. Drugs whose clearance is impaired in CYP2D6 PMs are cleared faster in UMs.

Whether the impact of CYP2D6 polymorphisms on the pharmacokinetics of a drug translate into changes in pharmacodynamic response depends on the nature of the polymorphism (ranging from PM to UMs), the magnitude of the PK response (which is determined by fm_{CYP2D6}, the fractional contribution of CYP2D6 to drug clearance [see Point 24 in the section "Introduction"]), and the pharmacological and toxicological properties of the metabolites. For example, the metabolites produced by CYP2D6 from the antiarrhythmic drug encainide are more potent than those of the parent drug; hence, QT prolongation is more apparent in CYP2D6 EMs than PMs. On the hand, propafenone is a more potent β-blocker than its metabolites; hence, PMs experience prolonged hypotension from a standard dose of propafenone. CYP2D6 status affects the pharmacokinetics of most β-blockers but many of them have active metabolites such that changes in pharmacokinetics have little or no effect on their overall pharmacological activity (Tucker, 1994; Turner *et al.*, 2001; Ingelman-Sundberg, 2005; Zhou, 2009a). CYP2D6 PMs are at increased risk from the hepatotoxic and other adverse effects (sedation, extrapyramidal, and psychomotor symptoms) of perhexiline, for which reason perhexiline joined sparteine and debrisoquine in being denied regulatory approval by the US FDA.

The analgesic codeine (which is *O*-demethylated to morphine) and the anticancer drug tamoxifen (which is hydroxylated and *N*-demethylated to endoxifen) are converted to pharmacologically active metabolites by CYP2D6. Consequently, CYP2D6 PMs derive less therapeutic benefit than CYP2D6 EMs. In contrast, in the case of codeine, CYP2D6 UMs are at increased risk from morphine toxicity. The death of an elderly man administered a recommended dose of codeine and the death of baby who was breastfed by a woman on codeine have been attributed to the CYP2D6 UM genotype that causes rapid conversion of codeine to morphine (which causes respiratory suppression) (Gasche *et al.*, 2004; Koren *et al.*, 2006). CYP2D6 converts the breast cancer drug tamoxifen to endoxifen (which is 30- to 100-fold more potent than tamoxifen in suppressing estrogen-dependent cell proliferation); hence, CYP2D6 PMs are at increased risk for breast cancer recurrence following tamoxifen adjuvant therapy (Goetz *et al.*, 2005; Schroth *et al.*, 2009). The effects of codeine in CYP2D6 UMs (who form too much active metabolite) and tamoxifen in PMs (who form too little active metabolite) represent examples of Type A and Type F toxicity, respectively.

The propensity for CYP2D6 to metabolize so many cardiovascular and CNS drugs (and other lipophilic amines) can be attributed in large part to the binding of the amine function to anionic residues (Glu216 and Asp301) in the substrate-binding site. Substrate oxidation usually occurs 5 to 7.5 Å from the basic nitrogen atom. Other substrate binding orientations are possible, which is why CYP2D6 can N-dealkylate drugs, even drugs that contain a single amine function (ie, drugs that appear to bind upside down in the active site) (Bonn et al., 2008; Unwalla et al., 2010).

Quinidine is a potent inhibitor of CYP2D6 because it interacts favorably with the anionic sites on CYP2D6 but it cannot be oxidized at a site 5 to 7.5 Å from its basic nitrogen atoms. Quinidine, paroxetine, and fluoxetine (and especially norfluoxetine, its N-demethylated metabolite) are strong CYP2D6 inhibitors in vivo, and a PM phenotype can be induced pharmacologically with these particular inhibitors. Quinine, the levorotatory diastereomer of quinidine, is not a potent inhibitor of CYP2D6, and neither drug is a potent inhibitor of the CYP2D enzymes expressed in rats. Compared with other SSRIs, fluoxetine causes surprisingly prolonged inhibition of CYP2D6; this is attributable in part to the long half-life of norfluoxetine (a primary amine), which also inhibits CYP2D6 (Liston et al., 2002). Paroxetine has a relatively short plasma half-life (16-24 hours) but causes prolonged inhibition of CYP2D6 because it contains a methylenedioxy (benzodioxole) moiety that causes MDI of CYP2D6 (Venkatakrishnan and Obach, 2005). Because of the low dose of paroxetine (20 mg), maximum inactivation of CYP2D6 activity is not achieved without 7 to 10 days of paroxetine treatment. Bupropion, a commonly used in vitro probe of CYP2B6 activity, causes clinically relevant inhibition of CYP2D6 even though it is a relatively weak inhibitor of the enzyme in vitro (in human liver microsomes) (Reese et al., 2008). Bupropion represents one of a handful of examples of system-dependent inhibition (Parkinson et al., 2010) (see the section "Inhibition of Cytochrome P450"). The ability of bupropion to inhibit CYP2D6 in vivo is attributable in large part to its reduction to inhibitory metabolites (erythrohydrobupropion and threohydrobupropion). Accordingly, the in vivo inhibition of CYP2D6 by bupropion is better predicted in human hepatocytes than in human liver microsomes (Parkinson et al., 2010).

The prominent determinants of CYP2D6 activity in vivo are genetic polymorphisms and treatment with inhibitory drugs. CYP2D6 is considered a noninducible enzyme, although its levels increase during pregnancy and decrease following renal impairment (Rostami-Hodjegan et al., 1999; Sit et al., 2010).

Compared with hepatic levels, low levels of CYP2D6 are present in several tissues including brain, kidney, lung, intestine, breast, and placenta (Zhou, 2009a,b). The metabolism of CNS drugs by CYP2D6 in the brain has attracted considerable interest, as has its ability to convert m- and p-tyramine to dopamine and to catalyze the 21-hydroxylation of certain steroid hormones such as progesterone.

Individuals lacking CYP2D6 have an unusually low incidence of some chemically induced neoplastic diseases (Idle, 1991). For example, CYP2D6 PMs appear to be relatively resistant to lung cancer, whereas CYP2D6 UMs appear to be at increased risk, although the effects are modest (Rostami-Hodjegan et al., 1998; Agundez et al., 2001). It has been hypothesized that CYP2D6 may play a role in the metabolic activation of chemical carcinogens, such as those present in the environment, in the diet, and/or in cigarette smoke. According to this hypothesis, CYP2D6 PMs have a low incidence of cancer because they fail to activate chemical carcinogens, whereas CYP2D6 UMs have an increased risk because they rapidly and/or extensively activate procarcinogens. However, CYP2D6 plays little or no role in the activation of known chemical carcinogens to DNA-reactive or mutagenic metabolites, with the notable exception of the tobacco-smoke-specific nitrosamine, NNK, which is also activated by numerous other CYP enzymes (see the section "CYP2A6, CYP2A7, and 2A13").

CYP2E1 As shown in Fig. 6-25, CYP2E1 was first identified as the microsomal ethanol oxidizing system (MEOS) (Lieber, 1999). It is now recognized as a key enzyme involved in the activation of acetaminophen (Tylenol) to its reactive metabolite NAPQI (see Fig. 6-35), a leading cause of DILI (Kaplowitz, 2005). CYP2E1 also biotransforms a large number of volatile halogenated alkanes (chloroform, carbon tetrachloride, vinyl chloride, and many more), halogenated anesthetics (halothane, enflurane, and others), small aromatic and nitrogen aromatic compounds (benzene, styrene, toluene, pyridine, pyrazole, and others), alkanes (ethane–hexane), alcohols (ethanol–pentanol), the colon carcinogen azoxymethane, and numerous mutagenic/carcinogenic nitrosamines (reviewed in Pohl and Scinicariello, 2011). In many cases CYP2E1 converts the aforementioned xenobiotics to reactive (toxic/mutagenic/carcinogenic) metabolites, as shown in Table 6-14 and as illustrated for carbon tetrachloride in Fig. 6-18, halothane in Fig. 6-19, benzene in Fig. 6-32, and N-nitrosamine, urethane (ethyl carbamate), trichloroethylene, and tetrachloroethylene in Fig. 6-50 (Guengerich, 1991). CYP2E1 activates acetylhydrazine, a metabolite formed following the N-acetylation of isoniazid, to a hepatotoxic metabolite. The severity of isoniazid hepatotoxicity is influenced by genetic polymorphisms that decrease N-acetyltransferases (NAT) and increase CYP2E1 activity, as discussed in the section "Acetylation."

Studies in CYP2E1 knockout mice have established an important role for CYP2E1 in the in vivo activation of some of the aforementioned xenobiotics. Compared with wild-type mice, CYP2E1 knockout mice are protected (partially or completely) from the hepatotumorigenic effects of urethane (ethyl carbamate), the preneoplastic changes induced in the colon by azoxymethane, the myelotoxicity of benzene, and the hepatotoxicity of acetaminophen (Gonzalez, 2003, 2007; Ghanayem, 2006). CYP2E1 is 1 of 3 enzymes that catalyze the conversion of acetaminophen to NAPQI, the others being CYP1A2 and CYP3A4. Double knockout mice, in which both CYP2E1 and CYP1A2 are deleted, are even more resistant to acetaminophen hepatotoxicity than CYP2E1 knockout mice (Gonzalez, 2007). These findings in mice are thought to translate to the situation in humans. It is interesting to note, however, that human CYP2E1 knockin mice (transgenic mice harboring human CYP2E1 in place of the mouse enzyme, also known as CYP2E1-humanized mice) are more resistant to acetaminophen hepatotoxicity than wild-type mice, suggesting mouse CYP2E1 may be more active than human CYP2E1 in converting acetaminophen to NAPQI (Cheung and Gonzalez, 2008). The role of CYP2E1 in acetaminophen hepatotoxicity is discussed later in this section.

The only orally administered drug (as opposed to volatile anesthetics) that is primarily metabolized by CYP2E1 is chlorzoxazone, an FDA-approved muscle relaxant (Paraflex®). The urinary excretion of 6-hydroxychlorzoxazone and the plasma ratio of 6-hydroxychlorzoxazone to chlorzoxazone have been used as in vivo probes of CYP2E1. In human liver microsomes, CYP2E1 activity can be conveniently measured by the 6-hydroxylation of chlorzoxazone and the hydroxylation of 4-nitrophenol (Table 6-13). The 6-hydroxylation of chlorzoxazone can also be catalyzed by CYP1A1, but this enzyme is rarely expressed in human liver and only low levels are present in extrahepatic tissues. CYP2E1 is one of the CYP enzymes that require cytochrome b_5, which lowers the K_m for certain substrates (Levin et al., 1986).

Table 6-14

Examples of Xenobiotics Activated by Human P450

CYP1A2
  Acetaminophen
  2-Acetylaminofluorene
  4-Aminobiphenyl
  2-Aminofluorene
  2-Naphthylamine
  NNK
  Amino acid pyrolysis products
    (DiMeQx, MeIQ, MeIQx, Glu P-2,
      IQ, PhIP, Trp P-1, Trp P-2)
  Tacrine

CYP2A6 and 2A13
  NNK and bulky nitrosamines
  N-Nitrosodiethylamine
  Aflatoxin B_1

CYP2B6
  6-Aminochrysene
  Cyclophosphamide
  Ifosfamide

CYP2C8, 9, 18, 19
  Tienilic acid
  Phenytoin
  Valproic acid

CYP2D6
  NNK

CYP2F1
  3-Methylindole
  Acetaminophen
  Valproic acid

CYP1A1 and 1B1
  Benzo[a]pyrene and other polycyclic
    aromatic hydrocarbons

CYP2E1
  Acetaminophen
  Acrylonitrile
  Benzene
  Carbon tetrachloride
  Chloroform
  Dichloromethane
  1,2-Dichloropropane
  Ethylene dibromide
  Ethylene dichloride
  Ethyl carbamate
  Halothane
  N-Nitrosodimethylamine
  Styrene
  Trichloroethylene
  Vinyl chloride

CYP3A4
  Acetaminophen
  Aflatoxin B_1 and G_1
  6-Aminochrysene
  Benzo[a]pyrene 7,8-dihydrodiol
  Cyclophosphamide
  Ifosfamide
  1-Nitropyrene
  Sterigmatocystin
  Senecionine
  $Tris$(2,3-dibromopropyl)phosphate

CYP4B1 (in animals but not humans)[*]
  Ipomeanol
  3-Methylindole
  2-Aminofluorene

NNK, 4-(methylnitrosamino)-1-(3-pyridyl)-1-butanone, a tobacco-specific nitrosamine. Data
    from Guengerich and Shimada (1991).
[*]Due to lack of heme incorporation human CYP4B1 is probably inactive.

The function and regulation of CYP2E1 are relatively well conserved across mammalian species. CYP2E1 is expressed constitutively in liver and several extrahepatic tissues, such as the kidney, pancreas, brain, lung, intestine, nasal epithelium, bone marrow, and lymphocytes. The levels of CYP2E1 in human liver microsomes do not show the high degree of interindividual variation characteristic of other enzymes, as shown in Table 6-12. Numerous genetic polymorphisms in the CYP2E1 gene have been identified but none impact function and/or expression in a manner that gives rise to a PM or UM phenotype (reviewed in Pohl and Scinicariello, 2011). In humans and most other mammalian species, CYP2E1 is moderately inducible (<5-fold) by ethanol, isoniazid, pyrazole, acetone, and other ketone bodies (which form during uncontrolled diabetes). In contrast to the induction of most other CYP enzymes, the induction of CYP2E1 often involves increased translation of preexisting mRNA and/or protein stabilization rather than transcriptional activation of the CYP2E1 gene; hence, induction of CYP2E1 often occurs in the absence of an increase in mRNA levels (Gonzalez, 2007). An exception to this general rule is the induction of CYP2E1 by diabetes, which involves transcriptional activation and a marked increase in CYP2E1 mRNA. CYP2E1 can be inhibited by 4-methylpyrazole (fomepizole), which also inhibits ADH (class I ADH), and by disulfiram (Antabuse), which also inhibits ALDH (ADH2).

Disulfiram is one of many sulfur-containing agents that competitively or irreversibly inhibit CYP2E1, such as chlormethiazole, diallylsulfide, diethyldithiocarbamate, and phenylethylisothiocyanate) (Pohl and Scinicariello, 2011).

Alcohol can potentiate the hepatotoxicity of acetaminophen. Several mechanisms have been proposed, including increased activation of acetaminophen due to the induction of CYP2E1, increased oxidative stress (ROS production), and decreased inactivation of NAPQI and ROS due to a lowering of GSH levels. Likewise fasting potentiates acetaminophen hepatotoxicity, presumably by inducing CYP2E1 (which is inducible by ketone bodies) and lowering UDPGA levels, which impairs the direct conjugation of acetaminophen and directs more drug toward the formation of NAPQI (Whitcomb and Block, 1994).

CYP2E1 is receiving considerable attention for several reasons that impact our understanding of its role in acetaminophen and alcohol toxicity. First, during its catalytic cycle CYP2E1 is prone to uncoupling (see Fig. 6-40), such that, during the metabolism of ethanol (alcohol) and acetaminophen, roughly 50% of its catalytic cycles result in the production of superoxide anion and related ROS instead of metabolite formation (Gonzalez, 2005; Lu and Cederbaum, 2008). Second, in rat liver, approximately 40% of CYP2E1 is phosphorylated and localized to the inner membrane

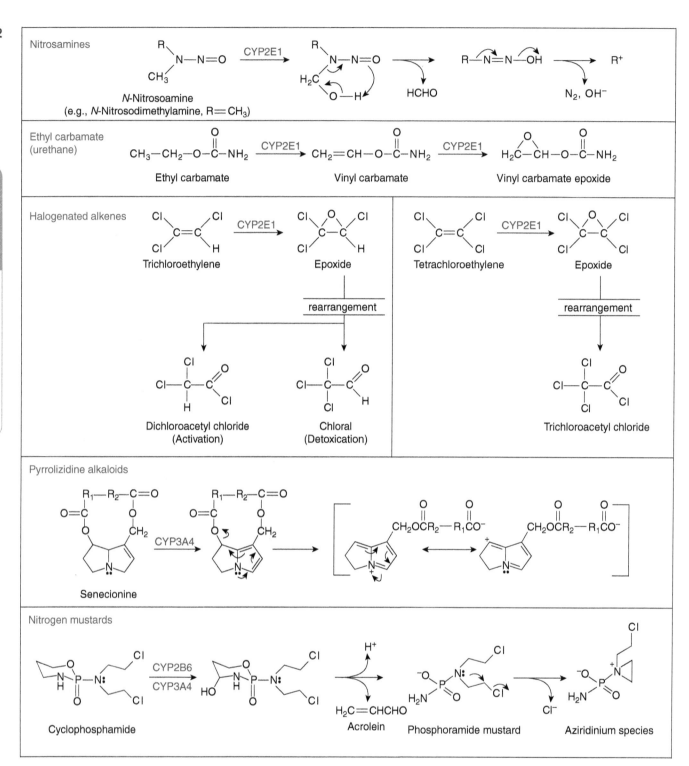

Figure 6-50. *Additional mechanisms of cytochrome P450–dependent activation of xenobiotics to reactive (electrophilic) metabolites.*

of mitochondria (Knockaert *et al.*, 2011a,b). Like all microsomal enzymes, CYP2E1 has a canonical N-terminal signal recognition peptide (SRP) that targets its translation to the rough endoplasmic reticulum (in ribosomes bound to the endoplasmic reticulum) but the process is relatively inefficient such that about half of CYP2E1 is transcribed by membrane-free ribosomes. CYP2E1 contains a mitochondrial targeting signal (2 positively charged amino acids, Lys$_{24}$ and Lys$_{25}$) and a serine residue (Ser$_{129}$) that, when phosphorylated by cAMP-dependent protein kinase A (PKA), complexes with heat-shock proteins (Hsp70 and Hsp90) and is translocated to the inner membrane of mitochondria (Knockaert *et al.*, 2011b). Cell culture

experiments in which CYP2E1 is expressed only in mitochondria or in both mitochondria and microsomes established that mitochondrial CYP2E1 is catalytically active (it is presumably supported by ferredoxin/ferredoxin reductase, the electron transporters that support endobiotic biotransformation by mitochondrial CYP enzymes) and is sufficient to cause oxidative stress, GSH depletion, and cell toxicity in response to acetaminophen or alcohol (Knockaert *et al.*, 2011a). A variety of evidence points to mitochondrial toxicity by NAPQI and ROS as the key event in acetaminophen hepatotoxicity (Jaeschke *et al.*, 2012). For example, studies with radioactive acetaminophen (4′-hydroxyacetanilide) and its nonhepatotoxic *meta* isomer 3′-hydroxyacetanilide show comparable levels of overall covalent binding to mouse liver proteins but covalent binding of acetaminophen is predominantly in mitochondria, whereas binding of the nonhepatotoxic regioisomer is in the cytoplasm (reviewed in Jaeschke *et al.*, 2012). The mitochondrial localization of CYP2E1 and its ability to form NAPQI and ROS in the mitochondrion appear to be important determinants of acetaminophen hepatotoxicity. It is of interest that several CYP enzymes in addition to CYP2E1 have been located inside mitochondria (Knockaert *et al.*, 2011a,b).

There is growing evidence that the potentially deleterious ROS produced by microsomal CYP2E1 and other CYP enzymes (notably CYP1A2; the other high-spin enzyme that, like CYP2E1, can produce ROS even in the absence of substrate) is actively inhibited during the process known as ER stress, which is triggered by the accumulation of unfolded proteins (the ER plays a key role in protein folding and posttranslational modification of proteins prior to their exit to the Golgi and other destinations), which occurs in response to ischemia/reperfusion injury and exposure to certain xenobiotics such as tunicamycin (an *N*-glycosylation inhibitor) and thapsigargin (an ER calcium ATPase inhibitor) (Rasheva and Domingos, 2009; Tabas and Ron, 2011). Extensive ER stress (ie, a prolonged unfolded protein response [UPR], which is mediated by PERK, ATF6, and IRE1) results in the activation of caspases and Bcl-2, which leads to apoptotic cell death. However, mild ER stress activates Nrf2 and the antiapoptotic factor BI-1. Both activation of Nrf2 (through its phosphorylation by PERK, one of the 3 main ER stress responders) and BI-1 protect the endoplasmic reticulum from further damage by inhibiting the production of ROS by CYP2E1 (and presumably other CYP enzymes such as CYP1A2) by 2 distinct mechanisms (Lee *et al.*, 2007; Kim *et al.*, 2009). In the case of Nrf2, this transcription factor causes a marked (~10-fold) induction of heme oxygenase (among other antioxidant defense enzymes), which inhibits CYP activity by competing for electrons from NADPH-cytochrome P450 reductase (which serves both enzymes) (Reed *et al.*, 2011). Heme oxygenase can also inactivate certain CYP enzymes by converting their heme moiety to biliverdin (Kutty *et al.*, 1988). BI-1 also inhibits CYP but does so by complexing with NADPH-cytochrome P450 reductase (the 2 proteins coimmunoprecipitate), which inhibits ROS production by CYP2E1 (Kim *et al.*, 2009). From these studies it is emerging that CYP2E1 and possibly CYP1A2, the 2 high-spin CYP enzymes, produce ROS and contribute to oxidative stress, processes that are augmented by xenobiotics such as acetaminophen and alcohol and processes that are particularly damaging during ER stress.

CYP2F1 CYP2F1 is a human enzyme; its homologs in mouse and rat are CYP2F2 and CYP2F4, respectively. These enzymes are expressed in the respiratory tract (lung and nasal mucosa), although CYP2F1 is expressed in human lung at much lower levels than CYP2F2 is expressed in mice. In mice CYP2F2 plays an important role in activating various pulmonary/nasal toxicants including 3-methylindole, naphthalene, 1-nitronaphthalene, styrene, benzene, B[*a*]P, dichloroethylene, and trichloroethylene. For example, CYP2F2 knockout mice are resistant to the toxic effects of naphthalene on the lung and nasal olfactory mucosa (Li *et al.*, 2011a) and they are similarly resistant to the toxic effects of styrene on lung Clara cells and terminal bronchial cells (Cruzan *et al.*, 2012). Studies on the metabolic activation of 3-methylindole (a constituent in tobacco smoke) are interesting for illustrating how 2 respiratory enzymes, CYP2F2 and CYP2A5 (the homologs of human CYP2F1 and CYP2A13), can make the same initial reactive metabolites with different subsequent fates (Zhou *et al.*, 2012). Both CYP2F2 and CYP2A convert 3-methylindole to a carbon radical and epoxide, but these are further converted by CYP2A5

to stable metabolites: the carbon radical is converted to indole-3-carbinol by oxygen rebound and the epoxide is converted to an amide (3-methyloxindole) by rearrangement. In contrast, CYP2F2 converts these intermediates to reactive metabolites: the carbon radical is converted by dehydrogenation to a Michael acceptor, 3-methyleneindolenine, whereas the epoxide is either released or converted to iminium ions, all of which react with GSH. In animals, the activation of 3-methylindole can also activated by another pulmonary enzyme, namely, CYP4B1, an enzyme that is thought to be functionally inactive in humans due to lack of heme incorporation (see the section "CYP4 Enzymes").

CYP2G1 CYP2G1 is not expressed in humans but it is expressed in the olfactory mucosa of rodents and other animals. Numerous xenobiotics cause nasal cytotoxicity and cancer in rodents (reviewed in Jeffrey *et al.*, 2006). Along with other CYP enzymes that are highly expressed in olfactory mucosa, such as CYP2A5 and CYP2F2 in mice and CYP2A3 and CYP2F4 in rats, CYP2G1 is a potential contributor to the formation of reactive metabolites in this target of xenobiotic toxicity in rodents.

CYP2J2 CYP2J2 is of interest for a number of reasons. First, it is expressed in vascular epithelium and high levels are found in the heart and many other tissues. CYP2J2 is the most abundant CYP expressed in heart and left ventricular levels are ~1.5-fold higher in women than in men (Michaud *et al.*, 2010). Based on mRNA levels (which may not reflect protein levels), the expression of CYP2J2 is highest in small intestine followed by heart > skeletal muscle > kidney > salivary gland > lung > liver. Second, CYP2J2 metabolizes many of the same drugs that are substrates for CYP3A4 (although not always to the same metabolites) and it is inhibited by many of the same drugs that inhibit CYP3A4 (Lee *et al.*, 2010a, 2012). Various derivatives of terfenadine have been identified as selective competitive or metabolism-dependent inhibitors of CYP2J2 (Lafite *et al.*, 2006, 2007). However, given the relatively low levels of intestinal and hepatic CYP2J2 compared with CYP3A4, Lee *et al.* (2010a) concluded that the contribution of CYP2J2 to presystemic clearance of drugs is probably low compared with that of CYP3A4. Furthermore, in contrast to CYP3A4, CYP2J2 is not inducible by CAR/PXR agonists (Neat *et al.*, 2009).

The third notable aspect is that CYP2J2 is the major enzyme in vascular endothelial cells responsible for the epoxidation of arachidonic acid to 4 EETs (5,6-, 8,9-, 11,12-, and 14,15-epoxyeicosatrienoic acid) with a minor contribution from CYP2C8 and CYP2C9 (Liu *et al.*, 2006a; Spiecker and Liao, 2006; Deng *et al.*, 2011; Xu *et al.*, 2011). EETs are endothelin-derived hyperpolarizing factors (EDHFs) (ie, vasodilators) that possess anti-inflammatory properties and protect tissues from ischemic injury. Hydrolysis of EETs by sEH terminates their vasodilatory and anti-inflammatory effects (see the section "Epoxide Hydrolases") (Fretland and Omiecinski, 2000; Morisseau and Hammock, 2005; Imig and Hammock, 2009). The acute vascular inflammatory response to endotoxin in transgenic mice can be attenuated either by overexpressing CYP2J2 (or CYP2C8) or by deleting sEH (sEH knockout mice) (Deng *et al.*, 2011).

The fourth and final notable aspect is that CYP2J2 is overexpressed in many human cancers and cancer-derived cell lines (Chen *et al.*, 2011a; Xu *et al.*, 2011). In human-derived tumor cell lines, overexpression of CYP2J2 (or direct application of EETs) stimulates cell proliferation and inhibits apoptosis, whereas the opposite effects are achieved by inhibiting CYP2J2 with terfenadine-like inhibitors or silencing CYP2J2 expression with antisense oligonucleotides (Chen *et al.*, 2009, 2011a; Xu *et al.*, 2011). Inhibitors of CYP2J2 are under consideration as anticancer agents, but by blocking EET formation in vascular endothelial cells they may potentially predispose to hypertension and CAD (Chen *et al.*, 2011a; Xu *et al.*, 2011), whereas inhibitors of sEH are under consideration as cardioprotective drugs, but by inhibiting the hydrolysis of EETs in cancer cells they may potentially predispose to tumor development and metastatic tumorigenesis (Imig and Hammock, 2009; Wang *et al.*, 2010c).

In addition to its role in arachidonic acid metabolism, CYP2J2 can also catalyze the 25-hydroxylation of vitamin D_1, D_2, and D_3, the first of 2 steps in the formation of the active metabolite $1\alpha,25$-dihydroxyvitamin D (Aiba *et al.*, 2006).

CYP2R1, 2S1, 2U1, and 2W1 CYP2R1, 2S1, 2U1, and 2W1 are 4 of the 8 members of the CYP1 and 2 families that are so well conserved from an evolutionary perspective that they have been given the same names across all mammalian species (the other members are CYP1A1, 1A2, 1B1, and 2E1). These enzymes have been conserved during evolution presumably because they perform an important but in some cases a poorly defined physiological function. The hepatic enzyme CYP2R1 was identified as a vitamin D 25-hydroxylating enzyme in 2004, but other CYP enzymes in human liver microsomes (CYP27A1, CYP2J2, and CYP3A4) have been implicated in catalyzing this first step in the activation of vitamin D to $1\alpha,25$-dihydroxyvitamin D (Cheng *et al.*, 2004; Schuster, 2011). However, based on an analysis of genetic determinants of vitamin D deficiency, 2 groups established that genetic polymorphism of CYP2R1 is associated with circulating 25-hydroxyvitamin D, which provides strong evidence that CYP2R1 is the main enzyme responsible for the critical first step in vitamin D activation (Ahn *et al.*, 2010; Wang *et al.*, 2010b).

CYP2U1 is highly expressed in brain and thymus and to a lesser extent in kidney, lung, and heart (Devos *et al.*, 2010). CYP2U1 metabolizes arachidonic acid, docosahexaenoic acid (DHA), and other long-chain fatty acids. CYP2U1 catalyzes the ω-1 and ω-hydroxylation of arachidonic acid 19- and 20-HETE. The latter metabolite, 20-HETE, is a powerful vasoconstrictor in kidney and brain, which suggests CYP2U1 may play a role in the regulation of blood flow in these tissues. However, several CYP4A and CYP4F enzymes can also catalyze the ω-1 and ω-hydroxylation of arachidonic acid to 19- and 20-HETE. Genetic polymorphisms in CYP2U1 have been identified but they do not appear to alter its function or expression (Devos *et al.*, 2010).

CYP2S1 and CYP2W1 are intriguing enzymes because they are expressed in certain tumors and because they have unusual catalytic properties. CYP2S1 is expressed in several extrahepatic tissues such as lung, trachea, stomach, small intestine, colon, spleen, bladder, and skin (Saarikoski *et al.*, 2005). It is also expressed in psoriatic skin, ovarian cancer, and colorectal tumors where its presence is associated with poor prognosis (Kumarakulasingham *et al.*, 2005). CYP2W1 is expressed in a large number of tumors including colorectal and adrenal tumors, but it does not appear to be expressed to a significant extent in normal (ie, noncancerous) hepatic or extrahepatic tissues (Karlgren *et al.*, 2006). Both enzymes are induced by hypoxia, which may account for their upregulation in tumors. CYP2S1 is also inducible by AhR agonists and joins CYP1A1, CYP1A2, and CYP1B1 as a TCDD-inducible enzyme (Saarikoski *et al.*, 2005). There is some evidence to suggest that, at least in certain cell lines, CYP2W1 is also inducible by AhR ligands (Tan *et al.*, 2011).

There is considerable controversy surrounding the catalytic function of CYP2S1, but this controversy has been resolved (at least in part) by understanding the importance of oxygen tension in the function of CYP2S1. Under aerobic conditions, CYP2S1 can catalyze the oxidative metabolism of several carcinogens (PAHs and

their diol epoxides, aflatoxin B_1, naphthalene, and styrene) but only if these reactions are supported by lipid peroxides or hydrogen peroxide (by the peroxide shunt) and not if the enzyme is supported by $NADPH/O_2$ together with NADPH-cytochrome P450 reductase (Wu *et al.*, 2006; Bui and Hankinson, 2009; Bui *et al.*, 2009). However, under anaerobic conditions, CYP2S1 can efficiently use NAPDH-cytochrome P450 reductase and NADPH to catalyze reductive reactions, as can CYP2W1 (discussed later in this section) (Nishida *et al.*, 2010). These reactions are inhibited by oxygen. The ability of CYP2S1-expressing cells to catalyze the oxidative metabolism of carcinogens is suspect of being due to the presence of intracellular lipid peroxides and hydrogen peroxide that support the peroxide shunt (Bui and Hankinson, 2009; Bui *et al.*, 2009).

CYP2W1 catalyzes the oxidative metabolism of a wide variety of PAHs and their diol epoxides, aflatoxin B_1, and indoline to cytotoxic/mutagenic metabolites (Wu *et al.*, 2006; Gomez *et al.*, 2010). CYP2W1 also hydroxylates and epoxidates a variety of lysophospholipids (Xiao and Guengerich, 2012). It is unusual, however, for being one of the few CYP enzymes to undergo glycosylation, which places CYP2W1 on the lumenal side of the endoplasmic reticulum, which is the wrong side for an interaction with NADPH-cytochrome P450 reductase, which faces the cytoplasmic side (Gomez *et al.*, 2010). Nevertheless, CYP2W1 expressed in cells is functional, either because it uses lipid peroxides/hydrogen peroxide (as does CYP2S1) or because it can use electron donors other than NADPH-cytochrome P450 reductase. As a result of its lumenal orientation in the endoplasmic reticulum (where it becomes glycosylated), approximately 8% of CYP2W1 is expressed on the plasma membrane (Gomez *et al.*, 2010).

Because of their presence and upregulation in hypoxic tumors, CYP2S1 and CYP2W1 have been targeted for their potential to activate anticancer drugs. AQ4N is a prodrug (a di-*N*-oxide) that undergoes *N*-oxide reduction to 4QA, a potent topoisomerase II inhibitor. The reaction is catalyzed by both CYP2S1 and CYP2W1 under anaerobic conditions. The reductive activation by CYP2S1 and CYP2W1 requires NADPH-cytochrome P450 reductase but the reaction is inhibited by oxygen.

Phortress (a prodrug) is representative of a new class of anticancer drugs that are derivatives of 2-(4-amino-3-methylphenyl)-5-fluorobenzothiazole, better known as 5F-203. Phortress is in clinical trials as an anticancer agent. It is an AhR agonist that induces CYP1A1 and induces its own activation to one or more cytotoxic metabolites (Brantley *et al.*, 2004). Like CYP1A1, CYP2W1 also activates 5F-203 (the active metabolite of Phortress) and the related fluorinated benzothiazole GW-610 to cytotoxic metabolites, whereas CYP2S1 converts 5F-203 and GW-610 to inactive metabolites (Tan *et al.*, 2011). 5F-203 and GW-610 are AhR agonists that induce CYP1A1, CYP2S1, and, in certain cell lines, CYP2W1 (Tan *et al.*, 2011).

CYP3A Enzymes In terms of the number of drugs it metabolizes, CYP3A4 is the most important CYP enzyme. Numerous drugs, herbals, and food constituents inhibit or induce CYP3A4, making the enzyme the center of many drug interactions. The high levels in the liver and small intestine (where it works in conjunction with P-glycoprotein [ABCB1] and BCRP [ABCG2]) allow CYP3A4 to play a key role in the presystemic elimination of drugs and other xenobiotics. CYP3A5 is a polymorphically expressed enzyme expressed in liver, small intestine, and kidney. It is unusual inasmuch as the CYP3A5*3 allele that gives rise to a common PM genotype is more prevalent than the wild-type enzyme (the *1 allele) in several ethnic groups such that most Caucasians, Asians, and Mexicans are CYP3A5 PMs. CYP3A5 plays a significant role in the disposition of tacrolimus but few (if any) other drugs. CYP3A7 is expressed in fetal liver. It is also expressed in adult liver and the levels increase with age (Ohtsuki *et al.*, 2012). Like CYP3A5, CYP3A43 plays an important role in the disposition of a select few drugs.

The function and regulation of the CYP3A enzymes is fairly well conserved among mammalian species, with some notable exceptions. For example, rifampin is an inducer of the CYP3A enzymes in humans and rabbits but not rats or mice, whereas the opposite is true of PCN. In adult rats, the levels of CYP3A2 in males are much greater (>10-fold) than in females (Waxman and Holloway, 2009). In humans, men do not have higher levels of CYP3A4 than women; in fact, there is evidence to suggest that the reverse is true—that women have slightly higher levels of CYP3A4 than men, although it should be noted that CYP3A4 levels vary widely in both men and women (Parkinson *et al.*, 2004; Soldin *et al.*, 2011).

CYP3A4 CYP3A4 is abundantly expressed in liver and small intestine, where it biotransforms an extraordinary array of xenobiotics and endobiotics (such as steroid hormones, sterols, and vitamin D), including drugs from numerous therapeutic classes as shown in Table 6-13. CYP3A4 metabolizes over half of all drugs (Gonzalez *et al.*, 2011). A large number of clinically significant drug–drug, drug–herbal, and drug–food interactions involve the inhibition or induction of hepatic and/or intestinal CYP3A4. Three victim drugs whose clearance is mainly determined by CYP3A4, namely, terfenadine (Seldane), cisapride (Propulsid), and astemizole (Hismanal), have been withdrawn from the market because of their potential to cause ventricular arrhythmias (and on rare occasions heart attacks) when their metabolism by CYP3A4 was inhibited by drugs such as ketoconazole and erythromycin (Huang *et al.*, 2008; Zhang *et al.*, 2009). One perpetrator drug, namely, mibefradil (Posicor), has been withdrawn from the market because of its ability to cause marked and prolonged inhibition of CYP3A4 by virtue of its ability to cause MDI of CYP3A4 (which persists after the inhibitory drug is withdrawn and until new enzyme is synthesized) (Foti *et al.*, 2011).

Intestinal CYP3A4 contributes significantly to the presystemic elimination of drugs because drugs in the small intestine are recycled by P-glycoprotein (ABCB1) and BCRP (ABCG2) on the lumenal surface of enterocytes, which delays absorption and increases the opportunity for xenobiotic biotransformation by CYP3A4 (Benet, 2009; Galetin *et al.*, 2010). Furanocoumarins in grapefruit juice inhibit intestinal but not hepatic CYP3A4 and yet grapefruit juice increases systemic exposure to felodipine and other drugs that undergo first-pass metabolism by CYP3A4 (Paine *et al.*, 2006). The impact of the CYP3A4 inhibitor ketoconazole on the disposition of the CYP3A4 substrate midazolam depends on whether midazolam is given orally or intravenously. When midazolam is given intravenously, such that its clearance is dependent only on hepatic metabolism, ketoconazole causes a 3- to 5-fold increase in the AUC. However, when midazolam is given orally, ketoconazole causes a 10- to 15-fold increase in AUC, the difference reflecting the significant role of intestinal metabolism to the presystemic clearance of midazolam. In rats, administration of the general CYP inhibitor 1-aminobenzotriazole (ABT) by the intravenous route (which inhibits only hepatic CYP enzymes) and the oral route (which inhibits both intestinal and hepatic CYP enzymes) can be used to assess the relative role of the intestine and liver to the first-pass metabolism of a drug or other xenobiotic (Strelevitz *et al.*, 2006).

The induction of CYP3A4 is mediated by CAR and PXR, agonists for which include several antibiotics, such as rifampin and rifabutin, several EIAEDs, such as phenobarbital, phenytoin, carbamazepine, and felbamate, and the herbal St. John's wort

(active inducer hyperforin), as shown in Table 6-13 (a more complete list of CYP3A4 inducers is given in the section "Induction of Cytochrome P450—Xenosensors"). The induction of intestinal and hepatic CYP3A4 (and conjugating enzymes, as outlined in the sections "Glucuronidation and Formation of Acyl-CoA Thioesters" and "Sulfonation") by these agents can result in a loss of therapeutic efficacy of oral contraceptive steroids, anti-HIV, and anti-organ rejection drugs. It is an important mechanism of drug–drug and drug–herbal interactions (Huang *et al.*, 2008). Prolonged induction of CYP3A4 also adversely impacts the metabolism of vitamin D, as discussed in the section "Induction of Cytochrome P450—Xenosensors."

CYP3A4 metabolizes more drugs than any other xenobiotic-biotransforming enzyme, which is apparent from the large list of CYP3A4 substrates listed in Table 6-13. Like CYP2C8, CYP3A4 can metabolize large substrates, such as paclitaxel (Taxol®), which is a substrate for both enzymes. The active site of CYP3A4 is sufficiently large to bind 2 drugs simultaneously (Ekroos and Sjögren, 2006), and individual drugs tend to bind to discrete regions, which has several consequences. First, the binding of 2 substrates to CYP3A4 allows for homotropic activation (where a substrate stimulates its own metabolism, as in the case of testosterone and diazepam) and heterotropic activation (where one compound, such as α-naphthoflavone, stimulates the metabolism of another). These effects give rise to non-Michaelis–Menten or atypical enzyme kinetics, which is characteristic of the metabolism of several drugs by CYP3A4 (Atkins, 2005). The binding of one ligand (substrate, inhibitor, or activator) to CYP3A4 can cause conformational changes that increase the size of the active site by 80% or more, which allows additional ligands to bind, possibly in a stacked or side-by-side configuration (Ekroos and Sjögren, 2006). Second, substrates can bind to relatively discrete sites within the active site. Testosterone and midazolam appear to bind to distinct sites (called the steroid and benzodiazepine binding site, respectively); consequently, these 2 prototypical substrates only weakly inhibit each other's metabolism by CYP3A4 (Schrag and Wienkers, 2001; Galetin *et al.*, 2003). As a result of these different substrate-binding sites or orientations, it is possible for a drug to inhibit CYP3A4 in a substrate-dependent manner (Schrag and Wienkers, 2001; Galetin *et al.*, 2003). However, inhibitors that coordinate directly with the heme moiety of CYP3A4 will inhibit the metabolism of all CYP3A4 substrates, as will most metabolism-dependent inhibitors of CYP3A4 (see the section "Inhibition of Cytochrome P450"). Although the active site of CYP3A4 is sufficiently large to bind substrates in apparently discrete sites and to bind 2 molecules simultaneously, it nevertheless often catalyzes reactions with a high degree of regioselectivity and stereoselectivity. In the case of testosterone, for example, CYP3A4 catalyzes hydroxylation at several sites on the β-face of the molecule (eg, 1β-, 2β-, 6β-, and 15β-hydroxylation) but none on the α-face.

More than 25 SNPs have been identified in the CYP3A4 gene, some of which contribute to the large interindividual variation in CYP3A4 activity (Staatz *et al.*, 2010). An individual with low CYP3A4 activity was found to be heterozygous for a null allele (CYP3A4*20) and was characterized as a genetically determined IM (Westlind-Johnsson *et al.*, 2006). The *20 variant was the first null allele identified for CYP3A4. A genetic polymorphism in intron 6 (CYP3A4*22; rs35599367, C > T) affects the expression and, hence, the activity of CYP3A4 such that individuals who are homozygous for the *1 allele (CC carriers) have 1.7 times more CYP3A4 activity than heterozygotes (*1/*22 or CT) and 2.5 times more CYP3A4 activity than individuals homozygous for the *22 allele (TT carriers) (Wang *et al.*, 2011a). Compared with *1/*1 (wild-type) carriers, individuals carrying 1 or 2 of the loss-of-function *22 alleles require lower doses (40%–80% less) of atorvastatin, simvastatin, and lovastatin for optimal lipid control (Wang et al., 2011a). The same genetic polymorphism impacts the disposition of cyclosporine and tacrolimus (Elens et al., 2011a,b). In individuals who lack CYP3A5 (the majority of Caucasians, for example), carriers of the *22/*22 (TT) genotype (low CYP3A4) and *1/*22 (TC) genotype (intermediate CYP3A4) have dose-adjusted concentrations of cyclosporine that are, respectively, 1.5- and 2.2-fold greater than in carriers of the *1/*1 (CC) genotype (high CYP3A4); in the case of tacrolimus they are 1.6- and 4.1-fold greater (Elens et al., 2011b).

The most widely studied CYP3A4 allelic variant (392A > G) is designated CYP3A4*1B. This allelic variant encodes a functional CYP3A4 enzyme that is expressed to the same extent (or perhaps to a slightly greater extent) than the wild-type enzyme (CYP3A4*1). The prevalence of the *1B allele varies from one ethnic group to the next as follows: 2% to 9.6% in Caucasians, 35% to 67% in black Africans, 9.3% to 11% in Hispanics, and 0% in Asians. This polymorphism is linked to the *1 genetic polymorphism in CYP3A5 such that CYP3A5 EMs tend to express the CYP3A4*1B variant, as discussed in the next section.

CYP3A5 CYP3A5 is a polymorphically expressed enzyme whose role in drug metabolism is a matter of considerable debate. The relative role of CYP3A4 versus CYP3A5 in the disposition of drugs is not easy to ascertain from in vitro or in vivo studies. Both enzymes are inducible by the same drugs; both enzymes metabolize the same drugs, and both are inhibited by the same drugs, although the 2 enzymes may differ in the affinity with which they bind to substrates and inhibitors. For example, when evaluated as inhibitors of recombinant human CYP3A enzymes, 14 out of 14 compounds inhibited CYP3A4 more potently than they inhibited CYP3A5 by a factor of 3.9- to 142-fold (Ekins et al., 2003). A large number of drugs are metabolized in vitro by both CYP3A4 and CYP3A5. Some drugs appear to be metabolized by CYP3A4 but not CYP3A5; however, no drug is known to be metabolized by CYP3A5 but not by CYP3A4. Accordingly, there is no in vitro or in vivo probe drug to selectively measure CYP3A5 activity.

Assessing the relative contribution of CYP3A4 and CYP3A5 to the metabolism of drugs is complicated by several factors. For example, studies with human liver microsomes are complicated by conflicting reports on the relative levels of CYP3A5 and CYP3A4; some reports indicate that the levels of CYP3A5 in human liver microsomes are uniformly low (Patki et al., 2003; Westlind-Johnsson et al., 2003), whereas others indicate that, in some liver samples, the levels of CYP3A5 can approach those of CYP3A4 (Lin et al., 2002). Analysis of the specific content of CYP enzymes by mass spectrometry indicates that, on average, CYP3A4 levels are considerably higher (>10 times) than the levels of CYP3A5, as shown in Table 6-12, but in individual livers the levels of CYP3A5 can approach those of CYP3A4 (Ohtsuki et al., 2012). There are also conflicting reports on the relative rate of drug and steroid metabolism by recombinant CYP3A5 and CYP3A4. Early studies with recombinant enzymes generally showed that CYP3A4 is considerably more active than CYP3A5 in the metabolism of a wide range of substrates. However, these studies were criticized later by Huang et al. (2004) on the basis that few of them were conducted with recombinant enzymes in the presence of both NADPH-cytochrome P450 reductase and cytochrome b_5. Under such conditions, the catalytic activity of CYP3A5 can rival or even surpass that of CYP3A4. Of the 8 substrates examined by Huang et al. (2004), midazolam represented the extreme case: in the presence of both

NADPH-cytochrome P450 reductase and cytochrome b_5, recombinant CYP3A5 was 3 times more active than CYP3A4 at catalyzing the 1'-hydroxylation of midazolam, based on estimates of in vitro intrinsic clearance (ie, V_{max}/K_m). However, when this same group evaluated the metabolism of the same 8 substrates in 2 pools ($n = 10$) of human liver microsomes each with the same levels of CYP3A4 but with markedly different levels of CYP3A5 (to mimic the CYP3A5 genetic polymorphism), it was found that CYP3A5 contributed nothing to the metabolism of testosterone, carbamazepine, lidocaine, terfenadine, dextromethorphan, or itraconazole, but contributed 27%, 26%, and 35% to the metabolism of midazolam, erythromycin, and flunitrazepam, respectively.

Huang et al. (2004) demonstrated that, under certain in vitro conditions, the catalytic activity of CYP3A5 can surpass that of CYP3A4 in a substrate-dependent manner, and they further predicted that CYP3A5 contributes to the in vivo metabolism of midazolam, a drug whose disposition is known to be highly dependent on CYP3A-catalyzed metabolism in the liver and small intestine. However, 2 clinical studies have shown that CYP3A5 genotype has no influence on the disposition of midazolam in vivo (Goh et al., 2002; Shih and Huang, 2002). Possible reasons for the discrepancy between the in vitro prediction of the contribution of CYP3A5 to drug metabolism and the in vivo observation have been reviewed by Williams et al. (2003a).

The relative role of CYP3A4 and CYP3A5 in the metabolism of the calcineurin inhibitors cyclosporine and tacrolimus has been studied in vitro (Staatz et al., 2010). These 2 antiorgan rejection drugs have a narrow therapeutic index and factors that affect their disposition are of great clinical interest. Studies with recombinant CYP3A4 and CYP3A5 and studies with human liver microsomes that contain both CYP3A4 and CYP3A5 or that contain only CYP3A4 suggest that the metabolism of cyclosporine is predominantly catalyzed by CYP3A4, whereas the metabolism of tacrolimus is predominantly catalyzed by CYP3A5 when this enzyme is present in human liver microsomes. Estimates of in vitro intrinsic clearance suggest that CYP3A4 contributes 2.3-fold more to the metabolism of cyclosporine than CYP3A5, whereas CYP3A5 contributes 2.0-fold more to the metabolism of tacrolimus than CYP3A4. Although these in vitro studies suggest a role for CYP3A5 in the metabolism of tacrolimus and, to a lesser extent, cyclosporine, it should be remembered that identical studies by Huang et al. (2004) predicted a role for CYP3A5 in the metabolism of midazolam, a prediction that subsequent clinical studies proved to be false.

In the case of CYP3A5, 11 SNPs have been identified, one of which (the *3 allele) causes a complete loss of CYP3A5 expression and, hence, a complete loss of CYP3A5 activity (Staatz et al., 2010). Individuals who are homozygous for the *3 allele can be classified as CYP3A5 PMs; they are genetically deficient in CYP3A5. Individuals with at least 1 wild-type allele (*1/*1 and *1/*3) are considered CYP3A5 EMs.

The *3 allele that gives rise to the CYP3A5 PM genotype is unusual in that it is more prevalent than the wild-type allele (*1), at least in most populations. The prevalence of the wild-type allele (CYP3A5*1) varies from one ethnic group to the next as follows: 5% to 15% in Caucasians, 55% to 73% in black Africans, ~25% in Mexicans, and 15% to 35% in Asians. In Caucasians, Mexicans, and Asians, most individuals are CYP3A5 PMs, which creates an atypical situation with respect to drug metabolism, one that contrasts sharply with genetic polymorphisms in other CYP enzymes where, to take CYP2D6 as an example, most Caucasians are EMs and only a minority (about 7%) are PMs. In the case of a drug that is largely cleared by CYP2D6, for example, the dose that confers therapeutic benefit to the largest number of people is a relatively *high* dose because most individuals are EMs. In the small number of individuals who are PMs (such as the 7% of Caucasians who lack CYP2D6), this dose may be too high; it may cause extended pharmacological effects (as seen with debrisoquine and sparteine) or adverse side effects (as seen with perhexiline). However, in the case of a drug that is primarily cleared by CYP3A5, the dose that confers therapeutic benefit to the largest number of people (in most ethnic populations) is a relatively *low* dose because most individuals are PMs. In the small number of individuals who are EMs (such as the 5%–15% of Caucasians who are CYP3A5 EMs), this dose may be too low; it may fail to confer a therapeutic benefit, which is a major concern for an antiorgan rejection drug such as tacrolimus.

Several studies have shown linkage disequilibrium between the CYP3A4*1B allelic variant and the CYP3A5*1 wild-type allele, as evidenced by the observation that 67% of Caucasians and 100% of black Africans expressing the CYP3A4*1B variant allele also express the CYP3A5*1 wild-type allele (Staatz *et al.*, 2010). There is also evidence of linkage disequilibrium between the P-glycoprotein 3435C > T variant allele and the CYP3A5*3 variant allele. Such linkages underscore the need for caution in attributing an effect to one allelic variant when in fact the effect may be caused by another allele in close linkage.

Numerous studies have been conducted to assess the impact of genetic polymorphisms of CYP3A4 and CYP3A5 (as well as P-glycoprotein [ABCB1]) on the pharmacokinetics of cyclosporine and tacrolimus. These studies were extensively reviewed by Staatz *et al.* (2010), and their findings can be summarized as follows:

1. The CYP3A4*1B allele has no effect on the disposition of cyclosporine.
2. The CYP3A4*1B allele increases the metabolism of tacrolimus, but this association likely reflects its linkage with CYP3A5*1 (the EM genotype).
3. The CYP3A5*3 allele has no consistent effect on the disposition of cyclosporine; some studies suggest the lack of functional CYP3A5 actually increases the rate of metabolism of cyclosporine, but others show no effect or a slight decrease.
4. The CYP3A5*3 allele impairs the metabolism of tacrolimus. The dose-adjusted trough level of tacrolimus in CYP3A5 PMs (*3/*3) is roughly twice that in CYP3A5 EMs (*1/*1 and *1/*3). Accordingly, to achieve the same blood levels, the dose of tacrolimus administered to CYP3A5 EMs is twice that administered to CYP3A5 PMs.

Overall, the results establish that the disposition of tacrolimus, but not cyclosporine, is affected by genetic polymorphisms of CYP3A5. Individuals with 1 or 2 copies of the wild-type *1 allele (EMs) metabolize tacrolimus twice as quickly as individuals with 2 copies of the *3 allele (PMs). In contrast, genetic polymorphisms of CYP3A4 (such as the loss-of-function *22 allele) impact the disposition of both cyclosporine and tacrolimus, as outlined in the section "CYP3A4".

CYP3A7 CYP3A7 is expressed in fetal liver where it may play a role in the activation of drugs and other xenobiotics to teratogenic metabolites (Li *et al.*, 1997; Pang *et al.*, 2012). This is a concern because the laboratory animals used in drug safety testing (rats, mice, dogs, and monkeys) do not express a fetal CYP3A enzyme, raising the possibility that teratogenic metabolites formed by CYP3A7 may go undetected during reproductive toxicity testing in animals. In the fetus CYP3A7 is also expressed in extrahepatic tissue such as intestine, endometrial, placenta, adrenal gland, prostate, and lung in the fetus.

CYP3A7 is also expressed in most adult human livers and the levels increase with age (Ohtsuki *et al.*, 2012). CYP3A7 shows high activity toward endobiotics such as dehydroepiandrosterone (DHEA), estrone, and retinoic acid but low activity toward the majority of drugs metabolized by CYP3A4 (Williams *et al.*, 2002; Pang *et al.*, 2012). The 16α-hydroxylation of DHEA is catalyzed by CYP3A7 but not by CYP3A4. A null allelic variant (CYP3A7*3, caused by a thymidine insertion [4011insT] that prematurely terminates translation) has been identified in a Korean subject (Lee *et al.*, 2010b).

CYP3A43 CYPA43 is expressed in human liver but higher levels are found in brain, testis, and ovary (Westlind *et al.*, 2001). It is upregulated in prostate, breast, and ovarian carcinomas. There are reports of an association between the loss-of-function CYP3A43*3 polymorphism (Pro$_{340}$Ala) and the risk of prostate cancer and the grade and size of benign prostatic hyperplasia but there is no association with breast cancer risk (Justenhoven *et al.*, 2010, and references therein). A genetic polymorphism (an intronic SNP) in CYP3A43 (rs472660) accounts for the long recognized ethnic difference in the metabolism of olanzapine, an antipsychotic drug associated with a high rate of discontinuation due to lack of efficacy or the prevalence of adverse effects. Although the functional consequences of the SNP remain to be determined, 67% of African Americans carry the A variant and have higher rates of olanzapine clearance than Caucasians, only 14% of whom carry the A variant. Among the AA carriers 89% are African Americans (compared with 11% of Caucasians), whereas 95% of GG carriers are Caucasians compared with only 5% of African Americans (Justenhoven *et al.*, 2010).

The expression CYP3A43 in brain impacts the metabolism of the antianxiety drug alprazolam (Agarwal *et al.*, 2008). In the liver, CYP3A4 mainly converts alprazolam to the pharmacologically inactive metabolite 4-hydroxy-alprazolam, whereas in the brain CYP3A43 converts alprazolam to both 4-hydroxy-alprazolam and the pharmacologically active metabolite α-hydroxy-alprazolam.

CYP4 Enzymes Humans express 11 members of the CYP4 family, namely, CYP4A11, 4A22, 4F2, 4F3, 4F8, 4F11, 4F12, 4F22, 4V2, 4X1, and 4Z1. CYP4B1 is often considered a 12th member but the human CYP4B1 gene, in contrast to that in other mammalian species, encodes a protein that does not incorporate heme; hence, human CYP4B1 is catalytically inactive (Baer and Rettie, 2006). For the most part, the CYP4 enzymes can be divided into 2 groups: a large group that is known to metabolize fatty acids and/or eicosanoids and a small group (CYP4A22 and CYP4X1) with no known function (so-called orphan enzymes), as shown in Table 6-10. The first group (CYP4A11, 4F2, 4F3, 4F8, 4F12, 4F22, 4V2, and 4Z1) is part of a larger group of fatty acid– and eicosanoid-metabolizing enzymes, which includes CYP2C8, 2C9, and 2J2. However, these latter enzymes are fatty acid/eicosanoid epoxygenases; they oxidize arachidonic acid to 4 regioisomers of EETs, which are vasodilators. In contrast, the CYP4 enzymes hydroxylate the terminal methyl group (ω-hydroxylation) of fatty acids and eicosanoids. In the case of arachidonic acid, ω-hydroxylation by CYP4 enzymes produces 20-HETE, which is a vasoconstrictor. Hydroxylation of the terminal methyl group (ω-hydroxylation) by CYP4 enzymes is thermodynamically unfavorable compared with hydroxylation of a methylene group (eg, ω-1 hydroxylation), which some CYP4 enzymes also catalyze (Baer and Rettie, 2006; Kalsotra and Strobel, 2006; Johnston *et al.*, 2011). Following ω-hydroxylation, the terminal hydroxymethyl group can be further oxidized to convert the original fatty acid/eicosanoid to a dicarboxylic acid. These dicarboxylic acids are then catabolized by fatty acid β-oxidation (chain shortening) and eliminated.

Unlike other CYP families, the majority of CYP4 enzymes have a covalently attached heme moiety in which the heme forms an ester bond with a conserved glutamic acid residue (Ortiz de Montellano, 2008). However, CYP4F8 and CYP4F12 are exceptions (and CYP4X1 probably also lacks a covalent heme because it lacks the critical glutamate residue). It is noteworthy that CYP4F8 and CYP4F12 preferentially hydroxylate fatty acids in the ω-1 or ω-2 position, which are more energetically favorable than ω-hydroxylation but which do not lead to the formation of dicarboxylic acids (Stark et al., 2005). It has been postulated that the purpose of the covalently bound heme in CYP4 ω-hydroxylases is to help restrict the orientation of the fatty acid in the active site to direct hydroxylation toward the ω-position (Ortiz de Montellano, 2008; Johnston et al., 2011).

Several CYP4 enzymes have been shown to metabolize drugs and other xenobiotics, but in nearly all cases the drugs that are metabolized by the CYP4 enzymes are also metabolized more extensively by CYP1, 2, or 3 family members. A notable exception is the antiparasitic prodrug pafuramidine (DB-289), which is O-demethylated in human liver microsomes by CYP4F2 and CYP4F3 with negligible contribution from CYP enzymes in the 1, 2, or 3 family (Wang et al., 2006). O-Demethylation converts pafuramidine (DB-289) to an amidoxime, which undergoes dehydroxylation by mARC/cytochrome b_5/NADH-cytochrome b_5 reductase as shown for other amidoxmimes in Fig. 6-22. Other examples of CYP4-mediated drug metabolism include the CYP4F12-dependent hydroxylation of ebastine and terfenadine (Cauffiez et al., 2004), and the CYP4F2-dependent ω-hydroxylation of fingolimod (FTY720, Gilenya), an FDA-approved immunosuppressive drug for the treatment of multiple sclerosis (Zollinger et al., 2011).

Another notable exception is CYP4B1, which is expressed in a wide range of extrahepatic tissues and which activates several protoxicants including the pneumotoxins ipomeanol and 3-methyllindole, the bladder carcinogen 2-AF, as well as aromatic amines in animals (Baer and Rettie, 2006). However, CYP4B1 appears to be inactive in humans due to a mutation that interferes with heme incorporation; the mutation is located in the meander region and encodes for a serine residue at amino acid 427. This amino acid is an evolutionarily conserved proline in other species where CYP4B1 is known to be active including cow, mouse, rat, rabbit, and dog. Introducing a $Pro_{427}Ser$ mutation into rabbit CYP4B1 interferes with heme incorporation, and reverting Ser_{427} to the conserved proline in the human CYP4B1 gene yields a functional enzyme that incorporates heme (Zheng et al., 1998). The $Pro_{427}Ser$ mutation likely explains why attempts to express human CYP4B1 in a recombinant system have yielded inactive enzyme lacking heme.

CYP4F2 has been implicated in the clearance of both vitamins K and E (Parker et al., 2004; Sontag and Parker, 2007; McDonald et al., 2009). Both of these compounds have phytyl-derived, long alkyl chains attached to a polar moiety (which makes them roughly structurally analogous to fatty acids). Urinary metabolites of vitamins K and E that lack the phytyl chain likely arise from CYP4F2-catalyzed ω-hydroxylation followed by further oxidation to the carboxylic acid with subsequent chain shortening by β-oxidation. A genetic polymorphism in CYP4F2 ($Val_{433}Met$) that impairs the metabolism of vitamin K_1 is clinically relevant because individuals with this loss-of-function allelic variant require a higher warfarin dose to compete with the increased levels of the vitamin K_1 in the liver (McDonald et al., 2009; Lurie et al., 2010).

Genetic defects in CYP4V2 and CYP4F22 have been linked to diseases with symptoms possibly caused by disruption of fatty acid homeostasis and/or disruption of eicosanoid signaling. Mutations in CYP4V2 are linked to Bietti crystalline corneoretinal dystrophy (Li et al., 2004), a late-onset eye disease characterized by night blindness and eventually blindness caused by crystalline deposits in the retinal epithelium and cornea. Mutations in CYP4F22 are associated with autosomal recessive congenital ichthyosis (Lefèvre et al., 2006), which is characterized by large dark scales on the skin without exfoliative dermatitis. CYP4F22 is likely involved in the metabolism of hepoxillins or trioxillins, signaling molecules that are part of the arachidonic acid cascade (Kelly et al., 2011).

Activation of Xenobiotics by Cytochrome P450

Biotransformation by CYP does not always lead to detoxication, and several examples have been given previously where the toxicity or tumorigenicity of a chemical depends on its activation by CYP. The role of individual human CYP enzymes in the activation of selected procarcinogens and protoxicants is summarized in Table 6-14 (adapted from Guengerich, 1991). A variety of CYP-dependent reactions are involved in the activation of the chemicals listed in Table 6-14. The conversion of PAHs to tumor-forming metabolites involves the formation of bay-region diol epoxides, as shown in Fig. 6-10, for the conversion of B[a]P to B[a]P 7,8-dihydrodiol-9,10-epoxide. Epoxidation generates hepatotoxic metabolites of chlorobenzene and coumarin (Fig. 6-43), and generates a hepatotumorigenic metabolite of aflatoxin B1 (Fig. 6-34).

The initial step in the conversion of aromatic amines and amides to tumor-forming metabolites involves N-hydroxylation, as shown for 2-amino-6-nitrobenzylalcohol (Fig. 6-12), 2-AF, and 2-AAF (Fig. 6-61). The aromatic amides phenacetin, a discontinued drug, undergoes N-hydroxylation by CYP (and peroxidases) to form a hydroxamic acid. Under acidic conditions (such as in urine), the hydroxamic acid can lose water to form reactive nitrenium ion, which is thought to contribute to the renal toxicity of phenacetin (Testa and Krämer, 2008, 2010). In the case of acetaminophen, activation to hepatotoxic metabolite involves dehydrogenation to NAPQI, as shown in Fig. 6-35. A similar reaction converts BHT to a toxic quinone methide, as shown in Fig. 6-36. The myelotoxicity of benzene depends on its conversion to phenol and hydroquinone (Fig. 6-32). The toxicity of several OP insecticides involves oxidative group transfer to the corresponding organophosphate, as shown for the conversion of parathion to paraoxon in Figs. 6-46 and 6-47. The hepatotoxicity of carbon tetrachloride involves reductive dechlorination to a trichloromethyl free radical, which binds to protein and initiates lipid peroxidation, as shown in Fig. 6-18. The hepatotoxicity and nephrotoxicity of chloroform involves oxidative dechlorination to phosgene (Fig. 6-18). Both oxidative and reductive dehalogenation play a role in the activation of halothane, although hepatotoxicity in rats is more dependent on reductive dehalogenation, whereas the immune hepatitis in humans is largely a consequence of oxidative dehalogenation, which leads to the formation of neoantigens (Pohl et al., 1989). Formation of neoantigens (by covalent binding to CYP2C9) is also the mechanism by which the uricosuric diuretic drug, tienilic acid, causes immune hepatitis (Lecoeur et al., 1994).

Some of the chemicals listed in Table 6-14 are activated to toxic or tumorigenic metabolites by mechanisms not mentioned previously. For example, N-nitrosodimethylamine, which is representative of a large class of tumorigenic nitrosamines, is activated to an alkylating electrophile by N-demethylation, as shown in Fig. 6-50. The activation of ethyl carbamate (urethane) involves 2 sequential reactions catalyzed by CYP (CYP2E1): dehydrogenation to vinyl carbamate followed by epoxidation, as shown in Fig. 6-50. CYP2E1 is one of several CYP enzymes that can catalyze the epoxidation of tetrachloroethylene. The rearrangement of this epoxide to a carbonyl is accompanied by migration of chlorine, which produces the highly reactive metabolite, trichloroacetyl chloride, as shown in Fig. 6-50. The toxic pyrrolizidine alkaloids, such as senecionine, are cyclic arylamines that are dehydrogenated by CYP (CYP3A4) to the corresponding pyrroles. Pyrroles themselves are nucleophiles, but electrophiles are generated through the loss of substituents on the pyrrolizidine nucleus, as shown in Fig. 6-50. Cyclophosphamide and ifosfamide are examples of chemicals designed to be activated to toxic electrophiles for the treatment of malignant tumors and other proliferative diseases. These drugs are nitrogen mustards, which have a tendency to undergo intramolecular nucleophilic displacement to form an electrophilic aziridinium species. In the case of cyclophosphamide and ifosfamide, the nitrogen mustard is stabilized by the presence of a phosphoryl oxygen, which delocalizes the lone pair of nitrogen electrons required for intramolecular nucleophilic displacement. For this reason, formation of an electrophilic aziridinium species requires hydroxylation by CYP, as shown in Fig. 6-50 for cyclophosphamide. Hydroxylation of the carbon atom next to the ring nitrogen leads spontaneously to ring opening and elimination of acrolein. In the resultant phosphoramide mustard, delocalization of the lone pair of nitrogen electrons to the phosphoryl oxygen is now disfavored by the presence of the lone pair of electrons on the oxygen anion; hence, the phosphoramide undergoes an intramolecular nucleophilic elimination to generate an electrophilic aziridinium species. This reaction is catalyzed by CYP2B6 and CYP3A4. Activation of cyclophosphamide by CYP enzymes in the skin would generate a cytotoxic metabolite at the base of hair follicles, which may be the reason why hair loss is one of the side effects of cyclophosphamide treatment.

Many of the chemicals listed in Table 6-14 are also detoxified by CYP by biotransformation to less toxic metabolites. In some cases, the same CYP enzyme catalyzes both activation and detoxication reactions. For example, CYP3A4 activates aflatoxin B_1 to the hepatotoxic and tumorigenic 8,9-epoxide, but it also detoxifies aflatoxin B_1 by 3-hydroxylation to aflatoxin Q_1. Similarly, CYP3A4 activates senecionine by converting this pyrrolizidine alkaloid to the corresponding pyrrole, but it also detoxifies senecionine through formation of an N-oxide (a reaction mainly catalyzed by FMO3). Epoxidation of trichloroethylene by CYP2E1 is both an activation and detoxication pathway, as shown in Fig. 6-50. Rearrangement of trichloroethylene epoxide can be accompanied by migration of chlorine, which produces chloral (trichloroacetaldehyde), or hydrogen, which produces dichloroacetylchloride. Chloral is much less toxic than dichloroacetylchloride; hence, migration of the chlorine during epoxide rearrangement is a detoxication reaction, whereas migration of the hydrogen is an activation reaction. These few examples serve to underscore the complexity of factors that determine the balance between xenobiotic activation and detoxication.

Structural alerts (functional groups) for the bioactivation of xenobiotics to reactive metabolites by CYP include the following: acetylenes, activated aromatics, 3-alkly indoles, anilines, cyclopropylamines, formamides, furans, hydrazines, polyaromatics, pyrroles, nitro aromatics, sulfonylureas, thiazolidinones, thioamides, thiophenes, and thioureas (Walsh and Miwa, 2011). As outlined more fully in Point 12 (see the section "Introduction"), the prominence of cytochrome P450 in converting xenobiotics to reactive and potentially harmful metabolites is illustrated by the widespread use of liver microsomes in the in vitro safety evaluation of drug candidates. Liver microsomes are used in (1) the Ames bacterial mutagenicity assay, (2) an assessment of the formation of reactive metabolites that bind covalently to protein or GSH (or a related nucleophile such as N-acetylcysteine [NAC]), and (3) an assessment of a drug candidate's potential to cause irreversible inhibition of the

major drug-metabolizing CYP enzymes. The latter application is the topic of the next section.

Inhibition of Cytochrome P450

Inhibition of CYP is a major cause of drug–drug interactions (and occasionally the withdrawal of regulatory approval), as illustrated by the examples cited earlier (terfenadine, cisapride, astemizole, cerivastatin, and mibefradil) in the sections "CYP3A4" and "CYP2C8" (Ogilvie et al., 2008). The magnitude of the drug–drug interaction depends on the degree of CYP inhibition by the perpetrator drug and the fractional metabolism (fm) of the victim drug by the affected enzyme. This principle is explained in Point 23 in the section "Introduction." In summary, complete inhibition of a CYP enzyme that contributed 50% to the clearance of Drug A (fm = 0.5) and 90% to the clearance of Drug B (fm = 0.9) would cause a 2-fold increase in systemic exposure (plasma AUC) to Drug A, and a 10-fold increase in exposure to Drug B. The concept of "maximum exposure," where 2 perpetrators inhibit 2 parallel pathways of clearance and cause dramatic increases in systemic exposure to the victim drug, was explained in Point 24 in the section "Introduction." Maximum exposure often occurs when a genetic polymorphism affects one pathway of clearance and a perpetrator drug inhibits a second, parallel pathway of clearance, as illustrated in Point 24 for the weak effect (~2-fold) of the CYP3A4 inhibitor ritonavir on voriconazole exposure in CYP2C19 EMs (individuals in whom CYP3A4 plays a minor role in voriconazole metabolism) and the dramatic (26-fold) increase in voriconazole AUC in CYP2C19 PMs (individuals who lack CYP2C19 and in whom CYP3A4 plays the major role in voriconazole clearance) (Collins et al., 2006; Ogilvie and Parkinson, in press). A single drug can inhibit multiple CYP enzymes and thereby inhibit 2 or more parallel pathways of drug clearance. An exceptional case is the interaction between fluvoamine and ramelteon. The 3 major enzymes involved in the clearance of ramelteon are CYP1A2, CYP2C19, and CYP3A4, all of which are inhibited by flovaxamine. The product label for ramelteon (Rozerem, Takeda Pharmaceuticals, Osaka, Japan) describes a drug–drug interaction study in which fluvoxamine caused a 190-fold increase in the plasma AUC of ramelteon, which is the largest drug interaction reported. Interestingly, the magnitude of the interaction surpasses that predicted from in vitro studies (Obach and Ryder, 2010).

Inhibitory drug interactions generally fall into 2 categories: direct inhibition (which can be competitive, noncompetitive, and uncompetitive) and metaboliism-dependent inhibition (MDI, which can be irreversible or quasi-irreversible). Direct inhibition can be subdivided into 2 types. The first involves competition between 2 drugs that are metabolized by the same CYP enzyme. The second type of direct inhibition is when the inhibitor is not a substrate for the affected CYP enzyme. The inhibition of dextromethorphan biotransformation by quinidine is a good example of this type of drug interaction. Dextromethorphan is O-demethylated by CYP2D6, and the clearance of dextromethorphan is impaired in individuals lacking this polymorphically expressed enzyme. The clearance of dextromethorphan is similarly impaired when this antitussive drug is taken with quinidine, a potent inhibitor of CYP2D6. However, quinidine is not biotransformed by CYP2D6, even though it binds to this enzyme with high affinity (K_i ~100 nM). Quinidine is actually biotransformed by CYP3A4, and is a weak competitive inhibitor of this enzyme (K_i >100 μM), although its effects are highly dependent on the CYP3A4 substrate employed.

As the name implies, MDI occurs when CYP converts a xenobiotic to a metabolite that is a more potent inhibitor than the parent compound. In some cases, the metabolite, once formed, functions as a potent, reversible inhibitor, as occurs when fluoxetine is

N-demethylated to norfluoxetine. The contribution of norfluoxetine to the inhibitory effects of fluoxetine illustrates a common finding that drug metabolites often function as reversible inhibitors of CYP and thereby contribute significantly to drug–drug interactions (Isoherranen *et al.*, 2009; Yeung *et al.*, 2011). In other cases, however, the metabolite functions as an irreversible inhibitor (which occurs when the metabolite alkylates the heme or apoprotein moiety of CYP) or a quasi-irreversible inhibitor (which occurs when the metabolite coordinates tightly but not covalently with the ferrous heme to form what is known as a metabolite-inhibitory complex [MIC]). Metabolism-dependent inhibitors that cause irreversible inactivation of CYP include 8-methoxypsoralen (CYP2A6), clopidogrel (CYP2B6), tienilic acid (CYP2C9), and ticlopidine (CYP2C19), all of which contain a furan or thiophene that is activated by CYP to a reactive metabolite that inactivates the enzyme (suicide inactivation). Metabolism-dependent inhibitors that form metabolite inhibitory complexes and cause quasi-irreversible inhibition include the CYP3A4 inhibitor troleandomycin, which contains a tertiary amine $(R\text{-}N(CH_3)_2)$ that is converted by several successive oxidative reactions to a putative nitroso metabolite $(R\text{-}N{=}O)$ that coordinately binds to the ferrous heme iron. This interaction resembles the binding of CO to the ferrous heme iron, and indeed compounds that form inhibitory metabolite complexes with CYP can be detected spectrophotometrically based on an absorbance peak at around 455 nm (which is similar to the peak at ~450 nm when CO binds to CYP). The chemical structures commonly associated with MDI of CYP are shown in Table 6-15.

In some cases, MDI involves metabolism by enzymes other than the affected CYP enzyme, which can give rise to system-dependent inhibition in in vitro studies (whereby the results obtained in human liver microsomes or recombinant enzymes do not predict as well as studies performed with human hepatocytes). For example, the inhibition of CYP2C8 by gemfibrozil requires the formation of gemfibrozil glucuronide by UGT, after which gemfibrozil glucuronide functions as a metabolism-dependent inhibitor of CYP2C8 (Ogilvie *et al.*, 2006). Likewise, the reduction of bupropion to erythrohydrobupropion and threohydrobupropion is largely responsible for its ability to cause clinically relevant inhibition of CYP2D6 (Reese *et al.*, 2008). Experiments with human liver microsomes and recombinant CYP enzymes underpredict the inhibition of CYP2C8 by gemfibrozil and the inhibition of CYP2D6 by bupropion, whereas hepatocytes do not because they support the necessary glucuronidation and reduction pathways, respectively (Parkinson *et al.*, 2010). Conversely, experiments with human liver microsomes and recombinant CYP enzymes overpredict the inhibition of CYP3A4 by ezetimibe. In the clinic (and in hepatocytes) rapid glucuronidation of ezetimibe protects CYP3A4 from MDI by ezetimibe (Parkinson *et al.*, 2010). Other issues that can arise during the in vitro evaluation of drug candidates as metabolism-dependent inhibitors of CYP enzymes are described by Parkinson *et al.* (2011). An extensive database on drug–drug interactions is available at the University of Washington Metabolism and Transport Drug Interaction Database (http://www.druginteractioninfo.org).

There are cases where inhibition of CYP has proved advantageous, as in the case of certain combinations of anti-HIV drugs. For example, by inhibiting CYP3A4, the HIV protease inhibitor ritonavir improves the pharmacokinetic profile of saquinavir and lopinavir, protease inhibitors that are otherwise cleared so rapidly by CYP3A4 that blood levels easily fall below therapeutically effective concentrations.

Induction of Cytochrome P450—Xenosensors The induction (upregulation) of xenobiotic-biotransforming enzymes and transporters is a receptor-mediated, adaptive process that augments xenobiotic elimination during periods of high xenobiotic exposure. It is not a toxicological or pathological response, but enzyme induction is often associated with liver enlargement (due to both hepatocellular hypertrophy and hyperplasia), and it may be associated with toxicological and pharmacological consequences, especially for the safety evaluation of drug candidates in laboratory animals and for clinical practice in humans. In animals and humans, enzyme induction may be associated with pharmacokinetic tolerance, whereby the xenobiotic induces its own elimination. Carbamazepine is one of many EIAEDs that induced its own metabolism. Because of autoinduction it is often necessary to increase the dose of carbamazepine at a rate of 200 mg every 1 to 2 weeks to achieve the desired seizure threshold. During safety testing in animals, autoinduction may require increasing dosages of drug candidate to achieve the same degree of systemic exposure. In rodents, lifetime exposure to enzyme inducers may be associated with liver or thyroid tumor formation, as discussed later in this section. In humans, enzyme induction may also be associated with pharmacokinetic tolerance (autoinduction). Long-term treatment of humans with enzyme inducers can cause osteomalacia due to increased inactivation of $1,25\text{-}(OH)_2\text{-}D_3$, the active metabolite of vitamin D (discussed later in this section), but it is not associated with liver or thyroid tumor formation. However, in humans, enzyme induction by one drug (the perpetrator) can augment the clearance of a concomitantly administered drug (the victim), which is a cause of drug–drug interactions.

As an underlying cause of serious adverse events, enzyme induction is generally less important than enzyme inhibition because the latter can cause a rapid and profound increase in blood levels of a victim drug, which can cause an exaggerated pharmacological or toxicological effect. In contrast, enzyme induction lowers blood levels, which usually does not cause an exaggerated pharmacological or toxicological response to the drug. However, enzyme induction may be associated with a loss of therapeutic effectiveness, which is a particular concern when it compromises the therapeutic effectiveness of drugs that have a narrow therapeutic index and are being used to treat a life-threatening illness, such as anti-HIV drugs, antirejection drugs (such as cyclosporine and tacrolimus), and oral anticoagulants (such as warfarin), or when it is used with drugs that exhibit a quantal (all-or-nothing) dose–response relationship, such as oral contraceptive steroids (which either block or do not block ovulation and thereby provide or do not provide protection against pregnancy).

CYP induction does not necessarily enhance the biotransformation of the inducer, in which case the induction is said to be gratuitous. Consequently, lack of autoinduction cannot be taken as evidence that a xenobiotic does not cause enzyme induction. For example, in humans, omeprazole induces CYP1A2, even though the disposition of this acid-suppressing drug is largely determined by CYP2C19 and, to a lesser extent, CYP3A4. Some of the most effective inducers of CYP are polyhalogenated aromatic hydrocarbons (PHAHs), such as polychlorinated derivatives of dibenzo-*p*-dioxin (PCDDs), dibenzofurans (PCDFs), azobenzenes and azoxybenzenes, biphenyl (PCBs), and naphthalene. In general, highly chlorinated compounds are resistant to biotransformation and cause a prolonged induction of CYP and other enzymes. Some inducers are potent direct-acting or metabolism-dependent inhibitors such that they mask the activity of one or more of the enzymes they induce. Such dual-acting xenobiotics include macrolide antibiotics (eg, erythromycin and troleandomycin), methylenedioxy-containing compounds (eg, tadalafil [Cialis®], safrole, isosafrole), and imidazole antimycotics (eg, clotrimazole, ketoconazole, and

Table 6-15

Structures Associated With Metabolism-Dependent Inhibition of Cytochrome P450 (CYP) Enzymes

CHEMICAL GROUPS (EXAMPLES)	STRUCTURES
Terminal (ω) and ω-1 acetylenes (gestodene)	
Furans and thiophenes (8-methoxypsoralen and tienilic acid)	
Epoxides (R-bergamottin-6′,7′-epoxide)	
Dichloroethylenes and trichloroethylenes (1,2,-dichloroethylene and trichloroethylene)	
Secondary amines (fluoxetine)	
Benzodioxoles (paroxetine)	
Isothiocyanates (phenethyl isothiocyanate)	
Thioamides (methimazole)	
Dithiocarbamates (disulfiram)	
Conjugated structures (rhapontigenin)	
Terminal alkenes (tiamulin)	
4-Alkyl-1,4-dihydropyridines (3,5-diethoxycarbonyl-1, 4-dihydro-2,6-dimethyl-4-ethylpyridine [DDEP])	
2-Alkyl-1H-imidazoles (furafylline)	

Data from Fontana et al. (2005) and Testa and Krämer (2008, 2010).

miconazole). In the case of dual-acting drugs (such as the induction/inhibition of CYP3A4 by ritonavir and several other HIV protease inhibitors, and the induction/inhibition of CYP2E1 by isoniazid), the initial effect—and often the effect observed during the period of drug treatment—is CYP inhibition, with induction becoming evident after prolonged drug treatment or following drug cessation. However, when ritonavir induces CYP3A4, for example, it also induces several other CYP enzymes, as well as conjugating enzymes and transporters that are regulated by CAR/PXR. Ritonavir does not inhibit all of the enzymes it induces. For

example, in the presence of 2 to 20 μM ritonavir for 72 hours, CYP2B6 activity is increased by 4- to 6-fold in primary cultures of human hepatocytes, conditions that cause CYP3A4 inhibition (Faucette *et al.*, 2004). Some dual-acting xenobiotics, such as allyl-isopropylacetamide, cause certain types of porphyria (a disorder of heme synthesis) because they induce CYP enzymes and destroy the CYP heme moiety, which greatly increases the demand for heme synthesis (discussed later in this section).

In general, CYP induction is mediated by four ligand-activated receptors, namely, AhR, CAR, PXR, and PPARα, as summarized in

Table 6-16

Receptors Mediating the Induction (or Suppression) of Cytochrome P450 Enzymes and Other Xenobiotic-Biotransforming Enzymes and Transporters

NUCLEAR RECEPTOR	RESPONSE ELEMENT(S)	RECEPTOR ACTIVATORS	REGULATED GENES[*]
AhR	XRE	PAHs, TCDD (other PHAHs), β-naphthoflavone, indigoids, tryptophan metabolites, omeprazole, lansoprazole	CYP1A1, 1A2, 1B1, 2S1, UGT1A1, UGT1A6, AKR1A1, AKR1C1-4
CAR	DR-3 DR-4 ER-6	Phenobarbital, phenytoin, carbamazepine, CITCO (human), TCPOBOP (mouse), clotrimazole, Yin Zhi Wuang (many PXR agonists are also CAR agonists, and vice versa)	CYP2A6, 2B6, 2C8, 2C9, 2C19, 3A4, UGT1A1, SULT1A1, AKR1D1, ALAS, MRP2, MRP3, MRP4
PXR	DR-3 DR-4 ER-6 ER-8	Amprenavir, avasimibe, bosentan, bile acids, carbamazepine, clindamycin, clotrimazole, cortisol, cyproterone acetate, dicloxacillin, efavirenz, etoposide, dexamethasone, griseofulvin, guggulsterone, hyperforin (SJW), indinavir, lovastatin, mifepristone, nafcillin, nelfinavir, nifedipine, omeprazole, paclitaxel, PCBs, phenobarbital, phthalate monoesters, 5β-pregnane-3,20-dione, rifabutin, rifampin, ritonavir, saquinavir, simvastatin, spironolactone, sulfinpyrazole, TAO, tetracycline, topotecan, transnanoclor, troglitazone, verapamil, vitamin E, vitamin K_2	CYP2A6, 2B6, 2C8, 2C9, 2C19, 3A4, 3A7, 4F12, 7A1↓, CES2, SULT2A1, UGT1A1, 1A3, 1A4, 1A6, GSTA1, AKR1D1, PAPSS2, ALAS, MDR1, MRP2, AhR
PPARα	DR-1	Fibrates, WY-14643, perfluorodecanoic acid	CYP4A, UGT1A9, 2B4
Nrf2	ARE	β-Naphthoflavone, oltipraz, phenolic antioxidants (eg, BHA and BHT), phenylisothiocyanate, and various glutathione depletors (diethyl maleate, phorone)	NQO1, mEH, AKR7A, UGTs, GSTA1, γ-GCL, MRP1
GR	GRE	Glucocorticoids (eg, dexamethasone)	CYP2C9, 2B6, 3A4, 3A5, CAR, PXR
FXR	IR-1	Bile acids, GW4064, AGN29, AGN31	BSEP, I-BABP, MDR3, UGT2B4, SULT2A1, OATP1B3, PPARα, SHP
LXRα	DR-4	GW3965, T0901317, paxiline, F_3methylAA,[†] acetylpodocarpic dimer (APD)	LRH1, SHP, CYP7A, LXRα, CYP3A4 ↓↓, 2B6 ↓
VDR	DR-3 ER-6 IR-0	1α,25-Dihydroxyvitamin D_3, lithocholate	CYP2B6, 2C9, 3A4, SULT2A1
HNF1α	‡		OATP1B1, OATP1B3, CYP7A1, UGT1A6, 1A8, 1A9, 1A10, HNF4α, PXR, kidney-specific expression of OAT1, OAT3, URAT1
HNF4α	DR		CYP2A6, 2B6, 2C9, 2D6, 3A4, DD4, MDR1, PXR, CAR, FXR, PPARα, HNF1α
LRH-1	DR-4		CYP7A, ASBT
SHP	None		Targets of PPARα ↓, AhR ↓, PXR ↓, CAR ↓, LRH-1 ↓, HNF4α ↓, LXRα ↓, GR ↓

Data from Tirona and Kim (2005), Penning and Drury (2007), and Jin et al. (2011).
[*]*A downward arrow indicates downregulation (suppression). All others are upregulated (induced).*
[†]*[3-Chloro-4-(3-(7-propyl-3-trifluoromethyl-6-(4,5)-isoxazolyl)propylthio)-phenylacetic acid].*
[‡]*The HNF1α consensus sequence is GTTTAATNATTAAC.*

Table 6-16 (adapted from Tirona and Kim, 2005). These so-called xenosensors resemble other nuclear receptors, such as steroid and TH receptors, which has consequences for receptor interactions (cross-talk among xenosensors and cross-talk between xenosensors and other nuclear receptors), the role that some xenosensors play in responding to endobiotics and regulating their metabolism (eg, bilirubin, bile acids, fatty acids, and 1,25-$(OH)_2$-D_3), and the role that some nuclear receptors (such as farnesoid X receptor [FXR], VDR, small heterodimer partner-1 [SHP], NF-κB) play in inducing or suppressing the expression of xenobiotic-biotransforming enzymes and transporters, as discussed later in this section. Details of the nomenclature system of this superfamily of DNA-binding transcriptional factors have been reviewed (Germain *et al.*, 2006). Xenosensors have a ligand-binding domain (LBD) and a highly conserved cysteine-rich DNA-binding domain (DBD). In general, CYP induction involves the following steps (with steps 2 and 3 reversed in the case of AhR): (1) binding of ligand (xenobiotic) to the receptor, which triggers conformational changes that promote its dissociation from accessory proteins (such as corepressors, chaperones, and cytoplasm retention proteins) and promote its association with coactivators; (2) dimerization of the ligand-bound receptor with a partner protein to form a DNA-binding heterodimer (which is analogous to the two halves of a clothes peg coming together to form a functional unit); (3) translocation of the functional receptor heterodimer from the cytoplasm to the nucleus; (4) binding of the functional receptor heterodimer to discrete regions of DNA (response elements) that are typically located in the 5′-promoter region of the gene (which is analogous to a clothes peg being fastened to a clothes line); (5) recruitment of other transcription factors and coactivators (such as histone and RNA methyltransferases, histone and chromatin deacetylases, and histone remodeling helicases) and RNA polymerase to form a transcription complex; and (6) gene transcription, which leads to increased levels of CYP mRNA and protein (as well as other xenobiotic-biotransforming enzymes and transporters). As is the case with all nuclear receptors, the details of the process of activating a xenosensor to its transcriptionally active form are complex and multifaceted. Over 200 coactivators/coregulators of nuclear receptor function have been identified (Lonard and O'Malley, 2006), some of which are known to play a critical but undefined role in xenosensor activation.

As shown in Table 6-16, the major ligand-activated receptors mediating CYP induction are (1) AhR, which partners with aryl hydrocarbon receptor nuclear translocator (ARNT) to induce CYP1A1, 1A2, 1B1, and 2S1; (2) CAR (aka the constitutively active receptor), which partners with RXRα (the retinoid X receptor, which binds 9-cis-retinoic acid) to induce several members of the CYP2A, 2B, 2C, and 3A subfamilies; (3) PXR (aka SXR, the steroid X receptor) that, like CAR, partners with RXRα and induces several members of the CYP2A, 2B, 2C, and 3A subfamilies; and (4) PPARα, which partners with RXRα and induces CYP4A enzymes. The response elements (aka consensus sequences) to which xenosensors bind are generally a pair of hexanucleotide sequences in a direct repeat (DR), inverted repeated (IR), or everted repeat (ER) orientation, separated by a 0 to 8 nucleotide spacer. As shown in Tables 6-16 and 6-17, activation of a xenosensor leads to the induction of multiple enzymes, which is called a pleiotypic response. However, in terms of fold induction, CYP enzymes tend to be the most inducible and, consequently, the most studied enzymes (although activation of PPARα has a more pronounced effect on the expression of peroxisomal enzymes involved in fatty acid oxidation). Like induction of CYP enzymes, induction of conjugating and other non-CYP enzymes is an important mechanism of drug–drug and drug–endobiotic interactions. For example, induction of various conjugating enzymes (both SULT and UGT enzymes) plays a key role in the metabolism of oral contraceptive steroids in humans, which is associated with a loss of therapeutic effect. In rodents induction of conjugating enzymes is responsible for increased metabolism of thyroid hormone, which is associated with thyroid follicular cell hyperplasia and tumor formation. As shown in Table 6-16, AhR, CAR, PXR, and PPARα are not the only receptors that regulate CYP expression in response to xenobiotics (or certain endobiotics). Nuclear factor erythroid 2-related factor 2 (Nrf2) plays a key role in regulating the induction of several enzymes in response to electrophilic metabolites, oxidative stress, or GSH depletion, as discussed previously (see Point 9 in the section "Introduction" and sections "Epoxide Hydrolases" and "Quinone Reduction—NQO1 and NQO2"). The enzymes regulated by Nrf2

include several conjugating but few CYP enzymes (notable exceptions are CYP2C55 and 2U1 in mice), whereas those regulated by AhR, CAR, PXR, and PPARα include both conjugating and CYP enzymes. A role for HNF1α in the kidney-specific expression of drug transporters, OAT1, OAT3, and URAT1, has been documented (Jin et al., 2011). Some of the other receptors listed in Table 6-16 are discussed later in this section. CYP induction can also involve mechanisms other than receptor-mediated transcriptional activation. Increased translation of mRNA is the mechanism by which several xenobiotics increase the levels of CYP2E1, and increased translational efficiency and protein stabilization play important roles in the induction of several CYP enzymes including CYP1A2, 2E1, and 3A enzymes (Gonzalez, 2007).

It might be assumed that xenobiotics can be divided into four categories of inducers represented by the xenosensors AhR, CAR, PXR, and PPARα. This is largely true of rats where 3-methylcholanthrene, phenobarbital, PCN, and clofibric acid are prototypical inducers of CYP1A, 2B, 3A, and 4A by virtue of their ability to activate AhR, CAR, PXR, and PPARα, respectively. In fact, rats have 5 classes of inducible CYP enzymes with the fifth class represented by CYP2E1, which is inducible by the prototypical inducer isoniazid. However, the situation in other species (including rats) on a xenobiotic-by-xenobiotic basis) is not so straightforward because (1) CAR and PXR have similar but not identical LBDs such that ligands that activate one receptor activate the other and vice versa (although they can do so with markedly different affinities) and (2) CAR and PXR have similar but not identical DBDs such that, once activated, CAR and PXR bind to some of the same response elements and induce the same enzymes. It was once thought that CYP2B induction was mediated only by CAR, and that CYP3A induction was mediated only by PXR. However, the PXR agonist dexamethasone can maximally induce both CYP2B10 and CYP3A11 in wild-type and CAR knockout mice, indicating that PXR can maximally induce both CYP2B and 3A enzymes in mice. Similarly, the CAR activator phenobarbital can maximally induce CYP2B10 and induce CYP3A11 (albeit submaximally) in wild-type and PXR knockout mice, indicating that CAR can also induce both CYP2B and 3A enzymes (Kodama and Negishi, 2006). The same is true of humans: PXR can maximally induce both CYP2B6 and CYP3A4, whereas CAR can maximally induce CYP2B6 and induce CYP3A4 submaximally due to its relatively weaker binding and functional activation of the CYP3A4 ER6 (Faucette et al., 2006). Furthermore, there are species and strain differences in the LBDs, the DBDs, and the DNA-response elements that give rise to species and strain differences in enzyme induction, and even interindividual differences in humans. Some species differences in enzyme induction reflect differences in the catalytic activity of CYP enzymes. For example, although 7-methoxyresorufin and 7-ethoxyresorufin are useful substrates to study CYP1A enzyme induction in all mammalian species, 7-pentoxyresorufin is useful for studying CYP2B only in mouse and rat (not hamster, dog, monkey, or humans). However, many species, strain, and individual differences in enzyme induction reflect differences in xenosensor function, as discussed below (this section). The following descriptions of the individual xenosensors focus largely on the mouse and human receptors; studies of the latter have been driven by the desire to investigate drug–drug interactions, whereas studies of the former have been facilitated by the ability to create transgenic mice in which a particular xenosensor has been deleted (so-called knockout or null mice) or replaced with the human receptor (so-called humanized mice).

Aryl Hydrocarbon Receptor AhR and ARNT are cytosolic and nuclear transcription factors, respectively, that are expressed in

Table 6-17

Examples of Agonists and Antagonists for the Receptors That Mediate Enzyme Induction (AhR, CAR, and PXR) and PXR/CAR Target Genes in Humans and Mice

	AGONISTS			ANTAGONISTS		
AhR	TCDD			CH-223191		
	Omeprazole			Omeprazole sulfide		
	Agonists	Human	Mouse	Inverse Agonists	Human	Mouse
CAR	Chlorpromazine	No	Yes	Chlorpromazine	Yes	No
	Meclizine	No	Yes	Meclizine	Yes	No
	Clotrimazole	No	Yes			
	CITCO	Yes	No			
	TCPOBOP	No	Yes			
	Indirect Activators					
	Phenobarbital	Yes	Yes			
	Phenytoin	Yes	Yes			
	Agonists	Human	Mouse	Antagonists	Human	Mouse
PXR	Artemisinin	Yes	No	Ketoconazole	Yes	Unknown
	Clotrimazole	Yes	No	Trabectedin (ET-743)	Yes	Unknown
	Hyperforin	Yes	Yes			
	Nicardipine	Yes	No			
	Nifedipine	Yes	No			
	Phenobarbital	Yes	Yes			
	PCN	Weak	Yes			
	Rifampin	Yes	No			
	TCPOBOP	Yes	Unknown			

XENOSENSOR	HUMAN PXR/CAR TARGET GENES[*]		MOUSE PXR/CAR TARGET GENES[*]	
PXR and CAR	CYP2A6		CYP2B10	SULT1E1
	CYP2B6		CYP3A11	SULT2A1
	CYP2C9		ALDH1	SULT2A2
	CYP2C19		AKR1B7	MDR1a
	CYP3A4		UGT1A1	MRP2
	UGT1A1		UGT1A9	MRP3
	MDR1		GSTA1/2	
	MRP2			
PXR only	CYP3A7	UGT1A3	CES6	
	CYP4F12	UGT1A6	UGT2B5	
	CYP7A1 $\downarrow$	GSTA1	GST (α, π, μ)	
	AKR1C1/2		MDR1b	
	CES2		OATP1A4	
CAR only	MRP3		CYP1A1	EST1
	MRP4		CYP1A2	UGT1A6
			CYP2A4	UGT2B1
			CYP2C29	MRP1
			CYP2C37	MRP4

PCN, pregnenolone-16α-carbonitrile; TCDD, 2,3,7,8-tetrachlorodibenzo-p-dioxin; CITCO, 6-(4-chloropheny)imidazo[2,1-b][1,3] thiazole-5-carbaldehyde O-(3,4-dichlorobenzyl)oxime; TCPOBOP, 1,4-bis[2-(3,5-dichloropyridyloxy)]benzene.
[*]Data from Tolson and Wang (2010).

most tissues and many cell lines. The binding of an agonist such as TCDD (the structure of which is shown in Table 6-17) to AhR initiates a number of changes (such as dissociation from heat-shock protein [hsp90] and other chaperones, dissociation from proteins that retain the unbound receptor in the cytoplasm, phosphorylation by tyrosine kinase) that culminate in (1) the translocation of AhR to the nucleus, (2) the dimerization of AhR with ARNT (which is somewhat misnamed as the *aryl hydrocarbon receptor nuclear translocator* because it is a nuclear, not a cytoplasmic protein that complexes with AhR after it translocates to the nucleus), (3) the binding of AhR–ARNT to DNA-response elements known as XRE, and (4) the increased transcription of CYP1A1 and numerous other genes listed in Table 6-16. Whereas members of the nuclear receptor superfamily (such as CAR, PXR, and PPARα) are "zinc finger" proteins, AhR and ARNT are "bHLH-PAS" proteins, so-named because they belong to the per-arnt-sim (PAS) class of receptors and they have a basic helix–loop–helix (bHLH) domain near their N-terminus, which is involved in protein–protein interactions.

TCDD is a high-affinity ligand for AhR (K_D values tend to be in the nanomolar-to-submicromolar range), and AhR mediates the toxicity of TCDD and related PHAHs (such as various chlorinated or brominated dibenzodioxins, dibenzofurans, and biphenyls), which is characterized by a wasting syndrome (progressive weight loss or cachexia resulting in death), immunosuppression (thymic atrophy), tumor promotion, fetal abnormalities (cleft palate and other teratogenic disorders), and, in some species, liver enlargement and a skin condition called chloracne. TCDD binds to AhR and induces CYP1A1 in all mammalian species, but it causes lethal cachexia in some species (such as guinea pig, where the LD_{50} is ~1 μg/kg) but not others (such as hamsters, where the LD_{50} exceeds 1000 μg/kg). This species difference in toxicity but not in CYP1A1 induction raised the possibility that AhR does not mediate the toxicity of TCDD, but several lines of evidence established that AhR does in fact mediate many, perhaps all, of the toxic effects of TCDD and related compounds. First, naturally occurring strain differences in the responsiveness of mice (such as so-called responsive C57 and nonresponsive DBA mice) and rats (such as responsive Long–Evans and nonresponsive Han/Wistar rats) to TCDD toxicity are associated with polymorphisms in AhR (Pohjanvirta *et al.*, 1999). Second, AhR knockout mice are resistant to TCDD-induced toxicity, whereas transgenic mice that express a constitutively active form of AhR (CA-AhR mice) spontaneously display numerous signs of TCDD toxicity (even though the CYP1A1 levels in the liver of CA-AhR mice are elevated to a lesser extent than those in TCDD-treated wild-type mice) (Brunnberg *et al.*, 2006). Third, the AhR antagonist CH-223191 (see Table 6-17) blocks the enzyme-inducing effects and various toxic effects of TCDD (Kim *et al.*, 2006). Nevertheless, it remains to be determined why prolonged activation of AhR by TCDD and related compounds causes an irreversible cachexia that leads to death after a certain time (after a latency period that varies from one species to the next but that cannot be shortened by administering "superlethal" doses of TCDD).

AhR agonists include PHAHs (such as TCDD), PAHs (such as 3-methylcholanthrene and B[*a*]P), flavonoids (such as β-naphthoflavone), and various acid-catalyzed condensation products or UV-induced derivatives of naturally occurring indoles (such as indole-3-carbinol and tryptophan). The indole derivative indirubin and indoxyl sulfate, the major metabolite of indole in mammals, and two metabolites of the indoleamine-2,3-dioxygenase pathway, namely, kynurenic acid and xanthurenic acid, are AhR agonists particularly of the human receptor (Omiecinski *et al.*, 2011b). In general, AhR agonists induce CYP1A1 and other enzymes across all mammalian and many nonmammalian species. A notable exception is a class of benzimidazole-containing compounds that includes the proton pump inhibitors omeprazole and lansoprazole. These drugs are not typical AhR agonists for 2 reasons. First, they do not bind to the LBD of AhR but activate AhR either directly (by binding to a second site on AhR) or indirectly (by activating a tyrosine kinase that phosphorylates AhR). Second, they activate AhR and induce CYP1A enzymes in humans but not in rats or mice, which is 1 of the few species differences in AhR activation by xenobiotics (Diaz *et al.*, 1990). An endogenous AhR ligand is suspected to exist because AhR function is so well conserved from fish to humans and because of developmental abnormalities observed in AhR knockout mice. In addition to agonists and antagonists there is a third class of AhR ligands known as selective AhR modulators (SAhRMs) as exemplified by SGA360. In contrast to AhR agonists that induce both XRE-driven transcriptional activity and repression of acute-phase gene expression, SAhRMs are only capable of mediating repression of acute-phase genes (Murray *et al.*, 2010). The SAhRM-mediated suppression of acute-phase genes is a non-XRE-driven, cytoplasmic event. This process illustrates an emerging role of AhR in the regulation of inflammatory process and liver homeostasis. AhR influences T-cell differentiation and influences the balance of T_H1 and T_H2 cells, as was established through the use of an AhR agonist M50367 that preferentially promotes the production of T_H1 over T_H2 cells. Exposure of mice to M50367 leads to a decrease in IgE synthesis and peritoneal eosinophilia in allergic experimental models (Negishi *et al.*, 2005).

Several compounds can disrupt AhR signaling at a variety of levels. CH-223191 (Table 6-17) and α-naphthoflavone are receptor antagonists that bind to the LBD of AhR without activating the receptor. Omeprazole sulfide (which forms by reduction of the sulfoxide group in omeprazole [see Table 6-17]) antagonizes CYP1A1 induction by omeprazole by stabilizing AhR in an inactive conformation (Gerbal-Chaloin *et al.*, 2006). After AhR is activated, its translocation to the nucleus is blocked by 3′-methoxy-4-nitroflavone, its binding to XRE is blocked by salicylamide, and its ability to recruit transcription factors and initiate gene transcription is blocked by resveratrol (an antioxidant in red wine) (Gerbal-Chaloin *et al.*, 2006). The presence of exogenous (and perhaps endogenous) AhR antagonists is one of the many factors that are known or suspected of causing clinically observed interindividual differences in CYP1A induction. These factors have been reviewed by Ma and Lu (2003), who have documented that differences in the magnitude of CYP1A induction in humans can be attributed to (1) genetic polymorphisms in AhR, ARNT, or XRE; (2) altered levels or function of accessory proteins (some of which are associated with inflammation and other disease states that activate NF-κB, as discussed later in this section); (3) gender differences in basal CYP1A2 activity (which tends to be lower in females compared with males); and (4) variation in the intracellular concentration of the inducing drug, as exemplified by variation in the metabolism of omeprazole. The clearance of omeprazole is largely determined by its rate of metabolism by the polymorphically expressed enzyme CYP2C19. Based on measurements of caffeine metabolism, a daily dose of 40 mg omeprazole causes CYP1A2 induction in CYP2C19 PMs but not in CYP2C19 EMs, which require higher doses (120 mg) to achieve CYP1A2 induction. In a clinical setting, the formation of omeprazole sulfide (an AhR antagonist) does not prevent CYP1A induction by omeprazole (an agonist). However, it is possible that the formation of rabeprazole sulfide, which occurs rapidly and extensively (by nonenzymatic means), explains why rabeprazole is one of the proton pump inhibitors that does not induce CYP1A.

Although strain differences in CYP1A inducibility have been linked to genetic polymorphisms in the mouse and rat AhR gene, species differences have been attributed either to the unusual interaction of AhR with benzimidazole-containing compounds such as omeprazole and lansoprazole or to species differences in the location of XRE. For example, rat UGT1A6 and 1A7 are highly inducible (>20-fold) enzymes because these conjugating genes are under the control of XRE in rats but in few other species.

Increased expression of AhR is correlated with tumor invasiveness of cigarette-smoke-associated urothelial carcinoma cells in vitro, presumably due to enhanced expression of MMP-1 and MMP-9, matrix metalloproteinases involved in tumor invasion (Ishida et al., 2010). The involvement of AhR signaling in tumor invasiveness is further supported by a positive correlation between nuclear localization of the receptor and histopathological characteristics of the neoplasm and long-term survival of urothelial carcinoma patients.

Constitutive Androstane Receptor and Pregnane X Receptor

CAR and PXR are members of the nuclear receptor family 1 (NR1I2 and NR1I3, respectively). In contrast to AhR, which is expressed in most tissues and numerous cell lines, CAR and PXR are expressed in relatively few organs—liver, small intestine, and colon—and in few cell lines. Both CAR and PXR are cytoplasmic nuclear receptors; both are activated by some of the same compounds, and both dimerize with RXRα to form DNA-binding proteins that recognize some of the same response elements, as shown in Tables 6-16 and 6-17. Consequently, there is considerable crosstalk between these two xenosensors, and it can sometimes be difficult to ascertain whether induction is mediated by CAR, PXR, or both receptors. Both humans and mice have drug-metabolizing enzymes and transporters that are regulated by CAR only, PXR only, and both xenosensors, but the enzymes/transporters are inducible in a species-dependent manner, as shown for humans and mice in Table 6-17 (Tolson and Wang, 2010).

As shown in Table 6-16, three factors combine to make CAR and PXR the most important human xenosensors in terms of drug–drug interactions. First, CAR and PXR regulate several CYP enzymes (eg, CYP2B6, 2C8, 2C9, 2C19, and 3A4), conjugating enzymes (several UGTs and SULTs), and transporters (such as P-glycoprotein [MDR1 or ABCB1], MRP2, and MRP4). Second, a large number of xenobiotics (drugs and the herbal preparations, St. John's wort, and Yin Zhi Huang) and certain endobiotics (such as bilirubin, bile acids, and 1,25-$(OH)_2$-D_3) activate CAR and/or PXR. Third, some of the genes regulated by CAR and PXR encode proteins with broad substrate specificities, such as CYP3A4 and P-glycoprotein, such that the induction mediated by CAR and PXR impacts the disposition of a large number of xenobiotics and certain endobiotics (see Table 6-13). In terms of drug–drug interactions, human xenosensors can be rank-ordered (from most important to least) as follows: CAR/PXR > AhR > "CYP2E1" > PPARα. PPARα is ranked last because its activation in humans, in contrast to its activation in rodents, does not lead to induction of CYP4 enzymes (a family of enzymes that plays a limited role in drug metabolism compared with CYP1, 2, and 3 enzymes). CYP2E1 is an inducible enzyme in humans (by mechanisms that do not appear to involve any of the xenosensors listed in Table 6-16), but relatively few drugs are inducers of—or substrates for—CYP2E1. AhR is less important than CAR/PXR because there are relatively few drugs that activate AhR and because the major hepatic enzyme regulated by AhR, namely, CYP1A2, plays a more limited role in drug metabolism than the hepatic and intestinal CYP enzymes regulated by CAR/PXR, namely, CYP2B6, 2C8, 2C9, 2C19, 3A4, and other enzymes (see Tables 6-16 and 6-17).

The activation of PXR follows the canonical steps outlined above (this section), beginning with (1) ligand binding to LBD, (2) dissociation of PXR from cytoplasmic retention protein and corepressors (such as nuclear receptor corepressor [NCOR] and silencing mediator for retinoid and thyroid hormone receptors [SMRT]), (3) association with coactivators (such as SRC1, GRIP-1, PGC-1, C/EBPα, and RAC3), (4) dimerization with RXRα, (5) translocation to the nucleus, and (6) binding to a set of core gene promoter elements within xenobiotic-responsive enhancer modules that typically contain DR-3 or ER-6 motifs, which culminates in transcriptional activation of multiple genes, as shown in Tables 6-16 and 6-17 (Chang and Waxman, 2006; Stanley et al., 2006; Gao and Xie, 2010; Tolson and Wang, 2010; Omiecinski et al., 2011a). Sequence variation in the LBD of PXR accounts for certain species differences in CYP3A induction. For example, PCN is a prototypical inducer of CYP3A in rats and mice, but not humans, whereas the opposite is true of rifampin. Transgenic mice with human PXR in place of mouse PXR (PXR-humanized mice) lose the ability to respond to PCN and gain the ability to respond to rifampin. Rifampin can also bind and activate rat PXR once the opening to the LBD is slightly widened (by changing a phenylalanine to a leucine residue). As shown in Table 6-17, rifampin, artemisinin, clotrimazole, nicardipine, and nifedipine are agonists for human PXR but not mouse PXR, which exemplifies why enzyme induction studies in rodents often fail to predict enzyme induction in humans. Some agonists bind to human PXR with relatively high affinity (with K_D values in the [sub]micromolar range), including rifampin and hyperforin, the inducing agent in St. John's wort. In general, activation of CAR/PXR shows little or no stereospecificity, although the C-cyclopropylalkylamide known as S20 is a rare exception: (−)-C20 preferentially activates mouse PXR, whereas (+)-C20 preferentially activates human PXR. This difference further underscores the lack of predictability of rodent data to the human situation.

Tang et al. (2005) have reviewed the factors that give rise to differences in the magnitude of enzyme induction by PXR/CAR agonists in humans; such differences can be attributed to (1) genetic polymorphisms or splicing variation in PXR or CAR and/or polymorphism in their DNA-response elements; (2) altered levels or function of accessory proteins (some of which are associated with inflammation and other disease states that activate NF-κB, as discussed later in this section); (3) gender differences in basal CYP3A4 activity (which tends to be lower in males compared with that in females); and (4) variation in the intracellular concentration of the inducing drug, as exemplified by variation in the metabolism of propafenone and celecoxib. Propafenone is metabolized by CYP2D6, 3A4, and 1A2. In CYP2D6 EMs, the clearance of propafenone is determined by CYP2D6, and treatment with rifampin causes no induction of propafenone metabolism. However, in CYP2D6 PMs, CYP3A4 plays a significant role in the clearance of propafenone, and treatment of CYP2D6 PMs with rifampin causes a doubling of propafenone clearance. The COX-2 inhibitor celecoxib is a PXR agonist whose in vivo clearance is largely determined by CYP2C9. At recommended clinical doses, celecoxib induces CYP3A4 in CYP2C9 PMs but not in CYP2C9 EMs due to the higher levels of celecoxib in the PMs (Rodrigues et al., 2006).

The activation of CAR is considerably more complex than that of PXR (Chang and Waxman, 2006; Kodama and Negishi, 2006; Stanley et al., 2006; Mutoh et al., 2009; Tolson and Wang, 2010; Omiecinski et al., 2011b; Osabe and Negishi, 2011). CAR is constitutively active, meaning that, in the absence of an exogenous ligand, it can complex with RXRα, translocate to the nucleus, bind to DNA-response elements (known as PBREM [for phenobarbital response elements] and containing DR4 and DR5 elements), and activate gene transcription, which is what generally happens when CAR is expressed in cell lines in vitro. In the in vivo situation (such as occurs in hepatocytes), CAR is prevented from

UNIT II

DISPOSITION OF TOXICANTS

296

being transcriptionally active by its retention in the cytoplasm by cytoplasmic CAR retention protein (CCRP) and chaperones such as hsp90, and possibly by its binding to an endogenous reverse agonist such as androstanol (5α-androstan-3α-ol) and androstenol (5α-androst-16-en-3α-ol), the androstanes for which CAR is named (reverse agonists are discussed later in this section). The retention of CAR in the cytoplasm is achieved by its phosphorylation (at threonine 38 in human CAR and threonine 48 in mouse CAR) by protein kinase C (PKC) (Mutoh *et al.*, 2009). Once phosphorylated, CAR complexes with P-ERK1/2, the phosphorylated (active) form of extracellular-signal-regulated kinase (also known as mitogen-activated protein kinase p42/p44), which binds to the so-called xenochemical response signal (XRS), a peptide sequence ([313]LGLLAEL[319]) near the C-terminus of the CAR receptor (Osabe and Negishi, 2011). Similar XRSs are present in RXR, VDR, peroxisome proliferator–activated receptors (PPARs), and estrogen receptor. Binding of P-ERK1/2 to XRS prevents the hydrolysis of the phosphate group at threonine 38 (human CAR) or threonine 48 (mouse CAR). The activation of CAR by xenobiotics involves the dephosphorylation of the threonine residue by protein phosphatase 2A, as evidenced by the observation that the protein phosphatase 2A inhibitor okadaic acid blocks CAR translocation in mouse hepatocytes (Mutoh *et al.*, 2009). How this dephosphorylation is triggered by xenobiotics is not fully understood and the situation is complicated by the fact that CAR activators can be divided into *direct activators*, which bind directly to the LBD of CAR, and *indirect activators*, which do not bind to CAR.

Because CAR is constitutively active but retained in the cytoplasm, ligands can function as agonists, reverse agonists, or antagonists. Agonists activate CAR by displacing endogenous reverse agonists (eg, androstanes) (Chang and Waxman, 2006; Kodama and Negishi, 2006; Stanley *et al.*, 2006; Mutoh *et al.*, 2009; Tolson and Wang, 2010; Omiecinski *et al.*, 2011b; Osabe and Negishi, 2011) or by promoting the dissociation of corepressors (such as P-ERK1/2 and NCOR) and the recruitment of coactivators (such as SRC-1, SP1, ASC-2, and PBP). Reverse agonists have the opposite effect: they promote the dissociation of coactivators and the recruitment of corepressors, and they may also decrease the transcriptional activity of CAR. Antagonists bind to the same LBD as agonists and reverse agonists; they neither activate nor deactivate CAR, but they block the binding of other ligands. Examples of agonists, reverse agonists, or antagonists of CAR are shown in Table 6-17.

Xenobiotics can function as CAR agonists or antagonists in a species-specific manner. For example, chlorpromazine and meclizine are agonists for mouse CAR, but they are inverse agonists for human CAR. TCPOBOP and CITCO are potent direct activators of CAR, but they function as CAR agonists in a species-specific manner: TCPOBOP is a potent agonist for mouse CAR, whereas CITCO is a potent agonist for human CAR (Table 6-17). These selective CAR agonists must be used in a species-specific manner, as underscored by the fact that the mouse CAR agonist TCPOBOP is *not* an agonist for human CAR but it *is* an agonist for human PXR. Phenobarbital is an indirect activator of mouse and human CAR, but it is also an activator of human PXR (but not mouse or rat PXR). In contrast, another enzyme-inducing antiepileptic drug phenytoin does not activate human PXR and, like CITCO, is a selective activator of human CAR. There are also species differences in the genes regulated specifically by CAR, specifically by PXR, and by both xenosensors, as shown for mouse and human in Table 6-17. These species differences in CAR, like those described earlier in this section for PXR, illustrate why, during the safety evaluation of drug candidates, enzyme induction studies in rodents are often of limited value in predicting enzyme induction in humans.

Alternative splicing of CAR mRNA gives rise to CAR2 and CAR3, which are not constitutively active but are ligand-activated forms of the receptor. CAR2 and CAR3 contain 4 and 5 amino acid inserts, respectively, within the LBD of the receptor. The inserts interfere with the ligand-binding pocket affinity of CAR2 but not CAR3. As a result, the ubiquitous plasticizer and environmental pollutant, di(2ethylhexyl)phthalate (DEHP), is a highly potent and selective CAR2 activator. Alternative splicing of CAR mRNA leads to the expression of tissue-specific variants, which can increase CAR's functional diversity and broaden the human receptor's repertoire of responses to xenobiotics (DeKeyser *et al.*, 2009, 2011). The splice variants detected for human CAR are not present in rats or mice, which further underscores why rodents may not be adequate to assess CAR-mediated events in humans.

Certain cofactors/enzymes are required for activation of CAR to its transcriptionally active form. For example, the coactivator PBP/MED1 (PPAR-binding protein/TRAP220/DRIP205/mediator subunit 1) is required for CAR activation (as well as PPARα activation) (Pyper *et al.*, 2010), as is AMP-activated protein kinase (AMPK) (Rencurel *et al.*, 2006). The ability of phenobarbital to induce CYP2B10 and CYP3A11 is abolished in transgenic mice lacking CAR, PBP/MED1, or the α-subunit of AMPK. However, the role of AMPK in CAR activation is not clear. Phenobarbital activates the upstream kinase LKB1, which in turn phosphorylates and activates AMPK. Once activated, AMPK does not appear to phosphorylate CAR directly but it does phosphorylate transcriptional coactivators such as p300 (a nuclear phosphoprotein with histone acetylase activity), TORC2 (transducer of regulated cAMP response element-binding protein [CREB]), and peroxisome proliferator–activated receptor γ coactivator-1α (PGC-1α) (Blättler *et al.*, 2007; Shindo *et al.*, 2007). Metformin, a drug used to lower fasting blood glucose levels in patients with noninsulin-dependent (Type 2) diabetes, also activates AMPK, and metformin induces CYP2B6 and 3A4 in human hepatocytes (Rencurel *et al.*, 2006). 5-Amino-4-carboxamide-1-β-ribofuranoside (AICAR) is another activator of AMPK that induces CYP2B enzymes in human and mouse hepatocytes (Rencurel *et al.*, 2006). However, AICAR does not induce CYP2B in rat hepatocytes (Kanno *et al.*, 2010) and metformin does not induce CYP2B in vivo in mice or rats (Shindo *et al.*, 2007). Furthermore, metformin does not cause clinically significant CYP2B6 or CYP3A4 induction in humans (Blättler *et al.*, 2007). Collectively these results establish that activation of AMPK is necessary for CYP2B induction by CAR activators but AMPK activation alone is not sufficient.

AMPK is sensitive to energy charge; consequently, it is activated by an increase in the ratio of AMP to ATP, which occurs, for example, during fasting. AMPK, PGC-1α, and CAR are all activated by fasting, which is associated with the induction of CYP2B10 and other CAR-regulated enzymes and transporters in mice (Ding *et al.*, 2006). Like metformin, phenobarbital also lowers glucose levels in patients with Type 2 diabetes and improves glucose tolerance and insulin sensitivity in mice (Rencurel *et al.*, 2006; Dong *et al.*, 2009). This glucose-lowering effect involves, at least in part, the following steps: (1) activation of AMPK by phenobarbital or metformin; (2) activation of CAR by dephosphorylation of threonine 38; (3) binding of activated CAR to forkhead box protein O1 (FOXO1), a transcription factor that binds to insulin-response sequences (IRS) in the promoter region of gluconeogenic genes such as phosphoenolpyruvate carboxykinase-1 (PEPCK1) and glucose-6-phosphatase (G6Pase); and (4) suppression of PEPCK1 and G6Pase leading to decreased gluconeogenesis (ie, decreased glucose synthesis) as a result of FOXO1 inactivation by CAR (Kodama and Negishi, 2006; Rencurel *et al.*, 2006). Consistent with this mechanism of action, phenobarbital decreases glucose levels in wild-type mice but not in CAR knockout mice. PXR agonists can also suppress gluconeogenesis either by the binding of activated PXR to FOXO1, which impairs the ability of FOXO1 to activate IRS-regulated gluconeogenic enzymes such as PEPCK1 and G6Pase, or by the binding of activated PXR to phosphorylated CREB that prevents CREB-dependent transcription of G6Pase (Kodama *et al.*, 2004; Gao and Xie, 2010). In addition to suppressing gluconeogenic enzymes (PEPCK1 and G6Pase), CAR activators also induce hexokinase and glucose metabolism by the pentose phosphate pathway, which supports drug metabolism by generating the NADPH required by CYP, FMO, and certain other xenobiotic-biotransforming enzymes (Kodama *et al.*, 2004; Dong *et al.*, 2009).

The interaction between CAR and transcription factor FOXO1 has opposing effects on each other's transcriptional activity: CAR is a *corepressor* of FOXO1, whereas FOXO1 is a *coactivator* of CAR. Activation of FOXO1 by diabetes increases CYP2B and 3A expression in rats and mice, and this effect is reversed by insulin treatment (which stimulates the phosphorylation of FOXO1 and thereby decreases its activity). By inactivating FOXO1 (which removes a coactivator for CAR), insulin blunts the induction of CYP2B enzymes by phenobarbital and represses the gluconeogenic pathway (Kodama and Negishi, 2006; Moreau *et al.*, 2008). The interactions between CAR and FOXO1 have also been described for PXR and FOXO1 (Kodama *et al.*, 2004; Gao and Xie, 2010).

In addition to playing a role in glucose homeostasis (by suppressing gluconeogenic enzymes), CAR also plays a role in lipid homeostasis (largely by suppressing lipogenic enzymes). Multiple mechanisms have been identified that contribute to the suppression of lipogenesis by CAR activators (Gao and Xie, 2010). CAR activation and its associated activation of AMPK lead to the induction of Insig-1, a microsomal protein that, together with Insig-2, plays a key role in the control of hepatic triglyceride and cholesterol synthesis (Roth *et al.*, 2008). Induction of Insig-1 results in repression of sterol regulatory element-binding protein-1 (SREBP-1), which in turn results in the downregulation of lipogenic enzymes and, hence, a decrease in hepatic triglyceride and, to a lesser extent, cholesterol levels. In addition to Insig-1 induction, the mechanism of SREBP-1 repression may also occur by an indirect mechanism that involves induction of CAR-regulated SULT2B enzyme(s) that sulfonate and inactivate the oxysterols that function as agonists for the liver X receptor-α (LXRα), which is an inducer of SREBP-1. This indirect pathway may play a significant role in suppressing SREBP-1 expression based on the observation that the ability of CAR activators to suppress triglyceride/cholesterol synthesis is substantially impaired in SULT1B1b knockout mice (Dong *et al.*, 2009). In addition to suppressing lipogenesis, CAR activators also induce fatty acid β-oxidation. The mechanism is distinct from the induction of fatty acid β-oxidation by PPARα agonists, which are the main regulators of lipid catabolism (discussed in the next section). CAR activators promote fatty acid β-oxidation by repressing the expression of acetyl-coenzyme A (acetyl-CoA) carboxylase (both ACC1 and ACC2; gene symbols ACACA and ACACB), which results in a decrease in the levels of malonyl-CoA, the initial intermediate in lipogenesis and an allosteric inhibitor of the carnitine-dependent transport of fatty acids into mitochondria for β-oxidation (Dong *et al.*, 2009). From the foregoing it can be appreciated that there is growing interest in CAR as a potential therapeutic target in Type 2 diabetes and fatty liver disease.

Just as activation of CAR suppresses lipogenesis so excess lipid in the liver suppresses CAR activity. Obesity, steatosis (fatty liver), and high-fat diets all suppress CAR activation and CYP2B induction (Blouin *et al.*, 1993; Gao and Xie, 2010). The effects are mediated, at least in part, by suppression of CAR (and PXR) by the key lipogenic factors SREBP-1 and LXRα presumably by competition for nuclear receptor coactivators. Although CAR and PXR have the same effect on gluconeogenesis (both of them suppress glucose synthesis), these xenosensors have opposing effects on lipid homeostasis: activation of CAR leads to repression of lipogenesis, whereas activation of PXR leads to the promotion of lipogenesis (Gao and Xie, 2010). Transgenic mice expressing a constitutively activated PXR develop hepatomegaly with marked steatosis, as do PXR-humanized mice treated with rifampin, albeit to a lesser extent (Zhou *et al.*, 2006c). PXR activation causes fatty liver by inducing CD36 (a transporter of free fatty acids), PPARγ (a lipogenic peroxisome proliferation activation receptor discussed in the next section), and several accessory lipogenic enzymes including stearoyl-CoA desaturase-1 (SDC-1) and long-chain fatty acid elongase and by suppressing enzymes involved in β-oxidation (Zhou *et al.*, 2006c). Both PXR and CAR agonists induce thyroid hormone-responsive spot 14 (gene symbol THRSP), the expression of which correlates with lipogenesis, which is consistent with the aforementioned role of PXR in lipogenesis and which suggests that the role of CAR in lipid homeostasis may be complex because paradoxically CAR appears to induce both lipid synthesis and catabolism. In the clinical setting, a number of PXR agonists (rifampin, nifedipine, and carbamazepine) and a number of CAR activators (phenobarbital, phenytoin, and valproic acid) have been shown to alter lipid homeostasis and/or cause steatosis (fatty liver) (reviewed in Zhou *et al.*, 2006c).

CAR and PXR are activated by certain endobiotics, and the enzymes regulated by these xenosensors play important roles in terminating the hormonal activity of 1,25-$(OH)_2$-D_3 and attenuating the toxicity of high levels of bilirubin and bile acids. The active form of vitamin D, namely, 1,25-$(OH)_2$-D_3, binds to the VDR to induce the synthesis of calbindin-D9K, a calcium-binding protein that facilitates the uptake of calcium from the intestinal lumen to blood. VDR also induces CYP enzymes that further hydroxylate and thereby inactivate 1,25-$(OH)_2$-D_3, which establishes a negative feedback loop. Two VDR-inducible CYP enzymes have been shown to inactivate 1,25-$(OH)_2$-D_3 by hydroxylating the active hormone in the 24-position and, to a lesser extent, the 23-position. The first is CYP24A1, which is expressed mainly in the kidney, and which catalyzes the 24 *R*-hydroxylation of 1,25-$(OH)_2$-D_3. The second is CYP3A4, which is expressed mainly in intestine and liver, and which catalyzes the 24 *S*-hydroxylation of 1,25-$(OH)_2$-D_3. The stereochemical differences in the 24-hydroxylation reaction helped to establish that CYP3A4 is the principal inactivator of 1,25-$(OH)_2$-D_3 in the intestine, with little or no contribution from CYP24A1. These findings are important for two reasons. First, the ability of VDR to mimic PXR/CAR and induce CYP3A4 is an example of the crosstalk that can occur between a xenosensor and other nuclear receptors. Second, the key role played by CYP3A4 in the inactivation of 1,25-$(OH)_2$-D_3 in the intestine provides an explanation for the clinical observation that long-term treatment of patients with rifampin, phenobarbital, phenytoin, or carbamazepine can lead to osteomalacia, a bone disorder that is symptomatic of vitamin D deficiency. These PXR/CAR agonists are thought to cause osteomalacia by inducing CYP3A4 in the intestine, which accelerates the inactivation of 1,25-$(OH)_2$-$D_3$and thereby impairs calcium absorption (Xu *et al.*, 2006; Zhou *et al.*, 2006a).

CAR plays an important role in detoxifying high levels of bilirubin, as might occur in patients with hemolytic anemia. Like phenobarbital, bilirubin is an indirect activator of CAR. When activated, CAR induces UGT1A1 and several SULTs, the major hepatic enzymes responsible for conjugating bilirubin, as well as transporters of bilirubin/bilirubin conjugates (MRP2 and MRP4).

When hemolytic anemia is induced by treating mice with phenylhydrazine, bilirubin levels rise to a greater extent in CAR knockout mice compared with wild-type mice, which demonstrates the important role CAR plays in responding to high levels of bilirubin. Phenobarbital was once used to treat neonatal jaundice, and the Chinese herbal Yin Zhi Huang is still used for this purpose. Phenobarbital and scoparone (6,7-dimethylesculetin), the active ingredient in Yin Zhi Huang, are CAR activators that, like bilirubin itself, induce the major bilirubin-conjugating enzyme UGT1A1 and related transporters (Chang and Waxman, 2006; Kodama and Negishi, 2006). In contrast, CAR appears to play a role in acetaminophen hepatotoxicity presumably by allowing acetaminophen to induce its own activation to a toxic quinoneimine. CAR knockout mice are relatively resistant to acetaminophen hepatotoxicity compared with both wild-type and CAR-humanized mice, which suggests early treatment with a CAR antagonist might be a useful adjunct treatment for acetaminophen overdose.

CAR, PXR, and the VDR appear to act as backup receptors to prevent bile acid accumulation and toxicity when the principal bile acid sensor, FXR, is overloaded. In the mouse ileum and colon, bile acid activation of FXR and, to a lesser extent, VDR and PXR promotes bile acid detoxication (by AKR1B7 and CYP3A11), intracellular binding (to ileal bile acid binding protein [IBABP]), and secretion (by organic solute transporters, OSTα/β) (Ballatori et al., 2009b; Degirolamo et al., 2011; Schmidt et al., 2011). FXR induces the expression of AKR1B7 in murine small intestine, colon, and liver by binding directly to a response element in the AKR1B7 promoter and this AKR metabolizes 3-keto bile acids to the corresponding 3β-hydroxy bile acids, which are less toxic than their 3α-hydroxy isomers. High concentrations of bile acids activate FXR, which suppresses the expression of CYP7A1, the cholesterol 7α-hydroxylase that catalyzes the rate-limiting step in bile acid synthesis, and which induces the expression of bile acid conjugating enzymes (UGT2B4 and SULT2A1) and bile acid transporters (such as the bile salt export pump [BSEP]). When hepatocytes contain low concentrations of bile acids, FXR is inactive and the expression of CYP7A1 is stimulated by liver receptor homolog-1 (LRH-1), a constitutively active nuclear receptor. When hepatocytes contain high concentrations of bile acids, FXR is activated, and it inactivates LRH-1 by inducing the synthesis of small heterodimer partner-1 (SHP), so named because it lacks a DNA-binding domain (hence its small size) and because it forms heterodimers with LRH-1 and numerous other nuclear receptors including AhR, CAR, PXR, LXRα, HNF4α, and the glucocorticoid receptor (GR). Because it lacks a DBD, SHP inactivates all of these receptors; in the case of LRH-1, this results in a loss of CYP7A1 expression and a decrease in bile acid synthesis, which represents a negative feedback loop. FXR knockout mice are more sensitive than wild-type mice to bile acid toxicity, and treatment with the FXR ligand GW4064 further protects wild-type mice against experimentally induced extrahepatic and intrahepatic cholestasis. Cholic acid is both an FXR and PXR agonist; it suppresses CYP7A1 expression by activating first FXR and then PXR. In contrast to the situation in wild-type or single receptor knockout mice, 1% dietary cholic acid is lethal to FXR/PXR double knockout mice. PXR and CAR play a similar role in attenuating the toxicity of lithocholic acid, which is both a PXR agonist and a substrate for many of the enzymes regulated by PXR, including CYP3A, SULT, and transporters involved in the hepatic uptake and efflux of lithocholic acid. In PXR/CAR double knockout mice, lithocholic acid causes lethal hepatotoxicity at doses that are well tolerated by wild-type mice. The mouse PXR agonist PCN can markedly suppress CYP7A1 expression and bile acid synthesis in mice, and the human PXR agonist rifampin can markedly suppress CYP7A1 expression in human hepatocytes. The ability of PXR/CAR to function as a backup system for FXR may be compromised by the expression of SHP, which represses the activity of these xenosensors. This complex interplay is one of the likely reasons why there are some conflicting results from studies of the role of PXR/CAR in bile acid detoxication. The overall role of FXR is to provide protection against the toxic and tumorigenic effects of bile acids in the liver and colon; consequently, agonists of this receptor are being considered as potential colon cancer chemotherapeutic agents (Degirolamo et al., 2011).

As the preceding examples in this section illustrate, there is a complex interplay between many of the nuclear receptors listed in Table 6-16. Some nuclear receptors, such as the hepatic nuclear factors HNF1α and HNF4α, and the coactivator PBP/MED1 (PPAR-binding protein/TRAP220/DRIP205/mediator subunit 1) play a critical permissive role in gene regulation by CAR, PXR, and other receptors, whereas others, such as SHP, play a widespread role in suppressing nuclear receptor activity. HNF1α is instrumental for the expression of high levels of CYP2E1 mRNA in liver, although it is not the only factor because disruption of the β-catenin gene in mice greatly reduces CYP2E1 mRNA levels in the liver in the absence of changes in HNF1α expression (Gonzalez, 2007). Interestingly, the cross-talk between transcription factors, particularly between HNF4α, CAR, and PXR, is markedly increased in tissues from patients with severe viral hepatitis with pronounced inflammation and fibrosis (Congiu et al., 2009).

The glucocorticoid receptor (GR) plays an important role in inducing the synthesis of CAR and PXR (and individual xenobiotic-biotransforming enzymes such as CYP2C9). The role of GR in regulating the synthesis of xenosensors and the interplay among nuclear receptors are instrumental to the mechanism by which infections and inflammatory diseases suppress the expression and blunt the induction of xenobiotic-biotransforming enzymes and, conversely, the mechanism by which PXR agonists cause immunosuppression.

The expression and induction of xenobiotic-biotransforming enzymes by AhR, CAR, PXR, and PPARα are all suppressed by infection (viral, bacterial, and parasitic), vaccination, inflammation, and treatment with endotoxin (lipopolysaccharide or LPS) or inflammatory cytokines such as interleukin-1β (IL-1β) and IL-6. The suppression involves (1) an increase in proinflammatory cytokines, (2) a decrease in the levels of PXR and CAR due to a decrease in GR activity, and (3) a decrease in the activity of GR, PXR, CAR, AhR, PPARα, and several other nuclear receptors including the androgen, estrogen, and mineralocorticoid receptors (De Bosscher et al., 2006; Pascual and Glass, 2006; Zhou et al., 2006b). The decrease in receptor activity is caused by NF-κB, which is activated during infection and inflammatory disease, and which induces the synthesis of COX-2, TNFα, ICAM-1, and several interleukins. NF-κB binds to the DBD of RXRα and thereby decreases the transcriptional activity of all nuclear receptors that form heterodimers with RXRα (such as PXR, CAR, PPARα, GR, etc.). It also decreases the transcriptional activity of AhR even though AhR forms heterodimers with ARNT, not RXRα. By lowering the levels and/or inhibiting the activity of the major xenosensors and numerous other nuclear factors, NF-κB mediates the widespread suppression of xenobiotic-biotransforming enzymes associated with infection and inflammatory disease. However, the converse is also true inasmuch as certain nuclear receptors, when activated, can complex NF-κB and thereby repress the expression of NF-κB-regulated genes (COX-2, TNFα, ICAM-1, interleukins). This is the basis, at least in part, for the immunosuppressive effect of corticosteroids, which activate GR, and the immunosuppressive effect of PXR ligands such as rifampin and mifepristone (RU-486). PXR plays a role in suppressing NF-κB activity in the small intestine. PXR knockout mice show signs of inflammation of the small intestine, and certain genetic polymorphisms and splicing variants of PXR are associated with inflammatory bowel disease. Common environmental AhR agonists can suppress the response to bacterial LPS, through downregulation of IL-6. This suppression occurs at the level of IL-6 gene transcription and may be regulated by NF-κB (Jensen *et al.*, 2003). The AhR can also attenuate cytokine-mediated induction of acute-phase response genes in liver in a XRE-independent manner. This function of the receptor suggests its role in maintaining liver homeostasis during inflammation. The role of PXR in regulating NF-κB activity, responding to high levels of bile acids, and terminating the actions of 1,25-(OH)$_2$-D$_3$, the role of CAR in responding to high level of bilirubin, and the role of CAR and PXR in glucose and lipid (energy) metabolism all illustrate that these so-called xenosensors do not simply respond to xenobiotics but play key roles in endobiotic homeostasis.

Peroxisome Proliferator–Activated Receptor-Alpha An increase in the size and number of rat hepatic peroxisomes was first observed in response to the hypolipidemic drug, clofibrate. Peroxisome proliferation is accompanied by hepatomegaly, induction of fatty acid oxidation in peroxisomes, mitochondria, and microsomes, and with long-term administration of hypolipidemic drugs, hepatocarcinogenicity. Induction of microsomal fatty acid oxidation is due to the induction of CYP4A enzymes that play a limited role in xenobiotic biotransformation but that convert fatty acids to dicarboxylic acids by ω-hydroxylation (see the section "CYP4 Enzymes"). Numerous xenobiotic "peroxisome proliferators" have been identified including hypolipidemic fibrate drugs (eg, clofibrate, fenofibrate, ciprofibrate, bezafibrate, nafenopin, methylcofenapate), various NSAIDs, aspirin, leukotriene receptor antagonists (MK-0571 and RG 7512), organic solvents (trichloroacetic acid), phthalate ester plasticizers, herbicides (haloxyfab, lactyofen, 2,4-dichlorophenoxyacetic acid [2,4-D]), perfluorodecanoic acid, nicotinic acid, cinnamyl anthranilate, and the potent and widely used experimental peroxisome proliferator-activated receptor α (PPARα) agonist Wy-14643 (Lake, 2009). Peroxisome proliferation by some of these xenobiotics occurs stereoselectively. The receptor that mediates peroxisome proliferation by these xenobiotics is the PPARα. PPARα (NR1C1) is one of a family of three nuclear receptors; the other members are PPARβ/δ (NR1C2) and PPARγ (NR1C3). All three are Type II nuclear receptors that reside in the nucleus (in contrast to AhR, CAR, and PXR, which reside in the cytoplasm) (Pyper *et al.*, 2010).

The distinction between xenobiotic- and endobiotic-sensing functions is particularly blurred in the case of PPARα, which is activated by the aforementioned xenobiotics and by several endogenous fatty acids (eg, notably the acyl-CoA and enoyl-CoA derivatives of long-chain fatty acid), dicarboxylic acids (such as those formed by CYP4-dependent ω-hydroxylation of long-chain fatty acids and arachidonic acid [HETEs]), LTB$_4$, products formed by fatty acid synthase (such as 1-palmityl-2-oleoyl-*sn*-glycerol-3-phosphocholine [16:0/18:1-GPC]), and DHEA sulfate. From this list of endogenous ligands it is apparent that fatty acids (generally in the form of acyl-CoA thioesters) can activate PPARα and induce their own metabolism. All three receptors play an important role in lipid (energy) metabolism. In general, PPARα and PPARβ/δ are regulators of fatty acid catabolism (catabolic energy metabolism) that are highly expressed in liver, heart, kidney, brown adipose tissue, muscle, and the small and large intestines (Issemann and Green, 1990; Braissant *et al.*, 1996; Bookout *et al.*, 2006). PPARγ, which is expressed in at least three forms (eg, PPARγ1, PPARγ2, and PPARγ3), regulates lipid synthesis and is abundant

in white and brown adipose tissues (Tontonoz *et al.*, 1994; Fajas *et al.*, 1998). The pattern of tissue expression of PPARα is similar in rodents and humans (Bookout *et al.*, 2006). PPARα exerts a dominant role in regulating fatty acid catabolism and ketone body synthesis in the liver. PPARβ/δ also participates in the regulation of fatty acid oxidation, but its effects are more prominent in muscle and heart; however, PPARβ/δ also regulates certain lipid-metabolizing enzymes in the liver (Sanderson *et al.*, 2009). PPARα functions as the major xenobiotic and lipid sensor to regulate fatty acid catabolism, hepatic steatosis, lipoprotein synthesis, inflammation, and hepatocarcinogenesis; hence, this xenosensor is the major focus of discussion here.

Activation of PPARα follows the canonical steps outlined earlier in this section. Binding of ligands to the LBD of PPARα results in (1) dissociation of corepressors (such as NCOR and SMRT), (2) dimerization with RXRα, (3) association with coactivators (p300, SRC/p160 family members, PBP/MED1, PGC-1α, and many others), and (4) binding of activated PPARα to response elements (PPREs) that usually reside in the promoter (5′-region) of target genes. The PPRE is a direct repeat (DR1) composed of two copies of the consensus hexamer sequence AGG(A)TCA separated by a single base pair. PPARα activity is increased by phosphorylation of serine residues 12 and 21. Insulin stimulates the phosphorylation and, hence, the transcriptional activity of PPARα. The expression of PPARα is increased by fasting/starvation to provide energy through the oxidation of fatty acids released from adipose tissue. During starvation, PPARα is essential for the upregulation of the genes necessary for fatty acid oxidation, although PPARβ/δ can also upregulate some of the same enzymes independently of PPARα (Sanderson *et al.*, 2009). The β-oxidation of fatty acids produces acetyl-CoA that either enters the mitochondrial tricarboxylic acid cycle or undergoes condensation reactions to form ketone bodies that are released into blood for energy (ATP) production in extrahepatic tissues. PPARα is also regulated by stress, growth hormone, leptin, and glucocorticoids. Direct binding of glucose to PPARα may be an important mechanism of stimulating fatty acid oxidation during uncontrolled diabetes (Pyper *et al.*, 2010).

Once activated, PPARα induces the expression of key enzymes involved in the oxidation of fatty acids in peroxisomes, mitochondria, and endoplasmic reticulum (the three major organelles involved in lipid catabolism). Oxidation of fatty acids in peroxisomes and mitochondria involves β-oxidation, whereas their oxidation in microsomes involves ω- and ω-1 hydroxylation by CYP (especially CYP4 enzymes). Peroxisomal β-oxidation targets very long straight-chain fatty acids, 2-methyl branched fatty acids, prostanoids, and dicarboxylic acids. The latter are formed by the ω-hydroxylation of fatty acids by CYP4 enzymes. Compared with their precursors (monocarboxylic acids), dicarboxylic acids are highly toxic; hence, the coordinate induction of microsomal ω-hydroxylation and peroxisomal β-oxidation is an important function of PPARα. There are two peroxisomal β-oxidation systems: system 1 targets long-chain fatty acids and is inducible by PPARα, with the initial step being catalyzed by the highly inducible enzyme peroxisomal acyl-coenzyme A oxidase 1 (ACOX1). The second is a noninducible system that targets 2-methyl-branched fatty acids (with the initial step catalyzed by ACOX2). Peroxisomal β-oxidation of long-chain fatty acids (C$_{20+}$) produces chain-shortened fatty acids (approximately C$_{10}$) that are transported to mitochondria for further β-oxidation. The three enzymes involved in peroxisomal β-oxidation of long-chain fatty acids, namely, ACOX1, the bifunctional enzyme L-PBE/MFP1 (enoyl-CoA hydratase/3-hydroxyacyl-CoA dehydrogenase), and PTL (3-ketoacyl-CoA thiolase), are all inducible by PPARα. PPARα also induces mitochondrial carnitine palmitoyl transferase-1, which facilitates the entry of fatty acyl carnitine into mitochondria, and long-chain acyl-CoA synthetases, which initiate β-oxidation of fatty acids.

Fatty liver is the most common liver disease. It encompasses steatosis and steatohepatitis, diseases that can progress to cirrhosis and hepatocellular carcinoma. Fatty liver disease is divided into *alcoholic fatty liver disease* (due to excessive alcohol consumption) and *nonalcoholic fatty liver disease* (due to obesity, which may occur with or without insulin resistance). During fasting PPARα knockout mice develop steatosis, hyperlipidemia, hypoketonemia, hypoglycemia, and hypothermia because they are unable to induce the peroxisomal, mitochondrial, and microsomal enzymes required to metabolize lipids released from adipose tissue. PPARα knockout mice also develop severe steatohepatitis if fed a choline- and methionine-deficient diet. Ethanol-fed PPARα knockout mice develop marked hepatomegaly, steatohepatitis, hepatocellular proliferation, and cell death. In wild-type mice and humans ethanol impairs PPARα function, which is thought to contribute to the mechanism by which alcohol causes alcoholic fatty liver disease (Pyper *et al.*, 2010).

In addition to playing a key role in protecting the liver against fatty liver disease, PPARα plays an important role in reducing inflammation. The proinflammatory eicosanoid LTB$_4$ is an activator of PPARα and induces its own metabolism by β- and ω-oxidation. PPARα ligands significantly reduce the levels of other proinflammatory cytokines/enzymes including interleukin-1 (IL-1), tumor necrosis factor-α (TNFα), COX-2, and inducible nitric oxide synthase (NOS-2) by inhibiting NF-κB and by decreasing phosphorylation of the c-Jun subunit of AP-1 (Pyper *et al.*, 2010).

Paradoxically, in addition to inducing peroxisomal, mitochondrial, and microsomal enzymes involved in fatty acid catabolism, PPARα can upregulate the expression of hepatic lipogenic genes by activating SREBP-1 and liver X receptor α (LXRα) (Browning and Horton, 2004; Hebbachi *et al.*, 2008). The situation is analogous to CAR that also upregulates lipid synthesis and catabolism (see the preceding section). The upregulation of lipogenic genes by PPARα is possibly a fail-safe mechanism to save fatty acids by incorporating them into triglycerides during starvation.

Species differences in PPARα and peroxisome proliferation are a complex issue. Activation of human PPARα in humans and other primates (and guinea pigs) is generally considered to cause little or no induction of microsomal CYP4A enzymes and minimal peroxisome proliferation (Lake, 2009). However, peroxisome proliferation does occur in rhesus and cynomolgus monkeys treated with supertherapeutic doses of ciprofibrate. The lack of hepatomegaly and peroxisome proliferation in humans administered PPARα agonists is attributed to dose and the levels of hepatic PPARα, which are about an order of magnitude lower in humans compared with those in rodents. PPARα-humanized mice (ie, mice harboring human PPARα instead of the mouse receptor) are resistant to peroxisome proliferation but the overexpression of human PPARα in mice restores peroxisome proliferation, the pleiotropic induction response, and cell proliferation (Pyper *et al.*, 2010). These findings are pertinent to the risk of hepatocellular carcinogenesis posed by fibrate drugs and other PPARα agonists, which is discussed in the next section.

Enzyme Induction and Chemical Carcinogenesis In humans, induction of CYP2E1 and the associated increased activation of acetaminophen to *N*-acetylbenzo-*p*-quinoneimine (NAPQI) is one of the mechanisms by which alcohol consumption and fasting potentiate acetaminophen hepatotoxicity (other contributing mechanisms include the impaired conjugation of acetaminophen

due to lowered levels of UDPGA and PAPS and the impaired detoxication of NAPQI due to lowered levels of GSH). By analogy, induction of CYP enzymes would be expected to increase the activation of procarcinogens to DNA-reactive metabolites, leading to increased tumor formation. However, contrary to expectation, treatment of rodents with a CYP inducer prior to treatment with a known proximate carcinogen (tumor initiators such as aflatoxin, various nitrosamines, or PAHs) is generally associated with a decrease, not an increase, in tumor incidence (Parkinson and Hurwitz, 1991; Nebert and Dalton, 2006; Shimada, 2006; Ma and Lu, 2007). The route of exposure to the carcinogen can affect the impact of enzyme induction; it protects against orally administered drugs but may increase the tumorigenicity of carcinogens applied directly to their site of action (Nebert *et al.*, 2004). Although treatment of rats and mice with a CYP inducer *before* treatment with an initiator (a genotoxic carcinogen) generally decreases tumor incidence, treatment with a CYP inducer *after* the initiator (such as diethylnitrosamine) generally increases tumor incidence because CYP inducers generally function as tumor promoters in rodents.

Phenobarbital is representative of a large number of compounds that appear to promote liver tumor formation in mice and, to a lesser extent, in rats by an epigenetic mechanism, including phenytoin, carbamazepine, chlordecone, butylated hydroxytoluene, DDT, dieldrin, hexachlorocyclohexane, certain polychlorinated and polybrominated biphenyls, loratadine, doxylamine, lansoprazole, musk xylene, and fenbuconazole (Williams and Iatropoulos, 2002; Juberg *et al.*, 2006). Although the exact mechanism of tumor formation remains unknown, it is critically dependent on CAR activation, as evidenced by the finding that phenobarbital and related compounds do not function as tumor promoters in CAR knockout mice (Gonzalez and Yu, 2006). Replicative DNA synthesis and possibly inhibition of apoptosis are mechanistically important. Phenobarbital does not function as a tumor promoter in Syrian hamsters (even following treatment with a genotoxic agent such as DMN, DEN, or methylazoxymethanol acetate). Phenobarbital is a CYP2B inducer in hamsters but it does not induce replicative DNA synthesis and does not inhibit apoptosis in hamster hepatocytes (either spontaneous or transforming growth factor-β1 [TGF-β1]–induced apoptosis) (Lake, 2009). In mice and rats phenobarbital and related compounds only cause liver tumors at doses that cause liver enlargement due to an increase in cell number (hepatocellular hyperplasia) and cell size (hepatocellular hypertrophy). The liver changes induced by phenobarbital, including an increase in DNA synthesis within 24 hours, a wave of mitotic activity after 1 to 3 days, enzyme induction (eg, CYP2B enzymes), and a progressive increase in liver weight, all exhibit nonlinear dose–response relationships, suggesting that there is a threshold dose below which no activation of CAR and no liver tumor promotion occur.

Although induction of CYP2B enzymes (and other xenobiotic-biotransforming enzymes and transporters) is a common feature of phenobarbital and related tumor-promoting chemicals, the two events do not appear to be mechanistically linked (Williams and Iatropoulos, 2002). Activation of CAR is critical to liver tumor development in mice, although upregulation of xenobiotic-biotransforming enzymes is less important than other xenosensor-dependent events, such as, in the cases of the indirect (phenobarbital) or direct mouse CAR-activator (TCPOBOP), altered DNA methylation of numerous genes, upregulation of GADD45B (an antiapoptotic factor) and Mdm2 (a negative regulator of the tumor suppressor p53), and the downregulation of gap junctional proteins (connexin 32), which diminishes cell–cell communication (Omiecinski *et al.*, 2011b). Although phenobarbital and other CAR activators induce CYP2B6 in human hepatocytes (both in vitro and in vivo), they neither cause replicative DNA synthesis nor inhibit spontaneous or TGF-β1-induced apoptosis (Lake, 2009).

Prolonged treatment of rodents with clofibrate, fenofibrate, ciprofibrate, bezafibrate, nafenopin, methylcofenapate, Wy-14643, DEHP, DEHA, cinnamyl anthranilate, or trichloroethylene is associated with hepatic peroxisome proliferation and liver tumor (adenoma and/or carcinoma) formation (Lake, 2009). PPARα plays a critical role in tumor formation by peroxisome proliferators as evidenced by the finding that Wy-14643 does not function as a tumor promoter in PPARα knockout mice (Gonzalez and Yu, 2006). Furthermore, there is excellent agreement between the potency with which agonists activate PPARα and the potency (in terms of latency period and tumor incidence) with which they promote liver tumor formation in rodents (which in turn is correlated with their ability to induce the proliferation of peroxisomes, induce peroxisomal enzymes involved in the β-oxidation of fatty acids, and induce microsomal CYP4A enzymes). Like CAR agonists, PPARα agonists are considered epigenetic (nongenotoxic) tumorigens because they are not mutagenic and they are not known to be converted to mutagenic metabolites. Another similarity with CAR agonists is that, in rodents, PPARα agonists cause replicative DNA synthesis in association with hepatomegaly (due to early hyperplastic and hypertrophic growth of hepatocytes) and they inhibit apoptosis. Just as it is sensitive to the enzyme-inducing/endoplasmic reticulum proliferative effects but not the tumor-promoting effects of CAR agonists, so the Syrian hamster is sensitive to the enzyme-inducing/peroxisome proliferating effects of PPARα agonists but is resistant to their tumor-promoting effects (Lake, 2009). PPARα agonists cause replicative DNA synthesis and inhibit apoptosis in rat and mouse hepatocytes but not in hepatocytes from hamsters, guinea pigs, monkeys, and humans (Lake, 2009). Treatment of mice with Wy-14643 represses the expression of let-7C microRNA, which results in increased expression (derepression) of c-myc oncogene expression (Shah et al., 2007). Interestingly, suppression of let-7C miRNA does not occur in PPARα-humanized mice treated with Wy-14643 (Yang et al., 2008).

Although PPARα agonists are not genotoxic, the dramatic (>20-fold) induction of peroxisomal ACOX1 by Wy-14643 and other peroxisome proliferators (dramatic when compared with the modest [2- to 5-fold] induction of peroxisomal catalase) leads to increased production of hydrogen peroxide, which can cause oxidative stress and DNA damage that possibly play a role in some of the downstream events leading to tumor promotion (Pyper et al., 2010). Oxidative DNA damage is evident from the fact that treatment of rodents with PPARα agonists leads to the induction of long-patch base excision DNA repair, the principal pathway for removing oxidized DNA bases (Rusyn et al., 2004).

Activation of PPARα is required but apparently not sufficient to lead to liver tumor formation. Other key events include increased oxidant production (such as increased peroxisomal H_2O_2 production), increased cell proliferation (which fixes mutations), and suppression of apoptosis (which prevents the removal of genetically damaged cells and permits clonal expansion) (Klaunig et al., 2003; Lai, 2004; Bosgra et al., 2005). Kupffer cells appear to play an important role in liver tumor formation by releasing mitogenic cytokines and possibly by contributing to oxidative stress by releasing superoxide anion, although it is not clear how PPARα agonists trigger these events. Inhibition of gap junctional intercellular communication plays an important role in liver tumor formation by PPARα agonists, just as it does in the promotion of liver tumors by phenobarbital-type inducers.

Epidemiological studies designed to assess the human cancer risk posed by PPARα agonists have produced inconclusive results.

Clofibrate has been reported to cause a statistically significant increase in cancer mortality rate during a 5- to 8-year treatment period. However, there was no significant increase in cancer rate in a follow-up study, which included a posttreatment period (Lai, 2004). Three compelling lines of evidence suggest that PPARα agonists will not cause liver tumors in humans. First, PPARα agonists do not cause peroxisome proliferation and microsomal CYP4A induction in human hepatocytes in vitro or in primates in vivo at therapeutic doses. Second, PPARα agonists do not cause replicative DNA synthesis or inhibit apoptosis in human hepatocytes (or in hepatocytes from hamsters and guinea pigs, two species that are resistant to the hepatocarcinogenic effects of PPARα agonists). Third, treatment of PPARα-humanized mice (transgenic mice with human PPARα in place of mouse PPARα) with Wy-14643 or fenofibrate neither results in the hepatocellular proliferation characteristic of wild type nor results in the repression of let-7C miRNA and the upregulation of the c-myc oncogene (Gonzalez and Yu, 2006; Yang et al., 2008; Lake, 2009; Pyper et al., 2010).

The mechanism of thyroid tumor formation is better understood. In rodents, CAR activators (as well as PXR and PPARα agonists) induce UGT and SULT enzymes and transporters that accelerate the conjugation and elimination of thyroid hormones, which triggers a compensatory increase in thyroid stimulating hormone (TSH). T4 is a substrate for UGT1A enzymes, whereas T3 is a substrate for UGT2B2 and an as yet unidentified UGT enzyme (van Raaij et al., 1993; Visser et al., 1993; Richardson and Klaassen, 2010). Induction of T3 glucuronidation, rather than induction of T4 glucuronidation, is strongly associated with a compensatory increase in TSH and thyroid follicular hyperplasia. The PXR agonist PCN induces T3 glucuronidation in both Sprague–Dawley rats and UGT2B2-deficient Fischer 344 rats, which establishes that at least two PCN-inducible UGTs are involved in T3 glucuronidation (Richardson and Klaassen, 2010).

Sustained stimulation of the thyroid gland by TSH leads to the development of thyroid follicular tumors, the development of which can be blocked by administering T4, which blocks the release of TSH and thereby abrogates the hormonal stimulation of the thyroid gland. It is not clear why sustained stimulation of the thyroid gland by TSH results in tumor formation in rodents, but such tumors develop in other rodent organs following prolonged hormonal stimulation: LH causes Leydig cell tumors, gastrin causes stomach tumors, and corticosteroids cause pancreatic tumors. In addition, just as proliferation of the hepatic endoplasmic reticulum and peroxisomes by phenobarbital and Wy-14643 is associated with liver tumor formation, so the proliferation of hepatic lysosomes by Ponceau S and the proliferation of mitochondria by methapyrilene are also associated with liver tumor formation (Grasso et al., 1991).

Epidemiological studies of epileptic patients treated for more than 35 years with phenobarbital or phenytoin have established that chronic liver microsomal enzyme induction in humans does not increase the incidence of thyroid tumor formation (Singh et al., 2005). Prolonged elevation of TSH in humans does not lead to tumor formation but causes goiter, a reversible enlargement of the thyroid gland associated with iodide deficiency and treatment with drugs that block TH synthesis. In humans and monkeys, circulating T4 is largely bound to thyroxine-binding globulin (TBG). This high-affinity binding protein is not present in rodents, for which reason T4 is rapidly conjugated and excreted in bile in rodents. Accordingly, the plasma half-life of T4 in rats (12–24 hours) is considerably shorter than in humans (5–9 days). Similar differences are observed for T3. To compensate for the increased turnover of thyroid hormones, the rat pituitary secretes more TSH. Whereas baseline plasma TSH levels in humans are ~2.2 μU/mL, TSH levels in rats range from 55.5 to 65 μU/mL in males and 36.5 to 41 μU/mL in females (Hill *et al.*, 1989). It is estimated that rats require a 10-fold higher rate of T4 production (on a per kilogram body weight basis) than do humans to maintain physiological T4 and T3 levels. These differences in plasma half-life, protein binding, thyroid hormone metabolism, and TSH secretion between rats and humans are thought to be reasons for the greater sensitivity of rats to developing hyperplastic and/or neoplastic nodules in response to chronic TSH stimulation (Capen, 1997).

Enzyme Induction and Porphyria Due to the increased demand for heme, persistent induction of CYP can lead to porphyria, a disorder characterized by excessive accumulation of intermediates in the heme biosynthetic pathway. In 1956, widespread consumption of wheat contaminated with the fungicide hexachlorobenzene caused an epidemic of porphyria cutanea tarda in Turkey. Another outbreak occurred in 1964 among workers at a factory in the United States manufacturing 2,4,5-trichlorophenoxyacetic acid (the active ingredient in several herbicides and in the defoliant, Agent Orange). The outbreak of porphyria cutanea tarda was caused not by the herbicide itself but by a contaminant, namely, TCDD. Drugs that cause P450 induction have not been shown to cause porphyria cutanea tarda under normal circumstances, but phenobarbital, phenytoin, and alcohol are recognized as *precipitating factors* because they cause episodes of porphyria in individuals with an inherited deficiency in the heme-biosynthetic enzyme, uroporphyrinogen decarboxylase. Studies conducted in mice suggest that the use of flurane-based anesthetics, such as enflurane and isoflurane, which affect heme metabolism, should be avoided in porphyria patients (Sampayo *et al.*, 2009).

Enzyme Suppression The suppression (downregulation) of drug-metabolizing enzymes and transporters is an adaptive process that reduces xenobiotic elimination during periods of inflammation, infection, and postvaccination or in response to certain therapeutic proteins. The phenomenon may be associated with pharmacological and toxicological consequences, especially in case of drugs with a narrow therapeutic index, and it can be a manifestation of a drug–disease interaction. Suppression of xenobiotic-biotransforming enzymes, a consequence of influenza infection, resulted in severe toxicity of theophylline, a CYP1A2 substrate with a narrow therapeutic index. A number of children infected with the influenza virus and receiving theophylline, a prophylactic asthma treatment, experienced convulsions and cardiac conduction anomalies associated with elevated plasma levels of the drug (which increased up to 5-fold in association with a prolongation of plasma half-life from 4 to up to 20 hours) (Kraemer *et al.*, 1982). Suppression of xenobiotic-biotransforming enzymes, as a result of vaccination or treatment with certain therapeutic protein, may cause drug–drug interactions involving a small drug molecule as victim and the biological drug as perpetrator. Blood trough levels of tacrolimus, a narrow therapeutic index immunosuppressant and a substrate of CYP3A4/5, increased by 63% in patients treated with basiliximab, a chimeric monoclonal antibody to the interleukin-2 (IL-2) receptor (Sifontis *et al.*, 2002). Similar effects of basiliximab on the calcineurin inhibitor cyclosporine A were observed in children following kidney transplantation. Within the first 10 days following transplantation, substantially less cyclosporine was required in the basiliximab treatment group than in controls, but it resulted in higher trough concentrations and was associated with liver enzymes and kidney toxicity (Strehlau *et al.*, 2000). The proposed mechanism of these interactions is an IL-2-mediated suppression of CYP3A4. This mechanism is in agreement with CYP suppression initiated by proinflammatory cytokines, such as IL-1β, IL-6,

interferon γ (INF-γ), or TNFα, released in response to infection or inflammation. These proinflammatory cytokines, in turn, modulate expression and activity of transcription factors and specific nuclear receptors determining the levels of CYP mRNA (Morgan, 2009). In the liver proinflammatory cytokines can induce NOS-2 and the increased production of NO can directly inhibit CYP enzymes. Accordingly infection and inflammation can both suppress and inhibit CYP enzymes (Morgan *et al.*, 2008; Zhou and Mascelli, 2011). Therapeutic proteins that are cytokines or cytokine modulators deserve special scrutiny during the drug development process because they can suppress CYP enzymes without stimulating the release of endogenous cytokines. All the major drug-metabolizing CYP enzymes, including the noninducible CYP2D6, are subject of suppression by cytokines (IL-1, IL-2, IL-6, IL-10, IFN-α, IFNα-2b, IFN-β, TNFα) or cytokine modulators (tocilizumab, basiliximab, muromonab-CD3) (Huang *et al.*, 2010). By reversing the disease process—such as lessening the inflammation associated with rheumatoid arthritis—some biologics, for example, tocilizumab (a humanized monoclonal antibody against the interleukin-6 receptor), can reverse the suppression of drug-metabolizing enzymes and restore their activity to normal levels (Morgan, 2009; Schmitt *et al.*, 2011).

CONJUGATION

Conjugation reactions include glucuronidation, sulfonation (often called sulfation), acetylation, methylation, conjugation with glutathione (GSH; mercapturic acid synthesis), and conjugation with Coenzyme A (CoA) followed by conjugation with amino acids such as glycine, taurine, and glutamine. The cofactors for these reactions, which are shown in Fig. 6-51, react with functional groups that are either present on the xenobiotic or introduced/exposed during oxidation, reduction, or hydrolysis. With the exception of methylation and acetylation, conjugation reactions result in a large increase in xenobiotic hydrophilicity and total polar surface area (TPSA), so they greatly promote the excretion of foreign chemicals (see Point 6 in the section "Introduction"). Because of their high water solubility, most xenobiotic conjugates cannot readily diffuse across the plasma membrane; hence, their exit from hepatocytes, for example, generally involves transport across the canalicular membrane into bile (for elimination in feces) or the sinusoidal membrane into blood (for elimination in urine) (see Point 6 in the section "Introduction"). Glucuronidation, sulfonation, acetylation, and methylation involve reactions with activated or "high-energy" cofactors, whereas conjugation with amino acids or GSH involves reactions with activated xenobiotics. Most conjugation enzymes are located in the cytosol; a notable exception is the UDP-glucuronosyltransferases (UGTs), which are microsomal enzymes (Table 6-1).

Glucuronidation and Formation of Acyl-CoA Thioesters

Glucuronidation is a major pathway of xenobiotic biotransformation in mammalian species except for members of the cat family (lions, lynxes, civets, and domestic cats) (Tukey and Strassburg, 2000). It requires primarily the cofactor UDP-glucuronic acid (UDPGA), but can also use UDP-glucose, UDP-xylose, and UDP-galactose. The reaction is catalyzed by UGTs, which are located predominantly in the endoplasmic reticulum of liver and other tissues, such as the kidney, gastrointestinal tract, lungs, prostate, mammary glands, skin, brain, spleen, and nasal mucosa (Fig. 6-52). Examples of xenobiotics that are

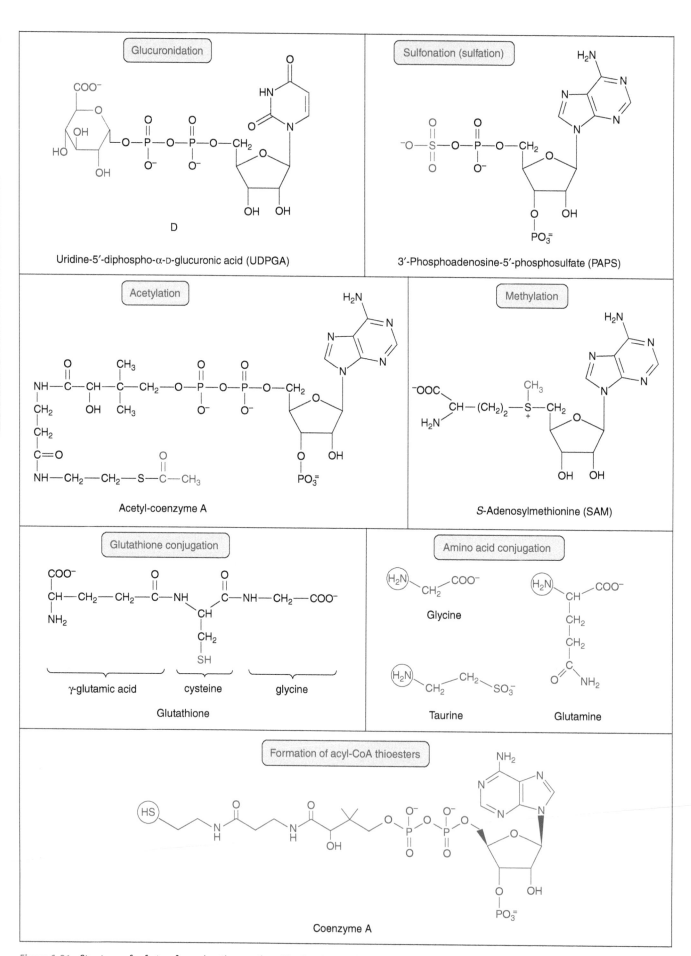

Figure 6-51. *Structures of cofactors for conjugation reactions.* The functional group that reacts with or is transferred to the xenobiotic is shown in red.

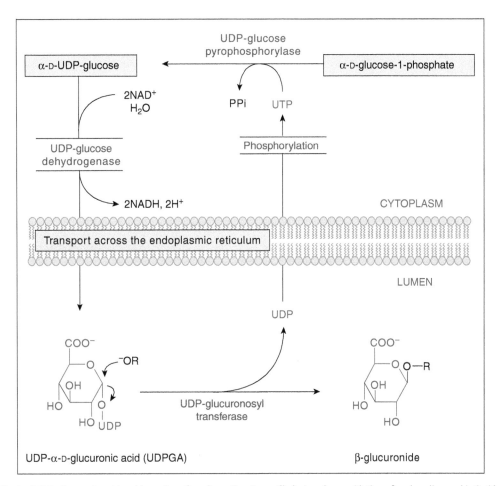

Figure 6-52. *Synthesis of UDP-glucuronic acid and inversion of configuration ($\alpha \rightarrow \beta$) during glucuronidation of a phenolic xenobiotic (designated RO$^-$).*

glucuronidated are shown in Fig. 6-53. The site of glucuronidation is generally an electron-rich (nucleophilic) O, N, or S heteroatom. Glucuronidation reactions mediated by UGTs are S_N2 substitution reactions where the nucleophilic heteroatom of the substrate attacks the C_1 atom of UDPGA which results in a xenobiotic glucuronide in the β-configuration (Yin *et al.*, 1994). Therefore, substrates for glucuronidation are typically small lipophilic compounds that contain functional groups such as aliphatic alcohols and phenols (which form *O*-glucuronide acetals), carboxylic acids (which form acyl glucuronides), primary and secondary aromatic and aliphatic amines (which form *N*-glucuronides), and free sulfhydryl groups (which form *S*-glucuronides). In humans and monkeys (but in few other species), numerous tertiary amines (including tripelennamine, cyclobenzaprine, and imipramine) are substrates for *N*-glucuronidation, which leads to the formation of positively charged quaternary glucuronides, some of which may be carcinogenic (see below in this section) (Hawes, 1998). Certain xenobiotics, such as phenylbutazone, sulfinpyrazone, suxibuzone, ethchlorvynol, Δ^6-tetrahydrocannabinol, and feprazone, contain carbon atoms that are sufficiently nucleophilic to form *C*-glucuronides. Coumarin and certain other carbonyl-containing compounds are glucuronidated to form arylenol-glucuronides.

In addition to the typical conjugation reactions above, UGTs can form unusual conjugates: (1) bisglucuronides (eg, bilirubin and morphine), where two different functional groups on the same molecule are glucuronidated; (2) diglucuronides (eg, 5α-*dihydroxytestosterone; DHT*), where two glucuronides are attached in tandem to a single site; (3) *N*-carbamoyl glucuronides (eg, sertraline and varenicline), where carbonate is incorporated in the glucuronide; and (4) glycosidation with UDP-sugars other

than UDPGA (eg, glucosidation of barbiturates). Two examples are shown in Fig. 6-54. These reactions will be covered in greater detail later in this section. In addition to numerous xenobiotics, substrates for glucuronidation include several endogenous compounds, such as bilirubin, steroid hormones, and thyroid hormones (THs). Table 6-18 provides examples of marker substrates for the major human UGTs. A listing of over 350 UGT substrates is available at http://arjournals.annualreviews.org/doi/suppl/10.1146/annurev.pharmtox.40.1.581 (Tukey and Strassburg, 2000). Reviews by Radominska-Pandya *et al.* (1999), Kiang *et al.* (2005), and Miners *et al.* (2010) also provide extensive descriptions of UGT substrates, K_m and V_{max} values, and specificity of substrates and inhibitors for individual UGT enzymes.

The cofactor for glucuronidation, UDPGA, is synthesized from glucose-1-phosphate, and the linkage between glucuronic acid and UDP has an α-configuration, as shown in Fig. 6-52. This configuration protects the cofactor from hydrolysis by β-glucuronidase. However, glucuronides of xenobiotics have a β-configuration. This inversion of configuration occurs because glucuronides are formed by nucleophilic attack by an electron-rich atom (usually O, N, or S) on UDPGA, and this attack occurs on the opposite side of the linkage between glucuronic acid and UDP, as shown in Fig. 6-52. In contrast to the UDPGA cofactor, xenobiotics conjugated with glucuronic acid are substrates for β-glucuronidase. Although present in the lysosomes of some mammalian tissues, considerable β-glucuronidase activity is present in the intestinal microflora. The intestinal enzyme can release the aglycone, which can be reabsorbed and thereby enter a cycle called *enterohepatic circulation*, which delays the elimination of xenobiotics. In general, *N*-glucuronides are hydrolyzed

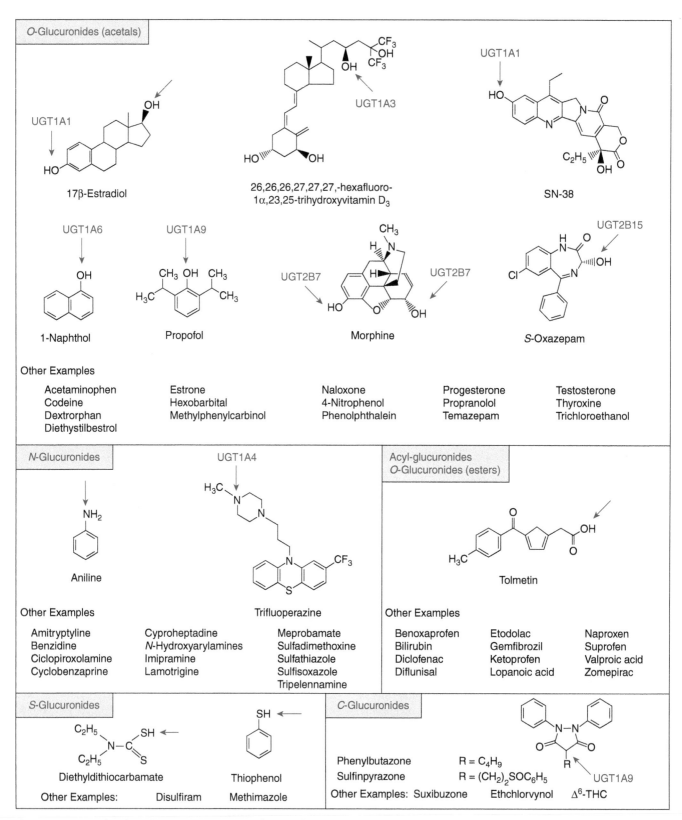

Figure 6-53. *Examples of xenobiotics and endogenous substrates that are glucuronidated.* The arrow indicates the site of glucuronidation, with the UGT enzyme if selective.

relatively slowly by β-glucuronidase (with some *N*-glucuronides being resistant to hydrolysis by β-glucuronidase) but some *N*-glucuronides undergo hydrolysis in acidic conditions (hence, some *N*-glucuronides are hydrolyzed in urine, which can give the impression that the parent compound was eliminated in urine

unchanged). In contrast, acyl glucuronides are stable under acidic conditions; unless the samples are acidified (to pH ~5), acyl glucuronides in plasma and other biological matrices can isomerize or hydrolyze to a significant extent. The instability of *N*-glucuronides under acidic conditions has implications for the tumorigenicity of

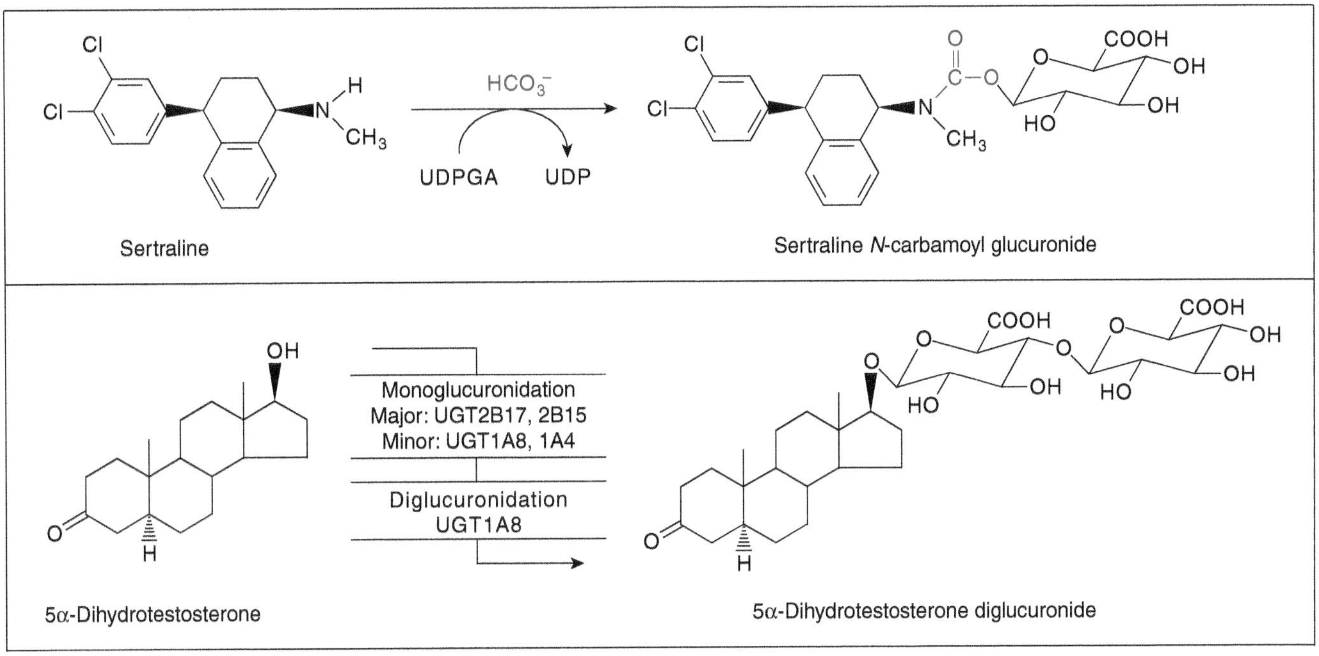

Figure 6-54. *Examples of unusual glucuronide conjugates.*

N-glucuronides of compounds such as benzidine (discussed later in this section).

Glucuronide conjugates of xenobiotics and endogenous compounds are polar (typically anionic with a pK_a of approximately 4), water-soluble metabolites that are eliminated from the body in urine or bile. Whether glucuronides are excreted from the body in bile (following their canalicular transport by MRP2) or urine (following their sinusoidal transport into blood by MRP3) depends, in part, on the size of the aglycone (ie, the parent compound or its unconjugated metabolite). In rat, glucuronides are preferentially excreted in urine if the molecular weight of the aglycone is less than 250, whereas glucuronides of larger molecules (aglycones with molecular weight >350) are preferentially excreted in bile. Molecular weight cutoffs for the preferred route of excretion vary among mammalian species. Yang *et al.* (2009) conducted a statistical analysis of the molecular weight cutoff for biliary excretion of anionic, cationic, zwitterionic, and neutral compounds and concluded that, for anionic compounds, the molecular weight cutoff was approximately 400 and 475 Da in rats and humans, respectively. The carboxylic acid moiety of glucuronic acid (pK_a 3–3.5), which is ionized at physiological pH, promotes excretion because (1) it increases the aqueous solubility and TPSA of the xenobiotic and (2) it is recognized by the biliary and renal organic anion transport systems, which enable glucuronides to be secreted into urine and bile. Furthermore, as anions, glucuronides generally bind extensively to albumin, which, in addition to their large TPSA, confines glucuronides to plasma (although some glucuronides are actively taken up by the liver, as described below).

As discussed above, glucuronide metabolites are often substrates of transmembrane transport proteins that mediate the vectoral transport of conjugates into systemic circulation or into bile for fecal excretion or enterohepatic circulation. These transport proteins efflux the glucuronide either across the canalicular membrane for biliary excretion or across the sinusoidal membrane into the blood for excretion in urine. Transport of glucuronides across the sinusoidal membrane into the blood is mediated largely by MRP3 (ABCC3) and, to a lesser extent, by MRP1 (ABCC1) and MRP4 (ABCC4). The transport of glucuronides across the canalicular membrane into bile is largely mediated by MRP2 (ABCC2) and, to a lesser extent, by BCRP (ABCG2). Glucuronides can also be taken up by hepatocytes through the action of OATP1B1 (SLCO1B1) and OATP1B3 (SLCO1B3) on the sinusoidal membrane (Giacomini and Sugiyama, 2006; Giacomini *et al.*, 2010).

Bilirubin monoglucuronide and diglucuronide, certain steroid conjugates (such as estradiol-17β-glucuronide), and certain bile acids are also substrates for MRP2 and MRP3, although bile acids are mainly effluxed into bile by the bile salt export pump (BSEP). The important role of MRP2 in transporting conjugated bilirubin into bile is evident from the observation that rats deficient in MRP2 (such as TR⁻/GY and EHBR rats) have high plasma levels of monoconjugated and diconjugated bilirubin. In humans, a deficiency of MRP2 also leads to conjugated hyperbilirubinemia, and this inherited disease is called Dubin–Johnson syndrome. When MRP2 function is impaired (due to a genetic deficiency or due to drug-induced cholestasis or bile duct ligation), MRP3 levels increase. In this way, when the biliary efflux of xenobiotics and endobiotics by MRP2 is impaired, their efflux into blood is increased (as if the back door is opened wider when the front door is closed). The upregulation of MRP3 in response to a loss of MRP2 augments the basolateral efflux of drug, steroid and bilirubin conjugates, and certain bile acids during cholestasis. MRP2 can be highly effective at transporting glucuronides and anionic compounds into bile as evidenced by bile-to-blood concentration ratios greater than 1 (and commonly between 10 and 1000) (Brauer, 1959). However, the elimination of drug conjugates in bile may not result in the elimination of the drug in feces because the conjugates may be hydrolyzed in the gut and the parent drug may be reabsorbed or eliminated in feces. For orally administered drugs, the former process (biliary excretion of conjugates, hydrolysis in the gut, and reabsorption of the parent drug) gives rise to the phenomenon of enterohepatic circulation, whereas the latter process (biliary excretion of conjugates, hydrolysis in the gut, and elimination of the parent drug in feces) can give the impression of incomplete intestinal absorption.

The mammalian UGT gene superfamily contains 4 families, UGT1, UGT2, UGT3, and UGT8. To date, at least 22 human UGT enzymes have been identified. The current UGT nomenclature may

Table 6-18

Major Human UDP-Glucuronosyltransferase Enzymes

UGT	PRESENT IN LIVER? (SPECIFIC CONTENT[*])	TISSUE	EXAMPLE SUBSTRATES
1A1	Yes (33.2 pmol/mg)	Liver, small intestine, colon	**Bilirubin, 17β-estradiol (3-glucuronidation), etoposide**, tranilast, raloxifene, ethinyl estradiol, carvedilol, levothyroxine, acetaminophen, SN-38 (active metabolite of irinotecan)
1A3	Yes (17.3 pmol/mg)	Liver, small intestine, colon	**Hexafluoro-1α,23(s),25-trihydroxyvitamin D$_3$, R-lorazepam**, beviramat, 17β-estradiol, zolosartan, ketotifen, naproxen, ketoprofen, ibuprofen, fenoprofen, valproic acid, ezetimibe, chenodeoxycholic acid, norbuprenorphine, tertiary amines, antihistamines
1A4	Yes	Liver, small intestine, colon	**Trifluoperazine, 1′-hydroxymidazolam**, tertiary amines, antihistamines, lamotrigine, amitriptyline, cyclobenzaprine, olanzapine
1A5	Yes	Liver	Unknown
1A6	Yes (114 pmol/mg)	Liver, small intestine, colon, stomach	**1-Naphthol, serotonin, deferiprone**, 4-nitrophenol, 4-methylumbelliferone, ibuprofen, acetaminophen, SN-38 (active metabolite of irinotecan), diclofenac
1A7	No	Esophagus, stomach, lung	Octylgallate, arylamines, 4-hydroxybiphenyl, 4-hydroxyestrone, mycophenolic acid, SN-38 (active metabolite of irinotecan)
1A8	No	Colon, small intestine, kidney	Entacapone, troglitazone, anthraquinone, 8-hydroxyquinoline, furosemide, raloxifene, niflumic acid, ciprofibric acid, clofibric acid, valproic acid, mycophenolic acid, diflunisal, furosemide
1A9	Yes (25.9 pmol/mg)	Liver, colon, kidney	**Propofol, mycophenolic acid, phenylbutazone, sulfinpyrazone**, thyroid hormones, entacapone, salicylic acid, scopoletin, fenofibrate, acetaminophen, ketoprofen, ibuprofen, fenoprofen, naproxen, furosemide, diflunisal, diclofenac, bumetanide
1A10	No	Stomach, small intestine, colon	**Dopamine**, 1-naphthol, mycophenolic acid, raloxifene, troglitazone, furosemide
2A1	No	Olfactory	Valproic acid, ibuprofen
2A2	Unknown	Unknown	Unknown
2A3	Yes	Liver, small intestine, colon, adipose tissue	Bile acids
2B4	Yes	Liver, small intestine	Hyodeoxycholate, estriol, codeine, androsterone, carvedilol
2B7	Yes (84.3 pmol/mg)	Kidney, small intestine, colon	**Zidovudine (AZT), morphine (6-glucuronidation[†])**, carbamazepine, epirubicin, hydroxyprogesterone (6a- and 21-), ibuprofen, ketoprofen, diclofenac, opioids, oxazepam, carvedilol, clofibric acid, naloxone, valproic acid, tiaprofenic, zomepirac, benoxaprofen, other NSAIDs, denopamine
2B10	Yes	Liver, ileum, prostate	Cotinine, imipramine, amiltryptiline, levomedetomidine
2B11	Yes	Mammary, prostate, others	4-Nitrophenol, naphthol, estriol, 2-aminophenol, 4-hydroxybiphenyl
2B15	Yes (61.8 pmol/mg)	Liver, small intestine, prostate	**S-Oxazepam, S-lorazepam**, androgens, flavonoids, 4-hydroxytamoxifen, estriol, entacapone, SN-38 (active metabolite of irinotecan), tolcapone, diclofenac
2B17	Yes	Liver, prostate	Androgens, eugenol, scopoletin, galangin, ibuprofen
2B28	Yes	Liver, mammary	17β-Estradiol, testosterone

Bold text represents selective substrates (or reactions) for hepatic UGTs. These compounds may be glucuronidated in extrahepatic tissues by other UGT enzymes. Data from Miners et al. (2006, 2010), Kaivosaari et al. (2011), Ohtsuki et al. (2012), Kiang et al. (2005), Williams et al. (2004), Fisher et al. (2000), and Court et al. (2008).

[*]*Specific content of UGT enzymes (pmol/mg protein) was determined in pooled human liver microsomes (n = 17) by LC–MS/MS (Ohtsuki et al., 2012).*

[†]*UGT2B7 also catalyzes the 3-glucuronidation of morphine, but this reaction is also catalyzed by other UGTs.*

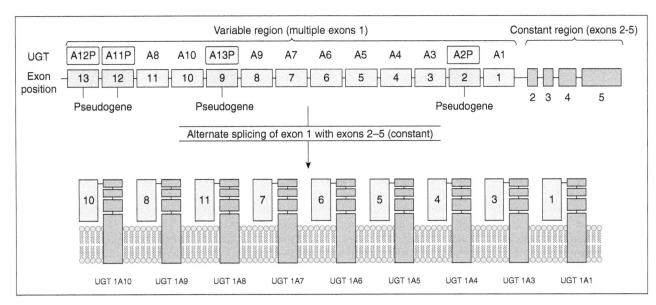

Figure 6-55. *Structure of the human UGT1 locus that encodes multiple forms of UDP-glucuronosyltransferase.* Note that these microsomal enzymes face the lumen of the endoplasmic reticulum.

be found at http://som.flinders.edu.au/FUSA/ClinPharm/UGT/index.html. Families 1 and 2 preferentially utilize UDPGA as the cofactor, but may use other UDP-sugars such as UDP-glucose and UDP-xylose (Mackenzie *et al.*, 2005). UGT3A1 and 3A2 were identified in the human genome, and are ~30% similar to UGT1 and 2 sequences but prefer *N*-acetylglucosamine as a cofactor (Mackenzie *et al.*, 2005; Meech and Mackenzie, 2010). UGT8A1 utilizes UDP-galactose and is involved in the synthesis of membrane components, which is beyond the scope of this chapter.

The major xenobiotic-metabolizing human UGT enzymes are products of either a single UGT1A gene locus (see Fig. 6-55) or multiple individual UGT2 genes (with the exception of UGT2A1 and 2A2, see below). The human UGT1A locus encodes 13 potential UGT enzymes (namely, UGT1A1, 1A2, 1A3, 1A4, 1A5, 1A6, 1A7, 1A8, 1A9, 1A10, 1A11, 1A12, and 1A13), 9 of which are expressed in vivo; the 4 transcripts that are not expressed are UGT1A2, 1A11, 1A12, and 1A13, which are pseudogenes because they lack an open reading frame (Mackenzie *et al.*, 2005). Each of the UGT1A enzymes is encoded by 5 exons, 4 of which (exons 2-5) are the same and encode the cofactor-binding site. Because of the cassette nature of the UGT1A locus, the individual UGT1A enzymes differ in only the first exon, which encodes the substrate-binding site. Because they share 4 out of 5 exons, all the UGT1A enzymes share extensive amino acid sequence identity. The UGT2 genes expressed in humans are UGT2A1, 2A2, 2A3, 2B4, 2B7, 2B10, 2B11, 2B15, 2B17, and 2B28. Human UGT2B24 to 27 and 2B29 are pseudogenes. The UGT2 genes are made up of 6 exons each, which are not shared between subfamily members, with the exception of UGT2A1 and 2A2, and these two genes are >70% similar (Mackenzie *et al.*, 2005). UGT2A1 and 2A2 share 5 exons with a variable first exon, similar to the UGT1A enzymes.

Meech and Mackenzie (2010) reviewed UGT3A expression, function, and cofactor preference (sugar donor). The UGT3 genes expressed in humans are UGT3A1 and 3A2. UGT3A1 mRNA is expressed in liver and, to a lesser extent, in kidney, stomach, duodenum, colon, and testes. UGT3A2 mRNA is expressed at high levels in kidney and testes. UGT3A1 utilizes *N*-acetylglucosamine as a sugar donor and is implicated in the formation of *N*-acetylglucosamide conjugates of various steroidal substrates, such as steroid hormones and bile acids.

The C-terminus of all UGTs contains a membrane-spanning domain that anchors the enzyme in the endoplasmic reticulum. The enzyme faces the lumen of the endoplasmic reticulum, which places UGTs on the opposite side of the endoplasmic reticulum from CYP. As outlined in Point 6 in the section "Introduction," biotransformation of xenobiotics by CYP generally results in a modest increase in TPSA and hydrophilicity; hence, metabolites formed by cytochrome can generally diffuse through the lipid bilayer of the endoplasmic reticulum to access UGTs on the lumenal side of the membrane. The lumenal orientation of UGT poses a problem because UDPGA is a water-soluble cofactor synthesized in the cytoplasm. Several nucleotide sugar transporters (NSTs) have been postulated to shuttle UDPGA from the cytoplasm to the lumen of the endoplasmic reticulum, and they may also shuttle UDP (the by-product of glucuronidation) back into the cytoplasm for synthesis of UDPGA, as shown in Fig. 6-52.

Historically, studies on the ontogeny and inducibility of various UGT enzyme activities in rats contributed considerably to our understanding of the multiplicity of UGT enzymes. These studies predated widespread gene sequencing and genomic analysis and they were reviewed in previous versions of this chapter. Today we know that the genes encoding the xenobiotic-metabolizing UGT enzymes in rats are organized like those in humans: multiple UGT1A enzymes are encoded in cassette fashion by a single gene locus and multiple UGT2B enzymes are encoded by numerous individual genes. Three historical findings in rats are worth noting. First, in contrast to the situation in humans, some of the rat UGT enzymes are highly inducible. For example, AhR ligands such as TCDD and 3-methylcholanthrene cause more than a 10-fold induction of UGT1A6 and 1A7 in rats but not in humans because the human UGT genes lack the XRE activated by AhR. Second, activators of rat PXR, such as dexamethasone and PCN, cause more than a 10-fold induction of a UGT enzyme that conjugates digitoxigenin monodigitoxoside (dt_1), a metabolite of digitoxin (dt_3) formed by CYP3A (see Fig. 6-48). The specific rat UGT1A enzyme responsible for glucuronidating dt_1 has not been identified. Third, all UGT1A enzymes are deficient in Gunn rats. In this hyperbilirubinemic rat, a mutation at codon 415 introduces a premature stop signal, so that all forms of UGT encoded by the UGT1 locus are truncated and functionally inactive. The UGTs known to be encoded by the rat UGT1 locus include the 3-methylcholanthrene-inducible enzyme that conjugates planar molecules such as 1-naphthol (UGT1A6 and UGT1A7), the phenobarbital- and clofibric acid–inducible enzyme that conjugates bilirubin (UGT1A1), and the PCN-inducible enzyme that conjugates dt_1. Whereas Gunn rats are genetically defective in all UGT1A enzymes, LA rats are selectively defective in UGT2B2, which allowed this enzyme to be identified as the principal enzyme responsible for glucuronidating androsterone and triiodothyronine (T_3) in rats (Burchell, 1999).

A summary of the current understanding of the tissue distribution and substrate specificity of the human UGT1 and UGT2 enzymes can be found in Table 6-18. Suffice it to say that these enzymes are expressed in a wide variety of tissues, and some enzymes—including UGT1A7, 1A8, 1A10, and 2A1—are expressed only in extrahepatic tissues, which has implications for the common practice of using human liver microsomes to investigate the role of glucuronidation in drug metabolism. Of the hepatically expressed UGT enzymes, UGT1A1, 1A3, 1A4, 1A6, 1A9, 2B7, 2B10, and 2B15 are considered to be the UGT enzymes most important for hepatic drug metabolism because UGT1A5, 2B4, 2B11, 2B17, and 2B28 are reported to have low or negligible activity toward xenobiotics (Miners *et al.*, 2006, 2010; Kaivosaari *et al.*, 2011). UGT1A7, 1A8, and 1A10 expressed in the gastrointestinal tract may also be important for prehepatic elimination of various orally administered drugs. Numerous UGT1 and UGT2 enzymes are expressed throughout the gastrointestinal tract, where they contribute significantly to the first-pass (presystemic) elimination of numerous xenobiotics. UGT2A1 is primarily expressed in nasal epithelia, whereas UGT2A3 is a polymorphic enzyme expressed in the liver, GI tract, and kidneys (Jedlitschky *et al.*, 1999; Court *et al.*, 2008). Several UGT2B enzymes are expressed in steroid-sensitive tissues, such as prostate and mammary gland, where they presumably terminate the effects of steroid hormones. The tissue distribution of human UGTs (largely based on mRNA levels) and the levels (specific content) of selected UGT enzymes in human liver microsomes (as determined by mass spectrometry) are described in Table 6-18.

Probe drugs have been identified for most but not all of the human UGTs, including UGT1A1 (bilirubin, etoposide, and 17β-estradiol 3-glucuronidation), UGT1A3 (hexafluoro-1α,25-trihydroxyvitamin D_3, *R*-lorazepam, and beviramat), UGT1A4 (trifluoperazine and 1′-hydroxymidazolam), UGT1A6 (serotonin, desferiprone, and 1-naphthol), UGT1A9 (propofol and mycophenolic acid), UGT2B7 (morphine 6-glucuronidation and zidovudine [AZT]), and UGT2B15 (*S*-oxazepam) (Miners *et al.*, 2010; Kaivosaari *et al.*, 2011). The glucuronidation of morphine by UGT2B7 involves conjugation of the phenolic 3-hydroxyl and the alcoholic 6-hydroxyl group in a 7:1 ratio. The 6-*O*-glucuronide is 600 times more potent an analgesic than the parent drug, whereas the 3-*O*-glucuronide is devoid of analgesic activity. UGT2B7 is present in the brain, where it might facilitate the analgesic effect of morphine through formation of the 6-*O*-glucuronide, which presumably does not readily cross the blood–brain barrier and may be retained in the brain longer than morphine (Tukey and Strassburg, 2000). Only UGT2B7 catalyzes the 6-glucuronidation of morphine, whereas several UGTs including UGT1A1, 1A3, 1A6, 1A8, 1A9, 1A10, as well as 2B7 can catalyze the 3-glucuronidation (Stone *et al.*, 2003). Whereas UGT1A4 catalyzes quaternary *N*-glucuronide formation with low affinity, UGT2B10 catalyzes *N*-glucuronidation of tertiary amines with high affinity; consequently, CYP2B10 is primarily responsible for the *N*-glucuronidation of some tricyclic antidepressants (eg, imipramine and amitriptyline) at low, pharmacologically relevant substrate concentrations (Zhou *et al.*, 2010a;

Kaivosaari *et al.*, 2011). Selective probe inhibitors have only been characterized for a few UGT enzymes. Those include UGT1A1 (erlotinib), UGT1A4 (hecogenin), 1A9 (niflumic acid), 2B7 (fluconazole), and 2B10 (nicotine) (Liu *et al.*, 2010; Miners *et al.*, 2010).

Despite their broad and overlapping substrate specificities, some generalities can be made regarding the types of substrates conjugated by certain UGT enzymes. For instance, UGT1A4 and 2B10 are largely responsible for glucuronidating tertiary amines (Kaivosaari *et al.*, 2011). For UGT1A1 and 1A4, the site of glucuronidation is always adjacent to a hydrophobic region of the substrate, with another hydrophobic region 6 to 8 Å from the site of glucuronidation (Smith *et al.*, 2004). UGT1A9 is similar, except that the distal hydrophobic region also contains a hydrogen-bond acceptor (Smith *et al.*, 2004). UGT1A6 prefers to glucuronidate less bulky phenolic substrates. Specifically, rat UGT1A6 enzyme has restricted selectivity toward planar phenols with a molecular thickness <4 Å and a total length of <6.3 Å (Smith *et al.*, 2004). In a series of 24 *para*-substituted phenols, a methyl or ether in any position increased the rate of glucuronidation in human liver (in vitro) compared with phenol itself (Temellini *et al.*, 1991). A hydrogen bond acceptor 10 Å from the nucleophile is common to UGT2B4 substrates (Sorich *et al.*, 2004). The *C*-glucuronidation of the enolic form of phenylbutazone is catalyzed specifically by UGT1A9 (Nishimura and Naito, 2006). Additionally, Sorich *et al.* (2008) reviewed a number of pharmacophores and their importance as determinants in enzyme-specific glucuronidation with in silico modeling.

Kaivosaari *et al.* (2011) reviewed *N*-glucuronidation of drugs and xenobiotics. Historically, UGT1A4 was considered the major UGT enzyme responsible for the formation of *N*-glucuronides of primary, secondary, and tertiary amines but it is now known that several UGT enzymes including UGT1A3, 1A9, 2B4, 2B7, and 2B10 can also form *N*-glucuronides (Zhou *et al.*, 2010a; Kaivosaari *et al.*, 2011). UGT1A4 and UGT2B10 are considered low- and high-affinity enzymes specific for *N*-glucuronidation in liver, especially for tertiary amines, which are converted to positively charged quaternary ammonium glucuronides. In vitro, many tertiary amine substrates, such as imipramine and amitriptyline, exhibit biphasic kinetics with UGTB10 as the high-affinity, low-capacity component and UGT1A4 as the low-affinity, high-capacity component (Zhou *et al.*, 2010a). Many in vitro studies that previously identified other UGT enzymes as key enzymes involved in *N*-glucuronidation may have overlooked the role of UGT2B10 because they employed substrate concentrations several times higher than those observed in vivo. *N*-Glucuronidation can be divided into 4 categories based on the structure of the aglycone: (1) primary amines and hydroxylamines, (2) amides and sulfonamides, (3) tertiary amines, and (4) aromatic *N*-heterocycles. In the case of primary amines, hydroxylamines, amides, and sulfonamides, UGT1A4 is the primary *N*-glucuronidating enzyme, with other enzymes such as UGT1A1, 1A3, 1A9, 1A10, and 2B7 playing a secondary role. In the case of tertiary amines and *N*-heterocycles, UGT2B10 and UGT1A4 are the primary high- and low-affinity enzymes, respectively, whereas several other enzymes have the potential to form *N*-glucuronides with these substrates, namely, UGT1A1, 1A3, and 2B7 (Kaivosaari *et al.*, 2011).

Kaivosaari *et al.* (2011) also summarized species differences in *N*-glucuronide formation based on the structure of the aglycone. Most species are capable of *N*-glucuronidating primary amines and hydroxylamines, although rats preferentially acetylate these compounds. Primary amine *N*-glucuronides are generally labile under acidic conditions and can undergo hydrolysis in urine (discussed in more detail later in this section). There are marked species differences in the *N*-glucuronidation of tertiary amines. Formation of quaternary *N*-glucuronides is observed in humans and higher primates but is generally not observed in rats, mice, guinea pigs, and dogs, presumably due to the negligible contribution of UGT1A4 (a pseudogene in rodents). *N*-Glucuronidation of *N*-heterocycles is variable between species. For instance, the pyridine derivative nicotine is *N*-glucuronidated in humans > rhesus and cynomolgus monkeys > guinea pigs >> undetectable levels in dogs, rats, mice, and rabbit. In most cases, heterocyclic amines form *N*-glucuronides in humans and certain higher primates but are highly variable among all other species, particularly rats and dogs, two species that are commonly used to conduct safety toxicology studies for new drug candidates.

N-Carbamoyl glucuronidation has been reported for relatively few primary amines, or the demethylated metabolites of secondary and tertiary amines, and includes drugs such as sertraline (Fig. 6-54), carvedilol, varenicline, mofegiline, garenoxacin, tocainide, and sibutramine (Gipple *et al.*, 1982; Tremaine *et al.*, 1989; Beconi *et al.*, 2003; Hayakawa *et al.*, 2003; Link *et al.*, 2006; Obach *et al.*, 2006). Marked species difference have been found in the formation of *N*-carbamoyl glucuronides, and humans have only been found to produce these conjugates from even fewer drugs, including sertraline, varenicline, and mofegiline. To form this type of conjugate in vitro, the incubation must be performed under a CO_2 atmosphere, in a carbonate buffer. Although not directly demonstrated, it has been hypothesized that a transient carbamic acid intermediate is formed by the interaction of the amine with the dissolved CO_2, followed by glucuronidation (Obach *et al.*, 2005). Because the intermediate is not stable, the hypothesis that UGT also catalyzes the formation of the carbamic acid cannot be disproved. However, in the case of sertraline and varenicline, it is predominantly UGT2B7 that forms the *N*-carbamoyl glucuronide, which also conjugates various carboxylic acids (Obach *et al.*, 2005, 2006). Given that the in vitro formation of *N*-carbamoyl glucuronides occurs only under special incubation conditions that are not typically employed, it is possible that many other primary and secondary amines or their oxidative metabolites can be converted to such conjugates but have not been detected because of the unusual incubation conditions required to support the formation of *N*-carbamoyl glucuronides.

As mentioned above and as shown in Fig. 6-54, UGTs can form unusual conjugates including bisglucuronides, diglucuronides, *N*-carbamoyl glucuronides, *N*-glucosides, and other glycoside conjugates. Bisglucuronides (ie, a glucuronide in which two separate functional groups on the aglycone are glucuronidated) are more common than diglucuronides, and include the bisglucuronides of bilirubin, morphine, octylgallate, diosmetin, phenolphthalein, and hydroxylated PAHs (such as hydroxylated chrysene and B[*a*]P) (Murai *et al.*, 2006). A diglucuronide is a glucuronide in which a single functional group on the aglycone is conjugated twice resulting in two glucuronosyl groups in tandem (Murai *et al.*, 2006). Diglucuronides of the xenobiotics nalmefene and 4-hydroxybiphenyl and of the endogenous steroids androsterone, DHT, 17β-estradiol, estriol, estrone, and testosterone have previously been detected in dogs. Rat liver microsomes do not form diglucuronides of these steroids, whereas monkey liver microsomes form detectable levels of the DHT, testosterone, and 17β-estradiol diglucuronides, with human liver microsomes forming only the diglucuronide of DHT (see Fig. 6-54) (Murai *et al.*, 2005). In all cases, it is the 2-hydroxyl group of the first glucuronide moiety that is subject to additional glucuronidation. In the case of DHT, only human UGT1A8 (an intestinal UGT) has been found to produce the diglucuronide from DHT itself, although UGT1A4, 2B15, and 2B17 can produce the monoglucuronide, and UGT1A1 and 1A9 can produce the diglucuronide when the monoglucuronide is the substrate (Murai *et al.*, 2006). Human intestinal microsomes form

the diglucuronide more efficiently than human liver microsomes, reflecting the fact that UGT1A8, an extrahepatic UGT, is the predominant enzyme involved in the diglucuronidation of DHT.

Although human UGTs typically are highly selective in the use of UDPGA as a sugar donor, they can accommodate the use of other sugar donors such as UDP-glucose, UDP-galactose, and UDP-xylose in an aglycone-dependent manner, as mentioned previously (Tang and Ma, 2005). For instance, recombinant human UGT1A1 can utilize UDPGA, UDP-xylose, or UDP-glucose to form glycosides, but only with bilirubin (Tang and Ma, 2005). Recombinant human UGT2B7 can glycosidate Compound A [(+)-(5*S*,6*R*,7*R*)-2-isopropylamino-7-[4-methoxy-2-((2*R*)-3-methoxy-2-methylpropyl)-5-(3,4-methylenedioxyphenyl)cyclopenteno[1,2-*b*]pyridine 6-carboxylic acid], an endothelin ET_A receptor antagonist, with UDPGA, UDP-glucose, and UDP-galactose, but can glycosidate diclofenac with only UDPGA (Tang and Ma, 2005). In the case of AS-3201, an aldose reductase inhibitor, Toide *et al.* (2004) found that UGT2B4, 2B7, and especially 2B15 all *preferentially* utilize UDP-glucose over UDPGA. Several other compounds have been found to be glucosidated in mammals, including 5-aminosalicylic acid, bromfenac, pranoprofen, pantothenic acid, hyodeoxycholic acid, mycophenolic acid, sulfadimidine, sulfamerazine, sulfamethoxazole, and various barbiturates (eg, phenobarbital and amobarbital) (Tang and Carro-Ciampi, 1980; Nakano *et al.*, 1986; Arima, 1990; Kirkman *et al.*, 1998; Toide *et al.*, 2004; Picard *et al.*, 2005). In the case of the carboxyl-containing amine, bromfenac, the aglycone was observed in rat bile after base hydrolysis, and it was concluded that it was formed by hydrolysis of an acyl glucuronide (Kirkman *et al.*, 1998). In later studies to characterize the stability of the putative acyl glucuronide, an *N*-glucoside was detected (Kirkman *et al.*, 1998). 5-Aminosalicylic acid is structurally similar to bromfenac in that both NSAIDs contain a primary amine near the carboxyl group, and both are converted to *N*-glucosides (Kirkman *et al.*, 1998). In the human metabolism of barbiturates, *N*-glucosides are the major metabolites found in urine, and glucuronides have not been detected. Accordingly, it was theorized that enzymes other than UGTs may be involved in the conjugation of barbiturates in humans (Toide *et al.*, 2004). This theory is interesting because liver homogenates from cats, which lack UGT activity, can *N*-glucosidate amobarbital (however, it should be noted that glucose conjugates can sometimes form nonenzymatically) (Carro-Ciampi *et al.*, 1985). However, Toide *et al.* (2004) have demonstrated that the *N*-glucosidation of amobarbital in human liver microsomes correlates highly with the *N*-glucosidation of AS-3201, but not its *N*-glucuronidation, indicating that UGT2B15 is probably the predominant human UGT responsible for the glucosidation of amobarbital.

In general, in vivo hepatic clearance is often estimated from kinetic parameters (K_m and V_{max}) determined in vitro with human hepatocytes, liver microsomes or S9 fraction. The process is commonly used for in vitro–in vivo extrapolation (IVIVE). However, for drugs that are primarily eliminated by glucuronidation, these in vitro studies conducted with liver microsomes and, to a lesser extent, hepatocytes consistently underpredict UGT-mediated clearance in vivo (Miners *et al.*, 2010). There are several intrinsic factors that influence the clearance of glucuronidated compounds in vitro, such as: (1) the permeability of the microsomal membranes to allow access of both the aglycone substrate and cofactor UDPGA, (2) the influence of long-chain unsaturated fatty acids released in microsomal incubations, and (3) the homodimerization and heterodimerization of UGT proteins in the ER membranes. Additionally, the kinetic properties of UGTs vary in vitro with changes in the incubation conditions (extrinsic factors), such as the concentration of cofactor, membrane composition, nonspecific binding to microsomes, type of buffer, ionic strength, pH, organic solvents (used for the addition of substrates), β-glucuronidase activity, and the stability of the glucuronide in the incubation buffer (Miners et al., 2010). Many of these extrinsic factors are minimized with appropriate experimental conditions. For instance, cofactor availability is overcome with saturating concentrations of UDPGA, typically 2 to 5 mM. However, Fujiwara et al. (2008) reported that UDP, the by-product of glucuronidation reactions, is a competitive inhibitor that blocks binding of UDGPA. Therefore, for in vitro experiments, the concentrations of cofactor must be maintained at very high levels (up to 20 mM UDPGA) to overcome competitive inhibition of the UDPGA binding site by free UDP produced during the incubation, especially for high-turnover UGT substrates such as 1-naphthol. Other common in vitro conditions for microsomal assays include the addition of the pore-forming peptide alamethicin or zwitterionic detergent CHAPS (described below), the addition of saccharic acid-1,4-lactone to inhibit β-glucuronidase, and the acidification (pH 5-6.8) of the organic solvent used to stop reactions when acyl glucuronide formation is expected (Miners et al., 2010).

In vitro intrinsic clearance (CL_{int}) values (measured as V_{max}/K_m) for zidovudine (AZT) glucuronidation in human liver microsomes were shown to vary 6-fold depending on incubation conditions, but even under conditions that produced the greatest CL_{int}, the in vivo clearance rate was underpredicted by 3- to 4-fold (Miners et al., 2006). This in vitro underprediction of the in vivo rate of clearance of drugs that are glucuronidated is typical when human liver microsomes are used to assess CL_{int}, and is likely due to a number of factors including the presence or absence of albumin, the effects of long-chain unsaturated fatty acids, correction for nonspecific binding, atypical in vitro kinetics, active uptake into hepatocytes, and significant extrahepatic expression of various UGTs (Miners et al., 2010). The prediction of the in vivo clearance of drugs that are glucuronidated by hepatocytes is generally more accurate than predictions made with microsomes, but underprediction is still the common outcome. Zidovudine is an exception to this rule because its in vivo clearance is accurately predicted from in vitro studies with hepatocytes (Miners et al., 2006). The use of either microsomes or recombinant UGT2B7 also underpredicts the in vivo magnitude of the inhibitory interaction between fluconazole and zidovudine by 5- to 10-fold (Miners et al., 2006). However, when 2% bovine serum albumin (BSA) is added to either systems, there is a decrease in the K_i value of 85% which results in a much improved prediction of the in vivo interaction (Miners et al., 2006). The effect of BSA is not due to nonspecific binding but rather the sequestration of inhibitory fatty acids released from membranes during the incubation. The BSA or "albumin" effect is also observed with fatty-acid-free human serum albumin (HSA-FAF) added to incubations. The K_m values of reactions catalyzed by UGT1A9 and 2B7 are markedly influenced by the presence of free fatty acids released from microsomal membranes (notably arachidonic, linoleic, and oleic acids) and albumin serves as a fatty acid scavenger. Similarly, the addition of intestinal fatty-acid binding protein (IFABP) to microsomal incubations decreased the K_m values for zidovudine glucuronidation, a UGT2B7 substrate (Rowland et al., 2009). Unsaturated long-chain fatty acids are potent competitive inhibitors of some, but not all, UGT enzymes and can lead to overestimation of K_m values and, therefore, underprediction of CL_{int}. Furthermore, the effect of fatty acids varies depending on the membrane composition of the enzyme source (recombinant vs microsomes vs hepatocytes) inasmuch as kinetic constants for a specific reaction may vary based on the test system. Unlike UGT1A9 and 2B7, fatty acids have little to no effect on reactions catalyzed by UGT1A1, 1A4, and 1A6 (Miners et al., 2010).

The glucuronidation of xenobiotics by liver microsomes in vitro displays a property known as latency inasmuch as it can be stimulated by detergents (eg, CHAPS and Brij-58) and the pore-forming peptide alamethicin, which disrupt the lipid bilayer of the endoplasmic reticulum and allow UGTs free access to UDPGA. High concentrations of detergent, especially nonionic detergents such as Brij, can inhibit certain UGTs, presumably by disrupting their interaction with phospholipids, which are important for catalytic activity (Fisher et al., 2000). Treatment of microsomes with detergents also virtually eliminates CYP activity; hence, detergents cannot be used to study the possible coupling of oxidation reactions catalyzed by CYP with conjugation reactions catalyzed by UGT. This is not a limitation of alamethicin which does not inhibit CYP. Furthermore, in contrast to certain detergents, alamethicin increases V_{max} without affecting K_m. From a review of the literature, Miners et al. (2006) report that alamethicin and nonionic detergents such as Brij-58 generally result in the highest UGT activity and that alamethicin is the preferred activator because the effects of detergents are not reproducible between substrates. However, in incubations designed strictly to measure UGT activity (and not both UGT and CYP activity), the zwitterionic detergent, CHAPS, can activate certain UGT activities to a comparable or even greater extent than alamethicin.

The kinetic properties of UGTs are possibly influenced by the formation of homodimers and heterodimers among UGT enzymes and by the formation of heterodimers with other microsomal enzymes such as various CYP enzymes, NADPH-cytochrome P450 reductase, or epoxide hydrolase (Ishii et al., 2010). For instance, it has been demonstrated that the ratio of morphine-3-glucuronide to morphine-6-glucuronide formed by UGT2B7 is altered by the presence of CYP3A4. The K_m of UGT2B7-catalyzed formation of morphine-3-glucuronide was increased 9.8-fold (0.38 to 3.7 µM) when coexpressed with CYP3A4 (Takeda et al., 2005; Ishii et al., 2010). Fremont et al. (2005) reported that UGT1A1, 1A6, and 2B7 coimmunoprecipitated with CYP3A4 in solubilized human liver microsomes. If there are functional consequences to the associations between different UGT enzymes and/or the association between UGT and CYP enzymes, then such associations would have implications for studies with recombinant UGT enzymes, which are invariably expressed individually. Additionally, there is historically no universally accepted method to quantify the amount (specific content) of UGTs in human liver microsomes and recombinant enzyme preparation, which precludes a meaningful comparison of rates of glucuronidation between these two in vitro systems as is done with CYP enzymes (through the application of relative activity factors [RAF] or intersystem extrapolation factors [ISEF]). However, advances in mass spectrometry have enabled the quantification of UGT proteins in samples of human liver microsomes and cultured hepatocytes (Table 6-18) (Ohtsuki et al., 2012). The role of heteromeric or homomeric expression of UGTs in vivo is largely undefined. Several publications have investigated the coexpression of UGT enzymes in vitro with cell lines overexpressing various UGTs with mixed results: enhancement of some activities and impairment of others (Ishii et al., 2010). Finally, posttranslational modifications to UGTs that occur in vivo in humans (eg, phosphorylation and N-glycosylation) may not occur in the cell expression system chosen to produce the recombinant UGTs (ie, bacterial systems), which can impact activity in a substrate-dependent manner (Miners et al., 2006). All of these findings suggest that the use of recombinant human UGT enzymes may not provide accurate indications of the extent to which a given UGT can glucuronidate a given substrate.

Glucuronidation can be impaired by cofactor availability, polymorphisms, drug–drug interactions, or the effects of endogenous or dietary compounds, any of which can result in toxicities due to decreased elimination of certain compounds (eg, bilirubin). Cofactor availability can limit the rate of glucuronidation of drugs that are administered in high doses and are conjugated extensively, such as aspirin and acetaminophen. In experimental animals, the glucuronidation of xenobiotics can be impaired in vivo by factors that reduce or deplete UDPGA levels, such as diethyl ether, borneol, and galactosamine. The lowering of UDPGA levels by fasting, such as might occur during a severe toothache or oral cancer, is thought to predispose individuals to the hepatotoxic effects of acetaminophen, although even then hepatotoxicity only occurs with higher-than-recommended doses of this analgesic (Whitcomb and Block, 1994; Rumack, 2004).

Drug–drug interactions that are at least partly due to inhibition of UGTs have been reported. For instance, plasma levels of indomethacin are increased about 2-fold upon coadministration of diflunisal, and in vitro studies indicate that this interaction is due in part to inhibition of indomethacin glucuronidation in the intestine (Gidal et al., 2003; Mano et al., 2006). Valproic acid coadministration increases the AUC of lorazepam and lamotrigine by 20% and 160%, respectively (Williams et al., 2004). In contrast to the situation with CYP enzymes, there are fewer inhibitory drug–drug interactions caused by the inhibition of UGT enzymes, and AUC increases are rarely greater than 2-fold (Williams et al., 2004), whereas dramatic AUC increases have been reported for CYP enzymes, such as the 190-fold increase in AUC reported for the CYP1A2 substrate ramelteon (Rozerem™) upon coadministration of fluvoxamine (Obach and Ryder, 2010). The low magnitude of UGT-based inhibitory interactions is partly due to the fact that most drugs that are primarily cleared by glucuronidation are metabolized by several UGTs. However, administration of drugs that inhibit UGT enzymes, particularly the bilirubin conjugating enzyme UGT1A1, can lead to toxicities by inhibiting clearance of endogenous substrates. For example, administration of the protease inhibitors atazanavir and indinavir to HIV patients is proposed to result in reversible hyperbilirubinemia caused by the inhibition of UGT1A1 (Zhang et al., 2005). Drug–drug interactions due to induction of UGT enzymes have also been observed. Rifampin coadministration increases mycophenolic acid clearance by 30%, and increases the AUC of its acyl glucuronide (formed by UGT2B7) and its 7-O-glucuronide (formed by various UGT1 enzymes) by more than 100% and 20%, respectively (Naesens et al., 2006). Similarly, rifampin coadministration in humans causes a decrease in the systemic AUC of some UGT substrates, including raltagravir (UGT1A1; decreases AUC by 40%) and zidovudine (UGT2B7; decreases AUC 30%–50%) (Gallicano et al., 1999; Wenning et al., 2009). Coadministration of other drugs, such as the enzyme-inducing antiepileptics (eg, phenobarbital), and certain physiological conditions (eg, increased levels of estrogens during pregnancy) can cause an increase of hepatic UGT enzymes and, therefore, the clearance of some UGT substrates. In general, the magnitude of drug–drug interactions due to UGT enzyme induction is less than those reported for CYP-mediated induction.

Human UGT1A6 glucuronidates acetaminophen. This reaction is enhanced by cigarette smoking and dietary cabbage and Brussels sprouts, which suggests that human UGT1A6 is inducible by PAHs and derivatives of indole 3-carbinol, but not to the extent observed in rats (Bock et al., 1994). Ligands for AhR, such as those present in cigarette smoke, induce CYP1A2, which would be expected to enhance the hepatotoxicity of acetaminophen. Increased acetaminophen glucuronidation may explain why cigarette smoking does not enhance the hepatotoxicity of acetaminophen. Conversely, decreased glucuronidation may explain why some individuals with

Gilbert syndrome are predisposed to the hepatotoxic effects of acetaminophen (de Morais et al., 1992). Low rates of glucuronidation predispose newborns to jaundice and to the toxic effects of chloramphenicol; the latter was once used prophylactically to prevent opportunistic infections in newborns until it was found to cause severe cyanosis and even death (gray baby syndrome).

Some glucuronide conjugates have been found to act as substrates for further biotransformation by oxidation or even by further conjugation. For instance, in male Wag/Rij rats, estradiol 17β-glucuronide can be sulfonated by one or more sulfotransferases (SULTs) to estradiol 3-sulfate-17β-glucuronide (Sun et al., 2006). In addition, the acyl glucuronide of 4-hydroxydiclofenac can be formed either by a combination of 4′-hydroxylation followed by acyl glucuronidation or by a combination of acyl glucuronidation followed by 4′-hydroxylation. In the former case, the 4′-hydroxylation of diclofenac is catalyzed by CYP2C9, whereas in the latter case the 4′-hydroxylation if diclofenac acyl glucuronide is catalyzed by CYP2C8 (Kumar et al., 2002). Glucuronidation converts several other CYP2C9 substrates into CYP2C8 substrates or inhibitors. For instance, CYP2C8 catalyzes the oxidation of several glucuronides, the aglycones of which are CYP2C9 substrates, including estradiol 17β-glucuronide and the acyl glucuronides of naproxen, the PPARα/ agonist MRL-C, and gemfibrozil (Delaforge et al., 2005; Kochansky et al., 2005; Ogilvie et al., 2006). In the case of gemfibrozil, the CYP2C8-mediated hydroxylation of its 1-O-β-glucuronide to the formation of a reactive product, presumably a benzyl radical intermediate, that alkylates the γ-meso position of the heme and causes irreversible inhibition of this enzyme (Baer et al., 2009). The inactivation of CYP2C8 by gemfibrozil glucuronide is responsible for drug–drug interactions between gemfibrozil and CYP2C8 substrates such as repaglinide and cerivastatin (Ogilvie et al., 2006). Similar to its inhibition of CYP2C8, gemfibrozil and its glucuronide are inhibitors (and substrates) of the organic anion transporter OATP1B1 on the sinusoidal membrane of hepatocytes. Inhibition of OATP1B1 by gemfibrozil and gemfibrozil glucuronide accounts, at least in part, for the pharmacokinetic drug–drug interaction between gemfibrozil and several statin drugs whose systemic clearance is predominately through OATP-mediated hepatic uptake, namely, pravastatin and rosuvastatin (Tornio et al., 2008). Although inactivation of CYP2C8 by gemfibrozil glucuronide is the only known example of CYP inactivation by the glucuronide of a clinically used drug, Kazmi et al. (2010) identified a carbamoyl-glucuronide of a drug candidate that caused irreversible metabolism-dependent inhibitor (MDI) of CYP2C8 in vitro, the clinical significance of which is unknown.

Glucuronidation is important for the conversion of atorvastatin acid to its pharmacologically inactive lactone form at physiological pH; however, the formation of atorvastatin lactone is also associated with dose-limiting toxicities (Riedmaier et al., 2011). Atorvastatin (Lipitor) is administered as a free acid but is found in systemic circulation at levels similar to its pharmacologically inactive lactone based on plasma AUC. The major cause of adverse events associated with atorvastatin therapy is myopathy (skeletal muscle toxicity) which, in severe cases, can result in rhabdomyolysis and fatal kidney failure. In vitro studies with the acid and lactone forms of atorvastatin in primary skeletal muscle cells established that the lactone form is 14 times more potent than the acid form at inducing cell death. Both atorvastatin acid and lactone can undergo oxidative metabolism by CYP3A4 and CYP3A5 to form ortho- and para-hydroxylated metabolites. Atorvastatin acid also undergoes glucuronidation to form atorvastatin acyl glucuronide. The conversion of atorvastatin acid to its pharmacologically inactive lactone occurs nonenzymatically at low pH (eg, intestine) or enzymatically at physiological pH (7.4); the latter is dependent on formation of the acyl glucuronide

(Riedmaier *et al.*, 2011). The glucuronide moiety is a good leaving group and is lost during the lactonization reaction. Based on in vitro and in vivo studies Riedmaier *et al.* (2010) identified UGT1A3 as the enzyme largely responsible for the lactonization of atorvastatin and further demonstrated that the paraoxonases PON1 and PON3 are responsible for the hydrolysis of atorvastatin lactone back to the acid form. Taken together, UGT1A3, PON1, and PON3 are important determinants of the atorvastatin acid–lactone ratio in vivo and, hence, the potential for atorvastatin myopathy and rhabdomyolysis.

Kumar and colleagues demonstrated that failure to take into account the formation of the acyl glucuronide of 4′-hydroxydiclofenac leads to an underestimation of hepatic clearance of diclofenac. It may also be that oxidation of glucuronide metabolites can lead to toxicity. A case report described the formation of an IgM antibody that bound erythrocytes, but only in the presence of the 4-hydroxydiclofenac acyl glucuronide in a patient who developed hemolysis (hemolytic anemia) during diclofenac treatment (Shipkova *et al.*, 2003). A determination of the absolute amount of diclofenac acyl glucuronide formed in vivo relative to the amount of 4-hydroxydiclofenac formed in vivo would be confounded by the rapid hydrolysis of the glucuronide to the aglycone, and it would therefore be likely that detection of 4-hydroxydiclofenac acyl glucuronide would be attributed to oxidative metabolism occurring prior to conjugation. Two recent reports suggest that direct glucuronidation with subsequent oxidation (by a combination of UGT2B7 and CYP2C8 in humans) may be the major determinants of diclofenac clearance in humans (possibly as high as 75%) and monkeys (>90%) (Kumar *et al.*, 2002; Prueksaritanont *et al.*, 2006), as opposed to earlier in vivo data that suggested oxidative metabolism by CYP2C9 alone is the major determinant of clearance (Stierlin and Faigle, 1979; Stierlin *et al.*, 1979). Prueksaritanont *et al.* (2006) further note that there are no clinical reports that implicate pharmacokinetic interactions between diclofenac and potent CYP2C9 inhibitors or inducers. Taken together, these observations suggest that the CYP-mediated oxidation of glucuronide metabolites has implications not only for the prediction of in vivo drug–drug interactions from in vitro data (ie, gemfibrozil) but also for the prediction of in vivo clearance (ie, diclofenac), and possibly also toxicity, as in the case of immune-mediated toxicity of diclofenac.

In humans, Crigler–Najjar syndrome (type I and II) and Gilbert disease are congenital defects in bilirubin conjugation. The diseases have historically been differentiated largely on the basis of the severity of symptoms and total plasma concentrations of bilirubin (eg, Crigler–Najjar Type I: 310-855 μM, Crigler–Najjar Type II: 100-430 μM, and Gilbert disease: 20-100 μM). The major bilirubin-conjugating enzyme in humans is UGT1A1. Genetic polymorphisms in exons 2 to 5 (which affect all enzymes encoded by the UGT1A locus), in exon 1 (which affect only UGT1A1), in the promoter regions, and in introns 1 and 3 have been identified in patients with Crigler–Najjar syndrome or Gilbert disease. More than 60 genetic polymorphisms are associated with these diseases. A current list of all UGT polymorphisms and phenotypes (when known) can be found at http://galien.pha.ulaval.ca/alleles/alleles.html. Some polymorphisms cause the introduction of a premature stop codon in one of the UGT1A common exons 2 to 5 (which causes a loss of all UGT1A enzymes, analogous to the Gunn rat) and are associated with type I Crigler–Najjar syndrome, a severe form of the disease characterized by a complete loss of bilirubin-conjugating activity and marked hyperbilirubinemia. Type I Crigler–Najjar syndrome is also associated with various frameshifts and deletions in exons 1 to 5, and in at least three cases with changes in introns 1 and 3 that affect splice donor or acceptor sites. Other polymorphisms are associated with the less severe type II Crigler–Najjar syndrome (ie, UGT1A1*7-9, 12, 26, 30, 33-38, 42, 48, 51, 52, 59, and 64).

Individuals with Gilbert disease have an occasionally transient, and generally mild, hyperbilirubinemia that is often caused by the addition of one "TA" segment in the TATA promoter region (ie, UGT1A1*28: $A(TA)_6TAA \rightarrow A(TA)_7TAA$). There is some overlap between Crigler–Najjar Type II and Gilbert disease, not only in terms of the plasma concentrations of bilirubin but also in the type of polymorphism that underlies the disease. In addition to the *28 allele, the *6, *27, *29, *60, and *62 alleles are associated with Gilbert disease, and some of these polymorphisms affect coding regions of the UGT1A1 gene. In addition, the UGT1A1*37 allele produces a $A(TA)_8TAA$ promoter defect that results in Crigler–Najjar Type II. A Korean individual heterozygous for three UGT1A1 alleles associated with Gilbert disease (ie, likely *6, *28, and *60) was found to have total bilirubin concentrations as high as 193 μM (Seo *et al.*, 2007), which is a concentration typically associated with Crigler–Najjar Type II. Crigler–Najjar Type II and Gilbert disease (in contrast to Crigler–Najjar Type I) typically respond to some extent to phenobarbital treatment, which stimulates bilirubin conjugation presumably by inducing UGT1A1. Type I Crigler–Najjar syndrome is also associated with impaired glucuronidation of propofol, ethinylestradiol, and various phenolic substrates for UGT1A enzymes. Polymorphisms that might affect the other UGT1A enzymes have not been thoroughly characterized in vivo, but there are data to suggest that polymorphisms in these enzymes may modify the risk of developing certain types of cancer (Nagar and Remmel, 2006).

The UGT1A1*28 allele has received widespread attention in recent years due to the impact this variant has on the toxicity of the topoisomerase I inhibitor, irinotecan, which is used primarily to treat colorectal cancer. The disposition of irinotecan is complex. Irinotecan (a prodrug) is administered intravenously with hydrolysis to the active metabolite, SN-38, occurring mainly by tissue carboxylesterases, namely, CES2, and hydrolytic enzymes in plasma. The active metabolite SN-38 is subsequently glucuronidated in the liver primarily by UGT1A1 after which the glucuronide conjugate is excreted into bile. Other UGT enzymes that contribute to glucuronidation, at least in part, include hepatic UGT1A6 and 1A9 and intestinal UGT1A7 and 1A10 (Nagar and Blanchard, 2006; Wallace *et al.*, 2010). The UGT1A1*28 variant has now been referenced in the Camptosar® prescribing information, which notes that patients with reduced UGT1A1 activity have a higher exposure to SN-38 (which is 50–100 times more toxic than the glucuronide), and that the dose of irinotecan should be adjusted downward accordingly (Nagar and Blanchard, 2006). The toxicity of SN-38 primarily manifests as severe diarrhea and myelosuppression (in the form of leucopenia, severe thrombocytopenia, severe anemia, or grade 3–4 neutropenia) (Nagar and Blanchard, 2006). Several studies have demonstrated grade 3 to 4 neutropenia and/or grade 3 to 4 diarrhea upon irinotecan administration in patients with at least one UGT1A1*28 or *27 allele, and one study implicated *high*-activity variants of UGT1A7 and 1A9 with diarrhea (Nagar and Blanchard, 2006).

Wallace *et al.* (2010) reported that inhibition of bacterial β-glucuronidase is a potential pharmacological approach to overcome the severe diarrhea associated with irinotecan (CPT-11) chemotherapy. Hydrolysis of SN-38-*O*-glucuronide (SN-38G) by bacterial β-glucuronidase in the gastrointestinal tract releases the pharmacologically active SN-38 into the intestinal lumen where it can be reabsorbed and cause dose-limiting diarrhea. The β-glucuronidase enzyme responsible for hydrolysis of SN-38G in the gut is found in the symbiotic microflora. Wallace *et al.* (2010) identified 4 compounds that potently (K_i values in the nanomolar range) and specifically inhibit *E. coli* β-glucuronidase, but not human β-glucuronidase activity, by targeting a 17-residue loop in the bacterial enzyme that is not present in mammalian forms. Inhibition of

E. coli–specific β-glucuronidase protected mice from the GI toxicity of irinotecan (Wallace *et al.*, 2010). Taken together, these results suggest that β-glucuronidase may be a potential pharmacological target to limit pharmacokinetic or toxicological concerns associated with hydrolysis of glucuronides in the GI tract, which may lead to reabsorption of, and prolonged exposure to, the aglycone.

Polymorphisms have been identified in UGT2B4, 2B7, 2B10, 2B15, 2B17, and 2B28. For example, oxazepam is glucuronidated by UGT2B15, which preferentially glucuronidates *S*-oxazepam over its *R*-enantiomer. Ten percent of the population appear to be poor glucuronidators of *S*-oxazepam, and one study has implicated the low-activity UGT2B15*2 allele as a possible determinant of such variation (Nagar and Remmel, 2006). Such polymorphisms also appear to be the underlying cause of alterations in hyodeoxycholate glucuronidation in gastric mucosa (Tukey and Strassburg, 2000). Glucuronidation of dihydrotestosterone, testosterone, and androsterone by UGT2B17 terminates androgen signaling in prostate and other androgen target cells. The UGT2B17 gene is deleted in some individuals and the role of this genetic polymorphism on circulating testosterone levels has gained importance in many areas, such as sports doping and some instances of an increased risk of prostate cancer, among others (Guillemette *et al.*, 2010).

In some cases, glucuronidation represents an important event in the toxicity of xenobiotics. For example, the aromatic amines that cause bladder cancer (such as benzidine, 2-aminonaphthalene, and 4-aminobiphenyl) undergo *N*-hydroxylation in the liver (*aryl*-NH$_2$ → *aryl*-NHOH) followed by *N*-glucuronidation (not *O*-glucuronidation) of the resultant hydroxylamine. Direct *N*-glucuronidation (prior to *N*-hydroxylation) also occurs, and is a competing pathway of hepatic metabolism. In the case of 4-aminobiphenyl, the competing pathways of ring hydroxylation and *O*-esterification (ie, *O*-glucuronidation, *O*-sulfonation, or *O*-acetylation) are detoxication pathways, whereas *N*-esterification catalyzed by UGTs, SULTs, or NATs represent activating pathways (see the section "Acetylation") (Cohen *et al.*, 2006). Benzidine and 2-aminonaphthalene are particularly tumorigenic. The risk of bladder cancer may increase by up to 100-fold in workers exposed to these substances in the course of their occupation in various manufacturing processes (Al-Zoughool *et al.*, 2006). The *N*-glucuronides of such carcinogens, which accumulate in the urine of the bladder, are unstable in acidic pH and thus are hydrolyzed to the corresponding unstable, tumorigenic hydroxylamines, as shown in Fig. 6-56. Under acidic condition, hydroxylamines can produce highly electrophilic aromatic nitrenium ions (*aryl*-NHOH + H$^+$ → *aryl*-N$^+$ + H$_2$O) that can bind to DNA and other macromolecules, or they can be converted to reactive acetoxy metabolites directly in the bladder epithelium by NAT-mediated *O*-acetylation (*aryl*-NH–O–CO–CH$_3$), which also leads to the formation of aromatic nitrenium ions

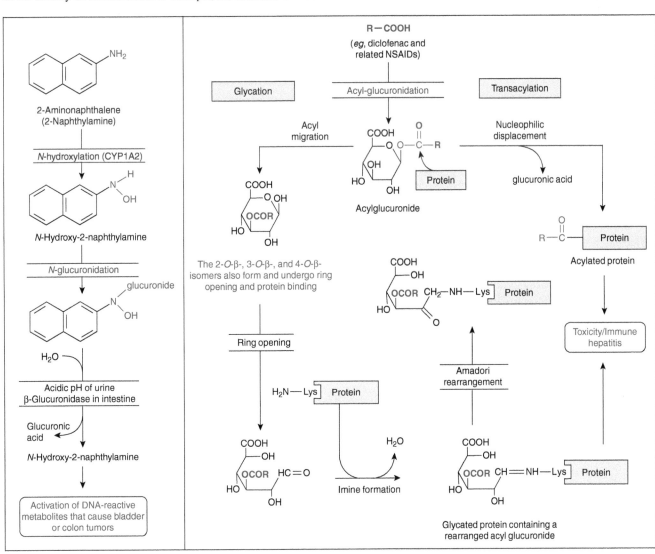

Figure 6-56. *Role of glucuronidation in the activation of xenobiotics to toxic metabolites.*

(Al-Zoughool *et al.*, 2006). Because *N*-glucuronidation of aromatic amines can also occur directly without a prior oxidation, this reaction competes with oxidation, and therefore a decrease in UGT activity in the liver would favor *N*-hydroxylation, with subsequent *O*-acetylation by NAT and spontaneous formation of aromatic nitrenium ions in the liver, rather than the bladder. In contrast, decreased acetylation with normal UGT activity would lead to a greater accumulation of *N*-glucuronides (of the parent aromatic amine and its hydroxylamine) in the bladder with increased bladder tumor formation. Concordant with this scenario, benzidine induces predominantly liver tumors in rats (fast acetylators) but bladder cancer in dogs (poor acetylators) (Al-Zoughool *et al.*, 2006). In humans, there are sex differences in aromatic amine carcinogenicity. Irrespective of ethnicity or race, men are 2.5 to 5 times more likely to develop bladder cancer than women in general, and in particular male smokers, hairdressers, and dye and textile workers who are exposed to aromatic amines have several times increased risk relative to their female counterparts. Male mice, which *N*-glucuronidate 4-aminobiphenyl faster than females, were found during the treatment with this carcinogen to have a 2.2-fold higher rate of DNA-adduct formation, and increased rates of bladder tumor formation relative to females, and female mice were found to have tumors only in the liver (Al-Zoughool *et al.*, 2006). In mice, coadministration of 4-aminobiphenyl with hecogenin, which in humans has been found to inhibit hepatic UGT1A4 (Uchaipichat *et al.*, 2006), was found to increase DNA-adduct formation in a statistically significant manner in the livers of male mice, and to slightly decrease adduct formation in the bladders of both male and female mice (Al-Zoughool *et al.*, 2006). The available literature regarding sex differences in human UGT activity is conflicting. On the one hand, glucuronidation of temazepam, oxazepam, propranolol, and salicylic acid was 20% to 60% higher in men than in women (Al-Zoughool *et al.*, 2006), whereas 4-methylumbelliferone glucuronidation in cryopreserved human hepatocytes was found to be an average of 40% higher in female samples ($n = 33$) than in male samples ($n = 31$). The carcinogenicity of aromatic amines is multifactorial, and involves not only hepatic *N*-glucuronidation but also hepatic oxidation, hepatic and bladder acetylation, and possibly peroxidation of *N*-hydroxy-*N*-acetyl aromatic amines in the bladder (Al-Zoughool *et al.*, 2006). Therefore, sex differences in UGT activity alone may not fully explain the sex differences observed in the carcinogenicity of aromatic amines. A similar mechanism may be involved in colon tumor formation by aromatic amines, although in this case hydrolysis of the *N*-glucuronide is probably catalyzed by β-glucuronidase in intestinal microflora. Aromatic amides (such as phenacetin) can also be *N*-hydroxylated by CYP (and peroxidases) to form hydroxamic acids: $aryl$-N(OH)–COCH$_3$. Under acidic conditions (such as in urine), these can lose water to form reactive nitrenium ions that are thought to contribute to the renal toxicity of phenacetin. The N–OH group can also be conjugated, which introduces a good leaving group. This represents a second pathway to nitrenium ion formation (Testa and Krämer, 2008, 2010).

Steroid hormones glucuronidated on the D-ring (but not the A-ring) cause cholestasis. For instance, 17β-estradiol-glucuronide causes cholestasis in rats by inhibition of MRP2 and BSEP, which are transporters located on the apical membrane of hepatocytes and are important for biliary efflux of endobiotic and xenobiotics and formation of bile (Huang *et al.*, 2000; Stieger *et al.*, 2000). Induction of UGT activity has been implicated as an epigenetic mechanism of thyroid tumor formation in rodents (McClain, 1989; Curran and DeGroot, 1991). Inducers of UGTs cause a decrease in plasma thyroid hormone (TH) levels, which triggers a compensatory increase in thyroid stimulating hormone (TSH). During sustained exposure to the enzyme-inducing agent, prolonged stimulation of the thyroid gland by TSH (>6 months) results in the development of thyroid follicular cell neoplasia. Glucuronidation followed by biliary excretion is a major pathway of thyroxine (T4) biotransformation in rodents, whereas deiodination is the major pathway (up to 85%) of T4 metabolism in humans. In contrast to the situation in rodents, prolonged stimulation of the thyroid gland by TSH in humans will result in malignant tumors only in exceptional circumstances and possibly only in conjunction with some thyroid abnormality. Therefore, chemicals that cause thyroid tumors in rats or mice by inducing UGT activity are unlikely to cause such tumors in humans. In support of this conclusion, extensive epidemiological data in epileptic patients suggest that phenobarbital and other anticonvulsants do not function as thyroid (or liver) tumor promoters in humans (Parkinson *et al.*, 2006).

Earlier in this chapter the metabolic activation of drugs to reactive metabolites was discussed on the basis of structural class (acidic vs neutral/basic) and is illustrated in Fig 6-57. In particular, acidic drugs (eg, NSAIDs) can undergo conjugation by UGTs to form acyl glucuronides and/or conjugation with amino acids through the formation of acyl-CoA thioesters catalyzed by mitochondrial acyl-CoA ligases (see the section "Amino Acid Conjugation"). Both conjugation pathways potentially lead to formation of chemically reactive metabolites that have the intrinsic ability to covalently modify proteins by glycation (acyl glucuronides) and/or transacylation (acyl glucuronides and acyl-CoA thioesters). Reactive acyl glucuronides glycate amine group of lysine residues through Schiff base formation (in which case the glucuronide moiety covalently modifies the protein) and they can also transacylate proteins by nucleophilic displacement reactions (in which case the glucuronic acid moiety serves as the leaving group and is not covalently bound to the protein), as shown in Fig. 6-57 (Regan *et al.*, 2010). Similarly, acyl-CoA thioesters can transacylate proteins at nucleophilic sites (such as lysine, serine, cysteine, and tyrosine residues), in which case the thio-CoA moiety is the leaving group (Grillo, 2011). An important difference between acyl glucuronides and acyl-CoA thioesters is that only the former are transported into bile where they can damage cholangiocytes and other bile duct cells (discussed later in this section). Several drugs, including the NSAIDs benoxaprofen, bromfenac, diclofenac, diflunisal, etodolac, fenoprofen, flurbiprofen, indoprofen, ketoprofen, ketorolac, loxoprofen, sulindac, suprofen (very similar to the diuretic, tienilic acid), tiaprofenic acid, tolmetin, and zomepirac, contain a carboxylic acid moiety that can be glucuronidated to form a reactive acyl glucuronide that can form covalent adducts with proteins. Acyl glucuronides vary widely in their reactivity, from the highly reactive zomepirac and tolmetin acyl glucuronides to the less reactive acyl glucuronides of ibuprofen and salicylic acid (Shipkova *et al.*, 2003). A relationship between the reactivity of acyl glucuronides and the substitution near the carboxylic acid has been found. In general, α-unsubstituted acetic acid derivatives such as zomepirac, tolmetin, and diclofenac exhibit the highest degree of covalent binding, while mono-α-substituted acetic acids such as fenoprofen show intermediate levels, and fully substituted α-acetic acids such as furosemide, ketoprofen, ibuprofen, and suprofen exhibit lower levels of covalent binding (Bolze *et al.*, 2002). The chemical reactivity of acyl glucuronides (as measured by glycation of albumin or a trapping agent such as the dipeptide phenylalanine-lysine) is highly correlated with its rate of isomerization whereby the xenobiotic sequentially migrates from the initial 1-*O*-β position to the 2-, 3-, and 4-positions (which can be in either the α- or β-configuration) (Wang *et al.*, 2004). It is only after the xenobiotic migrates from the 1-position that the glucuronide moiety can transiently open to its hemiacetal form and form a Schiff base with lysine residues. When

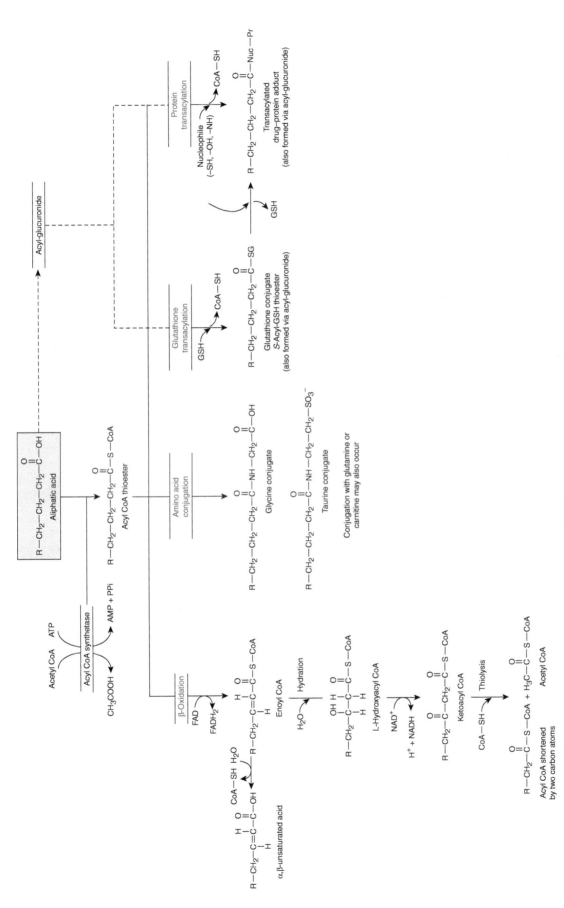

Figure 6-57. *Conversion of carboxylic acid–containing xenobiotics to acyl-CoA thioesters and their subsequent biotransformation by chain shortening by β-oxidation, conjugation with amino acid, and transacylation with glutathione and protein.*

incubated in protein-free phosphate buffer at pH 7.4, those acyl gluc-uronides with a half-life of less than 30 minutes (with the loss of the 1-O-β isomer occurring by a combination of isomerization and hydrolysis) include the acyl glucuronides of the particularly hepa-totoxic NSAIDs zomepirac and tolmetin. Isomerization is slowed by the addition of one or two substituents on the α-carbon (next to the carboxylic acid moiety) which correlates with their reduced toxicity. However, a direct correlation between the ability of acyl glucuronides to give rise to covalent adducts with proteins such as albumin and their ability to cause drug-related toxicity has not been firmly established, and other mechanisms may come into play. For instance, diclofenac is still a widely used drug in spite of the fact that its acyl glucuronide is very reactive, whereas zomepirac, which is less reactive than these other drugs, was withdrawn from the market in 1983 (Chen *et al.*, 2006; Regan *et al.*, 2010).

Neoantigens formed by binding of acyl glucuronides to protein might be the cause of rare cases of NSAID-induced immune hepa-titis. Covalent adducts with proteins in the liver, kidneys, colon, small intestine, skeletal muscle, and bladder were detected in rats administered diflunisal, and in the liver, lungs, and spleen of rats administered diclofenac of UGT activity (Shipkova *et al.*, 2003). Covalent binding of acyl glucuronides to proteins can be selective, with diclofenac acyl glucuronide forming adducts with dipeptidyl peptidase in rat liver, and with aminopeptidase N and sucrase-isomaltase in rat intestine (Shipkova *et al.*, 2003). Human and rat liver UGTs are themselves targets of adducts formed by ketoprofen acyl glucuronide, which may cause nonspecific irreversible inhibi-tion (Shipkova *et al.*, 2003). Both acyl glucuronides and acyl-CoA thioesters can transacylate proteins either directly or after their con-version to GSH adducts. Based on in vitro trapping studies with *N*-acetylcysteine (NAC) as the nucleophile, the reactivity of acyl-CoA thioesters is dependent on the substitution of the α-carbon and β-carbon of the xenobiotic (Grillo, 2011). The addition of methyl groups to the α-carbon and/or oxygen to the β-carbon decreases the reactivity of acyl-CoA thioesters just as it decreases the reactivity of acyl glucuronides. In terms of binding to NAC (an indicator of transacylation reactivity), acyl-CoA thioesters and their correspond-ing acyl-GSH thioesters can be orders of magnitude more reactive than acyl glucuronides, for which reason the formation of acyl-CoA thioesters may contribute to the hepatotoxicity of NSAIDs and other carboxylic acid–containing drugs (Grillo, 2011).

Knights *et al.* (2007) reviewed the ability of acyl-CoA conju-gates of acidic drugs to cause mitochondrial toxicity by interruption of the mitochondrial β-oxidation of fatty acids, which is dependent on their conversion to fatty acyl-CoA thioesters. Xenobiotic-CoA conjugates that are resistant to hydrolysis and are not conjugated with amino acids (*eg*, valproic acid) can sequester the pool of mito-chondrial CoA and disrupt fatty acid β-oxidation, which are key events in the hepatotoxicity of valproic acid. Valproic acid is metab-olized in mitochondria (major pathway) and microsomes (where it is dehydrogenated to 4-ene-valporic acid by CYP2C9 [Fig. 6-48]). In mitochondria valproic acid is converted to an acyl-CoA thioester that in turn is converted to metabolites that resemble intermediates in the β-oxidation of fatty acids, as shown in Fig. 6-57. Valproic acid is present in mitochondria primarily in the form of its acyl-CoA thioester, which is too polar to diffuse out of the mitochondrion. Taken together, these studies suggest that the conversion of car-boxylic acid–containing drugs to acyl-CoA thioesters can play an important role in cell toxicity by causing mitochondrial damage (by depleting CoA and disrupting fatty acid β-oxidation) or by binding covalently to proteins (either directly or following conversion to acyl-GSH thioesters) (Knights *et al.*, 2007; Grillo, 2011).

The intrinsic reactivity of acyl glucuronides and acyl-CoA thioesters is not the only factor that contributes to the toxicity of carboxylic acid–containing drugs and metabolites. Extrinsic fac-tors also influence the potential for toxicity, such as dose/exposure, disposition of the parent drug and its metabolites, hydrolysis of acyl glucuronides in the gut (or even in plasma), and reexposure to the aglycone via enterohepatic circulation, transport mechanisms for the efflux of acyl glucuronides from liver into bile or blood, and, perhaps most importantly, targets of these reactive species. Dose or daily body burden is a concern for many acidic drugs (eg, NSAIDs) because hundreds of milligrams—or even gram quantities—are consumed daily. The reactivity of these metabolites can be assessed with relatively simple in vitro techniques as described above. Intrinsic reactivity can be predicted, to some extent, with structural alerts; the substitution pattern of the α-carbon is particularly infor-mative. Transport proteins also play a crucial role in the disposition of acidic drugs and their acyl glucuronides. MRP2 and MRP3 play critical roles in the efflux of acyl glucuronides into bile and blood, respectively. Shifts in the vectoral transport of these acyl glucuro-nides may dictate whether toxicity is limited to the cells in which they are formed or whether these reactive metabolites enter bile where they can cause damage to biliary endothelial cells or enter the systemic circulation where they can cause damage to other tissues or blood. Just as efflux transporters are crucial for transporting these anionic compounds into blood, uptake transporters (OATPs) are involved in tissue-mediated uptake of acyl glucuronides as well as active renal elimination. Expression patterns of certain transporters may predispose or preclude certain cell types to toxicities caused by acyl glucuronides. It should be noted that unlike acyl glucuro-nides, acyl-CoA thioester metabolites are not transporter substrates and do not leave the cell in which they are formed. This suggests that toxicities caused by acylation of proteins by acyl-CoA thioester metabolites are restricted to the cell where the metabolite is formed (eg, formed in the hepatocyte and causes hepatotoxicity). In the case of acyl glucuronides and acyl-CoA thioesters, the identity of the protein adducted may determine whether or not these acidic drugs are toxic.

Sulfonation

Many of the xenobiotics and endogenous substrates that undergo *O*-glucuronidation also undergo sulfonation, as illustrated in Fig. 6-35 for acetaminophen (Mulder, 1981; Paulson *et al.*, 1986). Sulfonation generally produces a highly water-soluble sulfuric acid ester. The reaction is catalyzed by sulfotransferases (SULTs), a large multigene family of enzymes found primarily in the liver, kidney, intestinal tract, lung, platelets, and brain. In mammals, there are two major classes of SULTs: (1) membrane-bound SULTs in the Golgi apparatus and (2) soluble SULTs in the cytoplasm (Gamage *et al.*, 2006). The membrane-bound SULTs are respon-sible for the sulfonation of glycosaminoglycans, proteins, and pep-tides such as cholecystokinin, factors V and VIII, α-2-glycoprotein, gastrin, and p-selective glycoprotein ligand-1, thereby modulating their structure and function. At least 5 different Golgi-resident *N*-acetylglucosamine 6-*O*-sulfotransferases have been identified in humans. They are important for many biological processes includ-ing cell–cell adhesion, axon function, T-cell response, cell prolif-eration, and modulation of viral and bacterial infection (reviewed by Grunwell and Bertozzi, 2002), but they have no activity toward xenobiotics (Wang and James, 2006). Brachymorphic mice are undersized because the defect in PAPS synthesis prevents the nor-mal sulfonation of glycosaminoglycans and proteoglycans, such as heparin and chondroitin, which are important components of cartilage. These particular sulfonation reactions are catalyzed by membrane-bound SULTs, which are thought not to play a role in xenobiotic sulfonation. This section will focus on the cytosolic

SULTs, which are known for the sulfonation of various drugs, mutagens, flavonoids, and other xenobiotics, as well as endogenous substrates such as bile acids, thyroid hormones, catecholamine neurotransmitters, and steroids.

The cofactor for the sulfonation reaction is 3′-phosphoadenosine-5′-phosphosulfate (PAPS), the structure of which is shown in Fig. 6-51. The sulfonation of aliphatic alcohols and phenols, R-OH, proceeds as follows:

$$R-OH + \text{phospho-adenosine} -O-\overset{\overset{O}{\|}}{\underset{\underset{O}{\|}}{P}}-O-\overset{\overset{O}{\|}}{\underset{\underset{O}{\|}}{S}}-O^- \longrightarrow$$

$$R-O-\overset{\overset{O}{\|}}{\underset{\underset{O}{\|}}{S}}-O^- + \text{phospho-adenosine} -O-\overset{\overset{O^-}{|}}{\underset{\underset{O}{\|}}{P}}-O^- + H^+$$

Sulfonation involves the transfer of sulfonate, not sulfate (ie, SO_3^-, not SO_4^-) from PAPS to the xenobiotic. SULTs are single α/β globular proteins that contain a PAPS-binding site which is present on a characteristic 5-stranded β-sheet along with the core of the catalytic site. The central β-sheet is surrounded by α-helices (Wang and James, 2006). The sulfonate donor PAPS is synthesized from inorganic sulfate (SO_4^{2-}) and ATP in a 2-step reaction. The first reaction is catalyzed by ATP sulfurylase, which converts ATP and SO_4^{2-} to adenosine-5′-phosphosulfate (APS) and pyrophosphate. The second reaction is catalyzed by APS kinase, which transfers a phosphate group from ATP to the 3′-position of APS. The major source of sulfate required for the synthesis of PAPS is derived from cysteine through a complex oxidation sequence. Because the concentration of free cysteine is limited, the cellular concentrations of PAPS (4–80 μM) are considerably lower than those of UDPGA (200–350 μM) and GSH (5–10 mM). This topic has been thoroughly reviewed, and is outside the scope of this chapter (Klaassen and Boles, 1997). The relatively low concentration of PAPS limits the capacity for xenobiotic sulfonation. In general, sulfonation is a high-affinity but low-capacity pathway of xenobiotic conjugation, whereas glucuronidation is a low-affinity but high-capacity pathway. Acetaminophen is one of the several xenobiotics that are substrates for both SULTs and UGTs (see Fig. 6-35). The relative amount of sulfonate and glucuronide conjugates of acetaminophen is dependent on dose. At low doses, acetaminophen sulfonate is the main conjugate formed due to the high affinity of SULTs. As the dose increases, the proportion of acetaminophen conjugated with sulfonate decreases, whereas the proportion conjugated with glucuronic acid increases. In some cases, even the absolute amount of xenobiotic conjugated with sulfonate can decrease at high doses apparently because of substrate inhibition of SULT.

Sulfonation is not limited to phenols and aliphatic alcohols (which are often the products of oxidative or hydrolytic biotransformation), although these represent the largest groups of substrates for SULTs. Certain aromatic amines, such as aniline and 2-aminonaphthalene, can undergo sulfonation to the corresponding sulfamates. The primary amines in cisapride and DPC423 can also be directly N-sulfonated. The N-oxide group in minoxidil and the N-hydroxy group in N-hydroxy-2-aminonaphthalene and hydroxy-2-acetylaminofluorene (NOH-AAF) can also be sulfonated. In all cases, the conjugation reaction involves nucleophilic attack of oxygen or nitrogen on the electrophilic sulfur atom in PAPS with cleavage of the phosphosulfate bond. Table 6-19 lists some examples of xenobiotics and endogenous compounds that are sulfonated without prior biotransformation by oxidative enzymes. An even greater number of xenobiotics are sulfonated after a hydroxyl group is exposed or introduced during oxidative or hydrolytic biotransformation.

Carboxylic acids can be conjugated with glucuronic acid but not with sulfonate. However, a number of carboxylic acids, such as benzoic acid, naphthoic acid, naphthylacetic acid, salicylic acid, and naproxen, are inhibitors of SULTs (Rao and Duffel, 1991). Pentachlorophenol and 2,6-dichloro-4-nitrophenol are potent SULT inhibitors because they bind to the enzyme but cannot initiate a nucleophilic attack on PAPS due to the presence of electron-withdrawing substituents in the ortho- and para-positions on the aromatic ring.

Sulfonate conjugates of xenobiotics are excreted mainly in urine. Those excreted in bile may be hydrolyzed by aryl sulfatases present in gut microflora, which contributes to the enterohepatic circulation of certain xenobiotics. Sulfatases are also present in the endoplasmic reticulum and lysosomes, where they primarily hydrolyze sulfonates of endogenous compounds presumably in a manner analogous to that described for microsomal β-glucuronidase (Dwivedi et al., 1987) (see comments on egasyn in the section "Carboxylesterases"). Sulfonation facilitates the deiodination of T4 and triiodothyronine (T3) and can determine the rate of elimination of thyroid hormones in some species. Inhibition of SULTs can occur with exposure to drugs such as mefenamic acid, salicylic acid, clomiphene, danazol, environmental chemicals, such as hydroxylated PCBs, hydroxylated PAHs, pentachlorophenol, triclosan, and bisphenol A, and dietary constituents, such as catechins, colorants, phytoestrogens, and flavonoids. Adverse effects on human health can potentially result from SULT inhibition, such as the thyroid hormone disruption that occurs with exposure to hydroxylated PCBs (Wang and James, 2006). In contrast, given that some sulfonate conjugates are chemically reactive, inhibition of their formation may be protective. There are a few reports of drug–drug interactions due to SULT inhibition. It has been reported that the sulfonation rates of both acetaminophen and salicylamide are decreased when these drugs are coadministered, and dapsone and lamivudine have been found to decrease acetaminophen sulfonation (Wang and James, 2006). Coadministration of acetaminophen with ethinyl estradiol increases its AUC by up to 54% and decreases the AUC of ethinyl estradiol sulfate by ~40%, indicating that acetaminophen may directly inhibit one or more SULTs (Rogers et al., 1987). Drug–drug interactions involving induction of SULT are detailed later in this section.

Sulfonation may represent a benign metabolic pathway compared with competing pathways that can lead to the activation of promutagens and procarcinogens. For instance, sulfonation of hydroquinones, phenols, and aminophenols can prevent or reduce the formation of reactive quinones, semiquinones, and quinoneimines. Sulfonation of aromatic amines such as 2-amino-3,8-dimethylimidazo-[4,5-f]quinoxaline (MeIQx), which leads to sulfamate formation, can compete with activation by N-O-acetylation or N-O-sulfonation (Wang and James, 2006).

Like glucuronide conjugates, some sulfonate conjugates are substrates for further biotransformation. For instance, the 7- and 4-sulfates of daidzein and genistein can be sulfonated by SULT1E1 to disulfates (Nakano et al., 2004). Other examples include the oxidation of sulfonate conjugates of testosterone and estrogens. Dehydroepiandrosterone-3-sulfate is 16α-hydroxylated by CYP3A7, the major CYP enzyme expressed in human fetal liver (Ingelman-Sundberg et al., 1975; Kitada et al., 1987; Ohmori et al., 1998). CYP2C12, which is expressed in female but not male rats, catalyzes the oxidation of a steroid di-sulfate (namely, 5α-androstane-3α,17β-diol-3,17-disulfate) (Ryan et al., 1984).

Multiple SULTs have been identified in all mammalian species examined. An international workshop approved the abbreviation "SULT" for sulfotransferase (although ST remains a common abbreviation) and developed a nomenclature system based on amino acid sequences (and, to some extent, function). The SULTs are arranged

Table 6-19

Properties of the Human Cytosolic Sulfotransferases (SULTs)

HUMAN SULT	POLYMORPHIC?[*]	TISSUE DISTRIBUTION	MAJOR SUBSTRATES[†]
SULT1A1	Yes *1-*4	Liver (very high), platelets. placenta, adrenals, endometrium, colon, jejunum, leukocytes, brain (cerebellum, occipital and frontal lobes)	**4-Nitrophenol**, 4-ethylphenol, 4-cresol, 2-naphthol, other phenols, acetaminophen, minoxidil, N-hydroxy-PhIP, T2, T3, 17β-estradiol (and other phenolic steroids), dopamine, benzylic alcohols, 2-nitropropane, aromatic amines, hydroxylamines, hydroxamic acids, apomorphine, troglitazone, genestein, epinephrine
SULT1A2	Yes *1-*6	Liver, kidney, brain, GI tract, bladder tumors	4-Nitrophenol, N-hydroxy-2-acetylaminofluorene, 2-naphthol, various aromatic hydroxylamines and hydroxamic acids
SULT1A3	Yes *1-*4	Jejunum and colon mucosa (very high), liver (low), platelets, placenta, brain (superior temporal gyrus, hippocampus, and temporal lobe), leukocytes, fetal liver	**Dopamine**, 4-nitrophenol, 1-hydroxymethylpyrene, norepinephrine, salbutamol, dobutamine, vanillin, albuterol
SULT1A4		Liver, pancreas, colon, brain[‡]	Not characterized. Likely similar to SULT1A3
SULT1B1		Colon (highest), liver, leukocytes, small intestine	4-Nitrophenol, T2, T3, r-T3, T4, dopamine, benzylic alcohols
SULT1C2	Yes *1-*5	Fetal lung and kidney, kidney, stomach, thyroid gland	4-Nitrophenol, N-hydroxy-2-AAF, aromatic hydroxylamines, thyroid hormones
SULT1C4		Kidney, ovary, spinal cord, fetal kidney, fetal lung (highest)	4-Nitrophenol, N-hydroxy-2-AAF, 17β-estrone, bisphenol-A, 4-octylphenol, nonylphenol, diethylstilbestrol, 1-hydroxymethylpyrene
SULT1E1		Liver (highest), endometrium, jejunum, adrenals, mammary epithelial cells, fetal liver, fetal lung, fetal kidney	**17β-Estradiol**, estrone, ethinyl estradiol, 17β-estrone, equilenin, 2-hydroxy-estrone, 2-hydroxy-estradiol, 4-hydroxy-estrone, 4-hydroxy-estradiol, diethylstilbestrol, tamoxifen, thyroid hormones, 4-hydroxylonazolac, pregnenolone, dehydroepiandrosterone, 1-naphthol, naringenin
SULT2A1	Yes *1-*3	Liver (highest), adrenals, ovaries, prostate, jejunum, kidney, brain	**Dehydroepiandrosterone (DHEA)**, 1-hydroxymethylpyrene, 6-hydroxymethylbenzo[a]pyrene, hycanthone, bile acids, pregnenolone, testosterone, androgens, estrone, 17β-estradiol, other hydroxysteroids, budesonide
SULT2B1a (SULT2B_v1)		Placenta (highest), prostate, trachea, skin	Dehydroepiandrosterone, pregnenolone, oxysterols, other hydroxysteroids
SULT2B1b (SULT2B_v2)		Lung, spleen, thymus, kidney, prostate, ovary, adrenal gland, liver (low), GI tract (low)	**Cholesterol**, pregnenolone, dehydroepiandrosterone, other hydroxysteroids
SULT4A1a (SULT4A_v1)		Brain: cortex, globus pallidus, islands of Calleja, septum, thalamus, red nucleus, substantia nigra and pituitary	Endogenous: 4 unidentified compounds from mouse brain homogenate[§] Other: T3, T4, estrone, 4-nitrophenol, 2-naphthylamine, 2-naphthol[**]
SULT4A1b (SULT4A_v2)			
SULT6B1		Testis	

Substrates in bold are reported to be selective probe substrates for the SULT listed (Coughtrie and Fisher, 2003). Data from Coughtrie and Fisher (2003), Lindsay et al. (2008), Riches et al. (2009), Salman et al. (2009), Gamage et al. (2006), Wang and James (2006), and Blanchard et al. (2004).
[*]*Data from Lindsay et al. (2008).*
[†]*T4 is thyroxine. T2 and T3 are diiodothyronine and triiodothyronine. r-T3 is reverse triiodothyronine.*
[‡]*Data from Bradley and Benner (2005).*
[§]*Sakakibara et al. (2002) reported that recombinant human SULT4A1 expressed in E. coli (and subsequently purified) sulfonated 4 distinct endogenous substances from mouse brain homogenate.*
[**]*Sakakibara et al. (2002) reported that recombinant human SULT4A1 expressed in E. coli (and subsequently purified) sulfonated these prototypical SULT substrates.*

into gene families that share at least 45% amino acid sequence identity. The 9 gene families identified to date (vertebrate: SULT1-SULT6; insect: SULT101; and plant: SULT201-SULT202) are subdivided into subfamilies that are at least 60% identical (Blanchard et al., 2004; Gamage et al., 2006). For example, SULT1 is divided into 5 subfamilies designated SULT1A to SULT1E. Two SULTs that share more than 60% similarity are considered individual members of the same subfamily. For example, SULT1A1, SULT1A2, SULT1A3, and SULT1A4 are four individual members of the human SULT1A subfamily. In general, the first published sequence in a subfamily is designated as enzyme 1 and subsequent enzymes within that subfamily are assigned on the basis of percentage amino acid identity relative to the "1" enzyme (Blanchard et al., 2004). Exceptions to this rule have been made to maintain historical use of a name (eg, SULT2A1). Variant forms with different amino acid sequences encoded by the same gene are designated by "vn" at the end. For instance, the SULTs initially referenced as SULT2B1a and SULT2B1b are now called SULT2B1_v1 and SULT2B1_v2. Although 9 SULT gene families have been identified, these have not been identified in all mammalian species. Currently, SULT1 and SULT2 are the only gene families subdivided into multiple subfamilies (5 in the case of SULT1 [SULT1A-1E]; two in the case of SULT2 [SULT2A and SULT2B]).

Most of the SULTs cloned belong to one of the two families, SULT1 and SULT2. These two families are functionally different; the SULT1 enzymes catalyze the sulfonation of phenols, isoflavones, the procarcinogen N-OH-2-acetylaminofluorene, endogenous compounds such as 17β-estradiol (including its glucuronide conjugate; see the section "Glucuronidation and Formation of Acyl-CoA Thioesters"), and other steroids, iodothyronines, endogenous catecholamines, and eicosanoids. The SULT2 enzymes catalyze the sulfonation of the 3β-hydroxy groups of steroids with unsaturated A rings, bile acids, benzylic alcohols of PAHs, and other primary and secondary alcohols. A SULT that catalyzes the sulfonation of heterocyclic amines such as 2-naphthylamine, desipramine, and aniline (to form sulfamates) has been cloned from rabbit and mouse (SULT3A1).

SULT4A1 has been identified in rat, mouse, and human. These enzymes are expressed in the cerebral cortex, cerebellum, pituitary, and brainstem and do not sulfonate typical SULT substrates (Blanchard et al., 2004; Gamage et al., 2006). These SULTs share ~97% amino acid sequence identity across species, which suggests that SULT4A1 likely serves a critical endogenous function. The SULT4A1 sequence has also been identified as SULT5A1, but the 4A1 nomenclature has been retained. A separate gene, SULT5A1, has been cloned from mouse, but no information on its function is available. SULT6A1 has been cloned from chicken liver, and the recombinant enzyme was found to sulfonate 17β-estradiol and corticosterone (Blanchard et al., 2004). SULT6B1 has been cloned from human testis (Freimuth et al., 2004). SULT201 and 202 represent two families of plant SULTs. SULTT101A1 is an insect SULT cloned from Spodoptera frugiperda and converts retinol to anhydroretinol via a retinyl sulfate intermediate (Blanchard et al., 2004). SULT101A also exhibits SULT activity toward ethanol, dopamine, vanillin, 4-nitrophenol, serotonin, and hydroxybenzylhydrazine (Blanchard et al., 2004). Thirteen cytosolic SULTs have been cloned from rat, and they belong to the SULT1, SULT2, or SULT4 gene families. The individual rat enzymes are SULT1A1, 1B1, 1C1, 1C2, 1C3, 1D1, 1E1, 1E2, 2A1, 2A2, 2A3, 2A4, and 4A1.

Eleven genes encoding 13 cytosolic SULTs have been identified in humans, and they belong to the SULT1, SULT2, or SULT4 gene families. The individual human enzymes are listed in Table 6-19. Various SNPs have been reported in most of the SULT genes with rare single-base deletions in SULT1A2 and 4A1 (Glatt and Meinl,

2004a). With a few exceptions, the functional consequences of most of these polymorphisms remain unknown. Several of the human SULT genes have multiple initiation sites for transcription, which produces different mRNA transcripts. Consequently, in some cases, different versions of the same human SULT gene have been cloned several times. For example, there are 3 alternative first exons (exons 1a, 1b, and 1c) in the human SULT1A3 gene (none of which contains a coding region), and 5 SULT1A3 cDNAs have been cloned from various human tissues, each with a unique 5'-region (Nagata and Yamazoe, 2000).

Riches et al. (2009) quantified 5 of the major SULT enzymes (SULT1A1, 1B1, 1E1, 2A1, and 1A3) in human liver, small intestine, kidney, and lung cytosol with quantitative immunoblotting techniques. In human liver cytosol, the rank order of protein expression was as follows: SULT1A1 (53%) > 2A1 (27%) > 1B1 (14%) > 1E1 (6%) > 1A3 (0%). Kidney was similar to liver inasmuch as SULT1A1 was the major enzyme expressed (40%), followed by SULT1B1 (31%) > 1A3 (28%) > 2A1 (1%) > 1E1 (0%). In the small intestine, SULT1B1 and 1A3 were most highly expressed enzymes (36% and 31%, respectively), followed by SULT1A1 (19%) > 1E1 (8%) > 2A1 (6%). Lastly, SULT1E1 protein was most highly expressed in lung (40%), followed by SULT1A1 (20%) > 1A3 (19%) > 1B1 (12%) > 2A1 (9%). Further details on the tissue expression of SULTs are summarized in Table 6-19.

Historically, human liver cytosol was found to contain two phenol SULT activities (PST) that could be distinguished by their thermal stability; hence, they were known as TS-PST (thermally stable) and TL-PST (thermally labile) (Weinshilboum, 1992a; Weinshilboum et al., 1997). It is now known that TS-PST actually reflects the activity of two SULTs, namely, SULT1A1 and SULT1A2, which share 93% identity, whereas TL-PST reflects the activity of SULT1A3 (and likely SULT1A4), which is 60% similar to both SULT1A1 and 2 (Gamage et al., 2006). Hence, the 4 members of the SULT1A gene subfamily in human were represented functionally by TS-PST and TL-PST activity. SULT1A1 and SULT1A2 function as homodimers and heterodimers, and are coregulated. Although these two individual SULTs are not catalytically identical, they are sufficiently similar to consider them as the single activity traditionally known as TS-PST. Because of differences in their substrate specificity, SULT1A1/2 and 1A3 were also known as phenol-PST and monoamine-PST, respectively. SULT1A3 preferentially catalyzes the sulfonation of catecholamines such as dopamine, epinephrine, and levodopa, whereas SULT1A1 and 1A2 preferentially catalyze the sulfonation of simple phenols, such as phenol, 4-nitrophenol, minoxidil, and acetaminophen. SULT1A1 and 1A2 also catalyze the N-sulfonation of 2-aminonaphthalene. SULT1A1/2 and SULT1A3 can also be distinguished by differences in their sensitivity to the inhibitory effects of 2,6-dichloro-4-nitrophenol.

The expression of SULT1A1 and 1A2 in human liver is largely determined by genetic factors, which also determines the corresponding SULT activity in blood platelets. Inherited variation in platelet SULT1A1 and 1A2 largely reflects genetic polymorphisms in these enzymes. One allelic variant of SULT1A1 known as SULT1A1*2 ($Arg_{213} \rightarrow His_{213}$) is associated with decreased activity in platelets but not liver, and decreased thermal stability (Glatt and Meinl, 2004a). This particular genetic polymorphism is common in both Caucasians and Nigerians (with an allele frequency of 31% and 37%, respectively), and is correlated with interindividual variation in the sulfonation of acetaminophen. Low SULT1A1 and 1A2 activity predisposes individuals to diet-induced migraine headaches, possibly due to impaired sulfonation of unidentified phenolic compounds in the diet that cause such headaches. Interestingly, SULT1A1 has been implicated in the pharmacological effect of tamoxifen by sulfonation of the 4-hydroxymetabolite, which was shown to be a potent inducer of apoptosis in certain breast cancer cell lines. Contrary to expectation, the lower activity SULT1A1*2 allele did not improve the efficacy of tamoxifen in breast cancer patients by decreasing clearance of 4-hydroxytamoxifen. It was the wild-type allele that, paradoxically, was correlated with improved outcomes with tamoxifen therapy (Nowell and Falany, 2006). A fourth member of the human SULT1A subfamily, SULT1A4, has been described, which appears to be a duplication of SULT1A3, and these two enzymes share >99% sequence identity (Bradley and Benner, 2005; Gamage et al., 2006). The genes for both of these SULTs lie on chromosome 16p, which contains a segmental duplication that results in two nearly identical, transcriptionally active copies of SULT1A3 and SULT1A4. Each

copy shares exons with an adjacent copy of SULT1A1. Four nonsynonymous SNPs were reported for these genes, which show different enzyme activities (Gamage et al., 2006).

Human SULT1B1, like the corresponding enzyme in other species, catalyzes the sulfonation of thyroid hormones, 2-naphthol, and dopamine. SULT1B1 levels in human liver cytosol vary widely, possibly due to polymorphisms (eg, $Glu_{186} \rightarrow Gly_{186}$ and $Glu_{204} \rightarrow Asp_{204}$) (Glatt and Meinl, 2004a). SULT1B1 is also expressed in human colon, small intestine, and blood leukocytes. Humans have two SULT1C enzymes (SULT1C2 and SULT1C4). Their function has not been determined, although the corresponding rat enzyme (SULT1C1) catalyzes the sulfonation of NOH-AAF (see Fig. 6-58). SULT1C2 is expressed at high levels in the thyroid, stomach, and

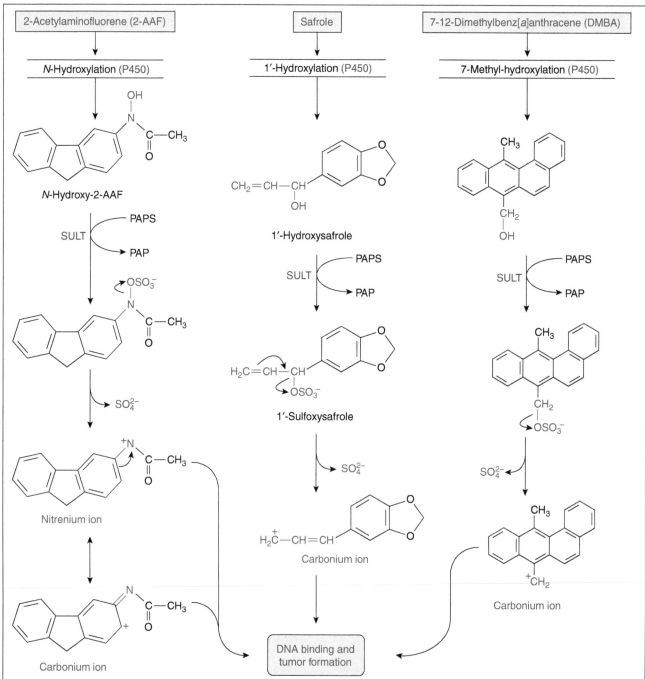

Figure 6-58. Role of sulfonation in the generation of tumorigenic metabolites (nitrenium or carbonium ions) of 2-acetylaminofluorene, safrole, and 7,12-dimethylbenz[a]anthracene (DMBA).

kidneys (Blanchard *et al.*, 2004). High levels of SULT1C4 are expressed in fetal liver and kidney, with hepatic levels declining in adulthood, but it is also present in adult ovary and brain.

Human SULT1E1 has been identified as a high-affinity estrogen SULT. SULT1A1 also catalyzes the sulfonation of estrogens, such as 17β-estradiol, but it does so with a much lower affinity than does SULT1E1. The sulfonation of ethinyl estradiol in human hepatocytes is inducible by rifampin (Li *et al.*, 1999), which raises the possibility that SULT1E1 is an inducible enzyme. In addition to human liver, SULT1E1 is expressed in placenta, breast, brain, testes, adrenal glands, and uterine tissue. SULT1E1 has been studied in SULT1E1-deficient mice, and it was shown that these mice had spontaneous fetal loss caused by placental thrombosis, which was reversible by administration of antiestrogens (Gamage *et al.*, 2006).

SULT2A1 is the human alcohol SULT, long known as DHEA-ST (for its ability to sulfonate dehydroepiandosterone [DHEA]). In addition to DHEA, substrates for SULT2A1 include steroid hormones, bile acids, and cholesterol. Furthermore, SULT2A1 converts several procarcinogens to electrophilic metabolites, including hydroxymethyl PAHs, NOH-AAF, and 1-hydroxysafrole, as shown in Fig. 6-58. The thermal stability of SULT2A1 is intermediate between that of the 4 phenol SULTs (SULT1A1/2 and 1A3/4), and the enzyme is resistant to the inhibitory effects of 2,6-dichloro-4-nitrophenol. In humans, SULT2A1 selectively catalyzes the *N*-sulfonation of quinolone drugs, such as ciprofloxacin, moxifloxacin, garenoxacin, and other amine drugs such as desipramine and metoclopramide (Senggunprai *et al.*, 2009). SULT2A1 is not expressed in blood platelets, but the activity of this enzyme has been measured in human liver cytosol. It is also expressed in adrenal cortex, brain, and intestine (Blanchard *et al.*, 2004). SULT2A1 is bimodally distributed, possibly due to a genetic polymorphism that apparently lies outside of the coding region, and perhaps outside of the SULT2A1 gene itself, with a high-activity group composed of ~25% of the population (Glatt and Meinl, 2004a). Several SULT2A1 SNPs have been identified, but the underlying basis for the high-activity group remains to be determined as these polymorphisms appear to be too rare to explain the bimodal distribution.

Human SULT2B1 is also a DHEA-sulfotransferase. It is expressed in placenta, prostate, and trachea. The SULT2B1 gene can be transcribed from one of the two exons, both of which contain coding sequences; hence, two forms of SULT2B1 (known as 2B1_v1 and 2B1_v2) with different N-terminal amino acid sequences can be transcribed by alternate splicing of precursor mRNA. This situation is analogous to the alternative splicing of multiple exons 1 in the UGT1 gene family (see Fig. 6-55). SULT2B1_v1 catalyzes the sulfonation of pregnenolone, and SULT2B1_v2 can catalyze the sulfonation of both pregnenolone and cholesterol (Blanchard *et al.*, 2004).

The SULT enzymes were previously categorized into 5 classes based on their catalytic activity. These 5 functional classes were: *arylsulfotransferase*, which sulfonates numerous phenolic xenobiotics; *alcohol SULT*, which sulfonates primary and secondary alcohols including nonaromatic hydroxysteroids (for which reason these enzymes are also known as hydroxysteroid SULTs); *estrogen SULT*, which sulfonates estrone and other aromatic hydroxysteroids; *tyrosine ester SULT*, which sulfonates tyrosine methyl ester and 2-cyanoethyl-*N*-hydroxythioacetamide; and *bile salt SULT*, which sulfonates conjugated and unconjugated bile acids. The *arylsulfotransferase* and *estrogen SULT* are composed largely of SULT1 enzymes, which catalyze the sulfonation of phenolic xenobiotics, catechols, and aromatic (phenolic) steroids. The *alcohol SULT* and *bile salt SULT* are composed largely of SULT2 enzymes,

which catalyze the sulfonation of a variety of primary and secondary alcohols, bile acids, and hydroxysteroids (such as DHEA).

In rats, SULT activity varies considerably with sex and age. In mature rats, phenol SULT activity (SULT1A activity) is higher in males, whereas alcohol SULT and bile acid SULT activities (SULT2 activities) are higher in females. Sex differences in the developmental expression of individual SULTs are the result of a complex interplay between gonadal, thyroidal, and pituitary hormones (particularly growth hormone), which similarly determine sex differences in CYP enzyme expression. However, compared with CYP enzymes, the SULTs are refractory or only marginally responsive to the enzyme-inducing effects of AhR and CAR activators such as 3-methylcholanthrene and phenobarbital, respectively, although one or more individual SULT2 enzymes are inducible by PXR agonists such as PCN. Likewise, SULT1A1, 2A1, or 2E1 expressed in Caco-2 cells are refractory to various PAHs, and 3-methylcholanthrene has no effect on SULT1A1 and 1A3 mRNA levels in primary human hepatocytes (Gamage *et al.*, 2006). From rodent studies, it is generally held that AhR agonists have suppressive effects on SULT regulation. 2-AAF, TCDD, 3-methylcholanthrene, and β-naphthoflavone markedly suppress SULT1A1 and 2A activities and mRNA levels in rat livers (Gamage *et al.*, 2006). In contrast, there is evidence that the rat liver hydroxysteroid SULTs (SULT2s) may be inducible by tamoxifen and estrogens (Gamage *et al.*, 2006). For mouse SULT2A2, a functional nuclear response element responsive for CAR has been reported (Gamage *et al.*, 2006). Human SULT2A1 has been reported to be regulated by FXR, PXR, VDR, and PPARα, whereas SULT1A1, 2A1, and 2A9 genes in mice are regulated by CAR (Tirona and Kim, 2005; Gamage *et al.*, 2006). There are conflicting data regarding the influence of CAR ligands on SULT1A1 and 1A3. One study reports an 11-fold increase in SULT1A1 mRNA in primary human hepatocytes by the CAR ligand, CITCO, whereas another study could not reproduce these results for either SULT1A1 or 1A3 (Gamage *et al.*, 2006). The glucocorticoid dexamethasone has been reported to induce both murine and human SULT2A1 through PXR and GR activation (Gamage *et al.*, 2006). Human SULT2A1 mRNA and protein have also been reported to be induced by rifampin, vitamin D_3, phenobarbital, TCPOBOP, and the PPARα-agonist, ciprofibrate (Runge-Morris and Kocarek, 2005).

Induction of SULTs by rifampin, on the other hand, may be clinically relevant. Rifampin (600 mg q.d.) has been reported to cause up to a 190% increase in the clearance of ethinyl estradiol (35 μg q.d.) (Barditch-Crovo *et al.*, 1999). The interaction between ethinyl estradiol–containing oral contraceptives and antibiotics such as rifampin is often attributed to the induction of CYP3A4, which is the major CYP involved in the *oxidative* metabolism of ethinyl estradiol (eg, Ortho-Evra® prescribing information). Several lines of evidence suggest that induction of CYP3A4 is not the predominant mechanism by which rifampin increases the clearance of ethinyl estradiol. First, Li *et al.* (1999) reported that treatment of primary cultures of human hepatocytes with rifampin (33.3 μM) caused up to a 3.3-fold increase in ethinyl estradiol 3-*O*-sulfate formation. Second, SULTs 1A1, 1A2, 1A3, 1E1, and 2A1 catalyze the 3-*O*-sulfonation of ethinyl estradiol with K_m values ranging from 6.7 to 4500 nM, nearer the pharmacologically relevant concentrations (Schrag *et al.*, 2004). Finally, it is known that ethinyl estradiol is predominantly excreted in bile and urine as the 3-sulfate and, to a lesser extent, the 3-glucuronide (Li *et al.*, 1999), which suggests that 3-sulfonation is the major pathway of ethinyl estradiol metabolism. Taken together, these data suggest that induction of SULTs can be clinically relevant at least for low-dose drugs that can be sulfonated with high affinity.

Extrapolation of animal data with regard to biotransformation by SULTs is confounded by the number of SULTs, the expression pattern of SULTs, and pronounced sexual dimorphisms in many rodents (Gamage *et al.*, 2006). For instance, expression of SULTs in humans is largely extrahepatic, whereas SULT expression in rodents is predominantly hepatic. For instance, based on RT-PCR measurements of mRNA levels in human tissues, SULT1A3 is expressed at the greatest level in the small intestine, 1B1 in the colon, 2B1 in the placenta, and 4A1 in the brain (Nishimura and Naito, 2006). Of the SULTs that have been characterized by RT-PCR in various human tissues, only SULT1A1, 1E1, and 2A1 are predominantly expressed in the liver (Nishimura and Naito, 2006).

Additionally, humans have 4 members of the SULT1A subfamily, whereas rodents have only one. In contrast, rats have 4 members of the SULT2A subfamily, whereas humans have only a single SULT2A gene. Human equivalents of mouse SULT3A1 and 5A1 have not yet been identified in humans (Gamage *et al.*, 2006). There are also significant differences between other mammalian species. For instance, SULT activity is low in pigs but high in cats. The high SULT activity in cats offsets their low capacity to conjugate xenobiotics with glucuronic acid.

In general, sulfonation is an effective means of decreasing the pharmacological and toxicological activity of xenobiotics. There are cases, however, in which sulfonation increases the toxicity of foreign chemicals because certain sulfonate conjugates are chemically unstable and degrade to form potent electrophilic species. As shown in Fig. 6-58, sulfonation plays an important role in the activation of aromatic amines, methyl-substituted PAHs, and safrole to tumorigenic metabolites. To exert its tumorigenic effect in rodents, safrole must be hydroxylated by CYP to 1′-hydroxysafrole, which is then sulfonated to the electrophilic and tumor-initiating metabolite, 1′-sulfooxysafrole (Boberg *et al.*, 1983). 1′-Hydroxysafrole is a more potent hepatotumorigen than safrole. Two lines of evidence support a major role for sulfonation in the hepatotumorigenic effect of 1′-hydroxysafrole. First, the hepatotumorigenic effect of 1′-hydroxysafrole can be inhibited by treating mice with the SULT inhibitor, pentachlorophenol. Second, the hepatotumorigenic effect of 1′-hydroxysafrole is markedly reduced in brachymorphic mice, which have a diminished capacity to sulfonate xenobiotics because of a genetic defect in PAPS synthesis. The sulfo-conjugates of benzylic and allylic alcohols, aromatic hydroxylamines, and hydroxamic acids (including those in cooked meat) are short-lived electrophiles capable of reacting with nucleophilic substances including proteins and DNA (Wang and James, 2006). Sulfonation can also convert procarcinogens and promutagens to electrophilic nitrenium or carbocation intermediates such as NOH-AAF, 1-hydroxymethylpyrene (1-HMP), 1′-hydroxysafrole, and the cooked food mutagen *N*-hydroxy-2-amino-1-methyl-6-phenylimidazo(4,5-*b*)pyridine (*N*-OH-PhIP) (Wang and James, 2006). The initial metabolite in 2-AAF activation is the hydroxamic acid formed by CYP1A2. Under acidic conditions (such as in urine), hydroxamic acids can lose water to form reactive nitrenium ions. This pathway is thought to contribute to the renal toxicity of phenacetin (Testa and Krämer, 2008, 2010).

Some drugs must be converted to a sulfonate conjugate to exert their desired effect, including triamterene, cicletanine, and minoxidil (Wang and James, 2006). Sulfonation (as well as glucuronidation) converts morphine to more potent analgesics than the parent, with morphine-6-sulfate being 30 times more potent and with morphine-6-glucuronide being 45 to 800 times more potent than morphine itself in rats (Wang and James, 2006). Similarly, several sulfonated steroids such as pregnenolone sulfate and DHEA sulfate interact directly with neurotransmitter receptors. It has been found that pregnenolone sulfate and DHEA sulfate enhance memory in mice. Prevention of hydrolysis of these sulfates by the steroid sulfatase inhibitor (*para-O*-sulfamoyl)-*N*-tetradecanoyl tyramine increases the memory enhancement caused by DHEA sulfate in rats, which suggests there is an important role of these sulfates in the central nervous system (Wang and James, 2006).

Polymorphisms with consequences for the bioactivation of xenobiotics have been reported. For instance, the human SULT1A*Arg (*1) allelozyme expressed in *S. typhimurium* is 12- to 350-fold more active in the sulfonation of 2-acetylamino-4-hydroxyaminotoluene, 2-nitropropoane, 2,4-dinitrobenzylalcohol, (−)-1-(α-hydroxyethyl) pyrene, and 1-hydroxymethlpyrene to mutagens than are cells expressing SULT1A1*His (Gamage *et al.*, 2006). Enantioselective sulfonation of promutagens has been reported, as in the case of 1-(α-hydroxyethyl) pyrene, for which SULT2A1 exhibits a 15-fold preference for the (+)-enantiomer, and SULT1E1 exhibits a 160-fold preference for the (−)-enantiomer (Gamage *et al.*, 2006).

Methylation

Methylation is a common but generally minor pathway of xenobiotic biotransformation. It differs from most other conjugation reactions because it often decreases the water solubility of xenobiotics and masks functional groups that might otherwise be metabolized by other conjugating enzymes. One exception to this rule is the *N*-methylation of pyridine-containing xenobiotics, such as nicotine, which produces quaternary ammonium ions that are water-soluble and readily excreted. Another exception is the *S*-methylation of thioethers to form positively charged sulfonium ions, a reaction catalyzed by thioether methyltransferase (TEMT), which has only been identified in mice (Weinshilboum *et al.*, 1999). The cofactor for methylation is *S*-adenosylmethionine (SAM), the structure of which is shown in Fig. 6-51. The methyl group bound to the sulfonium ion in SAM has the characteristics of a carbonium ion and is transferred to xenobiotics and endogenous substrates by nucleophilic attack from an electron-rich heteroatom (*O*, *N*, or *S*). Consequently, the functional groups involved in methylation reactions are phenols, catechols, aliphatic and aromatic amines, *N*-heterocyclics, and sulfhydryl-containing compounds. The conversion of benzo[*a*]pyrene (B[*a*]P) to 6-methylbenzo[*a*]pyrene is a rare example of *C*-methylation. Another reaction that appears to involve *C*-methylation, the conversion of cocaine to ethylcocaine, is actually a transesterification reaction catalyzed by CES1, as shown in Fig. 6-5. Metals can also be methylated. Both inorganic mercury and arsenic can be dimethylated, and inorganic selenium can be trimethylated. The selenium atom in ebselen is methylated following the ring opening of this anti-inflammatory drug. Some examples of xenobiotics and endogenous substrates that undergo *O*-, *N*-, or *S*-methylation are shown in Fig. 6-59. During these methylation reactions, SAM is converted to *S*-adenosyl-L-homocysteine (SAH). This section will cover the following methyltransferases: arsenic (III) methyltransferase (AS3MT), catechol-*O*-methyltransferase (COMT), glycine *N*-methyltransferase (GNMT), histamine *N*-methyltransferase (HNMT), indolethylamine *N*-methyltransferase (INMT), nicotinamide *N*-methyltransferase (NNMT), phenylethanolamine *N*-methyltransferase (PNMT), phenol *O*-methyltransferase (POMT) (thiol methyltransferase [TMT]), TEMT, and thiopurine methyltransferase (TPMT). Other methyltransferases that have been implicated as drug-metabolizing enzymes include guanidinoacetate *N*-methyltransferase (GAMT) and phosphatidylethanolamine *N*-methyltransferase (PEMT) (Nishimura and Naito, 2006).

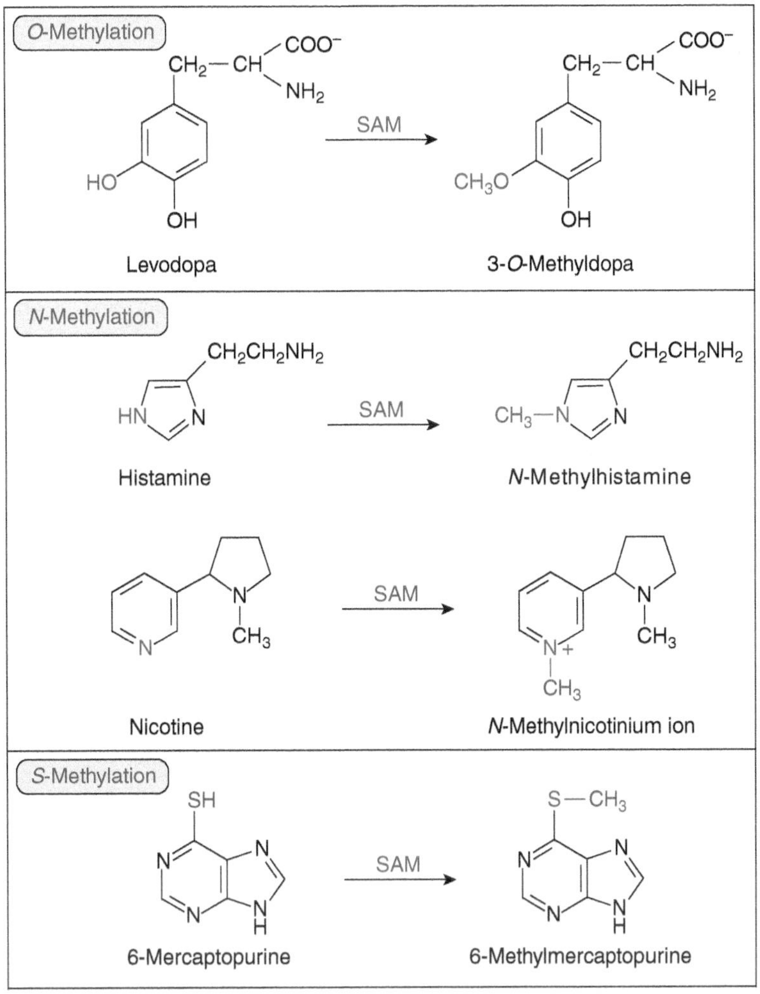

Figure 6-59. *Examples of compounds that undergo O-, N-, or S-methylation.*

The *O*-methylation of phenols and catechols is catalyzed by two different enzymes known as COMT and the enzyme historically termed POMT (Weinshilboum, 1989, 1992b). POMT is a microsomal enzyme that methylates phenols but not catechols, and COMT is both a cytosolic and microsomal enzyme with the converse substrate specificity, that is, an absolute requirement for catechol substrates (Weinshilboum, 2006). COMT plays a greater role in the biotransformation of catechols than POMT plays in the biotransformation of phenols. It should be noted that there is strong evidence to suggest that the membrane-bound POMT is the same enzyme as TMT (Weinshilboum, 2006). COMT was originally described as a cytosolic, Mg^{2+}-requiring, monomeric enzyme (Mr 25,000). However, in rats and humans, the enzyme is encoded by the COMT gene (on chromosome 22 in humans) with two different promoters and transcription initiation sites. Transcription at one site produces a cytosolic form of COMT, whereas transcription from the other site produces a membrane-bound form by adding 50 hydrophobic amino acids to the N-terminal of the microsomal COMT, which targets this form to the endoplasmic reticulum (Weinshilboum *et al.*, 1999; Weinshilboum, 2006). The microsomal COMT is expressed at high levels in the brain and lymphocytes (Weinshilboum, 2006). The cytosolic form of COMT is present in virtually all tissues, including erythrocytes, but the highest concentrations are found in liver and kidney. The membrane-bound form is more highly expressed in brain.

Substrates for COMT include several catecholamine neurotransmitters, such as epinephrine, norepinephrine, and dopamine;

and catechol drugs, such as the anti-Parkinson disease agent levodopa (L-3,4-dihydroxyphenylalanine) and the antihypertensive drug methyldopa (α-methyl-3,4-dihydroxyphenylalanine). Catechol estrogens, which are formed by 2- or 4-hydroxylation of the steroid A-ring, are substrates for COMT, as are drugs that are converted to catechols by two consecutive hydroxylation reactions (as in the case of phenobarbital, duloxetine, and diclofenac), by ring opening of a phenyl methylenedioxy (benzodioxole) group (as in the case of stiripentol and 3,4-methylenedioxymethamphetamine), or by hydrolysis of vicinal esters (as in the case of ibopamine). Formation of catechol estrogens, particularly 4-hydroxyestradiol, has been suggested to play an important role in estrogen-induced tumor formation in hamster kidney, rat pituitary, and mouse uterus (Zhu and Liehr, 1993) (see the section "CYP1B1"). These tissues contain high levels of epinephrine or dopamine, which inhibit the *O*-methylation of 4-hydroxyestradiol by COMT. Nontarget tissues do not contain high levels of catecholamines, which suggests that 4-hydroxyestradiol induces tumor formation in those tissues that fail to methylate and detoxify this catechol estrogen. These observations in animals are especially intriguing in view of subsequent epidemiological evidence demonstrating that low COMT activity appears to increase the risk of breast cancer, with odds ratios ranging from 1.7 to 3.0 (Weinshilboum, 2006).

In the 1970s, when COMT levels in erythrocytes (predominantly the cytosolic form) were measured in human subjects, it was apparent that there was a subpopulation that displayed low levels of this enzyme. Segregation analysis indicated that erythrocyte COMT activity was an autosomal codominant trait, and that erythrocyte levels correlated with relative COMT levels in liver and lymphocyte cytosol (Weinshilboum, 2006). It was subsequently found that COMT is encoded by a single gene with alleles for a low-activity form (COMT^L) and high-activity form (COMT^H) (Weinshilboum, 1989, 1992b, 2006; Weinshilboum et al., 1999). This polymorphism results from a single G → A transition in exon 4 that results in the substitution Val$_{108}$Met in cytosolic COMT and Val$_{158}$Met in microsomal COMT (Weinshilboum et al., 1999; Weinshilboum, 2006). The presence of methionine at position 108 in the cytosolic enzyme not only decreases the catalytic activity of COMT but also decreases the thermal stability of the enzyme, which has long been used to differentiate COMT^L (thermolabile) from COMT^H (thermostable). In Caucasians, these allelic variants are expressed with equal frequency, so that 25% of the population is homozygous for either the low- or high-activity enzyme, and 50% is heterozygous and has intermediate COMT activity. COMT activity is generally higher in Asians and African Americans due to a higher frequency of the COMT^H allele (~75% for Asians and African Americans compared with ~50% for Caucasians; McLeod et al., 1994). Subsequent resequencing of the COMT gene has revealed numerous SNPs, with at least 8 that occur with a frequency >10% in Caucasians, and 11 such SNPs in African Americans. Several of these SNPs are found in the intronic regions. A list of current COMT (and many other) alleles can be found at http://alfred.med.yale.edu/alfred/index.asp.

The genetically determined levels of COMT in erythrocytes correlate with individual differences in the proportion of levodopa converted to 3-O-methyldopa and the proportion of methyldopa converted to its 3-O-methyl metabolite. O-Methylation is normally a minor pathway of levodopa biotransformation, but 3-O-methyldopa is the major metabolite when levodopa is administered with a dopa decarboxylase inhibitor, such as carbidopa or benserazide, which is common clinical practice. High COMT activity, resulting in extensive O-methylation of levodopa to 3-O-methyldopa, has been associated with poor therapeutic management of Parkinson disease and an increased incidence of drug-induced toxicity (dyskinesia). A large number of epidemiological studies have been performed to examine the effects of the COMT Val$_{108/158}$Met polymorphism, and there is no evidence that the genetic polymorphism in COMT represents a risk modifier for the development of Parkinson disease (Weinshilboum et al., 1999). However, Egan et al. (2001) have demonstrated that COMT genotype was related in an allele-dosage manner to cognitive performance, with individuals homozygous for Met$_{108}$ (COMT^L phenotype) demonstrating increased executive cognition, as measured by the Wisconsin Card Sorting Test. The impact of the Met$_{108}$ allele was attributed to decreased dopamine catabolism in the prefrontal cortex, which results in enhanced neuronal function. Conversely, those individuals who are homozygous for Val$_{108}$ (COMT^H phenotype) appear to have decreased executive cognition, and may be at a slightly increased risk of developing schizophrenia (Egan et al., 2001).

Several N-methyltransferases have been described in humans and other mammals, including PNMT, which catalyzes the N-methylation of the neurotransmitter norepinephrine to form epinephrine; HNMT, which specifically methylates the imidazole ring of histamine and closely related compounds (Fig. 6-59); and NNMT, which methylates compounds containing a pyridine ring, such as nicotinamide, or an indole ring, such as tryptophan and serotonin (Weinshilboum, 1989, 1992b; Weinshilboum et al., 1999). PNMT is a cytosolic enzyme expressed at high levels in adrenal medullary chromafin cells, and in neurons of the medulla oblongata, hypothalamus, as well as in sensory nuclei of the vagus nerve and the retina, and is not thought to play a significant role

in the biotransformation of xenobiotics (Ji et al., 2005; Testa and Krämer, 2008, 2010).

HNMT is a cytosolic enzyme (Mr 33,000) that is highly expressed in kidney, liver, colon, prostate, ovary, and spinal cord cells (Horton et al., 2005). Its activity (which can be measured in erythrocytes) varies 6-fold among individuals due to a genetic polymorphism (C → T) that results in a point mutation, namely, Thr$_{115}$Ile. The latter allele (Ile$_{115}$) is quite common in Caucasians and Han Chinese (10% frequency) and encodes a variant of HNMT with decreased catalytic activity and thermal stability. HNMT may influence efficacy of some drugs by a mechanism that is not yet fully understood. For instance, individuals who are heterozygous for the Ile$_{115}$ allele have been found to exhibit significantly decreased methylprednisolone-induced cortisol suppression relative to (Thr$_{115}$)-homozygous individuals (Hon et al., 2006). Several other polymorphisms in the noncoding region of the HNMT gene have also been identified. HNMT can be inhibited by several antihistamines, quinacrine, amodiaquine, metoprine, and tacrine (Horton et al., 2005).

NNMT is a monomeric, cytosolic enzyme (Mr ~30,000) that appears to be a member of a family of methyltransferases that includes PNMT and TEMT (the thioether S-methyltransferase present in mouse lung). It catalyzes the N-methylation of nicotinamide and structurally related pyridine compounds (including pyridine itself) to form positively charged pyridinium ions. Nicotinic acid (niacin), a commonly used lipid-lowering agent, is converted to nicotinamide in vivo, which is then methylated by NNMT (or it is incorporated into nicotinamide adenine dinucleotide [NAD]). In contrast to many other methyltransferases, NNMT is not expressed in erythrocytes.

NNMT activity in human liver, like HNMT activity in erythrocytes, varies considerably from one individual to the next, and has a trimodal distribution dependent on variations in mRNA and protein levels, and up to 25% of the general population has high NNMT levels (Souto et al., 2005; Williams et al., 2005). It is not known to what extent genetic polymorphisms account for this variation. However, 10 SNPs in the untranslated regions of the gene have been detected in a Spanish population (Souto et al., 2005). A genome-wide scan for genes associated with plasma homocysteine levels determined that there was a statistically significant association with the NNMT gene, and, moreover, that 1 SNP (dbSNP ID#: rs694539) has a greater statistically significant association with homocysteine levels ($P = .017$) (Souto et al., 2005). Homocysteine plasma levels are an independent intermediate risk marker for osteoporotic fractures, congestive heart failure, venous thrombosis, myocardial infarction, stroke, and Alzheimer disease (Souto et al., 2005). In humans, the only source of homocysteine is from the demethylation of methionine in a multistep pathway that involves SAM-dependent methyltransferases to form S-adenosylhomocysteine, the immediate precursor to homocysteine. Taken together, these data suggest that high methyltransferase activity could contribute to hyperhomocysteinemia. Of the many SAM-dependent methyltransferase genes examined for an association with homocysteine levels, only NNMT (which is highly expressed in the liver) was found to show a significant association (Souto et al., 2005). NNMT is reported to be expressed in the brain and has been implicated as a component of the etiology of idiopathic Parkinson disease because it can convert 4-phenylpyridine to MPP$^+$, which is known to cause Parkinson disease symptoms due to its toxic effect on neuronal mitochondria (see the section "Amine Oxidases" and Fig. 6-29) (Williams et al., 2005).

There are numerous other human N-methyltransferases (as well as O-, S-, and C-methyltransferases) that appear to play relatively specific roles in the methylation of endogenous compounds, and most have not been well characterized with regard to their capability to methylate xenobiotics (there are at least 39 SAM-dependent methyltransferases in humans) (Souto *et al.*, 2005). For instance, INMT catalyzes the *N*-methylation of tryptamine and structurally related compounds (Thompson *et al.*, 1999). Other such enzymes that were initially thought to play a role only in the *N*-methylation of endogenous compounds were later found to play a role, albeit a minor one, in the *N*-methylation of one or more xenobiotics. Amine *N*-methyltransferase (AMNT, also called arylamine *N*-methyltransferase or nicotine *N*-methyltransferase), which is highly expressed in human thyroid and is also found in adrenal gland and lung, exhibits some activity toward tryptamine and has been also found to preferentially methylate the pyridine nitrogen of *R*-nicotine, which gives rise to nicotine isomethonium ions (Hukkanen *et al.*, 2005). GNMT is thought to play an important role in the regulation of methyl group metabolism in the liver and pancreas through regulation of the ratio between *S*-adenosyl-L-methionine and SAH. Rat data show that the tetrameric form of the GNMT has catalytic activity, and the dimeric form binds PAHs. There is also evidence that the dimeric form of human GNMT sequesters B[*a*]P, and thereby decreases its cytotoxic effects (Chen *et al.*, 2004b; Lee *et al.*, 2006).

The system that is used to classify human *N*-methyltransferases may not be appropriate for other species. In guinea pigs, for example, both nicotine and histamine are methylated by a common *N*-methyltransferase. Guinea pigs have an unusually high capacity to methylate histamine and xenobiotics. The major route of nicotine biotransformation in the guinea pig is methylation, although *R*-nicotine is preferentially methylated over its *S*-enantiomer (Cundy *et al.*, 1985). Guinea pigs also methylate the imidazole ring of cimetidine.

S-Methylation is an important pathway in the biotransformation of sulfhydryl-containing xenobiotics, such as the antihypertensive drug captopril, the antirheumatic agent D-penicillamine, the antineoplastic and immunosuppressive drugs 6-mercaptopurine, 6-thioguanine, and azathioprine, metabolites of the alcohol deterrent disulfiram, and the deacetylated metabolite of the antidiuretic, spironolactone. In humans, *S*-methylation is catalyzed by at least 2 enzymes, TPMT and TMT (which may be the same enzyme as POMT).

TPMT is a cytoplasmic enzyme that preferentially methylates aromatic and heterocyclic compounds such as the thiopurine drugs 6-mercaptopurine, 6-thioguanine, and azathioprine. TMT is a microsomal enzyme that preferentially methylates aliphatic sulfhydryl compounds such as captopril, D-penicillamine, and disulfiram derivatives. It has also been found to methylate the heterocyclic thiol-containing leaving groups of some cephalosporins (Wood *et al.*, 2002), the thiazolidinedione drug, MK-0767, a dual α/γ PPAR agonist (Karanam *et al.*, 2004), dithiothreitol (Weinshilboum, 2006), and some thiofuran flavoring agents (Lake *et al.*, 2003). Although a gene that encodes TMT has not yet been definitively identified, there is strong evidence to suggest that the membrane-bound POMT is the same enzyme as TMT, which means that TMT could also catalyze the *O*-methylation of phenols (Weinshilboum, 2006).

Both TMT and TPMT are present in erythrocytes at levels that reflect the expression of TPMT and TMT in liver and other tissues. Although TPMT and TMT are independently regulated, their expression in erythrocytes is largely determined by genetic factors. TPMT is encoded by a single gene with alleles for a low-activity form (TPMT^L) and for a high-activity form (TPMT^H). The allele frequencies of TPMT^L and TPMT^H are 0.06 and 0.94, respectively,

which produces a trimodal distribution of TPMT activity with low, intermediate, and high activity expressed in 0.3%, 11.1%, and 88.6% of Caucasians, respectively. At least 28 separate genetic polymorphisms have been identified and most are associated with low TPMT activity, with the *2, *3A, and *3C alleles accounting for greater than 95% of the TPMT^L phenotype (Weinshilboum, 2006; Ujiie *et al.*, 2008; Wang *et al.*, 2010a). In Caucasians, the allele that is most commonly associated with the TPMT^L phenotype is TPMT*3A (5%), which contains two nonsynonymous SNPs: Ala$_{154}$Thr and Tyr$_{240}$Cys (Wood *et al.*, 2006). These amino acid changes (and those in the TPMT*3B and *3C variants) lead to aggregation and rapid degradation of expressed TPMT by a ubiquitin/proteasome-dependent mechanism (Wang *et al.*, 2005). Another variant, TPMT*4, results in alternative TPMT mRNA splicing and reduced enzyme expression, leading to low TPMT activity in individuals carrying this allele (Wang *et al.*, 2010a).

Cancer patients with low TPMT activity are at increased risk for thiopurine-induced myelotoxicity, in contrast to the potential need for higher-than-normal doses to achieve therapeutic levels of thiopurines in patients with high TPMT activity (Weinshilboum, 1989, 1992b). The thiopurine drugs metabolized by TPMT have a relatively narrow therapeutic index, and are used to treat life-threatening illnesses such as acute lymphoblastic leukemia or organ-transplant patients. The thiopurines are also oxidized by xanthine oxidoreductase (XOR), but since there is extensive variation in TPMT activity and XOR is not present in hematopoietic tissues, TPMT activity in these tissues is more important in the avoidance of life-threatening myelosuppression at standard doses (Weinshilboum, 2006). Phenotyping for the TPMT genetic polymorphism represents one of the first examples in which testing for a genetic variant has entered standard clinical practice (Weinshilboum *et al.*, 1999). The clinical relevance of TPMT polymorphisms is reflected by the inclusion of TPMT as a "valid biomarker" for pharmacogenomics, along with CYP2D6 polymorphisms, in the FDA's 2005 "Guidance for Pharmacogenomic Data Submission." TPMT can be inhibited by benzoic acid derivatives, which also complicates therapy with drugs that are metabolized by TPMT. Patients with inflammatory bowel disorders such as Crohn disease are often treated with thiopurine drugs, which are metabolized by TPMT, and with sulfasalazine or olsalazine, which are potent TPMT inhibitors. The combination of these drugs can lead to thiopurine-induced myelosuppression.

A genetic polymorphism for TMT also has been described, but its pharmacological and toxicological significance remains to be determined. The molecular basis for the polymorphism has not been determined, but studies have shown that 98% of the 5-fold individual variation in erythrocyte TMT activity is due to inheritance, with an allele for high TMT activity having a frequency of 0.12. TMT is relatively specific for aliphatic sulfhydryl compounds such as 2-mercatoethanol, captopril, D-penicillamine, and NAC. It also rapidly methylates a dihydro metabolite of ziprasidone that is formed by AO as shown in Fig. 6-4 (Obach *et al.*, 2005). TMT is present at high levels in the colonic mucosa and is also expressed in liver microsomes and erythrocyte membranes. It is not inhibited by benzoic acid derivatives, but it is inhibited by the CYP inhibitor proadifen (aka SKE-525A) (Weinshilboum *et al.*, 1999).

Some of the hydrogen sulfide produced by anaerobic bacteria in the intestinal tract is converted by *S*-methyltransferases to methane thiol and then to dimethylsulfide. Another source of substrates for *S*-methyltransferases are the thioethers of GSH conjugates. GSH conjugates are hydrolyzed to cysteine conjugates, which can either be acetylated to form mercapturic acids or cleaved by cysteine-conjugate β-lyase (CCBL1). This β-lyase pathway converts the cysteine conjugate to pyruvate, ammonia, and a sulfhydryl-containing xeno-biotic, which is a potential substrate for *S*-methylation.

Methylation can also lead to increased toxicity. AS3MT is a methyltransferase (previously called Cyt19) that methylates inorganic arsenic to form methylarsonic and dimethylarsonic acids, which are more cytotoxic and genotoxic than arsenate and arsenite (Wood *et al.*, 2006). As many as 27 polymorphisms have been identified in this gene, with 2 rare alleles that cause markedly decreased activity and immunoreactive protein levels, and one frequent allele (ie, ~10% in both African Americans and Caucasians) that causes increased activity and immunoreactive protein levels (Wood *et al.*, 2006). Up to 1% of African Americans and Caucasians would be expected to be homozygous for the allele that encodes the high-activity AS3MT, and this may potentially lead to increased arsenic toxicity in such individuals.

Acetylation

N-Acetylation is a major route of biotransformation for xeno-biotics containing an aromatic amine (R-NH$_2$) or a hydrazine group (R-NH–NH$_2$), which are converted to aromatic amides (R-NH–COCH$_3$) and hydrazides (R-NH–NH–COCH$_3$), respectively (Evans, 1992). Xenobiotics containing primary aliphatic amines are rarely substrates for *N*-acetylation, a notable exception being cysteine conjugates, which are formed from GSH conjugates and converted to mercapturic acids by *N*-acetylation in the kidney (see the section "Glutathione Conjugation"). In rare cases, *N*-acetylation can occur on aliphatic basic amino groups as in the cases of the antibacterial agent trovafloxacin and the primary metabolite of the β-adrenoreceptor blocker propranolol (Testa and Krämer, 2008, 2010). In a few cases, the *N*-acetylation of aliphatic acidic amine groups (such as a sulfonamide) has also been documented, an example of which is the anticonvulsant agent zonisamide (Testa and Krämer, 2008, 2010). Like methylation, *N*-acetylation masks an amine with a nonionizable group, so that many *N*-acetylated metabolites are less water-soluble than the parent compound. An exception is the *N*-acetylation of the acidic amine (the sulfonamide) in zonisamide; in this case *N*-acetylation increases ionization (by lowering the pK_a from ~10 to ~5) and, hence, its water solubility. *N*-Acetylation of isoniazid also increases its water solubility and facilitates its urinary excretion.

The *N*-acetylation of xenobiotics is catalyzed by *N*-acetyltransferases (NATs) and requires the cofactor acetyl coenzyme A (acetyl-CoA), the structure of which is shown in Fig. 6-51. The reaction occurs in 2 sequential steps according to a *ping-pong Bi–Bi* mechanism (Hein, 1988). In the first step, the acetyl group from acetyl-CoA is transferred to a cysteine residue in the NAT active site with release of CoA (E-SH + CoA-SCOCH$_3$ → E-S-COCH$_3$ + CoA-SH). In the second step, the acetyl group is transferred from the acylated enzyme to the amino group of the substrate with regeneration of the enzyme. For strongly basic amines, the rate of *N*-acetylation is determined by the first step (acetylation of the enzyme), whereas the rate of *N*-acetylation of weakly basic amines is determined by the second step (transfer of the acetyl group from the acylated enzyme to the acceptor amine). In certain cases (discussed below), NATs can catalyze the *O*-acetylation of xenobiotics.

NATs are cytosolic enzymes found in liver and many other tissues of most mammalian species, with the notable exception of the dog, fox, and musk shrew (*Suncus marinus*) which are unable to acetylate xenobiotics (a notable exception being the ability of dogs to *N*-acetylate cyanamide, which contains an acidic amine group) (Nakura *et al.*, 1995; Trepanier *et al.*, 1997; Sim *et al.*, 2008; Testa and Krämer, 2008, 2010). In contrast to other xenobiotic-biotransforming enzymes, the number of NATs known to play a role in xenobiotic metabolism is limited (Vatsis *et al.*, 1995; Boukouvala and Fakis, 2005). NAT activities are distinguishable from other NATs such as those involved in melatonin synthesis and serotonin metabolism (arylalkylamine NATs) but are indistinguishable from the group of bacterial enzymes termed *N*-hydroxyarylamine *O*-acetyltransferases (Boukouvala and Fakis, 2005). Rabbits and hamsters express only 2 NAT enzymes, known as NAT1 and NAT2, whereas mice and rats express 3 enzymes, namely, NAT1, NAT2, and NAT3. The Human Genome Organisation (HUGO) Gene Nomenclature Committee (http://www.gene.ucl.ac.uk/nomenclature) has designated NAT as the official symbol for arylamine *N*-acetyltransferases. The two well-known and characterized xenobiotic-acetylating human enzymes are NAT1 and NAT2, which are encoded by two highly polymorphic genes located on chromosome 8. Other HUGO-approved human NAT gene symbols include NAT6, NAT8 to 10, NAT14, and NAT16, located on other chromosomes. The activities and expression pattern of these enzymes have not yet been definitively characterized, although some of these genes have been associated with atopic dermatitis or psoriasis (NAT9) and nasopharyngeal cancer (NAT6) (Helms *et al.*, 2003; Bowcock and Cookson, 2004; Duh *et al.*, 2004; Yamada and Ymamoto, 2005; Morar *et al.*, 2006). Individual NATs and their allelic variants were named in the order of their description in the literature, which makes for a somewhat confusing nomenclature system (Vatsis *et al.*, 1995). For example, in humans, the "wild-type" NAT1 and NAT2 alleles are designated NAT1*4 and NAT2*4, respectively, because they are the most common alleles in some but not all ethnic groups (Hein, 2006). For NAT enzymes, the term "wild type" may be somewhat arbitrary because it depends on ethnicity. The official Web site for maintaining and updating NAT allele nomenclature is http://www.louisville.edu/medschool/pharmacology/NAT.html. The frequency of some SNPs and alleles in various ethnic groups is available online from the National Cancer Institute's SNP500Cancer database (http://snp500cancer.nci.nih.gov).

In each species examined, NAT1 and NAT2 are closely related proteins (79%–95% identical in amino acid sequence) with an active-site cysteine residue (Cys$_{68}$) in the N-terminal region (Grant *et al.*, 1992; Vatsis *et al.*, 1995). In addition to the active-site cysteine residue, the presence of a histidine residue (His$_{107}$) and an aspartate residue (Asp$_{122}$) are required for activity, forming a catalytic triad necessary for the transfer of an acetyl group from acetyl-CoA to the substrate (Sandy *et al.*, 2005; Sim *et al.*, 2008). Human NAT1 and NAT2 genes are composed of intronless open reading frames of 870 bp on the same chromosome with a NAT pseudo-gene (NATP1) between them, and encode proteins of 290 amino acids that share 87% homology in the coding region (Boukouvala and Fakis, 2005; Hein, 2006). In spite of this apparently simple structure, NAT genes are fairly complex. For instance, comparisons of genomic and cDNA clones of the human NAT2 gene performed in the early 1990s revealed that the 5′ untranslated region is contained in a "noncoding exon," 8 kb upstream of the coding region (Boukouvala and Fakis, 2005). A similar type of unusual structure was later revealed for NAT2 genes in rabbit, hamster, mouse, and rat. More recent sequence alignments of expressed sequence tags (ESTs) with genomic sequences reveal that the presence of one or more upstream "noncoding exons" is typical for all vertebrate NAT genes, with the contiguous coding region contained in a single exon in the 3′ untranslated region (Boukouvala and Fakis, 2005). Furthermore, the splice site nearest the coding region is universally conserved at position 6, relative to the first codon. The primary transcript of both NAT1 and 2 genes is also subject to alternative intron splicing in human, rat, and possibly chicken, whereas alternative splicing for NAT2 has been observed in rabbit and hamster. Alternative splicing in the case of NATs generates mRNAs with variable 5′ untranslated regions. The presence of "noncoding exons" lying upstream of higher eukaryotic genes (especially intronless genes) is common, and their transcription is likely required for transport of the entire transcript to the cytoplasm (Boukouvala and Fakis, 2005). The differential transcription of upstream noncoding exons has been frequently associated with cell-specific regulation of transcription and translation, and recent studies show that certain noncoding NAT exons are present to different extents in different tissues (Boukouvala and Fakis, 2005). There is also evidence of differential utilization of multiple tandem poly-adenosine repeats in the 3′ untranslated regions in different species, but the precise effect of polyadenylation of NATs remains unknown (Boukouvala and Fakis, 2005).

Despite their coexistence on the same chromosome, NAT1 and NAT2 are independently regulated proteins. For instance, human NAT1 protein and/or mRNA have been detected in every tissue examined (eg, liver, gastrointestinal tract, leukocytes, erythrocytes, bladder, uroepithelial cells, mammary, lung, placenta, kidney, pineal gland, skeletal muscle, heart, brain, and pancreas) and are present from the blastocyst stage, whereas NAT2 is thought to be mainly expressed in liver and intestine. However, most (but not all) of the tissues that express NAT1 also appear to express low levels of NAT2, at least at the level of mRNA (Debiec-Rychter et al., 1999). Hein (2006) has also challenged the hypothesis that NAT2 is expressed mainly in the liver and intestine, and noted that the O-acetylation of N-hydroxy-4-aminobiphenyl in human urinary bladder cytosol did not correlate with NAT1 activity (4-aminobenzoic acid [PABA] N-acetylation), consistent with acetylation by both enzymes. Regulation of human NAT1 is complex, and involves a promoter region composed of an AP-1 box flanked by 2 TCATT boxes (Boukouvala and Fakis, 2005). The 3′ TCATT box is required for expression, whereas the 5′-box attenuates promoter activity. Transcription factors such as c-Fos/Fra, c-Jun, and YY1 bind to the NAT1 promoter (Boukouvala and Fakis, 2005). In addition, because transcription of human NAT1 can begin with different upstream "noncoding exons," it is likely that there are additional promoters that regulate expression.

NAT1 and NAT2 also have different but overlapping substrate specificities, although no substrate is exclusively N-acetylated by one enzyme or the other. Substrates preferentially N-acetylated by human NAT1 include 4-aminobenzoic acid (PABA), 4-aminosalicylic acid, sulfamethoxazole, and sulfanilamide, whereas substrates preferentially N-acetylated by human NAT2 include isoniazid, hydralazine, procainamide, dapsone, aminoglutethimide, and sulfamethazine. Some investigators have used PABA as a selective probe substrate for wild-type NAT1, and either sulfamethazine or sulfadiazine as selective probe substrate for wild-type NAT2 (Winter and Unadkat, 2005). Some xenobiotics, such as the carcinogenic aromatic amine, 2-aminofluorene (2-AF), are N-acetylated equally well by NAT1 and NAT2. The calcium-sensitizing agent levosimendan, developed for the treatment of congestive heart failure, has a pharmacologically active N-acetylated metabolite produced by NAT2 (Testa and Krämer, 2008, 2010). Other drugs that are substrates for either NAT1 or NAT2 include acebutolol, amantadine, amonafide, amrinone, benzocaine, declopramide, metamizole, and phenelzine (Gonzalez and Tukey, 2006; Sirot et al., 2006; Sim et al., 2008).

Several drugs are N-acetylated following their biotransformation by hydrolysis, reduction, or oxidation. For example, caffeine is N_3-demethylated by CYP1A2 to paraxanthine (Fig. 6-45), which

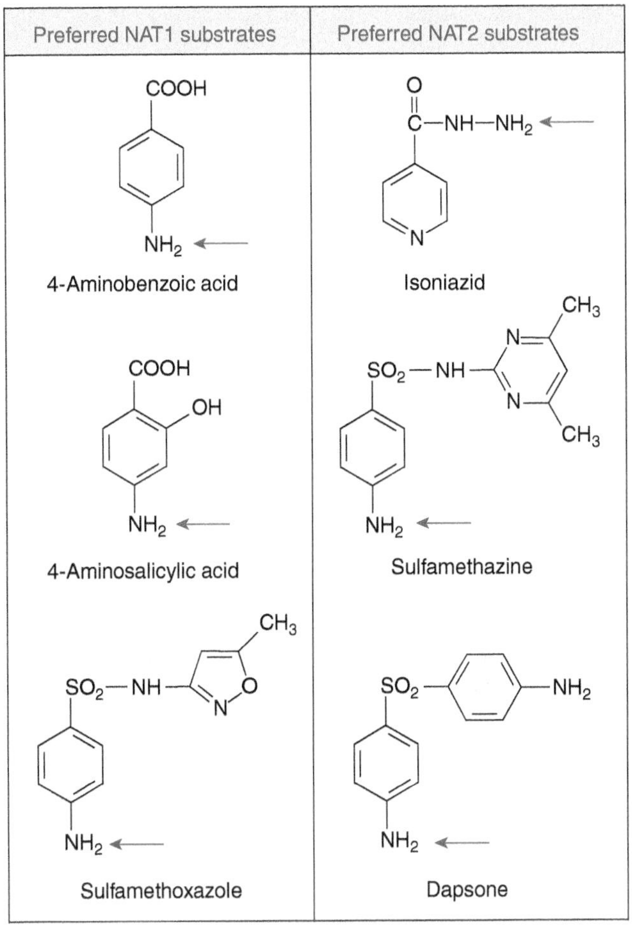

Preferred NAT1 substrates	Preferred NAT2 substrates
4-Aminobenzoic acid	Isoniazid
4-Aminosalicylic acid	Sulfamethazine
Sulfamethoxazole	Dapsone

Figure 6-60. Examples of substrates for the human N-acetyltransferases, NAT1, and the highly polymorphic NAT2.

is then N-demethylated to 1-methylxanthine and N-acetylated to 5-acetylamino-6-formylamino-3-methyluracil (AFMU) by NAT2. The ratio of AFMU to 1-methylxanthine can be used to determine acetylator phenotype (Testa and Krämer, 2008, 2010). Other drugs converted to metabolites that are N-acetylated by NAT2 include sulfasalazine, nitrazepam, and clonazepam. Examples of drugs that are N-acetylated by NAT1 and NAT2 are shown in Fig. 6-60. It should be noted, however, that there are species differences in the substrate specificity of NATs. For example, PABA is preferentially N-acetylated by NAT1 in humans and rabbits but by NAT2 in mice and hamsters.

Genetic polymorphisms for N-acetylation have been documented in humans, hamsters, rabbits, and mice (Evans, 1992; Vatsis et al., 1995; Hirvonen, 1999; Hein et al., 2000; Sim et al., 2008). A series of clinical observations in the 1950s established the existence of slow and fast acetylators of the antitubercular drug isoniazid. In general, ~50% of patients treated with isoniazid have adverse events such as peripheral neuropathy and hepatotoxicity. These adverse effects are more pronounced in slow acetylators (discussed later in this section). Slow acetylators also exhibit a higher incidence of adverse events with clonazepam, hydralazine, procainamide, and sulfonamides (Sirot et al., 2006). The incidence of the slow acetylator phenotype is high in Middle Eastern populations (eg, ~92% in Egyptians), intermediate in Caucasian and African populations (eg, ~50%–59% in Caucasian Americans, Australians, and Europeans; ~41% in African Americans; ~50%–60% in black Africans), and low in Asian populations (eg, <20% in Chinese; ~8%–10% in Japanese) (Sirot et al., 2006). Many studies have demonstrated the typical bimodal distribution of fast and slow acetylators with drugs such as isoniazid, but the use of other drugs such as caffeine or sulfamethazine exhibits slow, intermediate, and fast acetylators (Hein, 2006). Parkin *et al.* (1997) also demonstrated that isoniazid elimination is trimodal, and that phenotype and genotype were concordant.

The slow acetylator phenotype is caused by various mutations in the NAT2 gene that decrease either NAT2 activity or enzyme stability. At least 36 allelic variants of human NAT2 have been documented. For example, a point mutation $T_{341}C$ (which causes the amino acid substitution $Ile_{114}Thr$) decreases V_{max} for N-acetylation without altering the K_m for substrate binding or the stability of the enzyme. This mutation (which is the basis for the NAT2*5 allele) is the most common cause of the slow acetylator phenotype in Caucasians (eg, frequency >50% in the United Kingdom) but is rarely observed in Koreans (ie, <5%) (Hein, 2006). (*Note:* There are 10 known NAT2*5 alleles, designated NAT2*5A to NAT*5J.) The alleles containing only the $Ile_{114}Thr$ substitution are NAT2*5A (which also contains a silent $C_{481}T$ nucleotide change) and NAT2*5D. The others contain this and at least one other nucleotide and/or amino acid substitution, and NAT2*5B confers the "slowest acetylator" phenotype (Patin *et al.*, 2006). The NAT2*7 allele is more prevalent in Asians than Caucasians or Africans (Hein, 2006), and involves either a point mutation $G_{857}A$ (ie, NAT2*7A) or both this change and $C_{282}T$ (ie, NAT2*7B). Both of these changes cause the amino acid substitution $Gly_{286}Glu$, which decreases the stability, rather than the activity, of NAT2. NAT2*6 (more common in southern India) and NAT2*14 (present mainly in Africa and Spain) also result in one or more amino acid changes that lead to decreased NAT2 activity, whereas the amino acid change in NAT2*12 (present mainly in Africa and Spain) does not decrease activity (Hein, 2006). Within the slow NAT2 acetylator phenotype there is considerable variation in rates of xenobiotic N-acetylation. This is partly because different mutations in the NAT2 gene have different effects on NAT2 activity and/or enzyme stability, heterozygotes retain moderate NAT2 activity, and the N-acetylation of "NAT2-substrates" by NAT1 becomes significant in slow acetylators.

The slowest acetylator haplotype (NAT2*5B, which has the strongest association with bladder cancer) appears to have been positively selected for in only the last 6500 years in western and central Eurasians, which suggests that slow acetylation conferred an evolutionary advantage within this population, contrary to much of the recent epidemiological data (Patin *et al.*, 2006). Moreover, because most of the NAT2 polymorphisms that lead to slow acetylation are present at high frequencies in various populations, it would seem that varied rates of acetylation may be an important human adaptation to environmental variables. Because acetylation can be very important in the determination of the interaction between human populations and many xenobiotics in their particular environment (eg, through different diets and lifestyles), it is not surprising that they are recent targets for natural selection.

NAT1 and NAT2 used to be referred to as *monomorphic* and *polymorphic* NATs because only the latter enzyme was thought to be genetically polymorphic. However, at least 26 allelic variants have now been documented for the human NAT1 gene, although these variants are less prevalent than the NAT2 allelic variants; hence, there is less genetically determined variation in the metabolism of "NAT1 substrates." Nevertheless, there is evidence that phenotypic differences in the N-acetylation of 4-aminosalicylic acid are distributed bimodally, consistent with the existence of low- and high-activity forms of NAT1. Furthermore, an extremely slow acetylator of 4-aminosalicylic acid has been identified with mutations in both NAT1 alleles: one that decreases NAT1 activity and stability and one that encodes a truncated and catalytically inactive form

of the enzyme. Two NAT1 variants, NAT1*10 and NAT1*11, are gain-of-function polymorphisms that lead to increased efficiency of protein translation (Wang *et al.*, 2011b). Individuals homozygous for NAT1*10 or heterozygous for NAT1*11 are classified as fast acetylators, whereas those rare individuals who are homozygous for NAT1*11 have been classified as ultrafast acetylators (Wang *et al.*, 2011b). Both NAT*10 and NAT*11 alleles are risk modifiers of sulfamethoxazole-induced hypersensitivity in HIV/AIDS patients, such that individuals who are NAT1 *fast* acetylators but are also NAT2 *slow* acetylators are protected against this type of hypersensitivity (Wang *et al.*, 2011b). It has also been demonstrated that NAT1*16 but not NAT1*10 or NAT1*11 causes a 50% decrease in NAT1 activity and NAT1 protein levels in COS-1 cell cytosol (Soucek *et al.*, 2004). Cascorbi *et al.* (2001) found that individuals who express NAT1*10 and NAT2*4 (ie, intermediate NAT1 activity and normal NAT2 activity) were at a significantly lower risk of bladder cancer, especially when exposed to environmental carcinogens. It is therefore likely that the interplay between NAT1 and NAT2 phenotypes is relevant to the susceptibility to certain carcinogens.

Genetic polymorphisms in NAT2 have a number of pharmacological and toxicological consequences for drugs that are N-acetylated by this enzyme. The pharmacological effects of the antihypertensive drug hydralazine are more pronounced in slow NAT2 acetylators. Slow NAT2 acetylators are predisposed to several drug toxicities, including nerve damage (peripheral neuropathy) from isoniazid and dapsone, systemic lupus erythematosus from hydralazine and procainamide, and the toxic effects of coadministration of the anticonvulsant phenytoin with isoniazid. Slow NAT2 acetylators who are also deficient in glucose-6-phosphate dehydrogenase are particularly prone to hemolysis from certain sulfonamides. HIV-infected individuals of the slow acetylator phenotype suffer more often from adverse drug events and, among patients with Stevens Johnson syndrome, the overwhelming majority are slow acetylators. Fast NAT2 acetylators are predisposed to the myelotoxic effects of amonafide because N-acetylation retards the clearance of this antineoplastic drug.

Early epidemiological studies suggested that rapid NAT2 acetylators were at increased risk for the development of isoniazid-induced liver toxicity; however, the current consensus is that slow NAT2 acetylation is a risk modifier for isoniazid-induced hepatotoxicity while rapid acetylators are protected from toxicity. Following its acetylation by NAT2, isoniazid can be hydrolyzed to isonicotinic acid and acetylhydrazine ($CH_3CO-NHNH_2$). The latter metabolite can be N-hydroxylated by FMO or CYP to a reactive intermediate, as shown in Fig. 6-38. The generation of a reactive metabolite from acetylhydrazine would seem to provide a mechanistic basis for enhanced isoniazid hepatotoxicity in fast acetylators. However, acetylhydrazine can be further acetylated to diacetylhydrazine ($CH_3CO-NHNH-COCH_3$), and this detoxication reaction is also catalyzed by NAT2. Therefore, acetylhydrazine is both produced and detoxified by NAT2; hence, slow acetylation, not fast acetylation, becomes the risk modifier for isoniazid-induced hepatotoxicity, just as it is for isoniazid-induced peripheral neuropathy. Isoniazid can also be directly hydrolyzed to yield isonicotinic acid and hydrazine (H_2N-NH_2). Hydrazine (also a toxic substance used as rocket propellant) has been proposed to be the hepatotoxic metabolite of isoniazid as slow acetylators have significantly higher plasma concentrations of hydrazine relative to rapid acetylators (Testa and Krämer, 2008, 2010; Metushi *et al.*, 2011). Rifampin and alcohol have been reported to enhance the hepatotoxicity of isoniazid. These drug interactions are probably the result of increased N-hydroxylation of acetylhydrazine due to CYP induction

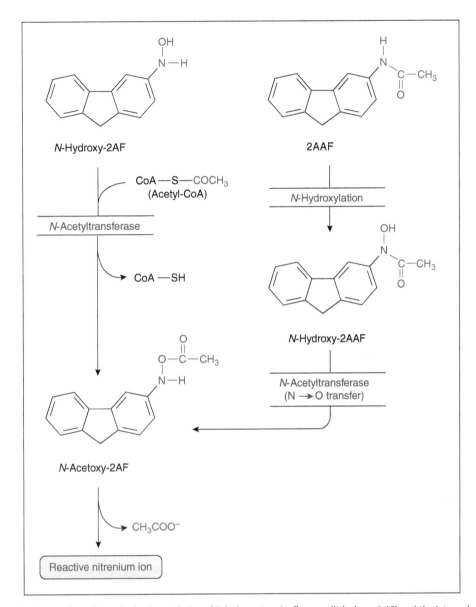

Figure 6-61. *Role of N-acetyltransferase in the O-acetylation of N-hydroxy-2-aminofluorene (N-hydroxy-2-AF) and the intramolecular rearrangement of N-hydroxy-2-acetylaminofluorene (N-hydroxy-2-AAF).*

rather than due to an alteration in NAT2 activity. This is further corroborated by studies in which slow acetylator patients who also carried the high-activity CYP2E1 c1/c1 genotype had more severe hepatotoxicity (Metushi *et al.*, 2011). Isoniazid is an antitubercular drug, and its inactivation by NAT2 is interesting from the perspective that several organisms, including *M. tuberculosis*, express a NAT2-like enzyme, which has implications for isoniazid-resistance in tuberculosis.

Aromatic amines can be both activated and deactivated by NATs (Kato and Yamazoe, 1994; Hirvonen, 1999; Hein *et al.*, 2000). The NATs detoxify aromatic amines by converting them to the corresponding amides because aromatic amides are less likely than aromatic amines to be activated to DNA-reactive metabolites by CYP, peroxidases such as PHS, and UGTs (see the section "Glucuronidation and Formation of Acyl-CoA Thioesters"). However, NATs can activate aromatic amines if they are first *N*-hydroxylated by CYP because NATs can also function as *O*-acetyltransferases and convert hydroxylamines to acetoxy esters (*aryl*-NHOH → *aryl*-NH-O-COCH$_3$). As shown in Fig. 6-12, the acetoxy esters of hydroxylamines, like the corresponding sulfonate

esters (Fig. 6-58), can break down to form highly reactive nitrenium and carbonium ions that bind to DNA. NATs catalyze the *O*-acetylation of *N*-hydroxyaromatic amines by two distinct mechanisms. The first reaction, which is exemplified by the conversion of *N*-hydroxyaminofluorene to *N*-acetoxyaminofluorene, requires acetyl-CoA and proceeds by the same mechanism previously described for *N*-acetylation. The second reaction is exemplified by the conversion of 2-acetylaminofluorene (2-AAF) to *N*-acetoxyaminofluorene, which does not require acetyl-CoA but involves an intramolecular transfer of the *N*-acetyl group from nitrogen to oxygen. These reactions are shown in Fig. 6-61.

Genetic polymorphisms in NAT2 have been reported to influence susceptibility to aromatic amine–induced bladder and colon cancer (see the section "Glucuronidation and Formation of Acyl-CoA Thioesters") (Evans, 1992; Kadlubar, 1994; Hirvonen, 1999; Hein *et al.*, 2000; Sim *et al.*, 2008). Bladder cancer is thought to be caused by bicyclic aromatic amines (benzidine, 2-aminonaphthalene, and 4-aminobiphenyl), whereas colon cancer is thought to be caused by heterocyclic aromatic amines, such as the products of amino acid pyrolysis (eg, 2-amino-6-methylimidazo[4,5-*b*] pyridine or PhIP, and others listed in Table 6-14). Epidemiological studies suggest that slow NAT2 acetylators are more likely than fast NAT2 acetylators to develop bladder cancer from cigarette smoking and from occupational exposure to bicyclic aromatic amines. The possibility that slow NAT2 acetylators are at increased risk for aromatic amine–induced cancer is supported by the finding that dogs, which are poor acetylators, are highly prone to aromatic amine–induced bladder cancer. By comparison, fast NAT2 acetylators appear to be at increased risk for colon cancer from heterocyclic aromatic amines.

The influence of acetylator phenotype on susceptibility to aromatic amine–induced cancer can be rationalized on the ability of NATs to activate and detoxify aromatic amines and by differences in the substrate specificity and tissues distribution of NAT1 and NAT2 (recall that NAT1 is expressed in virtually all tissues, whereas NAT2 is expressed mainly in the liver and intestinal tract). Both NAT1 and NAT2 catalyze the *O*-acetylation (activation) of *N*-hydroxy bicyclic aromatic amines, whereas the *O*-acetylation of *N*-hydroxy heterocyclic aromatic amines is preferentially catalyzed by NAT2. Bicyclic aromatic amines can also be *N*-acetylated (detoxified) by NAT1 and NAT2, but heterocyclic aromatic amines are poor substrates for both enzymes. Therefore, the fast acetylator phenotype protects against aromatic amine–induced bladder cancer because NAT2 (as well as NAT1) catalyzes the *N*-acetylation (detoxication) of bicyclic aromatic amines in the liver. In slow acetylators, a greater proportion of the bicyclic aromatic amines are activated through *N*-hydroxylation by CYP1A2. These *N*-hydroxylated aromatic amines can be activated by *O*-acetylation, which can be catalyzed in the bladder itself by NAT1. A high level of NAT1 in the bladder is a risk modifier for aromatic amine–induced bladder cancer. In addition, the fast acetylator phenotype potentiates the colon cancer–inducing effects of heterocyclic aromatic amines. These aromatic amines are poor substrates for NAT1 and NAT2, so that high levels of NAT2 in the liver do little to prevent their *N*-hydroxylation by CYP1A2. The *N*-hydroxylated metabolites of heterocyclic aromatic amines can be activated by *O*-acetylation, which can be catalyzed in the colon itself by NAT2. The presence of NAT2 (and NAT1) in the colons of fast acetylators probably explains why this phenotype is a risk modifier for the development of colon cancer.

Whether fast acetylators are protected from or predisposed to the cancer-causing effects of aromatic amines depends on the nature of the aromatic amine (bicyclic vs heterocyclic) and on other important risk modifiers. Both the activation of aromatic amines by *N*-glucuronidation and the activation of *N*-hydroxy aromatic amines by sulfonation are suspected of playing an important role in the incidence of bladder and colon cancer. These and other risk modifiers may explain why some epidemiological studies, contrary to expectation, have shown that slow NAT2 acetylators are at increased risk for aromatic amine–induced bladder cancer, as was demonstrated for benzidine manufacturers in China (Hayes *et al.*, 1993).

The *N*-acetylation of aromatic amines (a detoxication reaction) and the *O*-acetylation of *N*-hydroxy aromatic amines (an activation reaction) can be reversed by a microsomal enzyme called arylacetamide deacetylase (gene symbol AADAC) (Probst *et al.*, 1994). This enzyme is similar to but distinct from the microsomal carboxylesterases that hydrolyze esters and amides. AADAC can potentially alter the overall balance between detoxication and activation of aromatic amines.

Overall, it would appear that low NAT2 activity increases the risk of bladder, breast, liver, and lung cancers, and decreases the risk of colon cancer, whereas low NAT1 activity increases the

risk of bladder and colon cancers and decreases the risk of lung cancer (Hirvonen, 1999). The individual risks associated with particular NAT1 and/or NAT2 acetylator genotypes are small, but they increase when considered in conjunction with other susceptibility genes and/or exposure to carcinogenic aromatic and heterocyclic amines. Because of the relatively high frequency of allelic variants of NAT1 and NAT2, the attributable risk of cancer in the population may be high (Hein *et al.*, 2000).

Amino Acid Conjugation

There are two principal pathways by which xenobiotics are conjugated with amino acids, as illustrated in Fig. 6-62. The first involves conjugation of xenobiotics containing a carboxylic acid group with the *amino group* of amino acids such as glycine, glutamine, and taurine (see Fig. 6-51). This pathway involves activation of the xenobiotic by conjugation with coenzyme A (CoA), which produces a xenobiotic-CoA thioester that reacts with the *amino group* of an amino acid to form an amide linkage. The second pathway involves conjugation of xenobiotics containing an aromatic hydroxylamine (*N*-hydroxy aromatic amine) with the *carboxylic acid group* of such amino acids as serine and proline. This pathway involves activation of an amino acid by aminoacyl-tRNA-synthetase, which reacts with an aromatic hydroxylamine to form a reactive *N*-ester (Kato and Yamazoe, 1994).

The conjugation of benzoic acid with glycine to form hippuric acid (see Fig. 6-1) was discovered in 1842, making it the first biotransformation reaction discovered (Knights *et al.*, 2007). The first step in this conjugation reaction involves activation of benzoic acid to an acyl-CoA thioester. This reaction requires ATP and is catalyzed by acyl-CoA synthetase (ATP-dependent acid:CoA ligase [AMP forming]). The second step is catalyzed by acyl-CoA:amino acid *N*-acyltransferase, which transfers the acyl moiety of the xenobiotic to the amino group of the acceptor amino acid. The reaction proceeds by a *ping-pong Bi–Bi* mechanism, and involves transfer of the xenobiotic to a cysteine residue in the enzyme with release of CoA, followed by transfer of the xenobiotic to the acceptor amino acid with regeneration of the enzyme. The second step in amino acid conjugation is analogous to amide formation during the acetylation of aromatic amines by NAT. Substrates for amino acid conjugation are restricted to certain aliphatic, aromatic, heteroaromatic, cinnamic, and arylacetic acids.

The ability of xenobiotics to undergo amino acid conjugation depends on steric hindrance around the carboxylic acid group, and by substituents on the aromatic ring or aliphatic side chain. In rats, ferrets, and monkeys, the major pathway of phenylacetic acid biotransformation is amino acid conjugation. However, due to steric hindrance, diphenylacetic acid cannot be conjugated with an amino acid, so the major pathway of diphenylacetic acid biotransformation in these 3 species is acyl glucuronidation. Bile acids are endogenous substrates for glycine and taurine conjugation. However, the activation of bile acids to an acyl-CoA thioester is catalyzed by a microsomal enzyme, cholyl-CoA synthetase, and conjugation with glycine or taurine is catalyzed by the cytosolic enzyme, bile acid-CoA:amino acid *N*-acyltransferase (BACAT, gene symbol BAAT) (Falany *et al.*, 1994; Testa and Krämer, 2008, 2010). BACAT is expressed at high levels in the liver, kidney, gallbladder, and intestine, with lower levels in the adrenal gland, muscle, lung, and brain, which suggests that it may have substrates other than bile acids (O'Byrne *et al.*, 2003). In vitro studies show that BACAT can form glycine conjugates of long-chain fatty acids, and also possesses thioesterase activity toward the same substrates (O'Byrne *et al.*, 2003). In contrast to bile acids, the

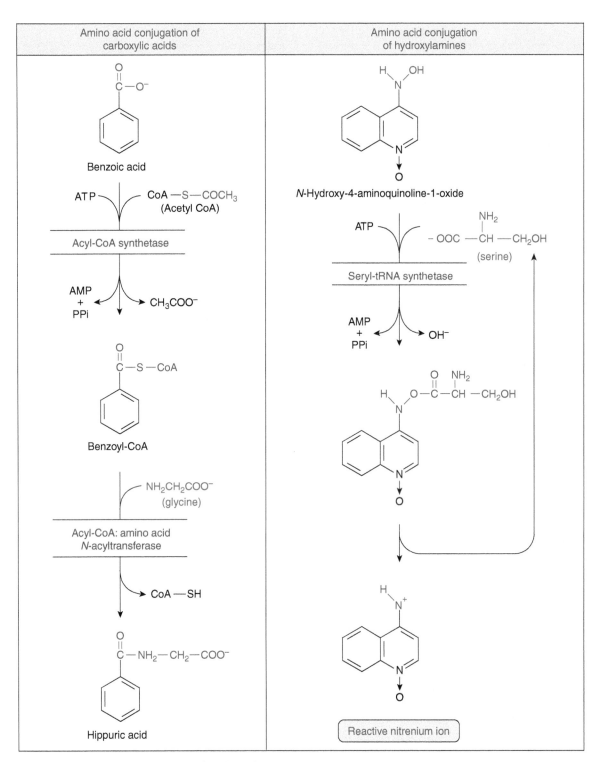

Figure 6-62. *Conjugation of xenobiotics with amino acids.*

activation of xenobiotics occurs mainly in mitochondria, which appear to contain multiple acyl-CoA ligases. There are 3 acid-thiol ligases that are involved in the formation of a xenobiotic acyl-CoA intermediate, namely, the short-, medium-, and long-chain acyl-CoA ligase (Testa and Krämer, 2008, 2010). These enzymes are also involved in endogenous fatty acid activation. Of particular importance to amino acid conjugation is the medium-chain [butyrate]-CoA ligase present in the mitochondrial matrix, which converts medium-chain fatty acids (C_4-C_{12}) to CoA thioesters to initiate β-oxidation (Knights *et al.*, 2007). In humans, two

distinct forms of medium-chain fatty acid CoA ligases have been characterized, HXM-A (48 kDa) and HXM-B (49 kDa), each of which has overlapping substrate specificities. Common substrates of HXM-A and HXM-B include benzoate, propionate, hexano-ate, octanoate, valproate, and salicylate (Knights *et al.*, 2007). The formation of xenobiotic acyl-CoA conjugates is interest-ing because of their potential to cause mitochondrial toxicity by inhibiting fatty-acid β-oxidation due to a combination of CoA sequestration and direct inhibition of acyl-CoA ligases (Knights *et al.*, 2007; Testa and Krämer, 2008, 2010). Some xenobiotic acyl-CoA conjugates can also act as reactive electrophiles and form protein adducts with immunogenic potential (see the section "Glucuronidation and Formation of Acyl-CoA Thioesters"). The second step in the conjugation of xenobiotics with amino acids is catalyzed by cytosolic and/or mitochondrial forms of N-acyltransferase, expressed primarily in the liver and kidney (Knights et al., 2007). Amino acid conjugation is apparently catalyzed by separate N-acyltransferases specific for each amino acid (Gopaul et al., 2003). Glycine-N-acyltransferase and glutamine-N-phenylacetyltransferase have been isolated from human hepatic mitochondria (Gopaul et al., 2003).

There are several examples of xenobiotics that undergo amino acid conjugation as a major metabolic pathway, such as the hypolipidemic drug nicotinic acid (niacin) that is conjugated with glycine to form nicotinuric acid (Iwaki et al., 1996; Testa and Krämer, 2008, 2010). In humans, over 90% of a dose of acetylsalicylic acid (aspirin) is hydrolyzed to salicylic acid, of which 75% is excreted in urine as the glycine conjugate, salicyluric acid (Knights et al., 2007; Testa and Krämer, 2008, 2010). Whereas benzoic acids and small analogs generally are conjugated with glycine, larger substrates such as 4-phenylbutanoic acid are generally conjugated with glutamine. 4-Phenylbutanoic acid is a drug used in the treatment of hyperammonemia caused by genetic errors in urea synthesis. Conjugation of 4-phenylbutanoic acid with glutamine contributes to nitrogen elimination under conditions of impaired urea synthesis (Kasumov et al., 2004; Testa and Krämer, 2008, 2010). Taurine (along with glycine) plays an important role in the conjugation of bile acids. The herbicide 4-chloro-2-methylphenoxyacetic acid (MCPA) forms both taurine and glycine conjugates in dogs, but only trace glycine conjugates in rats (Lappin et al., 2002; Testa and Krämer, 2008, 2010). The PPARα agonist MRL-II exhibits dose-dependent formation of acyl glucuronides and taurine conjugates, major biliary metabolites in dogs, with lower doses favoring the formation of the taurine conjugate (Kim et al., 2004; Testa and Krämer, 2008, 2010). While few reports of xenobiotic taurine conjugates in humans exist, taurine conjugation of the NSAID ibuprofen is a minor metabolite eliminated in urine almost solely as the S-enantiomer (Shirley et al., 1994; Testa and Krämer, 2008, 2010).

An important difference between the amino acid conjugates of xenobiotics and bile acids is their route of elimination: bile acids are secreted into bile, whereas amino acid conjugates of xenobiotics are eliminated primarily in urine. The addition of an endogenous amino acid to xenobiotics may facilitate this elimination by increasing their ability to interact with the tubular organic anion transport system in the kidney. The precursor to amino acid conjugation, namely, the xenobiotic acyl-CoA thioester, is not transported out of the cell and is not detected in bile, plasma, or urine, but it can be detected in tissue samples and in vitro test systems. The formation of xenobiotic acyl-CoA thioesters in adipose tissue (and their further metabolism to more complex lipid conjugates) can be a relatively long-lived repository for certain acidic drugs. Consequently, in mass balance studies (ie, in studies of the disposition of a radiolabeled drug) the formation of acyl-CoA thioesters and their lipid derivatives in adipose tissue can contribute to incomplete recovery of radioactivity in the case of acidic drugs and drugs that are extensively metabolized to one or more carboxylic acid–containing metabolites.

In addition to glycine, glutamine, and taurine, acceptor amino acids for xenobiotic conjugation include ornithine, arginine, histidine, serine, aspartic acid, and several dipeptides, such as glycylglycine, glycyltaurine, and glycylvaline. The acceptor amino acid used for conjugation is both species- and xenobiotic-dependent.

For benzoic, heterocyclic, and cinnamic acids, the acceptor amino acid is glycine, except in birds and reptiles, which use ornithine. Arylacetic acids are also conjugated with glycine except in primates, which use glutamine. In mammals, taurine is generally an alternative acceptor to glycine. Taurine conjugation is well developed in nonmammalian species and carnivores. Whereas most species conjugate bile acids with both glycine and taurine, cats and dogs conjugate bile acids only with taurine.

Amino acid conjugation of carboxylic acid–containing xenobiotics is an alternative to glucuronidation. Conjugation of carboxylic acid–containing xenobiotics with amino acids has long been considered a predominantly detoxication reaction. However, as outlined in the section "Glucuronidation and Formation of Acyl-CoA Thioesters," there is growing evidence that the toxicity of certain NSAIDs is due in part to the formation of reactive acyl-CoA thioesters (the precursors to amino acid conjugates), which represents an alternative activation pathway to the formation of reactive acyl glucuronides, as illustrated in Fig. 6-57. Amino acid conjugation of ibuprofen, ketoprofen, and related profens (2-substituted propionic acid NSAIDs) is significant for two reasons: it limits the formation of potentially toxic acyl glucuronides and it leads to chiral inversion (the interconversion of R- and S-enantiomers) (Shirley et al., 1994). The latter reaction requires conversion of the profen to its acyl-CoA thioester, which undergoes chiral inversion by 2-arylpropionyl-CoA epimerase (this involves the intermediacy of a symmetric, conjugated enolate anion). Chiral inversion may explain why the R- and S-enantiomers of several profen NSAIDs have comparable anti-inflammatory effects in vivo, even though the S-enantiomers are considerably more potent than their antipodes as in vitro inhibitors of cyclooxygenase (the target of NSAID therapy). There is also evidence that the acyl-CoA thioesters of the R-enantiomers are pharmacologically active and contribute to the therapeutic effect by inhibiting COX-2 (Neupert et al., 1997; Levoin et al., 2004; Testa and Krämer, 2008, 2010). In general, amino acid conjugation is a high-affinity–low-capacity reaction, whereas glucuronidation is a high-capacity–low-affinity reaction. At low substrate concentrations, amino acid conjugation can be the predominant reaction.

Amino acid conjugation of N-hydroxy aromatic amines (hydroxylamines) is an activation reaction because it produces N-esters that can degrade to form electrophilic nitrenium and carbonium ions (Anders, 1985; Kato and Yamazoe, 1994). Conjugation of hydroxylamines with amino acids is catalyzed by cytosolic aminoacyl-tRNA synthetases and requires ATP (Fig. 6-62). Hydroxylamines activated by aminoacyl-tRNA synthetases include N-hydroxy-4-aminoquinoline 1-oxide, which is conjugated with serine, and N-hydroxy-Trp-P-2, which is conjugated with proline. (N-Hydroxy-Trp-P-2 is the N-hydroxylated metabolite of Trp-P-2, a pyrolysis product of tryptophan [see Table 6-14].) It is now apparent that the hydroxylamines formed by the CYP-dependent N-hydroxylation of aromatic amines can potentially be activated by numerous reactions, including N-glucuronidation by UGTs (Fig. 6-56), O-acetylation by NAT (Fig. 6-12), O-sulfonation by SULT (Fig. 6-58), and conjugation with amino acids by seryl- or prolyl-tRNA synthetase (Fig. 6-62).

Various amino acid conjugates of valproic acid, including glutamine, glutamate, and glycine conjugates, have been detected in urine, plasma, and cerebrospinal fluid (CSF) of patients administered this antiepileptic (Gopaul et al., 2003). CSF concentrations of the glutamine and glutamate conjugates of valproic acid were 5 and 9 times higher than in plasma, which suggests that these conjugation reactions in the brain decrease levels of the excitatory neurotransmitter glutamic acid and decrease the incidence of seizure

(Gopaul *et al.*, 2003). Taken together, these data suggest that amino acid conjugation in the brain may play a role in the mechanism of action of valproic acid.

Glutathione Conjugation

The preceding section described the conjugation of xenobiotics with certain amino acids, including some simple dipeptides, such as glycyltaurine. This section describes the conjugation of xenobiotics with the tripeptide glutathione (GSH) in a reaction also known as glutathionylation, which is fundamentally different from other conjugation reactions. Whereas glucuronidation, sulfonation, and all of the other previously described conjugation reactions involve conjugation of nucleophilic xenobiotics or their nucleophilic metabolites, GSH conjugation occurs with electrophilic xenobiotics or their electrophilic metabolites. GSH is composed of glycine, cysteine, and glutamic acid (the latter being linked to cysteine via the γ-carboxyl group, not the usual α-carboxyl group, as shown in Fig. 6-51). Glutathione transferase (GST) activity was first discovered as the enzyme-catalyzed conjugation of GSH with halogenated compounds such as chloronitrobenzenes and bromosulfophthalein (Mannervik *et al.*, 2005; Higgins and Hayes, 2011). The activity was initially designated GSH *S*-aryltransferase, and GST activities toward other substrates such as alkyl halides and epoxides were called *S*-alkyl and *S*-epoxide transferases. The original names were later replaced with letter designations once the overlapping substrate specificity was described, and it was recognized that GSTs do not simply conjugate xenobiotics with GSH but also catalyze reactions such as hydroperoxide reduction (an example of which is shown in Fig. 6-18 as part of the metabolism of carbon tetrachloride), dehydrohalogenation (as shown in Figs. 6-20 [general mechanisms] and 6-21 [dechlorination of DDT]), thiolysis (the general mechanism for disulfide cleavage is shown in Fig. 6-14), disulfide interchange, and isomerization (Mannervik *et al.*, 2005; Higgins and Hayes, 2011). Although the abbreviation "GST" has survived to describe the enzyme family, the term "glutathione *S*-transferase" is technically incorrect because the glutathionyl group (GS-) is transferred rather than a single sulfur atom (Mannervik *et al.*, 2005) (the correct term is glutathione transferase). GSTs function endogenously as part of a defense mechanism against reactive oxygen species (ROS); GSTs reduce the formation of hydroperoxides of fatty acids, phospholipids, and cholesterol and protect against the redox cycling of many quinone-containing compounds by conjugating them with GSH (Hayes *et al.*, 2005; Testa and Krämer, 2010). GSTs also play a role in other endogenous functions such as the degradation of aromatic amino acids, steroid hormone synthesis, eicosanoid synthesis (leukotrienes are GSH conjugates), and modulation of signaling pathways (Hayes *et al.*, 2005; Higgins and Hayes, 2011; Oakley, 2011).

Substrates for glutathionylation include an enormous array of electrophilic xenobiotics, or xenobiotics that can be biotransformed to electrophiles. GSH conjugates are thioethers that form by nucleophilic attack of GSH thiolate anion (GS⁻) with an electrophilic carbon or heteroatom (*O*, *N*, and *S*) in the xenobiotic or its metabolite. Michael acceptors are also conjugated with GSH (discussed later in this section). The sulfhydryl group in GSH has a pK_a value of ~9.0; hence, at physiological pH, only ~1% of GSH is present in the thiolate anion (GS⁻) form. A primary function of GSTs is to lower the pK_a of GSH by more than 2 orders of magnitude (to pK_a 6–7), such that most (>50%) of the GSH bound to GST is in the reactive anionic form, which is stabilized by hydrogen bonding with a tyrosine, serine, or cysteine residue in the active site (Testa and Krämer,

2008, 2010). GSH, cysteine, *N*-acetylcysteine (NAC), and various analogs (esters and amides) are used in vitro to trap electrophilic metabolites formed by CYP in liver microsomes. In this system, which lacks the cytosolic GSTs, only ~1% of GSH is present in the thiolate anion (GS⁻), compared with 6% of cysteine and up to 16% for certain cysteine esters, which is why agents other than GSH are widely used to trap electrophilic metabolites formed by CYP in vitro (Reed, 1985). Cysteine has 6-fold greater ionization than GSH at physiological pH; however, the concentration of GSH in liver is ~50 times greater than that of cysteine, and its ionization is greatly increased by binding to GSTs.

The synthesis of GSH involves formation of the peptide bond between cysteine and glutamic acid, followed by peptide bond formation with glycine. The first and overall rate-limiting reaction is catalyzed by γ-glutamylcysteine synthetase (γ-GCL), the second by GSH synthetase. At each step, ATP is hydrolyzed to ADP and inorganic phosphate (Testa and Krämer, 2008, 2010). Due to the sheer multiplicity of GSTs, they cannot be collectively inhibited or induced; therefore, the importance of glutathionylation in xenobiotic toxicity in vivo is often assessed by altering levels of GSH. This can be achieved by (1) inhibiting GSH synthesis, (2) depleting GSH, or (3) increasing GSH levels through Nrf2 activation. Inhibition of GSH synthesis can be achieved with buthionine-*S*-sulfoximine (BSO), which inhibits γ-GCL, the enzyme that catalyzes the first reaction in GSH synthesis (Ballatori *et al.*, 2009a). Michael acceptors such as diethyl maleate (DEA) and phorone are commonly used in vivo to deplete GSH levels in experimental animals. Other agents, such as 2-cyclohexen-1-one and 2-cyclohepten-1-one, selectively decrease cerebral GSH levels in comparison with BSO treatment (Masukawa *et al.*, 1989; Yoneyama *et al.*, 2008). Lastly several agents can activate Nrf2, which induces γ-GCL, the rate-limiting step in GSH synthesis. Nrf2 activators include butylated hydroxytoluene (BHT), butylated hydroxyanisole (BHA), ethoxyquin, and low doses of acetaminophen (Higgins and Hayes, 2011).

The conjugation of xenobiotics with GSH is catalyzed by GSTs in cytosol, microsomes (ie, the membrane-associated proteins in eicosanoid and glutathione metabolism [MAPEG] family), and mitochondria (Hayes *et al.*, 2005; Higgins and Hayes, 2011; Oakley, 2011). Most GSTs were originally found in the soluble cell fraction, and they are referred to as cytosolic or soluble GSTs, even though they may also be found in the nucleus or peroxisomes (Mannervik *et al.*, 2005; Higgins and Hayes, 2011; Oakley, 2011). The only mitochondrial GST found to date has traditionally been referred to as Kappa GST (detailed later in this section), and although it dimerizes (as do the cytosolic GSTs), Kappa GST has a structure that is distinct from the cytosolic GSTs and is also present in peroxisomes, which suggests that it is involved in fatty acid β-oxidation (Hayes *et al.*, 2005; Mannervik *et al.*, 2005; Morel and Aninat, 2011). The microsomal GSTs (or MAPEGs) are an independent group of proteins which are integral microsomal and mitochondrial membrane components. It should also be noted that some GSTs have nonenzymatic functions such as binding of zeaxanthin in the retina and c-Jun N-terminal kinase 1 by GST P1-1, and were initially designated by other names (Mannervik *et al.*, 2005). There are also other proteins that are homologous to some GSTs but are not yet known to serve as detoxication enzymes, such as the chloride intracellular channels (CLIC) (Mannervik *et al.*, 2005; Littler *et al.*, 2010). Hence, proteins that are already characterized and named may eventually be designated as GSTs, as was the case with GSH-dependent hematopoietic prostaglandin D synthase (HPGDS), now determined to be GST S1-1 due to similarities with the Sigma class GSTs expressed in nonmammalian

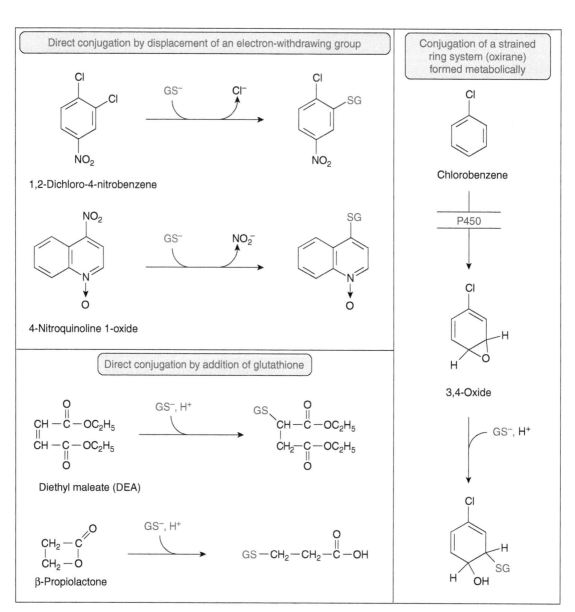

Figure 6-63. *Examples of glutathione conjugation of xenobiotics with an electrophilic carbon.* GS$^-$ represents the anionic form of glutathione.

organisms. The GSTs are present in most tissues, with high concentrations in the liver, intestine, kidney, testis, adrenal, and lung.

Substrates for GST share 3 common features: they are hydrophobic, they contain an electrophilic atom, and they react nonenzymatically with GSH at some measurable rate. The mechanism by which GST increases the rate of GSH conjugation involves deprotonation of GSH to GS$^-$ by an active-site tyrosine or serine, which functions as a general base catalyst (Atkins *et al.*, 1993; Dirr *et al.*, 1994). In the case of the Omega class GSTs, the active site contains a cysteine residue (Mukherjee *et al.*, 2006; Board, 2011). The concentration of GSH in liver is extremely high (5–10 mM) relative to plasma (0.5–10 μM); hence, the nonenzymatic conjugation of certain xenobiotics with GSH can be significant (Testa and Krämer, 2008, 2010). However, some xenobiotics are conjugated with GSH stereoselectively, indicating that the reaction is largely catalyzed by GST. Like GSH, the GSTs are themselves abundant cellular components, accounting for up to 10% of the total cellular protein. These enzymes bind, store, and/or transport a number of compounds that are not substrates for GSH conjugation. The cytoplasmic protein formerly known as ligandin, which binds heme, bilirubin, steroids,

azo-dyes, polycyclic aromatic hydrocarbons (PAHs), and thyroid hormones (THs), is an Alpha class GST (Oakley, 2011).

As shown in Fig. 6-63, substrates for GSH conjugation can be divided into two groups: those that are sufficiently electrophilic to be conjugated directly and those that must first be biotransformed to an electrophilic metabolite prior to conjugation. The second group of substrates for GSH conjugation includes reactive intermediates (often formed by CYP) such as oxiranes (arene oxides and alkene epoxides), nitrenium ions, carbonium ions, and free radicals. The conjugation reactions themselves can be divided into two types: *displacement reactions*, in which GSH displaces an electron-withdrawing group, and *addition reactions*, in which GSH is added to an activated double bond or strained ring system. Table 6-20 provides examples of typical substrates for each of the characterized GSTs.

The displacement of an electron-withdrawing group by GSH typically occurs when the substrate contains halide, sulfate, sulfonate, phosphate, or a nitro group (ie, good *leaving groups*) attached to an allylic or benzylic carbon atom. Displacement of an electron-withdrawing group from aromatic xenobiotics is decreased by the

Table 6-20

Human Glutathione Transferase Enzymes

GST FAMILY	CLASS	GENE	EXAMPLE ENZYMES	EXAMPLE SUBSTRATES
Cytosolic	Alpha	GSTA1	GST A1-1	Δ^5-ADD, BCDE, BPDE, busulfan, chlorambucil, DBADE, DBPDE, BPhDE, N-acetoxy-PhIP
		GSTA2	GST A2-2	CuOOH, DBPDE, 7-chloro-4-nitrobenz-2-oxa-1,3-diazole
		GSTA3	GST A3-3	Δ^5-ADD, Δ^5-pregnene-3,20-dione, DBPDE
		GSTA4	GST A4-4	COMC-6, EA, 4-hydroxynonenal, 4-hydroxydecenal
		GSTA5	GST A5-5	Unknown
	Mu	GSTM1	GST M1-1	trans-4-Phenyl-3-buten-2-one, BPDE, CDE, DBADE, trans-stilbene oxide, styrene-7,8-oxide
		GSTM2	GST M2-2	COMC-6, 1,2-dichloro-4-nitrobenzene, aminochrome, dopa O-quinone, $PGH_2 \rightarrow PGE_2$
		GSTM3	GST M3-3	BCNU, $PGH_2 \rightarrow PGE_2$
		GSTM4	GST M4-4	CDNB
		GSTM5	GST M5-5	CDNB
	Pi	GSTP1	GST P1-1	Acrolein, base propenals, BPDE, CDE, chlorambucil, COMC-6, EA, Thio-TEPA
	Sigma	HPGDS	GST S1-1*	$PGH_2 \rightarrow PGD_2$
	Theta	GSTT1	GST T1-1	BCNU, butadiene epoxide, CH_2Cl_2, EPNP, ethylene oxide
		GSTT2	GST T2-2	CuOOH, menaphthyl sulfonate
	Zeta	GSTZ1	GST Z1-1	Dichloroacetate, fluoroacetate, 2-chloropropionate, maleylacetoacetate
	Omega	GSTO1	GST O1-1	Monomethylarsonic acid, dehydroascorbic acid
		GSTO2	GST O2-2	Monomethylarsonic acid, dehydroascorbic acid
Mitochondrial	Kappa	GSTK1	GST K1-1	CDNB, CuOOH, (S)-15-hydroperoxy-5,8,11,13-eicosatetraenoic acid
Microsomal (MAPEGs)	Clan 1	MGST2	MGST2	CDNB, $LTA_4 \rightarrow LTC_4$, (S)-5-hydroperoxy-8,11,14-cis-6-trans-eicosatetraenoic acid
		MGST3	MGST3	CDNB, $LTA_4 \rightarrow LTC_4$, (S)-5-hydroperoxy-8,11,14-cis-6-trans-eicosatetraenoic acid
		LTC4S	LTC_4S	$LTA_4 \rightarrow LTC_4$
	Clan 2	PTGEs	PGES1	$PGH_2 \rightarrow PGE_2$
		MGST1	MGST1	CDNB, CuOOH, hexachlorobuta-1,3-diene
	Clan 3	ALOX5AP	FLAP	Arachidonic acid binding (nonenzymatic)

Δ^5-ADD, Δ^5-androstene-3,17-dione; BCDE, benzo[g]chrysene diol epoxide; BCNU, 1,3-bis(2-chloroethyl)-1-nitrosourea; BPDE, benzo[a]pyrene diol epoxide; BPhDE, benzo[c]phenanthrene diol epoxide; CDE, chrysene-1,2-diol 3,4-epoxide; CDNB, 1-chloro-2,4-dinitrobenzene; COMC-6, crotonyloxymethyl-2-cyclohexenone; CuOOH, cumene hydroperoxide; DBADE, dibenz[a,h]anthracene diol epoxide; DBPDE, dibenzo[a,l]pyrene diol epoxide; EA, ethacrynic acid; EPNP, 1,2-epoxy-3-(p-nitrophenoxy)propane; N-acetoxy-PhIP, N-acetoxy-2-amino-1-methyl-6-phenylimidazo[4,5-b] pyridine. Data from Hayes et al. (2005), Mannervik et al. (2005), and Higgins and Hayes (2011).
*GST S1-1 is also the glutathione-dependent prostaglandin D synthase.

presence of other substituents that donate electrons to the aromatic ring (–NH$_2$, –OH, –OR, and –R). Conversely, such displacement reactions are increased by the presence of other electron-withdrawing groups (–F, –Cl, –Br, –I, –NO$_2$, –CN, –CHO, and –COOR). This explains why 1,2-dichloro-4-nitrobenzene and 1-chloro-2,4-dinitrobenzene, each of which contains 3 electron-withdrawing groups, are commonly used as substrates for measuring GST activity in vitro, and one or more members of all 3 GST families can catalyze this conjugation reaction (Hayes *et al.*, 2005; Higgins and Hayes, 2011). GST can catalyze the O-demethylation of dimethylvinphos and other methylated organophosphorus compounds. The reaction is analogous to the interaction between methyliodide and GSH, which produces methylglutathione and iodide ion (GS$^-$ + CH$_3$I → GS–CH$_3$ + I$^-$). In this case, iodide is the leaving group. In the case of dimethylvinphos, the entire organophosphate molecule (minus the methyl group) functions as the leaving group.

The addition of GSH to a carbon–carbon double bond is also facilitated by the presence of a nearby electron-withdrawing group; hence, substrates for this reaction typically contain a double bond attached to –CN, –CHO, –COOR, or –COR (ie, they are Michael acceptors). The double bond in diethyl maleate (DEA) is attached to 2 electron-withdrawing groups and readily undergoes a Michael addition reaction with GSH, as shown in Fig. 6-63. The loop diuretic, ethacrynic acid, contains an α/β-unsaturated ketone that readily reacts with GSH and other sulfhydryls by Michael addition. The conversion of acetaminophen to a GSH conjugate involves addition of GSH to an activated double bond, which is formed during the CYP-dependent dehydrogenation of acetaminophen to NAPQI, as shown in Fig. 6-35.

An interesting feature of GSH conjugation is the potential for nonenzymatic GSH conjugation in xenobiotic metabolism. The mechanism for this nonenzymatic activity is based on electrophilicity or nucleophilicity of potential reactants (Testa and Krämer, 2008, 2010). Electrophiles and nucleophiles are scaled according to their hardness or softness, and this determines whether a nonenzymatic or GST-catalyzed enzymatic reaction will be favored. Hard electrophilic sites are highly localized positive charges that maintain a high charge density during the approach of a nucleophilic reactant (ie, they are not readily polarized). On the other hand, soft electrophilic sites have a low charge density (ie, a delocalized charge) and are easily polarized by an approaching nucleophilic reactant (Testa and Krämer, 2008, 2010). Since GSH acts as a soft nucleophile, it will react spontaneously with soft electrophiles, such as in the case of 1-4(nitrophenoxy)propane-2,3-oxide, which is a poor GST substrate, but reacts spontaneously with GSH (Testa and Krämer, 2008, 2010). Hard electrophiles are unlikely to react spontaneously with GSH and require the catalytic facilitation of GSTs (Testa and Krämer, 2008, 2010).

Arene oxides and alkene epoxides, which are often formed by CYP-dependent oxidation of aromatic hydrocarbons and alkenes, are examples of strained ring systems that open during the addition of GSH (Fig. 6-63). In many cases, conjugation of arene oxides with GSH proceeds stereoselectively, as shown in Fig. 6-64 for the 1,2-oxides of naphthalene. The GSH conjugates of arene oxides may undergo rearrangement reactions, which restore aromaticity and possibly lead to migration of the conjugate to the adjacent carbon atom (through formation of an episulfonium ion), as shown in Fig. 6-64. Conjugation of quinones and quinoneimines with GSH also restores aromaticity, as shown in Fig. 6-35 for NAPQI, the reactive metabolite of acetaminophen. Compared with glucuronidation and sulfonation, conjugation with GSH is a minor pathway of acetaminophen biotransformation, even though the liver contains high levels of both GSH and GSTs. The relatively low rate of GSH conjugation reflects the slow rate of formation of NAPQI, which is catalyzed by CYP (Fig. 6-35).

GSH can also conjugate xenobiotics with an electrophilic heteroatom (O, N, and S) as shown in Fig. 6-65. In each of the examples shown in Fig. 6-65, the initial conjugate formed between GSH and the heteroatom is cleaved by a second molecule of GSH to form oxidized GSH, which is also known as glutathione disulfide (GSSG). The initial reactions shown in Fig. 6-65 are catalyzed by GST, whereas the second reaction (which leads to GSSG formation) generally occurs nonenzymatically. Analogous reactions leading to the reduction and cleavage of disulfides have been described previously (see Fig. 6-14). Some of the reactions shown in Fig. 6-65, such as the reduction of hydroperoxides to alcohols, can also be catalyzed by glutathione peroxidase (GPX), which is a selenium-dependent enzyme. For their role in the reduction of hydroperoxides, the GSTs are sometimes called nonselenium-requiring GPXs. For instance, one or more members of the mammalian cytosolic, microsomal, and mitochondrial GSTs exhibit GPX activity toward cumene hydroperoxide (Hayes et al., 2005). Cleavage of the nitrate esters of nitroglycerin releases nitrite, which can be converted to the potent vasodilator, nitric oxide (NO). The ability of sulfhydryl-generating chemicals to partially prevent or reverse tolerance to nitroglycerin suggests that GSH-dependent denitration may play a role in nitroglycerin-induced vasodilation, although ALDH2 is recognized as the principal enzyme responsible for activating nitroglycerin as discussed in the section "Aldehyde Dehydrogenase" (Marchitti et al., 2008).

Cytosolic or mitochondrial GSTs catalyze two important isomerization reactions, namely, the conversion of the endoperoxide, PGH_2, to the prostaglandins PGD_2 and PGE_2 and the conversion of Δ^5 steroids to Δ^4 steroids, such as the formation of androstenedione from androst-5-ene-3,17-dione. Another physiological function of GST is the synthesis of leukotriene C_4, which is catalyzed by the microsomal GSTs, namely, MGST2, MGST3, and LTC_4S (see Table 6-20).

GSH conjugates formed in the liver can be effluxed into bile by MRP2 (ABCC2) on the canalicular membrane, or they can be transported into blood by various transporters on the sinusoidal membrane such as MRP1 (ABCC1), MRP3 (ABCC3), MRP4 (ABCC4), MRP5 (ABCC5), and MRP6 (ABCC6) (Giacomini and Sugiyama, 2006; Ballatori et al., 2009a; Klaassen and Aleksunes, 2010). MRP7 (ABCC10) and MRP8 (ABCC11)

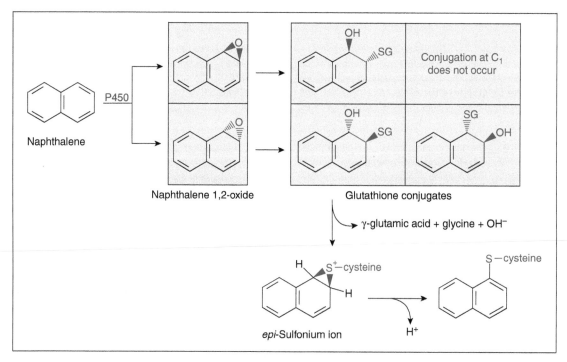

Figure 6-64. *Stereoselective conjugation of naphthalene 1,2-oxide and rearrangement of 2-naphthyl to 1-naphthyl conjugates.*

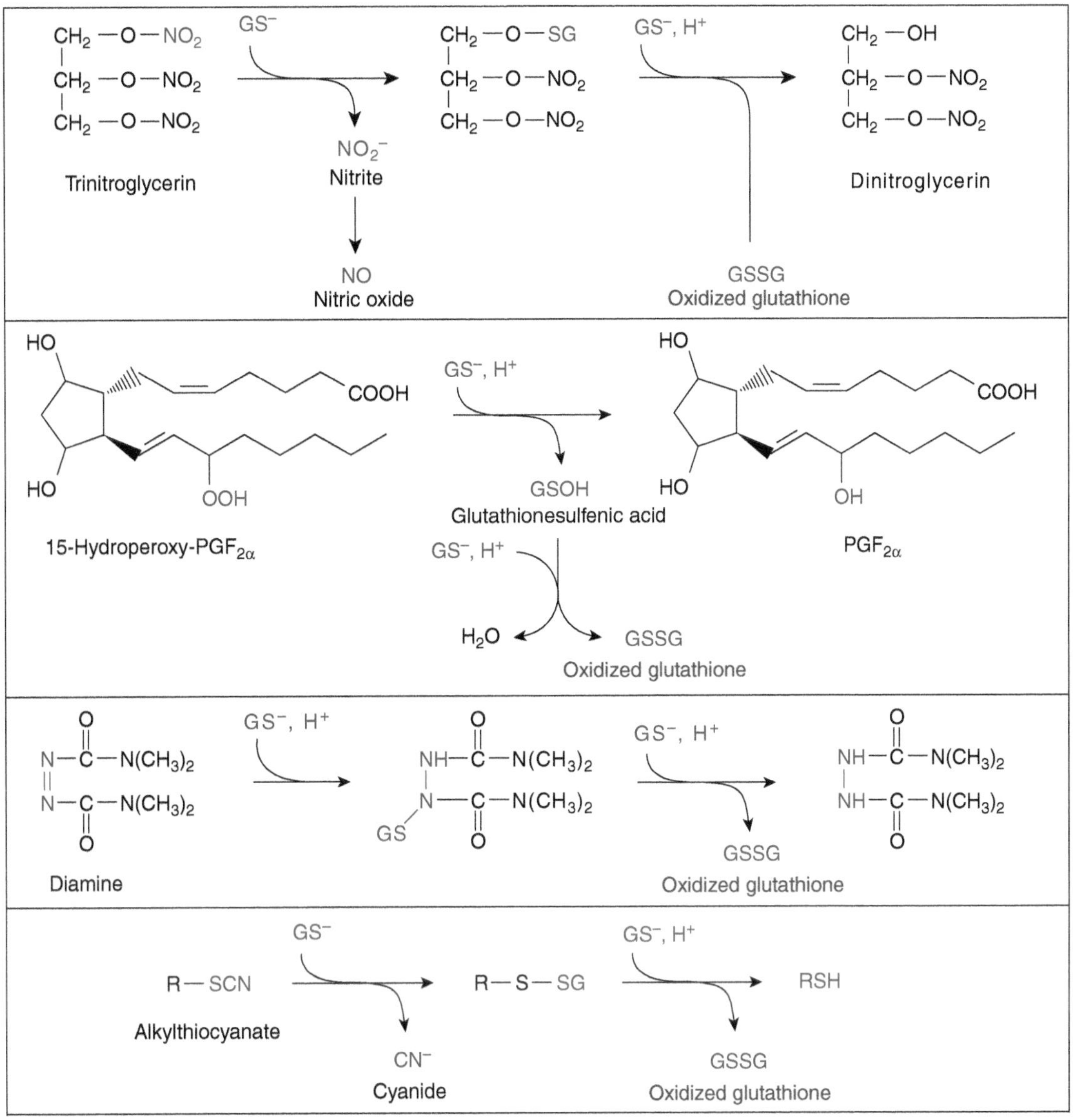

Figure 6-65. *Examples of glutathione conjugation of electrophilic heteroatoms.*

have also been implicated in the transport of GSH conjugates (Ballatori *et al.*, 2009a). GSH itself is often cotransported with other xenobiotics or xenobiotic metabolites, namely, by MRP2 into bile, and by MRP1, MRP4, and MRP5 into blood (Ballatori *et al.*, 2009a). This cotransport is exemplified by drugs such as vincristine, etoposide, and vinblastine, each of which stimulates MRP-mediated GSH transport (Ballatori *et al.*, 2009a). BCRP (ABCG2) is also involved in GSH transport (Brechbuhl *et al.*, 2010). Furthermore, GST and MRP overexpression can act synergistically to confer multiple-drug resistance in many cancers, and can affect the efficacy of chemotherapeutic drugs such as chlorambucil, etoposide, ethacrynic acid, vincristine, and doxorubicin (Sau *et al.*, 2010).

GSH conjugates can be converted to mercapturic acids (*N*-acetylcysteine conjugates) in the kidney and excreted in urine. As shown in Fig. 6-66, the conversion of GSH conjugates to mercapturic acids involves the sequential cleavage of glutamic acid and glycine from the GSH moiety, followed by *N*-acetylation of the resulting cysteine conjugate. The first 2 steps in mercapturic acid synthesis are catalyzed by γ-glutamyltransferase (GGT1; located primarily in the liver) and membrane alanyl aminopeptidase

(ANPEP; located in the kidney). The GSH conjugate, leukotriene C$_4$, is similarly hydrolyzed by GGT1 to form leukotriene E$_4$.

Cytosolic GSTs are dimers, typically composed of identical subunits (Mr 23-29 kDa), although some forms are heterodimers. Each subunit contains 199 to 244 amino acids and one catalytic site. The general structural features of cytosolic GSTs include an N-terminal thioredoxin-like domain (with βαβαββαα topology) and a C-terminal domain consisting of α-helices (Oakley, 2011). Mitochondrial GSTs are also dimeric with 226 amino acids per subunit. The microsomal GSTs vary in their ability to form complex aggregates across the 3 groups of human MAPEGs. Numerous GST subunits have been cloned and sequenced, which forms the basis of a nomenclature system (Mannervik *et al.*, 1992, 2005; Hayes and Pulford, 1995; Whalen and Boyer, 1998; Hayes *et al.*, 2005; Higgins and Hayes, 2011), as shown in Table 6-20. Each cytosolic and mitochondrial enzyme is assigned a two-digit number to designate its subunit composition. For example, the homodimers of subunits 1 and 2 are designated 1-1 and 2-2, respectively, whereas the heterodimer is designated 1-2. The soluble GSTs were initially arranged into 4 classes designated A, M, P, and T (which refer to Alpha, Mu, Pi, and Theta). Four additional

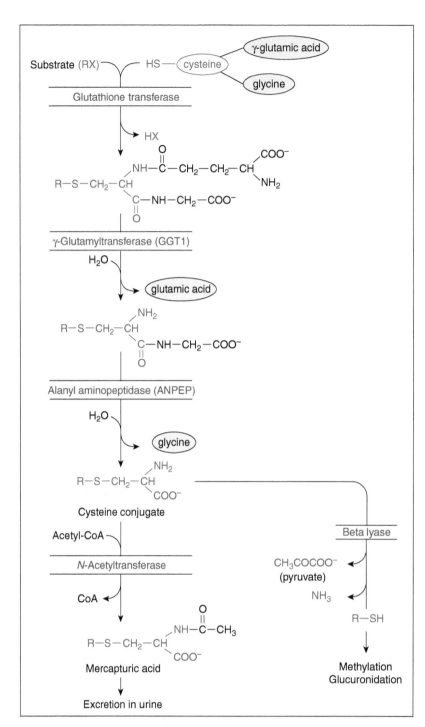

Figure 6-66. *Glutathione conjugation and mercapturic acid biosynthesis.*

classes were subsequently identified, namely, K (Kappa; the mitochondrial form), S (Sigma), Z (Zeta), and O (Omega) (Hayes and Pulford, 1995; Whalen and Boyer, 1998; Strange *et al.*, 2000; Hayes *et al.*, 2005; Higgins and Hayes, 2011; Oakley, 2011). None of these 8 gene classes corresponds to the microsomal GSTs, which appear to have evolved independently. By definition, the subunits in the different classes share less than 50% amino acid sequence identity. Generally, the subunits within a class are ~70% identical, but can share up to 90% sequence identity, and can form heterodimers, whereas the subunits in different classes are generally only ~30% identical. On the basis of structural similarity as well as the residues in the GSH-binding site that are involved in thiolate anion formation, the cytosolic GSTs can be divided

into two groups: the more recently evolved Alpha, Mu, Pi, and Sigma classes that use a tyrosine residue near the N-terminus to activate GSH; and the older Theta, Omega, and Zeta classes that use either an N-terminal proximate serine or cysteine residue to activate GSH (Higgins and Hayes, 2011). Members of the Alpha and Mu classes can also form heterodimers with each other (Hayes *et al.*, 2005). Affinity labeling studies with rat Alpha GSTs demonstrated the presence of a high-affinity, nonsubstrate binding site within the cleft between the two subunits of the dimer. Presumably, the cleft in heterodimers would be different from that in homodimers, which suggests the possibility that there is an evolutionary reason that the formation of heterodimers between Alpha and Mu subunits has been conserved (Hayes *et al.*, 2005).

Several GSTs are overexpressed in various cancers, such as Alpha, Mu, Theta, Pi, and microsomal GSTs, which can confer resistance against many chemotherapeutic agents. For example, GST Alpha overexpression has been correlated with resistance to alkylating agents (Sau et al., 2010). GST Mu overexpression is associated with chlorambucil resistance and a poor prognosis in childhood acute lymphoblastic leukemia (Sau et al., 2010). The microsomal GSTs have been shown to confer resistance to chlorambucil, melphalan, cisplatin, and doxorubicin treatment (Sau et al., 2010). GSTP1-1 overexpression, the most highly expressed GST in various cancers, is often associated with a poor prognosis and chemotherapeutic resistance in ovarian, non-small cell lung, breast, and colorectal cancers (Sau et al., 2010; Tew and Townsend, 2011). Two strategies have been adopted in the development of cancer therapies that specifically target cells that overexpress GSTs, namely (1) inhibition of GSTs and (2) activation of prodrugs by GSTs to form reactive metabolites. Telintra™ (TLK199: Ezatiostat—not yet approved) is a GSH-peptidomimetic prodrug that is activated by cellular esterases to the selective GSTP1-1 inhibitor TLK117 (Sau et al., 2010; Tew and Townsend, 2011). Although not commonly used due to its diuretic effects, ethacrynic acid inhibition of GSTs sensitizes cancer cells to chemotherapeutics (Sau et al., 2010). A synthetic GSH analog specifically inhibits GSTA1-1, whereas the 7-nitro-2,1,3-benzoxadiazole derivative, NBDHEX, is an inhibitor of GSTP1-1 that is not effluxed by transporters (Sau et al., 2010). Several other drugs have been shown to inhibit GSTs, such as drugs that act as NO donors (PABA/NO and oxathiazolylum-5-olate derivatives) and bombesin-sulfonamide derivatives (Sau et al., 2010). Telcyta™ (TLK286: canfosfamide—not yet approved) is a modified GSH analog that can be metabolized by GSTP1-1, which results in the release of two electrophilic fragments, GSH vinyl sulfone and a tetrakis (chloroethyl) phosphorodiamidate that leads to apoptosis (Townsend and Tew, 2003; Rosen et al., 2004; Gonzalez and Tukey, 2006; Tew and Townsend, 2011). Other drugs have also been developed to take advantage of activation by GSTs, such as 2-crotonyloxymethyl-2-cycloalkenone (COMC) derivatives, brostallicin and ethacraplatin (Sau et al., 2010).

As is the case with many of the other xenobiotic-metabolizing enzymes, all of the GST enzymes are polymorphic and this likely contributes to interindividual differences in drug response or toxicity. For example, the null phenotypes for GST Mu and GST Theta, GSTM1*0 and GSTT1*0, respectively, contribute to the drug-associated toxicities of several xenobiotics, such as carbamazepine, valproic acid, and troglitazone (Saruwatari et al., 2010; Ikeda, 2011). Therefore, individuals who are polymorphic for these enzymes (and also potentially for other GST allelic variants) are at an increased risk of toxicity by xenobiotics that are selectively biotransformed by specific GSTs.

The alpha GSTs are the major GSTs in liver and kidney. They have basic isoelectric points. The rat genome database (http://rgd.mcw.edu) indicates that rats express at least four GSTA genes, GSTA1, GSTA2, GSTA3, and GSTA4 (provisional). Humans express five subunits belonging to the Alpha class of GSTs, designated GSTA1 to GSTA5. Human GSTA1 and GSTA2 are polymorphic, with at least two and five alleles identified, respectively, which affect the amount or the activity of expressed protein (Hayes et al., 2005). GSTA1*A expression is higher than GSTA1*B, and individuals with the latter loss-of-function variant have improved rates of breast cancer survival, presumably due to increased efficacy of chemotherapeutic drugs (Ekhart et al., 2009). On the other hand, GSTA2 variants *A to *D do not show much difference in enzymatic activity, whereas GSTA2*E is a

loss-of-function variant (McIlwain et al., 2006). Rats express at least 7 functional Mu subunits, designated GSTM1 to 7. Humans express 5 subunits belonging to the Mu class of GSTs, designated GSTM1 to 5. Human GSTM1, 3, and 4 are known to be polymorphic. In the case of GSTM1, the *A and *B allelic variants differ by a single amino acid; *A is a "basic variant" with lysine at residue 173, whereas *B is an "acidic variant" with asparagine at the corresponding site. There is also a GSTM1 deletion (*0) and a duplication (*1 × 2) (Hayes et al., 2005). The incidence of the GSTM1 deletion is high in Pacific Islander and Malaysian populations (ie, 62%–100%), intermediate in several other populations (ie, 35%–62% in those of European descent; 32%–53% in those of Asian descent; 40%–53% in those of Hispanic descent), and low in those of African descent (ie, 23%–41%) (Geisler and Olshan, 2001; Piacentini et al., 2011). GSTM1*0 has only a modest effect on the incidence of lung, head, and neck cancers consistent with its high prevalence in various populations. The GSTM1*0 polymorphism has been linked to an increased susceptibility to certain inflammatory diseases (eg, asthma) (Hayes et al., 2005). At least two allelic variants of GSTM3 and GSTM4 have also been identified. Members of the Mu class of GSTs have neutral isoelectric points. Human GSTM2 and M3 are expressed in muscle and brain, respectively. The GSTM1*0 polymorphism is a risk factor for carbamazepine and valproic acid hepatotoxicity, whereas the double null phenotype of GSTM1*0 and GSTT1*0 is a risk factor for troglitazone hepatotoxicity (Saruwatari et al., 2010; Ikeda, 2011).

Humans and rats express one subunit belonging to the Pi class of GSTs, GSTP1, whereas mice have been found to express two Pi subunits, GSTP1 and GSTP2 (provisional). The human Pi enzyme is polymorphic, with at least 4 allelic variants reported (Hayes et al., 2005). The subunit encoded by GSTP1*B is 7 times more active than that encoded by GSTP1*A in conjugating diol epoxides of polycyclic aromatic hydrocarbons (PAHs) (Strange et al., 2000). GSTP polymorphisms are known to influence susceptibility to carcinogens (including some pesticides), affect the response to chemotherapy used in the treatment of metastatic colon cancer and multiple myeloma, and modify the risk of acute myeloid leukemia which results from the successful treatment of Hodgkin's disease, non-Hodgkin's lymphoma, breast, and ovarian cancer (Hayes et al., 2005; Liu et al., 2006b). GSTP polymorphisms that result in decreased activity have been implicated in an increased susceptibility to certain inflammatory diseases (eg, asthma) (Hayes et al., 2005). Members of the Pi class of GSTs have acidic isoelectric points. They are expressed in the placenta, lung, gut, and other extrahepatic tissues. In rats, GSTP1 is one of several proteins (so-called preneoplastic antigens) that are overexpressed in chemical-induced tumors.

The Sigma class of GSTs is widely distributed in nature, and is present in many species including humans, mice, rats, chickens, insects, flatworms, and mollusks (Flanagan and Smythe, 2011). Sigma GSTs, also known as hematopoietic prostaglandin D synthases (HPGDS), are involved in the synthesis of prostaglandin in mammals, and catalyze the conversion of the cyclooxygenase product PGH_2 to PGD_2. Sigma subunits are also capable of conjugating GSH to a variety of aryl halide substrates and organic isothiocyanates and also have GPX activity toward cumene hydroperoxide (Flanagan and Smythe, 2011). The human Sigma class GST (HPGDS) is different from other cytosolic GSTs in that it is activated by divalent metal ions, such as Mg^{2+} and Ca^{2+}, binding at the center of the dimer interface formed by a group of 6 conserved Asp residues (Inoue et al., 2003; Flanagan and Smythe, 2011). Rats and humans appear to express a single Sigma GST (GSTS1, also known as the GSH-dependent HPGDS). The tissue distribution of Sigma GST occurs in a species-specific manner. In mammals, high levels of Sigma GST are present in the spleen, bone marrow, placenta, lung, adipose, oviduct, and both dermal and epidermal layers of skin (Flanagan and Smythe, 2011). In rats, Sigma GST is highly expressed in bone marrow and spleen, whereas in humans it is highly expressed in adipose tissue, placenta, lung, and fetal liver (Flanagan and Smythe, 2011). Immunohistochemical studies of Sigma GST (ie, HPGDS) in rat, mouse, and human have shown that expression of the enzyme is limited to select cell types, namely, antigen-presenting cells, resident tissue and infiltrating mast cells, and T-helper (Th)-2 cells (Flanagan and Smythe, 2011). Sigma GST can play multiple roles in the immune response because the PGD_2 produced by Sigma GST (ie, by HPGDS) can exert both proinflammatory and anti-inflammatory effects (Flanagan and Smythe, 2011). To block PGD_2 production associated with allergic inflammation, drugs have been or are currently being developed as Sigma GST (HPGDS) inhibitors, such as tranilast (N-(3,4-dimethoxycinnamoyl) anthranilic acid), which is an inhibitor of both HPGDS and LPGDS (lipocalin prostaglandin D synthase) (Flanagan and Smythe, 2011). At least 2 allelic variants of Sigma GST (HPGDS) have been identified, but their functional significance remains to be elucidated (Hayes et al., 2005).

Humans express two subunits belonging to the Theta class of GSTs (GSTT1 and GSTT2), whereas rats and mice each express 4 subunits (GSTT1-4). GST Theta catalyzes the conjugation of mono and dihaloalkanes with GSH, in contrast to α-haloalkanoates and α,α-dihaloalkanoates which tend to be substrates of GST Zeta (Josephy, 2010). Due to the small active site of GST Theta, small xenobiotics are typical substrates of this enzyme, such as dichloromethane (Josephy, 2010). Additionally, analogous to the reaction shown in Fig. 6-20, GSTT-1 is involved in the bioactivation of ethylene dibromide (an insecticide and gasoline additive) to an electrophilic sulfonium ion that can form adducts with macromolecules (Josephy, 2010). A GSTT1 deletion has been identified (GSTT1*0), which has a modest effect on the incidence of lung, head, and neck cancers, and has also been implicated in an increased susceptibility to certain inflammatory diseases (eg, asthma) (Hayes et al., 2005). The incidence of the GSTT1*0 is present in several populations, at a low to intermediate frequency (10%–43%) in those of European and Mediterranean descent and a slightly higher frequency (20%–45%) in those of African descent (Piacentini et al., 2011). The GSTT1 null allele, in conjunction with GST Mu deficiency, predisposes to troglitazone hepatotoxicity (Ikeda, 2011). Human GSTT2-2 conjugates ethacrynic acid with GSH and catalyzes the GSH-dependent reduction of cumene hydroperoxide, as well as the GSH-dependent sulfatase activity of 1-menaphthyl sulfate (Higgins and Hayes, 2011).

Zeta class GSTs are found in many species, such as plants, fungi, and mammals. Within mammals, there is also a wide tissue distribution of the protein with high levels predominantly in the liver and kidney (Board and Anders, 2011). A single Zeta subunit is expressed in rats, mice, and humans (GSTZ1), which dimerizes to form the functional enzyme GSTZ1-1. GSTZ1-1 is the same enzyme as maleylacetoacetate isomerase (MAAI), the enzyme that catalyzes the isomerization of maleylacetoacetate to fumarylacetoacetate, the penultimate step in tyrosine and phenylalanine catabolism (Board and Anders, 2011). GSTZ1-1 also catalyzes the GSH-dependent biotransformation of dichloroacetate (DCA) to glyoxylate ($CHCl_2$–COOH → CHO–COOH) (Board and Anders, 2011). Although GSH is required for the biotransformation of DCA to glyoxylate, it is not consumed as the GSTZ1-1-catalyzed nucleophilic attack of GSH on DCA yields S-(α-chlorocarboxymethyl)glutathione (GS–CHClCOOH), which in turn undergoes dehalogenation and

facile hydrolysis to produce glyoxylate and GSH (Board and Anders, 2011). In rats, DCA irreversibly inhibits GSTZ1-1 through covalent modification of Cys_{16} by S-(α-chlorocarboxymethyl)glutathione (Board and Anders, 2011). While monohaloalkanes and dihaloalkanes tend to be substrates for GST Theta, a number of α-haloalkanoates and α,α-dihaloalkanoates have been identified as substrates for GSTZ1-1 (Board and Anders, 2011). At least 4 polymorphic variants of GSTZ1-1 have been identified in humans, with the haplotypes designated as GSTZ1A (Lys_{32}, Arg_{42}, Thr_{82}), GSTZ1B (Lys_{32}, Gly_{42}, Thr_{82}), GSTZ1C (Glu_{32}, Gly_{42}, Thr_{82}), and GSTZ1D (Glu_{32}, Gly_{42}, Met_{82}) (Board and Anders, 2011). GSTZ1C shows the highest allele frequency and has been designated the wild-type enzyme. GSTZ1A shows the highest rate of conversion of DCA to glyoxylate and is resistant to inactivation by DCA (Board and Anders, 2011). Genetically determined differences in DCA turnover may be significant if DCA is utilized in cancer therapy (Michelakis et al., 2010; Board and Anders, 2011). GSTZ1 knockout mice have increased levels of GSTA1, A2, M1, M5, P1, P2, and NQO1 in the liver, and undergo rapid weight loss, leucopenia, and death when provided 2% phenylalanine in drinking water (recall that GSTZ1-1 is the same enzyme as MAAI, the enzyme that catalyzes the isomerization of maleylacetoacetate to fumarylacetoacetate, the penultimate step in tyrosine and phenylalanine catabolism) (Board and Anders, 2011).

The Omega class of GST was initially identified through bioinformatics analysis of the expressed sequence tag (EST) database. Omega GSTs are present in many species including plants, yeast, nematodes, insects, and mammals (Board, 2011). Two Omega subunits have been identified in mice, rats, and humans (GSTO1 and GSTO2). GSTO1 and GSTO2 are also expressed strongly in mouse liver, heart, and kidney with wide distribution in other tissues (Board, 2011). The GSTOs differ from the other cytosolic GSTs in that they do not display the typical activity toward substrates such as 1-chloro-2,4-dinitrobenzene, dichloromethane, cumene hydroperoxide, or ethacrynic acid, but have some characteristics of glutaredoxins (GLRXs) (Mukherjee et al., 2006; Board, 2011). Interestingly, a mutation in GSTO1 (Cys_{32}Ala) significantly improves its GSH-conjugating activity with 1-chloro-2,4-dinitrobenzene (Board, 2011). Human GSTO1 shows thiol-transferase activity and can catalyze the reduction of S-phenacylglutathione (a metabolite of tear gas), dehydroascorbate, and methylated arsenic species (Board, 2011). The major component in tear gas 2-chloroacetophenone is converted to a GSH conjugate (phenyl-CO–CH_2Cl + GSH → phenyl-CO–CH_2–SG + HCl) that is further metabolized by GSTO1 to acetophenone (phenyl-CO–CH_2–SG + GSH → phenyl-CO–CH_3 + GSSG) (Board, 2011). Inasmuch as the reaction with S-phenacylglutathione is highly specific to GSTO1, a novel substrate was developed, namely, S-(4-nitrophenacyl)glutathione, that can be used in spectrophotometric assays to determine GSTO1 activity (Board, 2011). GSTO2 also exhibits thiol-transferase activity and can catalyze the reduction of monomethylarsenate and dehydroascorbate, but not S-phenacylglutathiones (Board, 2011). Sulfonylurea cytokine-release inhibitory drugs (CRIDS) can bind to GSTO1 and inhibit IL-1β activation, suggesting GSTO1 involvement in a proinflammatory response (Board, 2011). This suggests that inhibition of GSTO1 is a potential therapeutic target to treat inflammation (Board, 2011). Other agents have been shown to inhibit GSTO1 activity, such as tocopherol succinate, phenylsulfonate, omeprazole, and rifampicin (Bachovchin et al., 2009; Board, 2011). As Omega GSTs can reduce monomethylarsenic acid, they have been suggested to play a key role in arsenic biotransformation through the arsenic methylation pathway (Board, 2011). However, several studies have not supported a major role for GSTOs in overall arsenic biotransformation (Board, 2011). Whereas most GSTs have a tyrosine or serine at the active site, GSTOs have a cysteine and an additional 19 amino acids at the N-terminus (Mukherjee *et al.*, 2006; Board, 2011). Many polymorphisms have been detected in both GSTO1 and GSTO2, with 5 and 4 polymorphisms that result in amino acid changes, respectively (Mukherjee *et al.*, 2006; Board, 2011). GSTO genes have also been associated with several neurological diseases, suggesting that variation of these GSTs may modify disease susceptibility or age of onset through a common pathological mechanism (Board, 2011).

The Kappa class of GSTs is an ancient protein family and represents a separate evolutionary pathway that has significant differences in function, localization, and structure than other soluble GSTs (Morel and Aninat, 2011). Harris *et al.* (1991) initially discovered and isolated GST Kappa from rat liver mitochondrial matrix. The Kappa subunit is a soluble, dimeric protein with a 36% sequence identity to GST Theta, and localized to both the mitochondria and peroxisomes (Morel and Aninat, 2011). A single Kappa subunit is expressed in mouse, rat, and humans, with the gene designated as GSTK1 in each species. The 3-dimensional structure of the Kappa subunit is more similar to bacterial GSH-dependent and disulfide-bond-forming oxidoreductase (DsbA) than to the cytosolic GSTs. The Kappa subunit contains a thioredoxin-like domain but with a DsbA-like α-helical domain inserted between the α2 helix and the β3 strand (Oakley, 2011). GSTK1 is ubiquitously expressed in humans with kidney, liver, adrenal gland, and adipose tissue expressing the most abundant levels (Morel and Aninat, 2011). Differential expression of GSTK1 has been seen between fetal and adult liver and brain tissues, indicating possible ontogenic regulation of GST Kappa (Morel and Aninat, 2011). In rodents it is present at high levels in the liver and stomach; moderate levels in the kidney, heart, and lung; and subsequent decreasing levels in the duodenum, jejunum, and ileum (Thomson *et al.*, 2004; Knight *et al.*, 2007; Morel and Aninat, 2011). GSTK1 expression in the heart shows marked gender differences, with females expressing twice as much Kappa subunit than males (Knight *et al.*, 2007; Morel and Aninat, 2011).

Two human single nucleotide polymorphisms (SNPs) of GSTK1 have been identified in the 5′-flanking region of the GSTK1 gene located −1308 and −1032 bp from the transcription start site (Shield *et al.*, 2010; Morel and Aninat, 2011). The −1308 SNP corresponds to a G to T transition, whereas the −1032 SNP corresponds to an alteration in a CpG methylation site (Shield *et al.*, 2010; Morel and Aninat, 2011). The T allele variant (−1308 SNP) occurs with a 20% frequency in Asian populations (Morel and Aninat, 2011). The −1032 SNP has been demonstrated to cause a 38% decrease in GSTK1 promoter activity in HEK293 and HepG2 cells (Shield *et al.*, 2010; Morel and Aninat, 2011). GSTK1 expression has been correlated with obesity; hence, GST Kappa may represent a new target for xenobiotics in the treatment of insulin resistance and related metabolic disorders (Morel and Aninat, 2011).

The microsomal GSTs are distinct from the soluble enzymes and have been referred to as the membrane associated proteins in eicosanoid and glutathione metabolism (MAPEG) (Higgins and Hayes, 2011). Six human microsomal GSTs divided into 3 clans have been identified (see Table 6-20), which differ in their ability to form aggregates. For instance, MGST1 exists as a trimer, as does the other clan 2 MAPEG, namely, PGES1, whereas the clan 1 MAPEGs, LTC$_4$S and MGST2, as well as the clan 3 MAPEG 5-lipoxygenase-activating protein (FLAP), can function as monomers, dimers, trimers, or more complex aggregates (Hayes *et al.*, 2005; Martinez Molina *et al.*, 2008; Higgins and Hayes, 2011).

MGST1 conjugates xenobiotics with GSH and probably functions solely as a detoxication enzyme. It is a highly abundant microsomal protein (1% of total ER protein) in human liver and the outer mitochondrial membrane (5% of outer mitochondrial membrane protein) in rat liver (Morgenstern *et al.*, 2011). MGST1 plays a role in the biotransformation of certain lipophilic reactive electrophiles and the reduction of membrane-embedded hydroperoxides with substrates that include halogenated hydrocarbons and phospholipid hydroperoxides (Morgenstern *et al.*, 2011). The denitration of glyceryl trinitrate is another role for MGST1 (Morgenstern *et al.*, 2011). While no specific substrates for MGST1 have been found, this MAPEG can be selectively activated with N-ethylmaleimide to determine its contribution toward overall GST activity (Morgenstern *et al.*, 2011). Furthermore, MGST1 is the only GST that can utilize N-acetyl-L-cysteine as a cofactor instead of GSH (Morgenstern *et al.*, 2011). MGST1 is involved in the formation of the mitochondrial permeability transition (MPT), suggesting a role for MGST1 in mitochondria-mediated cell death (Aniya and Imaizumi, 2011). It is also upregulated in many tumor types, overexpressed in many stem cells and stem-cell-like tumor cells, where it may be playing a protective role for these cells (Morgenstern *et al.*, 2011). Other MAPEGs, such as MGST2 and 3, contribute to detoxication and synthesis of leukotriene C$_4$ (Hayes *et al.*, 2005). FLAP does not have catalytic activity, but binds arachidonic acid and is essential for leukotriene synthesis. LTC$_4$S and PGES1 do not appear to be involved in xenobiotic metabolism (Hayes *et al.*, 2005). Many SNPs have been identified in MGST1 and FLAP as well as diallelic variants in MGST3 in certain populations, but the biological significance has not yet been determined (Hayes *et al.*, 2005).

The conjugation of certain xenobiotics with GSH is catalyzed by most classes of GST. For example, members of the Alpha, Kappa, Mu, and Pi classes of human cytosolic GSTs, as well as several of the MAPEG GSTs, all catalyze the conjugation of 1-chloro-2,4-dinitrobenzene. Other reactions are fairly specific for one class of enzymes (Hayes and Pulford, 1995). For example, the Alpha GSTs preferentially isomerize Δ^5 steroids to Δ^4 steroids and reduce linoleate and cumene hydroperoxide to their corresponding alcohols. The Mu GSTs preferentially conjugate certain arene oxides and alkene epoxides, such as styrene-7,8-epoxide. The Pi GSTs preferentially conjugate ethacrynic acid. (For additional examples, see Table 6-20.) However, individual members within a class of GSTs can differ markedly in their substrate specificity. In mice, for example, the Alpha GSTs composed of GSTA3 subunits can rapidly conjugate aflatoxin B$_1$ 8,9-epoxide, whereas those composed of GSTA1 subunits are virtually incapable of catalyzing this reaction (Eaton and Gallagher, 1994).

In rodents, individual members of the Alpha and Mu classes of GSTs are inducible (generally 2- to 3-fold) by 3-methylcholanthrene, phenobarbital, corticosteroids, oltipraz, and various antioxidants (such as ethoxyquin and BHA). Several GST substrates (ie, Michael acceptors) are GST inducers, as are certain nonsubstrates, such as hydrogen peroxide and other ROS (Rushmore *et al.*, 1991; Daniel, 1993; Nguyen *et al.*, 1994; Hayes and Pulford, 1995; Hayes *et al.*, 2005; Higgins and Hayes, 2011). Induction is usually associated with increased levels of mRNA due to transcriptional activation of the gene encoding a subunit of GST. Not all subunits are induced to the same extent (Higgins and Hayes, 2011).

The enhancer regions of the genes encoding some of the rodent GSTs (such as rat GSTA2-2) have been shown to contain a xenobiotic-response element (XRE), a putative phenobarbital-responsive element, a glucocorticoid-responsive element (GRE), and an antioxidant-response element (ARE, which is also known as the electrophile-responsive element [see Point 9 in the section "Introduction"]). Accordingly, in rodents, certain GST subunits are regulated by both AhR and Nrf2 activators (ie, by both *monofunctional* and *bifunctional* agents), as described previously for DT-diaphorase (see the sections "Quinone Reduction—NQO1 and NQO2" and "Induction of Cytochrome P450—Xenosensors"). Induction of GSTs by the Nrf2 activator sulforaphane is thought to be responsible, at least in part, for the anticancer effects of broccoli (Zhang *et al.*, 1992; Higgins and Hayes, 2011). GSTA4 is induced in mice administered α-angeliclactone, butylated hydroxyanisole (BHA), ethoxyquin, indole-3-carbinol, limettin, and oltipraz (Hayes *et al.*, 2005; Higgins and Hayes, 2011). In addition to inducing one or more GSTs, activation of Nrf2 by oxidative stress or exposure to electrophiles induces γ-GCL, which increases GSH levels in response to an initial decrease in GSH levels (see Point 9 in the section "Introduction").

Factors that regulate the expression of GSTs in rodents may have similar effects in humans, but some differences have been noted. For example, the 5′ promoter region of Alpha GST in humans (GSTA1) lacks the ARE and XRE consensus sequences through which the corresponding rat enzyme is induced. However, such sequences appear to be present in the promoter region of human GSTM4 and GSTP1 genes (Hayes and Pulford, 1995; Whalen and Boyer, 1998; Higgins and Hayes, 2011). (A functional ARE is also present in the promoter region of human DT-diaphorase [NQO1].) Therefore, certain subunits of GSTs are inducible by a variety of mechanisms in rats, and other subunits appear to be inducible by similar mechanisms in humans. Species differences in GST regulation may also stem from differences in xenobiotic biotransformation, especially differences in the formation of electrophiles, Michael acceptors, and/or the production of oxidative stress. For example, coumarin is thought be an inducer of GSTP1 in rats because it is converted in rat liver to reactive metabolites, namely, coumarin 3,4-epoxide and *ortho*-hydroxyphenylacetaldehyde (see Fig. 6-43). In contrast, the major route of coumarin biotransformation in humans is by 7-hydroxylation, which would not be expected to be associated with GST induction.

Conjugation with GSH represents an important detoxication reaction because electrophiles are potentially toxic species that can bind to critical nucleophiles, such as proteins and nucleic acids, and cause cellular damage and genetic mutations. All the enzymes involved in xenobiotic biotransformation have the potential to generate reactive intermediates, most of which are detoxified to some extent by conjugation with GSH. GSH is also a cofactor for GPXs, which play an important role in protecting cells against lipid and hemoglobin peroxidation. Resistance to toxic compounds is often associated with an overexpression of GST. Examples include the resistance of insects to DDT (see Fig. 6-21), of corn to atrazine, and of cancer cells to chemotherapeutic agents.

GST is the major determinant of certain species differences in chemical-induced toxicity. For example, low doses of aflatoxin B_1 cause liver toxicity and tumor formation in rats but not mice, even though rats and mice convert aflatoxin B_1 to the highly reactive 8,9-epoxide at similar rates (this reaction is shown in Fig. 6-34). This species difference arises because mice express high levels of an Alpha class GST (GSTA3) enabling them to conjugate aflatoxin B_1 8,9-epoxide with GSH up to 50 times faster than rats (or humans, which are also considered a susceptible species) (Eaton and Gallagher, 1994). Mice become sensitive to the adverse effects of aflatoxin B_1 following treatment with chemicals that decrease GSH levels, such as diethyl maleate (DEA) (which depletes GSH) or buthionine-*S*-sulfoximine (BSO) (which inhibits GSH synthesis). Conversely, treatment of rats with inducers of certain GSTs, such

as ethoxyquin, BHA, oltipraz, and phenobarbital, protects them from the hepatotoxic/tumorigenic action of aflatoxin B_1 (Hayes *et al.*, 1994).

The conjugation of aflatoxin B_1 8,9-epoxide with GSH provides an interesting example of the stereospecificity with which certain GSH conjugation reactions can occur. CYP converts aflatoxin B_1 to a mixture of *exo*- and *endo*-8,9-epoxides (only a generic 8,9-epoxide is shown in Fig. 6-34, meaning the figure does not indicate whether the oxygen atom is above or below the plane of the ring system). Both enantiomeric epoxides are formed by liver microsomes from mice, rats, and humans, but only the *exo*-epoxide binds extensively to DNA (where it binds to the N^7 position of guanine). One or more mouse Alpha GSTs rapidly conjugate the *exo*-epoxide, which accounts for the resistance of this species to aflatoxin-induced hepatotoxicity and tumorigenicity (as described above). Rat and human GSTAs do not rapidly conjugate either the *exo*- or the *endo*-epoxide (with the exception of the inducible rat GST, which is not constitutively expressed in rats to any great extent). However, human GSTM1-1 can conjugate aflatoxin B_1 8,9-epoxide, but it preferentially conjugates the relatively innocuous *endo*-isomer (Wang *et al.*, 2000).

Species differences in the detoxication of aflatoxin B_1 8,9-epoxide suggest that individual differences in GST may determine susceptibility to the toxic effects of certain chemicals. In support of this interpretation, a genetic polymorphism for GSTM1 has been identified, and individuals who are homozygous for the null allele (ie, those with low GST activity due to complete deletion of the GSTM1 gene) appear to be at a moderately increased risk for cigarette-smoking-induced lung cancer, head and neck cancer, and possibly bladder cancer (Hayes and Pulford, 1995; Whalen and Boyer, 1998; Strange *et al.*, 2000; Hayes *et al.*, 2005). Depending on the ethnic group, 22% to 100% of the population is homozygous for the GSTM1 null genotype, which results in a complete lack of GSTM1 activity in all tissues. On the other hand, there is evidence that GSTM1 confers significant protection from breast cancer in individuals homozygous for a functional GSTM1 allele (Hayes *et al.*, 2005). GSTT1 activity is absent from 11% to 58% of the population (depending on ethnicity) due to deletion of the GSTT1 gene, which appears to increase susceptibility to development of astrocytoma, meningioma, and myelodysplasia. When examined for their individual effect, these null genotypes generally have a small effect on disease susceptibility, with an odds ratio of 2 or less. However, the odds ratio can increase dramatically when these null GST genotypes are examined in conjunction with other genotypes or with environmental factors (such as exposure to carcinogens). For example, when the GSTM1 null genotype is combined with cigarette smoking and a particular CYP1A1 allele, the odds ratio can increase to 8.9 (in one study) or 21.9 (in another study). Polymorphisms that result in amino acid substitutions have been reported for most human GST genes, some of which alter GST function. Some of these polymorphisms may also be risk modifiers for certain diseases in an analogous manner to the GSTM1 and GSTT1 null genotypes.

In some cases, conjugation with GSH enhances the toxicity of a xenobiotic (Monks *et al.*, 1990; Dekant and Vamvakas, 1993; Testa and Krämer, 2008, 2010). Five mechanisms of GSH-dependent activation of xenobiotics have been identified, with the first 4 shown in Fig. 6-67. These mechanisms are (1) formation of GSH conjugates of haloalkanes, organic thiocyanates, and nitrosoguanides that release a toxic metabolite; (2) formation of GSH conjugates of vicinal dihaloalkanes that are inherently toxic because they can form electrophilic sulfur mustards; (3) formation of GSH conjugates of halogenated alkenes that are degraded

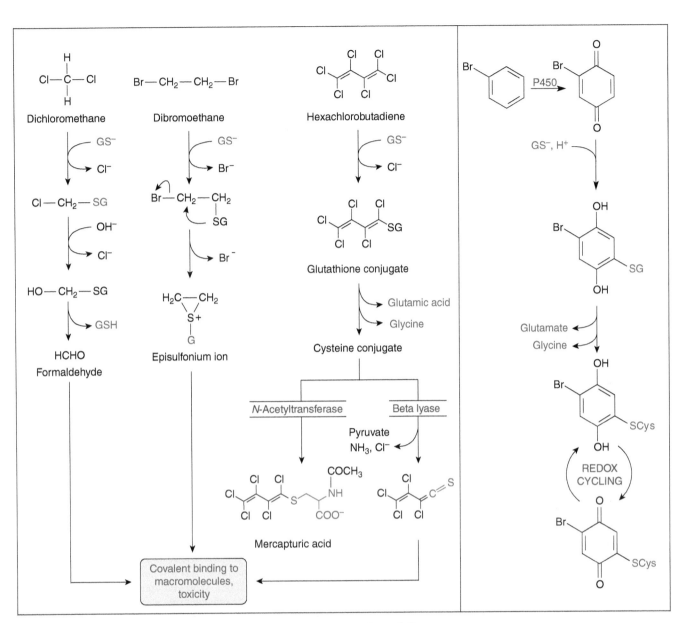

Figure 6-67. *Role of glutathione conjugation in the activation of xenobiotics to toxic metabolites.*

to toxic metabolites by β-lyase in the kidney; (4) formation of GSH conjugates of quinones, quinoneimines, and isothiocyanates that are degraded to toxic metabolites by GGT1 and ANPEP in the kidney; and (5) cyclic GSH conjugation that leads to GSH depletion.

The first mechanism is illustrated by dichloromethane, which is conjugated with GSH to form the highly unstable *S*-chloromethyl-glutathione, which then breaks down to formaldehyde. Both formaldehyde and the GSH conjugate are reactive metabolites, and either or both may be responsible for dichloromethane-induced tumorigenesis in sensitive species. The rate of conjugation of dichloromethane with GSH is considerably faster in mice, which are susceptible to dichloromethane-induced tumorigenesis, than in rats or hamsters, which are resistant species. Other examples include the 1,1,3,3,3-pentafluoro-2-(fluromethoxy)prop-1-ene breakdown product of the general anesthetic sevoflurane. This breakdown product and its derivatives are conjugated to GSH, biotransformed to cysteine conjugates and mercapturic acids, which are then converted through β-lyase cleavage and thiol rearrangement to the highly reactive thioacyl fluoride (Testa and Krämer,

2008, 2010). This highly reactive metabolite can form adducts with proteins and may explain its associated nephrotoxicity (Testa and Krämer, 2008, 2010).

The second mechanism accounts for the toxicity of dichloroethane and dibromoethane. These vicinal dihaloalkanes are converted to GSH conjugates that can rearrange to form mutagenic and nephrotoxic episulfonium ions (sulfur half-mustards) (Fig. 6-67). Dichloroethane and dibromoethane can also be oxidized by CYP to chloroacetaldehyde and bromoacetaldehyde (by reactions analogous to those shown in Fig. 6-50). Either pathway can potentially account for the toxic and tumorigenic effects of these dihaloalkanes. However, the toxicity and DNA binding of dihaloalkanes are increased by factors that decrease their oxidation by CYP and increase their conjugation with GSH.

The third mechanism accounts for the nephrotoxicity of several halogenated alkenes. Several halogenated alkenes, such as hexachlorobutadiene, cause damage to the kidney tubules in rats, which leads to carcinoma of the proximal tubules. These nephrotoxic halogenated alkenes are conjugated with GSH and transported to the kidney for processing to mercapturic acids. The cysteine conjugates, which form by removal of glutamic acid and glycine, are substrates for *N*-acetyltransferase (NAT), which completes the synthesis of mercapturic acids, and cysteine-conjugate β-lyase (CCBL1), which removes pyruvate and ammonia from the cysteine conjugate to produce thionylacyl halides, thiiranes, thiolactones, and thioketenes. The early damage to renal mitochondria caused by halogenated alkenes is probably because CCBL1 is a mitochondrial enzyme.

The fourth mechanism accounts for the nephrotoxicity of bromobenzene, which causes damage to the proximal tubules in rats. Bromobenzene is oxidized by CYP in the liver to bromohydroquinone, which is conjugated with GSH and transported to the kidney (Fig. 6-67). The GSH conjugate is converted to the cysteine derivative by GGT1 and membrane ANPEP. Substitution of bromohydroquinones with cysteine lowers their redox potential and thereby facilitates their oxidation to toxic quinones. The cysteine conjugates of bromohydroquinone are thought to undergo redox cycling and cause kidney damage through the generation of reactive oxygen species (ROS). 4-Aminophenol is thought to cause kidney damage by a similar mechanism, except a benzoquinoneimine is involved in conjugation with GSH and subsequent damage to proximal tubules of the kidney. Treatment of rats with the GSH depletor, buthionine-*S*-sulfoximine (BSO), protects them against the nephrotoxic effects of 4-aminophenol, which implicates GSH conjugation in the activation of this compound.

The fifth mechanism occurs with moderately toxic allyl-, benzyl-, and phenethyl isothiocyantes as well as sulforaphane formed from plant glucosinolates. These compounds are reversibly conjugated with GSH to form thiocarbamates which spontaneously degrade to their isothiocyanates upon export from the cell, which releases GSH. The isothiocyanate is then taken up by the cells again and the cycle can repeat until intracellular GSH is depleted. Once GSH levels are low, the compounds will tend to thiocarbamylate proteins, which can lead to cell death (Hayes *et al.*, 2005).

Thiosulfate Sulfurtransferase (Rhodanese)

Cyanide forms naturally in leucocytes and neural cells, and also as a result of vitamin B_{12} metabolism, and is also encountered as a xenobiotic in plants containing cyanogenic glycosides, such as cassava, and tobacco smoke (Billaut-Laden *et al.*, 2006). Thiosulfate sulfurtransferase is a mitochondrial enzyme encoded by the TST gene that converts cyanide to the far less toxic metabolite, thiocyanate. The reaction involves transfer of sulfur from thiosulfate (or another sulfur donor) as follows:

$$CN^- \;+\; S_2O_3^{2-} \;\longrightarrow\; SCN^- \;+\; SO_3^{2-}$$

Cyanide   Thiosulfate   Thiocyanate   Sulfite

The sulfite produced by this reaction can be converted to sulfate by the molybdoenzyme, sulfite oxidase (see the section "Molybdenum Hydroxylases (Molybdoenzymes)"). Cyanide can also be "detoxified" by binding to methemoglobin (the oxidized or ferric form of hemoglobin). 4-Dimethylaminophenol is used to induce methemoglobinemia as an antidote to cyanide poisoning because methemoglobin competes with cytochrome oxidase for the cyanide ion. However, 4-dimethylaminophenol is nephrotoxic to rats, presumably by a mechanism similar to that described above for the structural analog, 4-aminophenol (see preceding section and the section "Glutathione Conjugation").

In humans, TST is expressed at high levels in the colon, where it plays a major role in the detoxication of hydrogen sulfide (which can reach concentrations of >3 mM) produced by anaerobic bacteria (Billaut-Laden *et al.*, 2006). TST is also widely distributed in

the central nervous system and may also play a role in the import of 5S rRNA into mitochondria (Smirnov *et al.*, 2010). Six allelic variants of TST have been identified, namely, TST*1B to TST*1F and TST*2, with the latter showing significantly reduced intrinsic clearance for thiocyanate formation (Billaut-Laden *et al.*, 2006). TST polymorphisms that decrease cyanide and hydrogen sulfide detoxication may ultimately become important in understanding certain diseases, such as ulcerative colitis and ALS. For instance, hydrogen sulfide release has been found to be 3 to 4 times higher in patients with ulcerative colitis when compared with normal subjects, and is positively correlated with disease severity (Billaut-Laden *et al.*, 2006). Finally, it has been postulated that individuals with ALS display a disorder in cyanide metabolism because of the higher blood and urine levels of cyanide (Billaut-Laden *et al.*, 2006). Mimori *et al.* (1984) also reported significantly decreased TST activity in cervical and thoracic spinal cords of patients with ALS, compared with normal subjects.

Unusual Conjugation Reactions

In rare cases, xenobiotics can be biotransformed to unusual conjugates which can contribute to xenobiotic clearance. As shown in Fig. 6-68, the immunosuppressive drug, 6-mercaptopurine (as well as its precursor azathioprine), is converted to 6-thioinosine monophosphate (TIMP) by hypoxanthine guanine phophoribosyltransferase (HGPRT) with phophoribosyl pyrophosphate (PRPP) as the phophoribosyl donor (Wielinga *et al.*, 2002; Gearry *et al.*, 2010; Hofmann *et al.*, 2012). Similarly to 6-mercaptopurine, 6-thiopurine can also be converted to a thionucleotide monophosphate (TNMP) (Wielinga *et al.*, 2002). Whereas the 6-thioguanine nucleotides are responsible for immunosuppressant activity, 6-methylmercaptopurine nucleotides have been associated with hepatotoxicity at high doses (Gearry *et al.*, 2010). Thiopurine nucleosides have also been shown to be transported by the transporters MRP4 (ABCC4) and MRP5 (ABCC5) (Wielinga *et al.*, 2002). Another example of an unusual conjugate is that of the immunosuppressant macrolide everolimus, which forms a phosphocholine conjugate as a major metabolite (ATG181) in both animals and humans (Zollinger *et al.*, 2008). While phosphocholine esters of endogenous lipids, such as sphingomyelins or phosphatidylcholines, are common, phosphocholine conjugates of xenobiotics are very rare. Previously, only fluorescence-labeled endogenous lipids and an unnatural stereoisomer of dihydroceramide have been shown to form this type of conjugate (Zollinger *et al.*, 2008). The addition of activated phosphocholine is catalyzed by the enzymes cholinephosphotransferase found in the Golgi apparatus, as well as choline/ethanolaminephosphotransferase found in the endoplasmic reticulum and nuclear envelope; however, it is not known whether these enzymes also catalyze the phosphocholine conjugation of everolimus (Zollinger *et al.*, 2008). Furthermore, the tyrosine kinase inhibitor, imatinib, has also been shown to generate a novel ADP^+ adduct when incubated in vitro with rat liver microsomes and the cofactor NADPH (Ma *et al.*, 2008). This activity has been attributed to the enzyme NAD-glycohydrolase, which has been previously shown to be involved in the ADP^+ conjugation of many pyridine-containing compounds such as cotinine, nicotinic acid, 3-acetyl pyridine, nicotinic acid hydrazine, 6-aminocotinamide, and nitrosamines, and thiophenopyridine-containing IκB-kinase β inhibitors (Ma *et al.*, 2008). The conjugating enzyme, NAD-glycohydrolase, functions through the cleavage of the nicotinamide-ribose bond of $NADP^+$ which in turn generates an oxocarbenium ion intermediate with subsequent transfer of the ADP-ribosyl group to water, methanol, or pyridine-containing

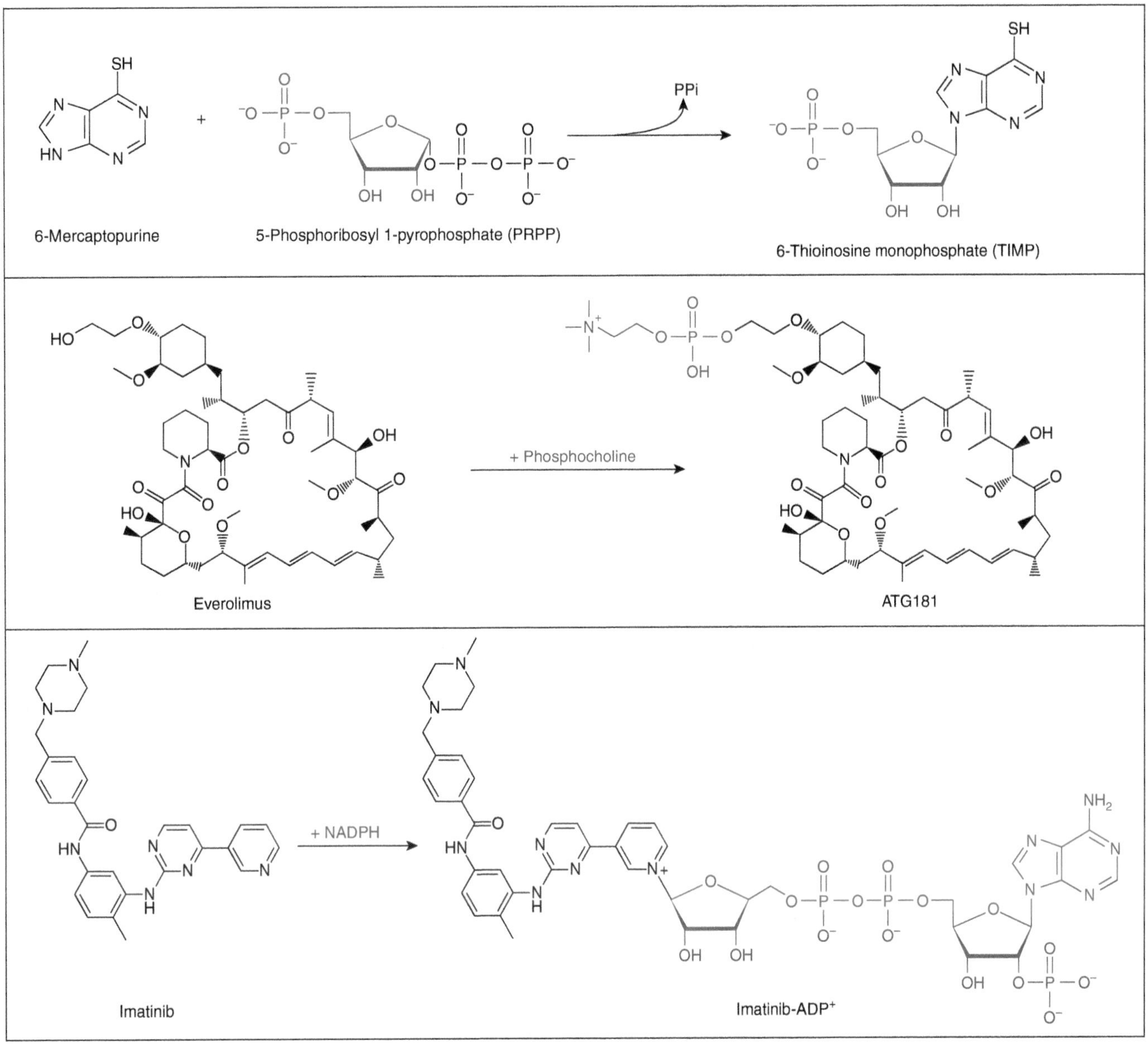

Figure 6-68. *Examples of unusual conjugation reactions.*

compounds (Ma *et al.*, 2008). NAD-glycohydrolase is ubiquitously expressed in many organisms, including mammals, and the implications of xenobiotic-ADP⁺ adducts formed by this enzyme are not well understood (Ma *et al.*, 2008).

Phosphorylation

Some drugs are intentionally designed to be phosphorylated by intracellular enzymes. For example, the anti-HIV drug zidovudine (AZT) is converted to a triphosphate nucleoside by enzymes in the salvage pathway (nucleoside kinase, nucleoside monophosphate kinase [NMK], and nucleoside diphosphate kinase [NDK]). However, phosphorylation of xenobiotics is the exception rather than the rule. All conjugation reactions ultimately require ATP, either to activate the xenobiotic for conjugation with GSH or amino acids or to synthesize high-energy cofactors such as UDPGA and PAPS. The process is inefficient in that several ATP molecules (or their equivalent) are used to synthesize each cofactor molecule. The question arises: why is ATP not used directly by conjugating enzymes? In other words, why are xenobiotics never phosphorylated directly (with the exception of drugs such as zidovudine), which would require less ATP and would achieve the goal of converting xenobiotics to water-soluble conjugates? It is difficult to be certain why this does not occur, but 4 reasons suggest themselves. First, if xenobiotics could be phosphorylated, high intracellular levels of a xenobiotic might consume so much ATP as to jeopardize cell viability, whereas UDPGA and PAPS can be depleted without killing cells. Second, phosphorylation of endogenous substrates, such as glucose, is a mechanism for trapping endogenous substrates inside a cell. This works because the plasma membrane of all cells is a barrier to the passage of polar compounds by virtue of its hydrophobic properties (lipid bilayer) and its general lack of transporters that efflux phosphorylated compounds out of the cell. The same is true for the phosphorylated metabolites of zidovudine and related antiviral drugs; they are retained inside the cell that forms them. A lipid bilayer is also a physical barrier to other water-soluble conjugates, such as glucuronides and sulfonates, but these are transported out of the cell by various transporters. Third, phosphorylation of both small molecules (such as inositol) and proteins (such as membrane-bound receptors and various transcription factors) plays an important role in intracellular and intranuclear signaling. It is possible that some xenobiotics, if they were phosphorylated, might interfere with these regulatory systems and thereby disrupt cellular homeostasis. Fourth, even if xenobiotics were phosphorylated in the liver and excreted in bile, they would be rapidly hydrolyzed by high levels of alkaline phosphatase lining the surface of enterocytes in the small intestine, which would promote reabsorption of the xenobiotic (by the very process exploited in the design of phosphorylated prodrugs such as fosamprenavir). Whatever the reason, there appears to be strong evolutionary pressure against the conjugation of xenobiotics with phosphoric acid.

REFERENCES

Adamson RH, Bridges JW, Evans ME, Williams RT. Species differences in the aromatization of quinic acid in vivo and the role of gut bacteria. *Biochem J.* 1970;116:437–443.

Agarwal DP. Pharmacogenetics of alcohol dehydrogenase. In: Kalow W, ed. *Pharmacogenetics of Drug Metabolism.* New York, NY: Pergamon; 1992:263–280.

Agarwal V, Kommaddi RP, Valli K, et al. Drug metabolism in human brain: high levels of cytochrome P4503A43 in brain and metabolism of anti-anxiety drug alprazolam to its active metabolite. *PLoS One.* 2008;3:e2337.

Agostinelli E, Arancia G, Vedova LD, et al. The biological functions of polyamine oxidation products by amine oxidases: perspectives of clinical applications. *Amino Acids.* 2004;27:347–358.

Agundez JA, Gallardo L, Ledesma MC, et al. Functionally active duplications of the CYP2D6 gene are more prevalent among larynx and lung cancer patients. *Oncology.* 2001;61:59–63.

Ahn J, Yu K, Stolzenberg-Solomon R, et al. Genome-wide association study of circulating vitamin D levels. *Hum Mol Genet.* 2010;19:2739–2745.

Aiba I, Yamasaki T, Shinki T, et al. Characterization of rat and human CYP2J enzymes as vitamin D 25-hydroxylases. *Steroids.* 2006;71:849–856.

Al-Zoughool M, Succop P, Desai P, Vietas J, Talaska G. Effect of *N*-glucuronidation on urinary bladder genotoxicity of 4-aminobiphenyl in male and female mice. *Environ Toxicol Pharmacol.* 2006;22:153–159.

Aldridge WN. Serum esterases. I. Two types of esterase (A and B) hydrolysing *p*-nitrophenyl acetate, propionate and butyrate, and a method for their determination. *Biochem J.* 1953;53:110–117.

Alfaro JF, Jones JP. Studies on the mechanism of aldehyde oxidase and xanthine oxidase. *J Org Chem.* 2008;73:9469–9472.

Alfirevic A, Pirmohamed M. Drug induced hypersensitivity and the HLA complex. *Pharmaceuticals.* 2010;4:69–90.

Amano T, Ochi N, Sato H, Sakaki S. Oxidation reaction by xanthine oxidase: theoretical study of reaction mechanism. *J Am Chem Soc.* 2007;129:8131–8138.

Anders MW. *Bioactivation of Foreign Compounds.* New York, NY: Academic Press; 1985.

Anders MW, Ratnayake JH, Hanna PE, Fuchs JA. Thioredoxin-dependent sulfoxide reduction by rat renal cytosol. *Drug Metab Dispos.* 1981;9:307–310.

Aniya Y, Imaizumi N. Mitochondrial glutathione transferases involving a new function for membrane permeability transition pore regulation. *Drug Metab Rev.* 2011;43:292–299.

Arima N. Acyl glucuronidation and glucosidation of pranoprofen, a 2-arylpropionic acid derivative, in mouse liver and kidney homogenates. *J Pharmacobiodyn.* 1990;13:724–732.

Armstrong RN. Kinetic and chemical mechanism of epoxide hydrolase. *Drug Metab Rev.* 1999;31:71–86.

Atkins WM. Non-Michaelis–Menten kinetics in cytochrome P450-catalyzed reactions. *Annu Rev Pharmacol Toxicol.* 2005;45:291–310.

Atkins WM, Wang RW, Bird AW, Newton DJ, Lu AYH. The catalytic mechanism of glutathione *S*-transferase (GST). Spectroscopic determination of the pKa of Tyr-9 in rat alpha 1-1 GST. *J Biol Chem.* 1993;268:19188–19191.

Augustinsson KB. The nature of an "anionic" site in butyrylcholinesterase compared with that of a similar site in acetylcholinesterase. *Biochim Biophys Acta.* 1966;128:351–362.

Ayesh R, Smith RL. Genetic polymorphism of trimethylamine *N*-oxidation. In: Kalow W, ed. *Pharmacogenetics of Drug Metabolism.* New York, NY: Pergamon; 1992:315–332.

Bachovchin DA, Brown SJ, Rosen H, Cravatt BF. Identification of selective inhibitors of uncharacterized enzymes by high-throughput screening with fluorescent activity-based probes. *Nat Biotechnol.* 2009;27:387–394.

Baer B, Rettie A. CYP4B1: an enigmatic P450 at the interface between xenobiotic and endobiotic metabolism. *Drug Metab Rev.* 2006;38:451–476.

Baer BR, DeLisle RK, Allen A. Benzylic oxidation of gemfibrozil-1-*O*-beta-glucuronide by P450 2C8 leads to heme alkylation and irreversible inhibition. *Chem Res Toxicol.* 2009;22:1298–1309.

Baillie TA, Rettie AE. Role of biotransformation in drug-induced toxicity: influence of intra- and inter-species differences in drug metabolism. *Drug Metab Pharmacokinet.* 2011;26:15–29.

Bains OS, Grigliatti TA, Reid RE, Riggs KW. Naturally occurring variants of human aldo-keto reductases with reduced in vitro metabolism of daunorubicin and doxorubicin. *J Pharmacol Exp Ther.* 2010;335:533–545.

Ballard JE, Prueksaritanont T, Tang C. Hepatic metabolism of MK-0457, a potent aurora kinase inhibitor: interspecies comparison and role of human cytochrome P450 and flavin-containing monooxygenase. *Drug Metab Dispos.* 2007;35:1447–1451.

Ballatori N, Krance SM, Marchan R, Hammond CL. Plasma membrane glutathione transporters and their roles in cell physiology and pathophysiology. *Mol Aspects Med.* 2009a;30:13–28.

Ballatori N, Li N, Fang F, Boyer JL, Christian WV, Hammond CL. OST alpha-OST beta: a key membrane transporter of bile acids and conjugated steroids. *Front Biosci.* 2009b;14:2829–2844.

Barditch-Crovo P, Trapnell CB, Ette E, et al. The effects of rifampin and rifabutin on the pharmacokinetics and pharmacodynamics of a combination oral contraceptive. *Clin Pharmacol Ther.* 1999;65:428–438.

Bauman JN, Kelly JM, Tripathy S, et al. Can in vitro metabolism-dependent covalent binding data distinguish hepatotoxic from nonhepatotoxic drugs? An analysis using human hepatocytes and liver S-9 fraction. *Chem Res Toxicol.* 2009;22:332–340.

Bayrak A, Bayrak T, Tokgozoglu SL, et al. Serum PON-1 activity but not Q192R polymorphism is related to the extent of atherosclerosis. *J Atheroscler Thromb.* 2012;19(4):376–384. doi: JST.JSTAGE/jat/11320.

Beconi MG, Mao A, Liu DQ, et al. Metabolism and pharmacokinetics of a dipeptidyl peptidase IV inhibitor in rats, dogs, and monkeys with selective carbamoyl glucuronidation of the primary amine in dogs. *Drug Metab Dispos.* 2003;31:1269–1277.

Beedham C, Miceli JJ, Obach RS. Ziprasidone metabolism, aldehyde oxidase, and clinical implications. *J Clin Psychopharmacol.* 2003;23:229–232.

Beetham J, Grant D, Arand M, et al. Gene evolution of epoxide hydrolases and recommended nomenclature. *DNA Cell Biol.* 1995;14:61–71.

Benedetti M, Dostert P. Contribution of amine oxidases to the metabolism of xenobiotics. *Drug Metab Rev.* 1994;26:507–535.

Benedetti MS. Biotransformation of xenobiotics by amine oxidases. *Fundam Clin Pharmacol.* 2001;15:75–84.

Benet LZ. The drug transporter–metabolism alliance: uncovering and defining the interplay. *Mol Pharmacol.* 2009;6:1631–1643.

Billaut-Laden I, Allorge D, Crunelle-Thibaut A, et al. Evidence for a functional genetic polymorphism of the human thiosulfate sulfurtransferase (Rhodanese), a cyanide and H$_2$S detoxification enzyme. *Toxicology.* 2006;225:1–11.

Bjornsson TD, Callaghan JT, Einolf HJ, et al. The conduct of in vitro and in vivo drug–drug interaction studies: a Pharmaceutical Research and Manufacturers of America (PhRMA) perspective. *Drug Metab Dispos.* 2003;31:815–832.

Blanchard RL, Freimuth RR, Buck J, Weinshilboum RM, Coughtrie MW. A proposed nomenclature system for the cytosolic sulfotransferase (SULT) superfamily. *Pharmacogenetics.* 2004;14:199–211.

Blättler SM, Rencurel F, Kaufmann MR, Meyer UA. In the regulation of cytochrome P450 genes, phenobarbital targets LKB1 for necessary activation of AMP-activated protein kinase. *Proc Natl Acad Sci U S A.* 2007;104:1045–1050.

Blouin RA, Bandyopadhyay AM, Chaudhary I, Robertson LW, Gemzik B, Parkinson A. Cytochrome P450 2B enzyme (CYP2B) induction defect following phenobarbital treatment in the fa/fa Zucker rat: molecular characterization. *Arch Biochem Biophys.* 1993;303:313–320.

Board PG. The omega-class glutathione transferases: structure, function, and genetics. *Drug Metab Rev.* 2011;43:226–235.

Board PG, Anders MW. Glutathione transferase zeta: discovery, polymorphic variants, catalysis, inactivation, and properties of Gstz1–/– mice. *Drug Metab Rev.* 2011;43:215–225.

Boberg E, Miller E, Miller J, Poland A, Liem A. Strong evidence from studies with brachymorphic mice and pentachlorophenol that 1′-sulfooxysafrole is the major ultimate electrophilic and carcinogenic metabolite of 1′-hydroxysafrole in mouse liver. *Cancer Res.* 1983;43:5163–5173.

Bock K, Schrenk D, Forster A, et al. The influence of environmental and genetic factors on CYP2D6, CYP1A2 and UDP-glucuronosyltransferases in man using sparteine, caffeine, and paracetamol as probes. *Pharmacogenetics.* 1994;4:209–218.

Bolton J, Trush M, Penning TM, Dryhurst G, Monks T. Role of quinones in toxicology. *Chem Res Toxicol.* 2000;13:135–160.

Bolze S, Bromet N, Gay-Feutry C, Massiere F, Boulieu R, Hulot T. Development of an in vitro screening model for the biosynthesis of acyl glucuronide metabolites and the assessment of their reactivity toward human serum albumin. *Drug Metab Dispos.* 2002;30:404–413.

Bonn B, Masimirembwa CM, Aristei Y, Zamora I. The molecular basis of CYP2D6-mediated N-dealkylation: balance between metabolic clearance routes and enzyme inhibition. *Drug Metab Dispos.* 2008;36:2199–2210.

Bookout AL, Jeong Y, Downes M, Yu RT, Evans RM, Mangelsdorf DJ. Anatomical profiling of nuclear receptor expression reveals a hierarchical transcriptional network. *Cell.* 2006;126:789–799.

Borst P, Zelcer N, van de Wetering K. MRP2 and 3 in health and disease. *Cancer Lett.* 2006;234:51–61.

Bosgra S, Mennes W, Seinen W. Proceedings in uncovering the mechanism behind peroxisome proliferator-induced hepatocarcinogenesis. *Toxicology.* 2005;206:309–323.

Boukouvala S, Fakis G. Arylamine N-acetyltransferases: what we learn from genes and genomes. *Drug Metab Rev.* 2005;37:511–564.

Boulton DW, Fawcett JP. Pharmacokinetics and pharmacodynamics of single oral doses of albuterol and its enantiomers in humans. *Clin Pharmacol Ther.* 1997;62:138–144.

Bouman HJ, Schomig E, van Werkum JW, et al. Paraoxonase-1 is a major determinant of clopidogrel efficacy. *Nat Med.* 2011;17:110–116.

Bowcock AM, Cookson WO. The genetics of psoriasis, psoriatic arthritis and atopic dermatitis. *Hum Mol Genet.* 2004;13(spec no 1):R43–R55.

Bradley ME, Benner SA. Phylogenomic approaches to common problems encountered in the analysis of low copy repeats: the sulfotransferase 1A gene family example. *BMC Evol Biol.* 2005;5:22–40.

Braissant O, Foufelle F, Scotto C, Dauca M, Wahli W. Differential expression of peroxisome proliferator-activated receptors (PPARs): tissue distribution of PPAR-alpha, -beta, and -gamma in the adult rat. *Endocrinology.* 1996;137:354–366.

Brantley E, Trapani V, Alley MC, et al. Fluorinated 2-(4-amino-3-methylphenyl) benzothiazoles induce CYP1A1 expression, become metabolized, and bind to macromolecules in sensitive human cancer cells. *Drug Metab Dispos.* 2004;32:1392–1401.

Brauer RW. Mechanisms of bile secretion. *JAMA.* 1959;169:1462–1466.

Brechbuhl HM, Gould N, Kachadourian R, Riekhof WR, Voelker DR, Day BJ. Glutathione transport is a unique function of the ATP-binding cassette protein ABCG2. *J Biol Chem.* 2010;285:16582–16587.

Brennan P, Lewis S, Hashibe M, et al. Pooled analysis of alcohol dehydrogenase genotypes and head and neck cancer: a HuGE review. *Am J Epidemiol.* 2004;159:1–16.

Browning JD, Horton JD. Molecular mediators of hepatic steatosis and liver injury. *J Clin Invest.* 2004;114:147–152.

Brunnberg S, Andersson P, Lindstam M, Paulson I, Poellinger L, Hanberg A. The constitutively active Ah receptor (CA-Ahr) mouse as a potential model for dioxin exposure—effects in vital organs. *Toxicology.* 2006;224:191–201.

Bui PH, Hankinson O. Functional characterization of human cytochrome P450 2S1 using a synthetic gene-expressed protein in *Escherichia coli. Mol Pharmacol.* 2009;76:1031–1043.

Bui PH, Hsu EL, Hankinson O. Fatty acid hydroperoxides support cytochrome P450 2S1-mediated bioactivation of benzo[a]pyrene-7,8-dihydrodiol. *Mol Pharmacol.* 2009;76:1044–1052.

Burchell B. Transformation reactions: glucuronidation. In: Woolf T, ed. *Handbook of Drug Metabolism.* New York, NY: Marcel Dekker Inc; 1999:153–173.

Burczynski ME, Penning TM. Genotoxic polycyclic aromatic hydrocarbon *ortho*-quinones generated by aldo-keto reductases induce CYP1A1 via nuclear translocation of the aryl hydrocarbon receptor. *Cancer Res.* 2000;60:908–915.

Burke MD, Mayer RT. Ethoxyresorufin: direct fluorimetric assay of a microsomal O-dealkylation which is preferentially inducible by 3-methylcholanthrene. *Drug Metab Dispos.* 1974;2:583–588.

Capen CC. Mechanistic data and risk assessment of selected toxic end points of the thyroid gland. *Toxicol Pathol.* 1997;25:39–48.

Carbone V, Hara A, El-Kabbani O. Structural and functional features of dimeric dihydrodiol dehydrogenase. *Cell Mol Life Sci.* 2008; 65:1464–1474.

Carro-Ciampi G, Jurima M, Kadar D, Tang BK, Kalow W. N-Glucosidation of amobarbital in the cat. *Can J Physiol Pharmacol.* 1985;63: 1263–1266.

Cascorbi I, Roots I, Brockmoller J. Association of NAT1 and NAT2 polymorphisms to urinary bladder cancer: significantly reduced risk in subjects with NAT1*10. *Cancer Res.* 2001;61:5051–5056.

Cashman JR. Structural and catalytic properties of the mammalian flavin-containing monooxygenase. *Chem Res Toxicol.* 1995;8:166–181.

Cashman JR. In vitro metabolism: FMO and related oxygenations. In: Woolf T, ed. *Handbook of Drug Metabolism.* New York, NY: Marcel Dekker Inc; 1999:477–505.

Cashman JR. Role of flavin-containing monooxygenase in drug development. *Expert Opin Drug Metab Toxicol.* 2008;4:1507–1521.

Cashman JR, Akerman BR, Forrest SM, Treacy EP. Population-specific polymorphisms of the human FMO3 gene: significance for detoxication. *Drug Metab Dispos.* 2000;28:169–173.

Cashman JR, Zhang J. Human flavin-containing monooxygenases. *Annu Rev Pharmacol Toxicol.* 2006;46:65–100.

Casida JE, Quistad GB. Serine hydrolase targets of organophosphorus toxicants. *Chem Biol Interact.* 2005;157–158:277–283.

Cauffiez C, Klinzig F, Rat E, et al. Human CYP4F12 genetic polymorphism: identification and functional characterization of seven variant allozymes. *Biochem Pharmacol.* 2004;68:2417–2425.

Cerf C, Mesguish M, Gabriel I, Amselem S, Duvaldestin P. Screening patients with prolonged neuromuscular blockade after succinylcholine and mivacurium. *Anesth Analg.* 2002;94:461–466.

Chalasani N, Björnsson E. Risk factors for idiosyncratic drug-induced liver injury. *Gastroenterology.* 2010;138:2246–2259.

Chalmers RA, Bain MD, Michelakakis H, Zschocke J, Iles RA. Diagnosis and management of trimethylaminuria (FMO3 deficiency) in children. *J Inherit Metab Dis.* 2006;29:162–172.

Chandrasena R, Vatsis K, Coon M, Hollenberg P, Newcomb M. Hydroxylation by the hydroperoxy-iron species in cytochrome P450 enzymes. *J Am Chem Soc.* 2004;126:115–126.

Chang TK, Waxman DJ. Synthetic drugs and natural products as modulators of constitutive androstane receptor (CAR) and pregnane X receptor (PXR). *Drug Metab Rev.* 2006;38:51–73.

Chen B, Qiu LX, Li Y, et al. The CYP1B1 Leu432Val polymorphism contributes to lung cancer risk: evidence from 6501 subjects. *Lung Cancer.* 2010;70:247–252.

Chen C, Li G, Liao W, et al. Selective inhibitors of CYP2J2 related to terfenadine exhibit strong activity against human cancers in vitro and in vivo. *J Pharmacol Exp Ther.* 2009;329:908–918.

Chen C, Wei X, Rao X, et al. Cytochrome P450 2J2 is highly expressed in hematologic malignant diseases and promotes tumor cell growth. *J Pharmacol Exp Ther.* 2011a;336:344–355.

Chen J, Lin Y, Zhang R, Huang ZJ, Pan XG. Contribution of NAD(P)H quinone oxidoreductase 1 (NQO1) Pro187Ser polymorphism and risks of colorectal adenoma and cancer for Caucasians: a meta-analysis. *Arch Med Res.* 2012;43(1):58–66. doi: 10.1016/j.arcmed.2012.01.005.

Chen J, Mannargudi BM, Xu L, Uetrecht J. Demonstration of the metabolic pathway responsible for nevirapine-induced skin rash. *Chem Res Toxicol.* 2008;21:1862–1870.

Chen Q, Doss GA, Tung EC, et al. Evidence for the bioactivation of zomepirac and tolmetin by an oxidative pathway: identification of glutathione adducts in vitro in human liver microsomes and in vivo in rats. *Drug Metab Dispos.* 2006;34:145–151.

Chen Q, Tan E, Strauss JR, et al. Effect of quinidine on the 10-hydroxylation of *R*-warfarin: species differences and clearance projection. *J Pharmacol Exp Ther.* 2004a;311:307–314.

Chen S, Wu K, Knox R. Structure–function studies of DT-diaphorase (NQO1) and NRH:quinone oxidoreductase (NQO2). *Free Radic Biol Med.* 2000;29:276–284.

Chen S-Y, Lin J-RV, Darbha R, Lin P, Liu T-Y, Chen Y-MA. Glycine *N*-methyltransferase tumor susceptibility gene in the benzo(a)pyrene-detoxification pathway. *Cancer Res.* 2004b;64:3617–3623.

Chen Y, Goldstein JA. The transcriptional regulation of the human CYP2C genes. *Curr Drug Metab.* 2009;10:567–578.

Chen Z, Li Z, Niu X, Ye X, Yu Y, Lu S. The effect of CYP1A1 polymorphisms on the risk of lung cancer: a global meta-analysis based on 71 case–control studies. *Mutagenesis.* 2011b;26:437–446.

Cheng JB, Levine MA, Bell NH, Mangelsdorf DJ, Russell DW. Genetic evidence that the human CYP2R1 enzyme is a key vitamin D 25-hydroxylase. *Proc Natl Acad Sci U S A.* 2004;101:7711–7715.

Cheung C, Gonzalez FJ. Humanized mouse lines and their application for prediction of human drug metabolism and toxicological risk assessment. *J Pharmacol Exp Ther.* 2008;327:288–299.

Chladek J, Martinkova J, Sispera L. An in vitro study on methotrexate hydroxylation in rat and human liver. *Physiol Res.* 1997;46:371–379.

Cohen S, Boobis A, (Bette) Meek M, Preston R, McGregor D. 4-Aminobiphenyl and DNA reactivity: case study within the context of the 2006 IPCS human relevance framework for analysis of a cancer mode of action for humans. *Crit Rev Toxicol.* 2006;36:803–819.

Cole TB, Jansen K, Park S, Li WF, Furlong CE, Costa LG. The toxicity of mixtures of specific organophosphate compounds is modulated by paraoxonase 1 status. *Adv Exp Med Biol.* 2010;660:47–60.

Collins C, Levy R, Ragueneau-Majlessi I, Hachad H. Prediction of maximum exposure in poor metabolizers following inhibition of nonpolymorphic pathways. *Curr Drug Metab.* 2006;7:295–299.

Congiu M, Mashford ML, Slavin JL, Desmond PV. Coordinate regulation of metabolic enzymes and transporters by nuclear transcription factors in human liver disease. *J Gastroenterol Hepatol.* 2009;24:1038–1044.

Conney AH. Induction of microsomal enzymes by foreign chemicals and carcinogenesis by polycyclic aromatic hydrocarbons. *Cancer Res.* 1982;42:4875–4917.

Coughtrie MW, Fisher MB. The role of sulfotransferases (SULTs) and UDP-glucuronosyltransferases (UGTs) in human drug clearance and bioactivation. In: Lee JS, Obach RS, Fisher MB, eds. *Drug Metabolizing Enzymes.* New York, NY: Marcel Dekker; 2003:541–575.

Court MH, Hazarika S, Krishnaswamy S, Finel M, Williams JA. Novel polymorphic human UDP-glucuronosyltransferase 2A3: cloning, functional characterization of enzyme variants, comparative tissue expression, and gene induction. *Mol Pharmacol.* 2008;74:744–754.

Crofts F, Taioli E, Trachman J, et al. Functional significance of different human CYP1A1 genotypes. *Carcinogenesis.* 1994;15:2961–2963.

Cronin A, Decker M, Arand M. Mammalian soluble epoxide hydrolase is identical to liver hepoxilin hydrolase. *J Lipid Res.* 2011;52:712–719.

Cruzan G, Bus J, Hotchkiss J, Harkema J, Banton M, Sarang S. CYP2F2-generated metabolites, not styrene oxide, are a key event mediating the mode of action of styrene-induced mouse lung tumors. *Regul Toxicol Pharmacol.* 2012;62:214–220.

Cundy K, Sato M, Crooks P. Stereospecific in vivo *N*-methylation of nicotine in the guinea pig. *Drug Metab Dispos.* 1985;13:175–185.

Curran P, DeGroot L. The effect of hepatic enzyme-inducing drugs on thyroid hormones and the thyroid gland. *Endocr Rev.* 1991;12:135–150.

Dahabreh IJ, Kitsios GD, Kent DM, Trikalinos TA. Paraoxonase 1 polymorphisms and ischemic stroke risk: a systematic review and meta-analysis. *Genet Med.* 2010;12:606–615.

Daily EB, Aquilante CL. Cytochrome P450 2C8 pharmacogenetics: a review of clinical studies. *Pharmacogenomics.* 2009;10:1489–1510.

Daly AK. Pharmacogenetics. In: Woolf T, ed. *Handbook of Drug Metabolism.* New York, NY: Marcel Dekker Inc; 1999:175–202.

Daniel V. Glutathione *S*-transferases: gene structure and regulation of expression. *Crit Rev Biochem Mol Biol.* 1993;28:173–207.

Dansette P, Rosi J, Bertho G, Mansuy D. Cytochromes P450 catalyze both steps of the major pathway of clopidogrel bioactivation, whereas paraoxonase catalyzes the formation of a minor thiol metabolite isomer. *Chem Res Toxicol.* 2012;25(2):348–356. doi: 10.1021/tx2004085.

Dawson JH. Probing structure–function relations in heme-containing oxygenases and peroxidases. *Science.* 1988;240:433–439.

De Bosscher K, Vanden Berghe W, Haegeman G. Cross-talk between nuclear receptors and nuclear factor kappaB. *Oncogene.* 2006;25:6868–6886.

de Morais SM, Uetrecht JP, Wells PG. Decreased glucuronidation and increased bioactivation of acetaminophen in Gilbert's syndrome. *Gastroenterology.* 1992;102:577–586.

de Morais SM, Wilkinson GR, Blaisdell J, Nakamura K, Meyer UA, Goldstein JA. The major genetic defect responsible for the polymorphism of *S*-mephenytoin metabolism in humans. *J Biol Chem.* 1994;269:15419–15422.

Debiec-Rychter M, Land SJ, King CM. Histological localization of acetyltransferases in human tissue. *Cancer Lett.* 1999;143:99–102.

Decker CJ, Cashman JR, Sugiyama K, Maltby D, Correia MA. Formation of glutathionyl-spironolactone disulfide by rat liver cytochromes P450 or hog liver flavin-containing monooxygenases: a functional probe of two-electron oxidations of the thiosteroid? *Chem Res Toxicol.* 1991;4:669–677.

Degirolamo C, Modica S, Palasciano G, Moschetta A. Bile acids and colon cancer: solving the puzzle with nuclear receptors. *Trends Mol Med.* 2011;17:564–572.

Dekant W, Vamvakas S. Glutathione-dependent bioactivation of xenobiotics. *Xenobiotica.* 1993;23:873–887.

DeKeyser JG, Laurenzana EM, Peterson EC, Chen T, Omiecinski CJ. Selective phthalate activation of naturally occurring human constitutive androstane receptor splice variants and the pregnane X receptor. *Toxicol Sci.* 2011;120:381–391.

DeKeyser JG, Stagliano MC, Auerbach SS, Prabhu KS, Jones AD, Omiecinski CJ. Di(2-ethylhexyl) phthalate is a highly potent agonist for the human constitutive androstane receptor splice variant CAR2. *Mol Pharmacol.* 2009;75:1005–1013.

Delaforge M, Pruvost A, Perrin L, Andre F. Cytochrome P450-mediated oxidation of glucuronide derivatives: example of estradiol-17beta-glucuronide oxidation to 2-hydroxy-estradiol-17beta-glucuronide by CYP 2C8. *Drug Metab Dispos.* 2005;33:466–473.

Deng Y, Edin ML, Theken KN, et al. Endothelial CYP epoxygenase overexpression and soluble epoxide hydrolase disruption attenuate acute vascular inflammatory responses in mice. *FASEB J.* 2011;25:703–713.

Devarajan A, Bourquard N, Hama S, et al. Paraoxonase 2 deficiency alters mitochondrial function and exacerbates the development of atherosclerosis. *Antioxid Redox Signal.* 2011;14:341–351.

Devos A, Lino Cardenas CL, Glowacki F, et al. Genetic polymorphism of CYP2U1, a cytochrome P450 involved in fatty acids hydroxylation. *Prostaglandins Leukot Essent Fatty Acids.* 2010;83:105–110.

Diaz D, Fabre I, Daujat M, et al. Omeprazole is an aryl hydrocarbon-like inducer of human hepatic cytochrome P450. *Gastroenterology.* 1990;99:737–747.

Dick RA, Kanne DB, Casida JE. Nitroso-imidacloprid irreversibly inhibits rabbit aldehyde oxidase. *Chem Res Toxicol.* 2007;20:1942–1946.

Ding S, Lake BG, Friedberg T, Wolf CR. Expression and alternative splicing of the cytochrome P-450 CYP2A7. *Biochem J.* 1995;306(pt 1):161–166.

Ding X, Lichti K, Kim I, Gonzalez FJ, Staudinger JL. Regulation of constitutive androstane receptor and its target genes by fasting, cAMP, hepatocyte nuclear factor alpha, and the coactivator peroxisome proliferator-activated receptor gamma coactivator-1alpha. *J Biol Chem.* 2006;281:26540–26551.

Dirr H, Reinemer P, Huber R. X-ray crystal structures of cytosolic glutathione S-transferases. *Eur J Biochem.* 1994;220:645–661.

Dolphin CT, Beckett DJ, Janmohamed A, et al. The flavin-containing monooxygenase 2 gene (FMO2) of humans, but not of other primates, encodes a truncated, nonfunctional protein. *J Biol Chem.* 1998;273: 30599–30607.

Dong B, Saha PK, Huang W, et al. Activation of nuclear receptor CAR ameliorates diabetes and fatty liver disease. *Proc Natl Acad Sci U S A.* 2009;106:18831–18836.

Draganov DI, La Du BN. Pharmacogenetics of paraoxonases: a brief review. *Naunyn Schmiedebergs Arch Pharmacol.* 2004;369:78–88.

Dragin N, Dalton TP, Miller ML, Shertzer HG, Nebert DW. For dioxin-induced birth defects, mouse or human CYP1A2 in maternal liver protects whereas mouse CYP1A1 and CYP1B1 are inconsequential. *J Biol Chem.* 2006;281:18591–18600.

Driscoll JP, Aliagas I, Harris JJ, et al. Formation of a quinoneimine intermediate of 4-fluoro-N-methylaniline by FMO1: carbon oxidation plus defluorination. *Chem Res Toxicol.* 2010;23:861–863.

Dubé C, Rostom A, Lewin G, et al. The use of aspirin for primary prevention of colorectal cancer: a systematic review prepared for the U.S. Preventive Services Task Force. *Ann Intern Med.* 2007;146: 365–375.

Duell EJ, Sala N, Travier N, et al. Genetic variation in alcohol dehydrogenase (ADH1A, ADH1B, ADH1C, ADH7) and aldehyde dehydrogenase (ALDH2), alcohol consumption, and gastric cancer risk in the European Prospective Investigation into Cancer and Nutrition (EPIC) cohort. *Carcinogenesis.* 2012;33(2):361–367. doi: 10.1093/carcin/bgr285.

Duh FM, Fivash M, Moody M, et al. Characterization of a new SNP c767A/T (Arg222Trp) in the candidate TSG FUS2 on human chromosome 3p21.3: prevalence in Asian populations and analysis of association with nasopharyngeal cancer. *Mol Cell Probes.* 2004;18:39–44.

Duysen EG, Koentgen F, Williams GR, et al. Production of ES1 plasma carboxylesterase knockout mice for toxicity studies. *Chem Res Toxicol.* 2011;24:1891–1898.

Duysen EG, Li B, Darvesh S, Lockridge O. Sensitivity of butyrylcholinesterase knockout mice to (−)-huperzine A and donepezil suggests humans with butyrylcholinesterase deficiency may not tolerate these Alzheimer's disease drugs and indicates butyrylcholinesterase function in neurotransmission. *Toxicology.* 2007;233:60–69.

Dwivedi C, Downie AA, Webb TE. Net glucuronidation in different rat strains: importance of microsomal beta-glucuronidase. *FASEB J.* 1987;1:303–307.

Eaton DL, Gallagher EP. Mechanisms of aflatoxin carcinogenesis. *Annu Rev Pharmacol Toxicol.* 1994;34:135–172.

Edenberg HJ. The genetics of alcohol metabolism: role of alcohol dehydrogenase and aldehyde dehydrogenase variants. *Alcohol Res Health.* 2007;30:5–13.

Edmondson DE, Mattevi A, Binda C, Li M, Hubalek F. Structure and mechanism of monoamine oxidase. *Curr Med Chem.* 2004;11: 1983–1993.

Egan MF, Goldberg TE, Kolachana BS, et al. Effect of COMT Val108/158 Met genotype on frontal lobe function and risk for schizophrenia. *Proc Natl Acad Sci U S A.* 2001;98:6917–6922.

Eichenbaum G, Skibbe J, Parkinson A, et al. Use of enzyme inhibitors to evaluate the conversion pathways of ester and amide prodrugs: a case study example with the prodrug ceftobiprole medocaril. *J Pharm Sci.* 2012;101:1242–1252.

Ekhart C, Rodenhuis S, Smits PH, Beijnen JH, Huitema AD. An overview of the relations between polymorphisms in drug metabolising enzymes and drug transporters and survival after cancer drug treatment. *Cancer Treat Rev.* 2009;35:18–31.

Ekins S, Stresser DM, Andrew Williams J. In vitro and pharmacophore insights into CYP3A enzymes. *Trends Pharmacol Sci.* 2003;24: 161–166.

Ekroos M, Sjögren T. Structural basis for ligand promiscuity in cytochrome P450 3A4. *Proc Natl Acad Sci U S A.* 2006;103:13682–13687.

Elens L, Bouamar R, Hesselink DA, et al. A new functional CYP3A4 intron 6 polymorphism significantly affects tacrolimus pharmacokinetics in kidney transplant recipients. *Clin Chem.* 2011a;57:1574–1583.

Elens L, van Schaik RH, Panin N, et al. Effect of a new functional CYP3A4 polymorphism on calcineurin inhibitors' dose requirements and trough blood levels in stable renal transplant patients. *Pharmacogenomics.* 2011b;12:1383–1396.

EMA (European Medicines Agency). *Guideline on the Investigation of Drug Interactions (Final).* 2012. Available at: www.ema.europa.eu/ema/pages/includes/document/open_document.jsp?webContentId=WC500129606.

Eriksson T, Björkman S, Roth B, Fyge Å, Höglun P. Enantiomers of thalidomide: blood distribution and the influence of serum albumin on chiral inversion and hydrolysis. *Chirality.* 1998;10:223–228.

Evans D. N-Acetyltransferase. In: Kalow W, ed. *Pharmacogenetics of Drug Metabolism.* New York, NY: Pergamon; 1992:95–178.

Evans MJ, Cravatt BF. Mechanism-based profiling of enzyme families. *Chem Rev.* 2006;106:3279–3301.

Fajas L, Fruchart JC, Auwerx J. PPARgamma3 mRNA: a distinct PPARgamma mRNA subtype transcribed from an independent promoter. *FEBS Lett.* 1998;438:55–60.

Falany CN, Johnson MR, Barnes S, Diasio RB. Glycine and taurine conjugation of bile acids by a single enzyme. Molecular cloning and expression of human liver bile acid CoA:amino acid N-acyltransferase. *J Biol Chem.* 1994;269:19375–19379.

Faucette SR, Sueyoshi T, Smith CM, Negishi M, Lecluyse EL, Wang H. Differential regulation of hepatic CYP2B6 and CYP3A4 genes by constitutive androstane receptor but not pregnane X receptor. *J Pharmacol Exp Ther.* 2006;317:1200–1209.

Faucette SR, Wang H, Hamilton GA, et al. Regulation of CYP2B6 in primary human hepatocytes by prototypical inducers. *Drug Metab Dispos.* 2004;32:348–358.

FDA (Food and Drug Administration). *Guidance for Industry. Drug Interaction Studies—Study Design, Data Analysis, Implications for Dosing, and Labeling Recommendations.* 2012. Available at: http://www.fda.gov/downloads/Drugs/GuidanceComplianceRegulatoryInformation/Guidances/UCM292362.pdf.

Feng C, Tollin G, Enemark JH. Sulfite oxidizing enzymes. *Biochim Biophys Acta.* 2007;1774:527–539.

Fisher MB, Campanale K, Ackermann BL, VandenBranden M, Wrighton SA. In vitro glucuronidation using human liver microsomes and the pore-forming peptide alamethicin. *Drug Metab Dispos.* 2000;28:560–566.

Flanagan JU, Smythe ML. Sigma-class glutathione transferases. *Drug Metab Rev.* 2011;43:194–214.

Fontana E, Dansette PM, Poli SM. Cytochrome p450 enzymes mechanism based inhibitors: common sub-structures and reactivity. *Curr Drug Metab.* 2005;6:413–454.

Foti RS, Rock DA, Pearson JT, Wahlstrom JL, Wienkers LC. Mechanism-based inactivation of cytochrome P450 3A4 by mibefradil through heme destruction. *Drug Metab Dispos.* 2011;39:1188–1195.

Francois AA, Nishida CR, de Montellano PR, Phillips IR, Shephard EA. Human flavin-containing monooxygenase 2.1 catalyzes oxygenation of the antitubercular drugs thiacetazone and ethionamide. *Drug Metab Dispos.* 2009;37:178–186.

Franks ME, Macpherson GR, Figg WD. Thalidomide. *Lancet.* 2004;363: 1802–1811.

Freimuth RR, Wiepert M, Chute CG, Wieben ED, Weinshilboum RM. Human cytosolic sulfotransferase database mining: identification of seven novel genes and pseudogenes. *Pharmacogenomics J.* 2004;4:54–65.

Fremont JJ, Wang RW, King CD. Coimmunoprecipitation of UDP-glucuronosyltransferase isoforms and cytochrome P450 3A4. *Mol Pharmacol.* 2005;67:260–262.

Fretland AJ, Omiecinski CJ. Epoxide hydrolases: biochemistry and molecular biology. *Chem Biol Interact.* 2000;129:41–59.

Frezza M, di Padova C, Pazzato G, Terpin M, Baraona E, Lieber CS. High blood alcohol levels in women. The role of decreased gastric alcohol dehydrogenase activity and first-pass metabolism. *N Engl J Med.* 1990;322:95–99.

Fujikawa Y, Satoh T, Suganuma A, et al. Extremely sensitive biomarker of acute organophosphorus insecticide exposure. *Hum Exp Toxicol.* 2005;24:333–336.

Fujiwara R, Nakajima M, Yamanaka H, Katoh M, Yokoi T. Product inhibition of UDP-glucuronosyltransferase (UGT) enzymes by UDP obfuscates the inhibitory effects of UGT substrates. *Drug Metab Dispos.* 2008;36:361–367.

Fung M, Thornton A, Mybeck A, Wu JH-H, Hornbuckle K, Muniz E. Evaluation of the characteristics of safety withdrawal of prescription drugs from worldwide pharmaceutical markets—1960 to 1999. *Drug Inf J.* 2001;35:293–317.

Furlong CE, Suzuki SM, Stevens RC, et al. Human PON1, a biomarker of risk of disease and exposure. *Chem Biol Interact.* 2010;187:355–361.

Furukawa M, Nishimura M, Ogino D, et al. Cytochrome P450 gene expression levels in peripheral blood mononuclear cells in comparison with the liver. *Cancer Sci.* 2004;95:520–529.

Furuta T, Shirai N, Sugimoto M, Nakamura A, Hishida A, Ishizaki T. Influence of CYP2C19 pharmacogenetic polymorphism on proton pump inhibitor-based therapies. *Drug Metab Pharmacokinet.* 2005;20:153–167.

Gaedigk A, Simon SD, Pearce RE, Bradford LD, Kennedy MJ, Leeder JS. The CYP2D6 activity score: translating genotype information into a qualitative measure of phenotype. *Clin Pharmacol Ther.* 2008;83:234–242.

Galetin A, Clarke SE, Houston JB. Multisite kinetic analysis of interactions between prototypical CYP3A4 subgroup substrates: midazolam, testosterone, and nifedipine. *Drug Metab Dispos.* 2003;31:1108–1116.

Galetin A, Gertz M, Houston JB. Contribution of intestinal cytochrome p450-mediated metabolism to drug–drug inhibition and induction interactions. *Drug Metab Pharmacokinet.* 2010;25:28–47.

Gallicano KD, Sahai J, Shukla VK, et al. Induction of zidovudine glucuronidation and amination pathways by rifampicin in HIV-infected patients. *Br J Clin Pharmacol.* 1999;48:168–179.

Gamage N, Barnett A, Hempel N, et al. Human sulfotransferases and their role in chemical metabolism. *Toxicol Sci.* 2006;90:5–22.

Gao J, Xie W. Pregnane X receptor and constitutive androstane receptor at the crossroads of drug metabolism and energy metabolism. *Drug Metab Dispos.* 2010;38:2091–2095.

Garattini E, Fratelli M, Terao M. Mammalian aldehyde oxidases: genetics, evolution and biochemistry. *Cell Mol Life Sci.* 2008;65:1019–1048.

Garattini E, Terao M. Increasing recognition of the importance of aldehyde oxidase in drug development and discovery. *Drug Metab Rev.* 2011;43:374–386.

Gasche Y, Daali Y, Fathi M, et al. Codeine intoxication associated with ultrarapid CYP2D6 metabolism. *N Engl J Med.* 2004;351:2827–2831.

Gearry RB, Day AS, Barclay ML, Leong RW, Sparrow MP. Azathioprine and allopurinol: a two-edged interaction. *J Gastroenterol Hepatol.* 2010;25:653–655.

Geisler SA, Olshan AF. GSTM1, GSTT1, and the risk of squamous cell carcinoma of the head and neck: a mini-HuGE review. *Am J Epidemiol.* 2001;154:95–105.

Gerbal-Chaloin S, Pichard-Garcia L, Fabre JM, et al. Role of CYP3A4 in the regulation of the aryl hydrocarbon receptor by omeprazole sulphide. *Cell Signal.* 2006;18:740–750.

Gerlach M, Riederer P, Przuntek H, Youdim MB. MPTP mechanisms of neurotoxicity and their implications for Parkinson's disease. *Eur J Pharmacol.* 1991;208:273–286.

Germain P, Staels B, Dacquet C, Spedding M, Laudet V. Overview of nomenclature of nuclear receptors. *Pharmacol Rev.* 2006;58:685–704.

Geshi E, Kimura T, Yoshimura M, et al. A single nucleotide polymorphism in the carboxylesterase gene is associated with the responsiveness to imidapril medication and the promoter activity. *Hypertens Res.* 2005;28:719–725.

Ghanayem BI. Inhibition of urethane-induced carcinogenicity in Cyp2e1−/− in comparison to Cyp2e1 +/+ mice. *Toxicol Sci.* 2006;95:331–339.

Giacomini KM, Huang SM, Tweedie DJ, et al. Membrane transporters in drug development. *Nat Rev Drug Discov.* 2010;9:215–236.

Giacomini KM, Sugiyama Y. Membrane transporters and drug response. In: Goodman LS, Gilman A, Brunton LL, Lazo JS, Parker KL, eds. *Goodman & Gilman's The Pharmacological Basis of Therapeutics.* New York, NY: McGraw-Hill; 2006:41–70.

Gidal BE, Sheth R, Parnell J, Maloney K, Sale M. Evaluation of VPA dose and concentration effects on lamotrigine pharmacokinetics: implications for conversion to lamotrigine monotherapy. *Epilepsy Res.* 2003;57:85–93.

Gipple KJ, Chan KT, Elvin AT, Lalka D, Axelson JE. Species differences in the urinary excretion of the novel primary amine conjugate: tocainide carbamoyl *O*-beta-ᴅ-glucuronide. *J Pharm Sci.* 1982;71:1011–1014.

Glatt H, Meinl W. Pharmacogenetics of soluble sulfotransferases (SULTs). *Naunyn Schmiedebergs Arch Pharmacol.* 2004a;369:55–68.

Glatt H, Meinl W. Use of genetically manipulated *Salmonella typhimurium* strains to evaluate the role of sulfotransferases and acetyltransferases in nitrofen mutagenicity. *Carcinogenesis.* 2004b;25:779–786.

Goedde HW, Agarwal D. Pharmacogenetics of aldehyde dehydrogenase. In: Kalow W, ed. *Pharmacogenetics of Drug Metabolism.* New York, NY: Pergamon; 1992:281–311.

Goetz MP, Rae JM, Suman VJ, et al. Pharmacogenetics of tamoxifen biotransformation is associated with clinical outcomes of efficacy and hot flashes. *J Clin Oncol.* 2005;23:9312–9318.

Goh BC, Lee SC, Wang LZ, et al. Explaining interindividual variability of docetaxel pharmacokinetics and pharmacodynamics in Asians through phenotyping and genotyping strategies. *J Clin Oncol.* 2002;20:3683–3690.

Gomez A, Nekvindova J, Travica S, et al. Colorectal cancer-specific cytochrome P450 2W1: intracellular localization, glycosylation, and catalytic activity. *Mol Pharmacol.* 2010;78:1004–1011.

Gonzalez FJ. Role of gene knockout and transgenic mice in the study of xenobiotic metabolism. *Drug Metab Rev.* 2003;35:319–335.

Gonzalez FJ. Role of cytochromes P450 in chemical toxicity and oxidative stress: studies with CYP2E1. *Mutat Res.* 2005;569:101–110.

Gonzalez FJ. The 2006 Bernard B. Brodie Award Lecture. Cyp2e1. *Drug Metab Dispos.* 2007;35:1–8.

Gonzalez FJ, Coughtrie MW, Tukey RH. Drug metabolism. In: Brunton L, Chabner B, Knollmann B, eds. *Goodman & Gilman's the Pharmacological Basis of Therapeutics.* New York, NY: McGraw-Hill; 2011:123–144.

Gonzalez FJ, Tukey RH. Drug metabolism. In: Goodman LS, Gilman A, Brunton LL, Lazo JS, Parker KL, eds. *Goodman & Gilman's the Pharmacological Basis of Therapeutics.* New York, NY: McGraw-Hill; 2006:71–91.

Gonzalez FJ, Yu A-M. Cytochrome P450 and xenobiotic receptor humanized mice. *Annu Rev Pharmacol Toxicol.* 2006;46:41–64.

Gonzalez-Covarrubias V, Ghosh D, Lakhman SS, Pendyala L, Blanco JG. A functional genetic polymorphism on human carbonyl reductase 1 (CBR1 V88I) impacts on catalytic activity and NADPH binding affinity. *Drug Metab Dispos.* 2007;35:973–980.

Gopaul VS, Tang W, Farrell K, Abbott FS. Amino acid conjugates: metabolites of 2-propylpentanoic acid (valproic acid) in epileptic patients. *Drug Metab Dispos.* 2003;31:114–121.

Gorell JM, Rybicki BA, Johnson CC, Peterson EL. Smoking and Parkinson's disease: a dose–response relationship. *Neurology.* 1999;52:115–119.

Grant DM, Blum M, Meyer UA. Polymorphisms of *N*-acetyltransferase genes. *Xenobiotica.* 1992;22:1073–1081.

Grasso P, Sharratt M, Cohen AJ. Role of persistent, non-genotoxic tissue damage in rodent cancer and relevance to humans. *Annu Rev Pharmacol Toxicol.* 1991;31:253–287.

Grillo MP. Drug-*S*-acyl-glutathione thioesters: synthesis, bioanalytical properties, chemical reactivity, biological formation and degradation. *Curr Drug Metab.* 2011;12:229–244.

Grose KR, Bjeldanes LF. Oligomerization of indole-3-carbinol in aqueous acid. *Chem Res Toxicol.* 1992;5:188–193.

Grunwell JR, Bertozzi CR. Carbohydrate sulfotransferases of the GalNAc/Gal/GlcNAc6ST family. *Biochemistry.* 2002;41:13117–13126.

Gu Z, Feng X, Dong X, Chan P. Smoking, genes encoding dopamine pathway and risk for Parkinson's disease. *Neurosci Lett.* 2010;482:31–34.

Guengerich FP. Reactions and significance of cytochrome P-450 enzymes. *J Biol Chem.* 1991;266:10019–10022.

Guengerich FP. Common and uncommon cytochrome P450 reactions related to metabolism and chemical toxicity. *Chem Res Toxicol.* 2001a;14:611–650.

Guengerich FP. Uncommon P450-catalyzed reactions. *Curr Drug Metab.* 2001b;2:93–115.

Guengerich FP. Mechanisms of cytochrome P450 substrate oxidation: mini review. *J Biochem Mol Toxicol.* 2007;21:163–168.

Guengerich FP, Shimada T. Oxidation of toxic and carcinogenic chemicals by human cytochrome P-450 enzymes. *Chem Res Toxicol.* 1991;4:391–407.

Guengerich FP, Tang Z, Salamanca-Pinzon SG, Cheng Q. Characterizing proteins of unknown function: orphan cytochrome P450 enzymes as a paradigm. *Mol Interv.* 2010;10:153–163.

Guillemette C, Levesque E, Harvey M, Bellemare J, Menard V. UGT genomic diversity: beyond gene duplication. *Drug Metab Rev.* 2010;42:24–44.

Gunes A, Dahl ML. Variation in CYP1A2 activity and its clinical implications: influence of environmental factors and genetic polymorphisms. *Pharmacogenomics.* 2008;9:625–637.

Gupta N, Gill K, Singh S. Paraoxonases: structure, gene polymorphism and role in coronary artery disease. *Indian J Med Res.* 2009;130:361–368.

Gupta RA, DuBois RN. Aspirin, NSAIDS, and colon cancer prevention: mechanisms? *Gastroenterology.* 1998;114:1095–1098.

Gutierrez PL. The role of NAD(P)H oxidoreductase (DT-Diaphorase) in the bioactivation of quinone-containing antitumor agents: a review. *Free Radic Biol Med.* 2000;29:263–275.

Hagihara K, Kazui M, Kurihara A, Kubota K, Ikeda T. Glutaredoxin and thioredoxin can be involved in producing the pharmacologically active metabolite of a thienopyridine antiplatelet agent, prasugrel. *Drug Metab Dispos.* 2011;39:208–214.

Hakkinen MR, Hyvonen MT, Auriola S, et al. Metabolism of *N*-alkylated spermine analogues by polyamine and spermine oxidases. *Amino Acids.* 2010;38:369–381.

Hamman M, Haehner-Daniels B, Wrighton S, Rettie A, Hall S. Stereoselective sulfoxidation of sulindac sulfide by flavin-containing monooxygenases. *Biochem Pharmacol.* 2000;60:7–17.

Han Y, Oota H, Osier MV, et al. Considerable haplotype diversity within the 23kb encompassing the ADH7 gene. *Alcohol Clin Exp Res.* 2005;29:2091–2100.

Harris JM, Meyer DJ, Coles B, Ketterer B. A novel glutathione transferase (13-13) isolated from the matrix of rat liver mitochondria having structural similarity to class theta enzymes. *Biochem J.* 1991;278(pt 1):137–141.

Hartmann T, Terao M, Garattini E, et al. The impact of SNPs on human aldehyde oxidase. *Drug Metab Dispos.* 2012;40(5):856–864. doi: 10.1124/dmd.111.043828.

Havemeyer A, Grunewald S, Wahl B, et al. Reduction of *N*-hydroxy-sulfonamides, including *N*-hydroxy-valdecoxib, by the molybdenum-containing enzyme mARC. *Drug Metab Dispos.* 2010;38:1917–1921.

Havemeyer A, Lang J, Clement B. The fourth mammalian molybdenum enzyme mARC: current state of research. *Drug Metab Rev.* 2011;43:524–539.

Hawes EM. *N*-Glucuronidation, a common pathway in human metabolism of drugs with a tertiary amine group. *Drug Metab Dispos.* 1998;26:830–837.

Hayakawa H, Fukushima Y, Kato H, et al. Metabolism and disposition of novel des-fluoro quinolone garenoxacin in experimental animals and an interspecies scaling of pharmacokinetic parameters. *Drug Metab Dispos.* 2003;31:1409–1418.

Hayes JD, Flanagan JU, Jowsey IR. Glutathione transferases. *Annu Rev Pharmacol Toxicol.* 2005;45:51–88.

Hayes JD, Nguyen T, Judah DJ, Petersson DG, Neal GE. Cloning of cDNAs from fetal rat liver encoding glutathione *S*-transferase Yc polypeptides. The Yc2 subunit is expressed in adult rat liver resistant to the hepatocarcinogen aflatoxin B1. *J Biol Chem.* 1994;269:20707–20717.

Hayes JD, Pulford DJ. The glutathione *S*-transferase supergene family: regulation of GST and the contribution of the isoenzymes to cancer chemoprotection and drug resistance. *Crit Rev Biochem Mol Biol.* 1995;30:445–600.

Hayes RB, Bi W, Rothman N, et al. *N*-Acetylation phenotype and genotype and risk of bladder cancer in benzidine-exposed workers. *Carcinogenesis.* 1993;14:675–678.

Hebbachi AM, Knight BL, Wiggins D, Patel DD, Gibbons GF. Peroxisome proliferator-activated receptor alpha deficiency abolishes the response of lipogenic gene expression to re-feeding: restoration of the normal response by activation of liver X receptor alpha. *J Biol Chem.* 2008;283:4866–4876.

Hein DW. Acetylator genotype and arylamine-induced carcinogenesis. *Biochim Biophys Acta.* 1988;948:37–66.

Hein DW. *N*-Acetyltransferase 2 genetic polymorphism: effects of carcinogen and haplotype on urinary bladder cancer risk. *Oncogene.* 2006;25:1649–1658.

Hein DW, Doll MA, Fretland AJ, et al. Molecular genetics and epidemiology of the NAT1 and NAT2 acetylation polymorphisms. *Cancer Epidemiol Biomarkers Prev.* 2000;9:29–42.

Helms C, Cao L, Krueger JG, et al. A putative RUNX1 binding site variant between SLC9A3R1 and NAT9 is associated with susceptibility to psoriasis. *Nat Genet.* 2003;35:349–356.

Higgins LG, Hayes JD. Mechanisms of induction of cytosolic and microsomal glutathione transferase (GST) genes by xenobiotics and proinflammatory agents. *Drug Metab Rev.* 2011;43:92–137.

Hill RN, Erdreich LS, Paynter OE, Roberts PA, Rosenthal SL, Wilkinson CF. Thyroid follicular cell carcinogenesis. *Fundam Appl Toxicol.* 1989;12:629–697.

Hines RN, Hopp KA, Franco J, Saeian K, Begun FP. Alternative processing of the human FMO6 gene renders transcripts incapable of encoding a functional flavin-containing monooxygenase. *Mol Pharmacol.* 2002;62:320–325.

Hinrichs AL, Murphy SE, Wang JC, et al. Common polymorphisms in FMO1 are associated with nicotine dependence. *Pharmacogenet Genomics.* 2011;21:397–402.

Hirvonen A. Polymorphic NAT's and cancer predisposition. In: Ryder W, ed. *Metabolic Polymorphisms and Susceptibility to Cancer (IARC).* Lyon: IARC Scientific Publications; 1999:251–270.

Hofmann U, Heinkele G, Angelberger S, et al. Simultaneous quantification of eleven thiopurine nucleotides by liquid chromatography–tandem mass spectrometry. *Anal Chem.* 2012;84(3):1294–1301. doi: 10.1021/ac2031699.

Holčapek M, Kolárová L, Nobilis M. High-performance liquid chromatography–tandem mass spectrometry in the identification and determination of phase I and phase II drug metabolites. *Anal Bioanal Chem.* 2008;391:59–78.

Holmes RS, Wright MW, Laulederkind SJ, et al. Recommended nomenclature for five mammalian carboxylesterase gene families: human, mouse, and rat genes and proteins. *Mamm Genome.* 2010;21:427–441.

Hon YY, Jusko WJ, Spratlin VE, Jann MW. Altered methylprednisolone pharmacodynamics in healthy subjects with histamine *N*-methyltransferase C314T genetic polymorphism. *J Clin Pharmacol.* 2006;46:408–417.

Horton JR, Sawada K, Nishibori M, Cheng X. Structural basis for inhibition of histamine *N*-methyltransferase by diverse drugs. *J Mol Biol.* 2005;353:334–344.

Hrycay EG, Bandiera SM. The monooxygenase, peroxidase, and peroxygenase properties of cytochrome P450. *Arch Biochem Biophys.* 2012;522(2):71–89. doi: 10.1016/j.abb.2012.01.003.

Hu R, Xu C, Shen G, et al. Identification of Nrf2-regulated genes induced by chemopreventive isothiocyanate PEITC by oligonucleotide microarray. *Life Sci.* 2006;79:1944–1955.

Huang L, Smit JW, Meijer DK, Vore M. Mrp2 is essential for estradiol-17beta(beta-D-glucuronide)-induced cholestasis in rats. *Hepatology.* 2000;32:66–72.

Huang SM, Strong JM, Zhang L, et al. New era in drug interaction evaluation: US Food and Drug Administration update on CYP enzymes, transporters, and the guidance process. *J Clin Pharmacol.* 2008;48:662–670.

Huang SM, Zhao H, Lee JI, et al. Therapeutic protein–drug interactions and implications for drug development. *Clin Pharmacol Ther.* 2010;87:497–503.

Huang W, Lin YS, McConn DJ II, et al. Evidence of significant contribution from CYP3A5 to hepatic drug metabolism. *Drug Metab Dispos.* 2004;32:1434–1445.

Hukkanen J, Jacob P III, Benowitz NL. Metabolism and disposition kinetics of nicotine. *Pharmacol Rev.* 2005;57:79–115.

Humphrey MJ, Ringrose PS. Peptides and related drugs: a review of their absorption, metabolism, and excretion. *Drug Metab Rev.* 1986;17:283–310.

Idle JR. Is environmental carcinogenesis modulated by host polymorphism? *Mutat Res.* 1991;247:259–266.

Ikeda T. Drug-induced idiosyncratic hepatotoxicity: prevention strategy developed after the troglitazone case. *Drug Metab Pharmacokinet.* 2011;26:60–70.

Imig JD, Hammock BD. Soluble epoxide hydrolase as a therapeutic target for cardiovascular diseases. *Nat Rev Drug Discov.* 2009;8:794–805.

Ingelman-Sundberg M. Genetic polymorphisms of cytochrome P450 2D6 (CYP2D6): clinical consequences, evolutionary aspects and functional diversity. *Pharmacogenomics J.* 2005;5:6–13.

Ingelman-Sundberg M, Rane A, Gustafsson JA. Properties of hydroxylase systems in the human fetal liver active on free and sulfoconjugated steroids. *Biochemistry.* 1975;14:429–437.

Inoue T, Irikura D, Okazaki N, et al. Mechanism of metal activation of human hematopoietic prostaglandin D synthase. *Nat Struct Biol.* 2003;10:291–296.

Ishida M, Mikami S, Kikuchi E, et al. Activation of the aryl hydrocarbon receptor pathway enhances cancer cell invasion by upregulating the MMP expression and is associated with poor prognosis in upper urinary tract urothelial cancer. *Carcinogenesis.* 2010;31:287–295.

Ishii Y, Takeda S, Yamada H. Modulation of UDP-glucuronosyltransferase activity by protein–protein association. *Drug Metab Rev.* 2010;42: 145–158.

Ishizuka T, Fujimori I, Nishida A, et al. Paraoxonase 1 as a major bioactivating hydrolase for olmesartan medoxomil in human blood circulation: molecular identification and contribution to plasma metabolism. *Drug Metab Dispos.* 2012;40:374–380.

Isin EM, Guengerich FP. Complex reactions catalyzed by cytochrome P450 enzymes. *Biochim Biophys Acta.* 2007;1770:314–329.

Iskander K, Jaiswal AK. Quinone oxidoreductases in protection against myelogenous hyperplasia and benzene toxicity. *Chem Biol Interact.* 2005;153–154:147–157.

Isoherranen N, Hachad H, Yeung CK, Levy RH. Qualitative analysis of the role of metabolites in inhibitory drug–drug interactions: literature evaluation based on the metabolism and transport drug interaction database. *Chem Res Toxicol.* 2009;22:294–298.

Issemann I, Green S. Activation of a member of the steroid hormone receptor superfamily by peroxisome proliferators. *Nature.* 1990;347:645–650.

Iwaki M, Ogiso T, Hayashi H, Tanino T, Benet LZ. Acute dose-dependent disposition studies of nicotinic acid in rats. *Drug Metab Dispos.* 1996;24:773–779.

Iwata H, Fujita K, Kushida H, et al. High catalytic activity of human cytochrome P450 co-expressed with human NADPH-cytochrome P450 reductase in *Escherichia coli*. *Biochem Pharmacol.* 1998;55: 1315–1325.

Jaeschke H, Williams CD, Ramachandran A, Bajt ML. Acetaminophen hepatotoxicity and repair: the role of sterile inflammation and innate immunity. *Liver Int.* 2012;32:8–20.

Jedlitschky G, Cassidy AJ, Sales M, Pratt N, Burchell B. Cloning and characterization of a novel human olfactory UDP-glucuronosyltransferase. *Biochem J.* 1999;340(pt 3):837–843.

Jeffrey AM, Iatropoulos MJ, Williams GM. Nasal cytotoxic and carcinogenic activities of systemically distributed organic chemicals. *Toxicol Pathol.* 2006;34:827–852.

Jensen BA, Leeman RJ, Schlezinger JJ, Sherr DH. Aryl hydrocarbon receptor (AhR) agonists suppress interleukin-6 expression by bone marrow stromal cells: an immunotoxicology study. *Environ Health.* 2003;2:16.

Jeong S, Woo MM, Flockhart DA, Desta Z. Inhibition of drug metabolizing cytochrome P450s by the aromatase inhibitor drug letrozole and its major oxidative metabolite 4,4′-methanol-bisbenzonitrile in vitro. *Cancer Chemother Pharmacol.* 2009;64:867–875.

Jez JM, Penning TM. The aldo-keto reductase (AKR) superfamily: an update. *Chem Biol Interact.* 2001;130–132:499–525.

Ji Y, Salavaggione OE, Wang L, et al. Human phenylethanolamine *N*-methyltransferase pharmacogenomics: gene re-sequencing and functional genomics. *J Neurochem.* 2005;95:1766–1776.

Jin L, Kikuchi R, Saji T, Kusuhara H, Sugiyama Y. Regulation of tissue-specific expression of renal organic anion transporters by hepatocyte nuclear factor 1 alpha/beta and DNA methylation. *J Pharmacol Exp Ther.* 2012;340(3):648–655. doi: 10.1124/jpet.111.187161.

Jin S, Bryson TA, Dawson JH. Hydroperoxoferric heme intermediate as a second electrophilic oxidant in cytochrome P450-catalyzed reactions. *J Biol Inorg Chem.* 2004;9:644–653.

Johnston JB, Ouellet H, Podust LM, Ortiz de Montellano PR. Structural control of cytochrome P450-catalyzed ω-hydroxylation. *Arch Biochem Biophys.* 2011;507:86–94.

Josephy PD. Genetic variations in human glutathione transferase enzymes: significance for pharmacology and toxicology. *Hum Genomics Proteomics.* 2010;2010:876940.

Josephy PD, Guengerich FP, Miners J. Phase I and phase II drug metabolism: terminology that we should phase out? *Drug Metab Rev.* 2005;37:575–580.

Juberg DR, Mudra DR, Hazelton GA, Parkinson A. The effect of fenbuconazole on cell proliferation and enzyme induction in the liver of female CD1 mice. *Toxicol Appl Pharmacol.* 2006;214:178–187.

Just W, Zeller J, Riegert C, Speit G. Genetic polymorphisms in the formaldehyde dehydrogenase gene and their biological significance. *Toxicol Lett.* 2011;207:121–127.

Justenhoven C, Winter S, Hamann U, et al. The frameshift polymorphism CYP3A43_74_delA is associated with poor differentiation of breast tumors. *Cancer.* 2010;116:5358–5364.

Kadlubar FF. Biochemical individuality and its implications for drug and carcinogen metabolism: recent insights from acetyltransferase and cytochrome P4501A2 phenotyping and genotyping in humans. *Drug Metab Rev.* 1994;26:37–46.

Kaitaniemi S, Elovaara H, Gron K, et al. The unique substrate specificity of human AOC2, a semicarbazide-sensitive amine oxidase. *Cell Mol Life Sci.* 2009;66:2743–2757.

Kaivosaari S, Finel M, Koskinen M. *N*-Glucuronidation of drugs and other xenobiotics by human and animal UDP-glucuronosyltransferases. *Xenobiotica.* 2011;41:652–669.

Kalsotra A, Strobel HW. Cytochrome P450 4F subfamily: at the crossroads of eicosanoid and drug metabolism. *Pharmacol Ther.* 2006;112:589–611.

Kamataki T, Fujieda M, Kiyotani K, Iwano S, Kunitoh H. Genetic polymorphism of CYP2A6 as one of the potential determinants of tobacco-related cancer risk. *Biochem Biophys Res Commun.* 2005;338:306–310.

Kanamitsu SI, Ito K, Okuda H, et al. Prediction of in vivo drug–drug interactions based on mechanism-based inhibition from in vitro data: inhibition of 5-fluorouracil metabolism by (*E*)-5-(2-bromovinyl) uracil. *Drug Metab Dispos.* 2000;28:467–474.

Kang SJ, Scott WK, Li YJ, et al. Family-based case–control study of MAOA and MAOB polymorphisms in Parkinson disease. *Mov Disord.* 2006;21:2175–2180.

Kanno Y, Inoue Y, Inouye Y. 5-Aminoimidazole-4-carboxamide-1-beta-ribofuranoside (AICAR) prevents nuclear translocation of constitutive androstane receptor by AMP-activated protein kinase (AMPK) independent manner. *J Toxicol Sci.* 2010;35:571–576.

Kaplowitz N. Idiosyncratic drug hepatotoxicity. *Nat Rev Drug Disc.* 2005;4:489–499.

Karanam BV, Hop CE, Liu DQ, et al. In vitro metabolism of MK-0767 [(+/−)-5-[(2,4-dioxothiazolidin-5-yl)methyl]-2-methoxy-*N*-[[(4-trifluoromethyl) phenyl]methyl]benzamide], a peroxisome proliferator-activated receptor alpha/gamma agonist. I. Role of cytochrome P450, methyltransferases, flavin monooxygenases, and esterases. *Drug Metab Dispos.* 2004;32:1015–1022.

Karlgren M, Gomez A, Stark K, et al. Tumor-specific expression of the novel cytochrome P450 enzyme, CYP2W1. *Biochem Biophys Res Commun.* 2006;341:451–458.

Kasumov T, Brunengraber LL, Comte B, et al. New secondary metabolites of phenylbutyrate in humans and rats. *Drug Metab Dispos.* 2004;32:10–19.

Kato R, Yamazoe Y. Metabolic activation of *N*-hydroxylated metabolites of carcinogenic and mutagenic arylamines and arylamides by esterification. *Drug Metab Rev.* 1994;26:413–429.

Kavanagh KL, Jornvall H, Persson B, Oppermann U. Medium- and short-chain dehydrogenase/reductase gene and protein families: the SDR superfamily: functional and structural diversity within a family of metabolic and regulatory enzymes. *Cell Mol Life Sci.* 2008;65: 3895–3906.

Kawakami H, Ohtsuki S, Kamiie J, Suzuki T, Abe T, Terasaki T. Simultaneous absolute quantification of 11 cytochrome P450 isoforms in human liver microsomes by liquid chromatography tandem mass spectrometry with in silico target peptide selection. *J Pharm Sci.* 2011;100:341–352.

Kazmi F, Smith B, Hvenegaard M, et al. Identification of a novel carbamoyl glucuronide as a metabolism-dependent inhibitor of CYP2C8. *Drug Metab Rev.* 2010;42:A105.

Kelly EJ, Nakano M, Rohatgi P, Yarov-Yarovoy V, Rettie AE. Finding homes for orphan cytochrome P450s: CYP4V2 and CYP4F22 in disease states. *Mol Interv.* 2011;11:124–132.

Kiang TKL, Ensom MHH, Chang TKH. UDP-glucuronosyltransferases and clinical drug–drug interactions. *Pharmacol Ther.* 2005;106:97–132.

Kim H-R, Lee G-H, Yi Cho E, Chae S-W, Ahn T, Chae H-J. Bax inhibitor 1 regulates ER-stress-induced ROS accumulation through the regulation of cytochrome P450 2E1. *J Cell Sci.* 2009;122:1126–1133.

Kim K-A, Kim M-J, Park J-Y, et al. Stereoselective metabolism of lansoprazole by human liver cytochrome P450 enzymes. *Drug Metab Dispos.* 2003;31:1227–1234.

Kim MS, Shen Z, Kochansky C, et al. Differences in the metabolism and pharmacokinetics of two structurally similar PPAR agonists in dogs: involvement of taurine conjugation. *Xenobiotica.* 2004;34:665–674.

Kim SH, Henry EC, Kim DK, et al. Novel compound 2-methyl-2H-pyrazole-3-carboxylic acid (2-methyl-4-*o*-tolylazo-phenyl)-amide (CH-223191) prevents 2,3,7,8-TCDD-induced toxicity by antagonizing the aryl hydrocarbon receptor. *Mol Pharmacol.* 2006;69:1871–1878.

Kimura M, Higuchi S. Genetics of alcohol dependence. *Psychiatry Clin Neurosci.* 2011;65:213–225.

Kinobe RT, Parkinson OT, Mitchell DJ, Gillam EMJ. P450 2C18 catalyzes the metabolic bioactivation of phenytoin. *Chem Res Toxicol.* 2005;18:1868–1875.

Kirkman SK, Zhang M-Y, Horwatt PM, Scatina J. Isolation and identification of bromfenac glucoside from rat bile. *Drug Metab Dispos.* 1998;26:720–723.

Kitada M, Kamataki T, Itahashi K, Rikihisa T, Kanakubo Y. P-450 HFLa, a form of cytochrome P-450 purified from human fetal livers, is the 16 alpha-hydroxylase of dehydroepiandrosterone 3-sulfate. *J Biol Chem.* 1987;262:13534–13537.

Klaassen CD, Aleksunes LM. Xenobiotic, bile acid, and cholesterol transporters: function and regulation. *Pharmacol Rev.* 2010;62:1–96.

Klaassen CD, Boles JW. Sulfation and sulfotransferases 5: the importance of 3′-phosphoadenosine 5′-phosphosulfate (PAPS) in the regulation of sulfation. *FASEB J.* 1997;11:404–418.

Klaunig JE, Babich MA, Baetcke KP, et al. PPARalpha agonist-induced rodent tumors: modes of action and human relevance. *Crit Rev Toxicol.* 2003;33:655–780.

Knight TR, Choudhuri S, Klaassen CD. Constitutive mRNA expression of various glutathione *S*-transferase isoforms in different tissues of mice. *Toxicol Sci.* 2007;100:513–524.

Knights KM, Sykes MJ, Miners JO. Amino acid conjugation: contribution to the metabolism and toxicity of xenobiotic carboxylic acids. *Expert Opin Drug Metab Toxicol.* 2007;3:159–168.

Knockaert L, Descatoire V, Vadrot N, Fromenty B, Robin M-A. Mitochondrial CYP2E1 is sufficient to mediate oxidative stress and cytotoxicity induced by ethanol and acetaminophen. *Toxicol In Vitro.* 2011a;25:475–484.

Knockaert L, Fromenty B, Robin MA. Mechanisms of mitochondrial targeting of cytochrome P450 2E1: physiopathological role in liver injury and obesity. *FEBS J.* 2011b;278:4252–4260.

Kochansky CJ, Xia Y-Q, Wang S, et al. Species differences in the elimination of a peroxisome proliferator-activated receptor agonist highlighted by oxidative metabolism of its acyl glucuronide. *Drug Metab Dispos.* 2005;33:1894–1904.

Kodama S, Koike C, Negishi M, Yamamoto Y. Nuclear receptors CAR and PXR cross talk with FOXO1 to regulate genes that encode drug-metabolizing and gluconeogenic enzymes. *Mol Cell Biol.* 2004;24:7931–7940.

Kodama S, Negishi M. Phenobarbital confers its diverse effects by activating the orphan nuclear receptor CAR. *Drug Metab Rev.* 2006;38:75–87.

Koivusalo M, Baumann M, Uotila L. Evidence for the identity of glutathione-dependent formaldehyde dehydrogenase and class III alcohol dehydrogenase. *FEBS Lett.* 1989;257:105–109.

Koren G, Cairns J, Chitayat D, Gaedigk A, Leeder SJ. Pharmacogenetics of morphine poisoning in a breastfed neonate of a codeine-prescribed mother. *Lancet.* 2006;368:704.

Kraemer MJ, Furukawa CT, Koup JR, Shapiro GG, Pierson WE, Bierman CW. Altered theophylline clearance during an influenza B outbreak. *Pediatrics.* 1982;69:476–480.

Kroetz DL, Loiseau P, Guyot M, Levy RH. In vivo and in vitro correlation of microsomal epoxide hydrolase inhibition by progabide. *Clin Pharmacol Ther.* 1993;54:485–497.

Krueger S, VanDyke J, Williams D, Hines R. The role of flavin-containing monooxygenase (FMO) in the metabolism of tamoxifen and other tertiary amines. *Drug Metab Rev.* 2006;38:139–147.

Kubo T, Kim SR, Sai K, et al. Functional characterization of three naturally occurring single nucleotide polymorphisms in the CES2 gene encoding carboxylesterase 2 (HCE-2). *Drug Metab Dispos.* 2005;33:1482–1487.

Kudo M, Sasaki T, Ishikawa M, Hirasawa N, Hiratsuka M. Kinetics of 6-thioxanthine metabolism by allelic variants of xanthine oxidase. *Drug Metab Pharmacokinet.* 2010;25:361–366.

Kuhl H, Wiegratz I. Can 19-nortestosterone derivatives be aromatized in the liver of adult humans? Are there clinical implications? *Climacteric.* 2007;10:344–353.

Kumar S, Samuel K, Subramanian R, et al. Extrapolation of diclofenac clearance from in vitro microsomal metabolism data: role of acyl glucuronidation and sequential oxidative metabolism of the acyl glucuronide. *J Pharmacol Exp Ther.* 2002;303:969–978.

Kumarakulasingham M, Rooney PH, Dundas SR, et al. Cytochrome P450 profile of colorectal cancer: identification of markers of prognosis. *Clin Cancer Res.* 2005;11:3758–3765.

Kurian JR, Chin NA, Longlais BJ, Hayes KL, Trepanier LA. Reductive detoxification of arylhydroxylamine carcinogens by human NADH cytochrome b_5 reductase and cytochrome b_5. *Chem Res Toxicol.* 2006;19:1366–1373.

Kutty RK, Daniel RF, Ryan DE, Levin W, Maines MD. Rat liver cytochrome P-450b, P-420b, and P-420c are degraded to biliverdin by heme oxygenase. *Arch Biochem Biophys.* 1988;260:638–644.

La Du B. Human serum paraoxonase/arylesterase. In: Kalow W, ed. *Pharmacogenetics of Drug Metabolism.* New York, NY: Pergamon; 1992:51–91.

Lafite P, Dijols S, Buisson D, et al. Design and synthesis of selective, high-affinity inhibitors of human cytochrome P450 2J2. *Bioorg Med Chem Lett.* 2006;16:2777–2780.

Lafite P, Dijols S, Zeldin DC, Dansette PM, Mansuy D. Selective, competitive and mechanism-based inhibitors of human cytochrome P450 2J2. *Arch Biochem Biophys.* 2007;464:155–168.

Lai DY. Rodent carcinogenicity of peroxisome proliferators and issues on human relevance. *J Environ Sci Health C Environ Carcinog Ecotoxicol Rev.* 2004;22:37–55.

Lai L, Xu Z, Zhou J, Lee KD, Amidon GL. Molecular basis of prodrug activation by human valacyclovirase, an alpha-amino acid ester hydrolase. *J Biol Chem.* 2008;283:9318–9327.

Lai WG, Farah N, Moniz GA, Wong YN. A Baeyer–Villiger oxidation specifically catalyzed by human flavin-containing monooxygenase 5. *Drug Metab Dispos.* 2011;39:61–70.

Lai XS, Yang LP, Li XT, Liu JP, Zhou ZW, Zhou SF. Human CYP2C8: structure, substrate specificity, inhibitor selectivity, inducers and polymorphisms. *Curr Drug Metab.* 2009;10:1009–1047.

Lake BG. Species differences in the hepatic effects of inducers of CYP2B and CYP4A subfamily forms: relationship to rodent liver tumour formation. *Xenobiotica.* 2009;39:582–596.

Lake BG, Price RJ, Walters DG, Phillips JC, Young PJ, Adams TB. Studies on the metabolism of the thiofurans furfuryl mercaptan and 2-methyl-3-furanthiol in rat liver. *Food Chem Toxicol.* 2003;41:1761–1770.

Lammert C, Björnsson E, Niklasson A, et al. Oral medications with significant hepatic metabolism at higher risk for hepatic adverse events. *Hepatology.* 2010;51:615–620.

Lammert C, Einarsson S, Saha C, et al. Relationship between daily dose of oral medications and idiosyncratic drug-induced liver injury: Search for signals. *Hepatology.* 2008;47:2003–2009.

Lappin GJ, Hardwick TD, Stow R, Pigott GH, Van Ravenzwaay B. Absorption, metabolism and excretion of 4-chloro-2-methylphenoxyacetic acid (MCPA) in rat and dog. *Xenobiotica.* 2002;32:153–163.

Largeron M. Amine oxidases of the quinoproteins family: their implication in the metabolic oxidation of xenobiotics. *Ann Pharm Fr.* 2011;69:53–61.

Lasser KE, Allen PD, Woolhandler SJ, Himmelstein DU, Wolfe SM, Bor DH. Timing of new black box warnings and withdrawals for prescription medications. *JAMA.* 2002;287:2215–2220.

Lawton MP, Cashman JR, Cresteil T, et al. A nomenclature for the mammalian flavin-containing monooxygenase gene family based on amino acid sequence identities. *Arch Biochem Biophys.* 1994;308:254–257.

Lazarou J, Pomeranz BH, Corey PN. Incidence of adverse drug reactions in hospitalized patients: a meta-analysis of prospective studies. *JAMA.* 1998;279:1200–1205.

Lecoeur S, Bonierbale E, Challine D, et al. Specificity of in vitro covalent binding of tienilic acid metabolites to human liver microsomes in relationship to the type of hepatotoxicity: comparison with two directly hepatotoxic drugs. *Chem Res Toxicol.* 1994;7:434–442.

Lee CA, Jones J, Katayama J, et al. Identifying a selective substrate and inhibitor pair for the evaluation of CYP2J2 activity. *Drug Metab Dispos.* 2012;40(5):943–951. doi: 10.1124/dmd.111.043505.

Lee CA, Neul D, Clouser-Roche A, et al. Identification of novel substrates for human cytochrome P450 2J2. *Drug Metab Dispos.* 2010a;38:347–356.

Lee CM, Chen SY, Lee YC, Huang CY, Chen YM. Benzo[a]pyrene and glycine N-methyltransferse interactions: gene expression profiles of the liver detoxification pathway. *Toxicol Appl Pharmacol.* 2006;214:126–135.

Lee G-H, Kim H-K, Chae S-W, et al. Bax inhibitor-1 regulates endoplasmic reticulum stress-associated reactive oxygen species and heme oxygenase-1 expression. *J Biol Chem.* 2007;282:21618–21628.

Lee JM, Johnson JA. An important role of Nrf2–ARE pathway in the cellular defense mechanism. *J Biochem Mol Biol.* 2004;37:139–143.

Lee SS, Jung HJ, Park JS, Cha IJ, Cho DY, Shin JG. Identification of a null allele of cytochrome P450 3A7: CYP3A7 polymorphism in a Korean population. *Mol Biol Rep.* 2010b;37:213–217.

Lefèvre C, Bouadjar B, Ferrand V, et al. Mutations in a new cytochrome P450 gene in lamellar ichthyosis type 3. *Hum Mol Genet.* 2006;15:767–776.

Lehman-McKeemanm LD, Caudill D, Vassallo JD, Pearce RE, Madan A, Parkinson A. Effects of musk xylene and musk ketone on rat hepatic cytochrome P450 enzymes. *Toxicol Lett.* 1999;111:105–115.

Levano S, Keller D, Schobinger E, Urwyler A, Girard T. Rapid and accurate detection of atypical and Kalow variants in the butyrylcholinesterase gene using denaturing high performance liquid chromatography. *Anesth Analg.* 2008;106:147–151.

Levin W, Thomas P, Oldfield N, Ryan D. N-Demethylation of N-nitrosodimethylamine catalyzed by purified rat hepatic microsomal cytochrome P-450: isozyme specificity and role of cytochrome b5. *Arch Biochem Biophys.* 1986;248:158–165.

Levitt MD. Review article: lack of clinical significance of the interaction between H2-receptor antagonists and ethanol. *Aliment Pharmacol Ther.* 1993;7:131–138.

Levoin N, Blondeau C, Guillaume C, et al. Elucidation of the mechanism of inhibition of cyclooxygenases by acyl-coenzyme A and acylglucuronic conjugates of ketoprofen. *Biochem Pharmacol.* 2004;68:1957–1969.

Li A, Jiao X, Munier FL, et al. Bietti crystalline corneoretinal dystrophy is caused by mutations in the novel gene CYP4V2. *Am J Hum Genet.* 2004;74:817–826.

Li AP, Hartman NR, Lu C, Collins JM, Strong JM. Effects of cytochrome P450 inducers on 17α ethinyloestradiol (EE2) conjugation by primary human hepatocytes. *Br J Clin Pharmacol.* 1999;48:733–742.

Li B, Sedlacek M, Manoharan I, et al. Butyrylcholinesterase, paraoxonase, and albumin esterase, but not carboxylesterase, are present in human plasma. *Biochem Pharmacol.* 2005;70:1673–1684.

Li C, Wu W, Cho KB, Shaik S. Oxidation of tertiary amines by cytochrome P450-kinetic isotope effect as a spin-state reactivity probe. *Chemistry.* 2009a;15:8492–8503.

Li DN, Seidel A, Pritchard MP, Wolf CR, Friedberg T. Polymorphisms in P450 CYP1B1 affect the conversion of estradiol to the potentially carcinogenic metabolite 4-hydroxyestradiol. *Pharmacogenetics.* 2000;10:343–353.

Li H, Gu S, Cai X, et al. Ethnic related selection for an ADH Class I variant within East Asia. *PLoS One.* 2008;3:e1881.

Li L, Wei Y, Van Winkle L, et al. Generation and characterization of a Cyp2f2-null mouse and studies on the role of CYP2F2 in naphthalene-induced toxicity in the lung and nasal olfactory mucosa. *J Pharmacol Exp Ther.* 2011a;339:62–71.

Li TK. Pharmacogenetics of responses to alcohol and genes that influence alcohol drinking. *J Stud Alcohol.* 2000;61:5–12.

Li X, He Y, Ruiz CH, Koenig M, Cameron MD, Vojkovsky T. Characterization of dasatinib and its structural analogs as CYP3A4 mechanism-based inactivators and the proposed bioactivation pathways. *Drug Metab Dispos.* 2009b;37:1242–1250.

Li X, Hu Z, Qu X, et al. Putative EPHX1 enzyme activity is related with risk of lung and upper aerodigestive tract cancers: a comprehensive meta-analysis. *PLoS One.* 2011b;6:e14749.

Li Y, Yokoi T, Katsuki M, Wang JS, Groopman JD, Kamataki T. In vivo activation of aflatoxin B1 in C57BL/6N mice carrying a human fetus-specific CYP3A7 gene. *Cancer Res.* 1997;57:641–645.

Li-Wan-Po A, Girard T, Farndon P, Cooley C, Lithgow J. Pharmacogenetics of CYP2C19: functional and clinical implications of a new variant CYP2C19*17. *Br J Clin Pharmacol.* 2010;69:222–230.

Lieber CS. Microsomal ethanol-oxidizing system (MEOS): the first 30 years (1968-1998)—a review. *Alcohol Clin Exp Res.* 1999;23:991–1007.

Lieber CS. The discovery of the microsomal ethanol oxidizing system. *Drug Metab Rev.* 2004;36:511–529.

Liederer BM, Borchardt RT. Enzymes involved in the bioconversion of ester-based prodrugs. *J Pharm Sci.* 2006;95:1177–1195.

Lillibridge J, Kalhorn T, Slattery J. Metabolism of lisofylline and pentoxifylline in human liver microsomes and cytosol. *Drug Metab Dispos.* 1996;24:1174–1179.

Lin YS, Dowling ALS, Quigley SD, et al. Co-regulation of CYP3A4 and CYP3A5 and contribution to hepatic and intestinal midazolam metabolism. *Mol Pharmacol.* 2002;62:162–172.

Lindberg RLP, Negishi M. Alteration of mouse cytochrome P450coh substrate specificity by mutation of a single amino-acid residue. *Nature.* 1989;339:632–634.

Lindsay J, Wang LL, Li Y, Zhou SF. Structure, function and polymorphism of human cytosolic sulfotransferases. *Curr Drug Metab.* 2008;9:99–105.

Link M, Hakala KS, Wsol V, Kostiainen R, Ketola RA. Metabolite profile of sibutramine in human urine: a liquid chromatography-electrospray ionization mass spectrometric study. *J Mass Spectrom.* 2006;41:1171–1178.

Liston HL, DeVane CL, Boulton DW, Risch SC, Markowitz JS, Goldman J. Differential time course of cytochrome P450 2D6 enzyme inhibition by fluoxetine, sertraline, and paroxetine in healthy volunteers. *J Clin Psychopharmacol.* 2002;22:169–173.

Littler DR, Brown LJ, Breit SN, Perrakis A, Curmi PM. Structure of human CLIC3 at 2Å resolution. *Proteins.* 2010;78:1594–1600.

Liu K-H, Kim M-G, Lee D-J, et al. Characterization of ebastine, hydroxyebastine, and carebastine metabolism by human liver microsomes and expressed cytochrome P450 enzymes: major roles for CYP2J2 and CYP3A. *Drug Metab Dispos.* 2006a;34:1793–1797.

Liu T, David SP, Tyndale RF, et al. Associations of CYP2A6 genotype with smoking behaviors in southern China. *Addiction.* 2011;106:985–994.

Liu Y, Ramirez J, House L, Ratain MJ. Comparison of the drug–drug interactions potential of erlotinib and gefitinib via inhibition of UDP-glucuronosyltransferases. *Drug Metab Dispos.* 2010;38:32–39.

Liu Y-J, Huang P-L, Chang Y-F, et al. GSTP1 genetic polymorphism is associated with a higher risk of DNA damage in pesticide-exposed fruit growers. *Cancer Epidemiol Biomarkers Prev.* 2006b;15:659–666.

Liu ZC, Uetrecht JP. Metabolism of ticlopidine by activated neutrophils: implications for ticlopidine-induced agranulocytosis. *Drug Metab Dispos.* 2000;28:726–730.

Lockley DJ, Howes D, Williams FM. Cutaneous metabolism of glycol ethers. *Arch Toxicol.* 2005;79:160–168.

Lockridge O. Genetic variants of human serum butyrylcholinesterase influence the metabolism of the muscle relaxant succinylcholine. In: Kalow W, ed. *Pharmacogenetics of Drug Metabolism.* New York, NY: Pergamon; 1992:15–50.

Löhle M, Reichmann H. Controversies in neurology: why monoamine oxidase B inhibitors could be a good choice for the initial treatment of Parkinson's disease. *BMC Neurol.* 2011;11:112.

Lonard DM, O'Malley BW. The expanding cosmos of nuclear receptor coactivators. *Cell.* 2006;125:411–414.

Long RM, Rickert DE. Metabolism and excretion of 2,6-dinitro [14C] toluene in vivo and in isolated perfused rat livers. *Drug Metab Dispos.* 1982;10:455–458.

Lu Y, Cederbaum AI. CYP2E1 and oxidative liver injury by alcohol. *Free Radic Biol Med.* 2008;44:723–738.

Lunam CA, Hall PM, Cousins MJ. The pathology of halothane hepatotoxicity in a guinea-pig model: a comparison with human halothane hepatitis. *Br J Exp Pathol.* 1989;70:533–541.

Lurie Y, Loebstein R, Kurnik D, Almog S, Halkin H. Warfarin and vitamin K intake in the era of pharmacogenetics. *Br J Clin Pharmacol.* 2010;70:164–170.

Ma Q, Lu AY. Origins of individual variability in P4501A induction. *Chem Res Toxicol.* 2003;16:249–260.

Ma Q, Lu AY. CYP1A induction and human risk assessment: an evolving tale of in vitro and in vivo studies. *Drug Metab Dispos.* 2007;35:1009–1016.

Ma S, Subramanian R, Xu Y, Schrag M, Shou M. Structural characterization of novel adenine dinucleotide phosphate conjugates of imatinib in incubations with rat and human liver microsomes. *Drug Metab Dispos.* 2008;36:2414–2418.

Mackenzie PI, Walter BK, Burchell B, et al. Nomenclature update for the mammalian UDP glycosyltransferase (UGT) gene superfamily. *Pharmacogenet Genomics.* 2005;15:677–685.

Madan A, Williams TD, Faiman MD. Glutathione- and glutathione-*S*-transferase-dependent oxidative desulfuration of the thione xenobiotic diethyldithiocarbamate methyl ester. *Mol Pharmacol.* 1994;46:1217–1225.

Maecker B, Sherr DH, Vonderheide RH, et al. The shared tumor-associated antigen cytochrome P450 1B1 is recognized by specific cytotoxic T cells. *Blood.* 2003;102:3287–3294.

Malatkova P, Maser E, Wsol V. Human carbonyl reductases. *Curr Drug Metab.* 2010;11:639–658.

Mannervik B, Awasthi YC, Board PG, et al. Nomenclature for human glutathione transferases. *Biochem J.* 1992;282:305–306.

Mannervik B, Board PG, Hayes JD, Listowsky I, Pearson WR. Nomenclature for mammalian soluble glutathione transferases. *Methods Enzymol.* 2005;401:1–8.

Mano Y, Usui T, Kamimura H. In *vitro* drug interaction between diflunisal and indometacin via glucuronidation in humans. *Biopharm Drug Dispos.* 2006;27:267–273.

Marchitti SA, Brocker C, Stagos D, Vasiliou V. Non-P450 aldehyde oxidizing enzymes: the aldehyde dehydrogenase superfamily. *Expert Opin Drug Metab Toxicol.* 2008;4:697–720.

Marchitti SA, Deitrich RA, Vasiliou V. Neurotoxicity and metabolism of the catecholamine-derived 3,4-dihydroxyphenylacetaldehyde and 3,4-dihydroxyphenylglycolaldehyde: the role of aldehyde dehydrogenase. *Pharmacol Rev.* 2007;59:125–150.

Marchitti SA, Orlicky DJ, Brocker C, Vasiliou V. Aldehyde dehydrogenase 3B1 (ALDH3B1): immunohistochemical tissue distribution and cellular-specific localization in normal and cancerous human tissues. *J Histochem Cytochem.* 2010;58:765–783.

Marill J, Capron CC, Idres N, Chabot GG. Human cytochrome P450s involved in the metabolism of 9-*cis*- and 13-*cis*-retinoic acids. *Biochem Pharmacol.* 2002;63:933–943.

Marill J, Cresteil T, Lanotte M, Chabot GG. Identification of human cytochrome P450s involved in the formation of all-*trans*-retinoic acid principal metabolites. *Mol Pharmacol.* 2000;58:1341–1348.

Martinez Molina D, Eshaghi S, Nordlund P. Catalysis within the lipid bilayer—structure and mechanism of the MAPEG family of integral membrane proteins. *Curr Opin Struct Biol.* 2008;18:442–449.

Masson P, Lockridge O. Butyrylcholinesterase for protection from organophosphorus poisons: catalytic complexities and hysteretic behavior. *Arch Biochem Biophys.* 2010;494:107–120.

Masukawa T, Sai M, Tochino Y. Methods for depleting brain glutathione. *Life Sci.* 1989;44:417–424.

Matsunaga T, Shintani S, Hara A. Multiplicity of mammalian reductases for xenobiotic carbonyl compounds. *Drug Metab Pharmacokinet.* 2006;21:1–18.

McClain R. The significance of hepatic microsomal enzyme induction and altered thyroid function in rats: implications for thyroid gland neoplasia. *Toxicol Pathol.* 1989;17:294–306.

McCormack M, Alfirevic A, Bourgeois S, et al. HLA-A*3101 and carbamazepine-induced hypersensitivity reactions in Europeans. *N Engl J Med.* 2011;364:1134–1143.

McDonald MG, Rieder MJ, Nakano M, Hsia CK, Rettie AE. CYP4F2 is a vitamin K1 oxidase: an explanation for altered warfarin dose in carriers of the V433M variant. *Mol Pharmacol.* 2009;75:1337–1346.

McGrath AP, Hilmer KM, Collyer CA, Dooley DM, Guss JM. A new crystal form of human diamine oxidase. *Acta Crystallogr Sect F Struct Biol Cryst Commun.* 2010;66:137–142.

McIlwain CC, Townsend DM, Tew KD. Glutathione *S*-transferase polymorphisms: cancer incidence and therapy. *Oncogene.* 2006;25:1639–1648.

McLaughlin LA, Ronseaux S, Finn RD, Henderson CJ, Roland Wolf C. Deletion of microsomal cytochrome b5 profoundly affects hepatic and extrahepatic drug metabolism. *Mol Pharmacol.* 2010;78:269–278.

McLeod HL, Fang L, Luo X, Scott EP, Evans WE. Ethnic differences in erythrocyte catechol-*O*-methyltransferase activity in black and white Americans. *J Pharmacol Exp Ther.* 1994;270:26–29.

Meech R, Mackenzie PI. UGT3A: novel UDP-glycosyltransferases of the UGT superfamily. *Drug Metab Rev.* 2010;42:45–54.

Metushi IG, Cai P, Zhu X, Nakagawa T, Uetrecht JP. A fresh look at the mechanism of isoniazid-induced hepatotoxicity. *Clin Pharmacol Ther.* 2011;89:911–914.

Meyer UA. The molecular basis of genetic polymorphisms of drug metabolism. *J Pharm Pharmacol.* 1994;46:409–415.

Michaud V, Frappier M, Dumas M-C, Turgeon J. Metabolic activity and mRNA levels of human cardiac CYP450s involved in drug metabolism. *PLoS One.* 2010;5:e15666.

Michelakis ED, Sutendra G, Dromparis P, et al. Metabolic modulation of glioblastoma with dichloroacetate. *Sci Transl Med.* 2010;2:31ra34.

Mimori Y, Nakamura S, Kameyama M. Regional and subcellular distribution of cyanide metabolizing enzymes in the central nervous system. *J Neurochem.* 1984;43:540–545.

Miners JO, Knights KM, Houston JB, Mackenzie PI. In vitro-in vivo correlation for drugs and other compounds eliminated by glucuronidation in humans: pitfalls and promises. *Biochem Pharmacol.* 2006;71:1531–1539.

Miners JO, Mackenzie PI, Knights KM. The prediction of drug-glucuronidation parameters in humans: UDP-glucuronosyltransferase enzyme-selective substrate and inhibitor probes for reaction phenotyping and in vitro–in vivo extrapolation of drug clearance and drug–drug interaction potential. *Drug Metab Rev.* 2010;42:196–208.

Mirsalis JC, Butterworth BE. Induction of unscheduled DNA synthesis in rat hepatocytes following in vivo treatment with dinitrotoluene. *Carcinogenesis.* 1982;3:241–245.

Mitchell SC. Flavin mono-oxygenase (FMO)—the 'other' oxidase. *Curr Drug Metab.* 2008;9:280–284.

Mitoma C, Posner HS, Leonard F. Aromatization of hexahydrobenzoic acid by mammalian liver mitochondria. *Biochim Biophys Acta.* 1958;27:156–160.

Miura M, Satoh S, Tada H, Habuchi T, Suzuki T. Stereoselective metabolism of rabeprazole-thioether to rabeprazole by human liver microsomes. *Eur J Clin Pharmacol.* 2006;62:113–117.

Molina MA, Sitja-Arnau M, Lemoine MG, Frazier ML, Sinicrope FA. Increased cyclooxygenase-2 expression in human pancreatic carcinomas and cell lines: growth inhibition by nonsteroidal anti-inflammatory drugs. *Cancer Res.* 1999;59:4356–4362.

Monks TJ, Anders MW, Dekant W, Stevens JL, Lau SS, van Bladeren PJ. Glutathione conjugate mediated toxicities. *Toxicol Appl Pharmacol.* 1990;106:1–19.

Moore TJ, Cohen MR, Furberg CD. Serious adverse drug events reported to the Food and Drug Administration, 1998-2005. *Arch Intern Med.* 2007;167:1752–1759.

358

Morar N, Bowcock AM, Harper JI, Cookson WO, Moffatt MF. Investigation of the chromosome 17q25 PSORS2 locus in atopic dermatitis. *J Invest Dermatol.* 2006;126:603–606.

Mordente A, Meucci E, Martorana GE, Giardina B, Minotti G. Human heart cytosolic reductases and anthracycline cardiotoxicity. *IUBMB Life.* 2001;52:83–88.

Moreau A, Vilarem MJ, Maurel P, Pascussi JM. Xenoreceptors CAR and PXR activation and consequences on lipid metabolism, glucose homeostasis, and inflammatory response. *Mol Pharm.* 2008;5:35–41.

Morel F, Aninat C. The glutathione transferase kappa family. *Drug Metab Rev.* 2011;43:281–291.

Morgan ET. Impact of infectious and inflammatory disease on cytochrome P450-mediated drug metabolism and pharmacokinetics. *Clin Pharmacol Ther.* 2009;85:434–438.

Morgan ET, Goralski KB, Piquette-Miller M, et al. Regulation of drug-metabolizing enzymes and transporters in infection, inflammation, and cancer. *Drug Metab Dispos.* 2008;36:205–216.

Morgenstern R, Zhang J, Johansson K. Microsomal glutathione transferase 1: mechanism and functional roles. *Drug Metab Rev.* 2011;43:300–306.

Morisseau C, Hammock BD. Epoxide hydrolases: mechanisms, inhibitor designs, and biological roles. *Annu Rev Pharmacol Toxicol.* 2005;45:311–333.

Mukherjee B, Salavaggione OE, Pelleymounter LL, et al. Glutathione *S*-transferase omega 1 and omega 2 pharmacogenomics. *Drug Metab Dispos.* 2006;34:1237–1246.

Mulder GJ. *Sulfation of Drugs and Related Compounds.* Boca Raton, FL: CRC Press; 1981.

Murai T, Iwabuchi H, Ikeda T. Repeated glucuronidation at one hydroxyl group leads to structurally novel diglucuronides of steroid sex hormones. *Drug Metab Pharmacokinet.* 2005;20:282–293.

Murai T, Samata N, Iwabuchi H, Ikeda T. Human udp-glucuronosyltransferase, UGT1A8, glucuronidates dihydrotestosterone to a monoglucuronide and further to a structurally novel diglucuronide. *Drug Metab Dispos.* 2006;34:1102–1108.

Murray IA, Krishnegowda G, DiNatale BC, et al. Development of a selective modulator of aryl hydrocarbon (Ah) receptor activity that exhibits anti-inflammatory properties. *Chem Res Toxicol.* 2010;23:955–966.

Mutoh S, Osabe M, Inoue K, et al. Dephosphorylation of threonine 38 is required for nuclear translocation and activation of human xenobiotic receptor CAR (NR1I3). *J Biol Chem.* 2009;284:34785–34792.

Naesens M, Kuypers DR, Streit F, et al. Rifampin induces alterations in mycophenolic acid glucuronidation and elimination: implications for drug exposure in renal allograft recipients. *Clin Pharmacol Ther.* 2006;80:509–521.

Nagar S, Blanchard R. Pharmacogenetics of uridine diphosphoglucuronosyltransferase (UGT) 1A family members and its role in patient response to irinotecan. *Drug Metab Rev.* 2006;38:393–409.

Nagar S, Remmel RP. Uridine diphosphoglucuronosyltransferase pharmacogenetics and cancer. *Oncogene.* 2006;25:1659–1672.

Nagata K, Yamazoe Y. Pharmacogenetics of sulfotransferase. *Annu Rev Pharmacol Toxicol.* 2000;40:159–176.

Nakajima M, Itoh M, Sakai H, et al. CYP2A13 expressed in human bladder metabolically activates 4-aminobiphenyl. *Int J Cancer.* 2006;119:2520–2526.

Nakano H, Ogura K, Takahashi E, et al. Regioselective monosulfation and disulfation of the phytoestrogens daidzein and genistein by human liver sulfotransferases. *Drug Metab Pharmacokinet.* 2004;19:216–226.

Nakano K, Ohashi M, Harigaya S. The beta-glucosidation and beta-glucuronidation of pantothenic acid compared with *p*-nitrophenol in dog liver microsome. *Chem Pharm Bull (Tokyo).* 1986;34:3949–3952.

Nakayama S, Atsumi R, Takakusa H, et al. A zone classification system for risk assessment of idiosyncratic drug toxicity using daily dose and covalent binding. *Drug Metab Dispos.* 2009;37:1970–1977.

Nakura H, Itoh S, Kusano K, Ishizone H, Deguchi T, Kamataki T. Evidence for the lack of hepatic *N*-acetyltransferase in suncus (*Suncus murinus*). *Biochem Pharmacol.* 1995;50:1165–1170.

Neat J, Simpson J, Brawner S, et al. In vitro evaluation of selected AhR, CAR, GR and PXR agonists as inducers of CYP2J2 activity and gene expression in cultured human hepatocytes. *Drug Metab Rev.* 2009;41:Abstract 195.

Nebert DW, Dalton TP. The role of cytochrome P450 enzymes in endogenous signalling pathways and environmental carcinogenesis. *Nat Rev Cancer.* 2006;6:947–960.

Nebert DW, Dalton TP, Okey AB, Gonzalez FJ. Role of aryl hydrocarbon receptor-mediated induction of the CYP1 enzymes in environmental toxicity and cancer. *J Biol Chem.* 2004;279:23847–23850.

Negishi T, Kato Y, Ooneda O, et al. Effects of aryl hydrocarbon receptor signaling on the modulation of TH1/TH2 balance. *J Immunol.* 2005;175:7348–7356.

Nelson DR. The cytochrome P450 homepage. *Hum Genomics.* 2009;4:59–65. Available at: http://drnelson.uthsc.edu/CytochromeP450.html.

Neupert W, Brugger R, Euchenhofer C, Brune K, Geisslinger G. Effects of ibuprofen enantiomers and its coenzyme A thioesters on human prostaglandin endoperoxide synthases. *Br J Pharmacol.* 1997;122:487–492.

Newcomb M, Chandrasena RE. Highly reactive electrophilic oxidants in cytochrome P450 catalysis. *Biochem Biophys Res Commun.* 2005;338:394–403.

Nguyen T, Rushmore TH, Pickett CB. Transcriptional regulation of a rat liver glutathione *S*-transferase Ya subunit gene. Analysis of the antioxidant response element and its activation by the phorbol ester 12-*O*-tetradecanoylphorbol-13-acetate. *J Biol Chem.* 1994;269:13656–13662.

Nigg HN, Knaak JB. Blood cholinesterases as human biomarkers of organophosphorus pesticide exposure. *Rev Environ Contam Toxicol.* 2000;163:29–111.

Nishida CR, Lee M, de Montellano PR. Efficient hypoxic activation of the anticancer agent AQ4N by CYP2S1 and CYP2W1. *Mol Pharmacol.* 2010;78:497–502.

Nishida CR, Ortiz de Montellano PR. Thermophilic cytochrome P450 enzymes. *Biochem Biophys Res Commun.* 2005;338:437–445.

Nishihara M, Sudo M, Kawaguchi N, et al. An unusual metabolic pathway of sipoglitazar, a novel antidiabetic agent: cytochrome P450-catalyzed oxidation of sipoglitazar acyl glucuronide. *Drug Metab Dispos.* 2012;40:249–258.

Nishimura M, Naito S. Tissue-specific mRNA expression profiles of human ATP-binding cassette and solute carrier transporter superfamilies. *Drug Metab Pharmacokinet.* 2005;20:452–477.

Nishimura M, Naito S. Tissue-specific mRNA expression profiles of human phase I metabolizing enzymes except for cytochrome P450 and phase II metabolizing enzymes. *Drug Metab Pharmacokinet.* 2006;21:357–374.

Nishimura M, Naito S, Yokoi T. Tissue-specific mRNA expression profiles of human nuclear receptor subfamilies. *Drug Metab Pharmacokinet.* 2004;19:135–149.

Nishimura M, Yaguti H, Yoshitsugu H, Naito S, Satoh T. Tissue distribution of mRNA expression of human cytochrome P450 isoforms assessed by high-sensitivity real-time reverse transcription PCR. *Yakugaku Zasshi.* 2003;123:369–375.

Nowell S, Falany CN. Pharmacogenetics of human cytosolic sulfotransferases. *Oncogene.* 2006;25:1673–1678.

Oakley A. Glutathione transferases: a structural perspective. *Drug Metab Rev.* 2011;43:138–151.

Obach RS. Potent inhibition of human liver aldehyde oxidase by raloxifene. *Drug Metab Dispos.* 2004;32:89–97.

Obach RS, Cox LM, Tremaine LM. Sertraline is metabolized by multiple cytochrome P450 enzymes, monoamine oxidases, and glucuronyl transferases in human: an in vitro study. *Drug Metab Dispos.* 2005;33:262–270.

Obach RS, Kalgutkar AS, Soglia JR, Zhao SX. Can in vitro metabolism-dependent covalent binding data in liver microsomes distinguish hepatotoxic from nonhepatotoxic drugs? An analysis of 18 drugs with consideration of intrinsic clearance and daily dose. *Chem Res Toxicol.* 2008;21:1814–1822.

Obach RS, Reed-Hagen AE, Krueger SS, et al. Metabolism and disposition of varenicline, a selective α4β2 acetylcholine receptor partial agonist, in vivo and in vitro. *Drug Metab Dispos.* 2006;34:121–130.

Obach RS, Ryder TF. Metabolism of ramelteon in human liver microsomes and correlation with the effect of fluvoxamine on ramelteon pharmacokinetics. *Drug Metab Dispos*. 2010;38:1381–1391.

O'Brien PJ. Peroxidases. *Chem Biol Interact*. 2000;129:113–139.

O'Byrne J, Hunt MC, Rai DK, Saeki M, Alexson SE. The human bile acid-CoA:amino acid *N*-acyltransferase functions in the conjugation of fatty acids to glycine. *J Biol Chem*. 2003;278:34237–34244.

Ogilvie BW, Parkinson A. Drugs as victims and perpetrators and the pharmacokinetic concept of maximum exposure. In: Lee PW, Aizawa H, Gan LL, Prakash C, Zhong D, eds. *Handbook of Metabolic Pathways of Xenobiotics*. Wiley. In press.

Ogilvie BW, Usuki E, Yerino P, Parkinson A. In vitro approaches for studying the inhibition of drug-metabolizing enzymes and identifying the drug-metabolizing enzymes responsible for the metabolism of drugs (reaction phenotyping) with emphasis on cytochrome P450. In: Rodrigues AD, ed. *Drug–Drug Interactions*. New York, NY: Informa Healthcare USA Inc; 2008:231–358.

Ogilvie BW, Yerino P, Kazmi F, et al. The proton pump inhibitor, omeprazole, but not lansoprazole or pantoprazole, is a metabolism-dependent inhibitor of CYP2C19: implications for coadministration with clopidogrel. *Drug Metab Dispos*. 2011;39:2020–2033.

Ogilvie BW, Zhang D, Li W, et al. Glucuronidation converts gemfibrozil to a potent, metabolism-dependent inhibitor of CYP2C8: implications for drug–drug interactions. *Drug Metab Dispos*. 2006;34:191–197.

Ogura K, Nishiyama T, Takubo H, et al. Suicidal inactivation of human dihydropyrimidine dehydrogenase by (*E*)-5-(2-bromovinyl)uracil derived from the antiviral, sorivudine. *Cancer Lett*. 1998;122:107–113.

Oguro A, Imaoka S. Lysophosphatidic acids are new substrates for the phosphatase domain of soluble epoxide hydrolase. *J Lipid Res*. 2012;53(3):505–512. doi: 10.1194/jlr.M022319.

Ohmori S, Fujiki N, Nakasa H, et al. Steroid hydroxylation by human fetal CYP3A7 and human NADPH-cytochrome P450 reductase coexpressed in insect cells using baculovirus. *Res Commun Mol Pathol Pharmacol*. 1998;100:15–28.

Ohtsuki S, Schaefer O, Kawakami H, et al. Simultaneous absolute protein quantification of transporters, cytochromes P450, and UDP-glucuronosyltransferases as a novel approach for the characterization of individual human liver: comparison with mRNA levels and activities. *Drug Metab Dispos*. 2012;40:83–92.

Okamoto K, Matsumoto K, Hille R, Eger BT, Pai EF, Nishino T. The crystal structure of xanthine oxidoreductase during catalysis: implications for reaction mechanism and enzyme inhibition. *Proc Natl Acad Sci U S A*. 2004;101:7931–7936.

Omiecinski CJ, Coslo DM, Chen T, Laurenzana EM, Peffer RC. Multi-species analyses of direct activators of the constitutive androstane receptor. *Toxicol Sci*. 2011a;123:550–562.

Omiecinski CJ, Vanden Heuvel JP, Perdew GH, Peters JM. Xenobiotic metabolism, disposition, and regulation by receptors: from biochemical phenomenon to predictors of major toxicities. *Toxicol Sci*. 2011;120 suppl 1:S49–S75.

Omura T. Recollection of the early years of the research on cytochrome P450. *Proc Jpn Acad Ser B Phys Biol Sci*. 2011;87:617–640.

Oppermann UCT, Filling C, Jornvall H. Forms and functions of human SDR enzymes. *Chem Biol Interact*. 2001;130–132:699–705.

Ortiz de Montellano PR. Mechanism and role of covalent heme binding in the CYP4 family of P450 enzymes and the mammalian peroxidases. *Drug Metab Rev*. 2008;40:405–426.

Osabe M, Negishi M. Active ERK1/2 protein interacts with the phosphorylated nuclear constitutive active/androstane receptor (CAR; NR1I3), repressing dephosphorylation and sequestering CAR in the cytoplasm. *J Biol Chem*. 2011;286:35763–35769.

Oshima M, Dinchuk JE, Kargman SL, et al. Suppression of intestinal polyposis in Apc[Delta]716 knockout mice by inhibition of cyclooxygenase 2 (COX-2). *Cell*. 1996;87:803–809.

Otto TC, Harsch CK, Yeung DT, Magliery TJ, Cerasoli DM, Lenz DE. Dramatic differences in organophosphorus hydrolase activity between human and chimeric recombinant mammalian paraoxonase-1 enzymes. *Biochemistry*. 2009;48:10416–10422.

Pacher P, Nivorozhkin A, Szabo C. Therapeutic effects of xanthine oxidase inhibitors: renaissance half a century after the discovery of allopurinol. *Pharmacol Rev*. 2006;58:87–114.

Paine MF, Widmer WW, Hart HL, et al. A furanocoumarin-free grapefruit juice establishes furanocoumarins as the mediators of the grapefruit juice–felodipine interaction. *Am J Clin Nutr*. 2006;83:1097–1105.

Pal D, Mitra AK. MDR- and CYP3A4-mediated drug–herbal interactions. *Life Sci*. 2006;78:2131–2145.

Pang X-Y, Cheng J, Kim J-H, Matsubara T, Krausz KW, Gonzalez FJ. Expression and regulation of human fetal-specific CYP3A7 in mice. *Endocrinology*. 2012.

Park BK, Boobis A, Clarke S, et al. Managing the challenge of chemically reactive metabolites in drug development. *Nat Rev Drug Discov*. 2011;10:292–306.

Parker RS, Sontag TJ, Swanson JE, McCormick CC. Discovery, characterization, and significance of the cytochrome P450 ω-hydroxylase pathway of vitamin E catabolism. *Ann N Y Acad Sci*. 2004;1031:13–21.

Parkin DP, Vandenplas S, Botha FJ, et al. Trimodality of isoniazid elimination: phenotype and genotype in patients with tuberculosis. *Am J Respir Crit Care Med*. 1997;155:1717–1722.

Parkinson A, Hurwitz A. Omeprazole and the induction of human cytochrome P-450: a response to concerns about potential adverse effects. *Gastroenterology*. 1991;100:1157–1164.

Parkinson A, Kazmi F, Buckley DB, Yerino P, Ogilvie BW, Paris BL. System-dependent outcomes during the evaluation of drug candidates as inhibitors of cytochrome P450 (CYP) and uridine diphosphate glucuronosyltransferase (UGT) enzymes: human hepatocytes versus liver microsomes versus recombinant enzymes. *Drug Metab Pharmacokinet*. 2010;25:16–27.

Parkinson A, Kazmi F, Buckley DB, et al. An evaluation of the dilution method for identifying metabolism-dependent inhibitors of cytochrome p450 enzymes. *Drug Metab Dispos*. 2011;39:1370–1387.

Parkinson A, Leonard N, Draper A, Ogilvie BW. On the mechanism of hepatocarcinogenesis of benzodiazepines: evidence that diazepam and oxazepam are CYP2B inducers in rats, and both CYP2B and CYP4A inducers in mice. *Drug Metab Rev*. 2006;38:235–259.

Parkinson A, Mudra DR, Johnson C, Dwyer A, Carroll KM. The effects of gender, age, ethnicity, and liver cirrhosis on cytochrome P450 enzyme activity in human liver microsomes and inducibility in cultured human hepatocytes. *Toxicol Appl Pharmacol*. 2004;199:193–209.

Parkinson A, Ogilvie BW. Biotransformation of xenobiotics. In: Klaassen CD, ed. *Casarett & Doull's Toxicology: The Basic Science of Poisons*. New York City, NY: McGraw-Hill Inc; 2008:161–304.

Pascual G, Glass CK. Nuclear receptors versus inflammation: mechanisms of transrepression. *Trends Endocrinol Metab*. 2006;17:321–327.

Patin E, Barreiro LB, Sabeti PC, et al. Deciphering the ancient and complex evolutionary history of human arylamine *N*-acetyltransferase genes. *Am J Hum Genet*. 2006;78:423–436.

Patki KC, von Moltke LL, Greenblatt DJ. In vitro metabolism of midazolam, triazolam, nifedipine, and testosterone by human liver microsomes and recombinant cytochromes P450: role of CYP3A4 and CYP3A5. *Drug Metab Dispos*. 2003;31:938–944.

Paulson GD, Caldwell J, Hutson DH, Menn JJ. *Xenobiotic Conjugation Chemistry*. Washington, DC: American Chemical Society; 1986.

Pearce RE, McIntyre CJ, Madan A, et al. Effects of freezing, thawing, and storing human liver microsomes on cytochrome P450 activity. *Arch Biochem Biophys*. 1996a;331:145–169.

Pearce RE, Rodrigues AD, Goldstein JA, Parkinson A. Identification of the human P450 enzymes involved in lansoprazole metabolism. *J Pharmacol Exp Ther*. 1996b;277:805–816.

Penning T. Molecular endocrinology of hydroxysteroid dehydrogenases. *Endocr Rev*. 1997;18:281–305.

Penning TM, Drury JE. Human aldo-keto reductases: function, gene regulation, and single nucleotide polymorphisms. *Arch Biochem Biophys*. 2007;464:241–250.

Phillips IR, Shephard EA. Flavin-containing monooxygenases: mutations, disease and drug response. *Trends Pharmacol Sci*. 2008;29:294–301.

Piacentini S, Polimanti R, Porreca F, Martinez-Labarga C, De Stefano GF, Fuciarelli M. GSTT1 and GSTM1 gene polymorphisms in European and African populations. *Mol Biol Rep*. 2011;38:1225–1230.

Picard N, Ratanasavanh D, Premaud A, Le Meur Y, Marquet P. Identification of the udp-glucuronosyl transferase isoforms involved in mycophenolic acid phase II metabolism. *Drug Metab Dispos.* 2005;33: 139–146.

Plaa GL. Chlorinated methanes and liver injury: highlights of the past 50 years. *Annu Rev Pharmacol Toxicol.* 2000;40:43–65.

Pohjanvirta R, Viluksela M, Tuomisto JT, et al. Physicochemical differences in the Ah receptors of the most TCDD-susceptible and the most TCDD-resistant rat strains. *Toxicol Appl Pharmacol.* 1999;155:82–95.

Pohl HR, Scinicariello F. The impact of CYP2E1 genetic variability on risk assessment of VOC mixtures. *Regul Toxicol Pharmacol.* 2011;59:364–374.

Pohl LR, Kenna JG, Satoh H, Christ D, Martin JL. Neoantigens associated with halothane hepatitis. *Drug Metab Rev.* 1989;20:203–217.

Poland A, Glover E. Comparison of 2,3,7,8-tetrachlorodibenzo-*p*-dioxin, a potent inducer of aryl hydrocarbon hydroxylase, with 3-methylcholanthrene. *Mol Pharmacol.* 1974;10:349–359.

Probst MR, Beer M, Beer D, Jeno P, Meyer UA, Gasser R. Human liver arylacetamide deacetylase. Molecular cloning of a novel esterase involved in the metabolic activation of arylamine carcinogens with high sequence similarity to hormone-sensitive lipase. *J Biol Chem.* 1994;269:21650–21656.

Prochaska HJ, Talalay P. Regulatory mechanisms of monofunctional and bifunctional anticarcinogenic enzyme inducers in murine liver. *Cancer Res.* 1988;48:4776–4782.

Proctor NJ, Tucker GT, Rostami-Hodjegan A. Predicting drug clearance from recombinantly expressed CYPs: intersystem extrapolation factors. *Xenobiotica.* 2004;34:151–178.

Prueksaritanont T, Li C, Tang C, Kuo Y, Strong-Basalyga K, Carr B. Rifampin induces the in vitro oxidative metabolism, but not the in vivo clearance of diclofenac in rhesus monkeys. *Drug Metab Dispos.* 2006;34:1806–1810.

Pryde DC, Dalvie D, Hu Q, Jones P, Obach RS, Tran TD. Aldehyde oxidase: an enzyme of emerging importance in drug discovery. *J Med Chem.* 2010;53:8441–8460.

Pyper SR, Viswakarma N, Yu S, Reddy JK. PPARalpha: energy combustion, hypolipidemia, inflammation and cancer. *Nucl Recept Signal.* 2010;8:e002.

Quinn LP, Perren MJ, Brackenborough KT, et al. A beam-walking apparatus to assess behavioural impairments in MPTP-treated mice: pharmacological validation with *R*-(−)-deprenyl. *J Neurosci Methods.* 2007;164: 43–49.

Racha JK, Rettie AE, Kunze KL. Mechanism-based inactivation of human cytochrome P450 1A2 by furafylline: detection of a 1:1 adduct to protein and evidence for the formation of a novel imidazomethide intermediate. *Biochemistry.* 1998;37:7407–7419.

Radominska-Pandya A, Czernik PJ, Little JM, Battaglia E, Mackenzie PI. Structural and functional studies of UDP-glucuronosyltransferases. *Drug Metab Rev.* 1999;31:817–899.

Rajagopalan KV. Xanthine oxidase and aldehyde oxidase. In: Jakoby WB, ed. *Enzymatic Basis of Detoxication.* New York, NY: Academic Press; 1980:295–306.

Ramchandani VA. Genetic aspects of alcohol metabolism. In: Watson RR, Preedy VR, eds. *Nutrition and Alcohol: Linking Nutrient Interactions and Dietary Intake.* Boca Raton, FL: CRC Press; 2004:187–199.

Ramkissoon A, Wells PG. Human prostaglandin H synthase (hPHS)-1 and hPHS-2 in amphetamine analog bioactivation, DNA oxidation, and cytotoxicity. *Toxicol Sci.* 2011;120:154–162.

Rao SI, Duffel MW. Inhibition of aryl sulfotransferase by carboxylic acids. *Drug Metab Dispos.* 1991;19:543–545.

Rasheva V, Domingos P. Cellular responses to endoplasmic reticulum stress and apoptosis. *Apoptosis.* 2009;14:996–1007.

Rasmussen BB, Brix TH, Kyvik KO, Brosen K. The interindividual differences in the 3-demthylation of caffeine alias CYP1A2 is determined by both genetic and environmental factors. *Pharmacogenetics.* 2002;12:473–478.

Ratnayake JH, Hanna PE, Anders MW, Duggan DE. Sulfoxide reduction. In vitro reduction of sulindac by rat hepatic cytosolic enzymes. *Drug Metab Dispos.* 1981;9:85–87.

Reed DJ. Cellular defense mechanisms against reactive metabolites. In: Anders MW, ed. *Bioactivation of Foreign Compounds.* Orlando: Academic Press; 1985:72–74.

Reed JR, Cawley GF, Backes WL. Inhibition of cytochrome P450 1A2-mediated metabolism and production of reactive oxygen species by heme oxygenase-1 in rat liver microsomes. *Drug Metab Lett.* 2011;5:6–16.

Reese MJ, Wurm RM, Muir KT, Generaux GT, St John-Williams L, McConn DJ. An in vitro mechanistic study to elucidate the desipramine/bupropion clinical drug–drug interaction. *Drug Metab Dispos.* 2008;36: 1198–1201.

Regan SL, Maggs JL, Hammond TG, Lambert C, Williams DP, Park BK. Acyl glucuronides: the good, the bad and the ugly. *Biopharm Drug Dispos.* 2010;31:367–395.

Reiss J, Hahnewald R. Molybdenum cofactor deficiency: mutations in GPHN, MOCS1, and MOCS2. *Hum Mutat.* 2010;32:10–18.

Reiss J, Johnson JL. Mutations in the molybdenum cofactor biosynthetic genes *MOCS1, MOCS2,* and *GEPH. Hum Mutat.* 2003;21:569–576.

Relling MV, Giacomini KM. Pharmacogenetics. In: Goodman LS, Gilman A, Brunton LL, Lazo JS, Parker KL, eds. *Goodman & Gilman's the Pharmacological Basis of Therapeutics.* New York, NY: McGraw-Hill; 2006:93–115.

Rencurel F, Foretz M, Kaufmann MR, et al. Stimulation of AMP-activated protein kinase is essential for the induction of drug metabolizing enzymes by phenobarbital in human and mouse liver. *Mol Pharmacol.* 2006;70:1925–1934.

Rettie AE, Fisher MB. Transformation enzymes: oxidative; non-P450. In: Woolf T, ed. *Handbook of Drug Metabolism.* New York, NY: Marcel Dekker Inc; 1999:131–151.

Rettie AE, Jones JP. Clinical and toxicological relevance of CYP2C9: drug–drug interactions and pharmacogenetics. *Annu Rev Pharmacol Toxicol.* 2005;45:477–494.

Richardson TA, Klaassen CD. Role of UDP-glucuronosyltransferase (UGT) 2B2 in metabolism of triiodothyronine: effect of microsomal enzyme inducers in Sprague Dawley and UGT2B2-deficient Fischer 344 rats. *Toxicol Sci.* 2010;116:413–421.

Riches Z, Stanley EL, Bloomer JC, Coughtrie MW. Quantitative evaluation of the expression and activity of five major sulfotransferases (SULTs) in human tissues: the SULT "pie". *Drug Metab Dispos.* 2009;37: 2255–2261.

Riedmaier S, Klein K, Hofmann U, et al. UDP-glucuronosyltransferase (UGT) polymorphisms affect atorvastatin lactonization in vitro and in vivo. *Clin Pharmacol Ther.* 2010;87:65–73.

Riedmaier S, Klein K, Winter S, Hofmann U, Schwab M, Zanger UM. Paraoxonase (PON1 and PON3) polymorphisms: impact on liver expression and atorvastatin-lactone hydrolysis. *Front Pharmacol.* 2011;2:41.

Rittle J, Green MT. Cytochrome P450 compound I: capture, characterization, and C–H bond activation kinetics. *Science.* 2010;330:933–937.

Robert J, Morvan VL, Smith D, Pourquier P, Bonnet J. Predicting drug response and toxicity based on gene polymorphisms. *Crit Rev Oncol Hematol.* 2005;54:171–196.

Roberts KM, Jones JP. Anilinic *N*-oxides support cytochrome P450-mediated *N*-dealkylation through hydrogen-atom transfer. *Chemistry.* 2010;16:8096–8107.

Rodrigues AD. Comparison of levels of aldehyde oxidase with cytochrome P450 activities in human liver in vitro. *Biochem Pharmacol.* 1994;48:197–200.

Rodrigues AD, Yang Z, Chen C, Pray D, Kim S, Sinz M. Is celecoxib an inducer of cytochrome P450 3A4 in subjects carrying the CYP2C9*3 allele? *Clin Pharmacol Ther.* 2006;80:298–301.

Rogers SM, Back DJ, Stevenson PJ, Grimmer SF, Orme ML. Paracetamol interaction with oral contraceptive steroids: increased plasma concentrations of ethinyloestradiol. *Br J Clin Pharmacol.* 1987;23:721–725.

Rosemond MJ, Walsh J. Human carbonyl reduction pathways and a strategy for their study in vitro. *Drug Metab Rev.* 2004;36:335–361.

Rosen LS, Laxa B, Boulos L, et al. Phase 1 study of TLK286 (Telcyta) administered weekly in advanced malignancies. *Clin Cancer Res.* 2004;10:3689–3698.

Ross D. Functions and distribution of NQO1 in human bone marrow: potential clues to benzene toxicity. *Chem Biol Interact.* 2005;153–154: 137–146.

Ross MK, Crow JA. Human carboxylesterases and their role in xenobiotic and endobiotic metabolism. *J Biochem Mol Toxicol.* 2007;21:187–196.

Rostami-Hodjegan A, Kroemer HK, Tucker GT. In-vivo indices of enzyme activity: the effect of renal impairment on the assessment of CYP2D6 activity. *Pharmacogenetics.* 1999;9:277–286.

Rostami-Hodjegan A, Lennard MS, Woods HF, Tucker GT. Meta-analysis of studies of the CYP2D6 polymorphism in relation to lung cancer and Parkinson's disease. *Pharmacogenetics.* 1998;8:227–238.

Roth A, Looser R, Kaufmann M, et al. Regulatory cross-talk between drug metabolism and lipid homeostasis: constitutive androstane receptor and pregnane X receptor increase Insig-1 expression. *Mol Pharmacol.* 2008;73:1282–1289.

Rowland A, Knights KM, Mackenzie PI, Miners JO. Characterization of the binding of drugs to human intestinal fatty acid binding protein (IFABP): potential role of IFABP as an alternative to albumin for in vitro–in vivo extrapolation of drug kinetic parameters. *Drug Metab Dispos.* 2009;37:1395–1403.

Rumack BH. Acetaminophen misconceptions. *Hepatology.* 2004;40:10–15.

Runge-Morris M, Kocarek TA. Regulation of sulfotransferases by xenobiotic receptors. *Curr Drug Metab.* 2005;6:299–307.

Rushmore TH, Morton MR, Pickett CB. The antioxidant responsive element. Activation by oxidative stress and identification of the DNA consensus sequence required for functional activity. *J Biol Chem.* 1991;266:11632–11639.

Rusyn I, Asakura S, Pachkowski B, et al. Expression of base excision DNA repair genes is a sensitive biomarker for in vivo detection of chemical-induced chronic oxidative stress: identification of the molecular source of radicals responsible for DNA damage by peroxisome proliferators. *Cancer Res.* 2004;64:1050–1057.

Ryan DE, Dixon R, Evans RH, et al. Rat hepatic cytochrome P-450 isozyme specificity for the metabolism of the steroid sulfate, 5α-androstane-3α, 17β-diol-3,17-disulfate. *Arch Biochem Biophys.* 1984;233: 636–642.

Saarikoski ST, Rivera SP, Hankinson O, Husgafvel-Pursiainen K. CYP2S1: a short review. *Toxicol Appl Pharmacol.* 2005;207:62–69.

Sakakibara Y, Suiko M, Pai TG, et al. Highly conserved mouse and human brain sulfotransferases: molecular cloning, expression, and functional characterization. *Gene.* 2002;285:39–47.

Sakamoto A, Matsumaru T, Ishiguro N, et al. Reliability and robustness of simultaneous absolute quantification of drug transporters, cytochrome P450 enzymes, and Udp-glucuronosyltransferases in human liver tissue by multiplexed MRM/selected reaction monitoring mode tandem mass spectrometry with nano-liquid chromatography. *J Pharm Sci.* 2011;100:4037–4043.

Salman ED, Kadlubar SA, Falany CN. Expression and localization of cytosolic sulfotransferase (SULT) 1A1 and SULT1A3 in normal human brain. *Drug Metab Dispos.* 2009;37:706–709.

Sampayo R, Lavandera JV, Batlle A, Buzaleh AM. Sevoflurane: its action on heme metabolism and phase I drug metabolizing system. *Cell Mol Biol (Noisy-le-grand).* 2009;55:140–146.

Sanderson LM, Degenhardt T, Koppen A, et al. Peroxisome proliferator-activated receptor beta/delta (PPARbeta/delta) but not PPARalpha serves as a plasma free fatty acid sensor in liver. *Mol Cell Biol.* 2009;29: 6257–6267.

Sandy J, Mushtaq A, Holton SJ, Schartau P, Noble ME, Sim E. Investigation of the catalytic triad of arylamine N-acetyltransferases: essential residues required for acetyl transfer to arylamines. *Biochem J.* 2005;390: 115–123.

Sano M, Ernesto C, Thomas RG, et al. A controlled trial of selegiline, alpha-tocopherol, or both as treatment for Alzheimer's disease. *N Engl J Med.* 1997;336:1216–1222.

Saruwatari J, Ishitsu T, Nakagawa K. Update on the genetic polymorphisms of drug-metabolizing enzymes in antiepileptic drug therapy. *Pharmaceuticals.* 2010;3:2709–2732.

Satoh T, Hosokawa M. The mammalian carboxylesterases: from molecules to functions. *Annu Rev Pharmacol Toxicol.* 1998;38:257–288.

Satoh T, Hosokawa M. Structure, function and regulation of carboxylesterases. *Chem Biol Interact.* 2006;162:195–211.

Sau A, Pellizzari Tregno F, Valentino F, Federici G, Caccuri AM. Glutathione transferases and development of new principles to overcome drug resistance. *Arch Biochem Biophys.* 2010;500:116–122.

Saulter JY, Kurian JR, Trepanier LA, et al. Unusual dehydroxylation of antimicrobial amidoxime prodrugs by cytochrome b5 and NADH cytochrome b5 reductase. *Drug Metab Dispos.* 2005;33:1886–1893.

Saunders MP, Patterson AV, Harris AL, Stratford IJ. NADPH:cytochrome c (P450) reductase activates tirapazamine (SR4233) to restore hypoxic and oxic cytotoxicity in an aerobic resistant derivative of the A549 lung cancer cell line. *Br J Cancer.* 2000;82:651–656.

Schmidt DR, Schmidt S, Holmstrom SR, et al. AKR1B7 is induced by the farnesoid X receptor and metabolizes bile acids. *J Biol Chem.* 2011;286:2425–2432.

Schmitt C, Kuhn B, Zhang X, Kivitz AJ, Grange S. Disease–drug–drug interaction involving tocilizumab and simvastatin in patients with rheumatoid arthritis. *Clin Pharmacol Ther.* 2011;89:735–740.

Schofield PC, Robertson IG, Paxton JW. Inter-species variation in the metabolism and inhibition of N-[(2′-dimethylamino)ethyl]acridine-4-carboxamide (DACA) by aldehyde oxidase. *Biochem Pharmacol.* 2000;59:161–165.

Schrag ML, Cui D, Rushmore TH, Shou M, Ma B, Rodrigues AD. Sulfotransferase 1E1 is a low km isoform mediating the 3-O-sulfation of ethinyl estradiol. *Drug Metab Dispos.* 2004;32:1299–1303.

Schrag ML, Wienkers LC. Covalent alteration of the CYP3A4 active site: evidence for multiple substrate binding domains. *Arch Biochem Biophys.* 2001;391:49–55.

Schroth W, Goetz MP, Hamann U, et al. Association between CYP2D6 polymorphisms and outcomes among women with early stage breast cancer treated with tamoxifen. *JAMA.* 2009;302:1429–1436.

Schuster I. Cytochromes P450 are essential players in the vitamin D signaling system. *Biochim Biophys Acta.* 2011;1814:186–199.

Scott SA, Sangkuhl K, Gardner EE, et al. Clinical Pharmacogenetics Implementation Consortium guidelines for cytochrome P450-2C19 (CYP2C19) genotype and clopidogrel therapy. *Clin Pharmacol Ther.* 2011;90:328–332.

Seitz J, Oneta C. Gastrointestinal alchohol dehydrogenase. *Nutr Rev.* 1998;56:52–60.

Senggunprai L, Yoshinari K, Yamazoe Y. Selective role of sulfotransferase 2A1 (SULT2A1) in the N-sulfoconjugation of quinolone drugs in humans. *Drug Metab Dispos.* 2009;37:1711–1717.

Senter PD, Marquardt H, Thomas BA, Hammock BD, Frank IS, Svensson HP. The role of rat serum carboxylesterase in the activation of paclitaxel and camptothecin prodrugs. *Cancer Res.* 1996;56:1471–1474.

Seo YS, Keum B, Park S, et al. Gilbert's syndrome phenotypically expressed as Crigler–Najjar syndrome type II. *Scand J Gastroenterol.* 2007;42:540–541.

Seto Y, Guengerich FP. Partitioning between N-dealkylation and N-oxygenation in the oxidation of N,N-dialkylarylamines catalyzed by cytochrome P450 2B1. *J Biol Chem.* 1993;268:9986–9997.

Shah YM, Morimura K, Yang Q, Tanabe T, Takagi M, Gonzalez FJ. Peroxisome proliferator-activated receptor alpha regulates a microRNA-mediated signaling cascade responsible for hepatocellular proliferation. *Mol Cell Biol.* 2007;27:4238–4247.

Sheng X, Zhang H, Hollenberg PF, Newcomb M. Kinetic isotope effects in hydroxylation reactions effected by cytochrome P450 compounds I implicate multiple electrophilic oxidants for P450-catalyzed oxidations. *Biochemistry.* 2009;48:1620–1627.

Shephard EA, Chandan P, Stevanovic-Walker M, Edwards M, Phillips IR. Alternative promoters and repetitive DNA elements define the species-dependent tissue-specific expression of the FMO1 genes of human and mouse. *Biochem J.* 2007;406:491–499.

Shi D, Yang J, Yang D, et al. Anti-influenza prodrug oseltamivir is activated by carboxylesterase human carboxylesterase 1, and the activation Is inhibited by antiplatelet agent clopidogrel. *J Pharmacol Exp Ther.* 2006;319:1477–1484.

Shield AJ, Murray TP, Cappello JY, Coggan M, Board PG. Polymorphisms in the human glutathione transferase kappa (GSTK1) promoter alter gene expression. *Genomics.* 2010;95:299–305.

Shih J, Chen K, Tidd M. Monamine oxidase: from genes to behavior. *Annu Rev Neurosci.* 1999;22:197–217.

Shih P-S, Huang J-D. Pharmacokinetics of midazolam and 1'-hydroxymidazolam in Chinese with different CYP3A5 genotypes. *Drug Metab Dispos.* 2002;30:1491–1496.

Shimada T. Xenobiotic-metabolizing enzymes involved in activation and detoxification of carcinogenic polycyclic aromatic hydrocarbons. *Drug Metab Pharmacokinet.* 2006;21:257–276.

Shimizu M, Denton T, Kozono M, Cashman JR, Leeder JS, Yamazaki H. Developmental variations in metabolic capacity of flavin-containing mono-oxygenase 3 in childhood. *Br J Clin Pharmacol.* 2011;71:585–591.

Shindo S, Numazawa S, Yoshida T. A physiological role of AMP-activated protein kinase in phenobarbital-mediated constitutive androstane receptor activation and CYP2B induction. *Biochem J.* 2007;401:735–741.

Shipkova M, Armstrong VW, Oellerich M, Wieland E. Acyl glucuronide drug metabolites: toxicological and analytical implications. *Ther Drug Monit.* 2003;25:1–16.

Shirley MA, Guan X, Kaiser DG, Halstead GW, Baillie TA. Taurine conjugation of ibuprofen in humans and in rat liver in vitro. Relationship to metabolic chiral inversion. *J Pharmacol Exp Ther.* 1994;269:1166–1175.

Sibbing D, Koch W, Gebhard D, et al. Cytochrome 2C19*17 allelic variant, platelet aggregation, bleeding events, and stent thrombosis in clopidogrel-treated patients with coronary stent placement. *Circulation.* 2010;121:512–518.

Siegel D, Yan C, Ross D. NAD(P)H:quinone oxidoreductase 1 (NQO1) in the sensitivity and resistance to antitumor quinones. *Biochem Pharmacol.* 2012;83(8):1033–1040. doi: 10.1016/j.bcp.2011.12.017.

Sifontis NM, Benedetti E, Vasquez EM. Clinically significant drug interaction between basiliximab and tacrolimus in renal transplant recipients. *Transplant Proc.* 2002;34:1730–1732.

Sim E, Walters K, Boukouvala S. Arylamine *N*-acetyltransferases: from structure to function. *Drug Metab Rev.* 2008;40:479–510.

Singh G, Driever PH, Sander JW. Cancer risk in people with epilepsy: the role of antiepileptic drugs. *Brain.* 2005;128:7–17.

Singh J, Petter RC, Baillie TA, Whitty A. The resurgence of covalent drugs. *Nat Rev Drug Discov.* 2011;10:307–317.

Sirot EJ, van der Velden JW, Rentsch K, Eap CB, Baumann P. Therapeutic drug monitoring and pharmacogenetic tests as tools in pharmacovigilance. *Drug Saf.* 2006;29:735–768.

Sit D, Perel JM, Luther JF, Wisniewski SR, Helsel JC, Wisner KL. Disposition of chiral and racemic fluoxetine and norfluoxetine across childbearing. *J Clin Psychopharmacol.* 2010;30:381–386.

Skarydova L, Wsol V. Human microsomal carbonyl reducing enzymes in the metabolism of xenobiotics: well-known and promising members of the SDR superfamily. *Drug Metab Rev.* 2012;44(2):173–191.

Sládek NE. Human aldehyde dehydrogenases: potential pathological, pharmacological, and toxicological impact. *J Biochem Mol Toxicol.* 2003;17:7–23.

Smirnov A, Comte C, Mager-Heckel AM, et al. Mitochondrial enzyme rhodanese is essential for 5 S ribosomal RNA import into human mitochondria. *J Biol Chem.* 2010;285:30792–30803.

Smith DA, Dalvie D. Why do metabolites circulate? *Xenobiotica.* 2012;42:107–126.

Smith PA, Sorich MJ, Low LSC, McKinnon RA, Miners JO. Towards integrated ADME prediction: past, present and future directions for modelling metabolism by UDP-glucuronosyltransferases. *J Mol Graph Model.* 2004;22:507–517.

Soldin OP, Chung SH, Mattison DR. Sex differences in drug disposition. *J Biomed Biotechnol.* 2011;2011:1–14.

Sontag TJ, Parker RS. Influence of major structural features of tocopherols and tocotrienols on their ω-oxidation by tocopherol-ω-hydroxylase. *J Lipid Res.* 2007;48:1090–1098.

Sorenson RC, Primo-Parmo SL, Kuo C, Adkins S, Lockridge O, Du BNL. Reconsideration of the catalytic center and mechanism of mammalian paraoxonase/arylesterase. *Proc Natl Acad Sci U S A.* 1995;92:7187–7191.

Sorich MJ, Miners JO, McKinnon RA, Smith PA. Multiple pharmacophores for the investigation of human UDP-glucuronosyltransferase isoform substrate selectivity. *Mol Pharmacol.* 2004;65:301–308.

Sorich MJ, Smith PA, Miners JO, Mackenzie PI, McKinnon RA. Recent advances in the in silico modelling of UDP glucuronosyltransferase substrates. *Curr Drug Metab.* 2008;9:60–69.

Soucek P, Skjelbred CF, Svendsen M, Kristensen T, Kure EH, Kristensen VN. Single-track sequencing for genotyping of multiple SNPs in the *N*-acetyltransferase 1 (NAT1) gene. *BMC Biotechnol.* 2004;4:28.

Souto JC, Blanco-Vaca F, Soria JM, et al. A genomewide exploration suggests a new candidate gene at chromosome 11q23 as the major determinant of plasma homocysteine levels: results from the GAIT project. *Am J Hum Genet.* 2005;76:925–933.

Spiecker M, Liao J. Cytochrome P450 epoxygenase CYP2J2 and the risk of coronary artery disease. *Trends Cardiovasc Med.* 2006;16:204–208.

Staatz CE, Goodman LK, Tett SE. Effect of CYP3A and ABCB1 single nucleotide polymorphisms on the pharmacokinetics and pharmacodynamics of calcineurin inhibitors: part I. *Clin Pharmacokinet.* 2010;49:141–175.

Stanley LA, Horsburgh BC, Ross J, Scheer N, Wolf CR. PXR and CAR: nuclear receptors which play a pivotal role in drug disposition and chemical toxicity. *Drug Metab Rev.* 2006;38:515–597.

Stark K, Wongsud B, Burman R, Oliw EH. Oxygenation of polyunsaturated long chain fatty acids by recombinant CYP4F8 and CYP4F12 and catalytic importance of Tyr-125 and Gly-328 of CYP4F8. *Arch Biochem Biophys.* 2005;441:174–181.

Stieger B, Fattinger K, Madon J, Kullak-Ublick GA, Meier PJ. Drug- and estrogen-induced cholestasis through inhibition of the hepatocellular bile salt export pump (Bsep) of rat liver. *Gastroenterology.* 2000;118:422–430.

Stierlin H, Faigle JW. Biotransformation of diclofenac sodium (Voltaren) in animals and in man. II. Quantitative determination of the unchanged drug and principal phenolic metabolites, in urine and bile. *Xenobiotica.* 1979;9:611–621.

Stierlin H, Faigle JW, Sallmann A, et al. Biotransformation of diclofenac sodium (Voltaren) in animals and in man. I. Isolation and identification of principal metabolites. *Xenobiotica.* 1979;9:601–610.

Stone AN, Mackenzie PI, Galetin A, Houston JB, Miners JO. Isoform selectivity and kinetics of morphine 3- and 6-glucuronidation by human UDP-glucuronosyltransferases: evidence for atypical glucuronidation kinetics by UGT2B7. *Drug Metab Dispos.* 2003;31:1086–1089.

Strange RC, Jones PW, Fryer AA. Glutathione *S*-transferase: genetics and role in toxicology. *Toxicol Lett.* 2000;112–113:357–363.

Strehlau J, Pape L, Offner G, Nashan B, Ehrich JH. Interleukin-2 receptor antibody-induced alterations of ciclosporin dose requirements in paediatric transplant recipients. *Lancet.* 2000;356:1327–1328.

Strelevitz TJ, Foti RS, Fisher MB. In vivo use of the P450 inactivator 1-aminobenzotriazole in the rat: varied dosing route to elucidate gut and liver contributions to first-pass and systemic clearance. *J Pharm Sci.* 2006;95:1334–1341.

Strickland KC, Krupenko NI, Dubard ME, Hu CJ, Tsybovsky Y, Krupenko SA. Enzymatic properties of ALDH1L2, a mitochondrial 10-formyltetrahydrofolate dehydrogenase. *Chem Biol Interact.* 2011;191:129–136.

Strolin-Benedetti M. FAD-dependent enzymes involved in the metabolic oxidation of xenobiotics. *Ann Pharm Fr.* 2011;69:45–52.

Strolin Benedetti M, Allievi C, Cocchiara G, Pevarello P, Dostert P. Involvement of FAD-dependent polyamine oxidase in the metabolism of milacemide in the rat. *Xenobiotica.* 1992;22:191–197.

Strolin Benedetti M, Tipton KF, Whomsley R. Amine oxidases and monooxygenases in the in vivo metabolism of xenobiotic amines in humans: has the involvement of amine oxidases been neglected? *Fundam Clin Pharmacol.* 2007;21:467–480.

Strom SC, Davila J, Grompe M. Chimeric mice with humanized liver: tools for the study of drug metabolism, excretion, and toxicity. *Methods Mol Biol.* 2010;640:491–509.

Subramanyam B, Woolf T, Castagnoli NJ. Studies on the in vitro conversion of haloperidol to a potentially neurotoxic pyridinium metabolite. *Chem Res Toxicol.* 1991;4:123–128.

Sugiura M, Iwasaki K, Kato R. Reduction of tertiary amine *N*-oxides by liver microsomal cytochrome P-450. *Mol Pharmacol.* 1976;12:322–334.

Sugiura M, Kato R. Reduction of tertiary amine *N*-oxides by rat liver mitochondria. *J Pharmacol Exp Ther.* 1977;200:25–32.

Sun H, Ehlhardt WJ, Kulanthaivel P, Lanza DL, Reilly CA, Yost GS. Dehydrogenation of indoline by cytochrome P450 enzymes: a novel "aromatase" process. *J Pharmacol Exp Ther.* 2007;322:843–851.

Sun H, Liu L, Pang KS. Increased estrogen sulfation of estradiol 17β-D-glucuronide in metastatic tumor rat livers. *J Pharmacol Exp Ther.* 2006;319:818–831.

Sun H, Moore C, Dansette PM, Kumar S, Halpert JR, Yost GS. Dehydrogenation of the indoline-containing drug 4-chloro-*N*-(2-methyl-1-indolinyl)-3-sulfamoylbenzamide (Indapamide) by CYP3A4: correlation with in silico predictions. *Drug Metab Dispos.* 2009;37:672–684.

Sun H, Yost GS. Metabolic activation of a novel 3-substituted indole-containing TNF-alpha inhibitor: dehydrogenation and inactivation of CYP3A4. *Chem Res Toxicol.* 2008;21:374–385.

Tabas I, Ron D. Integrating the mechanisms of apoptosis induced by endoplasmic reticulum stress. *Nat Cell Biol.* 2011;13:184–190.

Tafazoli S, O'Brien PJ. Peroxidases: a role in the metabolism and side effects of drugs. *Drug Discov Today.* 2005;10:617–625.

Tafazoli S, O'Brien PJ. Accelerated cytotoxic mechanism screening of hydralazine using an in vitro hepatocyte inflammatory cell peroxidase model. *Chem Res Toxicol.* 2008;21:904–910.

Takahashi RH, Grigliatti TA, Reid RE, Riggs KW. The effect of allelic variation in aldo-keto reductase 1C2 on the in vitro metabolism of dihydrotestosterone. *J Pharmacol Exp Ther.* 2009;329:1032–1039.

Takeda S, Ishii Y, Iwanaga M, et al. Modulation of UDP-glucuronosyltransferase function by cytochrome P450: evidence for the alteration of UGT2B7-catalyzed glucuronidation of morphine by CYP3A4. *Mol Pharmacol.* 2005;67:665–672.

Tan BS, Tiong KH, Muruhadas A, et al. CYP2S1 and CYP2W1 mediate 2-(3,4-dimethoxyphenyl)-5-fluorobenzothiazole (GW-610, NSC 721648) sensitivity in breast and colorectal cancer cells. *Mol Cancer Ther.* 2011;10:1982–1992.

Tang BK, Carro-Ciampi G. A method for the study of *N*-glucosidation in vitro—amobarbital-*N*-glucoside formation in incubations with human liver. *Biochem Pharmacol.* 1980;29:2085–2088.

Tang C, Lin JH, Lu AY. Metabolism-based drug–drug interactions: what determines individual variability in cytochrome P450 induction? *Drug Metab Dispos.* 2005;33:603–613.

Tang C, Ma B. Glycosidation of an endothelin ETA receptor antagonist and diclofenac in human liver microsomes: aglycone-dependent UDP-sugar selectivity. *Drug Metab Dispos.* 2005;33:1796–1802.

Tang M, Mukundan M, Yang J, et al. Antiplatelet agents aspirin and clopidogrel are hydrolyzed by distinct carboxylesterases, and clopidogrel is transesterificated in the presence of ethyl alcohol. *J Pharmacol Exp Ther.* 2006;319:1467–1476.

Tang W, Lu AY. Metabolic bioactivation and drug-related adverse effects: current status and future directions from a pharmaceutical research perspective. *Drug Metab Rev.* 2010;42:225–249.

Temellini A, Franchi M, Giuliani L, Pacifici GM. Human liver sulphotransferase and UDP-glucuronosyltransferase: structure–activity relationship for phenolic substrates. *Xenobiotica.* 1991;21:171–177.

Terao M, Kurosaki M, Demontis S, Zanotta S, Garattini E. Isolation and characterization of the human aldehyde oxidase gene: conservation of intron/exon boundaries with the xanthine oxidoreductase gene indicates a common origin. *Biochem J.* 1998;332:383–393.

Testa B, Krämer SD. *The Biochemistry of Drug Metabolism: Principles, Redox Reactions, Hydrolyses.* Zurich: Wiley-VCH; 2008.

Testa B, Krämer SD. *The Biochemistry of Drug Metabolism: Conjugations, Consequences of Metabolism, Influencing Factors.* Zurich: Wiley-VCH; 2010.

Tew KD, Townsend DM. Regulatory functions of glutathione *S*-transferase P1-1 unrelated to detoxification. *Drug Metab Rev.* 2011;43:179–193.

Thomas JA. "Black box" warning labels and drug withdrawals. *Toxicol Appl Pharmacol.* 2002;183:81–82.

Thompson MA, Moon E, Kim UJ, Xu J, Siciliano MJ, Weinshilboum RM. Human indolethylamine *N*-methyltransferase: cDNA cloning and expression, gene cloning, and chromosomal localization. *Genomics.* 1999;61:285–297.

Thomson RE, Bigley AL, Foster JR, et al. Tissue-specific expression and subcellular distribution of murine glutathione *S*-transferase class kappa. *J Histochem Cytochem.* 2004;52:653–662.

Tijet N, Boutros PC, Moffat ID, Okey AB, Tuomisto J, Pohjanvirta R. Aryl hydrocarbon receptor regulates distinct dioxin-dependent and dioxin-independent gene batteries. *Mol Pharmacol.* 2006;69:140–153.

Tinguely JN, Wermuth B. Identification of the reactive cysteine residue (Cys227) in human carbonyl reductase. *Eur J Biochem.* 1999;260:9–14.

Tirona RG, Kim RB. Nuclear receptors and drug disposition gene regulation. *J Pharm Sci.* 2005;94:1169–1186.

Tiwawech D, Srivatanakul P, Karalak A, Ishida T. Cytochrome P450 2A6 polymorphism in nasopharyngeal carcinoma. *Cancer Lett.* 2006;241:135–141.

Toide K, Terauchi Y, Fujii T, Yamazaki H, Kamataki T. Uridine diphosphate sugar-selective conjugation of an aldose reductase inhibitor (AS-3201) by UDP-glucuronosyltransferase 2B subfamily in human liver microsomes. *Biochem Pharmacol.* 2004;67:1269–1278.

Tolson AH, Wang H. Regulation of drug-metabolizing enzymes by xenobiotic receptors: PXR and CAR. *Adv Drug Deliv Rev.* 2010;62:1238–1249.

Tontonoz P, Hu E, Spiegelman BM. Stimulation of adipogenesis in fibroblasts by PPAR gamma 2, a lipid-activated transcription factor. *Cell.* 1994;79:1147–1156.

Tornio A, Niemi M, Neuvonen M, et al. The effect of gemfibrozil on repaglinide pharmacokinetics persists for at least 12 h after the dose: evidence for mechanism-based inhibition of CYP2C8 in vivo. *Clin Pharmacol Ther.* 2008;84:403–411.

Townsend DM, Tew KD. The role of glutathione-*S*-transferase in anti-cancer drug resistance. *Oncogene.* 2003;22:7369–7375.

Tremaine LM, Stroh JG, Ronfeld RA. Characterization of a carbamic acid ester glucuronide of the secondary amine sertraline. *Drug Metab Dispos.* 1989;17:58–63.

Trepanier LA, Ray K, Winand NJ, Spielberg SP, Cribb AE. Cytosolic arylamine *N*-acetyltransferase (NAT) deficiency in the dog and other canids due to an absence of NAT genes. *Biochem Pharmacol.* 1997;54:73–80.

Tsuchiya Y, Nakajima M, Takagi S, Taniya T, Yokoi T. MicroRNA regulates the expression of human cytochrome P450 1B1. *Cancer Res.* 2006;66:9090–9098.

Tucker GT. Clinical implications of genetic polymorphism in drug metabolism. *J Pharm Pharmacol.* 1994;46:417–424.

Tucker GT, Houston JB, Huang SM. Optimizing drug development: strategies to assess drug metabolism/transporter interaction potential—toward a consensus. *Pharm Res.* 2001;18:1071–1080.

Tukey RH, Strassburg C. Human UDP-glucuronosyltransferases: metabolism, expression, and disease. *Annu Rev Pharmacol Toxicol.* 2000;40:581–616.

Turner ST, Schwartz GL, Chapman AB, Hall WD, Boerwinkle E. Antihypertensive pharmacogenetics: getting the right drug into the right patient. *J Hypertens.* 2001;19:1–11.

Uchaipichat V, Mackenzie PI, Elliot DJ, Miners JO. Selectivity of substrate (trifluoperazine) and inhibitor (amitriptyline, androsterone, canrenoic acid, hecogenin, phenylbutazone, quinidine, quinine, and sulfinpyrazone) "probes" for human UDP-glucuronosyl transferases. *Drug Metab Dispos.* 2006;34:449–456.

Uetrecht J. Prediction of a new drug's potential to cause idiosyncratic reactions. *Curr Opin Drug Discov Dev.* 2001;4:55–59.

Ujiie S, Sasaki T, Mizugaki M, Ishikawa M, Hiratsuka M. Functional characterization of 23 allelic variants of thiopurine *S*-methyltransferase gene (TPMT*2-*24). *Pharmacogenet Genomics.* 2008;18:887–893.

Unwalla RJ, Cross JB, Salaniwal S, et al. Using a homology model of cytochrome P450 2D6 to predict substrate site of metabolism. *J Comput Aided Mol Des.* 2010;24:237–256.

Van Booven D, Marsh S, McLeod H, et al. Cytochrome P450 2C9-CYP2C9. *Pharmacogenet Genomics.* 2010;20:277–281.

van Kuilenburg A, Meinsma R, van Gennip A. Pyrimidine degradation defects and severe 5-fluorouracil toxicity. *Nucleosides Nucleotides Nucleic Acids.* 2004;23:1371–1375.

Van LM, Heydari A, Yang J, et al. The impact of experimental design on assessing mechanism-based inactivation of CYP2D6 by MDMA (Ecstasy). *J Psychopharmacol.* 2006;20:834–841.

van Raaij JA, Kaptein E, Visser TJ, van den Berg KJ. Increased glucuronidation of thyroid hormone in hexachlorobenzene-treated rats. *Biochem Pharmacol.* 1993;45:627–631.

Varaprath S, Salyers KL, Plotzke KP, Nanavati S. Identification of metabolites of octamethylcyclotetrasiloxane (D(4)) in rat urine. *Drug Metab Dispos.* 1999;27:1267–1273.

Vasiliou V, Pappa A, Estey T. Role of human aldehyde dehydrogenases in endobiotic and xenobiotic metabolism. *Drug Metab Rev.* 2004;36:279–299.

Vatsis KP, Weber WW, Bell DA, et al. Nomenclature for *N*-acetyltransferases. *Pharmacogenetics.* 1995;5:1–17.

Veeramah KR, Thomas MG, Weale ME, et al. The potentially deleterious functional variant flavin-containing monooxygenase 2*1 is at high frequency throughout sub-Saharan Africa. *Pharmacogenet Genomics.* 2008;18:877–886.

Venkatakrishnan K, Obach RS. In vitro–in vivo extrapolation of CYP2D6 inactivation by paroxetine: prediction of nonstationary pharmacokinetics and drug interaction magnitude. *Drug Metab Dispos.* 2005;33:845–852.

Visser TJ, Kaptein E, van Toor H, et al. Glucuronidation of thyroid hormone in rat liver: effects of in vivo treatment with microsomal enzyme inducers and in vitro assay conditions. *Endocrinology.* 1993;133:2177–2186.

Wahl B, Reichmann D, Niks D, et al. Biochemical and spectroscopic characterization of the human mitochondrial amidoxime reducing components hmARC-1 and hmARC-2 suggests the existence of a new molybdenum enzyme family in eukaryotes. *J Biol Chem.* 2010;285:37847–37859.

Walgren JL, Mitchell MD, Thompson DC. Role of metabolism in drug-induced idiosyncratic hepatotoxicity. *Crit Rev Toxicol.* 2005;35:325–361.

Wallace BD, Wang H, Lane KT, Scott JE, et al. Alleviating cancer drug toxicity by inhibiting a bacterial enzyme. *Science.* 2010;330:831–835.

Walsh JS, Miwa GT. Bioactivation of drugs: risk and drug design. *Annu Rev Pharmacol Toxicol.* 2011;51:145–167.

Walsky RL, Astuccio AV, Obach RS. Evaluation of 227 drugs for in vitro inhibition of cytochrome P450 2B6. *J Clin Pharmacol.* 2006;46:1426–1438.

Walsky RL, Obach RS. A comparison of 2-phenyl-2-(1-piperidinyl)propane (ppp), 1,1′,1″-phosphinothioylidynetrisaziridine (thioTEPA), clopidogrel, and ticlopidine as selective inactivators of human cytochrome P450 2B6. *Drug Metab Dispos.* 2007;35:2053–2059.

Walton MI, Wolf CR, Workman P. The role of cytochrome P450 and cytochrome P450 reductase in the reductive bioactivation of the novel benzotriazine di-*N*-oxide hypoxic cytotoxin 3-amino-1,2,4-benzotriazine-1,4-dioxide (SR 4233, WIN 59075) by mouse liver. *Biochem Pharmacol.* 1992;44:251–259.

Wang C, Bammler TK, Guo Y, Kelly EJ, Eaton DL. Mu-class GSTs are responsible for aflatoxin B1-8,9-epoxide-conjugating activity in the nonhuman primate *Macaca fascicularis* liver. *Toxicol Sci.* 2000;56:26–36.

Wang D, Guo Y, Wrighton SA, Cooke GE, Sadee W. Intronic polymorphism in CYP3A4 affects hepatic expression and response to statin drugs. *Pharmacogenomics J.* 2011a;11:274–286.

Wang D, Para MF, Koletar SL, Sadee W. Human *N*-acetyltransferase 1 *10 and *11 alleles increase protein expression through distinct mechanisms and associate with sulfamethoxazole-induced hypersensitivity. *Pharmacogenet Genomics.* 2011b;21:652–664.

Wang H, Tompkins LM. CYP2B6: new insights into a historically overlooked cytochrome P450 isozyme. *Curr Drug Metab.* 2008;9:598–610.

Wang J, Davis M, Li F, Azam F, Scatina J, Talaat RE. A novel approach for predicting acyl glucuronide reactivity via Schiff base formation: development of rapidly formed peptide adducts for LC/MS/MS measurements. *Chem Res Toxicol.* 2004;17:1206–1216.

Wang L, Christopher LJ, Cui D, et al. Identification of the human enzymes involved in the oxidative metabolism of dasatinib: an effective approach for determining metabolite formation kinetics. *Drug Metab Dispos.* 2008;36:1828–1839.

Wang L, Nguyen TV, McLaughlin RW, Sikkink LA, Ramirez-Alvarado M, Weinshilboum RM. Human thiopurine *S*-methyltransferase pharmacogenetics: variant allozyme misfolding and aggresome formation. *Proc Natl Acad Sci U S A.* 2005;102:9394–9399.

Wang L, Pelleymounter L, Weinshilboum R, et al. Very important pharmacogene summary: thiopurine *S*-methyltransferase. *Pharmacogenet Genomics.* 2010a;20:401–405.

Wang LQ, James MO. Inhibition of sulfotransferases by xenobiotics. *Curr Drug Metab.* 2006;7:83–104.

Wang MZ, Saulter JY, Usuki E, et al. CYP4F enzymes are the major enzymes in human liver microsomes that catalyze the *O*-demethylation of the antiparasitic prodrug DB289 [2,5-bis(4-amidinophenyl)furan-bis-*O*-methylamidoxime]. *Drug Metab Dispos.* 2006;34:1985–1994.

Wang TJ, Zhang F, Richards JB, et al. Common genetic determinants of vitamin D insufficiency: a genome-wide association study. *Lancet.* 2010b;376:180–188.

Wang YX, Ulu A, Zhang LN, Hammock B. Soluble epoxide hydrolase in atherosclerosis. *Curr Atheroscler Rep.* 2010c;12:174–183.

Wardman P, Dennis MF, Everett SA, Patel KB, Stratford MR, Tracy M. Radicals from one-electron reduction of nitro compounds, aromatic *N*-oxides and quinones: the kinetic basis for hypoxia-selective, bioreductive drugs. *Biochem Soc Symp.* 1995;61:171–194.

Watanabe A, Fukami T, Takahashi S, et al. Arylacetamide deacetylase is a determinant enzyme for the difference in hydrolase activities of phenacetin and acetaminophen. *Drug Metab Dispos.* 2010;38:1532–1537.

Watkins PB. Noninvasive tests of CYP3A enzymes. *Pharmacogenetics.* 1994;4:171.

Waxman DJ, Holloway MG. Sex differences in the expression of hepatic drug metabolizing enzymes. *Mol Pharmacol.* 2009;76:215–228.

Wei S, Liu Z, Zhao H, et al. A single nucleotide polymorphism in the alcohol dehydrogenase 7 gene (alanine to glycine substitution at amino acid 92) is associated with the risk of squamous cell carcinoma of the head and neck. *Cancer.* 2010;116:2984–2992.

Weil A, Martin P, Smith R, et al. Pharmacokinetics of vandetanib in subjects with renal or hepatic impairment. *Clin Pharmacokinet.* 2010;49:607–618.

Weinshilboum R. Methyltransferase pharmacogenetics. *Pharmacol Ther.* 1989;43:77–90.

Weinshilboum R. Sulfotransferase pharmacogenetics. In: Kalow W, ed. *Pharmacogenetics of Drug Metabolism.* New York, NY: Pergamon; 1992a:227–242.

Weinshilboum R, Otterness D, Szumlanski C. Methylation pharmacogenetics: catechol *O*-methyltransferase, thiopurine methyltransferase, and histamine *N*-methyltransferase. *Annu Rev Pharmacol Toxicol.* 1999;39:19–52.

Weinshilboum RM. Methylation pharmacogenetics: thiopurine methyltransferase as a model system. *Xenobiotica.* 1992b;22:1055–1071.

Weinshilboum RM. Pharmacogenomics: catechol *O*-methyltransferase to thiopurine *S*-methyltransferase. *Cell Mol Neurobiol.* 2006;4–6:539–561.

Weinshilboum RM, Otterness DM, Aksoy IA, Wood TC, Her C, Raftogianis RB. Sulfation and sulfotransferases 1: sulfotransferase molecular biology: cDNAs and genes. *FASEB J.* 1997;11:3–14.

Wen B, Coe KJ, Rademacher P, Fitch WL, Monshouwer M, Nelson SD. Comparison of in vitro bioactivation of flutamide and its cyano analogue: evidence for reductive activation by human NADPH:cytochrome P450 reductase. *Chem Res Toxicol.* 2008;21:2393–2406.

Wenning LA, Hanley WD, Brainard DM, et al. Effect of rifampin, a potent inducer of drug-metabolizing enzymes, on the pharmacokinetics of raltegravir. *Antimicrob Agents Chemother.* 2009;53:2852–2856.

Westlind A, Malmebo S, Johansson I, et al. Cloning and tissue distribution of a novel human cytochrome P450 of the CYP3A subfamily, CYP3A43. *Biochem Biophys Res Commun.* 2001;281:1349–1355.

Westlind-Johnsson A, Hermann R, Huennemeyer A, et al. Identification and characterization of CYP3A4*20, a novel rare CYP3A4 allele without functional activity. *Clin Pharmacol Ther.* 2006;79:339–349.

Westlind-Johnsson A, Malmebo S, Johansson A, et al. Comparative analysis of CYP3A expression in human liver suggests only a minor role for CYP3A5 in drug metabolism. *Drug Metab Dispos.* 2003;31:755–761.

Whalen R, Boyer TD. Human glutathione *S*-transferases. *Semin Liver Dis.* 1998;18:345–358.

Whitcomb D, Block G. Association of acetaminophen hepatoxicity with fasting and ethanol use. *JAMA.* 1994;272:1845–1850.

Whitfield JB, Pang D, Bucholz KK, et al. Monoamine oxidase: associations with alcohol dependence, smoking and other measures of psychopathology. *Psychol Med.* 2000;30:443–454.

Wielinga PR, Reid G, Challa EE, et al. Thiopurine metabolism and identification of the thiopurine metabolites transported by MRP4 and MRP5 overexpressed in human embryonic kidney cells. *Mol Pharmacol.* 2002;62:1321–1331.

Wilkinson GR, Guengerich FP, Branch RA. Genetic polymorphism of *S*-mephenytoin hydroxylation. *Pharmacol Ther.* 1989;43:53–76.

Williams AC, Cartwright LS, Ramsden DB. Parkinson's disease: the first common neurological disease due to auto-intoxication? *Q J Med.* 2005;98:215–226.

Williams GM, Iatropoulos MJ. Alteration of liver cell function and proliferation: differentiation between adaptation and toxicity. *Toxicol Pathol.* 2002;30:41–53.

Williams JA, Cook J, Hurst SI. A significant drug-metabolizing role for CYP3A5? *Drug Metab Dispos.* 2003a;31:1526–1530.

Williams JA, Hurst SI, Bauman J, et al. Reaction phenotyping in drug discovery: moving forward with confidence? *Curr Drug Metab.* 2003b;4:527–534.

Williams JA, Hyland R, Jones BC, et al. Drug–drug interactions for UDP-glucuronosyltransferase substrates: a pharmacokinetic explanation for typically observed low exposure (AUCI/AUC) ratios. *Drug Metab Dispos.* 2004;32:1201–1208.

Williams JA, Ring BJ, Cantrell VE, et al. Comparative metabolic capabilities of CYP3A4, CYP3A5, and CYP3A7. *Drug Metab Dispos.* 2002;30:883–891.

Williams RT. *Detoxication Mechanisms; The Metabolism and Detoxication of Drugs, Toxic Substances, and Other Organic Compounds.* New York, NY: Wiley; 1959.

Williams-Gray C, Goris A, Foltynie T, Compston A, Sawcer S, Barker RA. No evidence for association between an MAOA functional polymorphism and susceptibility to Parkinson's disease. *J Neurol.* 2009;256: 132–133.

Winter HR, Unadkat JD. Identification of cytochrome P450 and arylamine *N*-acetyltransferase isoforms involved in sulfadiazine metabolism. *Drug Metab Dispos.* 2005;33:969–976.

Wood AW, Swinney DC, Thomas PE, et al. Mechanism of androstenedione formation from testosterone and epitestosterone catalyzed by purified cytochrome P-450b. *J Biol Chem.* 1988;263:17322–17332.

Wood TC, Johnson KL, Naylor S, Weinshilboum RM. Cefazolin administration and 2-methyl-1,3,4-thiadiazole-5-thiol in human tissue: possible relationship to hypoprothrombinemia. *Drug Metab Dispos.* 2002;30:1123–1128.

Wood TC, Salavagionne OE, Mukherjee B, et al. Human arsenic methyltransferase (AS3MT) pharmacogenetics: gene resequencing and functional genomics studies. *J Biol Chem.* 2006;281:7364–7373.

Wu D, Li Y, Song G, Zhang D, Shaw N, Liu ZJ. Crystal structure of human esterase D: a potential genetic marker of retinoblastoma. *FASEB J.* 2009;23:1441–1446.

Wu WKK, Yiu Sung JJ, Lee CW, Yu J, Cho CH. Cyclooxygenase-2 in tumorigenesis of gastrointestinal cancers: an update on the molecular mechanisms. *Cancer Lett.* 2010;295:7–16.

Wu Z-L, Sohl CD, Shimada T, Guengerich FP. Recombinant enzymes overexpressed in bacteria show broad catalytic specificity of human cytochrome P450 2W1 and limited activity of human cytochrome P450 2S1. *Mol Pharmacol.* 2006;69:2007–2014.

Xiao Y, Guengerich FP. Metabolomic analysis and identification of a role for the orphan human cytochrome P450 2W1 in selective oxidation of lysophospholipids. *J Lipid Res.* 2012;53:1610–1617.

Xie W, Stribley JA, Chatonnet A, et al. Postnatal developmental delay and supersensitivity to organophosphate in gene-targeted mice lacking acetylcholinesterase. *J Pharmacol Exp Ther.* 2000;293:896–902.

Xu X, Zhang XA, Wang DW. The roles of CYP450 epoxygenases and metabolites, epoxyeicosatrienoic acids, in cardiovascular and malignant diseases. *Adv Drug Deliv Rev.* 2011;63:597–609.

Xu Y, Hashizume T, Shuhart MC, et al. Intestinal and hepatic CYP3A4 catalyze hydroxylation of 1alpha,25-dihydroxyvitamin D(3): implications for drug-induced osteomalacia. *Mol Pharmacol.* 2006;69:56–65.

Yamada R, Ymamoto K. Recent findings on genes associated with inflammatory disease. *Mutat Res.* 2005;573:136–151.

Yamano S, Tatsuno J, Gonzalez FJ. The CYP2A3 gene product catalyzes coumarin 7-hydroxylation in human liver microsomes. *Biochemistry.* 1990;29:1322–1329.

Yamazaki H, Johnson WW, Ueng YF, Shimada T, Guengerich FP. Lack of electron transfer from cytochrome b5 in stimulation of catalytic activities of cytochrome P450 3A4. Characterization of a reconstituted cytochrome P450 3A4/NADPH-cytochrome P450 reductase system and studies with apo-cytochrome b5. *J Biol Chem.* 1996;271:27438–27444.

Yamazaki H, Shimada T, Martin MV, Guengerich FP. Stimulation of cytochrome P450 reactions by apo-cytochrome b5: evidence against transfer of heme from cytochrome P450 3A4 to apo-cytochrome b5 or heme oxygenase. *J Biol Chem.* 2001;276:30885–30891.

Yan B, Yang D, Brady M, Parkinson A. Rat kidney carboxylesterase. Cloning, sequencing, cellular localization, and relationship to rat liver hydrolase. *J Biol Chem.* 1994;269:29688–29696.

Yang Q, Nagano T, Shah Y, Cheung C, Ito S, Gonzalez FJ. The PPAR alpha-humanized mouse: a model to investigate species differences in liver toxicity mediated by PPAR alpha. *Toxicol Sci.* 2008;101:132–139.

Yang X, Gandhi YA, Duignan DB, Morris ME. Prediction of biliary excretion in rats and humans using molecular weight and quantitative structure–pharmacokinetic relationships. *AAPS J.* 2009;11:511–525.

Yao K-S, Hageboutros A, Ford P, O'Dwyer PJ. Involvement of activator protein-1 and nuclear factor-kappa B transcription factors in the control of the DT-diaphorase expression induced by mitomycin C treatment. *Mol Pharmacol.* 1997;51:422–430.

Yeung CK, Fujioka Y, Hachad H, Levy RH, Isoherranen N. Are circulating metabolites important in drug–drug interactions? Quantitative analysis of risk prediction and inhibitory potency. *Clin Pharmacol Ther.* 2011;89:105–113.

Yin H, Bennett G, Jones JP. Mechanistic studies of uridine diphosphate glucuronosyltransferase. *Chem Biol Interact.* 1994;90:47–58.

Yoneyama M, Nishiyama N, Shuto M, et al. In vivo depletion of endogenous glutathione facilitates trimethyltin-induced neuronal damage in the dentate gyrus of mice by enhancing oxidative stress. *Neurochem Int.* 2008;52:761–769.

Yoshida A, Rzhetsky A, Hsu L, Chang C. Human aldehyde dehydrogenase gene family. *Eur J Biochem.* 1998;251:549–557.

Yraola F, Zorzano A, Albericio F, Royo M. Structure–activity relationships of SSAO/VAP-1 arylalkylamine-based substrates. *Chem Med Chem.* 2009;4:495–503.

Yumibe N, Huie K, Chen KJ, Snow M, Clement RP, Cayen MN. Identification of human liver cytochrome P450 enzymes that metabolize the nonsedating antihistamine loratadine. Formation of descarboethoxyloratadine by CYP3A4 and CYP2D6. *Biochem Pharmacol.* 1996;51:165–172.

Zhan P, Wang Q, Qian Q, Wei SZ, Yu LK. CYP1A1 MspI and exon7 gene polymorphisms and lung cancer risk: an updated meta-analysis and review. *J Exp Clin Cancer Res.* 2011;30:99.

Zhang D, Chando TJ, Everett DW, Patten CJ, Dehal SS, Humphreys WG. In vitro inhibition of UDP glucuronosyltransferases by atazanavir and other HIV protease inhibitors and the relationship of this property to in vivo bilirubin glucuronidation. *Drug Metab Dispos.* 2005;33: 1729–1739.

Zhang J, Cashman JR. Quantitative analysis of FMO gene mRNA levels in human tissues. *Drug Metab Dispos.* 2006;34:19–26.

Zhang L, Zhang YD, Zhao P, Huang SM. Predicting drug–drug interactions: an FDA perspective. *AAPS J.* 2009;11:300–306.

Zhang Y, Talalay P, Cho C, Posner GH. A major inducer of anticarcinogenic protective enzymes from broccoli: isolation and elucidation of structure. *Proc Natl Acad Sci U S A.* 1992;89:2399–2403.

Zheng Y-M, Fisher MB, Yokotani N, Fujii-Kuriyama Y, Rettie AE. Identification of a meander region proline residue critical for heme binding to cytochrome P450: Implications for the catalytic function of human CYP4B1. *Biochemistry.* 1998;37:12847–12851.

Zhi X, Chan EM, Edenberg HJ. Tissue-specific regulatory elements in the human alcohol dehydrogenase 6 gene. *DNA Cell Biol.* 2000;19:487–497.

Zhou C, Assem M, Tay JC, et al. Steroid and xenobiotic receptor and vitamin D receptor crosstalk mediates CYP24 expression and drug-induced osteomalacia. *J Clin Invest.* 2006a;116:1703–1712.

Zhou C, Tabb MM, Nelson EL, et al. Mutual repression between steroid and xenobiotic receptor and NF-kappaB signaling pathways links xenobiotic metabolism and inflammation. *J Clin Invest.* 2006b;116: 2280–2289.

Zhou D, Guo J, Linnenbach AJ, Booth-Genthe CL, Grimm SW. Role of human UGT2B10 in *N*-glucuronidation of tricyclic antidepressants, amitriptyline, imipramine, clomipramine, and trimipramine. *Drug Metab Dispos*. 2010a;38:863–870.

Zhou H, Mascelli MA. Mechanisms of monoclonal antibody–drug interactions. *Annu Rev Pharmacol Toxicol*. 2011;51:359–372.

Zhou J, Zhai Y, Mu Y, et al. A novel pregnane X receptor-mediated and sterol regulatory element-binding protein-independent lipogenic pathway. *J Biol Chem*. 2006c;281:15013–15020.

Zhou SF. Polymorphism of human cytochrome P450 2D6 and its clinical significance: part I. *Clin Pharmacokinet*. 2009a;48:689–723.

Zhou SF. Polymorphism of human cytochrome P450 2D6 and its clinical significance: part II. *Clin Pharmacokinet*. 2009b;48:761–804.

Zhou SF, Liu JP, Chowbay B. Polymorphism of human cytochrome P450 enzymes and its clinical impact. *Drug Metab Rev*. 2009a;41:89–295.

Zhou SF, Wang B, Yang LP, Liu JP. Structure, function, regulation and polymorphism and the clinical significance of human cytochrome P450 1A2. *Drug Metab Rev*. 2010b;42:268–354.

Zhou SF, Zhou ZW, Yang LP, Cai JP. Substrates, inducers, inhibitors and structure–activity relationships of human cytochrome P450 2C9 and implications in drug development. *Curr Med Chem*. 2009b;16:3480–3675.

Zhou X, D'Agostino J, Li L, Moore CD, Yost GS, Ding X. Respective roles of CYP2A5 and CYP2F2 in the bioactivation of 3-methylindole in mouse olfactory mucosa and lung: studies using Cyp2a5-null and Cyp2f2-null mouse models. *Drug Metab Dispos*. 2012;40(4):642–647.

Zhu BT, Liehr JG. Inhibition of the catechol-*O*-methyltransferase-catalyzed *O*-methylation of 2- and 4-hydroxyestradiol by catecholamines: implications for the mechanism of estrogen-induced carcinogenesis. *Arch Biochem Biophys*. 1993;304:248–256.

Zhu HJ, Markowitz JS. Activation of the antiviral prodrug oseltamivir is impaired by two newly identified carboxylesterase 1 variants. *Drug Metab Dispos*. 2009;37:264–267.

Ziegler DM. Recent studies on the structure and function of multisubstrate flavin-containing monooxygenases. *Annu Rev Pharmacol Toxicol*. 1993;33:179–199.

Ziegler DM. An overview of the mechanism, substrate specificities, and structure of FMOs. *Drug Metab Rev*. 2002;34:503–511.

Zineh I, Beitelshees AL, Gaedigk A, et al. Pharmacokinetics and CYP2D6 genotypes do not predict metoprolol adverse events or efficacy in hypertension. *Clin Pharmacol Ther*. 2004;76:536–544.

Zollinger M, Gschwind H-P, Jin Y, Sayer C, Zécri F, Hartmann S. Absorption and disposition of the sphingosine 1-phosphate receptor modulator fingolimod (FTY720) in healthy volunteers: a case of xenobiotic biotransformation following endogenous metabolic pathways. *Drug Metab Dispos*. 2011;39:199–207.

Zollinger M, Sayer C, Dannecker R, Schuler W, Sedrani R. The macrolide everolimus forms an unusual metabolite in animals and humans: identification of a phosphocholine ester. *Drug Metab Dispos*. 2008;36:1457–1460.

Zordoky BN, El-Kadi AO. Effect of cytochrome P450 polymorphism on arachidonic acid metabolism and their impact on cardiovascular diseases. *Pharmacol Ther*. 2010;125:446–463.

chapter 7

Toxicokinetics

Danny D. Shen

INTRODUCTION

Toxicokinetics is the quantitative study of the movement of an exogenous chemical from its entry into the body, through its distribution to organs and tissues via the blood circulation, and to its final disposition by way of biotransformation and excretion. The basic kinetic concepts for the absorption, distribution, metabolism, and excretion of chemicals in the body system initially came from the study of drug actions or pharmacology; hence, this area of study is traditionally referred to as pharmacokinetics. Toxicokinetics represents extension of kinetic principles to the study of toxicology and encompasses applications ranging from the study of adverse drug effects to investigations on how disposition kinetics of exogenous chemicals derived from either natural or environmental sources (generally refer to as xenobiotics) govern their deleterious effects on organisms including humans.

The study of toxicokinetics relies on mathematical description or modeling of the time course of toxicant disposition in the whole organism. The classic approach to describing the kinetics of drugs is to represent the body as a system of one or more compartments, even though the compartments do not have exact correspondence to anatomical structures or physiological processes. These empirical compartmental models are almost always developed to describe the kinetics of toxicants in readily accessible body fluids (mainly blood) or excreta (eg, urine, stool, and breath). This approach is particularly suited for human studies, which typically do not afford organ or tissue data. In such applications, extravascular distribution, which does not require detail elucidation, can be represented simply by lumped compartments. An alternate and newer approach,

physiologically based toxicokinetic modeling attempts to portray the body as an elaborate system of discrete tissue or organ compartments that are interconnected via the circulatory system. Physiologically based models are capable of describing a chemical's movements in body tissues or regions of toxicological interest. It also allows a priori predictions of how changes in specific physiological processes affect the disposition kinetics of the toxicant (eg, changes in respiratory status on pulmonary absorption and exhalation of a volatile compound) and the extrapolation of the kinetic model across animal species to humans.

It should be emphasized that there is no inherent contradiction between the classic and physiological approaches. The choice of modeling approach depends on the application context, the available data, and the intended utility of the resultant model. Classic compartmental model, as will be shown, requires assumptions that limit its application. In comparison, physiological models can predict tissue concentrations; however, it requires much more data input and often the values of the required parameters cannot be estimated accurately or precisely, which introduces uncertainty in its prediction.

We begin with a description of the classic approach to toxicokinetic modeling, which offers an introduction to the basic kinetic concepts for toxicant absorption, distribution, and elimination. This will be followed by a brief review of the physiological approach to toxicokinetic modeling that is intended to illustrate the construction and application of these elaborate models. Finally, we will address the application of toxicokinetic principles to biological monitoring for exposure assessments in industrial and environmental contexts.

CLASSIC TOXICOKINETICS

Ideally, quantification of xenobiotic concentration at the site of toxic insult or injury would afford the most direct information on exposure–response relationship and dynamics of response over time. Serial sampling of relevant biological tissues following dosing can be cost-prohibitive during in vivo studies in animals and is nearly impossible to perform in human exposure studies. The most accessible and simplest means of gathering information on absorption, distribution, metabolism, and elimination of a compound is to examine the time course of blood or plasma toxicant concentration over time. If one assumes that the concentration of a chemical in blood or plasma is in some describable dynamic equilibrium with its concentrations in tissues, then changes in plasma toxicant concentration should reflect changes in tissue toxicant concentrations and relatively simple kinetic models can adequately describe the behavior of that toxicant in the body system.

Classic toxicokinetic models typically consist of a central compartment representing blood and tissues that the toxicant has ready access and equilibration is achieved almost immediately following its introduction, along with one or more peripheral compartments that represent tissues in slow equilibrium with the toxicant in blood (Fig. 7-1). Once introduced into the central compartment, the toxicant distributes between central and peripheral compartments. Elimination of the toxicant, through biotransformation and/or excretion, is usually assumed to occur from the central compartment, which should comprise the rapidly perfused visceral organs capable of eliminating the toxicant (eg, kidneys, lungs, and liver). The obvious advantage of compartmental toxicokinetic models is that they do not require information on tissue physiology or anatomic structure. These models are useful in predicting the toxicant concentrations in blood at different doses or exposure levels, in establishing the time course of accumulation of the toxicant, either in its parent form or as biotransformed products during continuous or episodic exposures, in defining concentration–response (vs dose–response) relationships, and in

guiding the choice of effective dose and design of dosing regimen in animal toxicity studies (Rowland and Tozer, 2011).

One-Compartment Model

The most straightforward toxicokinetic assessment entails quantification of the blood or more commonly plasma concentrations of a toxicant at several time points after a bolus intravenous (iv) injection.

Often, the data obtained fall on a straight line when they are plotted as the logarithm of plasma concentration versus time; the kinetics of the toxicant is said to conform to a one-compartment model (Fig. 7-2). Mathematically, this means that the decline in plasma concentration over time profile follows a simple exponential pattern as represented by the following mathematical expressions:

$$C = C_0 \cdot e^{-k_{el} \cdot t} \tag{7-1}$$

or its logarithmic transform

$$\mathrm{Log}\, C = \mathrm{Log}\, C_0 - \frac{k_{el} \cdot t}{2.303} \tag{7-2}$$

where C is the plasma toxicant concentration at time t after injection, C_0 is the plasma concentration achieved immediately after injection, and k_{el} is the exponential constant or elimination rate constant with dimensions of reciprocal time (eg, $minute^{-1}$ or $hour^{-1}$). The constant 2.303 in Equation (7-2) is needed to convert natural logarithm into base-10 logarithm. It can be seen from Equation (7-2) that the elimination rate constant can be determined from the slope of the log C versus time plot (ie, $k_{el} = -2.303 \cdot$ slope).

The elimination rate constant k_{el} represents the overall elimination of the toxicant, which includes biotransformation, exhalation, and/or excretion pathways. When elimination of a toxicant from the body occurs in an exponential fashion, it signifies a first-order process, that is, the rate of elimination at any time is proportional to the amount of toxicant remaining in the body (ie, body load) at that time. This means that following an iv bolus injection, the absolute rate of elimination (eg, milligrams of toxicant eliminated per minute) continually changes over time. Shortly after introduction of the dose, the rate of toxicant elimination will be at the highest. As elimination proceeds and body load of the toxicant is reduced, the elimination rate will decline in step. As a corollary, it also means that at multiple levels of the toxicant dose, the absolute rate of elimination at corresponding times will be proportionately more rapid at the higher doses. This mode of elimination offers an obvious advantage for the organism to deal with increasing exposure to a toxicant. First-order kinetics occur at toxicant concentrations that are not sufficiently high to saturate either metabolic or transport processes.

In view of the nature of first-order kinetics, k_{el} is said to represent a constant fractional rate of elimination. Thus, if the fractional elimination rate is constant, for example, 0.3 $hour^{-1}$, the percentage of dose or plasma concentration remaining in the body ($C/C_0 \cdot 100$) and the percentage of the dose or concentration eliminated from the body after 1 hour, that is, $1 - (C/C_0 \cdot 100)$, are 74% and 26%, respectively, regardless of the dose administered (Table 7-1). The reason why the amount remaining at 1 hour is slightly more than 70%, or the amount eliminated is less than 30%, is because the amount in the body declined continually over the 1-hour period and thus the actual amount eliminated is less than anticipated based on the starting amount in the body. Again, this illustrates the fact that under first-order kinetics, the actual elimination rate declines with the depletion in body load, but the percentage eliminated over a given period of time is the same regardless of dose, that is, the

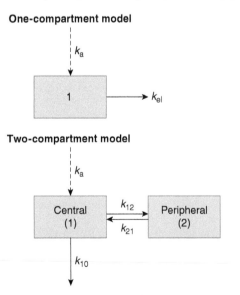

Figure 7-1. *Compartmental toxicokinetic models.* Symbols for 1-compartment model: k_a is the first-order absorption rate constant, and k_{el} is the first-order elimination rate constant. Symbols for 2-compartment model: k_a is the first-order absorption rate constant into the central compartment (1), k_{10} is the first-order elimination rate constant from the central compartment (1), k_{12} and k_{21} are the first-order rate constants for distribution between central (1) and peripheral (2) compartment.

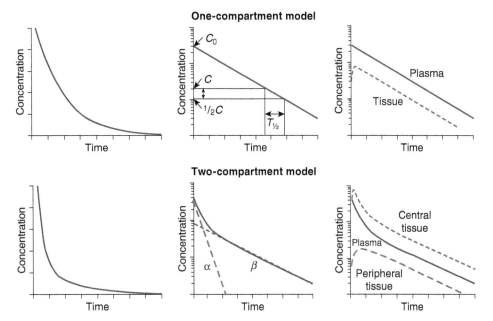

Figure 7-2. *Plasma concentration versus time curves of toxicants exhibiting kinetic behavior conforming to a 1-compartment model (top row) and a 2-compartment model (bottom row) following iv bolus injection. Left and middle panels show the plots on a rectilinear and semilogarithmic scale, respectively. Right panels illustrate the relationship between tissue (dash lines) and plasma (solid line) concentrations over time.* The right panel for the 1-compartment model shows the concentration–time profile for a typical tissue with a higher concentration than plasma. Note that tissue concentration can be higher, nearly the same, or lower than plasma concentration. Tissue concentration peaks almost immediately, and thereafter declines in parallel with plasma concentration. The right panel for the 2-compartment model shows concentration–time profiles for typical tissues associated with the central (1) and peripheral (2) compartments as represented by short and long dash lines, respectively. For tissues associated with the central compartment, their concentrations decline in parallel with plasma. For tissues associated with peripheral compartment, toxicant concentration rises, while plasma concentration declines rapidly during the initial phase; it then reaches a peak and eventually declines in parallel with plasma in the terminal phase. Elimination rate constant k_{el} for 1-compartment model and the terminal exponential rate constant β are determined from the slope of the log–linear concentration versus time curve. Half-life ($T_{1/2}$) is the time required for plasma toxicant concentration to decrease by one-half. C_0 is the concentration of a toxicant for a 1-compartment model at $t = 0$ determined by extrapolating the log–linear concentration–time curve to the Y-axis.

fractional rate of elimination of the toxicant remains constant over time after iv injection or any acute exposure. Because a constant percentage of toxicant present in the body is eliminated over a given time period regardless of dose or the starting concentration, it is more intuitive and convenient to refer to an elimination half-life ($T_{1/2}$), that is, the time it takes for the original blood or plasma concentration to fall by 50% or to eliminate 50% of the original body load. By substituting $C/C_0 = 0.5$ into Equation (7-1), we obtain the following relationship between $T_{1/2}$ and k_{el}:

$$T_{1/2} = \frac{0.693}{k_{el}} \qquad (7\text{–}3)$$

Table 7-1

Elimination of a Toxicant That Follows First-Order Kinetics ($k_{el} = 0.3$ h^{-1}) by 1 Hour After iv Administration at Four Different Dose Levels

DOSE (mg)	TOXICANT REMAINING (mg)	TOXICANT ELIMINATED (mg)	TOXICANT ELIMINATED (% of dose)
10	7.4	2.6	26
30	22	8	26
90	67	23	26
250	185	65	26

where 0.693 is the natural logarithm of 2. Simple calculations reveals that it would take about 4 half-lives for >90% (exactly 93.8%) of the dose to be eliminated, and about 7 half-lives for >99% (exactly 99.2%) elimination. Thus, given the elimination $T_{1/2}$ of a toxicant, the length of time it takes for near-complete washout of a toxicant after discontinuation of its exposure can easily be estimated. As will be seen in next section, the concept of $T_{1/2}$ is also applicable to toxicants that exhibit multiexponential kinetics.

We can infer from the monoexponential decline of blood or plasma concentration that the toxicant equilibrates very rapidly between blood and the various tissues relative to the rate of elimination, such that extravascular equilibration is achieved nearly instantaneously and maintained thereafter. Depiction of the body system by a one-compartment model does not mean that the concentration of the toxicant is the same throughout the body, but it does assume that the changes that occur in the plasma concentration reflect proportional changes in tissue toxicant concentrations (Fig. 7-2 upper, right panel). In other words, toxicant concentrations in tissues are expected to decline with the same elimination rate constant or $T_{1/2}$ as in plasma; tissue and plasma concentrations should decline in parallel.

Two-Compartment Model

After rapid iv administration of some toxicants, the semilogarithmic plot of plasma concentration versus time does not yield a straight line but a curve that implies more than one dispositional phase (Fig. 7-2). In these instances, it takes some time for the toxicant to be taken up into certain tissue groupings, and to then

Table 7-2

Prediction of Equilibration Half-Times for Tissues in the Groupings of Highly Perfused Visceral Tissues, Poorly Perfused Lean Tissues, and Adipose Tissues for a Lipid-Soluble, Organic Toxicant With Assumed Typical Tissue-to-Blood Partitioning Ratios (P)*

GROUPING	TISSUE	PERFUSION (L/min)[†]	VOLUME (L)[†]	EQUILIBRATION $T_{1/2}$ (Min)[‡]
Highly perfused viceral tissues, $P = 1$	Heart	0.20	0.28	0.97
	Lungs	5.0	1.1	0.15
	Liver, Gut	1.4	1.6	0.79
	Kidneys	1.1	0.35	0.22
	Brain	0.70	1.4	1.4
Poorly perfused tissues, $P = 0.5$	Muscle (resting)	0.75	30	14
	Skin (cool weather)	0.30	7.7	9.0
Adipose tissue, $P = 5$	—	0.20	14	243

[*]*Adapted from Rowland and Tozer (2011).*
[†]*Data taken from the compilation of Rowland and Tozer (2011), Table 4-4 on p. 88.*
[‡]*Equilibration half-time is the predicted time it takes to achieve 50% of the eventual equilibrated concentration in a tissue when arterial toxicant concentration is held constant and assuming that distribution is perfusion rate-limited. It is calculated by $(0.693 \cdot V \cdot P)/Q$, where Q is the blood perfusion rate of the tissue, V is the tissue volume, and P is the tissue-to-blood partition ratio.*
Note that the equilibration half-times for the highly perfused visceral tissues are predicted to be very short, <2 minutes. The equilibration half-times for poorly perfused lean tissues are estimated to be around 10 to 20 minutes. The equilibration half-time predicted for fat is the order of at least several hours. This tissue grouping in equilibration kinetics gives rise to multiphasic toxicokinetics that are describable by 2- or 3-compartment models.

reach an equilibration with the concentration in plasma; hence, a multicompartmental model is needed for the description of its kinetics in the body (Fig. 7-1). The concept of tissue groupings with distinct uptake and equilibration rates of toxicant becomes apparent when we consider the factors that govern the uptake of a lipid-soluble, organic toxicant. Table 7-2 presents data on the volume and blood perfusion rate of various organs and tissues in a standard size human. From these data and assuming reasonable partitioning ratios of a typical lipid-soluble, organic compound in the various tissue types, we can estimate the uptake equilibration half times of the toxicant in each organ or tissue region during constant, continuous exposure. The results suggest that the tissues can be grouped into rapid-equilibrating visceral organs, moderately slow-equilibrating lean body tissues (mainly skeletal muscle), and very slow-equilibrating body fat; these groupings give rise to three distinct uptake phases, that is, half times of <2 minutes for the rapid-equilibrating tissues, several tens of minutes for the moderately slow-equilibrating lean body tissues, and hours for the very slow-equilibrating body fat. By inference, three distinct phases of washout should also be evident following a brief exposure to the toxicant, such as after a bolus iv injection. The relative prominence of these distributional phases will vary depending on the average lipid solubility of the toxicant in each tissue grouping and any other sequestration and export mechanisms of a toxicant in particular tissues (eg, tight binding to tissue proteins, active influx into or efflux out of the tissue cell types), as well as the competing influence of elimination from the visceral organs. For example, very rapid metabolism or excretion at the visceral organs would limit distribution into the slow or very slow tissue groupings. Also, there are times when equilibration rates of a toxicant into visceral organs overlaps with lean body tissues, such that the distribution kinetics of a toxicant into these two tissue groupings become indistinct with respect to the exponential decline of plasma concentration, in which case two instead of three tissue groupings may be observed. The concept of tissue groupings with respect to uptake or washout kinetics serves

to justify the seemingly simplistic, yet pragmatic, mathematical description of extravascular distribution by the classic two- or three-compartment models.

Plasma concentration–time profile of a toxicant that exhibits multicompartmental kinetics can be characterized by multiexponential equations. For example, a two-compartment model can be represented by the following biexponential equation:

$$C = A \cdot e^{-\alpha \cdot t} + B \cdot e^{-\beta \cdot t} \qquad (7\text{–}4)$$

where A and B are coefficients in units of toxicant concentration, and α and β are the respective exponential constants for the initial and terminal phases in units of reciprocal time. The initial (α) phase is often referred to as the distribution phase, and terminal (β) phase as the postdistribution or elimination phase. The lower, middle panel of Fig. 7-2 shows a graphical resolution of the two exponential phases from the plasma concentration–time curve. It should be noted that the α constant is the slope of the residual log-linear plot and not the initial slope of the decline in the observed plasma toxicant concentration, that is, the initial rate of decline in plasma concentration approximates, but is not exactly equal, the α rate constant in Equation (7-4).

It should be noted that distribution into and out of the tissues and elimination of the toxicant are ongoing at all times, that is, elimination does occur during the "distribution" phase, and distribution between compartments is still ongoing during the "elimination" phase. As illustrated in Fig. 7-3, the dynamics of a multicompartmental system is such that the governing factor, that is, be it intercompartmental distribution or elimination, for each of the phases depends on the relative magnitude of the rate constants for intercompartmental exchange and the elimination process. In the usual case, that of rapid distribution and relatively slow elimination (left panel of Fig. 7-3), the initial rapid phase indeed reflects extravascular distribution, and the later, slow phase reflects elimination after a dynamic equilibrium between tissue and blood is attained. There are cases where distribution into some tissue group is much slower than elimination. Then, the initial phase could largely reflect

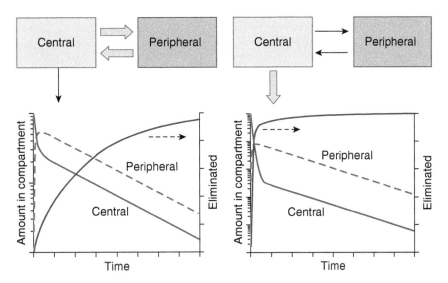

Figure 7-3. *Effects of interplay between kinetics of distribution and elimination processes on time course of exchange between body compart-ments and removal from the body for toxicants whose disposition conforms to a 2-compartment model.* Left panel depicts the more common scenario of rapid distribution between compartments relative to elimination, in which case elimination from the body occurs largely during the terminal phase when a dynamic equilibration between the central and peripheral compartment has been reached. Accordingly, half-life of the terminal phase is an appropriate measure of elimination. Right panel depicts the scenario of very slow distribution relative to elimination, in which case a substantial (>90% of dose) loss of toxicant occurs during the initial phase. The terminal phase reflects the slow redistribution of the toxicant sequestered in the peripheral site to the central site where it can be eliminated (ie, washout is rate-limited by redistribution). Under this scenario, the initial phase reflects elimination kinetics, whereas the terminal phase reflects tissue distribution kinetics. (Adapted from Tozer and Rowland, 2006.)

elimination, and the later phase is controlled by the slow redistribution of the toxicant from the tissues associated with the peripheral compartment to the central compartment, where it is eliminated (ie, washout in the terminal phase is rate-limited by redistribution from the peripheral compartment). The aminoglycoside antibiotic genta-micin is a case in point (Schentag and Jusko, 1977). Following an iv injection of gentamicin in patients with normal renal function, serum gentamicin concentration exhibits biphasic kinetics. Serum concentration of gentamicin initially falls very quickly with a half-life of around 2 hours reflecting rapid excretion by the kidneys; a slow terminal phase does not emerge until serum concentration has fallen to less than 10% of initial concentration. The terminal half-life of serum gentamicin is in the range of 4 to 7 days. This protracted terminal half-life reflects the slow turnover of gentami-cin sequestered in the kidneys. In fact, repeated administration of gentamicin leads to accumulation of gentamicin in the kidneys, which is a risk factor for its nephrotoxicity. Because of the inter-play of distribution and elimination kinetics, it has been recom-mended that multiphasic disposition should be simply described as consisting of early and late or rapid and slow phases; mechanistic labels of distribution and elimination should be applied with some caution. Lastly, the initial phase may last for only a few minutes or for hours. Whether multiphasic kinetics becomes apparent depends to some extent on how often and when the early blood samples are obtained, and on the relative difference in the exponential rate constants between the early and later phases. If the early phase of decline in toxicant concentration is considerably more rapid than the later phase or phases, the timing of blood sampling becomes critical in the ability to resolving two or more phases of washout.

Sometimes three or even 4 exponential terms are needed to fit a curve to the plot of log C versus time. Such compounds are viewed as displaying characteristics of three- or four-compartment open models. The principles underlying such models are the same as those applied to the two-compartment open model, but the math-ematics is more complex and beyond the scope of this chapter.

Apparent Volume of Distribution

For a one-compartment model, a toxicant is assumed to equilibrate between plasma and tissues immediately following its entry into the systemic circulation. Thus, a consistent relationship should exist between plasma concentration and the amount of toxicant in each tissue and, by extension, to the entire amount in the body or body burden. The apparent volume of distribution (V_d) is defined as the proportionality constant that relates the total amount of the tox-icant in the body to its concentration in plasma, and typically has units of liters or liters per kilogram of body weight (Rowland and Tozer, 2011). V_d is the apparent fluid space into which an amount of toxicant is distributed in the body to result in a given plasma concentration. As an illustration, envision the body as a tank con-taining an unknown volume (L) of well-mixed water. If a known amount (mg) of dye is placed into the water, the volume of that water can be calculated indirectly by determining the dye concen-tration (mg/L) that resulted after the dye has fully dispersed, that is, by dividing the amount of dye added to the tank by the resultant concentration of the dye in water. Analogously, the apparent vol-ume of distribution of a toxicant in the body is determined after iv bolus administration, and is mathematically defined as the quotient of the amount of toxicant in the body and its plasma concentration. V_d is calculated as

$$V_d = \frac{Dose_{iv}}{\beta \cdot AUC_0^\infty} \tag{7-5}$$

where $Dose_{iv}$ is the iv dose or known amount of toxicant in the body at time zero, β is the elimination rate constant, and AUC_0^∞ is the area under the toxicant concentration versus time curve from time zero to infinity. AUC_0^∞ is estimated by numerical methods, the most common one being the trapezoidal rule (Gibaldi and Perrier, 1982). The product, $\beta \cdot AUC_0^\infty$, in unit of concentration, is the theo-retical concentration of toxicant in plasma if dynamic equilibration were achievable immediately after introduction of the toxicant into the systemic circulation. For a 1-compartment model, immediate equilibration of the toxicant between plasma and tissues after an acute exposure does hold true, in which case V_d can be calculated by a simpler and more intuitive equation

$$V_d = \frac{Dose_{iv}}{C_0} \qquad (7\text{–}6)$$

where C_0 is the concentration of toxicant in plasma at time zero. C_0 is determined by extrapolating the plasma disappearance curve after iv injection to the zero time point (Fig. 7-2, upper, middle panel).

For the more complex multicompartmental models, V_d is calculated according to Equation (7-5) that involves the computation of area under the toxicant concentration–time curve. Moreover, the concept of an overall apparent volume of distribution is strictly applicable to the terminal exponential phase when equilibration of the toxicant between plasma and all tissue sites are attained. This has led some investigators to refer to the apparent volumes of distribution calculated by Equation (7-5) as V_β (for a two-compartment model) or V_z (for a general multicompartmental model); the subscript designation refers to the terminal exponential phase (Gibaldi and Perrier, 1982). It should also be noted that when Equation (7-6) is applied to the situation of a multicompartmental model, the resultant volume is the apparent volume of the central compartment, often times referred to as V_c. By definition, V_c is the proportionality constant that relates the total amount of the toxicant in the central compartment to its concentration in plasma. It has limited utility, for example, it can be used to calculate an iv dose of the toxicant to target an initial plasma concentration.

V_d is appropriately called the *apparent* volume of distribution because it does not correspond to any real anatomical volumes. The magnitude of the V_d term is toxicant-specific and represents the extent of distribution of toxicant out of plasma and into extravascular sites (Table 7-3). Equation (7-7) provides a more intuitive interpretation of an apparent volume of distribution:

$$V_d = V_p + \sum P_{t,i} \cdot V_{t,i} \qquad (7\text{–}7)$$

where V_p is the plasma volume and the Σ represents the summation of the apparent volume of each tissue region (t,i) as represented by the product of $P_{t,i}$ (ie, partition ratio or tissue-to-plasma concentration ratio at dynamic equilibrium) and $V_{t,i}$ (ie, anatomical volume of tissue). At one extreme, a toxicant that predominantly remains in the vasculature will have a low V_d that approximates the volume of blood or plasma, that is, the minimum V_d for any toxicant is the plasma volume. For toxicants that distribute extensively into extravascular tissues, V_d exceeds physiological fluid spaces, such as plasma or blood volume, interstitial fluid, or extracellular fluid. A toxicant that is highly sequestered in tissues (ie, high $P_{t,i}$) can have a volume of distribution larger than average body size (>1 L/kg). The mechanisms of tissue sequestration include partitioning of a toxicant into tissue fat, high-affinity binding to tissue proteins, trapping in specialized organelles (eg, pH trapping of amine compounds in acidic lysozomes), and concentrative uptake by active transporters. In fact, the equation below is an alternate form of Equation (7-7), which features the interplay of binding to plasma and tissue proteins in determining the partitioning of a toxicant in that only free or unbound drug can freely diffuse across membrane and cellular barriers.

$$V_d = V_p + \sum \left(\frac{f_{up}}{f_{ut,i}} \right) \cdot V_{t,i} \qquad (7\text{–}8)$$

Table 7-3

Volume of Distribution (V_d) and Unbound or Free Fraction in Plasma (f_{up}) for Several Drugs That Are of Clinical Toxicological Interest

CHEMICAL	V_d (L/kg)	f_{up}
Chloroquine	~200	~0.45
Nortriptyline	18	0.080
Oxycodone	2.0	0.55
	Body size = 1.0	
Acetaminophen	0.95	<0.20
	Total body water = 0.60	
Phenytoin	0.64	0.11
	Extracellular fluid = 0.27	
Warfarin	0.14	0.005
Epoetin alfa	0.05	–
	Plasma volume = 0.045	

Volumes of body fluid compartments in healthy human adults are included for comparison.
Data from Thummel et al. (2006).

where f_{up} is the unbound fraction of toxicant in plasma and $f_{ut,i}$ is the effective unbound fraction in a tissue region. Here, $P_{t,i}$ is governed by the ratio $f_{up} / f_{ut,i}$. Thus, a toxicant that has high affinity for plasma proteins (eg, albumin and/or α_1-acid glycoprotein) relative to tissue proteins has a restricted distribution volume; for example, the anticoagulant warfarin with a plasma-bound fraction of 0.995 or an f_{up} of 0.005 (Table 7-3). On the contrary, a toxicant that has a high affinity for tissue proteins and lesser affinity for plasma proteins can have a very high V_d. For example, the tricyclic antidepressant nortriptyline has a good affinity for plasma proteins with a bound fraction of 0.92 or an f_{up} of 0.08; however, binding of nortriptyline to tissues constituents is so much higher such that it has a V_d of 18 times the body weight in adult humans.

In addition to its value as a parameter to indicate the extent of extravascular distribution of a toxicant, V_d also has practical utility. Once the V_d for a toxicant is known, it can be used to estimate the amount of toxicant remaining in the body at any time when the plasma concentration at that time is known, that is,

$$X_B = V_d \cdot C \qquad (7\text{–}9)$$

where X_B is the amount of toxicant in the body or body burden, and C is the plasma concentration at a time after equilibration between tissue and plasma had been achieved.

Clearance

Toxicants are cleared from the body via various routes, for example, excretion by the kidneys into urine or via bile into the intestine ending in feces, biotransformation by the liver, or exhalation by the lungs. Clearance is an important toxicokinetic parameter that relates the rate of toxicant elimination from the whole body in relation to plasma concentration (Wilkinson, 1987). Although terminal $T_{1/2}$ is reflective of the rate of removal of a toxicant from plasma or blood, as was explained earlier, it is also subject to the influence of distributional processes, especially for toxicants exhibiting multicompartmental kinetics.

Clearance, on the contrary, is a parameter that solely represents the rate of toxicant elimination; it is not influenced by extravascular distribution.

A formal definition of total body clearance is the ratio of overall elimination rate of a toxicant divided by plasma concentration at any time after an acute exposure or during repetitive or continuous exposure (ie, elimination rate/C); in effect, clearance expresses the overall efficiency of the elimination mechanisms. Because this measure of elimination efficiency is in reference to blood or plasma toxicant concentration, it is also named blood or plasma clearance. High values of clearance indicate efficient and generally rapid removal, whereas low clearance values indicate slow and less efficient removal of a toxicant from the body. By definition, clearance has the units of flow (eg, mL/min or L/h). In the classic compartmental context, clearance is portrayed as the apparent volume containing the toxicant that is cleared per unit of time. After iv bolus administration, total body clearance (Cl) is calculated by

$$Cl = \frac{Dose_{iv}}{AUC_0^\infty} \qquad (7\text{–}10)$$

Clearance can also be calculated if the volume of distribution and elimination rate constants are known within the context of a compartmental model; that is, $Cl = V_d \cdot k_{el}$ for a 1-compartment model and $Cl = V_\beta \cdot \beta$ for a 2-compartment model. It should be noted that the preceding relationship is a mathematical derivation and does not imply that clearance is dependent on the distribution volume (see later section for further commenting). A clearance of 100 mL/min can be visualized as having 100 mL of blood or plasma completely cleared of toxicant in each minute during circulation.

The biological significance of total body clearance is better appreciated when it is recognized that it is the sum of clearances by individual eliminating organs (ie, organ clearances):

$$Cl = Cl_r + Cl_h + Cl_p + \ldots \qquad (7\text{–}11)$$

where Cl_r depicts renal, Cl_h hepatic, and Cl_p pulmonary clearance. Each organ clearance is in turn determined by blood perfusion flow through the organ (i) and the fraction of toxicant in the arterial inflow that is irreversibly removed, that is, the extraction fraction (E_i). Various organ clearance models have been developed to provide quantitative description of clearance that is related to blood perfusion flow (Q_i), free fraction in blood (f_{ub}), and intrinsic clearance ($Cl_{int,i}$) (Wilkinson, 1987). For example, for hepatic clearance (Cl_h), if the delivery of the toxicant to its intracellular site of removal is rate-limited by liver blood flow (Q_h) and the toxicant is assumed to have equal, ready access to all the hepatocytes within the liver (ie, the so-called well-stirred model):

$$Cl_h = Q_h \cdot E_h = \frac{Q_h \cdot f_{ub} \cdot Cl_{int,h}}{f_{ub} \cdot Cl_{int,h} + Q_h} \qquad (7\text{–}12)$$

where $Cl_{int,h}$ is the hepatic intrinsic clearance that embodies a combination of factors that determine the access of the toxicant to the enzymatic sites (eg, plasma protein binding and sinusoidal membrane transport) and the biochemical efficiency of the metabolizing enzymes (eg, V_{max}/K_M for an enzyme obeying Michaelis kinetics). $Cl_{int,h}$ would also embody canalicular transport activity if the toxicant is subject to biliary excretion. Equation (7–12) dictates that hepatic clearance of a toxicant from the blood is bounded by either liver blood flow or intrinsic clearance (ie, $f_{ub} \cdot Cl_{int,h}$). Note that when $f_{ub} \cdot Cl_{int,h}$ is very much higher than Q_h, E_h approaches

unity (ie, near-complete extraction during each passage of toxicant through the hepatic sinusoid or high extraction) and Cl_h approaches Q_h. Put in another way, hepatic clearance cannot exceed the hepatic blood flow rate even if the intrinsic rate of metabolism in the liver is more rapid than the rate of hepatic blood flow because the rate of overall hepatic clearance is limited by the delivery of the toxicant to the metabolic enzymes in the liver via the blood. At the other extreme, when $f_{ub} \cdot Cl_{int,h}$ is very much lower than Q_h, E_h becomes quite small (ie, low extraction) and Cl_h nearly equals $f_{ub} \cdot Cl_{int,h}$. In this instance, the intrinsic clearance is relatively inefficient; hence, alteration in liver blood flow would have little, if any, influence on liver clearance of the toxicant. Thus, the concept of clearance is grounded in the physiological and biochemical mechanisms of an eliminating organ.

Relationship of Elimination Half-Life to Clearance and Volume

Elimination half-life ($T_{1/2}$) is probably the most easily understood toxicokinetic concept and is an important parameter as it measures the persistence of a toxicant following discontinuation of exposure. As will be seen in a later section, elimination half-life also governs the rate of accumulation of a toxicant in the body during continuous or repetitive exposure. Elimination half-life is dependent on both volume of distribution and clearance. $T_{1/2}$ can be calculated from V_d and Cl:

$$T_{1/2} = \frac{0.693 \cdot V_d}{Cl} \qquad (7\text{–}13)$$

The above relationship among $T_{1/2}$, V_d, and Cl is another illustration that care should be exercised in interpretation of data when relying upon $T_{1/2}$ as the sole representation of elimination of a chemical in toxicokinetic studies, since $T_{1/2}$ is influenced by both the volume of distribution for the toxicant and the rate by which the toxicant is cleared from the blood. For a fixed V_d, $T_{1/2}$ decreases as Cl increases because the chemical is being removed from this fixed volume faster as clearance increases (Fig. 7-4). Conversely, as V_d increases, $T_{1/2}$ increases for a fixed Cl since the volume of fluid that must be cleared of chemical increases but the efficiency of clearance does not.

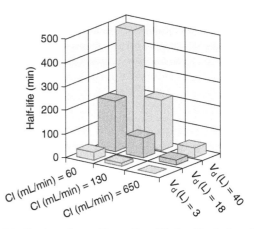

Figure 7-4. *The dependence of $T_{1/2}$ on V_d and Cl.* Consider the hypothetical case of a toxicant that is eliminated entirely by renal excretion. Renal **Cl** values of 60, 130, and 650 mL/min represent partial reabsorption, glomerular filtration, and tubular secretion, respectively. Values for **V_d** of 3, 18, and 40 L represent approximate volumes of plasma water, extracellular fluid and total body water, respectively, for an average-sized person. Note that **$T_{1/2}$** depends on both **Cl** and **V_d**.

Absorption and Bioavailability

For most chemicals in toxicology, exposure occurs mostly via extravascular routes (eg, inhalation, dermal, or oral), and absorption into the systemic circulation is often incomplete. The extent of absorption of a toxicant can be experimentally determined by comparing the plasma toxicant concentration after iv and extravascular dosing. Because iv dosing assures full (100%) delivery of the dose into the systemic circulation, the *AUC* ratio should equal the fraction of extravascular dose absorbed and reaches the systemic circulation in its intact form, and is called *bioavailability* (*F*). In acute toxicokinetic studies, bioavailability can be determined by using different iv and non-iv doses according to the following equation, provided that the toxicant does not display dose-dependent or saturable kinetics.

$$F = \frac{\left(AUC_{non\text{-}iv} / Dose_{non\text{-}iv}\right)}{\left(AUC_{iv} / Dose_{iv}\right)} \qquad (7\text{--}14)$$

where $AUC_{non\text{-}iv}$, AUC_{iv}, $Dose_{non\text{-}iv}$, and $Dose_{iv}$ are the respective area under the plasma concentration versus time curves and doses for non-iv and iv administration. Bioavailabilities for various chemicals range in value between 0 and 1. Complete availability of chemical to the systematic circulation is demonstrated by $F = 1$. When $F < 1$, less than 100% of the dose is able to reach the systemic circulation. Because the concept of bioavailability is judged by how much of the dose reaches the systemic circulation, it is often referred to as systemic availability. Systemic availability is determined by how well a toxicant is absorbed from its site of application and any intervening processes that could remove or inactivate the toxicant between its point of entry and the systemic circulation. Specifically, systemic availability of an orally administered toxicant is governed by its absorption at the gastrointestinal barrier, metabolism within the intestinal mucosa, and metabolism and biliary excretion during its first transit through the liver. Metabolic inactivation and excretion of the toxicant at the intestinal mucosa and the liver prior to its entry into the systemic circulation is called presystemic extraction or first-pass effect. The following equation accounts for the action of absorption and sequential first-pass extraction at the intestinal mucosa and the liver as determinants of the bioavailability of a toxicant taken orally:

$$F = f_{g} \cdot (1 - E_{m}) \cdot (1 - E_{h}) \qquad (7\text{--}15)$$

where f_{g} is the fraction of the applied dose that is released and absorbed across the mucosal barrier along the entire length of the gut, E_{m} is the extent of loss due to metabolism within the gastrointestinal mucosa, and E_{h} is the loss due to metabolism or biliary excretion during first-pass through the liver. Note that E_{h} in this equation is same as the hepatic extraction E_{h} defined in Equation (7-12), which refers to hepatic extraction of a toxicant during recirculation. This means that low oral bioavailability of a chemical can be attributed to multiple factors. The chemical may be absorbed to a limited extent because of low aqueous solubility preventing its effective dissolution in the gastrointestinal fluid or low permeability across the brush-border membrane of the intestinal mucosa. Extensive degradation by metabolic enzymes residing at the intestinal mucosa and the liver may also minimize entry of the chemical in its intact form into the systemic circulation.

The rate of absorption of a toxicant via an extravascular route of entry is another critical determinant of outcome, particularly in acute exposure situations. As shown in Fig. 7-5, slowing the absorption rate of a toxicant, while maintaining the same extent of absorption or bioavailability, leads to a delay in time to peak plasma

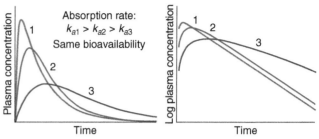

Figure 7-5. *Influence of absorption rate on the time to peak (T_p) and maximum plasma concentration (C_{max}) of a toxicant that exhibit 1-compartment kinetics.* The left panel illustrates the change in plasma concentration–time curves as the first-order absorption rate constant (k_a) decreases, while keeping the extent of absorption or bioavailability (*F*), hence the *AUC*, constant. The right panel displays the same curves in a semilogarithmic plot. Time to peak plasma concentration shows a progressive delay as k_a decreases, along with a decrease in C_{max}. In case 1 and 2, the terminal decline in plasma concentration is governed by elimination half-life; hence, the parallel decline in the semilogarithmic plot. In case 3 where $k_a \ll k_{el}$, the absorption becomes so slow that decline in plasma concentration in the terminal phase reflects the absorption half-life, that is, washout of toxicant is rate-limited by absorption. Accordingly, the terminal decline is slower than in case 1 and 2.

concentration (T_p) and a decrease in the maximum concentration (C_{max}) (compare case 2 to case 1). The converse is true; accelerating absorption shortens T_p and increases C_{max}. The dependence of T_p and C_{max} on absorption rate has obvious implication in the speed of onset and maximum toxic effects following exposure to a chemical. Case 3 in Fig. 7-5 illustrates the peculiar situation when the absorption rate is so much slower than the elimination rate (eg, $k_a \ll k_{el}$ for a one-compartment model). The terminal rate of decline in plasma concentration reflects the absorption rate constant, instead of the elimination rate constant; that is, the washout of toxicant is rate-limited by slow absorption until the applied dose is completely absorbed or removed, beyond which time the toxicant remaining in the body will be cleared according the elimination rate-constant. This means that continual absorption of a chemical can affect the persistence of toxic effect following an acute exposure, and that it is important to institute decontamination procedure quickly after overdose or accidental exposure to a toxicant. This is especially a consideration in occupational exposure via dermal absorption following skin contact with permeable industrial chemicals.

Metabolite Kinetics

The toxicity of a chemical is in some cases attributed to its biotransformation product(s). Hence, the formation and subsequent disposition kinetics of a toxic metabolite is at times of interest. In biological monitoring, urinary excretion of a signature metabolite often serves as a surrogate measure of exposure to the parent compound (see later section). As expected, the plasma concentration of a metabolite rises as the parent drug is transformed into the metabolite. Once formed, the metabolite is subject to further metabolism to a nontoxic byproduct or undergoes excretion via the kidneys or bile; hence at some point in time, the plasma metabolite concentration peaks and falls thereafter. Fig. 7-6 illustrates the plasma concentration–time course of a primary metabolite in relation to its parent compound under contrasting scenarios. The left panel shows the case when the elimination rate constant of the metabolite is much greater than the overall elimination rate constant of the parent compound (ie, $k_m \gg k_p$). The terminal decline of the metabolite parallels that of the parent compound; the metabolite is cleared as quickly as it is formed or its washout is rate-limited by

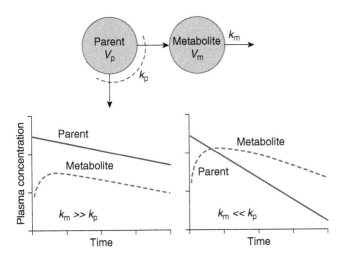

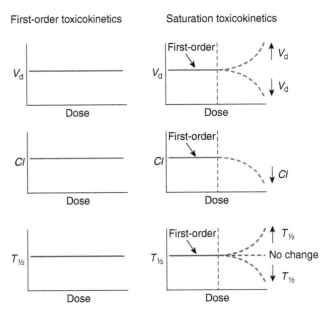

Figure 7-6. *Plasma concentration–time course of a primary metabolite and its parent compound under contrasting scenarios: when elimination of the metabolite is much more rapid than its formation ($k_m \gg k_p$ lower left panel) and when elimination of the metabolite is much slower than its formation ($k_m \ll k_p$, lower right panel). Semilogarithmic plots are shown to compare the slope of the terminal decline of parent compound and its metabolite.* The top panel shows the model for conversion of the parent compound to a single metabolite. Note that the elimination rate constant for the parent compound (k_p) includes both the rate constants for metabolism and extra-metabolic routes of elimination. k_m is the elimination rate constant for the derived metabolite. When $k_m \gg k_p$, the terminal decline of the metabolite parallels that of the parent compound, that is, metabolite washout is rate-limited by its formation. When $k_m \ll k_p$, the terminal decline of metabolite concentration is much slower than that of parent compound, that is, metabolite washout is rate-limited by its elimination.

conversion from the parent compound. The right panel shows the opposite case when the elimination rate constant of the metabolite is much lower than the overall elimination rate constant of the parent compound (ie, $k_m \ll k_p$). The slower terminal decline of the metabolite compared to the parent compound simply reflects a longer elimination half-life of the metabolite. It should also be noted that the AUC_0^∞ of the metabolite relative to the parent compound is dependent on the partial clearance of the parent drug to the metabolite and clearance of the derived metabolite. A biologically active metabolite assumes toxicological significance when it is the major metabolic product and is cleared much less efficiently than the parent compound.

Saturation Toxicokinetics

As already mentioned, the distribution and elimination of most chemicals occurs by first-order processes. Under first-order elimination kinetics, the elimination rate constant, apparent volume of distribution, clearance, and half-life are expected not to change with increasing or decreasing dose (ie, dose independent). As a result, a semilogarithmic display of plasma concentration versus time over a range of doses shows a set of parallel plots. Furthermore, plasma concentration at a given time or the AUC_0^∞ is strictly proportional to dose; for example, a 2-fold change in dose results in an exact 2-fold change in plasma concentration at a given time after dosing or AUC_0^∞. However, for some toxicants, as the dose of a toxicant increases, its volume of distribution and/or clearance may change, as shown in Fig. 7-7. This is generally referred to as nonlinear or dose-dependent kinetics. Biotransformation, active transport processes, and protein binding have finite capacities and can be saturated. For instance, most metabolic enzymes operate in accordance to Michaelis–Menten kinetics (Gibaldi and Perrier,

Figure 7-7. *Changes in V_d, Cl, and $T_{1/2}$ following first-order toxicokinetics (left panels) and following saturable toxicokinetics (right panels).* Vertical dashed lines in the right panels represent point of departure from first-order to saturation toxicokinetics. Pharmacokinetic parameters for toxicants that follow first-order toxicokinetics are independent of dose. When plasma protein binding or elimination mechanisms are saturated with increasing dose, pharmacokinetic parameter estimates become dose-dependent. V_d may increase, for example, when protein binding is saturated, allowing more free toxicant to distribute into extravascular sites. Conversely, V_d may decrease with increasing dose if tissue protein binding saturates. Then, toxicant may redistribute more freely back into plasma. When toxicant concentrations exceed the capacity for biotransformation by metabolic enzymes, overall clearance of the toxicant decreases. These changes may or may not have effects on $T_{1/2}$ depending upon the magnitude and direction of changes in both V_d and Cl.

1982). As the dose is escalated and concentration of a toxicant at the site of metabolism approaches or exceeds the K_M (substrate concentration at one-half V_{max}, the maximum metabolic capacity), the increase in rate of metabolism becomes less than proportional to the dose and eventually approaches a maximum at exceedingly high doses. The transition from first-order to saturation kinetics is important in toxicology because it can lead to prolonged persistence of a compound in the body after an acute exposure and excessive accumulation during repeated exposures. Some of the salient characteristics of nonlinear kinetics include the following: (1) the decline in the concentrations of the chemical in the body is not exponential; (2) AUC_0^∞ is not proportional to the dose; (3) V_d, Cl, k_{el} (or β), or $T_{1/2}$ change with increasing dose; (4) the composition of excretory products changes quantitatively or qualitatively with the dose; and (5) dose–response curves show an abruptly steeper change in response to an increasing dose, starting at the dose at which saturation effects become evident.

Inhaled methanol provides an example of a chemical whose metabolic clearance changes from first-order kinetics at low level exposures to zero-order kinetics at near toxic levels (Burbacher *et al.*, 2004). Fig. 7-8 shows predicted blood methanol concentration–time profiles in female monkeys followed a 2-hour controlled exposure in an inhalation chamber at 2 levels of methanol vapor, 1200 and 4800 ppm. Blood methanol kinetics at 1200 ppm exposure follows typical first-order kinetics. At 4800 ppm, methanol metabolism is fully saturated, such that the initial decline in blood methanol following the 2-hour exposure occurs at a constant rate (ie, a fixed decrease in concentration per unit time independent of blood

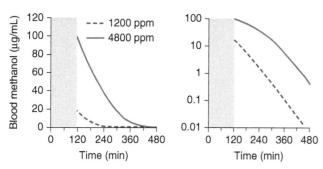

Figure 7-8. *Predicted time course of blood methanol concentration following a 120-minute exposure to 1200 and 4800 ppm of methanol vapor in the female monkey based on the toxicokinetic model reported by Burbacher et al. (2004) that features a saturable (Michaelis–Menten type) metabolic clearance.* The left panel is a rectilinear plot of the simulated blood methanol concentration–time curves at the 2 exposure levels. The right panel shows the same simulations in a semilogarithmic plot. The washout of blood methanol following the 120-minute inhalation exposure at 1200 ppm follows a typical concave or exponential pattern in the rectilinear plot (left panel) and is linear in a semilogarithmic plot (right panel). The postexposure profile at 4800 ppm shows a linear segment during the first 120 minutes of washout and becomes exponential thereafter in the rectilinear plot (left panel). The linear segment reflects saturation of alcohol dehydrogenase, which is the principal enzyme responsible for the metabolism of methanol. The in vivo K_M for this simulation was set at 32.7 μg/mL. At concentrations well above K_M, the kinetics approach zero-order kinetics. At concentrations below K_M, washout kinetics become first-order with a half-life of about 60 minutes. The right panel shows a characteristic convex semilogarithmic plot for the initial phase of zero-order kinetics and becomes linear as expected for first-order kinetics when the concentration falls below K_M. It should also be noted that the maximum blood methanol following 4800 ppm exposure is predicted to be 5.9-times higher than that following 1200 ppm. Also, the area under the blood concentration–time curve (*AUC*) from time zero to 480 minutes at 4800 ppm exposure is 8-fold higher than at 1200 ppm. Under linear kinetics, the increase in maximum blood methanol and *AUC* ought to be proportionate to the dose increase, that is, a 4-fold increment. Here, we observe a more than proportionate increase in blood methanol concentration in relation to the dose, which is another hallmark of saturation kinetics.

concentration), rather than a constant fractional rate. As a result, a rectilinear plot of blood methanol concentration versus time yields an initial linear decline, whereas a convex curve is observed in the semilogarithmic plot (compare left and right panels of Fig. 7-8). In time, methanol metabolism converts to first-order kinetics when blood methanol concentration falls below K_M (ie, the Michaelis constant for the dehydrogenase enzyme), at which time blood methanol shows an exponential decline in the rectilinear plot and a linear decline in the semilogarithmic plot. Moreover, Fig. 7-8 shows the greater than proportionate increase (ie, >4-fold) in C_{max} and AUC_0^∞ as the methanol vapor concentration is raised from 1200 to 4800 ppm. It should be noted that a constant $T_{1/2}$ or k_{el} does not exist during the saturation regimen; it varies depending upon the saturating methanol dose.

In addition to the complication of dose-dependent kinetics, there are toxicants whose clearance kinetics changes over time (ie, time-dependent kinetics). A common cause of time-dependent kinetics is autoinduction of xenobiotic metabolizing enzymes; that is, the substrate is capable of inducing its own metabolism through activation of gene transcription. The classic example of autoinduction is with the antiepileptic drug, carbamazepine. Daily administration of carbamazepine leads to a continual increase in clearance and shortening in elimination half-life over the first few weeks of therapy (Bertilsson *et al.*, 1986).

Accumulation During Continuous or Intermittent Exposure

It stands to reason that continual or chronic exposure to a chemical leads to its cumulative intake and accumulation in the body. For a chemical that follows first-order elimination kinetics, the elimination rate increases as the body burden increases. Therefore, at a fixed level of continuous exposure, accumulation of a toxicant in the body eventually reaches a point when the intake rate of the toxicant equals its elimination rate, from thereon the body burden stays constant. This is referred to as the steady state. Fig. 7-9 illustrates the rise of toxicant concentration in plasma over time during continuous exposure and the eventual attainment of a plateau or the steady state. Steady-state concentration of a toxicant in plasma (C_{ss}) is related to the intake rate (R_{in}) and clearance of the toxicant.

$$C_{ss} = \frac{R_{in}}{Cl} \qquad (7–16)$$

For a one-compartment model, an exponential rise in plasma concentration is expected during continuous exposure and the time it takes for a toxicant to reach steady state is governed by its elimination half-life. It takes 1 half-life to reach 50%, 4 half-lives to reach 93.8%, and 7 half-lives to reach 99.2% of steady state. Time to attainment of steady state is not dependent on the intake rate of the toxicant. The left panel of Fig. 7-9 shows the same time to 50% steady state at 3 different rates of intake; on the contrary, the steady-state concentration is strictly proportional to the intake rate. The change in clearance of a toxicant often leads to a corresponding

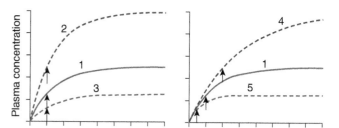

Figure 7-9. *Accumulation of plasma toxicant concentration over time during constant, continuous exposure as a function of exposure level (left panel) and elimination half-life (right panel).* These simulations are based on a 1-compartment model at a constant apparent volume of distribution. Case 1 serves as the reference with an elimination half-life set equal to 1 arbitrary time unit. In the left panel, which illustrates accumulation of toxicant as a function of exposure level, exposure level is raised by 2-fold in case 2 and lowered by 50% in case 3. The changes in eventual steady state concentration are proportional to the changes in exposure level, that is, increased by 2-fold in case 2 and decreased by 50% in case 3. During continuous exposure, 50% of steady state is achieved in 1 half-life. Near plateau or steady state (>90%) is reached after 4 half-lives. Since the elimination half-life is constant across cases 1–3 in the left panel, the time it takes to attain 50% of steady state concentration (see arrows) is the same, that is, 1 time unit. Right panel illustrates the influence of elimination half-life and clearance on accumulation at a fixed constant rate of exposure. Case 4 represents a 50% decrease in clearance and a corresponding 2-fold increase in elimination half-life compared to case 1. Case 5 represents a 2-fold increase in clearance and a corresponding 50% decrease in elimination half-life. Changes in both the time to attain steady state and the steady state concentration are evident. In case 4, the steady state concentration increased by 2-fold as a result of a 50% reduction in clearance, and the time to achieved 50% of steady state increased by 2-fold as a result of the prolonged elimination half-life. In case 5, the steady state concentration is reduced by 50%, while the time to reach 50% steady state is shortened by 50%.

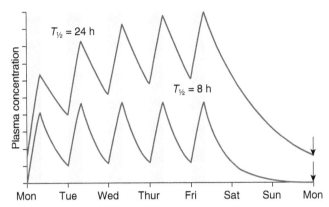

Figure 7-10. *Simulated accumulation of plasma concentration from occupational exposure over the cycle of a work week for 2 industrial chemicals with short and long elimination half-lives.* Shading represents the exposure period during the 8-hour workday, Monday through Friday. Intake of the chemical into the systemic circulation is assumed to occur at a constant rate during exposure. Exposure is negligible over the weekend. For the chemical with the short elimination half-life of 8 hours, minimal accumulation occurs from day to day over the workdays. Near-complete washout of the chemical is observed when work resumes on Monday (see arrow). For the chemical with the long elimination half-life of 24 hours, progressive accumulation is observed over the 5 workdays. Washout of the longer half-life chemical over the weekend is incomplete; a significant residual is carried into the next work week. Because of its lower clearance, the overall *AUC* of the long half-life chemical over the cycle of a week is higher by 3-fold.

change in elimination half-life (see right panel of Fig. 7-9), in which case both the time to reach and magnitude of steady state concentration are altered. The same steady state principle applies to toxicants that exhibit multicompartmental kinetics; except that, accumulation occurs in a multiphasic fashion reflective of the multiple exponential half-lives for intercompartmental distribution and elimination. Typically, the rise in plasma concentration is relatively rapid at the beginning, being governed by the early (distribution) half-life, and becomes slower at later times when the terminal (elimination) half-life takes hold.

The concept of accumulation applies to intermittent exposure as well. Fig. 7-10 shows a typical occupational exposure scenario to volatile chemicals at the workplace over the course of a week. Whether accumulation occurs from day to day and further from week to week depends on the intervals between exposure and the elimination half-life of the chemicals involved. For a chemical with relatively short half-life compared to the interval between work shifts and the "exposure holiday" over the weekend, little accumulation is expected. In contrast, for a chemical with elimination half-life approaching or exceeding the between-shift intervals (>12–24 hours), progressive accumulation is expected over the successive workdays. Washout of the chemical may not be complete over the weekend and result in a significant carry forward of body burden into the next week. It should also be noted that the overall internal exposure as measured by the *AUC* over the cycle of a week is dependent on the toxicant clearance.

Conclusion

For many chemicals, blood or plasma chemical concentration versus time data can be adequately described by a one- or two-compartment, classic pharmacokinetic model when basic assumptions are made (eg, instantaneous mixing within compartments and first-order kinetics). In some instances, more sophisticated models with increased numbers of compartments will

be needed to describe blood or plasma toxicokinetic data; for example, if the chemical is preferentially sequestered and turns over slowly in select tissues. The parameters of the classic compartmental models are usually estimated by statistical fitting of data to the model equations using nonlinear regression methods. A number of software packages are available for both data fitting and simulations with classic compartmental models; examples include WinNonlin (Pharsight Corp, Palo Alto, CA), SAAM II (The Epsilon Group, Charlottesville, VA), ADAPT II (University of Southern California, Los Angeles, CA), and PK Solutions (Summit Research Services, Montrose, CO).

Knowledge of toxicokinetic data and compartmental modeling are useful in deciding what dose or dosing regimen of chemical to use in the planning of toxicology studies (eg, targeting a toxic level of exposure), in choosing appropriate sampling times for biological monitoring, and in seeking an understanding of the dynamics of a toxic event (eg, what blood or plasma concentrations are achieved to produce a specific response, how accumulation of a chemical controls the onset and degree of toxicity, and the persistence of toxic effects following termination of exposure).

PHYSIOLOGICAL TOXICOKINETICS

The primary difference between physiological compartmental models and classic compartmental models lies in the basis for assigning the rate constants that describe the toxicant's movement into and out of the body compartments and its elimination (Andersen, 1991). In classic kinetics, the rate constants are defined by the data; thus, these models are often referred to as data-based models. In physiological models, the rate constants represent known or hypothesized biological processes, and these models are commonly referred to as physiologically based models. The concept of incorporating biological realism into the analysis of drug or xenobiotic distribution and elimination is not new. For example, one of the first physiological models was proposed by Teorell (1937). This model contained all the important determinants in xenobiotic disposition that are considered valid today. Unfortunately, the computational tools required to solve the underlying equations were not available at that time. With advances in computer technology, the software and hardware needed to implement physiological models are now well within the reach of toxicologists.

The advantages of physiologically based models compared with classic models are that (1) these models can describe the time course of distribution of toxicants to any organ or tissue, (2) they allow estimation of the effects of changing physiological parameters on tissue concentrations, (3) the same model can predict the toxicokinetics of toxicants across species by allometric scaling, and (4) complex dosing regimens and saturable processes such as metabolism and binding are easily accommodated (Gargas and Andersen, 1988). The disadvantages are that (1) much more information is needed to implement these models compared with classic models, (2) the mathematics can be difficult for many toxicologists to handle, and (3) values for parameters are often poorly defined in various species and pathophysiological states. Nevertheless, physiologically based toxicokinetic models are conceptually sound and are potentially useful tools for gaining rich insight into the kinetics of toxicants beyond what classic toxicokinetic models can provide.

Basic Model Structure

Physiological models are fundamentally complex compartmental models; it generally consists of a system of tissue or organ

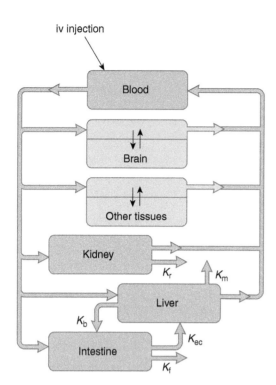

Figure 7-11. *Physiological model for a hypothetical toxicant that is soluble in water, has a low vapor pressure (not volatile), and has a relatively large molecular weight (MW > 100).* This hypothetical toxicant is injected into the blood stream and eliminated through metabolism in the liver (K_m), biliary excretion (K_b), renal excretion (K_r) into the urine, and fecal excretion (K_f). The toxicant can also undergo enterohepatic circulation (K_{ec}). Perfusion-limited compartments are noted in red and diffusion-limited compartments are noted in blue.

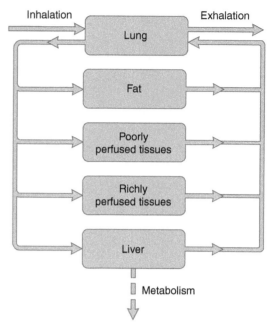

Figure 7-12. *Physiological model for a typical volatile organic chemical.* Chemicals for which this model would be appropriate have low molecular weights (*MW* < 100), are soluble in organic solvents, and have significant vapor pressures (volatile). The main route of its intake is via inhalation and absorption by the lungs. Transport of chemical throughout the body by blood is depicted by the arrows. Elimination of chemical as depicted by the model includes metabolism (*dashed arrow*) and exhalation (*arrows indicate ventilation of the lung*). All compartments are perfusion-limited.

compartments that are interconnected by the circulatory network. If necessary, each tissue or organ compartments can further be divided into extracellular and intracellular compartments to describe movement of toxicant at the cellular level. The exact model structure, or how the compartments are organized and linked together, depends on both the toxicant and the organism being studied. For example, a physiological model describing the disposition of a toxicant in fish would require a description of the gills (Nichols *et al.*, 1994), whereas a model for the same toxicant in mammals would require a lung compartment (Ramsey and Andersen, 1984). Model structures can also vary with the toxicants being studied. For example, a model for a nonvolatile, water-soluble chemical, which might be administered by iv injection (Fig. 7-11), has a structure different from that of a model for a volatile organic chemical for which inhalation is the likely route of exposure (Fig. 7-12). The route of administration is not the only difference between these 2 models. For example, the first model has a compartment for the intestines, because biliary excretion, fecal elimination, and enterohepatic circulation are presumed important in the disposition of this chemical. The second model has a compartment for fat because fat is an important storage organ for organics. However, the models are not completely different. Both contain a liver compartment because hepatic metabolism of each chemical is an important element of its disposition. It is important to realize that there is no generic physiological model. Models are simplifications of reality and should contain elements considered to represent the essential disposition features of a toxicant.

In view of the fact that physiological modeling requires more effort than does classic compartmental modeling, what then accounts for the popularity of this approach among toxicologists?

The answer lies in the potential predictive power of physiological models. Toxicologists are constantly faced with the issue of extrapolation in risk assessments—from laboratory animals to humans, from high to low doses, from acute to chronic exposure, and from single chemicals to mixtures. Because the kinetic constants in physiological models represent measurable biological or chemical processes, the resultant physiological models have the potential for extrapolation from observed data to predicted scenarios.

One of the best illustrations of the predictive power of physiological models is their ability to extrapolate kinetic behavior from laboratory animals to humans. For example, physiological models developed for styrene and benzene correctly simulate the concentration of each chemical in the blood of both rodents and humans (Ramsey and Andersen, 1984; Travis *et al.*, 1990). Simulations are the outcomes or results (such as a chemical's concentration in blood or tissue) of numerically solving the model equations over a time period of concern, using a set of initial (such as level of exposure) or input conditions (such as route of exposure) and parameter values appropriate for the species (such as organ weights and blood flow). Both styrene and benzene are volatile organic chemicals; thus, the model structures for the kinetics of both chemicals in rodents and humans are identical to that shown in Fig. 7-12. However, the parameter values for rodents and humans are different. Humans have larger body weights than rodents, and thus weights of organs such as the liver are larger. Because humans are larger, they also breathe more air per unit of time than do rodents, and a human heart pumps a larger volume of blood per unit of time than does that of a rodent, although the rodent's heart beats more times in the same period. The parameters that describe the chemical behavior of styrene and benzene, such as solubility in tissues, are similar in the rodents and human models. This is often the case because the composition of tissues in different species is similar.

For both styrene and benzene, there are experimental data for humans and rodents and the model simulations can be compared with the actual data to see how well the model has performed (Ramsey and Andersen, 1984; Andersen *et al.*, 1984; Travis *et al.*, 1990). The conclusion is that the same model structure is capable of describing the chemicals' kinetics in two different species. Because the parameters underlying the model structure represent measurable biological and chemical determinants, the appropriate values for those parameters can be chosen for each species, forming the basis for successful interspecies extrapolation. Even though the same model structure is used for both rodents and humans, the simulated and the observed kinetics of both chemicals differ between rats and humans. The terminal half-life of both organics is longer in humans compared with rats. This longer half-life for humans is due to the fact that clearance rates for smaller species are faster than those for larger ones. Even though the larger species breathes more air or pumps more blood per unit of time than does the smaller species, blood flows and ventilation rates per unit of body mass are greater for the smaller species. The smaller species has more breaths per minute or heartbeats per minute than does the larger species, even though each breath or stroke volume is smaller. The faster flows per unit mass result in a more efficient delivery of a chemical to organs responsible for elimination. Thus, a smaller species can eliminate the chemical faster than a larger one can. Because the parameters in physiological models represent real, measurable values, such as blood flows and ventilation rates; the same model structure can resolve such disparate kinetic behaviors among species.

Compartments

The basic unit of the physiological model is the lumped compartment, which is often depicted as a box in a graphical scheme (Fig. 7-13). A compartment represents a definable anatomical site or tissue type in the body that acts as a unit in effecting a measurable kinetic process (Rowland, 1984, 1985). A compartment may represent a particular structure or functional portion of an organ, a segment of blood vessel with surrounding tissue, an entire discrete organ such as the liver or kidney, or a widely distributed tissue type such as fat or skin. Compartments usually consist of three individual well-mixed regions, or subcompartments, that correspond

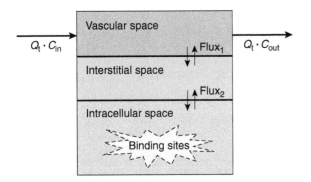

Figure 7-13. *Schematic representation of a lumped tissue compartment in a physiological model.* The blood capillary and cell barriers separating the vascular, interstitial, and intracellular subcompartments are depicted in heavy black lines. The vascular and interstitial subcompartments are often combined into a single extracellular subcompartment. Q_t is the blood perfusion flow, C_{in} is the toxicant's concentration in the blood entering the compartment, and C_{out} is the toxicant's concentration in the blood leaving the compartment.

to specific physiological spaces or regions of the organ or tissue. These subcompartments are (1) the vascular space through which the compartment is perfused with blood, (2) the interstitial space that surrounds the cells, and (3) the intracellular space representing the cells in the tissue (Gerlowski and Jain, 1983).

As shown in Fig. 7-13, the toxicant enters the vascular subcompartment at a certain rate in mass per unit of time (eg, mg/h). The rate of entry is a product of the blood flow rate to the tissue (Q_t in L/h) and the concentration of the toxicant in the blood entering the tissue (C_{in} in mg/L). Within the compartment, the toxicant moves from the vascular space to the interstitial space at a certain net rate (Flux$_1$) and moves from the interstitial space to the intracellular space at a different net rate (Flux$_2$). Some toxicants can bind to protein components; thus, within a compartment there may be both free and bound toxicants. The toxicant leaves the vascular space at a certain venous concentration (C_{out}). C_{out} is equal to the concentration of the toxicant in the vascular space assuming a well-mixed compartment.

Parameters

The most common types of parameters, or information required, in physiological models are anatomic, physiological, thermodynamic, and transport.

Anatomic Anatomic parameters are used to describe the physical size of various compartments. The size is generally specified as a volume (milliliters or liters) because a unit density is assumed even though weights of organs and tissues are most frequently obtained experimentally. If a compartment contains subcompartments such as those in Fig. 7-13, those volumes also must be known. Volumes of compartments often can be obtained from the literature or from specific toxicokinetic experiments. For example, kidneys, liver, brain, and lungs can be weighed. Obtaining precise data for volumes of compartments representing widely distributed tissues such as fat or muscle is more difficult. If necessary, these tissues can be removed by dissection and weighed. Among the numerous sources of general information on organ and tissue volumes across species, Brown *et al.* (1997) is a good starting point.

Physiological Physiological parameters encompass a wide variety of processes in biological systems. The most commonly used physiological parameters are blood flows and lung ventilation. The blood flow rate (Q_t in volume per unit time, such as mL/min or L/h) to individual compartments must be known. Additionally, information on the total blood flow rate or *cardiac output* (Q_c) is necessary. If inhalation is the route for exposure to the chemical or is a route of elimination, the alveolar ventilation rate (Q_p) also must be known. Blood flow rates and ventilation rates can be taken from the literature or can be obtained experimentally.

Parameters for renal excretion and hepatic metabolism are another subset of physiological parameters, and are required, if these processes are important in describing the elimination of a chemical. For example, glomerular filtration rate and renal tubular transport parameters are required to describe renal clearance. If a chemical is known to be metabolized via a saturable process, both V_{max} (the maximum rate of metabolism) and K_M (the concentration of chemical at one-half V_{max}) for each of the enzymes involved must be obtained so that elimination of the chemical by metabolism can be described in the model. In principle, these parameters can be determined from in vitro metabolism or transport studies with freshly isolated cells, cultured cells, or recombinant DNA expression systems; metabolic studies are also feasible with tissue homogenates or cellular fractions containing the metabolic enzymes (eg, microsomes for cytochrome P450 enzymes and uridine diphosphate glucuronosyltransferases). Appropriate in vitro–in vivo scaling is required (Iwatsubo *et al.*, 1997; MacGregor *et al.*, 2001; Miners *et al.*, 2006). Although there have been examples of remarkable success with quantitative prediction of in vivo hepatic clearance based on in vitro metabolic data, there are also notable failures. There is still very limited experience with in vitro–in vivo scaling of renal or hepatic transporter function. Unfortunately, estimation of metabolic or transport parameters from in vivo studies is also fraught with difficulties, especially when multiple metabolic pathways and enzymes are involved in the metabolic clearance of a substrate, or when parallel and/or sequential transport processes mediate the passage of a solute across a cellular barrier. Estimation of metabolic and excretory parameters remains a challenging aspect of physiologically based toxicokinetic modeling.

Thermodynamic Thermodynamic parameters relate the *total* concentration of a toxicant in a tissue (C_t) to the concentration of *free* toxicant in that tissue (C_f). Two important assumptions are that (1) total and free concentrations are in equilibrium with each other, and (2) only free toxicant can be exchanged between the tissue subcompartments (Lutz *et al.*, 1980). Most often, total concentration is measured experimentally; however, it is the free concentration that is available for diffusion across membrane barriers, binding to proteins, metabolism, or carrier-mediated transport. Various mathematical expressions describe the relationship between these two entities. In the simplest situation, the toxicant is a freely diffusible water-soluble chemical that does not bind to any molecules. In this case, free concentration of the chemical is equal to the total concentration of the chemical in the tissue: $C_t = C_f$. The affinity of toxicants for tissues of different composition varies. The extent to which a toxicant partitions into a tissue is directly dependent on the composition of the tissue and usually independent of the concentration of the toxicant. Thus, the relationship between free and total concentration becomes one of proportionality: $C_t = C_f \cdot P_t$; P_t is in effect the partition coefficient between total concentration in the tissue and freely diffusible concentration in the interstitial fluid or plasma water. Knowledge of the value of P_t permits an indirect calculation of the free concentration of toxicant in the tissue or $C_f = C_t/P_t$, assuming intracellular, interstitial and plasma concentrations of free drug are equal (ie, no concentrative transport across barriers in either direction). P_t is most often determined from tissue distribution studies in animals, preferably at steady state during continuous iv infusion of the toxicant. In some cases, it has been successfully estimated from in vitro binding studies with human or animal tissues or tissue fractions (Lin *et al.*, 1982; MacGregor *et al.*, 2001).

Table 7-4 compares the partition coefficients for a number of toxic volatile organic chemicals. The larger values for the fat-to-blood partition coefficients compared with those for other tissues suggest that these chemicals distribute into fat to a greater extent than they distribute into other tissues. This has been observed experimentally. Fat and fatty tissues, such as bone marrow, contain higher concentrations of benzene than do tissues such as liver and blood. Similarly, styrene concentrations in fatty tissue are higher than styrene concentrations in other tissues. It should be noted that lipophilic organic compounds often can bind to plasma proteins and/or blood cell constituents, in which case the observed tissue/blood partition coefficients will be a function of both the tissue and blood partition coefficient (ie, P_t/P_b). Hence, partitioning or binding to blood constituents (P_b) must be known in order to estimate the true thermodynamic partitioning coefficient for a tissue or the free toxicant concentration at equilibrium. P_b can be determined from in vitro studies of blood cells to plasma distribution and plasma protein binding of the toxicant.

A more complex relationship between the free concentration and the total concentration of a chemical in tissues is also possible. For example, the chemical may bind to saturable binding sites on tissue components. In these cases, nonlinear functions relating the free concentration in the tissue to the total concentration are necessary. Examples in which more complex binding has been used are physiological models for dioxin and *tertiary*-amyl methyl ether (Andersen *et al.*, 1993; Collins *et al.*, 1999).

Transport Passage of a toxicant across a biological membrane may occur by passive diffusion, carrier-mediated transport involving either facilitated or active transporters, or a combination thereof (Himmelstein and Lutz, 1979). The simplest of these processes—passive diffusion is a first-order process described by Fick's law of diffusion. Diffusion of a toxicant occurs during its passage across the blood capillary endothelium (Flux$_1$ in Fig. 7-13) and across cell barriers (Flux$_2$ in Fig. 7-13). Flux refers to the rate of transfer of a chemical across a boundary. For simple diffusion, the net flux (mg/h) from one side of a membrane to the other is governed by the barrier permeability and the toxicant concentration gradient.

$$\text{Flux} = PA \cdot (C_1 - C_2) = PA \cdot C_1 - PA \cdot C_2 \qquad (7\text{--}17)$$

The term *PA* is often called the *permeability–area product* for the membrane or cellular barrier in flow units (eg, L/h), and is a product of the barrier permeability coefficient (P in velocity units, eg, μm/h) for the toxicant and the total barrier surface area (A, in μm^2). The permeability coefficient takes into account the diffusivity of the specific toxicant and the thickness of the cell membrane. C_1 and C_2 are the respective *free* concentrations of the toxicant in the originating and receiving compartments. Diffusional flux is enhanced when the barrier thickness is small, the barrier surface area is large, and a large concentration gradient exists. Membrane transporters offer an additional route of entry into cells, and allow more effective tissue penetration for toxicants that have limited passive permeability. Alternately, the presence of efflux transporters at epithelial or endothelial barriers can limit toxicant penetration into critical organs, even for highly permeable toxicant (eg, P-glycoprotein-mediated efflux functions as part of the blood–brain barrier). For both transporter-mediated influx and efflux processes, the kinetics is saturable and can be characterized by T_{max} (the maximum transport rate) and K_T (the concentration of toxicant at one-half T_{max}) for each of the transporters involved. In principle, kinetic parameters for passive permeability or carrier-mediated transport can be estimated from in vitro studies with tissue slices (eg, with tetraethylammonium ion; Mintun *et al.*, 1980) or cultured cell monolayer systems. However, the predictability and applicability of such in vitro approaches for physiological modeling has not been systematically evaluated (MacGregor *et al.*, 2001). At this time, the transport parameters have to be estimated from in vivo data, which are at times difficult and carry a significant degree of uncertainty.

Table 7-4

Partition Coefficients for Four Volatile Organic Chemicals in Several Tissues

CHEMICAL	BLOOD/AIR	MUSCLE/BLOOD	FAT/BLOOD
Isoprene	3	0.67	24
Benzene	18	0.61	28
Styrene	40	1	50
Methanol	1350	3	11

There are two limiting conditions for the uptake of a toxicant into tissues: perfusion-limited and diffusion-limited. An understanding of the assumptions underlying the limiting conditions is critical because the assumptions change the way in which the model equations are written to describe the movement of a toxicant into and out of the compartment.

Perfusion-Limited Compartments

A perfusion-limited compartment, alternately referred to as blood flow-limited or simply flow-limited compartment, describes the situation when permeability across the cellular or membrane barriers (PA) for a particular toxicant is much greater than the blood flow rate to the tissue (Q_t), that is, $PA_1 \gg Q_t$. In this case, uptake of toxicant by tissue subcompartments is limited by the rate at which the toxicant is presented to the tissue via the arterial inflow, and not by the rate at which the toxicant penetrates through the vascular endothelium, which is fairly porous in most tissues, or gains passage across the cell membranes. As a result, equilibration of a toxicant between the blood in the tissue vasculature and the interstitial subcompartment is maintained at all times, and the two subcompartments are usually lumped together as a single extracellular compartment. An important exception to this vascular-interstitial equilibrium relationship is in the brain, where the capillary endothelium with its tight junctions poses a diffusional barrier between the vascular space and the brain interstitium. Furthermore, as indicated in Fig. 7-13, the cell membrane separates the extracellular compartment from the intracellular compartment. The cell membrane is the most crucial diffusional barrier in a tissue. Nonetheless, for molecules that are very small (molecular weight < 100) or lipophilic (log P > 2), cellular permeability generally does not limit the rate at which a molecule moves across cell membranes. For these molecules, flux across the cell membrane is fast compared with the tissue perfusion rate ($PA_2 \gg Q_t$), and the molecules rapidly distribute throughout the subcompartments. In this case, free toxicant in the intracellular compartment is always in equilibrium with the extracellular compartment, and these tissue subcompartments can be lumped as a single compartment. Such a flow-limited tissue compartment is shown in Fig. 7-14. Movement into and out of the entire tissue compartment can be described by a single equation.

$$V_t \cdot \frac{dC_t}{dt} = Q_t \cdot (C_{in} - C_{out}) \qquad (7\text{–}18)$$

where V_t is the volume of the tissue compartment, C_t is the toxicant concentration in the compartment ($V_t \cdot C$ equals the amount of toxicant in the compartment), $V_t \cdot dC_t/dt$ is the change in the amount of toxicant in the compartment with time, expressed as mass per unit of time, Q_t is blood flow to the tissue, C_{in} is the toxicant

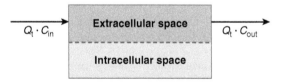

Figure 7-14. *Schematic representation of a tissue compartment that features blood flow–limited uptake kinetics.* Rapid exchange of toxicant between the extracellular space (*blue*) and intracellular space (*light blue*), unhindered by a significant diffusional barrier as symbolized by the dashed line, allows equilibrium to be maintained between the two subcompartments at all times. In effect, a single compartment represents the tissue distribution of the toxicant. Q_t is blood flow, C_{in} is the toxicant concentration entering the compartment via the arterial inflow, and C_{out} is the toxicant concentration leaving the compartment in the venous outflow.

concentration entering the compartment, and C_{out} is the toxicant concentration leaving the compartment. Equations of this type are called mass-balance differential equations. Differential refers to the term dC_t/dt. Mass balance refers to the requirement that the rate of change in the amount of toxicant in a compartment (left-hand side of Equation (7-18)) equals the difference in the rate of entry via arterial inflow and the rate of departure via venous outflow (right-hand side of Equation (7-18)).

In the perfusion-limited case, the concentration of toxicant in the venous drainage from the tissue is equal to the concentration of toxicant in the tissue when the toxicant is not bound to blood constituents (ie, $C_{out} = C_t = C_f$). As was noted previously, when there is binding of toxicant to tissue constituents, C_f (or C_{out}) can be related to the total concentration of toxicant in the tissue through a simple linear partition coefficient, $C_{out} = C_f = C_t/P_t$. In this case, the differential equation describing the rate of change in the amount of a toxicant in a tissue becomes

$$V_t \cdot \frac{dC_t}{dt} = Q_t \cdot \left[C_{in} - \frac{C_t}{P_t} \right] \qquad (7\text{–}19)$$

In the event the toxicant does bind to blood constituents, blood partitioning coefficient needs to be recognized in the mass-balance equation.

$$V_t \cdot \frac{dC_t}{dt} = Q_t \cdot \left[C_{in} - \frac{C_t}{P_t / P_b} \right] \qquad (7\text{–}20)$$

The physiological model shown in Fig. 7-12, which was developed for volatile organic chemicals such as styrene and benzene, is a good example of a model in which all the compartments are described as flow-limited. Distribution of a toxicant in all the compartments is described by using equations of the type noted above. In a flow-limited compartment, the assumption is that the concentrations of a toxicant in all parts of the tissue are in equilibrium. For this reason, the compartments are generally drawn as simple boxes (Fig. 7-12) or boxes with dashed partitioning lines that symbolize the equilibrium between the intracellular and extracellular subcompartments (Fig. 7-14). Additionally, with a flow-limited model, estimates of fluxes between subcompartments are not required to develop the mass-balance differential equation for the compartment. Given the challenges in measuring flux across the vascular endothelium and cell membrane, this is a simplifying assumption that significantly reduces the number of parameters required in the physiological model.

Diffusion-Limited Compartments

When uptake of a toxicant into a compartment is governed by its diffusion or transport across cell membrane barriers, the model is said to be diffusion-limited or barrier-limited. Diffusion-limited uptake or release occurs when the flux, or the transport of a toxicant across cell barriers, is slow compared with blood flow to the tissue. In this case, the permeability–area product is small compared with blood flow, that is, $PA \ll Q_t$. The distribution of large and/or polar molecules into tissue cells is likely to be limited by the rate at which the molecules pass through cell membranes. In contrast, entry into the interstitial space of the tissue through the leaky capillaries of the vascular space is usually rapid even for large molecules. Fig. 7-15 shows the structure of such a compartment. The toxicant concentrations in the vascular and interstitial spaces are in equilibrium and make up the extracellular subcompartment, where uptake from the incoming blood is flow-limited. The rate of toxicant uptake across the cell membrane from the extracellular space

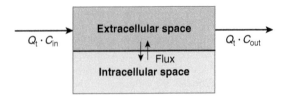

Figure 7-15. *Schematic representation of a tissue compartment that features membrane-limited uptake kinetics.* Perfusion of blood into and out of the extracellular compartment is depicted by thick arrows. Transmembrane transport (flux) from the extracellular to the intracellular subcompartment is depicted by thin arrows. Q_t is blood flow, C_{in} is toxicant concentration entering the compartment, and C_{out} is toxicant concentration leaving the compartment.

into the intracellular space is limited by membrane permeability. Two mass-balance differential equations are necessary to describe the events in these 2 subcompartments:

$$\text{Extracellular: } V_{t1} \cdot \frac{dC_{t1}}{dt} = Q_t \cdot (C_{in} - C_{out})$$
$$- PA_t \cdot \left(\frac{C_{t1}}{P_{t1}}\right) + PA_t \cdot \left(\frac{C_{t2}}{P_{t2}}\right) \quad (7\text{–}21)$$

$$\text{Intracellular: } V_{t2} \cdot \frac{dC_{t2}}{dt} = PA_t \cdot \left(\frac{C_{t1}}{P_{t1}}\right)$$
$$- PA_t \cdot \left(\frac{C_{t2}}{P_{t2}}\right) \quad (7\text{–}22)$$

Q_t is blood flow, and C is the toxicant concentration in the entering blood (in), exiting blood (out), tissue extracellular space (t1), or tissue intracellular space (t2). The subscript (ti) for the PA term acknowledges the fact that PA, reflecting either passive diffusion and/or carrier-mediated processes, can differ between tissues. Both equations feature fluxes or transfers across the cell membrane that are driven by free concentration. Hence, partition coefficients are needed to convert extracellular and intracellular tissue concentration to their corresponding free concentration. C_{out} in Equation (7-21) is related to $C_{t1}/(P_{t1}/P_b)$; the blood partitioning coefficient P_b is required if the toxicant binds to plasma proteins and blood cells. The physiological model in Fig. 7-11 is composed of two diffusion-limited compartments each of which contain two subcompartments—extracellular and intracellular space, and several perfusion-limited compartments.

Specialized Compartments

Lung The inclusion of a lung compartment in a physiological model is an important consideration because inhalation is a common route of exposure to many volatile toxic chemicals. Additionally, the lung compartment serves as an instructive example of the assumptions and simplifications that can be incorporated into physiological models while maintaining the overall objective of describing processes and compartments in biologically relevant terms. For example, although lung physiology and anatomy are complex, Haggard (1924) developed a simple approximation that sufficiently describes the uptake of many volatile chemicals by the lungs. A diagram of this simplified lung compartment is shown in Fig. 7-16. The assumptions inherent in this compartment description are as follows: (1) ventilation is continuous, not cyclic; (2) conducting airways (nasal passages, larynx, trachea, bronchi, and bronchioles) function as inert tubes, carrying the vapor to the alveoli where gas exchange occurs; (3) diffusion of vapor across the alveolar epithelium and capillary walls is rapid compared with

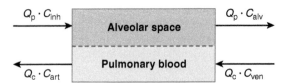

Figure 7-16. *Simple model for exchange of volatile chemicals in the alveolar region of the respiratory tract.* Rapid exchange of toxicant in the simplified lung compartment between the alveolar gas (*blue*) and the pulmonary blood (*light blue*) maintains an equilibrium between them as symbolized by the dashed line. Q_p is alveolar ventilation (L/h); Q_c is cardiac output (L/h); C_{inh} is inhaled vapor concentration (mg/L); C_{art} is concentration of chemical in the arterial blood; C_{ven} is concentration of chemical in the mixed venous blood. The equilibrium relationship between the chemical in the alveolar air (C_{alv}) and the chemical in the arterial blood (C_{art}) is determined by the blood/air partition coefficient $P_{b/a}$, that is, $C_{alv} = C_{art}/P_{b/a}$.

blood flow through the alveolar region; (4) all chemicals disappearing from the inspired air appears in the arterial blood (ie, there is no hold-up of chemical in the lung tissue and insignificant lung mass); and (5) vapor in the alveolar air and arterial blood within the lung compartment are in rapid equilibrium and are related by $P_{b/a}$, the blood/air partition coefficient (eg, $C_{alv} = C_{art}/P_{b/a}$). $P_{b/a}$ is a thermodynamic parameter that quantifies the equilibrium partitioning of a volatile chemical between blood and air.

In the lung compartment depicted in Fig. 7-16, the rate of inhalation of a volatile chemical is controlled by the ventilation rate (Q_p) and the inhaled concentration (C_{inh}). The rate of exhalation of the chemical is a product of the ventilation rate and the chemical's concentration in the alveoli (C_{alv}). Chemical also can enter the lung compartment via mixed venous blood returning from the heart, at a rate represented by the product of cardiac output (Q_c) and the concentration of chemical in venous blood (C_{ven}). Chemical leaves the lungs via the blood at a rate determined by both cardiac output and the concentration of chemical in arterial blood (C_{art}). Putting these four processes together, a mass-balance differential equation can be written for the rate of change in the amount of chemical in the lung compartment (L):

$$\frac{dL}{dt} = Q_p \cdot (C_{inh} - C_{alv}) + Q_c \cdot (C_{ven} - C_{art}) \quad (7\text{–}23)$$

Because of these assumptions, during continuous exposure at steady state the rate of change in the amount of chemical in the lung compartment becomes zero ($dL/dt = 0$). C_{alv} can be replaced by $C_{art}/P_{b/a}$, and the differential equation can be solved for the arterial blood concentration:

$$C_{art} = \frac{Q_p \cdot C_{inh} + Q_c \cdot C_{ven}}{Q_c + Q_p/P_{b/a}} \quad (7\text{–}24)$$

This algebraic equation is incorporated into physiological models for many volatile organics. In this case, the lung is viewed as a portal of entry and not as a target organ; the concentration of a chemical delivered to other organs by the arterial blood is of primary interest. The assumptions of continuous ventilation, rapid equilibration with arterial blood, and no hold-up in the lung tissues have worked extremely well with many volatile organics, especially relatively lipophilic volatile solvents. Indeed, the use of these assumptions simplifies and speeds model calculations and may be entirely adequate for describing the toxicokinetic behavior of relatively inert vapors with low water solubility.

Inspection of the equation for calculating the arterial concentration of the inhaled organic vapor indicates that $P_{b/a}$, the blood/air partition coefficient of the chemical, becomes an important term for simulating the uptake of various volatile organics. As the value for $P_{b/a}$ increases, the maximum concentration of the chemical in the blood increases. Additionally, the time to reach the steady state concentration and the time to clear the chemical also increase with increasing $P_{b/a}$. Fortunately, $P_{b/a}$ is readily measured by using in vitro techniques in which a volatile chemical in air is equilibrated with blood in a closed system, such as a sealed vial (Gargas and Andersen, 1988).

Liver The liver is almost always featured as a distinct compartment in physiological models because biotransformation is an important route of elimination for many toxicants and the liver is considered the major organ for biotransformation of xenobiotics. A simple compartmental structure for the liver is depicted in Fig. 7-17, where uptake into the liver compartment is assumed to be flow-limited. This liver compartment is similar to the general tissue compartment in Fig. 7-14, except that the liver compartment contains an additional process for metabolic elimination. Under first-order elimination, the rate of hepatic metabolism (R) by the liver can be presented as

$$R = Cl_1 \cdot C_f \qquad (7\text{–}25)$$

where C_f is the free concentration of toxicant in the liver (mg/L), and Cl_1 is the clearance of free toxicant within the liver (L/h). The latter parameter is conceptually the same as the intrinsic hepatic clearance term ($Cl_{int,h}$) in Equation (7-12). In the case of a single enzyme mediating the biotransformation and Michaelis–Menten kinetics are obeyed, Cl_1 is related to the maximum rate of metabolism, V_{max} (in mg/h) and the Michaelis constant, K_M (in mg/L) (Andersen, 1981). As a result, the rate of hepatic metabolism can be expressed in terms of the Michaelis parameters.

$$R = \left[\frac{V_{max}}{K_M + C_f} \right] \cdot C_f \qquad (7\text{–}26)$$

Under nonsaturating or first-order condition (ie, $C_f \ll K_M$), Cl_1 becomes equal to the ratio of V_{max}/K_M. Because many toxicants at high exposure levels display saturable metabolism, the above equation is often invoked for simulation of toxicant disposition across a wide range of doses.

Other, more complex expressions for metabolism also can be incorporated into physiological models. Bi-substrate

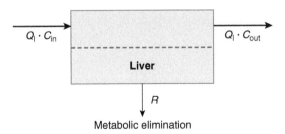

Figure 7-17. *Schematic representation of a flow-limited liver compartment in which metabolic elimination occurs.* **R**, in milligrams per hour, is the rate of metabolism. Q_1 is hepatic blood flow, C_{in} is toxicant concentration entering the liver compartment, and C_{out} is chemical concentration out of the liver compartment. It should be noted that the liver receives blood from 2 sources, arterial inflow via hepatic artery and outflow from the upper mesentery via portal vein. This dual inflow is featured in the physiological model featuring enterohepatic circulation in Fig. 7-11. Inflow via hepatic artery is often ignored, as in this case and in the physiological model shown in Fig. 7-12, because of its relatively small flow rate compared to portal flow.

second-order reactions, reactions involving the destruction of enzymes, inhibition of enzymes, or the depletion of cofactors, have been simulated using physiological models. Metabolism can be also included in other compartments in much the same way as described for the liver.

Blood In a physiological model, the tissue compartments are linked together by the circulatory network. Figs. 7-11 and 7-12 represent different approaches toward describing the circulatory network in physiological models. In general, the arterial system delivers a chemical into various tissues. Exceptions are the liver, which receives arterial and portal blood, and the lungs, which receive mixed venous blood from the right cardiac ventricle. In the body, the venous blood supplies draining from tissue compartments eventually merge in the vena cava and heart chambers to form mixed venous blood. In Fig. 7-11, a blood compartment is created in which the input is the sum of the toxicant outflow from each compartment ($Q_t \cdot C_{vt}$). Outflow from the blood compartment is a product of the blood concentration in the compartment and the total cardiac output ($Q_c \cdot C_{bl}$). The mass-balance differential equation for the blood compartment in Fig. 7-11 is as follows:

$$V_{bl} \cdot \frac{dC_{bl}}{dt} = (Q_{br} \cdot C_{vbr} + Q_{ot} \cdot C_{vot} + Q_k \cdot C_{vk} + Q_1 \cdot C_{vl})$$
$$- Q_c \cdot C_{bl} \qquad (7\text{–}27)$$

where V_{bl} is the volume of the blood compartment; C is concentration; Q is blood flow; bl, br, ot, k, and l represent the blood, brain, other tissues, kidney, and liver compartments, respectively; and vbr, vot, vk, and vl represent the venous blood leaving the organs. Q_c is the total blood flow equal to the sum of the venous blood flows from each organ.

In contrast, the physiological model in Fig. 7-12 does not feature an explicit blood compartment. For simplicity, the blood volumes of the heart and the major blood vessels that are not within organs are assumed to be negligible. The venous concentration of a chemical returning to the lungs is simply the weighted average of the concentrations in the venous blood emerging from the tissues.

$$C_v = (Q_1 \cdot C_{vl} + Q_{rp} \cdot C_{vrp} + Q_{pp} \cdot C_{vpp} + Q_f \cdot C_{vf})/Q_c \qquad (7\text{–}28)$$

where C is concentration; Q is blood flow; l, rp, pp, and f represent the liver, richly perfused, poorly perfused, and fat tissue compartments, respectively; and vl, vrp, vpp, and vf represent the venous blood leaving the corresponding organs. Q_c is the total blood flow equal to the sum of the blood flows exiting each organ.

In the physiological model in Fig. 7-12, the blood concentration entering each tissue compartment is the arterial concentration (C_{art}) that was calculated above for the lung compartment (Equation (7-24)). The decision to use one formulation as opposed to another to describe blood in a physiological model depends on the role the blood plays in disposition and the type of application. If the toxicokinetics after iv injection is to be simulated or if binding to or metabolism by blood components is suspected, a separate compartment for the blood that incorporates these additional processes is required. A blood compartment is obviously needed if the model were developed to explain a set of blood concentration–time data for a toxicant. However, if blood is simply a conduit to the other compartments, as in the case for inhaled volatile organics shown in Fig. 7-12, the algebraic solution is acceptable.

Fig. 7-18 shows the application of physiological modeling in elucidating the disposition fate of methylmercury and its

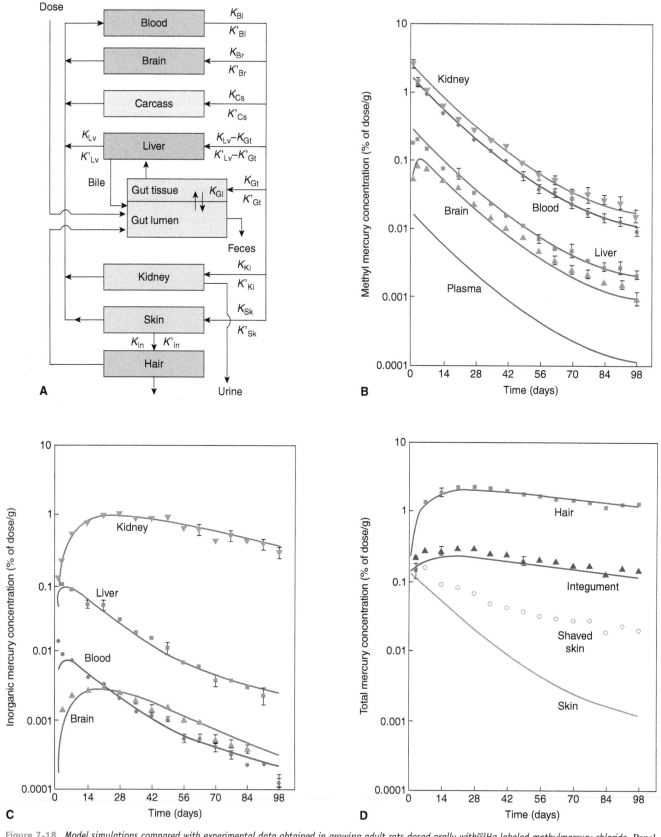

Figure 7-18. *Model simulations compared with experimental data obtained in growing adult rats dosed orally with*[203]*Hg-labeled methylmercury chloride.* Panel (**A**) shows the physiological model for methylmercury and its demethylated product, inorganic mercury. Primed symbols denote the parameters for inorganic mercury. Panels (**B**) and (**C**) show the respective time course of methylmercury and inorganic mercury concentration in blood, liver, kidneys, and the brain. Panel (**D**) shows the slow accumulation of total mercury in hair and skin, or the integument (skin plus hair). (Reprinted from Farris *et al.*, 1993, with permission from Elsevier.)

demethylated product, inorganic mercury following a single per-oral administration in the growing adult rat (Farris *et al.*, 1993). The model scheme presented in Panel A for both the organic and inorganic forms of mercury has the following unique features: (1) increase in compartment size due to growth over the long duration of the tissue washout experiment; (2) mercury enters the gut lumen via biliary excretion and secretory transport from gut tissue to lumen, some of which is reabsorbed; (3) uptake of methylmercury from blood into tissues, except for the brain, is assumed to be rate-limited by plasma flow because of sequestration of mercury in rat erythrocytes and its slow release; (4) uptake of methylmercury across the blood–brain barrier is rate-limited by transport; (5) uptake of inorganic mercury into all tissues, except the liver, is limited by permeability/transport; (6) mercury is transferred from skin into hair, where it is irreversibly bound; and (7) mercury in hair is either shed or ingested by the animal during grooming. The model simulations displayed in Panels B, C, and D show two prominent features of methylmercurcy disposition: (1) methylmercury is rapidly demethylated to inorganic mercury, which is slowly eliminated from the brain and the kidneys, two major sites of methylmercury toxicities; and (2) a significant portion of mercury is sequestered in hair and the ingestion of hair by the animal contributes to the remarkable persistence of mercury in the rat. This example illustrates the capability of physiological models to deal with the varied and complex disposition kinetics of toxicants from a wide range of sources under a multitude of experimental and environmental exposure scenarios.

Conclusions

The second section provides an introduction to the simpler elements of physiological models and the important assumptions that underlie model structures. For more detailed aspects of physiological modeling, the readers can consult several in-depth and well-annotated reviews on physiologically based toxicokinetic models (Clewell and Anderson, 1994, 1996; O'Flaherty, 1998; Krishnan and Anderson, 2001; Krishnan *et al.*, 2002; Andersen, 2003). Computer softwares are available for numerically integrating the system of differential equations that form the models. Investigators have successfully used Advanced Continuous Simulation Language (Pharsight Corp, Palo Alto, CA), Simulation Control Program (Simulation Resources, Inc, Berrien Springs, MI), MATLAB (The MathWorks, Inc, Natick, MA), and SAS software applications to name a few. Choice of software depends on prior experience, familiarity with the computer language used, and cost of the software package.

The field of physiological modeling continues to evolve as toxicologists and pharmacologists develop increasingly more sophisticated applications. Three-dimensional visualizations of xenobiotic transport in fish and vapor transport in the rodent nose, physiological models of a parent chemical linked in series with one or more active metabolites, models describing biochemical interactions among xenobiotics, and more biologically realistic descriptions of tissues previously viewed as simple lumped compartments are just a few of the more sophisticated applications. Finally, physiologically based toxicokinetic models are now being linked to biologically based toxicodynamic models to simulate the entire exposure → dose → response paradigm that is basic to the science of toxicology.

BIOLOGICAL MONITORING

This final section considers some of the basic toxicokinetic principles and methods underlying the practice of biological monitoring, which over the past several decades has become an important tool for assessment of environmental health risk, first in occupational exposure and more recently in general population exposure. Biological monitoring or biomonitoring is defined as the systematic sampling of body fluids, and at times body tissue, for the purpose of estimating an individual's internal dose from exposure to chemicals in the workplace or assessing the range of internal exposure within a select population to environmental pollutants (Manno and Viau, 2010; Paustenbach and Galbraith, 2006). The advantages of biomonitoring over traditional environmental monitoring, such as ambient or personal air sampling or dermal dosimetry, include the accounting of other unanticipated routes of exposure, individual differences in toxicant absorption and disposition, and critical personal or lifestyle variables, such as body size and composition, workload that affects pulmonary ventilation, or cigarette smoking that could affect the metabolic status of an individual. Linking environmental exposure or dose to measurements of concentration of the parent chemical or its metabolite(s) in a biological sample is essentially an exercise in toxicokinetics.

Biomonitoring Reference

Although biomonitoring provides a measure of internal exposure, in the final analysis the data obtained must be relatable to a probable degree of health risk. Hence, for each chemical of concern a reference value must be established that corresponds to a threshold limit, below which a reasonable assurance of safety exist and above which significant risk to the exposed individual or population becomes likely.

In the occupational setting, the concept of Biological Exposure Index (BEI) has been established by the American Conference of Governmental Industrial Hygienists (ACGIH) since early 1980s. BEI for a given chemical exposure represented "...the level of the determinant most likely to be observed in the specimens collected from a worker with an internal dose equivalent to that arising solely from inhalation exposure at the TLV" (Morgan, 1997). Threshold limit values (TLVs) are the reference values recommended by ACGIH for airborne chemical concentrations in the workplace, below which nearly all workers may be exposed repeatedly over a working lifetime without known adverse health effects. BEIs for various industrial chemicals have been established through controlled exposure studies in a laboratory setting and/or simultaneous ambient exposure and biological sampling in the workplace. BEIs have also been estimated through the use of physiologically based modeling and simulations (Leung, 1992). The modeling approach is particularly attractive as it can readily simulate a wide variety of exposure condition, along with the ability to vary personal variables such as the level of physical exertion in a hypothetical worker. The impact of interindividual variability in physiological parameters on the BEI can also be evaluated using physiological models coupled with Monte Carlo simulations (Thomas *et al.*, 1996).

A similar referencing concept, referred to as the Biomonitoring Equivalents (BEs) approach, has also been proposed in population environmental exposure context. For BEs, available toxicokinetic data are used to convert an existing exposure guidance value (eg, reference doses or concentrations—RfDs or RfCs, minimal risk levels—MRLs, tolerable daily intakes—TDIs, or a unit cancer risk—UCR) into an equivalent concentration in a biological sample (Hays and Aylward, 2009). As in the case of BEIs, the conversion can be accomplished using classic or physiological models (Hays *et al.*, 2007).

It should be noted that in both settings, the measurement of parent chemical and/or its metabolite in a chosen biological matrix serves as a biomarker for exposure, which in turn allows for health risk assessment based on generally accepted environmental exposure–risk data. It remains to be seen whether at some future time evidence providing a direct link between biological monitoring of internal dose and health risk will become available in both the occupational and general environmental settings.

Monitoring Strategy

The design of an optimal sampling strategy for biomonitoring is guided by three key considerations: (1) sampling matrix or site that includes blood, urine, exhaled breath, saliva, or hair; (2) choice of the determinant(s) (ie, parent compound and/or metabolites); and (3) sampling time relative to the exposure routine, especially when exposure is intermittent. In addition, normalization procedures have been proposed for some matrices to account for variation in individual physiological condition at the time of sampling. These issues are, in many cases, interrelated.

Decision on sampling time relative to the exposure pattern would be a straightforward matter if exposure was continuous and constant, in which case blood, urine, or other samples can be collected at any time after steady state is reached, that is, after 4 elimination half-lives have elapsed since the start of exposure. In reality, exposure is often episodic or intermittent, and in occupational setting exposure is dictated by the work shift.

Specific sampling times are recommended by ACGIH for each BEI. The commonly designated times include the end of shift, prior to start of a workday, the end of the last shift of the workweek, and the morning after returning from the weekend. The end-of-shift is a reasonable time to assess daily peak exposure for workplace chemicals that have reasonably short elimination half-lives (<6 hours) such that carryover from day to day is not significant (see Fig. 7-10). For chemicals that have elimination half-lives in the order of 12 to 24 hours (or longer), the end of the last shift of the week would be a better measure of peak exposure (see the 24-hour $T_{1/2}$ example in Fig. 7-10). For chemicals that have multiphasic washout kinetics (ie, kinetics conforming to a multicompartmental model), timing of sample collection relative to the end of exposure in the immediate after-shift period is critical when the early disposition half-life of the parent compound prevails and could be very short (eg, in the order of minutes). This renders the end-of-shift sampling imprecise because of the high degree of measurement variability, such is the case with blood or breath toluene samples taken at the end-of-shift (Morgan, 1997). One solution is to collect the sample just before the worker returns to the next shift on the day following or after a weekend, by which time washout kinetics has reached the terminal phase with an acceptably long half-life, so as to provide a more reproducible index. Finally, repeat sampling over days or weeks are often needed to firmly establish a representative exposure pattern in individual or groups of workers.

Systematically timed sampling is hardly feasible in a community population exposure study, where sampling is typically random, and exposure comes from diffuse sources and may not occur with any definable regularity. The only approach to overcome such shortcoming is to obtain samples at different times of a day to provide diurnal coverage, which introduces obvious logistical and cost challenges in a population surveillance program.

The choice of determinant or biomarker and the sampling matrix are interrelated. Monitoring of parent compound in blood or urine is preferred, particularly if toxicology of the chemical is attributed to the parent entity. In those instances where a metabolite is solely responsible for or contribute to the adverse effects of exposure, monitoring of the active metabolite, along with the parent compound, would be a logical approach. Inactive metabolite(s) is(are) often times monitored as a surrogate marker in place of the parent toxicant due to its relative abundance, ease of analysis, and desirable toxicokinetic properties. For many chemicals, urinary excretion is not a principal route of elimination. At the same time, polar metabolites are often removed by renal excretion; hence, metabolites are present at high concentrations in urine. For example, hippuric acid (glycine conjugate of the major oxidation metabolite of toluene, benzoic acid) in urine is an accepted BEI for toluene exposure. For chemicals that have inherently short elimination half-life or effectively short washout half-life due to a prominent distribution phase, metabolite(s) with longer elimination half-life may be a more suitable biomarker (ie, being less sensitive to sampling time variation). It should, however, be noted that metabolite levels are governed by both its formation kinetics from parent chemical and its own elimination kinetics; hence, individual differences in metabolite elimination represents an additional sources of variability for metabolite monitoring. Hence, the kinetic advantage of metabolite monitoring is not predictable and must be assessed on a case-by-case basis.

It is not often appreciated that the observed level of a determinant for a chemical exposure is a function not only of current exposure, but also what happened some time before (Droz et al., 1991). This is particular so when exposure is continuous or the interval between intermittent exposures is on the order of the chemical's elimination half-life (eg, an elimination $T_{1/2}$ of 24 hours or longer when exposure reoccurs on a daily basis). In other words, the elimination half-life of a biomarker or index compound dictates how far back in exposure history it reports. For example, exposure to the degreaser solvent, trichloroethylene results in urinary excretion of trichloroethanol (TCE) and trichloroacetic acid (TCA). The elimination $T_{1/2}$ of TCE is known to be 3 to 5 hours, whereas that of TCA ranges from 48 to 96 hours. Measuring these 2 metabolites in urine allows one to estimate the exposure of a worker to trichloroethylene during the current work shift with TEC and in the preceding workweek with TCA (Lowry, 1987). A corollary to this principle is the fact that short half-life biomarkers reflect more of the within day or day-to-day fluctuation in exposure, whereas daily fluctuation in exposure is dampened with long half-life biomarkers. Although the former cases may be viewed as undesirable because of variability in the measurement, it offers a better reflection of the oscillation in internal dose and particularly the transient peak exposures. The latter cases provide a less variable, time-averaged measure of exposure.

In addition to the above consideration of determinant abundance, the choice of sampling matrix is driven by ease of sampling and reliability in respect to inter- and intraindividual variations. The advantages and disadvantages for each of the common biological matrices are considered below.

Blood   Blood concentration of determinant(s) is the most representative biological sample, because it should be in equilibrium with all tissue concentrations in the postdistribution phase (Fig. 7-2, right panels). This consideration extends to the relationship of blood concentration to other biological fluids (eg, urine and saliva); as such, concentration of determinant in all other biological fluids (eg, urine and saliva) indirectly reflects the concentration in blood. The major drawbacks of blood sampling are its invasive nature, subject acceptance, and the need for qualified medical personnel to perform blood draw. For environmental pollutants that are sequestered in adipose tissue, fat-soluble fraction of blood has been proposed as a more practical substitute for adipose tissue sampling (Paustenbach and Galbraith, 2006).

Urine Ease in collection is often cited as a major advantage of sampling urine for biomonitoring; unfortunately, it belies the kinetic complexity involved in the analysis of urinary biomarker data. As mentioned earlier, monitoring of parent compound in urine only applies to a few chemicals that are excreted in significant amounts in urine; in most cases, metabolite(s) are measured in urine. Hence, the elimination kinetics of the marker metabolite need to be taken into account in data interpretation.

There are several types of urine collection: (1) timed collection over 24 hours or several hours; (2) spot urine usually from random collection; and (3) first morning specimen (Hill *et al.*, 1988). The timed urine collection should be performed according to the "double-void" protocol. Urine is collected after first emptying the bladder and then waiting until the next voiding. For extended collection, say over 24 hours, multiple in-between voids are collected and pooled with the final voiding at the end of the collection period. Timed urine collection affords a measure of the total amount of determinant excreted or the average excretion rate of the determinant over a defined time period. Spot urine, either from first morning sample or other times during the day, offers a measure of the urinary concentration of the determinant. The first morning sample has the advantage of being a concentrated overnight sample.

In order to appreciate the applicability and limitation of various urine collection methods in biomonitoring, a brief review of urinary excretion kinetics is in order. As was shown in the "Clearance" section, urinary excretion rate (dU_B/dt) of a biomarker or determinant is related to its concentration in blood or plasma concentration (C) by renal clearance (Cl_r).

$$\frac{dU_B}{dt} = Cl_r \cdot C \qquad (7\text{--}29)$$

It should be noted that dU_B/dt represents an average urinary excretion over a relatively short collection interval; C is the blood or plasma concentration at the mid-time point. The differential form of Equation (7-29) can be integrated over an extended collection period, say 24 hours, to yield a relationship between the total amount excreted in the collection period ($U_{B,24}$) and the corresponding area under the blood or plasma concentration–time curve (AUC_{0-24}, an integral measure of exposure).

$$U_{B,24h} = Cl_r \cdot AUC_{0-24} \qquad (7\text{--}30)$$

Hence, either excretion rate or cumulative excretion over a defined collection period of a urinary biomarker is the most appropriate index secondary to blood concentration measurement. Unfortunately timed urine collection is not widely adopted because of logistical difficulties in the occupational setting and cost issue in a population surveillance system.

Urinary excretion rate is in turn related to pooled urine concentration ($C_{UB,\Delta t}$) and urinary flow rate ($V_{\Delta t}/\Delta t$).

$$\frac{dU_B}{dt} = C_{UB,\Delta t} \cdot \left(\frac{V_{\Delta t}}{\Delta t} \right) \qquad (7\text{--}31)$$

Urinary concentration as measured from spot collection offers convenience and flexibility; however, it has the distinct disadvantage of being influenced by urine flow rate, which varies greatly from time to time depending on the hydration state of the individual. Several methods have been proposed to adjust for variation in urine flow rate. Urinary creatinine is most often used to normalize urinary concentration data. The following equation shows one such normalization (Garde *et al.*, 2011).

$$U_{B,24} = \left(\frac{C_{UB}}{C_{UCr}} \right) \cdot U_{Cr,24} \qquad (7\text{--}32)$$

where C_{UB} and C_{UCr} are the respective biomarker and creatinine concentration in the spot urine collection, and $U_{Cr,24}$ is the daily urinary output of creatinine. This method assumes that blood concentration of biomarker is reasonably constant throughout the day (eg, during stable, continuous exposure or for a chemical with very long elimination half-life). The daily urinary output of creatinine is assumed to be constant between individual; alternately, it can also be adjusted according to individual variables that are known to affect creatinine production: body mass, age, and sex (Boeniger *et al.*, 1993).

An alternate, more commonly adopted normalization is to simply express the amount of biomarker in the spot urine collection per mmol of creatinine. This simple normalization is valid for spot urine collection if we assume creatinine excretion is constant throughout the day and reproducible from individual to individual, which are often not true. It is not surprising that validity of normalizing urinary biomarker to per mmol creatinine has been questioned (Boeniger *et al.*, 1993). Other normalization methods including adjustment to a standard urine flow rate, specific gravity, or osmolality have also been proposed (Hill *et al.*, 1988; Boeniger *et al.*, 1993).

The performance of these various normalization procedures has not been subject to rigorous comparison. It is doubtful any of them could offer a facile solution to the inherently difficult problem posed by spot urine collection in face of the known physiological variability in diuresis and creatinine production and excretion.

Breath Breath sampling is applicable to biomonitoring of volatile organic compounds (VOCs) including many industrial solvents. In some instances, it can be extended to volatile metabolites of non-volatile organic chemicals. Breath sampling offers the advantages of being noninvasive and can be performed rapidly, especially when repeated sampling at short time intervals is needed.

The utility of breath sample as a biomarker rests on the assumption that during exposure, VOC in the inspired air reaches the alveoli where it undergoes equilibrium exchange with the arterial blood, which in theory is predicted by the blood/air partition coefficient in vitro (see "Specialized Compartment: Lung"). This alveolar equilibrium assumption is valid for VOCs that have blood/air partition coefficients exceeding 10 (Kelman, 1982). Likewise, in the postexposure situation, unmetabolized volatile compound in mixed venous blood comes into equilibrium exchange with alveolar air, which is exhaled and sampled. Hence, breath sampling can provide an estimate of arterial blood concentration of VOCs based on their known blood/air partition coefficients (Wallace *et al.*, 1996). Partition coefficients for a large number of VOCs have been determined from in vitro studies; most have been validated by blood/breath ratios observed in controlled exposure studies in human subjects at ppm levels that are encountered in occupational settings. There are data to suggest that blood/breath ratio of some VOCs may increase at low ppb exposure levels typically present in the general environment (see example with benzene, Perbellini *et al.*, 1988).

Only 350 mL of the 500 mL inspired volume (tidal volume) actually ventilate the alveoli and undergo gaseous exchange. About 150 mL of inspired air is held in the anatomical dead space between the nose or mouth and the respiratory bronchioles. As a result, expired air when collected in total is a mixture of alveolar air and dead space air. If sampling is done during exposure, the dead space air has a VOC concentration of the last inspired air. If sampling is done postexposure, the dead space air would have a near zero or background VOC concentration (Hill *et al.*, 1988). Therefore, total breath collection is not appropriate for biomonitoring. It has been suggested that mixed expired air concentration can be normalized to alveolar concentration using the observed CO_2 concentration (Wilson, 1986). However, this proposed method of normalization has not been sufficiently validated for VOCs of environmental interest.

Alveolar concentration is best measured by collecting the last part of an expiration (about 200 mL), that is, the end-expired or end-tidal air (Wilson, 1986; Hill *et al.*, 1988). Various devices for collection of end-expired air have been described (Wilson, 1986; Wilson and Monster, 1999). Breath holding and rebreathing techniques have also been proposed to promote equilibration of VOCs between alveolar air and blood in the pulmonary capillaries.

The major difficulty with breath as a biomonitoring matrix is achieving reproducible sampling. Success is critically dependent on strict adherence to a standardized breathing and collection protocol aimed at maintaining a consistent blood/breath ratio between occasions. It is well documented that variability is introduced when subjects breathe too quickly (hyperventilate) or breathe too slowly (hypoventilate) (Wilson, 1986; Hill *et al.*, 1988). Physical activity or workload, which affects ventilation–perfusion of the lungs, is known to alter end-expired air concentration of some VOCs (Wilson, 1986). Finally, standardization of volume and concentration from ambient condition during measurement to body temperature, pressure and water vapor saturation (Hill *et al.*, 1988), along with minor adjustment for contamination of dead space air in end-expired sample using CO_2 level have been proposed to improve the estimation of alveolar air concentration (Wallace *et al.*, 1996).

Saliva Saliva has drawn attention as a matrix for biomonitoring because of ease in its collection. Transfer of drugs and xenobiotics from blood into saliva occurs via diffusion across the salivary glands and is known to depend on the compound's lipophilicity and ionization (Caporossi *et al.*, 2010). Saliva contains a low concentration of proteins, mainly albumin derived from plasma and glycoproteins, which impart viscosity and protect the buccal epithelium. As a result, saliva/plasma ratio for neutral, nonprotein bound compounds is expected to be about one. Compounds that are highly bound to plasma proteins can have a saliva/plasma ratio well below one. Saliva pH is usually less than that of plasma; hence, in the absence of binding to plasma proteins, acidic compounds are predicted to have a saliva/plasma ratio less than one, whereas basic compounds could have saliva/plasma ratios greater than one due to pH trapping.

There are several ways to collect saliva. Most often whole saliva is collected, which is a complex mixture of oral fluids, including salivary gland secretions, gingival crevicular fluids, expectorated bronchial and nasal secretions, and even trace of serum and blood from oral bleeding. Whole saliva can be collected by spitting into a vial, wiping the oral cavity with a swap, or using commercially available collectors (eg, Salivette). Stimulants of salivary flow, such as citric acid and chewing gum, have been used to facilitate collection and increase the sample volume. Blood/saliva ratio could differ between stimulated and unstimulated collection condition; for example, change in saliva pH is associated with an increase in salivary flow, which may affect transfer of ionizable compounds into saliva. Direct collection of secretion from the parotid gland for therapeutic monitoring of drug level has been attempted using special collection devices.

In order to apply saliva sampling to biomonitoring, a consistent relationship between blood and saliva concentrations of the determinant is required. This has proven to be a problem for metals and industrial chemicals. For example, the use of saliva

for monitoring of Hg and Pb has been investigated in a number of studies. In many instances, Hg or Pb levels in saliva were below the limit of detection, or when detected poor correlations between concentrations in saliva and those in blood were observed. Use of saliva has also been evaluated for several pesticides, polychlorinated biphenyls (PCBs), polychlorinated dibenzo-*p*-dioxins (PCDDs), and industrial chemicals with mixed results (Esteban and Castaño, 2009; Caporossi *et al.*, 2010). More data will be required to assess the applicability of saliva in occupational and environmental biomonitoring.

Hair Hair is easy to collect, transport, and store. As hair grows out of the hair follicle, it carries with it a record of past exposure that stretch over weeks to many months. In fact, a temporal exposure pattern can be reconstructed by segmental analysis of a strand of hair. As such, hair is a unique biomonitor of cumulative exposure and is best suited for environmental pollutants that have long elimination half-lives in the order of days to weeks. The main disadvantages of hair as a biological matrix are the difficulty in differentiating external and internal exposure and the variable influence of hair pigmentation and hair care. Assay of biomarkers in the typical quantity of hair collected (50–200 mg) also requires highly sensitive analytical methodologies.

Hair has been used as a matrix for human biomonitoring of exposure to methylmercury for a number of years (Esteban and Castaño, 2009). A strong correlation exists between total Hg in hair and dietary intake of methylmercury, mainly through fish consumption. A predictable relation between hair Hg and blood Hg has also been documented; hence, hair Hg is an acceptable biomarker for the internal dose of Hg from methylmercury exposure. There are also adequate data to support the use of hair measurement as an indicator for occupational and environmental Pb exposure. In contrast, conflicting data exist on the relationship between hair Cd and body burden of Cd.

Much less is known in regards to hair as a biomonitor for organic pollutants (Appenzeller and Tsatsakis, 2012). Pesticides, particularly organochlorine pesticides, are the most investigated environmental pollutants in hair. Indeed hair sampling has been used to monitor workplace exposure to pesticides, as well as PCDDs, polychlorinated dibenzofurans (PCDFs), and coplanar PCBs; however, these reports offer mostly descriptive information (eg, percent of individuals being positive for presence of test pollutants in hair samples, levels of pollutants present in the hair) and have rarely evaluated the relationship of hair pollutant concentration to environmental levels or corresponding concentrations in blood and other biological matrices. Hence, the feasibility of hair sampling for occupational and environmental biomonitoring awaits further research.

Conclusions

The toxicokinetic principles that guide the design of biological monitoring have been established through more than two decades of occupational health research and are now being extended to assessment of population health risk from exposure to environmental pollutants. With the forthcoming of the wealth of environmental biomonitoring data that have recently been collected by public health agencies, such as the U.S. Centers for Disease Control and Prevention (CDC), much more will be learned in regards to biomonitoring strategy as it is applied to surveillance of low level environmental exposure in the various community settings. Even in the occupational health sector, more research is needed to improve the existing biomonitoring methods and technologies so that they become more cost-effective and in turn widen its adoption at the workplace.

REFERENCES

Andersen ME. A physiologically based toxicokinetic description of the metabolism of inhaled gases and vapors: analysis at steady state. *Toxicol Appl Pharmacol.* 1981;60:509–526.

Andersen ME. Physiological modeling of organic compounds. *Ann Occup Hyg.* 1991;35:309–321.

Andersen ME. Toxicokinetic modeling and its applications in chemical risk assessment. *Toxicol Lett.* 2003;138:9–27.

Andersen ME, Gargas ML, Ramsey JC. Inhalation pharmacokinetics: evaluating systemic extraction, total *in vivo* metabolism, and the time course of enzyme induction for inhaled styrene in rats based on arterial blood:inhaled air concentration ratios. *Toxicol Appl Pharmacol.* 1984;73:176–187.

Andersen ME, Mills JJ, Gargas ML, et al. Modeling receptor-mediated processes with dioxin: implications for pharmacokinetics and risk assessment. *Risk Anal.* 1993;13:25–36.

Appenzeller BM, Tsatsakis AM. Hair analysis for biomonitoring of environmental and occupational exposure to organic pollutants—state of the art, critical review and future needs. *Toxicol Lett.* 2012;210:119–140.

Bertilsson L, Tomson T, Tybring G. Pharmacokinetics: time-dependent changes—autoinduction of carbamazepine epoxidation. *J Clin Pharmacol.* 1986;26:459–462.

Boeniger MF, Lowry LL, Rosenberg J. Interpretation of urine results used to assess chemical exposure with emphasis on creatinine adjustments—a review. *Am Ind Hyg Assoc J.* 1993;54:615–627.

Brown RP, Delp MD, Lindstedt SL, et al. Physiological parameter values for physiologically based pharmacokinetic models. *Toxicol Ind Health.* 1997;13:407–484.

Burbacher TM, Shen DD, Lalovic B, et al. Chronic maternal methanol inhalation in nonhuman primates (*Macaca fascicularis*): exposure and toxicokinetics prior to and during pregnancy. *Neurotoxicol Teratol.* 2004;26:201–221.

Caporossi L, Santoro A, Papaleo B. Saliva as an analytical matrix: state of the art and application for biomonitoring. *Biomarkers.* 2010;15:475–487.

Clewell HJ IIIrd, Andersen ME. Physiologically-based pharmacokinetic modeling and bioactivation of xenobiotics. *Toxicol Ind Health.* 1994;10:1–24.

Clewell HJ IIIrd, Andersen ME. Use of physiologically based pharmacokinetic modeling to investigate individual versus population risk. *Toxicology.* 1996;111:315–329.

Collins AS, Sumner SCJ, Borghoff SJ, et al. A physiological model for tert-amyl methyl ether and *tert*-amyl alcohol: hypothesis testing of model structures. *Toxicol Sci.* 1999;49:15–28.

Droz PO, Berode M, Wu NN. Evaluation of concomitant biological and air monitoring results. *Appl Occup Environ Hyg.* 1991;6:465–474.

Esteban M, Castaño A. Non-invasive matrices in human biomonitoring—a review. *Environ Int.* 2009;35:438–449.

Farris FF, Dedrick RL, Allen P, et al. Physiological model for the pharmacokientics of methyl mercury in the growing rat. *Toxciol Appl Pharmacol.* 1993;119:74–90.

Garde H, Hansen A, Kristiansen J, et al. Comparison of uncertainties related to standardization of urine samples with volume and creatinine correction. *Ann Occup Hyg.* 2004;48:171–179.

Gargas ML, Andersen ME. Physiologically based approaches for examining the pharmacokinetics of inhaled vapors. In: Gardner DE, Crapo JD, Massaro EJ, eds. *Toxicology of the Lung.* New York: Raven Press; 1988:449–476.

Gerlowski LE, Jain RK. Physiologically based pharmacokinetic modeling: principles and applications. *J Pharm Sci.* 1983;72:1103–1127.

Gibaldi M, Perrier D. *Pharmacokinetics.* 2nd ed. New York: Marcel Dekker; 1982.

Haggard HW. The absorption, distribution, and elimination of ethyl ether: II. Analysis of the mechanism of the absorption and elimination of such a gas or vapor as ethyl ether. *J Biol Chem.* 1924;49:753–770.

Hays SM, Aylward LL. Using biomonitoring equivalents to interpret human biomonitoring data in a public health risk context. *J Appl Toxicol.* 2009;29:275–288.

Hays SM, Becker RA, Leung HW, et al. Biomonitoring equivalents: a screening approach for interpreting biomonitoring results from a public health risk perspective. *Regul Toxicol Pharmacol.* 2007;47:96–109.

Hill RH, Guillemin M, Droz PO. Sample collection. In Kneip TJ, Crable JV, eds. *Methods for Biological Monitoring.* Washington, DC: American Public Health Association; 1988:37–63, Chap. 6.

Himmelstein KJ, Lutz RJ. A review of the applications of physiologically based pharmacokinetic modeling. *J Pharmacokinet Biopharm.* 1979;7:127–145.

Iwatsubo T, Hirota N, Ooie T, et al. Prediction of in vivo drug metabolism in the human liver from in vitro metabolism data. *Pharmacol Ther.* 1997;73:147–171.

Kelman GR. Theoretical basis of alveolar sampling. *Br J Ind Med.* 1982;39:259–264.

Krishnan K, Anderson ME. Physiologically based pharmacokinetic modeling in toxicology. In: Hayes AW, ed. *Principles and Methods of Toxicology.* Philadelphia: Taylor & Francis; 2001:193–241.

Krishnan K, Haddad S, Beliveau M, et al. Physiological modeling and extrapolation of pharmacokinetic interactions from binary to more complex chemical mixtures. *Environ Health Perspect.* 2002;110(suppl 6):989–994.

Leung HW. Use of physiologically based pharmacokinetic models to establish biological exposure indexes. *Am Ind Hyg Assoc J.* 1992;53:369–374.

Lin JH, Sugiyama Y, Awazu S, et al. In vitro and in vivo evaluation of the tissue-to-blood partition coefficient for physiological pharmacokinetic models. *J Pharmacokinet Biopharm.* 1982;10:637–647.

Lowry LK. The biological exposure index: its use in assessing chemical exposures in the workplace. *Toxicology.* 1987;47:55–69.

Lutz RJ, Dedrick RL, Zaharko DS. Physiological pharmacokinetics: an in vivo approach to membrane transport. *Pharmacol Ther.* 1980;11:559–592.

MacGregor JT, Collins JM, Sugiyama Y, et al. In vitro human tissue models in risk assessment: report of a consensus-building workshop. *Toxicol Sci.* 2001;59:17–36.

Manno M, Viau C. Biomonitoring for occupational health risk assessment (BOHRA). *Toxicol Lett.* 2010;192:3–16.

Miners JO, Knights KM, Houston JB, et al. In vitro-in vivo correlation for drugs and other compounds eliminated by glucuronidation in humans: pitfalls and promises. *Biochem Pharmacol.* 2006;71:1531–1539.

Mintun M, Himmelstein KJ, Schroder RL, et al. Tissue distribution kinetics of tetraethylammonium ion in the rat. *J Pharmacokinet Biopharm.* 1980;8:373–409.

Morgan MS. The biological exposure indices: a key component in protecting workers from toxic chemicals. *Environ Health Perspect.* 1997;105 (suppl 1):105–115.

Nichols J, Rheingans P, Lothenbach D, et al. Three-dimensional visualization of physiologically based kinetic model outputs. *Environ Health Perspect.* 1994;102:952–956.

O'Flaherty EJ. Physiologically based models of metal kinetics. *Crit Rev Toxicol.* 1998;28:271–317.

Paustenbach D, Galbraith D. Biomonitoring and biomarkers: exposure assessment will never be the same. *Environ Health Perspect.* 2006;114:1143–1149.

Perbellini L, Faccini GB, Pasini F, et al. Environmental and occupational exposure to benzene by analysis of breath and blood. *Br J Ind Med.* 1988;45:345–352.

Ramsey JC, Andersen ME. A physiologically based description of the inhalation pharmacokinetics of styrene in rats and humans. *Toxicol Appl Pharmacol.* 1984;73:159–175.

Rowland M. Physiologic pharmacokinetic models: relevance, experience, and future trends. *Drug Metab Rev.* 1984;15:55–74.

Rowland M. Physiologic pharmacokinetic models and interanimal species scaling. *Pharmacol Ther.* 1985;29:49–68.

Rowland M, Tozer TN. *Clinical Pharmacokinetics and Pharmacodynamics–Concepts and Applications.* Philadelphia: Wolters Kluwer/Lippincott, Williams & Wilkins; 2011.

Schentag JJ, Jusko WJ. Renal clearance and tissue accumulation of gentamicin. *Clin Pharmacol Ther.* 1977;22:364–370.

CHAPTER 7

TOXICOKINETICS

Teorell T. Kinetics of distribution of substances administered to the body: I. The extravascular modes of administration. *Arch Int Pharmacodyn Ther.* 1937;57:205–225.

Thomas RS, Bigelow PL, Keefe TJ, et al. Variability in biological exposure indices using physiologically based pharmacokinetic modeling and Monte Carlo simulation. *Am Ind Hyg Assoc J.* 1996;57:23–32.

Thummel KE, Shen DD, Isoherranen N, Smith HE. Appendix II. Design and optimization of dosage regimens: pharmacokinetic data. In: Brunton LL, Parker KL, Buxton IOL, Blumenthal DK, eds. *Goodman & Gilman's: The Pharmacological Basis of Therapeutics.* 11th ed. The McGraw-Hill Companies; 2006.

Tozer NT, Rowland M. *Introduction to Pharmacokinetics and Pharmacodynamics: The Quantitative Basis of Drug Therapy.* Lippincott Williams & Wilkins; 2006:75.

Travis CC, Quillen JL, Arms AD. Pharmacokinetics of benzene. *Toxicol Appl Pharmacol.* 1990;102:400–420.

Wallace L, Buckley T, Pellizzari E, et al. Breath measurements as volatile organic compound biomarkers. *Environ Health Perspect.* 1996;104(suppl 5):861–869.

Wilkinson GR. Clearance approaches in pharmacology. *Pharmacol Rev.* 1987;39:1–47.

Wilson HK. Breath analysis: physiological basis and sampling techniques. *Scand J Work Environ Health.* 1986;12:174–192.

Wilson HK, Monster AC. New technologies in the use of exhaled breath analysis for biological monitoring. *Occup Environ Med.* 1999;56: 753–757.

Unit III

Non-Organ-Directed Toxicity

chapter 8

Chemical Carcinogenesis

James E. Klaunig

OVERVIEW

Cancer is a disease characterized by mutation, modified gene expression, cell proliferation, and aberrant cell growth. It ranks as one of the leading causes of death in the world. In the United States, cancer ranks as the second leading cause of death, with over one million new cases of cancer diagnosed and more than 1.5 million Americans dying from cancer annually. Multiple causes of cancer have been established including infectious agents, radiation, and chemicals. Estimates suggest that 70% to 90% of all human cancers have a linkage to environmental, dietary, and behavioral factors (Fig. 8-1). Although our understanding of the biology of the progression from a normal cell to a malignant one has advanced considerably in the past several decades, many aspects of the cause, prevention, and treatment of human cancer in particular the influence of lifestyle remain unresolved.

HISTORICAL BACKGROUND

A strong historical foundation for the linkage of the induction of cancer by chemicals has been documented (Table 8-1). Several excellent reviews of the historical background of carcinogenesis and cancer research have been published (Creech, 2000; Diamandopoulos, 1996; Shimkin, 2008). Studies over the last three centuries on chemically induced cancer are marked initially by epidemiological observations followed by experimental studies involving animal carcinogenesis models.

In 1775, Percival Pott described a linkage between the increased occurrence of scrotal and nasal cancer among chimney sweeps and their occupation. Pott concluded that chimney soot was the causative agent for cancer induction in these individuals (Pott, 1775). Other investigators also recognized an association between exposure to chemicals and the induction of human cancer.

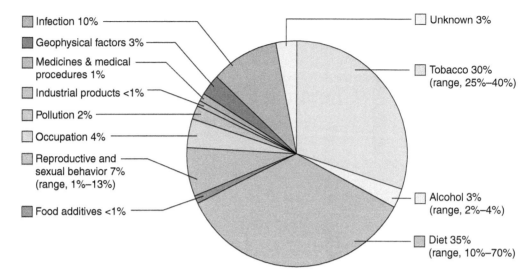

Figure 8-1. *Proportions of human cancer deaths attributed to various factors.* (Reproduced with permission from [no authors listed] Harvard reports on cancer prevention: causes of human cancer. Center for Cancer Prevention Harvard School of Public Health. *Cancer Causes and Control.* 1996;7 (Suppl 1):S3–S4, 1996.)

Thiersch (1875) described a relationship between sunlight exposure and skin cancer in humans. A linkage between an increased incidence of lung cancer and uranium mining was detected (Harting and Hesse, 1879). Butlin, in a follow-up of the Potts' observations, noted that scrotal cancer in chimney sweeps in the European continent was relatively rare on the continent compared to that seen in England (Butlin, 1892). He attributed this difference to better hygiene practices by the European sweeps as well as to the use of younger boys in England, suggesting that age of exposure and the duration of exposure influence the formation of the cancer. In

Table 8-1

Historical Events in Chemically Induced Cancer

DATE	INVESTIGATOR(S)	CAUSATIVE AGENT
1775	Pott	Soot and chimney sweeps
1822	Ayrton	Arsenic containing metal
1875	Thiersch	Sunlight
1876	Manourriez	Coal tar
1879	Harting and Hesse	Lung cancer and uranium
1892	Butlin	Soot and chimney sweeps
1895	Rehn	Manufacture of aniline dyes
1902	Frieben	X-rays
1915	Davis	Pipe smokers and betel nut chewers
1915	Yamagiwa, Ichikawa, and Tsusui	Induction of skin cancer in rabbits and mice by coal tar
1920	Leitch and Seguina	Radium radiation
1928	Delore and Bergamo	Benzene
1930	Kennaway and Hieger	Tumor induction by dibenz[a,h]anthracene
1932	Stephens	Nickel
1932	Alwens	Chromium compounds
1933	Cook, Hewett, and Hieger	Isolation of the carcinogen benzo[a]pyrene from coal tar
1936	Yoshida and Kinosita	Induction of liver cancer in rats by o-aminoazotoluene
1934	Wood and Gloyne	Arsenicals, beryllium, and asbestos
1934	Neitzel	Mineral oil mists and radiation
1936	Kawahata	Coal tar fumes
1938	Hueper, Wiley, and Wolfe	Induction of urinary cancer in dogs by 2-naphthylamine
1941	Berenblum, Rous, MacKenzie, and Kidd	Initiation and promotion stages in skin carcinogenesis with benzo[a]pyrene
1951	Miller and Miller	Carcinogen binding to cellular macromolecule
1956	Doll and Hill	Lung cancer and other causes of death in relation to smoking

1895, Rehn reported a linkage between the manufacturer of aniline dyes and the induction of bladder cancer in dye workers (Rehn, 1895). Due to the increase in demand for synthetic dyes in the 19th century, production of the aniline-based dyes increased, as did the development of skin and bladder cancer in exposed workers. The specific chemicals in the dyes related to the cause of skin and bladder cancer were later determined to be the aromatic compounds 2-naphthylamine and benzidine (Hueper *et al.*, 1938). Exposure of workers to metals, such as chromium (Alwens, 1938) and asbestos (Wood and Gloyne, 1934), was shown to be associated with an increased incidence of lung cancers in workers. Tobacco use and its linkage to lung cancer provide an excellent case study on the linkage between epidemiology and experimental carcinogenesis. As early as 1912, Adler noted an association between smokers and lung cancer (Spiro and Silvestri, 2005). Similarly, Lickint reported on the linkage between tobacco smoking and lung cancer in the 1920s and also associated the higher rate of lung cancer seen in males with tobacco smoking (Proctor, 2001). Subsequent investigations lead to the observation by Doll and colleagues, in a longitudinal epidemiology study, a direct cause and effect of smoking to lung cancer (Doll *et al.*, 2004).

Based on these human epidemiological observations, experimental investigations starting in the first half of the 20th century were performed to understand the biological mechanisms, nature of these chemical mixtures, and individual chemical compounds in the mixtures using animal models. Initial studies by Yamagiwa and co-workers examined the linkage between exposure to coal tar and its derivatives on cancer induction in humans by painting with coal tar on rabbit ears, which resulted in the formation of skin cancer (Yamagiwa *et al.*, 1915). Subsequently, Kennaway and Hieger purified dibenz(*a,h*)anthracene from this coal tar extract, and determined that dibenz(*a,h*)anthracene was at least one component of the coal tar mixture that was responsible for inducing skin cancer (Kennaway and Hieger, 1930). Cook and co-workers (1933) similarly extracted another polyaromatic hydrocarbon (PAH), benzo(*a*)pyrene, from the coal tar and showed this to also function as a carcinogen in rodents. In similar approaches with aromatic amines, Hueper and colleagues reported that 2-naphthylamine induced bladder tumors in dogs (Hueper *et al.*, 1938) and Yoshida (1933) and Kinosita (1936) found that feeding aminoazotoulene or aminoazobenzene to rodents induced liver cancer. James and Elizabeth Miller (and their students) in the last half of the 20th century established the role of chemical structure and metabolism in the "activation" of carcinogens to a macromolecular interactive form (Miller *et al.*, 1951; Miller and Miller, 1981; Miller *et al.*, 1983). Studies with the aromatic amine compounds in animal models correlated with the human epidemiological studies that had revealed an association between bladder cancer in humans and exposure to aniline dyes in the occupational setting and helped to define the specific chemicals in the dyes responsible for the cancer induction. Studies by investigators such as Harris and colleagues over the last 30 years have utilized the laboratory to examine the environmentally induced cancers reported in epidemiological finding, especially in the area of lung cancer and tobacco smoking (Greenblatt *et al.*, 1994). These epidemiological and experimental studies have shown a clear correlation between the induction of cancer in humans and rodents by chemical exposure.

An important historical event in the development of carcinogenesis testing was the development of a short-term bacterial-based mutagenesis bioassay in the early 1970s by Ames and colleagues. This Salmonella-based assay has become a stalwart in the early detection of mutagenic compounds that have the potential to be carcinogenic. A recent review of the historical aspects of the development and use of the Salmonella assay has been published (Claxton *et al.*, 2010). The success of the Ames Salmonella Assay spurred the use of in vitro assays for mutagenicity in bacteria and mammalian cells as predictors of potential rodent and human carcinogens (Tennant *et al.*, 1987), culminating in the current genetic toxicity test battery (Eastmond *et al.*, 2009). As we move into the second decade of the 21st century, the onus to further develop high-throughput and shortened bioassays for carcinogen detection (cell or molecular biology based) has been identified, is ongoing (NAS, Tox 21 National Toxicology Program [NTP/NIEHS]; Tox cast [USEPA]), and represents new approaches based on our current understanding of the molecular steps in cancer-dependent pathways.

Definitions

An understanding of the cellular and molecular aspects of the cancer process requires an understanding of the scientific terms involved in defining and describing the pathology of neoplasia (Table 8-2). Neoplasia is defined as new growth or autonomous growth of tissue. A neoplastic lesion is referred to as a neoplasm. A neoplasm can be either benign or malignant. Both types of lesions are induced by chemical carcinogens. Benign neoplasms (eg, adenomas) are lesions characterized by expansive growth, frequently exhibiting slow rates of proliferation that do not invade surrounding tissue or other organs. Benign neoplasms can impair and damage the normal function of an organ through its growth impeding of blood flow. A malignant neoplasm (eg, a carcinoma) demonstrates invasive growth characteristics, capable of spreading not only through the organ of origin but via metastasis to other organs. Metastases are secondary growths derived from the cells of the primary malignant neoplasm.

The term tumor is a general term that is frequently used synonymous with a neoplastic lesion and describes a grossly visible lesion prior to a histopathological examination can confirm the exact type, grade, and stage of the neoplasm. In classifying neoplasms,

Table 8-2

Terminology

Neoplasia	New growth or autonomous growth of tissue
Neoplasm	The lesion resulting from the neoplasia
Benign	Lesions characterized by expansive growth, frequently exhibiting slow rates of proliferation that do not invade surrounding tissues
Malignant	Lesions demonstrating invasive growth, capable of metastases to other tissues and organs
Metastases	Secondary growths derived from a primary malignant neoplasm
Tumor	Lesion characterized by swelling or increase in size, may or may not be neoplastic
Cancer	Malignant neoplasm
Carcinogen	A physical or chemical agent that causes or induces neoplasia
Genotoxic	Carcinogens that interact with DNA resulting in mutation
Nongenotoxic	Carcinogens that modify gene expression but do not damage DNA

Table 8-3

Neoplasm Nomenclature

TISSUE OF ORIGIN	BENIGN NEOPLASM	MALIGNANT NEOPLASM
Connective tissue		
Bone	Osteoma	Osteosarcoma
Fibrous	Fibroma	Fibrosarcoma
Fat Lipid	Lipoma	Liposarcoma
Blood cells and related cells		
Hematopoietic cells		Leukemias
Lymphoid tissue		Lymphomas
Muscle		
Smooth	Leiomyoma	Leiomyosarcoma
Striated	Rhabdomyoma	Rhabdomyosarcoma
Endothelium	Hemangioma	Angiosarcoma
Mesothelium		Mesothelioma
Epithelial		
Squamous	Squamous cell papilloma	Squamous cell or carcinoma
Respiratory	Bronchial adenoma	Bronchogenic carcinoma
Renal epithelium	Renal tubular adenoma	Renal cell carcinoma
Liver cells	Liver cell adenoma	Hepatocellular carcinoma
Urinary epithelium	Transitional cell papilloma	Transitional cell carcinoma
Testicular epithelium		Seminoma
Melanocytes		Malignant melanoma

the nomenclature reflects both the tissue or cell of origin, and the characteristics of the type of tissue involved (Table 8-3). For benign neoplasms, the tissue of origin is frequently followed by the suffix "oma"; for example, a benign fibrous neoplasm would be termed *fibroma*, and a benign glandular epithelium termed an *adenoma*. Malignant neoplasms from epithelial origin are called *carcinomas* (from with the term cancer has evolved) while those derived from mesenchymal origin are referred to as *sarcoma*. Thus, a malignant neoplasm of fibrous tissue would be a *fibrosarcoma* while that derived from bone would be an *ostoesarcoma*. Similarly, a malignant neoplasm from the liver would be a *hepatocellular carcinoma* while that derived from skin squamous epithelium is referred to as a *squamous cell carcinoma*. Preoplastic lesions have also been observed in a number of target organs both animal models and humans, and reflect an early reversible lesion in neoplasm progression. The characterization and study of preneoplastic cells have led to further understanding of the process of cancer formation.

The term *cancer* describes a subset of neoplasia that represents malignant neoplasms. A *carcinogen* is an agent, chemical or physical, that causes or induces a cancer, although it is often also used to describe an agent that produces benign neoplastic lesions in rodent bioassays. In regulatory science this has been further defined as an agent whose administration to previously untreated animals leads to a statistically significant increased incidence of neoplasia of one of more histogenetic types as compared with the incidence seen in untreated control animals (Pitot, 1986). Thus,

the induction of either or both benign and malignant neoplasms by a chemical or physical agent is included in the definition of a carcinogen. Carcinogens can be chemicals, viruses, hormones, radiation, or solid materials. Carcinogens either produce new neoplastic growth in a tissue or organ or increase the incidence and/or multiplicity of background spontaneous neoplastic formation in the target tissue.

The process of carcinogenesis is a multistage and multistep process involving modification and mutation to a number of normal cellular processes. An extensive literature base exists to describe the changes that cells undergo during the formation of neoplasia. Characteristics of cancers and the biological processes involved have been extensively reviewed (Hanahan and Weinberg, 2011). For regulatory classification purposes carcinogens have frequently been divided simplistically into two major categories based on their general mode of action: genotoxic and nongenotoxic. Genotoxic carcinogens are those agents that interact with DNA to damage or change its structure. They are frequently mutagenic in a dose-responsive manner, and for regulatory purposes, they are classified as exhibiting low-dose linear patterns, which approximates a straight line at very low doses without a threshold and a lack of reversibility of effect upon removal of the agent.

Nongenotoxic carcinogens are the agents that do not directly interact with nuclear DNA. Nongenotoxic carcinogens may change gene expression, modify normal cell function, bind to or modify cellular receptors, and increase cell growth. These agents work through epigenetic mechanisms and change DNA expression without modifying or directly damaging its structure. Nongenotoxic chemicals create a situation in a cell or tissue that makes it more susceptible to DNA damage from other sources (natural or xenobiotic). Nongenotoxic agents for regulatory purposes exhibit a nonlinear, threshold, and reversible dose response pattern in their carcinogenicity. Common features of genotoxic and nongenotoxic carcinogens are shown in Table 8-4.

This knowledge has led to continued efforts, using both epidemiological information and experimental animal models, to assess chemical carcinogenicity of occupational, industrial, and environmental agents, to gain an understanding of the mechanisms of action of these agents, and to determine the relevance of human exposure to cancer risk.

MULTISTAGE CARCINOGENESIS

Extensive experimental studies with animal models and pathological evaluation of human cancers, have demonstrated that the carcinogenesis process involves a series of definable stages and steps

Table 8-4

Features of Genotoxic and Nongenotoxic Carcinogens

Genotoxic carcinogens
Mutagenic
Can be complete carcinogens
Tumorigenicity is dose responsive
No theoretical threshold
Nongenotoxic carcinogens
Nonmutagenic
Threshold, reversible
Tumorigenicity is dose responsive
May function at tumor promotion stage
No direct DNA damage
Species, strain, tissue specificity

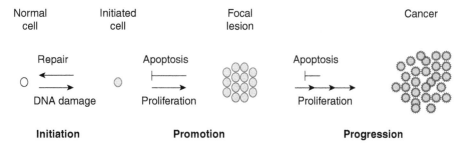

Figure 8-2. *Multistage model carcinogenesis.*

(Shih *et al.*, 2001; Osada and Takahashi, 2002). Operationally, three defined stages, initiation, promotion, and progression have been identified in rodent studies (initially in skin and liver tumors models) (Fig. 8-2). These steps follow a temporal sequence of events demonstrable by histopathology and observed in a wide variety of target tissues. The defining characteristics of each of these stages are outlined in Table 8-5.

Initiation

The first stage of the cancer process involves initiation, a process that is defined as a stable, heritable change. This stage is a rapid, irreversible process that results in a carcinogen-induced mutational event. Chemical and physical agents that function at this stage are referred to as initiators or initiating agents. Initiating agents lead to genetic changes including mutations and deletions. Chemical carcinogens that covalently bind to DNA and form adducts that result in mutations are initiating agents. Included among chemicals classified as initiating carcinogens are compounds such as polycyclic hydrocarbons and nitrosamines,

Table 8-5

Characteristics of the Stages of Carcinogenesis Process

Initiation
DNA modification
Mutation
Genotoxic
One cell division necessary to lock-in mutation
Modification is not enough to produce cancer
Nonreversible
Single treatment can induce mutation

Promotion
No direct DNA modification
Nongenotoxic
No direct mutation
Multiple cell divisions necessary
Clonal expansion of the initiated cell population
Increase in cell proliferation or decrease in cell death
  (apoptosis)
Reversible
Multiple treatments (prolonged treatment) necessary
Threshold

Progression
DNA modification
Genotoxic event
Mutation, chromosome disarrangement
Changes from preneoplasia to neoplasia benign/malignant
Irreversible
Number of treatments needed with compound unknown
  (may require only single treatment)

biological agents, certain viruses, and physical agents such as x-rays and ultraviolet (UV) light. Most chemical carcinogens that function at the initiation stage of the cancer process are indirect-acting genotoxic compounds that require metabolic activation in the target cell to produce the DNA-damaging event. For these compounds, the chemical must be taken into the target site and metabolized (in the case of an indirect genotoxic carcinogen). The ultimate form of the carcinogen is then able to bind to nuclear DNA, resulting in adduct formation. The initiating event becomes "fixed" when the DNA adducts or other damage to DNA is not correctly repaired or is incompletely repaired prior to DNA synthesis. This event can lead to inappropriate base pairing and formation of a mutation.

Initiation by itself does not appear to be sufficient for neoplastic formation. Once initiated cells are formed, their fate has multiple potential outcomes: (1) the initiated cell can remain in a static nondividing state through influences by growth control either via normal surrounding cells or through endocrine influence; (2) the initiated cell may possess mutations incompatible with viability or normal function and be deleted through apoptotic mechanisms; or (3) the cell, through stimuli such as intrinsic factors or from chemical exposure, may undergo cell division resulting in the growth in the proliferation of the initiated cell. Besides the production of an initiated cell through carcinogen binding and misrepair, additional evidence has come forth showing that induction of continual stress, resulting in continual cell proliferation, can also produce new mutated, initiated cells (Matthews *et al.*, 2009; Johnstone and Baylin, 2010) Therefore, modification of cell signaling and gene expression (while usually ascribed to the tumor promotion process and as an epigenic pathway [see below]) may indirectly through sustained cell proliferation also result in the formation of mutations (Lewandowska and Bartoszek, 2011). In some instances, typically following relatively high doses and/or repeated exposure to the genotoxic carcinogen, a chemical carcinogen may function as a complete carcinogen, that is, it is capable of progressing through all stages of the cancer process.

Promotion

The second stage of the carcinogenesis process, derived from either endogenous or exogenous stimuli of cell growth, involves the selective clonal expansion of initiated cells to produce a preneoplastic lesion. This is referred to as the promotion stage of the carcinogenesis process. Both exogenous and endogenous agents that function at this stage are referred to as tumor promoters. Tumor promoters are not mutagenic and generally are not able to induce tumors by themselves; rather they act though several mechanisms involving gene expression changes that result in sustained cell proliferation either through increases in cell proliferation and/or the inhibition of apoptosis. This stage involves the modulation of gene expression through receptor or non–receptor-mediated processes. Nongenotoxic carcinogens frequently function at the tumor promotion stage. The growth of preneoplastic lesions requires repeated applications or continuous exposure to tumor-promoting compounds. Although initial exposure to tumor promoters may result in an increase in cell proliferation and/or DNA synthesis in all tissues of the organ, this is usually a transient effect on the normal cells and with repeated applications of the tumor promoter only the initiated cells continue to clonally expand and divide (Fig. 8-2). Promotion is a reversible phenomenon whereby upon removal of the promotional agent, the focal cells may return back to the initiated cell. In addition, these agents demonstrate a well-documented threshold for their effects—below a certain dose or frequency of application; tumor promoters are unable to induce cell proliferation. Multiple chemical compounds as well as physical agents have been linked to the tumor promotion stage of the cancer process. Tumor promoters in general show organ-specific effects, for example, a tumor promoter of the liver, such as phenobarbital, will not function as a tumor promoter in the skin or other tissues.

Progression

The final stage of the carcinogenesis process, progression, involves the conversion of the benign preneoplastic lesions into a neoplastic cancer. In this stage, due to increase in DNA synthesis in cell proliferation in the preneoplastic lesions, additional genotoxic events may occur resulting in additional DNA damage including chromosomal damage such as aberrations and translocations. These events result in the transfer from preneoplastic, clonally derived cell populations into neoplastic cell populations. Cells accumulate a variety of mutations and epigenetic changes that cause them to outgrow the surrounding cells and to attract all of the necessary nutrients via angiogenesis. The tumor microenvironment has been also shown to be an important component of this process and the presence of "normal" cells and stroma within the lesion is critical for the neoplastic cells to survive and propagate. During the progression phase of the process the clonal nature of the neoplastic lesion is typically lost with a polyclonal appearance of cells within the lesion. Agents that impact on the progression stage are usually genotoxic agents although the acquisition of additional mutagenic events may occur through the continual stimulation of cell proliferation. By definition, the progression stage is an irreversible stage in that neoplasm formation, whether benign or malignant, occurs. With the formation of neoplasia, an autonomous growth and/or lack of growth control is achieved. Spontaneous progression can occur from spontaneous karyotypic changes that occur in mitotically active initiated cells during promotion. An accumulation of nonrandom chromosomal aberrations and karyotypic instability are hallmarks of progression. As such, chemicals that function as progressor agents are many times clastogenic and are capable of causing chromosomal abnormalities. Complete carcinogens have the ability to produce initiation, promotion and progression and hence by definition have genotoxic properties. In addition, a number of model systems are available to test for carcinogenicity and/or to study the multistep mechanisms involved in chemical carcinogenesis. The models are described in a later section of this chapter.

MECHANISMS OF ACTION OF CHEMICAL CARCINOGENS

The formation of a neoplasm is a multistage, multistep process that involves the ultimate release of the neoplastic cells from normal growth control processes and creating a tumor microenvironment.

Table 8-6

Hallmarks of Cancer

Eight properties of neoplastic cells that impart and contribute to their ability to independently growth and eventually metastasize
1. sustaining cell proliferation
2. resisting cell death (apoptosis)
3. inducing angiogenesis
4. enabling replicative immortality
5. activating invasion and metastasis
6. evading growth suppressors
7. reprogramming of energy metabolism
8. evading immune destruction

SOURCE: Data from Hanahan and Weinberg [2011].

In a highly regarded review, Hanahan and Weinberg (2000) initially defined the major characteristics of a neoplasm as it progresses into a malignant state. This review has recently been updated (Hanahan and Weinberg, 2011). These authors have proposed eight "hallmarks of cancer" that involve modifications to the homeostasis of normal cells imparting the growth and metastatic properties seen in the development of a neoplastic cell. These eight properties include (1) sustaining cell proliferation, (2) resisting cell death (apoptosis), (3) inducing angiogenesis, (4) enabling replicative immortality, (5) activating invasion and metastasis, (6) evading growth suppressors, (7) reprogramming of energy metabolism, and (8) evading immune destruction (Table 8-6). An important concept from this review is the fact that tumors are not just a collection of clonal neoplastic cells but a complex tissue with multiple cell populations and interact with one another and function as a unique tissue. This tumor microenvironment involves the recruitment of normal stromal and inflammatory cells that contribute to the growth the development of the neoplasm.

Although our understanding of the cancer process has expanded exponentially in the past several decades as is illustrated by the "hallmarks-of-cancer" concept, in its minimalist form two major processes are needed with regard to the induction of neoplasia by chemical agents: a mutational event and a selective proliferation of the mutated cell to form a neoplasm. Based on this supposition, chemicals that induce cancer have been classified into one of two broad categories (as noted above)—genotoxic or DNA-reactive agents, and nongenotoxic or epigenetic agents. This is admittedly a very simplistic approach to the complexities of the cancer process (as illustrated by the Hanahan and Weinberg's review [2011]); however, for the purposes of regulatory processes and risk assessment this categorization has for the most part continued.

Genotoxic/DNA-Reactive Compounds

Genotoxic compounds interact with nuclear DNA of a target cell producing unrepaired DNA damage that is inherited in subsequent daughter cells. Experimental and epidemiological observations made in the middle of the 20th century identified a number of chemicals that could cause cancer in humans or experimental animals. Coal tar carcinogens including benzo(*a*)pyrene, pesticides such as 2-acetylaminofluorene and azo dyes such as diaminobenzamide were among the first chemical carcinogens to be studied. DNA-reactive carcinogens can be further subdivided according to whether they are active in their parent form (ie, direct-acting: agents that can directly bind to DNA without being metabolized) and those that require metabolic activation (ie, indirect-acting carcinogens: compounds that require metabolism in order to react with

Table 8-7

Examples of Genotoxic Carcinogens

A. Direct-acting carcinogens
  Nitrogen or sulfur mustards
  Propane sulfone
  Methyl methane sulfonate
  Ethyleneimine
  B-Propiolactone
  1,2,3,4-Diepoxybutane
  Dimethyl sulfate
  Bis-(Chloromethyl) ether
  Dimethylcarbamyl chloride

B. Chemicals requiring activation (indirect-acting carcinogens)
  Polycyclic aromatic hydrocarbons and heterocyclic aromatics
  Aromatic amines
  N-Nitrosoamines
  Azo dyes
  Hydrazines
  Cycasin
  Safrole
  Chlorinated hydrocarbons
  Aflatoxin
  Mycotoxin
  Pyrrolizidine alkaloids
  Bracken fern
  Carbamates

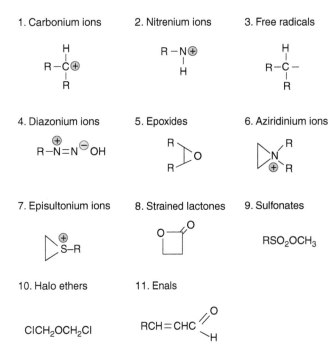

Figure 8-3. *Structures of reactive electrophiles.*

DNA). Examples of direct-acting and indirect-acting carcinogens are listed in Table 8-7.

Direct-Acting (Activation-Independent) Carcinogens A class of carcinogens that do not require metabolic activation or modification to induce cancer, are termed direct-acting or activation-independent carcinogens. These chemicals are also defined as ultimate carcinogens. Examination of the chemical structure of these chemicals reveals that they are highly reactive electrophilic molecules that can interact with and bind to nucleophiles such as cellular macromolecules including DNA. Some common electrophilic species in these groups are shown in Fig. 8-3. Generally these chemicals containing these moieties frequently cause tumor formation at the site of chemical exposure.

Direct-acting carcinogens include epoxides, imines, alkyl and sulfate esters, and mustard gasses (Fox and Scott, 1980; Sontag, 1981). Direct-acting electrophilic carcinogenic chemicals typically test positive in the Ames test without additional bioactivation with a liver metabolic fraction. The relative carcinogenic strength of direct-acting carcinogens depends in part on the relative rates of interaction between the chemical and genomic DNA, as well as competing reactions with the chemical and other cellular nucleophiles. The relative carcinogenic activity of direct-acting carcinogens is dependent upon such competing reactions and also on detoxification reactions. Chemical stability, transport, and membrane permeability determine the carcinogenic activity of the chemical. Direct-acting carcinogens are typically carcinogenic at multiple sites and in all species examined. A number of direct-acting alkylating agents, including a number of chemotherapeutic chemicals, are carcinogenic in humans (Marselos and Vainio, 1991).

Indirect-Acting Genotoxic Carcinogens An important discovery in the understanding of chemical carcinogenesis came from the investigations of the Millers who established that many carcinogens are not intrinsically carcinogenic, but require metabolic activation to be carcinogenic. They demonstrated that azo dyes covalently bind to proteins in liver, leading to the conclusion that carcinogens may bind to proteins that are critical for cell growth control (Miller and Miller, 1947). Work with benzo(*a*)pyrene showed covalent binding of benzo(*a*)pyrene or the metabolites of benzo(*a*)pyrene in rodents (Miller *et al.*, 1951). Subsequent investigations with other indirect-acting genotoxic carcinogens by other investigators confirmed that metabolism of the parent compound was necessary to produce a metabolite (activation) that was able to interact with DNA (Miller, 1970).

It has since been shown that the majority of DNA-reactive carcinogens are found as parent compounds, or procarcinogens. Procarcinogens are stable chemicals that require subsequent metabolism to be carcinogenic (Conney, 1982; Miller and Miller, 1981; Miller *et al.*, 1983; Weisburger and Williams, 1981 in Becker, 1982). The terms procarcinogen, proximate carcinogen, and ultimate carcinogen have been coined to define the parent compound (procarcinogen) and its metabolite form, either intermediate (proximate carcinogen) or final (ultimate carcinogen) that reacts with DNA (Fig. 8-4). The ultimate form of the carcinogen is most likely the chemical species that results in mutation and neoplastic transformation. The ultimate form of certain carcinogenic chemicals is not known, whereas for other chemicals there may be more than one ultimate carcinogenic metabolite depending on the metabolic pathway followed. It is important to note that besides activation of the procarcinogen to a DNA-reactive form, detoxification pathways may also occur inactivating the carcinogen.

Indirect-acting genotoxic carcinogens usually produce their neoplastic effects, not at the site of exposure (as seen with direct-acting genotoxic carcinogens) but at the target tissue where the metabolic activation of the chemical occurs. Indirect-acting genotoxic carcinogens include the polycyclic PAHs, nitrosamines, aromatic amines, and aflatoxin B1. Fig. 8-4 shows the parent

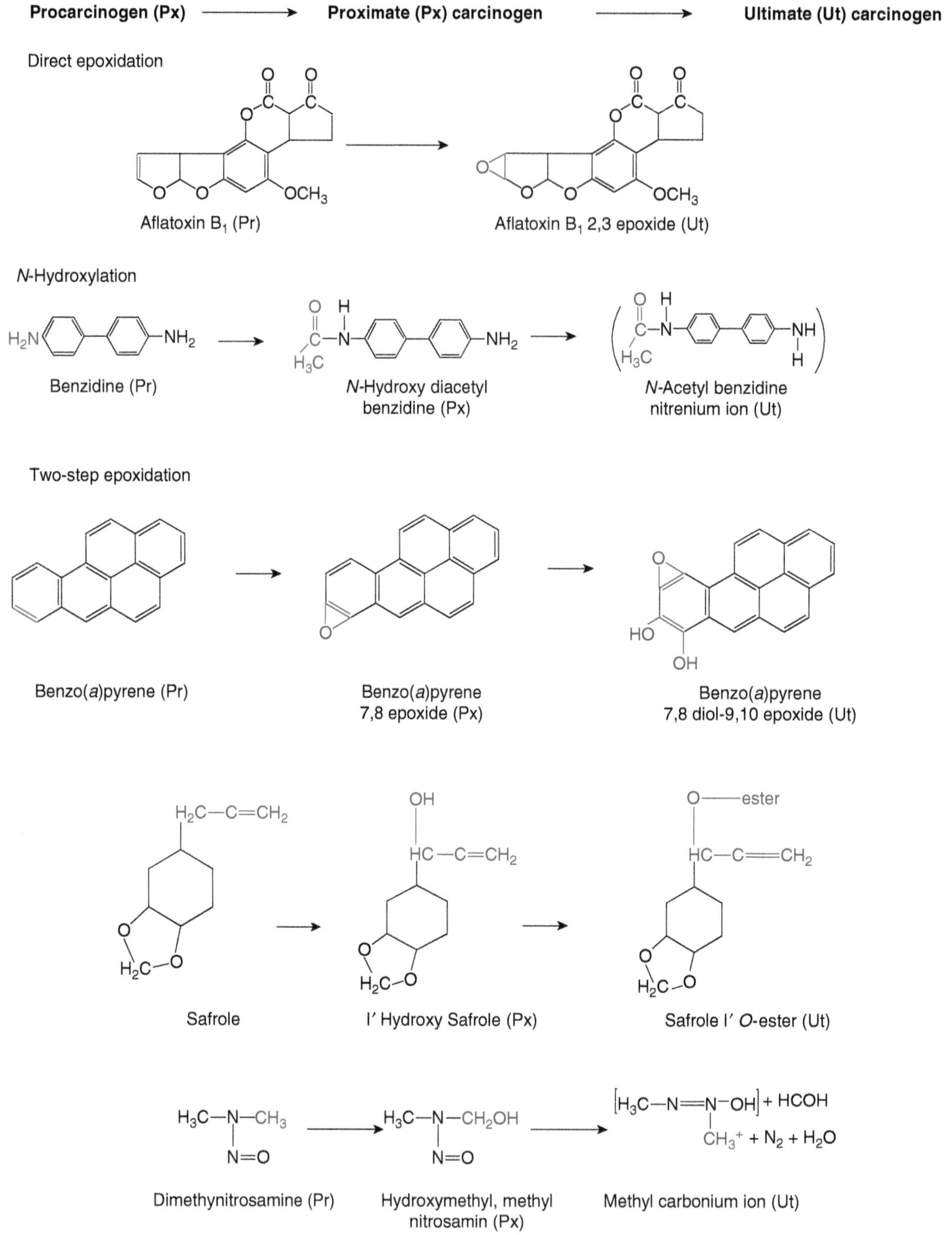

Procarcinogen (Px)   ⟶   Proximate (Px) carcinogen   ⟶   Ultimate (Ut) carcinogen

Direct epoxidation

Aflatoxin B$_1$ (Pr)   Aflatoxin B$_1$ 2,3 epoxide (Ut)

N-Hydroxylation

Benzidine (Pr)   *N*-Hydroxy diacetyl benzidine (Px)   *N*-Acetyl benzidine nitrenium ion (Ut)

Two-step epoxidation

Benzo(*a*)pyrene (Pr)   Benzo(*a*)pyrene 7,8 epoxide (Px)   Benzo(*a*)pyrene 7,8 diol-9,10 epoxide (Ut)

Safrole   I' Hydroxy Safrole (Px)   Safrole I' *O*-ester (Ut)

Dimethynitrosamine (Pr)   Hydroxymethyl, methyl nitrosamin (Px)   Methyl carbonium ion (Ut)

Figure 8-4. *Structures of representative indirect-acting carcinogens and their metabolic derivatives, the proximate (Px) and ultimate (Ut) carcinogenic form result from the metabolism of the procarcinogenic form (Pr).*

(procarcinogen) and metabolites for several representative indirect-acting genotoxic carcinogens.

Mutagenesis

The reaction of a carcinogen with genomic DNA either directly or indirectly may result in DNA adduct formation or DNA damage, and frequently produces a mutation. Several mechanisms of mutagenesis are known to occur. Modification of DNA by electrophilic

carcinogens can lead to a number of products. These events are dependent upon when in the cell cycle the adducts are formed, where the adducts are formed, and, the type of repair process used in response to the damage.

Transitions are a substitution of one pyrimidine by the other or one purine by the other (changes within a chemical class), whereas a transversion occurs when a purine is replaced by a pyrimidine or a pyrimidine is replaced by a purine (changes across a chemical class). Carcinogens can induce transitions and transversions several ways. In one scenario, when adducts (or apurinic or apyrimidinic sites) are encountered by the DNA replication processes, they may be misread. The polymerase may preferentially insert an adenine (A) in response to a noninformative site. Thus, the daughter strand of an A, C, G, or T adduct will have an adenine (A) and this change is fixed (mutation) and resistant to subsequent DNA repair. A second outcome, a shift in the reading frame (resulting in a frame shift mutation) may also result from carcinogen–DNA adducts formation. Most frame shift mutations are deletions and occur more frequently when the carcinogen–DNA adduct is formed on a nucleotide. In a third scenario, DNA strand breaks can also result from carcinogen–DNA adducts. These may arise either as a result of excision repair mechanisms that are incomplete during DNA replication or via direct alkylation of the phosphodiester backbone leading to backbone cleavage. Strand scission can lead to double-strand breaks, recombination, or loss of heterozyogosity.

Damage by Alkylating Electrophiles

As noted above, most chemical carcinogens require metabolic activation to exert a carcinogenic effect. The ultimate carcinogenic forms of these chemicals are frequently strong electrophiles (Fig. 8-3) that can readily form covalent adducts with nucleophilic targets. Because of their unpaired electrons, S:, O:, and N: atoms are nucleophilic targets of many electrophiles. The extent of adducts formed is limited by the structure of DNA where bulky electrophilic chemicals can bind, and size of the ultimate carcinogenic form. In general, the stronger electrophiles display a greater range of nucleophilic targets (ie, they can attack weak and strong nucleophiles), whereas weak electrophiles are only capable of alkylating strong nucleophiles (eg, S: atoms in amino acids). In addition, the metabolic capability of a target cell will dictate the extent and types of electrophiles generated from the procarcinogenic parent.

An important and abundant source of nucleophiles is contained not only in the DNA bases, but also in the phosphodiester backbone (Fig. 8-5). Although carcinogen–DNA adducts may be formed at all sites in DNA, the most common sites of alkylation include the N^7 of guanine, the N^3 of adenine, the N^1 of adenine, the N^3 of guanine, and the O^6 of guanine. Alkylations of phosphate may also occur at a high frequency. Selective examples of carcinogen interactions with proteins and nucleic acids are shown in Fig. 8-6. Different electrophilic carcinogens will often display different preferences for nucleophilic sites in DNA and different spectra of damage. Dimethylnitrosamine and diethylnitrosamine, for example, are metabolized by P450 oxidation to yield a methyl carbonium ion (CH_3^+) and an ethyl carbonium ion ($CH_3CH_3^+$), respectively. Despite the structural similarities of the ultimate electrophiles, they display significant differences in alkylation profiles (Pegg, 1984). The relative proportions of methylated bases present in DNA following reaction with carcinogen-methylating agents are shown in Table 8-8 (Pegg, 1984). The predominant adduct formed following exposure to methylating agents such as methylmethane sulfonate is 7-methylguanine. In contrast, ethylating agents produce adducts predominately in the phosphate backbone of DNA. The carcinogenic potential of the type of adducts formed is often debated; some believe that O^6-alkylguanine is the most carcinogenic adduct, whereas others report that O^4-alkylthymine is more important in the carcinogenic process due to its persistence relative to other adducts (Pegg, 1984; Swenberg et al., 1984).

Another common modification to DNA is the hydroxylation of DNA bases. Oxidative DNA adducts have been identified in all four DNA bases (Fig. 8-7); however, 8-hydroxyguanine is among

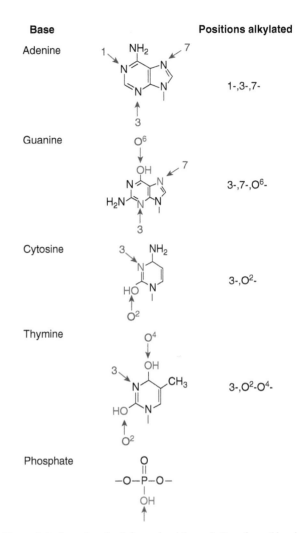

Figure 8-5. *Examples of cellular nucleophiles and sites of possible adduct formation.*

the most prevalent oxidative DNA adduct (Floyd, 1990). The source of oxidative DNA damage is typically formed from free radical reactions that occur endogenously in the cell or from exogenous sources (Klaunig and Kamendulis, 2004; Floyd, 1990; Ames and Shigenaga, 1993). Although a relatively large amount of oxidative DNA adducts have been proposed to be formed per day, repair mechanisms exist that maintain the cellular level at a low rate and keep endogenous mutations to a relatively low level. The role of oxidative damage and oxidative stress is discussed in greater detail later in this chapter.

Methylation of deoxycytidine residues is a well-studied DNA adduct. This reaction occurs by the transfer of a methyl group from S-adenosylmethionine by DNA methyltransferases (Holliday, 1989). Methylation of DNA results in heritable expression or repression of genes, with hypomethylation associated with active transcription of genes, whereas hypermethylated genes tend to be rarely transcribed. Chemical carcinogens may inhibit DNA methylation by several mechanisms including forming covalent adducts, single-strand breaks in the DNA, alteration of methionine pools, and inactivation of the DNA methyltransferase responsible for methylation (Riggs and Jones, 1983). The importance of DNA methylation in chemical carcinogenesis is discussed further later in this chapter.

Although a large number of adducts can be formed following exposure to chemicals, whether a particular DNA adduct will result in mutation and participate in the carcinogenesis process

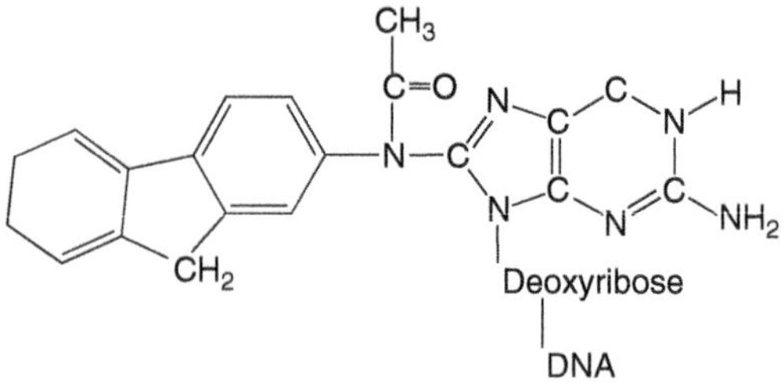

N-(deoxyguanosine-8-yl)-acetylaminofluorene in
DNA

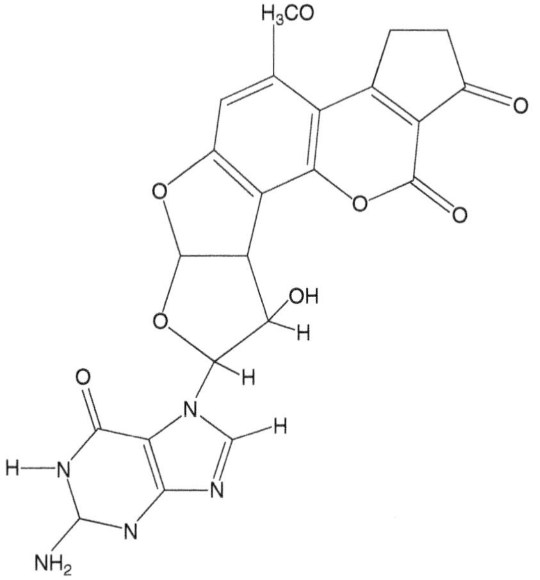

Aflatoxin B$_1$ N-^{7} guanine-adduct

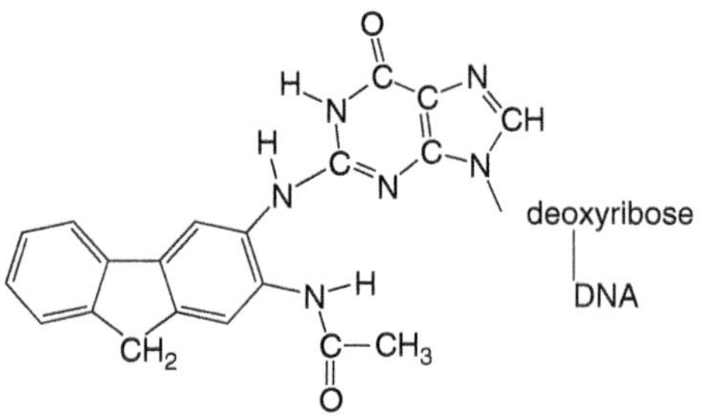

3-(Deoxyguanosine N$_2$-yl)-acetylaminofluorene
in DNA

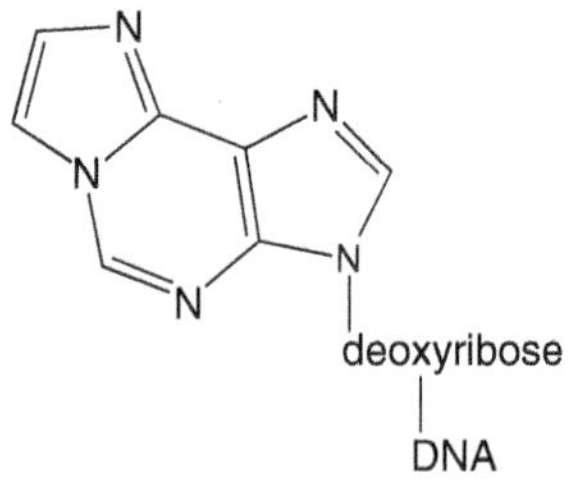

1, N^6-ethenoadenine in
DNA

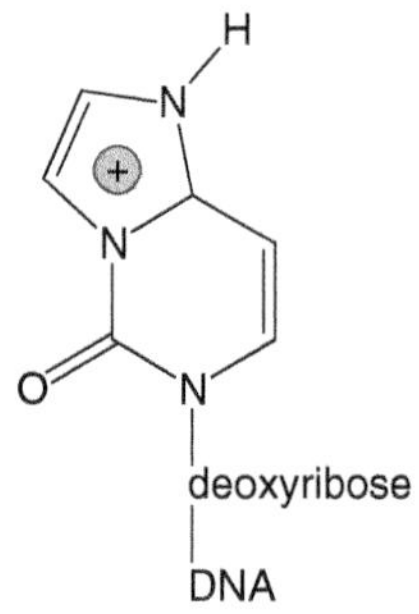

3, N^4-ethenocytosine in DNA

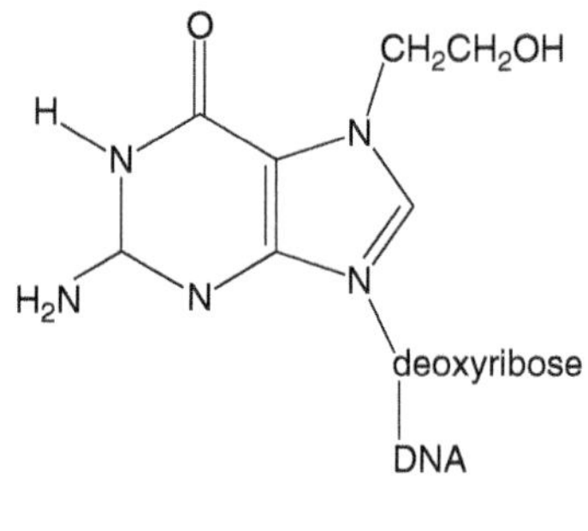

7-(2-Hydroxyethyl) guanosine
in DNA

Figure 8-6. *Select structures of protein- and nucleic acid–bound forms of certain chemical carcinogens.*

is dependent in part on the persistence of the adduct through the process of DNA replication, which is also in part dependent upon DNA repair.

DNA Repair

Following the formation of a carcinogen–DNA adduct, the persistence of the adduct is a major determinant of the outcome. This persistence depends on the ability of the cell to repair the altered DNA. The detection of unique DNA adducts has proven to be important in understanding the mechanism of action of specific carcinogens and has been correlated with carcinogenesis (Goth and Rajewsky, 1974; Swenberg *et al.*, 1985; Kadlubar *et al.*, 1981; Becker and Shank, 1985). However, the presence of a DNA adduct is not sufficient

for the carcinogenesis process to proceed. The relative rates or persistence of particular DNA adducts may be an important determinant of carcinogenicity, for example, O^4-ethylthymine is relatively stable in DNA whereas O^6-ethylguanine does not persist in DNA after continuous exposure to diethylnitrosamine (Swenberg *et al.*, 1984). The persistence of DNA adducts of *trans*-4-aminostilbene does not correlate with organ carcinogenicity and/or tissue susceptibility. Although the liver and kidney exhibited the greatest burden and persistence of the adduct and the Zymbals gland showed the least amount of DNA adducts, the latter tissue was more susceptible to carcinogenesis by this chemical (Neumann, 1983). As such, differences in susceptibility to carcinogenesis are likely the result of a number of factors, including DNA replication within a tissue and repair of a DNA adduct.

Table 8-8

Relative Proportions of Methylated Bases Present in DNA After Reaction With Carcinogenic Alkylating Agents

	PERCENT OF TOTAL ALKYLATION BY	
	DIMETHYL-NITROSAMINE, N-METHYL-N-NITROSOUREA, OR 1,2-DIMETHYL-HYDAZINE	DIETHYL-NITROSAMINE OR N-ETHYL-N-NITROSOUREA
1-Alkyladenine	0.7	0.3
3-Alkyladenine	8	4
7-Alkyladenine	1.5	0.4
3-Alkylguanine	0.8	0.6
7-Alkylguanine	68	12
O^6-Alkylguanine	7.5	8
3-Alkylcytosine	0.5	0.2
O^2-Alkylcytosine	0.1	3
3-Alkylthymine	0.3	0.8
O^2-Alkylthymine	0.1	7
O^4-Alkylthymine	0.1–0.7	1–4
Alkylphosphates	12	53

The quantitation of covalent DNA adducts in tissues has been used to demonstrate exposure of humans to carcinogenic chemicals and to assess the relative risk from exposure to carcinogenic chemicals. For example, DNA adducts of carcinogenic PAHs have been demonstrated at relatively high levels in tissues and blood of smokers and foundry workers compared with nonexposed individuals (Perera et al., 1991). In addition, DNA adducts of aflatoxin B1 were seen in samples of human placenta and cord blood in individuals in Taiwan, an area that demonstrates a high incidence of liver cancer (Hsieh and Hsieh, 1993). The presence of macromolecular carcinogen adducts may be important to their mechanism of carcinogenicity, the presence and persistence of the adducts is only one factor in the process of cancer development.

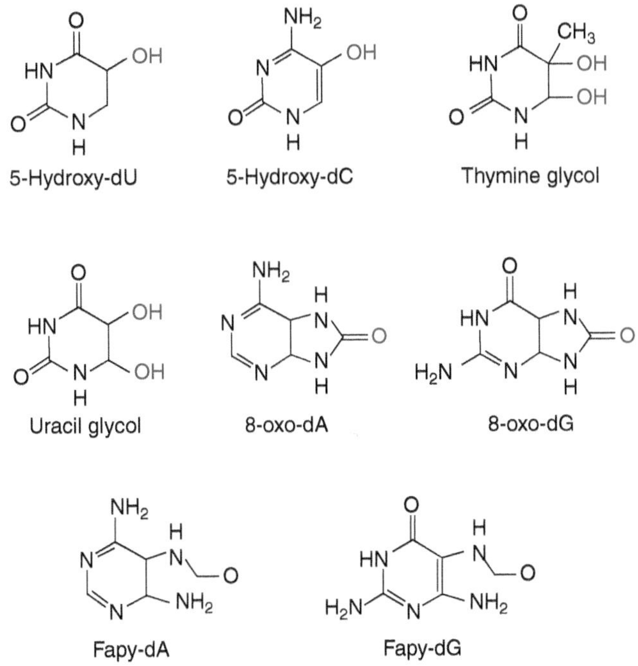

Experimental and epidemiological evidence indicates that the development of cancer following exposure to chemical carcinogens is a relatively rare event. This can be explained by the ability of a cell to recognize and repair DNA. The DNA region containing the adduct is removed and a new patch of DNA is synthesized, using the opposite intact strand as a template. The new DNA segment is then spliced into the DNA molecule in place of the defective one. To be effective in restoring a cell to normal, repair of DNA must occur prior to cell division; if repair is not complete prior to replication, the presence of the adducts can give rise to mispairing of bases and other genetic effects such as rearrangements and translocations of DNA segments. Thus, a chemical that alters the repair process or the rate of cell division can itself affect the frequency of mutation and neoplastic transformation.

DNA Repair Mechanisms

Although cells posses mechanisms to repair many types of DNA damage, these are not always completely effective, and residual DNA damage can lead to the insertion of an incorrect base during DNA replication, followed by transcription and translation of the mutated templates, ultimately leading to the synthesis of altered protein. Mutations in an oncogene, tumor-suppressor gene or gene that controls the cell cycle, can result in a clonal cell population with a proliferative or survival advantage. The development of a tumor requires many such events, occurring over a long period of time, and for this reason human cancer induction often takes place within the context of chronic exposure to chemical carcinogens.

A number of structural alterations may occur in DNA as a result of interaction with reactive chemicals or radiation, and the more frequent types of damage are depicted in Fig. 8-8. The reaction of chemical species with DNA can produce adducts within the bases, sugar and phosphate backbone of DNA. In addition, bifunctional alkylating agents (such as mustards) may cause DNA crosslinking between two opposing bases. Other structural changes such as pyrimidine dimmer formation are specific for exposure to UV light whereas double-stranded breaks in DNA are more commonly associated with ionizing radiation. A variety of mechanisms have evolved to effectively remediate and repair DNA damage. The more common types of DNA repair mechanisms seen in mammalians are listed in Table 8-9.

In addition to the proofreading activity of DNA polymerases that can correct miscopied bases during replication, cells have several mechanisms for repairing DNA damage. Repair of DNA damage does not always occur prior to cell replication, and, in addition, repair of DNA damage by some chemicals is relatively inefficient, as such, exposure to chemicals that cause DNA damage can increase the probability of acquiring mutations that ultimately lead to cancer development.

Mismatch Repair of Single-Base Mispairs Spontaneous mutations may occur through normal cellular DNA replication mistakes. Many spontaneous mutations are point mutations, a change in a single base pair in the DNA sequence, or a small insertion or deletion or a frame shift mutation of some modest size. The issue for mismatch repair is determining which is the normal DNA

Figure 8-7. *Structures of selected oxidative bases.*

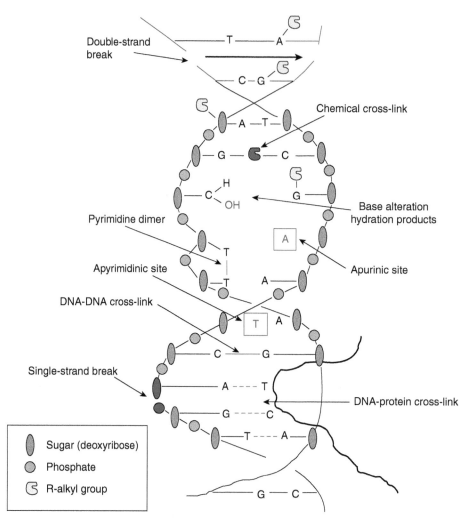

Figure 8-8. *Schematic representation of chemical and radiation-induced lesions in DNA.*

and which is the damaged DNA strand, and, therefore, repairing the mutated strand such that the correct base pairs are restored. Depurination is a fairly common occurrence and spontaneous event in mammals, and results in the formation of apurinic sites. If these lesions are left unrepaired, mutations are generated during DNA replication as DNA synthetic machinery is unable to determine the appropriate base with which to pair. All mammalian cells possess apurinic endonucleases that function to cut DNA near apurinic sites. The cut is then extended by exonucleases, and the resulting gap repaired by DNA polymerase and ligase.

Excision Repair DNA regions containing chemically modified bases, or DNA chemical adducts, are typically repaired by

Table 8-9

DNA Repair Pathways

1. Direct reversal of DNA damage
2. Excision repair systems
   Base excision repair
   Nucleotide excision repair
   Mismatch repair
3. Postreplicational repair (recombination repair)
4. Nonhomologous end-jointing (NHEJ): double-strand break repair

excision repair processes. DNA adducts cause a distortion in the normal shape of DNA. Proteins that slide along the surface of a double-stranded DNA molecule recognize the irregularities in the shape of the double helix, and affect the repair of the lesion. DNA lesions that are repaired by excision repair processes include thymine–thymine dimmers, produced following exposure to UV light, dimers that interfere with both replication and transcription of DNA. The repair of DNA regions containing bases altered by the attachment of large chemical adducts such as benzo(*a*)pyrene are also effectively repaired by excision repair processes (Fig. 8-9).

End-Joining Repair of Nonhomologous DNA A cell that has double-strand breaks can be repaired by joining the free DNA ends. The joining of broken ends from different chromosomes, however, will lead to the translocation of DNA pieces from one chromosome to another, translocations that have the potential to enable abnormal cell growth by placing a proto-oncogene next to, and, therefore, under the control of another gene promoter. Double-strand breaks can be caused by ionizing radiation and drugs such as anticancer drugs. Double-strand breaks are correctly repaired only when the free ends of DNA rejoin exactly. The repair of double-stranded DNA is therefore confounded by the absence of single-stranded regions that can signal the correct base pairing during the rejoining process. Homologous recombination is one of two mechanisms responsible for the repair of double-strand breaks. In this process, the double-strand break on one chromosome is repaired using the information on the homologous, intact chromosome.

The predominant mechanism for double-stranded DNA repair in multicellular organisms is nonhomologous repair and involves the rejoining the ends of the two DNA molecules. Although this process yields a continuous double-stranded molecule, several base pairs are lost at the joining point. This type of deletion may produce a possibly mutagenic coding change.

Classes of Genotoxic Carcinogens

Polyaromatic Hydrocarbons PAHs are found at high levels in charcoal-broiled foods, cigarette smoke, and in diesel exhaust. Representative chemicals belonging to this class are shown in Fig. 8-10A. A recent review of the causes of human cancer (*103 human carcinogens*) also lists those PAHs linked to human cancer by the International Agency for Research in Cancer

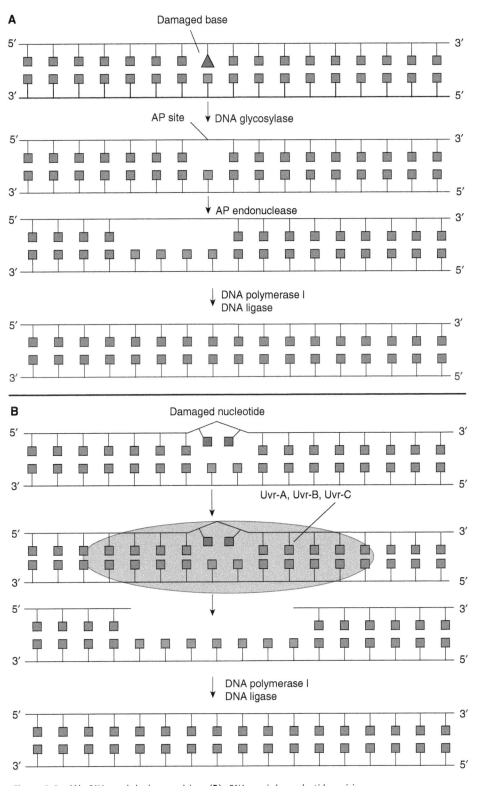

Figure 8-9. (**A**), DNA repair by base excision. (**B**), DNA repair by nucleotide excision.

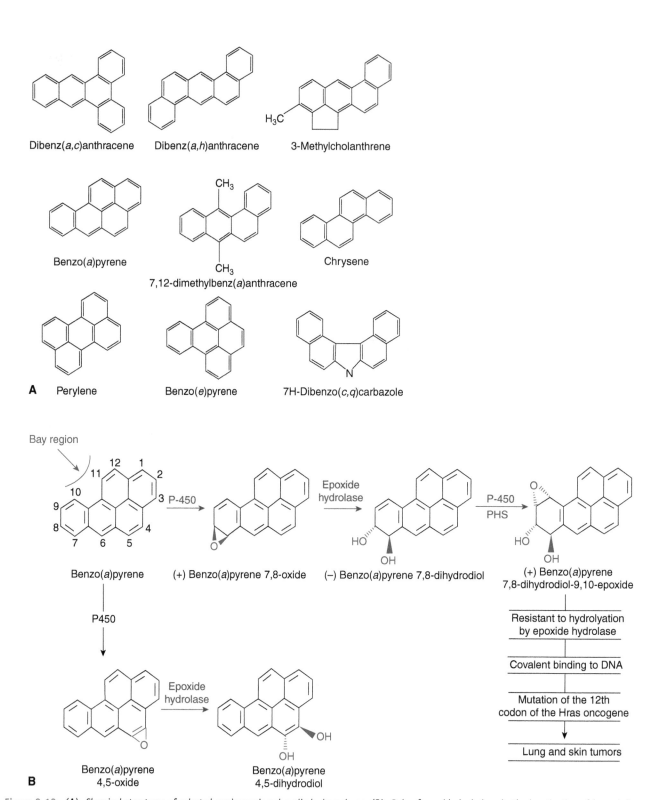

Figure 8-10. *(A), Chemical structures of selected carcinogenic polycyclic hydrocarbons. (B), Role of epoxide hydrolase in the inactivation of benzo[a]pyrene 4,5-oxide and in the conversion of benzo[a]pyrene to its tumorigenic Bay region diolepoxide.*

(IARC monographs [Vol. 100 A–F]). Benzo(a)pyrene is a representative polycyclic hydrocarbon that has been extensively studied. The metabolism and pathways that lead to tumor formation have been characterized through the work of a number of laboratories (Conney, 1982). The ultimate carcinogen is a diol epoxide of benzo(a)pyrene, formed following three separate enzymatic reactions (Sims *et al.*, 1974). Benzo[a]pyrene is first oxidized by cytochrome P4501A1 to form benzo[a]pyrene 7,8-oxide, further metabolized by epoxide hydrolase, yielding the 7,8-dihydrodiol.

And then further metabolism by cytochrome P4501A1 to yield the ultimate carcinogen, the 7,8-dihydrodiol-9,10-epoxide (Yang *et al.*, 1976; Lowe and Silverman, 1984). The Bay region or K region of the benzo(a)pyrene molecule is the site of metabolic targeting and DNA interaction (Fig. 8-10B). The importance of the Bay region (K region) of the benzo(a)pyrene molecule was demonstrated from the understanding of the metabolism of the benzo(a)pyrene to its ultimate DNA-reactive form. Similar regions (to the Bay region) have been identified in other carcinogenic polycyclic hydrocarbons and used to access and predict carcinogenic potential of other PAHs. Evidence has emerged that besides the P450 metabolism pathway, PAHs can also be metabolized through a peroxidase pathway and the aldo–keto reductase (AKR) pathway. The latter of which has been attributed to cancer risk in humans exposed to coal burning smoke in China (Lan *et al.*, 2004). Oxidative damage-related genes AKR1C3 and OGG2 also appear to modulate risks for lung cancer due to exposure to PAH-rich coal combustion emissions.

Alkylating Agents Alkylating agents represent an important class of chemical carcinogens. Although some aklylating agents are direct-acting genotoxic agents, many require metabolic activation to produce electrophilic metabolites that can react with DNA. Alkylating agents can be classified into several groups including the direct-acting alkylalkanesulfonates (methyl- and ethyl methanesulfonate) and nitrosamides (N-methyl-N-nitrosourea, N-ethyl-N-nitrosourea, N-methyl-N-nitro-N-nitrosoguanidine, and the indirect-acting nitrosamides (dimethyl- and diethylnitrosamines) (Fig. 8-11). The alkylating compounds (or in the case of diethylnitrosamine and dimethylnitrosamine and their metabolites) readily react with DNA at more than 12 sites. The N^7 position of guanine and the N^3 position of adenine are the most reactive sites for alkylating chemicals to find to DNA. DNA methylation reactions occur more readily and thus exhibit >20 more adduct formation compared with ethylation reactions. However, ethylation reactions have a greater affinity for oxygen centers, an event that appears to correlate with the mutagenicity and carcinogenicity of these compounds. Nitrosamines were initially used as solvents in chemistry. Their toxic effects were identified when workers using the nitrosamines

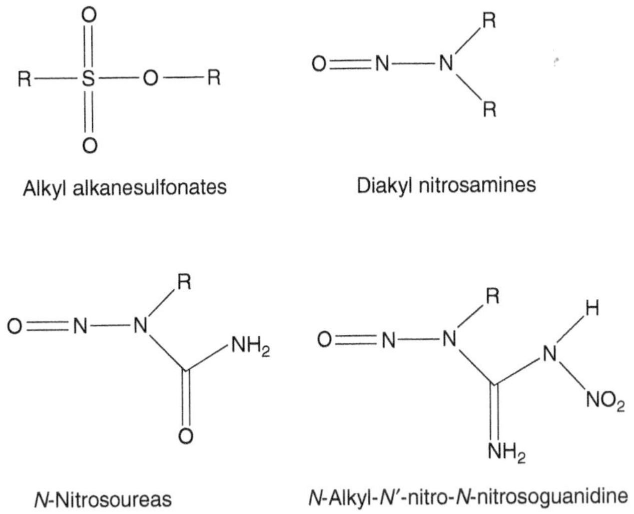

Figure 8-11. *Structures of representative methylating and ethylating agents.*

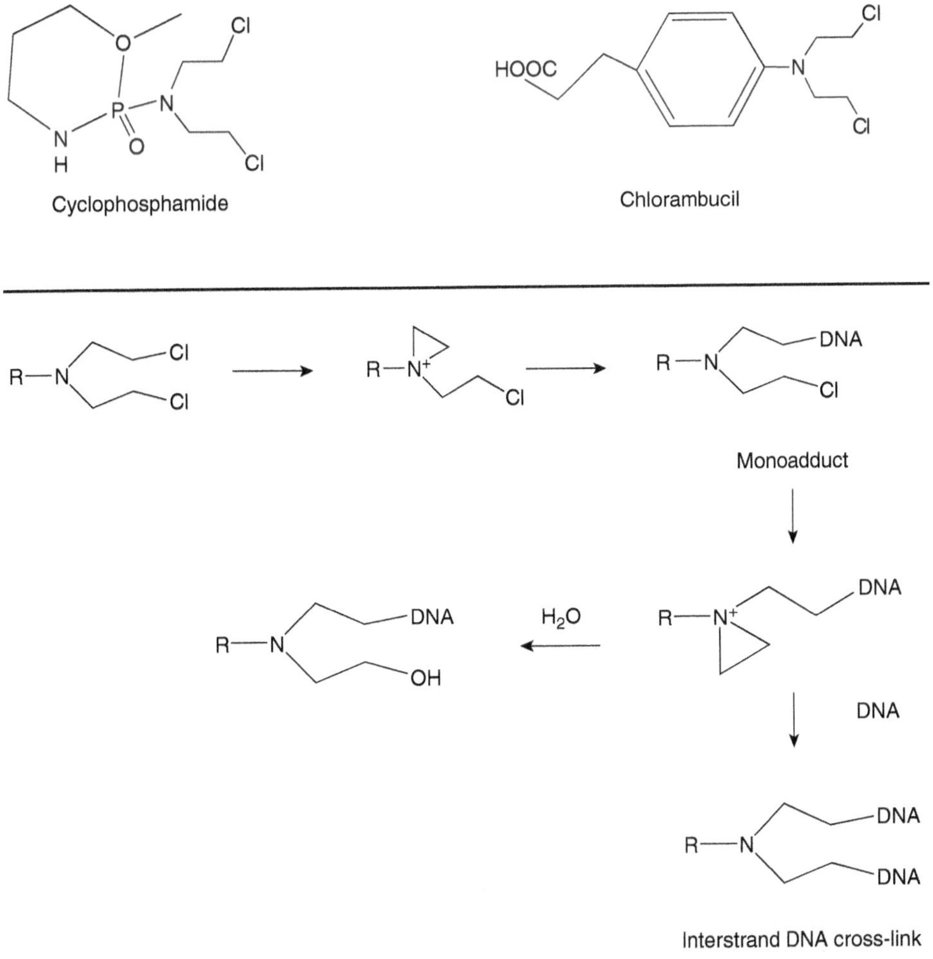

solvents developed jaundice and liver damage. Subsequent studies in animal models revealed that dimethylnitrosamine, and eventually diethylnitrosamine were highly hepatotoxic and hepatocarcinogenic.

Other alkylating chemicals including the nitrogen mustards (eg, chlorambucil, cyclophosphamide) have been used in cancer chemotherapy. They produce DNA adducts as well as induce the formation of DNA strand breaks. The alkylation of DNA by nitrogen mustards requires the formation of highly reactive N-alkylazirdinium ions (Fig. 8-12). Nitrogen mustards can produce

Cyclophosphamide

Chlorambucil

Figure 8-12. *Nitrogen mustards and proposed mechanism for the reactions of nitrogen mustards with DNA.*

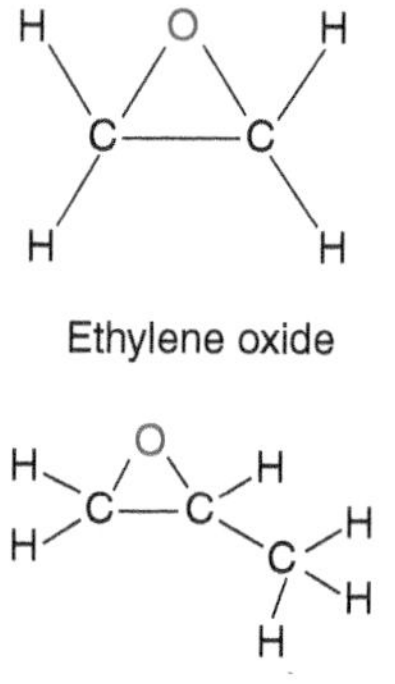

Figure 8-13. *Chemical structures for ethylene and propylene oxide.*

a wide spectrum of mutations including base pair substitutions (AT and GC) and deletions. In addition, nitrogen mustards are potent clastogens causing chromosomal aberrations and sister chromatid exchanges (SCEs), predominantly in GC-rich regions.

Ethylene oxide and propylene oxide are other examples of mutatgenic and carcinogenic alkylating agents (Fig. 8-13). Ethylene oxide is a direct-acting alkylating carcinogen in rodents and perhaps of human concern (Hogstedt *et al.*, 1986). Ethylene oxide is mutagenic in short-term in vitro assays and produces chromosomal aberrations and SCEs in eukaryotic cells (Ehrenberg and Hussain, 1981). Propylene oxide is also a mutagenic rodent carcinogen inducing nasal tumors in rodents following inhalation exposure (NTP, 1985). Alkylation of DNA by ethylene and propylene oxide occurs predominantly at the N^7 position of guanine, yielding 7-(2-hydroxyethyl) guanine and 7-(2-hydroxypropyl)guanine adducts, respectively. These adducts represent the major adducts formed following either in vitro or in vivo exposure (Walker *et al.*, 1992).

Vinyl chloride is another known rodent and human carcinogen, producing angiosarcomas in the liver and tumors in the lung and hematopoetic system in humans (Doll, 1988). Limited evidence also suggests that vinyl chloride exposure results in brain tumors. Vinyl chloride is mutagenic and is metabolized by cytochrome P450 to form chloroethylene oxide, which rearranges nonenzymatically to produce chloroacetaldehyde, both of which can alkylate DNA. Vinyl chloride and metabolites form several DNA adducts including 7-(2'-oxoethyl)guanine, N^2, 3-etheneoguanine, 3,N^4-ethenocytosine, and 1,N^6-ethenoadenine (Guengerich, 1994).

Aromatic Amines and Amides Aromatic amines and amides encompass a class of chemicals with varied structures (aromatic amines, eg, aniline dyes, 2-natphylamine, benzidine, 2-acetylaminofluofene) (Fig. 8-14). Because of their use in the dye industry and other industrial processes their carcinogen risk to humans was realized in the late 19th century. Exposure to these chemicals still occurs through cigarette smoke and environmental sources, even though proper industrial hygiene processes have considerably reduced the human exposure to aromatic amines and amides in the workplace. The aromatic amines undergo both phase I and phase II metabolism. Phase I reactions occur mainly by cytochrome P450-mediated reactions, yielding hydroxylated metabolites that are often associated with adduct formation in proteins and DNA, and produce liver and bladder carcinogenicity (Miller *et al.*, 1964). Metabolism of 2-acetylaminofluorene (AAF) results in the formation of *N*-hydroxy-AAF, which is a metabolite responsible for the liver tumorigenicity. Similarly, 1-napthylamine exhibits carcinogenic activity only in test systems capable of producing the *N*-hydroxy metabolite of napthylamine. Aromatic amines are capable of forming adducts with several DNA bases. Both heterocyclic amines (HCAs) and PAHs are formed when muscle meat, including beef, pork, fish, and poultry, is cooked using high-temperature

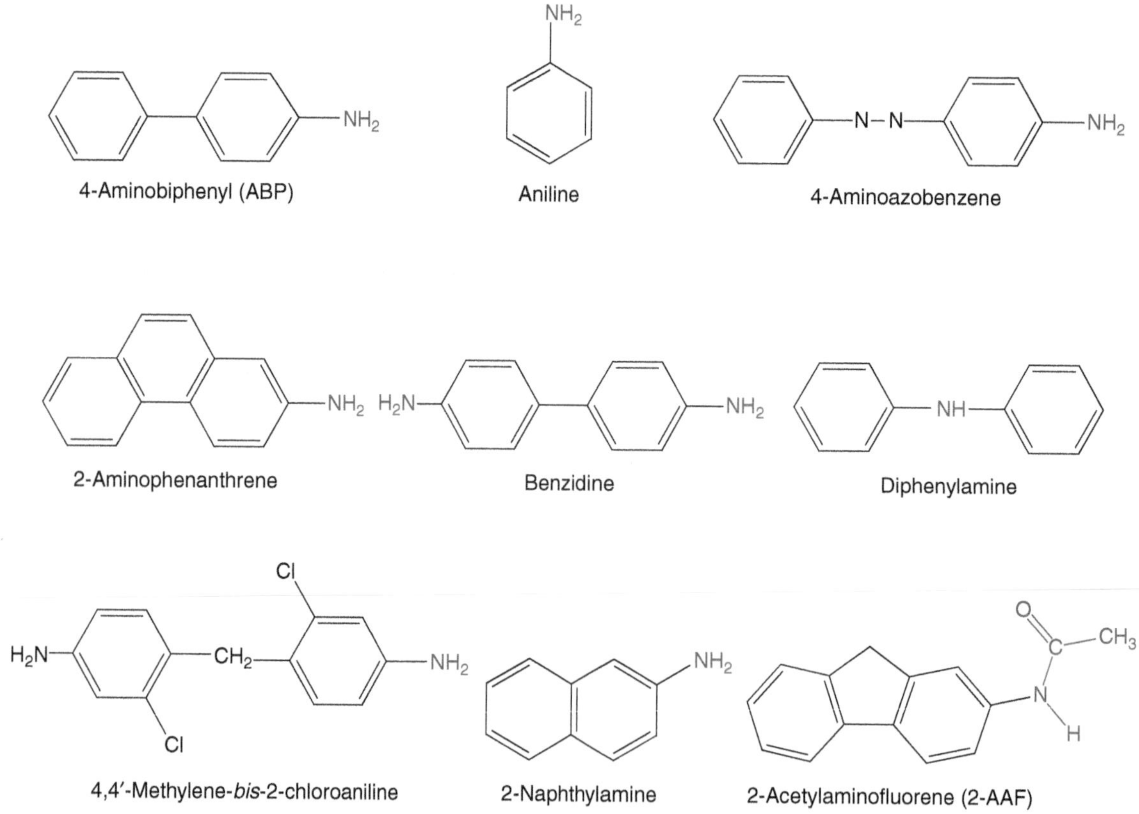

Figure 8-14. *Chemical structures of selected carcinogenic aromatic amines.*

methods, such as pan frying or grilling directly over an open flame. HCAs are also formed from fried foods, specifically fried meats (Turesky, 2007). Mutagenic activity of cooked meats at high temperature has been reported using the Ames Salmonella mutagenesis assay. In particular, an increase in HCAs (specifically MeIQx(2-amino-3,8-dimethylimidazo[4,5-*b*]quinoxaline), DiMeIQx (2-amino-3,4,8-dimethylimidazo [4,5-*f*]quinoxaline), and IQ (2-amino-3-methylimidazo [4,5-*f*]quinolone)) were found with increasing frying temperatures and cooking duration (Knize *et al.*, 1995). In support of these experimental studies epidemiology linkages between consumption of high-temperature cooked foods and human cancer have been reported (Cross and Sinha, 2004; Rohrmann *et al.*, 2007).

Classes and Mode of Action of Nongenotoxic (Epigenetic) Carcinogens

A number of chemicals that produce tumors in experimental animals following chronic treatment appear to act via mechanisms not involving direct binding, damage, or interaction of the chemical or its metabolites with DNA (Williams and Whysner, 1996). Based on the lack of genotoxicity, yet their ability to induce tumors in rodent models, these chemicals have been labeled nongenotoxic carcinogens. The organ and tissue targets induced by nongenotoxic carcinogens are many times in tissues where a significant incidence of background, spontaneous tumors is seen in the animal model. Prolonged exposure to relatively high levels of chemicals is usually necessary for the production of tumors. In addition, with nongenotoxic carcinogens, tumors are not theoretically expected to occur at exposures below a threshold at which relevant cellular effects are not observed. In contrast to DNA-reactive genotoxic effects, non–DNA-reactive mechanisms may be unique to the rodent species used for testing. Certain chemical carcinogens have been well studied and provide examples for the use of mechanistic information in risk assessment. Further, the biochemical modes of action for non–DNA-reactive carcinogens are diverse. Examples include chemicals that function via sustained cytotoxicity, receptor-mediated (eg, CAR, peroxisome proliferator–activated receptor alpha [PPARα], aryl hydrocarbon receptor [AhR]) effects, hormonal perturbation, as well as the induction of oxidative stress and modulation of methylation status (Table 8-10). Each of these potential mechanisms is discussed in greater detail in the following sections.

Cytotoxicity Cytotoxicity and consequent regenerative hyperplasia is well-documented mode of action for a variety of non–DNA-reactive chemical carcinogens (Dietrich and Swenberg, 1991). Chloroform-induced liver and kidney tumors and melamine-induced bladder tumors are classic examples of chemical carcinogens that are classified as functioning via a cytolethal mode of action (Andersen *et al.*, 1998; Bull *et al.*, 1986; Pereira, 1994; Larson *et al.*, 1994; Butterworth *et al.*, 1990). Chemicals that function through this mechanism produce sustained cell death, often related to metabolism of the chemical, that is accompanied by persistent regenerative growth, resulting in the potential for the acquisition of "spontaneous" DNA mutations and allowing mutated cells to accumulate and proliferate. This process then gives rise to preneoplastic focal lesions that upon further expansion can lead to tumor formation. Chloroform has been shown to induce mouse liver tumors only at doses of compound that produce liver necrosis, thus demonstrating an association between necrosis with compensatory hyperplasia and the resulting tumorigenicity, and also supports that a threshold for the induction of tumors is likely at doses that do not produce toxicity. It is important to note that the

Table 8-10

Proposed Modes of Action for Selected Nongenotoxic Chemical Carcinogens

MODE OF ACTION	EXAMPLE
Cytotoxicity	Chloroform
	Melamine
α2u-Globulin-binding	D-Limonene,
	1,4-dichlorobenzene
Receptor-mediated	
CAR	Phenobarbital
PPARα	Trichloroethylene
	Perchloroethylene
	Diethylhexylphthalate
	fibrates (eg, clofibrate)
AhR	2,3,7,8-Tetrachlorodibenzo-*p*-dioxin (TCDD)
	Polychlorinated biphenyls (PCBs)
	Polybrominates biphenyls (PBBs)
Hormonal	Biogenic amines
	steroid and peptide hormones
	DES
	Phytoestrogens (bisphenol-A)
	Tamoxifen
	Phenobarbital
Altered methylation	Phenobarbital
	Choline deficiency
	Diethanolamine
Oxidative stress inducers	Ethanol
	TCDD
	Lindane
	Dieldrin
	Acrylonitrile

DES, diethylstilbesterol.

induction of cytotoxicity may be observed with many carcinogens both genotoxic and nongenotoxic when high toxic exposures occur. Thus, the induction of cytotoxicity with compensatory hyperplasia may contribute to the observed tumorigenicity of many carcinogenic agents at high-dose levels.

α2u-Globulin-Binding Drugs The carcinogens D-limonene, 1,4-dichlorobenzene, and trimethylpentane (Fig. 8-15) induce renal tumors selectively in the male rat, and provide excellent examples of the species, sex, and tissue specificity of non–DNA-reactive carcinogens. The mechanism for the species and sex specificity is related to the ability of these compounds to bind to α2u-globulin, a protein synthesized by the male rat liver at the onset of puberty, as the mechanism of tumorigenesis. α2u-Globulin is, filtered through the glomerulus, and only partially excreted (~50%) in the urine. The reabsorbed fraction accumulates in lysosomes of the P2 segment of the proximal tubules, where it is hydrolyzed to amino acids (Melnick *et al.*, 1996). Chemicals with the ability to bind to α2u-globulin decrease the rate of digestion of α2u-globulin and results in the accumulation in the lysosomes, dysfunction of this organelle and subsequent release of digestive enzymes and cell necrosis. The greater loss of tubule cells leads to increased cell proliferation in the P2 segment, which may be responsible for the tumor development and malignant transformation (Dietrich and Swenberg, 1991).

CHAPTER 8   CHEMICAL CARCINOGENESIS

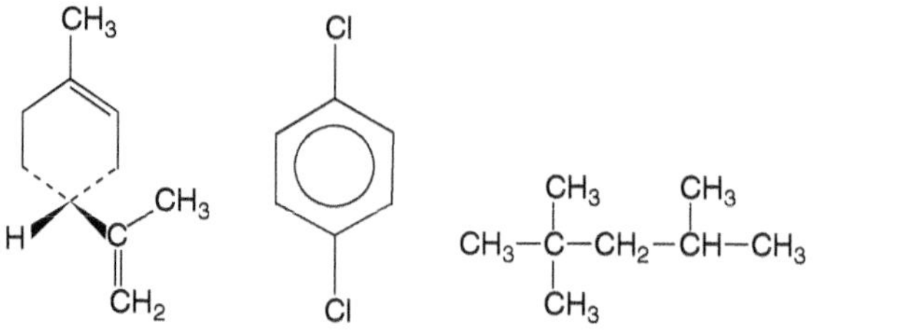

D-Limonene   1,4-Dichlorobenzene   2,2,4-Trimethylpentane C_8H_{18}

Figure 8-15. *Examples of selective α2u-globulin-binding chemicals.*

Receptor-Mediated

CAR Receptor-Mediated (Phenobarbital-Like Carcinogens)
Phenobarbital is a commonly studied non–DNA-reactive compound that is known to cause tumors by a nongenotoxic mechanism involving liver hyperplasia (Williams and Whysner, 1996). One feature seen following phenobarbital exposure is the induction of P450 enzymes, particularly Cyp2b (Nims and Lubet, 1996). Because a number of diverse chemicals are known to induce various members of the P450 system (eg, dieldrin, ethanol, 2,3,7,8-Tetrachlorodibenzo-*p*-dioxin [TCDD]), the specificity of this effect to the carcinogenesis has been questioned. Recent evidence has shown that the induction of Cyp2b is mediated by activation of the constitutive androstane receptor (CAR), a member of the nuclear receptor family (Ueda *et al.*, 2002; Kodama *et al.*, 2004; Honkakoski *et al.*, 1998). CAR-null mice show no induction of Cyp2b following phenobarbital exposure (Wei *et al.*, 2000). Other phenobarbital responses that are critical for tumor formation include increased cell proliferation, inhibition of apoptosis, inhibition of gap junctional communication, hypertrophy, and development of preneoplastic focal lesions in the liver (Whysner *et al.*, 1996), effects that have all been shown to be CAR-dependent (Wei *et al.*, 2000; Kodama *et al.*, 2004) (Fig. 8-16).

Peroxisome Proliferator–Activated Receptor α A wide array of chemicals are capable of increasing the number and volume of peroxisomes in the cytoplasm of cells. These agents, termed peroxisome proliferators, include chemicals such as herbicides, chlorinated solvents (eg, trichloroethylene and perchloroethylene) plasticizers (eg, diethylhexylphthalate and other phthalates), lipid-lowering fibrate drugs (eg, ciprofibrate, clofibrate), and natural products. In addition, many of the chemicals within this group produce liver enlargement and hepatocellular carcinoma in rats and mice through non–DNA-reactive mechanisms (Lake, 1995; Reddy and Rao, 1997). Two additional tumor types are also associated with exposure to peroxisome proliferating compounds: Leydig cell tumors and pancreatic acinar cell tumors in rats. Studies conducted either in vivo or in vitro in primary hepatocyte cultures have shown important interspecies differences in the hepatic peroxisome proliferation responses to chemicals within the class of compounds. The rat and the mouse were clearly revealed as responsive species, whereas primates and the guinea pig proved to be nonresponders. The Syrian hamster exhibits an intermediate response (Lake, 1995; Bentley *et al.*, 1993). Due to the wide structural diversity of this chemical class, the mechanism(s) involved in peroxisome proliferation and tumorigenesis went unrecognized for years. The currently accepted mode of action for this class of chemicals involves agonist binding to a nuclear hormone receptor, the PPARα. Largely through the use of PPARα knockout mice, it has been demonstrated that the activation of PPARα by agonists is needed for these chemicals to induce peroxisome proliferation and tumorigenesis in rodents (Issemann and Green, 1990; Lee *et al.*, 1995; Peters *et al.*, 1998, reviewed in Klaunig *et al.*, 2003). PPARα is highly expressed in cells that have active fatty acid oxidation capacity (eg, hepatocytes, cardiomyocytes, enterocytes). It is well documented that PPARα plays a central role in lipid metabolism and acts as a transcription factor to modulate gene expression following ligand activation. This latter effect arises through the heterodimerization of PPARα and RXRα, which results in binding to

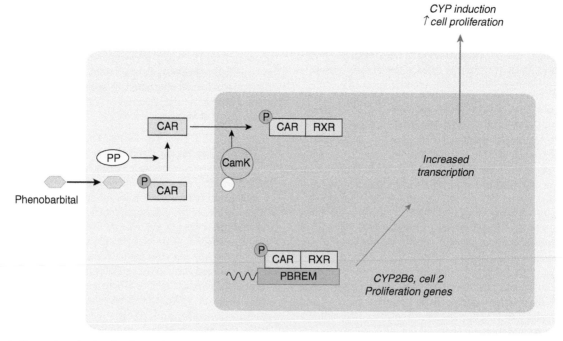

Figure 8-16. *Proposed mechanism for the involvement of the constitutive androstane receptor (CAR) in phenobarbital-induced gene expression changes.* PP, protein phosphatase; CamK, CaM Kinase; RXR, retinoic acid receptor; PBREM, phenobarbital response element. Following dephosphorylation of CAR by protein phosphatase, CAR crosses the cell membrane and becomes phosphorylated by CaM kinase. CAR then forms a dimer with RXR and binds to PBREMs, resulting in increased gene expression.

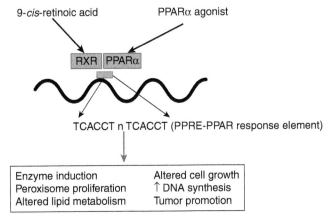

Figure 8-17. *Mechanism for altered gene expression by peroxisome proliferator activated receptor α (PPARα) agonist binding.* Following agonist binding to PPARα, the receptor dimerizes with the retinoic acid receptor (RXR). This complex then binds to PPREs, resulting in enhanced gene transcription.

response elements (PPREs) and subsequent modulation of target gene transcription (Fig. 8-17). Following this event is the induction of cell proliferation and suppression of apoptosis (Marsman *et al.*, 1992; Burkhardt *et al.*, 2001; James and Roberts, 1996). Both of these events would then be expected to affect tumor development as these effects would enhance the rate of fixation of DNA damage in the genome, leading to changes in gene expression, such as the silencing of tumor-suppressor genes or increased expression of oncogenes, or suppress apoptosis that may normally remove DNA-damaged, potentially tumorigenic, cells. Because humans are exposed to a number of these chemicals, the relevance of this mode of action to humans has been evaluated (Klaunig *et al.*, 2003). Although the same events would be expected to occur in exposed humans, several species differences have been noted including a lack of induction of cell proliferation in nonhuman primates (Pugh *et al.*, 2000), and the finding that PPARα in human liver is at least 10-fold lower compared with the rat or mouse (Palmer *et al.*, 1998; Tugwood *et al.*, 1998). Based on these kinetic and dynamic differences between species, it has been concluded that tumors are not likely to occur in humans by PPARα agonists (Klaunig *et al.*, 2003).

Aryl Hydrocarbon Receptor Activators of the AhR receptor including TCDD and selected polychlorinated- and brominated-biphenyl (PCBs and PBBs) compounds (Fig. 8-18) have been linked to tumor promotion in rodent livers (IARC, 1997a,b; 2011; Pitot *et al.*, 1982). The tumor response has been determined to be AhR-dependent (Knutson and Poland, 1982) (Fig. 8-19). Upon ligand binding to the AhR, the ligand bound AhR translocates to the nucleus, dimerizes with the Ah receptor nuclear translocator (ARNT) and binds to aryl hydrocarbon response elements (AREs also known as doxin response elements [DRE] and xenobiotic response elements [XRE]) (for review see Nebert *et al.*, 2000). AhR-ARNT–dependent genes include cytochrome P450 family members, NAD(P)H:quinone oxidoreductase, a cytosolic aldehyde dehydrogenase 3, a UDP-glucuronosyltransferase, and a glutathione transferase (Nebert *et al.*, 2000), genes that are involved in metabolic activation as well as detoxification of chemical agents. It has been hypothesized that there are additional AhR-ARNT–dependent genes (Nebert *et al.*, 2000). AhR knockout mice have a diminished response to tumor induction by AhR ligands (Nakatsuru *et al.*, 2004), and conversely, constitutively overexpressed AhR resulted in an increased incidence of liver tumors (Moennikes *et al.*, 2004).

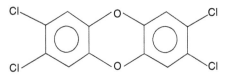

2,3,7,8-*p*-TCDD

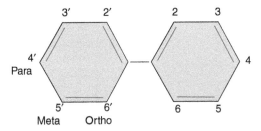

Figure 8-18. *Selective examples of aryl hydrocarbon receptor-binding chemicals.* Prototypical structure for PCBs or PBBs. PCBs and PBBs exhibit varying degrees of chlorination or bromination at positions 2-6 and 2′-6′ of the biphenyl molecule.

As seen with other hepatic tumor-promoting chemicals, TCDD also inhibits apoptosis in hepatic foci (Stinchcombe *et al.*, 1995).

Hormonal Mode of Action Hormonally active chemicals include steroids and peptide hormones that produce tissue-specific changes through interaction with a receptor. A number of non–DNA-reactive chemicals induce neoplasia through receptor-mediated mechanisms, and/or perturbation of hormonal balance. Trophic hormones are known to induce cell proliferation at their target organs. This action may lead to the development of tumors when the mechanisms of hormonal control are disrupted and some or other hormone shows persistently increased levels. Several well-studied examples include the induction of ovarian neoplasms via decreased estradiol and increased luteinizing hormone (LH) levels (Capen *et al.*, 1995), and the induction of thyroid tumors in rats by phenobarbital-type P450 inducers (which modulate T3 and T4) (McClain, 1994; Whysner *et al.*, 1996).

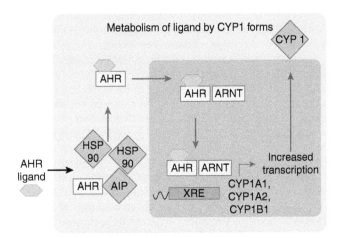

Figure 8-19. *Proposed mechanism of aryl hydrocarbon receptor (AhR) mediated gene expression.* ARNT, AhR nuclear transporter; XRE, xenobiotic response element. Non-ligand bound AhR is maintained in the cytoplasm via association with chaperone proteins (eg, AIP, Hsp90). Following ligand binding, chaperone proteins dissociate and AhR translocates to the nucleus where it binds with ARNT. The heterodimer binds to XREs resulting in an increase in gene transcription.

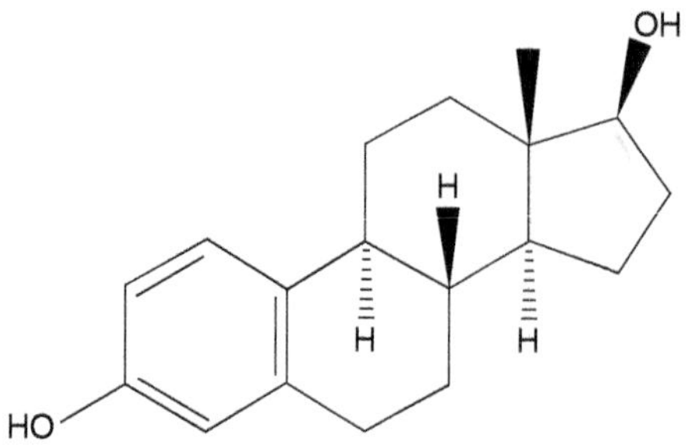

Figure 8-20. *Chemical examples of estrogenic agonists and antagonists.*

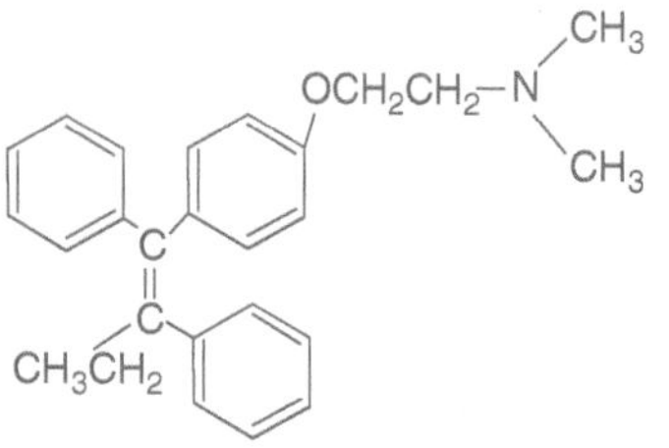

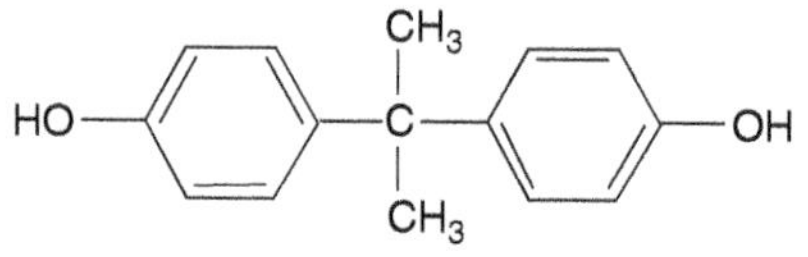

Estrogenic agents can induce tumors in estrogen-dependent tissue. Selective estrogenic agents (agonists and antagonists) are shown in Fig. 8-20. Oral administration of 17β-estradiol to female mice increases the incidence of mammary tumors (Welsch *et al.,* 1977; Highman *et al.,* 1978) whereas subcutaneous administration of estradiol to young female mice produced tumors of the cervix and vagina (Pan and Gardner, 1948). Evidence that estrogenic chemicals are carcinogenic to humans comes from epidemiological data on breast and ovarian cancer, which indicates that individuals with higher circulating estrogen levels and those with exposure to the potent estrogenic chemical diethylstilbesterol (DES) are at increased risk for cancer development. DES was first shown to induce mammary tumors in male mice following subcutaneous administration of the hormone. DES has been causally associated to the higher incidence of adenocarcinomas of the vagina and cervix in daughters of women treated with the hormone during pregnancy (Herbst and Scully, 1970; Herbst *et al.,* 1972; Noller *et al.,* 1972). The mechanism of action for DES is believed to function through its ability to induce aneuploidy (Tsutsui *et al.,* 1997; Li *et al.,* 1997). The effects of steroidal chemicals on the cell cycle (Sutherland *et al.,* 1995) and on microtubule assembly (Metzler *et al.,* 1996) may be important in the aneuploidy inducing effects of some hormonal agents (Li *et al.,* 1996).

Chronic exogenous administration of hormonally active chemicals including synthetic estrogens and anabolic steroids can increase hepatic adenoma incidence in rats (Li *et al.,* 1992) and in humans (IARC, 1997a,b). Women of childbearing age are sensitive to hepatic adenoma formation, which can be exacerbated by oral contraceptive use. These adenomas will regress upon hormone cessation (Edmondson *et al.,* 1977) and can progress with continued administration (Christopherson *et al.,* 1978). Chronic administration (>8 years) is required to detect this increased liver tumor risk from oral contraceptives (Tavani *et al.,* 1993).

Many substances in plants (phytoestrogens) have been described. These include compounds such as genestein, daidzein,

glycetein, equol, and their metabolites found in soy products and various lignan derivatives (Adlercreutz and Mazur, 1997). In addition, a number of environmental nonsteroidal synthetic compounds demonstrate apparent estrogenic activity (eg, nonyl-phenol, bisphenol-A, chlorinated hydrocarbons; Soto *et al.,* 1997). The potential for these chemicals to induce cancer in humans is an area of current investigation.

Species and tissue specificity in response to receptor- and hormone-mediated carcinogenesis is often observed. As an example, tamoxifen is antiestrogenic in the chick oviduct, estrogenic in the mouse uterus with acute administration, but antiestrogenic with chronic administration in the same tissue, whereas it is estrogenic in the rat uterus. Although this may be in part due to tissue and species differences in coactivator and corepressor levels and availability, many other pharmacokinetic and pharmacodynamic properties are likely to participate (Carthew *et al.,* 1995). To further exemplify the complexity of the role of estrogen in cancer development, estrogens have also been shown to act as a protective agent in prostate cancer.

Induction of ovarian tumors by dietary administration of nitrofurantoin in mice is an example of a tumorigenic effect secondary to drug-induced hormonal disturbance. Treatment resulted in ovarian atrophy with absence of graafian follicles and sterility. The reduction of follicles induced a reduction of sex steroid hormone by the ovary, resulting in increased production of gonadotrophins, notably LH, presumably due to the decreased negative feedback on the hypothalamus–pituitary axis by estrogens. Persistent stimulation by LH of the ovary cells resulted in development of tumors (Capen *et al.,* 1995). A similar effect is known to occur with dopamine agonists. The induction of hypoprolactinemia changes the number of LH receptors and leads to enhanced sensitivity to LH and a higher stimulation by LH similarly to nitrofurantoin.

A reduction of thyroid hormone concentrations (T4 and/or T3) and increased thyroid-stimulating hormone (TSH) have been

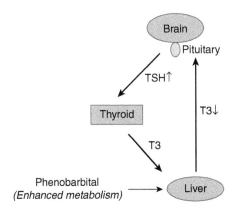

Figure 8-21. *Mechanism for phenobarbital-induced thyroid tumors.* Through alteration of gene expression, phenobarbital enhances metabolism of thyroid hormone (T3) resulting in enhanced TSH production. Increased TSH then leads to increased cell proliferation in the thyroid.

shown to induce neoplasia in the rodent thyroid. TSH increases proliferative activity in the thyroid. After chronic treatment chemical-induced TSH increases leading to follicular cell hypertrophy, hyperplasia, and eventually neoplasia. Inducers of metabolic enzymes in the liver, a classic and well-studied example being phenobarbital (Hood *et al.*, 1999), result in increased thyroid hormone metabolism and as such lead to increase in TSH levels (Fig. 8-21). It is this latter event that is associated with the development of thyroid tumors in rodents. Recent evidence suggests that the enhancement of metabolism and excretion of thyroid hormones by xenobiotics (via induction of phase II enzymes) is a consequence of CAR (and presumably PXR) activation. Qualitatively, thyroid gland function in rodents is much more susceptible to disturbances of the thyroid hormone levels than it is in humans. In contrast to humans, rodents lack the thyroid-binding globulin, which is the predominant plasma protein (at least in humans) responsible for

thyroxin binding and transport (McClain, 1995). A relatively higher level of functional activity is present in rat thyroid compared to humans.

DNA Methylation and Carcinogenesis Post-DNA synthetic methylation of the five position on cytosine (5-methyl-cytosine; 5mC) is a naturally occurring modification to DNA in higher eukaryotes that influences gene expression (Holliday, 1990) (Fig. 8-22). Under normal conditions, DNA is methylated symmetrically on both strands. Immediately following DNA replication, the newly synthesized double-stranded DNA contains hemimethylated sites that signal for DNA maintenance methylases to transfer methyl groups from S-adenosylmethionine to cytosine residues on the new DNA strand (Hergersberg, 1991). The degree of methylation within a gene inversely correlates with the expression of that gene; hypermethylation of genes is associated with gene silencing whereas hypomethylation results in an enhanced expression of genes. Several chemical carcinogens are known to modify DNA methylation, methyltransferase activity, and chromosomal structure. During carcinogenesis, both hypomethylation and hypermethylation of the genome have been observed (Counts and Goodman, 1995; Baylin, 1997). Increased methylation of CpG islands have been observed in bladder cancer and tumor-suppressor genes such as the retinoblastoma gene, *p16*[ink4a], and *p14*[ARF] have been reported to be hypermethylated in tumors (Salem *et al.*, 2000; Stirzaker *et al.*, 1997; Myöhänen *et al.*, 1998; Esteller *et al.*, 2001; Belinsky *et al.*, 1998). Hypomethylation has been associated with increased mutation rates. Most metastatic neoplasms in humans have significantly lower 5MeC than normal tissue (Gama-Sosa *et al.*, 1983); furthermore, many oncogenes are hypomethylated and their expression amplified.

Choline and methionine, which can be derived from dietary sources, provide a source of methyl groups used in methylation reactions. Rats exposed to choline and/or methionine-deficient diets resulted in hepatocellular proliferation and neoplasia (Abanobi

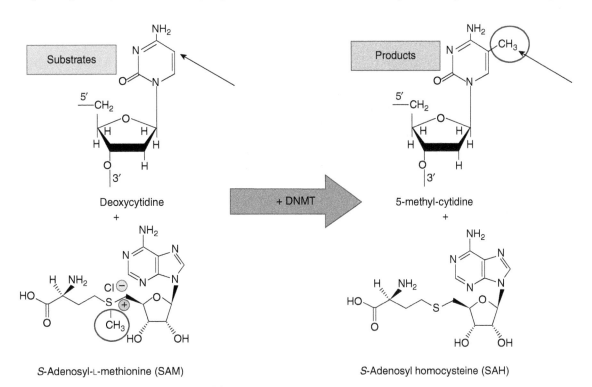

Figure 8-22. *Substrates and products involved in DNA methylation.* Methylation of DNA occurs through an enzymatic reaction catalyzed by DNA methyltransferases (DNMTs). DNA is methylated at the five-position of cytosine and requires the cofactor S-adenosyl methionine.

Table 8-11

Evidence for Choline Depletion in Hepatocarcinogenesis

CHOLINE	METHIONINE	FOLATE	HEPATOCELLULAR CARCINOMA (%)	DURATION (MONTHS)	REFERENCES
−	+	+	100	12	Nakae *et al.* (1992)
−	+	+	73	12	Lombardi *et al.* (1988)
−	Low	−	100	15	Henning *et al.* (1996)
−	−	+	51	13	Ghoshal *et al.* (1984)

et al., 1982; Wainfan and Poirier, 1992) (Table 8-11). In rodents fed choline or methyl donor groups deficient diets, the hepatic neoplasia is thought to arise from hypomethylation of *c-myc*, *c-fos*, and *c-H-ras* proto-oncogenes, due to the decreased availability of *S*-adenosylmethionine (Wainfan and Poirier, 1992; Newberne *et al.*, 1982). Chemicals such as diethanolamine result in hepatic neoplasia, in part, via a mechanism involving choline depletion, altered methylation and modulation of gene expression (Bachman *et al.*, 2006; Kamendulis and Klaunig, 2005). Reactive oxygen species have also been shown to modify DNA methylation resulting in changes in DNA methylation profiles through interfering with the ability of methyltransferases to interact with DNA, leading to hypomethylation of CpG sites (Weitzman *et al.*, 1994; Turk *et al.*, 1995). Also, the presence of 8-OHdG in DNA can lead to hypomethylation of DNA because this adduct, if present in CpCpGpGp sequences, will inhibit the methylation of adjacent C residues. Thus, oxidative DNA damage may be an important contributor to the carcinogenesis process brought about by the loss of DNA methylation, allowing the expression of normally quiescent genes. Also, the abnormal methylation pattern observed in cells transformed by chemical oxidants may contribute to an overall aberrant gene expression and promote the tumor process.

Oxidative Stress and Chemical Carcinogenesis   Experimental evidence has shown that increases in reactive oxygen in the cell, through either physiological modification or chemical carcinogen exposure, contribute to the carcinogenesis processes (Guyton and Kensler, 1993; Trush and Kensler, 1991; Vuillaume, 1987; Witz, 1991). Reactive oxygen species encompass a series of reactive compounds including the superoxide anion ($^{\bullet}O_2-$), hydroperoxyl radical ($HO_2^{\bullet}.$), hydrogen peroxide (H_2O_2), and the hydroxyl radical ($^{\bullet}OH$), all derived through the reduction of molecular oxygen (Table 8-12). Oxygen radicals can be produced by both endogenous and exogenous sources and are typically counterbalanced by antioxidants (Table 8-13). Antioxidant defenses are both enzymatic

(eg, superoxide dismutase, glutathione peroxidase, and catalase) and nonenzymatic (eg, vitamin E, vitamin C, β-carotene, and glutathione) (Betteridge, 2000; Abuja, 2001); importantly, many of these antioxidants are provided through dietary intake (Clarkson and Thompson, 2000).

Endogenous sources of reactive oxygen species include oxidative phosphorylation, P450 metabolism, peroxisomes, and inflammatory cell activation (Table 8-13). Within the mitochondria, a small percentage of oxygen is converted into the superoxide anion via 1-electron reduction of molecular oxygen. Superoxide can be dismutated by superoxide dismutase to yield hydrogen peroxide (Barber and Harris, 1994). In the presence of partially reduced metal ions hydrogen peroxide is converted into the highly reactive hydroxyl radical through Fenton and Haber–Weiss reactions (Betteridge, 2000). Neutrophils, eosinophils, and macrophages represent another intracellular source of reactive oxygen species. Activated macrophages, through a "respiratory burst," elicit a rapid increase in oxygen uptake that gives rise to a variety of reactive

Table 8-13

Reactive Oxygen Species Generation and Removal in the Cell

Cellular oxidants

Endogenous	Exogenous
Mitochondria	Redox Cycling Compounds
$\quad O_2^{\bullet}, H_2O_2, {}^{\bullet}OH$	$\quad O_2^{\bullet}$
Cytochrome P450	Metals (Fenton Reaction)
$\quad O_2^{\bullet}, H_2O_2$	$\quad H_2O_2 + Fe^{2+} \rightarrow OH^- +$
Macrophage/Inflammatory	$\quad {}^{\bullet}OH + Fe^{3+}$
Cells	Radiation
$\quad O_2^{\bullet}, {}^{\bullet}NO, H_2O_2, OCl^-$	$\quad {}^{\bullet}OH$
Peroxisomes	
$\quad H_2O_2$	

Cellular antioxidants

Enzymatic	Non-Enzymatic
Superoxide Dismutase	Vitamin E
Catalase	Glutathione
Glutathione Peroxidase	Vitamin C
Glutaredoxin	Catechins
Thioredoxin	

Oxidants > Antioxidants → Oxidative Damage (DNA, RNA, Lipid, Protein)

Oxidants can be produced via both endogenous and exogenous sources. Antioxidants function to maintain the cellular redox balancing. However, excess production of oxidants and/or inadequate supplies of antioxidants result in damage to cellular biomolecules and may impact on neoplastic development.

Table 8-12

Pathways for Intercellular Oxidant Generation

Generation of Reactive Oxygen Species via Reduction of Molecular Oxygen

$O_2 + e^- \rightarrow O_2^{\bullet}$ (superoxide anion)

$O_2^{\bullet} + H_2O \rightarrow HO_2^{\bullet}$ (hydroperoxyl radical)

$HO_2^{\bullet} + e^- + H \rightarrow H_2O_2$ (hydrogen peroxide)

$H_2O_2 + e^- \rightarrow OH^- + {}^{\bullet}OH$ (hydroxyl radical)

A series of oxygen radicals are produced by the reduction of molecular oxygen. Of the radicals produced, the hydroxyl radical, hydroperoxyl radical, and the superoxide anion are sufficiently reactive and may interact with biomolecules.

oxygen species including superoxide anion, hydrogen peroxide, and nitric oxide. The release of cytokines and reactive oxygen intermediates from activated Kupffer cells (the resident macrophage of the liver) has been implicated in hepatotoxicological and hepatocarcinogenic events (Rose *et al.*, 1999; Rusyn *et al.*, 1999); in particular, recent studies show that the Kupffer cell may function at the promotion stage of carcinogenesis. Reactive oxygen species can also be produced by cytochrome P450-mediated mechanisms including (1) redox cycling in the presence of molecular oxygen, (2) peroxidase-catalyzed single electron drug oxidations, and (3) "futile cycling" of cytochromes P450 (Parke, 1994; Parke and Sapota, 1996). Ethanol, phenobarbital, and a number of chlorinated and nonchlorinated compounds such as dieldrin, TCDD, and lindane are among the xenobiotics shown to increase reactive oxygen species through P450-mediated mechanisms (Eksrom and Ingleman-Sundberg, 1989; Rice *et al.*, 1994; Klaunig *et al.*, 1997). Chemicals classified as PPARα agonists (eg, clofibrate, phthalate esters) represent chemicals that induce cytochrome P4504A and increase the formation of peroxisomes. As such, an increase in H_2O_2 production often accompanies exposure to chemicals that stimulate the number and activity of peroxisomes (Rao and Reddy, 1991; Wade *et al.*, 1992). Through these or other currently unknown mechanisms, a number of chemicals that induce cancer (eg, chlorinated compounds, radiation, metal ions, barbiturates, and some PPARα agonists), induce reactive oxygen species formation and/or oxidative stress (Rice-Evans and Burdon, 1993; Klaunig *et al.*, 1997, 2011).

Oxidative DNA Damage and Carcinogenesis

Reactive oxygen species left unbalanced by antioxidants can result in damage to cellular macromolecules. In DNA, reactive oxygen species can produce single- or double-stranded DNA breaks, purine, pyrimidine, or deoxyribose modifications, and DNA cross-links (von Sonntag, 1987; Dizdaroglu, 1992; Demple and Harrison, 1994). Persistent DNA damage can result in either arrest or induction of transcription, induction of signal transduction pathways, replication errors, and genomic instability, events that are potentially involved in carcinogenesis. Oxidation of guanine at the C8 position, results in the formation of 8-hydroxydeoxyguanosine (8-OHdG; see Fig. 8-7). This oxidative DNA adduct is mutagenic in bacterial and mammalian cells, produces dose-related increases in cellular transformation, and causes G → T transversions that are commonly observed in mutated oncogenes and tumor-suppressor genes (Zhang *et al.*, 2000; Shibutani *et al.*, 1991; Moriya, 1993; Hussain and Haris, 1998). During DNA replication, 8-OHdG in the nucleotide pool can incorporate into the DNA template strand opposite dC or dA resulting in A:T to C:G transversions (Demple and Harrison, 1994; Cheng *et al.*, 1992). Oxidative damage to mitochondrial DNA and mutations in mitochondrial DNA have been identified in a number of cancers (Schumacher *et al.*, 1973; Cavalli and Liang, 1998; Tamura *et al.*, 1999; Horton *et al.*, 1996). Compared to nuclear DNA, the mitochondrial genome is relatively susceptible to oxidative base damage due to (1) close proximity to the electron transport system, a major source of reactive oxygen species (Barber and Harris, 1994); (2) mitochondrial DNA is not protected by histones; and (3) DNA repair capacity is limited in the mitochondria (Sawyer and Van Houten, 1999; Bohr and Dianov, 1999). Although many pathways exist that enable the formation of oxidative DNA damage, mammalian cells also possess specific repair pathways for the remediation of oxidative DNA damage (Tchou and Grollman, 1993; Fortini *et al.*, 1999).

Aside from oxidized nucleic acids, oxygen radicals can damage cellular biomembranes resulting in lipid peroxidation. Peroxidation of biomembranes generates a variety of products including reactive electrophiles such as epoxides and aldehydes, including malondialdehyde (MDA) (Janero, 1990). MDA is a highly reactive aldehyde and exhibits reactivity toward nucleophiles, and can form MDA–MDA dimers. Both MDA and the MDA–MDA dimers are mutagenic in bacterial assays and the mouse lymphoma assay (Riggins and Marnett, 2001).

Oxidative Stress and Cell Growth Regulation

Reactive oxygen species production and oxidative stress can affect both cell proliferation and apoptosis (Burdon, 1995; Slater *et al.*, 1995; Cerutti, 1985). H_2O_2 and superoxide anion can induce cell proliferation in several mammalian cell types (D'Souza *et al.*, 1993). Conversely, high concentrations of reactive oxygen species can initiate apoptosis (Dypbukt *et al.*, 1994). It has clearly been demonstrated that low levels of reactive oxygen species influence signal transduction pathways and alter gene expression (Fiorani *et al.*, 1995). Many xenobiotics, by increasing cellular levels of oxidants, alter gene expression through activation of signaling pathways including cAMP-mediated cascades, calcium-calmodulin pathways, and transcription factors such as AP-1 and NF-κB as well as signaling through mitogen-activated protein (MAP) kinases (extracellular signal-regulated kinases [ERK], c-Jun N-terminal kinases [JNK], and the p38 kinases) (Muller *et al.*, 1997; Kerr, 1992; Timblin *et al.*, 1997). Activation of these signaling cascades by reactive oxygen species induced by chemical carcinogens ultimately leads to altered gene expression for a number of genes including those affecting proliferation, differentiation, and apoptosis (Chang and Karin, 2001; Martindale and Holbrook, 2002; Brown *et al.*, 1998; Amstad *et al.*, 1992; Hollander and Fornace, 1989; Zawaski, 1993; Pinkus, 1993) (Fig. 8-23). Activation of NFκB, a ubiquitously expressed

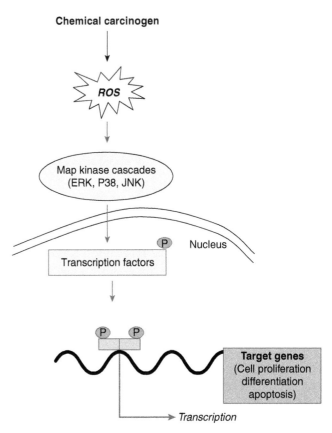

Figure 8-23. *Role of reactive oxygen species (ROS) on altered gene expression.* Many chemical carcinogens increase ROS and activate signaling cascades, such as the mitogen activated (MAP) kinase family. These serene/threonine kinases activate transcription factors, leading to DNA binding and gene expression changes.

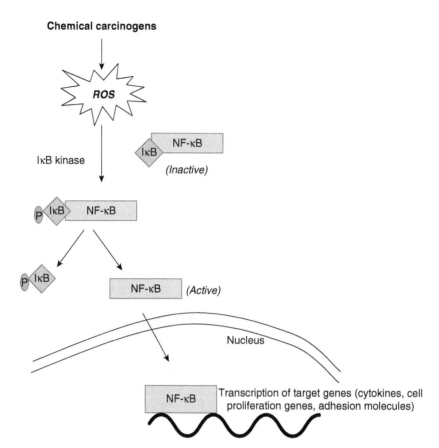

Figure 8-24. *Interaction between reactive oxygen species (ROS) and NFkB-induced gene expression.* A number of chemicals that increase ROS have been shown to activate NFkB. It is proposed that ROS enhance the dissociation of IkB from the NFkB/IkB complex leading to active NFkB. NFkB can then translocate into the nucleus where it binds DNA and increases gene transcription.

transcription factor, is regulated, in part, by reactive oxygen species and the cellular redox status. NFκB activation has been observed following a variety of extracellular stimuli including exposure to chemical carcinogens and physical agents that induce oxidative stress (Rusyn *et al.*, 2003; Glauert *et al.*, 2002; Beauerle *et al.*, 1988; Pahl, 1999; Li and Karin, 1998; Molina *et al.*, 2001; Schulze-Oshoff *et al.*, 1998; Nebreda and Porrai, 2000) (Fig. 8-24).

Gap Junctional Intercellular Communication and Carcinogenesis

Cells within an organism communicate in a variety of ways including through gap junctions, which are aggregates of connexin proteins that form a conduit between two adjacent cells (Lowenstein *et al.*, 1981) (Fig. 8-25). Gap junctional intercellular communication appears to play an important role in the regulation of cell growth and cell death, in part, through the ability to exchange small molecules (<1 kDa) between cells through gap junctions. Loss of gap junctions or decreased cell-to-cell communication is seen during liver regeneration following partial hepatectomy, a situation in which gap junction expression remains decreased until liver mass and lobular conformation are restored. Aberrant growth control is an essential feature of cancer cells, and because the absence or reduction in cell-to-cell communication has been observed between cancer cells, between cancer and normal cells, and in transformed cells, it has been speculated that altered gap junctional cell communication is involved in carcinogenesis (Trosko and Ruch, 1998). If cell communication is blocked between tumor and normal cells, the exchange of growth inhibitory signals from normal cells would be prevented from acting on initiated cells, thus allowing the potential for unregulated

growth and clonal expansion of initiated cell populations. This would therefore allow for the acquisition of additional genetic changes that may lead to neoplastic transformation (Klaunig and Ruch, 1990).

Intercellular communication is also decreased by growth factor administration and following exposure to a variety of tumor-promoting compounds (eg, phenobarbital, phthalates, dieldrin, phorbol esters). Tumor-promoting chemicals inhibit gap junctional intercellular communication in a number of cell types following

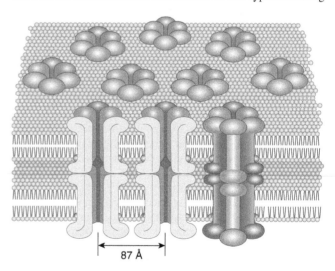

Figure 8-25. *Diagram of a gap junction traversing between two adjacent cells.* Connexons made up of six connexin proteins form the conduit between the two cells. (Reproduced with permission from Feldman RS, Quenzer LF. *Fundamentals of Neuropsychopharmacology.* Strauer Associates, Inc.; 1984.)

Table 8-14

Carcinogenicity of Metals

METAL	ANIMAL			HUMAN	
	SPECIES	TUMOR SITE	TUMOR TYPE	EXPOSURE	TUMOR TYPE
Arsenic	Mice, dogs, rats	None observed	None observed	Cu refinery As pesticides Chemical plants Drinking water (oral)	Pulmonary carcinoma Lymphoma, leukemia Dermal carcinoma Hepatic angiosarcoma
Beryllium	Mice, rats, monkeys	Bone Lung	Osteosarcoma Carcinoma	None observed	None observed
Cadmium	Mice, rats, chickens	Injection site Testes	Sarcoma Teratoma	Cd refinery	Pulmonary carcinoma
Chromium	Mice, rats, Rabbits	Injection site Lung	Sarcoma Carcinoma	Cr refinery Chrome plating Chromate pigments	Pulmonary carcinoma Gastrointestinal carcinoma
Cobalt	Rats, rabbits	Injection site	Sarcoma	None observed	None observed
Iron	Hamsters, mice, rats, rabbits	Injection site	Sarcoma	None observed	None observed
Lead	Mice, rats	Kidney	Carcinoma	None observed	None observed
Nickel	Mice, rats, cats, hamsters, rabbits Guinea pigs, rats	Injection site Lung Kidney	Carcinoma Carcinoma Carcinoma	Ni refinery	Pulmonary carcinoma Nasolaryngeal carcinoma Gastric and renal carcinoma Sarcoma (?)
Titanium	Rats	Injection site	Sarcoma	None observed	None observed
Zinc	Chickens, rats, hamsters	Testes Testes	Carcinoma Teratoma	None observed	None observed

exposure both in vivo and in vitro (Klaunig and Ruch, 1990). The ability of a tumor-promoting compound to block cell-to-cell communication in cultured cells correlates with its ability to induce rodent tumors (Klaunig and Ruch, 1987). In addition, the inhibition of gap junctional intercellular communication by tumor promoters appears to be tissue- and species-specific; they produced inhibition in target organs and sensitive species, whereas they do not inhibit cell-to-cell communication in nontarget tissues for carcinogenicity (Klaunig and Ruch, 1987). The mechanisms by which tumor promoters inhibit intercellular communication are not clear but may be due to decreased synthesis and/or enhanced degradation of gap junction proteins in the cell, reducing the number of channels in cell membranes, or other changes that modulate gap junction function and/or protein expression (Klaunig and Ruch, 1990; Sugie *et al.*, 1987).

Inorganic Carcinogens

Metals Several metals exhibit carcinogenicity in experimental animals and/or exposed humans. Table 8-14 provides a listing of some common metals and their corresponding carcinogenicity in animals and humans. A recent IARC review has examined in detail inorganic compounds deemed human carcinogens (IARC, 2010). Additional details on selected compounds are provided below.

Arsenic Arsenic compounds are poorly mutagenic in both bacterial and mammalian cell assays (Lofroth and Ames, 1978). Metallic arsenic, arsenic trioxide, sodium arsenite, sodium arsenate, potassium arsenite, lead arsenate, calcium arsenate, and pesticide mixtures containing arsenic have been tested for carcinogenicity in experimental animals (IARC, 1980, 1987). In the majority of

studies in experimental animals, including oral-exposure studies in mice, rats, and dogs, dermal-exposure studies in mice, inhalation-exposure studies in mice, injection studies in mice and rats, and intramedullary-injection studies in rats and rabbits, no tumors were observed or the results were inconclusive, and thus it has previously been concluded that limited evidence exists for the carcinogenicity of inorganic arsenic compounds in experimental animals (IARC, 1987).

In contrast, inorganic arsenic compounds are known human carcinogens based on sufficient evidence of carcinogenicity in humans. Epidemiological studies of humans exposed to arsenic compounds demonstrated that exposure to inorganic arsenic compounds increases the risk of cancer in the skin, lung, digestive tract, liver, bladder, kidney, and lymphatic and hematopoietic systems (IARC, 1973, 1980). Several of the epidemiological studies have reported dose–response relationships between arsenic in drinking water and several types of cancer, including bladder, kidney, lung, and skin cancer (Cantor, 1997; Ferreccio *et al.*, 2000). The mechanisms for cancer formation are unclear but are believed to possibly involve the induction of oxidative stress, altered cell signaling, modulation of apoptosis, and/or altered cell cycle (Hughes and Kitchin, 2006; Harris and Shi, 2003; Quian *et al.*, 2003). The latency period in humans of arsenic-related carcinogenesis is considered to be 30 to 50 years. The first signs of chronic exposure, frequently seen in water supplies contaminated with arsenic, are skin pigmentation, depigmentation, hyperkeratosis of palms and soles, and skin lesions. A unique peripheral vascular disease associated with chronic arsenic exposure is black foot disease, starting with numbness and ulceration of extremities and ending in gangrene and spontaneous amputations (Chen *et al.*, 1988).

Beryllium Beryllium and its salts are not mutagenic and do not appear to induce cellular transformation (IARC, 1993). Mechanistically, beryllium salts bind to nucleoproteins and inhibit enzymes involved in DNA synthesis, resulting in infidelity of DNA synthesis and also induce gene mutations in cultured cells (Leonard and Lauwerys, 1987). Studies in animal models have consistently reported increases in lung tumors in rodents and non-human primates exposed to beryllium or beryllium compounds (IARC, 1993; Finch *et al.*, 1996; NTP, 1998). Beryllium metal and several beryllium compounds (eg, beryllium-aluminum alloy, beryl ore, beryllium chloride, beryllium hydroxide, beryllium sulfate tetrahydrate, and beryllium oxide) induced lung tumors in rats. Beryllium oxide and beryllium sulfate produced lung cancer (anaplastic carcinoma) in monkeys after intrabronchial implantation or inhalation. In rabbits, osteosarcomas were reported after exposure to beryllium metal, beryllium carbonate, beryllium oxide, beryllium phosphate, beryllium silicate, or zinc beryllium silicate (IARC, 1993).

Beryllium and beryllium compounds have been classified as human carcinogens based on animal studies and evidence of carcinogenicity in humans. Epidemiological studies indicate an increased risk of lung cancer in occupational groups exposed to beryllium or beryllium compounds (Steenland and Ward, 1991; Ward *et al.*, 1992). Furthermore, an association with lung cancer has consistently been observed in occupational populations exposed to beryllium or beryllium compounds. Acute beryllium pneumonitis, a marker for exposure to beryllium, has been shown to be associated with higher lung cancer rates (Steenland and Ward, 1991).

Cadmium Animal studies have shown that cadmium and cadmium compounds induce tumor formation at various sites in multiple species of experimental animals, following multiple exposure routes, including the induction of prostate tumors in rats, testicular tumors in rats and mice, lymphoma in mice, adrenal gland tumors in hamsters and mice, and lung and liver tumors in mice (IARC, 1993; Waalkes *et al.*, 1994; 1999). It has been suggested that ionic cadmium, or compounds that release ionic cadmium, are the cause of genetic damage, and thus the carcinogenic species. Increased frequencies of chromosomal aberrations (changes in chromosome structure or number) have been observed in lymphocytes of workers occupationally exposed to cadmium. Many studies of cultured mammalian cells have shown that cadmium compounds cause genetic damage, including gene mutations, DNA strand breaks, chromosomal damage, cell transformation, and disrupted DNA repair (IARC, 1993).

Cadmium and cadmium compounds have been classified as known human carcinogens based on evidence of carcinogenicity in humans, including epidemiological and mechanistic information that indicate a causal relationship between exposure to cadmium and cadmium compounds and human cancer (9th RoC). Epidemiological studies of cadmium workers found that exposure to various cadmium compounds increased the risk of death from lung cancer (IARC, 1993). Follow-up analysis of some of these cohorts has confirmed that cadmium exposure is associated with elevated lung cancer risk under some industrial circumstances (Sorahan *et al.*, 1995; Sorahan and Lancashire, 1997). Some epidemiological evidence has also suggested an association between cadmium exposure and prostate (Shigematsu *et al.*, 1982; van der Gulden *et al.*, 1995), kidney (Mandel *et al.*, 1995), and bladder cancer (Siemiatycki *et al.*, 1994).

Chromium Chromium has multiple oxidation states—from −2 to +6; however, the most common forms are the trivalent (III) and hexavalent (VI) forms. With regard to carcinogenicity, chromium III does not exhibit carcinogenicity in laboratory animals whereas chromium VI has been shown to be positive for genotoxicity and carcinogenicity in a variety of bioassays (Langard, 1988; IARC, 1990). Chromium VI compounds cause genetic damage including gene mutations and DNA damage in bacteria. Several chromium VI compounds also caused mutations in yeast and insects. Many chromium VI compounds caused genetic damage in cultured human and other animal cells and in experimental animals exposed in vivo, including SCE, chromosomal aberrations, and cell transformation. Chromosomal aberrations, SCE, and aneuploidy were observed in workers exposed to chromium VI compounds (IARC, 1990). Chromium VI (calcium chromate, chromium trioxide, sodium dichromate, lead chromates, strontium chromate, or zinc chromates) exposure of rats following inhalation, intrabronchial, intrapleural, intratracheal, intramuscular, or subcutaneous administration resulted in benign and malignant lung tumors were observed in rats in a number of studies. In mice, calcium chromate caused benign lung tumors and chromium trioxide caused malignant lung tumors. Exposure of hamsters, guinea pigs, and rabbits to chromium (VI) compounds by intratracheal instillation did not cause lung tumors (IARC, 1980, 1990). Although the mechanisms for chromium VI carcinogenicity remain unresolved, it has been speculated that the reduction of chromium VI by glutathione is involved (Connett and Whtterhahn, 1985; Kortenkamp and O'Brien, 1994).

Hexavalent chromium (chromium VI) compounds have been classified as known human carcinogens based on data from animals studies and human epidemiological studies. Human epidemiological studies have consistently reported increased risks of lung cancer among chromate workers. Chromate workers are exposed to a variety of chromium compounds, including chromium (VI) and trivalent (III) compounds. In addition, an increased risk of a rare cancer of the sinonasal cavity was observed in these workers (IARC, 1990). Some studies suggested that exposure to chromium among workers such as chromium-exposed arc welders, chromate pigment workers, chrome platers, and chromium tanning workers may be associated with leukemia and bone cancer (Costa, 1997).

Nickel Many studies in cultured rodent and human cells have shown that a variety of nickel compounds, including both soluble and insoluble forms of nickel, exhibit genotoxicity, producing DNA strand breaks, mutations, chromosomal damage, cell transformation, and modulation of DNA repair. Soluble nickel salts can be complete carcinogens and/or initiators of carcinogenesis (Diwan *et al.*, 1992; Kasprzak *et al.*, 1990). In rats and mice, inhalation or intratracheal instillation of nickel subsulfide or nickel oxide produced dose-related increases of benign and malignant lung tumors (IARC, 1990; NTP, 1996). Inhalation of nickel compounds also caused malignant and benign pheochromocytoma in rats (NTP, 1996). Short-term intraperitoneal exposure during gestation to soluble nickel salt induced malignant pituitary tumors in the offspring. Additionally, exposure to nickel acetate through the placenta followed by exposure of the offspring to barbital (a known tumor promoter) produces tumors of the kidney (renal cortical and pelvic tumors) (Diwan *et al.*, 1992). In adult rats, injection of soluble nickel salts followed by exposure to a promoting carcinogen resulted in kidney cancer (renal cortical adenocarcinomas) that frequently metastasized to the lung, liver, and spleen (Kasprzak *et al.*, 1990). The carcinogenic properties of metallic nickel is believed to be due to ionic nickel, which can slowly dissolve in the body from nickel compounds.

Nickel compounds are classified as known human carcinogens (11th RoC) based on animal data and sufficient evidence of carcinogenicity from human studies. The IARC (1990, 2011) evaluation of nickel and nickel compounds concluded that nickel compounds are carcinogenic to humans based on sufficient evidence for the carcinogenicity of nickel compounds in the nickel refining industry and very strong evidence of carcinogenicity of a variety of nickel compounds in experimental studies in rodents. Several cohort studies of workers exposed to various nickel compounds showed an elevated risk of death from lung and nasal cancers (IARC, 1990). An excess risk of lung and nasal cancer was seen in nickel refinery workers exposed primarily to soluble nickel compounds (Andersen *et al.*, 1996).

Lead Lead compounds do not appear to cause genetic damage directly, but may do so through several indirect mechanisms, including inhibition of DNA synthesis and repair, oxidative damage, and interaction with DNA-binding proteins and tumor-suppressor proteins (NTP, 2003). Lead has exhibited conflicting results concerning its genotoxicity; it does not cause mutations in bacteria, but does cause chromosomal aberrations in vitro and in vivo, and causes DNA damage in vivo and in cell-free systems, whereas in mammalian systems, conflicting results were observed. Lead also inhibits the activity of DNA and RNA polymerase in cell-free systems and in mammalian cell cultures. Conflicting results were observed for SCE and micronucleus formation in mammalian test systems.

In studies with laboratory animals, carcinogenicity has been observed for soluble (lead acetate and lead subacetate) and insoluble (lead phosphate, lead chromate) inorganic lead compounds as well as for tetraethyl lead (an organic lead compound), following exposure via oral, injection, and in offspring exposed via the placenta or lactation. Although kidney tumors (including adenomas, carcinomas, and adenocarcinomas) were most frequently associated with lead exposure, tumors of the brain, hematopoietic system, and lung were reported in some studies (IARC, 1980; 1987, 2011; Waalkes *et al.*, 1995). Lead also appears to function as a tumor promoter, leading to increased incidence in kidney tumors initiated by *N*-ethyl-*N*-hydroxyethylnitrosamine and *N*-(4′-fluoro-4-biphenyl) acetamide) (IARC, 1980, 1987). The mechanisms by which lead causes cancer are not understood.

Lead and lead compounds are classified as reasonably anticipated to be human carcinogens based on limited evidence from studies in humans and sufficient evidence from studies in experimental animals. Lead exposure has been associated with increased risk of lung, stomach, and bladder cancer in diverse human populations (Fu and Boffetta, 1995; Steenland and Boffetta, 2000; NTP, 2003). Epidemiological studies link lead exposure to increased risk for lung and stomach cancer. However, most studies of lead exposure and cancer reviewed had limitations, including poor exposure assessment and failure to control for confounding factors.

Modifiers of Chemical Carcinogenic Effects

Genetic and environmental factors have a significant impact on the way in which individuals and/or organisms respond to carcinogen exposure. As with most genes, enzymes that metabolize carcinogens are expressed in a tissue-specific manner. Within tissues, the enzymatic profile can vary with cell type or display differential localization within cells. Further, carcinogen metabolizing enzymes are differentially expressed among species. These differences may represent an underlying factor explaining the differential responses to chemical carcinogens across species.

The expression of many carcinogen metabolizing enzymes is highly inducible by foreign chemicals. Compounds such as benzo(*a*)pyrene highly induce P450 isozymes CYP1A1 and 1A2,

enzymes that display catalytic activity toward a number of polycyclic aromatics. A number of other enzymes, for example, GST isozymes, Uridine Diphosphate Glucuronyltransferases (UDPGTs) are also induced by PAHs, thus the net result is enhanced metabolism of PAHs. Numerous other chemical carcinogens are potent inducers of drug metabolizing enzymes; examples include chemicals such as phenobarbital, dichlorodiphenyltrichloroethane (DDT), ethanol, 17β-estradiol, PPARα agonists, each of these results in the upregulation of a distinct set of phase I and phase II enzymes. Many chemicals produce inhibitory effects on drug metabolism enzymes, and could either increase the half-life of a chemical carcinogen or prevent or delay the formation of active metabolites of carcinogens.

Polymorphisms in Carcinogen Metabolism and DNA Repair

Genetic polymorphisms arise from human genetic variability. A genetic polymorphism is when a gene has more than one allele. In assessing variability in the human genome project it was found that base variations occurred at approximately once in every 1000 base pairs. Therefore, there may be over one million genetic variations between any two individuals. A single nucleotide polymorphism (SNP) is a variant in DNA sequence found in greater than 1% of the population (Fig. 8-26). Thus, by definition, changes in DNA sequence goes from mutation to polymorphism when a unique genotype is seen in over 1% of the population. Over three million candidate SNPs have been identified to date with up to 10 million being estimated to be present within the human genome. In carcinogenesis, genetic polymorphisms may account for the susceptibility of some individuals to certain cancers. In particular, SNPs of genes involved in carcinogen metabolism (activation and detoxification) and DNA repair, have received considerable attention. A number of polymorphisms have been described in carcinogen metabolizing enzymes, with certain alleles linked to altered risk of selective cancers (Boddy and Ratain, 1997; Naoe *et al.*, 2000). Glutathione-S-transferases (GSTs), which are involved in detoxification of many chemical carcinogens and also in the remediation of oxidative stress, are highly polymorphic in humans. Polymorphisms of the GSTM1 phenotype have been related to bladder, gastric, and lung cancer in humans (Welfare *et al.*, 1999; Tsuchida and Sato, 1992). Individuals expressing the GSTM1 null genotype have a 1.5-fold higher risk for bladder cancer and 1.7-fold increase risk for gastric cancer compared to individuals expressing the genotype (Risch

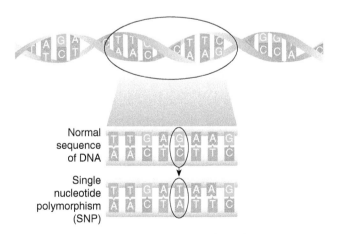

Figure 8-26. *Example of a single nucleotide polymorphism in DNA.* Single nucleotide polymorphisms are instances in which a single nucleotide is changed within a DNA sequence.

et al., 2001; Ates *et al.*, 2005). The GSTM1 isoform is of particular important in carcinogenesis because this isoform exhibits the highest reactivity toward epoxides. GSTT1 isoform null individuals show a three-fold increase risk in breast cancer, a 1.6-fold increase in gastric cancer, and a four-fold increase in liver cancer compared to individuals having the genotype (Bosch *et al.*, 2006).

Similarly in women (nonsmokers) with lung cancer, a higher level of PAH DNA adducts have been detected. Higher DNA adduct levels are also found to be associated with the expression of the cytochrome P4501A1 (*CYP1A1*) gene, which bioactivates PAHs (Han *et al.*, 2003). An increase in benzo(*a*)pyrene DNA adduct levels correlate with increased expression of the CYP1A1. DNA repair genes, in particular oxidative DNA repair, OGG1, involved in repair of 8-OHdG–induced damage, have been linked to an increase in lung cancer in individuals with lower OGG1 expression (Goode *et al.*, 2002; Klaunig *et al.*, 2011).

In the case of prostate cancer, studies have suggested roles for a number of candidate SNPs. Recent evidence suggests that the presence of a genetic variant that is more prevalent in African American men that is less effective of clearing reactive oxygen species. Examples of candidate genes that likely contribute to prostate cancer carcinogenesis include the androgen receptor gene, steroid synthesis, and metabolism genes (*CYP17*, *CYP1B1*, *CYP3A4*, *CYP3A5*, *CYP3A43*, *SD5A2*, *HSD3B1*, *HSD3B2*, *CYP19*), transmembrane drug efflux genes (*ABCG2*), and reactive oxygen species metabolizing genes (*MnSOD*, *APE1*, *XRCC1*, *GSTP1*; Dong, 2005). Individually, polymorphisms in each of these genes have been associated with an increased risk of prostate cancer.

The importance of SNPs, cancer susceptibility, and cancer risk are illustrated in Table 8-15. If exposure to a chemical carcinogen is low and the genetic susceptibility for genes related to the carcinogenic activity is low, then the risk for cancer will also be low. If exposure to a chemical carcinogen is high but the genetic susceptibility is low, then the risk for cancer development is likely to be low. However, if the genetic susceptibility is high, then exposure to a chemical carcinogen will result in a higher risk for cancer development.

Proto-Oncogenes and Tumor-Suppressor Genes

Proto-oncogenes and tumor-suppressor genes play a key role in cancer induction. These genes encode a wide array of proteins that function to control cell growth and proliferation. Common characteristics of oncogenes and tumor-suppressor genes are shown in Table 8-16. Mutations in both oncogenes and tumor-suppressor genes contribute to the progressive development of human cancers. Accumulated damage to multiple oncogenes and/or tumor-suppressor genes can result in altered cell proliferation, differentiation, and/or survival of cancer cells (Croce, 2008; Huff, 2011).

Table 8-15

Carcinogen Exposure and Cancer Risk in Humans

EXPOSURE	SUSCEPTIBILITY (GENOTYPE)	RESULT (DISEASE)
↓	↓	Low risk
↑	↓	Low risk
↓	↑	Mod risk
↑	↑	High risk

Table 8-16

Characteristics of Proto-Oncogenes, Cellular Oncogenes, and Tumor Suppressor Genes

PROTO-ONCOGENES	ONCOGENES	TUMOR SUPPRESSOR GENES
Dominant	Dominant	Recessive
Broad tissue specificity for cancer development	Broad tissue specificity for cancer development	Considerable tissue specificity for cancer development
Germline inheritance rarely involved in cancer development	Germline inheritance rarely involved in cancer development	Germline inheritance frequently involved in cancer development
Analogous to certain viral oncogenes	No known analogues in oncogenic viruses	No known analogues in oncogenic viruses
Somatic mutations activated during all stages of carcinogenesis	Somatic mutations activated during all stages of carcinogenesis	Germline mutations may initiate, but mutation to neoplasia occurs only during progression stage

Retroviruses Evidence that specific genes (oncogenes) could cause cancer first came from studies showing sarcomas could be produced in healthy chickens by injecting them with cell-free extracts derived from chicken tumors (Rous, 1911). The transforming agent in the filtrate eventually was shown to be an RNA-type tumor virus, the *Rous sarcoma virus* (RSV) that is capable of transforming a normal cell and produce sarcomas within weeks of injection (Temin and Rubin, 1958). The genome of RSV and other retroviruses consists of two identical copies of mRNA, which is then reverse transcribed into DNA and incorporated into the host-cell genome. Oncogenic transforming viruses such as RSV contain the v-*src* gene, a gene required for cancer induction. It was later demonstrated that normal cells from chickens and other species contain a gene closely related to v-*src* in RSV; the normal "proto-oncogene" commonly is distinguished from the viral gene by the prefix "c" (c-*src*; Oppermann *et al.*, 1979). This discovery showed that cancer may be induced by the action of normal, or nearly normal, genes.

DNA Viruses Six major classes of DNA tumor viruses have been identified: simian virus 40 (SV40), polyoma virus, hepatitis B virus, papilloma viruses, adenoviruses, herpes viruses, and poxviruses. Unlike retroviral oncogenes, which are derived from normal cellular genes and have no function for the virus, the known oncogenes of DNA viruses are integral parts of the viral genome required for viral replication. SV40 or polyoma viruses are not capable of inducing tumors in their natural host species (monkey and mice, respectively). Infection by small DNA viruses is lethal to most non-host animal cells; however, a small proportion integrates the viral DNA into the host-cell genome. The cells that survive infection become permanently transformed due to the presence of one or more oncogene in the viral DNA. For example, SV40 codes for the large T antigen, which alone is capable of inducing transformation (Fried and Privies, 1986). Both SV40 and polyoma viruses use the host-cells DNA synthetic apparatus for their own replication. Papilloma viruses can infect and cause tumors in rabbits, cows, and humans (Lancaster and Olsen, 1982). Of the human papilloma viruses, types 6, 10, and 11 are associated with genital warts whereas types 16, 18, 31, and 33 are associated with human cervical cancers (Vousden, 1989). Herpes viruses are complex and are capable of producing tumors in frogs, chickens, monkeys, and humans (Rapp, 1974). Included among this class is the Epstein–Barr virus, a causative agent in the development of Burkett B-cell lymphomas and in nasopharengyal carcinoma (de-Thé *et al.*, 1978), and is mediated by genes encoding *EBNA-1, EBNA-2,* and *latent membrane protein* (Fahreus *et al.*, 1990). Adenoviruses affect host and non-host cells differently; in host cells, infection causes lysis whereas in non-host cells, infection results in transformation via *E1A* and *E1B* genes (Pettersson and Roberts, 1986). Hepatitis B viruses specifically infect the liver of ducks, woodchucks, and squirrels, and are strongly associated with liver cancer development in humans; infected individuals exhibit a >100-fold risk for cancer development (Synder *et al.*, 1982). Hepatitis B gene X is thus far the main gene implicated in the transformation process (Kim *et al.*, 1991). Poxviruses (eg, Yaba monkey virus, Shope fibroma virus), replicate in the cytoplasm of infected cells and produce benign tumors (Niven *et al.*, 1961).

Proto-Oncogenes An oncogene is a gene encoding a protein that is capable of transforming cells in culture or inducing cancer in animals. Of the known oncogenes, the majority appear to have been derived from normal genes (ie, proto-oncogenes), and are involved in cell signaling cascades (Table 8-17). Because most proto-oncogenes are essential for maintaining viability, they are highly conserved evolutionarily. It has been clearly demonstrated that altered expression of these genes results in unregulated control of cell growth. Activation of proto-oncogenes arises through mutational events occurring within proto-oncogenes (Alitalo and Schwab, 1986; Bos, 1989). It has been recognized that a number of chemical carcinogens are capable of inducing mutations in proto-oncogenes (Balmain and Pragnell, 1983).

Several oncogene products are associated with growth factors. The *sis* oncogene encodes for platelet-derived growth factor (PDGF), which consists of type A and B chains. Active PDGF can consist of homo- or heterodimers of the A and B chains. Only cells that express the PDGF receptor are susceptible to transformation by the *sis* oncogene (Dooliter *et al.*, 1983). Fibroblast growth factor (FGF), epidermal growth factor (EGF), and the *wnt* family also have oncogenes that encode for their production (Burgess *et al.*, 1989; Nusse and Varmus, 1992). Enhanced expression of these growth factor genes leads to transformation of cultured cells. In addition, lung carcinomas and astrocytomas in humans express both PDGF and its receptor.

In order for the growth factors listed above to induce cell growth, the cell must also express the appropriate growth factor receptors. Ligand binding to receptors in many cases results in the activation of signaling cascades, of which a number have protein kinase activity. Protein kinases can phosphorylate at tyrosine, serine, or threonine residues. Several oncogene products have been identified that have tyrosine kinase activity (eg, *src, fps, fgr, fms, kit,* and *ros*; Collett and Erikson, 1978). Growth factor receptors including EGF, PDGF, insulin, insulin-like growth factor, and FGF have tyrosine activity (Wells, 1999). An extensive number of protein kinases are serine or threonine kinases, some of which can be activated in tumor cells and lead to transformation. The protein kinase C family consists of serine/threonine kinases (Nishizuka, 1988). This family of proteins participates in the inositol–phospholipid second messenger pathway and can be activated by calcium and diacylglycerol, and phorbol ester tumor promoters. The *raf* and

Table 8-17

Examples of Oncogenes and Cancer Association

	ONCOGENE	NEOPLASM
Tyrosine kinases	EGFR	Squamous cell carcinoma
	PDGF	Lung carcinoma
		Astrocytoma
	v-fms	Sarcoma
	v-kit	Sarcoma
	v-ros	Sarcoma
	v-fgr	Sarcoma
	v-fps	Sarcoma
	Src	Colon carcinoma
	Neu	Breast carcinoma
		Neuroblastoma
	Ret	Thyroid carcinoma
	Trk	Colon carcinoma
Serine/theronine kinases	v-raf	Sarcoma
	v-mos	Sarcoma
G proteins	H-Ras	Colon and lung carcinoma
	K-Ras	Melanoma, Acute myeloid leukemia (AML), and
	N-Ras	thyroid carcinoma
	NF-1	Carcinoma and melanoma Neurofibromas
Nuclear proteins	c-Myc	CML, Burkitt lymphoma
	N-Myc	AML, breast and lung carcinoma
	L-Myc	Neuroblastoma and lung carcinoma
	v-myb	Lung carcinoma
	v-jun	Sarcoma
	v-fos	Osteosarcoma
	v-rel	Leukemia
	v-ets	Myeloblastosis
	v-erbA	Erythroblastosis

mos oncogenes are other example of serine threonine kinases, that interact with mitogen activated kinase pathways, leading to enhance the expression of "immediate-early" genes such as Myc, and Fos/Jun heterodimers, and ultimately leads to enhanced cell growth (Su and Karin, 1996).

Guanine nucleotide binding proteins is a subset of the Guanosine-5′-triphosphate (GTP) superfamily. The primary oncogenic members of this family are the *ras* genes (eg, *Ha-, Ki-,* and *n-ras*), which were initially found in murine retroviruses, and are frequently activated in human tumors and in chemically induced tumors in rodent models (McCormick, 1994). The three ras forms differ by only 20 amino acids and have a conserved cytosine-186, which is a site for posttranslational modification by a farnesyl, isoprenyl group, a modification that is needed for membrane localization (Hancock *et al.*, 1989). Mutations in *ras* affect the association of the Ras with GTP, and because Ras is active when GTP is bound, constitutive Ras activation is often seen with mutated forms of *ras*. Many mutation sites are associated with activation of *ras* and include codons 12, 13, 61, 116, 117, 119, and 146 (de Vos *et al.*, 1988). Although a dominant gain-of-function mutation in the *ras* gene converts it into an oncogene, a recessive loss-of-function mutation in the *NF1* gene also leads to constitutive Ras activation. *NF1* encodes a GTPase-activating enzyme (GAP) that accelerates hydrolysis of GTP and the conversion of active GTP-bound Ras to inactive GDP-bound Ras. The loss of GAP leads to sustained Ras activation of downstream signal transduction proteins. Individuals with neurofibromatosis have inherited a single mutant *NF1* allele; subsequent somatic mutation in the other allele leads to formation of neurofibromas.

In addition to acting at the receptor level, some oncogene products are nuclear transcription factors and thus cause alteration of gene expression. One of the first to be identified was the erbA oncogene product, which is an altered form of the thyroid hormone receptor (Damm *et al.*, 1989). This altered form is unable to bind thyroid hormone and allows the oncogene protein to act in a dominant-negative manner, functioning as a constitutive repressor of normal expression of genes regulated by thyroid hormone. Another family of oncogenes encode for the AP-1 transcription factor, a complex consisting of *jun* and *fos*, as well as Jun family members with homology to c-jun (Jun B and Jun D) (Chiu *et al.*, 1988; Vogt, 2001). Phorbol esters and several other tumor-promoting compounds are able to rapidly induce gene expression of both *fos* and *jun*. Activation of both *fos* and *jun* results in the constitutive expression of the transcription factors and sustained stimulation of cell growth signals. The *myc* family (*c-myc, N-myc,* and *L-myc*) encode for transcription factors that are found activated in a number of tumor types (Marcu *et al.*, 1992).

Tumor-Suppressor Genes

Retinoblastoma (Rb) Gene In contrast to oncogenes, the proteins encoded by most tumor-suppressor genes act as inhibitors of cell proliferation or cell survival (Table 8-18). The prototype tumor-suppressor gene, *Rb*, was identified by studies of inheritance of retinoblastoma. Loss or mutational inactivation of *Rb* contributes to the development of a wide variety of human cancers. In its unphosphorylated form, Rb binds to the *E2F* transcription factors preventing E2F-mediated transcriptional activation of a number of genes whose products are required for DNA synthesis. In addition, the Rb–E2F complex acts as a transcriptional repressor for many of these same genes (Chellappan *et al.*, 1991). During the early G_1 phase of the cell cycle, Rb is an unphosphorylated state, but becomes phosphorylated during late G_1, causing dissociation from E2F—a process that allows E2F to induce synthesis of DNA replication enzymes, resulting in a commitment into the cell cycle. Rb phosphorylation is initiated by an active Cdk4–cyclin D complex and is completed by other cyclin-dependent kinases (Weinberg, 1995; Sherr, 1993). Most tumors contain an oncogenic mutation of one of the genes in this pathway such that cells enter the S phase of the cell cycle in the absence of the proper extracellular growth

signals that regulate Cdk activity. In addition, Rb is bound and inactivated by the E1A protein of the adenoviruses (Whyte *et al.*, 1988) and also by the large T antigen of SV40 and the E7 protein of the papilloma virus, suggesting that the elimination of Rb function may be an important mechanism in tumor development by viruses and/ or mutations induced by chemical carcinogens.

p53 Gene The p53 protein is a tumor-suppressor gene that is essential for the checkpoint control and arrests the cell cycle in cells with damaged DNA in G_1. Cells with functional p53 arrest in G_1 when exposed to DNA-damaging agents such as irradiation, whereas cells lacking functional p53 are unable to block the cell cycle. p53 is activated by a wide array of stressors including UV light, γ irradiation, heat, and several carcinogens. DNA damage by γ irradiation or by other stresses leads to the activation of certain kinases, including ataxia telangiectasia mutated (ATM), which is encoded by the gene mutated in ataxia telangiectasia and a DNA-dependent protein kinase. Phosphorylation of p53 by these and other kinases results in stabilization of p53 and an increase in cell content of this protein (Finlay *et al.*, 1989). The active form of p53 is a tetramer of four identical subunits. A missense point mutation in one *p53* of the two alleles in a cell can abrogate almost all p53 activity because virtually all the oligomers will contain at least one defective subunit and such oligomers cannot function as a transcription factor. Oncogenic *p53* mutations thus act as "dominant negatives," in contrast to tumor-suppressor genes such as *Rb*.

Virtually all p53 mutations abolish its ability to bind to specific DNA sequences and activate gene expression (El-Deiry *et al.*, 1992). The transcription of cyclin-kinase inhibitor p21, which binds to and inhibits mammalian G_1 Cdk–cyclin complexes, is induced by p53. As a result, cells with damaged DNA are arrested in G_1 until the damage is repaired and the levels of p53 and p21 fall; the cells then can progress into the S phase. In most cells, accumulation of p53 also leads to induction of proteins that promote apoptosis, and, therefore, would prevent proliferation of cells that are likely to accumulate multiple mutations. When the p53 checkpoint control does not operate properly, damaged DNA can replicate, producing mutations and DNA rearrangements that contribute to the development of transformed cells. Proteins that interact with and regulate p53 are also altered in many human tumors. The gene encoding one such protein, MDM2, is amplified in many sarcomas and other human tumors that maintain functional p53 (Leach *et al.*, 1993). Under normal conditions, MDM2 binds the N-terminus of p53, repressing the ability of p53 to activate transcription of *p21* and genes mediating p53 degradation. Thus, MDM2 normally inhibits the ability of p53 to block at G_1 or induce apoptosis. Enhanced MDM2 levels in tumor cells therefore results in decreased functional p53 and prevents p53 from growth arrest in response to irradiation or chemical carcinogens. For example, benzo(*a*)pyrene produces inactivating mutations at codons 175, 248, and 273 of the *p53* gene in cultured cells; these same positions are mutational hot spots in human lung cancer (Hollstein *et al.*, 1991). Aflatoxin exposure induces a G to T transversion at codon 249 of p53, and methyl-*N*′-nitro-*N*-nitrosoguanidine (MNNG) can alter methylation of DNA leading to inactivation of p53 (Bressac *et al.*, 1991).

BRCA1 Gene Genetic analysis of breast tumors has revealed a hereditary predisposition for breast cancer linked to *BRCA1,* a tumor-suppressor gene. Mutation of a single *BRCA1* allele results in a 60% probability of developing breast cancer by age 50. In families transmitting the mutant BRCA1 allele, the normal allele is often absent in tumors. A number of investigators have shown that germ line mutations lead to loss of function of the *BRCA1* gene, perhaps by acting as a transcription factor through binding at a zinc

---

Table 8-18

Examples of Tumor Suppressor Genes and Cancer Association

TUMOR SUPPRESSOR	DISORDER	NEOPLASM
Rb1	Retinoblastoma	Small-cell lung carcinoma
p53	Li–Fraumeni syndrome	Breast, colon, lung cancers
BRCA1	Unknown	Breast carcinoma
WT-1	Wilms tumor	Lung cancer
p16	Unknown	Melanoma

finger domain. However, no mutations have been observed in sporadic breast cancers (Futreal *et al.*, 1994), suggesting that *BRCA1* gene silencing may occur through nonmutational mechanisms.

Wilms Tumor Gene (WT1) Wilms tumor occurs in the developing kidney at a rate of approximately one per 10,000 children. The *WT1* gene is believed to be responsible for tumor development and is thought to function as a transcription factor (Hastie, 1994). The DNA-binding region of the *WT1* gene contains four zinc finger domains, and binds a consensus sequence shared with EGR1; however, *WT1* acts as a transcriptional repressor at this site (Rauscher *et al.*, 1990). Similar to *p53*, *WT1* mutant alleles act in a dominant-negative manner.

p16 Gene The group of proteins that function as cyclin-kinase inhibitors play an important role in cell cycle regulation. Mutations, especially deletions of the *p16* gene, that inactivate the ability of p16 to inhibit cyclin D–dependent kinase activity are common in several human cancers including a high percentage of melanomas (Kamb *et al.*, 1994). Loss of p16 would mimic cyclin D1 overexpression, leading to Rb hyperphosphorylation and release of active E2F transcription factor. Thus, p16 normally acts as a tumor suppressor. As with the *BRCA1* gene, relatively few mutations have been found in this gene, and some researchers have speculated that epigenetic mechanisms such as gene silencing by DNA methylation may occur during tumorigenesis (Merlo *et al.*, 1995).

Hormesis, Dose Response, and Carcinogenesis

Hormesis is defined as a dose–response curve in which a U, J, or inverted U-shaped dose–response is observed, with low-dose exposures often resulting in beneficial rather than harmful effects (Calabrese, 2002) (Fig. 8-27). One of the first reports establishing a hormetic response was observed with ionizing radiation, in which it was hypothesized to be due to adaptation to background radiation exposure, as well as enhanced metabolism and detoxification (Calabrese, 2002; Parsons, 2003). Numerous examples exist that provide evidence for U- and J-shape dose relationships to different biomarkers of carcinogenesis, both for initiating and promoting carcinogens. For example, low-dose styrene treatment resulted in a decrease of chromosomal aberrations (Camurri *et al.*, 1983). A reduction in DNA strand breaks in human keratinocytes was seen following low-dose exposure to *N*-methyl-*N'*-nitro-*N*-nitrosoguanidine, whereas high doses were greatly elevated compared to controls (Kleczkowska and Althaus, 1996). Several chronic bioassays for carcinogenicity in rats and mice have demonstrated a negative correlation between proliferative hepatocellular lesions and lymphomas at low- and medium-dose levels (Young and Gries, 1984). TCDD at hepatocarcinogenic doses resulted in a dose-dependent reduction in mammary and uterine tumors (Kociba *et al.*,

1978). TCDD also reduces tumor incidence after exposure to low doses of radiation and selenium (Pollycove *et al.*, 2001; Nordberg *et al.*, 1981). Evidence for a U-shaped dose–response curve has also been demonstrated for phenobarbital (Kitano *et al.*, 1998; Ito *et al.*, 2003; Kinoshita *et al.*, 2003). These investigators have shown that phenobarbital promoted the growth of diethylnitrosamine-induced hepatic lesions at doses between 60 and 500 ppm, whereas doses between one and 7.5 ppm decreased lesion growth, hepatocellular carcinoma, and tumor multiplicity.

Adaptive responses have been proposed to explain the hormetic effects observed by chemical carcinogens. When experimental animals are exposed to chemicals, the initial response is an adaptive response to maintain homeostasis (Calabrese, 2002). Adaptive responses usually involve actions of the chemical on cellular signaling pathways that lead to changes in gene expression, resulting in enhanced detoxification and excretion of the chemical as well as preserving the cell cycle and programmed cell death. It has been proposed that following very low doses of chemicals, the upregulation of these mechanisms overcompensates for cell injury such that a reduction in tumor promotion and/or tumor development is seen, and would explain the U- or J-shaped response curves obtained following carcinogen exposure.

A common feature of chemical carcinogens for which hormetic effects have been proposed is the formation of reactive oxygen species and the induction of cytochrome P450 isoenzymes. Inhibition of carcinogenesis by low levels of phenobarbital has been postulated to involve the suppression of 8-OHdG generation and cellular proliferation within areas of glutathione-*S*-transferase pi (GST-P) positive foci, possibly related to enhanced expression of the gene encoding the enzyme oxoguanine glycosylase one (Ogg1), which is responsible for the repair of 8-OHdG lesions (Kinoshita *et al.*, 2003). Another explanation for the suppressive effect of low-level phenobarbital on the development of preneoplastic lesions involves the stimulation of hepatic drug metabolizing enzymes, which detoxify carcinogens (Pitot *et al.*, 1987). In a low-dose phenobarbital study, cDNA microarray analysis resulted in a suppression of mRNA expression of MAP kinase p38, JNK1, 2, and other intracellular kinases (Kinoshita *et al.*, 2003). Thus, suppression of signal transduction modulators appears to be involved in the inhibitory effect of phenobarbital on cell proliferation.

Chemoprevention

The study of chemicals that prevent, inhibit, or slow down the process of cancer is referred to as chemoprevention. A number of chemicals, including drugs, antioxidants, foodstuffs, and vitamins have been found to inhibit or retard components of the cancer process (Table 8-19) in both in vitro and in vivo models (Stoner *et al.*, 1997). Cancer chemopreventive chemicals may function at one or more of the steps in the carcinogenesis process. Cancer chemoprevention involves the administration or inclusion in the diet of natural or synthetic chemicals in an attempt to prevent, halt, or reverse the process of carcinogenesis. A basic assumption in chemoprevention is that treating early stages of the malignant process will halt or delay the progression to neoplasia. Chemopreventive chemicals may function via one or several mechanisms; inhibitors of carcinogen formation, blocking agents, and/or as suppressing agents (Table 8-19). Blocking agents serve to prevent the metabolic activation of genotoxic or nongenotoxic carcinogens by either inhibiting its metabolism or enhancing the detoxification mechanisms. In the case of reactive oxygen species generation by a carcinogen, antioxidants, such as, *N*-acetylcysteine, or vitamins E, A, and C serve as blocking agents by trapping the oxidative species before it can induce cellular

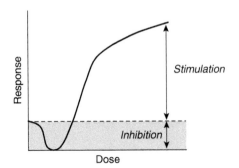

Figure 8-27. *Hormesis curve.*

Table 8-19

Classes of Chemopreventive Agents

INHIBITORS OF CARCINOGEN FORMATION	EXAMPLES
Reductive acids	Ascorbic acid
Phenols	Cafeic acid, ferulic acid, gallic acid
Sulfhydryl compounds	N-Acetylcysteine
Amino acids	Praline, thioproline
Blocking Agents	
Inhibition of cytochrome P450	Dithiocarbamates, ellagic acid, diallyl sulfide, isothiocyanates
Induction of cytochrome P450	Indole-3-carbinol, β-naphthoflavone
Induction of phase II enzymes	
Glutathione S-transferase	Allyl sulfides, dithiolethiones, isothiocyanates
UDP-glucuronyltransferase	Polyphenols
Glutathione peroxidase	Selenium
Scavenge electrophiles	Ellagic acid, N-acetylcysteine
Scavenge free radicals	Sodium thiosulfate, polyphenols, vitamin E
Increase overall levels of DNA repair	Vanillin
Increase poly(ADP-ribosyl) transferase	N-Acetylcysteine
Suppress error-prone DNA repair	Protease inhibitors
Suppressing Agents	
Inhibit polyamine metabolism	DRv10, polyphenols, substituted putrescines
Induce terminal cell differentiation	Calcium, retinoids, vitamin D_3
Modulate signal transduction	Glycyrrhetinic acid, nonsteroidal anti-inflammatory drugs (NSAIDs), polyphenols, retinoids
Modulate hormonal/growth factor activity	
Inhibit oncogene activity	NSAIDs, retinoids, tamoxifen
Promote intracellular communication	Genistein, NSAIDs, monoterpenes
Restore immune response	Carotenois, polyphenols, retinoids
Induce apoptosis	NSAIDs, selenium, vitamin E
Correct DNA methylation imbalances	Butyric acid, genistein, selenium, sulindac sulfone, retinoids
Inhibit basement membrance degradation	Folic acid, choline, methionine
Inhibit arachidonic acid metabolism	Protease inhibitors
	Glycyrrhetinic acid, N-acetylcysteine, NSAIDs, polyphenols

damage. The drug oltipraz induces phase two enzymes; in particular, glutathione-*S*-transferase has been shown to reduce the carcinogenicity of aflatoxin B1 by enhancing its detoxification (Jacobson *et al.*, 1997). Chemopreventive chemicals increase tissue resistance function on the target tissue, usually an early preneoplastic lesion by increasing tissue maturation and/or decreasing cell proliferation. Suppressing agents induce tissue differentiation, may counteract oncogenes, enhance tumor-suppressor gene activities, inhibit proliferation of premalignant cells, or modify the effect of the carcinogen on the target tissue. Retinoic acid is a classic agent that functions by inducing target tissue differentiation. Similarly, viral vectors containing wild-type p53 have been shown to negate the effects of tumor growth driven via p53 mutation. Extensive experimental evidence exists showing the inhibition or retarding of the cancer process by chemopreventive chemicals. These studies have been performed in animal models and cell systems. Although the human results of chemoprevention interventions are less convincing than the experimental models, considerable epidemiological evidence demonstrates an inverse relationship of some nutrient factors with cancer risks.

ASSESSING CARCINOGENICITY OF CHEMICALS

A number of in vivo and in vitro experimental systems are available to assess the potential carcinogenicity of chemicals. The types of tests available to identify chemicals with carcinogenic potential can be classified into general categories, based on the duration required

to conduct the test (Table 8-20). Short-term tests are typically of the duration of days to a few weeks, intermediate-term tests last from weeks up to a year, whereas chronic long-term tests usually encompass six months to two years exposure to a chemical. These bioassays use bacterial and mammalian targets.

Short-Term Tests for Mutagenicity

Short-term tests for mutagenicity were developed to identify potentially carcinogenic chemicals based on their ability to induce mutations in DNA either in vivo or in vitro. A variety of

Table 8-20

General Methods for Identification of Potential Carcinogens

METHOD	TIME FRAME
Short term	
Mutagenesis assays	Several weeks
Transformation in cell culture	1–3 months
Medium term	
Qualitative and quantitative analysis of preneoplasia	2–8 months
Long term	
Chronic bioassay in animals	18–24 months

Table 8-21

Short-Term Tests for Mutagenicity

TEST	ENDPOINT	REFERENCES
Gene mutation assays in vitro		
Prokaryote mutagenesis in vitro (Ames test, etc)	Back or forth mutations in specific bacterial strains	Maron and Ames (1983)
Mouse lymphoma thymidine kinase (TK)	Mutations in TK	Majeska and Matheson (1990)
Chinese hamster ovary (CHO) and V79 hypoxanthine guanine phosphoribosyltranferase (HGPRT)	Mutations in HGPRT	Li *et al.* (1987)
Gene mutation assays in vivo		
Dominant lethal assay	Death of fertilized egg in mammalian implanted species	Bateman (1973) Lockhart *et al.* (1992)
Sperm abnormality induction	Microscopically abnormal sperm	Wyrobek and Bruce (1975)
Mutation induction in transgenes in vivo		
LacZ mouse	Mutations in *LacZ* gene	Myhr (1991)
LacI mouse	Mutations in *LacI* gene	cf. Mirsalis *et al.* (1994)
LacI rat	Mutations in *LacI* gene	de Boer *et al.* (1996)
rpsL mouse	Mutations in *rpsL* gene	Gondo *et al.* (1996)
Chromosomal alterations in vivo		
Heritable translocation test (mice)	Translocations induced in germ cells	Generoso *et al.* (1980)
Rat bone marrow clastogenesis in vivo	Chromosomal aberrations in bone marrow cells in vivo	Ito *et al.* (1994)
Micronucleus test	Appearance of micronuclei in bone marrow cells in vivo	Tinwell and Ashby (1994) Heddle *et al.* (1983)
Chromosomal alterations in vitro		
Mitotic recombination, mitotic crossing over, or mitotic gene conversion in yeast	Conversion of heterozygous alleles to homozygous state	Wintersberger and Klein (1988)
Induced chromosomal aberrations in cell lines	Visible alterations in karyotype	Galloway *et al.* (1985)
Sister chromatid exchange	Visible exchange of differentially labeled sister chromatids	Latt (1981) Murphy *et al.* (1992)
Primary DNA damage		
DNA repair in vivo or in vitro	Unscheduled DNA synthesis and/or DNA strand breaks	Furihata and Matsushima (1987)
Rodent liver: unscheduled DNA synthesis induction	Unscheduled DNA synthesis in rodent cells in vivo and/or in vitro	Kennelly (1995) Steinmetz *et al.* (1988)

in vivo and in vitro short-term tests are available to test the potential carcinogenicity of a chemical (Table 8-21). The majority of these tests measure the mutagenicity of chemicals as a surrogate for carcinogenicity. Therefore, although they are usually very predictive of indirect acting and direct acting (if a metabolic source is provided), these tests routinely fail to detect nongenotoxic carcinogens.

In Vitro Gene Mutation Assays The most widely used short-term test is the Ames assay (Ames *et al.*, 1975; Mortelmans and Zeiger, 2000). The relative simplicity and low cost of the test make it a valuable screening tool for mutagenic carcinogens. *Salmonella typhimurium* strains, deficient in DNA repair and unable to synthesize histidine, are used. In the presence of a mutagenic chemical, the defective histidine gene can be mutated back to a functional state (*back mutation*), resulting in a restoration of bacterial growth in medium lacking histidine. The mutant colonies, which can make histidine, are referred to as "revertants." The Ames test in basic form can detect direct but not indirect genotoxic carcinogens. With the inclusion of a metabolic source, specifically the 9000g supernatant (S9) of a rat liver homogenate to promote metabolic conversion

of the chemical, the Ames can also detect indirect-acting genotoxic carcinogens. Fig. 8-28 describes the standard method used for performing the Ames assay.

Genetically unique strains of the *S typhimurium* bacterium have been developed for determining specific mutational targets. Strains TA100 and TA1535 are able to detect of point mutations whereas strains TA98, TA1537, and TA1538 are able to detect frame shift mutations. Chemicals are typically tested at several concentrations (usually five or more) and the mutation frequency (number of revertants) is calculated. Activation-independent (eg, sodium azide, methyl methanesulfonate) and activation-dependent (eg, 2-aminoanthracene) positive controls are included in each assay.

The mouse lymphoma assay is a mutagenicity assay used to determine whether a chemical is capable of inducing mutation in eukaryotic cells. Typically, mouse lymphoma L5178Y cells are used, and the ability of the cell cultures to acquire resistance to trifluorothymidine (the result of forward mutation at the thymidine kinase [TK] locus) is quantified. Another mammalian cell mutation assay, the Chinese hamster ovary (CHO) test, is also commonly used to assess the potential mutagenicity of chemicals. This assay uses the hypoxanthine–guanine phosphoribosyltransferase

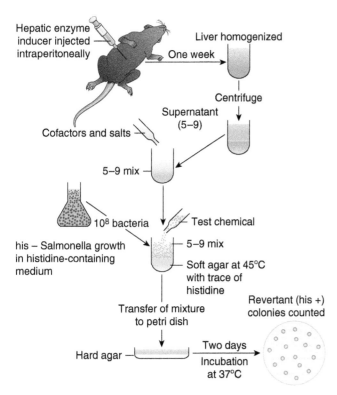

his – Salmonella growth in histidine-containing medium

Figure 8-28. *Scheme of the Ames test for mutagenesis of chemicals in Salmonella bacterial strains.*

(HGPRT) gene as the endpoint. The basis for these assays is shown in Fig. 8-29. Cells are treated with the test chemical and then placed into suspension with selective medium for replication and fixation of induced mutations. Cells are then plated for colony growth, and after several days, colony numbers and colony size are recorded. The number of mutant colonies is a measure of the ability of the test chemical to induce a genetic change at the TK or HGPRT loci in these transformed cells.

As with the Ames assay, these assays are frequently performed in the presence of an exogenous metabolic source (eg, irradiated epithelial cell feeder layer). Because not all carcinogens are mutagens and/or directly damage DNA, the concordance with the chronic in vivo bioassay for these mutagenicity assays is relatively low. For a historical perspective on the utilization of the Ames/Salmonella assay, a recent review by Claxton *et al.* (2010) provides more information on the use of the assay and the role of metabolic activation and mutagenicity testing with respect to genotoxic carcinogens.

In Vivo Gene Mutation Assays For the assessment of the carcinogenic potential of chemicals in vivo genotoxicity tests are important complement to in vitro mutagenicity tests. The in vivo tests have advantages over the in vitro test systems in that they take into account whole animal processes such as absorption, tissue distribution, metabolism, and excretion of chemicals and their metabolites. The commonly used in vivo models include transgenic rodent mutation assay systems based on the genes of the *lac* operon, MutaMouse (Gossen *et al.*, 1989) and Big Blue (Kohler *et al.*, 1991a,b). Some details of the *lac* operon are shown in Fig. 8-30).

The MutaMouse is a transgenic mouse in which a vector prepared from bacteriophage λDNA (λgt10) has been stably inserted

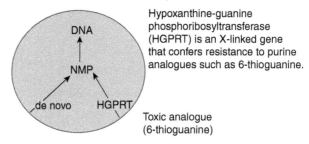

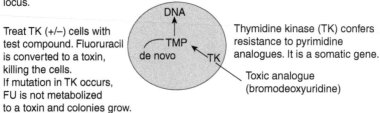

Figure 8-29. *Outline of chemically induced mutation in mouse cell lines with TK or HGPRT as the target gene.*

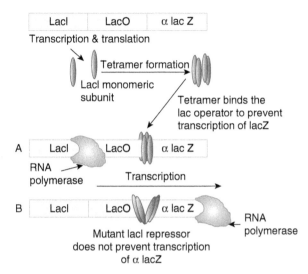

Figure 8-30. *Schematic representation of the lac operon in E coli.*

into the genome and exists within every cell. Within the λDNA sequence, the bacterial gene *lacZ*, which encodes for β-galactosidase, was inserted at the single *Eco*RI restriction site. The entire vector contains ~47,000 bp, of which the *lacZ* gene comprises 3126 bp. The construction and analysis of MutaMouse have been previously described (Gossen *et al.*, 1989). The Big Blue transgenic mouse was developed using a 47.6-kb λshuttle vector containing the bacterial *lacI* gene (1080 bp), which encodes the repressor protein of the *lacZ* gene. As with the MutaMouse, this vector is stably inserted into the genome and exists in every cell. Details on the Big Blue system are described elsewhere (Kohler *et al.*, 1991a,b).

To detect mutations, following exposure of mice to test chemicals, mutations are analyzed in high molecular DNA isolated from the tissue under investigation. The next step is to isolate a viable λphage for the analysis of mutations in the *lacZ* or *lacI* genes from the mouse. The infectious λparticles are detected as plaques that form on a bacterial (*Escherichia coli* strain) lawn grown on an agar surface. In the case of MutaMouse a positive selection system is used that involves the scoring of clear plaques on titration plates to determine the total number of plaque forming units and on selection plates to determine the number of mutants (Gossen and Vijg, 1993). For Big Blue, a nonselectable color screening assay is used, scoring blue mutant plaques among the nonmutant clear plaques (Kohler *et al.*, 1991a). In each case the ratio of mutants to the total population provides a mutation frequency for each chemical and each organ tested. As with the other short-term tests that have been discussed, it is unlikely that in vivo genotoxicity test systems will identify nongenotoxic/non–DNA-reactive compounds.

Chromosomal Alterations Chromosomal alterations are quite common in malignant neoplasms, as such, the detection of chromosomal abnormalities by test chemicals is considered an excellent test for the assessment of carcinogenic potential. Both in vivo and in vitro assays are available to assess chromosomal alterations. In mammalian cell lines, most of the test systems used the same lines as used in the mutation assay. To assess induction of chromosomal alterations, cells are harvested in their first mitotic division after the initiation of chemical exposure. Cells are stained with Giemsa, and scored for completeness of karyotype (21 ± 2 chromosomes). The classes of aberrations recorded include breaks and terminal deletions, rearrangements and translocations, as well as despiralized chromosomes, and cells containing 10 or more aberrations.

SCEs are a measure of DNA damage and increased levels of DNA damage, events that are associated with mutation induction and cancer. During metaphase, sister chromatids, each encompassing a complete copy of one chromosome, are bound together through specific protein interactions. SCEs are a reflection of an interchange of DNA between different chromatids at homologous loci within a replicating chromosome (Latt *et al.*, 1981). Differential staining of chromatids is therefore used to assess SCEs. Typically, 5-bromodeoxyuridine (BrdU) is added along with the test chemical for one cell replication followed by replacement of the medium with medium containing BrdU and colcemid, without test chemical. Cells are then harvested, stained and second-division metaphase cells scored to determine the frequency of SCE/cell for each dose level.

In vivo, analysis of chromosomal alterations has been described since the 1980s (Sasaki, 1980). Disruption of the DNA replication process or damage to chromosomes by chemicals can alter the genetic material distributed to either of the two daughter nuclei. When this occurs, the genetic material that is not incorporated into a new nucleus may form its own "micronucleus," which is clearly visible with a microscope. For this assay, animals are exposed to chemicals and the frequency of micronucleated cells is determined at some specified time after treatment. Micronucleus tests must be performed on cells that are dividing, most typically in cells from bone marrow samples (Heddle *et al.*, 1983). As with other short-term tests, the micronucleus test provides complementary information to gene mutation data but neither tests enhance the ability to detect genotoxic carcinogens, nor is capable of detecting non–DNA-reactive carcinogens. However, this assay does provide information on the ability of a chemical to disrupt mammalian chromosome structure and function.

DNA Damage Primary DNA damage represents possible premutational events that can be detected, either directly or indirectly, by a number of techniques using mammalian cells in culture or using rodent tissue. Unscheduled DNA synthesis (UDS) is a commonly used assay that measures the ability of a test article to induce DNA lesions by measuring the increase in DNA repair. Among the available techniques is the measurement of DNA strand breaks both in vivo and in vitro (Miyamae *et al.*, 1997). Although a wide array of assays are available to assess DNA damage, the Comet assay, or single cell gel electrophoresis, has become one of the standard methods for assessing DNA damage and repair at the individual cell level. Since its introduction 1988, the alkaline comet assay has been modified to increase the utility of this technique for detecting various forms of DNA damage (eg, single- and double-strand breaks, oxidative DNA base damage, and DNA–DNA/DNA–protein/DNA–Drug cross-linking) and DNA repair in virtually any eukaryotic cell. Through the use of lesion-specific endonucleases, the levels of UV-induced pyrimidine dimers, oxidized bases, and alkylation damage can be assessed in biological samples (Collins, 2004).

Short-Term Tests: Transformation Assays A variety of in vitro test systems have been developed to assess the carcinogenic potential of chemicals. The C3H/10T½ cell line has been widely used for the transformation assay. It was originally derived from fibroblasts taken from the prostate of a C3H mouse embryo. The cells are approximately tetraploid but the chromosome number in the cells varies widely. As such, these cells are chromosomally abnormal and have already passed through some of the stages that might be involved in the production of a cancerous cell. Upon plating these cells, they will stop growing when their density is

Table 8-22

Animal Models of Neoplastic Development

	ENDPOINT	REFERENCES
Chronic 2-year bioassay	Tumors in all organs	Sontag (1977)
Tissue-specific bioassays		
Liver, mouse	Hepatomas	Camichael *et al.* (1997)
Lung, mouse	Pulmonary adenomas	Shimkin and Stoner (1975)
Brain, rat	Gliomas	Kroh (1995)
Mammary gland, rat/mouse	Adenomas and carcinomas	Dunnick *et al.* (1995)
Medium-term bioassays		
Ito model	Hepatic adenomas and carcinomas	Ito *et al.* (1989)
Newborn mouse	Neoplasms in liver, lung, lymphoid organs	Fujii (1991)
Multistage models of neoplastic development		
Bladder, rat	Papillomas/carcinomas	Hicks (1980)
Colon, rat	Aberrant crypt polyp	Sutherland and Bird (1994)
Epidermis, mouse	Papillomas	DiGiovanni (1992)
Liver, rat	Altered hepatic foci	Pitot *et al.* (1996)
Transgenic mice		
Knockout of p53 tumor suppressor gene (p53[def])	Tumors in heterozygous animals having normal phenotype	Donehower (1996)
v-Ha-ras with zetaglobin promoter; tandem insertion on chromosome 11 (TG AC)	Induced transgene expression in skin leads to papilloma development	Spalding *et al.* (1993)

sufficiently high (contact growth inhibition). However, the contact inhibition can fail, resulting in cell piling forming a transformed colony. Therefore, following exposure to xenobiotics, this assay assesses carcinogenic potential based on the percentage of colonies that are transformed (Reznikoff *et al.*, 1973).

The most frequently used endpoint for cell transformation is morphological transformation of mammalian cell fibroblasts in culture. Transformation assays using BALB3T3 and Syrian hamster embryo (SHE) cells are available for the assessment of the carcinogenic potential of chemicals. BALB/3T3 transformation assay, however, has not gained full acceptance as a carcinogenic screening assay mainly due to issues regarding its relatively low sensitivity, low reproducibility and relatively long test period (Sakai and Sato, 1989; Schechtman, 1985). The SHE cell assay, a diploid cell transformation assay, measures carcinogenic potential of xenobiotics by assessing transformed colonies based on morphological criterion. The SHE cell assay has several features that make this an appealing method to evaluate the carcinogenic potential of xenobiotics: (1) The assay has a >85% concordance with the two-year rodent bioassay; (2) the stages involved in the clonal transformation of SHE cells (eg, morphological transformation, immortalization, and tumorogenicity) closely resemble those associated with the classic defined stages of carcinogenesis (eg, initiation, promotion and progression); and (3) non-genotoxic/non–DNA-reactive carcinogens elicit a positive response on morphological transformation in the SHE cell assay (Barrett and Lamb, 1985; LeBoeuf *et al.*, 1990; Isfort *et al.*, 1994, 1996). The SHE assay offers an alternative, regulatory approved, means to check the validity of the positive result before embarking on potentially unnecessary and expensive chronic or subchronic testing protocols.

Chronic Testing for Carcinogenicity

The majority of in vivo carcinogenicity testing is performed in rodent models. The administration of chemicals in the diet, often for extended periods, for assessment of their safety and/or toxicity

began in the 1930s (Sasaki and Yoshida, 1935). Animal testing today remains a standard approach for determining the potential carcinogenic activity of xenobiotics. In addition to the lifetime exposure rodent models, organ-specific model systems, multistage models, and transgenic models are being developed and used in carcinogen testing (Table 8-22).

Chronic (Two Year) Bioassay Two-year studies in laboratory rodents remain the primary method by which chemicals or physical agents are identified as having the potential to be hazardous to humans. The most common rodents used are the rat and mouse. Typically the bioassays are conducted over the lifespan of the rodents (two years). Historically, selective rodent strains have been used in the chronic bioassay; however, each strain has both advantages and disadvantages. For example, the NTP typically uses Fisher 344 (F344) rats and B6C3F1 mice. The F344 rat has a high incidence of testicular tumors and leukemias whereas the B6C3F1 mouse is associated with a high background of liver tumors (Table 8-23).

In the chronic bioassay, two or three dose levels of a test chemical and a vehicle control are administered to 50 males and 50 females (mice and rats), beginning at eight weeks of age, continuing throughout their lifespan. The route of administration can be via oral (gavage), dietary (mixed in feed), or inhalation (via inhalation chambers) exposure. Typically a number of short-term in vivo tests are conducted prior to the chronic bioassay to determine acute toxicity profiles, appropriate route of administration, and the maximum tolerated dose (MTD). Generally, the MTD is used to set the high dose in the chronic study. The use of the MTD as the upper dose level has been questioned by many investigators, as it is recognized that the doses selected represent those that are considered unrealistically high for human exposure. Pharmacokinetics and metabolism at high dose are frequently unrepresentative of those at lower doses; in addition, a general relationship between toxicity and carcinogenicity cannot be drawn for all classes of chemicals. During the study, food consumption and bodyweight gain should be monitored and the animals observed clinically on a regular basis;

Table 8-23

Spontaneous Tumor Incidence (Combined Benign and Malignant) in Selected Sites of the Two Species, B6C3F1 Mice and F344 Rats, Used in the NCI/NTP Bioassay

	B6C3F1 MICE		F344 RATS	
SITE	MALE	FEMALE	MALE	FEMALE
Liver				
Adenoma	10.3	4.0	3.4	3.0
Carcinoma	21.3	4.1	0.8	0.2
Pituitary	0.7	8.3	24.7	47.5
Adrenal	3.8	1.0	19.4	8.0
Thyroid	1.3	2.1	10.7	9.3
Hematopoietic	12.7	27.2	30.1	18.9
Mammary gland	0	1.9	2.5	26.1
Lung	17.1	7.5	2.4	1.2

at necropsy, the tumor number, location, and diagnosis for each animal is thoroughly assessed.

Organ-Specific Bioassays and Multistage Animal Models

Many tissue-specific bioassays have been developed with the underlying goal being to produce a sensitive and reliable assay that could be conduced in a time frame shorter in duration than the two-year chronic bioassay. These assays are commonly used to detect carcinogenic activity of chemicals in various target organs (Weisburger and Williams, 1984). Of the many models available, three models, the liver, skin, and lung models are more widely used.

Carcinogenicity Testing in the Liver The liver represents a major target organ for chemical carcinogens. It has been estimated that nearly half of the chemicals tested in the two-year chronic bioassay by the NTP showed an increased incidence of liver cancer. The rodent liver has been used as an animal model for carcinogenesis since the 1930s. Early pioneering work by Peraino and Pitot as well as Farber showed the multistaged process that occurs in the liver. The multistage nature of carcinogenesis is paralleled in the animal models; the system is characterized by well-defined changes including the formation of initiated cells by genotoxic agents that then progress to preoplastic focal lesions, which subsequently convert into neoplasms. The use of preneoplastic lesions as endpoints in carcinogenicity testing may shorten experiment from two years to a few months. Several rodent liver focus assays have been developed to assess the ability of a chemical to induce liver cancer and study the mechanisms involved in tumor development (Bannasch, 1986a,b; Williams, 1982). Liver carcinogenesis assays have been developed to study and distinguish chemicals that affect the initiation or promotion stage of hepatocarcinogenesis. During the assay for initiating activity of a chemical, the test substance is given prior to exposure to a promoting chemical. Although a single initiating dose can result in the induction of focal lesions, exposure over a several week period is often used to increase the sensitivity of the model (Parnell *et al.*, 1988; Williams, 1982). Phenobarbital is a commonly used tumor promoter; however, a wide range of chemicals have also been used as promoting agents (Solt and Farber, 1976; Oesterle and Deml, 1988). To assess the promoting activity of a chemical, the liver is initiated with a genotoxic chemical, often diethylnitrosamine. The test chemical is then administered for

a duration of weeks to several months, and chemicals with promoting activity may stimulate the proliferation of initiated cells or may inhibit the proliferation of the surrounding putatively normal cells. The dose of the initiating carcinogen should represent a dose that will not induce liver tumors during the course of the experiment.

Another method commonly used was developed in Japan by Ito and co-workers (Ogiso *et al.*, 1990; Shirai *et al.*, 1999; Ito *et al.*, 1994). The entire assay takes only eight weeks to perform. Rats are initiated with a single dose of diethylnitrosamine, followed by a two-week recovery period, after which point the animals are exposed to the test compound for eight weeks. After one week of exposure to the test substance, the animals are given a two-third partial hepatectomy. The control group receives the same initiation and partial hepatectomy, but is not exposed to the test chemical. Hepatic focal lesions, while individually are clonal in nature, express a number of phenotypic alterations in various enzyme markers. A common endpoint assessed is the formation of liver lesions that stain for GST-P, a marker that stains many focal lesions in the rat. Using this assay, these investigators demonstrated a significant correlation between the results obtained using this assay and medium- and long-term study results (Ogiso *et al.*, 1990). This group has also modified the original procedure to enable the detection of promoting agents. In this protocol, carcinogens are given over a four-week period to initiate the formation of focal lesion, after which, test chemicals are administered for an additional 24- to 36-week period (Ito *et al.*, 1996). In this manner, the ability of the test chemical to promote the growth of preneoplastic lesions can be assessed. The newborn mouse model originally described by Shubik and co-workers (Pietra *et al.*, 1959) has also been used as a model for hepatocarcinogenesis (Vesselinovitch *et al.*, 1978; Fujii, 1991). In this model, a single dose of diethylnitrosamine is administered to infant mice to initiate focal lesions. This step is then followed by exposure to test chemicals for several weeks to assess their potential to promote focal lesion development in the liver.

Identification of hepatic foci in H&E-stained sections is regarded as the most reliable approach for the diagnosis and quantification of preneoplastic liver lesions in rodents. Preneoplastic lesions are obligatory precursor lesions that can lead to liver tumors and will progress to benign and malignant liver cell tumors without further chemical exposure, and are used as endpoints in carcinogenicity testing (Ito *et al.*, 1989; Maronpot *et al.*, 1989; Pereira and Herren-Freund, 1988; Pitot *et al.*, 1987). In addition to the sensitive detection of these preneoplastic lesions in conventional H&E staining, a number of histochemically detectable phenotypic alterations have been used for their quantification; however, these markers are only useful in the rat model, as focal lesions in mice to not exhibit these same phenotypic markers.

Carcinogenicity Testing in the Skin The Mouse Skin model is one of the most extensively studied and used models for understanding multistage carcinogenesis. This model of carcinogenesis is an assay that has been used to dissect mechanisms of carcinogenesis and is also purported to be a useful intermediate-term cancer bioassay. The skin was the target organ of the first experimental induction of chemical carcinogenesis (Yamagiwa and Ichikawa, 1915). The early studies by Friedwald and Rous (1944) and Berenblub and Shubik (1947) introduced the two-stage concept of carcinogenesis in the skin (Fig. 8-31). This model exploits many of the unique properties of the mouse skin, one major being that the development of neoplasia can be followed visually. In addition, the number and relative size of papillomas and carcinomas can be quantified as the tumors progress.

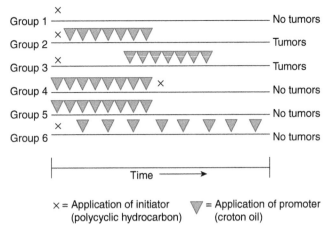

x = Application of initiator (polycyclic hydrocarbon)   ▽ = Application of promoter (croton oil)

Figure 8-31. *Experiments demonstrating the initiation and promotion phases of carcinogenesis in mice. Group 2: application of promoter repeated at twice-weekly intervals for several months. Group 3: application of promoter delayed for several months and then applied twice weekly. Group 6: promoter applied at monthly intervals.*

Both initiating and promoting activities of chemical carcinogens can be assessed using this model. In the promotion assay, a number of chemical carcinogens have been used to initiate cells in the mouse skin including urethane, UV light, benzo(*a*)pyrene, and dimethlybenzanthracene, with the latter of more common usage. The requirement for all initiating agents is to induce a genotoxic event that upon failure to repair DNA damage, results in the formation of a mutated cell. Grossly, initiated cells of the skin appear identical to normal skin. Initiation in skin is frequently linked with the mutation of the *CHr* gene. Because the terminally differentiated cells in the skin are no longer capable of undergoing cell division, only initiated cells retain their proliferative capacity and thus represent the cell populations that give rise to tumors. To assess promotion by a chemical, an initiating chemical is applied first and is followed by the administration of a test substance for several weeks on the shaved skin of mice (Slaga, 1984). The promotion of initiated karatinocytes is commonly assessed using the phorbol ester 12-*O*-tetradecanoylphorbol-13-acetate (TPA), which is routinely included as a positive control in this assay. The current hypothesis is that during the initiation stage the expansion or of initiated cells occurs as a result of inflammation and hyperplasia from either TPA or through mechanical wound healing mechanisms. Upon repeated application of tumor promoters, selective clonal expansion of initiated keratynocytes occurs, resulting in skin papillomas, which over time can progress to carcinomas. In the standard 2-stage protocol for mouse skin malignant progression is relatively rare with approximately 5% of the paillomas progressing to the carcinoma stage. For the detection of initiating activity, the test substance is applied to skin prior to promotion with phorbol esters. Several mouse models are available, including hairless mice, SENCAR mice, both of which have enhanced sensitivity to the induction of skin cancer (Brown and Balmain, 1995; Sundberg *et al.*, 1997).

Carcinogenicity Testing in the Lung Strain A mice are genetically susceptible to the development of lung tumors, with lung tumors being observed in control animals as early as three to four weeks of age with a steady increase to nearly 100% by 24 months of age (Shimkin and Stoner, 1975). Chemically induced tumors appear to be derived from hyperplastic lesions that progress to adenoma, carcinoma within adenoma, and ultimately, to carcinomas (Stoner *et al.*, 1993). In this model, carcinogenicity is typically assessed as an acceleration of tumor development rather than an increase in tumor incidence. The protocol currently used is that the chemical is administered for a period of eight weeks, after which the animals remain on test for four additional months without chemical exposure. The strain A mouse lung tumor assay is sensitive to particular classes of chemicals, such as PAHs, nitrosamines, nitrosoureas, carbamates, aflatoxin, certain metals, and hydrazines (Maronpot *et al.*, 1986; Stoner, 1991; Stoner and Shimkin, 1985).

Carcinogenicity Testing in Other Organs Test systems to examine the ability of a chemical to promote neoplastic development at organ sites other than liver, skin, and lung have also been developed. The available systems include animal models directed at examining carcinogenicity in the kidney, bladder, pancreas, stomach, colon, small intestine, and oral cavity. These models vary in the initiating carcinogen used, and frequency, duration, and site of application, as well as duration of promoting chemical exposure. Table 8-24 provides an overview of the animal models available for these target organs.

Transgenic Animals in Carcinogenicity Assessment

Due to the development of animal models with genetic alterations that invoke a susceptibility to carcinogenesis by chemical agents, the use of transgenic and knockout animals in carcinogenicity assessment is gaining more popularity. The common models that have been used include the Tg.AC and rasH2 transgenic mice and $p53^{+/-}$ and $XPA^{-/-}$ knockout mice (Gulezian *et al.*, 2000). Recently, the feasibility of the use of these animal models as alternative assays for the two-year chronic bioassay was assessed in a collaborative between the Health and Environmental Sciences Institute (HESI) branch of the International Life Sciences Institute (ILSI). In this assessment, 21 chemicals were evaluated, encompassing genotoxic, nongenotoxic, and noncarcinogenic chemicals. The conclusions drawn from the scientific review suggested that these models appear to have usefulness as screening models for assessment of chemical carcinogenicity; however, they do not provide definitive proof of potential human carcinogenicity. Further the scientific panel suggested that these models could be used in place of the mouse two-year bioassay (Cohen *et al.*, 2001; Blaauboer *et al.*, 1998). Coupled with information on genotoxicity, particularly DNA reactivity, structure–activity relationships, results from other bioassays, and the results of other mechanistic investigations including toxicokinetics, metabolism, and mechanistic information, these alternate mouse models for carcinogenicity appear to be useful models for assessing the carcinogenicity of chemicals. In general, replacement of the two-year rodent bioassay by transgenic mouse assay have not been as successful as originally planned (Boverhof, 2011). However, as models for studying the roles of specific pathways and mechanisms in the carcinogenesis process, these models remain an excellent resource.

New Approaches A major concern for the correct evaluation of the safety of chemicals, and as mixtures is the need to obtain reliable and pertinent scientific information on which to develop proper risk evaluation and assessment. Our current bioassays approaches have been criticized as being too time consuming and not pertinent to human health. Research during the last decade of the 20th century and the turn of the 21st century have resulted in a dramatic increase in our knowledge of the cellular and molecular pathways that contribute to the induction and prevention of cancer. This coupled with technological advances in high-throughput

Table 8-24

Target Organ Models for Studying Chemically Induced Carcinogenesis

ORGAN	SPECIES	INITIATING CARCINOGEN	INITIATOR DURATION	CARCINOGEN (PROMOTER) DURATION	REFERENCES
Kidney	Rat	N-Ethyl-N-hydroxyethylnitrosamine	Single exposure	20 weeks	Hiasa et al. (1991)
Bladder	Rat	N-Nitrosobutyl(4-hydroxybutyl)amine	4 weeks	32 weeks	Fukushima et al. (1983)
Pancreas	Rat, Syrian hamsters	N-nitrosobis(2-oxopropyl) amine, N-nitroso(2-hydroxypropyl)(2-oxopropyl) amine	Single exposure		Longnecker et al. (1985), Longnecker et al. (1984)
Stomach (forestomach)	Rat	Benzo(a)pyrene	1–2 times/week, 4 weeks	40 weeks	Silva et al. (1995)
Stomach (glandular)	Rat	N-Methyl-N'-nitro-N-nitronitrosoguanidine	Single exposure	40 weeks	Takahashi et al. (1986)
Colon	Rat	Azoxymethane	2 exposures	12 weeks	Yamashita et al. (1994)
Small intestine	Rat Mice	1,2-Dimethylhydrazine N-Ethyl-N'-nitro-N-nitrosoguanidine	2–9 weeks 4 weeks	16–20 weeks	Lindenschmidt et al. (1987), Jagadeesan et al. (1994)
Oral cavity (lip, oral, nasal)	Rat	4-Nitroquinoline N-oxide	4 weeks		Johansson et al. (1989)
Oral cavity (Tongue)	Rat	4-Nitroquinoline N-oxide	8 weeks		Tanaka et al. (1995)
Buccal cells (squamous cell carcinoma)	Syrian hamster	—	—	Repeated application 10–16 weeks	Solt et al. (1987)
Buccal cells (squamous cell carcinoma)	Syrian hamster	Dimethylbenz[a]anthracene	Single exposure	45 weeks	Gimenez-Conti and Slaga (1993)

assays, and computational science has raised the question if the current approaches for carcinogenesis evaluation of chemicals (and mixtures) should be reevaluated. Following a NRC report in 2007 (Toxicity Testing in the 21st Century: A Vision and a Strategy), several approaches have begun utilizing high-throughput and computational approaches to evaluating the effects of chemicals on biological processes and pathways that are important in toxicity (including cancer). These approaches are directed to using cells, cell lines and components of cells. Two approaches currently well underway include the USEPA Toxcast program and the NTP/NIEHS lead Tox 21 program (tox21 is a consortium of NIH, FDA, USEPA) utilizing this approach.

CHEMICAL CARCINOGENESIS IN HUMANS

Recently, the IARC (Vol 100) has reported a review of chemically induced cancer in humans. This body has identified and classified 103 compounds as carcinogenic in humans. This review is divided into four major categories of carcinogens deemed to be human carcinogens by the IARC. These include pharmaceuticals, metals, biologicals, and radiation. A number of factors have been implicated in the induction of cancer in humans. Infectious agents, lifestyle, medical treatments, environmental, and occupational exposure account either directly or indirectly to the majority of cancers seen

in humans. Of these, the component that contributes the most to human cancer induction and progression is lifestyle: tobacco use, alcohol use, and poor diet (Table 8-25). Tobacco usage either through smoking tobacco, chewing tobacco, or tobacco snuff-type products is estimated be responsible for 25% to 40% of all human cancers. In particular, a strong correlation between tobacco usage and mouth, larynx, lung, esophageal, and bladder cancer exists. It has been estimated (Doll and Peto, 1981) that 85% to 90% of all lung cancer cases in the United States are a direct result of tobacco

Table 8-25

Carcinogenic Factors Associated With Lifestyle

CHEMICAL(S)	NEOPLASM(S)
Alcohol beverage	Esophagus, liver, oropharynx, and larynx
Aflatoxins	Liver
Betel chewing	Mouth
Dietary intake (fat, protein, calories)	Breast, colon, endometrium, gallbladder
Tobacco smoking	Mouth, pharynx, larynx, lung, esophagus, bladder

Table 8-26

Occupational Human Carcinogens

AGENT	INDUSTRIAL PROCESS	NEOPLASMS
Asbestos	Construction, asbestos mining	Peritoneum, bronchus
Arsenic	Mining and smelting	Sking, bronchus, liver
Alkylating agents (mechloroethamine hydrochloride and bis[chloromethyl]ether)	Chemical manufacturing	Bronchus
Benzene	Chemical manufacturing	Bone marrow
Benzidine, β-naphthylamine	Dye and textile	Urinary bladder
Chromium and chromates	Tanning, pigment making	Nasal sinus, bronchus
Nickel	Nickel refining	Nasal sinus, bronchus
Polynuclear aromatic hydrocarbons	Steel making, roofing, chimney cleaning	Skin, scrotum, bronchus
Vinyl chloride monomer	Chemical manufacturing	Liver
Wood dust	Cabinet making	Nasal sinus
Beryllium	Aircraft manufacturing, electronics	Bronchus
Cadmium	Smelting	Bronchus
Ethylene oxide	Production of hospital supplies	Bone marrow
Formaldehyde	Plastic, textile, and chemical	Nasal sinus, bronchus
Polychlorinated biphenyls	Electrical-equipment production and maintenance	Liver

use. The induction of pancreatic cancer also appears to have a linkage to tobacco use. Alcohol consumption also contribute anywhere from 2% to 4% of cancers of the esophagus, liver, and larynx.

Poor diets whether high-fat, low-protein, high-calories or diets lacking in needed antioxidants and minerals account for anywhere from 10% to 70% of human cancers. Diet contaminated by molds such as *Aspergillus flavis* (which produces aflatoxin B1) have been linked epidemiologically to a higher incidence of liver cancer. It also appears that aflatoxin B1 exposure coupled with hepatitis B virus infection produces an increased incidence of liver cancer compared to aflatoxin B1 or hepatitis B exposure individually. Mold-contaminated foodstuffs have also been shown to produce nitroso compounds.

There is substantial evidence that overnutrition either through excess calories and/or high-fat diets contribute to a number of human cancers (Doll and Peto, 1981). In particular, high-fat and high-calorie diets have been linked to breast, colon, and gall bladder cancer in humans. Diets poor in antioxidants and/or vitamins such as vitamin A and vitamin E probably also contribute to the onset of cancer. The method of cooking may also influence the production of carcinogens produced in the cooking process. Carcinogenic HCAs and PAHs are formed during broiling and grilling of meat. Acrylamide, a suspected human carcinogen, has been found in fried foods at low concentrations.

A number of occupations have been associated with the development of specific cancers (Table 8-26). As noted earlier, the linkage between chimney sweeps who as young boys in England were exposed to PAHs through the constant exposure to soot developed scrotal cancer. The linkage between occupational exposure to asbestos and the development of bronchiogenic carcinoma and as well as malignant mesothelioma has been clearly established. The appearance of bronchiogenic carcinoma was much higher in shipyard workers who were exposed to both asbestos and cigarette

smoking. Muscat and Wynder (1995) noted no association between cigarette smoking and mesothelioma formation. Similarly, asbestos exposure by itself (without smoking) does not seem to increase the risk of bronchiogenic carcinoma. Aromatic amines used in the chemical and dye industries have been shown to produce or induce bladder cancer in humans. Prolonged high exposure to benzene in an occupational setting has been linked to the formation of acute myelogenous leukemia in humans.

A number of drugs and medical diagnostic tools have also been linked to the induction of human cancer (Table 8-27). Anticancer drugs such as the alkylating agent cyclophosphamide have been

Table 8-27

Human Carcinogenic Chemicals Associated With Medical Therapy and Diagnosis

CHEMICAL OR DRUG	ASSOCIATED NEOPLASMS
Alkylating agents (cyclophospamide, melphalan)	Bladder, leukemia
Azathioprine	Lymphoma, reticulum cell sarcoma, skin, Kaposi sarcoma
Chloramphenicol	Leukemia
Diethylstilbestrol	Vagina (clear cell carcinoma)
Estrogens	Liver cell adenoma, endometrium, skin
Phenacetin	Renal pelvis (carcinoma)
Phenytoin	Lymphoma, neuroblastoma
Thorotrast	Liver (angiosarcoma)

associated with bladder tumors and leukemia in patients receiving these treatments. The administration of the synthetic estrogenic compound diethylstibestrol to pregnant women in order to improve embryo implantation and prevent spontaneous abortion has been shown to result in the formation of clear cell carcinomas of the vagina in the female offspring of mothers treated with diethylstilbestrol during pregnancy. The use of oral contraceptives containing synthetic estrogens as their major or only component has been implicated in the induction of liver cell adenomas. In addition, an association exists between prolonged use of estrogenic oral contraceptives and an increase incidence of premenopausal breast cancer. Androgenic steroids and synthetic testosterone compounds have been implicated in hepatocellular carcinoma induction. Therapeutic immunosuppression given to transplant patients or arising secondary to selective diseases such as AIDS result in an increase in a variety of different neoplasms. These results further support the role of the immune system in identifying and removing early preneoplastic cells from the body. In addition, the previously used diagnostic tracer Thorotrast has been sufficiently linked to the formation of hemangiosarcomas.

CLASSIFICATION EVALUATION OF CARCINOGENICITY IN HUMANS

The assessment and designation of a chemical agent or a mixture of chemicals as carcinogenic in humans is evaluated by various agencies worldwide. The evaluation usually encompasses epidemiological, experimental animal, and in vitro data utilizing assays as described earlier in this chapter. One of the first schemes for the classification of an agent's carcinogenicity was devised by the IARC (Table 8-28). The IARC approach assigns the chemical or mixture to one of five groupings based upon strength of evidence for the agent's possible, probable, or definite carcinogenicity to humans. In Group one classification, the agent or mixture is classified as definitely carcinogenic to humans. The second grouping is Group 2A in which the agent is probably carcinogenic to humans. In Group 2B, the agent is classified as possibly carcinogenic to humans. Group 3, the agent is not classifiable. And in the last group, Group 4, the agent is not carcinogenic to humans. The IARC produces a series of monographs that describe the methodology for the evaluation of specific chemicals and the rationale for their final classification.

Table 8-28

IARC Classification of the Evaluation of Carcinogenicity for Human Beings

GROUP	EVIDENCE
1. Agent is carcinogenic to humans	Human data strong Animal data strong
2A. Agent is probably carcinogenic to humans	Human epidemiology data suggestive Animal data positive
2B. Agent is possibly carcinogenic to humans	Human epidemiology data weak Animal data positive
3. Agent is not classifiable as to carcinogenicity to humans	Human and animal data inadequate
4. Agent is probably not carcinogenic to humans	Human and animal data negative

Table 8-29

USEPA Cancer Guidelines Descriptors

Carcinogenic to humans:
- strong evidence of human carcinogenicity, including convincing epidemiological evidence of a causal association between human exposure and cancer
- the mode(s) of carcinogenic action and associated key precursor events have been identified in animals, and there is strong evidence that the key precursor events in animals are anticipated to occur in humans

Likely to be carcinogenic to humans:
- weight of the evidence is adequate to demonstrate carcinogenic potential to an agent in animal experiments in more than one species, sex, strain, site, or exposure route, with or without evidence of carcinogenicity in humans

Suggestive evidence of carcinogenic potential:
- the weight of evidence is suggestive of carcinogenicity; a concern for potential carcinogenic effects in humans is raised, but the data are judged not sufficient for a stronger conclusion

Inadequate information to assess carcinogenic potential:
- available data are judged inadequate for applying one of the other descriptors

Not likely to be carcinogenic to humans:
- this descriptor is appropriate when the available data are considered robust, there is no basis for human hazard concern, evidence in both humans and animals that the agent is not carcinogenic

Currently, 100 chemical agents or mixtures or exposure circumstances have been classified by IARC as falling in Group 1, which shows sufficient evidence for carcinogenicity to humans.

Similar classifications exist for the USEPA, the Food & Drug Administration, and the European Community (EC). The classification of agents with regard to human carcinogenicity can many times be very difficult in particular, when animal data and/or epidemiological data in humans are inconclusive or confounded.

New USEPA Guidelines for Cancer Risk Assessment (2005) uses descriptors for defining the relative carcinogenic risk to humans (Table 8-29). These descriptors include carcinogenic to humans, likely to be carcinogenic to humans, suggestive evidence of carcinogenic potential, inadequate information to access carcinogenic potential, and, not likely to be carcinogenic in humans. The EPA Guidelines take into account the understanding of the mode of carcinogenic action and associated key precursor events needed for the cancer to form (Table 8-30). Central to the USEPA Guidelines for Cancer Risk Assessment is the utilization of the mode of action framework to define the key events in rodents and assessment of

Table 8-30

USEPA Mode of Action Definitions

Mode of action: Key events and processes, starting with the interaction of an agent with a cell, through functional and anatomical changes, resulting in cancer or other health endpoints

Key event: Empirically observable precursor step that is itself a necessary element of the mode of action or is a biologically based marker for such an element

Table 8-31

USEPA Mode of Action Framework

Mode of action criteria

Summary description of the hypothesized mode of action
Identification of key events
Strength, consistency, specificity of association
Dose–response concordance
Temporal relationship
Biological plausibility and coherence
Consideration of the possibility of other MOAs
Is the mode of action sufficiently supported in the test animals?
Is the mode of action relevant to humans?
Which populations or life stages can be particularly susceptible to the mode of action?

whether those same key events and mode of action can occur in humans (Table 8-31). This approach is similar to that has been developed by the International Program on Chemical Safety and by panels in the International Life Sciences Institute.

The current listing of chemical, occupations, or behaviors deemed to be carcinogenic in humans by IARC and the NTP are noted in Tables 8-32 to 8-33, respectively.

SUMMARY

The induction of cancer by chemicals is well established in animal models as well as in humans. Linkages between chemicals found in human lifestyle, occupational exposure, and environmental exposure provides strong evidence for the induction or contribution to environmental occupational lifestyle carcinogens to human cancer. Cancer is a multistage process in its most reductive form involves initial mutational events followed by changes in gene expression leading to the selected clonal proliferation of the precancerous cell. Neoplasia appears to exhibit multiple characteristics including increase selective lesion growth (through sustained cell proliferation and /or resistance to apoptosis), the induction of angiogenesis, enabling replicative immortality, activation of factors that influence invasion and metastasis, evasion of normal growth suppression, modulation of energy metabolism, and the avoidance of attack by the immune system. The

Table 8-32

Known Human Carcinogens: International Agency for Research on Cancer

Acetaldehyde	Estrogen–progestogen therapy	Painter (workplace exposure)
Acid mists, strong inorganic	Estrogen–progestogen oral contraceptives (combined)	3,4,5,3′,4′-Pentachlorobiphenyl (PCB-126)
Aflatoxins		2,3,4,7,8-Pentachlorodibenzofuran
Alcoholic beverages	Ethanol in alcoholic beverages	Phenacetin (and mixtures containing it)
Aluminum production	Ethylene oxide	Phosphorus-32, as phosphate
4-Aminobiphenyl	Etoposide	Plutonium
Areca nut	Etoposide in combination with cisplatin and bleomycin Fission products, including strontium-90	Radioiodines, including iodine-131
Aristolochic acid		Radionuclides, α-particle-emitting
Arsenic and inorganic arsenic compounds		Radionuclides, β-particle-emitting,
Asbestos (all forms)	Formaldehyde	Radium-224 and its decay products
Auramine production	Haematite mining	Radium-226 and its decay products
Azathioprine	*Helicobacter pylori*	Radium-228 and its decay products
Benzene	Hepatitis B virus	Radon-222 and its decay products
Benzidine and dyes metabolized to benzidine	Hepatitis C virus	Rubber manufacturing industry
Benzo[a]pyrene	Human immunodeficiency virus type 1	Salted fish (Chinese-style)
Beryllium and beryllium compounds	Human papilloma virus (HPV)	Schistosoma haematobium (flatworm)
Betel quid, with or without tobacco	Human T-cell lymphotropic virus type I	Semustine (methyl-CCNU)
Bis(chloromethyl)ether and chloromethyl methyl ether	Ionizing radiation	Shale oils
	Iron and steel founding	Silica dust, crystalline (cristobalite)
Busulfan	Isopropyl alcohol	Solar radiation
1,3-Butadiene	Kaposi sarcoma herpesvirus	Soot (exposure of chimney sweeps)
Cadmium and cadmium compounds	Leather dust	Sulfur mustard
Chlorambucil	Magenta production	Tamoxifen
Chlornaphazine	Melphalan	2,3,7,8-Tetrachlorodibenzo-para-dioxin
Chromium (VI) compounds	Methoxsalen (8-methoxypsoralen) plus ultraviolet A radiation	Thiotepa
Clonorchis sinensis (infection with)		Thorium-232 and its decay products
Coal, household combustion	4,4′-Methylenebis(chloroaniline) (MOCA)	Tobacco, smokeless
Coal gasification	Mineral oils, untreated or mildly treated	Tobacco smoke, secondhand
Coal tar distillation	MOPP	Tobacco smoking
Coal tar pitch	2-Naphthylamine	ortho-Toluidine
Coke production	Neutron radiation	Treosulfan
Cyclophosphamide	Nickel compounds	Ultraviolet (UV) including UVA, UVB, and UVC
Cyclosporine	N′-Nitrosonornicotine (NNN) and 4-(N-Nitrosomethylamino)-1-(3-pyridyl)-1-butanone (NNK) Opisthorchis viverrini (liver fluke)	
Diethylstilbestrol		Ultraviolet-emitting tanning devices
Epstein–Barr virus (infection with)		Vinyl chloride
Erionite		Wood dust
Estrogen postmenopausal therapy		X- and γ-radiation

Table 8-33

Known to Be Human Carcinogens National Toxicology Program 12th Report on Carcinogens

Aflatoxins	Diethylstilbestrol (DES)	Tamoxifen
Alcoholic beverage consumption	Dyes metabolized to benzidine	TCDD; "dioxin"
4-Aminobiphenyl	Environmental tobacco smoke	Thiotepa
Analgesic mixtures containing phenacetin	Erionite	Thorium dioxide
Aristolochic acids	Estrogens, steroidal	Tobacco smoking
Arsenic compounds, inorganic	Ethylene oxide	Vinyl chloride
Asbestos	Formaldehyde	Ultraviolet radiation, broad spectrum
Azathioprine	Hepatitis B virus	UV radiation
Benzene	Hepatitis C virus	Wood dust
Benzidine	Human papilloma viruses: some genital-	X-radiation and γ-radiation
Beryllium and beryllium compounds	mucosal types	
1,3-Butadiene	Melphalan	
1,4-Butanediol dimethylsulfonate (busulfan, Myleran)	Methoxsalen with ultraviolet A therapy (PUVA)	
Cadmium and cadmium compounds	Mineral oils (untreated and mildly treated)	
Chlorambucil	Mustard gas	
1-(2-Chloroethyl)-3-(4-methylcyclohexyl)-1-nitrosourea (MeCCNU)	2-Naphthylamine	
	Neutrons	
bis(chloromethyl) ether and technical-grade chloromethyl methyl ether	Nickel compounds	
	Oral tobacco products	
Chromium hexavalent compounds	Radon	
Coal tar pitches	Silica, crystalline (respirable size)	
Coal tars	Solar radiation	
Coke oven emissions	Soots	
Cyclophosphamide	Strong inorganic acid mists containing sulfuric acid	
Cyclosporin A	Sunlamps or sun beds, exposure to	

multistage nature and characteristics of the process have been extensively examined with regard to molecular, cellular, tissue, and organ events.

REFERENCES

Abanobi SE, Lombardi B, Shinozuka H. Stimulation of DNA synthesis and cell proliferation in the liver of rats fed a choline-devoid diet and their suppression by phenobarbital. *Cancer Res.* 1982;41:412–415.

Abuja PM, Albertini R. Methods for monitoring oxidative stress, lipid peroxidation, and oxidation resistance of lipoproteins. *Clin Chim Acta.* 2001;306:1–17.

Adlercreutz H, Mazur W. Phyto-estrogens and western diseases. *Ann Med.* 1997;29:95–120.

Alitalo K, Schwab M. Oncogene amplication in tumor cells. *Adv Cancer Res.* 1986;47:235–281.

Alwens W, Jonas W. Chrome lung cancer. *Acta Unio Internationalis contra Cancrum.* 1938;3:1–114.

Ames BN, McCann J, Yamasaki E. Methods for detecting carcinogens and mutagens with the salmonella/mammalian-microsome mutagenicity test. *Mutat Res.* 1975;31:347–364.

Ames BN, Shigenaga MK. Oxidants are a major contributor to cancer and aging. In: Halliwell B, Aruoma O, eds. *DNA and Free Radicals.* London, UK: Ellis Horwood Ltd; 1993:1–15.

Amstad PA, Krupitza G, Cerutti PA. Mechanisms of c-fos induction by active oxygen. *Cancer Res.* 1992;52:3952–3960.

Andersen A, Berge SR, Engeland A, Norseth T. Exposure to nickel compounds and smoking in relation to incidence of lung and nasal cancer among nickel refinery workers. *Occup Environ Med.* 1996;53(10):708–713.

Andersen M, Brusick D, Cohen S, et al. U.S. Environmental Protection Agency's revised cancer guidelines for carcinogen risk assessment. *Toxicol Appl Pharmacol.* 1998;153:133–136.

Ates NA, Tamer L, Ates C, et al. Glutathione S-transferase M1, T1, P1 genotypes and risk for development of colorectal cancer. *Biochem Genet.* 2005;43(3–4):149–163.

Bachman AN, Kamendulis LM, Goodman JI. Diethanolamine and phenobarbital produce an altered pattern of methylation in GC-rich regions of DNA in B6C3F1 mouse hepatocytes similar to that resulting from choline deficiency. *Toxicol Sci.* 2006;90:317–325.

Balmain A, Pragnell IB. Mouse skin carcinomas induced in vivo by chemical carcinogens have a transforming Harvey-ras oncogene. *Nature.* 1983;303:72–74.

Bannasch P. Preoplastic lesions as end points in carcinogenicity testing I. Hepatic preneoplasia. *Carcinogenesis.* 1986a;7(5):689–695.

Bannasch P. Preneoplastic lesions as end points in carcinogenicity testing. II. Preneoplasia in various non-hepatic tissues. *Carcinogenesis.* 1986b;7(6):849–852.

Barber DA, Harris SR. Oxygen free radicals and antioxidants: a review. *Am Pharm.* 1994;NS34:26–35.

Barrett JC, Lamb PW. Tests with the Syrian hamster embryo cell transformation assay. In: Ashbey J, DeSerres FJ, Draper M, eds. *Progress in Mutation Research-Evaluation of Short Term Tests for Carcinogens.* Vol. 5. New York: Elsevier; 1985:623–628.

Bateman AJ. The dominant lethal assay in the mouse. *Agents Actions.* 1973;3(2):73–76.

Baylin SB. Tying it all together: epigenetics, genetics, cell cycle, and cancer. *Science.* 1997;277:1948–1949.

Beauerle PA, Lenardo M, Pierce JW, Baltimore D. Phorbol-ester-induced activation of the NF-$_\kappa$B transcription factor involved dissociation of an apparently cytoplasmic Nf-$_\kappa$B/Inhibitor complex. *Cold Springs Harb Symp Quant Biol.* 1988;53:789–798.

Becker RA, Shank RC. Kinetics of formation and persistence of ethyl-guanines in DNA of rats and hamsters treated with diethylnitrosamine. *Cancer Res.* 1985;45:2076–2084.

Belinsky SA, Nikula KJ, Palmisano WA, et al. Aberrant methylation of p16(INK4a) is an early event in lung cancer and a potential biomarker for early diagnosis. *Proc Natl Acad Sci U S A.* 1998;95:11891–11896.

Bentley P, Calder I, Elcombe C, Grasso P, Stringer D, Wiegand HJ. Hepatic peroxisome proliferation in rodents and its significance for humans. *Food Chem Toxicol.* 1993;31:857–907.

436

Berenblub J, Shubik P. A new quantitative approach to the study of the stages of chemical carcinogenesis in the mouse's skin. *Br J Cancer.* 1947;1:389–391.

Betteridge DJ. What is oxidative stress? *Metabolism.* 2000;49:3–8.

Blaauboer BJ, Balls M, Barratt M, et al. 13th meeting of the Scientific Group on Methodologies for the Safety Evaluation of Chemicals (SGOMSEC): alternative testing methodologies and conceptual issues. *Environ Health Perspect.* 1998;106(suppl 2):413–418.

Boddy AV, Ratain MJ. Pharmacogenetics in cancer etiology and chemotherapy. *Clin Cancer Res.* 1997;3:1025–1030.

Bohr VA, Dianov GL. Oxidative DNA damage processing in nuclear and mitochondrial DNA. *Biochimie.* 1999;81:155–160.

Bos JL. Ras oncogene in human cancer: a review. *Cancer Res.* 1989;49:4682–4689.

Bosch TM, Meijerman I, Beijnen JH, Schellens JHM. Genetic polymorphisms of drug metabolising enzymes and drug transporters in relation to cancer risk. *Curr Ther Rev.* 2006;2(2):137–155.

Boverhof DR. Transgenic animal models in toxicology: historical perspectives and future outlook. *Toxicol Sci.* 2011;121:207–233.

Bressac B, Kew M, Wands J, Ozturk M. Selective G to T mutations of p53 gene in hepatocellular carcinoma from southern Africa. *Nature.* 1991;350:429–431.

Brown JR, Nigh E, Lee RJ, et al. Fos family members induce cell cycle entry by activating Cyclin D1. *Mol Cell Biol.* 1998;18:55609–55619.

Brown K, Balmain A. Transgenic mice and squamous multistage skin carcinogenesis. *Cancer Metastasis Rev.* 1995;14:113–124.

Bull RJ, Brown JM, Meierhenry EA, Jorgenson TA, Robinson M, Stober JA. Enhancement of the hepatotoxicity of chloroform in B6C3F1 mice by corn oil: implications for chloroform carcinogenesis. *Environ Health Perspect.* 1986;69:49–58.

Burdon RH. Superoxide and hydrogen peroxide in relation to mammalian cell proliferation. *Free Radic Biol Med.* 1995;18:775–794.

Burgess WH, Maciag T, Jerome H. The heparin-binding (fibroblast) growth factor family of proteins. *Annu Rev Biochem.* 1989;58:575–606.

Burkhardt S, Mellert W, Reinacher M, Bahnenmann R. Zonal evaluation of proliferation and apoptosis in mice reveals new mechanistic data for PB, WY 14,643 and CH. *Toxicologist.* 2001;60:286.

Butlin HJ. Three lectures on cancer of the scrotum in chimney sweeps and others. I. Secondary cancer without primary cancer. II. Why foreign sweeps do not suffer from scrotal cancer. III. Tar and paraffin cancer. *Br Med J.* 1892;1:1341–1346, 2:1–6, 66–71.

Butterworth BE. Consideration of both genotoxic and nongenotoxic mechanisms in predicting carcinogenic potential. *Mutat Res.* 1990;239:117–132.

Calabrese EJ. Hormesis: changing view of the dose–response, a personal account of the history and current status. *Mutat Res.* 2002;511:181–189.

Camurri L, Codeluppi S, Pedroni C, Scarduelli L. Chromosomal aberrations and sister-chromatid exchanges in workers exposed to styrene. *Mutat Res.* 1983;119:361–369.

Cantor KP. Drinking water and cancer. *Cancer Causes Control.* 1997;8(3):292–308.

Capen CC, Dayan AD, Green S. Receptor-mediated mechanisms in carcinogenesis: an overview. *Mutat Res.* 1995;333(1–2):215–224.

Carmichael NG, Enzmann H, Pate I, Waechter F. The significance of mouse liver tumor formation for carcinogenic risk assessment: results and conclusions from a survey of ten years of testing by the agrochemical industry. *Environ Health Perspect.* 1997;105(11):1196–1203.

Carthew P, Martin EA, White IN, et al. Tamoxifen induces short-term cumulative DNA damage and liver tumors in rats: promotion by phenobarbital. *Cancer Res.* 1995;55(3):544–547.

Cavalli LR, Liang BD. Mutagenesis, tumorigenicity, and apoptosis: are the mitochondria involved? *Mutat Res.* 1998;398:19–26.

Cerutti PA. Prooxidant states and tumor promotion. *Science.* 1985;227:375–381.

Chandar N, Lombardi B. Liver cell proliferation and incidence of hepatocellular carcinomas in rats fed consecutively a choline-devoid and a choline supplemented diet. *Carcinogenesis.* 1988;9(2):259–263.

Chang L, Karin M. Mammalian MAP kinase signalling cascades. *Nature.* 2001;410:37–40.

Chellappan SP, Hiebert S, Mudryj M, Horowitz JM, Nevins JR. The E2F transcription factor is a cellular target for the RB protein. *Cell.* 1991;65:1053–1061.

Chen CJ, Wu MM, Lee SS, et al. Atherogenicity and carcinogenicity of high-arsenic artesian well water. Multiple risk factors and related malignant neoplasms of blackfoot disease. *Arteriosclerosis.* 1988;8:452–460.

Cheng KC, Cahill DS, Kasai H, Nishimura S, Loeb LA. 8-Hydroxyguanosine, an abundant form of oxidative DNA damage, causes G → T and A → C substitutions. *J Biol Chem.* 1992;267:166–172.

Chiu R, Boyle J, Meek J, et al. The c-Fos protein interacts with c-Jun/AP-1 to stimulate transcription of AP-1 responsive genes. *Cell.* 1988;54:541–552.

Christopherson W, Mays E, Barrows G. Hepatocellular carcinoma in young women on oral contraceptives. *Lancet.* 1978;2:38.

Clarkson PM, Thompson HS. Antioxidants: what role do they play in physical activity and health? *Am J Clin Nutr.* 2000;72:637–646.

Claxton LD, Umbuzeiro GdeA, DeMarini DM. The Salmonella mutagenicity assay: the stethoscope of genetic toxicology for the 21st century. *Environ Health Perspect.* 2010;118:1515–1522.

Cohen SM, Robinson D, MacDonald J. Alternative models for carcinogenicity testing. *Toxicol Sci.* 2001;64:14–19.

Collett MS, Erickson RL. Protein kinase activity associated with the avian sarcoma virus src gene product. *Proc Natl Acad Sci USA.* 1978;75, 2021–2024.

Collins AR. The Comet Assay for DNA damage and repair: principals, applications, and limitations. *Mol Biotech.* 2004;26:249–261.

Connett PH, Whtterhahn KE. In vitro reduction of the carcinogen chromate with cellular thiols and carboxylic acids. *J Am Chem Soc.* 1985;107:4282–4288.

Conney AH. Induction of microsomal enzymes by foreign chemicals and carcinogenesis by polycyclic aromatic hydrocarbons. *Cancer Res.* 1982;42:4875–4917.

Cook JW, Hewett CL, Hieger I. The isolation of a cancer-producing hydrocarbon from coal tar. *J Chem Soc.* 1933;24:395–405.

Costa M. Toxicity and carcinogenicity of Cr(VI) in animal models and humans. *Crit Rev Toxicol.* 1997;27(5):431–442.

Counts JL, Goodman JI. Alterations in DNA methylation may play a variety of roles in carcinogenesis. *Cell.* 1995;83:13–15.

Creech HJ. A brief history of the American Association for Cancer Research, Inc.: 1907–1995. In: *Directory of the American Association for Cancer Research.* Philadelphia: American Association for Cancer Research; 2000:viii–xi.

Croce CM. Molecular origins of cancer: oncogenes and cancer. *N Engl J Med.* 2008;358:502–511.

Cross AJ, Sinha R. Formation and biochemistry of carcinogenic heterocyclic aromatic amines in cooked meats and meat-related mutagens/carcinogens in the etiology of colorectal cancer. *Environ Mol Mutagen.* 2004;44(1):44–55.

D'Souza RJ, Philips EM, Jones PW, Strange RC, Aber GM. Interactions of hydrogen peroxide with interleukin-6 and platelet-derived growth factor in determining mesangial cell growth: effect of repeated oxidant stress. *Clin Sci.* 1993;86:747–751.

Damm K, Thompson CC, Evans RM. Proteinencoded by v-erbA functions as a thyroid-hormone receptor antagonist. *Nature.* 1989;339:593–597.

de Boer JG, Mirsalis JC, Provost GS, Tindall KR, Glickman BW. Spectrum of mutations in kidney, stomach, and liver from lacI transgenic mice recovered after treatment with tris(2,3-dibromopropyl)phosphate. *Environ Mol Mutagen.* 1996;28(4):418–423.

de Vos AM, Tong L, Milburn MV, et al. Three dimensional structure of an oncogene protein: catalytic domain of human C-H-ras p21. *Science.* 1988;239:888–893.

Demple B, Harrison L. Repair of oxidative damage to DNA. *Annu Rev Biochem.* 1994;63:915–948.

de-Thé G, Geser A, Day NE, et al. Epidemiological evidence for causal relationship between Epstein-Barr virus and Burkitt's lymphoma from Ugandan prospective study. *Nature.* 1978;274:756–761.

Diamandopoulos GT. Cancer: an historical perspective. *Anticancer Res.* 1996;16(4A):1595–1602.

Dietrich DR, Swenberg JA. Preneoplastic lesions in rodent kidney induced spontaneously or by non-genotoxic agents: predictive nature and comparison to lesions induced by genotoxic carcinogens. *Mutat Res.* 1991;248:239–260.

DiGiovanni J. Multistage carcinogenesis in mouse skin. *Pharmacol Ther.* 1992;54(1):63–128.

Diwan BA, Kasprzak KS, Rice JM. Transplacental carcinogenic effects of nickel(II) acetate in the renal cortex, renal pelvis and adenohypophysis in F344/NCr rats. *Carcinogenesis.* 1992;13(8):1351–1357.

Dizdaroglu M. Oxidative damage to DNA in mammalian chromatin. *Mutat Res.* 1992;275:331–342.

Doll R, Peto R. The causes of cancer: quantitative estimates of avoidable risks of cancer in the United States today. *J Natl Cancer Inst.* 1981;66(6):1191–1308.

Doll R. Effects of exposure to vinyl chloride. An assessment of evidence. *Scand J Work Environ Health.* 1988;14:61–78.

Doll R, Peto R, Boreham J, Sutherland I. Mortality in relation to smoking: 50 years' observations on male British doctors. *BMJ.* 2004;328(7455):1519.

Donehower LA. The p53-deficient mouse: a model for basic and applied cancer studies. *Semin Cancer Biol.* 1996;7(5):269–278.

Dong J-T. Prevalent mutations in prostate cancer. *J Cell Biochem.* 2005;97(3):433–447.

Dooliter RF, Hunkapiller MW, Hood LE, et al. Simian sarcoma virus oncogene, v-sis, is derived from the gene (or genes) encoding a platelet-derived growth factor. *Science.* 1983;221:275–277.

Dunnick JK, Elwell MR, Huff J, Barrett JC. Chemically induced mammary gland cancer in the National Toxicology Program's carcinogenesis bioassay. *Carcinogenesis.* 1995;16(2):173–179.

Dypbukt JM, Ankarcrona M, Burkitt M, et al. Different proxxidant levels stimulate growth, trigger apoptosis, or produce necrosis of insulin-secreting RINm5F cells. The role of intracellular polyamines. *J Biol Chem.* 1994;269:30533–30560.

Eastmond DA, Hartwig A, Anderson D, et al. Mutagenicity testing for chemical risk assessment: update of the WHO/IPCS Harmonized Scheme. *Mutagenesis.* 2009;24(4):341–349.

Edmondson H, Reynolds T, Henderson B, Benton B. Regression of liver cell adenomas associated with oral contraceptives. *Ann Intern Med.* 1977;86:180–182.

Ehrenberg L, Hussain S. Genetic toxicity of some important epoxides. *Mutat Res.* 1981;86:1–113.

Eksrom G, Ingleman-Sundberg M. Rat liver microsomal NADPH-supported oxidase activity and lipid peroxidation dependent on ethanol inducible cytochromes P-450. *Biochem Pharmacol.* 1989;38:1313–1319.

El-Deiry WS, Kern SE, Pietenpol JA, Kinzler KW, Vogelstein B. Definition of a consensus binding site for p53. *Nat Genet.* 1992;1:45–49.

Esteller M, Corn PG, Baylin SB, Herman JG. A gene hypermethylation profile of human cancer. *Cancer Res.* 2001;61:3225–3229.

Fahreus R, Rymo L, Rhim JS, et al. Morphological transformation of human keratinocytes expressing the LMP gene of Epstein-Barr virus. *Nature.* 1990;345:447–449.

Ferreccio C, González C, Milosavjlevic V, Marshall G, Sancha AM, Smith AH. Lung cancer and arsenic concentrations in drinking water in Chile. *Epidemiology.* 2000;11(6): 673–679.

Finch GL, Hoover MD, Hahn FF, et al. Animal models of beryllium-induced lung disease. *Environ Health Perspect.* 1996;104(suppl 5):973–979.

Final Report on Carcinogens Background Document for Beryllium and Beryllium Compounds December 16-17, 1999. Meeting of the NTP Board of Scientific Counselors Report on Carcinogens Subcommittee.

Finlay CA, Hinds PW, Levine AJ. The p53 proto-oncogene can act as a suppressor of transformation. *Cell.* 1989;57:1083–1093.

Fiorani M, Cantoni O, Tasinto A, Boscoboinik D, Azzi A. Hydrogen peroxide-and fetal bovine serum-induced DNA synthesis in vascular smooth muscle cells; positive and negative regulation by protein kinase C isoforms. *Biochem Biophys Acta.* 1995;1269:98–104.

Floyd RA. 8-Hydoxy-2′-deoxyguanosine in carcinogenesis. *Carcinogenesis.* 1990;11:1447–1450.

Fortini P, Parlanti E, Sidorkina OM, Laval J, Dogliotti E. The type of DNA glycosylase determines the base excision repair pathway in mammalian cells. *J Biol Chem.* 1999;274:230–236.

Fox M, Scott D. The genetic toxicology of nitrogen and sulphur mustard. *Mutat Res.* 1980;75(2):131–168.

Fried M, Prives C. In: Botchan M, Grodzicker T, Sharp PA, eds. *Cancer Cells 4: DNA Tumor Viruses.* New York: Cold Spring Harbor; 1986:1–16.

Friedwald WF, Rous P. Initiating and promoting elements in tumor production: analysis of effects of tar, benzpyrene and methylcholanthrene on rabbit skin. *J Exp Med.* 1944;80:101–126.

Fu H, Boffetta P. Cancer and occupational exposure to inorganic Lead compounds: a meta-analysis of published data. *Occup Environ Med.* 1995;52(2):73–81.

Fujii K. Evaluation of the newborn mouse model for chemical tumorigenesis. *Carcinogenesis.* 1991;12(8):1409–1415.

Fukushima S, Imaida K, Sakata T, Okamura T, Shibata M, Ito N. Promoting effects of sodium L-ascorbate on two-stage urinary bladder carcinogenesis in rats. *Cancer Res.* 1983;43(9):4454–4457.

Furihata C, Matsushima T. Use of in vivo/in vitro unscheduled DNA synthesis for identification of organ-specific carcinogens. *Crit Rev Toxicol.* 1987;17(3):245–277.

Futreal PA, Liu Q, Shattuck-Eidens D, et al. BRCA1 mutations in primary breast and ovarian carcinomas. *Science.* 1994;266(5182):120–122.

Galloway SM, Bloom AD, Resnick M, et al. Development of a standard protocol for in vitro cytogenetic testing with Chinese hamster ovary cells: comparison of results for 22 compounds in two laboratories. *Environ Mutagen.* 1985;7(1):1–51.

Gama-Sosa MA, Slagel VA, Trewyn RW, et al. The 5-methylcytosine content of DNA from human tumors. *Nucleic Acids Res.* 1983;11: 6883–6894.

Generoso WM, Cain KT, Krishna M, Sheu CW, Gryder RM. Heritable translocation and dominant-lethal mutation induction with ethylene oxide in mice. *Mutat Res.* 1980;73(1):133–142.

Ghoshal AK, Farber E. The induction of liver cancer by dietary deficiency of choline and methionine without added carcinogens. *Carcinogenesis.* 1984;5(10):1367–1370.

Gimenez-Conti IB, Slaga TJ. The hamster cheek pouch carcinogenesis model. *J Cell Biochem.* 1993;5283–5290.

Glauert HP, Robertson LW, Silberhorn EM. PCBs and tumor promotion. In: Robertson LW, Hansen LG, eds. *PCBs: Recent Advances in Environmental Toxicology and Health Effects.* Lexington, KY: University Press of Kentucky; 2001:355–371.

Gondo Y, Shioyama Y, Nakao K, Katsuki M. A novel positive detection system of in vivo mutations in rpsL (strA) transgenic mice. *Mutat Res.* 1996;360(1):1–14.

Goode EL, Ulrich CM, Potter JD. Polymorphisms in DNA repair genes and associations with cancer risk. *Cancer Epidemiol Biomarkers Prev.* 2002;11:1513–1530.

Gossen JA, de Leeuw WJF, Tan CHT, et al. Efficient rescue of integrated shuttle vectors from transgenic mice: a model for studying mutations in vivo. *Proc Natl Acad Sci U S A.* 1989;86:7971–7975.

Gossen JA, Vijg J. A selective system for lacZ− phage using a galactose-sensitive *E coli* host. *Biotechniques.* 1993;14:326–330.

Goth R, Rajewsky MF. Persistence of O6-ethylguanine in rat-brain DNA: correlation with nervous system-specific carcinogenesis by ethylnitrosourea. *Proc Natl Acad Sci U S A.* 1974;71(3):639–643.

Greenblatt MS, Bennett WP, Hollstein M, Harris CC. Mutations in the p53 tumor suppressor gene: clues to cancer etiology and molecular pathogenesis. *Cancer Res.* 1994;54(18):4855–4878.

Guengerich FP. Mechanisms of formation of DNA adducts from ethylene dihalides, vinyl halides, and arylamines. *Drug Metab Rev.* 1994;26:47–66.

Gulezian D, Jacobson-Kram D, McCullough CB, et al. Use of transgenic animals for carcinogenicity testing: considerations for risk assessment. *Toxicol Pathol.* 2000;28(3):482–499.

Guyton KZ, Kensler TW. Oxidative mechanisms in carcinogenesis. *Br Med Bul.* 1993;49:523–544.

438

Han W, Pentecost BT, Spivack SD. Functional evaluation of novel single nucleotide polymorphisms and haplotypes in the promoter regions of *CYP1B1* and *CYP1A1* genes. *Mol Carcinogen*. 2003;37(3):158–169.

Hanahan D, Weinberg RA. The hallmarks of cancer. *Cell*. 2000;100(1):57–70.

Hanahan D, Weinberg RA. Hallmarks of cancer: the next generation. *Cell*. 2011;144(5):646–674.

Hancock JF, Magee AI, Childs JE, et al. All ras proteins are polyisoprenylated but only some are palmitoylated. *Cell*. 1989;57:1167–1177.

Harris GK, Shi X. Signaling by carcinogenic metals and metal-induced reactive oxygen species. *Mutat Res*. 2003;533:183–200.

Harting FH, Hesse W. Der lungenkrebs, die Bergkrankheit in den Schneeberger gruben. *Vjschr Gerichtl Med Offentl Gesundheitswesen*. 1879;31:102–132, 313–337.

Hastie ND. The genetics of Wilms' tumor—a case of disrupted development. *Annu Rev Genet*. 1994;28:523–558.

Heddle JA, Hite M, Kirkhart B, et al. The induction of micronuclei as a measure of genotoxicity. A report of the US Environmental Protection Agency GENE-TOX program. *Mutat Res*. 1983;123:61–118.

Herbst AL, Kurman RJ, Scully RE, Poskanzer DC. Clear-cell adenocarcinoma of the genital tract in young females: registry report. *N Engl J Med*. 1972;287:1259–1264.

Henning SM, Swendseid ME, Coulson WF. Male rats fed methyl-and folate-deficient diets with or without niacin develop hepatic carcinomas associated with decreased tissue NAD concentrations and altered poly (ADP-ribose) polymerase activity. *J Nutr*. 1997;127:30–36.

Herbst AL, Scully RE. Adenocarcinoma of the vagina in adolescence: a report of 7 cases including 6 clear-cell carcinomas (so-called mesonephromas). *Cancer*. 1970;25:745–757.

Hergersberg M. Biological aspects of cytosine methylation in eukaryotic cells. *Experientia*. 1991;47:1171–1185.

Hiasa Y, Konishi N, Nakaoka S, et al. Possible application to medium-term organ bioassays for renal carcinogenesis modifiers in rats treated with N-ethyl-N-hydroxyethylnitrosamine and unilateral nephrectomy. *Jpn J Cancer Res*. 1991;82(12):1385–1390.

Hicks RM. Multistage carcinogenesis in the urinary bladder. *Br Med Bull*. 1980;36(1):39–46.

Highman B, Norvell MJ, Shellenberger TE. Pathological changes in female C3H mice continuously fed diets containining diethylstilbestrol or 17beta-estradiol. *J Environ Pathol Toxicol*. 1978;1:1–30.

Hogstedt C, Aringer L, Gustavsson A. Epidemiological support for ethylene oxide as a cancer-causing agent. *JAMA*. 1986;255:1575–1578.

Hollander MC, Fornace AJ Jr. Induction of fos RNA by DNA-damaging agents. *Cancer Res*. 1989;49:1687–1692.

Holliday R. Mechanisms for the control of gene activity during development. *Biol Rev*. 1990;65:431–471.

Hollstein M, Sidransky D, Vogelstein B, Harris CC. p53 mutations in human cancers. *Science*. 1991;253(5015):49–53.

Honkakoski P, Zelko I, Sueyoshi T, Negishi M. The nuclear orphan receptor CAR-retinoid X receptor heterodimer activates the phenobarbital-responsive enhancer module of the CYP2B gene. *Mol Cell Biol*. 1998;18:5652–5658.

Hood A, Liu J, Klaassen CD. Effects of phenobarbital, pregnenolone-16α-carbonitrile, and propylthiouracil on thyroid follicular cell proliferation. *Toxicol Sci*. 1999;50:45–53.

Horton TM, Petros JA, Heddi A, et al. Novel mitochondrial DNA deletion found in renal cell carcinoma. *Genes Chromosomes Cancer*. 1996;15:95–101.

Hsieh LL, Hsieh TT. Detection of aflatoxin B1-DNA adducts in human placenta and cord blood. *Cancer Res*. 1993;53:1278–1280.

Hueper WC, Wiley FH, Wolfe HD. Experimental production of bladder tumors in dogs by administration of beta-naphthylamine. *J Ind Hyg Toxicol*. 1938;20:46–84.

Huff V. Wilms' tumours: about tumour suppressor genes, an oncogene and a chameleon gene. *Nat Rev Cancer*. 2011;11:111–121.

Hughes MF, Kitchin KT. In: Singh KK, ed. *Arsenic, Oxidative Stress and Carcinogenesis Oxidative Stress, Disease and Cancer*. London: Imperial College Press; 2006.

Hussain SP, Haris CC. Molecular epidemiology of human cancer: contribution of mutation spectra studies of tumor suppressor genes. *Cancer Res*. 1998;58:4023–4037.

IARC. *Monographs on the Evaluation of Carcinogenic Risks to Humans Volume 100C. A Review of Human Carcinogens: Arsenic, Metals, Fibres, and Dusts*. IARC; 2012.

International Agency for Research on Cancer. Some Inorganic and organometallic compounds. *IARC Monographs on the Evaluation of Carcinogenic Risk of Chemicals to Humans*. Vol 2. Lyon, France: IARC; 1973:181.

International Agency for Research on Cancer. Some metals and metallic compounds. *IARC Monographs on the Evaluation of Carcinogenic Risk of Chemicals to Humans*. Vol 23. Lyon, France: International Agency for Research on Cancer; 1980:438.

International Agency for Research on Cancer. Overall evaluations of carcinogenicity. *IARC Monographs on the Evaluation of Carcinogenic Risk of Chemicals to Humans*. Suppl 7. Lyon, France: International Agency for Research on Cancer; 1987:440.

International Agency for Research on Cancer. Chromium, nickel and welding. *IARC Monographs on the Evaluation of Carcinogenic Risk of Chemicals to Humans*. Vol 49. Lyon, France: International Agency for Research on Cancer; 1990:677.

International Agency for Research on Cancer. Beryllium, cadmium, mercury and exposures in the glass manufacturing industry. *IARC Monographs on the Evaluation of Carcinogenic Risk of Chemicals to Humans*. Vol 58. Lyon, France: International Agency for Research on Cancer; 1993:444.

International Agency for Research on Cancer. Polychlorinated dibenzo-para-dioxins and polychlorinated dibenzofurans. *IARC Monographs on the Evaluation of the Carcinogenic Risks to Humans*. Vol 69. Lyon, France: IARC; 1997a.

International Agency for Research on Cancer. Polychlorinated dibenzofurans. *Monographs on the Evaluaiton of Carcinogenic Risks to Humans*. Vol 69. Lyon, France: IARC; 1997b.

Isfort RJ, Cody DB, Doersen CJ, Kerckaert GA, LeBoeuf RA. Alterations in cellular differentiation, mitogenesis, cytoskeleton and growth characteristics during Syrian hamster embryo cell multistep in vitro transformation. *Int J Cancer*. 1994;59:114–125.

Isfort RJ, Kerckaert GA, LeBoeuf RA. Comparison of the standard and reduced pH Syrian hamster embryo (SHE) cell in vivo transformation assays in predicting the carcinogenic potential of chemicals. *Mutat Res*. 1996;356:11–63.

Issemann I, Green S. Activation of a member of the steroid hormone receptor superfamily by peroxisome proliferators. *Nature*. 1990;347:645–650.

Ito N, Hasegawa R, Imaida K, et al. Medium-term rat liver bioassay for rapid detection of hepatocarcinogenic substances. *J Toxicol Pathol*. 1997;10:1–11.

Ito N, Hasegawa R, Imaida K, Takahashi S, Shirai T. Medium-term rat liver bioassay for rapid detection of carcinogens and modifiers of hepatocarcinogenesis. *Drug Metab Rev*. 1994;26:431–442.

Ito N, Imaida K, Hasegawa R, Tsuda H. Rapid bioassay methods for carcinogens and modifiers of hepatocarcinogenesis. *Crit Rev Toxicol*. 1989;19:386–415.

Ito N, Tamano S, Shirai T. A medium-term rat liver bioassay for rapid in vivo detection of carcinogenic potential of chemicals. *Cancer Sci*. 2003;94:3–8.

Jacobson LP, Zhang BC, Zhu YR, et al. Oltipraz chemoprevention trial in Qidong, People's Republic of China: study design and clinical outcomes. *Cancer Epidemiol Biomarkers Prev*. 1997;6(4):257–265.

Jagadeesan V, Rao JN, Sesikeran B. Effect of iron deficiency on DMH-induced gastrointestinal tract tumours and occurrence of hepatocyte abnormalities in Fischer rats. *Nutr Cancer*. 1994;22:285–291.

James NH, Roberts RA. Species differences in response to peroxisome proliferators correlate in vitro with induction of DNA synthesis rather than suppression of apoptosis. *Carcinogenesis*. 1996;17:1623–1632.

Janero DR. Malondialdehyde and thiobarbituric acid reactivity as diagnostic indices of lipid peroxidation and peroxidative tissue injury. *Free Radic Biol Med*. 1990;9:515–540.

Johansson SL, Hirsch JM, Larsson PA, Saidi J, Osterdahl BG. Snuff-induced carcinogenesis: effect of snuff in rats initiated with 4-nitroquinoline N-oxide. *Cancer Res*. 1989;49(11):3063–3069.

Johnstone SE, Baylin SB. Stress and the epigenetic landscape: a link to the pathobiology of human diseases? *Nat Rev*. 2010;11:806.

Jones PA, Baylin SB. The epigenomics of cancer. *Cell*. 2007;128:683–692.

Kadlubar FF, Unruh LE, Flammang TJ, Sparks D, Mitchum RK, Mulder GJ. Alteration of urinary levels of the carcinogen, N-hydroxy-2-naphthylamine, and its N-glucuronide in the rat by control of urinary pH, inhibition of metabolic sulfation, and changes in biliary excretion. *Chem Biol Interact*. 1981;33:129–147.

Kamb A, Gruis NA, Weaver-Feldhaus J, et al. A cell cycle regulator potentially involved in genesis of many tumor types. *Science* 1994;264(5151):436–440.

Kamendulis LM, Klaunig JE. Species differences in the induction of hepatocellular DNA synthesis by diethanolamine. *Toxicol Sci*. 2005;87(2):328–336.

Kasprzak KS, Diwan BA, Konishi N, Misra M, Rice JM. Initiation by nickel acetate and promotion by sodium barbital of renal cortical epithelial tumors in male F344 rats. *Carcinogenesis*. 1990;11(4):647–652.

Kennaway EL, Hieger I. Carcinogenic substances and their fluorescence spectra. *Br Med J*. 1930;1:1044–1046.

Kennelly JC. Design and interpretation of rat liver UDS assays. *Mutagenesis*. 199510(3):215–221.

Kerr LD. Signal transduction: the nuclear target. *Curr Opin Cell Biol*. 1992;4:496–501.

Kim CM, Koike K, Saito I, et al. HBx gene of hepatitis B virus induces liver cancer in transgenic mice. *Nature*. 1991;351:317–320.

Kinoshita A, Wanibuchi H, Morimura K, et al. Phenobarbital at low dose exerts hormesis in rat hepatocarcinogenesis by reducing oxidative DNA damage, altering cell proliferation, apoptosis and gene expression. *Carcinogenesis*. 2003;24:1389–1399.

Kinosita R. Researches on the carcinogenesis of the various chemical substances. *Gann*. 1936;30:423–426.

Kitano M, Ichihara T, Matsuda T, et al. Presence of a threshold for promoting effects of phenobarbital on diethylnitrosamine-induced hepatic foci in the rat. *Carcinogenesis*. 1998;19:1475–1480.

Klaunig JE, Babich MA, Baetcke KP, et al. PPARα agonist-induced rodent tumors: modes of action and human relevance. *Crit Rev Toxicol*. 2003;33:655–780.

Klaunig JE, Kamendulis LM. The role of oxidative stress in carcinogenesis. *Annu Rev Pharmacol Toxicol*. 2004;44:239–267.

Klaunig JE, Ruch RJ. Strain and species effects on the inhibition of hepatocyte intercellular communication by liver tumor promoters. *Cancer Lett*. 1987;36:161–168.

Klaunig JE, Ruch RJ. Role of inhibition of intercellular communication in carcinogenesis. *Lab Invest*. 1990;62(2):135–146.

Klaunig JE, Xu Y, Bachowski S, Jiang J. Free-radical oxygen-induced changes in chemical carcinogenesis. In: Wallace KB, ed. *Free Radical Toxicology*. London: Taylor & Francis; 1997:375–400.

Klaunig JE, Wang Z, Pu X, Zhou S. Oxidative stress and oxidative damage in chemical carcinogenesis. *Toxicol Appl Pharmacol*. 2011;254:86–99.

Kleczkowska HE, Althaus FR. Response of human keratinocytes to extremely low concentrations of N-methyl-N'-nitro-N-nitrosoguanidine. *Mutat Res*. 1996;367:151–159.

Knize MG, Dolbeare FA, Cunningham PL, Felton JS. Mutagenic activity and heterocyclic amine content of the human diet. *Princess Takamatsu Symp*. 1995;23:30–38.

Knutson JC, Poland A. Response of murine epidermis to 2,3,7,8-tetrachlorodibenzo-p-dioxin: Interaction of the Ah and hr loci. *Cell*. 1982;30:225–234.

Kociba RJ, Keyes DG, Beyer JE, et al. Results of a two-year chronic toxicity and oncogenicity study of 2,3,7,8-tetrachlorodibenzo-p-dioxin in rats. *Toxicol Appl Pharmacol*. 1978;46:279–303.

Kodama S, Koike C, Negishi M, Yamamoto Y. Nuclear receptors CAR and PXR cross talk with FOXO1 to regulate genes that encode drug-metabolizing and gluconeogenic enzymes. *Mol Cell Biol*. 2004;24:7931–7940.

Kohler SW, Provost GS, Fieck A, et al. Spectra of spontaneous and mutagen-induced mutations in the lacI gene in transgenic mice. *Proc Natl Acad Sci U S A*. 1991a;88:7958–7962.

Kohler SW, Provost GS, Fieck A, et al. Spectra of spontaneous and induced mutations using a lambda ZAP/lacI shuttle vector. *Environ Mol Mutagen*. 1991b;18:316–321.

Kortenkamp A, O'Brien P. The generation of DNA single-strand breaks during the reduction of chromate by ascorbic acid and/or glutathione in vitro. *Environ Health Perspect*. 1994;102(3):237–241.

Kroh H. Periphery of ethylnitrosourea-induced spinal gliomas in rats with special reference to the vascular structure. *Acta Neuropathol*. 1987;73(1):92–98.

Lake BG. Mechanisms of hepatocarcinogenicity of peroxisome-proliferating drugs and chemicals. *Annu Rev Pharmacol Toxicol*. 1995;35:483–507.

Lan Q, Zhang L, Li G, et al. Hematotoxicity in workers exposed to low levels of benzene. *Science*. 2004;306;1774–1776.

Lancaster WD, Olson C. Animal papilloma-viruses. *Microbiol Rev*. 1982;46:191–207.

Langard S. Chromium carcinogenicity: a review of experimental animal data. *Sci Total Environ*. 1988;71:341–350.

Larson JL, Wolf DC, Butterworth BE. Induced cytolethality and regenerative cell proliferation in the livers and kidneys of male B6C3F1 mice given chloroform by gavage. *Fundam Appl Toxicol*. 1994;23:537–543.

Latt SA, Allen J, Bloom SE, et al. Sister-chromatid exchanges: a report of the GENE-TOX program. *Mutat Res*. 1981;87(1):17–62.

Latt SA. Sister chromatid exchange formation. *Annu Rev Genet*. 1981;15:11–55.

Leach FS, Tokino T, Meltzer P, et al. Mutation and MDM2 amplification in human soft tissue sarcomas. *Cancer Res*. 1993;53 (10 suppl):2231–2234.

LeBoeuf RA, Kerckaert GA, Aardema MJ, Gibson DP. Multistage neoplastic transformation of Syrian hamster embryo cells cultured at pH 6.70. *Cancer Res*. 1990;50:3722–3729.

Lee SS, Pineau T, Drago J, et al. Targeted disruption of the alpha isoform of the peroxisome proliferators-activated receptor gene in mice results in abolishment of the pleiotropic effects of peroxisome proliferators. *Mol Cell Biol*. 1995;15:3012–3022.

Leonard A, Lauwerys R. Mutagenicity, carcinogenicity and teratogenicity of beryllium *Mutat Res*. 1987;186:35–42.

Lewandowska J, Bartoszek A. DNA methylation in cancer development, diagnosis and therapy—multiple opportunities for genotoxic agents to act as methylome disruptors or remediators. *Mutagenesis*. 2011;26:475–487.

Li AP, Carver JH, Choy WN, et al. A guide for the performance of the Chinese hamster ovary cell/hypoxanthine-guanine phosphoribosyltransferase gene mutation assay. *Mutation Res*. 1987;189:135–141.

Li J, Kirkman H, Li S. Synthetic estrogens and liver cancer: risk analysis of animal and human data. In: Li J, Nandi S, Li S, eds. *Hormonal Carcinogenesis*. New York: Springer-Verlag; 1992:217–224.

Li N, Karin M. Ionizing radiation and short wavelength UV activate NF-κB through two distinct mechanisms. *Proc Natl Acad Sci USA*. 1998;95:13012–13017.

Li R, Yerganian G, Duesberg P, et al. Aneuploidy correlated 100% with chemical transformation of Chinese hamster cells. *Proc Natl Acad Sci USA*. 1997;94:14506–14511.

Li S, Hou X, Li J. Estrogen carcinogenesis: a sequential, epi-genetoxic, multistage process. In: Li J, Nandi S, Li S, eds. *Hormonal Carcinogenesis*. New York: Springer-Verlag; 1996:200–208.

Lindenschmidt RC, Tryka AF, Witschi H. Modification of gastrointestinal tumour development in rats by dietary butylatedhydroxytoluene. *Fundam Appl Toxicol*. 1987;8(4):474–481.

Lockhart AM, Piegorsch WW, Bishop JB. Assessing overdispersion and dose-response in the male dominant lethal assay. *Mutat Res*. 1992;272(1):35–58.

Loewenstein WR. Junctional intercellular communication: the cell-to-cell membrane channel. *Physiol Rev*. 1981;61:829–913.

Lofroth G, Ames BN. Mutagenicity of inorganic compounds in *Salmonella typhimurium*: arsenic, chromium and selenium. *Mutat Res*. 1978;53:65–66.

Longnecker DS, Roebuck BD, Kuhlmann ET. Enhancement of pancreatic carcinogenesis by a dietary unsaturated fat in rats treated with saline or N-nitroso(2-hydroxypropyl)(2-oxopropyl)amine. *J Natl Cancer Inst*. 1985;74(1):219–222.

Longnecker DS, Wiebkin P, Schaeffer BK, Roebuck BD. Experimental carcinogenesis in the pancreas. *Int Rev Exp Pathol*. 1984;26:177–229.

Lowe JP, Silverman BD. Predicting the carcinogenicity of polycyclic aromatic hydrocarbons. *J Am Chem Soc.* 1994;106:5955–5958.

Mandel JS, McLaughlin JK, Schlehofer B, et al. International renal-cell cancer study. IV. Occupation. *Int J Cancer.* 1995;61(5): 601–605.

Majeska JB, Matheson DW. Development of an optimal S9 activation mixture for the L5178Y TK+/– mouse lymphoma mutation assay. *Environ Mol Mutagen.* 1990;16(4):311–319.

Marcu KB, Bossone SA, Patel AJ. Myc function and regulation. *Annu Rev Biochem.* 1992;61:809–860.

Maron DM, Ames BN. Revised methods for the Salmonella mutagenicity test. *Mutat Res.* 1983;113(3–4):173–215.

Maronpot RR, Pitot HC, Peraino C. Use of rat liver altered focus models for testing chemicals that have completed two-year carcinogenicity studies. *Toxicol Pathol.* 1989;17:651–662.

Maronpot RR, Shimkin MB, Witschi HP, Smith I, Cline JM. Strain A mouse pulmonary tumor test results for chemicals previously tested in National Cancer Institute carcinogenicity tests. *J Natl Cancer Inst.* 1986;76:1101–1112.

Marselos M, Vainio H. Carcinogenic properties of pharmaceutical agents evaluated in the IARC Monographs programme. *Carcinogenesis.* 1991;12:1751–1766.

Marsman DS, Goldsworthy TL, Popp JA. Contrasting hepatocytic peroxisome proliferation, lipofuscin accumulation and cell turnover for the hepatocarcinogens WY 14,643-14,643 and clofibric acid. *Carcinogenesis.* 1992;3:1011–1017.

Martindale JL, Holbrook NJ. Cellular response to oxidative stress: signaling for suicide and survival. *J Cell Physiol.* 2002;192:1–15.

Matthews LA, Crea F, Farrar WL. Epigenetic gene regulation in stem cells and correlation to cancer. *Differentiation.* 2009;78:1–17.

McClain RM. Mechanistic considerations for the relevance of animal data on thyroid neoplasia to human risk assessment. *Mutat Res.* 1995;333:131–142.

McCormick F. Activators and effectors of ras p21 proteins. *Curr Opin Genet Dev.* 1994;4:71–76.

Melnick RL, Kohn MC, Portier CJ. Implications for risk assessment of suggested nongenotoxic mechanisms of chemical carcinogenesis. *Environ Health Perspect.* 1996;104(S1):123–133.

Merlo A, Herman JG, Mao L, et al. 5′ CpG island methylation is associated with transcriptional silencing of the tumour suppressor p16/CDKN2/MTS1 in human cancers. *Nat Med.* 1995;1:686–692.

Metzler M, Pfeiffer E, Schuler M, Rosenberg B. Effects of estrogens on microtubule assembly: significance for aneuploidy. In: Li J, Li S, Gustafsson J-A, Nandi S, Seakely L, eds. *Hormonal Carcinogenesis II.* New York: Springer-Verlag; 1996:193–199.

Miller EC. Studies onthe formation of protein-bound derivatives of 3,4-benzpyrene in the epidermal fraction of mouse skin. *Cancer Res.* 1951;11;100–108.

Miller EC. Studies on the formation of protein-bound derivatives of 3,4-benzpyrene in the epidermal fraction of mouse skin. *Cancer Res.* 1951;11;100–108.

Miller EC, Miller JA. Searches for ultimate chemical carcinogens and their reactions with cellular macromolecules. *Cancer.* 1981;47(10):2327–2345.

Miller EC, Miller JA. The presence and significance of bound amino azodyes in the livers of rats fed p-dimethylaminoazobenzene. *Cancer Res.* 1947;7:468–480.

Miller EC, Miller JA, Enomoto M. The comparative carcinogenicities of 2-acetylaminofluorene and its N-hydroxy metabolite in mice, hamsters, and guinea pigs. *Cancer Res.* 1964;24:2018–2031.

Miller EC, Swanson AB, Phillips DH, Fletcher TL, Liem A, Miller JA. Structure-activity studies of the carcinogenicities in the mouse and rat of some naturally occurring and synthetic alkenylbenzene derivatives related to safrole and estragole. *Cancer Res.* 1983;43:1124–1134.

Miller JA. Carcinogenesis by chemicals: an overview—G. H. A. Clowes memorial lecture. *Cancer Res.* 1970;3:559–576.

Mirsalis JC, Monforte JA, Winegar RA. Transgenic animal models for measuring mutations in vivo. *Crit Rev Toxicol.* 1994;24(3):255–280.

Miyamae Y, Iwasaki K, Kinae N, et al. Detection of DNA lesions induced by chemical mutagens by the single cell gel electrophoresis (Comet) assay: relationship between DNA migration and alkaline conditions. *Mutat Res.* 1997;393:107–113.

Moennikes O, Loeppen S, Buchmann A, et al. Constitutively active dioxin/aryl hydrocarbon receptor promotes hepatocarcinogenesis in mice. *Cancer Res.* 2004;64(14):4707–4710.

Molina EP, Klatt P, Vasquez J, et al. Glutathionylation of the p50 subunit of NF-$_\kappa$B: a mechanism for redox-induced inhibition of DNA binding. *Biochemistry.* 2001;40:14134–14142.

Moriya M. Single-stranded shuttle phagemid for mutagenesis studies in mammalian cells: 8-oxoguanine in DNA induces targeted G:C → T:A transversions in simian kidney cells. *Proc Natl Acad Sci U S A.* 1993;90:1122–1126.

Mortelmans K, Zeiger E. The Ames salmonella microsome mutagenicity assay. *Mutat Res.* 2000;455:29–60.

Muller JM, Krauss B, Kaltschmidt C, Baeuerle PA, Rupec RA. Hypoxia induces c-fos transcription via mitogen-activated protein kinase-dependent pathway. *J Biol Chem.* 1997;272:23435–23439.

Muscat JE, Wynder EL. Diesel engine exhaust and lung cancer: an unproven association. *Environ Health Perspect.* 1995;103(9):812–818.

Myhr BC. Validation studies with Muta Mouse: a transgenic mouse model for detecting mutations in vivo. *Environ Mol Mutagen.* 1991;18(4):308–315.

Myöhänen SK, Baylin SB, Herman JG. Hypermethylation can selectively silence individual p16^{ink4a} alleles in neoplasia. *Cancer Res.* 1998;58:591–593.

Nakae D, Yoshiji H, Mizumoto Y, et al. High incidence of hepatocellular carcinomas induced by a choline deficient L-amino acid defined diet in rats. *Cancer Res.* 1992;52(18):5042–5045.

Nakatsuru Y, Wakabayashi K, Fuji-Kuriyama T, Kusuma K, Ide F. Dibenzo[A,L]pyrene-induced genotoxic and carcinogenic responses are dramatically suppressed in aryl hydrocarbon receptor-deficient mice. *Int J Cancer.* 2004;112(2):179–183.

Naoe T, Takeyama K, Yokozawa T, et al. Analysis of genetic polymorphism in *NQO1, GST-M1, GST-T1,* and *CYP3A4* in 469 Japanese patients with therapy-related leukemia/myelodysplastic syndrome and *de novo* acute myeloid leukemia. *Clin Cancer Res.* 2000;6:4091–4095.

Nebert DW, Roe AL, Dieter MZ, Solis WA, Yang Y, Dalton TP. Role of the aromatic hydrocarbon receptor and [Ah] gene battery in the oxidative stress response, cell cycle control, and apoptosis. *Biochem Pharmacol.* 2000;59:65–85.

Nebreda AR, Porrai A. P38 MAP kinases: beyond the stress response. *Trends Biochem Sci.* 2000;25:257–260.

Neumann HG. Role of extent and persistence of DNA modifications in chemical carcinogenesis by aromatic amines. *Recent Results Cancer Res.* 1983;84:77–89.

Newberne PM, deCanargo JLV, Clark AJ. Choline deficiency, partial hepatectomy, and liver tumors in rats and mice. *Toxicol Pathol.* 1982;10:95–106.

Nims RW, Lubet RA. The CYP2B subfamily. In: Ioannides C, ed. *Cytochromes P450: Metabolic and Toxicological Aspects.* Boca Raton, FL: CRC Press; 1996:135–160.

Nishizuka Y. The molecular heterogeneity of protein kinase C and its implications for cellular regulation. *Nature.* 1988;334:661–665.

Niven JSF, Armstrong JA, Andrews CH, et al. Subcutaneous "growths" in monkeys produced by a poxvirus. *J Pathol Bacteriol.* 1961;81:1–14.

Noller KL, Decker DG, Lanier AP, Kurkland LT. Clear-cell adenocarcinoma of the cervix after maternal treatment with synthetic estrogens. *Mayo Clin Proc.* 1972;47:629–630.

Nordberg GF, Andersen O. Metal interactions in carcinogenesis: enhancement, inhibition. *Environ Health Perspect.* 1981;40:65–81.

National Toxicology Program. *Toxicology and Carcinogenesis Studies of Propylene Oxide (CAS No. 75-569) in F344/N Rats and B6C3F$_1$ Mice (Inhalation Studies), TR-267.* Research Triangle Park, NC: National Toxicology Program; 1985.

National Toxicology Program. *Toxicology and Carcinogenesis Studies of Nickel Subsulfide (CAS No. 12035-72-2) in F344 Rats and B6C3F1 Mice (Inhalation Studies). Technical Report Series No 453.* Research Triangle Park, NC: National Toxicology Program; 1996:365.

National Toxicology Program. *Report on Carcinogens Background Document for Lead and Lead Compounds.* National Toxicology Program. http://ntp-server.niehs.nih.gov/newhomeroc/roc11/Lead-Public.pdf; 2003.

Nusse R, Varmus HE. Wnt genes. *Cell.* 1992;69:1073–1087.

Oesterle D, Deml E. Lack of initiating and promoting activity of thiourea in rat liver foci bioassay. *Cancer Letters.* 1988;41;245–249.

Ogiso T, Tatematsu M, Tamano S, Hasegawa R, Ito N. Correlation between medium-term liver bioassay system data and results of long-term testing in rats. *Carcinogenesis.* 1990;11:561–566.

Oppermann H, Levinson AD, Varmus HE, Levintow L, Bishop JM. Uninfected vertebrate cells contain a protein that is closely related to the product of the avian sarcoma virus transforming gene (src). *Proc Natl Acad Sci U S A.* 1979;76:1804–1808.

Osada H, Takahashi T. Genetic alterations of multiple tumor suppressors and oncogenes in the carcinogenesis and progression of lung cancer. *Oncogene.* 2002;21:7421–7434.

Pahl HL. Activators and target genes of Rel/NF-$_\kappa$B transcription factors. *Oncogene.* 1999;18:6853–6866.

Palmer CN, Hsu MH, Griffin KJ, Raucy JL, Johnson EF. Peroxisome proliferator activated receptor-alpha expression in human liver. *Mol Pharmacol.* 1998;53:14–22.

Pan SC, Gardner WU. Carcinomas of the uterine cervix and vagina in estrogen- and androgen-treated hybrid mice. *Cancer Res.* 1948;8:337–341.

Parke DV. The cytochromes P450 and mechanisms of chemical carcinogenesis. *Environ Health Perspect.* 1994;102:852–853.

Parke DV, Sapota A. Chemical toxicity and reactive oxygen species. *Int J Occ Med Environ Health.* 1996;9:331–340.

Parnell MJ, Exon JH, Koller LD. Assessment of hepatic initiation-promotion properties of trichloroacetic acid. *Arch Environ Contam Toxicol.* 1988;17:429–436.

Parsons PA. Energy, stress and the invalid linear no-threshold premise: a generalization illustrated by ionizing radiation. *Biogerontology.* 2003;4:227–231

Pegg AE. Methylation of the O6 position of guanine in DNA is the most likely initiating event in carcinogenesis by methylating agents. *Cancer Invest.* 1984;2(3):223–231.

Pereira MA. Route of administration determines whether chloroform enhances or inhibits cell proliferation in the liver of B6C3F1 mice. *Fundam Appl Toxicol.* 1994;23:87–92.

Pereira MA, Herren-Freund SL. In: Ashby J, de Serres FJ, Shelby MD, Margolin BH, Ishidate M, Becking GC, eds. *Liver Initiation Assay, the Rat Liver Foci Bioassay of Carcinogens and Noncarcinogens. Evaluation of Short-term Assays for Carcinogens.* Cambridge University Press; 1988:1.325–1.328.

Perera F, Mayer J, Santella RM, et al. Biological markers in risk assessment for environmental carcinogens. *Environ Health Perspect.* 1991;90:247–254.

Peters JM, Aoyama T, Cattley RC, Nobumitsu U, Hashimoto T, Gonzalez FJ. Role of peroxisome proliferator-activated receptor alpha in altered cell cycle regulation in mouse liver. *Carcinogenesis.* 1998;19:1989–1994.

Pettersson U, Roberts RJ. In: Botchan M, Grodzicker T, Sharp PA, eds. *Cancer Cells 4: DNA Tumor Viruses.* New York: Cold Spring Harbor; 1986:37–57.

Pietra G, Spencer K, Shubik P. Response of newly bornmice to a chemical carcinogen. *Nature.* 1959;183:1689.

Pinkus R. Phenobarbital induction of AP-1 binding activity mediate activation of glutathione S-transferase and quinine reductase gene expression. *Biochem J.* 1993;290:637–640.

Pitot HC. *Fundamentals of Oncology.* New York: Marcel Dekker, Inc; 1986.

Pitot HC, Goldsworthy T, Moran S, Sirica J. Properties of incomplete carcinogens and promoters in hepatocarcinogenesis. *Carcinogen Compr Surv.* 1982;7:85–98.

Pitot HC, Goldsworthy TL, Moran S, et al. A method to quantitate the relative initiating and promoting potencies of hepatocarcinogenic agents in their dose–response relationships to altered hepatic foci. *Carcinogenesis.* 1987;8:1491–1499.

Pitot HC. Multistage carcinogenesis. In: Bertino JR, ed. *Encyclopedia of Cancer.* Vol II. New York: Academic Press; 1997:1108–1119.

Pollycove M, Feinendegen LE. Biologic responses to low doses of ionizing radiation: Detriment versus hormesis. Part 2. Dose responses of organisms. *J Nucl Med.* 2001;42:26N–32N, 37N.

Pott P. The chirurgical works. In: *Chirurgical Observations Relative to the Cataract, the Polypus of the Nose, the Cancer of the Scrotum, the Different Kinds of Ruptures, and the Mortification of the Toes and Feet.* Ch. III. London: Hawes, W. Clarke, and R. Collins; 1775:60–68.

Proctor RN. Commentary: Schairer and Schoniger's forgotten tobacco epidemiology and the Nazi quest for racial purity. *Int J Epidemiol.* 2001;30(1):31–34.

Pugh G Jr, Isenberg JS, Kamendulis LM, et al. Effects of diisononyl phthalate, di-2-ethylhexyl phthalate, and clofibrate in cynomolgus monkeys. *Toxicol Sci.* 2000;56:181–188.

Quian Y, Luo J, Leonard SS, et al. Hydrogen peroxide formation and actin filament reorganization by Cdc42 are essential for ethanol-induced in vitro angiogenesis. *J Biol Chem.* 2003;278:16189–16197.

Rao MS, Reddy JK. An overview of peroxisome proliferator-induced hepatocarcinogenesis. *Environ Health Perspect.* 1991;93:205–209.

Rapp F. Herpesviruses and cancer. *Adv Cancer Res.* 1974;19;265–302.

Rauscher FJ III, Morris JF, Tournay OE, Cook DM, Curran T. Binding of the Wilms tumor locus zinc finger protein to the EGR-1 consensus sequence. *Science.* 1990;250:1259–1262.

Reddy JK, Rao MS. Malignant tumors in rats fed nafenopin, a hepatic peroxisome proliferator. *J Natl Cancer Inst.* 1997;59:1645–1650.

Rehn L. Blasengeschwülste bei Fuchsin-arbeitern. *Arch Klin Chir.* 1895;50:588–600.

Reznikoff CA, Brankow DW, Heidelberger C. Establishment and characterization of a cloned line of C3H mouse embryo cells sensitive to postconfluence inhibition of division. *Cancer Res.* 33:3231–3238.

Rice JM, Diwan BA, Hu H, Ward JM, Nims RW, Lubet RA. Enhancement of hepatocarcinogenesis and induction of specific cytochromes P450-dependent monooxygenase activities by the barbiturates allobarbital, aprobarbital, pentobarbital, secobarbital, and 5-phenyl- and 5-ethylbarbituric acids. *Carcinogenesis.* 1994;15:395–402.

Rice-Evans C, Burdon R. Free radical-lipid interactions and their pathological consequences. *Prog Lipid Res.* 1993;32:71–110.

Riggins JN, Marnett LJ. Mutagenicity of the Malondialdehyde oligerimerization products 2-(3'oxo-1'-propeneyl)-malondialdehyde and 2,4-dyhydroxymethylene-3-(2, 2-dimethoxyethyl)-gluteraldehyde in Salmonella. *Mutat Res.* 2001;497:153–157.

Riggs AD, Jones PA. 5-Methylcytosine, gene regulation and cancer. *Adv Cancer Res.* 1983;40:1–30.

Risch A, Wikman H, Thiel S, et al. Glutathione-S-transferase M1, M3, T1 and P1 polymorphisms and susceptibility to non-small-cell lung cancer subtypes and hamartomas. *Pharmacogenetics.* 2001;1(9):757–764.

Rohrmann S, Platz EA, Kavanaugh CJ, Thuita L, Hoffman SC, Helzlsouer KJ. Meat and dairy consumption and subsequent risk of prostate cancer in a US cohort study. *Cancer Causes Control.* 2007;18(1):41–50.

Rose ML, Rivera CA, Bradford BU, Graves LM, Cattley RC, Thurman RG. Kupffer cell oxidant production is central to the mechanism of peroxisome proliferators. *Carcinogenesis.* 1999;20:27–33.

Rous P. A sarcoma of the foul transmissible by an agent separable from the tumor cells. *J Exp Med.* 1911;13(4):397–411.

Rusyn I, Bradham CA, Cohn L, Schoonhoven R, Swenberg JA, Thurman, RG. Corn oil rapidly activates nuclear factor-$_\kappa$B in hepatic Kupffer cells by oxidant-dependant mechanisms. *Carcinogenesis.* 1999;20:2095–2100.

Sakai A, Sato M. Improvement of carcinogen identification in BALB/3T3 cell transformation by the application of a 2-stage method. *Mutat Res.* 1989;214:289–296.

Salem C, Liang G, Tsai YC, et al. Progressive increases in de novo methylation of CpG islands in bladder cancer. *Cancer Res.* 2000;60:2473–2476.

Sasaki MS. Chromosome aberration formation and sister chromatid exchange in relation to DNA repair in human cells. In: Generoso WM, Shelby MD, De Serres FJ, eds. *DNA Repair and Mutagenesis in Eukaryotes.* New York, NY: Plenum Press; 1980:285–313

Sasaki T, Yoshida T. Experimentelle Erzeugung des Lebercarcinoms durch Fütterung mit o-Amidoazotoluol. *Virchows Archiv, Pathologische Anatomie.* 1935;295:175–200

Sawyer DE, Van Houten B. Repair of DNA damage in mitochondria. *Mutat Res.* 1999;434:161–176.

Schechtman LM. BALB/3T3 cell transformation: protocols, problems and improvements. *IARC Sci Publ*. 1985;67:165–184.

Schulze-Oshoff K, Ferrari D, Los M, Wesselborg S, Peter ME. Apoptosis signaling by death receptors. *Eur J Biochem*. 1998;254:439–459.

Schumacher HR, Szelkely LE, Patel SB, Fisher DR. Mitochondria: a clue to oncogenesis? *Lancet*. 1973;2:327.

Sherr CJ. Mammalian G₁ cyclins. *Cell*. 1993;73:1059–1065.

Shibutani S, Takeshita M, Grollman AP. Insertion of specific bases during DNA synthesis past the oxidative-damage base 8-oxo-dG. *Nature*. 1991;349:431–434.

Shigematsu IS, Kitamaru J, Takeuchi M, et al. A retrospective mortality study on cadmium exposed populations in Japan. In: Wilson D, Volpe RA, eds. *Third International Cadmium Conference*. Cadmium Association/Cadmium Council; 1982.

Shih IM, Zhou W, Goodman SN, Lengauer C, Kinzler KW, Vogelstein B. Evidence that genetic instability occurs at an early stage of colorectal tumorigenesis. *Cancer Res*. 2001;61:818–822.

Shimkin M. *Some Classics of Experimental Oncology, 50 Selections, 1775–1965*. US Department of Health and Human Services; 1980.

Shimkin MB, Stoner GD. Lung tumors in mice: application to carcinogenesis bioassay. *Adv Cancer Res*. 1975;21:1–58.

Shirai T, Hirose M, Ito N. Medium-term bioassays in rats for rapid detection of the carcinogenic potential of chemicals. *IARC Scientific Publ*. 1999;146:251–272.

Siemiatycki J, Dewar R, Nadon L, Gerin M. Occupational risk factors for bladder cancer: results from a case-control study in Montreal, Quebec, Canada. *Am J Epidemiol*. 1994;140(12):1061–1080.

Silva RA, Muñoz SE, Guzmán CA, Eynard AR. Effects of dietary n-3, n-6 and n-9 polyunsaturated fatty acids on benzo(a)pyrene-induced forestomachtumorigenesis in C57BL6J mice. *Prostaglandins Leukot Essent Fatty Acids*. 1995;53(4):273-7

Sims P, Grover PL, Swaisland A, Pal K, Hewer A. Metabolic activation of benzo[a]pyrene proceeds by a diol-epoxide. *Nature*. 1974;252:326–328.

Slaga TJ. Multistage skin carcinogenesis, a useful model for the study of the chemoprevention of cancer. *Acta Pharmacol Toxicol*. 1984;55:107–124.

Slater AF, Stefan C, Nobel I, van den Dobbelsteen DJ, Orrenius S. Signalling mechanisms and oxidative stress in apoptosis. *Toxicol Lett*. 1995;82–83:149–153.

Solt D, Farber E. New principle for the analysis of chemical carcinogenesis. *Nature*. 1976;263:701–703.

Solt DB, Polverini PJ, Calderon L. Carcinogenic response of hamster buccal pouch epithelium to 4 polycyclic aromatic hydrocarbons. *J Oral Pathol Med*. 1987;6:294–302.

Sontag J. Carcinogenicity of substituted-benzenediamines (phenylenediamines). in rats and mice. *J Natl Cancer Inst*. 1981;66:591–602.

Sontag JM. Aspects in carcinogen bioassay. In: Origins of Human Cancer. Cold Spring Harbor; 1977:1327–1338.

Sorahan T, Lancashire RJ. Lung cancer mortality in a cohort of workers employed at a cadmium recovery plant in the United States: an analysis with detailed job histories. *Occup Environ Med*. 1997;54(3):194–201.

Sorahan T, Lister A, Gilthorpe MS, Harrington JM. Mortality of copper cadmium alloy workers with special reference to lung cancer and non-malignant diseases of the respiratory system, 1946–92. *Occup Environ Med*. 1995;52(12):804–812.

Soto AM, Fernandez MF, Luizzi MF, et al. Developing a marker of exposure to xenoestrogen mixtures in hmn serum. *Environ Health Perspec*. 1997;105:647–654.

Spalding JW, Momma J, Elwell MR, Tennant RW. Chemically induced skin carcinogenesis in a transgenic mouse line (TG.AC) carrying a v-Ha-ras gene. *Carcinogenesis*. 1993;14(7):1335–1341.

Spiro SG, Silvestri GA. One hundred years of lung cancer. Am J Respir Crit Care Med. 2005;172(5):523.

Steenland K, Boffetta P. Lead and cancer in humans: where are we now? *Am J Ind Med*. 2000;38(3):295–299.

Steenland K, Ward E. Lung cancer incidence among patients with beryllium disease: a cohort mortality study. *J Natl Cancer Inst*. 1991;83(19):1380–1385.

Steinmetz KL, Green CE, Bakke JP, Spak DK, Mirsalis JC. Induction of unscheduled DNA synthesis in primary cultures of rat, mouse, hamster, monkey, and human hepatocytes. *Mutat Res*. 1988;206(1):91–102.

Stinchcombe S, Buchmann A, Bock KW, Schwarz M. Inhibition of apoptosis during 2,3,7,8-tetrachlorodibenzo-p-dioxin-mediated tumour promotion in rat liver. *Carcinogenesis*. 1995;16(6):1271-1275.

Stirzaker C, Millar DS, Paul CL, et al. Extensive DNA methylation spanning the RB promoter in retinoblastoma tumors. *Cancer Res*. 1997;57:2229–2237.

Stoner GD. Lung tumors in strain A mice as a bioassay for carcinogenicity of environmental chemicals. *Exp Lung Res*. 1991;17:405–423.

Stoner GD, Adam-Rodwell G, Morse MA. Lung tumors in strain A mice: application for studies in cancer chemoprevention. *J Cell Biochem*. 1993;17F:95–103.

Stoner GD, Morse MA, Kelloff GJ. Perspectives in cancer chemoprevention. *Environ Health Perspect*. 1997;105(suppl 4):945–954.

Stoner GD, Shimkin MB. Lung tumors in strain A mice for carcinogenesis bioassays. In: Milman H, Weisburger EK, eds. *Handbook of Carcinogen Testing*. Park Rigde, NJ: Noyes Publications; 1985:179–214.

Su B, Karin M. Mitogen-activated protein kinase cascades and regulation of gene expression. *Curr Opin Immunol*. 1996;8:402–411.

Sugie S, Mori H, Takahashi M. Effect of in vivo exposure to the liver tumor promoters phenobarbital or DDT on the gap junctions of rat hepatocytes: a quantitative freeze-fracture analysis. *Carcinogenesis*. 1987;8:45–51.

Sundberg JP, Sundberg BA, Beamer WG. Comparison of chemical carcinogen skin tumor induction efficacy in inbred, mutant, and hybrid strains of mice: morphologic variations of induced tumors and absence of a papilloma virus. *Mol Carcinog*. 1997;20:19–32.

Sutherland LA, Bird RP. The effect of chenodeoxycholic acid on the development of aberrant crypt foci in the rat colon. *Cancer Lett*. 1994;76(2–3):101–107.

Sutherland RL, Hamilton J, Sweeney KJ, Watts CK, Musgrove EA. Steroidal regulation of cell cycle progression. *Ciba Found Symp*. 1995;191:218–228.

Swenberg JA, Dyroff MC, Bedell MA, et al. O⁴-Ethyldeoxythymidine, but not O⁶-ethyldeoxyguanosine, accumulates in hepatocyte DNA of rats exposed continuously to diethylnitrosamine. *Proc Nat Acad Sci USA*. 1984;81(6):1692–1695.

Swenberg JA, Richardson FC, Boucheron JA, Dyroff MC. Relationships between DNA adduct formation and carcinogenesis. *Environ Health Perspect*. 1985;62:177–183.

Synder RL, Tyler G, Summers J. Chronic hepatitis and hepatocellular carcinoma associated with woodchuck hepatitis virus. *Am J Pathol*. 1982;107:422–425.

Takahashi M, Hasegawa R, Furukawa F, Toyoda K, Sato H, Hayashi Y. Effects of ethanol, potassium metabisulfite, formaldehyde and hydrogen peroxide on gastric carcinogenesis in rats after initiation with N-methyl-N′-nitro-N-nitrosoguanidine. *Jpn J Cancer Res*. 1986;77(2):118–124.

Tamura G, Nishizuka S, Maesawa C, et al. Mutations in mitochondrial control region DNA in gastric tumors of Japanese patients. *Eur J Cancer*. 1999;35:316–19.

Tanaka T, Kawabata K, Kakumoto M, et al. Chemoprevention of 4-nitroquinoline 1-oxide-induced oral carcinogenesis by citrus auraptene in rats. *Carcinogenesis*. 1998;19:425–431.

Tavani A, Negri E, Parazzini F, Franceschi S, La Vecchia C. Female hormone utilisation and risk of hepatocellular carcinoma. *Br J Cancer*. 1993;67(3):635–637.

Tchou J, Grollman AP. Repair of DNA containing the oxidatively damaged base, 8-oxoguanine. *Mutat Res*. 1993;299:277–287.

Temin HM, Rubin H. Characteristics of an assay for Rous sarcoma virus and Rous sarcoma cells in tissue culture. *Virology*. 1958;6:669–688.

Tennant RW, Margolin BH, Shelby MD, et al. Prediction of chemical carcinogenicity in rodents from in vitro genetic toxicity assays. *Science*. 1987;236(4804):933–941.

Thiersch K. Der Epithelialkrebs, Namentliehlder Ausseren Haut. Leipzig, Germany; 1875.

Tinwell H, Ashby J. Comparative activity of human carcinogens and NTP rodent carcinogens in the mouse bone marrow micronucleus assay: an integrative approach to genetic toxicity data assessment. *Environ Health Perspect*. 1994;102(9):758–762.

Timblin CR, Janssen YMW, Mossman BT. Free-radical-mediated alterations of gene expression by xenobiotics. In: Wallace KB, ed. *Free Radical Toxicology*. London: Taylor & Francis; 1997:325–349.

Trosko JE, Ruch R. Cell-cell communication and carcinogenesis. *Front Biosci.* 1998;3:208–236.

Trush MA, Kensler TW. An overview of the relationship between oxidative stress and chemical carcinogenesis. *Free Radic Biol Med.* 1991;10:201–209.

Tsuchida S, Sato K. Glutathione transferases and cancer. *Crit Rev Biochem Mol Biol.* 1992;27:337–384.

Tsutsui T, Taguchi S, Tanaka Y, Barrett JC. 17beta-estradiol, diethylstilbesterol, tamoxifen, toremifene, and ICI 164384 induce morphological transformation and aneuploidy in cultured Syrian hamster cells. *Int J Cancer.* 1997;70:188–193.

Tugwood JD, Holden PR, James NH, Prince RA, Roberts RA. A PPAR alpha cDNA cloned from guinea pig liver encodes a protein with similar properties to the mouse PPAR alpha: implications for species differences in response to peroxisome proliferators. *Arch Toxicol.* 1998;72:169–177.

Turesky RJ. Formation and biochemistry of carcinogenic heterocyclic aromatic amines in cooked meats. *Toxicol Lett.* 2007;168(3):219–227.

Turk PW, Laayoun A, Smith SS, Weitzman SA. DNA adduct 8-hydroxy-2'-deoxyguanosine (8-hydroxy-guanosine) affects function of human DNA methyltransferase. *Carcinogenesis.* 1995;16:1253–1256.

Ueda A, Hamadeh HK, Webb HK, et al. Diverse roles of the nuclear orphan receptor car in regulating hepatic genes in response to phenobarbital. *Mol Pharmacol.* 2002;61:1–6.

van der Gulden JW, Kolk JJ, Verbeek AL. Work environment and prostate cancer risk. *Prostate.* 1995;27(5):250–257.

Vesselinovitch SD, Hacker HJ, Bannasch P. Histochemical characterization of focal hepatic lesions induced by single diethylnitrosamine treatment in infant mice. *Cancer Res.* 1985;45:2774–2780.

Vogt PK. Jun, the oncoprotein. *Oncogene.* 2001;20:2365–2377.

von Sonntag C. New aspects in the free-radical chemistry of pyrimidine nucleobases. *Free Radic Res Commun.* 1987;2:217–24.

Vousden KH. Human papillomavirus and cervical carcinoma. *Cancer Cells.* 1989;1:43–50.

Vuillaume M. Reduced oxygen species, mutation, induction and cancer initiation. *Mutat Res.* 1987;186:43–72.

Waalkes MP, Anver MR, Diwan BA. Chronic toxic and carcinogenic effects of oral cadmium in the Noble (NBL/Cr) rat: induction of neoplastic and proliferative lesions of the adrenal, kidney, prostate, and testes. *J Toxicol Environ Health.* 1999;58(4):199–214.

Waalkes MP, Diwan BA, Ward JM, Devor DE, Goyer RA. Renal tubular tumors and atypical hyperplasias in B6C3F1 mice exposed to lead acetate during gestation and lactation occur with minimal chronic nephropathy. *Cancer Res.* 1995;55(22):5265–5271.

Waalkes MP, Rehm S, Sass B, Kovatch R, Ward JM. Chronic carcinogenic and toxic effects of a single subcutaneous dose of cadmium in male NFS and C57 mice and male Syrian hamsters. *Toxic Subst J.* 1994;13:15–28.

Wade N, Marsman DS, Popp JA. Dose related effects of hepatocarcinogen Wy 14,263 on peroxisomes and cell replication. *Fundam Appl Toxicol.* 1992;18:149–154.

Wainfan E, Poirier LA. Methyl groups in carcinogenesis: effects on DNA methylation and gene expression. *Cancer Res.* 1992;52(suppl):S2071–S2077.

Walker VE, Fennell TR, Upton PB, et al. Molecular dosimetry of ethylene oxide: formation and persistence of 7-(2-hydroxyethyl) guanine in DNA following repeated exposures of rats and rice. *Cancer Res.* 1992;52:5328–4334.

Ward E, Okun A, Ruder A, Fingerhut M, Steenland K. A mortality study of workers at seven beryllium processing plants. *Am J Ind Med.* 1992;22(6):885–904.

Wei P, Zhang J, Egan-Hafley M, Liang S, Moore DD. The nuclear receptor CAR mediates specific xenobiotic induction of drug metabolism. *Nature.* 2000;407:920–923.

Weinberg RA. The retinoblastoma protein and cell cycle control. *Cell.* 1995;81:323–330.

Weisburger JH, Williams GM. Metabolism of chemical carcinogens. In: Becker FF, ed. *Cancer: A Comprehensive Treatise.* 2nd ed. New York: Plenum; 1981:241–333.

Weisburger JH, Williams GM. Bioassay of carcinogens: in vitro and in vivo tests. In: Searle CE, ed. *Chemical Carcinogens.* Vol 2. Washington, DC: American Chemical Society; 1984:1323–1373.

Weitzman SA, Turk PW, Milkowski DH, Kozlowski K. Free radical adducts induce alterations in DNA cytosine methylation. *Proc Natl Acad Sci U S A.* 1994;91:1261–1264.

Welfare M, Monesola Adeokun A, Bassendine MF, Daly AK. Polymorphisms in *GSTP1*, *GSTM1*, and *GSTT1* and susceptibility to colorectal cancer. *Cancer Epidemiol Biomarker Prev.* 1999;8:289–292.

Wells A. EGF receptor. *Int J Biochem Cell Biol.* 1999;31:637–643.

Welsch CW, Adams C, Lambrecht LK, Hassett CC, Brooks CL. 17b-Oestradiol and enovid mammary tumorigenesis in C3H/HeJ female mice: Counteraction by concurrent 2-bromo-a-ergocryptine. *Br J Cancer Res.* 1977;52:1–17.

Whysner J, Ross PM, Williams GM. Phenobarbital mechanistic data and risk assessment: enzyme induction, enhanced cell proliferation, and tumor promotion. *Pharmacol Ther.* 1996;71:153–191.

Whyte P, Buchkovich FJ, Horowitz JM, et al. Association between an oncogene and an anti-oncogene: the adenovirus E1A proteins bind to the retinoblastoma gene product. *Nature.* 1988;334:124–129.

Wintersberger U, Klein F. Yeast-mating-type switching: a model system for the study of genome rearrangements induced by carcinogens. *Ann N Y Acad Sci.* 1988;534:513–520.

Williams GM. In vivo and in vitro markers of liver cell transformation. In: Smith GJ, Stewart BW, eds. *In Vitro Epithelial Cell Differentiation and Neoplasia.* Cancer Forum;1982;6:166–172.

Williams GM, Whysner J. Epigenetic carcinogens: evaluation and risk assessment. *Exp Toxicol Pathol.* 1996;48:189–195.

Witz G. Active oxygen species as factors in multistage carcinogenesis. *Proc Soc Exp Biol Med.* 1991;198:675–682.

Wood WB, Gloyne SR. Pulmonary asbestosis. A review of one hundred cases. *Lancet.* 1934;2:1383–1385.

Wyrobek AJ, Bruce WR. Chemical induction of sperm abnormalities in mice. *Proc Natl Acad Sci U S A.* 1975;72(11):4425–4429.

Yamagiwa K, Ichikawa K. Experimentelle Studie über die Pathogenese der Epithelialgeschwülste. *Mitt Med Fak Kaiserl Univ Tokio.* 1915;15:295–344.

Yamashita N, Minamoto T, Ochia A, Onda M, Esumi H. Frequent and characteristic K-ras activation and absence of p53 protein accumulation in aberrant crypt foci of colon. *Gastroenterology.* 1995;108:434–440.

Yang SK, McCourt DW, Roller PP, Gelboin HV. Enzymatic conversion of benzo[a]pyrene leading predominantly to the diol-epoxide r-7,t-8-dihydroxy-t-9,10-oxy-7,8,9,10-tetrahydrobenzo[a]pyrene through a single enantiomer of r-7,t-8-dihydroxy-7,8-dihydrobenzo[a]pyrene. *Proc Nat Acad Sci USA.* 1976;73(8):2594–2598.

Yoshida T. über die serienweise Verfolgung der Veränderungen der Leber der experimentellen Hepatomerzeugung durch o-aminoazotoluol. *Trans Jap Path Soc.* 1933;23:636–638.

Young SS, Gries CL. Exploration of the negative correlation between proliferative hepatocellular lesions and lymphoma in rats and mice—establishment and implications. *Fundam Appl Toxicol.* 1984;4:632–640.

Zawaski K. Evidence for enhanced expression of c-fos, c-jun, and the CA^{2+}-activated neutral protease in rat liver following carbon tetrachloride administration. *Biochem Biophys Res Commun.* 1993;197:585–590.

Zhang H, Kamendulis LM, Xu Y, Klaunig JE. The role of 8-hydroxy-2'-deoxyguanosine in morphological transformation of Syrian hamster embryo (SHE) Cells. *Toxicol Sci.* 2000;56:303–312.

chapter 9

Genetic Toxicology

R. Julian Preston and George R. Hoffmann

WHAT IS GENETIC TOXICOLOGY?

Genetic toxicology is a branch of the field of toxicology that assesses the effects of chemical and physical agents on the hereditary material (DNA) and on the genetic processes of living cells. Such effects can be assessed directly by measuring the interaction of agents with DNA or more indirectly through the assessment of DNA repair or the production of gene mutations or chromosome alterations. Given the risk assessment framework of this chapter, it is important at the outset to distinguish between genotoxicity and mutagenicity. Genotoxicity covers a broader spectrum of endpoints than mutagenicity. For example, unscheduled DNA synthesis (UDS), sister chromatid exchanges (SCEs), and DNA strand breaks are measures of genotoxicity, not mutagenicity because they are not themselves transmissible from cell to cell or generation to generation. Mutagenicity on the other hand refers to the production of transmissible genetic alterations. In the last few years, there has been an increased emphasis on the role of epigenetic changes in the production of altered phenotypes. Such changes can be transmitted and so it is appropriate to include epigenetic changes such as alterations in DNA methylation or in histones involved in the control of gene expression as genotoxic endpoints. However, they are not mutations by definition because they do not involve changes in DNA sequence (Hamilton, 2011).

This chapter discusses the history of the development of the field of genetic toxicology, the use of genetic toxicology data in cancer and genetic risk assessments, the mechanisms underlying genetic toxicology assays, the assays that can be used for detecting genotoxic endpoints, the use of the same assays for better understanding mechanisms of mutagenesis, and new methods for the assessment of genetic alterations. The field is evolving rapidly, and a review of its past and present state will set the stage to allow for a consideration of what are likely next major landmarks.

HISTORY OF GENETIC TOXICOLOGY

The field of genetic toxicology can be considered to have its roots in the pioneering work of H.J. Muller (1927), who showed that x-rays could induce mutations in the fruit fly, *Drosophila*. In his studies he showed not only that radiation exposure could increase the overall frequencies of mutations but also that the types of mutations induced were exactly the same in effect, or phenotype, as those observed in the absence of radiation exposure. Thus, the induced mutagenic responses should be assessed in relation to background mutations. As a conclusion to this study of radiation-induced mutations, Muller predicted the utility of mutagenesis studies not only for the study of mutations themselves but also for gene mapping approaches.

Karl Sax (1938) built upon Muller's original studies of radiation-induced mutations by showing that X-rays could also induce structural alterations to chromosomes in *Tradescantia* pollen grains. Sax and his colleagues, notably in the absence of knowledge of DNA structure and chromosomal organization, showed that at least two critical lesions in a nuclear target are required for the production of an exchange within (intrachromosome) or between (interchromosome) chromosomes. We know now that the lesions identified by Sax are DNA double-strand breaks, base damages, or multiply damaged sites (reviewed by Ward, 1988). In addition, Sax and colleagues (Sax, 1939; Sax and Luippold, 1952) showed that the yield of chromosome aberrations was reduced if the total dose of x-rays was delivered over extended periods of time or split into two fractions separated by several hours. These observations led to the concept of restitution of radiation-induced damage, which was later recognized as involving specific DNA repair processes (see below).

Consideration of the genetic effects of exogenous agents on cells was expanded to include chemicals in 1946, when Charlotte Auerbach and colleagues reported that mustard gas could induce mutations in *Drosophila* and that these mutations were phenotypically similar to those induced by x-rays (Auerbach and Robson, 1946). Thus, the field of chemical mutagenesis was initiated to run in parallel with studies of radiation mutagenesis. These original studies of Auerbach (actually conducted in 1941) are placed in a historical and biological perspective by the delightful review of Geoffrey Beale (1993).

Although the scientific value of the analysis of mutations in *Drosophila* was clear, there was an impression that the extrapolation to predict similar effects in human populations was too wide a step. Thus, a research effort of great magnitude was initiated to attempt to assess radiation-induced mutations in mice. This effort resulted in the publication by William Russell (1951) of data on x-ray–induced mutations using a mouse-specific-locus mutation assay. These data clearly showed that the type of results obtained with *Drosophila* could be replicated in a mammalian system. The mouse tester strain developed for the specific-locus assay has recessive mutations at seven loci coding for visible mutations, such as coat color, eye color, and ear shape. This homozygous recessive tester strain can be used for identifying recessive mutations induced in wild type genes at the same loci in mice treated with radiation or chemical mutagens. It was noteworthy that the mutation rate for x-ray–induced mutations in germ cells was similar in mouse and *Drosophila*. Subsequent studies by Liane Russell and colleagues showed that chemicals could induce mutations at the same seven loci (Russell *et al.*, 1981).

Over the next 20 years, genetic toxicologists investigated the induction of mutations and chromosomal alterations in somatic and germ cells, largely following exposures to radiation, but increasingly using chemical mutagens as well. The ability to grow cells in vitro, either as primary cultures or as transformed cell lines, enhanced these quantitative studies. The in vitro culture of human lymphocytes, stimulated to reenter the cell cycle by phytohemagglutinin, greatly expanded the information on the assessment of chromosomal alterations in human cells (an excellent review by Hsu [1979] is recommended). It also became feasible to use cytogenetic alterations in human lymphocytes as a biodosimeter for assessing human exposures to ionizing radiations (Bender and Gooch, 1962).

Two events during the 1970s served to expand the utility of mutagenicity data into the realm of risk assessment. The Millers and their colleagues (Miller and Miller, 1977) showed that chemical carcinogens could react to form stable, covalent derivatives with DNA, RNA, and proteins both in vitro and in vivo. In addition, they reported that these derivatives could require the metabolism of the parent chemical to form reactive metabolites. This metabolism is required for some chemicals to become mutagens and carcinogens. Metabolic capability is endogenous in vivo, but most cell lines in vitro do not express this capacity. To overcome this for in vitro mutagenicity studies, Heinrich Malling and colleagues developed an exogenous metabolizing system based on a rodent liver homogenate (S9) (Malling and Frantz, 1973; Malling, 2004). Although this exogenous metabolism system has had utility, it does have drawbacks related to species and tissue specificity and loss of cellular compartmentalization. The development of transgenic cell lines containing P450 genes has overcome this drawback to some extent (Sawada and Kamataki, 1998; Crespi and Miller, 1999).

The second development in the 1970s that changed the field of genetic toxicology was the development by Bruce Ames *et al.* (1975) of a simple, inexpensive mutation assay with the bacterium *Salmonella typhimurium*. This assay can be used to detect chemically induced reverse mutations in several histidine genes and can include the exogenous metabolizing S9 system described above. The Ames assay, as it is generally called, has been expanded and modified to enhance its performance as discussed below (under section "Gene Mutations in Prokaryotes"). The assay has been used extensively, especially for hazard identification, as part of the cancer risk assessment process. This use was based on the assumption that carcinogens were mutagens and that cancer required mutation induction. This latter dogma proved to be somewhat inhibitory to the field of genetic toxicology because it provided a framework that was too rigid. Nonetheless, over the decade of the mid-1970s to mid-1980s somewhere on the order of 200 short-term genotoxicity and mutagenicity assays were developed for screening potentially carcinogenic chemicals. The screens included mutation induction, DNA damage, DNA repair, and cell killing or other genotoxic activities.

Several international collaborative studies were organized to establish the sensitivity and specificity of a select group of assays as well as to assess interlaboratory variation (International Program on Chemical Safety [IPCS], 1988). Most assays were able to detect carcinogens or noncarcinogens with an efficiency of about 70% as compared with the outcome of two-year cancer bioassays. There are a number of possible reasons for the imperfect correspondence, the most likely being that there is a group of chemical carcinogens that do not induce cancer by a direct mutagenic action. The latter point was addressed to some extent by Tennant *et al.* (1987), who compared the effectiveness of a small standard battery of well-characterized short-term assays to identify carcinogens. Again, this battery predicted about 70% of known carcinogens. Subsequently, the lack of a tight correlation between carcinogenicity and mutagenicity (and the converse, noncarcinogenicity and nonmutagenicity) was found to be due to the fact that some chemicals were not directly mutagenic but instead induced the damage necessary for tumor development indirectly by, for example, clonally expanding preexisting mutant cells (ie, tumor promotion) or through the production of reactive oxygen species. Such chemicals were given the rather unfortunate name of *nongenotoxic* to contrast them with genotoxic ones; the classification as *not directly mutagenic* is more appropriate. In the context of the mechanism of their mutagenicity, it is preferable to distinguish between DNA-reactivity and its correlate non-DNA-reactivity. Emphasis has recently been placed on identifying mechanisms whereby nondirectly mutagenic chemicals can be involved in tumor production. Those identified include cytotoxicity with regenerative cell proliferation, mitogenicity, receptor-mediated processes, changes in methylation status, and alterations in cell–cell communication.

In the last 10 years or so, the field of genetic toxicology has moved away from the short-term assay approach for assessing carcinogenicity to a much more mechanistic approach, fueled to quite an extent by the advances in molecular biology. The ability to manipulate and characterize DNA, RNA, and proteins and to understand basic cellular processes and how they can be perturbed has advanced enormously over this period. Knowing how to take advantage of these technical developments is paramount. This chapter addresses these changes in approach to genetic toxicology: the assays for qualitative and quantitative assessment of cellular changes induced by chemical and physical agents, the underlying molecular mechanisms for these changes, and how such information can be incorporated into cancer and genetic risk assessments. In addition, the way forward for the field is addressed in the form of an epilogue. Thus, the preceding historical overview sets the stage for the rest of the chapter.

HEALTH IMPACT OF GENETIC ALTERATIONS

The importance of mutations and chromosomal alterations for human health is evident from their roles in genetic disorders, including birth defects and cancer. Therefore, mutations in both germ cells and somatic cells need to be considered when an overall risk resulting from mutations is concerned.

Somatic Cells

An association between mutation and cancer has long been evident, such as through the correlation between the mutagenicity and carcinogenicity of chemicals, especially in biological systems that have the requisite metabolic activation capabilities. Moreover, human chromosome instability syndromes and DNA repair deficiencies are associated with increased cancer risk (Friedberg, 1985). Cancer cytogenetics has greatly strengthened the association in that specific chromosomal alterations, including deletions, translocations, inversions, and amplifications, have been implicated in many human leukemias and lymphomas as well as in some solid tumors (Rabbitts, 1994; Zhang et al., 2010).

Critical evidence that mutation plays a central role in cancer has come from molecular studies of oncogenes and tumor-suppressor genes. Oncogenes are genes that stimulate the transformation of normal cells into cancer cells (Bishop, 1991). They originate when genes called proto-oncogenes, involved in normal cellular growth and development, are genetically altered. Normal regulation of cellular proliferation requires a balance between factors that promote growth and those that restrict it. Mutational alteration of proto-oncogenes can lead to overexpression of their growth-stimulating activity, whereas mutations that inactivate tumor-suppressor genes, which normally restrain cellular proliferation, free cells from their inhibitory influence (Hanahan and Weinberg, 2000, 2011).

The action of oncogenes is genetically dominant in that a single active oncogene is expressed, even though its normal allele is present in the same cell. Proto-oncogenes can be converted into active oncogenes by point mutations or chromosomal alterations. Base pair substitutions in ras proto-oncogenes are found in many human tumors (Bishop, 1991; Barrett, 1993; Croce, 2008). Among chromosomal alterations that activate proto-oncogenes,

translocations are especially prevalent (Rabbitts, 1994, Croce, 2008; Zhang et al., 2010). For example, Burkitt lymphoma involves a translocation between the long arm of chromosome eight, which is the site of the c-MYC oncogene, and chromosome 14 (about 90% of cases), 22, or 2. A translocation can activate a proto-oncogene by moving it to a new chromosomal location, typically the site of a T-cell receptor or immunoglobulin gene, where its expression is enhanced. A similar translocation-based mechanism also applies to various other hematopoietic cancers. Alternatively, the translocation may join two genes, resulting in a protein fusion that contributes to cancer development. Fusions have been implicated in other hematopoietic cancers and some solid tumors (Rabbitts, 1994; Croce, 2008; Zhang et al., 2010). Like translocations, other chromosomal alterations can activate proto-oncogenes, and genetic amplification of oncogenes can magnify their expression (Bishop, 1991; Croce, 2008).

Mutational inactivation or deletion of tumor-suppressor genes has been implicated in many cancers. Unlike oncogenes, the cancer-causing alleles that arise from tumor-suppressor genes are typically recessive in that they are not expressed when they are heterozygous (Evans and Prosser, 1992). However, several genetic mechanisms, including mutation, deletion, chromosome loss, and mitotic recombination, can cause loss of heterozygosity (LOH), in which the normal dominant allele is inactivated or eliminated. LOH leads to the expression of the recessive cancer gene in a formerly heterozygous cell (Cavenee et al., 1983; Turner et al., 2003; Reliene et al., 2007). The inactivation of tumor-suppressor genes has been associated with various cancers, including those of the eye, kidney, colon, brain, breast, lung, and bladder (Fearon and Vogelstein, 1990; Marshall, 1991). Gene mutations in a tumor-suppressor gene called P53, located on chromosome 17, occur in many different human cancers, and molecular characterization of P53 mutations has linked specific human cancers to mutagen exposures (Harris, 1993; Aguilar et al., 1994; Royds and Iacopetta, 2006).

In the simplest model for the action of tumor-suppressor genes, two events are considered to be required for the development of retinoblastoma, a tumor of the eye, because both normal alleles must be inactivated or lost (Knudson, 1997). In sporadic forms of the cancer (ie, no family history), the two genetic events occur independently, but in familial forms (eg, familial retinoblastoma), the first mutation is inherited, leaving the need for only a single additional event for expression. The strong predisposition to cancer in the inherited disease stems from the high likelihood that a LOH will occur by mutation, recombination, or aneuploidy in at least one or a few cells in the development of the affected organ. The simple model involving two events and a single pair of alleles cannot explain all observations concerning tumor-suppressor genes because many cancers involve more than one tumor-suppressor gene. For example, the childhood kidney tumor called Wilms tumor can be caused by damage in at least three different genes (Marshall, 1991), and colorectal carcinomas are often found to have lost not only the wild-type P53 tumor-suppressor gene but also other tumor-suppressor genes (Fearon and Vogelstein, 1990; Stoler et al., 1999). Moreover, a single mutation in a tumor-suppressor gene, even though not fully expressed, may contribute to carcinogenesis. For example, a single P53 mutation in a developing colorectal tumor may confer a growth advantage that contributes to the development of the disease (Venkatachalam et al., 1998). Subsequent LOH will increase the growth advantage as the tumor progresses from benign to malignant (Fearon and Vogelstein, 1990). In this regard (mutation and selection), carcinogenesis has been likened to an evolutionary process, with genomic instability providing the substrate and with growth advantage as the selection pressure (Gatenby and Vincent, 2003; Fischer et al., 2004).

Many cancers involve both activation of oncogenes and inactivation of tumor-suppressor genes (Fearon and Vogelstein, 1990; Bishop, 1991; Croce, 2008). The observation of multiple genetic changes supports the view that cancer results from an accumulation of genetic alterations and that carcinogenesis is a multistep process (Kinzler and Vogelstein, 1996; Hahn *et al.*, 1999; Stoler *et al.*, 1999; Croce, 2008). At least three stages have been defined in carcinogenesis: initiation, promotion, and progression (Barrett, 1993). *Initiation* involves the induction of a genetic alteration, such as the mutational activation of a *ras* proto-oncogene by a mutagen. It is an irreversible step that starts the process toward cancer. *Promotion* involves cellular proliferation in an initiated cell population. Promotion can lead to the development of benign tumors such as papillomas. Agents called promoters stimulate this process. Promoters may be mutagenic but are not necessarily so. *Progression* involves the continuation of cell proliferation and the accumulation of additional irreversible genetic changes; it is marked by increasing genetic instability and malignancy. More recent studies are beginning to change this view, leading to the concept of acquired capabilities (Hanahan and Weinberg, 2000). In their *Hallmarks of Cancer*, Hanahan and Weinberg (2000) describe a set of six acquired characteristics that are essential for the formation of all tumors irrespective of tumor type and species. These characteristics are broadly described as follows: self-sufficiency in growth signals, insensitivity to antigrowth signals, evading apoptosis, limitless replicative potential, sustained angiogenesis, and tissue invasion and metastasis. It seems probable that there is no specific order for obtaining these characteristics. Hanahan and Weinberg have revisited their hallmarks concept, and, based on progress in the field over the past decade, they have added two emerging hallmarks of potential generality to their existing six (Hanahan and Weinberg, 2011). These are reprogramming of energy metabolism and evading immune destruction. In addition, they describe genome instability and inflammation as general features that underlie their now eight hallmarks (Hanahan and Weinberg, 2011).

Genomic instability is a feature of all cancers, with the great majority having a large number of chromosomal and gene mutations and aneuploidies. In fact, one of the difficulties in trying to unravel the mechanisms of formation of tumors is establishing which genetic alterations are informative and which are merely incidental and a product of the cancer process itself. The advent of ultrahigh throughput sequencing has allowed for the complete sequencing and subsequent characterization of genomic changes in a number of tumor types. The outcome has been an ability to classify the genomic changes as drivers and passengers, with the former being essential key events in tumor formation, and the latter basically "coming along for the ride" (Stratton *et al.*, 2009; Pleasance *et al.*, 2010).

Gene mutations, chromosome aberrations, and aneuploidy are all implicated in the development of cancer. Mutagens and clastogens (chromosome breaking agents) contribute to carcinogenesis as initiators. Their role does not have to be restricted to initiation, however, in that mutagens, clastogens and aneugens (agents that induce aneuploidy) may contribute to the multiple genetic alterations that characterize progression or the development of acquired capabilities. Other agents that contribute to carcinogenesis, such as promoters, need not be mutagens. However, the role of mutations is critical, and analyzing mutations and mutagenic effects is essential for understanding and predicting chemical carcinogenesis.

Germ Cells

The relevance of gene mutations to health is evident from the many disorders that are inherited as simple Mendelian characteristics (Mohrenweiser, 1991). About 1.3% of newborns suffer from autosomal dominant (1%), autosomal recessive (0.25%), or sex-linked (0.05%) genetic diseases (National Research Council [NRC], 2007a,b; Sankaranarayanan, 1998; Elespuru and Sankaranarayanan, 2007). Molecular analysis of the mutations responsible for Mendelian diseases has revealed that almost half of these mutations are base pair substitutions; of the remainder, most are small deletions (Sankaranarayanan, 1998; Elespuru and Sankaranarayanan, 2007).

Many genetic disorders (eg, cystic fibrosis, phenylketonuria, Tay-Sachs disease) are caused by the expression of recessive mutations. These mutations are mainly inherited from previous generations and are expressed when an individual inherits the mutant gene from both parents. New mutations make a larger contribution to the incidence of dominant diseases than to that of recessive diseases because only a single dominant mutation is required for expression. Thus, new dominant mutations are expressed in the first generation. If a dominant disorder is severe, its transmission between generations is unlikely because of reduced fitness. For dominants with a mild effect, reduced penetrance, or a late age of onset, the contribution from previous generations is undoubtedly larger than it is for mutations with severe early expression. Estimating the proportion of all Mendelian genetic diseases that can be ascribed to new mutations is not straightforward; a rough estimate is 20% (Shelby, 1994).

Besides causing diseases that exhibit Mendelian inheritance, gene mutations undoubtedly contribute to human disease through the genetic component of disorders with a complex etiology (Sankaranarayanan *et al.*, 1999; Sankaranarayanan, 2006). Some 3% (United Nations Scientific Committee on the Effects of Atomic Radiation [UNSCEAR], 2001) or 5% to 6% (Sankaranarayanan, 1998) of infants are affected by congenital abnormalities; if one includes multifactorial disorders that often have a late onset, such as heart disease, hypertension, and diabetes, the proportion of the population affected increases to more than 60% (Sankaranarayanan, 1998; UNSCEAR, 2001; Sankaranarayanan, 2006). Such frequencies are necessarily approximate because of differences among surveys in the reporting and classification of disorders. A higher prevalence would be found if less severe disorders were included in the tabulation. Nevertheless, such estimates provide a sense of the large impact of genetic disease.

Sensitive cytogenetic methods have led to the discovery of minor variations in chromosome structure that have no apparent effect. On the contrary, other relatively minor structural chromosome aberrations cause fetal death or serious abnormalities. Aneuploidy (gain or loss of one or more chromosomes) also contributes to fetal deaths and causes disorders such as Down syndrome. About four infants per 1000 live births have syndromes associated with chromosomal abnormalities, including translocations and aneuploidy. The majority of these syndromes (about 85%) result from trisomies (NRC, 2007a,b; Griffin, 1996; Nagaishi *et al.*, 2004). Most of the adverse effects of chromosomal abnormalities occur prenatally. It has been estimated that 5% of all recognized pregnancies involve chromosomal abnormalities, as do about 6% of infant deaths and 30% of all spontaneous embryonic and fetal deaths (Mohrenweiser, 1991; Nagaishi *et al.*, 2004). Among the abnormalities that have been observed, aneuploidy is the most common, followed by polyploidy. Structural aberrations constitute about 5% of the total. Unlike gene mutations, many of which are inherited from the previous generation, about 85% of the chromosomal anomalies observed in newborns arise de novo in the germ cells of the parents (Mohrenweiser, 1991). The frequency of aneuploidy assessed directly in human sperm, initially by standard karyotyping and more recently by fluorescence in situ hybridization

(FISH), is 3% to 4%; about 0.4% are sex chromosome aneuploidies (Martin *et al.*, 1991, 1996). The frequency of aneuploidy in human oocytes is about 18% (Martin *et al.*, 1991).

CANCER AND GENETIC RISK ASSESSMENTS

Cancer Risk Assessment

The formalized process for conducting a cancer risk assessment has many variations based on national requirements and regulations. A summary of some of the different approaches can be found in Moolenaar (1994). A recent approach developed by the European Commission under the acronym REACH (Registration, Evaluation, Authorisation and Restriction of Chemical Substances) aims to ensure that the necessary information is acquired to assess hazards and risks for human health for the very large number of chemicals for which little information is currently available (ec.europa.eu/environment/chemicals/reach/reach_intro.htm). There are also ongoing attempts, for example, by IPCS and the International Life Sciences Institute (ILSI) to develop a harmonized approach to cancer risk assessments. Although no totally unified approach is currently available, there is a framework that has been developed around a mode of action/human relevance concept that is discussed later in this section (Boobis *et al.*, 2006; Meek *et al.*, 2003). This framework, together with the formalized approach developed by the US Environmental Protection Agency (EPA) based on the paradigm presented by the National Research Council (NRC, 1983), is discussed here to depict the use of genetic toxicology in the risk assessment process.

Genetic toxicology data have been used until recently almost exclusively for hazard identification. Namely, if a chemical is DNA-reactive, then tumors are considered to be produced by this chemical via direct mutagenicity. This has led, in turn, to the use of the default linear extrapolation from the rodent bioassay tumor data to exposure levels consistent with human environmental or occupational exposures (EPA, 1986). The assessment of risk requires the application of a series of default options, for example, from laboratory animals to humans, from high to low exposures, from intermittent to chronic lifetime exposures, and from route to route of exposure. Default options are "generic approaches, based on general scientific knowledge and policy judgment that are applied to various elements of the risk assessment process when specific scientific information is not available" (NRC, 1994). The default options have been, in some ways, the Achilles heel of the cancer risk-assessment process because they have a very significant impact on low exposure risk but are based on an uncertain database. This concern led the EPA (1996) to develop a very different approach, initially described in the *Proposed Guidelines for Carcinogen Risk Assessment*, now released as the *Guidelines for Carcinogen Risk Assessment* (EPA, 2005). In these guidelines, the emphasis is on using mechanistic data, when available, to inform the risk assessment process, particularly for dose–response assessment and risk characterization. The goal is to develop biologically based or other forms of dose–response models for estimating cancer risk at low environmental exposures. This does, in general, bring the EPA approach into some harmony with those in other countries (Moolenaar, 1994), where a more narrative approach to risk assessment is preferred to a strictly quantitative one, and with the approaches described by IPCS (Boobis *et al.*, 2006) and ILSI (Meek *et al.*, 2003). The outcome of a more mechanistically based cancer risk assessment process is that there is a greater impetus to developing databases for key events in adverse outcome pathways and mechanisms of disease production

in addition to the yes/no output from genotoxicity assays in support of hazard identification. The same genotoxicity assays can be used for the collection of all these types of information, and the application of molecular biology techniques has certainly aided in the pursuit of mechanisms of mutagenicity and carcinogenicity. It is anticipated that the cancer risk assessment process will evolve as these new types of data are obtained.

Some of the issues that remain to be more firmly elucidated are (1) the relative sensitivities of different species (particularly rodent and human) to the induction of organ-specific mutations and tumors by chemicals and radiation; (2) the shape of the dose response for key events (eg, genetic alterations) in the formation of tumors and for the tumors themselves at low (environmental) exposure levels, especially for genotoxic chemicals; and (3) the relative sensitivity of susceptible subpopulations of all types. A better understanding of these major issues will greatly reduce the uncertainty in cancer risk assessments by, in part, replacing default options with biological data.

The most recent EPA guidelines for cancer risk assessment (EPA, 2005) provide a framework for cancer risk assessment that utilizes a mode-of-action (MoA) as the means of describing the "necessary but not sufficient" steps required for a chemical to produce a tumor. A particular MoA can further be defined by a set of key events that are required for tumor development (Preston and Williams, 2005). In addition, the key events can be used to establish whether or not a particular MoA described for a rodent model is plausible in humans (the so-called Human Relevance Framework, Meek *et al.*, 2003; Boobis *et al.*, 2006). This more defined approach based on the use of the best available science can possibly be extended to include noncancer health effects (Seed *et al.*, 2005; Boobis *et al.*, 2008).

Genetic Risk Assessment

The approach for conducting a genetic risk assessment is less well defined than that for cancer risk. In fact, only a handful of genetic risk assessments have been conducted. An in-depth discussion of the topic can be found in the book *Methods for Genetic Risk Assessment* (Brusick, 1994). The reader is also referred to the genetic risk for ethylene oxide developed by the EPA (Rhomberg *et al.*, 1990) and the discussion of this and a recalculation presented by Preston *et al.* (1995). These two articles serve to highlight the difficulties with and uncertainties in genetic risk assessments.

The general approach is to use rodent germ cell and somatic cell data for induced genetic alterations and human data for induced genetic alterations in somatic cells (when available) to estimate the frequency of genetic alterations in human germ cells. This is the "parallelogram approach" (Fig. 9-1) first used by Brewen and Preston (1974) for X-irradiation and subsequently more fully developed for chemical exposures by Sobels (1982). The aim of this approach is to develop two sensitivity factors: (1) somatic to germ cell in the rodent and (2) rodent to human using somatic cells. These factors can then be used to estimate genetic alterations in human germ cells. Of course, for a complete estimate of genetic risk, it is necessary to obtain an estimate of the frequency of genetic alterations transmitted to the offspring (UNSCEAR, 2001). In addition, separate genetic risk assessments need to be conducted for males and females, given the considerable difference in germ cell development and observed and predicted sensitivity differences. Of particular note with regard to genetic risk assessment, to date there has been no unequivocal demonstration of an effect that can be detected in the children following parental exposure for chemicals or ionizing radiation.

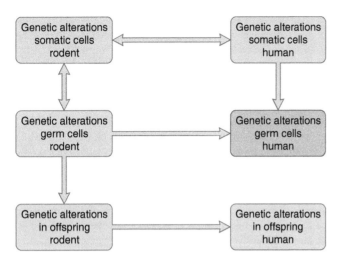

Figure 9-1. *Parallelogram approach for genetic risk assessment.* Data obtained for genetic alterations in rodent somatic and germ cells and human somatic cells are used to estimate the frequency of the same genetic alterations in human germ cells. The final step is to estimate the frequency of these genetic alterations that are transmitted to offspring.

MECHANISMS OF INDUCTION OF GENETIC ALTERATIONS

DNA Damage

The types of DNA damage produced by ionizing radiations, non-ionizing radiations, and chemicals are many and varied, including single- and double-strand breaks in the DNA backbone, cross-links between DNA bases or between DNA bases and proteins, and chemical addition to the DNA bases (adducts) (Fig. 9-2). The aim of this section is to introduce the topic of DNA damage because such damage is the substrate for the formation of genetic alterations and genotoxicity in general. However, much greater detail can be found in recent reviews that are referenced at the appropriate places within each section. It should be noted that endogenous processes and exogenous agents can produce DNA damage, but mutations themselves are produced by errors in DNA repair or replication that are a consequence of the induced DNA damage.

Ionizing Radiations Ionizing radiations such as x-rays, γ-rays, and α particles produce DNA single- and double-strand breaks and a broad range of base damages from oxidative processes (Goodhead, 1994; Wallace, 1994; Ward, 1994; Cadet *et al.*, 2010). In addition, recent evidence indicates that multiply damaged sites or clustered lesions can be formed that appear to be more difficult to repair (Eccles *et al.*, 2011). Such lesions consist of multi single lesions, including oxidized purine or pyrimidine bases, sites of base loss, and single-strand breaks. These multiple lesions can be formed in DNA from the same radiation energy deposition event (Blaisdell *et al.*, 2001). The relative proportions of these different classes of DNA damage vary with type of radiation. For example, single-strand breaks and base damages predominate with x-rays, for which ionization density is sparse, whereas the frequencies of single- and double-strand breaks are more similar with α particles, for which ionization is dense. The frequencies of individual base damages have been assessed using monoclonal antibodies, for example (Le *et al.*, 1998), but only a very few of the total spectrum of lesions have so far been studied. More recently, it has been demonstrated that the modified histone γ-H2AX can be used as a sensitive marker of DNA double-strand breaks (Nakamura *et al.*, 2006; Mah *et al.*, 2010).

Ultraviolet Light Ultraviolet light (a nonionizing radiation) induces two predominant lesions, cyclobutane pyrimidine dimers and 6,4-photoproducts. These lesions have been studied extensively because they can be quantitated by both chemical and immunological methods (Friedberg *et al.*, 1995). In part because of this feature, the repair of cyclobutane dimers and 6,4-photoproducts has been well characterized, as discussed below.

Chemicals Chemicals can produce DNA alterations either directly (DNA-reactive) by forming adducts or indirectly by intercalation of the chemical between the base pairs (see Heflich, 1991, for a review). Intercalation of acridine compounds (eg, 9-aminoacridine) and other planar molecules in repetitive DNA sequences has long been associated with the induction of frameshift mutations in which one or two base pairs have been gained or lost (Ferguson and Denny, 1990; Hoffmann *et al.*, 2003). Many electrophilic chemicals react with DNA, forming covalent addition products (adducts). The DNA base involved and the positions on DNA bases can be specific for a given chemical. Such specificity of DNA damage can result in a spectrum of mutations that is chemical specific, that is, a fingerprint of sorts (Dogliotti *et al.*, 1998; Jarabek *et al.*, 2009). Some alkylated bases can mispair, causing mutations when DNA is replicated. Alkylated bases can also lead to secondary alterations in DNA. For example, the alkyl group of an N^7-alkylguanine adduct, which is a major adduct formed by many alkylating agents, labilizes the bond that connects the base to deoxyribose, thereby stimulating base loss. Base loss from DNA leaves an apurinic or apyrimidinic site, commonly called an AP site. The insertion of incorrect bases into AP sites causes mutations (Laval *et al.*, 1990).

Bulky DNA adducts formed, for example, by metabolites of benzo(*a*)pyrene or *N*-2-acetylaminofluorene are recognized by the cell in a similar way to UV damages and are repaired similarly (see below). Such adducts can also hinder polymerases and cause mutation as a consequence of errors that they trigger in replication.

Endogenous Agents Endogenous agents are responsible for several hundred DNA damages per cell per day (Lindahl, 2000). The majority of these damages are altered DNA bases (eg, 8-oxoguanine and thymine glycol) and AP sites. The cellular processes that can lead to DNA damage are oxygen consumption that results in the formation of reactive oxygen species (eg, superoxide $O_2^{\cdot}$, hydroxyl free radicals $^{\cdot}OH$, and hydrogen peroxide) and deamination of cytosine and 5-methylcytosine leading to uracil and thymine, respectively. The process of DNA replication itself is somewhat error-prone, and an incorrect base can be added by replication polymerases (one in about 10^6 bases replicated). However, the frequency of misinserted bases in replication is not the sole determinant of the spontaneous mutation frequency. Living cells reduce the rate of polymerase error appreciably through error recognition and repair processes (Johnson, 2010). A high-fidelity polymerase may make one error in a million bases while copying roughly 300 base pairs per second, but polymerase proofreading and mismatch correction then lower the error rate as much as 1000-fold (Johnson, 2010). The result is a low spontaneous mutation rate. A recent study based on the sequencing of 19 *Escherichia coli* genomes in a 40,000-generation experiment estimated the rate of spontaneous base pair substitutions to be 8.9×10^{-11} per base pair per generation (Wielgoss *et al.*, 2011). Despite the fidelity of these biological processes, the frequencies of endogenously produced DNA damages can be increased by exogenous (genotoxic) agents (Swenberg *et al.*, 2011).

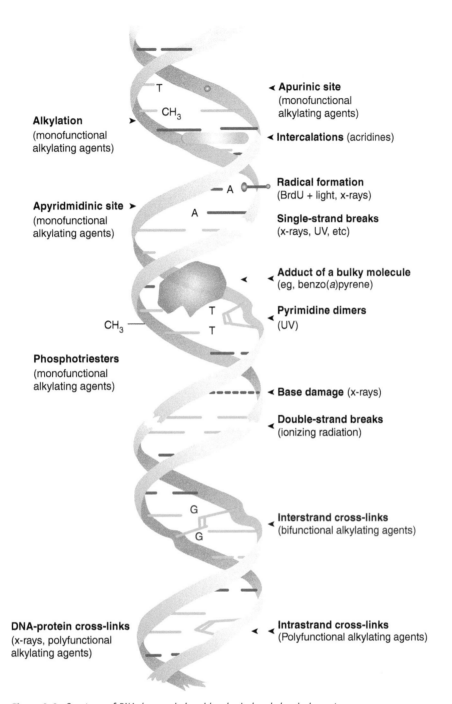

Alkylation
(monofunctional
alkylating agents)

Apyridmidinic site ➤
(monofunctional
alkylating agents)

Phosphotriesters
(monofunctional
alkylating agents)

DNA-protein cross-links
(x-rays, polyfunctional
alkylating agents)

◄ Apurinic site
(monofunctional
alkylating agents)

◄ Intercalations (acridines)

Radical formation
(BrdU + light, x-rays)

Single-strand breaks
(x-rays, UV, etc)

◄ Adduct of a bulky molecule
(eg, benzo(a)pyrene)

Pyrimidine dimers
(UV)

◄ Base damage (x-rays)

Double-strand breaks
(ionizing radiation)

Interstrand cross-links
(bifunctional alkylating agents)

Intrastrand cross-links
(Polyfunctional alkylating agents)

Figure 9-2. *Spectrum of DNA damage induced by physical and chemical agents.*

DNA Repair

The cell is faced with the problem of how to cope with the quite extensive DNA damage that it sustains. In a general sense, two processes are present to achieve this. If the damage is extensive, the cell can undergo apoptosis (programmed cell death), effectively avoiding its becoming a mutant cell (Evan and Littlewood, 1998). If the damage is less severe, it can be repaired by a range of processes that are part of a generalized cellular DNA damage response network that returns the DNA to its undamaged state (error-free repair) or to an improved but still altered state (error-prone repair). As a feature of this error-prone repair, it has been demonstrated that a family of polymerases, the eukaryotic translesion synthesis polymerases (eg, human Y-family polymerases eta, iota, kappa, and Rev1), can bypass lesions that otherwise would

block replication by the normal processive polymerases (Rattray and Strathern, 2003; Prakash *et al.*, 2005). These polymerases have the ability to bypass specific DNA lesions or groups of lesions. The result of the bypass can be an incorrect DNA sequence or a correct one depending on the induced lesion and the particular bypass polymerase. The basic principles underlying most repair processes (but not translesion synthesis) are damage recognition, followed by either direct reversal of the damage (eg, sealing of strand breaks or cleavage of pyrimidine dimers) or removal of the damage, repair DNA synthesis, and ligation. In order to achieve this for different types of DNA lesions, cells have modified the protein complexes used for other housekeeping processes (eg, transcription, replication, and recombination). This chapter presents a brief outline of the major classes of DNA repair; much greater detail can be found in the reviews provided for each section and general reviews by Van Houten and Albertini (1995), Friedberg (2000), Wood *et al.* (2005), and Bansbach and Cortez (2011).

Base Excision Repair The major pathways by which DNA base damages are repaired involve a glycosylase that removes the damaged base, causing the production of an apurinic or apyrimidinic site that can be filled by the appropriate base or processed further (Demple and Harrison, 1994; Seeberg *et al.*, 1995; Wood, 1996; McCullough *et al.*, 1999; Sung and Demple, 2006). The resulting gap from this further processing can be filled by a DNA polymerase, followed by ligation to the parental DNA. The size of the gap is dependent on the particular polymerase involved in the repair (ie, polymerase β for short patches; polymerase δ or ϵ for longer patches). Oxidative damage, either background or induced, are important substrates for base excision repair (Lindahl, 2000). The role of translesion bypass polymerases in the repair of DNA base alterations is discussed above.

Nucleotide Excision Repair The nucleotide excision repair (NER) system provides the cell's ability to remove bulky lesions from DNA. In the past decade the NER process has been studied extensively, and a complete characterization of the genes and proteins involved has been obtained (Reardon and Sancar, 2006; Reed, 2011). NER uses about 30 proteins to remove a damage-containing oligonucleotide from DNA. The basic steps are damage recognition, incision, excision, repair synthesis, and ligation. The characterization of these steps has been enhanced by the use of rodent mutant cell lines and cells from individuals with the UV-sensitivity, skin cancer-prone syndrome xeroderma pigmentosum (XP, for which there are at least seven distinct genetic complementation groups). Of particular interest is the link between NER and transcription, for which the DNA damage in actively transcribing genes, and specifically the transcribed strand, is preferentially and thus more rapidly repaired than the DNA damage in the rest of the genome (Lommel *et al.*, 1995; Jiang and Sancar, 2006). Thus, the cell protects the integrity of the transcription process. This link between transcription and repair appears to be provided by two factors: (1) when a bulky lesion is located on the transcribed strand of an active gene, RNA polymerase II is blocked, thus providing a signal for recruiting the NER complex, and (2) a major component of the NER complex is the TFII H basal transcription factor. The involvement of TFII H in repair also provides some specificity to the incisions in the DNA required to remove the damaged nucleotide. An incision on the 3′ side of the damage is made first by the XPG protein followed by 1 on the 5′ side by the XPF–ERRC1 complex. The lesion is removed in the 27- to 30-nucleotide segment formed by the two incisions. The gap is filled by polymerase δ or ϵ in the presence of replication factor C and proliferating cell nuclear antigen (PCNA). Ligation by DNA ligase I completes the process. This NER process has been reconstituted in vitro, allowing for complete characterization, kinetic studies, and estimates of fidelity (Aboussekhra *et al.*, 1995).

Double-Strand Break Repair Cell survival is seriously compromised by the presence in the cell of broken chromosomes. Unrepaired double-strand breaks trigger one or more DNA damage response systems to either check cell-cycle progression or induce apoptosis. In order to reduce the probability of persistent DNA double-strand breaks, cells have developed an array of specific repair pathways. These pathways are largely similar across a broad range of species from yeast to humans, although the most frequently used one is different among species. There are two general pathways for repair of DNA double-strand breaks: homologous recombination and nonhomologous end-joining. These two can be considered as being in competition for the double-strand break substrate (Haber, 2000; Sonoda *et al.*, 2006; Mladenov and Iliakis, 2011).

Homologous Recombination Eukaryotes undergo homologous recombination as part of their normal activities both in germ cells (meiotic recombination) and somatic cells (mitotic recombination) Zheng *et al.*, 2011. The repair of double-strand breaks (and single-strand gaps) basically uses the same process and complex of proteins, although some different protein–protein interactions are involved (Shinohara and Ogawa, 1995). In eukaryotes, the process has been characterized most extensively for yeast, but evidence is accumulating that a very similar process occurs in mammalian cells, including human (Johnson *et al.*, 1999; Cahill *et al.*, 2006). The basic steps in double-strand break repair are as follows. The initial step is the production of a 3′-ended single-stranded tail by exonucleases or helicase activity. Through a process of strand invasion, whereby the single-stranded tail invades an undamaged homologous DNA molecule, together with DNA synthesis, a so-called Holliday junction DNA complex is formed. By cleavage of this junction, two DNA molecules are produced (with or without a structural crossover), neither of which now contain a strand break. Additional models have been proposed but probably play a minor role in mammalian cells (Haber, 2000). A detailed description of the specific enzymes known to be involved can be found in Shinohara and Ogawa (1995), Cahill *et al.* (2006), and Hiom (2010).

Nonhomologous End-Joining The characterization of nonhomologous end-joining (NHEJ) in mammalian cells was greatly enhanced by the observation that mammalian cell lines that are hypersensitive to ionizing radiation are also defective in the V(D)J recombination process, which is the means by which the huge range of an antibody's antigen-binding sites and T-cell receptor proteins are generated during mammalian lymphoid cell development. V(D)J recombination requires the production of double-strand breaks, recombination of DNA pieces, and subsequent religation. A major component of the NHEJ repair complex is a DNA-dependent protein kinase (DNA-PK). This protein, a serine/threonine kinase, consists of a catalytic subunit (DNA-PK$_{cs}$) and a DNA-end-binding protein consisting of KU70 and KU80 subunits. The specific role of DNA-PK in the repair of double-strand breaks is unclear in mammalian cells; a detailed discussion of what is known and some possible models of NHEJ are presented in the reviews by Critchlow and Jackson (1998) and Burma *et al.* (2006). Perhaps the most viable role of DNA-PK is to align the broken DNA ends to facilitate their ligation. It also appears that DNA-PK helps in the selection of the specific repair pathway that is ultimately used for repair (Neal and Meek, 2011). In addition, DNA-PK might serve as a signal molecule for recruiting other repair proteins known to be involved in yeast and to some extent in mammalian cells. The final ligation step is performed by DNA ligase IV in human cells.

Mismatch Repair The study of DNA mismatch repair systems has received considerable attention over the past few years, in part, because an association has been demonstrated between genetic defects in mismatch repair genes and the genomic instability associated with cancer susceptibility syndromes and sporadic cancers. In general, DNA mismatch repair systems operate to repair mismatched bases formed during DNA replication, genetic recombination, and as a result of DNA damage induced by chemical and physical agents. Detailed reviews can be found in Kolodner (1995), Jiricny (1998), Modrich and Lahue (1996), and Jun *et al.* (2006).

The principal steps in all cells from prokaryotes to human are damage recognition by a specific protein that binds to the mismatch, stabilizing of the binding by the addition of one or more proteins, cutting the DNA at a distance from the mismatch, excision past the mismatch, resynthesis, and ligation. In some prokaryotes, the cutting of the DNA (for DNA replication mismatches) is directed to the strand that contains the incorrect base by using the fact that recently replicated DNA is unmethylated at N^6-methyladenine at a GATC sequence. The question of whether or not strand-specific mismatch repair occurs in mammalian cells has not been resolved, although evidence does point to its occurrence (Modrich, 1997; Mastrocola and Heinen, 2010). Strand specificity for DNA mismatches resulting from induced DNA damage has not been identified.

O^6-Methylguanine-DNA Methyltransferase Repair The main role for O^6-methylguanine-DNA methyltransferase (MGMT) is to protect cells against the toxic effects of simple alkylating agents. The methyl group is transferred from O^6-methylguanine in DNA to a cysteine residue in MGMT. The adducted base is reverted to a normal one by the enzyme, which is itself inactivated by the reaction. Details of the MGMT enzyme properties and the gene isolation and characterization can be found in Tano *et al.* (1990), Grombacher *et al.* (1996), and Margison *et al.* (2003).

The probability that induced DNA damage can be converted into a genetic alteration is influenced by the particular repair pathways recruited, the rate of repair of the damage, and the fidelity and completeness of the repair. The mechanisms of induction of gene mutations and chromosome alterations discussed in the following sections build upon the assessment of the probability of repair versus misrepair versus nonrepair that can be derived from a knowledge of the mechanism of action of the different DNA repair mechanisms. The preceding sections, together with the references provided, should assist in this assessment.

Formation of Gene Mutations

Somatic Cells Gene mutations are considered to be small DNA sequence changes confined to a single gene; larger genomic changes are considered below, under the section "Formation of Chromosomal Alterations." The general classes of gene mutations are base substitutions and small additions or deletions. More detailed classifications can be found in the review by Ripley (1991). Base substitutions are the replacement of the correct nucleotide by an incorrect one; they can be further subdivided as transitions where the change is purine for purine or pyrimidine for pyrimidine, and transversions where the change is purine for pyrimidine and vice versa. Frameshift mutations are strictly the addition or deletion of one or a few base pairs (not in multiples of three) in protein-coding regions. The definition is more generally expanded to include such additions and deletions in any DNA region. For the discussion of the mechanism of induction of gene mutations and chromosomal alterations, it is necessary to distinguish chemicals by their general mode of action. Chemicals that can produce genetic alterations with similar effectiveness in all stages of the cell cycle are called radiomimetic because they act like radiation in this regard. Chemicals that produce genetic alterations far more effectively in the S phase of the cell cycle are described as nonradiomimetic. The great majority of chemicals are nonradiomimetic; the radiomimetic group includes bleomycin, streptonigrin, neocarzinostatin, and 8-ethoxycaffeine.

Gene mutations can arise in the absence of specific exogenous exposures to radiation and chemicals. The great majority of so-called spontaneous (background) mutations arise from *replication* of an altered template. The DNA alterations that arise are either the result of oxidative damage or produced from the deamination

of 5-methylcytosine to thymine at CpG sites resulting in G:C → A:T transitions. Mutations induced by ionizing radiations tend to be deletions ranging in size from a few bases to multilocus events (Thacker, 1992). The rapid rate of repair of the majority of radiation-induced DNA damages greatly reduces the probability of DNA lesions being present at the time of DNA replication. Thus, mutations induced by ionizing radiations are generally the result of errors of *DNA repair* (Preston, 1992). The low frequencies of gene mutations are produced from any unrepaired DNA base damage present during DNA replication.

Gene mutations produced by a majority of chemicals and non-ionizing radiations are base substitutions, frameshifts, and small deletions. Of these mutations, a very high proportion is produced by errors of DNA *replication* on a damaged template. Thus, the probability of a DNA adduct, for example, being converted into a mutation is determined, to a significant extent by the number of induced DNA adducts that remain in the DNA at the time that it is replicated and by the nature of the adduct itself (Jarabek *et al.*, 2009). Thus, relative mutation frequency will be the outcome of the race between repair and replication, that is, in general terms, the more repair that takes place prior to replication, the lower the mutation frequency for a given amount of induced DNA damage. Significant regulators of the race are cell cycle checkpoint genes (eg, *P53*) because if the cell is checked from entering the S phase at a G_1/S checkpoint, more repair can take place prior to the cell starting to replicate its DNA (Mercer, 1998; Giglia-Mari *et al.*, 2011).

The proportion of chemically induced gene mutations that result from DNA repair errors is low, given that the DNA repair processes, unlike translesion synthesis, are typically error-free. Moreover, repair of chemically induced DNA damage is generally slower than for ionizing radiation damage, for which the balance tips toward replication prior to repair, especially for cells in the S phase at the time of exposure. In the case of translesion bypass, discussed above, gene mutations can be produced at relatively high frequencies.

Germ Cells The mechanism of production of gene mutations in germ cells is basically the same as in somatic cells. Ionizing radiations produce mainly deletions via errors of DNA repair; the majority of chemicals induce base substitutions, frameshifts, and small deletions by errors of DNA replication (Favor, 1999).

An important consideration for assessing gene mutations induced by chemicals in germ cells is the relationship between exposure and the timing of DNA replication. Fig. 9-3 depicts the stages in oogenesis and spermatogenesis. A few features are worthy of note. The spermatogonial stem cell in humans and rodents has a long cell cycle time, eight days or longer, with only a small fraction being occupied by the S phase. Thus, the probability of DNA repair taking place prior to DNA replication is high, for both acute and chronic treatments. However, for considerations of genetic risk, it is the spermatogonial stem cell that is the major contributor because it is present, in general, throughout the reproductive lifetime of an individual. Each time a spermatogonial stem cell divides it produces a differentiating spermatogonium and a stem cell. Thus, the stem cell can accumulate genetic damage from chronic exposures. Differentiating spermatogonia, as far as the induction of gene mutation is concerned, are the same as mitotically dividing somatic cells.

The first S phase after gametogenesis occurs in the zygote, formed by fertilization. This fact needs to be balanced by the lack of DNA repair in late spermatids and sperm. Thus, DNA damage induced in these stages will remain until the zygote. Postmeiotic germ cells are particularly sensitive to mutation induction by

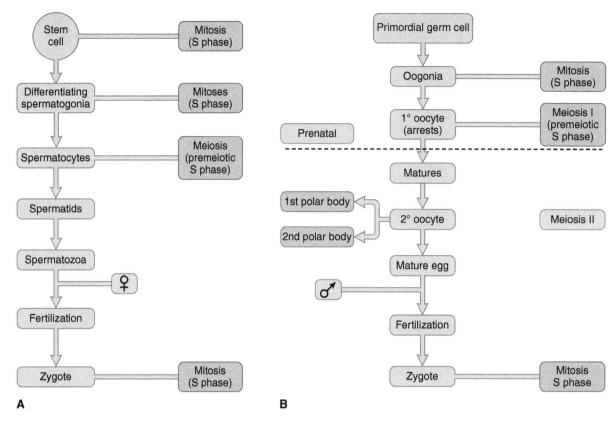

Figure 9-3. *The stages of spermatogenesis (**A**) and oogenesis (**B**) indicating the periods of cell division and DNA replication (S phase).*

nonradiomimetic chemicals, especially following acute exposures (Russell, 2004). The fairly short duration of this stage (approximately 21 days in the mouse) means that their contribution to genetic risk following chronic exposures is quite small.

For oogenesis (Fig. 9-3) similar observations on gene mutation induction and timing of S phase can be made. In this case the primary oocyte arrests prior to birth, and there is no further S phase until the zygote. For this reason, the oocyte is resistant to the induction of gene mutations by nonradiomimetic chemicals but not to radiation, for which DNA repair is the mode of formation of mutations, and DNA repair occurs in oocytes (Brewen and Preston, 1982).

These mechanistic aspects of the production of gene mutations (and chromosome alterations described in the following two sections) by chemicals and radiation in somatic and germ cells are most important for considerations of the design of genetic toxicology assays, the interpretation of the data generated, and the incorporation of the data into cancer and genetic risk assessments.

Formation of Chromosomal Alterations

Somatic Cells

Structural Chromosome Aberrations There are components of the formation of chromosome aberrations, SCEs (the apparently reciprocal exchange between the sister chromatids of a single chromosome), and gene mutations that are similar. In particular, damaged DNA serves as the substrate leading to all these events. However, chromosome aberrations induced by ionizing radiations are generally formed by errors of DNA repair, whereas those produced by nonradiomimetic chemicals are generally formed by errors of DNA replication on a damaged DNA template.

The DNA repair errors that lead to the formation of chromosome aberrations following ionizing radiation (and radiomimetic chemical) exposure arise from misligation of double-strand breaks or interaction of coincidentally repairing regions during NER of damaged bases. The details of the DNA damage types and their repair are described in the previous section. Thus, the overall kinetics and fidelity of DNA repair influence the sensitivity of cells to the induction of chromosomal aberrations produced by misrepair. The broad outcomes of misrepair are that incorrect rejoining of chromosomal pieces during repair leads to chromosomal exchanges within (eg, inversions and interstitial deletions) and between (eg, dicentrics and reciprocal translocations) chromosomes. In fact, using FISH, it can be shown that very complex rearrangements take place (Anderson *et al.*, 2000). Failure to rejoin double-strand breaks or to complete repair of other types of DNA damage leads to terminal deletions.

Acentric fragments arise from interstitial deletions, terminal deletions, and the formation of dicentric chromosomes and rings. The failure to incorporate an acentric fragment into a daughter nucleus at anaphase/telophase, or the failure of a whole chromosome to segregate at anaphase to the cellular poles, can result in the formation of a membrane-bound micronucleus that resides in the cytoplasm.

Errors of DNA replication on a damaged template can lead to a variety of chromosomal alterations. The majority of these involve deletion or exchange of individual chromatids (chromatid-type aberrations). Thus, nonradiomimetic chemicals induce only chromatid-type aberrations, whereas radiations and radiomimetic chemicals induce chromatid-type aberrations in the S and G_2 phases of the cell cycle, but chromosome-type aberrations affecting both chromatids in G_1. The reason for this latter observation is that the G_1 (or G_0) chromosome behaves as a single DNA molecule and aberrations formed in it will be replicated in the S phase and will involve both chromatids. This distinction is important for considerations of outcome of the aberrations and the probability of an effect on cells because for chromatid-type aberrations, one chromatid remains intact and genetically unaltered, in contrast to chromosome-type aberrations in which both chromatids are damaged (Preston *et al.*, 1995).

Numerical Chromosome Changes Numerical changes (eg, monosomies, trisomies, and ploidy changes) can arise from errors in chromosomal segregation. The complexity of the control and the mechanics of the mitotic process means that alteration of various cellular components can result in failure to segregate the sister chromatids to separate daughter cells or in failure to segregate a chromosome to either pole (Bickel and Orr-Weaver, 1996; Preston, 1996; Hunt, 2006). The mechanisms underlying chromosomal loss are pertinent to those involved in the formation of micronuclei.

A limited set of chemicals has been demonstrated to cause aneuploidy through interaction with components of the structures that facilitate chromosome movement (Preston, 1996; Aardema *et al.*, 1998). These include benomyl, griseofulvin, nocodazole, colchicine, colecemid, vinblastine, and paclitaxel. These chemicals affect tubulin polymerization or spindle microtubule stability. To date, other mechanisms of aneuploidy induction by chemicals have not been firmly identified.

Sister Chromatid Exchanges SCEs are produced during the S phase and are presumed to be a consequence of errors in the replication process, perhaps at the sites of stalled replication complexes (Painter, 1980; Heartlein *et al.*, 1983; Preston, 1991; Wilson and Thompson, 2007). Because SCEs are apparently reciprocal exchanges, it is quite possible that they result from a recombination process occurring at the site of the stalled replication fork. It is, in fact, this mode of action that makes assays for SCE less than ideal for detecting effects due directly to a chemical exposure. For example, the creation of intracellular conditions that slow the progress of DNA replication could lead to the formation of SCE.

Germ Cells The formation of chromosomal alterations in germ cells is basically the same as that for somatic cells, namely, via misrepair for ionizing radiations and radiomimetic chemicals for treatments in G_1 and G_2, and by errors of replication for all radiations and chemicals for DNA damage present during the S phase. Also, the restrictions on the timing of formation of chromosomal alterations induced by nonradiomimetic chemicals in germ cells is as described above for gene mutations, namely at the specific stages where DNA synthesis occurs, as depicted in Fig. 9-3.

The types of aberrations formed in germ cells are the same as those formed in somatic cells (eg, deletions, inversions, translocations), although their appearance in diplotene/diakinesis of meiosis I, where analysis is frequently conducted, is rather different because of the homologous chromosome pairing that takes place in meiotic cells (see the review by Léonard, 1973). The specific segregation of chromosomes during meiosis influences the probability of recovery of an aberration, particularly a reciprocal translocation, in the offspring of a treated parent. This is discussed in detail in Preston *et al.* (1995).

ASSAYS FOR DETECTING GENETIC ALTERATIONS

Introduction to Assay Design

Genetic toxicology assays are used to identify germ cell mutagens, somatic cell mutagens, and potential carcinogens. These assays can detect diverse kinds of genetic alterations (eg, gene mutations,

Table 9-1

Principal Assays in Genetic Toxicology

I. Pivotal assays
    A. A well-characterized assay for gene mutations
       The *Salmonella*/mammalian microsome assay (Ames test)
    B. A mammalian assay for chromosome damage in vivo: metaphase analysis in rodent bone marrow or micronucleus assay in rodent bone marrow or blood

II. Other assays offering an extensive database or unique genetic endpoint
    A. Assays for gene mutations
       E coli WP2 tryptophan reversion assay
       TK or *HPRT* forward mutation assays in cultured mammalian cells
       Drosophila sex-linked recessive lethal assay
       Gene-mutation assays in rodent somatic cells or transgenic animals
    B. Cytogenetic analysis in cultured Chinese hamster or human cells
       Assays for chromosome aberrations and micronuclei
       Assays for aneuploidy
    C. Other indicators of genetic damage
       Mammalian DNA damage and repair assays
       Mitotic recombination assays in yeast and *Drosophila*
    D. Mammalian germ cell assays
       Mouse specific-locus tests
       Cytogenetic analysis and heritable translocation assays
       DNA damage and repair in rodent germ cells
       Mutation analysis in tandem-repeat loci in mice

chromosome aberrations, and aneuploidy) that are relevant to the production of adverse human health outcomes. Over the last three decades, hundreds of chemicals and complex mixtures have been evaluated for genotoxic effects. Genetic toxicology assays serve two interrelated but distinct purposes in the toxicologic evaluation of chemicals: (1) identifying mutagens for purposes of hazard identification and (2) characterizing dose–response relationships and mutagenic mechanisms, both of which contribute to an understanding of genetic and carcinogenic risks.

A common experience when surveying the genetic toxicology literature is encountering a bewildering array of assays in viruses, bacteria, fungi, cultured mammalian cells, plants, insects, and mammals. More than 200 assays for mutagens have been proposed, and useful information has been obtained from many of them. Although most genetic toxicology testing and evaluation relies on relatively few assays, data from relatively obscure assays can sometimes contribute to a judgment about the genetic activity of a compound.

Table 9-1 lists key assays that have a prominent place in genetic toxicology. Table 9-2 is a more comprehensive list that provides literature citations to many of the assays that one might encounter in the genetic toxicology literature. Even this extensive table is not exhaustive, in that it emphasizes methods in applied genetic toxicology and not those assays whose use has been largely restricted to studies of mutational mechanisms. The commonly used assays rely on phenotypic effects as indicators of gene mutations or small deletions and on cytological methods for observing

Table 9-2

Overview of Genetic Toxicology Assays

ASSAYS	SELECTED LITERATURE CITATIONS
I. Prediction of genotoxicity	
A. Interpretation of chemical structure	
Structural alerts to genotoxicity	Ashby, (1994), Ashby and Tennant (1991), Ashby and Paton (1993)
B. In silico predictive models	
Computational and structural programs: MCASE, TOPKAT, DEREK	Snyder *et al.* (2004), Snyder and Smith (2005), Snyder (2009), Mahadevan *et al.* (2011)
Quantitative structure–activity relationship (QSAR) modeling	Votano *et al.* (2004), Snyder and Smith (2005), Mahadevan *et al.* (2011)
II. DNA damage and repair assays	
A. Direct detection of DNA damage:	
Alkaline elution assays for DNA strand breakage in hepatocytes	Storer *et al.* (1996), Gealy *et al.* (2007)
Comet assay (single-cell gel electrophoresis) for DNA strand breakage	Fairbairn *et al.* (1995), Singh (2000), Tice *et al.* (2000), Collins (2004), Olive (2009)
Comet-FISH assay for region-specific DNA damage and repair	Glei *et al.* (2009), Shaposhnikov *et al.* (2009)
Nonmammalian comets in ecotoxicology	Cotelle and Férard (1999), Lee and Steinert (2003), Jha (2004)
Assays for chemical adducts in DNA	Phillips *et al.* (2000), Farmer and Singh (2008), Himmelstein *et al.* (2009)
B. DNA repair, recombination, and genotoxic stress responses as indicators of damage:	
Differential killing of repair-deficient and wild type bacteria	Takigami *et al.* (2002)
Induction of the bacterial SOS system	Quillardet and Hofnung (1993), Yasunaga *et al.* (2004), Oda *et al.* (2009)
"Green Screen" for *GADD45a* gene induction in TK6 human cells	Hastwell *et al.* (2009), Jagger *et al.* (2009)
Unscheduled DNA synthesis (UDS) in isolated rat hepatocytes or rodents in vivo	Madle *et al.* (1994), Kirkland and Speit (2008)
Induction of mitotic recombination	Zimmermann (1992), Hoffmann (1994), Vogel and Nivard (2000), Turner *et al.* (2003), Reliene *et al.* (2007)
III. Prokaryote gene mutation assays	
A. Bacterial reverse mutation assays:	
Salmonella/mammalian microsome assay (Ames test)	Ames *et al.* (1975), Kier *et al.* (1986), Maron and Ames (1983), Gatehouse *et al.* (1994), Mortelmans and Zeiger (2000), Seifried *et al.* (2006), Claxton *et al.* (2010)
E coli WP2 tryptophan reversion assay	Gatehouse *et al.* (1994), Mortelmans and Riccio (2000)
Salmonella-specific base-pair substitution assay (Ames II assay)	Gee *et al.* (1994), Kamber *et al.* (2009)
E coli lacZ-specific reversion assay	Cupples and Miller (1989), Cupples *et al.* (1990), Josephy (2000), Hoffmann *et al.* (2003)
B. Bacterial forward mutation assays:	
E coli lacI assay	Calos and Miller (1981), Halliday and Glickman (1991)
Resistance to toxic metabolites or analogs in *Salmonella*	Jurado *et al.* (1994), Vlasakova *et al.* (2005)
IV. Assays in nonmammalian eukaryotes:	
A. Fungal assays:	
Forward mutations, reversion, and small deletions	Zimmermann *et al.* (1984), Crouse (2000)
Mitotic crossing over, gene conversion, and homology-mediated deletions in yeast	Zimmermann *et al.* (1984), Zimmermann (1992), Howlett and Schiestl (2000), Daigaku *et al.* (2004), Freeman and Hoffmann (2007)
Genetic detection of mitotic and meiotic aneuploidy in yeast	Zimmermann *et al.* (1984), Aardema *et al.* (1998), Howlett and Schiestl (2000), Nunoshiba *et al.* (2007)
B. Plant assays:	
Gene mutations affecting chlorophyll in seedlings, the *waxy* locus in pollen, or Tradescantia stamen-hair color	Ma *et al.* (2005), Grant and Owens (2006)

(continued)

Table 9-2

457

(*Continued*)

ASSAYS	SELECTED LITERATURE CITATIONS
Chromosome aberrations and micronuclei in mitotic and meiotic cells of corn, Tradescantia, and other plants	Ma *et al.* (2005), Grant and Owens (2006), Misík *et al.* (2011)
C. Drosophila assays:	
Sex-linked recessive lethal test in germ cells	Lee *et al.* (1983), Mason *et al.* (1987), Vogel *et al.* (1999)
Heritable translocation assays	Mason *et al.* (1987), Vogel *et al.* (1999)
Mitotic recombination and LOH in eyes or wings	Vogel *et al.* (1999), Vogel and Nivard (2000)
V. Mammalian gene mutation assays	
A. In vitro assays for forward mutations:	
tk mutations in mouse lymphoma or human cells	Clements (2000), Seifried *et al.* (2006), Wang *et al.* (2009), Moore *et al.* (2011)
hprt or x*prt* mutations in Chinese hamster or human cells	Li *et al.* (1988), DeMarini *et al.* (1989), Parry *et al.* (2005)
CD59 mutations in CHO-human hybrid A_L cells	Zhou *et al.* (2006), Ross *et al.* (2007)
B. In vivo assays for gene mutations in somatic cells:	
Mouse spot test (somatic cell specific-locus test)	Styles and Penman (1985), Lambert *et al.* (2005)
hprt mutations (6-thioguanine-resistance) in rodent lymphocytes	Cariello and Skopek (1993), Casciano *et al.* (1999), Lambert *et al.*, 2005
Pig-a mutations (immunological detection of mutations blocking glycosylphosphatidylinositol synthesis)	Dobrovolsky *et al.* (2010), Miura *et al.* (2011), Dobo *et al.* (2011)
C. Transgenic assays:	
Mutations in the bacterial *lacI* gene in "Big Blue" mice and rats	Lambert *et al.* (2005), Singer *et al.* (2006)
Mutations in the bacterial *lacZ* gene in the "Muta Mouse"	Lambert *et al.* (2005), Singer *et al.* (2006)
Mutations in the phage *cII* gene in *lacI* or *lacZ* transgenic mice	Swiger (2001), Lambert *et al.* (2005)
Point mutations and deletions in the *lacZ* plasmid mouse	Lambert *et al.* (2005), Singer *et al.* (2006)
Point mutations and deletions in *delta gpt* mice and rats	Okada *et al.* (1999), Lambert *et al.* (2005)
Forward mutations and reversions in ΦX174 transgenic mice	Valentine *et al.* (2010)
Inversions and deletions arising in pKZ1 mice by intrachromosomal recombination	Sykes *et al.* (2006)
VI. Mammalian cytogenetic assays	
A. Chromosome aberrations:	
Metaphase analysis in cultured Chinese hamster or human cells	Ishidate *et al.* (1988), Kirkland *et al.* (1990), Galloway *et al.* (1994), Galloway (2000), Corvi *et al.* (2008), Galloway *et al.* (2011)
Metaphase analysis of rodent bone marrow or lymphocytes in vivo	Preston *et al.* (1981), Kirkland *et al.* (1990), Tice *et al.* (1994)
Chromosome painting and other FISH applications in vitro and in vivo	Tucker *et al.* (1993b, 2005), Paccierotti and Sgura (2008)
B. Micronuclei:	
Cytokinesis-block micronucleus assay in human lymphocytes	Fenech *et al.* (2003), Corvi *et al.* (2008), Fenech (2008), Fenech *et al.* (2011a,b)
Micronucleus assay in mammalian cell lines	Kirsch-Volders *et al.* (2003), Corvi *et al.* (2008), Galloway *et al.* (2011)
In vivo micronucleus assay in rodent bone marrow or blood	Krishna and Hayashi (2000), Hayashi *et al.* (2007), Tweats *et al.* (2007), Dertinger *et al.* (2011)
In vivo micronucleus assay in tissues other than marrow or blood	Hayashi *et al.* (2007), Coffing *et al.* (2011), Morita *et al.* (2011)
C. Sister chromatid exchange:	
SCE in human cells or Chinese hamster cells	Tucker *et al.* (1993a), Wilson and Thompson (2007)
SCE in rodent tissues, especially bone marrow	Tucker *et al.* (1993a)

(*continued*)

Table 9-2

Overview of Genetic Toxicology Assays *(Continued)*

ASSAYS	SELECTED LITERATURE CITATIONS
D. Aneuploidy in mitotic cells:	
Hyperploidy detected by chromosome counting or FISH in cell cultures or bone marrow	Galloway and Ivett (1986), Natarajan (1993), Aardema *et al.* (1998), Paccierotti and Sgura (2008)
Micronucleus assay with centromere/kinetochore labeling in cell cultures	Lynch and Parry (1993), Natarajan (1993), Aardema *et al.* (1998), Fenech (2008), Paccierotti and Sgura (2008)
Altered parameters in flow-cytometric detection of micronuclei in CHO cells	Bryce *et al.* (2011)
Mouse bone marrow micronucleus assay with centromere labeling	Adler (1993), Aardema *et al.* (1998), Krishna and Hayashi (2000)
VII. Germ cell mutagenesis	
A. Measurement of DNA damage	
Molecular dosimetry based on mutagen adducts in reproductive cells	Russell and Shelby (1985), Olsen *et al.* (2010), Verhofsrad *et al.* (2011)
UDS in rodent germ cells	Bentley *et al.* (1994), Sotomayor and Sega (2000)
Alkaline elution assays for DNA strand breaks in rodent testes	Bentley *et al.* (1994)
Comet assay in sperm and gonadal tissue	Speit *et al.* (2009)
B. Gene mutations	
Mouse specific-locus test for gene mutations and deletions	Russell *et al.* (1981), Ehling (1991), Russell and Russell (1992), Favor (1999), Russell (2004), Singer *et al.* (2006)
Mouse electrophoretic specific-locus test	Lewis (1991)
Dominant mutations causing mouse skeletal defects or cataracts	Ehling (1991), Selby *et al.* (2004)
ESTR assay in mice	Yauk (2004), Dubrova (2005), Singer *et al.* (2006), Somers (2006)
Germ cell mutations in transgenic assays	Lambert *et al.* (2005), Singer *et al.* (2006)
C. Chromosomal aberrations	
Cytogenetic analysis of oocytes, spermatogonia, spermatocytes, or zygotes	Kirkland *et al.* (1990), Tease (1992), Russo (2000), Marchetti *et al.* (2001)
Direct detection in sperm by FISH	Marchetti *et al.* (2006, 2008)
Micronuclei in mouse spermatids	Russo (2000), Hayashi *et al.* (2007)
Mouse heritable translocation test	Russell and Shelby (1985), Singer *et al.* (2006)
D. Dominant lethal mutations	
Mouse or rat dominant lethal assay	Adler *et al.* (1994), Singer *et al.* (2006)
E. Aneuploidy	
Cytogenetic analysis for aneuploidy arising by nondisjunction	Allen *et al.* (1986), Adler (1993), Adler *et al.* (1994), Aardema *et al.* (1998), Russo (2000), Marchetti *et al.* (2001)
Sex chromosome loss test for nondisjunction or breakage	Russell and Shelby (1985)
Micronucleus assay in spermatids with centromere labeling	Aardema *et al.* (1998)
FISH with probes for specific chromosomes in sperm	Russo (2000), Marchetti *et al.* (2006, 2008)

gross chromosomal damage. Detailed information on assay design, testing data, controls, sample sizes, and other factors in effective testing is found in the references cited.

Some assays for gene mutations detect forward mutations whereas others detect reversion. Forward mutations, such as those detected in the thymidine kinase gene (*tk*) in the widely used assay in mouse lymphoma cells (Clements, 2000; Wang *et al.*, 2009), are genetic alterations in a wild type gene that are detected by a change in phenotype caused by the alteration or loss of gene function. In contrast, back mutations are mutations that restore gene function in a mutant, such as the histidine revertants detected in the Ames assay in Salmonella (Ames *et al.*, 1975; Mortelmans and Zeiger, 2000; Claxton *et al.*, 2010). Thus, a back mutation or reversion that restores gene function in a mutant brings about a return to the

wild type phenotype. In principle, forward-mutation assays should respond to a broad spectrum of mutagens because any mutation that interferes with gene expression should confer the detectable phenotype. A reversion assay might be expected to have a more restricted mutational response because only mutations that correct or compensate for the specific mutation in a particular mutant will be detected. In fact, some reversion assays respond to a broader spectrum of mutational changes than one might expect because mutations at a site other than that of the original mutation, either within the test gene or in a different gene (ie, a suppressor mutation), can sometimes confer the selected phenotype. Both forward mutation assays and reversion assays are used extensively in genetic toxicology.

The simplest gene mutation assays rely on selection techniques to detect mutations. A selection technique is a means of imposing experimental conditions under which only cells or organisms that have undergone mutation can grow. For example, only cells that have a mutation in the *tk* gene can grow in medium containing the inhibitory chemical trifluorothymidine (Seifried *et al.*, 2006; Wang *et al.*, 2009). Selection techniques greatly facilitate the identification of rare cells that have experienced mutation among the many cells that have not. Forward mutations (Clements, 2000; Vlasakova *et al.*, 2005) and reversions (Josephy, 2000; Mortelmans and Riccio, 2000; Mortelmans and Zeiger, 2000; Kamber *et al.*, 2009) can both be detected by selection techniques in microorganisms and cultured mammalian cells. Because of their speed, low cost, and ease of detecting events that occur at low frequency (ie, mutation), assays in microorganisms and cell cultures have figured prominently in genetic toxicology.

Studying mutagenesis in intact animals requires assays of more complex design than the simple selection methods used in microorganisms and cultured cells. Genetic toxicology assays therefore range from inexpensive short-term tests (Zeiger, 2010) that can be performed in a few days to complicated assays for mutations in mammalian germ cells (Favor, 1999; Russell, 2004; Singer *et al.*, 2006). Even in multicellular organisms, there has been an emphasis on designing assays that detect mutations with great efficiency (Vogel *et al.*, 1999; Casciano *et al.*, 1999; Lambert *et al.*, 2005; Dobrovolsky *et al.*, 2010). Nevertheless, there remains a gradation in which an increase in relevance for human risk entails more elaborate and costly tests (Table 9-2). The most expensive mammalian tests are typically reserved for agents of special importance in basic research or risk assessment, whereas the simpler assays can be applied more broadly.

Cytogenetic assays differ in design from typical gene mutation assays because of their reliance on cytological rather than genetic methods. The goal in cytogenetic methods is the unequivocal visual recognition of cells that have experienced genetic damage. The alterations measured include chromosome aberrations (Preston *et al.*, 1981; Ishidate *et al.*, 1988; Corvi *et al.*, 2008), micronuclei (Hayashi *et al.*, 2007; Corvi *et al.*, 2008; Fenech *et al.*, 2011a,b), SCEs (Tucker *et al.*, 1993a; Wilson and Thompson, 2007), and changes in chromosome number (Aardema *et al.*, 1998; Paccierotti and Sgura, 2008). The latter include ploidy changes (eg, polyploid cells) and aneuploidy, in which one or a few chromosomes have been gained (ie, hyperploidy) or lost (ie, hypoploidy) relative to the normal chromosome number. Aneuploidy is of great interest because of its implications for human health, but assays for aneuploidy are not yet as refined or systematically applied as those for other classes of chromosomal alterations.

In all mutagenicity testing, one must be aware of possible sources of error. Factors to consider in the application of mutagenicity assays are the choice of suitable organisms and growth conditions, appropriate monitoring of genotypes and phenotypes, effective experimental design and treatment conditions, inclusion of proper positive and negative controls, and sound methods of data analysis. The articles cited in Table 9-2 discuss these aspects of genetic toxicology testing.

Many compounds that are not themselves mutagenic or carcinogenic can be activated into mutagens and carcinogens by metabolism (Guenngerich, 2001; Malling, 2004). Such compounds are called promutagens and procarcinogens. Because microorganisms and mammalian cell cultures lack many of the metabolic capabilities of intact mammals, provision must be made for metabolic activation in order to detect promutagens in many genetic assays. Incorporating an in vitro metabolic activation system derived from a mammalian tissue homogenate is the most common means of adding metabolic activation to microbial or cell culture assays (Malling and Frantz, 1973; Ames *et al.*, 1975; Clements, 2000; Malling, 2004). For example, the promutagens dimethylnitrosamine and benzo[*a*]pyrene are not themselves mutagenic in bacteria, but they are mutagenic in bacterial assays if the bacteria are treated with the promutagen in the presence of a homogenate from mammalian liver.

The most widely used metabolic activation system in microbial and cell culture assays is a postmitochondrial supernatant from a rat liver homogenate, along with appropriate buffers and cofactors (Maron and Ames, 1983; Kirkland *et al.*, 1990). The standard liver metabolic activation system is called an S9 mixture, designating a supernatant from centrifugation at 9000*g* (Malling and Frantz, 1973; Maron and Ames, 1983). Most of the short-term assays in Table 9-2 require exogenous metabolic activation to detect promutagens. Exceptions are assays in intact mammals and a few simpler assays that have a high level of endogenous cytochrome P450 metabolism, such as the detection of UDS or DNA strand breakage in cultured hepatocytes (Madle *et al.*, 1994; Gealy *et al.*, 2007).

Rat liver S9 provides a broad assemblage of metabolic reactions, but they are not necessarily the same as those of hepatic metabolism in an intact rat. Metabolic activation systems based on homogenates from mice, guinea pigs, hamsters, or monkeys and preparations from organs other than liver have found some use in mutagenicity testing (Mortelmans and Zeiger, 2000). In some cases, these systems detect mutagenicity more efficiently than rat liver S9. However, like a homogenate from rat liver, these systems may differ from the species or organs of their origin. Therefore, alternative metabolic activation systems tend to be more useful if chosen for mechanistic reasons rather than simply testing another species or organ. Such systems include the use of intact hepatocytes (Madle *et al.*, 1994; Storer *et al.*, 1996; Gealy *et al.*, 2007) to preserve the cellular compartmentalization of reactions; an in vitro system that can carry out the reduction reactions needed to detect the activity of substances whose mutagenicity requires reductive metabolism, such as some azo compounds (Mortelmans and Zeiger, 2000; Seifried *et al.*, 2006); and the use of mammalian cells or bacteria engineered to express foreign genes that encode enzymes of metabolic activation (Sawada and Kamataki, 1998; Crespi and Miller, 1999; Josephy, 2000, 2002; Oda *et al.*, 2009).

Besides metabolic activation, some chemicals are subject to photochemical activation. The genotoxicity of such chemicals depends on the chemical being irradiated with ultraviolet or visible light. Many of the assays listed in Table 9-2, including gene-mutation assays in bacteria and cultured mammalian cells, cytogenetic assays, and the comet assay, have been adapted so that they can measure photogenotoxic effects (Brendler-Schwaab *et al.*, 2004; Lynch *et al.*, 2011).

Genes encoding enzymes of xenobiotic metabolism have been incorporated by recombinant DNA technology into microorganisms or cell cultures to expand their capacity for metabolic activation. The genes incorporated into bacteria may be derived from other bacteria or from humans (Josephy, 2002; Oda *et al.*, 2009). For example, bacterial genes that cause overexpression of N-acetyltranserase enhance the sensitivity of the bacteria to the mutagenicity of aromatic amines or nitroarenes (Josephy, 2002). The expression of human cytochrome P450 enzymes in Salmonella tester strains from the Ames assay (Josephy 2002; Yamazaki *et al.*, 2004), a Salmonella SOS-induction assay (Oda *et al.*, 2009), or *E coli* strains of the *lacZ* reversion assay (Josephy, 2000) permits the activation of such promutagens as 2-aminoanthracene and 2-aminofluorene without an S9 mixture. Mammalian cell lines have also been genetically engineered to express human Phase-I and Phase-II enzymes, including those catalyzing reactions of metabolic activation (Sawada and Kamataki, 1998). Many cell lines stably expressing a single form of P450 have been established. Mutagenesis can be measured through such endpoints as *HPRT* mutations and cytogenetic alterations, and the cells are well suited to analyzing the contribution of different enzymes to the activation of promutagens (Crespi and Miller, 1999).

Metabolic activation is so central to genetic toxicology that all mutagenicity testing programs must provide for it in the choice of assays and procedures. Despite their usefulness, in vitro metabolic activation systems, however well refined, cannot mimic mammalian metabolism perfectly. There are differences among tissues in reactions that activate or inactivate foreign compounds, and organisms of the normal flora of the gut can contribute to metabolism in intact mammals. Agents that induce enzyme systems or otherwise alter the physiological state can also modify the metabolism of toxicants, and the balance between activation and detoxication reactions in vitro may differ from that in vivo.

Structural Alerts and In Silico Assays

The first indication that a chemical is a mutagen often lies in chemical structure. Potential electrophilic sites in a molecule serve as an alert to possible mutagenicity and carcinogenicity because such sites confer reactivity with nucleophilic sites in DNA (Tennant and Ashby, 1991). Structural alerts in combination with critical interpretation are a valuable adjunct to mutagenicity testing (Tennant and Ashby, 1991; Ashby and Paton, 1993). Attempts to formalize the structural prediction through automated computer programs have not yet led to an ability to predict mutagenicity and carcinogenicity of new chemicals with great accuracy (Snyder *et al.*, 2004), but promising developmental work on such systems continues (Votano *et al.*, 2004; Snyder and Smith, 2005).

Computer-based systems for predicting genotoxicity based on chemical properties are sometimes called in silico assays. These assays include computational and structural programs (Knudsen *et al.*, 2011; Snyder and Smith, 2005; Snyder, 2009; Mahadevan *et al.*, 2011) and the modeling of quantitative structure–activity relationships (Votano *et al.*, 2004; Snyder and Smith, 2005; Mahadevan *et al.*, 2011). Although there is much skepticism that such approaches can replace biological testing, they hold promise of improving the efficiency of testing strategies and reducing current levels of animal use (Guha, 2011).

DNA Damage and Repair Assays

Some assays measure DNA damage itself, rather than mutational consequences of DNA damage. They may do so directly, through such indicators as chemical adducts or strand breaks in DNA, or indirectly, through the measurement of biological repair processes. Adducts in DNA are detected by ^{32}P-postlabeling, high-performance liquid chromatography (HPLC), fluorescence-based methods, mass spectrometry, immunological methods using antibodies against specific adducts, isotope-labeled DNA binding, and electrochemical detection (Phillips *et al.*, 2000; Farmer and Singh, 2008; Himmelstein *et al.*, 2009). The ^{32}P-postlabeling method is highly versatile, in that it is sensitive and can be applied to diverse mutagens, but it may fall short of other methods for quantitative accuracy (Farmer and Singh, 2008). Through a combination of methods, many classes of adducts, including those of such environmentally widespread compounds as polynuclear aromatic hydrocarbons, can be detected. The measurement of adducts after human chemical exposures has proven useful in human monitoring, molecular dosimetry, and risk assessment Phillips *et al.*, 2000; Farmer and Singh, 2008; Himmelstein *et al.*, 2009). Adducts in somatic cells are relevant to carcinogenesis

(Himmelstein *et al.*, 2009), whereas those in reproductive cells permit molecular dosimetry for germ cell mutagenesis (Olsen *et al.*, 2010; 2011; Verhofsrad *et al.*, 2011).

DNA strand breakage can be measured by alkaline elution (Storer *et al.*, 1996; Gealy *et al.*, 2007) and electrophoretic methods. Single-cell gel electrophoresis, also called the comet assay, is a widely used, rapid method of measuring DNA damage (Fairbairn *et al.*, 1995; Singh, 2000; Tice *et al.*, 2000; Collins, 2004; Olive, 2009). In this assay cells are incorporated into agarose on slides, lysed so as to liberate their DNA, and subjected to electrophoresis. The DNA is stained with a fluorescent dye for observation and image analysis. Because broken DNA fragments migrate more quickly than larger pieces of DNA, a blur of fragments (a "comet") is observed when the DNA is extensively damaged. The extent of DNA damage can be estimated from the length and other attributes of the comet tail (Collins, 2004). Variations in the procedure permit the general detection of DNA strand breakage under alkaline conditions (Fairbairn *et al.*, 1995; Singh, 2000; Tice *et al.*, 2000) or the preferential detection of double-strand breaks under neutral conditions (Fairbairn *et al.*, 1995; Olive, 2009). A recent development is the combination of the comet assay with FISH to detect damage in specific regions of the genome (Glei *et al.*, 2009; Shaposhnikov *et al.*, 2009). Although the comet assay is relatively new, it has proven to be a sensitive indicator of DNA damage with broad applicability. It has been used most commonly with human lymphocytes (Fairbairn *et al.*, 1995; Singh, 2000; Collins, 2004) and other mammalian cells (Tice *et al.*, 2000), but it can be adapted to diverse species, including plants, worms, mollusks, fish, and amphibians (Cotelle and Férard, 1999; Lee and Steinert, 2003; Jha, 2004). This adaptability makes it well suited to use in environmental genetic toxicology. The applicability of the comet assay and other DNA damage assays to rodent testes (Bentley *et al.*, 1994; Speit *et al.*, 2009) makes these methods helpful in interpreting risks to germ cells.

The occurrence of DNA repair can serve as an easily measured indicator of DNA damage. Repair assays have been developed in microorganisms, cultured mammalian cells, and intact mammals (Table 9-2). Greater toxicity of a chemical in DNA-repair-deficient strains than in their repair-proficient counterparts (eg, *rec*$^+$ and *rec*$^-$ in *Bacillus subtilis*) can serve as an indicator of DNA damage in bacteria (Takigami *et al.*, 2002). Bacterial repair assays find occasional application but are used less commonly today than historically. The measurement of UDS, which is a measure of excision repair, is a mammalian DNA repair assay. The occurrence of UDS indicates that DNA has been damaged (Madle *et al.*, 1994). The absence of UDS, however, does not provide evidence that DNA has not been damaged because some classes of damage are not readily excised, and some excisable damage may not be detected as a consequence of assay insensitivity (Kirkland and Speit, 2008). Despite these limitations, UDS assays continue to find some use because of their applicability to cultured hepatocytes with endogenous cytochrome P450 enzyme activities and to tissues of intact animals, including hepatocytes (Madle *et al.*, 1994) and germinal tissue (Bentley *et al.*, 1994; Sotomayor and Sega, 2000).

Besides specific DNA repair processes, the induction of general responses to genotoxic stress has been used as an indicator of genetic damage. The induction of SOS functions, indicated by phage induction or by colorimetry, can serve as an indicator of genetic damage in bacteria (Quillardet and Hofnung, 1993; Yasunaga *et al.*, 2004; Oda *et al.*, 2009). The GADD45a-GFP assay, also called "Green Screen," detects genotoxic stress in human lymphoblastoid TK6 cells (Hastwell *et al.*, 2009). The stress response is detected by a green-fluorescent protein reporter in the genetic construct, and the induction of fluorescence has been observed with mutagens, clastogens, and aneugens (Hastwell *et al.*, 2009). The assay can be conducted with S9 metabolic activation and lends itself to automated detection by flow cytometry (Jagger *et al.*, 2009).

Gene Mutations in Prokaryotes

The most common means of detecting mutations in microorganisms is selecting for reversion in strains that have a specific nutritional requirement differing from wild type members of the species; such strains are called auxotrophs. For example, the widely used assay developed by Bruce Ames and his colleagues is based on measuring reversion in several histidine auxotrophs in *Salmonella enterica* serovar Typhimurium, commonly called *S typhimurium* (Ames *et al.*, 1975).

In the Ames assay one measures the frequency of histidine-independent bacteria that arise in a histidine-requiring strain in the presence or absence of the chemical being tested. Auxotrophic bacteria are treated with the chemical of interest by one of several procedures (eg, the standard plate-incorporation assay) and plated on medium that is deficient in histidine (Ames *et al.*, 1975; Maron and Ames, 1983; Mortelmans and Zeiger, 2000). The assay is conducted using genetically different strains so that reversion by base pair substitutions and frameshift mutations in several DNA sequence contexts can be detected and distinguished. Because Salmonella does not metabolize promutagens in the same way as mammalian tissues, the assay is generally performed in the presence and absence of a rat liver S9 metabolic activation system. Hence, the Ames assay is also called the Salmonella/microsome assay.

The principal strains of the Ames test and their characteristics are summarized in Table 9-3. In addition to the histidine alleles that provide the target for measuring mutagenesis, the Ames tester strains contain other genes and plasmids that enhance the assay. Part I of the table gives genotypes, and Part II explains the rationale for including specific genetic characteristics in the strains. Part III summarizes the principal DNA target in each strain and the mechanisms of reversion. Taken together, the Ames strains detect a broad array of mutations, and they complement one another. For example, strains TA102 and TA104, which are sensitive to agents that cause oxidative damage in DNA, detect the A:T → G:C base pair substitutions that are not detected by *hisG46* strains (Mortelmans and Zeiger, 2000). TA102 also detects agents that cause DNA cross-links because it has an intact excision repair system whereas the other common tester strains do not.

The most common version of the Ames assay is the plate-incorporation test (Ames *et al.*, 1975; Maron and Ames, 1983; Mortelmans and Zeiger, 2000). In this procedure, the bacterial tester strain, the test compound (or solvent control), and the S9 metabolic activation system (or buffer for samples without S9) are added to 2 mL of molten agar containing biotin and a trace of histidine to allow a few cell divisions, mixed, and immediately poured onto the surface of a petri dish selective for histidine-independent revertants. For general testing it is recommended that at least three plates per dose and five doses be used with and without S9, along with appropriate concurrent positive and negative controls (Mortelmans and Zeiger, 2000). Variations on the standard plate-incorporation assay confer advantages for some applications. These include a preincubation assay that facilitates the detection of unstable compounds and short-lived metabolites, a desiccator assay for testing volatile chemicals and gases, a microsuspension assay for working with small quantities of test agent, assays incorporating reductive metabolism rather than the conventional S9 system, and assays under hypoxic conditions (Mortelmans and Zeiger, 2000).

Although simplicity is a great merit of microbial assays, it can also be deceptive. Even assays that are simple in design and application can be performed incorrectly. For example, in the Ames assay one may see very small colonies in the petri dishes at highly toxic doses (Maron and Ames, 1983; Kirkland *et al.*, 1990; Mortelmans and Zeiger, 2000). Counting such colonies as revertants would be an error because they may actually be nonrevertant survivors that grew on the low concentration of histidine in the plates. Were there millions of survivors, the amount of histidine would have been insufficient to allow any of them (except real revertants) to form colonies. This artifact is easily avoided by checking that there is a faint lawn of bacterial growth in the plates; one can also confirm that colonies are revertants by streaking them on medium without histidine to be sure that they grow in its absence. Such pitfalls exist in all mutagenicity tests. Therefore, anyone performing mutagenicity tests must have detailed familiarity with the laboratory application and literature of the assay and be observant about the responsiveness of the assay.

Although information from the Ames assay has become a standard in genetic toxicology testing, equivalent information can be obtained from other bacterial assays. Like the Ames assay, the WP2 tryptophan reversion assay in *E coli* (Kirkland *et al.*, 1990; Mortelmans and Riccio, 2000) incorporates genetic features that enhance assay sensitivity, can accommodate S9 metabolic activation, and performs well in many laboratories. Mutations are detected by selecting for reversion of a *trpE* allele from Trp⁻ to Trp⁺. Its responsiveness to mutagens most closely resembles TA102 among the Ames strains (Mortelmans and Riccio, 2000).

Bacterial reversion assays are commonly used for testing purposes, but they also provide information on molecular mechanisms of mutagenesis. The broader understanding of mutational mechanisms that comes from refined genetic assays and molecular analysis of mutations can contribute to the interpretation of mutational hazards. The primary reversion mechanisms of the Ames strains, summarized in Table 9-3, were initially determined by genetic and biochemical means (Maron and Ames, 1983). An ingenious method called allele-specific colony hybridization greatly facilitated the molecular analysis of revertants in the Ames assay (Koch *et al.*, 1994), and many spontaneous and induced revertants have been cloned or amplified by the polymerase chain reaction (PCR) and sequenced (Levine *et al.*, 1994; DeMarini, 2000).

Part III of Table 9-3 is by necessity a simplification with respect both to targets and mechanisms of reversion of the Ames strains. Some mutations that bring about reversion to histidine independence fall outside the primary target, and the full target has been found to be as much as 76 base pairs in *hisD3052* (DeMarini *et al.*, 1998). Other revertants can arise by suppressor mutations in other genes. It has been shown that *hisG46*, *hisG428*, *hisC3076*, *hisD6610*, and *hisD3052* all revert by multiple mechanisms and that the spectrum of classes of revertants may vary depending on the mutagen, experimental conditions, and other elements of the genotype (Cebula and Koch, 1990; Prival and Cebula, 1992; DeMarini *et al.*, 1998; Mortelmans and Zeiger, 2000).

The development of Salmonella strains that are highly specific with respect to mechanisms of reversion has made the identification of particular base pair substitutions more straightforward. These strains (TA7001–TA7006) each revert from *his⁻* to *his⁺* by a single kind of mutation (eg, G:C to T:A), and collectively they permit the specific detection of all six possible base pair substitutions (Gee *et al.*, 1994; Mortelmans and Zeiger, 2000; Kamber *et al.*, 2009). The assay is usually conducted using a fluctuation test in 24-well plates, rather than the plate-incorporation or preincubation method. The ability to discern mutagens and nonmutagens is comparable to the standard Ames assay (Kamber *et al.*, 2009).

Table 9-3

The Ames Assay: Tester Strains and Their Characteristics

I. STANDARD TESTER STRAINS OF *SALMONELLA TYPHIMURIUM*

STRAIN	TARGET ALLELE	CHROMOSOMAL GENOTYPE	PLASMIDS
TA1535	*hisG46*	*hisG46 rfa ΔuvrB*	None
TA100	*hisG46*	*hisG46 rfa ΔuvrB*	pKM101 (*mucAB* Ap^r)
TA1538	*hisD3052*	*hisD3052 rfa ΔuvrB*	None
TA98	*hisD3052*	*hisD3052 rfa ΔuvrB*	pKM101 (*mucAB* Ap^r)
TA1537	*hisC3076*	*hisC3076 rfa ΔuvrB*	None
TA97	*hisD6610*	*hisD6610 hisO1242 rf ΔuvrB*	pKM101 (*mucAB* Ap^r)
TA102	*hisG428*	*hisΔ(G)8476 rfa*	pKM101 (*mucAB* Ap^r); pAQ1 (*hisG428* Tc^r)
TA104	*hisG428*	*hisG428 rfa ΔuvrB*	pKM101 (*mucAB* Ap^r)

II. GENETIC CHARACTERISTICS OF THE AMES TESTER STRAINS

CHARACTERISTIC	RATIONALE FOR INCLUSION IN THE TESTER STRAIN
rfa	Alters the lipopolysaccharide wall, enhancing permeability to mutagens.
ΔuvrB	Deletes the excision repair system, increasing sensitivity to many mutagens; retention of excision in TA102 permits the detection of DNA cross-linking agents.
mucAB	Enhances sensitivity to some mutagens whose activity depends on the SOS system.
Ap^r	Permits selection for the presence of pKM101 by ampicillin resistance.
hisO1242	Affects regulation of histidine genes, enhancing revertibility of *hisD6610* in TA97.
His Δ(G)8476	Eliminates the chromosomal *hisG* gene, allowing detection of the reversion of *hisG428* on pAQ1 in TA102.
Tc^r	Permits selection for the presence of pAQ1 in TA102 by tetracycline resistance.

III. MECHANISMS OF REVERSION DETECTED BY THE AMES TESTER STRAINS

STRAIN	PRIMARY TARGET*	MUTATIONS DETECTED
TA1535, TA100	GGG/CCC	Base-pair substitutions, principally those beginning at G:C base pairs (G:C→A:T; G:C→T:A; G:C→C:G). These strains also detect A:T→C:G but not A:T→G:C.
TA1538, TA98	CGCGCGCG/GCGCGCGC	Frameshift mutations, especially −2 frameshifts (−GC or −CG), +1 frameshifts, other small deletions, and some complex mutations.
TA1537	GGGGG/CCCCC	Frameshift mutations, mainly −1 (−G or −C; less frequently −T), but also some +CG frameshifts.
TA97	GGGGGG/CCCCCC	Frameshift mutations, combining the specificity of TA1537 at the primary target and with some characteristics of TA98.
TA102, TA104	TAA/ATT	Base-pair substitutions, principally those beginning at A:T base pairs (A:T→G:C; A:T→T:A; A:T→C:G), but also G:C→T:A and G:C→A:T.

*The sequences before and after the backslash represent the 2 complementary strands of DNA.

Specific reversion assays are also available in *E coli*. A versatile system based on reversion of *lacZ* mutations in *E coli* permits the specific detection of all six possible base pair substitutions (Cupples and Miller, 1989; Josephy, 2000) and frameshift mutations for which one or two bases have been added or deleted in various sequence contexts (Cupples *et al.*, 1990; Josephy, 2000; Hoffmann *et al.*, 2003). The versatility of the *lacZ* assay has been expanded through the introduction of useful characteristics into the strains parallel to those incorporated into the Ames strains. Among the features added to the *lacZ* assay are DNA repair deficiencies, permeability alterations, plasmid-enhanced mutagenesis, and enzymes of mutagen metabolism (Josephy, 2000).

Bacterial forward mutation assays, such as selections for resistance to arabinose or to purine or pyrimidine analogs in Salmonella (Jurado *et al.*, 1994; Vlasakova *et al.*, 2005), are also used in research and testing, although less extensively than reversion assays. A versatile forward mutation assay that has contributed greatly to an understanding of mechanisms of mutagenesis is the *lacI* system in *E coli* (Calos and Miller, 1981; Halliday and Glickman, 1991). Mutations in the *lacI* gene, which encodes the repressor of the lactose operon, are easily identified by phenotype, cloned or amplified by PCR, and sequenced. The *lacI* gene is widely used as a target for mutagenesis both in *E coli* and in transgenic mice, and thousands of *lacI* mutants have been sequenced.

Genetic Alterations in Nonmammalian Eukaryotes

Gene Mutations and Chromosome Aberrations Many early studies of mutagenesis used yeasts, mycelial fungi, plants, and insects as experimental organisms. Even though well-characterized genetic systems permit the analysis of a diverse array of genetic alterations in these organisms (Table 9-2), they have been largely supplanted in genetic toxicology by bacterial and mammalian systems. Exceptions are to be found where the assays in nonmammalian eukaryotes permit the study of genetic endpoints that are not readily analyzed in mammals or where the organism has special attributes that fit a particular application.

The fruit fly, Drosophila, has long occupied a prominent place in genetic research. In fact, the first unequivocal evidence of chemical mutagenesis was obtained in Scotland in 1941 when Charlotte Auerbach and J.M. Robson demonstrated that mustard gas is mutagenic in Drosophila. Drosophila continues to be used in modern mutation research (Potter *et al.*, 2000) but its role in genetic toxicology is now more limited. The Drosophila assay of greatest historical importance is the sex-linked recessive lethal (SLRL) test. A strength of the SLRL test is that it permits the detection of recessive lethal mutations at 600 to 800 different loci on the X chromosome by screening for the presence or absence of wild type males in the offspring of specifically designed crosses (Mason *et al.*, 1987; Vogel *et al.*, 1999). The genetic alterations include gene mutations and small deletions. The spontaneous frequency of SLRL is about 0.2%, and a significant increase over this frequency in the lineages derived from treated males indicates mutagenesis. Although it requires screening large numbers of fruit fly vials, the SLRL test yields information about mutagenesis in germ cells, which is lacking in all microbial and cell culture systems. However, means of exposure, measurement of doses, metabolism, and gametogenesis in insects differ from those in mammalian toxicology, thereby introducing doubt about the relevance of Drosophila assays to human genetic risk. Drosophila assays are also available for studying the induction of chromosome abnormalities in germ cells, specifically heritable translocations (Mason *et al.*, 1987; Vogel *et al.*, 1999).

Genetic and cytogenetic assays in plants (Ma *et al.*, 2005; Grant and Owens, 2006; Misík *et al.*, 2011) also occupy a more restricted niche in modern genetic toxicology than they did years ago. However, plant assays continue to find use in special applications, such as in situ monitoring for mutagens and exploration of the metabolism of promutagens by agricultural plants. In situ monitoring entails looking for evidence of mutagenesis in organisms that are grown in the environment of interest. Natural plant populations can also be examined for evidence of genetic damage, but doing so requires utmost precaution when characterizing the environments and defining appropriate control populations.

Mitotic Recombination Assays in nonmammalian eukaryotes continue to be important in the study of induced recombination. Recombinogenic effects in yeast have long been used as a general indicator of genetic damage (Zimmermann *et al.*, 1984), and interest in the induction of recombination has increased as recombinational events have been implicated in the etiology of cancer (Sengstag, 1994; Reliene *et al.*, 2007). LOH is central to the expression of the mutant alleles of tumor-suppressor genes, and mitotic recombination is a major mechanism of LOH. Widely used assays for recombinogens detect mitotic crossing over and mitotic gene conversion in the yeast *Saccharomyces cerevisiae* (Zimmermann, 1992), and hundreds of chemicals have been tested for recombinogenic effects in straightforward yeast assays (Zimmermann *et al.*, 1984). In yeast strain D7, for example, mitotic crossing over involving the *ade2* locus is detected on the basis of pink and red colony color, mitotic gene conversion at the *trp5* locus by selection for growth without tryptophan, and gene mutations by reversion of the *ilv1-92* allele (Zimmermann, 1992; Freeman and Hoffmann, 2007). Newer yeast assays have been constructed to discern whether LOH has occurred by mitotic recombination or chromosome loss (Daigaku *et al.*, 2004; Nunoshiba *et al.*, 2007). Strategies have also been devised to detect recombinogenic effects in human lymphocytes (Turner *et al.*, 2003), other mammalian cells, mice, plants, and mycelial fungi (Hoffmann, 1994; Reliene *et al.*, 2007). At least 350 chemicals have been evaluated in Drosophila somatic cell assays in which recombinogenic effects are detected by examining wings or eyes for regions in which recessive alleles are expressed in heterozygotes (Vogel *et al.*, 1999; Vogel and Nivard, 2000).

Gene Mutations in Mammals

Gene Mutations In Vitro Mutagenicity assays in cultured mammalian cells have some of the same advantages as microbial assays with respect to speed and cost, and they use similar approaches. The most widely used assays for gene mutations in mammalian cells detect forward mutations that confer resistance to a toxic chemical. For example, mutations in the gene encoding hypoxanthine-guanine phosphoribosyltransferase (HPRT enzyme; *HPRT* gene) confer resistance to the purine analogue 6-thioguanine (Li *et al.*, 1988; Parry *et al.*, 2005), and thymidine kinase mutations (TK enzyme; *TK* gene) confer resistance to the pyrimidine analogue trifluorothymidine (Clements, 2000; Wang *et al.*, 2009). HPRT and TK mutations may therefore be detected by attempting to grow cells in the presence of purine analogues and pyrimidine analogues, respectively. For historical reasons, HPRT assays have most commonly been conducted in Chinese hamster cells or human cells, whereas TK assays have used mouse lymphoma cells or human cells. The mouse lymphoma assay, long used for detecting gene mutations, is now also used to detect other endpoints, including recombination, deletion, and aneuploidy (Wang *et al.*, 2009). Forward-mutation assays typically respond to diverse mechanisms of mutagenesis, but there are exceptions such as resistance to ouabain, which only occurs by a specific alteration (DeMarini *et al.*, 1989). Assays that do not detect various kinds of mutations are not useful for general mutagenicity testing. Genetic or molecular evidence that an assay is responsive to diverse mechanisms of mutagenesis is essential.

Instead of using selective media, flow cytometry can be used to detect gene mutations by immunological methods in mammalian cell cultures and intact animals. An in vitro assay for CD59 mutations is performed in CHO-human hybrid A_L cells (Zhou *et al.*, 2006). A_L cells contain a single human chromosome 11 along with the Chinese hamster chromosome complement of the Chinese hamster ovary (CHO) cells. CD59 is a cell-surface protein encoded by a gene on the human chromosome. Fluorescent anti-CD59 antibody is used to quantify CD59 cells by flow cytometry. Besides CD59 itself, mutations in other CD genes on chromosome 11 and in their glycosylphosphatidylinositol (GPI) anchor can be detected in the assay (Ross *et al.*, 2007). An assay for mutations in *Pig-a*, the GPI anchor gene, is discussed with in vivo assays.

Gene Mutations In Vivo In vivo assays involve treating intact animals and analyzing appropriate tissues for genetic effects. The choice of suitable doses, treatment procedures, controls, and sample sizes is critical in the conduct of in vivo tests. Mutations may be detected either in somatic cells or in germ cells. The latter are of special interest with respect to risk for future generations.

The mouse spot test is a traditional genetic assay for gene mutations in somatic cells (Styles and Penman, 1985; Lambert *et al.*, 2005). Visible spots of altered phenotype in mice heterozygous for coat-colored genes indicate mutations in the progenitor cells of the altered regions. Although straightforward in design, the spot test is less used today than other somatic cell assays or than its germ cell counterpart, the mouse specific-locus test.

Cells that are amenable to positive selection for mutants when collected from intact animals form the basis for efficient in vivo mutation-detection assays analogous to those in mammalian cell cultures. Lymphocytes with mutations in the *HPRT* gene are readily detected by selection for resistance to 6-thioguanine. The *hprt* assay in mice, rats, and monkeys (Casciano *et al.*, 1999) is of special interest because it permits comparisons to the measurement of *HPRT* mutations in humans in mutational monitoring (Cole and Skopek, 1994; Albertini and Hayes, 1997; Albertini, 2001).

The *Pig-a* assay is a newer assay that has versions suitable for human monitoring and laboratory studies. The assay detects mutations that block GPI synthesis (Dobrovolsky *et al.*, 2010). *Pig-a* is a sex-linked gene whose gene product functions as an anchor for cell-surface proteins. Mutations in *Pig-a* can be detected in red blood cells from rats, mice, monkeys, and humans by means of fluorescent antibodies against GPI-anchored cell-surface proteins, such as CD59. Using antibodies to more than one GPI-linked marker has been suggested as a means of making the assay specific to *Pig-a* rather than also detecting mutants for a particular cell-surface protein. Frequencies can be measured by clonal growth of *Pig-a* cells using proaerolysin (ProAER) selection or by flow cytometry (Dobrovolsky *et al.*, 2010; Miura *et al.*, 2011; Dobo *et al.*, 2011). The fact that the same assay can be performed in several species makes this a promising assay for comparisons of human monitoring and controlled exposures in laboratory animals.

Besides determining whether agents are mutagenic, mutation assays provide information on mechanisms of mutagenesis that contributes to an understanding of mutational hazards. Base pair substitutions and large deletions, which may be indistinguishable on the basis of phenotype, can be differentiated through the use of probes for the target gene and Southern blotting, in that base substitutions are too subtle to be detectable on the blots, whereas gross structural alterations are visible (Cole and Skopek, 1994; Albertini and Hayes, 1997). Molecular analysis has been used to determine proportions of mutations ascribable to deletions and other structural alterations in several assays, including the specific-locus test for germ cell mutations in mice (Favor, 1999) and the human *HPRT* assay (Cole and Skopek, 1994). Gene mutations have been characterized at the molecular level by DNA sequence analysis both in transgenic rodents (Lambert *et al.*, 2005; Singer *et al.*, 2006) and in endogenous mammalian genes (Cariello and Skopek, 1993). Many *HPRT* mutations from human cells in vitro and in vivo have been analyzed at the molecular level and classified with respect to base pair substitutions, frameshifts, small deletions, large deletions, and other alterations (Cole and Skopek, 1994).

Transgenic Assays Transgenic animals are products of DNA technology in which the animal contains foreign DNA sequences that have been added to the genome. The foreign DNA is represented in all the somatic cells of the animal and is transmitted in the germ line to progeny. Mutagenicity assays in transgenic animals combine in vivo metabolic activation and pharmacodynamics with simple microbial detection systems, and they permit the analysis of mutations induced in diverse mammalian tissues (Lambert *et al.*, 2005; Sykes *et al.*, 2006; Valentine *et al.*, 2010).

The transgenic animals that have figured most heavily in genetic toxicology are rodents that carry *lac* genes from *E coli*. The bacterial genes were introduced into mice or rats by injecting a vector carrying the genes into fertilized oocytes (Lambert *et al.*, 2005). The strains are commonly referred to by their commercial names—the "Big Blue mouse" and "Big Blue rat," which use *lacI* as a target for mutagenesis, and the "Muta Mouse," which uses *lacZ* (Lambert *et al.*, 2005). After mutagenic treatment of the transgenic animals, the *lac* genes are recovered from the animal, packaged in phage λ, and transferred to *E coli* for mutational analysis. Mutant plaques are identified on the basis of phenotype, and mutant frequencies can be calculated for different tissues of the treated animals. The *cII* locus may be used as a second target gene in both the *lacZ* and *lacI* transgenic assays (Swiger, 2001; Lambert *et al.*, 2005). Its use offers technical advantages as a small, easily sequenced target in which mutations are detected by positive selection, and it permits interesting comparisons both within and between assays.

A *lacZ* transgenic mouse that uses a plasmid-based system rather than a phage vector has the advantage that deletion mutants are more readily recovered than in the phage-based *lac* systems (Lambert *et al.*, 2005). Deletions may also be detected in the *gpt delta* mouse and rat using a phage vector system. These transgenic animals detect two kinds of genetic events in two targets—point mutations in *gpt* detected by resistance to 6-thioguanine and *spi* deletions that permit growth on P2 lysogens (Okada *et al.*, 1999; Lambert *et al.*, 2005). Other transgenic assays are under development and offer the prospect of expanding the versatility of such assays (Lambert *et al.*, 2005). These include pKZ1 mice in which inversions and deletions arising in various tissues by intrachromosomal recombination have been used to study effects of low doses of ionizing radiation (Sykes *et al.*, 2006) and an assay that detects both forward mutations and reversion in mice that carry the genome of phage ΦX174 (Valentine *et al.*, 2010).

Various mutagens, including alkylating agents, nitrosamines, procarbazine, cyclophosphamide, and polycyclic aromatic hydrocarbons have been studied in transgenic mouse assays, and mutant frequencies have been analyzed in such diverse tissues as liver, skin, spleen, kidney, bladder, small intestine, bone marrow, and testis (Lambert *et al.*, 2005). Mutation frequencies in transgenes in testes have been compared to results in standard germ cell mutagenesis assays (Singer *et al.*, 2006). Female germ cells are less amenable to study in transgenic assays because of the difficulty of collecting sufficient numbers of oocytes, but it has been suggested that granulosa cells from ovarian follicles may serve as a surrogate for the exposure of female germ cells to mutagens (Singer *et al.*, 2006). Mutant frequencies have been compared to the formation of adducts in various tissues and to the site specificity of carcinogenesis and DNA repair capacity (Lambert *et al.*, 2005). An important issue that remains to be resolved is the extent to which transgenes resemble endogenous genes. Although their mutational responses tend to be comparable (Lambert *et al.*, 2005), some differences have been noted (Burkhart and Malling, 1993; Lambert *et al.*, 2005), and questions have been raised about the relevance of mutations that might be recovered from dying or dead animal tissues (Burkhart and Malling, 1994). Therefore, transgenic animals offer promising models for the study of chemical mutagenesis, but they must be further characterized before their ultimate place in hazard assessment is clear.

Mammalian Cytogenetic Assays

Chromosome Aberrations Cytogenetic assays rely on the use of microscopy for the direct observation of the effects of interest. This approach differs sharply from the indirectness of traditional

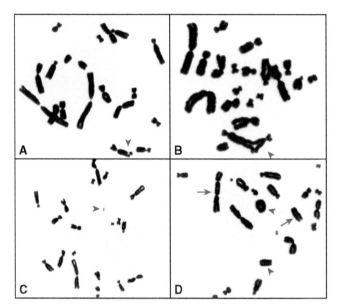

Figure 9-4. *Chromosome aberrations induced by x-rays in Chinese hamster ovary (CHO) cells.* (**A**) A chromatid deletion (▶). (**B**) A chromatid exchange called a triradial (▶). (**C**) A small interstitial deletion (▶) that resulted from chromosome breakage. (**D**) A metaphase with more than one aberration: a centric ring plus an acentric fragment (▶) and a dicentric chromosome plus an acentric fragment (→).

genetic assays in which one observes a phenotype and reaches conclusions about genes. It is only through the addition of DNA sequencing that genetic assays can approach the directness of cytogenetic assays.

In conventional cytogenetics, metaphase analysis is used to detect chromosomal anomalies, especially unstable chromosome and chromatid aberrations. A key factor in the design of cytogenetic assays is obtaining appropriate cell populations for treatment and analysis (Preston *et al.*, 1981; Ishidate *et al.*, 1988; Kirkland *et al.*, 1990; Galloway *et al.*, 1994). Cells with a stable, well-defined karyotype, short generation time, low chromosome number, and large chromosomes are ideal for cytogenetic analysis. For this reason, Chinese hamster cells have been used widely in cytogenetic testing. Other cells are also suitable, and human cells, especially peripheral lymphocytes, have been used extensively. Cells should be treated during a sensitive period of the cell cycle (typically S), and aberrations should be analyzed at the first mitotic division after treatment so that the sensitivity of the assay is not reduced by unstable aberrations being lost during cell division. Examples of chromosome aberrations are shown in Fig. 9-4.

Cytogenetic assays require careful attention to growth conditions, controls, doses, treatment conditions, and time intervals between treatment and the sampling of cells for analysis (Preston *et al.*, 1981; Ishidate *et al.*, 1988; Kirkland *et al.*, 1990; Galloway *et al.*, 2011). Data collection is a critical part of cytogenetic analysis. It is essential that sufficient cells be analyzed because a negative result in a small sample is inconclusive. Results should be recorded for specific classes of aberrations, not just an overall index of aberrations per cell. The need for detailed data is all the more important because of nonuniformity in the classification of aberrations and disagreement on whether small achromatic (ie, unstained) gaps in chromosomes are true chromosomal aberrations. Gaps should be quantified but not pooled with other aberrations.

In interpreting results on the induction of chromosome aberrations in cell cultures, one must be alert to the possibility of artifacts associated with extreme assay conditions because aberrations

induced under such circumstances may not be a reflection of a chemical-specific genotoxicity (Scott *et al.*, 1991; Galloway, 2000; Galloway *et al.*, 2011). Questionable positive results have been found at highly cytotoxic doses (Galloway *et al.*, 2011), high osmolality, and pH extremes (Scott *et al.*, 1991). The possibility that metabolic activation systems may be genotoxic also warrants scrutiny (Scott *et al.*, 1991). Although excessively high doses may lead to artifactual positive responses, the failure to test to a sufficiently high dose also undermines the utility of a test. Therefore, testing should be extended to a dose at which there is some cytotoxicity, such as a reduction in a replicative index or the mitotic index (the proportion of cells in division). If the chemical is nontoxic, testing dosages should extend up to an arbitrary limit of dosage (Galloway *et al.*, 2011). By a consensus of cytogeneticists and genetic toxicologists, a limit of 10 mM or 5 mg/mL, whichever is lower, has been recommended (Galloway *et al.*, 2011). Some have argued that the limit should be lowered, perhaps to 1 mM, but no consensus could be reached on this point (Galloway *et al.*, 2011).

In vivo assays for chromosome aberrations involve treating intact animals and later collecting cells for cytogenetic analysis (Preston *et al.*, 1981; Kirkland *et al.*, 1990; Tice *et al.*, 1994). The main advantage of in vivo assays is that they include mammalian metabolism, DNA repair, and pharmacodynamics. The target is typically a tissue from which large numbers of dividing cells are easily prepared for analysis. Bone marrow from rats, mice, or Chinese hamsters is most commonly used. Peripheral lymphocytes are another suitable target when stimulated to divide with a mitogen such as phytohemagglutinin. Effective testing requires dosages and routes of administration that ensure adequate exposure of the target cells, proper intervals between treatment and collecting cells, and sufficient numbers of animals and cells analyzed (Preston *et al.*, 1981; Kirkland *et al.*, 1990; Tice *et al.*, 1994).

An important development in cytogenetic analysis is FISH, in which a nucleic acid probe is hybridized to complementary sequences in chromosomal DNA (Tucker *et al.*, 1993b, 2005; Paccierotti and Sgura, 2008). The probe is labeled with a fluorescent dye so that the chromosomal location to which it binds is visible by fluorescence microscopy. Composite probes have been developed from sequences unique to specific human chromosomes, giving a uniform fluorescent label over the entire chromosome. Slides prepared for standard metaphase analysis are suitable for FISH after they have undergone a simple denaturation procedure. The use of whole-chromosome probes is commonly called "chromosome painting" (Tucker *et al.*, 1993b; Speicher and Carter, 2005; Paccierotti and Sgura, 2008). Another significant advantage of FISH methods is that the probes can be used with interphase cells/chromosomes making any tissue potentially available for analysis (Vorsanova *et al.*, 2010). Examples of cells showing chromosome painting and reciprocal translocations are shown in Figs. 9-5 and 9-6.

Chromosome painting facilitates cytogenetic analysis because aberrations are easily detected by the number of fluorescent regions in a painted metaphase. For example, if chromosome 4 were painted with a probe while the other chromosomes were counter-stained in a different color, one would see only the two homologues of chromosome 4 in the color of the probe in a normal cell. However, if there were a translocation or a dicentric chromosome and fragment involving chromosome 4, one would see three areas of fluorescence—one normal chromosome 4 and the two pieces involved in the chromosome rearrangement. Aberrations are detected only in the painted portion of the genome, but this disadvantage can be offset by painting a few chromosomes simultaneously with probes of different colors (Tucker *et al.*, 1993b). FISH reduces the time and technical skill required to detect chromosome aberrations, and

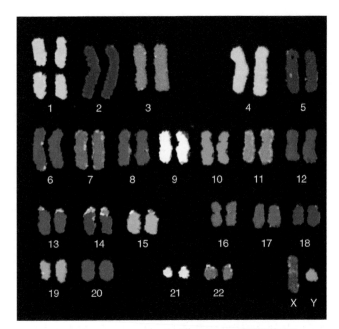

Figure 9-5. *Karyotype of human cell using FISH.* To produce a FISH-based karyotype of the type depicted here, appropriate chromosome probe sets are developed for each chromosome pair such that by using computer colorization each has a specific color for analysis. (Reproduced with permission from Schrock E, et al. Multicolor spectral karyotyping of human chromosomes. *Science.* 1996 Jul 26;273(5274):494–497.)

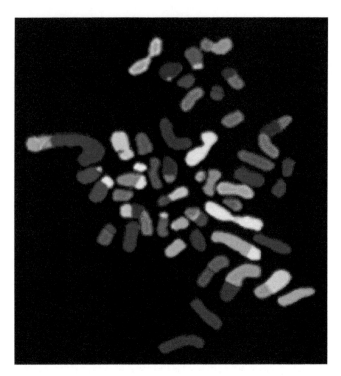

Figure 9-6. *Chromosome aberrations identified by FISH.* Human breast cancer cell with aneuploidy for some chromosomes and with reciprocal translocations (identified by color switches along a chromosome).

it permits the scoring of stable aberrations, such as translocations and insertions, that are not readily detected in traditional metaphase analysis without special labeling techniques. Using FISH, some chromosomal analysis can even be conducted in interphase cells (Paccierotti and Sgura, 2008; Vorsanova *et al.*, 2010). Although FISH is not routinely used in genotoxicity testing, it is a valuable research tool for studying clastogens and is having a substantial impact in monitoring human populations for chromosomal damage.

Micronuclei Metaphase analysis is time consuming and requires considerable skill, so simpler cytogenetic assays have been developed, of which micronucleus assays have become especially important. Micronuclei are membrane-bound structures that contain chromosomal fragments, or sometimes whole chromosomes, that were not incorporated into a daughter nucleus at mitosis. Because micronuclei usually represent acentric chromosomal fragments, they are most commonly used as simple indicators of chromosomal damage. However, the ability to detect micronuclei containing whole chromosomes has led to their use for detecting aneuploidy as well. Micronucleus assays may be conducted in primary cultures of human lymphocytes (Fenech *et al.*, 2003; Corvi *et al.*, 2008; Fenech, 2008; Fenech *et al.*, 2011b), mammalian cell lines (Kirsch-Volders *et al.*, 2003; Corvi *et al.*, 2008), or mammals in vivo (Krishna and Hayashi, 2000; Hayashi *et al.*, 2007; Dertinger *et al.*, 2011).

Micronucleus assays in lymphocytes have been greatly improved by the cytokinesis-block technique in which cell division is inhibited with cytochalasin B, resulting in binucleate and multinucleate cells (Fenech *et al.*, 2003, 2011b; Kirsch-Volders *et al.*, 2003; Fenech, 2008). In the cytokinesis-block assay in human lymphocytes, nondividing (G_0) cells are treated with ionizing radiation or a radiomimetic chemical and then stimulated to divide with the mitogen phytohemagglutinin. Alternatively, the lymphocytes may be exposed to the mitogen first, so that the subsequent mutagenic treatment with radiation or chemicals includes the S period of the cell cycle. In either case, cytochalasin B is added for the last part of

the culture period, and micronuclei are counted only in binucleate cells so as to ensure that the cells have undergone a single nuclear division that is essential for micronucleus development. The assay thereby avoids confusion owing to differences in cellular proliferation kinetics.

Although first devised using primary lymphocytes (Fenech *et al.*, 2003; Fenech, 2008; Fenech, 2011b), the cytokinesis-block micronucleus assay has since been adapted for use in continuous cell cultures, including the Chinese hamster and mouse lymphoma cells that are widely used in other genotoxicity assays (Kirsch-Volders *et al.*, 2003; Corvi *et al.*, 2008). Micronucleus assays should be conducted in such a way that cellular proliferation is monitored along with the micronucleus frequency, and this is facilitated by the cytokinesis block. Reliable data have been obtained in cultured cells both with and without cytokinesis block, but scoring results only in binucleate cells after blockage of cytokinesis with cytochalasin B confers advantages with respect to the measurement of proliferation, recognizing whether an agent is cytostatic, and obtaining clear dose–response relationships (Kirsch-Volders *et al.*, 2003).

Although micronuclei resulting from chromosome breakage comprise the principal endpoint in the cytokinesis-block micronucleus assay, the method can also provide evidence of aneuploidy, chromosome rearrangements that form nucleoplasmic bridges, inhibition of cell division, necrosis, apoptosis, and excision-repairable lesions (Fenech *et al.*, 2003; Fenech, 2008; Fenech *et al.*, 2011b). Micronuclei in a binucleate human lymphocyte are shown in Fig. 9-7. A recent review of the International Human Micronucleus (HUMN) Project provides a comprehensive description of standardized protocols for micronucleus assays in human lymphocytes and buccal cells together with a review of associations between micronucleus data and disease outcomes (Fenech *et al.*, 2011a).

The in vivo micronucleus assay is often performed by counting micronuclei in immature (polychromatic) erythrocytes in the bone marrow of treated mice, but it may also be based on peripheral blood

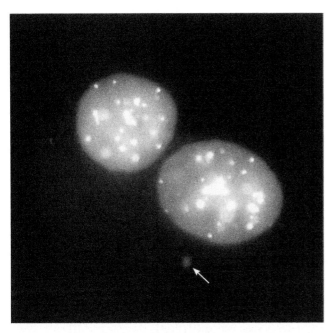

Figure 9-7. *Micronucleus in a human lymphocyte.* The cytochalasin B method was used to inhibit cytokinesis that resulted in a binucleate nucleus. The micronucleus (arrow) resulted from failure of an acentric chromosome fragment or a whole chromosome being included in a daughter nucleus following cell division. (Figure courtesy of James Allen, Jill Barnes, and Barbara Collins.)

(Krishna and Hayashi, 2000; Hayashi *et al.*, 2007). Micronuclei remain in the cell when the nucleus is extruded in the maturation of erythroblasts. In vivo micronucleus assays are increasingly used in genotoxicity testing as a substitute for bone marrow metaphase chromosome analysis. Micronucleus assays have been developed for mammalian tissues other than bone marrow and blood, including skin, duodenum, colon, liver, lung, spleen, testes, bladder, buccal mucosal cells, stomach, vagina, and fetal tissues (Coffing *et al.*, 2011; Morita *et al.*, 2011). Although assays in bone marrow and blood are the mainstay of genotoxicity testing, the new assays are important for mechanistic studies and research on the site specificity of genetic damage and carcinogenesis.

Micronuclei are most commonly visualized through microscopy, but automated means of detecting micronuclei are being developed through the application of flow cytometry. Flow cytometric detection is effective in micronucleus assays in rodent bone marrow or blood (Dertinger *et al.*, 2011). It can also be used to detect micronuclei in Chinese hamster CHO cells, where altered flow cytometric parameters can reveal whether the micronuclei arose primarily by chromosome breakage or by aneuploidy (Bryce *et al.*, 2011).

Sister Chromatid Exchanges SCE, in which there has been an apparently reciprocal exchange of segments between the two chromatids of a chromosome, are visible cytologically through differential staining of chromatids. Fig. 9-8 shows SCE in human cells. Many mutagens induce SCE in cultured cells and in mammals in vivo (Tucker *et al.*, 1993a; Wilson and Thompson, 2007). Despite the convenience and responsiveness of SCE assays, data on SCE are less informative than data on chromosome aberrations. There is uncertainty about the underlying mechanisms by which SCEs are formed and how DNA damage or perturbations of DNA synthesis stimulate their formation (Preston, 1991). SCE assays are therefore best regarded as general indicators of mutagen exposure, analogous to DNA damage and repair assays, rather than measures of a mutagenic effect.

Aneuploidy Although assays for the induction of aneuploidy are not yet as refined as those for gene mutations and chromosome aberrations, they are being developed (Aardema *et al.*, 1998). The targets of aneugens are often components of the mitotic or meiotic apparatus, rather than DNA. Therefore, aneugens should not be expected to overlap strongly with mutagens and clastogens. For example, a chemical that interferes with the polymerization of tubulin and thereby disrupts the formation of a mitotic spindle is likely to show specificity as an aneugen. Assays for chemicals that induce aneuploidy should therefore encompass all the relevant cellular targets that are required for the proper functioning of the mitotic and meiotic process. Means of detecting aneuploidy include chromosome counting (Galloway and Ivett, 1986; Natarajan, 1993; Aardema *et al.*, 1998; Pacchierotti and Sgura, 2008), the detection of micronuclei that contain kinetochores (Lynch and Parry, 1993; Natarajan, 1993; Aardema *et al.*, 1998; Fenech, 2008; Pacchierotti

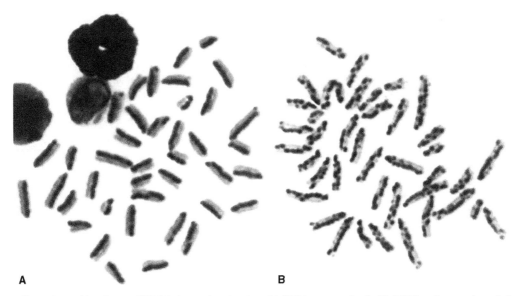

Figure 9-8. *Sister chromatid exchanges (SCEs) in human lymphocytes.* (**A**) SCE in untreated cell. (**B**) SCE in cell exposed to ethyl carbamate. The treatment results in a very large increase in the number of SCE. (Figure courtesy of James Allen and Barbara Collins.)

and Sgura, 2008), and the observation of abnormal spindles or spindle–chromosome associations in cells in which spindles and chromosomes have been differentially stained (Parry, 1998). FISH-based assays have also been developed for the assessment of aneuploidy in interphase somatic cells (Rupa *et al.*, 1997; Paccierotti and Sgura, 2008) and in sperm (Russo, 2000; Marchetti *et al.*, 2006, 2008).

A complication in chromosome counting is that a metaphase may lack chromosomes because they were lost during cell preparation for analysis, rather than having been absent from the living cell. To avoid this artifact, cytogeneticists generally use extra chromosomes (ie, hyperploidy) rather than missing chromosomes (ie, hypoploidy) as an indicator of aneuploidy in chromosome preparations from mammalian cell cultures (Galloway and Ivett, 1986; Aardema *et al.*, 1998) or mouse bone marrow (Adler, 1993). Techniques for counting chromosomes in intact cells may allow reliable measures of hypoploidy (Natarajan, 1993), but the detection of hyperploidy remains the norm in lieu of clear evidence that artifactual chromosome loss has been avoided. It has been suggested that counting polyploid cells, which is technically straightforward, may be an efficient way to detect aneugens (Aardema *et al.*, 1998), but there is disagreement on the point (Parry, 1998).

Micronucleus assays can detect aneugens as well as clastogens. Micronuclei that contain whole chromosomes tend to be somewhat larger than those containing chromosome fragments, but the two categories are not readily distinguished in typically stained preparations (Natarajan, 1993). However, one can infer that a micronucleus contains a whole chromosome if it is shown to contain a kinetochore or centromeric DNA. Aneuploidy may therefore be detected by means of antikinetochore antibodies with a fluorescent label or FISH with a probe for centromere-specific DNA (Lynch and Parry, 1993; Natarajan, 1993; Krishna and Hayashi, 2000; Fenech, 2008; Paccierotti and Sgura, 2008). Micronuclei containing kinetochores or centromeric DNA may be detected in cultured cells (Lynch and Parry, 1993; Aardema *et al.*, 1998; Fenech, 2008; Paccierotti and Sgura, 2008) and in mouse bone marrow in vivo (Adler, 1993; Krishna and Hayashi, 2000). Frequencies of micronuclei ascribable to aneuploidy and to clastogenic effects may therefore be determined concurrently by tabulating micronuclei with and without kinetochores.

Germ Cell Mutagenesis

Gene Mutations Germ cell mutagenesis assays are of special interest as indicators of genetic damage that can enter the gene pool and be transmitted through generations. Mammalian germ cell assays provide the best basis for assessing risks to human germ cells and therefore hold a central place in genetic toxicology despite their relative complexity and expense. The design of the test must compensate for the fact that mutations occur at low frequency, and even the simplest animal systems face the difficulty of their having a sufficiently large sample size. One can easily screen millions of bacteria or cultured cells by selection techniques, but screening large numbers of mice poses practical limitations. Therefore, a germ cell assay must offer a straightforward, unequivocal identification of mutants with minimal labor (Singer and Yauk, 2010).

The mouse specific-locus test detects recessive mutations that produce easily analyzed, visible phenotypes (coat pigmentation and ear size) conferred by seven genes (Russell and Shelby, 1985; Ehling, 1991; Russell and Russell, 1992; Favor, 1999; Russell, 2004; Singer *et al.*, 2006). Mutants may be classified as having point mutations or chromosomal alterations on the basis of genetic and molecular analysis (Favor, 1999). The assay has been important

in assessing genetic risks of ionizing radiation and has been used to study various chemical mutagens. Although they have been used less extensively, there are other gene mutation assays in mouse germ cells based on dominant mutations that cause skeletal abnormalities (Selby *et al.*, 2004) or cataracts (Ehling, 1991) and recessive mutations that cause electrophoretic changes in proteins (Lewis, 1991).

Mammalian assays permit the measurement of mutagenesis at different germ cell stages (Favor, 1999; Russell, 2004). Late stages of spermatogenesis are often found to be sensitive to mutagenesis, but effects in spermatocytes, spermatids, and spermatozoa are transitory. Mutagenesis in stem-cell spermatogonia and resting oocytes is of special interest in genetic risk assessment because of the persistence of these stages throughout reproductive life. Chemical mutagens show specificity with respect to germ cell stages. For example, ethylnitrosourea and chlorambucil are both potent mutagens in the mouse specific-locus test, but the former induces primarily point mutations in spermatogonia, whereas the latter mostly induces deletions in spermatids (Russell and Russell, 1992). The ratio of deletions to point mutations is not only a function of the nature of the mutagen but depends on germ cell stage, as some mutagens induce higher proportions of gross alterations in late stages of spermatogenesis than in spermatogonia (Lewis, 1991; Favor, 1999; Russell, 2004).

There is currently no unequivocal evidence of induced gene mutations in human germ cells, but studies in mice leave little doubt about the susceptibility of mammalian germ cells to mutagenesis by radiation and chemicals. New molecular methods, particularly those involving the assessment of changes in tandem repeat loci (Yauk, 2004; Dubrova, 2005; Singer *et al.*, 2006; Somers, 2006), hold great promise for the development of systems that will permit the efficient detection of genetic alterations in human germ cells. The development of methods based on expanded simple tandem repeat (ESTR) loci in mice and other species is important, in that it permits in situ monitoring for environmental mutagens and the quantification of mutagenesis after controlled exposures of laboratory animals using systems parallel to those being developed for human monitoring (Yauk, 2004; Dubrova, 2005; Wu *et al.*, 2006; Somers, 2006). Basic research on mechanisms underlying ESTR changes is essential, as it is still unclear how ESTR changes relate to the gene mutations that have been long studied by population geneticists and are detected in classical gene-mutation assays.

Chromosomal Alterations Cytogenetic assays in germ cells are not routinely included in mutagenicity testing, but they are an important source of information for assessing risks to future generations posed by the induction of chromosome aberrations. Metaphase analysis of germ cells is feasible in rodent spermatogonia, spermatocytes, or oocytes (Kirkland *et al.*, 1990; Tease, 1992; Russo, 2000; Marchetti *et al.*, 2001). A micronucleus assay has also been developed in which chromosomal damage induced in meiosis is measured by the observation of rodent germ cells, principally spermatids (Russo, 2000; Hayashi *et al.*, 2007).

Aneuploidy originating in mammalian germ cells may be detected cytologically through chromosome counting for hyperploidy (Allen *et al.*, 1986; Adler, 1993; Aardema *et al.*, 1998; Russo, 2000; Marchetti *et al.*, 2001) or genetically in the mouse sex-chromosome loss test (Russell and Shelby, 1985), but these methods are not widely used in toxicological testing. A promising development is the detection of aneuploidy in the sperm of mice or rats by FISH with chromosome-specific probes (Baumgarthner *et al.*, 1999; Russo, 2000; Marchetti *et al.*, 2006, 2008). The presence of two fluorescent spots indicates the presence of an extra copy of the chromosome identified by the probe; probes for several chromosomes are used simultaneously so that aneuploid sperm are distinguishable from diploid sperm.

Besides cytological observation, indirect evidence for chromosome aberrations is obtained in the mouse heritable translocation assay, which measures reduced fertility in the offspring of treated males (Russell and Shelby, 1985; Singer *et al.*, 2006). This presumptive evidence of chromosomal rearrangements can be confirmed through cytogenetic analysis. Data from the mouse heritable translocation test in postmeiotic male germ cells have been used in an attempt to quantify human germ cell risk for ethylene oxide, a mutagen used as a fumigant, sterilizing agent, and reactant in chemical syntheses (Rhomberg *et al.*, 1990; Preston *et al.*, 1995).

Dominant Lethal Mutations The mouse or rat dominant lethal assay (Adler *et al.*, 1994; Singer *et al.*, 2006) offers an extensive database on the induction of genetic damage in mammalian germ cells. In the most commonly used version of the assay, males are treated on an acute or subchronic basis with the chemical of interest and then mated with virgin females at appropriate intervals. The females are killed and necropsied during pregnancy so that embryonic mortality may be characterized and quantified. Most dominant lethal mutations, manifested as intrauterine deaths, are thought to arise from chromosomal anomalies.

Development of Testing Strategies

Concern about adverse effects of mutation on human health, principally carcinogenesis and the induction of transmissible damage in germ cells, has provided the impetus to identify environmental mutagens. Priorities must be set for testing because it is not feasible to conduct multiple tests of all chemicals to which people are exposed. Such factors as production volumes, intended uses, the extent of human exposure, environmental distribution, and effects that may be anticipated on the basis of chemical structure or previous testing must be considered in order to ensure that compounds with the greatest potential for adverse effects receive the most comprehensive study. The most obvious use of genetic toxicology assays is screening chemicals to detect mutagens, but they are also used to obtain information on mutagenic mechanisms and dose–responses that contribute to an evaluation of hazards. Besides testing pure chemicals, environmental samples are tested because many mutagens exist in complex mixtures (DeMarini 1998; Ohe *et al.*, 2003; White, 2004). The analysis of complex mixtures often requires a combination of mutagenicity assays and refined analytical methods (White, 2004; Hewitt and Marvin, 2005). Assessment of a chemical's genotoxicity requires data from well-characterized assays. Assays are said to be validated when they have been shown to perform reproducibly and reliably with many compounds from diverse chemical classes in several laboratories. An evaluation of test performance, however, sometimes extends beyond determining whether the assay effectively detects the specific endpoint that it actually measures to whether it is predictive of other endpoints of interest. For example, there is great interest in the ability of mutagenicity tests, which do not measure carcinogenicity per se, to predict whether chemicals are carcinogens.

Mutagenicity testing, combined with an evaluation of chemical structure, has been found to identify a large proportion of trans-species, multiple-site carcinogens (Tennant and Ashby, 1991; Gold *et al.*, 1993). In contrast, some carcinogens are not detected as mutagens. Putatively nongenotoxic carcinogens often give responses that are more specific with respect to species, sites, and conditions (Ashby and Paton, 1993; Gold *et al.*, 1993). In predicting carcinogenicity, one should consider both the sensitivity and the specificity of an assay. Sensitivity refers to the proportion of carcinogens that are positive in the assay, whereas specificity is the proportion of noncarcinogens that are negative (Tennant *et al.*, 1987; McGregor *et al.*, 1999). Sensitivity and specificity both contribute to the predictive reliability of an assay. The commonly held view that deficiencies in the sensitivity or specificity of individual assays may be circumvented by using assays in complementary combinations called tiers or batteries has fallen into disfavor because, rather than offsetting each other's strengths and weaknesses, genetic toxicology assays are often consistent with one another (Tennant *et al.*, 1987; Ashby and Tennant, 1991; Kim and Margolin, 1999).

Strategies for testing have evolved over the last few decades, such that data from a few well-chosen assays are now considered sufficient (MacGregor *et al.*, 2000). Rather than trying to assemble extensive batteries of complementary assays, it is prudent to emphasize mechanistic considerations in choosing assays. Such an approach makes a sensitive assay for gene mutations (eg, the Ames assay) and an assay for clastogenic effects in mammals pivotal in the evaluation of genotoxicity, and this is the basis for our highlighting these assays in Table 9-1. The Ames assay has performed reliably with hundreds of compounds in laboratories throughout the world. Other bacterial assays and mammalian cell assays also provide useful information on gene mutations. Beyond gene mutations, one should evaluate damage at the chromosomal level with a mammalian in vitro or in vivo cytogenetic assay. Cytogenetic assays in rodents are especially useful for this purpose because they combine a well-validated genetic assay with mammalian pharmacodynamics and metabolism. The other assays in Table 9-1 offer an extensive database on chemical mutagenesis (ie, Drosophila SLRL), a unique genetic endpoint (ie, aneuploidy; mitotic recombination), applicability to diverse organisms and tissues (ie, DNA damage assays, such as the comet assay), or special importance in the assessment of genetic risk (ie, germ cell assays). The more extensive listing of assays in Table 9-2 provides references that can be helpful in interpreting genetic toxicology data that can be found in the scientific literature.

HUMAN POPULATION MONITORING

For cancer risk assessment considerations, the human data utilized most frequently, in the absence of epidemiologic data, are those collected from genotoxicity/mutagenicity assessments in human populations. For this purpose, the studies conducted most frequently are for chromosome aberrations, micronuclei, mutations (for several loci), and SCEs in peripheral lymphocytes. Cytogenetic alterations have also been assessed in a small number of bone marrow samples. Mutations at the *HPRT* locus have been assessed in peripheral lymphocytes. Glycophorin A variants have been studied in red blood cells.

An important component of any population monitoring study is the selection of the study groups, namely those individuals who are potentially exposed and the matched unexposed controls. The size of each study group should be sufficiently large to avoid any confounder having undue influence. Certain characteristics should be matched among exposed and unexposed groups. These include age, sex, smoking status, and general dietary features. Certain characteristics are exclusionary, namely current or recent medication, radiation exposure, and certain illnesses. It is possible to develop a lengthy list of additional possible confounders of response that would make the selection of suitable study groups very difficult indeed. Study groups of 20 or more individuals can be used as a reasonable substitute for exact matching because confounders will be less influential on chromosome alteration or mutation frequency in larger groups (discussed in Au *et al.*, 1998; Battershill *et al.,* 2008)). In some instances, it might be informative to compare exposed groups with a historical control, as well as to a concurrent control.

The magnitude of different known confounders varies considerably among studies, based in part on the size of the study populations. Some general indication of the magnitude of the effects of age and smoking status on the frequencies of chromosome aberrations and SCE is presented to illustrate the importance of accounting for confounders in the design of a population monitoring study. The comparisons presented are for large studies only. For chromosome aberrations, the frequency of aberrations has been reported in one large study to be about 50% higher in smokers (1.5 aberrations per 100 cells in smokers vs 1.0 per 100 cells in the nonsmokers) (Galloway *et al.*, 1986) and in another no difference between smokers and nonsmokers (Bender *et al.*, 1988a,b). The complete data set has been reviewed by Au *et al.* (1998). In general, the frequency of SCE is increased by about one SCE per cell in smokers compared with nonsmokers (Bender *et al.*, 1988a,b; Barale *et al.*, 1998). The study by Barale *et al.* (1998) also reported a dose–response association between SCE frequency and smoking level. The differences among these studies might well be accounted for by differences among confounders in the respective groups, but it is virtually impossible to correct for these in this type of study.

The frequency of chromosome aberrations, particularly chromosome-type (reciprocal) exchanges, has been shown to increase with age of subject (Tucker and Moore, 1996). Galloway *et al.* (1986) reported an increase from 0.8 per 100 cells at about 25 years of age to about 1.5 at 60. Bender *et al.* (1988a,b) reported an increase with age only for chromosome-type dicentric aberrations, but the increase over a broad age range was small and just statistically significant. Ramsey *et al.* (1995), using chromosome painting techniques, reported that individuals 50 years and older had frequencies of stable aberrations, dicentrics, and acentric fragments that were 10.6-, 3.3-, and 2.9-fold, respectively, greater than the frequency in cord bloods. Bender *et al.* (1998a,b) did not find an increase in SCE frequency with the increasing age of the subject. The differences among the results from these large control studies emphasize the difficulty of adequately accounting for confounders (age and smoking presented here) when only a small control group is used, as is frequently the case.

Similar sources of variation have been identified for the monitoring of individuals for *HPRT* mutations. The data are reviewed in detail by Albertini and Hayes (1997). There is less information on sources of variation of glycophorin A (GPA) variants, although quite considerable interindividual variation exists (reviewed in Cole and Skopek, 1994; Kyoizumi *et al.*, 2005).

For cytogenetic assays (chromosome aberrations, SCEs, and micronuclei) the alterations are produced as a consequence of errors of DNA replication, as discussed in previous sections. From the nature of the alterations, assessed in traditional cytogenetic assays in which nontransmissible alterations are analyzed, it can be established that these alterations were produced at the first in vitro S phase. Irrespective of the duration of exposure, the frequency of cytogenetic alterations will be proportional to that fraction of the DNA damage that remains at the time of in vitro DNA replication. All the DNA damage induced by potent clastogens that results in chromosome alterations is repaired within a relatively short time after exposure for G_0 human lymphocytes. Thus, for chronic exposures the lymphocyte cytogenetic assay as typically conducted is insensitive.

It is now possible to analyze reciprocal translocations using FISH methods (reviewed in Tucker *et al.*, 1997; Kleinerman *et al.*, 2006; Beskid *et al.*, 2006), and because this aberration type is transmissible from cell generation to generation, its frequency can be representative of an accumulation over time of exposure. The importance of this is that stable chromosome aberrations observed in peripheral lymphocytes exposed in vivo, but assessed following in vitro culture, are produced in vivo in hematopoietic stem cells or other precursor cells of the peripheral lymphocyte pool. To date, population cytogenetic monitoring studies involving the analysis of reciprocal translocations in chemically exposed individuals or radiation-exposed individuals have been conducted quite rarely (Lucas *et al.*, 1992; Smith *et al.*, 1998; Kleinerman *et al.*, 2006). The overall sensitivity of the FISH analysis of reciprocal translocations for assessing effects of chronic, low levels of exposure to chemical clastogens has not been established. However, a cautionary note is provided by the study of Director *et al.* (1998), who showed that there was no increase in reciprocal translocations assessed by FISH following exposure to cyclophosphamide (0, 32, 64, or 96 ppm) or urethane (0, 5000, 10,000, or 15,000 ppm) for up to 12 weeks. In contrast, recent data on ethylene oxide (Donner *et al.*, 2010) have shown that exposure of male mice to ethylene oxide at concentrations of 0, 25, 50, 100, 200 ppm for 6, 12, 24, or 48 weeks resulted in a time and concentration-dependent increase in reciprocal translocations assessed by FISH.

Another factor that certainly affects the utility of population monitoring data with reciprocal translocations using FISH is that the frequency of reciprocal translocations increases significantly with increasing age (Ramsey *et al.*, 1995), but to a lesser extent for nontransmissible aberrations (Bender *et al.*, 1988a,b). Ramsey *et al.* (1995) provided data on the influence of other confounders on the frequency of reciprocal translocations in human groups. These confounders include smoking, consumption of diet drinks and/or diet sweeteners, exposure to asbestos or coal products, and having a previous major illness. This reemphasizes the point that the selection of study groups and accounting for confounders is essential for human population cytogenetic monitoring studies to be of utility.

Thus, very few of the published studies of cytogenetic population monitoring for individuals have analyzed the appropriate endpoint for detecting the genetic effects of long-term exposure to chemicals. It is quite surprising that positive responses have been reported for increases in unstable, chromatid aberrations because these are nontransmissible, and as noted above are induced at the first in vitro S phase. This anomaly is especially concerning when positive responses at very low levels of exposure are reported (reviewed for ethylene oxide in Preston, 1999b).

The *HPRT* mutation assay can assess the frequency of induced mutations in stem cells or other precursor cells because a proportion of the mutations are induced as nonlethal events. The transmissible proportion will be greater for chemicals that do not induce large deletions; this will include the majority of nonradiomimetic chemicals. Induction of mutations in lymphocyte precursor cells will lead to clonal expansion of mutations in the peripheral pool. However, assessment of the T-cell antigen receptor status of the mutant clones permits a correction for clonal expansion. The population of cells derived from any particular stem cell has a unique antigen receptor status (Albertini and Hayes, 1997). The GPA assay can similarly be used for the assessment of chronic exposures or for estimating exposures at some long time after exposure (Albertini and Hayes, 1997). The predictive value of the assay for adverse health outcome appears to be limited, but it can provide an estimate of exposure.

The potential for cytogenetic endpoints being predictive of relative cancer risk has been addressed in recent reports from the European Study Group on Cytogenetic Biomarkers and Health (Hagmar *et al.*, 1998a,b; Bonassi *et al.*, 2004; Norppa *et al.*, 2006). The groups selected for cytogenetic studies consisted of individuals with reported occupational exposure and unexposed controls. The association between cancer and the frequency of unstable chromosome aberrations in the study groups was not based on exposure status, but rather on the relative frequency of chromosome aberrations, namely, low (1–33 percentiles), medium (34–66 percentiles), and high (67–100 percentiles). In general, the higher the relative frequency of unstable aberrations, the greater the risk of cancer death for all tumors combined. The authors make it clear that there is insufficient information on exposure for it to be used as a predictor of cancer development. In fact, the data indicate that individuals with higher frequencies of chromosome aberrations for whatever reason (genetic or environmental) are *as a group* at greater risk of dying from cancer. This is very different from concluding that exposures to mutagens that result in a higher frequency of chromosome aberrations in peripheral lymphocytes leads to an increased risk of cancer, especially for specific tumor types. The relevance of exposure to mutagenic chemicals in these studies by Hagmar *et al.* (1998a,b) is uncertain because there was no association between increased SCE frequencies, which may be indicative of higher exposure levels, and increased cancer mortality.

This latter concern was addressed by the same group (Bonassi *et al.*, 2000) in a more recent study. The study again showed that there was a significantly increased risk for subjects with a high level of chromosome aberrations compared to those with a low level in both Nordic and Italian cohorts. Of particular relevance to risk assessment was the observation that the relationships were not affected by the inclusion of occupational exposure level or smoking. The risk for high versus low levels of chromosome aberrations was similar in individuals heavily exposed to carcinogens and in those who had never, to their knowledge, been exposed to any specific environmental carcinogen. These data highlight the need to use caution when considering the relevance of chromosome aberration data from human biomonitoring studies in cancer risk assessment.

NEW APPROACHES FOR GENETIC TOXICOLOGY

In the last 15 or so years, the field of genetic toxicology has moved into the molecular era. The potential for advances in our understanding of basic cellular processes and how they can be perturbed is enormous. The ability to manipulate and characterize DNA, RNA, and proteins has been at the root of this advance in knowledge. However, the development of sophisticated molecular biology does not in itself imply a corresponding advance in the utility of genetic toxicology and its application to risk assessment. Knowing the types of studies to conduct and knowing how to interpret the data remain as fundamental as always. Measuring finer and finer detail can perhaps complicate the utility of the various mutagenicity assays. There is a need for genetic toxicology to avoid the temptation to use more and more sophisticated techniques to address the same questions and in the end make the same mistakes as have been made previously. How successful we are in designing informative studies based on the most recent molecular techniques perhaps cannot be judged at this time. However, the following examples of recent approaches to obtaining data for enhancing our ability to use noncancer (genotoxicity) data in a mechanistically based cancer (and genetic) risk assessment process provide some encouragement. Several recent developments (eg, the refinement of FISH painting, the high-throughput adverse pathway detection approach, and the use of ultrahigh throughput DNA sequencing technologies) have already been described in the appropriate assay sections above because they are currently in general use.

Advances in Cytogenetics

Until quite recently, the analysis of chromosome alterations relied on conventional chromosome staining with DNA stains such as Giemsa or on the process of chromosome banding. Both approaches require considerable expenditure of time and a rather high level of expertise. However, chromosome banding does allow for the assessment of transmissible aberrations such as reciprocal translocations and inversions with a fairly high degree of accuracy. Knowing the induction frequency of such aberrations is very important, given that they are generally not lethal to the cell and constitute by far the major class observed in inherited genetic defects and a significant fraction of the alterations observed in tumors. In addition, because stable aberrations are transmissible from parent to daughter cell, they represent accumulated effects of chronic exposures. The more readily analyzed but cell-lethal, nontransmissible aberrations such as dicentrics and deletions reflect only recent exposures and then only when analyzed at the first division after exposure. A more detailed discussion of these factors can be found in Preston (1999b).

The relative ease with which specific chromosomes, specific genes, and chromosome alterations can be detected has been radically enhanced by the development of FISH (Trask *et al.*, 1993; Speicher and Carter, 2005). In principle, the technique relies on amplification of DNA from particular genomic regions such as whole chromosomes or gene regions and the hybridization of these amplified DNAs to metaphase chromosome preparations or interphase nuclei. Regions of hybridization can be determined by the use of fluorescent antibodies that detect modified DNA bases incorporated during amplification or by incorporating fluorescent bases themselves during amplification. The fluorescently labeled, hybridized regions are detected by fluorescence microscopy, and the signal can be increased in strength by computer-enhanced processes. The level of sophistication has increased so much that all 24 different human chromosomes (22 autosomes, X and Y) can be individually detected (Macville *et al.*, 1997), as can all mouse chromosomes (Liyanage *et al.*, 1996) (Figs. 9-5 and 9-6). Most recently, M-FISH (multicolor FISH) and M-BAND (multicolor banding) have been developed for defining chromosome abnormalities (Mackinnon and Chudoba, 2011) (Fig. 9-9). Alterations in tumors can also be detected on a whole-genome basis (Coleman *et al.*, 1997; Veldman *et al.*, 1997; Bridge and Cushman-Vokoun, 2011). The following example highlights the ability to construct breakpoint profiles of specific tumor types (Trost *et al.*, 2006). In this example, a detailed analysis by spectral karyotyping of specific breakpoints in a set of primary myelodysplastic syndrome and acute myeloid leukemia samples revealed recurrent involvement of specific chromosome bands that contained oncogenes or tumor-suppressor genes. The aim will be to attempt to reveal the possible prognostic significance of the subgroups linked to these specific markers.

There is an extensive literature on the use of FISH for karyotyping tumors and in gene mapping but less on its utility for genetic toxicology studies, especially the assessment of stable chromosome aberrations at long periods after exposure or after long-term exposures. Three particular studies do, however, serve to exemplify the use of FISH in genetic toxicology.

Lucas *et al.* (1992) demonstrated that stable chromosomal aberrations could be detected in individuals decades after exposure to atomic bombs in Japan. How these frequencies relate to frequencies at the time of exposure is not known with any certainty, given the fact that induced frequencies were not measured because appropriate techniques were not available at that time.

Studies by Tucker *et al.* (1997, 2005) provided some assessment of the utility of FISH for the analysis of radiation-induced,

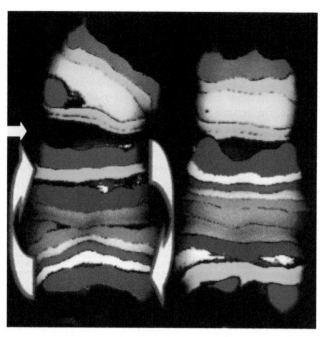

Figure 9-9. *Inversion identified by M-FISH.* Region of human chromosomes five stained by M-FISH; the left-hand segment has been inverted as can be seen when compared to the right-hand normal segment. (Reproduced with permission from Hande MP, et al. Past exposure to densely ionizing radiation leaves a unique permanent signature in the genome. *Am J Hum Genet.* 2003; May;72(5):1162–1170.)

stable chromosome alterations at various times after exposure. The frequency of reciprocal translocations induced by γ-rays in rat peripheral lymphocytes decreased with time after exposure, reaching a plateau at four days that was 55% to 65% of the induced frequency and with a dose dependency (Tucker *et al.*, 1997). Similar results were obtained for human samples (Tucker *et al.*, 2005). These results suggest that reciprocal translocations fall into two classes, stable and unstable (cell-lethal). It is quite possible that these "unstable" translocations are lost because of the presence of other cell-lethal damage in the same cell. Additional work is required to clarify this conclusion and to extend the studies to the effects of chemicals. In addition, a recent study by Tucker and Luckinbill (2011) demonstrated how FISH translocation analysis could be used to detect extremely low doses of ionizing radiation— a few centigray per year. Such analysis could be used to estimate responses at very low doses for utility in risk assessments at similarly low doses.

FISH methods have also allowed for an accurate and sensitive assessment of chromosomal alterations present in tumors. The particular advance that makes this assessment feasible is known as comparative genomic hybridization (CGH) (Kallioniemi *et al.*, 1992). CGH results in the ability to identify the role of chromosomal structural and numerical alterations in tumor development. The genomic instability present in all tumor types appears to have a specific genetic basis, as shown elegantly for colon cancer by Vogelstein and colleagues (Cahill *et al.*, 1998). For CGH, tumor and control DNAs are differentially labeled with fluorescence probes and cohybridized to normal metaphase chromosome preparations. The ratio of the fluorescence intensities of hybridized tumor and control DNA indicates regions of normal genomic content as well as those regions that are over- or underrepresented in tumors. The CGH method is being adapted for automated screening approaches using biochips (Solinas-Toldo *et al.*, 1997; Hosoya *et al.*, 2006). Assessing genetic alterations such as specific gene deletions in single metastatic tumor cells is feasible using a slightly different but complementary approach (Pack *et al.*, 1997, 2005).

The types of FISH approaches described here undoubtedly indicate the direction in which cytogenetic analysis will proceed. The types of data collected will affect our understanding of how tumors develop. Data on the dose–response characteristics for a specific chromosomal alteration as a proximate marker of cancer can enhance the cancer risk assessment process by describing effects of low exposures that are below those for which tumor incidence can be reliably assessed. Cytogenetic data of the types described above can also improve extrapolation from data generated with laboratory animals to humans.

Molecular Analysis of Mutations and Gene Expression

With the advent of molecular biology techniques, the exact basis of a mutation at the level of the DNA sequence can be established. In many cases, the genetic basis of human disease can be determined even though human genes have long DNA sequences and a complex genomic arrangement. Molecular biology techniques have also enabled a distinction to be made between background mutations and those induced by specific agents. The latter observations are addressed by analyzing the mutational spectra in target genes in laboratory organisms and in humans (DeMarini, 2000; Hemminki and Thilly, 2004). For reasons of inherent sensitivity of available methods, the genes analyzed for mutations are ones for which mutated forms can be selected. The confounding factor of many normal cells, which far outnumber a few mutant cells in an exposed cellular population, can be removed by mutant selection approaches. Methods to overcome the drawback of only being able to study selectable genes have been developed, and particular ones such as ligation-mediated PCR are close to the required sensitivity level (Albertini and Hayes, 1997; Makrigiorgos, 2004; Yeh *et al.*, 2006). For example, COLD-PCR (co-amplification at lower denaturation temperature-PCR) was developed to selectively amplify minority alleles from mixtures of wild-type and mutation-containing sequences (Li and Makrigiorgos, 2009).

A giant step forward in the ability to detect and characterize mutations at both the DNA and RNA level has been provided by the development of chip technology (Southern, 1996) and array-based assay systems (Wodicka *et al.*, 1997). With hybridization of test DNAs to oligonucleotide arrays, specific genetic alterations or their cellular consequences can be determined rapidly and automatically (Houlston and Peto, 2004; Vissers *et al.*, 2005). Cost remains a limiting factor, but the potential for assessing specific cellular changes following chemical exposure is enormous. Perhaps of even greater practical importance to the ability to detect mutations is that in the past few years the advent of second- and third-generation ultrahigh throughput DNA sequencing techniques has enormously enhanced the ability to assess mutations quantitatively at the whole genome level in a very short period of time. Such techniques have been used, for example, to characterize the genetic alterations in a number of tumor types (Stratton *et al.*, 2009). Until quite recently, alterations in gene expression following specific exposures or for specific genotypes were analyzed gene by gene. Such an approach makes it difficult to assess changes in gene expression that occur in a concerted fashion. Recent advances using cDNA microarray technologies have allowed the measurement of changes in expression of hundreds or even thousands of genes at one time (Harrington *et al.*, 2000; Elvidge, 2006). The level of expression at the mRNA level is measured by the amount of hybridization of isolated cDNAs to oligonucleotide fragments from known genes or expressed sequence tags (ESTs) on a specifically laid out grid. Although this technique holds great promise for establishing a cell's response to exposure to chemical or physical agents in the context of normal cellular patterns of gene expression, it remains to be established how to analyze the vast amounts of data that are being obtained and what magnitude of change in gene expression constitutes an adverse effect as far as cellular phenotype is concerned. Extrapolating the responses to organs and whole animals represents a challenge still to be addressed. These microarray-based techniques are now being replaced by massively parallel sequencing or ultrahigh throughput sequencing approaches that can quantitatively assess gene expression changes in response to exposures. Such sequencing-based techniques have the great advantage that they are based on molecule counting approaches rather than on hybridization, thereby making them more quantitative and able to detect very low level transcripts (Blencowe *et al.*, 2009). There are parallel efforts in the area of proteomics and metabolomics whereby changes in a broad range of cellular proteins can be assessed in response to endogenous or exogenous factors, potentially leading to the development of biomarkers of effect (Aebersold *et al.*, 2005; Robertson, 2005; Griffin, 2006; McGregor and Souza, 2006). The biggest hurdle currently is the relative paucity of sequence data available for the world of proteins and their multiple posttranslational modifications. Certainly progress is rapid, and so methodologies akin to gene expression assessment are likely to be close at hand (Xie *et al.*, 2011).

The move in the field of genetic toxicology is away from the "yes/no" approach to hazard identification and much more toward a mechanistic understanding of how a chemical or physical agent can produce adverse cellular and tissue responses. In turn such knowledge can be used for the development of informative bioindicators representing the key events along the pathway from initial interactions with cells to adverse outcome (Jarabek *et al.*, 2009). The move is clearly toward analysis at the whole genome level and away from single gene responses. The challenges are apparent and the solutions are being identified at a rapid pace.

CONCLUSIONS

The field of genetic toxicology has had an overall life of about 70 years and has undergone several rebirths during this period. Genetic toxicology began as a basic research field with demonstrations that ionizing radiations and chemicals could induce mutations and chromosome alterations in plant, insect, and mammalian cells. The development of a broad range of short-term assays for genotoxicity served to identify many mutagens and address the relationship between mutagens and cancer-causing agents, or carcinogens. The inevitable failure of the assays to be completely predictive resulted in the identification of nongenotoxic carcinogens. In the 1980s, genetic toxicology began to move more toward providing insights into a better understanding of the mutagenic mechanisms underlying carcinogenicity and heritable effects. With this improved understanding, genetic toxicology studies began to turn away from hazard identification alone and move toward quantitative risk assessment. Major advances in our knowledge of mechanisms of cancer formation have been fueled by truly amazing progress in molecular biology.

Genetic toxicology has begun to take advantage of the knowledge that cancer is a genetic disease with multiple steps, many of which require a mutation. The identification of chromosome alterations involved in tumor formation has been facilitated greatly by the use of FISH. The ability to distinguish between background and induced mutations, in some cases, can be achieved by mutation analysis at the level of DNA sequence. Second- and third-generation ultrahigh throughput sequencing technologies have allowed such whole genome mutation analysis to be accomplished in a very short time. Key cellular processes related to mutagenesis have been identified, including multiple pathways of DNA repair, cell cycle controls, and the role of checkpoints in ensuring that the cell cycle does not proceed until the DNA and specific cellular structures are checked for fidelity. These observations have enhanced our knowledge of the importance of genotype in susceptibility to cancer. Recent developments in genetic toxicology have greatly improved our understanding of basic cellular processes and alterations that can affect the integrity of the genetic material and its functions. The ability to detect and analyze mutations in mammalian germ cells continues to improve and can contribute to a better appreciation for the long-term consequences of mutagenesis in human populations. Improvements in the qualitative assessment of mutation in somatic cells and germ cells have been paralleled by advances in the ability to assess genetic alterations quantitatively, especially in ways that enhance the cancer and genetic risk assessment process (Preston, 2005).

ACKNOWLEDGMENTS

The authors thank Drs David DeMarini and Andrew Kligerman for their valuable comments as part of the review of this chapter.

This document has been reviewed in accordance with the USEPA policy and approved for publication but does not necessarily reflect EPA policy. Mention of trade names or commercial products does not constitute endorsement or recommendation for use.

REFERENCES

Aardema MJ, Albertini S, Arni P, et al. Aneuploidy: a report of an ECETOC task force. *Mutat Res.* 1998;410:3–79.

Aboussekhra A, Biggerstaff M, Shivji JA, et al. DNA nucleotide excision repair reconstituted with purified protein components. *Cell.* 1995;80:859–868.

Adler I-D. Synopsis of the in vivo results obtained with the 10 known or suspected aneugens tested in the CEC collaborative study. *Mutat Res.* 1993;287:131–137.

Adler I-D, Shelby MD, Bootman J, et al. Summary report of the working group on mammalian germ cell tests. *Mutat Res.* 1994;312:313–318.

Aebersold R, Anderson L, Caprioli R, et al. Perspective: a program to improve protein biomarker discovery for cancer. *Proteome Res.* 2005;4:1104–1109.

Aguilar F, Harris CC, Sun T, et al. Geographic variation of p53 mutational profile in nonmalignant human liver. *Science.* 1994;264:1317–1319.

Albertini RJ. *HPRT* mutations in humans; biomarkers for mechanistic studies. *Mutat Res.* 2001;489:1–16.

Albertini RJ, Hayes RB. Somatic cell mutations in cancer epidemiology. *IARC Sci Publ.* 1997;142:159–184.

Allen JW, Liang JC, Carrano AV, Preston RJ. Review of literature on chemical-induced aneuploidy in mammalian germ cells. *Mutat Res.* 1986;167:123–137.

Ames BN, McCann J, Yamasaki E. Methods for detecting carcinogens and mutagens with the Salmonella/mammalian-microsome mutagenicity test. *Mutat Res.* 1975;31:347–364.

Anderson RM, Marsden SJ, Wright EG, et al. Complex chromosome aberrations in peripheral blood lymphocytes as a potential biomarker of exposure to high-Let alpha-particles. *Int J Radiat Biol.* 2000;76:31–42.

Ashby J. Two million rodent carcinogens? The role of SAR and QSAR in their detection. *Mutat Res.* 1994;305:3–12.

Ashby J, Paton D. The influence of chemical structure on the extent and sites of carcinogenesis for 522 rodent carcinogens and 55 different human carcinogen exposures. *Mutat Res.* 1993;286:3–74.

Ashby J, Tennant RW. Definitive relationships among chemical structure, carcinogenicity and mutagenicity for 301 chemicals tested by the U.S. NTP. *Mutat Res.* 1991;257:229–306.

Au WW, Gajas-Salazar N, Salama S. Factors contributing to discrepancies in population monitoring studies. *Mutat Res.* 1998;400:467–478.

Auerbach C, Robson JM. Chemical production of mutations. *Nature.* 1946;157:302.

Bansbach CE, Cortez D. Defining genome maintenance pathways using functional genomic approaches. *Crit Rev Biochem Mol Biol.* 2011;46:327–341.

Barale R, Chelotti L, Davini T, et al. Sister chromatid exchange and micronucleus frequency in human lymphocytes of 1,650 subjects in an Italian population: II. Contribution of sex, age, and lifestyle. *Environ Mol Mutagen.* 1998;31:228–242.

Barrett JC. Mechanisms of multistep carcinogenesis and carcinogen risk assessment. *Environ Health Prospect.* 1993;100:9–20.

Battershill JM, Burnett K, Bull S. Factors affecting the incidence of genotoxicity biomarkers in peripheral blood lymphocytes: impact on design of biomonitoring studies. *Mutagenesis.* 2008;23:423–437.

Baumgarthner A, Van Hummelen P, Lowe XR, et al. Numerical and structural chromosomal abnormalities detected in human sperm with a combination of multicolor FISH assays. *Environ Mol Mutagen.* 1999;33:49–58.

Beale G. The discovery of mustard gas mutagenesis by Auerbach and Robson in 1941. *Genetics.* 1993;134:393–399.

Bender MA, Gooch PC. Persistent chromosome aberrations in irradiated human subjects. *Radiat Res.* 1962;16:44–53.

Bender MA, Preston RJ, Leonard RC, et al. Chromosomal aberration and sister-chromatid exchange frequencies in peripheral blood lymphocytes of a large human population sample. *Mutat Res.* 1988a;204:421–433.

Bender MA, Preston RJ, Leonard RC, et al. Chromosomal aberration and sister-chromatid exchange frequencies in peripheral blood lymphocytes of a large human population sample. II. Extension of age range. *Mutat Res.* 1988b;212:149–154.

Bentley KS, Sarrif AM, Cimino MC, Auletta AE. Assessing the risk of heritable gene mutation in mammals: *Drosophila* sex-linked recessive lethal test and tests measuring DNA damage and repair in mammalian germ cells. *Environ Mol Mutagen.* 1994;23:3–11.

Beskid O, Dusek Z, Solansky I, et al. The effects of exposure to different clastogens on the pattern of chromosomal aberrations detected by FISH whole chromosome painting in occupationally exposed individuals. *Mutat Res.* 2006;594:20–29.

Bickel SE, Orr-Weaver TL. Holding chromatids together to ensure they go their separate ways. *Bioessays.* 1996;18:293–300.

Bishop JM. Molecular themes in oncogenesis. *Cell.* 1991;64:235–248.

Blaisdell JO, Harrison L, Wallace SS. Base excision repair processing of radiation-induced clustered DNA lesions. *Radiat Prot Dosimetry.* 2001;97:25–31.

Blencowe BJ, Ahmad S, Lee LJ. Current-generation high-throughput sequencing: deepening insights into mammalian transcriptomes. *Genes Dev.* 2009;23:1379–1386.

Bonassi S, Hagmar L, Strömberg U, et al. Chromosomal aberrations in lymphocytes predict human cancer independently of exposure to carcinogens. *Cancer Res.* 2000;60:1619–1625.

Bonassi S, Znaor A, Norppa H, Hagmar L. Chromosomal aberrations and risk of cancer in humans: An epidemiologic perspective. *Cytogenet Genome Res.* 2004;104:376–382.

Boobis AR, Cohen S M, Dellarco V, et al. IPCS framework for analyzing the relevance of a cancer mode of action for humans. *Crit Rev Toxicol.* 2006;36:781–792.

Boobis AR, Doe JE, Heinrich-Hirsch B, et al. IPCS framework for analyzing the relevance of a noncancer mode of action for humans. *Crit Rev Toxicol.* 2008;38:87–96.

Brendler-Schwaab S, Czich A, Epe B, et al. Photochemical genotoxicity: principles and test methods. Report of a GUM task force. *Mutat Res.* 2004;566:65–91.

Brewen JG, Preston RJ. Cytogenetic effects of environmental mutagens in mammalian cells and the extrapolation to man. *Mutat Res.* 1974;26:297–305.

Brewen JG, Preston RJ. Cytogenetic analysis of mammalian oocytes in mutagenicity studies. In: Hsu TC, ed. *Cytogenetic Assays of Environmental Mutagens.* Totowa, NJ: Allanheld, Osmun; 1982:277–287.

Bridge JA, Cushman-Vokoun AM. Molecular diagnostics of soft tissue tumors. *Arch Pathol Lab Med.* 2011;135:588–601.

Brusick JD, ed. *Methods for Genetic Risk Assessment.* Boca Raton, FL: CRC Press; 1994.

Bryce SM, Avlasevich, SL, Bemis JC, et al. Miniaturized flow cytpmetry-basedCHO-K1 micronucleus assay discriminates aneugenic and clastogenic modes of action. *Environ Mol Mutagen.* 2011;52:280–286.

Burkhart JG, Malling HV. Mutagenesis and transgenic systems: perspective from the mutagen, N-ethyl-N-nitrosourea. *Environ Mol Mutagen.* 1993;22:1–6.

Burkhart JG, Malling HV. Mutations among the living and the undead. *Mutat Res.* 1994;304:315–320.

Burma S, Chen BP, Chen DJ. Role of non-homologous end joining (NHEJ) in maintaining genomic integrity. *DNA Repair.* 2006;5:1042–1048.

Cadet J, Douki T, Ravanat JL. Measurement of oxidatively generated base damage in cellular DNA. *Mutat Res.* 2011;711:3–12.

Cahill D, Connor B, Carney JP. Mechanisms of eukaryotic DNA double strand break repair. *Front Biosci.* 2006;11:1958–1976.

Cahill DP, Lengauer C, Yu J, et al. Mutations of mitotic checkpoint genes in human cancers. *Nature.* 1998;392:300–303.

Calos MP, Miller JH. Genetic and sequence analysis of frameshift mutations induced by ICR-191. *J Mol Biol.* 1981;153:39–66.

Cariello NF, Skopek TR. Analysis of mutations occurring at the human *hprt* locus. *J Mol Biol.* 1993;231:41–57.

Casciano DA, Aidoo A, Chen T, et al. *Hprt* mutant frequency and molecular analysis of *Hprt* mutations in rats treated with mutagenic carcinogens. *Mutat Res.* 1999;431:389–395.

Cavenee WK, Dryja TP, Phillips RA, et al. Expression of recessive alleles by chromosomal mechanisms in retinoblastoma. *Nature.* 1983;305:779–784.

Cebula TA, Koch WH. Sequence analysis of *Salmonella typhimurium* revertants. In: Mendelsohn ML, Albertini RJ, eds. *Mutation and the Environment*, Part D. New York: Wiley-Liss; 1990:367–377.

Claxton LD, Umbuzeiro GD, Demarini DM. The *Salmonella* mutagenicity assay: the stethoscope of genetic toxicology for the 21st century. *Environ Health Perspect.* 2010;118:1515–1522.

Clements J. The mouse lymphoma assay. *Mutat Res.* 2000;455:97–110.

Coffing S, Engel M, Dickinson D, et al. The rat gut micronucleus assay: a good choice for alternative in vivo genetic toxicology testing strategies. *Environ Mol Mutagen.* 2011;52:269–279.

Cole J, Skopek TR. Somatic mutant frequency, mutation rates and mutational spectra in the human population in vivo. *Mutat Res.* 1994;304:33–105.

Coleman AE, Schrock E, Weaver Z, et al. Previously hidden chromosome aberrations in t(12;15)-positive BALB/c plasmacytomas uncovered by multicolor spectral karyotyping. *Cancer Res.* 1997;57:4585–4592.

Collins AR. The comet assay for DNA damage and repair: principles, applications, and limitations. *Mol Biotechnol.* 2004;26:249–261.

Corvi R, Albertini S, Hartung T, et al. ECVAM retrospective validation of *in vitro* micronucleus test. *Mutagenesis.* 2008;23:271–283.

Cotelle S, Férard JF. Comet assay in genetic ecotoxicology. *Environ Mol Mutagen.* 1999;34:246–255.

Crespi CL, Miller VP. The use of heterologously expressed drug metabolizing enzymes—state of the art and prospects for the future. *Pharmacol Ther.* 1999;84:121–131.

Critchlow SE, Jackson SP. DNA end-joining from yeast to man. *Trends Biochem Sci.* 1998;23:394–398.

Croce CM. Oncogenes and cancer. *N Engl J Med.* 2008;358:502–511.

Crouse GF. Mutagenesis assays in yeast. *Methods.* 2000;22:116–119.

Cupples CG, Cabrera M, Cruz C, Miller JH. A set of *lacZ* mutations in *Escherichia coli* that allow rapid detection of specific frameshift mutations. *Genetics.* 1990;125:275–280.

Cupples CG, Miller JH. A set of *lacZ* mutations in *Escherichia coli* that allow rapid detection of each of the six base substitutions. *Proc Natl Acad Sci U S A.* 1989;86:5345–5349.

Daigaku Y, Endo K, Watanabe E, et al. Loss of heterozygosity and DNA damage repair in *Saccharomyces cerevisiae. Mutat Res.* 2004;556:183–191.

DeMarini DM. Mutation spectra of complex mixtures. *Mutat Res.* 1998;411:11–18.

DeMarini DM. Influence of DNA repair on mutation spectra in *Salmonella. Mutat Res.* 2000;450:5–17.

DeMarini DM, Brockman HE, de Serres FJ, et al. Specific-locus mutations induced in eukaryotes (especially mammalian cells) by radiation and chemicals: a perspective. *Mutat Res.* 1989;220:11–29.

DeMarini DM, Shelton ML, Abu-Shakra A, et al. Spectra of spontaneous frameshift mutations at the *his* D3052 allele of *Salmonella typhimurium* in four DNA repair backgrounds. *Genetics.* 1998;149:17–36.

Demple B, Harrison L. Repair of oxidative damage to DNA: enzymology and biology. *Annu Rev Biochem.* 1994;63:915–948.

Dertinger SD, Torous DK, Hayashi M, et al. Flow cytometric scoring of micronucleated erythrocytes: an efficient platform for assessing in vivo cytogenetic damage. *Mutagenesis.* 2011;26:139–145.

Director AE, Tucker JD, Ramsey MJ, Nath J. Chronic ingestion of clastogens by mice and the frequency of chromosome aberrations. *Environ Mol Mutagen.* 1998;32:139–147.

Dobrovolsky VN, Miura D, Heflich RH, et al. The in vivo *Pig-a* gene mutation assay, a potential tool for regulatory safety assessment. *Environ Mol Mutagen.* 2010;51:825–835.

Dobo KL, Fiedler RD, Gunther WC, et al. Defining EMS and ENU dose-response relationships using the Pig-a mutation assay in rats. *Mutat Res.* 2011;725:12–21.

Dogliotti E, Hainant P, Hernandez T, et al. Mutation spectra resulting from carcinogenic exposures: from model systems to cancer-related genes. *Recent Results Cancer Res.* 1998;154:97–124.

Donner EM, Wong BA, James RA, et al. Reciprocal translocations in somatic and germ cells of mice chronically exposed by inhalation to ethylene oxide: implications for risk assessment. *Mutagenesis.* 2010;25:49–55.

Dubrova YE. Radiation-induced mutation at tandem repeat DNA loci in the mouse germline: spectra and doubling doses. *Radiat Res.* 2005;163:200–207.

Eccles LJ, O'Neill P, Lomax ME. Delayed repair of radiation induced clustered DNA damage: friend or foe? *Mutat Res.* 2011;711:134–141.

Ehling UH. Genetic risk assessment. *Annu Rev Genet.* 1991;25:255–280.

Elespuru RK, Sankaranarayanan K. New approaches to assessing the effects of mutagenic agents on the integrity of the human genome. *Mutat Res.* 2007;616:83–89.

Elvidge G. Microarray expression technology: from start to finish. *Pharmacogenomics.* 2006;7:123–134.

EPA (US Environmental Protection Agency). Guidelines for carcinogen risk assessment. *Fed Reg.* 1986;51:33992–34003.

EPA (US Environmental Protection Agency). *Proposed Guidelines for Carcinogen Risk Assessment.* EPA/600P/P-92/003c. Office of Research and Development. Washington, DC: US Environmental Protection Agency; 1996.

EPA (US Environmental Protection Agency). *Guidelines for Carcinogen Risk Assessment.* Risk Assessment Forum. Washington, DC: US Environmental Protection Agency; 2005. www.epa.gov/cancerguidelines.

Evan G, Littlewood T. A matter of life and cell death. *Science.* 1998;281:1317–1322.

Evans HJ, Prosser J. Tumor-suppressor genes: cardinal factors in inherited predisposition to human cancers. *Environ Health Perspect.* 1992;98:25–37.

Fairbairn DW, Olive PL, O'Neill KL. The comet assay: a comprehensive review. *Mutat Res.* 1995;339:37–59.

Farmer PB, Singh R. Use of DNA adducts to identify human health risk from exposure to hazardous environmental pollutants: the increasing role of mass spectrometry in assessing biologically effective doses of genotoxic carcinogens. *Mutat Res.* 2008;659:68–76.

Favor J. Mechanisms of mutation induction in germ cells of the mouse as assessed by the specific-locus test. *Mutat Res.* 1999;428:227–236.

Fearon ER, Vogelstein B. A genetic model for colorectal tumorigenesis. *Cell.* 1990;61:759–767.

Fenech M, Chang WP, Kirsch-Volders M, et al. HUMN project: detailed description of the scoring criteria for the cytokinesis-block micronoucleus assay using isolated human lymphocyte cultures. *Mutat Res.* 2003;534:65–75.

Fenech M. The micronucleus assay determination of chromosomal level DNA damage. *Methods Mol Biol.* 2008;410:185–216.

Fenech M, Holland N, Zeiger E, et al. The HUMN and HUMNxL international collaboration projects on human micronucleus assays in lymphocytes and buccal cells—past, present and future. *Mutagenesis.* 2011a;26:239–245.

Fenech M, Kirsch-Volders M, Natarajan AT, et al. Molecular mechanisms of micronucleus, nucleoplasmic bridge and nuclear bud formation in mammalian and human cells. *Mutagenesis.* 2011b;26:125–132.

Ferguson LR, Denny WA. Frameshift mutagenesis by acridines and other reversibly-binding DNA ligands. *Mutagenesis.* 1990;5:529–540.

Fischer AH, Young KA, DeLellis RA. Incorporating pathologists' criteria of malignancy into the evolutionary model for cancer development. *J Cell Biochem.* 2004;93:28–36.

Freeman KM, Hoffmann GR. Frequencies of mutagen-induced coincident mitotic recombinationat unlinked loci in *Saccharomyces cerevisiae.* *Mutat Res.* 2007;616:119–132.

Friedberg EC. *DNA Repair.* New York: Freeman; 1985.

Friedberg EC. Biological responses to DNA damage: a perspective in the new millennium. *Cold Spring Harb Symp Quant Biol.* 2000;65:593–602.

Friedberg EC, Walker GC, Siede W. *DNA Repair and Mutagenesis.* Washington, DC: ASM Press; 1995.

Galloway SM. Cytotoxicity and chromosome aberrations in vitro: experience in industry and the case for an upper limit on toxicity in the aberration assay. *Environ Mol Mutagen.* 2000;35:191–201.

Galloway SM, Aardema MJ, Ishidate M Jr, et al. Report from working group on in vitro tests for chromosomal aberrations. *Mutat Res.* 1994;312:241–261.

Galloway SM, Berry PK, Nichols WW, et al. Chromosome aberrations in individuals occupationally exposed to ethylene oxide, and in a large control population. *Mutat Res.* 1986;170:55–74.

Galloway SM, Ivett JL. Chemically induced aneuploidy in mammalian cells in culture. *Mutat Res.* 1986;167:89–105.

Galloway S, Lorge E, Aardema MJ, et al. Workshop summary: top concentration for in vitro mammalian cell genotoxicity assays; and report from working group on toxicity measures and top concentration for in vitro cytogenetic assays (chromosome aberrations and micronucleus). *Mutat Res.* 2011;723:77–83.

Gatehouse D, Haworth S, Cebula T, et al. Recommendations for the performance of bacterial mutation assays. *Mutat Res.* 1994;312:217–233.

Gatenby RA, Vincent TL. An evolutionary model of carcinogenesis. *Cancer Res.* 2003;63:6212–6220.

Gealy R, Wright-Bourque JL, Kraynak AR, et al. Validation of a high-throughput in vitro alkaline elution/rat hepatocyte assay for DNA damage. *Mutat Res.* 2007;629:49–63.

Gee P, Maron DM, Ames BN. Detection and classification of mutagens: a set of base-specific *Salmonella* tester strains. *Proc Natl Acad Sci U S A.* 1994;91:11606–11610.

Giglia-Mari G, Zotter A, Vermeulen W. DNA damage response. *Cold Spring Harb Perspect Biol.* 2011;3:745–778.

Glei M, Hovhannisyan G, Pool-Zobel BL. Use of Comet-FISH in the study of DNA damage and repsir: review. *Mutat Res.* 2009;681:33–43.

Gold LS, Slone TH, Stern BR, Bernstein L. Comparison of target organs of carcinogenicity for mutagenic and non-mutagenic chemicals. *Mutat Res.* 1993;286:75–100.

Goodhead DT. Initial events in the cellular effects of ionizing radiations: clustered damage in DNA. *Int J Radiat Biol.* 1994;65:7–17.

Grant WF, Owens ET. *Zea mays* assays of chemical/radiation genotoxicity for the study of environmental mutagens. *Mutat Res.* 2006;613:17–64.

Griffin DK. The incidence, origin, and etiology of aneuploidy. *Int Rev Cytol.* 1996;167:263–296.

Griffin JL. Understanding mouse models of disease through metabolomics. *Curr Opin Chem Biol.* 2006;10:309–315.

Grombacher T, Mitra S, Kaina B. Induction of the alkyltransferase (MGMT) gene by DNA damaging agents and the glucocorticoid dexamethasone and comparison with the response of base excision repair. *Carcinogenesis.* 1996;17:2329–2336.

Guengerich FP. Forging the links between metabolism and carcinogenesis. *Mutat Res.* 2001;488:195–209.

Guha R. The ups and downs of structure-activity landscapes. *Methods Mol Biol.* 2011;672:101–117.

Haber JE. Partners and pathways: Repairing a double-strand break. *Trends Genet.* 2000;16:259–264.

Hagmar L, Bonassi S, Strömberg U, et al. Cancer predictive value of cytogenetic markers used in occupational health surveillance programs: a report from an ongoing study by the European Study Group on Cytogenetic Biomarkers and Health. *Mutat Res.* 1998a;405:171–178.

Hagmar L, Bonassi S, Strömberg U, et al. Chromosomal aberrations in lymphocytes predict human cancer: a report from the European Study Group on Cytogenetic Biomarkers and Health (ESCH). *Cancer Res.* 1998b;58:4117–4121.

Hahn WC, Counter CM, Lundberg AS, et al. Creation of human tumor cells with defined genetic elements. *Nature.* 1999;400:464–468.

Halliday JA, Glickman BW. Mechanisms of spontaneous mutation in DNA repair-proficient *Escherichia coli. Mutat Res.* 1991;250:55–71.

Hamilton JP. Epigenetics: principles and practice. *Dig Dis.* 2011;29:130–135.

Hanahan D, Weinberg RA. The hallmarks of cancer. *Cell.* 2000;100:57–70.

Hanahan D, Weinberg RA. Hallmarks of cancer: the next generation. *Cell.* 2011;144:646–674.

Harrington CA, Rosenow C, Retief J. Monitoring gene expression using DNA microarrays. *Curr Opin Microbiol.* 2000;3:285–291.

Harris CC. P53: at the crossroads of molecular carcinogenesis and risk assessment. *Science.* 1993;262:1980–1981.

Hastwell PW, Webster TW, Tate M, et al. Analysis of 75 marketed pharmaceuticals using the *GADD45a-GFP "GreenScreen HC"* genotoxicity assay. *Mutagenesis.* 2009;24:455–463.

Hayashi M, MacGregor JT, Gatehouse DG, et al. In vivo erythrocyte micronucleus assay III. Validation and regulatory acceptance of automated scoring and the use of rat peripheral blood reticulocytes, with discussion of non-hematopoietic target cells and a single dose-level limit test. *Mutat Res.* 2007;627:10–30.

Heartlein MW, O'Neill JP, Preston RJ. SCE induction is proportional to substitution in DNA for thymidine by CldU. *Mutat Res.* 1983;107:103–109.

Heflich RH. Chemical mutagens. In: Li AP, Heflich RH, eds. *Genetic Toxicology: A Treatise.* Boca Raton, FL: CRC Press; 1991:143–202.

Hemminki K, Thilly WG. Implications of results of molecular epidemiology on DNA adducts, their repair and mutations for mechanisms of human cancer. *IARC Sci Publ.* 2004;157:217–235.

Hewitt LM, Marvin CH. Analytical methods in environmental effects-directed investigations of effluents. *Mutat Res.* 2005;589:208–232.

Himmelstein MW, Boogaard PJ, Cadet J, et al. Creating context for the use of DNA adduct data in cancer risk assessment: II. Overview of methods of identification and quantitation of DNA damage. *Crit Rev Toxicol.* 2009;39:679–694.

Hiom K. Coping with DNA double strand breaks. *DNA Repair.* 2010;9:1256–1263.

Hoffmann GR. Induction of genetic recombination: consequences and model systems. *Environ Mol Mutagen.* 1994;23(suppl 24):59–66.

Hoffmann GR, Calciano MA, Lawless BM, Mahoney KM. Frameshift mutations induced by three classes of acridines in the *lacZ* reversion assay in *Escherichia coli*: potency of responses and relationship to slipped mispairing models. *Environ Mol Mutagen.* 2003;42:111–121.

Hosoya N, Sanada M, Nannya Y, et al. Genomewide screening of DNA copy number changes in chronic myelogenous leukemia with the use of high-resolution array-based comparative genomic hybridization. *Genes Chromosomes Cancer.* 2006;45:482–494.

Houlston RS, Peto J. The search for low-penetrance cancer susceptibility alleles. *Oncogene.* 2004;23:6471–6476.

Howlett NG, Schiestl RH. Simultaneous measurement of the frequencies of intrachromosomal recombination and chromosome gain using the yeast DEL assay. *Mutat Res.* 2000;454:53–62.

Hsu TC. Human and Mammalian Cytogenetics: A Historical Perspective. New York: Springer-Verlag; 1979.

Hunt PA. Meiosis in mammals: recombination, non-disjunction and the environment. *Biochem Soc Trans.* 2006;34:574–577.

International Program on Chemical Safety. In: Ashby J, de Serres FJ, Shelby MD, eds. *Evaluation of Short-Term Tests for Carcinogens,* Vols I and II. Cambridge, UK: Cambridge University Press; 1988.

Ishidate M Jr, Harnois MC, Sofuni T. A comparative analysis of data on the clastogenicity of 951 chemical substances tested in mammalian cell cultures. *Mutat Res.* 1988;195:151–213.

Jarabek AM, Pottenger LH, Andrews LS, et al. Creating context for the use of DNA adduct data in cancer risk assessment: I. Data organization. *Crit Rev Toxicol.* 2009;39:659–678.

Jagger C, Tate M, Cahill PA, et al. Assessment of the genotoxicity of S9-generated metabolites using the GreenScreenHC *GADD45a-GFP* assay. *Mutagenesis.* 2009;24:35–50.

Jha AN. Genotoxicological studies in aquatic organisms: an overview. *Mutat Res.* 2004;552:1–17.

Jiang G, Sancar A. Recruitment of DNA damage checkpoint proteins to damage in transcribed and nontranscribed sequences. *Mol Cell Biol.* 2006;26:39–49.

Jiricny J. Eukaryotic mismatch repair: an update. *Mutat Res.* 1998;409:107–121.

Johnson KA. The kinetic and chemical mechanism of high-fidelity DNA polymerases. *Biochim Biophys Acta.* 2010;1804:1041–1048.

Johnson RD, Liu N, Jasin M. Mammalian XRCC2 promotes the repair of DNA double-strand breaks by homologous recombination. *Nature.* 1999;401:397–399.

Josephy PD. The *Escherichia coli lacZ* reversion mutagenicity assay. *Mutat Res.* 2000;455:71–80.

Josephy PD. Genetically-engineered bacteria expressing human enzymes and their use in the study of mutations and mutagenesis. *Toxicology.* 2002;181–182:255–260.

Jun SH, Kim TG, Ban C. DNA mismatch repair system. Classical and fresh roles. *FEBS J.* 2006;273:1609–1619.

Jurado J, Alejandre-Durán E, Pueyo C. Mutagenicity testing in *Salmonella typhimurium* strains possessing both the His reversion and Ara forward mutation systems and different levels of classical nitroreductase or o-acetyltransferase activities. *Environ Mol Mutagen.* 1994;23:286–293.

Kallioniemi A, Kallioniemi O-P, Sudar D, et al. Comparative genomic hybridization for molecular cytogenetic analysis of solid tumors. *Science.* 1992;258:818–821.

Kamber M, Flückiger-Isler S, Engelhardt G, et al. Comparison of the Ames II and traditional Ames test responses with respect to mutagenicity, strain specificities, need for metabolism and correlation with carcinogenicity. *Mutagenesis.* 2009;24:359–366.

Kier LE, Brusick DJ, Auletta AE, et al. The *Salmonella typhimurium*/mammalian microsomal assay: a report of the U.S. Environmental Protection Agency Gene-Tox Program. *Mutat Res.* 1986;168:69–240.

Kim BS, Margolin BH. Prediction of rodent carcinogenicity utilizing a battery of in vitro and in vivo genotoxicity tests. *Environ Mol Mutagen.* 1999;34:297–304.

Kinzler KW, Vogelstein B. Lessons from hereditary colorectal cancer. *Cell.* 1996;87:159–170.

Kirkland DJ, Gatehouse DG, Scott D, et al., eds. *Basic Mutagenicity Tests: UKEMS Recommended Procedures.* New York: Cambridge University Press; 1990.

Kirkland D, Speit G. Evaluation of the ability of a battery of three in vitro genotoxicity tests to discriminate rodent carcinogens and non-carcinogens III. Appropriate follow-up testing in vivo. *Mutat Res.* 2008;654:114–132.

Kirsch-Volders M, Sofuni T, Aardema M, et al. Report from the in vitro micronucleus assay working group. *Mutat Res.* 2003;540:153–163.

Kleinerman RA, Romanyukha AA, Schauer DA, Tucker JD. Retrospective assessment of radiation exposure using biological dosimetry: chromosome painting, electron paramagnetic resonance and the glycophorin a mutation assay. *Radiat Res.* 2006;166:287–302.

Knudsen TB, Houck KA, Sipes NS, et al. Activity profiles of 309 ToxCast™ chemicals evaluated across 292 biochemical targets. *Toxicology.* 2011;282:1–15.

Knudson AG. Hereditary predisposition to cancer. *Ann NY Acad Sci.* 1997;833:58–67.

Koch WH, Henrikson EN, Kupchella E, Cebula TA. *Salmonella typhimurium* strain TA100 differentiates several classes of carcinogens and mutagens by base substitution specificity. *Carcinogenesis.* 1994;15:79–88.

Kolodner RD. Mismatch repair: mechanisms and relationship to cancer susceptibility. *Trends Biochem Sci.* 1995;20:397–401.

Krishna G, Hayashi M. In vivo rodent micronucleus assay: protocol, conduct and data interpretation. *Mutat Res.* 2000;455:155–166.

Kyoizumi S, Kusunoki Y, Hayashi T, et al. Individual variation of somatic gene mutability in relation to cancer susceptibility: prospective study on erythrocyte glycophorin a gene mutations of atomic bomb survivors. *Cancer Res.* 2005;65:5462–5469.

Lambert IB, Singer TM, Boucher SE, Douglas GR. Detailed review of transgenic rodent mutation assays. *Mutat Res.* 2005;590:1–280.

Laval J, Boiteux S, O'Connor TR. Physiological properties and repair of apurinic/apyrimidinic sites and imidazole ring-opened guanines in DNA. *Mutat Res.* 1990;233:73–79.

Le XC, Xing JZ, Lee J, et al. Inducible repair of thymine glycol detected by an ultrasensitive assay for DNA damage. *Science.* 1998;280:1066–1069.

Lee RF, Steinert S. Use of the single cell gel electrophoresis/comet assay for detecting DNA damage in aquatic (marine and freshwater) animals. *Mutat Res.* 2003;544:43–64.

Lee WR, Abrahamson S, Valencia R, et al. The sex-linked recessive lethal test for mutagenesis in *Drosophila melangoaster*: a report of the U.S. Environmental Protection Agency Gene-Tox Program. *Mutat Res.* 1983;123:183–279.

Léonard A. Observations on meiotic chromosomes of the male mouse as a test of the potential mutagenicity of chemicals in mammals. In: Hollaender A, ed. *Chemical Mutagens: Principles and Methods for Their Detection.* Vol 3. New York: Plenum Press; 1973:21.

Levine JG, Schaaper RM, DeMarini DM. Complex frameshift mutations mediated by plasmid pKM101: mutational mechanisms deduced from 4-aminobiphenyl-induced mutation spectra in *Salmonella. Genetics.* 1994;136:731–746.

Lewis SE. The biochemical specific-locus test and a new multiple-endpoint mutation detection system: considerations for genetic risk assessment. *Environ Mol Mutagen.* 1991;18:303–306.

Li AP, Gupta RS, Heflich RH, et al. A review and analysis of the Chinese hamster ovary/hypoxanthine guanine phosphoribosyl transferase assay to determine the mutagenicity of chemical agents. A report of the U.S. Environmental Protection Agency Gene-Tox Program. *Mutat Res.* 1988;196:17–36.

Li J, Makrigiorgos GM. COLD-PCR: a new platform for highly improved mutation detection in cancer and genetic testing. *Biochem Soc Trans.* 2009;37:427–432.

Lindahl T. Suppression of spontaneous mutagenesis in human cells by DNA base excision-repair. *Mutat Res.* 2000;462:129–135.

Liyanage M, Coleman A, duManoir S, et al. Multicolour spectral karyotyping of mouse chromosomes. *Nat Genet.* 1996;14:312–315.

Lommel L, Carswell-Crumpton C, Hanawalt PC. Preferential repair of the transcribed DNA strand in the dihydrofolate reductase gene throughout the cell cycle in UV-irradiated human cells. *Mutat Res.* 1995;366:181–192.

Lucas JN, Awa A, Straume T, et al. Rapid translocation analysis in humans decades after exposure to ionizing radiation. *Int J Radiat Biol.* 1992;62:53–63.

Lynch AM, Guzzie PJ, Bauer D, et al. Considerations on photochemical genotoxicity. II: report of the 2009 International Workshop on Genotoxicity Testing Working Group. *Mutat Res.* 2011;723:91–100.

Lynch AM, Parry JM. The cytochalasin-B micronucleus/kinetochore assay in vitro: studies with 10 suspected aneugens. *Mutat Res.* 1993;287:71–86.

Ma TH, Cabrera GL, Owens E. Genotoxic agents detected by plant bioassays. *Rev Environ Health.* 2005;20:1–13.

MacGregor JT, Casciano D, Muller L. Strategies and testing methods for identifying mutagenic risks. *Mutat Res.* 2000;455:3–20.

Mackinnon RN, Chudoba I. The use of M-FISH and M-BAND to define chromosome abnormalities. *Methods Mol Biol.* 2011;730:203–218.

Macville M, Veldman T, Padilla-Nash H, et al. Spectral karyotyping, a 24-colour FISH technique for the identification of chromosomal rearrangements. *Histochem Cell Biol.* 1997;108:299–305.

Madle S, Dean SW, Andrae U, et al. Recommendations for the performance of UDS tests in vitro and in vivo. *Mutat Res.* 1994;312:263–285.

Mah LJ, El-Osta A, Karagiannis TC. Gamma H2AX: a sensitive molecular marker of DNA damage and repair. *Leukemia.* 2010;24:679–686.

Mahadevan B, Snyder RD, Waters MD, et al. Genetic toxicology in the 21st century: reflections and future directions. *Environ Mol Mutagen.* 2011;52:339–354.

Makrigiorgos GM. PCR-based detection of minority point mutations. *Hum Mutat.* 2004;23:406–412.

Malling HV. Incorporation of mammalian metabolism into mutagenicity testing. *Mutat Res.* 2004;566:183–189.

Malling HV, Frantz CN. In vitro versus in vivo metabolic activation of mutagens. *Environ Health Prospect.* 1973;6:71–82.

Marchetti F, Bishop JB, Lowe X, et al. Etoposide induces heritable chromosomal aberrations and aneuploidy during male meiosis in the mouse. *Proc Natl Acad Sci U S A.* 2001;98:3952–3957.

Marchetti F, Cabreros D, Wyrobek AJ. Laboratory methods for the detection of chromosomal structural aberrations in human and mouse sperm by fluorescence in situ hybridization. *Methods Mol Biol.* 2008;410:241–271.

Marchetti F, Pearson FS, Bishop JB, et al. Etoposide induces chromosomal abnormalities in mouse spermatocytes and stem cell spermatogonia. *Hum Reprod.* 2006;21:888–895.

Margison GP, Povey AC, Kaina B, Santibanez Koref MF. Variability and regulation of O^6-alkylguanine-DNA alkyltransferase. *Carcinogenesis.* 2003;24:625–635.

Maron DM, Ames BN. Revised methods for the *Salmonella* mutagenicity test. *Mutat Res.* 1983;113:173–215.

Marshall CJ. Tumor suppressor genes. *Cell.* 1991;64:313–326.

Martin RH, Ko E, Rademaker A. Distribution of aneuploidy in human gametes: Comparison between human sperm and oocytes. *Am J Med Genet.* 1991;39:321–331.

Martin RH, Spriggs E, Rademaker AW. Multicolor fluorescence *in situ* hybridization analysis of aneuploidy and diploidy frequencies in 225,846 sperm from 10 normal men. *Biol Reprod.* 1996;54:394–398.

Mason JM, Aaron CS, Lee WR, et al. A guide for performing germ cell mutagenesis assays using *Drosophila melanogaster. Mutat Res.* 1987;189:93–102.

Mastrocola AS, Heinen CD. Nuclear reorganization of DNA mismatch repair proteins in response to DNA damage. *DNA Repair.* 2010;9:120–133.

McCullough AK, Dodson ML, Lloyd RS. Initiation of base excision repair: glycosylase mechanisms and structures. *Annu Rev Biochem.* 1999;68:255–285.

McGregor DB, Rice JM, Venitt S, eds. The Use of Short- and Medium-term Tests for Carcinogens and Data on Genetic Effects in Carcinogenic Hazard Evaluation. IARC Sci Pub No. 146. Lyon, France: IARC; 1999.

McGregor E, De Souza A. Proteomics and laser microdissection. *Methods Mol Biol.* 2006;333:291–304.

Meek ME, Bucher JR, Cohen SM, et al. A framework for human relevance analysis of information on carcinogenic modes of action. *Crit Rev Toxicol.* 2003;33:591–653.

Mercer WE. Checking on the cell cycle. *J Cell Biochem Suppl.* 1998;30–31:50–54.

Miller B, Pötter-Locher F, Seelbach A, et al. Evaluation of the in vitro micronucleus test as an alternative to the in vitro chromosomal aberration assay: position of the GUM working group on the in vitro micronucleus test. *Mutat Res.* 1998;410:81–116.

Miller JA, Miller EC. Ultimate chemical carcinogens as reactive mutagenic electrophiles. In: Hiatt HH, Watson JD, Winsten JA, eds. *Origins of Human Cancer.* Cold Spring Harbor, NY: Cold Spring Harbor Laboratory Press; 1977:605–628.

Misík M, Ma TH, Nersesyan A, et al. Micronucleus assays with *tradescantia* pollen tetrads: an update. *Mutagenesis.* 2011;26:215–221.

Miura D, Shaddock JG, Mittelstaedt RA, et al. Analysis of mutations in the Pig-a gene of spleen T-cells from N-ethyl-N-nitrosourea-treated Fischer 344 rats. *Environ Mol Mutagen.* 2011;52:419–423.

Mladenov E, Iliakis G. Induction and repair of DNA double strand breaks: the increasing spectrum of non-homologous end joining pathways. *Mutat Res.* 2011;711:61–72.

Modrich P, Lahue R. Mismatch repair in replication fidelity, genetic recombination, and cancer biology. *Annu Rev Biochem.* 1996;65:101–133.

Modrich P. Strand-specific mismatch repair in mammalian cells. *J Biol Chem.* 1997;272:24727–24730.

Mohrenweiser HW. Germinal mutation and human genetic disease. In: Li AP, Heflich RH, eds. *Genetic Toxicology: A Treatise.* Boca Raton, FL: CRC Press; 1991:67–92.

Moolenaar RJ. Carcinogen risk assessment: international comparison. *Regul Toxicol Pharmacol.* 1994;20:302–336.

Moore MM, Honma M, Clements J, et al. Suitable top concentration for tests with mammalian cells: mouse lymphoma assay workgroup. *Mutat Res.* 2011;723:84–86.

Morita T, Macgregor JT, Hayashi M. Micronucleus assays in rodent tissues other than bone marrow. *Mutagenesis.* 2011;26:223–230.

Mortelmans K, Riccio ES. The bacterial tryptophan reverse mutation assay with *Escherichia coli* WP2. *Mutat Res.* 2000;455:61–69.

Mortelmans K, Zeiger E. The Ames *Salmonella* /microsome mutagenicity assay. *Mutat Res.* 2000;455:29–60.

Muller HJ. Artificial transmutation of the gene. *Science.* 1927;66:84–87.

Nagaishi M, Yamamoto T, Iinuma K, et al. Chromosome abnormalities identified in 347 spontaneous abortions collected in Japan. *J Obstet Gynaecol Res.* 2004;30:237–241.

Nakamura A, Sedelnikova OA, Redon C, et al. Techniques for gamma-H2AX detection. *Methods Enzymol.* 2006;409:236–250.

Natarajan AT. An overview of the results of testing of known or suspected aneugens using mammalian cells in vitro. *Mutat Res.* 1993;287:113–118.

Neal JA, Meek A. Choosing the right path: does DNA-PK help make the decision? *Mutat Res.* 2011;711:73–86.

Norppa H, Bonassi S, Hansteen IL, et al. Chromosomal aberrations and SCEs as biomarkers of cancer risk. *Mutat Res.* 2006;600:37–45.

National Research Council. *Risk Assessment in the Federal Government: Managing the Process.* Washington, DC: The National Academy Press; 1983.

National Research Council. *Science and Judgment in Risk Assessment.* Washington, DC: National Academy Press; 1994.

National Research Council; Committee on the Biological Effects of Ionizing Radiations. *Health Effects of Exposure to Low Levels of Ionizing Radiation: BEIR VII.* Washington, DC: National Academy Press; 2007a.

National Research Council: *Toxicity Testing in the 21st Century—A Vision and a Strategy.* Washington, DC: The National Academies Press; 2007b.

Nunoshiba T, Watanabe E, Takahashi T, et al. Ames test-negative carcinogen, ortho-phenyl phenol, binds tubulin and causes aneuploidyin budding yeast. *Mutat Res.* 2007;617:90–97.

Oda Y, Hirayama T, Watanabe T. Genotoxic activation of the environmental pollutant 3,6-dinitrobenzo[e]pyrene in *Salmonella typhimurium umu* strains expressing human cytochrome P450 and N-acetyltransferase. *Toxicol Lett.* 2009;188:258–262.

Ohe T, White PA, DeMarini DM. Mutagenic characteristics of river waters flowing through large metropolitan areas in North America. *Mutat Res.* 2003;534:101–112.

Okada N, Masumura K, Nohmi T, Yajima N. Efficient detection of deletions induced by a single treatment of mitomycin C in transgenic mouse *gpt* delta using the Spi(-) selection. *Environ Mol Mutagen.* 1999;34:106–111.

Olive PL. Impact of the comet assay in radiobiology. *Mutat Res.* 2009;681:13–23.

Olsen AK, Andreassen A, Singh R, et al. Environmental exposure of the mouse germ line: DNA adducts in spermatozoa and formation of de novo mutations during spermatogenesis. *PLoS One.* 2010;5:e11349.

Paccierotti F, Sgura A. Fluorescence in situ hybridization for the detection of chromosome aberrations and aneuploidy induced by environmental toxicants. *Methods Mol Biol.* 2008;410:217–239.

Pack S, Vortmeyer AO, Pak E, et al. Detection of gene deletion in single metastatic tumor cells in lymph node tissue by fluorescent in-situ hybridization. *Lancet.* 1997;350:264–265.

Pack SD, Weil RJ, Vortmeyer AO, et al. Individual adult human neurons display aneuploidy: detection by fluorescence in situ hybridization and single neuron PCR. *Cell Cycle.* 2005;4:1758–1760.

Painter RB. A replication model for sister-chromatid exchange. *Mutat Res.* 1980;70:337–341.

Parry JM. Detecting and predicting the activity of rodent carcinogens. *Mutagenesis.* 1994;9:3–5.

Parry JM. Detecting chemical aneugens: a commentary to 'Aneuploidy: a report of an ECETOC task force.' *Mutat Res.* 1998;410:117–120.

Parry JM, Parry EM, Johnson G, et al. The detection of genotoxic activity and the qualitative assessment of the consequences of exposures. *Exp Toxicol Pathol.* 2005;57(suppl 1):205–212.

Phillips DH, Farmer PB, Beland FA, et al. Methods of DNA adduct determination and their application to testing compounds for genotoxicity. *Environ Mol Mutagen.* 2000;35:222–233.

Pleasance ED, Cheetham RK, Stephens DJ, et al. A comprehensive catalogue of somatic mutations from a human cancer genome. *Nature.* 2010;463:191–197.

Potter CJ, Turenchalk GS, Xu T: *Drosophila* in cancer research. *Trends Genet* 16:33–39, 2000.

Prakash S, Johnson RE, Prakash L. Eukaryotic translesion synthesis DNA polymerases: specificity of structure and function. *Annu Rev Biochem.* 2005;74:317–353.

Preston RJ. Mechanisms of induction of chromosomal alterations and sister chromatid exchanges. In: Li AP, Heflich RF, eds. *Genetic Toxicology: A Treatise.* Boca Raton, FL: CRC Press; 1991:41–66.

Preston RJ. A consideration of the mechanisms of induction of mutations in mammalian cells by low doses and dose rates of ionizing radiation. *Adv Radiat Biol.* 1992;16:125–135.

Preston RJ. Aneuploidy in germ cells: disruption of chromosome mover components. *Environ Mol Mutagen.* 1996;28:176–181.

Preston RJ. Chromosomal changes. In: McGregor DB, Rice JM, Venitt S, eds. *The Use of Short- and Medium-Term Tests for Carcinogens and Data on Genetic Effects in Carcinogenic Hazard Evaluation.* IARC Sci Pub 146. Lyon, France: IARC, 1999a:395–408.

Preston RJ. Cytogenetic effects of ethylene oxide, with an emphasis on population monitoring. *Crit Rev Toxicol.* 1999b;29:263–282.

Preston RJ. Mechanistic data and cancer risk assessment: the need for quantitative molecular endpoints. *Environ Mol Mutagen.* 2005;45:214–221.

Preston RJ, Au W, Bender MA, et al. Mammalian in vivo and in vitro cytogenetic assays: a report of the U.S. EPA's Gene-Tox Program. *Mutat Res.* 1981;87:143–188.

Preston RJ, Fennell TR, Leber AP, et al. Reconsideration of the genetic risk assessment for ethylene oxide exposures. *Environ Mol Mutagen.* 1995;26:189–202.

Preston RJ, Williams GM. DNA-reactive carcinogens: mode of action and human cancer hazard. *Crit Rev Toxicol.* 2005;35:673–683.

Prival MJ, Cebula TA. Sequence analysis of mutations arising during prolonged starvation of *Salmonella typhimurium.* *Genetics.* 1992;132:303–310.

Quillardet P, Hofnung M. The SOS chromotest: a review. *Mutat Res.* 1993;297:235–279.

Rabbitts TH. Chromosomal translocations in human cancer. *Nature.* 1994;372:143–149.

Ramsey MJ, Moore DH, Briner JF, et al. The effects of age and lifestyle factors on the accumulation of cytogenetic damage as measured by chromosome painting. *Mutat Res.* 1995;338:95–106.

Rattray AJ, Strathern JN. Error-prone DNA polymerases: when making a mistake is the only way to get ahead. *Annu Rev Genet.* 2003;37:31–66.

Reardon JT, Sancar A. Nucleotide excision repair. *Prog Nuclei Acid Res Mol Biol.* 2005;79:183–235.

Reed SH. Nucleotide excision repair in chromatin: damage removal at the drop of a HAT. *DNA Repair.* 2011;10:734–742.

Reliene R, Bishop AJR, Schiestl RH. Involvement of homologous recombination in carcinogenesis. *Adv Genet.* 2007;58:67–87.

Rhomberg L, Dellarco VL, Siegel-Scott C, et al. Quantitative estimation of the genetic risk associated with the induction of heritable translocations at low-dose exposure: ethylene oxide as an example. *Environ Mol Mutagen.* 1990;16:104–125.

Ripley LS. Mechanisms of gene mutations. In: Li AP, Heflich RH, eds. *Genetic Toxicology: A Treatise.* Boca Raton, FL: CRC Press; 1991:13–40.

Robertson DG. Metabonomics in toxicology: a review. *Toxicol Sci.* 2005;85:809–822.

Ross CD, French CT, Keysar SB, et al. Mutant spectra of irradiated CHO AL cells determined with multiple markers analyzed by flow cytometry. *Mutat Res.* 2007;624:61–70.

Royds JA, Iacopetta B. p53 and disease: when the guardian angel fails. *Cell Death Differ.* 2006;13:1017–1026.

Rupa DS, Schuler M, Eastmond DA. Detection of hyperdiploidy and breakage affecting the 1cen-1q12 region of cultured interphase human lymphocytes treated with various genotoxic agents. *Environ Mol Mutagen*. 1997;29:161–167.

Russell LB. Effects of male germ-cell stage on the frequency, nature, and spectrum of induced specific-locus mutations in the mouse. *Genetica*. 2004;122:25–36.

Russell LB, Russell WL. Frequency and nature of specific-locus mutations induced in female mice by radiations and chemicals: a review. *Mutat Res*. 1992;296:107–127.

Russell LB, Shelby MD. Tests for heritable genetic damage and for evidence of gonadal exposure in mammals. *Mutat Res*. 1985;154:69–84.

Russell LB, Selby PB, Von Halle E, et al. The mouse specific-locus test with agents other than radiations: interpretation of data and recommendations for future work. *Mutat Res*. 1981;86:329–354.

Russell WL. X-ray-induced mutations in mice. *Cold Spring Harb Symp Quant Biol*. 1951;16:327–336.

Russo A. In vivo cytogenetics: mammalian germ cells. *Mutat Res*. 2000;455:167–189.

Sankaranarayanan K. Ionizing radiation and genetic risks: IX. Estimates of the frequencies of mendelian diseases and spontaneous mutation rates in human populations: a 1998 perspective. *Mutat Res*. 1998;411:129–178.

Sankaranarayanan K. Estimation of the genetic risks of exposure to ioizing radiation in humans: current status and emerging perspectives. *J Radiat Res (Tokyo)*. 2006;47(suppl B):B57–B66.

Sankaranarayanan K, Chakraborty R, Boerwinkle EA. Ionizing radiation and genetic risks. VI. Chronic multifactorial diseases: a review of epidemiological and genetical aspects of coronary heart disease, essential hypertension and diabetes mellitus. *Mutat Res*. 1999;436:21–57.

Sawada M, Kamataki T. Genetically engineered cells stably expressing cytochrome P450 and their application to mutagen assays. *Mutat Res*. 1998;411:19–43.

Sax K. Induction by X-rays of chromosome aberrations in *Tradescantia* microspores. *Genetics*. 1938;23:494–516.

Sax K. The time factor in X-ray production of chromosome aberrations. *Proc Natl Acad Sci U S A*. 1939;25:225–233.

Sax K, Luippold H. The effects of fractional x-ray dosage on the frequency of chromosome aberrations. *Heredity*. 1952;6:127–131.

Scott D, Galloway SM, Marshall RR, et al. Genotoxicity under extreme culture conditions. *Mutat Res*. 1991;257:147–204.

Seeberg E, Eide L, Bjoras M. The base excision repair pathway. *Trends Biochem Sci*. 1995;20:391–397.

Seed J, Carney EW, Corley RA, et al. Overview: using mode of action and life stage information to evaluate the human relevance of animal toxicity data. *Crit Rev Toxicol*. 2005;35:674–672.

Seifried HE, Seifried RM, Clarke JJ, et al. A compilation of two decades of mutagenicity test results with the Ames *Salmonella typhimurium* and L5178Y mouse lymphoma cell mutation assays. *Chem Res Toxicol*. 2006;19:627–644.

Selby PB, Earhart VS, Garrison EM, et al. Tests of induction in mice by acute and chronic ionizing radiation and ethylnitrosourea of dominant mutations that cause the more common skeletal anomalies. *Mutat Res*. 2004;545:81–107.

Sengstag C. The role of mitotic recombination in carcinogenesis. *Crit Rev Toxicol*. 1994;24:323–353.

Shaposhnikov S, Frengen E, Collins AR. Increasing the resolution of the comet assay using fluorescent in situ hybridization—a review. *Mutagenesis*. 2009;24:383–389.

Shelby MD. Human germ cell mutagens. *Environ Mol Mutagen*. 1994;23(suppl 24):30–34.

Shinohara A, Ogawa T. Homologous recombination and the roles of double-strand breaks. *Trends Biochem Sci*. 1995;20:387–391.

Singer TM, Lambert IM, Williams A, et al. Detection of induced male germline mutation: correlations and comparisons between traditional germline mutation assays, transgenic rodent assays and expanded simple tandem repeat instability assays. *Mutat Res*. 2006;598:164–193.

Singer TM, Yauk CL. Germ cell mutagens: risk assessment challenges in the 21st century. *Environ Mol Mutagen*. 2010;51:919–928.

Singh NP. Microgels for estimation of DNA strand breaks, DNA protein crosslinks and apoptosis. *Mutat Res*. 2000;455:111–127.

Smith MT, Zhang L, Wang Y, et al. Increased translocations and aneusomy in chromosomes 8 and 21 among workers exposed to benzene. *Cancer Res*. 1998;58:2176–2181.

Snyder RD. An update on the genotoxicity and carcinogenicity of marketed pharmaceuticals with reference to in silico predictivity. *Environ Mol Mutagen*. 2009;50:435–450.

Snyder RD, Pearl GS, Mandakas G, et al. Assessment of the sensitivity of the computational programs DEREK, TOPKAT, and MCASE in the prediction of the genotoxicity of pharmaceutical molecules. *Environ Mol Mutagen*. 2004;43:143–158.

Snyder RD, Smith MD: Computational prediction of genotoxicity: room for improvement. *Drug Discov Today*. 2005;10:1119–1124.

Sobels FH. The parallelogram: an indirect approach for the assessment of genetic risks from chemical mutagens. In: Bora KC, Douglas GR, Nestman ER, eds. *Progress in Mutation Research*. Vol 3. Amsterdam: Elsevier Biomedical Press; 1982:323–327.

Solinas-Toldo S, Lampel S, Stilgenbauer S, et al. Matrix-based comparative genomic hybridization: biochips to screen for genomic imbalances. *Genes Chromosomes Cancer*. 1997;20:399–407.

Somers CM. Expanded simple tandem repeat (ESTR) mutation induction in the male germline: lessons learned from lab mice. *Mutat Res*. 2006;598:35–49.

Sonoda E, Hochegger H, Saberi A, Taniguchi Y, Takeda S. Differential usage of nonhomologous end-joining and homologous recombination in double strand break repair. *DNA Repair (Amst)*. 2006;5:1021–1029.

Sotomayor RE, Sega GA. Unscheduled DNA synthesis assay in mammalian spermatogenic cells: an update. *Environ Mol Mutagen*. 2000;36:255–265.

Southern EM. DNA chips: Analyzing sequence by hybridization to oligonucleotides on a large scale. *Trends Genet*. 1996;12:110–115.

Speicher MR, Carter NP. The new cytogenetics: blurring the boundaries with molecular biology. *Nat Rev Genet*. 2005;6:782–792.

Speit G, Vasquez M, Hartmann A. The comet assay as an indicator test for germ cell genotoxicity. *Mutat Res*. 2009;681:3–12.

Stoler DL, Chen N, Basik M, et al. The onset and extent of genomic instability in sporadic colorectal tumor progression. *Proc Natl Acad Sci USA*. 1999;96:15121–15126.

Storer RD, McKelvey TW, Kraynak AR, et al. Revalidation of the in vitro alkaline elution/rat hepatocyte assay for DNA damage: improved criteria for assessment of cytotoxicity and genotoxicity and results for 81 compounds. *Mutat Res*. 1996;368:59–101.

Stratton MR, Campbell PJ, Futreal PA. The cancer genome. *Nature*. 2009;458:719–724.

Styles JA, Penman MG. The mouse spot test: evaluation of its performance in identifying chemical mutagens and carcinogens. *Mutat Res*. 1985;154:183–204.

Sung JS, Demple B. Roles of base excision repair subpathways in correcting oxidized abasic sites in DNA. *FEBS J*. 2006;273:1620–1629.

Swenberg JA, Lu K, Moeller BC, et al. Endogenous versus exogenous DNA adducts: their role in carcinogenesis, epidemiology, and risk assessment. *Toxicol Sci*. 2011;120(suppl 1):S130–S145.

Swiger RR. Just how does the *cII* selection system work in Muta™Mouse? *Environ Mol Mutagen*. 2001;37:290–296.

Sykes PJ, Morley AA, hooker AM. The pKZ1 recombination mutation assay: a sensitive assay for low dose studies. *Dose-Response*. 2006;4:91–105.

Takigami H, Matsui S, Matsuda T, et al. The *Bacillus subtilis* rec-assay: a powerful tool for the detection of genotoxic substances in the water environment. Prospect for assessing potential impact of pollutants from stabilized wastes. *Waste Manag*. 2002;22:209–213.

Tano K, Shiota S, Collier J, et al. Isolation and structural characterization of a cDNA clone encoding the human DNA repair protein for O^6-alkylguanine. *Proc Natl Acad Sci U S A*. 1990;87:686–690.

Tease C. Radiation- and chemically-induced chromosome aberrations in mouse oocytes: a comparison with effects in males. *Mutat Res*. 1992;296:135–142.

Tennant RW, Ashby J. Classification according to chemical structure, mutagenicity to Salmonella and level of carcinogenicity of a further 39 chemicals tested for carcinogenicity by the U.S. National Toxicology Program. *Mutat Res*. 1991;257:209–227.

480

Tennant RW, Margolin BH, Shelby MD, et al. Prediction of chemical carcinogenicity in rodents from in vitro genetic toxicity assays. *Science.* 1987;236:933–941.

Thacker J. Radiation-induced mutation in mammalian cells at low doses and dose rates. *Adv Radiat Biol.* 1992;16:77–124.

Tice RR, Agurell E, Anderson D, et al. Single cell gel/comet assay: guidelines for in vitro and in vivo genetic toxicology testing. *Environ Mol Mutagen.* 2000;35:206–221.

Tice RR, Hayashi M, MacGregor JT, et al. Report from the working group on the in vivo mammalian bone marrow chromosomal aberration test. *Mutat Res.* 1994;312:305–312.

Trask BJ, Allen S, Massa H, et al. Studies of metaphase and interphase chromosomes using fluorescence in situ hybridizaiton. *Cold Spring Harb Symp Quant Biol.* 1993;58:767–775.

Trost D, Hildebrandt B, Beier M, et al. Molecular cytogenetic profiling of complex karyotypes in primary myelodysplastic syndromes and acute myeloid leukemia. *Cancer Genet Cytogenet.* 2006;165:51–63.

Tucker JD, Auletta A, Cimino M, et al. Sister-chromatid exchange: second report of the Gene-Tox program. *Mutat Res.* 1993a;297:101–180.

Tucker JD, Breneman JW, Briner JF, et al. Persistence of radiation-induced translocations in rat peripheral blood determined by chromosome painting. *Environ Mol Mutagen.* 1997;30:264–272.

Tucker JD, Cofield J, Matsumoto K, et al. Persistence of chromosome aberrations following acute radiation: I, PAINT translocations, dicentrics, rings, fragments, and insertions. *Environ Mol Mutagen.* 2005;45:229–248.

Tucker JD, Luckinbill LS. Estimating the lowest detectable dose of ionizing radiation by FISH whole-chromosome painting. *Radiat Res.* 2011;175:631–637.

Tucker JD, Moore DH 2nd. The importance of age and smoking in evaluating adverse cytogenetic effects of exposure to environmental agents. *Environ Health Perspect.* 1996;104:489–492.

Tucker JD, Ramsey MJ, Lee DA, Minkler JL. Validation of chromosome painting as a biodosimeter in human peripheral lymphocytes following acute exposure to ionizing radiation in vitro. *Int J Radiat Biol.* 1993b;64:27–37.

Turner DR, Dreimanis M, Holt D, Firgaira FA, Morley AA. Mitotic recombination is an important mutational event following oxidative damage. *Mutat Res.* 2003;522:21–26.

Tweats DJ, Blakey D, Heflich RH, et al. Report of the IWGT working group on strategies and interpretation of regulatory in vivo tests I. Increases in micronucleated bone marrow cells in rodents that do not indicate genotoxic hazards. *Mutat Res.* 2007;627:78–91.

United Nations Scientific Committee on the Effects of Atomic Radiation. Hereditary effects of radiation. *UNSCEAR 2001 Report to the General Assembly, With Scientific Annex.* New York: United Nations; 2001.

Valentine CR, Delongchamp RR, Pearce MG, et al. In vivo mutation analysis using the φX174 transgenic mouse and comparisons with other transgenes and endogenous genes. *Mutat Res.* 2010;705:205–216.

Van Houten B, Albertini R. DNA damage and repair. In: Craighead JE, ed. *Pathology of Environmental and Occupational Disease.* St. Louis: Mosby-Year Book; 1995:311–327.

Veldman T, Vignon C, Schrock E, et al. Hidden chromosome abnormalities in haematological malignancies detected by multicolour spectral karyotyping. *Nat Genet.* 1997;15:406–410.

Venkatachalam S, Shi YP, Jones SN, et al. Retention of wild-type p53 in tumors from p53 heterozygous mice: reduction of p53 dosage can promote cancer formation. *EMBO J.* 1998;17:4657–4667.

Verhofsrad N, van Oostrom CT, Zwart E, et al. Evaluation of benzo(a) pyrene-induced gene mutations in male germ cells. *Toxicol Sci.* 2011;119:218–223.

Vissers LE, Veltman JA, van Kessel AG, Brunner HG. Identification of disease genes by whole genome CGH arrays. *Hum Mol Genet.* 2005;14:R215–R223.

Vlasakova K, Skopek TR, Glaab WE. Induced mutation spectra at the *upp* locus in *Salmonella typhimurium*: response of the target gene in the FU assay to mechanistically different mutagens. *Mutat Res.* 2005;578:225–237.

Vogel EW, Graf U, Frei HJ, Nivara MM. The results of assays in *Drosophila* as indicators of exposure to carcinogens. *IARC Sci Publ.* 1999;146:427–470.

Vogel EW, Nivard MJ. Parallel monitoring of mitotic recombination, clastogenicity and teratogenic effects in eye tissue of *Drosophila*. *Mutat Res.* 2000;455:141–153.

Vorsanova SG, Yurov YB, Iourov IY. Human interphase chromosomes: a review of available molecular cytogenetic technologies. *Mol Cytogenet.* 2010;3:1–15.

Votano JR, Parham M, Hall LH, et al. Three new consensus OSAR models for the prediction of Ames genotoxicity. *Mutagenesis.* 2004;19:365–377.

Wallace SS. DNA damages processed by base excision repair: biological consequences. *Int J Radiat Biol.* 1994;66:579–589.

Wang J, Sawyer JR, Chen L, et al. The mouse lymphoma assay detects recombination, deletion, and aneuploidy. *Toxicol Sci.* 2009;109:96–105.

Ward JF. DNA damage produced by ionizing radiation in mammalian cells: identities, mechanisms of formation, and reparability. *Prog Nucl Acid Res Mol Biol.* 1988;35:95–125.

Ward JF. The complexity of DNA damage: relevance to biological consequences. *Int J Radiat Biol.* 1994;66:427–432.

White PA, ed. The sources and potential hazards of mutagens in complex environmental matrices. *Mutat Res.* 2004;567(2–3):105–479.

Wielgoss S, Barrick JE, Tenaillon O, et al. Mutation rate inferred from synonymous substitutions in a long-term evolution experiment with *Escherichia coli. G3.* 2011;1:183–186.

Wilson DM, Thompson LH. Molecular mechanisms of sister-chromatid exchange. *Mutat Res.* 2007;616:11–23.

Wodicka L, Dong H, Mittmann M, et al. Genome-wide expression monitoring in *Saccharomyces cerevisiae. Nat Biotech.* 1997;15:1359–1367.

Wood RD. DNA repair in eukaryotes. *Annu Rev Biochem.* 1996;65:135–167.

Wood RD, Mitchell M, Lindahl T. Human DNA repair genes, 2005. *Mutat Res.* 2005;577:275–283.

Wu J, Morimyo M, Hongo E, et al. Radiation-induced germline mutations detected by a direct comparison of parents and first-generation offspring DNA sequences containing SNPs. *Mutat Res.* 2006;596:1–11.

Xie F, Liu T, Qian WJ, et al. Liquid chromatography-mass spectrometry-based quantitative proteomics. *J Biol Chem.* 2011;286:25443–25449.

Yamazaki Y, Fujita K, Nakayama K, et al. Establishment of ten strains of genetically engineered *Salmonella typhimurium* TA1538 each co-expressing a form of human cytochrome P450 with NADPH-cytochrome P450 reductase sensitive to various promutagens. *Mutat Res.* 2004;562:151–162.

Yasunaga K, Kiyonari A, Oikawa T, et al. Evaluation of the Salmonella *umu* test with 83 NTP chemicals. *Environ Mol Mutagen.* 2004;44:329–345.

Yauk CL. Advances in the application of germline tandem repeat instability for in situ monitoring. *Mutat Res.* 2004;566:169.

Yeh HC, Ho YP, Shih IeM, Wang TH. Homogeneous point mutation detection by quantum dot-mediated two-color fluorescence coincidence analysis. *Nuclei Acids Res.* 2006;34:e35.

Zeiger E. Historical perspective on the development of the genetic toxicity test battery in the United States. *Environ Mol Mutagen.* 2010;51: 781–791.

Zhang Y, Gostissa M, Hildebrand DG, et al. The role of mechanistic factors in promoting chromosomal translocations found in lymphoid and other cancers. *Adv Immunol.* 2010;106:93–133.

Zheng X, Epstein A, Klein HL. Methods to study mitotic homologous recombination and genome stability. *Methods Mol Biol.* 2011; 745:3–13.

Zhou H, Xu A, Gillespie JA, et al. Quantification of CD59− mutants in human-hamster hybrid (AL) cells by flow cytometry. *Mutat Res.* 2006;594:113–119.

Zimmermann FK. Tests for recombinogens in fungi. *Mutat Res.* 1992;284:147–158.

Zimmermann FK, von Borstel RC, von Halle ES, et al. Testing of chemicals for genetic activity with *Saccharomyces cerevisiae*: a report of the U.S. Environmental Protection Agency Gene-Tox Program. *Mutat Res.* 1984;133:199–244.

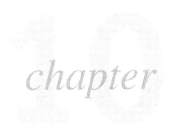

chapter

Developmental Toxicology

John M. Rogers

HISTORY

Developmental toxicology encompasses the study of developmental exposures, pharmacokinetics, mechanisms, pathogenesis, and outcomes potentially leading to adverse health effects. Manifestations of developmental toxicity include structural malformations, growth retardation, functional or metabolic impairment, and/or death of the organism. Developmental exposures may also alter the risk of diseases in adulthood. Developmental toxicology defined as such is a relatively new science, but teratology, the study of structural birth defects, as a descriptive science preceded written language. For example, a marble sculpture from southern Turkey dating to 6500 BC depicts conjoined twins (Warkany, 1983), and Egyptian wall paintings of human conditions such as cleft palate and achondroplasia date to as long as 5000 years ago. Conjecture has it that mythological figures such as the Cyclops and sirens took their origin in the birth of malformed infants (Thompson, 1930; Warkany, 1977). Ancient Babylonians, Greeks, and Romans believed that abnormal infants were reflections of celestial events and were considered to be portents of the future. Indeed, the Latin word *monstrum*, from *monstrare* (to show) or *monere* (to warn), connotes an ability to foretell the future. In turn, derivation of the word *teratology* is from the Greek word for monster, *teras*.

Hippocrates and Aristotle thought that abnormal development could originate in physical causes such as uterine trauma or pressure, but Aristotle also held a widespread belief that maternal impressions and emotions could influence the development of the child. He advised pregnant women to gaze at beautiful statuary to increase their child's beauty. Although this theory sounds fanciful, it is present in diverse cultures throughout recorded history. Indeed, we now know that maternal stress, depression, and anxiety during pregnancy can be deleterious to the developing conceptus and child (Dunkel Schetter and Tanner, 2012).

In 1649, the French surgeon Ambrois Paré expounded upon the theory of Aristotle and Hippocrates by writing that birth defects could result from narrowness of the uterus, faulty posture of the pregnant woman, or physical trauma such as a fall. Fetal limb amputations were thought to result from amniotic bands, adhesions, or twisting of the umbilical cord. This conjecture has proven to be accurate. With the blossoming of biology in the 16th and 17th centuries, scientific theories of causation of birth defects began to emerge. In 1651, William Harvey put forth the theory of developmental arrest, which stated that malformations resulted from incomplete development of an organ or structure. An example given by Harvey was harelip in humans, a congenital malformation that represents a normal developmental stage. Much later, the theory of developmental arrest was supported by the experiments of Stockard (1921) using eggs of the minnow, *Fundulus heteroclitus*. By manipulating the chemical constituents and temperature of growth media, he produced malformations in the embryos, the nature of which depended on the developmental stage at the time of the insult. He concluded that developmental arrest explained all malformations except those of hereditary origin (Barrow, 1971).

With the advent of the germplasm theory elucidated by Weissmann in the 1880s and the rediscovery of Mendel's laws in 1900, genetics as the basis for some birth defects was accepted. In 1894, Bateson published his treatise on the study of variations in animals as a tool for understanding evolution, inferring that inheritance of such variations could be a basis for speciation (Bateson, 1894). His study contains detailed descriptions and illustrations of such human birth defects as polydactyly and syndactyly, supernumerary cervical and thoracic ribs, duplicated appendages, and horseshoe (fused) kidneys. Bateson coined the term *homeosis* to denote morphological alterations in which one structure takes on the likeness of another. Studies of such alterations in mutants of the fruit fly *Drosophila melanogaster* and, more recently, vertebrates, have served as the basis for much of our present knowledge of the genetic control of development. *Homeobox genes* are found throughout the animal and plant kingdoms and direct embryonic pattern formation (Graham *et al.*, 1989; Deschamps and van Nes, 2005; Mallo *et al.*, 2010). Acceptance of a genetic basis of birth defects was furthered with studies of human inborn errors of metabolism in the first decade of the 20th century.

Modern experimental teratology began in the early 19th century with the work of Etienne Geoffrey Saint-Hilaire. Saint-Hilaire produced malformed chick embryos by subjecting eggs to various environmental conditions including physical trauma (jarring, inversion, pricking) and toxic exposures. In the latter part of the 19th century, Camille Dareste experimented extensively with chick embryos, producing a wide variety of malformations by administering noxious stimuli, physical trauma, or heat shock at various times during development. He found that timing was more important than the nature of the insult in determining the type of malformation produced. Among the malformations described and beautifully illustrated by Dareste (1877, 1891) were the neural tube defects (NTDs) anencephaly and spina bifida, cyclopia, heart defects, situs inversus, and conjoined twins. Many of the great embryologists of the 19th and 20th centuries, including Loeb, Morgan, Driesch, Wilson, Spemann, and Hertwig, performed teratological manipulations employing various physical and chemical probes to deduce principles of normal development.

In the early 20th century, a variety of environmental conditions (temperature, microbial toxins, drugs) were shown to perturb development in avian, reptilian, fish, and amphibian species. In contrast, mammalian embryos were at that time thought to be resistant to induction of malformations, protected from adverse environmental conditions by the maternal system. The first reports to the contrary were published in the 1930s and were the result of experimental maternal nutritional deficiencies. Hale (1935) produced malformations including anophthalmia and cleft palate in offspring of sows fed a diet deficient in vitamin A. Beginning in 1940, Josef Warkany and co-workers began a series of experiments in which they demonstrated that maternal dietary deficiencies and other environmental factors could affect intrauterine development in rats (Warkany and Nelson, 1940; Warkany, 1945; Warkany and Schraffenberger, 1944; Wilson *et al.*, 1953). These experiments were followed by many other studies in which chemical and physical agents, for example, nitrogen mustard, trypan blue, hormones, antimetabolites, alkylating agents, hypoxia, and x-rays, to name a few, were clearly shown to cause malformations in mammals (see Warkany, 1965).

The first recognized human epidemic of malformations induced by an environmental agent was reported by Gregg (1941), who linked an epidemic of rubella virus infection (German measles) in Australia to an elevation in the incidence of eye, heart, and ear defects, and mental retardation. The triad of deafness, cataracts, and cardiac disease is now recognized as the clinical signature of congenital rubella syndrome. Heart and eye defects predominated with maternal infection in the first or second months of pregnancy, whereas hearing and speech defects and mental retardation were most commonly associated with infection in the third month. Later, the risk of congenital anomalies associated with rubella infection in the first four weeks of pregnancy was estimated to be 61%; in weeks five to eight, 26%; and in weeks nine to 12, 8% (Sever, 1967). It has been estimated that in the United States alone approximately 20,000 children have been impaired as a consequence of prenatal rubella infections (Cooper and Krugman, 1966). Although maternal rubella is now uncommon in developed countries due to vaccination programs, there are still rubella outbreaks in developing countries (De Santis *et al.*, 2006; Chandy *et al.*, 2011), and some cases in developed countries as well (Vauloup-Fellous *et al.*, 2010).

Although embryos of mammals, including humans, were found to be susceptible to common external influences such as nutritional deficiencies and intrauterine infections, the impact of these findings was not fully appreciated at the time (Wilson, 1973). That changed, however, in 1961, when the association between thalidomide ingestion by pregnant women and the birth of severely malformed infants was established (see below).

SCOPE OF PROBLEM: THE HUMAN EXPERIENCE

The overall miscarriage rate in humans is estimated to be 15% to 20% of recognized pregnancies. However, with the development of highly sensitive tests, pregnancies can now be detected shortly after fertilization. When these tests are used early, recognized pregnancy loss increases to about 60% to 70%. Estimates of adverse outcomes include postimplantation pregnancy loss, 31%; major birth defects, 2% to 3% at birth and increasing to 6% to 7% at one year as more manifestations are diagnosed; minor birth defects, 14%; low birth weight, 7%; infant mortality (prior to one year of age), 1.4%; and abnormal neurological function, 16% to 17% (Schardein, 2000). Reasons for these adverse outcomes are largely unknown. Brent and Beckman (1990) attributed 15% to 25% of human birth defects to genetic causes, 4% to maternal conditions, 3% to maternal infections, 1% to 2% to *deformations* (eg, mechanical problems such as umbilical cord limb amputations), <1% to chemicals and other environmental influences, and 65% to unknown etiologies. These estimates are similar to those suggested by Wilson (1977). Regardless of etiology, the sum total represents a significant health burden in light of the over four million births annually in the United States.

It has been estimated that well over 4000 chemicals have been tested in animals for teratogenicity, with approximately 66% shown to be nonteratogenic, 7% teratogenic in more than one species, 18% teratogenic in most species tested, and 9% producing equivocal experimental results (Schardein, 2000). In contrast, only about 35 to 40 chemicals, chemical classes, or conditions (Table 10-1) have been documented to alter prenatal development in humans (Schardein and Keller, 1989; Shepard and Lemire, 2004). A brief review of selected human developmental toxicants provides both a

Table 10-1

Human Developmental Toxicants

Radiation	Drugs and chemicals
Atomic fallout	Aminoglycosides
Radioiodine	Androgenic hormones
Therapeutic	Angiotensin converting enzyme
	inhibitors: captopril, enalapril
Infections	Angiotensin receptor antagonists:
Cytomegalovirus	sartans
Herpes simplex	Anticonvulsants: Diphenylhydantoin,
virus I and II	trimethadione, valproic acid,
Parvovirus B-19	carbamazepine
(erythema	Busulfan
infectiosum)	Carbon monoxide
Rubella virus	Chlorambucil
Syphilis	Cocaine
Toxoplasmosis	Coumarins
Varicella virus	Cyclophosphamide
Venezuelan	Cytarabine
equine	Diethylstilbestrol
encephalitis	Danazol
virus	Ergotamine
	Ethanol
Maternal trauma	Ethylene oxide
and metabolic	Fluconazole
imbalances	Folate antagonists: aminopterin,
Alcoholism	methotrexate
Amniocentesis,	Iodides
early	Lead
Chorionic villus	Lithium
sampling	Mercury, organic
(before day 60)	Methimazole
Cretinism	Methylene blue
Diabetes	Misoprostal
Folic acid	Penicillamine
deficiency	Polychlorobiphenyls
Hyperthermia	Quinine (high dose)
Phenylketonuria	Retinoids: Accutane, isotretinoin,
Rheumatic	etretinate, acitretin
disease and	Tetracyclines
congenital	Thalidomide
heart block	Tobacco smoke
Sjogren syndrome	Toluene
Virilizing tumors	Vitamin A (high dose)

SOURCES: Data from Shepard (2004) and Schardein and Macina (2007).

historical view of developmental toxicology and an illustration of some of the key principles of the science.

Thalidomide

In 1960, a striking increase in newborns with rare limb malformations was recorded in West Germany. The affected individuals had amelia (absence of the limbs) or various degrees of phocomelia (reduction of the long bones of the limbs), usually affecting the arms more than the legs and usually involving both left and right sides, although to differing degrees. Congenital cardiac, ocular, otic, intestinal, and renal anomalies were also involved. However, the limb defects were pathognomonic, as limb reduction anomalies of this nature are exceedingly rare. At the university clinic

in Hamburg, for example, no cases of phocomelia were reported between 1940 and 1959. In 1959 there was a single case; in 1960, there were 30 cases; and in 1961, a total of 154 cases (Taussig, 1962). The unusual nature of the malformations was a key factor in unraveling the epidemic. In 1961, Lenz and McBride, working independently in Germany and Australia, respectively, identified the sedative thalidomide as the causative agent (McBride, 1961; Lenz, 1961, 1963). Thalidomide had been introduced in 1956 by Chemie Grunenthal as a sedative/hypnotic and was used throughout much of the world as a sleep aid and to treat nausea and vomiting in pregnancy. The drug was widely prescribed at an oral dose of 50 to 200 mg/day. There were a few reports of peripheral neuritis attributed to thalidomide, but only in patients with long-term use for up to 18 months (Fullerton and Kermer, 1961). Following the association with birth defects, thalidomide was withdrawn from the market by Grunenthal in November 1961, and case reports ended in mid-1962 as exposed pregnancies were completed. Estimates of the number of infants malformed by thalidomide worldwide during this period range from 5840 (Lenz, 1988) to over 10,000 in 46 countries (Bartlett et al., 2004). Quantitative estimates of malformation risks from exposure have been difficult to compile but are believed to be in the range of one in two to one in 10 (Newman, 1985). Due to concerns regarding the severity of the peripheral neuritis and subsequent questions with regard to safety in pregnancy, thalidomide did not receive marketing approval by the US Food and Drug Administration (FDA) prior to its removal from the world market following the epidemic. Much credit is due to Dr Frances Kelsey, who was a new FDA staff member at the time. She later received the highest honor that can be bestowed upon a US civilian, the medal for Distinguished Federal Civilian Service, from President John F. Kennedy, for her diligence in protecting the country.

As a result of the thalidomide catastrophe, regulatory agencies in many countries began developing animal testing requirements for evaluating the effects of drugs during pregnancy (Stirling et al., 1997). In the United States, the discussions ultimately led to the development of the Segment I, II, and III testing protocols of the FDA (Kelsey, 1988). Current regulatory testing guidelines for developmental toxicity are discussed later in this chapter.

It is both ironic and telling that the chemical largely responsible for the advent of modern regulation of potential developmental toxicants presents a complex pattern of effects in different animal species. It has been tested for prenatal toxicity in at least 19 laboratory species. Malformations and increased embryonic loss have been observed in some studies in rats, whereas generally no effects were reported in studies with hamsters or most mouse strains. Effects more or less similar to those observed in humans have been reported for several rabbit strains and in eight of nine primate species. The teratogenic potency of thalidomide ranges from approximately 1 to 100 mg/kg among sensitive species. In this ranking the human sensitivity was estimated to be 1 mg/kg (Schardein, 1993).

Studies of the relationship between timing of drug use and type of malformation revealed that thalidomide was teratogenic between 20 and 36 days after fertilization (Lenz and Knapp, 1962). Because of its short half-life, teratogenic potency, and good records/recall of prescribed drug use, fairly concise timetables of susceptibility have been constructed (Lenz and Knapp, 1962; Nowack, 1965; Neubert and Neubert, 1997; Miller and Stromland, 1999). During the susceptible period of 20 to 36 days postfertilization, anotia (missing ear) was the defect induced earliest, followed by thumb, upper extremity, lower extremity, and triphalangeal thumb (Miller and Stromland, 1999). Despite extensive effort, research to understand the species and strain differences in response to thalidomide has met with limited success until recently. Extensive structure–activity studies involving analogs of thalidomide found strict structural requirements (eg, an intact phthalimide or phthalimidine group) but shed little light on potential mechanisms (Jonsson, 1972; Schumacher, 1975; Helm et al., 1981). Stephens (1988) reviewed 24 proposed mechanisms, including biochemical alterations involving vitamin B, glutamic acid, acylation, nucleic acids, and oxidative phosphorylation; cellular mechanisms including cell death and cell–cell interactions; and tissue level mechanisms including inhibition of nerve and blood vessel outgrowth. None was considered sufficient by that reviewer. More recent hypotheses concerning the mechanism of thalidomide teratogenesis include effects on angiogenesis (D'Amato et al., 1994; Joussen et al., 1999; Sauer et al., 2000; Stephens et al., 2000; Therapontos et al., 2009), integrin regulation (Neubert et al., 1996), oxidative DNA damage (Parman et al., 1999), TNF-α inhibition (Argiles et al., 1998), growth factor antagonism (Stephens et al., 1998; Stephens and Fillmore, 2000), effects on glutathione and redox status (Hansen et al., 1999), and inhibition of ubiquitin-mediated protein degradation (Ito et al., 2011; Ito and Handa, 2012).

The idea that thalidomide exerts its teratogenicity in sensitive species by altering cellular redox status has been explored by Wells and colleagues (Parman et al., 1999), who compared the effects of thalidomide in the pregnant mouse (an insensitive species) and the pregnant rabbit (a sensitive species). First, they demonstrated a 380% increase in DNA oxidation in rabbit embryos. Pretreatment of pregnant rabbits with the spin-trapping (free-radical scavenging) agent α-phenyl-N-t-butylnitrone (PBN) reduced thalidomide-induced embryonal DNA oxidation by 73%. Thalidomide was teratogenic and embryotoxic in the rabbit, inducing characteristic limb defects as well as other malformations, embryo/fetal mortality, and reduced fetal weight. Almost all of these effects on the rabbit embryos were abolished by maternal pretreatment with PBN. These results indicate that, in the rabbit, thalidomide is activated to a free-radical intermediate that initiates the formation of reactive oxygen species that appear to be a key element of the mechanism of teratogenicity because both oxidation and teratogenicity are largely reduced by PBN. This group has recently demonstrated limb bud embryopathies in rabbit embryos cultured in medium containing thalidomide or two of its hydrolysis products, with concomitant DNA oxidation (Lee et al., 2011). Although oxidation of DNA may be part of the teratogenic mechanism of thalidomide, Hansen and Harris (2004) have provided strong evidence to support their hypothesis that the limb defects induced by thalidomide are due to misregulation of the expression of genes critical for the outgrowth of the limb. They too have shown that thalidomide causes oxidative stress in sensitive (rabbit) but not in resistant (rat) pregnant animals and their embryos, by comparing glutathione depletion following administration of thalidomide (Hansen et al., 2002). They further demonstrated that this shift in redox potential reduces binding of a key transcription factor, NF-κB, to its binding sites on DNA. Binding of NF-κB is required to turn on the expression of the genes twist and FGF-10 in the mesenchyme of the developing limb. Lack of expression of these two genes resulted in loss of FGF-8 expression in the apical ectodermal ridge of the developing limb bud. Given our understanding of the importance of these genes for normal limb development, ablation of their expression by thalidomide could be predicted to cause the limb defects seen in sensitive species. That these genes are under the control of the redox-sensitive NF-κB may be the basis for the differences in teratogenicity of thalidomide in the sensitive rabbit (and presumably human) and the resistant mouse and rat.

Research on alterations in immune function and angiogenesis has opened the possibility of expanded use of thalidomide in diseases including dermatological disorders, arthritis, multiple myeloma, diabetic retinopathy, and macular degeneration (Adler, 1994; Calabrese and Fleischer, 2000; Schwab and Jagannath, 2006; Chen et al., 2010). Thalidomide has been approved by the FDA for erythema nodosum leprosum, an inflammatory complication of Hansen disease (leprosy) and multiple myeloma. In addition, it is used off-label for a number of disorders. An unprecedented level of safeguards, embodied in the STEPS program (System of Thalidomide Education and Prescribing Safety: http://www.thalomid.com/steps_program.aspx), surrounds thalidomide use to prevent accidental exposure during pregnancy, including required registration of all prescribers, pharmacies, and patients, required use of contraception, and periodic pregnancy testing for patients of childbearing ability (Lary et al., 1999).

Diethylstilbestrol

Diethylstilbestrol (DES), a synthetic nonsteroidal estrogen, was widely used from the 1940s to the 1970s in the United States to prevent miscarriage by stimulating synthesis of estrogen and progesterone in the placenta. Between 1966 and 1969, seven young women between the ages of 15 and 22 were seen at Massachusetts General Hospital with clear cell adenocarcinoma of the vagina. This tumor had not previously been seen in patients younger than 30. An epidemiological case–control study subsequently found an association with first trimester DES exposure (reviewed in Poskanzer and Herbst, 1977). The Registry of Clear Cell Adenocarcinoma of the Genital Tract of Young Females was established in 1971 to track affected offspring. Maternal use of DES prior to the 18th week of gestation appeared to be necessary for induction of the genital tract anomalies in offspring. The incidence of genital tract tumors peaked at age 19 and declined through age 22, with absolute risk of clear cell adenocarcinoma of the vagina and cervix estimated to be 0.14 to 1.4 per 1000 exposed pregnancies (Herbst et al., 1977). However, the overall incidence of noncancerous alterations in the vagina, cervix, and uterus was estimated to be as high as 75% (Poskanzer and Herbst, 1977). Effects of developmental exposure on the female reproductive tract may be due to alterations in genetic pathways governing uterine differentiation (Huang et al., 2005). In male offspring of exposed pregnancies, epididymal cysts, hypotrophic testes, and capsular induration along with low ejaculated semen volume and poor semen quality have been observed (Bibbo et al., 1977). The realization of the latent and devastating manifestations of prenatal DES exposure has broadened our concept of the magnitude and scope of potential adverse outcomes of intrauterine exposures. Yet, recent studies suggest even broader developmental targets; a study in mice by Newbold et al. (2006) showed that the increased susceptibility to tumors and reproductive tract abnormalities conferred by DES exposure may be passed on to future generations (both males and females) of exposed mothers. Developmental exposure to DES has also been shown to cause obesity in mice (Newbold et al., 2009).

Ethanol

The developmental toxicity of ethanol has been a recurrent concern throughout history and can be traced to biblical times (eg, Judges 13: 3–4). Yet, only since the description of the Fetal Alcohol Syndrome (FAS) by Jones and Smith in the early 1970s (Jones and Smith, 1973; Jones et al., 1973) has there been a clear recognition and acceptance of alcohol's developmental toxicity. Since that time, there have been hundreds of clinical, epidemiological, and experimental studies of the effects of ethanol exposure during gestation, revealing an ever-widening array of effects of alcohol on development (for review, see Jones, 2011).

The FAS comprises craniofacial dysmorphology, intrauterine and postnatal growth retardation, retarded psychomotor and intellectual development, and other nonspecific major and minor abnormalities (Abel, 1982, 2006; Jones, 2011). The average IQ of FAS children has been reported to be 68 (Streissguth *et al.*, 1991a) and changes little over time (Streissguth *et al.*, 1991b). The craniofacial malformations as well as other morphological and anatomical effects of prenatal ethanol exposure may be due, at least in part, to interference with retinol metabolism in the early embryo, at a time when the anterior part of the embryo, including the brain, is just beginning to form (Yelin *et al.*, 2005). Oxidation of retinol to the signaling molecule, retinoic acid, is crucial for normal development of the embryo. However, the molecular mechanisms underlying FAS are still poorly understood, and the possible molecular and cellular targets are many (eg, Sulik, 2005; Smith, 2010; Zeisel, 2011).

Full-blown FAS has been observed primarily in children born to alcoholic mothers, and among alcoholics the incidence of FAS has been estimated at 25 per 1000 (Abel, 1984). Numerous methodological difficulties are involved in attempting to estimate the level of maternal ethanol consumption associated with FAS, but estimates of a minimum of 3 to 4 oz of alcohol per day have been made (Clarren *et al.*, 1987; Ernhart *et al.*, 1987).

Decades of research has demonstrated that FAS represents an extreme of the range of effects of developmental alcohol exposure, now termed fetal alcohol spectrum disorders (FASDs) (Koren *et al.*, 2003; Sokol *et al.*, 2003; Manning and Hoyme, 2007; Hellemans *et al.*, 2010). In utero exposure to lower levels of ethanol has been associated with a wide range of effects, including isolated components of FAS and effects on the developing brain leading to cognitive and behavioral deficits. Little (1977) studied 800 women prospectively to evaluate the effects of drinking on birth weight. After adjusting for smoking, gestational age, maternal height, age, parity, and sex of the child, it was found that for each ounce of absolute ethanol consumed per day during late pregnancy there was a 160-g decrease in birth weight. Effects of maternal alcohol consumption during pregnancy on attention, short-term memory, and performance on standardized tests have been noted in a longitudinal prospective study of 462 children (Streissguth *et al.*, 1994a,b). Alcohol intake was related to decrements in these measures, the number of drinks per drinking occasion being the strongest predictor. Streissguth and co-workers (Baer *et al.*, 2003) have also reported that prenatal alcohol exposure was significantly associated with alcohol drinking problems at age 21, independent of family history or other environmental factors. Later life vulnerability to stress, depression, and anxiety disorders after in utero exposure to alcohol are reviewed by Hellemans *et al.* (2010). For reviews of the neurotoxic effects of developmental ethanol exposure, see the special issue of *Neuropsychology Review* (June 2011;21(2)) on this topic.

One animal model of FAS in which pathogenesis of the craniofacial effects has been extensively studied involves intraperitoneal injection of ethanol to pregnant C57Bl/6J mice in early pregnancy when embryos are undergoing *gastrulation* (Sulik *et al.*, 1981; Sulik and Johnston, 1983). Following such exposures, term fetuses exhibit many of the features of FAS, including microcephaly, microphthalmia, short palpebral fissures, deficiencies of the philtral region, and a long upper lip. The specific set of craniofacial malformations produced in offspring depends on the time of exposure. Excess cell death in sensitive cell populations is a common finding (Kotch and Sulik, 1992; Sulik, 2005; Smith, 2010).

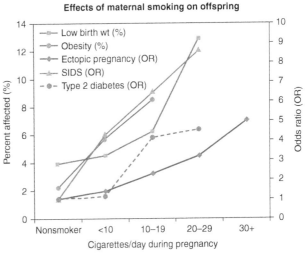

Figure 10-1. *Effects of maternal smoking on pregnancy and offspring.* These are effects for which dose–response relationships with maternal smoking have been established, but do not represent all of the effects of maternal smoking during pregnancy (see Rogers, 2008). (Plotted data are from: Preterm birth (spontaneous delivery at 33–36 weeks gestation), Kyrklund-Blomberg and Cnattingius (1998); small-for-gestational age (SGA, <10th percentile for gestational week) from Windham *et al.* (2000); stillbirth from Wisborg *et al.* (2001); ectopic pregnancy from Handler *et al.* (1989); sudden infant death syndrome (SIDS) from Fleming and Blair (2007); offspring type 2 diabetes from Montgomery and Ekbom (2002); offspring obesity (BMI > 97 percentile), Von Kries *et al.* (2002)).

Tobacco Smoke

Prenatal and early postnatal exposure to tobacco smoke or its constituents may well represent the leading cause of environmentally induced developmental disease and morbidity today (Rogers, 2008) (Fig. 10-1). Approximately 25% of women in the United States continue to smoke during pregnancy, despite public health programs aimed at curbing this behavior. Because of the high number of pregnant smokers and the relative accuracy of assessing smoking during pregnancy, results of epidemiological studies provide a well-characterized picture of the consequences of developmental tobacco smoke exposure. These include spontaneous abortions, perinatal deaths, sudden infant death syndrome (SIDS), learning, behavioral, and attention disorders, and lower birth weight (Slotkin, 1998; Fried *et al.*, 1998; Tuthill *et al.*, 1999; Haug *et al.*, 2000; Markussen Linnet *et al.*, 2006; Rogers, 2008). In a review of smoking and SIDS (Mitchell and Milerad, 2006), the relative risk associated with maternal smoking was 2.86 (95% confidence interval 2.77–2.95) before prone sleep-position intervention (putting infants on their backs for sleep reduces the overall risk of SIDS) and 3.93 (3.78–4.08) after intervention programs were started. The authors of the review estimated that about one-third of SIDS deaths might have been prevented if no fetuses had been exposed in utero to maternal smoking. Recent studies have found that offspring of smoking mothers have a higher risk of obesity, hypertension, and type 2 diabetes than offspring of nonsmokers (Oken *et al.*, 2008; Suzuki *et al.*, 2009; Bakker and Jaddoe, 2011; Cupul-Uicab *et al.*, 2012).

Maternal smoking has not been associated with a high risk of structural malformations. However, Hackshaw *et al.* (2011) performed a systematic review and meta-analysis of observational studies reporting odds ratios for having a nonchromosomal birth defect for women who smoked versus nonsmokers. There were 172 published articles comprising 173,687 malformed cases and 11.7 million controls considered in the review. Significant positive associations with maternal smoking were found for these defects [odds ratios]: cardiovascular [1.09], musculoskeletal [1.16], limb reduction [1.26], missing/extra digits [1.18], clubfoot [1.28], craniosynostosis [1.33], facial [1.19], eye [1.25], orofacial clefts [1.28], gastrointestinal [1.27], gastroschisis [1.5], anal atresia [1.20], hernia [1.40], and undescended testes [1.13]. Lammer and co-workers (Lammer *et al.*, 2005) found that maternal smoking was a risk factor for orofacial clefts, and increased risk is associated with particular genotypes indicating lack of enzymes involved in detoxification of smoking-derived chemicals. Gene–environment interactions may also be the basis for increased risk of other birth defects with maternal smoking (Shi *et al.*, 2008). Perinatal exposure to tobacco smoke can also affect branching morphogenesis and maturation of the lung, leading to altered physiological function (Pinkerton and Joad, 2000; Gilliland *et al.*, 2000; Maritz and Harding, 2011). In a genome-wide association study, two genes, TBK1 on chromosome 12 and ZNF236 on chromosome 18, showed multiple single nucleotide polymorphisms associated with higher risk of nonsyndromic cleft palate in the presence of maternal smoking (Beaty *et al.*, 2011). One component of tobacco smoke, nicotine, is a known neuroteratogen in experimental animals and can by itself produce many of the adverse developmental outcomes associated with tobacco smoke, including impaired fertility, neurobehavioral effects, respiratory dysfunction, obesity, hypertension, and type 2 diabetes (Slotkin, 1998; Bruin *et al.*, 2010).

It is important to state unequivocally that exposure to environmental (secondhand) tobacco smoke also represents a significant risk to the pregnant nonsmoker and her baby, and exposure to secondhand smoke has been associated with many of the effects caused by active maternal smoking (eg, Windham *et al.*, 2000; George *et al.*, 2006; Mitchell and Milerad, 2006). In a literature review with meta-analysis, Leonardi-Bee and co-workers (2008) found that exposure of nonsmoking pregnant women to secondhand smoke was associated with reduction of birth weight by 33 g or more, as well as a 22% increased risk of being of low birth weight (<2500 g). In a subsequent review and meta-analysis (Leonardi-Bee *et al.*, 2011), they found that nonsmoking pregnant women exposed to secondhand tobacco smoke were 23% more likely to experience stillbirth and 13% more likely to have a child with a congenital malformation.

Cocaine

Cocaine, a plant alkaloid derived from coca, is a local anesthetic with vasoconstrictor properties. Effects on the fetus are complicated and controversial and demonstrate the difficulty of monitoring the human population for adverse reproductive outcomes (reviewed in Scanlon, 1991; Volfe, 1992; Addis *et al.*, 2001; Ackerman *et al.*, 2010). Accurate exposure ascertainment is difficult, as many confounding factors, including socioeconomic status and concurrent use of cigarettes, alcohol, and other drugs of abuse, may be involved. In addition, reported effects on the fetus and infant (neurological and behavioral changes) are difficult to identify and quantify. Cocaine exposure during pregnancy in humans appears to be associated with abruptio placentae (Addis *et al.*, 2001), and preterm birth, low birth weight, and small-for-gestational age (SGA) infants (Gouin *et al.*, 2011). Congenital malformations of the genitourinary tract have also been reported (Lutiger *et al.*, 1991), and kidney and bladder function is diminished in fetuses of pregnant women using cocaine (Mitra, 1999). Moreover, fetal cocaine exposure has been associated with impaired neonatal auditory processing (Potter *et al.*, 2000). Fetal cocaine exposure can be estimated by chemical analysis of fetal meconium, which can provide a measure of developmental exposure to xenobiotic agents ranging from food additives to over-the-counter medications to drugs of abuse (Ostrea *et al.*, 1998).

Retinoids

The ability of excess vitamin A (retinol) to induce malformations has been known for at least 50 years (Cohlan, 1954). Effects on the developing embryo include malformations of the face, limbs, heart, central nervous system, and skeleton. Similar malformations were later shown to be induced by retinoic acid (RA) administration in the mouse (Kochhar, 1967) and hamster (Shenefelt, 1972). Since those observations, knowledge relating to the effects of retinol, RA, and structurally related chemicals that bind to and activate specific nuclear receptors has expanded rapidly (Chambon, 1994; Lohnes *et al.*, 1994; Mendelsohn *et al.*, 1994; Collins and Mao, 1999; Arafa *et al.*, 2000). The RXR-α receptor appears to play an important role in cleft palate induced by RA (Nugent *et al.*, 1999). The teratogenic effects of vitamin A and retinoids have been reviewed (Nau *et al.*, 1994; Collins and Mao, 1999).

Beginning in 1982, one retinoid, 13-*cis*-RA (isotretinoin or Accutane), was marketed as an effective treatment of cystic acne. Despite clear warnings against use in pregnancy on the label of this prescription drug (FDA pregnancy category X: proven fetal risks clearly outweigh any benefit), an extensive physician and patient education program, and restrictive requirements for prescription to women of childbearing potential, infants with pathognomonic malformations involving the ears, heart, brain, and thymus were reported as early as 1983 (Rosa, 1983; Lammer *et al.*, 1985). Among 115 exposed pregnancies not electively terminated, 18% ended in spontaneous abortion and 28% of live-born infants had at least one major malformation (Dai *et al.*, 1992). In another prospective study, there was nearly a doubling of the risk for premature delivery after first trimester exposure, and about 50% of the exposed children had full-scale IQ scores below 85 at age five (Lammer, 1992). Robertson *et al.* (2005) reported that almost 25% of women with an isotretinoin-exposed pregnancy did not recall having contraception counseling before starting their medication. Rates of recommended birth control and monthly pregnancy testing were low. Thus, voluntary pregnancy prevention programs for women receiving prescriptions for isotretinoin were not highly effective, resulting in fetal exposures to isotretinoin. Adams (2010) has reviewed the neurobehavioral teratology of retinoids over the last 50 years.

Antiepileptic Drugs

Clinical management of women of childbearing age who have epilepsy is difficult. Although control of seizures during pregnancy is crucial, most current antiepileptic drugs (AEDs) have been shown to carry risk of developmental toxicity including birth defects, cognitive impairment, and fetal death. As a class, including phenytoin, carbamazepine and valproic acid, AEDs are considered human teratogens. These drugs can be used as monotherapy or in combination. In general, the incidence of birth defects increases with the number of drugs used in combination. Newer AEDs such as gabapentin, lamotrigine, oxcarbazone, topiramate, and zonizamide have now been used for over a decade, and studies to date suggest that these alternatives may be safer than the older AEDs. The interested reader is directed to several recent reviews (Tatum, 2006; Tomson and Battino, 2005; Ornoy, 2006; Hansen, 2010).

Phenytoin (diphenylhydantoin) has been used as an AED for over 70 years and its antiepileptic effect occurs through inhibition of voltage-gated sodium channels. It is metabolized by the cytochrome P450 system to a reactive intermediate and then to an active metabolite that is excreted in the urine. The fetal hydantoin syndrome, described by Hanson and Smith (1975), includes craniofacial abnormalities, limb defects, growth deficiency, and mild-to-moderate mental retardation. This syndrome has been reported to occur in 5% to 10% of exposed offspring (Schardein, 2000). Proposed mechanisms involved in the teratogenicity of phenytoin include folic acid deficiency and the formation of reactive intermediates that damage tissue macromolecules (for review see Hansen, 2010).

Carbamazepine has been reported to be teratogenic in rats and mice (Schardein, 2000), and a report from the FDA (Rosa, 1991) linked the drug to NTDs in humans. A meta-analysis of 16 studies reported a 2.89-fold increased risk of a major birth defect in offspring of pregnant women treated with carbamazepine (Matalon *et al.*, 2002). An epoxide metabolite of carbamazepine was found to be teratogenic in mice in vivo (Bennett *et al.*, 1996) but not in mice or rats in vitro (Hansen *et al.*, 1996). The teratogenicity observed in mice may have been related to maternal toxicity or to a different metabolite.

Valproic acid, or 2-propylpentanoic acid, was first marketed in Europe in 1967 and in the United States in 1978. In 1982, Elizabeth Robert reported that, of 146 cases of spina bifida aperta recorded in Lyon, France, nine of the mothers had taken valproic acid during the first trimester of pregnancy. The odds ratio in a case–control study was 20.6, and the estimated risk of a valproate-exposed woman having a child with spina bifida was 1.2%, a risk similar to that for women with a previous child with an NTD (Centers for Disease Control and Prevention [CDC], 1982). The report was quickly confirmed in other areas of the world through the efforts of the International Clearinghouse of Birth Defect Registries (CDC, 1983). It was fortunate that several events came together to allow the determination of valproate as a human teratogen. These included the active birth defects registry, an interest by Robert in the genetics of spina bifida, a question on epilepsy and anticonvulsant use in a Robert survey, and the prevalence of valproate monotherapy for epilepsy in that region (Lammer *et al.*, 1987). These findings spurred a great deal of research on the effects of valproate in multiple species, including the effects of enantiomers of valproate analogs. Yet, the mechanism of action, as for most developmental toxicants, remains elusive (Nau *et al.*, 1991; Ehlers *et al.*, 1992a,b; Hauck and Nau, 1992). Use of inbred mouse strains differing in their sensitivity to valproate-induced teratogenesis has revealed several candidate genes conferring sensitivity (Finnell *et al.*, 1997, 2000; Craig *et al.*, 2000; Bennett *et al.*, 2000). Similar to phenytoin, some studies have indicated a possible role of interference with folate metabolism (Hansen, 2010). Valproic acid is also a histone deacetylase inhibitor, and this may play a role in its teratogenicity (Menegola *et al.*, 2006; Eikel *et al.*, 2006).

Angiotensin-Converting Enzyme Inhibitors and Angiotensin Receptor Antagonists

The renin–angiotensin system is a key controller of blood pressure. The active signaling messenger of this system is angiotensin II, which binds to angiotensin II (AT1) receptors to cause vasoconstriction and fluid retention, resulting in elevation of blood pressure. Antihypertensive agents acting on this system include the angiotensin-converting enzyme (ACE) inhibitors and the AT1 receptor blockers (collectively known as "sartans"). ACE inhibitors are widely prescribed and, when used in the second half of pregnancy, are known to cause oligohydramnios (low amniotic fluid volume), fetal growth retardation, pulmonary hypoplasia, joint contractures, hypocalvaria, neonatal renal failure, hypotension, and death. Angiotensin II receptor antagonists taken during the same period (second or third trimester) in pregnancy cause a similar spectrum of developmental toxicity (Friedman, 2006; Quan, 2006). These findings in the fetus can be related to the reduced amniotic fluid volume, a consequence of impaired fetal renal function (Tabacova, 2005). The developmental toxicity of first trimester use of ACE inhibitors and AT1 receptor antagonists has been somewhat controversial (Schaefer, 2003), although a recent study found an increased risk of major congenital malformations following first trimester exposure to ACE inhibitors (Cooper *et al.*, 2006). These authors studied a cohort of 29,507 infants born between 1985 and 2000. Of these, 209 infants had exposure to ACE inhibitors in the first trimester alone. These infants had an increased risk of major congenital malformations (relative risk = 2.71, 95% confidence interval 1.72–4.27). The risk ratio for malformations of the cardiovascular system and the central nervous system were 3.72 and 4.39, respectively. These authors concluded that exposure to ACE inhibitors during the first trimester should be avoided. However, a recent literature review and meta-analysis of studies of first trimester exposures to ACE inhibitors and AT1 blockers found that while there was a significant increase in risk of major malformations compared to healthy controls, the risk was similar to that of patients on other antihypertensives (Walfisch *et al.*, 2011). These results suggest that a first trimester exposure to antihypertensives in general may be teratogenic.

PRINCIPLES OF DEVELOPMENTAL TOXICOLOGY

Principles of teratology were put forth by James Wilson in 1959 and in his watershed monograph *Environment and Birth Defects* (Wilson, 1973) (Table 10-2). Much progress has been made in the ensuing decades, yet these principles have withstood the test of time and remain basic to developmental toxicology.

Critical Periods of Susceptibility and Endpoints of Toxicity

Familiarity with principles of normal development is a prerequisite to understanding abnormal development. Development is characterized by change: change in size, changes in biochemistry and physiology, and changes in form and functionality. These changes

Table 10-2

Wilson General Principles of Teratology

I. Susceptibility to teratogenesis depends on the genotype of the conceptus and the manner in which this interacts with adverse environmental factors.

II. Susceptibility to teratogenesis varies with the developmental stage at the time of exposure to an adverse influence.

III. Teratogenic agents act in specific ways (mechanisms) on developing cells and tissues to initiate sequences of abnormal developmental events (pathogenesis).

IV. The access of adverse influences to developing tissues depends on the nature of the influence (agent).

V. The four manifestations of deviant development are death, malformation, growth retardation, and functional deficit.

VI. Manifestations of deviant development increase in frequency and degree as dosage increases, from the no effect to the totally lethal level.

SOURCE: From Wilson (1959, 1973).

Table 10-3

Timing of Key Developmental Events in Some Mammalian Species*

	RAT	RABBIT	MONKEY	HUMAN
Blastocyst formation	3–5	2.6–6	4–9	4–6
Implantation	5–6	6	9	6–7
Organogenesis	6–17	6–18	20–45	21–56
Primitive streak	9	6.5	18–20	16–18
Neural plate	9.5	—	19–21	18–20
First somite	10	—	—	20–21
First branchial arch	10	—	—	20
First heartbeat	10.2	—	—	22
10 Somites	10–11	9	23–24	25–26
Upper limb buds	10.5	10.5	25–26	29–30
Lower limb buds	11.2	11	26–27	31–32
Testes differentiation	14.5	20	—	43
Heart septation	15.5	—	—	46–47
Palate closure	16–17	19–20	45–47	56–58
Urethral groove closed in male	—	—	—	90
Length of gestation	21–22	31–34	166	267

*Developmental ages are days of gestation.
SOURCE: Data from Shepard (2004).

are orchestrated by a cascade of factors regulating gene expression, the first of which are maternally inherited and present in the egg prior to fertilization. In turn, these maternal factors activate regulatory genes in the embryonic genome, and sequential gene activation continues throughout development. Intercellular and intracellular signaling pathways essential for normal development have been elucidated and rely on transcriptional, translational, and posttranslational controls.

Because of the rapid changes occurring during development, the nature of the embryo/fetus as a target for toxicity is also changing. Although the basic tenets of toxicology discussed elsewhere in this text also apply during development, the principle of critical periods of sensitivity based on developmental stage of the conceptus at the time of insult is a primary and somewhat unique consideration. In this section, normal developmental stages are discussed in the context of their known and potential susceptibility to toxicants. It should be emphasized, however, that development is a continuum; these stages are used for descriptive purposes and do not necessarily represent discrete developmental events. Timing of some key developmental events in humans and experimental animal species is presented in Table 10-3.

As a logical starting point, *gametogenesis* is the process of forming the haploid germ cells or gametes, the egg and sperm. These gametes fuse in the process of fertilization to form the diploid *zygote*, or one-celled embryo. Gametogenesis and fertilization are vulnerable to toxicants, but this is the topic of another chapter in this text. It is now known that the maternal and paternal genomes are not equivalent in their contributions to the zygotic genome. The process of *imprinting* occurs during gametogenesis, conferring to certain allelic genes a differential expressivity depending

on whether they are of maternal or paternal origin (Latham, 1999; Li and Sasaki, 2011). Because imprinting involves cytosine methylation and changes in chromatin conformation, this process may be susceptible to toxicants that affect these targets (Murphy and Jirtle, 2000). Jirtle and colleagues have demonstrated that both early nutrition (Waterland and Jirtle, 2003, 2004) and the estrogenic compound genistein (Dolinoy *et al.*, 2006) can modify the methylation patterns of specific genes and cause altered phenotypes in mice. Anway *et al.* (2006) demonstrated a transgenerational effect of the fungicide vinclozolin in rats, in which male offspring (F1) of treated F0 females had reduced spermatogenic capacity, which was transmitted to subsequent generations (F2–F4). For a review of transgenerational effects of environmental agents, the reader is referred to Skinner *et al.* (2011).

Epigenetics refers to the biochemical changes in chromatin that lead to changes in conformation and gene expression. Epigenetic changes include DNA methylation, histone modifications, and expression of microRNAs. Although epigenetics provides the basis for imprinting of genes, the role of epigenetics is much broader (Rogers *et al.*, 2010; Grace *et al.*, 2011). There are specific stages of the life cycle during which epigenetic marks may be erased and reestablished (Sasaki and Matsui, 2008), including two periods of development during which large-scale demethylations of the genome are known to occur. One is during migration and proliferation of the primordial gem cells (between embryonic days 10.5 and 12.5 in the mouse). It is during this period that imprinted genes are demethylated, with remethylation occurring in a gender-specific manner during gametogenesis in the offspring. The other period of widespread epigenetic reprogramming occurs shortly after formation of the zygote and in the early embryo, with total genomic methylation reaching a nadir at the blastocyst stage (Hales *et al.*, 2011). This process of epigenetic reprogramming represents a putative target for environmental chemicals, and examples of environmentally mediated epigenetic changes are emerging (Skinner *et al.*, 2011; Rogers *et al.*, 2010; Perera and Herbstman, 2011).

Following fertilization, the embryo moves down the fallopian tube (oviduct) and attaches to the wall of the uterus. The *preimplantation* period comprises mainly an increase in cell number through a rapid series of cell divisions with little growth in size (*cleavage* of the zygote) and cavitation of the embryo to form a fluid-filled blastocoele. This stage, termed the *blastocyst*, consisting of about a thousand cells, may contain as few as three cells destined to give rise to the embryo proper (Markert and Petters, 1978), and these cells are within a region called the *inner cell mass*. The remainder of the blastocyst cells gives rise to extraembryonic membranes and support structures (eg, trophoblast and placenta). However, the fates of the cells in the early embryo are not completely determined at this stage. The relatively undifferentiated preimplantation embryo has great restorative (regulative) growth potential (Snow and Tam, 1979). For example, experiments by Moore *et al.* (1968) demonstrated that single cells from eight-celled rabbit embryos are capable of producing normal offspring.

Toxicity during the preimplantation period is generally thought to result in either no or slight effect on growth (because of regulative growth) or in death (through overwhelming damage or failure to implant). Preimplantation exposure to dichlorodiphenyltrichloroethane (DDT), nicotine, or methyl-methane sulfonate results in body and/or brain weight deficits and embryo lethality, but not malformations (Fabro, 1973; Fabro *et al.*, 1984). However, there are a few examples of toxic exposures during the preimplantation period leading to fetal malformations. Exposure to toxicants during a brief period (approximately six hours) immediately following fertilization has been demonstrated to result in malformed fetuses for a few chemicals including ethylene oxide (Generoso *et al.*, 1987), ethylmethane sulfonate, ethylnitrosourea, and triethylene melamine (Generoso *et al.*, 1988). The mechanisms underlying these unexpected findings have not been elucidated but probably do not involve point mutations. Epigenetic changes were not examined, but given the time of the exposure, this is a plausible target. Treatment of pregnant mice with methylnitrosourea on days 2.5, 3.5, and 4.5 of gestation resulted in NTDs and cleft palate (Takeuchi, 1984). Cyproterone acetate and medroxyprogesterone acetate are capable of producing malformations when administered on day two of gestation (Eibs *et al.*, 1982). Rutledge and co-workers (Rutledge *et al.*, 1994) produced hind-limb and lower body duplications by treating pregnant mice with all-*trans* RA on gestation day 4.5 to 5.5, at which time the embryos are at the late blastocyst and proamniotic stages. Because of the rapid mitoses occurring during the preimplantation period, chemicals affecting DNA synthesis or integrity, or those affecting microtubule assembly, would be expected to be particularly toxic.

Following implantation, the embryo undergoes *gastrulation*. Gastrulation is the process of formation of the three primary germ layers—the *ectoderm*, *mesoderm*, and *endoderm*. During gastrulation, cells migrate through a midline structure called the *primitive streak*, and their movements set up basic morphogenetic fields in the embryo (Smith *et al.*, 1994). A prelude to *organogenesis*, the period of gastrulation is highly susceptible to teratogenesis. It is common for teratogens administered during gastrulation to produce malformations of the eye, brain, and face. These malformations are indicative of damage to the anterior *neural plate*, one of the regions defined by the cellular movements of gastrulation.

The formation of the neural plate in the ectoderm marks the onset of organogenesis, during which the rudiments of most bodily structures are established. This is a period of heightened susceptibility to malformations and extends from approximately the third to the eighth weeks of gestation in humans. Within this short period, the embryo undergoes rapid and dramatic changes. At three weeks of gestation, the human conceptus is in most ways indistinguishable from other mammalian and indeed other vertebrate embryos, consisting of only a few cell types in a trilaminar arrangement. By eight weeks, the conceptus, which can now be termed a fetus, has a form clearly recognizable as human. The rapid changes during organogenesis require cell proliferation and migration, cell–cell interactions, and morphogenetic tissue remodeling. These processes can be exemplified by the ontogeny of the *neural crest* cells. These cells originate at the border of the neural plate and migrate to form a wide variety of structures throughout the embryo. For example, neural crest cells derived from segments of the hindbrain (*rhombomeres*) migrate to form bone and connective tissues in the head (Krumlauf, 1993; Vaglia and Hall, 1999; Trainor and Krumlauf, 2001), while other neural crest cells form diverse structures including melanocytes, enteric ganglia, and adrenal medulla, and contribute to the cardiac outflow tract.

Within organogenesis, there are periods of peak susceptibility for each forming structure. This is nicely illustrated by the work of Shenefelt (1972), who studied the malformations caused by carefully timed doses of RA in pregnant hamsters. The incidences of some of the defects seen after RA administration at different times in pregnancy are shown in Fig. 10-2. The peak incidence of each malformation coincides with the timing of key developmental events in the affected structure. Thus, the specification of developmental fields for the eyes is established quite early, and microphthalmia has an early critical period. Establishment of rudiments of the long bones of the limbs occurs later, as does susceptibility to shortened limbs. The palate has two separate peaks of susceptibility, the first

corresponding to the early establishment of the palatal folds and the second to the later events leading to palatal closure. Notice also that the total incidence of malformations is lower prior to organogenesis but increases to 100% by gestation day 7¾. The processes underlying the development of normal structures are incompletely understood but involve a number of key events. A given toxicant may affect one or several developmental events, so the pattern of sensitivity of a structure can change depending on the nature of the toxic insult. Cleft palate can be induced in mouse fetuses following maternal exposure to methanol as early as day five of gestation, with a peak sensitivity at day seven and little or no sensitivity after day nine (Rogers and Mole, 1997). In contrast, the typical peak critical period for induction of cleft palate in the mouse for most teratogens is between gestation days 11 and 13, during the stages of growth, elevation, and fusion of the palatal shelves. In a large series of experiments in naval medical research institute (NMRI) mice, the day of peak sensitivity to the induction of cleft palate was day 11 for 2,3,7,8-tetrachlorodibenzodioxin (TCDD), day 12 for 2,4,5-trichlorophenoxyacetic acid, and day 13 for dexamethasone (Neubert *et al.*, 1973). Detection of unexpected critical periods like the early one for induction of cleft palate by methanol can provide clues to normal developmental processes not presently understood.

The end of organogenesis marks the beginning of the *fetal period* (from day ~57 to birth in humans), characterized primarily by tissue differentiation, growth, and physiological maturation. This is not to say that formation of the organs is complete, but rather that almost all organs are present and grossly recognizable. Further development of organs proceeds during the fetal period to attain requisite functionality prior to birth, including fine structural morphogenesis (eg, neural outgrowth and synaptogenesis, branching morphogenesis of the bronchial tree and renal cortical tubules) as well as biochemical maturation (eg, induction of tissue-specific enzymes and structural proteins). One of the latest organogenetic events is closure of the urethral groove in the male, which occurs at about gestation day 90. Failure of this event produces hypospadias, a ventral clefting of the penis.

Exposure during the fetal period is most likely to result in effects on growth and functional maturation. Functional anomalies of the central nervous system and reproductive organs—including behavioral, cognitive, and motor deficits as well as decreases in fertility—are among the possible adverse outcomes. These manifestations are not apparent prenatally and may require careful postnatal observation and testing. Such postnatal functional manifestations can be sensitive indicators of in utero toxicity, and reviews of postnatal functional deficits of the central nervous system (Rodier *et al.*, 1994; Miodovnik, 2011), immune system (Holladay and Luster, 1994; Dietert, 2008), and heart, lung, and kidneys (Lau and Kavlock, 1994) are available. Major structural alterations can occur during the fetal period, but these generally result from deformations (disruption of previously normal structures) rather than malformations. The extremities may be affected by amniotic bands, wrapping of the umbilical cord, or vascular disruptions, leading to loss of distal structures. Over the past two decades, the concept of "developmental programming" has emerged, in which the developmental environment is thought to influence the metabolic parameters of the offspring that will persist throughout life and may affect lifelong risk of disease (for review, see McMillen and Robinson, 2005; Gluckman *et al.*, 2011; Barouki *et al.*, 2012). Much of the work on fetal programming has focused on the role of maternal nutrition, and there is a paucity of data concerning the long-term effects of chemical exposure during the fetal and early postnatal periods (Lau and Rogers, 2004). Some effects could require years to become apparent (such as those noted

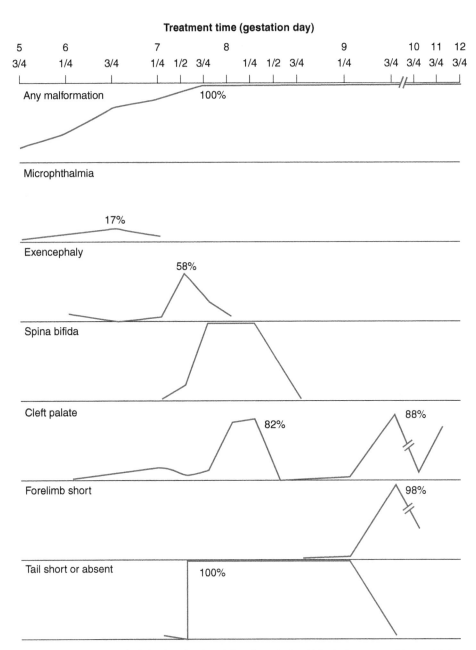

Figure 10-2. *Critical periods of sensitivity for induction of various defects by retinoic acid in the hamster.* Incidence of defects estimates for the embryo/fetal LD$_{50}$ maternal dosage. Note in the top panel that fewer malformations are induced on days five to six, prior to organogenesis, indicating that during this period embryos for the most part either die or recover. Likelihood of malformation increases rapidly during gastrulation and reaches 100% during organogenesis. Peak incidence for each defect is enumerated and reflect timing of critical events in the development of each structure. (Modified from Shenefelt (1972), with permission.)

above for DES), and others may even result in the premature onset of senescence and/or organ failure late in life. In rats, prenatal exposure to high dosages of ethanol during the second half of pregnancy shortens life span of the offspring, by about 20 weeks in females and 2.5 to seven weeks in males (Abel *et al.*, 1987).

Dose–Response Patterns and the Threshold Concept

The major effects of prenatal exposure, observed in fetuses near term in developmental toxicity studies, are growth retardation, malformations, and embryo death. The relationships among these effects are complex and vary with the chemical, the time of exposure, and the dose. For some chemicals these endpoints may represent a continuum of increasing toxicity, with low dosages producing growth retardation and increasing dosages producing malformations and then death. Malformations and/or death can occur without a concomitant effect on intrauterine growth, but this is unusual. Likewise, growth retardation and embryo lethality can occur without malformations. Chemicals producing the latter pattern of response would be considered embryotoxic or embryolethal but not teratogenic (unless it was established that death was due to a structural malformation). Effects on function in viable fetuses will usually require postnatal assessment. Transition to postnatal life is a rigorous test in itself, and severe functional effects may manifest as neonatal mortality.

Another key element of the dose–response relationship is the shape of the dose–response curve at low exposure levels. Because of the high restorative growth potential of the mammalian embryo, cellular homeostatic mechanisms, and maternal metabolic defenses, mammalian developmental toxicity has generally been considered to be a threshold phenomenon. Assumption of a threshold means that there is a maternal dosage below which no increase in an adverse outcome is elicited. Daston (1993) summarized two approaches for establishing the existence of a threshold. The first, exemplified by a large teratology study on 2,4,5-T (Nelson and Holson, 1978), suggests that no study is adequately capable of evaluating the dose–response at low response rates (eg, in this study it was calculated that 805 litters per dose would be necessary to detect a 5% increase in resorptions of embryos). The second approach is to determine whether a threshold exists for the molecular mechanism responsible for the observed effect. Although relatively few mechanisms of abnormal development have been thoroughly studied, it is clear that cellular and embryonic repair mechanisms and dose-dependent kinetics both support the plausibility of a mechanistic threshold. Lack of a threshold implies that exposure to any amount of a toxic chemical, even one molecule, has the potential to cause developmental toxicity. Hypothetically, a point mutation in a critical gene could be induced by a single hit or single molecule, leading to a deleterious change in a gene product and consequent abnormal development. This, of course, carries the large assumption that the molecule could traverse the maternal system and the placenta and enter a critical progenitor cell in the embryo. An effect on a single cell might result in abnormal development at the zygote (one-cell) stage, the blastocyst stage (when only a few cells in the inner cell mass are embryo progenitors), or during organogenesis, when organ rudiments may consist of only a few cells.

An apparent threshold for developmental toxicity based at least in part on cellular homeostatic mechanisms is demonstrated in studies of mechanisms underlying the teratogenicity of 5-fluorouracil (Shuey et al., 1994; see also "Safety Assessment" later in this chapter). This chemical inhibits the enzyme thymidylate synthetase (TS), thus interfering with DNA synthesis and cell proliferation. Significant embryonal TS inhibition is evident at maternal dosages an order of magnitude lower than those required to produce malformations and about fivefold below those affecting fetal growth (Fig. 10-3). The lack of developmental toxicity despite significant TS inhibition probably reflects an ability of the embryo to compensate for imbalances in cellular nucleotide pool sizes.

For human health risk assessment, it is also important to consider the distinction between individual thresholds and population thresholds. There is wide variability in the human population, and a threshold for a population can be defined as the threshold of the most sensitive individual in the population (Gaylor et al., 1988). Indeed, even though the biological target of a developmental toxicant may exhibit a threshold, background factors such as health status or concomitant exposures may render some individuals already at or even beyond the threshold for failure of that biological process. Any further toxic impact on that process, even one molecule, would theoretically increase risk. The concept of thresholds of adversity for reproductive toxicants has recently been reviewed by Piersma et al. (2011a).

MECHANISMS AND PATHOGENESIS OF DEVELOPMENTAL TOXICITY

The term *mechanisms* is used here to refer to cellular events that initiate a process leading to abnormal development. *Pathogenesis* comprises the cell-, tissue-, and organ-level sequelae that ultimately lead to abnormality. Mechanisms of teratogenesis listed by Wilson (1977) include mutations, chromosomal breaks, altered mitosis, altered nucleic acid integrity or function, diminished supplies of precursors or substrates, decreased energy supplies, altered

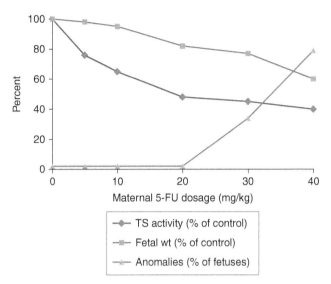

Figure 10-3. *Relationship between inhibition of embryonal thymidylate synthetase and adverse fetal outcome following maternal 5-fluorouracil (5-FU) administration on gestation day 14 in the rat.* 5-FU inhibits embryonal TS activity at low dosages, with most of the inhibition occurring below 20 mg/kg. Fetal weight is affected at 20 mg/kg and above, whereas incidence of anomalies increases only at 30 mg/kg and above. Anomalies include edema, skull dysmorphology, orbital hemorrhage, wavy ribs, cleft palate, brachygnathia and hindlimb defects. (Based on Shuey *et al.* (1994) and unpublished observations.)

membrane characteristics, osmolar imbalance, and enzyme inhibition. Although these cellular insults are not unique to development, they may relatively quickly trigger unique pathogenic responses in the embryo, such as reduced cell proliferation, cell death, altered cell–cell interactions, reduced biosynthesis, inhibition of morphogenetic movements, or mechanical disruption of developing structures.

Elucidating the mechanism(s) and pathogenesis of chemically induced developmental toxicity can be extremely challenging. Cyclophosphamide (CP), a chemotherapeutic and immunosuppressive drug, has been studied for its teratogenicity for 50 years, and is a good case study (Mirkes, 1985a; Ozolins, 2010). Because of its use as an immunosuppressive drug to treat lupus, at least nine cases of teratogenesis induced by inadvertent exposure to CP during early pregnancy have been recorded (Paladini et al., 2004). Efforts to understand the teratogenicity of this drug provide an example of approaches to understanding metabolic activation, teratogenic mechanisms, and pathogenesis. Much of this and other mechanistic work was made possible by the advent of rodent whole embryo culture (WEC), which involves removing rodent or rabbit embryos from the uterus at the beginning of organogenesis and growing them in serum-containing culture media (New, 1978; Sadler and Warner, 1984; Ellis-Hutchings and Carney, 2010; Robinson et al., 2012a,b,c,d; Lee et al., 2012). Embryos will grow normally for about 48 hours, completing most of organogenesis. The ability to grow embryos in isolation allows direct exposure, manipulation, and observation. The use of rodent WEC as a screening system for developmental toxicity will be discussed later in this chapter.

Using WEC, Fantel et al. (1979) and Sanyal et al. (1979) showed that hepatic S9 fractions and cofactors were required to elicit abnormal development by CP, demonstrating that it must be metabolically activated to be teratogenic. Activation of CP was inhibited by metyrapone or carbon monoxide, indicating involvement of P450 monooxygenases. Of the CP metabolites, 4-hydroxycyclophosphamide (4OHCP) and aldophosphamide (AP) are unstable. A stable derivative of 4OHCP, 4-hydroperoxy-cyclophosphamide (4OOHCP) was tested in vivo (Hales, 1982) and in WEC (Mirkes, 1987). In the latter study, the morphology of the treated embryos was indistinguishable from that of embryos cultured with CP plus an activating system. Spontaneous conversion of 4OOHCP to 4OHCP and then to phosphoramide mustard (PM) and acrolein (AC) occurs rapidly, and these further metabolites, as well as 4-ketocyclophosphamide (4-ketoCP) and carboxyphosphamide (CaP), have also been studied for their teratogenicity. It appears that 4OHCP is not teratogenic (Hales, 1983) and toxicity elicited by 4-ketoCP is dissimilar to that of activated CP (Mirkes *et al.*, 1981). Subsequent work centered on the two remaining metabolites, PM and AC. Mirkes *et al.* (1981) demonstrated that the effects of PM on cultured rat embryos were indistinguishable from those of activated CP. Hales (1982) administered CP, PM, or AC to gestation day 13 rat embryos by intraamniotic injection. CP and AC caused hydrocephaly, open eyes, cleft palate, micrognathia, omphalocele, and tail and limb defects, whereas PM produced only hydrocephaly and tail and limb defects. Thus, both PM and AC appear to be teratogenic metabolites of CP.

What are the cell and molecular targets of activated CP, and what is the nature of the interactions? Experiments with (^{3}H)CP showed that approximately 87% of bound radioactivity was associated with protein, 5% with DNA, and 8% with RNA (Mirkes, 1985b). Using alkaline elution, it was demonstrated that CP and PM produce single-strand DNA breaks and DNA–DNA and DNA–protein cross-linking. To determine whether DNA cross-linking is essential for teratogenicity, a monofunctional derivative of PM, capable of producing single-strand breaks but not cross-links in DNA, was tested. Although higher concentrations were needed, this derivative produced the same spectrum of effects as PM (Mirkes *et al.*, 1985). Later, Little and Mirkes (1990) showed that 4-hydroperoxydechlorocyclophosphamide, a CP analog that yields AC and a nonalkylating derivative of PM, did not produce DNA damage when embryos were exposed in serum-containing medium, but this analog retained teratogenicity. Using radiolabeled CP, they further found that AC preferentially binds to protein and shows high incorporation into the yolk sac, whereas PM binds preferentially to DNA. Hales (1989) showed that PM and AC have strikingly different effects on limb buds in culture. These results indicate that PM and AC have different targets in the embryo and that PM is responsible for CP-induced DNA damage.

How do chemical insults at the cell and molecular level translate to a birth defect? To illustrate pathogenesis, we will consider cell cycle perturbations and cell death, continuing our example of CP. Cell death plays a critical role in normal morphogenesis. The term *programmed cell death* refers to a specific type of cell death, *apoptosis*, under genetic control in the embryo (Lavin and Watters, 1993). Apoptosis is necessary for sculpting the digits from the hand plate, for instance (Hernandez-Martinez and Covarrubias, 2011), and for assuring appropriate functional connections between the central nervous system and distal structures. Cell proliferation is obviously essential for development. Cells within the primitive streak of the gastrula-stage rat embryo have the shortest known cell cycle time of any mammalian cell, three to 3.5 hours (MacAuley *et al.*, 1993). Cell proliferation rates change both spatially and temporally during ontogenesis, as can be demonstrated by examining the proportion of cells in S-phase over time in various tissues during mid-to late gestation (Fig. 10-4). There is a delicate balance between cell proliferation, cell differentiation, and apoptosis in the embryo, and one molecular mechanism discussed above, DNA damage, might lead to the cell cycle perturbations and cell death induced in specific cell populations by CP.

Maternal CP treatment on gestation day 10 in the rat causes an S-phase cell cycle block as well as widespread cell death in the

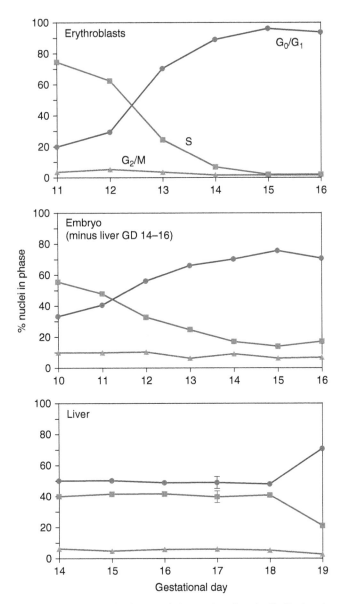

Figure 10-4. *Normal developmental changes in cell cycle distributions in erythroblasts, embryo (minus the liver after GD 13), and fetal liver. Percentages of cells in:* • G_0/G_1; ■ S; *and* ▲ G_2/M *are shown for rat embryos between gestation days 10 and 19 (note changing x-axis range). The proportion of cells in S-phase generally reflects proliferation rate, which decreases with developmental stage in the embryo and erythroblasts. The percentage of S-phase cells in the fetal liver remains fairly high and constant until near term, when a growth spurt occurs. (From Elstein et al. (1993), with permission.)*

embryo (Fig. 10-5). In agreement with the S-phase cell cycle block, cell death is observed in areas of rapid cell proliferation (Chernoff *et al.*, 1989; Francis *et al.*, 1990). Similar embryonal cell cycle blockage and cell death were observed using activated CP in WEC (Little and Mirkes, 1992). The embryonal neuroepithelium is quite sensitive to CP-induced cell death, whereas the heart is resistant; differences in cell cycle length may, in part, underlie this differential sensitivity. The neuroepithelium of the day 10 rat embryo has a cell cycle time of approximately 9.5 hours, whereas the cell cycle length in the heart was estimated to be 13.4 hours. This difference is due to a longer G0/G1 phase in the heart cells compared to the neuroepithelium (Mirkes *et al.*, 1989). Damage to DNA by PM occurs predominately during S-phase (Little and Mirkes, 1992), which constitutes a relatively smaller proportion of the cell cycle in the heart than in the neuroepithelium. Damage to DNA can inhibit

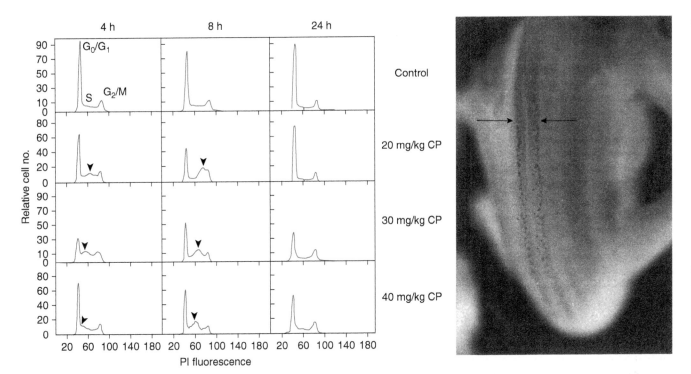

Figure 10-5. *Maternal cyclophosphamide (CP) administration on gestation day 10 in CD-1 mice produces perturbations of the embryonal cell cycle and cell death in areas of rapid proliferation.* Left: Cells are inhibited from progressing through the S (DNA synthetic) phase of the cell cycle, indicated by the abnormal population of cells (*arrowheads*) accumulating at progressively earlier stages of S phase four and eight hours after increasing maternal CP dosages. The upper panels show the normal GD 10-11 distributions, with the G_0/G_1, S, and G_2/M peaks identified in the upper left panel. By 24 hours postdosing, cell cycle distributions have returned to normal at 20 mg/kg, but remain abnormal at higher dosages. Right: Nile blue sulfate staining of a mouse embryo 24 hours after maternal CP dosing shows cell death (*stippling along either side of the midline, arrows*) in the neural tube, one of the most sensitive target sites for CP. (Adapted from Chernoff *et al.* (1989), with permission.)

cell cycle progression at the G1/S transition, through the S phase, and at the G2/M transition. If DNA damage is repaired, the cell cycle can return to normal, but if damage is too extensive or cell cycle arrest too long, apoptosis may be triggered. An increasing number of genes are being identified that play a role in apoptosis (White, 1993; Jurisicova and Acton, 2004). The *p53* gene, which functions as a tumor suppressor, can promote apoptosis or growth arrest. Apoptosis occurring during normal development does not require this gene, as p53-deficient embryos develop normally. However, p53 may be critical for induction of growth arrest or apoptosis in response to DNA damage. The incidence of benzo[*a*] pyrene-induced resorptions were increased 2.6-fold and 3.6-fold, respectively, in heterozygous and homozygous p53-deficient embryos compared to normal homozygous controls (Nicol *et al.*, 1995). Growth factors and some cytokines (eg, IL-3, IL-6) can prevent p53-dependent apoptosis. Expression of c-myc produces continued DNA synthesis, which may precipitate apoptosis in the face of DNA damage. Bcl-2 functions as a repressor of apoptosis and functions in conjunction with Bax, a homolog that dimerizes with itself or with Bcl-2. Bax homodimers favor cell death whereas Bcl-2/Bax heterodimers inhibit cell death (Oltvai and Korsmeyer, 1994; Boumela *et al.*, 2011).

A common approach to test a hypothesized mechanism of teratogenesis is to administer chemicals expected to ameliorate or exacerbate the effects based on the putative mechanism of action. Several investigators have taken this approach in studying CP. Because bioactivation of CP was hypothesized to be necessary for its teratogenicity, Gomes-Carneiro *et al.* (2003) treated rats with β-ionone, a known inhibitor of CYP2B1, the enzyme that activates CP, four minutes prior to CP injection. Severity and incidence of teratogenicity was reduced, supporting the hypothesis. Conversely,

licorice extract, an upregulator of CYP2B1 expression, exacerbated the teratogenicity of CP (Park *et al.*, 2011). Ginseng extract inhibits the CP-detoxifying enzyme CYP3A, and treatment with this extract also enhances the teratogenicity of CP. One hypothesis for the downstream teratogenic mechanism of the active CP metabolite(s) involves alkylation of cellular macromolecules. Thiol-containing molecules protect against alkylating agents, and the thiol molecules cysteine, glutathione, and Na-2-mercaptoethane sulfonate have been shown to ameliorate CP teratogenicity (Ashby *et al.*, 1976; Hales, 1981; Slott and Hales, 1986). However, these studies did not measure the degree of CP alkylation. Treatment with the antioxidant ascorbic acid attenuates CP-induced embryonic death and chromosomal damage (Kola *et al.*, 1989), whereas another antioxidant, butylated hydroxyanisole, protects against CP teratogenicity in rats (Kang *et al.*, 2003) and mice (Kim *et al.*, 2003).

Advances in the Molecular Basis of Dysmorphogenesis

Rapid advances in molecular biology, genomics, proteomics, and bioinformatics have brought new understanding of mechanisms of normal and abnormal development. A key approach, targeted gene disruption by homologous recombination (gene "knockout"; KO), has been used to study the function of many gene products in developing and adult animals. An example is the retinoic acid receptor (RAR) family of nuclear ligand-inducible transcription factors that bind RA and 9-*cis* RA. Chambon and colleagues have produced mice lacking several of these receptors either singly or as multiple KOs. Single-receptor isoform mutants were often unaffected, suggesting functional redundancy, whereas double mutants presented with widespread malformations of the skeleton and viscera (Lohnes *et al.*, 1994;

Mendelsohn *et al.*, 1994). The compound RARγ–RARβ null mouse exhibits syndactyly, indicating that RA plays a role in interdigital cell death (Dupe *et al.*, 1999). The rexinoid receptors (RXRα, β, and γ) bind 9-*cis* RA exclusively, and it is now understood that RAR/RXR heterodimers are involved in RA signaling via transcriptional control in the embryo (Mark *et al.*, 2006, 2009). A wide variety of spontaneous and genetically altered mouse strains are commercially available, and expanding compendia of mutants of other animals including zebrafish and frogs are available.

Synthetic antisense oligonucleotides have been used to ablate gene products in a temporally and spatially restricted manner. In this technique, 15 to 25 mer oligonucleotides are synthesized that are complimentary to the mRNA to be disrupted (Helene *et al.*, 1990). These probes can enter embryonal cells, and hybridization with cellular mRNA causes disruption of native message, such that gene function can be turned off at specific times. The proto-oncogenes Wnt-1 and Wnt-3a have been implicated in the development of the midbrain and hindbrain. Augustine *et al.* (1993) attenuated Wnt-1 expression using antisense oligonucleotide inhibition in mouse embryos developing in culture. Exposure during neurulation produced mid- and hindbrain malformations similar to those seen in Wnt-1 null mutant mice, as well as cardiac anomalies not observed in Wnt-1 KOs created by homologous recombination. Antisense attenuation of Wnt-3a caused anomalies of the forebrain, midbrain, and spinal cord. Simultaneously attenuating both Wnt-1 and Wnt-3a targeted all brain regions and worsened the effect on the spinal cord, suggesting that these genes may serve a complementary function in the development of the central nervous system. Morpholino antisense oligonucleotides contain nucleic acid analogs that resist breakdown, and morpholinos have been used extensively in the study of zebrafish biology (Bedell *et al.*, 2011). RNA interference is a more recent gene knockdown technique, exploiting the discovery of the RNA interference pathway. Small interference (Si)RNA, plasmid-, and virus-encoded small RNAs can be used to down regulate the expression of specific genes posttranscriptionally (Shan, 2010).

Gain of gene function can also be studied by engineering genetic constructs with an inducible promoter attached to the gene of interest. Ectopic gene expression can be made ubiquitous or site-specific depending on the choice of promoter to drive expression. Ectopic expression of the *Hoxa-7* gene induced in mouse embryos by attaching it to the chicken β-actin promoter resulted in a phenotype exhibiting multiple craniofacial and cervical vertebral malformations (Balling *et al.*, 1989; Kessel *et al.*, 1990). Transient overexpression of specific genes can be accomplished by adding extra copies using adenoviral transduction. In proof-of-concept, Hartig and Hunter (1998) injected an adenoviral vector containing either the bacterial β-galactosidase or green fluorescent protein reporter gene under the control of the human cytomegalovirus early gene promoter into the intra-amniotic space of neurulation-stage mouse embryos and achieved intense gene expression in the neuroepithelium.

Advances in gene targeting and transgenic strategies now allow modification of gene expression at specific points in development and in specific cell types. Conditional KOs or knockins, inducible gene expression and other techniques are being used to study the effects of specific gene products on development in great detail (Mikkola and Orkin, 2005).

Reporter transgenes contain a gene with a readily detectable product fused downstream of a selected regulatory region. The *Escherichia coli lacZ* (β-galactosidase) gene is commonly used for this purpose. Cell lineage studies can be carried out by fusing *lacZ* to a constitutive regulatory sequence and introducing the construct into a somatic cell early in ontogenesis. The reporter gene will then be expressed in and mark all progeny of the transfected cell. This method has been used to study postimplantation development in the mouse embryo (Sanes *et al.*, 1986), although intracellular injection of fluorescent dyes has also proven highly reliable for cell lineage studies (eg, Smith *et al.*, 1994). The pattern of expression of a particular gene of interest can be discriminated by fusing upstream regulatory elements of the gene to *lacZ*, which will then be transcribed under control of those upstream elements (Zakany *et al.*, 1990). RA can activate hox genes in vitro, and some hox genes have multiple RA response elements (RAREs). Evidence that RA-induced malformations in mouse embryos are related to changes in hox expression was first provided by staining of hox*lacZ* transgenic embryos (Marshall *et al.*, 1992). Within a few hours of RA treatment, hoxb-1 expression extended anteriorly, suggesting that hox genes could be direct targets of RA induction. Regions of altered hox expression could be manifest as abnormal cell fate and morphogenesis (Marshall *et al.*, 1996; Collins and Mao, 1999).

Reporter genes have recently been used to great advantage to study gene expression in zebrafish (eg, Saydmohammed *et al.*, 2011).

The use of modern biological techniques to elucidate a mechanism of developmental toxicity is exemplified by work on the perfluorinated alkyl acids (PFAAs), perfluorooctanoic acid (PFOA), and perfluorooctane sulfonate (PFOS). The PFAAs are a family of industrial chemicals that has been widely used as surfactants, hydrophobic and oleophobic treatments, and nonstick coatings. These chemicals are highly resistant to environmental degradation and are therefore persistent in the environment. Studies in experimental animals have demonstrated that developmental toxicity is among the most sensitive toxic effects of these chemicals (Lau *et al.*, 2004). Treatment of pregnant mice with either PFOS or PFOA resulted in dose-related increases in mortality of offspring in the first few days of life. Although the toxic endpoint is similar for PFOA and PFOS, their mechanisms of action may be different. PFAAs have varied affinity for the peroxisome proliferator-activated receptor alpha (PPARα), and activation of PPARα is a putative mechanism of action for the developmental toxicity of these chemicals. To explore the role of PPARα activation in the developmental toxicity of PFOA and PFOS, Abbott and colleagues tested the developmental toxicity of these chemicals in PPARα null mice. Exposure of pregnant wild-type and PPARα KO mice to PFOA revealed that neonatal mortality, the signature effect of developmental exposure to PFOA, was dependent on PPARα expression. The survival of PPAR null offspring was not affected by maternal PFOA exposure, whereas survival of wild-type offspring was significantly reduced (Abbott *et al.*, 2007). Somewhat surprisingly, when the same experiments were carried out with PFOS exposure, the PPARα null offsprings were not protected from neonatal mortality (Abbott *et al.*, 2009). Studies were undertaken to compare the ability of PFAAs to activate mouse and human PPARα in COS-1 cells (a commonly used cell line derived from kidney cells of the African green monkey) transiently transfected with either a mouse or human PPARα-luciferase reporter plasmid, such that activation of the receptor caused light emission that could be quantified on a luminometer (Wolf *et al.*, 2008). In agreement with the KO mouse studies, PFOA activated both the mouse and human PPARα at lower concentrations than did PFOS. Further evidence that PPARα activation was required for PFOA but not PFOS developmental toxicity came from studies of gene expression changes induced in fetal tissues by maternal treatment with PFOA or PFOS (Rosen *et al.*, 2007, 2009). Although both PFOA and PFOS activated PPARα downstream genes, PFOA did so in a more consistent and robust fashion. This could also be seen in livers from adult mice treated with PFOA or PFOS. Although PPARα KO mice did not upregulate certain PPARα–related genes

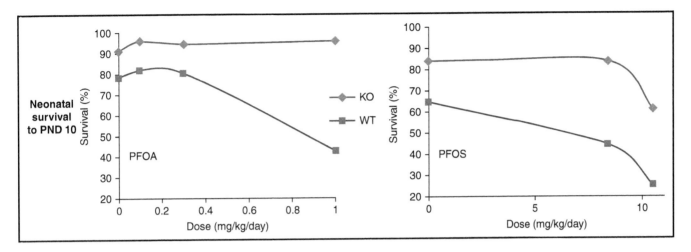

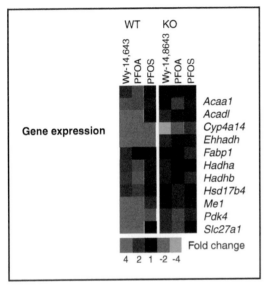

Figure 10-6. *Role of the peroxisome proliferator-activated receptor-α (PPARα) in the developmental toxicity of perfluorooctanoic acid (PFOA) and perfluoroctanesulfonate (PFOS).* *Top*: PFOA or PFOS was administered to pregnant wild-type (WT) and PPARα knockout (KO) mice throughout gestation. Neonatal survival of offspring of KO mice was not affected by PFOA, whereas survival of offspring of WT mice was greatly reduced at the high dose (left, data from Abbott *et al.*, 2007). In contrast, neonatal survival was affected by PFOS in both KO and WT offspring (right, data from Abbott *et al.*, 2009). These results suggest that PPARα plays a role in the toxicity of PFOA but not PFOS. *Bottom left*: Adult male KO or WT mice were treated for seven days with PFOA, PFOS, or the known PPARα agonist Wy-14,643. Expression of genes known to be upregulated by PPARα activation was increased by treatment with PFOA or Wy-14,643, but not PFOS (data from Rosen *et al.*, 2010; figure courtesy of Dr. Mitchell Rosen). *Bottom right*: PFOA or PFOS treatment of COS-1 cells transiently transfected with either a mouse or a human PPARα-luciferase reporter plasmid demonstrated that PFOA is a much stronger agonist of PPARα than is PFOS (data from Wolf *et al.*, 2008).

upon PFOA or PFOS treatment, the expression of other genes was changed by exposure to either of these PFAAs, indicating that the influence of either PFOA or PFOS may extend beyond activation of PPARα (Rosen *et al.*, 2010). This elegant set of experiments on the developmental toxicity of the PFAAs is illustrated in Fig. 10-6. It remains to be determined which of the pathways downstream of PPARα are involved in the developmental toxicity of PFOA, and which non-PPARα–related pathways might be perturbed by PFOS.

PHARMACOKINETICS AND METABOLISM IN PREGNANCY

The manner in which chemicals are absorbed during pregnancy and the extent to and form in which they reach the conceptus are important determinants of whether the chemical can impact development. The maternal, placental, and embryonic compartments are distinct but interacting systems that undergo profound changes during the course of pregnancy. Maternal adaptations to pregnancy include changes in hepatic metabolism, the gastrointestinal tract, cardiovascular system, excretory system, and the respiratory system (Hytten, 1984; Krauer, 1987; Mattison *et al.*, 1991). Although these changes are necessary to support the growing needs of the conceptus in terms of energy supply and waste elimination, they can have significant impact on the uptake, distribution, metabolism, and elimination of xenobiotics. For example, decreases in intestinal motility and increases in gastric emptying time result in longer retention of ingested chemicals in the upper gastrointestinal tract. Cardiac output in humans increases by 30% to 40% by the 27th week of pregnancy, whereas blood volume increases and plasma proteins and peripheral vascular resistance decrease. The relative increase in blood volume over red cell volume leads to borderline anemia and a generalized edema with a 70% elevation of extracellular space. Thus, the volume of distribution of a chemical and the amount bound by plasma proteins may change considerably during pregnancy. Renal blood flow and glomerular filtration rate also increase during pregnancy. Respiratory changes including increases in tidal volume, minute ventilation, and minute O_2 uptake can result in increased pulmonary distribution of gases and decreased time to reach alveolar steady state.

In addition to changes in maternal physiology, limited evidence suggests that relative rates of drug metabolizing enzymes also change during pregnancy (Juchau, 1981; Juchau and Faustman-Watts, 1983). Maternal hepatic P450 enzymes increase during pregnancy in humans, whereas decreased hepatic monooxygenase activity has been observed during pregnancy in rats, attributed to decreased enzyme levels and competitive inhibition by circulating steroids (Neims, 1976). Another factor that contributes to lower monooxygenase activity may be changes in inducibility—pregnant rats appear to be less responsive to induction of hepatic monooxygenases by phenobarbital (but not 3-methylcholanthrene) than are nonpregnant females (Guenther and Mannering, 1977). Maternal handling of a chemical bears considerable weight in determining the extent of embryotoxicity. In one of the few studies of its type, Kimmel and Young (1983) found that a linear combination of the 45-minute and the 24-hour maternal blood concentrations was able to predict the litter response rate for pregnant rats dosed with 500 mg/kg sodium salicylate on gestation day 11. These two kinetic parameters probably reflect the influence of peak drug concentration as well as cumulative area under the concentration–time curve on developmental toxicity.

The placenta plays a central role in influencing embryonic exposure by helping to regulate blood flow, by offering a transport barrier, and by metabolizing chemicals (Slikker and Miller, 1994). Functionally, the placenta acts as a lipid membrane that permits bidirectional transfer of substances between maternal and fetal compartments. The extent of transfer depends on three major elements: the type of placentation, the physicochemical properties of the chemical, and rates of placental metabolism. Although there are marked species differences in types of placentas, orientation of blood vessels, and numbers of exchanging layers (Carney et al., 2004), these do not seem to play a dominant role in placental transfer of most chemicals. It is important to note that virtually any substance present in the maternal plasma will cross the placenta to some extent. The passage of most drugs across the placenta seems to occur by simple passive diffusion, the rate of which is proportional to the diffusion constant of the drug, the concentration gradient between the maternal and embryonic plasma, the area of exchange, and the inverse of the membrane thickness (Nau, 1992). Important modifying factors to the rate and extent of transfer include lipid solubility, molecular weight, protein binding, the type of transfer (passive diffusion, facilitated or active transport), the degree of ionization, and placental metabolism. Weak acids appear to be rapidly transferred across the placenta during early pregnancy in rats and mice, due in part to the pH gradient between the maternal and embryonic plasma which can trap ionized forms of the drug in the slightly more basic embryonic compartment (Nau and Scott, 1986). In humans and rabbits, maternal serum is either similar to or slightly higher in pH than is the yolk sac fluid (Carney et al., 2005).

Quantifying the form, amount, and timing of chemical delivery to the embryonic compartment in the context of concurrent developmental processes is an important component of understanding mechanisms of embryotoxicity and species differences in embryonic sensitivity (Nau, 1986). The small size of the conceptus during organogenesis and the fact that the embryo is changing at a rapid rate during this period make assessment of toxicokinetics difficult. Nevertheless, there has been considerable progress in this area (Nau and Scott, 1987; Clark, 1993; Corley et al., 2003; Corley, 2010). Increasingly sensitive analytical methods are now providing

evidence to challenge the historical view, particularly for cytochrome P450-dependent monooxygenases, that the early embryo has low metabolic capabilities (Juchau et al., 1992). Using the WEC system, Juchau and co-workers demonstrated that the rat conceptus was able to generate sufficient amounts of metabolites of the proteratogen 2-acetylaminofluorene (2-AAF) to induce dysmorphogenesis, and that the proximate toxicant, the 7-hydroxy metabolite, was different from the metabolite responsible for 2-AAF mutagenesis and carcinogenesis. Prior exposure of the dams to 3-methylcholanthrene increased the sensitivity of the cultured embryos to 2-AAF, thus demonstrating the inducibility of at least some cytochromes in the conceptus. These investigators later showed that embryos could further metabolize the 7-hydroxy metabolite to an even more toxic catechol. No previous induction was necessary for this activation step, demonstrating the presence of constitutive metabolizing enzymes in the embryo. Although the rates of metabolism for these activation steps may be low relative to the maternal liver, they occur close to the target site of the embryo or even within it, and thus are significant in terms of inducing embryotoxicity.

Physiologically based pharmacokinetic models provide the framework to integrate what is known about physiological changes during pregnancy, both within and between species, with aspects of drug metabolism and embryonic development into a quantitative description of the events. Olanoff and Anderson (1980) described the kinetics of the antibiotic tetracycline in the pregnant rat and her fetuses. Importantly, growth of the fetus and placenta was incorporated into the model. Gabrielson and co-workers (Gabrielson and Paalkow, 1983; Gabrielson and Larsson, 1990) were among the early investigators to develop physiologically based models of pregnancy, and others (Fisher et al., 1989; O'Flaherty et al., 1992; Clark et al., 1993; Luecke et al., 1994, 1997; Young, 1998) have added to their comprehensiveness. The Fisher model included growth of several maternal tissues during pregnancy. The model of O'Flaherty and co-workers describes the entire period of gestation, and includes the uterus, mammary tissue, maternal fat, kidney, liver, other well-perfused maternal tissues, embryo/fetal tissues and yolk sac, and chorioallantoic placenta. It takes into account the growth of various compartments during pregnancy (including the embryo itself), as well as changes in blood flow and the stage-dependent pH gradients between maternal and embryonic plasma. Transfer across the placenta is diffusion limited in this model. The utility of the model was evaluated using 5,5-dimethyloxazolidine-2,4-dione (DMO), a weak acid that is not appreciably bound to plasma proteins and is eliminated by excretion in the urine. The model demonstrated that the whole body disposition of DMO, including distribution to the embryo, can be accounted for solely on the basis of its pKa and of the pH and volumes of body fluid spaces. Differences between the disposition of DMO by the pregnant mouse and rat are consistent simply with differences in fluid pH. Luecke and co-workers developed quantitative models for human embryofetal growth for use in models of human pregnancy (Luecke et al., 1994, 1997, 1999).

Chemical-specific PBPK models for pregnancy can range from simple to complex, with the degree of complexity often limited by lack of knowledge about mechanism of action or limited biological or chemical-specific data. One example is the solvent 2-methoxyethanol found to be embryotoxic and teratogenic in all species tested to date. The proximate teratogen appears to be the metabolite 2-methoxyacetic, acid (2-MAA). A physiologically based pharmacokinetic model has been developed for the pregnant mouse (Terry et al., 1995). Pharmacokinetics and tissue partition coefficients for 2-MAA were determined at different stages of embryonal development, and various models were tested based on the alternative hypotheses involving (1) blood flow limited delivery of 2-MAA to model compartments, (2) pH trapping of ionized 2-MAA within compartments, (3) active transport of 2-MAA into compartments, and (4) reversible binding of 2-MAA within compartments. Although the blood flow limited model best predicted gestation day eight dosimetry, the active transport models better described dosimetry on gestation days 11 and 13. Using published data on biotransformation of 2-methoxyethanol to ethylene glycol and 2-MAA in rats, Hays *et al.* (2000) adapted the pregnant mouse PBPK model to the pregnant rat and successfully predicted tissue levels of 2-MAA following oral or intravenous administration of 2-methoxyethanol. The next step was to extrapolate this model to the inhalation route of exposure, and to model both rats and humans (Gargas *et al.*, 2000). The extrapolation of the model enabled predictions of the exposures needed for pregnant women to reach blood concentrations (C_{max} or area under the curve [AUC]) equivalent to those in pregnant rats exposed to the no observed adverse effect level (NOAEL) or lowest observed adverse effect level (LOAEL) for developmental toxicity. The body of work on PBPK modeling of 2-methoxyethanol is exemplary of the power of these techniques for extrapolating across dose, developmental stage, route, and species. For a review of chemical-specific PBPK models, see Corley *et al.* (2003) and Corley (2010).

RELATIONSHIPS BETWEEN MATERNAL AND DEVELOPMENTAL TOXICITY

Although all developmental toxicity must ultimately result from an insult to the conceptus at the cellular level, in mammals the insult may occur through a direct effect on the embryo/ fetus, indirectly through toxicity of the agent to the mother and/ or the placenta, or a combination of direct and indirect effects. Maternal physiological conditions capable of adversely affecting the developing organism include decreased uterine blood flow, maternal anemia, under or malnutrition, toxemia, altered organ function, autoimmune states, diabetes, electrolyte or acid–base disturbances, decreased milk quantity or quality, elevated stress hormones, and abnormal behavior (Chernoff *et al.*, 1989; Daston, 1994). Induction or exacerbation of such maternal conditions by chemicals and the degree to which they manifest in abnormal development are dependent on maternal genetic background, age, parity, size, nutrition, disease, stress, and other health parameters and exposures (DeSesso, 1987; Chernoff *et al.*, 1989; Rogers *et al.*, 2005). These relationships are depicted in Fig. 10-7. In this section, we will discuss maternal conditions known to adversely affect the conceptus, as well as examples of xenobiotics whose developmental toxicity results completely or in large part from maternal or placental toxicity.

The distinction between direct and indirect developmental toxicity is important for interpreting results of standard developmental toxicity bioassays in pregnant animals, as the highest dosage levels in these experiments are deliberately chosen to produce measurable maternal toxicity (eg, decreased food or water intake, weight loss, clinical signs). However, maternal toxicity defined only by such overt manifestations provides little insight into the toxic actions of a xenobiotic. When developmental toxicity is observed only in the presence of maternal toxicity, the developmental effects may be indirect; however, an understanding of the physiological changes underlying the observed maternal toxicity and elucidation of their association with developmental

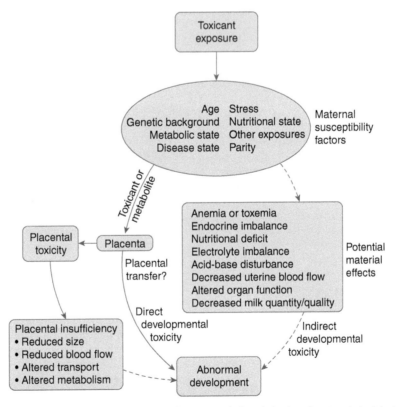

Figure 10-7. *Interrelationships between maternal susceptibility factors, metabolism, induction of maternal physiological or functional alterations, placental transfer and toxicity, and developmental toxicity.* A developmental toxicant can cause abnormal development through any one or a combination of these pathways. Maternal susceptibility factors determine the predisposition of the mother to respond to a toxic insult, and the maternal effects listed can adversely affect the developing conceptus. Most chemicals traverse the placenta in some form, and the placenta can also be a target for toxicity. In most cases, developmental toxicity is probably mediated through a combination of these pathways.

effects is needed before one can begin to address the relevance of the observations to human safety assessment. Many known human developmental toxicants, including ethanol and cocaine, adversely affect the embryo/fetus predominately at maternally toxic levels, and part of their developmental toxicity may be ascribed to secondary effects of maternal physiological disturbances. For example, the nutritional status of alcoholics is generally poor, and effects on the conceptus may be exacerbated by effects of alcohol on placental transfer of nutrients. Chronic alcohol abuse alters maternal folate and zinc metabolism, which may play a role in the induction of fetal alcohol syndrome (Dreosti, 1993). Carney (2010) has constructed a useful decision tree for interpreting developmental toxicity observed concomitantly with maternal toxicity (Fig. 10-8).

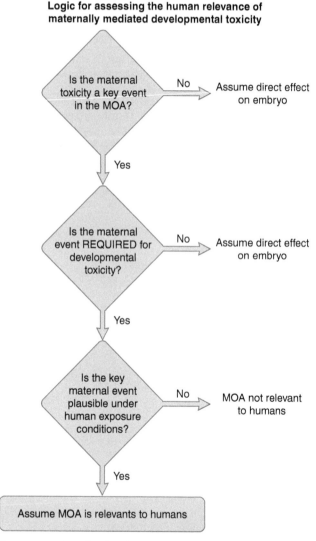

Logic for assessing the human relevance of maternally mediated developmental toxicity

Figure 10-8. *Assessing the relevance to humans of a maternally mediated mode of action.* Flow chart for considering whether a maternally mediated mode of action (MOA) in animal studies is relevant to humans. When developmental toxicity is observed only at maternally toxic dosages, the MOA for developmental toxicity may be direct or indirect (secondary to the maternal toxicity). Maternally mediated developmental toxicity is relevant to humans if expected human exposure conditions could plausibly trigger that MOA (redrawn from Carney, 2010, with permission). Knowledge of the MOA for developmental toxicity, which will likely require investigation beyond the dose–response study, is a prerequisite for using this approach.

MATERNAL FACTORS AFFECTING DEVELOPMENT

Genetics

The genetic makeup of the pregnant female has been well documented as a determinant of developmental outcome in both humans and animals. The incidence of cleft lip and/or palate [CL(P)], which occurs more frequently in whites than in blacks, has been investigated in offspring of interracial couples in the United States (Khoury *et al.*, 1983). Offspring of white mothers had a higher incidence of CL(P) than offspring of black mothers after correcting for paternal race, whereas offspring of white fathers did not have a higher incidence of CL(P) than offspring of black fathers after correcting for maternal race.

Among experimental animals, two related mouse strains, A/J and CL/Fr, produced spontaneous CL(P) at 8% to 10% and 18% to 26% frequencies, respectively. The incidence of CL(P) in offspring depends on the genotype of the mother rather than that of the embryo (Juriloff and Fraser, 1980). The response to vitamin A of mouse embryos heterozygous for the curly-tail mutation also depends on the genotype of the mother (Seller *et al.*, 1983). The teratogenicity of phenytoin has been compared in several inbred strains of mice. The susceptibility of offspring of crosses between susceptible A/J mice and resistant C57BL/6J mice was determined by the maternal, but not the embryonic genome (Hansen and Hodes, 1983).

Recent work has begun to identify genes associated with differential susceptibility of mouse strains to valproic acid (Finnell *et al.*, 1997; Craig *et al.*, 2000; Bennett *et al.*, 2000; Faiella *et al.*, 2000; Okada *et al.*, 2004, 2005). A recent study utilized inbred C57BL/6J (B6) and DBA/2J (D2) mice to examine the role of maternal genotype in sensitivity to valproic acid teratogenesis (Downing *et al.*, 2010). The B6 mice are more susceptible to valproate-induced digital and vertebral malformations, whereas D2 mice are more susceptible to rib malformations. In a reciprocal cross experiment between B6 and D2 mice, genetically identical F1 offspring responded in a manner consistent with the genotype of the mother: F1 carried in a B6 mother exhibited more vertebral and digital malformations, whereas F1 carried in a D2 mother exhibited more rib malformations. Such maternal effects clearly demonstrate the importance of the maternal milieu in determining outcomes of developmental exposures.

Disease

A number of maternal diseases can exert untoward effects on the conceptus. Chronic hypertension is a risk factor for the development of preeclampsia, eclampsia, and toxemia of pregnancy, and hypertension is a leading cause of pregnancy-associated maternal deaths. Uncontrolled maternal diabetes mellitus is a significant cause of prenatal morbidity. Certain maternal infections can adversely affect the conceptus (eg, rubella virus, discussed earlier), either through indirect disease-related maternal alterations or direct transplacental infection. Cytomegalovirus infection is associated with fetal death, microcephaly, mental retardation, blindness, and deafness (MacDonald and Tobin, 1978) and maternal infection with *Toxoplasma gondii* is known to induce hydrocephaly and chorioretinitis in infants (Alford *et al.*, 1974). One factor common to many disease states is hyperthermia. Hyperthermia is a potent experimental animal teratogen (Edwards, 1986), and there is a body of evidence associating maternal febrile illness during the first trimester of pregnancy with birth defects in humans, most notably malformations of the central nervous system (Warkany, 1986; Milunsky *et al.*, 1992; Edwards, 2006).

Nutrition

A wide spectrum of dietary insufficiencies ranging from protein-calorie malnutrition to deficiencies of vitamins, trace elements, and/or enzyme cofactors is known to adversely affect pregnancy (Keen *et al.*, 1993). Among the most significant findings related to human nutrition and pregnancy outcome in recent years are results of studies in which pregnant women at risk for having infants with NTDs were supplemented with folate (Wald, 1993; Czeizel, 2011). The largest and most convincing study is the Medical Research Council (MRC) Vitamin Study, in which supplementation with 4 mg of folic acid reduced NTD recurrence by over 70% (MRC, 1991; Bendich, 1993). Results of these studies prompted the US CDC to recommend folate supplementation for women of childbearing age and folate supplementation of some foodstuffs. In 1996, FDA mandated enrichment of cereal grain products with folate by 1998. One study has demonstrated more than a doubling of mean serum folate concentrations across all sex and age groups since then (Dietrich *et al.*, 2005). Yet, in the same population, less than 10% of women of childbearing age reached the recommended erythrocyte folate concentration of greater than 906 nmol/L that has been shown to be associated with a reduction in the risk of NTDs. The CDC (2004) estimated that the number of NTD-affected pregnancies in the United States declined from 4000 in 1995–1996 to 3000 in 1999–2000. Although this survey indicates partial success of the folate fortification program, women capable of becoming pregnant were urged to continue to follow the US Public Health Service recommendation to consume 400 µg folate daily. Mills and Signore (2004) compared the rates of antenatal detection of NTDs in the United States (incomplete ascertainment and underprediction of NTDs) and Canada (more complete antenatal ascertainment) and determined that the studies that best identify cases of NTDs show that folic acid fortification is preventing around 50% of NTDs. These authors estimate that the percentage of folate-preventable NTDs in the United States is about 50% to 60%, suggesting that we may be close to achieving optimum protection. However, recent studies using multivitamins containing folate have achieved even better results (Czeizel *et al.*, 2011).

Stress

Diverse forms of maternal toxicity may have in common the induction of a physiological stress response. Thus, understanding the potential effects of maternal stress on development may help interpret developmental toxicity observed in experimental animals at maternally toxic dosages. Various forms of physical stress have been applied to pregnant animals in attempts to isolate the developmental effects of stress. Subjecting pregnant rats or mice to noise stress throughout gestation can produce developmental toxicity (Kimmel *et al.*, 1976; Nawrot *et al.*, 1980, 1981). Restraint stress produces increased fetal death in rats (Euker and Riegle, 1973) and cleft palate (Barlow *et al.*, 1975), fused and supernumerary ribs, and encephaloceles in mice (Beyer and Chernoff, 1986).

Objective data on effects of stress in humans are difficult to obtain. Nevertheless, studies investigating the relationship of maternal stress and pregnancy outcome have indicated a positive correlation between stress and adverse developmental effects, including low birth weight and adverse mental health outcomes in offspring

(Stott, 1973; Gorsuch and Key, 1974; Beydoun and Saftlas, 2008; Entringer *et al.*, 2010; Dunkel Schetter and Tanner, 2012).

499

Placental Toxicity

The placenta is the interface between the mother and the conceptus, providing attachment, an immune interface, nutrition, gas exchange, and waste removal. The placenta also produces peptide and steroid hormones critical to the maintenance of pregnancy and the regulation of fetal and maternal metabolism. The placenta can also metabolize or store xenobiotics. Placental toxicity may compromise these functions and produce or contribute to adverse effects on the conceptus. Slikker and Miller (1994) listed 46 substances known to be toxic to the yolk sac or chorioallantoic placenta, including metals such as cadmium (Cd), arsenic or mercury, cigarette smoke, ethanol, cocaine, endotoxin, and sodium salicylate. Cd is among the best studied of these, and it appears that the developmental toxicity of Cd during mid-to-late gestation involves both placental toxicity (necrosis, reduced blood flow) and inhibition of nutrient transport across the placenta. Maternal injection of Cd during late gestation resulted in fetal death in rats, despite little cadmium entering the fetus (Parizek, 1964; Levin and Miller, 1980). Fetal deaths occurred concomitantly with reduced uteroplacental blood flow within 10 hours (Levin and Miller, 1980). The authors' conclusion that fetal death was caused by placental toxicity was supported by experiments in which fetuses were directly injected with Cd. Despite fetal Cd burdens almost 10-fold higher than those following maternal administration, only a slight increase in fetal death was observed.

Cd is a transition metal similar in physicochemical properties to the essential metal zinc (Zn). Cd interferes with Zn transfer across the placenta (Ahokas *et al.*, 1980; Sorrell and Graziano, 1990), possibly via metallothionein (MT), a metal-binding protein induced in the placenta by Cd. Because of its high affinity for Zn, MT may sequester Zn in the placenta, impeding transfer to the conceptus (induction of maternal hepatic MT by Cd or other agents can also induce fetal Zn deficiency, as discussed below). Cadmium inhibits Zn uptake by human placental microvesicles (Page *et al.*, 1992) suggesting that Cd may also compete directly with Zn for membrane transport. Cadmium may also competitively inhibit other Zn-dependent processes in the placenta. Coadministration of Zn ameliorates the developmental toxicity of administered Cd, further indicating that interference of Cd with Zn metabolism is a key to its developmental toxicity (Ferm and Carpenter, 1967, 1968; Daston, 1982).

In the last decade it has become evident that the placenta can undergo adaptive responses to the intrauterine milieu that can influence the metabolic "programming" of the fetus (Myatt, 2006). Adverse intrauterine conditions including hypoxia and nutritional deficiencies can lead to alterations in placental structure and function, including altered expression or activity of transporters and receptors. Placental morphometry has been proposed as a biomarker of fetal programming (Thornburg *et al.*, 2010). One role of the placenta that is key for fetal programming is as a regulator of glucocorticoid transfer between the mother and her fetus(es) (Seckl and Holmes, 2007). The enzyme 11β-hydroxysteroid dehydrogenase-2 (11β-HSD2) inactivates glucocorticoids; its activity in the placenta protects the fetus from over exposure to maternal stress hormone. In experimental animals, lowering the activity of 11β-HSD2 by nutritional deficiency or gene ablation leads to lower birth weight, and causes increases in adult blood pressure, circulating glucose concentrations and hypothalamic-pituitary-adrenal axis activity in offspring. In humans, babies with lower birth weight have higher levels of plasma cortisol throughout life.

Maternal Toxicity

A retrospective analysis of relationships between maternal toxicity and specific types of prenatal effects found species-specific associations. Yet, among rat, rabbit, and hamster studies, 22% failed to show any developmental toxicity in the presence of significant maternal toxicity (Khera, 1984, 1985). In a study designed to test the potential of maternal toxicity to affect development, Kavlock et al. (1985) administered 10 structurally unrelated compounds to pregnant mice at maternotoxic dosages. Developmental effects were agent-specific, ranging from complete resorption to lack of effect. An exception was an increased incidence of supernumerary ribs (ribs on the first lumbar vertebra), which occurred with seven of the 10 compounds. Chernoff et al. (1990) dosed pregnant rats for 10 days with a series of compounds chosen because they exhibited little or no developmental toxicity in previous studies. When these compounds were administered at higher dosages producing maternal toxicity (weight loss or a low incidence of death), varied adverse developmental outcomes were noted, including increased intrauterine death (two compounds), decreased fetal weight (two compounds), supernumerary ribs (two compounds), and enlarged renal pelves (two compounds). Two of the compounds produced no developmental toxicity despite substantial maternal toxicity. These diverse developmental responses led the authors to conclude that maternal toxicity characterized by weight loss or mortality was not associated with any consistent syndrome of developmental effects in the rat.

There have been a number of studies relating specific forms of maternal toxicity to developmental toxicity, including those in which the test chemical caused maternal effects that exacerbated the developmental toxicity of the chemical, and instances in which developmental toxicity was thought to be secondary to maternal effects. However, clearly delineating the relative role(s) of indirect maternal and direct embryo/fetal toxicity is difficult. What follows are examples of the kinds of experiments that may allow one to do so.

Acetazolamide inhibits carbonic anhydrase and is teratogenic in mice (Hirsch and Scott, 1983). Although maternal weight loss was not correlated with malformation frequency, maternal hypercapnia potentiated the teratogenicity of acetazolamide. In C57Bl/6J mice, maternal hypercapnia alone resulted in right forelimb ectrodactyly, the characteristic malformation induced by acetazolamide. Correction of maternal acidosis failed to reduce developmental toxicity, suggesting that the primary teratogenic factor was elevated maternal plasma CO_2 tension (Weaver and Scott, 1984a,b).

Diflunisal, an analgesic and anti-inflammatory drug, causes axial skeletal defects in rabbits. Developmentally toxic dosages resulted in severe maternal anemia (hematocrit = 20%–24% vs 37% in controls) and depletion of erythrocyte ATP levels (Clark et al., 1984). Teratogenicity, anemia, and ATP depletion were unique to the rabbit among the species studied. A single dose of diflunisal on day five of gestation produced maternal anemia that lasted through day 15. Concentration of the drug in the embryo was less than 5% of the peak maternal blood level, and diflunisal was cleared from maternal blood before day nine, the critical day for induction of similar axial skeletal defects by hypoxia. Thus, the teratogenicity of diflunisal in the rabbit was probably due to hypoxia resulting from maternal anemia.

Phenytoin, an anticonvulsant, can affect maternal folate metabolism in experimental animals, and these alterations may play a role in the teratogenicity of this drug (Hansen and Billings, 1985). Further, maternal heart rates were monitored on gestation day 10 after administration to susceptible A/J mice and resistant C57Bl/6J mice (Watkinson and Millikovsky, 1983). Heart rates were depressed by phenytoin in a dose-related manner in the A/J mice but not in C57Bl/6J mice. A mechanism of teratogenesis was proposed relating depressed maternal heart rate and embryonic hypoxia. Supporting studies have demonstrated that hyperoxia reduced the teratogenicity of phenytoin in mice (Millicovsky and Johnston, 1981).

Reduced uterine blood flow has been proposed as a mechanism of teratogenicity caused by hydroxyurea, which produces elevated systolic blood pressure, altered heart rate, decreased cardiac output, severely decreased uterine blood flow, and increased vascular resistance in pregnant rabbits (Millicovsky et al., 1981). Embryos exhibited craniofacial and pericardial hemorrhages immediately after treatment (Millicovsky and DeSesso, 1980a) and identical embryopathies were achieved by clamping the uterine vessels of pregnant rabbits for 10 minutes (Millicovsky and DeSesso, 1980b).

MT synthesis is induced by a wide variety of chemical and physical agents including metals, alcohols, urethane, endotoxin, alkylating agents, hyper- or hypothermia, and ionizing radiation (Daston, 1994). MT synthesis is also induced by endogenous mediators such as glucocorticoids and certain of the cytokines (Klaassen and Lehman-McKeeman, 1989). A mechanism common to the developmental toxicity of these diverse agents may be Zn deficiency of the conceptus secondary to induction of maternal MT. Induction of synthesis can produce hepatic MT concentrations over an order of magnitude higher than normal, leading to substantial sequestration of circulating Zn in maternal liver, lowered plasma Zn concentrations, and reduced Zn availability to the conceptus. Embryofetal zinc deficiency secondary to maternal hepatic MT induction has been demonstrated for diverse chemicals including valproic acid (Keen et al., 1989), 6-mercaptopurine (Amemiya et al., 1985, 1989), urethane (Daston et al., 1991), ethanol, and α-hederin (Taubeneck et al., 1994). In a study combining data for many of these compounds, Taubeneck and co-workers (1994) found a strong positive relationship between maternal hepatic MT induction and maternal hepatic [65]Zn retention, and a negative relationship between maternal MT induction and [65]Zn distribution to the litter. This is an example of a maternally mediated mechanism of exacerbating or directly causing developmental toxicity, one that is applicable to diverse maternal insults and for which direct exposure of the conceptus to the causative agent is not required.

Maternal ethanol exposure and the induction of FASD represent an excellent example of the interplay of indirect (maternally mediated) and direct toxic mechanisms of action (Fig. 10-9). Alcoholic mothers exhibit tolerance to alcohol such that their blood alcohol levels can be quite high and no doubt exert multiple direct effects on the embryo, including induction of cell death, altered neural crest cell migration, mitochondrial dysfunction, and effects on membrane integrity. At the same time, effects of chronic alcohol exposure on the mother include MT induction and secondary embrofetal zinc deficiency, as described above. Zn deficiency is teratogenic and exerts multiple adverse effects on the developing conceptus as shown in Fig. 10-9. Additional maternal effects that may exacerbate teratogenicity include hypoferremia, reduced circulating folate, reduced circulating vitamin A, and hypercupremia. Genetic polymorphisms in both the mother and the fetus likely play roles in manifestation of FASD as well, as evidenced by studies in humans and in animal models (Warren and Li, 2005). Thus, despite literally thousands of epidemiological, clinical, and laboratory studies, the complex interplay of factors involved in the teratogenicity of ethanol is still being elucidated.

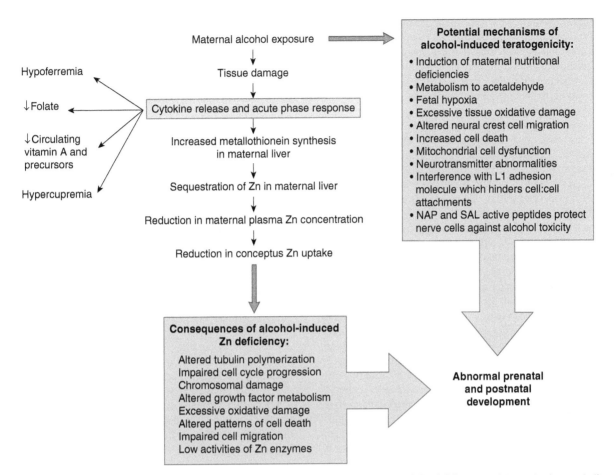

Figure 10-9. *Alcohol-induced acute phase response and sequence of events leading to conceptal zinc deficiency.* Multiple mechanisms underlie the teratogenicity of alcohol (box at upper right). Tissue damage in maternal tissues can initiate an acute phase response that includes induction of metallothionein in maternal liver, which removes available zinc from the maternal circulation, reducing availablility to the conceptus. In addition to contributing to zinc deficiency in the embryo/fetus, an acute phase response can affect the metabolism of other essential nutrients, including folate, Vitamin A, iron and copper. NAP: neuroprotective octapeptide NAPVSIPQ; SAL: neurotropic nonapeptide SALLRSIPA. (Redrawn from Keen *et al.* (2010), with permission).

DEVELOPMENTAL TOXICITY OF ENDOCRINE-DISRUPTING CHEMICALS

An "endocrine disruptor" has been broadly defined as "an exogenous chemical that interferes with the production, release, transport, metabolism, binding, action, or elimination of natural hormones responsible for the maintenance of homeostasis and the regulation of developmental processes" (Kavlock *et al.*, 1996). More recently, the Endocrine Society has stated: "an endocrine-disrupting substance is a compound, either natural or synthetic, which, through environmental or inappropriate developmental exposures, alters the hormonal and homeostatic systems that enable the organism to communicate with and respond to its environment" (Diamanti-Kandarakis *et al.*, 2009). Due to the critical role of hormones in directing differentiation in many tissues, the developing organism is particularly vulnerable to fluctuations in the timing or intensity of exposure to chemicals with hormonal (or antihormonal) activity. A wide variety of chemical classes (eg, pesticides, herbicides, fungicides, plasticizers, surfactants, organometals, halogenated polyaromatic hydrocarbons, phytoestrogens) have been shown to cause developmental toxicity via at least three modes of action involving the endocrine system: (1) by acting as hormone receptor ligands; (2) by altering steroid hormone synthetic and metabolic enzymes; and (3) by perturbing hypothalamic-pituitary release of tropic hormones. Interactions with the functions of estrogens, androgens, and

thyroid hormones have been the most studied, but the underlying principles apply to other hormones as well.

Laboratory Animal Evidence

Chemicals with estrogenic activity are a well-described class of developmental toxicants based on standard criteria of causing specific malformations during critical developmental periods of relatively short duration (Schardein, 2000). Estrogens induce pleiotropic effects, acting on diverse cell types with estrogen receptors, and can display cell and organ-specific agonist and antagonist actions. The pattern of outcomes is generally similar across different estrogens. DES provides one of the most well-characterized examples of the effects of a xenoestrogen on development. Manifestations include malformations and functional alterations of the male and female reproductive tract and brain. In the CD1 mouse, effective exposures are in the range of 0.1 to 100 μg/kg on gestation day (GD) nine to 16 (Newbold, 1995). At the higher end of the exposure range (10–100 μg/kg), total sterility of female offspring is noted, due in part to structural abnormalities of the oviduct, uterus, cervix, and vagina, and to depletion and abnormalities of ovarian follicles. In adulthood, male offspring show hypospadias, whereas females exhibit excessive vaginal keratinization and epidermoid tumors of the vagina. Vaginal adenocarcinoma is seen at dosages as low as 2.5 μg/kg maternal body weight, and benign uterine tumors (leiomyomas) are seen at as low as 0.1 µg/kg. In male offspring, sterility is observed at high doses, the result of retained rete testes and Mullerian duct remnants, abnormal sperm morphology and motility, cryptorchidism, abnormal reproductive tract secretions, and inflammation (Newbold, 1995). DES exposure of pregnant mice also causes obesity in female offspring (Newbold et al., 2009). Other estrogenic (or antiestrogenic) developmental toxicants include estradiol (Biegel et al., 1998; Cook et al., 1998), ethinyl estradiol, antiestrogenic drugs such as tamoxifen and clomiphene citrate (Branham et al., 1998), and pesticides and industrial chemicals such as methoxychlor (Gray et al., 1989; Hall et al., 1997; Amstislavsky et al., 2003, 2004, 2006), o,p-DDT (Heinrichs et al., 1971), kepone (Gellert, 1978; Guzelian, 1982), dioxins (Mably et al., 1992; Gray et al., 1997a,b), bisphenol A (Nagel et al., 1997), and phytoestrogens such as genistein and coumestrol (Medlock et al., 1995; Rozman et al., 2006). Female offspring are generally more sensitive than males and altered pubertal development, reduced fertility, and reproductive tract anomalies are common findings.

Although most studies on estrogens have indicated traditional dose–response patterns, vom Saal and co-workers (vom Saal et al., 1997; Nagel et al., 1997) have reported that unusual dose– response patterns may occur for endocrine effects on some endpoints. In their studies, a 50% elevation in fetal serum estradiol concentration resulting from implantation of estradiol-containing Silastic capsules on days 13 to 19 of gestation in mice caused a 30% increase in adult prostate weight in male offspring, whereas higher maternal serum concentrations were associated with decreased adult prostate weight. A similar U-shaped dose–response pattern was observed for DES given on days 11 to 17 of gestation, as increased adult prostate weights were seen between 0.02 and 20 ng/kg/day, whereas 200 ng/kg/day resulted in smaller prostates. Bisphenol A (2 or 20 µg/kg/day on gestation days 11–17) also increased adult prostate weight in these mice. However, the issue is controversial, as other researchers using similar testing paradigms have not seen this pattern (eg, Cagen et al., 1999). Vom Saal and colleagues (vom Saal and Hughes, 2005; Welshons et al., 2006) argue that bisphenol A exerts estrogenic effects at low doses and exhibits an inverted U-shaped dose response. Naciff et al. (2005) assessed changes in gene expression in response to in utero exposure to three estrogen receptor agonists, 17α-ethinyl estradiol, genistein, or bisphenol A. Expression of 50 genes was changed by all three chemicals, suggesting that these chemicals have a consistent mode of action. Further, the dose–response for these gene expression changes was monotonic, arguing against the existence of a U-shaped dose–response for these chemicals. Vandenberg and colleagues (Vandenberg et al., 2012) have recently reviewed the issue of low dose effects and nonmonotonic dose–response curves for endocrine disruptors.

Antiandrogens are another class of endocrine-disrupting chemicals. Effects of developmental exposure to an antiandrogen are generally restricted to males, and include hypospadias, retained nipples, reduced testes and accessory sex gland weights, and decreased sperm production. Examples of chemicals known to affect development via an antiandrogenic mechanism include pharmaceuticals such as the androgen receptor antagonist flutamide (Imperato-McGinley et al., 1992) and the 5α-reductase inhibitor finasteride (Clark et al., 1990), the fungicide vinclozolin (Gray et al., 1994) and the DDT metabolite p,p-dichlorodiphenyldichloroethylene (DDE) (Kelce et al., 1995; You et al., 1998); the latter two are androgen receptor antagonists. Dibutylphthalate has been shown to induce an antiandrogen phenotype in developing rats, but the effect does not appear to be mediated by direct interaction with the androgen receptor (Mylchreest et al., 1998, 1999). The critical developmental window for these effects of dibutylphthalate was

gestation days 16 to 18 in the rat (Carruthers and Foster, 2005). Dietary exposure of pregnant rats to dibutylphthalate from gestation days 12 to 19 resulted in dose-related decreases in androgen responsive gene expression and testicular testosterone content in male fetuses, and an antiandrogen phenotype in male offspring (Struve et al., 2009). A similar phenotype has been observed in offspring of dibutylphthalate treated rabbits (Higuchi et al., 2003). Importantly, recent studies have demonstrated that exposure of pregnant rats to mixtures of antiandrogenic chemicals can have a cumulative effect on development of the male offspring (Rider et al., 2009, 2010; Hotchkiss et al., 2010; Hannas et al., 2011).

Hypothyroidism during pregnancy and early postnatal development causes growth retardation, cognitive deficits, delayed eye opening, hyperactivity, and auditory defects in rodents. Polychlorinated biphenyls (PCBs) may act at several sites to lower thyroid hormone levels during development and cause body weight and auditory deficits (Goldey et al., 1995; Goldey and Crofton, 1998). PCBs also cause learning deficits and alter locomotor activity patterns in rodents (Eriksson et al., 1991; Schantz et al., 1995) and monkeys (Bowman, 1982; Schantz et al., 1991). The thyroid hormone synthesis inhibitor propylthiouracil (PTU) has been used to study the effects of chemically induced hypothyroidism on development of the brain in rats (Gilbert, 2011). Administration of 1 to 3 ppm PTU in the drinking water of female rats during pregnancy and lactation produced deficits of thyroxine (T4) in the offspring, but only modest reductions in triiodothyronine (T3, the active thyroid hormone) at the high dose. Excitatory postsynaptic transmission was reduced and long-term potentiation was impaired in adult offspring despite the modest and transient effect on T3 during treatment.

Human Evidence

Despite the biological plausibility of effects demonstrated in numerous laboratory studies, the extent to which human health is being adversely impacted from exposures to environmental endocrine disruptors is unclear. It is difficult to demonstrate cause and effect relationships in epidemiological studies where the signals may be weak, the effects may be evident only long after an exposure, and the endpoints are sensitive to other factors. Reports in humans which are or may be relevant are of two types: (1) Observations of adverse effects on reproductive system development and function following exposure to chemicals with known endocrine activities that are present in medicines, contaminated food, or the workplace. These have tended to involve relatively high exposures to chemicals with known endocrine effects (eg, DES). (2) Epidemiological evidence of increasing trends in adverse reproductive and developmental outcomes having an endocrine basis. With the exception of DES, evidence is either lacking to support a definitive link to an exposure, or is variable across studies. Secular trends have been reported for cryptorchidism (Toppari et al., 1996); hypospadias (Toppari et al., 1996; Paulozzi et al., 1997; Paulozzi, 1999); semen quality (Carlsen et al., 1992; Skakkebaek and Keiding, 1994; Olsen et al., 1995; Swan et al., 1997; Auger et al., 1995; de Mouzon et al., 1996; Irvine et al., 1996; Vierula et al., 1996; Bujan et al., 1996; Fisch and Goluboff, 1996), and testicular cancer (Toppari et al., 1996). Recently, connections between environmental exposures and cryptorchidism and hypospadias (Toppari et al., 2010), and early onset of puberty in girls (Mouritsen et al., 2010) have been suggested.

The most convincing evidence for effects of endocrine-disrupting chemicals in humans comes from reports of neurobehavioral changes and learning deficits in children exposed to PCBs in utero or lactationally, either through their mothers' consumption of PCB-contaminated fish (Jacobson *et al.*, 1990; Jacobson and Jacobson, 1996) or through exposure to background levels of PCBs in the United States (Rogan and Gladen, 1991) or the Netherlands (Koopman-Esseboom *et al.*, 1996). In addition, there have been two occurrences of high-level exposure to contaminated rice oil (in Japan in 1968 and in Taiwan in 1979) in which alterations in development of ectodermal tissues and delays in neurological development were seen (Hsu *et al.*, 1985; Yu *et al.*, 1991; Guo *et al.*, 1994; Schecter *et al.*, 1994). In these cases, there was coexposure to polychlorinated dibenzofurans and PCBs. The mode of action of the developmental neurotoxicity of PCBs is, however, not yet understood.

Impact on Screening and Testing Programs

The findings of altered reproductive development following early life stage exposures to endocrine-disrupting chemicals prompted revisions of traditional safety evaluation tests such as those issued by the EPA (USEPA, 1997). These include assessments of female estrous cyclicity, sperm parameters (total number, percent progressively motile and sperm morphology in both the parental and F1 generations), the age at puberty in the F1 (vaginal opening in the female, preputial separation in the males); an expanded list of organs for pathology and/or histopathology to identify and characterize effects at the target organ; as well as some triggered endpoints including anogenital distance in the F2 and primordial follicular counts in the parental and F1 generations. An important modification of prenatal developmental toxicity test guidelines aimed at improved detection of endocrine disruptors is the extension of the period of dosing to near the end of pregnancy in order to include the developmental period of urogenital tract differentiation.

MODERN SAFETY ASSESSMENT

Experience with chemicals that have the potential to induce developmental toxicity in humans indicates that laboratory animal testing, surveillance of the human population (ie, epidemiological studies), and alert clinical awareness (eg, Friedman, 2011) are all necessary to provide adequate public health protection. Laboratory animal investigations are guided by both regulatory requirements for drug or chemical marketing and the need to understand mechanisms of toxicity.

Regulatory Guidelines for In Vivo Testing

Prior to the thalidomide tragedy, safety evaluations for reproductive effects were limited in the types of chemicals evaluated and the sophistication of the endpoints. Subsequently, the FDA issued more extensive testing protocols (termed Segments I, II, and III) for application to a broader range of chemicals (USFDA, 1966). These testing protocols, with minor variations, were adopted by regulatory agencies around the world and remained similar for nearly 30 years. Several factors including the historical experience of testing thousands of chemicals, increased knowledge of basic reproductive processes, the ever-rising cost of testing, the acknowledged redundancy and overlap of required protocols, a growing divergence in study design requirements of various countries, and the expanding international presence of the pharmaceutical industry succeeded in producing new and streamlined testing protocols that have been accepted internationally (USFDA, 1994). These guidelines, the result of the International Conference of Harmonization of Technical Requirements for Registration of Pharmaceuticals for Human Use (ICH), allow considerable flexibility in implementation

depending on the particular circumstances of the agent under evaluation. Rather than specify study and technical details, they rely on the investigator to meet the primary goal of detecting and bringing to light any indication of toxicity to reproduction. Key elements of the FDA Segment I, II, and III studies, the ICH protocols, and the organisation for economic cooperation and development (OECD) equivalent of the FDA Segment II test are provided in Table 10-4. In each protocol, guidance is provided on species/strain selection, route of administration, number and spacing of dosage levels, exposure duration, experimental sample size, observational techniques, statistical analysis, and reporting requirements. Details are available in the original publications as well as in several reviews (eg, Manson, 1994; Claudio *et al.*, 1999; Reuter *et al.*, 2003). Variations of these protocols exist that include extensions of exposure to early or later time points in development and extensions of observations to postnatal ages with more sophisticated endpoints. For example, the Environmental Protection Agency's Developmental Neurotoxicity Protocol for the rat includes exposure from gestation day six though lactation day 10, and observation of postnatal growth, developmental landmarks of puberty (preputial separation, vaginal opening), motor activity, auditory startle, learning and memory, and neuropathology at various ages through postnatal day 60 (USEPA, 1998a,b).

In 2006, the Regulation on Registration, Evaluation, Authorization and restriction of Chemicals (REACH, 2006) was published. REACH requires that all chemicals marketed or manufactured in the European Union above one ton per year must be characterized as to their toxicity. The requirements are categorized by the annual tonnage of the chemical and are more extensive as the tonnage increases (Rovida *et al.*, 2011). Requirements for reproductive and developmental toxicity are included and are expected to be the largest user of live animals under REACH, which, although it encourages use of alternative toxicity tests to reduce animal use, does not currently deem screening tests for developmental toxicity sufficient to replace required whole animal tests (Scialli, 2008; Rovida *et al.*, 2011).

In part because of the development of new pharmaceuticals for use in children, a Workshop on Testing Strategies and Design of Juvenile Animal Studies was held in 2003 (Hurtt *et al.*, 2004). Subsequently, the FDA and the European Medicines Agency (EMA) have promulgated guidelines for determining the need for and the design of nonclinical studies in support of registering such drugs (USFDA, 2006; EMA, 2008). The design of such studies is flexible and would depend in part on the intended use of the drug (eg, age range, duration of treatment, drug target). To assess the value of such tests, juvenile animal data were compiled from over 200 studies and reviewed in a workshop (Bailey and Marien, 2011). The consensus was that the survey demonstrated the value of juvenile studies for the development of safe pediatric drugs.

The general goal of regulatory studies is to identify the NOAEL, which is the highest dosage level that does not produce a significant increase in adverse effects in the offspring or juvenile animals. These NOAELs are then used in the risk assessment process to assess the likelihood of effects in humans given certain exposure conditions. A preferable alternative, the Benchmark Dose approach, is discussed below.

Multigeneration Tests

Information pertaining to developmental toxicity can also be obtained from studies in which animals are exposed to the test substance continuously over one or more generations (eg, OECD Test Guideline 416 or USEPA 870.3800). For additional information

Table 10-4

Summary of In Vivo Regulatory Protocol Guidelines for Evaluation of Developmental Toxicity

STUDY	EXPOSURE	ENDPOINTS COVERED	COMMENTS
Segment I: Fertility and general reproduction study	Males: 10 week prior to mating Females: 2 week prior to mating through implantation	Gamete development, fertility, pre- and postimplantation viability, parturition, lactation	Assesses reproductive capabilities of male and female following exposure over one complete spermatogenic cycle or several estrous cycles.
Segment II: Teratogenicity test	Implantation (or mating) through end of organogenesis (or term)	Viability and anatomy (external, visceral, skeletal) of fetuses prior to birth	Shorter exposure prevents metabolic adaptation and provides high exposure during gastrulation and organogenesis. Earlier dosing option for bioaccumulative agents or those impacting maternal nutrition. Later dosing option covers reproductive tract development.
Segment III: Perinatal study	Last trimester of pregnancy through lactation	Postnatal survival, growth, and external morphology	Intended to observe effects on development of major organ functional competence during the perinatal period, and thus may be relatively more sensitive to adverse effects at this time.
ICH 4.1.1: Fertility protocol	Males: 4 week prior to mating Females: 2 week prior to mating through implantation	Males: Reproductive organ weights and histology, sperm counts and motility Females: Viability of conceptuses at mid-pregnancy or later	Improved assessment of male reproductive endpoints; shorter treatment duration than Segment I.
ICH 4.1.2: Effects on prenatal and postnatal development, including maternal function	Implantation through end of lactation	Relative toxicity to pregnant versus non-pregnant female; postnatal viability, growth, development, and functional deficits (behavior, maturation, reproduction)	Similar to Segment I study.
ICH 4.1.3: Effects on embryo/ fetal development	Implantation through end of organogenesis	Viability and morphology (external, visceral, skeletal) of fetuses prior to birth.	Similar to Segment II study. Usually conducted in two species (rodent and nonrodent).
OECD 4.1.4: Prenatal developmental	Implantation (or mating) through day prior to cesarean section	Viability and morphology (external, visceral, skeletal) of fetuses prior to birth.	Similar to Segment II study. Usually conducted in two species (rodent and nonrodent).

on this approach, see Chap. 20. A recent study (Piersma *et al.*, 2011b) has called into question the value of including a second generation on overall outcome of the assessment. These investigators conducted a retrospective analysis of 498 rat mulitgeneratonal studies, and found that the second-generation mating and offspring rarely provided critical information. These authors instead recommended adopting a proposed OECD extended one-generation test (Cooper, 2009; Vogel *et al.*, 2010) for risk assessment purposes. The extended one-generation test is flexible and could include a second generation if certain triggers were reached in the first generation. Others have argued that the triggers may be too lenient and will too frequently result in invoking production of the second generation (Beekhuijzen *et al.*, 2009).

Children's Health and the Food Quality Protection Act

In 1993, the National Academy of Sciences published a report entitled "Pesticides in the Diets of Infants and Children," which brought to light the fact that infants and children differ both qualitatively and quantitatively from adults in their exposure to pesticide residues in food because of different dietary composition and intake patterns and different activities (National Research Council [NRC], 1993). This report, along with the report from the International Life Sciences Institute entitled "Similarities and Differences Between Children and Adults" (Guzelian *et al.*, 1992) provided background and impetus for passage of the Food Quality Protection Act (FQPA) of 1996. The FQPA incorporates an additional 10-fold safety factor for children, cumulative effects of toxicants acting through a common mode of action, aggregate exposure (ie, same toxicant from different sources), and endocrine disruption. The inclusion (at the discretion of the EPA) of the 10-fold factor for calculating allowable intakes for children affects most strongly the pesticide industry, whose products can appear as residues in food. The application of this safety factor is controversial in part because its opponents' claim that developmental susceptibility is already considered in other tests, such as the Segment II test for prenatal toxicity, the two-generation test, and the developmental neurotoxicity test. On the other hand, proponents applaud the measure and point to the numerous factors that may increase the exposure of infants and children to environmental toxicants and their susceptibility to harm from these exposures. Children have different diets than adults and also have activity patterns that change their exposure profile compared to adults, such as crawling on the floor or ground, putting their hands and foreign objects in their mouths, and raising dust and dirt during play. Even the level of their activity (ie, closer to the ground) can affect their exposure to some toxicants. In addition to exposure differences, children are growing and developing, which makes them more susceptible to some types of insults. Effects of early childhood exposure, including neurobehavioral effects, obesity, diabetes, and cancer, may not be apparent until later in life. Debate continues over the approach to be used for risk assessment in consideration of infants and children.

A large prospective study on children's health in the United States, the National Children's Study (NCS) (Branum *et al.*, 2003; Needham *et al.*, 2005; Kimmel *et al.*, 2005; Landrigan and Miodovnic, 2011) was launched in 2009. For this longitudinal birth cohort, 100,000 children will be followed from before birth through 21 years of age. Among many parameters and endpoints to be assessed is exposure to environmental contaminants, including those present in breast milk. In this unique study, because the children will be followed to adulthood, the opportunity exists to assess the full range of potential adverse developmental consequences of environmental exposures. In addition to the National Children's Study, the US Environmental Protection Agency and the US National Institutes of Health support 14 Centers for Children's Environmental Health and Disease Prevention Research (Landrigan and Miodovnic, 2011).

Alternative Testing Strategies

A variety of alternative test systems have been proposed over several decades to refine, reduce, or replace the standard mammalian regulatory tests for assessing developmental toxicity. These assays are based on cell cultures, cultures of embryos in vitro, including those of worms, flies, frogs, fish, and mammals (Chapin *et al.*, 2008; Piersma *et al.*, 2010), and a short-term in vivo test (Chernoff and Kavlock, 1982). Daston (1996) has discussed the theoretical and empirical underpinnings supporting the use of a number of these systems. Yet, validation of these alternative tests was a major issue

(Neubert, 1989; Welsch, 1990). Although it was initially hoped that alternative approaches would become generally applicable to all chemicals, and help prioritize full-scale testing, this has not yet been accomplished. Given the complexity of embryogenesis and the multiple mechanisms and target sites of potential teratogens, it was perhaps unrealistic to have expected a single test, or even a small battery of tests, to accurately prescreen the activity of chemicals in general. Over the past decade, a validation study of three in vitro embryotoxicity assays, the rat embryo limb bud micromass assay, the mouse embryonic stem cell test (mEST), and the rat WEC test, has been carried out (Genschow *et al.*, 2000, 2002, 2004; Brown, 2002; Piersma *et al.*, 2004; Seiler *et al.*, 2004; Spielmann *et al.*, 2004). This study involved interlaboratory blind trials to validate these assays, and the approach involved the development of "prediction models," which mathematically combine assay endpoints to determine the combinations and formulations that are most predictive of mammalian in vivo results. More recently, the mEST and other approaches to using mouse embryonic stem cells have been further developed and tested, and the zebrafish embryo has gained prominence as a short-term test for developmental toxicity. Currently, developmental toxicity assays based on rodent WEC, mEST, and zebrafish embryos are receiving the bulk of research attention for use as teratogen screens (Fig. 10-10).

The rodent WEC has been discussed above as a tool for studies of chemical mechanism of action. For WEC, rodent or rabbit embryos are excised from the mother at an early stage of organogenesis with their yolk sacs intact and cultured for up to 48 hours (Ellis-Hutchings and Carney, 2010). During this time they continue to develop in a manner similar to in utero development. At the end of culture the embryos are scored for a number of growth and developmental parameters and assigned a developmental score (eg, rodents: Brown and Fabro, 1981; Van Maele-Fabry *et al.*, 1990;

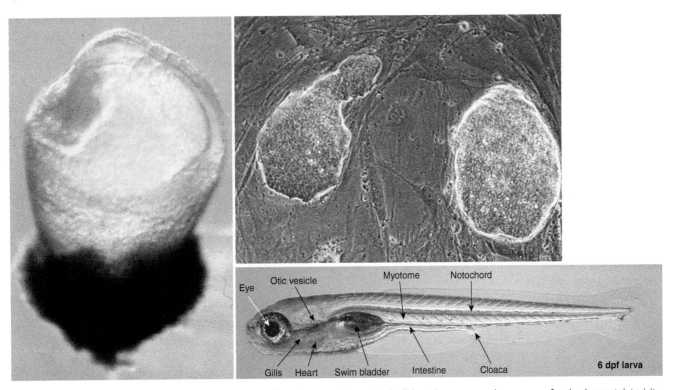

Figure 10-10. *Rodent whole embryos in culture, mouse embryonic stem cells, and zebrafish embryos are used as screens for developmental toxicity. Left*: A whole gestation day eight mouse embryo removed from the uterus with intact yolk sac and ectoplacental cone, ready to be cultured for up to 48 hours. (Picture courtesy of Dr E. Sidney Hunter.) *Top right*: Mouse embryonic stem cells (cell line J1) in pluripotent state maintained on a feeder layer of mitotically inactivated mouse embryonic fibroblasts. (Picture courtesy of Dr Kelly Chandler.) *Lower right*: Zebrafish larvae at six days postfertilization (dpf). Note the transparency of the larva, facilitating observation of internal structures such as those labeled. (From Airhart *et al.* (2007), with permission.)

rabbits: Carney *et al.*, 2007). As a screen for developmental toxicity, the WEC has the advantages of using mammalian embryos and being able to divide the many embryos in a litter into different treatment groups. Disadvantages include the technical difficult and time-consuming process of excising the embryos and scoring them at the end of culture, and the cost in animals for obtaining the embryos and the rat serum used as culture medium. As an alternative or in addition to morphological scoring, effects of chemicals on gene expression in the embryos have been studied to discern common patterns ("signatures") of transcriptomic effects (Luijten *et al.*, 2010; Robinson *et al.*, 2010, 2011a,b, 2012a,b,c,d).

The mEST uses established stem cell lines and examines the effects of test chemicals on viability and differentiation of the cells. The cells aggregate and form "embryoid bodies" when grown in hanging drop cultures. Cardiomyocyte differentiation in the cultures can be quantified by examining the cultures for beating cardiomyocytes. In a different version of the mEST, mouse embryonic stem cells are cultured to adherency in 96-well plates and test chemical applied for up to eight days (Barrier *et al.*, 2011; Chandler *et al.*, 2011). At the end of culture, cardiomyocyte differentiation is assessed by performing in-cell Westerns for cardiac myosin heavy chain and viability is assessed using a fluorescent dye technique. The mEST has the advantage of using established cell lines, therefore totally avoiding the use of live animals. It is also fairly rapid and inexpensive. A disadvantage is the limited developmental repertoire of the cells under the conditions of these tests. Human embryonic stem cell lines or induced pluripotent stem cells are also being developed for toxicity testing, with the obvious advantage of being human cells (Krtolica *et al.*, 2009; Vojnits and Bremer, 2010). However, at present these cells are less well characterized than are mouse embryonic stem cells, and they are generally less robust in culture.

Submammalian species have been used for many years in the study of normal developmental biology, and among these animal models, the African clawed frog, *Xenopus laevis* or *X tropicalis* (Bantle, 1995; Fort *et al.*, 2000, 2004; Fort and Paul, 2002), and the zebrafish, *Danio rerio* (Fraysse *et al.*, 2006; Love *et al.*, 2004; Ton *et al.*, 2006; Yang *et al.*, 2009; Brannen *et al.*, 2010; Sipes *et al.*, 2011a,b; McCollum *et al.*, 2011; Selderslaghs *et al.*, 2012), have been used for developmental toxicology to a number of advantages. Chief among the features of these species is the rapid external development of the embryos, the large historical and recent literature on their normal development, and the availability of genetic mutants and molecular biological tools for studying these embryos. In addition, these species can be bred to produce large numbers of embryos in a relatively short period and are easy and inexpensive to maintain.

The zebrafish has gained increased usage in a number of fields including developmental biology and cancer research. These small fish exhibit a great deal of homology to higher vertebrates in their development, anatomy, physiology, and behavior. Their rapidly developing embryos are transparent, allowing visualization of internal anatomy. Chemical toxicity studies in zebrafish have been comprehensively compiled and reviewed (McCollum *et al.*, 2011). Zebrafish developmental toxicity testing can be carried out in 96-well plates, an approach used for assessment in zebrafish of the Phase I chemical library in the US Environmental Protection Agency's ToxCast program (Padilla *et al.*, 2012). For a review of zebrafish development and use of zebrafish as a disease model, see *Birth Defects Research Part C: Embryo Today: Reviews* (2011;93(2)), an issue dedicated to this topic.

The ToxCast program at EPA (Kavlock *et al.*, 2012; http://actor.epa.gov/actor/faces/ToxCastDB/Home.jsp) includes hundreds of high-throughput assays directed at molecular and cellular targets of toxicity, a number of which are relevant to developmental

toxicity. Sipes *et al.* (2011a,b) have evaluated statistical associations of ToxCast assay data with the mammalian developmental toxicity data in EPA's Toxicity Reference Database, ToxRefDB (http://actor.epa.gov/toxrefdb/faces/Home.jsp). A high number of associations between the rat and rabbit in vivo data and the Toxcast data were discerned, and species-specific predictive models based on the ToxCast assays exhibited greater than 70% balanced accuracy.

A streamlined alternate in vivo test using rodents for prescreening for developmental toxicity was developed by Chernoff and Kavlock (1982), and is known as the Chernoff–Kavlock assay. Pregnant females are exposed during the period of major organogenesis to a limited number of dosage levels near those inducing maternal toxicity, and offspring are evaluated over a brief neonatal period for external malformations, growth, and viability. It has proven reliable over a large number of chemical agents and classes (Hardin *et al.*, 1987), and a regulatory testing guideline is available (USEPA, 1985).

Epidemiology

Reproductive epidemiology is the study of associations between specific exposures of the father or pregnant woman and her conceptus and the outcome of pregnancy (Chambers and Scialli, 2010). In rare situations, such as rubella, thalidomide, and isotretinoin, where a relatively high risk exists and the outcome is a rare event, formal studies may not be needed to identify causes of abnormal birth outcomes. The likelihood of linking a particular exposure with a series of case reports increases with the rarity of the defect, the rarity of the exposure in the population, a small source population, a short time span for study, and biological plausibility for the association (Khoury *et al.*, 1991). In other situations, such as those with ethanol and valproic acid, associations are sought through either a case–control or a cohort approach. Both approaches require accurate ascertainment of abnormal outcomes and exposures, and a large enough effect and study population to detect an elevated risk. Therein lies one of the difficulties for epidemiologists studying abnormal reproductive outcomes. For example, it has been estimated that the monitoring of more than one million births would have been necessary to detect a statistically significant increase in the frequency of spina bifida following the introduction of valproic acid in the United States, where the frequency of exposure was less than one in 1000 pregnancies and the risk was only a doubling over the background incidence (Khoury and Holtzman, 1987). Another challenge to epidemiologists is the high percentage of human pregnancy wastage, perhaps as much as 31% in the peri-implantation period (Wilcox *et al.*, 1988) and an additional 15% that are clinically recognized. Therefore, pregnancy failures related to a particular exposure may go undetected in the general population. Furthermore, with the availability of prenatal diagnostic procedures, some pregnancies with malformed embryos (particularly NTDs) are electively aborted. Thus, the incidence of abnormal outcomes at birth may not reflect the true rate of abnormalities, and the term prevalence, rather than incidence, is preferred when the denominator is the number of live births rather than total pregnancies.

Epidemiological studies of abnormal reproductive outcomes are usually undertaken with three objectives in mind: the first is scientific research into the causes of abnormal birth outcomes and usually involves analysis of case reports or clusters; a second aim is prevention and is targeted at broader surveillance of trends by birth defect registries around the world; and the last objective is informing the public and providing assurance. In this regard, it is informative to consider the review by Schardein (1993) of the method and year by which humans teratogens were detected.

For 23 of 28 chemicals reviewed (including nine cancer therapeutics, androgenic hormones, antithyroid drugs, aminoglycoside antibiotics, coumarin anticoagulants, DES, methylmercury, hydantoins, primidone, penicillamine, lithium, vitamin A, and RA), case reports presented the first evidence in humans. For two of these (DES and lithium), the case reports were soon followed by registries that provided confirmation, while for two others (methyl mercury and hydantoins) follow-up epidemiology studies added support. For only four chemicals, alcohol, PCBs, carbamazepine, and cocaine, did an analytical epidemiological study provide the first human evidence. Evidence for one chemical, valproic acid, was first obtained by analysis of a birth defect registry. For the 28 chemicals in that review, human evidence of developmental toxicity preceded published animal evidence in eleven instances. Cohort studies, with their prospective exposure assessment and ability to monitor both adverse and beneficial outcomes, may be the most methodologically robust approach to identifying human developmental toxicants. The lack of cohort studies demonstrating risk for pregnancy may be in part due to the difficulty in making such associations, but may also reflect the fact that use in pregnancy is not associated with increased risk for the majority of drugs (Irl and Hasford, 2000).

Assessment of the developmental toxicity of tobacco smoke has benefited greatly from the many epidemiological studies that have been carried out (see tobacco smoke under Scope of the Problem: The Human Experience). Reasons for this success include the prevalence of smoking and secondhand smoke exposure (allowing large studies), good recall of exposure, and biomarkers of exposure (eg, cotinine), and comprehensive assessment of effects in offspring. The large number of studies has allowed meta-analyses for selected effects.

Concordance of Data

There have been several reviews of the similarity of responses of laboratory mammals and humans to developmental toxicants. In general, these studies support the assumption that results from laboratory tests are predictive of potential human effects. Concordance is strongest when there are positive data from more than one test species. In a quantitative sense, the few comparisons that have been made suggest that humans tend to be more sensitive to developmental toxicants than is the most sensitive test species. Although concordance among species for chemicals reported as positive is high, often special steps must be taken retrospectively to produce an animal model that reflects the nature of outcome in humans (eg, valproic acid, Ehlers *et al.*, 1992 a,b).

Frankos (1985) reviewed data for 38 compounds having demonstrated or suspect developmental toxicity in humans; all except tobramycin, which caused otologic defects, were positive in at least one test species and 76% were positive in more than one test species. Predictiveness was highest in the mouse (85%) and rat (80%), with lower rates for rabbits (60%), and hamsters (40%). Frankos identified 165 chemicals with no evidence of human effects; only 29% were negative in all species tested while 51% were negative in more than one species. Schardein and Keller (1989) examined concordance by species and developmental manifestation for 51 potential human developmental toxicants that had adequate animal data (three human developmental toxicants did not). Thalidomide received the widest testing, with data from 19 species; 53% had data from three species, whereas 18% had data from four or five species. Across all chemicals, the most common findings in humans, rabbits, and monkeys were spontaneous abortion and fetal/neonatal death, followed by malformations and then growth retardation. In the rat, prenatal death, growth retardation, and then malformations was the typical pattern. All species showed at least one positive response for 64% of the human developmental toxicants and, with only one exception, all of the potential human developmental toxicants showed a positive response in at least one species. Overall, the match to the human, regardless of the nature of the developmental response, was rat, 98%; mouse, 91%; hamster, 85%; monkey, 82%; and rabbit, 77%. Jelovsek *et al.* (1989) reviewed the predictiveness of animal data for 84 negative human developmental toxicants, 33 with unknown activity, 26 considered suspicious, and 32 considered positive. Variables considered included the response of each species, the number of positive and negative species, percent positive and negative species, and mutagenicity and carcinogenicity. The compounds were correctly classified 63% to 91% of the time based on animal data, depending upon how the suspect and unknown human toxicants were considered. The various models had a sensitivity of 62% to 75%, a positive predictive value of 75% to 100%, and a negative predictive value of 64% to 91%. A summary comparison of rodent and rabbit results for 22 human developmental toxicants has recently been compiled by Daston and Knudsen (2010) (Table 10-5).

Table 10-5

Developmental Toxicity Findings in Rodents and Rabbits for Known Human Developmental Toxicants

CHEMICAL	RODENT	RABBIT	HUMAN
Cyclophosphamide	+	+	+
Diazepam	+		+
Diethylstilbestrol	+	+	+
Phenytoin/trimethadione	+	+	+
Ethanol	+		+
Lithium	+/−		+
Methylmercury	+		+
13-*cis*-Retinoic acid	+	+	+
Testosterone	+	+	+
Thalidomide	−	+	+
Valproic acid	+	+	+
Warfarin	+		+
Fumonisin B$_1$	+	−	+
Methimazole	+/−		+
Busufan	+		+
Enalapril/captopril	+		+
Polychlorinated biphenyls	+/−		+
Cocaine	+/−		+
Misoprostol	+	−	+
Penicillamine	+		+
Tetracycline	−		+
Toluene	+		+

+ indicates developmental toxicity in that species; − indicates negative findings; +/− indicates an equivocal response. Blank spaces indicate chemical not tested in that species. The type of positive finding is not necessarily the same in all species.
SOURCE: *Adapted from Daston and Knudsen (2010), with permission.*

Elements of Risk Assessment

The extrapolation of animal test data to predict human risk of developmental toxicity follows two basic directions, one for drugs where exposure is voluntary and usually to high dosages, the other for environmental chemicals where exposure is generally involuntary and to low levels. For drugs, a use-in-pregnancy rating has been utilized (USFDA, 1979). In this system the letters A, B, C, D, and X are used to classify the evidence that a chemical poses a risk to the human conceptus. For example, drugs are placed in category A if adequate, well-controlled studies in pregnant humans have failed to demonstrate a risk, and in category X (contraindicated for pregnancy) if studies in animals or humans, or investigational or post-marketing reports have shown fetal risk, which clearly outweighs any possible benefit to the patient. The default category is C (risks cannot be ruled out), assigned when there is a lack of human studies and animal studies are either lacking or are positive for fetal risk, but the benefits may justify the potential risk. Categories B and D represent areas of relatively lesser, or greater concern for risk, respectively. Manson (1994) reviewed the 1992 Physicians' Desk Reference and found 7% of the 1033 drugs belonged to category X, 66% to category C, and only 0.7% to category A. The FDA categorization procedure has been criticized (Teratology Society, 1994) as being too reliant on risk/benefit comparisons, especially given that the magnitude of risk is often unknown, or the benefits are not an issue (eg, after the drug in question has been taken during early pregnancy, the question is then directed to the management of the exposed pregnancy). The FDA system has also been criticized for demanding an unrealistically high quality of data for assignment to category A (negative controlled studies in pregnant women) and overuse of category C, interpreted as "risks cannot be ruled out" (Sannerstedt *et al.*, 1996). This is an important issue because presently the perception of teratogenic risk is strong among both patients and prescribers even for safe drugs (Pole *et al.*, 2000). The often necessary reliance on studies conducted in animals has also been criticized, and acceptance by clinicians of these studies as reflective of human risks/benefits may be limited (Doering *et al.*, 2002). The approach of FDA for informing physicians and patients about the risk of drugs for use in pregnancy is currently undergoing a complete overhaul. The proposed new system eliminates the letter categories and includes a risk summary and information about available data for the drug during pregnancy.

For environmental chemicals, the purpose of the risk assessment process for noncancer endpoints such as developmental toxicity is generally to define the dose, route, timing, and duration of exposure that induces effects at the lowest level in the most relevant laboratory animal model (USEPA, 1991a,b). The exposure associated with this "critical effect" is then subjected to a variety of safety or uncertainty factors in order to derive an exposure level for humans that is presumed to be relatively safe (see Chap. 4). The principal uncertainty factors include one for interspecies extrapolation and one for variability in the human population. The default value for each of these factors is 10. In the absence of firm evidence upon which to base decisions on whether or not to extrapolate animal test data, certain default assumptions are generally made. They include (1) a chemical that produces an adverse developmental effect in experimental animals will potentially pose a hazard to humans following sufficient exposure during development; (2) all four manifestations of developmental toxicity (death, structural abnormalities, growth alterations, and functional deficits) are of concern; (3) the specific types of developmental effects seen in animal studies are not necessarily the same as those that may be produced in humans; (4) the most appropriate species is used to estimate human risk when data are available (in the absence of such data, the most sensitive species

is appropriate); and (5) in general, a threshold is assumed for the dose–response curve for agents that produce developmental toxicity.

New Approaches

The Benchmark-Dose Approach The use of safety or uncertainty factors applied to an experimentally derived NOAEL to arrive at a presumed safe level of human exposure is predicated on the risk assessment assumption that a threshold for developmental toxicity exists (see "Principles of Developmental Toxicology"). A threshold should not be confused with the NOAEL, as the NOAEL is dependent entirely on the power of the study and is associated with risks perhaps on the order of 5% over the control incidence in typical studies. Also, the value obtained by the application of uncertainty factors to the NOAEL should not be confused with a threshold, as this exposure is only assumed to be without appreciable added risk.

The use of the NOAEL in the risk assessment process has been criticized for several reasons. Because it is dependent on statistical power to detect pairwise differences between a treated and a control group, the use of larger sample sizes and more dose groups (which might better characterize the dose–response relationship) can only yield lower NOAELs, and thus better experimental designs are actually penalized by this approach. In addition, the NOAEL is limited to an experimental dose level, and an experiment might need to be repeated to develop a NOAEL for risk assessment. A final point relates to the fact that, given varying experimental designs and variability of control values, NOAELs actually represent different levels of risk in different studies.

Crump (1984) proposed using a mathematical model to estimate the lower confidence bounds on a predetermined level of risk [the "benchmark dose" (BMD)] as a means of avoiding many of the disadvantages of the NOAEL. The application of this approach to a large compilation of Segment II type data sets (Faustman *et al.*, 1994; Allen *et al.*, 1994a,b; Kavlock *et al.*, 1995) demonstrated that a variety of mathematical models, including those that incorporate developmental-specific features such as litter size and intralitter correlations, can be readily applied to standard test results. On average, benchmark doses based on a 5% added risk of effect calculated on quantal endpoints (eg, whether an implant was affected or not) were approximately equivalent to traditionally determined NOAELs. When the litter was used as the unit of response (did it contain at least one affected implant?), benchmarks calculated for a 10% added risk were most similar to the correspondingly determined NOAEL. Discrepancies between the benchmark dose and the NOAEL were most pronounced when one or more of the following conditions were present: a shallow dose–response, small sample sizes, wide spacing of experimental dosage levels, or more than the typical number of dose levels. These features tend to make determination of the NOAEL more problematic (usually higher) and the confidence limits around the maximum likelihood estimate broader (resulting in lower BMDs). Software programs, including the USEPA's Benchmark Dose Software (BMDS), are available, helping to make the BMD approach the method of choice for many risk assessment organizations worldwide (Davis *et al.*, 2011).

Biologically Based Dose–Response Modeling The introduction of statistical dose–response models for noncancer endpoints is the first step in developing quantitative, mechanistic models that will help reduce the major uncertainties of high-to-low dose and species-to-species extrapolation of experimental data. These biologically based dose–response models integrate pharmacokinetic information on target tissue dosimetry with molecular/biochemical responses, cellular/tissue responses, and developmental toxicity (O'Flaherty, 1997; Lau and Setzer, 2000; Lau *et al.*, 2001; Setzer *et al.*, 2001).

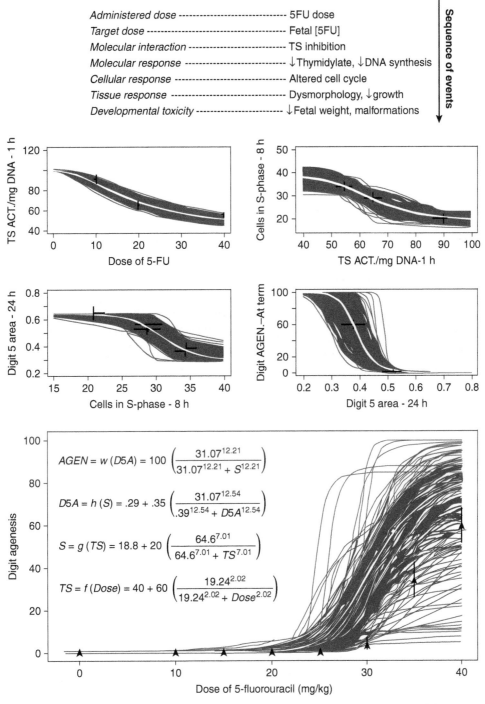

Figure 10-11. *Biologically based dose response modeling of the developmental toxicity of 5-fluorouracil (5-FU) following maternal administration on gestation day 14.* Top: Proposed model for the developmental toxicity of 5-FU based on thymidylate synthetase (TS) inhibition, decreased DNA synthesis, cell cycle alterations, and growth deficits and hind-limb dysmorphogenesis. Shaded events were measured experimentally. *Middle*: Relationships between successive endpoints are shown in these four panels (hind-limb bud TS activity versus 5-FU dose, S-phase accumulation versus TS activity, limb digit 5 area at 24 hours postdose versus proportion of cells in S phase, and digit agenesis at term versus limb digit 5 area at 24 hours). Data were fitted with Hill equations. The curves were generated by Monte-Carlo simulation to estimate variability around the predicted relationships. *Bottom*: Model for induction of hind-limb defects induced by 5-FU, generated by integration of the individual Hill equations describing the relationships between successive model endpoints as presented in the middle panels. These individual equations are listed here, and the curves were generated by Monte-Carlo simulation to estimate variability around the predicted relationship. The simulation results indicate that variability in the intermediate endpoints can account for differences between the predicted and actual dose response. AGEN: digit agenesis at term; D5A: digit 5 area; S: percent of cells in S-phase. (Adapted from Shuey *et al.* (1994), images courtesy of Dr. Woody Setzer.)

Gaylor and Razzaghi (1992) proposed a model that related induction of cleft palate to fetal growth inhibition, and Gaylor and Chen (1993) proposed a model relating fetal weight and the probability of fetal abnormality. Shuey *et al.* (1994) presented a model using the cancer chemotherapeutic 5-fluorouracil (Fig. 10-11). They postulated that the developmental toxicity observed in the term fetus was due to an active metabolite (FdUMP) inhibiting the enzyme TS, with subsequent depletion of thymidine, decreased DNA synthetic rates, reduced cell proliferation, and ultimately, reduced tissue growth and differentiation. Each step in the process was determined experimentally and the relationships were described by Hill equations. The individual equations were then linked in an integrated model to describe the entire relationship between administered dose and the incidence of hind-limb defects. Although this is still an empirically based model, the process clearly demonstrated the utility of the approach in understanding the relative importance of various pathways of abnormal development and in providing a basis for models that incorporate species-specific response parameters. Ultimately, biologically based dose-response (BBDR) models will need to be generalizable across dose, route of exposure, species, and perhaps even chemicals of similar mechanistic classes. Understanding the mode of action for any toxicant, including developmental toxicants, can greatly inform the human risk assessment process. Although the construction of BBDR models exemplifies the extent of sophistication and quantification to which such exercises can be pursued, even more qualitative information on modes of

action can have a great impact on the interpretation of developmental toxicity test results. For excellent examples of the utility of mode of action information, the reader is referred to an issue of *Critical Reviews in Toxicology* (September–October, 2005;35) devoted to this topic. Developmental toxicants for which mode of action is discussed include ethylene glycol (Corley *et al.*, 2005), nicotine (Slikker *et al.*, 2005), phthalate esters (Foster, 2005), vinclozolin (Kavlock and Cummings, 2005), valproic acid (Wiltse, 2005), hemoglobin-based oxygen carriers (Holson *et al.*, 2005), ACE inhibitors (Tabacova, 2005), and PTU (Zoeller and Crofton, 2005).

PATHWAYS TO THE FUTURE

In 2000, a committee assembled by the NRC released its report, "*Scientific Frontiers in Developmental Toxicology and Risk Assessment*" (NRC, 2000), which concluded that major

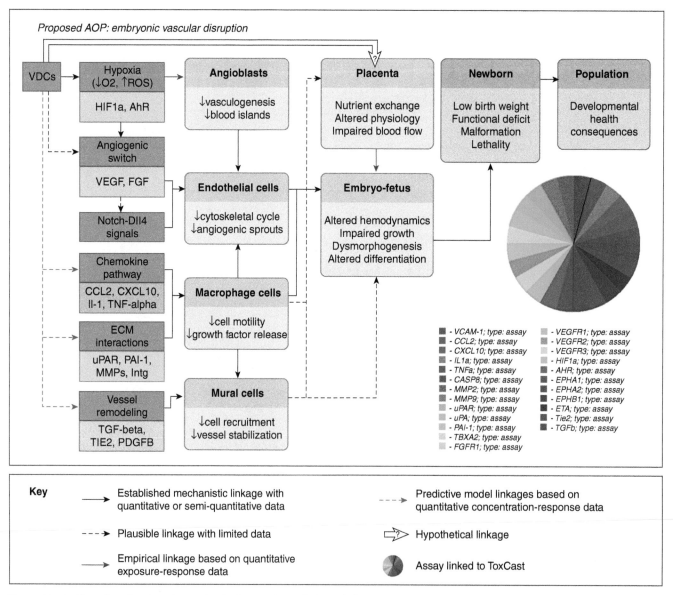

Figure 10-12. *Disruption of embryonic vascular development in predictive toxicology.* This model of an adverse outcome pathway (AOP) for embryonic vascular disruption was built using high-throughput screening data from the US Environmental Protection Agency's ToxCast database (http://actor.epa.gov/actor/faces/ToxCastDB/Home.jsp). Anchor 1 (red boxes on the left side) addresses macromolecular interactions of the toxicant with elements of the pathway. Anchor 2 (red boxes on the right) refer to relevant organismal and population responses. The middle columns address intervening cellular and organ responses. The color wheel indicates sectors for 25 ToxCast assays shown that had evidence of abnormal embryonic vascular development based on genetic mouse models and mapped to previously identified critical pathways (toxicity data were not applied to these pathways). VDC, vascular disrupting chemical. (From Knudsen and Kleinstreuer, 2011, with permission.)

discoveries have been made about mechanisms of normal development that have been conserved in diverse animals. Many of these animals have been used extensively in developmental biology and genetics, including the fruit fly, roundworm, zebrafish, frog, chick, and mouse. That these key pathways have been preserved over millions of years of evolution and speciation provides a strong scientific rationale for using these animal models for developmental toxicology. These organisms are advantageous for developmental toxicity studies due to their well-known genetics and embryology, their rapid generation time, and the ability to manipulate their genetics to probe specific developmental pathways or to incorporate human genes, such as those of drug metabolizing enzymes, to answer questions of interspecies extrapolation. As discussed above, there has been a great deal of progress over the past decade in using alternative approaches for evaluating developmental toxicity. A more recent NRC report entitled "Toxicity Testing in the 21st Century: A Vision and Strategy" (NRC, 2007) lays out an approach toward revolutionizing the way the toxicity is assessed, moving from expensive and time-consuming animal studies to high-throughput in vitro assays based on cellular toxicity pathways and analyzing outputs using a systems biology approach. This is the basis for EPA's ToxCast program discussed above, including assays relevant to developmental toxicity. Although full implementation of such approaches is probably years away, in the interim these assays should at least provide data for prioritizing chemicals for further study.

As our knowledge of the genetic control of normal development has advanced immensely in the past few years, so has the technology to examine gene expression and its control, networks of interrelated gene products, and changes in gene expression induced by alterations in the developmental environment. Advances in genomics, proteomics, metabolomics, and bioinformatics are being used to advance our understanding of health and disease, including normal and abnormal development. The ability to gather and analyze large amounts of biological data using databases and models of biological systems allows a more comprehensive approach to understanding pathways to developmental toxicity. Systems modeling and virtual tissues are among the nascent cutting-edge approaches being developed (Knudsen and Daston, 2010). An excellent example is the modeling of a proposed adverse outcome pathway for embryonic vascular disruption (Kleinstreuer et al., 2011; Knudsen and Kleinstreuer, 2011). The model includes a number of potentially responsive gene networks involved in responses to hypoxia, the angiogenic switch, extracellular matrix interactions and vessel remodeling, as well as predicted downstream consequences of disrupting these networks (Fig. 10-12).

Public sharing of data is a trend that is increasing in biology and toxicology. The ToxRefDB database at EPA mentioned above is a searchable public database of chemical toxicity results of regulatory guideline studies, and it includes data for developmental and reproductive toxicity. Knudsen et al. (2009) have extracted and analyzed rodent and rabbit maternal and developmental toxicity endpoints from ToxRefDB, providing a useful data set for comparison to tests in alternative species and other purposes. Another database, simply termed "Developmental Toxicity Database," (http://www.ilsi.org/ResearchFoundation/Pages/DevelopmentalToxicityDatabase.aspx) has recently been launched by the International Life Science Institute (ILSI) and includes maternal and developmental toxicity data from studies in rats, mice, rabbits, and hamsters. Databases such as these, along with advances in biology discussed above, will facilitate progress toward improving our ability to predict developmental toxicity reliably, quickly, and more economically.

Abbott BD, Wolf CJ, Das KP, et al. Developmental toxicity of perfluorooctane sulfonate (PFOS) is not dependent on expression of peroxisome proliferator activated receptor-alpha (PPAR alpha) in the mouse. *Reprod Toxicol.* 2009;27:258–265.

Abbott BD, Wolf CJ, Schmid JE, et al. Perfluorooctanoic acid induced developmental toxicity in the mouse is dependent on expression of peroxisome proliferator activated receptor-alpha. *Toxicol Sci.* 2007;98:571–581.

Abel EL. Consumption of alcohol during pregnancy: a review of effects on growth and development of offspring. *Hum Biol.* 1982;54:421–453.

Abel EL. Factors affecting the outcome of maternal alcohol exposure: I. Parity. *Neurobehav Toxicol Teratol.* 1984;3:49–51.

Abel EL. Fetal alcohol syndrome: a cautionary note. *Curr Pharm Des.* 2006;12:1521–1529.

Abel EL, Church MW, Dintcheff BA. Prenatal alcohol exposure shortens life span in rats. *Teratology.* 1987;36:217–220.

Ackerman JP, Riggins T, Black MM. A review of the effects of prenatal cocaine exposure among school-aged children. *Pediatrics.* 2010;125:554–565.

Adams J. The neurobehavioral teratology of retinoids: a 50-year history. *Birth Defects Res A Clin Mol Teratol.* 2010;88:895–905.

Addis A, Moretti ME, Ahmed Syed F, et al. Fetal effects of cocaine: an updated meta-analysis. *Reprod Toxicol.* 2001;15:341–369.

Adler T. The return of thalidomide. *Sci News.* 1994;146:424–425.

Ahokas RA, Dilts PV Jr, LaHaye EB. Cadmium-induced fetal growth retardation: protective effect of excess dietary zinc. *Am J Obstet Gynecol.* 1980;136:216–221.

Airhart MJ, Lee DH, Wilson TD, Miler BE, Miller MN, Skalko RG. Movement disorders and neurochemical changes in zebrafish larvae after bath exposure to fluoxetine (PROZAC). *Neurotoxicol Teratol.* 2007;29:652–664.

Alford CA, Stagno S, Reynolds DW. Perinatal infections caused by viruses, *Toxoplasma*, and *Treponema pallidum*. In: Aldjem S, Brown AK, eds. *Clinical Perinatology.* St. Louis: Mosby; 1974:31.

Allen BC, Kavlock RJ, Kimmel CA, Faustman EM. Dose response assessment for developmental toxicity: II. Comparison of generic benchmark dose models with No Observed Adverse Effect Levels. *Fundam Appl Toxicol.* 1994a;23:487–495.

Allen BC, Kavlock RJ, Kimmel CA, Faustman EM. Dose response assessment for developmental toxicity: III. Statistical models. *Fundam Appl Toxicol.* 1994b;23:496–509.

Amemiya K, Hurley LS, Keen CL. Effect of the anticarcinogenic drug 6-mercaptopurine on mineral metabolism in the mouse. *Toxicol Lett.* 1985;25:55–62.

Amemiya K, Hurley LS, Keen CL. Effect of 6-mercaptopurine on 65Zn distribution in the pregnant rat. *Teratology.* 1989;39:387–393.

Amstislavsky SY, Amstislavskaya TG, Amstislavsky VS, et al. Reproductive abnormalities in adult male mice following preimplantation exposures to estradiol or pesticide methoxychlor. *Reprod Toxicol.* 2006;21:154–159.

Amstislavsky SY, Kizilova EA, Eroschenko VP. Preimplantation mouse embryo development as a target of the pesticide methoxychlor. *Reprod Toxicol.* 2003;17:79–86.

Amstislavsky SY, Kizilova EA, Golubitsa AN, et al. Preimplantation exposures of murine embryos to estradiol or methoxychlor change postnatal development. *Reprod Toxicol.* 2004;18:103–108.

Anway MD, Memon MA, Uzumcu M, Skinner MK. Transgenerational effect of the endocrine disruptor vinclozolin on male spermatogenesis. *J Androl.* 2006;27:868–879.

Arafa HM, Elmazar MM, Hamada FM, et al. Selective agonists of retinoic acid receptors: comparative toxicokinetics and embryonic exposure. *Arch Toxicol.* 2000;73:547–556.

Argiles JM, Carbo N, Lopez-Soriano FJ. Was tumour necrosis factor-alpha responsible for the fetal malformations associated with thalidomide in the early 1960s? *Med Hypotheses.* 1998;50:313–318.

Ashby R, Davis L, Dewhurst BB, et al. Aspects of the teratology of cyclophosphamide (NSC-26271). *Cancer Treat Rep.* 1976;60:477–482.

Auger J, Kunstmann JM, Czyglik F, Jouannet P. Decline in semen quality among fertile men in Paris during the past 20 years. *N Engl J Med.* 1995;332:281–285.

Augustine K, Liu ET, Sadler TW. Antisense attenuation of Wnt-1 and Wnt-3a expression in whole embryo culture reveals roles for these genes in craniofacial, spinal cord, and cardiac morphogenesis. *Dev Genet.* 1993;14:500–520.

Baer JS, Sampson PD, Barr HM, Connor PD, Streissguth AP. A 21-year longitudinal analysis of the effects of prenatal alcohol exposure on young adult drinking. *Arch Gen Psychiatry.* 2003;60:377–385.

Bailey GP, Marien D. The value of juvenile animal studies "What have we learned from preclinical juvenile toxicity studies?" *Birth Defects Res B Dev Reprod Toxicol.* 2011;92:273–291.

Bakker H, Jaddoe VW. Cardiovascular and metabolic influences of fetal smoke exposure. *Eur J Epidemiol.* 2011;26:763–770.

Balling R, Mutter G, Gruss P, Kessel M. Craniofacial abnormalities induced by ectopic expression of the homeobox gene Hox-1.1 in transgenic mice. *Cell.* 1989;58:337–347.

Bantle JA. FETAX: a developmental toxicity assay using frog embryos. In: Rand G, ed. *Fundamentals of Aquatic Toxicology: Effects, Environmental Fate, Risk Assessment.* 2nd ed. Washington, DC: Taylor and Francis; 1995:207–230.

Barlow SM, McElhatton PR, Sullivan FM. The relation between maternal restraint and food deprivation, plasma corticosterone, and cleft palate in the offspring of mice. *Teratology.* 1975;12:97–103.

Barouki R, Gluckman PD, Grandjean P, et al. Developmental origins of non-communicable disease: implications for research and public health. *Environ Health.* 2012;11:42.

Barrier M, Jeffay S, Nichols HP, et al. Mouse embryonic stem cell adherent cell differentiation and cytotoxicity (ACDC) assay. *Reprod Toxicol.* 2011;31:383–391.

Barrow MV. A brief history of teratology to the early 20th century. *Teratology.* 1971;4:119–130.

Bartlett JB, Dredge K, Dalgleish AG. The evolution of thalidomide and its imid derivatives as anticancer agents. *Nat Rev Cancer.* 2004;4:314–322.

Bateson W. *Materials for the Study of Variation Treated With Especial Regard to Discontinuity in the Origin of Species.* London: Macmillan; 1894.

Beaty TH, Ruczinski I, Murray JC, et al. Evidence for gene-environment interaction in a genome wide study of nonsyndromic cleft palate. *Genet Epidemiol.* 2011;35:469–478.

Bedell VM, Westcot SE, Ekker SC. Lessons from morpholino-based screening in zebrafish. *Brief Funct Genomics.* 2011;10:181–188.

Beekhuijzen M, Zmarowski A, Emmen H, et al. To mate or not to mate: a retrospective analysis of two-generation studies for evaluation of criteria to trigger additional mating in the extended one-generation design. *Reprod Toxicol.* 2009;28:203–208.

Bendich A. Folic acid and neural tube defects. Introduction to Part II. *Ann NY Acad Sci.* 1993;678:108–111.

Bennett GD, Amore BM, Finnell RH, et al. Teratogenicity of carbamazepine-10,11-epoxide and oxcarbazepine in the SWV mouse. *J Pharmacol Exp Ther.* 1996;279:1237–1242.

Bennett GD, Wlodarczyk B, Calvin JA, et al. Valproic acid-induced alterations in growth and neurotrophic factor. *Reprod Toxicol.* 2000;14:1–11.

Beydoun H, Saftlas AF. Physical and mental health outcomes of prenatal maternal stress in human and animal studies: a review of recent evidence. *Paediatr Perinat Epidemiol.* 2008;22:438–466.

Beyer PE, Chernoff N. The induction of supernumerary ribs in rodents: role of maternal stress. *Teratogenesis Carcinog Mutagen.* 1986;6:419–429.

Bibbo M, Gill W, Azizi F, et al. Follow-up study of male and female offspring of DES-exposed mothers. *Obstet Gynecol.* 1977;49:1–8.

Biegel LB, Flaws JA, Hirshfield AN, et al. 90-day feeding and one-generation reproduction study in Crl:CD BR rats with 17 beta-estradiol. *Toxicol Sci.* 1998;44:116–142.

Boumela I, Assou S, Aouacheria A, et al. Involvement of BCL2 family members in the regulation of human oocyte and early embryo survival and death: gene expression and beyond. *Reproduction.* 2011;141:549–561.

Bowman RE. Behavioral sequelae of toxicant exposure during neurobehavioral development. In: Hunt VR, Smith MK, Worth D, eds. *Banbury Report 11: Environmental Factors in Human Growth and Development.* Cold Spring Harbor, NY: Cold Spring Harbor Laboratory Press; 1982: 283–294.

Branham WS, Zehr DR, Chen JJ, Sheehan DM. Uterine abnormalities in rats exposed neonatally to diethylstilbestrol, ethynyl estradiol, or clomiphene citrate. *Toxicology.* 1998;51:201–212.

Brannen KC, Panzica-Kelly JM, Danberry TL, et al. Development of a zebrafish embryo teratogenicity assay and quantitative prediction model. *Birth Defects Res B Dev Reprod Toxicol.* 2010;89:66–77.

Branum AM, Collman GW, Correa A, et al. The National Children's Study of environmental effects on child health and development. *Environ Health Perspect.* 2003;111:642–646.

Brent RL, Beckman DA. Environmental teratogens. *Bull NY Acad Med.* 1990;66:123–163.

Brown NA. Selection of test chemicals for the ECVAM international validation study on in vitro embryotoxicity tests. European Centre for the Validation of Alternative Methods. *Altern Lab Anim.* 2002;30:177–198.

Brown NA, Fabro S. Quantitation of rat embryonic development in vitro: a morphological scoring system. *Teratology.* 1981;24:65–78.

Bruin JE, Gerstein HC, Holloway AC. Long-term consequences of fetal and neonatal nicotine exposure: a critical review. *Toxicol Sci.* 2010;116:364–374.

Bujan L, Mansat A, Pontonnier F, Mieusset R. Time series analysis of sperm concentration in fertile men in Toulouse, France between 1977 and 1992. *Br Med J.* 1996;312:471–472.

Cagen SZ, Waechter JM, Dimond SS, et al. Normal reproductive organ development in CF-1 mice following prenatal exposure to Bisphenol A. *Toxicol Sci.* 1999;50:36–44.

Calabrese L, Fleischer AB. Thalidomide: current and potential clinical applications. *Am J Med.* 2000;108:487–495.

Carlsen E, Giwercman A, Keiding N, Skakkebaek NE. Evidence for decreasing quality of semen during past 50 years. *Br Med J.* 1992;305:609–613.

Carney EW. Maternally mediated developmental toxicity. In: McQueen CA, ed. *Comprehensive Toxicology.* 2nd ed., Vol 12. Daston GP, Knudsen TB, eds. *Developmental Toxicology,* New York: Elsevier; 2010:163–176.

Carney EW, Scialli AR, Watson RE, et al. Mechanisms regulating toxicant disposition to the embryo during early pregnancy: an interspecies comparison. *Birth Defects Res C Embryo Today.* 2004;72:345–360.

Carney EW, Sciali AR, Watson RE, DeSesso JM. Mechanisms regulating toxicant disposition to the embryo during early pregnancy: an interspecies comparison. *Birth Defects Res Part C.* 2005;72:345–360.

Carney EW, Tornesi B, Keller C, et al. Refinement of a morphological scoring system for postimplantation rabbit conceptuses. *Birth Defects Res B Dev Reprod Toxicol.* 2007;80:213–222.

Carruthers CM, Foster PM. Critical window of male reproductive tract development in rats following gestational exposure to di-n-butyl phthalate. *Birth Defects Res B Dev Reprod Toxicol.* 2005;74:277–285.

Centers for Disease Control and Prevention. Use of vitamins containing folic acid among women of childbearing age—United States, 2004. *MMWR Morb Mortal Wkly Rep.* 2004;36:847–850.

Centers for Disease Control and Prevention. *MMWR.* 1982;31(42):565–566.

Centers for Disease Control and Prevention. *MMWR.* 1983;32(33):438–439.

Chambers CD, Scialli A. Epidemiological factors in developmental toxicology. In: McQueen CA, ed. *Comprehensive Toxicology.* 2nd ed., Vol 12. Daston GP, Knudsen TB, eds. *Developmental Toxicology.* New York: Elsevier; 2010:135–144.

Chambon P. The retinoid signaling pathway: molecular and genetic analyses. *Semin Cell Biol.* 1994;5:115–125.

Chandler KJ, Barrier M, Jeffay S, et al. Evaluation of 309 environmental chemicals using a mouse embryonic stem cell adherent cell differentiation and cytotoxicity assay. *PLoS One.* 2011;6:e18540.

Chandy S, Abraham AM, Jana AK, et al. Congenital rubella syndrome and rubella in Vellore, South India. *Epidemiol Infect.* 2011;139:962–966.

Chapin R, Augustine-Rauch K, Beyer B, et al. State of the art in developmental toxicity screening methods and a way forward: a meeting report addressing embryonic stem cells, whole embryo culture, and zebrafish. *Birth Defects Res B Dev Reprod Toxicol.* 2008;83:446–456.

Chen M, Doherty SD, Hsu S. Innovative uses of thalidomide. *Dermatol Clin.* 2010;28:577–586.

Chernoff N, Kavlock RJ. An in vivo teratology screen utilizing pregnant mice. *J Environ Toxicol Health.* 1982;10:541–550.

Chernoff N, Rogers JM, Alles AJ, et al. Cell cycle alterations and cell death in cyclophosphamide teratogenesis. *Teratogenesis Carcinog Mutagen.* 1989;9:199–209.

Chernoff N, Setzer RW, Miller DM, et al. Effects of chemically-induced maternal toxicity on prenatal development in the rat. *Teratology.* 1990;42:651–658.

Clark DO. Pharmacokinetic studies in developmental toxicology: practical considerations and approaches. *Toxicol Meth.* 1993;3:223–251.

Clark DO, Elswick BA, Welsch F, Conolly R. Pharmacokinetics of 2-methoxyethanol and 2-methoxyacetic acid in the pregnant mouse: a physiologically based mathematical model. *Toxicol Appl Pharmacol.* 1993;121:239–252.

Clark RL, Antonello JM, Grosman SJ, et al. External genitalia abnormalities in male rats exposed in utero to finasteride, a 5α-reductase inhibitor. *Teratology.* 1990;42:91–100.

Clark RL, Robertson RT, Minsker DH, et al. Diflunisal-induced maternal anemia as a cause of teratogenicity in rabbits. *Teratology.* 1984;30:319–332.

Clarren SK, Sampson PD, Larsen J, et al. Facial effects of fetal alcohol exposure: assessment by photographs and morphometric analysis. *Am J Med Genet.* 1987;26:651–666.

Claudio L, Bearer CF, Wallinga D. Assessment of the US Environmental Protection Agency methods for identification of hazards to developing organisms: Part II. The developmental toxicity testing guideline. *Am J Ind Med.* 1999;35:554–563.

Cohlan SQ. Congenital anomalies in the rat produced by excessive intake of vitamin A during pregnancy. *Pediatrics.* 1954;13:556–567.

Collins MD, Mao GE. Teratology of retinoids. *Annu Rev Pharmacol Toxicol.* 1999;39:399–430.

Cook JC, Johnson L, O'Connor JC, et al. Effects of dietary 17β-estradiol exposure on serum hormone concentrations and testicular parameters in male Crl:CD BR rats. *Toxicol Sci.* 1998;44:155–168.

Cooper LZ, Krugman S. Diagnosis and management: congenital rubella. *Pediatrics.* 1966;37:335–342.

Cooper RL. Current developments in reproductive toxicity testing of pesticides. *Reprod Toxicol.* 2009;28:180–187.

Cooper WO, Hernandez-Diaz S, Arbogast PG, et al. Major congenital malformations after first-trimester exposure to ACE inhibitors. *N Engl J Med.* 2006;354:2443–2451.

Corley RA. Pharmacokinetics and PBPK models. In: McQueen CA, ed. *Comprehensive Toxicology.* 2nd ed., Vol 12. Daston GP, Knudsen TB, eds. *Developmental Toxicology.* New York: Elsevier; 2010:27–58.

Corley RA, Mast TJ, Carney EW, Rogers JM, Daston GP. Evaluation of physiologically based models of pregnancy and lactation for their application in children's health risk assessments. *Crit Rev Toxicol.* 2003;33:137–211.

Corley RA, Meek ME, Carney EW. Mode of action: oxalate crystal-induced renal tubule degeneration and glycolic acid-induced dysmorphogenesis—renal and developmental effects of ethylene glycol. *Crit Rev Toxicol.* 2005;35:691–702.

Craig JC, Bennett GD, Miranda RC, et al. Ribonucleotide reductase subunit R1: a gene conferring sensitivity to valproic acid-induced neural tube defects in mice. *Teratology.* 2000;61:305–313.

Crump KS. A new method for determining allowable daily intakes. *Fundam Appl Toxicol.* 1984;4:854–871.

Cupul-Uicab LA, Baird DD, Skjaerven R, Saha-Chaudhuri P, Haug K, Longnecker MP. In utero exposure to maternal smoking and women's risk of fetal loss in the Norwegian mother and child cohort (MoBa). *Environ Health Perspect.* 2012;120:355–360.

Czeizel AE. Periconceptional folic acid-containing multivitamin supplementation for the prevention of neural tube defects and cardiovascular malformations. *Ann Nutr Metab.* 2011;59:38–40.

Czeizel AE, Dudas I, Paput L, et al. Prevention of neural-tube defects with periconceptional folic acid, methylfolate, or multivitamins? *Ann Nutr Metab.* 2011;58:263–271.

D'Amato RJ, Loughman MS, Flynn E, Folkman J. Thalidomide is an inhibitor of angiogenesis. *Proc Natl Acad Sci.* 1994;91:4082–4085.

Dai WS, LaBraico JM, Stern RS. Epidemiology of isotretinoin exposure during pregnancy. *J Am Acad Dermatol.* 1992;26:599–606.

Dareste C. *Récherches sur la production artificielle des monstruosités, ou essais de tératogénie expérimentale.* Paris: Reinwald; 1877.

Dareste C. *Récherches sur la production artificielle des monstruosités, ou essais de tératogénie expérimentale.* 2nd ed. Paris: Reinwald; 1891.

Daston GP. Fetal zinc deficiency as a mechanism for cadmium-induced toxicity to the developing rat lung and pulmonary surfactant. *Toxicology.* 1982;24:55–63.

Daston GP. Do thresholds exist for developmental toxicants? A review of the theoretical and experimental evidence. In: Kalter H, ed. *Issues and Review in Teratology.* New York: Plenum Press; 1993:169–197.

Daston GP. Relationships between maternal and developmental toxicity. In: Kimmel CA, Buelke-Sam J, eds. *Developmental Toxicology.* 2nd ed. New York: Raven Press; 1994:189–212.

Daston GP. The theoretical and empirical case for in vitro developmental toxicity screens, and potential applications. *Teratology.* 1996;53:339–344.

Daston GP, Knudsen TB. Fundamental concepts, current regulatory design and interpretation. In: McQueen CA, ed. *Comprehensive Toxicology.* 2nd ed., Vol 12. Daston GP, Knudsen TB, eds. *Developmental Toxicology.* New York: Elsevier; 2010:3–9.

Daston GP, Overmann GJ, Taubeneck MW, Lehman-Mckeeman LD, Rogers JM, Keen CL. The role of metallothionein induction and altered zinc status in maternally mediated developmental toxicity: comparison of the effects of urethane and styrene in rats. *Toxicol Appl Pharmacol.* 1991;110:450–463.

Davis JA, Gift JS, Zhao QJ. Introduction to benchmark dose methods and U.S. EPA's benchmark dose software (BMDS) version 2.1.1. *Toxicol Appl Pharmacol.* 2011;254:181–191.

de Mouzon J, Thonneau P, Spira A, Multigner L. Semen quality has declined among men born in France since 1950. *Br Med J.* 1996;313:43.

De Santis M, Cavaliere AF, Straface G, Caruso A. Rubella infection in pregnancy. *Reprod Toxicol.* 2006;21:390–398.

Deschamps J, van Nes J. Developmental regulation of the Hox genes during axial morphogenesis in the mouse. *Development.* 2005;132:2931–2942.

DeSesso JM. Maternal factors in developmental toxicity. *Teratogenesis Carcinog Mutagen.* 1987;7:225–240.

Diamanti-Kandarakis E, Bourguignon JP, Giudice LC, et al. Endocrine-disrupting chemicals: an Endocrine Society scientific statement. *Endocr Rev.* 2009;30:293–342.

Dietert RR. Developmental immunotoxicology (DIT): windows of vulnerability, immune dysfunction and safety assessment. *J Immunotoxicol.* 2008;5:401–412.

Dietrich M, Brown CJ, Block G. The effect of folate fortification of cereal-grain products on blood folate status, dietary folate intake, and dietary folate sources among adult non-supplement users in the United States. *J Am Coll Nutr.* 2005;24:266–274.

Doering PL, Boothby LA, Cheok M. Review of pregnancy labeling of prescription drugs: is the current system adequate to inform of risks? *Am J Obstet Gynecol.* 2002;187:333–339.

Dolinoy DC, Weidman JR, Waterland RA, Jirtle RL. Maternal genistein alters coat color and protects Avy mouse offspring from obesity by modifying the fetal epigenome. *Environ Health Perspect.* 2006;114:567–572.

Downing C, Biers J, Larson C, et al. Genetic and maternal effects on valproic acid teratogenesis in C57BL/6J and DBA/2J mice. *Toxicol Sci.* 2010;116:632–639.

Dreosti IE. Nutritional factors underlying the expression of the fetal alcohol syndrome. *Ann NY Acad Sci.* 1993;678:193–204.

Dunkel Schetter C, Tanner L. Anxiety, depression and stress in pregnancy: implications for mothers, children, research, and practice. *Curr Opin Psychiatry.* 2012;25:141–148.

Dupe V, Ghyselinck NB, Thomazy V, et al. Essential roles of retinoic acid signaling in interdigital apoptosis and control of BMP-7 expression in mouse autopods. *Dev Biol.* 1999;208:30–43.

Edwards MJ. Hyperthermia as a teratogen: a review of experimental studies and their clinical significance. *Teratog Carcinog Mutag.* 1986;6:563–582.

Edwards MJ. Hyperthermia and fever during pregnancy. *Birth Defects Res A Clin Mol Teratol.* 2006;76:507–516.

Ehlers K, Sturje H, Merker HJ, et al. Valproic acid-induced spina bifida: a mouse model. *Teratology.* 1992a;45:145–154.

Ehlers K, Sturje H, Merker H-J, Nau H. Spina bifida aperta induced by valproic acid and by all-*trans*-retinoic acid in the mouse: distinct differences in morphology and periods of sensitivity. *Teratology*. 1992b;46: 117–130.

Eibs HG, Speilman H, Hagele M. Teratogenic effects of cyproterone acetate and medroxyprogesterone treatment during the pre- and postimplantation period of mouse embryos. *Teratology*. 1982;25:27–36.

Eikel D, Lampen A, Nau H. Teratogenic effects mediated by inhibition of histone deacetylases: evidence from quantitative structure activity relationships of 20 valproic acid derivatives. *Chem Res Toxicol*. 2006; 19:272–278.

Ellis-Hutchings RG, Carney EW. Whole embryo culture: a "New" technique that enabled decades of mechanistic discoveries. *Birth Defects Res B Dev Reprod Toxicol*. 2010;89:304–312.

Elstein KH, Zucker RM, Andrews JE, et al. Effects of developmental stage and tissue type on embryo/fetal DNA distributions and 5-fluorouracil-induced cell-cycle perturbations. *Teratology*. 1993;48:355–363.

Entringer S, Buss C, Wadhwa PD. Prenatal stress and developmental programming of human health and disease risk: concepts and integration of empirical findings. *Curr Opin Endocrinol Diabetes Obes*. 2010;17:507–516.

Eriksson P, Lundkvist U, Fredricksson A. Neonatal exposure to 3,4,3′,4′-tetrachlorobiphenyl: changes in spontaneous behavior and cholinergic muscarinic receptors in the adult mouse. *Toxicology*. 1991;69:27–34.

Ernhart CB, Sokol RJ, Martier S, et al. Alcohol teratogenicity in the human: a detailed assessment of specificity, critical period and threshold. *Am J Obstet Gynecol*. 1987;156:33–39.

Euker JS, Riegle GD. Effect of stress on pregnancy in the rat. *J Reprod Fertil*. 1973;34:343–346.

Fabro S. Passage of drugs and other chemicals into the uterine fluids and preimplantation blastocyst. In: Boreus L, ed. *Fetal Pharmacology*. New York: Raven Press; 1973:443–461.

Fabro S, McLachlan JA, Dames NM. Chemical exposure of embryos during the preimplantation stages of pregnancy: mortality rate and intrauterine development. *Am J Obstet Gynecol*. 1984;148:929–938.

Faiella A, Wernig M, Consalez GG, et al. A mouse model for valproate teratogenicity: parental effects, homeotic transformations, and altered HOX expression. *Hum Mol Genet*. 2000;9:227–236.

Fantel AG, Greenaway JC, Juchau MR, Shepard TH. Teratogenic bioactivation of cyclophosphamide in vitro. *Life Sci*. 1979;25:67–72.

Faustman EM, Allen BC, Kavlock RJ, Kimmel CA. Dose response assessment for developmental toxicity: I. Characterization of database and determination of No Observed Adverse Effect Levels. *Fundam Appl Toxicol*. 1994;23:478–486.

Ferm VH, Carpenter SJ. Teratogenic effect of cadmium and its inhibition by zinc. *Nature*. 1967;216:1123.

Ferm VH, Carpenter SJ. The relationship of cadmium and zinc in experimental mammalian teratogenesis. *Lab Invest*. 1968;18:429–432.

Finnell RH, Gelineau-van Waes J, Bennett GD, et al. Genetic basis of susceptibility to environmentally induced neural tube defects. *Ann NY Acad Sci*. 2000;919:261–277.

Finnell RH, Wlodarczyk BC, Craig JC, et al. Strain-dependent alterations in the expression of folate pathway genes following teratogenic exposure to valproic acid in a mouse model. *Am J Med Genet*. 1997;70:303–311.

Fisch H, Goluboff ET. Geographic variation in sperm counts: a potential cause of bias in studies of semen quality. *Fertil Steril*. 1996;65: 1044–1046.

Fisher JW, Whitaker TA, Taylor DH, et al. Physiologically based pharmocokinetic modeling of the pregnant rat: a multiroute exposure model for trichloroethylene and its metabolite, trichloroacetic acid. *Toxicol Appl Pharmacol*. 1989;99:395–414.

Fleming P, Blair PS. Sudden infant death syndrome and parental smoking. *Early Hum Dev*. 2007;83:721–725.

Fort DJ, Paul RR. Enhancing the predictive validity of Frog Embryo Teratogenesis Assay—Xenopus (FETAX). *J Appl Toxicol*. 2002;22: 185–191.

Fort DJ, Rogers RL, Thomas JH, Buzzard BO, Noll AM, Spaulding CD. Comparative sensitivity of *Xenopus tropicalis* and *Xenopus laevis* as test species for the FETAX model. *J Appl Toxicol*. 2004;24:443–457.

Fort DJ, Stover EL, Farmer DR, Lemen JK. Assessing the predictive validity of frog embryo teratogenesis assay—Xenopus (FETAX). *Teratogenesis Carcinog Mutagen*. 2000;20:87–98.

Foster PM. Mode of action: impaired fetal leydig cell function—effects on male reproductive development produced by certain phthalate esters. *Crit Rev Toxicol*. 2005;35:713–719.

Francis BM, Rogers JM, Sulik KK, et al. Cyclophosphamide teratogenesis: evidence for compensatory responses to induced cellular toxicity. *Teratology*. 1990;42:473–482.

Frankos VH. FDA perspectives on the use of teratology data for human risk assessment. *Fundam Appl Toxicol*. 1985;5:615–622.

Fraysse B, Mons R, Garric J. Development of a zebrafish 4-day embryo-larval bioassay to assess toxicity of chemicals. *Ecotoxicol Environ Saf*. 2006;63:253–267.

Fried PA, Watkinson B, Gray R. Differential effects on cognitive functioning in 9- to 12-year olds prenatally exposed to cigarettes and marihuana. *Neurotoxicol Teratol*. 1998;20:293–306.

Friedman JM. ACE inhibitors and congenital anomalies. *N Engl J Med*. 2006;354:2498–2500.

Friedman JM. How do we know if an exposure is actually teratogenic in humans? *Am J Med Genet C Semin Med Genet*. 2011;157: 170–174.

Fullerton PM, Kermer M. Neuropathy after intake of thalidomide. *Br Med J*. 1961;2:855–858.

Gabrielson JL, Larson KS. Proposals for improving risk assessment in reproductive toxicology. *Pharmacol Toxicol*. 1990;66:10–17.

Gabrielson JL, Paalkow LK. A physiological pharmacokinetic model for morphine disposition in the pregnant rat. *J Pharmacokinet Biopharm*. 1983;11:147–163.

Gargas ML, Tyler TR, Sweeney LM, et al. A toxicokinetic study of inhaled ethylene glycol monomethyl ether (2-ME) and validation of a physiologically based pharmacokinetic model for the pregnant rat and human. *Toxicol Appl Pharmacol*. 2000;165:53–62.

Gaylor DW, Chen JJ. Dose response models for developmental malformations. *Teratology*. 1993;47:291–297.

Gaylor DW, Razzaghi M. Process of building biologically based dose response models for developmental defects. *Teratology*. 1992;46: 573–581.

Gaylor DW, Sheehan DM, Young JF, Mattison DR. The threshold dose question in teratogenesis. *Teratology*. 1988;38:389–391.

Gellert RJ. Kepone, mirex, dieldrin and aldrin: estrogenic activity and the induction of persistent vaginal estrus and anovulation in rats following prenatal treatment. *Environ Res*. 1978;16:131–138.

Generoso WM, Rutledge JC, Cain KT, et al. Exposure of female mice to ethylene oxide within hours after mating leads to fetal malformations and death. *Mutat Res*. 1987;176:269–274.

Generoso WM, Rutledge JC, Cain KT, et al. Mutagen-induced fetal anomalies and death following treatment of females within hours after mating. *Mutat Res*. 1988;199:175–181.

Genschow E, Scholz G, Brown N, et al. Development of prediction models for three in vitro embryotoxicity tests in an ECVAM validation study. *In Vitro Mol Toxicol*. 2000;13:51–65.

Genschow E, Spielmann H, Scholz G, et al. The ECVAM international validation study on in vitro embryotoxicity tests: results of the definitive phase and evaluation of prediction models. European Centre for the Validation of Alternative Methods. *Altern Lab Anim*. 2002;30: 151–176.

Genschow E, Spielmann H, Scholz G, et al. Validation of the embryonic stem cell test in the international ECVAM validation study on three in vitro embryotoxicity tests. *Altern Lab Anim*. 2004;32:209–244.

George L, Granath F, Johansson AL, Anneren G, Cnattingius S. Environmental tobacco smoke and risk of spontaneous abortion. *Epidemiology*. 2006;17:500–505.

Gilbert ME. Impact of low-level thyroid hormone disruption induced by propylthiouracil on brain development and function. *Toxicol Sci*. 2011;124:432–445.

Gilliland FD, Berhane K, McConnell R, et al. Maternal smoking during pregnancy, environmental tobacco smoke exposure and childhood lung function. *Thorax*. 2000;55:271–276.

Gluckman PD, Hanson MA, Low FM. The role of developmental plasticity and epigenetics in human health. *Birth Defects Res C Embryo Today.* 2011;93:12–18.

Goldey ES, Crofton KM. Thyroxine replacement attenuates hypothyroxinemia, hearing loss and motor deficits following developmental exposure to Arochlor 1254 in rats. *Toxicol Sci.* 1998;45:94–105.

Goldey ES, Kehn LS, Lau C, et al. Developmental exposure to polychlorinated biphenyls (Arochlor 1254) reduces circulating thyroid hormone concentrations and causes hearing deficits in rats. *Toxicol Appl Pharmacol.* 1995;135:77–88.

Gomes-Carneiro MR, De-Oliveira AC, De-Carvalho RR, et al. Inhibition of cyclophosphamide-induced teratogenesis by beta-ionone. *Toxicol Lett.* 2003;138:205–213.

Gorsuch RL, Key MK. Abnormalities of pregnancy as a function of anxiety and life stress. *Psychosom Med.* 1974;36:352–362.

Gouin K, Murphy K, Shah PS, et al. Effects of cocaine use during pregnancy on low birth weight and preterm birth: systematic review and meta-analyses. *Am J Obstet Gynecol.* 2011;204:340e1–340e12.

Grace CE, Kim SJ, Rogers JM. Maternal influences on epigenetic programming of the developing hypothalamic-pituitary-adrenal axis. *Birth Defects Res A Clin Mol Teratol.* 2011;91:797–805.

Graham A, Papoalopulu N, Krumlauf R. The murine and *Drosophila* homeobox gene complexes have common features of organization and expression. *Cell.* 1989;57:367–378.

Gray LE, Ostby J, Ferrell J, et al. A dose–response analysis of methoxychlor-induced alterations of reproductive development and function in the rat. *Fundam Appl Toxicol.* 1989;12:92–108.

Gray LE, Ostby JS, Kelce WR. Developmental effects of an environmental anti-androgen: the fungicide vinclozolin alters sex differentiation of the male rat. *Toxicol Appl Pharmacol.* 1994;129:46–52.

Gray LE, Ostby J, Kelce WR. A dose–response analysis of the reproductive effects of a single gestational dose of 2,3,7,8-tetrachloro-p-dioxin (TCDD) in male Long Evans Hooded rat offspring. *Toxicol Appl Pharmacol.* 1997a;146:11–20.

Gray LE, Wold C, Mann P, Ostby JS. In utero exposure to low doses of 2,3,7,8-tetrachloro-p-dioxin (TCDD) alters reproductive development of female Long Evans Hooded rat offspring. *Toxicol Appl Pharmacol.* 1997b;146:237–244.

Gregg NM. Congenital cataract following German measles in the mother. *Trans Ophthalmol Soc Aust.* 1941;3:35–40.

Guenther TM, Mannering GT. Induction of hepatic monooxygenase systems of pregnant rats with phenobarbital and 3-methylcholanthrene. *Biochem Pharmacol.* 1977;26:577–584.

Guo YL, Lin CJ, Yao WJ, Ryan JJ, Hsu CC. Musculoskeletal changes in children prenatally exposed to polychlorinated biphenyls and related compounds (Yu-Cheng children). *J Toxicol Environ Health.* 1994;41:83–93.

Guzelian PS. Comparative toxicology of chlordecone (kepone) in humans and experimental animals. *Annu Rev Pharmacol Toxicol.* 1982;22:89–113.

Guzelian PS, Henry CJ, Olin SS, eds. *Similarities and Differences Between Children & Adults: Implications for Risk Assessment.* Washington, DC: ILSI Press; 1992.

Hackshaw A, Rodeck C, Boniface S. Maternal smoking in pregnancy and birth defects: a systematic review based on 173 687 malformed cases and 11.7 million controls. *Hum Reprod Update.* 2011;17:589–604.

Hale F. Pigs born without eyeballs. *J Hered.* 1935;27:105–106.

Hales B. Comparison of the mutagenicity of cyclophosphamide and its active metabolites, 4-hydroxycyclophosphamide, phosphoramide mustard and acrolein. *Cancer Res.* 1982;42:3018–3021.

Hales B. Relative mutagenicity and teratogenicity of cyclophosphamide and two of its structural analogs. *Biochem Pharmacol.* 1983;32:3791–3795.

Hales BF. Modification of the teratogenicity and mutagenicity of cyclophosphamide with thiol compounds. *Teratology.* 1981;23:373–381.

Hales BF. Effects of phosphoramide mustard and acrolein, cytotoxic metabolites of cyclophosphamide, on mouse limb development in vitro. *Teratology.* 1989;40:11–20.

Hales BF, Grenier L, Lalancette C, et al. Epigenetic programming: from gametes to blastocyst. *Birth Defects Res A Clin Mol Teratol.* 2011;91:652–665.

Hall DL, Payne LA, Putnam JM, et al. Effect of methoxychlor on implantation and embryo development in the mouse. *Reprod Toxicol.* 1997;11:703–708.

Handler A, Davis F, Ferre C, Yeko T. The relationship of smoking and ectopic pregnancy. *Am J Public Health.* 1989;79:1239–1242.

Hannas BR, Lambright CS, Furr J, et al. Dose-response assessment of fetal testosterone production and gene expression levels in rat testes following in utero exposure to diethylhexyl phthalate, diisobutyl phthalate, diisoheptyl phthalate, and diisononyl phthalate. *Toxicol Sci.* 2011;123:206–216.

Hansen DK. Developmental toxicity of antiepileptic drugs. In: McQueen CA, ed. *Comprehensive Toxicology.* 2nd ed., Vol 12. Daston GP, Knudsen TB, eds. *Developmental Toxicology.* New York: Elsevier; 2010:177–187.

Hansen DK, Billings RE. Phenytoin teratogenicity and effects on embryonic and maternal folate metabolism. *Teratology.* 1985;31:363–371.

Hansen DK, Dial SL, Terry KK, et al. In vitro embryotoxicity of carbamazepine and carbamazepine-10, 11-epoxide. *Teratology.* 1996;54:45–51.

Hansen DK, Hodes ME. Comparative teratogenicity of phenytoin among several inbred strains of mice. *Teratology.* 1983;28:175–179.

Hansen JM, Carney EW, Harris C. Differential alteration by thalidomide of the glutathione content of rat vs rabbit conceptuses in vitro. *Reprod Toxicol.* 1999;13:547–554.

Hansen JM, Harris C. A novel hypothesis for thalidomide-induced limb teratogenesis: redox misregulation of the NF-kappaB pathway. *Antioxid Redox Signal.* 2004;6:1–14.

Hansen JM, Harris KK, Philbert MA, Harris C. Thalidomide modulates nuclear redox status and preferentially depletes glutathione in rabbit limb versus rat limb. *J Pharmacol Exp Ther.* 2002;300:768–776.

Hanson JW, Smith DW. The fetal hydantoin syndrome. *J Pediatr.* 1975;87:285–290.

Hardin BD, Becker RJ, Kavlock RJ, et al. Overview and summary: workshop on the Chernoff/Kavlock preliminary developmental toxicity test. *Teratogenesis Carcinog Mutagen.* 1987;7:119–127.

Hartig PC, Hunter ES III. Gene delivery to the neurulating embryo during culture. *Teratology.* 1998;58:103–112.

Hauck R-S, Nau H. The enantiomers of the valproic acid analogue 2-*n*-propylpentyoic acid (4-yn-VPA): Asymmetric synthesis and highly stereoselective teratogenicity in mice. *Pharm Res.* 1992;9:850–854.

Haug K, Irgens LM, Skjaerven R, et al. Maternal smoking and birthweight: effect modification of period, maternal age and paternal smoking. *Acta Obstet Gynecol Scand.* 2000;79:485–489.

Hays SM, Elswick BA, Blumenthal GM, et al. Development of a physiologically based pharmacokinetic model of 2-methoxyethanol and 2-methoxyacetic acid disposition in pregnant rats. *Toxicol Appl Pharmacol.* 2000;163:67–74.

Heinrichs WL, Gellert RJ, Bakke JL, Lawrence NL. DDT administered to neonatal rats induces persistent estrus syndrome. *Science.* 1971;173:642–643.

Helene C, Toulme JJ. Specific regulation of gene expression by antisense, sense and antigene nucleic acids. *Biochim Biophys Acta.* 1990;1049:99–125.

Hellemans KG, Sliwowska JH, Verma P, et al. Prenatal alcohol exposure: fetal programming and later life vulnerability to stress, depression and anxiety disorders. *Neurosci Biobehav Rev.* 2010;34:791–807.

Helm FC, Frankus E, Friderichs E, et al. Comparative teratological investigation of compounds structurally related to thalidomide. *Arnz Forsch Drug Res.* 1981;31:941–949.

Herbst AL, Cole P, Colton T, et al. Age-incidence and risk of diethylstilbestrol-related clear cell adenocarcinoma of the vagina and cervix. *Am J Obstet Gynecol.* 1977;128:43–50.

Hernandez-Martinez R, Covarrubias L. Interdigital cell death function and regulation: new insights on an old programmed cell death model. *Dev Growth Differ.* 2011;53:245–258.

Higuchi TT, Palmer JS, Gray LE Jr, Veeramachaneni DN. Effects of dibutyl phthalate in male rabbits following in utero, adolescent, or postpubertal exposure. *Toxicol Sci.* 2003;72:301–313.

Hirsch KS, Scott WJ Jr. Searching for the mechanism of acetazolamide teratogenesis. In: Kalter H, ed. *Issues and Reviews in Teratology.* Vol 1. New York: Plenum Press; 1983:309–347.

Holladay SD, Luster MI. Developmental immunotoxicology. In: Kimmel CA, Buelke-Sam J, eds. *Developmental Toxicology.* 2nd ed. New York: Raven Press; 1994:93–117.

Holson JF, Stump DG, Pearce LB, Watson RE, DeSesso JM. Mode of action: yolk sac poisoning and impeded histiotrophic nutrition—HBOC-related congenital malformations. *Crit Rev Toxicol.* 2005;35: 739–745.

Hotchkiss AK, Rider CV, Furr J, et al. In utero exposure to an AR antagonist plus an inhibitor of fetal testosterone synthesis induces cumulative effects on F1 male rats. *Reprod Toxicol.* 2010;30:261–270.

Hsu S-T, Ma C-I, Hsu SK, et al. Discovery and epidemiology of PCB poisoning in Taiwan: a four-year followup. *Environ Health Perspect.* 1985;59:5–10.

Huang WW, Yin Y, Bi Q, et al. Developmental diethylstilbestrol exposure alters genetic pathways of uterine cytodifferentiation. *Mol Endocrinol.* 2005;19:669–682.

Hurtt ME, Daston G, Davis-Bruno K, et al. Juvenile animal studies: testing strategies and design. *Birth Defects Res B Dev Reprod Toxicol.* 2004;71:281–288.

Hytten FE. Physiologic changes in the mother related to drug handling. In: Krauer B, Hytten F, del Pozo E, eds. *Drugs and Pregnancy.* New York: Academic Press; 1984:7–17.

Imperato-McGinley J, Sanchez R, Spencer JR, Yee B, Vaughan ED. Comparison of the effects of the 5α-reductase inhibitor finasteride and the antiandrogen flutamide on prostate and genital differentiation: dose-response studies. *Endocrinology.* 1992;131:1149–1156.

Irl C, Hasford J. Assessing the safety of drugs in pregnancy: the role of prospective cohort studies. *Drug Saf.* 2000;22:169–177.

Irvine S, Cawood E, Richardson D, et al. Evidence of deteriorating semen quality in the United Kingdom: birth cohort study in 577 men in Scotland over 11 years. *Br Med J.* 1996;312:467–471.

Ito T, Ando H, Handa H. Teratogenic effects of thalidomide: molecular mechanisms. *Cell Mol Life Sci.* 2011;68:1569–1579.

Ito T, Handa H. Deciphering the mystery of thalidomide teratogenicity. *Congenit Anom (Kyoto).* 2012;52:1–7.

Jacobson J, Jacobson S, Humphrey H. Effects of exposure to PCBs and related compounds on growth and activity in children. *Neurotoxicol Teratol.* 1990;12:319–326.

Jacobson J, Jacobson S. Intellectual impairment in children exposed to polychlorinated biphenyls in utero. *N Engl J Med.* 1996;335: 783–789.

Jelovsek FR, Mattison DR, Chen JJ. Prediction of risk for human developmental toxicity: how important are animal studies for hazard identification? *Obstet Gynecol.* 1989;74:624–636.

Jones KL. The effects of alcohol on fetal development. *Birth Defects Res C Embryo Today.* 2011;93:3–11.

Jones KL, Smith DW. Recognition of the fetal alcohol syndrome in early infancy. *Lancet.* 1973;2:999–1001.

Jones KL, Smith DW, Ulleland CN, Streissguth AP. Pattern of malformation in offspring of chronic alcoholic mothers. *Lancet.* 1973;1: 1267–1271.

Jonsson NA. Chemical structure and teratogenic properties. *Acta Pharm Suecica.* 1972;9:521–542.

Joussen AM, Germann T, Kirchhof B. Effect of thalidomide and structurally related compounds on cornela angiogenesis is comparable to their teratological potency. *Graefes Arch Clin Exp Ophthalmol.* 1999;237: 952–961.

Juchau MR. Enzymatic bioactivation and inactivation of chemical teratogens and transplacental carcinogens/mutagens. In: Juchau MR, ed. *The Biochemical Basis of Chemical Teratogenesis.* New York: Elsevier/North Holland; 1981:63–94.

Juchau MR, Faustman-Watts EM. Pharmacokinetic considerations in the maternal-placental unit. *Clin Obstet Gynecol.* 1983;26:379–390.

Juchau MR, Lee QP, Fantel AG. Xenobiotic biotransformation/bioactivation in organogenesis-stage conceptual tissues: implications for embryotoxicity and teratogenesis. *Drug Metab Rev.* 1992;24: 195–238.

Juriloff DM, Fraser FC. Genetic maternal effects on cleft lip frequency in A/J and CL/Fr mice. *Teratology.* 1980;21:167–175.

Jurisicova A, Acton BM. Deadly decisions: the role of genes regulating programmed cell death in human preimplantation embryo development. *Reproduction.* 2004;128:281–291.

Kang H-G, Lee C-H, Lee K-C, et al. Effects of butylated hydroxyanisole on glutathione S-transferase activity and cyclophosphamide-induced teratogenicity in rats. *J Toxicol Pub Health.* 2003;19:181–187.

Kavlock R, Chandler K, Houck K, et al. Update on EPA's ToxCast program: providing high throughput decision support for chemical risk management. *Chem Res Toxicol.* 2012;25:1287–1302.

Kavlock R, Cummings A. Mode of action: inhibition of androgen receptor function—vinclozolin-induced malformations in reproductive development. *Crit Rev Toxicol.* 2005;35:721–726.

Kavlock RJ, Allen BC, Faustman EM, Kimmel CA. Dose response assessment for developmental toxicity: IV. Benchmark doses for fetal weight changes. *Fundam Appl Toxicol.* 1995;26:211–222.

Kavlock RJ, Chernoff N, Rogers EH. The effect of acute maternal toxicity on fetal development in the mouse. *Teratogenesis Carcinog Mutagen.* 1985;5:3–13.

Kavlock RJ, Daston GP, DeRosa D, et al. Research needs for the risk assessment of health and environmental effects of endocrine disruptors: a report of the US EPA-sponsored workshop. *Environ Health Perspect.* 1996;104(suppl 4):715–740.

Keen CL, Bendich A, Willhite CC, eds. *Maternal Nutrition and Pregnancy Outcome. Ann NY Acad Sci* 1993;678:1–372.

Keen CL, Peters JM, Hurley LS. The effect of valproic acid on ^{65}Zn distribution in the pregnant rat. *J Nutr.* 1989;119:607–611.

Keen CL, Uriu-Adams JY, Skalny A, et al. The plausibility of maternal nutritional status being a contributing factor to the risk for fetal alcohol spectrum disorders: The potential influence of zinc status as an example. *Biofactors.* 2010;36:125–135.

Kelce WR, Stone CR, Laws SC, et al. Persistent DDT metabolite p,p'-DDE is a potent androgen receptor antagonist. *Nature.* 1995;375:581–585.

Kelsey FO. Thalidomide update: regulatory aspects. *Teratology.* 1988; 38:221–226.

Kessel M, Balling R, Gruss P. Variations of cervical vertebrae after expression of a Hox-1.1 transgene in mice. *Cell.* 1990;61:301–308.

Khera KS. Maternal toxicity: a possible etiological factor in embryo/fetal deaths and fetal malformations of rodent-rabbit species. *Teratology.* 1985;31:129–153.

Khera KS. Maternal toxicity—a possible factor in fetal malformations in mice. *Teratology.* 1984;29:411–416.

Khoury MJ, Erickson JD, James LM. Maternal factors in cleft lip with or without palate: evidence from interracial crosses in the United States. *Teratology.* 1983;27:351–357.

Khoury MJ, Holtzman NA. On the ability of birth defects monitoring systems to detect new teratogens. *Am J Epidemiol.* 1987;126: 136–143.

Khoury MJ, James LM, Lynberg MC. Quantitative analysis of associations between birth defects and suspected human teratogens. *Am J Med Genet.* 1991;40:500–505.

Kim H-J, Lee J-E, Choi E-K, Kim Y-B. Effects of butylated hydroxyanisole on glutathione S-transferase activity and teratogenicity of cyclophosphamide in mice. *Korean J Lab Anim Sci.* 2003;19:120–125.

Kimmel CA, Collman GW, Fields N, Eskenazi B. Lessons learned for the National Children's Study from the National Institute of Environmental Health Sciences/U.S. Environmental Protection Agency Centers for Children's Environmental Health and Disease Prevention Research. *Environ Health Perspect.* 2005;113:1414–1418.

Kimmel CA, Cook RO, Staples RE. Teratogenic potential of noise in rats and mice. *Toxicol Appl Pharmacol.* 1976;36:239–245.

Kimmel CA, Young JF. Correlating pharmacokinetics and teratogenic endpoints. *Fundam Appl Toxicol.* 1983;3:250–255.

Klaassen CD, Lehman-McKeeman LD. Induction of metallothionein. *J Am Coll Toxicol.* 1989;8:1315–1321.

Kleinstreuer NC, Judson RS, Reif DM, et al. Environmental impact on vascular development predicted by high-throughput screening. *Environ Health Perspect.* 2011;119:1596–1603.

Kochhar DM. Teratogenic activity of retinoic acid. *Acta Pathol Microbiol Scand.* 1967;70:398–404.

Knudsen TB, Kleinstreuer NC. Disruption of embryonic vascular development in predictive toxicology. *Birth Defects Res C Embryo Today.* 2011;93:312–323.

Knudsen TB, Daston GP. Virtual tissues and developmental systems biology. In: McQueen CA, ed. *Comprehensive Toxicology.* 2nd ed., Vol 12. Daston GP, Knudsen TB, eds. *Developmental Toxicology.* New York: Elsevier; 2010:347–358.

Knudsen TB, Martin MT, Kavlock RJ, et al. Profiling the activity of environmental chemicals in prenatal developmental toxicity studies using the U.S. EPA's ToxRefDB. *Reprod Toxicol.* 2009;28:208–219.

Kola I, Vogel R, Spielmann H. Co-administration of ascorbic acid with cyclophosphamide (CPA) to pregnant mice inhibits the clastogenic activity of CPA in preimplantation murine blastocysts. *Mutagenesis.* 1989;4:297–301.

Koopman-Esseboom C, Weisglas-Kuperus N, de Ridder MAJ, et al. Effects of polychlorinated biphenyl/dioxin exposure and feeding type on infants mental and psychomotor development. *Pediatrics.* 1996;97: 700–706.

Koren G, Nulman I, Chudley AE, Loocke C. Fetal alcohol spectrum disorder. *CMAJ.* 2003;169:1181–1185.

Kotch LE, Sulik KK. Experimental fetal alcohol syndrome: proposed pathogenic basis for a variety of associated facial and brain anomalies. *Am J Med Genet.* 1992;44:168–176.

Krauer B. Physiological changes and drug disposition during pregnancy. In: Nau H, Scott WJ, eds. *Pharmacokinetics in Teratogenesis.* Vol 1. Boca Raton, FL: CRC Press; 1987:3–12.

Krtolica A, Ilic D, Genbacev O, et al. Human embryonic stem cells as a model for embryotoxicity screening. *Regen Med.* 2009;4:449–459.

Krumlauf R. *Hox* genes and pattern formation in the branchial region of the vertebrate head. *Trends Genet.* 1993;9:106–112.

Kyrklund-Blomberg NB, Cnattingius S. Preterm birth and maternal smoking: risks related to gestational age and onset of delivery. *Am J Obstet Gynecol.* 1998;179:1051–1055.

Lammer EJ, Chen DT, Hoar RM, et al. Retinoic acid induced embryopathy. *N Engl J Med.* 1985;313:837–841.

Lammer EJ, Sever LE, Oakley GP Jr. Teratogen update: valproic acid. *Teratology.* 1987;35:465–473.

Lammer EJ, Shaw GM, Iovannisci DM, Finnell RH. Maternal smoking, genetic variation of glutathione s-transferases, and risk for orofacial clefts. *Epidemiology.* 2005;16:698–701.

Lammer EJ. Retinoids: interspecies comparisons and clinical results. In: Sundwall A, Danielsson BR, Hagberg O, et al., eds. *Developmental Toxicology—Preclinical and Clinical Data in Retrospect.* Stockholm: Tryckgruppen; 1992:105–109.

Landrigan PJ, Miodovnik A. Children's health and the environment: an overview. *Mt Sinai J Med.* 2011;78:1–10.

Lary JM, Daniel KL, Erickson JD, et al. The return of thalidomide: can birth defects be prevented? *Drug Saf.* 1999;21:161–169.

Latham KE. Epigenetic modification and imprinting of the mammalian genome during development. *Curr Top Dev Biol.* 1999;43:1–49.

Lau C, Butenhoff JL, Rogers JM. The developmental toxicity of perfluoroalkyl acids and their derivatives. *Toxicol Appl Pharmacol.* 2004;198:231–241.

Lau C, Kavlock RJ. Functional toxicity in the developing heart, lung and kidney. In: Kimmel CA, Buelke-Sam J, eds. *Developmental Toxicology.* 2nd ed. New York: Raven Press; 1994:119–188.

Lau C, Mole ML, Copeland MF, et al. Toward a biologically based dose-response model for developmental toxicity of 5-fluorouracil in the rat: acquisition of experimental data. *Toxicol Sci.* 2001;59:37–48.

Lau C, Rogers JM. Embryonic and fetal programming of physiological disorders in adulthood. *Birth Defects Res C Embryo Today.* 2004;72:300–312.

Lau C, Setzer RW. Biologically based risk assessment models for developmental toxicity. In: Tuan RS, Lo CW, eds. *Developmental Biology Protocols.* Vol II. Totowa, NJ: Humana Press; 2000:271–281.

Lavin M, Watters D, eds. *Programmed Cell Death: The Cellular and Molecular Biology of Apoptosis.* Chur, Switzerland: Harwood Academic Publishers; 1993.

Lee CJ, Goncalves LL, Wells PG. Embryopathic effects of thalidomide and its hydrolysis products in rabbit embryo culture: evidence for a prostaglandin H synthase (PHS)-dependent, reactive oxygen species (ROS)-mediated mechanism. *FASEB J.* 2011;25:2468–2483.

Lee HY, Inselman AL, Kanungo J, et al. Alternative models in developmental toxicology. *Syst Biol Reprod Med.* 2012;58:10–22.

Lenz W. Kindliche Missbildungen nach Medikament-Einnahme während der Gravidität? *Dtsch Med Wochenschr.* 1961;86:2555–2556.

Lenz W. Das thalidomid-syndrom. *Fortschr Med.* 1963;81:148–153.

Lenz W. A short history of thalidomide embryopathy. *Teratology.* 1988;38:203–215.

Lenz W, Knapp K. Die thalidomide-embryopathie. *Dtsch Med Wochenschr.* 1962;87:1232–1242.

Leonardi-Bee J, Britton J, Venn A. Secondhand smoke and adverse fetal outcomes in nonsmoking pregnant women: a meta-analysis. *Pediatrics.* 2011;127:734–741.

Leonardi-Bee J, Smyth A, Britton J, et al. Environmental tobacco smoke and fetal health: systematic review and meta-analysis. *Arch Dis Child Fetal Neonatal Ed.* 2008;93:F351–F361.

Levin AA, Miller RK. Fetal toxicity of cadmium in the rat: maternal vs. fetal injections. *Teratology.* 1980;22:1–5.

Li Y, Sasaki H. Genomic imprinting in mammals: its life cycle, molecular mechanisms and reprogramming. *Cell Res.* 2011;21:466–473.

Little RE. Moderate alcohol use during pregnancy and decreased infant birth weight. *Am J Public Health.* 1977;67:1154–1156.

Little SA, Mirkes PE. Relationship of DNA damage and embryotoxicity induced by 4-hydroperoxydichlorocyclophosphamide in postimplantation rat embryos. *Teratology.* 1990;41:223–231.

Little SA, Mirkes PE. Effects of 4-hydroperoxycyclophosphamide (4-OOH-CP) and 4-hydroperoxydichlorocyclophosphamide (4-OOH-deClCP) on the cell cycle of postimplantation rat embryos. *Teratology.* 1992;45:163–173.

Lohnes D, Mark M, Mendelsohn C, et al. Function of the retinoic acid receptors (RARs) during development: I. Craniofacial and skeletal abnormalities in RAR double mutants. *Development.* 1994;120:2723–2748.

Love DR, Pichler FB, Dodd A, Copp BR, Greenwood DR. Technology for high-throughput screens: the present and future using zebrafish. *Curr Opin Biotechnol.* 2004;15:564–571.

Luecke RH, Wosilait WD, Pearce BA, Young JF. A physiologically based pharmacokinetic computer model for human pregnancy. *Teratology.* 1994;49:90–103.

Luecke RH, Wosilait WD, Young JF. Mathematical analysis for teratogenic sensitivity. *Teratology.* 1997;55:373–380.

Luecke RH, Wosilait WD, Young JF. Mathematical modeling of human embryonic and fetal growth rates. *Growth Dev Aging.* 1999;63:49–59.

Luijten M, van Beelen VA, Verhoef A, et al. Transcriptomics analysis of retinoic acid embryotoxicity in rat postimplantation whole embryo culture. *Reprod Toxicol.* 2010;30:333–340.

Lutiger B, Graham K, Einarson TR, Koren G. Relationship between gestational cocaine use and pregnancy outcome: a meta-analysis. *Teratology.* 1991;44:405–414.

Mably TA, Bjerke DL, Moore RW, et al. In utero and lactational exposure of male rats to 2,3,7,8-tetrachlorodibenzo-p-dioxin. 3. Effects on spermatogenesis and reproductive capability. *Toxicol Appl Pharmacol.* 1992;114:118–126.

MacAuley AM, Werb Z, Mirkes PE. Characterization of the unusually rapid cell cycles during rat gastrulation. *Development.* 1993;117:873–883.

MacDonald H, Tobin JOH. Congenital cytomegalovirus infection: a collaborative study on epidemiological, clinical and laboratory findings. *Dev Med Child Neurol.* 1978;20:271–282.

Mallo M, Wellik DM, Deschamps J. Hox genes and regional patterning of the vertebrate body plan. *Dev Biol.* 2010;344:7–15.

Manning MA, Hoyme EH. Fetal alcohol spectrum disorders: a practical clinical approach to diagnosis. *Neurosci Biobehav Rev.* 2007;31:230–238.

Manson JM. Testing of pharmaceutical agents for reproductive toxicity. In: Kimmel CA, Buelke-Sam J, eds. *Developmental Toxicology.* 2nd ed. New York: Raven Press; 1994:379–402.

Maritz GS, Harding R. Life-long programming implications of exposure to tobacco smoking and nicotine before and soon after birth: evidence for altered lung development. *Int J Environ Res Public Health.* 2011;8:875–898.

Mark M, Ghyselinck NB, Chambon P. Function of retinoid nuclear receptors: lessons from genetic and pharmacological dissections of the retinoic acid signaling pathway during mouse embryogenesis. *Annu Rev Pharmacol Toxicol.* 2006;46:451–480.

Mark M, Ghyselinck NB, Chambon P. Function of retinoic acid receptors during embryonic development. *Nucl Recept Signal.* 2009;7:e002.

Markert CL, Petters RM. Manufactured hexaparental mice show that adults are derived from three embryonic cells. *Science.* 1978;202:56–58.

Markussen Linnet K, Obel C, Bonde E, et al. Cigarette smoking during pregnancy and hyperactive-distractible preschoolers: a follow-up study. *Acta Paediatr.* 2006;95:694–700.

Marshall H, Morrison A, Studer M, et al. Retinoids and hox genes. *FASEB J.* 1996;10:969–978.

Marshall H, Nonchev S, Sham MH, et al. Retinoic acid alters hindbrain Hox code and induces transformation of rhombomeres 2/3 into a 4/5 identity. *Nature.* 1992;360:737–741.

Matalon S, Schechtman S, Goldzweig G, et al. The teratogenic effect of carbamazepine: a meta-analysis of 1255 exposures. *Reprod Toxicol.* 2002;16:9–17.

Mattison DR, Blann E, Malek A. Physiological alterations during pregnancy: impact on toxicokinetics. *Fundam Appl Toxicol.* 1991;16:215–218.

McBride WG. Thalidomide and congenital anomalies. *Lancet.* 1961;2:1358.

McCollum CW, Ducharme NA, Bondesson M, Gustafsson J-A. Developmental toxicity screening in zebrafish. *Birth Defects Res C Embryo Today.* 2011;93:67–114.

McMillen IC, Robinson JS. Developmental origins of the metabolic syndrome: prediction, plasticity, and programming. *Physiol Rev.* 2005;85: 571–633.

Medlock KL, Branham WS, Sheehan DM. Effects of coumestrol and equol on the developing reproductive tract of the rat. *Proc Soc Exp Biol Med.* 1995;208:67–71.

Mendelsohn C, Lohnes D, Décimo D, et al. Function of the retinoic acid receptors (RARs) during development: II. Multiple abnormalities at various stages of organogenesis in RAR double mutants. *Development.* 1994;120:2749–2771.

Menegola E, Di Renzo F, Broccia ML, et al. Inhibition of histone deacetylase as a new mechanism of teratogenesis. *Birth Defects Res C Embryo Today.* 2006;78:345–353.

Mikkola HK, Orkin SH. Gene targeting and transgenic strategies for the analysis of hematopoietic development in the mouse. *Methods Mol Med.* 2005;105:3–22.

Miller MT, Stromland K. Teratogen update: thalidomide: a review with a focus on ocular findings and new potential uses. *Teratology.* 1999;60: 306–321.

Millicovsky G, DeSesso JM, Kleinman LI, Clark KE. Effects of hydroxyurea on hemodynamics of pregnant rabbits: a maternally mediated mechanism of embryotoxicity. *Am J Obstet Gynecol.* 1981;140:747–752.

Millicovsky G, DeSesso JM. Cardiovascular alterations in rabbit embryos in situ after a teratogenic dose of hydroxyurea: an in vivo microscopic study. *Teratology.* 1980a;22:115–124.

Millicovsky G, DeSesso JM. Differential embryonic cardiovascular responses to acute maternal uterine ischemia: an in vivo microscopic study of rabbit embryos with either intact or clamped umbilical cords. *Teratology.* 1980b;22:335–343.

Millicovsky G, Johnston MC. Maternal hyperoxia greatly reduces the incidence of phenytoin-induced cleft lip and palate in A/J mice. *Science.* 1981;212:671–672.

Mills JL, Signore C. Neural tube defect rates before and after food fortification with folic acid. *Birth Defects Res A Clin Mol Teratol.* 2004;70: 844–845.

Milunsky A, Ulcickas M, Rothman KJ, et al. Maternal heat exposure and neural tube defects. *JAMA.* 1992;268:882–885.

Miodovnik A. Environmental neurotoxicants and developing brain. *Mt Sinai J Med.* 2011;78:58–77.

Mirkes PE, Fantel AG, Greenaway JC, Shepard TH. Teratogenicity of cyclophosphamide metabolites: phosphoramide mustard, acrolein, and 4-ketocyclophosphamide on rat embryos cultured in vitro. *Toxicol Appl Pharmacol.* 1981;58:322–330.

Mirkes PE, Greenaway JC, Hilton J, Brundrett R. Morphological and biochemical aspects of monofunctional phosphoramide mustard teratogenicity in rat embryos cultured in vitro. *Teratology.* 1985;32:241–249.

Mirkes PE, Ricks JL, Pascoe-Mason JM. Cell cycle analysis in the cardiac and neuroepithelial tissues of day 10 rat embryos and the effects of phosphoramide mustard, the major teratogenic metabolite of cyclophosphamide. *Teratology.* 1989;39:115–120.

Mirkes PE. Cyclophosphamide teratogenesis: a review. *Teratogenicity Carcinog Mutagen.* 1985a;5:75–88.

Mirkes PE. Molecular and metabolic aspects of cyclophosphamide teratogenesis. In: Welsch F, ed. *Approaches to Elucidate Mechanisms in Teratogenesis.* Washington, DC: Hemisphere; 1987:123–147.

Mirkes PE. Simultaneous banding of rat embryo DNA, RNA and protein in cesium trifluoroacetate gradients. *Anal Biochem.* 1985b;148: 376–383.

Mitchell EA, Milerad J. Smoking and the sudden infant death syndrome. *Rev Environ Health.* 2006;21:81–103.

Mitra SC. Effects of cocaine on fetal kidney and bladder function. *J Maternal Fetal Med.* 1999;8:262–269.

Montgomery SM, Ekbom A. Smoking during pregnancy and diabetes mellitus in a British longitudinal birth cohort. *BMJ.* 2002;324:26–27.

Moore NW, Adams CE, Rowson LEA. Developmental potential of single blastomeres of the rabbit egg. *J Reprod Fertil.* 1968;17:527–531.

Mouritsen A, Aksglaede L, Sørensen K, et al. Hypothesis: exposure to endocrine-disrupting chemicals may interfere with timing of puberty. *Int J Androl.* 2010;33:346–359.

MRC Vitamin Study Research Group [prepared by Wald N with assistance from Sneddon J, Frost C, Stone R]. Prevention of neural tube defects: results of the MRC vitamin study. *Lancet.* 1991;338:132–137.

Murphy SK, Jirtle RL. Imprinted genes as potential genetic and epigenetic toxicologic targets. *Environ Health Perspect.* 2000;108(suppl 1):5–11.

Myatt L. Placental adaptive responses and fetal programming. *J Physiol.* 2006;572:25–30.

Mylchreest E, Cattley RC, Foster PM. Male reproductive tract malformations in rats following gestational and lactational exposure to di(n-butyl) phthalate: an anti-androgenic mechanism? *Toxicol Sci.* 1998;43:47–60.

Mylchreest E, Sar M, Cattley RC, Foster PM. Disruption of androgen-regulated male reproductive development by di(*n*-butyl)phthalate during late gestation in rats is different from flutamide. *Toxicol Appl Pharmacol.* 1999;156:81–95.

Naciff JM, Hess KA, Overmann GJ, et al. Gene expression changes induced in the testis by transplacental exposure to high and low doses of 17{alpha}-ethynyl estradiol, genistein, or bisphenol A. *Toxicol Sci.* 2005;86:396–416.

Nagel SC, vom Saal FS, Thayer KA, et al. Relative binding affinity–serum modified access (RBA–SMA) assay predicts the relative in vivo bioactivity of the xenoestrogens bisphenol A and octylphenol. *Environ Health Perspect.* 1997;105:70–76.

National Research Council. *Pesticides in the Diets of Infants and Children.* Washington, DC: National Academy Press; 1993.

National Research Council. *Scientific Fromtiers in Developmental Toxicology and Risk Assessment.* Washington, DC: National Academy Press; 2000.

National Research Council. *Toxicity Testing in the Twenty-FirstCentury: A Vision and a Strategy.* Washington, DC: National Academies Press; 2007.

Nau H. Species differences in pharmacokinetics and drug teratogenesis. *Environ Health Perspect.* 1986;70:113–129.

Nau H. Physicochemical and structural properties regulating placenta drug transfer. In: Polin RA, Fox WW, eds. *Fetal and Neonatal Physiology.* Vol 1. Philadelphia: Saunders; 1992:130–149.

Nau H, Chahoud I, Dencker L, et al. Teratogenicity of vitamin A and retinoids. In: Blomhoff R, ed. *Vitamin A in Health and Disease.* New York: Marcel Dekker; 1994:615–664.

Nau H, Hauck R-S, Ehlers K. Valproic acid induced neural tube defects in mouse and human: aspects of chirality, alternative drug development, pharmacokinetics and possible mechanisms. *Pharmacol Toxicol.* 1991;69:310–321.

Nau H, Helge H, Luck W. Valproic acid in the perinatal period: decreased maternal serum protein binding results in fetal accumulation and neonatal displacement of the drug and some metabolites. *J Pediatr.* 1984;104:627–634.

Nau H, Scott WJ. Weak acids may act as teratogens by accumulating in the basic milieu of the early mammalian embryo. *Nature.* 1986;323:276–278.

Nau H, Scott WJ. *Pharmacokinetics in Teratogenesis.* Vols I and II. Boca Raton, FL: CRC Press; 1987.

Nawrot PS, Cook RO, Hamm CW. Embryotoxicity of broadband high-frequency noise in the CD-1 mouse. *J Toxicol Environ Health.* 1981;8:151–157.

Nawrot PS, Cook RO, Staples RE. Embryotoxicity of various noise stimuli in the mouse. *Teratology.* 1980;22:279–289.

Needham LL, Ozkaynak H, Whyatt RM, et al. Exposure assessment in the National Children's Study: introduction. *Environ Health Perspect.* 2005;113:1076–1082.

Neims AH, Warner M, Loughnan PM, Aranda JV. Developmental aspects of the hepatic cytochrome P_{450} monooxygenase system. *Annu Rev Pharmacol Toxicol.* 1976;16:427–444.

Nelson CJ, Holson JF. Statistical analysis of teratologic data: problems and recent advances. *J Environ Pathol Toxicol.* 1978;2:187–199.

Neubert D. In-vitro techniques for assessing teratogenic potential. In: Dayan AD, Paine AJ, eds. *Advances in Applied Toxicology.* London: Taylor and Francis; 1989:191–211.

Neubert R, Hinz N, Thiel R, Neubert D. Down-regulation of adhesion receptors on cells of primate embryos as a probable mechanism of the teratogenic action of thalidomide. *Life Sci.* 1996;58:295–316.

Neubert R, Neubert D. Peculiarities and possible mode of actions of thalidomide. In: Kavlock RJ, Daston GP, eds. *Drug Toxicity in Embryonic Development, II.* Berlin, Heidelberg: Springer-Verlag; 1997: 41–119.

Neubert D, Zens P, Rothenwallner A, Merker H-J. A survey of the embryotoxic effects of TCDD in mammalian species. *Environ Health Perspect.* 1973;5:63–79.

New DAT. Whole embryo culture and the study of mammalian embryos during organogenesis. *Biol Rev.* 1978;5:81–94.

Newbold RR, Padilla-Banks E, Jefferson WN. Adverse effects of the model environmental estrogen diethylstilbestrol are transmitted to subsequent generations. *Endocrinology.* 2006;147:S11–S17.

Newbold RR, Padilla-Banks E, Jefferson WN. Environmental estrogens and obesity. *Mol Cell Endocrinol.* 2009;304:84–89.

Newbold RR. Cellular and molecular effects of developmental exposure to diethylstilbestrol: implications for other environmental estrogens. *Environ Health Perspect.* 1995;103(suppl 7):83–87.

Newman CGH. Teratogen update: clinical aspects of thalidomide embryopathy—a continuing preoccupation. *Teratology.* 1985;32:133–144.

Nicol CJ, Harrison ML, Laposa RR, Gimelshtein IL, Wells PG. A teratologic suppressor role for p53 in benzo[a]pyrene-treated transgenic p53-deficient mice. *Nat Genet.* 1995;10:181–187.

Nowack E. The sensitive phase in thalidomide embryopathy. *Humangenetik.* 1965;1:516–536.

Nugent P, Sucov HM, Pisano MM, Greene RM. The role of RXR-alpha in retinoic acid–induced cleft palate as assessed with the RXR-alpha knock-out mouse. *Int J Dev Biol.* 1999;43:567–570.

O'Flaherty EJ, Scott WJ, Shreiner C, Beliles RP. A physiologically based kinetic model of rat and mouse gestation: disposition of a weak acid. *Toxicol Appl Pharmacol.* 1992;112:245–256.

O'Flaherty EJ. Pharmacokinetics, pharmacodynamics, and prediction of developmental abnormalities. *Reprod Toxicol.* 1997;11:413–416.

Okada A, Aoki Y, Kushima K, Kurihara H, Bialer M, Fujiwara M. Polycomb homologs are involved in teratogenicity of valproic acid in mice. *Birth Defects Res A Clin Mol Teratol.* 2004;70:870–879.

Okada A, Kushima K, Aoki Y, Bialer M, Fujiwara M. Identification of early-responsive genes correlated to valproic acid-induced neural tube defects in mice. *Birth Defects Res A Clin Mol Teratol.* 2005;73:229–238.

Oken E, Levitan EB, Gillman MW. Maternal smoking during pregnancy and child overweight: systematic review and meta-analysis. *Int J Obes (Lond).* 2008;32:201–210.

Olanoff LS, Anderson JM. Controlled release of tetracycline—III: a physiological pharmacokinetic model of the pregnant rat. *J Pharmacokinet Biopharm.* 1980;8:599–620.

Olsen GW, Bodner KM, Ramlow JM, Ross CE, Lipshultz LI. Have sperm counts been reduced 50 percent in 50 years? A statistical model revisited. *Fertility and Sterility.* 1995;63:887–893.

Oltvai ZN, Korsmeyer SJ. Checkpoints of dueling dimers foil death wishes. *Cell.* 1994;79:189–192.

Ornoy A. Neuroteratogens in man: an overview with special emphasis on the teratogenicity of antiepileptic drugs in pregnancy. *Reprod Toxicol.* 2006;22:214–226.

Ostrea EM Jr, Matias O, Keane C, et al. Spectrum of gestational exposure to illicit drugs and other xenobiotic agents in newborn infants meconium analysis. *J Pediatr.* 1998;133:513–515.

Ozolins TR. Cyclophosphamide and the Teratology Society: an awkward marriage. *Birth Defects Res B Dev Reprod Toxicol.* 2010;89: 289–299.

Padilla S, Corum D, Padnos B, et al. Zebrafish developmental screening of the ToxCast Phase I chemical library. *Reprod Toxicol.* 2012;33:174–187.

Page K, Abramovich D, Aggett P, et al. Uptake of zinc by the human placenta microvillus border membranes and characterization of the effects of cadmium on the process. *Placenta.* 1992;13:151–162.

Paladini D, Vassallo M, D'Armiento MR, et al. Prenatal detection of multiple fetal anomalies following inadvertent exposure to cyclophosphamide in the first trimester of pregnancy. *Birth Defects Res A Clin Mol Teratol.* 2004;70:99–100.

Parizek J. Vascular changes at sites of estrogen biosynthesis produced by parenteral injection of cadmium salts: the destruction of the placenta by cadmium salts. *J Reprod Fertil.* 1964;7:263–265.

Park D, Yang YH, Choi EK, et al. Licorice extract increases cyclophosphamide teratogenicity by upregulating the expression of cytochrome P-450 2B mRNA. *Birth Defects Res B Dev Reprod Toxicol.* 2011;92: 553–559.

Parman T, Wiley MJ, Wells PG. Free radical-mediated oxidative DNA damage in the mechanism of thalidomide teratogenicity. *Nat Med.* 1999;5:582–585.

Paulozzi LJ, Erickson JD, Jackson RJ. Hypospadias trends in two American surveillance systems. *Pediatrics.* 1997;100:831–834.

Paulozzi LJ. International trends in rates of hypospadias and cryptorchidism. *Environ Health Perspect.* 1999;107:297–302.

Perera F, Herbstman J. Prenatal environmental exposures, epigenetics, and disease. *Reprod Toxicol.* 2011;31:363–373.

Piersma AH, Genschow E, Verhoef A, et al. Validation of the postimplantation rat whole-embryo culture test in the international ECVAM validation study on three in vitro embryotoxicity tests. *Altern Lab Anim.* 2004;32:275–307.

Piersma AH, Hernandez LG, van Benthem J, et al. Reproductive toxicants have a threshold of adversity. *Crit Rev Toxicol.* 2011a;41:545–554.

Piersma AH, Rorije E, Beekhuijzen ME, et al. Combined retrospective analysis of 498 rat multi-generation reproductive toxicity studies: on the impact of parameters related to F1 mating and F2 offspring. *Reprod Toxicol.* 2011b;31:392–401.

Piersma AH, van Dartel DAM, van der Ven LTM. Alternative methods in developmental toxicology. In: McQueen CA, ed. *Comprehensive Toxicology.* 2nd ed., Vol 12. Daston GP, Knudsen TB, eds. *Developmental Toxicology.* New York: Elsevier; 2010:293–305.

Pinkerton KE, Joad JP. The mammalian respiratory system and critical windows of exposure for children's health. *Environ Health Perspect.* 2000;108(suppl 3):457–462.

Pole M, Einarson A, Pairaudeau N, et al. Drug labeling and risk perceptions of teratogenicity: a survey of pregnant Canadian women and their health professionals. *J Clin Pharmacol.* 2000;40:573–577.

Poskanzer D, Herbst AL. Epidemiology of vaginal adenosis and adenocarcinoma associated with exposure to stilbestrol in utero. *Cancer.* 1977;39:1892–1895.

Potter SM, Zelazo PR, Stack DM, Papageorgiou AN. Adverse effects of fetal cocaine exposure on neonatal auditory information processing. *Pediatrics.* 2000;105:E40.

Quan A. Fetopathy associated with exposure to angiotensin converting enzyme inhibitors and angiotensin receptor antagonists. *Early Hum Dev*. 2006;82:23–28.

Registration, Evaluation, Authorisation and Restriction of Chemicals. Regulation (EC) No 1907/2006 of the European Parliament and of the Council of 18 December 2006 concerning the Registration, Evaluation, Authorisation and Restriction of Chemicals (REACH), establishing a European Chemicals Agency, amending Directive 1999/45/EC and repealing Council Regulation (EEC) No 793/93 and Commission Regulation (EC) No 1488/94 as well as Council Directive 76/769/EEC and Commission Directives 91/155/EEC, 93/67/EEC, 93/105/EC and 2000/21/EC. *Official Journal of the European Union L*. 2006; 396:1–849. http://home.kpn.nl/reach/downloads/reachtestingneedsfinal.pdf. Accessed on May 11, 2011.

Reuter U, Heinrich-Hirsch B, Hellwig J, Holzum B, Welsch F. Evaluation of OECD screening tests 421 (reproduction/developmental toxicity screening test) and 422 (combined repeated dose toxicity study with the reproduction/developmental toxicity screening test). *Regul Toxicol Pharmacol*. 2003;38:17–26.

Rider CV, Furr JR, Wilson VS, et al. Cumulative effects of in utero administration of mixtures of reproductive toxicants that disrupt common target tissues via diverse mechanisms of toxicity. *Int J Androl*. 2010;33:443–462.

Rider CV, Wilson VS, Howdeshell KL, et al. Cumulative effects of in utero administration of mixtures of "antiandrogens" on male rat reproductive development. *Toxicol Pathol*. 2009;37:100–113.

Robertson J, Polifka JE, Avner M, et al. A survey of pregnant women using isotretinoin. *Birth Defects Res A Clin Mol Teratol*. 2005;73:881–887.

Robinson JF, Pennings JL, Piersma AH. A review of toxicogenomic approaches in developmental toxicology. *Methods Mol Biol*. 2012a;889:347–371.

Robinson JF, Theunissen PT, van Dartel DA, et al. Comparison of MeHg-induced toxicogenomic responses across in vivo and in vitro models used in developmental toxicology. *Reprod Toxicol*. 2011a;32: 180–188.

Robinson JF, Tonk EC, Verhoef A, Piersma AH. Triazole induced concentration-related gene signatures in rat whole embryo culture. *Reprod Toxicol*. 2012b;34:275–283.

Robinson JF, van Beelen VA, Verhoef A, et al. Embryotoxicant-specific transcriptomic responses in rat postimplantation whole-embryo culture. *Toxicol Sci*. 2010;118:675–685.

Robinson JF, Verhoef A, Pennings JL, et al. A comparison of gene expression responses in rat whole embryo culture and in vivo: time-dependent retinoic acid-induced teratogenic response. *Toxicol Sci*. 2012c;126: 242–254.

Robinson JF, Verhoef A, Piersma AH. Transcriptomic analysis of neurulation and early organogenesis in rat embryos: an in vivo and ex vivo comparison. *Toxicol Sci*. 2012d;126:255–266.

Robinson JF, Yu X, Moreira EG, et al. Arsenic- and cadmium-induced toxicogenomic response in mouse embryos undergoing neurulation. *Toxicol Appl Pharmacol*. 2011b;250:117–129.

Rodier PM, Cohen IR, Buelke-Sam J. Developmental neurotoxicology: neuroendocrine manifestations of CNS insult. In: Kimmel CA, Buelke-Sam J, eds. *Developmental Toxicology*. 2nd ed. New York: Raven Press; 1994:65–92.

Rogan WJ, Gladen BC. PCBs, DDE and child development at 18 and 24 months. *Am J Epidemiol*. 1991;1:407–413.

Rogers JM. Tobacco and pregnancy: overview of exposures and effects. *Birth Defects Res C Embryo Today*. 2008;84:1–15.

Rogers JM, Chernoff N, Keen CL, Daston GP. Evaluation and interpretation of maternal toxicity in Segment II studies: issues, some answers, and data needs. *Toxicol Appl Pharmacol*. 2005;207:367–374.

Rogers JM, Ellis-Hutchings RG, Lau C. Epigenetics and the developmental origins of health and disease. In: McQueen CA, ed. *Comprehensive Toxicology*. 2nd ed., Vol 12. Daston GP, Knudsen TB, eds. *Developmental Toxicology*. New York: Elsevier; 2010:69–88.

Rogers JM, Mole ML. Critical periods of sensitivity to the developmental toxicity of inhaled methanol in the CD-1 mouse. *Teratology*. 1997;55:364–372.

Rosa FW. Teratogenicity of isotretinoin. *Lancet*. 1983;2:513.

Rosa FW. Spina bifida in infants of women treated with carbamazepine during pregnancy. *N Engl J Med*. 1991;324:674–677.

Rosen MB, Schmid JE, Das KP, et al. Gene expression profiling in the liver and lung of perfluorooctane sulfonate-exposed mouse fetuses: comparison to changes induced by exposure to perfluorooctanoic acid. *Reprod Toxicol*. 2009;27:278–288.

Rosen MB, Schmid JR, Corton JC, et al. Gene expression profiling in wild-type and PPAR-alpha-null mice exposed to perfluorooctane sulfonate reveals PPAR-alpha-independent effects. *PPAR Res*. 2010; 2010:23.

Rosen MB, Thibodeaux JR, Wood CR, et al. Gene expression profiling in the lung and liver of PFOA-exposed mouse fetuses. *Toxicology*. 2007;239:15–33.

Rovida C, Longo F, Rabbit RR. How are reproductive toxicity and developmental toxicity addressed in REACH dossiers? *ALTEX*. 2011;28: 273–294.

Rozman KK, Bhatia J, Calafat AM, et al. NTP-CERHR expert panel report on the reproductive and developmental toxicity of soy formula. *Birth Defects Res B Dev Reprod Toxicol*. 2006;77:280–397.

Rutledge JC, Shourbaji AG, Hughes LA, et al. Limb and lower-body duplications induced by retinoic acid in mice. *Proc Natl Acad Sci U S A*. 1994;91:5436–5440.

Sadler TW, Warner CW. Use of whole embryo culture for evaluating toxicity and teratogenicity. *Pharmacol Rev*. 1984;36:145S–150S.

Sanes JR, Rubenstein LR, Nicolas JF. Use of a recombinant retrovirus to study postimplantation cell lineage in mouse embryos. *EMBO J*. 1986;5:3133–3142.

Sannerstedt R, Lundborg P, Danielsson BR, et al. Drugs during pregnancy: An issue of risk classification and information to prescribers. *Drug Saf*. 1996;14:69–77.

Sanyal MK, Kitchin KT, Dixon RL. Anomalous development of rat embryos cultured in vitro with cyclophosphamide and microsomes. *Pharmacologist*. 1979;21:A231.

Sasaki H, Matsui Y. Epigenetic events in mammalian germ-cell development: reprogramming and beyond. *Nat Rev Genet*. 2008;9:129–140.

Sauer H, Gunther J, Hescheler J, Wartenberg M. Thalidomide inhibits angiogenesis in embryoid bodies by the generation of hydroxyl radicals. *Am J Pathol*. 2000;56:151–158.

Saydmohammed M, Vollmer LL, Onuoha EO, et al. A high-content screening assay in transgenic zebrafish identifies two novel activators of fgf signaling. *Birth Defects Res C Embryo Today*. 2011;93:281–287.

Scanlon JW. The neuroteratology of cocaine: background, theory, and clinical implications. *Reprod Toxicol*. 1991;5:89–98.

Schaefer C. Angiotensin II-receptor-antagonists: further evidence of fetotoxicity but not teratogenicity. *Birth Defects Res A Clin Mol Teratol*. 2003;67:591–594.

Schantz SL, Levin ED, Bowman RE. Long-term neurobehavioral effects of perinatal PCB exposure in monkeys. *J Environ Toxicol Chem*. 1991;10:747–756.

Schantz SL, Moshtaghian J, Ness DK. Spatial learning deficits in adult rats exposed to ortho-substituted PCB congeners during gestation and lactation. *Fundam Appl Toxicol*. 1995;26:117–126.

Schardein JL. *Chemically Induced Birth Defects*. 2nd ed. New York: Marcel Dekker; 1993.

Schardein JL. *Chemically Induced Birth Defects*. 3nd ed. New York: Marcel Dekker; 2000.

Schardein JL, Keller KA. Potential human developmental toxicants and the role of animal testing in their identification and characterization. *CRC Crit Rev Toxicol*. 1989;19:251–339.

Schardein JL, Macina OT. *Human Developmental Toxicants: Aspects of Toxicology and Chemistry*. Boca Raton, FL: CRC Press, Taylor and Francis Group; 2007;427.

Schecter A, Ryan JJ, Masuda Y, et al. Chlorinated and brominated dioxins and dibenzofurans in human tissue following exposure. *Environ Health Perspect*. 1994;102(suppl 1):135–147.

Schumacher HJ. Chemical structure and teratogenic properties. In: Shepard T, Miller R, Marois M, eds. *Methods for Detection of Environmental*

Agents That Produce Congenital Defects. New York: American Elsevier; 1975:65–77.

Schwab C, Jagannath S. The role of thalidomide in multiple myeloma. *Clin Lymphoma Myeloma.* 2006;7:26–29.

Scialli AR. The challenge of reproductive and developmental toxicology under REACH. *Regul Toxicol Pharmacol.* 2008;51:244–250.

Seckl JR, Holmes MC. Mechanisms of disease: glucocorticoids, their placental metabolism and fetal 'programming' of adult pathophysiology. *Nat Clin Pract Endocrinol Metab.* 2007;3:479–488.

Seiler A, Visan A, Buesen R, Genschow E, Spielmann H. Improvement of an in vitro stem cell assay for developmental toxicity: the use of molecular endpoints in the embryonic stem cell test. *Reprod Toxicol.* 2004;18:231–240.

Selderslaghs IWT, Blust R, Witters HE. Feasibility study of the zebrafish assay as an alternative method to screen for developmental toxicity and embryotoxicity using a training set of 27 compounds. *Reprod Toxicol.* 2012;33:142–154.

Seller MJ, Perkins KJ, Adinolfi M. Differential response of heterozygous curly-tail mouse embryos to vitamin A teratogenesis depending on maternal genotype. *Teratology.* 1983;28:123.

Setzer RW, Lau C, Mole ML, Copeland MF, Rogers JM, Kavlock RJ. Toward a biologically based dose-response model for developmental toxicity of 5-fluorouracil in the rat: a mathematical construct. *Toxicol Sci.* 2001;59:49–58.

Sever JL. Rubella as a teratogen. *Adv Teratol.* 1967;2:127–138.

Shan G. RNA interference as a gene knockdown technique. *Int J Biochem Cell Biol.* 2010;42:1243–1251.

Shenefelt RE. Morphogenesis of malformations in hamsters caused by retinoic acid: Relation to dose and stage of treatment. *Teratology.* 1972;5:103–118.

Shepard TH, Lemire RJ. *Catalog of Teratogenic Agents.* 11th ed. Baltimore: The Johns Hopkins University Press; 2004.

Shi M, Wehby GL, Murray JC. Review on genetic variants and maternal smoking in the etiology of oral clefts and other birth defects. *Birth Defects Res C Embryo Today.* 2008;84:16–29.

Shuey DL, Lau C, Logsdon TR, et al. Biologically based dose–response modeling in developmental toxicology: biochemical and cellular sequelae of 5-fluorouracil exposure in the developing rat. *Toxicol Appl Pharmacol.* 1994;126:129–144.

Sipes NS, Martin MT, Reif DM, et al. Predictive models of prenatal developmental toxicity from ToxCast high-throughput screening data. *Toxicol Sci.* 2011a;124:109–127.

Sipes NS, Padilla S, Knudsen TB. Zebrafish: as an integrative model for twenty-first century toxicity testing. *Birth Defects Res C Embryo Today.* 2011b;93:256–267.

Skakkebaek NE, Keiding N. Changes in semen and the testis. *Br Med J.* 1994;309:1316–1317.

Skinner MK, Manikkam M, Guerrero-Bosagna C. Epigenetic transgenerational actions of endocrine disruptors. *Reprod Toxicol.* 2011;31:337–343.

Slikker W Jr, Xu ZA, Levin ED, Slotkin TA. Mode of action: disruption of brain cell replication, second messenger, and neurotransmitter systems during development leading to cognitive dysfunction—developmental neurotoxicity of nicotine. *Crit Rev Toxicol.* 2005;35:703–711.

Slikker W, Miller RK. Placental metabolism and transfer: role in developmental toxicology. In: Kimmel CA, Buelke-Sam J, eds. *Developmental Toxicology.* 2nd ed. New York: Raven Press; 1994:245–283.

Slotkin TA. Fetal nicotine or cocaine exposure: which one is worse? *J Pharmacol Exp Ther.* 1998;285:931–945.

Slott VL, Hales BF. Sodium 2-mercaptoethane sulfonate protection against cyclophosphamide-induced teratogenicity in rats. *Toxicol Appl Pharmacol.* 1986;82:80–86.

Smith SM. Alcohol and cell death. In: McQueen CA, ed. *Comprehensive Toxicology.* 2nd ed., Vol 12. Daston GP, Knudsen TB, eds. *Developmental Toxicology.* New York: Elsevier; 2010:223–238.

Smith JL, Gesteland KM, Schoenwolf GC. Prospective fate map of the mouse primitive streak at 7.5 days of gestation. *Dev Dynam.* 1994;201:279–289.

Snow MHL, Tam PPL. Is compensatory growth a complicating factor in mouse teratology? *Nature.* 1979;279:555–557.

Sokol RJ, Delaney-Black V, Nordstrom B. Fetal alcohol spectrum disorder. *JAMA.* 2003;290:2996–2999.

Sorrell TL, Graziano JH. Effect of oral cadmium exposure during pregnancy on maternal and fetal zinc metabolism in the rat. *Toxicol Appl Pharmacol.* 1990;102:537–545.

Spielmann H, Genschow E, Brown NA, et al. Validation of the rat limb bud micromass test in the international ECVAM validation study on three in vitro embryotoxicity tests. *Altern Lab Anim.* 2004;32:245–274.

Stephens TD. Proposed mechanisms of action in thalidomide embryopathy. *Teratology.* 1988;38:229–239.

Stephens TD, Bunde CJ, Fillmore BJ. Mechanism of action in thalidomide teratogenesis. *Biochem Pharmacol.* 2000;59:1489–1499.

Stephens TD, Bunde CJW, Torres RD, et al. Thalidomide inhibits limb development throught its antagonism of IFG-I+FGF-2+heparin (abstr). *Teratology.* 1998;57:112.

Stephens TD, Fillmore BJ. Hypothesis: thalidomide embryopathy: proposed mechanism of action. *Teratology.* 2000;61:189–195.

Stirling DI, Sherman M, Strauss S. Thalidomide: a surprising recovery. *J Am Pharmacol Assoc.* 1997;NS37:307–313.

Stockard CR. Developmental rate and structural expression: an experimental study of twins, "double monsters," and single deformities, and the interaction among embryonic organs during their origin and development. *Am J Anat.* 1921;28:115–277.

Stott DH. Follow-up study from birth of the effects of prenatal stress. *Dev Med Child Neurol.* 1973;15:770–787.

Streissguth AP, Aase JM, Clarren SK, et al. Fetal alcohol syndrome in adolescents and adults. *JAMA.* 1991a;265:1961–1967.

Streissguth AP, Barr HM, Olson HC, et al. Drinking during pregnancy decreases word attack and arithmetic scores on standardized tests: adolescent data from a population-based prospective study. *Alcohol Clin Exp Res.* 1994a;18:248–254.

Streissguth AP, Randels SP, Smith DF. A test-retest study of intelligence in patients with fetal alcohol syndrome: implications for care. *J Am Acad Child Adolesc Psychiatry.* 1991b;30:584–587.

Streissguth AP, Sampson PD, Olson HC, et al. Maternal drinking during pregnancy: attention and short-term memory in 14-year-old offspring: a longitudinal prospective study. *Alcohol Clin Exp Res.* 1994b;18:202–218.

Struve MF, Gaido KW, Hensley JB, et al. Reproductive toxicity and pharmacokinetics of di-n-butyl phthalate (DBP) following dietary exposure of pregnant rats. *Birth Defects Res B Dev Reprod Toxicol.* 2009;86:345–354.

Sulik KK. Genesis of alcohol-induced craniofacial dysmorphism. *Exp Biol Med.* 2005;230:366–375.

Sulik KK, Johnston MC. Sequence of developmental alterations following acute ethanol exposure in mice: craniofacial features of the fetal alcohol syndrome. *Am J Anat.* 1983;166:257–269.

Sulik KK, Johnston MC, Webb MA. Fetal alcohol syndrome: embryogenesis in a mouse model. *Science.* 1981;214:936–968.

Suzuki K, Ando D, Sato M, et al. The association between maternal smoking during pregnancy and childhood obesity persists to the age of 9-10 years. *J Epidemiol.* 2009;19:136–142.

Swann SH, Elkin EP, Fenster L. Have sperm counts declined? A reanalysis of global trend data. *Environ Health Perspect.* 1997;105:1228–1232.

Tabacova S. Mode of action: angiotensin-converting enzyme inhibition—developmental effects associated with exposure to ACE inhibitors. *Crit Rev Toxicol.* 2005;35:747–755.

Takeuchi IK. Teratogenic effects of methylnitrosourea on pregnant mice before implantation. *Experientia.* 1984;40:879–881.

Tatum WO. Use of antiepileptic drugs in pregnancy. *Expert Rev Neurother.* 2006;6:1077–1086.

Taubeneck MW, Daston GP, Rogers JM, Keen CL. Altered maternal zinc metabolism following exposure to diverse developmental toxicants. *Reprod Toxicol.* 1994;8:25–40.

Taussig HB. A study of the German outbreak of phocomelia: the thalidomide syndrome. *JAMA.* 1962;180:1106.

Teratology Society. FDA classification system of drugs for teratogenic risk. *Teratology.* 1994;49:446–447.

Terry KK, Elswick BA, Welsch F, et al. Development of a physiologically based pharmacokinetic model describing 2-methoxyacetic acid disposition in the pregnant mouse. *Toxicol Appl Pharmacol*. 1995;132:103–114.

Therapontos C, Erskine L, Gardner ER, et al. Thalidomide induces limb defects by preventing angiogenic outgrowth during early limb formation. *Proc Natl Acad Sci U S A*. 2009;106:8573–8578.

Thompson CJS. *Mystery and Lore of Monsters*. London: Williams and Norgate; 1930.

Thornburg KL, O'Tierney PF, Louey S. The placenta is a programming agent for cardiovascular disease. *Placenta*. 2010;31(suppl):S54–S59.

Tomson T, Battino D. Teratogenicity of antiepileptic drugs: state of the art. *Curr Opin Neurol*. 2005;18:135–140.

Ton C, Lin Y, Willett C. Zebrafish as a model for developmental neurotoxicity testing. *Birth Defects Res A Clin Mol Teratol*. 2006;76:553–567.

Toppari J, Larsen JC, Christiansen P, et al. Male reproductive health and environmental xenoestrogens. *Environ Health Perspect*. 1996;104 (suppl 4):741–776.

Toppari J, Virtanen HE, Main KM, Skakkebaek NE. Cryptorchidism and hypospadias as a sign of testicular dysgenesis syndrome (TDS): environmental connection. *Birth Defects Res A Clin Mol Teratol*. 2010;88:910–919.

Trainor PA, Krumlauf R. Hox genes, neural crest cells and branchial arch patterning. *Curr Opin Cell Biol*. 2001;13:698–705.

Tuthill DP, Stewart JH, Coles EC, et al. Maternal cigarette smoking and pregnancy outcome. *Paediatr Perinatol Epidemiol*. 1999;13:245–253.

US Environmental Protection Agency. *Health Effects Test Guidelines*. OPPTS 870.3700. Prenatal Developmental Toxicity Study. EPA 712-C-98-207; 1998a.

US Environmental Protection Agency. Endocrine Screening Program: Statement of Policy. *Fed Reg*. 1998b;63(248):71542–71568.

US Environmental Protection Agency. Guidelines for Developmental Toxicity Risk Assessment; Notice. *Fed Reg*. 1991a;56:63798–63826.

US Environmental Protection Agency. *Pesticide Assessment Guidelines, subdivision F, Hazard Evaluation: human and domestic animals, addendum 10: neurotoxicity*. Series 81, 82, and 83. EPA 540/09-91-123 PB 91-154617; 1991b.

US Environmental Protection Agency. *Special Report on Environmental Endocrine Disruption: An Effects Assessment and Analysis*. US Environmental Protection Agency, EPA/630/R-012. Washington, DC: USEPA; February 1997.

US Environmental Protection Agency. Toxic Substance Control Act Testing Guidelines. Final Rules: preliminary developmental toxicity screen. *Fed Reg*. 1985;50:39428–39429.

US Food and Drug Administration. *Guidelines for Reproduction Studies for Safety Evaluation of Drugs for Human Use*. Rockville, MD: USFDA; 1966.

US Food and Drug Administration. International Conference on Harmonization; Guideline on Detection of Toxicity to Reproduction for Medicinal Products; Availability; Notice. *Fed Reg*. 1994;59: 48746–48752.

US Food and Drug Administration. Labeling and prescription drug advertising: Content and format for labeling for human prescription drugs. *Fed Reg*. 1979;44:37434–37467.

US Food and Drug Administration. *Guidance document. Nonclinical safety Evaluation of Pediatric Drug Products*. Silver Spring, MD: FDA; 2006.

Vaglia JL, Hall BK. Regulation of neural crest cell populations: occurrence, distribution and underlying mechanisms. *Int J Dev Biol*. 1999;43: 95–110.

Van Maele-Fabry G, Delhaise F, Picard JJ. Morphogenesis and quantification of the development of post-implantation mouse embryos. *Toxicol In Vitro*. 1990;4:149–156.

Vandenberg LN, Colborn T, Hayes TB, et al. Hormones and endocrine-disrupting chemicals: low-dose effects and nonmonotonic dose responses. *Endocr Rev*. 2012;33:378–455.

Vauloup-Fellous C, Hubschen JM, Abernathy ES, et al. Phylogenetic analysis of rubella viruses involved in congenital rubella infections in France between 1995 and 2009. *J Clin Microbiol*. 2010;48:2530–2535.

Vierula M, Niemi M, Keiski A, et al. High and unchanged sperm counts of Finnish men. *Int J Androl*. 1996;19:11–17.

Vogel R, Seidle T, Spielmann H. A modular one-generation reproduction study as a flexible testing system for regulatory safety assessment. *Reprod Toxicol*. 2010;29:242–245.

Vojnits K, Bremer S. Challenges of using pluripotent stem cells for safety assessments of substances. *Toxicology*. 2010;270:10–17.

Volfe JJ. Effects of cocaine on the fetus. *N Engl J Med*. 1992;327:399–407.

vom Saal FS, Hughes C. An extensive new literature concerning low-dose effects of bisphenol A shows the need for a new risk assessment. *Environ Health Perspect*. 2005;113:926–933.

vom Saal FS, Timms BG, Montano MM, et al. Prostate enlargement in mice due to fetal exposure to low doses of estradiol or diethylstilbestrol and opposite effects at high doses. *Proc Natl Acad Sci U S A*. 1997;94:2056–2061.

Von Kries R, Toschke AM, Koletzko B, Slikker W Jr. Maternal smoking during pregnancy and childhood obesity. *Am J Epidemiol*. 2002;156:954–961.

Wald N. Folic acid and the prevention of neural tube defects. In: Keen CL, Bendich A, Willhite CC, eds. *Maternal Nutrition and Pregnancy Outcome*. Ann NY Acad Sci. 1993;678:112–129.

Walfisch A, Al-maawali A, Moretti ME, et al. Teratogenicity of angiotensin converting enzyme inhibitors or receptor blockers. *J Obstet Gynaecol*. 2011;31:465–472.

Warkany J. Manifestations of prenatal nutritional deficiency. *Vit Horm*. 1945;3:73–103.

Warkany J. Development of experimental mammalian teratology. In: Wilson JG, Warkany J, eds. *Teratology: Principles and Techniques*. Chicago: University of Chicago Press; 1965:1–11.

Warkany J. History of teratology. In: *Handbook of Teratology*. Vol 1. New York: Plenum Press; 1977:3–45.

Warkany J. Teratology: spectrum of a science. In: Kalter H, ed. *Issues and Reviews in Teratology*. Vol 1. New York: Plenum Press; 1983:19–31.

Warkany J. Teratogen update: hyperthermia. *Teratology*. 1986;33: 365–371.

Warkany J, Nelson RC. Appearance of skeletal abnormalities in the offspring of rats reared on a deficient diet. *Science*. 1940;92:383–384.

Warkany J, Schraffenberger E. Congenital malformations induced in rats by roentgen rays. *Am J Roentgenol Radium Ther*. 1944;57:455–463.

Warren KR, Li TK. Genetic polymorphisms: impact on the risk of fetal alcohol spectrum disorders. *Birth Defects Res A Clin Mol Teratol*. 2005;73:195–203.

Waterland RA, Jirtle RL. Transposable elements: targets for early nutritional effects on epigenetic gene regulation. *Mol Cell Biol*. 2003;23: 5293–5300.

Waterland RA, Jirtle RL. Early nutrition, epigenetic changes at transposons and imprinted genes, and enhanced susceptibility to adult chronic diseases. *Nutrition*. 2004;20:63–68.

Watkinson WP, Millicovsky G. Effects of phenytoin on maternal heart rate in A/J mice: possible role in teratogenesis. *Teratology*. 1983;28: 1–8.

Weaver TE, Scott WJ Jr. Acetazolamide teratogenesis: association of maternal respiratory acidosis and ectrodactyly in C57BL/6J mice. *Teratology*. 1984a;30:187–193.

Weaver TE, Scott WJ Jr. Acetazolamide teratogenesis: Interactions of maternal metabolic and respiratory acidosis in the induction of ectrodactyly in C57BL/6J mice. *Teratology*. 1984b;30:195–202.

Welsch F. Short term methods of assessing developmental toxicity hazard. In: Kalter H, ed. *Issues and Review in Teratology*. Vol 5. New York: Plenum Press; 1990:115–153.

Welshons WV, Nagel SC, vom Saal FS. Large effects from small exposures. III. Endocrine mechanisms mediating effects of bisphenol A at levels of human exposure. *Endocrinol*. 2006;147:S56–S69.

White E. Death defying acts: a meeting review on apoptosis. *Genes Dev*. 1993;7:2277–2284.

Wilcox AJ, Weinberg CR, O'Connor JF, et al. Incidence of early loss of pregnancy. *N Engl J Med*. 1988;319:189–194.

Wilson JG. Experimental studies on congenital malformations. *J Chron Dis*. 1959;10:111–130.

Wilson JG. *Environment and Birth Defects*. New York: Academic Press; 1973.

Wilson JG. Embryotoxicity of drugs in man. In: Wilson JG, Fraser FC, eds. *Handbook of Teratology*. New York: Plenum Press; 1977: 309–355.

Wilson JG, Roth CB, Warkany J. An analysis of the syndrome of malformations induced by maternal vitamin A deficiency: effects of restoration of vitamin A at various times during gestation. *Am J Anat*. 1953;92:189–217.

Wiltse J. Mode of action: inhibition of histone deacetylase, altering WNT-dependent gene expression, and regulation of beta-catenin—developmental effects of valproic acid. *Crit Rev Toxicol*. 2005;35:727–738.

Windham GC, Hopkins B, Fenster L, Swan SH. Prenatal active or passive tobacco smoke exposure and the risk of preterm delivery or low birth weight. *Epidemiology*. 2000;11:427–433.

Wisborg K, Kesmodel U, Henriksen TB, et al. Exposure to tobacco smoke in utero and the risk of stillbirth and death ain the first year of life. *Am J Epidemiol*. 2001;154:322–327.

Wolf CJ, Takacs ML, Schmid JE, et al. Activation of mouse and human peroxisome proliferator-activated receptor alpha by perfluoroalkyl acids of different functional groups and chain lengths. *Toxicol Sci*. 2008;106:162–171.

Yang L, Ho NY, Alshut R, et al. Zebrafish embryos as models for embryotoxic and teratological effects of chemicals. *Reprod Toxicol*. 2009;28:245–253.

Yelin R, Schyr RB, Kot H, et al. Ethanol exposure affects gene expression in the embryonic organizer and reduces retinoic acid levels. *Dev Biol*. 2005;279:193–204.

You L, Casanova M, Archibeque-Engel S, et al. Impaired male sexual development in perinatal Sprague-Dawley and Long-Evans Hooded rats exposed in utero and lactationally to pp'-DDE. *Toxicol Sci*. 1998;45:162–173.

Young JF. Physiologically-based pharmacokinetic model for pregnancy as a tool for investigation of developmental mechanisms. *Comput Biol Med*. 1998;28:359–364.

Yu M-L, Hsu C-C, Gladen B, Rogan WJ. In utero PCB/PCDF exposure: relation of developmental delay to dysmorphology and dose. *Neurotoxicol Teratol*. 1991;13:195–202.

Zakany J, Tuggle CK, Nguyen-Huu CM. The use of *lacZ* gene fusions in the studies of mammalian development: developmental regulation of mammalian homeobox genes in the CNS. *J Physiol Paris*. 1990;84:21–26.

Zeisel SH. What choline metabolism can tell us about the underlying mechanisms of fetal alcohol spectrum disorders. *Mol Neurobiol*. 2011;44:185–191.

Zoeller RT, Crofton KM. Mode of action: developmental thyroid hormone insufficiency—neurological abnormalities resulting from exposure to propylthiouracil. *Crit Rev Toxicol*. 2005;35:771–781.

Unit IV

Target Organ Toxicity

chapter

Toxic Responses of the Blood

John C. Bloom, Andrew E. Schade,
and John T. Brandt

BLOOD AS A TARGET ORGAN

Hematotoxicology is the study of adverse effects of drugs, nontherapeutic chemicals, and other chemicals in our environment on blood and blood-forming tissues. This subspecialty draws on the discipline of hematology and the principles of toxicology. Scientific understanding of the former began with the contributions of Leeuwenhoek and others in the 17th century with the microscopic examination of blood. Hematology was later recognized as an applied laboratory science but limited to quantitation of formed elements of the blood and the study of their morphology, along with that of bone marrow, spleen, and lymphoid tissues. It is now a diverse medical specialty, which—perhaps more than any other discipline—has made tremendous contributions to molecular medicine.

The vital functions that blood cells perform, together with the susceptibility of this highly proliferative tissue to intoxication, make the hematopoietic system unique as a target organ. Accordingly, it ranks with liver and kidney as among the most important considerations in the risk assessment of individual patient populations exposed to potential toxicants in the environment, workplace, and medicine cabinet.

The delivery of oxygen to tissues throughout the body, maintenance of vascular integrity, and provision of the many affector and effector immune functions necessary for host defense require a prodigious proliferative and regenerative capacity. Each of the various blood cells (erythrocytes, granulocytes, and platelets) is produced at a rate of approximately one to three million/s in a healthy adult and several times that rate in conditions where demand for these cells is high, as in hemolytic anemia or suppurative inflammation (Kaushansky, 2006). As with intestinal mucosa and gonads, this characteristic makes hematopoietic tissue a particularly sensitive target for cytoreductive or antimitotic agents, such as those used to treat cancer, infection, and immune-mediated disorders. This tissue is also susceptible to secondary effects of toxic agents that affect the supply of nutrients, such as iron; the clearance of toxins and metabolites, such as urea; or the production of vital growth factors, such as erythropoietin and granulocyte colony-stimulating factor (G-CSF).

The consequences of direct or indirect damage to blood cells and their precursors are predictable and potentially life-threatening. They include hypoxia, hemorrhage, and infection. These effects may be subclinical and slowly progressive or acute and fulminant, with dramatic clinical presentations. Hematotoxicity is usually assessed in the context of risk versus benefit. It may be used to define dosage in treatment modalities in which these effects are limiting, such as those employing certain anticancer, antiviral, and antithrombotic agents.

Hematotoxicity is generally regarded as unacceptable, however, in treatments for less serious illnesses, such as mild hypertension or arthritis, or following exposure to contaminated foods or environmental contaminants. Risk-versus-benefit decisions involving hematotoxicity may be controversial, especially when the incidence of these effects is very low. Irrespective of whether the effect is linked to the pharmacologic action of the drug, as with cytoreductive or thrombolytic agents, or unrelated to its intended action, the right balance between risk and benefit is not always clear.

Hematotoxicity may be regarded as *primary,* where one or more blood components are directly affected, or *secondary,* where the toxic effect is a consequence of other tissue injury or systemic disturbances. Primary toxicity is regarded as among the more common serious effects of xenobiotics, particularly drugs (Vandendries and Drews, 2006). Secondary toxicity is exceedingly common, due to the propensity of blood cells to reflect a wide range of local and systemic effects of toxicants on other tissues. These secondary effects on hematopoietic tissue are often more reactive or compensatory than toxic and provide the toxicologist and clinician with an important and accessible tool for monitoring and characterizing toxic responses.

HEMATOPOIESIS

The production of blood cells, or hematopoiesis, is a highly regulated sequence of events by which blood cell precursors proliferate and differentiate to meet the relentless needs of oxygen transport, host defense and repair, hemostasis, and other vital functions described previously. The bone marrow is the principal site of hematopoiesis in humans and most laboratory and domestic animals. The spleen has little function in blood cell production in the healthy human but plays a critical role in the clearance of defective or senescent cells, as well as in host defense. In the human fetus, hematopoiesis can be found in the liver, spleen, bone marrow, thymus, and lymph nodes. The bone marrow is the dominant hematopoietic organ in the latter half of gestation and the only blood-cell-producing organ at birth (Moore, 1975). All marrow is active, or "red marrow," at birth (Hudson, 2006). During early childhood, hematopoiesis recedes in long bones and, in adults, is confined to the axial skeleton and proximal humerus and femur (Custer and Ahlfeldt, 1932). The marrow in the distal long bones becomes "yellow" or fatty. When demand for blood cell production is great, as with certain disease states, fatty marrow can be reactivated as sites of hematopoiesis (Fig. 11-1). This can be useful in toxicology studies as a marker of sustained hematopoietic stress, as exemplified in studies on the hematopathology of cephalosporin toxicity in the dog (Bloom *et al.,* 1987). Under extreme conditions, embryonic patterns of hematopoiesis may reappear as *extramedullary hematopoiesis* (Young and Weiss, 1997).

While the central function of bone marrow is hematopoiesis and lymphopoiesis, bone marrow is also one of the sites of the mononuclear phagocyte system (MPS), contributing monocytes that differentiate into a variety of MPS cells located in liver (Kupffer cells), spleen (littoral cells), lymph nodes, and other tissues. Conventional histologic and cytologic sampling of bone marrow reveals a very limited picture of an exceedingly complex tissue containing erythroid, granulocytic, megakaryocytic, MPS, and lymphoid precursors in varied stages of maturation; stromal cells; and vasculature all encased by bone (Fig. 11-1). Routine examinations of such specimens in our pathology and toxicology laboratories cannot possibly reveal the sophisticated interactions that mediate lineage commitment, proliferation, differentiation, acquisition of functional characteristics, and trafficking that result in the delivery of mature cells to the circulation, as required in sickness and in health. Exactly how the process of hematopoietic progenitor cell differentiation and maturation and subsequent release into the peripheral circulation is so tightly regulated is not fully known. Early and elegant morphologic studies revealed a complex interplay of developing cells with stromal cells, extracellular matrix components, and cytokines that make up the *hematopoietic inductive microenvironment* (HIM) (Young and Weiss, 1997). More recent studies have shown that each lineage, and even stage of maturation, is supported within a specific niche that is maintained by the surrounding stromal cells (Heissig *et al.,* 2005). An array of cytokines and chemokines directs a particular progenitor cell to the appropriate niche (Lataillade *et al.,* 2004). Today's powerful research tools, which include the use of knockout mice, have begun to define how hematopoietic growth factors, cytokines, and chemokines interact with the HIM and other tissues to control the production and trafficking of blood cells (Kaushansky, 2006; Laurence, 2006). These tools also include the evolving applications of systems biology, which uses a combination of mathematical, engineering, and computational tools for constructing and validating models for studying complex biologic phenomena such as hematopoieses (Whichard *et al.,* 2010). These understandings are providing opportunities to develop promising therapies that are now presenting new pharmacologic and toxicologic challenges.

TOXICOLOGY OF THE ERYTHRON

The Erythrocyte

Erythrocytes (red blood cells [RBCs]) make up 40% to 45% of the circulating blood volume and serve as the principal vehicle of transportation of oxygen from the lungs to the peripheral tissues. In addition, erythrocytes are involved in the transport of carbon dioxide from tissues to the lung, maintenance of a constant pH in blood, and regulation of blood flow to tissues (Hsia, 1998; Kim-Shapiro *et al.,* 2005). Erythrocytes help modulate the inflammatory response through clearance of immune complexes containing complement components and through interaction with nitric oxide, a potent vasodilator (Kim-Shapiro *et al.,* 2005; Lindorfer *et al.,* 2001). An area of developing interest is the role of erythrocytes as a carrier and/or reservoir for drugs and toxins (Schrijvers *et al.,* 1999). The effect of xenobiotics on erythrocytes has been extensively evaluated, because of both the ready access to the tissue and the frequency with which xenobiotics cause changes in this critical tissue.

Xenobiotics may affect the production, function, and/or survival of erythrocytes. These effects are most frequently manifest as a change in the circulating red cell mass, usually resulting in a decrease (anemia). Occasionally, agents that increase oxygen affinity lead to an increase in red cell mass (erythrocytosis), but this is distinctly less common. Shifts in plasma volume can alter the relative concentration of erythrocytes/hemoglobin and can be easily confused with true anemia or erythrocytosis.

There are two general mechanisms that lead to true anemia—either decreased production or increased erythrocyte destruction. Both mechanisms may be operative in some disorders, or a combination may arise due to the imposition of a second disorder on a compensated underlying problem. For example, patients with compensated congenital hemolytic anemias are very susceptible to additional insults that may precipitate an acute drop in a previously stable red cell mass, such as parvovirus infection-associated suppression of erythropoiesis.

Evaluation of a peripheral blood sample can provide evidence for the underlying mechanism of anemia. The usual parameters

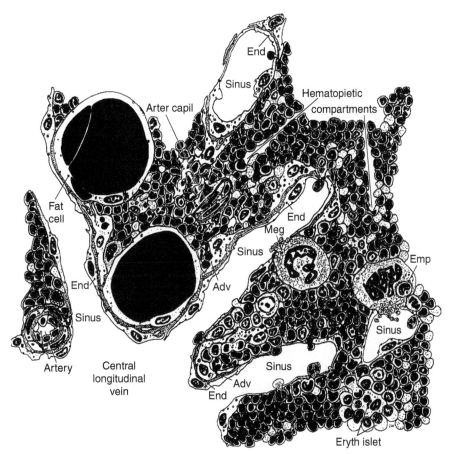

Figure 11-1. *Bone marrow schema.* Several venous sinuses (Sinus), cut longitudinally, drain into the central longitudinal vein, cut in cross-section. A branch of the nutrient artery (Artery) and an arterial capillary (Arter Capil) are present. The circulation in the bone marrow, as in the other tissues of the body save the spleen, is "closed," that is, there is endothelial continuity from artery into vein. Veins in bone marrow have in common with veins elsewhere the primary function of returning blood to the heart. Marrow veins, in addition, possess the distinctive function of receiving blood cells produced and stored in the marrow and carrying them to thymus or spleen, or into the general circulation, for further maturation, widespread distribution, and function. The hematopoietic compartments of the bone marrow consist of hematopoietic cells in varying stages of differentiation supported by a fibroblastic stroma. They lie between the most proximal veins, termed venous sinuses or vascular sinuses. When hematopoiesis is rather quiet and few nascent blood cells cross the wall of vascular sinuses, moving from hematopoietic compartments into the sinus lumen, the wall of the sinus tends to be trilaminar, consisting of endothelium (end), wispy basement membrane (in stipple), and adventitial reticular cells (adv) that form an incomplete outermost layer and branch out into the hematopoietic compartment, forming a scaffolding enclosing and supporting the hematopoietic cells. Thus, adventitial reticular cells are both vascular, as the outermost wall of the vascular sinus, and stromal, branching into the perivascular hematopoietic space, holding the vascular sinus in place and supporting hematopoietic cells. Where hematopoietic cell traffic across the wall of the venous sinus is heightened, the adventitial cell cover is retracted and a larger expanse of endothelium, covered only by wisps of basement membrane, is exposed to the hematopoietic cells, facilitating their transmural cell passage. Where transmural cell passage is greatly reduced, adventitial cells accumulate fat and become rounded and bulky, now termed adipocytes, impeding hematopoietic cell passage, and occupying space in the hematopoietic compartment that, when they transform again to adventitial cells flattened upon veins, yield to hematopoiesis. These fibroblastic stromal cells in the marrow of central bones can modulate readily to and from adventitial cell and adipocyte and retain their granulocyte inductive capacities in either form. In the distal limb and tail bones, where there is little hematopoiesis, they assume the adipocyte form in such large numbers that the marrow is grossly yellow. These adipocytes lose fat only in marked hematopoietic stress, as in spherocytic and other severe anemias where this marrow becomes hematopoietic and grossly red. In such stress, moreover, barrier cells may augment or replace adventitial reticular cells and even endothelial cells. Thus, adventitial cells/adipocytes, by their disposition and bulk, mechanically regulate hematopoiesis and blood cell delivery. In addition, they do so in a subtle manner, through paracrine secretion of several small-protein regulatory factors termed cytokines, which include interleukins. (Reprinted from Young and Weiss [1997], with permission from the authors and Elsevier Science.)

of a complete blood count (CBC)—including the RBC count, hemoglobin concentration (Hbg), and hematocrit (also referred to as packed cell volume [PCV])—can establish the presence of anemia. Two additional parameters helpful in classifying an anemia are the mean corpuscular volume (MCV) and the reticulocyte count. Increased destruction is usually accompanied by an increase in reticulocytes (young erythrocytes containing residual RNA), which are easily enumerated using appropriate stains. The introduction of automated methods has improved the precision of reticulocyte counting and introduced new parameters that aid in

characterization of red cell production. With these new methods, reticulocyte counting may also be useful in conditions associated with decreased production, particularly when assessing response to therapy. Other readily performed parameters helpful in the evaluation of the human erythron include erythrocyte morphology (eg, megaloblastic changes, erythrocyte fragmentation, sickled RBCs); serum concentration of haptoglobin, lactic dehydrogenase (LD), free hemoglobin, vitamin B_{12}, folate, iron, and ferritin; direct and indirect red cell antiglobulin tests; and bone marrow morphology (Prchal, 2006; Ryan, 2006).

Alterations in Red Cell Production

Erythrocyte production is a continuous process that is dependent on frequent cell division and a high rate of hemoglobin synthesis. Human adult hemoglobin (hemoglobin A), the major constituent of the erythrocyte cytoplasm, is a tetramer composed of two α-globin and two β-globin chains, each with a heme residue located in a stereospecific pocket of the globin chain. Synthesis of hemoglobin is dependent on coordinated production of globin chains and heme moieties. Abnormalities that lead to decreased hemoglobin synthesis are relatively common (eg, iron deficiency) and are often associated with a decrease in the MCV and hypochromasia (increased central pallor of RBCs on stained blood films due to the low hemoglobin concentration).

An imbalance between α- and β-chain production is the basis of congenital thalassemia syndromes and results in decreased hemoglobin production and microcytosis (Weatherall, 2006). Xenobiotics can affect globin chain synthesis and alter the composition of hemoglobin within erythrocytes. This is perhaps best demonstrated by hydroxyurea, which has been found to increase the synthesis of γ-globin chains. The γ-globin chains are a normal constituent of hemoglobin during fetal development, replacing the β chains in the hemoglobin tetramer (hemoglobin F, $\alpha_2\gamma_2$). Hemoglobin F has a higher affinity for oxygen than hemoglobin A and can protect against crystallization (sickling) of deoxyhemoglobin S in sickle cell disease (Steinberg, 2006).

Synthesis of heme requires incorporation of iron into a porphyrin ring (Fig. 11-2) (Napier *et al.*, 2005; Ponka, 1997). Iron

Table 11-1

Xenobiotics Associated with Sideroblastic Anemia

Ethanol	Chloramphenicol
Isoniazid	Copper chelation/deficiency
Pyrazinamide	Zinc intoxication
Cycloserine	Lead intoxication

deficiency is usually the result of dietary deficiency or increased blood loss. Drugs that contribute to blood loss, such as nonsteroidal anti-inflammatory agents, with their increased risk of gastrointestinal ulceration and bleeding, may potentiate the risk of developing *iron deficiency anemia.* Defects in the synthesis of porphyrin ring of heme can lead to *sideroblastic anemia,* with its characteristic accumulation of iron in bone marrow erythroblasts. The accumulated iron precipitates within mitochondria in a complex with mitochondrial ferritin, causing the characteristic staining pattern of ringed sideroblasts evident on iron stains such as Prussian blue (Cazzola *et al.*, 2003). A number of xenobiotics (Table 11-1) can interfere with one or more of the steps in erythroblast heme synthesis and result in sideroblastic anemia (Alcindor and Bridges, 2002; Beutler, 2006a,b,c; Fiske *et al.*, 1994).

Hematopoiesis requires active DNA synthesis and frequent mitoses. Folate and vitamin B_{12} are necessary to maintain synthesis of thymidine for incorporation into DNA (Fig. 11-3). Deficiency of folate and/or vitamin B_{12} results in *megaloblastic anemia,* with its

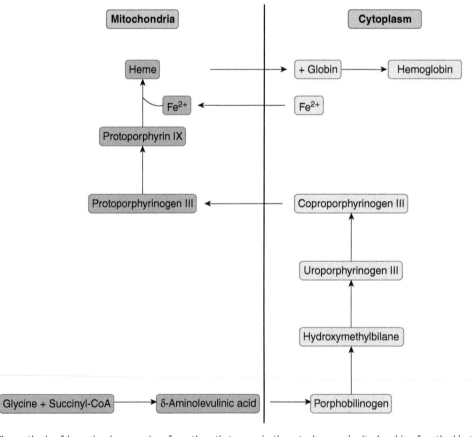

Figure 11-2. *The synthesis of heme involves a series of reactions that occur in the cytoplasm and mitochondria of erythroblasts.* The initial step in the pathway is the mitochondria synthesis of δ-aminolevulinic acid, a step that is commonly affected by xenobiotics, including lead. Ferrochelatase catalyzes the incorporation of ferrous iron into the tetrapyrrole protoporphyrin IX. Inhibition of the synthetic pathway leading to protoporphyrin IX, as occurs in the sideroblastic anemias, can cause an imbalance between iron concentration and ferrochelatase activity, resulting in iron deposition within mitochondria. Mitochondrial accumulation of iron is the hallmark lesion of the sideroblastic anemias.

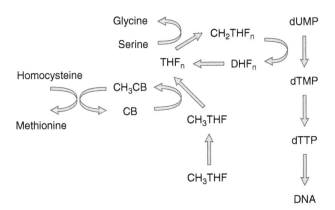

Figure 11-3. *Both tetrahydrofolate (THF) and cobalamin (CB, or vitamin B_{12}) are necessary for the synthesis of thymidine (dTMP) for incorporation into DNA.* Folate enters the cell as a monoglutamate (CH_3THF) but is transformed to a polyglutamate within the cell, a step that helps prevent leakage of folate back across the cell membrane. However, CH_3THF cannot be conjugated with glutamate. CB is necessary for demethylation of the folate, allowing formation of conjugated (polyglutamate) folate (THF_n). In the absence of CB, folate levels within the cell drop, causing a functional deficiency of folate and impairing synthesis of thymidine.

characteristic morphologic and biochemical changes (Table 11-2), which commonly affect erythroid, myeloid, and megakaryocytic lineages. A number of xenobiotics may contribute to a deficiency of vitamin B_{12} and/or folate (Table 11-3), leading to megaloblastic anemia (Babior, 2006).

Many of the antiproliferative drugs used in the treatment of malignancy predictably inhibit hematopoiesis, including erythropoiesis. The resulting bone marrow toxicity may be dose-limiting, as previously discussed. Drugs, such as amifostine, have been developed that may help protect against the marrow toxicity of these agents (Phillips, 2002). The development of recombinant forms of some of the growth factors that regulate hematopoiesis has helped shorten the duration of bone marrow suppression. As with other therapeutic proteins, there is a risk of antibody formation in response to administration of these proteins; if the antibody reacts with the endogenous growth factor, it may cause profound cytopenia (Bennett *et al.,* 2004; Li *et al.,* 2001).

Erythropoietin is commonly used to support red cell production in patients undergoing chemotherapy and with renal failure. Following a change in formulation, a series of cases of red cell aplasia associated with erythropoietin use was reported

Table 11-2

Laboratory Features of Megaloblastic Anemia

MORPHOLOGY	BIOCHEMISTRY
Peripheral blood	Peripheral blood
Pancytopenia	Decreased B_{12} and/or folate
Macrocytosis ($\uparrow$ MCV)	Increased LD
Oval macrocytes	Antiparietal cell antibodies
Hypersegmented	Antibody to intrinsic factor
neutrophils	Increased serum iron
Variation in RBC shape	Hypokalemia
Bone marrow	
Erythroid hyperplasia	
Megaloblastic anemia	
Giant band neutrophils	
Giant metamyelocytes	

Table 11-3

Xenobiotics Associated with Megaloblastic Anemia

B_{12} DEFICIENCY	FOLATE DEFICIENCY
Paraminosalicylic acid	Phenytoin
Colchicine	Primidone
Neomycin	Carbamazepine
Ethanol	Phenobarbital
Omeprazole	Sulfasalazine
Hemodialysis	Cholestyramine
Zidovudine	Triamterene
Fish tapeworm	Malabsorption syndromes
	Antimetabolites

(Bennett *et al.,* 2004). The etiology was antibodies to the synthetic protein that cross-reacted with endogenous erythropoietin. A change in formulation in combination with the nature of the storage container and route of administration is thought to have promoted the formation of protein aggregates, a phenomenon known to be associated with an increased risk of antibody formation (Koren *et al.,* 2002). The incidence of red cell aplasia appears to have diminished following a change in packaging and administration of erythropoietin by intravenous injection (Bennett *et al.,* 2004).

Drug-induced *aplastic anemia* may represent either a predictable or idiosyncratic reaction to a xenobiotic. This life-threatening disorder is characterized by peripheral blood pancytopenia, reticulocytopenia, and bone marrow hypoplasia (Vandendries and Drews, 2006; Young, 1999, 2000). Agents such as benzene and radiation have a *predictable* effect on hematopoietic progenitors, and the resulting aplastic anemia corresponds to the magnitude of the exposure to these agents. In contrast, idiosyncratic aplastic anemia does not appear to be related to the dose of the agent initiating the process. A long list of chemicals has been associated with the development of aplastic anemia (Table 11-4), many of which have been reported in only a few patients. The principal mechanisms of aplastic anemia, as with the more common agranulocytosis, are still debated. Immune mechanisms have long been thought to contribute to the development of both idiosyncratic disorders, as discussed in greater detail in the next section. However, it has been, up until recently, difficult to obtain definitive evidence for humoral and/or cellular mechanisms of marrow suppression (Vandendries and Drews, 2006; Young, 2000). Recent observations have strongly suggested that both toxicities are immune-mediated, often involving altered proteins through reactive metabolite–mediated damage (Zhang *et al.,* 2011).

Pure red cell aplasia is a syndrome in which the decrease in marrow production is limited to the erythroid lineage (Djaldetti *et al.,* 2003; Fisch *et al.,* 2000). It is an uncommon disorder that may be due to genetic defects, infection (parvovirus B19), immune-mediated injury, myelodysplasia, drugs, or other toxins. As pure red cell aplasia occurs sporadically and infrequently, the linkage between drug exposure and pathogenesis of the aplasia remains speculative for some agents. The drugs most clearly implicated and for which there are multiple case reports include isoniazid, phenytoin, and azathioprine. The mechanism of drug-induced pure red cell aplasia is unknown, but some evidence suggests that it may also be immune-mediated. Patients with drug-induced red cell aplasia should not be reexposed to the purported offending chemical. As noted above, pure red aplasia may also occur as a consequence of an immune response to therapeutic erythropoietin.

Table 11-4

Drugs and Other Chemicals Associated with the Development of Aplastic Anemia

Chloramphenicol	Organic arsenicals	Quinacrine
Methylphenylethylhydantoin	Trimethadione	Phenylbutazone
Gold	Streptomycin	Benzene
Penicillin	Allopurinol	Tetracycline
Methicillin	Sulfonamides	Chlortetracycline
Sulfisoxazole	Sulfamethoxypyridazine	Amphotericin B
Mefloquine	Ethosuximide	Felbamate
Carbimazole	Methylmercaptoimidazole	Potassium perchlorate
Propylthiouracil	Tolbutamide	Pyrimethamine
Chlorpropamide	Carbutamide	Tripelennamine
Indomethacin	Carbamazepine	Diclofenac
Meprobamate	Chlorpromazine	Chlordiazepoxide
Mepazine	Chlorophenothane	Parathion
Thiocyanate	Methazolamide	Dinitrophenol
Bismuth	Mercury	Chlordane
Carbon tetrachloride	Cimetidine	Metolazone
Azidothymidine	Ticlopidine	Isoniazid
Trifluoperazine	D-Penicillamine	

Alterations in the Respiratory Function of Hemoglobin

Hemoglobin is necessary for effective transport of oxygen and carbon dioxide between the lungs and tissues. The respiratory function of hemoglobin has been studied in detail, revealing an intricately balanced system for the transport of oxygen from the lungs to the tissues (Hsia, 1998). Electrostatic charges hold the globin chains of deoxyhemoglobin in a "tense" (T) conformation characterized by a relatively low affinity for oxygen. Binding of oxygen alters this conformation to a "relaxed" (R) conformation that is associated with a 500-fold increase in oxygen affinity. Thus, the individual globin units show cooperativity in the binding of oxygen, resulting in the familiar sigmoid shape to the oxygen dissociation curve (Fig. 11-4). The ability of hemoglobin to safely and efficiently transport oxygen is dependent on both intrinsic (homotropic) and extrinsic (heterotropic) factors that affect the performance of this system.

Homotropic Effects One of the most important homotropic properties of oxyhemoglobin is the slow but consistent oxidation of heme iron to the ferric state to form methemoglobin (Percy *et al.*, 2005). Methemoglobin is not capable of binding and transporting oxygen. In addition, the presence of methemoglobin in a hemoglobin tetramer has allosteric effects that increase the affinity of oxyhemoglobin for oxygen, resulting in a leftward shift of the oxygen dissociation curve (Fig. 11-4). The combination of decreased oxygen content and increased affinity may significantly impair delivery of oxygen to tissues when the concentration of methemoglobin rises beyond critical levels (Hsia, 1998; Percy *et al.*, 2005).

Not surprisingly, the normal erythrocyte has metabolic mechanisms for reducing heme iron back to the ferrous state; these mechanisms are normally capable of maintaining the concentration of methemoglobin at less than 1% of total hemoglobin (Percy *et al.*, 2005). The predominant pathway is cytochrome b_5 methemoglobin reductase, which is dependent on reduced nicotine adenine dinucleotide (NADH) and is also known as NADH diaphorase. An alternate pathway involves a reduced nicotine adenine dinucleotide phosphate (NADPH) diaphorase that reduces a flavin that in turn reduces methemoglobin. This pathway usually accounts for less

than 5% of the reduction of methemoglobin, but its activity can be greatly enhanced by methylene blue, which is reduced to leukomethylene blue by NADPH diaphorase. Leukomethylene blue then reduces methemoglobin to deoxyhemoglobin.

A failure of these control mechanisms leads to increased levels of methemoglobin, or *methemoglobinemia*. The most common cause of methemoglobinemia is exposure to an oxidizing xenobiotic that overwhelms the NADH diaphorase system. A large number of chemicals and therapeutic agents may cause methemoglobinemia

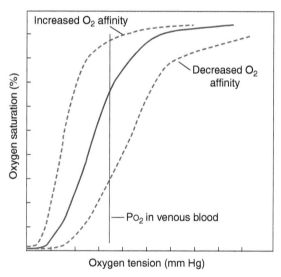

Figure 11-4. *The normal oxygen dissociation curve (solid line) has a sigmoid shape due to the cooperative interaction between the four globin chains in the hemoglobin molecule.* Fully deoxygenated hemoglobin has a relatively low affinity for oxygen. Interaction of oxygen with one heme-iron moiety induces a conformational change in that globin chain. Through surface interactions, that conformational change affects the other globin chains, causing a conformational change in all of the globin chains that increases their affinity for oxygen. Homotropic and heterotropic parameters also affect the affinity of hemoglobin for oxygen. An increase in oxygen affinity results in a shift to the left in the oxygen dissociation curve. Such a shift may decrease oxygen delivery to the tissues. A decrease in oxygen affinity results in a shift to the right in the oxygen dissociation curve, facilitating oxygen delivery to the tissues.

Table 11-5

Xenobiotics Associated with Methemoglobinemia

THERAPEUTIC AGENTS	ENVIRONMENTAL AGENTS
Benzocaine	Nitrites
Lidocaine	Nitrates
Prilocaine	Nitrobenzenes
Dapsone	Aniline dyes and aniline derivatives
Amyl nitrate	Butyl nitrite
Isobutyl nitrite	Potassium chlorate
Nitroglycerine	Gasoline additives
Primaquine	Aminobenzenes
Sulfonamide	Nitrotoluenes
Phenacetin	Trinitrotoluene
Nitric oxide	Nitroethane
Phenazopyridine	*ortho*-Toluidine
Metoclopramide	*para*-Toluidine
Flutamide	β-Naphthol disulfonate
Silver nitrate	
Quinones	
Methylene blue	

(Table 11-5) (Bradberry *et al.*, 2001; Bradberry, 2003; Coleman and Coleman, 1996). These chemicals may be divided into direct oxidizers, which are capable of inducing methemoglobin formation when added to erythrocytes in vitro or in vivo, and indirect oxidizers, which do not induce methemoglobin formation when exposed to erythrocytes in vitro but do so after metabolic modification in vivo. Nitrites appear to be able to interact directly with heme to facilitate oxidation of heme iron, but the precise mechanism that leads to methemoglobin formation is unknown for many of the other substances listed in Table 11-5.

The development of methemoglobinemia may be slow and insidious or abrupt in onset, as with the use of some topical anesthetics (Bradberry *et al.*, 2001; Bradberry, 2003; Khan and Kruse, 1999; Nguyen *et al.*, 2000). Most patients tolerate low levels (<10%) of methemoglobin without clinical symptoms. Cyanosis is often evident when the methemoglobin concentration exceeds 5% to 10%. Levels above 20% are generally clinically significant and some patients may begin to manifest symptoms related to tissue hypoxemia at methemoglobin levels between 10% and 20%. The severity of clinical manifestations increases as the concentration rises above 20% to 30%, with methemoglobin levels above 70% being life-threatening. Intravenous administration of one to two mg/kg methylene blue is effective in rapidly reversing methemoglobinemia through activation of the NADPH diaphorase pathway (Clifton and Leikin, 2003). The effect of methylene blue is dependent on an adequate supply of NADPH. Consequently, methylene blue is not effective in patients with glucose-6-phosphate dehydrogenase (G-6-PD) deficiency because of the decreased capacity to form NADPH (Bradberry, 2003; Coleman and Coleman, 1996).

Heterotropic Effects There are three major heterotropic effectors of hemoglobin function: pH, erythrocyte 2,3-bisphosphoglycerate (2,3-BPG, formerly designated 2,3-diphosphoglycerate) concentration, and temperature (Hsia, 1998). A decrease in pH (eg, lactic acid, carbon dioxide) lowers the affinity of hemoglobin for oxygen, that is, it causes a right shift in the oxygen dissociation curve, facilitating the delivery of oxygen to tissues (Fig. 11-4). As bicarbonate and carbon dioxide equilibrate in the lung, the hydrogen ion concentration decreases, increasing the affinity of hemoglobin for oxygen and facilitating oxygen uptake. Thus, the buffering capacity of hemoglobin also serves to improve oxygen uptake and delivery.

The binding site for 2,3-BPG is located in a pocket formed by the 2 β chains of a hemoglobin tetramer. Binding of 2,3-BPG to deoxyhemoglobin results in stabilization of the "T" conformation, with reduced oxygen affinity (a shift to the right of the oxygen dissociation curve). The conformational change induced by binding of oxygen alters the binding site for 2,3-BPG and results in release of 2,3-BPG from hemoglobin. This facilitates uptake of more oxygen for delivery to tissues. The concentration of 2,3-BPG increases whenever there is tissue hypoxemia but may decrease in the presence of acidosis or hypophosphatemia. Thus, hypophosphatemia may result in a left shift of the oxygen dissociation curve.

Clofibric acid and bezafibrate are capable of lowering the oxygen affinity of hemoglobin, analogous to 2,3-BPG (Poyart *et al.*, 1994). However, the association constant of bezafibrate for hemoglobin is too low for there to be a meaningful effect in vivo. Work continues on bezafibrate derivatives that may lower oxygen affinity and enhance tissue oxygenation. In contrast, some aromatic benzaldehydes have been shown to increase oxygen affinity and shift the dissociation curve to the left. It was thought that these compounds may be useful in preventing the sickling of deoxyhemoglobin S in patients with sickle cell disease. However, these and other chemicals evaluated for their effect on hemoglobin oxygen affinity have not progressed into clinical usage (Papassotiriou *et al.*, 1998; Poyart *et al.*, 1994).

The oxygen affinity of hemoglobin decreases as the body temperature increases (Hsia, 1998). This facilitates delivery of oxygen to tissues during periods of extreme exercise and febrile illnesses associated with increased temperature. Correspondingly, oxygen affinity increases during hypothermia, which may lead to decreased oxygen delivery under these conditions. This must be taken into consideration during surgical procedures during which there is induction of deep hypothermia.

The respiratory function of hemoglobin may also be impaired by blockade of the ligand binding site following interaction with other substances, most notably carbon monoxide (Hsia, 1998). Carbon monoxide has a relatively low rate of association with deoxyhemoglobin but has high affinity once bound. The affinity is about 200 times that of oxygen, and thus persistent exposure to a low level of carbon monoxide (eg, 0.1%) may lead to 50% saturation of hemoglobin. Binding of carbon monoxide also results in stabilization of the hemoglobin molecule in the high-affinity "R" conformation. Consequently, the oxygen dissociation curve is shifted to the left, further compromising oxygen delivery to the tissues. Carbon monoxide is produced at low levels by the body through the metabolism of heme and equilibrates across the pulmonary capillary/alveolar bed. Low concentrations of carboxyhemoglobin can be cytoprotective during inflammatory stress or ischemia/reperfusion injury and the therapeutic use of low concentrations of carbon monoxide is being explored (Kao and Nanagas, 2005; Ryter and Otterbein, 2004).

The major sources of significant exogenous exposure to carbon monoxide are smoking and burning of fossil fuels (including automobiles), particularly in enclosed spaces. Heavy smoking during pregnancy may result in significant levels of carboxyhemoglobin in fetal blood and diminished oxygenation of fetal tissues. Symptoms of carbon monoxide toxicity, such as dizziness, shortness of breath, and headache, begin to appear when carboxyhemoglobin levels reach 20%. Levels of 50% to 80% carboxyhemoglobin may be lethal. In addition to effects due to interaction with hemoglobin, CO may cause toxicity through effects on myoglobin, cytochromes, guanylate cyclase, or nitric oxide. The key to therapy is removal from the source of carbon monoxide and provision of an adequate supply of oxygen; hyperbaric hyperoxia may be used in serious cases (Kao and Nanagas, 2005; Ryter and Otterbein, 2004).

Methemoglobin can combine reversibly with a variety of chemical substances, including cyanide, sulfides, peroxides, fluorides, and azides. The affinity of methemoglobin for cyanide is utilized in two settings. First, nitrites are administered in cyanide poisoning to form methemoglobin, which then binds free cyanide, sparing other critical cellular respiratory enzymes (Cummings, 2004). Second, formation of cyanmethemoglobin by reaction of hemoglobin with potassium ferricyanide is a standard method for measurement of hemoglobin concentration.

Nitric oxide, an important vasodilator that modulates vascular tone, binds avidly to heme iron. An additional function of erythrocytes is related to this interaction, which can influence the availability of nitric oxide in parts of the circulation (Hsia, 1998; Lundberg and Weitzberg, 2005). Solutions of hemoglobin have been evaluated as a potential replacement for RBC transfusions. However, these trials have been halted due to the toxicity associated with administration of hemoglobin solutions. Vascular instability is one of the complications associated with infusion of hemoglobin solutions and is thought to be related to the scavenging of essential nitric oxide by the administered hemoglobin (Moore *et al.*, 2005; Rother *et al.*, 2005).

Alterations in Erythrocyte Survival

The normal survival of erythrocytes in the circulation is about 120 days (Dessypris, 1999). During this period the erythrocytes are exposed to a variety of oxidative injuries and must negotiate the tortuous passages of the microcirculation and the spleen. This requires a deformable cell membrane and energy to maintain the sodium–potassium gradients and repair mechanisms (Van Wijk and van Solinge, 2005). Very little protein synthesis occurs during this time, as erythrocytes are anucleate when they enter the circulation and residual mRNA is rapidly lost over the first one to two days in the circulation. Consequently, senescence occurs over time until the aged erythrocytes are removed by the spleen, where the iron is recovered for reutilization in heme synthesis. Any insult that increases oxidative injury, decreases metabolism, or alters the membrane may cause a decrease in erythrocyte concentration and a corresponding anemia.

Nonimmune Hemolytic Anemia

Microangiopathic Anemias Intravascular fragmentation of erythrocytes gives rise to the *microangiopathic hemolytic anemias* (Baker, 2006). The hallmark of this process is the presence of schistocytes (fragmented RBCs) in the peripheral blood. These abnormal cellular fragments are usually promptly cleared from the circulation by the spleen. Thus, their presence in peripheral blood samples indicates either an increased rate of formation or abnormal clearance function of the spleen. The formation of fibrin strands in the microcirculation is a common mechanism for RBC fragmentation. This may occur in the setting of disseminated intravascular coagulation, sepsis, the hemolytic-uremic syndrome (HUS), and thrombotic thrombocytopenic purpura (TTP). The erythrocytes are essentially sliced into fragments by the fibrin strands that extend across the vascular lumen and impede the flow of erythrocytes through the vasculature. Excessive fragmentation can also be seen in the presence of abnormal vasculature, as occurs with damaged cardiac valves, arteriovenous malformations, vasculitis, and widely metastatic carcinoma (Baker, 2006). The high shear associated with malignant hypertension may also lead to RBC fragmentation.

Other Mechanical Injuries March hemoglobinuria is an episodic disorder characterized by destruction of RBCs during vigorous exercise or marching (Abarbanel *et al.*, 1990; Sagov, 1970). The erythrocytes appear to be destroyed by mechanical trauma in the feet. Sufficient hemoglobin may be released to cause hemoglobinuria. The disorder should be distinguished from other causes of intermittent hemoglobinuria such as paroxysmal nocturnal hemoglobinuria. The introduction of improved footgear for athletes and soldiers has significantly decreased the incidence of this problem.

Major thermal burns are also associated with a hemolytic process. The erythrocyte membrane becomes unstable as the temperature increases. With major burns there can be significant heat-dependent lysis of erythrocytes. Small RBC fragments break off, with resealing of the cell membrane. These cell fragments usually assume a spherical shape and are not as deformable as normal erythrocytes. Consequently, these abnormal cell fragments are removed in the spleen, leading to an anemia. The burden of RBC fragments may impair the phagocytic function of the spleen, contributing to the increased susceptibility to endotoxic shock following major burns (Hatherill *et al.*, 1986; Schneidkraut and Loegering, 1984).

Infectious Diseases A variety of infectious diseases may be associated with significant hemolysis, by either direct effect on the erythrocyte or development of an immune-mediated hemolytic process (Berkowitz, 1991; Beutler, 2006a,b,c). The most common agents that directly cause hemolysis include malaria, babesiosis, clostridial infections, and bartonellosis. Erythrocytes are parasitized in malaria and babesiosis, leading to their destruction. Clostridial infections are associated with release of hemolytic toxins that enter the circulation and lyse erythrocytes. The hemolysis can be severe with significant hemoglobinuria, even with apparently localized infections. *Bartonella bacilliformis* is thought to adhere to the erythrocyte, leading to rapid removal from the circulation. The hemolysis can be severe and the mortality rate in this disorder (Oroya fever) is high.

Oxidative Hemolysis Molecular oxygen is a reactive and potentially toxic chemical species; consequently, the normal respiratory function of erythrocytes generates oxidative stress on a continuous basis. The major mechanisms that protect against oxidative injury in erythrocytes include NADH diaphorase, superoxide dismutase, catalase, and the glutathione pathway (Coleman and Coleman, 1996; Njalsson and Norgren, 2005). As indicated previously, a small amount of methemoglobin is continuously formed during the process of loading and unloading of oxygen from hemoglobin. Formation of methemoglobin is associated with formation of superoxide free radicals, which must be detoxified to prevent oxidative injury to hemoglobin and other critical erythrocyte components. Under physiologic conditions, superoxide dismutase converts superoxide into hydrogen peroxide, which is then metabolized by catalase and glutathione peroxidase (Fig. 11-5).

A number of xenobiotics, particularly compounds containing aromatic amines, are capable of inducing oxidative injury in erythrocytes (Table 11-6) (Bradberry, 2003; Percy *et al.*, 2005). These chemicals appear to potentiate the normal redox reactions and are capable of overwhelming the usual protective mechanisms. The interaction between these xenobiotics and hemoglobin leads to the formation of free radicals that denature critical proteins, including hemoglobin, thiol-dependent enzymes, and components of the erythrocyte membrane. In the presence of hydrogen peroxide and xenobiotics such as hydroxylamine, hydroxamic acid, and phenolic

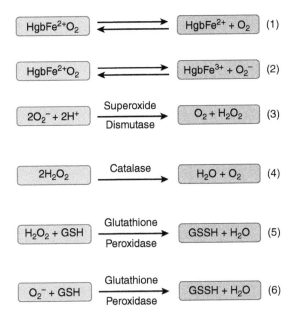

$$HgbFe^{2+}O_2 \rightleftharpoons HgbFe^{2+} + O_2 \quad (1)$$

$$HgbFe^{2+}O_2 \rightleftharpoons HgbFe^{3+} + O_2^- \quad (2)$$

$$2O_2^- + 2H^+ \xrightarrow{\text{Superoxide Dismutase}} O_2 + H_2O_2 \quad (3)$$

$$2H_2O_2 \xrightarrow{\text{Catalase}} H_2O + O_2 \quad (4)$$

$$H_2O_2 + GSH \xrightarrow{\text{Glutathione Peroxidase}} GSSH + H_2O \quad (5)$$

$$O_2^- + GSH \xrightarrow{\text{Glutathione Peroxidase}} GSSH + H_2O \quad (6)$$

Figure 11-5. *Oxygen normally exchanges with the ferrous iron of deoxyhemoglobin (Eq. (1)).* Oxygen can "capture" one of the iron electrons, resulting in the generation of methemoglobin (HgbFe^{3+}) and superoxide (O$_2^-$) (Eq. (2)). Superoxide must be detoxified or it can lead to oxidative injury within the cell. The pathways involved include superoxide dismutase (Eq. (3)), catalase (Eq. (4)), and glutathione peroxidase (Eqs. (5) and (6)). A supply of reduced glutathione (GSH) is necessary to prevent excessive oxidative injury.

compounds, a reactive ferryl (Fe^{4+}) hemoglobin intermediate may be formed according to the following reaction:

$$H_2O_2 + Hgb - Fe^{3+} \rightarrow H_2O + Hgb(\bullet+) - Fe^{4+} - O^-.$$

In this intermediate, referred to as compound 1, tyrosine may donate the extra electron, turning it into a reactive free radical. Compound 1 may undergo further reaction with organic compounds (AH$_2$ in the following equations) to yield additional free radicals according to the following reactions:

$$Hgb(\bullet+) - Fe^{4+} - O + AH_2 \rightarrow Hgb - Fe^{4+} - O^- + AH\bullet + H^+;$$

$$Hgb - Fe^{4+} - O^- + AH_2 + H^+ \rightarrow Hgb - Fe^{3+} + AH\bullet + H_2O.$$

Hemoglobin contains exposed free cysteines (β93) that are critical for the structural integrity of the molecule. Oxidation of these groups can denature hemoglobin and decrease its solubility. The oxidized, denatured hemoglobin species comprise what has been designated sulfhemoglobin. The denatured hemoglobin can

Table 11-6

Xenobiotics Associated with Oxidative Injury

Acetanilide	Phenylhydrazine
Naphthalene	Nitrobenzene
Nitrofurantoin	Phenacetin
Sulfamethoxypyridazine	Phenol
Aminosalicylic acid	Hydroxylamine
Sodium sulfoxone	Methylene blue
Dapsone	Toluidine blue
Phenazopyridine	Furazolidone
Primaquine	Nalidixic acid
Chlorates	Sulfanilamide
Sulfasalazine	

form aggregates that bind to the cell membrane to form inclusions called *Heinz bodies,* a hallmark of oxidative injury to erythrocytes (Jandl, 1987). Heinz bodies can be visualized by use of phase contrast microscopy or supravital stains such as crystal violet. These membrane-associated inclusions impair the deformability of the erythrocyte membrane and thus impede movement of erythrocytes through the microcirculation and the spleen. Heinz bodies are effectively removed from the erythrocyte by the spleen, so they are not often observed in peripheral blood samples from patients despite ongoing oxidative injury. However, the culling of Heinz bodies can alter the morphology of the affected cells, giving rise to what are called "bite" cells and "blister" cells, which may provide an important clue as to the ongoing process (Yoo and Lessin, 1992). These cells look as though a portion of the cytoplasm had been cut away. Heinz body formation can be induced by in vitro exposure to oxidizing agents and patients with oxidative hemolysis often show increased in vitro formation of Heinz bodies.

Oxidative denaturation of the globin chain decreases its affinity for the heme group, which may dissociate from the globin chain during oxidative injury (Kumar and Bandyopadhyay, 2005). Free heme itself is toxic to cells and can induce tissue injury through formation of reactive oxygen species. The ferric iron in the heme ring may react with chloride to form a complex called hemin. Hemin is hydrophobic and intercalates into the erythrocyte membrane from which it is removed by interaction with albumin. However, if the rate of hemin formation exceeds the rate of removal by albumin, hemin accumulates in the membrane, where it can cause rapid lysis of the erythrocyte.

The generation of free radicals may also lead to peroxidation of membrane lipids (Jandl, 1987; Kumar and Bandyopadhyay, 2005). This may affect the deformability of the erythrocyte and the permeability of the membrane to potassium. The alteration of the Na$^+$/K$^+$ gradient is independent of injury to the Na$^+$/K$^+$ pump and is potentially lethal to the affected erythrocyte. Oxidative injury also impairs the metabolic machinery of the erythrocyte, resulting in a decrease in the concentration of ATP (Tavazzi *et al.,* 2000). Damage to the membrane can also permit leakage of denatured hemoglobin from the cell. Such free denatured hemoglobin can be toxic on its own. Free hemoglobin may irreversibly bind nitric oxide, resulting in vasoconstriction. Released hemoglobin may form nephrotoxic hemoglobin dimers, leading to kidney damage.

Oxidative injury thus results in a number of changes that decrease the viability of erythrocytes. Protection against many of the free radical–induced modifications is mediated by reduced glutathione (Njalsson and Norgren, 2005). Formation of reduced glutathione is dependent on NADPH and the hexose monophosphate shunt (Fig. 11-6). Significant oxidative injury usually occurs when the concentration of the xenobiotic is high enough (due to either high exposure or decreased metabolism of the xenobiotic) to overcome the normal protective mechanisms, or, more commonly, when there is an underlying defect in the protective mechanisms.

The most common enzyme defect associated with oxidative hemolysis is G-6-PD deficiency, a relatively common sex-linked disorder characterized by alterations in the primary structure of G-6-PD that diminish its functional activity (Beutler, 1996). It is often clinically asymptomatic until the erythrocytes are exposed to oxidative stress. The stress may come from the host response to infection or exposure to xenobiotics. The level of G-6-PD normally decreases as the erythrocytes age. In the African type of G-6-PD deficiency, the enzyme is less stable than normal; thus, the loss of activity is accelerated compared with normals. In the Mediterranean type of G-6-PD deficiency, the rate of loss of enzyme activity is even higher. Consequently, the older erythrocytes with the lowest

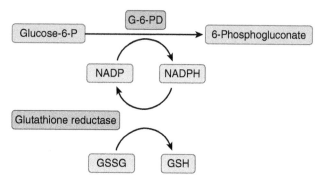

Figure 11-6. *The hexose monophosphate shunt in the erythrocyte is critical for generation of NADPH, which helps maintain an intracellular supply of reduced glutathione (GSH).* With a deficiency of glucose-6-phosphate dehydrogenase (G-6-PD), the rate-limiting step in this pathway, the cellular levels of GSH are reduced. Such cells show increased susceptibility to oxidative injury. Acute exposure of such cells to an oxidizing agent can result in rapid hemolysis.

levels of G-6-PD are most susceptible to hemolysis, with the degree of hemolysis affected by the residual amount of enzyme activity as well as the magnitude of the oxidative injury.

Erythrocyte-reduced glutathione is rapidly depleted on exposure to an oxidizing agent in patients with G-6-PD deficiency. This leads to the series of oxidative injuries described above with the development of intravascular and extravascular hemolysis. Oxidative hemolysis is usually reversible if the process is promptly recognized and the offending agent is removed. Occasionally the hemolysis may be sufficiently severe to result in death or serious morbidity (eg, renal failure). Hemolytic anemia may occur in patients with deficiency of glutathione synthetase due to the reduced intracellular concentration of glutathione (Njalsson and Norgren, 2005).

Nonoxidative Chemical-Induced Hemolysis Exposure to some xenobiotics is associated with hemolysis without significant oxidative injury (Beutler, 2006a,b,c). Arsenic hydride is a gas that is formed during several industrial processes. Inhalation of the gas can result in severe hemolysis, with anemia, jaundice, and hemoglobinuria. The mechanism of hemolysis in arsine toxicity is not understood. Lead poisoning is associated with defects in heme synthesis and a shortening of erythrocyte survival. The cause of the hemolysis is uncertain, but lead can cause membrane damage and interfere with the Na+/K+ pump. These effects may cause premature removal of erythrocytes from the circulation. Excess copper has been associated with hemolytic anemia. The pathogenesis may relate to inhibitory effects on the hexose monophosphate shunt and the Embden–Meyerhof pathway. Ingestion of excess chromium may result in hemolytic anemia and thrombocytopenia, although the mechanism is not known (Cerulli *et al.,* 1998). Significant hemolysis may also occur with biologic toxins found in insect and snake venoms (Beutler, 2006a,b,c).

Immune Hemolytic Anemia Immunologic destruction of erythrocytes is mediated by the interaction of IgG or IgM antibodies with antigens expressed on the surface of the erythrocyte. In the case of autoimmune hemolytic anemia the antigens are intrinsic components of the patient's own erythrocytes. A large number of drugs have been associated with enhanced binding of immunoglobulin to the erythrocyte surface and shortened RBC survival (Arndt and Garratty, 2005).

A number of mechanisms have been implicated in xenobiotic-mediated antibody binding to erythrocytes (Arndt and Garratty, 2005). Some drugs, of which penicillin is a prototype, appear to bind to the surface of the cell, with the "foreign" drug acting as a *hapten* and eliciting an immune response. The antibodies that arise in this type of response only bind to drug-coated erythrocytes. Other drugs, of which quinidine is a prototype, bind to components of the erythrocyte surface and induce a conformational change in one or more components of the membrane. This type of interaction can give rise to a confusing array of antibody specificities. Some of the antibodies recognize only the *drug–membrane component* complex; others are specific for the membrane component, but only when drug is present; while still others may recognize the membrane component in the presence or absence of the drug. A third mechanism, for which α-methyldopa is a prototype, results in production of a *drug-induced autoantibody* that cannot be distinguished from the antibodies arising in idiopathic autoimmune hemolytic anemia. The mechanism for induction of this group of antibodies is not understood, but may be related to development of an autoimmune response. A variant of this type of response is the augmentation of autoimmune hemolytic anemia that may occur during therapy of some lymphoproliferative disorders. Autoimmune phenomena, including autoimmune hemolytic anemia, are known to occur in lymphoproliferative disorders such as chronic lymphocytic leukemia (CLL). Treatment of these disorders with some drugs has been associated with worsening of the hemolytic anemia (Gonzalez *et al.,* 1998). It has been hypothesized that therapy further disrupts regulation of the autoimmune phenomenon, allowing increased antibody production.

Some xenobiotics are associated with *nonspecific deposition of proteins* on erythrocytes. This was first associated with cephalosporins but has also been seen with other drugs, including cisplatin and the β-lactamase inhibitors sulbactam and clavulanate (Arndt and Garratty, 2005). Immunoglobulin and complement proteins may be among the proteins deposited on the erythrocyte surface. These proteins may cause a positive direct antiglobulin test, suggesting a drug-induced antibody response. However, there is no evidence of a drug-dependent antibody in the patient's serum, and drug-treated erythrocytes may bind antibody from normal nondrug exposed serum. This form of antibody deposition is generally not associated with hemolysis, although the possibility of hemolysis related to this type of reaction has been raised.

Drug-induced intravascular hemolysis is often a dramatic clinical event and may be associated with fever, chills, back pain, hypotension, a rapid fall in hemoglobin concentration, a decrease in serum haptoglobin, a marked increase in serum LD, and hemoglobinuria (Arndt and Garratty, 2005). The clinical picture of extravascular hemolysis depends on the rate of hemolysis but is usually less dramatic. Often there is evidence of reticulocytosis, polychromasia, spherocytosis, a moderate increase in serum LD, and an increase in serum bilirubin. Serologic studies usually show evidence of IgG and/or complement on the surface of erythrocytes, although it may be difficult to document that antibody binding is drug-dependent. The mainstay of therapy in patients with drug-induced hemolytic anemia is removal of the offending agent and avoidance of reexposure.

TOXICOLOGY OF THE LEUKON

Components of Blood Leukocytes

The leukon consists of leukocytes, or white blood cells. They include granulocytes, which may be subdivided into neutrophils, eosinophils, and basophils; monocytes; and lymphocytes. Granulocytes and monocytes are nucleated ameboid cells that are phagocytic. They play a central role in the inflammatory response and host defense. Unlike the RBC, which resides exclusively within blood, granulocytes and monocytes generally pass through the blood on their way to the extravascular tissues, where they reside in large numbers, although it is now understood that senescent neutrophils that remain in the circulation return to the bone marrow through the stromal-derived factor-1 (SDF-1)α/CXCR4 chemokine axis (Martin *et al.,* 2003).

Granulocytes are defined by the characteristics of their cytoplasmic granules as they appear on a blood smear stained with a polychromatic (Romanovsky) stain. Neutrophils, the largest component of blood leukocytes, are highly specialized in the mediation of inflammation and the ingestion and destruction of pathogenic microorganisms. The turnover of neutrophils is enormous and increases dramatically in times of inflammation and infection, elevating the number of these cells released from the bone marrow. Eosinophils and basophils modulate inflammation through the release of various mediators and play an important role in other homeostatic functions. All these are influenced by cellular and humoral immune responses, as discussed in greater detail in Chap. 12.

In the world of clinical and experimental toxicology, the neutrophil is the focus of concern when evaluating granulocytes as possible targets for drug and nontherapeutic chemical effects. Eosinophils and basophils are far more difficult to study, with changes in these populations most frequently associated with reactions to other target organ or systemic toxicity. Examples include the eosinophilia observed with the toxic oil syndrome that resulted from exposure to rapeseed oil denatured in aniline utilized in northwestern Spain (Kilbourne *et al.,* 1991), and the eosinophilia–myalgia syndrome associated with λ-tryptophan preparations contaminated with 1,1-ethylidene-bis[tryptophan] (Varga *et al.,* 1992). Peripheral eosinophilia is often but not reliably observed with hypersensitivity reactions to drugs (Roujeau, 2005), while tissue eosinophilia can be diagnostic, in the context of a suggestive clinical course, in conditions such as drug-induced cutaneous vasculitis (Bahrami *et al.,* 2006) and eosinophilic pneumonia (Flieder and Travis, 2004). This variability in systemic response can be genetically predisposed, as demonstrated in studies using transgenic mice on genetic restrictions in people afflicted by the aforementioned toxic oil syndrome (Gallardo *et al.,* 2005). The time course of the reaction can also influence whether eosinophilia can be demonstrated in hypersensitivity disease (Roujeau, 2005).

Evaluation of Granulocytes

The most informative test to assess the neutrophil compartment is the blood neutrophil count. Accurate interpretation requires an understanding of neutrophil kinetics and the response of this tissue to physiologic and pathologic changes. In the blood, neutrophils are distributed between *circulating* and *marginated* pools, which are of equal size in humans and in constant equilibrium (Athens *et al.,* 1961). A blood neutrophil count assesses only the circulating pool, which remains between 1800 and 7500/μL in a healthy adult human (Dale, 2006).

This constancy is remarkable, considering that as many as 10^{11} neutrophils are released from the marrow daily, that this circulating pool represents only 1% of the total body neutrophils (Semerad *et al.,* 2002), and that the circulating half-life of these cells is only approximately six hours (Cartwright *et al.,* 1964). How this extraordinary regulation is achieved is only partially understood. Studies using knockout mice suggest that G-CSF is an essential regulator of both granulopoiesis and neutrophil release

from the bone marrow (Semerad *et al.,* 2002). It is induced by the T-cell-derived cytokine IL-17 that, in turn, is controlled by IL-23 that is provided by dendritic cells and macrophages (Stark *et al.,* 2005). The latter is downregulated by the phagocytosis of apoptotic neutrophils in the tissues, which provides an important negative feedback loop. The upregulation and downregulation of chemokine receptors further controls the release of neutrophils from the bone marrow (as discussed below) and their return following senescence (Martin *et al.,* 2003). Pharmaceutical companies are currently developing recombinant proteins that function as agonists and inhibitors of these mediators, which have great potential as exciting new therapies. Many will also be shown to cause unacceptable immunotoxicity and hematotoxicity, which portends exciting times for the academic and industrial hematopathologist and toxicologist.

Neutrophil kinetics and response to disease will vary substantially among animal species (Feldman *et al.,* 2006). Thus, a thorough understanding of these features in any animal model used in investigative toxicology is required before informed interpretations can be made. In humans, clinically significant neutropenia occurs when the blood neutrophil count is less than 1000/μL, but serious recurrent infections do not usually occur until counts fall below 500/μL (Dale, 2006). Morphologic assessment of peripheral blood granulocytes can be helpful in characterizing neutropenia. In humans and most healthy animal species, mature (segmented) and a few immature (band) neutrophils can be identified on blood films stained with Wright or Giemsa stain. During inflammation, a "shift to the left" may occur, which refers to an increased number of immature (nonsegmented) granulocytes in the peripheral blood, which may include bands, metamyelocytes, and occasionally myelocytes. During such times, neutrophils may also show "toxic" granulation, Döhle bodies, and cytoplasmic vacuoles. These morphologic changes may be prominent in sepsis or as a result of drug or chemical intoxication. In order to fully characterize such changes or understand the pathogenesis of the abnormality, bone marrow must be examined using marrow aspirates and biopsies. These provide information on rates of production, bone marrow reserves, and abnormalities in cell distribution, and occasionally specific clues as to etiology. In vitro stem cell assays may be used to assess the granulocyte progenitor cell compartment, which may include colony-forming-units granulocyte/monocyte (CFU-GM) performed in a semisolid medium, such as agar or methylcellulose, which contains appropriate growth factors, as discussed later in this chapter. Normal human marrow specimens contain approximately 50 to 1000 CFU-GM per 10^6 nucleated cells cultured (Liesveld and Lichtman, 1997). Marrow stem cell reserves can be assessed in vitro after administration of G-CSF (Demirer and Bensinger, 1995), which stimulates increased production and release of neutrophil precursors. Glucocorticoids (Peters *et al.,* 1972) and epinephrine (Babior and Golde, 1995) may also be used for this purpose but are rarely used in a clinical setting.

The recent understanding that the CXC chemokine ligand SDF-1/CXCR4 mediates the retention of granulopoietic stem cells within their bone marrow niche (Laurence, 2006; Sharma *et al.,* 2011), as well as mature neutrophils within the bone marrow pool (Semerad *et al.,* 2002), has led to the development of an inhibitor of this ligand that, when administered with G-CSF, can cause a transient release of neutrophils and CD34+ (stem) cells into the circulation (Liles *et al.,* 2005). The latter can be collected and re-engrafted to form new functioning bone marrow (Broxmeyer *et al.,* 2005). The homing and retention of such hematopoietic stem/progenitor cells is influenced by complex and highly coordinated interactions among adhesion molecules, cytokines, growth factors, and regulatory cofactors that are only partially understood (Sharma *et al.,* 2011). The ability to manipulate this system, as in the above experiments and through the many recombinant proteins under development, will continue to provide important research, diagnostic, and therapeutic tools for the hematologist, oncologist, and toxicologist.

The degree of proliferation in the granulocyte compartment can also be assessed using older techniques that employ ^{3}H-thymidine suicide assays or DNA-binding dyes with fluorescence-activated cell sorting analyses (Keng, 1986).

Toxic Effects on Granulocytes

The toxicologist is concerned with the effect of xenobiotics on granulocytes as relates to proliferation (granulopoiesis) and kinetics, the extent to which a drug or chemical contaminant can impair the vital functions these cells perform, and how neutrophils mediate or exacerbate inflammatory disease or other target organ toxicity. The last two areas are discussed in Chap. 12, as they relate to their role as important effector cells of the immune system. However, it is difficult to separate effects on granulopoiesis and neutrophil kinetics from that of function. Both are complex and highly regulated, as discussed above, through an array of growth factors, chemokines, cytokines, and interactions with monocytes, dendritic cells, and lymphocytes in a bidirectional, multicompartmental manner (Nathan, 2006). Such complexity is not surprising, given the daunting task these cells perform, which is elegantly described in a review by Nathan (2006): "The [neutrophil] must remain non-sticky as it hurtles through the arterial and arteriolar circulation; then it must squeeze through capillaries smaller in diameter than itself, without allowing collision, friction, or distortion to activate it. A fraction of the population must adhere tightly enough to the normal endothelium of post-capillary venules to resist being washed away in the circulation, but loosely enough to roll while scouting for evidence of tissue damage and microbial infection. If such evidence is received, the cell must crawl to a boundary between endothelial cells, penetrate the junctions and the underlying basement membrane without damaging these structures, move up the chemotactic gradient, and decide whether its original information remains valid. If the answer is negative, the cell must execute itself by apoptosis. If the answer is positive, the cell must attempt to engulf and destroy microbes. If it cannot locate microbes quickly, it must attempt to destroy them at a distance by releasing every weapon at its disposal." Many of the mediators and interactions that enable this feat have now become targets for the therapeutic dysregulation of these processes, which has led to the development of candidate drugs that may prove to be uniquely efficacious and/or toxic, as discussed below.

Effects on Proliferation and Kinetics As with other hematopoietic tissue, the high rate of proliferation of neutrophils makes their progenitor and precursor granulocyte pool particularly susceptible to inhibitors of mitosis. Such effects by cytotoxic drugs are generally nonspecific, as they similarly affect cells of the dermis, gastrointestinal tract, and other rapidly dividing tissues. Agents that affect both neutrophils and monocytes pose a greater risk for toxic sequelae, such as infection (Dale, 2006). Such effects tend to be dose-related, with mononuclear phagocyte recovery preceding neutrophil recovery (Arneborn and Palmblad, 1982).

Myelotoxicity in clinical medicine and preclinical safety studies today is most commonly seen with cytoreductive cancer chemotherapy agents. However, this is changing, as more cancer cell–targeted, normal-tissue-sparing anticancer agents are being developed. In fact, most published reviews today on drug-induced neutropenia and agranulocytosis do not even address that associated with such cytotoxic agents. Accordingly, the term commonly refers to *idiosyncratic reactions,* most often secondary to accelerated immune-mediated destruction of neutrophils and their progenitors, as discussed below. The toxicity associated with cytotoxic drugs, however, remains important in that it is often dose-limiting (even with some of the newer drugs) with serious manifestations that include febrile neutropenia associated with life-threatening infections (Kuderer *et al.,* 2002). These drugs vary in terms of their mechanism, the kinetics of the cytopenias they induce, and how individual patients or animals respond. Most act to inhibit DNA synthesis or directly attack its integrity through the formation of DNA adducts or enzyme-mediated breaks (Chabner *et al.,* 2006). While cytoreductive drugs such as alkylating agents, cisplatin, and nitrosureas can be toxic to both resting and actively dividing cells, nonproliferating cells such as metamyelocytes, bands, and mature neutrophils are relatively resistant (Friberg and Karlsson, 2003). Generally, stem cells cycle slowly and are therefore minimally affected by a single administration of a cytotoxic drug such as 5-fluorouricil; however, such exposure can stimulate cycling activity, making these cells more vulnerable to doses administered three to five days later (Harrison and Lerner, 1991). Cytokines have long been thought to enhance these effects by driving cells into the S phase (Smith *et al.,* 1994). Sustained exposure to drugs affecting slowly cycling stem cells is believed to cause more prolonged myelosuppression, similar to that observed with idiosyncratic toxic neutropenia (Tannock, 1986). Recent studies suggest that these features are shared by cancer stem cells, which is the basis for the more sophisticated cancer interventions and regimens under development today (Eramo *et al.,* 2008; Vermeulen *et al.,* 2010; Ricci-Vitiani *et al.,* 2010).

Finally, there is considerable variation among individuals as regards susceptibility to bone marrow toxicity; this can relate to how the drug is metabolized as with 5-fluorouracil (Sundman-Engberg *et al.,* 1998) and 6-mercaptopurine (Chabner *et al.,* 2006), gender (Huang *et al.,* 2007; Gamazon *et al.,* 2011), and other factors. Based on these and other data, including plasma drug concentrations, "semi-mechanistic" pharmacokinetic/pharmacodynamic models of myelosuppression have been developed to tailor doses and treatment regimens to individual patients (Friberg and Karlsson, 2003). Pharmacokinetic monitoring is now routinely performed with some anticancer treatment regimens, particularly high-dose methotrexate (Chabner *et al.,* 2006).

Two innovations have had a dramatic impact on cancer chemotherapy and the dose-limiting myelotoxicity associated with these drugs: (1) the aforementioned development of drugs with cancer cell–specific molecular targets that are relatively bone marrow sparing, such as those that target aberrant growth factor receptor signaling, apoptosis, angiogenesis, and other metabolic, immune, inflammatory, and mutation-promoting pathways that selectively advantage tumor cells (Hanahan and Weinberg, 2011); and (2) the use of hematopoietic growth factors, the cotreatment with which mitigates or successfully rescues patients from the effects of myelosuppression (Andres *et al.,* 2010). Most notable of the latter has been the development and application of the G-CSFs filgrastim and the longer acting pegfilgrastim, the action of which was discussed previously. Treatment with these recombinant proteins can substantially reduce the incidence, severity, and duration of neutropenia and its complications (Rader, 2006). Antagonists to the aforementioned chemokine ligand CXCR4 are also under development for treatment alone or in combination with G-CSF, which have been shown to be effective in mobilizing both stem cells and mature neutrophils (De Clercq, 2005; Larochelle *et al.*, 2006). Cytokine-induced differentiation therapy of leukemias is another exciting treatment modality (Leung *et al.*, 2005). The prospect of exaggerated pharmacology and off-target effects of these sophisticated interventions should provide the preclinical toxicologist and oncologist with interesting hematotoxicologic challenges.

Lindane, an insecticide used to treat seeds and soil, has been associated with leukopenia (Parent-Massin *et al.*, 1994). It is cytotoxic for human CFU-GMs at concentrations observed in blood and adipose tissue from exposed human subjects. An example of chemicals affecting mature cells is methyl methacrylate monomer, which has been used in orthopedic surgical procedures and is cytotoxic to both neutrophils and monocytes at clinically relevant concentrations (Dahl *et al.*, 1994).

Chemicals that affect granulocyte kinetics can cause neutropenia or neutrophilia that has variable toxicologic significance. The effects of epinephrine and glucocorticoids on granulocyte kinetics were discussed previously. Dexamethasone has long been known to cause neutrophilia through enhanced release of mature neutrophils from the bone marrow and demargination, with the latter being the largest contributor to the expanded circulating pool (Nakagawa *et al.*, 1998). It is now clear that the reduced margination of neutrophils is mediated by multiple effects, including altered chemotaxis, expression of adhesion molecules, and the release of mediators from other cells (Barnes, 2006; Caramori and Adcock, 2005). It is widely assumed that inhibition of margination and homing are among the important mechanisms of the anti-inflammatory and immunosuppressive effects of these widely used drugs. The development of drugs with more selective effects on neutrophils is among the most active areas of investigative pharmacology and toxicology today.

Inhibitors of the CXC chemokine ligands such as CXCR4 are under development as anticancer drugs and often associated with transient neutropenia (unpublished data). The commonly observed (yet remarkable) late-onset neutropenia (LAN) following treatment with rituximab, an anti-CD20 monoclonal antibody used to treat CD20-positive lymphoma and rheumatoid arthritis, is a good example of a common drug-induced neutropenia—in this case, typically self-limiting and thought to be of limited clinical significance. Informed hypotheses on the mechanism of LAN include perturbations of granulocyte homeostasis, mediated by the complex interaction between B-cell recovery and SDF-1 (Grant *et al.*, 2011) and polymorphisms in immunoglobulin Fc receptor genotypes, which enhance ADCC by rituximab, resulting in increased killing of malignant and normal B cells. The latter could lead to the release of lysosomal enzymes and the destruction of neutrophils as "bystanders" (Hincks *et al.*, 2011). Consistent with these hypotheses is the recent observation of LAN being a good prognostic indicator in lymphoproliferative disorders (Hincks *et al.*, 2011).

Effects on Function While there are a variety of disorders associated with defects in the parameters of neutrophil function discussed above, demonstrable in vivo effects associated with drugs and nontherapeutic chemicals are surprisingly few (Borregaard and Boxer, 2006). Examples include ethanol and glucocorticoids, which impair phagocytosis and microbe ingestion in vitro and in vivo (Brayton *et al.*, 1970). Iohexol and ioxaglate, components of radiographic contrast media, have also been reported to inhibit phagocytosis (Lillevang *et al.*, 1994). Superoxide production, required for microbial killing and chemotaxis, has been reported to be reduced in patients using parenteral heroin as well

as in former opiate abusers on long-term methadone maintenance (Mazzone *et al.*, 1994).

In addition to glucocorticoids, several drugs and nontherapeutic chemicals have been shown to inhibit neutrophil chemotaxis. Examples include macrolide antibiotics, which suppress the expression of the adhesion molecule ICAM (Tamaoki, 2004); zinc salts, which are found in antiacne preparations (Dreno *et al.*, 1992); the insecticide chlordane (Miyagi *et al.*, 1998); and mercuric chloride/methylmercuric chloride (Contrino *et al.*, 1988). More common is the activation of neutrophils with the potential for proinflammatory consequences, specifically through increased phagocytosis, O_2^- production, or both. Examples include the environmental contaminants sodium sulfite, mercuric chloride, chlordane, and toxaphene (Girard, 2003). This toxicologic potential of xenobiotics will be discussed in more detail in Chap. 12.

Idiosyncratic Toxic Neutropenia Of greater concern are chemicals that unexpectedly damage neutrophils and granulocyte precursors—particularly to the extent of inducing *agranulocytosis,* which is characterized by a profound depletion in blood neutrophils to less than 500/μL (Pisciotta, 1973). The term was first used by Schultz in 1922 in patients with severe sore throat associated with a marked reduction of granulocytes, followed by sepsis and death (Schultz, 1922). Drug association was first demonstrated through rechallenge experiments performed on two patients with aminopyrine-induced agranulocytosis, who developed leucopenia within two hours of reexposure (Madison and Squier, 1934). A later study demonstrated that blood transferred from an agranulocytosis patient to normal controls resulted in a rapid drop in neutrophil count, suggesting a role for a preformed blood factor(s) such as antibodies (Moeschlin and Wagner, 1952). Such toxicity occurs in specifically conditioned individuals, and is therefore termed "idiosyncratic." While rare, the seriousness of this disorder, as with aplastic anemia, makes it among the most important hematotoxicities, as regards regulatory scrutiny and risk:benefit considerations, which justifies the detailed discussion below. Acute agranulocytosis is attributed to drugs in >70% of cases (Garb, 2007).

Mechanisms of idiosyncratic damage often do not relate to pharmacologic properties of the parent drug, which makes managing this risk a particular challenge to hematologists and toxicologists, as discussed later in this chapter. Preclinical toxicology is rarely predictive of these effects, which are generally detected and characterized following exposure of a large population to the drug (Dieckhaus *et al.*, 2002; Szarfman *et al.*, 2002). Idiosyncratic drug-induced neutropenia may be dose-related and involve a nonselective disruption of protein synthesis or cell replication resulting in agranulocytosis, as discussed below. Alternatively, and more commonly, it may not be dose-dependent (as qualified below), in which case it is usually thought to be allergic or immunologic in origin. The latter has been observed with many drugs, and is more frequently observed in women, older patients, and patients with a history of allergies (Dale, 2006).

Idiosyncratic xenobiotic-induced agranulocytosis may involve a sudden depletion of circulating neutrophils concomitant with exposure, which may persist as long as the chemical or its metabolites persist in the circulation. Hematopoietic function is usually restored when the agent is detoxified or excreted. Suppression of granulopoiesis, however, is more prevalent than peripheral lysis of neutrophils and is asymptomatic unless sepsis supervenes (Pisciotta, 1973). The onset of leukopenia in the former is more gradual, but may be precipitous if lysis of circulating neutrophils also occurs. The pattern of the disease varies with the stage of granulopoiesis affected, which has been well defined for several drugs that cause

Table 11-7

Stages of Granulocytopoiesis: Site of Xenobiotic-Induced Cellular Damage

STAGE OF DEVELOPMENT	DISEASE	OFFENDING DRUGS
Uncommitted (totipotential) stem cell CFU-S	Aplastic anemia	Chloramphenicol Gold salts Phenylbutazone Phenytoin Mephenytoin Carbamazepine

Committed stem cell
 	
  CFU-G
 	
  CFU-E
  BFU-E
	Aplastic anemia
	Agranulocytosis
	
	Pure red cell aplasia
		Carbamazepine
		Chlorpromazine
		Carbamazepine
		Clozapine
		
		Phenytoin

Morphologically recognizable precursors	Hypoplastic marrow	Most cancer chemotherapy agents

Dividing pool
  Promyelocyte
  Myelocyte
	Hypoplastic marrow	Chloramphenicol
		Alcohol

Nondividing pool
  Metamyelocytes, bands
  PMNs
	Agranulocytosis	Clozapine
		Phenothiazines, etc

Peripheral blood lysis PMNs	Agranulocytosis	Clozapine, etc Aminopyrine
Tissue pool		

SOURCE: *Modified from Pisciotta (1997), with permission from Elsevier Science.*

bone marrow toxicity (Table 11-7). Toxicants affecting uncommitted stem cells induce total marrow failure, as seen in aplastic anemia, which generally carries a worse prognosis than chemicals affecting more differentiated precursors, such as CFU-G. It is thought that, in the latter case, surviving uncommitted stem cells eventually produce recovery, provided that the risk of infection is successfully managed during the leukopenic episodes (Pisciotta, 1973).

The incidence of drug-induced idiosyncratic agranulocytosis ranges from 2 to 15 cases per million patients exposed to drugs per year (Andres *et al.*, 2002). While all drugs may be causative, the most commonly incriminated drugs include antithyroid agents and antibiotics, particularly sulfonamides (Andres *et al.*, 2002; Berliner *et al.*, 2004). An extensive case–control study on drug-induced agranulocytosis in Barcelona, Spain, followed 177 community cases (representing 78.73 million person-years), which were compared with 586 sex-, age-, and hospital-matched control subjects previously treated with the same putative drugs (Ibanez *et al.*, 2005). The annual incidence was 3.46:1 million, which increased with age. The fatality and mortality rates were 7.0% and 0.24:1 million, respectively. The drugs most frequently implicated (in decreasing order of odds ratio) were ticlopidine hydrochloride, calcium dobesilate, antithyroid drugs, dipyrone, and spironolactone. Other drugs associated with significant risk were pyrithyldione, cinepazide, aprindine hydrochloride, carbamazepine, sulfonamides, phenytoin and phenytoin sodium, β-lactam antibiotics, erythromycin stearate and erythromycin ethylsuccinate, and diclofenac sodium. These drugs accounted for 68.6% of all cases. Some drugs commonly implicated in the past, such as phenylbutazone, chloramphenicol, and ticlopidine, are used less commonly today due to this and other toxicity. Curiously, the incidence of this idiosyncratic reaction has not

changed in the western hemisphere over the past 30 years, despite this evolution of putative drugs, suggesting that host factors are critical in the pathogenesis of the toxicity (Tesfa *et al.*, 2009).

The severity of the neutropenia often causes severe sepsis or localized infections, such as sore throat, pneumonia, or various cutaneous infections. Prior to the use of hematopoietic growth factors, the mortality was 10% to 20% (Julia *et al.*, 1991); with appropriate management it is now less than 5% (Andres *et al.*, 2010).

Clozapine-induced agranulocytosis is unique, as a genetic predisposition has been established (Turbay *et al.*, 1997; Yunis *et al.*, 1995). Prior to an aggressive risk management program that included careful screening of prospective patients and early detection through hematologic monitoring, the incidence of agranulocytosis with this highly efficacious atypical antipsychotic was as high as 1% to 2%. This measure reduced the incidence to 0.38% and the mortality by 90% (Honigfeld *et al.*, 1998).

Mechanisms of Toxic Neutropenia Because cases of drug-induced neutropenia are relatively rare, sporadic, or transient, studies on the pathogenesis of this hematotoxicity have been limited. Toxic neutropenia has historically been classified according to mechanism as *immune-mediated* or *nonimmune-mediated*. There has long been a debate in the literature as to whether the principal mechanism of idiosyncratic drug-induced neutropenia (including agranulocytosis) is immune-mediated, or subsequent to the generation of toxic metabolites—both involving "preconditioning" through genetically determined immune responses to, or metabolism of, the putative drug, respectively. Both are consistent with the aforementioned early observations of Madison and Squier (1934) where transfusion of blood from affected patients to normal subjects induced neutropenia, presumably involving a humoral factor—presumably an antibody. There is now consensus that the mechanism of most drug-induced idiosyncratic diseases, including hepatotoxicity, Stevens–Johnson syndrome, agranulocytosis, and aplastic anemia, usually is immune-mediated, often involving altered proteins through reactive metabolite–mediated damage (Zhang *et al.*, 2011). The Th-17 T lymphocyte is emerging as an important mediator of this through a cellular immune mechanism demonstrated in aplastic anemia (de Latour *et al.*, 2010; Platanias, 2010). Two hypotheses as to the mechanism (or alternative pathogeneses) for these idiosyncratic reactions that have emerged based on observations over the past 10 years include the *hapten hypothesis* and the *danger hypothesis* (Zhang *et al.*, 2011). The former involves a reactive metabolite binding to a protein making it "foreign," which in turn induces an immune response that leads to the toxicity. The latter has a reactive metabolite damaging a cell, which elicits an immune response against the drug or an autoimmune response. The "perfect storm" in the rare individual in which these reactions occur is thought to be caused by preconditioned (or individual-specific) circumstances that drive both the metabolism of the drug and the immune reactions to the altered proteins. Consistent with these hypotheses is the fact that aplastic anemia and the more common agranulocytosis can be induced by many of the same drugs, most of which can be oxidized to reactive metabolites by the myeloperoxidase system of neutrophils, macrophages, and/or their precursors (Uetrecht, 1990).

The incidence of xenobiotic-induced immune neutropenia is considerably less than that of immune hemolytic anemias (Vandendries and Drews, 2006). In immune-mediated neutropenia, antigen–antibody reactions lead to destruction of peripheral neutrophils, granulocyte precursors, or both. As with RBCs, an immunogenic xenobiotic can act as a hapten, where the chemical must be physically present to cause cell damage, or may induce immunogenic cells to produce antineutrophil antibodies that do not require the drug to be present (Salama *et al.*, 1989). Also like immune hemolytic anemia, drug-induced *autoimmune* neutropenia has been observed (Capsoni *et al.*, 2005). Examples of drugs that have been implicated include fludarabine (Stern *et al.*, 1999), propylthiouracil (Sato *et al.*, 1985), and rituximab (Voog *et al.*, 2003). Xenobiotic-induced immune-mediated damage may also be cell-mediated (Pisciotta, 1973).

Detection of xenobiotic-induced neutrophil antibodies is also considerably more difficult than that of RBCs or platelets. This is because the neutrophil is relatively fragile and short-lived, and becomes easily activated (Palmblad *et al.*, 2001). There is no good test for direct antigranulocyte antibodies comparable to the Coombs (antiglobulin) test. Several assays have been used, which can be grouped into four categories: those measuring end points of leukoagglutination, cytotoxic inhibition of neutrophil function, immunoglobulin binding, and those using cell-mediated mechanisms. Among the specific challenges these assays pose are the tendency of neutrophils to stick to each other in vitro, attract immunoglobulin nonspecifically to their surface, and reflect membrane damage through indirect and semiquantitative changes (Pisciotta, 1973). Most neutrophil-associated antibody assays applied clinically today employ flow cytometry, with the indirect granulocyte immunofluorescence test being the most promising (Sella *et al.*, 2010). The reader is referred elsewhere for a more detailed discussion of assays for immune-mediated neutrophil damage (Hagen *et al.*, 1993; Nifli *et al.*, 2006; Palmblad *et al.*, 2001; Sella *et al.*, 2010).

Some nonimmune-mediated toxic neutropenias have long been known to have a genetic predisposition (Pisciotta, 1973). Direct damage may cause inhibition of granulopoiesis or neutrophil

Table 11-8

Examples of Toxicants that cause Immune and Nonimmune Idiopathic Neutropenia

DRUGS ASSOCIATED WITH WBC ANTIBODIES	DRUGS NOT ASSOCIATED WITH WBC ANTIBODIES
Aminopyrine	INH
Propylthiouracil	Rifampicin
Ampicillin	Ethambutol
Metiamide	Allopurinol
Dicloxacillin	Phenothiazines/CPZ
Phenytoin	Flurazepam
Aprindine	HCTZ
Azulfidine	
Chlorpropamide	
CPZ/phenothiazines	
Procainamide	
Nafcillin	
Tolbutamide	
Lidocaine	
Methimazole	
Levamisole	
Gold	
Quinidine	
Clozapine	

SOURCE: *Modified from Pisciotta (1997), with permission from Elsevier Science.*

function. It may entail failure to detoxify or excrete a xenobiotic or its metabolites, which subsequently build up to toxic proportions (Gerson and Meltzer, 1992; Gerson *et al.*, 1983; Uetrecht, 1990). Some studies suggest that a buildup of toxic oxidants generated by leukocytes can result in neutrophil damage, as with the reactive intermediates derived from the interaction between clozapine and neutrophils. The resulting superoxide and hypochlorous acid production by the myeloperoxidase system are thought to contribute to clozapine-induced neutropenia (Uetrecht, 1990). Accumulation of nitrenium ion, a metabolite of clozapine that causes a depletion of ATP and reduced glutathione, rendering the neutrophil highly susceptible to oxidant-induced apoptosis, is now thought to be the principal mechanism of this disorder (Williams *et al.*, 2000).

Examples of agents associated with immune and nonimmune neutropenia/agranulocytosis are listed in Table 11-8.

LEUKEMOGENESIS AS A TOXIC RESPONSE

Human Leukemias

Leukemias are proliferative disorders of hematopoietic tissue that are monoclonal in origin and thus originate from individual bone marrow cells. Historically they have been classified as myeloid or lymphoid, referring to the major lineages for erythrocytes/granulocytes/thrombocytes or lymphocytes, respectively. Because the degree of leukemic cell differentiation has also loosely correlated with the rate of disease progression, poorly differentiated phenotypes have been designated as "acute," whereas well-differentiated ones are referred to as "chronic" leukemias. The classification of human leukemias proposed by the French–American–British (FAB) Cooperative Group, based on the above and other morphologic features (Bennett and Sanger, 1982; Bennett *et al.*, 1985; Levine and Bloomfield, 1992), has largely been replaced by the

WHO classification. The WHO classification of acute myelogenous leukemia (AML) incorporates some of the traditional features associated with AML subtyping while placing increasing significance on molecular features, particularly recurrent cytogenetic abnormalities such as t(8;21), inv(16), t(15;17), and 11q23. The revised *WHO Classification of Tumours of Haematopoietic and Lymphoid Tissues* provides the most up-to-date diagnostic framework for classifying CLL, chronic myelogenous leukemia (CML), acute lymphoblastic leukemia (ALL), AML, myeloproliferative neoplasms (MPN), and the myelodysplastic syndromes (MDS), along with various subtypes of these disorders (Swerdlow *et al.*, 2008). The result of the WHO classification is that hematologic diseases that are biologically homogenous are subtyped, leading to greater prognostic and therapeutic relevance (Altucci *et al.*, 2005). These early correlations imply that the biology and clinical features of these proliferative disorders relate to the stage of differentiation of the target cell, which is now being linked to individual gene alterations, as well as epigenetic factors such as cytokine stimulation (Altucci *et al.*, 2005; Look, 2005).

There is considerable evidence supporting the notion that leukemogenesis is a multievent progression (Look, 2005; Pedersen-Bjergaard *et al.*, 1995; Varmus and Weinberg, 1993; Vogelstein *et al.*, 1988; Williams and Whitaker, 1990). These studies suggest that factors involved in the regulation of hematopoiesis also influence neoplastic transformation. Such factors include cellular growth factors (cytokines), proto-oncogenes, and other growth-promoting genes, as well as additional genetic and epigenetic factors that govern survival, proliferation, and differentiation.

Secondary leukemia is a term used to describe patients with AML or MDS who have a history of environmental, occupational, or therapeutic exposure to hematotoxins or radiation. It also includes patients with AML evolving from antecedent myelodysplastic or other myeloid stem cell disorders. *Therapy-related AML and MDS* is a term applied to the former group; both are used to distinguish from features of AML that arise de novo. Various cytogenetic findings have been associated with prognosis and response to therapy. It has been suggested that secondary leukemias be redefined as any leukemia with a specific cytogenic or molecular poor prognostic feature due to a presumed predisposing factor (Rowe, 2002). While it is generally accepted that the incidence of secondary AML is increasing, the true incidence remains unknown (Preiss *et al.*, 2010).

Mechanisms of Toxic Leukemogenesis

The understanding that certain chemicals and radiation can dysregulate hematopoiesis, resulting in leukemogenesis, is a relatively recent one. While suggested by Hunter as early as 1939, following his observations on benzene exposure and AML (Hunter, 1939), it was not until the introduction of radiation and chemotherapy as treatments for neoplasia that these agents became associated with blood dyscrasias that included (or led to) AML (Andersen *et al.*, 1981; Casciato and Scott, 1979; Foucar *et al.*, 1979). The notion emerged that myelotoxic agents, under certain circumstances, can be leukemogenic.

Curiously, AML is the dominant leukemia associated with drug or chemical exposure, followed by MDS (Andersen *et al.*, 1981; Casciato and Scott, 1979; Irons, 1997). The evidence that this represents a continuum of one toxic response is compelling (Irons, 1997; Look, 2005). This has also been linked to cytogenetic abnormalities, particularly nonrandom deletions that include 7q⁻, 5q⁻, 20q⁻, 6q⁻, 11q⁻, and 13q⁻, which activate tumor suppressor genes required for normal myeloid cell development (Bench *et al.*, 1998), as well as translocations implicating the mixed lineage leukemia (MLL) gene located in the 11q23 region. Monosomal karyotype, including that for 5 and 7, together with the latter translocations, is associated with a highly adverse prognosis in secondary AML like those following treatment of acute promyelocytic leukemia (Sanz and Montesinos, 2011). The frequency of at least one of the aforementioned deletions in patients who develop MDS and/or AML after treatment with alkylating or other antineoplastic chemicals has historically run from 67% to 95%, depending on the study (Bitter *et al.*, 1987; Johansson *et al.*, 1991; Le Beau *et al.*, 1986; Pedersen-Bjergaard *et al.*, 1984; Rowley *et al.*, 1981). The cytogenetic classification known as *complex karyotypes*, or complex chromosomal aberrations (CCAs, defined as more than three aberrations), has been shown to occur in up to 50% of therapy-related AML and MDS cases (Mauritzson *et al.*, 2000; Rossi *et al.*, 2000). CAAs are also associated with the most unfavorable prognosis among the subtypes of MDS and AML (Look, 2005). These observations, together with the understandings on the pathogenesis of leukemia previously discussed, have further corroborated the model proposed by Irons 15 years ago for the evolution of toxic leukemogenesis, which is illustrated in Fig. 11-7 (Irons, 1997).

Hypothetical changes occuring during the evolution of secondary AML

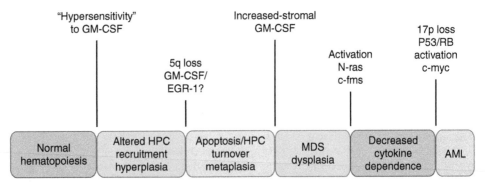

Figure 11-7. *Hypothetical model for the evolution of s-AML involving 5q-.* Schematic representation of one model for tumor progression consistent with frequently observed events in the development of AML secondary to drug or chemical exposure. Altered myeloid progenitor cell proliferation leads to increased division in the target cell population, which results in clonal loss of heterozygosity due to nondysjunction (eg, 5q⁻). The resulting haploinsufficiency of a gene, such as GM-CSF, results in increased cell turnover, abnormal maturation, and ineffective hematopoiesis (ie, MDS) in the abnormal clone. This is subsequently followed by activation of additional proto-oncogenes that result in progressive growth and survival independence in successive subclones and the development of overt AML. (Adapted from Irons (1997), with permission from Elsevier Science.)

The relatively low frequency of deletions in chromosomes 5 and 7 thought to occur in de novo, as compared with secondary AML, has led to using these cytogenetic markers to discriminate between toxic exposures and other etiologies of this leukemia. However, a recent population-based cytogenetic study of adult secondary AML and age- and sex-matched de novo AML patients showed that, with the exception of monosomy 7, the distributions of chromosomal abnormalities among the groups were comparable (Preiss *et al.*, 2010). The same study found a higher degree of genetic instability in the therapy-related AML patients, compared with secondary AML that evolved from antecedent stem cell disorders such as MDS, which was characterized by a more frequent combination of numerical and structural aberrations, complex karyotypes, abnormal mitoses only, and hypodiploidy.

Larson and LeBeau reported the results of cytogenetic analyses on 306 consecutive patients with therapy-related AML, which were largely consistent with the above understandings (Larson and Le Beau, 2005; Look, 2005). They went on, however, to perform gene expression profiling of CD34+ hematopoietic progenitor cells from these patients, through which they were able to identify distinct subtypes of AML with characteristic gene expressions. Not surprisingly, these early progenitor cells showed expression patterns typical of arrested differentiation. Through this work they positioned therapy-related AML as an important model that provides a unique opportunity to examine the effects of mutagens on carcinogenesis in humans, as well as the role of genetic susceptibility. The fact that therapy-related AML behaves differently than the de novo disease with the same chromosomal abnormalities suggests that there is indeed a fundamental difference on the genetic level. Tools such as next-generation transcriptome sequencing are now being used to identify perturbations in genetic and molecular pathways that are unique to therapy-related leukemias, which will have implications for interventions with the new sophisticated targeted agents under development today (Stoddart *et al.*, 2011).

Some of the same chromosomal deletion changes described with therapy-related AML have been observed in AML patients occupationally exposed to benzene (Bitter *et al.*, 1987; Cuneo *et al.*, 1992; Fagioli *et al.*, 1992; Golomb *et al.*, 1982; Mitelman *et al.*, 1978, 1981), who also show aneuploidy with a high frequency of involvement of chromosome 7 (Irons, 1997). However, more recent evidence suggests that chromosomes 5 and 7 are not preferential targets in benzene-related cases, which is consistent with the fact that benzene metabolites are actually very weak alkylating agents (Pyatt and Thirman, 2011). Molecular mechanisms for benzene-induced hematotoxicity, which include both leukemogenesis and aplastic anemia (Hoffmann *et al.*, 2001), are thought to include the bioactivation of reactive metabolites (Powley and Carlson, 2001), the formation of reactive oxygen species (Kolachana *et al.*, 1993), and activation of the aryl hydrocarbon receptor (AhR) and the oncogene C-Myb (Wan *et al.*, 2005). Studies have also suggested that polymorphisms in genes involved in DNA double strand break repair might influence susceptibility to these effects (Shen *et al.*, 2006).

Other forms of leukemia—including CML, CLL, ALL, and multiple myeloma—have shown weak correlations with occupational exposure or treatment with alkylating agents (Irons, 1997). The latter has been repeatedly associated with exposure to benzene, although a causal relationship has yet to be demonstrated (Bergsagel *et al.*, 1999).

Leukemogenic Agents

The overwhelming majority of toxic or secondary leukemias seen today are therapy-related (Godley and Larson, 2001), due, in part, to stricter workplace and environmental regulations that have limited exposure to potential carcinogens. Putative agents can be classified by mechanism, as discussed previously, and include alkylating agents, topoisomerase II inhibitors, antimetabolite, and antitubulin drugs. The clinical syndrome is a late complication of these cytotoxic therapies, with a latency period between primary diagnosis and treatment-related disease ranging from months to years. While the morphologic abnormalities may vary (Godley and Larson, 2001; Jaffe, 2001; Thirman and Larson, 1996), there is a continuum in the percentage of marrow blasts from a MDS to overt AML (Larson and Le Beau, 2005).

Most *alkylating agents* used in cancer chemotherapy can cause MDS and/or AML, including cyclophosphamide, melphalan, busulfan, chlorambucil, and nitrosurea compounds such as carmustine, or BCNU (Casciato and Scott, 1979; Greene *et al.*, 1986). Other oncolytic agents implicated include azathioprine, procarbazine, doxorubicin, and bleomycin (Carver *et al.*, 1979; Valagussa *et al.*, 1979; Vismans *et al.*, 1980). The risk these drugs pose varies considerably with the therapeutic regimen. The incidence of MDS/AML in patients treated with alkylating agents has been reported to be 0.6% to 17%, with an average of 100-fold relative risk. Moreover, treatment-related MDS is associated with a substantially higher rate of transformation to AML than is primary or spontaneous MDS (Bitter *et al.*, 1987; Kantarjian *et al.*, 1986).

Treatment with *topoisomerase II inhibitors*, particularly the epipodophyllotoxins etoposide and teniposide, can induce AML, the clinical course of which has the following distinguishing characteristics: (1) the absence of a preleukemic phase, (2) a short latency period, (3) frequent involvement of an M4/5 subtype, and (4) balanced chromosome aberrations involving chromosomes 11q23 and 21q22, among others (Larson and Le Beau, 2005; Murphy, 1993). Similar cytogenetic features have been observed following treatment with doxorubicin or dactinomycin (intercalating topoisomerase II inhibitors) in conjunction with alkylating agents and irradiation (Sandoval *et al.*, 1993).

Of the *aromatic hydrocarbons*, only benzene has been proven to be leukemogenic. While substituted aromatic hydrocarbons have long been suspected to be causative, due to the fact that preparations of xylene and toluene in the past contained as much as 20% benzene (Browning, 1965), clinical or experimental evidence for that is lacking (Irons, 1997).

Exposure to *high-dose γ- or x-ray radiation* has long been associated with ALL, AML, and CML, as demonstrated in survivors of the atom bombings of Nagasaki and Hiroshima (Cartwright *et al.*, 1964; Shimizu *et al.*, 1989). Less clear is the association of these diseases with low-dose radiation secondary to fallout or diagnostic radiographs (Cartwright *et al.*, 1964).

Other *controversial agents* include 1,3-butadiene, nonionizing radiation (electromagnetic, microwave, infrared, visible, and the high end of the ultraviolet spectrum), and cigarette smoking, for which published studies on the relationship to leukemia incidence is confusing, contradictory, or difficult to interpret based on dose response (Irons, 1997). Data suggesting that formaldehyde may be leukemogenic in humans have also been recently reviewed (Golden *et al.*, 2006). The results were similarly inconclusive.

TOXICOLOGY OF PLATELETS AND HEMOSTASIS

Hemostasis is a multicomponent system responsible for preventing the loss of blood from sites of vascular injury and maintaining circulating blood in a fluid state. Loss of blood is prevented by formation of stable hemostatic plugs mediated by the procoagulant arm of hemostasis. This procoagulant response is normally limited to sites of vascular injury by the multicomponent regulatory arm of hemostasis. The dynamically modulated balance between procoagulant and regulatory pathways permits a rapid, localized response to injury. The major constituents of the hemostatic system include circulating platelets, a variety of plasma proteins, and vascular endothelial cells. The role of other cells in hemostasis, especially leukocytes, has been documented (Lane *et al.,* 2005; Monroe and Hoffman, 2005). Alterations in these components or systemic activation of this system can lead to the clinical manifestations of deranged hemostasis, including excessive bleeding and thrombosis. The hemostatic system is a frequent target of therapeutic intervention as well as inadvertent expression of the toxic effect of a variety of xenobiotics. This section briefly reviews the inadvertent effects of xenobiotics on hemostasis and the toxic effects of chemicals used to manipulate the hemostatic system.

Toxic Effects on Platelets

The Thrombocyte Platelets are essential for formation of a stable hemostatic plug in response to vascular injury. They initially adhere to the damaged wall through binding of von Willebrand factor (vWF) with the platelet glycoprotein Ib/IX/V (GP Ib/IX/V) receptor complex (Jurk and Kehrel, 2005). Ligand binding to GP Ib/IX/V or interaction of other platelet agonists (eg, thrombin, collagen, ADP, thromboxane A_2) with their specific receptors initiates biochemical response pathways that lead to shape change, platelet contraction, platelet secretion of granule contents, activation of the GP IIb/IIIa receptor, and externalization of phosphatidylserine (Jurk and Kehrel, 2005). Activation of the GP IIb/IIIa receptor permits fibrinogen and other multivalent adhesive molecules to form cross-links between nearby platelets, resulting in platelet aggregation. Xenobiotics may interfere with the platelet response by causing thrombocytopenia or interfering with platelet function; some agents are capable of affecting both platelet number and function.

Thrombocytopenia Like anemia, thrombocytopenia may be due to decreased production or increased destruction. Thrombocytopenia is a common side effect of intensive chemotherapy, due to the predictable effect of antiproliferative agents on hematopoietic precursors, including those of the megakaryocytic lineage. It is a clinically significant component of idiosyncratic xenobiotic-induced aplastic anemia, as discussed previously. Indeed, the initial manifestation of aplastic anemia may be mucocutaneous bleeding secondary to thrombocytopenia.

Exposure to xenobiotics may cause increased immune-mediated platelet destruction through any one of several mechanisms (Table 11-9) (Aster, 2005; Aster and Bougie, 2007; Aster *et al.,* 2009; van den Bemt *et al.,* 2004). Some drugs function as haptens, binding to platelet membrane components and eliciting an immune response that is specific for the hapten. The responding antibody then binds to the hapten on the platelet surface, leading to removal of the antibody-coated platelet from the circulation. This type of antibody interaction can often be blocked in vitro by excess soluble drug that binds to the antibody and prevents its interaction with the platelet surface (van den Bemt *et al.,* 2004).

A second mechanism of immune thrombocytopenia is initiated by xenobiotic-induced exposure of a neoepitope on a platelet membrane glycoprotein. This elicits an antibody response, with the responding antibody binding to this altered platelet antigen in the presence of drug, resulting in removal of the platelet from the circulation by the mononuclear phagocytic system. The epitope specificity can be quite selective, as there is often little or no cross-reactivity between drugs having a very similar structure (eg, quinine and quinidine). This type of interaction is not inhibited in vitro by excess soluble drug, as the antibody target is a platelet-dependent epitope. Quinidine is a prototype of this type of mechanism and can induce antibodies directed at GP Ib/IX/V, GP IIb/IIIa, and/or platelet endothelial cell adhesion molecule-1 (PECAM-1) (van den Bemt *et al.,* 2004). Epitope heterogeneity has been described, regarding the binding site of these antibodies (Peterson *et al.,* 2008), which has been hypothesized to be due to the drug binding to and stabilizing denatured or nonnative conformations in these platelet receptors, which are then recognized as foreign and initiate a specific immune response (Li, 2010).

Table 11-9

Mechanism of Immune-Mediated Thrombocytopenia

MECHANISM	PROTOTYPIC AGENT	ANTIGEN/EPITOPE	PLATELET EFFECT	CLINICAL EFFECT
Hapten-directed antibody	Penicillin	Drug	Opsonization ↑ Clearance	Bleeding
Acquired antibody to drug-induced epitope	Quinidine	Drug–GP Ib/IX/V Drug–GP IIb/IIIa	Opsonization ↑ Clearance	Bleeding
Natural antibody to drug-induced epitope	Abciximab	GP IIb/IIIa	Opsonization ↑ Clearance	Bleeding
Induction of autoimmune antibodies	Gold	Platelet membrane	Opsonization ↑ Clearance	Bleeding
Immune complex	Heparin	PF 4–heparin complex	Platelet activation and aggregation ↑ Clearance	Thrombosis
Thrombotic thrombocytopenic purpura (TTP)	Ticlopidine	vWF-cleaving protease	Platelet activation Platelet aggregation ↑ Clearance	Microvascular thrombosis Microangiopathic hemolytic anemia
Hemolytic-uremic syndrome	Mitomycin	Unknown	Platelet activation and aggregation ↑ Clearance	Microvascular thrombosis Microangiopathic hemolytic anemia Renal failure

The diagnosis of drug-dependent antiplatelet antibodies can be quite difficult. Despite availability limited to specialized centers, flow cytometry is the most sensitive method for detecting drug-dependent antiplatelet antibodies. However, even this methodology has limitations, and must be interpreted with the clinical information. Therefore, these assays are not used in routine clinical practice. Consequently, the diagnosis is usually established by observing the resolution of thrombocytopenia following discontinuation of the offending drug. In most cases, the platelet count returns to normal within 5 to 10 days of drug discontinuation. Although a large number of chemicals have been implicated in the development of immune thrombocytopenia, the supporting evidence in many cases is weak (van den Bemt et al., 2004).

A recent survey was conducted using three methods for identifying drugs that are associated with immune thrombocytopenia: published case reports; analysis of serum samples from affected patients for drug-dependent, platelet-reactive antibodies; and the Food and Drug Administration's Adverse Event Reporting System (Reese et al., 2010). An astonishing 1444 drugs were found to have at least one report associated with thrombocytopenia, of which 573 demonstrated a statistically distinctive reporting association. Of 1468 drugs suspected as causal, 102 were evaluated by all three methods, of which 23 were found to have an association in all three.

Thrombocytopenia is an uncommon but serious complication of inhibitors of GP IIb/IIIa such as abciximab (Huxtable et al., 2006). The mechanism appears to be related to exposure of epitopes on GP IIb/IIIa that react with naturally occurring antibodies. Because the reaction is dependent on antibodies formed prior to exposure to drug, it may occur shortly after the first exposure to the drug. Ligand binding is known to alter the conformation of GP IIb/IIIa. The GP IIb/IIIa inhibitors bind at the ligand binding site and also cause a conformational change in GP IIb/IIIa, permitting naturally occurring antibodies to bind to and initiate clearance of platelets by the mononuclear phagocytic system.

Heparin-induced thrombocytopenia (HIT) represents another mechanism of immune-mediated platelet destruction. This disorder is due to the development of antibodies that react with a multimolecular complex formed by the interaction between heparin and a protein, usually platelet factor 4 (PF 4) (Davoren and Aster, 2006; Warkentin and Greinacher, 2004). When the relative concentration of heparin to PF 4 is appropriate, formation of this complex is associated with exposure of a neoepitope on PF 4 (or another target protein) and development of an IgG response to the neoepitope. The IgG then binds to the PF 4–heparin complex to form an immune complex that binds to the platelet Fc receptor, FcγRIIa. Clustering of platelet FcγRIIa by the immune complex activates biochemical signaling pathways mediated by the cytoplasmic domain of FcγRIIa. This results in platelet activation and aggregation. During the process of platelet activation, platelet microparticles that promote thrombin generation are released. Consequently, HIT is associated with both thrombocytopenia and an increased risk of arterial and venous thrombosis. Other drug–antibody complexes (eg, streptokinase–IgG) may trigger platelet activation and thrombocytopenia through a similar mechanism (Deckmyn et al., 1998; McRedmond et al., 2000).

TTP is a syndrome characterized by the sudden onset of thrombocytopenia, a microangiopathic hemolytic anemia, and multisystem organ failure, which often includes neurologic dysfunction. The syndrome tends to occur following an infectious disease but may also occur following administration of some drugs. The pathogenesis of TTP appears to be related to the ability of unusually large vWF multimers to activate platelets, even in the absence of significant vascular damage (Lian, 2005). Although these large multimers are normally secreted into blood by endothelial cells,

they are rapidly processed into smaller multimers by a protease (ADAMTS13) present in plasma. Acquired TTP is associated with the development of an antibody that inhibits this protease, permitting the very large vWF multimers to persist in the circulation (Lian, 2005; Veyradier and Meyer, 2005). Consequently, these multimers bind to platelet GP Ib/IX/V and induce platelet activation and aggregation. The organ failure and hemolysis in TTP is due to the formation of platelet-rich microthrombi throughout the circulation. The development of TTP or TTP-like syndromes has been associated with drugs such as ticlopidine, clopidogrel, cocaine, mitomycin, and cyclosporine (Veyradier and Meyer, 2005; Zakarija and Bennett, 2005). In some cases, drug-induced TTP is related to development of antibodies to ADAMTS13, whereas in other cases it may be due to direct endothelial cell toxicity from the drug.

The *HUS* is a disorder characterized by clinical features similar to those of TTP, with microangiopathic hemolytic anemia, thrombocytopenia, and renal failure (Zakarija and Bennett, 2005). Neurologic complications tend to be less severe, while renal failure often dominates the clinical picture. Sporadic cases of HUS have been linked to infection with verocytotoxin-producing *Escherichia coli*, but they may also occur during therapy with some drugs, including mitomycin. In contrast to TTP, the vWF-cleaving protease is normal in patients with HUS (Furlan et al., 1998). The pathogenesis of the thrombocytopenia and microangiopathic changes in HUS is still uncertain, but there is experimental evidence suggesting that it is related to endothelial cell injury, with subsequent platelet activation and thrombus formation (Delvaeye et al., 2009).

Desmopressin, a vasopressin analog, is an example of nonimmune-mediated increased platelet destruction. It induces a 2- to 5-fold increase in the plasma concentration of vWF and factor VIII. It is commonly used in the treatment of patients with von Willebrand disease and other mild bleeding syndromes. Desmopressin has been associated with the development or accentuation of thrombocytopenia in some patients with type 2B von Willebrand disease. The thrombocytopenia in such cases is related to the release of an abnormal vWF from endothelial cells. The abnormal vWF has enhanced affinity for GP Ib/IX/V and the interaction of the vWF with its receptor leads to platelet clearance from the circulation (Mannucci, 1998).

Toxic Effects on Platelet Function Platelet function is dependent on the coordinated interaction of a number of biochemical response pathways. A variety of drugs and foods have been found to inhibit platelet function, either in vivo or in vitro (Abrams, 2006). Major drug groups that affect platelet function include nonsteroidal anti-inflammatory drugs, β-lactam-containing antibiotics, cardiovascular drugs, particularly β-blockers, psychotropic drugs, anesthetics, antihistamines, and some chemotherapeutic agents. The effect of these drugs can vary between individuals, perhaps due to subclinical variations in underlying platelet function.

Xenobiotics may interfere with platelet function through a variety of mechanisms. Some drugs inhibit the phospholipase A_2/cyclooxygenase pathway and synthesis of thromboxane A_2 (eg, nonsteroidal anti-inflammatory agents). Other drugs appear to interfere with the interaction between platelet agonists and their receptors (eg, antibiotics, ticlopidine, clopidogrel). As the platelet response is dependent on a rapid increase in cytoplasmic calcium, any chemical that interferes with translocation of calcium may inhibit platelet function (eg, calcium channel blockers). Occasionally, drug-induced antibodies will bind to a critical platelet receptor and inhibit its function. The functional defect induced by such antibodies may potentiate the bleeding risk associated with the xenobiotic-induced thrombocytopenia. In some cases, the mechanism of inhibition is not known.

The effect of xenobiotics on platelet function can often be studied following in vitro exposure of platelets to the chemical of interest. However, evaluation following exposure is preferred, as metabolites of the parent compound may contain the platelet inhibitory activity. The most common method of assessing platelet function is turbidimetric platelet aggregation using platelet-rich plasma, but alternate techniques are available, including the PFA 100 analyzer, flow cytometry, and whole-blood impedance aggregometry (Cesar *et al.*, 2005; Matzdorff, 2005).

Toxic Effects on Fibrin Clot Formation

Coagulation   Fibrin clot formation is the result of sequential activation of a series of serine proteases that culminates in the formation of thrombin (Lane *et al.*, 2005; Monroe and Hoffman, 2005). Thrombin is a multifunctional enzyme that converts fibrinogen to fibrin; activates factors V, VIII, XI, XIII, protein C, and platelets; and interacts with a variety of cells (eg, leukocytes and endothelial cells), activating cellular signaling pathways (Lane *et al.*, 2005).

The most common toxic effect of xenobiotics on fibrin clot formation are related to a decreased level of one or more of the critical proteins necessary for this process. The decrease in clotting factor activity may be due to decreased synthesis of the protein(s) or increased clearance from the circulation. Decreased synthesis is most often a reflection of hepatocellular damage or interference with vitamin K metabolism, as discussed below, whereas increased clearance is usually associated with the development of an antibody to a specific coagulation factor.

Decreased Synthesis of Coagulation Proteins   The majority of proteins involved in the coagulation cascade are synthesized in the liver. Therefore, any chemical that impairs liver function may cause a decrease in production of coagulation factors. The common tests of the coagulation cascade, the prothrombin time (PT) and activated partial thromboplastin time (aPTT), may be used to screen for liver dysfunction and a decrease in clotting factors. These assays are often performed as part of the safety evaluation of a new chemical entity. The half-life of clotting factors in the circulation varies significantly, with factor VII having the shortest half-life (three–four hours). Therefore, with acute toxicity (eg, acetaminophen overdose), the effect on blood coagulation may be first seen as a decrease in the level of factor VII. Such a decrease would lead to prolongation of the PT with a normal aPTT. With a more chronic process, the PT, the aPTT, or both may be affected.

Factors II, VII, IX, and X are dependent on vitamin K for their complete synthesis (Stafford, 2005). Anything that interferes with vitamin K metabolism may lead to a deficiency of these factors and a bleeding tendency. This may occur with xenobiotics that interfere with absorption of vitamin K from the intestine or with chemicals that interfere with the reduction of vitamin K epoxide (Table 11-10). The

combination of antibiotic therapy and limited oral intake is a common cause of acquired deficiency of vitamin K–dependent proteins among hospitalized patients (Chakraverty *et al.*, 1996). The "super rodenticides" are another cause of acquired vitamin K deficiency (Berry *et al.*, 2000; Chua and Friedenberg, 1998). These agents have a very prolonged half-life in vivo; thus, the coagulation defect may persist for weeks or months following exposure. Rodenticide exposure may occur accidentally, as part of a Munchausen syndrome, in association with a suicide attempt, or as part of a homicide attempt. At times it may be important to distinguish between a true vitamin K deficiency and interference with the reduction of vitamin K epoxide. This is most readily accomplished by measuring the level of vitamin K and vitamin K epoxide in serum or plasma. In the case of vitamin K deficiency, both vitamin K and vitamin K epoxide are decreased, whereas in the case of inhibition of vitamin K reduction, vitamin K epoxide is significantly increased. Specific rodenticides may be measured using HPLC techniques, but it is important to specify which active agent (eg, brodifacoum) should be measured, as the assays may not show cross-reactivity between agents.

Increased Clearance of Coagulation Factors   Idiosyncratic reactions to xenobiotics include the formation of antibodies that react with coagulation proteins. These antibodies bind to the coagulation factor, forming an immune complex that is rapidly cleared from the circulation and resulting in deficiency of the factor. The antibody is often reversible over time if the initiating agent is withdrawn. However, during the acute phase, these patients may have life-threatening bleeding. The factors that are most often affected include factors VIII, V, and XIII, vWF, prothrombin, and thrombin (Table 11-11) (Lollar, 2004, 2005). Many of these antibodies

Table 11-10

Conditions Associated with Abnormal Synthesis of Vitamin K–Dependent Coagulation Factors

Warfarin and analogs	Intravenous α-tocopherol
Rodenticides (eg, brodifacoum)	Dietary deficiency Cholestyramine resin
Broad-spectrum antibiotics	Malabsorption syndromes
N-Methyl-thiotetrazole cephalosporins	

Table 11-11

Relationship between Xenobiotics and the Development of Specific Coagulation Factor Inhibitors

COAGULATION FACTOR	XENOBIOTIC
Thrombin	Topical bovine thrombin Fibrin glue
Factor V	Streptomycin Penicillin Gentamicin Cephalosporins Topical bovine thrombin
Factor VIII	Penicillin Ampicillin Chloramphenicol Phenytoin Methyldopa Nitrofurazone Phenylbutazone
Factor XIII	Isoniazid Procainamide Penicillin Phenytoin Practolol
von Willebrand factor	Ciprofloxacin Hydroxyethyl starch Valproic acid Griseofulvin Tetracycline Pesticides

inhibit the functional activity of the coagulation factor in addition to increasing the rate of clearance. Other antibodies have been demonstrated to have catalytic activity, resulting in proteolysis of the target coagulation factor (Ananyeva *et al.*, 2004).

Lupus anticoagulants are antibodies that interfere with in vitro phospholipid-dependent coagulation reactions (Bertolaccini *et al.*, 2004). Although it was once hypothesized that these antibodies were directed against phospholipid, it is now evident that lupus anticoagulants are directed against phospholipid-binding proteins, including prothrombin and β_2-glycoprotein 1. These antibodies usually do not cause a deficiency of any specific coagulation factor. However, in vivo, these antibodies can potentiate procoagulant mechanisms and interfere with the protein C system. Consequently, these antibodies have been associated with an increased risk of thrombosis (Bertolaccini *et al.*, 2004). The development of lupus anticoagulants has been seen in association with a variety of medications, including procainamide, chlorpromazine, and hydralazine.

Toxicology of Chemicals Used to Modulate Hemostasis

Patients with bleeding or thrombotic problems are commonly encountered in clinical practice. A variety of agents are available to treat such patients, ranging from recombinant hemostatic proteins to chemical entities that modulate the activity of the coagulation system. The major toxicologic reactions to plasma-derived products are infectious diseases (eg, hepatitis C) and allergic reactions, which can be severe. The use of some products, such as activated concentrates of vitamin K–dependent proteins (eg, Autoplex and FEIBA), has been associated with the development of disseminated intravascular coagulation and/or thrombosis in some patients (Mannucci, 1998).

Oral Anticoagulants Oral anticoagulants (warfarin) interfere with vitamin K metabolism by preventing the reduction of vitamin K epoxide, resulting in a functional deficiency of reduced vitamin K (Ansell *et al.*, 2004). These drugs are widely used for prophylaxis and therapy of venous and arterial thrombosis. The therapeutic window for oral anticoagulants is relatively narrow, and there is considerable interindividual variation in the response to a given dose. A number of factors, including concurrent medications and genetics, affect the individual response to oral anticoagulants (Ansell *et al.*, 2004; D'Andrea *et al.*, 2005; Rojas *et al.*, 2005). For these reasons, therapy with these drugs must be routinely monitored to maximize both safety and efficacy. This is routinely performed with the PT, with results expressed in terms of the international normalized ratio (INR).

A number of xenobiotics, including foods, have been found to affect the response to oral anticoagulants (Ansell *et al.*, 2004). Perhaps the most common mechanism for interference with oral anticoagulants is mediated by inhibition of CYP2C9 (Rojas *et al.*, 2005). Other mechanisms of interference include induction of CYP2C9, which tends to diminish the effect of warfarin by shortening its half-life; interference with absorption of warfarin from the gastrointestinal tract; displacement of warfarin from albumin in plasma, which temporarily increases the bioavailability of warfarin until equilibrium is reestablished; diminished vitamin K availability, due to either dietary deficiency or interference with the absorption of this lipid-soluble vitamin; and inhibition of the reduction of vitamin K epoxide, which potentiates the effect of oral anticoagulants.

Just as other drugs interfere with the action of oral anticoagulants, administration of oral anticoagulants may affect the activity of other medications, particularly those that are metabolized by

CYP2C9. Dicumarol administration prolongs the half-life of chlorpropamide and phenytoin, resulting in hypoglycemia in the case of chlorpropamide and an increased plasma drug concentration in the case of phenytoin. Bis-hydroxycoumarin, but not warfarin, potentiates the activity of tolbutamide, resulting in enhanced hypoglycemia (Harder and Thurmann, 1996).

Oral anticoagulants have been associated with the development of warfarin-induced skin necrosis (Ansell *et al.*, 2004). This disorder is due to the development of extensive microvascular thrombosis in the affected skin. This uncommon toxic effect is thought to be related to a rapid drop in protein C following administration of the drug, resulting in impaired protein C function. The risk of developing warfarin-induced skin necrosis increases with the dose of warfarin used to initiate therapy, particularly when the initial dose exceeds 10 mg per day; this is one of the reasons that loading doses of warfarin are no longer recommended.

Vitamin K is necessary for the synthesis of proteins other than the coagulation-related factors, including osteocalcin, a major component of bone. Perhaps because of this, long-term administration of warfarin has been associated with bone demineralization (Ansell *et al.*, 2004; Stafford, 2005). This effect can be important in patients with borderline bone density. Administration of warfarin during pregnancy, particularly the first 12 weeks of pregnancy, is associated with congenital anomalies in 25% to 30% of exposed infants (Bates *et al.*, 2004). Many of the anomalies are related to abnormal bone formation. It is thought that warfarin may interfere with synthesis of proteins critical for normal structural development.

Heparin Heparin is a widely used anticoagulant for both prophylaxis and therapy of acute venous thromboembolism (Hirsh and Raschke, 2004). In many hospitals, the majority of patients are exposed to this potent anticoagulant at some point during their hospitalization. The major complication associated with heparin therapy is bleeding, a direct manifestation of its anticoagulant activity. The risk of bleeding is related to the intensity of therapy, the patient's body mass and underlying condition, and the presence of other hemostatic defects (eg, thrombocytopenia).

As discussed in the section "Toxic Effects on Platelets," heparin administration is also associated with the development of HIT. For unknown reasons, this complication occurs more frequently with heparin derived from bovine sources than with that derived from porcine sources. The incidence of HIT is also significantly higher in patients receiving unfractionated heparin than it is in patients receiving low-molecular-weight heparin (Davoren and Aster, 2006; Warkentin and Greinacher, 2004).

Long-term administration of heparin is associated with an increased risk of clinically significant osteoporosis (Dinwoodey and Ansell, 2006; Hirsh and Raschke, 2004). The mechanism underlying the development of osteoporosis in these patients is not known. Patients may suffer from spontaneous vertebral fractures and demineralization of long bones of the arms and legs. The risk of osteoporosis may be less with low-molecular-weight heparin as compared with that with unfractionated heparin.

Heparin administration may also cause a transient rise in serum transaminases, suggesting significant liver dysfunction (Guevara *et al.*, 1993). However, the rise is rapidly reversible on discontinuation of heparin and may reverse even before heparin is discontinued. The elevation of serum transaminases has not been associated with chronic liver dysfunction. The mechanism of heparin-induced increase in transaminases is not known.

In 2008, serious injuries and deaths were associated with the use of heparin originating in China. It was determined that certain sources of heparin were contaminated with oversulfated chondroitin sulfate (OSCS). The presence of OSCS is believed to be responsible for the observed severe allergic reactions, gastrointestinal disturbances, and hypotension (Blossom *et al.,* 2008).

Fibrinolytic Drugs Fibrinolytic drugs are used in the treatment of acute thromboembolic disease with the goal of dissolving the pathogenic thrombus (Collen and Lijnen, 2005). Each of these drugs works by converting plasminogen, an inactive zymogen, to plasmin, an active proteolytic enzyme. Plasmin is normally tightly regulated and is not freely present in the circulation. However, administration of fibrinolytic drugs regularly results in the generation of free plasmin leading to systemic fibrin(ogen)olysis. The toxicology of the fibrinolytic drugs can be divided into toxic effects of systemic plasmin activation and toxic effects of the activators themselves.

Systemic fibrinolysis is associated with the development of a complex coagulopathy characterized by a decrease in fibrinogen, factors V and VIII, and α_2-antiplasmin; an increase in circulating fibrin split products; degradation of platelet GP Ib/IX/V and IIb/IIIa; degradation of endothelial cell glycoproteins; degradation of fibronectin and thrombospondin; and prolongation of the PT, aPTT, and thrombin time (Hajjar, 2006). All of these effects potentiate the risk of bleeding. Anatomic locations that are frequently involved in bleeding complications include the cerebral circulation and sites of recent vascular access. As systemic plasmin can lyse physiologic as well as pathologic thrombi, reactivation of bleeding from sites of vascular access is not uncommon. Platelet inhibitors and heparin are commonly used in conjunction with fibrinolytic therapy to prevent recurrent thrombosis. As one might expect, the concurrent use of anticoagulants with systemic fibrinolysis may contribute to the risk of bleeding (Menon *et al.,* 2004).

Another complication associated with fibrinolysis is recurrent thrombosis at the site of pathologic thrombosis. While rethrombosis may be related to underlying damage to the vascular wall, there is some evidence that fibrinolytic therapy may contribute to this process. For example, plasmin, in appropriate concentrations, can actually induce platelet activation (McRedmond *et al.,* 2000). This process may be mediated by plasmin or streptokinase/plasminogen cleavage of the platelet thrombin receptor (protease activated receptor-1). Cleavage of the receptor is associated with activation of the platelet biochemical signaling pathways. There is sufficient "cross-talk" between the fibrinolytic system and the contact system of coagulation that one could also anticipate increased thrombin generation occurring as a result of fibrinolytic therapy (Schmaier *et al.,* 1999).

Streptokinase is a protein derived from group C β-hemolytic streptococci and is antigenic in humans. Antibody formation to streptokinase occurs commonly in association with streptococcal infections as well as exposure to streptokinase. Acute allergic reactions may occur in 1% to 5% of patients exposed to streptokinase, and these allergic reactions may consist of minor symptoms such as hives and fever as well as major, life-threatening anaphylactic reactions. In addition, delayed hypersensitivity reactions associated with severe morbidity may occur (Curzen *et al.,* 1998; Siebert *et al.,* 1992). Allergic reactions also occur with other fibrinolytic agents containing streptokinase (eg, anisoylated plasminogen–streptokinase complex) or streptokinase-derived peptides. The immune complex formed by IgG and streptokinase is capable of binding to and clustering platelet FcγRIIa, initiating platelet activation and aggregation (McRedmond *et al.,* 2000).

Urokinase and recombinant tissue plasminogen activator (t-PA) are generally not associated with allergic reactions. However, work is progressing on a number of genetically engineered forms of t-PA. Whether or not such mutant forms of t-PA

are immunogenic has not been firmly established (Collen and Lijnen, 2005).

Inhibitors of Fibrinolysis Inhibitors of fibrinolysis are commonly used to control bleeding in patients with congenital abnormalities of hemostasis, such as von Willebrand disease. Tranexamic acid and ε-aminocaproic acid are small molecules that block the binding of plasminogen and plasmin to fibrin and other substrate proteins through interaction with lysine binding sites on plasmin(ogen). Although relatively well tolerated, there is some evidence that administration of these chemicals may increase the risk of thrombosis due to the inhibition of the fibrinolytic system (Mannucci, 1998). In a single case, intravenous infusion of ε-aminocaproic acid in a patient with chronic renal failure was associated with acute hyperkalemia (Perazella and Biswas, 1999).

Aprotinin is a naturally occurring polypeptide inhibitor of serine proteases. It is usually derived from bovine material and consequently is immunogenic when administered to humans. Aprotinin is given by intravenous infusion, as it is inactive when given orally. Allergic reactions in response to aprotinin have been reported, ranging from minor cutaneous manifestations to anaphylactic reactions (Peters and Noble, 1999). A more recent observational study compared clinical outcomes after cardiac surgery performed with aprotinin, tranexamic acid, or ε-aminocaproic acid with outcomes after cardiac surgery without an inhibitor of fibrinolysis (Mangano *et al.,* 2006). In this study, use of antifibrinolytics was associated with decreased blood loss. However, use of aprotinin was associated with a significant increase in end-organ damage, including renal, cardiac, and cerebral events. The design and results of this study have been questioned, with calls for prospective randomized comparator studies (Sedrakyan *et al.,* 2006). The results also point out the intricate balance within the hemostatic system and the potential for problems when modulating the activity of one portion of this system.

RISK ASSESSMENT

Assessing the risk that exposure to new drugs, chemical products, and other agents poses to humans—in terms of significant toxic effects on hematopoiesis and the functional integrity of blood cells and hemostatic mechanisms—can be logistically and intellectually challenging. This is due in part to the complexity of hematopoiesis and the range of important tasks that these components perform, as previously discussed. A central issue in drug and nontherapeutic chemical development is the *predictive value* of preclinical toxicology data and the expansive but inevitably limited preregistration clinical database for the occurrence of significant hematotoxicity on broad exposure to human populations. Appropriately, this area of well-resourced applied toxicology is highly regulated yet provides unique and exciting opportunities for sophisticated, well-controlled research (Bloom, 1993).

Preclinical Risk Assessment

Most preclinical studies that assess the potential for candidate drugs or nontherapeutic chemicals to induce hematotoxicity in humans are performed in industry as part of the routine safety evaluation of these molecules. These studies are largely prescribed by government regulatory bodies of the various countries and regions, including the United States, the European Union, and Japan (ICH, 2000; Hall, 1992, 1997). The unique accessibility of blood as a potential target organ, which allows direct ex vivo assessment of the tissue (compared with the indirect parameters used to detect effects on liver, kidney, etc), together with the use of hematologic monitoring to reflect systemic effects of other organ toxicity, enables more sensitive signal detection, and may account for the relatively high predictive value of these studies. In fact, earlier studies have shown that hematotoxicity that is preclinically identified predicts toxicity in human clinical trials with a 91% concordance (Olson *et al.,* 2000). It is doubtful, however, that preclinical animal studies are as predictive for today's candidate drug portfolios of highly targeted agents that include more human recombinant proteins, monoclonal antibodies, and targets that are specific to human tissue and disorders such as cancer and autoimmune disease. Another consequence is that more sophisticated biomarkers are increasingly required to demonstrate both pharmacodynamic and off-target effects in human and animal models, some of which provide opportunities for companion diagnostics and personalized medicine. Immunogenicity of heterologous proteins further complicates pharmacokinetic, pharmacodynamic, and safety assessment in animals. As a result, there is a greater sense of urgency to study these novel agents in humans. Accordingly, phase I clinical studies have become more important not only for safety assessment but also as a venue for early proof of concept experiments. Finally, as with other organ toxicity, the predictive value of preclinical studies for idiosyncratic iatrogenic disease in humans, such as aplastic anemia and agranulocytosis, is limited.

The issues relating to the assessment of blood as a target organ that confront the industrial toxicologist are largely similar to those of other target organs and include the selection of the appropriate animal model, how to best monitor for hematotoxicity, and the appreciation of species differences in responding to hematotoxic insults.

Animal Models and Hematologic Monitoring Selection of a species that is practical to study and predictive for hematotoxicity in humans is always a challenge. While this is driven in part by the aforementioned regulatory requirements, the selection is also influenced by other considerations, including having a pharmacokinetic profile comparable to that of humans, prior information on sensitivity of a particular species to a class of compounds, the ability to fully characterize effects on peripheral blood and bone marrow, and practical considerations, such as logistics and economics (Bloom, 1993). These become of particular importance in choosing a model to fully characterize the toxicity of a chemical known to have a hematotoxic potential.

Of the commonly used animal species, rats and mice offer the advantage of their small size, which favorably impacts test compound requirements and number of subjects that can be economically housed and tested. Both have been well characterized hematologically (Moore, 2000a,b; Valli and McGrath, 1997). Blood volume limitations, however, often prohibit the frequent, or serial, evaluation of blood and bone marrow required to characterize the progression of a hematotoxic effect. While this can be addressed in part through serial sacrifices, the inability to fully characterize individual animals poses a significant disadvantage. Test results will also vary in accordance with the phlebotomy site and method, particularly in rodents (Suber and Kodell, 1985), and with the physical and chemical restraint employed (Loomis *et al.,* 1980).

Serial blood and bone marrow sampling is practical in larger species, such as the dog and monkey. These models offer the additional advantage of being hematologically more similar to humans, as regards hematopoiesis and blood cell kinetics, which in the monkey extends to immunohematologic features (Ladiges *et al.,* 1990; Shifrine and Wilson, 1980). The latter species, however, presents more interanimal hematologic variability, particularly in

wild-caught primates, due to temperament, vascular access, and other influences, which include nutritional status and infection.

Tests used to assess blood and bone marrow in preclinical toxicology studies will vary with the phase or objective of the evaluation (acute, subacute, chronic), the intended use of the chemical, and what is understood or suspected regarding the toxicologic profile of the xenobiotic. Ideally, the studies in aggregate should provide information on the effects of single- and multiple-dose exposure on erythrocyte parameters (RBC, Hbg, PCV, MCV, MCHC), leukocyte parameters (WBC and absolute differential counts), thrombocyte counts, screening coagulation tests (PT, aPTT), peripheral blood cell morphology, and bone marrow cytologic and histologic features (Bloom, 1993; Lund, 2000; Weingand *et al.,* 1996). Notable are the applications of flow cytometry, which have been refined in recent years and recently reviewed regarding the advantages and disadvantages of these techniques in preclinical studies (Reagan *et al.,* 2011). Forward-angle scatter has been used to effectively type canine bone marrow hematopoietic cells (Weiss *et al.,* 2000), where that combined with side-angle scatter and the use of fluorochromes and lymphocyte-specific antibodies has been accurate and reproducible in rats (Chriswell *et al.,* 1998a). The latter correlates well with manual counts and has been used to characterize and quantitate the effects of phenylhydrazine, phlebotomy, cyclophosphamide, and various hematopoietic growth factors (Chriswell *et al.,* 1998b, 2000). Other techniques using cell surface markers have been used to enumerate subpopulations, which must be validated for each species due to variation in surface antigen expression and other preanalytical variables (Reagan *et al.,* 2011).

Additional tests should be employed in a problem-driven fashion, as required to better characterize findings from the aforementioned screening efforts or to more fully explore a class-specific effect or other hematotoxicologic potential of concern (Bloom, 1993). Examples of these tests are listed in Table 11-12. While much progress has been made in validating many of the more specialized assays in our principal animal models, additional validation that addresses laboratory- and species-specific preanalytical and analytical variables is often required.

Table 11-12
Examples of Problem-Driven Tests Used to Characterize Hematologic Observations in Preclinical Toxicology
Flow cytometry (see text)
Heinz body preparation
Cell-associated antibody assays (erythrocyte, platelet, neutrophil)
Erythrocyte osmotic fragility test
Erythrokinetic/ferrokinetic analyses
Cytochemical/histochemical staining
Electron microscopy
In vitro hematopoietic clonogenic assays
Platelet aggregation
Plasma fibrinogen concentration
Clotting factor assays
Thrombin time
Bleeding time

Despite the importance of bone marrow assessment in detecting and characterizing hematotoxicity, there is remarkably little regulatory guidance on indications, frequency, or preferred techniques. The Federal Drug Administration (FDA) Centers for Drug (CDER) and Biologic (CBER) Evaluation and Research, and the European Medicines Agency (EMA) have issued guidelines largely in the context of immunotoxicity risk assessment (Food and Drug Administration *et al.,* 2006; European Medicines Agency and Committee for Proprietary Medicinal Products, 2006). Limited guidance is also provided by Japan's Ministry of Health, Labor and Welfare, the FDA's Center for Veterinary Medicine, and the Environmental Protection Agency (Reagan *et al.,* 2011). To address this gap, a joint effort of the American Society for Veterinary Clinical Pathology and the Society of Toxicologic Pathology (Bone Marrow Working Group) has resulted in a recent publication on best practices for evaluation of bone marrow in nonclinical toxicity studies (Reagan *et al.,* 2011).

Because hematologic features and response to disease can vary substantially among animal species, it is essential that the toxicologist fully understands the hematology of the animal model used for preclinical risk assessment. While complete and accurate reference data are helpful, they do not provide information on pathophysiology that may be species-specific and required to accurately interpret the preclinical data. Examples of these features include the relative influence of preanalytical variables (blood collection technique, nutritional status, sample stability), response to blood loss or hemolysis, stress effects on the leukogram, susceptibility to secondary effects associated with other target organ toxicity, etc. It is beyond the scope of this chapter to fully discuss the comparative hematology of laboratory animals, which is provided in several excellent reviews (Feldman *et al.,* 2006; Valli and McGrath, 1997).

In Vitro Bone Marrow Assays As with other target organ risk assessment, in vitro methods for assessing potential hematotoxicity are attractive in that they are faster and less expensive than in vivo studies, while providing data that often suggest or clarify the mechanism of a toxic effect. Drug- or chemical-induced bone marrow suppression can result from effects on specific hematopoietic stem cells or on the hematopoietic microenvironment. These effects can be distinguished and confirmed using short-term clonogenic assays and long-term functional assays, respectively (Deldar, 1994; Naughton *et al.,* 1992; Williams *et al.,* 1988). The former include burst-forming-unit erythroid (BFU-E), colony-forming-unit erythroid (CFU-E), colony-forming-unit granulocyte/monocyte (CFU-GM), colony-forming-unit megakaryocyte (CFU-MK), and colony-forming-unit granulocyte, erythroid, megakaryocyte, monocyte (CFU-GEMM), which have been developed for several laboratory animal species (Deldar and Parchment, 1997; Pessina *et al.,* 2005). It is therefore possible to examine effects on the myeloid, erythroid, and megakaryocytic lineages in a fashion where concentrations of the chemical are tightly controlled, as is duration of exposure to it.

While the most commonly applied clonogenic techniques used to assess the above still employ viscous or semisolid matrices and culture supplements that promote differentiation of the hematopoietic cells (Erickson-Miller *et al.,* 1997; McMullin *et al.,* 1998), some newer techniques measure intracellular ATP, which is influenced by artifacts such as apoptosis, cytotoxicity, necrosis, and fibroblast contamination (Fan and Wood, 2007; Slater, 2001). Several commercial services are available that provide stem cells of human, canine, primate, and rodent origin to which are added cytokines and growth factors to support cell development (Reagan *et al.,* 2011).

In vitro clonogenic assays are best used in a preclinical setting in combination with in vivo testing. Used in this way, the predictive value of these assays is enhanced. This has been particularly true for anticancer and antiviral drugs, where the in vitro component of risk assessment has been used for therapeutic index-based screening to identify less myelosuppressive analogs, structure–toxicity relationships, and new-drug lead candidates (Deldar and Stevens, 1993; Parchment *et al.,* 1993; Pessina *et al.,* 2003). Other advantages of the in vitro hematopoietic stem cell assays include the opportunities they provide to test combinations of chemicals as well as their metabolites and effects of serum and other cell components, such as lymphocytes (Deldar and Parchment, 1997). Most important is the ability to test human hematopoietic cells directly in a preclinical setting, thus obviating extrapolation considerations. Concern for possible metabolic activation can be addressed by culturing the target cells in question with metabolizing systems in a cell-free extract (s9), with isolated hepatocytes, or with other CYP450-expressing cell types (Frazier, 1992; Negro *et al.,* 2001).

Perhaps the most interesting use of these in vitro clonogenic assays in risk assessment has been their role in making practical interspecies comparisons regarding sensitivity to a particular agent or group of drugs or chemicals. Comparisons to the sensitivity of human cells can be made that have implications for the relative predictive value of various animal models for hematotoxicity in humans. Examples include the resistance of murine CFU-GM to the anticancer drug topotecan relative to that of the canine and human cells (Deldar and Stevens, 1993). This is consistent with the early observations of Marsh—that the dog is a particularly predictive model for the myelosuppression associated with anticancer drugs in humans (Marsh, 1985). Thus, while some chemicals show comparable suppressive activity across species lines (doxorubicin, pyrazoloacridine, hepsulfan, cyclopentenyl cytosine), others, such as camptothecins, carboxyamidotriazole, and fostriecin, show differences of as much as three log concentrations (Du *et al.,* 1991; Horikoshi and Murphy, 1982; Reagan *et al.,* 1993).

Because myelotoxicity, and particularly suppression of granulopoiesis, is a major limitation in administering anticancer drugs, and is often used to determine the optimal dose, the clonogenic assay for CFU-GM has received the most attention as a preclinical tool for predicting this response. It is the only assay that has been validated by an international study supported by the European Centre for Validation of Alternative Methods (ECVAM) (Pessina *et al.,* 2003). Analytical validation was completed for the human and mouse assays, and a predictive model was developed to calculate the maximum tolerated dose (MTD) in humans using data from the mouse assay that is adjusted for the established interspecies variation (Pessina *et al.,* 2001). The model was applied in an international blind trial to 20 drugs that included 14 antineoplastic drugs, the antiviral drugs zidovudine and acyclovir, and the pesticide lindane (Pessina *et al.,* 2003). It predicted the MTD for all 20 chemicals, although extrapolation on the regression curve out of the range of the actual drug doses tested was required to derive the IC90 for 10 of these drugs. Since then, the Scientific Advisory Committee of the ECVAM endorsed the CFU-GM assay for predicting acute neutropenia in humans as a substitute to using a second species, such as the dog, for this purpose (24th meeting at ECVAM of the ECVAM Scientific Advisory Committee, European Commission, March 2006). Subsequent studies have confirmed the predictive value of this assay in both anticancer drugs (Masubuchi, 2006) and nononcology candidate drugs (Horn *et al.,* 2008). The latter study illustrates the species specificity encountered and the importance of integrating the in vivo and in vitro approaches required to fully characterize the hematotoxicity observed in pre-clinical safety assessment today.

While this discussion has focused on in vitro hematopoietic clonogenic assays in the context of risk assessment, these assays have also proven to be extraordinarily useful tools for investigating mechanisms of toxic cytopenia in humans (Deldar, 1994). Parchment and Murphy (1997) review the application of these to four categories of hematologic toxicity observed clinically: (1) the reversible cytopenia following acute exposure to a cytotoxic or cytostatic chemical; (2) the permanent loss in the production of a mature blood cell type(s); (3) cytosis, or the dramatic increase in blood cell counts following single or repeated toxicant exposure; and (4) the progressive loss of one or more blood cell lineages during chronic exposure to a toxicant. In all these circumstances, in vitro and ex vivo hematopoietic clonogenic assays have proven useful in understanding the mechanism(s) of these toxic effects and formulating strategies for risk management and treatment.

Emerging Technologies As discussed previously, the well-controlled and resource-intensive preclinical toxicology and safety studies prescribed for candidate drugs and nontherapeutic chemicals provide unique opportunities for studies on mechanisms of xenobiotic-induced hematotoxicity (Bloom, 1993; Deldar and Parchment, 1997). Together with the traditional biomarkers for toxicity, mechanism-based technologies such as toxicogenomics, proteomics, and metabonomics are now available to the toxicologist and are increasingly helpful in both predicting toxicity and determining whether a particular finding is relevant to humans (Todd and Ulrich, 1999). Challenges that the application of these tools presents relate to informatics, standardization, and validation (Reynolds, 2005).

Clinical Trials and Risk Assessment

As with preclinical risk assessment, most of the clinical research on hematotoxicity is driven by regulatory requirements and supported by the drug, cosmetic, and chemical industries. The challenges and opportunities this presents are similar to those in preclinical development with the following differences. Most clinical studies involve actual patients with the targeted disease, in contrast to the inbred, healthy, well-defined animals employed in preclinical studies. This presents additional variables and challenges to manage. Second, the scale of clinical trials, the volume of data produced, and the resources required exceed by orders of magnitude those of preclinical studies. Third, many clinical trials involve research cooperative groups that represent a network of clinical scientists from academic medical centers, such as the Eastern Cooperative Oncology Group (ECOG), the AIDS Clinical Trial Group (ACTG), Thrombolysis in Myocardial Infarction (TIMI), and others. Most of the information on drug- or chemical-induced hematotoxicity in humans is collected through this industry-sponsored and highly regulated clinical research.

It is well understood that the ways in which drugs and nontherapeutic chemicals affect the hematopoietic system are influenced by both the nature of the chemical and the response of the subject or target population. As discussed previously, many chemicals are known to induce dose-dependent hematotoxicity in a fashion that is highly predictable. Others cause toxicity in a small number of susceptible individuals, and these often include chemicals not otherwise hematotoxic in most individuals (Dieckhaus *et al.*, 2002; Patton and Duffull, 1994). These *idiosyncratic reactions* present the biggest challenge as regards detection and characterization before human patients or populations are broadly exposed. They include aplastic anemia, thrombocytopenia, hemolysis, and leukopenia, which may or may not be immune-mediated (Salama *et al.*, 1989).

Prevailing theories today, as regards mechanisms for these idiosyncratic reactions, have been discussed previously. The chemical structure can be a risk factor if it is similar to that of other known toxicants. Patient- or population-related risk factors include pharmacogenetic variations in drug metabolism and detoxification that lead to reduced clearance of the chemical or production of novel intermediate metabolites (Cunningham *et al.*, 1974; Gerson *et al.*, 1983; Mason and Fischer, 1992), histocompatibility antigens (Frickhofen *et al.*, 1990), interaction with drugs or other chemicals (West *et al.*, 1988), increased sensitivity of hematopoietic precursors to damage (Vincent, 1986), preexisting disease of the bone marrow, and metabolic defects that predispose to oxidative or other stresses associated with the chemical (Stern, 1989).

In drug development, the clinical evaluation of candidate molecules is usually performed in 3 phases: *phase I* examines the effect of single and multiple increasing doses in small numbers of normal and/or patient volunteers. Pharmacokinetic properties are usually addressed, as well as the routes of excretion and metabolism; and the assessment of active and inactive metabolites. The emphasis is usually on safety assessment. *Phase II* includes controlled studies in the target patient population that examine both safety and efficacy. They explore dose response and usually provide the first indication of benefit versus risk. *Phase III* entails larger studies designed to confirm efficacy in an expanded patient population and evaluate less frequent adverse effects, such as the aforementioned idiosyncratic blood dyscrasias.

Development of a demonstrably hematotoxic drug is usually stopped in phase I or II, unless the indication includes life-threatening conditions where toxicity is acceptable (eg, anticancer drugs). Thus, drugs tested in phase III generally show an acceptable safety profile in most subjects at the doses used. Even phase III studies, however, are not usually powered to detect the low incidence of idiosyncratic hematotoxicity previously discussed (Levine and Szarfman, 1996). In order to detect one adverse event affecting 1% of an exposed patient population at a 95% confidence level, a trial must include approximately 300 subjects (O'Neill, 1988). Clinical databases supporting new drug applications generally cannot be used to detect adverse events that occur below 1 per 1000 exposures (ICH, 2001), and most will not rule out events with a frequency of less than 1 per 500 (Szarfman *et al.*, 1997). Thus, rare, delayed, or cumulative toxicity is often missed in preregistration clinical trials.

Detection of low-incidence hematotoxicity is usually achieved through postmarketing surveillance, such as the MedWatch program introduced by the FDA in 1993 (Szarfman *et al.*, 1997). Other countries that practice comprehensive postmarketing surveillance include Canada, the United Kingdom, Sweden, Germany, France, Australia, and New Zealand. Adverse event data, including serious hematotoxicity, are provided to the WHO; this information is compiled by a computer-based recording system employing WHO terminology and system and organ classifications for adverse reactions (Edwards *et al.*, 1990). Examples of iatrogenic blood dyscrasias detected through postmarketing surveillance include the hemolysis and thrombocytopenia associated with the antibiotic temafloxacin, the aplastic anemia linked to the antiepileptic felbamate, the hemolysis caused by the antidepressant nomifensine, and the agranulocytosis associated with the antiarrhythmic aprindine.

The WHO has also established criteria for grading hematotoxicity (WHO, 1979), which are summarized in Table 11-13. These have been particularly useful in establishing and communicating treatment strategies and guidelines for chemicals known to suppress hematopoiesis (cytoreductive oncolytic, immunosuppressive, and

Table 11-13

WHO Grading Criteria for Subacute and Acute Hematotoxicity

HEMATOLOGIC PARAMETERS (ADULTS)	GRADE 0	GRADE 1	GRADE 2	GRADE 3	GRADE 4
Hemoglobin (g/dL) (nmol/L)	11.0 (6.8)	9.5–10.5 (6.5–6.7)	8.0–9.4 (4.95–5.8)	6.5–7.9 (4.0–4.9)	6.5 (4.0)
Leukocytes (1000/μL)	4.0	3.0–3.9	2.0–2.9	2.0–1.9	1.0
Granulocytes (1000/μL)	2.0	1.5–1.9	1.0–1.4	0.5–0.9	0.5
Platelets (1000/μL)	100	75–99	50–74	25–49	<25
Hemorrhage, blood loss	None	Petechiae	Mild	Gross	Debilitating

SOURCE: Data from WHO (1979).

antiviral agents, etc) and for which this limiting toxicity is used to establish MTDs for individual patients.

Greater risk is acceptable with these drugs due to the life-threatening conditions they are used to treat. Similar risk–benefit decisions are also made regarding the use of drugs that cause blood dyscrasias in an idiosyncratic fashion, as previously discussed. Some are used to treat nonmalignant or life-threatening conditions, the risk of which is managed through rigorous laboratory monitoring. Examples include felbamate, ticlopidine, and clozapine, as discussed previously. Postmarketing surveillance plays a critical role in measuring the effectiveness of such monitoring.

Critical to the effectiveness of such surveillance by manufacturers and government regulatory agencies is the ability to detect a "signal," such as that related to life-threatening idiosyncratic hematotoxicity. Over the past five years, regulatory agencies and drug monitoring centers have been developing computerized data mining methods to better identify reporting relationships in spontaneous reporting databases that have enabled and optimized such signal detection (Almenoff *et al.*, 2005). This includes the use of screening algorithms and computer systems that efficiently signal higher-than-expected combinations of drugs and events in the FDA's spontaneous reports database, such as aplastic anemia, agranulocytosis, and idiopathic thrombocytopenic purpura. Examples include the Multi-Item Gamma Poisson Shrinker (MGPS) program, which computes signal scores for pairs, and for higher-order (eg, triplet, quadruplet) combinations of xenobiotics and events that are significantly more frequent than their pairwise associations would predict (Szarfman *et al.*, 2002). Such tools provide an objective and unprecedented systematic and simultaneous view of these large databases and alert government and manufacturers to critically important new safety signals that inform the toxicologist.

REFERENCES

Abarbanel J, Benet AE, Lask D, et al. Sports hematuria. *J Urol.* 1990; 143:887–890.

Abrams CS. Acquired qualitative platelet disorders. In: Lichtman MA, Beutler E, Kipps TJ, Seligsohn U, Kaushansky K, Prchal JT, eds. *Williams Hematology.* 7th ed. New York: McGraw-Hill; 2006:1833–1855.

Alcindor T, Bridges KR. Sideroblastic anaemias. *Br J Haematol.* 2002;116:733–743.

Almenoff J, Tonning JM, Gould AL, et al. Perspectives on the use of data mining in pharmaco-vigilance. *Drug Saf.* 2005;28:981–1007.

Altucci L, Clarke N, Nebbioso A, et al. Acute myeloid leukemia: therapeutic impact of epigenetic drugs. *Int J Biochem Cell Biol.* 2005;37:1752–1762.

Ananyeva NM, Lacroix-Desmazes S, Hauser CA, et al. Inhibitors in hemophilia A: mechanisms of inhibition, management and perspectives. *Blood Coagul Fibrinolysis.* 2004;15:109–124.

Andersen RL, Bagby GC Jr, Richert-Boe K. Therapy-related preleukemic syndrome. *Cancer.* 1981;47:1867–1871.

Andres E, Kurtz JE, Martin-Hunyadi C, et al. Nonchemotherapy drug-induced agranulocytosis in elderly patients: the effects of granulocyte colony-stimulating factor. *Am J Med.* 2002;112:460–464.

Andres E, Maloisel F, Zimmer J. The role of haematopoietic growth factors granulocyte colony-stimulating factor and granulocyte-macrophage colony-stimulating factor in the management of drug-induced agranulocytosis. *Br J Haematol.* 2010;150(1):3–8.

Ansell J, Hirsh J, Poller L, et al. The pharmacology and management of the vitamin K antagonists: the seventh ACCP conference on antithrombotic and thrombolytic therapy. *Chest.* 2004;126:204S–233S.

Arndt PA, Garratty G. The changing spectrum of drug-induced immune hemolytic anemia. *Semin Hematol.* 2005;42:137–144.

Arneborn P, Palmblad J. Drug-induced neutropenia—a survey for Stockholm 1973–1978. *Acta Med Scand.* 1982;212:289–292.

Aster RH. Drug-induced immune cytopenias. *Toxicology.* 2005;209: 149–153.

Aster RH, Bougie DW. Drug-induced immune thrombocytopenia. *N Engl J Med.* 2007;357:580–587.

Aster RH, Curtis BR, McFarland JG, et al. Drug-induced immune thrombocytopenia: pathogenesis, diagnosis and management. *J Thromb Haemost.* 2009;7:911–918.

Athens JW, Haab OP, Raab SO, et al. Leukokinetic studies. IV. The total blood, circulating and marginal granulocyte pools and the granulocyte turnover rate in normal subjects. *J Clin Invest.* 1961;40:989–995.

Babior BM. Folate, cobalamin, and myeloblastic anemias. In: Lichtman MA, Beutler E, Kipps TJ, Seligsohn U, Kaushansky K, Prchal JT, eds. *Williams Hematology.* 7th ed. New York: McGraw-Hill; 2006:477–509.

Babior BM, Golde DW. Production, distribution and fate of neutrophils. In: Beutler E, Lichtman MA, Coller BS, Kipps TJ, eds. *Williams Hematology.* 5th ed. New York: McGraw-Hill; 1995:773–779.

Bahrami S, Malone JC, Webb KG, et al. Tissue eosinophilia as an indicator of drug-induced cutaneous small-vessel vasculitis. *Arch Dermatol.* 2006;142:155–161.

Baker KR. Hemolytic anemia resulting from physical injury to red cells. In: Lichtman MA, Beutler E, Kipps TJ, Seligsohn U, Kaushansky K, Prchal JT, eds. *Williams Hematology.* New York: McGraw-Hill; 2006:709–716.

Barnes PJ. Corticosteroids: the drugs to beat. *Eur J Pharmacol.* 2006;533: 2–14.

Bates SM, Greer IA, Hirsh J, et al. Use of antithrombotic agents during pregnancy: the seventh ACCP conference on antithrombotic and thrombolytic therapy. *Chest.* 2004;126:627S–644S.

Bench AJ, Nacheva EP, Champion KM, et al. Molecular genetics and cytogenetics of myeloproliferative disorders. *Baillieres Clin Haematol.* 1998;11:819–848.

Bennett A, Sanger GJ. Pinane thromboxane A2 analogues are non-selective prostanoid antagonists in rat and human stomach muscle. *Br J Pharmacol.* 1982;77:591–596.

Bennett CL, Luminari S, Nissenson AR, et al. Pure red-cell aplasia and epoetin therapy. *N Engl J Med.* 2004;351:1403–1408.

Bennett JM, Catovsky D, Daniel MT, et al. Proposed revised criteria for the classification of acute myeloid leukemia. A report of the

French–American–British Cooperative Group. *Ann Intern Med.* 1985;103: 620–625.

Bergsagel DE, Wong O, Bergsagel PL, et al. Benzene and multiple myeloma: appraisal of the scientific evidence. *Blood.* 1999;94:1174–1182.

Berkowitz FE. Hemolysis and infection: categories and mechanisms of their interrelationship. *Rev Infect Dis.* 1991;13:1151–1162.

Berliner N, Horwitz M, Loughran TP Jr. Congenital and acquired neutropenia. In: Broudy VC, Berliner N, Larson RA, Leung LL, eds. *American Society of Hematology Education Program Book.* Washington, DC: American Society of Hematology; 2004:63–79.

Berry RG, Morrison JA, Watts JW, et al. Surreptitious superwarfarin ingestion with brodifacoum. *South Med J.* 2000;93:74–75.

Bertolaccini ML, Hughes GR, Khamashta MA. Revisiting antiphospholipid antibodies: from targeting phospholipids to phospholipid binding proteins. *Clin Lab.* 2004;50:653–665.

Beutler E. G6PD: population genetics and clinical manifestations. *Blood Rev.* 1996;10:45–52.

Beutler E. Hemolytic anemias resulting from infections with microorganisms. In: Lichtman MA, Beutler E, Kipps TJ, Seligsohn U, Kaushansky K, Prchal JT, eds. *Williams Hematology.* 7th ed. New York: McGraw-Hill; 2006a:723–727.

Beutler E. Hemolytic anemias resulting from chemical and physical agents. In: Lichtman MA, Beutler E, Kipps TJ, Seligsohn U, Kaushansky K, Prchal JT, eds. *Williams Hematology.* 7th ed. New York: McGraw-Hill; 2006b:717–721.

Beutler E. Hereditary and acquired sideroblastic anemias. In: Lichtman MA, Beutler E, Kipps TJ, Seligsohn U, Kaushansky K, Prchal JT, eds. *Williams Hematology.* 7th ed. New York: McGraw-Hill; 2006c:823–828.

Bitter MA, Le Beau MM, Rowley JD, et al. Associations between morphology, karyotype, and clinical features in myeloid leukemias. *Hum Pathol.* 1987;18:211–225.

Bloom JC. Principles of hematotoxicology: laboratory assessment and interpretation of data. *Toxicol Pathol.* 1993;21:130–134.

Bloom JC, Lewis HB, Sellers TS, et al. The hematopathology of cefonicid- and cefazedone-induced blood dyscrasias in the dog. *Toxicol Appl Pharmacol.* 1987;90:143–155.

Blossom D, Kallen A, Patel PR, et al. Outbreak of adverse reactions associated with contaminated heparin. *N Engl J Med.* 2008;359:2674–2684.

Borregaard N, Boxer LA. Disorders of neutrophil function. In: Lichtman MA, Beutler E, Kipps TJ, Seligsohn U, Kaushansky K, Prchal JT, eds. *Williams Hematology.* 7th ed. New York: McGraw-Hill; 2006: 921–957.

Bradberry SM. Occupational methaemoglobinaemia. Mechanisms of production, features, diagnosis and management including the use of methylene blue. *Toxicol Rev.* 2003;22:13–27.

Bradberry SM, Aw TC, Williams NR, et al. Occupational methaemoglobinaemia. *Occup Environ Med.* 2001;58:611–615.

Brayton RG, Stokes PE, Schwartz MS, et al. Effect of alcohol and various diseases on leukocyte mobilization, phagocytosis and intracellular bacterial killing. *N Engl J Med.* 1970;282:123–128.

Browning E. *Toxicity and Metabolism of Industrial Solvents.* London: Elsevier; 1965.

Broxmeyer HE, Orschell CM, Clapp DW, et al. Rapid mobilization of murine and human hematopoietic stem and progenitor cells with AMD3100, a CXCR4 antagonist. *J Exp Med.* 2005;201:1307–1318.

Capsoni F, Sarzi-Puttini P, Zanella A. Primary and secondary autoimmune neutropenia. *Arthritis Res Ther.* 2005;7:208–214.

Caramori G, Adcock I. Anti-inflammatory mechanisms of glucocorticoids targeting granulocytes. *Curr Drug Targets Inflamm Allergy.* 2005;4:455–463.

Cartwright GE, Athens JW, Wintrobe MM. The kinetics of granulopoiesis in normal man. *Blood.* 1964;24:780–803.

Carver JH, Hatch FT, Branscomb EW. Estimating maximum limits to mutagenic potency from cytotoxic potency. *Nature.* 1979;279:154–156.

Casciato DA, Scott JL. Acute leukemia following prolonged cytotoxic agent therapy. *Medicine.* 1979;58:32–47.

Cazzola M, Invernizzi R, Bergamaschi G, et al. Mitochondrial ferritin expression in erythroid cells from patients with sideroblastic anemia. *Blood.* 2003;101:1996–2000.

Cerulli J, Grabe DW, Gauthier I, et al. Chromium picolinate toxicity. *Ann Pharmacother.* 1998;32:428–431.

Cesar JM, de Miguel D, Garcia AA, et al. Platelet dysfunction in primary thrombocythemia using the platelet function analyzer, PFA-100. *Am J Clin Pathol.* 2005;123:772–777.

Chabner BA, Wilson W, Supko J. Pharmacology and toxicity of antineoplastic drugs. In: Lichtman MA, Beutler E, Kipps TJ, Seligsohn U, Kaushansky K, Prchal JT, eds. *Williams Hematology.* 7th ed. New York: McGraw-Hill; 2006:247–274.

Chakraverty R, Davidson S, Peggs K, et al. The incidence and cause of coagulopathies in an intensive care population. *Br J Haematol.* 1996;93:460–463.

Chriswell KA, Bleavins MR, Zeilinski D, et al. Comparison of flow cytometric and manual bone marrow differentials in Wistar rats. *Cytometry.* 1998a;32:9–17.

Chriswell KA, Bleavins MR, Zeilinski D, et al. Flow cytometric evaluation of bone marrow differentials in rats with pharmacologically induced hematologic abnormalities. *Cytometry.* 1998b;32:18–27.

Chriswell KA, Sulkanen AP, Hochbaum AF, et al. Effects of phenylhydrazine or phlebotomy on peripheral blood, bone marrow and erythropoietin in Wistar rats. *J Appl Toxicol.* 2000;20:25–34.

Chua JD, Friedenberg WR. Superwarfarin poisoning. *Arch Intern Med.* 1998;158:1929–1932.

Clifton J, Leikin JB. Methylene blue. *Am J Ther.* 2003;10:289–291.

Coleman MD, Coleman NA. Drug-induced methaemoglobinaemia. Treatment issues. *Drug Saf.* 1996;14:394–405.

Collen D, Lijnen HR. Thrombolytic agents. *Thromb Haemost.* 2005;93: 627–630.

Contrino J, Marucha P, Ribaudo R, et al. Effects of mercury on human polymorphonuclear leukocyte function in vitro. *Am J Pathol.* 1988;132: 110–118.

Cummings TF. The treatment of cyanide poisoning. *Occup Med.* 2004;54:82–85.

Cuneo A, Fagioli F, Pazzi I, et al. Morphologic, immunologic and cytogenetic studies in acute myeloid leukemia following occupational exposure to pesticides and organic solvents. *Leuk Res.* 1992;16:789–796.

Cunningham JL, Leyland MJ, Delamore IW, et al. Acetanilide oxidation in phenylbutazone-associated hypoplastic anaemia. *Br Med J.* 1974;3:313–317.

Curzen N, Haque R, Timmis A. Applications of thrombolytic therapy. *Intensive Care Med.* 1998;24:756–768.

Custer RP, Ahlfeldt FE. Studies on the structure and function of bone marrow. *J Lab Clin Med.* 1932;17:960–962.

Dahl OE, Garvik LJ, Lyberg T. Toxic effects of methylmethacrylate monomer on leukocytes and endothelial cells in vitro. *Acta Orthop Scand.* 1994;65:147–153.

Dale DC. Neutropenia and neutrophilia. In: Lichtman MA, Beutler E, Kipps TJ, Seligsohn U, Kaushansky K, Prchal JT, eds. *Williams Hematology.* 7th ed. New York: McGraw-Hill; 2006:907–955.

D'Andrea G, D'Ambrosio RL, Di Perna P, et al. A polymorphism in the VKORC1 gene is associated with an interindividual variability in the dose-anticoagulant effect of warfarin. *Blood.* 2005;105:645–649.

Davoren A, Aster RH. Heparin-induced thrombocytopenia and thrombosis. *Am J Hematol.* 2006;81:36–44.

De Clercq E. Potential clinical applications of the CXCR4 antagonist bicyclam AMD3100. *Mini Rev Med Chem.* 2005;5:805–824.

de Latour RP, Visconte V, Takaku T, et al. Th17 immune responses contribute to the pathophysiology of aplastic anemia. *Blood.* 2010;116: 4175–4180.

Deckmyn H, Vanhoorelbeke K, Peerlinck K. Inhibitory and activating human antiplatelet antibodies. *Baillieres Clin Haematol.* 1998;11:343–359.

Deldar A. Drug-induced blood disorders: review of pathogenetic mechanisms and utilization of bone marrow cell culture technology as an investigative approach. *Curr Topics Vet Res.* 1994;1:83–101.

Deldar A, Parchment RE. Preclinical risk assessment for hematotoxicity: animal models and in vitro systems. In: Sipes IG MAGA, ed. *Comprehensive Toxicology.* Oxford: Pergamon Press; 1997:321–333.

Deldar A, Stevens CE. Development and application of in vitro models of hematopoiesis to drug development. *Toxicol Pathol.* 1993;21:231–240.

Delvaeye M, Noris M, de Vriese A, et al. Thrombomodulin mutations in atypical hemolytic-uremic syndrome. *N Engl J Med*. 2009;361: 345–357.

Demirer T, Bensinger WI. Optimization of peripheral blood stem cell collection. *Curr Opin Hematol*. 1995;2:219–226.

Dessypris EN. Erythropoiesis. In: Lee CR, Foerster J, Lukens J, Paraskevas P, Greer JP, Rodgers GM, eds. *Wintrobe's Clinical Hematology*. 10th ed. Philadelphia: Lippincott Williams & Wilkins; 1999:169–192.

Dieckhaus CM, Thompson CD, Roller SG, et al. Mechanisms of idiosyncratic drug reactions: the case of felbamate. *Chem Biol Interact*. 2002;142: 99–117.

Dinwoodey DL, Ansell JE. Heparins, low-molecular-weight heparins, and pentasaccharides. *Clin Geriatr Med*. 2006;22:1–15, vii.

Djaldetti M, Blay A, Bergman M, et al. Pure red cell aplasia—a rare disease with multiple causes. *Biomed Pharmacother*. 2003;57:326–332.

Dreno B, Trossaert M, Boiteau HL, et al. Zinc salts effects on granulocyte zinc concentration and chemotaxis in acne patients. *Acta Derm Venereol*. 1992;72:250–252.

Du DL, Volpe DA, Grieshaber CK, et al. Comparative toxicity of fostriecin, hepsulfam and pyrazine diazohydroxide to human and murine hematopoietic progenitor cells in vitro. *Invest New Drugs*. 1991;9:149–157.

Edwards IR, Lindquist M, Wiholm BE, et al. Quality criteria for early signals of possible adverse drug reactions. *Lancet*. 1990;336:156–158.

Eramo A, Lotti F, Sette G, et al. Identification and expansion of the tumorigenic lung cancer stem cell population. *Cell Death Differ*. 2008;15:504–514.

Erickson-Miller CL, May RD, Tomaszewski J, et al. Differential toxicity of camptothecin, topotecan and 9-aminocamptothecin to human, canine and murine myeloid progenitors (CFU-GM) in vitro. *Cancer Chemother Pharmacol*. 1997;39:467–472.

European Medicines Agency, Committee for Proprietary Medicinal Products. *Notes for Guidance of Immunotoxicity Studies for Human Pharmaceuticals*. London: European Medicines Agency; 2006:1–9.

Fagioli F, Cuneo A, Piva N, et al. Distinct cytogenetic and clinicopathologic features in acute myeloid leukemia after occupational exposure to pesticides and organic solvents. *Cancer*. 1992;70:77–85.

Fan F, Wood KV. Bioluminescent aasays for high-throughput screening. *Assay Drug Dev Technol*. 2007;5:127–136.

Feldman BF, Zinkle JG, Jain NC, eds. *Schalm's Veterinary Hematology*. 5th ed. Ames, IA: Blackwell Publishing; 2006.

Fisch P, Handgretinger R, Schaefer HE. Pure red cell aplasia. *Br J Haematol*. 2000;111:1010–1022.

Fiske DN, McCoy HE III, Kitchens CS. Zinc-induced sideroblastic anemia: report of a case, review of the literature, and description of the hematologic syndrome. *Am J Hematol*. 1994;46:147–150.

Flieder DB, Travis WD. Pathologic characteristics of drug-induced lung disease. *Clin Chest Med*. 2004;25:37–45.

Food and Drug Administration, Center for Drug Evaluation and Research, and Center for Biologics Evaluation and Research. S8 immunotoxicity studies for human pharmaceuticals. In: *Guidance for Industry*. Rockville, MD: Food and Drug Administration; 2006:1–13.

Foucar K, McKenna RW, Bloomfield CD, et al. Therapy-related leukemia: a panmyelosis. *Cancer*. 1979;43:1285–1296.

Frazier JM. In vitro toxicity testing: applications to safety evaluation. In: Frazier JM, ed. *In Vitro Toxicity Testing Applications to Safety Evaluation*. New York: Marcel Dekker; 1992:5–7.

Friberg LE, Karlsson MO. Mechanistic models for myelosuppression. *Invest New Drugs*. 2003;21:183–194.

Frickhofen N, Liu JM, Young NS. Etiologic mechanisms of hematopoietic failure. *Am J Pediatr Hematol Oncol*. 1990;12:385–395.

Furlan M, Robles R, Galbusera M, et al. von Willebrand factor-cleaving protease in thrombotic thrombocytopenic purpura and the hemolytic-uremic syndrome. *N Engl J Med*. 1998;339:1578–1584.

Gallardo S, Cardaba B, Posada M, et al. Toxic oil syndrome: genetic restriction and immunomodulatory effects due to adulterated oils in a model of HLA transgenic mice. *Toxicol Lett*. 2005;159:173–181.

Gamazon ER, Im HK, O'Donnell PF, et al. Comprehensive evaluation of the contribution of X chromosome genes to platinum sensitivity. *Mol Cancer Ther*. 2011;10(3):472–480.

Garb E. Non-chemotherapy drug-induced agranulocytosis. *Expert Opin Drug Saf*. 2007;6(3):323–335.

Gerson SL, Meltzer H. Mechanisms of clozapine-induced agranulocytosis. *Drug Saf*. 1992;7(suppl 1):17–25.

Gerson WT, Fine DG, Spielberg SP, et al. Anticonvulsant-induced aplastic anemia: increased susceptibility to toxic drug metabolites in vitro. *Blood*. 1983;61:889–893.

Girard D. Activation of human polymorphonuclear neutrophils by environmental contaminants. *Rev Environ Health*. 2003;18:75–89.

Godley LA, Larson RA. The syndrome of therapy-related myelodysplasia and myeloid leukemia. In: Bennett JM, ed. *The Myelodysplastic Syndromes: Pathobiology and Clinical Management*. New York: Dekker; 2001:139–176.

Golden R, Pyatt D, Shields PG. Formaldehyde as a potential human leukemogen: an assessment of biological plausibility. *Crit Rev Toxicol*. 2006;36:135–153.

Golomb HM, Alimena G, Rowley JD, et al. Correlation of occupation and karyotype in adults with acute nonlymphocytic leukemia. *Blood*. 1982;60:404–411.

Gonzalez H, Leblond V, Azar N, et al. Severe autoimmune hemolytic anemia in eight patients treated with fludarabine. *Hematol Cell Ther*. 1998;40:113–118.

Grant C, Wilson WH, Dunleavy K. Neutropenia associated with rituximab therapy. *Curr Opin Hematol*. 2011;18(1):49–54.

Greene MH, Harris EL, Gershenson DM, et al. Melphalan may be a more potent leukemogen than cyclophosphamide. *Ann Intern Med*. 1986;105:360–367.

Guevara A, Labarca J, Gonzalez-Martin G. Heparin-induced transaminase elevations: a prospective study. *Int J Clin Pharmacol Ther Toxicol*. 1993;31:137–141.

Hagen EC, Ballieux BE, van Es LA, et al. Antineutrophil cytoplasmic autoantibodies: a review of the antigens involved, the assays, and the clinical and possible pathogenetic consequences. *Blood*. 1993;81:1996–2002.

Hajjar A. Fibrinolysis and thrombolysis. In: Lichtman MA, Beutler E, Kipps TJ, Seligsohn U, Kaushansky K, Prchal JT, eds. *Williams Hematology*. 7th ed. New York: McGraw-Hill; 2006:1833–1855.

Hall RL. Clinical pathology for preclinical safety assessment: current global guidelines. *Toxicol Pathol*. 1992;20:472–476.

Hall RL. Evaluation and interpretation of hematologic data in preclinical toxicology. In: Sipes IG, McQueen AC, Gandolfi AJ, eds. *Comprehensive Toxicology*. Oxford: Pergamon Press; 1997:321–333.

Hanahan D, Weinberg R. Hallmarks of cancer: the next generation. *Cell*. 2011;144:646–674.

Harder S, Thurmann P. Clinically important drug interactions with anticoagulants. An update. *Clin Pharmacokinet*. 1996;30:416–444.

Harrison DE, Lerner CP. Most primitive hematopoietic stem cells are stimulated to cycle rapidly after treatment with 5-fluorouracil. *Blood*. 1991;78:1237–1240.

Hatherill JR, Till GO, Bruner LH, et al. Thermal injury, intravascular hemolysis, and toxic oxygen products. *J Clin Invest*. 1986;78:629–636.

Heissig B, Ohki Y, Sato Y, et al. A role for niches in hematopoietic cell development. *Hematology*. 2005;10:247–253.

Hincks I, Woodcock BE, Thachil J. Is rituximab-induced late-onset neutropenia a good prognostic indicator in lymphoproliferative disorders? *Br J Haematol*. 2011;153:402–416.

Hirsh J, Raschke R. Heparin and low-molecular-weight heparin: the seventh ACCP conference on antithrombotic and thrombolytic therapy. *Chest*. 2004;126:188S–203S.

Hoffmann MJ, Sinko PJ, Lee YH, et al. Pharmacokinetic studies in Tg.AC and FVB mice administered [14C] benzene either by oral gavage or intradermal injection. *Toxicol Appl Pharmacol*. 2001;174:139–145.

Honigfeld G, Arellano F, Sethi J, et al. Reducing clozapine-related morbidity and mortality: 5 years of experience with the Clozaril National Registry. *J Clin Psychiatry*. 1998;59(suppl 3):3–7.

Horikoshi A, Murphy MJ Jr. Comparative effects of chemotherapeutic drugs on human and murine hematopoietic progenitors in vitro. *Chemotherapy*. 1982;28:480–501.

Horn TL, Harder JB, Johnson WD, et al. Integration of in vivo and in vitro approaches to characterize the toxicity of antalarmin, a corticotropin-releasing hormone receptor antagonist. *Toxicology*. 2008;248:8–17.

Hsia CC. Respiratory function of hemoglobin. *N Engl J Med.* 1998;338:239–247.

Huang RS, Kistner EO, Bleibel WK, et al. Effect of population and gender on chemotherapeutic agent-induced cytotoxicity. *Mol Cancer Ther.* 2007;6(1):31–36.

Hudson G. Bone-marrow volume in the human foetus and newborn. *Br J Haematol.* 2006;11:446–452.

Hunter FT. Chronic exposure of benzene. II. The clinical effects. *J Ind Hyg Toxicol.* 1939;21:331–354.

Huxtable LM, Tafreshi MJ, Rakkar AN. Frequency and management of thrombocytopenia with the glycoprotein IIb/IIIa receptor antagonists. *Am J Cardiol.* 2006;97:426–429.

Ibanez L, Vidal X, Ballarin E, et al. Population-based drug-induced agranulocytosis. *Arch Int Med.* 2005;165(8):869–874.

ICH. Note for guidance on non-clinical safety studies for the conduct of human clinical trials for pharmaceuticals. *Fed Reg.* 2000.

ICH. Safety pharmacology studies for human pharmaceuticals. *Fed Reg.* 2001;66:36791–36792.

Irons RD. Leukemogenesis as a toxic response. In: Sipes IG, McQueen AC, Gandolfi AJ, eds. *Comprehensive Toxicology.* Oxford: Pergamon Press; 1997:175–199.

Jaffe ES. *World Health Organization Classification of Tumours: Tumours of Haematopoietic and Lymphoid Tissues Pathology and Genetics.* Lyon: IARC Press; 2001.

Jandl JH. *Blood.* Boston: Little Brown & Co; 1987.

Johansson B, Mertens F, Heim S, et al. Cytogenetics of secondary myelodysplasia (sMDS) and acute nonlymphocytic leukemia (sANLL). *Eur J Haematol.* 1991;47:17–27.

Julia A, Olona M, Bueno J, et al. Drug-induced agranulocytosis: prognostic factors in a series of 168 episodes. *Br J Haematol.* 1991;79:366–371.

Jurk K, Kehrel BE. Platelets: physiology and biochemistry. *Semin Thromb Hemost.* 2005;31:381–392.

Kantarjian HM, Keating MJ, Walters RS, et al. Therapy-related leukemia and myelodysplastic syndrome: clinical, cytogenetic, and prognostic features. *J Clin Oncol.* 1986;4:1748–1757.

Kao LW, Nanagas KA. Carbon monoxide poisoning. *Med Clin North Am.* 2005;89:1161–1194.

Kaushansky K. Lineage-specific hematopoietic growth factors. *N Engl J Med.* 2006;354:2034–2045.

Keng PC. Use of flow cytometry in the measurement of cell mitotic cycle. *Int J Cell Cloning.* 1986;4:295–311.

Khan NA, Kruse JA. Methemoglobinemia induced by topical anesthesia: a case report and review. *Am J Med Sci.* 1999;318:415–418.

Kilbourne EM, Posada de la Paz M, Abaitua B, I, et al. Toxic oil syndrome: a current clinical and epidemiologic summary, including comparisons with the eosinophilia–myalgia syndrome. *J Am Coll Cardiol.* 1991;18:711–717.

Kim-Shapiro DB, Gladwin MT, Patel RP, et al. The reaction between nitrite and hemoglobin: the role of nitrite in hemoglobin-mediated hypoxic vasodilation. *J Inorg Biochem.* 2005;99:237–246.

Kolachana P, Subrahmanyam VV, Meyer KB, et al. Benzene and its phenolic metabolites produce oxidative DNA damage in HL60 cells in vitro and in the bone marrow in vivo. *Cancer Res.* 1993;53:1023–1026.

Koren E, Zuckerman LA, Mire-Sluis AR. Immune responses to therapeutic proteins in humans—clinical significance, assessment and prediction. *Curr Pharm Biotechnol.* 2002;3:349–360.

Kuderer NM, Cosler L, Crawford J. Cost and mortality associated with febrile neutropenia in adult cancer patients. *Proc Am Soc Clin Oncol.* 2002;21:250a.

Kumar S, Bandyopadhyay U. Free heme toxity and its detoxification systems in human. *Toxicol Lett.* 2005;157:175–188.

Ladiges WC, Storb R, Thomas ED. Canine models of bone marrow transplantation. *Lab Anim Sci.* 1990;40:11–15.

Lane DA, Philippou H, Huntington JA. Directing thrombin. *Blood.* 2005;106:2605–2612.

Larochelle A, Krouse A, Metzger M, et al. AMD3100 mobilizes hematopoietic stem cells with long-term repopulating capacity in nonhuman primates. *Blood.* 2006;107:3772–3778.

Larson RA, Le Beau MM. Therapy-related myeloid leukaemia: a model for leukemogenesis in humans. *Chem Biol Interact.* 2005;153–154:187–195.

Lataillade JJ, Domenech J, Le Bousse-Kerdiles MC. Stromal cell-derived factor-1 (SDF-1)\CXCR4 couple plays multiple roles on haematopoietic progenitors at the border between the old cytokine and new chemokine worlds: survival, cell cycling and trafficking. *Eur Cytokine Netw.* 2004;15:177–188.

Laurence AD. Location, movement and survival: the role of chemokines in haematopoiesis and malignancy. *Br J Haematol.* 2006;132:255–267.

Le Beau MM, Albain KS, Larson RA, et al. Clinical and cytogenetic correlations in 63 patients with therapy-related myelodysplastic syndromes and acute nonlymphocytic leukemia: further evidence for characteristic abnormalities of chromosomes no. 5 and 7. *J Clin Oncol.* 1986;4:325–345.

Leung KN, Mak NK, Fung MC. Cytokines in the differentiation therapy of leukemia: from laboratory investigations to clinical applications. *Crit Rev Clin Lab Sci.* 2005;42:473–514.

Levine EG, Bloomfield CD. Leukemias and myelodysplastic syndromes secondary to drug, radiation, and environmental exposure. *Semin Oncol.* 1992;19:47–84.

Levine JG, Szarfman A. Standardized data structures and visualization tools: a way to accelerate the regulatory review of the integrated summary of safety of new drug applications. *Biopharm Rep.* 1996;4:12–17.

Li J, Yang C, Xia Y, et al. Thrombocytopenia caused by the development of antibodies to thrombopoietin. *Blood.* 2001;98:3241–3248.

Li R. A hypothesis that explains the heterogeneity of drug-induced immune thrombocytopenia. *Blood.* 2010;115:914.

Lian EC. Pathogenesis of thrombotic thrombocytopenic purpura: ADAMTS13 deficiency and beyond. *Semin Thromb Hemost.* 2005;31:625–632.

Liesveld JL, Lichtman MA. Evaluation of granulocytes and mononuclear phagocytes. In: Sipes IG, McQueen CA, Gandolfi AJ, eds. *Comprehensive Toxicology.* Oxford: Pergamon Press; 1997:123–144.

Liles WC, Rodger E, Broxmeyer HE, et al. Augmented mobilization and collection of CD34+ hematopoietic cells from normal human volunteers stimulated with granulocyte-colony-stimulating factor by single-dose administration of AMD3100, a CXCR4 antagonist. *Transfusion.* 2005;45:295–300.

Lillevang ST, Albertsen M, Rasmussen F, et al. Effect of radiographic contrast media on granulocyte phagocytosis of *Escherichia coli* in a whole blood flow cytometric assay. *Invest Radiol.* 1994;29:68–71.

Lindorfer MA, Hahn CS, Foley PL, et al. Heteropolymer-mediated clearance of immune complexes via erythrocyte CR1: mechanisms and applications. *Immunol Rev.* 2001;183:10–24.

Lollar P. Pathogenic antibodies to coagulation factors. Part one: factor VIII and factor IX. *J Thromb Haemost.* 2004;2:1082–1095.

Lollar P. Pathogenic antibodies to coagulation factors. Part II. Fibrinogen, prothrombin, thrombin, factor V, factor XI, factor XII, factor XIII, the protein C system and von Willebrand factor. *J Thromb Haemost.* 2005;3:1385–1391.

Look AT. Molecular pathogenesis of MDS. In: Berliner N, Lee SJ, Linenberger M, Vogelsang GB, eds. *American Society of Hematology Education Program Book.* Washington, DC: American Society of Hematology; 2005:156–160.

Loomis MR, Henrickson RV, Anderson JH. Effects of ketamine hydrochloride on the hemogram of rhesus monkeys (*Macaca mulatta*). *Lab Anim Sci.* 1980;30:851–853.

Lund JE. Toxicologic effects on blood and bone marrow. In: Feldman BF, Zinkl JG, Jain NC, eds. *Schalm's Veterinary Hematology.* 5th ed. Ames, IA: Blackwell Publishing; 2000:44–50.

Lundberg JO, Weitzberg E. NO generation from nitrite and its role in vascular control. *Arterioscler Thromb Vasc Biol.* 2005;25:915–922.

Madison FW, Squier T. The etiology of primary granulocytopenia (agranulocytic angina). *J Am Med Assoc.* 1934;102:755–763.

Mangano DT, Tudor IC, Dietzel C. The risk associated with aprotinin in cardiac surgery. *N Engl J Med.* 2006;354:353–365.

Mannucci PM. Hemostatic drugs. *N Engl J Med.* 1998;339:245–253.

Marsh JC. Correlation of hematologic toxicity of antineoplastic agents with their effects on bone marrow stem cells: interspecies studies using an in vivo assay. *Exp Hematol.* 1985;13(suppl 16):16–22.

Martin C, Burdon PC, Bridger G, et al. Chemokines acting via CXCR2 and CXCR4 control the release of neutrophils from the bone marrow and their return following senescence. *Immunity.* 2003;19:583–593.

Mason RP, Fischer V. Possible role of free radical formation in drug-induced agranulocytosis. *Drug Saf.* 1992;7(suppl 1):45–50.

Masubuchi N. Risk assessment of human myelotoxicity of anticancer drugs: a predictive model and the in vitro colony forming unit granulocyte/macrophage (CFU-GM) assay. *Pharmazie.* 2006;61:135–139.

Matzdorff A. Platelet function tests and flow cytometry to monitor antiplatelet therapy. *Semin Thromb Hemost.* 2005;31:393–399.

Mauritzson N, Johansson B, Albin M, et al. Survival time in a population-based consecutive series of adult acute myeloid leukemia—the prognostic impact of karyotype during the time period 1976–1993. *Leukemia.* 2000;14:1039–1043.

Mazzone A, Mazzucchelli I, Fossati G, et al. Granulocyte defects and opioid receptors in chronic exposure to heroin or methadone in humans. *Int J Immunopharmacol.* 1994;16:959–967.

McMullin MF, Buckley O, Magill MK, et al. Long-term bone marrow culture profiles in patients with myelodysplastic syndromes are not explicable by defective apoptosis. *Leuk Res.* 1998;22:735–740.

McRedmond JP, Harriott P, Walker B, et al. Streptokinase-induced platelet activation involves antistreptokinase antibodies and cleavage of protease-activated receptor-1. *Blood.* 2000;95:1301–1308.

Menon V, Harrington RA, Hochman JS, et al. Thrombolysis and adjunctive therapy in acute myocardial infarction: the seventh ACCP conference on antithrombotic and thrombolytic therapy. *Chest.* 2004;126:549S–575S.

Mitelman F, Brandt L, Nilsson PG. Relation among occupational exposure to potential mutagenic/carcinogenic agents, clinical findings, and bone marrow chromosomes in acute nonlymphocytic leukemia. *Blood.* 1978;52:1229–1237.

Mitelman F, Nilsson PG, Brandt L, et al. Chromosome pattern, occupation, and clinical features in patients with acute nonlymphocytic leukemia. *Cancer Genet Cytogenet.* 1981;4:197–214.

Miyagi T, Lam KM, Chuang LF, et al. Suppression of chemokine-induced chemotaxis of monkey neutrophils and monocytes by chlorinated hydrocarbon insecticides. *In Vivo.* 1998;12:441–446.

Moeschlin S, Wagner K. Agranulocytosis due to the occurrence of leukocyte-agglutinin; pyramidon and cold agglutinins. *Acta Haematol.* 1952;8:29–41.

Monroe DM, Hoffman M. What does it take to make the perfect clot? *Arterioscler Thromb Vasc Biol.* 2005;25:2463–2469.

Moore DM. Hematology of the mouse. In: Feldman BF, Zinkl JG, Jain NC, eds. *Schalm's Veterinary Hematology.* 5th ed. Ames, IA: Blackwell Publishing; 2000a:1219–1224.

Moore DM. Hematology of the rat. In: Feldman BF, Zinkl JG, Jain NC, eds. *Schalm's Veterinary Hematology.* 5th ed. Ames, IA: Blackwell Publishing; 2000b:1210–1218.

Moore EE, Johnson JL, Cheng AM, et al. Insights from studies of blood substitutes in trauma. *Shock.* 2005;24:197–205.

Moore MAS. Embryologic and phylogenetic development of the haematopoietic system. *Adv Biosci.* 1975;16:87–103.

Murphy SB. Secondary acute myeloid leukemia following treatment with epipodophyllotoxins. *J Clin Oncol.* 1993;11:199–201.

Nakagawa M, Terashima T, D'yachkova Y, et al. Glucocorticoid-induced granulocytosis: contribution of marrow release and demargination of intravascular granulocytes. *Circulation.* 1998;98:2307–2313.

Napier I, Ponka P, Richardson DR. Iron trafficking in the mitochondrion: novel pathways revealed by disease. *Blood.* 2005;105:1867–1874.

Nathan C. Neutrophils and immunity: challenges and opportunities. *Nat Rev Immunol.* 2006;6:173–182.

Naughton BA, Sibanda B, Azar L, et al. Differential effects of drugs upon hematopoiesis can be assessed in long-term bone marrow cultures established on nylon screens. *Proc Soc Exp Biol Med.* 1992;199:481–490.

Negro GD, Bonato M, Gribaldo L. In vitro bone marrow granulocyte-macrophage progenitor cultures in the assessment of hematotoxic potential of the new drugs. *Cell Biol Toxicol.* 2001;17:95–105.

Nguyen ST, Cabrales RE, Bashour CA, et al. Benzocaine-induced methemoglobinemia. *Anesth Analg.* 2000;90:369–371.

Nifli AP, Notas G, Mamoulaki M, et al. Comparison of a multiplex, bead-based fluorescent assay and immunofluorescence methods for the detection of ANA and ANCA autoantibodies in human serum. *J Immunol Methods.* 2006;311:189–197.

Njalsson R, Norgren S. Physiological and pathological aspects of GSH metabolism. *Acta Paediatr.* 2005;94:132–137.

Olson H, Betton G, Robinson D, et al. Concordance of the toxicity of pharmaceuticals in humans and animals. *Regul Toxicol Pharmacol.* 2000;32:56–67.

O'Neill R. Assessment of safety. In: Peace KE, ed. *Biopharmaceutical Statistics for Drug Development.* New York: Marcel Dekker; 1988:543–604.

Palmblad J, Papadaki HA, Eliopoulos G. Acute and chronic neutropenias. What is new? *J Intern Med.* 2001;250:476–491.

Papassotiriou I, Kister J, Griffon N, et al. Modulating the oxygen affinity of human fetal haemoglobin with synthetic allosteric modulators. *Br J Haematol.* 1998;102:1165–1171.

Parchment RE, Huang M, Erickson-Miller CL. Roles for in vitro myelotoxicity tests in preclinical drug development and clinical trial planning. *Toxicol Pathol.* 1993;21:241–250.

Parchment RE, Murphy MJ. Human hematopoietic stem cells: laboratory assessment and response to toxic injury. In: Sipes IG MAGA, ed. *Comprehensive Toxicology.* Oxford: Pergamon Press; 1997:303–320.

Parent-Massin D, Thouvenot D, Rio B, et al. Lindane haematotoxicity confirmed by in vitro tests on human and rat progenitors. *Hum Exp Toxicol.* 1994;13:103–106.

Patton WN, Duffull SB. Idiosyncratic drug-induced haematological abnormalities. Incidence, pathogenesis, management and avoidance. *Drug Saf.* 1994;11:445–462.

Pedersen-Bjergaard J, Pedersen M, Roulston D, et al. Different genetic pathways in leukemogenesis for patients presenting with therapy-related myelodysplasia and therapy-related acute myeloid leukemia. *Blood.* 1995;86:3542–3552.

Pedersen-Bjergaard J, Philip P, Pedersen NT, et al. Acute nonlymphocytic leukemia, preleukemia, and acute myeloproliferative syndrome secondary to treatment of other malignant diseases. II. Bone marrow cytology, cytogenetics, results of HLA typing, response to antileukemic chemotherapy, and survival in a total series of 55 patients. *Cancer.* 1984;54:452–462.

Perazella MA, Biswas P. Acute hyperkalemia associated with intravenous epsilon-aminocaproic acid therapy. *Am J Kidney Dis.* 1999;33:782–785.

Percy MJ, McFerran NV, Lappin TR. Disorders of oxidised haemoglobin. *Blood Rev.* 2005;19:61–68.

Pessina A, Albella B, Bayo M, et al. Application of the CFU-GM assay to predict acute drug-induced neutropenia: an international blind trial to validate a prediction model for the maximum tolerated dose (MTD) of myelosuppressive xenobiotics. *Toxicol Sci.* 2003;75:355–367.

Pessina A, Albella B, Bueren J, et al. Prevalidation of a model for predicting acute neutropenia by colony forming unit granulocyte/macrophage (CFU-GM) assay. *Toxicol In Vitro.* 2001;15:729–740.

Pessina A, Malerba I, Gribaldo L. Hematotoxicity testing by cell clonogenic assay in drug development and preclinical trials. *Curr Pharm Des.* 2005;11:1055–1065.

Peters DC, Noble S. Aprotinin: an update of its pharmacology and therapeutic use in open heart surgery and coronary artery bypass surgery. *Drugs.* 1999;57:233–260.

Peters WP, Holland JF, Senn H, et al. Corticosteroid administration and localized leukocyte mobilization in man. *N Engl J Med.* 1972;286:342–345.

Peterson JA, Nelson TN, Kanack AJ, et al. Fine specificity of drug-dependent antibodies reactive with a restricted domain of platelet GPIIIA. *Blood.* 2008;111:1234–1239.

Phillips GL. The potential of amifostine in high-dose chemotherapy and autologous hematopoietic stem cell transplantation. *Semin Oncol.* 2002;29:53–56.

Pisciotta AV. Immune and toxic mechanisms in drug-induced agranulocytosis. *Semin Hematol.* 1973;10:279–310.

Pisciotta AV. Response of granulocytes to toxic injury. In: Sipes IG, McQueen AC, Gandolfi AJ, eds. *Comprehensive Toxicology.* Oxford: Pergamon Press; 1997:145–158.

Platanias LC. Abnormalities in Th 17 cells in aplastic anemia. *Blood.* 2010;116:4039–4040.

Ponka P. Tissue-specific regulation of iron metabolism and heme synthesis: distinct control mechanisms in erythroid cells. *Blood.* 1997;89:1–25.

Powley MW, Carlson GP. Hepatic and pulmonary microsomal benzene metabolism in CYP2E1 knockout mice. *Toxicology.* 2001;169:187–194.

Poyart C, Marden MC, Kister J. Bezafibrate derivatives as potent effectors of hemoglobin. *Methods Enzymol.* 1994;232:496–513.

Prchal JT. Clinical manifestations and classification of erythrocyte disorders. In: Lichtman MA, Beutler E, Kipps TJ, Seligsohn U, Kaushansky K, Prchal JT, eds. *Williams Hematology.* 7th ed. New York: McGraw-Hill; 2006:411–418.

Preiss BS, Bergman OJ, Friis LS, et al. Cytogenetic findings in adult secondary acute myeloid leukemia (AML): frequency of favorable and adverse chromosomal aberrations do not differ from adult de novo AML. *Cancer Genet Cytogenet.* 2010;202:108–122.

Pyatt DW, Thirman M. Benzene as a leukemogenic agent: what do cytogenetics tell us? In: Proceedings of the 4th International Symposium on Secondary Leukemia and Leukemogenesis; March 24–26, 2011; Rome, Italy; p. 48.

Rader M. Granulocyte colony-stimulating factor use in patients with chemotherapy-induced neutropenia: clinical and economic benefits. *Oncology.* 2006;20:16–21.

Reagan WJ, Handy V, McKamey A, et al. Effects of doxorubicin on the canine erythroid and myeloid progenitor cells and bone marrow microenvironment. *Comp Haematol.* 1993;3:96–101.

Reagan WJ, Irizarry-Rovira A, Poitout-Belissent F, et al. Best practices for evaluation of bone marrow in nonclinical toxicity studies. *Toxicol Pathol.* 2011;39(2):435–448.

Reese JA, Li X, Hauben M, et al. Identifying drugs that cause acute thrombocytopenia: an analysis using 3 distinct methods. *Blood.* 2010;116:2127–2133.

Reynolds VL. Applications of emerging technologies in toxicology and safety assessment. *Int J Toxicol.* 2005;24:135–137.

Ricci-Vitiani L, Pallini R, Biffoni M, et al. Tumour vascularization via endothelial differentiation of glioblastoma stem-like cells. *Nature.* 2010;468:824–828.

Rojas JC, Aguilar B, Rodriguez-Maldonado E, et al. Pharmacogenetics of oral anticoagulants. *Blood Coagul Fibrinolysis.* 2005;16:389–398.

Rossi G, Pelizzari AM, Bellotti D, et al. Cytogenetic analogy between myelodysplastic syndrome and acute myeloid leukemia of elderly patients. *Leukemia.* 2000;14:636–641.

Rother RP, Bell L, Hillmen P, et al. The clinical sequelae of intravascular hemolysis and extracellular plasma hemoglobin: a novel mechanism of human disease. *JAMA.* 2005;293:1653–1662.

Roujeau JC. Clinical heterogeneity of drug hypersensitivity. *Toxicology.* 2005;209:123–129.

Rowe JM. Therapy of secondary leukemia. *Leukemia.* 2002;16:748–750.

Rowley JD, Golomb HM, Vardiman JW. Nonrandom chromosome abnormalities in acute leukemia and dysmyelopoietic syndromes in patients with previously treated malignant disease. *Blood.* 1981;58:759–767.

Ryan DH. Examination of the blood. In: Lichtman MA, Beutler E, Kipps TJ, Seligsohn U, Kaushansky K, Prchal JT, eds. *Williams Hematology.* 7th ed. New York: McGraw-Hill; 2006:11–19.

Ryter SW, Otterbein LE. Carbon monoxide in biology and medicine. *Bioessays.* 2004;26:270–280.

Sagov SE. March hemoglobinuria treated with rubber insoles: two case reports. *J Am Coll Health Assoc.* 1970;19:146.

Salama A, Schutz B, Kiefel V, et al. Immune-mediated agranulocytosis related to drugs and their metabolites: mode of sensitization and heterogeneity of antibodies. *Br J Haematol.* 1989;72:127–132.

Sandoval C, Pui CH, Bowman LC, et al. Secondary acute myeloid leukemia in children previously treated with alkylating agents, intercalating topoisomerase II inhibitors, and irradiation. *J Clin Oncol.* 1993;11: 1039–1045.

Sanz MA, Montesinos P. Secondary leukemia in patients treated for acute promyelocytic leukemia. In: Proceedings of the 4th International Symposium on Secondary Leukemia and Leukemogenesis; March 24–26, 2011; Rome, Italy; p. 21.

Sato K, Miyakawa M, Han DC, et al. Graves' disease with neutropenia and marked splenomegaly: autoimmune neutropenia due to propylthiouracil. *J Endocrinol Invest.* 1985;8:551–555.

Schmaier AH, Rojkjaer R, Shariat-Madar Z. Activation of the plasma kallikrein/kinin system on cells: a revised hypothesis. *Thromb Haemost.* 1999;82:226–233.

Schneidkraut MJ, Loegering DJ. Effect of extravascular hemolysis on the RES depression following thermal injury. *Exp Mol Pathol.* 1984;40:271–279.

Schrijvers D, Highley M, De Bruyn E, et al. Role of red blood cells in pharmacokinetics of chemotherapeutic agents. *Anticancer Drugs.* 1999;10:147–153.

Schultz W. About specific sore throat. *Dtsch Med Wochenschr.* 1922;48:1495–1496.

Sedrakyan A, Atkins D, Treasure T. The risk of aprotinin: a conflict of evidence. *Lancet.* 2006;367:1376–1377.

Sella R, Flomenbilt L, Goldstein I, et al. Detection of anti-neutrophil antibodies in autoimmune neutropenia of infancy: a multicenter study. *Isr Med Assoc J.* 2010;12:91–96.

Semerad CL, Liu F, Gregory AD, et al. G-CSF is an essential regulator of neutrophil trafficking from the bone marrow to the blood. *Immunity.* 2002;17:413–423.

Sharma M, Afrin F, Satija N, et al. Stromal-derived factor-1/CXCR4 signaling: indispensable role in homing and engraftment of hematopoietic stem cells in bone marrow. *Stem Cells Dev.* 2011;20(6):933–946.

Shen M, Lan Q, Zhang L, et al. Polymorphisms in genes involved in DNA double strand break repair pathway and susceptibility to benzene-induced hematotoxicity. *Carcinogenesis.* 2006;27:2083–2089.

Shifrine M, Wilson FD. *The Canine as a Biomedical Research Model: Immunological, Hematological and Oncological Aspects.* Springfield: US Department of Commerce Technical Information Center; 1980.

Shimizu Y, Kato H, Schull WJ, et al. Studies of the mortality of A-bomb survivors. 9. Mortality, 1950–1985: part 1. Comparison of risk coefficients for site-specific cancer mortality based on the DS86 and T65DR shielded kerma and organ doses. *Radiat Res.* 1989;118:502–524.

Siebert WJ, Ayres RW, Bulling MT, et al. Streptokinase morbidity—more common than previously recognised. *Aust N Z J Med.* 1992;22:129–133.

Slater K. Cytotoxicity tests for high-throughput drug discovery. *Curr Opin Biotechnol.* 2001;12:70–74.

Smith MA, Smith JG, Provan AB, et al. The effect of rh-cytokines on the sensitivity of normal human CFU-GM progenitors to Ara-C and on the S-phase activity of light density human bone marrow cells. *Leuk Res.* 1994;18:105–110.

Stafford DW. The vitamin K cycle. *J Thromb Haemost.* 2005;3:1873–1878.

Stark MA, Huo Y, Burcin TL, et al. Phagocytosis of apoptotic neutrophils regulates granulopoiesis via IL-23 and IL-17. *Immunity.* 2005;22:285–294.

Steinberg MH. Pathophysiologically based drug treatment of sickle cell disease. *Trends Pharmacol Sci.* 2006;27:204–210.

Stern A. Drug-induced oxidative denaturation in red blood cells. *Semin Hematol.* 1989;26:301–306.

Stern SC, Shah S, Costello C. Probable autoimmune neutropenia induced by fludarabine treatment for chronic lymphocytic leukaemia. *Br J Haematol.* 1999;106:836–837.

Stoddart A, McNerney M, Bartom E, et al. Genetic pathways leading to therapy-related myeloid neoplasms. In: Proceedings of the 4th International Symposium on Secondary Leukemia and Leukemogenesis; March 24–26, 2011; Rome, Italy; p. 3.

Suber RL, Kodell RL. The effect of three phlebotomy techniques on hematological and clinical chemical evaluation in Sprague–Dawley rats. *Vet Clin Pathol.* 1985;14:23–30.

Sundman-Engberg B, Tidefelt U, Paul C. Toxicity of cytostatic drugs to normal bone marrow cells in vitro. *Cancer Chemother Pharmacol.* 1998;42:17–23.

Swerdlow SH, Campo E, Harris NL, et al. WHO classification of tumours of the hematopoietic and lymphoid tissues. 4th ed. In: *WHO Classification of Tumours.* Vol. 2. Lyon, France: IACR Press; 2008:439.

Szarfman A, Machado SG, O'Neill RT. Use of screening algorithms and computer systems to efficiently signal higher-than-expected combinations of drugs and events in the US FDA's spontaneous reports database. *Drug Saf.* 2002;25:381–392.

Szarfman A, Talarick L, Levine JG. Analysis and risk assessment of hematological data from clinical trials. In: Sipes IG MAGA, ed. *Comprehensive Toxicology.* Oxford: Pergamon Press; 1997:363–379.

Tamaoki J. The effects of macrolides on inflammatory cells. *Chest.* 2004;125:41S–50S.

Tannock IF. Experimental chemotherapy and concepts related to the cell cycle. *Int J Radiat Biol Relat Stud Phys Chem Med.* 1986;49:335–355.

Tavazzi B, Di PD, Amorini AM, et al. Energy metabolism and lipid peroxidation of human erythrocytes as a function of increased oxidative stress. *Eur J Biochem.* 2000;267:684–689.

Tesfa D, Keisu M, Palmblad J. Idiosyncratic drug-induced agranulocytosis: possible mechanisms and management. *Am J Hematol.* 2009;84:428–434.

Thirman MJ, Larson RA. Therapy-related myeloid leukemia. *Hematol Oncol Clin North Am.* 1996;10:293–320.

Todd MD, Ulrich RG. Emerging technologies for accelerated toxicity evaluation of potential drug candidates. *Curr Opin Drug Disc Res.* 1999;2:58–68.

Turbay D, Lieberman J, Alper CA, et al. Tumor necrosis factor constellation polymorphism and clozapine-induced agranulocytosis in two different ethnic groups. *Blood.* 1997;89:4167–4174.

Uetrecht J. Drug metabolism by leukocytes and its role in drug-induced lupus and other idiosyncratic drug reactions. *Crit Rev Toxicol.* 1990;20:213–235.

Valagussa P, Kenda R, Fossati F, et al. Incidence of 2d malignancies in Hodgkin's-disease (HD) after various forms of treatment [abstract]. *Proc Am Soc Clin Oncol.* 1979;20:360.

Valli VE, McGrath JP. Comparative leukocyte biology and toxicology. In: Sipes IG MAGA, ed. *Comprehensive Toxicology.* Oxford: Pergamon Press; 1997:201–215.

van den Bemt PM, Meyboom RH, Egberts AC. Drug-induced immune thrombocytopenia. *Drug Saf.* 2004;27:1243–1252.

Van Wijk R, van Solinge WW. The energy-less blood cell is lost: erythrocyte enzyme abnormalities of glycolysis. *Blood.* 2005;106:4034–4042.

Vandendries ER, Drews RE. Drug-associated disease: hematologic dysfunction. *Crit Care Clin.* 2006;22:347–355.

Varga J, Uitto J, Jimenez SA. The cause and pathogenesis of the eosinophilia–myalgia syndrome. *Ann Intern Med.* 1992;116:140–147.

Varmus H, Weinberg RA. *Genes and the Biology of Cancer.* New York: Scientific American Library; 1993.

Vermeulen L, De Sousa F, Melo E, et al. Wnt activity defines colon cancer stem cells and is regulated by the microenvironment. *Nat Cell Biol.* 2010;12:468–476.

Veyradier A, Meyer D. Thrombotic thrombocytopenic purpura and its diagnosis. *J Thromb Haemost.* 2005;3:2420–2427.

Vincent PC. Drug-induced aplastic anaemia and agranulocytosis. Incidence and mechanisms. *Drugs.* 1986;31:52–63.

Vismans JJ, Briet E, Meijer K, et al. Azathioprine and subacute myelomonocytic leukemia. *Acta Med Scand.* 1980;207:315–319.

Vogelstein B, Fearon ER, Hamilton SR, et al. Genetic alterations during colorectal-tumor development. *N Engl J Med.* 1988;319:525–532.

Voog E, Morschhauser F, Solal-Celigny P. Neutropenia in patients treated with rituximab. *N Engl J Med.* 2003;348:2691–2694.

Wan J, Badham HJ, Winn L. The role of c-MYB in benzene-initiated toxicity. *Chem Biol Interact.* 2005;153–154:171–178.

Warkentin TE, Greinacher A. Heparin-induced thrombocytopenia: recognition, treatment, and prevention: the seventh ACCP conference on antithrombotic and thrombolytic therapy. *Chest.* 2004;126:311S–337S.

Weatherall D. Disorders of globin synthesis in the thalassemias. In: Lichtman MA, Beutler E, Kipps TJ, Seligsohn U, Kaushansky K, Prchal JT, eds. *Williams Hematology.* 7th ed. New York: McGraw-Hill; 2006:663–666.

Weingand K, Brown G, Hall R, et al. Harmonization of animal clinical pathology testing in toxicity and safety studies. *Fundam Appl Toxicol.* 1996;29:198–201.

Weiss DJ, Blauvelt M, Sykes J, et al. Flow cytometric evaluation of canine bone marrow differential cell counts. *Vet Clin Pathol.* 2000;29:97–104.

West BC, DeVault GA Jr, Clement JC, et al. Aplastic anemia associated with parenteral chloramphenicol: review of 10 cases, including the second case of possible increased risk with cimetidine. *Rev Infect Dis.* 1988;10:1048–1051.

Whichard ZL, Sarkar CA, Kimmel M, et al. Hematopoiesis and its disorders: a systems biology approach. *Blood.* 2010;115(12):2339–2347.

WHO. *World Health Organization Handbook for Reporting Results of Cancer Treatments.* Offset Publication No. 48. Geneva: WHO; 1979.

Williams CL, Whitaker MH. The molecular biology of acute myeloid leukemia. Proto-oncogene expression and function in normal and neoplastic myeloid cells. *Clin Lab Med.* 1990;10:769–796.

Williams DP, Pirmohamed M, Naisbitt DJ, et al. Induction of metabolism-dependent and -independent neutrophil apoptosis by clozapine. *Mol Pharmacol.* 2000;58:207–216.

Williams LH, Udupa KB, Lipschitz DA. Long-term bone marrow culture as a model for host toxicity: the effect of methotrexate on hematopoiesis and adherent layer function. *Exp Hematol.* 1988;16:80–87.

Yoo D, Lessin LS. Drug-associated "bite cell" hemolytic anemia. *Am J Med.* 1992;92:243–248.

Young KM, Weiss L. Hematopoiesis: structure–function relationships in bone marrow and spleen. In: Sipes IG, McQueen AC, Gandolfi AJ, eds. *Comprehensive Toxicology.* Oxford: Pergamon Press; 1997:11–34.

Young NS. Acquired aplastic anemia. *JAMA.* 1999;282:271–278.

Young NS. Hematopoietic cell destruction by immune mechanisms in acquired aplastic anemia. *Semin Hematol.* 2000;37:14.

Yunis JJ, Corzo D, Salazar M, et al. HLA associations in clozapine-induced agranulocytosis. *Blood.* 1995;86:1177–1183.

Zakarija A, Bennett C. Drug-induced thrombotic microangiopathy. *Semin Thromb Hemost.* 2005;31:681–690.

Zhang X, Liu F, Chen X, et al. Involvement of the immune system in idiosyncratic drug reactions. *Drug Metab Pharmacokinet.* 2011;26(1):47–59.

chapter 12

Toxic Responses of the Immune System

Barbara L.F. Kaplan, Courtney E.W. Sulentic, Michael P. Holsapple, and Norbert E. Kaminski

INTRODUCTION

Immunotoxicology can be most simply defined as the study of adverse effects on the immune system resulting from occupational, inadvertent, or therapeutic exposure to drugs, environmental chemicals, and, in some instances, biological materials. Studies in animals and humans have indicated that the immune system is comprised of potential target organs, and that damage to this system can be associated with morbidity and even mortality. Indeed, in some instances, the immune system can be compromised (decreased lymphoid cellularity, alterations in lymphocyte subpopulations, decreased host resistance, and altered specific immune function responses) in the absence of observed toxicity in other organ systems. These studies coupled with tremendous advances made in immunology and molecular biology have led to a steady and exponential growth in our understanding of immunotoxicology during the past 30 years. Recognition by regulatory agencies that the immune system is an important, as well as sensitive, target organ for chemical- and drug-induced toxicity is another indication of the growth of this subdiscipline of toxicology. With the availability of sensitive, reproducible, and predictive tests, it is now apparent that the inclusion of immunotoxicity testing represents a significant adjunct to routine safety evaluations for therapeutic agents, biological agents, and chemicals now in development.

Understanding the impact of toxic responses on the immune system requires an appreciation of its role, which may be stated succinctly as the preservation of integrity. It is a series of delicately balanced, complex, multicellular, and physiological mechanisms that allow an individual to distinguish foreign material (ie, "nonself") from "self," and to neutralize, eliminate, and/or coexist with the foreign matter. Examples of self are all the tissues, organs, and cells of the body. Examples of nonself are a variety of opportunistic pathogens, including bacteria and viruses, and transformed cells or tissues (ie, tumors). The immune system is characterized by a virtually infinite repertoire of specificities, highly specialized effectors, complex regulatory mechanisms, and an ability to travel throughout the body. The great complexity of the mammalian immune system is an indication of the importance, as well as the difficulty, of its role. If the immune system fails to recognize as nonself an infectious entity or neoantigens expressed by a newly arisen tumor, then the host is in danger of rapidly succumbing to the unopposed invasion. This aspect of immune competence is the reason why the immune system is often synonymous with "host defense." Alternatively, if some integral bodily tissue is not identified as self, then the immune system is capable of turning its considerable defensive capabilities against that tissue, and an autoimmune disease may be the end result. This aspect of immunocompetence emphasizes the tremendous destructive potential that is associated with the host defense mechanisms of the immune system. The cost to the host of these mistakes, made in either direction, may be quite high. The fact that mistakes can occur in either direction is an indication that immunotoxicology should be considered as a continuum (Fig. 12-1). At the center of the concept of the continuum is the recognition that immune responses in the normal human population can vary by more than two standard deviations (Luebke *et al.*, 2004), as described in greater detail in the subsection entitled "Approaches to the Assessment of Human Immunotoxicity." Because the cost of mistakes in immunocompetence can be so high, and because of

the tremendous diversity involved in the identification of self versus nonself, a complex array of organs, cells, soluble factors, and their interactions has evolved to regulate this system and minimize the frequency of errors in either direction. Due to the potentially profound effects resulting from disruption of the delicately balanced immune system, there is a need to understand the cellular, biochemical, and molecular mechanisms of xenobiotic-induced immune modulation.

This chapter provides (1) an overview of basic concepts in immunology (structure, components, and functions), which are important to the understanding of the impact that xenobiotics may have on the exposed individual; (2) a summary of selected current methods utilized to assess immune function; and (3) a brief review of current information on the immune modulation (immune suppression, immune enhancement, hypersensitivity, and autoimmunity) induced by a variety of xenobiotics. This chapter is not meant to be an immunology textbook, nor an exhaustive review of the mechanisms of immunotoxicity of a myriad of xenobiotics. For detailed information on immunology, the reader is referred to three texts: the first edited by Paul, *Fundamental Immunology* (6th edition, 2008), the second written by Delves, Martin, Burton, and Roitt, *Roitt's Essential Immunology* (12th edition, 2011), and the third written by Murphy, Travers, and Walport, *Janeway's Immunobiology* (7th edition, 2008). For a more comprehensive review of immunotoxicology, the reader is referred to two texts: the first edited by Vohr and colleagues, *Encyclopedic Reference of Immunotoxicology* (2005), and the second edited by Luebke, House, and Kimber, *Immunotoxicology and Immunopharmacology, Target Organ Toxicity Series* (3rd edition, 2007). The reader might also find the list of abbreviations in Table 12-1 helpful.

THE IMMUNE SYSTEM

Unlike most organ systems, the immune system has the unique quality of not being confined to a single site within the body. It comprises numerous lymphoid organs (Table 12-2) and many different cellular populations with a variety of functions. The bone marrow and thymus are referred to as primary lymphoid organs because they contain the microenvironments capable of supporting the production of mature B and T cells, respectively. Central tolerance (nonreactive to self-antigens) is also established in the primary lymphoid organs to prevent the maturation of lymphocytes that recognize self-antigens. In addition, the bone marrow is the site of origin of the pluripotent and self-renewing hematopoietic stem cell (HSC) from which all other hematopoietic cells are derived. While immunologists differ on how to define and identify the hematopoietic intermediates, Fig. 12-2 shows one model of hematopoiesis (adapted from Baltimore *et al.* 2008; Chaplin, 2010). During gestation, the HSC is found in the embryonic yolk sac and fetal liver; eventually, it migrates to the bone marrow. Within the bone marrow, the HSC developmentally commits to either the lymphoid or myeloid lineages by giving rise to the common lymphoid progenitor (CLP) or the common myeloid progenitor (CMP), which differentiate into various types of hematopoietic cells. CLP cells make a further commitment to become either T cells or B cells (Fig. 12-3). The maturation process for both T cells and B cells involves the establishment of central tolerance, but this process occurs at different primary lymphoid organs. For B cells, central tolerance occurs in the bone marrow and simply involves the removal of self-reactive cells. It is more complex for T cells and involves the migration of T-cell precursors from the bone marrow to the thymus where they undergo a process of both positive and negative selection resulting in mature T cells that recognize the host's cells

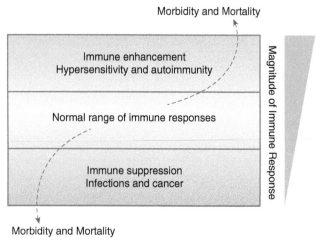

Morbidity and Mortality

Figure 12-1. *The continuum of immunotoxicology.* Immune toxicity results from xenobiotic-induced suppression or enhancement of immune function.

Table 12-1

Abbreviations

TERM	ABBREVIATION	TERM	ABBREVIATION
Antibody-dependent cell-mediated cytotoxicity	ADCC	Interleukin	IL
Antibody-forming cell	AFC	Keyhole limpet hemocyanin	KLH
Antigen-presenting cell	APC	Lipopolysaccharide	LPS
Aryl hydrocarbon receptor	AHR	Local lymph node assay	LLNA
B-cell receptor	BCR	Major histocompatibility complex	MHC
B-regulatory cell	Breg	Membrane attack complex	MAC
Carboxyfluorescein succinimidyl ester	CFSE	Mixed lymphocyte response	MLR
CD40 ligand	CD40L	National Toxicology Program	NTP
Cell-mediated immunity	CMI	Natural killer	NK
Central nervous system	CNS	NOD-like receptors	NRL
Cluster of differentiation	CD	Non-human primates	NHP
Colony stimulating factor	CSF	Pathogen-associated molecular patterns	PAMPs
Common lymphoid progenitor	CLP	Pattern recognition receptors	PRR
Common myeloid progenitor	CMP	Peripheral blood mononuclear cells	PBMC
Concanavalin-A	Con A	Phytohemagglutinin	PHA
Conventional dendritic cell	cDC	Plaque-forming cell	PFC
Cytotoxic T lymphocyte	CTL	Plasmacytoid dendritic cell	pDC
Danger-associated molecular patterns	DAMPs	Polymerase chain reaction	PCR
Delayed-type hypersensitivity	DTH	Pre/postnatal development	PPND
Dendritic cell	DC	RIG-like receptors	RLR
Developmental and reproductive toxicology	DART	Reverse transcriptase	RT
Developmental immunotoxicology	DIT	Sheep red blood cells	sRBC
Embryo fetal development	EFD	Single nucleotide polymorphism	SNP
Experimental allergic encephalomyelitis	EAE	Systemic lupus erythematosus	SLE
Hematopoietic stem cell	HSC	T-cell receptor	TCR
Human lymphocyte activation	HuLa	T cytotoxic cell	Tc
Human peripheral blood	HPB	T helper cell	Th
Inteferon	IFN	Toll-like receptor	TLR
Immunoglobulin	Ig	T-regulatory cell	Treg
Innate lymphoid cell	iLC	Transforming growth factor	TGF
		Tumor necrosis factor	TNF

(ie, positive selection) but not too strongly. T cells that recognize self too strongly are deleted from the T-cell repertoire (ie, negative selection). Recognition of self is essential for T cells to initiate and regulate immune responses.

Table 12-2

Organization of the Immune System: Lymphoid Tissue

CLASSIFICATION	LYMPHOID ORGANS
Primary	Bone marrow
	Thymus
Secondary	Spleen
	Lymph nodes
	Peyer's patches
	Skin-associated lymphoid tissue (SALT)
	Mucosal lamina propria (MALT)
	Gut-associated lymphoid tissue (GALT)
	Bronchial-associated lymphoid tissue (BALT)
	Nasal-associated lymphoid tissue (NALT)
	Cells lining the genitourinary tract
Tertiary	Lymphoid neogenesis in nonlymphoid organs

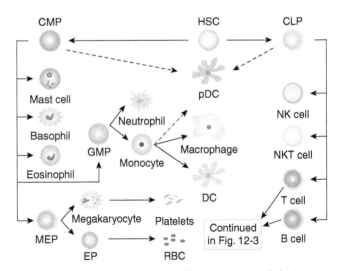

Figure 12-2. *Development of the cellular components of the immune system.* All immune cells initially develop in the bone marrow. The HSC differentiates into two main progenitors from which all other cells develop. The progenitor for pDCs is still unclear (dashed lines). HSC, hematopoietic stem cell; CMP, common myeloid progenitor; CLP, common lymphoid progenitor; GMP, granulocyte-macrophage progenitor; MEP, megakaryocyte-erythrocyte progenitor; DC, dendritic cell; pDC, plasmacytoid dendritic cell; EP, erythrocyte precursor; NK, natural killer; RBC, red blood cells.

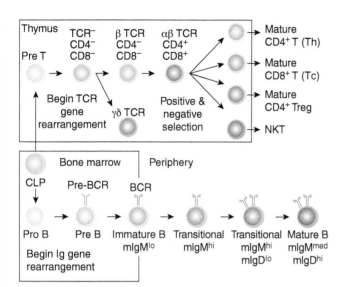

Figure 12-3. *Development and differentiation of T and B cells.* T cells develop in the thymus and B cells develop in the bone marrow. For T cells, an initial step is commitment to either αβ or γδ TCR. After positive and negative selection, T cells acquire either CD4 or CD8 to become Th or Tc, respectively, become natural Tregs (nTregs), or become NKT cells. The B-cell lineage depicted here is of the conventional B-2 lineage. B-1 cells are not depicted since these cells arise from a distinct precursor not found in the bone marrow, which might be a precursor that can generate B-1 or myeloid cells. m, membrane.

Mature, naive, or virgin lymphocytes (those T and B cells that have never undergone antigenic stimulation) are first brought into contact with exogenously derived antigens within the highly organized microenvironment of the spleen and lymph nodes, which are secondary lymphoid organs. These organs can be thought of as biological sieves. The spleen serves as a filter for the blood, removing both foreign antigens and any circulating dead cells and cellular debris. The lymph nodes are part of a network of lymphatic veins that filter antigens from the fluid surrounding the tissues of the body. In addition to the spleen and lymph nodes, other secondary lymphoid tissues associated with the skin, mucosal lamina propria, gut, bronchioles, or nasal cavity are referred to as associated lymphoid tissues (abbreviated SALT, MALT, GALT, BALT, and NALT, respectively). Included in the GALT are specialized structures in the small intestine called Peyer's patches that collect antigens from the gastrointestinal tract. The associated lymphoid tissues tend to have more exposure to antigen and greater plasticity (ie, increase or decrease in size and/or number) than lymph nodes. The plasticity of lymphoid organs is underscored by the detection of lymphoid neogenesis in nonlymphoid organs during chronic inflammation. The new lymphoid tissue is classified as tertiary lymphoid tissue, and its development is reversible if the inflammatory response is resolved. Although studies suggest that tertiary lymphoid tissues support transient, local immune responses, there is still much to learn regarding lymphoid neogenesis and its role in the immune response particularly with clinical and experimental evidence supporting an association between lymphoid neogenesis (ie, tertiary lymphoid tissues) and pathophysiological conditions such as autoimmune disease and cancer (Drayton *et al.*, 2006).

Antigen Recognition

Immunity Mammalian immunity can be classified into two functional divisions: innate immunity and acquired (adaptive) immunity (Table 12-3). Innate immunity has historically been characterized as a first-line defense response with little immunological memory.

Table 12-3

Innate versus Acquired Immunity

CHARACTERISTIC	INNATE IMMUNITY	ACQUIRED IMMUNITY
Cells involved	Neutrophils Macrophages NK/NKT cells DC	T cells B cells Macrophages (accessory cell) DC (accessory cell)
Primary soluble mediators	Complement Perforin/granzyme Acute-phase proteins IFN-α/β Other cytokines	Antibody Cytokines Perforin/granzyme
Specificity of response	Limited	Yes (very high specificity)
Receptors	TLR Complement receptors NLR Fc TCRγδ	TCRαβ TCRγδ Igαβ
Response enhanced by repeated antigen challenge	No	Yes

Therefore, in a normal healthy adult, the magnitude of the innate immune response to a foreign organism is similar for a secondary or a tertiary challenge as it is for the primary exposure. By contrast, acquired (adaptive) immunity is characterized by specificity and immunological memory. Thus, in a normal healthy adult, the speed and magnitude of the acquired immune response to a foreign organism is greater for a secondary challenge than it is for the primary challenge.

Antigen The primary determinant in either type of immune response is the ability of the immune system components to recognize self versus nonself. One definition of nonself, essentially, is anything other than that encoded in one's own germline genome (Nathan, 2006). Given this broad interpretation of nonself, this includes foreign DNA, RNA, protein, and carbohydrates, and may even include aberrantly expressed or mutated self-proteins, since those are likely not contained in one's own germline genome. A nonself substance that can be recognized by the immune system is called an antigen (also referred to as an immunogen or allergen). Antigens are usually (but not absolutely) biological molecules that can be cleaved and rearranged for presentation to other immune cells. Generally, antigens are about 10 kDa or larger in size. Smaller antigens are termed "haptens" and must be conjugated with carrier molecules (larger antigens) in order to elicit a specific response. However, once an initial response is made, the hapten can induce subsequent responses in the absence of the carrier.

Antibodies Antibodies are produced by B cells and are defined functionally by the antigen with which they react, and by their subtype, termed "isotypes" (IgM, IgG, IgE, IgD, and IgA; Table 12-4). Thus, an IgM antibody directed against sheep red blood cells (sRBCs) is called anti-sRBC IgM. Because the immune system

Table 12-4

Properties of Immunoglobulin Classes and Subclasses

CLASS	MEAN SERUM CONCENTRATION (MG/ML)	HUMAN HALF-LIFE (DAYS)	BIOLOGICAL PROPERTIES
IgG			Complement fixation (selected subclasses) Crosses placenta
IgG$_1$	9	21	
IgG$_2$	3	20	
IgG$_3$	1	7	
IgG$_4$	1	21	
IgA	3	6	Secretory antibody
IgM	1.5	10	Complement fixation Efficient agglutination
IgD	0.03	3	Possible role in antigen-triggered lymphocyte differentiation
IgE	0.0001	2	Allergic responses (mast-cell degranulation)

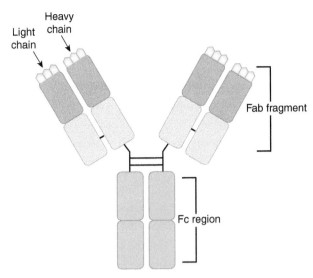

Figure 12-5. *Ig structure.* Igs are comprised of two heavy chains and two light chains, which are connected by disulfide bonds. Orange areas are variable regions and green areas at top are antigen recognition regions.

generates antibodies to thousands of antigens with which the host may or may not ever come into contact, antibodies of unknown specificity are referred to as immunoglobulin (eg, serum immunoglobulin or serum IgM) until they can be defined by their specific antigen (eg, anti-sRBC IgM).

The ability of the immune system to generate antibody to thousands of antigens is the result of somatic recombination, in which the germline DNA that encodes for antibodies is rearranged in B cells. All Igs are made up of heavy and light chains and of constant and variable regions. For the light chain genes, two separate gene segments (V and J) are combined to form the variable region, which is then joined to one constant region. For the heavy chain genes, three separate gene segments (V, D, and J) are combined to form the variable region, which is then joined to one constant region. There are several light chain V and J genes, and several heavy chain V, D, and J genes, which when rearranged in various combinations, contribute to the immense genetic diversity of the Ig genes (Fig. 12-4).

Finally, the five types of Ig are dependent on which heavy chain constant region is transcribed and translated (heavy chain genes μ, γ, ε, δ, or α encode for the IgM, IgG, IgE, IgD, or IgA heavy chain proteins, respectively).

The variable regions, which are contained within the Fab regions of the antibody molecule, determine antibody specificity and interact with antigen (Fig. 12-5). The Fc region mediates various effector functions, such as complement activation (IgM and some IgG subclasses) and phagocyte binding (via Fc receptors). Antibodies possess several functions: (1) opsonization, which is coating of a pathogen with antibody to enhance Fc receptor-mediated endocytosis by phagocytic cells; (2) initiation of the classic pathway of complement-mediated lysis; (3) neutralization of viral infection by binding to viral particles and preventing further infection; and (4) enhancement of the specificity of effectors of cell-mediated immunity (CMI) by binding to specific antigens on target cells, which are then recognized and eliminated by effector cells such as natural killer (NK) cells or cytotoxic T lymphocytes (CTLs).

Complement One of the consequences of antigen–antibody binding is initiation of the classical pathway of complement-mediated lysis (reviewed by Stoermer and Morrison, 2011). The complement system is a series of about 30 serum proteins whose primary functions are the destruction of membranes of infectious agents and the promotion of an inflammatory response (see the "Inflammation" section). Complement activation occurs with each component sequentially acting on others, in a manner similar to the blood-clotting cascade (Fig. 12-6). Proximal components of the cascade are often modified serine proteases, which activate the system but have limited substrate specificity. Several components are capable of binding to microbial membranes and serve as ligands for complement receptors associated with the membrane. The final components, which are related structurally, are also membrane-binding proteins that can enter into the membrane and disrupt membrane integrity, termed the membrane attack complex (MAC).

Specifically, three pathways have been identified in activation of the complement cascade. The classical complement pathway is initiated when antibody binds antigen on the microorganism. The classical pathway then proceeds by activating a C1 subunit serine protease, subsequently recruiting C4, C2, and C3. Various cleavages ultimately result in C3b surface binding to the microorganism and

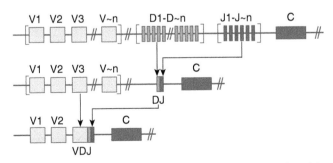

Figure 12-4. *Ig recombination.* An example of VDJ recombination that might occur for Ig heavy chain in B cells or TCR β chain in T cells. Ig light chain in B cells or TCR α chain in T cells is similar, but does not include D genes.

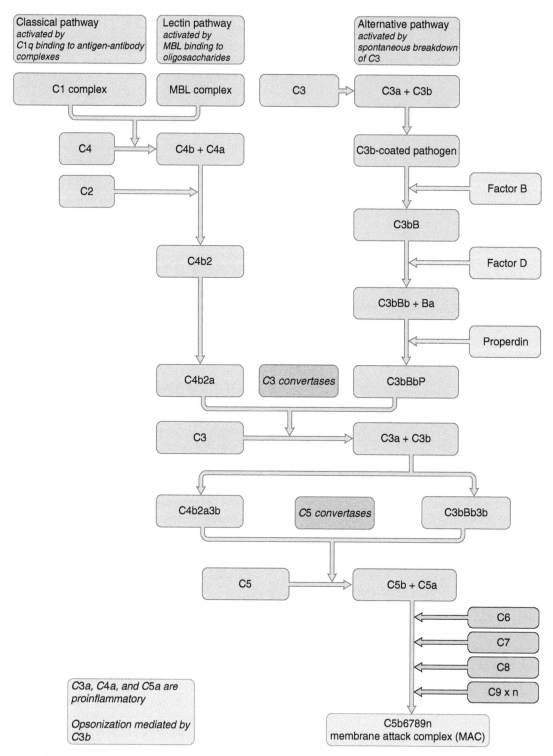

Figure 12-6. *The complement cascade.* The complement cascade can be activated in three different ways. Cytolysis occurs via generation of the MAC. Various complement proteins generated along the pathway are either proinflammatory mediators (C3a, C5a) or result in opsonization (C3b).

release of C3a, a proinflammatory mediator (see the "Inflammation" section). Microorganism-bound C3b can then be recognized by complement receptors on phagocytic cells, which engulf and destroy the microorganism. It is also at this point that the alternative pathway can be activated and amplifies the complement-mediated killing of the microorganism. Finally, C3b mediates recruitment of C5, which is cleaved, generating C5b on the surface and releasing C5a, another proinflammatory mediator (see the "Inflammation"

section). Microorganism-bound C5b recruits C6 and C7, the three of which form a complex and recruit C8. C9 is ultimately recruited, polymerizes, and forms a pore in the membrane of the microorganism, causing its death. In addition to the classical and alternative pathways, complement-mediated lysis is also activated through the lectin pathway, in which binding of mannin-binding lectin (MBL) to the surface of the microorganism activates the pathway and converges with the classical pathway at C4 (Fig. 12-6).

A functional outcome of complement activation, in addition to cytolysis and generation of proinflammatory mediators, is opsonization, the process by which microorganisms are altered by opsonins (predominantly IgM and IgG and C3b), rendering them vulnerable to phagocytosis by cells (usually macrophages and neutrophils) (Dunkelberger and Song, 2010). Complement activation results in microorganism-bound C3b. Therefore, in combination with IgG antibodies recognizing extracellular antigens and C3b opsonization, phagocytic cells efficiently engulf the microbe through Fc receptors specific for IgG or complement receptors.

Antigen Processing In order to elicit an acquired immune response to a particular antigen, that antigen must be taken up and processed by accessory cells for presentation to lymphocytes. Accessory cells that perform this function are termed antigen-presenting cells (APCs) and include macrophages, B cells, and dendritic cells (DCs). Of these, the most proficient APC is the DC. There are several subtypes of DC, including plasmacytoid (pDCs), conventional (cDCs; can be resident or migratory depending on whether they migrate to the site of infection), and specialized DCs in the skin called Langerhan's cells. In addition, there are follicular DCs, which predominantly mediate T-cell-independent stimulation of B cells in germinal centers (Vinuesa *et al.*, 2010) and will not be discussed further as they are beyond the scope of this chapter.

In most tissues in the absence of antigenic stimulation, DCs are in an immature state, during which they efficiently capture antigens. DCs can mature in response to antigen itself, toll-like receptor (TLR) agonists such as lipopolysaccharide (LPS), or cytokines (GM-CSF, tumor necrosis factor [TNF-α]) (Banchereau and Steinman, 1998). Upon maturation, DCs migrate to lymph nodes and present antigen to T cells. Thus, the DC–T cell interaction is critical for the development of an acquired immune response.

Immature DCs internalize the antigen either by phagocytosis, pinocytosis, or by receptor-mediated endocytosis (via antigen, Fc, or complement receptors), after which the DCs mature to express high levels of both classes of MHC (MHCI and MHCII), which can stimulate both innate and adaptive immune responses, and of costimulatory molecules to facilitate interaction with T cells (Banchereau and Steinman, 1998). Interestingly, Langerhan's cells express high levels of major histocompatibility complex class II (MHCII) even in a resting state (ie, nonactivated) (Kaplan, 2010). Following internalization, antigen is processed (intracellular denaturation and catabolism) through several cytoplasmic compartments, and a piece of the antigen (peptide fragments about 20 amino acids in length) becomes physically associated with MHCII (Fig. 12-7). This MHCII–peptide complex is then transported to the surface of the cell and can interact in a specific manner with T lymphocytes. For most APCs, an immunogenic determinant is expressed on the surface of the APC within an hour after internalization, although this is slightly longer for B cells (three–four hours). In addition to processing and presentation, pieces of processed antigen may be expelled into the extracellular space. These pieces of processed antigen can then bind in the peptide groove of empty MHCII on the surface of other APCs for the presentation of that peptide fragment to lymphocytes.

In addition to antigen processing and presentation via MHCII, some antigens may be processed and presented via MHCI. Although the pathways share some similarities in that short peptide fragments of antigens are generated, loaded onto MHCI, and presented on the surface of cells to T lymphocytes, major differences between the MHCI and MHCII pathways are

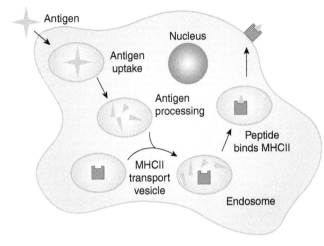

Figure 12-7. *Antigen processing by the MHCII pathway.* Antigen is engulfed by an APC (DC, macrophage, or B cell), degraded, and loaded onto MHCII. The MHCII–peptide complex is then expressed on the surface of the APC for presentation to CD4[+] Th cells.

(1) antigens processed and presented via MHCI are not limited to professional APC; (2) all nucleated cells express MHCI; (3) the mechanisms by which the antigen is processed and loaded onto MHCI are slightly different than MHCII; (4) the MHCI antigenic peptides are usually smaller, often 8 to 10 amino acids in length; (5) the MHCI antigens to be processed are usually aberrantly expressed proteins, such as viral-associated proteins or mutated proteins; (6) MHCI facilitates antigen presentation to CD8[+] T cells, whereas MHCII facilitates antigen presentation to CD4[+] T cells. MHCI antigen processing and presentation is the major pathway by which virally infected cells are detected and killed by the acquired immune system.

Regardless of the MHC utilized to present antigens to lymphocytes, T cells are able to recognize antigen in the context of MHC with their T-cell receptor (TCR). Similar to Ig, the ability of T cells to specifically recognize thousands of antigens is due to somatic recombination. All TCRs are comprised of two different subunits, each encoded from a distinct gene (most abundant T-cell population expresses αβ, but γδ also exist). All TCR subunits are made up of constant and variable regions. For α subunits, two separate gene segments (V and J) are combined to form the variable region, which is then joined to one constant region. For β subunits, three separate gene segments (V, D, and J) are combined to form the variable region, which is then joined to one of the two constant regions. Similar to the Ig genes, there are several light chain V and J genes, and several heavy chain V, D, and J genes (Fig. 12-4).

With regard to T and B cells, key events that occur following antigen encounter are (1) specific antigen recognition either in the context of MHCI or MHCII for T cells or through the Ig receptor for B cells; (2) cellular activation and initiation of intracellular signaling cascades that contribute to production and release of cytokines and other cellular mediators; (3) clonal expansion (proliferation) of antigen-specific cells; and (4) differentiation of antigen-stimulated lymphocytes into effector and memory cells.

Innate Immunity

As stated above, innate immunity acts as a first line of defense against anything nonself. With respect to infectious agents, the innate immune system eliminates most potential pathogens before significant infection occurs. The innate immune system includes physical and biochemical barriers both inside and outside the body, as well as immune cells designed for host defense responses.

Externally, the skin provides an effective barrier, as most organisms cannot penetrate intact skin. Most infectious agents enter the body through the respiratory system, gut, or genitourinary tract. Innate defenses present to combat infection from pathogens entering through the respiratory system include mucus secreted along the nasopharynx, the presence of lysozyme in most secretions, and cilia lining the trachea and main bronchi. In addition, reflexes such as coughing, sneezing, and elevation in body temperature are also a part of innate immunity. Pathogens that enter the body via the digestive tract are met with severe changes in pH (acidic) within the stomach and a host of microorganisms living in the intestines.

Cellular Components: Neutrophils, Macrophages, Dendritic Cells, Natural Killer Cells, NKT Cells, and γδ T Cells Several cell types are involved in innate immunity, and in fact, some also provide critical signals to initiate adaptive immune responses (Tables 12-3 and 12-5). Neutrophils (also known as polymorphonuclear cells or PMNs) are phagocytic cells that develop from the myeloid lineage of HSCs. Neutrophils enter the bloodstream where they circulate for about 10 hours and then enter the tissues where they perform effector functions for about one to two days. Neutrophils are capable of passing between (ie, extravasation) the endothelial cells of the blood vessels and thereby represent a primary line of defense against infectious agents. They are excellent phagocytic cells and can eliminate most microorganisms through the release of various reactive oxygen species (ROS), such as superoxide, singlet oxygen, ozone, hydrogen peroxide, and hydroxyl radicals. Their phagocytic activity is greatly enhanced by the presence of complement and antibody deposited on the surface of the foreign target. They are also important in the induction of an inflammatory response (see the "Inflammation" section).

Also important in the inflammatory response are macrophages. Macrophages are terminally differentiated monocytes, which develop from the myeloid lineage of HSCs. Upon exiting the bone marrow, monocytes circulate within the bloodstream for about one day. At that time, they begin to distribute to the various tissues where they can then differentiate into macrophage subsets. Tissue-specific macrophages include Kupffer cells (liver), alveolar macrophages (lung), microglial cells (CNS), and peritoneal and splenic macrophages. These tissue-specific macrophages have distinct properties and vary in the extent of surface receptors, oxidative metabolism, and expression of MHCII, due to the factors present within the microenvironment in which the monocyte differentiates. Macrophages can be classified as classically activated macrophages (M1), which are proinflammatory and participate in antigen presentation, or alternatively activated macrophages (M2), which do not present antigen well, but are efficient in apoptotic cell removal (reviewed by Martinez *et al.*, 2008). Thus, M1 macrophages are also considered APCs.

A more proficient APC is the DC, which was introduced above in the "Antigen Processing" section. DCs are a critical part of innate immunity since they survey their environment for pathogens, then mature to become highly efficient APCs. Thus, they provide a critical bridge between initial detection of an infectious

---

Table 12-5

Characteristics of Selected Immune Cells

PROPERTIES	MACROPHAGE	DC	T CELLS	B CELLS	NK CELLS
Phagocytosis	Yes	Yes	No	Yes	No
Adherence	Yes	Yes	No	No	No
Surface receptors:					
Antigen receptors	No	No	Yes	Yes	No
Complement	Yes	Yes	No	Yes	Yes
Fc region of Ig	Yes	Yes	Some	Yes	Yes
Surface markers	CD16	CD11c	CD4	Ig	CD16
	CD11b	CD11b	CD8	CD19	CD11b
	CD64		CD3	B220	
Proliferation in response to:					
Allogeneic cells (MLR)	No	No	Yes	No	No
LPS	No	No	No	Yes	No
PHA	No	No	Yes	No	No
Con A	No	No	Yes	No	No
Anti-Ig + IL-4	No	No	No	Yes	No
Anti-CD3 + IL-2	No	No	Yes	No	No
CD40L + cytokines	Yes	Yes	No	Yes	No
Effector functions:					
Antibody production	No	No	No	Yes	No
Cytokine production	Yes	Yes	Yes	Yes	Yes
Bactericidal activity	Yes	Yes	No	No	No
Tumor cell cytotoxicity	Yes	Yes	Yes	No	Yes
Immunological memory	No	No	Yes	Yes	No
Suppressor activity	Yes	No	Yes	Yes	No

agent and elicitation of T-cell responses. DCs can be classified into several subsets and it is thought that the various subsets develop from either CLPs or CMPs, although the exact details are still not clear (reviewed by Watowich and Liu, 2010). Although not reviewed here, part of the challenge with lineage definition is due to extensive heterogeneity of cell surface protein expression of DC subsets, including varying expression of CD11b, CD11c, MHCII, CD4, CD8, and CD205 (reviewed by Watowich and Liu, 2010). All DCs possess efficient APC activity and cytokine production (Watowich and Liu, 2010), but may also possess specialized functions (pDC, for instance, secrete large amounts of Type I interferons (IFNs), such as IFN-α, which is necessary for T-cell differentiation) (Sachdeva et al., 2008).

Like other immune cells, NK cells are derived from a HSC. NK cells are part of a larger family of cells defined as innate lymphoid cells (iLCs), which play roles in innate immunity and inflammation, particularly during the initial phases of inflammation prior to T-cell differentiation (Spits and Di Santo, 2011; Vanaudenaerde et al., 2011). There are two major NK functions: cytokine production and cytolysis. NK cells are a predominant producer of IFN-γ, which helps mature DC (Vivier et al., 2011). Thus, NK cells also facilitate the innate-adaptive immunity bridge. NK cells mediate both antibody-independent and antibody-dependent cellular cytotoxicity (ADCC) using a variety of mechanisms, including perforin and granzyme, Fas L, TRAIL, and TNF-α. ADCC occurs via the FcγRIIIA, which is present on most NK cell subsets. NKT cells are one such subset of NK cells that express both NK- and T-cell markers, including Cd1d, which allows the NKT cell to present self and exogenous antigenic glycolipids (Diana and Lehuen, 2009).

Another cell type that has recently been shown to facilitate the innate-adaptive immunity bridge is the γδ T cell. These cells migrate predominantly to "exposed" tissues, including skin, lung, gut, and reproductive organs, and are also expressed highly in the liver (Bonneville et al., 2010). In part through the expression of TLRs, which are discussed in more detail below, γδ T cells can acquire effector functions, which are not unlike NK cells (cytokine production and cytotoxicity). There is also a subpopulation of B cells (ie, CD5$^+$ or B-1 cells) that also bridge innate and adaptive immunity. Unlike the conventional B-2 cells, B-1 cells predominate in embryonic life and are later found mostly in the peritoneal and pleural cavities. B-1 cells are self-renewing and spontaneously produce polyspecific IgM antibodies (ie, natural antibodies) independent of T-cell help (Baumgarth, 2011).

Historically, innate immunity was defined as nonspecific. It is clear, however, that innate cells express receptors that respond to soluble components (eg, Fc or complement receptors) or to certain antigenic motifs. Pattern recognition receptors are a family of receptors that recognize pathogen-derived molecules or cell-derived molecules produced in response to cellular stress ("danger" molecules). Receptors that recognize pathogen-associated molecular patterns (PAMPs) are TLRs; receptors that recognize danger-associated molecular patterns (DAMPs) include NOD-like receptors (NLR) and RIG-like receptors (RLR) (Davis et al., 2011). Several TLRs are expressed extracellularly, and several are expressed intracellularly in endosomes. This diverse localization allows cells to respond to a variety of pathogenic components, such as bacterial cell wall lipids, single- and double-stranded nucleic acids, or fungal and parasitic products (Chang, 2010). Functional consequences of TLR engagement on cells include expression of adhesion molecules, chemokines or cytokines to stimulate T- or B-cell differentiation, enhance phagocytosis, or maturation of DC (Chang, 2010).

NLRs or RLRs that recognize DAMPs are expressed on many innate cells. Several family members of NLRs participate in a complex called the inflammasome, which activates inflammatory caspases to enhance production of mature interleukin (IL)-1β and IL-18 (Martinon et al., 2009).

A common effector mechanism for many immune cells, including innate cells, is cytokine or chemokine production. Although a partial list of cytokines and a brief description of the cell types that release and are acted upon by these various mediators is provided in Table 12-6, there are also several shared characteristics of cytokines, chemokines, and IFNs that merit discussion for the purposes of understanding immunotoxicological mechanisms. First, the primary function of cytokines, chemokines, and IFNs is cell–cell communication. The resulting actions by cells receiving messages in the form of cytokines, chemokines, or IFNs are diverse and include cellular activation, initiation or termination of intracellular signaling events, proliferation, differentiation, migration, trafficking, or effector functions. Second, although some of these molecules might be constitutively expressed, most are inducible in response to antigens, cellular stressors, or other cytokines. Thus, many cytokines, chemokines, and IFNs are not stored in the cell, but rather are tightly regulated, often at the transcriptional level, so that they are quickly generated on demand. An example of a cytokine important in innate immunity is IL-1, which is rapidly transcribed in response to various stimulants using the critical transcription factor nuclear factor kappa B (NF-κB). Third, many cytokines share common receptor subunits such that should one particular subunit of a receptor be adversely affected by an immunotoxic agent, the functional outcome might be amplified. An example would be the common γ chain, which is shared by the IL-2, IL-4, IL-7, IL-9, IL-13, IL-15, and IL-21 receptors. Although a compound might "only" affect transcription of the common γ chain, the immunological consequences of affecting this target could be quite destructive.

Other soluble components of innate immunity include the complement cascade, acute-phase proteins, granzyme and perforin, and various cytokines, chemokines and IFNs. Although the complement cascade is described elsewhere in this chapter (see "Antigen Recognition" and "Inflammation" sections), it is also important in innate immunity because of its activation through the lectin pathway. Furthermore, C3a and C5a, which are chemokines generated during the cascade, recruit phagocytic cells to the site of complement activation. Acute-phase proteins, such as serum amyloid A, serum amyloid P, and C-reactive protein, participate in an acute-phase response to infection by binding bacteria and facilitating complement activation. Granzyme and perforin work in conjunction, with perforin disrupting the target cell membrane, allowing granzyme to enter and mediate cell lysis by several mechanisms.

Acquired (Adaptive) Immunity

If the primary defenses against infection (innate immunity) are breached, the acquired arm of the immune system is activated and produces a specific immune response to each infectious agent, which usually eliminates the infection. This branch of immunity is also capable of remembering the pathogen and can protect the host from future infection by the same agent. Therefore, the two key features that define acquired immunity are specificity and memory. Acquired immunity may be further subdivided into humoral and CMI. Humoral immunity is directly dependent on the production of antigen-specific antibody by B cells and involves the coordinated

Table 12-6

Cytokines: Sources and Functions in Immune Regulation

CYTOKINE	SOURCE	PHYSIOLOGICAL ACTIONS
IL-1	Macrophages Epithelial cells	Activation and proliferation of T cells Proinflammatory Induces fever and acute-phase proteins Induces synthesis of proinflammatory cytokines
IL-2	T cells	Primary T-cell growth factor Growth factor for B cells and NK cells
IL-4	Th2 cells Mast cells	Proliferation of activated Th2 and B cells B-cell differentiation and IgE isotype switching Antagonizes IFN-γ Inhibits Th1 responses
IL-5	Th2 cells Mast cells	Proliferation and differentiation of eosinophils
IL-6	Macrophages Th2 cells B cells Endothelial cells	Enhances B-cell differentiation and Ig secretion Induction of acute-phase proteins by liver Proinflammatory Proliferation of T cells and increased IL-2 receptor expression
IL-10	Tregs Bregs Macrophages	Inhibits T-cell and macrophage responses
IL-12	DCs Macrophages	Activates NK cells Induces Th1 responses
IL-13	Th2 cells	Stimulates B-cell growth Inhibits Th1 responses
IL-17	Th17 cells NK cells $\gamma\delta$ T cells Neutrophils	Proinflammatory Inhibits Tregs
IFN-α/β (Type I IFN)	Leukocytes DCs Fibroblasts	Induction of MHCI expression Antiviral activity Stimulation of NK cells
IFN-γ	T cells NK cells	Induction of MHCI and MHCII Activates macrophages
TGF-β	Macrophages Megakaryocytes T cells	Enhances monocyte/macrophage chemotaxis Enhances wound healing: angiogenesis, fibroblast Proliferation, deposition of extracellular matrix Inhibits T- and B-cell proliferation Inhibits antibody secretion Primary inducer of isotype switch to IgA
GM-CSF	T cells Macrophages Endothelial cells Fibroblasts	Stimulates growth and differentiation of monocytes and granulocytes

SOURCE: *Data from Murphy K: Janeway's Immunobiology. Garland Science Group, LLC, 8th edition: Taylor and Francis (2012).*

interaction of APCs, T cells, and B cells. CMI is that part of the acquired immune system in which effector cells, such as phagocytic cells, helper T cells, regulatory T cells, APCs, cytotoxic T cells, or T memory cells, play the critical role(s) without antibody involvement.

Cellular Components: Antigen-Presenting Cells, T Cells, and B Cells
APCs, which were discussed previously in the "Antigen Processing" section, include professional APCs such as B cells, macrophages, and DC. Although all cells may act as APCs with internal antigen processing through the MHCI pathway, what distinguishes a professional APC from the others is the ability to internalize external antigens and process them through the MHCII pathway for presentation to T cells.

B cells are not only capable of serving as professional APCs, but they are also the effector cells of humoral immunity, producing a number of Ig isotypes with varying specificities and affinities.

Like other immune cells, the B cell develops in the bone marrow from the HSC and becomes committed to the B-cell lineage when the cell begins to rearrange its Ig genes, as described in the "Antigen Recognition" section (Figs. 12-3 and 12-4). Following successful Ig rearrangement, these cells express heavy chains in their cytoplasm and are termed pre-B cells. Expression of membrane IgM and IgD indicates a mature B cell. B cells expressing CD5 (termed B-1 cells) predominate in embryonic life and are later found mostly in the intestinal mucosa (Hardy, 2006). These cells are probably associated with innate immunity and are long-lived, self-renewing cells that produce high levels of polyspecific IgM, much of which are autoantibodies suggesting a possible role of B-1 cell subtype in autoimmunity (Baumgarth, 2011). Mature B cells of the conventional B-2 subset are found in the lymph nodes, spleen, and peripheral blood. Upon antigen binding to surface immunoglobulin (part of the B-cell receptor [BCR]), the mature B cell becomes activated and, after proliferation, undergoes differentiation into either a memory B cell or an antibody-forming cell ([AFC]; also known as a plaque-forming cell [PFC]) that actively secretes antigen-specific antibody. A broad description of several B-cell characteristics can be found in Table 12-5.

At a specified time following their commitment to the T-cell lineage, T-cell precursors migrate from the bone marrow to the thymus where, in a manner analogous to B cells, they begin to rearrange their TCRs, as described in the "Antigen Recognition" section (Fig. 12-3). The TCR consists of two chains, either $\alpha\beta$ or $\gamma\delta$. The majority of T cells express the $\alpha\beta$ TCR, which is critical for the recognition of antigens in the context of MHC. A much smaller population of T cells express a $\gamma\delta$ TCR. The $\gamma\delta$ T cells differ from $\alpha\beta$ T cells in that they do not require antigen processing or presentation by MHC but instead directly bind intact host and pathogen proteins. Like the B-1 lineage, the $\gamma\delta$ T cells are expressed first in embryonic development and may be associated with innate immunity (see the "Innate Immunity" section). T cells committed to the $\alpha\beta$ lineage will express the surface marker cluster of differentiation antigens (CD) 4 and 8. CD4 and CD8 are coreceptors expressed by $\alpha\beta$ T cells and are involved in the interaction of the T cell with MHC. T cells expressing $\alpha\beta$ TCR and both CD4 and CD8 are termed immature double-positive cells (CD4$^+$/CD8$^+$). These immature cells then undergo positive and negative selection to (1) eliminate cells that do not produce a functional TCR or produce TCRs with no affinity for self-MHC (positive selection); or (2) eliminate cells that strongly bind MHC plus self-peptide (negative selection). Double-positive cells that survive positive and negative selection will give rise to NKT cells or T cells that lose expression of either CD4 or CD8 and enter the periphery as mature single-positive cells (CD4$^+$ or CD8$^+$) with a high level of $\alpha\beta$ TCR expression. This rigorous selection process produces T cells that can recognize MHC plus foreign peptides and eliminates autoreactive T cells. Additionally, expression of CD4 or CD8 will determine to which MHC class the $\alpha\beta$ TCR will bind. CD4 will facilitate binding to MHCII expressed on APCs; T cells expressing CD4 (helper T cells, Th) help activate other cells of the adaptive immune response. CD8 will facilitate binding to MHCI, which is expressed on all nucleated cells; generally, T cells expressing CD8 mediate cell killing (CTL). A broad description of several T-cell characteristics (specific to $\alpha\beta$ T cells) can be found in Table 12-5. In contrast to $\alpha\beta$ T cells, the $\gamma\delta$ T cells do not express CD4 or CD8 and therefore do not interact with MHC and do not undergo positive or negative selection. Since $\gamma\delta$ T cells are not negatively selected for autoreactivity, these cells may be associated with the development of hypersensitivity and autoimmunity.

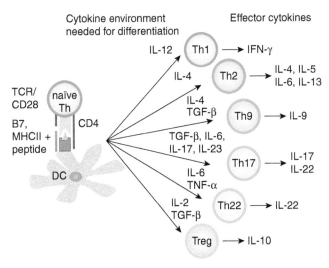

Cytokine environment needed for differentiation

Effector cytokines

Figure 12-8. *The cytokine environment drives different Th populations.* Various Th cells (and T regulatory cells, Tregs) are differentially induced in response to the cytokine milieu. Th1 cells drive CTL responses; Th2 cells drive humoral immune responses; Th9, Th17, and Th22 all produce proinflammatory cytokines; Tregs control other T-cell responses.

Mature T cells are found in the lymph nodes, spleen, and peripheral blood. Upon binding of the TCR to MHC plus antigen, the mature T cell becomes activated and, after proliferation, undergoes differentiation into either an effector cell or a memory T cell. Effector Th cells can subsequently differentiate into several phenotypes depending on the cytokine milieu (Fig. 12-8), two of which, Th1 and Th2, dictate whether CMI or humoral immunity will predominate, respectively. Th1 cells predominantly express IL-2, IFN-γ, and lymphotoxin, which promote CMI and humoral defense against intracellular invaders. Th2 cells predominantly express IL-3, IL-4, IL-5, IL-6, IL-10, and IL-13, which promote humoral defense against extracellular invaders. Although the two populations are not mutually exclusive, they do negatively regulate each other, such that a strong Th1 response suppresses a Th2 response and vice versa.

Th17, Th9, and Th22 cells have been shown to be critical for inflammatory responses (see the "Inflammation" section), and several studies including autoimmune models and clinical studies support a role of Th17 cells in inflammation and autoimmune diseases. Modulation of Th17 cellular function by xenobiotics may alter these disease states. Conversely, a better understanding of the relationship between Th17 and specific disease states may lead to new therapeutics in the treatment of autoimmune and inflammatory diseases (Hemdan *et al.*, 2010; Kimura and Kishimoto, 2011).

The ability of APCs, B cells, and T cells to communicate with each other is dependent on a variety of receptor–ligand interactions between cell types. These interactions also help dictate the type of immune response (ie, humoral vs. CMI) and the magnitude of the immune response. For example, TCR binding by antigen presented in the context of MHC is the major interaction that must occur between APCs and T cells to initiate an acquired immune response. Subsequent to this initial interaction, costimulatory molecules must be engaged on both the T cells and APCs to sustain and direct the immune response. One of the best-characterized interactions occurs between CD28 on the T cells and CD80 or CD86 (B7.1 and B7.2) on the APCs, which provides a more robust immune response as measured by clonal expansion and cytokine (eg, IL-2) production. Later in the response (two–three days), T cells express CTLA-4, which exhibits higher affinity for CD80/CD86 than does CD28, and

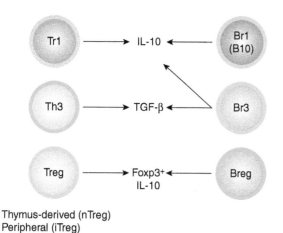

Thymus-derived (nTreg)
Peripheral (iTreg)

Figure 12-9. *Tregs and Bregs.* There are at least three different subpopulations of Tregs and Bregs, all of which suppress immune function via IL-10 or TGF-β. Tregs can be natural (thymus-derived) or induced in the periphery.

the CTLA-4–CD80/CD86 interaction serves to suppress the T-cell response. Other important interactions between APCs and T cells include CD40 and CD40 ligand (CD40L), which sustains clonal expansion and differentiation of the T cells and provides activation signals to the APC; inducible T-cell costimulator (ICOS [CD278], a member of the CD28-superfamily) and ligand for ICOS, which sustains clonal expansion and differentiation of the T cells and induces IL-10 production; and 4-1BB (CD137/Ly63, a member of the TNF receptor superfamily) and 4-1BB ligand, which sustains clonal expansion of the T cells and helps to activate the APC (CD40 ligand, ICOS, and 4-1BB are expressed on T cells). Therapeutic agents that bind some of these costimulatory surface molecules have been developed and utilized clinically to suppress immune function for transplantation and autoimmune therapy, which will be discussed in "Therapeutic Agents" under the "Immune Modulation by Xenobiotics" section. For simplicity, in figures throughout the chapter, only the CD28–B7 interaction is depicted.

The duration and extent of an acquired immune response is also controlled by specialized regulatory cells found in both the T-cell and B-cell lineages, and there are considerable functional similarities between the different regulatory subsets found within both lineages (reviewed by Noh and Lee, 2011) (Figs. 12-8 and 12-9). For the T-cell lineage, there is a small population of CD4+ cells that develop into T-regulatory cells (Tregs), which help to control various immune responses, including those directed against self. Tregs are generally identified as CD4+CD25+Foxp3+, which are defined as natural Tregs if they develop in the thymus (Lio and Hsieh, 2011), but can also be induced in the periphery in response to IL-2 and TGF-β (Horwitz *et al.*, 2008). Tregs can suppress CD4+ and CD8+ IL-2 production and proliferation, and in vivo have been shown to suppress autoimmune disease (Sakaguchi *et al.*, 2009). The mechanisms by which Tregs suppress immune responses involve direct Treg-cell contact since Tregs are unable to suppress immune function when separated from the target cell population by a semipermeable membrane or when Treg-conditioned medium is used (Takahashi *et al.*, 1998; Thornton and Shevach, 1998). Immune suppression by Tregs is likely a multistep process, which might involve direct cell killing via granzyme or perforin, induction of intracellular cAMP, or affecting cell surface expression of critical proteins, such as CD80/CD86. For instance, Foxp3 induces high levels of CTLA-4, which would interact with target cell CD80/CD86 and prevent target cell CD80/CD86 from interacting with CD28 on other stimulatory cells (reviewed by Sakaguchi *et al.*, 2009). It has also been suggested that the high expression level of CD25 on Tregs

might act as a reservoir for IL-2 in an immune synapse microenvironment, thereby preventing IL-2 from stimulating surrounding cells (Sakaguchi *et al.*, 2009). In addition to Tregs, other regulatory T-cell subsets have been identified such as the IL-10 producing Tr1 cells and the TGF-β producing Th3 cells; all three regulatory subsets appear to be involved in regulating immune responses (Noh and Lee, 2011). Regardless of the processes that direct Treg (or perhaps Tr1 and Th3) suppression of immune function, their induction has been identified as one mechanism by which drugs and xenobiotics might result in immune suppression (Marshall and Kerkvliet, 2010; Ohkura *et al.*, 2011). Like the regulatory T cells, several subsets of regulatory B cells are emerging and several recent reviews have been devoted to outlining the experimental evidence for specific regulatory B-cell subpopulations and their generally suppressive role in hypersensitivity and autoimmune diseases (DiLillo *et al.*, 2010; Mauri, 2010; Noh and Lee, 2011). Although phenotypically diverse, regulatory B cells appear to have arisen from the CD5 B-1 population (briefly described above). Noh and Lee (2011) have described three subsets of regulatory B cells based on cytokine or Foxp3 expression, which include Br1 or B10 cells that produce IL-10, Br3 that produce TGF-β, and Breg that express Foxp3. These subsets resemble the regulatory T-cell subsets, Tr1, Th3, and Treg, respectively (Fig. 12-9 adapted from Noh and Lee, 2011). The regulatory T- and B-cell subsets also appear to reciprocally activate or suppress each other and may cooperatively control immune responses. The interplay between regulatory T- and B-cell subsets and their impact on immune responses, including autoimmune and hypersensitivity diseases, are important areas of investigation that will likely lead to a better understanding of immune pathologies including those induced by drugs and other xenobiotics.

Humoral and Cell-Mediated Immunity As described earlier, there are two branches of acquired immunity, humoral immunity, and CMI. Humoral immunity is that part of the acquired immune system in which antibody is involved. In general, B cells produce antibodies specific to an antigen, which may act to opsonize or neutralize the invader, or the antibodies act to recruit other factors, such as the complement cascade. CMI is that part of the immune system in which various effector cells perform a wide variety of functions to eliminate invaders. Often, these two branches are coordinated, such as activation of Th cells that produce specific cytokines that enhance B-cell proliferation and differentiation to secrete more antibody. A general diagram of the cellular interactions involved in a humoral immune response is given in Fig. 12-10. The production of antigen-specific IgM requires three to five days after the primary (initial) exposure to antigen (Fig. 12-11). Upon secondary antigenic challenge, the B cells undergo isotype switching, producing primarily IgG antibody, which is of higher affinity for the activating antigen. In addition, there is a higher serum antibody titer associated with a secondary antibody response. CMI functions include delayed-type hypersensitivity (DTH) and cell-mediated cytotoxicity. Cell-mediated cytotoxicity responses may occur in numerous ways: (1) MHC-dependent recognition of specific antigens (such as viral particles or tumor proteins) by CTL (Fig. 12-12); (2) indirect antigen-specific recognition by the binding of Fc receptors on NK cells to antibodies coating target cells; and (3) receptor-mediated recognition of complement-coated foreign targets by macrophages. Many of these are described in more detail in "Hypersensitivity" under the section entitled "Immune-Mediated Disease"

In cell-mediated cytotoxicity, the CTL or NK effector cell binds in a specific manner to the target cell. The majority of CTLs express CD8 and recognize either foreign MHCI on the surface of allogeneic cells, or antigen in association with self-MHCI (eg, viral

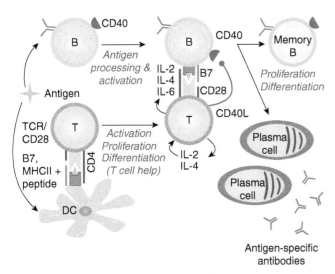

Figure 12-10. *Cellular interactions in the humoral immune response.* Antigen is engulfed by an APC (usually DC) and the antigenic peptide is presented to CD4⁺ T cells in the context of MHCII. CD4⁺ T cells then become activated, proliferate, and differentiate into Th cells, which release cytokines to help B cells that had also encountered the same antigen. B cells then become activated, proliferate, and differentiate into memory B cells or antigen-producing plasma cells.

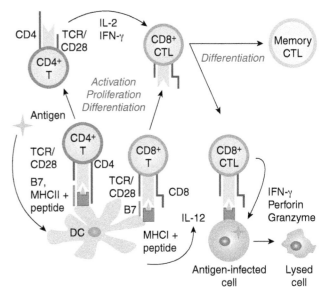

Figure 12-12. *Cellular interactions in the CTL response.* Antigen is engulfed by an APC (usually DC) and the antigenic peptide is presented to CD4⁺ and CD8⁺ T cells in the context of MHCII and I, respectively. CD4⁺ T cells then become activated, proliferate, and differentiate into Th cells, which release cytokines to help CD8⁺ T cells that had also encountered the same antigen. Especially in the presence of IL-12 produced by the DC, CD8⁺ T cells become activated, proliferate, and differentiate into CTL that can kill other antigen-infected cells.

particles). Fig. 12-12 shows the cell-mediated CTL response. NK cell recognition of target cells is also antigen-specific because the mechanism of recognition involves binding of Fc receptors on NK cells to the Fc portion of antigen-specific antibody that coats the target cell; a process referred to as ADCC. Once the CTL or NK cells interact with the target cell, the effector cell undergoes cytoplasmic reorientation so that cytolytic granules are oriented along the side of the effector, which is bound to the target. The effector cell then releases the contents of these granules onto the target cell. The target cell may be damaged by the perforins or enzymatic contents of the cytolytic granules. In addition, CTLs induce the target to undergo apoptosis through activation of the Fas and cytotoxic cytokine (ie, TNF and lymphotoxin) pathways. Once it has degranulated, the effector cell can release the dying target and move on to kill other target cells. Notably, many of the soluble factors critical to the innate immune system are also primary effectors in the acquired immune system, including ROS, granzyme, perforin, cytokines, and IFNs, again demonstrating the interplay among the various arms of the immune system.

Inflammation

Inflammation, simply defined, refers to a complex reaction to injury, irritation or foreign invaders characterized by pain, swelling, redness, and heat. Inflammation involves various stages, including release of chemotactic factors following the insult, increased blood flow, increased capillary permeability allowing for cellular infiltration, followed by either an acute resolution of tissue damage or persistence of the response that might contribute to fibrosis or subsequent organ failure (Serhan and Savill, 2005). It is important to emphasize that while inflammation is a natural reaction to repair tissue damage or attack foreign invaders, the process often results in destruction of adjacent cells and/or tissues. Thus, there is overwhelming evidence that inflammation plays a critical role in many diseases, including asthma, multiple sclerosis, cardiovascular disease, Alzheimer's disease, bowel disorders, and cancer. In addition, inflammation exacerbates idiosyncratic reactions to drugs and other chemicals (reviewed by Ganey *et al.*, 2004).

Cellular Components: Macrophages, Neutrophils, and T Cells Many of the cellular components described in the sections above are critical to initiation and maintenance of an inflammatory response. Major cellular contributors to an inflammatory response are macrophages, neutrophils, and T cells. Neutrophils are often the first, and most numerous, responders to sites of insult. In response to either host- or pathogen-derived signals, neutrophils secrete chemotactic factors to recruit other proinflammatory cells, such as macrophages, to the area. Recently, it has been demonstrated that IL-17 produced early by various sources, including NKT cells, is a critical proinflammatory cytokine that will rapidly induce neutrophil and macrophage influx to the area of insult (Vanaudenaerde *et al.*, 2011). Macrophages can be activated by a variety of mechanisms at the site of insult, such as activation via TLR, proinflammatory cytokines, or recognition of opsonized particles by Fc receptors or complement receptors. Macrophages and neutrophils also induce apoptosis of cells in the insult area

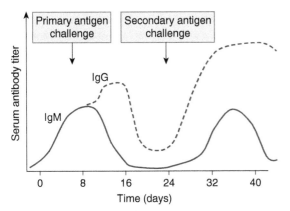

Figure 12-11. *Kinetics of humoral immune responses.* In response to primary antigen encounter, IgM is produced within several days. In response to secondary antigen encounter, IgG is produced more rapidly, and to a higher magnitude, than IgM.

through the release of nitric oxide and other ROS, resulting in disruption of extracellular structures that compromise tissue structure and function (reviewed by Duffield 2003). Both neutrophils and macrophages are phagocytic cells and can contribute to clearing of apoptotic cells. Later in the inflammatory response, T cells are critical for generating an adaptive immune response. T cells are attracted to the insult area by adhesion molecules and integrins, and are activated in response to antigen presented in the context of MHC, often by a DC. As described above, depending on the signals that the T cell receives from the cytokine milieu, distinct subpopulations of T cells are induced (Fig. 12-8). Chronic inflammatory states are maintained with activation and differentiation of Th2 and Th17, which drive chronic eosinophilic and neutrophilic inflammation, respectively (Jutel and Akdis, 2011). Th9 and Th22 cells also likely contribute to chronic inflammation, but their roles are not yet completely understood.

Of all Th subsets, Th17 cells have certainly been shown to play a critical role in inflammation (Kimura and Kishimoto, 2011). In contrast to cells involved in the innate response (NK or NKT cells, γδ T cells, or other iLCs) that produce IL-17, Th17 cells are part of the adaptive immune response, and produce IL-17, IL-22, and TNF-α (Vanaudenaerde et al., 2011). They are induced in the presence of IL-6 and TGF-β, conditions that are unfavorable for Tregs, thereby exacerbating the proinflammatory response through suppression of Treg differentiation and chronic neutrophilic infiltration (Awasthi and Kuchroo, 2009). Th17 cells are defined by expression of retinoid-related orphan receptors RORγ and RORα. Interestingly, Th17 cells also express high levels of aryl hydrocarbon receptor ([AHR]; Veldhoen et al., 2008), providing an additional cellular target for immune modulation by AHR ligands (see the subsection "Polychlorinated Dibenzodioxins" under "Immune Modulation by Xenobiotics").

There are several other soluble factors that contribute to inflammation that warrant discussion. In addition to ROS that are released from both macrophages and neutrophils to compromise membrane integrity, a plethora of cytokines and chemokines contribute to the inflammatory process. As mentioned above in the "Innate Immunity" section, some proinflammatory cytokines (IL-1β and IL-18) are produced in a mature form as a result of the activation of the inflammasome (Martinon et al., 2009). In fact, it has been demonstrated that inflammation as a result of disease (ie, influenza) or toxicity (ie, silicosis) depends on inflammasome activation (Cassel et al., 2008; Ichinohe et al., 2009). An additional discussion for the role of the inflammasome in immune responses to inhaled particles is provided in the subsection "Inhaled Substances" under "Immune Modulation by Xenobiotics" and in Fig. 12-22. The actions of various proinflammatory cytokines include inducing fever or activating T cells and macrophages (IL-1); stimulating B- or T-cell proliferation (IL-6); inducing neutrophilia (IL-17); and increasing vascular permeability or inducing apoptosis (TNF-α). Many proinflammatory cytokines also induce acute-phase proteins, such as C-reactive protein. C-reactive protein binds to several ligands, including phosphatidylcholine on the membranes of cells, Fc receptors, and C1q (part of the complement C1 complex), which activates the classical complement cascade (reviewed by Marnell et al., 2005). Complement participates in inflammation through inappropriate and sustained activation of the cascade, ultimately leading to destruction of cells through the MAC (Fig. 12-6). Furthermore, complement fragments, such as C3a and C5a, act as chemotactic factors to recruit other phagocytic cells to sites of insult (macrophages, neutrophils, eosinophils, or mast cells) or induce degranulation (basophils, eosinophils, or mast cells) (Dunkelberger and Song, 2010). Finally, prostaglandins and other eicosanoids possess various

proinflammatory actions, including increased blood flow and pain (prostaglandin E2), increase in vascular permeability (prostacyclin I2), and stimulation of endothelial inflammatory responses (thromboxane A2) (reviewed by Ricciotti and FitzGerald, 2011). Prostaglandins contribute to hyperalgesia and it is for this reason that cyclooxygenase-2, which converts arachidonic acid to other bioactive prostaglandins, is an attractive therapeutic target to reduce inflammation and pain (see the subsection "Anti-inflammatory Agents" under "Immune modulation by Xenobiotics").

As mentioned above, it is undisputed that chronic inflammation plays a critical role in many disease states, including asthma, multiple sclerosis, cardiovascular disease, Alzheimer's disease, bowel disorders, and cancer. Chronic inflammation could result in high circulating levels of proinflammatory cytokines, complement fragments, prostaglandins, and thromboxanes. An inflammatory cascade can be established because many of these mediators induce expression of others (ie, TNF-α induces expression of IL-1 and IL-6 or complement fragment C3a causes chemotaxis of phagocytic cells). Moreover, the sustained presence of proinflammatory cytokines could exacerbate ROS production from neutrophils and macrophages. As seen in the next section, the underlying proinflammatory response also plays a critical role in immune-mediated disease.

Immune-Mediated Disease

As stated earlier, the purpose of the immune system is to preserve the integrity of the individual from disease states, whether infectious, parasitic, or cancerous, through both cellular and humoral mechanisms. In so doing, the ability to distinguish self from nonself plays a predominant role. However, situations arise in which the individual's immune system responds in a manner producing tissue damage, resulting in a self-induced disease. These disease states fall into two categories: (1) hypersensitivity, or allergy, and (2) autoimmunity. Hypersensitivity reactions result from the immune system responding in an exaggerated or inappropriate manner after repeated exposure to the offending antigen. These reactions have been subdivided by Coombs and Gell (1975) into four types, which represent four different mechanisms leading to tissue damage. In the case of autoimmunity, mechanisms involve a break down in self-recognition resulting in the production of autoreactive antibodies and/or TCRs recognizing self-antigens as nonself, ultimately culminating in tissue damage and disease.

Hypersensitivity
Classification of Hypersensitivity Reactions One characteristic common to all four types of hypersensitivity reactions is the necessity of prior exposure leading to sensitization in order to elicit a reaction upon subsequent challenge. In the case of Types I, II, and III, prior exposure to antigen leads to the production of allergen-specific antibodies (IgE, IgM, or IgG) and, in the case of Type IV, the generation of allergen-specific memory T cells. Fig. 12-13 illustrates the mechanisms of hypersensitivity reactions as classified by Coombs and Gell. Although not completely understood, regulation of Ig production is dependent in part on the characteristics of the antigen, the genetics of the individual, and environmental factors. The mechanisms of antibody production in hypersensitivity reactions are identical to those described earlier in the chapter (Fig. 12-10). A brief description of the four types of hypersensitivity reactions is presented below.

Type I (Immediate or IgE-Mediated Hypersensitivity) Using penicillin as an example, Fig. 12-14 depicts the major events involved in a Type I hypersensitivity reaction (what most people

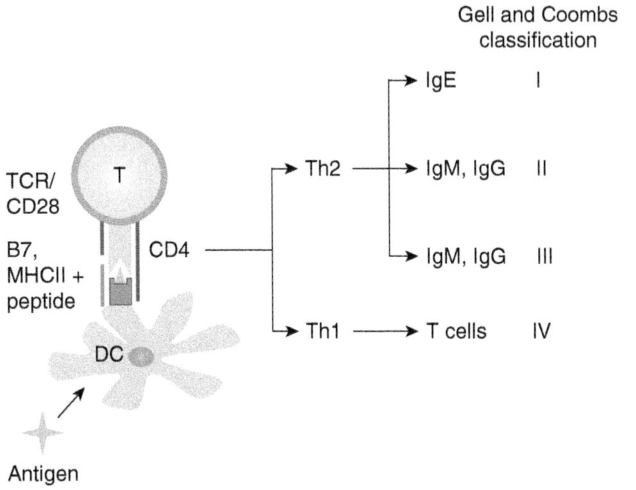

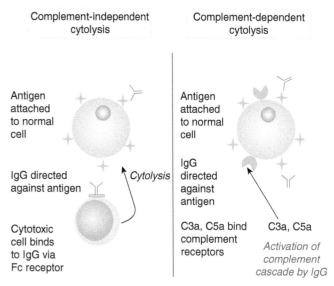

Figure 12-13. *Overview of classification of hypersensitivity reactions.* Hypersensitivity reactions are mediated via T cells and antibody production.

think of as "allergy" and is clinically referred to as "atopy"). Sensitization occurs as the result of dermal exposure to antigens or by exposure to antigens through the respiratory or gastrointestinal tract. Most people would mount an IgM, IgG, or IgA immune response to these antigens and clear them without causing any allergic symptoms. It is unclear why these antigens become allergens in certain individuals who respond by mounting an IgE immune response instead, but appears to involve genetic and/or environmental determinants and likely some type of triggering event (eg, acute pathogen exposure and emotional stress). IgE production is highest in lymphatic tissues that drain sites of exposure (ie, tonsils, bronchial lymph nodes, and intestinal lymphatic tissues, including Peyer's patches) and is low in the spleen. Compared to other Igs, IgE has a low serum concentration and a short serum half-life (Table 12-4). Once produced, soluble IgE not only binds to local tissue mast cells, but also enters the circulation, where it binds to circulating mast cells, basophils, and tissue mast cells at distant sites. Once an individual is sensitized, reexposure to the antigen results in

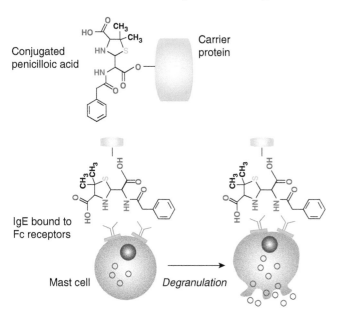

Figure 12-14. *Type I hypersensitivity reaction.* Metabolized penicillin is a hapten that conjugates with a protein. The conjugated hapten cross-links IgE antibodies on mast cells. IgE cross-linking causes mast-cell degranulation and releasing histamine and other proinflammatory mediators.

Figure 12-15. *Type II hypersensitivity reactions.* In complement-independent cytolysis, antigen becomes attached to a normal cell, which can be recognized by IgG. A cell capable of cytolysis (CTL, NK cell) binds to IgG via its Fc receptor and kills the antigen-coated cell. In complement-dependent cytolysis, antigen becomes attached to a normal cell, which can be recognized by IgG. Complement gets activated by the classical pathway (antigen–antibody complexes) and C3a and C5a bind complement receptors.

binding to IgE on local mast cells and degranulation with the release of preformed mediators and cytokines which recruit and activate circulating eosinophils, basophils, macrophages, and neutrophils leading to the synthesis and release of more cytokines and of leukotrienes and thromboxanes. These mediators promote vasodilation, bronchial constriction, and inflammation. Clinical manifestations can vary from urticarial skin reactions (wheals and flares) to signs of hay fever, including rhinitis and conjunctivitis, to more serious diseases, such as asthma and potentially life-threatening anaphylaxis. These responses may begin within minutes of reexposure to the offending antigen; therefore, Type I hypersensitivity is often referred to as immediate hypersensitivity.

Type II (Antibody-Dependent Cytotoxic Hypersensitivity)
Type II hypersensitivity is IgG or IgM-mediated. The antibody response may be mediated by a foreign antigen attached to the surface of a cell or tissue. Conversely, an antibody response could be mediated by an autoantibody due to a breakdown in tolerance and the resulting response would be part of an autoimmune disease (eg, autoimmune hemolytic anemias and Goodpasture's syndrome). Fig. 12-15 shows the mechanisms of action for complement-independent and complement-dependent cytotoxic reactions. Tissue damage may result from the direct action of cytotoxic cells, such as macrophages, neutrophils, or eosinophils, linked through the Fc receptor to antibody-coated target cells (complement-independent) or by antibody-induced activation of the classic complement pathway. Complement activation may result in C3b binding to the target cell surface with C3b acting as a recognition site for effector cells. Alternatively, the C5b-9 MAC may be bound to the target cell surface, resulting in direct cell lysis.

Type III (Immune Complex-Mediated Hypersensitivity) Type III hypersensitivity reactions also involve IgG or IgM. The distinguishing feature of Type III is that, unlike Type II, in which Ig production is against specific cellular or tissue-associated antigen, Ig production is against soluble antigen in the serum (Fig. 12-16). This allows for the formation of circulating immune complexes

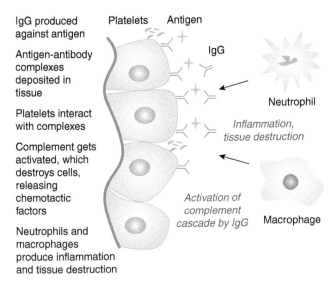

Figure 12-16. *Type III hypersensitivity reactions.* IgG is produced against an antigen and antigen–antibody complexes form, which can become deposited in tissue. Complement gets activated by the classical pathway (antigen–antibody complexes), and platelets also interact with complexes. Following complement-mediated cytolysis, released chemotactic factors attract neutrophils and macrophages, causing additional inflammation and tissue damage.

composed of a lattice of antigen and Ig, which may result in widely distributed tissue damage in areas where immune complexes are deposited. The most common location is the vascular endothelium in the lung, joints, and kidneys. The skin and circulatory systems may also be involved. Pathology results from the inflammatory response initiated by the activation of complement. Macrophages, neutrophils, and platelets attracted to the deposition site contribute to the tissue damage. As with Type II hypersensitivity, responses similar to Type III hypersensitivity can be induced in autoimmune diseases due to autoantibodies directed against soluble antigens such as double-stranded DNA or small nuclear proteins as seen with SLE.

Type IV (Cell-Mediated Hypersensitivity) Type IV, or DTH responses, can be divided into three classes: contact hypersensitivity, tuberculin-type hypersensitivity, and hypersensitivity pneumonitis. The following discussion is focused on contact hypersensitivity using the classical example of contact hypersensitivity seen following poison ivy exposure. Contact hypersensitivity is initiated by topical exposure, and the associated pathology is primarily epidermal. It is characterized clinically by an eczematous reaction at the site of allergen contact and, like Type I through III responses, consists of two phases: sensitization and elicitation. However, in this case sensitization is the result of the development of activated and memory T cells as opposed to antibody production (Figs. 12-17 and 12-18). Sensitization occurs when a hapten penetrates the epidermis and forms a complex with a protein carrier. The hapten–carrier complex is processed by Langerhan's DCs that migrate out of the epidermis to the local lymph nodes. There, the APC presents the processed antigen to CD4+ Th cells, leading to clonal expansion and the generation of memory T cells including memory CD8+ CTL, (Tc) which appear to play a major role in the elicitation phase.

Upon secondary contact, Langerhan's DCs present the processed hapten–carrier complex to memory CD8+ CTL in either the skin or the lymph nodes. These activated T cells then secrete cytokines that bring about further proliferation of T cells and generation of CTLs, as well as increased expression of adhesion molecules on the surface of keratinocytes and endothelial cells in the dermis.

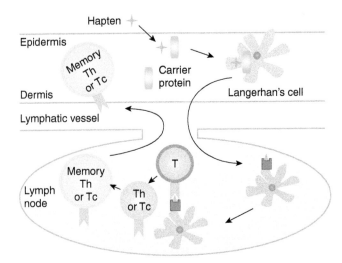

Figure 12-17. *Type IV hypersensitivity sensitization.* A hapten permeates the epidermis and forms a complex with a carrier protein. The conjugated hapten gets engulfed by Langerhan's cells, which migrate to the lymph node and present antigen to CD4+ T cells in the context of MHCII. CD4+ T cells activate, proliferate, and differentiate into Th or Tc cells and memory T cells.

Both the expression of adhesion molecules and the secretion of proinflammatory cytokines by T cells and keratinocytes facilitate the recruitment of inflammatory cells into the skin, resulting in erythema and the formation of papules and vesicles. In addition and under certain circumstances, intracellular proteins can be modified by lipid-soluble chemicals that might readily cross the cell membrane. These cells then present modified peptides on their cell surface in conjunction with MHCI molecules. CD8+ cytotoxic T cells recognize these foreign peptides and cause tissue damage by either direct cytotoxic action (CTL) or the secretion of cytokines that further promote the inflammatory response.

Autoimmunity Autoimmune disease occurs when the reactions of the immune system are directed against the body's own tissues, and, as with hypersensitivity, is characterized by a genetic susceptibility. Autoimmune diseases may be tissue-specific, where the damage is associated with a specific type of tissue or a specific organ, or tissue-nonspecific, where the signs and symptoms

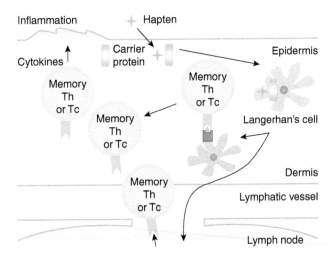

Figure 12-18. *Type IV hypersensitivity elicitation.* Upon secondary exposure to the hapten, Langerhan's cells either migrate to the lymph node or directly present antigen to memory T cells. Memory T cells become activated and produce cytokines to stimulate proinflammatory cytokine release from other cell types, such as keratinocytes.

are associated with several organs and tissues. The targets from the perspective of the primary sites of tissue damage in autoimmune disease are many and varied. The following organs, cells, and organelles have all been determined to be the site of autoimmune reactions: nuclei (specifically histones and/or single-stranded DNA—one of the hallmark indicators of certain types of autoimmune disease is the expression of antinuclear antibodies), red blood cells, lymphocytes, neutrophils, platelets, Igs (primarily IgG), striated muscle (cholinergic receptors), smooth muscle, mitochondria, skin (basement membranes), thyroid (thyroglobulin), kidney (glomerular and tubular basement membrane), CNS (myelin), connective tissue (synovial lining of joints), lung, and liver. Both humoral immunity and CMI can be involved as effector mechanisms in causing the damage in autoimmune conditions. Examples of autoimmune diseases include (1) myasthenia gravis, in which cholinergic receptors, especially those associated with neuromuscular junctions, are targeted; (2) multiple sclerosis, in which myelin is targeted; and (3) rheumatoid arthritis, in which connective tissue, especially the synovial lining of joints, is targeted. The terms "hypersensitivity" and "autoimmunity" are often confused and are certainly interrelated. Based on their definitions, a hypersensitivity response can be a mechanism by which an autoimmune disease is produced.

In the section on hypersensitivity presented above, two mechanisms by which host tissues are damaged by the host's own immune system were discussed (Types II and III), creating autoimmune-like disease. In these situations, unaltered self-antigens are not the target of the immune mechanisms, but damage occurs to cells bearing hapten on membranes or to innocent bystander cells in close proximity to antigen–antibody complexes. For example, damage produced in autoimmune Goodpasture's disease is similar to that seen in Type III hypersensitivity reactions in the lung due to trimellitic anhydride (TMA) exposure. Although the resulting pathology may be the same for autoimmune reactions and hypersensitivity, mechanisms of true autoimmune disease are distinguished from hypersensitivity. In cases of autoimmunity, self-antigens are the target, and in the case of chemical-induced autoimmunity, the disease state is induced by a modification of host tissues or immune cells by the chemical and not the chemical acting as an antigen/hapten as in hypersensitivity reactions.

Mechanisms of Autoimmunity As discussed earlier, the rearrangement and recombination of the genes that comprise Ig and TCR result in tremendous diversity in the potential antigen recognition of B cells and T cells, respectively. Ideally, during development those lymphocytes recognizing self-antigens will largely be deleted by negative selection as central tolerance is established. Autoreactive clones that escape central tolerance and migrate to the periphery are normally controlled by peripheral tolerance mediated by various mechanisms that ultimately induce anergy or clonal deletion. For autoimmune disease to occur, an autoreactive clone must escape central tolerance, pass into the periphery, and bind with specificity to its self-antigen then mechanisms of peripheral tolerance must fail and the autoreactive clone must induce a detrimental immunological response. Clearly, induction of autoimmunity is multifaceted and likewise has been associated with several mechanisms primarily related to insufficient peripheral tolerance. Conversely, defects in central tolerance are rarely encountered. However, an example of autoimmunity due to defective central tolerance is the disease autoimmune polyendocrinopathy candidiasis ectodermal dystrophy, which results from a defective transcriptional regulator called autoimmune regulator (AIRE). For the negative selection process in the thymus, AIRE induces the

expression of a wide variety of self-antigens normally found in the periphery. Loss of AIRE results in release of autoreactive T cells to the periphery. Several mechanisms have been associated with the breakdown of peripheral tolerance and prime events for the onset of autoimmune disease. These mechanisms include inflammation; molecular mimicry by pathogen antigens; inherent defects in T or B cells including regulatory subsets, APCs, cytokines, or complement; and epitope spreading. For example, increasing evidence supports a potential breakdown of peripheral tolerance during an inflammatory response, which may be mediated by the inappropriate maturation of immature DCs that process both pathogenic antigens and self-antigens released during the inflammatory response. Self-antigens could then be presented to naive autoreactive T cells via MHC. With molecular mimicry, a pathogen presents epitopes that resemble those on self-antigens and because the pathogen will induce a strong inflammatory response, peripheral tolerance may be overridden. Defects in immune system components, such as complement, could reduce C3b-mediated clearance of self-antigen and autoantibody immune complexes (described in Types II and III hypersensitivity). Additionally, interference of normal immune regulation by Tregs or Bregs could create an environment conducive to autoimmune disease. Finally, epitope spreading may occur during an immune response due to tissue damage and the release of new epitopes that were hidden either because they were sequestered from the immune system or their expression levels were insufficient to induce negative selection or peripheral tolerance mechanisms.

Effector mechanisms involved in autoimmune disease can be the same as those described earlier for Types II and III hypersensitivity or, in the case of pathology associated with solid tissues, including organs, they may involve CD8+ CTL. Tissue damage associated with CTL may be the result of direct cell membrane damage and lysis, or the result of cytokines produced and released by the T cell. TNF-β has the ability to kill susceptible cells, and IFN-γ may increase the expression of MHCI on cell surfaces, making them more susceptible to CD8+ cells. Cytokines may also be chemotactic for macrophages, which can cause tissue damage directly or indirectly through the release of proinflammatory cytokines. As is the case with hypersensitivity reactions, autoimmune disease is often the result of more than one mechanism working simultaneously. Therefore, pathology may be the result of direct or indirect effects of CTL, antibody-dependent cytotoxicity, or complement-dependent antibody-mediated lysis.

Developmental Immunology

A sequential series of carefully timed and coordinated developmental events, beginning early in embryonic/fetal life and continuing through the early postnatal period, is required to establish a functional immune system in all mammals, including humans. The immune system develops initially from a population of pluripotent HSCs that are generated early in gestation from uncommitted mesenchymal stem cells in the intraembryonic splanchnopleure surrounding the heart. This early population of HSCs gives rise to all circulating blood cell lineages, including cells of the immune system, via migration through an orderly series of tissues, and a dynamic process that involves continual differentiation of lineage-restricted stem cells. Lymphoid-hematopoietic progenitor cells are established via the migration of these cells from intraembryonic mesenchyme to fetal liver and fetal spleen, and ultimately, the relocation of these cells in late gestation to bone marrow and thymus. The latter two organs are the primary sites of lymphopoiesis and appear to be unique in providing the microenvironment factors necessary for the development of functionally competent immune cells. These lineage-restricted stem cells expand to form a pool of highly proliferative progenitor cells that are capable of continual renewal of short-lived functional immunocompetent cells, and that ultimately provide the necessary cellular capacity for effective immune responsiveness, and the necessary breadth of the immune repertoire (Good, 1995).

It is important to recognize that immune system development does not cease at birth, and that immunocompetent cells continue to be produced from proliferating progenitor cells in the bone marrow and thymus. Mature immunocompetent cells leave these primary immune organs and migrate via the blood to the secondary immune organs: spleen, lymph nodes, and mucosal lymphoid tissues. Because birth occurs at various stages of fetal maturity, the significance of parturition as a landmark in the development of the immune system can vary from species to species (Holsapple et al., 2003). As such, direct comparison of immune functional development between humans and animals is complicated by differences in the maturity of the immune system before and after parturition. This difference has been linked to the length of gestation (Holladay and Smialowicz, 2000) in that animals with short gestation periods (eg, mice, rats, rabbits, and hamsters) have relatively immature immune systems at birth compared to humans. The onset of functional immune competence depends on the specific parameter being measured, and varies across species with striking differences noted between rodents and humans (Holsapple et al., 2003). The consensus in the scientific and regulatory arenas is that the immune system of children continues to develop postnatally until 5 to 12 years of age (Miyawaki et al., 1981). Exposure to specific antigens during the perinatal period results in a rapidly expanding accumulation of lymphocyte specificities in the pool of memory cells in secondary lymphoid tissues. As thymic function wanes and thymocytes are no longer produced in that tissue, it is this pool of memory B and T cells that maintains immune competence for the life of the individual. Senescence of immunity is associated with reductions in both innate and acquired immune responses to antigens during the last quartile of life. This failure of the immune response is due, in part, to a continual reduction in the production of newly formed cells, and to the decreased survival of long-lived memory cells in lymphoid tissues. The concept of immune senescence is discussed further below.

One feature of the developing immune system that clearly distinguishes it from the mature immune system, especially during gestation, is the role played by organogenesis. Defects in the development of the immune system due to heritable changes in the lymphoid elements have provided clinical and experimental examples of the devastating consequences of impaired immune development (Rosen et al., 1995). Therefore, the effects of chemicals on the genesis of critical immune organs in the developing fetus may be more important than effects on these tissues after having been populated by hematopoietic and lymphoid cells. However, a chemical that induces this kind of developmental structural abnormality in the fetus would legitimately be classified as a teratogen, prompting the question as to how many known teratogens would have an impact on organs essential to the normal functioning of the immune system. Interestingly, immune organs, such as the thymus, spleen, and/ or bone marrow, are not typically assessed in routine developmental and reproductive toxicology studies, and it has been noted that this failure to assess developmental damage to the immune system in standard developmental and reproductive toxicology protocols should be reevaluated (Holsapple et al., 2003). Additional perspectives on the methods to assess developmental immunotoxicology (DIT) and on the emergence of regulatory guidelines that include developmental immunotoxicity testing strategies are included elsewhere in this chapter.

At the other end of the spectrum from the development of the immune system during gestation and the perinatal period is the status of the immune system in the aging population. Unlike DIT, there have been very few studies that have addressed the impact of specific xenobiotics on the aging immune system. Nonetheless, it is known that the immune system of older people is usually perceived as declining in fidelity and efficiency with age resulting in an increased susceptibility to infectious diseases and pathological conditions relating to inflammation (eg, cardiovascular disease and Alzheimer's disease) or autoreactivity (eg, rheumatoid arthritis) (Caruso et al., 2009). Immune senescence has been defined as the impairment in immunity as a result of age-associated changes in function in a variety of cell types. It is a phenomenon of decreased function, involving changes in both innate and adaptive immunity, and a disbalance between the two arms (Pawelec et al., 2010). Virtually, all components of the immune system are affected (Ongradi and Kovesdi, 2010). The decline in the B-cell compartment is responsible for the decreased effectiveness of vaccines in older people; and the decline in immune surveillance (eg, the T-cell compartment and NK-cell function) is associated with an increased incidence in malignancy. Additionally, aging has been associated with a shift from the Th1 to the Th2 cytokine profile in response to immune stimulation, and the overproduction of Th2 cytokines could augment B-cell production of autoreactive antibodies. Studies in humans and mice have shown that TLR expression and function decline with age resulting in the decreased production of proinflammatory cytokines and chemokines. From a mechanistic standpoint, a number of factors have been proposed as contributing to the onset and severity of immune senescence including: the accumulation of damage to lymphocytes by oxidative stress, persistent microbial infections with immunosuppressive viruses that establish latency, such as cytomegalovirus and Epstein–Barr virus, and lifestyle factors such as smoking, alcohol use, and poor nutrition. An improved understanding of immune dysfunction in human aging will increase the probability of discovering means to restore appropriate function and alleviate the burden of infectious disease later in life (Ongradi and Kovesdi, 2010).

Neuroendocrine Immunology

There is overwhelming evidence that cytokines, neuropeptides, neurotransmitters, and hormones, as well as their receptors, are an integral and interregulated part of the CNS, the endocrine system, and the immune system (reviewed by Sanders and Kohm, 2002). Because receptors for neuropeptides, neurotransmitters, and hormones are present on lymphoid cells, it is reasonable to suspect that some chemicals may exert their immunomodulatory effects indirectly on the immune system by acting to modulate the activity of the nervous or endocrine systems. In addition, immune cells are capable of secreting, and do secrete, peptide hormones and neurotransmitters, which can have autocrine (immune system) and paracrine (endocrine and nervous systems) effects. Similar to the complexity of the cytokine network, the effects of various hormones and neurotransmitters are too vast to discuss here. However, it is evident, even from this brief overview of the immune system and its potential interaction with other biological systems, that immune responses are complex processes involving multiple cell types and mediators. It is not difficult to imagine then, that perturbation of leukocyte functions including the mediators they produce by drugs or chemicals could contribute to the mechanisms by which a compound is immunotoxic.

CHAPTER 12

ASSESSMENT OF IMMUNOLOGICAL INTEGRITY

For many years, it has been widely established that xenobiotics can exert significant effects on the immune system as evidenced by changes in circulating and lymphoid organ-associated leukocyte number, proliferative capacity, and in effector functions including defense against a broad array of bacterial, parasitic, and viral pathogens. More recently, and during the establishment of the subdiscipline of immunotoxicology, a significant emphasis was placed on the development of a standardized battery of tests to evaluate immune competence. Among the unique features of the immune system is the ability of immune cells to be removed from the body and to function in vitro. This unique quality makes it possible to comprehensively evaluate the actions of xenobiotics on the immune system employing in vivo, ex vivo, and in vitro approaches to dissect the cellular, biochemical, and molecular mechanisms of action of xenobiotics. While standard toxicological endpoints such as organ weights, cellularity, and enumeration of cell populations are important components in assessing when an agent is capable of altering the immune system, by far the most sensitive indicators of immunotoxicity are the tests that challenge the various cell types within the immune system to respond functionally to exogenous stimuli (Descotes, 2004; White, 1992). Employing such a battery of functional assays whereby different cell types can be evaluated not only for their effector functions, but also in certain cases for their ability to participate as accessory cells in an immune response, can provide important mechanistic information concerning which cell type(s) within the immune system are, in fact, targeted by a xenobiotic. This section focuses on selected in vivo, ex vivo, and in vitro tests currently used for evaluating immunotoxicity, as well as models and approaches that can be utilized for elucidation of the mechanism of action.

Methods to Assess Immunocompetence

The current state-of-the-science of immunotoxicity testing was recently reviewed in a single volume of *Methods in Molecular Biology*. An overview of immunotoxicology testing: past and future was provided by Luster and Gerberick (2010).

General Assessment Central to any series of studies evaluating immune competence is the inclusion of standard toxicological studies, because any immunological finding should be interpreted in conjunction with effects observed on other target organs. Standard toxicological studies that are usually evaluated include body and selected organ weights, general observations of overall animal health, selected serum chemistries, hematological parameters, and status of the bone marrow (ability to generate specific colony-forming units). In addition, histopathology of lymphoid organs, such as the spleen, thymus, and lymph nodes, may provide insight into potential immunotoxicants. General guidelines for the histopathological examination of each of these lymphoid organs was recently reviewed (Elmore, 2010).

Because of the unique nature of the immune system, there are several experimental approaches that may be taken to assess immunotoxicity and to evaluate the mechanisms of action of xenobiotics. These are depicted in Fig. 12-19 and vary with respect to in vivo or in vitro exposure, immunological challenge (ie, the stimulus employed to induce an immune response), or immunological evaluation (immune assay). As an example, Fig. 12-19 (2) is an ex vivo assay where xenobiotic exposure and antigen challenge occur in vivo and the immune response is evaluated in vitro. In contrast, as depicted in Fig. 12-19 (3), splenocytes can be isolated after in vivo

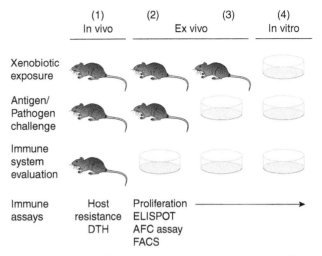

Figure 12-19. *Approaches for assessing the immunotoxicity of xenobiotics.* The ability to stimulate immune cells in vitro allows for much flexibility in the assessment of immunotoxicity of xenobiotics.

treatment with a xenobiotic, sensitized with an antigen in vitro and evaluated in vitro; or as depicted in Fig. 12-19 (4), splenocytes can be removed from a naive (untreated) animal, exposed to a xenobiotic and antigen in vitro, and evaluated in vitro. If splenocytes are sensitized in vitro with sRBC to generate AFC, this is known as the Mishell–Dutton assay (Mishell and Dutton, 1967).

Functional Assessment

Innate Immunity As described earlier, innate immunity encompasses all those immunological responses that are not induced through antigen receptors (ie, TCR or BCR) and for which there is no immunological memory. These responses include recognition of tumor cells by NK cells, phagocytosis of pathogens by macrophages, and the lytic activity of the components of the complement cascade.

To evaluate phagocytic activity, phagocytic cells, typically macrophages are harvested from the peritoneal cavity (peritoneal exudate cells) and are allowed to adhere either in a well of a tissue culture plate or in a chamber fabricated on a tissue culture slide. After adherence, macrophages are washed and incubated with fluorescently labeled latex covaspheres. At the end of incubation, cells are fixed in methanol and stained in methylene chloride. Macrophages containing five covaspheres or more are counted as positive for phagocytic activity and data are expressed as a percentage of phagocytosis (the ratio of macrophages with ≥5 covaspheres to total macrophages counted).

Phagocytosis assays are conducted in vitro after chemical exposure either in vivo or in vitro. If an in vivo assay to assess the ability of tissue macrophages to phagocytose a foreign antigen is required, the functional activity of the reticuloendothelial system can be evaluated. Intravenously injected radiolabeled sRBC (^{51}Cr-sRBCs) are removed from the circulation by the tissue macrophage and sequestered for degradation in organs such as the liver, spleen, lymph nodes, lung, and thymus. Clearance of the ^{51}Cr-sRBCs is monitored by sampling of the peripheral blood. When steady state has been attained, animals are euthanized and organs are removed and counted in a gamma counter to assess uptake of the ^{51}Cr-sRBCs.

When phagocytic cells encounter antigens, especially those associated with bacteria or a virus, they undergo activation, which is induced, in part, through interactions with TLRs. Extracellular antigens are processed and presented in association with MHCII, while intracellular antigens are processed and presented in association with MHCI, as described in the "Antigen Processing" section. Concomitantly with antigen encounter by the phagocyte, there is an increase in the expression of MHCI and/or MHCII as well as the costimulatory molecules CD80/CD86. The simultaneous increase in MHC molecules in combination with CD80 and CD86 is critically important in order for the phagocytic cell to drive T-cell effectors (CD4$^+$ and CD8$^+$ T cells). The upregulation of MHCI and/or II and CD80 and CD86 can be readily quantified by flow cytometry (see the "Flow Cytometric Analysis" section) after the activation of phagocytic cells, primarily those of the monocytic lineage, to further assess phagocytic cell function and the influence of an immunotoxicant. These measurements are especially informative when performed in combination with cell surface markers that are capable of identifying monocytic lineage subpopulations, for example such as tissue macrophages, conventional DC, and plasmacytoid DC because they provide information on whether the immunotoxicant interferes with the activation/differentiation of the phagocytic cell and its antigen-presenting capability. An overview of the types of macrophages, their hematopoietic origin, and a general discussion of the many different assays that are used to assess their functional status was recently provided by Barnett and Brundage (2010).

Evaluation of the ability of NK cells to lyse tumor cells is achieved using the YAC-1 cell line as a tumor target for an in vitro cytotoxicity assay. YAC-1 cells are radiolabeled with ^{51}Cr and incubated (in microtiter plates) in specific effector-to-target ratios with splenocytes from xenobiotic-exposed and nonexposed animals. During an incubation step, splenic NK cells (effectors) lyse the ^{51}Cr-YAC-1 cells, releasing ^{51}Cr into the supernatant. At the end of the incubation, plates are centrifuged and the supernatant is removed and counted on a gamma counter. After correcting for spontaneous release (which should be <10%), specific release of ^{51}Cr is calculated for each effector-to-target ratio and compared to the specific release from control animals. To avoid the use of radionucleotides, a number of flow cytometry based assays have been developed utilizing fluorescent stains to identify live and dead target cells. One such assay involves the coculture of NK cells with target cells that have been stained with the fluorescent green dye 3,3′-dioctadecyloxacarbocyanine perchlorate (DiO) (Kane et al., 1996). Utilizing DiO allows for readily discriminating between target and nontarget cells while propidium iodide is used to distinguish between live and dead cells. The various methods for NK assays used in immunotoxicity testing were recently reviewed (Li, 2010).

Acquired Immunity—Humoral The AFC assay is a sensitive indicator of immunological integrity for several reasons. It is a test of the ability of the host to mount an antibody response to a specific antigen. When a T-dependent antigen (an antigen that requires T cells to help B cells make antibody) like sRBC is used, this response requires the coordinated interaction of several different immune cells: APC (macrophages and DCs), T cells, and B cells. Therefore, an effect on any of these cell types (eg, antigen processing and presentation, cytokine production, proliferation, or differentiation) can have a profound impact on the ability of B cells to produce antigen-specific antibody. Other antigens, termed T-cell-independent antigens, such as dinitrophenyl-ficoll or trinitrophenyl-LPS, can also be used that bypass the requirement for T cells in eliciting antibody production by B cells. Although the AFC response assay was developed almost half a century ago, its sensitivity in identifying immunotoxicants has resulted in worldwide application for the purpose of hazard identification, which extends to present day (see the "Historical Perspective on Regulatory Guidance in Immunotoxicology" section).

A standard AFC assay involves immunizing control and xenobiotic-exposed mice either intravenously or intraperitoneally with sRBCs. The antigen is taken up in the spleen, and an anti-sRBC antibody response is induced. In the mouse, the peak day of antibody production is four days after immunization. Historically, the antibody response has been quantified by enumerating the number of plasma cells present in the spleen that are secreting anti-sRBC antibodies. This can be accomplished by removing the spleen, making a spleen cell suspension that is then mixed with sRBC, complement, and melted agar. This mixture is poured onto a petri dish and covered with a cover slip. After the agar hardens the petri dishes are incubated for three hours at 37°C. During this time, the B cells that have been appropriately activated by the antigen and have differentiated into plasma cells secrete anti-sRBC IgM antibody. When the complement and the secreted IgM coat the surrounding sRBCs, areas of hemolysis (plaques) appear against a lawn of sRBC that can be enumerated. At the center of each plaque is a single B cell (AFC). Data are usually presented as IgM AFC per million splenocytes. IgG AFC can also be enumerated by slight modifications of this same assay. This isotype switching (from IgM to IgG) is important in secondary responses in which memory B cells respond more quickly to an antigen. An overview of the T-cell-dependent antibody response to sRBCs was recently provided, in which this model is described as the "gold standard" for evaluating the potential adverse effects of xenobiotics on the immune system (White et al., 2010).

A second method to enumerate AFC cells is by ELISPOT. This method is similar to the plaque assay described above with the exception that the splenocytes isolated from sRBC-sensitized mice are incubated on ELISPOT mictotiter plates coated with either antimouse IgM or sRBC membranes to capture the secreted IgM. After incubation, the spleen cells are removed using a washing buffer followed by incubation with an enzyme-conjugated antimouse IgM antibody. A second washing step is used to remove unbound enzyme-conjugated antimouse IgM followed by addition of the chromogen substrate. The site at which each IgM secreting cell was present in the well of the ELISPOT microtiter plate is now visualized by the formation of a "spot" through the enzymatic conversion of the chromogen substrate. Typically, enumeration is performed using an ELISPOT reader that can rapidly quantify spot number (number of plasma cells) as well as the size and intensity (quantity of IgM being secreted) of the spots. It is noteworthy that in addition to enumeration of AFCs, the ELISPOT method can be applied to quantification of any secreted protein for which a suitable capture antibody exists. In evaluations of immunocompetent cells, the ELISPOT is especially useful for enumerating cytokine and chemokine secreting cells, and serves as an alternative to flow cytometry, where cell enumeration is critical.

A third way the anti-sRBC humoral immune response can be evaluated is ex vivo using serum from peripheral blood of immunized mice and an enzyme-linked immunosorbent assay or ELISA. Although the optimal response is delayed by one to two days (compared to the AFC assay), this approach takes into account antigen-specific antibody secreted by B cells in the spleen as well as B cells residing in the bone marrow. Like the AFC assay, mice (or other experimental animals) are immunized with sRBCs and six days postimmunization peripheral blood is collected. Serum from each sample is serially diluted and incubated in microtiter plates that have been coated with sRBC membranes. The membranes serve as the antigen to which sRBC-specific IgM or IgG will bind, as described above in the ELISPOT assay. After incubation of the test sera and a wash step, an enzyme-conjugated monoclonal antibody (the secondary antibody) against IgM (or IgG) is added. This antibody recognizes the IgM (or IgG) and binds specifically to that antibody. After incubation and a wash step, the enzyme substrate (chromogen) is added. Conversion of the substrate by the enzyme conjugated to the secondary antibody results in a color change, which can be quantified by measuring absorbance with a plate reader. Because this is a kinetic assay (color develops over time and is dependent on concentration of anti-sRBC antibody in the test sera), it is important to establish control concentration–response curves so that data can be evaluated in the linear range of the curve. Data are usually expressed in arbitrary optical density (OD) units. An advantage of the ELISA over the AFC assay and ELISPOT is the ability to attain a greater degree of flexibility, since serum samples can be stored frozen for analysis at a later date. In contrast, a disadvantage of the ELISA approach is that it provides no information on the actual number of plasma cells that were induced by sRBC sensitization. Other T-dependent antigens, including keyhole limpet hemocyanin (KLH), are routinely used to drive an antigen-specific antibody response and to assess the potential for immunotoxicity (Plitnick and Herzyk, 2010).

B cell to plasma cell differentiation can also be monitored by flow cytometry. This can be accomplished utilizing intracellular staining for IgM (or other Ig isotypes such as IgG) to identify IgM^{high} cells in combination with the transmembrane proteoglycan, CD138, also termed syndecan-1, which is a hallmark of a fully differentiated plasma cell (Costes *et al.*, 1999). It is noteworthy that even in resting nonactivated B cells, background levels of intracellular IgM are readily detectable because the monomeric form of IgM serves as the B-cell antigen receptor. For this reason, the designation IgM^{low} typically refers to a resting B cell versus IgM^{high}, which is indicative of high level IgM expression as exhibited by plasma cells.

One final assay measures the ability of B cells to undergo blastogenesis and proliferation, which are critical steps in the generation of an antibody response. Lymphocyte proliferation is most often quantified either using a radioisotope-based assay or by flow cytometry. Splenocytes are stimulated in microtiter plates with a monoclonal antibody to surface Ig in the presence of IL-4, or with a B-cell mitogen such as LPS. Proliferation is evaluated two to three days after stimulation. In the radioisotope-based assay, proliferation is quantified by quantifying the incorporation of ^{3}H-thymidine into the DNA of the cultured cells. Data are usually expressed as mean counts per minute (cpm) for each treatment group. In the flow cytometry-based assay, cells are stained with one of several membrane permeable dyes such as carboxyfluorescein succinimidyl ester (CFSE). CFSE is a colorless dye that passively diffuses into the cell. Once inside the cell, CFSE undergoes cleavage by intracellular esterases to yield carboxyfluorescein succinimidyl, which is highly fluorescent and covalently reacts with intracellular amines. As the cell divides, the intensity of staining in each of the two newly formed daughter cells decreases by approximately half, as well as in every subsequent cell division thereafter. The number of cell divisions each cell has undergone is inversely proportional to fluorescence intensity. T-cell proliferative responses can be quantified using the same methodologies as described above with the exception that T-cell-specific stimuli are used to induce T-cell proliferation. Often in broad-based immunotoxicological evaluations, B-cell proliferative responses are measured in conjunction with T-cell proliferation.

Acquired Immunity—Cell-Mediated While there are numerous assays used to assess CMI, three primary tests are used routinely in the National Toxicology Program (NTP, 2009) test battery (see the "The National Toxicology Program Tier Approach" section later in this chapter). The test battery includes the CTL assay, DTH response, and the T-cell proliferative responses to antigens

(anti-CD3 + IL-2), mitogens (phytohemaggluttinin [PHA] and concanavalin A [Con A]), and allogeneic cell antigens (mixed lymphocyte responses [MLR]).

The CTL assay measures the in vitro ability of splenic T cells to recognize allogeneic target cells (MHC mismatched) by evaluating the ability of the CTLs to proliferate and then lyse the target cells. Splenocytes are incubated with P815 mastocytoma cells, which serve as target cells. The target cells are pretreated with mitomycin C or irradiated, so that they cannot proliferate. During this sensitization phase, the CTLs recognize the targets and undergo proliferation. Five days after sensitization, the CTLs are harvested and incubated in microtiter plates with radiolabeled (^{51}Cr) P815 mastocytoma cells. During this elicitation phase, the CTLs that have acquired memory recognize the foreign MHCI on the P815 cells and lyse the targets. At the end of the incubation, the culture plates are centrifuged, the supernatant is removed, and radioactivity released into the supernatant is quantified on a gamma counter. After correcting for spontaneous release, the percent cytotoxicity is calculated for each effector-to-target ratio and compared to that from control animals. Several flow cytometry-based methods have also been developed to assay CTL activity that avoids the use of radionucleotides. One approach is similar to the one described for the NK cell assay above and involves the labeling of target cells with a fluorescent dye (eg, DiO or CFSE) in order to discern target cells from effectors. After coculture of target cells and CTL effectors, target cell viability is assessed by propidium iodide staining or using one of several other commercially available stains to assess viability. Another alternative nonradioactive surrogate assay widely used in place of measuring direct killing of target cells is quantification of IFNγ expressing CD8$^+$ T cells by flow cytometry using intracellular staining. An inherent limitation to this last approach is that direct target cell killing is not assessed and it is assumed that all IFNγ CD8$^+$ cells identified are CTL effectors (see the "Flow Cytometric Analysis" section). The current state-of-the-science of using the CTL assay to evaluate the effects of xenobiotics on CMI function was recently provided by Burleson *et al.* (2010).

The DTH response evaluates the ability of memory T cells to recognize foreign antigen, proliferate and migrate to the site of the antigen, and secrete cytokines and chemokines, which result in the influx of other inflammatory cells. The assay itself quantifies the influx of radiolabeled mononuclear cells into the sensitization site. During xenobiotic exposure, mice are sensitized twice with KLH subcutaneously between the shoulders. On the last day of exposure, mononuclear cells are labeled in vivo with an IV injection of ^{125}I-5-iododeoxyuridine. One day later, mice are challenged intradermally in one ear with KLH. Twenty-four hours after challenge, animals are euthanized, the ears are biopsied, and radiolabeled cells are counted in a gamma counter. Data are expressed as a stimulation index, which represents the cpm of ^{125}I activity in the challenged ear divided by the cpm in the unchallenged ear. As such, the DTH functional response may be influenced by disruption of either Th1-driven, antigen-dependent T-cell development or mobilization of sensitized T cells to a local site (Dietert *et al.*, 2010).

T cells play a central role in CMI and the ability of T cells to undergo blastogenesis and proliferation is critical to this role. Several mechanisms exist to evaluate proliferative capacity. The MLR measures the ability of T cells to recognize foreign MHCI and MHCII on splenocytes from an MHC-incompatible mouse (allogeneic cells) and undergo proliferation. For example, splenocytes from B6C3F1 mice (responders) are incubated with splenocytes from mitomycin C-treated (or irradiated) DBA/2 mice (stimulators). Proliferation is evaluated four to five days after stimulation by measuring uptake of ^{3}H-thymidine into the DNA of the cultured responder cells. Cells are collected from each well using a cell harvester and counted in a scintillation counter. Data may be expressed as either the mean cpm for each treatment group or as a stimulation index in which the index is calculated by dividing the cpm of wells containing responders and stimulators by the cpm of wells containing responders alone. Alternatively, cell proliferation can be quantified by flow cytometry using membrane permeable dyes such as CFSE (please see the following section "Flow Cytometric Analysis").

General T-cell proliferation can be evaluated in a manner similar to that described above for B cells (Table 12-5). Splenocytes are stimulated in microtiter plates with monoclonal antibodies directed to the CD3 complex of the TCR (anti-CD3) and the CD28 T-cell coreceptor (anti-CD28), or with the T-cell mitogens Con A or PHA. Proliferation is evaluated two to three days after stimulation by measuring uptake of ^{3}H-thymidine into the DNA of the cultured T cells. Data are usually expressed as mean cpm for each treatment group. As discussed above, proliferation can also be quantified by flow cytometry. These studies are usually done in conjunction with B-cell proliferative responses described above.

Flow Cytometric Analysis One of the most rapidly advancing areas and powerful tools in immunotoxicology has been the application of flow cytometry to investigations of immune modulation by xenobiotics. In the most general sense, flow cytometry is a method that employs light scatter, fluorescence, and absorbance measurements to analyze large numbers of cells (typically 5000-100,000/sample), on an individual basis. Most commonly, fluorochrome-conjugated monoclonal antibodies raised against a specific protein of interest are employed for detection. The strength of the approach is that a wide variety of measurements can be made on large numbers of cells, individually, rapidly, and with a high level of precision. In addition, methods are also available that allow for the analysis of specific proteins in cell-free preparations such as cell lysates, biological fluids, and culture supernatants. A broad selection of polyclonal and monoclonal antibodies is available to cell surface markers, intracellular proteins, and secreted proteins (Table 12-5).

The most common application of flow cytometry in immunotoxicology is to enumerate specific leukocyte populations and subpopulations. For example, antibodies are available to the T-cell surface proteins CD4, CD8, and CD3 (among others). Because flow cytometers can detect light emission of multiple wavelengths simultaneously, multiple-colored fluorochromes can be used concurrently facilitating an analysis of more than one protein simultaneously in a given sample (multicolor/parameter analysis). In this manner, the number of CD4$^+$ and CD8$^+$ cells can be determined simultaneously on a single sample of cells. In the thymus, dual staining can be used to assess T-cell maturation by determining the number of CD4$^+$/CD8$^+$ (double positive), CD4$^-$/CD8$^-$ (double negative), CD4$^+$/CD8$^-$ (single positive), and CD4$^-$/CD8$^+$ (single positive) cells residing in this organ (Fig. 12-20). This approach can be used to provide insight into which specific T-cell subsets are targeted after exposure to a xenobiotic and to identify putative effects on T-cell maturation. Similarly, antibodies are readily available to identify other leukocyte subpopulations including antibodies to surface Ig, CD19, and B220 (the CD45 phosphatase on B cells) for enumerating B cells, to Mac1 and F4/80 for macrophages, to CD16/CD56 for NK cells in humans, and to CD161 (NK-1.1) for NK cells in mice. Surface marker analysis of heterogeneous cell preparations can reveal significant alterations in lymphoid subpopulations, and in many instances, this is indicative of alterations in immunological integrity. Indeed, an indicator of disease progression in AIDS can be monitored by changes in CD4$^+$ T cell numbers. Luster and coworkers (1992) have reported that in conjunction with two or three functional tests, the enumeration of lymphocyte subsets can greatly enhance the detection of immunotoxic chemicals. However, it is important to emphasize that although surface marker analysis can identify changes in leukocyte populations, functional analysis of the immune system is more definitive for the detection of immunotoxicity since the ability of immunocompetent cells to mount an effector response is assessed directly.

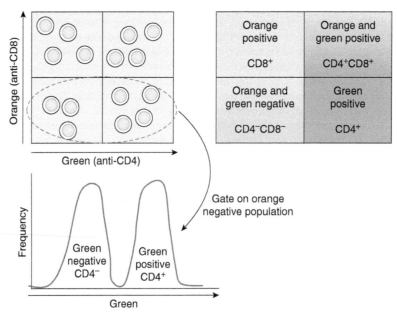

Figure 12-20. *Fluorescently activated cell sorting (FACS).* As an example, a mixed lymphocyte population expressing CD4$^+$ and CD8$^+$ (thymocytes) is assessed. Using antibodies directed against either CD4 or CD8 conjugated to different fluorophores ("colors"), the number of cells expressing CD4, CD8, both, or none can be quantified. In addition, differential gating can be used to quantify subpopulations of cells (bottom, the number of green positive and green negative within orange negative population).

With technical advancements of flow cytometers (ie, an increased number of wavelengths that can be simultaneously detected, enhanced sensitivity of detection, and more rapid analysis) coupled with a steady growth of applications, reagents, and methods, flow cytometry has become an integral tool in elucidating the cellular and molecular mechanisms of action produced by immunotoxicants by measuring their effects on a wide variety of cellular responses. Current applications go well beyond strictly evaluating cell surface markers and include measurements of cellular viability, cell cycle, cell proliferation, intracellular free calcium, induction of apoptosis, DNA strand breaks (TUNEL assay), intracellular proteins (cytosolic and nuclear), membrane potential, intracellular pH, oxidative stress, and membrane lipophilicity (reviewed by Burchiel et al., 1997, 1999; Hawley and Hawley 2004; Shapiro, 2003). Of particular utility in assessments of immune cell signaling and effector function has been the development of protocols and antibodies for intracellular staining of permeabilized cells. In the case of effector function, flow cytometry can be used to quantify the expression of multiple cytokines and/or chemokines simultaneously in individual cells by intracellular staining. Because activated leukocytes often secrete multiple regulatory factors simultaneously, termed "multifunctional," using intracellular staining in conjunction with extracellular staining for phenotypic markers to identify specific cell populations can provide important insights into the magnitude and profile of effects exerted by an immunotoxicant on specific cell types and populations. Measurements of regulatory factors in combination with phenotypic markers can be extended to also include markers of cell activation or differentiation to identify at which stage during effector cell generation an immunotoxicant is acting. For an example of intracellular cytokine staining, refer to the study of Karmaus et al. (2011). A second application of intracellular staining in flow cytometry has been for investigating cell signaling. The complex networks and pathways that control cellular activities can be studied on an individual cell basis to provide static or kinetic information in specific cell types. For example, by using intracellular staining, the abundance of specific signaling proteins, cytosolic and nuclear, can be quantified. In addition to signaling protein abundance, post-translational modifications of proteins represent an important mechanism for transducing regulatory signals. One of the most extensively studied is protein phosphorylation and dephosphorylation, which often results in the activation or inactivation of protein function. The development of antibodies capable of distinguishing the point at which proteins possess phospho-groups at specific regulatory sites has made it possible to study modulation of distinct regulatory pathways by immunotoxicants. Because basic flow cytometers have the ability to detect six to eight colors simultaneously, with more advanced instruments possessing 18 color capacity, it is possible to measure multiple signaling events and/or network interactions in single cells. This capability coupled with the fact that the flow cytometer can evaluate thousands of cells per second, allows for accurate and reproducible detection of even rare events occurring in small subsets of leukocytes. Moreover, flow cytometry has numerous advantages over other approaches such as Western blotting and immunoprecipitation because of the rapidity of analysis and that it is not a "bulk lysis" method in which all cells in a given sample are pooled for analysis to render results that are representative of the overall mean within the entire cell population rather than in individual cells. For examples of measurement of intracellular phosphoprotein and transcription factors by flow cytometry that can be applied to study mechanisms of immune modulation, see North et al. (2010) and Lu et al. (2011).

Another major advancement in flow cytometry-based analyses has been the development of fluorescent microspheres that are individually identified by the instrument. By coating the surface of microspheres with various concentrations of two fluorescent dyes, sets of microspheres can be generated with each set possessing a unique spectral signature. Subsequently, various materials (ie, proteins, antibodies, or nucleic acids) can be covalently conjugated to the surface of these microspheres in order to create unique detection systems. This technology is being widely applied for analyzing a broad variety of soluble cellular components including proteins in cell-free preparations by flow cytometry. For example, up to 15 different cytokines can be measured simultaneously in cell supernatants or biological fluids (eg, BALF). A major advantage of this method over more traditional approaches, such as ELISA-based assays, is that only small amounts of biological samples and reagents are required because multiple proteins are assayed simultaneously. The same technology is also being applied for analyzing cell lysates for changes in protein phosphorylation in investigations of cell signaling. In addition, flow cytometry is routinely used to purify and isolate leukocyte subpopulations from heterogeneous cellular preparations. Thus, flow cytometry has become a powerful tool for characterizing the cellular and molecular mechanisms associated with immunotoxicants.

For information concerning specific flow cytometry protocols and applications beyond those provided by commercial vendors, the reader is directed to several references including the 4th edition of Practical Flow Cytometry (Shapiro, 2003), the 2nd edition of Methods in Molecular Biology: Flow Cytometry Protocols (Hawley and Hawley, 2004), and the Purdue University Cytometry Laboratories website (www.cyto.purdue.edu), which hosts the "Discussion List," a blog to which one can submit questions to the broader community of flow cytometry users for technical assistance.

Measurements of Cytokines and Cytokine Profiling As discussed in the earlier part of this chapter, development, maturation, differentiation, and effector responses of the immune system are highly dependent on a multitude of small, secreted proteins termed cytokines. In most cases, these immunological processes are controlled by the production of multiple cytokines, some of which are released simultaneously while others are released in a very defined temporal sequence. Many of these cytokines are produced by T cells and are the mechanism by which a wide variety of functions by T cells are mediated. Due to the importance of cytokines in regulating the immune system, xenobiotics that alter the production and release of these mediators can significantly affect immune competence. Therefore, measurement of multiple cytokines, often referred to as cytokine profiling, has become routine in immunotoxicology and can provide significant insights into the mechanisms by which a xenobiotic produces its immunotoxicity. For example, cytokine profiling has been explored as an approach for identifying chemical allergens, either contact sensitizers, which typically induce a Th1 profile of cytokines (IL-2, IFN-γ, and TNF-β), or respiratory sensitizers, which typically produce a strong Th2 cytokine profile (IL-4, IL-5, IL-6, and IL-10) (Mosmann and Coffman, 1989; Mosmann et al., 1991). Cytokines can be measured in cell culture supernatants or biological fluids (ie, serum or BALF) by ELISA or by multiplex assays. Quantification of test samples is accomplished by comparison to a standard curve employing recombinant cytokine standards. The aforementioned method, the ELISPOT assay can also be used to quantify the number of cells producing the cytokine of interest. Likewise, flow cytometry can be used to identify cytokine producing cells by intracellular staining or to quantify cytokines in media or biological fluids with the main advantage being that the source of the cytokine(s) can be identified using the former approach and that many cytokines can be assayed simultaneously from one sample using the latter approach (see the "Flow Cytometric Analysis" section). Because cytokines are regulated transcriptionally and then actively synthesized by cells at the time they are secreted, rather than existing as stored proteins, measurements of cytokine mRNA levels have become another common approach of assessing which cytokines are being expressed at a given time and the putative effects xenobiotics exert on their regulation and expression. Real time polymerase chain reaction (PCR) is most commonly used for quantifying mRNA levels of specific cytokines as well as for other genes of interest in cells or tissues. For more global assessments of mRNA levels, low-density RNA arrays or microarrays can be applied. Major advantages to quantifying cytokine expression at the mRNA rather than the protein level include significantly greater sensitivity, the ability to quantify expression in solid tissues, and the capability to rapidly design appropriate reagents (PCR primers) specific for any cytokine. A major disadvantage is that changes at the mRNA level for a given cytokine may not necessarily correlate with changes in protein. Another disadvantage over flow cytometric determinations by intracellular staining is not knowing the cell type(s) from which the cytokines are being produced. One additional limitation to cytokine measurements by ELISA or via quantification of cytokine mRNA levels is that neither of these approaches provides information concerning the biological activity of the proteins being measured. As described by Corsini and House (2010), multicytokine analysis still needs to be standardized in terms of optimum sources for analysis, protocols, and quality control issues, such as the use of reference standards and the expression of results.

Host Resistance Assays Host resistance assays represent a way of assessing how xenobiotic exposure affects the ability of the host to combat infection by a variety of pathogens. Although host resistance studies provide significant insight into the mechanisms by which an immunotoxicant is acting, these assays are not used as a first or only choice for evaluating immune competence. The results from host resistance assays are typically more variable than other immune function assays already discussed and therefore require markedly greater numbers of animals in order to obtain statistical power. The increased number of animals required also raises ethical considerations as well as cost. In addition, as with other immune function tests, no single host resistance model can predict overall immune competence of the host, primarily because each model uses different mechanisms for elimination of various pathogens. A representative list of host resistance models is shown in Table 12-7. Typically, three challenge levels of pathogen (approximating the lethal dose 20 [LD_{20}], lethal dose 50 [LD_{50}], and lethal dose 80 [LD_{80}]) for each concentration of xenobiotic are used in order to be able to detect both increases and decreases in resistance. Endpoint analyses are lethality (for bacterial and viral pathogens), changes

Table 12-7

Models of Host Resistance

MODEL	PATHOGEN
Bacterial	*Listeria monocytogenes* *Streptococcus pneumoniae*
Parasite	*Trichinella spiralis*
Fungal	*Candida albicans*
Viral	Influenza A2
Tumor	B16F10 melanoma

SOURCE: From Burleson and Burleson (2010) and Luebke (2010).

in tumor burden, and increased or decreased parasitemia. In host resistance studies, it is also important to consider the following: (1) strain, route of administration, and challenge size of the pathogen; (2) strain, age, and sex of the host; (3) physiological state of the host and the pathogen; and (4) time of challenge with the pathogen (prior to, during, or after xenobiotic exposure). All of these can have significant effects on the results from any individual study.

A major advantage in applying host resistance models to investigations of immunotoxicity is the ability to study the effects of an immunotoxicant within the context of the intact immune system encompassing all its diversity as it acts to protect the host against a *bona fide* pathogen. It is important to emphasize that the immune system possesses significant redundancy (ie, multiple mechanisms to provide defense against invading microorganisms). Therefore, even if a particular cell type or effector response has been compromised by exposure to an immunotoxicant, other components of the immune system might provide partial or complete protection to the host from pathogen challenge. In addition, certain pathogens are restricted to specific tissues or anatomical sites, for example influenza, which is typically restricted to airways. Using host resistance models permits the study of immunotoxicants and their effects within the environment and context of the tissue targeted by the pathogen (Buchweitz *et al.*, 2007). The current state-of-the-science of a variety of host resistance models was recently reviewed including bacterial challenge models (Burleson and Burleson, 2010), viral host resistance models (Freebern, 2010), parasite challenge models (Luebke, 2010), and tumor challenge models (Ng *et al.*, 2010).

Assessment of Developmental Immunotoxicology Interest in DIT is predicated on the recognition that the developing immune system represents a novel target for xenobiotic-induced toxicity that presents some special considerations when it comes to assessment. The concept that any of a number of dynamic changes associated with the developing immune system might provide periods of unique susceptibility to chemical perturbation has been reviewed (Dietert *et al.*, 2000; Holladay and Smialowicz, 2000). This unique susceptibility may be manifested as a qualitative difference, in the sense that a chemical could affect the developing immune system without affecting the adult immune system, or as a quantitative difference, in the sense that a chemical could affect the developing immune system at lower doses than the adult immune system, or as a temporal difference, in the sense that a chemical could produce either a more persistent effect in younger animals than adults, or trigger a delayed effect (ie, the consequences of early exposure are not manifested until early adulthood). As a result, while effective assessment of DIT should certainly draw upon the prior experience gained from adult-exposure immunotoxicity assessments, it is important to examine the database of known immune changes that reflect the potential for unique susceptibility and are specific for the developing immune system (Dietert and Piepenbrink, 2006b).

One of the most comprehensive reports to date attempted to compare the immunotoxicity following developmental or adult exposure to the following compounds: diethylstilbestrol, diazepam, lead, 2,3,7,8-tetrachlorodibenzo-*p*-dioxin (TCDD), and tributyltin oxide (Luebke *et al.*, 2006a). The selection of these five compounds was reported to be based on the availability of some human data. The authors concluded that for all five chemicals, the developing immune system was found to be at greater risk than the adult, either because lower doses produced immunotoxicity, adverse effects were persistent, or both. However, it is noteworthy that no developmental immunotoxicants have been identified that have not also been immunomodulatory in the adult animal. Importantly, this observation may merely reflect the state-of-the-science—for example, all published DIT studies to-date have been conducted on known adult immunotoxicants, and systematic studies comparing the effects across multiple developmental windows are still uncommon.

A better understanding of the developing immune system, and in particular, an understanding of critical developmental hallmarks has prompted some to speculate about the existence of five critical windows of vulnerability (Dietert et al., 2000). The first window encompasses a period of HSC formation from undifferentiated mesenchymal cells. Exposure of the embryo to toxic chemicals during this period could result in failures of stem cell formation, abnormalities in production of all hematopoietic lineages, and altered immunocompetence. The second window is characterized by migration of hematopoietic cells to the fetal liver and thymus, differentiation of lineage-restricted stem cells, and expansion of progenitor cells for each leukocyte lineage. This developmental window is likely to be particularly sensitive to agents that interrupt cell migration, adhesion, and proliferation. The critical developmental events during the third window are the establishment of bone marrow as the primary hematopoietic site and the establishment of the bone marrow and the thymus as the primary lymphopoietic sites for B cells and T cells, respectively. The fourth window addresses the critical periods of immune system functional development, including the initial period of perinatal immunodeficiency, and the maturation of the immune system to adult levels of competence. The final window addresses the subsequent period during which mature immune responses are manifested, and functional pools of protective memory cells are established.

Most recently, considerable attention has been focused on the perinatal period (ie, prior to and just after birth) because this window of development is known to be replete with dynamic immune changes, many of which do not occur in adults (Dietert and Piepenbrink, 2006b). Indeed, one reality associated with DIT windows is that the developing immune system exists in an unbalanced state through the latter portion of gestation with certain functional CMI capacities deliberately impaired. In fact, Taylor and coworkers (2006) demonstrated that placentally induced immune skewing via the release of Fas-ligand-containing exosomes is one hallmark of a successful pregnancy brought to full term. Upon birth, restoring effective immune balance through the enhancement of Th1 capacity in the newborn is critical for protecting childhood health (Holt et al., 2005; Yun and Lee, 2005). Prenatal maturation and functional skewing of the fetal immune system followed by the rapid reversal of the imbalance at birth have features that are not effectively modeled using adult exposure-assessment (Dietert and Piepenbrink, 2006b), and DIT is best viewed as a continuum of alterations. Suppression of the developing immune system, manifested as increased susceptibility to infections and cancer, is not the only concern, and immunotoxic changes that increase the risk for allergic or autoimmune responses in later life should also be considered (Edwards and Cooper, 2006; Selgrade et al., 2006; Yeatts et al., 2006). Adding to the complexity is the demonstration that some DIT seem capable of inducing targeted immune suppression while at the same time elevating the risk of allergy and/or autoimmunity (Haggqvist et al., 2005). Because either significant immune suppression or disrupted immune regulation is a concern and needs to be detected, the most effective methodology for assessing DIT must also be capable of assessing significant changes in immune balance.

In spite of the increased interest in assessing the potential for developmental immunotoxicity, it must be emphasized that neither validated nor widely accepted methods currently exist for evaluating the effects of a chemical on the developing immune system. Several workshops have summarized consensus thinking concerning developmental immunotoxicity evaluation (Dietert et al.,

2000; Holsapple, 2002b; Holsapple et al., 2005; Ladics et al., 2005; Luster et al., 2003; van Loveren and Piersma, 2004) and a number of reviews have been written (Burns-Naas et al., 2008; Dietert and Burns-Naas, 2008; Dietert and Holsapple, 2007; Dietert and Piepenbrink, 2006b; Holsapple et al., 2003, 2004, 2007; Luebke et al., 2006a; Weinstock et al., 2010; Winans et al., 2011). Additionally, other reviews have dealt with issues concerning immunotoxicity evaluation across various life stages (Germolec et al., 2004; Holsapple et al., 2005; Ladics et al., 2005; Ravel and Descotes, 2005). In light of the fact that neither validated nor established protocols presently exist to comprehensively assess whether a xenobiotic is a developmental immunotoxicant, below is a brief discussion of critical issues requiring consideration in establishing a testing framework.

In constructing a DIT testing framework, one of the first points to consider is the selection of an animal model. Consistently, the rat has been identified as the preferred species for evaluations of DIT, largely due to the fact that the rat has been utilized extensively in guideline developmental and reproductive toxicology testing. The anatomical and functional differences in the immune systems of the mouse, rat, dog, primate and human, and their use as models for DIT testing have been reviewed (Holsapple et al., 2003). The review concluded that the developing immune systems of mice and humans have been best characterized to date. In addition, the review also concluded that immune ontogeny in the mouse and rat is likely similar. Another important consideration when selecting a species is that the development of the immune system in the rodent is delayed relative to the human, and how this differential maturation will impact data extrapolation for predicting human risk. For example, some developmental landmarks observed in utero in humans occur after parturition in the rat.

A second consideration when constructing a framework for assessing DIT concerns gender-specific effects. Results from perinatal exposure to xenobiotics suggest that significant sex-based differences in immunotoxic sensitivity are common and are at least as prevalent, if not more frequent, compared with the incidence observed following adult exposure-assessment (Dietert and Piepenbrink, 2006b; Luebke et al., 2006a). As such, for the evaluation of DIT, testing of both sexes may be critical.

A third major consideration in a DIT testing framework is consideration of exposure. There is general agreement that the best exposure protocol is one where exposure occurs across all nonadult developmental windows followed either by immediate assessment or assessment after a few weeks (Holsapple et al., 2005; Ladics et al., 2005; Luster et al., 2003). Exposure to pregnant dams has been a hallmark feature of most DIT protocols, and the maternal influences on exposure to the fetus/newborn pups would be dependent on transfer of the xenobiotic either across the placenta or via lactation. The gestational (eg, transplacental) and lactational periods in the rat would result in exposure from conception to early postweaning in the pup, approximately three weeks of age. Direct exposure of pups via the diet would generally commence at about three weeks after birth. An unresolved issue is whether direct exposure of the pups, which is generally accepted as a routine procedure at around postnatal Day seven, should occur during the lactational period as well (Ladics et al., 2005); however, any decisions concerning this issue will require consideration of how humans would be exposed and the specific properties of the chemical being studied. For example, if exposure is only oral and there is no reason to believe that the lactational transfer differs significantly for a class of compounds between rats and humans, then direct dosing of pups could be initiated postweaning. In addition, information on pharmacokinetic and dosimetry could be useful in determining whether any direct dosing of pups during lactation is necessary. However, it is important to emphasize that this type of information is not routinely available for most xenobiotics.

A fourth consideration in creating a DIT testing framework concerns which specific endpoints to measure. As discussed above, immune organs, such as the thymus, spleen, and/or bone marrow, are not typically assessed in routine developmental and reproductive toxicology studies, and it has been the consensus of a number of workshops that histopathological evaluation of these immune organs could be easily integrated into these existing protocols (Holsapple et al., 2005; Luster et al., 2003). However, presently, there is uncertainty whether routine histopathology is sufficiently sensitive to detect all potential immunotoxic effects, especially when the unique characteristics of the developing immune system, as discussed above, are considered. Indeed, there are examples where morphometric histopathological findings do not predict functional impairments due to toxicity produced on the developing immune system (Hussain et al., 2005). Ultimately, while the use of specific, rather than general, histopathology has been recommended, it has been also suggested that functional tests be employed in the assessment of DIT. Unfortunately, few, if any, functional assays have been validated for detection of DIT, even for routine assays like the T-cell-dependent antibody response, which has largely been confined to adult exposure protocols. Results published on several chemicals and drugs in recent years suggest that functional tests are a front-line priority for perinatal immunotoxicity detection and that a combination of at least two functional tests, such as a multiisotype T-cell-dependent antibody response, and a CMI response assay, such as the DTH assay and/or CTL or NK cytotoxicity assays, should be paired with histopathological analysis and phenotypic analysis of lymphocyte subsets using flow cytometry (Dietert and Piepenbrink, 2006b).

One final point regarding the evaluation of developmental immunotoxicity needs to be considered. As developmental immunotoxicity protocols are inserted into existing toxicology testing regimes, such as developmental and reproductive toxicology protocols, it is likely to be necessary to incorporate immunization protocols. This approach has raised concerns among those evaluating other physiological systems (eg, reproductive and neurological) in terms of potential immunization-induced changes. However, investigations addressing this potential by determining the impact of the incorporation of immunotoxicological functional assays on standard toxicological studies in rats have been largely negative. Ladics and colleagues (1995) showed that immunization did not significantly alter the weights or morphology of routine protocol tissues with the exception of the spleen (ie, which manifested the anticipated increases in the numbers and size of germinal centers). In a subsequent study by this same group, immunization did not alter any hematological or clinical chemistry parameters, or lymphocyte subset numbers (ie, measured on peripheral blood with a flow cytometer), and did not mask the anticipated hepatotoxic effects of subchronic exposure to carbon tetrachloride (Ladics et al., 1998). An additional component of this discussion is the reality that the species being modeled, the human, has immunizations as a routine lifelong component of preventative medicine. As such, to avoid all immunizations in animal evaluation protocols does not closely simulate the childhood experience. Additionally, until the immune system is asked to respond specifically to a foreign antigen, the capacity to detect immunotoxicity may be severely limited. Therefore, immunization and a range of functional T-cell-dependent immune response evaluations seem necessary as components of an effective DIT assessment.

Assessment of Hypersensitivity Responses As noted above, a primary role of the immune system is the discrimination of self versus nonself, and immunotoxicology can be thought of as a continuum with immunotoxic effects occurring in either direction (Fig. 12-1). The adverse consequences of exaggerated immune function would reflect an inability to recognize self, and are generally depicted as hypersensitivity and autoimmunity.

Drugs and chemicals that are capable of eliciting an immune response are generally low molecular weight substances possessing some inherent reactivity. There is a genetic susceptibility to hypersensitivity responses in that not all individuals react to the same drugs and chemicals. For the most part, the xenobiotic cannot be considered an antigen, simply because by itself it is not capable of stimulating an immune response. Instead, the xenobiotic often forms a hapten, which triggers the immune response in some tissue in the host. This property is called the sensitizing potential of the hapten and is associated with its inherent reactivity. Hapten-specific immune responses are therefore triggered only in the presence of the hapten–carrier complex and can be mediated either by humoral immunity or CMI. The damage associated with any type of hypersensitivity response can be directed against the tissue that is bound by the hapten. One of the most important and challenging problems in the field of immunotoxicology is determining the potential for chemicals to induce immune modulation and, in the current context, to demonstrate the sensitizing potential of xenobiotics. Thus, it becomes essential to have validated predictive animal models, and to understand the underlying mechanisms of action. The following is a discussion of the currently used methods of predicting the most frequently occurring hypersensitivity reactions to chemicals, Types I and IV, which are most often manifested as respiratory hypersensitivity and contact sensitization, respectively.

Assessment of Respiratory Hypersensitivity in Experimental Animals Methods for assessing the potential to induce respiratory hypersensitivity have been reviewed (Holsapple et al., 2006). The objectives of this review were to describe the appropriate methods for identifying and characterizing respiratory hazards and risks and to identify the key data gaps and related research needs. The review addressed these objectives from the perspectives of proteins, chemicals, and drugs; and emphasized the important roles played by IgE and Th2 cell-mediated responses, while recognizing that damage to the respiratory tract can be triggered either by nonspecific irritation or by other specific (ie, non-IgE/Th2) immune-mediated mechanisms.

The state-of-the-science of animal models for respiratory hypersensitivity was also reviewed (Pauluhn, 2005). Current assays utilize two phases: induction/sensitization and challenge/elicitation. The induction phase usually includes multiple exposures to the test compound (sensitization) via the respiratory tract (ie, intranasal or intratracheal instillations, or by inhalation) or by dermal contact. There are advantages and disadvantages to each. Inhalation more closely represents environmental exposure by allowing for chemical contact with the upper as well as the lower respiratory tract. However, the equipment required is expensive and difficult to maintain. Exposure via the intranasal route is easily accomplished and allows for distribution of antigen to the upper and lower respiratory tract; however, studies have shown that a large proportion of the material can be recovered from the stomach (Robinson et al., 1996). In contrast, intratracheal instillation results in exposure to the lower respiratory tract only. The observation that a predominant respiratory sensitizer would still trigger an IgE response when applied topically has suggested an important interplay between Type I hypersensitivity reactions, manifested primarily as respiratory sensitization, and

Type IV hypersensitivity reactions, manifested primarily as contact sensitization. The basis for this observation can be accounted for by a cytokine network model, which involves important cross talk between humoral immunity and CMI. Basically, a chemical with the capability of being a respiratory sensitizer will trigger an IgE response regardless of its route of exposure because it "selects" or supports the development of a Th2-dependent response, with the associated cytokine profile: IL-4, IL-5, IL-10, and IL-13. In contrast, a chemical which lacks the capability of being a respiratory sensitizer, but which can still trigger contact dermatitis, will select or support a Th1-dependent response, with the associated cytokine profile including IL-2 and IFN-γ.

The challenge (elicitation) phase involves exposure to the chemical (hapten), the homologous protein conjugate of the hapten, or the antigen. Endpoints to characterize a positive response range from the induction of Igs (ie, total IgE for chemicals or specific IgE for protein antigens), cytokines, or lymphokines in serum, to pathophysiological responses, including the influx of inflammatory cells and the onset of bronchoconstriction along with the associated changes in respiratory functional parameters. The latter may be accomplished by visual inspection of the animals' respiratory pattern or more quantitatively by plethysmography. With plethysmography, changes in the respiratory rate, tidal volume, and plethysmographic pressure can be measured. However, plethysmography in guinea pigs, rats, and mice can be technically challenging and labor intensive. In addition, there is some controversy over the interpretation of measurements made from whole body plethysmography, and whether these measurements truly reflect changes in airway mechanics (Lundblad et al., 2002; Mitzner and Tankersley, 2003).

None of the currently applied animal models duplicates all features of human asthma, and most of the current animal models were developed for studying specific hypersensitivity responses to high molecular weight protein allergens (Pauluhn, 2005). Fewer animal models have been developed for use in the area of chemically induced respiratory allergy, which was one of the key data gaps identified in the review by Holsapple et al. (2006). One of the limitations associated with low molecular weight models is that often these compounds must conjugate with body proteins to become antigenic (ie, form hapten–carrier complexes). Often, a challenge with the conjugated chemical is necessary to induce a pulmonary response. Adding this variable can make the analysis of test results more difficult. False-negative results may occur due to variability in test article conjugation; and chemical conjugates are also necessary to measure specific immunological responses.

The majority of the current animal models are based on antibody-mediated events occurring as a reflection of the induction phase (Pauluhn, 2005). In certain cases, immunological sensitization may be confirmed by the detection of antigen-specific antibody; however, subsequent challenge does not produce clinical signs of respiratory distress. It is also possible to detect pulmonary sensitization in animal models where there is no detectable antigen-specific antibody production. In these cases, CMI or other mechanisms may be involved, or there may be difficulty in antibody detection.

Guinea pig models have been most frequently used for detection of pulmonary reactions to chemicals, because this species is known to respond vigorously to appropriate stimuli by developing an asthmatic-like bronchial spasm. In the guinea pig, as in the human, the lung is the major shock organ for anaphylactic response. Like humans, the guinea pig also demonstrates immediate- and late-onset allergic reactions as well as bronchial hyperreactivity and eosinophil influx and inflammation. The major difference in the mechanism of pulmonary responses between humans and guinea pigs is that the antibody involved in Type I reactions in humans is IgE and in guinea pigs is predominantly IgG_1. The key features of this animal model involve protocols using single or repeated inhalation or cutaneous (ie, primarily topical or intradermal) exposures followed by a rest period until Day 21 (Pauluhn, 2005). After the rest period, an inhalation challenge with the hapten or antigen is performed thereby focusing on a measurement of the elicitation phase of the response (Karol et al., 1994). Respiratory patterns are often measured in whole-body plethysmographs, as discussed above. A common pathological accompaniment of increased airway hyperactivity is prolonged eosinophil-rich inflammatory leukocyte infiltration into the lungs of guinea pigs after inhalation challenge of the protein or hapten-conjugate. One of the disadvantages of using guinea pigs is the lack of reagents needed to identify cell types and mediators involved in respiratory allergy, which has hampered mechanistic studies.

Murine models, in which reagent availability is not an issue, have become more frequently utilized in the evaluation of respiratory hypersensitivity, and two approaches have been described. The first approach capitalizes on the fact that, like humans, IgE is the major anaphylactogenic antibody in mice, and focuses on the induction of total serum IgE (Dearman et al., 1998). The second approach capitalizes on the aforementioned cytokine network and has been referred to as cytokine profiling (Dearman et al., 2002, 2003; Plitnick et al., 2002, 2003). Both approaches have relied on dermal application of potential allergens/sensitizers, and on the theoretical foundation that chemical allergens induce divergent immune responses characteristic of the selective activation of discrete T-cell subpopulations (Pauluhn, 2005). Contact allergens, such as 2,4-dinitrochlorobenzene, are considered not to cause sensitization of the respiratory tract, and trigger an immune response in mice that is consistent with the preferential activation of Th1 cells (ie, little to no increase in total serum IgE and the production of IL-2 and IFN-γ in the draining lymph nodes). In contrast, topical sensitization to chemical respiratory allergens, such as TMA, triggers an immune response in mice that is consistent with the preferential activation of Th2 cells (ie, a moderate to marked increase in total serum IgE and the production of IL-4, IL-5, IL-10, and IL-13 in the draining lymph nodes). It is important to emphasize that while both the mouse total serum IgE test and cytokine profiling hold much promise, neither approach can be considered validated at this time.

Assessment of IgE-Mediated Hypersensitivity Responses in Humans Described below are methods of human Type I hypersensitivity testing. These test results, in conjunction with a relevant history and physical exam, can be diagnostic of IgE-mediated pulmonary disease. Two skin tests are available for immediate hypersensitivity testing. In both, the measured endpoint is a wheal and flare reaction (ie, the result of edema and erythema subsequent to the release of preformed inflammatory mediators). The prick–puncture test introduces very small amounts of antigen under the skin and, owing to the reduced chance of systemic reaction, is recommended as a screening test. For test compounds not eliciting a reaction, the intradermal test using dilute concentrations of antigen may be used, but there is a higher risk of systemic reactions. The reader is referred to an additional text for a more detailed description of testing methods (Demoly et al., 1998).

In vitro serological tests, ELISAs, and radioallergosorbent tests may also be used to detect the presence of antigen-specific antibody in the patient's serum. These tests do not pose a risk of adverse reactions and may be used in situations where standardized reagents for skin testing are not available. Serological testing is often used in population-based epidemiological studies. Additionally, bronchial provocation tests may be performed by having the patient inhale an antigen into the bronchial tree and evaluating his or her pulmonary response. In some cases, this may be the only way to demonstrate that a test article is capable of producing an asthmatic response. Care must be taken in these test situations in that it is possible to produce severe asthmatic reactions or anaphylaxis in sensitized individuals.

Assessment of Contact Hypersensitivity in Experimental Animals Classically, the potential for a chemical to produce contact hypersensitivity has been assessed by the use of guinea pig models. These tests vary in their method of application of the test article, in the dosing schedule, and in the utilization of adjuvants. For a description of methods employed in representative tests, refer to the study of Klecak (1987). The two most commonly utilized guinea pig models, the Buehler test (Buehler, 1965) and the guinea pig maximization test (Magnusson and Kligman, 1969), are described briefly below.

In the Buehler test, the test article is applied to the shaven flank and covered with an occlusive bandage for six hours. This procedure is repeated on Days 7 and 14. On Day 28, a challenge dose of the test article is applied to a shaven area on the opposite flank and covered with an occlusive dressing for 24 hours. At 24 and 48 hours after the patch is removed, test animals are compared with vehicle-treated controls for signs of edema and erythema. The guinea pig maximization test differs in that the test article is administered by intradermal injection, an adjuvant is employed, and irritating concentrations are used. Animals are given pairs of intradermal injections at a shaven area on the shoulders. One pair of injections contains adjuvant alone, one pair contains test article alone, and one pair contains the test article mixed with adjuvant. Seven days following injection, after the area is reshaven, the test article is applied topically and an occluded patch is applied for 48 hours. In cases where the test article at the given concentration is nonirritating, the area is pretreated with 10% sodium lauryl sulfate 24 hours before the patch is applied to produce a mild inflammatory response. Two weeks following topical application, the animals are challenged on the shaven flank with a nonirritating concentration of the test article, which remains under an occluded patch for 24 hours. Then, after 24 and 48 hours, the test site is examined for signs of erythema and edema, two well-recognized indicators of cutaneous inflammation and contact dermatitis. However, the endpoints for evaluation in the guinea pig assays are visual and subjective, and it is difficult to assess irritating or colored compounds using these models.

Over the past 20 years, efforts have been made to develop and establish more quantitative and immunologically based assay methods in other species, focusing mainly on the mouse, again primarily because of the availability of reagents and techniques to conduct mechanistic studies. Gad and coworkers (1986) developed the mouse ear swelling test, which uses a quantitative measurement of ear thickness as an endpoint. Animals are sensitized by topical application of the test article for four consecutive days to abdominal skin that has been prepared by intradermal injection of adjuvant and tape stripping. On Day 10, the animals are challenged by topical application of the test article to one ear and vehicle to the contralateral ear. Measurements are made of ear thickness 24 and 48 hours later. A positive response is considered anything above a 20% increase in thickness of the treated ear over the control ear. Thorne and colleagues (1991) showed that dietary supplementation with vitamin A enhanced the mouse ear swelling assay in the absence of adjuvants, injections, or occlusive patches.

The assays described above evaluate the elicitation phase of the response in previously sensitized animals. In contrast, the mouse local lymph node assay (LLNA) identifies contact allergens as a function of the events occurring during the induction (sensitization) phase of a hypersensitivity response. The origins, development, evaluation, and eventual validation of the LLNA have been described in a comprehensive review (Kimber *et al.*, 2002). In this assay, the induction phase of contact sensitization is measured by the incorporation of ^{3}H-thymidine into proliferating lymphocytes in lymph nodes draining the site where the test article has been applied. Animals are dosed by topical application of the test article to the ears for three consecutive days. The animals are rested for two days and then injected intravenously with 20 μCi of ^{3}H-thymidine. Five hours later, animals are sacrificed, the draining lymph nodes are dissected out, and single-cell suspensions are prepared and radioassayed. With consideration of dose–response and statistical significance, a threefold increase in ^{3}H-thymidine cpm in chemically exposed animals over vehicle control animals (ie, the stimulation index) is considered to be a positive response.

The LLNA offers several advantages over the guinea pig assays in that (1) it has the potential to reduce the number of animals required and reduces animal distress; (2) it provides quantitative data that allow for statistical analysis; and (3) it provides dose–response data. The latter qualities of the LLNA have facilitated its integration into comparisons of potency across individual chemicals and/or within a chemical class. These additional advantages of the LLNA have facilitated its integration into risk assessments for contact dermatitis (Felter *et al.*, 2003). Additionally, because the LLNA evaluates the induction phase of the immune response, it is more applicable to mechanistic studies. As an example, some compounds capable of producing contact sensitization also induce IgE production and subsequent respiratory hypersensitivity. Using three known allergenic diisocyanates—diphenylmethane-4,4'-diisocyanate, dicyclohexylmethane-4,4'-diisocyanate, and isophorone diisocyanate—Dearman and coworkers (1992) showed that all three known contact sensitizers induced lymphocyte proliferation in the draining lymph node but that only diphenylmethane-4,4'-diisocyanate, a known respiratory sensitizer, induced elevated levels of serum IgE and IgG2b. These types of results have prompted a number of investigators to propose that the LLNA could be considered as the first step in a safety evaluation process for allergenic potential (ie, as a method to identify sensitization potential of a chemical) with other methods being deployed to distinguish between skin and respiratory sensitizing activity (Holsapple *et al.*, 2006).

Assessment of Contact Hypersensitivity in Humans Human testing for contact hypersensitivity reactions is by skin patch testing. Patch testing allows for the diagnostic production of acute lesions of contact hypersensitivity by the application of a suspected allergen to the skin. Patches containing specified concentrations of the allergen in the appropriate vehicle are applied under an occlusive patch for 48 hours in most test protocols. Once the patch is removed and enough time elapses for the signs of mechanical irritation to resolve (approximately 30 minutes), the area is read for signs of erythema, papules, vesicles, and edema. Generally, the test is read again at 72 hours and, in some cases, signs may not appear for up to one week or more. Detailed information on patch testing has been reviewed (Mydlarski *et al.*, 1998).

Human repeat insult patch tests are available as predictive tests in humans. Like predictive testing in animal models, there are many variations in attempts to increase the sensitivity of these procedures. These include preparation of the induction site by either tape-stripping, the application of an irritating concentration of sodium lauryl sulfate, or use of high concentrations of the test article for induction of sensitization. In general, the application of multiple occlusive patches, up to ten for 48 hours each at the same site, is followed by a rest period and then a challenge takes place under an occlusive patch at a different site. Positive reactions are scored in the same manner as for diagnostic patch tests.

Assessment of Autoimmune Responses As described in the preceding section, exaggerated immune responses can be mediated by two entirely different types of interactions between the immune system and xenobiotics. One type of interaction was described in the preceding section in which the xenobiotic is a hapten, and the immune system plays an active role in eliciting a hypersensitivity response. The immune system can also be a passive target for the enhancing effects of drugs and chemicals, such as occurs when a xenobiotic mimics or causes the aberrant production of immuno-modulatory cytokines, or when a xenobiotic disrupts the regulatory mechanisms which serve to protect self (ie, disrupt a suppressor mechanism). Additional mechanisms were presented above in the subsection "Autoimmunity" under "Immune-Mediated Disease."

Another way that xenobiotics can enhance immune function is by acting as an adjuvant, which is defined as any substance that nonspecifically enhances the immune response to an antigen. The classic adjuvant is complete Freund's adjuvant, which is a water-in-oil emulsion containing killed mycobacteria. The effectiveness of adjuvants in enhancing immune responses can be demonstrated by the fact that animals are often injected with complete Freund's adjuvant to increase the production of antigen-specific antibodies, and by the desire to develop an adjuvant that is safe in humans (ie, complete Freund's adjuvant produces severe side effects) that could be used in conjunction with vaccines or immunotherapy. The specific mechanisms for the actions of adjuvants, including complete Freund's adjuvant, are not known. Moreover, the existence of environmental adjuvants is controversial and/or poorly studied.

In the context of testing strategies, the situation with autoimmunity is much more complex than with hypersensitivity responses. Animal models exist for a number of autoimmune diseases, and autoimmunity has been clearly demonstrated in humans. Therefore, the existence of autoimmune disease and the expected consequences cannot be denied. However, the ability of drugs and chemicals to exacerbate or trigger autoimmune disease in either animal models or humans is poorly understood. In fact, of all the possible consequences of immunotoxicity, autoimmunity is unquestionably the least understood. Primarily because of the strong genetic component in the susceptibility to autoimmunity, deciphering the exact role of xenobiotics in the induction of these conditions has proven to be very difficult. The following is a brief review of some of the currently used methods of predicting the potential of a xenobiotic to trigger or exacerbate autoimmunity leading to an inappropriate immune response to self-tissue antigens that can be associated with the generation of autoantibodies and/or autoreactive T cells.

As emphasized throughout this chapter, immunotoxicology has evolved to the point where an ever-increasing number of studies are being conducted to characterize the immunotoxicity of a variety of xenobiotics using standard immunotoxicological parameters. Depending on the specific drug/chemical, the exposure conditions, the species being tested and the immune parameter being measured, the outcomes can be manifested as decreases, increases, or no effect. While there is no question that the most frequent observation has been immune suppression, there is also no doubt that some examples of immune stimulation have been reported, a profile consistent with the concept of immunotoxicology existing as a continuum (Fig. 12-1). However, this observation can trigger some important questions. Should a treatment-related increase in an immune parameter such as the T-cell-dependent antibody response be considered

an adverse response? Should an increase in the antibody response to a neoantigen be considered a harbinger of autoimmune potential? There simply is no consensus regarding the correct way to interpret an increase in immune parameters such as the T-cell-dependent antibody response, which were primarily developed to characterize the immunosuppressive potential of xenobiotics.

An assay that was specifically developed to characterize the immunostimulatory capacity of low molecular weight compounds (ie, pharmaceuticals in particular) is the popliteal lymph node assay (PLNA) (Kammuller et al., 1989). The concept for this assay was originally proposed by Gleichmann and coworkers (1984), who speculated that graft-versus-host reactions might be the basis for the pathogenetic mechanisms behind the development of drug-induced allergy and autoimmunity. The primary approach to the PLNA is to inject compounds subcutaneously into the hind footpad of either mice or rats. After six to eight days, the draining popliteal lymph nodes (PLNs) are excised and compared with PLNs from vehicle-treated animals. Differences (eg, increase) in the weight or cellularity of the treated nodes are an indication of the immunostimulatory potential of the test compound. Over the past 20 to 25 years, more than 130 chemicals have been tested in the PLNA (Pieters and Albers, 1999), yet the assay can still not be considered to be validated. Intralaboratory studies with the PLNA concluded that this method might be able to detect drugs capable of causing human drug hypersensitivity with high prevalence; but that additional development is needed to increase the reproducibility of the PLNA and to increase detection of drugs that require metabolic activation to become allergenic, or drugs for which there is dose-limiting toxicity (Weaver et al., 2005). The interpretability of the PLNA was increased by the integration of reporter antigens, trinitrophenyl-ficoll and trinitrophenyl-ovalbumin (Albers et al., 1997; Gutting et al., 1999). The reporter antigen PLNA differs from the standard PLNA in two ways. First, the reporter antigens are injected with the test substance under investigation. Second, anti-trinitrophenyl-specific antibodies are measured via ELISPOT, in addition to the comparisons of the PLNs. The profile of antibody production against the T-cell-independent antigen, trinitrophenyl-ficoll, and against trinitrophenyl-ovalbumin, an antigen recognized by T cells and B cells, enables the discrimination between immuno-sensitizing, and mere adjuvant or irritant potential of compounds.

The state-of-the-science of animal models of autoimmune disease has been summarized (Germolec, 2005). This review emphasized that while a wide variety of animal species have been studied, rodents have been most common, and concluded that rodent models fall into three categories: genetically predisposed animal models; animal models in which the autoimmune disease is produced by immunization with specific antigens; and animal models in which the disease is chemically induced.

Examples of genetically predisposed animal models include the nonobese diabetic (NOD) mouse, the F1 cross between the New Zealand black (NZB) and New Zealand white (NZW) mouse, and the MRL/lpr mouse. The NOD model has been used to study type 1 diabetes, specifically the T-cell autoimmune response, the role of B-cell antigen presentation, and the role of cytokines in the disease progression. The NZB × NZW F1 and the MRL/lpr mouse models have been used to study human SLE. The NZB × NZW F1 model has been used to map the specific susceptibility loci and to assess the importance of B-cell hyperactivity and T-cell involvement in autoantibody production in the development of SLE (reviewed by Germolec, 2005), while the important role of apoptosis in negative selection has been studied in the MRL/lpr mouse model, in which a genetic defect results in a mutation in the *Fas* gene. While both models exhibit characteristics of human SLE including high levels of serum immunoglobulins (ie, antinuclear and anti-DNA antibodies), as well as the immune-mediated nephritis, the MRL/lpr mouse model also exhibits rheumatoid factor autoantibodies and inflammatory joint disease characteristic of an arthritic response.

Arthritis can also be induced in susceptible rat strains by immunization with complete Freund's adjuvant containing killed *Mycobacterium tuberculosis* in oil. Immunization of susceptible mouse strains (ie, those containing H-2^q or H-2^r alleles of the MHC) with type II collagen or cartilage glycoproteins, in the presence of adjuvant, can induce pathology similar to human rheumatoid arthritis. In collagen-induced models of arthritis, the immune response is directed against specific connective tissue antigens, while the complete Freund's adjuvant-induced response is directed against a mycobacterium heat shock protein, with the observed pathology resulting from cross-reactive destruction of a proteoglycan found in joints (Germolec, 2005). Experimental autoimmune encephalomyelitis can be induced in a number of species by immunization with myelin basic protein and complete Freund's adjuvant. This model has been used in rodents to characterize the role of T helper cell-mediated autoimmune disease characterized by perivascular lymphocyte infiltration of the CNS and the destruction of the myelin nerve sheath resulting in paralysis, similar to human multiple sclerosis.

One of the most commonly used models of chemically induced autoimmunity is the Brown Norway rat model, where animals are injected with mercuric chloride. While the selection of doses is such that exposure produces no overt signs of toxicity, Brown Norway rats develop an immunologically-mediated disease characterized by T-cell-mediated polyclonal B-cell activation, autoantibodies to laminin, collagen IV, and other components of the glomerular basement membrane similar to human autoimmune glomerulonephritis. Numerous mouse strains have also been used to evaluate the development of autoantibodies following exposure to mercury, gold, and cadmium (Selgrade *et al.*, 1999). Other examples of xenobiotics that have been demonstrated to be associated with autoimmune disease will be provided below.

Molecular Biology Approaches to Immunotoxicology As in all of the biological sciences, the continuing evolution of molecular biology-based methods and technologies have vastly expanded the tools available to immunotoxicologists. In general, molecular biology approaches have been thus far employed primarily in the investigation and elucidation of mechanisms of immunotoxicity rather than for identifying immunotoxicants. As these approaches become more refined and sophisticated with time, their application will surely expand. Presently, the primary application of molecular biology in immunotoxicology has been to identify genes whose expression has been altered by a xenobiotic, often termed gene expression profiling, and/or to quantify the magnitude to which gene expression has been changed due to some treatment. As already discussed, methods for assessing changes in gene expression have been particularly useful for studies of the immune system due to the fact that many of the immunological mediators produced by leukocytes (eg, cytokines, chemokines, and immunoglobulins) are regulated transcriptionally (ie, synthesized and secreted on demand) rather than being maintained in cells as stored products. Toward this end, quantitative reverse transcriptase-polymerase chain reaction (RT-PCR) has been the principal method currently used to assess changes in mRNA levels for specific genes in tissues and cells. With the development of real time RT-PCR, accurate quantification of gene-specific mRNA levels is readily achieved through the analysis of PCR kinetics by detecting products as they accumulate in "real time" through the application of fluorogenic

probes or double-stranded DNA binding dyes. Significant advantages of RT-PCR over traditional methods for analysis of mRNA levels, principally Northern blotting, includes accuracy, sensitivity, markedly less RNA required to conduct the analysis, and less time required to complete the analysis. Recent advances in thermocycler technology and the availability of commercial reagents currently permit the quantification of up to 384 genes from one RNA sample by employing what are termed "low-density" arrays. The technology takes advantage of plates comprised of 384 wells that have been precoated with primers for up to 384 specific genes of interest.

Another approach for conducting gene expression profiling by assessing changes in mRNA levels for multiple genes simultaneously has been through the use of cDNA microarrays. The approach facilitates the analysis of hundreds to tens of thousands of genes from a single RNA sample. The principal advantage of microarrays is the ability to assay mRNA levels for a large number of genes simultaneously. The primary disadvantages are the cost associated with microarray analysis, the complexity associated with data analysis and bioinformatics, and the sensitivity of the methodology to assess moderate changes in mRNA levels. In spite of these challenges, the application of microarray analysis in immunotoxicology has been increasing (Luebke *et al.*, 2006b).

A routinely employed methodology for characterizing effects on gene transcription has been the use of reporter assays. Reporter assays are being widely used to discern whether xenobiotic-induced changes in mRNA levels for specific genes are due to alterations at the level of transcription versus mRNA stability. Likewise, reporters can be used to characterize the effects of xenobiotics on specific transcription factors acting through defined regulatory elements. The approach involves construction of a DNA plasmid possessing the 5′ untranslated regulatory region of the gene of interest that has been ligated to the translated region of a reporter gene. Commonly used reporter genes are typically enzymes, since their expression can be easily assayed. Moreover, studies in mammalian systems commonly employ reporter genes of insect or bacterial origin, thus eliminating the need to differentiate between endogenous and ectopic expression. The most widely used reporter genes are firefly luciferase and bacterial β-galactosidase. Most often, reporter assays are performed by transient transfection into cell lines. This approach has been extensively used to study the effects of leukocyte activation stimuli and xenobiotics on the regulation of promoter and enhancer regions of cytokine and Ig genes. In spite of the important mechanistic information that can be gained from these types of studies, significant challenges often arise in utilizing reporter assays to study leukocytes. Transfection of primary leukocytes, especially lymphocytes, yielding both high transfection efficiency and good cell viability is extremely difficult. An additional complicating factor concerns the fact that lymphocytes can only be maintained viable in culture for short periods (approximately 24 hours) in the absence of activation, which limits the duration the cells can be given to recover after transfection. Likewise, it is not uncommon for T- and B-cell derived lines to be resistant to transfection in spite of the many commercial transfection reagents presently available and new refinements made to electroporation instruments. In most cases, transfection conditions must be optimized for transfection efficiency and cell viability for each cell line or preparation using a control plasmid (ie, a plasmid possessing strong constitutive expression).

RNA interference employing small interfering double-stranded RNAs (siRNA) to achieve posttranscriptional gene-specific silencing is widely applied to investigations aimed at elucidation of mechanism of immunotoxicity. RNA duplexes of 21 nucleotides possessing two nucleotide 3′ overhanging ends once transfected into the cell incorporate into a nuclease complex known as the RNA-induced silencing complex (RISC). Through an ATP-dependent mechanism, the duplexes are unwound and separated into their sense and antisense strands. RISC is directed by the unwound antisense siRNA strand homologous to the target mRNA, which then undergoes cleavage by an endonuclease termed "Slicer." The ensuing destruction of the target gene mRNA results in the posttranslational silencing of gene expression. This approach provides a rapid mechanism by which the involvement of a specific gene product can be linked to biochemical and functional events induced by a xenobiotic in a given cell type, including leukocytes (Sandy et al., 2005). Major challenges in the application of this methodology can exist. First, identification of an effective siRNA is critical, as not all sites of a given mRNA being targeted will result in gene silencing. Numerous strategies and criteria have been developed to assist in the rationale design of siRNA (Jia et al., 2006; Khvorova et al., 2003; Schwarz et al., 2003). Second, as with the transient transfection of reporters discussed above, leukocytes, and especially lymphocytes, are often resistant to transfection resulting either in poor delivery of the siRNA into the desired cell preparation or low viability. Since siRNA are most often used in cell lines, the doubling rate of the cells can significantly affect the level of knockdown achieved based on the fact that each time a cell undergoes replication, the cellular siRNA is diluted by half. The half-life of the protein can also significantly impact on the level of knockdown achieved even if large amounts of siRNA are delivered into the cells. Also, genes that are highly expressed can be difficult to effectively knockdown due to the large amount of mRNA that must be destroyed. Likewise, genes with very low expression can be difficult to silence as the odds of the RISC complex finding rare mRNAs in the cell may be low. Lastly, antibodies must be available to the gene product being targeted for knockdown so that the magnitude of knockdown can be confirmed at the protein level. In spite of these many potential challenges, the ability to effectively achieve gene-specific silencing, in some cases of a magnitude greater than 90%, is a remarkably powerful tool when elucidating biological mechanisms for which knockout mice are not available.

A relatively new area of research that has not yet had broad application to the field of immunotoxicology is proteomics. Proteomics can be defined as research that aims to identify, quantify, and classify the function of proteins produced by given genomes. In addition to the systematic identification and characterization of proteins, a potentially important application of proteomics is in the characterization of protein–protein interactions, especially as they relate to the elucidation of signal transduction mechanisms. Strategies have been proposed for the functional analysis of signal transduction, termed phosphoproteomics (Morandell et al., 2006). Unfortunately, a major drawback in the application of proteomics includes the lack of an experimental platform currently available to systematically measure the diverse properties of proteins in a high-throughput approach. Presently, most proteomic methods are based on mass spectrometry and require expensive instrumentation, information-technology infrastructure, and highly specialized personnel. In addition, the complexity of the proteome is enormous as illustrated by Aebersold when he compared the human genome, which is comprised of approximately 30,000 genes, to human serum, which alone has been estimated to contain approximately 500,000 different protein species (Aebersold, 2003). Nevertheless, the application of proteomics to study proteins is occurring routinely in cell-based systems.

As stated above, the use of molecular biology based methods in immunotoxicology to date has been primarily for understanding mechanisms of action of known immunotoxicants. Much research is currently focused on quantifying changes in mRNA levels (eg, cytokines) and elucidating mechanisms responsible for those xenobiotic-induced changes. Similarly, changes in mRNA expression profiles may be useful as possible biomarkers of exposure. Proteomics and genomics, combined with bioinformatics, are making it possible to evaluate chemically induced alterations in entire pathways and signaling networks. The utility of molecular biology tools such as proteomics and genomics in elucidating mechanisms of action is obvious. More challenging will be the application of these tools for identifying new or suspected immunotoxicants (Luebke et al., 2006b).

Mechanistic Approaches to Immunotoxicology Once an agent has been identified as being an immunotoxicant, it may be necessary to further characterize the mechanism by which it exerts its effects on the immune system. Toward this end, a unique aspect of the immune system that greatly facilitates investigations aimed at delineating the underlying mechanisms of action is the ability to study the immune system in the intact animal as well as remove immune cells from the intact animal and have them function in vitro. Using a combination of these two approaches, a general strategy has been successfully employed by a wide number of laboratories for characterizing mechanisms of immunotoxic action by xenobiotics and involves the following steps: (1) identifying the cell type(s) targeted by the agent; (2) determining whether the effects are mediated by the parent compound or by a metabolite of the parent; (3) determining whether the effects are mediated directly or indirectly by the xenobiotic; and (4) elucidating the molecular events responsible for altered leukocyte function. The significance of each and the experimental strategies typically employed are discussed below.

Identification of the Cell Type or Type(s) Targeted With few exceptions, the first objective toward elucidation of the mechanism(s) responsible for immunotoxicity is the identification of the cell type(s) affected by the xenobiotic. The rationale is that the immune system is comprised of a wide variety of cell types with broad, and often, overlapping effector functions. Therefore, identification of specific cell type(s) affected allows for the selection of appropriate approaches and techniques to employ to further elucidate the mechanism of action.

The approaches available for the identification of the cell types targeted by a specific agent are numerous but typically originate with the employment of one or more of the functional assays within the immunotoxicology tier testing battery (see the "The National Toxicology Program Tier Approach" section later in this chapter). Each of the functional assays in the immunotoxicology tier testing battery provides information on accessory and/or effector cell function. For example, the AFC response to the T-cell-dependent antigen, sRBC, requires macrophages and CD4+ T cells (Th cells) to function as accessory cells, and B cells to serve as the effector cells. Therefore, if any one of these three cell types is adversely affected by an immunotoxicant, changes in the magnitude of the AFC response would be observed as compared to control (ie, enhancement or suppression). Similarly, the CTL response requires APC and CD4+ T cells (Th cells) as the accessory cells and CD8+ T cells, which are the effector CTL. Functional assays can be further refined to provide additional information concerning the targeted cell types by employment of various defined antigens requiring different cellular cooperativity to elicit an effector response. The AFC response has been especially useful in this respect. In addition to using a T-cell-dependent sensitizing antigen such as sRBC, T-cell-independent antigens can be employed including dinitrophenyl-ficoll or trinitrophenyl-LPS, which require macrophages, but do not require T cells, to elicit an antibody response. Likewise, B cells can be driven to differentiate into AFC in the absence of accessory cells using polyclonal B-cell activators such as LPS. By employing the three different types of antigens in order to characterize a xenobiotic, a profile of activity emerges that can distinguish between affects on the B cell, T cell, and APC.

As described in the examples above, when accessory cells are required in the elicitation of an immune response, it is often difficult to discern whether alteration of an immune response is due to the xenobiotic targeting the effector cell population or one or more of the accessory cell populations. Under such circumstances, another strategy utilized for identifying the cellular targets is a cell fractionation–reconstitution approach. Specifically, leukocytes can be isolated from treated and vehicle control animals, typically mice, and fractionated into their respective populations. The fractioned cell populations from vehicle and treated animals can then be reconstituted in various combinations to be used in functional assays to determine the population of cells that has been altered. A comprehensive discussion of the various methods that can be used to fractionate leukocyte populations and subpopulations is beyond the scope of this chapter; however, two of the most common approaches to fractionate leukocyte populations are briefly described here. The first is by cell sorting using flow cytometry. The primary advantage of this approach is that it yields an exceptionally high purity of cell populations and subpopulations. The primary disadvantages include: (1) access to a high-end flow cytometer; (2) cost of reagents and trained personnel capable of operating a flow cytometer; (3) practical limitations concerning the total number of cells that can be collected within a reasonable period of time due to the rate at which the instrument analyzes and collects the cells; and (4) positive selection (ie, the cells are bound by a cell-specific antibody) is used for identifying the desired cell population being collected. The second and more commonly used approach utilizes antibodies directed at surface antigens unique to specific leukocyte populations and subpopulations that have been covalently conjugated to magnetic beads. Using the conjugated magnetic beads and a magnet, large numbers of highly pure cell populations can be isolated rapidly, by positive or negative selection, without requirements for expensive instrumentation. As with the cell sorting approach, purified population of cells isolated from vehicle and treated animals can be isolated and reconstituted in various combinations for evaluation in functional assays.

Determination of Whether Immunotoxicity is Mediated by the Parent or by a Metabolite of the Parent Compound A critical aspect in the elucidation of the mechanism of toxicity for any compound, regardless of the target or tissue is whether the adverse effects are mediated by the parent form of the compound or its metabolite. An understanding of the role of metabolism is especially critical when studying immunotoxicants as it will dictate the experimental approaches that can be utilized. In general, leukocytes possess very modest levels of drug-metabolizing enzymes, especially those within the cytochrome P450 family. Therefore, those agents that are metabolically bioactivated to an immunosuppressive form will in most cases not exhibit their immunotoxic profile of activity when added directly to cultured leukocytes. In fact, an important indication that metabolic activation may be a requisite mechanistic event is the observation that an agent is immunotoxic following in vivo administration while exhibiting no immunotoxic activity when added directly to cultured leukocytes. An example of such an agent is the therapeutic agent, cyclophosphamide. When administered in vivo, cyclophosphamide is a potent immunosuppressant that preferentially suppresses humoral immune responses while having no effect when directly added to cultured leukocytes.

In order to assess whether metabolic bioactivation is required for immunotoxicity, several different approaches can be employed. One approach is to determine whether pre- or co-treatment with either an inducer or an inhibitor of the enzymes known to be involved in the metabolism of the agent modify the immunotoxicity produced in vivo. Similarly, in vitro approaches have also been used to assess the role of metabolism for an immunotoxicant. Specifically, these approaches utilize various in vitro metabolic activation systems such as S9 liver homogenates or isolated liver microsomes, which can activate the xenobiotic when incorporated with leukocyte cultures. Alternatively, freshly isolated primary hepatocytes can be cocultured with leukocytes in the presence of the xenobiotic. Although primary hepatocytes most closely simulate the metabolic activity observed in vivo, this approach is also the most technically challenging since the approach is critically dependent on the isolation of viable and metabolically active hepatocytes. Cyclophosphamide is typically employed as a positive control in all three of the aforementioned in vitro activation systems to confirm metabolic activity. The metabolic activation systems discussed above can also be employed for conducting mechanistic studies in vitro that cannot be performed in the intact animal to further characterize immunotoxicants requiring metabolic bioactivation.

Determination of Whether the Effects are Mediated Directly or Indirectly by the Xenobiotic or a Metabolite of the Xenobiotic In most instances, immunotoxicants mediate their effects by interacting directly with the immune system. These direct actions may include structural alterations in lymphoid organs or on the cellular composition of lymphoid organs, on the expression of regulatory molecules on the immune cell surface, and/or by altering intracellular biochemical or molecular events (Table 12-8). However, some xenobiotics mediate changes in immune competence through an indirect action on the immune system. Under these circumstances, changes in immune competence are mediated through the release of an immunomodulatory factor resulting from the actions of the immunotoxicant on cells or tissues other than the immune system. One tissue most often implicated in indirectly modulating the immune system is the liver, as it is the source of a broad and extremely diverse group of proteins, including acute-phase proteins. Acute-phase proteins are a family of serum proteins produced by the liver in response to inflammation or infection (see the "Inflammation" section). Acute-phase proteins are believed to have evolved as part of an immediate survival response to systemic infection. In general, acute-phase proteins are associated with downregulation of the immune system and are therefore believed to play a role in maintaining immune homeostasis. The acute-phase proteins most extensively characterized with respect to immune-modulating properties include α-fetoprotein, serum amyloid A, and C-reactive protein. Another important group of regulatory proteins involved in indirectly modulating the immune system are those that contribute to the repair and regeneration of the liver after acute injury; specifically, TGF-β1 and hepatocyte growth factor. A second example of indirect actions on the immune system is stress as well as agents that alter the regulation of the hypothalamic–pituitary–adrenal axis, thus leading to changes in hormonal homeostasis. Deregulation of hormonal homeostasis, especially increased circulating levels of glucocorticoids, can markedly decrease immune competence.

The elucidation of indirect mechanisms of action by an immunotoxicant can be challenging by virtue that the effect is indirect

Table 12-8

Possible Mechanisms of Chemical-Induced Immune Modulation

TYPE OF EFFECT	MECHANISM	EXAMPLES
Direct	Functional changes	Altered antibody-mediated responses
		Altered cell-mediated responses
		Altered release of preformed mediators
		Altered host resistance
		Inability of one or more cell types to perform a required activity, for example:
		Production of antibody
		Release of cytokines
		Processing and presentation of antigen
		Proliferation and differentiation
		Receptor-mediated signal transduction
	Structural changes	Alterations in surface receptors or ligands
		Alteration in expression of receptors or ligands
		Histopathological changes in lymphoid organs
	Compositional Changes	Alterations in $CD3^+$, $CD4^+$, $CD8^+$, $B220^+$, and/or Ig^+ in spleen
		Alterations in $CD4^+$, $CD8^+$, $CD4^+/CD8^+$, and/or $CD4^-/CD8^-$ in thymus
		Changes in hematological cellular parameters
		Alterations in circulating Ig
		Alterations in CFU profile in bone marrow
	Metabolic activation	Conversion to a toxic metabolite
Indirect	Effects secondary to other target organ toxicity	Induction of acute-phase proteins as a result of liver injury
		Increased corticosteroid release from the adrenal gland
	Hormonal changes	Alteration in neuroendocrine regulation
		Alteration in autonomic output from the CNS
		Altered release of steroids from sex organs

and mediated by one or more circulating immunomodulatory serum factors. The involvement of an immunomodulatory serum factor can be partially deduced by two distinguishing features. First, the profile of immunotoxicity observed after in vivo administration of the causative agent is different from that produced by its direct addition to leukocytes in culture. Second, the profile of immunotoxicity observed after in vivo administration of the agent can be mimicked by direct addition of serum from the treated animal to naive leukocytes in culture. Third, the involvement of a metabolite of the parent form of the chemical has been ruled out. Confirmation of the involvement of a specific serum factor is most often accomplished in vitro by abrogating the immunotoxic activity produced by serum from treated animals using neutralizing antibodies directed against the suspected serum factor.

Elucidation of the Molecular Mechanism Numerous methodologies are available to evaluate cellular and molecular mechanisms of action and those continue to increase with the availability of new "omics" technologies, new animal models including transgenic and knockouts, and an ever-expanding list of reagents and molecular probes. Due to the broad nature of this topic area, this section is devoted to a general discussion of considerations and strategies aimed at the elucidation of molecular mechanisms. The discussion will be directed at B cells and T cells for illustrative purposes, but is certainly applicable to other cell types comprising the immune system.

When considering the molecular mechanism by which a xenobiotic alters the function of a mature lymphocyte, a practical strategy is to first identify at which stage of leukocyte function the agent is acting, antigen recognition/signaling through the antigen receptor, activation, proliferation, or differentiation. As discussed in the earlier sections of this chapter, lymphocytes have evolved

a number of specialized mechanisms by which B and T cells recognize antigen. Common to both cell types is that immediately after recognition of an antigen, there are a number of biochemical events triggered, including changes in protein phosphorylation and activation of a variety of kinases, fluxes in ions, and changes in the level of cyclic nucleotides. Because lymphocytes undergo a rapid and robust rise in intracellular calcium almost immediately after antigen–receptor binding, changes in calcium flux prior to and immediately following stimulation by an antigen provide important insights into whether an agent alters the most proximal stage of leukocyte function. Similarly, changes in the phosphorylation status of the intracellular domain of membrane-associated proteins (CD3 complex, CD4 and CD8 on T cells, and CD79, CD45, and CD22 on B cells) and the kinases that mediate the phosphorylation (eg, lyk and fyn) can be investigated to study the most proximal events associated with triggering of antigen receptors. Polyclonal activators are often employed to simultaneously activate large numbers of lymphocytes facilitating the evaluation of changes in these early biochemical events. For B cells, antibodies directed against the BCR in combination with CD40L can be used. Conversely, for T cells, antibodies directed against the TCR/CD3 complex and the coreceptor CD28.

The stage termed lymphocyte activation is functionally defined and refers to that period that begins when the T cell has initiated a response to an activation stimulus and ends when there is robust transcription of the T-cell autocrine/paracrine growth factor, IL-2 and upregulation of proteins on the cell surface including CD40L, CD69, and CD25 (alpha chain of the IL-2 receptor). In B cells, it is the period that begins with the cell responding to an activation signal culminating in the upregulation of activation markers CD80 (B7.1), CD86 (B7.2), CD69, and increased MHCII. All of the aforementioned changes associated with B-cell and T-cell activation, including IL-2 synthesis, can be readily monitored and quantified in individual cells by flow cytometry. Investigations directed at elucidating the molecular events deregulated by xenobiotics during lymphocyte activation represent one of the most intensively studied areas presently in immunotoxicology as many different immunotoxicants affect this stage of lymphocyte function.

Clonal expansion is a critical phase of the immune response as it insures that a sufficient number of antigen-specific B- and T-effector cells are generated to respond effectively to combat a pathogen. In light of the importance of clonal expansion in mounting an effective immune response, the effect xenobiotics exert on lymphocyte proliferation has been widely used to determine whether a xenobiotic has immunotoxic properties. As with measurements directed at other stages of the immune response, it is often convenient to employ polyclonal B- and T-cell activators for investigating effects on proliferative responses. Due to a significant increase in the understanding of the cell cycle, coupled with the availability of reagents for measuring specific proteins involved in the regulation of cell cycle, it is now possible to functionally characterize and dissect the mechanism and specific intracellular targets affected by xenobiotics that disrupt lymphocyte proliferation. Measurements of changes in cell-cycle-associated regulatory proteins are most commonly achieved by employing flow cytometric approaches.

The final stage of the immune response involves differentiation into a mature effector or memory cell. For B and T cells, terminal differentiation into effector cells can be best assessed by measurements of effector function in conjunction with the upregulation and downregulation of proteins on the cell surface. Antibody production and upregulation of CD138 (also known as syndecan-1) are most often used as indicators of B-cell differentiation into effector cells while either cytokine production (Th cells and CTL) or lysis of target cells expressing viral or tumor proteins (CTL) are used to indicate T-cell differentiation. A number of commonly used immune function methods for assessing B- and T-cell effector functions were described earlier in this section.

Once the specific stage of lymphocyte function being altered by a specific xenobiotic has been established, experiments can be designed to identify the specific intracellular proteins affected by the xenobiotic and the molecular mechanism by which it is modulated. Cell line models can be invaluable tools for studies involving cell signaling and gene regulation.

Cell Line Models in Immunotoxicology Cell line-based models are being widely used for identifying agents possessing the potential of producing immunotoxicity as well as for conducting in-depth investigations aimed at elucidating molecular mechanisms for immunotoxicity. Significant advantages and disadvantages exist when applying cell line-based models, some of which are unique to investigations of the immune system. A brief discussion of the strengths and limitations of cell line-based models in the context of studies of immunotoxicants is provided below.

Although there are many advantages to cell line-based models, the most important characteristic is that all of the cells are derived from the same clone thus providing a homogenous cellular preparation. The homogeneity of the model is especially useful for studies directed at characterizing signal transduction pathways as well as gene expression profiling due to the greater likelihood of obtaining reproducible results. There are a number of advantages of cell line-based models that are especially useful in immunotoxicology. Primary leukocytes whether isolated from blood or lymphoid organs are highly heterogeneous in their cellular composition. Purification of these primary cell preparations into specific cell types is expensive, can be labor intensive and with most isolation methods typically yielding 50% to 75% efficiency (ie, 25%–50% of the desired cells are lost during the purification process). Purification efficiency can become a critical issue when utilizing small rodents such as mice where the number of animals per assay can be significantly increased due to the loss of cells being recovered in the cell isolation procedure. When employing cell line models, typically there is no limitation on the number of cells available for a given study. Another important consideration in the case of primary lymphocytes is that they are only viable in culture for relatively brief periods of time (approximately 24 hours) in the absence of an activation signal. Therefore, extended preincubation periods in culture with an immunotoxicant or other response modifiers that do not activate primary lymphocytes cannot be performed. Primary leukocytes, especially lymphocytes, are also difficult to transfect, often yielding poor transfection efficiency and/or viability. The combination of poor transfection efficiency and limited culture duration in the absence of activation make reporter assays, transient ectopic gene expression, and utilization of siRNA to silence gene expression challenging in primary lymphocytes. Conversely, cell line-based models, especially of the lymphoid lineage, in most cases can be readily transfected with suitable efficiency and viability to conduct reporter assays, ectopic gene expression, and gene silencing with siRNA. It is noteworthy that primary cells of the myeloid lineage are more suited for long-term culture- and transfection-based experimental approaches as they have less stringent requirements for activation to be maintained in culture for extended periods. In such instances, it may be more advantageous to employ primary cells. Lastly, cell line-based models are also now being widely adapted for high-throughput screening due to the reproducibility of results obtained with these models and the ease in which cell lines can be maintained and manipulated.

In spite of the advantages discussed above, there are numerous disadvantages and limitations inherent in utilizing cell line models for characterizing immunotoxicants. The most important consideration when utilizing cell line models is that by definition, a cell line is an abnormal population of cells that has undergone a change rendering it capable of dividing indefinitely in culture. Since cell lines are continuously dividing, in most cases they are not good models for studying immunotoxicants that act by altering cell proliferation and/or regulators of the cell cycle. The aberrant nature of cell lines may also extend to a loss of function through one or more of its cognate receptors. Lastly, it is critical that cell lines are carefully monitored and characterized for changes in function and morphology after repeated passage in culture. Additional important considerations when selecting a cell line for mechanistic studies are the capacity of the cell line to perform a given effector function and the stimuli to which the model will respond. Toward this end, a number of cell lines have been extensively characterized and widely utilized that are capable of induced effector functions including cytokine production, antibody secretion, and release of a wide variety of mediators. Table 12-9 provides examples of some commonly used cell lines in immunotoxicology. As discussed above, with some cell lines, induction of an effector function may only be achievable by using pharmacological activators (eg, phorbol ester plus calcium ionophore) that bypass extracellular receptors or by agents that are polyclonal activators (eg, LPS) that do not activate directly through antigen receptors. Again these are characteristics of the models that need to be considered in the context of how the models will be used and for what specific purpose. In most cases, the utilization of cell line-based models can be extremely useful but results should always

Table 12-9

Cellular Models for Immunotoxicology

CELL LINE	CELL TYPE	SPECIES	EFFECTOR RESPONSE	STIMULUS
EL4	T cell	Mouse	IL-2	Phorbol ester
Jurkat E6	T cell	Human	IL-2	Phorbol ester + Ca ionophore or anti-CD3 + anti-CD28
CHI2.LX	B cell	Mouse	IgM	LPS
BCL-1	B cell	Mouse	IgM	LPS
SKW	B cell	Human	IgM	LPS or αIgM + CD40L
Daudi	B cell	Human	None (signal transduction)	αIgM
RAW 264.7	Macrophage	Mouse	Nitric oxide, IL-1	LPS
J774.1	Macrophage	Mouse	Nitric oxide, IFN-γ	LPS
U937	Macrophage	Human	TNF-α, IL-1α, IL-6, IL-8	LPS

be confirmed, when possible, in primary leukocytes since cell lines are aberrant models.

Animal Models: Transgenics, Knockouts, and Humanized/Severe Combined Immunodeficient The developments in molecular biology have not only permitted the evaluation of specific genes or arrays of genes but have also allowed for the manipulation of the embryonic genome, creating transgenic, and knockout mice (reviewed by IPCS, 1996). As a consequence of transgenic technology, complex immune responses can be dissected into their components. In this way, the mechanisms by which immunotoxicants act can be better understood. Mice engineered to express nonself genes (eg, human MHCI) or overexpress self genes (eg, constitutively active transcription factors) are termed "transgenic," and can be used to address the role of a certain protein in immunotoxicology. On the other hand, mice lacking certain proteins (eg, receptors, transcription factors, or cytokines) are termed "knockouts," and can be used for similar mechanistic studies. Numerous transgenic and knockout mice have been created and are available to investigators worldwide. Of particular interest and potential utility in the area of immunotoxicology is what has been termed "humanized" mice. Humanized mice refer to immune-deficient mice that have been reconstituted either with human HSC to support a fully human immune system, or with mature cells to evaluate immune regulation, hematopoiesis, hypersensitivity, and autoimmunity. Severe combined immunodeficient (SCID) mice, which are mouse T- and B-cell deficient due to a VDJ recombination defect, are a major strain into which human immune cells/system are established. In addition, SCID mice are backcrossed with other strains in order to eliminate various arms of the immune system (eg, β2M^{null}/SCID eliminate MHCI interactions) prior to reconstitution with human cells (reviewed by Thomsen *et al.*, 2005). Although their use in mechanistic studies is obvious, SCID/hu mice have also been utilized for evaluation of efficacy of antiviral drugs for HIV/AIDS (reviewed by Taggart *et al.*, 2004). There are still considerations, however, for broader application of these humanized mouse models for immunotoxicological assessment of compounds. For instance, one must consider how these animals compare with standard animal models with respect to time course of action, dose response, pharmacokinetics, and other factors of chemical toxicity. With the hope that these humanized mouse models can be used to identify new or suspected immunotoxicants, and mechanisms of action, one must also consider whether they are as sensitive, predictive, and/or cost-effective as traditional animal models.

Approaches to the Assessment of Human Immunotoxicity

As emphasized throughout this chapter, animal models have been extensively utilized to characterize immunotoxicity, and it is widely recognized that chemicals that produce immunotoxicity in animals have the potential to produce immune effects in the human population. The increasing emphasis on human risk assessment requires that those potential health hazards be identified whenever possible. In spite of the significant homology of the rodent and human immune systems which has facilitated our ability to make decisions on the immunotoxic potential of test materials based on the results of these experimental models (House, 1997), there is also an increasing recognition of distinct, although often subtle, differences in the composition of the immune system between animal species. These differences have primarily come to light in studies of leukocyte subpopulations, the phenotypic markers they express, and by the regulatory factors they secrete. Whether these differences in immune system composition result in significant differences across species in sensitivity to immunotoxicants is unclear. It is important to emphasize that to date there are no known cases of significant human immunotoxicity that has resulted due to false-negative results from rodent-based immunotoxicity testing. In contrast, there is extremely limited human immunotoxicology data on test materials other than those directly intended for human immunotherapy.

One of the obvious and most important goals of an experimental immunotoxicity testing strategy is to enable the best extrapolations between the results generated in the animal models and the potential risk of immunotoxicity in humans. A parallelogram approach has been used to assess relationships between animal data and human data (Selgrade, 1999; van Loveren *et al.*, 1995) and an adaptation of which is presented in Fig. 12-21. The overall strategy is to utilize in vivo and in vitro data from animal studies and in vitro data using human leukocytes in order to predict the in vivo effects of an immunotoxicant in humans. This approach has been used to extrapolate animal to human data in an initial quantitative assessment of the risk for deleterious effects of UV radiation (van Loveren *et al.*, 1995) and of the immunotoxicity associated with exposure to bis(tri-*n*-butyltin)oxide (van Loveren *et al.*, 1998). A parallelogram approach has also been used to propose that data for ozone suggest that effects of in vivo human exposure to phosgene on alveolar macrophages phagocytosis may be predicted based on effects of in vitro exposure and in vivo animal data (reviewed by Selgrade *et al.*, 1995).

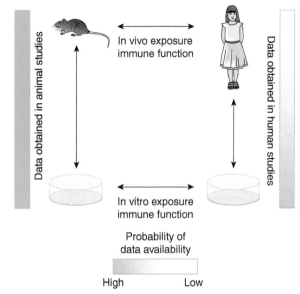

Figure 12-21. *Parallelogram approach in immunotoxicology for relating animal and human data.* Immune in vitro data are often available for animals and humans. However, much of human immunotoxicity risk must be estimated from human in vitro studies and animal in vivo studies.

In spite of these successful applications of the parallelogram approach, it is recognized that extrapolations of alterations in immune function observed in animals to human health is associated with various uncertainties (House, 1997). For example, experimental animals are often inbred, which certainly lessens interanimal variability thereby simplifying the statistical evaluation of observations. Additionally, laboratory studies in rodents are highly controlled for environment, diet, and health status. In contrast, humans are a highly outbred species with a high degree of interindividual variability in immune response, and any human study must take into account extreme variability in all of the controlled parameters. In fact, it has been estimated that the overall immunocompetence of the individual is affected by age, gender, genetic factors, use of certain medications, drug/alcohol use, smoking history, stress and nutritional status, and that these factors can account for variability of more than two standard deviations in the "normal" human population (Luebke *et al.*, 2004). Luster *et al.* (2007) have speculated that the major gap in clarifying the shape of the dose–response curve (ie, between immune response and disease) is a lack of large-scale epidemiological studies in populations with mild-to-moderate immunodeficiency that have been monitored for immune system parameters and clinical disease taking into account potential complications by nonimmune factors which can affect infectious disease incidences.

Nonetheless, there is a clear association between suppression of immune function and an increased incidence of infectious and neoplastic disease in humans (reviewed by Biagini, 1998). However as noted above, a major limitation of immunotoxicity risk assessment has been the lack of human data (Descotes, 2006). In the context of xenobiotics, the majority of such data comes from immunotherapeutic drugs, which were intentionally designed to influence the immune system. The aforementioned association has been established primarily with a standard battery of parameters used extensively in clinical immunology studies, including routine complete blood counts and differentials, phenotypic characterization of surface markers and more detailed analysis of cellular subsets using a flow cytometer, lymphoproliferative assays (ie, using a number of stimuli including mitogens such as Con A and PHA,

recall antigens such as tetanus toxoid, anti-CD3 monoclonal antibody, and allogeneic lymphocytes in an MLR), and DTH responses using a test panel of recall antigens. In contrast with the clear association demonstrated for drugs used to deliberately suppress immune function or treat cancer, the assessment of immunotoxicity in humans exposed to potentially immunotoxic chemicals is much more complicated than in experimental animals (reviewed by IPCS, 1996). One of the fallouts of this observation has been the recognition that the historic approaches that have been used in clinical immunology may not have much use in human immunotoxicology. While these endpoints are sufficient to detect immunodeficiencies associated with either congenital disorders or immunosuppressive drug therapy, they do not possess the necessary sensitivity to detect the more subtle consequences of xenobiotic-induced immunotoxicity. Interestingly, Luebke *et al.* (2004) noted that in contrast to individuals with severe forms of primary or secondary immunodeficiency in whom infections to opportunistic pathogens (ie, members of the herpes viruses family, certain protozoans, *Candida albicans*, a yeast, and *Pneumocystis carinii*, a fungus) are seen, humans with low to moderate suppression of immune function are more susceptible to infection with pathogens associated with infections common in the general population (ie, encapsulated bacteria like *Streptococcus*, and influenza viruses). As a result, several proposals have been put forth to reevaluate the way that we measure immune function in humans. Most of these testing strategies have incorporated plans to measure the primary response to a new antigen, and several of these testing strategies have recommended using newly developed vaccines as the new antigen (van Loveren *et al.*, 2001). Vaccine response rates have been successfully used to characterize the impact of chronic stress on human immunocompetence (Glaser *et al.*, 2000; Kiecolt-Glaser *et al.*, 1996). Importantly, in spite of the limitations in human data, there is no question that environmental chemicals are associated with immunotoxicity in humans (Selgrade, 2007; Veraldi *et al.*, 2006).

It is anticipated that the development, validation, and utilization of more predictive methods to assess immunotoxicology in humans will be increasingly important in the future. Notably, the application of the parallelogram approach—by definition—requires the ability to measure immunotoxic effects using in vitro approaches with human lymphocytes. As described in another section of this chapter, human lymphocytes have been previously applied to study the effects of dibenzo-*p*-dioxins (Lu *et al.*, 2011, 2010; Wood and Holsapple, 1993; Wood *et al.*, 1993). Partly because of the recognition that investigations conducted exclusively using in vitro and in vivo animals models may not always be predictive of toxicity in humans (Selgrade, 1999; Vos and van Loveren, 1998), and partly because of the tremendous increase in the development of new drugs that are known to, or suspected of targeting the human immune system as discussed elsewhere in this chapter, there has been increasing interest in establishing predictive in vitro methods using human lymphocytes. A polyclonal IgM AFC response model was developed using the combination of CD40 ligand (CD40L) plus recombinant cytokines because it effectively drives both primary human and mouse B cells in a physiologically relevant manner to mimic T-cell-dependent antibody responses in vivo (Lu *et al.*, 2009). A second assay, the human lymphocyte activation (HuLa) assay, was developed that measures an influenza antigen-specific response using frozen-stored human peripheral blood mononuclear cells (PBMC) (Collinge *et al.*, 2010). Although proliferation is the primary endpoint in the HuLa, flow cytometry approaches can be used to characterize the proliferating lymphocyte subsets (eg, CD4[+] and CD8[+] T lymphocytes and B lymphocytes), and ELISPOT can be used to measure influenza-specific AFC. A third in vitro model, termed MIMIC (Modular IMmune In vitro Construct), uses the circulating immune cells of individual donors to recapitulate each individual human immune response by maintaining the autonomy of the donor and represents a physiologically accurate model of the human immune system (Higbee et al., 2009). Interestingly, a version of MIMIC was recently used to investigate the immunopotency of a number of TLR agonists on DC generation, maturation, and antigen-presenting capacity (Ma et al., 2010). Importantly, all three of these models have been used to characterize the dose–response characteristics and potency of a number of immunosuppressive drugs and nondrug chemicals.

For illustrative purposes it is useful to briefly compare and contrast the in vitro T cell-dependent IgM AFC response, which uses mouse spleen cells and is often considered one of the "gold standard" assays for characterizing immunotoxicants, to the human CD40L-induced IgM AFC assay, which utilizes purified HPB B cells. Unlike the widely used T-cell-dependent IgM AFC response assay, which uses a heterogeneous leukocyte preparation from the mouse spleen and sRBC as the sensitizing antigen, the CD40L drives IgM production using purified HPB B cells or primary mouse B cells, thus allowing for direct comparisons of sensitivity of immunotoxicants between mouse and human B cells (Lu et al., 2009). It is important to emphasize that there are a number of significant and fundamental differences between the sRBC IgM AFC response and the CD40L-induced IgM AFC response. The most significant is that the CD40L response has no accessory cell involvement (ie, T cells or APC) since CD40L stimulation is provided either through the direct addition of rCD40L or by coculturing B cells with a genetically engineered CD40L-expressing fibroblast cell line (CD40L-L cells) plus recombinant T-cell cytokines. Therefore, the CD40L assay only provides information on B-cell function. In contrast, the sRBC IgM AFC response assay, in addition to B cells, requires functional T cells and APC for IgM production. From the perspective of hazard identification, the sRBC assay has greater capacity to detect immunotoxicants since in addition to B cells, the interactions of two other cell types and their consequent accessory cell functions are required in comparison to the CD40L assay. However, mechanistically, modulation of the CD40L-induced IgM response provides definitive identification of B-cell immunotoxicants and is an assay system in which mechanisms of B-cell immunotoxicology can be investigated in the absence of potential confounders associated with the presence of other cell types. In fact, using CD40L plus cytokines, the effects of immunotoxicants on B cells can be studied temporally throughout the entire continuum from activation to differentiation using flow cytometry. Another significant difference between the sRBC and the CD40L-induced IgM response is that the former is an antigen-specific response and the latter is not. In fact, presently there is no established antibody assay that employs human primary leukocytes to drive a primary, antigen-specific, T-cell-dependent antibody response. One of the major challenges in establishing such an assay is that there are very few circulating naive B cells present in peripheral blood and even fewer that possess BCRs specific for any given antigen. Because all B cells constitutively express CD40, the CD40L-induced IgM response circumvents the requirement for antigen specificity and induces a polyclonal B-cell response. Antigen-specific secondary antibody responses are more feasible, especially in response to recall antigens, such as tetanus toxoid. Because a large portion of the human population has undergone repeated and regular vaccination throughout their life (eg, tetanus), HPB B cells possessing BCRs specific for vaccine-associated antigens in these individuals have been clonally expanded and can

be readily activated and quantified in vitro. The disadvantage to this approach is that memory B cells, which are the cells that drive the secondary immune responses to recall antigens, have been found to be less sensitive to modulation by immunotoxicants. In light of this, even the CD40L-induced IgM response has been primarily conducted with naive HPB B cells after removal of memory B cells.

Recently, three extensively studied B-cell immunotoxicants in mice, arsenic, benzo[a]pyrene-7,8-dihydrodiol-9,10-epoxide (BPDE) and 2,3,7,8-tetrachlorodibenzo-p-dioxin (TCDD) were evaluated using the CD40L-induced IgM AFC response (Lu et al., 2009, 2010). All three immunotoxicants were found to suppress the CD40L-induced IgM AFC response in mouse splenic B cells with the magnitude of suppression being comparable to that previously reported using the sRBC IgM AFC response (Burns et al., 1991; Holsapple et al., 1986; Kawabata and White, 1989). BPDE and TCDD were also found to markedly suppress the CD40L-induced IgM AFC response in HPB B cells, and with a similar magnitude of suppression being observed between mouse and human B cells. In contrast, arsenic did not suppress the CD40L-induced IgM AFC response in HPB B cells. These limited results using only three B-cell immunotoxicants suggest that the mouse may not always serve as a reliable surrogate for predicting immune toxicity in humans.

As will be discussed in the section "The National Toxicology Program Tier Testing Approach," a cornerstone of immunotoxicological assessments using rodents has been a tier testing battery of immune function assays capable of evaluating the effects of xenobiotics on a host of different immunological parameters. Such an approach has been necessary due to the diversity of cell types and functions that are involved in maintaining immune competence (Luster et al., 1988). In fact, there is strong historical evidence, from examination of the NTP immunotoxicology database, that no immune function assay or endpoint can reliably identify all immunotoxicants. However, if expanded to two or three key assays, a significant increase in concordance with results from the expanded testing battery can be achieved (Luster et al., 1992). Toward this end, it is conceivable that a multiassay approach, analogous to that currently used for evaluations in the mouse, could be employed for immunotoxicity evaluations in conjunction with human primary leukocytes. Until recently, a significant obstacle to such a strategy has been the absence of an in vitro assay to assess B-cell effector function (Lu et al., 2009). In fact, a number of immune function assays using primary human leukocytes have historically been widely employed such as the MLR, which provides information on CD4[+] and CD8[+] T cell function, in the clinical setting to determine histocompatibility between donors and recipients for tissue transplantation. Similarly, B-cell and T-cell lymphoproliferative responses, which assess lymphocyte clonal expansion, have been used for the past several decades as a preliminary approach to assess human lymphocyte function. Collectively, these assays represent a potential foundation for a human leukocyte immunotoxicology testing battery. As described in the "Biomarkers in Immunotoxicology" section, the development of more predictive biomarkers for the immune system that can provide specific information on the impact of changes in human immunocompetence, and on the susceptibility for disease associated with drug or chemical exposure is another area of intense interest. The possibility of developing better translational biomarkers could facilitate the progression from preclinical studies to clinical studies in drug development.

Regulatory Approaches to the Assessment of Immunotoxicity The maturity and acceptance of any subdiscipline of toxicology can frequently be directly correlated to the level of interest being demonstrated by the regulatory community. This section will provide a brief review of the history of regulatory approaches to immunotoxicity. It is important to note that the regulatory approaches to immunotoxicity have evolved with the science, and the timing of the introduction of specific guidelines has generally reflected the state-of-the-science. Because of the importance of the evolution of the science, this section will begin with an overview of one of the most comprehensive databases for immunotoxicology.

The National Toxicology Program Tier Approach Although the concept of required immunotoxicity testing is a relatively recent development, the recognition that the immune system is a potential target organ has prompted a consideration of the need to assess the potential of immunotoxicity for some time. All testing strategies to date have recognized the complexity of the immune system as a target organ, and that no single immune parameter can be used with sufficient confidence to test for the hazard of immunotoxicity. Therefore, historically immunotoxicity has been assessed using a battery of assays, which are typically structured in a multi-tiered approach. Importantly, studies conducted by the NTP have indicated that immunotoxicity can be assessed with a finite number of assays. Luster and colleagues (1988) originally described the selection of a battery of tests used by the NTP to screen for potential immunotoxic agents. The result was a tier approach to assessing immunotoxicity, which is summarized in Table 12-10.

Tier I tests provide assessment of general toxicity (eg, immunopathology, hematology, body, and organ weights) as well as some assays to assess immune functional capability (eg, proliferative responses, the T-cell-dependent antibody response assay, measured as AFC, and the NK assay). Tier I was designed to detect potential immunotoxic compounds at concentrations that do not produce overt toxicity. Tier II tests were designed to further define an immunotoxic effect, and included functional tests for CMI (eg, CTL and DTH), secondary antibody responses, enumeration of lymphocyte populations, and host resistance models.

In the original NTP effort, over 50 chemicals were studied, and included a variety of chemical classes, such as catalysts, solvents, dyes, lubricants, pesticides, disinfectants, drugs, food additives, and natural products (Luster *et al.*, 1988). It is important to emphasize

Table 12-10

Tier Approach for Immunotoxicology Testing

TESTING LEVEL	PROCEDURES
Tier I	Hematology
	Body weight
	Organ weights (spleen, thymus, kidney, and liver)
	Spleen cellularity
	Bone marrow cellularity and CFU
	Immunopathology
	AFC assay
	Proliferative responses
	NK assay
Tier II	Surface marker analysis
	Secondary (IgG) AFC assay
	CTL assay
	DTH response
	Host resistance studies

Table 12-11

Suggested Testing Configurations: Three Tests with 100% Concordance

AFC	DHR	Surface markers
AFC	NK	DHR
AFC	NK	Thymus: body weight
AFC	DHR	Thymus: body weight
Surface markers	NK	DHR
Surface markers	DHR	T-cell mitogens
Surface markers	DHR	Thymus: body weight
Surface markers	DHR	LPS response

SOURCE: Luster et al. (1988), modified, with permission.

that the chemicals selected for study by the NTP were nominated for testing because of a suspicion that they would target the immune system. These studies were conducted in young adult rodents, principally the mouse, and involved comparative studies across multiple labs. The experimental design emphasized that regardless of the specific immune parameters included in a testing strategy, the interpretation for immunotoxicity could only be made in the context of a well-designed study from the perspective of the dose–response relationship. The approach by Luster and coworkers also emphasized the importance of avoiding high doses (ie, triggered less than a 10% reduction in body weight), because these types of exposures will increase the likelihood that indirect mechanisms of immunotoxicity may be involved.

Several testing configurations were ultimately defined that would minimize the number of immune tests needed, yet could still provide a high degree of sensitivity for detecting potential immunotoxicants. These configurations are depicted in Table 12-11. Specifically, the results indicated that none of the assays measured was 100% predictive alone. The top three assays in terms of detecting immunotoxicants were an assessment of lymphocyte subpopulations by flow cytometric analysis (eg, 83% concordance), the T cell-dependent antibody response (eg, 78% concordance), and an assessment of NK cell activity (eg, 69% concordance) (Luster *et al.*, 1992). With regards to the comparison between the two most sensitive assays, it is important to note that a change in flow cytometric analysis of any of the lymphocyte subsets measured, for example, total B cells, total T cells, CD4$^+$ T cells, or CD8$^+$ T cells, would be sufficient to establish the concordance of flow cytometry, while the concordance of the T-cell-dependent antibody response was determined solely by the number of AFCs. Subsequent analysis indicated that an application of the full extent of the tiered approach was not necessary. The NTP studies indicated that several combinations of only two tests could give >90% concordance, and that a number of combinations of just three tests gave 100% concordance. In this regard, it is important to note that flow cytometric analysis of lymphocyte subsets, and the-T cell-dependent antibody response were consistently involved in both the 2-test concordance of >90%, and in the 3-test concordance of 100%.

Subsequent results also indicated a good correlation between the results from functional tests and host resistance models (Luster *et al.*, 1993), which indicated that the latter were not necessary to adequately identify immunosuppressive potential. The impacts of the NTP database are clear, and one only needs to consider the structure of the immunotoxicity guidelines that have been established to see the impact of the NTP results. Specifically, after several years of international debate, the importance of including functional immunotoxicity assessments in regulatory studies has been emphasized, as opposed to relying solely on histopathology as an indicator of further testing needs. Moreover, as described further below, the specific immune functional tests in most, if not all, immunotoxicity regulatory guidelines reflect the concordance results described above, and include the T-cell-dependent antibody response, immune cell phenotyping by flow cytometry, and the NK cell assay.

While the original NTP studies in the 1980s were intended to develop and validate methods to evaluate modulation of immune function, the emphasis was clearly focused on immunosuppression. The NTP contract to assess the "Potential for Environmental and Therapeutic Agents to Induce Immunotoxicity" is still assessing chemicals for potential immunomodulation at the rate of four chemicals per year for screening (eg, rangefinding) studies and two chemicals per year for definitive (eg, full protocol) studies. Importantly, the current approaches by the NTP reflect the state-of-the-science of immunotoxicology, in that two developmental immunotoxicity studies, two contact hypersensitivity studies and one study assessing the potential of a xenobiotic-associated change in an autoimmune disease model are assessed each year.

In 2009, the NTP provided another critical component to our understanding of xenobiotic-induced immunotoxicity when they released their "Explanation of Levels of Evidence for Immune System Toxicity" (NTP, 2009) as an approach to judging the quality of results in a study purporting to establish xenobiotic-induced immunotoxicity. In the document, which was prepared by a panel of experts representing the academic, government, and industry sectors of the scientific community, the NTP emphasized the importance of recognizing that the "levels of evidence" statements that are described reflected only immunological *hazard*, and that the actual determination of *risk* to humans required *exposure* data that was not covered in the document. Five categories of evidence of immune system toxicity were used to summarize the strength of the evidence observed in each experiment being considered: two categories for positive results (*clear evidence* and *some evidence*); one category for uncertain findings (*equivocal evidence*); one category for no observable effects (*no evidence*); and one category for experiments that cannot be evaluated because of major design or performance flaws (*inadequate study*). Each category included one or more bullet points for additional clarification. The category for *clear evidence* is worthy of specific mention.

Clear Evidence of Toxicity to the Immune System:

- Is demonstrated by data that indicate a dose-related effect (considering the magnitude of the effect and the dose–response) on more than one functional parameter and/or a disease resistance assay that is not a secondary effect of overt systemic toxicity, or
- Is demonstrated by data that indicate dose-related effects on one functional assay and additional endpoints that indicate biological plausibility. (NTP, 2009)

The significance of this category is that clear evidence of immunotoxicity can be established without the need to conduct a disease resistance assay, and that mechanistic data to establish biological plausibility is weighed very heavily. The NTP report also indicates that negative results, in which the study animals do not exhibit evidence of immunotoxicity, do not necessarily imply that a test article is not an immune system toxicant, but only that the test article is not an immune system toxicant under the specified experimental conditions. Finally, the report indicates that positive results demonstrating that a test article causes immunotoxicity in laboratory animals under the conditions of the study are assumed to be relevant in humans, unless data are available which demonstrate otherwise.

Historical Perspective on Regulatory Guidance in Immunotoxicology The history of regulatory guidance in immunotoxicology was reviewed by House (2005). As noted above, the T-cell-dependent antibody response has been the consensus choice for a functional endpoint to identify immunotoxicity hazard in most, if not all regulatory guidelines. A reasonable question to address is what accounts for the sensitivity, predictivity, and (perceived) utility of the T-cell-dependent antibody response. The simplest answer is something that has been known within the immunology community for over 50 years. The T-cell-dependent antibody response requires the orchestrated coordination and cooperativity of multiple cell types (eg, APCs, Th cells, and B cells at the ultimate effector cell because of their ability to secrete antigen-specific antibodies) and the manifestation of most, if not all of the biological functions important to immunocompetence. As noted throughout this chapter, the discipline of immunotoxicology continues to evolve along with advances in immunology and molecular biology. However, in the context of providing an effective screen for immunotoxic hazard, nothing can compare to the time-tested and mechanistically understood specific antibody response to a well-characterized T-dependent antigen.

The Office of Prevention, Pesticides and Toxic Substances (OPPTS) of the US Environmental Protection Agency (EPA) published guidelines entitled, "*Biochemicals Test Guidelines: OPPTS 880.3550 Immunotoxicity*" in 1996. These guidelines described the preferred study design for an exceptionally thorough evaluation of the potential immunotoxicity in biochemical pest control agents. This guideline described a panel of tests that included standard toxicology tests as well as immune functional tests assessing both humoral immunity and CMI. OPPTS 880.3550 clearly presented a very comprehensive approach to immunotoxicity; but a second document, "*Biochemicals Test Guidelines: OPPTS 880.3800 Immune Response*," was needed to provide the rationale for when these studies should be conducted. The 880 series of immunotoxicity guidelines would arguably detect any type of immunotoxic potential by pesticides. However, the comprehensive nature of these guidelines rendered them prohibitively expensive and time-consuming. The EPA released the "*Health Effects Test Guidelines: OPPTS 870.7800 Immunotoxicity*" in 1998 (EPA, 1998). These guidelines described the approach to immunotoxicology testing for nonbiochemical agents regulated by the EPA. The testing approach in OPPTS 870.7800 reflected the continued evolution of the science of immunotoxicology and called for a more limited, case-by-case approach than previously described by the earlier more comprehensive guidelines. The cornerstone of OPPTS 870-7800 was a functional test, the primary T-cell-dependent antibody response. If the chemical was shown to produce significant suppression of the humoral response, then surface marker assessment by flow cytometry may be performed. If the chemical was not shown to produce suppression of the humoral response, then an assessment of innate immunity (eg, specifically, the NK cell activity assay) may be performed. The specific criteria for the conduct of these "optional" tests have never been identified. The tests do not represent a comprehensive assessment of immune function but are intended to complement assessment made in routine toxicity testing (eg, hematological assessments, lymphoid organ weights, and histopathology).

Internationally, the Organization for Economic Cooperation and Development (OECD) has not as yet adopted specific guidelines for immunotoxicity assessment. As reviewed by House (2005), the OECD Guideline 407, entitled *"Repeated Dose 28-day Oral Toxicity Study in Rodents"* while not specific for immunotoxicology, includes a variety of toxicological endpoints that can provide early evidence of immune system alterations. House (2005) also noted at the time that over 10 years earlier, an international immunology working group recommended that functional assessments be included in standard toxicology studies when desired or when suggested by expanded histopathological results on other standard toxicology studies. However, to date, the OECD Guideline 407 has not been modified in accord with these recommendations. Moreover, while the OECD published a template for immunotoxicity studies on its website in 2011, there are still no corresponding OECD Test Guidelines for immunotoxicity.

The earliest immunotoxicity guidelines from the Food and Drug Administration (FDA) were centered on food additives as the *"Draft Redbook II"* in 1993. This document, although never finalized, contained an extensive description of immunotoxicology testing. In general, the Redbook guidelines reflected the tiered approach to immunotoxicology (Fig. 12-10), as described in greater detail below. Specifically, the Redbook emphasized a stepwise approach that began with expanded studies utilizing data obtained in standard toxicology testing as initial indicators of immunotoxicity. Progressively more complicated immunological tests were prescribed using an approach that was very much case-by-case, with each new level of testing predicated on positive results in the preceding level. The FDA Center for Drug Evaluation and Research (CDER) released its document entitled, *"Guidance for Industry: Immunotoxicology Evaluation of Investigational New Drugs,"* in 2002 (FDA, 2002). This document is arguably the most comprehensive description of approaches to immunotoxicology. Not only does the FDA CDER *"Guidance for Industry"* describe the full spectrum of adverse events associated with the immunotoxicology continuum including immune suppression, immunogenicity, hypersensitivity, autoimmunity and adverse immune stimulation, but also provides approaches at the level of specific methodology for evaluating each event. As with the earlier document from the FDA, the new *"Guidance for Industry"* advocated the use of information derived from standard repeat-dose toxicity studies to provide the earliest indicators of immunotoxicity. The review by House (2005) also addressed the current status of regulatory guidance for biologicals, vaccines, devices, and radiological agents within the FDA.

Internationally, perhaps one of the most significant advances in our approach to the assessment of immunotoxicity with human pharmaceuticals has been a guidance entitled, *"S8 Immunotoxicity Studies for Human Pharmaceuticals,"* which was prepared under the auspices of the International Conference on Harmonization (ICH) of Technical Requirements for Registration of Pharmaceutical for Human Use (ICHS8, 2006). The objectives of this guideline are twofold: (1) to provide recommendations on nonclinical testing approaches to identify compounds which have the potential for immunotoxicity; and (2) to provide guidance on a weight-of-evidence decision-making approach for immunotoxicity testing. The guidance applies to unintended immune suppression and immune enhancement, excluding allergenicity or drug-specific autoimmunity. The ICH S8 guideline is based on a cause for concern approach using a review of factors such as the following: results from Standard Toxicity Studies (STS), pharmacological properties of the drug, the intended patient population, structural similarities to known immune modulators, the disposition of the drug, and clinical information.

As emphasized in the Introduction, immunotoxicity exists in a continuum (Fig. 12-1). By and large, more effort has been invested in the validation of studies to address the immunosuppressive part of the continuum, and there is no doubt that much attention is paid to immune suppression in the majority of guidance documents (House, 2005). Nonetheless, it is important to measure xenobiotic-induced changes in immune function in both directions. As noted by House (2005), it is hypersensitivity that is the most common type of immune modulation in humans resulting from exposure to xenobiotics. One of the most significant advances in our approach to assessing the potential of xenobiotics has been the LLNA. As discussed above, the LLNA was the first assay to be evaluated by the Interagency Coordinating Committee for the Validation of Alternative Methods (ICCVAM). The impact of this decision by ICCVAM is that the LLNA is now an accepted assay and discussed in considerable detail in the OECD 429 Guideline, *"Skin Sensitization: Local Lymph Node Assay,"* and the EPA document, *"OPPTS 870.2600 Skin Sensitization."*

Recent Advances in Regulatory Guidance on Immunotoxicology

There have been two areas over the last few years that have impacted the status of immunotoxicology testing which are either legislative demands or because of the continued evolution in the state-of-the-science.

As noted in the sections above on "Molecular Biology Approaches to Immunotoxicology" and "Mechanistic Approaches to Immunotoxicology", the use of in vitro and cell-based tissue culture methods have always played an important role in the science of immunotoxicology. Of course, it has always been recognized that the use of these alternative approaches are consistent with the 3Rs of reducing, replacing, and refining the use of whole animal studies. However, recent legislative actions, such as the implementation of *R*egistration, *E*valuation and *A*uthorization of *Ch*emicals (REACH) and of the Cosmetics Directive in Europe, have focused renewed and required attention on in vitro approaches to all types of toxicity assessment, including immunotoxicity, especially in Europe (Carfi *et al.*, 2007; Galbiati *et al.*, 2010; Lankveld *et al.*, 2010). Some recent specific examples of the utility of in vitro approaches to assess immunotoxicity include an improved in vitro cytokine release using human PBMC (Kooijman *et al.*, 2010), and some renewed interest (Fischer *et al.*, 2011) in the Mishell–Dutton culture system (Mishell and Dutton, 1967) that was described earlier in the subsection "General Assessment" under the "Methods to Assess Immunocompetence" section. Not too surprisingly, Fischer *et al.* (2011) conclude that the investigation of in vitro antibody responses is a sensitive and reliable approach for the detection of a compound-specific effect on the immune system. They also conclude that the implementation of this approach in routine toxicology would enable the refinement of existing in vivo studies by reducing the number of animals. However, somewhat surprising is their conclusion that the in vitro Mishell–Dutton culture system for measuring specific antibody responses of primary cells may replace the ex vivo T-cell-dependent antibody response in the future. A significant concern pertaining to the utilization of this strictly in vitro approach is that leukocytes possess remarkably limited drug-metabolizing capability and as such, agents that are activated by metabolism to an immunotoxic form would not be detected utilizing this strategy.

As described in another section of this chapter, the interest in DIT testing has increased significantly over the last few years, with considerable attention being devoted to this area of study by the scientific and regulatory communities on a global scale. While it is important to emphasize that there are currently no regulatory guidelines for either drugs or nondrug chemicals specifically focused on assessment of DIT, but there are some general guidelines included in both developmental and reproductive toxicity (DART) and general immunotoxicology guidance documents. Evaluations of DIT began to be required as part of the US Environmental Protection Agency's Office of Prevention, Pesticide and Toxic Substances (OPPTS) test guideline for the 2-generation reproductive toxicity study (EPA, 1998), which requires collection of spleen and thymus weights in one pup per sex per litter in F_1 and F_2 weanlings. Another example of this trend in the context of assessing the effects of chemicals on the developing immune system is the paper by Cooper et al. (2006), in which the authors described an expanded one-generation DART protocol that included the assessment of immunotoxicology—among other endpoints—following exposure during critical windows of development. More recently, Vogel et al. (2010) described a modular one-generation reproduction study—that included an immunotoxicity module—as a flexible testing system for regulatory safety assessment, and highlighted the application of such an approach to the EUs REACH program. Based on these kinds of proposed studies, the US EPA and the Dutch authorities convened a working group to revise the OECD 415 protocol to embrace some of the principles articulated by Cooper et al. (2006) and by Vogel et al. (2010). Indeed, in 2010, the OECD released a draft protocol for a revised OECD 415, extended one-generation study (OECD, 2010) that included three cohorts, with the third cohort devoted to an assessment of the potential impact of chemical exposure on developmental immunotoxicity.

In its 2002 guidance for industry, FDA noted that all drugs that are immunotoxic in adult animals and are to be given to pregnant women should be evaluated for DIT (FDA, 2002). Endpoints recommended to be assessed were hematology and lymphoid organ weights on F_1 pups in standard DART studies. More recently, a number of regulatory guidelines have also emerged to address the safety of drugs intended for pediatric indications, including the US FDA *Guidance for Industry Nonclinical Safety Evaluation of Pediatric Drug Products* (FDA, 2006; Tassinari et al., 2011), and the European Medicines Agency *Guideline on the Need for Nonclinical Testing in Juvenile Animals on Human Pharmaceuticals for Paediatric Indications* (Carleer and Karres, 2011; EMA, 2008). In Japan, the Ministry of Health, Labor, and Welfare (MHLW) started to prepare their *Guideline for Nonclinical Safety Studies in Juvenile Animals* in 2010 (Shimomura, 2011). In general, juvenile toxicity studies are conducted to identify potential latent signs of toxicity, to characterize the potential for chronic developmental toxicity that cannot be thoroughly assessed through standard DART protocols, and to ensure that children are not unnecessarily exposed to potentially adverse risk factors. The primary objective of juvenile animal toxicity studies of pharmaceuticals is to obtain safety data, including information on the potential for adverse effects on postnatal growth and development (Cappon et al., 2009). Indeed, the FDA Guidance from their CDER addresses "...*the role and timing of animal studies in the safety evaluation of therapeutics intended for the treatment of pediatric patients*," and emphasizes the following premise, "*It is thought that organ systems at highest risk for drug toxicity are those that undergo significant postnatal development*" (FDA, 2006). Importantly, the immune system was identified in the FDA Guidance as an important endpoint.

While the revised OECD 415 protocol described above has been designed to assess the effects of chemical exposure in rats, more recently, evaluations of DIT for pharmaceuticals in non-human primates have been conducted as part of embryofetal development (EFD), pre-/postnatal development (PPND), or juvenile studies. With regard to critical immune system "windows," the enhanced PPND (ePPND) study design in non-human primates (NHPs) appears optimal for DIT testing, and has been shown to have similar benefits to the testing of monoclonal antibodies (Stewart, 2009) and biopharmaceuticals (Martin et al., 2009). Additional perspective on

the state-of-the-science of juvenile immunotoxicology studies for pharmaceuticals is provided in a paper by Holsapple and O'Lone (2011).

Biomarkers in Immunotoxicology There are many potential definitions for a "biomarker." From a toxicological perspective, the most general definition of a biomarker is a substance that can be measured in a biological system or sample that reflects a xenobiotic-induced change in cellular or biochemical components or processes, structures, or function. From a clinical perspective, a biomarker is a term often used to refer to something that can be measured whose concentration reflects the severity or presence of some disease state. As such "true" biomarkers indicate exposure to a specific chemical or drug as well as susceptibility to an adverse effect, and/or are predictive of changes in a disease state associated with chemical or drug exposure. Although traditionally biomarkers are most often associated with proteins that can be measured in the blood, biomarkers can also be associated with changes in the expression of cell-surface proteins, and, in the new world of "omics" technologies, biomarkers can not only be identified through proteomics; but through transcriptomics and metabolomics (metabonomics), as well. Translational biomarkers are those that can be effectively used in multiple species, and that can be used to bridge the effects seen in two different species so that it would be possible to directly link responses between species. In the context of drug development, translational biomarkers that can be measured in both humans and non-human species are critical so that effects seen with a drug candidate can be followed in both preclinical and clinical settings.

Based on an understanding of the immune system, especially in the context of any type of immune response, it is easy to see the potential for biomarkers in immunotoxicology. Essentially, any xenobiotic-induced change in any parameter associated with an immune response—for example, a change in an antigen-specific antibody response, or a change in the expression of a surface marker, or a change in the numbers of a particular immune cell type, or a change in the levels of a cytokine or cytokines, or a change in the expression of an immune response-related gene—could be used as a biomarker for the immunotoxicity associated with that xenobiotic. As such, a chapter entitled, "The Promise of Genomics and Proteomics in Immunotoxicology and Immunopharmacology" (Pruett et al., 2007), emphasized that further implementation of these methods could move immunotoxicology into the area of systems biology, could be beneficial with regard to mechanistic and screening applications, and could reveal new insights about immune function. Similarly, an earlier report by the National Research Council's Committee on Biological Markers undertook to study the interrelationship of toxic exposure and immune system response at a time when the discipline of immunotoxicology was described as being "relatively young"—for example, the IL family ended with IL-8 (NRC, 1992). The NRC Subcommittee on Immunotoxicology reviewed research on currently known markers, and identified and evaluated promising technologies to find new markers.

In spite of this early effort by the NRC, and although the NTP Tier Approach for assessing whether a compound is immunotoxic has been used for many years and has served as the basis for most immunotoxicity regulatory guidelines, there is no consensus for an accepted panel of biomarkers that one can use to determine whether, and to what extent, exposure to an immunotoxic agent has occurred. Various studies have been conducted to ascertain the feasibility, predictability, and accuracy of various biomarkers of immune modulation (Karmaus et al., 2005; Luster et al., 2005; Schwab et al., 2005). Besides the potential biomarkers already mentioned, which include cytokine gene expression patterns, cell population quantification using flow cytometry, and serum antibody titers, the assessment for the presence of single nucleotide polymorphisms (SNPs) in various genes makes it possible to determine whether small populations of individuals might be more susceptible to immunotoxicants. These same approaches are being applied to the development of immuno-modulators and biologics, which are either designed to target the immune system, or are likely to do so because of their mechanisms of action. As such, it is more critical than ever that translational biomarkers for the immune system be developed and tested.

Finally, while it is clear from a number of studies currently available that biomarkers for the immune system can be predictive and accurate, there are limitations of their use, especially in the context of their application in human epidemiological studies. For example, suppression of CD4+ T cells certainly indicates immune suppression, but it would be challenging to determine which agent(s) correlate with the magnitude of suppression, and how the exposure to multiple agents affects that magnitude. Moreover, it should be noted that immunological biomarkers might be affected by other physiological processes, such as stress (Schwab *et al.*, 2005); and as described in the preceding subsection, "Approaches to the Assessment of Human Immunotoxicity," stress can affect immune responses to vaccines in humans (Glaser *et al.*, 2000; Kiecolt-Glaser *et al.*, 1996). Certainly, the complex interplay between different physiological processes is not unique to immunotoxicology; but it will need to be considered as the concept of biomarkers in immunotoxicology is developed.

IMMUNE MODULATION BY XENOBIOTICS

The very nature of the immune system with the different cell types, the presence of various cell types in every tissue of the body, the dependence on proliferation and differentiation for effector functions, and the necessity to maintain immune function homeostasis renders it susceptible to modulation by a wide variety of xenobiotics. Although many of the xenobiotics discussed below exhibit immunosuppressive actions, it is important to realize that many of these chemicals are actually immunomodulatory, that is, they might produce both immune suppression and immune enhancement (in the absence of true hypersensitivity or autoimmunity). Of course, one cannot ignore the chemicals that do produce true hypersensitivity and/or autoimmunity and some examples of these are discussed later in the section entitled, "Xenobiotic-Induced Hypersensitivity and Autoimmunity." Regardless of the end effect (immune suppression, immune enhancement, hypersensitivity, or autoimmunity) of a particular xenobiotic on the immune system, several common themes exist regarding the mechanisms by which these chemicals act. First, the mechanisms by which a xenobiotic affects immune function are likely to be multifaceted, involving several proteins, signaling cascades, or receptors. In fact, for several of the xenobiotics discussed below, there is evidence to suggest that immune system effects are both xenobiotic-specific receptor-dependent and -independent. Second, whether a xenobiotic produces a particular immune effect might depend on the concentration or dose of the xenobiotic, the mode and/or magnitude of cellular stimulation, and the kinetic relationship between exposure to the xenobiotic and exposure to the immune stimulant (ie, antigen, mitogen, and pharmacological agent). Third, xenobiotic exposures rarely occur one chemical at a time; thus, the effects and/or mechanisms observed might be attributable to several chemicals or classes of chemicals. Finally, determination of immune system effects and/or mechanisms by xenobiotics in humans might be further confounded by the physiological or immunological state of the individual. Despite these variables, the application of general, functional, and mechanistic tools discussed above have driven the determination of some of the effects and mechanisms for several xenobiotics.

Halogenated Aromatic Hydrocarbons

Few classes of xenobiotics have been as extensively studied for immunotoxicity as the halogenated aromatic hydrocarbons ([HAHs]; reviewed by Holsapple, 1996; Kerkvliet, 2002; Kerkvliet and Burleson, 1994). The prototypical and most biologically potent member of this family of chemicals, which includes the polychlorinated biphenyls (PCBs), the polybrominated biphenyls (PBBs), the polychlorinated dibenzofurans (PCDFs), and the polychlorinated dibenzodioxins (PCDDs), is 2,3,7,8-tetrachlorodibenzo-*p*-dioxin (TCDD; dioxin). Substantial evidence has demonstrated that the immune system is a sensitive target for toxicity by these chemicals. Derived from a variety of animal models, primarily rodents, this evidence includes thymic atrophy, pancytopenia, cachexia, immune suppression, and tumor promotion. There is also epidemiological evidence suggesting that immunotoxicity by the HAHs can also occur in humans (Weisglas-Kuperus *et al.*, 1995, 2000, and 2004); however, significant immune suppression has not been associated conclusively with specific alterations of human immune function.

The majority of the biochemical and toxic effects produced by the HAHs are mediated via HAH binding to the cytosolic AHR. The AHR is a 95 to 110 kDa basic helix-loop-helix type of ligand-activated transcription factor (Burbach *et al.*, 1992; Ema *et al.*, 1992), which is associated with two heat shock proteins (hsp90) (Denis *et al.*, 1988; Perdew, 1988; Pongratz *et al.*, 1992), prostaglandin E synthase 3 (p23) (Cox and Miller, 2004; Kazlauskas *et al.*, 1999) and AHR-activated 9 (ARA-9) (Carver *et al.*, 1998; LaPres *et al.*, 2000; Ma and Whitlock, 1997). Ligand binding induces conformational changes in the AHR, enabling the receptor–ligand complex to initially release p23 and ARA9 in the cytosol followed by nuclear translocation where it sheds its hsp90 and is transformed into a DNA-binding protein (Cuthill *et al.*, 1987; Denis *et al.*, 1988; Okey *et al.*, 1980; Perdew, 1988; Pollenz *et al.*, 1994; Pongratz *et al.*, 1992; Probst *et al.*, 1993). This transformation involves dimerization of the receptor–ligand complex with a structurally related 87 kDa basic helix-loop-helix protein termed the aryl hydrocarbon receptor nuclear translocator (ARNT) (Hoffman *et al.*, 1991; Probst *et al.*, 1993; Reyes *et al.*, 1992). The ligand–AHR/ARNT complex acts as a transcription factor by binding to DNA at the dioxin-responsive element (DRE), also termed xenobiotic response elements (XRE), in the promoter and enhancer region of sensitive genes such as cytochrome P4501A1, aldehyde dehydrogenase-3, glutathione *S*-transferase, and menadione oxidoreductase (Dunn *et al.*, 1988; Elferink *et al.*, 1990; Fujisawa-Sehara *et al.*, 1987; Hoffman *et al.*, 1991; Poland and Knutson, 1982; Reyes *et al.*, 1992; Sutter and Greenlee, 1992; Watson and Hankinson, 1992; Whitlock, 1990). Numerous lines of evidence have supported the involvement of the AHR in mediation of toxicity including immunotoxicity by HAHs. Structure–activity relationship studies have demonstrated that with few exceptions, high-affinity AHR ligands are more immunosuppressive than low-affinity ligands (Davis and Safe, 1988). In mice, allelic variation at the *Ah* locus has been described. These alleles code for AHR with differential binding affinities for TCDD. For example, the C57BL/6 mouse represents a strain of mice (*Ah*^bb), which is exquisitely sensitive to TCDD (TCDD responsive), while the DBA/2 mouse strain (*Ah*^dd) is much less sensitive to the toxic effects of TCDD (TCDD nonresponsive or TCDD low-responsive). More recently, AHR null mice and cell lines that do not express the AHR have collectively provided compelling evidence supporting the role of AHR in the toxicity mediated by HAHs including immunotoxicity (Sulentic et al., 2000; Vorderstrasse et al., 2001).

Polychlorinated Dibenzodioxins By far the majority of the investigations into the immunotoxic potential and mechanisms of action of the HAHs have focused on TCDD, primarily because this chemical is the most potent of the HAHs, binding the AHR with the highest affinity. The effects of TCDD on immune function have been demonstrated to be among the earliest and most sensitive indicators of TCDD-induced toxicity (reviewed by Holsapple, 1996; Holsapple et al., 1991a, b; Kerkvliet, 2002; Kerkvliet and Burleson, 1994). TCDD is not produced commercially, except in small amounts for research purposes. Rather, it is an environmental contaminant formed primarily as a by-product of the manufacturing process that uses chlorinated phenols or during the combustion of chlorinated materials. It is usually associated with the production of herbicides such as 2,4,5-trichlorophenoxyacetic acid (2,4,5-T), and Agent Orange (a 1:1 combination of 2,4-dichlorophenoxyacetic acid [2,4-D] and 2,4,5-T). Other sources include pulp and paper manufacturing (chlorine bleaching), automobile exhaust (leaded gasoline), combustion of municipal and industrial waste, and the production of PCBs.

Like other HAHs, exposure to TCDD results in severe lymphoid atrophy. Because thymus-derived cells play an integral role in tumor surveillance and host resistance, the earliest studies on TCDD-induced immunotoxicity focused on changes in CMI. Studies on CMI have shown that this branch of acquired immunity is sensitive to the toxic effects of TCDD after in vivo administration. CTL development and activity have been shown by numerous investigators to be significantly decreased after exposure to TCDD, an effect that appeared to be age dependent (eg, the younger the mice when exposed, the greater the sensitivity to TCDD). In an in vivo acute graft-versus-host model of T-cell immunity, the direct AHR-dependent effects of TCDD on T cells were demonstrated. In this model, T cells from C57BL/6 mice were injected into C57BL/6 × DBA/2 F1 host mice resulting in the generation of an antihost CTL response (Kerkvliet et al., 2002). By comparing the ability of TCDD to suppress the CTL response of T cells obtained from $AHR^{+/+}$ and $AHR^{-/-}$ C57BL/6 mice, the role for AHR expression in T cells was assessed. These studies showed that the CTL response was suppressed by TCDD through direct effects on $CD4^+$ and $CD8^+$ T cells via an AHR-dependent mechanism (Kerkvliet et al., 2002). The findings are consistent with the identification of AHR expression in T cells (Lawrence et al., 1996) and structure–activity relationship studies showing a positive correlation between AHR-binding affinity of dioxin-like PCBs and suppression of in vivo CTL responses (Kerkvliet et al., 1990). More recently using the same graft-versus-host model, TCDD treatment resulted in a significant increase in the percentage of donor $CD4^+$ cells that expressed high levels of CD25, low levels of CD62L as well as glucocorticoid-induced TNFR (GITR) and CTLA-4, a phenotype associated with some types of Tregs, suggesting that an important component of the immune suppression of the CTL response induced by TCDD might be the generation of Tregs (Funatake et al., 2005). In addition to suppression of CTL function, TCDD exposure also results in decreases in PHA- and Con A-induced proliferative responses, and DTH responses. Enhanced proliferative responses in juvenile mice have also been observed (Lundberg et al., 1990). Concordant with the aforementioned findings, more recently it has been reported that AHR activation by TCDD or by the tryptophan-derived endogenous AHR ligand, 2-(1′H-indole-3′carbonyl)-thiazole-4-carboxylic

acid methyl ester, induced the generation of Tregs in a model of experimental autoimmune encephalomyelitis (EAE), which produced a reduction in severity of disease (Quintana et al., 2008). These findings are somewhat in contrast to the observation that 6-formylindolo[3,2-b]carbazole, also a tryptophan-derived high-affinity AHR ligand, induced IL-17 production by Th17 cells and increased the severity of disease in the same EAE autoimmune model (Quintana et al., 2008; Veldhoen et al., 2008). Importantly, Th17 cells and Tregs negatively cross regulate each other, and this observation raises what appears to be a dichotomy in that AHR activation in the same model of autoimmunity can produce very different outcomes and may be in part explained by the ligand which activates the AHR. Moreover, transcriptome analysis showed that of four types of $CD4^+$ T cells (Th1, Th2, Tregs, and Th17 cells), AHR was only detected in Th17 cells suggesting that some of the effects produced by TCDD and dioxin-like compounds on T cells may occur indirectly (Veldhoen et al., 2008).

In light of the critical role DCs play in regulating T-cell-mediated responses by presenting antigen to $CD4^+$ and $CD8^+$ T cells as well as by providing costimulatory signals through surface expression of CD80 and CD86 to drive T-cell activation via CD28 (T-cell coreceptor), recent investigations have focused on characterizing the effects TCDD exerts on DC function. Indeed, differentiation of bone marrow-derived precursors into DCs in the presence of TCDD was found to influence the expression of several surface proteins on DCs known to play a critical role in T-cell antigen recognition and T-cell activation. Specifically, differentiation of bone marrow precursors in the presence of TCDD resulted in an increase in MHCII, CD80, and CD86 expression, when compared to vehicle controls (Bankoti et al., 2010; Simones and Shepherd, 2011), which occurred in an AHR-dependent manner. Interestingly, in spite of the dependence on the AHR these changes were not dependent on AHR-mediated changes in gene expression since DCs from mice possessing a mutation within the AHR nuclear localization signaling domain exhibited a similar profile of activity as those derived from wild-type mice. While significant TCDD-mediated increases in MHCII, CD80, and CD86 expression were observed, TCDD-treated DCs exhibited a similar capacity as vehicle-treated DCs to activate $CD8^+$ T cells, which would suggest that TCDD-mediated suppression of CTL responses does not involve altered DC function. In contrast, DCs differentiated in the presence of TCDD exhibited suppressed levels of TNF-α, IL-6, and IL-12 in response to TLR-mediated (LPS or CpG) activation suggesting altered cytokine regulation (Simones and Shepherd, 2011).

Consistent with the observation that mice exposed perinatally or postnatally are more sensitive to the effects of TCDD, it has been determined that thymic involution is a result of TCDD-induced terminal differentiation of the thymic epithelium and, thus, T cells do not have a proper nutrient-filled microenvironment in which to develop (Greenlee et al., 1984, 1985). This conclusion is consistent with observations that TCDD significantly decreased the number of immature T cells ($CD4^+/CD8^+$) in the thymus (Kerkvliet and Brauner, 1990). It was also reported that in vivo administration of TCDD-induced apoptosis in mouse thymocytes (Kamath et al., 1999) and that the mechanism involved a TCDD-induced increase in Fas ligand in thymic stromal, but not thymic, T cells (Camacho et al., 2005). In these experiments, it was demonstrated that when TCDD-exposed stromal cells were mixed with untreated thymic T cells, increased apoptosis was detected in T cells that involved Fas–Fas ligand interactions. In addition, the TCDD-mediated apoptosis of thymic T cells was demonstrated to occur via an AHR-dependent mechanism, which also involved NF-κB-mediated upregulation of Fas ligand promoter activity in the thymic stromal cells (Camacho *et al.*, 2005). It has also been shown that TCDD interferes with cell-cycle regulation during early thymocyte development, which may in part account for the profound sensitivity of thymocytes to AHR ligands (Laiosa *et al.*, 2003). More recently, differential TCDD-induced gene expression was observed during different stages of thymocyte development providing new insights into putative targets responsible for altered thymocyte differentiation in the presence of TCDD. Interestingly, this study also revealed that the cell cycle was unaffected at the earliest stages of thymocyte development prior to commitment to the $\alpha\beta$ T-cell lineage (Laiosa *et al.*, 2010).

Numerous investigations have demonstrated humoral immunity, and in particular, the IgM AFC response, to be exquisitely sensitive to the toxic effects of TCDD (Sulentic and Kaminski, 2011). This effect segregates with the *Ah* locus (Sulentic *et al.*, 2000; Vecchi *et al.*, 1983) and appears to be dependent on duration and conditions of exposure. Although TCDD induces profound changes in the AFC assay, no changes have been observed in splenic cellularity (numbers of Ig$^+$, CD4$^+$, or Thy-1$^+$ cells) either before or after antigen challenge. Cell fraction/reconstitution of splenocytes from in vivo TCDD and/or vehicle-treated mice identify the B cell as the primary cell type impaired in the AFC response, with only modest changes observed in T-cell accessory function (Dooley and Holsapple, 1988). Interestingly, unlike CMI-mediated responses, which were only affected when TCDD treatment was performed in vivo, direct addition of TCDD to leukocyte cultures was found to strongly suppress humoral immune responses to a variety of B-cell antigens and activators (ie, LPS, dinitrophenyl-ficoll, and sRBC) demonstrating the ability of TCDD to directly target B cells (Holsapple *et al.*, 1986). Investigations using AHR null mice and cell lines that differentially express AHR have demonstrated definitively that suppression of primary humoral immune responses by TCDD is dependent on AHR activation (Sulentic *et al.*, 2000; Vorderstrasse *et al.*, 2001). More recently, motif searches of regulatory regions of genes involved in controlling Ig expression led to the identification of DREs in a transcriptional regulatory region (termed 3'*Igh*RR) of the Ig heavy chain gene. The 3'*Igh*RR plays a crucial role in mediating high-level Ig heavy chain expression and Ig class switching. Electrophoretic mobility shift assays identified TCDD-induced AHR DNA binding, and transient transfection experiments demonstrated strong suppression of 3'*Igh*RR reporter activity by TCDD in a cell line model of B-cell differentiation (Henseler *et al.*, 2009; Sulentic *et al.*, 2000, 2004a, b). However, suppression of humoral immune responses by TCDD cannot be completely reconciled by altered regulation of the 3'*Igh*RR and the Ig heavy chain as TCDD-treatment also significantly suppresses expression of the Ig light chain and Ig J chain (Yoo *et al.*, 2004). Additional studies revealed that a bistable biological switch controlling B cell to plasma cell differentiation as formed by the transcriptional repressors, B-cell lymphoma-6 protein (BCL-6), B lymphocyte-induced maturation protein-1 (Blimp-1), and paired box protein 5 (Pax5) is significantly altered in the presence of TCDD (Bhattacharya *et al.*, 2010; Zhang *et al.*, 2010) resulting in elevated levels of Pax5 due to repression of Blimp-1 (North *et al.*, 2009; Schneider *et al.*, 2008, 2009). Importantly, Pax5 is highly expressed in resting B cells simultaneously repressing the Ig heavy chain, light chain, and J chain and is in turn repressed by Blimp-1 to allow plasma cell differentiation and Ig production. Deregulation of this bifunctional switch by TCDD is mediated in part through decreased AP-1 DNA binding within the Blimp-1 promoter (Schneider *et al.*, 2009) in combination with direct AHR-mediated induction of Bach2 (De Abrew *et al.*, 2011), which acts as a repressor of Blimp-1. Collectively, the aforementioned findings suggest that humoral immune responses are suppressed through the direct actions of TCDD on B cells via a

AHR-dependent mechanism through multiple related, but distinct, mechanisms acting in concert which include but are likely not limited to: (1) direct action of the AHR on the 3'*Igh*RR of the Ig heavy chain; (2) deregulation of a bifunctional switch controlling B-cell differentiation resulting in elevated Pax5 and repression of the Ig heavy chain, light chain, and J chain; and (3) impaired B-cell activation (North *et al.*, 2010).

The effects of TCDD on innate immunity are less well studied. TCDD has been shown to suppress some functions of neutrophils, including cytolytic and cytostatic activities. This suppression has been postulated as being related to neutrophil development in the bone marrow. Results by several investigators have shown TCDD-induced alterations in serum C3, indicating that soluble mediators of innate immunity may also be targeted (White and Anderson, 1985; White *et al.*, 1986). There have been no observed effects on macrophage-mediated cytotoxicity, NK function, or IFN production. In host resistance models, TCDD exposure has been shown to increase susceptibility to several bacterial, viral, and tumor models. The most extensively employed model of host resistance for assessing the effects of TCDD on immune competence has been influenza virus. Uniformly, all of these studies have shown impaired resistance to influenza after TCDD treatment as evidenced typically by increased mortality (Burleson *et al.*, 1996; Nohara *et al.*, 2002; Warren *et al.*, 2000). However, it is noteworthy that significant differences have been reported between laboratories concerning the magnitude of impairment produced by TCDD, which may be due in part to differences in the strain of influenza virus used. In this model of host resistance, lymphocyte migration to the lung and the production of virus-specific IgG$_{2a}$, IgG$_1$, and IgG$_{2b}$ antibodies were markedly diminished while IgA and neutrophilia were increased in TCDD-treated mice (Vorderstrasse *et al.*, 2003). Conversely, in this same study, no significant TCDD-associated effects were found on T-cell expansion in the lymph nodes and on the production of IFN-γ and IL-12. Collectively, the results suggested that the increase in mortality to influenza in TCDD-treated mice was due to decreased antibody production and increased pulmonary inflammation (Vorderstrasse *et al.*, 2003).

TCDD has also been identified as a potent immunohematopoietic toxicant with the ability to alter the number of Lin-Sca-1$^+$cKit$^+$ (LSK) bone marrow cells, a population enriched for murine HSCs. Assessment of bone marrow cells from TCDD-treated C57BL/6J mice for hematopoietic alterations revealed increases in the number of bone marrow LSK cells, relative to control, over 24 hours through 31 days following TCDD treatment. These findings suggest that proliferation and/or differentiation processes of HSCs are affected by TCDD and that these effects contribute to a reduced capacity of bone marrow to generate pro-T lymphocytes (Murante and Gasiewicz, 2000). Activation of the AHR by TCDD was also found to elicit disruptions in the circadian rhythms of hematopoietic precursors as evidenced by an abnormal in vivo rhythm of the percentage of the total number of LSK cells in G$_0$ phase of the cell cycle, suggesting disruption of stem cell quiescence (Garrett and Gasiewicz, 2006). In addition, expression of AHR and ARNT mRNA within enriched hematopoietic precursors oscillated with a circadian period. Taken together, these findings demonstrate that activation of the AHR by TCDD alters the profile of hematopoietic precursors as well as the circadian rhythms associated with these precursors.

There is little doubt that TCDD and related PCDDs are immunotoxic, particularly in mice. However, extrapolation to human exposure has proven to be difficult. There are a few instances in which accidental human exposure to TCDD and related congeners has afforded the opportunity to study exposure-related human immunological responses. In children exposed to PCDDs in Seveso, Italy (1976), nearly half of the exposed study group exhibited chloracne (a hallmark of high-level human exposure to PCDDs) three years after the accident. Immune parameters measured at that time were unaffected. In a second study conducted six years later on different subjects, there was an increase in complement, which correlated with the incidence of chloracne, an increase in circulating T and B cells, and an increase in PBMC mitogenic responses. In 2002, follow-up studies in which the population in the most highly exposed zone was randomly sampled, revealed modestly decreased median serum IgG but not IgM, IgA, C3, and C4 concentrations as compared to human subjects in the surrounding noncontaminated area (Baccarelli et al., 2002). A second incident occurred in 1971 in Times Beach, Missouri, when wastes containing TCDD were sprayed on roads to prevent dust formation. Both low-risk and high-risk individuals from this area were examined for DTH responses. Slight, but statistically nonsignificant alterations were observed in high-risk compared to low-risk individuals. In addition, there was a low-level increase in mitogenic responsiveness in high-risk persons. In a second study conducted 12 years later, no alterations were observed in DTH or mitogenic responses between exposed or control individuals. In studies undertaken to evaluate the in vitro effects of TCDD on human cells, TCDD suppressed IgM secretion by human B cells in response to the superantigen toxic shock syndrome toxin-1 and the proliferation and IgG secretion of human tonsillar B cells in response to LPS and cytokines (Wood and Holsapple, 1993; Wood et al., 1993). More recently, employing an in vitro CD40L B-cell activation model, HPB B cells were found to possess similar sensitivity to TCDD, as quantified by suppression of IgM AFC response, as mouse B cells expressing the high-affinity form of the AHR (C57BL/6) (Lu et al., 2010). In addition, HPB B cells also showed a marked impairment in the upregulation of activation markers, CD80, CD86, and CD69, and rapid attenuation (15–30 minutes postactivation) of protein phosphokinases including Akt as well as the mitogen-activated protein kinase, ERK, in the presence of TCDD (Lu et al., 2011). The impairment of CD80 and CD86 by TCDD on HPB B cells is in contrast to the increased upregulation of CD80 and CD86 by TCDD on mouse bone marrow DC discussed above (Bankoti et al., 2010; Simones and Shepherd, 2011) and may reflect species and/or cell-type related differences in the actions of TCDD within the immune system. Collectively, these results suggest that human B cells are sensitive to suppression by TCDD. Moreover, the effects of TCDD on human B cells are direct and involve, at least in part, attenuation of early B-cell activation events, which culminate in impairment of plasma cell formation. These results further suggest that TCDD-mediated suppression of B-cell function, although AHR-dependent, likely involves transcriptional as well as nontranscriptional mechanisms.

Polychlorinated Dibenzofurans Like the PCDDs, polychlorinated dibenzofurans (PCDFs) are not produced commercially but are true environmental contaminants associated with the production of chlorophenoxy acids, pentachlorophenol, and other PCB mixtures. Although higher concentrations are required to achieve observable effects, the immunotoxic profile of the PCDFs is similar in nature to that described for TCDD. In fact, most of what is known regarding the immunotoxicity of the PCDFs in animal models has been learned with structure–activity relationship studies comparing TCDD to congeners of the dibenzofurans. Tetrachlorodibenzofuran (TCDF) exposure in most species is associated with thymic atrophy and, in guinea pigs, it has been shown to suppress the DTH and lymphoproliferative responses to PHA and LPS. Suppression of the AFC response to SRBC after exposure to several PCDF

congeners has also been reported. In a more recent study of simple mixtures, dose–response studies comparing TCDD to either a mixture of PCDDs and PCDFs or to a mixture of PCDFs, PCDDs, and PCBs showed that each of the two mixtures produces strikingly similar suppression of the mouse in vivo anti-sRBC IgM AFC responses as TCDD alone when normalized to the total TCDD equivalents administered (Smialowicz et al., 2008). It is noteworthy that although the immunotoxicology database is extensive for TCDD and other PCDDs, it remains limited for PCDFs.

Two important case studies of human immunotoxicology involved populations accidentally exposed to HAHs. There is evidence that the PCDFs were the primary contributors to the observed toxic effects. Greater than 1850 individuals in Japan (in 1968) and in excess of 2000 people in Taiwan (in 1979) were affected when commercial rice oil was found to be contaminated with HAHs. PCDFs were observed in the tissues of the exposed populations, and subsequent studies on immune status revealed a decrease in total circulating T cells, decreased DTH response, and enhanced lymphoproliferative responses to PHA and pokeweed mitogen. In addition, many of the exposed individuals suffered from recurring respiratory infections, suggesting that host resistance mechanisms had been compromised.

Polychlorinated Biphenyls PCBs have seen extensive commercial use for over half a century. Their unique physical and chemical properties make PCB mixtures ideal for use as plasticizers, adhesives, and as dielectric fluids in capacitors and transformers. Mixtures of PCBs (eg, Aroclors) have been commonly used to evaluate the immunotoxicity of PCBs and have been reported to suppress immune responses and decrease host resistance (reviewed by Holsapple, 1996). The first indication that PCBs produced immunotoxic effects was the observation of severe atrophy of the primary and secondary lymphoid organs in general toxicity tests and the subsequent demonstration of the reduction in numbers of circulating lymphocytes. Studies to characterize the immunotoxic action of the PCBs have primarily focused on the antibody response. This parameter is by far the one most consistently affected by PCB exposure, and effects on antibody response have been demonstrated in guinea pigs, rabbits, mice, and rhesus monkeys. PCB-exposed monkeys exhibit chloracne, alopecia, and facial edema, all classical symptoms of HAH toxicity. In an extensive characterization of the effects of PCBs on non-human primates, Tryphonas and colleagues (1991a, b) exposed rhesus monkeys to Aroclor 1254 for 23 to 55 months. The only immune parameter consistently suppressed was the AFC response to sRBC (both IgM and IgG). In addition, after 55 months of exposure, lymphoproliferative responses were dose-dependently suppressed and serum complement levels were significantly elevated. The observed elevation in serum complement has also been reported in PCDD-exposed children from Seveso, Italy (Tognoni and Boniccorsi, 1982) and in PCDD-exposed mice (White et al., 1986).

The effects of PCBs on CMI are far less clear and both suppression and enhancement have been reported. Exposure to Aroclor 1260 has been demonstrated to suppress DTH responses in guinea pigs, whereas exposure to Aroclor 1254 was reported to enhance lymphoproliferative responses in rats. In a similar study in Fischer 344 rats (Aroclor 1254), thymic weight was decreased, NK cell activity was suppressed, PHA-induced proliferative responses were enhanced, and there was no effect on the MLR proliferative response or CTL activity. Other investigators (Silkworth and Loose, 1978, 1979) have reported enhancement of graft-versus-host reactivity and the MLR proliferative response. The augmentation of selected CMI assays may reflect a PCB-induced change in T-cell subsets (as discussed above with TCDD), which contributes to immune regulation.

Studies on host resistance following exposure to PCBs indicate that the host defenses against herpes simplex virus, *Plasmodium berghei*, *Listeria monocytogenes*, and *Salmonella typhimurium* in mice are suppressed (reviewed by Dean *et al.*, 1985). PCB-induced changes in tumor defenses have not been well defined, and both augmentation and suppression have been reported. This probably reflects the variability in the observed CMI responses.

The immunotoxicological effects of PCBs in humans are unclear. There are four separate reports of a longitudinal study in a cohort of Dutch children suggesting that the developing human immune system may be susceptible to immunotoxic alterations from exposure to Western European environmental levels of dioxin-like compounds, primarily PCBs (ten Tusscher *et al.*, 2003; Weisglas-Kuperus *et al.*, 1995, 2000, 2004). Three industrial areas were compared to a rural area with about 20% less PCBs in maternal plasma. In above studies of Dutch children, the major PCB congeners were measured in plasma in the mother and the newborn, and all dioxin-like compounds in maternal breast milk at two weeks after birth. The results showed an association between dioxin-like compound exposure and immunological changes, which included an increased number of lymphocytes, $\gamma\delta$ T cells, $CD3^+HLA-DR^+$ (activated) T cells, $CD8^+$ cells, $CD4^+CD45RO^+$ (memory T cells), and lower antibody levels to mumps and measles vaccination at preschool age (Weisglas-Kuperus *et al.*, 1995, 2000, 2004). In addition, an association was found between dioxin/PCB prenatal exposure and decreased shortness of breath with wheeze, and the PCB burden was associated with a higher prevalence of recurrent middle-ear infections and chicken pox and a lower prevalence of allergic reactions (Weisglas-Kuperus *et al.*, 2000). It is notable that although an association between dioxin/PCB exposure and changes in immune status was observed, all infants were found to be in the normal range. In a second study, modest but persistent changes in immune status were reported in children with perinatal exposure to dioxin-like compounds, as evidenced by a decrease in allergy and increased $CD4^+$ T cells and increased $CD45RA^+$ cell counts in a longitudinal subcohort of 27 healthy eight-year-old children with documented perinatal dioxin exposure (ten Tusscher *et al.*, 2003). The original cohort at 42 months demonstrated an association among reduced vaccine titers, increased incidence of chicken pox, and increased incidence of otitis media with higher exposure to toxicity equivalents of dioxin. However, by eight years of age the more frequent recurrent ear infections were still apparent (overall), although the chicken pox frequency showed an inverse correlation with PCB/dioxin levels.

Polybrominated Biphenyls The polybrominated biphenyls (PBBs) have been used primarily as flame retardants (Firemaster BP-6 and FF-1). While it is assumed that their profile of activity is similar to that of the PCBs, few studies have actually evaluated the action of the PBBs on immunocompetence. In Michigan (in 1973), Firemaster BP-6 was inadvertently substituted for a nutrient additive in cattle feed, resulting in widespread exposure of animals and humans to PBBs. Studies conducted on livestock following the incident indicated little if any PBB-induced alterations in immunocompetence (Kately and Bazzell, 1978; Vos and Luster, 1989). Like CMI observations involving PCBs, CMI responses in PBB-exposed individuals are not conclusive, showing both a reduction in circulating numbers of T and B cells and a suppression of selected CMI parameters or no effect on CMI at all. In a recent birth cohort study of 384 mother–infant pairs in Eastern Slovakia, PBB concentrations for selected PBB congeners were quantified in maternal and cord serum and infant blood at six months of age. Although the PBB concentrations in the Eastern Slovakia birth cohort were several-fold higher than those found in the United States, no association was observed between PBB levels, sum total or congener specific, and total serum IgG, IgA, IgM, and IgE (Jusko *et al.*, 2011).

Polycyclic Aromatic Hydrocarbons The polycyclic aromatic hydrocarbons (PAHs) are a ubiquitous class of environmental contaminants. They enter the environment through many routes including the burning of fossil fuels and forest fires. In addition to being carcinogenic and mutagenic, the PAHs have been found to be potent immunosuppressants. Effects have been documented on immune system development, humoral immunity, CMI, and host resistance. The most extensively studied PAHs are 7,12-dimethylbenz[*a*] anthracene (DMBA) and benzo[*a*]pyrene (BaP).

Early immunotoxicology studies of PAHs such as BaP, DMBA, and 3-methylcholanthrene demonstrated suppression of the antibody response to a variety of T-cell-dependent and T-cell-independent antigens. In addition, mice treated with BaP exhibited suppressed lymphoproliferative responses to mitogens, but not alloantigens (Dean *et al.*, 1983). In Dean's studies, host resistance to the PYB6 tumor and to *L. monocytogenes* were unaffected by BaP exposure, as was the DTH response and allograft rejection, suggesting that T cells and CMI were only minimally affected by BaP. In contrast to BaP, DMBA (the more potent PAH) significantly suppressed, not only AFC responses, but also NK cell activity, CTL responses, DTH responses, and alloantigen-induced lymphoproliferative responses. Therefore, DMBA exposure appears to result in long-lasting immune suppression of humoral immunity, CMI, and tumor resistance mechanisms in mice. In addition, both BaP and DMBA also produced significant effects on the bone marrow as evidenced by suppression of pre-B cell formation. A recent comprehensive immunotoxicological evaluation of 1,2:5,6-dibenzanthracene (DBA) demonstrated that a single dose via pharyngeal aspiration at doses up to 30 mg/kg had no effect on NK cell activity, anti-CD3 antibody-mediated T lymphocyte proliferation, the MLR, or B lymphocyte proliferation. In contrast, suppression of the anti-sRBC IgM AFC response was observed at 1.0 mg/kg DBA and the DTH response to *C. albicans* was significantly decreased at 3.0 mg/kg DBA (Smith *et al.*, 2010). In another study, the immunosuppressive activity of various PAHs was greatly enhanced, in vitro, when combined with arsenic, a second common environmental contaminant (Li *et al.*, 2010). Interestingly, in this same study it was observed that PAH metabolites were more potent in inducing p53 than their parent compounds.

Significant progress has been made toward elucidation of the mechanism(s) by which PAHs exert their toxicological effects including those on the immune system. Biological and toxicological activity of PAHs is generally dependent on two factors, AHR activation and the metabolism of PAHs to active metabolites by cytochrome P450 isozymes, CYP1A1, CYP1A2 and CYP1B1, which are transcriptionally induced by AHR binding to DREs in the promoter region of the genes that code for the aforementioned isozymes. Although leukocytes, in general, possess modest cytochrome P450 drug-metabolizing activity, in in vitro studies, splenocytes from naive untreated mice were found to metabolize exogenously added DMBA via P450 enzymes (Ladics *et al.*, 1991). In addition, Ladics and colleagues (1992a, b) demonstrated that macrophages were the primary cell type in a splenic leukocyte preparation capable of metabolizing BaP to 7,8-dihydroxy-9,10-epoxy-7,8,9,10-benzo[*a*]pyrene (BPDE), the reactive metabolite proposed to be the ultimate carcinogenic and immunotoxic form of BaP. These data are consistent with other studies demonstrating the presence and inducibility of CYP1A1, CYP1A2, and most importantly in leukocytes, CYP1B1 (Gao *et al.*, 2005a).

PAHs, including BaP, have also been shown to induce AHR-independent biochemical changes in lymphocytes leading to oxidative stress, activation of tyrosine kinases, and increased intracellular calcium (Mounho and Burchiel, 1998; Pessah et al., 2001). The elevation in intracellular calcium in B and T lymphocytes was shown to be mediated by BaP-7,8-dione and blocked by high concentrations of ryanodine suggesting the involvement of ryanodine receptors (Gao et al., 2005b).

Progress has also been made on the elucidation of the mechanism by which BaP and DMBA mediate bone marrow toxicity, specifically suppression of pre-B-cell formation. In vitro models demonstrated that BaP and DMBA rapidly induced apoptosis in primary pre-B cells and in the pro/pre-B cell line, BU-11 (Yamaguchi et al., 1997). The mechanism for pre-B-cell apoptosis by PAHs was shown to be dependent on bone marrow-derived stromal cells (Yamaguchi et al., 1997), CYP1B1 metabolism (Heidel et al., 1998), and the AHR (Yamaguchi et al., 1997) as well as coinciding with the induction of p53 (Yamaguchi et al., 1997). It has been demonstrated that DMBA-mediated bone marrow cytotoxicity was absent in p53 null mice and that apoptosis of primary bone marrow progenitor B cells cocultured with bone marrow stromal cells and DMBA was p53-dependent (Page et al., 2003). Collectively, these and other studies suggest that PAHs are metabolized by bone marrow stromal cells, which in turn release active PAH metabolites as part of a metabolite protein complex that induces apoptosis in pre-B cells (Allan et al., 2003).

Pesticides

Pesticides include all xenobiotics whose specific purpose is to kill another form of life, including insects (insecticides), small rodents (rodenticides), or even vegetation (herbicides). As such, these chemicals have clear biological activity and many pesticides have been studied for their effects on the immune system (Galloway and Handy, 2003). While there is much evidence that pesticides produce alterations in immune function in a variety of mammalian, amphibian, and fish animal models, the studies described here will focus on those that provide mechanistic information related to epidemiological effects in humans (reviewed by Colosio et al., 2005). Exposure to pesticides occurs most often in occupational settings, in which manufacturers, those applying the pesticides, or those harvesting treated agricultural products, are exposed. In the United States, the most widely used class of pesticides (through 2007) were the organophosphates (Grube et al., 2011), although effects of organochlorines, organotins, carbamates, and the herbicide atrazine will also be discussed.

Organophosphates Organophosphates include malathion, parathion, methyl parathion, diazinon, and chlorpyrifos. Although the neurotoxic effects of organophosphates are well understood to occur via the inhibition of acetylcholinesterase (see Chap. 22, "Toxic Effects of Pesticides"), the mechanism by which these compounds suppress the immune system is not as well defined.

Malathion exhibits both immune suppressive and immune enhancing effects (Rodgers and Ellefson, 1990). Malathion has been shown to suppress humoral immunity as measured by the AFC response to sRBC following a subacute exposure in mice (Casale et al., 1983). In vitro exposure of either human PBMC or murine splenocytes to malathion results in decreased lymphoproliferative responses, suppressed CTL generation, and a decrease in the stimulus-induced respiratory burst in peritoneal cells (Rodgers and Ellefson, 1990). The mechanisms by which malathion is immunotoxic has been attributed to induction of oxidative stress in unstimulated mouse thymocytes (Olgun et al., 2004) or human PBMC

(Ahmed et al., 2011). Parathion has attracted more attention than malathion, probably because it is more acutely toxic. This pesticide also produces mixed responses, which might depend on strain or dose (Casale et al., 1983; Crittenden et al., 1998). A comprehensive screen of various classes of pesticides that exhibit binding affinity to, and activation of, the pregnane X receptor (PXR) demonstrated that parathion activates PXR (Kojima et al., 2011), which has been shown to suppress inflammatory responses through inhibition of NF-κB (Zhou et al., 2006).

Fewer studies exist that describe the immunotoxicity of diazinon. Recently, it has been shown that diazinon produced gross changes in the spleen and thymus in response to acute doses in mice (Handy et al., 2002; Neishabouri et al., 2004). Diazinon also suppressed humoral immunity as measured by the AFC response to sRBC and CMI as measured by the DTH response following subchronic exposure to mice (Neishabouri et al., 2004).

Chlorpyrifos is one of the most widely used pesticides in the United States (Grube et al., 2011). Similar to other pesticides, its effects on immune function vary. An examination of humans exposed to chlorpyrifos demonstrated suppressed proliferative responses to Con A or PHA, but an increase in autoantibodies (Thrasher et al., 2002). Using human PBMC, it was demonstrated that chlorpyrifos modestly enhanced or suppressed IFN-γ production in response to LPS at low (1–100 μg/mL) or high (1000 μg/mL) concentrations, respectively (Duramad et al., 2006). The mechanism by which chlorpyrifos modulates immunity likely involves ERα, PXR, and AHR, as it induced reporter activity in receptor-activation assays (Kojima et al., 2004, 2011; Takeuchi et al., 2008).

Organochlorines The organochlorines include chemicals such as chlordane, dichlorodiphenyltrichloroethane (DDT), mirex, pentachlorophenol, aldrin, dieldrin, and hexachlorobenzene. Although technically this class of compounds also includes the herbicides 2,4-D and 2,4,5-T, these compounds are considered separately under "Halogenated Aromatic Hydrocarbons." The organochlorines are among the longer-lived pesticides and they have an increased propensity for contamination of soil and ground water, thus providing an additional route of exposure to the general population. Many organochlorine compounds also have been shown to mediate their effects via ERα (DDT, dieldrin, and chlordane), ERβ (DDT) (Kojima et al., 2004), or PXR (DDT, dieldrin, and chlordane) (Kojima et al., 2011).

Although DDT has been banned in several countries, it is still used to control malaria, typhoid, and dengue infections in some places of the world. DDT suppresses both humoral immunity and CMI. Early studies demonstrated suppression of humoral immunity following oral gavage in mice (Wiltrout et al., 1978). More recently, DDT has been shown to suppress IL-2 production from a human T-cell line and that the mechanism involved suppression of the critical transcription factor NF-κB (Ndebele et al., 2004). In another study in which occupationally exposed individuals were evaluated for cytokine levels, DDE, a primary metabolite of DDT, was associated with suppression of IL-2 and IFN-γ, and enhancement of IL-4, suggesting an imbalance of Th1/Th2 populations (Daniel et al., 2002). Finally, a correlation between DDE levels in breast milk and incidence of infant ear infections was observed, suggesting increased susceptibility to infection following DDT exposure (Dewailly et al., 2000). An increased susceptibility to infection might also involve suppression of macrophage function by DDT (Nunez et al., 2002), increased apoptosis of macrophages, reduced complement function (Dutta et al., 2008), or suppression of NK cell function (Udoji et al., 2010).

Dieldrin was used from the 1950s until 1987 when its use was banned due to environmental and human health concerns. The humoral immune response to both T-cell-dependent and T-cell-independent antigens is suppressed following exposure to dieldrin (Bernier *et al.*, 1987), and macrophage function from dieldrin-exposed animals are depressed. The apparent effect of dieldrin on macrophages correlates with the increased susceptibility of dieldrin-exposed animals to murine hepatitis virus, which targets macrophages (Krzystyniak *et al.*, 1985). CMI was also suppressed in mice following dieldrin exposure as measured by a suppression of the MLR and graft-versus-host disease (Hugo *et al.*, 1988a, b). Dieldrin is also immunostimulatory under certain conditions as dieldrin enhanced the proinflammatory cytokine IL-8 in vitro and induced neutrophilic inflammation in vivo (Pelletier *et al.*, 2001).

Chlordane refers to a group of structurally related chemicals used to control termites. The principle constituents of chlordane are heptachlor, α-chlordane, γ-chlordane, α-nonachlor, β-nonachlor, α-chlordene, β-chlordene, and γ-chlordene. Definitive immune suppression produced by chlordane was first reported by Spyker-Cranmer and colleagues (1982). In utero exposure resulted in decreased DTH responses in mice with no deficit in antibody production to sRBC. This effect correlated with an increase in resistance to influenza infection because DTH contributes to the pathology of the infection (Menna *et al.*, 1985). In contrast to observations from mice exposed in utero, exposure of adult mice to chlordane did not result in any changes to several immune parameters, including AFC response to sRBC, MLR, DTH response, or mitogenic lymphoproliferation. In rats, immunomodulatory effects of three constituents of chlordane were noted following 28-day oral dosing (technical chlordane, *cis*-nonachlor, and *trans*-nonachlor), the most profound being increased lymphocyte numbers with decreased NK cell activity and proliferation in response to *S. typhimurium* (Tryphonas *et al.*, 2003). The increase in cell numbers was consistent with a study conducted in Japan in which high concentrations of chlordane in breast milk increased CD3$^+$ and CD8$^+$ T-cell percentages in infants measured at approximately 10 months of age (Nagayama *et al.*, 2007).

Many organochlorine pesticides have also been associated with increased cancer incidence (reviewed by Dich *et al.*, 1997). The mechanism by which this occurs is unclear but is likely multifaceted, including, in part, organochlorine-induced modulation of the immune system. For instance, chlordane suppressed expression of the tumor suppressor, retinoblastoma protein, in a human B-cell/T-cell hybrid cell line (Rought *et al.*, 1999). Furthermore, several organochlorine pesticides were demonstrated in vitro to suppress NK cell activity, which plays a role in defense against tumor formation (Reed *et al.*, 2004). An analysis of the influence of organochlorine exposure and immune gene variants demonstrated increased risk of non-Hodgkin's lymphoma in chlordane-exposed individuals with certain SNPs in IL-10 (Wang *et al.*, 2007), IFN-γ, and IL-4 (Colt *et al.*, 2009).

Organotins Trisubstituted organotins such as tributyltin oxide are widely used as biocides and have recently been recognized as producing some immunotoxic effects. The most prominent action of tributyltin oxide is the induction of profound but reversible thymic atrophy. Studies by Vos and colleagues (1984) demonstrated a decrease in cellularity in the spleen, bone marrow, and thymus. The decrease in splenic cellularity was associated with a concomitant loss of T lymphocytes. In Jurkat T cells, tributyltin oxide increased intracellular calcium and nuclear factor of activated T cells (NFAT) translocation to the nucleus, but the increase in proliferation was not sustained, and at later times, there was decreased proliferation

and increased expression of several apoptotic genes (Katika *et al.*, 2011). In mouse thymocytes, there were increased annexin-V$^+$ and Fas ligand-expressing cells following oral administration of tributyltin chloride (Chen *et al.*, 2011), providing additional evidence that thymic atrophy is due to apoptosis.

Another sensitive target of organotin compounds is the NK cell. van Loveren and colleagues (1990) observed suppressed lung NK cytotoxicity in rats exposed orally to tributyltin oxide. The mechanism by which NK cell activity was suppressed has been investigated using human NK cells. Studies have demonstrated an increase in intracellular calcium and increased expression of various AP-1 transcription factors (Lane *et al.*, 2009; Person and Whalen, 2010). However, overall, there was decreased AP-1 binding activity, which the authors suggested was due to increased prevalence of jun–jun homodimers, which exhibit lower affinity for the AP-1 site than other complexes, such as jun–fos heterodimers (Person and Whalen, 2010). Moreover, the mechanism by which di- and tributyltin suppressed NK cell activity might be due to its ability to interact with sulfhydryl groups since glutathione treatment reversed the suppression (Powell *et al.*, 2009).

Carbamates Carbamates, which include carbaryl (Sevin), aldicarb, mancozeb, and sodium methyldithiocarbamate, are used primarily as insecticides. Similar to the organophosphates, the mechanism of action for the neurotoxic effects involves inhibition of acetylcholinesterase. In an evaluation of humoral immunity following a two-week exposure to carbaryl in rats, suppression of the IgM AFC response to sRBC was observed following inhalation exposure, but not oral or dermal exposure (Ladics *et al.*, 1994). Following oral exposure in rats, carbaryl suppressed splenic proliferative responses, but enhanced pulmonary inflammation and IgE, in response to house dust mite, suggesting that carbaryl exhibits tissue-specific effects (Dong *et al.*, 1998). The mechanism by which carbaryl is suppressive involves inhibition of LPS-induced signaling in macrophages (Ohnishi *et al.*, 2008).

Pruett and coworkers (1992a) evaluated the immunotoxicity of sodium methyldithiocarbamate, and observed decreased thymus weight, depletion of the CD4$^+$/CD8$^+$ population of thymocytes, and profound suppression of NK cell activity following both oral and dermal exposure. They also determined that the mechanism by which sodium methyldithiocarbamate altered cytokine production from peritoneal macrophages involves inhibition of MAP kinase activity via TLR4 (Pruett *et al.*, 2005). Pruett and coworkers (2006) further determined that the mechanism of cytokine alteration involved depletion of glutathione, alteration of copper-dependent proteins, and induction of stress.

Atrazine Atrazine is an herbicide applied to various agricultural crops to control broad leaf weeds. It is widely used in the United States, and it has been detected in soils and ground water because of its resistance to degradation. Similar to other agents discussed, atrazine exhibits immunomodulatory effects. Using offspring of dams treated with atrazine and challenged with antigen, atrazine induced elevations in T-cell proliferation, cytolytic activity, and antigen-specific B cells in male offspring (Rowe *et al.*, 2006). In contrast, young mice directly administered atrazine orally for 14 days exhibited suppressed thymic weight, spleen and thymic cellularity, and B cell fractions, although CD4$^+$ T cell numbers increased (Filipov *et al.*, 2005). Similarly, in adult mice, it was confirmed that atrazine suppressed thymic weight, and also suppressed splenic weight and decreased the host resistance of the mice to B16F10 melanoma tumors (Karrow *et al.*, 2005). In vitro, atrazine suppressed cell surface expression of MHCII, CD86, CD11b, and CD11c using a mouse DC line (Pinchuk *et al.*, 2007). Although the exact mechanism by which atrazine-induced immune suppression occurred is unclear, atrazine treatment of mice does induce corticosterone levels, indicating that activation of the hypothalamic–pituitary–adrenal axis might be involved (Pruett *et al.*, 2003).

Metals

Generally speaking, metals target multiple organ systems and exert their toxic effects via an interaction of the free metal with targets, such as enzyme systems, membranes, or cellular organelles. In considering the immunotoxicity of most metals, it is important to remember that at high concentrations, metals usually exert immunosuppressive effects; however, at lower concentrations, immune enhancement is often observed (Koller, 1980; Vos, 1977). Furthermore, as with most immunotoxic agents, it is important to note that exposures to metals are likely not single exposures, although one metal might dominate depending on the exposure conditions (eg, high levels of mercury in fish or high levels of lead from paint).

Similar to pesticides, there is certainly a large body of literature describing the metal-induced immune alterations in mammalian, amphibian, and fish animal models, but again, the studies described here will focus on those that provide mechanistic information related to epidemiological effects in humans. Moreover, there has been a substantial increase in efforts to understand immune alterations following exposures to metal-containing nanomaterials; for these, the reader is referred to Chap. 28, "Nanotoxicology" or Chap. 23, "Toxic Effects of Metals." Specific immunotoxic consequences of metal exposure have been reviewed (Zelikoff and Thomas, 1998), but this section focuses on the four best-studied immunotoxic metals: lead, arsenic, mercury, and cadmium.

Lead By far the most consistent finding in studies evaluating the effects of metals on immune responses is increased susceptibility to pathogens. For lead, decreased resistance to the bacterial pathogens *S. typhimurium, Escherichia coli*, and *L. monocytogenes* has been observed (reviewed by Kasten-Jolly *et al.*, 2010). In mechanistic studies (reviewed by Dietert and Piepenbrink, 2006a), an alteration in the ability of the macrophage to process and present antigen to antigen-primed T cells confirmed the previous observation and suggested that lead alters immune recognition. Both suppression and enhancement of the AFC response by lead has been reported.

The enhanced AFC response could be due to the observation that lead shifts the T-cell balance from Th1 to Th2 (reviewed by Dietert and Piepenbrink, 2006a). Interestingly, it has been hypothesized that lead exposure might contribute to the development of asthma (Dietert and Piepenbrink, 2006a), a predominantly Th2-mediated disease. This theory is consistent with the observation that there is increased IgE production and asthma incidence in lead-exposed children (Lutz *et al.*, 1999) and that lead inhibits IFN-γ production, a Th1 cytokine (Heo *et al.*, 2007). The mechanism by which lead induces a Th2 switch has been suggested to involve lead-induced alterations in bone marrow-derived DC populations that preferentially stimulate Th2 differentiation (Gao *et al.*, 2007). Additional evidence for lead-induced alteration of APC function comes from the observation that lead-treated APCs stimulated CD4+ T-cell proliferation, likely via reduction of myeloid suppressor cell function (myeloid suppressor cells are macrophages that control T-cell proliferation) (Farrer *et al.*, 2005, 2008).

Arsenic A challenge in understanding the mechanisms by which arsenic is immunotoxic is that in addition to inconsistencies that arise from route of administration, concentrations/doses, and species/strain differences, the speciation of arsenic plays a significant role in arsenic toxicity. Moreover, early studies demonstrated the intricate interplay among the host, the pathogen, and the xenobiotic. Following exposure to the semiconductor material gallium arsenide, there was modest protection against infection of either *S. pneumoniae* or *L. monocytogenes*, but resistance to the B16F10 melanoma was reduced. It was subsequently determined that the arsenic concentrations in the blood of these animals was high enough to offer a chemotherapeutic effect against the bacterial pathogens (Burns *et al.*, 1993).

Arsenic compounds affect human immune function. For instance, in environmentally exposed children, there was a correlation between total arsenic in urine (inorganic and arsenic metabolites) and superoxide anion production from stimulated monocytes (Luna *et al.*, 2010) and in adult smelter workers, higher levels of urinary arsenic correlated with increased lipid peroxidation and lower vitamin E levels in blood (Escobar *et al.*, 2010). These results suggest that arsenic exposure causes oxidative stress and in fact, using the THP-1 monocytic cell line, it was shown that arsenic trioxide decreased glutathione levels and induced heme oxygenase, which is often induced to combat oxidative stress (Wang *et al.*, 2011).

There are also several studies in which human PBMC from unexposed individuals were treated in vitro with arsenic compounds. The percentage of IL-2-producing T cells in human PBMC was suppressed following treatment with sodium arsenite (Galicia *et al.*, 2003). An additional study showed that sodium arsenite suppressed IL-2 production while also stimulating heme oxygenase in purified T cells, indicating that the direct T-cell impairment by arsenic occurs in parallel with oxidative stress (Martin-Chouly *et al.*, 2011). B-cell and accessory cell (ie, macrophage) function is also compromised by arsenic compounds, as suggested by early anti-sRBC AFC responses in mice (Sikorski *et al.*, 1991). Interestingly, in spite of a fairly extensive database showing suppression of antibody responses in murine models, in purified human B cells stimulated with CD40L, sodium arsenite did not suppress IgM production (Lu *et al.*, 2009). Finally, treatment of primary human macrophages with arsenic trioxide resulted in decreased expression of CD14 (a PRR and coreceptor of TLRs), and altered the morphology thereby suppressing adhesion (Lemarie *et al.*, 2006). The alterations in macrophage function were dependent on arsenic trioxide-induced activation of RhoA (small GTPase and Ras homolog) (Lemarie *et al.*, 2006). At higher concentrations, arsenic trioxide also induced apoptosis of macrophages through inhibition of NF-κB signaling (Lemarie *et al.*, 2006). Induction of macrophage apoptosis is the basis for the therapeutic use of arsenic trioxide to treat acute promyelocytic leukemia.

Mercury Mercury compounds include organic (ie, methyl mercury) or inorganic forms. Mercury compounds not only suppress immunological responses, but also induce autoimmunity (see Mercury discussion under the "Autoimmunity" section). Interestingly, in one genetically susceptible mouse model of autoimmunity, subcutaneous administration of methyl mercury reduced T and B cell numbers prior to autoimmunity induction, demonstrating the immunomodulatory actions of mercury in vivo (Haggqvist *et al.*, 2005).

Similar to arsenic, the mechanism by which mercury compounds are immunotoxic might be induction of apoptosis. Mercury also induces oxidative stress as evidenced by glutathione depletion (Mondal *et al.*, 2005). Several studies have examined the effect of in vitro treatment of human PBMC with mercury compounds. Using mercuric chloride in PBMC stimulated with either anti-CD3/CD28/CD40 or bacterial antigen demonstrated that mercury differentially affects Th1/Th2 cytokines depending on the mode of T-cell activation (Hemdan *et al.*, 2007). Using LPS to stimulate inflammatory cytokines, mercuric chloride enhanced an inflammatory response (Gardner *et al.*, 2009). The induction of proinflammatory cytokines was also observed in Brazilian gold miners using mercury as an amalgam. Mercury-exposed miners demonstrated higher levels of IL-1β, TNF-α, and IFN-γ (Gardner *et al.*, 2010). The mechanism for cytokine induction could be due to mercury-induced phosphorylation of ERK and p38 MAPKs as demonstrated using mercuric chloride in Jurkat T cells. This was due, in part, to ROS since mercury-induced phosphorylation of ERK and p38 MAPKs was abrogated by *N*-acetylcysteine (Haase *et al.*, 2011).

Cadmium Like other metals, cadmium exhibits immunomodulatory effects. Early studies demonstrated that oral administration of cadmium to mice increased susceptibility to herpes simplex type 2 virus, suppressed T and B cell proliferation, but enhanced macrophage phagocytosis (Thomas *et al.*, 1985). As with many other immunotoxic agents, it has been suggested that the stress response, a shift to a Th2 cell population, induction of oxidative stress and induction of apoptosis all contribute to the mechanism by which cadmium suppresses humoral immunity and CMI (Hemdan *et al.*, 2006; Lall and Dan, 1999; Pathak and Khandelwal, 2006, 2008). Using human HSCs isolated from umbilical cord blood, it was shown that in vitro treatment with cadmium chloride activated autophagy, an internal cellular degradation pathway allowing clearance of damaged cellular components (Di Gioacchino *et al.*, 2008). Cadmium-induced oxidative stress was confirmed in PBMC isolated from a Japanese population of women living in a cadmium polluted area in which higher blood and urinary cadmium correlated with increased expression of several genes involved in oxidative stress signaling (Dakeshita *et al.*, 2009).

It has long been known that cadmium (and other metals, such as mercury) bind to a protein called metallothionein, which is a small, cysteine-rich protein that complexes normally with divalent cations, such as copper and zinc. The role of metallothionein in metal-induced immunotoxicity has been recently reviewed (Klaassen *et al.*, 2009), and there are several mechanisms by which the cadmium–metallothionein complex might contribute to immune modulation. The binding of cadmium to metallothionein could displace copper or zinc, altering the availability of the latter cations for biochemical processes. Alternatively, metallothionein is induced in response to several stimuli, including metals, and it has been demonstrated that metallothionein influences lymphocyte proliferation, differentiation, and various effector functions. Finally, since metallothionein is a cysteine-rich protein, it also plays a role in the oxidative homeostasis of the cell, which could be compromised under conditions of oxidative stress.

Solvents and Related Chemicals

There is limited but substantive evidence that exposure to organic solvents and their related compounds can produce immune suppression. Chemicals included in this section are aromatic hydrocarbons, such as benzene, haloalkanes and haloalkenes, glycols and glycol ethers, and nitrosamines.

Aromatic Hydrocarbons By far the best-characterized immunotoxic effects by an organic solvent are those produced by benzene. In animal models, benzene induces anemia, lymphocytopenia, and hypoplastic bone marrow. In addition, it has been suggested that this myelotoxicity may be a result of altered differentiative capacity in bone marrow-derived lymphoid cells. Benzene (oral and inhaled) exposure has been reported to alter both humoral and

CMI parameters including suppression of the anti-sRBC antibody response, decreased T- and B-cell lymphoproliferative responses (mitogens and alloantigens), and suppression of CTL activity. Benzene exposure also appears to increase the production of both IL-1 and TNF-α and to suppress the production of IL-2. With these dramatic effects on immune responses, it is not surprising that animals exposed to benzene exhibit reduced resistance to a variety of pathogens. In terms of a possible mechanism of action, Pyatt *et al.* (1998) demonstrated that hydroquinone, a reactive metabolite of benzene, inhibited the activity of NF-κB, a transcription factor known to regulate the expression of a number of genes critical for normal T-cell function. The authors concluded that NF-κB might be an important molecular mediator of the immunotoxicity of hydroquinone (and benzene).

A number of compounds structurally related to benzene have also been studied for their potential effects on the immune system. For example, nitrobenzene (an oxidizing agent used in the synthesis of aniline and benzene compounds) has been reported to produce immunotoxic effects (Burns *et al.*, 1994b), with the primary targets being erythrocytes and bone marrow. Immunomodulating activity has also been observed for toluene, although most effects occur at markedly high concentrations. When compared with benzene, toluene has little to no effect on immunocompetence. However, it is noteworthy that toluene exposure effectively attenuates the immunotoxic effects of benzene (probably because of competition for metabolic enzymes). In contrast to the parent toluene, the monosubstituted nitrotoluenes (*para*- and *meta*-nitrotoluene) do significantly alter the immune system (Burns *et al.*, 1994a, c). Exposure to *p*-nitrotoluene has been demonstrated to suppress the antibody response to sRBC, to decrease the number of CD4$^+$ splenic T cells, and to suppress the DTH response to KLH. In addition, host resistance to *L. monocytogenes* was impaired, suggesting the T cell as a primary target. Similarly, *m*-nitrotoluene suppresses the antibody response to sRBC, the DTH response to KLH, T-cell mitogenesis, and host resistance to *L. monocytogenes*, again suggesting the T cell as the cellular target. The disubstituted nitrotoluene (2,4-dinitrotoluene) is also immunosuppressive (Burns *et al.*, 1994a), with exposure resulting in suppressed humoral immunity, NK cell activity, and phagocytosis by splenic macrophages. Host resistance to bacterial challenge was also impaired. This profile of activity following exposure to 2,4-dinitrotoluene is consistent with a perturbation of the differentiation and maturation of leukocytes.

Haloalkanes and Haloalkenes Carbon tetrachloride is widely recognized as hepatotoxic. Studies in mice revealed that carbon tetrachloride is also immunosuppressive. Mice exposed for 7 to 30 days to carbon tetrachloride (orally or intraperitoneally) exhibited a decreased T-cell-dependent antibody response (sRBC), suppressed MLR response, and lower lymphoproliferative capacity (T and B cells) (Kaminski *et al.*, 1989a). Ex vivo activation of splenic T cells isolated from carbon tetrachloride-treated mice revealed a marked enhancement in IL-2 production. Moreover, the effect on IL-2 by carbon tetrachloride was associated with a serum factor in treated animals as direct addition of serum from carbon tetrachloride-treated mice also produced strong enhancement of IL-2 in naive activated splenic T cells. Further characterization demonstrated that exposure to carbon tetrachloride caused the induction and release of TGF-β_1 from the liver. The timing and conditions for the carbon tetrachloride-induced releases of TGF-β_1 was concomitant with the onset of immune suppression. Addition of anti-TGF-β_1 neutralizing antibodies abrogated IL-2 enhancement by serum isolated from carbon tetrachloride-treated mice, suggesting that the enhancing effects on IL-2 were mediated indirectly through

TGF-β_1 released from the liver (Delaney *et al.*, 1994; Jeon *et al.*, 1997). Induction or inhibition of liver cytochrome P450 activity augmented and blocked, respectively, the immunotoxic actions of carbon tetrachloride, suggesting a requirement for metabolism in order for carbon tetrachloride to be immunosuppressive (Kaminski *et al.*, 1990). Subsequently, it was demonstrated that TGF-β_1 produces profound effects on IL-2 regulation. Specifically, results in mouse spleen cells showed that TGF-β_1 exerts bifunctional effects on IL-2 and lymphoproliferation as evidenced by the fact that TGF-β_1 stimulates IL-2 production at low concentrations (0.1–1 pg/mL) and conversely suppresses IL-2 production at high concentrations (1–10 ng/mL), when activated using monoclonal antibodies directed against the CD3 complex and CD28 (McKarns and Kaminski, 2000). Additionally, concentrations of TGF-β_1 that stimulated IL-2 production concomitantly suppressed splenocyte proliferation under similar conditions. Studies have revealed that IL-2 regulation by TGF-β_1 is mediated, at least in part, via a mechanism dependent on SMAD3, a transcription factor involved in signaling through the TGF-β receptor (McKarns *et al.*, 2004). In studies comparing acute versus subchronic carbon tetrachloride administration, acute carbon tetrachloride treatment enhanced phagocytosis and NK cell activity while subchronic treatment significantly impaired phagocytosis and NK cell activity (Jirova *et al.*, 1996). In contrast, Fischer 344 rats exposed orally for 10 days showed no immunotoxic effects, despite signs of liver toxicity (Smialowicz *et al.*, 1991c). The difference in sensitivity between studies in the mouse and rat may represent differences in the metabolic capabilities between these two species as well as the degree of liver injury induced, and hence the magnitude of TGF-β_1 production.

There is relatively little information on solvents and other chemicals structurally related to carbon tetrachloride. Some early studies were conducted to assess the potential immunotoxicity of a number of drinking water contaminants. Exposure to dichloroethylene (in drinking water for 90 days) has been reported to suppress the anti-sRBC antibody response in male CD-1 mice and to inhibit macrophage function in females (Shopp *et al.*, 1985). Similarly, exposure to trichloroethylene (in the drinking water for four–six months) was reported to inhibit both humoral immunity and CMI and bone marrow colony-forming activity (Sanders *et al.*, 1982). In those experiments, females were more sensitive than males. Exposure to 1,1,2-trichloroethane resulted in suppression of humoral immunity in both sexes. In addition, macrophage function was suppressed (males only) (Sanders *et al.*, 1985). Inhalation studies with dichloroethane, dichloromethane, tetrachloroethane, and trichloroethene indicated that the pulmonary host resistance to *Klebsiella pneumoniae* was suppressed (Aranyi *et al.*, 1986; Sherwood *et al.*, 1987), suggesting that alveolar macrophages may be affected. More recent work with this series of solvents indicated that exposure to trichloroethylene may be an effective developmental immunotoxicant in B6C3F1 mice, suggesting that additional studies are required to determine the health risks associated with developmental exposure to this chemical (Peden-Adams *et al.*, 2006).

Glycols and Glycol Ethers Exposure to glycol ethers has been associated with adverse effects in laboratory animals, including thymic atrophy and mild leukopenia. Oral administration of ethylene glycol monomethyl ether for one to two weeks (House *et al.*, 1985; Kayama *et al.*, 1991) or its metabolite methoxyacetic acid for two weeks (House *et al.*, 1985) produced decreased thymic weight, thymic atrophy, and a selective depletion of immature thymocytes in mice. No alterations in humoral immunity, CMI, macrophage function, or host resistance to *L. monocytogenes* were observed (House *et al.*, 1985). It has also been suggested that perinatal exposure to ethylene glycol monomethyl ether may produce thymic hypocellularity and inhibition of thymocyte maturation, and that it may affect prolymphocytes in fetal liver (Holladay *et al.*, 1994).

Oral studies (5–10 days) on the glycol ether 2-methoxyethanol have consistently shown a decrease in thymus weight in the rat (Smialowicz *et al.*, 1991a; Williams *et al.*, 1995). This decrease is often accompanied by alterations in lymphoproliferative responses, although suppression is seen in some cases and stimulation in others, with no clear reason for the differences in response. Alterations in spleen weight and splenic cell populations have also been observed, as well as suppression of trinitrophenyl-LPS and anti-sRBC AFC responses. Similar results have been obtained following dermal exposure to 2-methoxyethanol (Williams *et al.*, 1995). A decrease in IL-2 production has also been reported (Smialowicz *et al.*, 1991a). Studies using the metabolites of 2-methoxyethanol (methoxyacetaldehyde and methoxyacetic acid) or specific metabolic pathway inhibitors have shown that methoxyacetaldehyde and methoxyacetic acid are more immunotoxic than 2-methoxyethanol alone (methoxyacetaldehyde > methoxyacetic acid > 2-methoxyethanol) (Kim and Smialowicz, 1997; Smialowicz *et al.*, 1991a, b), suggesting a role for metabolism in the observed alterations in immunocompetence. Although there was no effect following 10-day oral exposures to 2-methoxyethanol (50–200 mg/kg per day) (Smialowicz *et al.*, 1991a), subchronic exposure for 21 days to 2000 to 6000 ppm (males) or 1600 to 4800 ppm (females) did produce an enhanced NK cell response (Exon *et al.*, 1991) in addition to suppression of the AFC response and a decrease in IFN-γ production.

Nitrosamines The nitrosamine family of chemicals comprises the nitrosamines, nitrosamides, and *C*-nitroso compounds. Exposure to nitrosamines, especially *N*-nitrosodimethylamine (eg, also known as dimethylnitrosamine or DMN; and the most prevalent nitrosamine) comes primarily through industrial and dietary means, and minimally through environmental exposure. DMN is used commonly as an industrial solvent in the production of dimethylhydrazine. It has been used as an antioxidant, as an additive for lubricants and gasolines, and as a softener of copolymers. The toxicity and immunotoxicity of DMN have been extensively reviewed (Myers and Schook, 1996). Single or repeated exposure to DMN inhibits T-dependent humoral immune responses (IgM and IgG), but not T-independent responses. Other symmetrical nitrosamines, such as diethylnitrosamine, dipropylnitrosamine, and dibutylnitrosamine, demonstrated similar effects on humoral immunity but were not as potent as DMN (Kaminski *et al.*, 1989b). In fact, as the length of the aliphatic chain increased, the dose required to suppress the anti-sRBC AFC response by 50% (ED_{50}) also increased. In contrast, nonsymmetrical nitrosamines suppressed humoral immunity at comparable concentrations. Overall, the rank order of ED_{50} values paralleled their LD_{50} values. T-cell-mediated lymphoproliferative responses (mitogens or MLR) and DTH response were also suppressed following DMN exposure. In vivo exposure to DMN followed by challenge with several pathogens did not produce a consistent pattern of effects: decreased resistance to *Streptococcus zooepidemicus* and influenza, no effects on resistance to herpes simplex types 1 or 2 or *Trichinella spiralis*, and increased resistance to *L. monocytogenes*. In contrast, anti-tumor activity in DMN-exposed animals was consistently enhanced. DMN-exposed animals also have altered development of hematopoietic cells (increased macrophage precursors). Taken together, these data suggest the macrophage (or its developmental precursors) as a primary target. Mechanistic studies have demonstrated that DMN-induced alterations in CMI are associated with enhanced macrophage activity, increased myelopoietic activity, and alterations in TNF-α transcriptional activity. It has been postulated that DMN may cause the enhanced production of GM-CSF, which can have autocrine (enhanced tumoricidal and bactericidal activity) and paracrine (induced secretion of T-cell-suppressing cytokines by macrophages) activities.

Mechanistic studies have also indicated a critical role for metabolism in the immune suppression by DMN (Haggerty and Holsapple, 1990; Johnson et al., 1987; Kim et al., 1988). It is known that DMN is metabolized by the liver cytochrome P450 system to a strong alkylating agent, and studies have shown that there is a relationship between DMN-induced immune suppression and the anticipated hepatotoxicity. Interestingly, a molecular dissection of DMN-induced hepatotoxicity by mRNA differential display demonstrated an increase in transcripts for the complement protein C3 and serum amyloid A (Bhattacharjee et al., 1998). Previous work by Kaminski and Holsapple (1987) had demonstrated the potential immune suppression associated with an increase in serum amyloid A.

Mycotoxins

Mycotoxins are structurally diverse secondary metabolites of fungi that grow on feed. This class of chemicals comprises such toxins as aflatoxin, ochratoxin, and the trichothecenes, notably T-2 toxin and deoxynivalenol (vomitoxin). As a class, these toxins can produce cellular depletion in lymphoid organs, alterations in T- and B-lymphocyte function, suppression of antibody responses, suppression of NK cell activity, decreased DTH responses, and an apparent increase in susceptibility to infectious disease (reviewed by Bondy and Pestka, 2000; IPCS, 1996). T-2 toxin has also been implicated as a developmental immunotoxicant, targeting fetal lymphocyte progenitors leading the thymic atrophy often observed with these mycotoxins (Holladay et al., 1993). For ochratoxin, at least, the dose, the route of administration, and the species appear to be critical factors in results obtained in immunotoxicity studies. Past studies with aflatoxin B1 suggest that CMI and phagocytic cell functions are affected as evidenced by decreased proliferative responses to PHA and suppression of DTH responses (Raisuddin et al., 1993). In addition, in vitro experiments demonstrated that aflatoxin B1 required metabolic bioactivation in order to produce suppression of antibody responses and of mitogen-induced lymphoproliferation (Yang et al., 1986). Studies in laboratory animals have also shown increased risk to secondary infection after aflatoxin B1 treatment. The effects of aflatoxins on the human immune system have not been characterized but are of concern in light of the fact that in many parts of the world, such as in West Africa, exposure to aflatoxins is widespread as studies in Benin and Togo found that 99% of children possessed measurable aflatoxin-albumin adducts in blood (Gong et al., 2003).

For the extensively studied trichothecenes, the mechanism of immune impairment is related in part to inhibition of protein synthesis. Interestingly, trichothecenes at high doses induce leukocyte apoptosis concomitantly with immune suppression (Pestka et al., 1994). Conversely, at low doses, trichothecenes promote expression of a diverse array of cytokines including IL-1, IL-2, IL-5, and IL-6. In addition, trichothecenes activate mitogen-activated protein kinases in vivo and in vitro via a mechanism known as the ribotoxic stress response (Chung et al., 2003; Moon and Pestka, 2002; Zhou et al., 2003). Prolonged consumption of deoxynivalenol by mice was shown to induce elevation of IgA and IgA immune complex formation, and kidney mesangial IgA deposition (Pestka, 2003). It has been postulated that the enhancement in IgA production induced by deoxynivalenol may be associated with the increase in

cytokine production described above. The trichothecenes are currently considered among the most potent small-molecule inhibitors of protein synthesis in eukaryotic cells, which is dichotomous to the observed increase in IgA secretion.

Adverse health effects have been associated with damp indoor environments following building envelope breech resulting from heavy rains and/or flooding, as occurred during Hurricanes Katrina and Rita in the Gulf Coast of the United States. The adverse health effects have been attributed, at least in part, to the presence of molds, most notably *Stachybotrys chartarum*, also known as black mold. *S. chartarum* produces the macrocyclic trichothecene toxin, satratoxin G, which like many of the trichothecenes is a potent inhibitor of protein synthesis. In a recent study, satratoxin G exposure of mice, 100 μg/kg for five consecutive days by intranasal instillation, induced apoptosis of olfactory sensory neurons and neutrophilic rhinitis (Islam et al., 2006). Elevated mRNA levels for proinflammatory cytokines TNF-α, IL-6, and IL-1, and the chemokine, MIP-2, were detected in nasal airways and the adjacent olfactory bulb of the brain. By Day seven, marked atrophy of the olfactory nerve and glomerular layer of the olfactory bulb was detected. These findings suggest that neurotoxicity and inflammation within the nose may be potential adverse health effects associated with *Stachybotrys* exposure in indoor air.

Natural and Synthetic Hormones

It is well established that a sexual dimorphism exists in the immune system. Females have higher levels of circulating Igs, a greater antibody response, and a higher incidence of autoimmune disease than males. Males appear to be more susceptible to the development of sepsis and the mortality associated with soft tissue trauma and hemorrhagic shock. Specific natural sex hormones in this dichotomy have been implicated. Immune effects of androgens and estrogens appear to be very tightly controlled within the physiological range of concentrations, and profound changes in immune activity can result from very slight changes in concentrations of hormones.

Estrogens Diethylstilbestrol is a synthetic nonsteroidal compound possessing estrogenic activity. Diethylstilbestrol was used in men to treat prostate cancer and in women to prevent threatened abortions, as an estrogen replacement, and as a contraceptive drug. Extensive functional and host resistance studies on diethylstilbestrol (mg/kg per day range) have indicated that exposure to this chemical results in alterations in CMI and/or macrophage function and are believed to be mediated by the presence of the estrogen receptor on immune cells (Brown et al., 2006a,b; Holsapple et al., 1983; Kalland, 1980; Lai et al., 2000; Luster et al., 1980, 1984). Targeted sites of action include the thymus (thymic depletion, alteration in T-cell maturation process), T cells (decreased MLR, DTH, and lymphoproliferative responses), and macrophage (enhanced phagocytic, antitumor, and suppressor function). Pre- and neonatal exposures (mg/kg per day dose range) have also demonstrated immunotoxic effects related to T-cell dysfunction. DTH and inflammatory responses associated with diethylstilbestrol exposure in adult mice have been shown to be reversible upon cessation of exposure (Holsapple et al., 1983; Luster et al., 1980). However, effects from in utero and neonatal exposures appear to have more lasting, possibly permanent effects on immune responses (Kalland et al., 1979; Luster et al., 1979; Ways et al., 1980).

Exposure of human PBMC from men and women to 17β-estradiol (E2) increased basal IgM, IgG, and IL-10 production with no effect on IL-1α, IL-1β, IL-2, IL-4, and IL-6. Interestingly, addition of IL-10 enhanced the effect of E2 on IgM and IgG production (Kanda et al., 1999). IL-10 appears to have both positive and negative effects on immune function since in mouse models IL-10 is the mediator of a Breg subset (ie, B10 or Br1). Similar to the above results, E2 enhanced the induction of IgM and IgA AFCs from PBMC stimulated with pokeweed mitogen (testosterone had no effect) (Paavonen et al., 1981). In an autoimmune disease state, basal IgG production was more markedly induced by E2 in patients with active systemic lupus erythematosus (SLE) as compared to normal donors. In addition to an increase in total IgG, E2 also induced anti-dsDNA antibody (absent in normal donors). The profile was somewhat different for inactive SLE patients in that E2 increased total IgG production to a similar degree as SLE patients, but E2 did not induce anti-dsDNA antibody, which had a lower basal level than active SLE (Kanda et al., 1999). Furthermore, microarray analysis of T cells purified from human PBMC demonstrated E2-altered gene expression for cellular signaling proteins in activated T cells from SLE patients versus controls (Walters et al., 2009). Isoflavones ("isoflavone intervention") administered for 16 weeks to postmenopausal women through soy milk or supplemental tablets resulted in higher frequency of B cells in peripheral blood with no effect on the frequency of CD4$^+$, CD8$^+$, or NK subsets. The isoflavone intervention had no effect on IL-2 or TNFα plasma levels, but IFN-γ trended toward an almost twofold nonsignificant increase (Ryan-Borchers et al., 2006). Other studies demonstrated an increase in plasma IL-6 with isoflavone diets (73 mg per day) (Jenkins et al., 2002) and increased cytotoxicity of human PBMC NK cells with isoflavone metabolites (0.1 μmol/L) (Zhang et al., 1999). In contrast to the human results with E2, in vivo administration of the phytoestrogen, genistein, suppressed anti-KLH IgG titers in mice (Yellayi et al., 2002). However, mouse cells treated with E2, diethylstilbestrol, or bisphenol A (discussed below) enhanced IgG anti-DNA antibody production and IgG immune complex deposition in the kidney, which may be a result of increased autoantibody secretion from B-1 cells (Yurino et al., 2004). Additionally, E2 has been shown to drive the expansion of the mouse Treg cell compartment and to increase Treg activity (Luo et al., 2011; Polanczyk et al., 2004). E2 was also shown in mice to inhibit recruitment and activation of inflammatory cells resulting in inhibition of TNF-α and IFN-γ production and of the inflammatory response (Salem et al., 2000). These discrepancies in the effects of E2 (activation vs. inhibition) may be due to species differences, different cellular targets, or a lack of disease state. Taken together, it is clear that E2 and phytoestrogens alter the human antibody response, an effect that is more marked in an autoimmune disease state.

A potential mechanism for the effects by estrogen and estrogenic compounds is activation of the nuclear estrogen receptor (ER, α, or β isoform), which is ubiquitously expressed in most tissues. Binding of ligand stabilizes ER dimers, which then bind to estrogen response elements (ERE) in target genes leading to transcriptional activation or inhibition. A recent and in-depth review outlines the studies demonstrating ER expression and ER-mediated effects in T cells, B cells, and APCs as well as a role of ER in murine models of autoimmunity (Cunningham and Gilkeson, 2011). In resting and activated human PBMC, CD4$^+$ T cells expressed higher levels of ERα than B cells which expressed higher levels of ERβ. CD8$^+$ cells express ERα and ERβ equally, but at low levels (Phiel et al., 2005). ERα and ERβ are differentially expressed in APCs (Cunningham and Gilkeson, 2011) and in human secondary lymphoid tissues (Shim et al., 2006). Additionally, estrogen and the ER appear to play a significant role in autoimmunity. Ovariectomy before sexual maturation resulted in a significant suppression in a murine model of SLE, which could be reversed by supplementary estrogen treatment (Talal, 1981). ER knockout studies have primarily corroborated this finding with knockout of ERα in three

different mouse models of SLE showing attenuation of the disease and prolonged survival (Bynote et al., 2008; Svenson et al., 2008). This effect was selective for ERα since ERβ did not alter the disease state (Svenson et al., 2008). In contrast to these results, ERα (but not ERβ) knockout in a mildly autoimmune prone mouse strain led to signs of autoimmunity and spontaneous (no antigen challenge) formation of germinal centers in the spleen (Shim et al., 2004). An additional consideration in elucidating the mechanisms by which the ER mediates biological effects is the extensive cross talk that can occur between the ER and other receptor signaling pathways (eg, AHR and PPAR) and transcription factors (eg, AP-1 and NF-κB) that may be independent of the ERE.

Bisphenol A, a monomer in polycarbonate plastics and a constituent of epoxy and polystyrene resins possessing weak binding affinity for the estrogen receptor, has been recently evaluated by a number of laboratories for its potential to affect various aspects of immune function. The majority of studies to date demonstrate that leukocytes cultured in the presence of very high concentrations (>1 μM) of bisphenol A exhibit a number of alterations primarily in innate immune function responses including suppression of LPS-induced nitric oxide production and TNF-α secretion by macrophages (Kim and Jeong, 2003). The effects on nitric oxide production were shown to be correlated with a decrease in NF-κB DNA binding activity, a transcription factor critically involved in the regulation of inducible nitric oxide synthase and TNF-α. In this study, suppression by bisphenol A of LPS-induced nitric oxide production was blocked by the estrogen receptor antagonist, ICI 182,780. Bisphenol A (10–50 μM) has also been reported to enhance IL-4 production in a model of a secondary immune response (Lee et al., 2003). In vivo treatment of mice with bisphenol A (2.5 mg/kg) for seven days produced a decrease in ex vivo Con A-induced proliferation and IFN-γ secretion, but had no effect on the number of CD4$^+$, CD8$^+$, and CD19$^+$ cells in the spleen (Sawai et al., 2003). Additional studies corroborate these findings by demonstrating an augmentation of Th1 immune responses (ie, cytokine profile and increased expression of antigen-specific IgG$_{2a}$ and IgA) with one study showing increased Th1 and Th2 immune responses. In these studies, bisphenol A was administered either by i.p. injection (0.1 mg/g) four times every second day (Alizadeh et al., 2006) in drinking water (10 mg/L, ad libitum) for two weeks (Goto et al., 2007) or through maternal dosing (3–3000 μg/kg) for 18 days (Yoshino et al., 2004). Presently, the putative effects of bisphenol A on immune function are poorly defined and based on the current literature, it is unclear whether the majority of the immunomodulatory effects reported are mediated through an ER-dependent mechanism. Additionally, the relatively high potential for human exposure to bisphenol A due to its wide use in plastics and other products has been of considerable concern to the public and government regulators. Despite the large number of safety-related studies published on bisphenol A, there is considerable controversy regarding its safety and the current tolerable daily intake value (0.05 mg/kg body weight per day) (Hengstler et al., 2011; Sekizawa, 2008; Vandenberg et al., 2009).

Androgens Oxymetholone is a synthetic androgen structurally related to testosterone and was used in the past in the treatment of pituitary dwarfism and as an adjunctive therapy in osteoporosis. Its current use is limited to treatment of certain anemias. Oxymetholone was administered orally to male mice daily for 14 consecutive days (50–300 mg/kg per day) resulting in a minimal decrease in CMI (MLR and CTL response) but without altering the ability of the animals to resist infection in host resistance assays (Karrow et al., 2000). In contrast, anabolic androgenic steroids have been shown to significantly suppress the sRBC AFC response and to increase the production of proinflammatory cytokines from human PBMC.

No comprehensive studies evaluating the effects of testosterone on immune parameters have been conducted. However, it is clear that testosterone is capable of contributing to the suppression of immune function; in particular, CMI responses and macrophage activity. There are numerous reports in the clinical literature that males are more susceptible than females to infection following soft tissue trauma and hemorrhagic shock (reviewed by Catania and Chaudry, 1999). Treatment of males with agents that block testosterone (eg, flutamide) can prevent the trauma- and hemorrhage-induced depression of immunity. Similarly, treatment of females with dihydrotestosterone prior to trauma-hemorrhage results in depression of CMI similar to that of males. Furthermore, gonadectomized mice of either sex have elevated immune responses to endotoxin, which can be attenuated in either sex by the administration of testosterone. The mechanisms in these cases, including influences by the neuroendocrine system, are not clear. Other investigators have reported that, like estrogenic agents, testosterone and other androgens are capable of influencing host defense by altering lymphocyte trafficking in the body and altering the ability of the macrophage to participate in immune responses. It is uncertain if these responses are mediated by the cytosolic androgen receptor, which like the ER, is part of the nuclear receptor superfamily and regulates gene transcription by binding androgen response elements in target genes.

Glucocorticoids The immunosuppressive actions of corticosteroids have been known for years. Following binding to a cytosolic receptor, these agents produce profound lymphoid cell depletion in rodent models. In non-human primates and humans, lymphopenia associated with decreased monocytes and eosinophils and increased neutrophils are seen. Corticosteroids induce apoptosis in rodents, and T cells are particularly sensitive. In addition, these agents suppress macrophage accessory cell function, the production of IL-1 from the macrophages, and the subsequent synthesis of IL-2 by T cells. In general, corticosteroids suppress the generation of CTL responses, MLR, NK cell activity, and lymphoproliferation. While it is clear that these drugs suppress T-cell function, their effects on B cells are not completely clear. Corticosteroids suppress humoral responses, but this appears to be due to effects on T cells, as antigen-specific antibody production by B cells to T-independent antigens does not appear to be affected by corticosteroid treatment.

In spite of the wide therapeutic use of glucocorticoids, the mechanism of action by which glucocorticoids mediate their anti-inflammatory/immunosuppressive activity is not well understood. Several mechanisms have been proposed all of which involve activation of the glucocorticoid receptor. Binding of glucocorticoids to the cytosolic glucocorticoid receptor (member of the nuclear receptor superfamily) induces the receptor to function as a ligand-activated transcription factor that undergoes homodimerization and DNA binding to glucocorticoid response elements (GREs) in the regulatory regions of glucocorticoid-responsive genes. Depending on the gene, GRE can either positively or negatively regulate transcription. For example, glucocorticoids induce annexin 1 (lipocortin 1), a calcium and phospholipid binding protein, which acts to inhibit PLA2 (Goulding and Guyre, 1992; Taylor et al., 1997). Inhibition of PLA2 results in a decrease in arachidonate formation, the precursor in the biosynthesis of inflammatory prostaglandins and leukotrienes. Similarly, glucocorticoids induce transcription of IκB, which is the endogenous inhibitor of the transcription factor, NF-κB (Auphan et al., 1995; Scheinman et al., 1995). Since transcription of many key inflammatory cytokines is regulated positively by NF-κB, induction of IκB results in retention of NF-κB in the cytosol and thus suppression of inflammatory cytokine production. Ligand-activated glucocorticoid receptors have also been found to physically interact with other transcription factors including AP-1 (Schule et al., 1990) and NF-κB (Ray and Prefontaine, 1994), to inhibit DNA binding and/or their transcriptional activity. Cross talk between the glucocorticoid receptor and other nuclear receptors may also play a role in mediating the effects of glucocorticoid ligands. Presently, it is believed that all of the above mechanisms contribute to the anti-inflammatory and immunosuppressive properties of glucocorticoids.

Therapeutic Agents

Historically speaking, very few drugs used today as immunosuppressive agents were actually developed for that purpose. In fact, if one looks closely enough, nearly all therapeutic agents possess some degree of immunomodulatory activity at some doses (Descotes, 1986). The recent explosion of knowledge regarding the function and regulation of the immune system (at the cellular, biochemical, and molecular levels) has provided investigators with a relatively new avenue for specific drug development. The following discussion focuses on those drugs used primarily for modulating the immune system: immunosuppressants (corticosteroids are described in the section "Natural and Synthetic Hormones"), AIDS therapeutics, biologics (ie, monoclonal antibodies, recombinant cytokines, and IFNs), and anti-inflammatory drugs.

Immunosuppressive Agents Several immunosuppressive drugs are efficacious simply due to their ability to impair cellular proliferation, since proliferation is required for lymphocyte clonal expansion and, subsequently, differentiation. Other drugs inhibit specific intracellular proteins that are critical in the activation of the immune response.

Originally developed as an antineoplastic agent, cyclophosphamide (Cytoxan, CYP) is the prototypical member of a class of drugs known as alkylating agents. Upon entering the cell, the inactive drug is metabolically cleaved into phosphoramide mustard, a powerful DNA alkylating agent that leads to blockade of cell replication, and acrolein, a compound known to primarily bind to sulfhydral groups. Clinically, CYP has found use in reducing symptoms of autoimmune disease and in the pretreatment of bone marrow transplant recipients. Experimentally, this drug is often used as a positive immunosuppressive control in immunotoxicology studies because it can suppress both humoral and CMI responses. There appears to be preferential suppression of B-cell responses, possibly due to decreased production and surface expression of Igs. CMI activities that are suppressed include the DTH response, CTL, graft-versus-host disease, and the MLR. Administration of low doses of CYP prior to antigenic stimulation can produce immune enhancement of cell-mediated and humoral immune responses, which has been attributed, in part, to an inhibition of suppressor T-cell activity (Limpens et al., 1990; Limpens and Scheper, 1991). The immune-enhancing properties of CYP were demonstrated to be mediated by only one of the two major metabolites, acrolein, but not phosphoramide mustard (Kawabata and White, 1988).

Azathioprine (Imuran), one of the antimetabolite drugs, is a purine analog that is more potent than the prototype, 6-mercaptopurine, as an inhibitor of cell replication. Immune suppression likely occurs because of the ability of the drug to inhibit purine biosynthesis. It has found widespread use in the suppression of allograft rejection. It can also act as an anti-inflammatory drug and can reduce the number of neutrophils and monocytes. Clinical use of the drug is limited by bone marrow suppression and leukopenia.

Azathioprine inhibits humoral immunity, but secondary responses (IgG) appear more sensitive than primary responses (IgM). Several CMI activities are also reduced by azathioprine treatment, including DTH response, MLR, and graft-versus-host disease. Although T-cell functions are the primary targets for this drug, inhibition of NK function and macrophage activities has also been reported.

Leflunomide (Arava), an isoxazole derivative, is another agent that suppresses cellular proliferation, which has been used in the treatment of rheumatic disease and transplantation (Xiao *et al.*, 1994). Leflunomide inhibits de novo pathways of pyrimidine synthesis, thereby blocking progression from G_1 to S of the cell cycle. Thus, direct inhibition of B-cell proliferation may account for the drug's ability to inhibit both T-cell-dependent and T-cell-independent specific antibody production. Leflunomide can also directly inhibit T-cell proliferation induced by mitogens, anti-CD3, or IL-2.

Cyclosporin A (CsA, Sandimmune) is a cyclic undecapeptide isolated from fungal organisms found in the soil. Important to its use as an immunosuppressant is the relative lack of secondary toxicity (eg, myelotoxicity) at therapeutic concentrations (Calne *et al.*, 1981). However, hepatotoxicity and nephrotoxicity are limiting side effects. CsA acts preferentially on T cells by inhibiting the biochemical signaling pathway emanating from the TCR (reviewed by Ho *et al.*, 1996). The result is inhibition of IL-2 gene transcription and subsequent inhibition of T-cell proliferation and clonal expansion of effector T cells. More specifically, CsA interacts with the intracellular molecule cyclophilin, an intracellular protein with peptidyl proline isomerase activity (although this enzymatic activity has nothing to do with the immunosuppressive effect of CsA). The CsA–cyclophilin complex inhibits the serine/threonine phosphatase activity of a third molecule, calcineurin. The function of calcineurin is to dephosphorylate the cytoplasmic form of the transcription factor, NFAT, therefore facilitating the transport of NFAT into the nucleus, where it can couple with nuclear components and induce the transcription of the IL-2 gene. Inhibition of calcineurin phosphatase activity by the CsA–cyclophilin complex prevents nuclear translocation of NFAT and the resulting IL-2 gene transcription.

FK506 (Tacrolimus or Prograf) is a cyclic macrolide which is structurally distinct from CsA, but which possesses a nearly identical mechanism of action (reviewed by Ho *et al.*, 1996). Like CsA, FK506 binds intracellularly to proteins with peptidyl proline isomerase activity, the most abundant of which is FK506 binding protein-12 (FKBP12). The FK506–FKBP12 complex also binds to and inhibits calcineurin activity, thereby inhibiting IL-2 gene transcription. Clinically, FK506 inhibits T-cell proliferation, lacks myelotoxicity (although, like CsA, it does cause nephrotoxicity), and induces transplantation tolerance. In addition, the minimum effective dose appears to be approximately 10-fold lower than that of CsA.

Rapamycin (RAP, Sirolimus or Rapamune) is also a cyclic macrolide, which is structurally related to FK506. However, the mechanism by which it produces inhibition of proliferation is strikingly distinct. Unlike CsA and FK506, RAP does not inhibit TCR-dependent signaling events and IL-2 gene transcription. Rather, this compound inhibits IL-2-stimulated T-cell proliferation by blocking cell-cycle progression from late G_1 into S phase (Morice *et al.*, 1993; Terada *et al.*, 1993). Like FK506, RAP binds to the intracellular protein FKBP12. However, this RAP–FKBP12 complex does not bind calcineurin. Rather, the RAP–FKBP12 complex binds to the target of rapamycin, mTOR (Sabers *et al.*, 1995), inhibiting its function. Inhibition of mTOR results in reduced cell growth and suppression of cell cycle progression and proliferation (reviewed by Fingar and Blenis, 2004). Unlike both CsA and FK506, RAP does not appear to be nephrotoxic. Due to its mechanisms of action,

a significant advantage of RAP over CsA and FK506 is that it is an effective immune suppressant even after T cells have been activated, due to the fact that it blocks signaling through the IL-2 receptor. Conversely, for CsA and FK506 to be effective, T cells must encounter the drug prior to activation because once IL-2 transcription begins, neither therapeutic will provide effective suppression of the already activated T cells and IL-2 production.

AIDS Therapeutics Traditionally, antiviral therapies have not been extremely successful in their attempt to rid the host of viral infection. This may be due to the fact that these pathogens target the DNA of the host. Thus, eradication of the infection means killing infected cells, which for HIV, are primarily CD4+ T cells. Numerous strategies have been developed to combat HIV, including targeting viral reverse transcriptase (nucleoside and nonnucleoside reverse transcriptase inhibitors), viral protease, viral fusion and entry, virus–T-cell interaction proteins, and stimulating immune responses (reviewed by Broder, 2010). The multidrug therapy used currently is referred to as highly active antiretroviral therapy (HAART) (reviewed by Este and Cihlar, 2010). However, eradication of this virus, and subsequently AIDS, remains a challenge because the very nature of the infection has significant immunosuppressive consequences. In addition, some of the current therapies also exhibit immunosuppressive actions. One such antiviral drug is zidovudine (Retrovir).

Zidovudine (3′-azido-3′-deoxythymidine) is a pyrimidine analog that inhibits viral reverse transcriptase. It was the first drug shown to have any clinical efficacy in the treatment of HIV-1 infection. Unfortunately, its use is limited by myelotoxicity (macrocytic anemia and granulocytopenia) (Luster *et al.*, 1989). Early studies confirmed that the primary action of zidovudine is on innate immunity, although changes in both humoral immunity and CMI have also been observed (reviewed by Feola *et al.*, 2006). In addition, it was shown that oral administration of high doses of zidovudine caused thymic involution and decreased responsiveness of T cells to the HIV protein, gp120 (McKallip *et al.*, 1995). Clinically, zidovudine increases the number of circulating CD4+ cells and can transiently stimulate cell-mediated immune responses (lymphoproliferation, NK cell activity, and IFN-γ production). A final consideration for the immunotoxicity associated with AIDS therapeutics like zidovudine is that they are rarely administered alone and thus, drug interactions likely contribute to various immune effects.

Abacavir (ABC), a purine analog, is also an inhibitor of viral reverse transcriptase, but it has less adverse effects than zidovudine. However, in contrast to the immunosuppressive adverse effects of zidovudine, ABC induces hypersensitivity reactions in approximately 5% to 9% of patients initiating antiretroviral therapy with ABC. This adverse effect has been associated with the expression of the HLA haplotype HLA-B*5701 and elevated CD8+ CTL at the initiation of ABC treatment as well as an increase in CD8+ (not CD4+) T-cell proliferation in patients testing positive for ABC hypersensitivity (Easterbrook *et al.*, 2003; Phillips *et al.*, 2005). Based on these studies, a large study (1956 patients) was conducted to determine the effectiveness of prospective HLA-B*5701 screening in preventing hypersensitivity reactions to ABC (Mallal *et al.*, 2008). Screening eliminated hypersensitivity reactions to ABC, and the introduction of screening prior to therapy has made a hypersensitivity reaction to ABC a rare event.

Biologics Biologics refers to those therapies that are derived in some manner from living organisms and include monoclonal antibodies, recombinant proteins, and adoptive cell therapies. By its very nature, the immune system is often both the intended therapeutic target and unintended toxicological target of various biologics. Overall, manifestations of toxicity may include exaggerated pharmacology, effects due to biochemical cross talk, and disruptions in immune regulation by cytokine networks. Monoclonal antibodies can bind normal as well as targeted tissues, and any foreign protein may elicit the production of neutralizing antibodies against the therapeutic protein (ie, the therapeutic protein may be immunogenic). While certainly many biologics are being utilized safely, the immunotoxicological aspects of a monoclonal antibody (anti-CD3), TNF blockers, and a recombinant protein (IFN-α) will be discussed.

Monoclonal antibodies have been designed in general to suppress immune function, and include antibodies directed against certain molecules that are critical for inducing or sustaining an immune response and can be divided into the following mechanistic categories: (1) bind and neutralize specific cytokines (TNF-α; IL-6); (2) bind cell-surface molecules to trigger lysis by the adaptive immune response (CD3 on T cells; CD25, α subunit of IL-2 receptor; CD20 on mature B cells; CD52 on B cells, T cells, NK cells, monocytes, and macrophages); (3) bind cell-surface molecules and block costimulation signals from other cells (CD2 on T cells; CD80/CD86 on APCs, soluble BLyS/BAFF, CD40L on T cells); and (4) bind cell adhesion molecules and block lymphocyte trafficking (LFA-1 or α4 on leukocytes). Monoclonal antibodies directed against CD3 (Muromonab-CD3, OKT3), part of the TCR complex, have been used for acute transplant rejection. All T cells express CD3 and binding by anti-CD3 Ig opsonizes T cells for depletion by complement activation and immune clearance. Since CD3 is part of the TCR signaling complex, binding of OKT3 to CD3 can acutely induce a "cytokine release syndrome" due to a transient activation and release of cytokines, which soon after initial administration, flu-like symptoms, pulmonary edema, and hematological disorders have been reported (reviewed by Sgro, 1995). Anaphylactic reactions (Type I hypersensitivity) to the antibody can also occur. Additionally, OKT3 is a murine monoclonal antibody, therefore the therapeutic efficacy and duration of action may be decreased due to host recognition and clearance. The establishment of immunological memory will lead to more rapid clearance on subsequent administration.

Etanercept (Enbrel), adalimumab (Humira), and infliximab (Remicade) are disease-modifying antirheumatic drugs (DMARD) that block TNF to prevent (1) induction of other proinflammatory cytokines such as IL-1, IL-6, and IL-8; (2) macrophage and neutrophil activation; (3) fibroblast and endothelial activation; (4) induction of other acute-phase proteins; and (5) leukocyte migration to inflammation sites. Etanercept is a recombinant protein consisting of a dimer of the extracellular ligand-binding portion of the human 75 kD TNF receptor (TNFR2) fused to the Fc portion of human IgG1. Because TNFR2 is not selective, etanercept binds both circulating TNF-α and TNF-β preventing binding to the endogenous TNFR1 (55 kDa, TNF-α selective) and TNFR2 receptors. Adalimumab and infliximab, however, are recombinant monoclonal antibodies directed against TNF-α, which neutralize circulating TNF-α and prevent interaction with either TNFR1 or TNFR2. Hypersensitivity is a potential adverse effect of these drugs. Other immune-related adverse effects include opportunistic infections, malignancy, and autoimmune disorders which are a potential problem for all drugs that suppress the immune system. Of particular concern for TNF-α inhibitors is an association with a greater risk of tuberculosis; patients are now evaluated for tuberculosis risk factors and for latent tuberculosis infection prior to starting TNF-α inhibitor therapy (Toussirot and Wendling, 2007).

The majority of recombinant proteins have been used as immunostimulants, including IFN-α, IFN-γ, GM-CSF, erythropoietin, IL-2, and IL-12. Recombinant proteins used as immunosuppressants include IL-1 receptor antagonist (IL-1RA) and the abovementioned etanercept which is a hybrid of the extracellular ligand-binding portion of TNFR2 fused to the Fc portion of human IgG1. IFN-α, which is used as an antiviral agent, is used to treat hepatitis C and other chronic viral illnesses. The mechanism of the antiviral action of IFN-α involves, in part, direct suppression of viral replication, activation of NK cells, and enhanced expression of MHCI on virally infected cells thus increasing the likelihood of recognition by virus-specific T cells. Administration of IFN-α has been associated with autoimmune diseases, including autoimmune hypothyroidism and lupus (Vial and Descotes, 1995) and hematological disorders stemming from bone marrow suppression.

Anti-inflammatory Agents Anti-inflammatory agents include nonselective and selective nonsteroidal anti-inflammatory drugs (NSAIDs), which suppress the production of proinflammatory soluble factors, such as prostaglandins and thromboxanes. Nonselective NSAIDs are a large class of drugs that reversibly inhibit both isoforms of cyclooxygenase (COX-1 and COX-2). The COX-2 enzyme, in particular, is induced in response to inflammatory cytokines and mediators and therefore, represents an attractive target to combat inflammatory diseases. However, due to an increased risk of cardiovascular effects in some patients (reviewed by Grosser et al., 2006), which is a side effect to varying degrees for all NSAIDs, the only COX-2 selective inhibitor currently approved for clinical use is celecoxib (celebrex). Aspirin, like nonselective NSAIDs, inhibits COX-1 and 2 enzymes, but inhibition is irreversible due to covalent binding of aspirin by acetylation to a serine residue in the COX enzyme. Aspirin is especially effective as an antiplatelet since platelets possess little biosynthesizing capacity and therefore, aspirin will inhibit COX for the life of the platelet (8–11 days).

Drugs of Abuse

Drug abuse is a social issue with extensive pathophysiological effects on the abuser. Drugs of abuse exhibit immunosuppressive actions, and in fact it has been suggested that in addition to the direct risk of HIV contraction via needle sharing or judgment lapses, abuse of some drugs has been associated with disease progression to AIDS (Rogers, 2011). Several classes of drugs will be discussed, including cannabinoids, opioids, cocaine, methamphetamine, and ethanol. Reports regarding the immune system effects of many of these drugs are often contradictory, so it should be noted that the mechanisms by which drugs of abuse suppress immune function might depend on the development of tolerance or addiction to the drugs; the immune, withdrawal, and pain status of the individual; and levels of endogenous molecules (ie, endorphins or endocannabinoids).

Cannabinoids Much attention has been focused on the immunomodulatory effects of the cannabinoids, which can be defined as plant-derived (ie, from the marijuana plant), synthetic, or endogenous. Therapeutically, the primary psychoactive congener of marijuana, Δ⁹-tetrahydrocannabinol, is approved for use as an antiemetic in patients undergoing cancer chemotherapy and as an appetite stimulant for cachexia associated with advanced AIDS disease. Cannabinoids have also recently been approved for use in the treatment of symptoms associated with autoimmune disease, such as multiple sclerosis (Lakhan and Rowland, 2009). In addition, several states in the United States have legalized marijuana for medical use thereby increasing its use (Joffe and Yancy, 2004).

The mechanism by which Δ⁹-tetrahydrocannabinol produces psychotropic effects is through a G protein-coupled cannabinoid receptor, CB1 (Varvel *et al.*, 2005). Peripheral tissues also express CB1, in addition to a second cannabinoid receptor, CB2. Although both receptors are expressed on immune system cells and are coupled to suppression of adenylate cyclase activity (Schatz *et al.*, 1997), it is not entirely clear the extent to which the receptors and/or suppression of adenylate cyclase activity contributes to immune system effects by cannabinoids.

Many studies have shown that exposure to Δ^9-tetrahydrocannabinol decreases host resistance to bacterial and viral pathogens (reviewed by Cabral and Staab, 2005). Cannabinoids alter both humoral and CMI responses as evidenced by suppression of the T-cell-dependent AFC response both in vivo and in vitro (Schatz *et al.*, 1993) and direct suppression of T-cell function (Condie *et al.*, 1996). With respect to the mechanism of T-cell suppression, many plant-derived compounds suppress IL-2 at the transcriptional level which is due, in part, to suppression of transcription factor activation (AP-1, NFAT, NF-κB) and ERK MAPK activity (Condie *et al.*, 1996; Faubert and Kaminski, 2000; Herring *et al.*, 1998). Although both cannabinoid receptors are expressed on T cells (Galiegue *et al.*, 1995), many of the direct T-cell effects of cannabinoids have been demonstrated to occur independently of either cannabinoid receptor (Kaplan *et al.*, 2003). On the other hand, B-cell suppression by Δ^9-tetrahydrocannabinol was CB1 and/or CB2 receptor-dependent (Springs *et al.*, 2008).

Cannabinoid suppression of other APC, such as macrophages and DCs, is also mediated through the CB1 and/or CB2 receptors. Δ^9-Tetrahydrocannabinol exposure impaired lysosomal or cytochrome *c* processing in macrophages (Matveyeva *et al.*, 2000; McCoy *et al.*, 1995) likely via the CB2 receptor (Buckley *et al.*, 2000; Chuchawankul *et al.*, 2004). IL-12 production from DC and subsequent Th1 activation was suppressed by Δ^9-tetrahydrocannabinol in a CB1 and/or CB2 receptor-dependent manner (Lu *et al.*, 2006a, b). Taken together, these studies demonstrate that cannabinoid compounds alter immune function, and the mechanisms involve both cannabinoid receptor-dependent and -independent actions.

Opioids Similar to cannabinoids, opioids refer to plant-derived, synthetic, or endogenous (endorphins) compounds that bind opioid receptors. Although technically "opioid" refers to drugs derived from the poppy plant, and "opiate" refers to agonists and antagonists with morphine-like activity (including plant-derived and synthetic compounds), they are often used interchangeably. It is well established that opioids suppress immune responses and the mechanism often involves one of the G_i-coupled opioid receptors (μ, κ, and δ receptors), but there are opioid receptor-independent mechanisms as well (Roy *et al.*, 2011).

Early studies evaluating the immune competence of heroin addicts revealed a decrease in total T cells, which was reversed with the general opioid receptor antagonist, naloxone, suggesting a role for an opioid receptor in mediating immune suppression (McDonough *et al.*, 1980). Later studies demonstrated that although morphine suppressed several immune parameters, there was no dose–response, suggesting that the effects were not receptor mediated, but were the result of increased circulating corticosteroids (which were significantly elevated in those animals) (LeVier *et al.*, 1994). This conclusion is supported by the findings of other investigators as well (Pruett *et al.*, 1992b).

Several investigators have reported decreased host resistance to viral and bacterial infections in opioid-treated animals or heroin addicts. In one study, morphine treatment of mice infected with *S. pneumoniae* demonstrated increased bacterial burden in the lungs and increased mortality. The mechanism by which the

immune response was compromised involved, in part, suppression of NF-κB gene transcription, which likely contributes to decreased expression of inflammatory mediators, such as chemokines, reducing recruitment of neutrophils to the infection site (Wang *et al.*, 2005a). There is also evidence that opioid use increases susceptibility to HIV infection. Although morphine and/or heroin use is associated with risk of HIV infection through shared needles, opioid use may contribute to progression of AIDS through immune suppression. Specifically, there is evidence that morphine treatment increases CCR5 expression, which is a primary receptor for HIV entry into macrophages (Guo *et al.*, 2002). In addition, chronic morphine treatment shifts the T-cell balance toward Th2 (Azarang *et al.*, 2007; Roy *et al.*, 2004). Further evidence for compromised immunity toward HIV is the observation that morphine inhibited anti-HIV activity in CD8$^+$ cells in an opioid receptor-dependent manner (Wang *et al.*, 2005b).

Opioids also modulate innate immunity. Consistent with the observations that morphine and/or heroin use contributes to the progression of AIDS, Kupffer cells infected with HIV maintained in vitro in the presence of morphine resulted in a higher number of viral particles relative to untreated HIV-infected cells (Schweitzer *et al.*, 1991). More recent studies demonstrate either suppression (Sacerdote, 2003) or enhancement (Peng *et al.*, 2000) of cytokine production from macrophages. The differences might be due to the agonist used, in vitro versus in vivo administration, and the dosing regimen (ie, whether tolerance was induced or not). Overall, it is clear that opioids suppress immune function and that the mechanism by which this occurs is complex and likely involves the CNS, the autonomic nervous system, the hypothalamic–pituitary–adrenal axis, and one or more opioid receptors (Alonzo and Bayer, 2002).

Cocaine Cocaine is a potent local anesthetic and central nervous system stimulant. This drug and its derivatives have been shown to alter several measures of immune competence, including humoral and cell-mediated immune responses and host resistance (Watson *et al.*, 1983; Ou *et al.*, 1989; Starec *et al.*, 1991). Jeong *et al.* (1996) evaluated the effect of acute in vivo cocaine exposure on the generation of the anti-sRBC AFC, and determined that immune suppression was due to a cytochrome P450 metabolite of cocaine. Further studies demonstrated that sex, strain, and age differences can be detected in cocaine-induced immunodulation as assessed by the anti-SRBC AFC response (Matulka *et al.*, 1996). Similar to other immunotoxic agents, the mechanism by which cocaine alters immune function involves a disruption of the Th1/Th2 balance and the stress response (Jankowski *et al.*, 2010; Stanulis *et al.*, 1997a, b). Cocaine also induces the secretion of TGF-β, which has been linked to the observation that cocaine exposure enhances replication of the HIV-1 virus in human PBMC (Chao *et al.*, 1991; Peterson *et al.*, 1991). A proteomic analysis was conducted in human DCs treated ex vivo with cocaine for 48 hours and demonstrated increased expression of NF-κB (Reynolds *et al.*, 2009b), which could contribute to increased expression of various cytokines or chemokines. Cocaine was demonstrated to cause an increased HIV viral burden in a human PBL-SCID animal model, which was mediated through sigma 1 (σ1) receptors, which are informally referred to as psychoactive drug receptors (Roth *et al.*, 2005). Although the function and role of σ1 receptors still remain to be elucidated, additional studies also suggest that cocaine effects are mediated through these receptors (Cabral, 2006; Maurice and Romieu, 2004).

Methamphetamine Methamphetamine is a stimulant that is similar to amphetamine, although highly addictive and its use has been growing over the past several years. Relatively recently, the immunotoxicity of methamphetamine was explored (In *et al.*, 2005). Following oral administration to mice, methamphetamine suppressed the anti-sRBC AFC response, IgG production, and mitogenic stimulation of T-cell proliferation. Even more striking was the suppression of GM-CSF-stimulated bone marrow colony growth by methamphetamine. These results indicate suppression of both CMI and humoral immunity in vivo following methamphetamine administration.

In human T cells, methamphetamine treatment ex vivo induced ROS and increased intracellular calcium (Potula *et al.*, 2010). Consistent with this, ex vivo treatment of human DCs with methamphetamine induced MEK, which activate MAPKs (Reynolds *et al.*, 2009a). Both of these studies demonstrate that in the absence of immune stimulation, acute methamphetamine treatment causes biochemical changes consistent with cellular activation. On the other hand, in mice treated in vivo with methamphetamine or in methamphethamine-using patients, plasma IL-6 was suppressed and IL-10 was increased, suggesting immune suppression following chronic methamphetamine use (Loftis *et al.*, 2011).

Ethanol Ethanol exposure has been studied both in alcoholic patients and in animal models of binge drinking. In humans, alcoholism is associated with an increased incidence of, and mortality from, pulmonary infection (reviewed by Happel and Nelson, 2005). There is also an increased incidence of bacterial infection and spontaneous bacteremia in alcoholics with cirrhosis of the liver (reviewed by Leevy and Elbeshbeshy, 2005). A consistent finding in abusers of ethanol is the significant change in PBMC. In animal models, this is observed as depletion of T and B cells in the spleen and the T cells in the thymus, particularly $CD4^+/CD8^+$ cells. The latter effect may be related in part to increased levels of corticosteroids, particularly in females (Glover *et al.*, 2011; Han *et al.*, 1993). In a binge-drinking animal model, ethanol suppresses innate immunity through impairment of TLR3 signaling in peritoneal macrophages. The authors also demonstrated suppression of proinflammatory cytokines (Pruett *et al.*, 2004b). In addition to suppression of TLR3, ethanol suppresses signaling through other TLRs, contributing to pleiotropic effects of ethanol on innate immunity (Pruett *et al.*, 2004a). Moreover, signaling alterations via TLRs depend on whether the alcohol exposure is acute or chronic (Dai and Pruett, 2006).

Inhaled Substances

Pulmonary defenses against inhaled gases and particulates are dependent on both physical and immunological mechanisms. Immune mechanisms primarily involve the complex interactions between neutrophils and alveolar macrophages and their abilities to phagocytize foreign material and produce cytokines, which not only act as local inflammatory mediators, but also serve to attract other cells into the airways.

Oxidant Gases It is clear that exposure to oxidant gases—such as ozone (O_3), sulfur dioxide (SO_2), nitrogen dioxide (NO_2), and phosgene—alters pulmonary immunological responses and might increase the susceptibility of the host to bacterial infections (reviewed by Selgrade and Gilmour, 1994). Infiltration of both neutrophils and macrophages has been observed, resulting in the release of cellular enzyme components and free radicals, which contribute to pulmonary inflammation, edema, and vascular changes. Exposure to O_3 has been demonstrated to impair the phagocytic function of alveolar macrophages and to inhibit the clearance of bacteria from the lung. These changes were correlated with decreased resistance to *S. zooepidemicus* and suggest

that other extracellular bacteriostatic factors may be impaired following exposure to these oxidant gases. Short-term NO_2 exposure decreases killing of several bacterial pathogens and, like O_3, this decreased resistance is probably related to changes in pulmonary macrophage function. A role for the products of arachidonic acid metabolism (specifically, the prostaglandins) has recently been implied and is supported by the fact that decreased macrophage function is associated with increased PGE_2 production and that pretreatment with indomethacin inhibits O_3-induced pulmonary hyperresponsiveness and related inflammatory responses. In humans, O_3 challenge produced a decrease in the number of macrophages in airway sputum; however, the recovered macrophages exhibited evidence of activation and enhanced antigen-presenting capability as demonstrated by increased CD80, CD86, and HLA-DR (Lay *et al.*, 2007). In controlled studies, allergic asthmatic volunteers challenged with O_3 were found to have increased levels of inflammatory cytokines, IL-1β and IL-6, while levels of the anti-inflammatory cytokine, IL-10, were decreased in airway sputum. O_3 has also been associated with increased airway neutrophilia and eosinophilia (Peden, 2011).

It is clear that exposure to oxidant gases can also augment pulmonary allergic reactions. This may be a result of increased lung permeability (leading to greater dispersion of the antigen) and to the enhanced influx of antigen-specific IgE-producing cells in the lungs. In studies involving O_3 exposure and challenge with *L. monocytogenes*, decreased resistance to the pathogen correlated not only with changes in macrophage activity, but also with alterations in T-cell-derived cytokine production (which enhances phagocytosis). In support of an effect on T cells, other cell-mediated changes were observed including changes in the T- to B-cell ratio in the lung, decreased DTH response, enhanced allergic responses, and changes in T-cell proliferative responses.

Particles: Asbestos, Silica, and nanoparticles It is believed that alterations in both humoral immunity and CMI occur in individuals exposed to asbestos and exhibiting asbestosis. Decreased DTH response and fewer T cells circulating in the periphery as well as decreased T-cell proliferative responses have been reported to be associated with asbestosis (reviewed by Miller and Brown, 1985; Warheit and Hesterberg, 1994). Autoantibodies and increased serum Ig levels have also been observed. Within the lung, alveolar macrophage activity has been implicated as playing a significant role in asbestos-induced changes in immune competence. Fibers of asbestos that are deposited in the lung are phagocytized by macrophages, resulting in macrophage lysis and release of lysosomal enzymes and subsequent activation of other macrophages. It has been hypothesized that the development of asbestosis in animal models occurs by the following mechanism: fibers of asbestos deposited in the alveolar space recruit macrophages to the site of deposition. Some fibers may migrate to the interstitial space where the complement cascade becomes activated, releasing C5a, a potent macrophage activator and chemoattractant for other inflammatory cells. Recruited interstitial and resident alveolar macrophages phagocytize the fibers and release cytokines, which cause the proliferation of cells within the lung and the release of collagen. A sustained inflammatory response could then contribute to the progressive pattern of fibrosis, which is associated with asbestos exposure.

The primary adverse consequence of silica exposure, like that to asbestos, is the induction of lung fibrosis (silicosis). However, several immune alterations have been associated with silica exposure in experimental animals, including decreased antibody-mediated and CMI parameters (reviewed by IPCS, 1996). Alterations in both T- and B-cell parameters have been reported, although T-cell-dependent responses appear to be more affected than B-cell-dependent responses. Dose and route of antigen exposure appear to be important factors in determining silica-induced immunomodulation. Silica is toxic to macrophages and neutrophils, and exposure is correlated with increased susceptibility to infectious pathogens. The significance of these immunological alterations for the pathogenesis of silicosis remains to be determined. The association of this disease with the induction of autoantibodies is discussed in the subsection "Silica" under "Xenobiotic-Induced Hypersensitivity and Autoimmunity."

More recently, there has been growing interest in the effects of nanomaterials, especially airborne nanoparticles on lung-related diseases and the role of the immune system in the etiology of these diseases. The term "nanomaterial" is extremely broad and only signifies that the material is less than 100 nm in size. Among these nanomaterials, nanosized silicas are members. Although much is known concerning the toxicity of crystalline silica, little is known about the toxicity of nanosized silicas, as is the case for the majority of other nanosized materials. Significant effort is currently being directed toward understanding the influence of shape, charge, composition, specific functional groups, catalytic activity, and other properties on the biological and toxicological potential of these nanomaterials. In more recent studies, it has been reported that airway exposure to nanoparticles can induce a number of proinflammatory cytokines including IL-1β, MCP-1, MIP-2, GM-CSF, and MIP-1α. The mechanism by which exposure to nanoparticles results in induction of proinflammatory cytokines is presently poorly understood, but is believed, in part, to involve induction of oxidative stress (Di Gioacchino *et al.*, 2011) and, in part, through the activation of the NALP3-inflammasome (Martinon *et al.*, 2009). The NALP3-inflammasome is a cytosolic multiprotein complex, which when activated promotes the production of inflammatory cytokines (Fig. 12-22). In fact, pulmonary inflammation is a common response induced by nanoparticles in airways that cannot be explained by their surface chemistry and composition (Sager *et al.*, 2008). A concern with exposure to nanoparticles is the possibility they can enhance immune responses to airborne antigens due to their ability to induce pulmonary inflammation. Indeed, several recent studies have demonstrated with a number of different nanoparticles, including multiwalled carbon nanotubes and titanium oxide, that when administered to experimental animals in combination with ovalbumin, the inflammatory and immunological responses, as measured by cytokine production, cellular infiltrate, and ovalbumin-specific antibodies, were significantly increased when compared to ovalbumin alone (Larsen *et al.*, 2010; Ryman-Rasmussen *et al.*, 2009). Exposure to nanoparticles can occur in the occupational setting, or through environmental exposure to ultra-fine particles, which are, for example, by-products of combustion engines and common constituents of urban air pollutants. Further investigation is needed to understand the risks associated with exposure to nanoparticles, especially on respiratory disease.

Pulmonary Irritants Chemicals such as formaldehyde, silica, and ethylenediamine have been classified as pulmonary irritants and may produce hypersensitivity-like reactions. Macrophages from mice exposed to formaldehyde vapor exhibit increased synthesis of hydroperoxide (Dean *et al.*, 1984). This may contribute to enhanced bactericidal activity and potential damage to local tissues. Although silica is usually thought of for its potential to induce silicosis in the lung (a condition similar to asbestosis), its immunomodulatory effects have also been documented (Levy and Wheelock, 1975). Silica decreased reticuloendothelial system clearance and suppressed both humoral immunity (AFC response) and the CMI response (CTL) against allogeneic fibroblasts. Both local and serum factors were found to play a role in silica-induced alterations in T-cell proliferation. Silica exposure may also inhibit phagocytosis of bacterial antigens (related to reticuloendothelial system clearance) and inhibit tumoricidal activity (Thurmond and Dean, 1988).

Ultraviolet Radiation

Ultraviolet radiation (UVR), especially midrange UVB (290–340 nm), is an important environmental factor affecting human health with both beneficial effects including vitamin D production, tanning, and adaptation to UV, and adverse effects including sunburn, skin cancer, and ocular damage. Most, if not all of the chemicals, drugs and other materials discussed in this chapter were selected because they have been associated with immunotoxic effects, and because there is the chance for human exposure. And indeed, UVR has also been demonstrated to modulate immune responses in animals and humans. In fact, UVR is cited elsewhere in this chapter as one of the examples of where the parallelogram approach has been effectively used for a human risk assessment (van Loveren *et al*, 1995). It is important to emphasize that all humans encounter lifetime exposure to this ubiquitous environmental immunotoxicant (Ullrich, 2007a). The effects of UV exposure on the immune system have been reviewed (Garssen and van Loveren, 2001). While UV-induced immunomodulation has been shown to have some beneficial effects on some skin diseases, such as psoriasis, and has been demonstrated to impair some allergic and autoimmune diseases in both animals and humans, UV-induced immunomodulation can also lead to several adverse health consequences, including a pivotal role during the process of skin carcinogenesis. Kripke (1981) provided the first evidence that UVR was immunosuppressive. UV-induced skin tumors were removed and transplanted into normal age- and sex-matched syngeneic recipient mice. Interestingly, the tumors did not grow in normal mice, and progressive tumor growth was only seen when the tumors were transplanted into recipient mice that were immunosuppressed. These results were explained by proposing that exposure to UVR had two effects: induction of skin tumors and induction of immune suppression. Studies have shown that these two events are related

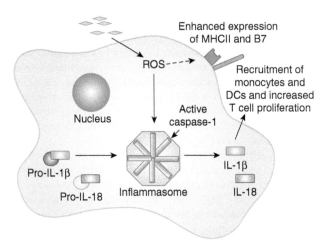

Figure 12-22. *Activation of the inflammasome by nanomaterials.* Nanomaterials can be adjuvants through effects in APCs. For example, in a macrophage, nanomaterials can induce reactive oxygen species (ROS) to enhance expression of MHCII or B7 proteins or activate the inflammasome. Upon activation, the inflammasome produces active IL-1β and IL-18, which can recruit other monocytes or DCs, or enhance T-cell proliferation.

(Ullrich, 2007b) based on a series of observations. First, UVR-induced keratinocyte-derived platelet activating factor was shown to play a role in the induction of immunosuppression. Second, *cis*-urocanic acid, a skin-derived immunosuppressive compound, mediates immune suppression by binding to serotonin receptors on target cells. Finally, studies showed that blocking the binding of these compounds to their receptors not only suppresses UVR-induced immune suppression, but that this approach also interferes with skin cancer induction.

There have been a number of studies to further characterize the mechanism of action for UV-induced immunomodulation. The first step is the absorption of UV photons by chromophores, so-called "photoreceptors," such as DNA and urocanic acid (Garssen *et al.*, 1997). As a consequence of UV absorption by chromophores, epidermal and dermal cells, including keratinocytes, melanocytes, Langerhan's cells, mast cells, dermal fibroblasts, endothelial cells, as well as skin-infiltrating cells (ie, granulocytes and macrophages), produce and/or release many immunoregulatory mediators, including cytokine, chemokines, and neurohormones (Sleijffers *et al.*, 2004). The mediators include both pro- and anti-inflammatory cytokines, such as TNF-α, IL-1, IL-6, and IL-10, which can modify directly or indirectly the function of APCs. Langerhan's cells, the major APC in the skin, change phenotypically and functionally, which ultimately impacts the activity of T cells at the time of antigen presentation, both locally and systemically. One early explanation for UV-induced immunomodulation is that UVR induced a switch from a predominantly Th1 response (favoring DTH responses) to a Th2 response (favoring antibody responses). This hypothesis was supported by findings of altered cytokine secretion patterns indicative of a Th1 to Th2 switch (Araneo *et al.*, 1989; Simon *et al.*, 1990). Indeed, the majority of studies dealing with the effects of UVR indicated that Th1-mediated immune responses are especially sensitive to UV exposure. However, as noted above, UVR has been demonstrated to be associated with a suppression of certain allergic and autoimmune reactions. Indeed, more recent studies have demonstrated that Ig isotypes that are linked to either Th1 or Th2 cells can be suppressed by UVR and that UV exposure not only impairs Th1 responses; but also some Th2 responses (Sleijffers *et al.*, 2004).

Schwartz (2008) summarized 25 years of studies by noting that in contrast to the general immunosuppression associated with the use of conventional immunosuppressive drugs, UVR suppresses the immune system in an antigen-specific fashion via the induction of immunotolerance. Several investigators have noted that this effect is mostly mediated via Tregs induced by UVR, and that induction of Tregs, expressing CD4 and CD25, is an active process, which requires antigen presentation by UV damage. Once activated in an antigen-specific manner, these Tregs can suppress immune responses in a general fashion via the release of IL-10. Ullrich (2007a) noted that this model is consistent with the fact that UVR is absorbed in the upper layers of the skin, does not penetrate into the underlying tissues and internal organs, and that T cells are not directly targeted by UVR in vivo because few T cells are found in normal skin.

XENOBIOTIC-INDUCED HYPERSENSITIVITY AND AUTOIMMUNITY

When an individual's immune system responds in a manner producing tissue damage, it could result in hypersensitivity or autoimmunity, which could be exacerbated, or even induced by, a xenobiotic.

Fig. 12-23 is a schematic delineating the possible cascade of effects that can occur when a chemical produces an immune-mediated disease.

Hypersensitivity

Polyisocyanates Polyisocyanates have a widespread use in industry and are responsible for occupationally related lung disease. These chemicals are used in the production of adhesives, paint hardeners, elastomers, and coatings. Occupational exposure is by inhalation and skin contact. Polyisocyanates are known to induce all four types of hypersensitivity responses.

Compounds in this group include toluene diisocyanate, methylene diphenyl diisocyanate, and hexamethylene diisocyanate. They are highly reactive compounds that readily conjugate with endogenous proteins, such as albumin, forming neoantigens responsible for hypersensitivity (Wisnewski *et al.*, 2011). Pulmonary sensitization to these compounds can occur through either topical or inhalation exposure. In murine models employing intranasal or intratracheal sensitization and challenge with toluene diisocyanate, significant induction of Th2 cytokines, IgE, and eosinophilia has been demonstrated (Ban *et al.*, 2006; Matheson *et al.*, 2005; Plitnick *et al.*, 2005). It has also been demonstrated that albumin-conjugated methylene diphenyl diisocyanate challenge via intranasal instillation following initial dermal exposure caused increased airway inflammation as characterized by eosinophil and lymphocyte infiltration into the BALF (Wisnewski *et al.*, 2011).

In humans diagnosed with occupational asthma associated with diisocyanate exposure, there was increased production of IL-8, MCP-1, TNF-α, and RANTES (chemokine ligand CCL5) in PBMC stimulated ex vivo with albumin-conjugated diisocyanate (Lummus *et al.*, 1998). Moreover, an examination of humans exposed to various diisocyanates demonstrated an association between incidence of occupational asthma from hexamethylene diisocyanate and specific SNPs in genes encoding IL-4 receptor α, IL-13, and CD14 (Bernstein *et al.*, 2006, 2011). It has also been shown that diisocyanate-induced IgE is not as robust as that observed in allergic asthma, suggesting that distinct pathophysiological mechanisms control occupational versus allergic asthma (Bernstein *et al.*, 2002). In a mouse model in which toluene diisocyanate plus ovalbumin was used to induce asthma, PI3 kinase was critical for the upregulation of IL-17 and pulmonary inflammation (Kim *et al.*, 2007). The mechanism by which cytokines and chemokines are upregulated also likely involves activation of p38 MAPK (Mitjans *et al.*, 2008).

Acid Anhydrides The acid anhydrides are reactive organic compounds used in the manufacturing of paints, varnishes, coating materials, adhesives, and casting and sealing materials. Trimellitic acid anhydride (TMA) is one of the most widely used compounds in this group, and it causes all four hypersensitivity reactions. Similar to the diisocyanates, acid anhydrides bind to serum proteins, such as albumin (Valstar *et al.*, 2006).

In an attempt to understand mechanisms by which TMA induced asthma following occupational exposure, a comparison between topical versus intranasal sensitization with TMA was conducted (Farraj *et al.*, 2006). Intranasal challenge with TMA in mice that were either topically or intranasally sensitized with TMA produced a marked allergic rhinitis of similar severity, characterized by an influx of eosinophils and lymphocytes. Both the topical and intranasal routes of sensitization also produced significant increases in total serum IgE after intranasal challenge with TMA. In addition, both the topical and intranasal routes of sensitization induced significant increases in the mRNA expression of the Th2 cytokines IL-4, IL-5, and IL-13 (Farraj *et al.*, 2006). These findings are significant

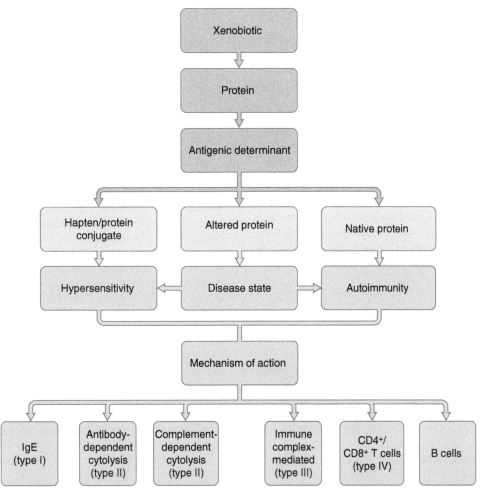

Figure 12-23. *Schematic diagram of xenobiotic induction of hypersensitivity or autoimmunity.* The mechanisms by which xenobiotics induce hypersensitivity or autoimmunity can overlap, although IgE production is most often associated with hypersensitivity.

as they suggest that dermal exposure represents a potential route of sensitization of the respiratory tract to chemical allergens.

Toxicogenomic analyses have been conducted in an attempt to identify gene expression profiles for TMA-induced occupational asthma and/or contact dermatitis (Regal *et al.*, 2007). In one study, although overlap between genes induced in response to ovalbumin (allergic asthma model) or TMA (occupational asthma model) in mice occurred, over 100 unique TMA-induced genes were identified (Regal *et al.*, 2007). Another study examined the gene expression profile in auricular lymph nodes following dermal exposure to TMA to determine changes in gene expression that correlated with the LLNA (Boverhof *et al.*, 2009). Over 1000 genes were expressed in response to the highest dose of TMA following dermal exposure, including IL-4, IL-21, Mki67 (involved in cell division), and Aicda (involved in B cell class switch recombination) (Boverhof *et al.*, 2009).

Cellular assays are also being developed to identify respiratory sensitizers, particularly to determine if low dose exposures contribute to occupational asthma. For instance, in response to a low dose of intratracheal administration of TMA, IgE+ and MHCII+ B cells were identified in the lung-associated lymph nodes (Fukuyama *et al.*, 2010). The increase in IgE+MHCII+ B cells correlated with increased serum and BALF IgE and IgG1, and increased inflammatory cells in the BALF (eosinophils, neutrophils) (Fukuyama *et al.*, 2010).

Metals Metals and metallic substances, including metallic salts and metal-containing nanomaterials, are responsible for producing contact and pulmonary hypersensitivity reactions. For additional information on the mechanisms by which metal-containing nanomaterials induce hypersensitivity, the reader is referred to "Chap. 28, Nanotoxicology." Exposure to these compounds may occur via inhalation or due to their solubility in aqueous media. Although many metals induce contact dermatitis (Forte *et al.*, 2008), platinum, cobalt, chromium, nickel, and beryllium will be discussed here.

Platinum Exposure to platinum-group elements occurs occupationally in the mining, dentistry, and jewelry industries. There may also be acute hypersensitivity to platinum-containing chemotherapeutics in up to 20% of patients (Syrigou *et al.*, 2010). Platinum salts are allergenic and induce Type 1 and IV hypersensitivity reactions such as contact dermatitis and occupational asthma.

Exposure to the platinum salt sodium hexachloroplatinate by intradermal sensitization followed by intranasal challenge as a model of platinum-induced occupational asthma demonstrated that IL-4, IL-5, and IL-13 were modestly induced following ex vivo stimulation of lung-associated lymph nodes with Con A (Ban *et al.*, 2010). Serum IgE levels and BALF neutrophils and eosinophils were also increased. These results are consistent with increased IgE in peripheral blood of platinum-sensitized patients (Raulf-Heimsoth *et al.*, 2000).

Cobalt Cobalt exposure comes from metal-on-metal replacement prostheses, or occupationally in superalloy production and pigment manufacturing. Cobalt also induces Type 1 and IV hypersensitivity reactions such as contact dermatitis, DTH in peri-implant areas in hip replacement patients, and occupational asthma (Thyssen and Menne, 2010).

There are several studies in which hip replacement patients who received metal-on-metal arthroplasty had increased metal-reactive T-cell responses. In one study, 7 out of 16 hip replacement patients demonstrated skin reactivity to cobalt, and of those 7 patients, 3 had elevated serum IgE (Thomas *et al.*, 2009). Moreover, PBMC from 7 out of 16 patients proliferated ex vivo in response to cobalt chloride stimulation (Thomas *et al.*, 2009). Part of this mechanism might involve creation of metal–protein complexes, which act as haptens (Mabilleau *et al.*, 2008).

In workers exposed to hard metal dust (a cobalt-containing alloy), there was increased incidence of asthma and higher serum IgE levels (Shirakawa *et al.*, 1992), indicating cobalt-induced occupational asthma. In a mouse model in which control or hypoxia inducible factor-1α (HIF-1α) was postnatally deleted in the lung, oropharyngeal aspiration of cobalt chloride induced a robust Th2-mediated asthma-like response characterized by eosinophilia, mucus cell metaplasia, and altered cytokine profile (Saini *et al.*, 2010a, b). These results suggest that hypoxia signaling via HIF-1α might contribute to cobalt-induced occupational asthma.

Chromium Chromium is another metal in which exposure occurs either from metal-on-metal prosthesis, or occupationally in the electroplating, leather tanning, and paint, cement, and paper pulp production industries. Chromium predominantly elicits contact dermatitis (Shelnutt *et al.*, 2007), a Type IV hypersensitivity reaction, but can also induce hypersensitivity in patients with metal-on-metal hip arthroplasty, similar to those observed in response to cobalt (Thomas *et al.*, 2009). Chromium exists in several oxidation states, including chromium (III) or chromium (VI), but chromium (VI) more readily permeates the skin barrier (Forte *et al.*, 2008). However, once absorbed, chromium (VI) is reduced to chromium (III), which is most likely responsible for chromium toxicity (Shelnutt *et al.*, 2007).

Upon the reduction of chromium (VI) to chromium (III), ROS are produced. Production of ROS is one mechanism by which hypersensitivity reactions are exacerbated (Roychowdhury and Svensson, 2005). Indeed, chromium has been shown to increase ROS production in several cell types. In human dermal fibroblasts treated with potassium dichromate, heme oxygenase-1 expression (HMO-1) was induced in a MAPK-dependent manner (Joseph *et al.*, 2008). Similarly, in a HaCT keratinocyte cell line, potassium dichromate increased ROS formation, and activated Akt, NF-κB, and MAPK, ultimately contributing to the induction of IL-1α and TNF-α (Wang *et al.*, 2010).

Nickel Exposure to nickel occupationally occurs in the mining, milling, smelting, and refinishing industries. Consumers are exposed through clothing fasteners or body piercings, with adult women having the highest prevalence of nickel allergy (up to 17%) (Thyssen and Menne, 2010). Nickel causes both Type I and IV hypersensitivity. Similar to chromium, higher oxidation states of nickel have greater potential to sensitize individuals (Kasper-Sonnenberg *et al.*, 2011), which could also be due to higher potential to generate ROS when reduced in vivo.

Most people are sensitized to nickel dermally; however, there have been reports that exposure of children to relatively high ambient air nickel concentrations was associated with a positive skin test for nickel (Kasper-Sonnenberg *et al.*, 2011). Nickel sulfate treatment of human DC isolated from PBMC demonstrated robust induction of IL12, which was due to nickel sulfate activation of NF-κB, p38 MAPK, and IFN regulatory factor-1 (IRF-1) (Antonios *et al.*, 2010). Induction of IL-12 helps to stimulate T cells and in

fact, nickel-reactive T cells can be isolated from PBMC of nickel-sensitized individuals (Moed *et al.*, 2004). However, a recent study demonstrated that nickel chloride treatment of purified CD3+ T cells activated with anti-CD3/CD28 impaired T-cell activation likely through inhibition of intracellular calcium concentration and NFAT activation (Saito *et al.*, 2011). The authors suggested that the discrepancy in T-cell effects by nickel is either due to differences in nickel concentrations and/or differences in the ability of nickel to target different transcription factors (Saito *et al.*, 2011).

Beryllium Beryllium exposure occurs most frequently in high-technology ceramics and dental alloy manufacturing, and in the electronics, nuclear, and aerospace industries. Although its use in the manufacturing of fluorescent bulbs has been discontinued, chronic beryllium disease (CBD) was originally identified in 1946 in a group of fluorescent lamp manufacturing workers (Forte *et al.*, 2008). Beryllium produces Type IV hypersensitivity reactions. Skin contact has been found to produce lesions of contact hypersensitivity, whereas lesions produced by penetration of splinters of beryllium under the skin are granulomatous in nature. Inhalation of beryllium can result in acute beryllium disease (ABD such as pneumonitis, tracheobronchitis), CBD, and increased risk of lung cancer (Cummings *et al.*, 2009; McCleskey *et al.*, 2009).

CBD is a pulmonary disease characterized by granulomas. Most patients with CBD also possess lymphocytes that proliferate in response to ex vivo beryllium treatment (Rosenman *et al.*, 2011). One possible mechanism for the sensitization and subsequent development of disease is that beryllium can alter peptide binding to MHC molecules. In fact, it has been reported that there is a glutamic acid substitution in one of the MHCII molecules in humans both sensitized to beryllium and those diagnosed with CBD, indicating a genetic susceptibility to beryllium-induced hypersensitivity (Rosenman *et al.*, 2011).

Therapeutic Agents Hypersensitivity responses to therapeutic drugs are among the major types of unpredictable drug reactions, accounting for up to 10% of all adverse effects. Drugs that commonly induce hypersensitivity include sulfa drugs, barbiturates, anticonvulsants, insulin, iodine (used in many X-ray contrast dyes), and platinum-containing chemotherapeutics. Penicillin is the most common agent involved in drug allergy and is discussed here as an example. The high incidence of allergic reaction to penicillin is in part due to widespread exposure to the compound. Not only has there been indiscriminant use of the drug, but exposure occurs through food products including milk from treated animals and the use of penicillin as an antimicrobial in the production of vaccines. Efforts are still being made to reduce unnecessary exposure.

The mechanism by which hypersensitivity to penicillin occurs is through the formation of a neoantigen. The formation of the primary penicillin neoantigen occurs during the breakdown of penicillin, in which the β-lactam ring opens, forming a reactive intermediate that reacts with other proteins. The resultant penicilloylated protein now acts as a hapten to which the immune system mounts a response. As is the case with other haptens, subsequent exposures to penicillin may not absolutely require the formation of penicilloylated proteins to elicit secondary responses.

Reactions to penicillin are varied and may include any of the four types of hypersensitivity reactions (reviewed by Chang *et al.*, 2011). The most commonly seen clinical manifestation of Type I reactions is urticaria; however, anaphylactic reactions occur in about 10 to 40 of every 100,000 patients receiving injections. Clinical signs of rhinitis and asthma are much less frequently observed. Blood dyscrasias can occur due to the production of IgG against penicillin metabolites bound to the surface of red blood cells (Type II reaction). Penicillin has also been implicated in Type III reactions leading to serum-sickness-like symptoms. Owing to the high frequency of Type IV reactions when penicillin is applied topically, especially to inflamed or abraded skin, products are no longer available for topical application. Type IV reactions generally result in an eczematous skin reaction, but a rare, life-threatening form of dermal necrosis may result. In these cases, there is severe erythema and a separation of the epidermis at the basal layer. This reaction, which gives the clinical appearance of severe scalding, is thought to be a severe delayed reaction.

Latex Natural rubber latex is derived from the rubber tree *Hevea brasiliensis* and is used in the manufacture of over 40,000 products including examination and surgical gloves, among other medical products. Allergic reactions to natural rubber latex products have become an important occupational health concern with increased use of universal precautions, particularly latex gloves, to combat the spread of bloodborne pathogens. Hypersensitivity to latex usually occurs via a Type I or Type IV reaction. Dermatological reactions to latex include irritant dermatitis due to chemical additives or mechanical abrasion and the occlusive conditions caused by wearing gloves; contact dermatitis due to the chemical additives used in the glove manufacturing (eg, thiurams, carbamates, mercapto compounds, and phenylenediamines), and potentially more serious IgE-mediated responses due to residual latex proteins that remained in the finished products (reviewed by Shah and Chowdhury, 2011). The IgE responses may manifest as urticaria, asthma, or life-threatening anaphylaxis. Several latex proteins have been identified, and antibodies to most can be detected in latex-allergic individuals (Ahmed *et al.*, 2004; Lehto *et al.*, 2007).

Food and Genetically Modified Organisms Awareness of hypersensitivity reactions to foods and genetically modified organisms (or crops; GMOs) has increased in the last several years. The most common food allergens are milk, egg, peanuts and other tree nuts, fish, shellfish, soy, and wheat. Peanut allergies are relatively common, can be severe, thus, current information regarding the mechanism of peanut hypersensitivity is provided as an example. Hypersensitivity to peanuts occurs primarily via a Type I reaction, and the IgE responses may include shortness of breath, asthma, and anaphylaxis. At least 11 peanut proteins have been identified and antibodies to most can be detected in peanut-allergic patients (reviewed by Finkelman, 2010). More recent studies have shown that peanut extract treatment of mouse or human plasma induced complement C3a, which could contribute to anaphylaxis (Khodoun *et al.*, 2009). In addition, peanut-reactive T cells have been isolated from the blood of peanut-allergic individuals, suggesting that the hypersensitivity to peanuts also involves a Type IV reaction (de Jong *et al.*, 1996; DeLong *et al.*, 2011).

Exposure to GMOs is becoming more widespread as biotechnological advances in food production are used, for example, to confer insect resistance or provide desired nutrients. Allergenic determinants in GMOs result from the expression of novel proteins that might be recognized as nonself by the immune system. There are several considerations in determining potential hypersensitivity to a GMO. Bioinformatic tools are being developed in order to establish whether the introduced protein is allergenic and/ or whether its amino acid sequence is similar enough to known allergens to be considered potentially allergenic (Goodman and Tetteh, 2011; Ladics *et al.*, 2011). In addition, the appropriate test must be selected (eg, radioallergosorbent tests and Ig levels) in order to avoid false positives or false negatives. Finally,

ideally, hypersensitivity to GMOs will be tested on subjects prior to release, but it is also important to survey reactions in the general public following widespread availability (reviewed by Germolec *et al.*, 2003).

Formaldehyde Formaldehyde is used as a preservative, sterilant, and fumigant. Additional exposures come from the textile industry, where it is used to improve wrinkle resistance, and in the furniture, auto upholstery, and resins industries. This low molecular weight compound is extremely soluble in water and forms haptens with human proteins easily (Maibach, 1983). Human predictive testing with 1% to 10% formalin (formalin is 37% formaldehyde) for induction and 1% formalin for challenge showed sensitization rates of 4.5% to 7.8% (Marzulli and Maibach, 1987), and Basketter *et al.* examined 10 aldehydes of varying degrees of allergenicity in humans using the LLNA. The results confirmed that formaldehyde was the strongest allergen and is a contact sensitizer (Basketter *et al.*, 2001).

Occupational exposure to formaldehyde has been associated with the occurrence of asthma (Thompson and Grafstrom, 2008) and increased formaldehyde exposure has now also been associated with increased incidence of childhood asthma (McGwin *et al.*, 2010). Formaldehyde can enhance the respiratory allergic response to other stimuli. For example, Sadakane and coworkers (2002) showed that formaldehyde exposure (0.5% mist once a week for four weeks) in ICR mice enhanced the eosinophilic airway inflammation following the intratracheal instillation with a dust mite allergen. Fujimaki and colleagues (2004) exposed C3H/He mice to formaldehyde at 0, 80, 400, or 2000 ppb formaldehyde for 12 weeks. When mice were immunized with ovalbumin and then exposed to formaldehyde, the total number of BALF cells, macrophages, and eosinophils were significantly increased at the highest concentration. Exposure to 400 ppb formaldehyde induced significant decreases in antiovalbumin IgG1 and IgG3 antibodies, but there was no effect on antiovalbumin IgE antibody. In contrast, in response to a two-week formaldehyde exposure in the absence of another stimulation, total IgE was increased in the serum of C57BL/6 mice (Jung *et al.*, 2007). Lung and liver IL-1β, IL-4, and IL-5 were also increased, and histopathology showed eosinophil infiltration, and inflammatory cell influx (Jung *et al.*, 2007). It has been postulated that part of the mechanism for formaldehyde-increased pulmonary inflammation involves disruption of airway thiol levels, which could affect levels of reactive oxygen and nitrogen species (Staab *et al.*, 2008; Thompson and Grafstrom, 2008).

Autoimmunity

There are numerous reports of xenobiotics that have been associated with autoimmunity; however, firm evidence for their involvement is difficult to obtain. Presently, there are very few instances of human autoimmune diseases for which an environmental trigger has been definitely identified (Rose, 2005). These relationships may be causative through direct mechanisms, or they may be indirect, acting as an adjuvant. In the area of xenobiotic-induced autoimmunity, exact mechanisms of action are not always known. Chemical exposure may also serve to exacerbate a preexisting autoimmune state (Coleman and Sim, 1994; Kilburn and Warshaw, 1994). Table 12-12 lists chemicals known to be associated with autoimmunity and identifies the proposed self-antigenic determinant for each chemical except for silica, which most likely acts as an adjuvant. Table 12-13 shows chemicals that have been implicated in autoimmune reactions, but in these cases the mechanism of autoimmunity has not been as clearly defined or confirmed. The list includes both

Table 12-12

Chemical Agents Known to be Associated with Autoimmunity

PROPOSED ANTIGENIC CHEMICAL	CLINICAL MANIFESTATIONS	DETERMINANT	REFERENCE
Drugs			
Methyl dopa	Hemolytic anemia	Rhesus antigens	Murphy and Kelton (1991)
Hydralazine	SLE-like syndrome	Myeloperoxidase	Cambridge et al. (1994)
Isoniazid	SLE-like syndrome	Myeloperoxidase	Jiang et al. (1994)
Procainamide	SLE-like syndrome	DNA	Totoritis et al. (1988)
Halothane	Autoimmune hepatitis	Liver microsomal proteins	Kenna et al. (1987)
Nondrug chemicals			
Vinyl chloride	Scleroderma-like syndrome	Abnormal protein synthesized in liver	Ward et al. (1976)
Mercury	Glomerular neuropathy	Glomerular basement membrane protein	Pelletier et al. (1994)
Silica	Scleroderma	Most likely acts as an adjuvant	Pernis and Paronetto (1962)

drug and nondrug chemicals. The heterogeneity of these structures and biological activities illustrate the breadth of potential for the induction of chemically mediated autoimmune disease. A number of recent papers have reviewed some specific examples of xenobiotics associated with autoimmune disease (Pollard et al., 2010), including drugs/immunotherapeutics (D'Cruz, 2000; Pichler, 2003; Vial et al., 2002), vaccines (Descotes et al., 2002; Vial and Descotes, 2004), environmental chemicals (D'Cruz, 2000; Hess, 2002), and pesticides (Holsapple, 2002a). A brief discussion of selected drug and nondrug chemicals is provided.

Therapeutic Agents

Methyldopa Methyldopa is a centrally acting sympatholytic drug that has been widely used for the treatment of essential hypertension; but with the advent of newer antihypertensive drugs, the use of methyldopa has declined. Platelets and erythrocytes are targeted by the immune system in individuals treated with this drug (Garratty, 2010). In the case of thrombocytopenia, antibodies are detected against platelets, which are indicative of immune recognition of a self- or altered self-antigen. Hemolytic anemia occurs in at least 1% of individuals treated with methyldopa, and

up to 30% of these individuals develop antibodies to erythrocytes as manifest in a positive Coombs test. Interestingly, the antibodies are not directed against the chemical or a chemical membrane conjugate.

Hydralazine, Isoniazid, and Procainamide Hydralazine is a direct-acting vasodilator drug used in the treatment of hypertension. Isoniazid is an antimicrobial drug used in the treatment of tuberculosis. Procainamide is a drug that selectively blocks sodium channels in myocardial membranes, making it useful in the treatment of cardiac arrhythmias. All three drugs produce autoimmunity, which is manifested as a SLE-like syndrome. Indeed, procainamide represents one of the best examples for a clear association between exposure to a xenobiotic and the onset or progression of an autoimmune disease. The association between procainamide and the SLE-like condition is based on the finding that the disease remits when the drug is discontinued and recurs when the drug is re-administered. Antibodies to DNA have been detected in individuals showing this syndrome. Studies with hydralazine and isoniazid indicate that the antigenic determinant is myeloperoxidase. Although the actual mechanism by which these drugs induce autoimmunity requires further elucidation, studies suggest a breakdown of central tolerance to low affinity self-antigens in the thymus and altered peripheral tolerance due to inhibition of DNA methylation (reviewed by Chang and Gershwin, 2010). There is no evidence indicating that the immune system is recognizing the chemical or a chemical conjugate. In addition, these drugs have also been shown to produce hypersensitivity responses not associated with the SLE syndrome.

Halothane Halothane, one of the most widely studied of the drugs inducing autoimmunity, is an inhalation anesthetic that can induce autoimmune hepatitis (Reichle and Conzen, 2003). The incidence of this iatrogenic disease in humans is about 1 in 20,000. The pathogenesis of the hepatitis results from the chemical altering a specific liver protein to such a degree that the immune system recognizes the altered protein and antibodies are produced. Studies using rat microsomes show that halothane has to be oxidized by cytochrome P450 enzymes to trifluoroacetylhalide before it binds to the protein. Investigations indicate that in affected individuals antibodies to specific microsomal proteins are produced.

Vinyl Chloride Vinyl chloride, which is used in the plastics industry as a refrigerant and in the synthesis of organic chemicals, is a known carcinogen and is also associated with a scleroderma-like

Table 12-13

Chemicals Implicated in Autoimmunity

MANIFESTATION	IMPLICATED CHEMICAL	REFERENCE
Scleroderma	Solvents (toluene, xylene)	Walder (1983)
	Tryptophan	Silver et al. (1990)
	Silicones	Fock et al. (1984)
Systemic lupus erythematosus	Phenothiazines	Canoso et al. (1990)
	Penicillamine	Harpey et al. (1971)
	Propylthiouracil	DeSwarte (1985)
	Quinidine	Jiang et al. (1994)
	L-DOPA	DeSwarte (1985)
	Lithium carbonate	Ananth et al. (1989)
	Trichloroethylene	Kilburn and Warshaw (1992)
	Silicones	Fock et al. (1984)

syndrome. The disease affects multisystemic collagenous tissues, manifesting itself as pulmonary fibrosis, skin sclerosis, and/or fibrosis of the liver and spleen. Ward *et al.* reported on 320 exposed workers, showing that 58 (18%) had a scleroderma-like syndrome (Ward *et al.*, 1976). The individuals who showed the disease were in a group genetically similar (ie, HLA-DR5) to patients with classic idiopathic scleroderma. Although the exact mechanism whereby this chemical produces autoimmunity is unclear, it is presumed that vinyl chloride acts as an amino acid and is incorporated into protein. Because this would produce a structurally abnormal protein, which would be antigenic, an immune response would be directed against tissues with the modified protein present.

Other occupational exposures suspected to induce scleroderma-like reactions include solvents, particularly organic solvents; but the evidence is still limited. For example, several epidemiological studies found an increased relative risk for scleroderma-like reactions following exposure to solvents when compared to the general population. However, the association was weak and not reproduced in other studies, and these studies frequently assessed exposure to solvents in general without providing details on specific solvents (Garabrant and Dumas, 2000; Garabrant *et al.*, 2003).

Mercury This widely used metal is known to have several target systems, including the CNS and renal system. Mercury also has two different actions with respect to the immune system. The first action is direct injury, described previously in the subsection "Metals" under "Immunomodulation by Xenobiotics." The second action is mercury-induced autoimmune disease that is manifested as glomerular nephropathy. Antibodies produced to laminin are believed to be responsible for damage to the basement membrane of the kidney. Mice and rats exposed to mercury also show antinuclear antibodies. The role of these antibodies in the autoimmune disease is not clear; however, they represent a known biomarker of autoimmunity. Studies in the brown Norway rat point to a mercury-induced autoreactive CD4$^+$ cell as being responsible for the polyclonal antibody response. Mercury chloride induces an increase in the expression of MHCII molecules on B lymphocytes as well as shifting the T helper cell population along the Th2 line. It is the Th2 cell that promotes antibody production. The imbalance between Th1 and Th2 cells is believed to be caused by the depletion of cysteine and the reduced form of glutathione in Th1 cells. Reduced glutathione is known to be important in the synthesis of and responsiveness to IL-2 in T cells. Thus, Th1 cells that synthesize and respond to IL-2 would be at a greater risk than Th2 cells.

Mercury-induced autoimmunity has a strong genetic component. This has been extensively studied in the rat and mouse. For example, some strains of rats, such as the Lewis rat, are completely resistant, while others, such as the brown Norway, are exquisitely sensitive. Susceptibility appears to be linked to 3 or 4 genes, one of which is the MHC. A number of reviews addressing the role of mercury in autoimmunity have been prepared (Bigazzi, 1999; Pelletier *et al.*, 1994; Schiraldi and Monestier, 2009).

Silica Crystalline silica (silicon dioxide) is a primary source of elemental silicon and is used commercially in large quantities as a constituent of building materials, ceramics, concretes, and glasses. Experimental animals as well as humans exposed to silica may have perturbations in the immune system. Depending on the length of exposure, dose, and route of administration of silica, it may kill macrophages or may act as an immunostimulant. Silica has been shown to be associated with an increase in scleroderma in silica-exposed workers (Kilburn and Warshaw, 1994). This effect

is believed to be mediated via an adjuvant mechanism. Adjuvancy as a mechanism of causing autoimmunity has been implicated with a number of other chemicals, including paraffin and silicones. Inherent in adjuvancy as a mechanism of producing autoimmunity is that the population affected by these chemicals must already be at risk for the autoimmune disease. This is supported by the data indicating a genetic component to many autoimmune diseases.

Brown and colleagues (2004) developed a model in which apoptosis plays a critical role in silica-induced autoimmune diseases. As described by the authors, inhalation of crystalline silica results in concurrent activation and apoptosis of the alveolar macrophage resulting in an environment of inflammation and apoptosis. This environment may provide excess self-antigen that is further ingested by activated macrophages or DCs that are able to migrate to local lymph nodes. Within these local lymph nodes, these APCs, laden with apoptotic material, activate T cells and B cells thereby inducing an autoimmune response.

Hexachlorobenzene As noted above, autoimmunity induced by pesticides has been previously reviewed (Holsapple, 2002a). There is little doubt that the pesticide most extensively studied in the context of autoimmunity is hexachlorobenzene. Hexachlorobenzene is a low molecular weight compound that was used in the past as a fungicide for seed grains. Even though its use as a pesticide was prohibited in most countries in the 1970s, it is still generated as a by-product of several industrial processes and trace amounts of hexachlorobenzene are present as contaminants in some chlorine-containing pesticides. Although emissions of hexachlorobenzene have decreased dramatically compared to the 1970s, residues can still be found throughout the environment due to its stability and persistence.

One of the drivers for including hexachlorobenzene in this brief presentation of xenobiotics associated with autoimmune disease is based on an accidental poisoning incident that occurred in Turkey in 1955 to 1959. Approximately, 3000 to 5000 people ingested seed grain contaminated with hexachlorobenzene. Patients developed a disease characterized by hepatic porphyria, called *porphyria turcica*, which was manifested as bullous skin lesions, mainly in sun-exposed skin that ultimately healed with severe scars. The skin lesions have been attributed to the phototoxicity associated with the elevated levels of porphyrins. In addition to the dermatological changes, other clinical manifestations included neurological symptoms, hepatomegaly, enlarged thyroid, splenomegaly, hyperpigmentation, hirsutism, enlarged lymph nodes, and painful arthritis of the hands. For many of the clinical symptoms exhibited by the victims, an immune etiology was considered.

Indeed, the autoimmunogenic potential of hexachlorobenzene has been characterized in a number of laboratory studies, which have been reviewed (Ezendam *et al.*, 2004; Michielsen *et al.*, 1999). The former review emphasized a striking difference in the profile of activity in rats, where the predominant effect was immune enhancement, and in mice, where the predominant effect was immune suppression (Michielsen *et al.*, 1999). Only the former results will be discussed further in this section. Exposure to a variety of strains of rats produced increases in the following types of parameters: peripheral blood counts, serum IgM and IgG levels, autoantibodies, spleen and lymph node weights, marginal zones and follicles of spleens, and primary and secondary antibody responses to tetanus toxoid. Interestingly, exposure to hexachlorobenzene caused opposite effects on two induced autoimmune models in Lewis rats, causing an increase in the severity of experimental allergic encephalomyelitis, and a decrease in the severity of adjuvant arthritis (Michielsen *et al.*, 1999). These findings suggest that comparative studies using different genetically autoimmune-prone models may be needed to investigate the role of xenobiotics in the onset and progression of autoimmunity.

Concerning a possible mechanism of action, Ezendam *et al.* (2005), proposed that after exposure to hexachlorobenzene, its deposition can directly induce cell damage or elicit damage by interfering with the integrity of cell membranes due to its lipophilic nature. Ultimately, hexachlorobenzene exposure triggers proinflammatory mediators, such as TNF-α, IL-1, IL-6, ROS, and chemokines. These proinflammatory mediators serve as adjuvant signals that induce a systemic inflammatory response with influxes of neutrophils and macrophages into various nonimmune and immune organs. Subsequently, this leads to polyclonal activation of T and B cells, eosinophilia, and eventually to visible clinical effects.

NEW FRONTIERS AND CHALLENGES IN IMMUNOTOXICOLOGY

As noted throughout this chapter, the immune system has unquestionably been identified as a potential target organ for drugs and chemicals. With the demonstration that (1) chemicals can perturb the immune system of animals; (2) perturbation of immune function is correlated with an increased risk of infectious disease; and (3) perturbations in immune function can occur in the absence of any clinically observable effect, attention has focused, and will continue to focus, on the risk to the human population following exposure to chemicals that can alter immune function in animals. In fact, the characterization of the risk associated with xenobiotic-induced immunotoxicity arguably represents one of the key challenges for this discipline in the immediate future.

Risk can be defined as the probability that an adverse event/effect will manifest itself. Risk must also incorporate the hazard, including dose–response relationships, and exposure. Exposure is a function of the amount of chemical involved and the time of its interaction with people and/or the environment. As such, assessment of risk is often an assessment of the probability for exposure. However, most papers in the immunotoxicology literature that are identified as "risk assessment" papers have focused on just one of the above components, most often, hazard identification. Thus, risk assessment in immunotoxicology remains a "New Frontier."

The science of immunotoxicology continues to evolve, and any overview, including this chapter, must consider the discipline as a "snapshot" in time. Just during the period of time since this chapter was last published, immunotoxicology has experienced significant advancement. This, in part, has been driven by the tremendous growth in knowledge within immunology and cell biology coupled with an explosion in methodological and technological capabilities. New tests reflecting a variety of potential impacts of immunotoxicity have emerged, and traditional tests have been improved. In light of the aforementioned, there are several specific areas within the subdiscipline of immunotoxicology that are currently on the forefront, but will likely see significant advancements and changes. The first, as emphasized earlier in this chapter, will be the continued evolution and application of human primary leukocytes in mechanistic studies of immunotoxicology. In spite of the similarities between the human immune system and that of other animal species, there is an increasing appreciation that often subtle but potentially important differences exist. Advancements in technology, especially flow cytometry have already and will continue to greatly facilitate the application of human primary leukocytes in studies of immunotoxicology. A second area which will see significant changes will be the application of human-derived cell lines, and validation of assays using these cell lines for the purpose of evaluating and screening potential immunotoxicants. A significant driver for broader employment of cell lines in immunotoxicity testing are cost, ethical considerations to reduce the use of animals in toxicity testing, and a fundamental belief that toxicants which alter one or more of the major signaling pathways regulating cell function can be identified in this manner. A recent report by a National Academy of Sciences committee on "Toxicology in the 21st Century" as well as recent initiatives with US Federal agencies such as ToxCast have brought the strategy of using cell line for hazard identification to the forefront. It is highly likely that a significant shift toward the employment of cell lines in immunotoxicology from current strategies utilizing in vivo animal models will require the establishment of a panel of well-characterized cell lines and probably the development of new cell lines in order to make up such a cell line panel. The third area of emphasis in immunotoxicology, as well in other areas of toxicology, will be the application of computational biology to better understand and describe the underlying molecular mechanisms by which an immunotoxicant alters immune function. The application of computational biology has tremendous potential in estimating the potential risk from exposure to immunotoxicants as well as predicting the risk associated with exposure to multiple immunotoxicants simultaneously. The last area on the forefront of immunotoxicology, and in all biomedical disciplines, is increased use of transcriptome analysis. This change will be primarily driven by major advancements and applications of next generation sequencing which will likely make microarrays obsolete due to the significantly greater sensitivity of this technology, decreased cost, and open platform (ie, capable of quantifying the entire transcriptome and not restricted to the DNA tiled on a chip). Moreover, the applications of next generation sequencing beyond studies of the transcriptome are considerable and span uses such as identification of SNPs associated with sensitive subpopulations, and applications in personalized medicine to identification and analysis of DNA methylation for studies of epigenetics.

In spite of these advances, significant challenges remain to be addressed within the discipline of immunotoxicology and include: (1) how to interpret the significance of minor or moderate immunotoxic effects in animal models in relation to human risk assessment; (2) how to better integrate a consideration of exposure, especially to multiple agents simultaneously, into immunotoxicological risk assessment; (3) how to design better human studies to assess the impact on the immune system in the context of risk assessment; (4) how to identify and establish sensitive translational biomarkers of immunotoxicity that can be used to bridge studies conducted in preclinical species to studies in humans; and (5) how to gain a better understanding of the role of genetics in identifying sensitive subpopulations to immune-altering agents. Many of the challenges identified above are not unique to immunotoxicology, but nevertheless are critical, and will need to be addressed through concerted and systematic efforts to improve human immune testing strategies.

REFERENCES

Aebersold R. Constellations in a cellular universe. *Nature.* 2003;422: 115–116.

Ahmed SM, Aw TC, Adisesh A. Toxicological and immunological aspects of occupational latex allergy. *Toxicol Rev.* 2004;23:123–134.

Ahmed T, Pathak R, Mustafa M, et al. Ameliorating effect of *N*-acetylcysteine and curcumin on pesticide-induced oxidative DNA damage in human peripheral blood mononuclear cells. *Environ Monit Assess.* 2011;179: 293–299.

Albers R, Broeders A, van der Pijl A, et al. The use of reporter antigens in the popliteal lymph node assay to assess immunomodulation by chemicals. *Toxicol Appl Pharmacol*. 1997;143:102–109.

Alizadeh M, Ota F, Hosoi K, et al. Altered allergic cytokine and antibody response in mice treated with bisphenol A. *J Med Invest*. 2006;53:70–80.

Allan LL, Mann KK, Matulka RA, et al. Bone marrow stromal–B cell interactions in polycyclic aromatic hydrocarbon-induced pro/pre-B cell apoptosis. *Toxicol Sci*. 2003;76:357–365.

Alonzo NC, Bayer BM. Opioids, immunology, and host defenses of intravenous drug abusers. *Infect Dis Clin North Am*. 2002;16:553–569.

Ananth J, Johnson R, Kataria P, et al. Immune dysfunctions in psychiatric patients. *Psychiatr J Univ Ott*. 1989;14:542–546.

Antonios D, Rousseau P, Larange A, et al. Mechanisms of IL-12 synthesis by human dendritic cells treated with the chemical sensitizer $NiSO_4$. *J Immunol*. 2010;185:89–98.

Araneo BA, Dowell T, Moon HB, et al. Regulation of murine lymphokine production in vivo. Ultraviolet radiation exposure depresses IL-2 and enhances IL-4 production by T cells through an IL-1-dependent mechanism. *J Immunol*. 1989;143:1737–1744.

Aranyi C, O'Shea WJ, Graham JA, et al. The effects of inhalation of organic chemical air contaminants on murine lung host defenses. *Fundam Appl Toxicol*. 1986;6:713–720.

Auphan N, DiDonato JA, Rosette C, et al. Immunosuppression by glucocorticoids: inhibition of NF-kappa B activity through induction of I kappa B synthesis. *Science*. 1995;270:286–290.

Awasthi A, Kuchroo VK. Th17 cells: from precursors to players in inflammation and infection. *Int Immunol*. 2009;21:489–498.

Azarang A, Mahmoodi M, Rajabalian S, et al. T-helper 1 and 2 serum cytokine assay in chronic opioid addicts. *Eur Cytokine Netw*. 2007;18:210–214.

Baccarelli A, Mocarelli P, Patterson DG Jr, et al. Immunologic effects of dioxin: new results from Seveso and comparison with other studies. *Environ Health Perspect*. 2002;110:1169–1173.

Baltimore D, Boldin MP, O'Connell RM, et al. MicroRNAs: new regulators of immune cell development and function. *Nat Immunol*. 2008;9:839–845.

Ban M, Langonne I, Goutet M, et al. Simultaneous analysis of the local and systemic immune responses in mice to study the occupational asthma mechanisms induced by chromium and platinum. *Toxicology*. 2010;277:29–37.

Ban M, Morel G, Langonne I, et al. TDI can induce respiratory allergy with Th2-dominated response in mice. *Toxicology*. 2006;218:39–47.

Banchereau J, Steinman RM. Dendritic cells and the control of immunity. *Nature*. 1998;392:245–252.

Bankoti J, Rase B, Simones T, et al. Functional and phenotypic effects of AhR activation in inflammatory dendritic cells. *Toxicol Appl Pharmacol*. 2010;246:18–28.

Barnett JB, Brundage KM. Evaluating macrophages in immunotoxicity testing. *Methods Mol Biol*. 2010;598:75–94.

Basketter DA, Wright ZM, Warbrick EV, et al. Human potency predictions for aldehydes using the local lymph node assay. *Contact Dermatitis*. 2001;45:89–94.

Baumgarth N. The double life of a B-1 cell: self-reactivity selects for protective effector functions. *Nat Rev Immunol*. 2011;11:34–46.

Bernier J, Hugo P, Krzystyniak K, et al. Suppression of humoral immunity in inbred mice by dieldrin. *Toxicol Lett*. 1987;35:231–240.

Bernstein DI, Cartier A, Cote J, et al. Diisocyanate antigen-stimulated monocyte chemoattractant protein-1 synthesis has greater test efficiency than specific antibodies for identification of diisocyanate asthma. *Am J Respir Crit Care Med*. 2002;166:445–450.

Bernstein DI, Kissling GE, Khurana Hershey G, et al. Hexamethylene diisocyanate asthma is associated with genetic polymorphisms of CD14, IL-13, and IL-4 receptor alpha. *J Allergy Clin Immunol*. 2011;128:418–420.

Bernstein DI, Wang N, Campo P, et al. Diisocyanate asthma and gene–environment interactions with IL4RA, CD-14, and IL-13 genes. *Ann Allergy Asthma Immunol*. 2006;97:800–806.

Bhattacharjee A, Lappi VR, Rutherford MS, et al. Molecular dissection of dimethylnitrosamine (DMN)-induced hepatotoxicity by mRNA differential display. *Toxicol Appl Pharmacol*. 1998;150:186–195.

Bhattacharya S, Conolly RB, Kaminski NE, et al. A bistable switch underlying B-cell differentiation and its disruption by the environmental contaminant 2,3,7,8-tetrachlorodibenzo-*p*-dioxin. *Toxicol Sci*. 2010;115:51–65.

Biagini RE. Epidemiology studies in immunotoxicity evaluations. *Toxicology*. 1998;129:37–54.

Bigazzi PE. Metals and kidney autoimmunity. *Environ Health Perspect*. 1999;107(suppl 5):753–765.

Bondy GS, Pestka JJ. Immunomodulation by fungal toxins. *J Toxicol Environ Health B Crit Rev*. 2000;3:109–143.

Bonneville M, O'Brien RL, Born WK. Gammadelta T cell effector functions: a blend of innate programming and acquired plasticity. *Nat Rev Immunol*. 2010;10:467–478.

Boverhof DR, Gollapudi BB, Hotchkiss JA, et al. Evaluation of a toxicogenomic approach to the local lymph node assay (LLNA). *Toxicol Sci*. 2009;107:427–439.

Broder S. The development of antiretroviral therapy and its impact on the HIV-1/AIDS pandemic. *Antiviral Res*. 2010;85:1–18.

Brown JM, Pfau JC, Pershouse MA, et al. Silica, apoptosis, and autoimmunity. *J Immunotoxicol*. 2004;1:177–188.

Brown N, Nagarkatti M, Nagarkatti PS. Diethylstilbestrol alters positive and negative selection of T cells in the thymus and modulates T-cell repertoire in the periphery. *Toxicol Appl Pharmacol*. 2006a;212:119–126.

Brown N, Nagarkatti M, Nagarkatti PS. Induction of apoptosis in murine fetal thymocytes following perinatal exposure to diethylstilbestrol. *Int J Toxicol*. 2006b;25:9–15.

Buchweitz JP, Karmaus PW, Harkema JR, et al. Modulation of airway responses to influenza A/PR/8/34 by Delta9-tetrahydrocannabinol in C57BL/6 mice. *J Pharmacol Exp Ther*. 2007;323:675–683.

Buckley NE, McCoy KL, Mezey E, et al. Immunomodulation by cannabinoids is absent in mice deficient for the cannabinoid CB(2) receptor. *Eur J Pharmacol*. 2000;396:141–149.

Buehler EV. Delayed contact hypersensitivity in the guinea pig. *Arch Dermatol*. 1965;91:171–177.

Burbach CM, Poland A, Bradfield CA. Cloning of the Ah-receptor cDNA reveals a distinctive ligand-activated transcription factor. *Proc Natl Acad Sci USA*. 1992;89:8185–8189.

Burchiel SW, Kerkvliet NL, Gerberick GF, et al. Assessment of immunotoxicity by multiparameter flow cytometry. *Fundam Appl Toxicol*. 1997;38:38–54.

Burchiel SW, Lauer FT, Gurule D, et al. Uses and future applications of flow cytometry in immunotoxicity testing. *Methods*. 1999;19:28–35.

Burleson FG, Burleson GR. Host resistance assays including bacterial challenge models. *Methods Mol Biol*. 2010;598:97–108.

Burleson GR, Burleson FG, Dietert RR. The cytotoxic T lymphocyte assay for evaluating cell-mediated immune function. *Methods Mol Biol*. 2010;598:195–205.

Burleson GR, Lebrec H, Yang YG, et al. Effect of 2,3,7,8-tetrachlorodibenzo-*p*-dioxin (TCDD) on influenza virus host resistance in mice. *Fundam Appl Toxicol*. 1996;29:40–47.

Burns LA, Bradley SG, White KL Jr, et al. Immunotoxicity of mononitrotoluenes in female B6C3F1 mice: I. *Para*-nitrotoluene. *Drug Chem Toxicol*. 1994a;17:317–358.

Burns LA, Bradley SG, White KL Jr, et al. Immunotoxicity of nitrobenzene in female B6C3F1 mice. *Drug Chem Toxicol*. 1994b;17:271–315.

Burns LA, McCay JA, Brown R, et al. Arsenic in the sera of gallium arsenide-exposed mice inhibits bacterial growth and increases host resistance. *J Pharmacol Exp Ther*. 1993;265:795–800.

Burns LA, Sikorski EE, Saady JJ, et al. Evidence for arsenic as the immunosuppressive component of gallium arsenide. *Toxicol Appl Pharmacol*. 1991;110:157–169.

Burns LA, White KL Jr, McCay JA, et al. Immunotoxicity of mono-nitrotoluenes in female B6C3F1 mice: II. *Meta*-nitrotoluene. *Drug Chem Toxicol*. 1994c;17:359–399.

Burns-Naas LA, Hastings KL, Ladics GS, et al. What's so special about the developing immune system? *Int J Toxicol*. 2008;27:223–254.

Bynote KK, Hackenberg JM, Korach KS, et al. Estrogen receptor-alpha deficiency attenuates autoimmune disease in (NZB × NZW)F1 mice. *Genes Immun*. 2008;9:137–152.

Cabral GA. Drugs of abuse, immune modulation, and AIDS. *J Neuroimmune Pharmacol.* 2006;1:280–295.

Cabral GA, Staab A. Effects on the immune system. *Handb Exp Pharmacol.* 2005;385–423.

Calne RY, Rolles K, White DJ, et al. Cyclosporin-A in clinical organ grafting. *Transplant Proc.* 1981;13:349–358.

Camacho IA, Singh N, Hegde VL, et al. Treatment of mice with 2,3,7,8-tetrachlorodibenzo-*p*-dioxin leads to aryl hydrocarbon receptor-dependent nuclear translocation of NF-kappaB and expression of Fas ligand in thymic stromal cells and consequent apoptosis in T cells. *J Immunol.* 2005;175:90–103.

Cambridge G, Wallace H, Bernstein RM, et al. Autoantibodies to myeloperoxidase in idiopathic and drug-induced systemic lupus erythematosus and vasculitis. *Br J Rheumatol.* 1994;33:109–114.

Canoso RT, de Oliveira RM, Nixon RA. Neuroleptic-associated autoantibodies. A prevalence study. *Biol Psychiatry.* 1990;27:863–870.

Cappon GD, Bailey GP, Buschmann J, et al. Juvenile animal toxicity study designs to support pediatric drug development. *Birth Defects Res B Dev Reprod Toxicol.* 2009;86:463–469.

Carfi M, Gennari A, Malerba I, et al. In vitro tests to evaluate immunotoxicity: a preliminary study. *Toxicology.* 2007;229:11–22.

Carleer J, Karres J. Juvenile animal studies and pediatric drug development: a European regulatory perspective. *Birth Defects Res B Dev Reprod Toxicol.* 2011;92(4):254–260.

Caruso C, Buffa S, Candore G, et al. Mechanisms of immunosenescence. *Immun Ageing.* 2009;6:10.

Carver LA, LaPres JJ, Jain S, et al. Characterization of the Ah receptor-associated protein, ARA9. *J Biol Chem.* 1998;273:33580–33587.

Casale GP, Cohen SD, DiCapua RA. The effects of organophosphate-induced cholinergic stimulation on the antibody response to sheep erythrocytes in inbred mice. *Toxicol Appl Pharmacol.* 1983;68:198–205.

Cassel SL, Eisenbarth SC, Iyer SS, et al. The Nalp3 inflammasome is essential for the development of silicosis. *Proc Natl Acad Sci USA.* 2008;105:9035–9040.

Catania RA, Chaudry IH. Immunological consequences of trauma and shock. *Ann Acad Med Singapore.* 1999;28:120–132.

Chang C, Gershwin ME. Drugs and autoimmunity—a contemporary review and mechanistic approach. *J Autoimmun.* 2010;34:J266–J275.

Chang C, Mahmood MM, Teuber SS, Gershwin ME. Overview of penicillin allergy. *Clin Rev Allergy Immunol.* 2011;43:84–97.

Chang ZL. Important aspects of toll-like receptors, ligands and their signaling pathways. *Inflamm Res.* 2010;59:791–808.

Chao CC, Molitor TW, Gekker G, et al. Cocaine-mediated suppression of superoxide production by human peripheral blood mononuclear cells. *J Pharmacol Exp Ther.* 1991;256:255–258.

Chaplin DD. Overview of the immune response. *J Allergy Clin Immunol.* 2010;125:S3–S23.

Chen Q, Zhang Z, Zhang R, et al. Tributyltin chloride-induced immunotoxicity and thymocyte apoptosis are related to abnormal Fas expression. *Int J Hyg Environ Health.* 2011;214:145–150.

Chuchawankul S, Shima M, Buckley NE, et al. Role of cannabinoid receptors in inhibiting macrophage costimulatory activity. *Int Immunopharmacol.* 2004;4:265–278.

Chung YJ, Zhou HR, Pestka JJ. Transcriptional and posttranscriptional roles for p38 mitogen-activated protein kinase in upregulation of TNF-alpha expression by deoxynivalenol (vomitoxin). *Toxicol Appl Pharmacol.* 2003;193:188–201.

Coleman JW, Sim E. Autoallergic responses to drugs: mechanistic aspects, in Dean JH, Luster MI, Munson AB, Kimber I, eds. *Immunotoxicology and Immunopharmacology.* New York: Raven Press; 1994:553–572.

Collinge M, Cole SH, Schneider PA, et al. Human lymphocyte activation assay: an in vitro method for predictive immunotoxicity testing. *J Immunotoxicol.* 2010;7:357–366.

Colosio C, Birindelli S, Corsini E, et al. Low level exposure to chemicals and immune system. *Toxicol Appl Pharmacol.* 2005;207:320–328.

Colt JS, Rothman N, Severson RK, et al. Organochlorine exposure, immune gene variation, and risk of non-Hodgkin lymphoma. *Blood.* 2009;113:1899–1905.

Condie R, Herring A, Koh WS, et al. Cannabinoid inhibition of adenylate cyclase-mediated signal transduction and interleukin 2 (IL-2) expression in the murine T-cell line, EL4.IL-2. *J Biol Chem.* 1996;271:13175–13183.

Coombs RRA, Gell PGH. Classification of allergic reactions responsible for clinical hypersensitivity and disease, in Gell PGH, Coombs RRA, Lachmann PJ, eds. *Clinical Aspects of Immunology.* Oxford: Oxford University Press; 1975:761.

Cooper RL, Lamb JC, Barlow SM, et al. A tiered approach to life stages testing for agricultural chemical safety assessment. *Crit Rev Toxicol.* 2006;36:69–98.

Corsini E, House RV. Evaluating cytokines in immunotoxicity testing. *Methods Mol Biol.* 2010;598:283–302.

Costes V, Magen V, Legouffe E, et al. The Mi15 monoclonal antibody (anti-syndecan-1) is a reliable marker for quantifying plasma cells in paraffin-embedded bone marrow biopsy specimens. *Hum Pathol.* 1999;30:1405–1411.

Cox MB, Miller CA, 3rd. Cooperation of heat shock protein 90 and p23 in aryl hydrocarbon receptor signaling. *Cell Stress Chaperones.* 2004;9:4–20.

Crittenden PL, Carr R, Pruett SB. Immunotoxicological assessment of methyl parathion in female B6C3F1 mice. *J Toxicol Environ Health A.* 1998;54:1–20.

Cummings KJ, Stefaniak AB, Virji MA, et al. A reconsideration of acute beryllium disease. *Environ Health Perspect.* 2009;117:1250–1256.

Cunningham M, Gilkeson G. Estrogen receptors in immunity and autoimmunity. *Clin Rev Allergy Immunol.* 2011;40:66–73.

Cuthill S, Poellinger L, Gustafsson JA. The receptor for 2,3,7,8-tetrachlorodibenzo-*p*-dioxin in the mouse hepatoma cell line Hepa 1c1c7. *J Biol Chem.* 1987;262:3477–3481.

D'Cruz D. Autoimmune diseases associated with drugs, chemicals and environmental factors. *Toxicol Lett.* 2000;112–113:421–432.

Dai Q, Pruett SB. Different effects of acute and chronic ethanol on LPS-induced cytokine production and TLR4 receptor behavior in mouse peritoneal macrophages. *J Immunotoxicol.* 2006;3:217–225.

Dakeshita S, Kawai T, Uemura H, et al. Gene expression signatures in peripheral blood cells from Japanese women exposed to environmental cadmium. *Toxicology.* 2009;257:25–32.

Daniel V, Huber W, Bauer K, et al. Associations of dichlorodiphenyltrichloroethane (DDT) 4.4 and dichlorodiphenyldichloroethylene (DDE) 4.4 blood levels with plasma IL-4. *Arch Environ Health.* 2002;57:541–547.

Davis BK, Wen H, Ting JP. The inflammasome NLRs in immunity, inflammation, and associated diseases. *Annu Rev Immunol.* 2011;29:707–735.

Davis D, Safe S. Immunosuppressive activities of polychlorinated dibenzofuran congeners: quantitative structure activity relationships and interactive effects. *Toxicol Appl Pharmacol.* 1988;94:141–149.

De Abrew KN, Phadnis AS, Crawford RB, et al. Regulation of Bach2 by the aryl hydrocarbon receptor as a mechanism for suppression of B-cell differentiation by 2,3,7,8-tetrachlorodibenzo-*p*-dioxin. *Toxicol Appl Pharmacol.* 2011;252:150–158.

de Jong EC, Spanhaak S, Martens BP, et al. Food allergen (peanut)-specific TH2 clones generated from the peripheral blood of a patient with peanut allergy. *J Allergy Clin Immunol.* 1996;98:73–81.

Dean JH, Lauer LD, House RV, et al. Studies of immune function and host resistance in B6C3F1 mice exposed to formaldehyde. *Toxicol Appl Pharmacol.* 1984;72:519–529.

Dean JH, Luster MI, Boorman GA, et al. Selective immunosuppression resulting from exposure to the carcinogenic congener of benzopyrene in B6C3F1 mice. *Clin Exp Immunol.* 1983;52:199–206.

Dean JH, Luster MI, Munson AE, et al. *Immunotoxicology and Immunopharmacology.* New York: Raven Press; 1985.

Dearman RJ, Basketter DA, Blaikie L, et al. The Mouse IgE test: interlaboratory evaluation and comparison of BALB/c and C57BL/6 strain mice. *Toxicol Meth.* 1998;8:69–85.

Dearman RJ, Betts CJ, Humphreys N, et al. Chemical allergy: considerations for the practical application of cytokine profiling. *Toxicol Sci.* 2003;71:137–145.

Dearman RJ, Spence LM, Kimber I. Characterization of murine immune responses to allergenic diisocyanates. *Toxicol Appl Pharmacol.* 1992;112:190–197.

Dearman RJ, Warbrick EV, Skinner R, et al. Cytokine fingerprinting of chemical allergens: species comparisons and statistical analyses. *Food Chem Toxicol.* 2002;40:1881–1892.

Delaney B, Strom SC, Collins S, et al. Carbon tetrachloride suppresses T-cell-dependent immune responses by induction of transforming growth factor-beta 1. *Toxicol Appl Pharmacol.* 1994;126:98–107.

DeLong JH, Simpson KH, Wambre E, et al. Ara h 1-reactive T cells in individuals with peanut allergy. *J Allergy Clin Immunol.* 2011;127:1211–1218.

Demoly P, Michel F, Bousquet J. In vivo methods for study of allergy skin tests, techniques and interpretation, in Middleton EJ, Reed C, Ellis E, eds. *Allergy Principles and Practice.* St. Louis: Mosby; 1998:430–439.

Denis M, Cuthill S, Wikstroem AC, et al. Association of the dioxin receptor with the Mr 90,000 heat shock protein. *Biochem Biophys Res Commun.* 1988;155:801–807.

Descotes J. *Immunotoxicology and Drugs and Chemicals.* Amsterdam: Elsevier; 1986.

Descotes J. *Immunotoxicology of Drugs and Chemicals: An Experimental and Clinical Approach.* Amsterdam: Elsevier; 2004.

Descotes J. Methods of evaluating immunotoxicity. *Expert Opin Drug Metab Toxicol.* 2006;2:249–259.

Descotes J, Ravel G, Ruat C. Vaccines: predicting the risk of allergy and autoimmunity. *Toxicology.* 2002;174:45–51.

DeSwarte RD. Drug allergy, in Patterson R, ed. *Allergic Diseases, Diagnosis and Management.* Philadephia, PA: Lippincott Williams & Wilkins; 1985:505–661.

Dewailly E, Ayotte P, Bruneau S, et al. Susceptibility to infections and immune status in Inuit infants exposed to organochlorines. *Environ Health Perspect.* 2000;108:205–211.

Di Gioacchino M, Petrarca C, Lazzarin F, et al. Immunotoxicity of nanoparticles. *Int J Immunopathol Pharmacol.* 2011;24:65S–71S.

Di Gioacchino M, Petrarca C, Perrone A, et al. Autophagy as an ultrastructural marker of heavy metal toxicity in human cord blood hematopoietic stem cells. *Sci Total Environ.* 2008;392:50–58.

Diana J, Lehuen A. NKT cells: friend or foe during viral infections? *Eur J Immunol.* 2009;39:3283–3291.

Dich J, Zahm SH, Hanberg A, et al. Pesticides and cancer. *Cancer Causes Control.* 1997;8:420–443.

Dietert R, Burns-Naas LA. Developmental immunotoxicity in rodents, in Herzyk DJ, Bussiere JL eds. *Immunotoxicology Strategies for Pharmaceutical Safety Assessment.* Hoboken, NJ: John Wiley and Sons, Inc.; 2008:273–297.

Dietert RR, Bunn TL, Lee JE. The delayed type hypersensitivity assay using protein and xenogeneic cell antigens. *Methods Mol Biol.* 2010;598:185–194.

Dietert RR, Etzel RA, Chen D, et al. Workshop to identify critical windows of exposure for children's health: immune and respiratory systems work group summary. *Environ Health Perspect.* 2000;108(suppl 3):483–490.

Dietert RR, Holsapple MP. Methodologies for developmental immunotoxicity (DIT) testing. *Methods.* 2007;41:123–131.

Dietert RR, Piepenbrink MS. Lead and immune function. *Crit Rev Toxicol.* 2006a;36:359–385.

Dietert RR, Piepenbrink MS. Perinatal immunotoxicity: why adult exposure assessment fails to predict risk. *Environ Health Perspect.* 2006b;114:477–483.

DiLillo DJ, Matsushita T, Tedder TF. B10 cells and regulatory B cells balance immune responses during inflammation, autoimmunity, and cancer. *Ann N Y Acad Sci.* 2010;1183:38–57.

Dong W, Gilmour MI, Lambert AL, et al. Enhanced allergic responses to house dust mite by oral exposure to carbaryl in rats. *Toxicol Sci.* 1998;44:63–69.

Dooley RK, Holsapple MP. Elucidation of cellular targets responsible for tetrachlorodibenzo-p-dioxin (TCDD)-induced suppression of antibody responses: I. The role of the B lymphocyte. *Immunopharmacology* 1988;16:167–180.

Drayton DL, Liao S, Mounzer RH, et al. Lymphoid organ development: from ontogeny to neogenesis. *Nat Immunol.* 2006;7:344–353.

Duffield JS. The inflammatory macrophage: a story of Jekyll and Hyde. *Clin Sci (Lond).* 2003;104:27–38.

Dunkelberger JR, Song WC. Complement and its role in innate and adaptive immune responses. *Cell Res.* 2010;20:34–50.

Dunn TJ, Lindahl R, Pitot HC. Differential gene expression in response to 2,3,7,8-tetrachlorodibenzo-p-dioxin (TCDD). *J Biol Chem.* 1988;263:10878–10886.

Duramad P, Tager IB, Leikauf J, et al. Expression of Th1/Th2 cytokines in human blood after in vitro treatment with chlorpyrifos, and its metabolites, in combination with endotoxin LPS and allergen Der p1. *J Appl Toxicol.* 2006;26:458–465.

Dutta R, Mondal AM, Arora V, et al. Immunomodulatory effect of DDT (bis[4-chlorophenyl]-1,1,1-trichloroethane) on complement system and macrophages. *Toxicology.* 2008;252:78–85.

Easterbrook PJ, Waters A, Murad S, et al. Epidemiological risk factors for hypersensitivity reactions to abacavir. *HIV Med.* 2003;4:321–324.

Edwards CJ, Cooper C. Early environmental factors and rheumatoid arthritis. *Clin Exp Immunol.* 2006;143:1–5.

Elferink CJ, Gasiewicz TA, Whitlock JP. Protein–DNA interactions at a dioxin-responsive enhancer. *J Biol Chem.* 1990;265:20708–20712.

Elmore SA. Enhanced histopathology evaluation of lymphoid organs. *Methods Mol Biol.* 2010;598:323–339.

EMA. *Guideline on the Need for Non-clinical Testing in Juvenile Animals of Pharmaceuticals for Paediatric Indications.* London, UK: European Medicines Agency, Committee for Human Medicinal Products; 2008.

Ema M, Sogawa K, Watanabe N, et al. cDNA cloning and structure of mouse putative Ah receptor. *Biochem Biophys Res Commun.* 1992;184:246–253.

EPA. *EPA Health Effects Guidelines: OPPTS 870.3800—Reproduction and Fertility Effects.* Office of Prevention, Pesticides and Toxic Substances; 1998.

Escobar J, Varela-Nallar L, Coddou C, et al. Oxidative damage in lymphocytes of copper smelter workers correlated to higher levels of excreted arsenic. *Mediators Inflamm.* 2010;2010:403830.

Este JA, Cihlar T. Current status and challenges of antiretroviral research and therapy. *Antiviral Res.* 2010;85:25–33.

Exon JH, Mather GG, Bussiere JL, et al. Effects of subchronic exposure of rats to 2-methoxyethanol or 2-butoxyethanol: thymic atrophy and immunotoxicity. *Fundam Appl Toxicol.* 1991;16:830–840.

Ezendam J, Vos JG, Pieters R. Mechanisms of hexachlorobenzene-induced adverse immune effects in brown Norway rats. *J Immunotoxicol.* 2004;1:167–176.

Ezendam J, Vos JG, Pieters R. Research articles mechanisms of hexachlorobenzene-induced adverse immune effects in brown Norway rats. *J Immunotoxicol.* 2005;1:167–175.

Farraj AK, Harkema JR, Kaminski NE. Topical application versus intranasal instillation: a qualitative comparison of the effect of the route of sensitization on trimellitic anhydride-induced allergic rhinitis in A/J mice. *Toxicol Sci.* 2006;92:321–328.

Farrer DG, Hueber S, Laiosa MD, et al. Reduction of myeloid suppressor cell derived nitric oxide provides a mechanistic basis of lead enhancement of alloreactive CD4(+) T cell proliferation. *Toxicol Appl Pharmacol.* 2008;229:135–145.

Farrer DG, Hueber SM, McCabe MJ Jr. Lead enhances CD4+ T cell proliferation indirectly by targeting antigen presenting cells and modulating antigen-specific interactions. *Toxicol Appl Pharmacol.* 2005;207:125–137.

Faubert BL, Kaminski NE. AP-1 activity is negatively regulated by cannabinol through inhibition of its protein components, c-fos and c-jun. *J Leukoc Biol.* 2000;67:259–266.

FDA. *Guidance for Industry—Immunotoxicology Evaluation of Investigational New Drugs.* Center for Drug Evaluation and Research, Department of Health and Human Services; 2002.

FDA. *Guidance for Industry—Nonclinical Safety Evaluation of Pediatric Drug Products.* Office of Training and Communication, Division of Drug Information, Center for Drug Evaluation and Research, Department of Health and Human Services; 2006.

Felter SP, Ryan CA, Basketter DA, et al. Application of the risk assessment paradigm to the induction of allergic contact dermatitis. *Regul Toxicol Pharmacol.* 2003;37:1–10.

Feola DJ, Thornton AC, Garvy BA. Effects of antiretroviral therapy on immunity in patients infected with HIV. *Curr Pharm Des.* 2006;12:1015–1022.

Filipov NM, Pinchuk LM, Boyd BL, et al. Immunotoxic effects of short-term atrazine exposure in young male C57BL/6 mice. *Toxicol Sci*. 2005;86:324–332.

Fingar DC, Blenis J. Target of rapamycin (TOR): an integrator of nutrient and growth factor signals and coordinator of cell growth and cell cycle progression. *Oncogene*. 2004;23:3151–3171.

Finkelman FD. Peanut allergy and anaphylaxis. *Curr Opin Immunol*. 2010;22:783–788.

Fischer A, Koeper LM, Vohr HW. Specific antibody responses of primary cells from different cell sources are able to predict immunotoxicity in vitro. *Toxicol In Vitro*. 2011;25(8):1966–1973.

Fock KM, Feng PH, Tey BH. Autoimmune disease developing after augmentation mammoplasty: report of 3 cases. *J Rheumatol*. 1984;11:98–100.

Forte G, Petrucci F, Bocca B. Metal allergens of growing significance: epidemiology, immunotoxicology, strategies for testing and prevention. *Inflamm Allergy Drug Target*. 2008;7:145–162.

Freebern WJ. Viral host resistance studies. *Methods Mol Biol*. 2010;598:109–117.

Fujimaki H, Kurokawa Y, Kunugita N, et al. Differential immunogenic and neurogenic inflammatory responses in an allergic mouse model exposed to low levels of formaldehyde. *Toxicology*. 2004;197:1–13.

Fujisawa-Sehara A, Sogawa K, Yamane M, et al. Characterization of xenobiotic responsive elements upstream from the drug metabolizing cytochrome P450c gene: a similarity to glucocorticoid response elements. *Nucleic Acids Res*. 1987;15:4179–4191.

Fukuyama T, Tajima Y, Ueda H, et al. A method for measuring mouse respiratory allergic reaction to low-dose chemical exposure to allergens: an environmental chemical of uncertain allergenicity, a typical contact allergen and a non-sensitizing irritant. *Toxicol Lett*. 2010;195:35–43.

Funatake CJ, Marshall NB, Steppan LB, et al. Cutting edge: activation of the aryl hydrocarbon receptor by 2,3,7,8-tetrachlorodibenzo-*p*-dioxin generates a population of CD4+ CD25+ cells with characteristics of regulatory T cells. *J Immunol*. 2005;175:4184–4188.

Gad SC, Dunn BJ, Dobbs DW, et al. Development and validation of an alternative dermal sensitization test: the mouse ear swelling test (MEST). *Toxicol Appl Pharmacol*. 1986;84:93–114.

Galbiati V, Mitjans M, Corsini E. Present and future of in vitro immunotoxicology in drug development. *J Immunotoxicol*. 2010;7:255–267.

Galicia G, Leyva R, Tenorio EP, et al. Sodium arsenite retards proliferation of PHA-activated T cells by delaying the production and secretion of IL-2. *Int Immunopharmacol*. 2003;3:671–682.

Galiegue S, Mary S, Marchand J, et al. Expression of central and peripheral cannabinoid receptors in human immune tissues and leukocyte subpopulations. *Eur J Biochem*. 1995;232:54–61.

Galloway T, Handy R. Immunotoxicity of organophosphorous pesticides. *Ecotoxicology*. 2003;12:345–363.

Ganey PE, Luyendyk JP, Maddox JF, et al. Adverse hepatic drug reactions: inflammatory episodes as consequence and contributor. *Chem Biol Interact*. 2004;150:35–51.

Gao D, Mondal TK, Lawrence DA. Lead effects on development and function of bone marrow-derived dendritic cells promote Th2 immune responses. *Toxicol Appl Pharmacol*. 2007;222:69–79.

Gao J, Lauer FT, Dunaway S, et al. Cytochrome P450 1B1 is required for 7,12-dimethylbenz(a)-anthracene (DMBA) induced spleen cell immunotoxicity. *Toxicol Sci*. 2005a;86:68–74.

Gao J, Voss AA, Pessah IN, et al. Ryanodine receptor-mediated rapid increase in intracellular calcium induced by 7,8-benzo(a)pyrene quinone in human and murine leukocytes. *Toxicol Sci*. 2005b;87:419–426.

Garabrant DH, Dumas C. Epidemiology of organic solvents and connective tissue disease. *Arthritis Res*. 2000;2:5–15.

Garabrant DH, Lacey JV Jr, Laing TJ, et al. Scleroderma and solvent exposure among women. *Am J Epidemiol*. 2003;157:493–500.

Gardner RM, Nyland JF, Evans SL, et al. Mercury induces an unopposed inflammatory response in human peripheral blood mononuclear cells in vitro. *Environ Health Perspect*. 2009;117:1932–1938.

Gardner RM, Nyland JF, Silva IA, et al. Mercury exposure, serum antinuclear/antinucleolar antibodies, and serum cytokine levels in mining populations in Amazonian Brazil: a cross-sectional study. *Environ Res*. 2010;110:345–354.

Garratty G. Immune hemolytic anemia associated with drug therapy. *Blood Rev*. 2010;24:143–150.

Garrett RW, Gasiewicz TA. The aryl hydrocarbon receptor agonist 2,3,7,8-tetrachlorodibenzo-*p*-dioxin alters the circadian rhythms, quiescence, and expression of clock genes in murine hematopoietic stem and progenitor cells. *Mol Pharmacol*. 2006;69:2076–2083.

Garssen J, van Loveren H. Effects of ultraviolet exposure on the immune system. *Crit Rev Immunol*. 2001;21:359–397.

Garssen J, Vandebriel RJ, van Loveren H. Molecular aspects of UVB-induced immunosuppression. *Arch Toxicol Suppl*. 1997;19:97–109.

Germolec D. Autoimmune disease, animal models, in vohr H-W, ed. *Encyclopedic Reference of Immunotoxicology*. Heidelberg: Springer, 2005:75–79.

Germolec DR, Kashon M, Nyska A, et al. The accuracy of extended histopathology to detect immunotoxic chemicals. *Toxicol Sci*. 2004;82:504–514.

Germolec DR, Kimber I, Goldman L, et al. Key issues for the assessment of the allergenic potential of genetically modified foods: breakout group reports. *Environ Health Perspect*. 2003;111:1131–1139.

Glaser R, Sheridan J, Malarkey WB, et al. Chronic stress modulates the immune response to a pneumococcal pneumonia vaccine. *Psychosom Med*. 2000;62:804–807.

Gleichmann E, Pal ST, Rolink AG, et al. Graft versus host reactions: clues to the etiopathology of a spectrum of immunological diseases. *Immunol Today*. 1984;5.

Glover M, Cheng B, Deng X, et al. The role of glucocorticoids in the immediate vs. delayed effects of acute ethanol exposure on cytokine production in a binge drinking model. *Int Immunopharmacol*. 2011;11:755–761.

Gong YY, Egal S, Hounsa A, et al. Determinants of aflatoxin exposure in young children from Benin and Togo, West Africa: the critical role of weaning. *Int J Epidemiol*. 2003;32:556–562.

Good RA. Organization and development of the immune system. Relation to its reconstruction. *Ann N Y Acad Sci*. 1995;770:8–33.

Goodman RE, Tetteh AO. Suggested improvements for the allergenicity assessment of genetically modified plants used in foods. *Curr Allergy Asthma Rep*. 2011;11:317–324.

Goto M, Takano-Ishikawa Y, Ono H, et al. Orally administered bisphenol A disturbed antigen specific immunoresponses in the naive condition. Biosci Biotechnol Biochem. 2007;71:2136–2143.

Goulding NJ, Guyre PM. Regulation of inflammation by lipocortin 1. *Immunol Today*. 1992;13:295–297.

Greenlee WF, Dold KM, Irons RD, et al. Evidence for direct action of 2,3,7,8-tetrachlorodibenzo-*p*-dioxin (TCDD) on thymic epithelium. *Toxicol Appl Pharmacol*. 1985;79:112–120.

Greenlee WF, Dold KM, Osborne R. A proposed model for the actions of TCDD on epidermal and thymic epithelial target cells in Poland A, inKR D, ed. *Banbury Report 18: Biological Mechanisms of Dioxin Action*. New York: Cold Harbor Spring Laboratory; 1984:435ff.

Grosser T, Fries S, FitzGerald GA. Biological basis for the cardiovascular consequences of COX-2 inhibition: therapeutic challenges and opportunities. *J Clin Invest*. 2006;116:4–15.

Grube A, Donaldson D, Kiely T, et al. *Pesticides Industry Sales and Usage: 2006 and 2007 Market Estimates*. USA: Biological and Economic Analysis Division Office of Pesticide Programs Office of Chemical Safety and Pollution Prevention US Environmental Protection Agency; 2011. http://www.epa.gov/pesticides/pestsales/07pestsales/market_esti mates2007.pdf

Guo CJ, Li Y, Tian S, et al. Morphine enhances HIV infection of human blood mononuclear phagocytes through modulation of beta-chemokines and CCR5 receptor. *J Investig Med*. 2002;50:435–442.

Gutting BW, Schomaker SJ, Kaplan AH, et al. A comparison of the direct and reporter antigen popliteal lymph node assay for the detection of immunomodulation by low molecular weight compounds. *Toxicol Sci*. 1999;51:71–79.

Haase H, Engelhardt G, Hebel S, et al. Mercuric ions inhibit mitogen-activated protein kinase dephosphorylation by inducing reactive oxygen species. *Toxicol Appl Pharmacol*. 2011;250:78–86.

Haggerty HG, Holsapple MP. Role of metabolism in dimethylnitrosamine-induced immunosuppression: a review. *Toxicology*. 1990;63:1–23.

Haggqvist B, Havarinasab S, Bjorn E, et al. The immunosuppressive effect of methylmercury does not preclude development of autoimmunity in genetically susceptible mice. *Toxicology*. 2005;208:149–164.

Han YC, Lin TL, Pruett SB. Thymic atrophy caused by ethanol in a mouse model for binge drinking: involvement of endogenous glucocorticoids. *Toxicol Appl Pharmacol*. 1993;123:16–25.

Handy RD, Abd-El Samei HA, Bayomy MF, et al. Chronic diazinon exposure: pathologies of spleen, thymus, blood cells, and lymph nodes are modulated by dietary protein or lipid in the mouse. *Toxicology*. 2002;172:13–34.

Happel KI, Nelson S. Alcohol, immunosuppression, and the lung. *Proc Am Thorac Soc*. 2005;2:428–432.

Hardy RR. B-1 B cell development. *J Immunol*. 2006;177:2749–2754.

Harpey JP, Caille B, Moulias R, et al. Lupus-like syndrome induced by D-penicillamine in Wilson's disease. *Lancet* 1971;1:292.

Hawley TS, Hawley H, eds. *Methods in Molecular Biology: Flow Cytometry Protocols*. Totowa, NJ: Humana Press Inc; 2004.

Heidel SM, Czuprynski CJ, Jefcoate CR. Bone marrow stromal cells constitutively express high levels of cytochrome P4501B1 that metabolize 7,12-dimethylbenz[*a*]anthracene. *Mol Pharmacol*. 1998;54:1000–1006.

Hemdan NY, Birkenmeier G, Wichmann G, et al. Interleukin-17-producing T helper cells in autoimmunity. *Autoimmun Rev*. 2010;9:785–792.

Hemdan NY, Emmrich F, Sack U, et al. The in vitro immune modulation by cadmium depends on the way of cell activation. *Toxicology*. 2006;222:37–45.

Hemdan NY, Lehmann I, Wichmann G, et al. Immunomodulation by mercuric chloride in vitro: application of different cell activation pathways. *Clin Exp Immunol*. 2007;148:325–337.

Hengstler JG, Foth H, Gebel T, et al. Critical evaluation of key evidence on the human health hazards of exposure to bisphenol A. *Crit Rev Toxicol*. 2011;41:263–291.

Henseler RA, Romer EJ, Sulentic CE. Diverse chemicals including aryl hydrocarbon receptor ligands modulate transcriptional activity of the 3′ immunoglobulin heavy chain regulatory region. *Toxicology*. 2009;261:9–18.

Heo Y, Mondal TK, Gao D, et al. Posttranscriptional inhibition of interferon-gamma production by lead. *Toxicol Sci*. 2007;96:92–100.

Herring AC, Koh WS, Kaminski NE. Inhibition of the cyclic AMP signaling cascade and nuclear factor binding to CRE and kappaB elements by cannabinol, a minimally CNS-active cannabinoid. *Biochem Pharmacol*. 1998;55:1013–1023.

Hess EV. Environmental chemicals and autoimmune disease: cause and effect. *Toxicology*. 2002;181–182:65–70.

Higbee RG, Byers AM, Dhir V, et al. An immunologic model for rapid vaccine assessment—a clinical trial in a test tube. *Altern Lab Anim*. 2009;37(suppl 1):19–27.

Ho S, Clipstone N, Timmermann L, et al. The mechanism of action of cyclosporin A and FK506. *Clin Immunol Immunopathol*. 1996;80:S40–S45.

Hoffman EC, Reyes H, Chu FF, et al. Cloning of a factor required for activity of the Ah (dioxin) receptor. *Science*. 1991;252:954–958.

Holladay SD, Blaylock BL, Comment CE, et al. Fetal thymic atrophy after exposure to T-2 toxin: selectivity for lymphoid progenitor cells. *Toxicol Appl Pharmacol*. 1993;121:8–14.

Holladay SD, Comment CE, Kwon J, et al. Fetal hematopoietic alterations after maternal exposure to ethylene glycol monomethyl ether: prolymphoid cell targeting. *Toxicol Appl Pharmacol*. 1994;129:53–60.

Holladay SD, Smialowicz RJ. Development of the murine and human immune system: differential effects of immunotoxicants depend on time of exposure. *Environ Health Perspect*. 2000;108(suppl 3):463–473.

Holsapple MP. Autoimmunity by pesticides: a critical review of the state of the science. *Toxicol Lett*. 2002a;127:101–109.

Holsapple MP. Developmental immunotoxicology and risk assessment: a workshop summary. *Hum Exp Toxicol*. 2002b;21:473–478.

Holsapple MP. Immunotoxicity of halogenated aromatic hydrocarbons, in Smialowicz RJ, Holsapple MP, eds. *Experimental Immunotoxicology*. Boca Raton, FL: CRC Press; 1996:257–297.

Holsapple MP, Burns-Naas LA, Hastings KL, et al. A proposed testing framework for developmental immunotoxicology (DIT). *Toxicol Sci*. 2005;83:18–24.

Holsapple MP, Dooley RK, McNerney PJ, et al. Direct suppression of antibody responses by chlorinated dibenzodioxins in cultured spleen cells from (C57BL/6 × C3H)F1 and DBA/2 mice. *Immunopharmacology*. 1986;12:175–186.

Holsapple MP, Jones D, Kawabata TT, et al. Assessing the potential to induce respiratory hypersensitivity. *Toxicol Sci*. 2006;91:4–13.

Holsapple MP, Morris DL, Wood SC, et al. 2,3,7,8-tetrachlorodibenzo-*p*-dioxin-induced changes in immunocompetence: possible mechanisms. *Annu Rev Pharmacol Toxicol*. 1991a;31:73–100.

Holsapple MP, Munson AE, Munson JA, et al. Suppression of cell-mediated immunocompetence after subchronic exposure to diethylstilbestrol in female B6C3F1 mice. *J Pharmacol Exp Ther*. 1983;227:130–138.

Holsapple MP, O'Lone R. Juvenile immunotoxicology. *Toxicol Pathol*. 2012;40(2):248–258.

Holsapple MP, Paustenbach DJ, Charnley G, et al. Symposium summary: children's health risk—what's so special about the developing immune system? *Toxicol Appl Pharmacol*. 2004;199:61–70.

Holsapple MP, Snyder NK, Wood SC, et al. A review of 2,3,7,8-tetrachlorodibenzo-*p*-dioxin-induced changes in immunocompetence: 1991 update. *Toxicology*. 1991b;69:219–255.

Holsapple MP, van der Laan JW, van Loveren H. Development of a framework for developmental immunotoxicity testing, in Luebke R, House R, Kimber I, eds. *Immunotoxicology and Immunopharmacology*. Boca Raton, FL: CRC Press; 2007:347–361.

Holsapple MP, West LJ, Landreth KS. Species comparison of anatomical and functional immune system development. *Birth Defects Res B*. 2003;68:321–334.

Holt PG, Upham JW, Sly PD. Contemporaneous maturation of immunologic and respiratory functions during early childhood: implications for development of asthma prevention strategies. *J Allergy Clin Immunol*. 2005;116:16–24; quiz 25.

Horwitz DA, Zheng SG, Gray JD. Natural and TGF-beta-induced Foxp3(+) CD4(+) CD25(+) regulatory T cells are not mirror images of each other. *Trends Immunol*. 2008;29:429–435.

House R. Immunotoxicology methods, in Massaro E, ed. *Handbook of Human Toxicology*. Boca Rotton, FL: CRC Press; 1997:677–708.

House R. Regulatory guidance in immunotoxicology, in Vohr H-W ed. *Encyclopedic Reference of Immunotoxicology*. Heidelberg: Springer, 2005, pp. 551–555.

House RV, Laurer LD, Murray MJ. Immunological studies in B6C3F1 mice following exposure to ethylene glycol monomethyl ether and its principal metabolite methoxyacetic acid. *Toxicol Appl Pharmacol*. 1985;77:358–362.

Hugo P, Bernier J, Krzystyniak K, et al. Transient inhibition of mixed lymphocyte reactivity by dieldrin in mice. *Toxicol Lett*. 1988a;41:1–9.

Hugo P, Bernier J, Krzystyniak K, et al. Abrogation of graft-versus-host reaction by dieldrin in mice. *Toxicol Lett*. 1988b;41:11–22.

Hussain I, Piepenbrink MS, Fitch KJ, et al. Developmental immunotoxicity of cyclosporin-A in rats: age-associated differential effects. *Toxicology*. 2005;206:273–284.

Ichinohe T, Lee HK, Ogura Y, et al. Inflammasome recognition of influenza virus is essential for adaptive immune responses. *J Exp Med*. 2009;206:79–87.

ICHS8: *International Conference on Harmonization, Immunotoxicity Studies for Human Pharmaceuticals*; 2006. http://www.ema.eurpoa.eu/pdfs/human/ich/16723504en.pdf

In SW, Son EW, Rhee DK, et al. Methamphetamine administration produces immunomodulation in mice. *J Toxicol Environ Health A*. 2005;68:2133–2145.

IPCS. *Environmental Health Criteria 180: Principles and Methods for Assessing Direct Immunotoxicity Associated with Exposure to Chemicals*. Geneva, Switzerland: Safety IPoC, World Health Organization; 1996.

Islam Z, Harkema JR, Pestka JJ. Satratoxin G from the black mold *Stachybotrys chartarum* evokes olfactory sensory neuron loss and inflammation in the murine nose and brain. *Environ Health Perspect*. 2006;114:1099–1107.

Jankowski MM, Ignatowska-Jankowska B, Glac W, et al. Cocaine administration increases CD4/CD8 lymphocyte ratio in peripheral blood despite lymphopenia and elevated corticosterone. *Int Immunopharmacol*. 2010;10:1229–1234.

Jenkins DJ, Kendall CW, Connelly PW, et al. Effects of high- and low-isoflavone (phytoestrogen) soy foods on inflammatory biomarkers and proinflammatory cytokines in middle-aged men and women. *Metabolism* 2002;51:919–924.

Jeon YJ, Han SH, Yang KH, et al. Induction of liver-associated transforming growth factor beta 1 (TGF-beta 1) mRNA expression by carbon tetrachloride leads to the inhibition of T helper 2 cell-associated lymphokines. *Toxicol Appl Pharmacol.* 1997;144:27–35.

Jeong TC, Jordan SD, Matulka RA, et al. Immunosuppression induced by acute exposure to cocaine is dependent on metabolism by cytochrome P450. *J Pharmacol Exp Ther.* 1996;276:1257–1265.

Jia P, Shi T, Cai Y, et al. Demonstration of two novel methods for predicting functional siRNA efficiency. *BMC Bioinform.* 2006;7:271.

Jiang X, Khursigara G, Rubin RL. Transformation of lupus-inducing drugs to cytotoxic products by activated neutrophils. *Science.* 1994;266:810–813.

Jirova D, Sperlingova I, Halaskova M, et al. Immunotoxic effects of carbon tetrachloride—the effect on morphology and function of the immune system in mice. *Cent Eur J Public Health.* 1996;4:16–20.

Joffe A, Yancy WS. Legalization of marijuana: potential impact on youth. *Pediatrics.* 2004;113:e632–e638.

Johnson KW, Munson AE, Kim DH, et al. Role of reactive metabolites in suppression of humoral immunity by *N*-nitrosodimethylamine. *J Pharmacol Exp Ther.* 1987;240:847–855.

Joseph P, He Q, Umbright C. Heme-oxygenase 1 gene expression is a marker for hexavalent chromium-induced stress and toxicity in human dermal fibroblasts. *Toxicol Sci.* 2008;103:325–334.

Jung WW, Kim EM, Lee EH, et al. Formaldehyde exposure induces airway inflammation by increasing eosinophil infiltrations through the regulation of reactive oxygen species production. *Environ Toxicol Pharmacol.* 2007;24:174–182.

Jusko TA, De Roos AJ, Schwartz SM, et al. Maternal and early postnatal polychlorinated biphenyl exposure in relation to total serum immunoglobulin concentrations in 6-month-old infants. *J Immunotoxicol.* 2011;8:95–100.

Jutel M, Akdis CA. T-cell subset regulation in atopy. *Curr Allergy Asthma Rep.* 2011;11:139–145.

Kalland T. Alterations of antibody response in female mice after neonatal exposure to diethylstilbestrol. *J Immunol.* 1980;124:194–198.

Kalland T, Strand O, Forsberg JG. Long-term effects of neonatal estrogen treatment on mitogen responsiveness of mouse spleen lymphocytes. *J Natl Cancer Inst.* 1979;63:413–421.

Kamath AB, Camacho I, Nagarkatti PS, et al. Role of Fas–Fas ligand interactions in 2,3,7,8-tetrachlorodibenzo-*p*-dioxin (TCDD)-induced immunotoxicity: increased resistance of thymocytes from Fas-deficient (lpr) and Fas ligand-defective (gld) mice to TCDD-induced toxicity. *Toxicol Appl Pharmacol.* 1999;160:141–155.

Kaminski NE, Barnes DW, Jordan SD, et al. The role of metabolism in carbon tetrachloride-mediated immunosuppression: in vivo studies. *Toxicol Appl Pharmacol.* 1990;102:9–20.

Kaminski NE, Holsapple MP. Cell type responsible for SAA-induced immunosuppression in casein-treated preamyloid mice. *J Immunol.* 1987;139:1804–1811.

Kaminski NE, Jordan SD, Holsapple MP. Suppression of humoral and cell-mediated immune responses by carbon tetrachloride. *Fundam Appl Toxicol.* 1989a;12:117–128.

Kaminski NE, Jordan SD, Page D, et al. Suppression of humoral immune responses by dialkylnitrosamines: structure–activity relationships. *Fundam Appl Toxicol.* 1989b;12:321–332.

Kammuller ME, Thomas C, De Bakker JM, et al. The popliteal lymph node assay in mice to screen for the immune disregulating potential of chemicals—a preliminary study. *Int J Immunopharmacol.* 1989;11:293–300.

Kanda N, Tsuchida T, Tamaki K. Estrogen enhancement of anti-double-stranded DNA antibody and immunoglobulin G production in peripheral blood mononuclear cells from patients with systemic lupus erythematosus. *Arthritis Rheum.* 1999;42:328–337.

Kane KL, Ashton FA, Schmitz JL, et al. Determination of natural killer cell function by flow cytometry. *Clin Diagn Lab Immunol.* 1996;3:295–300.

Kaplan BL, Rockwell CE, Kaminski NE. Evidence for cannabinoid receptor-dependent and -independent mechanisms of action in leukocytes. *J Pharmacol Exp Ther.* 2003;306:1077–1085.

Kaplan DH. In vivo function of Langerhans cells and dermal dendritic cells. *Trends Immunol.* 2010;31:446–451.

Karmaus PW, Chen W, Crawford RB, et al. Deletion of cannabinoid receptors 1 and 2 exacerbates APC function to increase inflammation and cellular immunity during influenza infection. *J Leukoc Biol.* 2011;90(5):983–995.

Karmaus W, Brooks KR, Nebe T, et al. Immune function biomarkers in children exposed to lead and organochlorine compounds: a cross-sectional study. *Environ Health.* 2005;4:5.

Karol MH, Cormier Y, Donham KJ, et al. Animal models. *Am J Ind Med.* 1994;25:135–138.

Karrow NA, McCay JA, Brown R, et al. Oxymetholone modulates cell-mediated immunity in male B6C3F1 mice. *Drug Chem Toxicol.* 2000;23:621–644.

Karrow NA, McCay JA, Brown RD, et al. Oral exposure to atrazine modulates cell-mediated immune function and decreases host resistance to the B16F10 tumor model in female B6C3F1 mice. *Toxicology.* 2005;209:15–28.

Kasper-Sonnenberg M, Sugiri D, Wurzler S, et al. Prevalence of nickel sensitization and urinary nickel content of children are increased by nickel in ambient air. *Environ Res.* 111:266-273, 2011.

Kasten-Jolly J, Heo Y, Lawrence DA. Impact of developmental lead exposure on splenic factors. *Toxicol Appl Pharmacol.* 2010;247:105–115.

Kately JR, Bazzell SJ. Immunological studies in cattle exposed to polybrominated biphenyl. *Environ Health Perspect.* 1978;23:750.

Katika MR, Hendriksen PJ, van Loveren H, et al. Exposure of Jurkat cells to bis (tri-*n*-butyltin) oxide (TBTO) induces transcriptomics changes indicative for ER- and oxidative stress, T cell activation and apoptosis. *Toxicol Appl Pharmacol.* 2011;254:311–322.

Kawabata TT, White KL Jr. Benzo(a)pyrene metabolism by murine spleen microsomes. *Cancer Res.* 1989;49:5816–5822.

Kawabata TT, White KL Jr. Enhancement of in vivo and in vitro murine immune responses by the cyclophosphamide metabolite acrolein. *Cancer Res.* 1988;48:41–45.

Kayama F, Yamashita U, Kawamoto T, et al. Selective depletion of immature thymocytes by oral administration of ethylene glycol monomethyl ether. *Int J Immunopharmacol.* 1991;13:531–540.

Kazlauskas A, Poellinger L, Pongratz I. Evidence that the co-chaperone p23 regulates ligand responsiveness of the dioxin (aryl hydrocarbon) receptor. *J Biol Chem.* 1999;274:13519–13524.

Kenna JG, Neuberger J, Williams R. Identification by immunoblotting of three halothane-induced liver microsomal polypeptide antigens recognized by antibodies in sera from patients with halothane-associated hepatitis. *J Pharmacol Exp Ther.* 1987;242:733–740.

Kerkvliet NI. Recent advances in understanding the mechanisms of TCDD immunotoxicity. *Int Immunopharmacol.* 2002;2:277–291.

Kerkvliet NI, Baecher-Steppan L, Smith BB, et al. Role of the Ah locus in suppression of cytotoxic T lymphocyte activity by halogenated aromatic hydrocarbons (PCBs and TCDD): structure–activity relationships and effects in C57Bl/6 mice congenic at the Ah locus. *Fundam Appl Toxicol.* 1990;14:532–541.

Kerkvliet NI, Brauner JA. Flow cytometric analysis of lymphocyte subpopulations in the spleen and thymus of mice exposed to an acute immunosuppressive dose of 2,3,7,8-tetrachlorodibenzo-*p*-dioxin (TCDD). *Environ Res.* 1990;52:146–154.

Kerkvliet NI, Burleson GR. Immunotoxicity of TCDD and related halogenated aromatic hydrocarbons, in Dean JH, Luster MI, Munson AE, et al., eds. *Immunotoxicology and Immunopharmacology.* New York: Raven Press, 1994, pp. 97–121.

Kerkvliet NI, Shepherd DM, Baecher-Steppan L. T lymphocytes are direct, aryl hydrocarbon receptor (AhR)-dependent targets of 2,3,7,8-tetrachlorodibenzo-*p*-dioxin (TCDD): AhR expression in both CD4+ and CD8+ T cells is necessary for full suppression of a cytotoxic T lymphocyte response by TCDD. *Toxicol Appl Pharmacol.* 2002;185:146–152.

Khodoun M, Strait R, Orekov T, et al. Peanuts can contribute to anaphylactic shock by activating complement. *J Allergy Clin Immunol.* 2009;123:342–351.

Khvorova A, Reynolds A, Jayasena SD. Functional siRNAs and miRNAs exhibit strand bias. *Cell.* 2003;115:209–216.

Kiecolt-Glaser JK, Glaser R, Gravenstein S, et al. Chronic stress alters the immune response to influenza virus vaccine in older adults. *Proc Natl Acad Sci USA.* 1996;93:3043–3047.

Kilburn KH, Warshaw RH. Chemical-induced autoimmunity, in Dean JH, Luster MI, Munson AE, et al. eds. *Immunotoxicology and Immunopharmacology.* New York: Raven Press; 1994:523–538.

Kilburn KH, Warshaw RH. Prevalence of symptoms of systemic lupus erythematosus (SLE) and of fluorescent antinuclear antibodies associated with chronic exposure to trichloroethylene and other chemicals in well water. *Environ Res.* 1992;57:1–9.

Kim BS, Smialowicz RJ. The role of metabolism in 2-methoxyethanol-induced suppression of in vitro polyclonal antibody responses by rat and mouse lymphocytes. *Toxicology.* 1997;123:227–239.

Kim DH, Yang KH, Johnson KW, et al. Role of the transfer of metabolites from hepatocytes to splenocytes in the suppression of in vitro antibody response by dimethylnitrosamine. *Biochem Pharmacol.* 1988;37:2765–2771.

Kim J, Jeong H. Suppression of inducible nitric oxide synthase and tumor necrosis a expression by bisphenol A via nuclear factor kappa B inactivation in macrophages. *Toxicol Sci.* 2003;71:153–154.

Kim SR, Lee KS, Park SJ, et al. PTEN down-regulates IL-17 expression in a murine model of toluene diisocyanate-induced airway disease. *J Immunol.* 2007;179:6820–6829.

Kimber I, Dearman RJ, Basketter DA, et al. The local lymph node assay: past, present and future. *Contact Dermatitis.* 2002;47:315–328.

Kimura A, Kishimoto T. Th17 cells in inflammation. *Int Immunopharmacol.* 2011;11:319–322.

Klaassen CD, Liu J, Diwan BA. Metallothionein protection of cadmium toxicity. *Toxicol Appl Pharmacol.* 2009;238:215–220.

Klecak G. Identification of contact allergens: predictive tests in animals, in Marzulli FN, Maibach HI, eds. *Dermatotoxicology.* New York: Hemisphere; 1987:227–290.

Kojima H, Katsura E, Takeuchi S, et al. Screening for estrogen and androgen receptor activities in 200 pesticides by in vitro reporter gene assays using Chinese hamster ovary cells. *Environ Health Perspect.* 2004;112:524–531.

Kojima H, Sata F, Takeuchi S, et al. Comparative study of human and mouse pregnane X receptor agonistic activity in 200 pesticides using in vitro reporter gene assays. *Toxicology.* 2011;280:77–87.

Koller LD. Immunotoxicology of heavy metals. *Int J Immunopharmacol.* 1980;2:269–279.

Kooijman R, Devos S, Hooghe-Peters E. Inhibition of in vitro cytokine production by human peripheral blood mononuclear cells treated with xenobiotics: implications for the prediction of general toxicity and immunotoxicity. *Toxicol In Vitro.* 2010;24:1782–1789.

Kripke ML. Immunologic mechanisms in UV radiation carcinogenesis. *Adv Cancer Res.* 1981;34:69–106.

Krzystyniak K, Hugo P, Flipo D, et al. Increased susceptibility to mouse hepatitis virus 3 of peritoneal macrophages exposed to dieldrin. *Toxicol Appl Pharmacol.* 1985;80:397–408.

Ladics GS, Chapin RE, Hastings KL, et al. Developmental toxicology evaluations—issues with including neurotoxicology and immunotoxicology assessments in reproductive toxicology studies. *Toxicol Sci.* 2005;88:24–29.

Ladics GS, Cressman RF, Herouet-Guicheney C, et al. Bioinformatics and the allergy assessment of agricultural biotechnology products: industry practices and recommendations. *Regul Toxicol Pharmacol.* 2011;60:46–53.

Ladics GS, Kawabata TT, Munson AE, et al. Generation of 7,8-dihydroxy-9,10-epoxy-7,8,9,10-tetrahydrobenzo[a]pyrene by murine splenic macrophages. *Toxicol Appl Pharmacol.* 1992a;115:72–79.

Ladics GS, Kawabata TT, Munson AE, et al. Metabolism of benzo[a]pyrene by murine splenic cell types. *Toxicol Appl Pharmacol.* 1992b;116:248–257.

Ladics GS, Kawabata TT, White KL Jr. Suppression of the in vitro humoral immune response of mouse splenocytes by 7,12-dimethylbenz[a]anthracene metabolites and inhibition of immunosuppression by alpha-naphthoflavone. *Toxicol Appl Pharmacol.* 1991;110:31–44.

Ladics GS, Smith C, Elliott GS, et al. Further evaluation of the incorporation of an immunotoxicological functional assay for assessing humoral immunity for hazard identification purposes in rats in a standard toxicology study. *Toxicology.* 1998;126:137–152.

Ladics GS, Smith C, Heaps K, et al. Evaluation of the humoral immune response of CD rats following a 2-week exposure to the pesticide carbaryl by the oral, dermal, or inhalation routes. *J Toxicol Environ Health.* 1994;42:143–156.

Ladics GS, Smith C, Heaps K, et al. Possible incorporation of an immunotoxicological functional assay for assessing humoral immunity for hazard identification purposes in rats on standard toxicology study. *Toxicology.* 1995;96:225–238.

Lai ZW, Fiore NC, Hahn PJ, et al. Differential effects of diethylstilbestrol and 2,3,7,8-tetrachlorodibenzo-p-dioxin on thymocyte differentiation, proliferation, and apoptosis in bcl-2 transgenic mouse fetal thymus organ culture. *Toxicol Appl Pharmacol.* 2000;168:15–24.

Laiosa MD, Mills JH, Lai ZW, et al. Identification of stage-specific gene modulation during early thymocyte development by whole-genome profiling analysis after aryl hydrocarbon receptor activation. *Molecular Pharmacol.* 2010;77:773–783.

Laiosa MD, Wyman A, Murante FG, et al. Cell proliferation arrest within intrathymic lymphocyte progenitor cells causes thymic atrophy mediated by the aryl hydrocarbon receptor. *J Immunol.* 2003;171:4582–4591.

Lakhan SE, Rowland M. Whole plant cannabis extracts in the treatment of spasticity in multiple sclerosis: a systematic review. *BMC Neurol.* 2009;9:59.

Lall SB, Dan G. Role of corticosteroids in cadmium induced immunotoxicity. *Drug Chem Toxicol.* 1999;22:401–409.

Lane R, Ghazi SO, Whalen MM. Increases in cytosolic calcium ion levels in human natural killer cells in response to butyltin exposure. *Arch Environ Contam Toxicol.* 2009;57:816–825.

Lankveld DP, van Loveren H, Baken KA, et al. In vitro testing for direct immunotoxicity: state of the art. *Methods Mol Biol.* 2010;598:401–423.

LaPres JJ, Glover E, Dunham EE, et al. ARA9 modifies agonist signaling through an increase in cytosolic aryl hydrocarbon receptor. *J Biol Chem.* 2000;275:6153–6159.

Larsen ST, Roursgaard M, Jensen KA, et al. Nano titanium dioxide particles promote allergic sensitization and lung inflammation in mice. *Basic Clin Pharmacol Toxicol.* 2010;106:114–117.

Lawrence BP, Leid M, Kerkvliet NI. Distribution and behavior of the Ah receptor in murine T lymphocytes. *Toxicol Appl Pharmacol.* 1996;138:275–284.

Lay JC, Alexis NE, Kleeberger SR, et al. Ozone enhances markers of innate immunity and antigen presentation on airway monocytes in healthy individuals. *J Allergy Clin Immunol.* 2007;120:719–722.

Lee MH, Chung SW, Kang BY, et al. Enhanced interleukin-4 production in CD4+ T cells and elevated immunoglobulin E levels in antigen-primed mice by bisphenol A and nonylphenol, endocrine disruptors: involvement of nuclear factor-AT and Ca²⁺. *Immunology.* 2003;109:76–86.

Leevy CB, Elbeshbeshy HA. Immunology of alcoholic liver disease. *Clin Liver Dis.* 2005;9:55–66.

Lehto M, Kotovuori A, Palosuo K, et al. Hev b 6.01 and Hev b 5 induce proinflammatory cytokines and chemokines from peripheral blood mononuclear cells in latex allergy. *Clin Exp Allergy.* 2007;37:133–140.

Lemarie A, Morzadec C, Bourdonnay E, et al. Human macrophages constitute targets for immunotoxic inorganic arsenic. *J Immunol.* 2006;177:3019–3027.

LeVier DG, McCay JA, Stern ML, et al. Immunotoxicological profile of morphine sulfate in B6C3F1 female mice. *Fundam Appl Toxicol.* 1994;22:525–542.

Levy MH, Wheelock EF. Effects of intravenous silica on immune and nonimmune functions of the murine host. *J Immunol.* 1975;115:41–48.

Li Q. NK cell assays in immunotoxicity testing. *Methods Mol Biol.* 2010;598:207–219.

Li Q, Lauer FT, Liu KJ, et al. Low-dose synergistic immunosuppression of T-dependent antibody responses by polycyclic aromatic hydrocarbons and arsenic in C57BL/6J murine spleen cells. *Toxicol Appl Pharmacol.* 2010;245:344–351.

Limpens J, Garssen J, Scheper RJ. Local administration of cytostatic drugs enhances delayed-type hypersensitivity to Sendai virus in mice. *Clin Immunol Immunopathol.* 1990; 54:161–165.

Limpens J, Scheper RJ. Inhibition of T suppressor cell function by local administration of an active cyclophosphamide derivative at the sensitization site. *Clin Exp Immunol.* 1991;84:383–388.

Lio CW, Hsieh CS. Becoming self-aware: the thymic education of regulatory T cells. *Curr Opin Immunol*. 2011;23:213–219.

Loftis JM, Choi D, Hoffman W, et al. Methamphetamine causes persistent immune dysregulation: a cross-species, translational report. *Neurotox Res*. 2011;20:59–68.

Lu H, Crawford RB, Kaplan BL, et al. 2,3,7,8-Tetrachlorodibenzo-*p*-dioxin-mediated disruption of the CD40 ligand-induced activation of primary human B cells. *Toxicol Appl Pharmacol*. 2011;255(3):251–260.

Lu H, Crawford RB, North CM, et al. Establishment of an immunoglobulin m antibody-forming cell response model for characterizing immunotoxicity in primary human B cells. *Toxicol Sci*. 2009;112:363–373.

Lu H, Crawford RB, Suarez-Martinez JE, et al. Induction of the aryl hydrocarbon receptor-responsive genes and modulation of the immunoglobulin M response by 2,3,7,8-tetrachlorodibenzo-*p*-dioxin in primary human B cells. *Toxicol Sci*. 2010;118:86–97.

Lu T, Newton C, Perkins I, et al. Cannabinoid treatment suppresses the T helper cell polarizing function of mouse dendritic cells stimulated with *Legionella pneumophila* infection. *J Pharmacol Exp Ther*. 2006a;319(1):269–276.

Lu T, Newton C, Perkins I, et al. Role of cannabinoid receptors in Delta-9-tetrahydrocannabinol suppression of IL-12p40 in mouse bone marrow-derived dendritic cells infected with *Legionella pneumophila*. *Eur J Pharmacol*. 2006b;532:170–177.

Luebke RW. Parasite challenge as host resistance models for immunotoxicity testing. *Methods Mol Biol*. 2010;598:119–141.

Luebke RW, Chen DH, Dietert R, et al. The comparative immunotoxicity of five selected compounds following developmental or adult exposure. *J Toxicol Environ Health B Crit Rev*. 2006a;9:1–26.

Luebke RW, Holsapple MP, Ladics GS, et al. Immunotoxicogenomics: the potential of genomics technology in the immunotoxicity risk assessment process. *Toxicol Sci*. 2006b;94(1):22–27.

Luebke RW, Parks C, Luster MI. Suppression of immune function and susceptibility to infections in humans: association of immune function with clinical disease. *J Immunotoxicol*. 2004;1:15–24.

Lummus ZL, Alam R, Bernstein JA, et al. Diisocyanate antigen-enhanced production of monocyte chemoattractant protein-1, IL-8, and tumor necrosis factor-alpha by peripheral mononuclear cells of workers with occupational asthma. *J Allergy Clin Immunol*. 1998;102:265–274.

Luna AL, Acosta-Saavedra LC, Lopez-Carrillo L, et al. Arsenic alters monocyte superoxide anion and nitric oxide production in environmentally exposed children. *Toxicol Appl Pharmacol*. 2010;245:244–251.

Lundberg K, Grovnick K, Goldschmidt TJ. 2,3,7,8-tetrachlorodibenzo-*p*-dioxin (TCDD) alters intrathymic T cell development in mice. *Chem Biol Interact*. 1990;74:179.

Lundblad LK, Irvin CG, Adler A, et al. A reevaluation of the validity of unrestrained plethysmography in mice. *J Appl Physiol*. 2002;93:1198–1207.

Luo CY, Wang L, Sun C, et al. Estrogen enhances the functions of CD4(+)CD25(+)Foxp3(+) regulatory T cells that suppress osteoclast differentiation and bone resorption in vitro. *Cell Mol Immunol*. 2011;8:50–58.

Luster MI, Boorman GA, Dean JH. Effect of in utero exposure of diethylstilbestrol on the immune response in mice. *Toxicol Appl Pharmacol*. 1979;47:287–293.

Luster MI, Boorman GA, Dean JH, et al. The effect of adult exposure to diethylstilbestrol in the mouse: alterations in immunological functions. *J Reticuloendothel Soc*. 1980;28:561–569.

Luster MI, Dean JH, Germolec DR. Consensus workshop on methods to evaluate developmental immunotoxicity. *Environ Health Perspect*. 2003;111:579–583.

Luster MI, Gerberick GF. Immunotoxicology testing: past and future. *Methods Mol Biol*. 598:3–13, 2010.

Luster MI, Germolec DR, White KL Jr, et al. A comparison of three nucleoside analogs with anti-retroviral activity on immune and hematopoietic functions in mice: in vitro toxicity to precursor cells and microstromal environment. *Toxicol Appl Pharmacol*. 1989;101:328–339.

Luster MI, Hayes HT, Korach K, et al. Estrogen immunosuppression is regulated through estrogenic responses in the thymus. *J Immunol*. 1984;133:110–116.

Luster MI, Johnson VJ, Yucesoy B, et al. Biomarkers to assess potential developmental immunotoxicity in children. *Toxicol Appl Pharmacol*. 2005;206:229–236.

Luster MI, Munson AE, Thomas PT, et al. Development of a testing battery to assess chemical-induced immunotoxicity: National Toxicology Program's guidelines for immunotoxicity evaluation in mice. *Fundam Appl Toxicol*. 1988;10:2–19.

Luster MI, Parks CG, Germolec DR. Interpreting immunotoxicology data for risk assessment, in Luebke R, House R, Kimber I, eds. *Immunotoxicology and Immunopharmacology*. Boca Rotton, FL: CRC Press; 2007:35–47.

Luster MI, Portier C, Pait DG, et al. Risk assessment in immunotoxicology. I. Sensitivity and predictability of immune tests. *Fundam Appl Toxicol*. 1992;18:200–210.

Luster MI, Portier C, Pait DG, et al. Risk assessment in immunotoxicology. II. Relationships between immune and host resistance tests. *Fundam Appl Toxicol*. 1993;21:71–82.

Lutz PM, Wilson TJ, Ireland J, et al. Elevated immunoglobulin E (IgE) levels in children with exposure to environmental lead. *Toxicology*. 1999;134:63–78.

Ma Q, Whitlock JP Jr. A novel cytoplasmic protein that interacts with the Ah receptor, contains tetratricopeptide repeat motifs, and augments the transcriptional response to 2,3,7,8-tetrachlorodibenzo-*p*-dioxin. *J Biol Chem*. 1997;272:8878–8884.

Ma Y, Poisson L, Sanchez-Schmitz G, et al. Assessing the immunopotency of toll-like receptor agonists in an in vitro tissue-engineered immunological model. *Immunology*. 2010;130:374–387.

Mabilleau G, Kwon YM, Pandit H, et al. Metal-on-metal hip resurfacing arthroplasty: a review of periprosthetic biological reactions. *Acta Orthop*. 2008;79:734–747.

Magnusson B, Kligman AM. The identification of contact allergens by animal assay. The guinea pig maximization test. *J Invest Dermatol*. 1969;52:268–276.

Maibach H. Formaldehyde: effects on animal and human skin, in Gibson J, ed. *Formaldehyde Toxicity*. New York: Hemisphere; 1983:166–174.

Mallal S, Phillips E, Carosi G, et al. HLA-B*5701 screening for hypersensitivity to abacavir. *N Engl J Med*. 2008;358:568–579.

Marnell L, Mold C, Du Clos TW. C-reactive protein: ligands, receptors and role in inflammation. *Clin Immunol*. 2005;117:104–111.

Marshall NB, Kerkvliet NI. Dioxin and immune regulation: emerging role of aryl hydrocarbon receptor in the generation of regulatory T cells. *Ann N Y Acad Sci*. 2010;1183:25–37.

Martin PL, Breslin W, Rocca M, et al. Considerations in assessing the developmental and reproductive toxicity potential of biopharmaceuticals. *Birth Defects Res B Dev Reprod Toxicol*. 2009;86:176–203.

Martin-Chouly C, Morzadec C, Bonvalet M, et al. Inorganic arsenic alters expression of immune and stress response genes in activated primary human T lymphocytes. *Mol Immunol*. 2011;48:956–965.

Martinez FO, Sica A, Mantovani A, et al. Macrophage activation and polarization. *Front Biosci*. 2008;13:453–461.

Martinon F, Mayor A, Tschopp J. The inflammasomes: guardians of the body. *Annu Rev Immunol*. 2009;27:229–265.

Marzulli FN, Maibach HI. Contact allergy: predictive testing in humans, in Marzulli FN, Maibach HI, ed. *Dermatotoxicology*. New York: Hemisphere; 1987:319–340.

Matheson JM, Johnson VJ, Vallyathan V, et al. Exposure and immunological determinants in a murine model for toluene diisocyanate (TDI) asthma. *Toxicol Sci*. 2005;84:88–98.

Matulka RA, Jordan SD, Stanulis ED, et al. Evaluation of sex- and strain-dependency of cocaine-induced immunosuppression in B6C3F1 and DBA/2 mice. *J Pharmacol Exp Ther*. 1996;279:12–17.

Matveyeva M, Hartmann CB, Harrison MT, et al. Delta(9)-tetrahydrocannabinol selectively increases aspartyl cathepsin D proteolytic activity and impairs lysozyme processing by macrophages. *Int J Immunopharmacol*. 2000;22:373–381.

Mauri C. Regulation of immunity and autoimmunity by B cells. *Curr Opin Immunol*. 2010;22:761–767.

Maurice T, Romieu P. Involvement of the sigma1 receptor in the appetitive effects of cocaine. *Pharmacopsychiatry*. 2004;37(suppl 3):S198–S207.

McCleskey TM, Buchner V, Field RW, et al. Recent advances in understanding the biomolecular basis of chronic beryllium disease: a review. *Rev Environ Health*. 2009;24:75–115.

McCoy KL, Gainey D, Cabral GA. delta 9-Tetrahydrocannabinol modulates antigen processing by macrophages. *J Pharmacol Exp Ther.* 1995;273:1216–1223.

McDonough RJ, Madden JJ, Falek A, et al. Alteration of T and null lymphocyte frequencies in the peripheral blood of human opiate addicts: in vivo evidence for opiate receptor sites on T lymphocytes. *J Immunol.* 1980;125:2539–2543.

McGwin G, Lienert J, Kennedy JI. Formaldehyde exposure and asthma in children: a systematic review. *Environ Health Perspect.* 2010;118: 313–317.

McKallip RJ, Nagarkatti M, Nagarkatti PS. Immunotoxicity of AZT: inhibitory effect on thymocyte differentiation and peripheral T cell responsiveness to gp120 of human immunodeficiency virus. *Toxicol Appl Pharmacol.* 1995;131:53–62.

McKarns SC, Kaminski NE. TGF-beta 1 differentially regulates IL-2 expression and [3H]-thymidine incorporation in CD3 epsilon mAb- and CD28 mAb-activated splenocytes and thymocytes. *Immunopharmacology.* 2000;48:101–115.

McKarns SC, Schwartz RH, Kaminski NE. Smad3 is essential for TGF-beta 1 to suppress IL-2 production and TCR-induced proliferation, but not IL-2-induced proliferation. *J Immunol.* 2004;172:4275–4284.

Menna JH, Barnett JB, Soderberg LS. Influenza type A virus infection of mice exposed in utero to chlordane; survival and antibody studies. *Toxicol Lett.* 1985;24:45–52.

Michielsen CC, van Loveren H, Vos JG. The role of the immune system in hexachlorobenzene-induced toxicity. *Environ Health Perspect.* 1999;107(suppl 5):783–792.

Miller K, Brown RC. The immune system and asbestos-associated disease, in Dean JH, Luster MI, Munson AE, et al., eds. *Immunotoxicology and Immunopharmacology.* New York: Raven Press; 1985:429–440.

Mishell RI, Dutton RW. Immunization of dissociated mouse spleen cell culture from normal mice. *J Exp Med.* 1967;126:423–442.

Mitjans M, Viviani B, Lucchi L, et al. Role of p38 MAPK in the selective release of IL-8 induced by chemical allergen in naive THp-1 cells. *Toxicol In Vitro.* 2008;22:386–395.

Mitzner W, Tankersley C. Interpreting Penh in mice. *J Appl Physiol.* 2003;94:828–831; author reply 831–822.

Miyawaki T, Moriya N, Nagaoki T, et al. Maturation of B-cell differentiation ability and T-cell regulatory function in infancy and childhood. *Immunol Rev.* 1981;57:61–87.

Moed H, Boorsma DM, Stoof TJ, et al. Nickel-responding T cells are CD4+ CLA+ CD45RO+ and express chemokine receptors CXCR3, CCR4 and CCR10. *Br J Dermatol.* 2004;151:32–41.

Mondal TK, Li D, Swami K, et al. Mercury impairment of mouse thymocyte survival in vitro: involvement of cellular thiols. *J Toxicol Environ Health A.* 2005;68:535–556.

Moon Y, Pestka JJ. Vomitoxin-induced cyclooxygenase-2 gene expression in macrophages mediated by activation of ERK and p38 but not JNK mitogen-activated protein kinases. *Toxicol Sci.* 2002;69:373–382.

Morandell S, Stasyk T, Grosstessner-Hain K, et al. Phosphoproteomics strategies for the functional analysis of signal transduction. *Proteomics.* 2006;6(14):4047–4056.

Morice WG, Brunn GJ, Wiederrecht G, et al. Rapamycin-induced inhibition of p34cdc2 kinase activation is associated with G1/S-phase growth arrest in T lymphocytes. *J Biol Chem.* 1993;268:3734–3738.

Mosmann TR, Coffman RL. Heterogeneity of cytokine secretion patterns and functions of helper T cells. *Adv Immunol.* 1989;46:111–147.

Mosmann TR, Schumacher JH, Street NF, et al. Diversity of cytokine synthesis and function of mouse CD4+ T cells. *Immunol Rev.* 1991;123:209–229.

Mounho BJ, Burchiel SW. Alterations in human B cell calcium homeostasis by polycyclic aromatic hydrocarbons: possible associations with cytochrome P450 metabolism and increased protein tyrosine phosphorylation. *Toxicol Appl Pharmacol.* 1998;149:80–89.

Murante FG, Gasiewicz TA. Hemopoietic progenitor cells are sensitive targets of 2,3,7,8-tetrachlorodibenzo-p-dioxin in C57BL/6J mice. *Toxicol Sci.* 2000;54:374–383.

Murphy K, Travers P, Walport M. *Janeway's Immunobiology.* New York: Taylor and Francis; 2007.

Murphy WG, Kelton JG. Immune haemolytic anaemia and thrombocytopenia: drugs and autoantibodies. *Biochem Soc Trans.* 1991;19:183–186.

Mydlarski P, Katz A, Sauder D. Contact dermatitis, in Middleton EJ, Reed C, Ellis E, eds. *Allergy Principles and Practice.* St. Louis: Mosby; 1998:1141–1143.

Myers MJ, Schook LB. Immunotoxicity of nitrosamines, in Smialowicz RJ, Holsapple MP, eds. *Experimental Immunotoxicology.* Boca Rotton, FL: CRC Press; 1996:351–366.

Nagayama J, Tsuji H, Iida T, et al. Immunologic effects of perinatal exposure to dioxins, PCBs and organochlorine pesticides in Japanese infants. *Chemosphere.* 2007;67:S393–S398.

Nathan C. Neutrophils and immunity: challenges and opportunities. *Nat Rev Immunol.* 2006;6:173–182.

Ndebele K, Tchounwou PB, McMurray RW. Coumestrol, bisphenol-A, DDT, and TCDD modulation of interleukin-2 expression in activated CD+4 Jurkat T cells. *Int J Environ Res Public Health.* 2004;1:3–11.

Neishabouri EZ, Hassan ZM, Azizi E, et al. Evaluation of immunotoxicity induced by diazinon in C57BL/6 mice. *Toxicology.* 2004;196:173–179.

Ng S, Yoshida K, Zelikoff JT. Tumor challenges in immunotoxicity testing. *Methods Mol Biol.* 2010;598:143–155.

Noh G, Lee JH. Regulatory B cells and allergic diseases. Allergy Asthma Immunol Res 2011;3:168–177.

Nohara K, Izumi H, Tamura S, et al. Effect of low-dose 2,3,7,8-tetrachlorodibenzo-p-dioxin (TCDD) on influenza A virus-induced mortality in mice. *Toxicology.* 2002;170:131–138.

North CM, Crawford RB, Lu H, et al. 2,3,7,8-tetrachlorodibenzo-p-dioxin-mediated suppression of toll-like receptor stimulated B-lymphocyte activation and initiation of plasmacytic differentiation. *Toxicol Sci.* 2010;116:99–112.

North CM, Crawford RB, Lu H, et al. Simultaneous in vivo time course and dose response evaluation for TCDD-induced impairment of the LPS-stimulated primary IgM response. *Toxicol Sci.* 2009;112:123–132.

NRC. Biologic Markers in Immunotoxicology. Washington, DC: National Academies Press; 1992. ISBN 0-309-04389-1.

NTP. *Explanation of Levels of Evidence for Immune System Toxicity.* National Toxicology Program; 2009. http://ntp.niehs. gov/?objectid+CC5E017E-F1F6-975E-7D86DAA5256F6AB8

Nunez GM, Estrada I, Calderon-Aranda ES. DDT inhibits the functional activation of murine macrophages and decreases resistance to infection by *Mycobacterium microti. Toxicology.* 2002;174:201–210.

OECD. *OECD Guideline for the Testing of Chemicals—Extended One-generation Reproductive Toxicity Study.* France: Organization for Economic Cooperation and Development; 2010. http://www.oecd.org/dataoecd/23/10/46466062.pdf

Ohkura N, Hamaguchi M, Sakaguchi S. FOXP3+ regulatory T cells: control of FOXP3 expression by pharmacological agents. *Trends Pharmacol Sci.* 2011;32:158–166.

Ohnishi T, Yoshida T, Igarashi A, et al. Effects of possible endocrine disruptors on MyD88-independent TLR4 signaling. *FEMS Immunol Med Microbiol.* 2008;52:293–295.

Okey AB, Bondy GP, Mason M, et al. Temperature-dependent cytosol-to-nuclear translocation of the Ah receptor for 2,3,7,8-tetrachlorodibenzo-p-dioxin in continuous cell culture lines. *J Biol Chem.* 1980;255:11415–11422.

Olgun S, Gogal RM Jr, Adeshina F, et al. Pesticide mixtures potentiate the toxicity in murine thymocytes. *Toxicology.* 2004;196:181–195.

Ongradi J, Kovesdi V. Factors that may impact on immunosenescence: an appraisal. *Immun Ageing.* 2010;7:7.

Ou DW, Shen ML, Luo YD. Effects of cocaine on the immune system of Balb/C mice. *Clin Immunol Immunopathol.* 1989;52:305–312.

Paavonen T, Andersson LC, Adlercreutz H. Sex hormone regulation of in vitro immune response. Estradiol enhances human B cell maturation via inhibition of suppressor T cells in pokeweed mitogen-stimulated cultures. *J Exp Med.* 1981;154:1935–1945.

Page TJ, O'Brien S, Holston K, et al. 7,12-Dimethylbenz[*a*]anthracene-induced bone marrow toxicity is p53-dependent. *Toxicol Sci.* 2003;74:85–92.

Pathak N, Khandelwal S. Impact of cadmium in T lymphocyte subsets and cytokine expression: differential regulation by oxidative stress and apoptosis. *Biometals.* 2008;21:179–187.

Pathak N, Khandelwal S. Oxidative stress and apoptotic changes in murine splenocytes exposed to cadmium. *Toxicology*. 2006;220:26–36.

Pauluhn J. Animal models for respiratory hypersensitivity, in Vohr H-W, ed. *Encyclopedic Reference of Immunotoxicology*. Heidelberg: Springer, 2005:15–21.

Pawelec G, Akbar A, Beverley P, et al. Immunosenescence and cytomegalovirus: where do we stand after a decade? *Immun Ageing*. 2010;7:13.

Peden DB. The role of oxidative stress and innate immunity in O(3) and endotoxin-induced human allergic airway disease. *Immunol Rev*. 2011;242:91–105.

Peden-Adams MM, Eudaly JG, Heesemann LM, et al. Developmental immunotoxicity of trichloroethylene (TCE): studies in B6C3F1 mice. *J Environ Sci Health A Tox Hazard Subst Environ Eng*. 2006;41:249–271.

Pelletier L, Castedo M, Bellon B, et al. Mercury and autoimmunity, in Dean JH, Luster MI, Munson AE, et al., eds. *Immunotoxicology and Immunopharmacology*. New York: Raven Press; 1994:539–552.

Pelletier M, Roberge CJ, Gauthier M, et al. Activation of human neutrophils in vitro and dieldrin-induced neutrophilic inflammation in vivo. *J Leukoc Biol*. 2001;70:367–373.

Peng X, Mosser DM, Adler MW, et al. Morphine enhances interleukin-12 and the production of other pro-inflammatory cytokines in mouse peritoneal macrophages. *J Leukoc Biol*. 2000;68:723–728.

Perdew GH. Association of the Ah receptor with the 90-kDa heat shock protein. *J Biol Chem*. 1988;263:13802–13805.

Pernis B, Paronetto F. Adjuvant effect of silica (tridymite) on antibody production. *Proc Soc Exp Biol Med*. 1962;110:390–392.

Person RJ, Whalen MM. Effects of butyltin exposures on MAP kinase-dependent transcription regulators in human natural killer cells. *Toxicol Mech Methods*. 2010;20:227–233.

Pessah IN, Beltzner C, Burchiel SW, et al. A bioactive metabolite of benzo[*a*]pyrene, benzo[*a*]pyrene-7,8-dione, selectively alters microsomal Ca^{2+} transport and ryanodine receptor function. *Mol Pharmacol*. 2001;59:506–513.

Pestka JJ. Deoxynivalenol-induced IgA production and IgA nephropathy-aberrant mucosal immune response with systemic repercussions. *Toxicol Lett*. 2003;140–141:287–295.

Pestka JJ, Yan D, King LE. Flow cytometric analysis of the effects of in vitro exposure to vomitoxin (deoxynivalenol) on apoptosis in murine T, B and IgA+ cells. *Food Chem Toxicol*. 1994;32:1125–1136.

Peterson PK, Gekker G, Chao CC, et al. Cocaine potentiates HIV-1 replication in human peripheral blood mononuclear cell cocultures. Involvement of transforming growth factor-beta. *J Immunol*. 1991;146:81–84.

Phiel KL, Henderson RA, Adelman SJ, et al. Differential estrogen receptor gene expression in human peripheral blood mononuclear cell populations. *Immunol. Lett*. 2005;97:107–113.

Phillips EJ, Wong GA, Kaul R, et al. Clinical and immunogenetic correlates of abacavir hypersensitivity. *AIDS* 2005;19:979–981.

Pichler WJ. Drug-induced autoimmunity. *Curr Opin Allergy Clin Immunol*. 2003;3:249–253.

Pieters R, Albers R. Screening tests for autoimmune-related immunotoxicity. *Environ Health Perspect*. 1999;107(suppl 5):673–677.

Pinchuk LM, Lee SR, Filipov NM. In vitro atrazine exposure affects the phenotypic and functional maturation of dendritic cells. *Toxicol Appl Pharmacol*. 2007;223:206–217.

Plitnik LM, Herzyk DJ. The T-dependent antibody response to keyhole limpet hemocyanin in rodents. *Methods Mol Biol*. 2010;598:159–171.

Plitnick LM, Loveless SE, Ladics GS, et al. Cytokine profiling for chemical sensitizers: application of the ribonuclease protection assay and effect of dose. *Toxicol Appl Pharmacol*. 2002;179:145–154.

Plitnick LM, Loveless SE, Ladics GS, et al. Cytokine mRNA profiles for isocyanates with known and unknown potential to induce respiratory sensitization. *Toxicology*. 2005;207:487–499.

Plitnick LM, Loveless SE, Ladics GS, et al. Identifying airway sensitizers: cytokine mRNA profiles induced by various anhydrides. *Toxicology*. 2003;193:191–201.

Polanczyk MJ, Carson BD, Subramanian S, et al. Cutting edge: estrogen drives expansion of the CD4+CD25+ regulatory T cell compartment. *J Immunol*. 2004;173:2227–2230.

Poland A, Knutson JC. 2,3,7,8-tetrachlorodibenzo-*p*-dioxin and related aromatic hydrocarbons: examination of the mechanism of toxicity. *Annu Rev Pharmacol Toxicol*. 1982;22:517–554.

Pollard KM, Hultman P, Kono DH. Toxicology of autoimmune diseases. *Chem Res Toxicol*. 2010;23:455–466.

Pollenz RS, Sattler CA, Poland A. The aryl hydrocarbon receptor and aryl hydrocarbon receptor nuclear translocator protein show distinct subcellular localizations in Hepa 1c1c7 cells by immunfluorescence microscopy. *Mol Pharmacol*. 1994;45:428–438.

Pongratz IG, Masson GF, Poellinger L. Dual roles of the 90-kDa heat shock protein hsp90 in modulating functional activities of the dioxin receptor. *J Biol Chem*. 1992;267:13728–13734.

Potula R, Hawkins BJ, Cenna JM, et al. Methamphetamine causes mitochondrial oxidative damage in human T lymphocytes leading to functional impairment. *J Immunol*. 2010;185:2867–2876.

Powell JJ, Davis MV, Whalen MM. Glutathione diminishes tributyltin- and dibutyltin-induced loss of lytic function in human natural killer cells. *Drug Chem Toxicol*. 2009;32:9–16.

Probst MP, Reisz-Porszasz S, Agbunag RV, et al. Role of the aryl hydrocarbon receptor nuclear translocator protein in aryl hydrocarbon (Dioxin) receptor action. *Mol Pharmacol*. 1993;44:511–518.

Pruett S, Holladay SD, Prater MR, et al. The promise of genomics and proteomics in immunotoxicology and immunopharmacology, in Luebke R, House R, Kimber I, eds. *Immunotoxicology and Immunopharmacology*. New York: Raven Press; 2007:79–95.

Pruett SB, Barnes DB, Han YC, et al. Immunotoxicological characteristics of sodium methyldithiocarbamate. *Fundam Appl Toxicol*. 1992a;18:40–47.

Pruett SB, Fan R, Zheng Q. Involvement of three mechanisms in the alteration of cytokine responses by sodium methyldithiocarbamate. *Toxicol Appl Pharmacol*. 2006;213:172–178.

Pruett SB, Fan R, Zheng Q, et al. Modeling and predicting immunological effects of chemical stressors: characterization of a quantitative biomarker for immunological changes caused by atrazine and ethanol. *Toxicol Sci*. 2003;75:343–354.

Pruett SB, Han YC, Fuchs BA. Morphine suppresses primary humoral immune responses by a predominantly indirect mechanism. *J Pharmacol Exp Ther*. 1992b;262:923–928.

Pruett SB, Schwab C, Zheng Q, et al. Suppression of innate immunity by acute ethanol administration: a global perspective and a new mechanism beginning with inhibition of signaling through TLR3. *J Immunol*. 2004a;173:2715–2724.

Pruett SB, Zheng Q, Fan R, et al. Acute exposure to ethanol affects toll-like receptor signaling and subsequent responses: an overview of recent studies. *Alcohol*. 2004b;33:235–239.

Pruett SB, Zheng Q, Schwab C, et al. Sodium methyldithiocarbamate inhibits MAP kinase activation through toll-like receptor 4, alters cytokine production by mouse peritoneal macrophages, and suppresses innate immunity. *Toxicol Sci*. 2005;87:75–85.

Pyatt DW, Stillman WS, Irons RD. Hydroquinone, a reactive metabolite of benzene, inhibits NF-kappa B in primary human CD4+ T lymphocytes. *Toxicol Appl Pharmacol*. 1998;149:178–184.

Quintana FJ, Basso AS, Iglesias AH, et al. Control of T(reg) and T(H)17 cell differentiation by the aryl hydrocarbon receptor. *Nature*. 2008;453:65–71.

Raisuddin S, Singh KP, Zaidi SI, et al. Immunosuppressive effects of aflatoxin in growing rats. *Mycopathologia*. 1993;124:189–194.

Raulf-Heimsoth M, Merget R, Rihs HP, et al. T-cell receptor repertoire expression in workers with occupational asthma due to platinum salt. *Eur Respir J*. 2000;16:871–878.

Ravel G, Descotes J. Popliteal lymph node assay: facts and perspectives. *J Appl Toxicol*. 2005;25:451–458.

Ray A, Prefontaine KE. Physical association and functional antagonism between the p65 subunit of transcription factor NF-kappa B and the glucocorticoid receptor. *Proc Natl Acad Sci USA*. 1994;91:752–756.

Reed A, Dzon L, Loganathan BG, et al. Immunomodulation of human natural killer cell cytotoxic function by organochlorine pesticides. *Hum Exp Toxicol*. 2004;23:463–471.

Regal JF, Greene AL, Regal RR. Mechanisms of occupational asthma: not all allergens are equal. *Environ Health Prev Med*. 2007;12:165–171.

Reichle FM, Conzen PF. Halogenated inhalational anaesthetics. *Best Pract Res Clin Anaesthesiol*. 17:29–46.

Reyes H, Reisz-Porszasz S, Hankinson O. Identification of the Ah receptor nuclear translocator protein (ARNT) as a component of the DNA binding form of the Ah receptor. *Science*. 1992;256:1193–1195.

Reynolds JL, Mahajan SD, Aalinkeel R, et al. Modulation of the proteome of peripheral blood mononuclear cells from HIV-1-infected patients by drugs of abuse. *J Clin Immunol*. 2009a;29:646–656.

Reynolds JL, Mahajan SD, Aalinkeel R, et al. Proteomic analyses of the effects of drugs of abuse on monocyte-derived mature dendritic cells. *Immunol Invest*. 2009b;38:526–550.

Ricciotti E, FitzGerald GA. Prostaglandins and inflammation. *Arterioscler Thromb Vasc Biol*. 2011;31:986–1000.

Robinson MK, Babcock LS, Horn PA, et al. Specific antibody responses to subtilisin Carlsberg (Alcalase) in mice: development of an intranasal exposure model. *Fundam Appl Toxicol*. 1996;34:15–24.

Rodgers KE, Ellefson DD. Modulation of respiratory burst activity and mitogenic response of human peripheral blood mononuclear cells and murine splenocytes and peritoneal cells by malathion. *Fundam Appl Toxicol*. 1990;14:309–317.

Rogers TJ. Immunology as it pertains to drugs of abuse, AIDS and the neuroimmune axis: mediators and traffic. *J Neuroimmune Pharmacol*. 2011;6:20–27.

Rose NR. Autoimmunity, autoimmune diseases, in Vohr H-W, ed. *Encyclopedic Reference of Immunotoxicology*. Heidelberg: Springer; 2005:79–82.

Rosen F, Cooper M, Wedgewood R. The primary immunodeficiencies. *N Engl J Med*. 1995;333:431–440.

Rosenman KD, Rossman M, Hertzberg V, et al. HLA class II DPB1 and DRB1 polymorphisms associated with genetic susceptibility to beryllium toxicity. *Occup Environ Med*. 2011;68:487–493.

Roth MD, Whittaker KM, Choi R, et al. Cocaine and sigma-1 receptors modulate HIV infection, chemokine receptors, and the HPA axis in the huPBL-SCID model. *J Leukoc Biol*. 2005;78:1198–1203.

Rought SE, Yau PM, Chuang LF, et al. Effect of the chlorinated hydrocarbons heptachlor, chlordane, and toxaphene on retinoblastoma tumor suppressor in human lymphocytes. *Toxicol Lett*. 1999;104:127–135.

Rowe AM, Brundage KM, Schafer R, et al. Immunomodulatory effects of maternal atrazine exposure on male Balb/c mice. *Toxicol Appl Pharmacol*. 2006;214:69–77.

Roy S, Ninkovic J, Banerjee S, et al. Opioid drug abuse and modulation of immune function: consequences in the susceptibility to opportunistic infections. *J Neuroimmune Pharmacol*. 2011;6(4):442–465.

Roy S, Wang J, Gupta S, et al. Chronic morphine treatment differentiates T helper cells to Th2 effector cells by modulating transcription factors GATA 3 and T-bet. *J Neuroimmunol*. 2004;147:78–81.

Roychowdhury S, Svensson CK. Mechanisms of drug-induced delayed-type hypersensitivity reactions in the skin. *AAPS J*. 2005;7:E834–E846.

Ryan-Borchers TA, Park JS, Chew BP, et al. Soy isoflavones modulate immune function in healthy postmenopausal women. *Am J Clin Nutr*. 2006;83:1118–1125.

Ryman-Rasmussen JP, Cesta MF, Brody AR, et al. Inhaled carbon nanotubes reach the subpleural tissue in mice. *Nat Nanotechnol*. 2009;4:747–751.

Sabers CJ, Martin MM, Brunn GJ, et al. Isolation of a protein target of the FKBP12-rapamycin complex in mammalian cells. *J Biol Chem*. 1995;270:815–822.

Sacerdote P. Effects of in vitro and in vivo opioids on the production of IL-12 and IL-10 by murine macrophages. *Ann N Y Acad Sci*. 2003;992:129–140.

Sachdeva N, Asthana V, Brewer TH, et al. Impaired restoration of plasmacytoid dendritic cells in HIV-1-infected patients with poor CD4 T cell reconstitution is associated with decrease in capacity to produce IFN-alpha but not proinflammatory cytokines. *J Immunol*. 2008;181:2887–2897.

Sadakane K, Takano H, Ichinose T, et al. Formaldehyde enhances mite allergen-induced eosinophilic inflammation in the murine airway. *J Environ Pathol Toxicol Oncol*. 2002;21:267–276.

Sager TM, Kommineni C, Castranova V. Pulmonary response to intratracheal instillation of ultrafine versus fine titanium dioxide: role of particle surface area. *Part Fibre Toxicol*. 2008;5:17.

Saini Y, Greenwood KK, Merrill C, et al. Acute cobalt-induced lung injury and the role of hypoxia-inducible factor 1alpha in modulating inflammation. *Toxicol Sci*. 2010a;116:673–681.

Saini Y, Kim KY, Lewandowski R, et al. Role of hypoxia-inducible factor 1{alpha} in modulating cobalt-induced lung inflammation. *Am J Physiol Lung Cell Mol Physiol*. 2010b;298:L139–L147.

Saito R, Hirakawa S, Ohara H, et al. Nickel differentially regulates NFAT and NF-kappaB activation in T cell signaling. *Toxicol Appl Pharmacol*. 2011;254:245–255.

Sakaguchi S, Wing K, Onishi Y, et al. Regulatory T cells: how do they suppress immune responses? *Int Immunol*. 2009;21:1105–1111.

Salem ML, Hossain MS, Nomoto K. Mediation of the immunomodulatory effect of beta-estradiol on inflammatory responses by inhibition of recruitment and activation of inflammatory cells and their gene expression of TNF-alpha and IFN-gamma. *Int Arch Allergy Immunol*. 2000;121:235–245.

Sanders VM, Kohm AP. Sympathetic nervous system interaction with the immune system. *Int Rev Neurobiol*. 2002;52:17–41.

Sanders VM, Tucker AN, White KL Jr, et al. Humoral and cell-mediated immune status in mice exposed to trichloroethylene in the drinking water. *Toxicol Appl Pharmacol*. 1982;62:358–368.

Sanders VM, White KL Jr, Shopp GM Jr, et al. Humoral and cell-mediated immune status of mice exposed to 1,1,2-trichloroethane. *Drug Chem Toxicol*. 1985;8:357–372.

Sandy P, Ventura A, Jacks T. Mammalian RNAi: a practical guide. *Biotechniques*. 2005;39:215–224.

Sawai C, Anderson K, Walser-Kuntz D. Effect of bisphenol A on murine immune function: modulation of interferon-gamma, IgG2a, and disease symptoms in NZB X NZW F1 mice. *Environ Health Perspect*. 2003;111:1883–1887.

Schatz AR, Koh WS, Kaminski NE. Delta 9-tetrahydrocannabinol selectively inhibits T-cell dependent humoral immune responses through direct inhibition of accessory T-cell function. *Immunopharmacology*. 1993;26:129–137.

Schatz AR, Lee M, Condie RB, et al. Cannabinoid receptors CB1 and CB2: a characterization of expression and adenylate cyclase modulation within the immune system. *Toxicol Appl Pharmacol*. 1997;142:278–287.

Scheinman RI, Cogswell PC, Lofquist AK, et al. Role of transcriptional activation of I kappa B alpha in mediation of immunosuppression by glucocorticoids. *Science*. 1995;270:283–286.

Schiraldi M, Monestier M. How can a chemical element elicit complex immunopathology? Lessons from mercury-induced autoimmunity. *Trends Immunol*. 2009;30:502–509.

Schneider D, Manzan MA, Crawford RB, et al. 2,3,7,8-Tetrachlorodibenzo-p-dioxin (TCDD)-mediated impairment of B cell differentiation involves dysregulation of paired box 5 (Pax5) isoform, Pax5a. *J Pharmacol Exp Ther*. 2008;326:463–474.

Schneider D, Manzan MA, Yoo BS, et al. Involvement of Blimp-1 and AP-1 dysregulation in the 2,3,7,8-Tetrachlorodibenzo-p-dioxin-mediated suppression of the IgM response by B cells. *Toxicol Sci*. 2009;108:377–388.

Schule R, Umesono K, Mangelsdorf DJ, et al. Jun-Fos and receptors for vitamins A and D recognize a common response element in the human osteocalcin gene. *Cell*. 1990;61:497–504.

Schwab CL, Fan R, Zheng Q, et al. Modeling and predicting stress-induced immunosuppression in mice using blood parameters. *Toxicol Sci*. 2005; 83:101–113.

Schwartz T. 25 years of UV-induced immunosuppression mediated by T cells—from disregarded T suppressor cells to highly respected regulatory T cells. *Photochem Photobiol*. 2008;84:10–18.

Schwarz DS, Hutvagner G, Du T, et al. Asymmetry in the assembly of the RNAi enzyme complex. *Cell*. 2003;115:199–208.

Schweitzer C, Keller F, Schmitt MP, et al. Morphine stimulates HIV replication in primary cultures of human Kupffer cells. *Res Virol*. 1991;142:189–195.

Sekizawa J. Low-dose effects of bisphenol A: a serious threat to human health? *J Toxicol Sci*. 2008;33:389–403.

Selgrade MK. Immunotoxicity: the risk is real. *Toxicol Sci*. 2007;100:328–332.

Selgrade MK. Use of immunotoxicity data in health risk assessments: uncertainties and research to improve the process. *Toxicology*. 1999;133:59–72.

Selgrade MK, Cooper GS, Germolec DR, et al. Linking environmental agents and autoimmune disease: an agenda for future research. *Environ Health Perspect*. 1999;107(suppl 5):811–813.

Selgrade MK, Cooper KD, Devlin RB, et al. Immunotoxicity—bridging the gap between animal research and human health effects. *Fundam Appl Toxicol*. 1995;24:13–21.

Selgrade MK, Gilmour MI. Effects of gaseous air pollutants on immune responses and susceptibility to infectious and allergic diseases, in Dean JH, Luster MI, Munson AE, et al., ed,. *Immunotoxicology and Immunopharmacology*. New York: Raven Press, 1994, pp. 395–411.

Selgrade MK, Lemanske RF Jr, Gilmour MI, et al. Induction of asthma and the environment: what we know and need to know. *Environ Health Perspect*. 2006;114:615–619.

Serhan CN, Savill J. Resolution of inflammation: the beginning programs the end. *Nat Immunol*. 2005;6:1191–1197.

Sgro C. Side-effects of a monoclonal antibody, muromonab CD3/ orthoclone OKT3: bibliographic review. *Toxicology*. 1995;105:23–29.

Shah D, Chowdhury MM. Rubber allergy. *Clin Dermatol*. 2011;29:278–286.

Shapiro HM. *Practical Flow Cytometry*. Hoboken, NJ: John Wiley & Sons, Inc; 2003.

Shelnutt SR, Goad P, Belsito DV. Dermatological toxicity of hexavalent chromium. *Crit Rev Toxicol*. 2007;37:375–387.

Sherwood RL, O'Shea W, Thomas PT, et al. Effects of inhalation of ethylene dichloride on pulmonary defenses of mice and rats. *Toxicol Appl Pharmacol*. 1987;91:491–496.

Shim GJ, Gherman D, Kim HJ, et al. Differential expression of oestrogen receptors in human secondary lymphoid tissues. *J Pathol*. 2006;208:408–414.

Shim GJ, Kis LL, Warner M, et al. Autoimmune glomerulonephritis with spontaneous formation of splenic germinal centers in mice lacking the estrogen receptor alpha gene. *Proc Natl Acad Sci USA* 2004;101:1720–1724.

Shimomura K. The value of juvenile animal studies: a Japanese industry perspective. *Birth Defects Res B Dev Reprod Toxicol*. 2011;92(4):266–268.

Shirakawa T, Kusaka Y, Morimoto K. Specific IgE antibodies to nickel in workers with known reactivity to cobalt. *Clin Exp Allergy*. 1992;22:213–218.

Shopp GM Jr, Sanders VM, White KL Jr, et al. Humoral and cell-mediated immune status of mice exposed to *trans*-1,2-dichloroethylene. *Drug Chem Toxicol*. 1985;8:393–407.

Sikorski EE, Burns LA, Stern ML, et al. Splenic cell targets in gallium arsenide-induced suppression of the primary antibody response. *Toxicol Appl Pharmacol*. 1991;110:129–142.

Silkworth JB, Loose LD. Cell-mediated immunity in mice fed either Aroclor 1016 or hexachlorobenzene. *Toxicol Appl Pharmacol*. 1978;45:326–327.

Silkworth JB, Loose LD. PCB and HCB induced alteration of lymphocyte blastogenesis. *Toxicol Appl Pharmacol*. 1979;49:86.

Silver RM, Heyes MP, Maize JC, et al. Scleroderma, fasciitis, and eosinophilia associated with the ingestion of tryptophan. *N Engl J Med*. 1990;322:874–881.

Simon JC, Cruz PD Jr, Bergstresser PR, et al. Low dose ultraviolet B-irradiated Langerhans cells preferentially activate CD4+ cells of the T helper 2 subset. *J Immunol*. 1990;145:2087–2091.

Simones T, Shepherd DM. Consequences of AhR activation in steady-state dendritic cells. *Toxicol Sci*. 2011;119:293–307.

Sleijffers A, Garssen J, Vos JG, et al. Ultraviolet light and resistance to infectious diseases. *J Immunol*. 2004;1:3–14.

Smialowicz RJ, DeVito MJ, Williams WC, et al. Relative potency based on hepatic enzyme induction predicts immunosuppressive effects of a mixture of PCDDS/PCDFS and PCBS. *Toxicol Appl Pharmacol*. 2008;227:477–484.

Smialowicz RJ, Riddle MM, Luebke RW, et al. Immunotoxicity of 2-methoxyethanol following oral administration in Fischer 344 rats. *Toxicol Appl Pharmacol*. 1991a;109:494–506.

Smialowicz RJ, Riddle MM, Rogers RR, et al. Evaluation of the immunotoxicity of orally administered 2-methoxyacetic acid in Fischer 344 rats. *Fundam Appl Toxicol*. 1991b;17:771–781.

Smialowicz RJ, Simmons JE, Luebke RW, et al. Immunotoxicologic assessment of subacute exposure of rats to carbon tetrachloride with comparison to hepatotoxicity and nephrotoxicity. *Fundam Appl Toxicol*. 1991c;17:186–196.

Smith DC, Smith MJ, White KL. Systemic immunosuppression following a single pharyngeal aspiration of 1,2:5,6-dibenzanthracene in female B6C3F1 mice. *J Immunotoxicol*. 2010;7:219–231.

Spits H, Di Santo JP. The expanding family of innate lymphoid cells: regulators and effectors of immunity and tissue remodeling. *Nat Immunol*. 2011;12:21–27.

Springs AE, Karmaus PW, Crawford RB, et al. Effects of targeted deletion of cannabinoid receptors CB1 and CB2 on immune competence and sensitivity to immune modulation by Delta9-tetrahydrocannabinol. *J Leukoc Biol*. 2008;84:1574–1584.

Spyker-Cranmer JM, Barnett JB, Avery DL, et al. Immunoteratology of chlordane: cell-mediated and humoral immune responses in adult mice exposed in utero. *Toxicol Appl Pharmacol*. 1982;62:402–408.

Staab CA, Alander J, Brandt M, et al. Reduction of *S*-nitrosoglutathione by alcohol dehydrogenase 3 is facilitated by substrate alcohols via direct cofactor recycling and leads to GSH-controlled formation of glutathione transferase inhibitors. *Biochem J*. 2008;413:493–504.

Stanulis ED, Jordan SD, Rosecrans JA, et al. Disruption of Th1/Th2 cytokine balance by cocaine is mediated by corticosterone. *Immunopharmacology*. 1997a;37:25–33.

Stanulis ED, Matulka RA, Jordan SD, et al. Role of corticosterone in the enhancement of the antibody response after acute cocaine administration. *J Pharmacol Exp Ther*. 1997b;280:284–291.

Starec M, Rouveix B, Sinet M, et al. Immune status and survival of opiate- and cocaine-treated mice infected with Friend virus. *J Pharmacol Exp Ther*. 1991;259:745–750.

Stewart J. Developmental toxicity testing of monoclonal antibodies: an enhanced pre- and postnatal study design option. *Reprod Toxicol*. 2009;28:220–225.

Stoermer KA, Morrison TE. Complement and viral pathogenesis. *Virology*. 2011;411:362–373.

Sulentic CE, Holsapple MP, Kaminski NE. Putative link between transcriptional regulation of IgM expression by 2,3,7,8-tetrachlorodibenzo-*p*-dioxin and the aryl hydrocarbon receptor/dioxin-responsive enhancer signaling pathway. *J Pharmacol Exp Ther*. 2000;295:705–716.

Sulentic CE, Kaminski NE. The long winding road toward understanding the molecular mechanisms for B-cell suppression by 2,3,7,8-tetrachlorodibenzo-*p*-dioxin. *Toxicol Sci*. 2011;120(suppl 1):S171–S191.

Sulentic CE, Kang JS, Na YJ, et al. Interactions at a dioxin responsive element (DRE) and an overlapping kappaB site within the hs4 domain of the 3′ alpha immunoglobulin heavy chain enhancer. *Toxicology*. 2004a;200:235–246.

Sulentic CE, Zhang W, Na YJ, et al. 2,3,7,8-tetrachlorodibenzo-*p*-dioxin, an exogenous modulator of the 3′ alpha immunoglobulin heavy chain enhancer in the CH12.LX mouse cell line. *J Pharmacol Exp Ther*. 2004b;309:71–78.

Sutter TR, Greenlee WF. Classification of members of the Ah gene battery. *Chemosphere*. 1992;25:223.

Svenson JL, EuDaly J, Ruiz P, et al. Impact of estrogen receptor deficiency on disease expression in the NZM2410 lupus prone mouse. *Clin Immunol*. 2008;128:259–268.

Syrigou E, Triantafyllou O, Makrilia N, et al. Acute hypersensitivity reactions to chemotherapy agents: an overview. *Inflamm Allergy Drug Targets*. 2010;9:206–213.

Taggart BR, Harrington P, Hollingshead M. HIV hollow fiber SCID model for antiviral therapy comparison with SCID/hu model. *Antiviral Res*. 2004;63:1–6.

Takahashi T, Kuniyasu Y, Toda M, et al. Immunologic self-tolerance maintained by CD25+CD4+ naturally anergic and suppressive T cells: induction of autoimmune disease by breaking their anergic/suppressive state. *Int Immunol*. 1998;10:1969–1980.

Takeuchi S, Iida M, Yabushita H, et al. In vitro screening for aryl hydrocarbon receptor agonistic activity in 200 pesticides using a highly sensitive reporter cell line, DR-EcoScreen cells, and in vivo mouse liver cytochrome P450-1A induction by propanil, diuron and linuron. *Chemosphere*. 2008;74:155–165.

Talal N. Sex steroid hormones and systemic lupus erythematosus. *Arthritis Rheum*. 1981;24:1054–1056.

Tassinari MS, Benson K, Elayan I, et al. Juvenile animal studies and pediatric drug development retrospective review: use in regulatory decisions and labeling. *Birth Defects Res B Dev Reprod Toxicol*. 2011;92(4):261–265.

Taylor AD, Christian HC, Morris JF, et al. An antisense oligodeoxynucleotide to lipocortin 1 reverses the inhibitory actions of dexamethasone on the release of adrenocorticotropin from rat pituitary tissue in vitro. *Endocrinology*. 1997;138:2909–2918.

Taylor DD, Akyol S, Gercel-Taylor C. Pregnancy-associated exosomes and their modulation of T cell signaling. *J Immunol*. 2006;176:1534–1542.

ten Tusscher GW, Steerenberg PA, van Loveren H, et al. Persistent hematologic and immunologic disturbances in 8-year-old Dutch children associated with perinatal dioxin exposure. *Environ Health Perspect*. 2003;111:1519–1523.

Terada N, Lucas JJ, Szepesi A, et al. Rapamycin blocks cell cycle progression of activated T cells prior to events characteristic of the middle to late G1 phase of the cycle. *J Cell Physiol*. 1993;154:7–15.

Thomas P, Braathen LR, Dorig M, et al. Increased metal allergy in patients with failed metal-on-metal hip arthroplasty and peri-implant T-lymphocytic inflammation. *Allergy*. 2009;64:1157–1165.

Thomas PT, Ratajczak HV, Aranyi C, et al. Evaluation of host resistance and immune function in cadmium-exposed mice. *Toxicol Appl Pharmacol*. 1985;80:446–456.

Thompson CM, Grafstrom RC. Mechanistic considerations for formaldehyde-induced bronchoconstriction involving *S*-nitrosoglutathione reductase. *J Toxicol Environ Health A*. 2008;71:244–248.

Thomsen M, Yacoub-Youssef H, Marcheix B. Reconstitution of a human immune system in immunodeficient mice: models of human alloreaction in vivo. *Tissue Antigens*. 2005;66:73–82.

Thorne PS, Hawk C, Kaliszewski SD, et al. The noninvasive mouse ear swelling assay. I. Refinements for detecting weak contact sensitizers. *Fundam Appl Toxicol*. 1991;17:790–806.

Thornton AM, Shevach EM. CD4+CD25+ immunoregulatory T cells suppress polyclonal T cell activation in vitro by inhibiting interleukin 2 production. *J Exp Med*. 1998;188:287–296.

Thrasher JD, Heuser G, Broughton A. Immunological abnormalities in humans chronically exposed to chlorpyrifos. *Arch Environ Health*. 2002;57:181–187.

Thurmond LM, Dean JH. Immunological responses following inhalation exposure to chemical hazards, in Gardner EE, Crapo JD, Massaro EJ, eds. *Toxicology of the Lung*. New York: Raven Press; 1988:375–406.

Thyssen JP, Menne T. Metal allergy—a review on exposures, penetration, genetics, prevalence, and clinical implications. *Chem Res Toxicol*. 2010;23:309–318.

Tognoni G, Boniccorsi A. Epidemiological problems with TCDD. A critical review. *Drug Metab Rev*. 1982;13:447–469.

Totoritis MC, Tan EM, McNally EM, et al. Association of antibody to histone complex H2A-H2B with symptomatic procainamide-induced lupus. *N Engl J Med*. 1988;318:1431–1436.

Toussirot E, Wendling D. The use of TNF-alpha blocking agents in rheumatoid arthritis: an update. *Expert Opin Pharmacother*. 2007;8:2089–2107.

Tryphonas H, Bondy G, Hodgen M, et al. Effects of *cis*-nonachlor, *trans*-nonachlor and chlordane on the immune system of Sprague–Dawley rats following a 28-day oral (gavage) treatment. *Food Chem Toxicol*. 2003;41:107–118.

Tryphonas H, Luster MI, Schiffman G, et al. Effect of chronic exposure of PCB (Aroclor 1254) on specific and nonspecific immune parameters in the rhesus (*Macaca mulatta*) monkey. *Fundam Appl Toxicol*. 1991a;16:773–786.

Tryphonas H, Luster MI, White KL Jr, et al. Effects of PCB (Aroclor 1254) on non-specific immune parameters in rhesus (*Macaca mulatta*) monkeys. *Int J Immunopharmacol*. 1991b;13:639–648.

Udoji F, Martin T, Etherton R, et al. Immunosuppressive effects of triclosan, nonylphenol, and DDT on human natural killer cells in vitro. *J Immunotoxicol*. 2010;7:205–212.

Ullrich SE. Mechanisms by which ultraviolet radiation, a ubiquitous environmental toxin, suppresses the immune response, in Luebke R, House R, Kimber I, eds. *Immunotoxicology and Immunopharmacology*. Boca Rotton, FL: CRC Press; 2007a:259–275.

Ullrich SE. Sunlight and skin cancer: lessons from the immune system. *Mol Carcinog*. 2007b;46:629–633.

Valstar DL, Schijf MA, Arts JH, et al. Alveolar macrophages suppress non-specific inflammation caused by inhalation challenge with trimellitic anhydride conjugated to albumin. *Arch Toxicol*. 2006;80:561–571.

van Loveren H, De Jong WH, Vandebriel RJ, et al. Risk assessment and immunotoxicology. *Toxicol Lett*. 1998;102–103:261–265.

van Loveren H, Goettsch W, Slob W, et al. Risk assessment of the harmful effects of UVB radiation on the immunological resistance to infectious diseases. *Arch Toxicol Suppl*. 1995;18:21–28.

van Loveren H, Krajnc EI, Rombout PJ, et al. Effects of ozone, hexachlorobenzene, and bis(tri-*n*-butyltin)oxide on natural killer activity in the rat lung. *Toxicol Appl Pharmacol*. 1990;102:21–33.

van Loveren H, Piersma A. Immunotoxicological consequences of perinatal chemical exposures. *Toxicol Lett*. 2004;149:141–145.

van Loveren H, Van Amsterdam JG, Vandebriel RJ, et al. Vaccine-induced antibody responses as parameters of the influence of endogenous and environmental factors. *Environ Health Perspect*. 2001;109:757–764.

Vanaudenaerde BM, Verleden SE, Vos R, et al. Innate and adaptive interleukin-17-producing lymphocytes in chronic inflammatory lung disorders. *Am J Respir Crit Care Med*. 2011;183:977–986.

Vandenberg LN, Maffini MV, Sonnenschein C, et al. Bisphenol-A and the great divide: a review of controversies in the field of endocrine disruption. *Endocr Rev*. 2009;30:75–95.

Varvel SA, Bridgen DT, Tao Q, et al. Delta9-tetrahydrocannbinol accounts for the antinociceptive, hypothermic, and cataleptic effects of marijuana in mice. *J Pharmacol Exp Ther*. 2005;314:329–337.

Vecchi A, Sironi M, Canegrati MA, et al. Immunosuppressive effects of 2,3,7,8-tetrachlorodibenzo-*p*-dioxin in strains of mice with different susceptibility to induction of aryl hydrocarbon hydroxylase. *Toxicol Appl Pharmacol*. 1983;68:434–441.

Veldhoen M, Hirota K, Westendorf AM, et al. The aryl hydrocarbon receptor links TH17-cell-mediated autoimmunity to environmental toxins. *Nature*. 2008;453:106–109.

Veraldi A, Costantini AS, Bolejack V, et al. Immunotoxic effects of chemicals: a matrix for occupational and environmental epidemiological studies. *Am J Ind Med*. 2006;49:1046–1055.

Vial T, Choquet-Kastylevsky G, Descotes J. Adverse effects of immunotherapeutics involving the immune system. *Toxicology*. 2002;174:3–11.

Vial T, Descotes J. Autoimmune diseases and vaccinations. *Eur J Dermatol*. 2004;14:86–90.

Vial T, Descotes J. Immune-mediated side-effects of cytokines in humans. *Toxicology*. 1995;105:31–57.

Vinuesa CG, Linterman MA, Goodnow CC, et al. T cells and follicular dendritic cells in germinal center B-cell formation and selection. *Immunol Rev*. 2010;237:72–89.

Vivier E, Raulet DH, Moretta A, et al. Innate or adaptive immunity? The example of natural killer cells. *Science*. 2011;331:44–49.

Vogel R, Seidle T, Spielmann H. A modular one-generation reproduction study as a flexible testing system for regulatory safety assessment. *Reprod Toxicol*. 2010;29:242–245.

Vorderstrasse BA, Bohn AA, Lawrence BP. Examining the relationship between impaired host resistance and altered immune function in mice treated with TCDD. *Toxicology*. 2003;188:15–28.

Vorderstrasse BA, Steppan LB, Silverstone AE, et al. Aryl hydrocarbon receptor-deficient mice generate normal immune responses to model antigens and are resistant to TCDD-induced immune suppression. *Toxicol Appl Pharmacol*. 2001;171:157–164.

Vos JG. Immune suppression as related to toxicology. *CRC Crit Rev Toxicol*. 1977;5:67–101.

Vos JG, de Klerk A, Krajnc EI, et al. Toxicity of bis(tri-*n*-butyltin)oxide in the rat. II. Suppression of thymus-dependent immune responses and of parameters of nonspecific resistance after short-term exposure. *Toxicol Appl Pharmacol*. 1984;75:387–408.

Vos JG, Luster MI. Immune alterations, in Kimbrough RD, Jensen AA, eds. *Halogenated Biphenyls, Terphenyls, Naphthalenes, Dibenzodioxins, and Related Products*. New York: Elsevier; 1989:295–322.

Vos JG, van Loveren H. Experimental studies on immunosuppression: how do they predict for man? *Toxicology*. 1998;129:13–26.

Walder BK. Do solvents cause scleroderma? *Int J Dermatol*. 1983;22:157–158.

Walters E, Rider V, Abdou NI, et al. Estradiol targets T cell signaling pathways in human systemic lupus. *Clin Immunol*. 2009;133:428–436.

Wang BJ, Sheu HM, Guo YL, et al. Hexavalent chromium induced ROS formation, Akt, NF-kappaB, and MAPK activation, and TNF-alpha and IL-1alpha production in keratinocytes. *Toxicol Lett*. 2010;198:216–224.

Wang J, Barke RA, Charboneau R, et al. Morphine impairs host innate immune response and increases susceptibility to *Streptococcus pneumoniae* lung infection. *J Immunol*. 2005a ;174:426–434.

Wang L, Weng CY, Wang YJ, et al. Lipoic acid ameliorates arsenic trioxide-induced HO-1 expression and oxidative stress in THP-1 monocytes and macrophages. *Chem Biol Interact*. 2011;190:129–138.

Wang SS, Cozen W, Cerhan JR, et al. Immune mechanisms in non-Hodgkin lymphoma: joint effects of the TNF G308A and IL10 T3575A polymorphisms with non-Hodgkin lymphoma risk factors. *Cancer Res*. 2007;67:5042–5054.

Wang X, Tan N, Douglas SD, et al. Morphine inhibits CD8+ T cell-mediated, noncytolytic, anti-HIV activity in latently infected immune cells. *J Leukoc Biol*. 2005b;78:772–776.

Ward AM, Udnoon S, Watkins J, et al. Immunological mechanisms in the pathogenesis of vinyl chloride disease. *Br Med J*. 1976;1:936–938.

Warheit DB, Hesterberg TW. Asbestos and other fibers in the lung, in Dean JH, Luster MI, Munson AE, et al., eds. *Immunotoxicology and Immunopharmacology*. New York: Raven Press; 1994:363–376.

Warren TK, Mitchell KA, Lawrence BP. Exposure to 2,3,7,8-tetrachlorodibenzo-*p*-dioxin (TCDD) suppresses the humoral and cell-mediated immune responses to influenza A virus without affecting cytolytic activity in the lung. *Toxicol Sci*. 2000;56:114–123.

Watowich SS, Liu YJ. Mechanisms regulating dendritic cell specification and development. *Immunol Rev*. 2010;238:76–92.

Watson AJ, Hankinson O. Dioxin and Ah receptor-dependent protein binding to xenobiotic responsive elements and G-rich DNA studied by in vivo footprinting. *J Biol Chem*. 1992;266:6874–6878.

Watson ES, Murphy JC, ElSohly HN, et al. Effects of the administration of coca alkaloids on the primary immune responses of mice: interaction with delta 9-tetrahydrocannabinol and ethanol. *Toxicol Appl Pharmacol*. 1983;71:1–13.

Ways SC, Blair PB, Bern HA, et al. Immune responsiveness of adult mice exposed neonatally to diethylstilbestrol, steroid hormones, or vitamin A. *J Environ Pathol Toxicol*. 1980;3:207–220.

Weaver JL, Chapdelaine JM, Descotes J, et al. Evaluation of a lymph node proliferation assay for its ability to detect pharmaceuticals with potential to cause immune-mediated drug reactions. *J Immunotoxicol*. 2005;2:11–20.

Weinstock D, Lewis DB, Parker GA, et al. Toxicopathology of the developing immune system: investigative and development strategies. *Toxicol Pathol*. 2010;38:1111–1117.

Weisglas-Kuperus N, Patandin S, Berbers GA, et al. Immunologic effects of background exposure to polychlorinated biphenyls and dioxins in Dutch preschool children. *Environ Health Perspect*. 2000;108:1203–1207.

Weisglas-Kuperus N, Sas TC, Koopman-Esseboom C, et al. Immunologic effects of background prenatal and postnatal exposure to dioxins and polychlorinated biphenyls in Dutch infants. *Pediatr Res*. 1995;38:404–410.

Weisglas-Kuperus N, Vreugdenhil HJ, Mulder PG. Immunological effects of environmental exposure to polychlorinated biphenyls and dioxins in Dutch school children. *Toxicol Lett*. 2004;149:281–285.

White KL Jr. Specific immune function assays, in Miller K, Turk JL, Nicklin S, eds. Principles and Practice of Immunotoxicology. Oxford: Blackwell; 1992:304–323.

White KL Jr., Anderson AC. Suppression of mouse complement activity by contaminants of technical grade pentachlorophenol. *Agents Actions*. 1985;16:385.

White KL Jr., Lysy HH, McCay JA, et al. Modulation of serum complement levels following exposure to polychlorinated dibenzo-*p*-dioxins. *Toxicol Appl Pharmacol*. 1986;84:209–219.

White KL, Musgrove DL, Brown RD. The sheep erythrocyte T-dependent antibody response (TDAR). *Methods Mol Biol*. 2010;598:173–184.

Whitlock JP Jr. Genetic and molecular aspects of 2,3,7,8-tetrachlorodibenzo-*p*-dioxin action. *Annu Rev Pharmacol Toxicol*. 1990;30:251–277.

Williams WC, Riddle MM, Copeland CB, et al. Immunological effects of 2-methoxyethanol administered dermally or orally to Fischer 344 rats. *Toxicology*. 1995;98:215–223.

Wiltrout RW, Ercegovich CD, Ceglowski WS. Humoral immunity in mice following oral administration of selected pesticides. *Bull Environ Contam Toxicol*. 1978;20:423–431.

Winans B, Humble MC, Lawrence BP. Environmental toxicants and the developing immune system: a missing link in the global battle against infectious disease? *Reprod Toxicol*. 2011;31:327–336.

Wisnewski AV, Xu L, Robinson E, et al. Immune sensitization to methylene diphenyl diisocyanate (MDI) resulting from skin exposure: albumin as a carrier protein connecting skin exposure to subsequent respiratory responses. *J Occup Med Toxicol*. 2011;6:6.

Wood SC, Holsapple MP. Direct suppression of superantigen-induced IgM secretion in human lymphocytes by 2,3,7,8-TCDD. *Toxicol Appl Pharmacol*. 1993;122:308–313.

Wood SC, Jeong HG, Morris DL, et al. Direct effects of 2,3,7,8-tetrachlorodibenzo-*p*-dioxin (TCDD) on human tonsillar lymphocytes. *Toxicology*. 1993;81:131–143.

Xiao F, Chong AS-F, Bartlett RR, et al. A promising immunosuppressant in transplantation, in Thomas AW, Starzyl TE, eds. *Immunosuppressive Drugs: Developments in Anti-Rejection Therapy*. London:Edward Arnold; 1994:203–212.

Yamaguchi K, Matulka RA, Shneider AM, et al. Induction of PreB cell apoptosis by 7,12-dimethylbenz[*a*]anthracene in long-term primary murine bone marrow cultures. *Toxicol Appl Pharmacol*. 1997;147:190–203.

Yang KH, Kim BS, Munson AE, et al. Immunosuppression induced by chemicals requiring metabolic activation in mixed cultures of rat hepatocytes and murine splenocytes. *Toxicol Appl Pharmacol*. 1986;83:420–429.

Yeatts K, Sly P, Shore S, et al. A brief targeted review of susceptibility factors, environmental exposures, asthma incidence, and recommendations for future asthma incidence research. *Environ Health Perspect*. 2006;114:634–640.

Yellayi S, Naaz A, Szewczykowski MA, et al. The phytoestrogen genistein induces thymic and immune changes: a human health concern? *Proc Natl Acad Sci USA*. 2002;99:7616–7621.

Yoo BS, Boverhof DR, Shnaider D, et al. 2,3,7,8-Tetrachlorodibenzo-*p*-dioxin (TCDD) alters the regulation of Pax5 in lipopolysaccharide-activated B cells. *Toxicol Sci*. 2004;77:272–279.

Yoshino S, Yamaki K, Li X, et al. Prenatal exposure to bisphenol A up-regulates immune responses, including T helper 1 and T helper 2 responses, in mice. *Immunology*. 2004;112:489–495.

Yun AJ, Lee PY. The link between T helper balance and lymphoproliferative disease. *Med Hypotheses*. 2005;65:587–590.

Yurino H, Ishikawa S, Sato T, et al. Endocrine disruptors (environmental estrogens) enhance autoantibody production by B1 cells. *Toxicol Sci*. 2004;81:139–147.

Zelikoff JT, Thomas P. *Immunotoxicology of Environmental and Occupational Metals*. Bristol, PA: Taylor & Francis; 1998.

Zhang Q, Bhattacharya S, Kline DE, et al. Stochastic modeling of B lymphocyte terminal differentiation and its suppression by dioxin. *BMC Syst Biol*. 2010;4:40.

Zhang Y, Song TT, Cunnick JE, et al. Daidzein and genistein glucuronides in vitro are weakly estrogenic and activate human natural killer cells at nutritionally relevant concentrations. *J. Nutr*. 1999;129:399–405.

Zhou C, Tabb MM, Nelson EL, et al. Mutual repression between steroid and xenobiotic receptor and NF-kappaB signaling pathways links xenobiotic metabolism and inflammation. *J Clin Invest*. 2006;116:2280–2289.

Zhou HR, Islam Z, Pestka JJ. Rapid, sequential activation of mitogen-activated protein kinases and transcription factors precedes proinflammatory cytokine mRNA expression in spleens of mice exposed to the trichothecene vomitoxin. *Toxicol Sci*. 2003;72:130–142.

chapter 13

Toxic Responses of the Liver

Hartmut Jaeschke

INTRODUCTION

The liver is the main organ where exogenous chemicals are metabolized and eventually excreted. As a consequence, liver cells are exposed to significant concentrations of these chemicals, which can result in liver dysfunction, cell injury, and even organ failure. If an industrial chemical, for example carbon tetrachloride, bromobenzene, or vinyl chloride, is identified as a hepatotoxicant, the use of the chemical may be restricted, the exposure may be minimized by mandating protective clothing and respirators, and attempts are made to replace it with a safer alternative. In the pharmaceutical industry, adverse effects on the liver are one of the most frequently cited reasons for discontinuing the development of drug candidates. In addition, hepatotoxicity recognized during the postmarketing phase is one of the main causes for withdrawing drugs from the market (Temple and Himmel, 2002). Troglitazone (Rezulin®), a new antidiabetic drug, was removed from the market after close to 100 of the 1.9 million patients treated with the drug suffered from liver failure (Chojkier, 2005). Thus, predictable and idiosyncratic hepatotoxicities severely restrict drug discovery efforts and drug development (Lee and Senior, 2005). Furthermore, the increasing popularity of herbal medicines, which are generally plant extracts, enhances the incidence of drug-induced liver injury and liver failure (Stickel et al., 2011). Since these medicines are mixtures of sometimes hundreds of compounds, it remains a difficult task to identify the causative chemical and the mechanism of injury (Lee and Senior, 2005). Basic science and clinical aspects of drug- and chemical-induced liver injury were discussed in detail in several monographs and reviews (Zimmerman, 1999; Jaeschke et al., 2002, 2012a, b; Kaplowitz and DeLeve, 2002; Boyer et al., 2006b; Grattagliano et al., 2009; Roth and Ganey, 2010; Jones et al., 2010).

Given the unprecedented speed of drug discovery and the increasing demand and use of "natural products" as food supplements and medicine, the early identification of hepatotoxicants remains a formidable challenge for the future. The liver, with its multiple cell types and numerous functions, can respond in many different ways to acute and chronic insults. To recognize potential liver cell dysfunction and injury, it is necessary to have a general knowledge of basic liver functions, the structural organization of the liver, the processes involved in the excretory functions of the liver, and mechanisms of cell and organ injury. Each of these aspects can contribute to mechanisms of drug- and chemical-induced hepatotoxicities.

LIVER PHYSIOLOGY

Hepatic Functions

The liver's strategic location between the intestinal tract and the rest of the body facilitates the performance of its enormous task of maintaining metabolic homeostasis of the body (Table 13-1). Venous blood from the stomach and intestine flows into the portal vein and then through the liver before entering the systemic circulation. Thus, the liver is the first organ to encounter ingested nutrients, vitamins, metals, drugs, and environmental toxicants as well as waste products of bacteria that enter portal blood. Efficient scavenging or uptake processes extract these absorbed materials from the blood for catabolism, storage, and/or excretion into bile.

All the major functions of the liver can be detrimentally altered by acute or chronic exposure to toxicants (Table 13-1). When toxicants inhibit or otherwise impede hepatic transport and synthetic processes, dysfunction can occur without appreciable cell damage. Loss of function also occurs when toxicants kill an appreciable number of cells and when chronic insult leads to replacement of cell mass by nonfunctional scar tissue. Alcohol abuse is the major cause of liver disease in most western countries (Crawford, 1999); thus ethanol provides a highly relevant example of a toxicant with multiple functional consequences (Gao and Bataller, 2011). Early stages of ethanol abuse are characterized by lipid accumulation (fatty liver) due to diminished use of lipids as fuels and impaired ability to synthesize the lipoproteins that transport lipids out of the liver. As alcohol-induced liver disease progresses, appreciable cell death occurs, the functioning mass of the

Table 13-1

Major Functions of Liver and Consequences of Impaired Hepatic Functions

TYPE OF FUNCTION	EXAMPLES	CONSEQUENCES OF IMPAIRED FUNCTIONS
Nutrient homeostasis	Glucose storage and synthesis Cholesterol uptake	Hypoglycemia, confusion Hypercholesterolemia
Filtration of particulates	Products of intestinal bacteria (eg, endotoxin)	Endotoxemia
Protein synthesis	Clotting factors Albumin Transport proteins (eg, very low density lipoproteins)	Excess bleeding Hypoalbuminemia, ascites Fatty liver
Bioactivation and detoxification	Bilirubin and ammonia Steroid hormones Xenobiotics	Jaundice, hyperammonemia-related coma Loss of secondary male sex characteristics Diminished drug metabolism Inadequate detoxification
Formation of bile and biliary secretion	Bile acid-dependent uptake of dietary lipids and vitamins Bilirubin and cholesterol Metals (eg, Cu and Mn) Xenobiotics	Fatty diarrhea, malnutrition, Vitamin E deficiency Jaundice, gallstones, hypercholesterolemia Mn-induced neurotoxicity Delayed drug clearance

liver is replaced by scar tissue, and hepatic capacity for biotransformation of certain drugs progressively declines. People with hepatic cirrhosis due to chronic alcohol abuse frequently become deficient at detoxifying both the ammonia formed by catabolism of amino acids and the bilirubin derived from breakdown of hemoglobin. Uncontrollable hemorrhage due to inadequate synthesis of clotting factors is a common fatal complication of alcoholic cirrhosis. A consequence of liver injury that merits emphasis is that loss of liver functions can lead to aberrations in other organ systems and to death (Gao and Bataller, 2011).

Structural Organization

Two concepts exist for organization of the liver into operational units, namely, the lobule and the acinus (McCuskey, 2006b). Classically, the liver was divided into hexagonal lobules oriented around terminal hepatic venules (also known as central veins). At the corners of the lobule are the portal triads (or portal tracts), containing a branch of the portal vein, a hepatic arteriole, and a bile duct (Fig. 13-1). Blood entering the portal tract via the portal vein and hepatic artery is mixed in the penetrating vessels, enters the sinusoids, and percolates along the cords of parenchymal cells (hepatocytes), eventually flows into terminal hepatic venules, and exits the liver via the hepatic vein. The lobule is divided into three regions known as centrilobular, midzonal, and periportal. The acinus is the preferred concept for a functional hepatic unit. The terminal branches of the portal vein and hepatic artery, which extend out from the portal tracts, form the base of the acinus. The acinus has three zones: zone 1 is closest to the entry of blood, zone 3 abuts the terminal hepatic vein, and zone 2 is intermediate. Despite the utility of the acinar concept, lobular terminology is still used to describe regions of pathological lesions of hepatic parenchyma. Fortunately, the three zones of the acinus roughly coincide with the three regions of the lobule (Fig. 13-1).

Acinar zonation is of considerable functional consequence regarding gradients of components both in blood and in hepatocytes (Jungermann and Kietzmann, 2000). Blood entering the acinus consists of oxygen-depleted blood from the portal vein

(60%–70% of hepatic blood flow) plus oxygenated blood from the hepatic artery (30%–40%). Enroute to the terminal hepatic venule, oxygen rapidly leaves the blood to meet the high metabolic demands of the parenchymal cells. Approximate oxygen concentrations in zone 1 are 9% to 13%, compared with only 4% to 5% in zone 3 (Kietzmann and Jungermann, 1997). Therefore, hepatocytes in zone 3 are exposed to substantially lower concentrations of oxygen than hepatocytes in zone 1. In comparison to other tissues, zone 3 is hypoxic. Another well-documented acinar gradient is that of bile salts (Groothuis *et al.*, 1982). Physiological concentrations

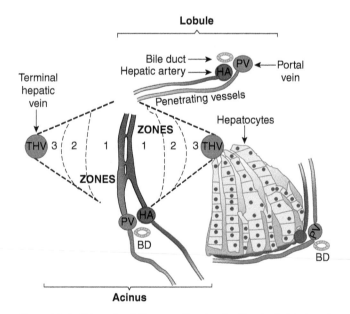

Figure 13-1. *Schematic of liver operational units, the classic lobule and the acinus.* The lobule is centered around the terminal hepatic vein (central vein), where the blood drains out of the lobule. The acinus has as its base the penetrating vessels, where blood supplied by the portal vein and hepatic artery flows down the acinus past the cords of hepatocytes. Zones 1, 2, and 3 of the acinus represent metabolic regions that are increasingly distant from the blood supply.

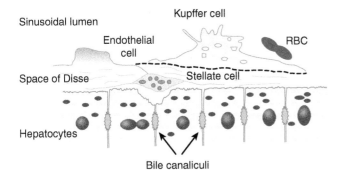

Sinusoidal lumen

Endothelial cell

Kupffer cell

RBC

Space of Disse

Stellate cell

Hepatocytes

Bile canaliculi

Figure 13-2. *Schematic of liver sinusoidal cells.* Note that the Kupffer cell resides within the sinusoidal lumen. The stellate cell is located in the space of Disse between the thin, fenestrated endothelial cells, and the cord of hepatocytes.

of bile salts are efficiently extracted by zone 1 hepatocytes with little bile acids left in the blood that flows past zone 3 hepatocytes. There is difference in bile acid transporter expression between different zones (Baier *et al.*, 2006).

Heterogeneities in protein levels of hepatocytes along the acinus generate gradients of metabolic functions. Hepatocytes in the mitochondria-rich zone 1 are predominant in fatty acid oxidation, gluconeogenesis, and ammonia detoxification to urea. Gradients of enzymes involved in the bioactivation and detoxification of xenobiotics have been observed along the acinus by immunohistochemistry (Jungermann and Katz, 1989; Gebhardt *et al.*, 1994). Notable gradients for hepatotoxins are the higher levels of glutathione (GSH) in zone 1 and the greater amounts of cytochrome P450 proteins in zone 3, particularly the CYP2E1 isozyme inducible by ethanol (Tsutsumi *et al.*, 1989; Niemelä *et al.*, 2000).

Hepatic sinusoids are the channels between cords of hepatocytes where blood percolates on its way to the terminal hepatic vein. Sinusoids are larger and more irregular than normal capillaries. The three major types of cells in the sinusoids are endothelial cells, Kupffer cells, and stellate cells (Fig. 13-2) (McCuskey, 2006b). In addition, the liver contains a substantial number of lymphocytes, especially natural killer (NK) and NKT cells (Gao *et al.*, 2009). Sinusoids are lined by thin, discontinuous endothelial cells with numerous fenestrae (or pores) that allow molecules smaller than 250 kDa to cross the interstitial space (known as the space of Disse) between the endothelium and hepatocytes. Sinusoidal endothelial cells are separated from the hepatocytes by a basement membrane-like matrix, which is not as electron-dense as a regular basement membrane (Friedman, 2000). However, this subendothelial extracellular matrix is important for the normal function of all resident liver cells (Friedman, 2000). The numerous fenestrae and the lack of basement membrane facilitate exchanges of fluids and molecules, such as albumin, between the sinusoid and hepatocytes, but hinder movement of particles larger than chylomicron remnants. Endothelial cells are important in the scavenging of lipoproteins via the apo E receptor and of denatured proteins and advanced glycation endproducts by the scavenger receptor (Enomoto *et al.*, 2004; Elvevold *et al.*, 2008). Hepatic endothelial cells also secrete cytokines, prostanoids, nitric oxide, and endothelins and express intercellular adhesion molecule-1 (ICAM-1) and vascular cell adhesion molecule-1 (VCAM-1) on the cell surface (Jaeschke, 1997).

Kupffer cells are the resident macrophages of the liver and constitute approximately 80% of the fixed macrophages in the body (McCuskey, 2006b). Kupffer cells are situated within the lumen of the sinusoid. The primary function of Kupffer cells is to ingest and degrade particulate matter. Also, Kupffer cells are a major source

of cytokines and eicosanoids and can act as antigen-presenting cells (APCs; Laskin, 2009). Hepatic stellate cells (HSCs; also known as Ito cells or by the more descriptive terms of *fat-storing cells*) are located between endothelial cells and hepatocytes (Friedman, 2008). Stellate cells are the major sites for vitamin A storage in the body (Friedman, 2008). Upon activation, these cells can synthesize and excrete collagen and other extracellular matrix proteins and express smooth muscle actin (Friedman, 2000; Lee and Friedman, 2011).

Bile Formation

Bile is a yellow fluid containing bile acids, GSH, phospholipids, cholesterol, bilirubin and other organic anions, proteins, metals, ions, and xenobiotics (Klaassen and Watkins, 1984). Formation of this fluid is a specialized function of the liver. Adequate bile formation is essential for uptake of lipid nutrients from the small intestine (Table 13-1), for protection of the small intestine from oxidative insults (Aw, 1994), and for excretion of endogenous and xenobiotic compounds. Hepatocytes begin the process of bile formation by transporting bile acids, GSH, and other osmotically active compounds including xenobiotics and their metabolites into the canalicular lumen. These molecules are the major driving force for the passive movement of water and electrolytes across the tight junctions and the hepatocyte epithelium. The canalicular lumen is a space formed by specialized regions of the plasma membrane between adjacent hepatocytes (Fig. 13-2). The canaliculi are separated from the intercellular space between hepatocytes by tight junctions, which form a barrier permeable only to water, electrolytes, and to some degree to small organic cations. Under physiological conditions, tight junctions are impermeable to organic anions allowing the high concentrations of bile acids, GSH, bilirubin diglucuronide, and other organic anions in bile. The structure of the biliary tract is analogous to the roots and trunk of a tree, where the tips of the roots equate to the canalicular lumens. Canaliculi form channels between hepatocytes that connect to a series of larger and larger channels or ducts within the liver. The large extrahepatic bile ducts merge into the common bile duct. Bile can be stored and concentrated in the gallbladder before its release into the duodenum. However, the gallbladder is not essential to life and is absent in several species, including the horse, whale, and rat.

With the identification of specific transporters, substantial progress has been made in the understanding of the molecular mechanisms of bile formation (reviewed by Jansen and Groen, 2006; Pauli-Magnus and Meier, 2006). On the basal (sinusoidal) side of the hepatocytes, there are sodium-dependent and sodium-independent uptake systems. Most conjugated bile acids (taurine and glycine conjugates) and some of the unconjugated bile acids are transported into hepatocytes by sodium/taurocholate cotransporting polypeptide (NTCP) (Fig. 13-3) (Trauner and Boyer, 2003; Hagenbuch and Dawson, 2004; Stieger *et al.*, 2007). Sodium-independent uptake of conjugated and unconjugated bile acids is performed by members of the organic anion transporting polypeptides (OATPs) (Hagenbuch and Meier, 2004; Csanaky *et al.*, 2011). OATP1B1 and OATP1B3 are predominantly expressed in liver and are capable of transporting conjugated and unconjugated bile acids and steroids, bromosulfophthalein, and many other organic anions. Furthermore, the OATPs are transporting numerous drugs and also some hepatotoxins, for example, phalloidin, microcystin, and amanitin (Hagenbuch and Gui, 2008; Roth *et al.*, 2011). In addition to the uptake systems, there are ATP-dependent efflux pumps located on the basolateral membrane of hepatocytes. These carriers are members of the multidrug resistance-associated proteins (MRPs;

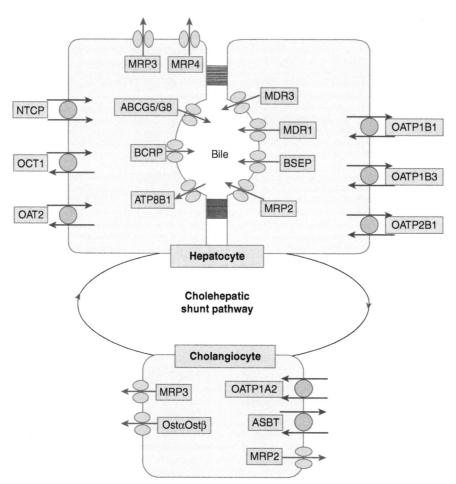

Figure 13-3. *Transport proteins in human hepatocytes and cholangiocytes.* Efflux transporters (blue symbols): BSEP, bile salt export pump; MDR, multidrug resistance protein; MRP, multidrug resistance-associated protein; ABCG5/8; BCRP, breast cancer resistance protein; Ostα/ Ostβ. Uptake transporters (red symbols): ASBT, apical sodium-dependent bile salt transporter; NTCP, sodium taurocholate cotransporting polypeptide; OATP, organic anion-transporting polypeptide; OCT, organic cation transporter; OAT, organic anion transporter. Transporters localized to the sinusoidal membrane extract solutes from the blood. Exporters localized to the canalicular membrane move solutes into the lumen of the canaliculus. Exporters of particular relevance to canalicular secretion of toxic chemicals and their metabolites are the canalicular multiple organic anion transporter (MOAT) system and the family of multiple-drug resistant (MDR) P-glycoproteins. Note: MDR3(ABCB4) flops phosphatidylcholine from the inner to the outer leaflet of the canalicular membrane. Phosphatidylcholine can then be extracted by bile salts. ATP8B1 together with the accessory protein CDC50A flips phosphatidylserine from the outer to the inner membrane to maintain the lipid asymmetry of the canalicular membrane and to protect against bile acids (Groen *et al.*, 2011). (Adapted from Pauli-Magnus and Meier (2006). Reprinted with permission of John Wiley & Sons, Inc.)

ABCC), which are multispecific transporters for many different anions (Homolya *et al.*, 2003) (Fig. 13-3).

All unconjugated bile acids in hepatocytes are conjugated before being transported by the bile salt export pump (BSEP) across the canalicular membrane. Bile acid excretion is a major driving force of bile formation (bile salt-dependent bile flow). Other constituents of bile are transported by members of the multidrug resistance (MDR) P-glycoprotein family such as MDR3 (ABCC2), which transports phospholipids, and the heterodimeric transporters ABCG5/ABCG8, which transport cholesterol and plant sterols into bile (Pauli-Magnus and Meier, 2006). In addition, MRP2 (a member of the multidrug resistance-associated proteins) transports GSH, which is the main compound responsible for the bile salt-independent bile flow, as well as sulfated and glucuronidated bile acids, glutathione disulfide and glutathione conjugates, bilirubin diglucuronide, and many other conjugated drugs and chemicals (Gerk and Vore, 2002; Borst *et al.*, 2000). Other transport systems of the canalicular membrane include the breast cancer resistance protein (BCRP; ABCG2), which can contribute to the biliary excretion of bile acids and xenobiotics.

Metals are excreted into bile by a series of processes that include (1) uptake across the sinusoidal membrane by facilitated diffusion or receptor-mediated endocytosis; (2) storage in binding proteins or lysosomes; and (3) canalicular secretion via lysosomes, a GSH-coupled event, or use of specific canalicular membrane transporter, for example MRP2 (Ballatori, 2002). Biliary excretion is important in the homeostasis of multiple metals, notably copper, manganese, cadmium, selenium, gold, silver, and arsenic (Klaassen, 1976; Gregus and Klaassen, 1986). Species differences are known for biliary excretion of several toxic metals; for example, dogs excrete arsenic into bile much more slowly than rats. Inability to export copper into bile is a central problem in Wilson's disease, a rare autosomal recessive inherited disorder characterized by a defect or the absence of a copper transporting P-type ATPase (ATP7B). This carrier is located in the trans-Golgi network and transports copper into the secretory pathway for binding to ceruloplasmin and then excretion into bile (Loudianos and Gitlin, 2000). Because biliary excretion is the only way to eliminate copper, a defect in ATP7B results in excessive copper accumulation in hepatocytes, which causes chronic hepatitis and cirrhosis (Loudianos and Gitlin, 2000).

Canalicular lumen bile is propelled forward into larger channels by dynamic, ATP-dependent contractions of the pericanalicular cytoskeleton (Watanabe *et al.*, 1991). Bile ducts, once regarded as passive conduits, modify bile by absorption and secretion of solutes (Lira *et al.*, 1992). Bile acids are taken up into biliary epithelial cells (cholangiocytes) by OATP1A2 (sodium-independent uptake) and by the sodium-dependent bile acid transporter ASBT (Hagenbuch and Dawson, 2004; Hagenbuch and Meier, 2004). These bile acids are then excreted on the basolateral side mainly by MRP3 and heterodimeric organic solute transporter (OSTα/OSTβ) (Ballatori *et al.*, 2005). The bile acids excreted from cholangiocytes return to the portal circulation via the peribiliary plexus (cholehepatic shunt pathway). Biliary epithelial cells also express a variety of phase I and phase II enzymes, which may contribute to the biotransformation of chemical toxicants present in bile (Lakehal *et al.*, 1999).

Secretion into biliary ducts is usually but not always a prelude to toxicant clearance by excretion in feces or urine. Exceptions occur when compounds such as arsenic are repeatedly delivered into the intestinal lumen via bile, efficiently absorbed from the intestinal lumen, and then redirected to the liver via portal blood, a process known as *enterohepatic cycling*. A few compounds, such as methyl mercury, are absorbed from the biliary tract; the extensive reabsorption of methyl mercury from the gallbladder is thought to contribute to the long biological half-life and toxicity of this toxicant (Dutczak *et al.*, 1991). Alternatively, secretion into bile of toxicant metabolites can be a critical prelude to the development of injury in extrahepatic tissues. A clinically relevant example of bile as an important delivery route for a proximate toxicant is that of diclofenac, a widely prescribed nonsteroidal anti-inflammatory drug (NSAID) that causes small intestinal ulceration. Experiments with mutant rats lacking a functional MRP2 exporter (Fig. 13-3) have shown that these mutants secrete little of the presumptive proximate toxicant metabolite into bile and are resistant to the intestinal toxicity of diclofenac (Seitz and Boelsterli, 1998).

Toxicant-related impairments of bile formation are more likely to have detrimental consequences in populations with other conditions where biliary secretion is marginal. For example, neonates exhibit delayed development of multiple aspects of bile formation, including synthesis of bile acids and the expression of sinusoidal and canalicular transporters (Arrese *et al.*, 1998). Neonates are more prone to develop jaundice when treated with drugs that compete with bilirubin for biliary clearance. Individuals with genetic deficiency of certain transporters are not only at risk for chronic liver injury and fibrosis, but may also be more susceptible to drugs and hepatotoxicants (Jansen and Sturm, 2003; Jansen and Groen, 2006). Patients with sepsis frequently develop cholestasis, which is mainly caused by downregulation of multiple canalicular transport systems (Geier *et al.*, 2006). In addition, direct inhibition of BSEP, as was shown for the endothelin receptor antagonist bosentan, can lead to retention of bile acids in the liver and potentially cell injury (Fattinger *et al.*, 2001).

LIVER PATHOPHYSIOLOGY

Mechanisms and Types of Toxicant-Induced Liver Injury

The response of the liver to chemical exposure depends on the intensity of the insults, the cell population affected, and the duration of the chemical exposure (acute vs chronic). Milder stresses may just cause reversible cellular dysfunction, for example, temporary cholestasis after exposure to estrogens, and could cause an adaptive response (conditioning). However, acute poisoning with acetaminophen (APAP) or carbon tetrachloride triggers parenchymal cell necrosis. Exposure to ethanol induces steatosis, which may enhance the susceptibility to subsequent inflammatory insults (Table 13-2). Note that the representative hepatotoxins listed in Table 13-2 include pharmaceuticals (valproic acid, cyclosporin A, diclofenac, APAP, and tamoxifen), recreational drugs (ethanol, ecstasy), a vitamin (vitamin A), metals (Fe, Cu, and Mn), hormones (estrogens, androgens), industrial chemicals (dimethylformamide, methylene dianiline), compounds found in teas (germander) or foods (phalloidin, pyrrolidine alkaloids), and toxins produced by fungi (sporidesmin) and algae (microcystin).

Cell Death Based on morphology, liver cells can die by two different modes, oncotic necrosis ("necrosis") or apoptosis. Necrosis is characterized by cell swelling, leakage of cellular contents, nuclear disintegration (karyolysis), and an influx of inflammatory cells. Because necrosis is generally the result of an exposure to a toxic chemical or other traumatic conditions, for example, ischemia, large numbers of contiguous hepatocytes and nonparenchymal cells may be affected. Cell contents released during oncotic necrosis include proteins such a high-mobility group box-1 (HMGB1) and other alarmins, which are a subset of the larger class of damage-associated molecular patterns (DAMPs) (Bianchi, 2007). These molecules are recognized by cells of the innate immune system including Kupffer cells through their toll-like receptors trigger cytokine formation, which orchestrate the inflammatory response after tissue injury. Thus, an ongoing oncotic necrotic process can be identified by the release of liver-specific enzymes such as alanine (ALT) or aspartate (AST) aminotransferase into the plasma and by

Table 13-2

Types of Hepatobiliary Injury

TYPE OF INJURY OR DAMAGE	REPRESENTATIVE TOXINS
Fatty liver	Amiodarone, CCl$_4$, ethanol, fialuridine, tamoxifen, valproic acid
Hepatocyte death	Acetaminophen, allyl alcohol, Cu, dimethylformamide, ethanol
Immune-mediated response	Diclofenac, ethanol, halothane, tienilic acid
Canalicular cholestasis	Chlorpromazine, cyclosporin A, 1,1-dichloroethylene, estrogens, Mn, phalloidin
Bile duct damage	Alpha-naphthylisothiocyanate, amoxicillin, methylenedianiline, sporidesmin
Sinusoidal disorders	Anabolic steroids, cyclophosphamide, microcystin, pyrrolizidine alkaloids
Fibrosis and cirrhosis	CCl$_4$, ethanol, thioacetamide, vitamin A, vinyl chloride
Tumors	Aflatoxin, androgens, arsenic, thorium dioxide, vinyl chloride

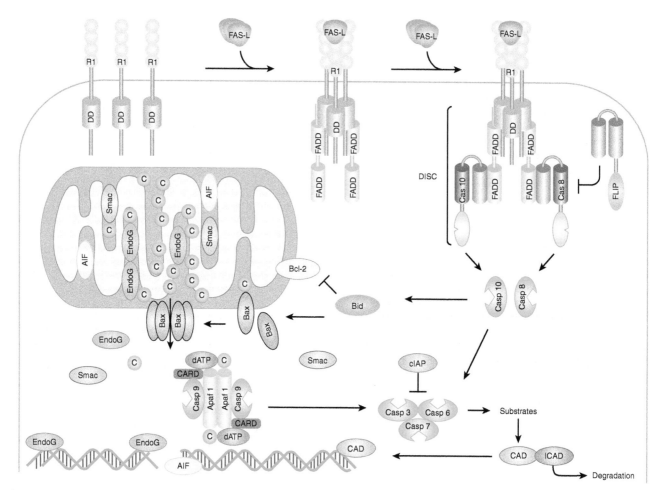

Figure 13-4. *Fas receptor-mediated apoptotic signaling pathways in hepatocytes.* AIF, apoptosis-inducing factor; Apaf1, apoptosis protease-activating factor-1; CARD, caspase-activating and -recruiting domain; Casp, caspase; c, cytochrome *c*; cIAP, cellular inhibitor of apoptosis proteins; DD, death domain; Smac, second mitochondria-derived activator of caspases; DISC, death-inducing signaling complex; EndoG, endonuclease G; FADD, Fas-associated death domain; FAS-L, Fas-ligand; FLIP, FLICE-inhibitory protein. (Adapted from Jaeschke, 2006a.)

histology, where areas of necrosis with loss of nuclei and inflammatory infiltrates are easily detectable in H&E sections. In contrast, apoptosis is characterized by cell shrinkage, chromatin condensation, nuclear fragmentation, formation of apoptotic bodies, and, generally, a lack of inflammation. The characteristic morphological features of apoptosis are caused by the activation of caspases, which trigger the activation of enzymes such as caspase-activated DNase (CAD) responsible for internucleosomal DNA fragmentation (Nagata *et al.*, 2003). In addition, caspases can directly cleave cellular and nuclear structural proteins (Fischer *et al.*, 2003). Apoptosis is always a single cell event with the main purpose of removing cells no longer needed during development or eliminating aging cells during regular tissue turnover. Under these conditions, apoptotic bodies are phagocytosed by Kupffer cells or taken up by neighboring hepatocytes. In the absence of cell contents release, the remnants of apoptotic cells disappear without causing an inflammatory response. Because of effective regeneration, apoptotic cell death during normal tissue turnover or even a moderately elevated rate of apoptosis is of limited pathophysiological relevance in the liver. However, if the rate of apoptosis is substantially increased, the apoptotic process cannot be completed. In this case, cells undergo secondary necrosis with breakdown of membrane potential, cell swelling, and release of cell contents (Ogasawara *et al.*, 1993; Bajt *et al.*, 2000). The fundamental difference between oncotic necrosis and secondary necrosis is the fact that during secondary necrosis many apoptotic cells can still be identified based

on morphology, many apoptotic characteristics such as activation of various caspases are present, and the process can be completely inhibited by potent pancaspase inhibitors (Jaeschke *et al.*, 2004). Oncotic necrosis does not involve relevant caspase activation and is not inhibitable by caspase inhibitors.

In recent years, signaling mechanisms of apoptosis were elucidated in great detail (Fig. 13-4) (reviewed by Jaeschke, 2006a; Malhi *et al.*, 2006; Schulze-Bergkamen *et al.*, 2006). In the extrinsic pathway of apoptosis, ligands (eg, Fas ligand, TNF-α) bind to their respective death receptor (Fas receptor, TNF receptor type I), which triggers the trimerization of the receptor followed by recruitment of various adapter molecules and procaspases to the cytoplasmic tail of the receptor. The assembly of this death-inducing signaling complex (DISC) leads to the activation of initiator caspases (caspase-8 or -10). In hepatocytes, the active initiator caspase cleaves Bid, a member of the Bcl-2 family of proteins, and the truncated Bid (tBid) translocates together with other Bcl-2 family members such as Bax to the mitochondria. These proteins form pores in the outer membrane of the mitochondria and cause the release of intermembrane proteins such as cytochrome *c* and the second mitochondria-derived activator of caspases (Smac). Cytochrome *c*, together with apoptosis protease activating factor-1 (APAF-1), ATP, and procaspase-9, forms the apoptosome causing the activation of caspase-9, which then processes (and activates) downstream effector caspases, for example caspase-3. The effector caspases can propagate the apoptosis signal by activating CAD to initiate nuclear DNA fragmentation and by cleaving numerous cellular proteins critical to cellular function and the structural integrity of the cell and the nucleus (Fischer et al., 2003; Nagata et al., 2003). In addition to downstream substrates, caspase-3 can also process more procaspase-8 and further amplify the apoptotic signal. Although hepatocytes constitutively express Fas and TNF receptors, the death signal generated with ligation of the receptor is in most cases insufficient to trigger apoptosis. Inhibitor studies and experiments with gene-deficient mice support the hypothesis that only the amplification of the receptor-derived signal through multiple mitochondrial cycles can successfully induce apoptosis in hepatocytes (Yin et al., 1999; Bajt et al., 2000). In addition to the direct propagation of the apoptosis signal by mitochondrial cytochrome c release, the simultaneous release of Smac ensures that the cytosolic inhibitors of apoptosis proteins (IAPs) are inactivated and do not interfere with the promotion of apoptosis (Li et al., 2002). Thus, mitochondria are an important part of the extrinsic (receptor-mediated) apoptotic signal transduction pathway in liver cells after most stimuli (type II cells). However, it was recently recognized that under conditions of strong Fas receptor activation (MegaFas ligand), hepatocytes can act as type I cells where downstream caspases are activated without involvement of mitochondria (Schüngel et al., 2009).

In contrast to the extrinsic pathway, the intrinsic or mitochondrial pathway of apoptosis is initiated independent of the TNF receptor family, caspase-8 activation, and formation of the DISC. Despite the upstream differences, the postmitochondrial effects are largely similar to the extrinsic pathway. The intrinsic pathway is generally triggered by a cytotoxic stress or DNA damage, which activates the tumor suppressor p53 (Sheikh and Fornace, 2000). This protein acts as a transcription factor to promote the formation of proapoptotic Bcl-2 family members, for example, Bax. The increased Bax translocation to the mitochondria induces the release of mitochondrial intermembrane proteins including cytochrome c, Smac, endonuclease G, and apoptosis-inducing factor (AIF) (Saelens et al., 2004). An intrinsic mechanism of apoptosis has been discussed for cell death in aging livers (Zhang et al., 2002), prolonged treatment with alcohol (Ishii et al., 2003), or toxicity of benzo(a)pyrene and APAP in hepatoma cells (Boulares et al., 2002; Ko et al., 2004). For other hepatotoxic chemicals, such as carbon tetrachloride (Cai et al., 2005), galactosamine (Gomez-Lechon et al., 2002), and microcystin (Ding et al., 2000), evidence for mitochondria-dependent apoptosis has been reported in cultured hepatocytes and relevant apoptotic cell death was observed after in vivo exposure to these chemicals (Shi et al., 1998; Hooser, 2000; Gujral et al., 2003b).

The dramatically increased knowledge of the signaling mechanisms of apoptotic cell death in hepatocytes lead to the identification of many biochemical "apoptosis" parameters, most of which turned out to be not as specific for apoptosis as originally thought. Prominent examples of these tests are the DNA ladder on agarose gels and the terminal deoxynucleotidyl transferase-mediated dUTP nick-end labeling (TUNEL) assay, which demonstrate internucleosomal DNA fragmentation and DNA strandbreaks, respectively. Originally thought to specifically identify apoptotic cells, both assays are positive for most mechanisms of necrotic cell death (Grasl-Kraupp et al., 1995; Gujral et al., 2002; Jaeschke and Lemasters, 2003). As a result of the misinterpretation of many of these assays, the contribution of apoptosis to the overall pathophysiology processes and toxicological liver injuries is controversially debated (Jaeschke and Lemasters, 2003; Jaeschke et al., 2004; Malhi et al., 2006; Schulze-Bergkamen et al., 2006). However, the controversy can be avoided if the decision to label the process as apoptosis is based primarily on the morphological features of the dying cells. Because the characteristic morphology is caused by the caspase-mediated cleavage of structural proteins within the cell, relevant caspase activation, especially of downstream effector caspases such as caspase-3 or -6, is another hallmark of apoptosis. As a result, pancaspase inhibitors can effectively prevent apoptosis-induced liver injury in vivo and in isolated hepatocytes. It should be emphasized that liver cells contain enough procaspases to execute apoptosis if properly stimulated. Thus, changes in caspase gene or protein expression are not evidence for apoptosis, only a relevant increase of enzyme activity. Once the process is identified as apoptosis, additional parameters can be used to further characterize the signaling mechanism. In addition, the use of positive controls, for example, Fas ligand- or TNF-mediated hepatocellular apoptosis, can be helpful in assessing qualitative and quantitative changes of many parameters relative to a proven apoptotic process (Jaeschke et al., 2004). Another critical issue to consider is the model system that is being used. For example, both the antidiabetic drug troglitazone and the analgesic APAP clearly induce apoptosis in hepatoma cell lines (Yamamoto et al., 2001; Boulares et al., 2002). However, there is no evidence for a relevant role of apoptotic cell death in animals or patients for both drugs (Gujral et al., 2002; Chojkier, 2005; Antoine et al., 2012; McGill et al., 2012b). Thus, characterization of cell death after chemical exposure has to be primarily based on morphology and a number of additional biochemical parameters, which need to quantitatively correlate with the number of apoptotic cells. In addition, the relevance of the model system for the human pathophysiology needs to be considered.

The mechanisms of oncotic necrosis are more diverse and depend on the chemical insult to the cell (a detailed example of the mechanism of APAP-induced hepatocellular necrosis is discussed later). However, a general trend is emerging. Independent of the initial insult and signaling pathways, mitochondria are almost always involved in the pathophysiology (Jaeschke et al., 2012a; Pessayre et al., 2012). The opening of the mitochondrial membrane permeability transition (MPT) pore with collapse of the membrane potential and depletion of cellular ATP is a common final step of the mechanism of necrotic cell death (Kim et al., 2003). The loss of ATP inhibits ion pumps of the plasma membrane resulting in the loss of cellular ion homeostasis, which causes the characteristic swelling of oncotic necrosis. A special form of cell death is the more recently described programmed necrosis (necroptosis) (Vandenabeele et al., 2010). Necroptosis is generally initiated by death receptors, for example TNF receptor 1, and the formation of complex 1 with various adapter molecules including receptor-interacting protein 1 and 3 (RIP1 and -3). If caspase-8 is activated, it will cleave RIP1 and -3 and apoptosis will be initiated. However, if caspase-8 is inhibited, RIP1 and -3 activate a caspase-independent execution mechanism involving mitochondrial oxidant stress and mitochondrial dysfunction (Vandenabeele et al., 2010). Although some of these signaling mechanisms of necroptosis have been described for various cell lines, the importance for liver cell death, especially in vivo, remains unclear.

Canalicular Cholestasis This form of liver dysfunction is defined physiologically as a decrease in the volume of bile formed or an impaired secretion of specific solutes into bile (Padda et al., 2011). Cholestasis is characterized biochemically by elevated serum levels of compounds normally concentrated in bile, particularly bile salts and bilirubin. When biliary excretion of the yellowish bilirubin pigment is impaired, this pigment accumulates in skin and eyes, producing jaundice, and spills into urine, which becomes bright yellow or dark brown. Because drug-induced jaundice reflects a more generalized liver dysfunction, it is considered a more serious warning sign in clinical trials than mild elevations of liver enzymes (Zimmerman, 1999). The histological features of cholestasis can be very subtle and difficult to detect without ultrastructural studies. Structural changes include dilation of the bile canaliculus and the presence of bile plugs in bile ducts and canaliculi. Toxicant-induced cholestasis can be transient or chronic; when substantial, it is associated with cell swelling, cell death, and inflammation. Cell injury is generally caused by the accumulation of chemicals in the liver, that is, the cholestasis-causing chemical and, as a consequence, potentially cytotoxic bile acids, bilirubin, and other bile constituents. Many different types of chemicals, including metals, hormones, and drugs, cause cholestasis (Table 13-2) (Zimmerman, 1999).

The molecular mechanisms of cholestasis are related to expression and function of transporter systems in the basolateral and canalicular membranes (reviewed by Pauli-Magnus and Meier, 2006; Padda et al., 2011) (Fig. 13-3). In principle, an increased hepatic uptake, decreased biliary excretion, and increased biliary reabsorption (cholehepatic shunting) of a drug may contribute to its accumulation in the liver. Although no case of drug toxicity has been reported in response to modifications of basolateral uptake, OATPs can contribute to the liver injury potential of toxins. The hepatotoxicity of phalloidin, microcystin, and amanitin is facilitated by the uptake through OATPs (Pauli-Magnus and Meier, 2006; Lu et al., 2008). Furthermore, there is a growing list of drugs including rifampicin, bosentan, and troglitazone, which are known to directly inhibit BSEP (Stieger et al., 2000; Fattinger et al., 2001). However, estrogen and progesterone metabolites inhibit BSEP from the canalicular side after excretion by MRP2 (Stieger et al., 2000). A substantial inhibition of bile salt excretion can lead to accumulation of these compounds in hepatocytes and may directly cause cell injury (Palmeira and Rolo, 2004). However, more recent findings indicate that most of the bile acids accumulating in the liver after obstructive cholestasis are nontoxic (Zhang et al., 2012) and instead of cell death cause proinflammatory gene expression in hepatocytes (Allen et al., 2011). Thus, liver injury after obstructive cholestasis is caused mainly by inflammatory cells (Gujral et al., 2003a). However, the increased bile acid levels can trigger compensatory mechanisms, which limit the injury potential of cholestasis (Zollner et al., 2006; Zhang et al., 2012). Bile acids are substrates for the nuclear receptor farnesoid X receptor (FXR). FXR activation stimulates the small heterodimeric partner 1 (SHP1), which downregulates NTCP and limits bile acid uptake (Denson et al., 2001). In addition, FXR activation causes the increased expression of BSEP and MDR3, which enhances the transport capacity for bile acids and phospholipids, respectively, at the canalicular membrane (Ananthanarayanan et al., 2001; Huang et al., 2003). Furthermore, the FXR-independent upregulation of the basolateral transporters MRP3 and MRP4 reduces intracellular bile acid and drug concentrations (Schuetz et al., 2001; Wagner et al., 2003; Fickert et al., 2006). Recent findings indicate that agonists of the nuclear xenobiotic receptors constitutive androstane receptor (CAR) and pregnane X receptor (PXR) can not only induce MRP3 and -4 expression, but also induce bile acid hydroxylation by Cyp3a11 and Cyp2b10 resulting in improved export and detoxification of bile acids during cholestasis (Wagner et al., 2005). In cholangiocytes, OSTα/OSTβ is upregulated at the basolateral membrane during cholestasis (Boyer et al., 2006a). This response, which is dependent on FXR, mediates the enhanced return of bile acids from bile to the plasma (Boyer et al., 2006a). Thus, the pharmacological modulation of transporter expression may counteract some of the detrimental effects of cholestasis with various etiologies (Zollner et al., 2006).

Bile Duct Damage   Another name for damage to the intrahepatic bile ducts is *cholangiodestructive cholestasis* (Cullen and Ruebner, 1991; Zimmerman, 1999). A useful biochemical index of bile duct damage is a sharp elevation in serum activities of enzymes localized to bile ducts, particularly alkaline phosphatase. In addition, serum levels of bile acids and bilirubin are elevated, as observed with canalicular cholestasis. Initial lesions following a single dose of cholangiodestructive chemicals include swollen biliary epithelium, debris of damaged cells within ductal lumens, and inflammatory cell infiltration of portal tracts. Chronic administration of toxicants that cause bile duct destruction can lead to biliary proliferation and fibrosis resembling primary biliary cirrhosis (PBC). A number of drugs have been implicated to cause prolonged cholestasis with features of PBC (Zimmerman, 1999). However, only in rare cases will there be permanent damage or even loss of bile ducts, a condition known as *vanishing bile duct syndrome*. Cases of this persisting problem have been reported in patients receiving antibiotics (Davies et al., 1994), anabolic steroids, contraceptive steroids, or the anticonvulsant carbamazepine (Zimmerman, 1999).

Sinusoidal Damage   The sinusoid is, in effect, a specialized capillary with numerous fenestrae for high permeability (Braet and Wisse, 2002). The functional integrity of the sinusoid can be compromised by dilation or blockade of its lumen or by progressive destruction of its endothelial cell wall. Dilation of the sinusoid will occur whenever efflux of hepatic blood is impeded. The rare condition of primary dilation, known as *peliosis hepatis*, has been associated with exposure to anabolic steroids and the drug danazol. Blockade will occur when the fenestrae enlarge to such an extent that red blood cells become caught in them or pass through with entrapment in the interstitial space of Disse. Endothelial cell gaps and injury have been shown after exposure to APAP (Ito et al., 2005), galactosamine/endotoxin (Ito et al., 2006), or an anti-Fas antibody (Ogasawara et al., 1993). These gaps can be caused by direct injury to endothelial cells by APAP (DeLeve et al., 1997) and the Fas antibody (Bajt et al., 2000) or could be just the result of detachment from the extracellular matrix (Ito et al., 2006). In general, matrix metalloproteinase inhibitors prevent the gap formation (McCuskey, 2006a). A consequence of endothelial cell injury is the loss of barrier function with extensive blood accumulation in the liver resulting in hypovolemic shock. Microcystin produces this effect within hours in rodents (Hooser et al., 1989). Microcystin dramatically deforms hepatocytes by altering cytoskeleton actin filaments, but it does not affect sinusoidal cells (Hooser et al., 1991). Thus, the deformities that microcystin produces on the cytoskeleton of hepatocytes likely produce a secondary change in the structural integrity of the sinusoid owing to the close proximity of hepatocytes and sinusoidal endothelial cells (Fig. 13-2).

Progressive destruction of the endothelial wall of the sinusoid will lead to gaps and then ruptures of its barrier integrity, with entrapment of red blood cells. These disruptions of the sinusoid are considered the early structural features of the vascular disorder known as veno-occlusive disease (DeLeve et al., 1999). Well established as a cause of veno-occlusive disease are the pyrrolizidine alkaloids (eg, monocrotaline, retrorsine, and seneciphylline) found in some plants used for herbal teas and in some seeds that contaminate food grains. Numerous episodes of human and animal poisoning by pyrrolizidine alkaloids have been reported around the world, including massive problems affecting thousands of people in Afghanistan in 1976 and 1993 (Huxtable, 1997). Veno-occlusive disease is also a serious complication in about 15% of the patients given high doses of chemotherapy (eg, cyclophosphamide) as part of bone-marrow transplantation regimens (DeLeve et al., 1999).

Selective depletion of GSH within sinusoidal endothelial cells and activation of matrix metalloproteinases are critical events in the mechanism of endothelial cell injury in the pathophysiology of veno-occlusive disease (Wang *et al.*, 2000; DeLeve *et al.*, 2003b). Endothelial cell gap formation and injury and the resulting microcirculatory disturbances have been well established as the cause of veno-occlusive disease (DeLeve *et al.*, 2003a).

Disruption of the Cytoskeleton Phalloidin and microcystin disrupt the integrity of hepatocyte cytoskeleton by affecting proteins that are vital to its dynamic nature. The detrimental effects of these two potent hepatotoxicants are independent of their biotransformation and are exclusive for hepatocytes, because there is no appreciable uptake of either toxin into other types of cells. Tight binding of phalloidin to actin filaments prevents the disassembly phase of the normally dynamic rearrangement of the actin filament constituent of the cytoskeleton. Phalloidin uptake into hepatocytes leads to striking alterations in the actin-rich web of cytoskeleton adjacent to the canalicular membrane; the actin web becomes accentuated and the canalicular lumen dilates (Phillips *et al.*, 1986). Experiments using time-lapse video microscopy have documented dose-dependent declines in the contraction of canalicular lumens between isolated hepatocyte couplets after incubation with a range of phalloidin concentrations (Watanabe and Phillips, 1986).

Microcystin uptake into hepatocytes leads to hyperphosphorylation of cytoskeletal proteins secondary to this toxicant's covalent binding to the catalytic subunit of serine/threonine protein phosphatases (Runnegar *et al.*, 1995b). Reversible phosphorylations of cytoskeletal structural and motor proteins are critical to the dynamic integrity of the cytoskeleton. Extensive hyperphosphorylation produced by large amounts of microcystin leads to marked deformation of hepatocytes due to a unique collapse of the microtubular actin scaffold into a spiny central aggregate (Hooser *et al.*, 1991). Lower doses of microcystin, insufficient to produce the gross structural deformations, diminish uptake and secretory functions of hepatocytes in association with preferential hyperphosphorylation of the cytoplasmic motor protein dynein (Runnegar *et al.*, 1999). Dynein is a mechanicochemical protein that drives vesicles along microtubules using energy from ATP hydrolysis; central to the hydrolysis of the dynein-bound ATP is a cycle of kinase phosphorylation and phosphatase dephosphorylation. Thus, hyperphosphorylation of dynein freezes this motor pump. Chronic exposure to low levels of microcystin has raised new concerns about the health effects of this water contaminant. Specifically, low levels of microcystin promote liver tumors and kill hepatocytes in the zone 3 region, where microcystin accumulates (Solter *et al.*, 1998).

Information about the binding of phalloidin and microcystin to specific target molecules is valuable for two reasons. First, the linkages of specific binding to loss of target protein functions provide compelling evidence that such a binding constitutes a defined molecular mechanism of injury. Second, the demonstrations of high-affinity binding to a target molecule without confounding effects on other processes or tissues have *translated* into applications of these toxins as tools for cell biology research. For example, phalloidin complexed with a fluorochrome (eg, rhodamine phalloidin or Texas Red phalloidin) is used to visualize the actin polymer component of the cytoskeleton in all types of permeabilized cells. The collapse of actin filaments into spiny aggregates after microcystin treatment was visualized by fluorescence microscopy of cells stained with rhodamine phalloidin (Hooser *et al.*, 1991). Low levels of microcystin are being used to discriminate the roles of dynein from other cytoskeletal motor proteins (Runnegar *et al.*, 1999).

Fatty Liver Fatty liver (steatosis) is defined biochemically as an appreciable increase in the hepatic lipid (mainly triglyceride) content, which is <5 wt% in the normal human liver. Histologically, in standard paraffin-embedded and solvent-extracted sections, hepatocytes containing excess fat appear to have multiple round, empty vacuoles that displace the nucleus to the periphery of the cell. Use of frozen sections and special stains is needed to document the contents of the vesicles as fat. Based on the size of the fat droplets, one can distinguish between macrovesicular and microvesicular steatosis.

Currently, the most common cause of hepatic steatosis is insulin resistance due to central obesity and sedentary lifestyle. However, acute exposure to many hepatotoxins, for example, carbon tetrachloride and drugs can induce steatosis (Zimmerman, 1999). Compounds that produce prominent steatosis associated with lethality include the antiepileptic drug valproic acid (Scheffner *et al.*, 1988) and the antiviral drug fialuridine (Honkoop *et al.*, 1997). Ethanol is by far the most relevant drug or chemical leading to steatosis in humans and in experimental animals. Often, drug-induced steatosis is reversible and does not lead to death of hepatocytes. The metabolic inhibitors ethionine, puromycin, and cycloheximide cause fat accumulation without causing cell death. Although steatosis alone may be benign, it can develop into steatohepatitis (alcoholic or nonalcoholic), which is associated with significant liver injury (Farrell, 2002; Pessayre *et al.*, 2002; Stravitz and Sanyal, 2003; Saito *et al.*, 2007; Neuschwander-Tetri, 2010). Steatohepatitis can progress to fibrosis and even hepatocellular carcinoma (Farrell and Larter, 2006). Livers with steatosis can be more susceptible to additional insults such as hepatotoxins (Donthamsetty *et al.*, 2007) or hepatic ischemia (Selzner and Clavien, 2001).

Free fatty acids (FFAs) can be newly synthesized in hepatocytes (mainly from carbohydrate-derived acetyl-coenzyme A). FFAs released from adipose tissue can be taken up into hepatocytes, or they are generated in the liver from hydrolysis of absorbed fat (chylomicrons). Once in the cytosol, FFAs can be imported into mitochondria for degradation (β-oxidation), or esterified into triglycerides for incorporation into very low density lipoproteins (VLDL), which transports the FFAs to the peripheral adipose tissue. FFA uptake into mitochondria depends on the activity of the mitochondrial enzyme carnitine palmitoyl transferase 1, which can be downregulated by malonyl-coenzyme A, the first intermediate of FFA synthesis. Thus, FFA synthesis, consumption, and storage are in a state of equilibrium with no relevant accumulation of triglycerides in the liver (Pessayre *et al.*, 2002). However, if there is chronic excess food consumption with obesity and insulin resistance, excess uptake of FFAs derived from adipose tissue and food into hepatocytes leads to an overload of FFAs, which cannot be degraded and are therefore esterified to triglycerides. One part of the excess triglycerides is incorporated into VLDL, and the other part is stored in the liver gradually leading to steatosis (Pessayre *et al.*, 2002). Drug-induced steatosis is mainly caused by compounds such as 4,4′-diethylaminoethoxyhexestrol, amiodarone, tamoxifen, perhexiline, amineptine, doxycycline, tetracycline, tianeptine, and pirprofen, which accumulate in mitochondria and inhibit β-oxidation and mitochondrial respiration (Berson *et al.*, 1998; Larosche *et al.*, 2007, Pessayre *et al.*, 2012). This effect does not only lead to steatosis, but also to increased reactive oxygen formation and lipid peroxidation. In addition, amineptine, amiodarone, tetracycline, pirprofen, and tianeptine can inhibit directly microsomal triglyceride transfer protein, which lipidates apolipoprotein B to form triglyceride-rich VLDL particles (Letteron *et al.*, 2003). Drugs with this dual effect on β-oxidation and VLDL secretion are generally most steatogenic.

The previously preferred hypothesis of nonalcoholic steato-hepatitis (NASH) considered triglyceride accumulation in hepato-cytes as the first hit and any additional stress (oxidant stress, lipid peroxidation) as a second hit leading to the progression from steato-sis to steatohepatitis (Day and James, 1998a). However, more recent data have clearly demonstrated that triglyceride accumulation does neither cause insulin resistance nor cell injury (Neuschwander-Teri, 2010). A new hypothesis postulates that nonalcoholic fatty liver dis-ease (NAFLD) is mainly caused by lipotoxicity of nontriglycer-ide fatty acid metabolites (Neuschwander-Tetri, 2010). Although the specific fatty acids or their metabolites causing NAFLD in patients have not been identified, the emerging evidence suggests that the excessive burden of fatty acids in the liver from either inappropriate lipolysis in adipose tissue or synthesis in the liver may cause liver injury (Neuschwander-Tetri, 2010). Mechanisms of lipotoxicity elucidated in cell culture experiments include endoplasmic reticulum stress, activation of the mitochondrial cell death pathway, and lysosomal dysfunction (Ibrahim *et al.*, 2011). Thus, it is likely that the typical histological phenotype of NAFLD may be caused by a variety of different lipotoxicity mechanisms (Neuschwander-Tetri, 2010).

Fibrosis and Cirrhosis Hepatic fibrosis (scaring) occurs in response to chronic liver injury and is characterized by the accu-mulation of excessive amounts of fibrous tissue, specifically fibril-forming collagens type I and III, and a decrease in normal plasma membrane collagen type IV (reviewed by Bataller and Brenner, 2005; Rockey and Friedman, 2006; Gutierrez-Ruiz and Gomez-Quiroz, 2007). Fibrosis can develop around central veins and por-tal tracts or within the space of Disse. The excessive extracellular matrix protein deposition and the loss of sinusoidal endothelial cell fenestrae and of hepatocyte microvilli limit exchange of nutrients and waste material between hepatocytes and sinusoidal blood. With continuing collagen deposition, the architecture of the liver is disrupted by interconnecting fibrous scars. When the fibrous scars subdivide the remaining liver mass into nodules of regenerating hepatocytes, fibrosis has progressed to cirrhosis and the liver has limited residual capacity to perform its essential functions. The primary cause of hepatic fibrosis/cirrhosis in humans worldwide is viral hepatitis. However, biliary obstruction and, in particular, alcoholic and NASH are of growing importance for the develop-ment of hepatic fibrosis (Bataller and Brenner, 2005). In addition, fibrosis can be induced by chronic exposure to drugs and chemicals including ethanol and by heavy metal overload (Gutierrez-Ruiz and Gomez-Quiroz, 2007). Repeated treatment with carbon tetra-chloride, thioacetamide, dimethylnitrosamine, aflatoxin, or other chemicals has been associated with hepatic fibrosis in experimental animals and humans (Zimmerman, 1999).

Central to the development of fibrosis is the activation of HSC (Fig. 13-2), which are the main cell type producing extra-cellular matrix proteins (Bataller and Brenner, 2005; Gressner and Weiskirchen, 2006; Rockey and Friedman, 2006). Products formed during liver cell injury initiate HSC activation. Activating signals can be reactive oxygen species and lipid peroxidation products generated in injured hepatocytes. In addition, Kupffer cells can release reactive oxygen and proinflammatory cytokines during the phagocytosis of cell debris or apoptotic bodies, thereby recruit-ing more inflammatory cells and enhancing the injury and oxidant stress (Tsukamoto, 2002). Damaged sinusoidal endothelial cells contribute to the activation of HSC by generating a splice variant of cellular fibronectin and by release of the urokinase-type plasmino-gen activator, which processes latent transforming growth factor-β1 (TGF-β1) (Friedman, 2000). Furthermore, accumulating platelets at the site of injury can produce TGF-β1 and growth factors such as platelet-derived growth factor (PDGF) (Rockey and Friedman, 2006). Together these stimuli cause the activation of HSC, which undergo phenotypic changes including proliferation, fibrogenesis and matrix remodeling, chemotaxis and proinflammatory media-tor formation, and contractility (Rockey and Friedman, 2006). The proliferation of HSC is induced by the formation of mitogens such as PDGF. In addition, it also involves the upregulation of the PDGF receptor, which further enhances the responsiveness of HSC to this mitogen (Pinzani, 2002). Another hallmark of HSC activation is enhanced contractility due to the increased expression of α-smooth muscle actin. Increased expression of endothelin-1 receptors on HSC together with the general imbalance between vasodilator (nitric oxide, carbon monoxide) and vasoconstrictor (ET-1) forma-tion contributes to the development of portal hypertension during fibrosis (Rockey, 2003). The increased accumulation of HSC at sites of injury is caused by migration and proliferation of HSC. PDGF, monocyte chemotactic protein 1 (MCP-1), and other chemokines have been shown to be HSC chemoattractants (Marra, 2002). One of the central events in HSC activation is the excessive formation of extracellular matrix proteins induced mainly by TGF-β1. The effects of TGF-β1, which is generated to a large degree by HSCs, are amplified by the increased expression of TGF-β receptors on HSC (Gressner and Weiskirchen, 2006). However, during fibro-genesis there is not only an overall increase in extracellular matrix deposition, but also a change from the basement membrane-like matrix dominated by nonfibril-forming collagens (types IV, VI, and XIV) to a basement membrane-type matrix involving fibril-forming collagen types I and III. The effect is caused by the differ-ential expression and release of matrix metalloproteinases (MMPs) and their inhibitors (TIMPs) from HSC and Kupffer cells. TIMP1 and TIMP2 are upregulated and MMP1 (collagenase I) is down-regulated during fibrogenesis leading to the reduced degradation of fibril-forming collagens, for example, type I. At the same time, MMP2 and -9 (collagenase IV) are activated causing the acceler-ated degradation of nonfibril-forming collagens (Arthur, 2000). Previously, it was assumed that fibrotic changes, especially the state of cirrhosis, were irreversible. However, more recent insight into the pathophysiology indicated the possibility for reversal of fibrosis. Stimulation of apoptosis in activated HSC and the expression of dif-ferent MMPs and TIMPs can reduce matrix deposition and enhance degradation resulting in a gradual reversal of fibrosis (Arthur, 2000; Bataller and Brenner, 2005; Rockey and Friedman, 2006). This area is of considerable interest for pharmaceutical intervention.

Tumors Chemically induced neoplasia can involve tumors that are derived from hepatocytes, bile duct progenitor cells, the ductu-lar "bipolar" progenitor cells, and the periductular stem cells (Sell, 2002). The rare, highly malignant angiosarcomas are derived from sinusoidal lining cells. Hepatocellular cancer has been linked to chronic abuse of androgens, alcohol, and a high prevalence of aflatoxin-contaminated diets. In addition, viral hepatitis, metabolic diseases such as hemochromatosis and α1-antitrypsin deficiency, and NASH are major risk factors for hepatocellular carcinoma (Zimmerman, 1999; McKillop *et al.*, 2006; Wands and Moradpour, 2006). The synergistic effect of coexposure to aflatoxin and hepati-tis virus B is well recognized (Henry *et al.*, 2002). The prevalence of hepatitis B and C viruses and environmental factors make hepa-tocellular carcinoma one of the most common malignant tumors worldwide (Bosch *et al.*, 2005). Angiosarcomas have been asso-ciated with occupational exposure to vinyl chloride and arsenic (Zimmerman, 1999). Exposure to Thorotrast (radioactive thorium dioxide used as contrast medium for radiology) has been linked to tumors derived from hepatocytes, sinusoidal cells, and bile duct cells (cholangiocarcinoma) (Zimmerman, 1999). The compound accumulates in Kupffer cells and emits radioactivity throughout its extended half-life. One study of Danish patients exposed to Thorotrast found that the risk for bile duct and gallbladder cancers was increased 14-fold and that for liver cancers more than 100-fold (Andersson and Storm, 1992). Furan is the only chemical known to cause cholangiocarcinomas experimentally in rats (Hickling *et al.*, 2010).

The molecular pathogenesis of hepatocellular carcinoma is complex and poorly understood. The malignant transformation of hepatocytes occurs as a result of increased cell turnover due to chronic liver injury, persistent inflammation, regeneration, and cirrhosis (Wands and Moradpour, 2006). Direct DNA binding of carcinogens or their reactive metabolites (eg, aflatoxin metabolites) or indirect DNA modifications by reactive oxygen species generated during inflammation and cell injury can lead to genetic alterations in hepatocytes resulting in impaired DNA repair, the activation of cellular oncogenes, and inactivation of tumor suppressor genes. An overall imbalance between stimulation of proliferation and inhibition of apoptosis in the liver leads to the survival and expansion of these preneoplastic cells (Fabregat *et al.*, 2007). This concept is supported by the observation that 30% of hepatocellular carcinomas show mutations in the tumor suppressor gene p53; the mutation rate is up to 70% in areas with high aflatoxin exposure (Wands and Moradpour, 2006). The functional inactivation of p53 by mutations prevents the induction of apoptosis. Because most chemotherapeutic agents require p53 to induce apoptosis in these cancer cells, hepatocellular carcinomas are mostly resistant to conventional chemotherapy (Bruix *et al.*, 2006). However, p53 mutations alone are not sufficient to initiate carcinogenesis. It was shown that telomere dysfunction and chromosomal instability in combination with p53 mutations are critical for the progression from neoplasms to malignant carcinomas (Farazi *et al.*, 2006). Because telomere dysfunction (shortening) limits the capacity of cancer cells to proliferate, the activity of the telomere-synthesizing enzyme telomerase is activated in advanced hepatocellular carcinomas (Satyanarayana *et al.*, 2004). Stabilization and repair of telomeres promote the expansion of the tumor. Additional tumor cell survival mechanisms include the disruption of TGF-β apoptosis signaling and

activation of phosphatidylinositol-3-kinase/AKT survival pathways (Thorgeirsson *et al.*, 1998). Furthermore, NF-κB activation during inflammation is responsible for induction of prosurvival genes such as Bcl-X$_L$ and XIAP, the downregulation of the Fas receptor on hepatocytes, and the reduced expression of the proapoptotic Bax gene (Fabregat *et al.*, 2007). These effects are combined with the overexpression and dysregulated signaling of promitogenic and antiapoptotic growth factors such as insulin-like growth factor (IGF), hepatocyte growth factor (HGF), wingless (Wnt), and transforming growth factor-α (TGF-α)/epidermal growth factor (EGF) (Breuhahn *et al.*, 2006). Many of these pathways may offer novel therapeutic targets to prevent or eliminate hepatocellular carcinoma (Aravalli *et al.*, 2008).

Critical Factors in Toxicant-Induced Liver Injury

Why is the liver the target site for many chemicals of diverse structure? Why do many hepatotoxicants preferentially damage one type of liver cell? Our understanding of these fundamental questions is incomplete. Influences of several factors are of obvious importance (Table 13-3). Location and specialized processes for uptake and biliary secretion produce higher exposure levels in the liver than in other tissues of the body, and strikingly high levels within certain types of liver cells. Then, the abundant capacity for bioactivation reactions influences the rate of exposure to proximate toxicants. Subsequent events in the pathogenesis appear to be critically influenced by responses of sinusoidal cells and the immune system. Discussion of the evidence for the contributions of these factors to the hepatotoxicity of representative compounds requires commentary about mechanistic events.

In vitro systems using tissue slices, the isolated perfused liver, primary isolated cultured liver cells, and cell fractions allow observations at various levels of complexity without the confounding influences of other systems. Some hepatoma cell lines with maintained drug metabolizing enzyme expression can be useful to study mechanisms of drug hepatotoxicity (Guguen-Guillouzo *et al.*, 2010; McGill *et al.*, 2011). Models using cocultures or chemicals that inactivate a given cell type can document the contributions and interactions between cell types. A limitation of these in vitro systems is the

Table 13-3

Factors in the Site-Specific Injury of Representative Hepatotoxicants

SITE	REPRESENTATIVE TOXICANTS	POTENTIAL EXPLANATION FOR SITE-SPECIFICITY
Zone 1 hepatocytes (vs zone 3)	Fe (overload) Allyl alcohol	Preferential uptake and high oxygen levels Higher oxygen levels for oxygen-dependent bioactivation
Zone 3 hepatocytes (vs zone 1)	CCl$_4$ Acetaminophen Ethanol	More P450 isozyme for bioactivation More P450 isozyme for bioactivation and less GSH for detoxification More hypoxic and greater imbalance in bioactivation/detoxification reactions
Bile duct cells	Methylenedianiline, sporidesmin	Exposure to the high concentration of reactive metabolites in bile
Sinusoidal endothelium (vs hepatocytes)	Cyclophosphamide, monocrotaline	Greater vulnerability to toxic metabolites and less ability to maintain glutathione levels
Kupffer cells	Endotoxin, GdCl$_3$	Preferential uptake and then activation
Stellate cells	Vitamin A Ethanol (chronic)	Preferential site for storage and then engorgement Activation and transformation to collagen-synthesizing cell

fact that the artificial cell culture conditions will modify the basal gene expression profile (Boess *et al.*, 2003) and may influence or even dominate the response of cells to a chemical. In particular, the generally high oxygen concentrations used during cell culture (room air, 21% oxygen) compared to physiologically relevant oxygen levels (4%–10% oxygen) can affect the mechanism of drug-induced cell injury (Yan *et al.*, 2010). Whole animal models are essential for assessment of the progression of injury and responses to chronic insult and the confirmation of in vitro results. Use of chemicals that induce, inhibit, deplete, or inactivate gene products can define roles of specific processes, although potential influences of nonspecific actions can confound interpretations. Application of molecular biology techniques for gene transfection or repression attenuates some of these interpretive problems. Gene knockout animals are extremely useful models to study complex aspects of hepatotoxicity. However, it is critical that the relevance of in vivo systems for the human pathophysiology is being established. In addition, compensatory responses due to the loss of a specific gene always need to be considered when using gene knockout animals (Ni *et al.*, 2012b).

Uptake and Concentration Hepatic "first pass" uptake of ingested chemicals is facilitated by the location of the liver downstream of the portal blood flow from the gastrointestinal tract. Lipophilic compounds, particularly drugs and environmental pollutants, readily diffuse into hepatocytes because the fenestrated epithelium of the sinusoid enables close contact between circulating molecules and hepatocytes. Thus, the membrane-rich liver concentrates lipophilic compounds. Other toxins are rapidly extracted from blood because they are substrates for transporters located on the sinusoidal membrane of hepatocytes (Hagenbuch and Gui, 2008; Roth *et al.*, 2011).

Phalloidin and microcystin are illustrative examples of hepatotoxins that target the liver as a consequence of extensive uptake into hepatocytes by sinusoidal transporters (Frimmer, 1987; Runnegar *et al.*, 1995a). Ingestion of the mushroom *Amanita phalloides* is a common cause of severe, acute hepatotoxicity in continental Europe and North America. Microcystin has produced numerous outbreaks of hepatotoxicity in sheep and cattle that drank pond water containing the blue-green alga *Microcystis aeruginosa*. An episode of microcystin contamination of the water source used by a hemodialysis center in Brazil led to acute liver injury in 81% of the 124 exposed patients and the subsequent death of 50 of these patients (Jochimsen *et al.*, 1998). Microcystin contamination was verified by analysis of samples from the water-holding tank at the dialysis center and from the livers of patients who died. This episode indicates the vulnerability of the liver to toxicants regardless of the route of administration. Because of its dual blood supply from both the portal vein and the hepatic artery, the liver is presented with appreciable amounts of all toxicants in the systemic circulation.

An early clue to preferential uptake as a factor in phalloidin's target-organ specificity was the observation that bile duct ligation, which elevates systemic bile acid levels, protects rats against phalloidin-induced hepatotoxicity in association with an 85% decrease in hepatic uptake of phalloidin (Walli *et al.*, 1981). Subsequent studies found that cotreatment with substrates (eg, cyclosporin A, rifampicin) known to prevent the in vivo hepatotoxicity of phalloidin or microcystin would also inhibit their uptake into hepatocytes by sinusoidal transporters for bile acids and other organic anions (Ziegler and Frimmer, 1984; Runnegar *et al.*, 1995a). Recently, conclusive evidence utilizing Oatp1b2-null mice has demonstrated that the OATP transporter family is responsible for the hapatic uptake and toxicity of phalloidin (Lu *et al.*, 2008).

Accumulation within liver cells by processes that facilitate uptake and storage is a determining factor in the hepatotoxicity of

vitamin A and several metals. Vitamin A hepatotoxicity initially affects stellate cells, which actively extract and store this vitamin. Early responses to high-dose vitamin A therapy are stellate cell engorgement, activation, increase in number, and protrusion into the sinusoid (Geubel *et al.*, 1991). Cadmium hepatotoxicity becomes manifest when the cells exceed their capacity to sequester cadmium as a complex with the metal-binding protein, metallothionein (MT). This protective role for MT was definitively documented by observations with MT transgenic and knockout mice. Overexpression of MT in the transgenic mice rendered them more resistant than wild-type animals to the hepatotoxicity and lethality of cadmium poisoning (Liu *et al.*, 1995). In contrast, MT gene knockout mice were dramatically more susceptible to cadmium heptatotoxicity (Liu *et al.*, 1996).

Iron poisoning produces severe liver damage. Hepatocytes contribute to the homeostasis of iron by extracting this essential metal from the sinusoid by a receptor-mediated process and maintaining a reserve of iron within the storage protein ferritin. Acute Fe toxicity is most commonly observed in young children who accidentally ingest iron tablets (Chang and Rangan, 2011). The cytotoxicity of free iron is attributed to its function as an electron donor for the Fenton reaction, where hydrogen peroxide is reductively cleaved to the highly reactive hydroxyl radical, an initiator of lipid peroxidation. Accumulation of excess iron beyond the capacity for its safe storage in ferritin is initially evident in the zone 1 hepatocytes, which are closest to the blood entering the sinusoid. Thus, the zone 1 pattern of hepatocyte damage after iron poisoning is attributable to location for (1) the preferential uptake of iron and (2) the higher oxygen concentrations that facilitate the injurious process of lipid peroxidation (Table 13-3). Chronic hepatic accumulation of excess iron in cases of hemochromatosis is associated with a spectrum of hepatic disease including a greater than 200-fold increased risk for liver cancer (Ramm and Ruddell, 2005).

Bioactivation and Detoxification One of the vital functions of the liver is to eliminate exogenous chemicals and endogenous intermediates. Therefore, hepatocytes contain high levels of phase I enzymes, which have the capacity to generate reactive electrophilic metabolites. Hepatocytes also have a wide variety of phase II enzymes, which enhance the hydrophilicity by adding polar groups to lipophilic compounds and target these conjugates to certain carriers in the canalicular or plasma membrane for excretion. Generally, phase II reactions yield stable, nonreactive metabolites. Although electrophiles may be effectively conjugated and excreted, if the intermediate is highly reactive, some of these compounds can react with proteins and other target molecules before an interaction with a phase II enzyme is possible. In contrast, if the amount of the reactive metabolite exceeds the capacity of the hepatocyte to detoxify it, covalent binding to cellular macromolecules will occur and potentially result in cell injury (Park *et al.*, 2011). Thus, the balance between phase I reactions, which generate the electrophile, and conjugating phase II reactions determines whether a reactive intermediate is safely detoxified or may cause cell dysfunction or injury. Because the expression of phase I and II enzymes and of the hepatic transporters can be influenced by genetics (eg, polymorphism of drug-metabolizing enzymes) and lifestyle (eg, diet, consumption of other drugs and alcohol), the susceptibility to potential hepatotoxicants can vary markedly between individuals. Several prominent and important examples are discussed.

Acetaminophen One of the most widely used analgesics, acetaminophen (APAP) is a safe drug when used at therapeutically recommended doses. However, an overdose can cause severe liver injury and even liver failure in experimental animals and in humans (Lee, 2004). About half of all overdose cases are caused by suicide

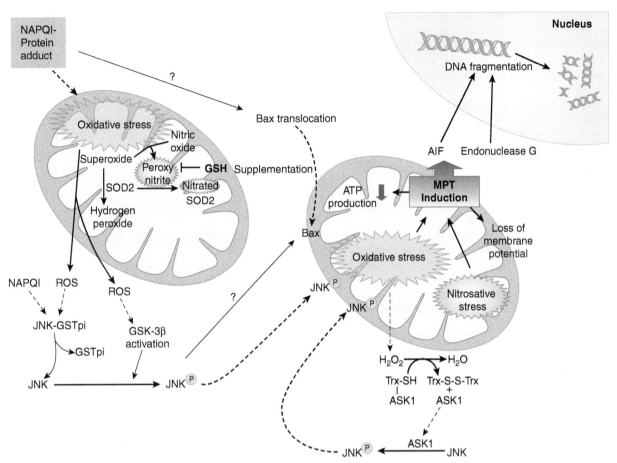

Figure 13-5. *Acetaminophen-induced mitochondrial oxidant stress and its influence on cellular signaling.* Metabolism of APAP results in the generation of the reactive intermediate, NAPQI, which forms protein adducts and induces mitochondrial oxidative stress. The increased generation of superoxide and its reaction with NO results in the production of peroxynitrite. The superoxide can be scavenged by SOD2 and converted into hydrogen peroxide, although the generation of peroxynitrite can interfere in this process by the nitration of SOD2. Mitochondrial oxidative stress and hydrogen peroxide can also activate the mitogen-activated protein kinase, JNK, by multiple pathways, resulting in its phosphorylation and translocation to the mitochondria. This then amplifies the mitochondrial oxidant stress, which, subsequently, leads to activation of the mitochondrial permeability transition, and translocation of mitochondrial proteins, such as AIF and endonuclease G, to the nucleus. This results in DNA fragmentation and, finally, oncotic necrosis. (From Jaeschke *et al.*, 2012a.)

attempts, but an increasing number of cases are reported with unintentional overdosing (Larson *et al.*, 2005). Although the toxicity is a rare event compared to the millions of patients taking the drug daily, APAP-mediated liver injury represents a significant clinical problem. During the last 10 years, APAP-induced hepatotoxicity became the most frequent cause of drug-induced liver failure in the United States and in the United Kingdom (Lee, 2004; Larson *et al.*, 2005).

Because >90% of a therapeutic dose of APAP is conjugated with sulfate or glucuronide, the limited formation of a reactive metabolite, that is, *N*-acetyl-*p*-benzoquinone imine (NAPQI), poses no risk for liver injury. In fact, long-term studies with APAP in osteoarthritis patients did not reveal any evidence of liver dysfunction or cell injury even in patients consuming the maximal recommended daily dose of APAP for 12 months (Kuffner *et al.*, 2006; Temple *et al.*, 2006). In contrast, after an overdose, the formation of large amounts of NAPQI leads first to depletion of cellular GSH stores and subsequently causes covalent binding of NAPQI to intracellular proteins (Jollow *et al.*, 1973; Mitchell *et al.*, 1973) (Fig. 13-5). The generally higher levels of P450 enzymes combined with the lower GSH content in centrilobular hepatocytes are the main reasons for the predominant centrilobular necrosis observed after APAP poisoning. Consistent with the critical role of protein binding for cell injury are the findings that APAP protein adducts are located predominantly in centrilobular hepatocytes undergoing

necrosis (Roberts *et al.*, 1991) and that no APAP hepatotoxicity is observed without protein binding (Nelson, 1990). Because protein binding can be prevented by conjugation of NAPQI with GSH, any manipulation that reduces hepatic GSH levels, for example, fasting or protein malnutrition, potentially enhances the toxicity of APAP. In contrast, interventions such as the supply of cysteine, the rate-limiting amino acid for GSH synthesis, promote the detoxification of NAPQI and limit cell injury (Mitchell *et al.*, 1973). Based on this fundamental insight into the mechanism of APAP hepatotoxicity, *N*-acetylcysteine was introduced in the clinic as intervention therapy (Smilkstein *et al.*, 1988). This highly successful approach, which saved the lives of many patients who took an APAP overdose, is still the most effective treatment available (Lee, 2004). More recent evidence indicates that *N*-acetyl cysteine treatment not only promotes cytosolic GSH synthesis to detoxify NAPQI, but also replenishes the depleted mitochondrial GSH content, which scavenges reactive oxygen and peroxynitrite. In addition, excess *N*-acetyl cysteine is degraded and supports the mitochondrial energy metabolism (Saito *et al.*, 2010b).

A significant factor in APAP hepatotoxicity can be the consumption of alcoholic beverages. In addition to potential malnutrition in alcoholics, ethanol is a potent inducer of CYP2E1, which is the main enzyme responsible for the metabolic activation of APAP in humans (Gonzalez, 2007). Whereas the simultaneous exposure of ethanol and APAP competitively inhibits NAPQI formation and therefore prevents APAP-induced toxicity (Sato and Lieber, 1981), the increased expression of CYP2E1 can enhance APAP toxicity after ethanol metabolism (Gonzalez, 2007). In addition, the presence of higher-chain alcohols, for example, isopentanol, in alcoholic beverages can induce additional P450 isoenzymes such as CYP3A, which can significantly enhance APAP hepatotoxicity (Sinclair et al., 2000; Guo et al., 2004). Despite the clear experimental evidence that alcohol consumption can increase the susceptibility to APAP (Sato et al., 1981) and the clinical observation of severe APAP hepatotoxicity in alcoholics, it remains controversial whether alcohol can actually induce hepatotoxicity at therapeutic doses of APAP as suggested by some case reports (Zimmerman and Maddrey, 1995). However, an extensive review of the literature involving APAP consumption in alcoholics suggests no relevant risk for APAP hepatotoxicity at therapeutic levels in this patient population (Dart et al., 2000). In addition, a randomized, double-blind, placebo-controlled trial with multiple therapeutic doses of APAP showed no evidence of liver dysfunction or cell injury in alcoholics (Kuffner et al., 2001). Thus, alcohol consumption does not increase the risk for liver injury after therapeutic doses of APAP. This finding may apply to the potential interaction with other drugs and dietary chemicals. Nevertheless, consistent with experimental data and clinical experience, inducers of CYPs aggravate liver injury after a hepatotoxic dose of APAP.

Although the focus of early mechanistic investigations was on the role of covalent binding in APAP-induced hepatotoxicity, it became apparent during the last decade that protein adduct formation is an important biomarker for APAP overdose (Davern et al., 2006), but protein binding alone was not sufficient to explain cell injury (Fig. 13-5). In fact, low levels of protein adducts are even observed after therapeutic doses of APAP in mice (McGill et al., 2012a) and humans (Heard et al., 2011). Because no APAP-induced cell injury is observed without covalent binding of NAPQI to cellular proteins, in particular mitochondrial proteins, it is considered a critical initiating event of the toxicity that requires amplification (Jaeschke et al., 2003, 2012a). Mitochondrial protein binding causes inhibition of mitochondrial respiration, a selective mitochondrial oxidant stress, mitochondrial peroxynitrite formation, and declining ATP levels in the liver (Jaeschke and Bajt, 2006). The early mitochondrial translocation of Bax and Bid, members of the Bcl-2 family of proteins, triggers the release of mitochondrial intermembrane proteins including endonuclease G and AIF (Jaeschke and Bajt, 2006). These endonucleases, which translocate to the nucleus after APAP exposure, cause the initial nuclear DNA fragmentation after mitochondrial Bax pore formation (Jaeschke et al., 2012a). However, the continued exposure of GSH-depleted mitochondria to peroxynitrite results in nitration of mitochondrial proteins and mitochondrial DNA modifications (Cover et al., 2005). The continued oxidant stress will eventually trigger the MPT pore opening with breakdown of the membrane potential, mitochondrial swelling, and rupture of the outer membrane (Kon et al., 2004; Ramachandran et al., 2011). These events lead to the loss of mitochondrial ATP synthesis capacity, more extensive nuclear DNA fragmentation due to the amplified release of intermembrane proteins after the MPT, and eventually oncotic necrotic cell death (Gujral et al., 2002). Because of the central role of the mitochondrial oxidant stress in APAP hepatotoxicity, its regulation could be an important therapeutic target. Once initiated by early protein binding, the mitochondrial oxidant stress triggers activation (phosphorylation) of c-jun-N-terminal kinase (JNK), which then translocates to the mitochondria and amplifies the mitochondrial oxidant stress (Han et al., 2010; Jaeschke et al., 2012a). JNK is phosphorylated by apoptosis signal regulating kinase-1 (ASK-1), which is

liberated from the ASK-1-thioredoxin-1 complex in the cytosol after oxidation of thioredoxin-1 by the mitochondrial oxidant stress (Han et al., 2010; Jaeschke et al., 2012a) (Fig. 13-5).

In addition to these intracellular signaling mechanisms leading to cell death, additional events may expand the area of necrosis. The release of calpains, which are Ca^{2+}-activated proteases, during necrosis can promote further cell injury in neighboring cells (Mehendale and Limaye, 2005). Likewise, the release of DNase-1 enhances nuclear DNA fragmentation in adjacent cells and aggravates the injury after APAP overdose. Also, the release of intracellular proteins such as the nuclear protein HMGB-1 from necrotic cells can stimulate macrophages to produce proinflammatory cytokines. This way, the necrotic cell death during APAP hepatotoxicity can promote an innate immune response with recruitment of neutrophils and other inflammatory leukocytes, which may clear cell debris and prepare for regeneration of the lost tissue (Jaeschke et al., 2012b) but, under certain conditions, may cause additional injury (see the "Inflammation" section).

Although many details of the mechanism still remain to be elucidated, the newly gained insight into signaling events in response to APAP overdose suggests two fundamentally new developments. First, necrotic cell death is in most cases not caused by a single catastrophic event but can be the result of a cellular stress, which is initiated by metabolic activation and triggers sophisticated signaling mechanisms culminating in cell death (Fig. 13-5). Second, the multitude of events following the initial stress offers many opportunities for therapeutic interventions at later time points. Because these events are not occurring in all cells to the same degree and at the same time, delayed interventions may not completely prevent cell damage but limit the area of necrosis enough to prevent liver failure. Delayed treatment with GSH to accelerate the recovery of mitochondrial GSH levels effectively scavenged peroxynitrite, reduced the area of necrosis, and promoted regeneration resulting in improved survival after APAP overdose (Bajt et al., 2003). Overexpression of calpastatin, an inhibitor of calpains, attenuated APAP-induced liver injury and enhanced survival (Limaye et al., 2006). Delayed treatment with a JNK inhibitor attenuated the mitochondrial oxidant stress and prevented the MPT and tissue injury (Hanawa et al., 2008; Saito et al., 2010a). Further support for the central role of mitochondrial dysfunction in APAP toxicity in hepatocytes comes from the recent observation that removal of damaged mitochondria by autophagy (mitophagy) limits APAP-induced liver injury in vivo and in cultured cells (Ni et al., 2012a). Together these findings underscore the concept that the later stages of APAP-induced liver injury can be potentially affected at the level of intracellular signaling in hepatocytes and during the propagation of the injury to neighboring cells.

Ethanol   Morbidity and mortality associated with the consumption of alcohol is mainly caused by the toxic effects of ethanol on the liver (Stewart and Day, 2006). This targeted toxicity is due to the fact that >90% of a dose of ethanol is metabolized in the liver. Three principal pathways of ethanol metabolism are known (Fig. 13-6). Alcohol dehydrogenase (ADH) oxidizes ethanol to acetaldehyde with a Km of 1 mM; the electrons are transferred to NAD^+, which leads to the production of NADH. Acetaldehyde is further oxidized to acetate in a NAD-dependent reaction by acetaldehyde dehydrogenase (ALDH). This pathway is mainly regulated by the mitochondrial capacity to utilize NADH and regenerate NAD^+ (Stewart and Day, 2006). The formation of excess reducing equivalents and acetate stimulates fatty acid synthesis and is a major factor in the development of alcohol-induced steatosis. Both ADH and ALDH exhibit genetic polymorphisms and ethnic variations, which play a role in

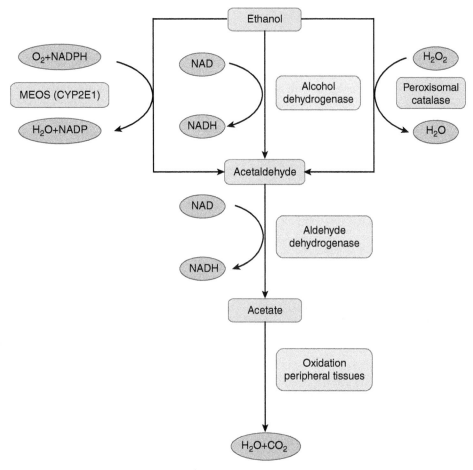

Figure 13-6. *Three pathways of alcohol oxidation: ADH, MEOS, and catalase.* ADH, alcohol dehydrogenase; MEOS, microsomal ethanol-oxidizing system; NADPH, nicotinamide-adenine dinucleotide phosphate. (From Stewart and Day, 2006.)

the development of alcoholism and liver damage (Agarwal, 2001; Day, 2006). A toxicologically relevant polymorphism involves the mitochondrial ALDH2, where the ALDH2*2 form shows little or no catalytic activity. The increased levels of acetaldehyde present in individuals that carry this polymorphism is thought to cause the "flushing" syndrome after ethanol exposure. The inactive form of ALDH is found in 50% of Asians but is absent in Caucasians. This may be the reason for the overall reduced incidence of alcoholism in Asia compared to Europe and North America (Chen *et al.*, 1999). However, heterozygotes of ALDH2*2 were found to develop more severe liver injury in response to lower alcohol consumption, suggesting a higher susceptibility to alcoholic liver disease (Enomoto *et al.*, 1991). These findings underscore the importance of acetaldehyde in the pathophysiology.

The second major pathway involves the alcohol-inducible enzyme CYP2E1, which oxidizes ethanol to acetaldehyde (Fig. 13-6). The enzyme is located predominantly in hepatocytes of the centrilobular region and requires oxygen and NADPH. Because the Km of CYP2E1 for ethanol is >10 mM, this reaction is most relevant for high doses of ethanol and, due to the enzyme's inducibility, for chronic alcoholism (Stewart and Day, 2006). The third pathway involves catalase in peroxisomes. In this reaction, ethanol functions as an electron donor for the reduction of hydrogen peroxide to water. Thus, the capacity of this pathway is limited due to the low levels of hydrogen peroxide. It is estimated that <2% of an ethanol dose is metabolized through this pathway (Stewart and Day, 2006).

The mechanisms of alcohol-induced liver disease are complex and still incompletely understood. Steatosis is a common feature of chronic alcohol consumption. It is caused by the excessive supply of acetate and NADH, which promotes fatty acid synthesis. In addition, ethanol and acetaldehyde inhibit the DNA binding of peroxisome proliferator-activated receptor-α (PPAR-α), which regulates constitutive and inducible expression of mitochondrial and peroxisomal fatty acid metabolizing enzymes (Aoyama *et al.*, 1998). In addition to the enhanced synthesis and reduced consumption of fatty acids, ethanol exposure inhibits the transfer of triglycerides from liver to adipose tissue. Acetaldehyde inhibits the microsomal triglyceride transfer protein, which incorporates triglycerides into VLDL (Lin *et al.*, 1997), and disrupts the export mechanism of VLDL by interfering with microtubular function (Kannarkat *et al.*, 2006). These effects of ethanol and its metabolites can be compounded in the presence of a high-fat diet. Although steatosis alone does generally not develop into more severe liver disease, it has been hypothesized that it plays a critical role in the advancement of the disease process (Day and James, 1998a, b). Steatosis is considered the "first hit," which requires a "second hit" to progress to severe alcoholic liver disease (Day and James, 1998a, b). However, more recent data support the concept of lipotoxicity as a critical determinant of disease progression (Neuschwander-Tetri, 2010). CYP2E1 is a relevant source of reactive oxygen formation during ethanol metabolism (Dey and Cederbaum, 2006). This intracellular oxidant stress in hepatocytes can ultimately induce mitochondrial dysfunction and cell death of hepatocytes, but also activate stellate cells and promote fibrosis (Dey and Cederbaum, 2006). In addition to the intracellular events, alcohol exposure causes an inflammatory response, which contributes to the oxidant stress (Arteel, 2003;

Hines and Wheeler, 2004). Gut-derived endotoxin and other bacteria-derived products can activate Kupffer cells through toll-like receptor activation to produce reactive oxygen species and cytokines such as TNF-α (Seki and Schnabl, 2012). The formation of these mediators can be further amplified by feedback loops, which enhance cytokine and chemokine formation through priming of the redox-sensitive transcription factor NF-κB in Kupffer cells (Arteel, 2003). In addition, TNF-α can induce the inducible nitric oxide synthase (iNOS, NOS2) leading to the formation of peroxynitrite, a potent oxidant and nitrating species (Arteel, 2003). TNF-α can also directly promote cell death by acting on hepatocytes, which are primed by ethanol-induced depletion of mitochondrial GSH (Colell et al., 1998). Inhibition of the proteasome pathway, a well-recognized feature of chronic alcohol exposure, can enhance chemokine formation in hepatocytes and promote inflammatory liver injury (McClain et al., 2005). Additional proinflammatory mediators and immune responses can be triggered by protein adducts of acetaldehyde and malondialdehyde (Freeman et al., 2005) and the release of other DAMPs (Miller et al., 2011). Interestingly, ethanol inhibits hepatic NK cells. As NK cells can kill HSC, the major cell type promoting hepatic fibrosis, ethanol can indirectly support fibrogenesis by preventing the elimination of activated stellate cells (Miller et al., 2011). Another defense mechanism that is activated during alcoholic liver disease is autophagy, which can remove damaged cell organelles and modified proteins (Ding et al., 2011) and thereby reduce the activation of the innate immune response. Thus, alcoholic liver disease is a complex interplay between the activation of pro-cell death mechanisms (reactive metabolite formation, oxidant stress, protein adducts, and stimulation of proinflammatory and profibrotic innate immune responses) and activation of defense mechanisms (antioxidants, autophagy, and NK cell activation) (Gao and Bataller, 2011).

Allyl Alcohol An industrial chemical used in the production of resins, plastics, and fire retardants, allyl alcohol is also used as a model hepatotoxin due to its preferential periportal (zone 1) hepatotoxicity. The alcohol is metabolized by ADH to acrolein, a highly reactive aldehyde, which is then further oxidized by ALDH to acrylic acid. The fact that the toxicity depends on depletion of hepatic GSH levels is prevented by inhibitors of ADH but enhanced by inhibitors of ALDH suggests that acrolein formation is the critical event in liver injury (Jaeschke et al., 1987; Rikans, 1987). Age and gender differences in allyl alcohol hepatotoxicity can be explained by variations in the balance between ADH and ALDH expression (Rikans and Moore, 1987). The preferential occurrence of allyl alcohol injury in zone 1 hepatocytes (Table 13-3) is caused by the predominant uptake of allyl alcohol in the periportal region and the oxygen dependence of the toxicity (Badr et al., 1986). Although protein binding of the reactive metabolite acrolein and subsequent adduct formation appears to be the main cause of liver cell death (Kaminskas et al., 2004), lipid peroxidation can become a relevant mechanism of cell injury under conditions of a compromised antioxidant status (Jaeschke et al., 1987). Lipid peroxidation is caused by a reductive stress where the excessive NADH formation leads to mobilization of redox-active iron from storage proteins (Jaeschke et al., 1992).

Carbon Tetrachloride Cytochrome P450-dependent conversion of CCl_4 to $\bullet CCl_3$ and then to $CCl_3OO\bullet$ is the classic example of xenobiotic bioactivation to a free radical that initiates lipid peroxidation by abstracting a hydrogen atom from the polyunsaturated fatty acid of a phospholipid (Recknagel et al., 1989; Weber et al., 2003). The metabolic activation of CCl_4 involves primarily CYP2E1 in vivo as indicated by the absence of toxicity in CYP2E1

knockout mice (Wong et al., 1998). CCl_4-induced lipid peroxidation increases the permeability of the plasma membrane to Ca^{2+}, leading to severe disturbances of the calcium homeostasis and necrotic cell death (Weber et al., 2003). Recent research indicates that CCl_4 also induces significant mitochondrial damage, which is dependent on lipid peroxidation events and on CYP2E1 activity (Knockaert et al., 2012). In addition, the $\bullet CCl_3$ radical can directly bind to tissue macromolecules and some of the lipid peroxidation products are reactive aldehydes, for example, 4-hydroxynonenal, which can form adducts with proteins (Weber et al., 2003). In addition to the intracellular events, Kupffer cell activation can contribute to liver injury (elSisi et al., 1993). Kupffer cells may enhance the injury by oxidant stress (elSisi et al., 1993) or TNF-α generation, which may lead to apoptosis (Shi et al., 1998). In support of these different components of the mechanism of CCl_4-mediated cell and organ damage, beneficial effects were shown with inhibition of CYPs, preservation of Ca^{2+} homeostasis, antioxidants, and anoxia (Weber et al., 2003). In contrast, treatments with chemicals that induce CYP2E1, for example, ethanol or acetone, enhance the injury. This was confirmed in humans. A case report showed the higher vulnerability of workers with a history of alcohol abuse to CCl_4 vapors compared to similarly exposed moderately drinking coworkers (Manno et al., 1996). Although the use of CCl_4 is restricted and human exposure is limited, it is still a popular model hepatotoxin to study mechanisms of cell injury and fibrosis.

Regeneration The liver has a high capacity to restore lost tissue and function by regeneration. Loss of hepatocytes due to hepatectomy or cell injury triggers proliferation of all mature liver cells. This process is capable of restoring the original liver mass (Michalopoulos and DeFrances, 1997; Fausto, 2000). However, if hepatocyte replication is blocked, hepatic stem cells or oval cells may proliferate to replace the lost parenchyma (Michalopoulos and DeFrances, 1997; Fausto, 2000). This effect is caused by the reduced sensitivity of oval cells to the proliferation-inhibiting cytokine transforming growth factor-β (TGF-β) (Nguyen et al., 2007). Hepatocytes are normally quiescent, that is, they are in G_0 phase of the cell cycle. In order to proliferate, they need to enter the cell cycle. The process is initiated by cytokines (TNF-α, IL-6), which prime hepatocytes to respond to essential growth factors such as HGF and TGF-α (Fausto, 2000). In contrast to Fausto's priming/progression hypothesis, Michalopoulos (2007) argues that hepatocytes do not fit the two stage model but there are primary direct mitogens for hepatocytes (eg, HGF) and secondary proregenerative substances (TNF-α), which enhance the effect of the primary mitogen (Michalopoulos, 2007). Both cytokines and growth factors are involved in the activation of transcription factors and ultimately expression of cell cycle-regulating proteins, that is, cyclins, the activators of cyclin-dependent kinases (CDKs), and p18, p21, and p27, inhibitors of CDKs (Trautwein, 2006). The coordinated expression of individual cyclins and inhibitors of CDKs guides the cell through the different phases of the cell cycle including DNA synthesis (S phase) and mitosis (M phase). For details on the intracellular signal mechanisms of hepatocyte regeneration, the reader is referred to excellent reviews on this subject (Trautwein, 2006; Michalopoulos, 2007).

In recent years, work from Mehendale and coworkers demonstrated extensively that regeneration is not just a response to cell death but is a process that actively determines the final injury after exposure to hepatotoxic chemicals such as thioacetamide, APAP, chloroform, bromobenzene, trichloroethylene, CCl_4, galactosamine, and allyl alcohol (Mehendale, 2005; Anand et al., 2005). Inhibition of mitosis with colchicine prevented tissue repair and aggravated liver injury after thioacetamide (Mangipudy *et al.*, 1996) and other chemicals (Mehendale, 2005). In contrast, stimulation of repair by exposure to a moderate dose of a hepatotoxicant strongly attenuates tissue damage of a subsequent high dose of the same chemical (autoprotection) or a different hepatotoxin (heteroprotection) (Mehendale, 2005). Tissue repair follows a dose–response up to a threshold where the injury is getting too severe and cell proliferation is inhibited (Mangipudy *et al.*, 1995). In addition to the dose of the hepatotoxicant, other factors such as age, nutritional status, and disease state may influence tissue repair (Mehendale, 2005). Of particular interest is the potential increased susceptibility of diabetic animals to hepatotoxicants. Streptozotocin-induced diabetes reduced liver injury after APAP overdose in rats (Price and Jollow, 1982) and in mice (Shankar *et al.*, 2003). The mechanism of protection included the faster clearance of APAP due to enhanced sulfation and glucuronidation and stimulated tissue repair (Price and Jollow, 1982; Shankar *et al.*, 2003). However, it remains to be evaluated if the reduced susceptibility is caused by the chemical streptozotocin rather than diabetes. In a genetic model of diabetes and obesity, APAP hepatotoxicity is actually enhanced (Kon *et al.*, 2010). This may have been caused by the increased oxidant stress in these steatotic livers (Kon *et al.*, 2010).

Inflammation The activation of resident macrophages (Kupffer cells), NK and NKT cells, and the migration of activated neutrophils, lymphocytes, and monocytes into regions of damaged liver is a well-recognized feature of the hepatotoxicity produced by many chemicals. The main reason for an inflammatory response is to remove dead and damaged cells. However, under certain circumstances, these inflammatory cells can aggravate the existing injury by release of directly cytotoxic mediators or by formation of pro- and anti-inflammatory mediators (Fig. 13-7).

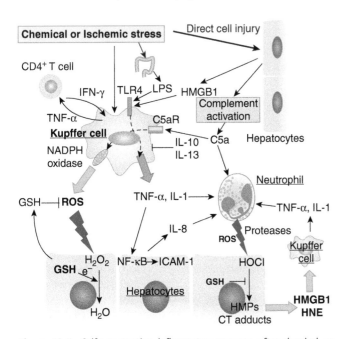

Figure 13-7. *Self-perpetuating inflammatory response after chemical or ischemic stress.* C5aR, C5a complement receptor; CT, chlorotyrosine protein adducts; GSH, reduced glutathione; HMGB1, high-mobility group box-1; HMPs, hypochlorous acid modified proteins; HNE, hydroxynonenal; HOCl, hypochlorous acid; ICAM-1, intercellular adhesion molecule-1; IFN-γ, interferon-γ; IL-1, interleukin-1; LPS, lipopolysaccharide; NF-κB, nuclear factor-κB; ROS, reactive oxygen species; TLR4, toll-like receptor-4; TNF, tumor necrosis factor.

Kupffer cells and neutrophils are potent phagocytes, which have a vital function in host defense and removal of cell debris. Formation of reactive oxygen species by NADPH oxidase is a critical tool for these cells. Upon activation, Kupffer cells generate mainly hydrogen peroxide, which can diffuse into neighboring liver cells and create an intracellular oxidant stress leading to cellular stress and injury (Bilzer *et al.*, 1999). Kupffer cells can be activated by bacterial products, opsonized particles, and activated complement factors to cause oxidant stress and cell injury (Bilzer *et al.*, 2006). A detrimental role of Kupffer cells in the pathogenesis of toxicant-induced liver injury has been suggested for a number of chemicals including ethanol, APAP, CCl$_4$, and 1,2-dichlorobenzene (Laskin, 2009) although the detrimental role Kupffer cells in APAP hepatotoxicity has been questioned (Ju *et al.*, 2002). Despite the capacity to directly cause cell damage, a prominent function of Kupffer cells is to generate inflammatory mediators (Decker, 1990). Recent evidence suggests that not only bacterial products but also intracellular proteins, for example, HMGB-1, which are released during necrotic cell death, can bind to toll-like receptors on Kupffer cells and trigger cytokine and chemokine formation (Schwabe *et al.*, 2006). These mediators may aggravate injury by recruiting cytotoxic neutrophils into the liver (Bajt *et al.*, 2001), directly cause apoptotic cell death in susceptible hepatocytes (Nagai *et al.*, 2002), or promote cytotoxic mechanisms such as induction of iNOS during APAP hepatotoxicity (Bourdi *et al.*, 2002). However, Kupffer cells can also generate anti-inflammatory mediators such as prostaglandin E$_2$ and interleukin-10 (Decker, 1990), which downregulate formation of proinflammatory cytokines and attenuate toxin-induced liver injury (Bourdi *et al.*, 2002; Ju *et al.*, 2002). Thus, Kupffer cells can promote or inhibit an injury process and assist in removal of cell debris and apoptotic bodies. In addition, newly recruited mononuclear cells (macrophages) can function in a similar way as Kupffer cells in liver. Although there is a capacity for additional damage by these cells, in general, the recruitment of macrophages into the damaged liver and even the formation of proinflammatory mediators are important signals for inducing regeneration and repair of the damaged tissue (Holt *et al.*, 2008; Laskin, 2009; Adams *et al.*, 2010).

Neutrophils are activated and accumulate in the liver vasculature in response to extensive cell injury or bacterial infection (Fig. 13-7). The main purpose of hepatic neutrophil recruitment is to remove bacteria and cell debris, at least in part through interactions with the resident macrophages (Gregory and Wing, 2002). Neutrophils generate the aggressive oxidant and chlorinating species hypochlorous acid through NADPH oxidase and myeloperoxidase (El-Benna *et al.*, 2005). In addition, neutrophils can release a large number of proteolytic enzymes and bacteriocidal proteins (Wiedow and Meyer-Hoffert, 2005). The capability of neutrophils to migrate out of the vasculature, adhere to and generate potent cytotoxins in close proximity to its target makes this leukocyte an effective killer of invading microorganisms and a remover of dead or dying cells. However, if the cytotoxicity is directed against still viable liver cells, this can cause additional tissue injury or even liver failure (Jaeschke, 2006b). Recent insight into the pathomechanisms revealed that neutrophil-induced liver cell injury is a multistep process (Jaeschke and Hasegawa, 2006; Ramaiah and Jaeschke, 2007) (Fig. 13-7). It requires exposure to inflammatory mediators, which upregulate adhesion molecules such as Mac-1 (CD11b/CD18) on the surface, prime the neutrophils for reactive oxygen formation, and cause their accumulation in vascular beds of the liver. If a chemotactic signal is received from the parenchyma, neutrophils will extravasate and adhere to the target. In contrast to other vascular beds, in the liver this process can take place in both sinusoids (capillaries) and venules (portal and/or postsinusoidal venules). However, extravasation from sinusoids is most critical for parenchymal cell injury (Chosay et al., 1997). At this time, the neutrophil becomes fully activated, that is, initiates a prolonged adherence-dependent oxidant stress and releases proteolytic enzymes (Jaeschke and Hasegawa, 2006). Cell killing is predominantly caused by hypochlorous acid diffusing into the target cell and causing an intracellular oxidant stress (Jaeschke, 2006b). Although proteases can also be directly involved in the injury process, the main function of neutrophil-derived proteases appears to be the promotion of the inflammatory process by generation of inflammatory mediators and facilitation of neutrophil migration (Jaeschke and Hasegawa, 2006). It has previously been assumed that the killing of "innocent bystanders" mainly caused the aggravation of liver injury by neutrophils during the attack on dying hepatocytes. More recent findings suggest that neutrophils only attack distressed or damaged, but not healthy cells (Gujral et al., 2004). Thus, the aggravation of liver injury by neutrophils is mainly caused by the killing of distressed cells, which would actually survive the original insult (Jaeschke, 2006b). Neutrophils have been shown to be involved in the injury process during hepatic ischemia-reperfusion, alcoholic hepatitis, alpha-naphthylisothiocyanate hepatotoxicity, obstructive cholestasis, and halothane-induced liver injury (Ramaiah and Jaeschke, 2007). The involvement of neutrophils in APAP hepatotoxicity is controversial but most of the experimental evidence in animals and humans support the hypothesis that neutrophils do not actively contribute to the injury process (Jaeschke et al., 2012b). Although many chemicals cause liver injury without neutrophil participation or do not cause injury at moderate doses, initiation of an inflammatory response with endotoxin triggers a neutrophil-induced injury or aggravates the existing injury after ethanol, allyl alcohol, aflatoxin B_1, monocrotaline, ranitidine, diclofenac, and trovafloxacin (Ganey and Roth, 2001; Shaw et al., 2010). Thus, a detrimental effect of neutrophils only occurs when activated neutrophils are recruited to the site of injury and if a relevant number of distressed cells, which are killed by neutrophils, would survive without the neutrophil attack (Jaeschke, 2006b).

Identification of the NALP3 inflammasome and its role in inflammation and autoimmunity (Agostini et al., 2004) has again led to resurgence in studies of inflammation as a critical factor in drug hepatotoxicity (Jaeschke et al., 2012b). The inflammasome forms in response to NALP1/2/3, forming an oligomer with the linker protein ASC and caspase 1 to cleave pro-IL-1β or pro-IL-18, thereby forming the active cytokine (Agostini et al., 2004). Activation of the NALP3 inflammasome has been associated with APAP-induced liver injury (Imaeda et al., 2009). However, detailed studies into NALP3 inflammasome-dependent caspase-1 activation and the role of IL-1β in the pathophysiology confirmed caspase-1 activation and formation of active IL-1β, but could not demonstrate a relevant impact of these inflammatory mediators in the injury mechanism (Williams et al., 2010; 2011). A risk of using interventions that target the immune response in drug hepatotoxicity are off-target effects modulating drug metabolism and disposition, which can impact the injury process independent of the assumed immune mechanism (Jaeschke et al., 2012b).

Immune Responses In addition to the activation of an inflammatory response, immune-mediated reactions may also lead to severe liver injury (Ju, 2005; Adams et al., 2010). Drugs and chemicals that have been suggested to cause immune-mediated injury mechanisms in the liver include halothane, tienilic acid, and dihydralazine (Ju, 2005; Uetrecht, 2007). A delay in onset of the injury or the requirement for repeated exposure to the drug and the

formation of antibodies against drug-modified hepatic proteins are characteristic features of immune reactions (Ju, 2005; Zhang et al., 2011). However, the mechanisms of these immune-mediated liver injuries are not well understood. The *hapten hypothesis* assumes that a reactive metabolite covalently binds to cellular proteins and the drug-modified protein is taken up by APCs, cleaved to peptide fragments, which are then presented within the major histocompatibility complex (MHC) to T cells (Ju, 2005; Uetrecht, 2007). In support of the hapten hypothesis, antibodies against drug-modified proteins were detected in the serum of patients with halothane hepatitis (Vergani et al., 1980; Satoh et al., 1989) or with liver injury caused by ethanol, tienilic acid, and dihydralazine (Bourdi et al., 1994; Lecoeur et al., 1996; Tuma, 2002). However, the hapten hypothesis does not explain why other drugs (eg, APAP), which also form reactive metabolites and drug-modified proteins, do not trigger an immune response. This suggests that additional activating factors may be necessary to induce immune-mediated liver injury. The *danger hypothesis* (Fig. 13-8) postulates that damaged cells release danger signals, which induce the upregulation of B7 on APCs and, the interaction of B7 with CD28 on T cells generates a costimulatory signal (Uetrecht, 2007). A cytotoxic immune response occurs only when the T-cell receptor stimulation with the antigen is accompanied by an independent costimulation of the T cell. In the absence of this costimulatory signal, the antigens derived from drug-modified proteins induce immune tolerance (Ju, 2005; Uetrecht, 2007). Both liver sinusoidal endothelial cells and Kupffer cells can function as APCs in the liver and can be inducers of tolerance to hapten-induced immunological responses (Knolle et al., 1999; Ju et al., 2003). More recently another mechanism of tolerance has been proposed. Hepatotoxic doses of APAP caused a loss of lymphocytes from spleen, thymus, and draining hepatic lymph node and immunesuppression (Masson et al., 2007). These mechanisms could be the reason that tolerance appears to be the default reaction to drug-induced protein modifications in most people. However, impairment of these mechanisms in a limited number of patients can make them susceptible to the immune-mediated liver disease (Ju, 2005; Uetrecht, 2007; Zhang et al., 2011).

Idiosyncratic Liver Injury Idiosyncratic drug hepatoxicity is a rare but potentially serious adverse event, which is not clearly dose-dependent, is at this point unpredictable, and affects only very few of the patients exposed to a drug or other chemicals. However, idiosyncratic toxicity is a leading cause for failure of drugs in clinical testing and it is the most frequent reason for posting warnings, restricting use, or even withdrawal of the drug from the market (Li, 2002; Kaplowitz, 2005) (Table 13-4). In addition, idiosyncratic hepatotoxicity is observed after consumption of herbal remedies and food supplements (Stickel et al., 2011). There are no known mechanisms of cell injury specific for idiosyncratic hepatotoxins. A number of drugs including halothane (anesthetic), nitrofurantoin (antibiotic), and phenytoin (anticonvulsant) are thought to cause injury mainly by immune (allergic) mechanisms as described in the previous paragraph (Kaplowitz, 2005; Uetrecht, 2007). Other drugs, for example, isoniazid (antituberculosis), disulfiram (alcoholism), valproic acid (anticonvulsant), or troglitazone (antidiabetic), are considered nonimmune (nonallergic) idiosyncratic hepatotoxins (Kaplowitz, 2005); however, some immune mechanisms might be involved (Metushi et al., 2011). Diclofenac (analgesic) can elicit allergic and nonallergic mechanisms of toxicity (Boelsterli, 2003). Because only very few patients (1 in 10,000 or less) treated with these drugs actually experience significant hepatotoxicity, the prevailing opinion at the present time is that an enhanced individual susceptibility with the failure to adapt to a mild adverse drug

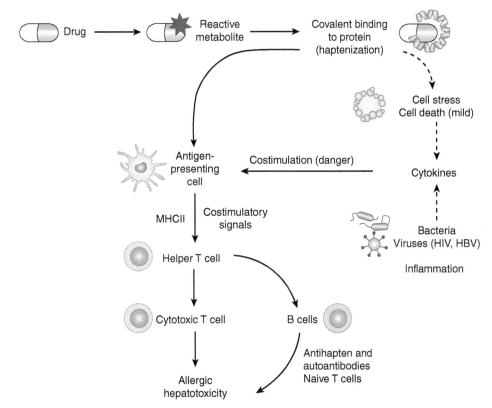

Figure 13-8. *The danger hypothesis for immune-mediated idiosyncratic hepatotoxicity.* Hapten formation leading to major histocompatibility complex class II (MHCII) presentation of haptenized peptide by antigen-presenting cells (APCs) along with costimulation of APC signalling molecules by mild injury, inflammation, or infection promotes helper T-cell activation leading to T-cell responses to the antigen. The cytotoxic T cells are then targeted against hepatocytes that express haptenized protein or MHCI presentation of haptenized peptides on the cell surface. Antibody to haptenized protein or concomitant autoantibodies could theoretically mediate and promote antibody-dependent cell-mediated hepatotoxicity. (From Kaplowitz, 2005.)

reaction is a key factor in the pathogenesis (Watkins, 2005). Thus, only small subsets of patients who show elevated plasma ALT levels during drug treatment actually develop severe tissue damage or liver failure (Watkins, 2005). In support of this concept, it was

Table 13-4

Examples of Drugs with Known Idiosyncratic Hepatotoxicity

A. *Immune-mediated (allergic) idiosyncratic hepatotoxicity*
   Diclofenac (analgesic)
   Halothane (anesthetic)
   Nitrofurantoin (antibiotic)
   Phenytoin (anticonvulsant)
   Tienilic acid (diuretic)

B. *Nonimmune-mediated (nonallergic) idiosyncratic hepatotoxicity*
   Amiodarone (antiarrhythmic)
   Bromfenac (analgesic)—withdrawn from market
   Diclofenac (analgesic)
   Disulfiram (alcoholism)
   Isoniazid (antituberculosis)
   Ketoconazole (antifungal)
   Rifampicin (antimicrobial)
   Troglitazone (antidiabetes)—withdrawn from market
   Valproate (anticonvulsant)

SOURCE: Data from Kaplowitz (2005) and Zimmerman (1999).

reported that 10% to 20% of patients treated with isoniazid show increased levels of plasma ALT levels as an indicator of hepatocellular injury (Mitchell *et al.*, 1975). However, only a small subgroup of these patients develops severe hepatotoxicity (Mitchell *et al.*, 1975). This raises the possibility that one or several gene defects, which prevent effective adaption to drug-induced cellular stress, may be involved in idiosyncratic reactions (Watkins, 2005). Recent findings appear to support this hypothesis. The antidiabetic drug troglitazone (Rezulin®) was withdrawn from the market due to idiosyncratic hepatotoxicity. In preclinical studies, troglitazone did not cause any relevant liver toxicity and despite extensive investigations since withdrawal of the drug, the mechanism of toxicity remains unclear (Chojkier, 2005). Several studies suggest that very high concentrations of troglitazone can induce mitochondrial dysfunction in vitro (Haskins *et al.*, 2001; Tirmenstein *et al.*, 2002). Because the conditions applied in these studies are not relevant for human exposure, the proposed mechanism cannot explain the idiosyncratic toxicity in humans. However, the data suggest that troglitazone can cause a subclinical mitochondrial stress, which could sensitize hepatocytes to troglitazone. In fact, mice partially deficient in mitochondrial manganese superoxide dismutase (Mn-SOD; SOD2) showed mitochondrial dysfunction and mild liver injury after treatment with 30 mg/kg troglitazone for 28 days (Ong *et al.*, 2007). Although the animals did not develop severe hepatic injury as observed in humans, the injury in mice occurred also after a lag time, which is consistent with the hypothesis that a certain threshold of mitochondrial stress has to be reached to cause cell injury (Ong *et al.*, 2007). Overall, these findings support the concept that a clinically silent genetic deficiency in individuals can trigger the hepatotoxicity of a drug, which by itself may only cause a mild and clinically silent cellular stress. This recent insight indicates the need for a paradigm shift for preclinical toxicity studies (Jaeschke, 2007). The assumption in traditional toxicity studies is that an adverse effect of a drug can be detected by progressively increasing the dose. The experience with troglitazone suggests that this is not always the case. It may be necessary to include experiments with genetically deficient animals in these studies if there is any evidence for clinically silent adverse effects of these drugs. In addition to the genetic makeup, which may render individuals more susceptible to stress induced by the metabolism of drugs or chemicals, a second "hit" such as a systemic inflammatory response can also contribute to the unmasking of the toxicity at least in experimental models (Ganey and Roth, 2001; Shaw *et al.*, 2010). A major argument against the systemic inflammatory hypothesis is the fact that neutrophils are prominent players in animal models (Shaw *et al.*, 2010) but not in humans (Zhang *et al.*, 2011). Because idiosyncratic hepatotoxicity is a rare event for most drugs, it is likely that a combination of gene defects and adverse events need to be present simultaneously in an individual to trigger the severe liver injury. A detailed genomic analysis of patients with idiosyncratic responses to drug exposure may give additional insight what gene expression profile renders a patient susceptible (Watkins, 2005).

FUTURE DIRECTIONS

Continued progress in the understanding of drug- and chemical hepatotoxicity will depend on the use of relevant in vivo and in vitro models including human hepatocytes and analysis of human liver tissue. Traditional mechanistic investigations in combination with genomic and proteomic approaches have the greatest potential to yield important new insight into pathomechanisms. Progress in the understanding of the liver's response to known hepatotoxins and other adverse conditions will not only aid in the development of therapies to limit and reverse acute and chronic liver injury, but also improve the predictability of the potential hepatotoxicity of new drugs and other chemicals (Guengerich and MacDonald, 2007; O'Connell and Watkins, 2010).

REFERENCES

Adams DH, Ju C, Ramaiah SK, et al. Mechanisms of immune-mediated liver injury. *Toxicol Sci.* 2010;115:307–321.

Agarwal DP. Genetic polymorphisms of alcohol metabolizing enzymes. *Pathol Biol (Paris).* 2001;49:703–709.

Agostini L, Martinon F, Burns K, et al. NALP3 forms an IL-1beta-processing inflammasome with increased activity in Muckle–Wells auto-inflammatory disorder. *Immunity.* 2004;20:319–325.

Allen K, Jaeschke H, Copple BL. Bile acids induce inflammatory genes in hepatocytes: a novel mechanism of inflammation during obstructive cholestasis. *Am J Pathol.* 2011;178:175–186.

Ananthanarayanan M, Balasubramanian N, Makishima M, et al. Human bile salt export pump promoter is transactivated by the farnesoid X receptor/bile acid receptor. *J Biol Chem.* 2001;276:28857–28865.

Andersson M, Storm HH. Cancer incidence among Danish Thorotrast exposed patients. *J Natl Cancer Inst.* 1992;84:1318–1325.

Anand SS, Mumtaz MM, Mehendale HM. Dose-dependent liver regeneration in chloroform, trichloroethylene and allyl alcohol ternary mixture hepatotoxicity in rats. *Arch Toxicol.* 2005;79:671–682.

Antoine DJ, Jenkins RE, Dear JW, et al. Molecular forms of HMGB1 and Keratin-18 as mechanistic biomarkers for mode of cell death and prognosis during clinical acetaminophen hepatotoxicity. *J Hepatol.* 2012;56:1070–1079.

Aoyama T, Peters JM, Iritani N, et al. Altered constitutive expression of fatty acid-metabolizing enzymes in mice lacking the peroxisome proliferator-activated receptor alpha (PPARalpha). *J Biol Chem.* 1998;273:5678–5684.

Aravalli RN, Steer CJ, Cressman EN. Molecular mechanisms of hepatocellular carcinoma. *Hepatology.* 2008;48:2047–2063.

Arrese M, Ananthanarayanan M, Suchy FJ. Hepatobiliary transport: molecular mechanisms of development and cholestasis. *Pediatr Res.* 1998;44:141–147.

Arteel GE: Oxidants and antioxidants in alcohol-induced liver disease. *Gastroenterology.* 2003;124:778–790.

Arthur MJ. Fibrogenesis II. Metalloproteinases and their inhibitors in liver fibrosis. *Am J Physiol Gastrointest Liver Physiol.* 2000;279:G245–G249.

Aw TY. Biliary glutathione promotes the mucosal metabolism of lumenal peroxidized lipids by rat small intestine in vivo. *J Clin Invest.* 1994;94:1218–1225.

Badr MZ, Belinsky SA, Kauffman FC, et al. Mechanism of hepatotoxicity to periportal regions of the liver lobule due to allyl alcohol: role of oxygen and lipid peroxidation. *J Pharmacol Exp Ther.* 1986;238:1138–1142.

Baier PK, Hempel S, Waldvogel B, et al. Zonation of hepatic bile salt transporters. *Dig Dis Sci.* 2006;51:587–593.

Bajt ML, Farhood A, Jaeschke H. Effects of CXC chemokines on neutrophil activation and sequestration in hepatic vasculature. *Am J Physiol Gastrointest Liver Physiol.* 2001;281:G1188–G1195.

Bajt ML, Knight TR, Farhood A, et al. Scavenging peroxynitrite with glutathione promotes regeneration and enhances survival during acetaminophen-induced liver injury in mice. *J Pharmacol Exp Therap.* 2003;307:67–73.

Bajt ML, Lawson JA, Vonderfecht SL, et al. Protection against Fas receptor-mediated apoptosis in hepatocytes and nonparenchymal cells by a caspase-8 inhibitor in vivo: evidence for a postmitochondrial processing of caspase-8. *Toxicol Sci.* 2000;58:109–117.

Ballatori N. Transport of toxic metals by molecular mimicry. *Environ Health Perspect.* 2002;110(suppl 5):689–694.

Ballatori N, Christian WV, Lee JY, et al. OSTalpha-OSTbeta: a major basolateral bile acid and steroid transporter in human intestinal, renal, and biliary epithelia. *Hepatology.* 2005;42:1270–1279.

Bataller R, Brenner DA. Liver fibrosis. *J Clin Invest.* 2005;115:209–218.

Berson A, De Beco V, Letteron P, et al. Steatohepatitis-inducing drugs cause mitochondrial dysfunction and lipid peroxidation in rat hepatocytes. *Gastroenterology.* 1998;114:764–774.

Bianchi ME. DAMPs, PAMPs and alarmins: all we need to know about danger. *J Leukoc Biol.* 2007;81:1–5.

Bilzer M, Jaeschke H, Vollmar AM, et al. Prevention of Kupffer cell-induced oxidant injury in rat liver by atrial natriuretic peptide. *Am J Physiol.* 1999;276:G1137–G1144.

Bilzer M, Roggel F, Gerbes AL. Role of Kupffer cells in host defense and liver disease. *Liver Int.* 2006;26:1175–1186.

Boelsterli UA. Diclofenac-induced liver injury: a paradigm of idiosyncratic drug toxicity. *Toxicol Appl Pharmacol.* 2003;192:307–322.

Boess F, Kamber M, Romer S, et al. Gene expression in two hepatic cell lines, cultured primary hepatocytes, and liver slices compared to the in vivo liver gene expression in rats: possible implications for toxicogenomics use of in vitro systems. *Toxicol Sci.* 2003;73:386–402.

Borst P, Evers R, Kool M, et al. A family of drug transporters: the multidrug resistance-associated proteins. *J Natl Cancer Inst.* 2000;92:1295–1302.

Bosch FX, Ribes J, Cleries R, Diaz M. Epidemiology of hepatocellular carcinoma. *Clin Liver Dis.* 2005;9:191–211.

Boulares AH, Zoltoski AJ, Stoica BA, et al. Acetaminophen induces a caspase-dependent and Bcl-XL sensitive apoptosis in human hepatoma cells and lymphocytes. *Pharmacol Toxicol.* 2002;90:38–50.

Bourdi M, Masubuchi Y, Reilly TP, et al. Protection against acetaminophen-induced liver injury and lethality by interleukin 10: role of inducible nitric oxide synthase. *Hepatology.* 2002;35:289–298.

Bourdi M, Tinel M, Beaune PH, et al. Interactions of dihydralazine with cytochromes P4501A: a possible explanation for the appearance of anticytochrome P4501A2 autoantibodies. *Mol Pharmacol.* 1994;45:1287–1295.

Boyer JL, Trauner M, Mennone A, et al. Upregulation of a basolateral FXR-dependent bile acid efflux transporter OSTalpha-OSTbeta in cholestasis in humans and rodents. *Am J Physiol Gastrointest Liver Physiol.* 2006a;290:G1124–G1130.

Boyer TD, Wright TL, Manns M. *Zakim and Boyer's Hepatology*. 5th ed. Philadelphia: Saunders-Elsevier; 2006b.

Braet F, Wisse E. Structural and functional aspects of liver sinusoidal endothelial cell fenestrae: a review. *Comp Hepatol*. 2002;1:1.

Breuhahn K, Longerich T, Schirmacher P. Dysregulation of growth factor signaling in human hepatocellular carcinoma. *Oncogene*. 2006;25: 3787–3800.

Bruix J, Hessheimer AJ, Forner A, et al. New aspects of diagnosis and therapy of hepatocellular carcinoma. *Oncogene*. 2006;25:3848–3856.

Cai Y, Gong LK, Qi XM, et al. Apoptosis initiated by carbon tetrachloride in mitochondria of rat primary cultured hepatocytes. *Acta Pharmacol Sin*. 2005;26:969–975.

Chang TP, Rangan C. Iron poisoning: a literature-based review of epidemiology, diagnosis, and management. *Pediatr Emerg Care*. 2011;27: 978–985.

Chen CC, Lu RB, Chen YC, et al. Interaction between the functional polymorphisms of the alcohol-metabolism genes in protection against alcoholism. *Am J Hum Genet*. 1999;65:795–807.

Chojkier M. Troglitazone and liver injury: in search of answers. *Hepatology*. 2005;41:237–246.

Chosay JG, Essani NA, Dunn CJ, et al. Neutrophil margination and extravasation in sinusoids and venules of liver during endotoxin-induced injury. *Am J Physiol*. 1997;272:G1195–G1200.

Colell A, Garcia-Ruiz C, Miranda M, et al. Selective glutathione depletion of mitochondria by ethanol sensitizes hepatocytes to tumor necrosis factor. *Gastroenterology*. 1998;115:1541–1551.

Cover C, Mansouri A, Knight TR, et al. Peroxynitrite-induced mitochondrial and endonuclease-mediated nuclear DNA damage in acetaminophen hepatotoxicity. *J Pharmacol Exp Therap*. 2005;315:879–887.

Crawford JM. The liver and the biliary tract, in Cotran RS, Kumar V, Collins T, eds. *Robbins: Pathologic Basis of Disease*. 6th ed. Philadelphia: WB Saunders; 1999:845–901.

Csanaky IL, Lu H, Zhang Y, Ogura K, Choudhuri S, Klaassen CD. Organic anion-transporting polypeptide 1b2 (Oatp1b2) is important for the hepatic uptake of unconjugated acids: studies in Oatp1b2-null mice. *Hepatology*. 2011;53:272–281.

Cullen JM, Ruebner BH. A histopathologic classification of chemical-induced injury of the liver, in Meeks RG, Harrison SD, Bull RJ, eds. *Hepatotoxicology*. Boca Raton, FL: CRC Press; 1991:67–92.

Dart RC, Kuffner EK, Rumack BH. Treatment of pain or fever with paracetamol (acetaminophen) in the alcoholic patient: a systematic review. *Am J Ther*. 2000;7:123–134.

Davern TJ 2nd, James LP, Hinson JA, et al. Measurement of serum acetaminophen–protein adducts in patients with acute liver failure. *Gastroenterology*. 2006;130:687–694.

Davies MH, Harrison RF, Elias E, et al. Antibiotic-associated acute vanishing bile duct syndrome: a pattern associated with severe, prolonged intrahepatic cholestasis. *J Hepatol*. 1994;20:112–116.

Day CP. Genes or environment to determine alcoholic liver disease and nonalcoholic fatty liver disease. *Liver Int*. 2006;26:1021–1028.

Day CP, James OF. Steatohepatitis: a tale of two "hits"? *Gastroenterology*. 1998a;114:842–845.

Day CP, James OF. Hepatic steatosis: innocent bystander or guilty party? *Hepatology*. 1998b;27:1463–1466.

Decker K. Biologically active products of stimulated liver macrophages (Kupffer cells). *Eur J Biochem*. 1990;192:245–261.

DeLeve LD, Ito Y, Bethea NW, et al. Embolization by sinusoidal lining cells obstructs the microcirculation in rat sinusoidal obstruction syndrome. *Am J Physiol Gastrointest Liver Physiol*. 2003a;284:G1045–G1052.

DeLeve LD, McCuskey RS, Wang X, et al. Characterization of a reproducible rat model of hepatic veno-occlusive disease. *Hepatology*. 1999;29:1779–1791.

DeLeve LD, Wang X, Kaplowitz N, et al. Sinusoidal endothelial cells as a target for acetaminophen toxicity. Direct action versus requirement for hepatocyte activation in different mouse strains. *Biochem Pharmacol*. 1997;53:1339–1345.

DeLeve LD, Wang X, Tsai J, et al. Sinusoidal obstruction syndrome (veno-occlusive disease) in the rat is prevented by matrix metalloproteinase inhibition. *Gastroenterology*. 2003b;125:882–890.

Denson LA, Sturm E, Echevarria W, et al. The orphan nuclear receptor, SHP, mediates bile acid-induced inhibition of the rat bile acid transporter, NTCP. *Gastroenterology*. 2001;121:140–147.

Dey A, Cederbaum AI. Alcohol and oxidative liver injury. *Hepatology*. 2006;43(2 suppl 1):S63–S74.

Donthamsetty S, Bhave VS, Mitra MS, et al. Nonalcoholic fatty liver sensitizes rats to carbon tetrachloride hepatotoxicity. *Hepatology*. 2007;45:391–403.

Ding WX, Manley S, Ni HM. The emerging role of autophagy in alcoholic liver disease. *Exp Biol Med (Maywood)*. 2011;236:546–556.

Ding WX, Shen HM, Ong CN. Critical role of reactive oxygen species and mitochondrial permeability transition in microcystin-induced rapid apoptosis in rat hepatocytes. *Hepatology*. 2000;32:547–555.

Dutczak WJ, Clarkson TW, Ballatori N. Biliary-hepatic recycling of a xenobiotic: gallbladder absorption of methyl mercury. *Am J Physiol*. 1991;260:G873–G880.

El-Benna J, Dang PM, Gougerot-Pocidalo MA, et al. Phagocyte NADPH oxidase: a multicomponent enzyme essential for host defenses. *Arch Immunol Ther Exp (Warsz)*. 2005;53:199–206.

elSisi AE, Earnest DL, Sipes IG. Vitamin A potentiation of carbon tetrachloride hepatotoxicity: role of liver macrophages and active oxygen species. *Toxicol Appl Pharmacol*. 1993;119:295–301.

Elvevold K, Smedsrød B, Martinez I. The liver sinusoidal endothelial cell: a cell type of controversial and confusing identity. *Am J Physiol Gastrointest Liver Physiol*. 2008;294:G391–G400.

Enomoto K, Nishikawa Y, Omori Y, et al. Cell biology and pathology of liver sinusoidal endothelial cells. *Med Electron Microsc*. 2004;37:208–215.

Enomoto N, Takase S, Takada N, et al. Alcoholic liver disease in heterozygotes of mutant and normal aldehyde dehydrogenase-2 genes. *Hepatology*. 1991;13:1071–1075.

Fabregat I, Roncero C, Fernandez M. Survival and apoptosis: a dysregulated balance in liver cancer. *Liver Int*. 2007;27:155–162.

Farazi PA, Glickman J, Horner J, et al. Cooperative interactions of p53 mutation, telomere dysfunction, and chronic liver damage in hepatocellular carcinoma progression. *Cancer Res*. 2006;66:4766–4773.

Farrell GC. Drugs and steatohepatitis: *Semin Liver Dis*. 2002;22:185–194.

Farrell GC, Larter CZ. Nonalcoholic fatty liver disease: from steatosis to cirrhosis. *Hepatology*. 2006;43(suppl 1):S99–S112.

Fattinger K, Funk C, Pantze M, et al. The endothelin antagonist bosentan inhibits the canalicular bile salt export pump: a potential mechanism for hepatic adverse reactions. *Clin Pharmacol Ther*. 2001;69:223–231.

Fausto N: Liver regeneration. *J Hepatol*. 2000;32(1 suppl):19–31.

Fickert P, Fuchsbichler A, Marschall HU, et al. Lithocholic acid feeding induces segmental bile duct obstruction and destructive cholangitis in mice. *Am J Pathol*. 2006;168:410–422.

Fischer U, Janicke RU, Schulze-Osthoff K. Many cuts to ruin: a comprehensive update of caspase substrates. *Cell Death Differ*. 2003;10: 76–100.

Freeman TL, Tuma DJ, Thiele GM, et al. Recent advances in alcohol-induced adduct formation. *Alcohol Clin Exp Res*. 2005;29:1310–1316.

Friedman SL. Molecular regulation of hepatic fibrosis, an integrated cellular response to tissue injury. *J Biol Chem*. 2000;275:2247–2250.

Friedman SL. Hepatic stellate cells: protean, multifunctional, and enigmatic cells of the liver. *Physiol Rev*. 2008;88:125–172.

Frimmer M. What we have learned from phalloidin. *Toxicol Lett*. 1987;35:169–182.

Ganey PE, Roth RA. Concurrent inflammation as a determinant of susceptibility to toxicity from xenobiotic agents. *Toxicology*. 2001;169:195–208.

Gao B, Bataller R: Alcoholic liver disease: pathogenesis and new therapeutic targets. *Gastroenterology*. 2011;141:1572–1585.

Gao B, Radaeva S, Park O. Liver natural killer and natural killer T cells: immunobiology and emerging roles in liver diseases. *J Leukoc Biol*. 2009;86:513–528.

Gebhardt R, Alber J, Wegner H, et al. Different drug metabolizing capacities in cultured periportal and pericentral hepatocytes. *Biochem Pharmacol*. 1994;48:761–766.

Geier A, Fickert P, Trauner M. Mechanisms of disease: mechanisms and clinical implications of cholestasis in sepsis. *Nat Clin Pract Gastroenterol Hepatol*. 2006;3:574–585.

Gerk PM, Vore M. Regulation of expression of the multidrug resistance-associated protein 2 (MRP2) and its role in drug disposition. *J Pharmacol Exp Ther.* 2002;302:407–415.

Geubel AP, De Galocsy C, Alves N, et al. Liver damage caused by therapeutic vitamin A administration: Estimate of dose-related toxicity in 41 cases. *Gastroenterology.* 1991;100:1701–1709.

Gomez-Lechon MJ, O'Connor E, Castell JV, et al. Sensitive markers used to identify compounds that trigger apoptosis in cultured hepatocytes. *Toxicol Sci.* 2002;65:299–308.

Gonzalez FJ. The 2006 Bernard B. Brodie Award Lecture. Cyp2e1. *Drug Metab Dispos.* 2007;35:1–8.

Grasl-Kraupp B, Ruttkay-Nedecky B, Koudelka H, et al. In situ detection of fragmented DNA (TUNEL assay) fails to discriminate among apoptosis, necrosis, and autolytic cell death: a cautionary note. *Hepatology.* 1995;21:1465–1468.

Grattagliano I, Bonfrate L, Diogo CV, et al. Biochemical mechanisms in drug-induced liver injury: certainties and doubts. *World J Gastroenterol.* 2009;15:4865–4876.

Gregory SH, Wing EJ. Neutrophil–Kupffer cell interaction: a critical component of host defenses to systemic bacterial infections. *J Leukoc Biol.* 2002;72:239–248.

Gregus Z, Klaassen CD. Disposition of metals in rats: a comparative study of fecal, urinary, and biliary excretion and tissue distribution of eighteen metals. *Toxicol Appl Pharmacol.* 1986;85:24–38.

Gressner AM, Weiskirchen R. Modern pathogenetic concepts of liver fibrosis suggest stellate cells and TGF-beta as major players and therapeutic targets. *J Cell Mol Med.* 2006;10:76–99.

Groen A, Romero MR, Kunne C, et al. Complementary functions of the flippase ATP8B1 and the floppase ABCB4 in maintaining canalicular membrane integrity. *Gastroenterology.* 2011;141:1927–1937. e1–1927–1937.e14.

Groothuis GMM, Hardonk MJ, Keulemans KPT, et al. Autoradiographic and kinetic demonstration of acinar heterogeneity of taurocholate transport. *Am J Physiol.* 1982;243:G455–G462.

Guengerich FP, MacDonald JS. Applying mechanisms of chemical toxicity to predict drug safety. *Chem Res Toxicol.* 2007;20:344–369.

Guguen-Guillouzo C, Corlu A, Guillouzo A. Stem cell-derived hepatocytes and their use in toxicology. *Toxicology.* 2010;270:3–9.

Gujral JS, Farhood A, Bajt ML, et al. Neutrophils aggravate acute liver injury during obstructive cholestasis in bile duct-ligated mice. *Hepatology.* 2003a;38:355–363.

Gujral JS, Farhood A, Jaeschke H. Oncotic necrosis and caspase-dependent apoptosis during galactosamine-induced liver injury in rats. *Toxicol Appl Pharmacol.* 2003b;190:37–46.

Gujral JS, Hinson JA, Farhood A, et al. NADPH oxidase-derived oxidant stress is critical for neutrophil cytotoxicity during endotoxemia. *Am J Physiol Gastrointest Liver Physiol.* 2004;287:G243–G252.

Gujral JS, Knight TR, Farhood A, et al. Mode of cell death after acetaminophen overdose in mice: apoptosis or oncotic necrosis? *Toxicol Sci.* 2002;67:322–328.

Guo GL, Moffit JS, Nicol CJ, et al. Enhanced acetaminophen toxicity by activation of the pregnane X receptor. *Toxicol Sci.* 2004;82:374–380.

Gutierrez-Ruiz MC, Gomez-Quiroz LE. Liver fibrosis: searching for cell model answers. *Liver Int.* 2007;27:434–439.

Hagenbuch B, Dawson P. The sodium bile salt cotransport family SLC10. *Pflugers Arch.* 2004;447:566–570.

Hagenbuch B, Gui C. Xenobiotic transporters of the human organic anion transporting polypeptides (OATP) family. *Xenobiotica.* 2008;38:778–801.

Hagenbuch B, Meier PJ. Organic anion transporting polypeptides of the OATP/SLC21 family: phylogenetic classification as OATP/SLCO super-family, new nomenclature and molecular/functional properties. *Pflugers Arch.* 2004;447:653–665.

Han D, Shinohara M, Ybanez MD, et al. Signal transduction pathways involved in drug-induced liver injury. *Handb Exp Pharmacol.* 2010;196:267–310.

Hanawa N, Shinohara M, Saberi B, et al. Role of JNK translocation to mitochondria leading to inhibition of mitochondria bioenergetics in acetaminophen-induced liver injury. *J Biol Chem.* 2008;283:13565–13577.

Haskins JR, Rowse P, Rahbari R, et al. Thiazolidinedione toxicity to isolated hepatocytes revealed by coherent multiprobe fluorescence microscopy and correlated with multiparameter flow cytometry of peripheral leukocytes. *Arch Toxicol.* 2001;75:425–438.

Heard KJ, Green JL, James LP, et al. Acetaminophen–cysteine adducts during therapeutic dosing and following overdose. *BMC Gastroenterol.* 2011;11:20.

Henry SH, Bosch FX, Bowers JC. Aflatoxin, hepatitis and worldwide liver cancer risks. *Adv Exp Med Biol.* 2002;504:229–233.

Hickling KC, Hitchcock JM, Chipman JK, et al. Induction and progression of cholangiofibrosis in rat liver injured by oral administration of furan. *Toxicol Pathol.* 2010;38:213–229.

Hines IN, Wheeler MD. Recent advances in alcoholic liver disease III. Role of the innate immune response in alcoholic hepatitis. *Am J Physiol Gastrointest Liver Physiol.* 2004;287:G310–G314.

Holt MP, Cheng L, Ju C. Identification and characterization of infiltrating macrophages in acetaminophen-induced liver injury. *J Leukoc Biol.* 2008;84:1410–1421.

Homolya L, Varadi A, Sarkadi B. Multidrug resistance-associated proteins: export pumps for conjugates with glutathione, glucuronate or sulfate. *Biofactors.* 2003;17:103–114.

Honkoop P, Scholte HR, de Man RA, Schalm SW. Mitochondrial injury: lessons from the fialuridine trial. *Drug Saf.* 1997;17:1–7.

Hooser SB. Fulminant hepatocyte apoptosis in vivo following microcystin-LR administration to rats. *Toxicol Pathol.* 2000;28:726–733.

Hooser SB, Beasley VR, Lovell RA, et al. Toxicity of microcystin-LR, a cyclic heptapeptide hepatotoxin from *Microcystis aeruginosa*, to rats and mice. *Vet Pathol.* 1989;26:246–252.

Hooser SB, Beasley VR, Waite LL, et al. Actin filament alterations in rat hepatocytes induced in vivo and in vitro by microcystin-LR, a hepatotoxin from the blue green alga *Microcystis aeruginosa*. *Vet Pathol.* 1991;28:259–266.

Huang L, Zhao A, Lew JL, et al. Farnesoid X receptor activates transcription of the phospholipid pump MDR3. *J Biol Chem.* 2003;278:51085–51090.

Huxtable RJ. Pyrrolizidine alkaloids, in Sipes IG, McQueen CA, Gandolfi AJ, eds. *Comprehensive Toxicology*, vol. 9. New York: Pergamon Press; 1997:423–431.

Ibrahim SH, Kohli R, Gores GJ. Mechanisms of lipotoxicity in NAFLD and clinical implications. *J Pediatr Gastroenterol Nutr.* 2011;53:131–140.

Imaeda AB, Watanabe A, Sohail MA, et al. Acetaminophen-induced hepatotoxicity in mice is dependent on Tlr9 and the Nalp3 inflammasome. *J Clin Invest.* 2009;119:305–314.

Ishii H, Adachi M, Fernandez-Checa JC, et al. Role of apoptosis in alcoholic liver injury. *Alcohol Clin Exp Res.* 2003;27:1207–1212.

Ito Y, Abril ER, Bethea NW, et al. Inhibition of matrix metalloproteinases minimizes hepatic microvascular injury in response to acetaminophen in mice. *Toxicol Sci.* 2005;83:190–196.

Ito Y, Abril ER, Bethea NW, et al. Mechanisms and pathophysiological implications of sinusoidal endothelial cell gap formation following treatment with galactosamine/endotoxin in mice. *Am J Physiol Gastrointest Liver Physiol.* 2006;291:G211–G218.

Jaeschke H. Cellular adhesion molecules: regulation and role in the pathogenesis of liver disease. *Am J Physiol Gastrointest Liver Physiol.* 1997;273:G602–G611.

Jaeschke H. Mechanisms of liver cell destruction, in Boyer TD, Wright TL, Manns M, eds. *Zakim and Boyer's Hepatology.* 5th ed. Philadelphia: Saunders-Elsevier; 2006a:37.

Jaeschke H. Mechanisms of liver injury. II. Mechanisms of neutrophil-induced liver cell injury during hepatic ischemia-reperfusion and other acute inflammatory conditions. *Am J Physiol Gastrointest Liver Physiol.* 2006b;290:G1083–G1088.

Jaeschke H. Troglitazone Hepatotoxicity: are we getting closer to understanding idiosyncratic liver injury? *Toxicol Sci.* 2007;97:1–3.

Jaeschke H, Bajt ML. Intracellular signaling mechanisms of acetaminophen-induced liver cell death. *Toxicol Sci.* 2006;89:31–41.

Jaeschke H, Gores GJ, Cederbaum AI, et al. Mechanisms of hepatotoxicity. *Toxicol Sci.* 2002;65:166–176.

Jaeschke H, Gujral JS, Bajt ML. Apoptosis and necrosis in liver disease. *Liver Int.* 2004;24:85–89.

Jaeschke H, Hasegawa T. Role of neutrophils in acute inflammatory liver injury. *Liver Int.* 2006;26:912–919.

Jaeschke H, Kleinwaechter C, Wendel A. The role of acrolein in allyl alcohol-induced lipid peroxidation and liver cell damage in mice. *Biochem Pharmacol.* 1987;36:51–57.

Jaeschke H, Kleinwaechter C, Wendel A. NADH-dependent reductive stress and ferritin-bound iron in allyl alcohol-induced lipid peroxidation in vivo: the protective effect of vitamin E. *Chem Biol Interact.* 1992;81:57–68.

Jaeschke H, Knight TR, Bajt ML. The role of oxidant stress and reactive nitrogen species in acetaminophen hepatotoxicity. *Toxicol Lett.* 2003;144:279–288.

Jaeschke H, Lemasters JJ. Apoptosis versus oncotic necrosis in hepatic ischemia/reperfusion injury. *Gastroenterology.* 2003;125:1246–1257.

Jaeschke H, McGill MR, Ramachandran A. Oxidant stress, mitochondria, and cell death mechanisms in drug-induced liver injury: lessons learned from acetaminophen hepatotoxicity. *Drug Metab Rev.* 2012a;44:88–106.

Jaeschke H, Williams CD, Ramachandran A. Acetaminophen hepatotoxicity and repair: the role of sterile inflammation and innate immunity. *Liver Int.* 2012b;32:8–20.

Jansen PL, Groen AK. Mechanisms of bile secretion, in Boyer TD, Wright TL, Manns M, eds. *Zakim and Boyer's Hepatology.* 5th ed. Philadelphia: Saunders-Elsevier; 2006:67.

Jansen PL, Sturm E. Genetic cholestasis, causes and consequences for hepatobiliary transport. *Liver Int.* 2003;23:315–322.

Jochimsen EM, Carmichael WW, An J, et al. Liver failure and death after exposure to microcystins at a hemodialysis center in Brazil. *N Engl J Med.* 1998;338:873–878.

Jollow DJ, Mitchell JR, Potter WZ, et al. Acetaminophen-induced hepatic necrosis. II. Role of covalent binding in vivo. *J Pharmacol Exp Ther.* 1973;187:195–202.

Jones DP, Lemasters JJ, Han D, et al. Mechanisms of pathogenesis in drug hepatotoxicity putting the stress on mitochondria. *Mol Interv.* 2010;10:98–111.

Ju C. Immunological mechanisms of drug-induced liver injury. *Curr Opin Drug Discov Dev.* 2005;8:38–43.

Ju C, McCoy JP, Chung CJ, et al. Tolerogenic role of Kupffer cells in allergic reactions. *Chem Res Toxicol.* 2003;16:1514–1519.

Ju C, Reilly TP, Bourdi M, et al. Protective role of Kupffer cells in acetaminophen-induced hepatic injury in mice. *Chem Res Toxicol.* 2002;15:1504–1513.

Jungermann K, Katz N. Functional specialization of different hepatocyte populations. *Physiol Rev.* 1989;69:708–764.

Jungermann K, Kietzmann T. Oxygen: modulator of metabolic zonation and disease of the liver. *Hepatology.* 2000;31:255–260.

Kaminskas LM, Pyke SM, Burcham PC. Strong protein adduct trapping accompanies abolition of acrolein-mediated hepatotoxicity by hydralazine in mice. *J Pharmacol Exp Ther.* 2004;310:1003–1010.

Kannarkat GT, Tuma DJ, Tuma PL. Microtubules are more stable and more highly acetylated in ethanol-treated hepatic cells. *J Hepatol.* 2006;44:963–970.

Kaplowitz N. Idiosyncratic drug hepatotoxicity. *Nat Rev Drug Discov.* 2005;4:489–499.

Kaplowitz N, DeLeve LD. *Drug-induced Liver Disease.* New York: Marcel Dekker, Inc.; 2002.

Kietzmann T, Jungermann K. Modulation by oxygen of zonal gene expression in liver studied in primary rat hepatocyte cultures. *Cell Biol Toxicol.* 1997;13:243–255.

Kim JS, He L, Lemasters JJ. Mitochondrial permeability transition: a common pathway to necrosis and apoptosis. *Biochem Biophys Res Commun.* 2003;304:463–470.

Klaassen CD. Biliary excretion of metals. *Drug Metab Rev.* 1976;5:165–193.

Klaassen CD, Watkins JB. Mechanisms of bile formation, hepatic uptake, and biliary excretion. *Pharmacol Rev.* 1984;36:1–67.

Knockaert L, Berson A, Ribault C, et al. Carbon tetrachloride-mediated lipid peroxidation induces early mitochondrial alterations in mouse liver. *Lab Invest.* 2012;92:396–410.

Knolle PA, Schmitt E, Jin S, et al. Induction of cytokine production in naive CD4(+) T cells by antigen-presenting murine liver sinusoidal endothelial cells but failure to induce differentiation toward Th1 cells. *Gastroenterology.* 1999;116:1428–1440.

Ko CB, Kim SJ, Park C, et al. Benzo(a)pyrene-induced apoptotic death of mouse hepatoma Hepa1c1c7 cells via activation of intrinsic caspase cascade and mitochondrial dysfunction. *Toxicology.* 2004;199:35–46.

Kon K, Ikejima K, Okumura K, et al. Diabetic KK-A(y) mice are highly susceptible to oxidative hepatocellular damage induced by acetaminophen. *Am J Physiol Gastrointest Liver Physiol.* 2010;299:G329–G337.

Kon K, Kim JS, Jaeschke H, et al. Mitochondrial permeability transition in acetaminophen-induced necrotic and apoptotic cell death to cultured mouse hepatocytes. *Hepatology.* 2004;40:1170–1179.

Kuffner EK, Dart RC, Bogdan GM, et al. Effect of maximal daily doses of acetaminophen on the liver of alcoholic patients: a randomized, double-blind, placebo-controlled trial. *Arch Intern Med.* 2001;161:2247–2252.

Kuffner EK, Temple AR, Cooper KM, et al. Retrospective analysis of transient elevations in alanine aminotransferase during long-term treatment with acetaminophen in osteoarthritis clinical trials. *Curr Med Res Opin.* 2006;22:2137–2148.

Lakehal F, Wendum D, Barbu V, et al. Phase I and phase II drug-metabolizing enzymes are expressed and heterogeneously distributed in the biliary epithelium. *Hepatology.* 1999;30:1498–1506.

Larosche I, Letteron P, Fromenty B, et al. Tamoxifen inhibits topoisomerases, depletes mitochondrial DNA, and triggers steatosis in mouse liver. *J Pharmacol Exp Ther.* 2007;321:526–535.

Larson AM, Polson J, Fontana RJ, et al. Acetaminophen-induced acute liver failure: results of a United States multicenter, prospective study. *Hepatology.* 42:1364–1372.

Laskin DL. Macrophages and inflammatory mediators in chemical toxicity: a battle of forces. *Chem Res Toxicol.* 2009;22:1376–1385.

Lecoeur S, Andre C, Beaune PH. Tienilic acid-induced autoimmune hepatitis: anti-liver and -kidney microsomal type 2 autoantibodies recognize a three-site conformational epitope on cytochrome P4502C9. *Mol Pharmacol.* 1996;50:326–333.

Lee WM. Acetaminophen and the U.S. Acute Liver Failure Study Group: lowering the risks of hepatic failure. *Hepatology.* 2004;40:6–9.

Lee WM, Senior JR. Recognizing drug-induced liver injury: current problems, possible solutions. *Toxicol Pathol.* 33:155–164.

Lee UE, Friedman SL. Mechanisms of hepatic fibrogenesis. *Best Pract Res Clin Gastroenterol.* 2011;25:195–206.

Letteron P, Sutton A, Mansouri A, et al. Inhibition of microsomal triglyceride transfer protein: another mechanism for drug-induced steatosis in mice. *Hepatology.* 2003;38:133–140.

Li AP. A review of the common properties of drugs with idiosyncratic hepatotoxicity and the "multiple determinant hypothesis" for the manifestation of idiosyncratic drug toxicity. *Chem Biol Interact.* 2002;142:7–23.

Li S, Zhao Y, He X, et al. Relief of extrinsic pathway inhibition by the Bid-dependent mitochondrial release of Smac in Fas-mediated hepatocyte apoptosis. *J Biol Chem.* 2002;277:26912–26920.

Limaye PB, Bhave VS, Palkar PS, et al. Upregulation of calpastatin in regenerating and developing rat liver: Role in resistance against hepatotoxicity. *Hepatology.* 2006;44:379–388.

Lin MC, Li JJ, Wang EJ, et al. Ethanol down-regulates the transcription of microsomal triglyceride transfer protein gene. *FASEB J.* 1997;11:1145–1152.

Lira M, Schteingart CD, Steinbach JH, et al. Sugar absorption by the biliary ductular epithelium of the rat: evidence for two transport systems. *Gastroenterology.* 1992;102:563–571.

Liu Y, Liu J, Iszard MB, et al. Transgenic mice that overexpress metallothionein-1 are protected from cadmium lethality and hepatotoxicity. *Toxicol Appl Pharmacol.* 1995;135:222–228.

Liu J, Liu Y, Michalska AE, et al. Metallothionein plays less of a protective role in cadmium–metallothionein-induced nephrotoxicity than in cadmium chloride-induced hepatotoxicity. *J Pharmacol Exp Ther.* 1996;276:1216–1223.

Loudianos G, Gitlin JD. Wilson's disease. *Semin Liver Dis.* 2000;20:353–364.

Lu H, Choudhuri S, Ogura K, et al. Characterization of organic anion transporting polypeptide 1b2-null mice: essential role in hepatic uptake/toxicity of phalloidin and microcystin-LR. *Toxicol Sci.* 2008;103:35–45.

Malhi H, Gores GJ, Lemasters JJ. Apoptosis and necrosis in the liver: a tale of two deaths? *Hepatology*. 2006;43(2 suppl 1):S31–S44.

Mangipudy RS, Chanda S, Mehendale HM. Tissue repair response as a function of dose in thioacetamide hepatotoxicity. *Environ Health Perspect*. 1995;103:260–267.

Mangipudy RS, Rao PS, Mehendale HM. Effect of an antimitotic agent colchicine on thioacetamide hepatotoxicity. *Environ Health Perspect*. 1996;104:744–749.

Manno M, Rezzadore M, Grossi M, et al. Potentiation of occupational carbon tetrachloride toxicity by ethanol abuse. *Hum Exp Toxicol*. 1996;15:294–300.

Marra F. Chemokines in liver inflammation and fibrosis. *Front Biosci*. 2002;7:d1899–d1914.

Masson MJ, Peterson RA, Chung CJ, et al. Lymphocyte loss and immuno-suppression following acetaminophen-induced hepatotoxicity in mice as a potential mechanism of tolerance. *Chem Res Toxicol*. 2007;20:20–26.

McClain C, Barve S, Joshi-Barve S, et al. Dysregulated cytokine metabolism, altered hepatic methionine metabolism and proteasome dysfunction in alcoholic liver disease. *Alcohol Clin Exp Res*. 2005;29(11 suppl):180S–188S.

McCuskey RS. Sinusoidal endothelial cells as an early target for hepatic toxicants. *Clin Hemorheol Microcirc*. 2006a;34:5–10.

McCuskey RS. Anatomy of the liver, in Boyer TD, Wright TL, Manns M, eds. *Zakim and Boyer's Hepatology*. 5th ed. Philadelphia: Saunders-Elsevier; 2006b:37.

McGill MR, Lebofsky M, Murray GJ, et al. Changing paradigms in acetaminophen toxicity: studies of plasma protein adducts and liver glutathione levels in mice (abstract). *Toxicol Sci*. 2012a;126(suppl 1):114.

McGill MR, Sharpe MR, Williams CD, et al. Mechanisms of acetaminophen hepatotoxicity in humans and mice involves mitochondrial damage and nuclear DNA fragmentation. *J Clin Invest*. 2012b;122:1574–1583.

McGill MR, Yan HM, Ramachandran A, et al. HepaRG cells: a human model to study mechanisms of acetaminophen hepatotoxicity. *Hepatology*. 2011;53:974–982.

McKillop IH, Moran DM, Jin X, et al. Molecular pathogenesis of hepatocellular carcinoma. *J Surg Res*. 2006;136:125–135.

Mehendale HM. Tissue repair: an important determinant of final outcome of toxicant-induced injury. *Toxicol Pathol*. 2005;33:41–51.

Mehendale HM, Limaye PB. Calpain: a death protein that mediates progression of liver injury. *Trends Pharmacol Sci*. 2005;26:232–236.

Metushi IG, Cai P, Zhu X, et al. A fresh look at the mechanism of isoniazid-induced hepatotoxicity. *Clin Pharmacol Ther*. 2011;89:911–914.

Michalopoulos GK. Liver regeneration. *J Cell Physiol*. 2007;213:286–300.

Michalopoulos GK, DeFrances MC. Liver regeneration. *Science*. 1997;276:60–66.

Miller AM, Horiguchi N, Jeong WI, et al. Molecular mechanisms of alcoholic liver disease: innate immunity and cytokines. *Alcohol Clin Exp Res*. 2011;35:787–793.

Mitchell JR, Jollow DJ, Potter WZ, et al. Acetaminophen-induced hepatic necrosis. IV. Protective role of glutathione. *J Pharmacol Exp Ther*. 1973;187:211–217.

Mitchell JR, Thorgeirsson UP, Black M, et al. Increased incidence of isoniazid hepatitis in rapid acetylators: possible relation to hydranize metabolites. *Clin Pharmacol Ther*. 1975;18:70–79.

Nagai H, Matsumaru K, Feng G, et al. Reduced glutathione depletion causes necrosis and sensitization to tumor necrosis factor-alpha-induced apoptosis in cultured mouse hepatocytes. *Hepatology*. 2002;36:55–64.

Nagata S, Nagase H, Kawane K, et al. Degradation of chromosomal DNA during apoptosis. *Cell Death Differ*. 2003;10:108–116.

Nelson SD. Molecular mechanisms of the hepatotoxicity caused by acetaminophen. *Semin Liver Dis*. 1990;10:267–278.

Neuschwander-Tetri BA. Hepatic lipotoxicity and the pathogenesis of non-alcoholic steatohepatitis: the central role of nontriglyceride fatty acid metabolites. *Hepatology*. 2010;52:774–788.

Nguyen LN, Furuya MH, Wolfraim LA, et al. Transforming growth factor-beta differentially regulates oval cell and hepatocyte proliferation. *Hepatology*. 2007;45:31–41.

Ni HM, Bockus A, Boggess N, et al. Activation of autophagy protects against acetaminophen hepatotoxicity in mice. *Hepatology*. 2012a;55:222–231.

Ni HM, Boggess N, McGill MR, et al. Liver specific loss of Atg5 causes persistent activation of Nrf2 and protects against acetaminophen-induced liver injury. *Toxicol Sci*. 2012b;127:438–450.

Niemelä O, Parkkila S, Juvonen RO, et al. Cytochromes P450 2A6, 2E1, and 3A and production of protein–aldehyde adducts in the liver of patients with alcoholic and non-alcoholic liver diseases. *J Hepatol*. 2000;33:893–901.

O'Connell TM, Watkins PB. The application of metabonomics to predict drug-induced liver injury. *Clin Pharmacol Ther*. 2010;88:394–399.

Ogasawara J, Watanabe-Fukunaga R, Adachi M, et al. Lethal effect of the anti-Fas antibody in mice. *Nature*. 1993;364:806–809.

Ong MM, Latchoumycandane C, Boelsterli UA: Troglitazone-induced hepatic necrosis in an animal model of silent genetic mitochondrial abnormalities. *Toxicol Sci*. 2007;97:205–213.

Padda MS, Sanchez M, Akhtar AJ, et al. Drug-induced cholestasis. *Hepatology*. 2011;53:1377–1387.

Palmeira CM, Rolo AP. Mitochondrially-mediated toxicity of bile acids. *Toxicology*. 2004;203:1–15.

Park BK, Laverty H, Srivastava A, et al. Drug bioactivation and protein adduct formation in the pathogenesis of drug-induced toxicity. *Chem Biol Interact*. 2011;192:30–36.

Pauli-Magnus C, Meier PJ. Hepatobiliary transporters and drug-induced cholestasis. *Hepatology*. 2006;44:778–787.

Pessayre D, Fromenty B, Berson A, et al. Central role of mitochondria in drug-induced liver injury. *Drug Metab Rev*. 2012;44:34–87.

Pessayre D, Mansouri A, Fromenty B. Nonalcoholic steatosis and steatohepatitis. V. Mitochondrial dysfunction in steatohepatitis. *Am J Physiol Gastrointest Liver Physiol*. 2002;282:G193–G199.

Phillips MJ, Poucell S, Oda M. Mechanisms of cholestasis. *Lab Invest*. 1986;54:593–608.

Pinzani M. PDGF and signal transduction in hepatic stellate cells. *Front Biosci*. 2002;7:d1720–d1726.

Price VF, Jollow DJ. Increased resistance of diabetic rats to acetaminophen-induced hepatotoxicity. *J Pharmacol Exp Ther*. 1982;220:504–513.

Ramachandran A, Lebofsky M, Baines CP, et al. Cyclophilin D deficiency protects against acetaminophen-induced oxidant stress and liver injury. *Free Radic Res*. 2011;45:156–164.

Ramaiah SK, Jaeschke H. Role of neutrophils in the pathogenesis of acute inflammatory liver injury. *Toxicol Pathol*. 2007;35:757–766.

Ramm GA, Ruddell RG. Hepatotoxicity of iron overload: mechanisms of iron-induced hepatic fibrogenesis. *Semin Liver Dis*. 2005;25:433–449.

Recknagel RO, Glende EA Jr, Dolak JA, et al. Mechanisms of carbon tetrachloride toxicity. *Pharmacol Ther*. 1989;43:139–154.

Rikans LE. The oxidation of acrolein by rat liver aldehyde dehydrogenases. Relation to allyl alcohol hepatotoxicity. *Drug Metab Dispos*. 1987;15:356–362.

Rikans LE, Moore DR. Effect of age and sex on allyl alcohol hepatotoxicity in rats: role of liver alcohol and aldehyde dehydrogenase activities. *J Pharmacol Exp Ther*. 1987;243:20–26.

Roberts DW, Bucci TJ, Benson RW, et al. Immunohistochemical localization and quantification of the 3-(cystein-S-yl)-acetaminophen protein adduct in acetaminophen hepatotoxicity. *Am J Pathol*. 1991;138:359–371.

Rockey DC. Vascular mediators in the injured liver. *Hepatology*. 2003;37:4–12.

Rockey DC, Friedman SL. Hepatic fibrosis and cirrhosis, in Boyer TD, Wright TL, Manns M, eds. *Zakim and Boyer's Hepatology*. 5th ed. Philadelphia: Saunders-Elsevier; 2006:87.

Roth M, Obaidat A, Hagenbuch B. OATPs, OATs and OCTs: the organic anion and cation transporters of the SLCO and SLC22A gene superfamilies. *Br J Pharmacol*. 2012;165:1260–1287.

Roth RA, Ganey PE. Hepatic toxicology, in McQueen CA, ed. *Comprehensive Toxicology*. 2nd ed. Vol 9. Oxford: Academic Press; 2010.

Runnegar MT, Berndt N, Kaplowitz N. Microcystin uptake and inhibition of protein phosphatases: effects of chemoprotectants and self-inhibition in relation to known hepatic transporters. *Toxicol Appl Pharmacol*. 1995a;134:264–272.

Runnegar MT, Berndt N, Kong S-M, et al. In vivo and in vitro binding of microcystin to protein phosphatases 1 and 2A. *Biochem Biophys Res Commun*. 1995b;216:162–169.

Runnegar MT, Wei X, Hamm-Alvarez SF. Increased protein phosphorylation of cytoplasmic dynein results in impaired motor function. *Biochem J.* 1999;342:1–6.

Saelens X, Festjens N, Vande Walle L, et al. Toxic proteins released from mitochondria in cell death. *Oncogene.* 2004;23:2861–2874.

Saito C, Lemasters JJ, Jaeschke H. c-Jun N-terminal kinase modulates oxidant stress and peroxynitrite formation independent of inducible nitric oxide synthase in acetaminophen hepatotoxicity. *Toxicol Appl Pharmacol.* 2010a;246:8–17.

Saito C, Zwingmann C, Jaeschke H. Novel mechanisms of protection against acetaminophen hepatotoxicity in mice by glutathione and *N*-acetylcysteine. *Hepatology.* 2010b;51:246–254.

Saito T, Misawa K, Kawata S. 1. Fatty liver and non-alcoholic steatohepatitis. *Intern Med.* 2007;46:101–103.

Sato C, Matsuda Y, Lieber CS. Increased hepatotoxicity of acetaminophen after chronic ethanol consumption in the rat. *Gastroenterology.* 1981;80:140–148.

Sato C, Lieber CS. Mechanism of the preventive effect of ethanol on acetaminophen-induced hepatotoxicity. *J Pharmacol Exp Ther.* 1981;218:811–815.

Satoh H, Martin BM, Schulick AH, et al. Human anti-endoplasmic reticulum antibodies in sera of patients with halothane-induced hepatitis are directed against a trifluoroacetylated carboxylesterase. *Proc Natl Acad Sci U S A.* 1989;86:322–326.

Satyanarayana A, Manns MP, Rudolph KL. Telomeres and telomerase: a dual role in hepatocarcinogenesis. *Hepatology.* 2004;40:276–283.

Scheffner D, Konig S, Rauterberg-Ruland I, et al. Fatal liver failure in 16 children with valproate therapy. *Epilepsia.* 1988;29:530–542.

Schuetz EG, Strom S, Yasuda K, et al. Disrupted bile acid homeostasis reveals an unexpected interaction among nuclear hormone receptors, transporters, and cytochrome P450. *J Biol Chem.* 2001;276:39411–39418.

Schulze-Bergkamen H, Schuchmann M, Fleischer B, et al. The role of apoptosis versus oncotic necrosis in liver injury: facts or faith? *J Hepatol.* 2006;44:984–993.

Schüngel S, Buitrago-Molina LE, Nalapareddy P, et al. The strength of the Fas ligand signal determines whether hepatocytes act as type 1 or type 2 cells in murine livers. *Hepatology.* 2009;50:1558–1566.

Schwabe RF, Seki E, Brenner DA. Toll-like receptor signaling in the liver. *Gastroenterology.* 2006;130:1886–1900.

Seitz S, Boelsterli UA. Diclofenac acyl glucuronide, a major biliary metabolite, is directly involved in small intestinal injury in rats. *Gastroenterology.* 1998;115:1476–1482.

Seki E, Schnabl B. Role of innate immunity and the microbiota in liver fibrosis—crosstalk between the liver and gut. *J Physiol.* 2012;590:447–458.

Sell S: Cellular origin of hepatocellular carcinomas. *Semin Cell Dev Biol.* 2002;13:419–424.

Selzner M, Clavien PA. Fatty liver in liver transplantation and surgery. *Semin Liver Dis.* 2001;21:105–113.

Shankar K, Vaidya VS, Apte UM, et al. Type 1 diabetic mice are protected from acetaminophen hepatotoxicity. *Toxicol Sci.* 2003;73:220–234.

Shaw PJ, Ganey PE, Roth RA. Idiosyncratic drug-induced liver injury and the role of inflammatory stress with an emphasis on an animal model of trovafloxacin hepatotoxicity. *Toxicol Sci.* 2010;118:7–18.

Sheikh MS, Fornace AJ Jr. Role of p53 family members in apoptosis. *J Cell Physiol.* 2000;182:171–181.

Shi J, Aisaki K, Ikawa Y, et al. Evidence of hepatocyte apoptosis in rat liver after the administration of carbon tetrachloride. *Am J Pathol.* 1998;153:515–525.

Sinclair JF, Szakacs JG, Wood SG, et al. Acetaminophen hepatotoxicity precipitated by short-term treatment of rats with ethanol and isopentanol: protection by triacetyloleandomycin. *Biochem Pharmacol.* 2000;59:445–454.

Smilkstein MJ, Knapp GL, Kulig KW, et al. Efficacy of oral *N*-acetylcysteine in the treatment of acetaminophen overdose. Analysis of the national multicenter study (1976 to 1985). *N Engl J Med.* 1988;319:1557–1562.

Solter PF, Wollenberg, GK, Huang X, et al. Prolonged sublethal exposure to the protein phosphatase inhibitor microcystin-LR results in multiple dose-dependent hepatotoxic effects. *Toxicol Sci.* 1998;44: 87–96.

Stewart SF, Day CP. Alcoholic liver disease, in Boyer TD, Wright TL, Manns M, eds. *Zakim and Boyer's Hepatology.* 5th ed. Philadelphia: Saunders-Elsevier; 2006:579.

Stickel F, Kessebohm K, Weimann R, et al. Review of liver injury associated with dietary supplements. *Liver Int.* 2011;31:595–605.

Stieger B, Fattinger K, Madon J, et al. Drug- and estrogen-induced cholestasis through inhibition of the hepatocellular bile salt export pump (BSEP) of rat liver. *Gastroenterology.* 2000;118:422–430.

Stieger B, Meier Y, Meier PJ. The bile salt export pump. *Pflugers Arch.* 2007;453:611–620.

Stravitz RT, Sanyal AJ. Drug-induced steatohepatitis. *Clin Liver Dis.* 2003;7:435–451.

Temple AR, Benson GD, Zinsenheim JR, et al. Multicenter, randomized, double-blind, active-controlled, parallel-group trial of the long-term (6–12 months) safety of acetaminophen in adult patients with osteoarthritis. *Clin Ther.* 2006;28:222–235.

Temple RJ, Himmel MH. Safety of newly approved drugs: implications for prescribing. *J Am Med Assoc.* 2002;287:2273–2275.

Thorgeirsson SS, Teramoto T, Factor VM. Dysregulation of apoptosis in hepatocellular carcinoma. *Semin Liver Dis.* 1998;18:115–122.

Tirmenstein MA, Hu CX, Gales TL, et al. Effects of troglitazone on HepG2 viability and mitochondrial function. *Toxicol Sci.* 2002;69:131–138.

Trauner M, Boyer JL. Bile salt transporters: molecular characterization, function, and regulation. *Physiol Rev.* 2003;83:633–671.

Trautwein C. Liver regeneration, in Boyer TD, Wright TL, Manns M, eds. *Zakim and Boyer's Hepatology.* 5th ed. Philadelphia: Saunders-Elsevier; 2006:23.

Tsukamoto H. Redox regulation of cytokine expression in Kupffer cells. *Antioxid Redox Signal.* 2002;4:741–748.

Tsutsumi M, Lasker JM, Shimizu M, et al. The intralobular distribution of ethanol-inducible P450IIE1 in rat and human liver. *Hepatology.* 1989;10:437–446.

Tuma DJ. Role of malondialdehyde-acetaldehyde adducts in liver injury. *Free Radic Biol Med.* 2002;32:303–308.

Uetrecht J. Idiosyncratic drug reactions: current understanding. *Annu Rev Pharmacol Toxicol.* 2007;47:513–539.

Vandenabeele P, Galluzzi L, Vanden Berghe T, et al. Molecular mechanisms of necroptosis: an ordered cellular explosion. *Nat Rev Mol Cell Biol.* 2010;11:700–714.

Vergani D, Mieli-Vergani G, Alberti A, et al. Antibodies to the surface of halothane-altered rabbit hepatocytes in patients with severe halothane-associated hepatitis. *N Engl J Med.* 1980;303:66–71.

Wagner M, Fickert P, Zollner G, et al. Role of farnesoid X receptor in determining hepatic ABC transporter expression and liver injury in bile duct-ligated mice. *Gastroenterology.* 2003;125:825–838.

Wagner M, Halilbasic E, Marschall HU, et al. CAR and PXR agonists stimulate hepatic bile acid and bilirubin detoxification and elimination pathways in mice. *Hepatology.* 2005;42:420–430.

Walli AK, Wieland E, Wieland TH. Phalloidin uptake by the liver of cholestatic rats in vivo, in isolated perfused liver and isolated hepatocytes. *Naunyn-Schmiedebergs Arch Pharmacol.* 1981;316:257–261.

Wands JR, Moradpour D. Molecular pathogenesis of hepatocellular carcinoma, in Boyer TD, Wright TL, Manns M, eds. *Zakim and Boyer's Hepatology.* 5th ed. Philadelphia: Saunders-Elsevier; 2006:165.

Wang X, Kanel GC, DeLeve LD. Support of sinusoidal endothelial cell glutathione prevents hepatic veno-occlusive disease in the rat. *Hepatology.* 2000;31:428–434.

Watanabe S, Phillips MJ. Acute phalloidin toxicity in living hepatocytes: evidence for a possible disturbance in membrane flow and for multiple functions for actin in the liver cell. *Am J Pathol.* 1986;122:101–111.

Watanabe N, Tsukada N, Smith CR, et al. Permeabilized hepatocyte couplets: adenosine triphosphate-dependent bile canalicular contractions and a circumferential pericanalicular microfilament belt demonstrated. *Lab Invest.* 1991;65:203–213.

Watkins PB. Idiosyncratic liver injury: challenges and approaches. *Toxicol Pathol.* 2005;33:1–5.

Weber LW, Boll M, Stampfl A. Hepatotoxicity and mechanism of action of haloalkanes: carbon tetrachloride as a toxicological model. *Crit Rev Toxicol.* 2003;33:105–136.

Wiedow O, Meyer-Hoffert U. Neutrophil serine proteases: potential key regulators of cell signalling during inflammation. *J Intern Med.* 2005;257(4):319–328.

Williams CD, Antoine DJ, Shaw PJ, et al. Role of the Nalp3 inflammasome in acetaminophen-induced sterile inflammation and liver injury. *Toxicol Appl Pharmacol.* 2011;252:289–297.

Williams CD, Farhood A, Jaeschke H. Role of caspase-1 and interleukin-1beta in acetaminophen-induced hepatic inflammation and liver injury. *Toxicol Appl Pharmacol.* 2010;247:169–178.

Wong FW, Chan WY, Lee SS. Resistance to carbon tetrachloride-induced hepatotoxicity in mice which lack CYP2E1 expression. *Toxicol Appl Pharmacol.* 1998;153:109–118.

Yamamoto Y, Nakajima M, Yamazaki H, et al. Cytotoxicity and apoptosis produced by troglitazone in human hepatoma cells. *Life Sci.* 2001;70:471–482.

Yan HM, Ramachandran A, Bajt ML, et al. The oxygen tension modulates acetaminophen-induced mitochondrial oxidant stress and cell injury in cultured hepatocytes. *Toxicol Sci.* 2010;117:515–523.

Yin XM, Wang K, Gross A, et al. Bid-deficient mice are resistant to Fas-induced hepatocellular apoptosis. *Nature.* 1999;400:886–891.

Zhang X, Liu F, Chen X, et al. Involvement of the immune system in idiosyncratic drug reactions. *Drug Metab Pharmacokinet.* 2011;26:47–59.

Zhang Y, Chong E, Herman B. Age-associated increases in the activity of multiple caspases in Fisher 344 rat organs. *Exp Gerontol.* 2002;37:777–789.

Zhang Y, Hong JY, Rockwell CE, et al. Effect of bile duct ligation on bile acid composition in mouse serum and liver. *Liver Intern.* 2012;32:58–69.

Ziegler K, Frimmer M. Cyclosporin A protects liver cells against phalloidin: potent inhibition of the inward transport by cholate and phallotoxins. *Biochim Biophys Acta.* 1984;805:174–180.

Zimmerman HJ. *Hepatotoxicity.* 2nd ed. Philadelphia: Lippincott, Williams & Wilkins; 1999.

Zimmerman HJ, Maddrey WC. Acetaminophen (paracetamol) hepatotoxicity with regular intake of alcohol: analysis of instances of therapeutic misadventure. *Hepatology.* 1995;22:767–773.

Zollner G, Marschall HU, Wagner M, et al. Role of nuclear receptors in the adaptive response to bile acids and cholestasis: pathogenetic and therapeutic considerations. *Mol Pharm.* 2006;3:231–251.

chapter 14

Toxic Responses of the Kidney

Rick G. Schnellmann

The functional integrity of the mammalian kidney is vital to total body homeostasis because the kidney plays a principal role in the excretion of metabolic wastes and in the regulation of extracellular fluid volume, electrolyte composition, and acid–base balance. In addition, the kidney synthesizes and releases hormones, such as renin and erythropoietin, and metabolizes vitamin D_3 to the active 1,25-dihydroxy vitamin D_3 form. A toxic insult to the kidney therefore could disrupt any or all of these functions and could have profound effects on total body metabolism. Fortunately, the kidneys are equipped with a variety of detoxification mechanisms and have considerable functional reserve and regenerative capacities. Nonetheless, the nature and severity of the toxic insult may be such that these detoxification and compensatory mechanisms are overwhelmed, and kidney injury ensues. The outcome of renal failure can be profound; permanent renal damage may result, requiring chronic dialysis treatment or kidney transplantation.

FUNCTIONAL ANATOMY

Gross examination of a sagittal section of the kidney reveals three clearly demarcated anatomic areas: the cortex, medulla, and papilla (Figs. 14-1 and 14-2). The cortex constitutes the major portion of the kidney and receives a disproportionately higher percentage (90%) of blood flow compared to the medulla (~6%–10%) or papilla (1%–2%). Thus, when a blood-borne toxicant is delivered to the kidney, a high percentage of the material will be delivered to the cortex and will have a greater opportunity to influence cortical rather than medullary or papillary functions. However, medullary and papillary tissues are exposed to higher luminal concentrations of toxicants for prolonged periods of time, a consequence of the more concentrated tubular fluid and the more sluggish flow of blood and filtrate in these regions.

The functional unit of the kidney, the nephron, may be considered in three portions: the vascular element, the glomerulus, and the tubular element.

Renal Vasculature and Glomerulus

The renal artery branches successively into interlobar, arcuate, and interlobular arteries (Fig. 14-1). The last of these give rise to the afferent arterioles, which supply the glomerulus; blood then leaves the glomerular capillaries via the efferent arteriole. Both the afferent and efferent arterioles, arranged in a series before and after the glomerular capillary tuft, respectively, are ideally situated to control glomerular capillary pressure and glomerular plasma flow rate. Indeed, these arterioles are innervated by the sympathetic nervous system and contract in response to nerve stimulation, angiotensin II, vasopressin, endothelin, adenosine, and norepinephrine, affecting glomerular pressures and blood flow. The efferent arterioles draining the cortical glomeruli branch into a peritubular capillary network, whereas those draining the juxtamedullary glomeruli form a capillary loop, the vasa recta, supplying the medullary structures. These postglomerular capillary loops provide an efficient arrangement for

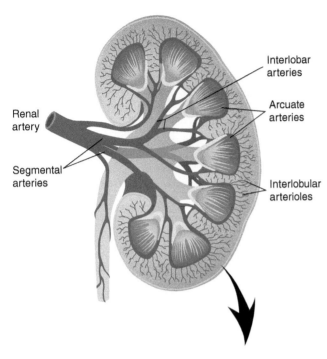

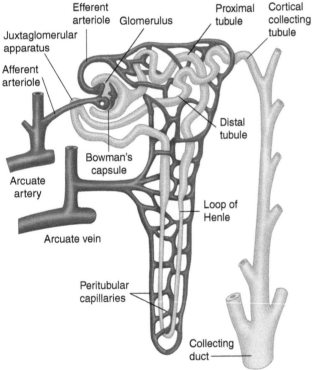

Figure 14-1. *Schematic of the human kidney showing the major blood vessels and the microcirculation and tubular components of each nephron.* (From Guyton AC, Hall JE, eds. Textbook of Medical Physiology. Philadelphia: WB Saunders; 1996:318, with permission from Elsevier.)

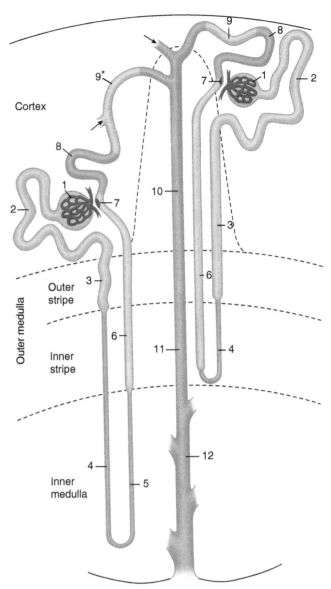

Figure 14-2. *Schematic of short- and long-looped nephrons and the collecting system.* A medullary ray is delineated by a dashed line within the cortex. (1) Renal corpuscle including Bowman's capsule and the glomerulus; (2) proximal convoluted tubule; (3) proximal straight tubule; (4) descending thin limb; (5) thin ascending limb; (6) thick ascending limb; (7) macula densa, located within the final portion of the thick ascending limb; (8) distal convoluted tubule; (9) connecting tubule; (9*) connecting tubule of the juxtamedullary nephron, which forms an arcade; (10) cortical collecting duct; (11) outer medullary collecting duct; (12) inner medullary collecting duct. (From Kriz W. Standard nomenclature for structures of the kidney. *Am J Physiol.* 1988;254:F1–F8, with permission.)

delivery of nutrients to the postglomerular tubular structures, delivery of wastes to the tubule for excretion, and return of reabsorbed electrolytes, nutrients, and water to the systemic circulation.

The glomerulus is a complex, specialized capillary bed composed primarily of endothelial cells that are characterized by an attenuated and fenestrated cytoplasm, visceral epithelial cells characterized by a cell body (podocyte) from which many trabeculae and pedicles (foot processes) extend, and a glomerular basement membrane (GBM), which is a trilamellar structure sandwiched

between the endothelial and epithelial cells (Fig. 14-3). A portion of the blood entering the glomerular capillary network is fractionated into a virtually protein-free and cell-free ultrafiltrate, which passes through Bowman's space and into the tubular portion of the nephron. The formation of such an ultrafiltrate is the net result of the Starling forces that determine fluid movement across capillary beds, that is, the balance between transcapillary hydrostatic pressure and colloid oncotic pressure (Maddox and Brenner, 1991). Filtration is therefore favored when transcapillary hydrostatic pressure exceeds plasma oncotic pressure. An additional determinant of ultrafiltration is the effective hydraulic permeability of the glomerular capillary wall, in other words, the ultrafiltration coefficient (K_f), which is determined by the total surface area available for filtration and the

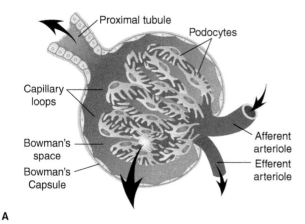

A

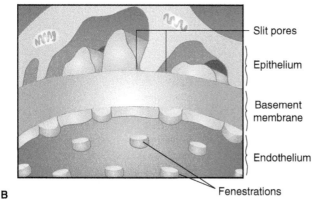

B

Figure 14-3. (A), Schematic of the ultrastructure of the glomerular capillaries. (B), Cross-section of the glomerular capillary membrane with the capillary endothelium, basement membrane, and epithelium podocytes. (From Guyton AC, Hall JE, eds. Textbook of Medical Physiology. Philadelphia: WB Saunders; 1996:32, with permission from Elsevier.)

hydraulic permeability of the capillary wall. Consequently, chemically induced decreases in glomerular filtration rate (GFR) may be related to decreases in transcapillary hydrostatic pressure and glomerular plasma flow due to increased afferent arteriolar resistance or to decreases in the surface area available for filtration, resulting from decreases in the size and/or number of endothelial fenestrae or detachment or effacement of foot processes.

Although the glomerular capillary wall permits a high rate of fluid filtration (approximately 20% of blood entering the glomerulus is filtered), it provides a significant barrier to the transglomerular passage of macromolecules. Experiments using a variety of charged and neutral tracers have established that this barrier function is based on the ability of the glomerulus to act as a size-selective and charge-selective filter (Brenner *et al.*, 1977). In general, the filtration of macromolecules is inversely proportional to the molecular weight of a substance; thus, small molecules, such as inulin (molecular weight [MW] ~5,500), are freely filtered, whereas large molecules, such as albumin (MW 56,000–70,000), are restricted. Filtration of anionic molecules tends to be restricted compared to that of neutral or cationic molecules of the same size. These permselective properties of the glomerulus appear to be directly related to the physicochemical properties of the different cell types within the glomerulus (Kanwar *et al.*, 1991). In particular, charge-selective properties of the glomerulus appear to be related to the anionic groups of the GBM coupled with the anionic coating of the epithelial and endothelial cells (Fig. 14-3). These highly anionic components produce electrostatic repulsion and hinder the circulation of polyanionic macromolecules, thereby markedly retarding passage of these molecules across the filtration barrier. Toxicants that neutralize or reduce the number of fixed anionic charges on glomerular structural elements therefore will impair the charge- and/or size-selective properties of the glomerulus, resulting in urinary excretion of polyanionic and/or high-molecular-weight proteins.

Proximal Tubule

The proximal tubule consists of three discrete segments: the S_1 (pars convoluta), S_2 (transition between pars convoluta and pars recta), and S_3 (the pars recta) segments (Fig. 14-2). The S_1 segment is the initial portion of the proximal convoluted tubule and is characterized by a tall brush-border and a well-developed vacuolar lysosomal system. The basolateral membrane is extensively interdigitated and many long mitochondria fill the basal portion of the cell, characteristic of Na^+-transporting epithelia. The S_2 segment comprises the end of the convoluted segment and the initial portion of the straight segment. These cells possess a shorter brush-border, fewer apical vacuoles and mitochondria, and less basolateral interdigitation compared to the S_1 cells. The S_3 segment comprises the distal portion of proximal segments and extends to the junction of the outer and inner stripe of the outer medulla. The S_3 cells have a well-developed brush border but fewer and smaller lysosomes and mitochondria than S_1 and S_2 cells.

The formation of urine is a highly complex and integrated process in which the volume and composition of the glomerular filtrate is progressively altered as fluid passes through each of the different tubular segments. The proximal tubule is the workhorse of the nephron, as it reabsorbs approximately 60% to 80% of solute and water filtered at the glomerulus. Toxicant-induced injury to the proximal tubule therefore will have major consequences to water and solute balance. Water reabsorption is through a passive iso-osmotic process, driven primarily by Na^+ reabsorption, mediated by the Na^+, K^+-ATPase localized in the basolateral plasma membrane. In addition to active Na^+ reabsorption, the proximal tubule reabsorbs other electrolytes, such as K^+, HCO_3^-, Cl^-, PO_4^{3-}, Ca^{2+}, and Mg^{2+}. The proximal tubule contains numerous transport systems capable of driving concentrative transport of many metabolic substrates, including amino acids, glucose, and citric acid cycle intermediates. The proximal tubule also reabsorbs virtually all the filtered low-molecular-weight proteins by specific endocytotic protein reabsorption processes. In addition, small linear peptides may be hydrolyzed by peptidases associated with the proximal tubular brush border. An important excretory function of the proximal tubule is secretion of weak organic anions and cations by specialized transporters that drive concentrative movement of these ions from postglomerular blood into proximal tubular cells, followed by secretion into tubular fluid. Toxicant-induced interruptions in the production of energy for any of these active transport mechanisms or the function of critical membrane-bound enzymes or transporters can profoundly affect proximal tubular and whole-kidney function.

The various segments of the proximal tubule exhibit marked biochemical and physiologic heterogeneity (Goldstein, 1993). For example, filtered HCO_3^-, low-molecular-weight proteins, amino acids, and glucose are primarily reabsorbed by the S_1 segment. Transport capacities for these substances in the S_2 and S_3 segments are appreciably less; for example, glucose reabsorption in the S_2 and S_3 segments is about 50% and 10% of that in the S_1 segment, respectively. In contrast, the principal site of organic anion and cation secretion is in the S_2 and S_1/S_2 segments, respectively. Oxygen consumption, Na^+, K^+-ATPase activity, and gluconeogenic capacity are greater in the S_1 and S_2 segments than in the S_3 segment. Catabolism and apical transport of glutathione (GSH) occur to a

Table 14-1

Filtration, Reabsorption, and Excretion Rates of Different Substances by the Kidneys*

	FILTERED (meq/24 h)	REABSORBED (meq/24 h)	EXCRETED (meq/24 h)	REABSORBED (%)
Glucose (g/day)	180	180	0	100
Bicarbonate (meq/day)	4320	4318	2	>99.9
Sodium (meq/day)	25,560	25,410	150	99.4
Chloride (meq/day)	19,440	19,260	180	99.1
Water (L/day)	169	167.5	1.5	99.1
Urea (g/day)	48	24	24	50
Creatinine (g/day)	1.8	0	1.8	0

*Glomerular filtration rate: 125 mL/min = 180 L/24 h.

much greater extent in the S_3 segment, where the brush-border enzyme γ-glutamyl transpeptidase is present in greater amounts. Chemically induced injury to distinct proximal tubular segments therefore may be related in part to their segmental differences in biochemical properties (see "Site-Selective Injury").

Loop of Henle

The thin descending and ascending limbs and the thick ascending limb of the loop of Henle are critical to the processes involved in urinary concentration (Fig. 14-2). Approximately 25% of the filtered Na^+ and K^+ and 20% of the filtered water are reabsorbed by the segments of the loop of Henle. The tubular fluid entering the thin descending limb is iso-osmotic to the renal interstitium; water is freely permeable and solutes, such as electrolytes and urea, may enter from the interstitium. In contrast, the thin ascending limb is relatively impermeable to water and urea, and Na^+ and Cl^- are reabsorbed by passive diffusion. The thick ascending limb is impermeable to water, and active transport of Na^+ and Cl^- is mediated by the Na^+/K^+–$2Cl^-$ cotransport mechanism, with the energy provided by the Na^+, K^+-ATPase. The relatively high rates of Na^+, K^+-ATPase activity and oxygen demand, coupled with the meager oxygen supply in the medullary thick ascending limb, are believed to contribute to the vulnerability of this segment of the nephron to hypoxic injury. The close interdependence between metabolic workload and tubular vulnerability has been demonstrated, revealing that selective damage to the thick ascending limb in the isolated perfused kidney can be blunted by reducing tubular work and oxygen consumption (via inhibition of the Na^+, K^+-ATPase with ouabain) or by increasing oxygen supply (via provision of an oxygen carrier, hemoglobin) (Brezis and Epstein, 1993). Conversely, increasing the tubular workload (via the ionophore amphotericin B) exacerbates hypoxic injury to this segment (Brezis et al., 1984).

Distal Tubule and Collecting Duct

The macula densa comprises specialized cells located between the end of the thick ascending limb and the early distal tubule, in close proximity to the afferent arteriole (Fig. 14-2). This anatomic arrangement is ideally suited for a feedback system whereby a stimulus received at the macula densa is transmitted to the arterioles of the same nephron. Under normal physiologic conditions, increased solute delivery or concentration at the macula densa triggers a signal resulting in afferent arteriolar constriction leading to decreases in GFR (and hence decreased solute delivery). Thus, increases in fluid/solute out of the proximal tubule, due to impaired

tubular reabsorption, will activate this feedback system, referred to as tubuloglomerular feedback (TGF) and resulting in decreases in the filtration rate of the same nephron. This regulatory mechanism is viewed as a powerful volume-conserving mechanism, designed to decrease GFR in order to prevent massive losses of fluid/electrolytes due to impaired tubular reabsorption. Humoral mediation of TGF by the renin–angiotensin system has been proposed, and evidence suggests that other substances may be involved. The distal tubular cells contain numerous mitochondria but lack a well-developed brush border and an endocytotic apparatus characteristic of the pars convoluta of the proximal tubule. The early distal tubule reabsorbs most of the remaining intraluminal Na^+, K^+, and Cl^- but is relatively impermeable to water.

The late distal tubule, cortical collecting tubule, and medullary collecting duct perform the final regulation and fine-tuning of urinary volume and composition. The remaining Na^+ is reabsorbed in conjunction with K^+ and H^+ secretion in the late distal tubule and cortical collecting tubule. The combination of medullary and papillary hypertonicity generated by countercurrent multiplication and the action of antidiuretic hormone (ADH, vasopressin) serve to enhance water permeability of the medullary collecting duct. Chemicals that interfere with ADH synthesis, secretion, or action therefore may impair concentrating ability. Additionally, because urinary concentrating ability is dependent upon medullary and papillary hypertonicity, chemicals that increase medullary blood flow may impair concentrating ability by dissipating the medullary osmotic gradient.

Table 14-1 illustrates the efficiency of the nephrons in the conservation of electrolytes, substrates, and water and excretion of nitrogenous wastes (urea). The reader may refer to *Brenner and Rector's The Kidney* (2011) and *Diseases of the Kidney and Urinary Tract* (2011) for further review of renal physiology.

PATHOPHYSIOLOGIC RESPONSES OF THE KIDNEY

Acute Kidney Injury

One of the most common manifestations of nephrotoxic damage is acute renal failure or acute kidney injury (AKI). AKI is a group of syndromes that comprises multiple causative factors and occurs in a variety of settings with varied clinical manifestations ranging from a minimal elevation in serum creatinine to anuric renal failure. Considering that AKI is a complex disorder, the Acute Dialysis Quality Initiative developed the RIFLE (Risk, Injury, Failure, Loss, and End-stage renal disease) classification of AKI (Bellomo et al.,

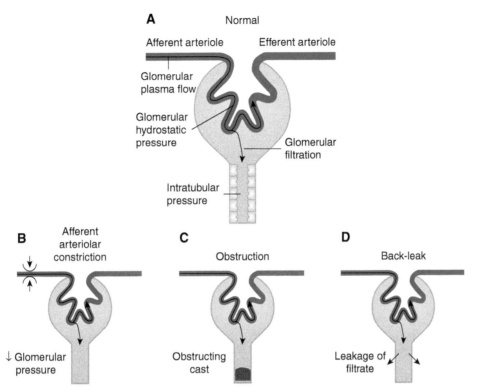

Figure 14-4. *Mechanisms of reduction of the GFR.* (**A**), GFR depends on 4 factors: (1) adequate blood flow to the glomerulus; (2) adequate glomerular capillary pressure; (3) glomerular permeability; and (4) low intratubular pressure. (**B**), Afferent arteriolar constriction decreases GFR by reducing blood flow, resulting in diminished capillary pressure. (**C**), Obstruction of the tubular lumen by cast formation increases tubular pressure; when tubular pressure exceeds glomerular capillary pressure, filtration decreases or ceases. (**D**), Back-leak occurs when the paracellular space between cells increases and the glomerular filtrate leaks into the extracellular space and bloodstream. (From Molitoris BA, Bacallao R. Pathophysiology of ischemic acute renal failure: cytoskeletal aspects. In: Berl T, Bonventre JV, eds. *Atlas of Diseases of the Kidney.* Philadelphia: Current Medicine; 1999:13.5, with permission.)

2004) and the AKI Network proposed minor modifications (Mehta *et al.*, 2007). In both cases, AKI classification is based on the extent of serum creatinine increases or changes in urine output.

Any decline in GFR is complex and may result from prerenal factors (renal vasoconstriction, intravascular volume depletion, and insufficient cardiac output), postrenal factors (ureteral or bladder obstruction), and intrarenal factors (glomerulonephritis, tubular cell injury, death, and loss resulting in back leak; renal vasculature damage, interstitial nephritis) (Fig. 14-4). Fig. 14-5 illustrates the pathways that lead to diminished GFR following chemical exposure. As discussed above, pre- and postrenal factors can lead to decreased GFR. If a chemical causes tubular damage directly, then tubular casts can cause tubular obstruction, increased tubular pressure, and decreased GFR. The tubular damage may result in epithelial cell death/loss, leading to back leak of glomerular filtrate and a decrease in GFR. If a chemical causes intrarenal vascular damage with hemodynamic alterations that lead to vasoconstriction, the resulting medullary hypoxia may cause tubular damage and/or decreases in perfusion pressure, glomerular hydrostatic pressure, and GFR. If a chemical causes intrarenal inflammation, then tubular and vascular damage may follow with decreases in GFR. Finally, a chemical may disrupt glomerular function, resulting in decreased glomerular ultrafiltration and GFR. It has been estimated that prerenal factors are responsible for AKI in 55% to 60% of patients, intrarenal factors are responsible for AKI in 35% to 40% of patients, and postrenal factors are responsible for AKI in <5% of patients (Brady *et al.*, 2004). Further, it is thought that more than 90% of AKI mediated by intrarenal factors is the result of ischemia/reperfusion injury or nephrotoxicity. Table 14-2 provides a partial list of chemicals that produce AKI through these different mechanisms.

The maintenance of tubular integrity is dependent on cell-to-cell and cell-to-matrix adhesion; these interactions are mediated in part by integrins and cell adhesion molecules (Fig. 14-6). It has been hypothesized that after a chemical or hypoxic insult, adhesion of nonlethally damaged, apoptotic, and oncotic cells to the basement membrane is compromised, leading to their detachment from the basement membrane and appearance in the tubular lumen (Goligorsky *et al.*, 2010). Morphologically, such an event would lead to gaps in the epithelial cell lining, potentially resulting in back leak of filtrate and diminished GFR. These detached cells may aggregate in the tubular lumen (cell-to-cell adhesion) and/or adhere or reattach to adherent epithelial cells downstream, resulting in tubular obstruction. Further, the loss of expression of integrins on the basolateral membrane may be responsible for the exfoliation of tubular cells, and the redistribution of integrins from the basolateral to the apical membrane facilitates adhesion of detached cells to the in situ epithelium.

Extensive evidence supports the idea that endothelial injury and inflammatory cells play a role in ischemia-induced AKI (Kinsey *et al.*, 2008). Injury to the renal vasculature endothelium results in chemokine and proinflammatory cytokine production and neutrophil adhesion (Fig. 14-7). Neutrophils respond rapidly to injury and adhesion to the vascular endothelium leads to capillary damage/leakage and vascular congestion. Macrophages infiltrate the kidney shortly after neutrophils and act through phagocytosis and the production of proinflammatory cytokines that stimulate other leukocytes. Rabb and colleagues provided evidence that T cells and B cells play a role in AKI (Rabb *et al.*, 2000; Burne *et al.*, 2001; Burne-Taney *et al.*, 2003; Ikeda *et al.*, 2006). Although significant advances have been made in the past few years concerning the roles of inflammatory cells in AKI, the specific role of each

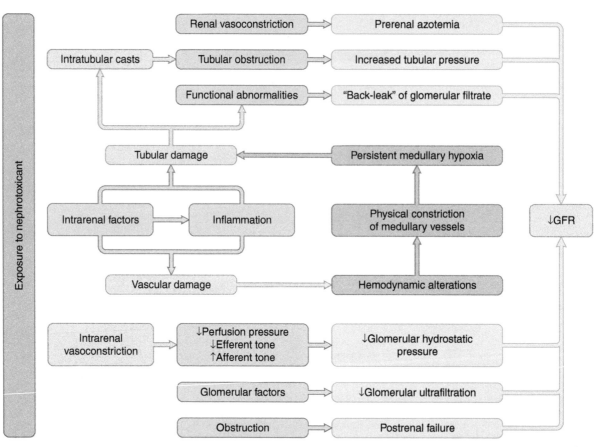

Figure 14-5. *Mechanisms that contribute to decreased GFR in acute renal failure.* After exposure to a nephrotoxicant, one or more mechanisms may contribute to a reduction in the GFR. These include renal vasoconstriction resulting in prerenal azotemia and obstruction due to precipitation of a drug or endogenous compound within the kidney. Intrarenal factors include direct tubular obstruction and dysfunction, with or without inflammation, resulting in tubular back-leak and increased tubular pressure. Vascular damage, with or without inflammation, leading to hemodynamic changes. Alterations in the levels of a variety of vasoactive mediators may result in decreased renal perfusion pressure or efferent arteriolar tone and increased afferent arteriolar tone, leading to decreased glomerular hydrostatic pressure. (Modified from Schnellmann RG, Kelly KJ. Pathophysiology of nephrotoxic acute renal failure. In: Berl T, Bonventre JV, eds. *Atlas of Diseases of the Kidney.* Philadelphia: Current Medicine; 1999:15.4, with permission.)

Table 14-2

Mechanisms of Chemically Induced Acute Renal Failure

PRERENAL	VASOCONSTRICTION	CRYSTALLURIA	TUBULAR TOXICITY	ENDOTHELIAL INJURY	GLOMERULOPATHY	INTERSTITIAL NEPHRITIS
Diuretics	Nonsteroidal anti-inflammatory drugs	Sulfonamides	Aminoglycosides	Cyclosporine	Gold	Antibiotics
Angiotensin receptor antagonists		Methotrexate	Cisplatin	Mitomycin C	Penicillamine	Nonsteroidal anti-inflammatory drugs
Angiotensin-converting enzyme inhibitors	Radiocontrast agents	Acyclovir	Vancomycin	Tacrolimus	Nonsteroidal anti-inflammatory drugs	
Antihypertensive agents	Cyclosporine Tacrolimus	Triamterene Ethylene glycol	Pentamidine Radiocontrast agents	Cocaine Conjugated estrogens		Diuretics
	Amphotericin B	Protease inhibitors	Heavy metals	Quinine		
			Haloalkane- and Haloalkene-cysteine conjugates			

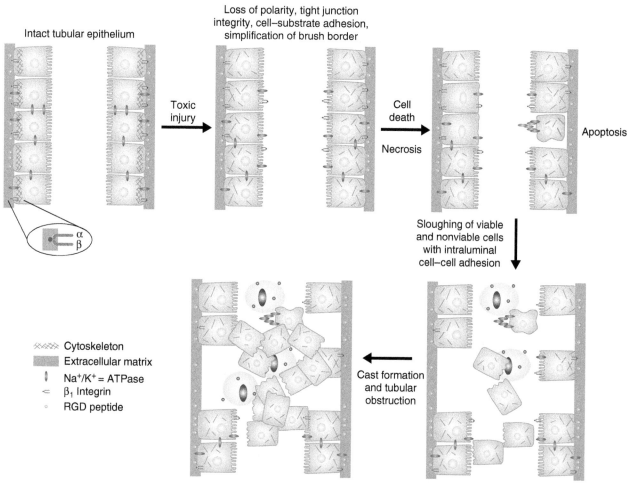

Figure 14-6. *After injury, alterations can occur in the cytoskeleton and in the normal distribution of membrane proteins such as Na⁺, K⁺-ATPase, and β₁ integrins in sublethally injured renal tubular cells.* These changes result in loss of cell polarity, tight junction integrity, and cell–substrate adhesion. Lethally injured cells undergo oncosis or apoptosis, and both dead and viable cells may be released into the tubular lumen. Adhesion of released cells to other released cells and to cells remaining adherent to the basement membrane may result in cast formation, tubular obstruction, and further compromise the GFR. (From Schnellmann RG, Kelly KJ. Pathophysiology of nephrotoxic acute renal failure. In: Berl T, Bonventre JV, eds. *Atlas of Diseases of the Kidney.* Philadelphia: Current Medicine; 1999:15.5, with permission.)

inflammatory cell and the interplay between innate and adaptive immunity remains to be elucidated. It should be noted that the role of inflammatory cells in chemical-induced AKI has received little attention.

Although chemically induced AKI can be initiated by proximal tubular cell injury, nephrotoxicants may also delay the recovery of renal function by inhibiting cellular repair and regeneration. For example, Leonard *et al.* (1994) demonstrated that cisplatin impaired tubular regeneration resulting in prolonged renal dysfunction, effects that were in contrast to the regenerative response and renal functional recovery following tobramycin-induced nephrotoxicity. Using an in vitro model, Counts *et al.* (1995) reported that following mechanically induced injury to a proximal tubular monolayer, proliferation and migration were inhibited by the heavy metal HgCl₂, the mycotoxin fumonisin B₁, and dichlorovinyl-L-cysteine (DCVC), suggesting that nephrotoxicants may inhibit/delay the regenerative process.

Adaptation Following Toxic Insult

Fortunately, the kidney has a remarkable ability to compensate for a loss in renal functional mass. Micropuncture studies have revealed that following unilateral nephrectomy, GFR of the remnant kidney

increases by approximately 40% to 60%, an effect associated with early compensatory increases in glomerular plasma flow rate and glomerular hydraulic pressure. Compensatory increases in single-nephron GFR are accompanied by proportionate increases in proximal tubular water and solute reabsorption; glomerulotubular balance is therefore maintained and overall renal function appears normal by standard clinical tests. Consequently, chemically induced changes in renal function may not be detected until these compensatory mechanisms are overwhelmed by significant nephron loss and/or damage.

There are a number of cellular and molecular responses to a nephrotoxic insult. After a population of tubular epithelial cells is exposed to a toxicant, a fraction of the cells will be severely injured and will undergo cell death by apoptosis or oncosis (see below). Those cells that are nonlethally injured may undergo cell repair and/or adaptation, and contribute to the recovery of the nephron (Fig. 14-8). In addition, there is a population of cells that are uninjured and may undergo compensatory hypertrophy, adaptation, and proliferation. Current evidence supports the hypothesis that tubular epithelial cells are primarily responsible for the structural and functional recovery of the nephron following injury and that bone marrow-derived stem cells do not play a significant role (see Humphreys *et al.*, 2008, 2011). Surviving tubular epithelial cells

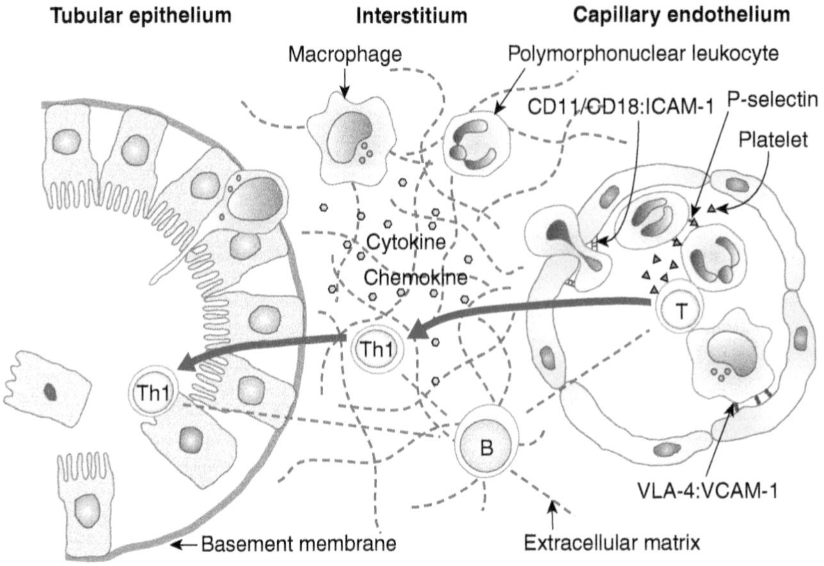

Tubular epithelium   **Interstitium**   **Capillary endothelium**

Macrophage   Polymorphonuclear leukocyte

CD11/CD18:ICAM-1   P-selectin

Platelet

Cytokine

Chemokine

Th1

Th1

T

B

VLA-4:VCAM-1

← Basement membrane   Extracellular matrix

Figure 14-7. *Ischemia acute tubular injury and inflammatory cells.* Initially ischemia causes injury of endothelial cells, followed by leukocyte activation and formation of platelet–leukocyte plugs. Chemokines and cytokines produced by both leukocytes and tubular cells lead to the recruitment of inflammatory cells from the microvasculature to the interstitium, allowing inflammatory cells to be able to interact with tubular epithelial cells. Renal inflammation is associated with the shortened microvilli of tubular epithelial cells and to the denuded epithelium. The sloughed cells adhere to each other and in turn form intratubule casts. Abbreviations: B, B cells; ICAM-1, intercellular adhesion molecule-1; T, CD4+ T cells; Th1, T helper 1 cells; VCAM-1, vascular cell adhesion molecule-1; VLA-4, very late antigen-4. (From Ikeda, *et al.* Ischemic acute tubular necrosis models and drug discovery: a focus on cellular inflammation. *Drug Discov Today.* 2006;11:364–370, with permission from Elsevier.)

replace dead and detached cells through dedifferentiation, proliferation, migration, and redifferentiation. Growth factors delivered to tubular epithelial cells from local and systemic sources may help orchestrate the proliferative response of the nephron. Although several growth factors such as epidermal growth factor (EGF), heparin-binding epidermal growth factor (HB-EGF), insulin-like growth factor-1 (IGF-1), hepatocyte growth factor (HGF), fibroblast growth factors, and transforming growth factors α and β have been implicated in proximal tubular regeneration (Hammerman and Miller, 1994), it appears that the EGF receptor is required for this

process (Wang *et al.*, 2003; Zhuang *et al.*, 2004; Hallman *et al.*, 2008). Interestingly, exogenous administration of EGF, HGF, or IGF-1 accelerates renal repair following ischemic-, gentamicin-, bromohydroquinone-, and/or $HgCl_2$-induced AKI. However, it is not clear which endogenous growth factors are required for tubular regeneration.

Two of the most notable cellular adaptation responses are metallothionein induction (see "Cadmium") and stress protein induction. HSPs and glucose-regulated proteins are two examples of stress protein families that are induced in response to a number

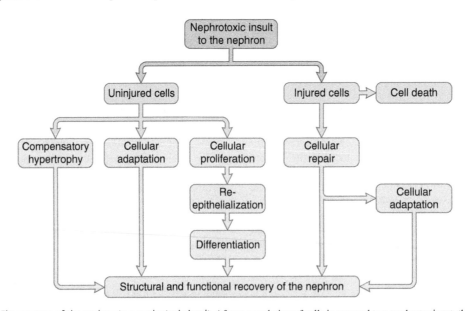

Figure 14-8. *The response of the nephron to a nephrotoxic insult.* After a population of cells is exposed to a nephrotoxicant, the cells respond; ultimately the nephron recovers function or, if cell death and loss are extensive, nephron function ceases. Terminally injured cells undergo cell death through oncosis or apoptosis. Cells injured sublethally undergo repair and adaptation in response to the nephrotoxicant. Cells not injured and adjacent to the injured area may undergo dedifferentiation, proliferation, migration or spreading, and differentiation. Cells not injured may also undergo compensatory hypertrophy in response to the cell loss and injury. Finally the uninjured cells also may undergo adaptation in response to a nephrotoxicant exposure. (From Schnellmann RG, Kelly KJ. Pathophysiology of nephrotoxic acute renal failure. In: Berl T, Bonventre JV, eds. *Atlas of Diseases of the Kidney.* Philadelphia: Current Medicine; 1999:15.4, with permission.)

of pathophysiologic states such as heat shock, anoxia, oxidative stress, toxicants, heavy metal exposure, and tissue trauma (Kelly, 2005; van de Water *et al.*, 2006). The distribution of individual stress proteins varies between different cell types in the kidney and within subcellular compartments (Goering *et al.*, 2000). These proteins play important roles in protein folding, translocation of proteins across organelle membranes, prevention of aggregation of damaged proteins, repair and degradation of damaged proteins, and thereby provide a defense mechanism against toxicity and/or for the facilitation of recovery and repair. HSP induction in renal tissue has been demonstrated following treatment with nephrotoxicants such as gentamicin (Komatsuda *et al.*, 1993), haloalkane cysteine conjugates (Chen *et al.*, 1992), and HgCl$_2$ (Goering *et al.*, 1992). Interestingly, proximal tubular HSP60 and mitochondrial HSP70 and HSP27 have been identified as molecular targets of the reactive metabolites of the haloalkane cysteine conjugate tetrafluoroethyl-L-cysteine (TFEC) and DCVC, respectively, an effect that could alter the normal housekeeping functions of the proximal tubule and thereby potentially contribute to and exacerbate nephrotoxicity (Bruschi *et al.*, 1993; van de Water *et al.*, 2006). HSP70 induction in the kidney is cytoprotective and renoprotective following injury and HSP70 blocks apoptosis upstream of mitochondrial events.

Chronic Kidney Disease

It is generally believed that progression to chronic kidney disease (CKD) and end-stage renal failure is not simply a function of a primary renal insult per se but rather is related to secondary pathophysiologic processes triggered by the initial injury. Animal studies have begun to define a relationship between AKI and CKD. For example, Basile *et al.* (2001) reported that rats subjected to ischemia undergo renal dysfunction followed by morphologic recovery and return to normal serum creatinine levels. However, 16 weeks following ischemia, protein and albumin excretion increased and microvessel density decreased, markers of CKD. Consequently, a low level of injury or inflammation may exist following AKI that ultimately leads to CKD and/or may sensitize the kidney to a second insult.

Progressive deterioration of renal function may occur with long-term exposure to a variety of chemicals (eg, analgesics, lithium, and cyclosporine). The progression of chronic renal disease, for example, has been postulated to be a consequence of the glomerular hemodynamic response to renal injury (Brenner *et al.*, 1982). That is, following nephron loss, there are adaptive increases in glomerular pressures and flows that increase the single-nephron GFR of remnant viable nephrons. Although these compensatory mechanisms serve to maintain whole-kidney GFR, evidence has accumulated to suggest that, with time, these alterations are mal-adaptive and foster the progression of renal failure. Focal glomerulosclerosis eventually develops and may lead to tubular atrophy and interstitial fibrosis. Consequently, glomerulosclerosis in these nephrons will perpetuate the cycle of triggering further compensatory increases in the hemodynamics of less damaged nephrons, contributing, in turn, to their eventual destruction. Although the underlying mechanisms are not precisely known, compensatory increases in glomerular pressures and flows of the remnant glomeruli may result in mechanical damage to the capillaries due to increased shear stress on the endothelium and damage to the glomerular capillary wall, leading to altered permeabilities, and mesangial thickening due to increased transcapillary flux and local deposition of macromolecules (Dunn *et al.*, 1986). Other factors likely to play a role in the pathogenesis of chronic renal failure include growth promoters and inhibitors, increased extracellular matrix deposition, reactive oxygen species (ROS), lipid accumulation, and tubulointerstitial injury.

SUSCEPTIBILITY OF THE KIDNEY TO TOXIC INJURY

Incidence and Severity of Toxic Nephropathy

A wide variety of drugs, environmental chemicals, and metals can cause nephrotoxicity (Table 14-2). As stated above, it has been estimated that ischemia/reperfusion and nephrotoxicants are responsible for 35% of AKI. Nephrotoxicity is a recognized clinical liability of certain classes of drugs, in particular, antibiotics, angiotensin-converting enzyme (ACE) inhibitors and angiotensin receptor blockers, analgesics and nonsteroidal anti-inflammatory drugs (NSAIDs), radiocontrast media, and anti-cancer agents. Approximately 70% of the patients presenting with drug-induced AKI were nonoliguric; the pathologic findings revealed acute tubular necrosis in 60%. Approximately 50% recovered completely. A myriad of risk factors appear to contribute to the incidence/severity of AKI, including genetic/hereditary factors, volume depletion, septic shock, hypotension, multiple chemical insults, age, diabetes, and preexisting renal disease. The consequences of AKI can be profound, as permanent renal damage may result and dialysis or renal transplantation may be required.

Chronic renal failure leading to end-stage renal failure has been associated with long-term abuse of analgesics. The incidence of analgesic nephropathy has been reported to be as high as 20% to 25% in certain countries (eg, Switzerland). Other agents, such as lithium, cyclosporine, NSAIDs, lead, and cadmium, may produce chronic tubulointerstitial nephropathy with progressive loss of renal function.

Reasons for the Susceptibility of the Kidney to Toxicity

The unusual susceptibility of the mammalian kidney to the toxic effects of noxious chemicals can be attributed in part to the unique physiologic and anatomic features of this organ. Although the kidneys constitute only 0.5% of total body mass, they receive about 20% to 25% of the resting cardiac output. Consequently, any drug or chemical in the systemic circulation will be delivered to these organs in relatively high amounts. The processes involved in forming concentrated urine also serve to concentrate potential toxicants in the tubular fluid. As water and electrolytes are reabsorbed from the glomerular filtrate, chemicals in the tubular fluid may be concentrated, thereby driving passive diffusion of toxicants into tubular cells. Therefore, a nontoxic concentration of a chemical in the plasma may reach toxic concentrations in the kidney. Progressive concentration of toxicants along the nephron may result in intraluminal precipitation of relatively insoluble compounds, causing AKI secondary to tubular obstruction. Finally, renal transport, accumulation, and metabolism of xenobiotics contribute significantly to the susceptibility of the kidney (and specific nephron segments) to toxic injury (see "Site-Selective Injury").

In addition to intrarenal factors, the incidence and/or severity of chemically induced nephrotoxicity may be related to the sensitivity of the kidney to circulating vasoactive substances. Under these conditions, vasoconstrictors such as angiotensin II or vasopressin are increased. Normally, the actions of high circulating levels of vasoconstrictor hormones are counterbalanced by the actions of increased vasodilatory prostaglandins; thus, renal blood flow (RBF) and GFR are maintained. However, when prostaglandin synthesis is suppressed by NSAIDs, RBF declines markedly and AKI ensues, due to the unopposed actions of vasoconstrictors. Another example of predisposing risk factors relates to the clinical use of ACE inhibitors. ACE inhibitors have been reported to produce AKI in patients with severe hypertension, due to either bilateral renal artery stenosis or renal artery stenosis in a solitary kidney. Under these conditions, glomerular filtration pressure is dependent on angiotensin II-induced efferent arteriolar constriction. ACE inhibitors will block this vasoconstriction, resulting in a precipitous decline in filtration pressure and AKI.

Site-Selective Injury

Many nephrotoxicants have their primary effects on discrete segments or regions of the nephron. For example, the proximal tubule is the primary target for most nephrotoxic antibiotics, antineoplastics, halogenated hydrocarbons, mycotoxins, and heavy metals, whereas the glomerulus is the primary site for immune complexes, the loop of Henle/collecting ducts for fluoride ions, and the medulla/papilla for chronically consumed analgesic mixtures. The reasons underlying this site-selective injury are complex but can be attributed in part to site-specific differences in blood flow, transport and accumulation of chemicals, physicochemical properties of the epithelium, reactivity of cellular/molecular targets, balance of bioactivation/detoxification reactions, cellular energetics, and/or regenerative/repair mechanisms. See Sweet (2010) and Lock (2010) for extensive reviews of the transporters and xenobiotic metabolizing enzymes in the kidney.

Glomerular Injury

The glomerulus is the initial site of chemical exposure within the nephron, and a number of nephrotoxicants produce structural injury to this segment. In certain instances, chemicals alter glomerular permeability to proteins by altering the size- and charge-selective functions. Both puromycin aminonucleoside and doxorubicin target glomerular epithelial cells, resulting in changes in size and charge selectivity and proteinuria. The decrease in charge selectivity is thought to result from a decrease in negatively charged sites, while the loss of size selectivity is thought to result from focal detachment of podocytes from the GBM.

Cyclosporine, amphotericin B, and gentamicin are examples of chemicals that impair glomerular ultrafiltration without significant loss of structural integrity and decrease GFR. Amphotericin B decreases GFR by causing renal vasoconstriction and decreasing the glomerular capillary ultrafiltration coefficient (K_f), an effect probably mediated through the endothelial cells. Because of its polycationic nature, the aminoglycoside gentamicin interacts with the anionic sites on the endothelial cells, decreasing K_f, and GFR. Finally, cyclosporine not only causes renal vasoconstriction and vascular damage but is injurious to the glomerular endothelial cell.

Chemically induced glomerular injury may also be mediated by extrarenal factors. Circulating immune complexes may be trapped within the glomeruli; binding of complement, attraction of neutrophils, and phagocytosis may result. Neutrophils and macrophages are commonly observed within glomeruli in membranous glomerulonephritis, and the local release of cytokines and ROS may contribute to glomerular injury. Heavy metals (eg, $HgCl_2$, gold, cadmium), hydrocarbons, penicillamine, and captopril can produce this type of glomerular injury. A chemical may function as a hapten attached to some native protein (eg, tubular antigens released secondary to toxicity) or as a complete antigen—particularly if it is sequestered within the glomerulus via electrostatic interactions—and elicit an antibody response. Antibody reactions with cell-surface antigens (eg, GBM) lead to immune deposit formation within the glomeruli, mediator activation, and subsequent injury to glomerular tissue. Volatile hydrocarbons, solvents, and $HgCl_2$ have been implicated in this type of glomerulonephritis. See Bikbov et al. (2010) for more information of glomerular injury.

Proximal Tubular Injury

The proximal tubule is the most common site of toxicant-induced renal injury. The reasons for this relate in part to the selective accumulation of xenobiotics into this segment of the nephron. For example, in contrast to the distal tubule, which is characterized by a relatively tight epithelium with high electrical resistance, the proximal tubule has a leaky epithelium, favoring the flux of compounds into proximal tubular cells. More importantly, tubular transport of organic anions and cations, low-molecular-weight proteins and peptides, GSH conjugates, and heavy metals is localized primarily if not exclusively to the proximal tubule. Thus, transport of these molecules will be greater in the proximal tubule than in other segments, resulting in proximal tubular accumulation and toxicity. Indeed, segmental differences in transport and accumulation appear to play a significant role in the onset and development of proximal tubular toxicity associated with certain drugs such as aminoglycosides, β-lactam antibiotics, and cisplatin; environmental chemicals such as ochratoxin, haloalkene S-conjugates, D-limonene, and 2,4,4-trimethylpentane; and metals such as cadmium and mercury. Although correlations between proximal tubular transport, accumulation, and toxicity suggest that the site of transport is a crucial determinant of the site of toxicity, transport is unlikely to be the sole criterion. For example, the S_2 segment is the primary site of transport and toxicity of cephaloridine, and several lines of evidence suggest a strong correlation between the transport, accumulation, and nephrotoxicity of this antibiotic. However, when a variety of cephalosporins are considered, the rank order of accumulation does not follow the rank order of nephrotoxicity; for example, renal cortical concentrations of the potent nephrotoxicant cephaloglycin are comparable to those of the relatively nontoxic cephalexin. Thus, site-specific transport and accumulation are necessary but not sufficient to cause proximal tubular toxicity of cephalosporins. Once taken up and sequestered by the proximal tubular cell, the nephrotoxic potential of these drugs ultimately may be dependent upon the intrinsic reactivity of the drug with subcellular or molecular targets.

In addition to segmental differences in transport, segmental differences in cytochrome P450 and cysteine conjugate β-lyase activity also are contributing factors to the enhanced susceptibility of the proximal tubule. Both enzyme systems are localized almost exclusively in the proximal tubule, with negligible activity in the glomerulus, distal tubules, or collecting ducts. Thus, nephrotoxicity requiring P450 and β-lyase-mediated bioactivation will most certainly be localized in the proximal tubule. Indeed, the site of proximal tubular bioactivation contributes at least in part to the proximal tubular lesions produced by chloroform (via cytochrome P450) and by haloalkene S-conjugates (via cysteine β-lyase).

Finally, proximal tubular cells appear to be more susceptible to ischemic injury than distal tubular cells. Therefore, the proximal tubule will likely be the primary site of toxicity for chemicals that interfere with RBF, cellular energetics, and/or mitochondrial function.

Loop of Henle/Distal Tubule/ Collecting Duct Injury

Chemically induced injury to the more distal tubular structures, compared to the proximal tubule, is an infrequent occurrence. Functional abnormalities at these sites manifest primarily as impaired concentrating ability and/or acidification defects. Drugs that have been associated with acute injury to the more distal tubular structures include amphotericin B, cisplatin, and methoxyflurane. Each of these drugs induces an ADH-resistant polyuria, suggesting that the concentrating defect occurs at the level of the medullary thick ascending limb and/or the collecting duct. However, the mechanisms mediating these drug-induced concentrating defects appear to be different. Amphotericin B is highly lipophilic and interacts with lipid sterols such as cholesterol, resulting in the formation of transmembrane channels or pores and disrupting membrane permeability (Bernardo and Branch, 1997). Thus, amphotericin effectively transforms the tight distal tubular epithelium into one that is leaky to water and ions and impairs reabsorption at these sites. The mechanisms mediating cisplatin-induced polyuria are not completely understood, but the first phase is responsive to vasopressin and inhibitors of prostaglandin synthesis (Safirstein and Deray, 1998). The second phase is not responsive to vasopressin or prostaglandin synthesis inhibitors but is associated with decreased papillary solute content. Methoxyflurane nephrotoxicity is associated with the inhibitory effects of the metabolite fluoride on solute and water reabsorption (Jarnberg, 1998). Fluoride inhibits sodium chloride reabsorption in the thick ascending limb and inhibits ADH-mediated reabsorption of water, possibly due to disruption in adenylate cyclase.

Papillary Injury

The renal papilla is susceptible to the chronic injurious effects of abusive consumption of analgesics. The initial target is the medullary interstitial cells, followed by degenerative changes in the medullary capillaries, loops of Henle, and collecting ducts (Bach, 1997). Although the exact mechanisms underlying selective damage to the papilla by analgesics are not known, the intrarenal gradient for prostaglandin H synthase activity has been implicated as a contributing factor. This activity is highest in the medulla and least in the cortex, and the prostaglandin hydroperoxidase component metabolizes phenacetin to reactive intermediates capable of covalent binding to cellular macromolecules. Other factors may contribute to this site-selective injury, including high papillary concentrations of potential toxicants and inhibition of vasodilatory prostaglandins, compromising RBF to the renal medulla/papilla and resulting in tissue ischemia. The lack of animal models that mimic the papillary injury observed in humans has limited mechanistic research in this area (Schnellmann, 1998).

ASSESSMENT OF RENAL FUNCTION

Evaluation of the effects of a chemical on the kidney can be accomplished using a variety of both in vivo and in vitro methods. Initially, nephrotoxicity can be assessed by evaluating serum and urine chemistries following treatment with the chemical in question. The standard battery of noninvasive tests includes measurement of urine volume and osmolality, pH, and urinary composition (eg, electrolytes, glucose, and protein). Although specificity is often lacking in such an assessment, urinalysis provides a relatively easy and noninvasive assessment of overall renal functional integrity and can provide some insight into the nature of the nephrotoxic insult. For example, chemically induced increases in urine volume accompanied by decreases in osmolality may suggest an impaired concentrating ability, possibly via a defect in ADH synthesis, release, and/or action. To determine whether the impaired concentrating ability is due to an altered tubular response to ADH, concentrating ability can be determined before and after an exogenous ADH challenge. Glucosuria may reflect chemically induced defects in proximal tubular reabsorption of sugars; however, because glucosuria also may be secondary to hyperglycemia, measurement of serum glucose concentrations also must be evaluated. Urinary excretion of high-molecular-weight proteins, such as albumin, is suggestive of glomerular damage, whereas excretion of low-molecular-weight proteins, such as β_2-microglobulin, suggests proximal tubular

injury. Urinary excretion of enzymes localized in the brush-border (eg, alkaline phosphatase, γ-glutamyl transpeptidase) may reflect brush-border damage, whereas urinary excretion of other enzymes (eg, lactate dehydrogenase) may reflect more generalized cell damage. Enzymuria is often a transient phenomenon, as chemically induced damage may result in an early loss of most of the enzyme available. Thus, the absence of enzymuria does not necessarily reflect an absence of damage. In vivo methodologies used to assess renal function and injury have recently been reviewed (Hart, 2010).

The simultaneous analysis of cellular metabolites in sera and urine using nuclear magnetic analysis (metabonomics) has matured over the past few years and may provide an additional technology to identify and monitor nephrotoxicity (Coen et al., 2008). For example, rats treated with the nephrotoxicant $HgCl_2$ exhibited increased levels of threonine, isobutyric acid, glutamate, and lysine in renal cortical tissue (Wang et al., 2006) and increased levels of isoleucine and lysine and decreased levels of fumarate in the urine. These changes were associated with renal dysfunction (Holmes et al., 2006). However, this technology will require further development and validation using different species and renal insults in the presence and absence of underlying diseases prior to greater use.

GFR can be measured directly by determining creatinine or inulin clearance. Creatinine is an endogenous compound released from skeletal muscle at a constant rate under most circumstances. Further, it is completely filtered with limited secretion. Inulin is an exogenous compound that is completely filtered with no reabsorption or secretion. Following the injection of inulin, inulin serum and urinary concentrations and urine volume are determined over time. If creatinine is being used, then serum and urinary creatinine concentrations and urine volume are determined over time. Creatinine or inulin clearance is determined by the following formula:

Inulin clearance (mL/min) =

$$\frac{\text{inulin concentration in urine (mg/L)} \times \text{urine volume (mL/min)}}{\text{inulin concentration in serum (mg/L)}}$$

Indirect markers of GFR are serial blood urea nitrogen (BUN) and serum creatinine concentrations. However, both serum creatinine and BUN are rather insensitive indices of GFR; a 50% to 70% decrease in GFR must occur before increases in serum creatinine and BUN develop (Fig. 14-9). Chemically induced increases

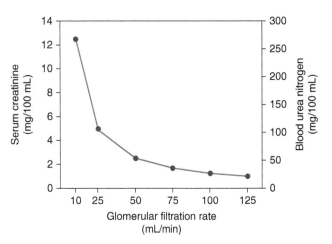

Figure 14-9. *Relationships among GFR, serum creatinine, and BUN concentrations in the determination of renal function.* In general, approximately 50% of renal function must be lost before serum creatinine or BUN increases. (From Tarloff JB, Kinter LB. In vivo methodologies used to assess renal function. In: Sipes IG, McQueen CA, Gandolfi AJ, eds. *Comprehensive Toxicology.* Vol 7. Oxford, UK: Elsevier; 1997:99–120, with permission.)

in BUN and/or serum creatinine may not necessarily reflect renal damage but rather may be secondary to dehydration, hypovolemia, and/or protein catabolism. These extrarenal events should be taken into consideration in evaluating BUN/serum creatinine as potential endpoints of renal toxicity and/or when correlating these endpoints with renal histopathology.

Cystatin C, a 13-kDa endogenous protein that inhibits cysteine proteases, is a viable candidate to replace creatinine in the measurement of GFR (Filler *et al.*, 2005; Stevens and Levey, 2005; Hart and Kinter, 2005). It is produced at a constant rate by all tissues, freely filtered by the glomerulus and catabolized by the tubular epithelial cells; thus, its use is limited to serum levels and not urinary levels. Serum cystatin C levels appear to be independent of height, gender, age, muscle mass, and coexisting diseases, and are more sensitive than creatinine in mildly impaired GFR.

The lack of sensitivity of current biomarkers of renal dysfunction has resulted in extensive searches for better biomarkers of AKI. Better biomarkers would not only advance the timely diagnosis of AKI but would also allow for a better prediction of severity and greatly advance safety assessment during drug development. Vaidya *et al.* (2010) have recently reviewed site-specific biomarkers for common nephrotoxicants and mechanisms of injury (Fig. 14-10). At this time kidney injury molecule-1 (KIM-1), neutrophil gelatinase-associated lipocalin (NGAL), *N*-acetyl-β-glucosaminidase (NAG), fatty acid-binding protein (FABP), hepatocyte growth factor (HGF), and albumin are promising biomarkers of AKI.

Histopathologic evaluation of the kidney following treatment is crucial in identifying the site, nature, and severity of a nephrotoxic lesion. Assessment of chemically induced nephrotoxicity therefore should include urinalysis, serum clinical chemistry, and histopathology to provide a reasonable profile of the functional and

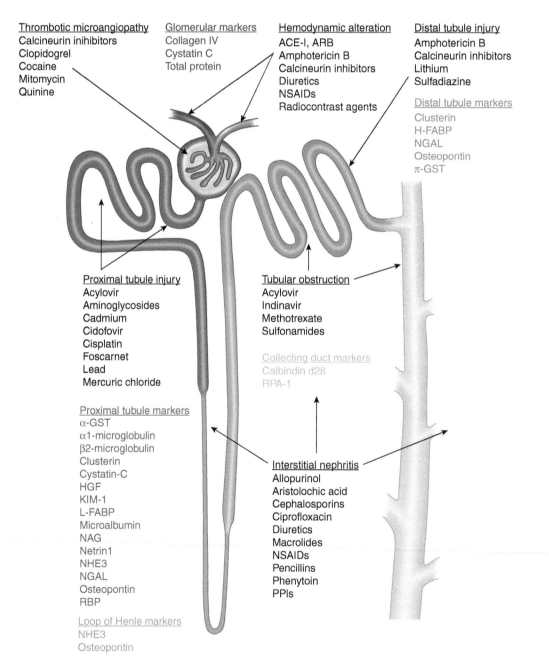

Figure 14-10. *Site-specific biomarkers, common nephrotoxicants, and mechanisms of injury.* (From Vaidya VS, Bonventre JV, Ferguson MA. Biomarkers of acute kidney injury. In: McQueen CA, Schnellmann RG, eds. *Comprehensive Toxicology.* Vol 7. Oxford, UK: Elsevier; 2010:197–211.)

Table 14-3

Models to Study Renal Function

In Vivo
    Continuous microperfusion
    Stopped-flow microperfusion
    Free-flow micropuncture
    Confocal microscopy
Ex Vivo
    Isolated perfused kidney
    Isolated perfused tubules
In Vitro
    Renal slices
    Freshly isolated and purified glomeruli
    Freshly isolated and purified tubular segments
    Freshly isolated and purified proximal tubular
        epithelial cells
    Primary cultures of renal cells
        Tubular epithelial cells
        Glomerular cells
        Fibroblasts
    Immortalized renal epithelial cell lines
        LLC-PK1
        MDCK
        NRK-52E
        OK
        HK-2

morphologic effects of a chemical on the kidney. Further, information on the biotransformation and toxicokinetics of the chemical should be used to direct further in vivo and in vitro studies; in particular, what metabolites are found in the kidney and what are the concentrations of parent compound and metabolites in the kidney over time.

Once a chemical has been identified as a nephrotoxicant in vivo, a variety of in vitro techniques may be used to elucidate underlying mechanisms (Table 14-3). Tissue obtained from naive animals may be used in the preparation of isolated perfused kidneys, kidney slices, isolated suspensions of renal tubules, cells, or subcellular organelles, primary cultures of renal cells, and established renal cell lines. For example, freshly prepared isolated perfused kidneys, kidney slices, and renal tubular suspensions and cells exhibit the greatest degree of differentiated functions and similarity to the in vivo situation. However, these models have limited lifespans of 2 to 24 hours. In contrast, primary cultures of renal cells and established renal cell lines exhibit longer lifespans (>2 weeks), but—by comparison to the in vivo condition—exhibit differentiated functions and similarity to a lesser degree; this is particularly true of immortalized renal cell lines. The reader is referred to several excellent reviews for further details on the utility and limitations of these preparations (Tarloff and Kinter, 1997; Ford, 1997, 2005; Hart and Kinter, 2005; Kirkpatrick and Gandolfi, 2005). Such approaches may be used to distinguish between an effect on the kidney due to a direct chemical insult and one caused by extrarenal effects such as extrarenally generated metabolites, hemodynamic effects, immunologic effects, and so forth. Care must be taken to ensure that the cell type affected in the in vitro model is the same as that affected in vivo. In addition, concentrations of the nephrotoxicant to be used in the in vitro preparations must be comparable to those observed in vivo, as different mechanisms of toxicity may be operative at concentrations that saturate metabolic pathways or overwhelm detoxification mechanisms. Once a

mechanism has been identified in vitro, the postulated mechanism must be tested in vivo. Thus, appropriately designed in vivo and in vitro studies should provide a complete characterization of the biochemical, functional, and morphologic effects of a chemical on the kidney and an understanding of the underlying mechanisms in the target cell population(s).

BIOCHEMICAL MECHANISMS/ MEDIATORS OF RENAL CELL INJURY

Cell Death

In many cases, renal cell injury may culminate in cell death. In general, cell death is thought to occur through either oncosis or apoptosis (Levin *et al.*, 1999). The morphologic and biochemical characteristics of oncosis ("necrotic cell death") and apoptosis are very different. For example, apoptosis is a tightly controlled, organized process that usually affects scattered individual cells. The organelles retain integrity while cell volume decreases. Ultimately, the cell breaks into small fragments that are phagocytosed by adjacent cells or macrophages without producing an inflammatory response. Caspases, a class of cysteine proteases, are primary mediators of apoptosis. In contrast, oncosis often affects many contiguous cells; the organelles swell, cell volume increases, and the cell ruptures with the release of cellular contents, followed by inflammation. The receptor interacting protein (RIP) kinase family has recently been reported to be mediators of oncosis (Declercq *et al.*, 2009). The reader is encouraged to see Chapter 3 for additional details of apoptosis and oncosis. With many toxicants, lower but injurious concentrations produce cell death through apoptosis. As the concentration of the toxicant increases, oncosis plays a predominant role. However, because apoptosis is an ATP-dependent process, for those toxicants that target the mitochondrion, oncosis may be the predominant pathway with only limited apoptosis occurring. In general, nephrotoxicants produce cell death through apoptosis and oncosis, and it is likely that both forms of cell death contribute to AKI.

Mediators of Toxicity

A chemical can initiate cell injury by a variety of mechanisms. In some cases the chemical may initiate toxicity due to its intrinsic reactivity with cellular macromolecules. For example, amphotericin B reacts with plasma membrane sterols, increasing membrane permeability; fumonisin B_1 inhibits sphinganine (sphingosine) N-acyltransferase; and Hg^{2+} binds to sulfhydryl groups on cellular proteins. In contrast, some chemicals are not toxic until they are biotransformed to a reactive intermediate. Biologically reactive intermediates, also known as alkylating agents, are electron-deficient compounds (electrophiles) that bind to cellular nucleophiles (electron-rich compounds) such as proteins and lipids. For example, acetaminophen and chloroform are metabolized in the mouse kidney by cytochrome P450 to the reactive intermediates, N-acetyl-*p*-benzoquinoneimine and phosgene, respectively (see "Chloroform" and "Acetaminophen"). The covalent binding of the reactive intermediate to critical cellular macromolecules is thought to interfere with the normal biological activity of the macromolecule and thereby initiate cellular injury. In other instances, extrarenal biotransformation may be required prior to the delivery of the penultimate nephrotoxic species to the proximal tubule, where it is metabolized further to a reactive intermediate.

Finally, chemicals may initiate injury indirectly by inducing oxidative stress via increased production of ROS, such as superoxide anion, hydrogen peroxide, and hydroxyl radicals. ROS can react with a variety of cellular constituents to induce toxicity. For example, ROS are capable of inducing lipid peroxidation, which may result in altered membrane fluidity, enzyme activity, and membrane permeability and transport characteristics; inactivating cellular enzymes by directly oxidizing critical protein sulfhydryl or amino groups; depolymerizing polysaccharides; and inducing DNA strand breaks and chromosome breakage. Each of these events could lead to cell injury and/or death. Oxidative stress has been proposed to contribute, at least in part, to the nephrotoxicity associated with ischemia/reperfusion injury, gentamicin, cyclosporine, cisplatin, and haloalkene cysteine conjugates.

Although nitric oxide is an important second messenger in a number of physiologic pathways, recent studies suggest that in the presence of oxidative stress, nitric oxide can be converted into reactive nitrogen species that contribute to cellular injury and death. For example, in the presence of superoxide anion, nitric oxide can be transformed into peroxynitrite ($ONOO^-$), a strong oxidant and nitrating species. Proteins, lipids, and DNA are all targets of peroxynitrite. The primary evidence for a role of peroxynitrite in renal ischemia/reperfusion injury is the formation of nitrotyrosine–protein adducts and the attenuation of renal dysfunction through the inhibition of the inducible form of nitric oxide synthase.

Cellular/Subcellular and Molecular Targets

A number of cellular targets have been identified to play a role in cell death. It is generally thought that an intracellular interaction (eg, an alkylating agent or ROS with a macromolecule) initiates a sequence of events that leads to cell death. In the case of oncosis, a "point of no return" is reached in which the cell will die regardless of any intervention. The idea of a single sequence of events is probably simplistic for most toxicants, given the extensive number of targets available for alkylating species and ROS. Rather, multiple pathways, with both distinct and common sequences of events, may lead to cell death. In the following paragraphs examples of molecular targets will be discussed and a more conclusive list can be found in Lash and Cummings (2010).

Many cellular processes depend on mitochondrial ATP and thus become compromised simultaneously with inhibition of respiration. Conversely, mitochondrial dysfunction may be a consequence of some other cellular process altered by the toxicant. Numerous nephrotoxicants cause mitochondrial dysfunction (Schnellmann and Griner, 1994). For example, following an in vivo exposure, $HgCl_2$ altered isolated renal cortical mitochondrial function and mitochondrial morphology prior to the appearance of tubular necrosis (Weinberg et al., 1982a). Furthermore, $HgCl_2$ produced similar changes in various respiratory parameters when added to isolated rat renal cortical mitochondria (Weinberg et al., 1982b). Various toxicants also produce different types of mitochondrial dysfunction. For example, pentachlorobutadienyl-L-cysteine initially uncouples oxidative phosphorylation in renal proximal tubular cells by dissipating the proton gradient, whereas TFEC does not uncouple oxidative phosphorylation but rather inhibits state three respiration by inhibiting sites I and II of the electron transport chain (Schnellmann et al., 1987, 1989; Wallin et al., 1987; Hayden and Stevens, 1990).

Whether toxicants target mitochondria directly or indirectly, it is clear that mitochondria play a critical role in determining whether cells die by apoptosis or oncosis. The mitochondrial permeability transition (MPT) is characterized by the opening of a high-conductance pore that allows solutes of <1500 molecular weight to pass (Lemasters et al., 1999). It is thought that the MPT occurs during cell injury and ultimately progresses to apoptosis if sufficient ATP is available, or oncosis if ATP is depleted. Further, the release of apoptotic proteins, such as apoptosis inducing factor, cytochrome c, Smac/Diablo, Omi and Endonuclease G following MPT play a key role in activating downstream caspases and executing apoptosis.

Ca^{2+} is a second messenger and plays a critical role in a variety of cellular functions. Sustained elevations or abnormally large increases in cytosolic free Ca^{2+} can exert a number of detrimental effects on the cell. For example, an increase in cytosolic free Ca^{2+} can activate a number of degradative Ca^{2+}-dependent enzymes, such as phospholipases and proteinases (eg, calpains), and can produce aberrations in the structure and function of cytoskeletal elements. Release of endoplasmic reticulum (ER) Ca^{2+} stores may be a key step in initiating the injury process and increasing cytosolic free Ca^{2+} concentrations, because prior depletion of ER Ca^{2+} stores protects renal proximal tubules from extracellular Ca^{2+} influx and cell death produced by mitochondrial inhibition and hypoxia (Waters et al., 1997b; Harriman et al., 2002). Further, the release of ER Ca^{2+} activates calpains that leads to further disruption of ion homeostasis, cleavage of cytoskeleton proteins, cell swelling, and, ultimately oncosis (Waters et al., 1997a; Liu and Schnellmann, 2003). Mitochondria are known to accumulate Ca^{2+} in lethally injured cells through a low-affinity, high-capacity Ca^{2+} transport system. Although this system plays a minor role in normal cellular Ca^{2+} regulation, under injurious conditions the uptake of Ca^{2+} may facilitate ROS formation and damage.

Caspases are another class of cysteine proteinases that play a role in the initiation and execution of renal cell apoptosis. A number of caspases have been identified in the rat kidney (eg, caspases 1, 2, 3, 6, 9), and rat kidneys subjected to ischemia/reperfusion injury exhibit differential expression of caspases with marked increases in caspases 1 and 3 (Kaushal et al., 1998, 2004). The administration of a pan-caspase inhibitor blocked the increase in caspase activities and renal injury following ischemia/reperfusion injury (Daemen et al., 1999).

Signaling kinases such as protein kinase C, mitogen-activated protein kinases (eg, ERK1/2, p38, JNK/SAPK), protein kinase B (Akt), src, and phosphoinositide-3-kinase phoshorylate other proteins and, thereby, alter their activity, expression, or localization. Numerous recent studies reveal critical roles for signaling kinases in renal cell death and in the recovery of renal cells after toxicant injury (Table 14-4). For example, PKC mediates fumonision-B1- and TNF-induced toxicity in human renal cells and in LLC-PK1 cells (Nowak, 2002; Gopee et al., 2003; Woo et al., 1996). However, the exact role of PKC in renal cell death depends on the toxicant and the specific isoform(s) involved (Nowak, 2002, 2003; Nowak et al., 2004, 2011). Activation of PKCα contributes to mitochondrial dysfunction and cell death in rabbit RPTC exposed to cisplatin whereas PKCε mediates mitochondrial dysfunction and cell death after exposure. Interestingly, cisplatin- and oxidant-induced PKC activation was followed by ERK1/2 activation, which decreased mitochondrial membrane potential and caused caspase 3 activation and apoptosis. Using LLC-PK1 cells exposed to 2,3,5-tris-(glutathion-S-yl)hydroquinone (TGHQ) and in vivo studies in mice exposed to cisplatin support a role for ERK in renal cell death (Ramachandiran et al., 2002; Arany et al., 2004; Dong et al., 2004; Sheikh-Hamad et al., 2004; van de Water et al., 2006). Other examples of signaling kinases that play a role in nephrotoxicant injury are found in Table 14-4.

Cell volume and ion homeostasis are tightly regulated and are critical for the reabsorptive properties of the tubular epithelial cells. Toxicants can disrupt cell volume and ion homeostasis by interacting directly with the plasma membrane and increasing ion permeability or by inhibiting energy production. The loss of ATP during oncosis, for example, results in the inhibition of

Table 14-4

Selected Signaling Kinases Involved in Renal Cell Injury, Survival, or Repair*

KINASE	LOCATION	NEPHROTOXICANT	REFERENCES
Protein kinase C (PKC)			
Conventional PKC			
PKCα	Proximal tubules	Cisplatin, DCVC[†]	Nowak (2002), Liu *et al.* (2004)
Novel PKC			
PKCε	Proximal tubules	TBHP[‡]	Nowak *et al.* (2004, 2011)
Mitogen-activated protein kinase (MAPK)			
ERK1/2	Proximal tubules	Cisplatin, H_2O_2, TBHP, TGHQ[§]	Nowak (2002), Arany *et al.* (2004), Ramachandiran *et al.* (2002), Dong *et al.* (2004), Zhuang *et al.* (2004), Nowak *et al.* (2006), Zhuang *et al.* (2007, 2008)
JNK/SAPK[†]	Proximal tubules	Cisplatin	Arany *et al.* (2004)
P38	Proximal tubules	Cisplatin, H_2O_2, TGHQ[§]	Arany *et al.* (2004), Ramachandiran *et al.* (2002), Dong *et al.* (2004), Zhuang *et al.* (2005)
Other kinases			
Protein kinase B	LLC-PK1, Proximal tubules	Cisplatin, mechanical injury, H_2O_2, DCVC	Zhuang *et al.* (2004), Shaik *et al.* (2007, 2008)

Data from Schnellmann and Cummings (2006).
[†] *S-(1,2)-Dichlorovinyl-L-cysteine.*
[‡] *t-Butylhyroperoxide*
[§] *2,3,5-tris-(Glutathion-S-yl)hydroquinone.*
Protein kinase B is also known as AKT.

membrane transporters that maintain the internal ion balance and drive transmembrane ion movement. Following ATP depletion, Na⁺, K^+-ATPase activity decreases, resulting in K^+ efflux, Na⁺ and Cl⁻ influx, cell swelling, and ultimately cell membrane rupture (Miller and Schnellmann 1993, 1995). In contrast, the cell shrinkage that occurs during apoptosis is mediated by K^+ and Cl⁻ efflux through respective channels and inhibition of these channels is cytoprotective (Okada *et al.*, 2004).

SPECIFIC NEPHROTOXICANTS

Heavy Metals

Many metals, including cadmium, chromium, lead, mercury, platinum, and uranium, are nephrotoxic (Fowler, 2010; Zalups, 2010). It is important to recognize that the nature and severity of metal nephrotoxicity varies with respect to its form. For example, salts of inorganic mercury produce a greater degree of renal injury and a lesser degree of neurotoxicity than do organic mercury compounds; the neurotoxicity is associated with the higher lipophilicity of organic mercury compounds (Conner and Fowler, 1993; Zalups and Lash, 1994). In addition, different metals have different primary targets within the kidney. For example, potassium dichromate and cadmium primarily affect the S_1 and S_2 segments of the proximal tubule, whereas mercuric chloride affects the S_2 and S_3 segments (Zalups and Lash, 1994; Zalups and Diamond, 2005).

Metals may cause toxicity through their ability to bind to sulfhydryl groups. For example, the affinity of mercury for sulfhydryl groups is very high and is about 10 orders of magnitude higher than the affinity of mercury for carbonyl or amino groups (Ballatori, 1991). Thus, metals may cause renal cellular injury through their ability to bind to sulfhydryl groups of critical proteins within the cells and thereby inhibit their normal function.

Mercury Humans and animals are exposed to elemental mercury vapor, inorganic mercurous and mercuric salts, and organic mercuric compounds through the environment. Administered elemental mercury is rapidly oxidized in erythrocytes or tissues to inorganic mercury, and thus the tissue distribution of elemental and inorganic mercury is similar. Due to its high affinity for sulfhydryl groups, virtually all of the Hg^{2+} found in blood is bound to cells—albumin, other sulfhydryl-containing proteins, glutathione, and cysteine.

The kidneys are the primary target organs for accumulation of Hg^{2+}, and the S_3 segment of the proximal tubule is the initial site of toxicity. As the dose or duration of treatment increases, the S_1 and S_2 segments may be affected. Renal uptake of Hg^{2+} is very rapid with as much as 50% of a nontoxic dose of Hg^{2+} found in the kidneys within a few hours of exposure. Considering the fact that virtually all of the Hg^{2+} found in blood is bound to an endogenous ligand, it is likely that the luminal and/or basolateral transport of Hg^{2+} into the proximal tubular epithelial cell is through cotransport of Hg^{2+} with an endogenous ligand such as glutathione, cysteine, or albumin, or through some plasma membrane Hg^{2+}-ligand complex (Zalups and Diamond, 2005). Current evidence indicates that at least two mechanisms are involved in the proximal tubular uptake of Hg^{2+} (Fig. 14-11) (Zalups and Diamond, 2005). One mechanism appears to involve the apical activity of γ-glutamyl transpeptidase, cysteinylglycinase, and the transport of Cys–S–Hg–S–Cys through one of more amino acid transporters. Basolateral membrane transport is likely to be mediated by the organic anion transport system.

The acute nephrotoxicity induced by $HgCl_2$ is characterized by proximal tubular necrosis and AKI within 24 to 48 hours after

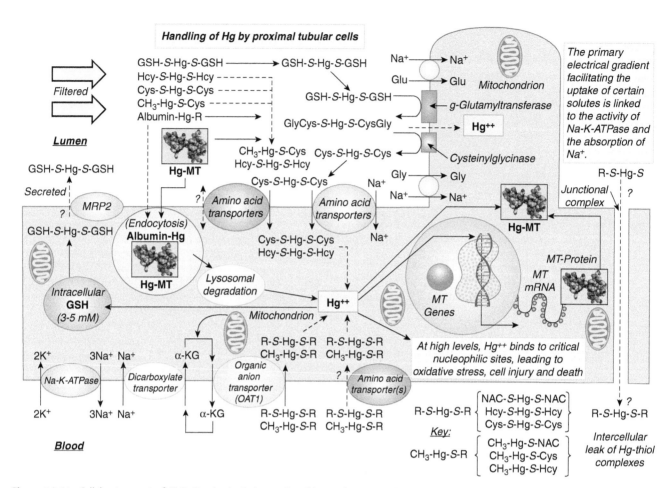

Figure 14-11. *Cellular transport of Hg²⁺.* Proximal tubular uptake of inorganic mercury is thought to be the result of the transport of Hg²⁺ conjugates (eg, diglutathione-Hg²⁺ conjugate [GSHHg-GSH], dicysteine-Hg²⁺ conjugate [CYS-HG-CYS]). At the luminal membrane, GSH-Hg-GSH is metabolized by γ-GT and a dipeptidase to form CYS-HG-CYS. CYS-HG-CYS may be taken up by amino acid transporters. It is not clear whether albumin-Hg-R conjugates are transported across the liminal membrane in vivo. At the basolateral membrane, Hg²⁺-conjugates appear to be transported by organic anion transporters OAT1 and OAT3. (Courtesy of Dr R. K. Zalups.) (From Zalups RK, Diamond GL. Nephrotoxicology of metals. In: Tarloff JB, Lash LH, eds. *Toxicology of the Kidney.* 3rd ed. Boca Raton: CRC Press; 2005:954, with permission.)

administration (Zalups, 1997). Early markers of HgCl₂-induced renal dysfunction include an increase in the urinary excretion of brush-border enzymes such as alkaline phosphatase and γ-GT, suggesting that the brush border may be an initial target of HgCl₂. As injury progresses, tubular reabsorption of solutes and water decreases and there is an increase in the urinary excretion of glucose, amino acids, albumin, and other proteins. Associated with the increase in injured proximal tubules is a decrease and progressive decline in the GFR. For example, GFR was reduced 35% in rats within six hours of HgCl₂ administration and continued to decline to 32% and 16% of controls at 12 and 24 hours, respectively (Eknoyan *et al.*, 1982). The reduction in GFR results from the glomerular injury, tubular injury, and/or vasoconstriction. Interestingly, there is an early decrease in RBF secondary to the vasoconstriction. RBF may return to normal within 24 to 48 hours, whereas GFR continues to decline. If the decline in renal function is not too severe, the remaining proximal tubular cells undergo a proliferative response and renal function returns over time. Chelation therapy with 2,3-dimercaptopropane-1-sulfonate or 2,3-mesodimercaptosuccinic acid is used for the treatment for mercury-induced nephrotoxicity (Zalups and Diamond, 2005).

As stated above, inorganic mercury has a very high affinity for protein sulfhydryl groups, and this interaction is thought to play an important role in the toxicity of mercury at the cellular level. Changes in mitochondrial morphology and function are

very early events following HgCl₂ administration, supporting the hypothesis that mitochondrial dysfunction is an early and important contributor to inorganic mercury-induced cell death along the proximal tubule. Other studies have suggested that oxidative stress and disregulation of Ca²⁺ homeostasis plays an important role in HgCl₂-induced renal injury (Fukino *et al.*, 1984; Smith *et al.*, 1987; Lund *et al.*, 1993).

Several animal studies have shown that chronic exposure to inorganic mercury results in an immunologically mediated membranous glomerular nephritis secondary to the production of antibodies against the GBM and the deposition of immune complexes (Zalups and Diamond, 2005). See Zalups (2010) for additional information.

Cadmium Chronic exposure of nonsmoking humans and animals to cadmium is primarily through food and results in nephrotoxicity (Kido and Nordberg, 1998; Zalups and Diamond, 2005). In the workplace, inhalation of cadmium-containing dust and fumes is the major route of exposure. Cadmium has a half-life of greater than 10 years in humans and thus accumulates in the body over time. Approximately 50% of the body burden of cadmium can be found in the kidney and nephrotoxicity can be observed when Cd concentrations exceed 50 μg/g kidney wet weight (Zalups and Diamond, 2005). Lauwerys and coworkers (1994) suggested that tubular dysfunction is associated with urinary cadmium concentrations greater than 5 and 2 nmol/mmol creatinine in adult male workers and in the general population, respectively, are associated with tubular dysfunction. Cadmium produces proximal tubule dysfunction (S_1 and S_2 segments) and injury characterized by increases in urinary excretion of glucose, amino acids, calcium, and cellular enzymes. This injury may progress to a chronic interstitial nephritis.

A very interesting aspect of cadmium nephrotoxicity is the role of metallothioneins (Klaassen *et al.*, 1999). Metallothioneins are a family of low-molecular-weight, cysteine-rich metal-binding proteins that have a high affinity for cadmium and other heavy metals. In general, the mechanism by which metallothionein is thought to play a role in cadmium and heavy metal toxicity is through its ability to bind to a heavy metal and thereby render it biologically inactive. This assumes that the unbound or "free" concentration of the metal is the toxic species. Metallothionein production can be induced by low, nontoxic concentrations of metals. Subsequently, animals challenged with a higher dose of the metal will not exhibit toxicity compared to naive animals.

Following an oral exposure to $CdCl_2$, Cd^{2+} is thought to reach the kidneys both as Cd^{2+} and as a Cd^{2+}-metallothionein complex formed and released either from intestinal cells or hepatocytes. The Cd^{2+}-metallothionein complex is freely filtered by the glomerulus and reabsorption by the proximal tubule is probably by endocytosis and is limited (Zalups and Diamond, 2005). Inside the tubular cells, it is thought that lysosomal degradation of the Cd^{2+}-metallothionein results in the release of "free" Cd^{2+}, which, in turn, induces renal metallothionein production. Once the renal metallothionein pool is saturated, "free" Cd^{2+} initiates injury. It is also likely that Cd is reabsorbed luminally and basolaterally as a cysteine conjugate (Zalups and Diamond, 2005). The mechanism by which Cd^{2+} produces injury at the cellular level is not clear; however, low concentrations of Cd^{2+} have been shown to interfere with the normal function of several cellular signal transduction pathways.

Chemically Induced α2u-Globulin Nephropathy

A diverse group of chemicals, including unleaded gasoline, jet fuels, D-limonene, 1,4-dichlorobenzene, tetrachloroethylene, decalin, and lindane, cause α_{2u}-globulin nephropathy or hyaline droplet nephropathy (Lehman-McKeeman, 2010). This nephropathy occurring in male rats is characterized by the accumulation of protein droplets in the S_2 segment of the proximal tubule, and results in single-cell necrosis, the formation of granular casts at the junction of the proximal tubule and the thin loop of Henle, and cellular regeneration. Chronic exposure to these compounds results in progression of these lesions and ultimately in chronic nephropathy. With compounds such as unleaded gasoline, chronic exposure results in an increased incidence of renal adenomas/carcinomas by nongenotoxic mechanisms.

As the name implies, the expression of this nephropathy requires the presence of the α_{2u}-globulin protein. α_{2u}-Globulin is synthesized in the liver of male rats and is under androgen control. Due to its low molecular weight (18.7 kDa), α_{2u}-globulin is freely filtered by the glomerulus with approximately half being re-absorbed via endocytosis in the S_2 segment of the proximal tubule. Many of the compounds that cause α_{2u}-globulin nephropathy bind to α_{2u}-globulin in a reversible manner and decrease the ability of lysosomal proteases in the proximal tubule to breakdown α_{2u}-globulin. This results in the accumulation of α_{2u}-globulin in the proximal tubule with an increase in the size and number of lysosomes and the characteristic protein-droplet morphology. A proposed mechanism of α_{2u}-globulin nephropathy is that cellular necrosis secondary to lysosomal overload leads to a sustained increase in cell proliferation, which, in turn, results in the promotion of spontaneously or chemically initiated cells to form preneoplastic and neoplastic foci (Lehman-McKeeman, 2010; Melnick, 1992).

α_{2u}-Globulin nephropathy appears to be sex- and species-specific. That is, it occurs in male rats but not female rats and in male or female mice, rabbits, or guinea pigs because they do not produce α_{2u}-globulin (Lehman-McKeeman, 2010). Furthermore, it does not occur in male Black Reiter rats that lack α_{2u}-globulin. Considering the diversity of compounds that cause α_{2u}-globulin nephropathy and renal tumors and the fact that humans are exposed to these compounds regularly, the question arises whether humans are at risk for α_{2u}-globulin nephropathy and renal tumors when exposed to these compounds. Current data suggest that humans are not at risk because (1) humans do not synthesize α_{2u}-globulin, (2) humans secrete less proteins in general and in particular less low-molecular-weight proteins in urine than the rat, (3) the low-molecular-weight proteins in human urine are either not related structurally to α_{2u}-globulin, do not bind to compounds that bind to α_{2u}-globulin, or are similar to proteins in female rats, male Black Reiter rats, rabbits, or guinea pigs that do not exhibit α_{2u}-globulin nephropathy, and (4) mice excrete a low-molecular-weight urinary protein that is 90% homologous to α_{2u}-globulin, but they do not exhibit α_{2u}-globulin-nephropathy and renal tumors following exposure to α_{2u}-globulin-nephropathy-inducing agents.

Halogenated Hydrocarbons

Halogenated hydrocarbons are a diverse class of compounds and are used extensively as chemical intermediates, solvents, and pesticides. Consequently, humans are exposed to these compounds not only in the workplace but also through the environment. Numerous toxic effects have been associated with acute and chronic exposure to halogenated hydrocarbons, including nephrotoxicity (Mehendale, 2011). The two examples provided below illustrate the importance of biotransformation in the nephrotoxicity of halogenated hydrocarbons (Dekant, 2005; Rankin and Valentovic, 2005).

Chloroform Chloroform produces nephrotoxicity in a variety of species, with some species being more sensitive than others. The primary cellular target is the proximal tubule, with no primary damage to the glomerulus or the distal tubule. Proteinuria, glucosuria, and increased BUN levels are all characteristic of chloroform-induced nephrotoxicity. The nephrotoxicity produced by chloroform is linked to its metabolism by renal cytochrome P450 and the formation of a reactive intermediate that binds covalently to nucleophilic groups on cellular macromolecules. Cytochrome P450 biotransforms chloroform to trichloromethanol, which is unstable and releases HCl to form phosgene. Phosgene can react with (1) water to produce $2HCl + CO_2$, (2) two molecules of glutathione to produce diglutathionyl dithiocarbonate, (3) cysteine to produce 2-oxothizolidine-4-carboxylic acid, or (4) cellular macromolecules to initiate toxicity. The sex differences observed in chloroform nephrotoxicity appear to be related to differences in renal cytochrome P450 isozyme contents. For example, castration of male mice decreased renal cytochrome P450 and chloroform-induced nephrotoxicity (Smith *et al.*, 1984). Likewise, testosterone pretreatment of female mice increased cytochrome P450 content and rendered female mice susceptible to the nephrotoxic effects of chloroform. Cytochrome P450 isozyme 2E1 is present in male mice and expressed in female mice treated with testosterone (Lock

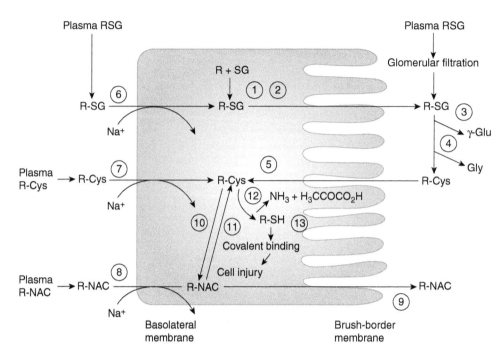

Figure 14-12. *Renal tubular uptake and metabolism of GSH conjugates.* (1) Intracellular formation of GSH conjugates (R-SG) catalyzed by renal GSH S-transferase(s); (2) Secretion of the R-SG into the lumen; (3) γ-GT-mediated catabolism of R-SG and formation of the corresponding cysteinylglycine conjugate; (4) formation of the corresponding cysteine conjugate (R-Cys); (5) Na$^+$-coupled transport of R-Cys into the renal proximal tubular cell; (6) Na$^+$-coupled transport of RSG across the basolateral membrane; (7) Na$^+$-coupled transport of R-Cys across the basolateral membrane; (8) Na$^+$-coupled and probenecid-sensitive transport of the mercapturate (RNAC) across the basolateral membrane; (9) secretion of R-NAC into the lumen; (10) deacetylation of R-NAC to R-Cys and (11) acetylation of RCys to R-NAC; (12) reactive thiol formation via β-lyase; (13) binding of the reactive thiol to cellular macromolecules and initiation of cell injury. (From TJ Monks, SS Lau. Renal transport processes and glutathione conjugate-mediated nephrotoxicity. *Drug Metab Dispos.* 1987;15:437–441, with permission.)

and Reed, 1997). Thus, these isozymes may play a role in chloroform-induced nephrotoxicity.

Tetrafluoroethylene Tetrafluoroethylene is metabolized in the liver by GSH-S-transferases to S-(1,1,2,2-tetrafluoroethyl)-glutathione. The GSH conjugate is secreted into the bile and small intestine where it is degraded to the cysteine S-conjugate (TFEC), reabsorbed, and transported to the kidney. The mercapturic acid may also be formed in the small intestine and reabsorbed. Alternatively, the glutathione conjugate can be transported to the kidney and biotransformed to the cysteine conjugate by γ-GT and a dipeptidase located on the brush border (Fig. 14-12). The mercapturic acid is transported into the proximal tubule cell by the organic anion transporter, whereas cysteine conjugates are transported by the organic anion transporter and the sodium-independent L and T transport systems. The cysteine S-conjugate of these compounds is thought to be the penultimate nephrotoxic species. Following transport into the proximal tubule, which is the primary cellular target for haloalkenes and haloalkanes, the cysteine S-conjugate is a substrate for the cytosolic and mitochondrial forms of the enzyme cysteine conjugate β-lyase. In the case of the N-acetyl-cysteine S-conjugate, the N-acetyl group must be removed by a deacetylase for it to be a substrate for cysteine conjugate β-lyase. The products of the reaction are ammonia, pyruvate, and a reactive thiol that is capable of binding covalently to cellular macromolecules. There is a correlation between the covalent binding of the reactive thiol of the cysteine conjugate with renal protein and nephrotoxicity. Hayden and colleagues (1991) and Bruschi and coworkers (1993) have shown that biotransformation of TFEC results in difluorothioamidyl-L-lysine-protein adducts in mitochondria and that two of the targeted proteins may belong to the heat shock family of proteins. Hayden and colleagues (1992) have also shown that halogenated thioamide

adducts of phosphatidylethanolamine are formed in mitochondria following cysteine conjugate β-lyase biotransformation of TFEC.

The nephrotoxicity produced by haloalkenes is characterized morphologically by proximal tubular necrosis, primarily affecting the S$_3$ segment, and functionally by increases in urinary glucose, protein, cellular enzymes, and BUN. Following in vivo and in vitro exposures to TFEC, the mitochondrion appears to be a primary target. In rabbit renal proximal tubules and isolated mitochondria, there is a marked decrease in state three respiration (respiration associated with maximal ATP formation) following TFEC exposure (Groves *et al.*, 1993). Furthermore, the decrease in mitochondrial function occurs prior to the onset of cell death. Oxidative stress may also play a contributing role in TFEC-induced cell death because lipid peroxidation products were formed prior to the onset of cell death, and antioxidants and iron chelators decreased cytotoxicity (Chen *et al.*, 1990; Groves *et al.*, 1991).

Aristolochic Acid and Fungal Toxins

Mycotoxins are products of molds and fungi and a number of mycotoxins produce nephrotoxicity such as aflatoxin B$_1$, citrinin, ochratoxins, fumonisins, and patulin (Dickman and Grollman, 2010). Three examples of nephrotoxic mycotoxins will be discussed. Citrinin nephrotoxicity is characterized by decreased urine osmolality, GFR and RBF, glycosuria, and increased urinary enzyme excretion. Interestingly, the location of citrinin-induced tubular vacuolization and necrosis (proximal, distal) varies among species. Whereas the mechanism of citrinin toxicity to the tubules remains unresolved, citrinin enters the cells through the organic anion transporter and causes mitochondrial dysfunction.

Fumonisins B$_1$ and B$_2$ are commonly found on corn and corn products, and produce nephrotoxicity in numerous species, some species are very sensitive (eg, rabbits) whereas others are more resistant (eg, mice) (Bucci *et al.*, 1998). Histologic examination of the kidney revealed disruption of the basolateral membrane, mitochondrial swelling, increased numbers of clear and electron-dense vacuoles, and apoptosis in proximal tubular cells at the junction of the cortex and medulla. Changes in renal function included increased urine volume, decreased osmolality, and increased excretion of low- and high-molecular-weight proteins. The fumonisins are structurally similar to sphingoid bases and are thought to produce their toxicity through the inhibition of sphinganine (sphingosine) *N*-acyltransferase. Inhibition of this enzyme results in an increase in the ratio of free sphinganine to free sphingosine and a decrease in complex sphingolipids. The toxicity of fumonisins may be through increased sphinganine, reactive oxygen species, and apoptosis.

Aristolochic acids (AAs) and aristolactams are natural products found in the *Aristolochia* and *Asarum* genera (Dickman and Grollman, 2010). Despite the extensive use of *Aristolochia* as a herbal remedy for thousands of years, its human renal toxicity was not reported until 1993 (Vanherweghem *et al.*, 1993). Since then AAs have been shown to play a role in Balkan endemic nephropathy and Chinese herb nephropathy, now known as AA nephropathy. In both cases the renal dysfunction is characterized by tubular dysfunction, proteinuria, and interstitial fibrosis.

AAs are a mixture of compounds that form covalent DNA adducts, and are genotoxic and carcinogenic. Renal uptake of penultimate toxicant, AA-I, is through mOat-mediated transport, and is bioactivated through nitroreduction to produce DNA and protein adducts (Fig. 14-13). The nephrotoxicity of AA has been studied in rabbits, rats, and mice, and in cell culture. Shibutani *et al.* (2007) reported that AA-I produced renal proximal tubule necrosis and interstitial fibrosis whereas AA-II did not. Interestingly, both AA-I and AA-II produced similar levels of DNA adducts. Thus, the nephrotoxicity of AA-I may not be due to DNA adducts and damage.

Therapeutic Agents

Acetaminophen Large doses of the antipyretic and analgesic acetaminophen (APAP) are commonly associated with hepatoxicity (Tarloff, 2010). However, large doses of APAP can also cause nephrotoxicity in humans and animals. APAP nephrotoxicity is characterized by proximal tubular necrosis with increases in BUN and plasma creatinine; decreases in GFR and clearance of *para*-aminohippurate; increases in the fractional excretion of water, sodium, and potassium; and increases in urinary glucose, protein, and brush-border enzymes. There appears to be a marked species difference in the nature and mechanism of APAP nephrotoxicity (Emeigh Hart *et al.*, 1994; Tarloff, 1997). Morphologically, the primary targets in the mouse kidney are the S_1 and S_2 segments of the proximal tubule, whereas in the rat kidney the S_3 segment is the target. In the mouse, renal cytochrome P450 2E1 has been associated with APAP biotransformation to a reactive intermediate, *N*-acetyl-*p*-amino-benzoquinoneimine, that arylates proteins in the proximal tubule and initiates cell death. Two of the proteins that are targets of *N*-acetyl-*p*-amino-benzoquinoneimine are a selenium-binding protein and a glutamine synthetase (Emeigh Hart *et al.*, 1994; Tarloff, 1997). However, the mechanism by which protein adducts initiate proximal tubular cell death and ultimately nephrotoxicity remains to be determined. Although renal cytochrome P450 plays a role in APAP activation and nephrotoxicity, glutathione conjugates of APAP may also contribute to APAP nephrotoxicity. Evidence for this pathway was provided by experiments in which γ-GT or

organic anion transport was inhibited and APAP-induced nephrotoxicity decreased (Emeigh Hart *et al.*, 1990). In contrast to its effects in the mouse, a critical and early step in APAP nephrotoxicity in the rat is the conversion of APAP to *para*-aminophenol (PAP) (Tarloff, 1997). The steps following PAP formation and the expression of nephrotoxicity are less clear.

Nonsteroidal Anti-Inflammatory Drugs NSAIDs such as aspirin, ibuprofen, naproxen, indomethacin, and cyclooxygenase-2 inhibitors (eg, celecoxib) are extensively used as analgesics and anti-inflammatory drugs and produce their therapeutic effects through the inhibition of prostaglandin synthesis. At least three different types of nephrotoxicity have been associated with NSAID administration (Tarloff, 2010). AKI may occur within hours of a large dose of a NSAID, is usually reversible upon withdrawal of the drug, and is characterized by decreased RBF and GFR and by oliguria. When the normal production of vasodilatory prostaglandins (eg, PGE_2, PGI_2) is inhibited by NSAIDs, vasoconstriction induced by circulating catecholamines and angiotensin II is unopposed, resulting in decreased RBF and ischemia. A number of risk factors (eg, renal insufficiency, congestive heart failure, hepatic cirrhosis, hemorrhage, hypertension, sepsis, diabetes) are known to facilitate the development of AKI following NSAIDs consumption.

In contrast, chronic consumption of combinations of NSAIDs and/or APAP (>3 years) results in an often irreversible form of nephrotoxicity known as analgesic nephropathy (Palmer and Heinrich, 2004; Tarloff, 2010; De Broe, 2005). The incidence of analgesic nephropathy varies widely in the western world, ranging from less than 2% to 5% of all end-stage renal disease patients in countries where analgesic consumption is low (eg, USA, Canada), and up to 20% of all end-stage renal disease patients in countries with the highest analgesic consumption (eg, Australia, Sweden). Impaired urinary concentration and acidification are the earliest clinical manifestations. The primary lesion in this nephropathy is papillary necrosis with chronic interstitial nephritis. Initial changes are to the medullary interstitial cells and are followed by degenerative changes to the medullary loops of Henle and medullary capillaries. Well-defined clinical signs have been associated with analgesic nephropathy and are helpful in the diagnosis thereof. De Broe (2005) and colleagues have developed an effective computed tomography (CT) protocol that does not use contrast media to diagnose analgesic nephropathy. Although analgesic nephropathy is associated with a number of well-defined effects, the mechanism by which NSAIDs produce analgesic nephropathy is not known, but may result from chronic medullary/papillary ischemia secondary to renal vasoconstriction. Other studies have suggested that a reactive intermediate is formed in the cells that, in turn, initiates an oxidative stress, or binds covalently to critical cellular macromolecules.

The third, even though rare, type of nephrotoxicity associated with NSAIDs is an interstitial nephritis with a mean time of NSAID exposure to development of approximately five months (Tarloff, 2010). This nephrotoxicity is characterized by a diffuse interstitial edema with mild-to-moderate infiltration of inflammatory cells. Patients normally present with elevated serum creatinine, proteinuria, and nephritic syndrome. If NSAIDs are discontinued, renal function improves in one to three months.

Aminoglycosides The aminoglycoside antibiotics are so named because they consist of two or more amino sugars joined in a glycosidic linkage to a central hexose nucleus. Although they are drugs of choice for many gram-negative infections, their use is primarily limited by their nephrotoxicity. The incidence of renal dysfunction following aminoglycoside administration ranges from 0% to 50%,

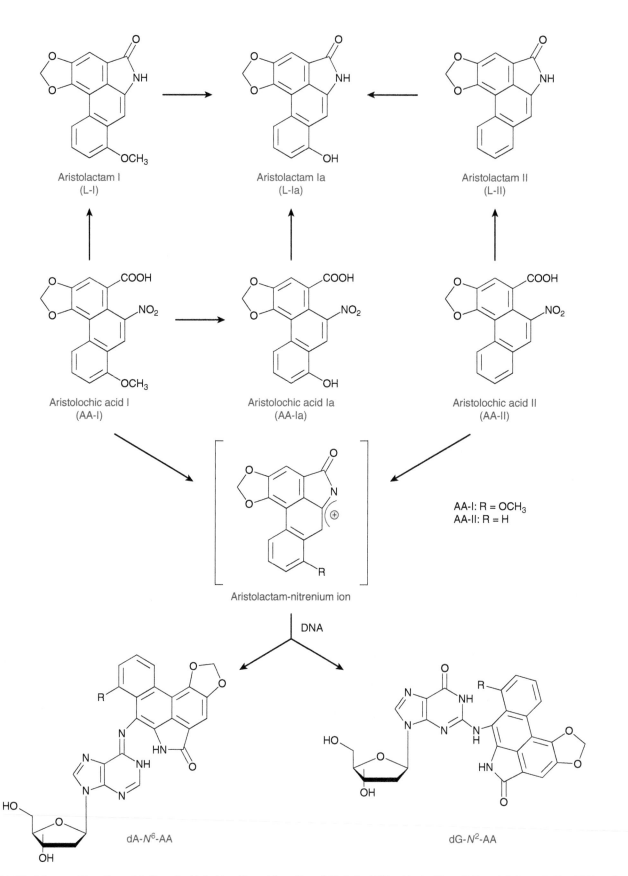

Figure 14-13. *Scheme outlines the metabolism of aristolochic acids and formation of AA-derived DNA adducts.* (From Shibutani S, Dong H, Suzuki N, et al. Selective toxicity of aristolochic acids I and II. Drug Metab Dispos, 2007;35(7):1217–1222.)

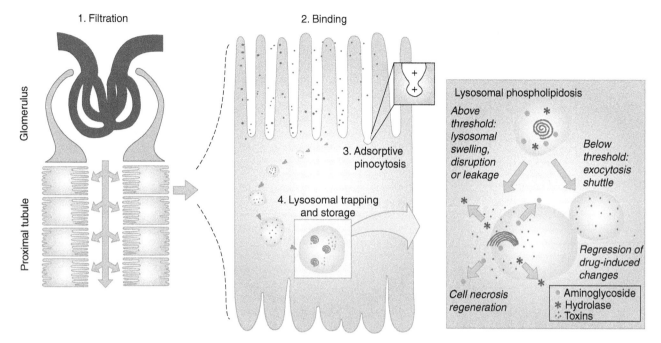

1. Filtration

2. Binding

Glomerulus

Proximal tubule

3. Adsorptive pinocytosis

4. Lysosomal trapping and storage

Lysosomal phospholipidosis

Above threshold: lysosomal swelling, disruption or leakage

Below threshold: exocytosis shuttle

Regression of drug-induced changes

Cell necrosis regeneration

• Aminoglycoside
∗ Hydrolase
∴ Toxins

Figure 14-14. *Renal handling of aminoglycosides: (1) glomerular filtration, (2) binding to the brush-border membranes of the proximal tubule, (3) pinocytosis, and (4) storage in the lysosomes.* (From De Broe ME. Renal injury due to environmental toxins, drugs, and contrast agents. In: Berl T, Bonventre JV, eds. Atlas of Diseases of the Kidney. Philadelphia: Current Medicine; 1999:11.4, with permission.)

but seldom leads to a fatal outcome (Servais *et al.*, 2005; Palmer and Heinrich, 2004; Decker and Molitoris, 2010).

Renal dysfunction by aminoglycosides is characterized by a nonoliguric renal failure with reduced GFR and an increase in serum creatinine and BUN. Polyuria is an early event following aminoglycoside administration and may be due to inhibition of chloride transport in the thick ascending limb (Kidwell *et al.*, 1994). Within 24 hours, increases in urinary brush-border enzymes, glucosuria, aminoaciduria, and proteinuria are observed. Histologically, lysosomal alterations are noted initially, followed by damage to the brush border, ER, mitochondria, and cytoplasm, ultimately leading to tubular cell necrosis. Interestingly, proliferation of renal proximal tubule cells can be observed early after the onset of nephrotoxicity.

Aminoglycosides are highly polar cations; they are almost exclusively filtered by the glomerulus and excreted unchanged. Filtered aminoglycosides undergo proximal tubular reabsorption by binding to anionic phospholipids in the brush border, followed by endocytosis and sequestration in lysosomes of the S_1 and S_2 segments of proximal tubules (Fig. 14-14). Basolateral membrane binding and uptake also may occur, but this is a minor contribution to the total proximal tubular uptake of aminoglycosides. The earliest lesion observed following clinically relevant doses of aminoglycosides is an increase in the size and number of lysosomes. These lysosomes contain *myeloid bodies*, which are electron-dense lamellar structures containing undergraded phospholipids. The renal phospholipidosis produced by the aminoglycosides is thought to occur through their inhibition of lysosomal hydrolases, such as sphingomyelinase and phospholipases. Although phospholipidosis plays an important role in aminoglycoside nephrotoxicity, the steps between the phospholipid accumulation in the lysosomes and tubular cell death are less clear. One hypothesis suggests that the lysosomes become progressively distended until they rupture, releasing lysosomal enzymes and high concentrations of aminoglycosides into the cytoplasm (Fig. 14-14). The released lysosomal contents can interact with various membranes and organelles and trigger

cell death. Another mechanism of aminoglycoside nephrotoxicity includes a decrease in K_f and GFR (see above).

Amphotericin B Amphotericin B is a very effective antifungal agent whose clinical utility is limited by its nephrotoxicity (Bernardo and Branch, 1997; Palmer and Heinrich, 2004; Ulozas, 2010). Renal dysfunction associated with amphotericin B treatment is dependent on cumulative dose and is due to both hemodynamic and tubular effects. With respect to hemodynamics, Amphotericin B administration is associated with decreases in RBF and GFR secondary to renal arteriolar vasoconstriction or activation of TGF. Amphotericin B nephrotoxicity is characterized by ADH-resistant polyuria, renal tubular acidosis, hypokalemia, and either acute or chronic renal failure. Amphotericin B nephrotoxicity is unusual in that it impairs the functional integrity of the glomerulus and of the proximal and distal portions of the nephron.

Some of the renal tubular cell effects of amphotericin B are due to the ability of this polyene to bind to cholesterol in the plasma membrane and form aqueous pores. In the presence of amphotericin B, cells of the turtle and rat distal tubule do not produce a normal net outward flux of protons, due to an increase in proton permeability (Steinmetz and Husted, 1982; Gil and Malnic, 1989). This results in impaired proton excretion and renal tubular acidosis. The hypokalemia observed with amphotericin B may be due to an increase in luminal potassium ion permeability in the late distal tubule and the cortical collecting duct and the loss of potassium ions in the urine.

Cyclosporine Cyclosporine is an important immunosuppressive agent and is widely used to prevent graft rejection in organ transplantation (Charney *et al.*, 2005; Palmer and Heinrich, 2004; Naesens *et al.*, 2009). Cyclosporine is a fungal cyclic polypeptide and acts by selectively inhibiting cyclophylin and, in turn, calcineurin and T-cell activation. Nephrotoxicity is a critical side effect of cyclosporine, with nearly all patients who receive the drug exhibiting some form of nephrotoxicity. Clinically, calcineurin inhibitor (CNI)-induced nephrotoxicity may manifest as (1) acute reversible renal dysfunction, (2) acute vasculopathy, and (3) chronic CNI nephrotoxicity with interstitial fibrosis.

Acute renal dysfunction is characterized by dose-related decreases in RBF and GFR and increases in BUN and serum creatinine. These effects are lessened by reducing the dosage or by cessation of therapy. The decrease in RBF and GFR is related to marked vasoconstriction induced by cyclosporine; and it is probably produced by a number of factors, including an imbalance in vasoconstrictor and vasodilatory prostaglandin production, increased production of the vasoconstrictor thromboxane and endothelin, and activation of the rennin–angiotensin system. Endothelin may contribute to constriction of the afferent arteriole because endothelin receptor antagonists inhibit cyclosporine-induced vasoconstriction (Lanese and Conger, 1993). Although cyclosporine can produce proximal tubular epithelial changes (many small equally sized vacuoles in the cytosol), it is still not clear whether a direct effect of cyclosporine on tubular cells plays a significant role in the nephrotoxicity.

Acute vasculopathy or thrombotic microangiopathy is a rather unusual nephrotoxic lesion that affects arterioles and glomerular capillaries, without an inflammatory component, following cyclosporine treatment. The lesion consists of fibrin-platelet thrombi and fragmented red blood cells occluding the vessels (Charney et al., 2005). The pathogenesis of this lesion is poorly understood. Although the characteristics of this lesion differ from the vascular changes of acute rejection, a variety of factors may contribute to this lesion in the clinical transplant setting.

Long-term treatment with cyclosporine can result in chronic nephropathy with interstitial fibrosis and tubular atrophy. Modest elevations in serum creatinine and decreases in GFR occur along with hypertension, proteinuria, and tubular dysfunction. Histologic changes are profound; they are characterized by arteriolopathy, global and segmental glomerular sclerosis, striped interstitial fibrosis, and tubular atrophy. These lesions may not be reversible if cyclosporine therapy is discontinued and may result in end-stage renal disease. Although the mechanism of chronic cyclosporine nephropathy is not known, vasoconstriction probably plays a contributing role. Studies by Wang and Salahudeen (1994, 1995) indicated that rats treated with cyclosporine and an antioxidant lazaroid for 30 days exhibited increased GFR and RBF and less tubulointerstitial fibrosis and lipid peroxidation than rats treated with cyclosporine alone, suggesting that oxidative stress plays a role in cyclosporine nephrotoxicity in rats. The marked interstitial cell proliferation and increased procollagen secretion that occurs following cyclosporine administration may contribute to the interstitial fibrosis (Racusen and Solez, 1993).

Tacrolimus (FK-506) is a newer immunosuppressive agent that also exhibits nephrotoxicity. At this time, the degree and incidence of nephrotoxicity and morphologic changes associated with tacrolimus exposure are similar to that exhibited with cyclosporine, suggesting similar modes of toxic action.

Cisplatin Cisplatin is a valuable drug in the treatment of solid tumors, with nephrotoxicity limiting its clinical use. The kidney is not only responsible for the majority of cisplatin excreted but is also the primary site of accumulation. The effects of cisplatin on the kidney are several, including acute and chronic renal failure, renal magnesium wasting, and polyuria and patients treated with cisplatin regimens permanently lose 10% to 30% of their renal function (Bonegio and Lieberthal, 2005; Sanchez-Gonzalez et al., 2011). The nephrotoxicity of cisplatin can be grouped as (1) tubular toxicity, (2) vascular damage, (3) glomerular injury, and (4) interstitial injury.

Early effects of cisplatin are decreases in RBF and polyuria that is concurrent with increased electrolyte excretion (Clifton et al., 1982). GFR produced by vasoconstriction and is followed by tubular injury with enzymuria. Although the primary cellular target associated with AKI is the proximal tubule S_3 segment in the rat, in humans the S_1 and S_2 segments, distal tubule, and collecting ducts can also be affected.

The mechanism by which cisplatin produces cellular injury is not known but may involve metabolites of cisplatin. For example, in a mouse model of cisplatin-induced nephrotoxicity the inhibition of γ-glutamyl transpeptidase or cysteine S-conjugate β-lyase blocked toxicity, suggesting that cisplatin–glutathione conjugates may be important in targeting cisplatin to the kidney and its resulting nephrotoxicity (Townsend and Hanigan, 2002). Uptake of cisplatin into tubular cells is thought to be mediated by organic cation transporter 2. Interestingly, the *trans* isomer of cisplatin is not nephrotoxic even though similar concentrations of platinum are observed in the kidney after dosing. Thus, it is not the platinum atom per se that is responsible for the toxicity but rather the geometry of the complex or a metabolite. The antineoplastic and perhaps the nephrotoxic effects of cisplatin may be due to its intracellular hydrolysis to the reactive mono-chloro-mono-aquodiammine-platinum or diaquo-diammine-platinum species and the ability of these metabolites to alkylate purine and pyrimidine bases.

In vitro studies using primary cultures of mouse proximal tubular cells revealed that the type of cell death produced by cisplatin is dependent on the concentration (Lieberthal et al., 1996). At cisplatin concentrations less than 100 μM, the primary form of cell death is apoptosis. As the concentration increases above 100 μM, a greater percentage of the cells die by oncosis. Cisplatin produces inter and intrastrand cross-links in renal genomic DNA. Using rabbit renal proximal tubule cells, Courjault et al. (1993) showed that while DNA synthesis, protein synthesis, glucose transport, Na^+, K^+-ATPase activity, and cell viability were all inhibited by cisplatin, DNA synthesis was the most sensitive. These results suggest that cisplatin may produce nephrotoxicity through its ability to inhibit DNA synthesis as well as transport functions. In addition, cisplatin is known to induce mitochondrial dysfunction and activates numerous pathways in the mitogen-activated protein kinase family (Francescato et al., 2009; Pabla and Dong, 2008). Finally, primarily through the use of antioxidants, in vivo and in vitro studies support a role for oxidative stress in cisplatin-induced nephrotoxicity (Bonegio and Lieberthal, 2005). The lack of complete return of renal function following cisplatin treatment in vivo may result from the interference of cisplatin with the normal proliferative response that occurs after injury.

Radiocontrast Agents Iodinated contrast media are used for the imaging of tissues, with two major classes of compounds currently in use. The ionic compounds, diatrizoate derivatives, are (1) ionized at physiologic pH, (2) not significantly bound to protein, (3) restricted to the extracellular space, (4) almost entirely eliminated by the kidney, and (5) freely filtered by the glomerulus and neither secreted nor reabsorbed. These agents have a very high osmolality (>1200 mOsm/L) and are potentially nephrotoxic, particularly in patients with existing renal impairment, diabetes, or heart failure or who are receiving other nephrotoxic drugs. The newer contrast agents (eg, iotrol, iopamidol) are nonionic owing to the addition of an organic side chain, their low osmolality, and their lower nephrotoxicity. The nephrotoxicity of these agents is due to both hemodynamic alterations (vasoconstriction) and proximal tubular injury (Koyner et al., 2010). The vasoconstriction is prolonged and is probably produced by more than one mediator while ROS are thought to play a role in the proximal tubular injury.

REFERENCES

Arany I, Megyesi JK, Kaneto H, et al. Cisplatin-induced cell death is EGFR/src/ERK signaling dependent in mouse proximal tubule cells. *Am J Physiol Renal Physiol.* 2004;87:F543.

Bach PH. The renal medulla and distal nephron toxicity. In: Sipes IG, McQueen CA, Gandolfi AJ, eds. *Comprehensive toxicology.* Vol 7. Oxford, UK: Elsevier; 1997:279–298.

Ballatori N. Mechanisms of metal transport across liver cell plasma membrane. *Drug Metab Rev.* 1991;23:83–132.

Basile DP, Donohoe D, Roethe K, Osborn JL. Renal ischemic injury results in permanent damage to peritubular capillaries and influences long-term function. *Am J Physiol Renal Physiol.* 2001;281:F887–F899.

Bellomo R, Ronco C, Kellum J, et al. Acute renal failure—definition, outcome measures, animal models, fluid therapy and information technology needs: the Second International Consensus Conference of the Acute Dialysis Quality Initiative (ADQI) Group. *Crit Care.* 2004;8(4):R204–R212.

Bernardo JF, Branch RA. Amphotericin B. In: Sipes IG, McQueen CA, Gandolfi AJ, eds. *Comprehensive Toxicology.* Vol 7. Oxford, UK: Elsevier; 1997:475–494.

Bikbov B, Perico N, Abbate M, et al. The glomerulus: mechanisms of injury. In: McQueen CA, Schnellmann RG, eds. *Comprehensive Toxicology.* Vol 7. Oxford, UK: Elsevier; 2010:245–261.

Bonegio R, Lieberthal W. Cisplatin-induced nephrotoxicity. In: Tarloff JB, Lash LH, eds. *Toxicology of the Kidney.* 3rd ed. Boca Raton, FL: CRC Press; 2005:779–815.

Brady HR, Clarkson W, Lieberthal W. Acute renal failure. In: Brenner BM, ed. *Brenner and Rector's The Kidney.* 7th ed. Philadelphia: WB Saunders; 2004:1215–1292.

Brenner BM, Bohrer MP, Baylis C, Deen WM. Determinants of glomerular permselectivity: insights derived from observations in vivo. *Kidney Int.* 1977;12:229–237.

Brenner BM, Meyer TH, Hotstetter TH. Dietary protein intake and the progressive nature of kidney disease: the role of hemodynamically mediated glomerular injury in the pathogenesis of glomerular sclerosis in angina, renal ablation and intrinsic renal disease. *N Engl J Med.* 1982;307:652–659.

Brezis M, Epstein FH. Pathophysiology of acute renal failure. In: Hook JB, Goldstein RS, eds. *Toxicology of the Kidney.* 2nd ed. New York: Raven Press; 1993:129–152.

Brezis M, Rosen S, Silva P. Transport activity modifies thick ascending limb damage in isolated perfused kidney. *Kidney Int.* 1984;25:65–72.

Bruschi SA, West K, Crabb JW, et al. Mitochondrial HSP60 (P1 protein) and a HSP-70 like protein (mortalin) are major targets for modification during *S*-(1,1,2,2-tetrafluorethyl)-L-cysteine induced nephrotoxicity. *J Biol Chem.* 1993;268:23157–23161.

Bucci TJ, Howard PC, Tolleson WH, et al. Renal effects of fumonisin mycotoxins in animals. *Toxicol Pathol.* 1998;26:160–164.

Burne MJ, Daniels F, El Ghandour A, et al. Identification of the CD4(+) T cell as a major pathogenic factor in ischemic acute renal failure. *J Clin Invest.* 2001;108:1065–1073.

Burne-Taney MJ, Ascon DB, Daniels F, Racusen L, Baldwin W, Rabb H. B cell deficiency confers protection from renal ischemia reperfusion injury. *J Immunol.* 2003;171:3210–3215.

Charney D, Solez K, Racusen LC. Nephrotoxicity of cyclosporine and other immunosuppressive and immunotherapeutic agents. In: Tarloff JB, Lash LH, eds. *Toxicology of the Kidney.* 3rd ed. Boca Raton, FL: CRC Press; 2005:687–777.

Chen Q, Jone1s TW, Brown PC, Stevens JL. The mechanism of cysteine conjugate cytotoxicity in renal epithelial cells. *J Biol Chem.* 1990;265:21603–21611.

Chen Q, Yu K, Stevens JL. Regulation of the cellular stress response by reactive electrophiles: the role of covalent binding and cellular thiols in transcriptional activation of the 70-kDa heat shock protein gene by nephrotoxic cysteine conjugates. *J Biol Chem.* 1992;267:24322–24327.

Clifton GG, Pearce C, O'Neill WM Jr, Wallin JD. Early polyuria in the rat following single-dose *cis*-dichlorodiammineplatinum (II): effects on plasma vasopressin concentration and posterior pituitary function. *J Lab Clin Med.* 1982;100:659–670.

Coen M, Holmes E, Lindon JC, Nicholson JK. NMR-based metabolic profiling and metabonomic approaches to problems in molecular toxicology. *Chem Res Toxicol.* 2008;21(1):9–27.

Conner EA, Fowler BA. Mechanisms of metal-induced nephrotoxicity. In: Hook JB, Goldstein RS, eds. *Toxicology of the Kidney.* 2nd ed. New York: Raven Press; 1993:437–457.

Counts RS, Nowak G, Wyatt RD, Schnellmann RG. Nephrotoxicants inhibition of renal proximal tubule cell regeneration. *Am J Physiol.* 1995:269:F274–F281.

Courjault F, Leroy D, Coquery I, Toutain H. Platinum complex-induced dysfunction of cultured renal proximal tubule cells. *Arch Toxicol.* 1993;67:338–346.

Daemen MARC, van 'tVeer C, Denecker G, et al. Inhibition of apoptosis induced by ischemia-reperfusion prevents inflammation. *J Clin Invest.* 1999;104:541–549.

De Broe ME. Anagesic nephropathy. In: Tarloff JB, Lash LH, eds. *Toxicology of the Kidney.* 3rd ed. Boca Raton, FL: CRC Press; 2005:619–634.

Decker B, Molitoris BA. Aminoglycoside-induced nephrotoxicity. In: McQueen CA, Schnellmann RG, eds. *Comprehensive Toxicology.* Vol 7. Oxford, UK: Elsevier; 2010:329–346.

Declercq W, Vanden Berghe T, Vandenabeele P. RIP kinases at the crossroads of cell death and survival. *Cell.* 2009;138(2):229–232.

Dekant W. Chemical-induced nephrotoxicity mediated by glutathione S-conjugate formation. In: Tarloff JB, Lash LH, eds. *Toxicology of the Kidney.* 3rd ed. Boca Raton, FL: CRC Press; 2005:995–1020.

Dickman KG, Grollman AP. Nephrotoxicity of natural products: aristolochic acid and fungal toxins. In: McQueen CA, Schnellmann RG, eds. *Comprehensive Toxicology.* Vol 7. Oxford, UK: Elsevier; 2010:433–458.

Dong J, Ramachandiran S, Tikoo K, Jia Z, Lauu SS, Monks TJ. EGFR-independent activation of p38 MAPK and EGFR-dependent activation of ERK1/2 are required for ROS-induced renal cell death. *Am J Physiol Renal Physiol.* 2004;287:F1049–F1058.

Dunn RB, Anderson S, Brenner B. The hemodynamic basis of progressive renal disease. *Semin Nephrol.* 1986;6:122–138.

Eknoyan G, Bulger RE, Dobyan DC. Mercuric chloride-induced acute renal failure in the rat: I. Correlation of functional and morphologic changes and their modification by clonidine. *Lab Invest.* 1982;46:613–620.

Emeigh Hart SGE, Wyand DS, Khairallah EA, Cohen SD. A role for the glutathione conjugate and renal cytochrome P450 in acetaminophen (APAP) induced nephrotoxicity in the CD-1 mouse. *Toxicologist.* 1990;11:57.

Emeigh Hart SGE, Beierschmitt WP, Wyand DS, et al. Acetaminophen nephrotoxicity in CD-1 Mice. I. Evidence of a role for in situ activation in selective covalent binding and toxicity. *Toxicol Appl Pharmacol.* 1994;126:267–275.

Filler G, Bokenkamp A, Hofmann W, Le Bricon T, Martinez-Bru C, Grubb A: Cystatin C as a maker of GFR-history, indications and future research. *Clin Biochem.* 2005;38:1–8.

Fowler BA. Other nephrotoxic metals and nanometallic particles. In: McQueen CA, Schnellmann RG, eds. *Comprehensive Toxicology.* Vol 7. Oxford, UK: Elsevier; 2010:495–506.

Ford SM. In vitro toxicity systems. In: Sipes IG, McQueen CA, Gandolfi AJ, eds. *Comprehensive Toxicology.* Vol 7. Oxford, UK: Elsevier; 1997:121–142.

Ford SM. In vitro techniques in screening and mechanistic studies: cell culture, cell-free systems, and molecular and cell biology. In: Tarloff JB, Lash LH, eds. *Toxicology of the Kidney.* 3rd ed. Boca Raton, FL: CRC Press; 2005:191–213.

Francescato HD, Costa RS, Junior FB, Coimbra TM. Effect of NK inhibition on cisplatin-induced renal damage. *Nephrol Dial Transplant.* 2007;22:2138–2148.

Fukino H, Hirai M, Hsueh YM, Yamane Y. Effect of zinc pretreatment on mercuric chloride-induced lipid peroxidation in the rat kidney. *Toxicol Appl Pharmacol.* 1984;73:395–401.

Gil FZ, Malnic G. Effect of amphotericin B on renal tubular acidification in the rat. *Pflugers Arch.* 1989;413:280–286.

Goering PL, Fisher BR, Chaudhary PP, Dick CA. Relationship between stress protein induction in rat kidney by mercuric chloride and nephrotoxicity. *Toxicol Appl Pharmacol.* 1992;113:184–191.

Goering PL, Fisher BR, Noren BT, et al. Mercury induces regional and cell-specific stress protein expression in rat kidney. *Toxicol Sci.* 2000;53:447–457.

Goldstein RS. Biochemical heterogeneity and site-specific tubular injury. In: Hook JB, Goldstein RS, eds. *Toxicology of the Kidney.* 2nd ed. New York: Raven Press; 1993:201–248.

Goligorsky MS, Patschan D, Kuo M-C, et al. Cell adhesion molecules in renal injury. In: McQueen CA, Schnellmann RG, eds. *Comprehensive Toxicology.* Vol 7. Oxford, UK: Elsevier; 2010:213–244.

Gopee NV, He Q, Sharma RP. Fumonisin B1-induced apoptosis is associated with delayed inhibition of protein kinase C, nuclear factor-kappaB and tumor necrosis factor alpha in LLC-PK1 cells. *Chem Biol Interact.* 2003;146:131–145.

Groves CE, Hayden PJ, Lock EA, Schnellmann RG. Differential cellular effects in the toxicity of haloalkene and haloalkane cysteine conjugates to rabbit renal proximal tubules. *J Biochem Toxicol.* 1993;8:49–56.

Groves CE, Lock EA, Schnellmann RG. The role of lipid peroxidation in renal proximal tubule cell death induced by haloalkene cysteine conjugates. *J Toxicol Appl Pharmacol.* 1991;107:54–62.

Hallman MA, Zhuang S, Schnellmann RG. Regulation of dedifferentiation and redifferentiation in renal proximal tubular cells by the epidermal growth factor receptor. *J Pharmacol Exp Ther.* 2008;325(2):520–528.

Hammerman MR, Miller SB. Therapeutic use of growth factors in renal failure. *J Am Soc Nephrol.* 1994;5:1–11.

Harriman JF, Liu XL, Aleo MD, Machaca K, Schnellmann RG. Endoplasmic reticulum Ca^{2+} signaling and calpains mediate renal cell death. *Cell Death Differ.* 2002;9:734–741.

Hart SE, Kinter LB. Assessing renal effects of toxicants in vivo. In: Tarloff JB, Lash LH, eds. *Toxicology of the Kidney.* 3rd ed. Boca Raton, FL: CRC Press; 2005:81–147.

Hart SGE. In vivo methodologies used to assess renal function and injury. In: McQueen CA, Schnellmann RG, eds. *Comprehensive Toxicology.* Vol 7. Oxford, UK: Elsevier; 2010:263–303.

Hayden PJ, Stevens JL. Cysteine conjugate toxicity, metabolism and binding to macro-molecules in isolated rat kidney mitochondria. *Mol Pharmacol.* 1990;37:468–476.

Hayden PJ, Welsh CJ, Yang Y, et al. Formation of mitochondrial phospholipid adducts by nephrotoxic cysteine conjugate metabolites. *Chem Res Toxicol.* 1992;5:231–237.

Hayden PJ, Yang Y, Ward AJ, et al. Formation of diflourothionoacetyl-protein adducts by *S*-(1,1,2,2-tetrafluoroethyl)-L-cysteine metabolites: nucleophilic catalysis of stable lysyl adduct formation by histidine and tyrosine. *Biochemistry.* 1991;30:5935–5943.

Holmes E, Cloarec O, Nicholson JK. Probing latent biomarker signatures and in vivo pathway activity in experimental disease states via statistical total correlation spectroscopy (STOCSY) of biofluids: application to HgCl$_2$ toxicity. *J Proteome Res.* 2006;5:1313–1320.

Humphreys BD, Czerniak S, DiRocco DP, Hasain W, Cheema R, Bonventre JV. Repair of injured proximal tubule does not involve specialized progenitors. *Proc Natl Acad Sci U S A.* 2011;108(22):9226–9231.

Humphreys BD, Valerius MT, Kibayashi A, et al. Intrinsic epithelial cells repair the kidney after injury. *Cell Stem Cell.* 2008;2(3):284–291.

Ikeda M, Prachasilchai W, Burner-Taney MJ, Rabb H, Yokota-Ikeda N. Ischemic acute tubular necrosis models and drug discovery: a focus on cellular inflammation. *Drug Discov Today.* 2006;11:364–370.

Jarnberg P. Renal toxicity of anesthetic agents. In: DeBroe ME, Porter GA, Bennett AM, Verpooten GA, eds. *Clinical Nephrotoxicants, Renal Injury from Drugs and Chemicals.* The Netherlands: Kluwer; 1998:413–418.

Kanwar YS, Liu ZZ, Kashihara N, Wallner EI. Current status of the structural and functional basis of glomerular filtration and proteinuria. *Semin Nephrol.* 1991;11:390–413.

Kaushal GP, Basnakian AG, Shah SV. Apoptotic pathways in ischemic acute renal failure. *Kidney Int.* 2004;66(2):500–506.

Kaushal GP, Singh AB, Shah SV. Identification of gene family of caspases in rat kidney and altered expression in ischemia-reperfusion injury. *Am J Physiol.* 1998;274:F587–F595.

Kelly KJ. Heat shock (stress response) proteins and renal ischemia/reperfusion injury. *Contrib Nephrol.* 2005;148:86–106.

Kido T, Nordberg G. Cadmium-induced renal effects in the general environment. In: DeBroe ME, Porter GA, Bennett AM, Verpooten GA, eds. *Clinical Nephrotoxicants, Renal Injury from Drugs and Chemicals.* The Netherlands: Kluwer; 1998:345–362.

Kidwell DT, KcKeown JW, Grider JS, et al. Acute effects of gentamicin on thick ascending limb function in the rat. *Eur J Pharmaco Environ Toxicol Pharmacol Section.* 1994;270:97–103.

Kinsey GR, Li L, Okusa MD. Inflammation in acute kidney injury. *Nephron Exp Nephrol.* 2008;109(4):e102–e107.

Kirkpatrick DS, Gandolfi AJ. In vitro techniques in screening and mechanistic studies: organ perfusion, slices, and nephron components. In: Tarloff JB, Lash LH, eds. *Toxicology of the Kidney.* 3rd ed. Boca Raton, FL: CRC Press; 2005:149–189.

Klaassen CD, Liu J, Choudhuri S. Metallothionein: an intracellular protein to protect cadmium toxicity. *Ann Rev Pharmacol Toxicol.* 1999;39:267–294.

Komatsuda A, Wakui H, Satoh K, et al. Altered localization of 73-kilodalton heat shock protein in rat kidneys with gentamicin–induced acute tubular injury. *Lab Invest.* 1993;68:687–695.

Koyner JL, Murray PT, Bakris GK. The pathogenesis and prevention of radiocontrast medium-induced renal dysfunction. In: McQueen CA, Schnellmann RG, eds. *Comprehensive Toxicology.* Vol 7. Oxford, UK: Elsevier; 2010:359–386.

Lanese DM, Conger JD. Effects of endothelin receptor antagonist on cyclosporine-induced vasoconstriction in isolated rat renal arterioles. *J Clin Invest.* 1993;91:2144–2149.

Lash LH, Cummings BS. Mechanisms of toxicant-induced acute kidney injury. In: McQueen CA, Schnellmann RG, eds. *Comprehensive Toxicology.* Vol 7. Oxford, UK: Elsevier; 2010:81–115.

Lauwerys RR, Bernard AM, Roels HA, Buchet JP. Cadmium: exposure markers as predictors of nephrotoxic effects. *Clin Chem.* 1994;40:1391–1394.

Lehman-McKeeman LD. α2u-Globulin nephropathy. In: McQueen CA, Schnellmann RG. eds. *Comprehensive Toxicology.* Vol 7. Oxford, England: Elsevier; 2010:507–521.

Lemasters JJ, Qian T, Bradham CA, et al. Mitochondrial dysfunction in the pathogenesis of necrotic and apoptotic cell death. *J Bioenerg Biomembr.* 1999;31:305–319.

Leonard I, Zanen J, Nonclercq D, et al. Modification of immunoreactive EGF and EGF receptor after acute tubular necrosis induced by tobramycin or cisplatin. *Ren Fail.* 1994;16(5):583–608.

Levin S, Bucci TJ, Cohen SM, et al. The nomenclature of cell death: recommendations of an *ad hoc* committee of the society of toxicologic pathologists. *Toxicol Pathol.* 1999;27:484–490.

Lieberthal W, Triaca V, Levine J. Mechanisms of death induced by cisplatin in proximal tubular epithelial cells: apoptosis vs. necrosis. *Am J Physiol.* 1996;270:F700–F708.

Liu X, Schnellmann RG. Calpain mediates progressive plasma membrane permeability and proteolysis of cytoskeleton-associated paxillin, talin, and vinculin during renal cell death. *J Pharmacol Exp Ther.* 2003;304: 63–70.

Liu X, Godwin ML, Nowak G. Protein kinase C-alpha inhibits the repair of oxidative phosphorylation after S-(1,2-dichlorovinyl)-L-cysteine injury in renal cells. *Am J Physiol Renal Physiol.* 2004;287(1):F64–F73.

Lock EA. Renal xenobiotic metabolism. In: McQueen CA, Schnellmann RG, eds. *Comprehensive Toxicology.* Vol 7. Oxford, UK: Elsevier; 2010:55–79.

Lock EA, Reed CJ. Renal xenobiotic metabolism. In: Sipes IG, McQueen CA, Gandolfi AJ, eds. *Comprehensive Toxicology.* Vol 7. Oxford, UK: Elsevier; 1997:77–98.

Lund BO, Miller DM, Woods JS. Studies in Hg(II)-induced H$_2$O$_2$ formation and oxidative stress in vivo and in vitro in rat kidney mitochondria. *Biochem Pharmacol.* 1993;45:2017–2024.

Maddox DA, Brenner BM. Glomerular ultrafiltration. In: Brenner BM, Rector FC, eds. *The Kidney.* 4th ed. Philadelphia: WB Saunders; 1991: 205–244.

Mehendale HM. Halogenated hydrocarbons. In: McQueen CA, Schnellmann RG, eds. *Comprehensive Toxicology.* Vol 7. Oxford, UK: Elsevier; 2010:459–474.

Mehta RL, Kellum JA, Shah SV, et al. Acute Kidney Injury Network: report of an initiative to improve outcomes in acute kidney injury. *Crit Care.* 2007;11(2): R31.

Melnick R. An alternative hypothesis on the role of chemically induced protein droplet (α_{2u}-globulin) nephropathy in renal carcinogenesis. *Regul Toxicol Pharmacol.* 1992;16:111–125.

Miller GW, Schnellmann RG. Cytoprotection by inhibition of chloride channels: the mechanism of action of glycine and strychnine. *Life Sci.* 1993;53:1211–1215.

Miller GW, Schnellmann RG. Inhibitors of renal chloride transport do not block toxicant-induced chloride influx in the proximal tubule. *Toxicol Lett.* 1995;76:179–184.

Naesens M, Kuypers DR, Sarwal M. Calcineurin inhibitor nephrotoxicity. *Clin J Am Soc Nephrol.* 2009;4(2):481–508.

Nowak G. Protein kinase C-alpha and ERK1/2 mediate mitochondrial dysfunction, decreases in active Na$^+$ transport, and cisplatin-induced apoptosis in renal cells. *J Biol Chem.* 2002;277:43377–43388.

Nowak G. Protein kinase C mediates repair of mitochondrial and transport functions after toxicant-induced injury in renal cells. *J Pharmacol Exp Ther.* 2003;306:157–165.

Nowak G, Bakajsova D, Clifton GL. Protein kinase C-{*epsilon*} modulates mitochondrial function and active Na$^+$ transport after oxidant injury in renal cells. *Am J Physiol Renal Physiol.* 2004;286:F307.

Nowak G, Bakajsova D, Samarel AM. Protein kinase C-{*varepsilon*} activation induces mitochondrial dysfunction and fragmentation in renal proximal tubules. *Am J Physiol Renal Physiol.* 2011;301:F197–F208.

Nowak G, Clifton, GL, Godwin ML, Bakajsova D. Activation of ERK1/2 pathway mediates oxidant-induced decreases in mitochondrial function in renal cells. *Am J Physiol Renal Physiol.* 2006;291: 5840–5855.

Okada Y, Maeno E, Shimizu T, Manabe K, Mori S, Nabekura T. Dual roles of plasmalemmal chloride channels in induction of cell death. *Pflugers Arch.* 2004;448:287–295.

Pabla N, Dong Z. Cisplatin nephrotoxicity: mechanisms and renprotective strategies. *Kidney Int.* 2008;73:994–1007.

Palmer BF, Heinrich WL. Toxic nephropathy. In: Brenner BM, ed. *Brenner and Rector's The Kidney.* 7th ed. Philadelphia: WB Saunders; 2004:1625–1658.

Rabb H, Daniels F, O'Donnell M, et al. Pathophysiological role of T lymphocytes in renal ischemia-reperfusion injury in mice. *Am J Physiol.* 2000;279:F525–F531.

Racusen LC, Solez K. Nephrotoxicity of cyclosporine and other immunotherapeutic agents. In: Hook JB, Goldstein RS, eds. *Toxicology of the Kidney.* 2nd ed. New York: Raven Press; 1993:319–360.

Ramachandiran S, Huang Q, Dong J, Lau SS, Monks TJ. Mitogen-activated protein kinases contribute to reactive oxygen species-induced cell death in renal proximal tubule epithelial cells. *Chem Res Toxicol.* 2002; 15:1635.

Rankin GO, Valentovic MA. Role of xenobiotic metabolism. In: Tarloff JB, Lash LH, eds. *Toxicology of the Kidney.* 3rd ed. Boca Raton, FL: CRC Press; 2005:217–243.

Safirstein R, Deray G. Anticancer, cisplatin/carboplatin. In: DeBroe ME, Porter GA, Bennett AM, Verpooten GA, eds. *Clinical Nephrotoxicants, Renal Injury from Drugs and Chemicals.* The Netherlands: Kluwer; 1998:261–272.

Sanchez-Gonzalez PD, Lopez-Hernandez FJ, Lopez-Novoa JM, Morales AI. An integrative view of the pathophysiological events leading to cisplatin nephrotoxicity. *Crit Rev Toxicol.* 2011;41:803–821.

Schnellmann RG. Analgesic nephropathy in rodents. *J Toxicol Environ Health, Part B.* 1998;1:81–90.

Schnellmann RG, Cross TJ, Lock EA. Pentachlorabutadienyl-L-cysteine uncouples oxidative phosphorylation by dissipating the proton gradient. *Toxicol Appl Pharmacol.* 1989;100:498–505.

Schnellmann RG, Griner RD. Mitochondrial mechanisms of tubular injury. In: Goldstein RS, ed. *Mechanisms of Injury in Renal Disease and Toxicity.* Boca Raton, FL: CRC Press; 1994:247–265.

Schnellmann RG, Lock EA, Mandel LJ. A mechanism of *S* -(1,2,3,4,4-pentachloro-1,3-butadienyl)-L-cysteine toxicity to rabbit renal proximal tubules. *Toxicol Appl Pharmacol.* 1987;90:513–521.

Servais H, Mingeot-Leclercq M-P, Tulkens PM. Antibiotic-induced nephrotoxicity. In: Tarloff JB, Lash LH, eds. *Toxicology of the Kidney.* 3rd ed. Boca Raton, FL: CRC Press; 2005:635–685.

Shaik SP, Fifer EK, Nowak G. Protein kinase B/Akt modulates nephrotoxicant-induced necrosis in renal cells. *Am J Physiol Renal Physiol.* 2007;292:F292–F303.

Shaik SP, Fifer EK, Nowak G. Akt activation improves oxidative phosphorylation in renal proximal tubular cells following nephrotoxicant injury. *Am J Physiol Renal Physiol.* 2008;294:F423–F432.

Sheikh-Hamad D, Cacini W, Buckley AR, et al. Cellular and molecular studies on cisplatin-induced apoptotic cell death in rat kidney. *Arch Toxicol.* 2004;78:147–155.

Shibutani S, Dong H, Suzuki N, et al. Selective toxicity of aristolochic acids I and II. *Drug Metab Dispos.* 2007;35(7):1217–1222.

Smith JH, Maita K, Sleight SD, Hook JB. Effect of sex hormone status on chloroform nephrotoxicity and renal mixed function oxidases in mice. *Toxicology.* 1984;30:305–316.

Smith MW, Ambudkar IS, Phelps PC, et al. HgCl$_2$-induced changes in cytosolic Ca^{2+} of cultured rabbit renal tubular cells. *Biochem Biophys Acta.* 1987;931:130–142.

Steinmetz PR, Husted RF. Amphotericin B toxicity for epithelial cells. In: Porter GA, ed. *Nephrotoxic Mechanisms of Drugs and Environmental Toxins.* New York, London: Plenum Press; 1982:95–98.

Stevens LA, Levey AS. Measurement of kidney function. *Med Clin North Am.* 2005;89:457–473.

Sweet DH. Renal organic cation and anion transport: from physiology to genes. In: McQueen CA, Schnellmann RG, eds. *Comprehensive Toxicology.* Vol 7. Oxford, UK: Elsevier; 2010:23–53.

Taal MW, Chertow GM, Marsden PA, Skorecki K, Yu ASL, Brenner BM. *Brenner and Rector's The Kidney.* 9th ed. Elsevier Health Sciences; 2011.

Tarloff JB. Analgesics and nonsteroidal anti-inflammatory drugs. In: Sipes IG, McQueen CA, Gandolfi AJ, eds. *Comprehensive Toxicology.* Vol. 7. Oxford, UK: Elsevier; 1997:583–600.

Tarloff JB. Analgesics and nonsteroidal anti-inflammatory drugs. In: McQueen CA, Schnellmann RG, eds. *Comprehensive Toxicology.* Vol. 7. Oxford, UK: Elsevier; 2010:387–403.

Tarloff JB, Kinter LB. *In vivo* methodologies used to assess renal function. In: Sipes IG, McQueen CA, Gandolfi AJ, eds. *Comprehensive Toxicology.* Vol. 7. Oxford, UK: Elsevier; 1997:99–120.

Townsend DM, Hanigan MH. Inhibition of γ tglutamyl transpeptidase or cysteine S-conjugate β-lyase activity blocks the nephrotoxicity of cisplain in mice. *J Pharmacol Exp Ther.* 2002;300:142–148.

Ulozas E. Amphotericin B-induced nephrotoxicity. In: McQueen CA, Schnellmann RG, eds. *Comprehensive Toxicology.* Vol 7. Oxford, UK: Elsevier; 2010:347–357.

Vaidya VS, Bonventre JV, Ferguson MA. Biomarkers of acute kidney injury. In: McQueen CA, Schnellmann RG, eds. *Comprehensive Toxicology.* Vol 7. Oxford, UK: Elsevier; 2010:197–211.

van de Water B, de Graauw M, Le Devedec S, Alderliesten M. Cellular stress responses and molecular mechanisms of nephrotoxicity. *Toxicol Lett.* 2006;162:83–93.

Vanherweghem JL, Depierreux M, Tielemans C, et al. Rapidly progressive interstitial renal fibrosis in young women: association with slimming regimen including Chinese herbs. *Lancet.* 1993;341(8842): 387–391.

Wallin A, Jones TW, Vercesi AE, et al. Toxicity of *S*-pentachorobutadienyl-L-cysteine studied with isolated rat renal cortical mitochondria. *Arch Biochem Biophys.* 1987;258:365–372.

Wang C, Salahudeen AK. Cyclosporine nephrotoxicity: attenuation by an antioxidant-inhibitor of lipid peroxidation in vitro and in vivo. *Transplantation.* 1994;58:940–946.

Wang C, Salahudeen AK. Lipid peroxidation accompanies cyclosporine nephrotoxicity: effects of vitamin E. *Kidney Int.* 1995;47:927–934.

Wang Y, Bollard ME, Nicholson JK, Holmes E. Exploration of the direct metabolic effects of mercury II chloride on the kidney on Sprague-Dawley rats using high-resolution magic angle spinning 1H NMR spectroscopy of intact tissue and patter recognition. *J Pharm Biomed Anal.* 2006;40:375–381.

Wang Z, Chen JK , Moeckel G, Harris RC. Importance of functional EGF receptors in recovery from acute nephrotoxic injury. *J Am Soc Nephrol*. 2003;14(12):3147–3154.

Waters SL, Sarang SS, Wang KKW, Schnellmann RG. Calpains mediate calcium and chloride influx during the late phase of cell injury. *J Pharmacol Exp Ther*. 1997a;283:1177–1184.

Waters SL, Wong JK, Schnellmann RG. Depletion of endoplasmic reticulum calcium stores protects against hypoxia- and mitochondrial inhibitor-induced cellular injury and death. *Biochem Biophys Res Commun*. 1997b;240:57–60.

Weinberg JM, Harding PG, Humes HD. Mitochondrial bioenergetics during the initiation of mercuric chloride-induced renal injury: II. Functional alterations of renal cortical mitochondria isolated after mercuric chloride treatment. *J Biol Chem*. 1982a;257:68–74.

Weinberg JM, Harding PG, Humes HD. Mitochondrial bioenergetics during the initiation of mercuric chloride-induced renal injury: I. Direct effects of in vitro mercuric chloride on renal cortical mitochondrial function. *J Biol Chem*. 1982b;257:60–67.

Woo KR, Shu WP, Kong L, Liu BC. Tumor necrosis factor mediates apoptosis via Ca^{2+}/Mg^{2+} dependent endonuclease with protein kinase C as a possible mechanism for cytokine resistance in human renal carcinoma cells. *J Urol*. 1996;155:1779–1783.

Zalups RK. Renal toxicity of mercury. In: Sipes IG, McQueen CA, Gandolfi AJ, eds. *Comprehensive Toxicology*. Vol 7. Oxford, UK: Elsevier; 1997:633–652.

Zalups RK. Renal handling and toxicity of mercury. In: McQueen CA, Schnellmann RG, eds. *Comprehensive Toxicology*. Vol 7. Oxford, UK: Elsevier; 2010:475–493.

Zalups RK, Diamond GL. Nephrotoxicology of metal. In: Tarloff JB, Lash LH, eds. *Toxicology of the Kidney*. 3rd ed. Boca Raton, FL: CRC Press; 2005:937–994.

Zalups RK, Lash LH. Advances in understanding the renal transport and toxicity of mercury. *J Toxicol Environ Health*. 1994;42:1–44.

Zhuang S, Dang Y, Schnellmann RG. Requirement of the epidermal growth factor receptor in renal epithelial cell proliferation and migration. *Am J Physiol Renal Physiol*. 2004;287(3):F365–F372.

Zhuang S, Yan Y, Han J, Schnellmann RG. p38 kinase-mediated transactivation of the epidermal growth factor receptor is required for dedifferentiation of renal epithelial cells after oxidant injury. *J Biol Chem*. 2005;280(22):21036–21042.

Zhuang S, Yan Y, Daubert RA, Han J, Schnellmann RG. ERK promotes hydrogen peroxide-induced apoptosis through caspase-3 activation and inhibition of Akt in renal epithelial cells. *Am J Physiol Renal Physiol*. 2007;292:F440–F447.

Zhuang S, Kinsey GR, Yan Y, Han J, Schnellmann RG. Extracellular signal-regulated kinase activation mediates mitochondrial dysfunction and necrosis induced by hydrogen peroxide in renal proximal tubular cells. *J Pharmacol Exp Ther*. 2008;325(3):732–740.

chapter 15

Toxic Responses of the Respiratory System

George D. Leikauf

"Since the time of Hippocrates the growth of scientific medicine has in reality been based on the study of the manner in which what he called 'Nature' of the living body expresses itself in response to changes in the environment, and reasserts itself in face of disturbances and injury"
    —*John Scott Haldane (Haldane, 1922)*

HISTORICAL PERSPECTIVE

Toxic substances can disrupt the respiratory system and distant organs after chemicals enter the body by means of inhalation. Pathological changes in the respiratory tract also can be a target of blood-borne agents. Inhalation toxicology refers to the route of exposure, whereas respiratory toxicology refers to target organ toxicity. This chapter reviews the toxic responses of the respiratory system and is an update of the previous chapter (Witschi *et al.*, 2008).

Historically, respiratory toxicology is a keystone of medicine, dating back to Hippocrates. In his medical thesis *On Airs, Waters, and Places*, Hippocrates recommended that physicians evaluate local atmospheres to discover the causes of diseases (Adams, 1849). In 1661, John Evelyn appealed to the English King and Parliament for relief from the poor air quality of London that was a result of the burning of "sea-coale" (a brown coal likely enriched in sulfur that washed up on the banks of the River Thames (Evelyn, 1661). This situation continued and became worse in the 19th century when the Industrial Revolution quickened awareness of respiratory toxicology due to air pollutions (see Chap. 29).

Later, Bernardino Ramazzini proposed that clinicians evaluate the relationships between occupational atmospheres and disease pathogenesis, starting a long history of respiratory toxicology role in occupational medicine. He observed that "corruption of the atmosphere" can be at the origin of many respiratory diseases. In his work *De Morbis Artificum Diatriba* (*Diseases of Workers*) (1713), he stated, "Miners who maintain an almost daily contact with evil powders in the earth's depths... have lungs which absorb mineral exhalations and must be the first to suffer the attack of poisonous fumes.... The mortality rate of miners is very high and, as a proof of this, we remember that their wives re-marry many times." Supporting the concept of exposure, he writes: "It is not only miners working in mines who run the risk of dying from diseases due to metals: so do many others working around mines". He also supported the concept of prevention over treatment stating "Prevention is better than cure, just as it is better, on seeing storm arrive, to get under cover than to suffer its damages" (Bisetti, 1988).

During the 19th century the relationship between dusty trades and bronchitis (Thackrah, 1832), silica dust and pneumoconiosis (Holland, 1843) became well recognized. In 1873, excessive bronchitis deaths were attributed to London fogs (smog) (British Medical Journal, 1880). In a report on London fogs (smog) in 1880 that lead to 1817 excessive deaths, Russell states "And smoke in London has continued probably for many years to shorten the lives of thousands, but only lately has the sudden, palpable rise of the death-rate in an unusually dense and prolonged fog attracted much attention to the depredations of this quiet and despised destroyer." He goes on to note: "A London fog is brown, reddish-yellow, or greenish, darkens more than a white fog, has a smoky, or sulphurous smell, is often somewhat dryer than a country fog, and produces, when thick, a choking sensation. Instead of diminishing while the sun rises higher, it often increases in density, and some of the most lowering London fogs occur about midday or late in the afternoon. Sometimes the brown masses rise and interpose a thick curtain at a considerable elevation between earth and sky. A white cloth spread out on the ground rapidly turns dirty, and particles of soot attach themselves to every exposed object." In 1884, John Aitken proposed that particles contribute to the haze and alter the color of the sunset (Aitken, 1884).

Also toward the end of the 19th century John Scott Haldane identified carbon monoxide as the lethal constituent of "afterdamp," a gas mixture created by combustion in mines, after examining many bodies of miners killed in pit explosions (Haldane, 1896). He noted skin was colored cherry-pink from carboxyhemoglobin and studied carbon monoxide's ability to displace oxygen. An experimentalist, he had investigated the effect of carbon monoxide on his own breathing in a chamber (Haldane, 1895). In the late 1800s, he supported efforts to improved mine safety by introducing gas masks for rescue workers and the use of small animals (canaries and white mice) to detect dangerous levels of carbon monoxide.

By the start of the 20th century, respiratory toxicology became even more inseparable from occupational medicine in which coal workers' pneumoconiosis (black lung), silicosis, and byssinosis were noted in specific trades, even in the absence of bacterial infection (tuberculosis) (Oliver, 1902; Hoffman, 1918; Blanc, 2005).

During World War I respiratory toxicology turned to the dark side. Efforts of Fritz Haber (Germany) (Witschi, 2000) and Victor Grignard (France) (Hodson, 1987) lead to the development and use of chlorine, phosgene, and other gases in chemical warfare. This was accompanied by toxicological studies of poison gases in laboratory animals, in which Haber noted that exposure to a low concentration of a poisonous gas for an extended time could produce the same effect (death) as exposure to a high concentration for a short time. The so-called "Haber's rule" is $C \times t = k$, where C is the gas concentration (mass/volume), t is the exposure time producing a given toxic effect, and k is a constant. Although sometimes useful, this rule has many exceptions and should be applied with caution.

In the 1920s, Yandell Henderson and Howard Haggard began testing numerous noxious chemicals and culminated a compendium of dose–response analysis and median lethal concentration (LC_{50}) of a number of noxious chemicals (Henderson and Haggard, 1943). Although a simple test of lethality clearly has limitation in understanding the mechanism of toxicity, it still has value today. The results from Henderson and Haggard's efforts are often referred to in assessments of Immediately Dangerous to Life or Health concentrations, which can be informative following accidental inhalation exposures.

From the 1920s to 1950, CN Davies (1949), Lucien Dautrebande (Dautrebande *et al.*, 1948), Phillip Drinker (Drinker *et al.*, 1928), Lars Friberg (Friberg, 1948), Theodore Hatch (Hatch, 1937; Hatch and Hemeon, 1948), Earl King (Robson *et al.*, 1934) Frank Patty (Patty, 1949), HD Landahl (Landahl and Black, 1947), Leslie Silverman (Silverman and Lee, 1946; Silverman and Whittenberger, 1949), Henry Smyth Jr (Smyth, 1946), Herbert Stokinger (Stokinger, 1949; Stokinger *et al.*, 1950), and many others advanced exposure science (ie, measure of concentrations of gas and particles in workplace and ambient atmospheres), began controlled inhalation exposure of laboratory animals, and made recommendations for human occupational exposure limits (threshold limit values [TLV]).

These investigations provided the foundation for the modern era of respiratory toxicology lead by Yves Alarie (Alarie *et al.*, 1961), Roy Albert (Albert and Arnett, 1955), Mary Amdur (Amdur *et al.*, 1952), David Bates (Young *et al.*, 1964), Eula Bingham (Bingham *et al.*, 1968), Joe Brain (Brain, 1970), Louis Casarett (Casarett, 1960), David Coffin (Coffin *et al.*, 1968), John Craighead (Tegtmeyer and Craighead, 1968), Carol Cross (DeLucia *et al.*, 1972), Tore Dalhamn (Dalhamn and Rodin, 1956), Robert Drew (Drew and Eisenbud, 1970), Juraj Ferin (Ferin *et al.*, 1965), Robert Frank (Frank, 1970), Gustav Freeman (Freeman and Haydo, 1964), Donald Gardner (Gardner *et al.*, 1969), Bernard Goldstein (Goldstein and Balchum, 1967), Elliot Goldstein (Goldstein *et al.*, 1969), Gareth Green (Green and Carolin, 1967), Paul Gross (Gross *et al.*, 1952), Theodore Hatch (Palm *et al.*, 1956), Harold Hodge (Hodge *et al.*, 1956), Sidney Laskin (Laskin *et al.*, 1963), Morton Lippmann (Lippmann and Albert, 1968), Paul Morrow (Morrow *et al.*, 1958), J. Brian Mudd (Mudd *et al.*, 1969), Shelton Murphy (Murphy *et al.*, 1963), Jay Nadel (Nadel and Comroe, 1961), Norton Nelson (Nelson, 1955), Ed Palmes (Palmes *et al.*, 1959), Otto Raabe (Raabe, 1967), Verald Rowe (Rowe *et al.*, 1952), Ragnar Rylander (Rylander, 1968), Irving Selikoff (Selikoff *et al.*, 1965), Norman Staub (Kato and Staub, 1966), Walter Tyler (Tyler and Pearse, 1965), and Hanspeter Witschi (Witschi and Aldridge, 1968). These individuals and many others enable a better understanding of the deposition and effects of gases and particles on the respiratory tract.

RESPIRATORY TRACT STRUCTURE AND FUNCTION

Oronasal Passages

Structure The respiratory tract is divided into the upper respiratory tract (extrathoracic airway passages above the neck) and lower respiratory track (airway passages and lung parenchyma below the pharynx) (Harkema *et al.*, 2006) (Fig. 15-1). The upper respiratory track reaches from the nostril or mouth to the pharynx and functions to conduct, heat, humidify, filter, and chemosense incoming air. Leaving the nasal passage, air is warmed to about 33°C and humidified to about 98% water saturation. Air is filtered in the nasal passages with highly water-soluble gases being absorbed efficiently. The nasal passages also filter particles, which may be deposited by impaction or diffusion on the nasal mucosa. Many species, particularly mice and rats, are obligate nose breathers in

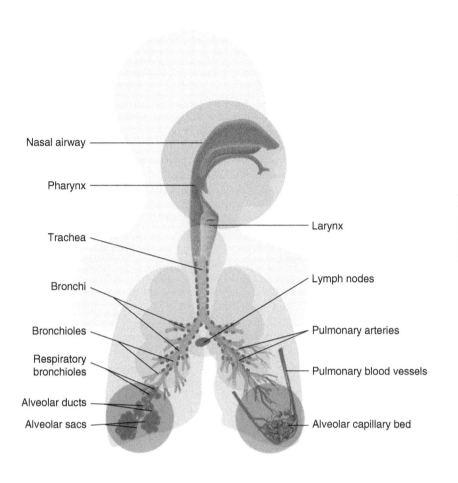

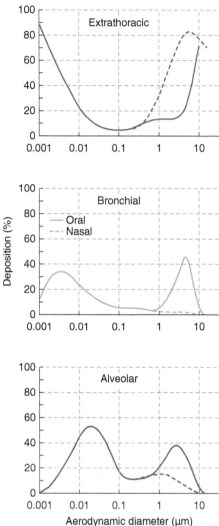

Figure 15-1. *Major regions of the respiratory tract and predicted fractional deposition of inhaled particles in the extrathoracic, bronchial, and alveolar region of the human respiratory tract during (solid line) oral or (dashed) nasal breathing.* (Adapted from Fig. 8 in Oberdörster *et al.* (2005) with drawing courtesy of J. Harkema and data from ICRP [1994].)

which air passes almost exclusively through the nasal passages. Other species, including humans, monkeys, and dogs, inhale air through both the nose and the mouth (oronasal breathers).

The surface area of oronasal region has been estimated to be 4700 cm². In mammals, the nasal passages are separated by a cartilaginous septum and the hard and soft palates form the base. Filtration, heating, and humidification are greatly aided by aqueous layer lining the mucosa and turbinates, which are perturbed from the lateral nasal walls. To warm the air, blood flow in the turbinates is retrograde to the inward direction of the air and can be modulated by pterygopalatine ganglion innervation of the venous plexus.

Turbinates vary in size and shape with the anterior being simple and the posterior being more complex. The airflow through the nasal passage is complex, and the narrowest region (smallest cross-sectional area) is located in the anterior aspect of the anterior turbinate. This region has the highest airflow and can be viewed as a nasal valve (ostium internum). The resistance of this region limits the amount of air that can be inhaled through the nose. In oronasal breathers, oral breathing can be initialed and will vary based on the workload, speech, and nasal congestion.

In humans, three flat turbinates are fairly simple structures. The inferior turbinates are the largest (~8 cm long) and are responsible for the majority of the control of airflow direction, humidification,

heating, and filtering of air inhaled through the nose. The smaller middle turbinates (~4–6 cm) project downward over the openings of the maxillary and ethmoid sinuses, and protect the sinuses from pressurized nasal airflow. Most of the inhaled air travels between the inferior turbinate and the middle turbinate. The superior turbinates are smaller structures and serve to protect the olfactory bulb. In rodents, the anterior portion of the nasal cavity contains a dorsal nasal turbinate and a ventral maxilloturbinate, both with simple scroll structures. Posterior to these turbinates are complex multiscrolled ethmoturbinates, which contain ~50% of the surface area of the rodent nasal passage. However, the amount of airflow over the ethmoturbinates region has been estimated to be only 10% to 15% of the air passing through the nose, and thus the complexity of this structure in rodents may contribute little additional risk of contact or damage.

The nasal passages are lined with stratified squamous epithelium in the anterior vestibule, nonciliated cuboidal/columnar epithelium in the anterior chamber, and ciliated pseudostratified respiratory epithelium in the remainder of the passage including the turbinates. The cell types of the nasal respiratory epithelium are similar to the cell types of the conducting airways. The turbinates also contain airflow pressure- and temperature-sensing neural receptors linked to the trigeminal nerve.

Sensory Functions In addition to conducting, conditioning, and filtering air to the lower respiratory tract, a major function of the oronasal passage is chemosensory (Morris, 2001; Feron *et al.*, 2001). Nasal epithelia can metabolize many foreign compounds by cytochrome P450 and other enzymes. Humans can distinguish between more than 5000 odors. The detection of odor can be protective and can induce avoidance behaviors. Odorant can be added to the otherwise colorless and almost odorless gas used by consumers (eg, mercaptans to methane), to assist in detecting leaks and thereby preventing fires or explosions.

Although the detection threshold concentrations can be low, a concentration only 10 to 50 times above the detection threshold value often is the maximum intensity that can be detected by humans. In contrast, the maximum intensity of sight or hearing is about 500,000 times and 1 to 10 trillion times that of the threshold intensity. For this reason, smell often identifies the presence or absence of odor rather than quantifies concentration. In addition, odor thresholds vary greatly between individuals (>1000 fold) and can be altered by allergies or nasal infections, and individuals can acclimate to odors. Some individuals cannot smell certain odors, for example, 0.1% cannot detect mercaptans in natural gas. Olfactory acuity also decreases with age (decreasing by 20%, 60%, and 70% at age of 20, 60, and 80 years). Therefore, about 30% of the elderly cannot detect mercaptans in natural gas. Lastly, odor thresholds for many compounds (eg, chlorinated solvents) are often higher than the Occupational Safety and Health Administration (OSHA) Permissible Exposure Limits (PELs). Therefore, odor should not be used as a measure of safety.

Chemosensory function of the nasal passages is accomplished by a wide variety of specialized receptors in major subtypes including (1) olfactory, (2) trace amine–associated receptors (TAARs), (3) membrane guanylyl cyclase GC-D, (4) vomeronasal, and (5) formyl peptide receptors (FPRs) (Table 15-1).

The olfactory epithelium contains specialized chemosensory olfactory neurons located above superior turbinates. Airflow in this region of the nasal passage is typical low, thus sniffing can increase perception. This may enable the assessment of multiple odors and strength of a smell through intermediate sampling. Capable of regeneration, olfactory neurons form the first cranial nerve and directly lead to the olfactory bulb in the brain. These cells have surface olfactory receptor proteins in cilia that interact with odorant molecules (DeMaria and Ngai, 2010). Olfactory receptors are 7-transmembrane domain G-protein–coupled receptors that mediate transduction of odorant signals through formation of cyclic adenosine monophosphate (cAMP) (Fleischer *et al.*, 2009). The olfactory receptor gene family is one of the largest in the genome, with over 400, 850, 1100, and 1200 members in humans, dogs, mice, and rats, respectively. Olfactory receptors are also involved in developmental

events, including the patterning of the olfactory sensory neuron synaptic connections in the brain.

Also in the olfactory region and originally identified because of activation by amine, TAARs detect trace amine (including 2-phenylethylamine, tyramine, tryptamine, and octopamine) and other substances (Fleischer *et al.*, 2009). Low-molecular-weight amines have a fishy or putrid odor. These odorants can be found in foods (including fish, chocolate, alcoholic beverages, cheese, soy sauce, sauerkraut, and processed meat) and can be generated during fermentation or decay. Certain trace amines are neurotransmitters and are found in the brain. Compared to olfactory receptors, the number of distinct TAAR subtypes is low (15 in mice and 6 in humans). In mouse urine, trace amine concentration varies by gender or during stress, suggesting that TAARs might be involved in the detection of "urine-borne" signals.

Another olfactory sensory neuron receptor is the membrane guanylyl cyclase GC-D receptor, which contains a cyclic guanosine monophosphate (cGMP)-dependent phosphodiesterase PDE2A and a cGMP-sensitive cyclic nucleotide-gated ion channel (Fleischer *et al.*, 2009). These receptors are localized to olfactory sensory neuron apical cilia and detect the natriuretic peptides: uroguanylin (which is also found in urine) and guanylin. In mice, GC-D receptors also can detect carbon dioxide by conversion into bicarbonate via carbonic anhydrase. In contrast to rodents, carbon dioxide is odorless to humans, and the GC-D gene is a pseudogene (ie, a gene that is present but does not yield a functional protein) in humans and other primates.

The main olfactory bulb is accompanied by the accessory olfactory bulb. Neurons from these two systems do not interconnect and the two systems function separately in the integration of specific chemicals. In rodents, the accessory olfactory bulb contains olfactory neurons that lead to the vomeronasal organ in the nose. Vomeronasal neurons can respond to olfactory stimuli that can be of higher molecular weight including nonvolatile chemicals (Touhara and Vosshall, 2009). Vomeronasal receptors exist in two protein families, VN1R and VN2R. These receptors are similar to pheromone receptors. Pheromones are chemical signals that elicit specific physiological and behavioral responses in recipients of the same species. Similar to olfactory receptor genes several vomeronasal genes exist in rodents, with few in humans, that is, 2, 8, 163, and 226 members in human, dogs, rats, and mice, respectively. Humans have not been demonstrated to generate or respond to pheromones. Expressed only during fetal gestation, vomeronasal receptors are thought to be merely vestigial in humans.

In addition, the vomeronasal organ contains FPRs that are activated by bacterial or mitochondrial formylated peptides (Fleischer *et al.*, 2009). These receptors were initially identified in leukocytes in which *N*-formyl-methionyl-leucyl-phenylalanine (fMLP)

Table 15-1

Oronasal Sensory Receptors I

RECEPTOR PROTEIN FAMILY	SYMBOL	LIGAND	HUMAN	MOUSE
Olfactory receptor	OR	Odorants	>400	>1200
Trace amine-associated receptor	TAAR	Amines	6	15
Guanylatecyclase, type D	GUCY	Natriuretic peptides	1	2
Vomeronasal receptor	VN1R/VN2R	Pheromones	2*	226
Formyl peptide receptors	FPR	*N*-Formyl-peptides	3	8

*Only expressed in fetus and may be vestigial.

Table 15-2

Oronasal Irritant, Thermo-, and Mechanosensory Receptors

RECEPTOR PROTEIN FAMILY	SYMBOL	LIGAND
Transient receptor potential channels	TRP	
Subfamily A (ANKTM1)	TRPA	Natural ingredients: allyl isothiocyanate (wasabi), cinamaldehyde, allicin and allyl sulfides (garlic), carvacrol, isovelleral, and polygodial
		Pain
		Cold (<17°C)
		Mechosenstory (Strech)
		Irritants (acrolein, isocyanates, tear gas, ozone, etc)
Subfamily C (Canonical)	TRPC	Mechanosensory
Subfamily M (Melastain)	TRPM2	Hydrogen peroxide
		Heat (>38°C)
	TRPM8	Menthol, eucaliptol
		Cold (<17°C)
Subfamily ML (Mucolipins)	MCOLN	Acid (low pH)
Subfamily P (Polycystic kidney disease)	PKD	Mechanosensory
		Acid (low pH)
Subfamily V (Vanilloid)	TRPV1	Capascin, allicin, and allyl sulfides (garlic)
		Moderate heat (≥43°C)
	TRPV2	High heat (>52°C)
Taste receptors	TAS	
Subfamily 1R	TAS1R	Umami (glutamate)
		Irritants (acrolein, isocyanates, tear gas, ozone, etc)
Subfamily 2R	TAS2R	Bitter
		Irritants (acrolein, isocyanates, tear gas, ozone, etc)
Subfamily 3R	TAS3R	Umami (glutamate)

mediates chemotaxis and cell activation. In the mouse vomeronasal epithelium, FPRs are activated by fMLP and other compounds (including lipoxin A4 and cathelicidin antimicrobial peptide) indicating that vomeronasal cells are likely to perform olfactory functions associated with the identification of pathogens or of pathogenic states, thereby enhancing detection of infected cells or contaminated food.

Two evolutionary hypotheses have been proposed to explain the large interspecies difference in the number of chemosensory receptor genes. One states that humans have developed full trichromatic vision and therefore do not need as many chemosensory receptor genes for finding food, mates, or supportive environments. The other is that the number of chemosensory receptor genes has expanded in the rodent lineage because rodents probably need a higher level of olfaction to survive in heterogeneous environments. However, dogs known for a good sense of smell have a smaller number of functional chemosensory receptor genes than mice or rats. This suggests that the relationship between the number of olfactory receptor genes and the sense of smell may not be straightforward. Even more complexity is suggested in that humans can detect certain odors at concentrations equal to or even below those detected by dogs or mice. One reason for this may be that olfactory perception also involves the brain. With a better memory, humans may have better olfactory ability from the small number of genes, particularly in detecting fine differences in food flavors.

Irritant, Thermosensory, and Mechanosensory Functions

In addition to the detection of odor, the detection of irritant chemicals, cold and hot temperatures, or mechanical stress can be a protective mechanism that may limit exposure. The main nerve endings that perceive irritants, the chemical nociceptors also discern temperature and mechanical stress. Two protein families, the transient receptor potential (TRP) channels and the taste (TAS) receptors, perform these functions in the upper respiratory tract (Table 15-2).

TRP channels are ion channels that are permeable to cations, including calcium, magnesium, and sodium. In mammals, 28 genes encode the TRP ion channel proteins that are divided into six subfamilies including TRPA (ANKTM1), TRPC (canonical), TRPM (melastatin), mucolipins (TRPML also known as [aka] MCOLN), polycystic kidney disease (autosomal dominant) (PCK or TRPP), and TRPV (vanilloid) families. TRPA1 and TRPV1 are the major irritant receptors in the nasal passage and are primarily within the trigeminal nerve (Bessac and Jordt, 2008). TRPA1 is responsive to a variety of natural ingredients including allyl isothiocyanate (in mustard and wasabi), cinnamaldehyde (in cinnamon), allicin and allyl sulfides (in garlic and onion), carvacrol (in oregano), isovelleral (a fungal deterrent), and polygodial (in Dorrigo pepper). TRPA1 is also responsive to pain stimuli, cold (≤17°C), stretch, and a wide range of chemical irritants. TRPV1 is responsive to capsaicin (in chili pepper) or moderate heat (≥43°C), whereas TRPV2 is responsive to higher heat (≥52°C). TRPM8 is responsive to menthol (in peppermint and cigarettes) and cold (≤28°C). Lysosomal protein, mucolipins are involved in the late endocytic pathway and in the regulation of lysosomal exocytosis. TRPC proteins are mainly located in the central nervous system and to a lesser extent in peripheral tissues. PCK1, TRPV5, and TRPV6 are calcium entry channels mainly found in the kidney and intestine.

Other chemonsensory receptors are taste receptors (TAS), which are divided into two types (Chandrashekar *et al.*, 2006). Taste buds determine salt, sour, sweet, umami (glutamates and nucleotides), and bitter. In the mouth, salt may be perceived by sodium ion channels, but this is controversial. Sour also may be perceived by hydrogen ion channels and possibly a TRP channel (polycystic kidney disease 2-like 1). Sweet and umami are perceived by type 1 receptors, which consist of three members (TAS1R1, TAS1R2, and TAS1R3). Taste variety is achieved by formation heterodimers of these proteins, for example, umami is detected by TAS1R1 and TAS1R3 heterodimers and through metabotropic glutamate receptors 1 and 4. Bitter taste is detected by type 2 receptors (TAS2Rs), which is a larger subfamily having over 35 members. Single solitary chemosensory cells (SCCs) are present in the nasal cavity and throughout the airways. In the mouse nose, SCCs contain both TAS1R and TAS2R, which can detect irritants and foreign substances that trigger trigeminally mediated protective airway reflexes.

Conducting Airways

Structure At the beginning of the lower respiratory track is the larynx, which is responsible for speech (phonation). The conducting airways of the lower respiratory tract can be divided into proximal (trachea and bronchi) and distal regions (bronchioles). Conducting airways have a bifurcating structure, with successive airway generations containing about twice the number of bronchi progressively decreasing in internal diameter. In humans, this branching pattern is referred to as irregular dichotomous (because some branches have more or less than two daughters) and resembles the pattern of an oak tree. In laboratory animals, the branching pattern is more monopodial and resembles the pattern of a pine tree. Successive branching has two consequences—it increases total surface area of the airway epithelium, and it increases the cumulative cross-section diameter of the airways. Thus, airflow is faster in the larger diameter proximal airways, whereas airflow is slower in the smaller distal airways. The latter is somewhat counterintuitive because flow through a smaller diameter increases in many incidences (as in a weir), but flow is slower because the larger number of small airways have a much larger cumulative diameter. Thus, the bifurcations of proximal airways are flow dividers and as airway bending points they serve as sites of impaction for particles. Successively narrower diameters ultimately lead to very slow airflows and thereby favor the collection of gases and particles on airway walls by radial diffusion. Eventually a transition zone is reached where cartilaginous airways (bronchi) give way to non-cartilaginous airways (bronchioles), which in turn give way to gas exchange regions, respiratory bronchioles, and alveoli. In the bronchiolar epithelium, mucus-producing cells and glands give way to bronchiolar secretoglobin cells (BSCs). The airflow is also altered by airway smooth muscle that surrounds the airways and is under autonomic innervation via the vagus nerve.

Mucociliary Clearance and Antimicrobial Functions In humans, the proximal airway and a portion of the nasal passage are covered by a pseudostratified respiratory epithelium that contains a number of specialized cells including ciliated, mucous, and basal cells (Fig. 15-2). These cells work together to form a mucous layer that traps and removes inhaled material via mucociliary clearance (Fahy and Dickey, 2010). The epithelial cells are covered by an upper mucus layer (a gel-like polymer network of high-molecular-weight mucins) and a lower periciliary liquid layer that separates the epithelial cell surface from the mucus layer. For mucociliary clearance in the airways to function optimally, regulation of ion transport, fluid, and mucus must be coordinated. To move fluid into the airway lumen, the large diameter airway epithelium can secrete chloride ion via chloride channels (Patel *et al.*, 2009) and

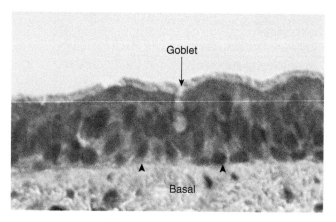

Figure 15-2. *Pseudo stratified respiratory epithelium lines the nasal cavity, trachea, and bronchi.* The surface includes mainly ciliated epithelial cells that may or may not touch the basement membrane, (arrow) surface mucous (goblet) cell, and (arrowhead) basal cells. Photomicrograph modified from the Human Protein Atlas (www.proteinatlas.org) (Uhlen *et al.*, 2010).

the cystic fibrosis transmembrane regulator (Chen *et al.*, 2010). To move water out of the lumen or alveolus, sodium ion is absorbed via sodium channels. These ionic gradients permit water movement that can travel pericellulary or through specialized proteins called aquaporins.

Ciliated cells have microtubule-based protrusions, cilia (Sanderson and Sleigh, 1981; Salathe, 2007). There are two general types of cilia: motile and primary. Motile cilia exert mechanical force through continuous motion to propel harmful inhaled material out of the nose and lung. Primary cilia often serve as sensory organelles. Motile cilia are ~6 to 10 μm in length with a tubulin-based axoneme motor. The axoneme of each cilia consists of nine outer doublets of microtubules and a single central pair of microtubules (9 + 2 structure) formed by heterodimers of α and β tubulin. In motile cilium, dynein heavy chains on one microtubule interact with an adjacent microtubule that enables ciliary movement through energy generated by ATPase. Primary cilium lack dynein and have 9 + 0 structure.

Ciliary beat frequency is about 12 to 15 Hz, which can change in response to cholinergic (acetylcholine) or purinergic (adenosine or ATP) stimuli that changes in the phosphorylation state of ciliary targets, in intracellular $[Ca^{2+}]$ and in intracellular pH. In addition to controlling ciliary beat frequency, calcium is also involved in synchronizing the beat among cilia of a single cell and between cilia on different cells (Schmid and Salathe, 2011). Adenosine acts through the adenosine A2b receptor (ADORA2B) (Allen-Gipson *et al.*, 2011). Motile cilia of the mammalian respiratory epithelium also exhibit both mechanosensory (via TRPV4) and chemosensory (via TAS2Rs) functions. TRPV4 channels respond to mechanical stress, heat, acidic pH, endogenous, and synthetic agonists, and activation leads to increases in intracellular calcium and ciliary beat frequency (Lorenzo *et al.*, 2008). In response to bitter compounds, TAS2Rs also increase the intracellular calcium and stimulate ciliary beat frequency (Shah *et al.*, 2009).

Mucus cells are full of lucid mucus granules. These granules increase in size as they move toward the apical cytoplasm, which produces a goblet shape and thus surface mucus cells are also called Goblet cells. Mucus consists mainly of water (95%) combined with salts, lipids, proteins, and mucin glycoproteins (Kesimer *et al.*, 2009; Ali *et al.*, 2011). Mucin glycoproteins provide the gel-like viscoelastic properties of mucus. Of the 20 identified membrane-associated or secretory mucin gene products, 16 have been identified in the airways (Leikauf, 2002b; Ali and Pearson, 2007).

Of these proteins, mucin 5, subtypes A and C (MUC5AC), and MUC5B are the predominant mucins and to a lesser extent MUC2, 7, 8, 11, 13, 19, and 20 are produced by goblet cells on the surface epithelium and mucus cells from submucosal glands (Rose and Voynow, 2006). Membrane-associated mucins in the airways include MUC1, MUC4, and MUC16. Mucus cells can secrete antimicrobial proteins including bactericidal permeablility increasing (BPI) protein, BPI fold containing family A, member 1 (BPIF1A) (aka palate, lung, and nasal epithelium associated 1 [PLUNC1]) and BPIF3 (Bingle and Bingle, 2011).

The pseudostratified epithelium also contains a basal cell with an apical membrane that does not make contact with the airway lumen (Evans *et al.*, 2001). These cells have desmosomal and hemidesmosomal attachments to other columnar cells and thereby anchor the respiratory epithelium. Positioned on basal lamina, basal cells can also interact with neurons, basement membrane, underlying mesenchymal cells, lymphocytes, and dendritic cells. Moreover, they can divide and differentiate into ciliated, goblet, or BC cells (Rock and Hogan, 2011).

Serous cells contain and secrete a less viscous fluid, and are also enriched in antimicrobial proteins including lysozyme and lactotransferin. In addition to surface epithelial cells, mucus and serous cells are contained in the submucosal glands limited mainly to the cartilaginous airways. The glands contain multiple branching tubules arranged with the proximal tubules contain mucus cells and the distal ascini contain serous cells. Submucosal glands secrete MUC5B, and MUC8, with MUC5B being predominate in submucosal glands, whereas surface mucus cells secrete mainly MUC5AC. Submucosal glands are contained in the cartilaginous airways (bronchi) in humans, but are minimal in rodents (especially mice). Serous cells contain the antimicrobial protein, BPIF2 (aka SPLUNC2). Secretory leukocyte proteinase inhibitor (SLPI) is a serine proteinase inhibitor that is produced locally in the lung by cells of the submucosal bronchial glands and by nonciliated epithelial cells. The main function of SLPI is the inhibition of neutrophil elastase and other proteinases, and may also have antimicrobial functions. Neutrophil elastase (ELANE) enhances SLPI mRNA levels while decreasing SLPI protein release in airway epithelial cells. In addition, glucocorticoids (which are used to treat airway inflammation) increase both constitutive and ELANE-induced SLPI mRNA levels (Abbinante-Nissen *et al.*, 1993; Sallenave, 2010). Other submucosal gland/nonciliated epithelial cell antiproteinase/antimicrobial proteins include peptidase 3, skin-derived (aka elafin), and whey acidic protein-type (WAF) 4-disulfide core domain 2.

Another airway secretory cell is the bronchiolar secretoglobin cell (BSC), previously called the Clara cell (Winkelmann and Noack, 2010). BSCs have an extensive endoplasmic reticulum and secretory granules containing secretoglobins including SCGB1A1 (aka CCSP or CC10). The roles of secretoglobins are not fully understood, but in the lung, SCGB1A1 can inhibit phospholipase A2 and limit inflammation. In humans, BSCs are found mainly in the distal airways and can act as tissue stem cells (Rock and Hogan, 2011). In mouse, BSCs are found throughout the airways and can become ciliated cells (Rawlins *et al.*, 2009) or mucus-producing cells (Chen *et al.*, 2009) and can express chitinases following inflammation (Homer *et al.*, 2006).

Neuroendocrine cells are contained in neuroepithelial bodies or separately in the proximal airways (Van Lommel, 2001) and contact can stimulate underlying sensory nerve fibers. They synthesize, store, and release bioactive substances including 5-hydroxytryptamine (aka serotonin), calcitonin-related polypeptide α (aka calcitonin), and gastrin-releasing peptide (aka bombesin). These cells express cholinergic receptor, nicotinic, α polypeptide 7 (Chrna7) and release serotonin in response to nicotine. Serotonin can also be released following hypoxia or mechanical strain. The release of these bioactive substances can redistribute pulmonary blood flow, and alter bronchomotor tone and immune responses (Cutz *et al.*, 2007). Pulmonary neuroendocrine cells and neuroepithelial bodies in the fetal and neonatal lung modulate airway development and these cells are linked to specific types of lung cancer.

Gas Exchange Region

Structure The gas exchange region consists of terminal bronchioles, respiratory bronchioles, alveolar ducts, alveoli, blood vessels, and lung interstitium (Fig. 15-3). Human lung has five lobes: the superior and inferior left lobes and the superior, middle, and inferior right lobes. In rat, mouse, and hamster, the left lung consists of a single lobe and the right lung is divided into four lobes: cranial, middle, caudal, and ancillary. A ventilatory unit is defined as an anatomical region that includes all alveolar ducts and alveoli distal to each bronchiolar–alveolar duct junction (Mercer and Crapo, 1991). Gas exchange occurs in the alveoli, which comprise ~85% of the total parenchymal lung volume. Adult human lungs contain an estimated 300 to 500 million alveoli. The ratio of total capillary

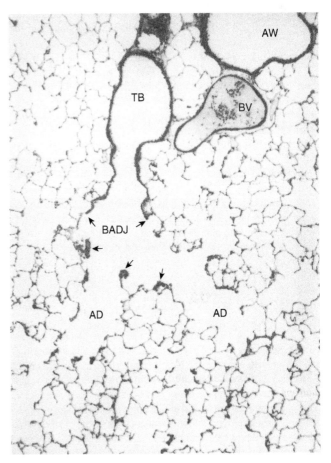

Figure 15-3. *Centriacinar region (ventilatory unit) of the lung.* An airway (AW) and a blood vessel (BV) (arteriole) are in close proximity to the terminal bronchiole (TB). The terminal bronchiole leads to the bronchiole–alveolar duct junction (BADJ) the alveolar duct (AD). A number of the (arrows) alveolar septal tips close to the BADJ are thickened after a brief (four-hour) exposure to asbestos fibers, indicating localization of fiber deposition. Other inhalants, such as ozone, produce lesions in the same locations. (Photograph courtesy of Dr Kent E. Pinkerton, University of California, Davis.)

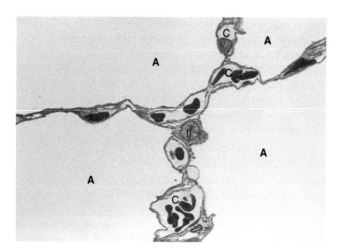

Figure 15-4. *Alveolar region of the lung.* The (A) alveolus is separated by the thin air-to-blood tissue barrier of the alveolar septal wall, which is composed of flat alveolar type I cells and occasional rounded (II) alveolar type II cells. A small interstitial space separates the epithelium and endothelium that form the (C) capillary wall. During lung injury the interstitial space enlarges and interferes with gas exchange. (Photograph courtesy of Dr Kent E. Pinkerton, University of California, Davis.)

surface to total alveolar surface is slightly less than one. Capillaries, blood plasma, and formed blood elements are separated from the air space by a thin layer of tissue formed by epithelial, interstitial, and endothelial components.

The alveolar epithelium consists of two cells, the alveolar type I and type II cell (Fig. 15-4). Alveolar type I cells cover ~95% of the alveolar surface and therefore are susceptible to damage by noxious agents that penetrate to the alveolus (Williams, 2003). Alveolar type I cells have an attenuated cytoplasm to enhance gas exchange. Alveolar type II cells are cuboidal and have abundant perinuclear cytoplasm, extensive secretory capacity, and contain secretory vesicles called lamellar bodies (Whitsett *et al.*, 2010). They produce surfactant, a mixture of lipids, and four surfactant associated proteins and can undergo mitotic division and replace damaged type I cells (Rock and Hogan, 2011). Surfactant protein B and C are amphipathic and aide in spreading secreted lipids which form a monolayer that reduces surface tension. Surfactant protein A1, A2, and D are members of the subfamily of C-type lectins called collectins, which defend against pathogens. Surfactant protein A1 and A2 do not alter lipid structure but do bind lipopolysaccharides (LPS) and various microbial pathogens, enhancing their clearance from the lung. Surfactant protein D is also necessary in the suppression of pulmonary inflammation and in host defense against viral, fungal, and bacterial pathogens. Like surfactant protein B and C, surfactant protein D does influence the structural form of pulmonary surfactant. Surfactant protein D also influences alveolar surfactant pool sizes and reuptake. The shape of type I and type II cells is independent of alveolar size and is remarkably similar in different species. A typical rat alveolus (14,000 μm² surface area) contains two type I cells and three type II cells, whereas a human alveolus with a surface area of 300,000 μm² contains ~30 type I cells and ~50 type II cells (Pinkerton *et al.*, 1991).

The mesenchymal interstitial cell population consists of fibroblasts and myofibroblasts that produce collagen and elastin as well as other cell matrix components and various effector molecules. Pericytes, monocytes, and lymphocytes also reside in the interstitium, as do macrophages before they enter the alveoli. Endothelial cells have a thin cytoplasm and cover about one-fourth of the area covered by type I cells.

Function

Ventilation The principal function of the lung is gas exchange, which consists of ventilation, perfusion, and diffusion. The lung is superbly equipped to handle its main task: bringing essential oxygen to the organs and tissues of the body and eliminating its most abundant waste product, CO_2 (Weibel, 1983).

During inhalation, fresh air is moved into the lung through the upper respiratory tract and conducting airways and into the terminal respiratory units when the thoracic cage enlarges and the diaphragm moves downward; the lung passively follows this expansion. The thoracic cage enlarges by the constriction of external intercostal and internal intercondral muscles, which elevate the sternum and ribs and thus increase the width of the thoracic cavity. When the parenchyma of the lung expands during inhalation, force is transferred to the airways (especially the small diameter distal airways), which increases the airway diameter and diminishes obstruction to airflow. After diffusion of oxygen into the blood and that of CO_2 from the blood into the alveolar spaces, the air (now enriched in CO_2) is expelled by exhalation. Relaxation of the chest wall and diaphragm diminishes the internal volume of the thoracic cage, the elastic fibers of the lung parenchyma recoil, and air is expelled from the alveolar zone through the airways. Any interference with the elastic properties of the lung, for example, the alteration of elastic fibers that occurs in emphysema, adversely affects ventilation, as do the decrease in the diameters of, or blockage of, the conducting airways, as in asthma.

Lung function changes with age and disease and can be measured with a spirometer (Fig. 15-5). The total lung capacity (TLC) is the total volume of air in an inflated human lung, 4 to 5 L (women) and 6 to 7 L (men) (American Thoracic Society [ATS], 1991). After a maximum expiration, the lung retains 1.1 L (women) and 1.2 L (men), which is the residual volume (RV). The functional residual capacity and residual volume cannot be measured with spirometry and are determined by several other methods including nitrogen washout, in which the concentration of nitrogen is measured in expired air following inhalation of 100% oxygen. The vital capacity is the air volume moved into and out of the lung during maximal

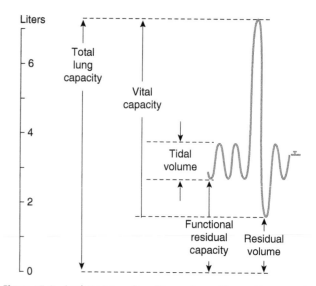

Figure 15-5. *A spirometer reading of lung volumes.* The total lung capacity is the total volume of air in an inflated human lung. After a maximum expiration, the lung retains a small volume of air, which is the residual volume. The air volume moved into and out of the lung during maximal inspiratory and expiratory movement, which is called the vital capacity. The tidal volume is typically moved into and out of the lung during each breathe. The functional residual capacity and residual volume cannot be measured with spirometer.

inspiratory and expiratory movement and typical is 3.1 L (women) and 4.8 L (men). Only a small fraction of the VC, the tidal volume (TV), is typically moved into and out of the lung during quiet breathing. In resting humans, the TV measures ~0.5 L with each breath. The respiratory frequency, or the number of breaths per minute, is 12 to 20 (thus the resting ventilation is about 6–8 L/min). During exercise, both the TV and the respiratory rate can increase markedly. The amount of air moved into and out of the human lung may increase from 12 to 15 L/min to 40 to 60 L/min with light and moderate exercise, respectively. Increased ventilation in a polluted atmosphere increases the deposition of inhaled toxic material. Thus, susceptible individuals, particularly children and the elderly, should not exercise during episodes of heavy air pollution.

Lung function changes with age and disease and can be measured by a forced expiratory maneuver with a spirometer. In this test, an individual first inhales maximally and then exhales as rapidly as possible. The volume of air expired in one second, called the forced expiratory volume 1 second (FEV1), and the total amount expired, forced vital capacity (FVC), and the ratio of FEV1/FVC, are good measures of the recoil capacity and airway obstruction of the lung. In a healthy individual the FEV1/FVC = ~80%. In chronic obstructive pulmonary disease (COPD), the parenchyma recoil is compromised, small airways close during exhalation obstructing airflow, and more air is trapped in the lung (Fletcher and Peto, 1977). Although the FVC may stay the same or may even increase slightly, narrowed small airways slow airflow at low lung volumes and thereby decrease FEV1. Thus, the FEV1/FVC is also decreased and airflow is considered obstructed when FEV1/FVC is >70% of predicted value (based on sex, height, and age). The decreased FVC is accompanied by an increase in RV. If part of the lung collapses, becomes filled with edema fluid, or is restricted due to altered lung collagen (fibrosis), FEV1, and FVC are equally reduced.

Perfusion The lung receives the entire output from the right ventricle, ~75 mL of blood per heartbeat. Blood with high CO_2 and low O_2 travels to the lung via the pulmonary artery and leaves the lung with high O_2 and low CO_2 via the pulmonary vein. The bronchi also have independent circulation with O_2-enriched blood supplied by an artery. Substantial amounts of toxic chemicals carried in the blood can be delivered to the lung. A chemical placed onto or deposited under the skin (subcutaneous injection) or introduced directly into a peripheral vein (intravenous injection) travels through the venous system to the right ventricle and then comes into contact with the pulmonary capillary bed before distribution to other organs or tissues in the body.

Diffusion Gas exchange takes place across the entire alveolar surface. Contact with an airborne toxic chemical thus occurs over a surface of ~140 m². This surface area is second only to the small intestine (~250 m²) and is considerably larger than the skin (~2 m²), two other organs that are in direct contact with the outside world. A variety of abnormal processes may severely compromise the unhindered diffusion of oxygen to the erythrocytes. Acute events may include collection of liquid in the alveolar or interstitial space and disruption of pulmonary surfactant system. Chronic toxicity can impair diffusion due to abnormal alveolar architecture or abnormal formation and deposition of extracellular substances such as collagen in the interstitium.

BIOTRANSFORMATION IN THE RESPIRATORY TRACT

Often overlooked as an organ involved in metabolism of chemicals, in favor of the liver, the lung has substantial capabilities for biotransformation (see Chap. 6). Total lung cytochrome P450 (CYP) activity is roughly one-tenth to one-third of that in the liver. However, when specific activity in a few cell types is considered, the difference is only twofold for many enzymes, and in the case of nasal mucosa, higher enzyme activity is reported per cell (Buckpitt and Cruikshank, 1997). Metabolic competence in the lung and nasal tissues is concentrated in a few cell types and these have a defined, and sometimes limited, the distribution in the respiratory tract that can vary substantially by species (Table 15-3). The balance of activation and inactivation is a critically important determinant of lung protection from injury. Protection from oxidation is another important function of enzymes in high tissue oxygen concentration that occurs in the respiratory tract. Other factors that can influence the role of phase I and phase II systems in lung toxicity include age, sex, diet, local inflammation, and the history of prior exposure (Plopper *et al.*, 2001). Interestingly, many xenobiotic metabolizing enzymes have different patterns of induction (less) in the respiratory tract than in the liver, leading to the concept that regulation of these systems may be different depending on where they are located (Buckpitt and Cruikshank, 1997).

Table 15-3

Distribution of Xenobiotic Metabolizing Enzymes in the Respiratory Tract

	EPITHELIUM					
ENZYME	NASAL TISSUE	PROXIMAL AIRWAY	DISTAL AIRWAY	ALVEOLAR	MACROPHAGE	ENDOTHELIUM
Cytochrome P450 monooxygenases	+++	++	+++	++	++	++
Microsomal epoxide hydrolases	+++	++	+++	++	+	++
Flavin monooxygenases	+	++	+++	++	−	+
Prostaglandin-endoperoxide synthase 1	++	++	++	±	++	−
Prostaglandin-endoperoxide synthase 2	++	+	++	±	+++	++
Gluthathione-S-transferases	+	++	+++	+	Unknown	Unknown
Glucuronsyl transferases	+	Unknown	++	+	Unknown	Unknown
Sulfotransferases	++	+	+	±	Unknown	Unknown

Code: +++, most isoforms highly expressed; ++, some isoforms highly expressed; +, low expression; ±, low expression found in some studies but not others.

The major phase I enzyme system, the CYP monooxygenases (Nebert and Dalton, 2006), is concentrated into a few lung cells: BSCs, alveolar type II cells, macrophages, and endothelial cells. Of these cell types, BSCs have the most CYP, followed by the type II cells. The amount of total lung CYP contributed by BSCs is species-dependent, with humans having less CYP in their lungs from BSCs than mice or rats. Furthermore, the CYP isoforms present and their location in the respiratory tract also vary by species. For an extrahepatic tissue, CYPs are expressed at high levels in the nasal mucosa and this pattern of expression varies by nasal region and cell type (Thorton-Manning and Dahl, 1997; Ding and Kaminsky, 2003; Harkema et al., 2006). Most species have CYPs in nasal tissue and some are predominantly expressed in the olfactory mucosa (eg, CYP2G1, CYP2A3, and CYP2A13) (Ling et al., 2004). Metabolism by the olfactory epithelium may play a role in providing or preventing access of inhalants directly to the brain; for example, inhaled xylene may be converted into metabolites that move to the brain by axonal transport (Ghantous et al., 1990). The presence of the following CYP isozymes in the respiratory tract of at least one species has been reported: CYP1A1, CYP1A2, CYP1B1, CYP2A3, CYP2A6, CYP2A10/2A11, CYP2B1/4, CYP2B6, CYP2B7, CYP2E1, CYP2F1/2/4, CYP2S1, CYP2J2, CYP2G1, CYP3A4, CYP3A5, CYP3A7, and CYP4B1 (Hukkanen et al., 2002; Anttila et al., 2011).

Other phase I enzymes found in lung tissue include epoxide hydrolases, flavin monooxygenases, prostaglandin (PG)-endoperoxide synthases, carbonyl reductases, and NAD(P)H:quinone oxidoreductase 1 (NQO1). The only constant feature of the expression of these enzymes is lack of uniformity in their expression by cell type and region throughout the lung and their tendency to concentrate in epithelia. Both microsomal (EPHX1) and cytosolic (EPHX2) epoxide hydrolases are found in the lung and nasal tissues, and the activity of microsomal epoxide hydrolase can be higher in the distal airways of the lung than in the liver (Bond et al., 1988). Functional variants of EPHX1 have been associated with respiratory diseases including lung cancer (Kiyohara et al., 2006), childhood asthma (Salam et al., 2007), and possibly COPD (Hu et al., 2008; Lee et al., 2011). Flavin monooxygenase activity (FMO1 and FMO2) is found in rodent and human lung and nasal tissue. The isoforms present in the lung (FMO2) are different from those found in the liver (FMO1). FMO1 is the predominant isoform in the nasal mucosa (Shehin-Johnson et al., 1995; Henderson et al., 2008). The gene for FMO2 in human lung contains a premature stop codon encoding production of an inactive protein, but some ethnic groups have at least one copy of an allele that expresses the full-length protein (Whetstine et al., 2000). PG-endoperoxide synthases (aka cyclooxygenases) oxidize substrates at a much lower rate than CYP monooxygenases but may have a role in human pulmonary metabolism due to the relatively lower CYP activity in human lung tissue compared to rodents (Smith et al., 1991).

Carbonyl reductase (especially carbonyl reductase 2) enables pulmonary metabolism of endogenous carbonyl compounds, such as aliphatic aldehydes and ketones, 3-ketosteroids, fatty aldehydes, and PGs (converting PGE2 to PGF2α). NQO1 reduces quinones to hydroquinones, which then can be acted upon by NADH CYP reductase to generate semiquinone free radicals. In the lung, NQO1 activates carcinogenic heterocyclic amines found in cigarette smoke (De Flora et al., 1994), whereas NQO1 prevents formation of benzo[a]pyrene–quinone DNA adducts (Joseph and Jaiswal, 1994). Genetic polymorphisms in NQO1 are associated with lung cancer (Kiyohara et al., 2005) and susceptibility to ozone (Minelli et al., 2011).

Phase II enzymes include glutathione-S-transferases (GSTs) (alpha, mu, and pi), glucuronsyl transferases, and sulfotransferases (SULTs). GSTs (and glutathione) and play a major role in the modulation of both acute and chronic chemical toxicity in the lung

(West et al., 2000). A key point to keep in mind is that these enzyme systems work in concert with one another (ie, a decrease in one enzyme may result in a concomitant increase in another) and it is the combined action of all of these enzymes, and their location, that determines toxicity. The regulation of many of these enzymes is under coordinated control of the transcription factor nuclear factor, erythroid derived 2, like 2 (aka NRF2) (Slocum and Kensler, 2011).

A major determinant of the potential for detoxification may also be the cellular localization of, and ability to synthesize, glutathione in the lung. Pulmonary GST activity is 5% to 15% that of the liver in rodents and about 30% of that in human liver (Buckpitt and Cruikshank, 1997). The distribution of the isoforms of glutathione S-transferase varies by lung region with the alpha, mu, and pi isoforms (the most abundant), and the alpha and pi classes predominate in the airway epithelium of human lung. In nasal tissue, glutathione S-transferases are found in the olfactory mucosa. The mu isoform has a zonal pattern of expression increased in the lateral olfactory turbinates of the mouse (Whitby-Logan et al., 2004). Polymorphisms in glutathione transferases genes have been associated with a possible increase in risk of developing lung cancer, particularly in smokers (Jourenkova-Mironova et al., 1998). The GSTM1 genotype is one of the most widely analyzed genetic variants for lung cancer and an increased risk has been noted among null carriers (Shi et al., 2008).

The activity of glucuronosyl transferase has been reported in both rodent and human nasal and pulmonary tissue. Glucoronosyl transferase (UGT2A1) is thought to have a role in termination of odorant signals (Lazard et al., 1991). The detoxification enzyme in the metabolism of polycyclic aromatic hydrocarbons (PAHs) within target tissues for tobacco carcinogens and functional polymorphisms in UGT2A1 may play a role in tobacco-related cancer risk (Bushey et al., 2011). Sulfotransferase activity has been demonstrated in human bronchoscopy samples (Gibby and Cohen, 1984) and SULT2B1 is immunochemically localized to the olfactory epithelium and conducting airway epithelium (He et al., 2005). Sulfotransferases have been localized to the sustentacular cells of the olfactory epithelium and some isoforms may be specific to the olfactory epithelium (Tamura et al., 1998). In lung endothelial and epithelial cells, SULT1A3 could play a role in the inactivation and/or disposal of excess chlorotyrosine (Yasuda et al., 2011).

GENERAL PRINCIPLES IN THE PATHOGENESIS OF LUNG DAMAGE CAUSED BY CHEMICALS

Toxic Inhalants, Gases, and Dosimetry

In inhalation toxicology, exposure is measured as a concentration (compound mass per unit of air). Typically highly toxic compounds can produce adverse effects in a concentration of mg/m^3 or $\mu g/m^3$. A m^3 is 1000 L. For gases, concentration may also be expressed as volume to volume of air, that is, parts per million (ppm) or parts per billion (ppb). This can be calculated from the mass per unit air by using the ideal gas law to determine the gas's volume. Concentration is useful because it can be measured by many air-sampling methods that rely on many chemical analytical methods. Large volumes of air can be collected so that low levels (ie, ppb) can be detected. Exposure does not equate to dose (compound mass per unit), which requires a measure of mass of the organ, cell, or subcellular target.

The sites of deposition of gases in the respiratory tract define the pattern of toxicity of those gases. Solubility, diffusivity, and metabolism/reactivity in respiratory tissues and breathing rate are the critical factors in determining how deeply a given gas penetrates into the lung (Asgharian et al., 2011; Gloede et al., 2011). Highly soluble gases such as SO_2 or formaldehyde do not penetrate farther than the nose (during nasal breathing) unless doses are very high, and are therefore relatively nontoxic to the lung of rats (which are obligatory nasal breathers). However, formaldehyde causes cancer in the rat nasal passages (Albert *et al.*, 1982). Relatively insoluble gases such as ozone and NO_2 penetrate deeply into the lung and reach the smallest airways and the alveoli (centriacinar region), where they can elicit toxic responses. Mathematical models of gas entry and deposition in the lung predict sites of lung lesions fairly accurately. These models may be useful for extrapolating findings made in laboratory animals to humans (Asgharian *et al.*, 2011; Gloede *et al.*, 2011). Very insoluble gases such as CO and H_2S efficiently pass through the respiratory tract and are taken up by the pulmonary blood supply to be distributed throughout the body.

Regional Particle Deposition

Because of the architecture of the airways that modulate airflow, particle size is a critical factor in determining the region of the respiratory tract in which a particle will be deposited. Deposition of particles on the airway mucosal surface is brought about by a combination of aerodynamic forces and particle characteristics (Lippmann *et al.*, 1980; International Commission on Radiological Protection [ICRP], 1994; Lippmann and Leikauf, 2009). The efficiency of particle deposition in various regions of the respiratory tract depends mainly on particle size.

Aerosols are dispersed solids or liquids. Particles in air are classified by particle size (Lippmann and Leikauf, 2009). Size controls particle shape and thus influences light-scattering properties or deposition by interception. Size also controls particle mass and thus influences the probability for coagulation, dispersion, sedimentation, and impaction. Aerosols are a population of particles that can be monodispersed (essential of one size like pollens) or more typically, heterodispersed (many difference sizes). Particles generated from a single source typically have diameters that are lognormal (Poisson) distributed. This distribution will become Gaussian when plotted on a log scale and the distribution's central tendency is expressed as the mass median diameter (MMD). This measure of central tendency is accompanied by the measure of variability called the geometric standard deviation (σ_g). Monodispersed aerosols are typically defined as having a low σ_g (typically <1.2). Because the density (eg, plutonium) and the shape (eg, asbestos fibers) of aerosols can vary greatly, MMD is normalized to a unit-density sphere and is referred to as the mass median aerodynamic diameter (MMAD). In the following discussion the particle size are MMADs. Particle surface area is of special importance when toxic materials are adsorbed on particles and thus are carried into the lung.

In respiratory toxicology, aerosols (particles dispersed into air) include any of the following: (1) dusts (≥1.0 μm particles generated by mechanical division as in grinding), (2) fumes (≤0.1 μm particles generated by condensation of vapors as in heat metals or oils), (3) smoke (≤0.5 μm complex carbon particles generated condensation of products from combustion), (4) mists (2–50 μm water droplet or solutions generated by mechanical shearing of bulk liquid as in spraying), (5) fog (≤1.0 μm water droplets generated by water vapor condensation on atmospheric nuclei), or (6) smog (≥0.01–50 μm air pollution generated by stationary and mobile pollution source) (Lippmann and Leikauf, 2009). Haze has been used to describe either a dilute fog (at lower humidity) or smog. Smaller aerosols include submicrometer particles ($0.1 \leq x \leq 1.0$ μm), nanometer particles or nanoparticles (≤0.1 μm). All these distinguishing forms are included in the term "aerosol" or "particle."

Aerosols are typically dynamic and change by processes including dilution, dispersion, coagulation, and chemical reaction

(Pandis, 2004). Atmospheric particles originate either as primary particles—by direct emission from a source—or as secondary particles—through atmospheric formation from the gas phase constituents (nucleation) (Fig. 15-6). Atmospheric particles are typically distributed into two modes and five submodes (John *et al.*, 1990).

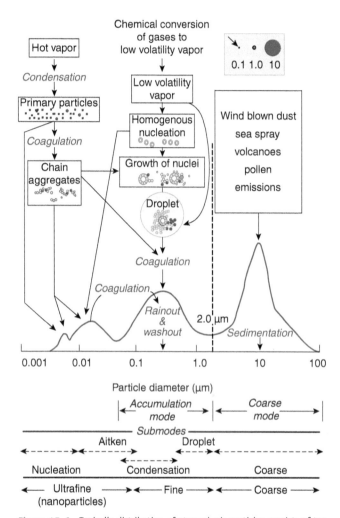

Figure 15-6. *Typically distribution of atmospheric particles consists of two major modes and five submodes.* The Accumulation and Coarse modes dominate the particle mass and Nucleation and Aitken submodes dominate the particle number. Nucleation particles are generated from gas phase emissions. Condensation can occur as plumes cool and particles and gases emitted together interact. Particles in the first two submodes typically have very short half-lives as singlet primary particles. The condensation submode is formed from the coagulation of smaller solid particles and condensation of gases including sulfates, nitrates, and organics on the particles' surface. They can be formed from chain aggregates of numerous particles of smaller diameter or also can be spherical with liquid surfaces. Particles move from the smaller submodes into the accumulation mode and these larger particles can have very long half-lives (hours to days) in the atmosphere and can travel over long distances. When the atmospheric relative humidity is very high (near 100%), particles in the accumulation mode seed rain droplets and are removed from the atmosphere. The coarse particles consist of particles >2.0 μm that are generated by mechanical processes or suspension of surface dust. Many of the particles in this range can be from natural sources (eg, wind blown desert sand). Particles larger than 50 μm readily settle and are removed from the atmosphere within minutes. Human exposure to these large particles is typically occupational (eg, dust from grinding wheels or wood sanding that is inhaled due to proximity to the source). Inset: The volume and therefore mass is to the cubed root of the radius is illustrated for difference in three orders of magnitude. This and the physical forces that maintain particles in the atmosphere are why the mass is mainly in the accumulation and coarse modes.

The two modes are the accumulation and coarse mode, which dominate the particle volume (and therefore mass) distribution.

Dominating the particle number distribution are the nucleation and Aitken submodes. The smallest nucleation submode particles are generated from gas phase emissions. This mode is dominated by a large number of nanoparticles ≤0.01 μm, but because they are so small they do not add much to the cumulative volume and therefore have little mass. For example, typical urban atmospheres can have 100,000 nucleation submode particles per cubic meter of air, but the total weight of all these particles is only about 50 ng (which is less than 0.5% of a typical urban atmosphere). The second submode is the Aitken nucleus submode, which also consists of nanoparticles $(0.01 \leq x \leq 0.1 \, \mu m)$. Like the nucleation submode, particles in the Aitken nucleus submode can be formed by chemical conversion of gases from combustion processes or can be freshly generated as primary particles. This mode is named after John Aitken, an atmospheric scientist interested in cloud physics (Aitken, 1880). Most Aitken particles are primary particles that have grown due to material condensing on their surface as they move through the atmosphere. Condensation can occur as plumes cool and particles and gases emitted together interact. Particles in the first two submodes typically have very short half-lives as singlet primary particles. This is because their motion is influenced by collision with gas molecules and other particles that lead them to coagulate, especially around larger, slower moving particles.

The next largest submode is the condensation submode $(0.05 \leq x \leq 0.5 \, \mu m)$. These particles are formed from the coagulation of smaller solid particles and condensation of gases including sulfates, nitrates, and organics on the particles' surface. They can be formed from chain aggregates of numerous particles of smaller diameter or also can be spherical with liquid surfaces. When these particles are hydroscopic and in a humid atmosphere, the size can increase to about 0.5 to 2.0 μm and become the droplet submode. Particles in the condensation and droplet submode contribute to the accumulation mode. These particles can have very long half-lives (hours to days) in the atmosphere and can travel over long distances from sources because they are too few in number for rapid coagulation and too small for gravitational sedimentation. Particles in this mode can travel from one state to another (eg, from the Ohio River Valley to the eastern seaboard), or even across oceans (from China to California). When the atmospheric relative humidity is very high (near 100%), particles in the accumulation mode seed rain droplets and are removed from the atmosphere. In addition, submicrometer particles have high light scattering properties that contribute to low visibility during pollution episodes. The second mode is the coarse particle and contains the coarse submode, which are particles >2.0 μm that are generated by mechanical processes or suspension of surface dust. Many of the particles in this range can be from natural sources (eg, wind blown desert sand). Particles larger than 50 μm settle readily and are removed from the atmosphere within minutes. Human exposure to these large particles is typically occupational (eg, dust from grinding wheels or wood sanding that is inhaled due to proximity to the source).

The upper respiratory tract is very efficient in removing particles that are very large (>10 μm) or very small (<0.01 μm) (Fig. 15-1). During nasal breathing, 1 to 10 μm particles are usually deposited in the upper nasopharyngeal region or the first five generations of large conducting airways. During oral breathing, deposition of these particles can increase in the tracheobronchial airways and alveolar region. Smaller particles (0.001–0.1 μm) can also be deposited in the trancheobronchial region. Particles ranging from 0.003 to 5 μm can be transported to the smaller airways and deposited in the alveolar region. Patterns of breathing can change the site of deposition of a particle of a given size. It must be kept in mind that the size of a particle may change during inspiration before deposition in the respiratory tract. Materials that are hygroscopic, such as sodium chloride, sulfuric acid, and glycerol, take on water and grow in size in the warm, saturated atmosphere of the upper and lower respiratory tract. Because adverse health effects of ambient particles have been associated with particles that were <10 μm, and subsequently <2.5 μm particles, the United States Environmental Protection Agency standard for ambient particulate matter (PM) is set at <2.5 μm particles, which is called $PM_{2.5}$ (see Chap. 29).

Deposition Mechanisms

In the respiratory tract, particles deposit by impaction, interception, sedimentation, diffusion (Brownian movement), and electrostatic deposition (for positively charged particles only) (Lippmann *et al.*, 1980; ICRP, 1994; Lippmann and Leikauf, 2009) (Fig. 15-7). Impaction occurs in the upper respiratory tract and large proximal airways where the airflow is faster than in the small distal airways because the cumulative diameter is smaller in the proximal airways. Fast airflow imparts momentum to the inhaled particle, and it is the particle's inertia that causes it to continue to travel along its original path. In airstream bends, such as an airway bifurcation, larger diameter particles deviate from the airflow and impact on the surface. In humans, most >10 μm particles are deposited in the nose or oral pharynx and cannot penetrate tissues distal to the larynx. For 2.5 to 10 μm particles, impaction continues to be the mechanism of deposition in the first generations of the tracheobronchial region.

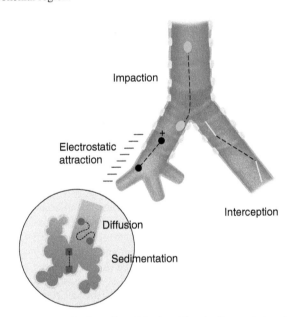

Figure 15-7. *Mechanism of particle deposition in the respiratory tract.* Impaction occurs in the upper respiratory tract and large proximal airways where fast airflow imparts momentum to the inhaled particle. The particle's inertia causes it to continue to travel along its original path and deposit on the airway surface. Interception occurs when the trajectory of a particle brings it near enough to a surface so that an edge of the particle contacts the airway surface. Sedimentation controls deposition in the smaller bronchi, the bronchioles, and the alveolar spaces, where the airways are small and the velocity of airflow is low. Sedimentation is dependent on the time a particle is in a compartment (ie, an alveolus) and can be increased by breath holding. Diffusion is an important factor in the deposition of submicrometer particles. Electrostatic deposition is a minor deposition mechanism for positively charged particles. The surface of the airways is negatively charged and attracts positively charged particles (adapted from Lippmann and Leikauf, 2009).

Interception occurs when the trajectory of a particle brings it near enough to a surface so that an edge of the particle contacts the airway surface. Interception is important for all particles but is particularly important in the deposition of fibers. Although fiber diameter determines the probability of deposition by impaction and sedimentation, interception is dependent on fiber length. Thus, a fiber with a diameter of 1 μm and a length of 200 μm will be deposited in the bronchial tree primarily by interception rather than impaction. Interception is also important for submicrometer particles in the tracheobronchial region where inertial airflow directs a disproportionately large fraction of the flow volume toward the surface of small airway bifurcations.

Sedimentation controls deposition in the smaller bronchi, the bronchioles, and the alveolar spaces, where the airways are small and the velocity of airflow is low. Indeed, in the alveoli, there is no bulk airflow. As a particle moves through air, buoyancy and the resistance of air act on the particle in an upward direction while gravitational force acts on the particle in a downward direction. Eventually, the gravitational force equilibrates with the sum of the buoyancy and the air resistance, and the particle continues to settle with a constant velocity known as the terminal settling velocity. Sedimentation is not a significant route of particle deposition when the aerodynamic diameter is ≤0.5 μm. Sedimentation is dependent on the time a particle is in a compartment (ie, an alveolus) and can be increased by breath holding.

Diffusion is an important factor in the deposition of submicrometer particles. A random motion is imparted to these particles by collisions with gas molecules. Thus, the ratio of a particle's mass to the momentum of the colliding gas molecules controls the distance the particle will travel. Larger particles are hardly moved by a gas molecule, whereas nanometer particles can be moved extensively. Diffusion is an important deposition mechanism in the nose, airways, and alveoli for particles ≤0.5 μm. Nanometer particles (0.1 μm and smaller) are also trapped relatively efficiently in the upper airways by diffusion. Particles that penetrate beyond the upper airways are available to be deposited in the bronchial region and the deep-lying airways. Therefore, the alveolar region has significant deposition efficiencies for particles smaller than 5 μm and larger than 0.01 μm.

During quiet breathing, in which the TV is only two to three times the volume of the anatomic dead space (ie, the volume of the conducting airways where gas exchange does not occur), a large proportion of the inhaled particles may be exhaled. During exercise, when larger volumes are inhaled at higher velocities, impaction in the large airways and sedimentation and diffusion in the smaller airways and alveoli increase. Breath holding also increases deposition from sedimentation and diffusion. Cigarette smoke is hydroscopic aerosol of nicotine-laden particles that grow to a median diameter of about 0.5 to 1.0 μm. Thus, a smoker's respiratory pause at the end of inhalation increases alveolar sedimentation and thereby nicotine delivery to the alveolar surface and to the blood upon absorption.

Electrostatic deposition is a minor deposition mechanism for positively charged particles. The surface of the airways is negatively charged and attracts positively charged particles. Freshly fractured mineral dust particles and laboratory-generated aerosols from evaporation of aqueous droplets can have substantial electrostatic mobilities.

Factors that modify the diameter of the conducting airways can alter particle deposition. In patients with chronic bronchitis or pneumonia, the airway lining fluid can greatly thicken and may partially block the airways in some areas. Sonic jets (eg, during wheezing and rales) formed by high air flowing through such partially occluded airways have the potential to increase the deposition of particles by impaction and diffusion in the small airways. Irritant materials that produce bronchoconstriction tend to increase the proximal tracheobronchial deposition of particles.

Nanoparticles are particles with at least one dimension of ≤100 nm. They are made from a variety of materials including carbon (eg, 60 carbon $[C_{60}]$ fullerenes, nanotubes, or nanowires), metals (eg, gold, silver, or quantum dots), or metal oxides (eg, cerium oxide, titanium dioxide, or zinc oxide). Engineered biological nanoparticles include liposomes and viruses designed for gene or drug delivery. These particles can be generated in a wide array of dimensions and physicochemical properties. For example, carbon nanotubes can be single-walled (ie, SWCNT) or multiwalled (ie, MWCNT) and generated at various lengths (>1.0 μm). Carbon nanotubes can have many surface modifications (eg, metal coat) or can be core loaded. In addition, nanoparticles make up a portion (small by mass, but large by number and surface area) of emissions from vehicle engines, especially diesel engines, and industrial furnaces and burners. The toxicity of nanoparticles may be enhanced over large particles because of an increased surface area that can provide a biological reactive surface that can generate secondary reaction products (eg, reactive oxygen species) or may provide an inert surface that carries adsorbed copollutants (Oberdörster *et al.*, 2005). Commercial nanoparticles are often rod shaped with lengths of 5 to 10 μm and thereby share aspect properties with asbestos (see below) (Donaldson *et al.*, 2010). Additional concern about potential toxicity of nanoparticles is triggered by epidemiological studies that associate increased mortality in sensitive populations with increased ambient PM exposure (see Chap. 29). Lastly, nanoparticles may have increased toxicity because normal host defenses may have limited effectiveness against these particles. These particles may be too small to be recognized by macrophage and because nanoparticles can move through membranes, these particles can escape from phagosomes (see Chap. 28).

Particle Clearance

Lung defense is dependent on particle clearance (Table 15-4). Rapid removal lessens the time available to cause damage to the pulmonary tissues or permit local absorption (Lippmann *et al.*, 1980). However, it is important to remember that particle clearance is not equivalent to complete protection for many reasons. An inert particle that can penetrate to the alveolar region can be a vehicle carrying adsorbed toxic gases. Once deposited in the lung, the adsorbed materials may dissolve from the surfaces of particles and enter the epithelium, endothelium, bloodstream, or lymphatics. Small particles (eg, nanoparticles) may directly penetrate cell membranes and evade clearance. Moreover, particle clearance from the respiratory tract is not equivalent to clearance from the body. The only mechanisms by which deposited particles can be removed from the body are nasal wiping and coughing.

Nasal Clearance Particles deposited in the nose are cleared depending on their site of deposition and solubility in mucus. Particles deposited in the anterior portion of the nose are removed by extrinsic actions such as wiping and blowing. Particles deposited in the posterior portion of the nose are entrapped in mucus and removed by mucociliary clearance that propels mucus toward the glottis, where the particles are swallowed. Insoluble particles are generally cleared from this region in healthy adults and swallowed within an hour of deposition. Particles that are soluble in mucus may dissolve and enter the epithelium and/or blood before they can be mechanically removed.

Tracheobronchial Clearance Particles deposited in the tracheobronchial tree are also removed by mucociliary clearance.

Table 15-4

Respiratory System Structures, Histology, Functions, and Particle Deposition and Clearance

REGION	HISTOLOGY	CELL TYPES	FUNCTIONS	NUMBER	SURFACE AREA EXPOSED TO AIR (m²)	VOLUME OF BREATH (l)	DEPOSITION MECHANISM	CLEARANCE MECHANISM
Nares and anterior nasal passage	Anterior vestibule: Stratified squamous epithelium Anterior chamber: Nonciliated cuboidal/ columnar epithelium with nasal hair	Anterior vestibule: Squamous epithelium Anterior chamber: Cuboidal epithelium, ciliated cells, mucus cells, serous cells, brush cells, neuroendocrine cells, basal cells, subcutaneous hair follicles	Conduct, heat, humidify, and filter air	2	2×10^{-2}	0.175	Impaction and interception	Sneeze
Posterior nasal passage	Ciliated pseudostratified respiratory epithelium, submucosal glands	Ciliated cells, mucus cells, serous cells, brush cells, neuroendocrine cells, basal cells, smooth muscle cells, submucosal glands (mucus and serous cells)	Conduct, heat, humidify, and filter air	2	4.5×10^{-2}			Sneeze and mucociliary clearance
Olfactory bulb	Olfactory epithelium, Bowman glands	Olfactory cells, supporting cells, basal cells, brush cells	Smell	2	2×10^{-4}			Sneeze
Mouth	Nonkertinized stratified squamous epithelium	Stratified squamous epithelium	Conduct, heat, humidify, and filter air	1	2.2×10^{-2}			Cough, Swallowing
Teeth and gingiva	Tooth: Bone with enamel, dentin, cenetum, pulp Gingiva: Gingival, junctional, and subcular epithelium	Tooth: Odontoblasts, fibroblasts, preodontoblasts Gingiva: Nonkertinized stratified squamous epithelium	Mastication	20 (primary) 32 (permanent)	5×10^{-3}			Swallowing
Tongue	Fungiform, filiform, foliate, circumvallate papillae	Supporting cells, gustatory cells	Taste, food manipulation	1	1×10^{-2}			Cough, swallowing
Salivary glands (partoid, submaxilary, sublingual, and minor)	Lobular secretory glands with adenomeres	Serous and mucous secretory epithelial cells	Moisten food, amylase digestion, lysozyme secretion	6 major 600 minor	*			Saliva secretion

Region	Structure	Cells	Function				Clearance
Pharynx	Nonkertinized stratified squamous epithelium, adenoid tissue, tonsils	Nonkertinized stratified squamous epithelium, adenoid and tonsils: mucosal associated lymphoid tissue	Conduct, heat, humidify, and filter air Adenoid, Immunoglobin A secretion	1	1×10^{-2}		Sneeze, cough, and mucociliary clearance
Larynx	Vocal folds (cords), 3 single (thyroid, cricoid, and epiglottic), and 3 paired (arytenoid, corniculate, and cuneiform) cartilages	Stratified squamous epithelium (true folds), respiratory epithelium (false fold), chondroblasts (cartilage)	Phonation	1	5×10^{-4}		Cough and mucociliary clearance
Trachea	Ciliated pseudostratified respiratory epithelium, submucosal glands, cartilage rings	Ciliated cells, mucus cells, serous cells, brush cells, neuroendocrine cells, basal cells, smooth muscle cells, submucosal glands (mucus and serous cells)	Conduct, heat, humidify, and filter air	1	7.5×10^{-3}		
Bronchi	Ciliated pseudostratified respiratory epithelium, cartilage plates, airway smooth muscle	Ciliated cells, mucus cells, serous cells, brush cells, neuroendocrine cells, basal cells, smooth muscle cells, submucosal glands (mucus and serous cells)	Conduct and filter air	510	0.26		
Bronchioles	Transition from ciliated pseudostratified to cuboidal ciliated respiratory epithelium (no cartilage and no submucosal glands)	Ciliated cells, clara cells, few or no mucus cells	Conduct and filter air	6.5×10^{4}	7.5		Mucocilary clearance
Respiratory bronchioles	Cuboidal nonciliated respiratory epithelium with alveoli in a portion of the wall	Cuboidal epithelium and alveolar epithelium	Conduct and filter air	4.6×10^{5}	*	0.2	Sedimentation, diffusion, and electrostatic attraction; Macrophage phagocytosis and migration
Alveolar duct and sac	Cuboidal nonciliated respiratory epithelium with alveoli in a portion of the wall	Some low cuboidal cells and mostly type I (squamous nonsecretory), type II (secretory cuboidal) alveolar epithelial cells, macropahge	Conduct and filter air, gas exchange	$3–5 \times 10^{8}$	140	4.5	
Pleural cavity and diaphragm	Mesothelium and skeletal muscle	Mesothelial cells, skeletal muscle cells, nerves	Generation of negative pleural pressure for inhalation	1	1.8	0	Translocation; Macrophage lymphatic migration

In addition to deposited particles, particle-laden macrophages are also moved upward to the oropharynx, where they are swallowed. Mucociliary clearance is relatively rapid in healthy individuals and is completed within 24 to 48 hours for particles deposited in the lower airways. Infection and other injuries can greatly impair clearance.

Alveolar Clearance Particles deposited in the alveolar region are removed by specialized cells, the alveolar macrophage. Lung defense involve both the innate and adaptive and immune systems. The innate immune system confers immediate recognition, phagocytosis, and killing of bacteria and microbes that are in the airway or alveolus. It is nonspecific and does not confer longer-term memory of the invading pathogenic stimuli. Alveolar macrophages are major effectors of innate immunity in the lung. Other innate immune cells include polymorphonuclear leukoctyes (aka neutrophils) that can augment this capacity but are typically present only when the lung is inflamed. The adaptive immune system confers long-lasting or protective immunity to the host that is specificity to a foreign microbe or material (antigen). Adaptive immunity involves dendritic cells that take up and present antigens to T lymphocytes (T cells) or antibody-producing B lymphocytes (B cells). Dendritic cells are derived from monocytes and reside in the airway epithelium. Lymphocytes reside in the hilar or mediastinal lymph nodes, lymphoid aggregates, and lymphoepithelial nodules, as well as in aggregates or as single cells throughout the airways. Ideally, the antibody generated by the B cell is recognizes a single molecular signature on the antigen and initiates other cells to evoke responses that protect the host (see Chap. 12).

Macrophage phagocytosis depends on the recognition of foreign or damage cells by a variety of macrophage surface macromolecules and receptors. Phagocytosis requires (1) particle binding to the membrane specifically via recognition molecule–receptor interactions or nonspecifically by electrostatic forces (inert materials), (2) receptor activation that initiates cell signaling, (3) actin polymerization and coordinated cytoskeletal movements that leads to extension of membranes, and (4) vesicular membrane closure closely apposed to the particle or the fiber ingested forming a phagosome shaped by the material ingested (Bowden, 1987).

Particles in the formed phagosome fuse with a lysosome to create a phagolysosome, where the ingested material is eventually degraded. Degradation can be oxygen-dependent (involving the respiratory burst) or oxygen-independent. Oxygen-independent degradation requires the fusion of granules containing proteolytic enzymes such as defensins, lysozyme, and cationic proteins. Additional antimicrobial peptides are present in these granules, including lactoferrin, which sequesters iron to provide unfavorable growth conditions for bacteria. Inhaled nanoparticles deposit along the entire respiratory tract, but are not efficiently engulfed by surface macrophages or may escape from phagosomes (Geiser, 2010).

Following alveolar deposition, macrophages rapidly engulf particles (≥50% within three hours and nearly 100% by 24 hours) (Alexis *et al.*, 2006). After several days or weeks, most macrophages then move to the airways and are removed mainly by mucociliary clearance. A small portion of insoluble particles may be phagocytized by alveolar macrophages and removed via lymphatic drainage. A portion of deposited particles not cleared by macrophages can be found in epithelial and interstitial cells or may be found in the lymphatic system with clearance time of months or years. Insoluble particles, especially long narrow fibers, may be sequestered in the lung for very long periods, often in macrophages located in the interstitium.

ALVEOLAR MACROPHAGE RECEPTORS

Alveolar Macrophage Receptors and Innate Immunity

Several receptors are involved in the phagocytic uptake of micrometer-sized particles (Geiser, 2010). Among these are Fc receptor and pattern-recognition receptors (PRRs) including complement, mannose, scavenger receptors (Table 15-5), and other PRRs (Table 15-6). These receptors differ in pathogen recognition motifs and are opsonin-dependent or -independent. Opsonins are binding enhancers (eg, antibodies), which coat the negatively charged molecules, especially those on bacterial membranes. Molecules that activate the complement system also are considered opsonins.

Phagocytosis of particles is mediated by various Fc receptors, which recognize immunoglobulin-coated particles. Macrophage Fc receptors recognize Fc fragments of the antibodies immunoglobin (Ig) A, E, and G. Fc receptors are classified based on the type of antibody they recognize, for example, Fc fragment of IgA, receptor for (FCAR aka CD89) recognizes IgA. Other macrophage Fc receptors include FCER1A/G, FCER2 (aka CD23) that recognize IgE, and FCGR1A/B/C (aka CD64), FCGR2A/B/C (aka CD32), and FCGR3A/B (aka CD16) that recognize IgG. The main receptors associated with alveolar macrophage phagocytosis are the IgA (FCAR) and IgG (FCGR1, 2, 3 types) receptors. Phagocytic cells do not have a FC receptor for IgM, making IgM ineffective in assisting phagocytosis. However, IgM efficiently activates complement and is therefore considered an opsonin. Clustering and activation of the low-affinity receptor FCGR2 by uncoated quartz has been demonstrated in vitro (Haberzettl *et al.*, 2008).

Once activated, FCAR modulates the respiratory burst (Ouadrhiri *et al.*, 2002). The respiratory burst involves the freshly generated reactive oxygen species produced by the phosphorylation, assembly, and activation of the reduced nicotinamide adenine dinucleotide phosphate (NADPH) oxidase (Iles and Forman, 2002). Assembly of the NADPH oxidase complex that includes cytochrome b-245 and β polypeptide ([CYBB] aka NADPH oxidase 2 [NOX2]) involves Ras-related C3 botulinum toxin substrate 1 (RAC1), neutrophil cytosolic factors (NCFs) 1, 2, and 4 (aka p47PHOX, p67PHOX, and p40PHOX, respectively), and CYBA (aka p22PHOX). Activation requires phosphorylation of the NCF2 subunit of the NADPH oxidase complex that activates the oxidase, which utilizes cytosolic NADPH to reduce extracellular oxygen to superoxide. Superoxide is converted to hydrogen peroxide by superoxide dismutase (SOD), hydrogen peroxide (H_2O_2), and diatomic oxygen. H_2O_2 can be combined with chlorine by myeloperoxidase to produce hypochorite (chlorine bleach), which plays a role in destroying bacteria. There are three types of SODs: SOD1 (containing Cu/Zn) is the cytoplasmic isoform, SOD2 (containing Mn/Fe) is the mitochondrial isoform, and SOD3 (containing Cu/Zn) is the extracellular isoform (Zelko *et al.*, 2002). The latter is particular abundant in the lung's extracellular matrix (ECM).

Under ideal conditions, superoxide anion is released totally into the phagosome and thereby held inside the cell. However, it can be released and react with NO. The oxidation of L-arginine produces NO endogenously by a reaction catalyzed by NO synthase. The enzyme exists in constitutive neuronal (NOS1), inducible (NOS2), and endothelial (NOS3) isoforms. In aqueous solution, freshly generated NO persists for several minutes in micromolar concentrations before it can react with O_2 to form much stronger oxidants such as NO_2. Nonetheless, in the body the half-life of NO is only seconds because NO diffuses

Table 15-5

Major Alveolar Macrophage Receptors

RECEPTOR PROTEIN FAMILY	SYMBOL	SYNONYMS	LIGAND
Fc receptors			
Subfamily A (FCAR)			
Fc fragment of IgA, receptor for	FCAR	CD89	Immunoglobin A
Subfamily E (FCER)			
Fc fragment of IgE, high affinity I, receptor for; alpha polypeptide	FCER1A		Immunoglobin E
Fc fragment of IgE, high affinity I, receptor for; gamma polypeptide	FCER1G		Immunoglobin E
Fc fragment of IgE, low affinity II, receptor for (CD23)	FCER2	CD23	
Subfamily G FCGR)			
Fc fragment of IgG, high affinity Ia, receptor (CD64)	FCGR1A	CD64a	Immunoglobin G
Fc fragment of IgG, high affinity Ib, receptor (CD64)	FCGR1B	CD64b	Immunoglobin G
Fc fragment of IgG, high affinity Ic, receptor (CD64)	FCGR1C	CD64c	Immunoglobin G
Fc fragment of IgG, low affinity IIa, receptor (CD32)	FCGR2A	CD32A	Immunoglobin G, quartz
Fc fragment of IgG, low affinity IIb, receptor (CD32)	FCGR2B	CD32B	Immunoglobin G, quartz
Fc fragment of IgG, low affinity IIc, receptor (CD32)	FCGR2C	CD32C	Immunoglobin G, quartz
Fc fragment of IgG, low affinity IIIa, receptor (CD16a)	FCGR3A	CD16a	Immunoglobin G
Fc fragment of IgG, low affinity IIIb, receptor (CD16b)	FCGR3B	CD16b	Immunoglobin G
Complement receptors			
integrin, alpha M (complement component 3 receptor 3 subunit)	ITGAM as a dimer with ITGBM	CD11b	Complement component 3 (iC3b), beta glucan, intercellular adhesion molecule I (ICAM1 aka CD54)
integrin, beta 2 (complement component 3 receptor 3 and 4 subunit)	ITGBM as a dimer with ITGAM	CD18	Complement component 3 (iC3b), beta glucan, intercellular adhesion molecule I (ICAM1 aka CD54)
Mannose receptor			
mannose receptor, C type 1	MRC1	CD206	Microbial mannose structures
Scavenger receptors			
macrophage scavenger receptor 1	MSR1	CD204	Acetylated LDL, oxidized LDL, advanced glycation end products-modified, maleylated-bovine serum albumin, lipoteichoic acid (LTA), lipid A component of LPS
macrophage receptor with collagenous structure	MARCO	SCARA2	Titanium dioxide, iron oxide and polystyrene latex particles. Acetylated LDL, oxidized LDL, advanced glycation end products-modified, maleylated-bovine serum albumin, LTA, lipid A component of LPS

(>100 μm) from the tissue and enters red blood cells and reacts with oxyhemoglobin. The direct toxicity of endogenous NO is modest but is greatly enhanced by reacting with superoxide to form peroxynitrite (ONOO−) (Beckman, 2009; Ferrer-Sueta and Radi, 2009). Most NO formed in the lung is excreted as nitrate in the urine within 48 hours or it can be exhaled (Meyer and Piiper, 1989). Other metabolites include nitrogen gas, ammonia, and urea (Yoshida and Kasama, 1987; Kosaka et al., 1989). Nonetheless,

NO is produced in sufficiently high concentrations to outcompete SOD for superoxide. Compared to other reactive oxygen and nitrogen species, peroxynitrite reacts relatively slowly with most biological molecules, making peroxynitrite a selective oxidant. Peroxynitrite mainly modifies tyrosine in proteins to create nitrotyrosines, leaving a biological signature. Nitration of structural proteins, including neurofilaments and actin, can disrupt filament assembly with major pathological consequences. Nitrotyrosines

Table 15-6

Major Alveolar Pattern Recognition Receptors

RECEPTOR PROTEIN FAMILY	SYMBOL	SYNONYMS	LIGAND
Toll-like receptors (TLRs)			
toll-like receptor 1	TLR1		Bacterial PAMPs (lipoproteins, lipoteichoic acid [LTA], peptidoglycan), Fungal PAMPs, beta-glucan, zymosan, mannan
toll-like receptor 2	TLR2		Bacterial PAMPs [Lipoproteins, lipoteichoic acid (LTA), peptidoglycan], Fungal PAMPs, beta-glucan, zymosan, mannan
toll-like receptor 3	TLR3		Viral PAMPs (double-stranded [ds] RNA)
toll-like receptor 4	TLR4		Gram-negative bacterial lipopolysacchrides (LPS), mannan
toll-like receptor 5	TLR5		Bacterial flaggen
toll-like receptor 6	TLR6		Bacterial PAMPs (Lipoproteins, LTA, peptidoglycan) Fungal PAMPs, beta-glucan, zymosan
toll-like receptor 7	TLR7		Bacterial or viral PAMPs (single-stranded [ss] RNA)
toll-like receptor 8	TLR8		Bacterial or viral PAMPs (ssRNA)
toll-like receptor 9	TLR9		Bacterial, viral, fungal, or parasitic DNA, unmethylated CpG motifs
toll-like receptor 10	TLR10		Lipoproteins, lipoteichoic acid (LTA), peptidoglycan (possibly)
toll-like receptor 11	TLR11		Parasitic PAMPs (profilin)
C-type lectin receptors (CLRs)			
C-type lectin domain family 4, member E	CLEC4E	Mincle	Cord factor (trehalose-6,6′-dimycolate (tuberculosis)
C-type lectin domain family 7, member A	CLEC7A	Dectin-1	Bacterial PAMPs (beta-glucans, zymosan)
Nucleotide binding oligomerization domain (NOD)-like receptors (NLRs)			
Caspase activation and recruitment domain (CARD) subtype			
nucleotide-binding oligomerization domain containing 1	NOD1	CARD4	*Legionella pneumophilia, Pseudomonas aeruginosa,* and *Staphylococcus aureus,* and other gram-negative and some gram-positive bacterial peptidoglycan: muropeptides (iE-DAPs)
nucleotide-binding oligomerization domain containing 2	NOD2	CARD15	Muramyl dipeptide in all peptidoglycan types
Pyrin domain (PYD) (aka death fold domain) subtype			
NLR family, pyrin domain containing 1	NLRP1	CARD7	Inflammasome initiators
NLR family, pyrin domain containing 3	NLRP3	NALP3	Inflammasome initiators
NLR family, CARD domain containing 4	NLRC4	IPAF	Inflammasome initiators
PYD and CARD domain containing	PYCARD	ASC	Inflammasome initiators
RNA helicase retinoic acid-inducible gene I-like receptors (RLRs)			
DEAD (Asp-Glu-Ala-Asp) box polypeptide 58	DDX58	RIG-I	Shorter dsRNA fragments, influenza A/B, respiratory syncyntial virus, and sendia virus
interferon induced with helicase C domain 1	IFIH1	MDA5	Longer nucleotide fragments poly(I:C) motifs and picoaviral ssRNA
DEXH (Asp-Glu-X-His) box polypeptide 58	DHX58	LPG2	Regulator of DDX58/IFIH signaling

have been detected in acute lung injury and several other inflammatory diseases (Beckman *et al.*, 1990; Freeman *et al.*, 1995; Squadrito and Pryor, 1998).

In addition, H_2O_2 produced by the respiratory burst also functions as a second messenger and activates signaling pathways in alveolar macrophage (Iles and Forman, 2002; Gwinn and Vallyathan, 2006). A major event is the activation of nuclear factor of kappa light polypeptide gene enhancer in B cells 1 (NFKB1)

by H_2O_2. Activated NFKB1 translocates into the nucleus and stimulates the expression of genes involved in a wide variety of biological functions, especially cytokines and chemokines that modulate the inflammatory response. Cytokines are intercellular mediators of inflammation that activate other inflammatory cells. Chemokines are intercellular mediators that attract other leukocytes through chemotaxis. The main cytokines generated by classically activated macrophages (aka M1 macrophages) include tumor necrosis factor (TNF), and interleukin (IL) 1, β (IL1B), IL6, and IL12. Interferon-γ (IFNG) released from activated macrophages or T cells (especially the Th1 subtype lymphocyte) drive immature macrophages toward the classically activated phenotype. Classically activated macrophages also express increased nitric oxide synthase 2, inducible (NOS2), which generate nitric oxide that can react with superoxide to form the more stable peroxynitrite, a reactive nitrogen species (Pacher *et al.*, 2007). H_2O_2 also activates the mitogen-activated protein kinase (MAPK) pathways that phosphorylate transcription factors including MAPK1/3 (aka extracellular-regulated kinase [ERK]) and the MAPK8 (aka c-Jun N-terminal kinase [JNK]). Phosphorylation of MAPK1/3 also modulates the expression of genes via phosphorylation of the transcription factor ELK1, member of ETS oncogene family (ELK1) that controls the production of the FBJ osteosarcoma oncogene (FOS) transcription factor.

Complement receptors recognize complement-coated particles (van Lookeren Campagne *et al.*, 2007). Macrophage complement receptors include integrin, α M (complement component 3 receptor 3 subunit) (ITGAM aka CD11b) and integrin, β 2 (complement component 3 receptor 3 and 4 subunit) (ITGBM aka CD18). Complement component C3 is central to opsonization and its first cleavage product, C3b, forms the multisubunit enzyme, C3bBb, that proteolytically cleaves additional C3 molecules on the pathogen surface. C3b is further degraded to iC3b, C3c and C3dg. These receptors dimerize to form the ITGAM/ITGBM (aka CD11b/CD18) complex, which recognizes multiple ligands including iC3b, β-glucans, and intercellular adhesion molecule 1 (ICAM1 aka CD54). β-Glucans are glucose polymers found in the cell walls of plants, fungi, and some bacteria (Palma *et al.*, 2006). Because cell walls are actively remodeled during bacterial cell growth and division, the constant release of these ligands from bacteria allows the innate immune system to survey its surroundings for the presence of active bacteria. ICAM1 is also a ligand for integrin α L (antigen CD11A (p180), lymphocyte function-associated antigen 1; α polypeptide) (aka CD11a) when complexed with ITGBM.

Macrophage mannose receptor, namely mannose receptor C type 1 (MRC1 aka CD206), is a C-type lectin receptor (CLR) that recognizes high-mannose structures on the surface of potentially pathogenic viruses, bacteria, and fungi (Gazi and Martinez-Pomares, 2009). Unlike other CLRs that elicit microbicidal effector functions (see below), MRC1 expression and its endocytic function are selectively decreased by IFNG, but increased by IL4 and IL13. IL4 and IL13 are cytokines generated by Th2 lymphocytes that increase in parasitic infections (eg, Helminthic infections) or acquired allergies (eg, allergic asthma). The induction of MRC1 is a marker of the alternatively activated macrophage (aka M2 macrophage) (Gordon and Martinez, 2010). Alternatively activated macrophages are thought to be immunesuppressive because they release IL10, do not produce IL12, and have decreased Th1-attracting chemokine, chemokine (C–C motif) ligand 3 (CCL3 aka MIP1A). However, alternatively activated macrophages express increased levels of arginase 1 (ARG1), resistin-like alpha (RETNLA), and chitinase 3-like 3 and 4 (CHI3L3 and CHI3L4). ARG1 can reduce NO production. RETNLA can modulate inflammation. CHI3L3/4 can bind chitins in insects, Helminth eggs, and Nematode pharynx. MRC1 also can interact with tumor cell mucin glycoproteins (eg, MUC16 aka CA125 and TAG-72), which induces MRC1 internalization and thereby modulate (perhaps suppress) cytokine production (Allavena *et al.*, 2010).

Macrophage scavenger receptors, macrophage scavenger receptor 1 (MSR1 aka CD204), and macrophage receptor with collagenous structure (MARCO) recognize a range of modified host polyanionic molecules and apoptotic cells (Bowdish and Gordon,

2009). Ligands for MSR1 shared for the most part with other SR, include acetylated low-density lipoprotein (LDL), oxidized LDL, advanced glycation end products (AGEs)-modified, and maleylated-bovine serum albumin. Other ligands include lipoteichoic acid (LTA) and the lipid A component of LPS. Three MSR1 protein isoforms can be generated from the *MSR1* gene. The isoform type 3 does not internalize modified LDL (acetyl-LDL) despite having the domain that mediates this function in type 1 and 2 isoforms. Isoform 3 has an altered intracellular processing and is trapped within the endoplasmic reticulum, rendering the macrophage unable to complete endocytosis. The isoform type 3 can inhibit the function of isoforms type 1 and type 2 when coexpressed, indicating a dominant negative effect and suggesting a mechanism for regulation of scavenger receptor activity in macrophages. MARCO is also involved in uptake of unopsonized particles such as titanium dioxide (TiO_2), iron oxide (Fe_2O_3), and polystyrene latex (PSL) (Arredouani *et al.*, 2005). These particles were about 1 mm in diameter.

Alveolar Macrophage Pattern-Recognition Receptors

PRRs have various ectodomains that recognize pathogen-associated molecular patterns (PAMPs) present on microbial surfaces. PRRs include Toll-like receptors (TLRs), C-type lectin receptors (CLRs), nucleotide-binding oligomerization domain (NOD)-like receptors (NLRs), and the RNA helicase retinoic acid-inducible gene I (RIG-I) (Table 15-6).

TLR proteins contain three major domains, a leucine-rich repeat motif containing ectodomaim, a transmembrane region, and a cytosolic Toll-IL1 receptor (TIR) domain (Kawai and Akira, 2011). Expressed either on the cell surface or associated with intracellular vesicles, 10 and 13 functional TLRs have been identified in human and mouse, respectively. TLR1, TLR2, TLR4, TLR5, TLR6, and TLR11 are expressed on the plasma membrane and mainly recognize microbial membrane components; TLR3, TLR7, TLR8, and TLR9 are expressed in the endosome and mainly recognize nucleic acids. Membrane-associated TLRs detect distinct PAMPs with the leading example being LPS, an endotoxin in the cell membrane of gram-negative bacteria, which is specifically recognized by TLR4. Other bacterial PAMPs include lipoproteins, LTA from gram-positive bacteria, and peptidoglycan (PGN) that are recognized by heterodimeric TLR2/TLR1 or TLR2/TLR6 and possibly TLR10, whereas bacterial flagellin is recognized by TLR5. Fungal PAMPs, β-glucan, and zymosan are recognized by TLR2 and TLR6, and mannan is recognized by TLR2 and TLR4. Parasitic PAMPs include profilin of *Toxoplasma gondii* recognized by TLR11. Viral PAMPs include nucleic acid variants of double-stranded (ds) RNA recognized by endosomal TLR3 with bacterial or viral single-stranded (ss) RNA being recognized by endosomal TLR7 and TLR8. Bacterial, viral, fungal, or parasitic DNA and unmethylated CpG motifs are recognized by endosomal TLR9. Alveolar macrophages express all the known TLRs, but most prominently TLR2, TLR3, TLR4, TLR5, TLR6 (Maris *et al.*, 2006), and TLR9 (Juarez *et al.*, 2010). In addition to TLRs, other membranes and cytosolic PRRs are found in the lung.

Other macrophage membrane PRRs include CLRs that recognize β-glucan and mannose structural molecules (Osorio and Reis e Sousa, 2011). For example, C-type lectin domain family 7, member A (CLEC7A aka Dectin-1) binds β-glucans and zymosan present in lung bacterial pathogens such as *Mycobacterium tuberculosis*, *Aspergillus* spp, and *Pneumocystis* spp. Another important macrophage CLR is CLEC4E, which recognizes trehalose-6,6′-dimycolate (aka cord factor), a major cell wall glycolipid of *M tuberculosis* (Ishikawa *et al.*, 2009). *M tuberculosis* produces several other molecules that are recognized via MRC1, TLR2, and TLR9.

Other cytosolic PRRs are NOD-like receptors (NLRs). NLR proteins are characterized by a shared domain architecture that includes a nucleotide-binding domain (NBD) and, like TLRs, a leucine-rich repeat (LRR) domain (Elinav *et al.*, 2011). NLRs can be grouped into two subfamilies based on additional domains, which can be either a caspase activation and recruitment domain (CARD) or a pyrin domain (PYD aka death-fold domain). The major CARD NLRs are NOD containing 1 (NOD1) and NOD2. NOD1 and NOD2 are cytosolic receptors that recognize distinct PGN subunits contained in gram-positive bacteria cell walls. NOD1 recognizes muropeptides (iE-DAPs) that are found in the PGN of gram-negative bacteria and only some gram-positive bacteria, whereas NOD2 recognizes a minimal motif of muramyl dipeptide that is found in all PGNs. In the lung, NOD1 is important because it recognizes and participates in regulating inflammatory responses to *Legionella pneumophila* (Berrington *et al.*, 2010), *Staphylococcus aureus* (Travassos *et al.*, 2004), and *Pseudomonas aeruginosa* (Travassos *et al.*, 2005).

PYD NLR proteins along with other members of the NLR protein family can form multiprotein complexes called inflammasomes (Sutterwala *et al.*, 2007). Inflammasomes are composed of one of several NLR and Pyhin proteins (Schattgen and Fitzgerald, 2011), including NLR family, pyrin domain containing 1 (NLRP1), NLRP3, and NLR family, CARD domain containing 4 (NLRC4 aka IPAF) sense endogenous or exogenous PAMPs (Sutterwala *et al.*, 2007). Inflammasomes are assembled through homophilic CARD–CARD and PYD–PYD interactions between NLRs, PYD, and CARD domains containing (PYCARD aka apoptosis-associated speck-like protein containing a CARD [ASC]) (Elinav *et al.*, 2011). Inflammasome assembly initiates the activation of inflammatory caspases, cysteine proteases that are synthesized as inactive prozymogens. Upon activation, caspases trigger cellular programs that lead to inflammation or cell death. Caspase 1, apoptosis-related cysteine peptidase (IL1, β, convertase (CASP1), which joins the inflammasome and is regulated in a signal-dependent manner, is the most prominent member of proinflammatory caspases. Other proinflammatory capases include CASP4, CASP5, CASP11, and CASP12. CASP1 catalytic activity is tightly regulated and essential for pro-IL1B and pro-IL18 processing and secretion. Inflammasomes require two signals to accomplish their biological function. Signal I initiates transcriptional activation of inflammasome components and is often provided through TLR and NFKB1 signaling, whereas signal II is required to initiate inflammasome assembly. For example, during influenza infection, signal I requires TLR7 viral RNA recognition and signal II activation of inflammasomes requires an acidified Golgi compartment (Ichinohe *et al.*, 2010).

Additional cytosolic PRRs are the RIG-I–like receptors (RLRs), a 3-protein family of DExD/H box RNA helicases that function as cytoplasmic sensors of viral PAMPs. The RLRs signal downstream transcription factor activation to drive type 1 IFN production and antiviral gene expression that elicits responses to control virus infection (Loo and Gale, 2011). The founding member of the family is DEAD (Asp–Glu–Ala–Asp) box polypeptide 58 (DDX58 aka RIG-I: retinoic acid-inducible gene I), which recognizes viral dsRNA. Lung pathogens recognized by DDX58 include influenza A, influenza B, respiratory syncyntial virus, and Sendai virus. The second member is IFN induced with helicase C domain 1 (IFIH1 aka MDA5 melanoma differentiation associated factor 5). IFIH was originally named MDA5 because it increases in response

to β-IFN, β1, fibroblast (IFNB), and mezerein, a protein kinase C-activating compound, which causes melanoma differentiation. These proteins contain an N-terminal region consisting of tandem CARD domains, a DExD/H box RNA helicase domain with the capacity to hydrolyze ATP and to bind and possibly unwind RNA, and a C-terminal repressor domain embedded within the C-terminal domain that in the case of RIG-I is involved in autoregulation. DDX58 preferentially associates with influenza's shorter RNA fragments (eg, 50 triphosphorylated ends-RNA sequence motifs) and some dsRNA regions (Baum *et al.*, 2010). In contrast, IFIH interacts with and preferentially recognizes high-molecular-weight fragments (eg, picornaviral ssRNA or longer synthetic poly(I:C) motif). The third member is DEXH (Asp–Glu–X–His) box polypeptide 58 (DHX58 aka LGP2: laboratory of genetics and physiology 2 and a homolog of mouse D11gp2). Although similar to DDX58 and IFIH in structure, DHX58 lacks the N-terminal CARD domains and may function as a regulator of DDX58/IFIH signaling.

Upon PAMP recognition, PRR proteins recruit a specific set of adaptor molecules that share a cytoplasmic domain that helps to initiate the cell signaling that actives antimicrobial responses and transcription of intra- and intercellular signaling molecules. For example, the TIR domains of TLR4 interact with the TIR-domain containing adaptor proteins, including the myeloid differentiation primary response gene (88) (MyD88) or TLR adaptor molecule 1 (TICAM1 aka TRIF), and initiate downstream signaling events (Kawai and Akira, 2010). The TLR4–TICAM1–MyD88 complex activates the IL1-receptor–associated kinase 1 (IRAK1) and TNF-receptor–associated factor 6 (TRAF6) complex, which in turn, activates transforming growth factor (TGF)-beta–activated kinase 1 (TAK1). This leads to the activation of NFKB1 by removal of the inhibitory protein, nuclear factor of kappa light polypeptide gene enhancer in B cells inhibitor, α (NFKBIA), and other members of an inhibitory complex that prevents NFKB1 movement to the nucleus. Nuclear NFKB1 increases transcription of a wide array of cytokines and chemokines. The secretion of inflammatory the newly generated cytokines attract and activate other leukocytes and structural cells. Alternatively, when TLR4 is internalized within the phagosome, it can form a complex with RAB11A, member RAS oncogene family (RAB11A), TICAM1, and TICAM2 (aka TRAM). This initiating step can either activate TRAF6 or add to a late NFKB1 response that causes additional recruitment of neutrophils and activation of macrophages. In addition, phagosomal TLR4 can activate TRAF3 that leads to IFN regulatory factor 3 (IRF3) activation. IRF3 translocates to the nucleus and activates the transcription of type I IFN (eg, *IFNA1* and *IFNB1*) genes, as well as other IFN-induced genes. This can result in direct killing of infected pathogens. Moreover, activation of TLR signaling leads to maturation of dendritic cells, a macrophage that presents antigens to lymphocytes, contributing to the induction of adaptive immunity (see below).

ACUTE RESPONSES OF THE LUNG TO INJURY

Trigeminally Mediated Airway Reflexes

Inhaled toxic chemicals or particles can come into contact with cells lining the respiratory tract from the nostrils to the gas-exchanging region. The sites of deposition in the respiratory tract have important implications in evaluating the risks posed by inhalants. For example, rats have more nasal surface on a per body weight basis than do humans. Measurement of DNA–protein cross-links formed in nasal tissue by formaldehyde has demonstrated that rats, which readily develop nasal tumors, have many more DNA cross-links per unit of exposure (concentration of formaldehyde × duration of exposure) than monkeys. Because the breathing pattern of humans resembles that of monkeys more than that of rats, extrapolation of tumor data from rats to humans on the basis of formaldehyde concentration may overestimate nasal doses of formaldehyde to humans. Patterns of animal activity can affect dose to the lung; nocturnally active animals such as rats receive a greater dose per unit of exposure at night than during the day, whereas humans show the opposite diurnal relationships of exposure concentration to dose.

Nasal and airway irritation represents a common response to inspired toxic compounds (Lanosa et al., 2010). Nasal irritation is mediated by irritant receptors (eg, TRPA1) that trigger trigeminal nerves characterized by tickling, itching, and painful nasal sensations (Alarie, 1973; Nielsen et al., 2007). TRPA1 is sensitive to several irritants including acrolein, allyl isothiocyanate, chlorine, 4-hydroxynonenal, and hydrogen peroxide (Bautista et al., 2006; Bessac and Jordt, 2008; Bessac et al., 2009). Nasal tissues of rodents express high levels of cytochromes P450 (CYP450) (Morris, 2000; Ding and Kaminsky, 2003), and biotransformation enzymes that can result in the formation of electrophilic metabolites from volatile organic compound vapors that activate TRPA1 (Lanosa et al., 2010). For example, styrene (Morris, 2000) and naphthalene (Morris and Buckpitt, 2009) are extensively metabolized by CYP2F isozymes within nasal mucosa. When the concentration of an inhaled substance exceeds the biotransformation capacity of the nasal passages, it can penetrate on to the lower respiratory tract (Morris, 2001).

Nasal irritation has been used as a basis for occupational exposure levels and is a common component in sick building syndrome resulting from poor indoor air quality (Hall et al., 1993; Hodgson, 2002). One of the consequences of nasal irritation is nasal mucus secretion that can dilute the irritant. In some cases, severe irritation that limits exposure can occur at concentrations below those that induce toxic response upon chronic exposure. These can be viewed as protective mechanisms. However, because the threshold dose of an irritant response can vary greatly among individuals (much like olfactory acuity), nasal irritation is not a reliable method for occupational safety. In mice, sensory irritation can lead to decreased breathing frequency during irritant exposure or increased pause at the onset of expiration, which can be highly quantifiable (Alarie, 1973; Vijayaraghavan et al., 1993; Morris et al., 2003). If continued exposure cannot be avoided, many irritants will produce cell necrosis and increase permeability of the airway epithelium.

Bronchoconstriction, Airway Hyperreactivity, and Neurogenic Inflammation

Substances that penetrate the nasal passage or are inhaled orally (with less efficient deposition) can trigger irritant receptors in the airways. Large diameter airways are surrounded by collagen and bronchial smooth muscle, which helps maintain airway tone and diameter during expansion and contraction of the lung. Bronchoconstriction can be evoked by irritants (acrolein, etc), cigarette smoke, or air pollutants, and by cholinergic drugs such as acetylcholine. Bronchoconstriction causes a decrease in airway diameter and a corresponding increase in resistance to airflow. Bronchoconstriction can also be due to an accumulation of thick mucus. Characteristics associated with signs include coughing, wheezing, and rapid shallow breathing, and those associated with symptoms include a sensation of chest tightness, substernal pain,

and dyspnea (a feeling of breathlessness). Dyspnea is a normal consequence of exercise, which potentiates these problems as well as leads to more mouth breathing. Because the major component of airway resistance usually is contributed by large bronchi, inhaled chemicals that cause bronchoconstriction are generally irritant gases with moderate solubility.

Bronchial smooth muscle tone is regulated by the autonomic nervous system. Postganglionic parasympathetic fibers will release acetylcholine to the smooth muscle layer surrounding the bronchi. These smooth muscle cells have membrane cholinergic receptors, muscarinic 3 (CHRM3). The activation of these receptors by acetylcholine activates an intracellular Gq protein domain, which increases cGMP. The increase in cGMP in turn activates a phospholipase C (PLC) pathway that increases intracellular calcium concentrations $[Ca^{2+}]_i$. Increased $[Ca^{2+}]_i$ leads to contraction of the smooth muscle cells. The actions of cGMP can be antagonized by increased cAMP evoked by protein kinase A (PKA). Increased cAMP can be accomplished by agents that bind to β-adrenergic receptors on the cell surface. The latter can be stimulated by inhaled bronchodilators (β-adrenergic agonists such as albuterol) or by injected epinephrine (adrenaline).

In addition to inducing an acute bronchoconstriction, irritants can prime the autonomic response by lowering the threshold dose of acetylcholine needed to induce bronchoconstriction. A lower threshold of acetylcholine-mediated bronchoconstriction is called airway hyperreactivity (or hyperresponsiveness). This response serves as the basis for a sensitive measure of whether a toxicant can cause bronchoconstriction in animals or humans primed by a prior dose of an acetylcholine-like chemical (bronchoprovocation testing). These tests are performed by measuring airway resistance following inhalation of increasing doses of a methacholine aerosol. Methacholine is used because it is more stable than acetylcholine. Other important bronchoconstrictive substances include histamine, various eicosanoids (including PGs [mainly $PGF_2\alpha$ and PGD_2], thromboxane A_2, leukotrienes C_4 and D_4), and adenosine. The bronchial smooth muscles of individuals with asthma contract at a lower threshold dose during provocation than do those of individuals without asthma (see Asthma).

In addition to bronchoconstriction, cough, and airway hyperreactivity, irritants can stimulate TRP channels (especially TRPA1 and TRPV1) that cause neurogenic inflammation. Mediated by neuropeptides (including tachykinins) released from nociceptive nerve terminals, neurogenic inflammation also includes vasodilatation, plasma protein extravasation, and leukocyte adhesion to the vascular endothelium (Geppetti et al., 2006). Tachykinins including substance P (aka neurokinin 1) activate tachykinin receptors (TACRs) on airway tissues. Tachykinins stimulate airway smooth muscle TACR2s and TACR1s to mediate bronchoconstriction, submucosal gland TACR1s to mediate mucin secretion, and cholinergic nerve TACR3s to mediate terminal stimulation. TRPV1 mediates the tussive action (cough) of capsaicin, which is widely used in cough provocation studies. TRPA1 is targeted by acrolein, 4-hydroxy-2-nonenal, and hydrogen peroxide. TRPV1 and TRPA1 antagonists may therefore represent potential antitussive and anti-inflammatory therapeutics for respiratory airway diseases.

Acute Lung Injury (Pulmonary Edema)

Initiated by numerous factors, acute lung injury (aka adult or infant respiratory distress syndrome) is marked by alveolar epithelial and endothelial cell perturbation and inflammatory cell influx that leads to surfactant disruption, pulmonary edema, and atelectasis (Ware and Matthay, 2000). Pulmonary edema produces a thickening of the alveolar capillary barrier and thereby limits O_2 and CO_2 exchange. Matching ventilation to vascular perfusion is critical to efficient gas exchange and is disrupted during acute lung injury. Alterations in coagulation and fibrinolysis accompany lung injury. Pulmonary edema may not only induce acute compromise of lung structure and function but also cause abnormalities that remain after resolution of the edematous process. Alveolar and interstitial exudates are resolved via fibrogenesis, an outcome that may be beneficial or damaging to the lung. Accumulation and turnover of inflammatory cells and related immune responses in an edematous lung probably play a role in eliciting both mitogenic activity and fibrogenic responses. During acute lung injury, profibrotic growth factors, TGFB1 (Wesselkamper et al., 2005) and platelet-derived growth factor (PDGF) (Bellomo, 1992) are activated and can initiate epithelial–mesenchymal transition (EMT) (see Pulmonary Fibrosis).

When inhaled in high concentrations, acrolein, HCl, NO_2, NH_3, or phosgene may produce immediate alveolar damage leading to a rapid death. However, these gases inhaled in lower concentrations may produce very little apparent damage in the respiratory tract. After a latency period of several hours, exposure to these compounds may compromise alveolar barrier function that leads to delayed pulmonary edema that is often fatal. In addition, acute lung injury can result from systemic effects including sepsis, transfusion, and blunt trauma to other organs. In several animal studies, neutrophil depletion can be protective; however, acute lung injury can develop in the absence of circulating neutrophils.

During acute lung injury, innate immunity is activated through activation PRRs (Xiang and Fan, 2010). In addition, a number of damage-associated molecular pattern proteins (DAMPs) are formed and include AGEs, high-mobility group protein B1 (HMGB1), amyloid β-peptide, and members of the S100 calcium binding protein (especially S100A8 [aka calgranulin A], S100A9 [aka calgranulin B], and S100A12 [aka ENRAGE]). These ligands bind to the ectodomain of AGE receptor (AGER aka RAGE) and initiate intracellular signaling leading to NFKB1-mediated induction of inflammatory cytokines and through positive feedback, AGER expression. In particular, HMGB1 is a potent mediator of acute lung injury and can induce PMN accumulation, edema formation, and production of proinflammatory mediators in the lung. HMGB1 is also a mediator of lethality during endotoxemia and sepsis in mice. In humans with severe trauma, plasma HMGB1 levels correlate positively with severity of injury and progression to acute lung injury. Activated macrophages and other inflammatory cells produce excessive reactive oxygen (superoxide anion, hydroxyl radicals, hydrogen peroxide) and nitrogen (nitric oxide, peroxynitrate) species. Because these oxidant species are potentially cytotoxic, they may mediate or promote the actions of various respiratory toxicants. Such mechanisms have been proposed for paraquat- and nitrofurantoin-induced lung injury. In this regard, the lung is well equipped with antioxidant enzymes, especially SOD3, extracellular, which converts superoxide anion to hydrogen peroxide. Hydrogen peroxide is the mediator of the extracellular cytotoxic mechanism of activated phagocytes. In addition, hydrogen peroxide is a potent intracellular signaling molecule that readily crosses cell membranes, and can thereby amplify cell damage. Phagocytic production of reactive oxygen species causes activation of proteinase enzyme and inactivation of proteinase inhibitors. Platelets (and platelet microthrombi) also have the ability to generate activated O_2 species.

Pulmonary edema is customarily quantified in experimental animals by measurement of lung water content. Lung water content can be expressed as the wet (undesiccated) weight of the whole lung or that of a single lung lobe. This value is often normalized to the weight of the animal or to the weight of the lung after complete drying in a desiccator or oven. The latter is typically expressed as lung wet weight:dry weight ratio.

CHRONIC RESPONSES OF THE LUNG TO INJURY

Chronic Obstructive Pulmonary Disease

Characterized by a progressive airflow obstruction, COPD involves an airway (bronchitis) and an alveolar (emphysema) pathology. With more than 200 million cases worldwide, COPD is the fourth leading cause of death (Pauwels and Rabe, 2004). The major risk factor for COPD is tobacco smoking and about 20% of smokers will develop COPD. Indoor air pollution from burning biomass fuels is associated with an increased risk of COPD in developing countries (Salvi and Barnes, 2009).

Chronic bronchitis is defined by the presence of sputum production and cough for at least three months in each of two consecutive years. Bronchitis in COPD involves airway inflammation with excessive mucus production from surface epithelial (goblet) cell and submucosal glands (Leikauf et al., 2002a; Rogers, 2007). The number of goblet cells increases, the number of ciliated cells decreases, and the size of the submucosal glands increase markedly. The latter are the major source of mucus and thereby sputum in the disease (Reid, 1960). The associated decreased mucociliary clearance and mucus retention may obstruct the airways and contribute to COPD exacerbations and possibly mortality (Miravitlles, 2011). Acrolein can increase mucin overproduction and can be formed endogenously in the airways during COPD (Bein, 2011).

COPD is almost characterized by chronic cough. A cough starts with activation of the sensory terminals of cough receptors located in the airway mucosa that triggers a deep inhalation and a forced respiratory exhalation against a closed glottis. It ends with the opening of the glottis that produces a rapid acceleration of air from the lungs accompanied by a distinct sound (Chung and Pavord, 2008). Frequent coughing in COPD can be exacerbated by respiratory infections, and many viruses and bacteria induce cough to move from host to host. Respiratory mechanical and ligand-gated cough receptors on rapidly adapting receptors, C fibers, and slowly adapting fibers provide input to the brainstem medullary central cough generator through the intermediary relay neurons in the nucleus tractus solitarius. As noted above, cough can be evoked by thermal, osmotic, and chemical (especially capsaicin) stimuli that engage the TRP channel (especially TRPV1) protein family. In addition, respiratory ligand-gated receptors are the degenerin/epithelial sodium channel proteins that include nonvoltage-gated sodium channels (eg, SCNN1A) and amiloride-sensitive cation channels (ACCN2 aka acid-sensing ion channel 1) (Kollarik and Undem, 2006). Members of both families have been implicated in the transduction of mechanical and acidic stimuli. Cough can also be evoked by stimuli of other ligand-gated receptors including 5-hydroxytryptamine activation of 5-hydroxytryptamine (serotonin) receptor 3A (HTR3A), ATP activation of purinergic receptor P2X, ligand-gated ion channels, and nicotine activation of chloinergic receptors, nicotinic subtypes. The central cough generator then establishes and coordinates the output to the muscles that cause cough, bronchoconstriction, and mucus secretion. Cough is effective in removing mucus in the first five to eight bronchial generations but as the cumulative diameter of the airways increases the acceleration of airflow is diminished.

Emphysema is physiologically defined by airflow obstruction that leads to dyspnea (especially on excursion) (Fig. 15-8) accompanied by diminished FEV1. The diagnosis of COPD is made by decreased FEV1:FVC ratio (which is not reversible by administration of a bronchodilator) and includes mild (<80% of normal; GOLD: I), moderate (50%–57%; GOLD: II), severe (30%–49%; GOLD: III), and very severe (<30% or chronic respiratory failure; GOLD: IV) (Rabe *et al.*, 2007). Emphysema is pathologically defined by an abnormal enlargement of the airspaces distal to the terminal bronchiole accompanied by destruction of the walls without obvious fibrosis (Snider *et al.*, 1985). Destruction of the gas-exchanging surface area results in a distended, hyperinflated lung that no longer effectively exchanges oxygen and carbon dioxide as a result of both loss of tissue and air trapping. Pathologically, emphysema can be (a) centriacinar emphysema that begins in the respiratory bronchioles and spreads peripherally (typically starting in the apical lung and is associated with cigarette smoking), (b) panacinar emphysema that destroys the entire alveolus uniformly (typically in the lower half of the lungs), and (c) paraseptal emphysema that forms giant bullae.

The pathogenesis of emphysema involves a proteinase–antiproteinase imbalance that leads to the remodeling of the supportive connective tissue in the parenchyma and separate lesions that coalesce to destroy lung tissue (Shapiro and Ingenito, 2005). This mechanism was proposed following the associated of serpin peptidase inhibitors, clade A (α-1 antiproteinase, antitrypsin), member 1 (SERPINA1) deficiency with early-onset emphysema (Laurell and Eriksson, 1963) and the ability to induce emphysema in rodents instilled with proteinase, for example, papain (Gross *et al.*, 1965) or neutrophil elastase (ELANE) (Janoff *et al.*, 1977). SERPINA1 inhibits serine proteinases including trypsin and ELANE and protects against cigarette smoke–induced alveolar enlargement in mice (Churg *et al.*, 2003; Churg, 2003). ELANE-deficient mice are partially protected against emphysema (Shapiro *et al.*, 2003) and macrophage matrix metalloproteinase 12 (MMP12 aka macrophage elastase)–deficient mice do not develop cigarette smoke–induced alveolar enlargement (Hautamaki *et al.*, 1997). In addition to MMP12, MMP1 (D'Armiento *et al.*, 1992), MMP2, MMP9 (Senior *et al.*, 1991), proteinase 3 (PRTN3) (Kao *et al.*, 1988), and plasminogen activator tissue (PLAT) (Chapman *et al.*, 1984) can mediate alveolar enlargement and MMP14, and ADAM metallopeptidase domain 17 (ADAM17) can mediate mucus overproduction. Both have been demonstrated in laboratory animals or human cells in culture. These changes can be accompanied by decreases in antiproteinases, for example, tissue inhibitor of metalloproteinase 3 (TIMP3) decreases when MMP9 increases in mucus overproduction (Deshmukh *et al.*, 2008).

In all individuals, elastolytic events accumulate with time and can cause a decline in lung function that is normally associated with aging. Toxicants that activate macrophages or cause inflammatory cell influx (which increases the burden of ELANE) can accelerate this process. Macrophages also can be activated by endogenous intracellular DAMPs released by activated or necrotic cells and degraded ECM molecules that increased following tissue damage. For example, ECM elastin fragments have been implicated in cigarette smoke–induced emphysema in mice (Houghton *et al.*, 2006).

In addition to macrophage and neutrophil activation, COPD involves cytotoxic T-cell lymphocytes (CTLs) that express a killer cell lectin-like receptor subfamily K, member 1 (KLRK1 aka natural killer cell group 2D) receptor, which recognizes MHC class I polypeptide-related sequence A (MICA) and MICB, and the related UL16-binding proteins (ULBP1, ULPB2, and ULBP3)

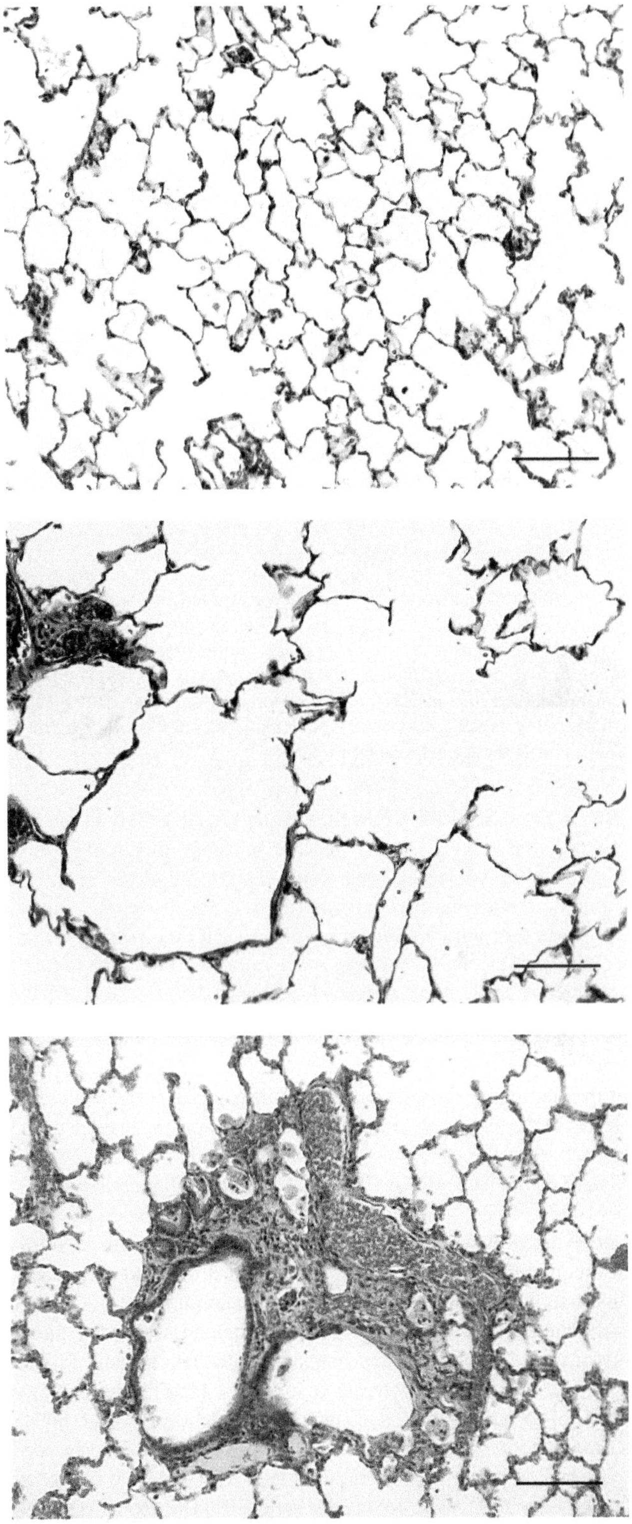

Figure 15-8. *Airspace enlargement induced by tobacco smoke and pulmonary fibrosis induced by asbestos in rat lung.* Top panel: Normal rat lung. Middle panel: Extensive distention of the alveoli (emphysema) in rat lung following inhalation of tobacco smoke (90 mg/m³ of total suspended particulate material). Bottom panel: Lung of a rat one year after exposure to chrysotile asbestos. Note accumulation of connective tissue around blood vessel and airways (fibrosis). Bar length: 100 μm. (Photograph courtesy of Dr Kent E. Pinkerton, University of California, Davis.)

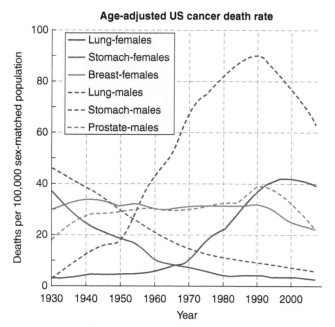

Figure 15-9. *Trends in age-adjusted United States cancer death rates for stomach, lung, breast (females), and prostate (males) cancers.* Solid line: females; dashed line: males. (From US Mortality Volumes 1930 to 1959, US Mortality Data, 1960 to 2007. National Center for Health Statistics, Centers for Disease Control and Prevention.)

(Borchers *et al.*, 2009). Respiratory epithelial cells undergoing toxicant stress (eg, caused by cigarette smoke or infection) express MICA on the cell surface and emphysema results from epithelial expression of the murine homolog (retinoic acid early transcript 1, α). These receptors are recognized by KLRK1 expressing CTLs, which then selectively perform cell cytolysis on the targeted cell and thereby remove damage or infected cells.

Lung Cancer

At the beginning of the 20th century, lung cancer was a rare disease. Because of cigarette smoking, lung cancer is now the leading cause of death from cancer among men and women in the United States (Siegel *et al.*, 2011) (Fig. 15-9). In addition to inducing COPD, retrospective and, more conclusively, prospective epidemiological studies unequivocally associated tobacco smoking with this epidemic in lung cancer. Currently, ~75% to 85% of lung cancer cases (and many cases of cancer of the bladder, esophagus, oral cavity, and pancreas) are caused by cigarette smoking. The main factor responsible for smoking dependence is nicotine, a ligand for the nicotinic acetylcholine receptor α subunit, which makes up 0.3% to 5% of tobacco plant and accumulates in the tobacco leaf during curing. The increased risk of developing lung cancer for average smokers compared with nonsmokers is 8- to 10-fold and for heavy smokers about 20- to 40-fold (Pope *et al.*, 2011). Stopping smoking reduces the risk of developing lung cancer or COPD (International Agency for Research on Cancer [IARC], 2004). The global burden is ~1.2 million cancer deaths per year, with 85% of lung cancer cases in men and 47% of lung cancer cases in women being attributable to tobacco use.

The development of lung cancer is likely to be a result of multiple genetic and gene–environment interactions because not all smokers develop lung cancer and nonsmokers develop lung cancer (Sun *et al.*, 2007). Single-nucleotide polymorphisms (SNPs) located on chromosomal regions 5p15.33 and 15q25.1 have been consistently identified by genome-wide association studies (GWAS)

as significant predictors of lung cancer risk, and an SNP in 6p22.1 has been associated with survival time in small-cell lung cancer (SCLC) patients (Xun *et al.*, 2011). Others have used transcription signatures to predict prognosis and therapeutic options in lung cancer (Chen *et al.*, 2007; Kadara *et al.*, 2011).

Many chemical exposures encountered in industrial settings also pose a lung cancer risk. Arsenic, asbestos, beryllium, cadmium, chromium, and nickel have been associated with cancer of the respiratory tract (IARC, 1993). Workers exposed to chloromethyl ether, mustard gas, or effluent gases from coke ovens have an increased lung cancer risk. First noted among radium miners and then in homes, radon gas is a known human lung carcinogen. Formaldehyde is a probable human respiratory carcinogen. Silica, human-made fibers, and welding fumes are suspected carcinogens. Smokers who inhale radon or asbestos fibers increase their risk for developing lung cancer several fold, suggesting a synergistic interaction between the carcinogens. For example, working with asbestos increases the risk about twofold and for persons who smoke moderately the risk is eightfold. However, asbestos workers who smoke moderately have an associated risk of 16-fold.

Lung cancer in never-smokers is the seventh leading cause of cancer death worldwide (Sun *et al.*, 2007). In addition to radon, indoor environmental tobacco smoke increases the risk of developing lung cancer in nonsmokers (IARC, 2004). In addition, biomass cooking, high-temperature oil cooking, and coal heating especially in poor-ventilated households are associated with lung cancer, COPD, and pneumonia, together leading to over 2 million deaths per year worldwide (World Health Organization [WHO], 2006). Ambient $PM_{2.5}$ has been associated with increased lung cancer risk (Beeson *et al.*, 1998; Pope *et al.*, 2002).

Human lung cancers may have a latency period of 20 to 40 years, making the relationship to specific exposures difficult to establish. The two major forms of lung cancer are non–small-cell lung cancer (NSCLC; which accounts for ~85% of all lung cancer cases) and SCLC (which accounts for ~15% of all lung cancer cases) (Herbst *et al.*, 2008). NSCLC can be subdivided into three major histological subtypes: squamous-cell carcinoma, adenocarcinoma, and large-cell lung cancer. Smoking causes all types of lung cancer but is most strongly linked with SCLC and squamous-cell carcinoma. Adenocarcinoma is the most common type in patients who have never smoked (Sun *et al.*, 2007). Large-cell lung is really rare and makes up less than 10% of the NSCLC cases.

Compared with lung cancer, cancer in the upper respiratory tract is less common in humans but can occur frequently in experimental animals exposed to inhaled carcinogens (Harkema *et al.*, 2006). Nonetheless, head and neck cancers are still a major cause of cancer deaths worldwide. Upper respiratory cancers are associated occupational exposures to chromium, nickel, mustard gas, and isopropyl alcohol. Nasal cancers also are associated with wood dust, textile dust, and possibly leather dust or formaldehyde. Buccal carcinogens are associated with tobacco smoke, smokeless tobacco, betel quid chewing, and alcohol consumption.

Epithelial lung cancers develop in a sequence of distinct morphological changes. Initially, cell numbers in the epithelium lining the airways increase (hyperplasia) and eventually display abnormal nuclei and changes in shape (dysplasia), often assuming squamous-cell characteristics (squamous metaplasia). The lesions then progress to first carcinoma in situ, an accumulation of cancerous cells in small foci and then into large tumor masses. Eventually tumor cells invade adjacent local tissues, blood vessels, and lymphatics, leading to the formation of distant metastases. The histologically visible sequential development is accompanied by multiple molecular lesions (Wistuba and Gazdar, 2003).

The potential mechanisms of lung carcinogenesis have been studied extensively by means of analysis of tumors and human bronchial cells maintained in culture. A key component is DNA damage induced by reactions with an activated carcinogen or its metabolic product, such as PAHs (eg, benzo[*a*]pyrene: BaP) or alkyldiazonium ions derived from tobacco specific *N*-nitrosamines (TSNAs). Formed from nicotine in the tobacco curing process, TNSAs include a potent carcinogen, nitrosoaminoketone (NNK) (ie, 4-(methylnitrosamino)-1-(3-pyridyl)-1-butanone) (Ter-Minassian *et al.*, 2011). Found in unburned tobacco and tobacco smoke, NNK is metabolized to 4-(methylnitrosamino)-1-(3-pyridyl)-1-butanol (NNAL) and its glucuronide metabolites (NNAL-Gluc). NNK and NNAL form DNA adducts, which are found in lung tumors in mice treated with NNK. Urinary levels of total NNAL (NNAL plus NNAL-Gluc) are associated with lung cancer in a dose-dependent manner in a cigarette smoker (Yuan *et al.*, 2009).

Persistence of O^6-alkyl-deoxyguanosine mutations in DNA appears to correlate with carcinogenicity (Hecht, 1999). However, tumors do not always develop when adducts are present, and adduct formation may be a necessary but not sufficient condition for carcinogenesis. DNA damage caused by reactive oxygen species is another potentially important mechanism. Ionizing radiation leads to the formation of superoxide, which is converted through the action of SOD to hydrogen peroxide. In the presence of Fe and other transition metals, hydroxyl radicals may be formed, which then cause DNA strand breaks. Cigarette smoke contains high quantities of reactive oxygen species (Pryor, 1997) and acrolein (Bein, 2011). Additional oxidative stress may be placed on the lung tissue of smokers by the release of reactive oxygen/nitrogen species formed by activated macrophages and other inflammatory leukocytes. In addition, diminished DNA repair and loss of enzymes that maintain chromosomal integrity (eg, aberrant telomere homeostasis that evades senescence) are critical events in many cancers, including lung cancer (Buch *et al.*, 2011).

Genomic instability is a hallmark of lung cancer (Sato *et al.*, 2007). Critical genetic and epigenetic changes include DNA mutations, loss of heterozygosity, and promoter methylation and global transcriptome changes that can include stimulation of mitogenic pathways and suppression of apoptosis pathways. Loss of heterozygosity is the loss of normal function of one allele of a gene in which the other allele was already inactivated. In the context of lung cancer, an inactivated allele of a tumor suppressor gene could be inherited from a parent's germline cell that was passed on to the offspring. The offspring would thereby be heterozygous for that allele and subsequent exposure to a mutagen during the offspring's life could then inactivate the functional allele. Genetic and epigenetic changes can persist over years and eventually lead to aberrant cellular function to produce premalignant changes, including dysplasia and clonal patches.

Many molecular changes in earliest-stage cancer also occur in advanced disease (Herbst, 2008). Premalignant patches contain clones and subclones, which often involve mutations in tumor protein p53 (TP53 aka p53) and epidermal growth factor receptor (EGFR). Lung cancers unrelated and related to smoking have different molecular profiles, mutation in EGFR being more common in never-smokers, and v-Ki-ras2 Kirsten rat sarcoma viral oncogene homolog (KRAS) being more common in smokers. Mutation TP53 are found in both smokers and nonsmokers; however, TP53 are more frequent in never-smokers (Sun *et al.*, 2007). In addition, the TP53 mutational signature (ie, relative amounts of specific transitions, transversions, or deletions), and spectrum (ie, specific mutation within the gene) differ between smokers and never-smokers.

In response to diverse cellular stresses, TP53 regulates target genes that induce cell cycle arrest, apoptosis, senescence, DNA repair, or changes in metabolism. TP53 is a DNA-binding protein containing transcription activation, DNA-binding, and oligomerization domains. Normally, TP53 can bind to a consensus DNA-binding site and activate expression of downstream genes that inhibit growth and/or invasion, and thus it functions as a tumor suppressor. Found in both NSCLCs and SCLCs, mutant TP53 protein fails to bind these sites, and hence lacks tumor suppressor activity. Acrolein (Tang *et al.*, 2011) and BaP (Denissenko *et al.*, 1996) adducts of TP53 are common in lung cancers.

A receptor tyrosine kinase (RTK), EGFR is a receptor for a number of growth factor ligands (including EGF and transforming growth factor α) and subsequently can stimulate downstream signaling pathways of mitogen-activated protein kinase and phosphatidylinositol-3 kinase. Amplications of *EGFR* are more common in squamous-cell carcinoma, whereas a kinase domain mutation is more common in adenocarcinoma. The latter occurs more frequently in women, persons of Han decent, and nonsmokers who develop lung cancer. This kinase is critical because it is the target of the RTK inhibitors gefitinib and erlotinib, which have been particularly successfully in treatment of this type of lung cancer. Also a member of the EGFR family, v-erb-b2 erythroblastic leukemia viral oncogene homolog 2, neuro/glioblastoma-derived oncogene homolog (avian) (ERBB2 aka HER2) protein lacks a ligand-binding domain and therefore cannot bind growth factors. However, it does bind tightly to other ligand-bound EGF receptor family members to form a heterodimer, stabilizing ligand binding and enhancing kinase-mediated activation of downstream signaling pathways that stimulate cell proliferation. Mutations in this gene are associated with adenocarcinoma.

KRAS is a guanine nucleotide (GDP/GTP)-binding protein that acts as a self-inactivating signal transducer. Normal KRAS can be transiently activated by signals from cell surface receptors that promote the exchange of bound GDP for GTP. The transient nature of this response is ensured by the intrinsic ability of KRAS to hydrolyze GTP, and thereby to switch itself off. Single point mutations produce KRAS proteins with amino acid substitutions that have reduced GTPase activity. Mutant KRAS proteins are thereby locked in a constitutively activated GTP-bound state. KRAS mutations are more common among or are associated with adenocarcinomas among smokers and activated NNK and BaP for KRAS bulky adducts. Mutation or amplification of *TP53*, *EGFR*, *ERBB2*, or *KRAS* thus provides a proliferative advantage to tumor cells.

Other RTKs mutated in lung cancer include Met protooncogene (hepatocyte growth factor receptor) (MET) and anaplastic lymphoma RTK (ALK). The ligand for MET is hepatocyte growth factor, HGF, which despite its name is a growth factor in the lung and important in repair (Ware and Matthay, 2002). ALK belongs to the insulin receptor superfamily. A chromosomal rearrangement of the *ALK* gene that leads to fusion with echinoderm microtubule-associated protein like 4 (*EML4*) can be found in about 7% of adenocarcinomas. Other fusion proteins can be generated with the ALK protein. A specific RTK inhibitor of MET and ALK, Crizotinib, has been effective against NSCLC cell lines that express oncogenic ALK fusion proteins and has been useful in an initial clinical trial for lung cancers of this type (Rodig and Shapiro, 2010).

Serine/threonine kinase 11 (STK11 aka liver kinase B1 homolog or LKB1) regulates cell polarity and other cellular functions. Normally, STK11 protein activates AMP-activated protein kinase (AMPK), which leads to growth suppression. However, mutant STK11 proteins lack the ability to phosphorylate AMPK and to interact with TP53 that diminish transcription of target genes.

Mutations in *STK11* are associated with smoking and are common in adenocarcinoma and squamous-cell carcinoma in persons of European decent, whereas it is uncommon in adenocarcinoma in persons of Hun decent. *STK11* mutations often are present in tumors with *KRAS* mutations, but are not found in tumors with *EGFR* mutations.

Other mutations common in lung cancer occur in NK2 homeobox 1 (NKX2-1 aka thyroid transcription factor 1: TITF1), and phosphoinositide-3-kinase, catalytic, α polypeptide (PIK3CA). Cancer stem cells (CSCs) are a subset of cancer cells with the ability to initiate cancer when injected into mice (Martelli *et al.*, 2011). CSCs are thought to be responsible for tumor onset, self-renewal/maintenance, mutation accumulation, and metastasis. The existence of CSCs could explain the high frequency of neoplasia relapse and resistance to therapies. Critical for alveolar type II cell development, NKX2-1 may have a role in modulating stem cell functions and *NKX2-1* amplication (with increased copy number) is common in adenocarcinoma. PIK3CA is the catalytic subunit of PI-3-kinase (PI3K), which is a member of the v-akt murine thymoma viral oncogene homolog 1 (AKT1) and mechanistic target of rapamycin (serine/threonine kinase) (MTOR) survival pathway. The PI3K–AKT1–MTOR pathway is downstream of EGFR and mutation in this pathway protects against apoptosis in tumor cells. Pharmaceuticals that inhibit PI3K/AKT1/MTOR can induce apoptosis in tumors and is a new target for eliminating CSCs.

Another common alteration is increased v-myc myelocytomatosis viral oncogene homolog (avian) (MYC aka c-Myc). MYC is frequently amplified in SCLC cell lines in a higher frequency than tumors, suggesting that MYC is more related to tumor progression and a relatively late event in lung cancer development. A transcription factor, MYC may contribute to the production of multiple growth factors that can promote and inhibit the proliferation via paracrine and autocrine loops via specific receptors.

In toxicological testing, lung tumors or cancers in laboratory animals do not always mimic those in humans. Most lung tumors in mice are peripherally located adenomas and adenocarcinomas, even after tobacco or NNK exposure. Rarely do mice or rats develop bronchial squamous-cell carcinoma found in humans that smoke. Rats on occasion develop lung tumors that are characterized by an epithelium surrounding a space filled with keratin. The mass may compress the adjacent lung parenchyma and occasionally invades it. These lesions are classified by some pathologists as bona fide tumors, whereas other pathologists characterize this type of lesion as a cyst filled with keratin. Classification of such a lesion is important because these lesions often are found in long-term tests in animals that have been exposed to agents that are not considered carcinogens, such as carbon black, titanium dioxide, and certain human-made fibers (ILSI, 2000). In other animal tests, a large particle number or mass is instilled into the trachea as a single exposure, which is used to mimic a daily or a lifetime exposure burden. These instillations may not be evenly distributed in the lung and histological examination often demonstrates focal accumulations of a large number of particles almost never observed in humans even after a lifetime of exposure. A unifying hypothesis postulates that because clearance mechanisms in the deep lung depend predominantly on phagocytosis and migration of pulmonary alveolar macrophages, such large doses overwhelm clearance mechanism and elicit irresolvable inflammation (called particle overload) (Morrow, 1992). As a consequence, lung burdens of these dusts persist for months or years, and may evoke unique mechanisms of disease pathogenesis not applicable to human experience with inhaled chemicals or particles. The issue of whether particle overload is useful in defining a toxicity threshold in such experiments remains unresolved.

Asthma

Asthma is defined by sporadic bouts of airflow obstruction, leading to dyspnea. Airflow obstruction is measured as increased airway resistance (or decreased predicted FEV1). In asthma, resting levels of airway resistance can be normal or slightly increased, which typically is reversible with bronchodilators. The hallmark of asthma is a persistent or recurrent airway hyperreactivity. As noted above, airway hyperreactivity is defined by a lower threshold to acetylcholine- or methacholine-mediated increased airway resistance. Airway hyperreactivity can be specific, as in allergic asthma, and induced by exposure to a single known irritant or antigen. Knowledge of the causal agent is extremely valuable because avoidance can reduce the frequency of or even eliminate bronchospasm. Airway hyperreactivity can also be nonspecific, and bronchoconstriction can result from a wide range of triggers including irritants, cold-dry air, or exercise. Therapy for nonspecific airway hyperreactivity is therefore more difficult.

Responses to a methacholine or histamine challenge can vary with severity of the disease. The response in mild asthma is marked by a greater sensitivity (ie, the dose–response curve is shifted to the left) but may not include a greater maximal airway resistance (Woolcock *et al.*, 1984). This may be caused by altered neural control, inflammation, mediator metabolism, or epithelial damage (Sterk and Bel, 1989). In more severe asthma, greater sensitivity is accompanied by a greater maximal response than observed in healthy subjects. This may be due to additional increases in airway smooth contractility, thickening of the airway wall, and decreased lung elastic load. Airway inflammation is typically marked by activation of receptor and epithelial injury that leads to an influx of eosinophils, which are rarely present in a healthy lung. During exacerbations, the inflammation involves eosinophils, mast cells, lymphocytes, and neutrophils.

The pathogenesis of asthma involves the adaptive and innate immune systems. In allergic asthma, previous exposure to an antigen typically leads to the generation of immunoglobin E (IgE) molecules that have molecular recognition sites specific to the antigen. Upon reexposure, the antigen causes cross-linking of IgE molecules and activation of lymphocytes, eosinophils, macrophages, and mast cells, with elaboration and release of an array of cytokines, chemokines, eicosanoids, histamine, tachykinins, and other mediators. Together, these mediators induce smooth muscle constriction, vascular leakage, mucus secretion, and inflammatory cell recruitment. These processes lead to airway obstruction, airway edema, formation of intraluminal mucus and plugging, and neutrophil recruitment with additional mediator release, respectively. Severe airway obstruction and ventilation-vascular perfusion mismatching lead to impaired gas exchange and hypoxemia. In irritant-induced (nonallergic) asthma, the inflammatory cascade is not initiated by an inhaled antigen but many of the same mediators and effector pathways are activated. Persistent inflammation and epithelial damage contribute to airway hyperreactivity. In laboratory animals, short-term airway hyperreactivity can be induced by many irritant stimuli but this response is likely to be reservable (lasting a few hours or days after a single exposure). It can also be induced by antigen sensitization (typically ovalbumin injections) and subsequent antigen challenges (typically an aerosol of albumin in saline). This is followed by a determination of airway resistance following increasing doses of methacholine or histamine.

Asthma has been associated with a number of occupations (Malo and Chan-Yeung, 2009). Occupational asthma can involve adaptive immunity induced by high-molecular-weight and some low-molecular-weight substances. High-molecular-weight agents including flour-, cereals-, latex- or animal-derived proteins and enzymes cause sensitization through an IgE-mediated mechanism, such as in common atopic asthma. Occupational asthma, for example, is common among laboratory technicians and veterinarians who become sensitized to proteins excreted in rodent urine. Many low-molecular-weight agents that induce occupational asthma include acid anhydrides and platinum salts that induce asthma through an IgE mechanism, but most low-molecular-weight agents involve an uncertain mechanism of induction. Many of the low-molecular-weight agents can cross-link biological macromolecules (Jarvis *et al.*, 2005). The latter low-molecular-weight agents include metals (eg, nickel, vanadium, chromium, cobalt, zinc, cadmium, and aluminum), diisocyanates (eg, toluene diisocyanate), cleaning agents, wood dusts, soldering fluxes, pesticides, pharmaceuticals, and reactive dyes. Low-molecular-weight agents may act as haptens that combine with endogenous proteins to form a complex that is recognized as an antigen by the immune system. A subtype of asthma (aka reactive airways dysfunction syndrome) or persistent cough can be a sequele to accidental high-level irritant (eg, chlorine or ammonia) exposure that can also induce acute lung injury (Brooks *et al.*, 1985). It is unclear whether the acute exposure alone causes asthma or uncovers existing asthma. Nonetheless, it is clear that persons with asthma may be susceptible to lower doses of irritants (such as sulfur dioxide) (Sheppard *et al.*, 1980). In addition, because ambient particle matter and other air pollutants contain many of the metals and other chemicals that are associated with asthma in the workplace, it is likely that these irritants can exacerbate asthma (Leikauf, 2002b).

Pulmonary Fibrosis

The pathological hallmark of pulmonary fibrosis is increased focal staining of collagen fibers in the alveolar interstitium. Excess lung collagen is usually observed not only in the alveolar interstitium but also throughout the centriacinar region, including the alveolar ducts and respiratory bronchioles (Fig. 15-8). The foci can coalesce to form large masses of noncompliant lung. The pleural surface of the lung may also become fibrotic and together with parenchymal stiffening prevent full lung inflation. Ultimately the lung is unable to inflate or deflate properly and thus is restricted. Restrictive lung disease can be detected by a decrease in the predicted FVC, with or without change in the FEV1.

The pathogenesis of pulmonary fibrosis involves epithelial cell injury and macrophage activation produced by a wide range of toxic insults (Wynn, 2011). For example, macrophages can be activated by phagocytosis of crystalline silica or crocidolite asbestos, which activate inflammasome receptor-mediated TNF and IL1B formation. Epithelial cells and macrophages also release chemokines that recruit and activate other inflammatory cells including neutrophils and T cells. These cells combine to produce excessive TGFB1, TNF, IL1B, IL13, and IL17. Of these, TNF and TGFB1 are major mediators in pulmonary fibrosis because fibrosis can be diminished experimentally by inhibition of TNF (Piguet *et al.*, 1990) or TGFB1 (Sheppard, 2004; Gharaee-Kermani *et al.*, 2009) activity. Importantly, TGFB1 and other TGFB family members (TGFB2 and TGFB3) are secreted in inactive complexes with a latency-associated peptide (LAP), a protein derived from the N-terminal of the region of the gene product. LAP is a ligand for the integrins, heterodimeric proteins consisting of α and β subunits that bind matrix molecules or cellular counterreceptors. In the lung, integrin α v β 6 (through cell–cell contact) and integrin α v β 8 (through a proteolytic process) can activate extracellular latent TGFB1 and TGFB3.

Repeated injury and the inability to resolve macrophage activation lead to areas of focal hypoxia. The consequence of the combined TGFB1/3, cytokine release, and hypoxia leads to epithelial-to-mesenchymal transition in which lung epithelial cells transdifferentiate into fibroblast-like cells (Chapman, 2011). These cells contribute to a larger population of myofibroblasts that arise from local mesenchymal cells, and bone marrow–derived fibrocytes. The migration, proliferation, and activation of myofibroblasts contribute to excessive excellular matrix deposition that has altered collagen cross-linking. The consequence of this process is disorderly repair and sustained fibrogeneis, which leads to progressive stiffness of the fibrotic lung.

AGENTS KNOWN TO PRODUCE LUNG INJURY IN HUMANS

Currently, the American Chemical Society (ACS) lists over 50 million chemicals with a unique Chemical Abstracts Service (CAS) Registry Number and over 280,000 are listed as inventoried/regulated chemicals by CHEMLIST, but only ~7900 compounds are listed as commonly used by industry (ACS, 2011). Many of these compounds represent hazards to the respiratory tract. For example, the American Conference of Governmental Industrial Hygienists (ACGIH) lists over 700 TLVs for atmospheric exposures (ACGIH, 2011). TLVs refer to occupational airborne concentrations of substances "that nearly all workers may be repeatedly exposed day after day without adverse health effects." These values and other exposure limits have been developed because prevention of exposure is one of the most effective approaches to prevent lung injury and disease. Nonetheless, given the large morbidity and mortality associated with current acute and chronic lung disease, a great need exists to develop additional preventative and therapeutic strategies based on the knowledge of the cellular and molecular events that determine lung injury and repair. Table 15-7 lists a portion of the respiratory toxicants that can produce acute and chronic lung injury in humans. In the following sections, a few examples of our current understanding of lung injury at the mechanistic level are discussed, with emphasis on agents directly responsible for human lung disease.

Inhalation Hazards

Acrolein As an α–β-unsaturated aldehyde, acrolein (2-propenal) is volatile at room temperature and is highly irritating to upper and lower respiratory tract (Bein, 2011). Acrolein can be formed by heating cooking oils and fats above 300°C (eg, wok cooking), and thus its name refers to the pungent "acrid" (from Latin stem: acer meaning sharp or sour) smell that is produced from "oleum" (Latin meaning "oil"). Acrolein also can be formed in cigarette smoke, environmental tobacco smoke, domestic cooking with biomass fuels (WHO, 2006), smoke from fires, and automotive and diesel exhaust. Additional human exposure can result from acrolein use as a biocide or chemical feedstock.

Acrolein contains a reactive carbonyl group and an electrophilic α-carbon and thus is highly reactive (often forming cross-links) with biological macromolecules. Irritant stimuli, of which acrolein is one of the most potent, activate respiratory sensory nerve endings, especially TRPA1 (Bautista *et al.*, 2006; Andre *et al.*, 2008). More plentiful in cigarette smoke than PAHs, acrolein can adduct tumor suppressor p53 (TP53) DNA (Tang *et al.*, 2011). Acrolein is also generated endogenously at sites of lung injury, and excessive breath levels (sufficient to activate metalloproteinases and increase mucin transcripts) (Deshmukh *et al.*, 2009) have been detected in persons with COPD or asthma (Deshmukh *et al.*, 2008). Because of its high reactivity, acrolein alters gene regulation, increases inflammation, decreases mucociliary transport, and

Table 15-7

Agents That Produce Lung Injury and Disease

TOXICANT	DISEASE	EXPOSURE	ACUTE EFFECT	CHRONIC EFFECT
Acrolein	Acute lung injury, chronic obstructive pulmonary disease	Biomass or hot oil cooking, fire fighters, environmental tobacco smoke, biocide water treatment	Cough, shortness of breath, extreme oronasal irritation, pulmonary edema, airway hyperreactivity	Chronic obstructive pulmonary disease, possibly asthma or lung cancer
Aluminum abrasives	Shaver disease, corundum smelter's lung, bauxite lung	Abrasives manufacturing, smelting	Alveolar edema	Interstitial fibrosis, emphysema
Aluminum dust	Aluminosis	Aluminum, firework, ceramic, paint, electrical good, and abrasive manufacturing	Cough, shortness of breath	Interstitial fibrosis
Ammonia		Farming, refrigeration operations, ammonia, fertilizer, chemical, and explosive manufacturing	Oronasal and bronchial irritation, pulmonary edema	Acute lung injury, chronic bronchitis
Arsenic		Pesticide, pigment, glass, and alloy manufacturing	Bronchitis	Laryngitis, bronchitis, and lung cancer
Asbestos	Asbestosis	Mining, construction, shipbuilding, brake repair, vermiculite contaminant		Fibrosis, pleural calcification, lung cancer, mesothelioma
Aspergillus	Framer lung, composte lung, malt worker's lung	Working with moldy hay, compost, or barley	Bronchoconstriction, cough, chest tightness	Extrinc allergic alveolitis (hypersensitivity pneumonitis)
Avian protein	Bird fancier's lung	Bird handling and farming with exposure to bird droppings	Bronchoconstriction, cough, chest tightness	Extrinc allergic alveolitis (hypersensitivity pneumonitis)
Beryllium	Berylliosis	Mining, alloy, and ceramic manufacturing, Milling beryllium	Pulmonary edema, pneumonia	Interstitial granulomatosis, progressive dyspnea, cor pulmonarle, fibrosis, and lung cancer
Cadmium		Welding, smelting, and electrical equipment, battery, alloy, and pigment manufacturing	Cough, pneumonia	Emphysema, cor pulmonale
Carbides of tungsten, titanium, or tantalum	Hard metal disease	Metal cutting and manufacturing	Bronchial epithelial hyper- and metaplasia	Peribronchial and perivascular fibrosis
Chlorine		Paper, plastics, chlorinated product manufacturing	Cough, hemoptysis, dyspnea, bronchitis, pneumonia	
Chromium (VI)		Chromium compound, paint, pigment, chromite ore reduction manufacturing	Oronasal and bronchial irritation	Fibrosis, lung cancer
Coal dust	Coal worker's pneumoconiosis	Coal mining		Fibrosis with emphysema
Cotton dust	Byssinosis	Textile manufacturing	Chest tightness, wheezing, dyspnea	Restrictive lung disease, chronic bronchitis

Agent	Associated disease/condition	Industry/process	Acute effect	Chronic effect
Hydrogen fluoride		Chemical, photograph film, solvent and plastic manufacturing	Airway irritation, hemorrhagic pulmonary edema	
Iron oxides	Siderotic lung disease, silver finisher's lung, hematite miner's lung, arc welder's lung	Welding, steel and jewelry manufacturing, foundry work, hematite mining	Cough	Silver finisher's lung with subpleural and perivascular macrophage aggregates; Hematite miner's lung with diffuse fibrosis-like pneumoconiosis; Arc welder's lung with bronchitis
Isocyanates		Auto painting, and plastic and chemical manufacturing	Airway irritation, cough, dyspnea	Asthma
Kaolin	Kaolinosis	Pottery making		Fibrosis
Manganese	Manganese pneumonia	Chemical and metal manufacturing	Acute pneumonia (often fatal)	Recurrent pneumonia
Nickel		Nickel mining, smelting, electroplating, battery manufacturing, fossil fuel combustion	Delayed pulmonary edema, skin allergy	Acute lung injury, chronic bronchitis, non-small-cell lung cancer, nasal cancer
Nitrogen oxides	Silo-filler's diseases	Silo filling, welding, explosive manufacturing	Immediate or delayed pulmonary edema	Bronchiolitis obliterans, emphysema in experimental animals
Nontuberculous mycobacteria	Metalworking fluid hypersensitivity	Working with metal cutting fluid contain water and contaminated with mycobacteria	Bronchoconstriction, cough, chest tightness	Extrinc allergic alveolitis (hypersensitivity pneumonitis)
Organic (sugar cane) dust (possibly contaminated with thermophilic actinomycete)	Bagassosis	Sugar cane and molasses manufacturing (bagasse is the fibrosis residue from sugar extraction)	Bronchoconstriction, cough, chest tightness	Extrinc allergic alveolitis (hypersensitivity pneumonitis)
Ozone		Welding, photocopying, bleaching flour, water treatment, deordorizing	Substernal pain, exacerbation of asthma, bronchitis, pulmonary edema	Fibrosis (including airways)
Perchloroethylene		Dry cleaning, metal degreasing, grain fumigation	Edema	Hepatic and lung cancer
Phosgene		Plastic, pesticide, and chemical manufacturing	Severe pulmonary edema	Bronchitis and fibrosis
Silica	Silicosis, pneumoconiosis	Mining, stone cutting, sand blasting, farming, quarry mining, tunneling	Acute silicosis (inflammation)	Fibrosis, silicotuberculosis
Sulfur dioxide		Chemical manufacturing, refrigeration, bleaching, fumigation	Bronchoconstriction, cough, chest tightness	Chronic bronchitis
Talc	Talcosis	Mining, rubber manufacturing, cosmetics	Cough	Fibosis
Thermophilic actinomycete	Farmer lung, mushroom worker's lung, penguin humidifier lung	Farming (hay or grain degradation)	Bronchoconstriction, cough, chest tightness	Extrinc allergic alveolitis (hypersensitivity pneumonitis)
Tin		Mining, tin processing		Widespread mottling in chest x-ray often without clinical impairment
Vanadium		Metal cutting and manufacturing, specialty steel manufacturing	Airway irritation and mucus production	Chronic bronchitis

diminishes alveolar-capillary barrier integrity (Jang *et al.*, 2011). In laboratory animals, high acrolein exposures have lead to acute lung injury and pulmonary edema (Leikauf *et al.*, 2011) similar to that produced by smoke inhalation, whereas lower concentrations have produced bronchial hyperreactivity (Leikauf *et al.*, 1989), excessive mucus production (Deshmukh *et al.*, 2005), and alveolar enlargement (Borchers *et al.*, 2007). Susceptibility to acrolein exposure is associated with differential regulation of cell surface receptor, transcription factor, and ubiquitin–proteasome genes (Fabisiak *et al.*, 2011; Leikauf *et al.*, 2011). Thus, acrolein contributes to the morbidly and mortality associated with acute lung injury and COPD, and possibly asthma and lung cancer. Although irritant-induced sensory responses can serve as warning signs and promote avoidance behavior or protective measures, acrolein exposure remains a global health problem because its release is closely linked to basic human needs (eg, cooking), emergencies (eg, fire fighting), or personal habits (eg, smoking).

Asbestos Asbestos refers to a group of silicate minerals in fiber form. The most commonly mined and commercially used asbestos fibers include the serpentine chrysotile asbestos and the amphiboles crocidolite, anthophyllite, amosite, actinolite, and tremolite asbestos. Exposure to asbestos fibers occurs in mining operations and in the construction and shipbuilding industries, where asbestos was at one time widely used for its insulating and fireproofing properties. Concern about asbestos in older buildings has led to the removal of asbestos-based insulating material; abatement workers may now represent an additional population at risk.

Asbestos causes three forms of lung disease: asbestosis, lung cancer, and malignant mesothelioma (Mossman *et al.*, 2011). Asbestosis is a form of pulmonary fibrosis with characteristically diffuse collagen foci and the presence of asbestos fibers, either free or coated with a proteinaceous material (asbestos bodies). Alveolar macrophage clearance is critical to the prevention of asbestosis and depends on fiber length, biopersistance, and dose (Churg *et al.*, 2003; Churg, 2003). Lung cancer develops in workers in the asbestos mining industry and smoking of cigarettes greatly enhances risk. Malignant mesothelioma is a rare form of cancer that develops mainly in the pleural mesothelium, the protective lining that covers the lungs, diaphragm, and interior of the chest wall. Unlike lung cancer, mesothelioma is not associated with smoking history.

Observations in humans sometimes differ from those in laboratory animals. In animal experiments, chrysotile produces mesothelioma much more readily than do the amphibole fibers. In humans, amphibole fibers are implicated more often even when the predominant exposure is to chrysotile asbestos. Chrysotile breaks down much more readily than do the amphiboles. One possibility is that in laboratory animals, the chrysotile fibers, even if broken down, are retained longer relative to the life span of the animal than they are in humans, thus explaining the higher rate of mesothelioma developed.

Health hazards associated with asbestos exposure depend on fiber shape, length, and surface properties (Lippmann, 1994; Oberdörster *et al.*, 2005; Donaldson *et al.*, 2010). Chrysolite asbestos are curved fibers and tend to be less toxic than crocidolite fibers that are long and thin, straight fibers. Fibers 2 μm in length may produce asbestosis; mesothelioma is associated with fibers ≥5 μm long, and lung cancer with fibers ≥10 μm. Fiber diameter is another critical feature. Fibers with diameters larger than ~3 μm do not readily penetrate into the peripheral lung. Only fibers ≥0.15 μm in diameter are likely to produce asbestosis or lung cancer. Mesothelioma, however, is more often associated with fiber diameter <0.5 μm because thinner fibers may be translocated from their site of deposition via the lymphatics to other organs, including the pleural surface (Oberdörster *et al.*, 2005). The surface properties of asbestos fibers also contribute

to toxicity (Upadhyay and Kamp, 2003; Mossman *et al.*, 2011). Crocidolite contains more iron (including ferrous iron (Fe^{2+}) that may participate in Fenton chemistry to generate reactive oxygen species) than chrysolite. The interaction of iron on the surface of asbestos fibers with oxygen may lead to the production of hydrogen peroxide and the highly reactive hydroxyl radical—events that have been associated with asbestos toxicity (Upadhyay and Kamp, 2003). The protection afforded by SOD or free radical scavengers in asbestos-related cell injury in vitro support a role of reactive oxygen species and concomitant oxidized lipids as a mechanism of asbestos toxicity.

Once asbestos fibers have been deposited in the lung, they may become phagocytized by alveolar macrophages (Churg *et al.*, 2003; Churg, 2003). Short fibers are completely ingested and subsequently removed via the mucociliary escalator. Longer fibers are incompletely ingested, and the macrophages become unable to leave the alveoli. Activated by the fibers, macrophages release mediators such as cytokine, chemokines, and growth factors, which in turn attract immunocompetent cells or stimulate collagen production. Asbestos-related lung disease thus may be mediated through the triggering of an epithelial injury and macrophage activation, and inflammatory events or through the production of changes that eventually lead to the initiation (DNA damage caused by reactive molecular species) or promotion (increased rate of cell turnover in the lung) of the carcinogenic process (Mossman *et al.*, 2011).

Silica Inhaled particles of silicon dioxide (silica) cause a characteristic human lung disease—silicosis. Crystalline silica is a major component of the earth's crust; silicon is only second to oxygen as the most common element. Mineral forms of silicon exist primarily as crystalline SiO_2 with a central silicon atom forming a tetrahedron with four shared oxygen atoms. The three principal crystalline isomeric forms are quartz, tridymite, and cristobalite. The tetrahedral structure is biopersisent and linked to fibrogenic potential. Stishovite, a rare crystalline variant without the tetrahedral conformation, is biologically inert. Amorphous forms of silica (eg, kieselguhr and vitreous silica) also have low fibrogenic potential. The ubiquitous presence of silica has made it an occupational hazard ever since tools were cut from stone, and silicosis remains a significant industrial hazard throughout the world in occupations such as mining and quarrying, sandblasting, and foundry work.

In addition to its structure, particle size, concentration, and surface properties affect the pathogenicity of silica both in vivo and in vitro. In humans, the most fibrogenic particle size appears to be about 1 μm (range 0.5–3 μm). In animal experiments (rats, hamsters), the comparable values appear to be 1 to 2 μm (range 0.5–5 μm). In animals, the concentration of silica dust is directly related to the intensity and rapidity of the histological reaction in the lung. When compared with stored silica or coated silica, freshly fractured silica particles produce more free radicals from their surface, increasing the respiratory burst when phagocytized and more pulmonary inflammation (Vallyathan *et al.*, 1995).

Silicosis may be acute or chronic with distinct pathological consequences. Acute silicosis occurs only in subjects exposed to a very high level silica (most often quartz or sand) small enough to be respirable (usually <5 μm) over a relatively short period, generally a few months or years. These patients have worsening dyspnea, fever, cough, and weight loss that can rapidly progress to respiratory failure, usually ending in death within two years. No known therapeutic strategy controls the relentless course of acute silicosis.

Chronic silicosis has a long latency period, usually >10 years and can be divided into simple and complicated silicosis. Even after radiographic changes, simple silicosis may be asymptomatic (ie, no dyspnea) with little change in pulmonary function. The x-ray presents fibrotic nodules, generally in the apical portion of lung. The hilar lymph nodes have peripheral calcifications known as egg-shell calcifications. Simple silicosis may progress into complicated silicosis, which is defined as the presence of conglomerate nodules larger than 1 cm in diameter. These nodules usually occur in the upper and mid-lung zones. In advanced stages, the nodules may be surrounded by emphysematous bullae. Chronic silicosis is associated with an increased incidence of tuberculosis.

The pathophysiological basis of pulmonary fibrosis in chronic silicosis is probably better understood than is the etiology of any other form of pulmonary fibrosis (Huaux, 2007). The role of pulmonary alveolar macrophages in the ingestion of silica is an initiating event. Macrophages phagocytose silica particles into phagosomes that fuse with endosomes during the internalization process (Costantini et al., 2011). Similar to the fate of microorganisms, macrophages experience phagosomal destabilization (Hornung et al., 2008) and activate pathways including the NALP3 inflammasome (Cassel et al., 2008; Dostert et al., 2008), PRRs, and antiviral pathways to release inflammatory cytokines (Giordano et al., 2010). In contrast to microorganisms, silica particles cannot be degraded and macrophages undergo cell death, releasing these particles that are engulfed by other macrophages, thus perpetuating the process of phagocytosis and cell death (Huaux, 2007). This leads to elevated mediator release (TGFB1, TNF, etc) (Di Giuseppe et al., 2009), EMT (Chapman, 2011), and initiates and maintains myofibroblast collagen (Munger and Sheppard, 2011).

Naphthalene Naphthalene occurs in cigarette smoke, tars, petroleum and is a precursor in the chemical synthesis of tanning agents, phthalic acid anhydride, carbaryl, and 2-naphthol. In laboratory animals, inhaled or parenterally administered naphthalene produces extensive necrosis in the bronchiolar epithelium of the mouse but much less necrosis in the airways of rats, hamsters, or monkeys (Buckpitt et al., 2002). The primary target in the surface epithelium is the bronchiolar secretoglobin cells. These cells were thought to be very important because they contain a stem cell subpopulation. They were once thought to be capable of cellular maintenance of the epithelium in bronchi, bronchioles, and alveolar regions. However, recent evidence suggests that these cells are only involved in the long-term maintenance and repair of airways but not alveolar epithelium (Rawlins et al., 2009). In mice, naphthalene is metabolized to naphthalene oxide primarily through CYP2F enzymes (Shultz et al., 1999; Baldwin et al., 2005). In rats and other species, including monkeys, conversion of naphthalene is less stereospecific and the rates of formation of the epoxide are much slower than in mice (Buckpitt et al., 2002). Naphthalene epoxides may subsequently be conjugated with glutathione and form adducts that are eliminated as mercapturic acids. The epoxide can undergo rearrangement to 1-naphthol with subsequent metabolism to quinones, which are potentially toxic compounds. Naphthalene metabolites bind covalently to cellular proteins that are important in normal cellular homeostasis and protein folding and this may be related to the mechanism of toxicity by this chemical. Interestingly, in both mice and rhesus monkeys the total amount of adducted protein is similar (Lin et al., 2006).

Blood-Borne Agents That Cause Pulmonary Toxicity in Humans

A number of compounds administered systematically can enter the lung through pulmonary circulation and cause lung injury and disease. For example, intraparenteral napthalene has marked lung toxicity in the mouse, probably due to an enrichment of an activating enzyme (CYP2F) in a specific cell in the lung epithelium (Buckpitt et al., 2002). Another example is that the ingestion of arsenic has

been associated with lung cancer (Putila and Guo, 2011). Below are two more examples that have had toxicological significance in clinical settings.

Bleomycin Bleomycin is a cancer chemotherapeutic drug with a major complication—pulmonary fibrosis that can be fatal (Jules-Elysee and White, 1990). Bleomycin produces a sequence of injury and necrosis capillary endothelial cells, alveolar type I cell, edema formation and hemorrhage, delayed (after one–two weeks) proliferation and apoptosis of alveolar type II cells, and eventually thickening of the alveolar walls by fibrotic changes. In many tissues, the cytosolic enzyme bleomycin hydrolase inactivates bleomycin (Schwartz et al., 1999). In lung and skin, two target organs for bleomycin toxicity, the activity of this enzyme is low compared with that in other organs. Bleomycin stimulates the production of collagen in the lung. Before increased collagen biosynthesis, steady-state levels of mRNA coding for fibronectin and procollagens are increased, subsequent to a bleomycin-mediated release of cytokines such as TGFB1 and TNF (Ortiz et al., 1999). In mice, bleomycin-induced TGFB1 is critical because mice deficiency in its receptor TGFBR2 in alveolar epithelial cells have attenuated fibrosis and increased survival following bleomycin treatment (Degryse et al., 2011). Bleomycin also combines with Fe(II) and molecular oxygen; when it combines with DNA, single- and double-strand breaks are produced by a free radical reaction. Animal models of belomycin-induced pulmonary fibrosis have been used to study the efficacy of promising antifibrotic drugs (Giri, 2003) and stem cell therapy (Ortiz et al., 2003).

Cyclophosphamide and 1,3 Bis (2-Chloroethyl)-1-Nitrosourea (BCNU) A number of chemotherapeutic drugs can produce lung damage and pulmonary toxicity in patients treated with these drugs and can be a significant problem (Meadors et al., 2006). Cyclophosphamide is widely used as an anticancer and immunosuppressive drug. The undesirable side effects include hemorrhagic cystitis and pulmonary fibrosis (Fraiser et al., 1991). Cyclophosphamide is metabolized by the cytochrome P450 system to two highly reactive metabolites: acrolein and phosphoramide mustard. In the lung, cooxidation with the PGH synthase system, which has high activity in the lung, is a possibility. Although the exact mechanism of action for causing lung damage has not been established, studies with isolated lung microsomes have shown that cyclophosphamide and its metabolite acrolein initiate lipid peroxidation (Patel and Block, 1985).

Another chemotherapeutic drug that has pulmonary fibrosis as a complication is carmustine (BCNU) BCNU exerts its antitumor properties by reacting with cellular macromolecules and forms inter- and intrastrand cross-links with DNA. In humans, a dose-related pulmonary toxicity is often noticed first by a decrease in diffusion capacity, which can develop into fatal pulmonary fibrosis (Weiss et al., 1981). The mechanism of action is not entirely clear (Wu et al., 2001). It is possible that BCNU inhibits pulmonary glutathione disulfide reductase, an event that may lead to a disturbed GSH/GSSG state in pulmonary cells. Eventually, this state leaves the cell unable to cope with oxidant stress. High concentrations of oxygen in the inspired air may enhance the pulmonary toxicity of BCNU and also that of the other anticancer drugs known to affect lung tissue: cyclophosphamide and bleomycin.

EVALUATION OF TOXIC LUNG DAMAGE

Humans Studies

Although the lung is susceptible to multiple toxic injuries, it is also amenable to a number of tests that allow evaluation of proper functioning (Utell and Frampton, 2000; Rennard and Spurzen, 2006;

Huang and Ghio, 2009). Commonly used tests include measurement of FEV1, FVC, and airway resistance. Additional tests evaluate the maximal flow rates and different lung volumes, diffusion capacity, oxygen, and carbon dioxide content of the arterial and venous blood, distribution of ventilation, and lung and chest wall compliance. Many pulmonary function tests (eg, FEV1 and FVC) require active collaboration by the subject examined. This noninvasive test is easy to administer to adults (ATS, 1991) and children (Beydon *et al.*, 2007), and does not require sophisticated equipment or a hospital setting. The subject is asked first to inhale deeply and then to exhale the air as quickly as possible. The test is repeated typically three times and the result of the best effort is recorded. The test is often used in epidemiological studies or controlled clinical studies designed to assess the potential adverse effects of air pollutants. A reduction in FEV1 is usually indicative of impaired ventilation such as that found in restrictive (increased lung stiffness) or obstructive (obstructed airflow) lung disease.

To accomplish proper oxygenation of venous blood and elimination of CO_2, the gases have to diffuse across the air–blood barrier (Macintyre *et al.*, 2005). The structural properties that control gas exchange include the lung gas volume, the path length for diffusion in the gas phase; the thickness and area of the alveolar capillary membrane, and the volume of blood in capillaries supplying ventilated alveoli. The functional properties that control gas exchange include the uniformity of ventilation and perfusion with respect to each other, the diffusion characteristics of the alveolar membrane; the binding properties of hemoglobin (Hb) in the alveolar capillaries, and the gas tensions in blood in the pulmonary vascular bed that exchanges gas with the alveoli. Gas exchange may be hindered by the accumulation of fluids or cellular elements in the alveoli (edema, pneumonic infiltrates), thickening of the alveolar wall (fibrosis), insufficient ventilation of the alveolar region (emphysema), ventilation–perfusion mismatching, or insufficient presence of oxygen transport elements (reduced alveolar blood volume or reduced amount of Hb in the blood). Gas exchange can be evaluated by measuring the arterial partial pressure of both oxygen and CO_2. In general, blood gas analysis is a comparatively insensitive assay for disturbed ventilation because of the organisms' buffering and reserve capacities, but may be a useful tool in clinical medicine. Measurement of diffusion capacity with CO, a gas that binds with 250 times higher affinity to Hb than does oxygen, is more sensitive. The test is easy to perform in humans and laboratory animals and is widely used in clinical studies.

Proper lung function in humans can be evaluated with several additional techniques. Computed tomography provides detailed roentgenographic information of airways and lung parenchyma and has been useful in screening high-risk patients for lung cancer (National Lung Screening Trial, 2011). Increased concentrations of nitric oxide are often found in exhaled air when inflammatory processes have led to induction of iNOS (Barnes *et al.*, 2010). As an experimental method, exhaled breath or induced sputum analysis may also be useful in assessing other inflammatory indicators in exhaled breath condensate such as oxidative stress markers (eg, hydrogen peroxide and isoprostanes), nitric oxide derivatives (eg, nitrate and nitrates), arachidonic acid metabolites (eg, prostanoids, leukotrienes, and epoxides), adenosine, and cytokines (Popov, 2011). Fiberoptic bronchoscopy has become one of the most valuable tools for the detection of toxic lung injury (Reynolds, 2011). The procedure allows direct visual inspection of the major lobar and segmental airways; the depth of penetration is limited by the external diameter of the bronchoscope, usually 5 mm. Bronchoscopy also allows the introduction and retrieval of saline solutions into the lung and subsequent analysis for cellular and molecular constituents

(broncholveolar lavage). Excision of small tissue samples (biopsies) during bronchoscopy is an additional diagnostic tool, most helpful in the evaluation and staging of precancerous and cancerous lesions.

Animals Studies

The toxicology of inhaled materials has been and continues to be extensively studied in experimental animals (Mauderly, 1996). In such studies, selection of animals with a respiratory system similar to that of humans is particularly desirable (Phalen *et al.*, 2008). The respiratory system of monkeys most closely resembles that of humans. However, the availability and cost of these animals and the necessity for special facilities for housing monkeys and performing long-term exposures, along with ethical considerations, including the confinement of primates in small exposure chambers for prolonged periods, severely limits the use of primates. Rats and mice are widely used, although fundamental differences in respiratory anatomy (eg, lack of respiratory bronchioles) and function (rats and mice are obligate nose breathers) can complicate the extrapolation of effects to humans. Experimental studies with guinea pigs and rabbits provided the first conclusive evidence that sulfuric acid and SO_2 may damage human lungs (Amdur, 1989). The following techniques are used to study the effects of inhaled toxicants in animals.

Inhalation Exposure Systems In inhalation studies, animals are kept within a chamber that is ventilated with a defined test atmosphere (Phalen, 1976; Wong, 2007). Generation of such an atmosphere is comparatively easy for gases that are available in high purity in a compressed tank, for example, SO_2, O_2, or NO_2. Metering and dilution produce appropriate concentrations for exposure. Final concentrations within the chamber monitored continuously with direct reading detectors (eg, UV for ozone or infrared for CO_2) that are calibrated. Exposure should be within 5% of the targeted concentration. Alternatively, wet chemical analysis procedures are applied after sampled gases from the chambers are bubbled through traps. Such sampling yields a time-weighted average for the concentration. More challenging is the generation of particles or complex mixtures (eg, tobacco smoke, diesel, and gasoline exhaust or residual oil fly ash), particularly because of the possibility of interactions between individual mixture constituents and the possibility of formation of artifacts (Pauluhn, 2005).

Exposure chambers must allow for the rapid attainment of the desired concentrations of toxicants, maintenance of desired toxicant levels homogeneously throughout the chamber, adequate capacity for experimental animals, and minimal accumulation of undesired products associated with animal occupancy (usually ammonia, dander, heat, and carbon dioxide). As a general rule, the total body volume of the animals should not exceed 5% of the chamber volume. Nose-only exposure chambers avoid some of these problems (Phalen *et al.*, 1984). However, nose-only exposure systems create different problems, including a great deal of stress on the animals due to confinement during exposure, and the very labor-intensive handling that is required for exposures by this route. The proper selection of exposure techniques for a given chemical is ultimately a decision that must be made on a case-by-case basis. Finally, concern for the environment and the safety of facility personnel suggest prudence in how chambers are exhausted.

Pulmonary Function Tests in Experimental Animals Conducting pulmonary function tests in experimental animals poses distinct challenges, especially in small rodents (Reinhard *et al.*, 2005). Experimental animals cannot be made to maximally inhale or exhale at the investigator's will. For example, FEV_1 can be obtained in experimental animals only under anesthesia. Expiration is forced by applying external pressure to the thorax or negative pressure to the airways (Vinegar *et al.*, 1979). Alternatively, analysis of pressure–volume curves is a comparatively easy test to perform in animals, not requiring a specialized apparatus (Alarie *et al.*, 1961; Sinnett *et al.*, 1981). The test provides some indication of lung compliance. Compliance (volume/pressure) is calculated as the slope of the volume–pressure curve. The volume–pressure curve involves deflating the lung and then inflating the lung with incremental volumes and recording the pressure, and can be obtained from lungs filled with air and/or physiological saline. The lung is then deflated with incremental volumes and pressure again recorded. Compliance provides an indication of the intrinsic elastic properties of the lung parenchyma and, when measured in vivo, the thoracic cage. In emphysema, compliance of the lung increases because elatic recoil is decreased. When the inflation and deflation are performed with air, the curves will not match and this hysteresis is an indication of surfactant function. The use of saline is sensitive to structural changes in lung parenchyma, as the effects of surfactant are eliminated in a saline-filled lung.

Another pulmonary function test is the analysis of airway resistance, which can be measured in laboratory animals by restrained plethysmography (Amdur and Mead, 1958), unrestrained video-assisted plethysmography (Bates *et al.*, 2008), or unrestrained acoustic plethysmography (Reynolds *et al.*, 2008). An increase in airway resistance is a measure of bronchoconstriction inasmuch as the airway smooth muscle contraction or airway mucosal edema narrows the airway lumen and obstructs airflow. Airway resistance also can be measured after a challenge of incremental doses of inhaled methacholine (or histamine) (Bates and Irvin, 2003) or infused acetylcholine (Swiecichowski *et al.*, 1993). This challenge provides a measure of airway hyperreactivity, a distinguishing feature of asthma in humans. In asthma, resting airway resistance is typically normal but when challenged, airway resistance will increase at a lower threshold dose of methacholine. Analysis of breathing pattern can also be used and may differentiate between upper airway and lower airway irritants (Alarie *et al.*, 1988; Bates *et al.* 2004). In rodents, upper airway ("sensory") irritants produce a breathing pattern of decreased respiratory frequency with increased tidal volume, whereas lower airway ("pulmonary") irritants produce a breathing pattern of increased respiratory frequency and decreased minute volume (ie, the total volume of air breathed in 1 minute).

Morphological Techniques The pathology of acute and chronic injury may be examined by gross inspection and under the microscope and should include the nasal passages, larynx, major bronchi, and the lung parenchyma.

Regional distribution of lesions in nasal passages can be assessed after fixation and decalcification. Various regions of the nasal passages can then be examined by obtaining cross sections at multiple levels. Proper fixation of the lung is done by vascular perfusion with fixative through the pulmonary artery or by instillation of fixative through the trachea. Perfusion fixation does not dislodge material (lining fluid, deposited particles) or cells in the lumen of the airways or the alveoli from their original position. Fixation by intratracheal instillation can be done under controlled pressure (usually 30 cm H_2O in rodents), which preserves alveolar architecture. This permits semiquantitative or quantitative measurements to be made. The choice of fixative depends on how the lung will be further analyzed. Formalin-based fixatives are satisfactory for routine histopathology, whereas the use of more sophisticated techniques such as electron microscopy, immunohistochemistry, and in situ hybridization require careful selection of the fixative.

Paraffin sections of respiratory tract tissue are suitable for routine histopathological analysis of gross pathological changes, for example, inflammation, fibrosis, or lung tumors. The tissue can be stained with (a) hematoxylin and eosin stain for routine assessment (Llewellyn, 2009), (b) periodic acid-Shiff's Alcian blue stain for glycoproteins (mucus cells) (Jeffery *et al.*, 1982), or (c) Masson trichrome stain for collagen (Goldner, 1938). Plastic or Epon sections 1-μm thick are required for proper identification of additional cell types or recognition of cytoplasmic changes as in damaged BSCs. Other structural alterations, such as degenerative changes or necrosis of type I epithelial cells or capillary endothelial cells, usually are detected by transmission electron microscopy (TEM). TEM is essential for an unequivocal identification of cells in the alveolar interstitium and is used mainly in morphometric analysis of the lung. Scanning electron microscopy allows visualization of the surface of interior lung structures, reveals alterations in the tissue surface, and detects rearrangement of the overall cell population. Confocal microscopy, consisting of a laser microscope coupled to a computer, allows examination of thick sections and discovery of specific cell types deep within the tissue labeled with fluorescent markers; it is an ideal tool for three-dimensional reconstruction of normal and damaged lung.

Morphometry, the quantitative description of structure, refers to a quantitative analysis of tissue (Gehr *et al.*, 1993). Measurements made in two dimensions on photographs taken under the microscope allow one to measure areas, the thickness of a structure, and numerical density. Using the appropriate formula, values such as the volume occupied by a specific cell population in the entire lung parenchyma can be calculated (Hyde *et al.*, 2007).

Additional tools for the study of toxic lung injury include immunohistochemistry, in situ hybridization, and analysis of cell kinetics. Transcriptome (Mohr *et al.*, 2002), proteomic (Miller *et al.*, 2008), and metabolome (Fabisiak *et al.*, 2011) profiling are additional value tools to assess the lung in health and disease. Antibodies to a variety of enzymes, mediators, and other proteins are available. It is possible to identify cell types that carry certain enzymes and their anatomic locations. In situ hybridization allows one to visualize anatomic sites where a specific gene product is expressed, for example, collagen production in a fibrotic lung. Two useful sites to obtain lung-specific expression include the Human Protein Atlas (Uhlen *et al.*, 2010) and GenePaint (Visel *et al.*, 2004). Ascribing a given metabolic capability to a specific cell type requires evaluation of gene expression and/or protein production in specific cells in situ. The normal adult lung is an organ for which under normal circumstances very few cells appear to die and to be replaced. When damaged by a toxic insult, the lung parenchyma is capable of repairing itself in an efficient manner. Type I cell damage is followed by proliferation of type II epithelial cells, which eventually transform into new type I cells (Adamson and Bowden, 1974; Fujino *et al.*, 2011); in the airways, the BSCs proliferate and divide following injury to ciliated cells (Rock and Hogan, 2011; Delgado *et al.*, 2011). Quantitative data can be obtained by either injection of the DNA precursors (tritated thymide, bromodeoxyuridine) or visualization of proliferating cell nuclear antigen (PCNA). Flow cytometry is valuable in the study of cell populations prepared from the lung.

Pulmonary Lavage and Pulmonary Edema Pulmonary edema and/or pulmonary inflammation are early events in acute and chronic lung injury. The fluid lining the pulmonary epithelium can be recovered by bronchoalveolar lavage. Analysis of the lavage fluid is a useful tool to detect respiratory tract toxicity (Henderson, 2005; Reynolds, 2011). Influx of neutrophils or other leukocytes such as lymphocytes or eosinophils into the lavage fluid is the most sensitive sign of inflammation. Measurements of lung injury include total protein and/or albumin. Additional measurements include secretory products of macrophages and epithelial cells include fribronectin, chemokines, and other cytokines (eg, TNF or IL1B). Reduced glutathione levels may be an indicator of oxidative stress. Lactate dehydrogenase activity (and its substituent isoenzymes), *N*-acetylglucosaminidase, acid or alkaline phosphatase, other lysosomal hydrolases, and sialic acid add additional information. In addition pulmonary edema can be assessed by determining lung wet:dry ratio or injection of Evan blue dye albumin (Patterson *et al.*, 1992; Li *et al.*, 2010).

In Vitro Studies

Isolated Perfused Lung In vitro systems with materials originally obtained from either human tissues or experimental animals are particularly suited for the study of mechanisms that cause lung injury (Aufderheide, 2005; Bakand and Hayes, 2010). The methods include isolated perfused lung, microdissection/organotypic tissue culture systems, and cell type–specific cell culture. The isolated perfused lung method is applicable to lungs from many laboratory species (eg, mouse, rat, guinea pig, or rabbit) (Mehendale *et al.*, 1981). The lung is perfused with blood or a blood substitute through the pulmonary arterial bed. At the same time, the lung is actively (through rhythmic inflation–deflation cycles with positive pressure) or passively (by creating negative pressure with an artificial thorax in which the lung is suspended) ventilated. Toxic agents can be introduced into the perfusate or the inspired air (Rhoades, 1984). Repeated sampling of the perfusate allows one to determine the rate of metabolism of drugs and the metabolic activity of the lung.

Airway Microdissection and Organotypic Tissue Culture Systems Many inhalants act in specific regions of the respiratory tract. For example, the terminal bronchioles, a region especially rich in the highly metabolically competent BSCs, is often a target of gases with low water solubility. Microdissection of the nasal passage (Fanucchi *et al.*, 1999) and airways (Plopper *et al.*, 1991) consists of stripping away surrounding tissue or parenchyma while maintaining the airway structure and exposing the epithelium. Microdissected airways can be studied in culture for up to one week, can be used to study site-specific gene expression, morphological changes in toxicant injury and repair, or can be used for biochemical analyses including enzyme activity measurements and determination of antioxidant concentrations (such as glutathione). This facilitates study of the metabolically active BSCs found in the airways (Plopper *et al.*, 2001). Tissue culture systems have been developed in which epithelial cells maintain their polarity, differentiation, and normal function similar to what is observed in vivo. Epithelial cell surfaces are exposed to air (or a gas phase containing an airborne toxic agent), while the basal portion is bathed by a tissue culture medium (Widdicombe and Welsh, 1980).

Lung Cell Culture Many lung-specific cell types have been isolated and can be maintained as cell culture. Human (Reynolds, 2011) and animal (Kobzik *et al.*, 1988) alveolar or interstitial macrophages can be obtained from lavage or lung tissue. Their function can be examined in vitro with or without exposure to appropriate toxic stimuli (Brain, 1986; Brain *et al.*, 1994). Type II alveolar epithelial cells can be isolated and primary cell cultures maintained in culture for short periods (Dobbs *et al.*, 1997; Wang *et al.*, 2007). Direct isolation of type I epithelial cells has also been successful (Williams, 2003).

Maintenance of the epithelial cells at the air–liquid interface is important to maintain polarity and differentiation. Epithelial cells may be seeded on top of a suitable supporting material (eg, collagen or nitrocellulose membranes) with mesenchymal cells seeded on the other side to observe epithelial cell–fibroblast interactions. Systems are available for the isolation and culture of human bronchial epithelial cells (Lechner *et al.*, 1982; Lechner and LaVeck, 1985) and BSCs (Belinsky *et al.*, 1995). These cells can be differentiated into ciliated and mucin-producing cell by growth in air–liquid interface systems (Whitcutt *et al.*, 1988; de Jong *et al.*, 1994). Serous and mucus cells can be obtained from submucosal glands and maintained as primary cell culture (Finkbeiner *et al.*, 2010). Lung fibroblasts are easily grown (Baglole *et al.*, 2005) and have been studied in coculture with epithelial cells (Delgado *et al.*, 2011). Primary cell cultures have been transformed (Gruenert *et al.*, 1988) and/or immortalized (Reddel *et al.*, 1988; Vaughan *et al.*, 2006) and can be passaged and maintained for long periods in the laboratory. Cell lines established from lung tumors have been extensively used by investigators and have yield many novel insights into lung cancer (Gazdar *et al.*, 2010).

ACKNOWLEDGMENTS

The author thanks Sara Gillooly for editorial assistance and mentors (especially Morton Lippmann and Jay Nadel), postdoctoral fellows, students, and colleagues for their continued interest and inspiration. This study was funded in part by NIH grants: ES015675, HL077763, and HL085655.

REFERENCES

Abbinante-Nissen JM, Simpson LG, Leikauf GD. Neutrophil elastase increases secretory leukocyte protease inhibitor transcript levels in airway epithelial cells. *Am J Physiol.* 1993;265:L286–L292.

Adams FA. On air, water, and places. In: *The Genuine Works of Hippocrates.* Vol 1. London: Sydenham Society; 1849:179–222.

Adamson IY, Bowden DH. The type 2 cell as progenitor of alveolar epithelial regeneration. A cytodynamic study in mice after exposure to oxygen. *Lab Invest.* 1974;30:35–42.

Aitken J. On dust, fogs, and clouds. *Nature.* 1880;23:195–197.

Aitken J. The remarkable sunsets. *Proc Roy Soc Edinb.* 1884;12:448–450.

Alarie Y. Sensory irritation by airborne chemicals. *CRC Crit Rev Toxicol.* 1973;2:299–363.

Alarie Y, Schaper M, Nielsen GD, Abraham MH. Structure-activity relationships of volatile organic chemicals as sensory irritants. *Arch Toxicol.* 1988;72:125–140.

Alarie Y, Stone H, Latour R, Robillard E, Dautrebande L. New studies on aerosols. XV. Influence of constricting and dilating microaerosols on "pressure-volume" curves of isolated atelectactic rats' lung. *Arch Int Pharmacodyn Ther.* 1961;133:470–480.

Albert RE, Arnett LC. Clearance of radioactive dust from the human lung. *AMA Arch Ind Health.* 1955;12:99–106.

Albert RE, Sellakumar AR, Laskin S, Kuschner M, Nelson N, Snyder CA. Gaseous formaldehyde and hydrogen chloride induction of nasal cancer in the rat. *J Natl Cancer Inst.* 1982;68:597–603.

Alexis NE, Lay JC, Zeman KL, Geiser M, Kapp N, Bennett WD. In vivo particle uptake by airway macrophages in healthy volunteers. *Am J Respir Cell Mol Biol.* 2006;34:305–313.

Ali M, Lillehoj EP, Park Y, Kyo Y, Kim KC. Analysis of the proteome of human airway epithelial secretions. *Proteome Sci.* 2011;9:4.

Ali MS, Pearson JP. Upper airway mucin gene expression: a review. *Laryngoscope.* 2007;117:932–938.

Allavena P, Chieppa M, Bianchi G, et al. Engagement of the mannose receptor by tumoral mucins activates an immune suppressive phenotype in human tumor-associated macrophages. *Clin Dev Immunol.* 2010;2010:547179.

Allen-Gipson DS, Blackburn MR, Schneider DJ, et al. Adenosine activation of A2B receptor(s) is essential for stimulated epithelial ciliary motility and clearance. *Am J Physiol Lung Cell Mol Physiol.* 2011;301:L171–L180.

Amdur MO. Sulfuric acid: the animals tried to tell us. 1989 Herbert Stokinger Lecture. *Appl Ind Hyg.* 1989;4:189–197.

Amdur MO, Mead J. Mechanics of respiration in unanesthetized guinea pigs. *Am J Physiol.* 1958;192:364–368.

Amdur MO, Schulz RZ, Drinker P. Toxicity of sulfuric acid mist to guinea pigs. *AMA Arch Ind Hyg Occup Med.* 1952;5:318–329.

American Chemical Society Chemical Abstract Service. CAS Registry Numbers. Available at: http://www.cas.org/expertise/cascontent/registry/regsys.html. Accessed October 1, 2011.

American Conference of Governmental Industrial Hygienists. *Documentation of the Threshold Limit Values and Biological Exposure Indices.* 7th ed. ACGIH Publication No. 0100Doc, Cincinnati, OH; 2011.

American Thoracic Society. Lung function testing: selection of reference values and interpretative strategies. American Thoracic Society. *Am Rev Respir Dis.* 1991;1144:1202–1218.

Andre E, Campi B, Materazzi S, et al. Cigarette smoke-induced neurogenic inflammation is mediated by alpha, beta-unsaturated aldehydes and the TRPA1 receptor in rodents. *J Clin Invest.* 2008;118:2574–2582.

Anttila S, Raunio H, Hakkola J. Cytochrome P450-mediated pulmonary metabolism of carcinogens: regulation and cross-talk in lung carcinogenesis. *Am J Respir Cell Mol Biol.* 2011;44:583–590.

Arredouani MS, Palecanda A, Koziel H, et al. MARCO is the major binding receptor for unopsonized particles and bacteria on human alveolar macrophages. *J Immunol.* 2005;175:6058–6064.

Asgharian B, Price OT, Schroeter JD, Kimbell JS, Jones L, Singal M. Derivation of mass transfer coefficients for transient uptake and tissue disposition of soluble and reactive vapors in lung airways. *Ann Biomed Eng.* 2011;39:1788–1804.

Aufderheide M. Direct exposure methods for testing native atmospheres. *Exp Toxicol Pathol.* 2005;57(suppl 1):213–226.

Baglole CJ, Reddy SY, Pollock SJ, et al. Isolation and phenotypic characterization of lung fibroblasts. *Methods Mol Med.* 2005;117:115–127.

Bakand S, Hayes A. Troubleshooting methods for toxicity testing of airborne chemicals in vitro. *J Pharmacol Toxicol Methods.* 2010;61:76–85.

Baldwin RM, Schultz MA, Buckpitt AR. Bioactivation of the pulmonary toxicants naphthalene and 1-nitronaphthalene by rat CYP2F4. *J Pharmacol Exp Ther.* 2005;312:857–865.

Barnes PJ, Dweik RA, Gelb AF, et al. Exhaled nitric oxide in pulmonary diseases: a comprehensive review. *Chest.* 2010;138:682–692.

Bates J, Irvin C, Brusasco V, et al. The use and misuse of Penh in animal models of lung disease. *Am J Respir Cell Mol Biol.* 2004;31:373–374.

Bates JH, Irvin CG. Measuring lung function in mice: the phenotyping uncertainty principle. *J Appl Physiol.* 2003;94:1297–1306.

Bates JH, Thompson-Figueroa J, Lundblad LK, Irvin CG. Unrestrained video-assisted plethysmography: a noninvasive method for assessment of lung mechanical function in small animals. *J Appl Physiol.* 2008;104:253–261.

Baum A, Sachidanandam R, García-Sastre A. Preference of RIG-I for short viral RNA molecules in infected cells revealed by next-generation sequencing. *Proc Natl Acad Sci U S A.* 2010;107:16303–16308.

Bautista DM, Jordt SE, Nikai T, et al. TRPA1 mediates the inflammatory actions of environmental irritants and proalgesic agents. *Cell.* 2006;124:1269–1282.

Beckman JS. Understanding peroxynitrite biochemistry and its potential for treating human diseases. *Arch Biochem Biophys.* 2009;484:114–116.

Beckman JS, Beckman TW, Chen J, Marshall PA, Freeman BA. Apparent hydroxyl radical production by peroxynitrite: implications for endothelial injury from nitric oxide and superoxide. *Proc Natl Acad Sci USA.* 1990;87:1620–1624.

Beeson WL, Abbey DE, Knutsen SF. Long-term concentrations of ambient air pollutants and incident lung cancer in California adults: results from the ASHMOG study. Adventist Health Study on Smog. *Environ Health Perspect.* 1998;106:813–822.

Bein K, Leikauf GD. Acrolein—a pulmonary hazard. *Mol Nutr Food Sci.* 2011;55:1342–1360.

Belinsky SA, Lechner JF, Johnson NF. An improved method for the isolation of type II and Clara cells from mice. *In Vitro Cell Dev Biol Anim.* 1995;31:361–366.

Bellomo R. The cytokine network in the critically ill. *Anaesth Intensive Care.* 1992;20:288–302.

Berrington WR, Iyer R, Wells RD, Smith KD, Skerrett SJ, Hawn TR. NOD1 and NOD2 regulation of pulmonary innate immunity to *Legionella pneumophila. Eur J Immunol.* 2010;40:3519–3527.

Bessac BF, Jordt SE. Breathtaking TRP channels: TRPA1 and TRPV1 in airway chemosensation and reflex control. *Physiology (Bethesda).* 2008;23:360–370.

Bessac BF, Sivula M, von Hehn CA, Caceres AI, Escalera J, Jordt SE. Transient receptor potential ankyrin 1 antagonists block the noxious effects of toxic industrial isocyanates and tear gases. *FASEB J.* 2009;23:1102–1114.

Beydon N, Davis SD, Lombardi E, et al. An official American Thoracic Society/European Respiratory Society statement: pulmonary function testing in preschool children. *Am J Respir Crit Care Med.* 2007;175:1304–1345.

Bingham E, Pfitzer EA, Barkley W, Radford EP. Alveolar macrophages: reduced number in rats after prolonged inhalation of lead sesquioxide. *Science.* 1968;162:1297–1299.

Bingle L, Bingle CD. Distribution of human PLUNC/BPI fold-containing (BPIF) proteins. *Biochem Soc Trans.* 2011;39:1023–1027.

Bisetti AA. Bernardino Ramazzini and occupational lung medicine. *Ann N Y Acad Sci.* 1988;534:1029–1037.

Blanc PD. Occupational and environmental medicine: the historical perspective (Chapter 2). In: Rosenstock L, Cullen MR, Brodlin CA, Redlich CA, eds. *Textbook of Clinical Occupational and Environmental Medicine.* 2nd ed. Philadelphia: Elsevier Saunders; 2005:17–27.

British Medical Journal. Fog fatality in London. *Br Med J.* 1880;1:254.

Bond JA, Harkema JR, Russell VI. Regional distribution of xenobiotic metabolizing enzymes in respiratory airways of dogs. *Drug Metab Dispos.* 1988;16:116–124.

Borchers MT, Wesselkamper SC, Curull V, et al. Sustained CTL activation by murine pulmonary epithelial cells promotes the development of COPD-like disease. *J Clin Invest.* 2009;119:636–649.

Borchers MT, Wesselkamper SC, Harris NL, et al. CD8+ T cells contribute to macrophage accumulation and airspace enlargement following repeated irritant exposure. *Exp Mol Pathol.* 2007;83:301–310.

Bowden DH. Macrophages, dust and pulmonary diseases. *Exp Lung Res.* 1987;12:89–107.

Bowdish DM, Gordon S. Conserved domains of the class A scavenger receptors: evolution and function. *Immunol Rev.* 2009;227:19–31.

Brain JD. The effects of increased particles on the number of alveolar macrophages. *Inhaled Part.* 1970;1:209–225.

Brain JD. Toxicological aspects of alterations of pulmonary macrophage function. *Annu Rev Pharmacol Toxicol.* 1986;26:547–565.

Brain JD, Godleski J, Kreyling W. In vivo evaluation of chemical biopersistence of nonfibrous inorganic particles. *Environ Health Perspect.* 1994;102(suppl 5):119–125.

Brooks SM, Weiss MA, Bernstein IL. Reactive airways dysfunction syndrome (RADS). Persistent asthma syndrome after high level irritant exposures. *Chest.* 1985;88:376–384.

Buch SC, Diergaarde B, Nukui T, et al. Genetic variability in DNA repair and cell cycle control pathway genes and risk of smoking-related lung cancer. *Mol Carcinog.* 2011 [Epub ahead of print] PMID: 21976407.

Buckpitt A, Boland B, Isbell M, et al. Naphthalene-induced respiratory tract toxicity: metabolic mechanisms of toxicity. *Drug Metab Rev.* 2002;34:791–820.

Buckpitt AR, Cruikshank MK. Biochemical function of the respiratory tract: metabolism of xenobiotics. In: Sipes IG, McQueen CA, Gandolfi JA, eds. *Comprehensive Toxicology, Vol 8, Toxicology of the Respiratory System.* Oxford: Elsevier Science; 1997:159–186.

Bushey RT, Chen G, Blevins-Primeau AS, Krzeminski J, Amin S, Lazarus P. Characterization of UDP-glucuronosyltransferase 2A1 (UGT2A1) variants and their potential role in tobacco carcinogenesis. *Pharmacogenet Genomics.* 2011;21:55–65.

Casarett LJ. Some physical and physiological factors controlling the fate of inhaled substances. II. Retention. *Health Phys.* 1960;2:379–386.

Cassel SL, Eisenbarth SC, Iyer SS, et al. The Nalp3 inflammasome is essential for the development of silicosis. *Proc Natl Acad Sci USA.* 2008;105:9035–9040.

Chandrashekar J, Hoon MA, Ryba NJ, Zuker CS. The receptors and cells for mammalian taste. *Nature.* 2006;444:288–294.

Chapman HA. Epithelial-mesenchymal interactions in pulmonary fibrosis. *Annu Rev Physiol.* 2011;73:413–435.

Chapman HA Jr, Stone OL, Vavrin Z. Degradation of fibrin and elastin by intact human alveolar macrophages in vitro. Characterization of a plasminogen activator and its role in matrix degradation. *J Clin Invest.* 1984;73;806–815.

Chen G, Korfhagen TR, Xu Y, et al. SPDEF is required for mouse pulmonary goblet cell differentiation and regulates a network of genes associated with mucus production. *J Clin Invest.* 2009;119:2914–2924.

Chen HY, Yu SL, Chen CH, et al. A five-gene signature and clinical outcome in non-small-cell lung cancer. *N Engl J Med.* 2007;356:11–20.

Chen JH, Stoltz DA, Karp PH, et al. Loss of anion transport without increased sodium absorption characterizes newborn porcine cystic fibrosis airway epithelia. *Cell.* 2010;143:911–923.

Chung KF, Pavord ID. Prevalence, pathogenesis, and causes of chronic cough. *Lancet.* 2008;371:1364–1374.

Churg A. Interactions of exogenous or evoked agents and particles: the role of reactive oxygen species. *Free Radic Biol Med.* 2003;34:1230–1235.

Churg A, Wang RD, Xie C, Wright JL. Alpha-1-Antitrypsin ameliorates cigarette smoke-induced emphysema in the mouse. *Am J Respir Crit Care Med.* 2003;168:199–207.

Coffin DL, Gardner DE, Holzman RS, Wolock FJ. Influence of ozone on pulmonary cells. *Arch Environ Health.* 1968;16:633–636.

Costantini LM, Gilberti RM, Knecht DA. The phagocytosis and toxicity of amorphous silica. *PLoS One.* 2011;6:e14647.

Cutz E, Yeger H, Pan J. Pulmonary neuroendocrine cell system in pediatric lung disease-recent advances. *Pediatr Dev Pathol.* 2007;10:419–435.

Dalhamn T, Rodin J. Mucous flow and ciliary activity in the trachea of rats exposed to pulmonary irritant gas. *Br J Ind Med.* 1956;13:110–113.

D'Armiento J, Dalal SS, Okada Y, Berg RA, Chada K. Collagenase expression in the lungs of transgenic mice causes pulmonary emphysema. *Cell.* 1992;7:955–961.

Dautrebande L, Highman B, Alford WC. Studies on aerosols; reduction of dust deposition in lungs of rabbits by aqueous aerosols. *J Ind Hyg Toxicol.* 1948;30:103–107.

Davies CN. Dust particles and aqueous aerosols; a critical review. *J Ind Hyg Toxicol.* 1949;31:169.

De Flora S, Bennicelli C, D'Agostini F, Izzotti A, Camoirano A. Cytosolic activation of aromatic and heterocyclic amines. Inhibition by dicoumarol and enhancement in viral hepatitis B. *Environ Health Perspect.* 1994;102(suppl 6):69–74.

de Jong PM, van Sterkenburg MA, Hesseling SC, et al. Ciliogenesis in human bronchial epithelial cells cultured at the air-liquid interface. *Am J Respir Cell Mol Biol.* 1994;10:271–277.

Degryse AL, Tanjore H, Xu XC, et al. TGFβ signaling in lung epithelium regulates bleomycin-induced alveolar injury and fibroblast recruitment. *Am J Physiol Lung Cell Mol Physiol.* 2011;300:L887–L897.

Delgado O, Kaisani AA, Spinola M, et al. Multipotent capacity of immortalized human bronchial epithelial cells. *PLoS One.* 2011;6:e22023.

DeLucia AJ, Hoque PM, Mustafa MG, Cross CE. Ozone interaction with rodent lung: effect on sulfhydryls and sulfhydryl-containing enzyme activities. *J Lab Clin Med.* 1972;80:559–566.

DeMaria S, Ngai J. The cell biology of smell. *J Cell Biol.* 2010;191:443–452.

Denissenko MF, Pao A, Tang M, Pfeifer GP. Referential formation of benzo[a]pyrene adducts at lung cancer mutational hotspots in P53. *Science.* 1996;274:430–432.

Deshmukh HS, Case LM, Wesselkamper SC, et al. Metalloproteinases mediate mucin 5AC expression by epidermal growth factor receptor activation. *Am J Respir Crit Care Med.* 2005;171:305–314.

Deshmukh HS, McLachlan A, Atkinson JJ, et al. Matrix metalloproteinase-14 mediates a phenotypic shift in the airways to increase mucin production. *Am J Respir Crit Care Med.* 2009;180:834–845.

Deshmukh HS, Shaver C, Case LM, et al. Acrolein-activated matrix metalloproteinase 9 contributes to persistent mucin production. *Am J Respir Cell Mol Biol.* 2008;38:446–454.

Di Giuseppe M, Gambelli F, Hoyle GW, et al. Systemic inhibition of NF-kappaB activation protects from silicosis. *PLoS One.* 2009;4:e5689.

Ding X, Kaminsky LS. Human extrahepatic cytochromes P450: function in xenobiotic metabolism and tissue-selective chemical toxicity in the respiratory and gastrointestinal tracts. *Annu Rev Pharmacol Toxicol.* 2003;43:149–173.

Dobbs LG, Pian MS, Maglio M, Dumars S, Allen L. Maintenance of the differentiated type II cell phenotype by culture with an apical air surface. *Am J Physiol.* 1997;273:L347–L354.

Donaldson K, Murphy FA, Duffin R, Poland CA. Asbestos, carbon nanotubes and the pleural mesothelium: a review of the hypothesis regarding the role of long fibre retention in the parietal pleura, inflammation and mesothelioma. *Part Fibre Toxicol.* 2010;7:5.

Dostert C, Pétrilli V, Van Bruggen R, Steele C, Mossman BT, Tschopp J. Innate immune activation through Nalp3 inflammasome sensing of asbestos and silica. *Science.* 2008;320:674–677.

Drew RT, Eisenbud M. The pulmonary dose from 220Rn received by indigenous rodents of the Morro Do Ferro, Brazil. *Radiat Res.* 1970;42:270–281.

Drinker P, Thomson RM, Finn JL. Quantitative measurements of the inhalation, retention and exhalation of dusts and fumes by man. I. Concentrations of 50 to 450 mg. per cubic meter. *J Indust Hyg Toxicol.* 1928;10:13.

Elinav E, Strowig T, Henao-Mejia J, Flavell RA. Regulation of the antimicrobial response by NLR proteins. *Immunity.* 2011;34:665–679.

Evans MJ, Van Winkle LS, Fanucchi MV, Plopper CG. Cellular and molecular characteristics of basal cells in airway epithelium. *Exp Lung Res.* 2001;27:401–415.

Evelyn J. *Fumifugium: or The Inconvenience of the Aer and Smoak of London Dissipated. Together With Some Remedies Humbly Proposed by JE Esq, to his Sacred Majesty and to the Parliament Now Assembled.* London: His Majesty's Command; 1661. (Reprinted by the National Society for Clean Air in 1961. Dorset Press, Dorchester. 1961.)

Fabisiak JP, Medvedovic M, Alexander DC, et al. Integrative metabolome and transcriptome profiling reveals discordant energetic stress between mouse strains with differential sensitivity to acrolein-induced acute lung injury. *Mol Nutr Food Res.* 2011;55:1423–1434.

Fahy JV, Dickey BF. Airway mucus function and dysfunction. *N Engl J Med.* 2010;363:2233–2247.

Fanucchi MV, Plopper CG, Harkema JR, Hotchkiss JA. In vitro culture of microdissected rat nasal airway tissues. *Am J Respir Cell Mol Biol.* 1999;20:1274–1285.

Ferin J, Urbánková G, Vlcková A. Influence of tobacco smoke on the elimination of particles from the lungs. *Nature.* 1965;206:515–516.

Feron VJ, Arts JH, Kuper CF, Slootweg PJ, Woutersen RA. Health risks associated with inhaled nasal toxicants. *Crit Rev Toxicol.* 2001;31:313–347.

Ferrer-Sueta G, Radi R. Chemical biology of peroxynitrite: kinetics, diffusion, and radicals. *ACS Chem Biol.* 2009;4:161–177.

Finkbeiner WE, Zlock LT, Mehdi I, Widdicombe JH. Cultures of human tracheal gland cells of mucous or serous phenotype. *In Vitro Cell Dev Biol Anim.* 2010;46:450–456.

Fleischer J, Breer H, Strotmann J. Mammalian olfactory receptors. *Front Cell Neurosci.* 2009;3:9.

Fletcher C, Peto R . The natural history of chronic airflow obstruction. *Br Med J.* 1977;1:1645–1648.

Fraiser LH, Kanekal S, Kehrer JP. Cyclophosphamide toxicity. Characterising and avoiding the problem. *Drugs.* 1991;42:781–795.

Frank R. The effects of inhaled pollutants on nasal and pulmonary flow-resistance. *Ann Otol Rhinol Laryngol.* 1970;79:540–546.

Freeman FA, Gutierrez H, Rubbo H. Nitric oxide: a central regulatory species in pulmonary oxidant reactions. *Am J Physiol Lung Cell Mol Physiol.* 1995;268:L697–L698.

Freeman G, Haydon GB. Emphysema after low-level exposure to NO2. *Arch Environ Health.* 1964;8:125–128.

Friberg L. Proteinuria and kidney injury among workmen exposed to cadmium and nickel dust; preliminary report. *J Ind Hyg Toxicol.* 1948;30:32–36.

Fujino N, Kubo H, Suzuki T, et al. Isolation of alveolar epithelial type II progenitor cells from adult human lungs. *Lab Invest.* 2011;91:363–378.

Gardner DE, Holzman RS, Coffin DL. Effects of nitrogen dioxide on pulmonary cell population. *J Bacteriol.* 1969;98:1041–1043.

Gazdar AF, Girard L, Lockwood WW, Lam WL, Minna JD. Lung cancer cell lines as tools for biomedical discovery and research. *J Natl Cancer Inst.* 2010;102:1310–1321.

Gazi U, Martinez-Pomares L. Influence of the mannose receptor in host immune responses. *Immunobiology*. 2009;214:554–561.

Gehr P, Geiser M, Stone KC, Crapo JD. Morphometric analysis of the gas exchange region of the lung. In: Gardner DE, Crapo JD, McClellan RO, eds. *Toxicology of the Lung*. 2nd ed. New York: Raven Press; 1993:111–154.

Geiser M. Update on macrophage clearance of inhaled micro- and nanoparticles. *J Aerosol Med Pulm Drug Deliv*. 2010;23:207–217.

Geppetti P, Materazzi S, Nicoletti P. The transient receptor potential vanilloid 1: role in airway inflammation and disease. *Eur J Pharmacol*. 2006;533:207–214.

Ghantous H, Dencker L, Gabrielsson J, Danielsson BR, Bergman K. Accumulation and turnover of metabolites of toluene and xylene in nasal mucosa and olfactory bulb in the mouse. *Pharmacol Toxicol*. 1990;66:87–92.

Gharaee-Kermani M, Hu B, Phan SH, Gyetko MR. Recent advances in molecular targets and treatment of idiopathic pulmonary fibrosis: focus on TGFbeta signaling and the myofibroblast. *Curr Med Chem*. 2009;16:1400–1417.

Gibby EM, Cohen GM. Conjugation of 1-naphthol by human bronchus and bronchoscopy samples. *Biochem Pharmacol*. 1984;33:739–743.

Giordano G, Van den Brúle S, Re SL, et al. Type I interferon signaling contributes to chronic inflammation in a murine model of silicosis. *Toxicol Sci*. 2010;116(2):682–692.

Giri SN. Novel pharmacological approaches to manage interstitial lung fibrosis in the twenty-first century. *Annu Rev Pharmacol Toxicol*. 2003;43:73–95.

Gloede E, Cichocki JA, Baldino JB, Morris JB. A validated hybrid computational fluid dynamics-physiologically based pharmacokinetic model for respiratory tract vapor absorption in the human and rat and its application to inhalation dosimetry of diacetyl. *Toxicol Sci*. 2011;123:231–246.

Goldner J. A modification of the masson trichrome technique for routine laboratory purposes. *Am J Pathol*. 1938;14:237–243.

Goldstein BD, Balchum OJ. Effect of ozone on lipid peroxidation in the red blood cell. *Proc Soc Exp Biol Med*. 1967;126:356–358.

Goldstein E, Green GM, Seamans C. The effect of silicosis on the antibacterial defense mechanisms of the murine lung. *J Infect Dis*.1969;120:210–216.

Gordon S, Martinez FO. Alternative activation of macrophages: mechanism and functions. *Immunity*. 2010;32:593–604.

Green GM, Carolin D. The depressant effect of cigarette smoke on the in vitro antibacterial activity of alveolar macrophages. *N Engl J Med*. 1967;276:421–427.

Gross P, Brown JH, Hatch TF. Experimental endogenous lipoid pneumonia. *Am J Pathol*. 1952;28:211–221.

Gross P, Pfitzer EA, Tolker E, Babyak MA, Kaschak M. Experimental emphysema: its production with papain in normal and silicotic rats. *Arch Environ Health*. 1965;11:50–58.

Gruenert DC, Basbaum CB, Welsh MJ, Li M, Finkbeiner WE, Nadel JA. Characterization of human tracheal epithelial cells transformed by an origin-defective simian virus 40. *Proc Natl Acad Sci USA*. 1988;85:5951–5955.

Gwinn MR, Vallyathan V. Respiratory burst: role in signal transduction in alveolar macrophages. *J Toxicol Environ Health B Crit Rev*. 2006;9:27–39.

Haberzettl P, Schins RP, Hohr D, Wilhelmi V, Borm PJ, Albrecht C. Impact of the FcgammaII-receptor on quartz uptake and inflammatory response by alveolar macrophages. *Am J Physiol Lung Cell Mol Physiol*. 2008;294:L1137–L1148.

Haldane JS. The action of carbonic oxide on man. *J Physiol*. 1895;18: 430–462.

Haldane JS. The causes of death in colliery explosions. *Trans Fed Inst Mining Eng*. 1896;11:502–513.

Haldane JS. Preface. *Respiration*. New Haven: Yale University Press; 1922:viii.

Hall H, Leaderer B, Cain W, Fidler A. Personal risk factors associated with mucosal symptom prevalence in office workers. *Indoor Air*. 1993;3:206–209.

Harkema JR, Carey SA, Wagner JG. The nose revisited: a brief review of the comparative structure, function, and toxicologic pathology of the nasal epithelium. *Toxicol Pathol*. 2006;34:252–269.

Hatch T. Progress in industrial sanitation: with special reference to the control of industrial dust. *Am J Public Health Nations Health*. 1937;27:671–679.

Hatch T, Hemeon WC. Influence of particle size in dust exposure. *J Ind Hyg Toxicol*. 1948;30:172–180.

Hautamaki RD, Kobayashi DK, Senior RM, Shapiro SD. Requirement for macrophage elastase for cigarette smoke-induced emphysema in mice. *Science*. 1997;277:2002–2004.

He D, Frost AR, Falany CN. Identification and immunohistochemical localization of Sulfotransferase 2B1b (SULT2B1b) in human lung. *Biochim Biophys Acta*. 2005;1724:119–126.

Hecht SS. Tobacco smoke carcinogens and lung cancer. *J Natl Cancer Inst*. 1999;91:1194–1210.

Henderson MC, Siddens LK, Morré JT, Krueger SK, Williams DE. Metabolism of the anti-tuberculosis drug ethionamide by mouse and human FMO1, FMO2 and FMO3 and mouse and human lung microsomes. *Toxicol Appl Pharmacol*. 2008;233:420–427.

Henderson RF. Use of bronchoalveolar lavage to detect respiratory tract toxicity of inhaled material. *Exp Toxicol Pathol*. 2005;57 (suppl 1):155–159.

Henderson Y, Haggard HW. *Noxious Gases*. 2nd ed. New York, NY: Reinhold Pub Corp; 1943.

Herbst RS, Heymach JV, Lippman SM. Molecular origins of cancer: lung cancer. *N Engl J Med*. 2008;359:1367–1380.

Hodge HC, Leach LJ, Scott JK Spiegl CJ, Steinhardt H. Acute inhalation toxicity of lithium hydride. *AMA Arch Ind Health*. 1956;14: 468–470.

Hodgson M. Indoor environmental exposures and symptoms. *Environ Health Perspect*. 2002;110(suppl 4):663–667.

Hodson D. Victor Grignard (1871-1935). *Chem Br*. 1987;23:141–142.

Hoffman FL. Mortality from respiratory diseases in dusty trades (inorganic dusts). *Bulletin of the United States Bureau of Labor Statistics*. Washington: United States Bureau of Labor Statistics; 1918.

Holland CG. *Diseases of the Lungs From Mechanical Causes*. London: John Churchill; 1843.

Homer RJ, Zhu Z, Cohn L, et al. Differential expression of chitinases identify subsets of murine airway epithelial cells in allergic inflammation. *Am J Physiol Lung Cell Mol Physiol*. 2006;291:L502–L511.

Hornung V, Bauernfeind F, Halle A, et al. Silica crystals and aluminum salts activate the NALP3 inflammasome through phagosomal destabilization. *Nat Immunol*. 2008;9:847–856.

Houghton AM, Quintero PA, Perkins DL, et al. Elastin fragments drive disease progression in a murine model of emphysema. *J Clin Invest*. 2006;116:753–759.

Hu G, Shi Z, Hu J, Zou G, Peng G, Ran P. Association between polymorphisms of microsomal epoxide hydrolase and COPD: results from meta-analyses. *Respirology*. 2008;13:837–850.

Huang YC, Ghio AJ. Controlled human exposures to ambient pollutant particles in susceptible populations. *Environ Health*. 2009;8:33.

Huaux F. New developments in the understanding of immunology in silicosis. *Curr Opin Allergy Clin Immunol*. 2007;7:168–173.

Hukkanen J, Pelkonen O, Hakkola J, Raunio H. Expression and regulation of xenobiotic-metabolizing cytochrome P450 (CYP) enzymes in human lung. *CRC Crit Rev Toxicol*. 2002;32:391–411.

Hyde DM, Tyler NK, Plopper CG. Morphometry of the respiratory tract: avoiding the sampling, size, orientation, and reference traps. *Toxicol Pathol*. 2007;35:41–48.

Ichinohe T, Pang IK, Iwasaki A. Influenza virus activates inflammasomes via its intracellular M2 ion channel. *Nat Immunol*. 2010;11: 404–410.

Iles KE, Forman HJ. Macrophage signaling and respiratory burst. *Immunol Res*. 2002;26:95–105.

ILSI Risk Science Institute Workshop. The relevance of the rat lung response to particle overload for human risk assessment. *Inhal Toxicol*. 2000;12:1–148.

International Agency for Research on Cancer. IARC monographs on the evaluation of carcinogenic risks to humans. In: *Beryllium, Cadmium, Mercury and Exposures in the Glass Manufacturing Industry*. Vol 58. Lyon, France: IARC; 1993.

International Agency for Research on Cancer. IARC monographs on the evaluation of the carcinogenic risk of chemicals to humans. In: *Tobacco Smoke and Involuntary Smoking.* Vol 83. Lyon, France: IARC; 2004.

International Commission on Radiological Protection. *Human Respiratory Tract Model for Radiological Protection.* ICRP Publication 66; Ann. ICRP 24 (Nos. 1–3). Oxford, UK: Elsevier; 1994.

Ishikawa E, Ishikawa T, Morita YS, et al. Direct recognition of the mycobacterial glycolipid, trehalose dimycolate, by C-type lectin Mincle. *J Exp Med.* 2009;206:2879–2888.

Jang AS, Concel VJ, Bein K, et al. Endothelial dysfunction and claudin 5 regulation during acrolein-induced lung injury. *Am J Respir Cell Mol Biol.* 2011;44:483–490.

Janoff A, Sloan B, Weinbaum G, et al. Experimental emphysema induced with purified human neutrophil elastase: tissue localization of the instilled protease. *Am Rev Respir Dis.* 1977;115:461–478.

Jarvis J, Seed MJ, Elton R, Sawyer L, Agius R. Relationship between chemical structure and the occupational asthma hazard of low molecular weight organic compounds. *Occup Environ Med.* 2005;62:243–250.

Jeffery PK, Ayers M, Rogers D. The mechanisms and control of bronchial mucous cell hyperplasia. *Adv Exp Med Biol.* 1982;144:399–409.

John W, Wall SM, Ondo JL, Winklmayr W. Modes in the size distributions of atmospheric inorganic aerosol. *Atmos Environ.* 1990;24A:2349–2359.

Joseph P, Jaiswal AK. NAD(P)H:quinone oxidoreductase1 (DT diaphorase) specifically prevents the formation of benzo[a]pyrenequinone-DNA adducts generated by cytochrome P4501A1 and P450 reductase. *Proc Natl Acad Sci U S A.* 1994;91:8413–8417.

Jourenkova-Mironova N, Wikman H, Bouchardy C, et al. Role of glutathione S-transferase GSTM1, GSTM3, GSTP1 and GSTT1 genotypes in modulating susceptibility to smoking-related lung cancer. *Pharmacogenetics.* 1998;8:495–502.

Juarez E, Nuñez C, Sada E, Ellner JJ, Schwander SK, Torres M. Differential expression of Toll-like receptors on human alveolar macrophages and autologous peripheral monocytes. *Respir Res.* 2010;11:2.

Jules-Elysee K, White DA. Bleomycin-induced pulmonary toxicity. *Clin Chest Med.* 1990;11:1–20.

Kadara H, Behrens C, Yuan P, et al. A five-gene and corresponding protein signature for stage-I lung adenocarcinoma prognosis. *Clin Cancer Res.* 2011;17:1490–1501.

Kao RC, Wehner NG, Skubitz KM, Gray BH, Hoidal JR. Proteinase 3. A distinct human polymorphonuclear leukocyte proteinase that produces emphysema in hamsters. *J Clin Invest.* 1988;82:1963–1973.

Kato M, Staub NC, Response of small pulmonary arteries to unilobar hypoxia and hypercapnia. *Circ Res.* 1966;19:426–440.

Kawai T, Akira S. The role of pattern-recognition receptors in innate immunity: update on Toll-like receptors. *Nat Immunol.* 2010;11:373–384.

Kawai T, Akira S. Toll-like receptors and their crosstalk with other innate receptors in infection and immunity. *Immunity.* 2011;34:637–650.

Kesimer M, Kirkham S, Pickles RJ, et al. Tracheobronchial air-liquid interface cell culture: a model for innate mucosal defense of the upper airways? *Am J Physiol Lung Cell Mol Physiol.* 2009;296:L92–L100.

Kiyohara C, Yoshimasu K, Takayama K, Nakanishi Y. NQO1, MPO, and the risk of lung cancer: a HuGE review. *Genet Med.* 2005;7:463–478.

Kiyohara C, Yoshimasu K, Takayama K, Nakanishi Y. EPHX1 polymorphisms and the risk of lung cancer: a HuGE review. *Epidemiology.* 2006;17:89–99.

Kobzik L, Godleski JJ, Barry BE, Brain JD. Isolation and antigenic identification of hamster lung interstitial macrophages. *Am Rev Respir Dis.* 1988;138:908–914.

Kollarik M, Undem BJ. Sensory transduction in cough-associated nerves. *Respir Physiol Neurobiol.* 2006;152:243–254.

Kosaka H, Uozumi M, Tyuma I. The interaction between nitrogen oxides and hemoglobin and endothelium-derived relaxing factor. *Free Radic Biol Med.* 1989;7:653–658.

Landahl HD, Black S. Penetration of air-borne particulates through the human nose. 1. *Indust Hyg Toxicol.* 1947;29:269–277.

Lanosa MJ, Willis DN, Jordt S, Morris JB. Role of metabolic activation and the TRPA1 receptor in the sensor irritation response to styrene and naphthalene. *Toxicol Sci.* 2010;115:589–595.

Laskin S, Kuschner M, Nelson N, Altshuler B, Harley JH, Daniels M. Carcinoma of the lung in rats exposed by the beta-radiation of intrabronchial ruthenium pellets. I. Dose-response relationships. *J Natl Cancer Inst.* 1963;31:219–231.

Laurell CB, Eriksson S. The electrophoretic alpha-1-globulin pattern of serum in alpha-1-antitrypsin deficiency. *Scand J Clin Invest.* 1963;15:132–140.

Lazard D, Zupko K, Poria Y, et al. Odorant signal termination by olfactory UDP glucuronosyl transferase. *Nature.* 1991;349:790–793.

Lechner JF, Haugen A, McClendon IA, Pettis EW. Clonal growth of normal adult human bronchial epithelial cells in a serum-free medium. *In Vitro.* 1982;18:633–642.

Lechner JF, LaVeck MA. A serum-free method for culturing normal bronchial epithelial cells at clonal density. *Meth Cell Sci.* 1985;9:43–48.

Lee J, Nordestgaard BG, Dahl M. EPHX1 polymorphisms, COPD and asthma in 47,000 individuals and in meta-analysis. *Eur Respir J.* 2011;37:18–25.

Leikauf GD. Hazardous air pollutants and asthma. *Environ Health Perspect.* 2002;110(suppl 4):505–526.

Leikauf GD, Borchers MT, Prows DR, Simpson LG. Mucin apoprotein expression in COPD. *Chest.* 2002;121:166S–182S.

Leikauf GD, Concel VJ, Liu P, et al. Haplotype association mapping of acute lung injury in mice implicates activin a receptor, type 1. *Am J Respir Crit Care Med.* 2011;183:1499–1509.

Leikauf GD, Leming LM, O'Donnell JR, Doupnik CA. Bronchial responsiveness and inflammation in guinea pigs exposed to acrolein. *J Appl Physiol.* 1989;66:171–178.

Li H, Su X, Yan X, et al. Toll-like receptor 4-myeloid differentiation factor 88 signaling contributes to ventilator-induced lung injury in mice. *Anesthesiology.* 2010;113:619–629.

Lin CY, Boland BC, Lee YJ, et al. Identification of proteins adducted by reactive metabolites of naphthalene and 1-nitronaphthalene in dissected airways of rhesus macaques. *Proteomics.* 2006;6:972–982.

Ling G, Gu J, Genter MB, Zhuo X, Ding X. Regulation of cytochrome P450 gene expression in the olfactory mucosa. *Chem Biol Interact.* 2004;147:247–258.

Lippmann M. Deposition and retention of inhaled fibres: effects on incidence of lung cancer and mesothelioma. *Occup Environ Med.* 1994;51:793–798.

Lippmann M, Albert RE. Use of monodisperse aerosols for studies on respiratory tract deposition and clearance. *J Air Pollut Control Assoc.* 1968;18:672–674.

Lippmann M, Leikauf GD. Introduction and background (Chapter 1). In: Lippmann M, ed. *Environmental Toxicants Human Exposures and Their Health Effects.* New York: Wiley; 2009:3–18.

Lippmann M, Yeates DB, Albert RE. Deposition, retention, and clearance of inhaled particles. *Br J Ind Med.* 1980;37:337–362.

Llewellyn BD. Nuclear staining with alum hematoxylin. *Biotech Histochem.* 2009;84:159–177.

Loo YM, Gale M Jr. Immune signaling by RIG-I-like receptors. *Immunity.* 2011;34:680–692.

Lorenzo IM, Liedtke W, Sanderson MJ, Valverde MA. TRPV4 channel participates in receptor-operated calcium entry and ciliary beat frequency regulation in mouse airway epithelial cells. *Proc Natl Acad Sci USA.* 2008;105:12611–12616.

Macintyre N, Crapo RO, Viegi G, et al. Standardisation of the single-breath determination of carbon monoxide uptake in the lung. *Eur Respir J.* 2005;26:720–735.

Malo JL, Chan-Yeung M. Agents causing occupational asthma. *J Allergy Clin Immunol.* 2009;123:545–550.

Maris NA, Dessing MC, de Vos AF, et al. Toll-like receptor mRNA levels in alveolar macrophages after inhalation of endotoxin. *Eur Respir J.* 2006;28:622–626.

Martelli AM, Evangelisti C, Follo MY, et al. Targeting the phosphatidylinositol 3-kinase/Akt/mammalian target of rapamycin signaling network in cancer stem cells. *Curr Med Chem.* 2011;18(18):2715–2126.

Mauderly JL. Usefulness of animal models for predicting human responses to long-term inhalation of particles. *Chest.* 1996;109(3 suppl):65S–68S.

Meadors M, Floyd J, Perry MC. Pulmonary toxicity of chemotherapy. *Semin Oncol*. 2006;33:98–105.

Mehendale HM, Angevine LS, Ohmiya Y. The isolated perfused lung—a critical evaluation. *Toxicology*. 1981;21:1–36.

Mercer RR, Crapo JD. Architecture of the acinus. In: Parent RA, ed. *Treatise on Pulmonary Toxicology: Comparative Biology of the Normal Lung*. Boca Raton, FL: CRC Press; 1991:109–120.

Meyer M, Piiper J. Nitric oxide (NO), a new test gas for study of alveolar-capillary diffusion. *Eur Respir J*. 1989;2:494–496.

Miller I, Eberini I, Gianazza E. Proteomics of lung physiopathology. *Proteomics*. 2008;8:5053–5073.

Minelli C, Wei I, Sagoo G, Jarvis D, Shaheen S, Burney P. Interactive effects of antioxidant genes and air pollution on respiratory runction and airway disease: a HuGE Review. *Am J Epidemiol*. 2011;173:603–620.

Miravitlles M. Cough and sputum production as risk factors for poor outcomes in patients with COPD. *Respir Med*. 2011;105:1118–1128.

Mohr S, Leikauf GD, Keith G, Rihn BH. Microarrays as cancer keys: an array of possibilities. *J Clin Oncol*. 2002;20:3165–3175.

Morris JB. Uptake of styrene in the upper respiratory tract of the CD mouse and Sprague-Dawley rat. *Toxicol Sci*. 2000;54:222–228.

Morris JB. Overview of upper respiratory tract vapor uptake studies. *Inhal Toxicol*. 2001;13:335–345.

Morris JB, Buckpitt AR. Upper respiratory tract uptake of naphthalene. *Toxicol Sci*. 2009;111:383–391.

Morris JB, Symanowicz PT, Olsen JE, Thrall RS, Cloutier MM, Hubbard AK. Immediate sensory nerve-mediated respiratory responses to irritants in healthy and allergic airway-diseased mice. *J Appl Physiol*. 2003;94:1563–1571.

Morrow PE. Dust overloading in the lungs: update and appraisal. *Toxicol Appl Phamacol*. 1992;113:1–12.

Morrow PE. Mehrhof E, Casarett LJ, Morken DA. An experimental study of aerosol deposition in human subjects. *AMA Arch Ind Health*. 1958;18:292–298.

Mossman BT, Lippmann M, Hesterberg TW, Kelsey KT, Barchowsky A, Bonner JC. Pulmonary endpoints (lung carcinomas and asbestosis) following inhalation exposure to asbestos. *Toxicol Environ Health B Crit Rev*. 2011;14:76–121.

Mudd JB, Leavitt R, Ongun A, McManus TT. Reaction of ozone with amino acids and proteins. *Atmos Environ*. 1969;3:669–682.

Murphy SD, Klingshirn DA, Ulrich DE Respiratory response of guinea pigs during acrolein inhalation and its modification by drugs. *J Pharmacol Exp Ther*. 1963;141:79–83.

Munger JS, Sheppard D. Cross talk among TGF-β signaling pathways, integrins, and the extracellular matrix. *Cold Spring Harb Perspect Biol*. 2011;3:a005017.

Nadel JA, Comroe JH Jr. Acute effects of inhalation of cigarette smoke on airway conductance. *J Appl Physiol*. 1961;16:713–716.

Nebert DW, Dalton TP. The role of cytochrome P450 enzymes in endogenous signalling pathways and environmental carcinogenesis. *Nat Rev Cancer*. 2006;6:947–960.

Nelson N. Some toxicologic aspects of atmospheric pollution. *Am J Public Health Nations Health*. 1955;145:1289–1301.

Nielsen GD, Wolkoff P, Alarie Y. Sensory irritation: risk assessment approaches. *Regul Toxicol Pharmacol*. 2007;48:6–18.

National Lung Screening Trial Research Team; Aberle DR, Adams AM, Berg CD, et al. Reduced lung-cancer mortality with low-dose computed tomographic screening. *N Engl J Med*. 2011;365:395–409.

Oberdörster G, Oberdörster E, Oberdörster J. Nanotoxicology: an emerging discipline evolving from studies of ultrafine particles. *Environ Health Perspect*. 2005;113:823–839.

Oliver T. Dust as a cause of occupational disease (Chapter 17). In: Oliver T, ed. *Dangerous Trades. The Historical, Social, Legal Aspects of Industrial Occupations as Affecting Health, by a Number of Medical Experts*. London: John Murray; 1902.

Ortiz LA, Gambelli F, McBride C, et al. Mesenchymal stem cell engraftment in lung is enhanced in response to bleomycin exposure and ameliorates its fibrotic effects. *Proc Natl Acad Sci USA*. 2003;100:8407–8011.

Ortiz LA, Lasky J, Lungarella G, et al. Upregulation of the p75 but not the p55 TNF-alpha receptor mRNA after silica and bleomycin exposure and protection from lung injury in double receptor knockout mice. *Am J Respir Cell Mol Biol*. 1999;20:825–833.

Osorio F, Reis e Sousa C. Myeloid C-type lectin receptors in pathogen recognition and host defense. *Immunity*. 2011;34(5):651–664.

Ouadrhiri Y, Pilette C, Monteiro RC, Vaerman JP, Sibille Y. Effect of IgA on respiratory burst and cytokine release by human alveolar macrophages: role of ERK1/2 mitogen-activated protein kinases and NF-kappaB. *Am J Respir Cell Mol Biol*. 2002;26:315–332.

Pacher P, Beckman JS, Liaudet L. Nitric oxide and peroxynitrite in health and disease. *Physiol Rev*. 2007;87:315–424.

Palm PE, McNernery JM, Hatch T. Respiratory dust retention in small animals; a comparison with man. *AMA Arch Ind Health*. 1956;13:355–365.

Palma AS, Feizi T, Zhang Y, et al. Ligands for the beta-glucan receptor, Dectin-1, assigned using "designer" microarrays of oligosaccharide probes (neoglycolipids) generated from glucan polysaccharides. *J Biol Chem*. 2006;281:5771–5779.

Palmes ED, Nelson N, Laskin S, Kuschner M. Inhalation toxicity of cobalt hydrocarbonyl. *Am Ind Hyg Assoc J*. 1959;20:453–468.

Pandis S. Atmospheric aerosol processes (Chapter 3). In: McMurry PH, Shepard M, Vickery JS, eds. *Particulate Matter Science for Policy Makers: A NARSTO Assessment*. Cambridge, UK: Cambridge University Press; 2004:103–107.

Patel AC, Brett TJ, Holtzman MJ. The role of CLCA proteins in inflammatory airway disease. *Annu Rev Physiol*. 2009;71:425–449.

Patel JM, Block ER. Cyclophosphamide-induced depression of the antioxidant defense mechanisms of the lung. *Exp Lung Res*. 1985;8:153–165.

Patterson CE, Rhoades RA, Garcia JG. Evans blue dye as a marker of albumin clearance in cultured endothelial monolayer and isolated lung. *J Appl Physiol*. 1992;72:865–873.

Patty FA. Industrial hygiene and its relation to medicine. *Ind Med Surg*. 1949;18:225–228.

Pauluhn J. Overview of inhalation exposure techniques: strengths and weaknesses. *Exp Toxicol Pathol*. 2005;57(suppl 1):111–128.

Pauwels R, Rabe K. Burden and clinical features of chronic obstructive pulmonary disease (COPD). *Lancet*. 2004;364:613–620.

Phalen RF, Mannix RC, Drew RT. Inhalation exposure methodology. *Environ Health Perspect*. 1984;56:23–34.

Phalen RF, Oldham MJ, Wolff RK. The relevance of animal models for aerosol studies. *J Aerosol Med Pulm Drug Deliv*. 2008;21:113–124.

Phalen RF. Inhalation exposure of animals. *Environ Health Perspect*. 1976;16:17–24.

Piguet PF, Collart MA, Grau GE, Sappino AP, Vassalli P. Requirement of tumour necrosis factor for development of silica-induced pulmonary fibrosis. *Nature*. 1990;344:245–247.

Pinkerton KE, Gehr P, Crapo JD. Architecture and cellular composition of the air-blood barrier. In: Parent RA, ed. *Treatise on Pulmonary Toxicology: Comparative Biology of the Normal Lung*. Boca Raton, FL: CRC Press; 1991:121–128.

Plopper CG, Chang AM, Pang A, Buckpitt AR. Use of microdissected airways to define metabolism and cytotoxicity in murine bronchiolar epithelium. *Exp Lung Res*. 1991;17:197–212.

Plopper CG, Van Winkle LS, Fanucchi MV, et al. Early events in naphthalene-induced acute Clara cell toxicity: II. Comparison of glutathione depletion and histopathology by airway location. *Am J Resp Cell Mol Biol*. 2001;24:272–281.

Pope CA 3rd, Burnett RT, Thun MJ, et al. Lung cancer, cardiopulmonary mortality, and long-term exposure to fine particulate air pollution. *JAMA*. 2002;287:1132–1141.

Pope CA 3rd, Burnett RT, Turner MC, et al. Lung cancer and cardiovascular disease mortality associated with ambient air pollution and cigarette smoke: shape of the exposure-response relationships. *Environ Health Perspect*. 2011;119:1616–1621.

Popov TA. Human exhaled breath analysis. *Ann Allergy Asthma Immunol*. 2011;106:451–456.

Pryor WA. Cigarette smoke radicals and the role of free radicals in chemical carcinogenicity. *Environ Health Perspect*. 1997;105(suppl 4):875–882.

Putila JJ, Guo NL. Association of arsenic exposure with lung cancer incidence rates in the United States. *PLoS One.* 2011;6:e25886.

Raabe OG. Some important considerations in use of power functions to describe clearance data. *Health Phys.* 1967;13:293–295.

Rabe KF, Hurd S, Anzueto A, et al. Global Initiative for Chronic Obstructive Lung Disease. Global strategy for the diagnosis, management, and prevention of chronic obstructive pulmonary disease: GOLD executive summary. *Am J Respir Crit Care Med.* 2007;176:532–555.

Rawlins EL, Okubo T, Xue Y, et al. The role of Scgb1a1+ Clara cells in the long-term maintenance and repair of lung airway, but not alveolar, epithelium. *Cell Stem Cell.* 2009;4:525–534.

Reddel RR, Ke Y, Gerwin BI, et al. Transformation of human bronchial epithelial cells by infection with SV40 or adenovirus-12 SV40 hybrid virus, or transfection via strontium phosphate coprecipitation with a plasmid containing SV40 early region genes. *Cancer Res.* 1988;48:1904–1909.

Reid L. Measurement of the bronchial mucous gland layer: a diagnostic yardstick in chronic bronchitis. *Thorax.* 1960;15:132–141.

Reinhard C, Meyer B, Fuchs H, et al. Genomewide linkage analysis identifies novel genetic Loci for lung function in mice. *Am J Respir Crit Care Med.* 2005;171:880–888.

Rennard SI, Spurzen JR. Methods for evaluating the lung in human subjects. In: Gardner DE, ed. *Toxicology of the Lung.* 4th ed. Boca Raton, FL: CRC Press, Taylor & Francis; 2006:1–28.

Reynolds HY. Bronchoalveolar lavage and other methods to define the human respiratory tract milieu in health and disease. *Lung.* 2011;189:87–99.

Reynolds JS, Johnson VJ, Frazer DG. Unrestrained acoustic plethysmograph for measuring specific airway resistance in mice. *J Appl Physiol.* 2008;105:711–717.

Rhoades RA. Isolated perfused lung preparation for studying altered gaseous environments. *Environ Health Perspect.* 1984;56:43–50.

Robson WD, Irwin DA, King EJ. Experimental silicosis: quartz, sericite and irritating gases. *Can Med Assoc J.* 1934;31:237–245.

Rock JR, Hogan BL. Epithelial progenitor cells in lung development, maintenance, repair, and disease. *Annu Rev Cel Dev Biol.* 2011;27:4.1–4.20.

Rodig SJ, Shapiro GI. Crizotinib, a small-molecule dual inhibitor of the c-Met and ALK receptor tyrosine kinases. *Curr Opin Investig Drugs.* 2010;11:1477–1490.

Rogers DF. Mucoactive agents for airway mucus hypersecretory diseases. *Respir Care.* 2007;52:1176–1193.

Rose MC, Voynow JA. Respiratory tract mucin genes and mucin glycoproteins in health and disease. *Physiol Rev.* 2006;86:245–278.

Rowe VK, McCollister DD, Spencer HC, Adams EM, Irish DD. Vapor toxicity of tetrachloroethylene for laboratory animals and human subjects. *AMA Arch Ind Hyg Occup Med.* 1952;5:566–579.

Russell R. *London Fogs.* London: Edward Stanford; 1880.

Rylander R. Environmental air pollutants and lung defense to airborne bacteria. *Aspen Emphysema Conf.* 1968;11:297–304.

Salam MT, Lin PC, Avol EL, Gauderman WJ, Gilliland FD. Microsomal epoxide hydrolase, glutathione S-transferase P1, traffic and childhood asthma. *Thorax.* 2007;62:1050–1057.

Salathe M. Regulation of mammalian ciliary beating. *Annu Rev Physiol.* 2007;69:401–422 .

Sallenave JM. Secretory leukocyte protease inhibitor and elafin/trappin-2: versatile mucosal antimicrobials and regulators of immunity. *Am J Respir Cell Mol Biol.* 2010;42:635–643.

Salvi SS, Barnes PJ. Chronic obstructive pulmonary disease in nonsmokers. *Lancet.* 2009;374:733–743.

Sanderson MJ, Sleigh MA. Ciliary activity of cultured rabbit tracheal epithelium: beat pattern and metachrony. *J Cell Sci.* 1981;47:331–347.

Sato M, Shames DS, Gazdar AF, Minna JD. A translational view of the molecular pathogenesis of lung cancer. *J Thorac Oncol.* 2007;2:327–343.

Schattgen SA, Fitzgerald KA. The PYHIN protein family as mediators of host defenses. *Immunol Rev.* 2011;243:109–118.

Schmid A, Salathe M. Ciliary beat co-ordination by calcium. *Biol Cell.* 2011;103:159–169.

Schwartz DR, Homanics GE, Hoyt DG, Klein E, Abernethy J, Lazo JS. The neutral cysteine protease bleomycin hydrolase is essential for epidermal integrity and bleomycin resistance. *Proc Natl Acad Sci USA.* 1999;96:4680–4685.

Selikoff IJ, Churg J, Hammond EC. Relation between exposure to asbestosis and mesothelioma. *N Engl J Med.* 1965;272:560–565.

Senior RM, Griffin GL, Fliszar CJ, Shapiro SD, Goldberg GI, Welgus HG. Human 92- and 72-kilodalton type IV collagenases are elastases. *J Biol Chem.* 1991;266:7870–7875.

Shah AS, Ben-Shahar Y, Moninger TO, Kline JN, Welsh MJ. Motile cilia of human airway epithelia are chemosensory. *Science.* 2009;325:1131–1134.

Shapiro SD, Goldstein NM, Houghton AM, et al. Neutrophil elastase contributes to cigarette smoke-induced emphysema in mice. *Am J Pathol.* 2003;163:2329–2335.

Shapiro SD, Ingenito EP. The pathogenesis of chronic obstructive pulmonary disease: advances in the past 100 years. *Am J Respir Cell Mol Biol.* 2005;32:367–372.

Shehin-Johnson SE, Williams DE, Larsen-Su S, Stresser DM, Hines RN. Tissue specific expression of flavin-containing monooxygenase (FMO) forms 1 and 2 in the rabbit. *J Pharmacol Exp Ther.* 1995;272:1293–1299.

Sheppard D, Wong WS, Uehara CF, Nadel JA, Boushey HA. Lower threshold and greater bronchomotor responsiveness of asthmatic subjects to sulfur dioxide. *Am Rev Respir Dis.* 1980;122:873–878.

Sheppard D. Roles of alphav integrins in vascular biology and pulmonary pathology. *Curr Opin Cell Biol.* 2004;16:552–557.

Shi X, Zhou S, Wang Z, Zhou Z, Wang Z. CYP1A1 and GSTM1 polymorphisms and lung cancer risk in Chinese populations: a meta-analysis. *Lung Cancer.* 2008;59:155–163.

Shultz MA, Choudary PV, Buckpitt AR. Role of murine cytochrome P-450 2F2 in metabolic activation of naphthalene and metabolism of other xenobiotics. *J Exp Ther.* 1999;290:281–288.

Siegel R, Ward E, Brawley O, Jemal A. Cancer statistics, 2011: the impact of eliminating socioeconomic and racial disparities on premature cancer deaths. *CA Cancer J Clin.* 2011;61:212–236.

Silverman L, Lee RC. A low-resistance valve and indicating flowmeter for respiratory measurements. *Science.* 1946;103:537–539.

Silverman L, Whittenberger JL. Blood changes due to ammonia inhalation? *Science.* 1949;109:121–122.

Sinnett EE, Jackson AC, Leith DE, Butler JP. Fast integrated flow plethysmograph for small mammals. *J Appl Physiol.* 1981;50:1104–1110.

Slocum SL, Kensler TW. Nrf2: control of sensitivity to carcinogens. *Arch Toxicol.* 2011;85:273–284.

Smith BJ, Curtis JF, Eling TE. Bioactivation of xenobiotics by prostaglandin H synthase. *Chem Biol Interact.* 1991;79:245–264.

Smyth HF Jr. Solving the problem of the toxicity of new chemicals in industry. *W V Med J.* 1946;42:177.

Snider GL, Kleinerman J, Thurlbeck WM, Bengali ZH. The definition emphysema: report of a National Heart, Lung, and Blood Institute workshop. *Am Rev Respir Dis.* 1985;132:182–185.

Squadrito GL, Pryor WA. Oxidative chemistry of nitric oxide: the roles of superoxide, peroxynitrite, and carbon dioxide. *Free Radic Biol Med.* 1998;25:392–403.

Sterk PJ, Bel EH. Bronchial hyperresponsiveness: the need for a distinction between hypersensitivity and excessive airway narrowing. *Eur Respir J.* 1989;2:267–274.

Stokinger HE. Air pollution and the particle size-toxicity problem. *Nucleonics.* 1949;5:50.

Stokinger HE, Sprague GF 3rd, Hall Rh, Ashenburg JJ, Scott JK, Steadman LT. Acute inhalation toxicity of beryllium: four definitive studies of beryllium sulfate at exposure concentrations of 100, 50, 10, and 1 mg per cubic meter. *Arch Ind Hyg Occup Med.* 1950;1:379–397.

Sun S, Schiller JH, Gazadar AF. Lung cancer in never smokers—a different disease. *Nat Rev Cancer.* 2007;7:778–790.

Sutterwala FS, Ogura Y, Flavell RA. The inflammasome in pathogen recognition and inflammation. *J Leukoc Biol.* 2007;82:259–264.

Swiecichowski AL, Long KJ, Miller ML, Leikauf GD. Formaldehyde-induced airway hyperreactivity in vivo and ex vivo in guinea pigs. *Environ Res.* 1993;61:185–199.

Tamura HO, Harada Y, Miyawaki A, Mikoshiba K, Matsui M. Molecular cloning and expression of a cDNA encoding an olfactory-specific mouse phenol sulphotransferase. *Biochem J.* 1998;331:953–958.

Tang MS, Wang HT, Hu Y, et al. Acrolein induced DNA damage, mutagenicity and effect on DNA repair. *Mol Nutr Food Res.* 2011;55:1291–1300.

Tegtmeyer PJ, Craighead JE. Infection of adult mouse macrophages in vitro with cytomegalovirus. *Proc Soc Exp Biol Med*. 1968;129:690–694.

Ter-Minassian M, Asomaning K, Zhao Y, et al. Genetic variability in the metabolism of the tobacco-specific nitrosamine 4-(methylnitrosamino)-1-(3-pyridyl)-1-butanone (NNK) to 4-(methylnitrosamino)-1-(3-pyridyl)-1-butanol (NNAL). *Int J Cancer*. 2011;130:1338–1346.

Thackrah C. *The Effects of Arts, Trades, and Professions, and of Civic States and Habits of Living, on Health and Longevity*. 2nd ed. London: Longman; 1832.

Thorton-Manning JR, Dahl AR. Metabolic capacity of nasal tissue inter-species comparisons of xenobiotic-metabolizing enzymes. *Mutat Res*. 1997;380:43–59.

Touhara K, Vosshall LB. Sensing odorants and pheromones with chemosensory receptors. *Annu Rev Physiol*. 2009;71:307–332.

Travassos LH, Carneiro LA, Girardin SE, et al. Nod1 participates in the innate immune response to *Pseudomonas aeruginosa*. *J Biol Chem*. 2005;280:36714–36718.

Travassos LH, Girardin SE, Philpott DJ, et al. Toll-like receptor 2-dependent bacterial sensing does not occur via peptidoglycan recognition. *EMBO Rep*. 2004;5:1000–1006.

Tyler WS, Pearse AG. Oxidative enzymes of the interalveolar spetum of the rat. *Thorax*. 1965;20:149–152.

Uhlen M, Oksvold P, Fagerberg L, et al. Towards a knowledge-based Human Protein Atlas. *Nat Biotechnol*. 2010;28:1248–1250.

Upadhyay D, Kamp DW. Asbestos-induced pulmonary toxicity: role of DNA damage and apoptosis. *Exp Biol Med*. 2003;228:650–659.

Utell MJ, Frampton MW. Toxicologic methods: controlled human exposures. *Environ Health Perspect*. 2000;108(suppl 4):605–613.

Vallyathan V, Castranova V, Pack D, et al. Freshly fractured quartz inhalation leads to enhanced lung injury and inflammation. Potential role of free radicals. *Am J Respir Crit Care Med*. 1995;152:1003–1009.

Van Lommel A. Pulmonary neuroendocrine cells (PNEC) and neuroendocrine bodies (NEB): chemoreceptors and regulators of lung development. *Paediatr Respir Res*. 2001;2:171–176.

van Lookeren Campagne M, Wiesman C, Brown EJ. Macrophage complement receptors and pathogen clearance. *Cell Microbiol*. 2007;9:2095–2102.

Vaughan MB, Ramirez RD, Wright WE, Minna JD, Shay JW. A three-dimensional model of differentiation of immortalized human bronchial epithelial cells. *Differentiation*. 2006;74:141–148.

Vijayaraghavan R, Schapper M, Thompson R, Stock MF, Alarie Y. Characteristic modification of the breathing pattern of mice to evaluate the effects of airborne chemicals on the respiratory tract. *Arch Toxicol*. 1993;67:478–490.

Vinegar A, Sinnett EE, Leith DE. Dynamic mechanisms determine functional residual capacity in mice. *Mus musculus J Appl Physiol*. 1979;46:867–871.

Visel A, Thaller C, Eichele G. GenePaint.org: an atlas of gene expression patterns in the mouse embryo. *Nucleic Acids Res*. 2004;32(database issue):D552–D556.

Wang J, Edeen K, Manzer R, et al. Differentiated human alveolar epithelial cells and reversibility of their phenotype in vitro. *Am J Respir Cell Mol Biol*. 2007;36:661–668.

Ware LB, Matthay MA. The acute respiratory distress syndrome. *N Engl J Med*. 2000;342:1334–1339.

Ware LB, Matthay MA. Keratinocyte and hepatocyte growth factors in the lung: roles in lung development, inflammation, and repair. *Am J Physiol Lung Cell Mol Physiol*. 2002;282:L924–L940.

Weibel ER. Is the lung built reasonably? The 1983 J. Burns Anderson lecture. *Am Rev Respir Dis*. 1983;128:752–760.

Weiss RB, Poster DS, Penta JS. The nitrosoureas and pulmonary toxicity. *Cancer Treat Rev*. 1981;8:111–124.

Wesselkamper SC, Case LM, Henning LN, et al. Gene expression changes during the development of acute lung injury: role of transforming growth factor beta. *Am J Respir Crit Care Med*. 2005;172:1399–1411.

West JA, Chichester CH, Buckpitt AR, et al. Heterogeneity of clara cell glutathione: a possible basis for differences in cellular responses to pulmonary cytotoxicants. *Am J Respir Cell Mol Biol*. 2000;23:27–36.

Whetstine JR, Yueh MF, McCarver DG, et al. Ethnic differences in human flavin-containing monooxygenase 2 (FMO2) polymorphisms: detection of expressed protein in African-Americans. *Toxicol Appl Pharmacol*. 2000;168:216–224.

Whitby-Logan GK, Weech M, Walters E. Zonal expression and activity of glutathione S-transferase enzymes in the mouse olfactory mucosa. *Brain Res*. 2004;995:151–157.

Whitcutt MJ, Adler KB, Wu R. A biphasic chamber system for maintaining polarity of differentiation of cultured respiratory tract epithelial cells. *In Vitro Cell Dev Biol*. 1988;24:420–428.

Whitsett JA, Wert SE, Weaver TE. Alveolar surfactant homeostasis and the pathogenesis of pulmonary disease. *Annu Rev Med*. 2010;61:105–119.

Widdicombe JH, Welsh MJ. Ion transport by dog tracheal epithelium. *Fed Proc*. 1980;39:3062–3066.

Williams MC. Alveolar type I cells: molecular phenotype and development. *Annu Rev Physiol*. 2003;65:669–695.

Winkelmann A, Noack T. The Clara cell: a "third reich eponym"? *Eur Respir J*. 2010;36:722–727.

Wistuba II, Gazdar AF. Characetristic genetic alterations in lung cancer. In: Driscoll B, ed. *Lung Cancer Volume 1: Molecular Pathology Methods and Reviews*. Totowa, NJ: Humana Press; 2003:3–28.

Witschi H. Fritz Haber: December 9, 1868-January 29, 1934. *Toxicology*. 2000;149:3–15.

Witschi HP, Aldridge WN. Uptake, distribution and binding of beryllium to organelles of the rat liver cell. *Biochem J*. 1968;106:811–820.

Witschi HR, Pinkerton KE, Van Winkle LS, Last JA. Toxic responses of the respiratory tract (Chapter 15). In: Klaassen CD, ed. *Casarett and Doull's Toxicology: The Basic Science of Poisons*. 7th ed. New York: McGraw Hilll; 2008:609–630.

Wong BA. Inhalation exposure systems: design, methods and operation. *Toxicol Pathol*. 2007;35:3–14.

Woolcock AJ, Salome CM, Yan K. The shape of the dose-response curve to histamine in asthmatic and normal subjects. *Am Rev Respir Dis*. 1984;130:71–75.

World Health Organization. *Fuel for Life: Household Energy and Health*. Geneva, Switzland: WHO Press; 2006.

Wu M, Kelley MR, Hansen WK, Martin WJ. Reduction of BCNU toxicity to lung cells by high-level expression of O(6)-methylguanine-DNA methyltransferase. *Am J Physiol Lung Cell Mol Physiol*. 2001;280:L755–L761.

Wynn TA. Integrating mechanisms of pulmonary fibrosis. *J Exp Med*. 2011;208:1339–1350.

Xiang M, Fan J. Pattern recognition receptor-dependent mechanisms of acute lung injury. *Mol Med*. 2010;16:69–82.

Xun WW, Brennan P, Tjonneland A, et al. Single-nucleotide polymorphisms (5p15.33, 15q25.1, 6p22.1, 6q27 and 7p15.3) and lung cancer survival in the European Prospective Investigation into Cancer and Nutrition (EPIC). *Mutagenesis*. 2011;26:657–666.

Yasuda S, Yasuda T, Liu MY, et al. Sulfation of chlorotyrosine and nitrotyrosine by human lung endothelial and epithelial cells: role of the human SULT1A3. *Toxicol Appl Pharmacol*. 2011;251:104–109.

Yoshida K, Kasama K. Biotransformation of nitric oxide. *Environ Health Perspect*. 1987;73:201–206.

Young WA, Shaw DB, Bates DV. Effects of low concentration of ozone on pulmonary function in man. *J Appl Physiol*. 1964;19:765–768.

Yuan JM, Koh WP, Murphy SE, et al. Urinary levels of tobacco-specific nitrosamine metabolites in relation to lung cancer development in two prospective cohorts of cigarette smokers. *Cancer Res*. 2009;69:2990–2995.

Zelko IN, Mariani TJ, Folz RJ. Superoxide dismutase multigene family: a comparison of the CuZn-SOD (SOD1), Mn-SOD (SOD2), and EC-SOD (SOD3) gene structures, evolution, and expression. *Free Radic Biol Med*. 2002;33:337–349.

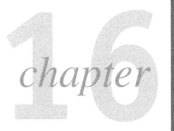

chapter 16

Toxic Responses of the Nervous System

Virginia C. Moser, Michael Aschner,
Rudy J. Richardson, and Martin A. Philbert

OVERVIEW OF THE NERVOUS SYSTEM

Neurotoxicants and toxins have been extensively studied because of their toxic effects on humans and their utility in the study of the nervous system (NS). Many insights into the organization and function of the NS are based on observations derived from the action of neurotoxicants. The binding of exogenous compounds to membranes has been the basis for the definition of specific receptors within the brain; an understanding of the roles of different cell types in the function of the NS has stemmed from the selectivity of certain toxicants in injuring specific cell types while sparing others, and important differences in basic metabolic requirements of different subpopulations of neurons have been inferred from the effects of toxicants.

It is estimated that millions of people worldwide are exposed to known neurotoxicants each year, a fact underscored by repeated outbreaks of neurological disease (Federal Register, 1994). An even larger potential problem stems from the incomplete information on many compounds that may have neurotoxic effects. Unknown is the extent to which neurological disability maybe related to chronic low-level exposures, nor do we understand the overall impact of environmental contaminants on brain function.

In order to study neurotoxicological consequences of chemical exposures, one must understand the structure, function, and development of the NS. These features can be quite complex, with differential anatomy, physiology, and cell types specific for location

and function. Several general aspects modulate the NS response to chemicals, including (1) the privileged status of the NS with the maintenance of a biochemical barrier between the brain and the blood, (2) the importance of the high energy requirements of the brain, (3) the spatial extensions of the NS as long cellular processes and the requirements of cells with such a complex geometry, (4) the maintenance of an environment rich in lipids, (5) the transmission of information across extracellular space at the synapse, (6) the distances over which electrical impulses must be transmitted, coordinated, and integrated, and (7) development and regenerative patterns of the NS. Each of these features of the NS carries with it specialized metabolic/physiological requirements and unique vulnerabilities to toxic compounds.

Blood–Brain Barrier

The NS is protected from the adverse effects of many potential toxicants by an anatomic barrier. In 1885, Ehrlich noticed that dyes did not distribute into the brain and spinal cord, whereas other tissues became stained. Conversely, when injected into the brain, the dye did not appear in the periphery. This observation pointed to the existence of an interface between the blood and the brain, or a "blood–brain barrier." Most of the brain, spinal cord, retina, and peripheral NS (PNS) maintain this barrier with the blood, with selectivity similar to the interface between cells and the extracellular space. The principal basis of the blood–brain barrier is thought to be specialized endothelial cells in the brain's microvasculature, aided, at least in part, by interactions with glia (Kniesel and Wolburg, 2000). In addition to this interface with blood, the brain, spinal cord, and peripheral nerves are also completely covered with a continuous lining of specialized cells that limits the entry of molecules from adjacent tissue. In the brain and spinal cord, this is the meningeal surface; in peripheral nerves, each fascicle of nerve is surrounded by perineurial cells.

Among the unique properties of endothelial cells in the NS is the presence of tight junctions between cells (Kniesel and Wolburg, 2000; Rubin and Staddon, 1999). Thus, molecules must pass through membranes of endothelial cells, rather than between them, as they do in other tissues. The blood–brain barrier also contains transporters, such as the multidrug-resistant protein, which transport some xenobiotics that have diffused through endothelial cells back into the blood. If not actively transported into the brain, the penetration of toxicants is largely related to their lipid solubility and to their ability to pass through the plasma membranes of the cells forming the barrier (Pardridge, 1999; Stewart, 2000). There are, however, important exceptions to this general rule. In the mature NS, the spinal and autonomic ganglia as well as a small number of other sites within the brain, called *circumventricular organs*, do not contain specialized endothelial tight junctions and are not protected by blood–tissue barriers. Rather, a somewhat less tight barrier is provided by several layers of overlapping astrocytic foot processes. Indeed, it is this cellular anatomical arrangement that allows the endocrine-regulating components of the circumventricular organs to sense changes in blood hormone levels and respond accordingly. This discontinuity of the barrier allows entry of some chemicals, for example, the anticancer drug doxorubicin, into the sensory ganglia. This is the basis for the selective neurotoxicity of this compound to ganglionic neurons (Spencer, 2000). The blood–brain barrier is incompletely developed at birth and even less so in premature infants. This predisposes the premature infant to brain injury by toxicants, such as unconjugated bilirubin or hexachlorophene, that later in life are excluded from the NS (Lucey *et al.*, 1964; Mullick, 1973).

Energy Requirements

Neurons and cardiac myocytes share the property of conduction of electrical impulses, and their critical dependence on aerobic respiration is due to the high metabolic demand associated with the maintenance and repetitive reinstitution of ion gradients. Neuronal cells are also postmitotic, making energy homeostasis critical to normal functioning of the NS. Membrane depolarizations and repolarizations occur with such frequency that these cells must be able to produce large quantities of high-energy phosphates even in a resting state. That the energy requirements of the brain are related to membrane depolarizations is supported by the fact that hyperactivity, as in epileptic foci, increases the energy requirements by as much as fivefold (Plum and Posner, 1985). The dependence on a continual source of energy, in the absence of energy reserves, places the neuron in a vulnerable position. To meet these high-energy requirements, the brain utilizes aerobic glycolysis and, therefore, is extremely sensitive to even brief interruptions in the supply of oxygen or glucose.

Exposure to toxicants that inhibit aerobic respiration (eg, cyanide) or to conditions that produce hypoxia (eg, carbon monoxide, or CO, poisoning) leads to the early signs of dysfunction in the myocardium and neurons. Damage to the NS under these conditions is a combination of direct toxic effects on neurons and secondary damage from systemic hypoxia or ischemia. For example, acute CO poisoning damages those structures in the central nervous system (CNS) that are most vulnerable to hypoxia: the

neurons in specific regions of the basal ganglia and hippocampus, certain layers of the cerebral cortex, and the cerebellar Purkinje cells. Experiments utilizing several different laboratory animal species have shown that systemic hypotension is the best predictor of these lesions following CO poisoning; however, CO poisoning also may produce white matter damage, and this leukoencephalopathy may result from a primary effect of CO in the CNS (Penny, 1990). As with CO, survivors of cyanide poisoning may develop lesions in the CNS that are characteristic of systemic hypoxic or ischemic injury, and experiments in rats and monkeys have led to the conclusion that global hypoperfusion, rather than direct histotoxicity, is the major cause of CNS damage (Auer and Benveniste, 1997). 3-Nitropropionic acid (3-NP), a naturally occurring mycotoxin, is an irreversible inhibitor of succinate dehydrogenase that results in adenosine triphosphate (ATP) depletion in cerebral cortical explants and is associated with motor disorders in livestock and humans that have ingested contaminated food (Ludolph *et al.*, 1991, 1992). Some investigators removed the complication of systemic toxicity by directly injecting 3-NP into specific regions of the brain. They have observed neuron degeneration mediated in part by excitotoxic mechanisms (Brouillet *et al.*, 1993a). These examples demonstrate the exquisite sensitivity of neurons to energy depletion and also underscore the complex relationships between direct neurotoxicity and the effects of systemic toxicity on the NS.

Axonal Transport

In the NS, impulses are conducted over great distances at rapid speed, and provide information about the environment to the organism in a coordinated manner that allows an organized response to be carried out at a specific site. However, the intricate organization of such a complex network places an unparalleled demand on the cells of the NS. Single cells, rather than being spherical and a few micrometers in diameter, are elongated and may extend over a meter in length.

The anatomy of such a complex cellular network creates features of metabolism and cellular geometry that are peculiar to the NS. The two immediate demands placed on the neuron are the maintenance of a larger cellular volume and the transport of intracellular materials over great distances. The length of neurons may exceed 200,000 times the dimensions of most other cells. For example, the cell body of a lower motor neuron is located in the spinal cord and the axon extends to the site of innervation of a muscle at a distant location. In spite of the smaller diameter of the axon, the length of the axon translates to an axonal volume that is hundreds of times greater than that of the cell body itself (Schwartz, 1991). The cellular machinery that provides protein synthesis to maintain this volume is readily visible in large neurons through the light microscope, as the Nissl substance, which is formed by clusters of ribosomal complexes for the synthesis of proteins (Parent, 1996). In fact, neurons are the only cell type with such a Nissl substance, reflecting the unusual demand for protein synthesis. Axonal microtubules are essential for transport of materials to and from the synapse, and the stability of microtubules is maintained by the binding of the microtubule-associated protein tau (Cleveland *et al.*, 1977).

In addition to the increased burden of protein synthesis, the neuron is dependent on the ability to distribute materials over the distances encompassed by its processes. Protein synthesis occurs in the cell body, and the products are then transported to the appropriate site through the process of axonal transport. The assembly of the cytoskeleton at tremendous distances from their site of synthesis in the cell body represents a formidable challenge (Nixon, 1998). Through studies of the movement of radiolabeled amino

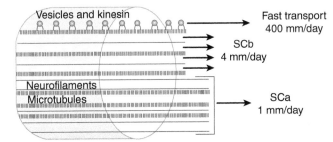

Figure 16-1. *Axonal transport.* Fast axonal transport is depicted as spherical vesicles moving along microtubules with intervening microtubule-associated motors. The slow component A (SCa) represents the movement of the cytoskeleton, composed of neurofilaments and microtubules. Slow component b (SCb) moves at a faster rate than SCa and includes soluble proteins, which are apparently moving between the more slowly moving cytoskeleton.

acid precursors, several major components of axonal transport are known (Grafstein, 1995). The fastest component, known as *fast axonal transport*, carries a large number of proteins, many of which are associated with vesicles (Grafstein, 1995). This ATP-dependent process reaches a rate of 400 mm/day (Fig. 16-1) and is dependent on microtubule-associated ATPase activity and motor proteins. These proteins, kinesin and dynein being the prototypes of a class of microtubule-associated motors, provide both the mechanochemical force in the form of a microtubule-associated ATPase and the interface between microtubules as the track and vesicles as the cargo. Vesicles are transported rapidly in an anterograde direction by kinesin and in a retrograde direction by dynein (Schnapp and Reese, 1989). In the axon, multiple waves of transport can be detected in the fast component of axonal transport (Mulugeta *et al.*, 2000).

The transport of some organelles, including mitochondria, constitutes an intermediate component of axonal transport, moving at 50 mm/day (Grafstein, 1995). As with the fast component, the function is apparently the continuous replacement of organelles within the axon. The slowest component of axonal transport represents the movement of the cytoskeleton itself (Fig. 16-1). The cytoskeleton is composed of structural elements, including microtubules formed by the association of tubulin subunits and neurofilaments formed by the association of three neurofilament protein subunits. Dynamic exchange of subunits of the filamentous structure has now been observed with high-resolution microscopy of living cells, indicating that stationary filamentous structures exchange subunits that move rapidly once dissociated (Wang *et al.*, 2000).

Neurofilaments and microtubules move at a rate of approximately 1 mm/day and make up the majority of slow component a (SCa), which is the slowest-moving component of axonal transport (Hoffman and Lasek, 1975). Subunit structures appear to migrate and reassemble in a process that is dependent on nucleoside triphosphates, kinases, and phosphatases (Koehnle and Brown, 1999; Nixon, 1998). Moving at only a slightly more rapid rate of 2 to 4 mm/day in an anterograde direction is slow component b (SCb) (Grafstein, 1995). Included in SCb are several structural proteins, such as the component of microfilaments (actin) and several microfilament-associated proteins (M2 protein and fodrin), as well as clathrin and many soluble proteins.

This continual transport of proteins from the cell body through the various components of axonal transport is the mechanism through which the neuron provides the distal axon with its complement of functional and structural proteins. Some vesicles are also moving in a retrograde direction and provide the cell body with information concerning the status of the distal axon. The evidence for such a dynamic interchange of materials and information stems

from not only the biochemical detection of these components of axonal transport but also the observations of the effects of terminating this interchange by severing the axon from its cell body. The result of transection of an axon is that the distal axon is destined to degenerate, a process known as axonal degeneration, which is unique to the NS. The cell body of the neuron responds to the transection of the axon as well and undergoes a process of chromatolysis. Notably, defects in components of the retrograde transport pathway have been linked to neurodegenerative diseases demonstrating that disruption of the dynein–dynactin motor complex that drives retrograde transport causes motor neuron loss and muscle denervation in a transgenic mouse model (LaMonte *et al.*, 2002). Studies in mice with either point mutations or a small deletion of the dynein heavy chain corroborate the hypothesis that neurons are preferentially susceptible to defects in dynein function, establishing that mutations in the dynein cofactor dynactin cause neurodegenerative sequalae (Perlson *et al.*, 2010).

Axonal Degeneration

Current concepts of axonal degeneration were initially derived from nerve transections reported by Augustus Waller over a hundred years ago. Accordingly, the sequence of events that occurs in the distal stump of an axon following transection is referred to as *Wallerian degeneration.* Because the axonal degeneration associated with chemicals and some disease states is thought to occur through a similar sequence of events, it is often referred to as *Wallerian-like* axonal degeneration.

Following axotomy, there is degeneration of the distal nerve stump, followed by generation of a microenvironment supportive of regeneration and involving the distal axon, ensheathing glial cells and the blood nerve barrier. Initially there is a period during which the distal stump survives and maintains relatively normal structural, transport, and conduction properties. The duration of survival is proportional to the length of the axonal stump (Chaudry and Cornblath, 1992), and this relationship appears to be maintained across species.

Wallerian degeneration was long thought to be a passive process that proceeded inexorably after separating the axon from the trophic support provided by the cell body. This thinking was changed by the discovery of the *Wld^S* mouse, in which the rate of axonal degeneration triggered by a variety of insults is retarded by about 10-fold (Beirowski *et al.*, 2005). We now know from several lines of evidence that Wallerian degeneration is an active process mediated by the axon itself, and that it is possible to slow or even halt its progression. Moreover, although axonal degeneration can be initiated by many different means, including physical, genetic, or toxic, the mechanisms of degeneration converge into common regulated pathways that are potentially subject to pharmacological intervention (Coleman, 2005; Stys, 2005).

The dynamic relationships between the neuronal cell body and its axon are important in understanding the basic pathological responses to some axonal and neuronal injuries caused by neurotoxicants (Fig. 16-2). When the neuronal cell body has been lethally injured, it degenerates, in a process called *neuronopathy.* This is characterized by the loss of the cell body and all of its processes, with no potential for regeneration. However, when the injury is at the level of the axon, the axon may degenerate while the neuronal cell body continues to survive, a condition known as an *axonopathy.* In this setting, there is a potential for regeneration and recovery from the toxic injury as the axonal stump sprouts and regenerates.

Terminating the period of survival is an active proteolysis that digests the axolemma and axoplasm, leaving only a myelin sheath

A   B   C   D   E

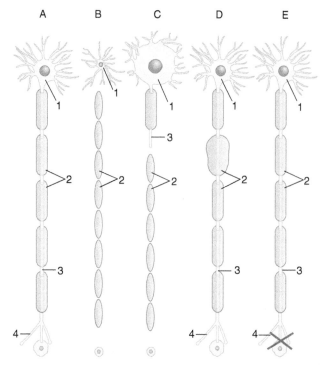

Figure 16-2. *Patterns of neurotoxic injury.* (**A**) Normal neuron showing (1) cell body and dendrites, (2) myelinating cells, encircling the (3) axon, and (4) synapse. (**B**) A neuronopathy resulting from the death of the entire neuron. Astrocytes often proliferate in response to the neuronal loss, creating both neuronal loss and gliosis. (**C**) An axonopathy occurs when the axon is the primary site of injury, the axon degenerates, and the surviving neuron shows only chromatolysis with margination of its Nissl substance and nucleus to the cell periphery. (**D**) Myelinopathy resulting from disruption of myelin or selective injury to the myelinating cells. To prevent cross-talk between adjacent axons, myelinating cells divide and cover the denuded axon rapidly; however, the process of remyelination is much less effective in the CNS than in the PNS. (**E**) Some forms of toxicity are due to interruption of the process of neurotransmission, either through blocking excitation or by excessive stimulation, rather than actual cell death.

surrounding a swollen degenerate axon. Digestion of the axon appears to be an all-or-none event effected through endogenous proteases (Schlafer and Zimmerman, 1984) that are activated through increased levels of intracellular free Ca^{2+} (George *et al.*, 1995). Although it is established that degeneration of the most terminal portion of the axon occurs first, whether degeneration of the remainder of the stump occurs from proximal to distal, distal to proximal, or simultaneously along its entire length remains a matter of debate. The active proteolysis phase occurs so rapidly in mammals that it has been difficult to define a spatial distribution.

In the PNS, Schwann cells respond to loss of axons by decreasing synthesis of myelin lipids, downregulating genes encoding myelin proteins, and dedifferentiating to a premyelinating mitotic Schwann cell phenotype (Stoll and Muller, 1999). The proliferating Schwann cells align along the original basal lamina, which creates a tubular structure referred to as a band of Bungner. In addition to providing physical guidance for regenerating axons, these tubes provide trophic support from nerve growth factor, brain-derived nerve growth factor, insulin-like growth factor, and corresponding receptors produced by the associated Schwann cells. Resident macrophages distributed along the endothelium within the endoneurium and the denervated Schwann cells assist in clearing myelin debris, but the recruitment of hematogenous macrophages accounts for the removal of the majority of myelin. Infiltrating macrophages express complement receptor 3, and the presence of complement 3 on the

surface of degenerating myelin sheaths facilitates opsonization. Another essential role of recruited circulating macrophages is the secretion of interleukin-1, which is responsible for stimulating production of nerve growth factor by Schwann cells. In contrast to the proteolysis of the axon, processing of myelin breakdown products proceeds in an established proximal-to-distal progression.

Investigations have shown that degeneration of the distal axonal stump after transection is an active, synchronized process that can be delayed experimentally through decreasing temperature, preventing the entry of extracellular Ca^{2+}, or inhibiting proteolysis by calpain II (George *et al.*, 1995). Accompanying events in glial cells and macrophages direct and facilitate the sprouting neurite originating from the surviving proximal axon that also undergoes changes in protein expression resembling a less differentiated state. The facilitation of regeneration in the PNS by Schwann cells distinguishes it from the CNS, in which oligodendrocytes secrete inhibitory factors that impede neurite outgrowth. Eventually, though, even in the PNS, if axonal contact is not restored, Schwann cell numbers will decrease, bands of Bungner will disappear, and increased fibroblast collagen production will render regeneration increasingly unlikely.

Thus, a critical difference exists in the significance of axonal degeneration in the CNS compared with that in the PNS: peripheral axons can regenerate, whereas central axons cannot. In the PNS, glial cells and macrophages create an environment supportive of axonal regeneration, and Schwann cells transplanted to the CNS maintain this ability. In the CNS, release of inhibitory factors from damaged myelin and astrocyte scarring actually interfere with regeneration (Qiu *et al.*, 2000). Interestingly, when this glial interference is removed through transplantation of CNS neurons to the PNS, the neurons are capable of extending neurites. There appears, however, to be more than just glial interference to account for the lack of CNS regeneration. The observation that embryonic neurons can overcome glial interference when placed into the adult NS is consistent with the development of an intrinsic sensitivity to inhibitory factors during maturation. Therefore, the inability of the CNS to regenerate appears to be due to both unfavorable environmental glial factors and properties of the mature neuron. The clinical relevance of the disparity between the CNS and PNS is that partial recovery—or, in mild cases, complete recovery—can occur after axonal degeneration in the PNS, whereas the same event is irreversible in the CNS.

Myelin Formation and Maintenance

Myelin is formed in the CNS by oligodendrocytes and in the PNS by Schwann cells. Both of these cell types form concentric layers of lipid-rich myelin by the progressive wrapping of their cytoplasmic processes around the axon in successive loops (Fig. 16-3). Ultimately, these cells exclude cytoplasm from the inner surface of their membranes to form the major dense line of myelin (Quarles *et al.*, 1997; Monuki and Lemke, 1995; Parent, 1996). In a similar process, the extracellular space is reduced on the extracellular surface of the bilayers, and the lipid membranes stack together, separated only by a proteinaceous intraperiod line existing between successive layers.

The formation and maintenance of myelin requires metabolic and structural proteins that are unique to the NS. Myelin basic protein, an integral protein of CNS myelin, is closely associated with the intracellular space (at the major dense line of myelin) (Quarles *et al.*, 1997; Monuki and Lemke, 1995), and an analogous protein, P1 protein, is located in the PNS. On the extracellular surface of the lipid bilayers is the CNS protein, proteolipid protein, at the intraperiod line of myelin. Mutation of this protein in several species,

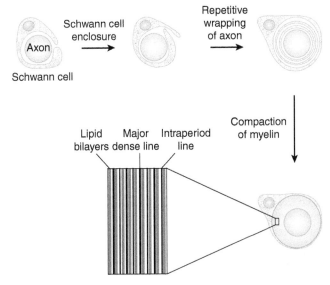

Figure 16-3. *Process of myelination.* Myelination begins when a myelinating cell encircles an axon, either Schwann cells in the peripheral nervous system or oligodendrocytes in the CNS. Simple enclosure of the axon persists in unmyelinated axons. Myelin formation proceeds by a progressive wrapping of multiple layers of the myelinating cell around the axon, with extrusion of the cytoplasm and extracellular space to bring the lipid bilayers into close proximity. The intracellular space is compressed to form the major dense line of myelin, and the extracellular space is compressed to form the intraperiod line.

including humans, or overexpression of the wild-type gene in transgenic mice, results in disorders in which myelin of the CNS does not form normally (Pham-Dinh *et al.*, 1991; Readhead *et al.*, 1994).

There are a variety of hereditary disorders where myelin is either poorly formed from the outset or maintained after its formation. In addition to mutation of proteolipid protein, there are a variety of inherited abnormalities of myelin proteins and myelin-specific lipid catabolism. These genetic defects have provided some insight into the special processes required to maintain the lipid-rich environment of myelin. It is now known that the maintenance of myelin is dependent on a number of membrane-associated proteins and on metabolism of specific lipids present in myelin bilayers. Some toxic compounds interfere with this complex process of the maintenance of myelin and result in the toxic "myelinopathies" (Fig. 16-2). In general, the loss of myelin with the preservation of axons is referred to as *demyelination*.

Neurotransmission

Intercellular communication is achieved in the NS through the synapse. Neurotransmitters released from one axon to another act as the first messenger. Binding of the transmitter to the postsynaptic receptor is followed by modulation of an ion channel or activation of a second messenger system, leading to changes in the responding cell. In the case of neuromuscular transmission, acetylcholine crosses the synaptic cleft to bind the cholinergic receptor of the myocyte and leads to muscle contraction. Chemically induced dysfunction of neurotransmission may occur in the absence of altered cellular structures; rather, the neurotoxicity expresses itself in terms of altered conduction and propagation of nerve impulses and changes in functions such as behavior, performance, and conditioning.

Chemicals acting on neurotransmission may interrupt the transmission of impulses, block or accentuate transsynaptic communication, block reuptake of neurotransmitters or precursors, or interfere with second-messenger systems. The structural similarity

of many compounds with similar actions has led to the recognition of specific categories of drugs and toxins. For example, some drugs mimic the process of neurotransmission of the sympathetic NS and are termed sympathomimetic compounds. As the targets of these drugs are located throughout the body, the responses are not localized; however, the responses are stereotyped in that each member of a class tends to have similar biological effects. At times, altered neurotransmission is beneficial to an individual, for example, by stabilizing a disease-induced imbalance, and it is this aspect of biological response that is studied in the field of neuropharmacology. However, excessive or inappropriate exposure to compounds that alter neurotransmission may result in responses considered as neurotoxic. The therapeutic index is a measure of the margin between the desirable (therapeutic) and toxic effects of a chemical.

In terms of toxicity, many side effects of neurological drugs may be viewed as short-term interactions that are reversible with time or that may be counteracted by the use of appropriate antagonists. However, some of the toxicity associated with long-term exposures may be irreversible. For example, phenothiazines, which have been used to treat chronic schizophrenia for long periods of time, may lead to the condition of tardive dyskinesia, in which the patient is left with a permanent disability of prominent facial grimaces (DeVeaugh-Geiss, 1982). Excessive stimulation of neurotransmitter systems may also have long-term consequences; for example, excitatory systems (eg, glutamate) produces excitotoxicity manifest as CNS diseases and nerve cell death (Wang and Qin, 2010).

Development of the Nervous System

The NS begins development during gestation (first month in humans, Day 7 in mice, Day 9.5 in rats) and continues through adolescence (Bayer *et al.*, 1993; Rice and Barone, 2000). Proliferation, migration, differentiation, synaptogenesis, apoptosis, and myelination are the basic processes that underlie development of the NS, and these occur in a tightly choreographed sequence that depends on the region, cell type, and neurotrophic signals. Both neuronal and glial precursors replicate in a discrete zone near the inner surface of the neural tube. The proliferation and migration of these cells occur in waves that are specific for brain regions, but in general, the brain develops in a caudal to rostral direction (with cerebellar development being a notable exception). During differentiation (phenotype expression) and synaptogenesis (formation of functional synaptic connections), the circuitry of the NS is established. Chemicals such as nerve growth factors, adhesive molecules, and neurotransmitters serve as morphogenic signals; neurotransmitter developmental signals are separate from their synaptic transmission function (Lauder, 1993). Selected cells are also removed during ontogeny via apoptosis (programmed cell death), which results in the appropriate cell types in the correct regions. The glial supportive cells develop last, and myelination is protracted. The period of rapid proliferation of glial cells is known as the brain growth spurt, during which time it is particularly vulnerable to insult (Dobbing and Sands, 1979; Dobbing and Smart, 1974). Although the order of neurogenesis is conserved across species, the rate of maturation and timing of specific events relative to birth vary; however, consideration of these data impact extrapolation of developmental consequences from laboratory animals to humans (Bayer *et al.*, 1993; Clancy *et al.*, 2007; Dobbing and Sands, 1973).

The immature NS is especially vulnerable to certain chemicals (Bondy and Campbell, 2005; Rodier, 1995), and there are several factors that make the developing NS uniquely susceptible. Cell sensitivity differs with the developmental stage, leading to critical windows of vulnerability (Adams *et al.*, 2000; Bayer *et al.*, 1993; Selevan *et al.*, 2000). Chemicals that alter the timing and formation of neural connections could result in permanent malformations, the consequences of which may be quite unlike the chemical's effects in the adult NS (Barone *et al.*, 2000). Furthermore, while synaptogenesis can continue throughout life, proliferation cannot; therefore, the CNS is unique in that damaged neural cells are not readily replaced. Finally, there are physiological and kinetic differences in the developing organism that may profoundly influence its sensitivity, including the slow formation of the blood–brain barrier and lack of key metabolic enzymes to protect the brain and eliminate toxicants (Bearer, 1995; Makri *et al.*, 2004).

Although the developing NS is often more sensitive to insult (depending on the stage of development), the high rate of proliferation and regeneration in the developing NS may also lead to greater recovery or plasticity (an ability of one portion of the NS to assume the function of an injured area), which could attenuate some injuries (Goldberger and Murray, 1985). An example is the faster recovery from organophosphorous (OP) pesticide-induced acetylcholinesterase (AChE) inhibition observed in younger laboratory rats, which is probably due to the rapid formation of the esterase enzyme and replacement of the phosphorylated form (Moser and Padilla, 1998). Some developmental changes may appear transient due to this plasticity and compensation, but underlying changes in the NS development could become manifest with aging or some form of challenge (eg, Barone *et al.*, 1995, 2000; Bondy and Campbell, 2005; Rice, 1996).

In evaluating developmental neurotoxicity, chemical exposure or treatment may occur during critical windows of susceptibility, or may cover the entire developmental process (ie, during gestation, lactation, and adolescence). In general, injurious exposures early in gestation impact development of major brain regions whereas later exposures alter biochemical, morphological, or functional features of the neural systems. Functional, neurochemical, morphometric, or neuroanatomical endpoints are often used to assess the impact of developmental exposures; multiple measures are often needed to assess the wide array of potential outcomes. The ontogeny of specific behaviors, reflexes, and motor functions has been established for laboratory rats and mice, and compared to human developmental patterns (eg, Altman and Sudarshan, 1975; Fox, 1965; Wood *et al.*, 2003). Markers of synaptic proteins, assays of synaptic enzymes, or challenges with pharmacologically specific chemicals are but a few methods by which to test synaptic function. Although frank neuropathology is not as common with developmental neurotoxicants, measurements of layer widths in synaptic zones may reflect physical malformations.

Environmental Factors Relevant to Neurodegenerative Diseases

Individuals exposed to insufficient 1-methyl-4-phenyl-1,2,3,6-tetrahydropyridine (MPTP) to result in immediate parkinsonism have developed early signs of the disease years later (Calne *et al.*, 1985). This observation presents the possibility that the onset of a neurotoxic problem may follow toxic exposure by many years (Landigan *et al.*, 2005). It does not seem likely that an early sublethal injury to dopaminergic (DAergic) neurons later becomes lethal. Rather, smaller exposures to MPTP may cause a decrement in the population of DAergic neurons within the substantia nigra (SN). Such a loss would most likely be silent because the symptoms of Parkinson disease (PD) do not develop until approximately 80% to 90% of the SN neurons are lost. These individuals with a diminished number of neurons may be more vulnerable to further loss of DAergic neurons. The neurological picture of PD develops at an earlier age than

in unexposed individuals, as a further loss of catecholaminergic neurons occurs during the process of aging.

The relationship between MPTP intoxication and parkinsonism has stimulated investigations into the role that environmental and occupational exposures may play in the pathogenesis of PD. Although several families with early-onset PD demonstrate autosomal dominant inheritance, with identification of candidate genes (Polymerpoulos *et al.*, 1997; Agundez *et al.*, 1995; Kurth and Kurth, 1993), twin studies indicate that environmental exposures play a more significant role than genetics in the vast majority of PD patients, particularly those with late-onset disease (Tanner *et al.*, 1999; Kuopio *et al.*, 1999). Epidemiological studies implicate exposure to herbicides, pesticides, and metals as risk factors for PD (Gorell *et al.*, 1998, 1999; Liou *et al.*, 1997). Several studies suggest that dithiocarbamates also play an important role (Miller, 1982; Ferraz *et al.*, 1988; Bachurin *et al.*, 1996). Some studies suggest that cigarette smoking may have a protective effect against both Alzheimer disease and PD, but alternative explanations have been offered (Riggs, 1992).

An epidemic of dialysis-related dementia with some pathological resemblance to Alzheimer disease appears to have been related to aluminum in the dialysate, and its removal has prevented further instances of dialysis dementia. However, there is no substantial evidence to date that aluminum is in any way related to sporadic Alzheimer disease in the general population (Letzel *et al.*, 2000).

The expanding field of the excitotoxic amino acids embodies many of the same attributes that characterize the entire discipline of neurotoxicology. Neurotoxicology is generally viewed as the study of compounds that are deleterious to the NS, and the effects of glutamate and kainate may be viewed as examples of this type of deleterious toxicity. Exposure to these excitotoxic amino acids leads to neuronal injury and—when of sufficient degree—may kill neurons. Many of these neurotoxic compounds have become tools for neurobiologists who seek to explore the anatomy and function of the NS. Kainate, through its selective action on neuronal cell bodies, has provided a greater understanding of the functions of cells within a specific region of the brain, while previous lesioning techniques addressed only regional functions. Finally, the questions surrounding domoic acid poisoning and the Guamanian neurodegenerative complex serve to remind the student of neurotoxicology that the causes of many neurological diseases remain unknown. This void in understanding and the epidemiological evidence that some neurodegenerative diseases may have environmental contributors provide a heightened desire to appreciate more fully the effects of elements of our environment on the NS.

It also needs to be recognized that environmental chemicals may cause heritable alterations in gene expression in the absence of changes in genome sequences. The study of epigenetics has established two categories of mechanisms affecting gene expression. These are referred to as DNA methylation and histone posttranslational modifications. The former is a naturally occurring modification characterized by addition of a methyl group to the 5′ position of the cytosine ring in the context of CpG dinucleotides to form 5-methylcytosine (5-MeC) (Arita and Costa, 2009). In most instances, promoter region methylation results in transcriptional repression of the gene. In histones, epigenetic information is stored by posttranslational modifications at well-conserved amino acid residues of its N- and C-terminal tails. Histone posttranslational modifications are characterized by lysine acetylation, arginine and lysine methylation, serine phosphorylation, lysine ubiquitylation, as well as others. Acetylation of histone lysines commonly results in transcriptional activation. Since it is now well established that epigenetics can control and modify neurological disorders, recent focus has been directed at the role of environmental chemicals in regulating heritable alterations in gene expression and the etiology of neurodegenerative diseases, absent changes in genome sequences. Epigenetic alterations have been implied in both neurodevelopmental and neurodegenerative disorders (Portela and Esteller, 2010). For example, *FMR1* promoter hypermethylation has been described in Fragile X syndrome patients, whereas promoter hypomethylated with an ensuing overexpression of tumor necrosis factor alpha (TNFα) has been reported in the SN of PD patients.

Finally, it is necessary to recognize that microRNAs (miRNAs) provide regulatory control over gene expression (Krichevsky *et al.*, 2006). miRNAs are noncoding transcripts of 18–25 nucleotides (nt) that are incorporated into the RNA-induced silencing complex (RISC), an RNA–protein complex that mediates target mRNA cleavage or regulates its translation. mRNAs can control developmental timing, cell proliferation, cell death, and patterning of the NS, thus providing an extensive regulatory networks with a complexity comparable to that of transcription factors. More than 250 miRNAs have been already identified, but their mRNA targets and functions have yet to be fully appreciated. Emerging studies also suggest that miRNAs may be targeted by neurotoxicants, thus potentially affecting a broad spectrum of functions, encompassing cell differentiation and migration, neurogenesis, as well as synaptic function, to name a few.

FUNCTIONAL MANIFESTATIONS OF NEUROTOXICITY

Although knowledge of a toxicant's complete biochemical or molecular mechanism(s) is the ultimate goal of neurotoxicology, a full understanding of the toxicity also requires knowledge of the functional outcomes of those changes. Being the final output or manifestation of the NS, function includes motor, sensory, autonomic, and cognitive capabilities. The strength of functional assessments has been exploited by many investigators and regulatory agencies, and they are now routinely used in the assessment of the neurological effects of chemicals. Tilson (1993) has proposed two distinct tiers of functional testing of neurotoxicants: a first tier in which observational batteries or motor activity tests may be used to identify the presence of a neurotoxic substance, and a second tier that involves more refined tests to allow better characterization of the effects.

An overall assessment of function may be described using a series, or battery, of tests. These tests typically evaluate a variety of neurological functions, and are sometimes used to screen for potential neurotoxicity in regulatory and safety pharmacology testing (Tilson and Moser, 1992; Moser, 2000). Specific behavioral methods include functional observational batteries (FOBs), Irwin screens, tests of motor activity, and expanded clinical observations. These tests have the advantage over biochemical and pathological measures in that they permit evaluation of a single animal over longitudinal studies to determine the onset, progression, duration, and reversibility of a neurotoxic injury. Comparisons of defined protocols of FOBs with limited numbers of compounds (Moser *et al.*, 1997a,b) suggest that these methods can identify neurotoxic compounds reliably.

Some functional tests are more specific than observations and motor activity, and may be used to more fully characterize neurotoxic effects. Many of these functions have a clinical or behavioral correlate in humans, thus improving extrapolation of the outcomes. Electrophysiological tests provide sensory-specific information on nerve conduction velocity and integrity, and have been used to complement behavioral evaluations (Dyer, 1985; Mattsson *et al.*, 1989). Measures of sensory function tap specific neuronal pathways that

govern stimuli-dependent reflexes. For example, the acoustic startle response is a sensory-evoked motor reflex with a defined neuronal pathway (Davis *et al.*, 1982). Treatment effects could indicate sensory, motor, or muscle fiber alterations with little or no central involvement. Autonomic function includes evaluations of cardiovascular status and cholinergic/adrenergic balance.

Deficits in cognitive function, especially in the context of developmental toxicity, represent an endpoint of great public concern and rhetoric. Behavioral toxicologists have incorporated methodologies from behavioral pharmacology and psychology to develop a range of tests of learning and memory for laboratory animals. These procedures include spatial navigation of mazes, associations with shock, conditioned responses, and appetite-motivated operant responses. In most cases, deficits in human cognitive function may be detected in laboratory animals as well, although the affected cognitive domain may vary. For example, in humans, exposure to lead in early childhood is known to lower IQ and alter behavioral control. Studies in rats have reported deficits in spatial learning, sustained attention, activity levels, and other behaviors (eg, Moreira *et al.*, 2001; Morgan *et al.*, 2001; Nihei *et al.*, 2000). Detailed assessments such as these provide valuable insights into the damage caused by neurotoxicants. Ultimately, neurotoxicants identified by behavioral methods are evaluated at a cellular and molecular level to provide an understanding of the events in the NS that cause the neurological dysfunction.

MECHANISMS OF NEUROTOXICITY

Efforts to understand the mechanism of action of individual neurotoxic compounds have begun with the identification of the cellular target. In the NS, this has most often been one of four targets: the neuron, the axon, the myelinating cell, or the neurotransmitter system. As a result, neurotoxic compounds may be identified which cause neuronopathies, axonopathies, myelinopathies, or neurotransmitter-associated toxicity (Fig. 16-2). This is the classification system that is utilized here to organize the discussion of neurotoxic compounds and their mechanisms of action.

Neuronopathies

Certain toxicants are specific for neurons, or sometimes a particular group of neurons, resulting in their injury or, when intoxication is severe enough, their death. The loss of a neuron is irreversible and includes degeneration of all of its cytoplasmic extensions, dendrites and axons, and of the myelin ensheathing the axon (Fig. 16-2). Although the neuron is similar to other cell types in many respects, some features of the neuron are unique, placing it at risk for the action of cellular toxicants. Some of the unique features of the neuron include a high metabolic rate, a long cellular process that is supported by the cell body, and an excitable membrane that is rapidly depolarized and repolarized. Because many neurotoxic compounds act at the site of the cell body, when massive loss of axons and myelin are discovered in the PNS or CNS, the first question is whether the neuronal cell bodies themselves have been destroyed.

Although a large number of compounds are known to produce toxic neuronopathies (Table 16-1), all of these toxicants share certain features. Each toxic condition is the result of a cellular toxicant that has a predilection for neurons, most likely due to one of the neuron's peculiar vulnerabilities. The initial injury to neurons is followed by apoptosis or necrosis, leading to permanent loss of the neuron. These chemicals tend to diffuse in their action, although they may show some selectivity in the degree of injury

Table 16-1

Compounds Associated with Neuronal Injury (Neuronopathies)

NEUROTOXICANT	NEUROLOGICAL FINDINGS	CELLULAR BASIS OF NEUROTOXICITY	REFERENCES
Aluminum	Dementia, encephalopathy (humans), learning deficits	Spongiosis cortex, neurofibrillary aggregates, degenerative changes in cortex	Chang and Dyer (1995), Graham and Lantos (1997), Spencer and Schaumburg (2000)
6-Amino-nicotinamide	Not reported in humans; hind limb paralysis (experimental animals)	Spongy (vacuolar) degeneration in spinal cord, brainstem, cerebellum; axonal degeneration of the peripheral nervous system (PNS)	Graham and Lantos (1997), Spencer and Schaumburg (2000)
Arsenic	Encephalopathy (acute), peripheral neuropathy (chronic)	(PNS) Brain swelling and hemorrhage (acute), axonal degeneration in PNS (chronic)	Graham and Lantos (1997), Spencer and Schaumburg (2000)
Azide	Insufficient data (humans); convulsions, ataxia (primates)	Neuronal loss in cerebellum and cortex	Graham and Lantos (1997), Spencer and Schaumburg (2000)
Bismuth	Emotional disturbances, encephalopathy, myoclonus	Neuronal loss, basal ganglia and Purkinje cells of cerebellum	Spencer and Schaumburg (2000)
Carbon monoxide	Encephalopathy, delayed parkinsonism/dystonia	Neuronal loss in cortex, necrosis of globus pallidus, focal demyelination; blocks oxygen binding site of hemoglobin and iron-binding sites of brain	Spencer and Schaumburg (2000)
Carbon tetrachloride	Encephalopathy (secondary to liver failure)	Enlarged astrocytes in striatum, globus pallidus	Spencer and Schaumburg (2000)
Chloramphenicol	Optic neuritis, peripheral neuropathy	Neuronal loss (retina), axonal degeneration (PNS)	Graham and Lantos (1997), Spencer and Schaumburg (2000)
Cyanide	Coma, convulsions, rapid death; delayed parkinsonism/dystonia	Neuronal degeneration, cerebellum and globus pallidus; focal demyelination; blocks cytochrome oxidase/adenosine triphosphate production	Graham and Lantos (1997), Spencer and Schaumburg (2000)
Doxorubicin	Insufficient data (humans); progressive ataxia (experimental animals)	Degeneration of dorsal root ganglion cells, axonal degeneration (PNS)	Graham and Lantos (1997), Spencer and Schaumburg (2000)
Ethanol	Mental retardation, hearing deficits (prenatal exposure)	Microcephaly, cerebral malformations	Graham and Lantos (1997)
Lead	Encephalopathy (acute), learning deficits (children), neuropathy with demyelination (rats)	Brain swelling, hemorrhages (acute), axonal loss in PNS (humans)	Chang and Dyer (1995), Graham and Lantos (1997), Spencer and Schaumburg (2000)
Manganese	Emotional disturbances, parkinsonism/dystonia	Degeneration of striatum, globus pallidus	Chang and Dyer (1995), Graham and Lantos (1997)
Mercury, inorganic	Emotional disturbances, tremor, fatigue	Insufficient data in humans (may affect spinal tracts; cerebellum)	Chang and Dyer (1995), Graham and Lantos (1997), Spencer and Schaumburg (2000)
Methanol	Headache, visual loss or blindness, coma (severe)	Necrosis of putamen, degeneration of retinal ganglion cells	Graham and Lantos (1997), Spencer and Schaumburg (2000)
Methylazoxymethanol acetate (MAM)	Microcephaly, retarded development (rats)	Developmental abnormalities of fetal brain (rats)	Abou-Donia (1993)
Methyl bromide	Visual and speech impairment; peripheral neuropathy	Insufficient data	Spencer and Schaumburg (2000)
Methyl mercury (organic mercury)	Ataxia, constriction of visual fields, paresthesias (adult) Psychomotor retardation (fetal exposure)	Neuronal degeneration, visual cortex, cerebellum, ganglia Spongy disruption, cortex and cerebellum	Chang and Dyer (1995), Graham and Lantos (1997), Spencer and Schaumburg (2000) Graham and Lantos (1997), Spencer and Schaumburg (2000)

(continued)

Table 16-1

(Continued)

NEUROTOXICANT	NEUROLOGICAL FINDINGS	CELLULAR BASIS OF NEUROTOXICITY	REFERENCES
1-Methyl-4-phenyl-1,2,3,6-tetrahydropyridine (MPTP)	Parkinsonism, dystonia (acute exposure) Early-onset parkinsonism (late effect of acute exposure)	Neuronal degeneration in substantia nigra Neuronal degeneration in substantia nigra	Graham and Lantos (1997), Spencer and Schaumburg (2000) Graham and Lantos (1997), Spencer and Schaumburg (2000)
3-Nitropropionic acid	Seizures, delayed dystonia/grimacing	Necrosis in basal ganglia	Graham and Lantos (1997), Spencer and Schaumburg (2000)
Phenytoin (diphenyl-hydantoin)	Nystagmus, ataxia, dizziness	Degeneration of Purkinje cells (cerebellum)	Graham and Lantos (1997), Spencer and Schaumburg (2000)
Quinine	Constriction of visual fields	Vacuolization of retinal ganglion cells	Spencer and Schaumburg (2000)
Streptomycin (aminoglycosides)	Hearing loss	Degeneration of inner ear (organ of Corti)	Spencer and Schaumburg (2000)
Thallium	Emotional disturbances, ataxia, peripheral neuropathy	Brain swelling (acute), axonal degeneration in PNS	Graham and Lantos (1997), Spencer and Schaumburg (2000)
Trimethyltin	Tremors, hyperexcitability (experimental animals)	Loss of hippocampal neurons, amygdala pyriform cortex	Graham and Lantos (1997)

of different neuronal subpopulations or at times an exquisite selectivity for such a subpopulation. The expression of these cellular events is often a diffuse encephalopathy, with global dysfunctions; however, the symptomatology reflects the injury to the brain, so neurotoxicants that are selective in their action and affect only a subpopulation of neurons may lead to interruption of only a particular functionality.

Doxorubicin Doxorubicin (Adriamycin), a quinone-containing anthracycline antibiotic, is one of the most effective antimitotics in cancer chemotherapy. Unfortunately, clinical application of doxorubicin is greatly limited by its acute and chronic cardiotoxicity. In addition to its cardiac toxicity that limits the quantity of doxorubicin that can be given to cancer patients, doxorubicin also injures neurons in the PNS, specifically those of the dorsal root ganglia and autonomic ganglia (Spencer, 2000). This selective vulnerability of peripheral ganglion cells is particularly dramatic in experimental animals. Doxorubicin's antineoplastic properties derive from its ability to intercalate into grooves of DNA, interfering with transcription. Other important mechanisms of action of doxorubicin include its interaction with topoisomerase II, which forms a DNA-cleavable complex (Chuang and Chuang, 1979; Cheng *et al.*, 1992) and generation of reactive oxygen species (ROS) by enzymatic electron reduction of doxorubicin by variety of oxidases, reductases, and dehydrogenases (Gutierrez, 2000; Kappus, 1987). The neurotoxicity of doxorubicin is quite limited in its extent, despite the fact that all neurons are dependent on the ability to transcribe DNA. The particular vulnerability of sensory and autonomic neurons appears to reflect the lack of protection of these neurons by a blood–tissue barrier within ganglia. If the blood–brain barrier is temporarily opened by the use of mannitol, the toxicity of doxorubicin is expressed in a much more diffuse manner, with injury of neurons in the cortex and subcortical nuclei of the brain (Spencer, 2000).

Methyl Mercury The neuronal toxicity of organomercurial compounds, such as methyl mercury (MeHg), was tragically revealed in large numbers of poisonings in Japan and Iraq. The residents of Minamata Bay in Japan, whose diet was largely composed of fish from the bay, were exposed to massive amounts of MeHg when mercury-laden industrial effluent was rerouted into the bay (Kurland *et al.*, 1960; Takeuchi *et al.*, 1962). MeHg injured even more people in Iraq, with more than 400 deaths and 6000 people hospitalized. In this epidemic, as well as in several smaller ones, the effects occurred after the consumption of grain that had been dusted with MeHg as an inexpensive pesticide (Bakir *et al.*, 1973). Typically, environmental exposure to mercury occurs via the food chain due to accumulation of MeHg in fish. Latest statistics in the United States indicate that 46 states have fish consumption advisories covering 40% of the nation's rivers, lakes, and streams. In addition, mercury is a common pollutant in hazardous waste sites in the nation (USEPA, 2001). It is estimated that three to four million children live within one mile of at least one of the 1300+ active hazardous waste sites in the USA (USEPA, 2001).

The clinical picture of MeHg poisoning varies with both the severity of exposure and the age of the individual at the time of exposure. In adults, the most dramatic sites of injury are the neurons of the visual cortex and the small internal granular cell neurons of the cerebellar cortex, whose massive degeneration results in blindness and marked ataxia. In children, developmental disabilities, retardation, and cognitive deficits occur. Such age-related differences are seen also in other mammals, although the specific areas damaged may differ. It has been suggested that these differences are caused by an immature blood–brain barrier causing a more generalized distribution of mercury in the developing brain. Recent studies in rats show that the neurons that are most sensitive to the toxic effects of MeHg are those that reside in the dorsal root ganglia, perhaps again reflecting the vulnerability of neurons not shielded by blood–tissue barriers (Schionning *et al.*, 1998).

The mechanism of MeHg toxicity has been the subject of intense investigation. However, it remains unknown whether the ultimate toxicant is MeHg or the liberated mercuric ion. Although Hg^{2+} is known to bind strongly to sulfhydryl groups, it is not clear that MeHg results in cell death through sulfhydryl binding.

UNIT IV TARGET ORGAN TOXICITY

A variety of aberrations in cellular function have been noted, including impaired glycolysis, nucleic acid biosynthesis, aerobic respiration, protein synthesis (Cheung and Verity, 1985), and neurotransmitter release (Atchison and Hare, 1994). In addition, there is evidence for enhanced oxidative injury (LeBel *et al.*, 1992; Shanker *et al.*, 2002) and altered calcium homeostasis (Marty and Atchison, 1997). Exposure to MeHg leads to widespread neuronal injury and subsequently to a diffuse encephalopathy. However, there is relative selectivity of the toxicant for some groups of neurons over others. The distribution of neuronal injury does not appear to be related to the tissue distribution of either MeHg or ionic mercury but rather to particular vulnerabilities of these neurons. Susceptibility of different brain regions or cell types to MeHg (Clarkson, 1997) may also be dependent on factors such as the intracellular reduced glutathione (GSH) concentration and the ability to increase glycolytic flux in the face of mitochondrial damage. These observations are consistent with morphological observations in which astrocytes that accumulate MeHg appear normal, whereas neurons that are found in their proximity and are void of MeHg undergo cell death (Garman *et al.*, 1975). It seems likely that MeHg toxicity is mediated by numerous reactions and that no single critical target will be identified. As these toxic events occur, the injured neurons eventually die.

Trimethyltin Organotins are used industrially as plasticizers, antifungal agents, or pesticides. Intoxication with trimethyltin has been associated with a potentially irreversible limbic-cerebellar syndrome in humans and similar behavioral changes in primates (Besser *et al.*, 1987; Reuhl *et al.*, 1985). Trimethyltin gains access to the NS where, by an undefined mechanism, it leads to diffuse neuronal injury. Trimethyltin triggers selective apoptosis in specific subregions of the mammalian CNS and specific subsets of immune system cells (Balaban *et al.*, 1988; Patanow *et al.*, 1997). The hippocampus is particularly vulnerable to this process. Following acute intoxication, the cells of the fascia dentata degenerate; with chronic intoxication, the cells of the corpus ammonis are lost. Ganglion cells and hair cells of the cochlea are similarly sensitive (Liu and Fechter, 1996). Several hypotheses are suggested for the mechanism of trimethyltin neurotoxicity, including energy deprivation and excitotoxic damage. Evidence to date suggests that organotins, such as trimethyltin, interact with the CXC region of stannic, and that trimethyltin treatment significantly alters its expression (Toggas *et al.*, 1993). Stannic is located on human chromosome 16p13, and has a syntenic relationship to the murine chromosomal homolog (Dejneka *et al.*, 1998).

Axonopathies

The neurotoxic disorders termed *axonopathies* are those in which the primary site of toxicity is the axon itself. The axon degenerates, and with it the myelin surrounding that axon; however, the neuron cell body remains intact (Fig. 16-2). John Cavanagh coined the term *dying-back neuropathy* as a synonym for *axonopathy* (Cavanagh, 1964). The concept of "dying back" postulated that the focus of toxicity was the neuronal cell body itself and that the distal axon degenerated progressively from the synapse, back toward the cell body with increasing injury. It now appears that, in the best-studied axonopathies, a different pathogenetic sequence occurs; the toxicant results in a "chemical transection" of the axon at some point along its length, and the axon distal to the transection, biologically separated from its cell body, degenerates in a Wallerian fashion.

Because longer axons have more targets for toxic damage than shorter axons, one would predict that longer axons would be more affected in toxic axonopathies. Indeed, such is the case. The

involvement of long axons of the CNS, such as ascending sensory axons in the posterior columns or descending motor axons, along with long sensory and motor axons of the PNS, prompted Spencer and Schaumburg (1976) to suggest that the toxic axonopathies in which the distal axon was most vulnerable be called *central peripheral distal axonopathies*, which, though cumbersome, accurately depicts the pathological sequence.

Axonopathies can be considered to result from a chemical transection of the axon. The number of axonal toxicants is large and increasing in number (Table 16-2); however, they may be viewed as a group, all of which result in the pathological loss of distal axons with the survival of the cell body. Because the axonopathies pathologically resemble the actual physical transection of the axon, axonal transport appears to be a likely target in many of the toxic axonopathies. Furthermore, as these axons degenerate, the result is most often the clinical condition of peripheral neuropathy, in which sensations and motor strength are first impaired in the most distal extent of the axonal processes, the feet and hands. With time and continued injury, the deficit progresses to involve more proximal areas of the body and the long axons of the spinal cord. The potential for regeneration is great when the insult is limited to peripheral nerves and may be virtually complete in axonopathies in which the initiating event can be determined and removed.

Gamma-Diketones It was first noted in the late 1960s that humans with chronic high exposures to *n*-hexane, a simple alkane, in a work setting develop a progressive sensorimotor distal axonopathy (Yamamura, 1969). Intentional inhalation of materials containing *n*-hexane is also common, and produces the same neurotoxic effects. An identical axonopathy was also produced by methyl *n*-butyl ketone (2-hexanone), leading to the discovery of the mechanism by which these two compounds are similarly metabolized. The carbon chain undergoes ω-1 oxidation, resulting in 2,5-hexanedione, a γ-diketone. This metabolite is ultimately the toxic species produced from *n*-hexane and 2-hexanone. Other γ-diketones or precursors also produced the same axonopathy, whereas α- or β-diketones are not toxic to the NS (Krasavage *et al.*, 1980).

γ-Diketones, including 2,5-hexanedione, react with amino groups on all proteins, forming pyrrole adducts. This is an important step in development of axonopathy, as evidenced by the inability of 3,3-dimethyl-2,5-hexanedione, a γ-diketone that is unable to form pyrrole adducts, to cause neurotoxicity (Sayre *et al.*, 1986). After forming, these pyrroles are oxidized and cross-linking occurs between neurofilament subunits. The inability of 3-acetyl-2,5-hexanedione to cross-link prevents toxicity, suggesting that pyrrole oxidation and cross-linking is a necessary step in the development of axonopathy (St. Clair *et al.*, 1988). Neurofilaments accumulate in the distal axon, usually just proximal to a node of Ranvier, and form massive axonal swellings leading to retraction of myelin from the nodes (Graham *et al.*, 1982). In addition to swelling, axonal atrophy is also a pathological feature of γ-diketone neurotoxicity.

This axonal atrophy was previously thought to occur secondary to swelling; however, more recent studies have suggested that it may be the more relevant pathophysiological feature. In one study, rats dosed at a lower rate (100–250 mg/kg/day) developed axonal swelling and atrophy, and rats given a higher dose rate (400 mg/kg/day) failed to consistently develop swellings, while atrophy and behavioral alterations were nearly universal. These data suggest that axonal atrophy is the pathological change that leads to nerve dysfunction and behavioral changes (Lehning *et al.*, 2000). The mechanism responsible for axonal atrophy is still unknown;

Table 16-2

Compounds Associated with Axonal Injury (Axonopathies)

NEUROTOXICANT	NEUROLOGICAL FINDINGS	BASIS OF NEUROTOXICITY	REFERENCES
Acrylamide	Peripheral neuropathy (often sensory)	Axonal degeneration, axon terminal affected in earliest stages	Graham and Lantos (1997), Spencer and Schaumburg (2000)
p-Bromophenylacetyl urea	Peripheral neuropathy	Axonal degeneration in the peripheral nervous system (PNS) and central nervous system (CNS)	Spencer and Schaumburg (2000)
Carbon disulfide	Psychosis (acute), peripheral neuropathy (chronic)	Axonal degeneration, early stages include neurofilamentous swelling	Graham and Lantos (1997), Spencer and Schaumburg (2000)
Chlordecone (Kepone)	Tremors, in coordination (experimental animals)	Insufficient data (humans); axonal swelling and degeneration	Spencer and Schaumburg (2000)
Chloroquine	Peripheral neuropathy, weakness	Axonal degeneration, inclusions in dorsal root ganglion cells; also vacuolar myopathy	Graham and Lantos (1997), Spencer and Schaumburg (2000)
Clioquinol	Encephalopathy (acute), subacute myelooptic neuropathy (subacute)	Axonal degeneration, spinal cord, PNS, optic tracts	Graham and Lantos (1997), Spencer and Schaumburg (2000)
Colchicine	Peripheral neuropathy	Axonal degeneration, neuronal perikaryal filamentous aggregates; vacuolar myopathy	Graham and Lantos (1997), Spencer and Schaumburg (2000)
Dapsone	Peripheral neuropathy, predominantly motor	Axonal degeneration (both myelinated and unmyelinated axons)	Graham and Lantos (1997)
Dichlorophenoxyacetate	Peripheral neuropathy (delayed)	Insufficient data	Spencer and Schaumburg (2000)
Dimethylaminopropionitrile	Peripheral neuropathy, urinary retention	Axonal degeneration (both myelinated and unmyelinated axons)	Spencer and Schaumburg (2000)
Ethylene oxide	Peripheral neuropathy	Axonal degeneration	Graham and Lantos (1997)
Glutethimide	Peripheral neuropathy (predominantly sensory)	Insufficient data	Spencer and Schaumburg (2000)
Gold	Peripheral neuopathy (may have psychiatric problems)	Axonal degeneration, some segmental demyelination	Graham and Lantos (1997), Spencer and Schaumburg (2000)
n-Hexane	Peripheral neuropathy, severe cases have spasticity	Axonal degeneration, early neurofilamentous swelling, PNS and spinal cord	Graham and Lantos (1997), Spencer and Schaumburg (2000)
Hydralazine	Peripheral neuropathy	Insufficient data	Spencer and Schaumburg (2000)
β,β′-Iminodipropionitrile	No data in humans; excitatory movement disorder (rats)	Proximal axonal swellings, degeneration of olfactory epithelial cells, vestibular hair cells	Graham and Lantos (1997)
Isoniazid	Peripheral neuropathy (sensory), ataxia (high doses)	Axonal degeneration	Graham and Lantos (1997), Spencer and Schaumburg (2000)
Lithium	Lethargy, tremor, ataxia (reversible)	Insufficient data	Spencer and Schaumburg (2000)
Methyl n-butyl ketone	Peripheral neuropathy	Axonal degeneration, early neurofilamentous swelling, PNS and spinal cord	Graham and Lantos (1997), Spencer and Schaumburg (2000)
Metronidazole	Sensory peripheral neuropathy, ataxia, seizures	Axonal degeneration, mostly affecting myelinated fibers; lesions of cerebellar nuclei	Graham and Lantos (1997), Spencer and Schaumburg (2000)
Misonidazole	Peripheral neuropathy	Axonal degeneration	Graham and Lantos (1997), Spencer and Schaumburg (2000)

(continued)

Table 16-2

(Continued)

NEUROTOXICANT	NEUROLOGICAL FINDINGS	BASIS OF NEUROTOXICITY	REFERENCES
Nitrofurantoin	Peripheral neuropathy	Axonal degeneration	Spencer and Schaumburg (2000)
Organophosphorous compounds (neurotoxic esterase inhibitors)	abdominal pain (acute); Peripheral neuropathy	Axonal degeneration	Chang and Dyer (1995), Graham and Lantos (1997), Spencer and Schaumburg (2000)
Paclitaxel (taxoids)	Delayed peripheral neuropathy (motor), spasticity	Axonal degeneration (delayed after single exposure), PNS and spinal cord	Chang and Dyer (1995), Graham and Lantos (1997), Spencer and Schaumburg (2000), Abou-Donia (1993)
Platinum (cisplatin)	Peripheral neuropathy	Axonal degeneration; microtubule accumulation in early stages	Graham and Lantos (1997), Spencer and Schaumburg (2000)
Pyridinethione (pyrithione)	Movement disorders (tremor, choreoathetosis)	Axonal degeneration (variable)	Chang and Dyer (1995), Spencer and Schaumburg (2000)
Vincristine (vinca alkaloids)	Cranial (most often trigeminal) neuropathy Peripheral neuropathy, variable autonomic symptoms	Insufficient data Axonal degeneration (PNS), neurofibrillary changes (spinalcord, intrathecal route)	Spencer and Schaumburg (2000) Graham and Lantos (1997), Spencer and Schaumburg (2000)

however, a depletion of tubulin subunits has been reported, and is a likely contributor to the overall neuropathological picture (LoPachin *et al.*, 2005).

The dimethyl analog of HD, 3,4-dimethyl-2,5-hexanedione (DMHD), produces a similar neuropathy. However, due to the methyl groups, DMHD forms the cyclic adduct much more rapidly than HD, forming pyrrole adducts that oxidize and lead to cross-linking faster than HD. The faster rate of adduct formation results in DMHD producing proximal axonal swellings similar to those seen with β,β′-iminodipropionitrile (IDPN) (Anthony *et al.*, 1983).

Carbon Disulfide The most significant exposures of humans to CS_2 have occurred in the vulcan rubber and viscose rayon industries. Manic psychoses were observed in the former setting and were correlated with very high levels of exposure (Seppaleinen and Haltia, 1980). In recent decades, interest in the human health effects has been focused on the NS and the cardiovascular system, where injury has been documented in workers exposed to much higher levels than those that are allowed today.

What is clearly established is the capacity of CS_2 to cause a distal axonopathy that is identical pathologically to that caused by *n*-hexane. There is growing evidence that covalent cross-linking of neurofilaments also underlies CS_2 neuropathy through a series of reactions that parallel the sequence of events in *n*-hexane neuropathy. Although *n*-hexane requires metabolism to 2,5-hexanedione, CS_2 is itself the ultimate toxicant, reacting with protein amino groups to form dithiocarbamate adducts (Lam and DiStefano, 1986). The dithiocarbamate adducts of lysyl amino groups undergo decomposition to isothiocyanate adducts, electrophiles that then react with protein nucleophiles to yield covalent cross-linking (Fig. 16-4). The reaction of the isothiocyanate adducts with cysteinyl sulfhydryls to form *N,S*-dialkyldithiocarbamate ester cross-links is reversible, whereas the reaction with protein amino functions forms thiourea cross-links irreversibly. Over time, the thiourea cross-links predominate and are most likely the most biologically significant (Amarnath *et al.*, 1991; Valentine *et al.*, 1992, 1995; Graham *et al.*, 1995).

As with hexane neuropathy, it has been postulated that the stability and long transport distance of the neurofilament determine that this protein is the toxicologically relevant target in chronic CS_2 intoxication. Nonetheless, proteins throughout the organism are derivatized and cross-linked as well. Cross-linking has been identified in erythrocyte-associated proteins including spectrin and globin as well as in the putative neurotoxic target neurofilament subunits (Valentine *et al.*, 1993, 1997). Analysis of cross-linking in erythrocyte proteins has verified that cross-linking occurs through thiourea bridges that accumulate with continuing exposure (Erve *et al.*, 1998a,b). Neurofilament cross-linking involves all three subunits and also demonstrates a cumulative dose–response and temporal relationship consistent with a contributing event in the development of the axonal neurofilamentous swellings. The correlation of protein cross-linking in erythrocyte proteins and axonal proteins together with the ability to detect covalent modifications on peripheral proteins at subneurotoxic levels and at preneurotoxic time points suggests that modifications on peripheral proteins can be used as biomarkers of effect for CS_2 exposure. These biomarkers, together with morphological changes, have been used to establish CS_2 as the ultimate neurotoxic species in the peripheral neuropathy produced by oral administration of *N,N*-diethyldithiocarbamate (Johnson *et al.*, 1998).

The clinical effects of exposure to CS_2 in the chronic setting are very similar to those of hexane exposure, with the development of sensory and motor symptoms occurring initially in a stocking-and-glove distribution. In addition to this chronic axonopathy, CS_2 can also lead to aberrations in mood and signs of diffuse encephalopathic disease. Some of these are transient at first and subsequently become more long lasting, a feature that is common in vascular insufficiency in the NS. This fact, in combination with the knowledge that CS_2, may accelerate the process of atherosclerosis, suggests that some of the effects of CS_2 on the CNS are vascular in origin.

β,β′-Iminodipropionitrile IDPN is a synthetic, bifunctional nitrile that causes a "waltzing syndrome" in rats and other mammals, although human exposure has never been documented. Features of this "waltzing syndrome" include excitement, circling, head twitching, and overalertness, and are observed after a single large intraperitoneal injection to a rat (1.5–2.0 g/kg) (Chou and Hartmann, 1964). Although the cause of this behavior has not been

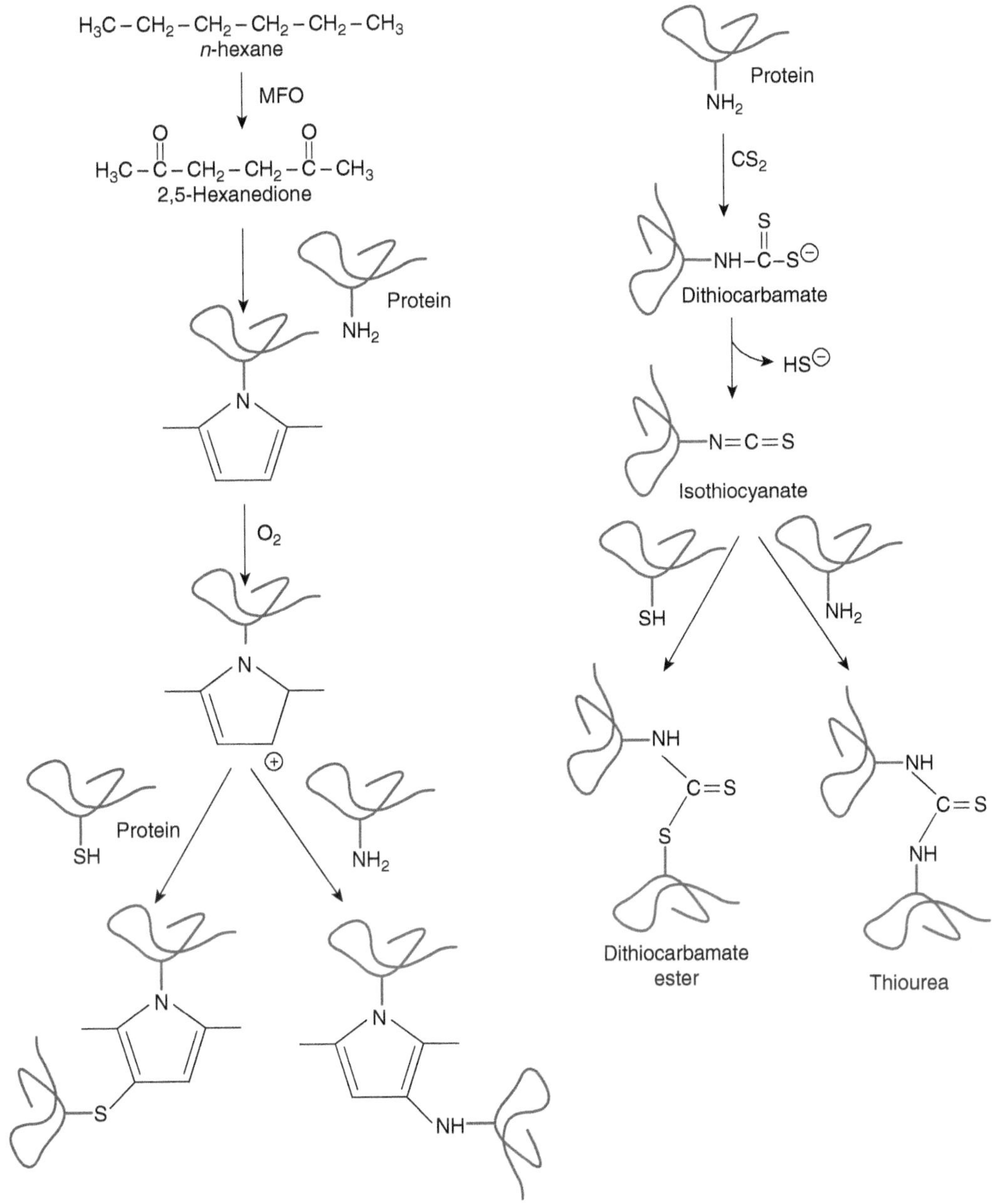

Figure 16-4. *Molecular mechanisms of protein cross-linking in the neurofilamentous neuropathies.* Both 2,5-hexanedione, produced from hexane via ω-1 oxidation function of mixed function oxidase (MFO), and CS2 are capable of cross-linking proteins. Pyrrole formation from 2,5-hexanedione is followed by oxidation and reaction with adjacent protein nucleophiles. Dithiocarbamate formation from CS2 is followed by formation of the protein-bound isothiocyanate and subsequent reaction with adjacent protein nucleophiles.

conclusively determined, it has been suggested that degeneration of vestibular sensory hair cells is responsible (Llorens *et al.*, 1993).

Pathological changes also follow administration of IDPN, most notably in large caliber axons, the primary target of neurotoxicity. The accumulation of neurofilaments in the proximal axon occurs, leading to swelling without degeneration in most animals (Gold, 2000). Quails deficient in neurofilaments demonstrate no swellings when administered IDPN, suggesting that the toxicity is due to a selective effect on neurofilaments (Mitsuishi *et al.*, 1993). These neurofilament swellings are similar to those observed in carbon disulfide or γ-diketones toxicity. Repeated exposure to IDPN leads to demyelination and onion bulb formation, and eventually can produce distal axonal atrophy due to a reduction in anterograde neurofilament transport to the distal axon (Clark *et al.*, 1980).

This impairment of axonal transport results from the disruption of the association between microtubules and neurofilaments by

IDPN, causing neurofilament accumulation (Griffin *et al.*, 1983). This leads to complete disturbance of the cytoskeleton of the axon. Although unclear, the mechanism responsible for this interference is hypothesized to result from the direct alteration of neurofilament proteins by IDPN, possibly by changing their chemical properties and causing aggregation (Anderson *et al.*, 1991).

Acrylamide Acrylamide is a man-made vinyl monomer used widely in water purification, paper manufacturing, mining, and waterproofing. It is also used extensively in biochemical laboratories, and is present in many foods prepared at high temperatures. Although it can be dangerous if not handled carefully, most toxic events in humans have been observed as peripheral neuropathies in factory workers exposed to high doses (Garland and Peterson, 1967; Kesson *et al.*, 1977; Collins *et al.*, 1989; Myers and Macun, 1991).

Early studies of acrylamide neuropathy revealed a distal axonopathy characterized by multiple axonal swellings (Spencer and Schaumburg, 1976). Although a single large dose is enough to produce toxicity, the process appears the same in multiple smaller doses, suggesting that acrylamide neurotoxicity is not due to an accumulation of the toxicant in the brain (Crofton *et al.*, 1996). Repeated dosing results in a more proximal axonopathy, in a "dying back" process. The first changes are seen in Pacinian corpuscles, followed by muscle spindles and the nerve terminal. These changes are caused by accumulations of neurofilaments at the nerve terminal. Paranodal swellings develop, leading to the retraction of myelin (Schaumburg *et al.*, 1974; Spencer and Schaumburg, 1974). A decrease in the number of synaptic vesicles and mitochondria at the nerve terminal is also characteristic, probably due to inhibition of retrograde and anterograde axonal transport (DeGrandchamp *et al.*, 1990; Padilla *et al.*, 1993; Harris *et al.*, 1994). It has also been observed that nerve terminal degeneration occurs prior to development of axonopathy, suggesting that this degeneration is the primary lesion (LoPachin *et al.*, 2002).

Many early studies investigating acrylamide neurotoxicity noted nerve terminal degeneration, but for three decades the distal axonopathy was believed to be the lesion responsible for neurological signs and symptoms (eg, ataxia and numbness in extremities). However, in more recent studies, neurological symptoms and nerve terminal degeneration were similarly observed in both short-term high-dose and long-term low-dose animals in the rat PNS, while axonal degeneration occurred only in low-dose studies subsequent to neurological alteration (LoPachin *et al.*, 2002).

Organophosphorus Compounds OP compounds are used not only as insecticides and chemical warfare agents, but also as chemical intermediates, flame retardants, fuel additives, hydraulic fluids, lubricants, pharmaceuticals, and plasticizers. The OP insecticides and nerve agents are designed to inhibit AChE, thereby causing accumulation of acetylcholine in cholinergic synapses resulting in cholinergic toxicity and death (Richardson, 2010; Thompson and Richardson, 2004). However, apart from the insecticides, nerve agents, and some of the pharmaceuticals, OP compounds produced for other applications often have little or no anti-AChE activity (Richardson, 2005).

Some OP compounds, such as tri-*o*-cresyl phosphate (TOCP), are neuropathic and can cause a severe sensorimotor central peripheral distal axonopathy called OP compound-induced delayed neurotoxicity (OPIDN) without inducing cholinergic poisoning. This condition is also referred to as a delayed neuropathy or delayed polyneuropathy (OPIDP) (Lotti and Moretto, 2005). However, *neuropathy* usually connotes peripheral nerve disease, whereas OPIDN also involves degeneration of ascending and descending spinal cord tracts (Richardson, 2005).

An OPIDN epidemic of massive proportions occurred during Prohibition in the United States, when Jamaica Ginger extract (Ginger Jake), a popular source of alcohol, was adulterated with TOCP. Another outbreak occurred in Morocco where olive oil was contaminated with TOCP. Human cases have also occurred after exposure to certain formerly used OP insecticides, such as EPN (*O*-ethyl-*O*-4-nitrophenyl phenylphosphonothioate) and leptophos [*O*-(4-bromo-2,5-dichlorophenyl)-*O*-methyl phenylphosphonothionate] (Lotti and Moretto, 2005).

Many OP compounds are lipophilic and readily enter the NS. If the parent compound or a metabolite has suitable reactivity, they can phosphorylate neural target proteins, such as various serine hydrolases (Casida and Quistad, 2005). When the principal target is AChE, cholinergic toxicity can ensue, either because

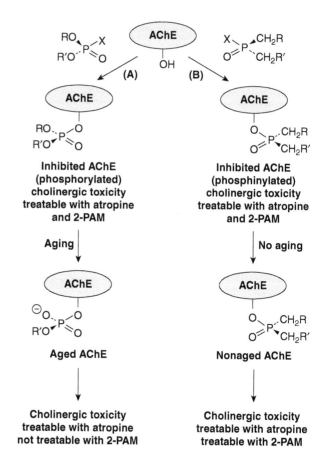

Figure 16-5. *AChE and cholinergic toxicity.* (**A**) Inhibition by an ageable organophosphate produces cholinergic toxicity, treatable with atropine and 2-PAM. Aging does not alter the type of toxicity, but it obviates 2-PAM therapy. (**B**) Inhibition by a nonageable phosphinate produces cholinergic toxicity, treatable with atropine and 2-PAM. R, R′: substituted or unsubstituted alkyl or aryl groups; X: primary leaving group displaced by the AChE active site serine.

of suprathreshold levels of inhibition or inhibition plus aging (Fig. 16-5). A substantial level of AChE inhibition on its own is sufficient to produce cholinergic toxicity and death. When *aging* of inhibited AChE also occurs (net loss of a ligand from the phosphorus of the OP-enzyme conjugate, leaving a negatively charged phosphoryl moiety attached to the active site), the qualitative nature of the toxicity does not change. Instead, the inhibited AChE becomes intractable to reactivation, rendering therapy with oximes, such as 2-pralidoxime methiodide (2-PAM) ineffective (Fig. 16-5) (Richardson, 2010; Thompson and Richardson, 2004).

When the principal target is neuropathy target esterase (neurotoxic esterase, NTE), OPIDN can result only if both suprathreshold (>70%) inhibition occurs *and* the inhibited enzyme undergoes aging. Thus, in the case of NTE and OPIDN, inhibition alone is insufficient to precipitate toxicity. It appears that the biochemical lesion is not simply a blockade of the active site. Instead, axonopathy is triggered by specific chemical modification of the NTE protein (Fig. 16-6). Neuropathic (aging) inhibitors of NTE include compounds from the phosphate, phosphonate, and phosphoramidate classes of OP compounds (Richardson, 1992; Kropp *et al.*, 2004; Wijeyesakere and Richardson, 2010) (Fig. 16-7).

Certain NTE inhibitors—including members of the phosphinate, carbamate, and sulfonylfluoride classes—do not age and do not cause OPIDN (Fig. 16-7). However, pretreatment with a nonaging NTE inhibitor prevents OPIDN from occurring after a challenge dose of a neuropathic (aging) NTE inhibitor. It has been

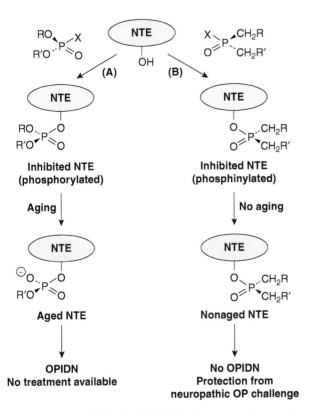

Figure 16-6. *NTE and OPIDN.* (**A**) Inhibition by an ageable organophosphate; rapid aging yields a negatively charged phosphoryl conjugate resulting in OPIDN. (**B**) Inhibition by a nonageable phosphinate does not produce OPIDN but provides protection against neuropathic (ageable) NTE inhibitors. R, R′: substituted or unsubstituted alkyl or aryl groups. X: primary leaving group displaced by the NTE active site serine.

proposed that these nonaging compounds protect against OPIDN by blocking the active site of NTE and preventing inhibition, and aging by a subsequent dose of an neuropathic (aging) inhibitor (Richardson, 2005) (Fig. 16-6).

In contrast, when protective NTE inhibitors are administered following exposure to a near-threshold subclinical dose of a neuropathic OP compound, OPIDN is fully expressed (Pope *et al.*, 1993). Because the initial treatment involves a compound that can produce OPIDN on its own and the disease is likely to be incipient rather than absent, this effect should be called *potentiation*; however, some authors refer to the phenomenon as *promotion* (Lotti, 2002). Although the potentiating agents inhibit NTE, this enzyme

is not thought to be the target of potentiation. The level of NTE inhibition produced by the potentiator is not related to the level of potentiation observed, and these potentiators appear to exacerbate axonopathies from other causes as well, such as trauma and 2,5-hexanedione exposure. These results have been interpreted to indicate that potentiation enhances progression of the axonopathic process, inhibits repair, or both (Lotti, 2002; Randall *et al.*, 1997).

Axonal degeneration does not commence immediately after acute exposure to a neuropathic OP compound but is delayed for at least eight days between the acute high-dose exposure and clinical signs of axonopathy. Some effective regeneration of axons occurs in the PNS, for example, excitatory inputs to skeletal muscle from lower motor neurons in the spinal cord. In contrast, axonal degeneration is progressive and persistent in long tracts of the spinal cord, for example, inhibitory pathways from upper motor neurons in the motor cortex to lower motor neurons in the spinal cord anterior horn. Accordingly, the clinical picture of OPIDN changes from flaccid to spastic paralysis during a course of months to years (Lotti and Moretto, 2005; Richardson, 2005).

Fortunately, studies of the initiation steps of OPIDN and structure–activity relationships of neuropathic OP compounds have led to highly accurate prediction of the neuropathic potential of these chemicals. Consequently, human cases of OPIDN are now rare and usually arise from intentional ingestion of massive doses of OP insecticides in suicide attempts. Nevertheless, the fact remains that OPIDN is a debilitating and incurable condition. Moreover, although the mechanism linking aged NTE to axonopathy is unknown, mutations affecting the catalytic domain of NTE produce motor neuron disease (Hein *et al.*, 2010; Rainier *et al.*, 2011). Accordingly, research continues in order to enhance mechanistic understanding that could be applied to improving biosensors and biomarkers of exposure, high-throughput testing of new compounds, prophylaxis and treatment for OPIDN, and understanding of motor neuron diseases (Richardson, 2005; Richardson *et al.*, 2009; Wijeyesakere and Richardson, 2010).

The foregoing discussion has been limited to organic compounds of pentacovalent phosphorus, which are by far the most common and best studied of the OP compounds. However, organic compounds of trivalent phosphorus, such as triphenylphosphine (TPPn) and triphenylphosphite (TPPi), have relatively widespread use, particularly as antioxidants, chemical intermediates, and polymer enhancers. Both TPPn and TPPi produce axonal degeneration in the CNS and PNS, but the spatial–temporal distributions of lesions are different from that of classical OPIDN produced by organic pentacovalent phosphorous compounds and the pathogenic

(A) Neuropathic (ageable)			
	Phosphate	Phosphonate	Phosphoramidate
(B) Nonneuropathic (nonageable) pretreatment: protection posttreatment: potentiation			
	Phosphinate	Sulfonate	Carbamate

Figure 16-7. *NTE inhibitors.* (**A**) Neuropathic (ageable). (**B**) Nonneuropathic (nonageable). R, R′: substituted or unsubstituted alkyl or aryl groups; X: primary leaving group displaced by the NTE active site serine.

mechanisms are unknown (Abou-Donia, 1992). In particular, it appears that the mechanism of initiation of axonopathy by TTPn is independent of NTE inhibition and aging (Davis *et al.*, 1999), and this relationship is unclear for TPPi (Padilla *et al.*, 1987; Richardson *et al.*, 2009).

Pyridinethione This compound is a chelating agent that is usually encountered as the zinc complex. Two molecules of pyridinethione are complexed with zinc to form bis[1-hydroxy-2(1*H*)-pyridine-thionato] zinc, commonly known as zinc pyridinethione or zinc pyrithione (ZPT) (Bond *et al.*, 2002; Lewis *et al.*, 2005).

ZPT is a biocide that has antibacterial and antifungal properties. It is the active ingredient in shampoos and other preparations for the treatment of seborrheic dermatitis and dandruff. ZPT is also used as an antifouling agent for ship paints, drywall, and tarps, and as an antibacterial agent for incorporation into cleaning sponges. Thus, the intended uses of ZPT can lead to human exposures through direct dermal contact and potential exposure to biota through leaching into marine and freshwater environments (Grunnet and Dahllof, 2005; Pierard-Franchimont *et al.*, 2002).

Because the compound is directly applied to the human scalp in antidandruff shampoos, the finding that ZPT produced limb weakness and peripheral neuropathy in rodents after oral administration raised concern about potential neurotoxicity in humans (Sahenk and Mendell, 1979). Rats, rabbits, and guinea pigs all develop a distal axonopathy when exposed to ZPT in the diet. Fortunately, however, dermal absorption of ZPT is minimal, and there have been no reports of neurological findings in humans attributable to occupational or consumer ZPT exposures (Sahenk and Mendell, 2000).

Although the zinc ion appears to be an important component of the therapeutic action of ZPT, only the pyridinethione moiety is absorbed following ingestion, with the majority of zinc eliminated in the feces. In addition, oral sodium pyridinethione is also neurotoxic, indicating that the pyridinethione moiety is responsible for the neurotoxicity. Pyridinethione chelates zinc, copper, and other metal ions and, once oxidized to the disulfide, may lead to the formation of protein–pyridinethione mixed disulfides. However, which of these properties, if any, is responsible for the molecular mechanism of its neurotoxicity remains unknown (Sahenk and Mendell, 2000).

Although these molecular issues remain to be resolved, pyridinethione appears to interfere with the fast axonal transport systems. Although the fast anterograde system is less affected, pyridinethione impairs the turnaround of rapidly transported vesicles and slows their retrograde transport (Sahenk and Mendell, 1980). This aberration of the fast axonal transport systems is the most likely physiological basis of the accumulation of tubulovesicular structures in the distal axon. As these materials accumulate in one region of the axon, they distend the axonal diameter, resulting in axonal swellings filled with membranous profiles. As in many other distal axonopathies, the axon degenerates in its more distal regions beyond the accumulated structures. The earliest signs are diminished grip strength and electrophysiological changes of the axon terminal, with normal conduction along the proximal axon in the early stages of exposure (Ross and Lawhorn, 1990).

Microtubule-Associated Neurotoxicity A number of plant alkaloids alter the assembly and depolymerization of microtubules in nerve axons, causing neurotoxicity. The oldest known of these are colchicine and the vinca alkaloids, which bind to tubulin and cause depolymerization of microtubules. Colchicine is an alkaloid pharmaceutical used in the treatment of gout, familial Mediterranean fever, and other disorders. A common side effect of treatment in patients with abnormal renal function is a peripheral axonal neuropathy. Although this neuropathy is generally mild, it

is often accompanied by a disabling myopathy that can lead to the inability to walk (Riggs *et al.*, 1986).

A number of vinca alkaloids, including vincristine and vinblastine—both chemotherapeutic agents—produce a peripheral axonopathy very similar to that induced by colchicine. Vincristine is commonly used to treat leukemias and lymphomas, and also has greater potential for adverse toxic effects than vinblastine. The chemical binds to tubulin subunits and prevents the polymerization into microtubules (Prakash and Timasheff, 1992). Nearly all evidence of vincristine-induced neuropathy has been observed in humans. Most treated patients develop neurotoxicity to some extent, beginning with parasthesias of the fingers. General weakness and clumsiness is common, but this improves quickly with removal of treatment. Parasthesias may persist, however, and some distal sensory loss may be permanent (Schaumburg, 2000).

More recently paclitaxel (Taxol), another plant alkaloid, has become a popular chemotherapeutic drug used to treat a variety of neoplasms. However, side effects include a predominantly sensory neuropathy, beginning in the hands and feet (Sahenk *et al.*, 1994). Like colchicine and the vinca alkaloids, paclitaxel binds to tubulin; however, instead of leading to depolymerization, it promotes the formation of microtubules. Once formed, these microtubules remain stabilized by paclitaxel even in conditions that normally lead to dissociation of tubulin subunits, including cold temperatures or the presence of calcium (Schiff and Horowitz, 1981). When paclitaxel is injected directly into the sciatic nerve of rats, microtubules aggregate along the axon, causing demyelination, axonal degeneration, and impairment of regeneration (Lipton *et al.*, 1989; Mielke *et al.*, 2006).

The pathologies of the axon induced by these drugs are different. Although colchicine leads to atrophy of the axon and a decrease in the number of microtubules, paclitaxel causes the aggregation to form a matrix that may inhibit fast axonal transport, which has been demonstrated with both colchicine and paclitaxel. A change in the number of microtubules has been observed in some reports and absent from others (Roytta *et al.*, 1984; Nakata and Yorifuji, 1999). Although the mechanisms may differ slightly, both exposures result in a peripheral neuropathy that must be taken into account in medical treatments.

Myelinopathies

Myelin provides electrical insulation of neuronal processes, and its absence leads to a slowing of and/or aberrant conduction of impulses between adjacent processes, so-called ephaptic transmission. Toxicants exist that result in the separation of the myelin lamellae, termed *intramyelinic edema*, and in the selective loss of myelin, termed *demyelination*. Intramyelinic edema may be caused by alterations in the transcript levels of myelin basic protein-mRNA (Veronesi *et al.*, 1991) and early in its evolution is reversible. However, the initial stages may progress to demyelination, with loss of myelin from the axon. Demyelination may also result from direct toxicity to the myelinating cell. Remyelination in the CNS occurs to only a limited extent after demyelination. However, Schwann cells in the PNS are capable of remyelinating the axon after a demyelinating injury. Interestingly, remyelination after segmental demyelination in peripheral nerve involves multiple Schwann cells and results, therefore, in internodal lengths (the distances between adjacent nodes of Ranvier) that are much shorter than normal and a permanent record of the demyelinating event.

The compounds in Table 16-3 all lead to a myelinopathy. Some of these compounds have created problems in humans, and many have been used as tools to explore the process of myelination of the NS and the process of remyelination following toxic disruption of

Table 16-3

Compounds Associated with Injury of Myelin (Myelinopathies)

NEUROTOXICANT	NEUROLOGICAL FINDINGS	BASIS OF NEUROTOXICITY	REFERENCES
Acetylethyltetramethyl tetralin (AETT)	Not reported in humans; hyperexcitability, tremors (rats)	Intramyelinic edema; pigment accumulation in neurons	Graham and Lantos (1997), Spencer and Schaumburg (2000)
Amiodarone	Peripheral neuropathy	Axonal degeneration and demyelination; lipid-laden lysosomes in Schwann cells	Graham and Lantos (1997), Spencer and Schaumburg (2000)
Cuprizone	Not reported in humans; encephalopathy (experimental animals)	Status spongiosis of white matter, intramyelinic edema (early stages); gliosis (late)	Graham and Lantos (1997), Spencer and Schaumburg (2000)
Disulfiram	Peripheral neuropathy, predominantly sensory	Axonal degeneration, swellings in distal axons	Graham and Lantos (1997)
Ethidium bromide	Insufficient data (humans)	Intramyelinic edema, status spongiosis of white matter	Spencer and Schaumburg (2000)
Hexachlorophene	Irritability, confusion, seizures	Brain swelling, intramyelinic edema in CNS and PNS, late axonal degeneration	Graham and Lantos (1997), Spencer and Schaumburg (2000)
Lysolecithin	Effects only on direct injection into PNS or CNS (experimental animals)	Selective demyelination	Graham and Lantos (1997)
Perhexilene	Peripheral neuropathy	Demyelinating neuropathy, membrane-bound inclusions in Schwann cells	Graham and Lantos (1997), Spencer and Schaumburg (2000)
Tellurium	Hydrocephalus, hind-limb paralysis (experimental animals)	Demyelinating neuropathy, lipofuscinosis (experimental animals)	Graham and Lantos (1997)
Triethyltin	Headache, photophobia, vomiting, paraplegia (irreversible)	Brain swelling (acute) with intramyelinic edema, spongiosis of white matter	Chang and Dyer (1995), Graham and Lantos (1997), Spencer and Schaumburg (2000)

myelin. In general, the functional consequences of demyelination depend on the extent of the demyelination and whether it is localized within the CNS or the PNS or is more diffuse in its distribution. Those toxic myelinopathies in which the disruption of myelin is diffuse generate a global neurological deficit, whereas those that are limited to the PNS produce the symptoms of peripheral neuropathy.

Hexachlorophene Hexachlorophene, or methylene 2,2′-methylenebis(3,4,6-trichlorophenol), resulted in human neurotoxicity when newborn infants, particularly premature infants, were bathed with the compound to avoid staphylococcal skin infections (Mullick, 1973). Following skin absorption of this hydrophobic compound, hexachlorophene enters the NS and results in intramyelinic edema, splitting the intraperiod line of myelin in both the CNS and the PNS. The intramyelinic edema leads to the formation of vacuoles, creating a "spongiosis" of the brain (Purves *et al.*, 1991). Experimental studies with erythrocyte membranes show that hexachlorophene binds tightly to cell membranes, resulting in the loss of ion gradients across the membrane (Flores and Buhler, 1974). This loss of the ability to exclude ions from between the layers of myelin leads to water and ion entry, which separates the myelin layers as "edema." Another, perhaps related, effect is the uncoupling of mitochondrial oxidative phosphorylation by hexachlorophene (Cammer and Moore, 1972) because this process is dependent on a proton gradient. Intramyelinic edema is reversible in the early stages, but with increasing exposure, hexachlorophene

causes segmental demyelination. Swelling of the brain causes increased intracranial pressure, which may be fatal. With high-dose exposure, axonal degeneration is seen, along with degeneration of photoreceptors in the retina. It has been postulated that the pressure from severe intramyelinic edema may also injure the axon, leading to axonal degeneration; endoneurial pressure measurements support this idea (Myers *et al.*, 1982). The toxicity of hexachlorophene expresses itself functionally in diffuse terms that reflect the diffuse process of myelin injury. Humans exposed acutely to hexachlorophene may have generalized weakness, confusion, and seizures. Progression may occur, to include coma and death.

Tellurium Although human exposures have not been reported, neurotoxicity of tellurium has been demonstrated in animals. Young rats exposed to tellurium in their diet develop a severe peripheral neuropathy. Within the first two days of dietary exposure, the synthesis of myelin lipids in Schwann cells displays striking changes (Harry *et al.*, 1989). These include decreased synthesis of cholesterol and cerebrosides (lipids richly represented in myelin), and downregulated myelin protein mRNA (Morell *et al.*, 1994). On the contrary, the synthesis of phosphatidylcholine, a more ubiquitous membrane lipid, is unaffected. The synthesis of free fatty acids and cholesterol esters increases to some degree, and there is a marked elevation of squalene, a precursor of cholesterol. These biochemical findings demonstrate a variety of lipid abnormalities, and the simultaneous increase in squalene and decrease in cholesterol suggests that tellurium or one of its derivatives may interfere with the normal conversion of squalene to cholesterol. Squalene epoxidase, a microsomal monooxygenase that utilizes NAPDH cytochrome P450 reductase, has been strongly implicated as the target of tellurium, because its inhibition by tellurium as well as certain other oranotellurium compounds shows a correlation between the potency of enzyme inhibition and demyelination in vivo (Goodrum, 1998).

In conjunction with these biochemical changes, lipids accumulate in Schwann cells within intracytoplasmic vacuoles; shortly afterward, these Schwann cells lose their ability to maintain myelin. Axons and the myelin of the CNS are impervious to the effects of tellurium. However, individual Schwann cells in the PNS disassemble their concentric layers of myelin membranes, depriving the adjacent intact axon of its electrically insulated status. Not all Schwann cells are equally affected by the process; rather, those Schwann cells that encompass the greatest distances appear to be the most affected. These cells are associated with the largest-diameter axons, encompass the longest intervals of myelination, and provide the thickest layers of myelin. Thus, it appears that the most vulnerable cells are those with the largest volume of myelin to support (Bouldin et al., 1988).

As the process of remyelination begins, several cells cooperate to reproduce the myelin layers that were previously formed by a single Schwann cell. Perhaps this diminished demand placed upon an individual cell is the reason that remyelination occurs even in the presence of continued exposure to tellurium (Bouldin et al., 1988). The expression of the neurological impairment is also short in duration, reflecting the transient cellular and biochemical events. The animals initially develop severe weakness in the hind limbs but then recover their strength after two weeks on the tellurium-laden diet.

Lead Lead exposure in animals results in a peripheral neuropathy with prominent segmental demyelination, a process that bears a strong resemblance to tellurium toxicity (Dyck et al., 1977). However, the neurotoxicity of lead is much more variable in humans than in rats, and there are also a variety of manifestations of lead toxicity in other organ systems.

The neurotoxicity of lead has been appreciated for centuries. In current times, adults are exposed to lead in occupational settings through lead smelting processes and soldering and in domestic settings through lead pipes or through the consumption of "moonshine" contaminated with lead. In addition, some areas contain higher levels of environmental lead, resulting in higher blood levels in the inhabitants. Children, especially those below five years of age, have higher blood levels of lead than adults in the same environment, due to the mouthing of objects and the consumption of substances other than food. In addition, children absorb lead more readily, and the very young do not have the protection of the blood–brain barrier. The most common acute exposure in children, however, has been through the consumption of paint chips containing lead pigments (Perlstein and Attala, 1966), a finding that has led to public efforts to prevent the use of lead paints in homes with children.

In young children, acute massive exposures to lead result in severe cerebral edema, perhaps from damage to endothelial cells. Children seem to be more susceptible to this lead encephalopathy than adults (Johnston and Goldstein, 1998); however, adults may also develop an acute encephalopathy in the setting of massive lead exposure.

Chronic lead intoxication in adults results in peripheral neuropathy, often accompanied by manifestations outside the NS, such as gastritis, colicky abdominal pain, anemia, and the prominent deposition of lead in particular anatomic sites, creating lead lines in the gums and in the epiphyses of long bones in children. The

effects of lead on the peripheral nerve of humans (lead neuropathy) are not entirely understood. Electrophysiological studies have demonstrated a slowing of nerve conduction. Although this observation is consistent with the segmental demyelination that develops in experimental animals, pathological studies in humans with lead neuropathy typically have demonstrated an axonopathy. Another finding in humans is the predominant involvement of motor axons, creating one of the few clinical situations in which patients present with predominantly motor symptoms. The basis for the effect on the brain (lead encephalopathy) is also unclear, although an effect on the membrane structure of myelin and myelin membrane fluidity has been shown (Dabrowski-Bouta et al., 1999). The etiologies associated with the pathogenesis of peripheral neuropathy are, like that of central neuropathy, rather speculative. One hypothesis postulates that the effects of lead on the blood–nerve barrier are similar to those on the blood–brain barrier, providing a unitary mechanism for lead's effects on both the PNS and CNS. Another theory on the mechanisms associated with lead-induced effects on the PNS suggests a toxic effect on Schwann cells, and the ensuing demyelination of nerves (Powell et al., 1982). Although the manifestations of acute and chronic exposures to lead have been long established, the effects of low-level exposures on infants and children have become realized. Initial reports noted a relationship between mild elevations of blood lead in children and school performance; more recently, correlations between elevated lead levels in decidual teeth and performance on tests of verbal abilities, attention, and behavior (nonadaptive) have been demonstrated (Needleman and Gatsonis, 1990; Needleman, 1994). Although there is a clear association between lead level and intellectual performance, there has been some discussion as to whether lead is causal. Children with higher blood levels tend to share certain other environmental factors, such as socioeconomic status and parental educational level. However, in spite of these complex social factors, it appears that lead exposure has an adverse effect on the intellectual abilities of children (Needleman, 1994), although a threshold for these effects has not yet been determined.

Astrocytes

Rather than being the passive glue described by Virchow and other pathologists, astrocytes are now known to perform and regulate a wide range of physiological functions in the CNS. Perturbations in the function of these important cells are frequently reflected in abnormal neuronal physiology, even in the absence of altered nerve cell morphology. Indeed, the astrocyte appears to be a primary means of defense in the CNS following exposure to neurotoxicants, as a spatial buffering system for osmotically active ions and as a depot for the sequestration and metabolic processing of endogenous molecules and xenobiotics. Although in its relative infancy, investigations into the role of astrocytes in normal/abnormal function of the NS will be crucial to a better understanding of neurotoxicity and its pathological sequelae.

Ammonia Hepatic encephalopathy (HE) and congenital and acquired hyperammonemia lead to excessive brain ammonia (ammonium, NH_4^+) accumulation. The condition results from liver failure. The effects of ammonia on the CNS vary with its concentration. At high CNS concentrations ammonia produces seizures, resulting from its depolarizing action on cell membranes, whereas, at lower concentrations, ammonia produces stupor and coma, consistent with its hyperpolarizing effects. Ammonia intoxication is associated with astrocytic swelling and morphological changes, yielding the so-called Alzheimer type II astrocytes, which precede any other morphological change (Mossakowski et al., 1970). The exclusive site for brain detoxification of glutamate to glutamine occurs within the astrocytes. This process requires ATP-dependent amidation of glutamate to glutamine, and it is mediated by the astrocyte-specific enzyme, glutamine synthetase (GS) and catalyzed by ammonia. Increased intracellular ammonia concentrations have also been implicated in the inhibition of neuronal glutamate precursor synthesis, resulting in diminished glutamatergic neurotransmission, changes in neurotransmitter uptake (glutamate), and changes in receptor-mediated metabolic responses of astrocytes to neuronal signals (Albrecht, 1996).

Nitrochemicals The therapeutic potential of organic nitrates has been recognized for more than a century and began with the use of nitroglycerine for the management of acute anginal episodes. The resulting peripheral vasodilation and reduction in blood pressure, while useful in treating cardiovascular disease, have recently been shown to be only one of the pharmacological properties of this class of chemical. The mitochondrion features prominently as a target for nitrochemicals; however, the causal relationship between mitochondrial dysfunction and initiation of the neurotoxic state remains to be established for many of the chemicals.

The dinitrobenzenes are important synthetic intermediates in the industrial production of dyes, plastics, and explosives. The neurotoxic compound, 1,3-dinitrobenzene (DNB), produces gliovascular lesions that specifically target astrocytes in the periaqueductal gray matter of the brainstem and deep cerebellar roof nuclei (Philbert et al., 1987). Although the molecular basis for the remarkable sensitivity of this cell population is unclear, it has been proposed that bioactivation of DNB by NADPH-dependent cytochrome c reductase (Hu et al., 1997; Romero et al., 1991) and subsequent induction of oxidative stress underlies its toxicity (Romero et al., 1995; Ray et al., 1992, 1994; Hu et al., 1999). Brainstem nuclei with high glucose requirements, such as the vestibular and deep cerebellar roof nuclei, are affected more severely than forebrain and mesencephalic structures that have similar or higher requirements for glucose and oxygen (Calingasan et al., 1994; Bagley et al., 1989; Mastrogiacomo et al., 1993). The molecular basis of the susceptibility of brainstem astrocytes is unknown but growing evidence suggests that differences in mitochondrial respiratory capacity, cellular antioxidant levels, and the expression of proteins that regulate the mitochondrial permeability transition pore (mtPTP) all contribute to the observed regional and cellular differences in susceptibility. In vitro studies indicate that DNB is a potent inducer of the mtPTP (for reviews of the mtPTP see Lemasters et al., 1998; Crompton, 1999) in cultured C6 glioma cells (Tjalkens et al., 2000). Mitochondrial inner membrane permeabilization in an in vitro model of DNB exposure is dependent on generation of ROS, in agreement with the reported capacity of DNB to deplete reduced pyridine nucleotides and GSH due to redox-cycling (Romero et al., 1995).

Metronidazole, a 5-nitroimidazole [1-(2-hydroxyethyl)-2-methyl-5-nitroimidazole], is an antimicrobial, antiprotozoal agent that is commonly used for the treatment of a wide variety of infections. Prolonged treatment with metronidazole is associated with a peripheral neuropathy characterized by paraesthesias, dysaesthesias, headaches, glossitis, urticaria, and pruritus in addition to other somatosensory disorders. Long-term administration of metronidazole produces an irreversible sensorimotor deficit in the lower extremities of humans (Kapoor et al., 1999). Metronidazole is readily reduced to the highly reactive and toxic hydroxylamine intermediate and binds to cellular macromolecules including proteins and DNA (Coxon and Pallis, 1976). Use of higher intravenous doses of metronidazole for extended periods results in the expression of epileptiform seizures, hallucination, and attendant encephalopathy. The distribution of lesions is similar to preceding descriptions for

DNB with the exception that both neurons and glia appear to be equally susceptible to the effects of metronidazole (Schentag, 1982). The mechanism of toxicity is well linked to the fact that metronidazole and its reduced metabolites bear close structural resemblance to the antineuritic nutrient, thiamine. Thiamine triphosphate (Vitamin B1) is an essential coenzyme in the mitochondrial metabolism of α-ketoglutarate, pyruvate, and also modulates the activity of sodium channels. Given the similarity in the lesions produced by metronidazole and pyrithiamine, a common antimetabolite mode of action has been proposed as the primary mechanism of neurotoxicity (Evans et al., 1975; Watanabe and Kanabe, 1978; Kapoor et al., 1999).

Methionine Sulfoximine Methionine sulfoximine (MSO) is an irreversible inhibitor of the astrocyte-specific enzyme, GS (Albrecht and Norenberg, 1990). Ingestion of large amounts of MSO leads to neuronal cell loss in the hippocampal fascia dentata and pyramidal cell layer, in the short association fibers and lower layers of the cerebral cortex, and in cerebellar Purkinje cells. MSO also leads to large increases of glycogen levels (Folbergrova, 1973), primarily within astrocytic cell bodies (Phelps, 1975), as well as swollen and damaged astrocytic mitochondria (Hevor, 1994). Although it is generally accepted that MSO inhibits GS, it remains unclear whether this inhibition represents the primary mechanism of MSO neurotoxicity. The relationship between inhibition of GS by MSO and seizure generation is also not well understood but is believed to be associated with inhibition of glutamate and GABA in seizure generation, since glutamine provides the precursor for these neurotransmitters. Rothstein and Tabakoff (1986) have demonstrated that the calcium-dependent, potassium-stimulated release of glutamate and aspartate is inhibited in striatal tissue after intracerebroventricular injection of MSO, and that their release correlates over time with the inhibition of GS.

Fluroacetate and Fluorocitrate The Krebs cycle inhibitor fluorocitrate (FC) and its precursor fluoroacetate (FA) are preferentially taken up by glia. FA occurs naturally in a number of plants, and is available commercially as a rodenticide (Compound, 1080). It is prevalent in the South African plant *Dichapetalum cymosum*, commonly referred to as the Gifblaar plant. Exposure to FA may also occur via exposure to the anti-cancer drug 5-fluorouracil (Okeda et al., 1990). Ingestion of large amounts of FA results in ionic convulsions. Animals consuming FA commonly seize within minutes, and those surviving these episodes frequently die later on due to respiratory arrest or heart failure. The actions of FC and FA have been attributed both to the disruption of carbon flux through the Krebs cycle and to impairment of ATP production (Swanson and Graham, 1994). FA can be metabolized to fluoroacetyl CoA, followed by condensation with oxaloacetate to form FC by citrate synthase. A second hypothesis implies that FA toxicity is associated with the inhibition of a bidirectional citrate carrier in mitochondrial membranes, which leads to elevated intramitochondrial citrate and could affect citrate-dependent ATP synthesis (Kirsten et al., 1978). Finally, it has been suggested that elevated citrate, secondary to inhibition of aconitase, is associated with the cytotoxicity of these compounds. FA selectively lowers the level of glutamine and inhibits glutamine formation in the brain, not by depleting glial cells of ATP, but by causing a rerouting of 2-oxoglutarate from glutamine synthesis into the TCA cycle during inhibition of aconitase (Hassel et al., 1994). After the inhibition of aconitase, citrate accumulates, whereas the levels of isocitrate and α-ketoglutarate decrease. The reversible enzyme glutamate dehydrogenase begins to work in the opposite direction feeding more α-ketoglutarate into the TCA cycle (Martin and Waniewski, 1996).

Neurotransmission-Associated Neurotoxicity

A wide variety of naturally occurring toxins, as well as synthetic chemicals, alter specific mechanisms of intercellular communication. Some chemicals that have neurotransmitter-associated toxicity are listed in Table 16-4.

Although neurotransmitter-associated actions may be well understood for some agents, the specificity of the mechanisms should not be assumed. OP and carbamate pesticides produce their insecticidal actions by inhibiting AChE, the catalytic enzyme that ends the postsynaptic action of acetylcholine. The resultant cholinergic overstimulation produces signs of acute toxicity ranging from flu-like symptoms to gastrointestinal distress, ataxia, twitching, convulsions, coma, and death. These effects are not as well-correlated with AChE inhibition as might be expected for all such pesticides, leading to suggestions of additional mechanisms of actions that have since been verified in animal and in vitro studies. These include direct actions on pre- and postsynaptic cholinergic receptors and altered reuptake of choline; such actions serve to modulate the downstream impact of cholinergic overstimulation (reviewed in Pope, 1999). Thus, multiple neurotransmitter targets may be more common than was once expected.

Nicotine Widely available in tobacco products and in certain pesticides, nicotine has diverse pharmacological actions and may be the source of considerable toxicity. These toxic effects range from acute poisoning to more chronic effects. Nicotine exerts its effects by binding to a subset of cholinergic receptors, the nicotinic receptors. These receptors are located in ganglia, at the neuromuscular

Table 16-4

Compounds Associated with Neurotransmitter-Associated Toxicity

NEUROTOXICANT	NEUROLOGICAL FINDINGS	BASIS OF NEUROTOXICITY	REFERENCES
Amphetamine and methamphetamine	Tremor, restlessness (acute); cerebral infarction and hemorrhage; neuropsychiatric disturbances	Bilateral infarcts of globus pallidus, abnormalities in dopaminergic, serotonergic, cholinergic systems; Acts at adrenergic receptors	Spencer and Schaumburg (2000), Hardman et al. (1996)
Atropine	Restlessness, irritability, hallucinations	Block cholinergic receptors (anticholinergic)	Spencer and Schaumburg (2000), Hardman et al. (1996)
Cocaine	Increased risk of stroke and cerebral atrophy (chronic users); increased risk of sudden cardiac death; movement and psychiatric abnormalities, especially during withdrawal
Decreased head circumference (fetal exposure)	Infarcts and hemorrhages; alteration in striatal dopamine neurotransmission
Structural malformations in newborns	Spencer and Schaumburg (2000), Hardman et al. (1996)
Domoic acid	Headache, memory loss, hemiparesis, disorientation, seizures	Neuronal loss, hippocampus and amygdala, layers 5 and 6 of neocortex
Kainate-like pattern of excitotoxicity	Graham and Lantos (1997), Spencer and Schaumburg (2000)
Kainate	Insufficient data in humans; seizures in animals (selective lesioning compound in neuroscience)	Degeneration of neurons in hippocampus, olfactory cortex, amygdala, thalamus
Binds α-amino-3-hydroxy-5-methylisoxazole-4-propionic acid (AMPA)/kainate receptors	Graham and Lantos (1997)
β-N-Methylamino-L-alanine (BMAA)	Weakness, movement disorder (monkeys)	Degenerative changes in motor neurons (monkeys)
Excitotoxic probably via N-methyl-D-aspartate receptors	Graham and Lantos (1997), Spencer and Schaumburg (2000)
Muscarine (mushrooms)	Nausea, vomiting, headache	Binds muscarinic receptors (cholinergic)	Hardman et al. (1996)
Nicotine	Nausea, vomiting, convulsions	Binds nicotinic receptors (cholinergic) low-dose stimulation; high-dose blocking	Spencer and Schaumburg (2000), Hardman et al. (1996)
β-N-Oxalylamino-L-alanine (BOAA)	Seizures	Excitotoxic probably via AMPA class of glutamate receptors	Graham and Lantos (1997), Spencer and Schaumburg (2000)

junction, and also within the CNS, where the psychoactive and addictive properties most likely reside. Smoking and "pharmacological" doses of nicotine accelerate heart rate, elevate blood pressure, and constrict blood vessels within the skin. Because the majority of these effects may be prevented by the administration of α- and β-adrenergic blockade, these consequences may be viewed as the result of stimulation of the ganglionic sympathetic NS (Benowitz, 1986). At the same time, nicotine leads to a sensation of "relaxation" and is associated with alterations of electroencephalographic (EEG) recordings in humans. These effects are probably related to the binding of nicotine with nicotinic receptors within the CNS, and the EEG changes may be blocked with mecamylamine, a nicotinic antagonist.

Acute overdose of nicotine has occurred in children who accidentally ingest tobacco products, in tobacco workers exposed to wet tobacco leaves (Gehlbach et al., 1974), and in workers exposed to nicotine-containing pesticides. In each of these settings, the rapid rise in circulating levels of nicotine leads to excessive stimulation of nicotinic receptors, a process that is followed rapidly by ganglionic paralysis. Initial nausea, rapid heart rate, and perspiration are followed shortly by marked slowing of heart rate with a fall in blood pressure. Somnolence and confusion may occur, followed by coma; if death results, it is often the result of paralysis of the muscles of respiration.

Such acute poisoning with nicotine fortunately is uncommon. Exposure to lower levels for longer duration, in contrast, is very common, and the health effects of this exposure are of considerable epidemiological concern. In humans, however, it has been difficult to separate the effects of nicotine from those of other components of cigarette smoke. The complications of smoking include cardiovascular disease, cancers (especially malignancies of the lung and upper airway), chronic pulmonary disease, and attention deficit disorders in children of women who smoke during pregnancy. Nicotine may be a factor in some of these problems. For example, an increased propensity for platelets to aggregate is seen in smokers, and this platelet abnormality correlates with the level of nicotine. Nicotine also places an increased burden on the heart through its acceleration of heart rate and blood pressure, suggesting that nicotine may play a role in the onset of myocardial ischemia (Benowitz, 1986). In addition, nicotine also inhibits apoptosis and may play a direct role in tumor promotion and tobacco-related cancers (Wright et al., 1993).

Cocaine and Amphetamines Although nicotine is a legal and readily available addictive compound, cocaine and amphetamines are illegal, though still widely used. The number of adults using these drugs in the United States was approximately nine million in 1972. This number grew to near 33 million in 1982, and in the 2001 National Household Survey on Drug Abuse it was reported that just over 10% of those surveyed had ever used cocaine, while approximately 2.6% claimed to have used it in the last 12 months (Fishburne et al., 1983; US Department of Health and Human Services, 2001). Cocaine use is abundant in urban settings. It is estimated that from 10% to 45% of pregnant women take cocaine (Volpe et al., 1992), and metabolites can be detected in up to 6% of newborns in suburban hospitals (Schutzman et al., 1991).

Cocaine blocks the reuptake of dopamine (DA), norepinephrine, and serotonin at the nerve terminal in the CNS, and also causes release of DA from storage vesicles. The primary event responsible for the addictive properties and euphoric feeling when intoxicated is a block on the DA reuptake transporter (DAT) (Giros et al., 1996). This leads to enhanced DAergic transmission, and can result in a

variety of symptoms in the user. Many individuals report a euphoric feeling and increased self-confidence, in addition to racing thoughts and a feeling of pressure. In other users, a period of paranoid psychosis ensues. The mechanism of altered neurotransmission has been linked to the DA D1 receptor, as mice lacking this receptor fail to exhibit many of the same characteristic behaviors as wild-type mice (Xu et al., 2000).

Cocaine abuse also puts individuals at risk for cerebrovascular defects. Habitual users exhibit a greater degree of cerebral atrophy, compared by CT scan, and are more at risk of stroke and intracranial hemorrhage (Berliner, 2000). Cerebrovascular resistance has also been found to be higher in cocaine abusers than controls using Doppler sonography (Herning et al., 1999). In chronic cocaine users, neurodegenerative disorders have been observed, similar to those observed with amphetamine use.

Amphetamines affect catecholamine neurotransmission in the CNS and have the potential to damage monoaminergic cells directly. Amphetamines, including methylenedioxymethamphetamine (MDMA, or "ecstasy"), have become popular with young adults in recent decades due to the belief that it is a "safe" drug, and its ability to increase energy and sensation in adults. However, they also exert serious side effects. Similar to cocaine, the most pronounced effect of amphetamines is on the DAergic neurons, but they can also damage 5-HT axons and axon terminals (McCann and Ricaurte, 2004). The result is a distal axotomy of DA and 5-HT neurons.

The exact mechanism of amphetamine neurotoxicity is still unknown, but several clues have emerged recently. It seems that oxidative stress plays a key role in toxicity. Following amphetamine-triggered DA release from the neuron, the DA is oxidized to produce free radicals (Lotharius and O'Malley, 2001). Chronic use can affect superoxide dismutase (SOD) and catalase balance in rodents (Frey et al., 2006), and amphetamine neurotoxicity is attenuated by antioxidants (DeVito and Wagner, 1989). It also induces hyperthermia when given at ambient temperatures, and it has been shown that increasing environmental temperature increases the associated neurotoxicity (Miller and O'Callaghan, 2003).

Because drug use and HIV infection have been linked, the effect of cocaine and amphetamine use on toxicity induced by HIV-1 proteins Tat and gp120 has also been investigated. HIV-associated dementia (HAD) is a neurological disorder afflicting many AID patients. Exposure to cocaine and amphetamines in AIDS patients results in a synergistic neurotoxicity, which is attenuated by β-estradiol (Turchan et al., 2001). Oxidative stress has been implicated in this mechanism as well. When a normally nontoxic dose of cocaine is administered, Tat-induced oxidative stress is enhanced (Aksenov et al., 2006).

Excitatory Amino Acids Glutamate and certain other acidic amino acids are excitatory neurotransmitters. The discovery that these excitatory amino acids can be neurotoxic at concentrations that can be achieved in the brain has generated a great amount of interest in these "excitotoxins." In vitro systems have established that the toxicity of glutamate can be blocked by certain glutamate antagonists (Rothman and Olney, 1986), and the concept has emerged that the toxicity of excitatory amino acids may be related to such divergent conditions as hypoxia, epilepsy, and neurodegenerative diseases (Meldrum, 1987; Choi, 1988; Lipton and Rosenberg, 1994; Beal, 1992, 1995, 1998).

Glutamate is the main excitatory neurotransmitter of the brain, and its effects are mediated by several subtypes of receptors (Fig. 16-8) called *excitatory amino acid receptors* (EAARs) (Schoepfer et al., 1994; Hollmann and Heinemann, 1994; Lipton

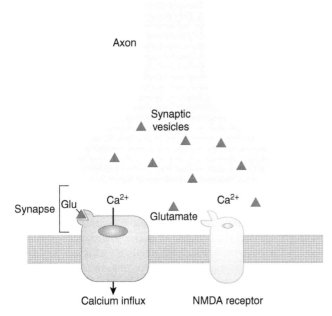

Figure 16-8. *Excitatory synapse.* Synaptic vesicles are transported to the axonal terminus, and released across the synaptic cleft to bind to the postsynaptic receptors. Glutamate, as an excitatory neurotransmitter, binds to its receptor and opens a calcium channel, leading to the excitation of the postsynaptic cell.

and Rosenberg, 1994). The two major subtypes of glutamate receptors are those that are ligand-gated directly to ion channels (ionotropic) and those that are coupled with G proteins (metabotropic). Ionotropic receptors may be further subdivided by their specificity for binding kainate, quisqualate, α-amino-3-hydroxy-5-methylisoxazole-4-propionic acid (AMPA), and N-methyl-D-aspartate (NMDA). The entry of glutamate into the CNS is regulated at the blood–brain barrier and, following an injection of a large dose of glutamate in infant rodents, glutamate exerts its effects in the area of the brain in which the blood–brain barrier is least developed, the circumventricular organ. Within this site of limited access, glutamate injures neurons, apparently by opening glutamate-dependent ion channels, ultimately leading to neuronal swelling and neuronal cell death (Olney, 1978; Coyle, 1987). The toxicity affects the dendrites and neuronal cell bodies but seems to spare axons. The only known related human condition is the "Chinese restaurant syndrome," in which consumption of large amounts of monosodium glutamate as a seasoning may lead to a burning sensation in the face, neck, and chest in sensitive individuals.

The cyclic glutamate analog kainate was initially isolated in Japan from seaweed as the active component of an herbal treatment of ascariasis. Kainate is extremely potent as an excitotoxin, being a hundredfold more toxic than glutamate and is selective at a molecular level for the kainate receptor (Coyle, 1987). Like glutamate, kainate selectively injures dendrites and neurons and shows no substantial effect on glia or axons. As a result, this compound has found use in neurobiology as a tool. Injected into a region of the brain, kainate can destroy the neurons of that area without disrupting the fibers that pass through the same region. Neurobiologists, with the help of this neurotoxic tool, are able to study the role of neurons in a particular area independent of the axonal injuries that occur when similar lesioning experiments are performed by mechanical cutting.

Development of permanent neurological deficits in individuals accidentally exposed to high doses of an EAAR agonist has underscored the potential importance of excitatory amino acids in disease (Perl *et al.*, 1990; Teitelbaum *et al.*, 1990). A total of 107 individuals

in the Maritime Provinces of Canada were exposed to domoic acid, an analog of glutamate, and suffered an acute illness that most commonly presented as gastrointestinal disturbance, severe headache, and short-term memory loss. A subset of the more severely afflicted patients was subsequently shown to have chronic memory deficits and motor neuropathy. Neuropathological investigation of patients who died within four months of intoxication showed neurodegeneration that was most prominent in the hippocampus and amygdala but also affected regions of the thalamus and cerebral cortex.

Other foci of unusual neurodegenerative diseases also have been evaluated for being caused by dietary exposure to EAARs. Perhaps the best known of these is the complex neurodegenerative disease in the indigenous population of Guam and surrounding islands that shares features of amyotrophic lateral sclerosis (ALS), PD, and Alzheimer disease. Early investigations of this Guamanian neurodegenerative complex suggested that the disorder might be related to an environmental factor, perhaps consumption of seeds of *Cycas circinalis* (Kurland, 1963). Subsequently, α-amino-methylaminopropionic acid (or B-N-methylamino-L-alanine, BMAA) was isolated from the cycad and was shown to be neurotoxic in model systems. The toxicity of BMAA is similar to that of glutamate in vitro and can be blocked by certain EAAR antagonists (Nunn *et al.*, 1987). Studies in vivo, however, have not demonstrated a relationship between BMAA and the Guamanian neurodegenerative complex (Spencer *et al.*, 1987; Hugon *et al.*, 1988; Seawright *et al.*, 1990; Duncan, 1992). Therefore, it remains unresolved what role cycad consumption and environmental factors play in this cluster of atypical neurodegenerative disease.

Models of Neurodegenerative Disease

1-Methyl-4-Phenyl-1,2,3,6-Tetrahydropyridine Because of an error on the part of a so-called designer chemist, people who injected themselves with a meperidine derivative that was intended to serve as a substitute for heroin also received a contaminant, MPTP (Fig. 16-9) (Langston *et al.*, 1983). Over hours to days, dozens of these patients developed the signs and symptoms of irreversible PD, some becoming immobile with rigidity (Langston and Irwin, 1986). Autopsy studies demonstrated marked degeneration

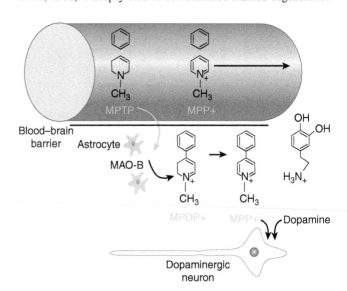

Figure 16-9. *MPTP toxicity.* MPP+, either formed elsewhere in the body following exposure to MPTP or injected directly into the blood, is unable to cross the blood–brain barrier. In contrast, MPTP gains access and is oxidized in situ to MPDP+ and MPP+. The same transport system that carries dopamine into the dopaminergic neurons also transports the cytotoxic MPP+.

of DAergic neurons in the SN, with degeneration continuing many years after exposure (Langston *et al.*, 1999).

It was initially surprising to find not only that MPTP is neurotoxic, but also that it is a substrate for the B isozyme of monoamine oxidase (MAO-B) (Gerlach *et al.*, 1991). MPTP, an uncharged species at physiological pH, crosses the blood–brain barrier (BBB) and diffuses into cells, including astrocytes. The MAO-B of astrocytes catalyzes a two-electron oxidation to yield MPDP$^+$, the corresponding dihydropyridinium ion. A further two-electron oxidation yields the pyridinium ion, MPP$^+$ (Fig. 16-9). MPP$^+$ enters DAergic neurons of the SN via the DA uptake system, resulting in injury or death of the neuron. Noradrenergic neurons of the locus ceruleus are also vulnerable to repeated exposures of MPTP (Langston and Irwin, 1986), although they are less affected by single exposures than the DAergic neurons are. Once inside neurons, MPP$^+$ acts as a general mitochondrial toxin, blocking respiration at complex I (Di Monte and Langston, 2000). MPP$^+$ may also lead to the production of ROS and the release of DA from vesicles due to the higher pH environment of the cytosol, where the neurotransmitter undergoes autoxidation (Lotharius and O'Malley, 2000).

Consistent with the role of MAO-B in the bioactivation of MPTP to MPP$^+$, inhibitors of this enzyme, such as L-(−)-deprenyl (selegiline) protect against MPTP neurotoxicity. However, the protection afforded by deprenyl does not appear to arise from its inhibition of MAO-B alone, but also upon other properties, including its ability to act as an antioxidant and free radical scavenger (Ebadi *et al.*, 2002; Magyar and Szende, 2004; Mandel *et al.*, 2003; Muralikrishnan *et al.*, 2003). Thus, mice deficient in Cu,Zn-SOD or GSH peroxidase show increased vulnerability to MPTP neurotoxicity (Zhang *et al.*, 2000), whereas overexpression of Mn-SOD attenuates the toxicity (Klivenyi *et al.*, 1998).

It should be noted that the general toxicity of the proximate neurotoxicant, MPP$^+$, is considerable when it is administered to animals, although systemic exposure to MPP$^+$ does not result in neurotoxicity because it does not cross the BBB. Moreover, compared to primates, rats are relatively resistant to DAergic neurotoxicity from systemic administration of the parent compound, MPTP, even when the compound is injected directly in the cerebral circulation via the carotid artery. This resistance appears to be conferred, at least in part, by a high level of biotransformation of MPTP by rat endothelial cells to MPP$^+$ and other polar metabolites, such as MPTP-N-oxide, that are retained in endothelial cells and do not readily traverse the BBB (Mushiroda *et al.*, 2001; Riachi *et al.*, 1990; Scriba and Borchardt, 1989).

Although not identical, MPTP neurotoxicity and PD are strikingly similar. The symptomatology of each reflects a disruption of the nigrostriatal pathway. Thus, masked facies, difficulties in initiating and terminating movements, resting "pill-rolling" tremors, rigidity (including characteristic "cogwheel rigidity"), and bradykinesias are all features of both conditions. Pathologically, there is an unusually selective degeneration of neurons in the SN and depletion of striatal DA in both diseases (Di Monte and Langston, 2000). However, positron emission tomography (PET) scanning studies employing the DAergic probe, [^{18}F]-fluorodopa, show that although patients with idiopathic PD demonstrate greater loss of DAergic function in the putamen than the caudate nucleus, the loss from these two nuclei was the same in patients who had taken MPTP (Snow *et al.*, 2000).

The discovery of the relationship between MPTP intoxication and parkinsonism provided researchers with a new model for studying the pathogenic mechanism of PD and prompted investigations to reveal environmental and occupational exposures that might be associated with the disease (Dauer and Przedborski, 2003). Thus, epidemiological studies have implicated exposures to herbicides,

other pesticides, or metals as risk factors for PD (Ferraz *et al.*, 1988; Gorell *et al.*, 1997, 1998, 1999; Liou *et al.*, 1997). Accordingly, the scope of neurotoxicants employed in experimental studies of PD has been enlarged beyond 6-hydroxydopamine (6-OHDA) and MPTP to include agricultural chemicals such as maneb, paraquat, and rotenone (Bove *et al.*, 2005; Uversky, 2004).

Epidemiological studies have also found apparent protective effects of cigarette smoking or coffee consumption on the development of PD (Lai *et al.*, 2002; Logroscino, 2005), and experimental studies indicate that nicotine and caffeine are protective in animal models of PD (Quik, 2004; Quik *et al.*, 2006; Ross and Petrovitch, 2001). It is interesting that PET studies of smokers show a marked reduction in brain MAO-B activity, similar to that produced by administration of the MAO-B inhibitor, L-deprenyl (Fowler *et al.*, 1996). Other MAO-B inhibitors are being developed as anti-PD drugs (Mandel *et al.*, 2005), and MAO-B inhibitors have been isolated from tobacco smoke (Khalil *et al.*, 2006). However, it appears that MAO-B inhibition is not essential for the neuroprotective activity of these chemicals; instead, their effectiveness stems from their overall ability to preserve mitochondrial integrity and function.

Although several families with early-onset PD demonstrate autosomal dominant inheritance and candidate genes have been identified (Agundez *et al.*, 1995; Kurth *et al.*, 1993; Polymerpoulos *et al.*, 1997), environmental exposures play a more significant role than genetics in the vast majority of PD patients, particularly those with late-onset disease (Kuopio *et al.*, 1999; Tanner *et al.*, 1999). Nevertheless, the delineation of specific genes involved in familial forms of PD (eg, those encoding α-synuclein, parkin, ubiquitin C-terminal hydrolase L1, DJ-1, Phosphatase and tensin homolog (PTEN)-induced putative kinase 1, and leucine-rich repeat kinase 2) have provided a rational basis for research concerning gene–environment interactions in the etiology of sporadic PD (Benmoyal-Segal and Soreq, 2006; Gosal *et al.*, 2006).

Several hypotheses on the loss of DAergic neurons in PD suggest that mitochondrial damage is a primary cause of DAergic neuronal death (Mandel *et al.*, 2005; Abou-Slieman *et al.*, 2005). These including the following: (1) mitochondria of DAergic neurons are selectively vulnerable to environmental contaminants that cause mitochondrial dysfunction (Przedborski *et al.*, 2004; Amiry-Moghaddam *et al.*, 2005), (2) DAergic neurons produce an endogenous mitochondrial toxin (Naoi *et al.*, 2002), and (3) mitochondria harbor defects in enzymes, such as complex I, that lead to impaired energy metabolism (Greene *et al.*, 2005; Gu *et al.*, 1998). The centrality of mitochondria in these hypotheses arises primarily from findings that mitochondrial poisons, such as (MPP$^+$) and rotenone can induce a Parkinson-like syndrome in humans, nonhuman primates, and rodents. These neurotoxicants are all capable of inhibiting mitochondrial complex I and appear to model the pathology of PD. Moreover, neuropathological studies reveal a ~30% decrease in complex I function in deceased PD patients, as compared with age-matched controls (Adam-Vizi, 2005).

Mitochondrial complex I inhibitors, such as MPP$^+$ and rotenone, damage nigral neurons by mechanisms involving oxidation. Oxidative damage also plays a significant role in DAergic neuronal cell death induced by intracranial injection of 6-OHDA, another experimental model of PD (Cannon *et al.*, 2006). Both enzymatic and auto-oxidation of 6-OHDA generate ROS, including H_2O_2, superoxide ions, and hydroxyl radicals (ROS). These ROS and the direct inhibition of complex I lead to lipid peroxidation, protein denaturation, and a decrease in reduced GSH: all hallmark features of postmortem PD (Jenner, 2003).

It is remarkable that the poisoning of drug addicts by MPTP has led to major advances in our understanding of PD, which is the second most prevalent neurodegenerative disorder in the western world (Alzheimer disease being first) (Landigan *et al.*, 2005). Although much remains to be done, knowing that most cases of PD arise from environmental exposures that promote mitochondrial dysfunction and oxidative damage provides us with promising avenues for prevention and treatment of this debilitating disease.

Manganese Manganese (Mn) is an essential metal in both humans and animals. Although Mn is present in almost all diets, animals maintain stable tissue Mn levels by tightly regulating absorption and excretory processes. As an essential trace metal that is found in all tissues, Mn is required for normal metabolism of amino acids, proteins, lipids, and carbohydrates. Mn acts as a cofactor for a variety of enzymes, such as manganese metalloenzymes and Mn-dependent enzyme families. Mn metalloenzymes include arginase, GS, phosphoenolpyruvate decarboxylase, and Mn-SOD. Mn-dependent enzymes include oxidoreductases, transferases, hydrolases, lyases, isomerases, and ligases. Therefore, Mn is necessary for the function of many organ systems. In rare Mn deficiencies, clinical manifestations can be seizures, impaired growth, skeletal abnormalities, and impaired reproductive function (Critchfield *et al.*, 1993; Wedler, 1993).

At the other end of the spectrum, it is well established that excessive exposure to Mn causes neurotoxicity (McMillan, 1999; Aschner *et al.*, 2005). The most common commercial sources of Mn include the fuel additive methylcyclopentadienyl manganese tricarbonyl (MMT), pesticides such as Maneb, steel factories, welding, and mining plants. Occupational exposure to toxic levels of Mn in industrial workers results in psychological and neurological disturbances, including delusions, hallucinations, depression, disturbed equilibrium, compulsive or violent behavior, weakness, and apathy, followed by extrapyramidal motor system defects such as tremors, muscle rigidity, ataxia, bradykinesia, and dystonia. Although Mn toxicity has been under investigation for many years, the underlying primary molecular mechanisms of its neurotoxicity remain to be elucidated. Very few potential biomarkers have been established with no early detection markers available.

The epidemiological associations and similarities in symptoms between Mn neurotoxicity and DA neuropathology suggest that exposure and accumulation of this metal may be an environmental factor that contributes to idiopathic Parkinson disease (IPD). Mn toxicity causes a loss of DA neurons in the SN, and as in PD, oxidative stress appears to play a significant role in the disorder (Oestreicher *et al.*, 1994; Kienzl *et al.*, 1995; Montgomery, 1995). The brain area most susceptible to Mn injury is also highly sensitive to oxidative stress. Many metabolically active cell types, particularly tonically active motor neurons in the SN, require high levels of ATP for optimal function and survival. Mn accumulates in the SN, globus pallidus (GP), and striatum and interferes with ATP synthesis, analogous to effects seen with mitochondrial inhibitors or ischemia. Appraisal of the literature strongly suggests that in addition to targeting similar brain areas, DAergic neurodegeneration associated with PD and Mn exposure shares multiple common mechanisms, namely mitochondrial dysfunction, aberrant signal transduction, oxidative stress, protein aggregation, and the activation of cell death pathways. The accumulation of Mn in the striatum causes damage to the SN, reduction in tyrosine hydroxylase (TH) activity, and loss of DA neurons (Parenti *et al.*, 1988; Tomas-Camardiel *et al.*, 2002). Intracellular Mn is sequestered by mitochondria through the Ca^{2+} uniporter (Gavin *et al.*, 1999). Intrastriatal injections of Mn result in excitotoxic brain injury similar to that caused by mitochondrial poisons, such as aminooxyacetic acid and 1-methyl-4-phenyl-pyridinium (Brouillet *et al.*, 1993b). The specificity for Mn accumulation in GP and striatum likely correlates with Mn transporter distribution and the metabolic activity of these basal ganglia nuclei.

Guamanian Cycad-Induced Parkinsonism/Amyotrophic Lateral Sclerosis Syndrome

An unusual prevalence of "hereditary paralysis" among the native Guam Chamorros was first reported in the early 1900s. This led to the formation of the National Institute of Neurological and Communicative Disorders and Stroke Research Center on Guam in 1939 (Rodgers-Johnson *et al.*, 1986). In the mid-1950s the incidence of ALS and parkinsonism–dementia complex (PDC) was up to 100 times higher on Guam than anywhere else in the world (Hirano *et al.*, 1961a). Although Guam ALS is clinically indistinguishable from ALS that occurs elsewhere in the world, Guam PDC is a distinct neurodegenerative disorder where parkinsonism and dementia may occur simultaneously in affected Chamorros.

Hirano and colleagues first described the clinical features and pathology in 1961 (Hirano *et al.*, 1961a,b). The main clinical features included mental deterioration, parkinsonism, and evidence of motor neuron involvement. The duration of clinical symptoms was about four years with the average age of diagnosis being approximately 52 years and a higher incidence in men. The main macroscopic neuropathological features are the presence of cortical atrophy and depigmentation of the SN. Microscopic evaluations revealed widespread ganglion cell degeneration and neurofibrillary tangles throughout the CNS. The lack of uniformity in the clinical presentation of these diseases has made it difficult to determine a possible causative agent.

Throughout the years, the focus has shifted from a genetic to an environmental causative agent. Due to the formation of the case registrar, established in 1958, entire pedigrees have been developed using Chamorros from the same village as controls. Although several investigators have reported a high degree of familial occurrence, no definitive inheritance pattern has been established (Plato *et al.*, 2002). Support for an environmental hypothesis includes a decrease in the incidence of the diseases and an increase in the age of onset with the Westernization of Guam (Plato *et al.*, 2003).

Cycads are primitive plants that contain several toxins, including cycasin and L-β-methylaminoalanine (BMAA) (Schneider *et al.*, 2002). Cycasin, which is metabolized to methylazoxymethanol (MAM), is known to be carcinogenic and cause hepatotoxicity (Sieber *et al.*, 1980). BMAA is a nonprotein amino acid that functions as a glutamate excitotoxin (Rakonczay *et al.*, 1991). In 1987, Spencer and colleagues reported that BMAA, when fed to primates in high concentrations (>100 mg/kg), produced a syndrome that closely resembled the neurological disorder observed on Guam. Traditionally, native Chamorros prepare food from cycads by washing the seeds several times, then grinding them into flour (Kisby *et al.*, 1992). However, it appears that the washing process is sufficient to remove the cycad toxins (Duncan *et al.*, 1990).

In 2002, Cox and Sacks suggested "the Chamorro population of Guam ingested large quantities of cycad toxins indirectly by eating flying foxes." This study demonstrated that the sharp decrease in the flying fox population was followed by a sharp decrease in the incidence of ALS. The flying fox, *Pteropus mariannus*, is a fruit bat with a wing span of three feet and is known to eat three times its weight in fruit, cycad seeds, or beetles, which are known to bioaccumulate cycad toxins for protective purposes (Schneider *et al.*, 2002). The consumption of the flying foxes by the Chamorros is not only included in social, but ceremonial settings (Banack and Cox, 2003).

Traditionally, the men consume the animal in its entirety, whereas the women only consume the breast meat.

Accumulation of the neurotoxin, BMAA, in the flying fox, *P mariannus*, may result in concentrations that are sufficient to cause behavioral and neuropathological changes in primates similar to those observed in the Guam ALS–PDC. Furthermore, BMAA-induced neurodegeneration may occur by an excitotoxic mechanism involving the mitochondria permeability transition pore (mtPTP). It has been shown that BMAA increases the intracellular calcium concentration through the formation of a β-carbamate intermediate (Brownson *et al.*, 2002). This intermediate can act as a glutamate agonist and induce glutamate excitotoxicity. Studies have also demonstrated that an increase in intracellular calcium (Dubinsky and Levi, 1998) and glutamate excitotoxicity are able to induce mtPTP (Schinder *et al.*, 1996).

Developmentally Neurotoxic Chemicals

Replication, migration, differentiation, myelination, and synapse formation are the basic processes that occur in specific spatial and temporal patterns and underlie development of the NS. There are a variety of insults known to disrupt NS development, the outcomes of which may be very different depending on the time of exposure, including exposures to certain metals, solvents, antimetabolites, persistent organic pollutants, pesticides, pharmaceuticals, and ionizing radiation. Multiple mechanisms of action may be present, producing a wide array of effects in the offspring. The impact on the developing NS may be very different, and often cannot be predicted, from effects observed in adults. A number of neurodevelopmental disorders have been, at least partially, attributed to exposures to neurotoxicological agents during the fetal, infant, or childhood periods. Although the number of chemicals shown to be developmentally neurotoxic in human populations is relatively small, the number of suspected toxicants from laboratory animal and other studies may be in the hundreds (Grandjean and Landrigan, 2006; Miodovnik, 2011).

Ethanol exposure during pregnancy can result in abnormalities in the fetus, including abnormal neuronal migration and facial development, and diffuse abnormalities in the development of neuronal processes, especially the dendritic spines (Stoltenburg-Didinger and Spohre, 1983). Although the exposure may be of little consequence to the mother, it can be devastating to the fetus. There is an effect on NMDA glutamate receptors and excessive activation of GABA receptors, with induction of apoptosis throughout the brain (Ikonomidou *et al.*, 2000). The clinical result of fetal alcohol exposure is often mental retardation, with malformations of the brain and delayed myelination of white matter (Riikonen *et al.*, 1999). Although there remains a great deal of uncertainty concerning the molecular basis of this developmental aberration, it occurs in a variety of experimental animals, and it appears that acetaldehyde, a product of ethanol catabolism, can produce migration defects in developing animals similar to those that occur in the fetal alcohol syndrome (O'Shea and Kaufman, 1979).

Some developmental neurotoxicants have been revealed by human studies or tragic poisoning occurrences. The contamination of fish in Minamata Bay, Japan, with MeHg led to developmental disabilities, including cerebral palsy, mental retardation, and seizures, in many children at birth. Children exposed to MeHg in utero show widespread neuronal loss, disruption of cellular migration, profound mental retardation, and paralysis (Costa *et al.*, 2004; Reuhl and Chang, 1979). Studies using primates exposed in utero also have demonstrated abnormal social development (Burbacher *et al.*, 1990). The earlier the exposure, the more generalized the damage that is observed. As with MeHg, ethanol and lead are known to produce frank neuropathology in highly exposed populations.

In recent years the concept has emerged that extremely low levels of exposure to these substances in "asymptomatic" children may have an effect on their behavioral and cognitive development. This has led to the suspicion that the number of chemically induced neurological disorders is larger than generally assumed. For example, the association between lead exposure and brain dysfunction has received experimental support in animal models and has prompted screening for lead in children (Benjamin and Platt, 1999). There is no proven safe lower limit for lead, and recent studies have associated lower IQ scores with blood lead levels less than 2 to 10 μg/dL (Bellinger, 2008; Canfield *et al.*, 2003; Gilbert and Weiss, 2006; Winneke *et al.*, 1994). Similarly, the debate regarding "safe" level of drinking during pregnancy is ongoing, with recent reports of no threshold for subtle cognitive effects (Sampson *et al.*, 2000). Analyses of epidemiological data have suggested that the incidence of low-level MeHg-induced neurotoxicity has been greatly underestimated (Grandjean and Herz, 2011).

There is considerable evidence that chronic exposure to nicotine has effects on the developing fetus (reviewed in Slikker *et al.*, 2005). Along with decreased birth weights, attention deficit disorders are more common in children whose mothers smoke cigarettes during pregnancy, and nicotine has been shown to lead to analogous neurobehavioral abnormalities in animals exposed prenatally to nicotine (Lichensteiger *et al.*, 1988). Nicotinic receptors are expressed early in the development of the NS, beginning in the developing brainstem and later expressed in the diencephalon. The role of these nicotinic receptors during development is unclear; however, it appears that prenatal exposure to nicotine alters the development of nicotinic receptors in the CNS (Van de Kamp and Collins, 1994)—changes that may be related to subsequent attention and cognitive disorders in animals and children.

Cocaine use during pregnancy is a major concern, especially in urban areas, where use can lead to a variety of acute and chronic adverse events in offspring. Cocaine is able to cross the placental barrier and the fetal blood–brain barrier, and also causes reduced blood flow in the uterus. In severe events at large doses taken by the mother, the fetus may develop hypoxia, leading to a higher rate of birth defects (Woods *et al.*, 1987). Maternal cocaine use is associated with low–birth weight and behavioral defects, including a decreased awareness of the surroundings and altered response to stress and pain sensitivity (Chasnoff *et al.*, 1985; Huber *et al.*, 2001).

Several epidemiological studies have reported deficits in neurodevelopment and psychological performance in children exposed to polychlorinated hydrocarbons (PCBs) and/or dioxins (Seegal, 1996). Research in animals has shown that these persistent pollutants produce endocrine disruptions, cognitive deficits, and changes in activity levels in exposed offspring; however, the specific outcomes depend on the congener or mixture tested as well as the timing of exposure. Changes in estrogen or thyroid hormone, neurotransmitter function, and second messenger systems have been proposed as cellular bases for PCB toxicity (Seegal, 1996; Tilson and Kodavanti, 1998). Recent studies with another persistent class of hydrocarbons, polybrominated diphenyl ethers (PBDEs), have shown similarities in altering thyroid hormone metabolism and cholinergic function, and it has thus been proposed that this chemical class would also be developmentally neurotoxic (Branchi *et al.*, 2003; Costa and Giordano, 2007). Thyroid hormone is critical to NS development, and animal studies have suggested that the developing brain may be vulnerable to environmental thyrotoxicants of all sorts (Porterfield, 1994, 2000). Finally, it has been shown that even reversible changes in neurotransmission, such as those produced by nicotine or cholinesterase inhibitors, may alter specific growth processes and produce long-lasting deficits (Slotkin, 2004).

CHEMICALS THAT INDUCE DEPRESSION OF NERVOUS SYSTEM FUNCTION

The CNS maintains balance via interplay between inhibitory and excitatory influences. With general depressant chemicals, initial suppression of inhibitory systems at low doses produces excitation, such as intoxication observed with ethanol. Thus, acutely, CNS depressants produce a continuum of effects from excitation to sedation, motor impairment, coma, and ultimately death by depression of respiratory centers. Therapeutic indications of drugs causing CNS depression include anxiety, insomnia, epilepsy, and muscle relaxation.

Generalized depression of CNS function is produced by a variety of volatile solvents, including ethanol, organics, and anesthetics. These solvents include several chemical classes—aliphatic and aromatic hydrocarbons, halogenated hydrocarbons, ketones, esters, alcohols, and ethers—that are small, lipophilic molecules. They are widely found in industry, medicine, and commercial products. Human exposure ranges from chronic low level to occupational to high levels occurring with solvent abuse.

There are several theories as to the mechanism of this generalized depression, but none are fully explanatory. Solvent potency correlates well with the olive oil:water or octanol:water partition coefficients, leading to the once-popular Meyer–Overton hypothesis that CNS depressants exert their actions through nonspecific disruption of the lipid portions of cell membranes (eg, Janoff et al., 1981). Anesthesia could occur as a consequence of membrane expansion or perturbations of mitochondrial calcium transport. More recent research has implicated interactions with ligand-gated ion channels as well as voltage-gated calcium channels. Specific receptors regulating these channels include gamma-aminobutyric acid type A ($GABA_A$), NMDA, and glycine receptors. These actions relate the effects of solvents to those of pharmaceutical agents such as barbiturates and benzodiazepines. Although these targets have been demonstrated mostly for ethanol (Davies, 2003), recent in vitro studies have extended this generality to other volatile solvents (eg, Cruz et al., 2000).

A syndrome known as solvent-induced chronic toxic encephalopathy has been described for some populations with long-term and/or high-level exposure. Somewhat vague presenting symptoms include irritability, fatigue, impaired memory, or concentration, leading to the need for widely accepted diagnostic criteria (Van der Hoek et al., 2000). The absence of corroborating animal studies have prevented studies of molecular changes, which may underlie these long-term effects, and indeed, have raised doubt as to the existence of such a syndrome (Ridgway et al., 2003). Specific solvents also produce other neurotoxicological actions, such as peripheral neuropathy, which are described elsewhere in this text.

IN VITRO AND OTHER ALTERNATIVE APPROACHES TO NEUROTOXICOLOGY

In its report, entitled "Toxicity Testing in the 21st Century: A Vision and a Strategy," the National Research Council (NRC, 2007) calls for innovative experimental in vitro approaches for the assessment and characterization of chemical toxicity, including key initiating molecular events. The long-term vision of the 2007 NRC report is to use high-throughput cell-based assays and quantitative structure–activity relationships (QSARs) to predict adverse outcomes. This will require the development of high-throughput approaches that

can screen thousands of chemicals for these key events using time- and cost-effective models, in addition to determining the predictive effectiveness of these methods using complementary approaches. The replacement of standard in vivo neurotoxicity assessments with QSAR and high-throughput in vitro methods will require a long-term research effort (Bal-Price et al., 2010; Smith, 2009). In the meantime, we cannot rely on standard in vivo approaches that have been used successfully in the past to assess the backlog of thousands of untested chemicals.

The use of tiered testing schemes has been proposed, where the first tiers rely on high-throughput methods that test for chemical actions on key biological receptors that initiate pathways of changes that lead to adverse outcomes, in order to identify chemicals for future testing. Second tier tests could involve the use of alternative species, such as small fish or invertebrate species, that will allow more moderate throughput, but in an intact or developing NS. Chemicals identified as having neurotoxic properties could then be tested in intact mammalian models as necessary. The mammalian models would be modified based on existing data; for example, if lower-tier data suggest effects on myelin formation, then mammalian models appropriate to test myelin-related endpoints (eg, histopathology) should be used.

In order to develop these new testing strategies in the field of neurotoxicology, new approaches for screening and characterizing the neurotoxic potential of chemicals must be established, driven by basic research of how xenobiotics interfere with basic neurobiological processes. Critical to this process are complementary approaches that will allow assessment of the impact of chemical-induced alterations on key events in intact multicellular organisms. The extraordinary conservation of both genomic/epigenomic elements and differentiation processes between mammals and non-mammalians, which has been revealed during the last two decades, makes more feasible the use of these alternative models. Finally, the results of these methods should inform and refine how, when, or if, the classical mammalian model approach are used. Each method of analysis will contribute unique information to the overall picture of neurotoxicity and inform the process and interpretation of the other avenues of investigation.

Cell-based assays can provide critical new information regarding toxicant effects on intracellular signaling and cell lifecycle processes. Nonmammalian whole animal models can provide important understanding of effects on intercellular and systemwide signaling in an anatomically and temporally intact biological system. Emerging high-throughput and complementary models can help direct the best use of the classic mammalian models (eg, thyroid or estrogenic effects). The integrated and tiered use of the spectrum of neurotoxicity approaches thus provides a rationale approach to decreasing the vast uncertain risk posed by thousands of chemicals with no available hazard information.

Emerging alternative test species, such as Caenorhabditis elegans (C elegans), Zebrafish (Danio rerio), and Drosophila melanogaster (D melanogaster), are making it possible to assess the effects of small molecules rapidly, inexpensively, and on a miniaturized scale. Such model systems provide an approach to study toxicity in an intact organism where cell–cell interactions and complex metabolic milieus influence and modify xenobiotic-induced neurotoxic potential, not possible in in vitro systems (Peterson et al., 2008). These and other species provide powerful model organisms for dissecting the components of neurodevelopment and degeneration. Moreover, these organisms are readily amenable to genetic manipulation. Embryonic stages of many of these species are optically transparent, allowing for easy real-time examination of the neuronal morphology and direct viewing of protein expression patterns.

The genomic sequencing of *C elegans*, *D rerio*, and *D melanogaster* has been completed, which allows for performance of whole animal PCR and provides a high-density polymorphism map of related strains. High-throughput approaches include genome-wide screening for molecular targets or mediators in toxicity and rapid, high-content chemical screens to detect potential toxicants. Genomewide screening is important for studying any toxicant with a poorly understood mechanism of action. This screening has been accomplished using RNA interference (RNAi), DNA microarrays, and gene expression analysis.

Evaluation of cytotoxicity, particularly in a heterogeneous system such as the brain, is difficult in the intact animal because numerous factors (neural, hormonal, and hemodynamic) are not under experimental control. Simplified models, such as tissue culture, have been therefore indispensable as tools for understanding of basic physiology and molecular mechanisms that govern neurotoxic responses. Neural cultures offer numerous advantages over in vivo techniques. Cell morphology, protein synthesis and release, energy metabolism, receptor interaction, neurotransmitter uptake and release, as well as electrolyte and nonelectrolyte uptake and release can be directly studied. Dispersion of cells in culture permits access to clean membrane surfaces for electrophysiological studies utilizing patch clamping. Furthermore, direct effects of chemicals on a relatively homogeneous population allows for the study of specific aspects of the growth and differentiation of cells. The culture model also makes it possible to study regional specialization, and can be extended to study cellular interactions by coculturing various cell types. There are, however, limitations of the culture systems that should also be considered. For example, cells can undergo varying degrees of differentiation, lose heterogeneous cell–cell interactions, and hence lose auto- and paracrine signaling processes that modulate form and function of the cell. In addition, a number of different, sometimes competing, processes can influence the ability of a toxicant to damage specific cells. The reductionist approach where one removes many cell types and barriers to focus on a single cell type can facilitate diffusion or even active transport of a given toxic compound or its metabolite, limiting or enhancing toxicity. The ability of a cell to repair or replace damaged organelles or enzymes can also be critical in determining cell survival. This effect may also be dependent on neighboring cells and physical barriers, which may altogether be absent in a culture system.

Despite the caveats and limitations of the "Tox 21" approach (NRC, 2007), emerging advances in analytical techniques, imaging, sensing, and massively parallel computational capabilities will permit new insights into the function and chemically induced dysfunction of the brain, spinal cord, and PNS. Systems approaches in a scalable fashion that link the molecular to organic and whole body, for example, brain–renal, brain–hepatic, or brain–immune system, are currently under development and will soon revolutionize the science of neurotoxicology. Nevertheless, the rudiments of the discipline remain inviolable. That is to say, considerations of dose, pharmacokinetics and dynamics, absorption, distribution, metabolism, and excretion must not be lost in the estimation of hazard and risk from exposure to neurotoxic chemicals.

REFERENCES

Abou-Donia MB. Triphenyl phosphite: a type II organophosphorus compound-induced delayed neurotoxic agent. In: Chambers JE, Levi PE, eds. *Organophosphates: Chemistry, Fate, and Effects*. San Diego: Academic Press; 1992:327–351.

Abou-Donia MB, ed. *Neurotoxicology*. Boca Raton, FL: CRC Press; 1993.

Abou-Slieman PM, Mugit MM, Wood NW. Expanding insights of mitochondrial dysfunction in Parkinson's disease. *Nat Rev Neurosci*. 2005;7:207–219.

Adam-Vizi V. Production of reactive oxygen species in brain mitochondria: contribution by electron-transport chain and non-electron transport chain sources. *Antioxid Redox Signal*. 2005;7:1140–1149.

Adams J, Barone S Jr, LaMantia A, et al. Workshop to identify critical windows of exposure for children's health: neurobehavioral work group summary. *Environ. Health Perspect*. 2000;108(suppl 3):535–544.

Agundez JA, Jimenex JF, Luengo A, et al. Association between the oxidative polymorphism and early onset of Parkinson's disease. *Clin Pharmacol Ther*. 1995;57:291–298.

Aksenov MY, Aksenov MV, Nath A, et al. Cocaine-mediated enhancement of Tat toxicity in rat hippocampal cell cultures: the role of oxidative stress and D1 dopamine receptor. *Neurotoxicology*. 2006;27:217–228.

Albrecht J. Astrocytes and ammonia neurotoxicity. In: Aschner M, Kimelberg HK, eds. *The Role of Glia in Neurotoxicity*. Boca Raton: CRC Press; 1996:137–153.

Albrecht J, Norenberg MD. L-Methionine-DL-sulfoximine induces massive efflux of glutamine from cortical astrocytes in primary culture. *Eur J Pharmacol*. 1990;182:587–599.

Altman J, Sudarshan K. Postnatal development of locomotion in the laboratory rat. *Anim Behav*. 1975;23:896–920.

Amarnath V, Anthony DC, Valentine WM, et al. The molecular mechanism of the carbon disulfide mediated crosslinking of proteins. *Chem Res Toxicol*. 1991;4:148–150.

Amiry-Moghaddam M, Lindland H, Zelenin S, et al. Brain mitochondria contain aquaporin water channels: evidence for the expression of a short AQP9 isoform in the inner mitochondrial membrane. *FASEB J*. 2005;19:1459–1467.

Anderson JP, Carroll Z, Smulowitz M, et al. A possible mechanism of action of the neurotoxic agent iminodipropionitrile (IDPN): a selective aggregation of the medium and heavy neurofilament polypeptides (NF-M and NF-H). *Brain Res*. 1991;547:353–357.

Anthony DC, Boekelheide K, Graham DG. The effect of 3,4-dimethyl substitution on the neurotoxicity of 2,5-hexanedione: I. Accelerated clinical neuropathy is accompanied by more proximal axonal swellings. *Toxicol Appl Pharmacol*. 1983;71:362–371.

Arita A, Costa M. Epigenetics in metal carcinogenesis: nickel, arsenic, chromium and cadmium. *Metallomics*. 2009;1:222–228.

Aschner M, Erikson KM, Dorman DC. Manganese dosimetry: species differences and implications for neurotoxicity. *Crit Rev Toxicol*. 2005;35:1–32.

Atchison WD, Hare MF. Mechanisms of methylmercury-induced neurotoxicity. *FASEB J*. 1994;8:622–629.

Auer RN, Benveniste H. Hypoxia and related conditions. In: Graham DI, Lantos PL, eds. *Greenfield's Neuropathology*. 6th ed. New York: Arnold; 1997:263–314.

Bachurin SO, Shevtzove EP, Lermontova NN, et al. The effect of dithiocarbamates on neurotoxic action of 1-methyl-4-phenyl-1,2,3,6-tetrahydropyridine (MPTP) and on mitochondrial respiration chain. *Neurotoxicology*. 1996;17:897–903.

Bagley PR, Tucker SP, Nolan C, et al. Anatomical mapping of glucose transporter protein and pyruvate dehydrogenase in rat brain: an immunogold study. *Brain Res*. 1989;499:214–224.

Bakir F, Damluji SF, Amin-Zaki L, et al. Methylmercury poisoning in Iraq. *Science*. 1973;181:230–241.

Bal-Price AK, Hogberg HT, Buzanska L, Coecke S. Relevance of in vitro neurotoxicity testing for regulatory requirements: challenges to be considered. *Neurotoxicol Teratol*. 2010;32:36–41.

Balaban CD, O'Callaghan JP, Billingsley ML. Trimethyltin-induced neuronal damage in the rat brain: comparative studies using silver degeneration stains, immunocytochemistry and immunoassay for neuronotypic and gliotypic proteins. *Neuroscience*. 1988;26:337–361.

Banack SA, Cox PA. Biomagnification of cycad neurotoxins in flying foxes: implications for ALS-PDC in Guam. *Neurology*. 2003;61:387–389.

Barone S Jr, Das KP, Lassiter TL, White LD. Vulnerable processes of nervous system development: a review of markers and methods. *Neurotoxicology*. 2000;21:15–36.

Barone S Jr, Stanton ME, Mundy WR. Neurotoxic effects of triethyltin (TET) exposure are exacerbated with aging. *Neurobiol Aging*. 1995;16:723–735.

Bayer SA, Altman J, Russo RJ, et al. Timetables of neurogenesis in the human brain based on experimentally determined patterns in the rat. *Neurotoxicology*. 1993;14:83–144.

Beal MF. Does impairment of energy metabolism result in excitotoxic neuronal death in neurodegenerative illnesses? *Ann Neurol*. 1992;31:119–130.

Beal MF. Aging, energy, and oxidative stress in neurodegenerative diseases. *Ann Neurol*. 1995;38:357–366.

Beal MF. Excitotoxity and nitric oxide in Parkinson's disease pathogenesis. *Ann Neurol*. 1998;44:S110–S114.

Bearer CF. How are children different from adults? *Environ Health Perspect*. 1995;103(suppl 6):7–12.

Beirowski B, Adalbert R, Wagner D, et al. The progressive nature of Wallerian degeneration in wild-type and slow Wallerian degeneration (WldS) nerves. *BMC Neurosci*. 2005;6:6.

Bellinger DC. Very low lead exposures and children's neurodevelopment. *Curr Opin Pediatr*. 2008;20:172–177.

Benjamin JT, Platt C. Is universal screening for lead in children indicated? An analysis of lead results in Augusta, Georgia in 1997. *J Med Assoc Georgia*. 1999;88:24–26.

Benmoyal-Segal L, Soreq H. Gene-environment interactions in sporadic Parkinson's disease. *J Neurochem*. 2006;97:1740–1755.

Benowitz NL. Clinical pharmacology of nicotine. *Annu Rev Med*. 1986;37:21–32.

Berliner R. Cocaine. In: Spencer PS, Schaumburg HH, eds. *Experimental and Clinical Neurotoxicology*. New York: Oxford University Press; 2000:408–413.

Besser R, Kramer G, Thumler R, et al. Acute trimethyltin limbic-cerebellar syndrome. *Neurology*. 1987;37:945–950.

Bond AD, Benevellit F, Jones W. Modification of the solid-state structure of bis(1-hydroxy-2(1H)-pyridine-S²,O)zinc(II): synthesis and characterization of a molecular solid solution incorporating 3-hydroxy-4-methyl-2-3H)-thiazolethione. *J Mater Chem*. 2002;12:324–332.

Bondy SC, Campbell A. Developmental neurotoxicology. *J Neurosci Res*. 2005;81:605–612.

Bouldin TW, Samsa G, Earnhardt TS, et al. Schwann cell vulnerability to demyelination is associated with internodal length in tellurium neuropathy. *J Neuropathol Exp Neurol*. 1988;47:41–47.

Bove J, Prou D, Perier C, et al. Toxin-induced models of Parkinson's disease. *NeuroRx*. 2005;2:484–494.

Branchi I, Capone F, Alleva E, et al. Polybrominated diphenyl ethers: neurobehavioral effects following developmental exposure. *Neurotoxicology*. 2003;24:449–462.

Brouillet E, Jenkins BG, Hyman BT, et al. Age-dependent vulnerability of the striatum to the mitochondrial toxin 3-nitropropionic acid. *J Neurochem*. 1993a;60:356–359.

Brouillet EP, Shinobu L, McGarvey U, et al. Manganese injection into the rat striatum produces excitotoxic lesions by impairing energy metabolism. *Exp Neurol*. 1993b;120:89–94.

Brownson DM, Mabry TJ, Leslie SW. The cycad neurotoxic amino acid, beta-N-methylamino-L-alanine (BMAA), elevates intracellular calcium levels in dissociated rat brain cells. *J Ethnopharmacol*. 2002;82:159–167.

Burbacher TM, Sackett GP, Mottet NK. Methylmercury effects on the social behavior of Macaca fascicularis. *Neurotoxicol Teratol*. 1990;12:65–71.

Calingasan NY, Baker H, Sheu KF, et al. Selective enrichment of cholinergic neurons with the alpha-ketoglutarate dehydrogenase complex in rat brain. *Neurosci Lett*. 1994;168:209–212.

Calne DB, Langston JW, Martin WR, et al. Positron emission tomography after MPTP: observations relating to the cause of Parkinson's disease. *Nature*. 1985;317:246–248.

Cammer W, Moore CL. The effect of hexachlorophene on the respiration of brain and liver mitochondria. *Biochem Biophys Res Commun*. 1972;46:1887–1894.

Canfield RL, Henderson CR Jr, Cory-Slechta DA, et al. Intellectual impairment in children with blood lead concentrations below 10 microg per deciliter. *N Engl J Med*. 2003;348:1517–1526.

Cannon JR, Keep RF, Schallert T, et al. Protease-activated receptor-1 mediates protection elicited by thrombin preconditioning in a rat 6-hydroxy-dopamine model of Parkinson's disease. *Brain Res*. 2006;1116:177–186.

Casida JE, Quistad GB. Serine hydrolase targets of organophosphorus toxicants. *Chem Biol Interact*. 2005;157–158:277–283.

Cavanagh JB. The significance of the "dying-back" process in experimental and human neurological disease. *Int Nat Rev Exp Pathol*. 1964;7:219–267.

Chang LW, Dyer RS. *Handbook of Neurotoxicology*. New York: M. Dekker; 1995.

Chasnoff IJ, Burns WJ, Schnoll SH, et al. Cocaine use in pregnancy. *N Engl J Med*. 1985;313:666–669.

Chaudry V, Cornblath DR. Wallerian degeneration in human nerves: serial electrophysiological studies. *Muscle Nerve*. 1992;15:687–693.

Cheng KC, Cahill DS, Kasai H, et al. 8-Hydroxyguanine, an abundant form of oxidative DNA damage, causes G–T and A–C substitutions. *J Biol Chem*. 1992;267:166–172.

Cheung MK, Verity MA. Experimental methyl mercury neurotoxicity: locus of mercurial inhibition of brain protein synthesis in vivo and in vitro. *J Neurochem*. 1985;44:1799–1808.

Choi DW. Glutamate neurotoxicity and diseases of the nervous system. *Neuron*. 1988;1:623–634.

Chou S-M, Hartmann HA. Axonal lesions and waltzing syndrome after IDPN administration in rats: with a concept "axostasis". *Acta Neuropathol*. 1964;3:428–450.

Chuang RY, Chuang LF. Inhibition of chicken myeloblastosis RNA polymerase II activity by adriamycin. *Biochemistry*. 1979;18:2069–2073.

Clancy B, Finlay BL, Darlington RB, Anand KJS. Extrapolation brain development from experimental species to humans. *Neurotoxicology*. 2007;28:931–937.

Clark AW, Griffin JW, Price DL. The axonal pathology in chronic IDPN intoxication. *J Neuropathol Exp Neurol*. 1980;39:42–55.

Clarkson TW. The toxicology of mercury. *Crit Rev Clin Lab Sci*. 1997;34:369–403.

Cleveland DW, Hwo SY, Kirschner MW. Physical and chemical properties of purified tau factor and the role of tau in microtubule assembly. *J Mol Biol*. 1977;116:227–247.

Coleman M. Axon degeneration mechanisms: commonality amid diversity. *Nat Rev*. 2005;6:889–898.

Collins JJ, Swaen GMH, Marsh GM, et al. Mortality patterns among workers exposed to acrylamide. *J Occup Med*. 1989;31:614–617.

Costa LG, Aschner M, Vitalone A, et al. Developmental neuropathology of environmental agents. *Ann Rev Pharmacol Toxicol*. 2004;44:87–110.

Costa LG, Giordano G. Developmental neurotoxicity of polybrominated diphenyl ether (PBDE) flame retardants. *Neurotoxicology*. 2007; 28:1047–1067.

Cox PA, Sacks OW. Cycad neurotoxins, consumption of flying foxes, and ALS-PDC disease in Guam. *Neurology*. 2002;58:956–959.

Coxon A, Pallis CA. Metronidazole neuropathy. *J Neurol Neurosurg Psychiatr*. 1976;36:403–405.

Coyle JT. Kainic acid: insights into excitatory mechanisms causing selective neuronal degeneration. In: Bock G, O'Connor M, eds. *Selective Neuronal Death*. New York: Wiley; 1987:186–203.

Critchfield JW, Carl FG, Keen CL. Anticonvulsant-induced changes in tissue manganese, zinc, copper, and iron concentrations in Wistar rats. *Metabolism*. 1993;42:907–910.

Crofton KM, Padilla S, Tilson HA, et al. The impact of dose rate on the neurotoxicity of acrylamide: the interaction of administered dose, target tissue concentrations, tissue damage, and functional effects. *Toxicol Appl Pharmacol*. 1996;139:163–176.

Crompton M. The mitochondrial permeability transition pore and its role in cell death. *Biochem J*. 1999;341:233–249.

Cruz SL, Balster RL, Woodward JJ. Effects of volatile solvents on recombinant N-methyl-D-aspartate receptors expressed in Xenopus oocytes. *Br J Pharmacol*. 2000;131:1303–1308.

Dabrowski-Bouta G, Sulkowski G, Bartosz G, et al. Chronic lead intoxication affects the myelin membrane status in the central nervous system of adult rats. *J Mol Neurosci*. 1999;13:127–139.

Dauer W, Prezedborski S. Parkinson's disease: mechanisms and models. *Neuron*. 2003;39:889–909.

Davies M. The role of GABAA receptors in mediating the effects of alcohol in the central nervous system. *J Psychiatry Neurosci*. 2003;28:263–274.

Davis M, Gendelman DS, Tischler MD, et al. A primary acoustic startle circuit: lesion and stimulation studies. *J Neurosci.* 1982;2:791–805.

Davis SL, Tanaka D Jr, Aulerich RJ, et al. Organophosphorus-induced neurotoxicity in the absence of neuropathy target esterase inhibition: the effects of triphenyl phosphine in the European ferret. *Toxicol Sci.* 1999;49:78–85.

DeGrandchamp RL, Reuhl KR, Lowndes HE. Synaptic terminal degeneration and remodeling at the rat neuromuscular junction resulting from a single exposure to acrylamide. *Toxicol Appl Pharmacol.* 1990;105:422–433.

Dejneka NS, Polavarapu R, Deng X, et al. Chromosomal localization and characterization of the stannin (Snn) gene. *Mamm Genome.* 1998;9:556–564.

DeVeaugh-Geiss J. Tardive dyskinesia: phenomenology, pathophysiology, and pharmacology. In: *Tardive Dyskinesia and Related Involuntary Movement Disorders.* Boston: John Wright PSG; 1982:1–18.

DeVito MJ, Wagner GC. Methamphetamine-induced neuronal damage: a possible role for free radicals. *Neuropharmacology.* 1989;28:1145–1150.

Di Monte DA, Langston JW. MPTP and analogs. In: Spencer PS, Schaumburg HH, eds. *Experimental and Clinical Neurotoxicology.* New York: Oxford University Press; 2000:812–818.

Dobbing J, Sands J. Quantitative growth and development of human brain. *Arch Dis Child.* 1973;48:757–767.

Dobbing J, Sands J. Comparative aspects of the brain growth spurt. *Early Human Dev.* 1979;3:79–83.

Dobbing J, Smart JL. Vulnerability of developing brain and behaviour. *Br Med Bull.* 1974;30:164–168.

Dubinsky JM, Levi Y. Calcium-induced activation of the mitochondrial permeability transition in hippocampal neurons. *J Neurosci Res.* 1998;53:728–741.

Duncan MW. β-Methylamino-L-alanine (BMAA) and amyotrophic lateral sclerosis-parkinsonism dementia of the western Pacific. *Ann NY Acad Sci.* 1992;648:161–168.

Duncan MW, Steele JC, Kopin IJ, et al. 2-Amino-3-(methylamino)-propanoic acid (BMAA) in cycad flour: an unlikely cause of amyotrophic lateral sclerosis and parkinsonism-dementia of Guam. *Neurology.* 1990;40:767–772.

Dyck PJ, O'Brien PC, Ohnishi A. Lead neuropathy: 2. Random distribution of segmental demyelination among "old internodes" of myelinated fibers. *J Neuropathol Exp Neurol.* 1977;36:570–575.

Dyer RS. The use of sensory evoked potentials in toxicology. *Fundam Appl Toxicol.* 1985;5:24–40.

Ebadi M, Sharma S, Shavali S, et al. Neuroprotective actions of selegiline. *J Neurosci Res.* 2002;67:285–289.

Erve JCL, Amarnath V, Graham D, et al. Carbon disulfide and *N,N*-diethyldithiocarbamate generate thiourea cross-links on erythrocyte spectrin. *Chem Res Toxicol.* 1998a;11:544–549.

Erve JCL, Amarnath V, Sills RC, et al. Characterization of a valine-lysine thiourea cross-link on rat globin produced by carbon disulfide or *N,N*-diethyldithiocarbamate in vivo. *Chem Res Toxicol.* 1998b;11:1128–1136.

Evans WC, Evans IA, Humphreys DJ, et al. Induction of thiamine deficiency in sheep with lesions similar to those of cerebro-cortical necrosis. *J Comp Pathol.* 1975;85:253–267.

Federal Register. *Principles of Neurotoxicity Risk Assessment. Environmental Protection Agencyfinal Report.* Vol 59, No 158. Washington, DC: US Government Printing Office; 1994:42360–42404.

Ferraz HB, Bertolucci PH, Pereira JS, et al. Chronic exposure to the fungicide maneb may produce symptoms and signs of CNS manganese intoxication. *Neurology.* 1988;38:550–553.

Fishburne PM, Abelson HI, Cisin I. *National Household Survey on Drug Abuse: National Institute of Drug and Alcohol Abuse Capsules, 1982.* Washington, DC: Department of Health and Human Services; 1983.

Flores G, Buhler DR. Hemolytic properties of hexachlorophene and related chlorinated biphenols. *Biochem Pharmacol.* 1974;23:1835–1843.

Folbergrova J. Glycogen and glycogen phosphorylase in the cerebral cortex of mice under the influence of methionine sulfoximine. *J Neurochem.* 1973;20:547–557.

Fowler JS, Volkow ND, Wang GJ, et al. Inhibition of monoamine oxidase B in the brains of smokers. *Nature.* 1996;379:733–736.

Fox WM. Reflex-ontogeny and behavioural development of the mouse. *Anim Behav.* 1965;13:234–241.

Frey BN, Valvassori SS, Reus GZ, et al. Changes in antioxidant defense enzymes after D-amphetamine exposure: implications as an animal model of mania. *Neurochem Res.* 2006;31:699–703.

Garland TO, Paterson MWH. Six cases of acrylamide poisoning. *Br Med J.* 1967;4:134–138.

Garman RH, Weiss B, Evans HL. Alkylmercurial encephalopathy in the monkey: a histopathologic and autoradiographic study. *Acta Neuropathol (Berlin).* 1975;32:61–74.

Gavin CE, Gunter KK, Gunter TE. Manganese and calcium transport in mitochondria: implications for manganese toxicity. *Neurotoxicology.* 1999;20:445–453.

Gehlbach SH, Williams WA, Perry LD, et al. Green-tobacco sickness: an illness of tobacco harvesters. *JAMA.* 1974;229:1880–1883.

George EB, Glass JD, Griffin JW. Axotomy-induced axonal degeneration is mediated by calcium influx through ion-specific channels. *J Neurosci.* 1995;15:6445–6452.

Gerlach M, Riederer P, Przuntek H, et al. MPTP mechanisms of neurotoxicity and their implications for Parkinson's disease. *Eur J Pharmacol.* 1991;12:273–286.

Gilbert SG, Weiss B. A rationale for lowering the blood lead action level from 10 to 2 microg/dL. *Neurotoxicology.* 2006;27:693–701.

Giros B, Jaber SR, Wightman RM, et al. Hyperlocomotion and indifference to cocaine and amphetamine in mice lacking the dopamine transporter. *Nature.* 1996;379:606–612.

Gold BG. β,β'-Iminodipropionitrile. In: Spencer PS, Schaumburg HH, eds. *Experimental and Clinical Neurotoxicology.* New York: Oxford University Press; 2000:678–679.

Goldberger ME, Murray M. Recovery of function and anatomical plasticity after damage to the adult and neonatal spinal cord. In: Cotman CW, ed. *Synaptic Plasticity.* New York: Guilford Press; 1985:77–110.

Goodrum JF. Role of organotellurium species in tellurium neuropathy. *Neurochem Res.* 1998;23:1313–1319.

Gorell JM, Johnson CC, Rybicki BA, et al. Occupational exposures to metals as risk factors for Parkinson's disease. *Neurology.* 1997;48:650–658.

Gorell JM, Johnson CC, Rybicki BA, et al. The risk of Parkinson's disease with exposure to pesticides, farming, well water and rural living. *Neurology.* 1998;59:1346–1350.

Gorell JM, Johnson CC, Rybicki BA, et al. Occupational exposure to manganese copper, lead, iron, mercury and zinc and the risk of Parkinson's disease. *Neurotoxicology.* 1999;20:239–247.

Gosal D, Ross OA, Toft M. Parkinson's disease: the genetics of a heterogeneous disorder. *Eur J Neurol.* 2006;13:616–627.

Grafstein B. Axonal transport: function and mechanisms. In: Waxman SG, Kocsis JD, Stys PK, eds. *The Axon: Structure, Function, and Pathophysiology.* New York: Oxford University Press; 1995:185–199.

Graham DG, Amarnath V, Valentine WM, et al. Pathogenetic studies of hexane and carbon disulfide neurotoxicity. *CRC Crit Rev Toxicol.* 1995;25:91–112.

Graham DG, Anthony DC, Boekelheide K, et al. Studies of the molecular pathogenesis of hexane neuropathy. II. Evidence that pyrrole derivatization of lysyl residues leads to protein crosslinking. *Toxicol Appl Pharmacol.* 1982;64:415–422.

Graham DI, Lantos PL, eds. *Greenfield's Neuropathology.* 6th ed. New York: Arnold; 1997.

Grandjean P, Herz KT. Methylmercury and brain development: imprecision and underestimation of developmental neurotoxicity in humans. *Mt Sinai J Med.* 2011;78:107–118.

Grandjean P, Landrigan PJ. Developmental neurotoxicity of industrial chemicals. *Lancet.* 2006;368:2167–2178.

Greene JG, Dingledine R, Greenmyre JT. Gene expression profiling of rat midbrain dopamine neurons: implications for selective vulnerability in parkinsonism. *Neurobiol Dis.* 2005;18:19–31.

Griffin JW, Fahnestock KE, Price DL, et al. Microtubule-neurofilament segregation produced by β,β'-iminodipropionitrile: evidence for the association of fast axonal transport with microtubules. *J Neurosci.* 1983;3:557–566.

Grunnet KS, Dahllof I. Environmental fate of the antifouling compound zinc pyrithione in seawater. *Environ Toxicol Chem.* 2005;24:3001–3006.

Gu M, Cooper JM, Taanman JW, et al. Mitochondrial DNA transmission of the mitochondrial defect in Parkinson's disease. *Ann Neurol.* 1998;44:177–186.

Gutierrez PL. The role of NAD(P)H oxidoreductase (DT-Diaphorase) in the bioactivation of quinone-containing antitumor agents: a review. *Free Radic Biol Med.* 2000;29:263–275.

Hardman JG, Limbird LE, Molinoff PB, Ruddon RW, eds. *Goodman and Gilman's The Pharmacological Basis of Therapeutics.* 9th ed. New York: McGraw-Hill; 1996.

Harris CH, Gulati AK, Friedman MA, et al. Toxic neurofilamentous axonopathies and fast axonal transport: V. Reduced bidirectional vesicle transport in cultured neurons by acrylamide and glycidamide. *J Toxicol Environ Health.* 1994;42:343–456.

Harry GJ, Goodrum JF, Bouldin TW, et al. Tellurium-induced neuropathy: metabolic alterations associated with demyelination and remyelination in rat sciatic nerve. *J Neurochem.* 1989;52:938–945.

Hassel B, Sonnewald U, Unsgard G, et al. NMR spectroscopy of cultured astrocytes: effects of glutamine and the gliotoxin fluorocitrate. *J Neurochem.* 1994;62:2187–2194.

Hein ND, Stuckey JA, Rainier SR, Fink JK, Richardson RJ. Constructs of human neuropathy target esterase catalytic domain containing mutations related to motor neuron disease have altered enzymatic properties. *Toxicol Lett.* 2010;196:67–73.

Herning R, King D, Better W, et al. Neurovascular deficits in cocaine abusers. *Neuropsychopharmacology.* 1999;21:110–118.

Hevor TK. Some aspects of carbohydrate metabolism in the brain. *Biochimie.* 1994;76:111–120.

Hirano A, Kurland LT, Krooth RS, et al. Parkinsonism-dementia complex, an endemic disease on the island of Guam. I. Clinical features. *Brain.* 1961a;84:642–661.

Hirano A, Malamud N, Kurland LT. Parkinsonism-dementia complex, an endemic disease on the island of Guam. II. Pathological features. *Brain.* 1961b;84:662–679.

Hoffman PN, Lasek RJ. The slow component of axonal transport: identification of major structural polypeptides of the axon and their generality among mammalian neurons. *J Cell Biol.* 1975;66:351–366.

Hollmann M, Heinemann S. Cloned glutamate receptors. *Ann Rev Neurosci.* 1994;17:31–108.

Hu HL, Bennett N, Holton JL, et al. Glutathione depletion increases brain susceptibility to m-dinitrobenzene neurotoxicity. *NeuroToxicology.* 1999;20:83–90.

Hu HL, Bennett N, Lamb JH, et al. Capacity of rat brain to metabolize m-dinitrobenzene: an in vitro study. *NeuroToxicology.* 1997;18:363–370.

Huber JD, Darling SF, Park K, et al. The role of NMDA receptors in neonatal cocaine-induced neurotoxicity. *Pharmacol Biochem Behav.* 2001;69:451–459.

Hugon J, Ludolph A, Roy DN, et al. Studies on the etiology and pathogenesis of motor neuron diseases: II. Clinical and electrophysiologic features of pyramidal dysfunction in macaques fed *Lathyrus sativus* and IDPN. *Neurology.* 1988;38:435–442.

Ikonomidou C, Bittigau P, Ishimaru MJ, et al. Ethanol-induced apoptotic neurodegeneration and fetal alcohol syndrome. *Science.* 2000;287:1056–1060.

Janoff AS, Pringle MJ, Miller KW. Correlation of general anesthetic potency with solubility in membranes. *Biochim Biophys Acta.* 1981;649:125–128.

Jenner P. Oxidative stress in Parkinson's disease. *Ann Neurol.* 2003;53 (suppl 3):S26–S36.

Johnson DJ, Graham DG, Amarnath V, et al. Release of carbon disulfide is a contributing mechanism in the axonopathy produced by *N,N*-diethyldithiocarbamate. *Toxicol Appl Pharmacol.* 1998;148:288–296.

Johnston MV, Goldstein GW. Selective vulnerability of the developing brain to lead. *Curr Opin Neurol.* 1998;11:689–693.

Kapoor K, Chandra M, Nag D, et al. Evaluation of metronidazole toxicity: a prospective study. *Int J Clin Pharm Res.* 1999;19:83–88.

Kappus H. Oxidative stress in chemical toxicity. *Arch Toxicol.* 1987;60:144–149.

Kesson CM, Baird AW, Lawson DH. Acrylamide poisoning. *Postgrad Med J.* 1977;53:16–17.

Khalil AA, Davies B, Castagnoli N Jr. Isolation and characterization of a monoamine oxidase B selective inhibitor from tobacco smoke. *Bioorg Med Chem.* 2006;14:3392–3398.

Kienzl E, Puchinger L, Jellinger K, et al. The role of transition metals in the pathogenesis of Parkinson's disease. *J Neurol Sci.* 1995;134:69–78.

Kirsten E, Sharma ML, Kun E. Molecular toxicology of (-)erythro-fluorocitrate: selective inhibition of citrate transport I mitochondria and the binding of fluorocitrate to mitochondrial proteins. *Mol Pharmacol.* 1978;14:172–184.

Kisby GE, Ellison M, Spencer PS. Content of the neurotoxins cycasin (methylazoxymethanol beta-D-glucoside) and BMAA (beta-N-methylamino-L-alanine) in cycad flour prepared by Guam Chamorros. *Neurology.* 1992;42:1336–1340.

Klivenyi P, Clair D, Wermer M, et al. Manganese superoxide dismutase overexpression attenuates MPTP toxicity. *Neurobiol Dis.* 1998;5:253–258.

Kniesel U, Wolburg H. Tight junctions of the blood-brain barrier. *Cell Mol Neurobiol.* 2000;20:57–76.

Koehnle TJ, Brown A. Slow axonal transport of neurofilament protein in cultured neurons. *J Cell Biol.* 1999;144:447–458.

Krasavage WJ, O'Donoghue JL, DiVincenzo GD, et al. The relative neurotoxicity of MnBk, *n*-hexane, and their metabolites. *Toxicol Appl Pharmacol.* 1980;52:433–441.

Krichevsky AM, Sonntag KC, Isacson O, Kosik KS. Specific microRNAs modulate embryonic stem cell-derived neurogenesis. *Stem Cells.* 2006;24:857–864.

Kropp TJ, Glynn P, Richardson RJ. The mipafox-inhibited catalytic domain of human neuropathy target esterase ages by reversible proton loss. *Biochemistry.* 2004;43:3716–3722.

Kuopio AM, Marttila RJ, Helenius H, et al. Changing epidemiology of Parkinson's disease in southwestern Finland. *Neurology.* 1999;52:302–308.

Kurland LT, Faro SN, Siedler J. Minamata disease. *World Neurol.* 1960;1:370–395.

Kurland LT. Epidemiological investigations of neurological disorders in the Mariana islands. In: Pemberton J, ed. *Epidemiology Reports on Research and Teaching.* Oxford and New York: Oxford University Press; 1963:219–223.

Kurth JH, Kurth MC, Poduslo SC, Schwankhaus JD. Association of a monoamine oxidase B allele with Parkinson's disease. *Ann Neurol.* 1993;33:368–372.

Kurth MC, Kurth JH. Variant cytochrome P450 CYP2D6 allelic frequencies in Parkinson's disease. *Am J Med Genet.* 1993;48:166–168.

Lai BC, Marion SA, Teschke K, et al. Occupational and environmental risk factors for Parkinson's disease. *Parkinsonism Relat Disord.* 2002;8:297–309.

Lam G-W, DiStefano V. Characterization of carbon disulfide binding in blood and to other biological substances. *Toxicol Appl Pharmacol.* 1986;86:235–242.

LaMonte BH, Wallace KE, Holloway BA, et al. Disruption of dynein/dynactin inhibits axonal transport in motor neurons causing late-onset progressive degeneration. *Neuron.* 2002;34:715–727.

Landigan PJ, Sonawane B, Butler RN, et al. Early environmental origins of neurodegenerative disease in later life. *Environ Health Perspect.* 2005;113:1230–1233.

Langston JW, Ballard P, Tetrud JW, et al. Chronic Parkinsonism in humans due to a product of meperidine-analog synthesis. *Science.* 1983;219:979–980.

Langston JW, Forno LS, Tetrud J, et al. Evidence of active nerve cell degeneration in the substantia nigra of humans years after 1-methyl-4-phenyl-1,2,3,6-tetrahydropyridine exposure. *Ann Neurol.* 1999;46:598–605.

Langston JW, Irwin I. MPTP. Current concepts and controversies. *Clin Neuropharmacol.* 1986;9:485–507.

Lauder JM. Neurotransmitters as growth regulatory signals: role of receptors and second messengers. *Trends Neurosci.* 1993;16:233–240.

LeBel CP, Ali SF, Bondy SC. Deferoxamine inhibits methyl mercury-induced increases in reactive oxygen species formation in rat brain. *Toxicol Appl Pharmacol.* 1992;112:161–165.

Lehning EJ, Jortner BS, Fox JH, et al. γ-Diketone peripheral neuropathy. I. Quantitative morphometric analyses of axonal atrophy and swelling. *Toxicol Appl Pharmacol*. 2000;165:127–140.

Lemasters JJ, Nieminen AL, Qian T, et al. The mitochondrial permeability transition in cell death: a common mechanism in necrosis, apoptosis and autophagy. *Biochim Biophys Acta*. 1998;366:177–196.

Letzel S, Lang CJ, Schaller KH, et al. Longitudinal study of neurotoxicity with occupational exposure to aluminum dust. *Neurology*. 2000;54: 997–1000.

Lewis JA, Tran BL, Puerta DT, et al. Synthesis, structure and spectroscopy of new thiopyrone and hydroxypyridine transition-metal complexes. *Dalton Trans*. 2005;7:2588–2596.

Lichensteiger W, Ribary U, Schlumpf M, et al. Prenatal adverse effects of nicotine on the developing brain. In: Boer GJ, Feenstra MGP, Mirmiran M, et al., eds. *Progress in Brain Research*. Vol 73. Amsterdam: Elsevier; 1988:137–157.

Liou HH, Tsai MC, Chen CJ, et al. Environmental risk factors and Parkinson's disease: a case-control study in Taiwan. *Neurology*. 1997;48:1583–1588.

Lipton RB, Apfel SC, Dutcher JP, et al. Taxol produces a predominantly sensory neuropathy. *Neurology*. 1989;39:368–373.

Lipton SA, Rosenberg PA. Excitatory amino acids as a final common pathway for neurologic disorders. *N Engl J Med*. 1994;330:613–622.

Liu Y, Fechter LD. Comparison of the effects of trimethyltin on the intracellular calcium levels in spiral ganglion cells and outer hair cells. *Acta Otolaryngol*. 1996;116:417–421.

Llorens J, Dememes D, Sans A. The behavioral syndrome caused by 3,3'-iminodipropionitrile and related nitriles in the rat is associated with degeneration of the vestibular sensory hair cells. *Toxicol Appl Pharmacol*. 1993;123:199–210.

Logroscino G. The role of early life environmental risk factors in Parkinson disease: what is the evidence? *Environ. Health Perspect*. 2005;113:1234–1238.

LoPachin RM, Jortner BS, Reid ML, et al. γ-Diketone central neuropathy: quantitative analyses of cytoskeletal components in myelinated axons of the rat rubrospinal tract. *Neurotoxicology*. 2005;26:1021–1030.

LoPachin RM, Ross JF, Reid ML, et al. Neurological evaluation of toxic axonopathies in rats: acrylamide and 2,5-hexanedione. *Neurotoxicology*. 2002;23:95–110.

Lotharius J, O'Malley KL. The parkinsonian-inducing drug 1-methyl-4-phenylpyridinium triggers intracellular dopamine oxidation. *J Biol Chem*. 2000;275:38581–38588.

Lotharius J, O'Malley KL. Role of mitochondrial dysfunction and dopamine-dependent oxidative stress in amphetamine-induced toxicity. *Ann Neurol*. 2001;49:79–89.

Lotti M. Promotion of organophosphate induced delayed polyneuropathy by certain esterase inhibitors. *Toxicology*. 2002;181–182:245–248.

Lotti M, Moretto A. Organophosphate-induced delayed polyneuropathy. *Toxicol Rev*. 2005;24:37–49.

Lucey JF, Hibbard E, Behrman RE, et al. Kernicterus in asphyxiated newborn rhesus monkeys. *Exp Neurol*. 1964;9:43–58.

Ludolph AC, He F, Spencer PS, et al. 3-Nitropropionic acid: exogenous animal neurotoxin and possible human striatal toxin. *Can J Neurol Sci*. 1991;18:492–498.

Ludolph AC, Seelig M, Ludolf A, et al. 3-Nitropropionic acid decreases cellular energy levels and causes neuronal degeneration in cortical explants. *Neurodegeneration*. 1992;1:155–161.

Magyar K, Szende B. (−)-Deprenyl, a selective MAO-B inhibitor, with apoptotic and anti-apoptotic properties. *Neurotoxicology*. 2004;25:233–242.

Makri A, Goveia M, Balbus J, et al. Children's susceptibility to chemicals: a review by developmental stage. *J Toxicol Environ Health Part B*. 2004;7:417–435.

Mandel S, Grunblatt E, Riederer P, et al. Neuroprotective strategies in Parkinson's disease: an update on progress. *CNS Drugs*. 2003;17: 729–762.

Mandel S, Weinreb O, Amit T, et al. Mechanism of neuroprotective action of the anti-Parkinson drug rasagiline and its derivatives. *Brain Res Brain Res Rev*. 2005;48:379–387.

Martin DL, Waniewski RA. Precursor synthesis and neurotransmitter uptake by astrocytes as targets of neurotoxicants. In: Aschner M, Kimelberg HK, eds. *The Role of Glia in Neurotoxicity*. Boca Raton: CRC Press; 1996:335–357.

Marty MS, Atchison WD. Pathways mediating Ca²⁺ entry in rat cerebellar granule cells following in vitro exposure to methyl mercury. *Toxicol Appl Pharmacol*. 1997;147:319–330.

Mastrogiacomo F, Bergeron C, Kish SJ. Brain alpha-ketoglutarate dehydrogenase complex activity in Alzheimer's disease. *J Neurochem*. 1993;61:2007–2014.

Mattsson JL, Albee RR, Eisenbrandt DL. Neurological approach to neurotoxicological examination in laboratory animals. *Int J Toxicol*. 1989;8:271–286.

McCann UD, Ricaurte GA. Amphetamine neurotoxicity: accomplishments and remaining challenges. *Neurosci Behav Rev*. 2004;27:821–826.

McMillan DE. A brief history of the neurobehavioral toxicity of manganese: some unanswered questions. *Neurotoxicology*. 1999;20: 499–507.

Meldrum B. Excitatory amino acid antagonists as potential therapeutic agents. In: Jenner P, ed. *Neurotoxins and Their Pharmacological Implications*. New York: Raven Press; 1987:33–53.

Mielke S, Sparreboom A, Mross K. Peripheral neuropathy: a persisting challenge in paclitaxel-based regimes. *Eur J Cancer*. 2006;42:24–30.

Miller DB. Neurotoxicity of the pesticidal carbamates. *Neurobehav Toxicol Teratol*. 1982;4:779–787.

Miller DB, O'Callaghan JP. Elevated environmental temperature and methamphetamine neurotoxicity. *Environ Res*. 2003;92:48–53.

Miodovnik A. Environmental neurotoxicants and developing brain. *Mt Sinai J Med*. 2011;78:58–77.

Mitsuishi K, Takahashi A, Mizutani M, et al. Beta, beta'-iminodipropionitrile toxicity in normal and congenitally neurofilament-deficient Japanese quails. *Acta Neuropathol*. 1993;86:578–581.

Montgomery EB Jr. Heavy metals and the etiology of Parkinson's disease and other movement disorders. *Toxicology*. 1995;97:3–9.

Monuki ES, Lemke G. Molecular biology of myelination. In: Waxman SG, Kocsis JD, Stys PK, eds. *The Axon: Structure, Function, and Pathophysiology*. New York: Oxford University Press; 1995:144–163.

Moreira EG, Vassilieff I, Vassilieff VS. Developmental lead exposure: behavioral alterations in the short and long term. *Neurotoxicol Teratol*. 2001;23:489–495.

Morell P, Toews AD, Wagner M, et al. Gene expression during tellurium-induced primary demyelination. *Neurotoxicology*. 1994;15:171–180.

Morgan RE, Garavan H, Smith EG, et al. Early lead exposure produces lasting changes in sustained attention, response initiation, and reactivity to errors. *Neurotoxicol Teratol*. 2001;23:519–531.

Moser VC, Becking GC, Cuomo V, et al. The IPCS collaborative study on neurobehavioral screening methods: V. Results of chemical testing. *Neurotoxicology*. 1997a;18:969–1055.

Moser VC, Becking GC, Cuomo V, et al. The IPCS collaborative study on neurobehavioral screening methods. III. Results of proficiency studies. *Neurotoxicology*. 1997b;18:939–946.

Moser VC, Padilla S. Age- and gender-related differences in the time-course of behavioral and biochemical effects produced by oral chlorpyrifos in rats. *Toxicol Appl Pharmacol*. 1998;149:107–119.

Moser VC. Observational batteries in neurotoxicity testing. *Int J Toxicol*. 2000;19:407–411.

Mossakowski MJ, Renkawek K, Krasnicka Z, et al. Morphology and histochemistry of Wilsonian and hepatic gliopathy in tissue culture. *Acta Neuropathol. (Berlin)* 1970;16:1–16.

Mullick FG. Hexachlorophene toxicity: human experience at the AFIP. *Pediatrics*. 1973;51:395–399.

Mulugeta S, Ciavarra RP, Maney RK, et al. Three subpopulations of fast axonally transported retinal ganglion cell proteins are differentially trafficked in the rat optic pathway. *J Neurosci Res*. 2000;59: 247–258.

Muralikrishnan D, Samantaray S, Mohanakumar KP. D-Deprenyl protects nigrostriatal neurons against 1-methyl-4-1,2,3,6-tetrahydropyridine-induced dopaminergic neurotoxicity. *Synapse*. 2003;50:7–13.

Mushiroda T, Ariyoshi N, Yokoi T, et al. Accumulation of the 1-methyl-4-pyridinium ion in suncus (*Suncus murinus*) brain: implication for flavin-containing monooxygenase activity in brain microvessels. *Chem Res Toxicol.* 2001;14:228–232.

Myers JE, Macun I. Acrylamide neuropathy in a South African factory: an epidemiologic investigation. *Am J Indust Med.* 1991;19:487–493.

Myers RR, Mizisin AP, Powell HC, et al. Reduced nerve blood flow in hexachlorophene neuropathy: relationship to elevated endoneurial pressure. *J Neuropathol Exp Neurol.* 1982;41:391–399.

Nakata T, Yorifuji H. Morphological evidence of the inhibitory effect of taxol on the fast axonal transport. *Neurosci Res.* 1999;35:113–122.

Naoi M, Maruyama W, Akao Y, et al. Dopamine-derived endogenous *N*-methyl-(*R*)-solsolinol: its role in Parkinson's disease. *Neurotoxicol Teratol.* 2002;24:579–591.

National Research Council (NRC). *Toxicity Testing in the 21ˢᵗ Century: A Vision and a Strategy.* Washington, DC: National Academies Press; 2007.

Needleman HL. Childhood lead poisoning. *Curr Opin Neurol.* 1994;7:187–190.

Needleman HL, Gatsonis CA. Low-level lead exposure and the IQ of children. A meta-analysis of modern studies. *JAMA.* 1990;263:673–678.

Nihei MK, Desmond NL, McGlothan JL, et al. *N*-Methyl-D-aspartate receptor subunit changes are associated with lead-induced deficits of long-term potentiation and spatial learning. *Neuroscience.* 2000;99:233–242.

Nixon RA. Dynamic behavior and organization of cytoskeleton proteins in neurons: reconciling old and new findings. *Bioessays.* 1998;20:798–807.

Nunn PB, Seelig M, Zagoren JC, et al. Stereospecific acute neurotoxicity of "uncommon" plant amino acids linked to human motor system diseases. *Brain Res.* 1987;410:375–379.

O'Shea KS, Kaufman MH. The teratogenic effect of acetaldehyde: implications for the study of fetal alcohol syndrome. *J Anat.* 1979;128:65–76.

Oestreicher E, Sengstock GJ, Riederer P, et al. Degeneration of nigrostriatal dopaminergic neurons increases iron within the substantia nigra: a histochemical and neurochemical study. *Brain Res.* 1994;660:8–18.

Okeda R, Shibutani M, Matsuo T, et al. Experimental neurotoxicity of 5-fluorouracil and its derivatives is due to poisoning by the monofluorinated organic metabolites, monofluoroacetic acid and alpha-fluoro-beta-alanine. *Acta Neuropathol. (Berlin)* 1990;81:66–73.

Olney JW. Neurotoxicity of excitatory amino acids. In: McGeer EG, Olney JW, McGeer PL, eds. *Kainic Acid as a Tool in Neurobiology.* New York: Raven Press; 1978:95–122.

Padilla S, Atkinson MB, Breuer AC. Direct measurement of fast axonal organelle transport in the sciatic nerve of rats treated with acrylamide. *J Toxicol Environ Health.* 1993;39:429–445.

Padilla S, Grizzle TB, Lyerly D. Triphenyl phosphite: in vivo and in vitro inhibition of rat neurotoxic esterase. *Toxicol Appl Pharmcol.* 1987;87:249–256.

Pardridge WM. Blood-brain barrier biology and methodology. *J Neurovirol.* 1999;5:556–569.

Parent A. *Carpenter's Human Neuroanatomy.* 9th ed. Baltimore: Williams & Wilkins; 1996:131–198.

Parenti M, Rusconi L, Cappabianca V, et al. Role of dopamine in manganese neurotoxicity. *Brain Res.* 1988;473:236–240.

Patanow CM, Day JR, Billingsley ML. Alterations in hippocampal expression of SNAP-25, GAP-43, stannin and glial fibrillary acidic protein following mechanical and trimethyltin-induced injury in the rat. *Neuroscience.* 1997;76:187–202.

Penny DG. Acute carbon monoxide poisoning: animal models: a review. *Toxicology.* 1990;62:123–160.

Perl TM, Bedard L, Kosatsky T, et al. An outbreak of toxic encephalopathy caused by eating mussels contaminated with domoic acid. *N Engl J Med.* 1990;322:1775–1780.

Perlson E, Maday S, Fu MM, Moughamian AJ, Holzbaur EL. Retrograde axonal transport: pathways to cell death? *Trends Neurosci.* 2010;33:335–344.

Perlstein MA, Attala R. Neurologic sequelae of plumbism in children. *Clin Pediatr.* 1966;5:292–298.

Peterson RT, Nass R, Boyd WA, Freedman JH, Dong K, Narahashi T. Use of non-mammalian alternative models for neurotoxicological study. *Neurotoxicology.* 2008;29:546–555.

Pham-Dinh D, Popot JL, Boespflug-Tanguy O, et al. Pelizaeus-Merzbacher disease: a valine to phenylalanine point mutation in a putative extracellular loop of myelin proteolipid. *Proc Natl Acad Sci USA.* 1991;88:7562–7566.

Phelps CH. An ultrastructural study of methionine sulphoximine-induced glycogen accumulation in astrocytes of the mouse cerebral cortex. *J Neurocytol.* 1975;4:479–490.

Philbert MA, Nolan CC, Cremer JE, et al. 1,3-Dinitrobenzene-induced encephalopathy in rats. *Neuropathol Appl Neurobiol.* 1987;13:371–389.

Pierard-Franchimont C, Goffin V, Decroix J, et al. A multicenter randomized trial of ketoconazole 2% and zinc pyrithione 1% shampoos in severe dandruff and seborrheic dermatitis. *Skin Pharmacol Appl Skin Physiol.* 2002;15:434–441.

Plato CC, Galasko D, Garruto R, et al. ALS and PDC of Guam: forty-year follow-up. *Neurology.* 2002;58:765–773.

Plato CC, Garruto RM, Galasko D, et al. Amyotrophic lateral sclerosis and parkinsonism-dementia complex of Guam: changing incidence rates during the past 60 years. *Am J Epidemiol.* 2003;157:149–157.

Plum F, Posner JB. Neurobiologic essentials. In: Smith LH Jr, Thier SO, eds. *Pathophysiology: The Biological Principles of Disease.* Philadelphia: Saunders; 1985:1009–1036.

Polymerpoulos MH, Lavedan C, Leroy E, et al. Mutation in the alphasynuclein gene identified in families with Parkinson's disease. *Science.* 1997;276:2045–2047.

Pope CN. Organophosphorus pesticides: do they all have the same mechanism of toxicity? *J Toxicol Environ Health B.* 1999;2:161–181.

Pope CN, Tanaka D Jr, Padilla S. The role of neurotoxic esterase (NTE) in the prevention and potentiation of organophosphorus-induced delayed neurotoxicity (OPIDN). *Chem Biol Interact.* 1993;87:395–406.

Portela A, Esteller M. Epigenetic modifications and human disease. *Nat Biotechnol.* 2010;28:1057–1068.

Porterfield SP. Vulnerability of the developing brain to thyroid abnormalities: environmental insults to the thyroid system. *Environ Health Perspect.* 1994;102(suppl 2):125–130.

Porterfield SP. Thyroidal dysfunction and environmental chemicals—potential impact on brain development. *Environ Health Perspect.* 2000;108(suppl 3):433–438.

Powell HC, Myers RR, Lampert PW. Changes in Schwann cells and vessels in lead neuropathy. *Am J Pathol.* 1982;109:193–205.

Prakash V, Timasheff SN. Aging of tubulin at neutral pH: the destabilizing effect of Vinca alkaloids. *Arch Biochem Biophys.* 1992;295:137–145.

Przedborski S, Tieu K, Perier C, et al. MPTP as a mitochondrial neurotoxic model of Parkinson's disease. *J Bioenerg Biomembr.* 2004;36:375–379.

Purves DC, Garrod IJ, Dayan AD. A comparison of spongiosis induced in the brain by hexachlorophene, cuprizone, and triethyl tin in the Sprague-Dawley rat. *Hum Exp Toxicol.* 1991;10:439–444.

Qiu J, Cai D, Filbin MT. Glial inhibition of nerve regeneration in mature mammalian CNS. *Glia.* 2000;29:166–174.

Quarles RH, Farrer RG, Yim SH. Structure and function of myelin, an extended and biochemically modified cell surface membrane. In: Juurlink BHJ, Devon RM, Doucette JR, et al., eds. *Cell Biology and Pathology of Myelin: Evolving Biological Concepts and Therapeutic Approaches.* New York: Plenum Press; 1997:1–12.

Quik M. Smoking, nicotine and Parkinson's disease. *Trends Neurosci.* 2004;27:561–568.

Quik M, Parameswaran N, McCallum SE, et al. Chronic oral nicotine treatment protects against striatal degeneration in MPTP-treated primates. *J Neurochem.* 2006;98:1866–1875.

Rainier S, Albers JW, Dyck PJ, et al. Motor neuron disease due to neuropathy target esterase gene mutation: clinical features of the index families. *Muscle Nerve.* 2011;43:19–25.

Rakonczay Z, Matsuoka Y, Giacobini E. Effects of L-beta-N-methylamino-L-alanine (L-BMAA) on the cortical cholinergic and glutamatergic systems of the rat. *J Neurosci Res.* 1991;29:121–126.

Randall JC, Yano BL, Richardson RJ. Potentiation of organophosphorus compound-induced delayed neurotoxicity (OPIDN) in the central and peripheral nervous system of the adult hen: distribution of axonal lesions. *J Toxicol Environ Health.* 1997;51:571–590.

Ray DE, Abbott NJ, Chan MW, et al. Increased oxidative metabolism and oxidative stress in m-dinitrobenzene neurotoxicity. *Biochem Soc Trans.* 1994;22:407S.

Ray DE, Brown AW, Cavanagh JB, et al. Functional/metabolic modulation of the brain stem lesions caused by 1,3-dinitrobenzene in the rat. *Neurotoxicology.* 1992;13:379–388.

Readhead C, Schneider A, Griffiths I, et al. Premature arrest of myelin formation in transgenic mice with increased proteolipid protein gene dosage. *Neuron.* 1994;12:583–595.

Reuhl KR, Chang LW. Effects of methylmercury on the development of the nervous system: a review. *Neurotoxicology.* 1979;1:21–55.

Reuhl KR, Gilbert SG, Mackenzie BA, et al. Acute trimethyltin intoxication in the monkey *(Macaca fascicularis). Toxicol Appl Pharmacol.* 1985;79:436–452.

Riachi NJ, Dietrich WD, Harik SI. Effects of internal carotid administration of MPTP on rat brain and blood-brain barrier. *Brain Res.* 1990;533:6–14.

Rice D, Barone S Jr. Critical periods of vulnerability for the developing nervous system: evidence from humans and animal models. *Environ Health Perspect.* 2000;108(suppl 3):511–533.

Rice DC. Evidence for delayed neurotoxicity produced by methylmercury. *Neurotoxicology.* 1996;17:583–596.

Richardson RJ. Interactions of organophosphorus compounds with neurotoxic esterase. In: Chambers JE, Levi PE, eds. *Organophosphates: Chemistry, Fate, and Effects.* San Diego: Academic Press; 1992:299–323.

Richardson RJ. Organophosphate poisoning, delayed neurotoxicity. In: Wexler P, ed. *Encyclopedia of Toxicology.* 2nd ed. Oxford: Elsevier; 2005:302–306.

Richardson RJ. Anticholinesterase insecticides. In: McQueen C. ed. *Comprehensive Toxicology.* Vol 13, 2nd ed. Oxford: Academic Press; 2010: 433–444.

Richardson RJ, Worden RM, Makhaeva GF. Biomarkers and biosensors of delayed neuropathic agents. In: Gupta RC, ed. *Handbook of Toxicology of Chemical Warfare Agents.* Amsterdam: Academic Press/Elsevier; 2009:859–876.

Ridgway P, Nixon TE, Leach JP. Occupational exposure to organic solvents and long-term nervous system damage detectable by brain imaging, neurophysiology or histopathology. *Food Chem Toxicol.* 2003;41:153–187.

Riggs JE. Cigarette smoking and Parkinson's disease: the illusion of a neuroprotective effect. *Clin Neuropharmacol.* 1992;15:88–99.

Riggs JE, Schochet SS, Gutmann L, et al. Chronic human colchicine neuropathy and myopathy. *Arch Neurol.* 1986;43:521–523.

Riikonen R, Salonen I, Partanen K, et al. Brain perfusion SPECT and MRI in foetal alcohol syndrome. *Dev Med Child Neurol.* 1999;41:652–659.

Rodgers-Johnson P, Garruto RM, Yanagihara R, et al. Amyotrophic lateral sclerosis and parkinsonism-dementia on Guam: a 30-year evaluation of clinical and neuropathologic trends. *Neurology.* 1986;36:7–13.

Rodier PM. Developing brain as a target of toxicity. *Environ Health Perspect.* 1995;103(suppl 6):73–76.

Romero I, Brown AW, Cavanagh JB, et al. Vascular factors in the neurotoxic damage caused by 1,3-dinitrobenzene in the rat. *Neuropathol Appl Neurobiol.* 1991;17:495–508.

Romero IA, Lister T, Richards HK, et al. Early metabolic changes during m-dinitrobenzene neurotoxicity and the possible role of oxidative stress. *Free Radic Biol Med.* 1995;18:311–319.

Ross GW, Petrovitch H. Current evidence for neuroprotective effects of nicotine and caffeine against Parkinson's disease. *Drugs Aging.* 2001;18:797–806.

Ross JF, Lawhorn GT. ZPT-related distal axonopathy: behavioral and electrophysiologic correlates in rats. *Neurotoxicol Teratol.* 1990;12:153–159.

Rothman SM, Olney JM. Glutamate and the pathophysiology of hypoxic-ischemic brain damage. *Ann Neurol.* 1986;19:105–111.

Rothstein JD, Tabakoff B. Regulation of neurotransmitter aspartate metabolism by glial glutamine synthetase. *J Neurochem.* 1986;46:1923–1928.

Roytta M, Horwitz SB, Raine CS. Taxol-induced neuropathy: short-term effects of local injection. *J Neurocytol.* 1984;13:685–701.

Rubin LL, Staddon JM. The cell biology of the blood-brain barrier. *Annu Rev Neurosci.* 1999;22:11–28.

Sahenk Z, Barohn R, New P, et al. Taxol neuropathy: electrodiagnostic and sural nerve biopsy findings. *Arch Neurol.* 1994;51:726–729.

Sahenk Z, Mendell JR. Ultrastructural study of zinc pyrdinethione-induced peripheral neuropathy. *J Neuropathol Exp Neurol.* 1979;38:532–550.

Sahenk Z, Mendell JR. Axoplasmic transport in zinc pyridinethione neuropathy: evidence for an abnormality in distal turn-around. *Brain Res.* 1980;186:343–353.

Sahenk Z, Mendell JR. Pyrithione. In: Spencer PS, Schaumburg HH, eds. *Experimental and Clinical Neurotoxicology.* New York: Oxford University Press; 2000:1050–1054.

Sampson PD, Streissguth AP, Bookstein FL, et al. On categorizations in analyses of alcohol teratogenesis. *Environ Health Perspect.* 2000;108(suppl 3):421–428.

Sayre LM, Shearson CM, Wongmongkolrit T, et al. Structural basis of γ-diketone neurotoxicity: non-neurotoxicity of 3,3-dimethyl-2,5-hexanedione a γ-diketone incapable of pyrrole formation. *Toxicol Appl Pharmacol.* 1986;84:36–44.

Schaumburg HH. Vinca alkaloids. In: Spencer PS, Schaumburg HH, eds. *Experimental and Clinical Neurotoxicology.* New York: Oxford University Press; 2000:1232–1236.

Schaumburg HH, Wisniewski HM, Spencer PS. Ultrastructural studies of the dying-back process I. Peripheral nerve terminal and axon degeneration in systemic acrylamide intoxication. *J Neuropathol Exp Neurol.* 1974;33:260–284.

Schentag JJ. Mental confusion in a patient treated with metronidazole—a concentration-related effect? *Pharmacotherapy.* 1982;2:384–387.

Schiff PB, Horwitz SB. Taxol assembles tubulin in the absence of exogenous guanosine 59-triphosphate or microtubule-associated proteins. *Biochemistry.* 1981;20:3242–3252.

Schinder AF, Olson EC, Spitzer NC, et al. Mitochondrial dysfunction is a primary event in glutamate neurotoxicity. *J Neurosci.* 1996;16: 6125–6133.

Schionning JD, Larsen JO, Tandrup T, et al. Selective degeneration of dorsal root ganglia and dorsal nerve roots in methyl mercury–intoxicated rats: a stereological study. *Acta Neuropathol.* 1998;96:191–201.

Schlafer WW, Zimmerman U-JP. Calcium-activated protease and the regulation of the axonal cytoskeleton. In: Elam JS, Cancalon P, eds. *Advances in Neurochemistry.* New York: Plenum Press; 1984:261–273.

Schnapp BJ, Reese TS. Dynein is the motor for retrograde axonal transport of organelles. *Proc Natl Acad Sci USA.* 1989;86:1548–1552.

Schneider D, Wink M, Sporer F, et al. Cycads: their evolution, toxins, herbivores and insect pollinators. *Naturwissenschaften.* 2002;89:281–294.

Schoepfer R, Monyer H, Sommer B, et al. Molecular biology of glutamate receptors. *Prog Neurobiol.* 1994;42:353–357.

Schutzman DL, Frankenfield-Chernicoff M, Clatterbaugh HE, et al. Incidence of intrauterine cocaine exposure in a suburban setting. *Pediatrics.* 1991;88:825–827.

Schwartz JH. The cytology of neurons. In: Kandel ER, Schwartz JH, Jessell TM, eds. *Principles of Neural Science.* 3nd ed. Norwalk, CT: Appleton & Lange; 1991:37–48.

Scriba GK, Borchardt RT. Metabolism of 1-methyl-4-phenyl-1,2,3,6-tetrahydropyridine (MPTP) by bovine brain microvessel endothelial cells. *Brain Res.* 1989;501:175–178.

Seawright AA, Brown AW, Nolan CC, et al. Selective degeneration of cerebellar cortical neurons caused by cycad neurotoxin, L-beta-methylaminoalanine (L-BMAA), in rats. *Neuropathol Appl Neurobiol.* 1990;16:153–164.

Seegal RF. Epidemiological and laboratory evidence of PCB-induced neurotoxicity. *Crit Rev Toxicol.* 1996;26:709–737.

Selevan SG, Kimmel CA, Mendola P. Identifying critical windows of exposure for children's health. *Environ Health Perspect.* 2000:108 (suppl 3):451–455.

Seppaleinen AM, Haltia M. Carbon disulfide. In: Spencer PS, Schaumburg HH, eds. *Experimental and Clinical Neurotoxicology.* Baltimore: Williams & Wilkins; 1980:356–373.

Shanker G, Mutkus LA, Walker S, et al. Methylmercury enhances arachidonic acid release and cytosolic phospholipase A_2 expression in primary cultures of neonatal astrocytes. *Mol Brain Res.* 2002;106:1–11.

Sieber SM, Correa P, Dalgard DW, et al. Carcinogenicity and hepatotoxicity of cycasin and its aglycone methylazoxymethanol acetate in nonhuman primates. *J Natl Cancer Inst.* 1980;65:177–189.

Slikker W Jr, Xu ZA, Levin ED, et al. Mode of action: disruption of brain cell replication, second messenger, and neurotransmitter systems during development leading to cognitive dysfunction—developmental neurotoxicity of nicotine. *Crit Rev Toxicol.* 2005;35:703–711.

Slotkin TA. Cholinergic systems in brain development and disruption by neurotoxicants: nicotine, environmental tobacco smoke, organophosphates. *Toxicol Appl Pharmacol.* 2004;15:132–151.

Smith RA. Twenty-first century challenges for in vitro neurotoxicity. *Altern Lab Anim.* 2009;37:367–375.

Snow BJ, Vingerhoets FJ, Langston JW, et al. Pattern of dopaminergic loss in the striatum of humans with MPTP induced parkinsonism. *J Neurol Neurosurg Psychiatry.* 2000;68:313–316.

Spencer PS. Doxorubicin and related anthracyclines. In: Spencer PS, Schaumburg HH, eds. *Experimental and Clinical Neurotoxicology.* New York: Oxford University Press; 2000:529–533.

Spencer PS, Nunn PB, Hugon J, et al. Guam amyotrophic lateral sclerosis-parkinsonism-dementia linked to a plant excitant neurotoxin. *Science.* 1987;237:517–522.

Spencer PS, Schaumburg HH. Ultrastructural studies of the dying-back process III. The evolution of experimental peripheral giant axonal degeneration. *J Neuropathol Exp Neurol.* 1974;36:276.

Spencer PS, Schaumburg HH. Central-peripheral distal axonopathy: The pathology of dying-back polyneuropathies. In: Zimmerman H, ed. *Progress in Neuropathology.* Vol 3. New York: Grune & Stratton; 1976:253–295.

Spencer PS, Schaumburg HH, eds. *Experimental and Clinical Neurotoxicology.* 2nd ed. New York: Oxford University Press; 2000.

St. Clair MBG, Amarnath V, Moody MA, et al. Pyrrole oxidation and protein crosslinking are necessary steps in the development of γ-diketone neuropathy. *Chem Res Toxicol.* 1988;1:179–185.

Stewart PA. Endothelial vesicles in the blood-brain barrier: are they related to permeability? *Cell Mol Neurobiol.* 2000;20:149–163.

Stoll G, Muller HW. Nerve injury, axonal degeneration and neural regeneration: basic insights. *Brain Pathol.* 1999;9:313–325.

Stoltenburg-Didinger G, Spohr HL. Fetal alcohol syndrome and mental retardation: spine distribution of pyramidal cells in prenatal alcohol exposed rat cerebral cortex. *Brain Res.* 1983;11:119–123.

Stys P. General mechanisms of axonal damage and its prevention. *J Neurol Sci.* 2005;233:3–13.

Swanson RA, Graham SH. Fluorocitrate and fluoroacetate effects on astrocyte metabolism in vitro. *Brain Res.* 1994;664:94–100.

Takeuchi T, Morikawa H, Matsumoto H, et al. A pathological study of Minamata disease in Japan. *Acta Neuropathol.* 1962;2:40–57.

Tanner CM, Ottman R, Goldman SM, et al. Parkinson disease in twins: an etiologic study. *JAMA.* 1999;281:341–346.

Teitelbaum JS, Zatorre RJ, Carpenter S, et al. Neurologic sequelae of domoic acid intoxication due to the ingestion of contaminated mussels. *N Engl J Med.* 1990;322:1781–1787.

Thompson CM, Richardson RJ. Anticholinesterase insecticides. In: Marrs TC, Ballantyne B, eds. *Pesticide Toxicology and International Regulation.* Chichester: John Wiley & Sons, Ltd; 2004:89–127.

Tilson HA. Neurobehavioral methods used in neurotoxicological research. *Toxicol Lett.* 1993;68:231–240.

Tilson HA, Kodavanti PR. The neurotoxicity of polychlorinated biphenyls. *Neurotoxicology.* 1998;19:517–525.

Tilson HA, Moser VC. Comparison of screening approaches. *Neurotoxicology.* 1992;13:1–14.

Tjalkens RB, Ewing MM, Philbert MA. Differential cellular regulation of the mitochondrial permeability transition in an in vitro model of 1,3-dinitrobenzene-induced encephalopathy. *Brain Res.* 2000;874:165–177.

Toggas SM, Krady JK, Thompson TA, et al. Molecular mechanisms of selective neurotoxicants: studies on organotin compounds. *Ann NY Acad Sci.* 1993;679:157–177.

Tomas-Camardiel M, Herrera AJ, Venero JL, et al. Differential regulation of glutamic acid decarboxylase mRNA and tyrosine hydroxylase mRNA expression in the aged manganese-treated rats. *Brain Res Mol Brain Res.* 2002;103:116–129.

Turchan J, Anderson C, Hauser KF, et al. Estrogen protects against the synergistic toxicity by HIV proteins, methamphetamine and cocaine. *BMC Neurosci.* 2001;2:3–13.

US Department of Health and Human Services, Substance Abuse and Mental Health Services Administration, Office of Applied Studies. *National Household Study on Drug Abuse, 2001.* Washington, DC: USDHHS.

US Environmental Protection Agency. *Water Quality Criterion for the Protection of Human Health: Methyl Mercury.* EPA-823-R-01-001. Washington, DC: Office of Science and Technology, Office of Water, Environmental Protection Agency; 2001.

Uversky VN. Neurotoxicant-induced animal models of Parkinson's disease: understanding the role of rotenone, maneb and paraquat in neurodegeneration. *Cell Tissue Res.* 2004;318:225–241.

Valentine WM, Amarnath V, Amarnath K, et al. Carbon disulfide-mediated protein cross-linking by N,N-diethyldithiocarbamate. *Chem Res Toxicol.* 1995;8:96–102.

Valentine WM, Amarnath V, Graham DG, et al. Covalent cross-linking of proteins by carbon disulfide. *Chem Res Toxicol.* 1992;5:254–262.

Valentine WM, Amarnath V, Graham DG, et al. CS_2 mediated cross-linking of erythrocyte spectrin and neurofilament protein: dose response and temporal relationship to the formation of axonal swellings. *Toxicol Appl Pharmacol.* 1997;142:95–105.

Valentine WM, Graham DG, Anthony DC. Covalent cross-linking of erythrocyte spectrin in vivo. *Toxicol Appl Pharmacol.* 1993;121:71–77.

Van de Kamp JL, Collins AC. Prenatal nicotine alters nicotinic receptor development in the mouse brain. *Pharmacol Biochem Behav.* 1994;47:889–900.

Van der Hoek JA, Verberk MM, Hageman G. Criteria for solvent-induced chronic toxic encephalopathy: a systematic review. *Int Arch Occup Environ Health.* 2000;73:362–368.

Veronesi B, Jones K, Gupta S, et al. Myelin basic protein-messenger RNA (MBP-mRNA) expression during triethyltin-induced myelin edema. *Neurotoxicology.* 1991;12:265–276.

Volpe JJ. Effect of cocaine use on the fetus. *N Engl J Med.* 1992;327:399–407.

Wang L, Ho CL, Sun D, et al. Rapid movement of axonal neurofilaments interrupted by prolonged pauses. *Nat Cell Biol.* 2000;2:137–141.

Wang Y, Qin ZH. Molecular and cellular mechanisms of excitotoxic neuronal death. *Apoptosis.* 2010;15:1382–1402.

Watanabe I, Kanabe S. Early edematous lesion of pyrithiamine-induced acute thiamine deficient encephalopathy in the mouse. *J Neuropath Exp Neurol.* 1978;37:401–413.

Wedler FC. Biological significance of manganese in mammalian systems. *Prog Med Chem.* 1993;30:89–133.

Wijeyesakere SJ, Richardson RJ. Neuropathy target esterase. In: Krieger R, ed. *Hayes' Handbook of Pesticide Toxicology.* 3rd ed. San Diego: Elsevier/Academic Press; 2010:1435–1478.

Winneke G, Altmann L, Kramer U, et al. Neurobehavioral and neurophysiological observations in six-year-old children with low lead levels in East and West Germany. *Neurotoxicology.* 1994;15:705–713.

Wood SL, Beyer BK, Cappon GD. Species comparison of postnatal CNS development: functional measures. *Birth Defects Res. (Part B)* 2003;68:391–407.

Woods JR, Plessinger MA, Clark KE. Effect of cocaine on uterine blood flow and fetal oxygenation. *JAMA.* 1987;257:957–961.

Wright SC, Zhong J, Zheng H, et al. Nicotine inhibition of apoptosis suggests a role in tumor production. *FASEB J.* 1993;7:1045–1051.

Xu M, Guo Y, Vorhees CV, et al. Behavioral responses to cocaine and amphetamine administration in mice lacking the dopamine D1 receptor. *Brain Res.* 2000;852:198–207.

Yamamura Y. n-Hexane polyneuropathy. *Folia Psychiatr Neurol.* 1969;23:45–57.

Zhang J, Graham DG, Montine TS, et al. Enhanced N-methyl-4-tetrahydropyridine toxicity in mice deficient in CuZn-superoxide dismutase or glutathione peroxidase. *J Neuropathol Exp Neurol.* 2000;59:53–61.

Toxic Responses of the Ocular and Visual System

Donald A. Fox and William K. Boyes

INTRODUCTION TO OCULAR AND VISUAL SYSTEM TOXICOLOGY

Environmental and occupational exposure to toxic chemicals, gases, and vapors, and side effects of systemic and ocular therapeutic drugs may result in structural and functional alterations to the eye and central visual system (Anger and Johnson, 1985; Grant and Schuman, 1993; Otto and Fox, 1993; Fox, 1998; Santaella and Fraunfelder, 2007; Bartlett and Jaanus, 2008). Almost half of all neurotoxic chemicals affect some aspect of sensory function (Crofton and Sheets, 1989). The most frequently reported sensory system alterations occur in the visual system (Anger and Johnson, 1985; Crofton and Sheets, 1989; Fox, 1998; Grant and Schuman, 1993). Approximately 3000 substances are toxic to the eye and visual system (Grant and Schuman, 1993). In many cases, alterations in retinal and visual function are the initial symptoms following chemical exposure (Hanninen *et al.*, 1978; Damstra, 1978; Baker *et al.*, 1984; Anger and Johnson, 1985; Mergler *et al.*, 1987; Iregren *et al.*, 2002). This suggests that sensory systems, and in particular the retina and central visual system, may be especially vulnerable to toxic insult. Alterations in the structure and/or function of the eye or central visual system are among the criteria utilized for setting permissible occupational or environmental exposure levels for many different chemicals in the United States (http://www.cdc.gov/niosh/npg/; http://www.epa.gov/iris/index.html). New or existing drugs may have visual side effects (Grant and Schuman, 1993; Novack, 2003; Brigell *et al.*, 2005; Santaella and Fraunfelder, 2007). Subtle alterations in visual processing of information (eg, visual perceptual, visual motor) can have profound immediate, long-term, and delayed effects on the mental, social, and physical health and performance of an individual. Among the elderly, reduced visual function is a major factor contributing to decreased ability to conduct routine activities of daily living, decreased ability to live independently, and increased risk of falls, car crashes, and other hazards. Ocular and visual system impairments can lead to increased occupational injuries, loss of productive work time, costs for providing medical and social services, lost productivity, and a distinct decrease in the overall quality of life.

The overall goals of this chapter are to provide essential information on ocular pharmacodynamics, pharmacokinetics, and drug

Table 17-1

Ocular and Central Visual System Sites of Action of Selected Xenobiotics Following Systemic Exposure

XENOBIOTIC	CORNEA	LENS	OUTER RETINA: RPE	OUTER RETINA: RODS AND CONES	INNER RETINA: BCS, ACS, IPCS	RGCS, OPTIC NERVE OR TRACT	LGN, VISUAL CORTEX
Acrylamide				−	−	++	++
Amiodarone	+	+				+	
Carbon disulfide				+	−	++	+
Chloroquine	+		+	+		+	
Chlorpromazine	+	+	+	+			
Corticosteroids		++				+	
Digoxin and digitoxin	+	+	+	++		+	+
Ethambutol				+		++	
Hexachlorophene				+			++
Indomethacin	+		+	+			
Isotretinoin	+						
Lead	+		+	++	+	+	+
Methanol			+	++	−	++	+
Methyl mercury, mercury			+	−	−	++	+
n-Hexane			+	+		+	
Naphthalene		+		+			
Organic solvents				+			+
Organophosphates			+	+		+	+
Sildenafil/tadalafil	−	−	−	+	+	+	−
Styrene				+			
Tamoxifen	+			+		+	
Vigabatrin	−	−	−	+	+	+	−

RPE, retinal pigment epithelium; BC, bipolar cell; AC, amacrine cell; IPC, interplexiform cell; RGC, retinal ganglion cell; LGN, lateral geniculate nucleus. "+" indicates that this site of action was cited in one or more case reports, review articles, clinical or animal studies. "−" indicates that this site of action showed no adverse effect as cited in one or more case reports, review articles, clinical or animal studies. productivity, and a distinct decrease in the overall quality of life.

metabolism; review the procedures for testing visual function; and evaluate and review the structural and functional alterations in the mammalian eye and central visual system produced by environmental and workplace chemicals, gases, and vapors, and major therapeutic drugs. Except where noted, all these compounds are referred to as chemicals and drugs. The adverse effects of these agents on the different compartments of the eye (ie, cornea, lens, retina, and retinal pigment epithelium [RPE]), central visual pathway (ie, optic nerve and optic tract), and the central processing areas (ie, lateral geniculate nucleus [LGN], visual cortex) are addressed (Table 17-1). To further understand the potential effects of these chemicals and drugs on the eye, the distribution of Phase I and Phase II drug metabolizing enzymes in ocular tissues are presented in Table 17-2. Table 17-3 provides examples of common signs, symptoms, and potential pathophysiological mechanisms of visual dysfunction associated with acute or chronic exposure to toxic compounds and selected drugs. Some of the symptoms are very nonspecific (eg, "blurred vision") whereas others are more definitive.

The ophthalmological evaluation of the eye and the testing of visual function are discussed in this chapter, as the results from clinical, behavioral, and electrophysiological studies form the basis of diagnosis and understanding of adverse visual system effects. Many of the chemicals discussed below initially appear to have a single site and, by inference, mechanism of action, whereas others have several sites and corresponding mechanisms of action. However, a more in-depth examination reveals that, depending upon dose (concentration), many of these chemicals have multiple sites of action. A few examples illustrate the point. First, as described below in more detail, carbon disulfide produces optic nerve and optic tract degeneration and also adversely affects the neurons and vasculature of the retina, resulting in photoreceptor and retinal ganglion cell (RGC) structural and functional alterations (Raitta *et al.*, 1974, 1981; Palacz *et al.*, 1980; Seppalainen and Haltia, 1980; De Rouck *et al.*, 1986; Eskin *et al.*, 1988; Merigan *et al.*, 1988; Fox, 1998). Second, gestational and postnatal exposure to inorganic lead clearly affects rod photoreceptors in developing and adult mammals, resulting in rod-mediated (scotopic) vision deficits; however, structural and functional deficits

Table 17-2

Distribution of Ocular Xenobiotic-Biotransforming Enzymes

	ENZYMES	TEARS	CORNEA	IRIS/CILIARY	LENS	RETINA	CHORIOD
Phase I reactions	Acetylcholinesterase (AChE)	+		+		+	+
	Alcohol dehydrogenase		+		−	+	+
	Aldehyde dehydrogenase		+		+	+	+
	Aldehyde reductase		+	+	+	+	+
	Aldose reductase		+		+	+	
	Carboxylesterase	+	+	+		+	+
	Catalase	−	+	+	+	+	+
	Cu/Zn superoxide dismutase	+	+	−	±	+	
	MAO-A or MAO-B	+		+		+	+
	CYP1A1 or CYP1A2	+	+	+	−	+	+
	CYP1B1		+	+	+	+	
	CYP2B1 or CYP2B2				+	+	
	CYP2C11				+		
	CYP3A1				+	+	
	CYP4A1 or CYP4B2		+	+		+	
	CYP27A1					+	
Phase II reactions	Glutathione peroxidase	−	+	+	+	+	+
	Glutathione reductase		+		+	+	
	Glutathione-S-transferase		+	+	+	+	
	Sulfotransferases				+	+	
	UDP-glucuronosyl transferases				+	+	
	N-Acetyltransferase		+	+	+	+	+

"+" and "−" indicate that the enzyme was present (localized by immunohistochemistry, immunogold electron microscopy, Western blot or gene expression) or absent, respectively, in human, monkey, or rodent tissues.

at the level of the RGCs, visual cortex, and oculomotor system also are observed (Fox and Sillman, 1979; Fox, 1984; Glickman *et al.*, 1984; Otto and Fox, 1993; Lilienthal *et al.*, 1988, 1994; Reuhl *et al.*, 1989; Ruan *et al.*, 1994; Fox *et al.*, 1997, 2011; Rice, 1998; Rice and Hayward, 1999; He *et al.*, 2000, 2003; Rothenberg *et al.*, 2002; Nagpal and Brodie, 2009; Giddabasappa *et al.*, 2011). Although both gestational and postnatal lead exposure produce scotopic electroretinographic (ERG) deficits, the amplitude changes are in opposite directions and their underlying mechanisms are distinctly different. Finally, some environmental and occupational neurotoxicants (eg, acrylamide, lead) have been utilized for in vivo and in vitro animal models to examine the pathogenesis of selected retinal, neuronal, or axonal diseases; the basic functions of the retinocortical pathways; and/or the molecular mechanisms of apoptosis (Fox and Sillman, 1979; Vidyasagar, 1981; Lynch *et al.*, 1992; He *et al.*, 2000, 2003).

The conceptual approach, format, and overall organization of this chapter on ocular and visual system toxicology for this edition of Casarett and Doull's *Toxicology: The Basic Science of Poisons* were designed in anticipation that the main audience would be graduate and medical school students, ophthalmologists and occupational physicians, basic and applied science researchers interested in ocular and visual system toxicology, and those interested in having a basic reference source. To write this chapter, information was synthesized and condensed from several excellent resources on different aspects of ocular, retinal, and visual system anatomy, biochemistry, cell and molecular biology, histology, pharmacology, physiology, and toxicology (Dayhaw-Barker *et al.*, 1986; Grant and Schuman, 1993; Albert *et al.*, 2008; Bartlett and Jaanus, 2008; Wässle, 2004; Banh *et al.*, 2005; Wu, 2010). The interested reader should consult these sources for more detail than is provided below. We gratefully acknowledge the use of the information in these sources as well as those cited in the text below.

EXPOSURE TO THE EYE AND VISUAL SYSTEM

Ocular Pharmacodynamics and Pharmacokinetics

Toxic chemicals and systemic drugs can affect all parts of the eye (Fig. 17-1; Table 17-1). Several factors determine whether a chemical can reach a particular ocular site of action, including the

Table 17-3

Common Signs and Symptoms of Visual System Dysfunction

COMMON SIGNS AND SYMPTOMS	POSSIBLE PATHOPHYSIOLOGICAL BASIS	EXAMPLES OF CHEMICALS PRODUCING THIS EFFECT
Cornea		
Pigment deposits in corneal epithelium (verticillate keratopathy)	Intralysosomal accumulation of lipids	Amphiphilic medications such as amiodarone, chloroquine, clofazimine, phenothiazines, suramin
Lens		
Cataracts anterior cortical, (AC), posterior subcapsular, (PSC)	Chemical deposition, photochemical oxidation	Long-term systemic use of phenothiazine (AC), corticosteroids (PSC)
Pupil		
Pupil constriction (miosis)	Anticholinesterases	Organophosphate and carbamate insecticides, nerve gas agents such as sarin, soman, and tabun
Pupil dilation (mydriasis) and photophobia	Cholinergic antagonists	Atropine or belladona
	Adrenergic agonists	Amphetamine, cocaine, phenylephrine
Ocular motility		
Diplopia (double vision), nystagmus	Oculomotor impairment, Damage or dysfunction in vestibular/oculomotor reflex pathways	Acute alcohol intoxication, barbiturate toxicity, acute solvent exposure
Retinal pigment epithelium		
Loss of central vision (central scotoma)	Degeneration of retinal pigment epithelium and underlying photoreceptors	Carbon disulfide, chloroquine
Retina		
Poor night (scotopic) vision and impaired dark adaptation	Damage to and apoptosis of rod photoreceptors,	Lead, methyl mercury, vigabatrin
	Acetylcholinesterase inhibitors	Organophosphate and carbamate insecticides, nerve gas agents
Altered color perception, central scotoma	Inhibition of cone photoreceptor sodium-pumps	Digitalis/digitoxin
Altered color perception	Inhibition of cone photoreceptor cGMP-phosphodiesterase	Sildenafil and tadalafil
Impaired color discrimination (Blue/Yellow)	Damage to cone photoreceptors and inner retina	Chronic exposure to styrene and organic solvents, trimethadione, chronic high dose antibiotics
Impaired color discrimination (Red/Green)	Acquired damage to cone photoreceptors, neural retina and/or afferent visual pathway	Higher level chronic exposure to organic solvents, carbon disulfide or hexane, chronic carbon monoxide, chronic alcoholism, ethambutol
Loss of peripheral vision (tunnel vision, peripheral scotoma, visual field constriction)	Degeneration of peripheral retina and nerve fiber layer	Methyl mercury, vigabatrin
Reduced contrast sensitivity and visual acuity	Degeneration of the retinal ganglion cells and optic tract, microaneurysms and retinal vasculopathy	Acrylamide, carbon disulfide
Optic nerve and optic tract		
Reduced contrast sensitivity and visual acuity	Optic neuritis and/or degeneration of the optic tract, generally affecting mitochondrial ATP production	Higher level chronic exposure to organic solvents such as carbon disulfide or hexane, ethambutol, ethylene glycol, isoniazid, linezolid and chloramphenicol, methanol, vigabatrin
Monocular and/or binocular visual loss	Nonarteretic anterior ischemic optic neuropathy	Amiodarone, sildenafil and tadalafil
Lateral geniculate and visual cortex		
Central scotoma	Degeneration of calcarine fissure of visual cortex	Methyl mercury
Visuomotor deficits and reduced contrast sensitivity	Visual and motor cortex dysfunction	Lead, chronic exposure to carbon disulfide, hexane and other solvents, toluene

Inclusion in this table indicates that this drug, chemical or toxicant was cited in one or more case reports, review articles, clinical or animal studies. The pathophysiological causes and chemicals listed are provided as examples and are not exhaustive.

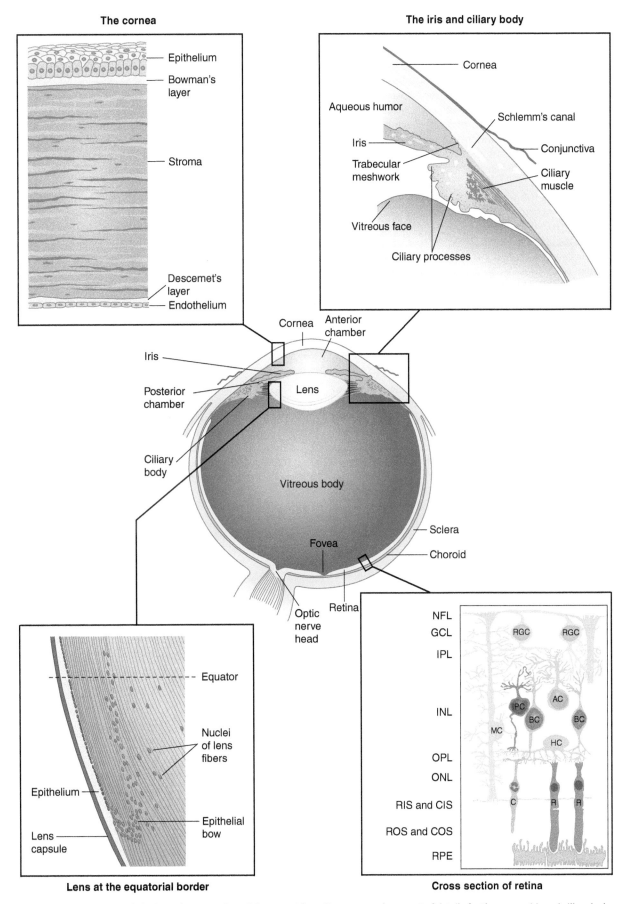

The cornea

- Epithelium
- Bowman's layer
- Stroma
- Descemet's layer
- Endothelium

The iris and ciliary body

- Cornea
- Aqueous humor
- Schlemm's canal
- Iris
- Conjunctiva
- Trabecular meshwork
- Ciliary muscle
- Vitreous face
- Ciliary processes

- Cornea
- Anterior chamber
- Iris
- Lens
- Posterior chamber
- Ciliary body
- Vitreous body
- Sclera
- Fovea
- Choroid
- Optic nerve head
- Retina

Lens at the equatorial border

- Equator
- Nuclei of lens fibers
- Epithelium
- Epithelial bow
- Lens capsule

Cross section of retina

- NFL
- GCL — RGC   RGC
- IPL
- INL — IPC   BC   AC   BC   MC   HC
- OPL
- ONL
- RIS and CIS — C   R   R
- ROS and COS
- RPE

Figure 17-1. *Diagrammatic horizontal cross section of the eye, with medium-power enlargement of details for the cornea, iris and ciliary body, lens, and retina.* The morphological features, their role in ocular pharmacodynamics, pharmacokinetics, drug metabolism, and the adverse effects of drugs and chemical agents on these sites are discussed in the text.

physiochemical properties of the chemical, concentration and duration of exposure/treatment, route of exposure, and the movement of the chemical into and across the different ocular compartments and barriers. The cornea and external adnexa of the eye, including the conjunctiva (the delicate membranes covering the inner surface of the eyelids and the exposed surface of the sclera) and eyelids are often exposed directly to chemicals (ie, acids, bases, solvents), gases, and particles, and drugs. The first site of action is the tear film: a three-layered structure with both hydrophobic and hydrophilic properties. The outermost tear film layer is a thin (0.1 μm) hydrophobic layer that is secreted by the meibomian (sebaceous) glands. This superficial lipid layer protects the underlying thicker (7 μm) aqueous layer that is produced by the lacrimal glands. The third layer, which has both hydrophobic and hydrophilic properties, is the very thin (0.02–0.05 μm) mucoid layer. It is secreted by the goblet cells of the conjunctiva and acts as an interface between the hydrophilic layer of the tears and the hydrophobic layer of the corneal epithelial cells. Thus, the aqueous layer is the largest portion of the tear film, and therefore water-soluble chemical compounds more readily mix with the tears and gain access to the cornea. However, a large proportion of the compounds that are splashed into the eyes is washed away by the tears and thus not absorbed.

The cornea, an avascular tissue, is considered the external barrier to the internal ocular structures. Once a chemical interacts with the tear film and subsequently contacts the cornea and conjunctiva, the majority of what is absorbed locally enters the anterior segment by passing across the cornea. In contrast, a greater systemic absorption and higher blood concentration occur through contact with the vascularized conjunctiva (Edelhauser, 2006; Fig. 17-2). The human cornea, which is approximately 500-μm thick, has several distinct layers, or barriers, through which a chemical must pass in order to reach the anterior chamber (see discussion on Cornea). The first is the corneal epithelium. It is a stratified squamous, nonkeratinized, and multicellular hydrophobic layer. These cells have a relatively low ionic conductance through apical cell membranes, and due to the tight junctions (desmosomes), they have a high-resistance paracellular pathway. The primary barrier to chemical penetration of

the cornea is the set of tight junctions at the superficial layer of the corneal epithelial cells. Thus, the permeability of the corneal epithelium as a whole is low and only lipid-soluble chemicals readily pass through this layer. Bowmann membrane separates the epithelium from the stroma. The corneal stroma makes up 90% of the corneal thickness and is composed of water, collagen, and glycosaminoglycans. It contains approximately 200 lamellae, each about 1.5- to 2.0-μm thick. Due to the composition and structure of the stroma, hydrophilic chemicals easily dissolve in this thick layer, which can also act as a reservoir for these chemicals. The inner edge of the corneal stroma is bounded by a thin, limiting basement membrane, called Descemet membrane, which is secreted by the corneal endothelium. The innermost layer of the cornea, the corneal endothelium, is composed of a single layer of large-diameter hexagonal cells connected by terminal bars and surrounded by lipid membranes. The endothelial cells have a relatively low ionic conductance through apical cell surface and a high-resistance paracellular pathway. Although, the permeability of the corneal endothelial cells to ionized chemicals is relatively low, it is still 100 to 200 times more permeable than the corneal epithelium. The Na^+,K^+-pump is located on the basolateral membrane while the energy-dependent Na^+,HCO_3^--transporter is located on the apical membrane (Edelhauser, 2006).

There are two separate vascular systems in the eye (Flammer and Mozaffarieh, 2008; Nickla and Wallman, 2010): (1) the uveal blood vessels, which include the vascular beds of the iris, ciliary body, and choroid, and (2) the retinal vessels. In humans, the ocular vessels are derived from the ophthalmic artery, which is a branch of the internal carotid artery. The ophthalmic artery branches into (1) the central retinal artery, which enters the eye and then further branches into four major vessels serving each of the retinal quadrants; (2) two posterior ciliary arteries; and (3) several anterior arteries. In the anterior segment of the eye, there is a blood–aqueous barrier that has relatively tight junctions between the endothelial cells of the iris capillaries and nonpigmented cells of the ciliary epithelium. The major function of the ciliary epithelium is the production of aqueous humor from the plasma filtrate present in the stroma of the ciliary processes.

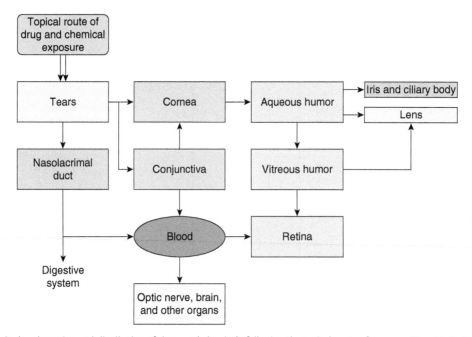

Figure 17-2. *Ocular absorption and distribution of drugs and chemicals following the topical route of exposure.* The details for movement of drugs and chemicals between compartments of the eye and subsequently to the optic nerve, brain, and other organs are discussed in the text. The conceptual idea for this figure was obtained from Lapalus and Garaffo (1992).

In humans and several widely used experimental animals (eg, monkeys, pigs, dogs, rats, mice), the retina has a dual circulatory supply: choroidal and retinal. The retinal blood vessels are distributed within the inner or proximal portion of the retina, which consists of the outer plexiform layer (OPL), inner nuclear layer (INL), inner plexiform layer (IPL), and ganglion cell layer (GCL). The endothelial cells of capillaries of the retinal vessels have tight junctions similar to those that form the blood–brain barrier in the cerebral capillaries. These capillaries form the blood–retinal barrier, and under normal physiological conditions, they are largely impermeable to chemicals such as glucose and amino acids. However, at the level of the optic disc, the blood–retinal barrier lacks these tight-junction types of capillaries and thus hydrophilic molecules can enter the optic nerve head by diffusion from the extravascular space (Flammer and Mozaffarieh, 2008; Nickla and Wallman, 2010) and cause selective damage at this site of action. The outer or distal retina, which consists of the RPE, rod, and cone photoreceptor outer segments (ROS, COS) and inner segments (RIS, CIS), and the photoreceptor outer nuclear layer (ONL), are avascular. These areas of the retina are supplied by the choriocapillaris: a dense, one-layered network of fenestrated vessels formed by the short posterior ciliary arteries and located next to the RPE. Consistent with their known structure, these capillaries have loose endothelial junctions and abundant fenestrae; they are highly permeable to large proteins. Thus, the extravascular space contains a high concentration of albumin and γ-globulin (Sears, 1984).

Following systemic exposure to drugs and chemicals by the oral, inhalation, dermal, or parenteral route, these compounds are distributed to all parts of the eye by the blood in the uveal blood vessels and retinal vessels (Fig. 17-3). Most of these drugs and chemicals rapidly equilibrate with the extravascular space of the choroid where they are separated from the retina and vitreous body by the RPE and endothelial cells of the retinal capillaries, respectively. Hydrophilic molecules with molecular weights less than 200 to 300 Da can cross the ciliary epithelium and iris capillaries and enter the aqueous humor (Sears, 1984). Thus, the corneal endothelium, the cells responsible for maintaining normal hydration and transparency of the corneal stroma, could be exposed to chemical compounds by the aqueous humor and limbal capillaries. Similarly, the anterior surface of the lens can also be exposed as a result of its contact with the aqueous humor. The most likely retinal target sites following systemic drug and chemical exposure appear to be the RPE and photoreceptors in the distal retina because the endothelial cells of the choriocapillaris are permeable to proteins smaller than 50 to 70 kDa. However, the cells of the RPE are joined on their basolateral surface by tight junctions, zonula occludens, that limit the passive penetration of large molecules into the neural retina (Strauss, 2005; Mecklenburg and Schraemeyer, 2007).

The presence of intraocular melanin plays a special role in ocular toxicology. First, it is found in several different locations in the eye: pigmented cells of the iris, ciliary body, RPE, and uveal tract. Second, it has a high binding affinity for polycyclic aromatic hydrocarbons, electrophiles, calcium, and toxic heavy metals such as aluminum, iron, lead, and mercury (Meier-Ruge, 1972; Potts and Au, 1976; Dräger, 1985; Ulshafer et al., 1990; Eichenbaum and Zheng, 2000). Although this initially may play a protective role, it also results in the excessive accumulation, long-term storage, and slow release of numerous drugs and chemicals from melanin. For example, atropine binds more avidly to pigmented irides and thus its duration of action is prolonged (Bartlett and Jaanus, 2008). In addition, the accumulation of chloroquine in the RPE produces an 80-fold higher concentration of chloroquine in the retina relative to liver (Meier-Ruge, 1972). Similarly, lead accumulates in the human retina such that its concentration is 5 to 750 times that in other ocular tissues (Eichenbaum and Zheng, 2000).

Nanoparticles and Ocular Drug Delivery

Ocular drug delivery and targeting create significant challenges and obstacles for most drugs that must enter the eye and reach their site of action. The main ocular target sites of importance for disease treatment and neuroprotection are the anterior segment and posterior retina. As noted above, there are numerous superficial barriers, blood–retina barriers, transporters, depot sites, and the like that restrict bioavailability, decrease therapeutic efficacy, and increase side effects. One new approach involves development of nanoscale preparations for drug delivery, which can substantially enhance penetration from the cornea, deliver a wide variety of drugs and molecules, and increase the concentration and contact time of drugs with these tissues (Diebold and Calonge, 2010). A wide variety of

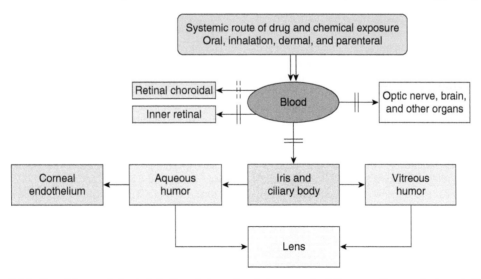

Figure 17-3. *Distribution of drugs and chemicals in the anterior and posterior segments of the eye, optic nerve, brain, and other organs following the systemic route of exposure.* The details for movement of drugs and chemicals between compartments of the eye are discussed in the text. The conceptual idea for this part of the figure was obtained from Lapalus and Garaffo (1992). The solid and dotted double lines represent the different blood–tissue barriers present in the anterior segment of the eye, retina, optic nerve, and brain. The solid double lines represent tight endothelial junctions, whereas the dotted double lines represent loose endothelial junctions.

nanoformulations have been considered including matrix-embedded materials and membrane-bound reservoirs (nanoencapsulation). Formulations being developed are solid lipid nanoparticles containing lipids, phospholipids, and/or metals; liposomes; nanosuspensions, and emulsions; and the use of biocompatible coatings such as chitosan (Diebold and Calonge, 2010; Nagpal et al., 2010; Seyfoddin et al., 2010). Metallic particles that enable remote magnetic targeting of drug delivery also are under development. The preparations being developed as pharmaceutical vehicles for ocular drug delivery should have low toxicity to ocular tissues (Prow, 2010). For a wide variety of nonocular purposes, many engineered nanomaterials are being developed. Among the thousands of materials being developed and incorporated into hundreds of consumer products, to date almost no attention has focused on their potential for ocular toxicity other than in vitro assessments of potential phototoxicity (discussed elsewhere).

Ocular Drug Metabolism

Metabolism of xenobiotics occurs in all compartments of the eye by well-known Phase I and II xenobiotic-biotransforming enzymes. Drug metabolizing enzymes such as acetylcholinesterase, carboxylesterase (also known as pseudocholinesterase: see Chap. 6), alcohol and aldehyde dehydrogenase, aldehyde and aldose reductase, catalase, monoamine oxidase A and/or B, and Cu^{2+}/Zn^{2+} superoxide dismutase as well as several types of proteases are present in the tears, iris–ciliary body, choroid, and retina of many different species (Shanthaverrappa and Bourne, 1964; Waltman and Sears, 1964; Bausher, 1976; Atalla et al., 1998; Crouch et al., 1991; Watkins et al., 1991; Gondhowiardjo and van Haeringen, 1993; Downes and Holmes, 1995; Gaudet et al., 1995; Behndig et al., 1998; King et al., 1999; Nakamura et al., 2005; Choudhary et al., 2006; Fox et al., 2011; Table 17-2).

Cytochrome P450 (CYP) is a superfamily of hemoproteins involved with xenobiotic and endogenous metabolism. There are age-, gender-, and region-specific differences (ie, cornea, ciliary and lens epithelium, and retina) in CYP expression in the developing and adult human and rodent eye (Nakamura et al., 2005; Choudhary et al., 2006; Doshi et al., 2006; Lee et al., 2006). Mutations or alterations in CYP expression (eg, CYP1B1) during development can produce ocular diseases and defects such as primary congenital glaucoma and corneal opacity (Choudhary et al., 2006). Numerous other CYP family members are located in the eye and respond to different drugs and toxicants. For example, CYP1A1 and CYP1A2 are found in all bovine and mouse ocular tissues except the lens and can be induced by 3-methylcholanthrene and β-naphthoflavone (Shichi and Nebert, 1982; Zhao and Shichi, 1995). Moreover, CYP4A1 in the mouse and CYP4B1 in the rabbit are present in corneal epithelium and can be induced by phenobarbital and the peroxisome proliferator clofibrate (Shichi, 1996; Zhao et al., 1996; Mastyugin et al., 1999). This corneal epithelial CYP monooxygenase metabolizes arachidonic acid to two of its major metabolites: 12(R)-HETE [12(R)-hydroxy-5,8,10,14-eicosatrienoic acid] and 12(R)-HETrE [12(R)-hydroxy-5,8,14-eicosatrienoic acid] (Schwartzman, 1997; Asakura et al., 1994; Mastyugin et al., 1999). In the corneal epithelium, 12(R)-HETE is a potent inhibitor of Na^{+},K^{+}-ATPase, whereas 12(R)-HETrE is a potent angiogenic and chemotactic factor (Schwartzman, 1997).

The Phase II conjugating enzymes found in bovine, rabbit, and rat ocular tissues include UDP glucuronosyltransferase, glutathione peroxidase, glutathione reductase, glutathione-S-transferase, and N-acetyltransferase (Awasthi et al., 1980; Shichi and Nebert, 1982; Penn et al., 1987; Watkins et al., 1991; Srivastava et al., 1996; Singh and Shichi, 1998; Nakamura et al., 2005; see Table 17-2). Although

the activity of these enzymes varies between species and ocular tissues, the whole lens appears to have low biotransformational activity. Metabolically, the lens is a heterogeneous tissue, with glutathione-S-transferase activity found in the lens epithelium and not in the lens cortex or nucleus (Srivastava et al., 1996). Overall, these findings suggest that ocular tissues that contact the external environment have a blood supply possessing both CYPs and Phase II conjugating enzymes, especially those enzymes related to glutathione conjugation. The presence and need for a competent glutathione conjugation system is clearly understandable in ocular tissues that directly interact with UV radiation, light, and xenobiotics. Further work is still needed to determine the presence and activity of other CYP family members in ocular tissue, the various factors (ie, age, gender, tissue-specific, xenobiotics, etc) that regulate their expression, and their endogenous and exogenous substrates.

Central Visual System Pharmacokinetics

The penetration of potentially toxic compounds into visual areas of the central nervous system (CNS) is governed, like other parts of the CNS, by the blood–brain barrier (Fig. 17-3). The blood–brain barrier is formed through a combination of tight junctions in brain capillary endothelial cells and foot processes of astrocytic glial cells that surround the brain capillaries. Together these structures serve to limit the penetration of blood-borne compounds into the brain and in some cases actively exclude compounds from brain tissue. The concept of an absolute barrier is not correct, however, because the blood–brain barrier is differentially permeable to compounds depending on their size, charge, and lipophilicity. Compounds that are large, highly charged, or otherwise not very lipid soluble tend to be excluded from the brain, whereas smaller, uncharged, and lipid-soluble compounds more readily penetrate into the brain tissue. In addition to entering the CNS through this nonspecific semipermeable diffusion barrier, some specific nutrients including ions, amino acids, and glucose enter the CNS through selective transport mechanisms. In some cases, toxic compounds may be actively transported into the brain by mimicking the natural substrates of active transport systems. A few areas of the brain lack a blood–brain barrier; consequently, blood-borne compounds readily penetrate into the brain tissue in these regions.

Light and Phototoxicity

The most important oxidizing agents are visible light and UV radiation, particularly UV-A (320–400 nm) and UV-B (290–320 nm), and other forms of electromagnetic radiation. Light- and UV-induced photooxidation leads to generation of reactive oxygen species, and oxidative damage that can accumulate over time. Higher-energy UV-C (100–290 nm) is even more damaging. Fortunately, at sea level the atmosphere filters out virtually all UV-C and all but a small fraction of UV-B derived from solar radiance (AMA Report, 1989). The cornea absorbs about 45% of light with wavelengths below 280 nm, but only about 12% between 320 and 400 nm. The lens absorbs much of the light between 300 and 400 nm and transmits 400 nm and above to the retina (Banh et al., 2005). Absorption of light energy in the lens triggers a variety of photoreactions, including the generation of fluorophores and pigments that lead to the yellow–brown coloration of the lens. Sufficient exposure to infrared radiation, as occurs to glassblowers, or microwave radiation will also produce cataracts through direct heating of the ocular tissues.

Drugs and other chemicals can serve as mediators of photoinduced toxicity in the cornea, lens, or retina (Dayhaw-Barker et al., 1986; Roberts, 2001, 2002; Glickman, 2002). This occurs when the chemical structure allows absorption of light energy in the UV or visible spectrum and the subsequent generation of activated intermediates, free radicals and reactive oxygen species. Chemical structures likely to participate in such phototoxic mechanisms include those with tricyclic, heterocyclic, or porphyrin ring structures because, with light, they produce stable triplet reactive molecules leading to free radicals and reactive oxygen species. The propensity of chemicals to cause phototoxic reactions can be predicted using photophysical and in vitro procedures (Roberts, 2001; Glickman, 2002).

The phototoxic properties of chemicals are being exploited for photodynamic therapies where photoactive chemicals are delivered to pathological tissues such as cancerous tumors or inappropriate angiogenic vessels in age-related macular degeneration. Wavelength-specific light is introduced to the tissue causing the photoactive chemical to activate thereby initiating a free-radical cascade that kills the pathological tissues. These agents also are being developed to utilize long wavelengths near the red/infrared end of the spectrum where the irradiation penetrates deeper into the tissue. A high-throughput screening assay has been developed to rapidly screen candidate chemicals for phototoxicity (Butler et al., 2010). However, photoactive chemicals that are not intentionally introduced for photodynamic therapy also can generate phototoxic reactions. Two examples, which exhibit in vitro ocular phototoxicity, are fullerene (Roberts et al., 2008) and titanium dioxide nanomaterials (Sanders et al., 2012).

EVALUATING OCULAR TOXICITY AND VISUAL FUNCTION

Testing for potential toxic effects of compounds on the eye and visual system can be divided into tests of ocular toxicity and tests of visual function. Alternatively, such tests could be grouped according to the professional training of the individual conducting the evaluation. Such a categorization might include tests of contact irritancy or toxicity akin to dermatological procedures, ophthalmological evaluations, neurophysiological studies of the function of the visual system, and behavioral or psychophysical evaluations of visual thresholds and aspects of perception.

Evaluation of Ocular Irritancy and Toxicity

Topical injury to the eye, especially the cornea, can result from contact with household and workplace products and chemicals. Accidents involving common household products produce over 100,000 eye injuries per year (McGwin et al., 2006; Peate, 2007). Regulatory agencies require ocular irritancy testing to determine whether chemicals and/or products can produce eye damage as well as the type and degree of damage. Based on this information, agents are classified as ocular hazard and appropriately labeled. Since 1944, the standard procedures for evaluating ocular irritation have been based on the Draize method (Draize et al., 1944). Over this time, the Draize test with some additions and revisions formed the basis of safety evaluations in data submitted to several government regulatory bodies including the European Economic Community and several federal agencies within the United States. Traditionally, albino rabbits were the subjects evaluated in the Draize test, although the Environmental Protection Agency (EPA) protocol allows different test species to be used if sufficient justification is provided. The standard procedure involves instillation of 0.1 mL of a liquid or 100 mg of a solid into the conjunctival sac of one eye and then gently holding the eye closed for one second.

The untreated eye serves as a control. Both eyes are evaluated at 1, 24, 48, and 72 hours after treatment. If there is evidence of damage in the treated eye at 72 hours, the examination time may be extended. The cornea, iris, and conjunctiva are evaluated and scored according to a weighted scale. The cornea is scored for both the degree of opacity and the area of involvement, with each measure having a potential range from 0 (none) to 4 (most severe). The iris receives a single score (0–2) for irritation, including degree of swelling, congestion, and degree of reaction to light. The conjunctiva is scored for the redness (0–3), chemosis (swelling 0–4), and discharge (0–3). The individual scores are then multiplied by a weighting factor: five for the cornea, two for the iris, and five for the conjunctiva. The results are summed for a maximum total score of 110. Photographic examples of lesions receiving each score are provided in Datson and Freeberg (1991). In this scale, the cornea accounts for 80 (73%) of the total possible points, in accordance with the severity associated with corneal injury.

The Draize test has been criticized due to its high interlaboratory variability, subjective nature of scoring, poor predictive value for human irritants, and most significantly for causing undue pain and distress to the tested animals. Recently, the Interagency Coordinating Committee on the Validation of Alternative Methods (ICCVAM), a committee representing 14 agencies of the US Federal government, recommended the routine use of topical anesthetics, systemic analgesics, and humane endpoints to avoid or minimize pain and distress in in vivo ocular safety testing (ICCVAM, 2010a: NIH Publication No. 10-7514). Moreover, ICCVAM recently evaluated the validation status of five different test methods to identify substances that cause reversible eye injuries or do not cause sufficient eye damage to require hazard labeling. These were the bovine corneal opacity and permeability (BCOP), Cytosensor Microphysiometer (CM), hen's egg test-chorioallantoic membrane (HET-CAM), isolated chicken eye (ICE), and isolated rabbit eye (IRE) test methods (ICCVAM, 2010b: NIH Publication No. 10-7553). These in vitro tests can be used to predict the extent of ocular damage that might occur in vivo so as to obviate using live animals. The report summarizes the validation status of each test method, provides test method protocols and future recommendations. Interested readers should consult the original documents as well as the ICCVAM website, which has continuous updates.

Ophthalmological Evaluations

There are many ophthalmological procedures for evaluating the health of the eye. These should be conducted by a trained ophthalmologist or optometrist experienced in evaluating the species of interest. The procedures available range from routine clinical screening evaluations to sophisticated techniques for targeted purposes: the latter are beyond the scope of this chapter. A clinical evaluation of the eye addresses the adnexa and both the anterior and posterior structures in the eye. Examination of the adnexa includes evaluating the eyelids, lacrimal apparatus, and palpebral (covering the eyelid) and bulbar (covering the eye) conjunctiva. The anterior structures or anterior segment include the cornea, iris, lens, and anterior chamber. The posterior structures, referred to as the ocular fundus, include the retina, retinal vasculature, choroid, optic nerve, and sclera. The adnexa and surface of the cornea can be examined initially with the naked eye and a hand-held light. Closer examination requires a slit-lamp biomicroscope, using a mydriatic drug (causes pupil dilation) if the lens is to be observed. The width of the reflection of a thin beam of light projected from the slit lamp is an indication of the thickness of the cornea and may be used to evaluate corneal edema. Lesions of the cornea can be better visualized with the use of fluorescein dye, which is retained where there is an ulceration of the corneal epithelium.

Examination of the fundus requires use of a mydriatic drug. These and other ocular examinations are described in several publications (Harroff, 1991; Peiffer *et al.*, 2000; Albert *et al.*, 2008). An ophthalmological examination of the eye may also involve, prior to introducing mydriatics, an examination of the pupillary light reflex. The direct pupillary reflex involves shining a bright light into the eye and observing the reflexive pupil constriction in the same eye. The consensual pupillary reflex is observed in the eye not stimulated. Both the direct and consensual pupillary light reflexes are dependent on function of a reflex arc involving cells in the retina, which travel through the optic nerve, optic chiasm, and optic tract to project to neurons in the pretectal area. Pretectal neurons project to ipsilateral (for the direct reflex) and contralateral (for the consensual reflex) parasympathetic neurons of the midbrain accessory oculomotor (Edinger–Westphal) nucleus. Preganglionic neurons from the Edinger–Westphal nucleus project through the oculomotor nerve to the ciliary ganglion. Postganglionic neurons from the ciliary ganglion then innervate the smooth muscle fibers of the iridal pupillary sphincter. The absence of a pupillary reflex is indicative of damage somewhere in the reflex pathway, and differential impairment of the direct or consensual reflexes can indicate the location of the lesion. The presence of a pupillary light reflex, however, is not synonymous with normal visual function. Pupillary reflexes can be maintained even with substantial retinal damage. In addition, lesions in visual areas outside of the reflex pathway, such as in the visual cortex, may also leave the reflex function intact.

Electrophysiological Techniques

Many electrophysiological or neurophysiological procedures are available for testing visual function in a toxicological context. In a simple sense, most of these procedures involve stimulating the eyes with visual stimuli and electrically recording potentials generated by visually responsive neurons. Different techniques and stimuli are used to selectively study the function of specific retinal or visual cortical neurons. In the study of the effects of potential toxic substances on visual function, the most commonly used electrophysiological procedures are electroretinograms (ERGs), visual-evoked potentials (VEPs), and, less often, electrooculograms (EOGs). Each of these procedures has numerous variations of stimulation and recording protocols depending on the specific aspects of visual function being evaluated.

ERGs are typically elicited with a brief flash of light and recorded from an electrode placed in contact with the cornea. A typical ERG waveform (Fox and Farber, 1988; Rosolen *et al.*, 2005) includes an initial negative-going waveform, called the a-wave, that reflects the activation of photoreceptors, and a following positive b-wave that reflects the activity of retinal ON-bipolar cells (Abd-El-Barr *et al.*, 2009). In addition, a series of oscillatory potentials can be observed overriding the b-wave, of which the neural generators are somewhat uncertain, but they presumably reflect various stages of intraretinal signal processing. A standard set of ERG procedures has been recommended for screening assessments of human clinical patients (Marmor and Zrenner, 1995). These procedures include the recording of (1) a response reflective of only rod photoreceptor function in the dark-adapted eye, (2) the maximal response in the dark-adapted eye, (3) a response developed by cone photoreceptors, (4) oscillatory potentials, and (5) the response to rapidly flickered light. These recommendations were used to create a protocol for screening the retinal function of dogs in toxicological

studies (Jones *et al.*, 1994). For testing retinal function beyond a screening level evaluation, ERG amplitude and latency versus log stimulus intensity functions are very useful (Fox and Farber, 1988; Rosolen *et al.*, 2005). Although flash-evoked ERGs do not reflect the function of the RGC layer, ERGs elicited with pattern-reversal stimuli (PERGs) do reflect the activation of RGCs. To date, PERGs have not been used widely in toxicological evaluations.

VEPs are elicited with stimuli similar to those used to evoke ERGs; however, VEPs are recorded from electrodes overlying the visual (striate) cortex. Consequently, VEPs reflect the activity of the retinogeniculostriate pathway and the activity of cells in the visual cortex. Flash-elicited VEPs have been used in a number of studies of potentially neurotoxic compounds in laboratory animals (Fox *et al.*, 1977; Herr and Boyes, 1995). Pattern-elicited VEPs are more widely used in human clinical evaluations because of their diagnostic value. However, they are infrequently used in laboratory animals because albino rats do not produce usable pattern VEPs (Boyes and Dyer, 1983). Recording pattern VEPs and conducting psychophysical studies with pigmented Long–Evans hooded rats, Fox (1984) found that the spatial frequency functions yielded almost the same visual acuity values (1.4 cycles per degree) as the psychophysically determined spatial resolution limit values (1.8 cycles per degree). These values are in good agreement with those obtained by others using single-cell electrophysiological and behavioral techniques (Birch and Jacobs, 1979). Moreover, pattern and flash-elicited VEPs have exhibited differential sensitivity to some neurotoxic agents (Boyes and Dyer, 1984; Fox, 1984). The USEPA published guidelines for conducting VEP testing in a toxicological context, along with analogous sensory-evoked potential procedures for evaluating auditory and somatosensory function (EPA, 1998a).

The EOG is generated by a potential difference between the front and back of the eye, which originates primarily within the RPE (Arden and Constable, 2006). Metabolic activity in the RPE generates a light-insensitive potential (the standing potential) and a light-sensitive potential; the difference in amplitude between these two potentials is easily measured as the EOG. The magnitude of the EOG is a function of the level of illumination and health status of the RPE. Electrodes placed on the skin on a line lateral or vertical to the eye measure potential changes correlated with eye movements as the relative position of the ocular dipole changes. Thus, the EOG finds applications in assessing both RPE status and measuring eye movements. The EOG is also used in monitoring eye movements during the recording of other brain potentials, so that eye movement artifacts are not misinterpreted as brain generated electrical activity (Arden and Constable, 2006). In addition, EOG measurements have been used to detect eye movement deficits caused by exposures to chemicals, such as those altering the function of the cerebellum (Geller *et al.*, 1995).

Visual Toxicity Screening Procedures

As noted in the introduction to this chapter, there is a clear need for testing visual function as a component of the toxicological evaluation of commercial chemicals. The magnitude of the potential threat posed by visual system toxicity is not known because sensory function has not been evaluated in a systematic fashion. Currently, the EPA screening batteries for neurotoxicological evaluation of laboratory animals include only minimal evaluations of visual function. Standard screening procedures such as those included in EPA's neurotoxicity screening battery (EPA, 1998b) include a functional observational battery (FOB): an automated measurement of motor activity and neuropathology. Of the screening procedures, only the FOB evaluates visual function and the extent of these measures is very limited. The entire assessment of visual function includes observing the animal's response to an approaching object such as a pencil and observing the pupil's response to a light. These procedures are limited in not exploring responsiveness over a range of stimulus features such as luminance, color, spatial frequency, and temporal frequency. In addition, they do not evaluate rod or cone sensory thresholds, nor do they isolate potential motor or integrative contributions to task performance. Despite these shortcomings, the FOB has been successful at detecting visual deficits produced by exposure to 3,3-iminodipropionitrile (Moser and Boyes, 1993) or carbon disulfide (Moser *et al.*, 1998), which illustrates the importance of conducting at least this level of visual function screening in routine testing programs. Some studies include ophthalmological and/or ocular pathological evaluations. Comprehensive visual toxicity studies should include ophthalmological and pathological evaluation of ocular tissues and assessments of visual function.

Another potentially limiting problem in product safety testing is the routine use of albino animals, whose capacity for visual function is limited at best. The toxicity of many polycyclic aromatic compounds is mediated through interactions with melanin (Potts, 1964; Meier-Ruge, 1972; see discussion of the retina below), which is absent in the eyes of albino strains. Furthermore, light-related ocular lesions, including cataracts and retinal degeneration, are often observed in control albino rats and mice used in two-year product-safety evaluations. The retinas of albino rats and mice are particularly susceptible to light-induced damage (Rapp *et al.*, 1990). For example, one study showed that the proportion of Fisher 344 rats in the control group with photoreceptor lesions ranged from less than 10% of rats housed on the bottom row of the cage racks to over 55% of rats housed on the top row, where the luminance was greater (Rao, 1991). Even under reduced light levels, the incidence of these effects was as high as 15%. If albino animals are used as the test subjects, it is important to control the overall level of illumination in the animal colony and also to periodically rotate the animals among the rows of the cage racks. Even under these conditions, it is extremely difficult to interpret pathological changes in albino rats and mice exposed to test compounds against such high rates of background retinal lesions.

Sensory dysfunction can confound other measures of neurotoxicity. Many behavioral and observational evaluations of neurotoxicity involve presentation of sensory stimuli to human or animal subjects followed by the observation or measurement of a behavioral or motor response. In many cases, the inferences drawn from such measures are stated in terms of the cognitive abilities of the test subject, such as whether learning or memory have been compromised as a function of exposure to the test compound. If the subject was unable to clearly and precisely perceive the test stimuli, which are often complex patterns or contain color, task performance may be affected independently of any effect on cognition. Controlling for visual deficits may alter the interpretation of performance or cognitive tasks (Anger *et al.*, 1994; Hudnell *et al.*, 1996; Walkowiak *et al.*, 1998; Cestnick and Coltheart, 1999).

Behavioral and Psychophysical Techniques

Behavioral and psychophysical testing procedures typically vary the parameters of the visual stimulus and then determine whether the subject can discriminate or perceive the stimulus (Woodhouse and Barlow, 1982; Maurissen, 1995). Many facets of visual function in humans and laboratory animals have been studied using these procedures. Often, the goal of these procedures is to resolve the spatial or temporal limits of visual discrimination; however, most visual scenes and targets in our daily life involve discrimination of objects with low to middle spatial and temporal frequencies (Woodhouse and Barlow, 1982). Contrast sensitivity functions are used to assess these parameters. In addition, as discussed below, other visual parameters also have been investigated using psychophysical procedures.

Contrast sensitivity refers to the ability to resolve small differences in luminance contrast, such as the difference between subtle shades of gray. Contrast sensitivity should be measured for a series of visual patterns that differ in pattern size. Typically, such patterns are a series of sine-wave gratings (striped patterns where the luminance changes across the pattern in a sinusoidal profile) where the spatial frequency of the sinusoidal pattern (ie, the width of the bars in the pattern) varies in octave steps. The patterns vary in contrast (ie, the difference between the brightest and darkest parts of the pattern that is adjusted for mean luminance). The resulting data, when plotted on log/log coordinates, forms a contrast sensitivity function that is representative of the ability to detect visual patterns over the range of visible pattern sizes. Contrast sensitivity functions are dependent primarily on the neural as opposed to the optical properties of the visual system. The contrast sensitivity functions generally form an inverted U-shaped profile with highest sensitivity to contrast at intermediate spatial frequencies. Sensitivity to high spatial frequencies is equivalent to a measure of visual acuity, whereas sensitivity to mid-range spatial frequencies is important for facial recognition (Ginsburg, 2003). The peak of the function as well as the limits of resolution on both the spatial frequency and contrast axes varies across species. For example, at relatively mesopic (rod- and cone-mediated) luminance levels, the peak of the spatial contrast sensitivity function for the albino rat, hooded rat, cat, and human are 0.1, 0.3, 0.3, and 2 cycles per degree, respectively (Birch and Jacobs, 1979; Fox, 1984).

Some of the visual parameters that have been investigated include (1) the absolute luminance threshold, which is the threshold value for detecting an illuminated target by a dark-adapted subject in a dark-adapted environment; (2) visual acuity, which is the spatial resolution of the visual system (approximately 50 cycles per degree in humans [Woodhouse and Barlow, 1982] and 1.1 to 1.8 cycles per degree in albino and hooded rats [Fox, 1984; Birch and Jacobs, 1979; Dean, 1981]); (3) color and spectral discriminations (Porkony *et al.*, 1979); (4) critical flicker fusion frequency, which is the threshold value for detecting a flickering light at different luminance intensities; and (5) the peak of the spatial and temporal contrast sensitivity functions at different luminance levels (Woodhouse and Barlow, 1982). Most of these tests are dependent upon the quality of the ocular optics and the ability to obtain a sharply focused visual image on the retina. Thresholds for detecting luminance, contrast, flicker, and color are primarily dependent on retinal and central mechanisms of neural function, although optical impairments (eg, cataracts) interfere with these functions. The assessment of visual acuity and contrast sensitivity has been recommended for field studies of humans potentially exposed to neurotoxic substances (Agency for Toxic Substances and Disease Registry [ATSDR], 1992).

Color Vision Testing

Color vision deficits are either inherited or acquired. Hereditary red–green color deficits occur in about 8% of males (X-linked) whereas only about 0.5% of females show similar congenital deficits (Porkony *et al.*, 1979). Inherited color deficiencies take two common forms: protan, a red–green confusion caused by abnormality or absence of the long-wavelength (red) sensitive cones (L-type cones); and deutan caused by abnormality or absence of the middle-wavelength sensitive (green) cones (M-type cones). Dutanopes demonstrate a concomitant confusion of red–green and blue–yellow due to the lack of M-type cones. Congenital loss of short-wavelength cones, resulting in a blue–yellow confusion (tritanopia, or type III), is extremely rare. Most acquired color vision deficits, such as those caused by drug and chemical exposure, begin with a reduced ability to perform blue–yellow discriminations (Porkony *et al.*, 1979; Bartlett and Jaanus, 2008). With increased or prolonged low-level exposure, the color confusion can progress to the red–green axis as well. Because of the rarity of inherited tritanopia, it is generally assumed that blue–yellow deficits, when observed, are acquired deficits. Köllner rule of thumb states that disorders of the outer retina produce blue–yellow deficits, whereas disorders of the inner retina and optic nerve produce red–green perceptual deficits (Porkony *et al.*, 1979). Bilateral lesions in the area V4 of visual cortex can also lead to color blindness (prosopagnosia). A recent review discusses the effects of drugs and chemicals on color vision (Bartlett and Jaanus, 2008).

Color vision has been evaluated in multiple occupationally and environmentally exposed populations (Iregren *et al.*, 2002). Color vision may be evaluated using several different testing procedures. Commonly used procedures in human toxicological evaluations include the Ishihara color plates and chip arrangement tests such as the Farnsworth-Munson 100 Hue (FM-100) test and the simplified 15-chip tests using either the saturated hues of the Farnsworth D-15 or the desaturated hues of the Lanthony Desaturated Panel D-15. The Ishihara plates involve a series of colored spots arranged in patterns that take advantage of perceived difference in shades resulting from congenital protan or deutan anomalies. Normal observers perceive different sets of embedded numbers than do those with color vision deficits. The Farnsworth-Munson procedure involves arrangement of 85 chips in order of progressively changing color. The relative chromatic value of successive chips induces those with color perception deficits to abnormally arrange the chips. The pattern is indicative of the nature of the color perception anomaly. The FM-100 is considered more diagnostically reliable but takes considerably longer to administer than the similar but more efficient Farnsworth and Lanthony tests. The desaturated hues of the Lanthony D-15 are designed to better identify subtle acquired color vision deficits. For this reason, and because it requires only a few minutes to administer, the Lanthony D-15 was recommended as the procedure for color vision screening of potentially occupationally and environmentally exposed populations (ATSDR, 1992). A critical review of this procedure, its test–retest reliability and its use in toxicological applications should be consulted prior to its use (Geller and Hudnell, 1997; Good *et al.*, 2005).

TARGET SITES AND MECHANISMS OF ACTION: CORNEA

The cornea provides the anterior covering of the eye and as such must provide three essential functions. First, it must provide a clear refractive surface. The air-to-fluid/tissue interface at the cornea is the principal refractive surface of the eye, providing approximately 48 diopters of refraction. The curvature of the cornea must be correct for the visual image to be focused at the retina. Second, the cornea provides tensile strength to maintain the appropriate shape of the globe. Third, the cornea protects the

eye from external factors, including potentially toxic chemicals. The anatomy is reviewed in the discussion of ocular pharmacodynamics and pharmacokinetics above.

The cornea is transparent to wavelengths of light ranging between 310 nm (UV) to 2500 nm (IR) in wavelengths. Exposure to UV light below this range can damage the cornea. It is most sensitive to wavelengths of approximately 270 nm. Excessive UV exposure leads to photokeratitis and corneal pathology, the classic example being welder's arc burns.

The cornea can be damaged by topical or systemic exposure to drugs and chemicals. Reports of such adverse reactions have been catalogued and reviewed by Diamante and Fraunfelder (1998). One summary analysis, of approximately 600 agricultural and industrial chemicals (raw materials, intermediates, formulation components, and sales products), evaluated using the Draize procedure, reported that over half of the materials tested caused no (18%–31%) or minimal (42%–51%) irritation. Depending on the chemical category, 9% to 17% of compounds were graded as slightly irritant, whereas 1% to 6% were graded as strong or extreme irritants (Kobel and Gfeller, 1985).

Direct chemical exposure to the eye requires emergency medical attention. Acid and alkali chemicals that come into contact with the cornea can be extremely destructive. Products at pH extremes ≤2.5 or ≥11.5 are considered as extreme ocular irritants. They can cause severe ocular damage and permanent loss of vision. Damage that extends to the corneal endothelium is associated with poor repair and recovery. The most important therapy is immediate and adequate irrigation with large amounts of water or saline, whichever is most readily available. The extent of damage to the eye and the ability to achieve a full recovery are dependent upon the nature of the chemical, the concentration and duration of exposure, and the speed and magnitude of the initial irrigation.

Acids

Strong acids with a pH ≤ 2.5 can be highly injurious. Among the most significant acidic chemicals in terms of the tendency to cause clinical ocular damage are hydrofluoric acid, sulfurous acid, sulfuric acid, chromic acid, hydrochloric acid, nitric acid, and acetic acid (McCulley, 1998). Injuries may be mild if contact is with weak acids or with dilute solutions of strong acids. Compounds with a pH between 2.5 and 7, produce pain or stinging; but with only brief contact, they will cause no lasting damage (Grant and Schuman, 1993). Following mild burns, the corneal epithelium may become turbid as the corneal stroma swells. Mild burns are typically followed by rapid regeneration of the corneal epithelium and full recovery. In more severe burns, the epithelium of the cornea and conjunctiva become opaque and necrotic and may disintegrate over the course of a few days. In severe burns, there may be no sensation of pain because the corneal nerve endings are destroyed (Grant and Schuman, 1993).

Acid chemical burns of the cornea occur through hydrogen ion-induced denaturing and coagulation of proteins. As epithelial cell proteins coagulate, glycosaminoglycans precipitate and stromal collagen fibers shrink. These events cause the cornea to become cloudy. The protein coagulation and shrinkage of the collagen is protective in that it forms a barrier and reduces further penetration of the acid. The collagen shrinkage, however, contracts the eye and can lead to a dangerous acute increase in intraocular pressure. The pH of the acid is not the only determinant of the severity of injury; however, as equimolar solutions of several chemicals adjusted to the same pH of 2 produce a wide range of outcomes. Both the hydrogen ion and anionic portions of the acid molecules contribute to protein coagulation and precipitation. The tissue proteins also tend to act as buffers (Grant and Schuman, 1993).

Bases or Alkalies

Compounds with a basic pH are potentially even more damaging to the eye than are strong acids. Among the compounds of clinical significance in terms of frequency and severity of injuries are ammonia or ammonium hydroxide, sodium hydroxide (lye), potassium hydroxide (caustic potash), calcium hydroxide (lime), and magnesium hydroxide (McCulley, 1998). One of the reasons that caustic chemicals are so dangerous is their ability to rapidly penetrate the ocular tissues. This is particularly true for ammonia, which has been measured in the aqueous humor just seconds after application to the cornea. The toxicity of these substances is a function of their pH, being more toxic with increasing pH values. As with acid burns, the concentration of the solution and the duration of contact with the eye are important determinants of the eventual clinical outcome. Rapid and extensive irrigation after exposure and removal of particles, if present, is the immediate therapy of choice (Grant and Schuman, 1993).

A feature of caustic burns that differentiates them from acid burns is that two phases of injury may be observed. There is an acute phase from exposure up to one week. Depending on the extent of injury, direct damage from exposure is observed in the cornea, adnexia, and possibly in the iris, ciliary body, and lens. The presence of strong hydroxide ions causes rapid necrosis of the corneal epithelium and, if sufficient amounts are present, penetration through and/or destruction of the successive corneal layers. Strong alkali substances attack membrane lipids, causing necrosis and enhancing penetration of the substance to deeper tissue layers. The cations also react with the carboxyl groups of glycosaminoglycans and collagen, the latter reaction leading to hydration of the collagen matrix and corneal swelling. The cornea may appear clouded or become opaque immediately after exposure as a result of stromal edema and changes to, or precipitation of, proteoglycans. The denaturing of the collagen and loss of protective covering of the glycosoaminoglycans is thought to make the collagen fibrils more susceptible to subsequent enzymatic degradation. Intraocular pressure may increase as a result of initial hydration of the collagen fibrils and later through the blockage of aqueous humor outflow. Conversely, if the alkali burn extends to involve the ciliary body, the intraocular pressure may decrease due to reduced formation of aqueous humor. The acute phase of damage is typically followed by initiation of corneal repair. The repair process may involve corneal neovascularization along with regeneration of the corneal epithelium. Approximately, two to three weeks after alkali burns, however, damaging ulceration of the corneal stroma often occurs. The formation of these lesions is related to the inflammatory infiltration of polymorphonuclear leukocytes and fibroblasts and the release of degratory proteolytic enzymes. Clinically, anti-inflammatory therapy limits ulcerative damage. Stromal ulceration usually stops when the corneal epithelium is restored (Grant and Schuman, 1993).

Organic Solvents

When organic solvents are splashed into the eye, the result is typically a painful immediate reaction. As in the case of acids and bases, exposure of the eye to solvents should be treated rapidly with abundant water irrigation. Highly lipophilic solvents can damage the corneal epithelium and produce swelling of the corneal stroma. Most organic solvents do not have a strongly acid or basic pH and therefore cause little in the way of chemical burns to the cornea. In most cases, the corneal epithelium will be repaired over the course of a few days and there will be no residual damage. Exposure to solvent vapors may produce small transparent vacuoles in the corneal epithelium, which may be asymptomatic or associated with moderate irritation and tearing (Grant and Schuman, 1993).

Surfactants

These compounds have water-soluble (hydrophilic) properties at one end of the molecule and lipophilic properties at the other end that help to dissolve fatty substances in water and also serve to reduce water surface tension. The widespread use of these chemicals in soaps, shampoos, detergents, cosmetics, and similar consumer products leads to abundant opportunities for exposure to ocular tissues. Many of these chemicals may be irritating or injurious to the eye. The hydrophilic portion of these compounds may be anionic, cationic, or neutral. In general, the cationic substances tend to be stronger irritants and more injurious than the other types, and anionic compounds more so than neutral ones (Grant and Schuman, 1993). Because these compounds are by design soluble in both aqueous and lipid media, they readily penetrate the sandwiched aqueous and lipid barriers of the cornea (see discussion of ocular pharmacodynamics and pharmacokinetics, above). This property has implications in drug delivery; for example, low concentrations of the preservative benzalkonium chloride to ophthalmic solutions enhance ocular penetration of topically applied medications (Bartlett and Jaanus, 2008), but also add to their corneal toxicity (Liang *et al.*, 2011).

TARGET SITES AND MECHANISMS OF ACTION: LENS

The lens of the eye plays a critical role in focusing the visual image on the retina. Although the cornea is the primary refractive surface for bending incoming light rays, the lens is capable of being reshaped to adjust the focal point to adapt for the distance of visual objects. The lens is a biconvex transparent body, encased in an elastic capsule, and located between the pupil and the vitreous humor (Fig. 17-1). The mature lens has a dense inner nuclear region surrounded by the lens cortex. The high transparency of the lens to visible wavelengths of light is a function of its chemical composition, approximately two-thirds water and one-third protein, and the special organizational structure of the lenticular proteins. The water-soluble crystallins are a set of proteins particular to the lens that, through their close intermolecular structure, give the lens both transparency and the proper refractive index. The lens fibers are laid down during development, as the epithelial cells grow and elongate along meridian pathways between the anterior and posterior poles of the lens. As the epithelial cells continue to grow, the nuclei recede and, in the central portions of the lens, disappear, such that the inner lens substance is composed of nonnucleated cells that form long proteinaceous fibers. The lens fibers are arranged within the lens in an onion-like fashion of concentric rings that have a prismatic arrangement in cross section. The regular geometric organization of the lens fibers is essential for the refractive index and transparency of the lens. At birth, the lens has no blood supply and no innervation. Nutrients are provided from the aqueous and vitreous fluids, and are transported into the lens substance through a system of intercellular gap-type junctions. The lens is a metabolically active tissue that maintains careful electrolyte and ionic balance. The lens continues to grow throughout life, with new cells added to the epithelial margin of the lens as the older cells condense into a central nuclear region. The growth of the lens is reflected in its weight, increasing from approximately 150 mg at

20 years of age to approximately 250 mg at 80 years of age (Banh *et al.*, 2005).

Cataracts are decreases in the optical transparency of the lens that can lead to functional visual disturbances. They are the leading cause of blindness worldwide, affecting an estimated 30 to 45 million people. In the United States, approximately 400,000 people develop cataracts each year. This accounts for about 35% of existing visual impairments (Banh *et al.*, 2005). Cataracts can occur at any age; they can also be congenital (Rogers and Chernoff, 1988). However, they are much more frequent with advancing age. Senile cataracts develop most frequently in the cortical or nuclear regions of the lens and less frequently in the posterior subcapsular region. Senile cataracts in the cortical region of the lens are associated with disruptions of water and electrolyte homeostasis, whereas nuclear cataracts are characterized by an increase in the water-insoluble fraction of lens proteins (Banh *et al.*, 2005).

Both genetic and environmental factors contribute to cataracts and several different mechanisms are involved (Hammond *et al.*, 2000; Ottonello *et al.*, 2000; Spector, 2000). Risk factors for the development of cataracts include aging, diabetes, low antioxidant levels, and exposure to a variety of environmental factors. Environmental factors include exposure to UV radiation and visible light, trauma, smoking, and exposure to a large variety of topical and systemic drugs and chemicals (Leske *et al.*, 1991; Grant and Schuman, 1993; Taylor and Nowell, 1997; Delcourt *et al.*, 2000; Spector, 2000). Several different mechanisms of action have been hypothesized to account for the development of cataracts. These include the disruption of lens energy metabolism, hydration and/or electrolyte balance, oxidative stress due to the generation of free radicals and reactive oxygen species, and the occurrence of oxidative stress due a decrease in antioxidant defense mechanisms such as glutathione, superoxide dismutase, catalase, ascorbic acid, or vitamin E (Giblin, 2000; Ottonello *et al.*, 2000; Spector, 2000). The generation of reactive oxygen species leads to oxidation of lens membrane proteins and lipids. A critical pathway is oxidation of protein thiol groups, particularly in methionine or cysteine amino acids, leading to the formation of polypeptide links through disulfide bonds, and in turn, high-molecular-weight protein aggregates (Ottonello *et al.*, 2000; Spector, 2000; Banh *et al.*, 2005). These large aggregations of proteins can attain a size sufficient to scatter light, thus reducing lens transparency. Oxidation of membrane lipids and proteins may also impair membrane transport and permeability.

Corticosteroids

Systemic treatment with corticosteroids causes cataracts (Urban and Cotlier, 1986). Observable opacities begin in the posterior subcapsular region of the lens and progress into the cortical region as the size of the lesion increases. Development of cataracts in individuals varies as a function of total dose of the drug, age, and the nature of the individual's underlying disease. It was estimated that 22% of patients receiving corticosteroid immunosuppressive therapy for renal transplants experienced cataracts as a side effect of therapy (Veenstra *et al.*, 1999). The use of inhaled corticosteroids—commonly prescribed asthma therapy—was once thought to be without this risk, but subsequent epidemiological evidence documented a significant association between inhaled steroidal therapy and development of nuclear and posterior subcapsular cataracts (Cumming *et al.*, 1997; Cumming and Mitchell, 1999). Epidemiological studies and meta-analysis indicate that higher doses and longer durations of use of inhaled steroid therapy are associated with an increased risk of cataracts (Smeeth *et al.*, 2003;

Weatherall *et al.*, 2009), although no significantly increased risks were observed in a population of chronic obstructive pulmonary disease (COPD) patients reporting inhaled corticosteroid use for 12 months or less (Miller *et al.*, 2011).

Naphthalene

Accidental exposure to naphthalene results in cortical cataracts and retinal degeneration (Grant and Schuman, 1993). Naphthalene itself is not cataractogenic; instead, the metabolite 1,2-dihydro-1,2-dihydroxynaphthalene (naphthalene dihydrodiol) is the cataract-inducing agent (van Heyningen and Pirie, 1967). Subsequent studies using biochemical and pharmacological techniques, in vitro assays, and transgenic mice showed that aldose reductase in the rat lens is a major protein associated with naphthalene dihydrodiol dehydrogenase activity and that lens aldose reductase is the enzyme responsible for the formation of naphthalene dihydrodiol (Sato, 1993; Lee and Chung, 1998; Sato *et al.*, 1999). In addition, in vivo and in vitro studies have shown that aldose reductase inhibitors prevent naphthalene-induced cataracts (Lou *et al.*, 1996; Sato *et al.*, 1999). Finally, there is a difference in naphthalene-induced cataract formation between albino and pigmented rats, with the latter showing a faster onset and more uniform cataract (Murano *et al.*, 1993).

Phenothiazines

It has been known since the 1950s that schizophrenics receiving phenothiazine drugs as antipsychotic medication develop pigmented deposits in their eyes and skin (Grant and Schuman, 1993). The pigmentation begins as tiny deposits on the anterior surface of the lens and progresses, with increasing dose, to involve the cornea as well. The phenothiazines combine with melanin to form a photosensitive product that reacts with sunlight, causing formation of the deposits. The amount of pigmentation is related to the dose of the drug, with the annual yearly dose being the most predictive dose metric (Thaler *et al.*, 1985). Epidemiological evidence suggests a dose-related increase in the risk of cataracts from use of phenothiazine-like drugs, including both antipsychotic drugs such as chlorpromazine and nonantipsychotic phenothiazines (Isaac *et al.*, 1991).

TARGET SITES AND MECHANISMS OF ACTION: RETINA

The adult mammalian retina is a highly differentiated tissue containing eight distinct layers plus the RPE, 10 major types of neurons, and a Müller glial cell (Fig. 17-1). The eight layers of the neural retina, which originate from the cells of the inner layer of the embryonic optic cup, are the nerve fiber layer (NFL), GCL, IPL, INL, OPL, ONL, rod and cone photoreceptor inner segment layer (RIS; CIS), and the rod and cone photoreceptor outer segment layer (ROS; COS). The RPE, which originates from the cells of the outer layer of the embryonic optic cup, is a single layer of cuboidal epithelial cells that lies on Bruch membrane adjacent to the vascular choroid. Between the RPE and photoreceptor outer segments lies the subretinal space, which is similar to the brain ventricles. The 10 major types of neurons are the rod and cone photoreceptors, (depolarizing) ON-rod and ON-cone bipolar cells, (hyperpolarizing) OFF-cone bipolar cells, horizontal cells, numerous subtypes of amacrine cells, an interplexiform cell, and ON-RGCs and OFF-RGCs. The Müller glial cell (MGC) is the only glial cell in the retina. The somas of the MGCs are in the INL. The end feet of the MGCs in the proximal or inner retina along with a basal lamina form the internal limiting membrane of the retina, which is similar to the pial surface of the brain. In the distal retina, the MGC end feet join with the photoreceptors and zonula adherens to form the external limiting membrane, which is located between the ONL and RIS/CIS. The interested reader is referred to the excellent references in the Introduction section as well as to numerous outstanding websites devoted exclusively to the retina (http://webvision.med.utah.edu; http://cvs.anu.edu.au; http://retina.anatomy.upenn.edu) for basic information on the anatomic, biochemical, cell and molecular biological, and physiological aspects of retinal structure and function.

The mammalian retina is highly vulnerable to toxicant-induced structural and/or functional damage due to (1) the presence of a highly fenestrated choriocapillaris that supplies the distal or outer retina as well as a portion of the inner retina; (2) the very high rate of oxidative mitochondrial metabolism, especially in photoreceptors (Ahmed et al., 1993; Medrano and Fox, 1995; Braun et al., 1995; Winkler, 1995; Shulman and Fox, 1996); (3) high daily turnover of rod and cone outer segments (LaVail, 1976); (4) high susceptibility of the rod and cones to degeneration due to inherited retinal dystrophies as well as associated syndromes and metabolic disorders (van Soest et al., 1999; Jones and Marc, 2005); (5) presence of specialized ribbon synapses and synaptic contact sites (Wässle, 2004; tom Dieck and Brandstätter, 2006); (6) presence of numerous neurotransmitter and neuromodulatory systems, including extensive glutamatergic, GABAergic and glycinergic systems (Kalloniatis and Tomisich, 1999; Wässle, 2004); (7) presence of numerous and highly specialized gap junctions used in the information signaling process (Bloomfield and Völgyi, 2009); (8) presence of melanin in the choroid, RPE, uvea, and iris (Meier-Ruge, 1972; Potts and Au, 1976); (9) a very high choroidal blood flow rate, as high as 10 times that of the gray matter of the brain (Nickla and Wallman, 2010); and (10) the additive or synergistic toxic action of certain chemicals with light (Dayhaw-Barker et al., 1986; Backstrom et al., 1993; Roberts, 2001, 2002; Glickman, 2002).

The retina is also an excellent model system for studying the effects of chemicals on the developing and mature CNS. Its structure–function relations are well established. The histogenic steps of development of the neurons and glial components are well characterized. The development of the CNS and most retinal cells occurs early during gestation in humans (Hendrickson, 1992; Hendrickson and Drucker, 1992) and continues for an additional seven to 14 days postnatally in the rat (Dobbing and Sands, 1979; Raedler and Sievers, 1975). Therefore, toxicological effects in the rodent retina have relevance for chemical exposure during the early gestation period in humans as well as during early postnatal development. The retina contains a wide diversity of synaptic transmitters and second messengers whose developmental patterns are well described. Moreover, the rodent retina is easily accessible, it has most of the same anatomical and functional features found in the developing and mature human retina, and the rat rod pathway is similar to that in other mammals (Finlay and Sengelbaub, 1989; Chun et al., 1993). Finally, rat rods have similar dimensions, photochemistry, and photocurrents as human and monkey rods (Baylor et al., 1984; Schnapf et al., 1988). These general and specific features underscore the relevance and applicability of using the rodent retina to investigate the effects of chemicals on this target site as well as a model to investigate the neurotoxic effects of chemicals during development.

Each retinal layer can undergo specific as well as general toxic effects. These alterations and deficits include, but are not limited to visual field deficits, scotopic vision deficits such as night blindness and increases in the threshold for dark adaptation, cone-mediated (photopic) deficits such as decreased color perception, decreased visual acuity, macular and general retina edema, retinal hemorrhages

and vasoconstriction, and pigmentary changes. The list of drugs and other chemicals that cause retinal alterations is extensive, as evidenced by an examination of Table 17-1, Grant's *Toxicology of the Eye* (Grant and Schuman, 1993), Bartlett and Jaanus (2008) discussion of the adverse retinal effects of therapeutic systemic drugs and a review by Wolfensberger (1998) that addresses the adverse effects of drugs on the RPE. The overall aim of this section is to discuss in detail several chemicals, solvents, and drugs: (1) that are used as drugs or that are environmentally relevant neurotoxicants; (2) whose behavioral, physiological, and/or pathological effects on the retina are known; and (3) whose retinal site(s) and/or mechanism of action are well characterized.

The chemical- and drug-induced alterations in retinal structure and function are grouped into two major categories. The first category focuses on retinotoxicity of systemically administered therapeutic drugs. Six major drugs are discussed in detail: chloroquine/hydroxychloroquine, digoxin/digitoxin, indomethacin, sildenafil, tamoxifen, and vigabatrin. The second category focuses on well-known neurotoxicants that produce retinotoxicity: inorganic lead, methanol, selected organic solvents, and organophosphates. See Chap. 16 and 23 for information on the effects of lead on the brain and other target organs and Chap. 24 for additional information on methanol and the organic solvents discussed below.

Retinotoxicity of Systemically Administered Therapeutic Drugs

Cancer Chemotherapeutics Ocular toxicity is a common side effect of cancer chemotherapy (Imperia et al., 1989; Schmid et al., 2006). Symptoms include blurred vision, diplopia, decreased color vision, decreased visual acuity, optic/retrobular neuritis, transient cortical blindness, and demyelination of the optic nerves (Imperia et al., 1989; Schmid et al., 2006). The retina due to its high metabolic activity and choroidal circulation (vide infra) appears to be particularly vulnerable to numerous cytotoxic drugs such as the alkylating agents cisplatin, carboplatin, and carmustine; the antimetabolites cytosine arabinoside, 5-fluorouracil, and methotrexate; and the mitotic inhibitors such as docetaxel. The ocular toxicity of different drugs is dependent upon the dose, duration of dosage, and route of administration. However, if not detected at an early stage of toxicity, the ocular complications are often irreversible even after chemotherapy is discontinued (Imperia et al., 1989; Schmid et al., 2006). One strategy to avoid such retinal complications is to conduct prospective ophthalmological examinations as well as scotopic and photopic ERG testing prior to the onset and during chemotherapy. The ocular side effects of tamoxifen, an estrogen antagonist used in oncology, are discussed below.

Chloroquine and Hydroxychloroquine Two of the most extensively studied retinotoxic drugs are chloroquine (Aralen) and hydroxychloroquine (Plaquenil). The first case of chloroquine-induced retinopathy was reported more than 40 years ago (Bartlett and Jaanus, 2008). These 4-aminoquinoline derivatives are used as antimalarial and anti-inflammatory drugs. The low-dose therapy used for malaria is essentially free from toxic side effects; however, the chronic, high-dose therapy used for rheumatoid arthritis, and discoid and systemic lupus erythematosus (initially 400–600 mg/day for four to 12 weeks and then 200–400 mg/day; Ellsworth et al., 1999) can cause irreversible loss of retinal function. Chloroquine, its major metabolite desethylchloroquine, and hydroxychloroquine have high affinity for melanin, which results in very high concentrations of these drugs accumulating in the choroid and RPE, ciliary body, and iris during and following drug administration (Rosenthal *et al.*, 1978). Prolonged exposure of the retina to these drugs, especially chloroquine, may lead to an irreversible retinopathy. In fact, small amounts of chloroquine and its metabolites were excreted in the urine years after cessation of drug treatment (Bernstein, 1967). Approximately, 20% to 30% of patients who received high doses of chloroquine exhibited some type of retinal abnormality, whereas 5% to 10% showed severe changes in retinal function (Burns, 1966; Shearer and Dubois, 1967; Sassaman *et al.*, 1970; Krill *et al.*, 1971). Hydroxychloroquine is now the drug of choice for treatment of rheumatic diseases because it has fewer side effects and less ocular toxicity. Doses less than 400 mg/day appear to produce little or no retinopathy even after prolonged therapy (Johnson and Vine, 1987).

The clinical findings accompanying chloroquine retinopathy can be divided into early and late stages. The early changes include (1) the pathognomonic "bull's-eye retina" visualized as a dark, central pigmented area involving the macula, surrounded by a pale ring of depigmentation, which is surrounded by another ring of pigmentation; (2) a diminished EOG; (3) possible granular pigmentation in the peripheral retina; and (4) visual complaints such as blurred vision and problems discerning letters or words. Late-stage findings, which can occur during or even following cessation of drug exposure, include (1) a progressive scotoma, (2) constriction of the peripheral fields commencing in the upper temporal quadrant, (3) narrowing of the retinal artery, (4) color and night blindness, (5) absence of a typical retinal pigment pattern, and (6) very abnormal EOGs and ERGs. These late-stage symptoms are irreversible. Interestingly, dark adaptation is relatively normal even during the late stages of chloroquine retinopathy, which helps distinguish the peripheral retinal changes from those observed in patients with retinitis pigmentosa (Bernstein, 1967).

In humans and monkeys, long-term chloroquine administration results in sequential degeneration of the RGCs, photoreceptors, and RPE and the eventual migration of RPE pigment into the ONL and OPL. In addition, in the RPE there is a thickening of the RPE layer, an increase in the mucopolysaccharide and sulfhydryl group content, and a decrease in activity of several enzymes (Ramsey and Fine, 1972; Rosenthal *et al.*, 1978). Although the molecular mechanism of action is unknown, it has been suggested that the primary biochemical mechanism is inhibition of protein synthesis (Bernstein, 1967).

Digoxin and Digitoxin The cardiac glycosides digoxin and digitoxin are digitalis derivatives used in the treatment of congestive heart disease and in certain cardiac arrhythmias. As part of the extract of the plant foxglove, digitalis was recommended for heart failure (dropsy) over 200 years ago. Digitalis-induced visual system abnormalities such as decreased vision, flickering scotomas, and altered color vision were documented during that time (Withering, 1785). Approximately, 20% to 60% of patients with cardiac glycoside serum levels in the therapeutic range and 50% to 80% of the patients with cardiac glycoside serum levels in the toxic range complain of visual system disturbances within two weeks after the onset of therapy (Robertson *et al.*, 1966; Haustein *et al.*, 1982; Duncker *et al.*, 1994). Digoxin produces more toxicity than digitoxin due to its greater volume of distribution and plasma protein binding (Haustein and Schmidt, 1988). The most frequent visual complaints are color vision impairments and hazy or snowy vision, although complaints of flickering light, colored spots surrounded by bright halos, blurred vision, and glare sensitivity also are reported. The color vision disturbances have been confirmed with the Farnsworth-Munsell 100 Hue Test (Haustein *et al.*, 1982; Haustein and Schmidt, 1988; Duncker and Krastel, 1990). Clinical examinations show that these patients have decreased visual acuity

and central scotomas but no funduscopic changes. ERG analysis revealed reduced rod and cone amplitudes, increased rod and cone implicit times, and elevated rod and cone thresholds (Robertson *et al.*, 1966; Alken and Belz, 1984; Duncker and Krastel, 1990; Madreperla *et al.*, 1994). Taken together, these ophthalmological, behavioral, and electrophysiological findings demonstrate that the photoreceptors are a primary target site of the cardiac glycosides digoxin and digitoxin.

The above results suggest that cone photoreceptors are more susceptible to the effects of cardiac glycosides than rod photoreceptors. Electrophysiological experiments by Madreperla *et al.* (1994) showed that cones were ~50 times more sensitive to digoxin and were impaired to a greater degree at the same digoxin concentration than the rods. Following short-duration saturating light flashes, rods appear to recover faster and more completely than cones. However, neither recover to their dark-adapted baseline response level. This latter finding correlates with the slow recovery of the ERG seen in patients following termination of digoxin exposure (Duncker and Krastel, 1990; Madreperla *et al.*, 1994) and is most likely due to the high affinity and slow off-rate of digoxin binding to the cardiac glycoside site located on the extracellular side of the catalytic α-subunit of the Na$^+$,K$^+$-ATPase enzyme (Sweadner, 1989).

Digitalis glycosides, like ouabain, are potent inhibitors of retinal Na$^+$,K$^+$-ATPase (Winkler and Riley, 1977; Fox *et al.*, 1991b; Shulman and Fox, 1996). Digoxin-binding studies show that the retina has the highest number of Na$^+$,K$^+$-ATPase sites of any ocular tissue, even higher than those of brain (Lissner *et al.*, 1971). There are three different isoforms of the α subunit of Na$^+$,K$^+$-ATPase (ie, α1, α2, and α3), and they differ significantly in their sensitivity to cardiac glycoside inhibition (Sweadner, 1989). In the rat retina, the α1-low and α3-high ouabain affinity isoforms of the enzyme account for ≥97% of the Na$^+$,K$^+$-ATPase mRNA. The α3 isoform is localized to rat photoreceptors, horizontal cells, and bipolar cells. Photoreceptors predominantly express the α3 mRNA (approximately 85%), a small amount of α1 mRNA (approximately 15%), and almost no detectable α2 mRNA. Electron microscopic immunocytochemistry studies reveal that the α3 isoform is localized exclusively to the plasma membrane of the rat photoreceptor inner segments (McGrail and Sweadner, 1989; Schneider *et al.*, 1991). The α3 isozyme accounts for most of the rod Na$^+$,K$^+$-ATPase activity (Shulman and Fox, 1996). The rat rod photoreceptor Na$^+$,K$^+$-ATPase specific activity is approximately threefold higher than whole retinal (Fox *et al.*, 1991b; Shulman and Fox, 1996) or whole brain values (Marks and Seeds, 1978). This also is reflected in the two- to threefold greater ouabain-sensitive oxygen consumption in the dark-adapted outer retina relative to the whole or inner retina, respectively (Medrano and Fox, 1995; Shulman and Fox, 1996).

Indomethacin Indomethacin is a nonsteroidal anti-inflammatory drug with analgesic and antipyretic properties that is frequently used for the management of arthritis, gout, and musculoskeletal discomfort. It inhibits prostaglandin synthesis by inhibiting cyclooxygenase. The first cases of indomethacin-induced retinopathy were reported approximately 30 years ago (Bartlett and Jaanus, 2008). Chronic administration of 50 to 200 mg/day of indomethacin for one to two years has been reported to produce corneal opacities, discrete pigment scattering of the RPE perifoveally, paramacular depigmentation, decreases in visual acuity, altered visual fields, increases in the threshold for dark adaptation, blue–yellow color deficits, and decreases in ERG and EOG amplitudes (Burns, 1966, 1968; Henkes *et al.*, 1972; Koliopoulos and Palimeris, 1972). Decreases in the ERG a- and b-wave amplitudes, with larger changes observed under scotopic dark-adapted than light-adapted conditions, have been reported. Upon cessation of drug treatment, the ERG waveforms and color vision changes return to near normal, although the pigmentary changes are irreversible (Burns, 1968; Henkes et al., 1972). The mechanism of retinotoxicity is unknown; however, it appears likely that the RPE is a primary target site.

Sildenafil Citrate Sildenafil citrate (Viagra) is a cGMP-specific phosphodiesterase (PDE) type 5 inhibitor that is utilized in the treatment of erectile dysfunction (Corbin et al., 2002). Sildenafil is also a weak cGMP PDE type 6 inhibitor, which is present in rod and cone photorecepotrs (Corbin et al., 2002; Zhang et al., 2005). Transient visual symptoms such as a blue tinge to vision, increased brightness of lights and blurry vision as well as alterations in scotopic and photopic ERGs have been reported following sildenafil usage (Laties and Zrenner, 2002; Jagle et al., 2004). More recently, sildenafil has been associated with the occurrence of nonarteritic anterior ischemic optic neuropathy (NAION) in at-risk patients (ie, those with small cup-to-disc ratios and/or arteriosclerotic risk profiles) within minutes to hours after the ingestion of the drug (Fraunfelder et al., 2006). However, available data suggest that the risk of occurrence of NAION in patients taking sildenafil or tadalafil is not significantly different from the general population (Fraunfelder et al., 2006; Gorkin et al., 2006; Laties, 2009).

Tamoxifen Tamoxifen (Nolvadex, Tamoplex), a triphenylethylene derivative, is a nonsteroidal antiestrogenic drug that competes with estrogen for its receptor sites. It is a highly effective antitumor agent used for the treatment of metastatic breast carcinoma in postmenopausal women. Tamoxifen-induced retinopathy following chronic high-dose therapy (180–240 mg/day for approximately two years) was first reported 20 years ago (Kaiser-Kupfer et al., 1981). At this dose, there is widespread axonal degeneration in the macular and perimacular area, as evidenced by the presence of different sized yellow–white refractile opacities in the IPL and NFL observed during fundus examination. Macular edema may or may not be present. Clinical symptoms include a permanent decrease in visual acuity and abnormal visual fields, as the axonal degeneration is irreversible (Ah-Song and Sasco, 1997; Bartlett and Jaanus, 2008). Several prospective studies, with sample sizes ranging from 63 to 303 women with breast cancer, have shown that chronic low-dose tamoxifen (20 mg/day) can result in a small but significant increase in the incidence (≤10%) of keratopathy (Pavlidis et al., 1992; Gorin et al., 1998; Lazzaroni et al., 1998; Noureddin et al., 1999). In addition, these studies showed that retinopathy is much less frequently observed than with high-dose therapy and, except for a few reports of altered color vision and decreased visual acuity, there were no significant alterations in visual function. Following cessation of low-dose tamoxifen therapy, most of the keratopathy and retinal alterations except the corneal opacities and retinopathy were reversible (Pavlidis et al., 1992; Gorin et al., 1998; Noureddin et al., 1999).

Vigabatrin Vigabatrin is an inhibitor of GABA-transaminase that is used to treat refractory complex partial seizures and infantile spasms (Tolman and Faulkner, 2009). After 20 years of use in Europe, it was approved in 2009 by the FDA for use in the USA despite its risk of retinopathy characterized by irreversible bilateral, concentric peripheral visual constriction, and decreased retinal nerve fiber thickness (Maguire et al., 2010; Clayton et al., 2011; Plant and Sergott, 2011). Clinical and meta-analysis studies reveal that the prevalence of the asymptomatic visual field loss is ~50% (Maguire et al., 2010; Clayton et al., 2011; Plant and Sergott, 2011). Onset of the visual field loss is variable as it has been observed as soon as six weeks of exposure, but generally requires a couple of

years (Maguire et al., 2010; Clayton et al., 2011; Plant and Sergott, 2011). In addition, rod and cone ERGs as well as flicker responses are altered, indicating that retinal damage also occurs (Daneshvar et al., 1999; Wang et al., 2008). Recent dose–response studies in mice revealed disorganization of the photoreceptors and OPL retinal synaptic following one month of vigabatrin exposure (Wang et al., 2008). The drug is recommended only for epileptic patients with no alternative choices.

Retinotoxicity of Known Neurotoxicants

Inorganic Lead Inorganic lead is probably the oldest known and most studied environmental toxicant. For almost 100 years, it has been known that overt lead poisoning (mean blood lead [BPb] ≥80 µg/dL) in man produces visual system pathology and overt visual symptoms (Otto and Fox, 1993; Fox, 1998). Clinical manifestations include amblyopia, blindness, optic neuritis or atrophy, peripheral and central scotomas, paralysis of eye muscles, and decreased visual function. Moderate to high level lead exposure produces scotopic and temporal visual system deficits in occupationally exposed factory workers and developmentally lead-exposed monkeys and rats (Bushnell et al., 1977; Betta et al., 1983; Signorino et al., 1983; Campara et al., 1984; Fox and Farber, 1988; Fox et al., 1991a; Fox and Katz, 1992; Otto and Fox, 1993; Lilienthal et al., 1994; Rice, 1998). Early work in monkeys exposed to moderate to high levels of lead during and following gestation reveal that this lead exposure regimen produces irreversible retinal deficits (Lilienthal et al., 1988, 1994; Kohler et al., 1997). A prospective epidemiological study in seven- to 10-year-old children revealed that low-level gestational lead exposure produces long-lasting scotopic supernormal ERG deficits (Rothenberg et al., 2002). Similar results were found in a rodent model of low-level gestational lead exposure (Fox et al., 2008). Recently, a case report with similar findings was published (Nagpal and Brodie, 2009). However, relatively little effort has been made to understand the impact of lead-induced alterations on retinal and central visual information processing on learning and memory in children. These types of visual deficits can adversely affect learning and memory as well as experimental procedures used to assess these cognitive parameters (Anger et al., 1994; Hudnell et al., 1996; Walkowiak et al., 1998; Cestnick and Coltheart, 1999).

Studies in Occupationally Exposed Lead Workers Clinical and electrophysiological studies in lead-exposed factory workers have assessed both the site of action and extent of injury. Several cases of retrobulbar optic neuritis and optic nerve atrophy have been observed following chronic moderate-level or acute high-level lead exposure (Baghdassarian, 1968; Baloh et al., 1979; Karai et al., 1982). Most of these cases presented with fundus lesions, peripheral or paracentral scotomas whereas the most severe cases also had a central scotoma. Generally, the scotomas were not observed until approximately five years of continuous lead exposure. Interestingly, the earliest observable scotomas were not detected under standard photopic viewing conditions but became evident only under scotopic or mesopic (rod- and cone-mediated) viewing conditions. These ophthalmological findings correlate directly with the ERG data observed in similarly exposed lead workers. No alterations in the critical flicker fusion threshold (ie, temporal resolution) were observed when the test was conducted under photopic conditions or when using red lights. However, consistent decreases in temporal resolution were observed when the test was conducted under scotopic conditions or when green lights were used (Cavelleri et al., 1982; Betta et al., 1983; Signorino et al., 1983; Campara et al., 1984). Moreover, in occupationally lead-exposed workers with or without visual acuity deficits or no observable alterations following ophthalmological examination, the sensitivity, and amplitude of the a-wave and/or b-wave of the dark-adapted ERG were decreased (Scholl and Zrenner, 2000). In other lead-exposed workers, one funduscopic study noted the presence of a grayish lead pigmentary deposit in the area peripheral to the optic disc margins (Sonkin, 1963).

In addition to the retinal deficits, oculomotor deficits occur in chronically lead-exposed workers who have no observable ophthalmological abnormalities. Results from three independent studies, including a follow-up, show that the mean accuracy of saccadic eye movements is lower in lead-exposed workers and the number of overshoots is increased (Baloh et al., 1979; Spivey et al., 1980; Specchio et al., 1981; Glickman et al., 1984). In addition, these studies also revealed that the saccade maximum velocity was decreased. Moreover, one study also observed abnormal smooth pursuit eye movements in lead-exposed workers (Specchio et al., 1981). Although the site and mechanism of action underlying these alterations are unknown, they most likely result from CNS-mediated deficits.

In summary, these results suggest that occupational lead exposure produces concentration- and time-dependent alterations in the retina such that higher levels of lead directly and adversely affect both the retina and optic nerve, whereas lower levels of lead appear to primarily affect the rod photoreceptors and their pathway. Interestingly, these latter clinical findings showing preferential lead-induced rod-selective deficits in sensitivity and temporal resolution are observed in both in vivo and in vitro animal studies (see below). Furthermore, these retinal and oculomotor alterations were, in most cases, correlated with the blood lead levels and occurred in the absence of observable ophthalmological changes, CNS symptoms, and abnormal performance test scores. Thus, these measures of temporal visual function may be among the most sensitive for the early detection of the neurotoxic effects of inorganic lead.

In Vivo and in Vitro Animal Studies with Lead Lead exposure to adult animals and postnatally developing animals produces retinal damage and functional deficits. The degree and extent of these alterations depends upon the dose, age, and duration of lead exposure. High-level lead exposure to adult rabbits for 60 to 300 days (Hass et al., 1964; Brown, 1974; Hughes and Coogan, 1974) and to newborn rats for 60 days (Santos-Anderson et al., 1984) resulted in focal necrosis of the rod inner and outer segments, necrosis in the INL and Müller cells, and lysosomal inclusions in the RPE. In addition, high-level lead exposure to mice and rats from birth to weaning resulted in hypomyelination of the optic nerve and a reduction in its diameter; but, interestingly, there were no changes in the sciatic nerve (Tennekoon et al., 1979; Toews et al., 1980). Newborn monkeys exposed to high levels of lead for six years had no changes in optic nerve diameter or myelination, although visual cortex neuronal volume and branching were decreased (Reuhl et al., 1989). Rhesus monkeys exposed prenatally and postnatally to moderate or high levels of lead for nine years, followed by almost two years of no lead exposure, had decreased tyrosine hydroxylase immunoreactivity in the large dopaminergic amacrine cells and a complete loss of tyrosine hydroxylase immunoreactivity in small subset of amacrine cells (Kohler et al., 1997). These results suggest that long-term lead exposure produces a decrease in tyrosine hydroxylase synthesis, a finding consistent with other studies (Lasley and Lane, 1988; Jadhav and Ramesh, 1997), and/or a loss of a subset of tyrosine hydroxylase-positive amacrine cells, a finding consistent with recent in vitro work (Scortegagna and Hanbauer, 1997). In contrast to these studies, six weeks of moderate-level lead exposure

to adult rats (Fox et al., 1997) and three weeks of low- or moderate-level lead exposure to neonatal rats from birth to weaning produced rod- and bipolar cell-selective apoptotic cell death (Fox and Chu, 1988; Fox et al., 1997). Moreover, recent results reveal that brief (15 minutes) exposure of isolated adult rat retinas to nanomolar to micromolar Pb^{2+}, concentrations regarded as pathophysiologically relevant (Cavalleri et al., 1984; Al-Modhefer et al., 1991), resulted in rod-selective apoptosis (He et al., 2000, 2003). By extension, these results suggest that the triggering event (initiating phase) and the execution phase of rod and bipolar cell death share common underlying biochemical mechanisms.

Results from several studies suggest that an elevated level of rod photoreceptor Ca^{2+} and/or Pb^{2+} plays a key role in the process of apoptotic rod cell death in humans and animals during inherited retinal degenerations, retinal diseases and injuries, chemical exposure, and lead exposure. These include patients with retinitis pigmentosa and cancer-associated retinopathy (Thirkill et al., 1987; van Soest et al., 1999), mice with retinal degeneration (rd) (Chang et al., 1993; Fox et al., 1999), rats injected with antirecoverin monoclonal antibodies (Adamus et al., 1998), rats with hypoxic–ischemic injury (Crosson et al., 1990), rats with light-induced damage (Edward et al., 1991), and lead-exposed rats (Fox and Chu, 1988; Fox et al., 1997, 1999). In addition, moderate level Pb^{2+} exposure produces apoptotic neuronal cell death in primary cultured cells (Oberto et al., 1996; Scortegagna and Hanbauer, 1997). In vivo and in vitro data suggest that Pb^{2+} produces a dose (concentration)-dependent inhibition of rod cGMP PDE, a resultant elevation of rod cGMP (Fox and Farber, 1988; Fox et al., 1991a; Srivastava et al., 1995a,b; Fox et al., 1997), which gates the nonselective cation channel of the rod photoreceptor outer segments (Yau and Baylor, 1989), and an elevation of the rod Ca^{2+} concentration (Fox and Katz, 1992; Medrano and Fox, 1994; He et al., 2000, 2003). Detailed kinetic analysis revealed that picomolar Pb^{2+} competitively and directly inhibits rod cGMP PDE relative to millimolar concentrations of Mg^{2+} (Srivastava et al., 1995a,b). In addition, nanomolar Pb^{2+} can elevate the rod Ca^{2+} (and Pb^{2+}) concentration via its competitive inhibition of retinal Na^+,K^+-ATPase relative to MgATP (Fox et al., 1991b). Once inside the rod, both Ca^{2+} and Pb^{2+} enter the mitochondria via the ruthenium red-sensitive Ca^{2+} uniporter and induce mitochondrial depolarization, swelling, and cytochrome c release (He et al., 2000, 2003). The effects of Ca^{2+} and Pb^{2+} were additive and blocked completely by the mitochondrial permeability transition pore inhibitor cyclosporin A. Following cytochrome c release, caspase-9 and caspase-3 are sequentially activated. There was no evidence of caspase-8, oxidative stress or lipid peroxidation in this model. These results demonstrate that rod mitochondria are the target site for Ca^{2+} and Pb^{2+}. This is consistent with numerous studies from different tissues demonstrating that lead is preferentially associated with mitochondria and particularly with the inner membrane and matrix fractions (Barltrop et al., 1971; Bull, 1980; Pounds, 1984). Taken together, the results suggest that Ca^{2+} and Pb^{2+} bind to the internal divalent metal binding site of the mitochondrial permeability transition pore (Szabo et al., 1992) and subsequently open it, which initiates the cytochrome c-caspase cascade of apoptosis in rods (He et al., 2000, 2003).

In vitro extracellular and intracellular electrophysiological recordings in isolated whole retinas or photoreceptors reveal that nanomolar to micromolar Pb^{2+} selectively depress the amplitude and absolute sensitivity of the rod but not cone photoreceptor potential (Fox and Sillman, 1979; Sillman et al., 1982; Tessier-Lavigne et al., 1985; Frumkes and Eysteinsson, 1988). These electrophysiological results are similar to the ERG alterations observed in occupationally lead-exposed workers (Cavelleri et al., 1982; Betta *et al.*, 1983; Signorino *et al.*, 1983; Campara *et al.*, 1984) and in adult rats exposed to low and moderate levels of lead only during development (Fox and Farber, 1988; Fox and Rubinstein, 1989; Fox *et al.*, 1991a; Fox and Katz, 1992). In addition, these postnatally lead-exposed rats exhibit rod-mediated increases in dark and light adaptation time, decreases in critical flicker fusion frequency (ie, temporal resolution), decreases in relative sensitivity, and increases in a- and b-wave latencies (Fox and Farber, 1988; Fox and Rubinstein, 1989; Fox *et al.*, 1991a; Fox and Katz, 1992) and decreases in the temporal response properties of both sustained (X-type) and transient (Y-type) RGCs, such as decreased optimal temporal frequency and temporal resolution (Ruan *et al.*, 1994). By extension, these results suggest that there is a common underlying biochemical mechanism responsible for these rod-mediated deficits. In vivo and in vitro data suggest that lead-induced inhibition of cGMP PDE and resultant elevation of rod Ca^{2+} underlies the ERG deficits (Fox and Katz, 1992; Medrano and Fox, 1994; Fox *et al.*, 1997; He *et al.*, 2000, 2003). Finally, rod-mediated alterations in dark adaptation and b-wave amplitude are also observed in adult rats and monkeys with prenatal and lifetime moderate- and high-level lead exposure (Hennekes *et al.*, 1987; Lilienthal *et al.*, 1988, 1994). In the gestationally and postnatally lead-exposed monkeys and children, the amplitude of the scotopic b-wave was increased (Lilienthal *et al.*, 1988, 1994; Rothenberg *et al.*, 2002; Nagpal and Brodie, 2009): an effect hypothesized to result from the loss of dopaminergic amacrine cells or their processes (Kohler *et al.*, 1997). If rods and blue-sensitive cones in humans exhibit the same sensitivity to a lead-induced inhibition of cGMP-PDE as they do to the drug-induced inhibition of cGMP-PDE (Zrenner and Gouras, 1979; Zrenner *et al.*, 1982; Fox and Farber, 1988) predicted that blue-cone (short wavelength or S-cones) color vision deficits as well as scotopic deficits may be found in adults and children exposed to lead. S-cone deficits have been observed in an occupationally lead-exposed worker (Scholl and Zrenner, 2000).

Methanol Methanol is a low-molecular-weight (32 Da), colorless, and volatile liquid that is widely used as an industrial solvent; a chemical intermediate; a fuel source for picnic stoves, racing cars, and soldering torches; an antifreeze agent; and an octane booster for gasoline. The basic toxicology and references can be found in a thorough review (Eells, 1992). Briefly, methanol is readily and rapidly absorbed from all routes of exposure (dermal, inhalation, and oral), easily crosses all membranes, and thus is uniformly distributed to organs and tissues in direct relation to their water content. Following different routes of exposures, the highest concentrations of methanol are found in the blood, aqueous, and vitreous humors, and bile as well as the brain, kidneys, lungs, and spleen. In the liver, methanol is oxidized sequentially to formaldehyde by alcohol dehydrogenase in human and nonhuman primates or by catalase in rodents and then to formic acid. It is excreted as formic acid in the urine or oxidized further to carbon dioxide and then excreted by the lungs. Formic acid is the toxic metabolite that mediates the metabolic acidosis as well as the retinal and optic nerve toxicity observed in humans, monkeys, and rats with a decreased capacity for folate metabolism (Murray *et al.*, 1991; Eells, 1992; Lee *et al.*, 1994; Garner *et al.*, 1995a, 1995b; Eells *et al.*, 1996; Seme *et al.*, 1999).

Human and nonhuman primates are highly sensitive to methanol-induced neurotoxicity due to their limited capacity to oxidize formic acid. The toxicity occurs in several stages. It first occurs as a mild CNS depression, followed by an asymptomatic 12- to 24-hour latent period, then by a syndrome consisting of formic acidemia, uncompensated metabolic acidosis, ocular and visual toxicity, coma, and possibly death (Eells, 1992). The treatment of methanol poisoning involves both combating acidosis and preventing methanol oxidation, but it is not discussed further here. Experimental rats were made as sensitive to acute methanol exposure as primates by using two different, but related, procedures that effectively reduce the levels of hepatic tetrahydrofolate. One study acutely inhibited methionine synthase and reduced the level of hepatic tetrahydrofolate (Murray *et al.*, 1991; Eells *et al.*, 1996; Seme *et al.*, 1999), whereas the other fed rats a folate-deficient diet for 18 weeks (Lee *et al.*, 1994). Administration of methanol to rats with a decreased capacity for folate metabolism resulted in toxic blood formate concentrations of 8 to 16 mM (Murray *et al.*, 1991; Lee *et al.*, 1994; Garner *et al.*, 1995a,b; Eells *et al.*, 1996; Seme *et al.*, 1999). Permanent visual damage occurred in humans and monkeys when the blood folate levels exceeded 7 mM (Eells, 1992).

Acute methanol poisoning in humans, monkeys, and experimental rats resulted in profound and permanent structural alterations in the retina and optic nerve and visual impairments ranging from blurred vision to decreased visual acuity and light sensitivity to blindness. Ophthalmological studies of exposed humans and monkeys reveal varying degrees of edema of the papillomacular bundle and optic nerve head (Benton and Calhoun, 1952; Potts, 1955; Baumbach *et al.*, 1977; Hayreh *et al.*, 1980). Histopathological and ultrastructural investigations in methanol-exposed monkeys and folate-modified rats showed retinal edema, swollen and degenerated photoreceptors, degenerated RGCs, swollen retinal pigment epithelial cells, axonal (optic nerve) swelling, and mitochondrial swelling and disintegration in each of these cells but especially in the photoreceptors and optic nerve (Baumbach *et al.*, 1977; Hayreh *et al.*, 1980; Murray *et al.*, 1991; Seme *et al.*, 1999). Considering the differences in species, methanol exposures, time course of analysis, and procedures utilized, the overall data for the acute effects of methanol on the ERG are remarkably consistent. Following methanol exposure, the ERG b-wave amplitude in humans, monkeys, and folate-modified rats starts to decrease significantly when the blood formate concentration exceeded 7 mM (Potts, 1955; Ruedeman, 1961; Ingemansson, 1983; Murray *et al.*, 1991; Lee *et al.*, 1994). These ERG b-wave alterations, as well as flicker-evoked ERG alterations (Seme *et al.*, 1999), occur at lower formate concentrations than those associated with structural changes in the retina and optic nerve, as discussed above. Decreases in the a-wave amplitude are delayed, relative to the b-wave and occur when blood formate concentrations further increase (Ruedeman, 1961; Ingemansson, 1983; Murray *et al.*, 1991; Eells *et al.*, 1996). In addition, it has been shown that intraretinal metabolism of methanol is necessary for the formate-mediated alterations in the ERG (Garner *et al.*, 1995a), although intravenous infusion of formate in monkeys does induce optic nerve edema (Martin-Amat *et al.*, 1978). Finally, in the folate-modified rats, it appears that photoreceptors that respond to a 15-Hz flicker/510-nm wavelength mesopic–photopic stimulus (ie, rods and middle wavelength-sensitive [M] cones) are more sensitive to methanol than the ultraviolet-sensitive (UV) cones (Seme *et al.*, 1999).

The retinal sources of the ERG a-wave and b-wave were previously discussed. Thus, the data from the ERG b-wave methanol studies suggest that the initial effect of formate is directly on the ON-type rod bipolar cells, MGCs, and/or synaptic transmission between the photoreceptors and bipolar cells. A well-designed series of pharmacological, ERG, and potassium-induced Müller cell depolarization studies using several controls and folate-modified rats revealed a direct toxic effect of formate on MGC function (Garner *et al.*, 1995a,b). These studies also provided evidence that formate does not directly affect depolarizing rod bipolar cells or synaptic transmission between the photoreceptors and bipolar cells. Formate also appears to directly and adversely affect the rod and cone photoreceptors as evidenced by the markedly decreased ERG a-wave and flicker response data (Ruedeman, 1961; Ingemansson, 1983; Murray *et al.*, 1991; Eells *et al.*, 1996; Seme *et al.*, 1999).

Although there are no direct data on the underlying molecular mechanism responsible for the toxic effects of formate on MGCs and photoreceptors, several findings suggest that the mechanism involves a disruption in oxidative energy metabolism. First, the whole retinal ATP concentration is decreased in folate-deficient rats 48 hours following methanol exposure, the time point when the b-wave was lost (Garner *et al.*, 1995b). Second, both formate (10–200 mM) and formaldehyde (0.5–5 mM) inhibited oxygen consumption in isolated ox retina, and formaldehyde was considerably more potent (Kini and Cooper, 1962). Third, similar concentrations of formaldehyde inhibited oxidative phosphorylation of isolated ox retinal mitochondria, with greater effects observed using FAD-linked than NADH-linked substrates (Kini and Cooper, 1962). Unfortunately, the effects of formate were not examined. Fourth, and consistent with the above results, formate inhibits succinate-cytochrome c reductase and cytochrome oxidase activity ($K_i = 5$–30 mM), but not NADH-cytochrome c reductase activity in isolated beef heart mitochondria and/or submitochondrial particles (Nicholls, 1976). Fifth, ultrastructural studies reveal swollen mitochondria in rat photoreceptor inner segment and optic nerve 48 to 72 hours after nitrous oxide/methanol exposure (Murray *et al.*, 1991; Seme *et al.*, 1999). To date, there are no such studies conducted on the MGCs. Taken together, these results suggest formate is a mitochondrial poison that inhibits oxidative phosphorylation of photoreceptors, MGCs, and optic nerve. The evidence for this hypothesis and establishment of subsequent steps resulting in retinal and optic nerve cell injury and death remain to be elucidated.

Organic Solvents

n-Hexane, Perchloroethylene, Styrene, Toluene, Trichloroethylene, Xylene, and Mixtures The neurotoxicity of organic solvents is well established. In addition, exposure to organic solvents and other volatile hydrocarbons are associated with deficits in color vision, contrast sensitivity and visual-motor performance. Similar deficits have been reported after occupational, residential and recreational exposures: the latter among inhalant drug abusers. However, there is a paucity of mechanistic studies on the adverse effects of organic solvents on the retina and visual system.

Loss of color vision (acquired dyschromatopsia) and contrast sensitivity have been reported in workers exposed to organic solvents and related compounds such as alcohols, *n*-hexane, toluene, trichloroethylene, styrene, xylene, and solvent mixtures (Mergler *et al.*, 1987, 1988, 1991; Iregren *et al.*, 2002; Paramei *et al.*, 2004; Benignus *et al.*, 2005; Attarchi *et al.*, 2010). Workers in microelectronic plants, print shops, and paint manufacturing facilities, and painters who were exposed to concentrations of solvents that exceeded the threshold limit values, had acquired dyschromatopsia as assessed by the Lanthony D-15 desaturated color arrangement panel (Mergler *et al.*, 1987, 1988, 1991; Iregren *et al.*, 2002). These workers had no observable clinical abnormalities as assessed by biomicroscopy, funduscopy, and peripheral visual field tests. The color vision losses were characterized initially as an increase in blue–yellow confusion errors, although more severe red–green deficits were reported with extended duration or higher concentrations of exposure. As a general rule, acquired blue–yellow losses may result from lens opacification or outer retinal alterations, whereas red–green losses are traditionally associated with retrobular, or central visual pathway alterations (Porkony *et al.*, 1979). In addition, many of the occupationally exposed workers also exhibited lower contrast sensitivity at intermediate spatial frequencies, which likely reflects

alterations in neural function (Mergler *et al.*, 1991; Broadwell *et al.*, 1995). The data from Mergler *et al.* (1987, 1988, 1991) appear to show gender differences in these adverse visual effects. A study of female workers, where the Lanthony D-15 desaturated test was used to assess color vision, showed a trend toward increased prevalence of color vision impairment following exposure to low to moderate concentrations of toluene (Zavalic *et al.*, 1996). The neuropathic compounds, *n*-hexane, its metabolite 2,5-hexanedione and carbon disulfide have been associated with macular changes (Raitta *et al.*, 1974, 1978, 1981) and rod and cone degeneration (Backstrom and Collins, 1992; Backstrom *et al.*, 1993). Photoreceptor damage and retinal pathology have not been reported for other hydrocarbon solvents. Clearly more detailed, well-designed, and well-executed studies are needed to determine the (1) specific solvents that cause alterations in color vision, (2) vulnerability of spatial and temporal contrast sensitivity, (3) dose (concentration)–response relations between exposures and effects, (4) possible gender differences, (5) potential reversibility of deficits if exposure is terminated, and (6) pathophysiological basis for these changes. Prospective occupational studies would be particularly helpful given the difficulties in obtaining appropriately matched control populations in cross-sectional study designs.

Perchloroethylene (Tetrachloroethylene) Deficits in visual function such as contrast sensitivity have been observed in residents of neighborhoods containing dry cleaners using perchloroethylene (Altmann *et al.*, 1995) and in residents of apartment buildings with co-located dry cleaners (Schreiber *et al.*, 2002). For both of these residential studies, the atmospheric concentrations of perchloroethylene were below those typical of occupational settings. Laboratory experiments with human subjects exposed to perchloroethylene for four hours for four days revealed increased peak latency delays in the N75, P100, and N150 of the VEP as well as decreases in contrast sensitivity at low and intermediate spatial frequencies (Altmann *et al.*, 1990). Acute perchloroethylene inhalation exposure also reduced pattern VEP amplitudes in rats (Boyes *et al.*, 2009). Moreover, gestational exposure to perchloroethylene produced clinical red–green color loss and decreased visual acuity in the children of occupationally exposed mothers (Till *et al.*, 2003). Recently, a study by the New York State Department of Health reported mild, but statistically significant, deficits of contrast sensitivity in children living in apartment buildings with co-located perchloroethylene drycleaners in comparison to residents of control buildings without drycleaners (Storm *et al.*, 2011). The above results reveal that perchloroethylene is toxic to both the developing and adult visual system.

Styrene Six independent studies report that workers exposed to mean atmospheric concentrations of styrene ranging from 20 to 70 ppm exhibit concentration-dependent alterations in color vision (Gobba *et al.*, 1991; Fallas *et al.*, 1992; Chia *et al.*, 1994; Eguchi *et al.*, 1995; Campagna *et al.*, 1995; Iregren *et al.*, 2005). A combined data analysis from two of the above studies (Gobba *et al.*, 1991; Campagna *et al.*, 1995) suggests that the threshold for color visual impairments is ≤4 ppm styrene (Campagna *et al.*, 1996). This was well below the threshold limit value-time-weighted average (TLV–TWA) value for any country: range 20 to 50 ppm. The similarity of the styrene-induced blue–yellow color vision deficits observed by five independent groups demonstrates the reproducibility of these color vision deficits. In addition, two meta-analysis studies of solvent exposure and color vision are consistent with these results. Paramei *et al.* (2004) evaluated the color confusion index (CCI) scores from 15 studies of workers exposed to toluene, styrene, or mixed solvents. They concluded that while 13 of the original 15 studies reported CCI values indicative of impaired performance in the solvent-exposed group, the large variations among the effect sizes across studies obscured an overall statistically significant association between exposure and CCI values for all the substances except styrene, which was significantly associated with impaired color discrimination. Benignus *et al.* (2005) focused on only reports of styrene exposure from the six independent studies and also observed a statistically significant relationship between cumulative styrene exposure and increased CCI scores. The slope of the function observed suggested that the magnitude of decrement in CCI scores for a worker exposed to 20 ppm styrene for eight years would be equivalent to an additional 1.7 years of aging (Benignus *et al.*, 2005). The reversibility of these impairments has not been thoroughly studied, although in one study no recovery was found after a one-month period of no exposure (Gobba *et al.*, 1991). Rats exposed to styrene for 13 weeks showed lower retinal dopamine content and fewer tyrosine hydroxylase immunoreactive retinal amacrine cells (Vettori *et al.*, 2000). In summary, there is a concordance of evidence that styrene exposure is associated with retinal toxicity in experimental animals and color vision deficits in occupationally exposed workers.

Toluene Toluene is one of the most widely used substances in industry and commerce. It is used as a solvent, degreaser, constituent of products such as paints and glues, and is a substantial component of gasoline and other fuels. Among the neurotoxic consequences of occupational toluene exposure are impaired color vision (Campagna *et al.*, 2001; Cavalleri *et al.*, 2000) and reduced visual contrast sensitivity (Donoghue *et al.*, 1995). Acute toluene exposure impaired oculomotor function (Niklasson *et al.*, 1995) and reduced pattern VEP amplitudes in proportion to estimated concentration of toluene in the brain (Boyes *et al.*, 2007). Moreover, toluene has a relatively low irritancy and a high euphoric potential making it a favored selection among inhalant drug abusers; many are young and expose themselves repeatedly to very high toluene concentrations. Abuse of toluene is associated with poor visual acuity, altered or unrecordable pattern VEPs, optic neuropathy, abnormal MRI signals in visual cortex, decreased perfusion of thalamus and cerebral cortex, and visual hallucinations (Ryu *et al.*, 1998; Kamran and Bakshi, 1998; Kiyokawa *et al.*, 2005).

Organophosphates The neurotoxicity of organophosphates is well established (see Chap. 16); however, the link between organophosphate exposure and retinotoxicity is unresolved. Clinical studies conducted in Japan, report on ocular toxicity from laboratory animals exposed to organophosphates, and reports to the EPA by pesticide manufacturers suggest that various organophosphates produce retinotoxicity and chronic ocular damage (Ishikawa, 1973; Dementi, 1994). However, many of the early clinical reports were poorly designed and remain unconfirmed. The evidence for organophosphate-induced retinal toxicity is strongest for fenthion (dimethyl 3-methyl-4-methylthiophenyl phosphorothionate) (Imai *et al.*, 1983; Misra *et al.*, 1985; Boyes *et al.*, 1994; Tandon *et al.*, 1994). Two epidemiological studies of licensed pesticide applicators and their spouses did not find a statistically increased risk of retinal degeneration from use of organophosphate insecticides as a class, but risks were increased for some individual organophosphate chemicals (Kamel *et al.*, 2000; Kirrane *et al.*, 2005). Interestingly, both studies identified an increased risk of retinal degeneration in individuals exposed to fungicides. There were also reports that Japanese children exposed to organophosphates had a high incidence of myopia (Ko *et al.*, 1988). Experimentally, the visual control of ocular growth, which is cholinergically mediated,

was impaired in the eyes of chicks exposed to the organophosphate insecticide chlorpyrifos (Geller *et al.*, 1998). Embryonic chick retinal cells did not develop normally when exposed to diazinon in vitro (Paraoanu *et al.*, 2006). Currently, the mechanisms of ocular toxicity, sites of action, and whether the effects are restricted to some specific organophosphates such as fenthion or are more general to the chemical class are unknown. The use of organophosphate insecticides has been restricted (but not eliminated) in North America and Europe in recent years, but continues in much of the developing world. Thus, it is important to resolve the potential risks of ocular toxicity for this class of agents.

TARGET SITES AND MECHANISMS OF ACTION: OPTIC NERVE AND TRACT

The optic nerve consists primarily of RGC axons carrying visual information from the retina to several distinct anatomic destinations in the CNS. Both myelinated and nonmyelinated axons are present and grouped into bundles of axons that maintain a topographic distribution with respect to the site of origin in the retina. At the optic chiasm, the fibers split, so that, in humans and other primates, those fibers originating from the temporal retina continue in the optic tract toward the ipsilateral side of the brain, while those fibers originating in the nasal half of the retina, cross the midline and project to the contralateral side of the brain. In species with sideward-facing eyes such as the rat, a larger proportion of the optic nerve fibers (up to 90%) cross the midline. Fibers from the optic nerve terminate in the dorsal LGN, the superior colliculus, and pretectal areas. Information passing through the LGN to the visual cortex gives rise to conscious visual perception. Information traveling to the superior colliculus is used to generate eye movements. Pathways leading to the pretectal areas subserve the pupil response. The LGN of primates contains six histological layers that are alternately innervated by cells from the contralateral and ipsilateral eyes. The cells projecting to and from the ventral two layers of the LGN have large cell bodies, and consequently, this pathway is referred to as the magnocellular system. RGCs projecting to the magnocellular layers of the LGN are referred to as either M-type or Pα cells. Magnocellular neurons are sensitive to fast moving stimuli and to low levels of luminance contrast, but are insensitive to differences in color. The cells from the magnocellular pathway are involved in motion perception. On the dorsal side of the LGN, the cells are smaller and form the parvocellular pathway. RGCs projecting to the parvocellular layers of the LGN are referred to as P-type or Pβ cells. Parvocellular neurons are sensitive to color and to fine detailed patterns, have slower conduction velocities, and are involved in perception of color and form (Kaplan and Benardette, 2001).

Disorders of the optic nerve may be termed optic neuritis, optic neuropathy, or optic nerve atrophy, referring to inflammation, damage, or degeneration, respectively, of the optic nerve. Retrobulbar optic neuritis refers to inflammation of the portion of the optic nerve posterior to the globe. Among the symptoms of optic nerve disease are reduced visual acuity, contrast sensitivity, and color vision. Toxic effects observed in the optic nerve may originate from damage to the optic nerve fibers themselves or to the RGC somas that provide axons to the optic nerve. A number of nutritional disorders can adversely affect the optic nerve. Deficiency of thiamine, vitamin B$_{12}$, or zinc results in degenerative changes in optic nerve fibers. Nutritional and toxic factors can interact to produce optic nerve damage. A condition referred to as alcohol–tobacco amblyopia or simply as toxic amblyopia is observed in habitually heavy users of these substances and is associated nutritional deficiency. Dietary supplementation with vitamin B_{12} is therapeutically helpful, even when patients continue to consume large amounts of alcohol and tobacco (Grant and Schuman, 1993).

Acrylamide

Acrylamide monomer is used in a variety of industrial and laboratory applications, where it serves as the basis for the production of polyacrylamide gels and other polyacrylamide products. Exposure to acrylamide produces a distal axonopathy in large-diameter axons of the peripheral nerves and spinal cord that is well documented in humans and laboratory animals (Spencer and Schaumburg, 1974a,b). Visual effects of acrylamide exposure occur at dose levels sufficient to cause substantial peripheral neuropathy, but the selective nature of the visual deficits and associated neuropathology is very instructive. Although the large-diameter and long axons are most vulnerable to acrylamide in the peripheral nerve and spinal cord, this is not the case in the optic tract. The middle diameter axons of the P_β-type RGCs that project to the parvocellular layers of the LGN of New- and Old-World primates degenerate after prolonged treatment with acrylamide (Eskin and Merigan, 1986; Lynch et al., 1989). The larger-diameter P_α-type RGCs that project to the magnocellular layers of the LGN are apparently spared. Visual function testing in these primates, without a functional parvocellular system, revealed selective perceptual deficits in detecting visual stimuli with high spatial–frequency components (ie, fine visual patterns) and low temporal–frequency components (ie, slowly modulating sine waves) (Merigan and Eskin, 1986). However, the monkeys' perception of larger visual patterns, modulated at higher temporal rates, was not impaired. These toxicological experiments helped elucidate the functional differentiation of primate parvocellular and magnocellular visual systems. Why the axons of the optic nerve and tract show a different size-based pattern of vulnerability than do axons of the peripheral nerve and spinal cord is not understood. Norwegian tunnel workers examined two to 10 years after using acrylamide and n-methylolacrylamide, for grouting operations, had altered color discrimination, light sensitivity and VEP latencies (Goffeng, 2008a,b). This indicates the sensitivity of and persistent adverse effects on the human visual system to occupational acrylamide exposure.

Carbon Disulfide

Carbon disulfide (CS_2) is used in industry to manufacture viscose rayon, carbon tetrachloride, and cellophane. The neurotoxicity of CS_2 is well known and involves damage to the peripheral and CNSs as well as profound effects on vision (Beauchamp et al., 1983). The peripheral neuropathy results from a distal axonal degeneration of the large-caliber and long axons of the peripheral nerves and spinal cord, probably through the reactions with the sulfhydryl groups of axonal neurofilament proteins, yielding covalent cross linkages that lead to filamentous tangles and axonal swellings (Graham and Valantine, 2000). The mechanism of action through which inhalation of high concentrations of CS_2 vapors leads to psychotic mania is not currently established but may result from alterations in catecholamine synthesis or neuronal degeneration in several brain areas (Beauchamp et al., 1983). Workers exposed to CS_2 experience loss of visual function accompanied by observable lesions in the retinal vasculature. Among the changes in visual function reported in viscose rayon workers are central scotoma, depressed visual sensitivity in the peripheral visual field, optic atrophy, pupillary disturbances, blurred vision, and disorders of color perception. A workplace

study of 123 Belgian viscose rayon workers found a statistical association between a weighted cumulative CS_2 exposure score, deficits in color vision measured using the Farnsworth-Munsell 100-HUE test, and observations of excess microaneurysms observed ophthalmoscopically and in fundus photographs (Vanhoorne et al., 1996). This association was not observed in the 42 workers who were never exposed to levels above the TLV value of 31 mg/m³. The coexistence of retinal microaneurysms with functional loss has led to the presumption that the visual deficits were a secondary consequence of vascular disease and perhaps of retinal hemorrhages. This association was addressed in carbon disulfide-exposed macaque monkeys used in visual psychophysical, fluorescein angiography, and fundus photography studies as well as postmortem neuropathological evaluations (Merigan et al., 1988; Eskin et al., 1988). They observed markedly decreased contrast sensitivity functions, decreased visual acuity, and degeneration of the RGCs, all of which occurred in the absence of retinal microaneurysms or hemorrhages. There was little evidence of effects on the other retinal neurons. These findings indicate that the retinal and optic nerve pathology produced by CS_2 are likely a direct neuropathological action and not the indirect result of vasculopathy. Interestingly, and importantly, after cessation of exposure, the visual acuity measures recovered temporarily in two of the CS_2-treated monkeys; however, the contrast sensitivity measures did not recover. This demonstrates the independence of these two measures and the utility and importance of independent evaluations of contrast sensitivity and visual acuity.

Cuban Epidemic of Optic Neuropathy

During 1992 and 1993, an epidemic occurred in Cuba in which over 50,000 people suffered from optic neuropathy, sensory and autonomic peripheral neuropathy, high-frequency neural hearing loss, and myelopathy. This is the largest epidemic of neurological disease in the 20th century (Roman, 1998). The affected individuals were characterized as having bilateral low visual acuity, impaired color perception, impaired visual contrast sensitivity, central scotoma, optic disc pallor, and, in particular, loss of nerve fibers from the papillomacular bundle (Sadun et al., 1994a; Hedges et al., 1997). Individuals with neurological findings demonstrated stocking-glove sensory deficits, leg cramps, sensory ataxia, altered reflexes, and complaints of memory loss (Mojon et al., 1997). Various authors noticed similarities between the Cuban cases and nutritional or alcohol–tobacco amblyopia, Leber hereditary optic neuropathy, and Strachan disease (Sadun et al., 1994b; Mojon et al., 1997). The optic neuropathy resembled methanol poisoning (Roman, 1998; Sadun, 1998). The outbreak of the epidemic was linked to nutritional deficiencies (Hedges et al., 1997; Mojon et al., 1997; Roman, 1998). In most cases, aggressive supplementation of the diet with B vitamins and folic acid led to a significant clinical improvement (Mojon et al., 1997). Nutritional deficiencies were a primary contributor to the epidemic; however, it was not clear whether they were solely responsible or whether dietary insufficiency served to make individuals more susceptible to other factors. One likely contributing factor was coexposure to low levels of neurotoxic compounds that would otherwise have been tolerated (Sadun, 1998). In addition to low food intake, risk factors for the development of optic neuropathy included use of tobacco, in particular the frequent smoking of cigars, and high cassava consumption (Roman, 1998). The mitochondrial toxicant cyanide may be a contaminant of both cassava and tobacco products. Moderate to severe folic acid deficiency was observed in more than half of the cases (Roman, 1998). Samples of local home-brewed rum showed approximately one percent contamination with methanol, a level that would not produce optic nerve toxicity in normal healthy individuals (Sadun *et al.*, 1994a,b). However, one-quarter of the Cuban patients showed elevated serum formate concentrations, probably a result of folic acid deficiency. The maximum serum formate concentrations observed (approximately 4 mM) were similar to levels that produce retinal and optic nerve toxicity in a rodent model of methanol toxicity (Eells *et al.*, 1996). Sadun (1998) postulated that mitochondrial impairment, created by the combination of low nutritional status and toxic exposures, was responsible for the neurological impairments. The nutritional deficiency would lead to ATP depletion. Exposure to either cyanide or formic acid, the toxic metabolite of methanol, causes inhibition of cytochrome oxidase, which further depletes ATP levels (Nicholls, 1976; see above for details). Because axoplasmic transport of new mitochondria from nerve cell bodies to distal axonal segments is energy-dependent (Vale *et al.*, 1992), the lowered ATP levels would be expected to impair mitochondrial transport and start a cycle of further ATP depletion and reduced mitochondrial transport to the nerve terminal regions. Sadun proposed that the nerve fibers most sensitive to this type of damage would be the long peripheral nerve axons, which have high transport demands, and the small caliber fibers of the optic nerve, in particular at the papillomacular bundle, which have physical constrictions to transporting mitochondria. Exposure to toxicants could not be documented in most of the people identified late in the epidemic, suggesting nutritional deficit as the principal cause. However, coexposure to low levels of mitochondrial toxicants or other factors may have pushed individuals over a threshold for causing nerve damage.

Ethambutol

The dextro isomer of ethambutol is widely used as an antimycobacterial drug for the treatment of tuberculosis. It is well known that ethambutol produces dose-related alterations in the visual system, such as blue–yellow and red–green dyschromatopsias, decreased contrast sensitivity, reduced visual acuity, and visual field loss. The earliest visual symptoms appear to be a decrease in contrast sensitivity and color vision, although impaired red–green color vision is the most frequently observed and reported complaint. However, the loss of contrast sensitivity may explain why some patients with normal visual acuity and color perception still complain of visual disturbance. These visual system alterations can occur with a few weeks of doses equal to or greater than 20 mg/kg body weight; however, they usually become manifest after several months of treatment (Koliopoulos and Palimeris, 1972; Polak *et al.*, 1985; Salmon *et al.*, 1987; Bartlett and Jaanus, 2008). The symptoms are primarily associated with one of two forms of retrobulbar optic neuritis (ie, optic neuropathy). The most common form, seen in almost all cases, involves the central optic nerve fibers and typically results in a central or paracentral scotoma in the visual field and is associated with impaired red–green color vision and decreased visual acuity, whereas the second form involves the peripheral optic nerve fibers and typically results in a peripheral scotoma and visual field loss (Lessell, 1998; Bartlett and Jaanus, 2008).

In experimental animals, ethambutol causes RGC and optic nerve degeneration, discoloration of the tapetum lucidum (in dogs), retinal detachment (in cats), and possibly amacrine and bipolar cell alterations (van Dijk and Spekreijse, 1983; Grant and Schuman, 1993; Sjoerdsma *et al.*, 1999). Although the mechanism responsible for producing the RGC and optic nerve degeneration is unknown, recent in vivo studies in rats and in vitro rat RGC cell culture experiments suggest that ethambutol causes RGC death secondary to glutamate-induced excitotoxicity (Heng *et al.*, 1999). Pharmacological studies, using the in vivo and in vitro models, show that although

ethambutol is not a direct NMDA-receptor agonist, it makes RGCs more sensitive to endogenous levels of glutamate. Using the fluorescent Ca^{2+} dyes calcium green 1-AM and rhod-2, Heng *et al.* (1999) showed that following application of ethambutol in the presence, but not absence, of glutamate to isolated RGCs, there was a decrease in cytosolic Ca^{2+} and a subsequent increase in mitochondrial Ca^{2+}. Interestingly, the increase in mitochondrial Ca^{2+} resulted in an increase in the mitochondrial membrane potential as measured by the mitochondrial membrane potential sensitive dye JC-1. The authors (Heng *et al.*, 1999) postulate that this latter phenomenon occurs as a result of an ethambutol-mediated chelation of Zn^{2+} from the mitochondrial ATPase inhibitor protein IF1 (Rouslin *et al.*, 1993) that subsequently results in the inhibition of mitochondrial ATP synthesis and elevation of mitochondrial membrane potential. These intriguing ideas have merit; however, many additional experiments will be needed to prove this hypothesis. In addition, the authors suggest that some glutamate antagonists may be useful in decreasing the side effects of ethambutol—a practical suggestion that appears worthy of clinical investigation.

TARGET SITES AND MECHANISMS OF ACTION: THE CENTRAL VISUAL SYSTEM

Many areas of the cerebral cortex are involved in the perception of visual information. The primary visual cortex (V1), Brodmann area 17, or striate cortex: receives the primary projections of visual information from the LGN and also from the superior colliculus. Neurons from the LGN project to the visual cortex maintaining a topographic representation of the receptive field origin in the retina. The receptive fields in the left and right sides of area 17 reflect the contralateral visual world and representations of the upper and lower regions of the visual field are separated below and above, respectively, the calcarine fissure. Cells in the posterior aspects of the calcarine fissure have receptive fields located in the central part of the retina. Cortical cells progressively deeper in the calcarine fissure have retinal receptive fields that are located more and more peripherally in the retina. The central part of the fovea has tightly packed photoreceptors for resolution of fine detailed images, and the cortical representation of the central fovea is proportionately larger than the peripheral retina in order to accommodate a proportionately larger need for neural image processing. The magnocelluar and parvocellular pathways project differently to the histologically defined layers of primary striate visual cortex and then to extrastriate visual areas. The receptive fields of neurons in the visual cortex are more complex than the circular center-surround arrangement found in the retina and LGN. Cortical cells respond better to lines of a particular orientation than to simple spots. The receptive fields of cortical cells are thought to represent computational summaries of a number of simpler input signals. As the visual information proceeds from area V1 to extrastriate visual cortical areas, the representation of the visual world reflected in the receptive fields of individual neurons becomes progressively more complex (Kaplan and Benardete, 2001).

Lead

In addition to the well-documented retinal effects of lead (see above), lead exposure during adulthood or perinatal development produces structural, biochemical, and functional deficits in the visual cortex of humans, nonhuman primates, and rats (Fox *et al.*, 1977; Winneke, 1979; Costa and Fox, 1983; Fox, 1984; Otto *et al.*, 1985; Lilienthal *et al.*, 1988; Reuhl *et al.*, 1989; Murata *et al.*,

1993; Otto and Fox, 1993; Altmann *et al.*, 1994, 1998; Winneke *et al.*, 1994). Quantitative morphometric studies in monkeys exposed to either high levels of lead from birth or infancy to six years of age revealed a decrease in visual cortex (areas V1 and V2), cell volume density, and a decrease in the number of initial arborizations among pyramidal neurons (Reuhl *et al.*, 1989). The former results may be due to an absolute decrease in total cell numbers, possibly resulting from lead-induced apoptosis as observed in the retina (Fox *et al.*, 1997; He *et al.*, 2000, 2003). This may also account for the decreased density of cholinergic muscarinic receptors found in the visual cortex of adult rats following moderate level developmental lead exposure (Costa and Fox, 1983). The morphometric results on neuronal branching are reminiscent of earlier findings in the neocortex of rats following high level developmental lead exposure (Petit and LeBoutillier, 1979), and recent findings in the somatosensory cortex of rats following low or moderate level developmental lead exposure (Wilson *et al.*, 2000). These alterations could partially contribute to the decreases in contrast sensitivity observed in lead-exposed rats and monkeys (Fox, 1984; Rice, 1998), the alterations in the amplitude and latency measures of the flash and pattern-reversal–evoked potentials in lead-exposed children, workers, monkeys, and rats (Fox *et al.*, 1977; Winneke, 1979; Otto *et al.*, 1985; Lilienthal *et al.*, 1988; Murata *et al.*, 1993; Altmann *et al.*, 1994, 1998; Winneke *et al.*, 1994), and the alterations in tasks assessing visual function in lead-exposed children (Winneke *et al.*, 1983; Hansen *et al.*, 1989; Muñoz *et al.*, 1993).

Methyl Mercury

Methyl mercury became notorious in two episodes of mass poisoning (see Chap. 16). In the 1950s, industrial discharges of mercury into Minamata Bay in Japan became biomethylated to form methyl mercury, which then accumulated in the food chain and reached toxic concentrations in the fish and shellfish consumed in the surrounding communities. Hundreds of people were poisoned, showing a combination of sensory, motor, and cognitive deficits. A more widespread episode of methyl mercury poisoning affected thousands of Iraqi citizens who mistakenly ground wheat grain into flour that had been treated with methyl mercury as a fungicide and that was intended for planting and not for direct human consumption.

Visual deficits are a prominent feature of methyl mercury intoxication in adult humans, along with several other neurological manifestations such as difficulties with sensation, gait, memory, and cognition. Methyl mercury poisoned individuals experienced a striking and progressive constriction of the visual field (peripheral scotoma) as patients became progressively less able to see objects in the visual periphery (Iwata, 1977). The narrowing of the visual field gives impression of looking through a long tunnel, hence the term tunnel vision. Visual field constrictions also have been observed in methyl mercury-poisoned monkeys (Merigan, 1979). On autopsy of some of the Minamata patients, focal neurological degeneration was observed in several brain regions including motor cortex, cerebellum, and calcarine fissure of visual cortex (Takeuchi and Eto, 1977). The histopathological feature was a destruction of the cortical neural and glial cells, with sparing of the subcortical white matter, optic radiations, and LGN. Monkeys and dogs that were treated experimentally with methyl mercury showed greater damage in the calcarine fissure, associated with higher regional concentrations of protein-bound mercury, than in other brain regions (Yoshino *et al.*, 1966; Berlin *et al.*, 1975). In the Minamata patients, there was a regional distribution of damage observed within striate cortex, such that the most extensive damage occurred deep in the

calcarine fissure and was progressively less in the more posterior portions. Thus, the damage was most severe in the regions of primary visual cortex that subserved the peripheral visual field, with relative sparing of the cortical areas representing the central vision. This regional distribution of damage corresponded with the progressive loss of peripheral vision while central vision was relatively preserved. Methyl mercury-poisoned individuals also experienced poor night vision (ie, scotopic vision deficits), also attributable to peripheral visual field losses. Similar changes were observed in adult monkeys exposed to methyl mercury (Berlin *et al.*, 1975). Mercury also accumulates in the retina of animals exposed to methyl mercury (DuVal *et al.*, 1987). Acute exposure of isolated retinas to mercury or methyl mercury produces rod-selective electrophysiological and morphological alterations (Fox and Sillman, 1979; Braekevelt, 1982), whereas subacute dosing with methyl mercury alters the photopic ERG prior to the scotopic ERG (Goto *et al.*, 2001). The neurological damage in adult cases of Minamata disease was focally localized in the calcarine cortex and other areas but was more globally distributed throughout the brain in those developmentally exposed.

The levels of methyl mercury exposure experienced by people in Minamata Bay were undoubtedly high. Studies of visual function in nonhuman primates exposed to methyl mercury during perinatal development demonstrate a decrease in visual contrast sensitivity, visual acuity, and temporal flicker resolution at dose levels lower than those associated with constriction of the visual fields (Rice and Gilbert, 1990; Rice, 1996). Monkeys exposed to methyl mercury from birth onward or in utero plus postnatally exhibited spatial vision deficits under both high and low luminance conditions, although the deficits were greater under scotopic illumination (Rice, 1998). The effects on temporal vision were different. That is, monkeys exposed from birth displayed superior low-luminance temporal vision, whereas high-luminance temporal vision was not impaired. In contrast, monkeys exposed to methyl mercury in utero plus postnatally exhibited deficits in low-frequency high-luminance temporal vision, whereas low-luminance temporal vision was superior to that of control monkeys (Rice, 1998). These data indicate that the spatial and temporal vision deficits produced by developmental exposure to methyl mercury are different from those produced during adulthood. The underlying mechanisms have yet to be determined.

ACKNOWLEDGMENTS

This chapter has been reviewed by the National Health and Environmental Effects Research Laboratory, USEPA, and approved for publication. Mention of trade names and commercial products does not constitute endorsement or recommendation for use.

REFERENCES

Abd-El-Barr MM, Pennesi ME, Saszik SM, et al. Genetic dissection of rod and cone pathways in the dark-adapted mouse retina. *J Neurophysiol.* 2009;102:1945–1955.

Adamus G, Machnicki M, Elerding H, et al. Antibodies to recoverin induce apoptosis of photoreceptor and bipolar cells in vivo. *J Autoimmun.* 1998;11:523–533.

Agency for Toxic Substances and Disease Registry. *Neurobehavioral Test Batteries for Use in Environmental Health Field Studies.* Atlanta, GA: U.S. Department of Health, Public Health Service; 1992.

Ahmed J, Braun RD, Dunn R Jr, Linsenmeier RA. Oxygen distribution in the macaque retina. *Invest Ophthalmol Vis Sci.* 1993;34:516–521.

Ah-Song R, Sasco AJ. Tamoxifen and ocular toxicity. *Cancer Detect Prev.* 1997;21:522–531.

Albert D, Miller JW, Azar DT, Blodi BA. *Albert & Jakobiec's Principles & Practice of Ophthalmology.* 3rd ed. New York: Saunders; 2008.

Alken RG, Belz GG. A comparative dose-effect study with cardiac glycosides assessing cardiac and extracardiac responses in normal subjects. *J Cardiovasc Pharmacol.* 1984;6:634–640.

Altmann L, Bottger A, Wiegand H. Neurophysiological and psychophysical measurements reveal effects of acute low-level organic solvent exposure in humans. *Int Arch Occup Environ Health.* 1990;62:493–499.

Altmann L, Florian Neuhann H, Kramer U, Witten J, Jermann E. Neurobehavioral and neurophysiological outcomes of chronic low-level tetrachloroethene exposure measured in neighborhoods of dry cleaning shops. *Environ Res.* 1995;69:83–89.

Altmann L, Gutowski M, Wiegand H. Effects of maternal lead exposure on functional plasticity in the visual cortex and hippocampus of immature rats. *Brain Res Dev Brain Res.* 1994;81:50–56.

Altmann L, Sveinsson K, Kramer U, et al. Visual functions in 6-year-old children in relation to lead and mercury levels. *Neurotoxicol Teratol.* 1998;20:9–17.

Al-Modhefer AJA, Bradbury MWB, Simons TJB. Observations on the chemical nature of lead in human blood serum. *Clin Sci.* 1991;81:823–829.

American Medical Association. Harmful effects of ultraviolet radiation. Council on Scientific Affairs. *JAMA.* 1989;262:380–384.

Anger WK, Johnson BL. Chemicals affecting behavior. In: O'Donoghue JL, ed. *Neurotoxicity of Industrial and Commercial Chemicals.* Boca Raton, FL: CRC Press; 1985:51–148.

Anger WK, Letz R, Chrislip DW, et al. Neurobehavioral test methods for environmental health studies of adults. *Neurotoxicol Teratol.* 1994;16:489–497.

Arden GB, Constable PA. The elecro-oculogram. *Prog Retin Eye Res.* 2006;25:207–248.

Asakura T, Matsuda M, Matsuda S, Shichi H. Synthesis of 12(R)- and 12(S)-hydroxyeicosatetraenoic acid by porcine ocular tissues. *J Ocul Pharmacol.* 1994;10:525–535.

Atalla LR, Sevanian A, Rao NA. Immunohistochemical localization of glutathione peroxidase in ocular tissue. *Curr Eye Res.* 1988;7:1023–1027.

Attarchi MS, Labbafinejad Y, Mohammadi S. Occupational exposure to different levels of mixed organic solvents and colour vision impairment. *Neurotox Teratol.* 2010;32:558–562.

Awasthi YC, Saneto RP, Srivastava SK. Purification and properties of bovine lens glutathione *S*-transferase. *Exp Eye Res.* 1980;30:29–39.

Backstrom B, Collins VP. The effects of 2,5-hexanedione on rods and cones of the retina of albino rats. *Neurotoxicology.* 1992;13:199–202.

Backstrom B, Nylen P, Hagman M, et al. Effect of exposure to 2,5-hexanediol in light or darkness on the retina of albino and pigmented rats. I. Morphology. *Arch Toxicol.* 1993;67:277–283.

Baghdassarian SA. Optic neuropathy due to lead poisoning. *Arch Ophthalmol.* 1968;80:721–723.

Baker EL, Feldman RG, White RA, et al. Occupational lead neurotoxicity: a behavioral and electrophysiological evaluation. *Br J Ind Med.* 1984; 41:352–361.

Baloh RW, Langhofer L, Brown CP, Spivey GH. Quantitative tracking tests in lead workers. *Am J Med.* 1979;1:109–113.

Baloh RW, Spivey GH, Brown CP, et al. Subclinical effects of chronic increased lead absorption—a prospective study. II. Results of baseline neurologic testing. *J Occup Med.* 1979;21:490–496.

Banh A, Bantseev V, Choh V, Moran KL, Sivak JG. The lens as a focusing device and its response to stress. *Prog Retin Eye Res.* 2005;25:189–206.

Barltrop D, Barrett AJ, Dingle JT. Subcellular distribution of lead in the rat. *J Lab Clin Med.* 1971;77:705–712.

Bartlett JD, Jaanus SD. *Clinical Ocular Pharmacology.* 5th ed. Boston: Butterworth-Heinemann; 2008.

Baumbach GL, Cancilla PA, Martin-Amat G, et al. Methyl alcohol poisioning: IV. Alterations of the morphological findings of the retina and optic nerve. *Arch Ophthalmol.* 1977;95:1859–1865.

Bausher LP. Identification of A and B forms of monoamine oxidase in the iris-ciliary body, superior cervical ganglion, and pineal gland of albino rabbits. *Invest Ophthalmol.* 1976;15:529–537.

Baylor DA, Nunn BJ, Schnapf JL. The photocurrent, noise and spectral sensitivity of rods of the monkey *Macaca fascicularis. J Physiol.* 1984; 357:575–607.

Beauchamp RO Jr, Bus JS, Popp JA, et al. A critical review of the literature on carbon disulfide toxicity. *CRC Crit Rev Toxicol.* 1983;11:168–277.

Behndig A, Svensson B, Marklund SL, Karlsson K. Superoxide dismutase isoenzymes in the human eye. *Invest Ophthalmol Vis Sci.* 1998; 39:471–475.

Benignus VA, Geller AM, Boyes WK, Bushnell PJ. Human neurobehavioral effects of long-term exposure to styrene: a meta-analysis. *Environ Health Perspect.* 2005;113:532–538.

Benton CD, Calhoun FP. The ocular effects of methyl alcohol poisioning: Report of a catastrophe involving three hundred and twenty persons. *Trans Am Acad Ophthalmol.* 1952;56:875–883.

Berlin M, Grant CA, Hellberg J, et al. Neurotoxicity of methyl mercury in squirrel monkeys. Cerebral cortical pathology, interference with scotopic vision, and changes in operant behavior. *Arch Environ Health.* 1975; 30:340–348.

Bernstein HN. Chloroquine ocular toxicity. *Surv Ophthalmol.* 1967;12: 415–477.

Betta A, De Santa A, Savonitto C, D'Andrea F. Flicker fusion test and occupational toxicology performance evaluation in workers exposed to lead and solvents. *Hum Toxicol.* 1983;2:83–90.

Birch D, Jacobs GH. Spatial contrast sensitivity in albino and pigmented rats. *Vision Res.* 1979;19:933–937.

Bloomfield SA, Völgyi B. The diverse roles and regulation of neuronal gap junctions in the retina. *Nat Rev Neurosci.* 2009;10:496–506.

Boyes WK, Bercegeay M, Krantz QT, et al. Acute toluene exposure and rat visual function in proportion to momentary brain concentration. *Toxicol Sci.* 2007;99:572–581.

Boyes WK, Bercegeay M, Oshiro WM, et al. Acute perchloroethylene exposure alters rat visual-evoked potentials in relation to brain concentrations. *Toxicol Sci.* 2009;108:159–172.

Boyes WK, Dyer RS. Pattern reversal visual evoked potentials in awake rats. *Brain Res Bull.* 1983;10:817–823.

Boyes WK, Dyer RS. Chlordimeform produces profound but transient changes in visual evoked potentials of hooded rats. *Exp Neurol.* 1984; 86:434–447.

Boyes WK, Tandon P, Barone S Jr, Padilla S. Effects of organophosphates on the visual system of rats. *J Appl Toxicol.* 1994;14:135–143.

Braekevelt CR. Morphological changes in rat retinal photoreceptors with acute methyl mercury intoxication. In: Hollyfield JG, ed. *The Structure of the Eye.* New York: Elsevier; 1982:123–131.

Braun RD, Linsenmeier RA, Goldstick TK. Oxygen consumption in the inner and outer retina of the cat. *Invest Ophthalmol Vis Sci.* 1995;36:542–554.

Brigell M, Dong CJ, Rosolen S, Tzekov R. An overview of drug development with special emphasis on the role of visual electrophysiological testing. *Doc Ophthalmol.* 2005;110:3–13.

Broadwell DK, Darcey DJ, Hudnell HK, et al. Worksite clinical and neurobehavioral assessment of solvent-exposed workers. *Am J Indust Med.* 1995;27:677–698.

Brown DVL. Reaction of the rabbit retinal pigment epithelium to systemic lead poisoning. *Tr Am Ophthalmol Soc.* 1974;72:404–447.

Bull RJ. Lead and energy metabolism. In: Singhal RL, Thomas JA, eds. *Lead Toxicity.* Baltimore: Urban and Schwarzenberg; 1980:119–168.

Burns CA. Ocular effects of indomethacin. Slit lamp and electroretinographic: ERG study. *Invest Ophthalmol.* 1966;5:325–331.

Burns CA. Indomethacin, reduced retinal sensitivity and corneal deposits. *Am J Ophthalmol.* 1968;66:825–835.

Bushnell PJ, Bowman RE, Allen JR, Marlar RJ. Scotopic vision deficits in young monkeys exposed to lead. *Science.* 1977;196:333–335.

Butler MC, Itotia PN, Sullivan JM. A high-throughput biophotonics instrument to screen for novel ocular photosensitizing therapeutic agents. *Invest Ophthalmol Vis Sci.* 2010;51:2705–2720.

Campagna D, Gobba F, Mergler D, et al. Color vision loss among styrene-exposed workers: neurotoxicological threshold assessment. *Neurotoxicology.* 1996;17:367–373.

Campagna D, Mergler D, Huel G, et al. Visual dysfunction among styrene-exposed workers. *Scand J Work Environ Health.* 1995;21:382–390.

Campagna D, Stengel B, Mergler D, et al. Color vision and occupational toluene exposure. *Neurotoxicol Teratol.* 2001;23:473–480.

Campara P, D'Andrea F, Micciolo R, et al. Psychological performance of workers with blood-lead concentration below the current threshold limit value. *Int Arch Occup Environ Health.* 1984;53:233–246.

Cavalleri A, Gobba F, Nicali E, Fiocchi V. Dose-related color vision impairment in toluene-exposed workers. *Arch Environ Health.* 2000; 55:399–404.

Cavalleri A, Minoia C, Ceroni A, et al. Lead in cerebrospinal fluid and its relationship to plasma lead in humans. *J Appl Toxicol.* 1984;4:63–65.

Cavelleri A, Trimarchi F, Gelmi C, et al. Effects of lead on the visual system of occupationally exposed subjects. *Scand J Work Environ Health.* 1982;8(suppl 1):148–151.

Cestnick L, Coltheart M. The relationship between language-processing and visual-processing deficits in developmental dyslexia. *Cognition.* 1999;71:231–255.

Chang GQ, Hao Y, Wong F. Apoptosis: final common pathway of photoreceptor death in rd, rds, and rhodopsin mutant mice. *Neuron.* 1993;11: 595–605.

Chia SE, Jeyaratnam J, Ong CN, et al. Impairment of color vision among workers exposed to low concentrations of styrene. *Am J Ind Med.* 1994; 26:481–488.

Chun MH, Han SH, Chung JW, Wässle H. Electron microscopic analysis of the rod pathway of the rat retina. *J Comp Neurol.* 1993;332:421–432.

Choudhary D, Jansson I, Sarfarazi M, Schenkman JB. Physiological significance and expression of P450s in the developing eye. *Drug Metab Rev.* 2006;38:337–52.

Clayton LM, Dévilé M, Punte T, et al. Retinal nerve fiber layer thickness in vigabatrin-exposed patients. *Ann Neurol.* 2011;69:845–854.

Corbin JD, Francis SH, Webb DJ. Phosphodiesterase type 5 as a pharmacologic target in erectile dysfunction. *Urology.* 2002;60:4–11.

Costa LG, Fox DA. A selective decrease in cholinergic muscarinic receptors in the visual cortex of adult rats following developmental lead exposure. *Brain Res.* 1983;276:259–266.

Crofton KM, Sheets LP. Evaluation of sensory system function using reflex modification of the startle response. *J Am Coll Toxicol.* 1989;8:199–211.

Crosson CE, Willis JA, Potter DE. Effect of the calcium antagonist, nifedipine, on ischemic retinal dysfunction. *J Ocul Pharmacol.* 1990;6: 293–299.

Crouch RK, Goletz P, Snyder A, Coles WH. Antioxidant enzymes in human tears. *J Ocul Pharmacol.* 1991;7:253–258.

Cumming RG, Mitchell P. Inhaled corticosteroids and cataract: prevalence, prevention and management. *Drug Safety.* 1999;20:77–84.

Cumming RG, Mitchell P, Leeder SR. Use of inhaled corticosteroids and the risk of cataracts. *N Engl J Med.* 1997;337:8–14.

Damstra T. Environmental chemicals and nervous system dysfunction. *Yale J Biol Med.* 1978;51:457–468.

Daneshvar H, Racette L, Coupland SG, Kertes PJ, Guberman A, Zackon D. Symptomatic and asymptomatic visual loss in patients taking vigabatrin. *Ophthalmology.* 1999;106:1792–1798.

Datson GP, Freeberg FE. Ocular irritation testing. In: Hobson DW, ed. *Dermal and Ocular Toxicity: Fundamentals and Methods.* Boca Raton, FL: CRC Press; 1991:509–539.

Dayhaw-Barker P, Forbes D, Fox DA, et al. Drug photoxicity and visual health. In: Waxler M, Hitchins VM, eds. *Optical Radiation and Visual Health.* Boca Raton, FL: CRC Press; 1986:147–175.

Dean P. Visual pathways and acuity hooded rats. *Behav Brain Res.* 1981; 3:239–271.

Delcourt C, Carriere I, Ponton-Sanchez A, et al. Light exposure and the risk of cortical, nuclear, and posterior subcapsular cataracts: the Pathologies Oculaires Liees a l'Age (POLA) study. *Arch Ophthalmol.* 2000;118:385–392.

Dementi B. Ocular effects of organophosphates: a historical perspective of Saku disease. *J Appl Toxicol.* 1994;14:119–129.

De Rouck A, De Laey JJ, Van Hoorne M, et al. Chronic carbon disulfide poisoning: a 4-year follow-up study of the ophthalmological signs. *Int Ophthalmol.* 1986;9:17–27.

Diamante GG, Fraunfelder FT. Adverse effects of therapeutic agents on cornea and conjunctiva. In: Leibowitz HM, Waring GO, eds. *Corneal Disorders, Clinical Diagnosis and Management,* 2nd ed. Philadelphia: Saunders; 1998:736–769.

Diebold Y, Calonge M. Applications of nanoparticles in ophthalmology. *Prog Retin Eye Res.* 2010;29:596–609.

Dobbing J, Sands J. Comparative aspects of the brain growth spurt. *Early Hum Dev.* 1979;3:79–91.

Donoghue AM, Dryson EW, Wynn-Williams G. Contrast sensitivity in organic-solvent-induced chronic toxic encephalopathy. *J Occup Environ Med.* 1995;37:1357–1363.

Doshi M, Marcus C, Bejjani BA, Edward DP. Immunolocalization of CYP1B1 in normal, human, fetal and adult eyes. *Exp Eye Res.* 2006; 82:24–32.

Downes JE, Holmes RS. Purification and properties of murine corneal alcohol dehydrogenase. Evidence for class IV ADH properties. *Adv Exp Med Biol.* 1995;372:349–354.

Dräger UC. Calcium binding in pigmented and albino eyes. *Proc Natl Acad Sci U S A.* 1985;82:6716–6720.

Draize JH, Woodard G, Calvery HO. Methods for the study of irritation and toxicity of substances applied topically to the skin and mucous membranes. *J Pharmacol Exp Ther.* 1944;82:377–389.

Duncker G, Krastel H. Ocular digitalis effects in normal subjects. *Lens Eye Tox Res.* 1990;7:281–303.

Duncker GI, Kisters G, Grille W. Prospective, randomized, placebo-controlled, double-blind testing of colour vision and electroretinogram at therapeutic and subtherapeutic digitoxin serum levels. *Ophthalmologica.* 1994;208:259–261.

DuVal G, Grubb BR, Bentley PJ. Mercury accumulation in the eye following administration of methyl mercury. *Exp Eye Res.* 1987;44:161–164.

Edelhauser HF. The balance between corneal transparency and edema: the Proctor Lecture. *Invest Ophthalmol Vis Sci.* 2006;47:1754–1767.

Edward DP, Lam TT, Shahinfar S, et al. Amelioration of light-induced retinal degeneration by a calcium overload blocker: flunarizine. *Arch Ophthalmol.* 1991;109:554–562.

Eells JT. Methanol. In: Thurman RG, Kauffman FC, eds. *Browning's Toxicity and Metabolism of Industrial Solvents: Alcohols and Esters.* Vol 3. Amsterdam: Elsevier; 1992:3–20.

Eells JT, Salzman MM, Lewandowski MF, Murray TG. Formate-induced alterations in retinal function in methanol-intoxicated rats. *Toxicol Appl Pharmacol.* 1996;140:58–69.

Eguchi T, Kishi R, Harabuchi I, et al. Impaired colour discrimination among workers exposed to styrene: relevance of a urinary metabolite. *Occup Environ Med.* 1995;52:534–538.

Eichenbaum JW, Zheng W. Distribution of lead and transthyretin in human eyes. *Clin Toxicol.* 2000;38:371–381.

Ellsworth AJ, Witt DM, Dugdale DC, Oliver LM. *Mosby's 1999-2000 Medical Drug Reference.* St Louis: Mosby; 1999:184–185.

Eskin TA, Merigan WH. Selective acrylamide-induced degeneration of color opponent ganglion cells in macaques. *Brain Res.* 1986;378:379–384.

Eskin TA, Merigan WH, Wood RW. Carbon disulfide effects on the visual system: II. Retinogeniculate degeneration. *Invest Ophthalmol Vis Sci.* 1988;29:519–527.

Fallas C, Fallas J, Maslard P, Dally S. Subclinical impairment of colour vision among workers exposed to styrene. *Br J Ind Med.* 1992;49:679–682.

Finlay BL, Sengelaub DR. *Development of the Vertebrate Retina.* New York: Plenum Press; 1989.

Flammer J, Mozaffarieh M. Autoregulation, a balancing act between supply and demand. *Can J Ophthalmol.* 2008;43:317–321.

Fox DA. Psychophysically and electrophysiologically determined spatial vision deficits in lead-exposed rats have a cholinergic component. In: Narahashi T, ed. *Cellular and Molecular Basis of Neurotoxicity.* New York: Raven Press; 1984:123–140.

Fox DA. Sensory system alterations following occupational exposure to chemicals. In: Manzo L, Costa LG, eds. *Occupational Neurotoxicology.* Boca Raton, FL: CRC Press; 1998:169–184.

Fox DA, Campbell ML, Blocker YS. Functional alterations and apoptotic cell death in the retina following developmental or adult lead exposure. *Neurotoxicology.* 1997;18:645–665.

Fox DA, Chu LWF. Rods are selectively altered by lead: II. Ultrastructure and quantitative histology. *Exp Eye Res*. 1988;46:613–625.

Fox DA, Farber DB. Rods are selectively altered by lead: I. Electrophysiology and biochemistry. *Exp Eye Res*. 1988;46:579–611.

Fox DA, Hamilton RW, Johnson JE, et al. Gestational lead exposure selectively decreases retinal dopamine amacrine cells and dopamine content in adult mice. *Toxicol Appl Pharmacol Toxicol*. 2011;256:258–267.

Fox DA, Kala SV, Hamilton WR, Johnson JE, O'Callaghan JP. Low-level human equivalent gestational lead exposure produces supernormal scotopic electroretinograms, increased retinal neurogenesis and decreased dopamine utilization in rats. *Environ Health Perspect*. 2008;116:618–625.

Fox DA, Katz LM. Developmental lead exposure selectively alters the scotopic ERG component of dark and light adaptation and increases rod calcium content. *Vision Res*. 1992;32:249–252.

Fox DA, Katz LM, Farber DB. Low-level developmental lead exposure decreases the sensitivity, amplitude and temporal resolution of rods. *Neurotoxicology*. 1991a;12:641–654.

Fox DA, Lewkowski JP, Cooper GP. Acute and chronic effects of neonatal lead exposure on the development of the visual evoked response in rats. *Toxicol Appl Pharmacol*. 1977;40:449–461.

Fox DA, Poblenz AT, He L. Calcium overload triggers rod photoreceptor apoptotic cell death in chemical-induced and inherited retinal degenerations. *Ann NY Acad Sci*. 1999;893:282–286.

Fox DA, Rubinstein SD. Age-related changes in retinal sensitivity, rhodopsin content and rod outer-segment length in hooded rats following low level lead exposure during development. *Exp Eye Res*. 1989;48:237–249.

Fox DA, Rubinstein SD, Hsu P. Developmental lead exposure inhibits adult rat retinal, but not kidney, Na⁺,K⁺-ATPase. *Toxicol Appl Pharmacol*. 1991b;109:482–493.

Fox DA, Sillman AJ. Heavy metals affect rod, but not cone photoreceptors. *Science*. 1979;206:78–80.

Fraunfelder FW, Pomeranz HD, Egan RA. Nonarteritic anterior ischemic optic neuropathy and sildenafil. *Arch Ophthalmol*. 2006;124:733–734.

Frumkes TE, Eysteinsson T. The cellular basis for suppressive rod-cone interaction. *Vis Neurosci*. 1988;1:263–273.

Garner CD, Lee EW, Louis-Ferdinand RT. Muller cell involvement in methanol-induced retinal toxicity. *Toxicol Appl Pharmacol*. 1995b;130:101–107.

Garner CD, Lee EW, Terzo TS, Louis-Ferdinand RT. Role of retinal metabolism in methanol-induced retinal toxicity. *J Toxicol Environ Health*. 1995a;44:43–56.

Gaudet SJ, Razavi P, Caiafa GJ, Chader GJ. Identification of arylamine *N* acetyltransferase activity in the bovine lens. *Curr Eye Res*. 1995;14:873–877.

Geller AM, Abdel-Rahman AA, Peiffer RL, et al. The organophosphate pesticide chlorpyrifos affects form deprivation myopia. *Invest Ophthalmol Vis Sci*. 1998;39:1290–1294.

Geller AM, Hudnell HK. Critical issues in the use and analysis of the Lanthony desaturate color vision test. *Neurotoxicol Teratol*. 1997;19:455–465.

Geller AM, Osborne C, Peiffer RL. The ERG, EOG and VEP in rats. In: Weisse I, et al., eds. *Ocular Toxicology*. New York, NY: Plenum Press; 1995:7–25.

Giblin FJ. Glutathione: a vital lens antioxidant. *J Ocul Pharmacol Ther*. 2000;16:121–135.

Giddabasappa A, Hamilton WR, Chaney S, et al. Gestational lead exposure selectively increases the proliferation and number of late-born rod photoreceptors and bipolar cells. *Environ Health Perspect*. 2011;119:71–77.

Ginsburg AP. Contrast sensitivity and functional vision. *Int Ophthalmol Clin*. 2003;43:5–15.

Glickman L, Valciukas JA, Lilis R, Weisman I. Occupational lead exposure. Effects on saccadic eye movements. *Int Arch Occup Environ Health*. 1984;54:115–125.

Glickman RD. Phototoxicity to the retina: mechanisms of damage. *Int J Toxicol*. 2002;21:473–490.

Gobba F, Galassi C, Imbriani M, et al. Acquired dyschromatopsia among styrene-exposed workers. *J Occup Med*. 1991;33:761–765.

Goffeng LO, Kjuus H, Heier MS, Alvestrand M, Ulvestad B, Skaug V. Colour vision and light sensitivity in tunnel workers previously exposed to acrylamide and N-methylolacrylamide containing grouting agents. *Neurotoxicology*. 2008a;29:31–39.

Goffeng LO, Heier MS, Kjuus H, Sjoholm H, Sorensen KA, Skaug V. Nerve conduction, visual evoked responses and electroretinography in tunnel workers previously exposed to acrylamide and N-methylolacrylamide containing grouting agents. *Neurotoxicol Teratol*. 2008b;30:186–194.

Gondhowiardjo TD, van Haeringen NJ. Corneal aldehyde dehydrogenase, glutathione reductase, and glutathione-S-transferase in pathologic corneas. *Cornea*. 1993;12:310–314.

Good GW, Schepler A, Nichols JJ. The reliability of the Lanthony Desaturated D-15 test. *Optom Vis Sci*. 2005;82:1054–1059.

Gorin MB, Day R, Costantino JP, et al. Long-term tamoxifen citrate use and potential ocular toxicity. *Am J Ophthalmol*. 1998;125:493–501.

Gorkin L, Hvidsten K, Sobel RE, Siegel R. Sildenafil citrate use and the incidence of nonarteritic anterior ischemic optic neuropathy. *Int J Clin Pract*. 2006;60:500–503.

Goto Y, Shigematsu J, Tobimatsu S, Sakamoto T, Kinukawa N, Kato M. Different vulnerability of rat retinal cells to methylmercury exposure. *Curr Eye Res*. 2001;23:171–178.

Graham DG, Valentine WM. Carbon disulfide. In: Spencer PS, Schaumburg HH, eds. *Experimental and Clinical Neurotoxicology*. 2nd ed. New York: Oxford University Press; 2000:315–317.

Grant WM, Schuman JS. *Toxicology of the Eye*, 4th ed. Springfield, IL: Charles C Thomas; 1993.

Hammond CJ, Snieder H, Spector TD, Gilbert CE. Genetic and environmental factors in age-related nuclear cataracts in monozygotic twins. *N Engl J Med*. 2000;342:1786–1790.

Hanninen H, Nurminen M, Tolonen M, Martelin T. Psychological tests as indicators of excessive exposure to carbon disulfide. *Scand J Work Environ*. 1978;19:163–174.

Hansen ON, Trillingsgaard A, Beese I, et al. A neuropsychological study of children with elevated dentine lead level: assessment of the effect of lead in different socioeconomic groups. *Neurotoxicol Teratol*. 1989;11:205–213.

Harroff HH. Pathological processes of the eye related to chemical exposure. In: Hobson DW, ed. *Dermal and Ocular Toxicity: Fundamentals and Methods*. Boca Raton, FL: CRC Press; 1991:493–508.

Hass GM, Brown DVL, Eisenstein R, Hemmens A. Relation between lead poisoning in rabbit and man. *Am J Pathol*. 1964;45:691–727.

Haustein KO, Oltmanns G, Rietbrock N, Alken RG. Differences in color vision impairment caused by digoxin, digitoxin, or pengitoxin. *J Cardiovasc Pharmacol*. 1982;4:536–541.

Haustein KO, Schmidt C. Differences in color discrimination between three cardioactive glycosides. *Int J Clin Pharmacol Ther Toxicol*. 1988;26:517–520.

Hayreh MM, Hayreh SS, Baumbach GL, et al. Ocular toxicity of methanol: an experimental study. In: Merigan WH, Weiss B, eds. *Neurotoxicity of the Visual System*. New York: Raven Press; 1980:33–53.

He L, Perkins GA, Poblenz AT, et al. Bcl-xL overexpression blocks bax-mediated mitochondrial contact site formation and apoptosis in rod photoreceptors of lead-exposed mice. *Proc Nat'l Acad Sci U S A*. 2003;100:1022–1027.

He L, Poblenz AT, Medrano CJ, Fox DA. Lead and calcium produce photoreceptor cell apoptosis by opening the mitochondrial permeability transition pore. *J Biol Chem*. 2000;275:12175–12184.

Hedges TR III, Hirano M, Tucker K, Caballero B. Epidemic optic and peripheral neuropathy in Cuba: a unique geopolitical public health problem. *Surv Ophthalmol*. 1997;41:341–353.

Hendrickson A. A morphological comparison of foveal development in man and monkey. *Eye*. 1992;6:136–144.

Hendrickson A, Drucker D. The development of parafoveal and mid-peripheral human retina. *Behav Brain Res*. 1992;49:21–31.

Heng JE, Vorwerk CK, Lessell E, et al. Ethambutol is toxic to retinal ganglion cells via an excitotoxic pathway. *Invest Ophthalmol Vis Sci*. 1999;40:190–196.

Henkes HE, van Lith GHM, Canta LR. Indomethacin retinopathy. *Am J Ophthalmol*. 1972;73:846–856.

Hennekes R, Janssen K, Munoz C, Winneke G. Lead-induced ERG altera-tions in rats at high and low levels of exposure. *Concepts Toxicol.* 1987;4:193–199.

Herr DW, Boyes WK. Electrophysiological analysis of complex brain sys-tems: sensory evoked potentials and their generators. In: Chang LW, Slikker W, eds. *Neurotoxicology: Approaches and Methods.* New York: Academic Press; 1995:205–221.

Hudnell HK, Otto DA, House DE. The influence of vision on computer-ized neurobehavioral test scores: a proposal for improving test protocols. *Neurotoxicol Teratol.* 1996;18:391–400.

Hughes WF, Coogan PS. Pathology of the pigment epithelium and retina in rabbits poisoned with lead. *Am J Pathol.* 1974;77:237–254.

Interagency Coordinating Committee on the Validation of Alternative Methods. *ICCVAM Test Method Evaluation Report: Recommendations for Routine Use of Topical Anesthetics, Systemic Analgesics, and Humane Endpoints to Avoid or Minimize Pain and Distress in Ocular Safety Testing.* NIH Publication No. 10-7514. Research Triangle Park, NC: National Institute of Environmental Health Sciences; 2010a.

Interagency Coordinating Committee on the Validation of Alternative Methods. *ICCVAM Test Method Evaluation Report: Current Validation Status of In Vitro Test Methods Proposed for Identifying Eye Injury Hazard Potential of Chemicals and Products.* NIH Publication No. 10-7553. Research Triangle Park, NC: National Institute of Environmental Health Sciences; 2010b.

Imai H, Miyata M, Uga S, Ishikawa S. Retinal degeneration in rats exposed to an organophosphate pesticide (fenthion). *Environ Res.* 1983;30:453–465.

Ingemansson SO. Studies on the effect of 4-methylpyrazole on retinal activ-ity in the methanol poisoned monkey by recording the electroretinogram. *Acta Ophthalmol.* 1983;(suppl 158):1–24.

Imperia PS, Lazarus HM, Lass JH. Ocular complications of systemic cancer chemotherapy. *Surv Ophthalmol.* 1989;34:209–230.

Iregren A, Andersson M, Nylén P. Color vision and occupational chemical exposures: I. An overview of tests and effects. *Neurotoxicology.* 2002;23:719–733.

Iregren A, Johnson, A-C, Nylén, P. Low-level styrene exposure and color vision in Swedish styrene workers. *Environ Toxicol Pharmacol.* 2005;19:511–516.

Isaac NE, Walker AM, Jick H, Gorman M. Exposure to phenothiazine drugs and risk of cataract. *Arch Ophthalmol.* 1991;109:256–260.

Ishikawa S. Chronic optica-neuropathy due to environmental exposure of organophosphate pesticides (Saku disease): clinical and experimental study. *Nippon Ganka Gakkai Zasshi.* 1973;77:1835–1886.

Iwata K. Neuro-ophthalmological findings and a follow-up study in the Agano area, Niigata Pref. In: Tsubaki T, Irukayama K, eds. *Minamata Disease: MethylMercury poisoning in Minamata and Niigata, Tokyo.* Tokyo: Kodansha; 1977:166–185.

Jadhav AL, Ramesh GT. Pb-induced alterations in tyrosine hydroxylase activity in rat brain. *Mol Cell Biochem.* 1997;175:137–141.

Jagle H, Jagle C, Serey L, et al. Visual short-term effects of Viagra: double-blind study in healthy young subjects. *Am J Ophthalmol.* 2004;137:842–849.

Johnson MW, Vine AK. Hydroxychloroquine therapy in massive total doses without retinal toxicity. *Am J Ophthalmol.* 1987;104:139–144.

Jones RD, Brenneke CJ, Hoss HE, Loney ML. An electroretinogram protocol for toxicological screening in the canine model. *Toxicol Lett.* 1994;70:223–234.

Jones BW, Marc RE. Retinal remodeling during retinal degeneration. *Exp Eye Res.* 2005;81:123–137.

Kaiser-Kupfer MI, Kupfer C, Rodriques MM. Tamoxifen retinopathy. A clinocopathologic report. *Ophthalmology.* 1981;88:89–93.

Kalloniatis M, Tomisich G. Amino acid neurochemistry of the vertebrate retina. *Prog Retinal Eye Res.* 1999;18:811–866.

Kamel F, Boyes WK, Gladen BC, et al. Retinal degeneration in licensed pesticide applicators. *Am J Ind Med.* 2000;37:618–628.

Kamran S, Bakshi R. MRI in chronic toluene abuse: low signal in the cerebral cortex on T2-weighted images. *Neuroradiology.* 1998;40:519–521.

Kaplan E, Benardete E. The dynamics of primate retinal ganglion cells. *Prog Brain Res.* 2001;134:17–34.

Karai I, Horiguchi SH, Nishikawa N. Optic atrophy with visual field defect in workers occupationally exposed to lead for 30 years. *J Toxicol Clin Toxicol.* 1982;19:409–418.

King G, Hirst L, Holmes R. Human corneal and lens aldehyde dehydroge-nases. Localization and function(s) of ocular ALDH1 and ALDH3 iso-zymes. *Adv Exp Med Biol.* 1999;463:189–198.

Kini MM, Cooper JR. Biochemistry of methanol poisoning. 4. The effect of methanol and its metabolites on retinal metabolism. *Biochem J.* 1962;82:164–172.

Kirrane EF, Hoppin JA, Kamel F, et al. Retinal degeneration and other eye disorders in wives of farmer pesticide applicators enrolled in the Agricultural Health Study. *Am J Epidemiol.* 2005;161:1020–1029.

Kiyokawa M, Mizota A, Takasoh M, Adachi-Usami E. Pattern visual evoked cortical potentials in patients with toxic optic neuropathy caused by toluene abuse. *Jpn J Ophthalmol.* 2005;43:438–442.

Ko LS, Shum JT, Chen YL, Wang YS. Pesticides and myopia, a working hypothesis. *Acta Ophthalmol Suppl.* 1988;185:145–146.

Kobel W, Gfeller W. Distribution of eye irritation scores of industrial chem-icals. *Food Chem Toxicol.* 1985;23:311–312.

Kohler K, Lilienthal H, Guenther E, et al. Persistent decrease of the dopamine-synthesizing enzyme tyrosine hydroxylase in the rhesus monkey retina after chronic lead exposure. *Neurotoxicology.* 1997;18:623–632.

Koliopoulos J, Palimeris G. On acquired colour vision disturbances during treatment with ethambutol and indomethacin. *Mod Probl Ophthalmol.* 1972;11:178–184.

Krill AE, Potts AM, Johanson CE. Chloroquine retinopathy. Investigation of discrepancy between dark adaptation and electroretinographic findings in advanced stages. *Am J Ophthalmol.* 1971;71:530–543.

Lapalus P, Garaffo RG. Ocular pharmacokinetics. In: Hockwin O, Green K, Rubin LF, eds. *Manual of Oculotoxicity Testing of Drugs.* Stuttgart, Germany: Gustav Fischer Verlag; 1992:119–136.

Lasley SM, Lane JD. Diminished regulation of mesolimbic dopaminer-gic activity in rat after chronic inorganic lead exposure. *Toxicol Appl Pharmacol.* 1988;95:474–483.

Laties A. Vision disorders and phosphodiesterase 5 inhibitors: a review of the evidence to date. *Druf Saf.* 2009;32:1–18.

Laties A, Zrenner E. Viagra (sildenafil citrate) and ophthalmology. *Prog Retin Eye Res.* 2002;21:485–506.

LaVail MM. Rod outer segment disk shedding in rat retina: relationship to cyclic lighting. *Science.* 1976;194:1071–1074.

Lazzaroni F, Scorolli L, Pizzoleo CF, et al. Tamoxifen retinopathy: does it really exist? *Graefes Arch Clin Exp Ophthalmol.* 1998;236:669–673.

Lee EW, Garner CD, Terzo TS. A rat model manifesting methanol-induced visual dysfunction suitable for both acute and long-term exposure stud-ies. *Toxicol Appl Pharmacol.* 1994;128:199–206.

Lee JW, Fuda H, Javitt NB, Strott CA, Rodriguez IR. Expression and local-ization of sterol 27-hydroxylase (CYP27A1) in monkey retina. *Exp Eye Res.* 2006;83:465–469.

Lee AY, Chung SS. Involvement of aldose reductase in naphthalene cata-ract. *Invest Ophthalmol Vis Sci.* 39:193–197.

Leske MC, Chylack LT Jr, Wu SY. The lens opacities case-control study. Risk factors for cataract. *Arch Ophthalmol.* 1991;109:244–251.

Lessell S. Toxic and deficiency optic neuropathies. In: Miller NR, Newman NJ, eds. *Walsh and Hoyt's Clinical Neuro-Ophthalmology.* 5th ed. Baltimore: Williams & Wilkins; 1998.

Liang H, Pauly A, Riancho L, Baudouin C, Brignole-Baudouin F. Toxicological evaluation of preservative-containing and preservative-free topical prostaglandin analogues on a three-dimensional-reconstituted corneal epithelium system. *Br J Ophthalmol.* 2011;95:869–875.

Lilienthal H, Kohler K, Turfeld M, Winneke G. Persistent increases in sco-topic b-wave amplitudes after lead exposure in monkeys. *Exp Eye Res.* 1994;59:203–209.

Lilienthal H, Lenaerts C, Winneke G, Hennekes R. Alteration of the visual evoked potential and the electroretinogram in lead-treated monkeys. *Neurotoxicol Teratol.* 1988;10:417–422.

Lissner W, Greenlee JE, Cameron JD, Goren SB. Localization of tritiated digoxin in the rat eye. *Am J Ophthalmol.* 1971;72:608–614.

Lou MF, Xu GT, Zigler S Jr, York B Jr. Inhibition of naphthalene cataract in rats by aldose reductase inhibitors. *Curr Eye Res.* 1996;15:423–432.

Lynch JJ III, Eskin TA, Merigan WH. Selective degeneration of the parvocellular-projecting retinal ganglion cells in a New World monkey, Saimiri sciureus. *Brain Res.* 1989;499:325–332.

Lynch JJ III, Silveira LC, Perry VH, Merigan WH. Visual effects of damage to P ganglion cells in macaques. *Vis Neurosci.* 1992;8:575–583.

Madreperla SA, Johnson MA, Nakatani K. Electrophysiological and electroretinographic evidence for photoreceptor dysfunction as a toxic effect of digoxin. *Arch Ophthalmol.* 1994;112:807–812.

Maguire MJ, Hemming K, Wild JM, et al. Prevalence of visual field loss following exposure to vigabatrin therapy: a systematic review. *Epilepsia.* 2010;51:2423–2431.

Marks MJ, Seeds NW. A heterogeneous ouabain-ATPase interaction in mouse brain. *Life Sci.* 1978;23:2735–2744.

Marmor MF, Zrenner E. Standard for clinical electroretinography (1994 update). *Doc Ophthalmol.* 1995;89:199–210.

Martin-Amat G, McMartin KE, Hayreh SS, et al. Methanol poisoning: ocular toxicity produced by formate. *Toxicol Appl Pharmacol.* 1978;45:201–208.

Mastyugin V, Aversa E, Bonazzi A, et al. Hypoxia-induced production of 12-hydroxyeicosanoids in the corneal epithelium: involvement of a cytochrome P-4504B1 isoform. *J Pharmacol Exp Ther.* 1999;289:1611–1619.

Maurissen JPJ. Neurobehavioral methods for the evaluation of sensory functions. In: Chang LW, Slikker W, eds. *Neurotoxicology: Approaches and Methods.* New York: Academic Press; 1995:239–264.

McCulley JP. Chemical injuries of the eye. In: Leibowitz HM, Waring GO. eds. *Corneal Disorders, Clinical Diagnosis and Management.* 2nd ed. Philadelphia: Saunders; 1998:770–790.

McGrail KM, Sweadner KJ. Complex expression patterns for Na$^+$, K$^+$-ATPase isoforms in retina and optic nerve. *Eur J Neurosci.* 1989;2:170–176.

McGwin G Jr, Hall TA, Seale J, Xie A, Owsley C. Consumer product-related eye injury in the United States, 1998-2002. *J Safety Res.* 2006;37:501–506.

Mecklenburg L, Schraemeyer U. An overview on the toxic morphological changes in the retinal pigment epitheliu after systemic compound administration. *Toxicol Pathol.* 2007;35:252–267.

Medrano CJ, Fox DA. Oxygen consumption in rat outer and inner retina: light- and pharmacologically induced inhibition. *Exp Eye Res.* 1995;61:273–284.

Medrano CJ, Fox DA. Substrate-dependent effects of calcium on rat retinal mitochondria respiration: physiological and toxicological studies. *Toxicol Appl Pharmacol.* 1994;125:309–321.

Meier-Ruge W. Drug-induced retinopathy. *CRC Toxicol.* 1972;1:325–360.

Mergler D, Belanger S, Grosbois S, Vachon N. Chromal focus of acquired chromatic discrimination loss and slovent exposure among printshop workers. *Toxicology.* 1988;49:341–348.

Mergler D, Blain L, Lagace JP. Solvent related colour vision loss: an indicator of damage? *Int Arch Occup Environ Health.* 1987;59:313–321.

Mergler D, Huel G, Bowler R, et al. Visual dysfunction among former microelectronics assembly workers. *Arch Environ Health.* 1991;46:326–334.

Merigan WH. Effects of toxicants on visual systems. *Neurobehav Toxicol.* 1979;1(suppl 1):15–22.

Merigan WH, Eskin TA. Spatio-temporal vision of macaques with severe loss of P beta retinal ganglion cells. *Vision Res.* 1986;26:1751–1761.

Merigan WH, Wood RW, Zehl D, Eskin TA. Carbon disulfide effects on the visual system: I. Visual thresholds and ophthalmoscopy. *Invest Ophthalmol Vis Sci.* 1988;29:512–518.

Miller DP, Watkins SE, Sampson T, Davis KJ. Long-term use of fluticasone propionate/salmeterol fixed-dose combination and incidence of cataracts and glaucoma among chronic obstructive pulmonary disease patients in the UK General Practice Research Database. *Int J COPD.* 2011;6:467–476.

Misra UK, Nag D, Misra NK, et al. Some observations on the macula of pesticide workers. *Hum Toxicol.* 1985;4:135–145.

Mojon DS, Kaufmann P, Odel JG, et al. Clinical course of a cohort in the Cuban epidemic optic and peripheral neuropathy. *Neurology.* 1997;48:19–22.

Moser VC, Boyes WK. Prolonged neurobehavioral and visual effects of short-term exposure to 3,3-iminodipropionitrile (IDPN) in rats. *Fund Appl Toxicol.* 1993;21:277–290.

Moser VC, Phillips PM, Morgan DL, Sills RC. Carbon disulfide neurotoxicity in rats: VII. Behavioral evaluations using a functional observational battery. *Neurotoxicology.* 1998;19:147–158.

Muñoz H, Romiew I, Palazuelos E, et al. Blood lead level and neurobehavioral development among children living in Mexico City. *Arch Environ Health.* 1993;48:132–139.

Murano H, Kojima M, Sasaki K. Differences in naphthalene cataract formation between albino and pigmented rat eyes. *Ophthalm Res.* 1993;25:16–22.

Murata K, Araki S, Yokoyama K, et al. Assessment of central, peripheral, and autonomic nervous system functions in lead workers: neuroelectrophysiological studies. *Environ Res.* 1993;61:323–336.

Murray TG, Burton TC, Rajani C, et al. Methanol poisoning. A rodent model with structural and functional evidence for retinal involvement. *Arch Ophthalmol.* 1991;109:1012–1016.

Nagpal AG, Brodie SE. Supranormal electroretinogram in a 10-year-old girl with lead toxicity. *Doc Ophthalmol.* 2009;118:163–166.

Nagpal K, Singh SK, Mishra DN. Chitosan nanoparticles: a promising system in novel drug delivery. *Chem Pharm Bull.* 2010;58:1423–1430.

Nakamura K, Fujiki T, Tamura HO. Age, gender and region-specific differences in drug metabolising enzymes in rat ocular tissues. *Exp Eye Res.* 2005;81:710–715.

Nicholls P. The effect of formate on cytochrome aa3 and on electron transport in the intact respiratory chain. *Biochim Biophys Acta.* 1976;430:13–29.

Nickla DL, Wallman J. The multifunctional choroid. *Prog Retin Eye Res.* 2010;29:144–168.

Niklasson M, Stengard K, Tham R. Are the effects of toluene on the vestibulo and opto-ocular motor system inhibited by the action of GABAB antagonist CGP 35348? *Neurotoxicol Teratol.* 1995;17:351–357.

Noureddin BN, Seoud M, Bashshur Z, et al. Ocular toxicity in low-dose tamoxifen: a prospective study. *Eye.* 1999;13:729–733.

Novack GD. Emerging drugs for ophthalmic diseases. *Expert Opin Emerg Drugs.* 2003;8:251–266.

Oberto A, Marks N, Evans HL, Guidotti A. Lead promotes apoptosis in newborn rat cerebellar neurons: pathological implications. *J Pharmacol Exp Ther.* 1996;279:435–442.

Otto DA, Fox DA. Auditory and visual dysfunction following lead exposure. *Neurotoxicology.* 1993;14:191–208.

Otto DA, Robinson G, Baumann S, et al. 5-Year follow-up study of children with low-to-moderate lead absorption: electrophysiological evaluation. *Environ Res.* 1985;38:168–186.

Ottonello S, Foroni C, Carta A, et al. Oxidative stress and age-related cataract. *Ophthalmologica.* 2000;214:78–85.

Palacz O, Szymanska K, Czepita D. Studies on the ERG in subjects with chronic exposure to carbon disulfide: I. Assessment of the condition of the visual system taking into account ERG findings depending on the duration of exposure to CS2. *Klin Oczna.* 1980;82:65–68.

Paramei GV, Meyer-Baron M, Seeber A. Impairments of colour vision induced by organic solvents: a meta-analysis study. *Neurotoxicology.* 2004;25:803–816.

Paraoanu LE, Mocko JB, Becker-Roeck M, et al. Exposure to diazinon alters in vitro retinogenesis: retinospheroid morphology, development of chicken retinal cell types, and gene expression. *Toxicol Sci.* 2006;89:314–324.

Pavlidis NA, Petris C, Briassoulis E, et al. Clear evidence that long-term, low-dose tamoxifen treatment can induce ocular toxicity. A prospective study of 63 patients. *Cancer.* 1992;69:2961–2964.

Peate WF. Work-related eye injuries and illnesses. *Am Fam Physician.* 2007;75:1017–1022.

Peiffer RL, McCary B, Bee W, et al. Contemporary methods in ocular toxicology. *Toxicol Methods.* 2000;10:17–39.

Penn JS, Naash MI, Anderson RE. Effect of light history on retinal antioxidants and light damage susceptibility in the rat. *Exp Eye Res.* 1987;44:779–788.

Petit TL, LeBoutillier JC. Effects of lead exposure during development on neocortical dendritic and synaptic structure. *Exp Neurol.* 1979;64:482–492.

Plant GT, Sergott RC. Understanding and interpreting vision safety issues with vigabatrin therapy. *Acta Neurol Scand Suppl.* 2011;192:57–71.

Polak BC, Leys M, van Lith GH. Blue-yellow colour vision changes as early symptoms of ethambutol oculotoxicity. *Ophthalmologica.* 1985; 191:223–226.

Potts AM. The reaction of uveal pigment in vitro with polycyclic compounds. *Invest Ophthalmol.* 1964;3:405–416.

Potts AM. The visual toxicity of methanol: VI. The clinical aspects of experimental methanol poisoning treated with base. *Am J Ophthalmol.* 1955;39:76–82.

Potts AM, Au PC. The affinity of melanin for inorganic ions. *Exp Eye Res.* 1976;22:487–491.

Pounds JG. Effect of lead intoxication on calcium homeostasis and calcium-mediated cell function: a review. *Neurotoxicology.* 1984;5:295–332.

Porkony J, Smith VS, Verriest G, Pinckers A. *Congenital and Acquired Color Vision Defects.* New York: Grune & Stratton; 1979.

Prow TW. Toxicity of nanomaterials to the eye. *Wiley Interdiscip Rev Nanomed Nanobiotechnol.* 2010;2:317–333.

Raedler A, Sievers J. The development of the visual system of the albino rat. *Adv Anat Embryol Cell Biol.* 1975;50:7–87.

Raitta C, Seppalainen AN, Huuskonen MS. *n*-hexane maculopathy in industrial workers. *Von Graefes Arch Klin Exp Ophthalmol.* 1978;209:99–110.

Raitta C, Teir H, Tolonen M, Nurminen M, Helpio E, Malmstrom S. Impaired color discrimination among viscose rayon workers exposed to carbon disulfide. *J Occup Med.* 1981;23:189–192.

Raitta C, Tolonen M, Nurminen M. Microcirculation of ocular fundus in viscose rayon workers exposed to carbon disulfide. *Arch Klin Exp Ophthalmol.* 1974;191:151–164.

Ramsey MS, Fine BS. Chloroquine toxicity in the human eye. Histopathologic observations by electron microscopy. *Am J Ophthalmol.* 1972;73:229–235.

Rao GN. Light intensity-associated eye lesions of Fisher 344 rats in long-term studies. *Toxicol Pathol.* 1991;19:148–155.

Rapp LM, Tolman BL, Koutz CA, Thum LA. Predisposing factors to light-induced photoreceptor cell damage: retinal changes in maturing rats. *Exp Eye Res.* 1990;51:177–184.

Reuhl KR, Rice DC, Gilbert SG, Mallett J. Effects of chronic developmental lead exposure on monkey neuroanatomy: visual system. *Toxicol Appl Pharmacol.* 1989;99:501–509.

Rice DC. Effects of lifetime lead exposure on spatial and temporal visual function in monkeys. *Neurotoxicology.* 1998;19:893–902.

Rice DC. Sensory and cognitive effects of developmental methylmercury exposure in monkeys, and a comparison to effects in rodents. *Neurotoxicology.* 1996;17:139–154.

Rice DC, Gilbert SG. Effects of developmental exposure to methylmercury on spatial and temporal visual function in monkeys. *Toxicol Appl Pharmacol.* 1990;102:151–163.

Rice DC, Hayward S. Comparison of visual function at adulthood and during aging in monkeys exposed to lead or methylmercury. *Neurotoxicology.* 1999;20:767–784.

Roberts JE. Ocular phototoxicity. *J Photochem Photobiol B.* 2001;64: 136–143.

Roberts JE. Screening for ocular phototoxicity. *Int J Toxicol.* 2002; 21:491–500.

Roberts JE, Wielgus AR, Boyes WK, Andley U, Chignell CF. Phototoxicity and cytotoxicity of fullerol in human lens epithelial cells. *Toxicol Appl Pharmacol.* 2008;228:49–58.

Robertson DM, Hollenhorst RW, Callahan JA. Ocular manifestations of digitalis toxicity. *Arch Ophthalmol.* 1966;76:640–645.

Rogers JM, Chernoff N. Chemically induced cataracts in the fetus and neonate. In: Kacew S, Lock S, eds. *Toxicologic and Pharmacologic Principles in Pediatrics.* New York: Hemisphere; 1988:255–275.

Roman G. Tropical myeloneuropathies revisited. *Curr Opin Neurol.* 1998;11:539–544.

Rosenthal AR, Kolb H, Bergsma D, et al. Chloroquine retinopathy in the Rhesus monkey. *Invest Ophthalmol Vis Sci.* 1978;17:1158–1175.

Rosolen SG, Rigaudiere F, Le Gargasson JF, Brigell MG. Recommendations for a toxicological screening ERG procedure in laboratory animals. *Doc Ophthalmol.* 2005;110:57–66.

Rothenberg SJ, Schnaas L, Salgado-Valladares M, et al. Increased ERG a-and b-wave amplitudes in 7-10 year old children resulting from prenatal lead exposure. *Invest Ophthalmol Vis Sci.* 2002;43:2036–2044.

Rouslin W, Broge CW, Chernyak BV. Effects of Zn^{2+} on the activity and binding of the mitochondrial ATPase inhibitor protein, IF1. *J Bioenerg Biomembr.* 1993;25:297–306.

Ruan DY, Tang LX, Zhao C, Guo YJ. Effects of low-level lead on retinal ganglion sustained and transient cells in developing rats. *Neurotoxicol Teratol.* 1994;16:47–53.

Ruedeman AD. The electroretinogram in chronic methyl alcohol poisoning in human beings. *Trans Am Ophthalmol Soc.* 1961;59:480–529.

Ryu YH, Lee JD, Yoon PH, Jeon P, Kim DI, Shin DW. Cerebral perfusion impairment in a patient with toluene abuse. *J Nucl Med.* 1998;39: 632–633.

Sadun AA. Acquired mitochondrial impairment as a cause of optic nerve disease. *Trans Am Ophthalmol Soc.* 1998;96:881–923.

Sadun AA, Martone JF, Muci-Mendoza R, et al. Epidemic optic neuropathy in Cuba. Eye findings. *Arch Ophthalmol.* 1994a;112:691–699.

Sadun AA, Martone JF, Reyes L, et al. Optic and peripheral neuropathy in Cuba. *JAMA.* 1994b;271:663–664.

Salmon JF, Carmichael TR, Welsh NH. Use of contrast sensitivity measurement in the detection of subclinical ethambutol toxic optic neuropathy. *Br J Ophthalmol.* 1987;71:192–196.

Sanders K, Degn LL, Mundy WR, et al. In vitro phototoxicity and hazard identification of nano-scale titanium dioxide. *Toxicol App Pharmacol.* 2012;258:226–236.

Santaella RM, Fraunfelder FW. Ocular adverse effects associated with systemic medications: recognition and management. *Drugs.* 2007;67:75–93.

Santos-Anderson RM, Tso MOM, Valdes JJ, Annau Z. Chronic lead administration in neonatal rats. Electron microscopy of the retina. *J Neuropathol Exp Neurol.* 1984;43:175–187.

Sassaman FW, Cassidy JT, Alpern M, Maaseidvaag F. Electroretinography in patients with connective tissue diseases treated with hydroxychloroquine. *Am J Ophthalmol.* 1970;70:515–523.

Sato S. Aldose reductase the major protein associated with naphthalene dihydrodiol dehydrogenase activity in rat lens. *Invest Ophthalmol Vis Sci.* 1993;34:3172–3178.

Sato S, Sugiyama K, Lee YS, Kador PF. Prevention of naphthalene-1,2-dihydrodiol-induced lens protein modifications by structurally diverse aldose reductase inhibitors. *Exp Eye Res.* 1999;68:601–608.

Schmid KE, Kornek GV, Scheithauer W, Binder S. Update on ocular complications of systemic cancer chemotherapy. *Surv Ophthalmol.* 2006;51:19–40.

Schnapf JL, Kraft TW, Nunn BJ, Baylor DA. Spectral sensitivity of primate photoreceptors. *Vis Neurosci.* 1988;1:255–261.

Schneider BG, Shygan AW, Levinson R. Co-localization and polarized distribution of Na, K-ATPase: $\alpha3$ and $\beta2$ subunits in photoreceptor cells. *J Histochem Cytochem.* 1991;39:507–517.

Scholl HPN, Zrenner E. Electrophysiology in the investigation of acquired retinal disorders. *Surv Ophthalmol.* 2000;45:29–47.

Schreiber JS, Hudnell HK, Geller AM, et al. Apartment residents' and day care workers' exposures to tetrachloroethylene and deficits in visual contrast sensitivity. *Environ Health Perspect.* 2002;110:655–664.

Schwartzmann ML. Cytochrome P450 and arachidonic acid metabolism in the corneal epithelium. In: Green K, Edelhauser HF, Hackett RB, et al., eds. *Advances in Ocular Toxicology.* New York: Plenum Press; 1997:3–20.

Scortegagna M, Hanbauer I. The effect of lead exposure and serum deprivation on mesencephalic primary cultures. *Neurotoxicology.* 1997;18:331–340.

Sears ML. *Pharmacology of the Eye.* Berlin: Springer-Verlag; 1984.

Seme MT, Summerfelt P, Henry MM, et al. Formate-induced inhibition of photoreceptor function in methanol intoxication. *J Pharmacol Exp Ther.* 1999;289:361–370.

Seppalainen AM, Haltia M. Carbon disulfide. In: Spencer PS, Schaumberg HH, eds. *Experimental and Clinical Neurotoxicology.* Baltimore: William & Wilkins; 1980:356–373.

Seyfoddin A, Shaw J, Al-Kassas R. Solid lipid nanoparticles for ocular drug delivery. *Drug Delivery.* 2010;17:467–489.

Shanthaverrappa TR, Bourne GH. Monoamine oxidase distribution in the rabbit eye. *J Histochem Cytochem.* 1964;12:281–287.

Shearer RV, Dubois EL. Ocular changes induced by long-term hydroxy-chloroquine (Plaqenil) therapy. *Am J Ophthalmol.* 1967;64:245–252.

Shichi H. Immunocytochemical study of cytochrome P4504A induction in mouse eye. *Exp Eye Res.* 1996;63:747–751.

Shichi H, Nebert DW. Genetic differences in drug metabolism associated with ocular toxicity. *Environ Health Perspect.* 1982;44:107–117.

Shulman LM, Fox DA. Dopamine inhibits mammalian photoreceptor Na$^+$,K$^+$-ATPase activity via a selective effect on the α3 isozyme. *Proc Natl Acad Sci U S A.* 1996;93:8034–8039.

Signorino M, Scarpino O, Provincialli L, et al. Modification of the electro-retinogram and of different components of the visual evoked potentials in workers exposed to lead. *Ital Electroencephalogr J.* 1983;10:51P.

Singh AK, Shichi H. A novel glutathione peroxidase in bovine eye. Sequence analysis, mRNA level, and translation. *J Biol Chem.* 1998; 273:26171–26178.

Sillman AJ, Bolnick DA, Bosetti JB, et al. The effects of lead and cadmium on the mass photoreceptor potential the dose-response relationship. *Neurotoxicology.* 1982;3:179–194.

Sjoerdsma T, Kamermans M, Spekreijse H. Effect of the tuberculostaticum ethambutol and stimulus intensity on chromatic discrimination in man. *Vision Res.* 1999;39:2955–2962.

Smeeth L, Boulis M, Hubbard R, Fletcher AE. A population based case-control study of cataract and inhaled corticosteroids. *Br J Ophthalmol.* 2003;87:1247–1251.

Sonkin N. Stippling of the retina: A new physical sign in the early dignosis of lead poisoning. *N Engl J Med.* 1963;269:779–780.

Specchio LM, Bellomo R, Dicuonzo F, et al. Smooth pursuit eye move-ments among storage battery workers. *Clin Toxicol.* 1981;18:1269–1276.

Spector A. Oxidative stress and disease. *J Ocul Pharmacol Ther.* 2000;16:193–201.

Spencer PS, Schaumburg HH. A review of acrylamide neurotoxicity: Part I. Properties, uses and human exposure. *Can J Neurol Sci.* 1974a;1:145–150.

Spencer PS, Schaumburg HH. A review of acrylamide neurotoxicity: Part II. Experimental animal neuorotoxicity and pathologic mechanisms. *Can J Neurol Sci.* 1974b;1:152–169.

Spivey GH, Baloh RW, Brown CP, et al. Subclinical effects of chronic increased lead absorption—a prospective study: III. Neurologic findings at follow-up examination. *J Occup Med.* 1980;22:607–612.

Srivastava D, Fox DA, Hurwitz RL. Effects of magnesium on cyclic GMP hydrolysis by the bovine retinal rod cyclic GMP phosphodiesterase. *Biochem J.* 1995a;308:653–658.

Srivastava D, Hurwitz RL, Fox DA. Lead- and calcium-mediated inhibition of bovine rod cGMP phosphodiesterase: interactions with magnesium. *Toxicol Appl Pharmacol.* 1995b;134:43–52.

Srivastava SK, Singhal SS, Awasthi S, et al. A glutathione S-transferases iso-zyme (bGST 5.8) involved in the metabolism of 4-hydroxy-2-transnonenal is localized in bovine lens epithelium. *Exp Eye Res.* 1996;63:329–337.

Storm JE, Mazor KA, Aldous KM, Blount BC, Brodie SE, Serle JB. Visual contrast sensitivity in children exposed to tetrachloroethylene. *Arch Environ Occup Health.* 2011;66:166–177.

Strauss O. The retinal pigment epithelium in visual function. *Physiol Rev.* 2005;85:845–881.

Sweadner KJ. Isozymes of Na$^+$/K$^+$-ATPase. *Biochem Biophys Acta.* 1989; 989:185–220.

Szabo I, Bernardi P, Zoratti M. Modulation of the mitochondrial megachan-nel by divalent cations and protons. *J Biol Chem.* 1992;267:2940–2946.

Takeuchi T, Eto K. Pathology and pathogenesis of Minamata disease. In: Tsubaki T, Irukayama K, eds. *Minamata Disease: Methylmercury poi-soning in Minamata and Niigata, Japan.* Tokyo; Kodansha; Amsterdam: Elsevier; 1977;103–141.

Tandon P, Padilla S, Barone S Jr, et al. Fenthion produces a persistent decrease in muscarinic receptor function in the adult rat retina. *Toxicol Appl Pharmacol.* 1994;125:271–280.

Taylor A, Nowell T. Oxidative stress and antioxidant function in relation to risk for cataract. *Adv Pharmacol.* 1997;38:515–536.

Tessier-Lavigne M, Mobbs P, Attwell D. Lead and mercury toxic-ity and the rod light response. *Invest Ophthalmol Vis Sci.* 1985;26: 1117–1123.

Thaler JS, Curinga R, Kiracofe G. Relation of graded ocular anterior chamber pigmentation to phenothiazine intake in schizophrenics—Quantification procedures. *Am J Optom Physiol Ophthalmol.* 1985;62:600–604.

Thirkill CE, Roth AM, Keltner JL. Cancer-associated retinopathy. *Arch Ophthalmol.* 1987;105:372–375.

Till C, Rovet JF, Koren G, Westall CA. Assessment of visual functions following prenatal exposure to organic solvents. *Neurotoxicology.* 2003;24:725–731.

Toews AD, Krigman MR, Thomas DJ, Morell P. Effect of inorganic lead exposure on myelination in the rat. *Neurochem Res.* 1980;5: 605–616.

Tolman JA, Faulkner MA. Vigabatrin: a comprehensive review of drug properties including clinical updates following recent FDA approval. *Expert Opin Pharmacother.* 2009;10:3077–3089.

tom Dieck S, Brandstätter JH. Ribbon synapses of the retina. *Cell Tiss Res.* 2006;326:339–346.

Ulshafer RJ, Allen CB, Rubin ML. Distributions of elements in the human retinal pigment epithelium. *Arch Ophthalmol.* 1990;108:113–117.

United States Environmental Protection Agency. *Prevention, Pesticides and Toxic Substances* (7101). EPA 712-C-98-242. *Health Effects Test Guideline.* OPPTS 870.6855. *Neurophysiology: Sensory Evoked Potentials.* August 1998a. Available at: http://www.epa.gov/docs/ OPPTS Harmonized/870 Health Effects Test Guidelines/Series/.

United States Environmental Protection Agency. *Prevention, Pesticides and Toxic Substances* (7101). EPA 712-C-98-238. *Health Effects Test Guideline.* OPPTS 870.6200. *Neurotoxicity Screening Battery.* August 1998b. Available at: http://www.epa.gov/docs/OPPTS Harmonized/870 Health Effects Test Guidelines/Series/.

Urban RC, Cotlier E. Corticosteroid-induced cataracts. *Surv Ophthalmol.* 1986;31:102–110.

Vale RD, Banker G, Hall ZW. The neuronal cytoskeleton. In: Hall ZW, ed. *An Introduction to Molecular Neurobiology.* Sunderland, MA: Sinauer; 1992:247–280.

van Dijk BW, Spekreijse H. Ethambutol changes the color coding of carp retinal ganglion cells reversibly. *Invest Ophthalmol Vis Sci.* 1983;24: 128–133.

van Heyningen R, Pirie A. The metabolism of naphthalene and its toxic effect on the eye. *Biochem J.* 1967;102:842–852.

Vanhoorne M, De Rouck A, Bacquer D. Epidemiological study of the sys-temic ophthalmological effects of carbon disulfide. *Arch Environ Health.* 1996;51:181–188.

van Soest S, Westerveld A, de Jong PT, et al. Retinitis pigmentosa: defined from a molecular point of view. *Surv Ophthalmol.* 1999;43:321–334.

Veenstra DL, Best JH, Hornberger J, et al. Incidence and long-term cost of steroid-related side effects after renal transplantation. *Am J Kidney Dis.* 1999;33:829–839.

Vettori MV, Corradi D, Coccini T, et al. Styrene-induced changes in ama-crine retinal cells: an experimental study in the rat. *Neurotoxicology.* 2000;21:607–614.

Vidyasagar TR. Optic nerve components may not be equally susceptible to damage by acrylamide. *Brain Res.* 1981;224:452–455.

Walkowiak J, Altmann L, Kramer U, et al. Cognitive and sensorimotor functions in 6-year-old children in relation to lead and mercury levels: adjustment for intelligence and contrast sensitivity in computerized test-ing. *Neurotoxicol Teratol.* 1998;20:511–521.

Waltman S, Sears ML. Catechol-O-methyltransferase and monoamine oxi-dase activity in the ocular tissues of albino rabbits. *Invest Ophthalmol.* 1964;3:601–605.

Wang QP, Jammoul F, Duboc A, et al. Treatment of epilepsy: the GABA-transaminase inhibitor, vigabatrin, induces neuronal plasticity in the mouse retina. *Eur J Neurosci.* 2008;27:2177–2187.

Wässle H. Parallel processing in the mammalian retina. *Nat Rev Neurosci.* 2004;5:747–757.

Watkins JB III, Wirthwein DP, Sanders RA. Comparative study of Phase II biotransformation in rabbit ocular tissues. *Drug Metab Dispos.* 1991;19:708–713.

Weatherall M, Clay J, James K, Perrin K, Shirtcliffe P, Beasley R. Dose-response relationship of inhaled corticosteroids and cataracts: a systematic review and meta-analysis. *Respirology.* 2009;14:983–990.

Wilson MA, Johnston MV, Goldstein GW, Blue ME. Neonatal lead exposure impairs development of rodent barrel field cortex. *Proc Natl Acad Sci U S A.* 2000;97:5540–5545.

Winkler BS. A quantitative assessment of glucose metabolism in the rat retina. In: Christen Y, Doly M, Droy-Lefaix MT, eds. *Vision and Adaptation, Les Seminaires Ophtamologiques d'IPSEN.* Vol 6. Paris: Elsevier; 1995:78–96.

Winkler BS, Kapousta-Bruneau N, Arnold MJ, Green DG. Effects of inhibiting glutamine synthetase and blocking glutamate uptake on b-wave generation in the isolated rat retina. *Vis Neurosci.* 1995;16:345–353.

Winkler BS, Riley MV. Na$^+$,K$^+$ and HCO3 ATPase activity in retina: dependence on calcium and sodium. *Invest Ophthalmol Vis Sci.* 1977;16:1151–1154.

Winneke G. Modification of visual evoked potentials in rats after long-term blood lead elevation. *Act Nerv Sup (Praha).* 1979;4:282–284.

Winneke G, Altmann L, Krämer U, et al. Neurobehavioral and neurophysiological observations in six year old children with low lead levels in East and West Germany. *Neurotoxicology.* 1994;15:705–713.

Winneke G, Beginn U, Ewert T, et al. Study to determine the subclinical effects of lead on the nervous system in children with known prenatal exposure in Nordenham. *Schr-Reine Verein Wabolu.* 1994;59:215–230.

Winneke G, Kramer U, Brockhaus A, et al. Neuropsychological studies in children with elevated tooth-lead concentrations: II. Extended study. *Int Arch Occup Environ Health.* 1983;51:231–252.

Withering W. *An Account of the Foxglove and Some of Its Medicinal Uses: With Practical Remarks on Dropsy and Other Diseases.* London: Broomsleigh Press, 1785.

Wolfensberger TJ. Toxicology of the retinal pigment epithelium. In: Marmor MF, Wolfensberger TJ, eds. *The Retinal Pigment Epithelium Function and Disease.* New York, NY: Oxford University Press; 1998:621–647.

Woodhouse JM, Barlow HB. Spatial and temporal resolution and analysis. In: Barlow HB, Mollon JD, eds. *The Senses.* Cambridge: Cambridge University Press; 1982:133–164.

Wu SM. Synaptic organization of the vertebrate retina: general principles and species-specific variations: the Friedenwald lecture. *Invest Ophthalmol Vis Sci.* 2010;51:1263–1274.

Yau KW, Baylor DA. Cyclic GMP-activated conductance of retinal photoreceptor cells. *Annu Rev Neurosci.* 1989;12:289–327.

Yoshino Y, Mozai T, Nako K. Distribution of mercury in the brain and its subcellular units in experimental organic mercury poisonings. *J Neurochem.* 1966;13:397–406.

Zavalic M, Turk R, Bogadi-Sare A, Skender L. Colour vision impairment in workers exposed to low concentrations of toluene. *Arh Hig Rada Toksikol.* 1996;47:167–175.

Zhao C, Schwartzman ML, Shichi H. Immunocytochemical study of cytochrome P450 4A induction in mouse eye. *Exp Eye Res.* 1996;63:747–751.

Zhao C, Shichi H. Immunocytochemical study of cytochrome P450 (1A1/1A2) induction in murine ocular tissues. *Exp Eye Res.* 1995;60:143–152.

Zhang X, Feng Q, Cote RH. Efficacy and selectivity of phosphodiesterase-targeted drugs in inhibiting photoreceptor phosphodiesterase (PDE6) in retinal photoreceptors. *Invest Ophthalmol Vis Sci.* 2005;46:3060–3066.

Zrenner E, Gouras P. Blue-sensitive cones of the cat produce a rod like electroretinogram. *Invest Ophthalmol Vis Sci.* 1979;18:1076–1081.

Zrenner E, Kramer W, Bittner C, et al. Rapid effects on colour vision following intravenous injection of a new, non-glycoside positive ionotropic substance (AR-L 115BS). *Doc Ophthalmol Proc Ser.* 1982;33:493–507.

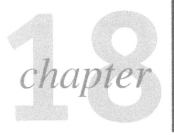

18 chapter

Toxic Responses of the Heart and Vascular System

Y. James Kang

INTRODUCTION

Cardiovascular toxicology is concerned with the adverse effects of extrinsic and intrinsic stresses on the heart and vascular system. Extrinsic stress involves exposure to therapeutic drugs, natural products, and environmental toxicants. Intrinsic stress refers to exposure to toxic metabolites derived from nontoxic compounds such as those found in food additives and supplements. The intrinsic exposures also include secondary neurohormonal disturbance such as overproduction of inflammatory cytokines derived from pressure overload of the heart and counter-regulatory responses to hypertension. These toxic exposures result in alterations in biochemical pathways, defects in cellular structure and function, and pathogenesis of the affected cardiovascular system. The manifestations of toxicological response of the heart include cardiac arrhythmia, hypertrophy, and overt heart failure. The responses of the vascular system include changes in blood pressure and lesions in blood vessels in the form of atherosclerosis, hemorrhage, and edema.

This chapter is divided into two parts: the heart and the vascular system. For a better understanding of the toxic manifestations of the cardiovascular system, an overview of the physiology and biochemistry of the heart and the vascular system is presented in relation to toxicological concerns. The toxicological responses of the heart and the vascular system and the mechanisms of these responses are the major focus of this chapter. This chapter also presents a brief discussion of chemicals that affect the heart and the vascular system.

OVERVIEW OF THE HEART

Overview of Cardiac Structural and Physiological Features

Cardiac muscle, along with nerve, skeletal muscle, and smooth muscle, is one of the excitable tissues of the body. It shares many bioelectrical properties with other excitable tissues, and also has unique features associated with cardiac structural and physiological specificities. Fig. 18-1 illustrates the basic anatomy of the heart. With regard to cardiac toxicology, this section will only review some features of cardiac physiology and structures. There are many textbooks of cardiac anatomy and physiology that provide extensive knowledge basis of cardiac physiology and structural properties, which will not be repeated in this section.

Review of Cardiac Structure The primary contractile unit within the heart is the cardiac muscle cell, or cardiac myocyte.

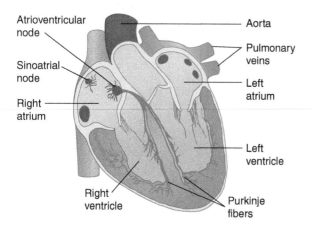

Figure 18-1. *Diagram illustrating the basic anatomy of the heart.*

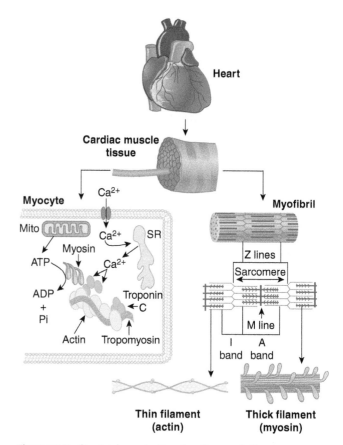

Figure 18-2. *Structural organization of cardiac muscle tissue.*

Cardiac myocytes are composed of several major structural features and organelles, as illustrated in Fig. 18-2. A primary component is the contractile elements known as the myofibril. Each myofibril consists of a number of smaller filaments (the thick and thin myofilaments). The thick filaments are special assemblies of the protein myosin, whereas the thin filaments are made up primarily of the protein actin. Cardiac myosin is a hexamer composed of one pair of myosin heavy chains (MHCs) and two pairs of myosin light chains (MLCs). Two isoforms of MHC, α and β, are expressed in cardiac muscle; the expression of these is under developmental control and may be altered by a variety of physiological, pathological, and pharmacological stimuli (Martin *et al.*, 1996; Metzger *et al.*, 1999). In addition, the predominant isoform expressed in normal adult cardiac tissue also depends on the species examined. Similarly, two isoforms of actin are expressed in the heart (cardiac and skeletal α-actin), and, as with MHC, actin isoform expression is influenced by developmental, physiological, pathological, and pharmacological stimuli, and the primary isoform of actin found in normal adult cardiac muscle also depends on the species examined.

Under electron microscopy, these essential structural components of myocardial contractile proteins display alternating dark bands (A bands, predominantly composed of myosin) and light bands (I bands, predominantly composed of actin). Visible in the middle of the I band is a dense vertical Z line. The area between two Z lines is called a sarcomere, the fundamental unit of muscle contraction. Although cardiac and skeletal muscle share many similarities, a major difference lies in the organization of cardiac myocytes into a functional syncytium where cardiac myocytes are joined end-to-end by dense structures known as intercalated disks. Within these, there are tight gap junctions that facilitate action potential propagation and intercellular communication. About 50% of each cardiac myocyte is composed of myofibrils. The rest of the

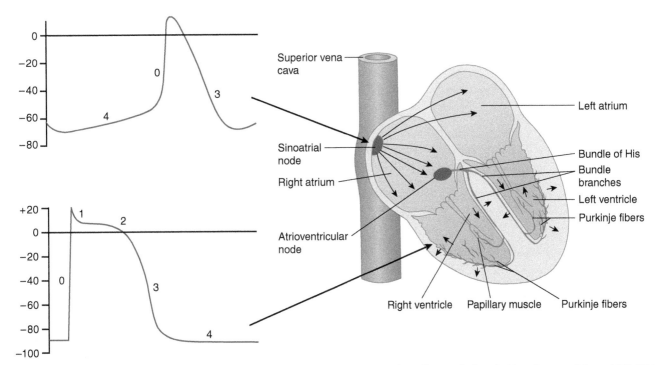

Figure 18-3. *Characteristic cardiac action potential recorded from sinoatrial node and Purkinje fibers as indicated.* (From Berne and Levy, 1983. With permission from Elsevier.)

intracellular space contains the remaining major components of the cell: mitochondria (33%), one or more nuclei (5%), the sarcoplasmic reticulum (SR) (2%), lysosomes (very low), glycogen granules, a Golgi network, and cytosol (12%) (Opie, 1996).

Cardiac myocytes are the largest cells in the heart and contributes to the majority of cardiac mass. However, cardiac myocytes make up only about one-quarter of all the cells in the heart. Cardiac fibroblasts, vascular cells, Purkinje cells, and other connective tissue cells make up the majority of cell number in the heart. Cardiac fibroblasts make up approximately 90% of these "nonmuscle" cells. Cardiac myocytes are generally considered to be terminally differentiated, although this view has been challenged recently (Anversa *et al.*, 2006). These cells may be multinucleated, but they may not divide after birth unless under certain circumstances in some species such as mice (Anversa et al., 2006). The heart undergoes a significant increase in size and mass throughout growth of the organism, but the increase in heart size and mass is produced by enlargement (or hypertrophy) of preexisting cardiac myocytes (Li *et al.*, 1996). With regard to this developmental period, cardiac hypertrophy is considered to be a normal physiological process. Under pathological conditions, hypertrophy of remaining cardiac myocytes is a hallmark of cardiac remodeling following myocardial injuries, such as myocardial infarction. Cardiac fibroblasts may continue to proliferate after birth, particularly in response to injury. Cardiac fibroblasts also contribute to cardiac remodeling following myocardial infarction and are believed to promote fibrosis and scarring of injured cardiac tissue. Thus, from a toxicological perspective, the heart is vulnerable to injury because of limited proliferative capacity of cardiac myocytes, and promotion of cardiac fibroblast proliferation and remodeling following injury.

Electrophysiology The electrophysiology of the heart is concerned with bioelectricity and its related cardiac physiological function. Bioelectricity is the result of charge generated from the movement of positively and negatively charged ions in tissues.

In cardiac myocytes, three major positively charged ions make a significant contribution to the bioelectricity of the heart; calcium (Ca^{2+}), sodium (Na^+), and potassium (K^+). Each of the ions has specific channels and transporters (pumps) on the membrane of cardiac myocytes. Through the movement of these ions across the cell membrane, an action potential is generated and propagated from one cell to another, so that electric conductance is produced in the heart.

Action Potential Cardiac myocytes produce an action potential when activated. In the resting state, the resting potential of a myocyte is about −60 to −90 mV relative to the extracellular fluid potential. A sudden depolarization changes the membrane potential from negative inside to positive inside, followed by a repolarization to reset the resting potential. The process of an action potential from depolarization to the completion of repolarization is divided into five phases in cardiac Purkinje fibers as shown in Fig. 18-3. Phase 0 represents a rapid depolarization due to the inward current of Na^+. Phase 1 is associated with an immediate rapid repolarization, during which the Na^+ inward current is inactivated and a transient K^+ outward current is activated, followed by an action potential plateau or phase 2, which is dominated by slowly decreasing inward Ca^{2+} current and a slow activation of an outward K^+ current. Phase 3 reflects a fast K^+ outward current and inactivation of the plateau Ca^{2+} inward current, and phase 4 is the diastolic interval for the resetting of the resting potential.

Automaticity A group of specialized cells in the heart are capable of repetitively spontaneous self-excitation, which generate and distribute each impulse through the heart in a highly coordinated manner to control the normal heartbeat. These cells include the sinus node P cells and Purkinje fibers in the ventricles. Other cells such as the atrial-specialized fibers under normal conditions do not have automaticity, but can become automatic under abnormal conditions. The sinus node P cells or pacemaker cells have only three distinct phases of action potential (Fig. 18-3): phase 0, rapid depolarization; phase 3, plateau and repolarization; and phase 4, slow depolarization or often referred to as *pacemaker potential*.

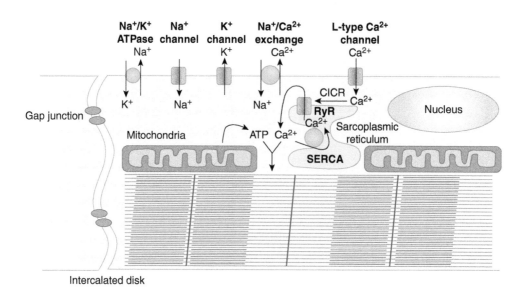

Figure 18-4. *Overview of excitation–contraction coupling in cardiac myocytes.* Upon rapid depolarization (rapid influx of Na^+ through fast channels; phase 0 of the action potential), L-type Ca^{2+} channels are opened allowing a slower but sustained influx of Ca^{2+} down the electrochemical gradient (phase 2 of the action potential). During the process of Ca^{2+}-induced Ca^{2+} release (CICR), slight elevation in intracellular-free Ca^{2+} stimulates Ca^{2+} release from the sarcoplasmic reticulum (SR) through ryanodine receptors (RyR). The SR provides the majority of Ca^{2+} required for contraction. The mitochondria provide energy for contraction in the form of ATP. Repolarization of the cell occurs largely by activation of K^+ channels and efflux of K^+ (phase 3 of the action potential). For relaxation, the SR Ca^{2+} ATPase (SERCA) actively pumps Ca^{2+} back into the SR, although some Ca^{2+} may be removed by the Na^+/Ca^{2+} exchanger or by sarcolemmal Ca^{2+} pumps.

It is the pacemaker potential that brings the membrane potential to a level near the threshold for activation of the inward Ca^{2+} current, which triggers the phase 0 rapid depolarization and makes the pacemaker cells of automaticity. In pacemaker cells, phase 0 is mediated almost entirely by increased conductance of Ca^{2+} ions.

Contractility Cardiac myocytes like other muscle cells have a unique functional feature, contractility. Myocyte contraction occurs when an action potential causes the release of Ca^{2+} from the SR as well as the entry of extracellular Ca^{2+}into the cell. This action potential-triggered Ca^{2+} increase in the plasma and myocyte contraction is called *excitation–contraction coupling* (Fig. 18-4). The increase in Ca^{2+} concentrations in the cell allows Ca^{2+} to bind to troponin and tropomysin leading to some conformational change in the contractile unit of the cardiac myocyte, thin filament. This conformational change permits interaction between the actin and myosin filaments through the crossbridges (myosin heads). ATP is hydrolyzed by ATPase present in the crossbridges to release energy for the movement of the crossbridges in a ratchet-like fashion. This action increases the overlap of the actin and myosin filaments, resulting in shortening of the sarcomeres and contraction of the myocardium.

Electrotonic Cell-to-Cell Coupling Myocardium as a whole has to synchronize the contraction and relaxation of individual myocytes in order to perform its pump function. This is achieved by a special structural feature of cell-to-cell interaction, electrotonic cell-to-cell coupling via the gap junction. Through the gap junction, major ionic fluxes between adjacent cardiomyocytes are spread, thus allowing electrical synchronization of contraction. Each single gap junction is composed of 12 connexin 43 (Cx43) units, assembled in two hexametric connexons (hemichannels) that are contributed, one each, by the two participating cells. The connexins interact with other proteins within the cell so that connexons are not only important for cell-to-cell coupling, but also involved in cell signaling and volume regulation. An important feature of the connexon-controlled electrotonic

cell-to-cell coupling is the electrotonic current flow that attenuates the differences in action potential duration of individual cardiac myocytes.

Electrocardiograph The electrophysiological features of cardiac myocytes and the electrotonic cell-to-cell coupling give rise to charge at any given locus in the heart with a magnitude and a direction. Therefore, at any given moment in the cardiac cycle, there is a complex pattern of electrical charges across the membranes of myriad cells in the heart. The sum of all the individual cells that exist at any given time within the heart is the *resultant cardiac vector*. The changes in the resultant cardiac vector throughout the cardiac cycle can be recorded as a *vector cardiograph*. Lead systems are used to record certain projections of the resultant cardiac vector. The potential difference between two recoding electrodes represents the projection of the vector on the line between the two leads. Components of vectors projected on such lines eliminate their directions and have a sum of magnitude, being scalar quantities. Thus, a recording of the changes with time in the potential differences between two points on the surface of the skin is the so-called *scalar electrocardiograph*.

In general, the pattern of the scalar electrocardiograph consists of P, QRS, and T waves, as shown in Fig. 18-5. The PR interval is a measure of the time from the onset of atrial activation to the onset of ventricular activation. The QRS complex represents the conduction pathways through the ventricles. The ST segment is the interval during which the entire ventricular myocardium is depolarized, and lies on the isoelectric line under normal conditions. The QT interval is sometimes referred to as the period of "electrical systole" of the ventricles, and reflects the action potential duration. The QT interval prolongation is recognized as a major life-threatening factor of drug cardiac toxicity, which is brought about by a reduction of outward currents and/or enhanced inward currents during phase 2 and 3 of the action potential.

Neurohormonal Regulation Although the heartbeat is governed by the automaticity of the sinus node P cells, neurohormonal

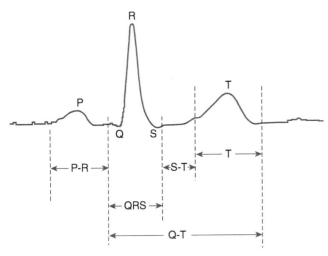

Figure 18-5. *A typical electrocardiogram (ECG) with the illustration of important deflections and intervals.*

regulation of cardiac electrophysiology and contraction controls cardiac function under normal and abnormal conditions. Toxicants often exert their effects on the cardiac system through interference with the neurohormonal regulation, thus this regulatory system is of significant relevance to cardiac toxicology. There are many neurohormonal systems that have significant impact on the heart. A detailed description of the regulatory system will be provided in the following sections in association with specific discussion of cardiac functional regulation, compensatory, and maladaptive responses to toxic exposures.

Overview of Cardiac Energy Metabolism and Biochemistry

ATP and the Heart It is easy to understand that the need of energy for the heart is high. The chemical energy in the form of ATP is absolutely needed to support the systolic and diastolic work of the heart (Ventura-Clapier *et al.*, 2004). In the heart, the primary ATP-utilizing reactions are catalyzed by actomyosin ATPase in the myofibril, the Ca^{2+}-ATPase in the SR, and the Na^+,K^+-ATPase in the sarcolemma (Ingwall and Weiss, 2004). ATP is also needed for molecular synthesis and degradation in the heart as in other organ systems. ATP synthesis by oxidative phosphorylation in the mitochondria is usually sufficient to support the normal needs of the heart, even when the work output of the heart increases three- to fivefold (Ingwall and Weiss, 2004). In addition, the glycolytic pathway and the tricarboxylic acid cycle also make small contributions to ATP synthesis. The concentration of ATP does not define the energetic state of the heart. The amount of ATP made and used at any given time is many times greater than the size of the measurable ATP pool (Ingwall and Weiss, 2004). Thus, cardiac myocytes contain high concentrations of mitochondria, which ensure that ATP remains constant through oxidation of a variety of carbon-based fuels for ATP synthesis under different conditions.

Phosphocreatine and the Heart A unique feature in energy metabolism of the heart is the use of energy reserve systems, such as phosphocreatine (PCr), to maintain a high phosphorylation potential to drive ATPase reactions under highly demanding conditions (Ingwall *et al.*, 1985). PCr exists in the heart at twice the ATP concentration (Bittl and Ingwall, 1985). The enzyme creatine kinase (CK) transfers the phosphoryl group between ATP and PCr at a rate about 10 times faster than the rate of ATP synthesis by oxidative phosphorylation. The reaction catalyzed by CK is:

$PCr + ADP + H^+ \leftrightarrow$ creatine $+ ATP$. Under the conditions when ATP demand exceeds ATP supply, the use of PCr is a major pathway to maintain a constant supply of ATP. The CK reaction is also important to maintain low ADP and Pi concentrations, thereby retaining high phosphorylation potential (Saupe *et al.*, 2000). Creatine is not made in the heart but accumulates against a large concentration gradient facilitated by a creatine transporter. In the normal heart, about two-thirds of the total creatine pool is phosphorylated through the CK reaction to form PCr (Wallimann *et al.*, 1998; Neubauer *et al.*, 1999).

Metabolic Pathways The continuous synthesis of ATP via mitochondrial oxidative phosphorylation is mandatory for the work of the heart (Huss and Kelly, 2005). Under normal conditions, the oxidation of fatty acids (FA) is the major pathway, providing about 65% of the total energy demand. In contrast, the oxidation of glucose provides about 30% of the total energy demand (Shipp *et al.*, 1961; Wisneski *et al.*, 1987). In hypertrophic and failing hearts, there is a metabolic shift from FA- to glucose-dependent energy supply. Thus, decreased FA oxidation and increased glucose utilization in association with depressed FA deposition and increased glucose uptake are observed in hypertrophic and failing hearts (van Bilsen *et al.*, 2004). This shift enhances the glycolytic pathway, and thus increases the anaerobic metabolism. However, it remains debated whether this metabolic shift to the so-called "fetal phenotype" is adaptive or maladaptive. It is important to note that the "shift" is only partial, and even when the proportion of ATP synthesized from glucose increases many fold, aerobic metabolism still remains dominant (van Bilsen *et al.*, 2004). With regard to the concern of cardiac toxicology, the metabolic shift is often observed with mitochondrial dysfunction. In response to toxic exposure, mitochondrial damage leads to impaired oxidative phosphorylation and a metabolic shift from aerobic to anaerobic and a reliance on glucose utilization.

Calcium and Calcineurin The role of calcium in cardiac toxic responses has been extensively investigated. However, our understanding of the role of calcium in cardiac toxicity remains superficial. When carefully examining the current literature, one can find that there are very few mechanistic studies that specifically probe the role of calcium in cardiac toxicity, although numerous studies have implicated intracellular Ca^{2+} as a signal for cardiac responses to environmental toxic insults (Shier and Dubourdieu, 1992; Toraason *et al.*, 1997; Buck *et al.*, 1999). In response to myocardial stress by environmental toxic exposures, calcium concentrations are increased in the myocardial cells (Sleight, 1996). This is consistent with the speculation that Ca^{2+} coordinates physiological responses to stresses. There are many other speculations that are derived from the studies examining the role of calcium in toxicological responses in other systems. The unique action of calcium in cardiac toxicity, however, has to be studied specifically.

The role of calcium in mediating myocardial hypertrophic signals has been extensively studied (Stemmer and Klee, 1994). A sustained increase in intracellular Ca^{2+} concentrations activates calcineurin. Calcineurin is a ubiquitously expressed serine/threonine phosphatase that exists as a heterodimer, comprises a 59 kDa calmodulin (CaM)-binding catalytic A subunit and a 19 kDa Ca^{2+}-binding regulatory B subunit (Molkentin *et al.*, 1998). Activation of calcineurin is mediated by binding of Ca^{2+} to the regulatory subunit and CaM to the catalytic subunit (Fig. 18-6). Of toxicological relevance is that calcineurin is activated by a sustained increase in Ca^{2+} concentration and is insensitive to transient Ca^{2+} fluxes, such as in response to cardiomyocyte contraction (Stemmer and Klee, 1994).

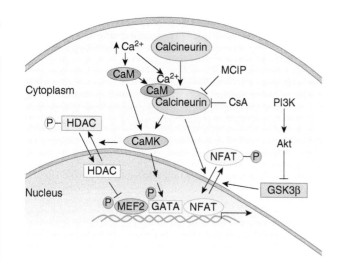

Figure 18-6. *Calcineurin signal transduction pathways in regulation of transcription factors involved in hypertrophic growth of cardiac myocytes.* Sustained increases in intracellular Ca^{2+} concentrations, along with calmodulin (CaM), activate calcineurin, which in turn causes dephosphorylation of nuclear factor of activated T cells (NFAT), enabling NFAT to translocate to the nucleus where it interacts with GATA4 to regulate gene expression. Phosphorylation of NFAT is stimulated by glycogen synthase kinase 3β (GSK3β), whose activity is inhibited by activation of the phosphoinositide 3-kinase (PI3K)/Akt pathway. Calcineurin also regulates CaM activation of CaM-dependent kinase (CaMK), which activates GATA transcription factor. CaMK also phosphorylates histone deacetylases (HDAC), leading to HDAC translocation from nucleus to cytoplasm. Otherwise, HDAC in the nucleus inhibits myocyte-enhancer factor 2 (MEF2) transcription activity. Cyclosporine A (CsA) and modulatory calcineurin-interacting protein (MCIP) inhibit calcineurin activation.

Numerous studies have demonstrated important roles for Ras, mitogen-activated protein kinase (MAPK), and protein kinase C (PKC) signaling pathways in myocardial responses to hypertrophic stimuli (Jalili *et al.*, 1999). All of these signal transduction pathways are associated with increase in intracellular Ca^{2+} concentrations (Ho *et al.*, 1998). The coordinating role of calcium in cardiac hypertrophic response has been demonstrated (Stemmer and Klee, 1994) as follows. Hypertrophic stimuli, such as angiotensin II and phenylephrine, cause an elevation of intracellular Ca^{2+} that results in activation of calcineurin. A series of reactions occur through activated calcineurin, including dephosphorylation of nuclear factor of activated T cell (NFAT) and its translocation to nucleus, where it interacts with GATA4 (Fig. 18-6). Calcineurin also acts through an NFAT-independent mechanism to regulate hypertrophic gene expression.

AMP-Activated Protein Kinase Activation of AMP-activated protein kinase (AMPK) often occurs when the myocardial metabolic phenotype shifts to the fetal form. Activation of AMPK occurs with changes in high-energy phosphate metabolism in hypertrophic and failing hearts. The increase in AMP/ATP ratio occurs when the PCr/ATP ratio decreases due to a decrease in PCr, with or without a concomitant decrease in ATP. The decrease in PCr/ATP ratio is an index of decreased energy reserve and correlates with the severity of heart failure and is of prognostic value (Neubauer *et al.*, 1997). Activation of AMPK leads to translocation of the insulin-dependent glucose transporter (GLUT4) from intracellular stores to the sarcolemma (Russell *et al.*, 1999). Mice overexpressing an active form of AMPK suffer from pathological cardiac glucogen accumulation (Arad *et al.*, 2003). Furthermore, the AMPK-dependent phosphorylation of the enzyme 6-phosphofructo-2-kinase stimulates

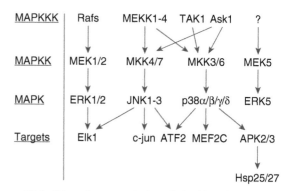

Figure 18-7. *Schematic representation of the hierarchy constituents of the MAPK signaling pathways.* MAPK, mitogen-activated protein kinase; MAPKK, MAPK kinase; MAPKKK, MAPK kinase kinase.

glycolysis (Marsin *et al.*, 2000). These pathways indicate the importance of AMPK activation for the cardiac metabolic shift to the energy supply reliance on glucose metabolism.

Mitogen-Activated Protein Kinases MAPKs play a major role in cardiac response to toxic insults. A generalized diagram for MAPK signaling is presented in Fig. 18-7. The MAPKs consist of a series of successively acting kinases and three major branches are involved in the classic MAKP signaling pathway. These branches are divided based on their terminal effector kinases: the extracellular signal-regulated protein kinases (ERK), the c-jun NH$_2$-terminal kinases (JNK), and p38 MAPKs (Sugden and Clerk, 1998). Each branch of the MAPKs has a hierarchy control system beginning at the MAPK kinase kinase (MAPKKK), as shown in Fig. 18-7. Among the MAPKs, p38 MAPKs have been extensively studied in myocardial apoptosis. This subfamily consists of p38α, p38β, p38γ, and p38δ (Sugden and Clerk, 1998). Several studies have identified p38 MAPKs as an important group of signaling molecules that mediate environmental stress responses in various cell types (Tibbles and Woodgett, 1999). In noncardiac cells, p38 MAPKs have been implicated in gene expression, morphological changes, and cell death in response to endotoxin, cytokines, physical stress, and chemical insults (Tan *et al.*, 1996; Wang and Ron, 1996). In cardiac cells, p38 MAPKs are associated with the onset of apoptosis in ischemia–reperfusion (Yin *et al.*, 1997). In particular, transfection experiments using primary cultures of neonatal rat cardiomyocytes have shown that p38α is critically involved in myocyte apoptosis (Wang *et al.*, 1998).

Adriamycin is a cardiac toxicant and two observations indicate that the p38 MAPK is involved in Adriamycin-induced myocyte apoptosis (Kang *et al.*, 2000a). First, a time-course analysis revealed that p38 MAPK activation preceded the onset of apoptosis. As early as 30 minutes after Adriamycin administration, myocyte apoptosis occurs, detected by a sensitive method of fluorescein isothiocyanate (FITC) conjugation of Annexin V (Annexin V-FITC). However, p38 MAPK activation detected by the FITC-conjugated anti-phosphop38 antibody and confocal microscopy is observed 20 minutes after Adriamycin treatment (Kang *et al.*, 2000a). Second, SB203580, a specific inhibitor of p38 MAPKs, inhibits Adriamycin-induced myocyte apoptosis (Kang *et al.*, 2000a). Because SB203580 acts as a specific inhibitor of p38α and p38β, but not p38γ and p38δ, the involvement of the former specific isoforms of the p38 MAPK in the Adriamycin-induced myocyte apoptosis is implicated. p38α is involved in apoptosis of neonatal rat cardiomyocytes in primary cultures and p38β mediates hypertrophy of these cells (Wang *et al.*, 1998).

Protein Kinase C PKC is among the most extensively studied signaling molecules in the heart. Many cardiac toxicological studies have examined the role of PKC in mediating toxic signals. Several excellent reviews on PKC in myocardial signaling pathways leading to cardiac hypertrophy and heart failure are available (Puceat and Vassort, 1996). PKC is a ubiquitously expressed serine/threonine kinase, which is activated predominantly by G_q/G_{11}-coupled receptors. The PKC family consists of 11 isoforms, which are divided into three subgroups: conventional PKCs (cPKCs) including α, β (I and II), and γ; novel PKCs (nPKCs) including ε, δ, η, ζ, and θ; and atypical PKCs (aPKCs) including ι, λ, and μ (Newton, 1995). The cPKCs are activated by Ca^{2+} and diacylglycerol (DAG), as well as phorbol esters. The nPKCs do not bind Ca^{2+}, but respond to DAG and phorbol ester stimulation. The aPKCs do not respond to either Ca^{2+}, DAG, or phorbol esters. PKC has been demonstrated to participate in the regulation of transcription, the maintenance of cell growth and membrane structure, and modulation of immune responses. Disturbances in PKC signaling pathways lead to cardiac hypertrophy and heart failure, which is of toxicological significance.

Transcription Factors Transcription factors activate or deactivate myocardial gene expression, which affects the function and phenotype of the heart. Many transcription factors have been studied in myocardial tissue. Several of them are of toxicological significance as described below.

Activator Protein-1 Activator Protein-1 (AP-1) is a transcription factor composed of *Jun* and *Fos* gene family members (McMahon and Monroe, 1992). The AP-1-binding site is the TRE (12-*O*-tetradecanoyl phorbol 13-acetate response element), and the binding of AP-1 to the TRE initiates transcription of the target genes (Diamond *et al.*, 1990). Elevated levels of c-Jun are seen in cardiomyocytes with ischemia–reperfusion (Brand *et al.*, 1992). In volume-overload hypertrophy, AP-1 plays an important role in the regulation of Fas and FasL activities (Wollert *et al.*, 2000). Overstretching of myocardium induces Fas expression (Cheng *et al.*, 1995). Subsequently, Fas-dependent signaling pathways can lead to myocardial cell apoptosis. However, there are other studies that indicate activation of AP-1 is not associated with the induction of apoptosis (Lenczowski *et al.*, 1997). AP-1 has been implicated in transcriptional regulation of several genes associated with a hypertrophic response (Paradis *et al.*, 1996).

Myocyte-Enhancer Factor-2 Myocyte-Enhancer Factor-2 (MEF-2) is a transcription factor that binds to A-/T-rich DNA sequences within the promoter regions of a number of cardiac genes, including muscle CK gene, β-MHC, MLC1/3, MLC2v, skeletal α-actin, SR Ca^{2+}-ATPase, cardiac troponin T, C, and I, desmin, and dystrophin (Black and Olson, 1998). MEF2 is critically involved in the regulation of inducible gene expression during myocardial hypertrophy. The activation of MEF2 involves phosphorylation of the transcription factor by p38 MAPK or ERK5-MAPK. The ERK5-MEF2 pathway has been observed in the generation of cardiac hypertrophy. An important function of MEF2 is the convergence in the binary downstream pathway of Ca^{2+} signaling. Increased intracellular Ca^{2+} binds to and activates Ca^{2+}-binding proteins including CaM, which regulates calcineurin and Ca^{2+}/CaM-dependent protein kinase (CaMKs). Activation of either calcineurin or CaMKs induces cardiac hypertrophy. CaMKs stimulate MEF2 through phosphorylation of the transcriptional suppressor, histone deacetylases (HDACs). CaMK is considered as HDAC kinase whose activity is enhanced by calcineurin. Thus, MEF2 converges the stimulating signaling of both CaMKs and calcineurin leading to activation of hypertrophic gene expression (Fig. 18-6).

Nuclear Factor of Activated T Cells 3 Nuclear Factor of Activated T Cells 3 (NFAT3) is a member of a multigene family that contains four members, NFATc, NFATp, NFAT3, and NFAT4 (Rao *et al.*, 1997). These transcription factors bind to the consensus DNA sequence GGAAAAT as monomers or dimers through a Rel homology domain (Rooney *et al.*, 1994). Unlike the other three members that are restricted in their expression to T cells and skeletal muscle, NFAT3 is expressed in a variety of tissues including the heart. NFAT3 plays a major role in cardiac hypertrophy (Pu *et al.*, 2003). Hypertrophic stimuli, such as angiotensin II and phenylephrine, cause an increase in intracellular Ca^{2+} levels in myocardial cells. This elevation in turn results in activation of calcineurin. NFAT3 is localized within the cytoplasm and is dephosphorylated by the activated calcineurin. This dephosphorylation enables NFAT3 to translocate to the nucleus where it interacts with GATA4 (Fig. 18-6). NFAT3 can also activate some hypertrophic responsive genes through mechanisms independent of GATA4.

GATA GATA factors are a family of nuclear transcriptional regulatory proteins that are related structurally within a central DNA-binding domain, but are restricted in expression to distinct sets of cell types (Yamamoto *et al.*, 1990). Currently, six different family members have been characterized in vertebrate species. They are GATA1, 2, 3, 4, 5, and 6. Each protein contains two similar repeats of a highly conserved zinc finger of the form $CXNCX_6LWRRX_7CNAC$. The C-terminal repeat constitutes a minimal DNA-binding domain sufficient for sequence-specific recognition of a "GATA" *cis*-element, usually (A/T)GATA(A/G) or a related DNA sequence, present in promoters and/or enhancers of target genes (Evans *et al.*, 1988). It has been shown that GATA-1/2/3 regulate various aspects of hematopoiesis (Orkin, 1992), whereas GATA-4/5/6 regulates cardiogenesis (Yamamoto *et al.*, 1990). The significance of GATA-4 in regulation of hypertrophic response in myocardial cells has been demonstrated (Evens, 1997). Cardiac hypertrophy induced by angiotensin II is mediated by an angiotensin II type$_{1\alpha}$ receptor ($AT_{1\alpha}R$). A GATA motif exists in the $AT_{1\alpha}R$ promoter. Mutations introduced to the consensus-binding site for GATA factor abolished the pressure overload response (Evens, 1997). Moreover, interactions between AP-1 and GATA-4, and between NFAT3 and GATA-4 are essential in myocardial hypertrophic responses.

CARDIAC TOXIC RESPONSES

Basic Concepts and Definitions

The ultimate functional effect of cardiac toxic manifestations is decreased cardiac output and peripheral tissue hypoperfusion, resulting from alterations in biochemical pathways, energy metabolism, cellular structural and function, electrophysiology, and contractility of the heart. These morphological and functional alterations induced by toxic exposure are referred to as toxicological cardiomyopathy. The critical cellular event leading to toxicological cardiomyopathy is myocardial cell death and extracellular matrix (ECM) remodeling. The recognition of the role of apoptosis in the development of heart failure during the last decade has significantly enhanced our knowledge of myocardial cell death (James, 1994; Haunstetter and Izumo, 1998; Sabbah and Sharov, 1998).

Manipulation of genes responsible for cardiac function began in the mid-1990s (Robbins, 2004). The most important conclusion of these studies is that a sustained expression of any single mutated functional gene, either in the form of gain-of-function or loss-of-function, can lead to a significant phenotype, often in the form of cardiac hypertrophy and heart failure (Robbins, 2004; Olson, 2004).

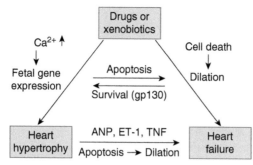

Figure 18-8. *Triangle analytical model of cardiac responses to drugs and xenobiotics.* Drugs or xenobiotics can directly cause both heart failure and heart hypertrophy. Under severe acute toxic insults, myocardial cell death becomes the predominant response leading to cardiac dilation and heart failure. In most cases, myocardial survival mechanisms can be activated so that myocardial apoptosis is inhibited. The survived cardiomyocytes often become hypertrophy through activation of calcium-mediated fetal gene expression and other hypertrophic program. If toxic insult continues, the counter-regulatory mechanisms against heart hypertrophy such as activation of cytokine-mediated pathways eventually lead to myocardial cell death through apoptosis or necrosis, dilated cardiomyopathy, and heart failure.

However, it is difficult to apply this knowledge to patients: first, acquired cardiac disease such as heart failure is the result of interaction between environmental factors and genetic susceptibility, indicating the role of polymorphisms. Second, extrinsic and intrinsic stresses produce lesions that cannot be explained by a single gene or a single pathway, suggesting complexity between deleterious factors and the heart. Cardiac toxicity is the critical link between environmental factors and myocardial pathogenesis.

For a better understanding of cardiac toxicology, a triangle model of cardiac toxicity is presented in Fig. 18-8. In this model, complexity of the interaction between environmental stresses and the heart, and the balance between myocardial protection and deleterious dose and time effects are considered. First, it is important to recognize that chemicals can lead to heart failure without heart hypertrophy. Second, a chemical can lead to activation of both protective and destructive responses in the myocardium. Third, long-term toxicological responses often result in maladaptive hypertrophy, which primes the heart for malignant arrhythmia, leading to sudden cardiac death or transition to heart failure.

In the study of cardiac toxicology, the manifestations of cardiac toxicity in human patients and animal models are critical parameters serving as indices of cardiac toxicity. These manifestations are expressed in the forms of cardiac arrhythmia, hypertrophy, and heart failure. These abnormal changes reflect myocardial functional alterations resulting from both acute and chronic cardiac toxicity. Although some changes including cardiac hypertrophy were viewed as a compensatory response to hemodynamic changes in the past, more recent studies suggest that cardiac hypertrophy is a maladaptive process of the heart in response to intrinsic and extrinsic stresses (van Empel and De Windt, 2004; Berenji *et al.*, 2005; Dorn and Force, 2005). Cardiac hypertrophy is a risk factor for sudden cardiac death and has a high potential to progress to overt heart failure. Therefore, a distinction between compensatory and maladaptive responses is critical for treatment of patients with toxicological cardiomyopathy.

Cardiac Arrhythmia Cardiac rhythms under physiological conditions are set by pacemaker cells that are normally capable of developing spontaneous depolarization and responsible for generating the cardiac rhythm, the so-called automatic rhythm. A cardiac rhythm that deviates from the normal automatic rhythm is called

cardiac arrhythmia, often manifested in the form of tachycardia (fast heart rate). There are several classes of tachycardia, including sinus tachycardia, atrial tachycardia, ventricular tachycardia, and torsades de pointes (TdP) (a life-threatening ventricular tachycardia). In addition, subclasses such as atrial fibrillation, atrial flutter, and accelerated idioventricular rhythm provide further description of the manifestations of arrhythmia. Mechanisms for different classes of arrhythmia will be discussed in the section "QT prolongation and sudden cardiac death." According to the cause of the tachycardia, it is divided into abnormal automatic arrhythmia and triggered arrhythmia, which will be discussed in other sections.

Cardiac Hypertrophy There are two basic forms of cardiac hypertrophy: concentric hypertrophy, which is often observed during pressure overload and is characterized by new contractile-protein units assembled in parallel resulting in a relative increase in the width of individual cardiac myocytes (De Simone, 2003). By contrast, eccentric hypertrophy is characterized by the assembly of new contractile-protein units in series resulting in a relatively greater increase in the length than in the width of individual myocytes, occurring in human patients and animal models with dilated cardiomyopathy (Kass *et al.*, 2004). Toxicological cardiomyopathy is often manifested in the form of eccentric hypertrophy. The development of cardiac hypertrophy can be divided into three stages: developing hypertrophy, during which period the cardiac workload exceeds cardiac output; compensatory hypertrophy, in which the workload/mass ratio is normalized and normal cardiac output is maintained; decompensatory hypertrophy, in which ventricular dilation develops and cardiac output progressively declines, and overt heart failure occurs (Richey and Brown, 1998).

Heart Failure A traditional definition of heart failure is the inability of the heart to maintain cardiac output sufficient to meet the metabolic and oxygen demands of peripheral tissues. This definition has been modified to include changes in systolic and diastolic function that reflect specific alterations in ventricular function and abnormalities in a variety of subcellular processes (Piano *et al.*, 1998). Therefore, a detailed analysis to distinguish right ventricular from left ventricular failure can provide a better understanding of the nature of the heart failure and predicting the prognosis.

Acute Cardiac Toxicity Acute cardiac toxicity is referred to as cardiac response to a single exposure to a high dose of cardiac toxic chemicals. It is often manifested by cardiac arrhythmia. However, myocardial apoptosis is also involved in acute cardiac toxicity. It is not difficult to define acute cardiac toxicity; however, it sometimes is technically difficult to measure acute cardiac toxicity. In particular, the impact of acute cardiac toxicity on the ultimate outcome of cardiac function is not often easily recognized. For instance, a single high dose of arsenic can lead to cardiac arrhythmia and sudden cardiac death, which is easy to measure (Goldsmith and From, 1980). However, that a single oral dose of monensin (20 mg/kg) leads to a diminished cardiac function progressing to heart failure in calves requires a long-term observation; often a few months for clinical signs of heart failure (van Vleet, *et al.*, 1983; Litwak *et al.*, 2005), which is difficult to measure. As shown in Fig. 18-8, toxic exposure can directly lead to heart failure, which is different from an often-observed hypertrophic response, which may or may not progress to heart failure.

Chronic Cardiac Toxicity Chronic cardiac toxicity is the cardiac response to long-term exposure to chemicals, which is often manifested by cardiac hypertrophy and the transition to heart failure. About 25% of human patients with cardiomyopathy are categorized as having idiopathic cardiomyopathy. At least a portion of these patients with idiopathic cardiomyopathy are due to chemical exposure. Environmental exposure to particulate matters (PMs) in the air can lead to cardiomyopathy, which has only been recognized a decade ago (Dockery, 2001; Gordon and Reibman, 2000). Recognition of chronic cardiac toxicity in the pathogenesis of cardiomyopathy is of clinical relevance, and this knowledge can be used to prevent and treat patients with toxicological cardiomyopathy.

Myocardial Degeneration and Regeneration

Myocardial degeneration is the ultimate response of the heart to toxic exposure, which can be measured by both morphological and functional degenerative phenotypes. However, myocardial degeneration should not be considered an irreversible toxic response. In the past, the heart has been considered incapable of regenerating, so that cardiac injury in the form of cell loss or scar tissue formation was considered permanent damage to the heart. However, evidence now indicates myocardial regeneration and recovery from cardiomyopathy. Cardiac toxic responses or damage are now divided into reversible and irreversible.

Myocardial Degenerative Responses Myocardial cell death, fibrosis (scar tissue formation), and contractile dysfunction are considered as degenerative responses, which can result in cardiac arrhythmia, hypertrophy, and heart failure. If acute cardiac toxicity does not affect the capacity of myocardial regeneration, the degenerative phenotype is reversible. Both acute and chronic toxic stresses can lead to irreversible degeneration, depending on whether or not the cardiac repair mechanisms are overwhelmed. Cell death is the most common phenotype of myocardial degeneration. Both apoptosis and necrosis occur in the process of myocardial cell death, which will be discussed in the next section. Myocardial cell death is accompanied by hypertrophy of the remaining cardiac myocytes so that in the hypertrophic heart, the total number of cardiac myocytes is reduced but the size or volume of individual cells is increased.

During myocardial remodeling after cell death, not only is there an increase in the size of cardiac myocytes, but also cardiac fibrosis occurs. Myocardial fibrosis results from excess accumulation of ECM, which is mainly composed of collagens. The net accumulation of ECM connective tissue results from enhanced synthesis or diminished break down of the matrix, or both. Collagens, predominately types I and III, are the major fibrous proteins in ECM and their synthesis may increase in response to toxic insults. The degradation of ECM is dependent on the activity of matrix metalloproteinases (MMPs). According to their substrate specificity, MMPs fall into five categories: collagenases (MMP-1, MMP-8, and MMP-13), gelatinases (MMP-2 and MMP-9), stromelysins (MMP-3, MMP-7, MMP-10, and MMP-11), membrane-type MMPs (MMP-14, MMP-15, MMP-16, MMP-17, MMP-24, and MMP-25), and metalloelastase (MMP-12). These MMPs are organ specific so that not all are present in the heart. The activities of these enzymes are altered during the processes of fibrogenesis and fibrinolysis. Under toxic stress conditions, the imbalance between fibrogenesis and fibrinolysis leads to enhanced fibrogenesis and excess collagen accumulation—fibrosis.

The MMPs are inhibited by specific endogenous tissue inhibitor of metalloproteinases (TIMPs), which comprise a family of four protease inhibitors: TIMP-1, TIMP-2, TIMP-3, and TIMP-4. In general, during heart remodeling the concentration of TIMPs increases. Synthetic inhibitors generally contain a chelating group that binds the catalytic zinc atom at the MMP active site tightly. Common chelating groups include hydroxamates, carboxylates, thiols, and phosphinyls. Hydroxymates are particularly potent inhibitors of MMPs and other zinc-dependent enzymes, due to their bidentate

chelation of the zinc atom. Other substituents of TIMPs are usually designed to interact with various binding pockets on the MMP of interest, making the inhibitor more or less specific for a given MMP.

Toxic Effect on Myocardial Regeneration The mainstay of cardiac medicine and therapy has centered on the concept that the heart is a terminally differentiated organ and that cardiac myocytes are incapable of proliferating. Thus, cell death would lead to a permanent loss of the total number of cardiac myocytes. However, this view has been challenged recently due to the identification of cardiac progenitor cells (Anversa et al., 2006). These cells are characterized and proposed to be responsible for cardiac repair because these cells can make myocytes and vascular structures. These cells possess the fundamental properties of stem cells; therefore, they are also called cardiac stem cells. They are self-renewing, clonogenic, and multipotent, as demonstrated by reconstitution of infarcted heart by intramyocardial injection of cardiac progenitor cells or the local activation of these cells by growth factors. It is important to note that toxicological studies of the cardiac progenitor cells have not been done, and it is important to determine the potential of cardiac stem cells to help recover from toxic insults. The effect of chemicals on the cardiac progenitor cells is unknown. One speculation is that when severe damage to cardiac progenitor cells occurs, the potential for recovery from severe cardiac injury would be limited.

The removal of scar tissue or fibrosis in the myocardium in the past has been considered impossible. Although there are no studies that have shown scar tissue is removable in humans, there are observations in animal models of hypertensive heart disease that myocardial fibrosis is recoverable (Weber, 2005).

Myocardial vascularization is required for myocardial regeneration. Many toxic insults affect the capacity of angiogenesis in the myocardium, so that cardiac ischemia occurs. The combination of cardiac ischemia and the direct toxic insults to cardiomyocytes constitute synergistic damage to the heart. During regeneration, coronary arterioles and capillary structures are formed to bridge the dead tissue (scar tissue) and supply nutrients for the survival of the regenerated cardiomyocytes. There is an orderly organization of myocytes within the myocardium and a well-defined relationship between the myocytes and the capillary network. This proportion is altered under cardiac toxic conditions; either toxicological hypertrophy or diminished capillary formation can lead to hypoperfusion of myocytes in the myocardium. Unfortunately, our understanding of the toxic effects on myocardial angiogenesis is limited.

Reversible and Irreversible Toxic Responses Cardiomyopathy was viewed not to be recoverable in the past, but there is cumulative evidence that demonstrates reversibility of cardiomyopathy. The issue related to whether or not toxicological cardiac lesions are reversible has not been explored. However, it can be speculated that there would be reversible and irreversible manifestations of the cardiac response to toxic insults. With regard to this, toxic effect on the capacity of myocardial regeneration is a major concern and myocardial regenerative toxicity determines the fate of toxicological cardiomyopathy reversible or irreversible.

Myocardial Cell Death and Signaling Pathways

Apoptosis and Necrosis Toxic insults trigger a series of reactions in cardiac cells leading to measurable changes. Mild injuries can be repaired. However, severe injuries will lead to cell death in the modes of apoptosis and necrosis. If the cell survives the insults, structural and functional adaptations will take place.

Apoptosis Apoptosis was found to be involved in cardiomyopathy in 1994 (Gottlieb *et al.*, 1994). The loss of cardiac myocytes is a fundamental component of myocardial injury, which initiates and aggravates cardiomyopathy. An important mode of myocardial cell loss is apoptosis, which has been demonstrated in heart failure patients (Olivetti *et al.*, 1997). Myocardial apoptosis has been shown to play an important role in cardiac toxic effects induced by Adriamycin (Kang *et al.*, 2000a; Wang *et al.*, 2001a), an important anticancer drug whose clinical application is limited by its cardiotoxicity. Exposure of primary cultures of cardiomyocytes to cadmium also induces apoptosis (El-Sherif *et al.*, 2000).

Many in vivo studies have shown that only a very small percentage of myocardial cell populations undergo apoptosis under pathological conditions. For example, less than 0.5% of cells appeared apoptotic in myocardial tissue under the stress of dietary copper deficiency in mice (Kang *et al.*, 2000b). At first glance, this number seems to be too insignificant to account for myocardial pathogenesis. In a carefully designed time-course study (Kajstura *et al.*, 1996), it was estimated that cardiomyocyte apoptosis is completed in less than 20 hours in rats. Myocytes that undergo apoptosis are lost and may not be replaced under toxicological conditions. Although the possibility of myocardial regeneration has been identified (Anversa *et al.*, 2006), xenobiotics often cause degenerative effect through apoptosis as well as inhibitory effect on regeneration. Adriamycin-induced cardiomyopathy is a good example for the pathogenesis resulting from both degeneration and inhibition of regeneration. If apoptosis occurs at a constant rate of about 0.5% myocytes a day (Kang *et al.*, 2000b), the potential contribution of apoptosis to the overall loss of myocytes over a long period of time is significant under Adrimycin toxic exposure.

Necrosis Necrosis is a term that had been widely used to describe myocardial cell death in the past. Myocardial infarction, in particular, had been considered as a consequence of necrosis (Eliot *et al.*, 1977). It is now recognized that apoptosis contributes significantly to myocardial infarction (Yaoita *et al.*, 2000). However, the importance of necrosis in myocardial pathogenesis cannot be underestimated. The contribution of necrosis to cardiomyopathy induced by environmental toxicants and pollutants is particularly important. A critical issue is how to distinguish apoptosis from necrosis.

Apoptosis and necrosis were originally described as two distinct forms of cell death that can be clearly distinguished (Wyllie, 1994). However, these two modes of cell death can occur simultaneously in tissues and cultured cells. The intensity and duration of insults may determine the outcome. Triggering events can be common for both types of cell death. A downstream controller, however, may direct cells toward a programmed execution of apoptosis. If the apoptotic program is aborted before this control point and the initiating stimulus is severe, cell death may occur by necrosis (Leist *et al.*, 1997).

To distinguish apoptosis from necrosis, specific oligonucleotide probes have been developed to recognize different aspects of DNA damage (Didenko *et al.*, 1998), and have been successfully applied, in combination with confocal microscopy, to identify apoptotic and necrotic cell death in the heart with different pathogenic challenges.

Single-Strand DNA Breaks

A monoclonal mouse anti-ssDNA antibody has been developed that is specifically reactive with ssDNA, but does not recognize dsDNA. An immunohistochemical assay for detection of ssDNA using this antibody in combination with a terminal deoxynucleotidyl-transferase-mediated dUTP nick end labeling (TUNEL) assay can distinguish repairable ssDNA breaks from apoptotic DNA damage in the heart.

Apoptotic DNA Damage This produces end products that are fragments of double-strand DNA cleavage with three overhangs (Didenko *et al.*, 1998), which can be specifically identified by *Tag* polymerase-generated probe (Didenko *et al.*, 1998). The specificity of this molecular probe to identify apoptosis has been confirmed by other methods such as dual labeling of TdT and caspase-3 (Frustaci *et al.*, 2000). In addition, this apoptotic specific probe in combination with fluorescence labeling of different cellular components allows quantitative detection of apoptotic cells, with the possibility of identifying the origin of the apoptotic cells, such as myocytes (stained with α-sarcomeric actin), endothelial cells (stained with factor VIII), and fibroblasts (stained with vimentin) in the heart (Anversa, 2000).

Necrotic DNA Damage This is characterized by double-strand DNA cleavage with blunt ends. That is because during necrosis, the release of lysosomal proteases degrades histones, resulting in loss of DNA protection and exposure to endonucleases and exonucleases. Endonucleases produce double-strand DNA cleavage with three overhangs, but exonucleases remove terminal nucleotides, leading to a blunt end of the damaged DNA. A probe generated by *pfu* polymerase can specifically recognize these blunt-end DNAs (Anversa, 2000). Its specific reaction with necrotic DNA has been confirmed by other methods such as the permeability of myosin antibody into necrotic cells (Guerra *et al.*, 1999), and the disruption of the sarcolemma by vinculin staining, which can clearly define the continuity of the sarcolemmal surface (Yamashita *et al.*, 2001).

Proportion of Apoptotic and Necrotic Cell Death in the Heart This can be estimated by the combination of the above procedures. First, a conventional TUNEL procedure can be used to identify the total TUNEL-positive cells. Second, the procedure to define double-strand DNA breaks with blunt ends can be used to quantify the proportion of necrotic cells in the total TUNEL-positive population. Finally, the combination of the procedure to identify double-strand DNA breaks with 3′ overhangs, and the specific antibody to identify total ssDNA breaks can distinguish the proportion of apoptotic cells from those with ssDNA breaks only.

Distinguishing Apoptotic Myocytes from Nonmyocytes in the Myocardium This is another problem to overcome. An in situ TUNEL assay in combination with a dual immunohistochemical detection of α-sarcomeric actin has been used to distinguish apoptotic myocytes from nonmyocytes (Kang *et al.*, 2000a). Apoptotic myocytes are dually stained by TUNEL and α-sarcomeric actin, and apoptotic nonmyocytes are stained only by TUNEL. Another procedure is immuno-gold TUNEL and electron microscopic examination of the apoptotic cells (Kang *et al.*, 2000a). The gold standard for identification of apoptotic cells is morphological examination by electron microscopy. The immuno-gold TUNEL and electron microscopic procedure defines the cell type and morphological characteristics of apoptotic cells.

Mitochondrial Control of Cell Death

The role of mitochondria in myocardial response to toxicants as well as therapeutic drugs has long been a focus of investigation. Mitochondrial control of cell death is an important topic of apoptotic research. Factors affecting mitochondrial control of cell death are presented in Fig. 18-9. These factors have the same target effect: modification of mitochondrial permeability transition (MPT).

Mitochondrial Permeability Transition MPT occurs under toxic insults (Kroemer *et al.*, 1997). This MPT behaves like a membrane pore that allows diffusion of solutes <1500 Da in size. Although MPT can occur as a temporary event, it can rapidly become irreversible, with the resulting loss of mitochondrial

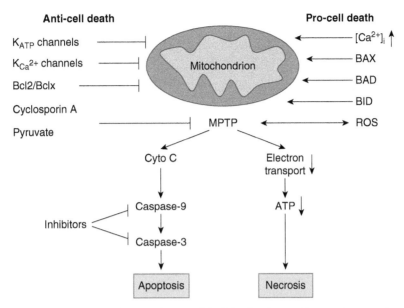

Figure 18-9. *Major factors affecting mitochondrial MPTP and myocardial cell death.* Mitochondrial cytochrome *c* release is a critical factor controlling cardiomyocyte apoptosis. Mitochondrial permeability transition pore (MPTP) opening is a determinant factor for cytochrome *c* release, as well as for electron transport collapsing leading to decreases in ATP production. The factors affecting MPTP thus are classified as pro-cell death and anti-cell death. Many other factors also affect cell death programs such as apoptosis inducing factor (AIF) released from mitochondria, but the involvement of MPTP is not evidenced.

homeostasis and high-amplitude mitochondrial swelling. Because the inner membrane has a larger surface area than the outer membrane, mitochondrial swelling can cause the rupture of the outer membrane, releasing intermembrane proteins into the cytosol (Reed *et al.*, 1998). Among the intermembrane proteins is cytochrome *c*. Another possible mechanism that leads to mitochondrial cytochrome *c* release is the action of Bax, a proapoptotic protein of the Bcl-2 family (Adams and Cory, 1998). Overexpression of Bax under oxidative stress conditions has been observed in a number of studies in different tissues including the heart (Cook *et al.*, 1999). It has been shown that Bax is translocated from cytosol to mitochondria and forms pores in mitochondrial outer membranes, leaving the inner membranes intact (Jurgensmeier *et al.*, 1998). This mechanism implies that Bax-mediated cytochrome *c* release is independent of MPT (Saikumar *et al.*, 1998). The release of cytochrome *c* from mitochondria into the cytosol is a critical initiation step in myocardial apoptosis. Cytochrome *c* aggregates with apoptotic protease activating factor-1 (apaf-1, another factor released from mitochondria under oxidative stress), procaspase-9, and dATP, and subsequently activates caspase-9, which activates caspase-3. The apoptotic pathway involving mitochondrial cytochrome *c* release and caspase-3 activation is presented in Fig. 18-10. To determine the significance of the caspase-3-activated apoptotic pathway in the pathogenesis of toxicological cardiomyopathy, a caspase-3-specific inhibitor, Ac-DEVD-cmk, is often used. For instance, treatment of cultured cardiomyocytes isolated from neonatal mice with Ac-DEVD-cmk efficiently suppressed caspase-3 activity and reduced the number of apoptotic cells in cultures under treatment with Adriamycin (Wang *et al.*, 2001a).

Defective Mitochondrial Oxidative Phosphorylation This has been extensively investigated ever since the identification of mitochondrial oxidative phosphorylation. The link between defective oxidative phosphorylation and pathogenesis of cardiomyopathy has been revealed recently. The early phase of defects in oxidative phosphorylation increases mitochondrial outer membrane permeability, leading to cytochrome *c* release, thus resulting in cytochrome *c*-mediated caspase-9 activation and thereby caspase-3

activation, leading to apoptosis (Fosslien, 2001). The defective oxidative phosphorylation also leads to depletion of cellular ATP levels, resulting in necrosis (Fosslien, 2001). Fig. 18-11 presents a generalized mitochondrial oxidative phosphorylation process, including electron-transferring complexes and ATP production. Detection of mutated or otherwise defective components in oxidative phosphorylation is important for understanding the myocardial cell death by xenobiotics.

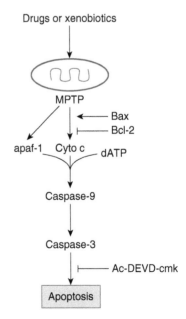

Figure 18-10. *Mitochondrial control of myocardial apoptotic pathway.* Exposure to drugs or xenobiotics can cause mitochondrial MPTP opening and cytochrome *c* release, which in association with apaf-1 and in the presence of dATP activates caspase-9. Caspase-9 consequently activates caspase-3 leading to apoptosis. Factors regulating the apoptotic pathway include those listed in Fig. 18-9, such as Bax and Bcl-2. Ac-DEVD-cml is a selective inhibitor of caspase-3.

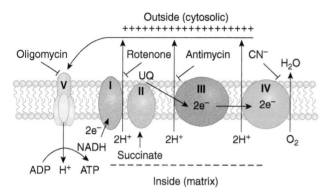

Figure 18-11. *Diagram of the electron-transferring complexes I, II, III, and IV and the ATPase (V) present in the inner mitochondrial membrane.* The respective complexes are I, NADH: ubiquinone oxidoreductase; II, succinate: ubiquinone oxidoreductase; III, ubiquinol: ferrocytochrome *c* oxidoreductase; IV, ferrocytochrome *c*: oxygen oxidoreductase; V, ATP synthesase. UQ 5 ubiquinone or coenzyme Q. The mitochondrial electron transport chain is coupled at three points so that the electron transfer between carriers is sufficiently exergonic to drive the transport of protons and to establish an electrochemical proton gradient upon which ATP formation depends. Various inhibitors and their sites are also noted.

Abnormal Mitochondrial Biosynthesis This is also linked to myocardial pathogenesis. Both nuclear and mitochondrial DNA encode mitochondrial proteins. Therefore, nuclear DNA damage can lead to mutated products and abnormal mitochondrial biosynthesis. However, mitochondrial DNA encodes essential elements for mitochondrial function. Mitochondrial DNA is subjected to far more oxidative injury than nuclear DNA due to the lack of histones and high exposure to reactive oxygen species (ROS) generated by the electron transport chain. Mitochondrial DNA repair mechanism exists, although the repair is not as efficient as that of nuclear DNA repair. Due to these unique characteristics of mitochondrial DNA, cumulative mitochondrial DNA damage under oxidative stress conditions such as Adriamycin treatment leads to irreversible mitochondrial dysfunction in the heart (Zhou *et al.*, 2001). This cumulative and relatively irreversible oxidative mitochondrial dysfunction concept has an important impact on our understanding of chronic as well as late-onset cardiomyopathy of anthracyclines. These drugs cause cardiomyopathy sometimes months to years after cessation of the drug therapy. During this time period, subtle pathological changes that may not be detectable but may continue to accumulate and lead to an overt toxic event. The cumulative and irreversible mitochondrial dysfunction might explain such a phenomenon, and may contribute to the delayed myocardial pathogenesis by Adriamycin.

Generation of Reactive Oxygen Species Generation of ROS has been ascribed as an "unwanted" function of mitochondria. Drugs and other chemicals have been studied individually to determine how they produce ROS; however, debate continues regarding the importance of each identified pathway as well as the site of ROS generation in mitochondria. In general, it is accepted that changes in mitochondrial membrane potential are critically involved in ROS generation. There are two important potassium channels that play important roles in mitochondrial membrane permeability. The first is the mitochondrial ATP-sensitive potassium channel (Akao *et al.*, 2001), and the second is the Ca^{2+}-activated potassium channel in the cardiac inner mitochondrial membrane (Xu *et al.*, 2002). It has been shown that diazoxide opens mitochondrial ATP-sensitive potassium channels and preserves mitochondrial integrity, as well as suppresses hydrogen peroxide-induced apoptosis in cardiomyocytes (Akao *et al.*, 2001). The Ca^{2+}-activated potassium

channels, in contrast, contribute to mitochondrial potassium uptake of myocytes, and opening of these channels protects the heart from infarction (Xu *et al.*, 2002).

Death Receptors and Signaling Pathways Death receptor-mediated apoptotic signaling pathway has been one of the focuses of cardiotoxicity research. In this regard, cytokines that trigger the death receptor signaling pathways have been studied. Among these cytokines is tumor necrosis factor-α (TNF-α) (Kubota *et al.*, 2001), the most studied cytokine in myocardial cell death signaling pathways. The pathway leading to TNF-α-induced myocardial apoptosis is mediated by TNF receptors, TNFR1, and TNFR2. TNF-α-binding of these receptors leads to activation of caspase 8, which in turn cleaves BID, a BH3 domain-containing proapoptotic Bcl2 family member. The truncated BID is translocated from cytosol to mitochondria, inducing first the clustering of mitochondria around the nuclei and release of cytochrome *c*, and then the loss of mitochondrial membrane potential, cell shrinkage, and nuclear condensation, that is, apoptosis. Caspase 8 also directly activates caspase-3, leading to apoptosis (Fig. 18-12). Besides TNF-α, Fas ligand is also able to induce apoptosis of cardiomyocytes through the death receptor-mediated signaling pathway (Hayakawa *et al.*, 2002).

The death receptor-mediated apoptosis thus can be divided into mitochondrion-dependent and mitochondrion-independent signaling pathways. There is a bewildering diversity of programmed cell death paradigms related to the mitochondrion-controlled process, eventually leading to caspase-3 activation and apoptosis. Under chronic toxic insults, the relative importance of mitochondrial MPT pore opening, cytochrome *c* release, and electron transport defects needs to be critically examined in order to understand the process or mode of cell death.

There are two important questions that need to be carefully addressed. First, how important is apoptosis in the overall pathogenesis of cardiomyopathy under different conditions? It essentially is a universal observation that apoptosis is involved in the

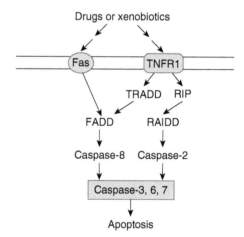

Figure 18-12. *Simplified presentation of death receptors-mediated myocardial apoptosis.* The cardiotoxicity-related death receptors include Fas and tumor necrotic factor receptor 1 (TNFR1), as shown. Other death receptors such as DR3 and DR4/5 are not included in the figure. Both Fas- and TNFR1-activated apoptotic pathways can be altered by drugs and xenobiotics directly or indirectly through changes in the production of Fas ligand (FasL) or TNF-α. Fas activation activates caspase-8 through Fas-associated death domain (FADD). TNFR1 activates TNF-R1-associated death domain (TRADD), leading to activation of FADD. TNFR1 also activates a receptor-interacting protein (RIP), which activates caspase-2 through the adaptor protein, RIP-associated ICH-1/CED-3 homologous protein with a death domain (RAIDD). Both caspase-8 and caspase-3 activate the apoptosis executor proteins, caspase-3, -6, and -7.

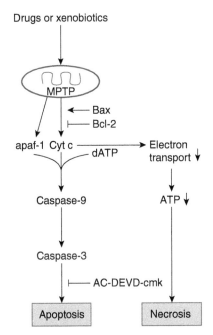

Drugs or xenobiotics

MPTP

Bax
Bcl-2

apaf-1 Cyt c — dATP → Electron transport ↓

Caspase-9   ATP ↓

Caspase-3

AC-DEVD-cmk

Apoptosis   Necrosis

Figure 18-13. *Interchange between apoptotic and necrotic cell death pathways regulated by mitochondrial MPTP.* Mitochondrial MPTP opening leads to cytochrome *c*-mediated activation of apoptotic pathway, which is ATP dependent. However, MPTP formation also leads to electron transport collapse and reduced ATP production, which eventually leads to necrosis. Inhibition of caspase-3 also potentially switches the cell death program from apoptotic to necrotic if the exposure to drugs or xenobiotics is persistent.

cardiotoxicity of drugs and chemicals; however, there is very limited information regarding its significance in a quantitative manner in contribution to cardiomyopathy. This concern is followed by the second important question: can caspase inhibitors offer long-term protection against myocardial cell death leading to prevention of cardiomyopathy? It is important to note that apoptosis and necrosis are linked phenomena sharing common triggers, such as MPT pore opening, as depicted in Fig. 18-13. For instance, some studies have shown that caspase inhibitors effectively inhibit apoptosis, but cell death occurred by necrosis instead of apoptosis (Suzuki *et al.*, 2001). It is thus important to define the most efficient approach to blocking myocardial cell death rather than inhibiting a particular cell death program (Kang, 2001).

It is important to note that apoptosis is an energy-dependent process and that the switch in the decision between apoptosis and necrosis depends on ATP concentrations (Eguchi *et al.*, 1997), as depicted in Fig. 18-13. In particular, conditions causing ischemia by many drug and chemical exposures to myocardial cells result in significant reduction and eventual depletion of adenine nucleotides. Loss of more than 70% of the total ATP pool present in myocardial cells results in a switch from apoptosis to necrosis (Leist *et al.*, 1999). This extent of ATP depletion is observed in myocardial infarction.

Mitochondrial Dynamics and Autophagy

The importance of mitochondria in cardiac response to toxic insults and in the process of toxicological cardiomyopathy is related not only to the control of cell death, but also to autophagy, the tightly regulated cellular "housekeeping" process responsible for the degradation of damaged and dysfunctional cellular organelles and protein aggregates.

Autophagy occurs in all eukaryotic cells under the stress of starvation, hypoxia, and toxic insults, as well as under physiological

stimulation such as hormones and developmental signals. There are selective autophagy and nonselective autophagy. Selective autophagy of mitochondria is termed mitophagy, which is triggered by MPT pore opening and loss of mitochondrial membrane potential (Tolkovsky, 2009). In cardiomyocytes and other terminally differentiated cells, mitophagy is a continuous process of mitochondrial turnover, but the rate of this turnover is influenced by stresses and makes a critical contribution to myocardial pathogenesis. Nonselective autophagy has been observed in response to nutrient starvation; the degradation of cytosolic components including mitochondria via autophagy provides amino acids and lipid substrates for intermediate metabolism (Tolkovsky, 2009).

Mitochondrial Dynamics The well-known and comprehensively depicted function of mitochondria is the generation of adenosine triphosphate (ATP) through oxidative phosphorylation. However, it has been known that mitochondria also carry out other critical functions, including regulation of programmed cell death or apoptosis, the synthesis and degradation of essential metabolites, heme and steroid synthesis, regulation of cell proliferation, maintenance of plasma membrane potential, and calcium signaling. These diverse functions demand mitochondrial biogenesis and turnover highly regulated. In cardiomyocytes and other terminally differentiated cells, this regulation is far more important for the vital function of the cell.

Mitochondria are dynamic organelles and the morphology of mitochondria undergoes interchange between two distinct arrangements: elongated interconnected mitochondrial networks and discrete fragments. The former is accomplished by mitochondrial fusion and the latter by mitochondrial fission. In the heart, mitochondrial fusion and fission constitute a major response of cardiomyocytes to stresses. For instance, sustained pressure overload promotes structural, functional and metabolic remodeling of cardiomyocyte mitochondria to compensate for changes in energy demands and to remove damaged organelles. This process ultimately determines the fate of a cardiomyocyte: survival versus death. The changes in mitochondrial morphology are orchestrated by a group of mitochondrial fusion and fission proteins. These proteins were first identified in yeast or *Drosophila*, and the function of these proteins has been a major focus in the study of mitochondrial dynamics. But the identification of these proteins in the mammalian heart has made a significant impact on the role of mitochondrial dynamics in the pathogenesis of cardiac disease.

Mitochondrial Fusion Mitochondrial fusion is a process of an elongated interconnected mitochondrial network formation. This is a fundamental process in the life of eukaryotic cells. Mitochondrial fusion requires coordinated joining of both the outer mitochondrial membrane (OMM) and the inner mitochondrial membrane (IMM). In this process, the constituents in the matrix and intermembrane space are secured—not to be released or mixed. Therefore, the fusion machinery involves OMM and IMM fusion, and their coordination.

OMM fusion is directed by mitofusins 1 and 2 (MFN1 and MFN2), large GTPase located in the OMM. They contain two transmembrane regions in the OMM, with a short loop in the intermembrane space and the major parts of the protein facing the cytosol. In mammalian cells, early during fusion two mitochondria approach each other in a tethered docking step. The carboxy-terminal heptad repeats of MFN1 have been shown to form an intermolecular antiparallel coiled coil that may tether adjacent mitochondria before fusion (Koshiba *et al.*, 2004). The coiled coil formation by mitofusins thus draws the membranes close together and initiates lipid bilayer mixing, and the GTPase provides biomechanical energy for outer membrane fusion. It has been shown that mutation of the GTPase domain of MFN2 results in an accumulation of tethered but unfused mitochondria (Eura *et al.*, 2003).

IMM fusion is governed by Mgm1, a dynamin-related large GTPase that is essential for inner membrane fusion in yeast (Meeusen *et al.*, 2006). The mammalian Mgm1 ortholog, optic atrophy 1 (OPA1) protein, is tethered to the IMM and in the inter-membrane space (Olichon *et al.*, 2002). Differential splicing of *Opa1* transcripts generates multiple variants (Song *et al.*, 2007). A number of proteases localized in mitochondria cleave OPA1 disrupting OPA1 function and inhibiting fusion. Mutations in OPA1 selectively block inner membrane fusion. After the completion of outer membrane fusion, OPA1 is required in *trans* on both inner membranes of the fusion parteres. A normal membrane potential is required for fusion of IMM. Loss of membrane potential promotes cleavage of OPA1, causing that outer membrane fusion proceeds in the absence of inner membrane fusion.

Mitochondrial Fission   Mitochondrial fusion is a process of the fragmented discrete mitochondrial morphogenesis. This process is regulated by dynamin-related protein 1 (DRP1) in mammals. This protein is soluble and contains an N-terminal GTPase, a middle domain, and a C-terminal GTPase effector, which is involved in self-assembly. Cells lacking DRP1 contain highly interconnected mitochondrial networks (Smirnova *et al.*, 1998). During fission, DRP1 is recruited from the cytoplasm to mitochondria. Mammalian fission protein 1 (FIS1) in the OMM interacts with DRP1. FIS1 overexpression promotes mitochondrial fragmentation and FIS1 depletion stimulates interconnected mitochondrial networks (Yoon *et al.*, 2003; James *et al.*, 2003). In yeast, a mitochondrial division protein 1 (Mdv1) has been shown to coexist with Fis1 and interact with DRP1, but its metazoan homologs have not been identified, indicating a significant difference between metazoan and yeast mitochondrial fission machineries.

The function of mitochondrial fission machinery has been extensively understood in yeast, but less comprehensively in meta-zoans. In yeast, the fis1–Mdv1–Dnm1 complex is important for mitochondrial fission, but the lack of Mdv1 in metazoans makes a different mitochondrial fission machinery. It has been shown that knockdown of human FIS1 does not affect the distribution of DRP1 in mitochondria (Lee *et al.*, 2004). A mitochondrial fission factor (MFF) has been found in mammalians, but not in yeast (Gandre-Babbe and van der Bliek, 2008). MFF is a tail-anchored protein containing heptad repeats and a C-terminal transmembrane domain that is embedded in the OMM. Depletion of MFF suppresses mitochondrial fission in mammalian cells. However, MFF and FIS1 exist in separate complexes, suggesting that they may act differently in mitochondrial fission (Gandre-Babbe and van der Bliek, 2008).

Regulation of Mitochondrial Dynamics   This is subjected to multiple factors that affect mitochondrial fusion and fission. However, a single factor-regulated mitochondrial dynamics rarely occurs because under most circumstances several factors are often coexisting. Therefore, whether or not mitochondria eventually undergo fusion or fission depends on the ultimate balance between the actions induced by several factors. On the other hand, it cannot be judged whether or not mitochondrial fusion or fission is beneficial or detrimental; only can the ultimate effect of mitochondrial fusion or fission be the judgment under certain conditions.

Cell cycle control of mitochondrial dynamics is often observed in mitotically active cells. Mitochondrial fusion is found during G1-S phase, but mitochondrial fission is necessary in cell division. In differentiated cells such as cardiomyocytes, the cell cycle control of mitochondrial dynamics is less important. However, reactivation of fetal gene program in adult cardiomyocytes in cardiac hypertrophy and heart failure would affect mitochondrial dynamics, which has not been understood.

Oxidative and nitrosative stress often induces mitochondrial fission. Mitochondria are the major site for the production of ROS in the heart. The process not only affects mitochondrial dynamics, but generates ROS-induced damage to proteins, lipids, and DNA. Studies have shown overexpression of MFN inhibits ROS-induced mitochondrial fission and protects cardiomyocytes from oxidative injury (Yu *et al.*, 2011).

Ca^{2+} regulation of mitochondrial dynamics is more related to the role of mitochondria in Ca^{2+} transport and homeostasis. Activation of calcineurin (CaN) and calmodulin-dependent protein kinase 1 (CaMK1) by Ca^{2+} affects the recruitment of DRP1 and mitochondrial translocation. Inhibition of mitochondrial Ca^{2+} uptake attenuates mitochondrial fission, indicating the importance of intermitochondrial Ca^{2+} concentrations in the regulation of mito-chondrial dynamics.

Metabolic regulation of mitochondrial dynamics is the funda-mental process of mitochondrial biological function. Mitochondrial dynamics and energy substrate metabolism are tightly linked. Increased metabolic rates upregulate mitochondrial fusion and dense packing of cristae. Downregulation of OPA1 or MFN leads to fragmented mitochondria with reduced membrane potential and oxygen consumption. Glucose concentrations play a critical role in the regulation of mitochondrial dynamics. Changes in fusion-related proteins have been observed in animal models and patients with type 2 diabetes (Zorzano *et al.*, 2010). High glucose levels stimulate mitochondrial fragmentation in H9c2 cardiomyoblasts and neonatal rat cardiomyocytes (Yu *et al.*, 2008).

Toxicological Significance of Mitochondrial Dynamics   Toxico-logical significance of mitochondrial dynamics in the heart can be observed under a diversity of exogenous and endogenous stress conditions. Mitochondrial dynamics is a physiological process as well as a feature of pathogenesis. Under physiological conditions, mitochondrial fusion and fission are essential to maintain meta-bolic homeostasis and the balance between energy production and consumption. Disruption of this physiological process under stress conditions or toxicological exposures leads to overwhelming of mitochondrial fusion or fission. Under these conditions, cell death and maladaptation occur, leading to toxicological pathogenesis.

Autophagy   Intricately regulated degradation and turnover of sub-cellular components ensure normal cellular function, growth, and development. The major catabolic pathway responsible for the dis-posal of damaged organelles and protein aggregates is autophagy, is a lysosome-dependent proteolytic pathway capable of process-ing cellular components, including damaged organelles and protein aggregates. During this process, damaged organelles and proteins are encircled in a double-membrane vesicle, so-called autophago-some, delivered to lysosomes. The contents in the autophagosome are hydrolyzed to yield amino acids, fatty acids, and substrates for ATP generation that can be recycled to synthesize new pro-teins, high energy phosphates, and renewed cellular components. Autophagy is a conserved mechanism for cell survival under condi-tions of starvation and stress. Therefore, autophagy has been recog-nized to play an important role in maintaining cellular homeostasis, and upregulation of autophagy under stress conditions may serve as an adaptive process.

Autophagy can be subdivided into three different processes: macroautophagy, microautophagy, and chaperone-mediated autophagy. Macroautophagy is often referred to as autophagy that is characterized by the sequestration of organelles and proteins within an autophagosome, as described above. Microautophagy refers to protrusion of the lysosomal membranes per se around a region of cytoplasm. Chaperone-mediated autophagy is defined as that degradation is restricted only to those proteins with a consensus peptide sequence recognized by specific chaperone complexes. Current mechanistic understanding mostly focuses on macroautophagy or autophagy.

There are multiple proteins and interrelated signaling pathways involved in autophagy. This complex process can be divided into four distinct but consecutive steps: (1) induction of autophagy; (2) assembly of autophagosomes; (3) docking and fusion of autophagosome with lysosomal membrane; and (4) breakdown of the autophagic body.

The induction of autophagy requires the participation of three different protein complexes: autophagy-specific gene 1 (Atg1) complex, target of rapamycin (TOR) complex 1 (TORC1), and class III phosphatidylinositol-1 kinase (PI3K) complex. In this step, TORC1 acts as a sensor of cellular nutrient status. Nutrient stress leads to the partial dephosphorylation of Atg13, which in turn increases the binding affinity of Atg13 to Atg1, a pivotal precursor for subsequent autophagosome formation.

The autophagosome assembly and formation is the most complex phase of autophagy. The Atg5 complex and microtubule-associated protein 1 light chain 1 (LC3)-II work in concert to initiate elongation or expansion of the isolated membrane that will eventually form the matured autophagosome. There are several Atg genes involved in this phase and they work sequentially. It has been shown that Atg5 is essential for autophagy. Mice with a cardiac-specific disruption of *Atg-5* develop premature age-related heart failure, indicating that autophagy is an essential regulatory mechanism for normal cardiac function over the course of a life (Taneike *et al.*, 2010).

Autophagosome docking and fusion have been studied in yeast and found to involve multiple vesicle trafficking and membrane fusion proteins. The final stage of autophagy, breakdown of autophagic body and its content, generates substances for protein synthesis, lipid turnover, and ATP production.

Cardiac Hypertrophy and Heart Failure

Adaptive and Maladaptive Responses Myocardial adaptation refers to the general process by which the ventricular myocardium changes in structure and function. This process is often referred to as "remodeling." During maturation, myocardial remodeling is a normal feature for adaptation to increased demands. However, in response to pathological stimuli, such as exposure to environmental toxicants, myocardial remodeling is adaptive in the short term, but is maladaptive in the long term, and often results in further myocardial dysfunction. The central feature of myocardial remodeling is an increase in myocardial mass associated with a change in the shape of the ventricle (Frey and Olson, 2003).

At the cellular level, the increase in myocardial mass is reflected by cardiac myocyte hypertrophy, which is characterized by enhanced protein synthesis, heightened organization of the sarcomere, and the eventual increase in cell size. At the molecular level, the phenotype changes in cardiac myocytes are associated with reintroduction of the so-called fetal gene program, characterized by the patterns of gene expression mimicking those seen during embryonic development. These cellular and molecular changes are observed in both adaptive and maladaptive responses, thus distinguishing adaptive from maladaptive responses is difficult.

Adaptive Response There are both physiological hypertrophy and pathological hypertrophy of the heart. Physiological hypertrophy is considered an adaptive response, which is an adjustment of

cardiac function for an increased demand of cardiac output. Such an adaptive hypertrophy is the increase in cardiac mass after birth and in response to exercise. A biochemical distinction of the adaptive hypertrophy is that myocardial accumulation of collagen does not accompany the hypertrophy. Functionally, the increased mass is associated with enhanced contractility and cardiac output. In response to toxicological stresses, the heart also often increases its mass, which has been viewed as an adaptive response as well. However, most recent evidence suggests that cardiac hypertrophy is a maladaptive process of the heart in response to intrinsic and extrinsic stresses.

Maladaptive Response Although toxic stress-induced hypertrophy can normalize wall tension, it is a risk factor for sudden cardiac death and has a high potential to progress to overt heart failure. A distinction between adaptive and maladaptive hypertrophy is whether the hypertrophy is necessary for the compensatory function of the heart under physiological and pathological stress conditions. Many studies using genetically manipulated mouse models, either in the form of gain-of-function or loss-of-function, have supported the hypothesis that cardiac hypertrophy is neither required nor necessarily compensatory. For instance, forced expression of a dominant-negative calcineurin mutant confers protection against hypertrophy and fibrosis after abdominal aortic construction (Zou *et al.*, 2001). Also, the elimination of hypertrophy in animals by calcineurin suppression did not cause compromised hemodynamic changes over a period of several weeks (Hill *et al.*, 2000). Therefore, in these experimental approaches, hypertrophic growth could be abolished in the presence of continuous pressure overload, but the compensatory response could not be compromised. An interesting observation is that an almost complete lack of cardiac hypertrophy in response to aortic banding in a transgenic mouse model was accompanied with a significant slower pace of deterioration of systolic function (Esposito *et al.*, 2002). These observations indicate that cardiac hypertrophy in response to extrinsic and intrinsic stresses is not a compensatory response. However, cardiac hypertrophy increases the risk for malignant arrhythmia and heart failure, and thus is now viewed as a maladaptive response.

Hypertrophic Signaling Pathways Extrinsic and intrinsic stresses activate signaling transduction pathways leading to fetal gene program activation, enhanced protein synthesis of adult cardiomyocytes, and the eventual hypertrophic phenotype. The signaling pathways include several components: G-protein-coupled receptors, protein kinases including MAPK, PKC, and AMPK, calcium and calcineurin, and phosphoinositide 3-kinase (PI3K)/glycogen synthase kinase 3β (GSK3β), and transcription factors. Activation of each of the components is sufficient to induce myocardial hypertrophic growth. These components also affect each other through cross talk. The diagram presented in Fig. 18-14 briefly summarizes these pathways and their interactions. Among these pathways, protein kinases, calcium/calcineurin, and transcription factors have been discussed above. A brief summary for the G-protein-coupled receptors and the PI3K/GSK3 pathway is presented as follows.

G-Protein-Coupled Receptors Myocardial adrenergic, angiotensin, and endothelin (ET-1) receptors belong to G-protein-coupled receptors, which are coupled to three major classes of heterotrimeric GTP-binding proteins, $G_{\alpha s}$, $G_{\alpha q}/G_{\alpha 11}$, and $G_{\alpha i}$. Activation of $G_{\alpha q}$-coupled receptors is sufficient to induce myocyte hypertrophy in vitro (Adams *et al.*, 1998). Cardiac-specific ablation of $G_{\alpha q}/G_{\alpha 11}$ in adult animals causes an almost complete lack of cardiac hypertrophy in response to aortic banding (Wettschureck *et al.*, 2001).

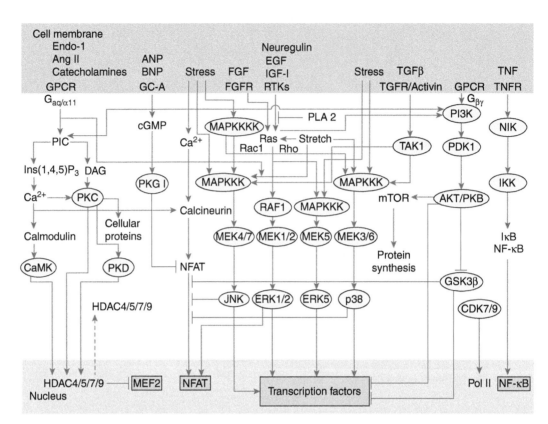

Figure 18-14. *Overview of signaling transduction pathways involved in cardiac hypertrophic growth and their cross-talk interactions.* The signaling that occurs at the sarcolemmal membrane is shown at the top and the intermediate transduction of signals by various kinases and phosphatases is shown in the middle. The nucleus is shown at the bottom. ANP, atrial natriuretic peptide; Ang II, angiotensin II; BNP, B-type natriuretic peptide; CaMK, calmodulin-dependent kinase; CDK, cyclin-dependent kinase; DAG, diacylglycerol; EGF, epidermal growth factor; Endo-1, endothelin-1; ERK, extracellular signal-regulated kinase; FGF, fibroblast growth factor; FGFR, FGF receptor; GC-A, guanyl cyclase-A; GPCR, G-protein-coupled receptors; GSK3β, glycogen synthase kinase-3β; HDAC, histone deacetylases; IκB, inhibitor of NF-κB; IGF-I, insulin-like growth factor-I; IKK; inhibitor of NF-κB kinase; Ins(1,4,5)P$_3$, inositol-1,4,5-trisphosphate; JNK, c-Jun N-terminal kinase; MAPKKK, mitogen-activated protein kinase kinase kinase; MAPKKKK, MAPKKK kinase; MEF, myocyte-enhancer factor; MEK, mitogen-activated protein kinase kinase; mTOR, mammalian target of rapamycin; NFAT, nuclear factor of activated T cells; NF-κB, nuclear factor-κB; NIK, NF-κB-inducing kinase; PDK, phosphoinositide-dependent kinase; PI3K, phosphatidylinositol 3-kinase; PKB, protein kinase B; PKC, protein kinase C; PKD, protein kinase D; PLA2, phospholipase A2; PLC, phospholipase C; Pol II, RNA polymerase II; RTK, receptor tyrosine kinase; TAK, TGFβ-activated kinase; TGF-β, transforming growth factor-beta; TGFR, TGF receptor; TNFα, tumor necrosis factor-α; TNFR, TNFα receptor (Copied from Heineke, 2006).

Overexpression of a dominant-negative mutant of G$_{αq}$ in transgenic mouse hearts suppresses pressure-overload hypertrophy (Akhter *et al.*, 1998). Cardiac overexpression of G$_{αs}$, the downstream effector of β1-adenergic receptors in the heart, initially increases contractility, but eventually results in cardiac hypertrophy, fibrosis, and heart failure (Bisognano *et al.*, 2000).

Phosphoinositide 3-Kinase/Glycogen Synthase Kinase 3β Pathway Activation of PI3K is found in both physiological and pathological hypertrophy. Insulin-like growth factor (IGF) is involved in the growth of the heart after birth (Shioi *et al.*, 2002). Overexpression of IGF induces cardiac hypertrophy (Delaughter *et al.*, 1999). IGF signals through PI3K to the serine/threonine kinase Akt or protein kinase B. Both PI3K and the Akt induce hypertrophic growth of adult hearts. Overexpression of constitutively active PI3K mutant in the heart leads to increased heart size in mice, and expression of dominant-negative PI3K results in a small heart (Shioi *et al.*, 2000). Overexpression of Akt induces cardiac hypertrophy in transgenic mice without adverse effects on systolic function (Matsui *et al.*, 2002). Akt phosphorylates GSK3β, and thus inhibits the activation of GSK3β. Otherwise, the activated GSK3β phosphorylates transcription factors of the NFAT family (Fig. 18-14). As discussed above, activation of calcineurin dephosphorylates NFAT3 in the cytoplasm, which enables NFAT3 to translocate to the nucleus where it can activate

hypertrophic gene expression dependent on or independent of GATA4. Phosphorylation of NFAT3 in the nucleus by GSK3β promotes NFAT3 translocation to the cytoplasm, becoming inactive. Hypertrophic stimuli such as β-adrenergic agonist isoproterenol, ET-1, and phenylepherine all induce GSK3β phosphorylation in a PI3K-dependent fashion, indicating possible requirement of inactivation of GSK3β through phosphorylation in hypertrophic growth of the heart.

Transition from Cardiac Hypertrophy to Heart Failure Pathological hypertrophy is a risk factor for malignant arrhythmia and heart failure. The link of heart hypertrophy to malignant arrhythmia will be discussed in the next section. The critical cellular event of this transition is myocardial apoptosis triggered by inflammatory cytokines, such as TNF-α, and neurohormonal factors, such as atrial natriuretic peptide (ANP), which leads to dilated cardiomyopathy and deterioration of cardiac function. Toxicological exposures may cause dilated cardiomyopathy or heart failure without an intermediate hypertrophic stage. Myocardial cell death also plays an essential role in direct cardiac dilation pathogenesis. Fig. 18-15 illustrates the process of xenobiotic-induced transition from cardiac hypertrophy to heart failure.

Alterations of biochemical reactions in the myocardium are often seen soon after exposure to environmental toxicants. These include alterations in ionic homeostasis, such as changes in

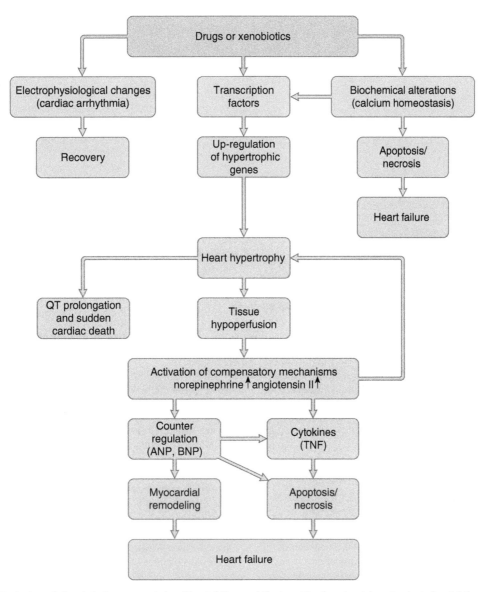

Figure 18-15. *Acute and chronic toxic exposure-induced heart failure and the transition from heart hypertrophy to heart failure.* Acute exposure to drugs or xenobiotics can cause cardiac arrhythmia, which is often observed. But if the toxic insult is so severe, myocardial apoptosis and necrosis become predominant leading to dilated cardiomyopathy and heart failure. However, the heart often survives from toxic insults through adaptive mechanisms involving upregulation of hypertrophic genes and heart hypertrophy. Heart hypertrophy increases the risk for QT prolongation and sudden cardiac death, and also activates neurohormonal regulatory mechanisms including elevation of plasma concentration of sympathetic neural transmitters and angiotensins. These compensatory mechanisms in turn activate counter-regulatory mechanisms such as ANP, BNP, and TNF-α. A long-term action of the counter-regulatory mechanisms leads to myocardial remodeling and the transition from heart hypertrophy to heart failure.

intracellular calcium concentrations, which occur in most exposures to environmental toxicants (Symanski and Gettes, 1993). Aberrant energy metabolism is another early response to environmental toxicants in the heart, resulting in decreased production and/or enhanced consumption of ATP (Abas *et al.*, 2000). Alterations in enzymatic reactions are often described in cardiac toxic responses (Depre and Taegtmeyer, 2000). The early signaling pathways leading to myocardial toxic responses are the focus of current cardiac toxicology research (Piano, 1994). Detailed descriptions of these pathways and their role in cardiotoxicity are yet to be explored. It is likely that activation of signaling pathways is a critical response of myocardial cells to environmental toxic insults (Cheng *et al.*, 1999a). The cross talk between signaling pathways determines the ultimate outcome of myocardial responses to chemicals.

Physiological alterations occur both as early responses to environmental toxicants and as subsequent events in the late development of cardiomyopathy. The most obvious myocardial dysfunction that occurs in the early responses to toxicants is cardiac arrhythmia (Peters *et al.*, 2000), which often results from the changes in intracellular calcium concentrations and other biochemical alterations, leading to miscommunication between cells and misconduction of electricity (Rosen, 1995). These changes, if not accompanied by cardiomyopathy, do not involve myocardial cell death and are reversible. In contrast, the late phase of cardiac dysfunction and arrhythmia, however, often result from cardiomyopathy.

Changes in myocardial morphology take place when extensive toxic insults are imposed on the heart and/or toxic exposures persist (He *et al.*, 1996). Cardiac hypertrophy is often observed as a consequence of long-term toxic insults. From cardiac hypertrophy to heart failure, activation of compensatory mechanisms, including the sympathetic nervous system and the renin–angiotensin system, occurs (Holtz, 1993). The compensatory response in turn activates counter-regulatory mechanisms such as upregulation of ANP expression (Francis and Chu, 1995) and increases in cytokines, such as TNF-α production. Extensive biochemical, physiological, and molecular changes result in myocardial remodeling (Swynghedauw, 1999) and remarkable cell death, ultimately leading to heart failure.

QT Prolongation and Sudden Cardiac Death

Recognition of QT prolongation and its associated adverse effects on the heart has been a major focus in drug discovery and development during the last decade. A number of drugs have been found to cause QT prolongation and TdP, and thus were removed from the market or relabeled for restricted use. It has been known for a long time that quinidine causes sudden cardiac death; however, the severe and lethal side effect of QT prolongation did not draw sufficient attention until the last decade, due to the lack of knowledge and experimental approaches to obtain a comprehensive understanding of QT prolongation. Knowledge on QT prolongation has accumulated and regulatory guidelines for a battery of preclinical tests to assess QT liability of a potential drug are recommended.

Definition of QT Prolongation A simple definition for QT prolongation is that the length of QT interval observed from a typical electrocardiogram is prolonged. Clinically, long QT syndrome is defined when the QT interval is longer than 460 milliseconds. However, TdP occurs with an average increase in QT interval by approximately 200 milliseconds (a normal QT interval is about 300 milliseconds). A human study has found that TdP does not occur with a QT interval shorter than 500 milliseconds (Joshi *et al.*, 2004). In general, the long QT syndrome can be divided into two classes: congenital and acquired. Congenital long QT syndrome is rare and acquired is the major concern of drug cardiac toxicity in pharmaceutical discovery and development.

Molecular Basis of QT Prolongation Prolongation of the QT interval on the electrocardiogram is caused by prolongation of the action potential of ventricular myocytes. In cardiac action potential, phase 0 represents depolarization of myocytes and the depolarization of all ventricular myocytes is measurable as the QRS complex on the electrocardiogram. Phase 1 of the cardiac action potential is recognized as a partial repolarization of the membrane due to inactivation of cardiac sodium channels, and activation of transit outward potassium channels. Phase 2 of the action potential is generated primarily by slowly decreasing inward calcium currents through L-type calcium channels, and gradually increasing outward currents through several types of potassium channels. This phase is sensitive to small changes in ion currents and is a critical determinant of the duration of the action potential. At this point, the cardiac cycle of the electrocardiogram has returned to baseline. Phase 3 of the cardiac action potential represents myocardial cell repolarization due to outward potassium currents. There are two critical potassium channels that terminate the plateau phase (phase 2) and initiate the final repolarization phase 3: I_{Kr} and I_{Ks}. I_{Kr} is the rapidly activating delayed rectifier potassium current, and I_{Ks} is the slowly activating delayed rectifier potassium current. The repolarization phase correlates with the T wave on the electrocardiogram. Therefore, the duration of the QT interval is related to the length of the ventricular action potentials.

A reduction in net outward current and/or an increase in inward current are potential contributors to the prolongation of cardiac action potential, thereby QT prolongation on the electrocardiogram. Although many channels are potentially involved in the prolongation of the cardiac action potential, current studies have identified three important channels that play a critical role in the plateau phase (phase 2) of the cardiac action potential, sodium inward channels, and potassium outward channels (I_{Kr} and I_{Ks}).

Sodium Channel Dysfunction Sodium channel dysfunction in congenital long QT syndrome is related to mutations in *SCN5A* gene that encodes the α-subunits of sodium channels. Mutational analyses have found 14 distinct mutations of *SCN5A* associated with long QT syndrome (Splawski *et al.*, 2000). It has been hypothesized that gain-of-function mutations in *SCN5A* would cause long QT syndrome because reopening of the sodium channels during the plateau phase of action potential, even in a small inward current, would lengthen the duration of the cardiac action potential. Sodium channel inactivation immediately following depolarization (phase 1) is important for the transition to phase 2 of the action potential. A mutation of *SCN5A* has been found to destabilize the inactivation gate (Bennett *et al.*, 1995). Activation of these mutant sodium channels is normal and the rate of inactivation appears slightly faster than normal, but these mutant channels can reopen during the plateau phase of the action potential, leading to a prolonged plateau phase.

The I_{Kr} *potassium channels* critically affect the length of the plateau phase of the cardiac action potential. The human *ether-à-go-go*-related gene (*HERG*) is expressed primarily in the heart and encodes the α-subunit of the cardiac I_{Kr} potassium channel. There are 94 mutations of *HERG*, which have been identified to represent 45% of the total number of mutations related to long QT syndrome to date (Splawski *et al.*, 2000). The HERG α-subunits assemble with MiRP1 β-subunits to form cardiac I_{Kr} channels. The I_{Kr} potassium channel is one of the two channels that are primarily responsible for termination of the plateau phase of the action potential. During the repolarization of the action potential, the I_{Kr} channels open, resulting in an increase in the magnitude of I_{Kr} current during the first-half of phase 3 repolarization. Many *HERG* mutations occur around the membrane-spanning domains and the pore region of the channel. Most of these mutations have a loss-of-function effect and many long QT syndrome-associated mutations in *HERG* are missense mutations, which lead to a dominant-negative effect on I_{Kr} channels because the functional I_{Kr} potassium channels are composed of heteromultimers including several HERG subunits. Therefore, the loss-of-function mutations in *HERG* make a critical contribution to the long QT syndrome due to the prolonged plateau phase of cardiac potential.

The I_{Ks} *potassium channel* is the other one of the two channels primarily responsible for the termination of the plateau phase of the action potential. The I_{Ks} potassium channel is assembled from KVLQT1 α-subunits and the minK β-subunits. There are two molecular mechanisms that possibly account for reduced KVLQT1 function in the long QT syndrome (Wollnik *et al.*, 1997). First, intragenic deletions of one *KVLQT1* allele result in synthesis of abnormal α-subunits that do not assemble with normal subunits, leading to a 50% reduction in the number of the functional channels. Second, missense mutations result in synthesis of KVLQT1 subunits with structural abnormalities, which can assemble with normal subunits. Channels formed from the mutant KVLQT1 subunits have reduced or no function. Both of these mutations result in a dominant-negative effect. Interestingly, both *KVLQT1* and *minK* are expressed in the inner ear, in which the channels function to produce a potassium-rich fluid known as endolymph that bathes the organ of Corti, the cochlear organ responsible for hearing. Individuals with Jervell and Lange-Nielsen syndrome have homozygous mutations of *KVLQT1* or minK, thus having no functional

I_{Ks} channels. These individuals have severe arrhythmia susceptibility and congenital neural deafness.

Therefore, the molecular basis of the QT prolongation on the electrocardiogram is the prolongation of cardiac action potential. In this regard, the inward sodium channels and outward potassium channels play an important role in increasing the length of the plateau phase of action potentials. Congenital long QT syndrome is related to gain-of-function mutations in sodium channels and/or loss-of-function mutations in potassium channels. Acquired long QT syndrome is also related to altered function of these channels; however, many other factors that affect the phenotype of long QT syndrome and the clinical manifestations.

Torsade De Pointes and Sudden Cardiac Death

The abnormalities of different channels in different regions of the heart at varying levels result in channel dysfunction with regional variability. The regional abnormalities of cardiac repolarization or conductance provide a substrate for arrhythmia. Under these conditions, arrhythmia is induced if a trigger mechanism is implanted. The trigger for arrhythmia in the long QT syndrome is believed to be spontaneous secondary depolarization that arises during or just following the plateau of the action potential. This small action potential is the so-called early afterdepolarization, which occurs preferentially in M cells and Purkinje cells due to reactivation of the L-type calcium channels and/or activation of the sodium–calcium exchange current. When the spontaneous depolarization is accompanied by a marked increase in dispersion of repolarization, the likelihood to trigger an arrhythmia is increased. Once triggered, the arrhythmia is maintained by a regenerative circuit of electrical activity around relatively inexcitable tissue, a phenomenon known as reentry. The development of multiple reentrant circuits within the heart causes ventricular arrhythmia, or TdP, leading to sudden cardiac death. Drugs causing TdP are considered severe cardiac toxic agents. There are several drugs that were removed from the market due to their TdP effect. These drugs include those recently removed cyclooxygenase-2 (COX-2) inhibitors, Vioxx and Bextra, which will be discussed in the "Cardiac Toxic Chemicals" section. QT prolongation effect is now a required test by the US Food and Drug Administration for drug development.

Parameters Affecting QT Prolongation and Torsadogenesis

Alterations in the function of cardiac channels or "cardiac channelopathies" occur at the cellular level. However, electrotonic cell-to-cell coupling influences the dispersion of repolarization. If myocardial cells with intrinsically different duration of action potential are well coupled, electrotonic current flow attenuates the differences in action potential duration in individual cardiomyocytes. Therefore, torsadogenesis results from not only cardiomyocytes, but also other types of cells and the interaction among these cells. There are many factors that affect the clinical manifestations of QT prolongation and torsadogenesis. Genetic polymorphisms and female gender are two distinct risk factors. The mechanism of the polymorphisms and the rationale for high susceptibility of females to QT prolongation and torsadogenesis are yet to be determined.

Drugs and Environmental Toxicants

Drug-induced QT prolongation is a major acquired long QT syndrome. Selective blockers of potassium channels, including the drugs so-called class III antiarrhythmics, have been developed for the treatment of various atrial arrhythmias. However, these drugs predictably produce long QT syndrome, which is sufficient to cause TdP in 5%–7% of recipients. Environmental exposure to PM pollution in air is a risk factor for QT prolongation in elders, children, and individuals with compromised hearts.

Disturbances in Ion Homeostasis

Hypokalemia in combination with torsadogenic drugs is a most recognized risk factor for QT prolongation and TdP. It is also shown that sodium supplementation can diminish the long QT syndrome due to the gain-of-function mutations in sodium channels. Stress-induced Ca^{2+} overload in myocardial cells increases the likelihood of arrhythmia. The electrode imbalance exerts more effect on compromised hearts.

Abnormal Gap Junction

Gap junction-mediated intercellular communication is essential in the propagation of electrical impulse in the heart. The gap junction is composed of connexons, as described in the overview of cardiac structural and physiological features section. Under normal conditions, the gap junction electrotonic current flow attenuates the differences in action potential duration of myocardial cells. Toxicological exposures cause damage to connexons leading to disruption of electrotonic cell-to-cell coupling, thus the differences in the action potential duration would be dominant, in particular under the influence of torsadogenic drugs or conditions.

Myocardial Ischemic Injury

Acute myocardial ischemia can cause immediate arrhythmia due to disturbance in ionic homeostasis, which is often transient. However, acute ischemia induces myocardial infarction that can lead to the block of cardiac conductance. Under the myocardial infarction, the areas separated by the scar tissue would be uncoupled, making the differences in the duration of action potential of myocardial cells in different regions apparent. The infarct heart thus is more susceptible to drug-induced QT prolongation and TdP.

Cardiac Hypertrophy

Purkinje fibers are derived from myogenic precursors during embryonic development. The normal distribution of Purkinje fibers in the myocardium is proportional to the mass of the heart. Cardiac hypertrophy resulting from the hypertrophic growth of cardiac myocytes would lead to unbalanced distribution of Purkinje fibers in the remodeling heart. The conduction of pacemaker potentials would thus be interrupted.

Myocardial Fibrosis

Dilated cardiomyopathy in alcoholics often involves myocardial fibrosis, which simulates the effect of myocardial infarction on the electrical conduction in the heart and block of cardiac conductance.

Heart Failure

Most individuals with failing hearts die suddenly of cardiac arrhythmias. Heart failure presents a common, acquired form of the long QT syndrome. In human heart failure, selective downregulation of two potassium channels, I_{to1} and I_{K1}, has been shown to be involved in action potential prolongation. The I_{to1} current is involved in phase 1 of the action potential and opposes the depolarization. The increase in depolarization may be adaptive in the short term because it provides more time for excitation–contraction coupling, mitigating the decrease in cardiac output. However, downregulation of potassium channels becomes maladaptive in the long term because it predisposes the individual to early afterdepolarization, inhomogeneous repolarization, and polymorphic ventricular tachycardia.

Biomarkers for Cardiac Toxicity

Myocardial injury can be divided into two major classes: structural and nonstructural injuries. The structural damage of the heart includes cell death and the associated histopathological changes such as myocardial infarction. Functional deficits often accompany the structural injury. Nonstructural damage represents functional deficits without apparent structural alterations.

Myocardial adaptation to intrinsic and extrinsic stresses leading to myocardial structural changes such as hypertrophy should be in the category of structural damage because the progression of hypertrophy leads to heart failure in which cell death is a major determinant factor. Myocardial structural changes and functional alterations can be indirectly measured by echocardiography and electrocardiogram in combination with stress testing. The data generated from these measurements can be considered in a broad sense as biomarkers. However, in clinical practice and experimental approach, biomarkers are referred to as indexes of myocardial injury measured from blood samples. The fundamental principle of the biomarkers is that molecules that are released from the myocardium under various injury conditions are readily detectable from blood samples.

Validation of Biomarkers

For a biomarker to be indicative of myocardial damage, an important question needs to be addressed is what characteristics are required for a valid biomarker. In 2000, an Expert Working Group (EWG) on biomarkers of drug-induced cardiac toxicity was established under the Advisory Committee for Pharmaceutical Sciences of the Center for Drug Evaluation and Research of the US Food and Drug Administration. The report from this EWG has summarized the characteristics of ideal cardiac toxic injury biomarkers (Wallace *et al.*, 2004). These characteristics include cardiac specificity, sensitivity, predictive value, robust, bridge preclinical to clinical, and noninvasive procedure/accessibility. These characteristics are adapted as a standard for development and validation of a biomarker of myocardial injury.

Availability of Biomarkers

Currently, validated biomarkers that are included in clinical diagnostic testing guidelines are all related to myocardial structural injury. Developing biomarkers for nonstructural injury is most challenging and demands implantation of more advanced technologies such as functional genomics and proteomics. In addition, currently available biomarkers have limitations, although they are useful.

Creatine Kinase There are three major CK isoenzymes identified; CK-MM is the principal form in skeletal muscle, CK-MB presents in myocardium in which CK-MM is also found, and CK-BB is the predominant form in brain and kidney. Elevation of serum CK-MB is considered a reasonably specific marker of acute myocardial infarction.

Myoglobin Myoglobin is found in all muscle types and its value as a biomarker of myocardial injury is based on the fact that serum concentrations of myoglobin increase rapidly following myocardial tissue injury, with peak values observed one to four hours after acute myocardial infarction. Elevation of serum myoglobin is likely reflective of the extent of myocardial damage.

B-Type Natriuretic Peptide BNP is a cardiac neurohormone secreted by the ventricular myocardium in response to volume and pressure overload, and the release of BNP appears to be directly correlated with the degree of ventricular wall tension. BNP is now accepted as a biomarker for congestive heart failure and is included in the European guidelines for the diagnosis of chronic heart failure.

C-Reactive Protein The acute phase reactant CRP is a marker of systemic and vascular inflammation, which appears to predict future cardiac events in asymptomatic individuals. In particular, inflammation has been shown to play a pivotal role in the inception, progression, and destabilization of atheromas. A predictive value of CRP for the prognosis of coronary heart disease is thus proposed. The measurement of CRP appears to provide additional prognostic information when cTnT is measured at the same time.

Cardiac Troponins Cardiac troponin T (cTnT) and I (cTnI) are constituents of the myofilaments and expressed exclusively in cardiomyocytes. It is thus of absolute myocardial tissue specificity. In healthy persons, serum cTnT or cTnI are rarely detectable. Therefore, any measurable concentrations of serum cTnT or cTnI reflect irreversible myocardial injury such as myocardial infarction. The clinical experience has arrived at a recommendation that cTn measurement becomes the "gold standard" for diagnosis of acute myocardial infarction.

Biomarker Applications and Limitations All the biomarkers described above have been used as indices of myocardial injury in clinical practice and experimental studies. The major concern of most of the biomarkers is their specificity. CK-MB is present in small quantities in skeletal muscle and other tissues, thus elevations of CK-MB occur in some diseases involving skeletal muscle injury. Myoglobin is found in all muscle types and its concentrations vary significantly between species and even within species. BNP has been proposed to use as a prognostic indicator of disease progression and outcome of congestive heart failure. However, the actual utility of this biomarker is untested. BNP is involved in the counter-regulation of heart hypertrophy, thus the changes in serum BNP concentrations as a function of time in the transition from cardiac hypertrophy to heart failure need to be understood comprehensively. Higher levels of BNP may not necessarily indicate more severity of the heart disease, indicating that more scrutiny to analysis is needed. CRP is a biomarker of inflammation, and its use in myocardial injury is more supplementary to other tests than having independently predictive value.

Considering all of the limitations above, more reliable biomarkers are needed. A significant advance in the development and validation of biomarkers for myocardial injury is the promising clinical experience with cTn, which has absolute myocardial tissue specificity and high sensitivity. cTn is now accepted by the clinical community as the biomarker of choice for assessing myocardial damage in humans. Its preclinical value for monitoring drug cardiac toxicity and in drug development needs to be evaluated.

CARDIAC TOXIC CHEMICALS

Many substances can cause cardiac toxic responses directly or indirectly. However, only chemicals that primarily act on the heart or whose cardiac toxicity is the primary concern should be categorized as cardiac toxic chemicals. Clinically, the most recognized toxicological cardiomyopathy is found in alcoholic heart muscle disease, which is often referred to as alcoholic cardiomyopathy (ACM). In this section, ACM will be discussed as a prototype of toxicological cardiomyopathy. However, cardiomyopathy induced by therapeutic drugs is also well recognized, but it is often referred to as cardiomyopathy induced by specific chemicals, such as anthracycline cardiomyopathy. In this context, the chemicals that cause cardiac toxicity can be classified in multiple ways, however, this chapter will category them into (1) pharmaceutical chemicals, (2) natural products, and (3) environmental and industrial chemicals. Because general mechanisms of cardiotoxicity have been discussed above, these cardiac toxic chemicals will be briefly discussed.

Alcohol and Alcoholic Cardiomyopathy

ACM has been recognized for a long time (Klatsky, 1998), and the prevalence of ACM in selected populations ranges from 23%

to 40% (Fauchier *et al.*, 2000; Mckenna *et al.*, 1998). Alcohol is believed to be the causal chemical in up to 40% of all patients with nonischemic, dilated cardiomyopathy (Gavazzi *et al.*, 2000). ACM is characterized by an increase in myocardial mass, dilation of the ventricles, wall thinning, ventricular dysfunction, and heart failure (Piano, 2002).

The pathogenesis of ACM is not completely understood. However, it is clear that the duration of heavy alcohol use in patients is a critical factor. Clinical data have shown that ACM typically is seen after a long term of consistent consumption of at least 80 g of alcohol per day (Regan, 1990; Lazarevic *et al.*, 2000). In general, asymptomatic ACM patients with changes in cardiac structure and function had a history of consuming >90 g per day of alcohol for more than 5 years (Lazarevic *et al.*, 2000). For the symptomatic ACM, some limited data have shown that more than 10 years of excessive alcohol consumption in alcoholics produces congestive heart failure (Mathews *et al.*, 1981).

The pathogenesis of heart failure begins after an index event such as alcohol-induced cardiac muscle injury that produces an initial decline in pumping capacity of the heart. Following this initial decline, a variety of compensatory mechanisms are activated, including the adrenergic nervous system, the renin–angiotensin system, and the cytokine system. Some of these compensatory changes have been detected in alcoholic patients (Adams and Hirst, 1986). However, with time, the sustained activation of these systems can lead to secondary end-organ damage within the ventricle by activating and accelerating the left ventricle remodeling and subsequent cardiac decompensation, resulting in the transition from asymptomatic to symptomatic heart failure (Mathews *et al.*, 1981).

It was proposed that the metabolite acetaldehyde is responsible for some of the cardiac injury associated with ethanol consumption. The metabolic enzyme responsible for the conversion of ethanol to acetaldehyde is alcohol dehydrogenase, which is absent in cardiac myocytes. Studies have indicated that the impaired liver function of alcoholics may be sufficient to generate quantities of acetaldehyde that can reach the heart. The direct effects of acetaldehyde on the myocardium include inhibition of protein synthesis, inhibition of Ca^{2+} sequestration by the SR, alterations in mitochondrial respiration, and disturbances in the association of actin and myosin. The exact mechanism of ACM is unresolved. It has been suggested that a combination of multiple factors is involved, including malnutrition, cigarette smoking, systemic hypertension, and beverage additives, in addition to a long-term consumption of alcohol in the ACM patients (Ahmed and Regan, 1992).

The generation of reactive oxidative metabolites from the biotransformation of ethanol has been suggested to be a major contributing factor for ACM, because these metabolites lead to lipid peroxidation of cardiac myocytes or oxidation of cytosolic and membraneous protein thiols (Ribiere *et al.*, 1992; Kannan *et al.*, 2004). Most experimental approaches involve alcohol-containing liquid diet feeding to rodent models of ACM for several weeks to several months. However, a key factor for the development of ACM in humans is the duration of excessive consumption of alcohol. The simulation of daily excessive amount of alcohol consumption in rodents without disturbances in food intake to produce nutritional deficiency is a constant challenge. One of the difficulties in using rodent models is that the short life span of the animals does not allow a sufficient long period of alcohol exposure to produce some of the critical pathological changes such as myocardial fibrosis observed in humans.

A recent study using a mouse model in which alcohol-induced heart hypertrophy and fibrosis were all produced may have been a breakthrough. In this mouse model, a zinc-regulatory protein,

metallothionein (MT), is genetically deleted and when zinc was exogenously added to the alcohol-containing liquid diet, alcohol-induced cardiac fibrosis, but not heart hypertrophy, in the MT knockout (MTKO) mice was prevented (Wang *et al.*, 2005). Zinc deficiency is an important feature in alcoholic patients and animal models (McClain and Su, 1983; Bogden *et al.*, 1984). Zinc homeostasis within the cell is dependent on MT, which under physiological conditions binds seven atoms of zinc (Kagi, 1991). The role of MT in the regulation of zinc homeostasis has been revealed only recently (Maret, 2000; Kang, 2006). The most important feature of MT is that under oxidative stress conditions, it releases zinc (Maret, 2000; Kang, 2006). In the MT-KO mice, alcohol-induced myocardial pathological changes are either accelerated or severely altered relative to those in WT mice. These pathological changes, in particular the myocardial fibrosis, resemble the pathology observed in patients with ACM.

There are several interesting clues that have been provided from the MT-KO mouse studies. First, the link between the deficiency in endogenously stored zinc due to the lack of MT and the alcohol-induced myocardial fibrosis is suggested by the fact that supplementation with zinc inhibits alcoholic myocardial fibrosis. Second, the dissociation between alcohol-induced heart hypertrophy and myocardial fibrosis is suggested by the fact that supplementation with zinc only inhibits fibrosis but not heart hypertrophy. Third, possible involvement of oxidative stress in the fibrogenesis is suggested by the fact that MT functions as an antioxidant (Kang, 1999) and zinc release from MT is an essential response of MT to oxidative stress (Maret, 2000; Kang, 2006), suggesting that oxidative stress is involved in the fibrogenesis. Further studies following the same direction will provide more comprehensive insights into the pathogenesis of ACM.

Pharmaceutical Chemicals

Cardiac toxicity of pharmaceutical chemicals is a major problem in drug development and their clinical application. The pharmaceutical chemicals that cause cardiac toxic responses can be simply classified as drugs that are used to treat cardiac disease, and others that are used to treat noncardiac disease. In the category of drugs used to treat cardiac disease, cardiac toxicity is often produced by overexpression of the principal pharmaceutical effects. Although overdosing of these drugs can be a major factor for untoward effects, cardiac toxicity is often inevitable for this group of drugs. Drugs such as digitalis, quinidine, and procainamide often cause acute cardiac toxicity in the form of arrhythmia, which is reversible upon cessation of their use. Other cardiac drugs may cause cardiac toxicity by mechanisms different from that of the therapeutic action. For instance, catecholamines may cause cardiac toxicity through oxidative stress, rather than by their pharmaceutical action on the sympathetic nervous system. The other category is noncardiac drugs that produce cardiac toxicity. For instance, anthracyclines, such as Adriamycin, are effective anticancer drugs, but their ability to produce severe cardiac toxicity limits their use in cancer patients. Vioxx is a selective COX-2 inhibitor used as an anti-inflammatory drug, but it causes QT prolongation and increases the risk for sudden cardiac death.

Antiarrhythmic Agents Antiarrhythmic drugs have historically been classified based upon a primary mechanism of action: Na^+ channel blockers (class I), β-adrenergic blockers (class II), drugs that prolong action potential duration, especially K^+ channel blockers (class III), and Ca^{2+} channel blockers (class IV). However, this classification is artificial because most of the drugs have multiple mechanisms of action.

Class I Antiarrhythmic Agents These are primarily Na$^+$ channel blockers, including disopyramide, encainide, flecainide, lidocaine, mexiletine, moricizine, phenytoin, procainamide, propafenone, quinidine, and tocainide. Blockade of cardiac Na$^+$ channels results in reduction of conduction velocity, prolonged QRS duration, decreased automaticity, and inhibition of triggered activity from delayed afterdepolarizations or early afterdepolarizations (Roden, 1996). The primary concern of Na$^+$ channel blocker toxicity is that proarrhythmic effects are seen at a much higher incidence in those patients with a previous history of myocardial infarction or with acute myocardial ischemia (Nattel, 1998). The proarrhythmic effects of these drugs would also be more prevalent in patients with other cardiac complications.

Class II Antiarrhythmic Drugs These are β-adrenergic receptor-blocking drugs, including acebutolol, esmolol, propranolol, and sotalol. The catecholamines increase contractility, heart rate, and conduction through activation of β-adrenergic receptors in the heart. These effects can be explained by increased adenylyl cyclase activity, increased cyclic AMP, activation of protein kinase A, and phosphorylation and activation of L-type Ca^{2+} channels, thereby increasing intracellular Ca^{2+}, and particularly the amplitude of the Ca^{2+} transient. Therefore, antagonists of β-adrenergic receptors in the heart lead to effects that are opposite that of catecholamines, and are useful for the treatment of supraventricular tachycardia. The main adverse cardiovascular effect of β-adrenergic receptor antagonists is hypotension. These drugs may also exacerbate AV conduction deficits (eg, heart block) and promote arrhythmias during bradycardia.

Class III Antiarrhythmic Drugs These are primarily K$^+$ channel blockers. These drugs include amiodarone, bretylium, dofetilide, ibutilide, quinidine, and sotalol. Blockade of K$^+$ channels increases action potential duration and increases refractoriness. Prolonged action potential duration contributes to the development of early afterdepolarizations and promotion of tachycardia, especially polymorphic ventricular tachycardia (TdP). The most noticeable adverse effect of these drugs is QT prolongation and torsadogenesis. Most of the drugs in this class also affect other ion channels and/or receptors. Amiodarone and quinidine also block Na$^+$ channels, whereas sotalol inhibits β-adrenergic receptors in the heart. Amiodarone prolongs action potential duration and effective refractory period of Purkinje fibers and ventricular myocytes, and the most common adverse cardiovascular effect of amiodarone is bradycardia. Amiodarone may also have cardiotoxic effects by stimulating excessive Ca^{2+} uptake, especially in the presence of procaine (Gotzsche and Pedersen, 1994).

Class IV Antiarrhythmic Drugs These are Ca^{2+} channel blockers and include diltiazem and verapamil. The dihydropyridine Ca^{2+} channel blockers are not used to treat arrhythmias because they have a greater selectivity for vascular cells; however, these drugs may also alter cardiac ion homeostasis when plasma concentrations of the drugs are elevated. The dihydropyridines interact with Ca^{2+} channels in the inactivated state of the channel, and because vascular smooth muscle resting potentials are lower than cardiac cells, the time spent in the inactivated state is relatively longer in vascular smooth muscle, thus providing some preference of dihydropyridines for the vasculature (Galan *et al.*, 1998). Bepridil, verapamil, and diltiazem exert negative inotropic and chronotropic effects. These drugs also exert a negative chronotropic effect, thus they may produce bradycardia. In contrast, the dihydropyridine Ca^{2+} channel blockers typically induce a reflex tachycardia subsequent to peripheral vascular dilation and baroreceptor reflex leading to increased sympathetic outflow from the medulla.

Inotropic Drugs Drugs involved in this category include the cardiac glycosides, Ca^{2+} sensitizing agents, catecholamines, and other sympathomimetic drugs. As with the antiarrhythmic drugs, inotropic drugs may exert cardiotoxic effects through extensions of their pharmacological action.

Cardiac Glycosides These (digoxin and digitoxin) are inotropic drugs used for the treatment of congestive heart failure. Ouabain is a cardiac glycoside commonly used in the laboratory for electrophysiological experiments in cardiac myocytes. The mechanism of inotropic action of cardiac glycosides involves inhibition of Na$^+$, K$^+$-ATPase, elevation of intracellular Na$^+$, activation of Na$^+$/Ca^{2+} exchange, and increased availability of intracellular Ca^{2+} for contraction. Consequently, cardiotoxicity may result from Ca^{2+} overload, potentially including reduction in resting membrane potential (less negative), delayed afterdepolarizations, and premature ventricular contraction or ectopic beats. Cardiac glycosides also exhibit parasympathomimetic activity through vagal stimulation and facilitation of muscarinic transmission; however, at higher doses, sympathomimetic effects may occur as sympathetic outflow is enhanced. The principal adverse cardiac effects of cardiac glycosides include slowed AV conduction with potential block, ectopic beats, and bradycardia. During overdose, when the resting membrane potential is significantly altered and ectopic beats are prevalent, ventricular tachycardia may develop and can progress to ventricular fibrillation. A wide variety of drug interactions with digoxin have been reported, including both pharmacokinetic interactions (drugs that alter serum concentrations of digoxin) and pharmacodynamic interactions (drugs that alter the cardiac effects of digoxin).

Ca^{2+}-Sensitizing Drugs Ca^{2+}-sensitizing drugs including adibendan, levosimendan, and pimobendan are useful as inotropic drugs for the treatment of heart failure. In contrast to the main mechanism by which many other inotropic drugs act through elevating intracellular-free Ca^{2+} ([Ca^{2+}]$_i$) during the Ca^{2+} transient (ie, increase the amplitude of the Ca^{2+} transient), these Ca^{2+}-sensitizing drugs increase Ca^{2+} sensitivity of cardiac myocytes, thereby avoiding Ca^{2+} overload (Lee and Allen, 1997). Although cardiotoxicity resulting from Ca^{2+} overload would not be expected following administration of these new drugs, some experimental data suggest that they may still exert proarrhythmic effects (Lee and Allen, 1997). The possibility that such Ca^{2+}-sensitizing drugs interfere with diastolic function (relaxation) requires further investigation but may contribute to the ventricular arrhythmias associated with these drugs. Other Ca^{2+}-sensitizing drugs include the xanthine oxidase inhibitors allopurinol and oxypurinol, which have been shown to increase contractile force but decrease Ca^{2+} transient amplitude (Perez *et al.*, 1998).

Catecholamines and Sympathomimetics Catecholamines represent a chemical class of neurotransmitters synthesized in the adrenal medulla (epinephrine and norepinephrine) and in the sympathetic nervous system (norepinephrine). These neurotransmitters exert a wide variety of cardiovascular effects. Because of their ability to activate α- and β-adrenergic receptors, especially in the cardiovascular system, a number of synthetic catecholamines have been developed for the treatment of cardiovascular disorders and other conditions such as asthma and nasal congestion. Inotropic and chronotropic catecholamines used to treat bradycardia, cardiac decompensation following surgery, or to increase blood pressure (eg, hypotensive shock) include epinephrine, isoproterenol, and dobutamine, and these drugs typically display nonselective activation of adrenergic receptors. More selective β$_2$-adrenergic receptor agonists used for bronchodilatory effects in asthma include albuterol, bitolterol, fenoterol, formoterol, metaproterenol, pirbuterol, procaterol, salmeterol, and terbutaline. High oral doses of albuterol or terbutaline or inhalation doses (ie, enhanced delivery to the stomach instead of the lungs with subsequent systemic absorption) of these drugs may lead to nonselective activation of β_1-adrenergic receptors in the heart with subsequent tachycardia.

Sympathomimetic drugs that are more selective for α-adrenergic receptors include the nasal decongestants ephedrine, phenylephrine, phenylpropanolamine, and pseudoephedrine. As with the asthma drugs, at high doses these nasal decongestants can produce tachycardia, and a number of deaths have been reported. Of particular interest is the high concentration of ephedra alkaloids that may be present in some herbal remedies or "neutraceuticals," especially in products containing ma huang (Gurley *et al.*, 1998). Tachycardia may occur from the consumption of large amounts of ephedra alkaloids, which may predispose the myocardium to ventricular arrhythmias.

High circulating concentrations of epinephrine (adrenaline) and norepinephrine (noradrenaline) and high doses of synthetic catecholamines, such as isoproterenol, may cause cardiac myocyte death. Many of the catecholamines and related drugs have been shown to induce cardiac myocyte hypertrophic growth in vitro. Catecholamine-induced cardiotoxicity involves pronounced pharmacological effects, including increased heart rate, enhanced myocardial oxygen demand, and an overall increase in systolic arterial blood pressure.

Other possible mechanisms for the cardiotoxicity of high concentrations of catecholamines include coronary insufficiency resulting from coronary vasospasm, decreased levels of high-energy phosphate stores caused by mitochondrial dysfunction, increased sarcolemmal permeability leading to electrolyte alterations, altered lipid metabolism resulting in the accumulation of FAs, and intracellular Ca^{2+} overload (Dhalla *et al.*, 1992).

Central Nervous System Acting Drugs Some of central nervous system (CNS)-acting drugs have considerable effects on the cardiovascular system, including tricyclic antidepressants (TCAs), general anesthetics, some of the opioids, and antipsychotic drugs.

TCAs including amitriptyline, desipramine, doxepin, imipramine, and protriptyline have significant cardiotoxic effects, particularly in cases of overdose. The effects of TCAs on the heart include ST segment elevation, QT prolongation, supraventricular and ventricular arrhythmias (including TdP), and sudden cardiac death. In addition, as a result of peripheral α-adrenergic blockade, TCAs cause postural hypotension—the most prevalent cardiovascular effect. Although many of these adverse effects are related to the quinidine-like actions, anticholinergic effects, and adrenergic actions of these drugs, the tricyclics also have direct actions on cardiac myocytes and Purkinje fibers, including depression of inward Na^+ and Ca^{2+} and outward K^+ currents (Pacher *et al.*, 1998). Furthermore, the risk of TCA-induced cardiotoxicity is significantly enhanced in children and by concomitant administration of other drugs that alter ion movement or homeostasis in the heart (eg, the Na^+ channel-blocking class I antiarrhythmic agents), or use in patients with cardiovascular disease.

Antipsychotic Drugs These include the phenothiazines (acetophenazine, chlorpromazine, fluphenazine, mesoridazine, perphenazine, thioridazine, and trifluoperazine), chlorprothixene, thiothixene, and other heterocyclic compounds (clozapine, haloperidol, loxapine, molindone, pimozide, and risperidone). As with TCAs, the most prominent adverse cardiovascular effect of antipsychotic drugs is orthostatic hypotension. However, the phenothiazines (eg, chlorpromazine and thioridazine) may exert direct effects on the myocardium, including negative inotropic

actions and quinidine-like effects (Baldessarini, 1996). Some ECG changes induced by these drugs include prolongation of the QT and PR intervals, blunting of T waves, and depression of the ST segment. Through anticholinergic actions, clozapine can produce substantial elevations in heart rate (tachycardia).

General Anesthetics General anesthetics as exemplified by enflurane, desflurane, halothane, isoflurane, methoxyflurane, and sevoflurane have adverse cardiac effects, including reduced cardiac output by 20%–50%, depression of contractility, and production of arrhythmias (generally benign in healthy myocardium but more serious in cardiac disease). These anesthetics may sensitize the heart to the arrhythmogenic effects of endogenous epinephrine or to β-receptor agonists. Halothane has been found to block the L-type Ca^{2+} channel by interacting with dihydropyridine-binding sites, to disrupt Ca^{2+} homeostasis associated with the SR, and to modify the responsiveness of the contractile proteins to activation by Ca^{2+} (Bosnjak, 1991). Propofol is an intravenously administered general anesthetic that also decreases cardiac output and blood pressure. In addition, propofol causes a negative inotropic effect by its direct action on cardiac myocytes. Propofol has been shown to antagonize β-adrenergic receptors, inhibit L-type Ca^{2+} current, and reduce Ca^{2+} transients (Zhou *et al.*, 1997, 1999; Guenoun *et al.*, 2000).

Local Anesthetics In general, local anesthetics have few undesirable cardiac effects. However, when high systemic concentrations of cocaine and procainamide are attained, these chemicals may have prominent adverse effects on the heart.

Cocaine This acts as a local anesthetic agent by blocking conduction in nerve fibers through reversibly inhibiting Na^+ channels and stopping the transient rise in Na^+ conductance. In the heart, cocaine decreases the rate of depolarization and the amplitude of the action potential, slows conduction speed, and increases the effective refractory period. The other major pharmacological action of cocaine is its ability to inhibit the reuptake of norepinephrine and dopamine into sympathetic nerve terminals (sympathomimetic effect). Cocaine also, indirectly through its actions on catecholamine reuptake, stimulates β- and α-adrenergic receptors, leading to increased cyclic AMP and inositol triphosphate levels. These second messengers will, in turn, provoke a rise in cytosolic Ca^{2+}, which causes sustained action potential generation and extrasystoles. The net effect of these pharmacological actions is to elicit and maintain ventricular fibrillation. In addition, cocaine causes cardiac myocyte death and myocardial infarction, but the mechanism of action remains to be elucidated.

Other Local Anesthetic Drugs These include benzocaine, bupivacaine, etidocaine, lidocaine, mepivacaine, pramoxine, prilocaine, procaine, procainamide, proparacaine, ropivacaine, and tetracaine. Lidocaine and procainamide are also used as antiarrhythmic drugs. Extremely high doses of these drugs cause decreases in electrical excitability, conduction rate, and force of contraction likely through inhibition of cardiac Na^+ channels (Catterall and Mackie, 1996).

Anthracyclines and Other Antineoplastic Agents Cardiotoxicity is recognized as a serious side effect of chemotherapy for malignant cancers, especially with well-known antitumor agents such as doxorubicin, daunorubicin, 5-fluorouracil, and cyclophosphamide (Havlin, 1992).

Anthracyclines These (doxorubicin or Adriamycin and daunorubicin) are widely used antineoplastic drugs for the treatment of breast cancer, leukemias, and a variety of other solid tumors. Unfortunately, the clinical usefulness of these drugs is limited because of acute and chronic cardiotoxic effects. The acute effects mimic anaphylactic-type responses, such as tachycardia and various arrhythmias. These effects are usually manageable and most likely are due to the potent release of histamine from mast cells sometimes observed in acute dosing. In addition, large acute doses can also cause left ventricular failure. The greatest limiting factor of the anthracyclines is associated with long-term exposure, which usually results in the development of cardiomyopathies and, in severe cases, congestive heart failure (Havlin, 1992).

Two new anthracyclines were introduced to the US market in 1999, and a lipid formulation of doxorubicin (liposomal doxorubicin) is under development. *Valrubicin* is a semisynthetic derivative of doxorubicin approved for treatment of carcinoma in situ of the bladder. It is administered locally for bladder cancer and therefore induces only mild systemic toxicities; however, systemic absorption from the bladder may occur, but valrubicin seems to exhibit a lower propensity for cardiotoxicity than doxorubicin (Hussar, 2000). *Epirubicin* is a semisynthetic derivative of daunorubicin approved for treatment of breast cancer. Like doxorubicin, epirubicin is given systemically and may induce cardiotoxicity. However, epirubicin is more lipophilic than doxorubicin and is biotransformed by conjugative pathways in the liver, resulting in a shorter half-life and a lower incidence of cardiotoxicity than with doxorubicin (Hussar, 2000).

Several major hypotheses have been suggested to account for the onset of anthracycline-induced cardiomyopathy: (1) oxidative stress from redox cycling or mitochondrial Ca^{2+} cycling, (2) defects in mitochondrial integrity and subsequent deterioration of myocardial energetics, (3) alterations in both SR Ca^{2+} currents and mitochondrial Ca^{2+} homeostasis, and (4) altered cardiac myocyte gene expression and induction of apoptosis. The cause-and-effect relationships of the proposed mechanisms of cardiotoxicity have not been determined, and no single theory adequately explains the exact mechanism for anthracycline-induced cardiomyopathy.

The free radical hypothesis has received the most attention in the understanding of anthrocycline-induced cardiotoxicity. The formation of ROS by doxorubicin (Fig. 18-16) has been attributed to redox cycling of the drug (Powis, 1989). Doxorubicin can undergo futile redox cycling that results in the production of oxygen free radicals; these ROS may then oxidize proteins, lipids, and nucleic acids and potentially cause DNA strand scission. The quinone-like structure of doxorubicin permits this molecule to accept an electron and form a semiquinone radical. Oxidation of the semiquinone back to the parent quinone by molecular oxygen results in the formation of superoxide radical ions that are believed to initiate oxidative stress. The enzymatic reduction that is believed to be responsible for the generation of superoxide by doxorubicin has been proposed to occur between complexes I and III of the mitochondrial respiratory chain. Doxorubicin has high affinity for cardiolipin, a phospholipid found on the inner mitochondrial membrane, where NADH dehydrogenase converts the drug to a semiquinone radical (Marcillat *et al.*, 1989). In the presence of oxygen, this radical is responsible for the generation of ROS, which then may peroxidize unsaturated membrane lipids and initiate myocardial cell injury.

Several alternate hypotheses to explain the cardiotoxicity of doxorubicin have been proposed and tested. For example, several studies have tested the hypothesis that doxorubicin induces a cycling of mitochondrial Ca^{2+} that is associated with the production of ROS and dissipation in the mitochondrial membrane potential, which in turn may result in depletion of cellular ATP (Chacon and Acosta, 1991; Solem *et al.*, 1994). It is important to note that the

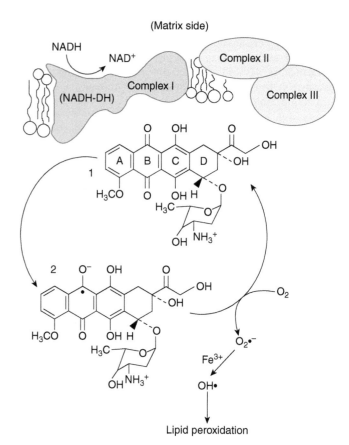

Figure 18-16. *Production of superoxide anions by oxidation–reduction cycling of doxorubicin at the level of the mitochondria.* NADH dehydrogenase (NAD-DH), which is located within complex I, has been proposed as the enzyme that catalyzes the one-electron reduction of doxorubicin (1) to a semiquinone radical (2). The semiquinone then may be reoxidized back to the parent compound by means of the reduction of molecular oxygen (O_2) to the superoxide anion (O_2^-).

observed changes in ROS accumulation, disruption of Ca^{2+} homeostasis, and mitochondrial damage are not isolated, but rather these changes occur sequentially or simultaneously. It is extremely difficult to dissect the sequences of these changes, leading to several alternate hypotheses, which may in fact occur sequentially. One of the ultimate consequences of these changes is myocardial cell death. Many studies have demonstrated that anthracycline-induced cardiotoxicity includes induction of apoptosis (Kang *et al.*, 2000a; Wang *et al.*, 2001a; Sawyer *et al.*, 1999; Andrieu-Abadie *et al.*, 1999; Arola *et al.*, 2000).

5-Fluorouracil Clinical evidence of 5-fluorouracil cardiotoxicity ranges from mild precordial pain and ECG abnormalities (ST segment elevation, high peaked T waves, T-wave inversions, and sinus tachycardia) to severe hypotension, atrial fibrillation, and abnormalities of ventricular wall motion. The mechanism of cardiotoxicity of fluorouracil is unknown, but it may relate to impurities present in commercial products of the drug, one of which is metabolized to fluoroacetate, a compound that might participate in fluorouracil-induced cardiotoxicity.

Cyclophosphamide High doses of cyclophosphamide given to cancer or transplant patients may lead to severe hemorrhagic cardiac necrosis. The mechanism of the cardiotoxicity of this drug is not clear, but there is suggestive evidence that the toxic metabolite of cyclophosphamide, 4-hydroperoxycyclophosphamide, may alter the ion homeostasis in cardiac myocytes, resulting in increased Na^+ and Ca^{2+} content and reduced K^+ levels (Levine *et al.*, 1993).

Antimicrobial and Antiviral Agents Cardiotoxicity associated with the clinical use of antimicrobial and antiviral drugs is often observed in overdosage and in patients with preexisting cardiovascular dysfunction.

Aminoglycosides These include amikacin, gentamicin, kanamycin, netilmicin, streptomycin, and tobramycin. Gentamicin is a representative aminoglycoside and has an inhibitory action on slow inward Ca^{2+} channels in heart muscle. Aminoglycosides inhibit the uptake or binding of Ca^{2+} at sarcolemmal sites, thus reducing the concentration of membrane-bound Ca^{2+} available for movement into the myoplasm during depolarization of the sarcolemma. The principle mechanism of cardiodepression by gentamicin is the dislocation of Ca^{2+} from slow-channel-binding sites on the external surface of the sarcolemma, which results in a blockade of the channels (Hino *et al.*, 1982).

Macrolides These include azithromycin, clarithromycin, dirithromycin, and erythromycin. Erythromycin is associated with QT prolongation and cardiac dysrhythmias characterized by polymorphic ventricular tachycardia (TdP). These effects occur primarily in patients with underlying cardiac disease.

Fluoroquinolones Fluoroquinolones are a group of rapid growing antibacterial chemicals in terms of numbers of new drugs released into the market in the United States. Fluoroquinolone antibacterial drugs include ciprofloxacin, enoxacin, gatifloxacin, gemifloxacin, grepafloxacin, levofloxacin (levorotatory isomer of ofloxacin), lomefloxacin, moxifloxacin, norfloxacin, ofloxacin, sparfloxacin, and trovafloxacin (Pickerill *et al.*, 2000). Grepafloxacin, moxifloxacin, and sparfloxacin are associated with QT prolongation in perhaps a higher incidence than macrolides. In fact, grepafloxacin was voluntarily removed from the US market because of the relatively high incidence of QT prolongation and risk of TdP.

Tetracycline and Chloramphenicol Tetracycline and Chloramphenicol have been reported to depress myocardial contractility by direct cardiac myocyte interaction or an indirect effect that lowers Ca^{2+} concentrations in the plasma or extracellular spaces. Tetracyclines are Ca^{2+} chelating agents, which explain the action of tetracyclines on myocardial contractility.

Antifungal Agents Antifungal agents, such as amphotericin B, may depress myocardial contractility by blocking activation of slow Ca^{2+} channels and inhibiting the influx of Na^+. Ventricular tachycardia and cardiac arrest have been reported in patients treated with amphotericin B. Flucytosine is another antifungal drug that has been associated with cardiotoxicity. In fungal cells, flucytosine is converted to 5-fluorouracil, which then exerts antifungal effects. However, flucytosine may be converted to 5-fluorouracil by gastrointestinal microflora in humans, which then may be absorbed systemically and induce cardiotoxicity as discussed above. Cardiac arrest has been reported in individuals receiving flucytosine.

Antiviral Drugs Antiviral drugs that are potentially cardiotoxic include the nucleoside analog reverse transcriptase inhibitors used for the treatment of human immunodeficiency virus (HIV) infections. Clinical studies of direct cardiotoxicity of these drugs in HIV patients are complicated by cardiomyopathy related to disease progression. The direct evidence for cardiotoxicity of zidovudine (AZT) has been obtained from a study using transgenic mice expressing replication-incompetent HIV (Lewis *et al.*, 2000). AZT-induced cardiotoxicity in this model is related to alteration in Ca^{2+} homeostasis and/or mitochondrial toxicity. The mitochondrial toxicity of AZT has also been shown in skeletal muscle biopsy samples from AIDS patients (Dalakas *et al.*, 1990).

Although cardiotoxicity of individual antiviral drugs is rare in clinical setting, the combination of several antiviral drugs for highly active antiretroviral therapy (HAART) has generated a major concern of cardiotoxicity (Bozkurt, 2004). HAART has dramatically improved the life expectancy of patients with HIV. The majority of the studies examining the incidence of cardiac effects demonstrated an increase in cardiac adverse event rate with HAART in the HIV-infected population. Overall, the cardiotoxicity risk appears to be greater in the HIV-infected population than in the general population, and the increased cardiac risk is associated with HAART, particularly with protease inhibitor use. However, there is general consensus that the benefits of HAART far outweigh toxicity-related risks of the treatment with HAART.

Anti-Inflammatory Agents Nonsteroidal anti-inflammatory drugs (NSAIDs) include aspirin, Motrin, and Naprosyn, which are classified as nonselective NSAIDs because they are inhibitors for both COX-1 and COX-2. Inhibition of COX-1 is associated with gastrointestinal toxicity because COX-1 exerts a protective effect on the lining of the stomach. A newer class of NSAIDs has been developed including rofecoxib (Vioxx), celecoxib (Celebrex), and valdecoxib (Bextra), which are selective inhibitors of COX-2. In September 2004, Vioxx was voluntarily withdrawn from the market based upon the data from a clinical trial that showed after 18 months of use Vioxx increased the relative risk for cardiovascular events, such as heart attack and stroke (Arellano, 2005). In April 2005, Bextra was removed from the market based on the potential increased risk for serious cardiovascular adverse events and increased risk of serious skin reactions (eg, toxic epidermal necrolysis, Stevens–Johnson syndrome, erythema multiforme) (Talhari *et al.*, 2005). Emerging information indicates the risk of cardiovascular events may be increased in patients receiving Celebrex (Solomon *et al.*, 2005). The cardiovascular events induced by COX-2 inhibitors are presumably related to thrombotic events. Studies have also indicated the link of Vioxx to long QT syndrome and the increased risk for TdP and sudden cardiac death (Arellano 2005; Fitzgerald 2004).

Antihistamines The most severe adverse effect of the second-generation histamine H_1 receptor antagonists (antihistamines) is their association with life-threatening ventricular arrhythmias and sudden cardiac death (Simons, 1994). Terfenadine and astemizole cause altered repolarization, notched inverted T waves, prominent TU waves, prolonged QT interval, first- and second-degree AV block, ventricular tachycardia or fibrillation, and TdP. These antihistamines produce cardiac arrhythmias by blocking the delayed rectifier K^+ channel and prolonging action potential duration in cardiac myocytes. The prolonged action potential duration promotes early afterdepolarizations and predisposes the myocardium to ventricular arrhythmias. However, terfenadine also inhibits L-type Ca^{2+} channels in rat ventricular myocytes at concentrations near or below that required to inhibit delayed rectifier K^+ current (Liu *et al.*, 1997). Therefore, both inhibition of Ca^{2+} and inhibition of K^+ current likely contribute to the cardiotoxic actions of terfenadine. As a result of cardiotoxicity, both astemizole and terfenadine have been removed from the US market. However, the understanding of astemizole- and terfenadine-induced cardiotoxicity continues to be an important consideration in drug development, and other drugs have demonstrated similar clinical limitations (eg, cisapride and fluoroquinolone antibacterial agents).

Immunosuppressants Rapamycin and tacrolimus may produce adverse cardiovascular effects, including hypertension, hypokalemia, and hypomagnesemia. Rapamycin and tacrolimus (FK506) interact with a protein that associates with ryanodine receptors (RyRs), and the protein carries the tacrolimus- or FK506-binding protein (FKBP). When rapamycin or tacrolimus binds to FKBP in cardiac myocytes, RyR becomes destabilized, resulting in Ca^{2+} leak from the SR (Marks, 1997). Tacrolimus has been shown to be associated with hypertrophic cardiomyopathy in pediatric patients, a condition that was reversed by discontinuation of tacrolimus and administration of cyclosporin A; some of these patients developed severe heart failure (Atkison *et al.*, 1995).

Miscellaneous Drugs Several drugs that are not included in the categories discussed above have significant cardiotoxic concerns and are briefly discussed below, including cisapride, methylxanthines, and sildenafil.

Cisapride Cisapride is a chemical that has been used as a prokinetic drug for gastrointestinal hypomotility. However, cisapride has been removed from the US market because of risk of potentially life-threatening arrhythmias (TdP) associated with its use. Like astemizole and terfenadine, cisapride inhibits delayed rectifier K^+ current, prolongs action potential duration, prolongs the QT interval, and predisposes the heart to ventricular arrhythmias.

Methylxanthines Methylxanthines (including caffeine, theobromine, and theophylline) can be found in significant quantities in coffee, tea, chocolate, soft drinks, and other foods. Theophylline has been used for many decades for the treatment of asthma, although the mechanism of action has not been fully understood. Overdose of theophylline or rapid intravenous administration of therapeutic doses of aminophylline (theophylline complexed with ethylenediamine to increase water solubility) may produce life-threatening ventricular arrhythmias; these effects may in part be explained by direct actions of theophylline on cardiac myocyte SR or by inhibition of phosphodiesterase and elevation of cyclic AMP. The cardiac effects of methylxanthines observed in vivo (including increases in cardiac output and heart rate) may also be explained by elevated catecholamines, as theophylline has been shown to increase plasma epinephrine concentrations (Vestal *et al.*, 1983). High concentrations of caffeine stimulate massive release of Ca^{2+} from the SR, an effect that is often utilized experimentally to determine SR function. Although it rarely occurs, caffeine-associated ventricular arrhythmias have been reported.

Sildenafil Sildenafil is a relatively specific inhibitor of phosphodiesterase-5, which is responsible for the degradation of cyclic guanosine monophosphate (cGMP; a vasodilatory second messenger). Interestingly, sildenafil was originally developed as a potential drug for treating angina; however, it was not very effective for this purpose and was subsequently developed for treatment of erectile dysfunction, where it produces vasodilation and filling of the corpus cavernosum. The primary concern regarding adverse effects of sildenafil is nonspecific inhibition of PDE3 in the heart and vasculature (Hussar, 1999). In vitro studies have revealed that sildenafil increases cyclic AMP in cardiac tissue without significant effects on cGMP (Stief *et al.*, 2000); however, whether these effects are associated with cardiotoxicity is not known.

Natural Products

Natural products include naturally occurring catecholamines, hormones, and cytokines, as well as animal and plant toxins. Many of these products have been shown to cause cardiac toxic responses. However, it is difficult to define whether or not the cardiac toxicity results directly from the action of these products in vivo, although these products cause deleterious effects on cultured cardiomyocytes. The exposure levels of these chemicals tested in vitro in general are much higher than the concentration reached in cardiac tissue under in vivo exposure conditions. Therefore, extrapolation

of in vitro data related to cardiac toxicity of natural products to in vivo conditions is challenging. However, there are some products that have clearly demonstrated cardiac toxic effects, and mechanisms of action of these products have been determined.

Catecholamines The naturally occurring sympathomimetic amines, such as epinephrine and norepinepherine, are potent and can cause deleterious effects to the heart. The synthetic catecholamine, isoproterenol, is able to cause massive necrotic changes in the myocardium and is often used as a prototype compound for the study of catecholamine cardiotoxicity, which has been discussed in the therapeutic drugs that cause cardiotoxicity.

Steroids and Related Hormones Estrogens, progestins, androgens, and adrenocortical steroids are major steroid hormones produced by mammals including humans. Myocardial tissue contains steroid receptors; therefore, the heart serves as a target organ for steroid effects. It also has been shown that cardiac tissue can synthesize steroid hormones, although the capacity for synthesis may be much lower than more classic steroid synthesizing tissues. There are two major mechanisms of action of the hormones: the first is to alter gene expression and the second is to change signaling transduction pathways.

Estrogens Estrogens are synthesized in ovaries, testes, and adrenal glands, and estrogen is an active metabolite of testosterone. Endogenous estrogens include 17β-estradiol (E_2), estrone, and estriol. Synthetic estrogens include diethylstilbestrol (nonsteroidal), equilin, esterified versions of E_2, ethinyl estradiol, mestranol, and quinestrol. In addition, many other synthetic chemicals have been shown to exert estrogenic activity, including the pesticides DDT and methoxychlor, the plasticizer bisphenol A, other industrial chemicals including polychlorinated biphenyls, and some compounds found in soybeans and tofu (eg, phytoestrogens). Estrogens (frequently in combination with progestins) have been used for over 40 years as oral contraceptive drugs. The older versions of estrogenic oral contraceptives that contained high amounts of estrogens were associated with increased risk of coronary thrombosis and myocardial infarction; however, lower doses of estrogens have been found by numerous investigators to impart protective effects on the cardiovascular system, including antiapoptotic effects, and beneficial effects on lipid metabolism such as decreased low-density lipoproteins (LDL cholesterol) and increased high-density lipoproteins (HDL cholesterol). Estrogens alter cardiac fibroblast proliferation, but they can either increase or decrease proliferation of these cells.

Progestins Progestins are also synthesized in the ovaries, testes, and adrenal glands. Naturally occurring and synthetic progestins include desogestrel, hydroxyprogesterone, medroxyprogesterone, norethindrone, norethynodrel, norgestimate, norgestrel, and progesterone. As part of hormone replacement therapy, progestins serve an opposing role to estrogens. Unfortunately, estrogen treatment opposed with progestins may negate the cardiovascular benefits of estrogens on lipid metabolism (Kalin and Zumoff, 1990). Very little is known about the direct effects of progestins on the heart. Although progestins could exert deleterious effects on the heart, more studies are required to investigate mechanisms.

Androgens Androgens cause adverse cardiovascular effects (Rockhold, 1993; Melchert and Welder, 1995). The principal androgens are testosterone and its active metabolite dihydrotestosterone. Testosterone is synthesized in the testes, ovaries, and adrenal glands, and dihydrotestosterone mediates most androgen actions. Synthetic anabolic-androgenic steroids include the alkylated and orally available drugs danazol, fluoxymesterone, methandrostenolone, methenolone, methyltestosterone, oxandrolone, oxymetholone, and stanozolol. The nonalkylated drugs with poor oral bioavailability include androstenedione and dehydroepiandrosterone (both sold in various "nutraceutical" formulations), boldenone (veterinary product), nandrolone (19-nortestosterone), and testosterone. Nearly all of these chemicals have received significant illicit use, particularly in extremely high doses with attempts to improve physical appearance or performance. Anabolic-androgenic steroids have been associated with alterations in lipid metabolism, including increased LDL cholesterol and decreased HDL cholesterol; therefore, these chemicals may predispose individuals to atherosclerosis (Melchert and Welder, 1995). Evidence indicating the direct cardiac toxic effect of anabolic-androgenic steroids includes alteration of Ca^{2+} fluxes in cardiac myocytes induced by testosterone (Koenig et al., 1989), hypertrophic growth of neonatal rat cardiac myocytes stimulated by testosterone and dihydrotestosterone (Marsh et al., 1998), and mitochondrial abnormalities and myofibrillar lesions induced by methandrostenolone given intramuscularly to rats (Behrendt and Boffin, 1977). In humans, high-dose anabolic-androgenic steroid use has been associated with cardiac hypertrophy and myocardial infarction. However, the mechanisms responsible for the cardiotoxic effects of anabolic-androgenic steroids remain poorly understood.

Glucocorticoids and Mineralocorticoids Glucocorticoids and mineralocorticoids are primarily synthesized in the adrenal glands. Naturally occurring glucocorticoids include corticosterone, cortisone, and hydrocortisone (cortisol), and the mineralocorticoid is aldosterone. A large number of synthetic glucocorticoids are used for treatment of various autoimmune and inflammatory diseases. These drugs include alclometasone, amcinonide, beclomethasone, betamethasone, clobetasol, desonide, desoximetasone, dexamethasone, diflorasone, fludrocortisone, flunisolide, fluocinolone, fluocinonide, fluorometholone, flurandrenolide, halcinonide, medrysone, methylprednisolone, mometasone, paramethasone, prednisolone, prednisone, and triamcinolone. Most of these drugs are primarily used topically, intranasally, or inhalationally. The primary glucocorticoids used systemically include cortisone, hydrocortisone, dexamethasone, methylprednisolone, prednisolone, and prednisone. The mineralocorticoid aldosterone is not used clinically; however, the aldosterone receptor antagonist spironolactone has been used for years to treat hypertension and is now thought to decrease morbidity and mortality associated with congestive heart failure. Both aldosterone and glucocorticoids appear to stimulate cardiac fibrosis by regulating cardiac collagen expression independently of hemodynamic alterations (Young et al., 1994; Robert et al., 1995). Furthermore, aldosterone and glucocorticoids induce hypertrophic growth and alter expression of Na^+, K^+-ATPase, Na^+/H^+ antiporter, and chloride/bicarbonate exchanger of cardiac myocytes in vitro. Clinically relevant cardiac hypertrophy has been observed in premature infants undergoing dexamethasone treatment. The mechanisms responsible for the direct effects of these chemicals remain poorly understood.

Thyroid Hormones These include thyroxine (T_4) and triiodothyronine (T_3). These hormones exert profound effects on the cardiovascular system. Hypothyroid states are associated with decreased heart rate, contractility, and cardiac output; whereas hyperthyroid states are associated with increased heart rate, contractility, cardiac output, ejection fraction, and heart mass. Patients with underlying cardiovascular disease may display arrhythmias under the treatment of thyroid hormones. Thyroid hormones also alter expression of cardiac SR Ca^{2+} handling proteins including increased expression of SR Ca^{2+} ATPase (SERCA) and decreased expression of phospholamban, an inhibitory protein of SERCA (Kaasik et al., 1997).

Cytokines More than 100 different cytokines have been found, and the cardiovascular effects of these substances can be classified as proinflammatory, anti-inflammatory, or cardioprotective (Pulkki, 1997). Members of the proinflammatory class include TNF-α; interleukin-1β (IL-1β), interleukin-2 (IL-2), interleukin-6 (IL-6), interleukin-8 (IL-8), Fas ligand, and chemokines (eg, CC chemokines such as MCP-1, macrophage chemoattractant protein-1; MIP-1α, macrophage inflammatory protein-1α; and RANTES, regulated on activation normally T-cell-expressed and secreted). Members of the anti-inflammatory class typically downregulate expression of proinflammatory cytokines and include interleukin-4 (IL-4), interleukin-10 (IL-10), interleukin-13 (IL-13), and transforming growth factor-beta (TGF-β). The cardioprotective cytokines include cardiotrophin-1 (CT-1) and leukemia inhibitor factor, which have been shown to inhibit cardiac myocyte apoptosis from a number of different stimuli. Many of these cytokines are elevated during cardiovascular diseases such as I/R injury, myocardial infarction, and congestive heart failure.

IL-1β IL-1β is known to exert negative inotropic actions and induce apoptosis of cardiac myocytes. The effects of IL-1β on cardiac myocytes are likely mediated through induction of nitric oxide synthase (NOS) and/or increased production of nitric oxide (NO) (Arstall et al., 1999). Superoxide anion and peroxynitrite formation was associated with reduced left ventricular ejection fraction in dogs treated with microspheres containing IL-1β, suggesting that involvement of peroxynitrite in IL-1β cardiotoxicity (Cheng et al., 1999b).

TNF-α TNF-α induces apoptotic cell death in myocardium (Krown et al., 1996). The mechanisms responsible for TNF-α-induced apoptosis of cardiac myocytes are not entirely clear. TNF-α also exerts negative inotropic effects on cardiac myocytes at least potentially through increased production of sphingosine (Sugishita et al., 1999). However, it has been shown that TNF-α is essential for the cardiac protective response to stresses such as ischemic cardiac injury (Kurrelmeyer et al., 2000).

IL-6 IL-6 has been shown to induce negative inotropic effects on cardiac myocytes, possibly through induction of NOS expression and increased NO production (Sugishita et al., 1999).

IL-2 IL-2 may decrease the mechanical performance and metabolic efficiency of the heart, and these myocardial effects may be related to changes in NO synthesis and Na^+/H^+ exchange.

Interferon Interferon may result in cardiac arrhythmias, dilated cardiomyopathy, and signs of myocardial ischemia. Interferon-γ acts synergistically with IL-1β to increase NO formation in the heart, and induce Bax expression and apoptosis in cardiac myocyte cultures (Arstall et al., 1999).

Animal and Plant Toxins Animal toxins in the venom of snakes, spiders, scorpions, and marine organisms have profound effects on the cardiovascular system. There are also a number of plants—such as foxglove, oleander, and monkshood—that contain toxic constituents and have adverse effects on the cardiovascular system.

Environmental Pollutants and Industrial Chemicals

There are many chemicals classified in this category that cause cardiac toxicity. Metals and metalloids can be found both in environmental pollutants and industrial chemicals. Some heavy metals, such as cadmium, block calcium channels that affect cardiac rhythm leading to arrhythmia, others such as arsenic have high affinity for sulfhydryl groups, and interfere with sulfhydryl-containing proteins, such as receptors, regulatory proteins, and transporters. During the last decade, epidemiological and experimental studies have identified an association of air pollution of PMs and cardiac toxicity, however, mechanistic insights into cardiac toxicity induced by PM remain elusive. In this section, a brief discussion of selected industrial agents with their prominent cardiotoxic effects and proposed mechanisms of cardiotoxicity is presented. For a more comprehensive review of industrial chemicals and their cardiotoxic potential, the reader is referred to the study of Zakhari (1992).

Particulate Matters There are several obstacles in the systemic study of cardiac toxicity caused by particulate air pollution. One of the major challenges is the complexity of the particulate components of air pollution. Current consensus in the field is to divide the airborne particulates into classes according to aerodynamic diameters. There are three major classes: coarse (PM_{10}, 2.5–10 μm), fine ($PM_{2.5}$, <2.5 μm), and ultrafine ($PM_{0.1}$, <0.1 μm). However, ambient air PM consists of a mixture of combustive by-products and resuspended crystal materials, of which the contents are highly related to geographic regions. Thus studying mechanisms by which particulate air pollution causes cardiovascular toxicity is extremely challenging, although attempts have been made to provide insights into the mechanistic link between particulate air pollution and cardiac toxicity. The documented cardiac toxic effects of particulate air pollution have been limited to electrocardiographic changes, including arrhythmia, decreased heart rate variability, and the exacerbation of ST-segment changes in experimental models of myocardial infarction.

Solvents Industrial solvents can exert adverse effects on the heart directly or indirectly; both are related to their inherent lipophilicity. Solvents may affect cardiac physiological functions such as contraction and energy production by directly dispersing into plasma membranes. However, the effects of solvents on the heart would be more related to their actions on the neurohormonal regulation of cardiac function. Solvents may disrupt sympathetic and parasympathetic control of the heart as well as cause release of circulating hormones such as catecholamines, vasopressin, and serotonin, which in turn affects cardiac function.

Alcohols and Aldehydes On a molar basis, there is a relationship between increased carbon chain length of the alcohol and cardiotoxicity. Metabolic oxidation of alcohols yields aldehydes. Aldehydes have sympathomimetic activity as a result of their effect on releasing catecholamines. Unlike alcohols, the sympathomimetic activity of aldehydes decreases with increased chain length. The acute cardiodepressant effects of alcohols and aldehydes may be related to inhibition of intracellular Ca^{2+} transport and/or generation of oxidative stress. Chronic alcoholic cardiotoxicity is more related to a long-term consumption of alcohol, referred to as ACM, which was discussed above. The environmental exposure to alcohols is more related to acute cardiotoxicity, including a negative dromotropic effect (reduced conductivity) and a decreased threshold for ventricular fibrillation. The common industrial alcohols include methanol (methyl alcohol or wood alcohol) and isopropyl alcohol (isopropanol). Methanol is metabolized by alcohol dehydrogenase and aldehyde dehydrogenase to formaldehyde and formic acid, and often causes reduction in heart rate. Isopropanol is metabolized to acetone, and both isopropanol and its metabolite are potent CNS depressants. Acetone is metabolized to formic acid and acetic acid, which have the potential to induce mild acidosis. Tachycardia is the most prominent clinical finding of isopropanol exposure.

Halogenated Alkanes The highly lipophilic nature of halogenated alkanes allows them to cross the blood–brain barrier readily. This action, coupled with their CNS-depressant activity, makes these compounds ideally suited for anesthetics (halothane, methoxyfluorane, and enflurane). Halogenated hydrocarbons depress heart rate, contractility, and conduction. In addition, some of these agents sensitize the heart to the arrhythmogenic effects of β-adrenergic receptor agonists such as endogenous epinephrine. Fluorocarbons (freons) have been reported to have this sensitizing effect on the myocardium. Chronic exposure to halogenated hydrocarbons may cause myocardial degenerative response.

Metals and Metalloids The most common heavy metals that have been associated with cardiotoxicity are cadmium, lead, and cobalt. These metals exhibit negative inotropic and dromotropic effects and can also produce structural changes in the heart. Chronic exposure to cadmium has been reported to cause cardiac hypertrophy. Lead has an arrhythmogenic sensitizing effect on the myocardium. In addition, lead has been reported to cause degenerative changes in the heart. Cobalt has been reported to cause cardiomyopathy. The cardiotoxic effects of heavy metals are attributed to their ability to form complexes with intracellular macromolecules and their ability to antagonize intracellular Ca^{2+}.

Other metals that have been reported to affect cardiac function are manganese, nickel, and lanthanum. Their mechanism of action appears to block Ca^{2+} channels. However, high concentrations are required to block Ca^{2+} channels (eg, millimolar range). Barium is another metal that can affect cardiac function. Barium chloride given intravenously in high doses to laboratory animals has been reported to induce arrhythmias. This arrhythmogenic effect of barium chloride has been utilized to screen antiarrhythmic agents.

Arsenic is a metalloid, which has been shown to cause cardiotoxicity directly. Arsenic has a high affinity for sulfhydryl proteins, which are involved in multiple cellular metabolism and function. Besides environmental exposure to arsenic such as through drinking water contamination, therapeutic use of arsenic in the form of arsenic trioxide for the treatment of acute promyelocytic leukemia (APL) is another important route of exposure. Clinical reports have shown serious ventricular tachycardia at the therapeutic doses of arsenic trioxide in APL patients. Experimental studies using a dose regiment that has been shown to produce plasma concentrations of arsenic within the range of those present in arsenic-treated APL patients have shown that arsenic causes myocardial cell death through apoptosis, and results in decreased systolic and diastolic function of the heart (Li *et al.*, 2002).

OVERVIEW OF VASCULAR SYSTEM

Vascular Physiology and Structural Features

The vascular system consists of blood vessels of varying size and different cellular composition. Blood vessels can be divided into arterial, venous, and capillary systems. In addition, the lymphatic system belongs to the vascular system, but it only carries plasma. Although blood is the content of the vascular system and changes in the status of blood and circulation are associated with the functional alteration and toxicity of the vascular system, the blood is not included in this chapter because Chap. 11 specifically addresses the toxic responses of the blood. The main function of the vascular system is to provide oxygen and nutrients to and remove carbon dioxide and metabolic products from organ systems (Fig. 18-17). In addition, the vascular system is a conduit that delivers hormones and cytokines to target organs. The vascular system also has regulatory functions to manipulate organ system responses under certain

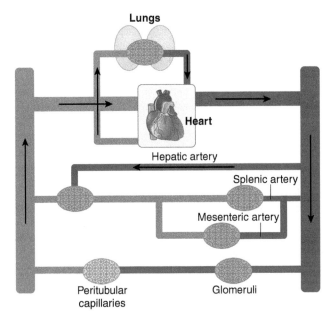

Figure 18-17. *Schematic diagram of vascular supply to selected organs.* The capillary beds represented by a meshwork connecting the arteries (right) with the veins (left); the distribution of the vasculature in several organs (liver, kidney, and lung) indicates the importance of the vascular system in toxicology.

toxicological conditions. For instance, endothelins produced by vascular endothelial cells alter cardiac rhythm and affect myocardial contractility. Many regulatory systems control the physiological function of the vascular system, so that the changes in the vascular system reflect either local action of chemicals or disruption of the regulatory systems, or both. The distinction between primary and secondary vascular toxic responses is challenging. To better understand the toxic responses of the vascular system, the following presents an overview of physiology and regulatory mechanism of the vascular system.

Arterial System and Physiological Function The arterial system is composed of the aorta, major arteries, and small arterioles. The aorta and major arteries are thick-walled structures with vascular smooth muscle, elastic, and connective tissues (Fig. 18-18). Blood flow within the arterial system is initiated by contraction of the heart and begins at the ascending aorta. The ascending aorta receives all of the output of the heart with the exception of the coronary blood flow. Blood is distributed to the organ systems of the

body through the major arteries that branch from the aorta. All these arteries further branch to give rise to smaller arteries and become arterioles that connect to capillaries for the delivery of oxygen and nutrients to target tissues.

The Aorta and Large Arteries The aorta and the large arteries provide supporting structures and maintain the blood flow from the heart to the target organs. Therefore, these vessels function primarily as conduits. The driving force for the blood flow is derived from the contraction of the heart and the elasticity of the aorta and large arteries under the regulation of the neurohormonal system and the resistance of the target organs. Chemicals can affect directly the arterial systems leading to alterations in blood flow or indirectly act through the regulatory system to change the blood flow.

Arterioles and Vascular Resistance The arterioles are composed of a tube of endothelial cells, surrounded by connective tissue basement membrane, a single or double layer of vascular smooth muscle cells, and a thin outer adventitial layer. The vascular smooth muscle cells are critical for the regulation of vascular resistance. The tension developed by the vascular smooth muscle cells alters the vessel diameter. Therefore, arterioles are primarily responsible for regulation of peripheral vascular resistance and blood flow. Chemicals affecting the structure and function of the vascular smooth muscle cells can thus change the physiological regulation of the vascular resistance, leading to excess dilation or restriction.

Coronary Arteries and Circulation Coronary arteries branch from the aorta immediately past the mitral valve. Supply of oxygen and nutrients to the heart is primarily supported by the coronary arteries. The coronary blood flow can increase about fourfold to supply additional oxygen needed by the heart muscle under demanding conditions, such as during exercise. However, even when the body is at rest, the oxygen supply through the coronary arteries to the heart is more than the supply to an equal mass of skeletal muscle during vigorous exercise. Heart tissue extracts most of the oxygen from blood during resting conditions, and the coronary blood flow increases with the workload demands on the heart. The increase in blood flow is the major mechanism of the heart to increase energy production. Coronary vasculature disruption both anatomically and physiologically leads to reduction in cardiac blood flow and cardiac work, which is an important effect of xenobiotics. In fact, pathology of the coronary vasculature is the cause of death in about one-third of the population in industrialized societies. Recent studies indicate that PMs in the air are associated with coronary heart disease (Dockery, 2001; Gordon and Reibman, 2000).

Capillaries and Microcirculation Capillaries directly connect to the distal portion of the arterioles serving as the communication site between blood and tissues, and constitute the major part of the microcirculation where nutrients, water, gases, hormones, cytokines, and waste products are exchanged between blood and tissues. In other parts of the vascular system, blood is separated from tissues by the walls of arterial and venous vessels. In contrast, capillaries are only one cell layer thick. The passage of molecules through the capillary wall can occur both between and through the endothelial cells. Lipid-soluble molecules such as oxygen and carbon dioxide readily pass through the endothelial cell membranes. Water-soluble molecules diffuse between endothelial cells. The other pathway for water-soluble molecules is the cell membrane vesicle formation via pinocytosis (inward) and exocytosis (outward) on both the luminal and the tissue side of the capillary wall. This pathway can transfer even the largest molecules. The endothelial cells are targets of xenobiotics, whose effects can be measured by accumulation of toxic metabolites

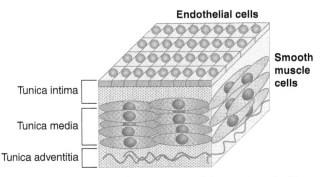

Figure 18-18. *Cross-sectional representation of the vascular wall of large and medium-size blood vessels.* The tunica intima is composed of endothelial cells, facing the vessel lumen, which rest on a thin basal lamina. The tunica media consists mainly of vascular smooth muscle cells interwoven with collagen and elastin. The tunica adventia is a layer of fibroblasts, collagen, elastin, and glycosaminoglycans.

in the target organs and the pathophysiological changes in the microcirculation.

In general, there is some capillary reserve in tissues so that a particular area of a tissue can be perfused by more than one capillary, but not all of the capillaries open up at any given time. This capillary reserve serves two important functions: one is to meet the increase in metabolic demands. Under the condition that metabolic demands increase, more capillaries can open up. The other is to compensate for lesions or disruption of certain capillaries. For instance, if an occlusion occurs due to a thrombus, capillaries in close proximity can open to provide perfusion to the vulnerable area. However, in the brain, this capillary reserve appears absent so that any occlusion may result in damage.

Venous System and Physiological Function The venous system is composed of venules, veins, and vena cava. The blood flow in the venous system starts from the thin-walled venules that collect the blood from the target tissues of the body. These vessels have a relatively large surface area facilitating the reabsorption of filtered plasma from the tissue. The venules merge to veins and eventually drain into the vena cava, returning blood to the heart. Therefore, the important physiological function of the venous system is collecting blood from organ systems of the body and returning the blood to the heart. The other important function of the venous system is the capacitance of the circulatory system. This is an important protective mechanism of the circulatory system. The large veins contain vascular smooth muscle cells that can increase the blood return to the heart by constriction and increase the capacitance by dilation. If hemorrhage occurs, the circulatory system can rapidly adjust the capacitance and maintain perfusion of the tissues. Xenobiotics can exert adverse effects on the vascular smooth muscle cells so that the capacitance function of the venous system can be compromised.

Lymphatic System and Physiological Function Lymphatic vessels are endothelial tubes within tissues. The lymphatic system begins as blind-ended lymphatic end bulbs that drain into a meshwork of interconnected lymphatic vessels. This is a low-pressure system that collects excess tissue water and plasma proteins that have not been reabsorbed by the venous system. In general, in all organ systems with the exception of the CNS, more fluid is filtered than reabsorbed by the venous system. Therefore, removal of the excess fluid as well as plasma proteins that diffuse into the interstitial spaces by the lymphatic system is essential. All the lymphatics ultimately drain into the vena cava. Therefore, the physiological function of the lymphatic system is to maintain a negative interstitial pressure by removing any excess fluid and plasma proteins. Toxic insults to the lymphatic system can lead to elevated interstitial pressures and subsequent tissue edema.

Regulatory Mechanisms of the Vascular System

The vascular system includes conduits and microcirculation. This system under physiological conditions is regulated by the demands of tissue metabolism. The mechanisms controlling vascular physiology can be divided into neural, hormonal, and local controls. However, this categorization is artificial because the performance of the vascular system at any given time is the result of the integration of all three controlling mechanisms, and each of the three mechanisms affects the other two. The controlling mechanisms can be divided into remote or systemic, and local regulation. The remote regulation includes both neural and hormonal mechanisms.

Neurohormonal Regulation Most arteries, arterioles, venules, and veins, with the exception of those of the external genitalia, receive sympathetic innervation only. Norepinephrine is the usual transmitter that binds to α_1-adrenergic receptors. These receptors are distributed to vascular smooth muscle cells, and activation of the receptors leads to contraction of the vascular smooth muscle and thus the constriction of blood vessels. There are also β_2-adrenergic receptors in vascular smooth muscle cells, to which binds the circulating epinephrine released from the adrenal medulla. Activation of the β_2-adrenergic receptors leads to vascular smooth muscle relaxation and vasodilation. Coronary and skeletal muscle arteries are highly responsive to the epinephrine-induced vasodilation. In addition, the blood vessels of skeletal muscles receive sympathetic cholinergic innervation in addition to their sympathetic adrenergic innervation, whose activation leads to vascular smooth muscle relaxation and vasodilation. The CNS regulates the activity of the autonomic nerves at several levels. Interactions between the central and autonomic nerves take place in the spinal cord, medulla, and hypothalamus. These central nervous regulations are reviewed in many physiology textbooks and not covered in this chapter.

There are many hormones that control the vascular system. Catecholamines, renin–angiotensin–aldosterone, antidiuretic hormone (ADH), and atrial natriuretic peptide (ANP) are important hormones that affect the vascular system and will be briefly reviewed.

Catecholamines *Catecholamines* are primarily secreted from the adrenal medulla. During the activation of the sympathetic nervous system, the adrenal medulla releases epinephrine (>90%) and norepinephrine (<10%) into the blood. As discussed above, the increase in circulating epinephrine activates the β_2-adrenergic receptors localized in the coronary and skeletal muscle arteries leading to vascular smooth muscle relaxation and vasodilation. This occurs during defense and exercise.

The Renin–Angiotensin–Aldosterone System This is critically involved in the regulation of blood pressure and volume. Renin is released from the kidney in response to reduced arterial pressure and blood volume, which catalyzes the conversion of a plasma protein angiotensinogen to angiotensin I. Angiotensin I is further converted to angiotensin II by an angiotensin-converting enzyme. Angiotensin II is a powerful arteriolar vasoconstrictor and also causes the release of aldosterone from the adrenal cortex. One of the important actions of the aldosterone is to reduce renal sodium excretion, resulting in retention of water and increase in blood volume.

ADH ADH is released from the posterior pituitary gland under the control of the hypothalamus. ADH is a vasoconstrictor but is not present in plasma in high concentrations under physiological conditions. However, ADH release is increased under the conditions of hemorrhage, decreased atrial stretch receptor firing, and increased plasma osmolarity. The effect of ADH on the vascular system is to increase the retention of water by the kidney, and thus increasing blood volume.

ANP is released from atrial muscle cells when they are stimulated by stretch. ANP increases the excretion of sodium so that it decreases the blood volume. Therefore, ANP regulation of blood volume is a counter-regulatory mechanism of the renin–angiotensin–aldosterone system and ADH.

Local Metabolic Regulation The local regulation of the vascular system is primarily referred to as the control of microcirculation. The microcirculation is also controlled by the above neurohormonal system. This section will focus on the local metabolic regulation of microcirculation. In addition, chemicals released from endothelial cells are major local regulators of microcirculation and highly toxicologically relevant.

Oxygen is a major regulator of microcirculation. Oxygen is not stored in the end organs, and has to be replenished constantly from the blood flow. Therefore, change in metabolic rate in the end organ will require a parallel change in oxygen supply from the blood flow. The change in oxygen tension signals vascular muscles to relax or constrict. The vascular smooth muscle is not sensitive enough to respond to changes in oxygen tension except for extremely low or high oxygen tensions. However, decrease in oxygen tension along with increases in metabolic rate causes the release of adenine nucleotides, free adenosine, and Krebs cycle intermediates. In addition, lactic acid accumulates under hypoxia conditions. All these cause vasodilation at physiological concentrations.

An important mechanism of local regulation of microcirculation is the substance released by endothelial cells, endothelium-derived relaxing factor. This substance is NO generated from arginine by NOS. The mechanism of action of the endothelium-derived relaxing factor involves the increase in cGMP and the subsequent activation of intracellular signaling pathways leading to relaxation of vascular smooth muscle cells. The endothelium-derived relaxing factor also suppresses platelet activation and reduces adhesion of leukocytes to endothelial cells.

VASCULAR SYSTEM TOXIC RESPONSES
Mechanisms of Vascular Toxicity

The effects of chemicals on the vascular system have been studied for some time, but the significance of the toxic responses of this system in affecting physiological function and pathogenesis of other organ systems is not fully understood. The potential effects of vascular toxicity on overall health and disease status are most likely underestimated. All chemicals, after absorption, contact the vascular system. Vascular endothelial cells are the immediate targets of the chemicals and are of the most frequent risk for toxic insults. These cells are the major component of the microcirculation system. Vascular smooth muscle cells are the next important targets of the chemicals.

Responses of Vascular Endothelial Cells to Toxic Insults
Vascular endothelial cells play a critical role in both vascular protection from toxic insults and triggering detrimental cascade in response to toxic insults. Damage to vascular endothelial cells is a critical starting point for vascular injury. In response to toxic insults, production of NO and ROS increases in endothelial cells. Substances mimicking agonists activate the receptors on the endothelial cells and trigger intracellular signaling transduction, leading to activation of nuclear factor kappa-B (NFκB) and MAPK activity. The downstream signaling transduction pathways triggered by NFκB, MAPK, NO, and ROS then activate gene expression and regulate posttranslational modification of proteins leading to cytoprotective action against toxic insults, or the production of cytokines, chemokines, and adhesion molecules to protect the circulatory system and the affected organ systems.

Angiogenesis is an adaptive response to damages that follow toxic insults. This process helps form new blood vessels and deliver nutrients and oxygen to damaged tissue to repair the lesion. Vascular endothelial cells are both central to initiating and promoting the formation of new blood vessels and essential for blood vessel formation by forming initial tube-like structures. Xenobiotics can both promote and suppress angiogenesis, and the primary target is the vascular endothelial cell. Apoptosis is a major mechanism for cell death of the vascular endothelial cells and mechanisms and molecular signaling pathways leading to apoptosis are basically the same as described for cardiomyocytes. Until recently, it was thought that preexisting endothelial cells are the sole cellular source for angiogenesis in adults. Recent results indicate the existence of endothelial progenitor cells. The injured endothelial monolayer can be regenerated by circulating bone marrow-derived endothelial progenitor cells, which accelerates re-endothelialization and limits atherosclerotic lesion formation. These endothelial progenitor cells may be important targets of xenobiotics, although no data are available.

Lesions to endothelial cells can result in atherosclerosis. Injury to endothelial cells results in increased production of endothelin-1 (ET-1) and increased release of prostacyclins. The endothelial cells are also involved in the recruitment of inflammatory cells to the lesion site. Activated lymphocytes secrete cytokines, such as TGF-β, which leads to a cascade of signaling transduction and a series of injurious responses including deposition of collagen.

ET-1 secreted by endothelial cells is a major mediator of vascular toxicity. ET is a peptide composed of 21 amino acids, derived from a large precursor, the big-ET, by the action of the endothelin-converting enzyme family. There are three isoforms of ET that have been identified, ET-1, ET-2, and ET-3. ET-1 is produced mainly by vascular endothelial cells and acts through two receptor subtypes, ET-A and ET-B. The ET receptors belong to the G-protein-coupled family. ET-1 is a potent vasoconstrictive chemical and plays an important role in the maintenance of vascular tone and blood pressure in healthy subjects. ET-1 contributes to the pathogenesis of myocardial disease. In failing hearts, activation of the ET system occurs; myocardial tissue levels of ET-1 are increased along with increased density of ET receptors, mainly in the form of ET-A due to upregulation in the myocardium (Ito et al., 1993). In addition, circulating levels of both ET-1 and big-ET-1 are elevated in the patients with failing hearts. The elevation in serum levels of ET-1 thus has been used as an important marker of heart failure in humans (Monge, 1998). ET-1 mediated myocardial response is involved in air pollution PM-induced cardiac toxicity (Bouthillier et al., 1998).

Responses of Smooth Muscle Cells to Toxic Insults
The consequence of damage to vascular smooth muscle cells involves changes in the vascular tone and atherosclerosis. Receptors localized on the plasma membrane of smooth muscle cells mediate the environmental changes and change the contractility of the blood vessels. The activation of these receptors leads to signaling transduction and changes in calcium conductance. Elevation of intracellular calcium activates the contractile apparatus, leading to alteration of vascular tone. Toxic substances influence calcium homeostasis in multiple ways. Calcium homeostasis is regulated by several regulatory mechanisms as well as affects many downstream actions. Toxic targets include the calcium-binding proteins, the calcium homeostasis regulatory proteins, the calcium-activated proteins such as calcineurin, and the calcium storing and releasing process.

Proliferation and migration of medial smooth muscle cells are primarily responsible for the formation of sclerosis. Under certain circumstances, smooth muscle cells lose most of their contractility and become transformed smooth muscle cells. In most cases, this transformation is reversible. This new form of smooth muscle cells synthesize collagen and accumulate low-density lipoproteins along with a loss in the number of myofilaments. This phenotype transformation of the smooth muscle cells occurs in atherosclerosis. The mechanism and factors involved in the transformation are not fully understood, but the involvement of platelet activation has been indicated. Toxic substances affect the phonotype transformation of smooth muscle cells through multiple pathways. However, the growth-promoting effect is apparently a major action involved in the atherosclerotic lesion.

Oxidative Stress and Vascular Injury Many xenobiotics generate ROS during their biotransformation. Both endothelial and smooth muscle cells are capable of producing ROS and the subsequent oxidative injury (Gurtner and Burke-Wolin, 1991). The mechanism of ROS generation from xenobiotics involves enzymatic and nonenzymatic reactions. Enzymes involved in the generation of ROS in vascular cells include amine oxidase, cytochrome $P450$ monooxygenases, and prostaglandin synthetase. These enzymes use a diversity of substrates to produce ROS. The nonenzymatic reaction involves free iron and copper in the circulation system, which catalyze the Fenton reaction to produce ROS.

An increase in ROS in endothelial cells is related to the stimulation by angiotensin II, as well as other neurohormonal factors and cyctokines. Angiotensin II binds to the AT1 receptor on the plasma membrane of endothelial cells. In response to receptor activation, cGMP production increases, leading to activation of endothelial CaM-dependent NOS and the production of NO. Stimulation of the AT1 receptor also leads to release of superoxide anion ($O_2^{\bullet-}$), through activation of a tyrosine phosphatase pathway. The release of both NO and ($O_2^{\bullet-}$) is a major oxidative stress response of endothelial cells. The NO and ($O_2^{\bullet-}$) production and release cause damage not only to endothelial cells, but also to other cells in the vascular system.

Vascular smooth muscle cells in response to angiotensin II markedly increase the production of ($O_2^{\bullet-}$). The source of ($O_2^{\bullet-}$) in these cells likely comes from NADPH oxidase, although NADH is also indicated in the production of ($O_2^{\bullet-}$) in these cells. Xenobiotics, as discussed in the "Vascular System Toxic Chemicals" section, can activate the enzyme system and lead to more extensive production of ($O_2^{\bullet-}$), or inhibit the antioxidant system including superoxide dismutase, catalase, glutathione peroxidase, and glutathione reductase resulting in accumulation of ROS in the cells.

Inflammatory Lesions Inflammatory lesions of the vascular system are a common response of the vascular system. Inflammatory lesions are also called vasculitis. The pathogenesis of vasculitis has been studied both in vivo and in vitro, but the causes of many types of vasculitis are unknown. The initial injury to endothelial cells and the release of chemicals from the injured cells are responsible for the initiation of the inflammatory response, including recruitment of inflammatory cells to the injured site. Cytokines released from the activated inflammatory cells further propagate the inflammatory response leading to the eventual lesion or vasculitis.

Toxic Responses of Blood Vessels

Hypertension and Hypotension The vasculature pressure change is a major phenotype of vascular injury. Hypertension results from excessive constriction of the arterial vasculatures and/or increased resistance of the microcirculation system. However, the primary problem of sustained hypertension is an elevated vascular resistance in all organs. Once hypertension is established, it becomes a disease of the microvasculature, particularly the arteriolar microvasculature. An increased incidence of temporary or, in some cases, permanent closure of small arterioles is associated with increased resistance of the end organs. The vascular smooth muscle cells become hypertrophied. However, the most predominant change is that all vascular smooth muscle cells are exceptionally

responsive to norepinephrine. Sustained hypertension is a major complication of primary cardiovascular diseases. Complications include accelerated atherosclerosis and overload of the left ventricular muscle due to high arterial pressure. Toxic substances may directly or indirectly affect the sympathetic nervous system or alter the turnover of catecholamines in the circulation, resulting in hypertension. However, sustained hypertension by xenobiotics may involve more complicated metabolic changes in the end organs and thus changes in microcirculation also take place. For example, chemicals may enhance the renin–angiotensin system as well as renal toxicity, which may cause hypertension.

Hypotension is practically defined as the symptoms caused by low blood pressure. There are several regulatory mechanisms in the vascular system and the integration of these regulations that maintain blood flow and blood pressure within the normal range. Baroreceptors, volume receptors, chemoreceptors, and pain receptors are all involved in the integrated regulatory action to maintain adequate blood pressure. During chemical exposure, these mechanisms may be affected individually or jointly resulting in a disturbance in the integration of the regulatory mechanisms. Both transient and sustained hypotension can be produced by xenobiotics. The most common adverse effect of antihypertension drugs is hypotension. Another major cause of hypotension is hemorrhage. Alcohol overdose also causes hypotension.

Atherosclerosis The most frequent vascular structural injury is atherosclerosis. The primary problem is the mechanical occlusion of the blood vessels so that blood flow is inadequate for the metabolic demands of the organs. As discussed above, activation of vascular smooth muscle cells is critically involved in atherosclerosis. Once stimulated, the vascular smooth muscle cells proliferate and migrate to the lesion site. These cells undergo phenotype transformation and increase the production of type I and II collagen, dermatan sulfate, proteoglycan, and stromelysins. In addition, the smooth muscle cells produce cytokines including macrophage colony-stimulating factor, TNF-α, and monocyte chemoattractant protein-1. The recruitment of inflammatory cells to the lesion site is the perpetuation process of atherosclerosis.

The classic definition of atherosclerotic plaque is a combination of changes in the intima of arteries consisting of local accumulation of lipids, complex carbohydrates, blood and blood products, fibrous tissue, and calcium deposits. However, this classic definition does not sufficiently describe the advanced atherosclerotic plaques that invade the media and produce bulging or enlarged arteries, cellular infiltration, and neovascularization. During the early development of atherosclerotic plaques, the lipid core has been described as the starting step of atherosclerosis. A lipid core develops and accumulates in the deep layer of the lesions before fibrous plaque formation begins. Inflammation and immune response are involved in both the early deposition of the lipid core and the late stage of fibrous accumulation. The inflammatory response includes cytokines, such as IL-6 and TNF-α. These cytokines are produced by vascular smooth muscle cells and infiltrated inflammatory cells. Many chemicals affect the oxidative metabolism of lipids in the circulatory system to trigger the formation and development of the lipid core of atherosclerosis. Toxic effects on smooth muscle cells can also initiate the formation of atherosclerotic plaques, which may be different from the lipid core mediated atherosclerosis. In addition, macrophages and monocytes are also targets for xenobiotics and have been shown to be importantly involved in the progression of atherosclerosis.

Hemorrhage A direct mechanical injury to blood vessels causes bleeding. Chemical-induced hemorrhages are seen when damage to capillaries takes place. In addition, toxic effects on blood clotting increase the probability of hemorrhage. A classic example of chemical-induced hemorrhage is observed in snake venom poisoning. Zinc-dependent metalloproteinases are major components of snake venom and responsible for the hemorrhage. Snake venom metalloproteinases degrade various components of the basement membrane and hydrolyze endothelial cell membrane proteins, such as integrins and cadherins, involved in cell–matrix and cell–cell adhesion. These actions weaken the capillary wall and perturb the interactions between endothelial cells and the basement membrane. Thus, the transmural pressure acting on the weakened capillary wall causes distention. As a consequence, endothelial cells become very thin and eventually, the integrity of the capillary wall is lost. In addition, endothelial cells become more susceptible to blood flow-dependent shear stress, further contributing to the capillary wall disruption.

Edema The capillary exchange of fluid is bidirectional and capillaries and venules may alter the balance of hydrostatic and colloid osmotic pressure. Filtration occurs most likely at the arteriolar end of capillaries, where filtration forces exceed absorption forces. The absorption of water occurs in the venular end of the capillary and small venules. The capillary pressure is determined by both the resistance of, and the blood pressure in arterioles and venules. Xenobiotics can change the pressure gradient and cause more filtration than reabsorption of the extracellular liquid by the capillary system. In addition, more fluid is filtered than is reabsorbed by the venous system under physiological conditions. Therefore, the removal of excess fluid as well as plasma proteins that diffuse into the interstitial space is essential. This is accomplished by the lymphatic system. The lymphatics ultimately drain into the vena cava. Toxic insults to the lymphatic system can lead to elevated interstitial pressures and the subsequent tissue edema.

VASCULAR SYSTEM TOXIC CHEMICALS

Chemicals that cause vascular toxicity can also be classified into pharmaceutical chemicals, natural products, and environmental pollutants and industrial chemicals. Blood vessels are the target organ of these chemicals. However, some of these chemicals affect both the blood vessels and the heart. For instance, blood vessels in the heart belong to the vascular system, so that the toxicity of vascular toxic chemicals may express their toxicity in the form of cardiac toxic manifestations. Endothelial cells are major target cells of the chemicals affecting the vascular system, which are also found in the heart and make a contribution to cardiac toxicity. The same principle applies to other organ systems. Due to the distribution of vascular system in the end organs, vascular toxicity affects the organs in which the vessels are localized and is often accompanied with functional defects of the organ.

Pharmaceutical Chemicals

Vascular toxicity of pharmaceutical chemicals that are used to treat vascular disease or used to treat nonvascular disease is well known clinically. The major manifestation and mechanisms of action of selected therapeutic agents are briefly discussed below.

Sympathomimetic Amines The sympathomimetic amines, including epinephrine, norepinephrine, dopamine, and isoproterenol, can damage the arterial vasculature by a variety of mechanisms. Large doses of norepinephrine produce toxic effects on the endothelium of the thoracic aorta of rabbits, including degenerative

changes in the aortic arch in the form of increased numbers of microvilli and many focal areas of unusual endothelial cytoarchitecture. Repeated exposure to catecholamines induces atherosclerotic lesions in several animal species. Experimental data suggest that catecholamines cause the proliferative disturbances in vascular cells via α-receptors because prazocin, an α-receptor antagonist, effectively prevents the toxic response (Nakaki et al., 1990). Smooth muscle cells subjected to increased stress by diabetes, hypertension, and balloon injury are more susceptible to the effects of catecholamines. Thus, the formation of arteriosclerotic lesions in certain forms of hypertension may be initiated and/or potentiated by high levels of circulating catecholamines.

Nicotine Nicotine is an alkaloid found in various plants and mimics the actions of acetylcholine at nicotinic receptors throughout the body. At pharmacological concentrations, nicotine increases heart rate and blood pressure as a result of stimulation of sympathetic ganglia and the adrenal medulla. Epidemiological and experimental studies have suggested that nicotine is a causative or aggravating factor in myocardial and cerebral infarction, gangrene, and aneurysm. The effects of nicotine are related to competitive inhibition of cyclooxygenase.

Cocaine The central actions of cocaine are to increase the circulating levels of catecholamines and cause a generalized state of vasoconstriction. Hypertension and cerebral strokes are common vascular complications. In pregnant women, cocaine-induced vascular changes have been associated with abortions and abruptio placentae. Studies have shown that cocaine enhances leukocyte migration across the cerebral vessel wall during inflammatory conditions. This effect is exerted through a cascade of augmented expression of inflammatory cytokines and endothelial adhesion molecules and may in fact underlie the cerebrovascular complications associated with cocaine abuse (Gan et al., 1999).

Psychotropic Agents Trifluoperazine and chlorpromazine among the psychotropic drugs have been shown to cause intracellular cholesterol accumulation in cultured cells of the aortic intima (Iakushkin et al., 1992). Enalapril has been shown to cause angioedema in humans. Aside from the atherogenic effects, postural hypotension has been identified as the most common cardiovascular side effect of TCAs.

Antineoplastic Agents The vasculotoxic responses elicited by antineoplastic drugs range from asymptomatic arterial lesions to thrombotic microangiopathy. Pulmonary veno-occlusive disease has been reported after the administration of various drugs, including 5-fluorouracil, doxorubicin, and mitomycin. Cyclophosphamide causes cerebrovascular and viscerovascular lesions, resulting in hemorrhages. Chronic infusions of 5-fluoro-2-deoxyuridine into the hepatic artery in dogs resulted in gastrointestinal hemorrhage and portal vein thrombosis.

Analgesics and Nonsteroidal Anti-Inflammatory Agents Aspirin can produce endothelial damage as part of a pattern of gastric erosion. Studies in rats have shown early changes in the basement membrane of endothelial cells of the capillaries and postcapillary venules, leading to obliteration of small vessels and ischemic infarcts in the large intestine. Regular use of analgesics containing phenacetin has been associated with an increased risk of hypertension and cardiovascular morbidity. NSAIDs may induce glomerular and vascular renal lesions.

Oral Contraceptives Oral contraceptive steroids can produce thromboembolic disorders. Epidemiological studies have shown that oral contraceptive users have an increased risk of myocardial infarction relative to nonusers, a correlation that is markedly exacerbated by smoking, and oral contraceptive users experience an increased risk of cerebral thrombosis, hemorrhage, venous thrombosis, and pulmonary embolism (Stolley *et al.*, 1989). However, the mechanism by which oral contraceptives increase the risk of vascular disease is unclear.

Natural Products

Natural products that cause vascular toxicity include those discussed for drugs causing cardiotoxicity. In addition, many other drugs also cause vascular lesions and toxicity such as bacterial endotoxins and homocysteines, which have unique vascular toxic effects.

Bacterial Endotoxins Bacterial endotoxins are potent toxic agents to vascular system and cause a variety of toxic effects in many vascular beds. In the liver, they cause swelling of endothelial cells and adhesion of platelets to sinusoid walls. In the lung, endotoxins produce increased vascular permeability and pulmonary hypertension. Infusion of endotoxin into experimental animals produces thickening of endothelial cells and the formation of fibrin thrombi in small veins. The terminal phase of the effects of endotoxin on the systemic vasculature results in marked hypotension. The ability of vitamin E to prevent disseminated intravascular coagulation induced by bacterial endotoxins in the rat suggests that action of these agents is somehow related to oxidative stress mechanisms.

Homocysteine Moderately elevated levels of homocysteine have been associated with atherosclerosis and venous thrombosis. Conditions including increases in the circulating homocysteine involve cardiac complications such as hypertrophic cardiomyopathy and heart failure. Toxicity may involve oxidative injury to vascular endothelial and/or smooth muscle cells, leading to deregulation of vascular smooth muscle growth, synthesis and deposition of matrix proteins, and adverse effects on anticoagulant systems (Harpel, 1997).

Hydrazinobenzoic Acid Hydrazinobenzoic acid is a nitrogen–nitrogen bonded chemical that is present in the cultivated mushroom *Agaricus bisporus*. This hydrazine derivative causes smooth muscle cell tumors in the aorta and large arteries of mice when administered over the life span of the animals (Mcmanus *et al.*, 1987). These tumors have the characteristic appearance and immunocytochemical features of vascular leiomyomas and leiomyosarcomas. Smooth muscle cell lysis with vascular perforation apparently precedes malignant transformation.

T-2 Toxin Trichothecene mycotoxins, commonly classified as tetracyclic sesquiterpenes, are naturally occurring cytotoxic metabolites of *Fusarium* species. These mycotoxins, including T-2 toxin [4β,15-diacetoxy-8α-(3-methylbutyryloxy)-3α-hydroxy-12,13-epoxytrichothec-9-ene], are major contaminants of foods and animal feeds and may cause illness in animals and humans. Intravenous infusion of T-2 toxin in rats causes an initial decrease in heart rate and blood pressure, followed by tachycardia and hypertension and finally by bradycardia and hypotension (Mcmanus *et al.*, 1987). Acute T-2 toxin exposure causes extensive destruction of myocardial capillaries, while repeated dosing promotes thickening of large coronary arteries.

Vitamin D The toxic effects of vitamin D may be related to its structural similarity to 25-hydroxycholesterol, a potent vascular toxin. The manifestations of vitamin D hypervitaminosis include medial degeneration, calcification of the coronary arteries, and smooth muscle cell proliferation in laboratory animals.

β-Amyloid Accumulation of β-amyloid is a major lesion in the brain of Alzheimer's patients. Studies have shown that administration of β-amyloid produces extensive vascular disruption, including endothelial and smooth muscle damage, adhesion and migration of leukocytes across arteries and venules (Thomas *et al.*, 1997). Most importantly, the vascular actions of β-amyloid appear to be distinct from the neurotoxic properties of the peptide. It appears that vascular toxicity of β-amyloid makes contributions to Alzheimer's dementia.

Environmental Pollutants and Industrial Chemicals

The environmental pollutants and industrial chemicals discussed in cardiac toxicity section all have toxic effects on the vascular system. As discussed above, the cardiac effect of some of these agents and pollutants may result primarily from the vascular effect. The by-products of vascular tissue damage or the secreted substances, such as cytokines derived from vascular injury, can affect the heart either directly because of the residual of the vascular system in the heart, or indirectly through blood circulation. In this context, some of the chemicals discussed in the cardiotoxicity will not be further described. Some unique vascular toxicity will be presented.

Carbon Monoxide Carbon monoxide induces focal intimal damage and edema in laboratory animals at a concentration (180 ppm) to which humans may be exposed from environmental sources such as automobile exhaust, tobacco smoke, and fossil fuels. However, it is difficult to distinguish the direct effects of carbon monoxide from those of chemicals such as sulfur oxides, nitrogen oxides, aldehydes, and hydrocarbons on humans because most sources of carbon monoxide are complex mixtures of chemicals. Degenerative changes of myocardial arterioles have been produced experimentally in dogs forced to smoke. Similar changes have also been detected in humans who were heavy smokers and died of noncardiac causes (Wald and Howard, 1975). Tobacco smoke not only exerts a direct atherogenic effect (endothelial injury, changes in lipid profiles, and proliferation of smooth muscle cells), but also facilitates thrombosis by modulation of platelet function and vascular spasm.

Short-term exposure to carbon monoxide is associated with direct damage to vascular endothelial and smooth muscle cells. Injury to endothelial cells increases intimal permeability and allows the interaction of blood constituents with underlying components of the vascular wall. This response may account in part for the ability of carbon monoxide to induce atherosclerotic lesions in several animal species. The toxic effects of carbon monoxide have been attributed to its reversible interaction with hemoglobin. As a result of this interaction, carboxyhemoglobin decreases the oxygen-carrying capacity of blood, eventually leading to functional anemia. In addition, carbon monoxide interacts with cellular proteins such as myoglobin and cytochrome *c* oxidase and elicits a direct vasodilatory response of the coronary circulation.

Carbon Disulfide Carbon disulfide (dithiocarbonic anhydride) occurs in coal tar and crude petroleum and is commonly used in the manufacture of rayon and soil disinfectants. This chemical has been identified as an atherogenic agent in laboratory animals. The mechanism for carbon disulfide-atheroma production may involve direct injury to the endothelium coupled with hypothyroidism, because thiocarbamate (thiourea), a potent antithyroid substance, is a principal urinary metabolite of carbon disulfide. Carbon disulfide also modifies low-density lipoprotein in vitro and enhances arterial fatty deposits induced by a high-fat diet in mice (Lewis *et al.*, 1999).

1,3-Butadiene Studies have shown that 1,3-butadiene, a chemical used in the production of styrene–butadiene, increases the incidence of cardiac hemangiosarcomas, which are tumors of endothelial origin (Miller and Boorman, 1990). Although hemangiosarcomas have also been observed in the liver, lung, and kidney, cardiac tumors are a major cause of death in animals exposed to this chemical. The toxic effects of 1,3-butadiene are dependent on its metabolic activation by cytochrome *P*450 to toxic epoxide metabolites. The ultimate outcomes of exposure probably are influenced by the rates of glutathione-mediated detoxification of oxidative metabolites.

Metals and Metalloids The vascular toxicity of food- and water-borne elements (selenium, chromium, copper, zinc, cadmium, lead, and mercury) as well as airborne elements (vanadium and lead) involves reactions of metals with sulfhydryl, carboxyl, or phosphate groups. Metals such as cobalt, magnesium, manganese, nickel, cadmium, and lead also interact with and block calcium channels. Intracellular calcium-binding proteins, such as CaM, are biologically relevant targets of heavy metals, including cadmium, mercury and lead, although the contribution of this mechanism to the toxic effects of metals has been fully understood.

Cadmium Cadmium effects on the vascular system have been studied in the greatest detail. Although cadmium is not preferentially localized in blood vessels relative to other tissues, when present, cadmium is localized in the elastic lamina of large arteries, with particularly high concentrations at arterial branching points (Perry *et al.*, 1989). A large portion of the cadmium that accumulates in the body is tightly bound to hepatic and renal MT. The low MT levels in vascular tissue may actually predispose a person to the toxic effects of cadmium (Perry *et al.*, 1989). Long-term exposure of laboratory animals to low levels of cadmium has been associated with the development of atherosclerosis and hypertension in the absence of other toxic effects. Selenium and zinc inhibit, whereas lead potentiates the hypertensive effects of cadmium. Calcium has antagonistic effect on cadmium-induced high blood pressure. Cadmium increases sodium retention, induces vasoconstriction, increases cardiac output, and produces hyperreninemia. Any one of these mechanisms could account for the putative hypertensive effects of cadmium.

Lead Lead has been shown from epidemiological studies to be associated with essential hypertension in a large percentage of patients (Batuman *et al.*, 1983). Elevated blood pressure has also been observed during childhood lead poisoning. The direct vasoconstrictor effect of lead may be related to the putative hypertensive response. This effect can be complemented by the ability of lead to activate the renin–angiotensin–aldosterone system. Lead also directly affects vascular endothelial and smooth muscle cells. For instance, lead inhibits the repair process in damaged endothelial cells (Fujiwara *et al.*, 1997) and modulates spontaneous release of fibrinolytic proteins from subendothelial cells through intracellular calcium-independent pathways (Yamamoto *et al.*, 1997). Acute lead-induced neuropathy may be due to cerebral capillary dysfunction. Inorganic lead alters arterial elasticity and causes sclerosis of renal vessels.

Mercury Mercury produces vasoconstriction of preglomerular vessels and disrupts the integrity of the blood–brain barrier. The opening of the blood–brain barrier results in extravasation of plasma protein across vascular walls into adjoining brain tissues. Mercury added to platelet-rich plasma causes a marked increase in platelet thromboxane B_2 production and platelet responsiveness to arachidonic acid.

Arsenic Arsenic poisoning causes vasodilation and capillary dilation. These actions have been associated with extravasation, transudation of plasma, and decreased intravascular volume. A severe form of arteriosclerosis, blackfoot disease, in Taiwan has been shown to be associated with high levels of arsenic in the soil and water. Blackfoot disease is an endemic peripheral vascular occlusive disease that exhibits arteriosclerosis obliterans and thromboangiitis. The ability of arsenic to induce these changes has been attributed to its effects on vascular endothelial cells. Arsenic has been reported to cause noncirrhotic portal hypertension in humans.

Aromatic Hydrocarbons Aromatic hydrocarbons, including polycyclic aromatic hydrocarbons and polychlorinated dibenzop-dioxins, are persistent toxic environmental contaminants. Aromatic hydrocarbons have been identified as vascular toxins that can initiate and/or promote the atherogenic process in experimental animals (Ou and Ramos, 1992). The atherogenic effect is associated with cytochrome *P*450-mediated conversion of the parent compound to toxic metabolic intermediates, but aromatic hydrocarbons can also initiate the atherogenic process. However, studies have also shown that treatment with several polycyclic hydrocarbons increases the size but not the frequency of atherosclerotic lesions (Albert *et al.*, 1977; Penn and Snyder, 1988), suggesting that polycyclic aromatic hydrocarbons act as promoters of the atherosclerotic process. Although additional studies are required to define the "initiating" versus "promotional" actions of polycyclic aromatic hydrocarbons, their ability to readily associate with plasma lipoproteins may play a critical role in vascular toxicity.

Particulate Air Pollution Recent epidemiological studies have provided a strong body of evidence that elevated levels of ambient particulate air pollution (PM) are associated with increased cardiovascular and respiratory morbidity and mortality. Besides the PM effects on cardiomyocytes such as alterations in ion channel function leading to cardiac malfunction, available clinical and experimental evidence lend support to the vascular effects of inhaled ambient particles, including endothelial dysfunction and promotion of atherosclerotic lesions. Importantly, these lesions lead to release or secretion of cytokines and chemokines, worsening cardiac complications. For instance, PM exposure significantly increases serum total endothelin concentrations and worsens premature ventricular complexes of the electrocardiograms that occur in the myocardial infarct rats (Kang *et al.*, 2002). The PM effects on the vascular system and the consequences are important health-related topics and further studies are needed to substantiate our current understanding of mechanisms for PM adverse vascular effects.

REFERENCES

Abas L, Bogoyevitch MA, Guppy M. Mitochondrial ATP production is necessary for activation of the extracellular-signal-regulated kinases during ischaemia/reperfusion in rat myocyte-derived H9c2 cells. *Biochem J.* 2000;349(pt 1):119–126.

Adams JM, Cory S. The Bcl-2 protein family: arbiters of cell survival. *Science.* 1998;281(5381):1322–1326.

Adams JW, Sakata Y, Davis MG, et al. Enhanced Galphaq signaling: a common pathway mediates cardiac hypertrophy and apoptotic heart failure. *Proc Natl Acad Sci USA.* 1998;95(17):10140–10145.

Adams MA, Hirst M. Ethanol-induced cardiac hypertrophy: correlation between development and the excretion of adrenal catecholamines. *Pharmacol Biochem Behav.* 1986;24(1):33–38.

Ahmed SS, Regan TJ. Cardiotoxicity of acute and chronic ingestion of various alcohols, In: Acosta D, ed. *Cardiovascular Toxicology,* 2nd ed. New York: Raven Press; 1992:345–407.

Akao M, Ohler A, O'Rourke B, et al. Mitochondrial ATP-sensitive potassium channels inhibit apoptosis induced by oxidative stress in cardiac cells. *Circ Res.* 2001;88(12):1267–1275.

Akhter SA, Luttrell LM, Rockman HA, et al. Targeting the receptor-Gq interface to inhibit in vivo pressure overload myocardial hypertrophy. *Science.* 1998;280(5363):574–577.

Albert RE, Vanderlaan M, Burns FJ, et al. Effect of carcinogens on chicken atherosclerosis. *Cancer Res.* 1977;37(7 pt 1):2232–2235.

Andrieu-Abadie N, Jaffrezou JP, Hatem S, et al. L-Carnitine prevents doxorubicin-induced apoptosis of cardiac myocytes: role of inhibition of ceramide generation. *FASEB J.* 1999;13(12):1501–1510.

Anversa P. Myocyte death in the pathological heart. *Circ Res.* 2000;86(2):121–124.

Anversa P, Leri A, Kajstura J. Cardiac regeneration. *J Am Coll Cardiol.* 2006;47(9):1769–1776.

Arad M, Moskowitz IP, Patel VV, et al. Transgenic mice overexpressing mutant PRKAG2 define the cause of Wolff–Parkinson–White syndrome in glycogen storage cardiomyopathy. *Circulation.* 2003;107(22):2850–2856.

Arellano FM. The withdrawal of rofecoxib. *Pharmacoepidemiol Drug Saf.* 2005;14:213–217.

Arola OJ, Saraste A, Pulkki K, et al. Acute doxorubicin cardiotoxicity involves cardiomyocyte apoptosis. *Cancer Res.* 2000;60(7):1789–1792.

Arstall MA, Sawyer DB, Fukazawa R, et al. Cytokine-mediated apoptosis in cardiac myocytes: the role of inducible nitric oxide synthase induction and peroxynitrite generation. *Circ Res.* 1999;85(9):829–840.

Atkison P, Joubert G, Barron A, et al. Hypertrophic cardiomyopathy associated with tacrolimus in paediatric transplant patients. *Lancet.* 1995;345(8954):894–896.

Baldessarini RJ. Drugs and the treatment of psychiatric disorders. In: Hardman JG, Limbird LE, Molinoff PB, et al. eds. *Goodman & Gilman's The Pharmacological Basis of Therapeutics*, 9th ed. New York: McGraw-Hill; 1996:399–430.

Batuman V, Landy E, Maesaka JK, et al. Contribution of lead to hypertension with renal impairment. *N Engl J Med.* 1983;309(1):17–21.

Behrendt H, Boffin H. Myocardial cell lesions caused by an anabolic hormone. *Cell Tissue Res.* 1977;181(3):423–426.

Bennett PB, Yazawa K, Makita N, et al. Molecular mechanism for an inherited cardiac arrhythmia. *Nature.* 1995;376(6542):683–685.

Berenji K, Drazner MH, Rothermel BA, et al. Does load-induced ventricular hypertrophy progress to systolic heart failure? *Am J Physiol Heart Circ Physiol.* 2005;289(1):H8–H16.

Berne RM, Levy MN. *Physiology.* St. Louis: Mosby; 1983.

Bisognano JD, Weinberger HD, Bohlmeyer TJ, et al. Myocardial-directed overexpression of the human beta(1)-adrenergic receptor in transgenic mice. *J Mol Cell Cardiol.* 2000;32(5):817–830.

Bittl JA, Ingwall JS. Reaction rates of creatine kinase and ATP synthesis in the isolated rat heart. A 31P NMR Magnetization Transfer Study. *J Biol Chem.* 1985;260(6):3512–3517.

Black BL, Olson EN. Transcriptional control of muscle development by myocyte enhancer factor-2 (MEF2) proteins. *Annu Rev Cell Dev Biol.* 1998;14:167–196.

Bogden JD, Al Rabiai S, Gilani SH. Effect of chronic ethanol ingestion on the metabolism of copper, iron, manganese, selenium, and zinc in an animal model of alcoholic cardiomyopathy. *J Toxicol Environ Health.* 1984;14(2–3):407–417.

Bosnjak ZJ. Cardiac effects of anesthetics. In: Blank TJJ, Wheeler DM, eds. *Mechanisms of Anesthetic Action in Skeletal, Cardiac and Smooth Muscle.* New York: Plenum Press; 1991:91–96.

Bouthillier L, Vincent R, Goegan P, et al. Acute effects of inhaled urban particles and ozone: lung morphology, macrophage activity, and plasma endothelin-1. *Am J Pathol.* 1998;153(6):1873–1884.

Bozkurt B. Cardiovascular toxicity with highly active antiretroviral therapy: review of clinical studies. *Cardiovas Toxicol.* 2004;4:243–260.

Brand T, Sharma HS, Fleischmann KE, et al. Proto-oncogene expression in porcine myocardium subjected to ischemia and reperfusion. *Circ Res.* 1992;71(6):1351–1360.

Buck ED, Lachnit WG, Pessah IN. Mechanisms of delta-hexachlorocyclohexane toxicity: I. Relationship between altered ventricular myocyte contractility and ryanodine receptor function. *J Pharmacol Exp Ther.* 1999;289(1):477–485.

Catterall W, Mackie K. Local anesthetics. In: Hardman JG, Limbird LE, Molinoff PB, et al., eds. *Goodman & Gilman's The Pharmacological Basis Of Therapeutics*, 9th ed. New York: McGraw-Hill; 1996:331–347.

Chacon E, Acosta D. Mitochondrial regulation of superoxide by Ca²⁺: an alternate mechanism for the cardiotoxicity of doxorubicin. *Toxicol Appl Pharmacol.* 1991;107(1):117–128.

Cheng TH, Shih NL, Chen SY, et al. Reactive oxygen species modulate endothelin-I-induced c-fos gene expression in cardiomyocytes. *Cardiovasc Res.* 1999a;41(3):654–662.

Cheng W, Li B, Kajstura J, et al. Stretch-induced programmed myocyte cell death. *J Clin Invest.* 1995;96(5):2247–2259.

Cheng XS, Shimokawa H, Momii H, et al. Role of superoxide anion in the pathogenesis of cytokine-induced myocardial dysfunction in dogs in vivo. *Cardiovasc Res.* 1999b;42(3):651–659.

Cook SA, Sugden PH, Clerk A. Regulation of Bcl-2 family proteins during development and in response to oxidative stress in cardiac myocytes: association with changes in mitochondrial membrane potential. *Circ Res.* 1999;85(10):940–949.

Dalakas MC, Illa I, Pezeshkpour GH, et al. Mitochondrial myopathy caused by long-term zidovudine therapy. *N Engl J Med.* 1990;322(16):1098–1105.

De Simone G. Left ventricular geometry and hypotension in end-stage renal disease: a mechanical perspective. *J Am Soc Nephrol.* 2003;14(10):2421–2427.

Delaughter MC, Taffet GE, Fiorotto ML, et al. Local insulin-like growth factor I expression induces physiologic, then pathologic, cardiac hypertrophy in transgenic mice. *FASEB J.* 1999;13(14):1923–1929.

Depre C, Taegtmeyer H. Metabolic aspects of programmed cell survival and cell death in the heart. *Cardiovasc Res.* 2000;45(3):538–548.

Dhalla NS, Yates JC, Maimark B, et al. Cardiotoxicity of catecholamines and related agents. In Acosta D, ed. *Cardiovascular Toxicology*, 2d ed. New York: Raven Press; 1992:239–282.

Diamond MI, Miner JN, Yoshinaga SK, et al. Transcription factor interactions: selectors of positive or negative regulation from a single DNA element. *Science.* 1990;249(4974):1266–1272.

Didenko VV, Tunstead JR, Hornsby PJ. Biotin-labeled hairpin oligonucleotides: probes to detect double-strand breaks in DNA in apoptotic cells. *Am J Pathol.* 1998;152(4):897–902.

Dockery DW. Epidemiologic evidence of cardiovascular effects of particulate air pollution. *Environ Health Perspect.* 2001;109(suppl 4):483–486.

Dorn GW, Force T. Protein kinase cascades in the regulation of cardiac hypertrophy. *J Clin Invest.* 2005;115(3):527–537.

Eguchi Y, Shimizu S, Tsujimoto Y. Intracellular ATP levels determine cell death fate by apoptosis or necrosis. *Cancer Res.* 1997;57(10):1835–1840.

EL-Sherif L, Wang GW, Kang YJ. Suppression of cadmium-induced apoptosis in metallothionein-overexpressing transgenic mouse cardiac myocytes. *FASEB J.* 2000;14:1193.

Eliot RS, Clayton FC, Pieper GM, et al. Influence of environmental stress on pathogenesis of sudden cardiac death. *Fed Proc.* 1977;36(5):1719–1724.

Esposito G, Rapacciuolo A, Naga Prasad SV, et al. Genetic alterations that inhibit in vivo pressure-overload hypertrophy prevent cardiac dysfunction despite increased wall stress. *Circulation.* 2002;105(1):85–92.

Eura Y, Ishihara N, Yokota S, Mihara K. Two mitofusin proteins, mammalian homologues of FZO, with distinct functions are both required for mitochondrial fusion. *J Biochem.* 2003;134(3):333–344.

Evans T, Reitman M, Felsenfeld G. An erythrocyte-specific DNA-binding factor recognizes a regulatory sequence common to all chicken globin genes. *Proc Natl Acad Sci U S A.* 1988;85(16):5976–5980.

Evens T. Regulation of cardiac gene expression by GATA-4/5/6. *Trends Cardiovasc Med.* 1997;7:75–83.

Fauchier L, Babuty D, Poret P, et al. Comparison of long-term outcome of alcoholic and idiopathic dilated cardiomyopathy. *Eur Heart J.* 2000;21(4):306–314.

Fitzgerald GA. Coxibs and cardiovascular disease. *N Engl J Med.* 2004;351:1709–1711.

Fosslien E. Mitochondrial medicine—molecular pathology of defective oxidative phosphorylation. *Ann Clin Lab Sci.* 2001;31(1):25–67.

Francis GS, Chu C. Compensatory and maladaptive responses to cardiac dysfunction. *Curr Opin Cardiol*. 1995;10(3):260–267.

Frey N, Olson EN. Cardiac hypertrophy: the good, the bad, and the ugly. *Annu Rev Physiol*. 2003;65:45–79.

Frustaci A, Kajstura J, Chimenti C, et al. Myocardial cell death in human diabetes. *Circ Res*. 2000;87(12):1123–1132.

Fujiwara Y, Kaji T, Sakurai S, et al. Inhibitory effect of lead on the repair of wounded monolayers of cultured vascular endothelial cells. *Toxicology*. 1997;117(2–3):193–198.

Galan L, Talavera K, Vassort G, et al. Characteristics of Ca^{2+} channel blockade by oxodipine and elgodipine in rat cardiomyocytes. *Eur J Pharmacol*. 1998;357(1):93–105.

Gan X, Zhang L, Berger O, et al. Cocaine enhances brain endothelial adhesion molecules and leukocyte migration. *Clin Immunol*. 1999;91(1):68–76.

Gandre-Babbe S, van der Bliek AM. The novel tail-anchored membrane protein Mff controls mitochondrial and peroxisomal fission in mammalian cells. *Mol Biol Cell*. 2008;19(6):2402–2412.

Gavazzi A, De Maria R, Parolini M, et al. Alcohol abuse and dilated cardiomyopathy in men. *Am J Cardiol*. 2000;85(9):1114–1118.

Goldsmith S, From AH. Arsenic-induced atypical ventricular tachycardia. *N Engl J Med*. 1980;303(19):1096–1098.

Gordon T, Reibman J. Cardiovascular toxicity of inhaled ambient particulate matter. *Toxicol Sci*. 2000;56:2–4.

Gottlieb RA, Burleson KO, Kloner RA, et al. Reperfusion injury induces apoptosis in rabbit cardiomyocytes. *J Clin Invest*. 1994;94(4):1621–1628.

Gotzsche LS, Pedersen EM. Dose-dependent cardiotoxic effect of amiodarone in cardioplegic solutions correlates with loss of dihydropyridine binding sites: in vitro evidence for a potentially lethal interaction with procaine. *J Cardiovasc Pharmacol*. 1994;23(1):13–23.

Guenoun T, Montagne O, Laplace M, et al. Propofol-induced modifications of cardiomyocyte calcium transient and sarcoplasmic reticulum function in rats. *Anesthesiology*. 2000;92(2):542–549.

Guerra S, Leri A, Wang X, et al. Myocyte death in the failing human heart is gender dependent. *Circ Res*. 1999;85(9):856–866.

Gurley BJ, Gardner SF, White LM, et al. Ephedrine pharmacokinetics after the ingestion of nutritional supplements containing *Ephedra Sinica* (Ma Huang). *Ther Drug Monit*. 1998;20(4):439–445.

Gurtner GH, Burke-Wolin T. Interactions of oxidant stress and vascular reactivity. *Am J Physiol*. 1991;260(4 pt 1):L207–L211.

Harpel PC. Homocysteine, atherogenesis and thrombosis. *Fibrinolysis Proteolysis*. 1997;11(suppl 1):77–80.

Haunstetter A, Izumo S. Apoptosis: basic mechanisms and implications for cardiovascular disease. *Circ Res*. 1998;82(11):1111–1129.

Havlin KA. Cardiotoxicity of anthracyclines and other antineoplastic agents. In: Acosta D, ed. *Cardiovascular Toxicology*, 2nd ed. New York: Raven Press; 1992:143–164.

Hayakawa K, Takemura G, Koda M, et al. Sensitivity to apoptosis signal, clearance rate, and ultrastructure of Fas ligand-induced apoptosis in in vivo adult cardiac cells. *Circulation*. 2002;105(25):3039–3045.

He SY, Matoba R, Sodesaki K, et al. Morphological and morphometric investigation of cardiac lesions after chronic administration of methamphetamine in rats. *Nippon Hoigaku Zasshi*. 1996;50(2):63–71.

Heineke J, Molkentin JD. Regulation of cardiac hypertrophy by intracellular signalling pathways. *Nat Rev Mol Cell Biol*. 2006;7(8):589–600.

Hill JA, Karimi M, Kutschke W, et al. Cardiac hypertrophy is not a required compensatory response to short-term pressure overload. *Circulation*. 2000;101(24):2863–2869.

Hino N, Ochi R, Yanagisawa T. Inhibition of the slow inward current and the time-dependent outward current of mammalian ventricular muscle by gentamicin. *Pflugers Arch*. 1982;394(3):243–249.

Ho PD, Zechner DK, He H, et al. The Raf-MEK-ERK Cascade represents a common pathway for alteration of intracellular calcium by Ras and protein kinase C in cardiac myocytes. *J Biol Chem*. 1998;273(34):21730–21735.

Holtz J. Pathophysiology of heart failure and the renin–angiotensin–system. *Basic Res Cardiol*. 1993;88(suppl 1):183–201.

Huss JM, Kelly DP. Mitochondrial energy metabolism in heart failure: a question of balance. *J Clin Invest*. 2005;115(3):547–555.

Hussar DA. New drugs of 1998. *J Am Pharm Assoc (Wash)*. 1999;39(2):151–206.

Hussar DA. New drugs of 1999. *J Am Pharm Assoc (Wash)*. 2000;40(2):181–221.

Iakushkin VV, Baldenkov GN, Tertov VV, et al. Atherogenic properties of phenothiazine drugs manifesting in cultured cells of the human aortic intima. *Kardiologiia*. 1992;32(6):66–68.

Ingwall JS, Kramer MF, Fifer MA, et al. The creatine kinase system in normal and diseased human myocardium. *N Engl J Med*. 1985;313(17):1050–1054.

Ingwall JS, Weiss RG. Is the failing heart energy starved? On using chemical energy to support cardiac function. *Circ Res*. 2004;95(2):135–145.

Ito H, Hirata Y, Adachi S, et al. Endothelin-1 is an autocrine/paracrine factor in the mechanism of angiotensin II-induced hypertrophy in cultured rat cardiomyocytes. *J Clin Invest*. 1993;92(1):398–403.

Jalili T, Takeishi Y, Walsh RA. Signal transduction during cardiac hypertrophy: the role of G alpha Q, PLC Beta I, and PKC. *Cardiovasc Res*. 1999;44(1):5–9.

James TN. Normal and abnormal consequences of apoptosis in the human heart. From postnatal morphogenesis to paroxysmal arrhythmias. *Circulation*. 1994;90(1):556–573.

James DI, Parone PA, Mattenberger Y, Martinou JC. hFis1, a novel component of the mammalian mitochondrial fission machinery. *J Biol Chem*. 2003;278(38):36373–36379.

Joshi A, Dimino T, Vohra Y, et al. Preclinical strategies to assess QT liability and torsadogenic potential of new drugs: the role of experimental models. *J Electrocardiol*. 2004;37(suppl):7–14.

Jurgensmeier JM, Xie Z, Deveraux Q, et al. Bax directly induces release of cytochrome *c* from isolated mitochondria. *Proc Natl Acad Sci U S A*. 1998;95(9):4997–5002.

Kaasik A, Minajeva A, Paju K, et al. Thyroid hormones differentially affect sarcoplasmic reticulum function in rat atria and ventricles. *Mol Cell Biochem*. 1997;176(1–2):119–126.

Kagi JH. Overview of metallothionein. *Methods Enzymol*. 1991;205:401–414.

Kajstura J, Cheng W, Reiss K, et al. Apoptotic and necrotic myocyte cell deaths are independent contributing variables of infarct size in rats. *Lab Invest*. 1996;74(1):86–107.

Kalin MF, Zumoff B. Sex hormones and coronary disease: a review of the clinical studies. *Steroids*. 1990;55(8):330–352.

Kang YJ. The antioxidant function of metallothionein in the heart. *Proc Soc Exp Biol Med*. 1999;222:263–273.

Kang YJ. Molecular and cellular mechanisms of cardiotoxicity. *Environ Health Perspect*. 2001;109(suppl 1):27–34.

Kang YJ. Metallothionein redox cycle and function. *Exp Biol Med (Maywood)*. 2006;231(9):1459–1467.

Kang YJ, Li Y, Zhou Z, et al. Elevation of serum endothelins and cardiotoxicity induced by particulate matter (PM 2.5) in rats with acute myocardial infarction. *Cardiovasc Toxicol*. 2002;2(4):253–261.

Kang YJ, Zhou ZX, Wang GW, et al. Suppression by metallothionein of doxorubicin-induced cardiomyocyte apoptosis through inhibition of P38 mitogen-activated protein kinases. *J Biol Chem*. 2000a;275(18):13690–13698.

Kang YJ, Zhou ZX, Wu H, et al. Metallothionein inhibits myocardial apoptosis in copper-deficient mice: role of atrial natriuretic peptide. *Lab Invest*. 2000b;80(5):745–757.

Kannan M, Wang L, Kang YJ. Myocardial oxidative stress and toxicity induced by acute ethanol exposure in mice. *Exp Biol Med (Maywood)*. 2004;229(6):553–559.

Kass DA, Saavedra WF, Sabbah HN. Reverse remodeling and enhanced inotropic reserve from the cardiac support device in experimental cardiac failure. *J Card Fail*. 2004;10(6 suppl):S215–S219.

Klatsky AL. Alcohol and cardiovascular diseases: a historical overview. *Novartis Found Symp*. 1998;216:2–12.

Koenig H, Fan CC, Goldstone AD, et al. Polyamines mediate androgenic stimulation of calcium fluxes and membrane transport in rat heart myocytes. *Circ Res*. 1989;64(3):415–426.

Koshiba T, Detmer SA, Kaiser JT, Chen H, McCaffery JM, Chan DC. Structural basis of mitochondrial tethering by mitofusin complexes. *Science.* 2004;305(5685):858–862.

Kroemer G, Zamzami N, Susin SA. Mitochondrial control of apoptosis. *Immunol Today.* 1997;18(1):44–51.

Krown KA, Page MT, Nguyen C, et al. Tumor necrosis factor alpha-induced apoptosis in cardiac myocytes. Involvement of the sphingolipid signaling cascade in cardiac cell death. *J Clin Invest.* 1996;98(12):2854–2865.

Kubota T, Miyagishima M, Frye CS, et al. Overexpression of tumor necrosis factor-alpha activates both anti- and pro-apoptotic pathways in the myocardium. *J Mol Cell Cardiol.* 2001;33(7):1331–1344.

Kurrelmeyer KM, Michael LH, Baumgarten G, et al. Endogenous tumor necrosis factor protects the adult cardiac myocote against ischemic-induced apoptosis in a murine model of acute myocardial infarction. *Proc Natl Acad Sci U S A.* 2000;97:5456–5461.

Lazarevic AM, Nakatani S, Neskovic AN, et al. Early changes in left ventricular function in chronic asymptomatic alcoholics: relation to the duration of heavy drinking. *J Am Coll Cardiol.* 2000;35(6):1599–1606.

Lee JA, Allen DG. Calcium sensitisers: mechanisms of action and potential usefulness as inotropes. *Cardiovasc Res.* 1997;36(1):10–20.

Lee YJ, Jeong SY, Karbowski M, Smith CL, Youle RJ. Roles of the mammalian mitochondrial fission and fusion mediators Fis1, Drp1, and Opa1 in apoptosis. *Mol Biol Cell.* 2004;15(11):5001–5011.

Leist M, Single B, Castoldi AF, et al. Intracellular adenosine triphosphate (ATP) concentration: a switch in the decision between apoptosis and necrosis. *J Exp Med.* 1997;185(8):1481–1486.

Leist M, Single B, Naumann H, et al. Inhibition of mitochondrial ATP generation by nitric oxide switches apoptosis to necrosis. *Exp Cell Res.* 1999;249(2):396–403.

Lenczowski JM, Dominguez L, Eder AM, et al. Lack of a role for jun kinase and AP-1 in Fas-induced apoptosis. *Mol Cell Biol.* 1997;17(1):170–181.

Levine ES, Friedman HS, Griffith OW, et al. Cardiac cell toxicity induced by 4-hydroperoxycyclophosphamide is modulated by glutathione. *Cardiovasc Res.* 1993;27(7):1248–1253.

Lewis JG, Graham DG, Valentine WM, et al. Exposure of C57BL/6 mice to carbon disulfide induces early lesions of atherosclerosis and enhances arterial fatty deposits induced by a high fat diet. *Toxicol Sci.* 1999;49(1):124–132.

Lewis W, Grupp IL, Grupp G, et al. Cardiac dysfunction occurs in The HIV-1 transgenic mouse treated with zidovudine. *Lab Invest.* 2000;80(2):187–197.

Li F, Wang X, Capasso JM, et al. Rapid transition of cardiac myocytes from hyperplasia to hypertrophy during postnatal development. *J Mol Cell Cardiol.* 1996;28(8):1737–1746.

Li Y, Sun X, Wang L, et al. Myocardial toxicity of arsenic trioxide in a mouse model. *Cardiovasc Toxicol.* 2002;2(1):63–73.

Litwak KN, Mcmahan A, Lott KA, et al. Monensin toxicosis in the domestic bovine calf: a large animal model of cardiac dysfunction. *Contemp Top Lab Anim Sci.* 2005;44(3):45–49.

Liu S, Melchert RB, Kennedy RH. Inhibition of L-type Ca^{2+} channel current in rat ventricular myocytes by terfenadine. *Circ Res.* 1997;81(2):202–210.

Marcillat O, Zhang Y, Davies KJ. Oxidative and non-oxidative mechanisms in the inactivation of cardiac mitochondrial electron transport chain components by doxorubicin. *Biochem J.* 1989;259(1):181–189.

Maret W. The function of zinc metallothionein: a link between cellular zinc and redox state. *J Nutr.* 2000;130(5S suppl):1455S–1458S.

Marks AR. Intracellular calcium-release channels: regulators of cell life and death. *Am J Physiol.* 1997;272(2 Pt 2):H597–H605.

Marsh JD, Lehmann MH, Ritchie RH, et al. Androgen receptors mediate hypertrophy in cardiac myocytes. *Circulation.* 1998;98(3):256–261.

Marsin AS, Bertrand L, Rider MH, et al. Phosphorylation and activation of heart PFK-2 by AMPK has a role in the stimulation of glycolysis during ischaemia. *Curr Biol.* 2000;10(20):1247–1255.

Martin XJ, Wynne DG, Glennon PE, et al. Regulation of expression of contractile proteins with cardiac hypertrophy and failure. *Mol Cell Biochem.* 1996;157(1–2):181–189.

Mathews EC Jr, Gardin JM, Henry WL, et al. Echocardiographic abnormalities in chronic alcoholics with and without overt congestive heart failure. *Am J Cardiol.* 1981;47(3):570–578.

Matsui T, Li L, Wu JC, et al. Phenotypic spectrum caused by transgenic over-expression of activated Akt in the heart. *J Biol Chem.* 2002;277(25):22896–22901.

Mcclain CJ, Su LC. Zinc deficiency in the alcoholic: a review. *Alcohol Clin Exp Res.* 1983;7(1):5–10.

Mckenna CJ, Codd MB, Mccann HA, et al. Alcohol consumption and idiopathic dilated cardiomyopathy: a case control study. *Am Heart J.* 1998;135(5 Pt 1):833–837.

Mcmahon SB, Monroe JG. Role of primary response genes in generating cellular responses to growth factors. *FASEB J.* 1992;6(9): 2707–2715.

Mcmanus BM, Toth B, Patil KD. Aortic rupture and aortic smooth muscle tumors in mice. Induction by *p*-hydrazinobenzoic acid hydrochloride of the cultivated mushroom *Agaricus Bisporus. Lab Invest.* 1987;57(1):78–85.

Meeusen S, DeVay R, Block J, et al. Mitochondrial inner-membrane fusion and crista maintenance requires the dynamin-related GTPase Mgm1. *Cell.* 2006;127(2):383–395.

Melchert RB, Welder AA. Cardiovascular effects of androgenic-anabolic steroids. *Med Sci Sports Exerc.* 1995;27(9):1252–1262.

Metzger JM, Wahr PA, Michele DE, et al. Effects of myosin heavy chain isoform switching on Ca^{2+}-activated tension development in single adult cardiac myocytes. *Circ Res.* 1999;84(11):1310–1317.

Miller RA, Boorman GA. Morphology of neoplastic lesions induced by 1,3-butadiene in B6C3F1 mice. *Environ Health Perspect.* 1990;86: 37–48.

Molkentin JD, Lu JR, Antos CL, et al. A calcineurin-dependent transcriptional pathway for cardiac hypertrophy. *Cell.* 1998;93(2):215–228.

Monge JC. Neurohormonal markers of clinical outcome in cardiovascular disease: is endothelin the best one? *J Cardiovasc Pharmacol.* 1998;32(suppl 2):S36–S42.

Nakaki T, Nakayama M, Yamamoto S, et al. Alpha 1-adrenergic stimulation and beta 2-adrenergic inhibition of DNA synthesis in vascular smooth muscle cells. *Mol Pharmacol.* 1990;37(1):30–36.

Nattel S. Experimental evidence for proarrhythmic mechanisms of antiarrhythmic drugs. *Cardiovasc Res.* 1998;37(3):567–577.

Neubauer S, Horn M, Cramer M, et al. Myocardial phosphocreatine-to-ATP ratio is a predictor of mortality in patients with dilated cardiomyopathy. *Circulation.* 1997;96(7):2190–2196.

Neubauer S, Remkes H, Spindler M, et al. Downregulation of the Na(+)-creatine cotransporter in failing human myocardium and in experimental heart failure. *Circulation.* 1999;100(18):1847–1850.

Newton AC. Protein kinase C: structure, function, and regulation. *J Biol Chem.* 1995;270(48):28495–28498.

Olichon A, Emorine LJ, Descoins E, et al. The human dynamin-related protein OPA1 is anchored to the mitochondrial inner membrane facing the inter-membrane space. *FEBS Lett.* 2002;523(1–3):171–176.

Olivetti G, Abbi R, Quaini F, et al. Apoptosis in the failing human heart. *N Engl J Med.* 1997;336(16):1131–1141.

Olson EN. A decade of discoveries in cardiac biology. *Nat Med.* 2004;10(5):467–474.

Opie L. Heart cells and organells. In: Opie L, ed. *The Heart.* New York: Harcourt Brace Jovanovich; 1996:15–29.

Orkin SH. GATA-binding transcription factors in hematopoietic cells. *Blood.* 1992;80(3):575–581.

Ou X, Ramos KS. Modulation of aortic protein phosphorylation by benzo(A)pyrene: implications in PAH-induced atherogenesis. *J Biochem Toxicol.* 1992;7(3):147–154.

Pacher P, Ungvari Z, Kecskemeti V, et al. Review of cardiovascular effects of fluoxetine, a selective serotonin reuptake inhibitor, compared to tricyclic antidepressants. *Curr Med Chem.* 1998;5(5):381–390.

Paradis P, Maclellan WR, Belaguli NS, et al. Serum response factor mediates AP-1-dependent induction of the skeletal alpha-actin promoter in ventricular myocytes. *J Biol Chem.* 1996;271(18):10827–10833.

Penn A, Snyder C. Arteriosclerotic plaque development is "promoted" by polynuclear aromatic hydrocarbons. *Carcinogenesis.* 1988;9(12):2185.

Perez NG, Gao WD, Marban E. Novel myofilament Ca^{2+}-sensitizing property of xanthine oxidase inhibitors. *Circ Res.* 1998;83(4): 423–430.

Perry HM Jr, Erlanger MW, Gustafsson TO, et al. Reversal of cadmium-induced hypertension by D-myo-inositol-1,2,6-trisphosphate. *J Toxicol Environ Health*. 1989;28(2):151–159.

Peters A, Liu E, Verrier RL, et al. Air pollution and incidence of cardiac arrhythmia. *Epidemiology*. 2000;11(1):11–17.

Piano MR. Cellular and signaling mechanisms of cardiac hypertrophy. *J Cardiovasc Nurs*. 1994;8(4):1–26.

Piano MR. Alcoholic cardiomyopathy: incidence, clinical characteristics, and pathophysiology. *Chest*. 2002;121(5):1638–1650.

Piano MR, Bondmass M, Schwertz DW. The molecular and cellular pathophysiology of heart failure. *Heart Lung*. 1998;27(1):3–19.

Pickerill KE, Paladino JA, Schentag JJ. Comparison of the fluoroquinolones based on pharmacokinetic and pharmacodynamic parameters. *Pharmacotherapy*. 2000;20(4):417–428.

Powis G. Free radical formation by antitumor quinones. *Free Radic Biol Med*. 1989;6(1):63–101.

Pu WT, Ma Q, Izumo S. NFAT transcription factors are critical survival factors that inhibit cardiomyocyte apoptosis during phenylephrine stimulation in vitro. *Circ Res*. 2003;92(7):725–731.

Puceat M, Vassort G. Signalling by protein kinase C isoforms in the heart. *Mol Cell Biochem*. 1996;157(1–2):65–72.

Pulkki KJ. Cytokines and cardiomyocyte death. *Ann Med*. 1997;29(4):339–343.

Rao A, Luo C, Hogan PG. Transcription factors of the NFAT family: regulation and function. *Annu Rev Immunol*. 1997;15:707–747.

Reed JC, Jurgensmeier JM, Matsuyama S. Bcl-2 family proteins and mitochondria. *Biochim Biophys Acta*. 1998;1366(1–2):127–137.

Regan TJ. Alcohol and the cardiovascular system. *JAMA*. 1990;264(3):377–381.

Ribiere C, Hininger I, Rouach H, et al. Effects of chronic ethanol administration on free radical defence in rat myocardium. *Biochem Pharmacol*. 1992;44(8):1495–1500.

Richey PA, Brown SP. Pathological versus physiological left ventricular hypertrophy: a review. *J Sports Sci*. 1998;16(2):129–141.

Robbins J. Genetic modification of the heart: exploring necessity and sufficiency in the past 10 years. *J Mol Cell Cardiol*. 2004;36(5):643–652.

Robert V, Silvestre JS, Charlemagne D, et al. Biological determinants of aldosterone-induced cardiac fibrosis in rats. *Hypertension*. 1995;26(6 pt 1):971–978.

Rockhold RW. Cardiovascular toxicity of anabolic steroids. *Annu Rev Pharmacol Toxicol*. 1993;33:497–520.

Roden DM. Antiarrhythmic drugs. In: Hardman JG, Limbird LE, Molinoff PB, et al., eds. *Goodman & Gilman's The Pharmacological Basis of Therapeutics*, 9th ed. New York: McGraw-Hill;1996:839–874.

Rooney JW, Hodge MR, Mccaffrey PG, et al. A common factor regulates both th1- and th2-specific cytokine gene expression. *EMBO J*. 1994;13(3):625–633.

Rosen MR. Cardiac arrhythmias and antiarrhythmic drugs: recent advances in our understanding of mechanism. *J Cardiovasc Electrophysiol*. 1995;6(10 pt 2):868–879.

Russell RR, III, Bergeron R, Shulman GI, et al. Translocation of myocardial GLUT-4 and increased glucose uptake through activation of AMPK by AICAR. *Am J Physiol*. 1999;277(2 pt 2):H643–H649.

Sabbah HN, Sharov VG. Apoptosis in heart failure. *Prog Cardiovasc Dis*. 1998;40(6):549–562.

Saikumar P, Dong Z, Patel Y, et al. Role of hypoxia-induced bax translocation and cytochrome *c* release in reoxygenation injury. *Oncogene*. 1998;17(26):3401–3415.

Saupe KW, Spindler M, Hopkins JC, et al. Kinetic, thermodynamic, and developmental consequences of deleting creatine kinase isoenzymes from the heart. Reaction kinetics of the creatine kinase isoenzymes in the intact heart. *J Biol Chem*. 2000;275(26):19742–19746.

Sawyer DB, Fukazawa R, Arstall MA, et al. Daunorubicin-induced apoptosis in rat cardiac myocytes is inhibited by dexrazoxane. *Circ Res*. 1999;84(3):257–265.

Shier WT, Dubourdieu DJ. Sodium- and calcium-dependent steps in the mechanism of neonatal rat cardiac myocyte killing by ionophores. I. The sodium-carrying ionophore, monensin. *Toxicol Appl Pharmacol*. 1992;116(1):38–46.

Shioi T, Kang PM, Douglas PS, et al. The conserved phosphoinositide 3-kinase pathway determines heart size in mice. *EMBO J*. 2000;19(11):2537–2548.

Shioi T, Mcmullen JR, Kang PM, et al. Akt/protein kinase B promotes organ growth in transgenic mice. *Mol Cell Biol*. 2002;22(8):2799–2809.

Shipp JC, Opie LH, Challoner D. Fatty acid and glucose metabolism in the perfused heart. *Nature*. 1961;189(4769):1018–1019.

Simons FE. The therapeutic index of newer H1-receptor antagonists. *Clin Exp Allergy*. 1994;24(8):707–723.

Sleight P. Calcium antagonists during and after myocardial infarction. *Drugs*. 1996;51(2):216–225.

Smirnova E, Shurland DL, Ryazantsev SN, van der Bliek AM. A human dynamin-related protein controls the distribution of mitochondria. *J Cell Biol*. 1998;143(2):351–358.

Solem LE, Henry TR, Wallace KB. Disruption of mitochondrial calcium homeostasis following chronic doxorubicin administration. *Toxicol Appl Pharmacol*. 1994;129(2):214–222.

Solomon SD, McMurray JJ, Pfeffer MA, et al. Cardiovascular risk associated with celecoxib in a clinical trual for colorectal adenoma prevntion. *N Engl J Med*. 2005;352:1071–1080.

Song Z, Chen H, Fiket M, Alexander C, Chan DC. OPA1 processing controls mitochondrial fusion and is regulated by mRNA splicing, membrane potential, and Yme1L. *J Cell Biol*. 2007;178(5):749–755.

Splawski I, Shen J, Timothy KW, et al. Spectrum of mutations in long-QT syndrome genes. KVLQT1, HERG, SCN5A, KCNE1, and KCNE2. *Circulation*. 2000;102(10):1178–1185.

Stemmer PM, Klee CB. Dual calcium ion regulation of calcineurin by calmodulin and calcineurin B. *Biochemistry*. 1994;33(22):6859–6866.

Stief CG, Uckert S, Becker AJ, et al. Effects of sildenafil on camp and cGMP levels in isolated human cavernous and cardiac tissue. *Urology*. 2000;55(1):146–150.

Stolley PD, Strom BL, Sartwell PE. Oral contraceptives and vascular disease. *Epidemiol Rev*. 1989;11:241–243.

Sugden PH, Clerk A. "Stress-responsive" mitogen-activated protein kinases (C-Jun N-terminal kinases and P38 mitogen-activated protein kinases) in the myocardium. *Circ Res*. 1998;83(4):345–352.

Sugishita K, Kinugawa K, Shimizu T, et al. Cellular basis for the acute inhibitory effects of IL-6 and TNF-alpha on excitation–contraction coupling. *J Mol Cell Cardiol*. 1999;31(8):1457–1467.

Suzuki K, Kostin S, Person V, et al. Time course of the apoptotic cascade and effects of caspase inhibitors in adult rat ventricular cardiomyocytes. *J Mol Cell Cardiol*. 2001;33(5):983–994.

Swynghedauw B. Molecular mechanisms of myocardial remodeling. *Physiol Rev*. 1999;79(1):215–262.

Symanski JD, Gettes LS: Drug effects on the electrocardiogram. A review of their clinical importance. *Drugs*. 1993;46(2):219–248.

Talhari C, lauceviciute I, Enderlein E, et al. COX-2-selective inhibitor valdecoxib induces severe allergic skin reactions. *J Allergy Clin Immunol*. 2005;115:1089–1090.

Tan Y, Rouse J, Zhang A, et al. FGF and stress regulate CREB and ATF-1 via A pathway involving P38 MAP kinase and MAPKAP kinase-2. *EMBO J*. 15(17):4629–4642, 1996.

Taneike M, Yamaguchi O, Nakai A, et al. Inhibition of autophagy in the heart induces age-related cardiomyopathy. *Autophagy*. 2010;6(5):600–606.

Thomas T, Sutton ET, Bryant MW, et al. In vivo vascular damage, leukocyte activation and inflammatory response induced by beta-amyloid. *J Submicrosc Cytol Pathol*. 1997;29(3):293–304.

Tibbles LA, Woodgett JR. The stress-activated protein kinase pathways. *Cell Mol Life Sci*. 1999;55(10):1230–1254.

Tolkovsky AM. Mitophagy. *Biochim Biophys Acta*. 2009;1793(9):1508–1515.

Toraason M, Wey HE, Richards DE, et al. Altered Ca²⁺ Mobilization during excitation–contraction in cultured cardiac myocytes exposed to antimony. *Toxicol Appl Pharmacol*. 1997;146(1):104–115.

van Bilsen M, Smeets PJ, Gilde AJ, et al. Metabolic remodelling of the failing heart: the cardiac burn-out syndrome? *Cardiovasc Res*. 2004;61(2):218–226.

van Empel VP, De Windt LJ. Myocyte hypertrophy and apoptosis: a balancing act. *Cardiovasc Res*. 2004;63(3):487–499.

van Vleet JF, Amstutz HE, Weirich WE, et al. Clinical, clinicopathologic, and pathologic alterations in acute monensin toxicosis in cattle. *Am J Vet Res.* 1983;44(11):2133–2144.

Ventura-Clapier R, Garnier A, Veksler V. Energy metabolism in heart failure. *J Physiol.* 2004;555(pt 1):1–13.

Vestal RE, Eiriksson CE Jr, Musser B, et al. Effect of intravenous aminophylline on plasma levels of catecholamines and related cardiovascular and metabolic responses in man. *Circulation.* 1983;67(1):162–171.

Wald N, Howard S. Smoking, carbon monoxide and arterial disease. *Ann Occup Hyg.* 1975;18(1):1–14.

Wallace KB, Hausner E, Herman E, et al. Serum troponins as biomarkers of drug-induced cardiac toxicity. *Toxicol Pathol.* 2004;32(1):106–121.

Wallimann T, Dolder M, Schlattner U, et al. Some new aspects of creatine kinase (CK): compartmentation, structure, function and regulation for cellular and mitochondrial bioenergetics and physiology. *Biofactors.* 1998;8(3–4):229–234.

Wang GW, Klein JB, Kang YJ. Metallothionein inhibits doxorubicin-induced mitochondrial cytochrome *c* release and caspase-3 activation in cardiomyocytes. *J Pharmacol Exp Ther.* 2001a;298(2):461–468.

Wang GW, Zhou Z, Klein JB, et al. Inhibition of hypoxia/reoxygenation-induced apoptosis in metallothionein-overexpressing cardiomyocytes. *Am J Physiol Heart Circ Physiol.* 2001b;280(5):H2292–H2299.

Wang L, Zhou Z, Saari JT, et al. Alcohol-induced myocardial fibrosis in metallothionein-null mice: prevention by zinc supplementation. *Am J Pathol.* 2005;167(2):337–344.

Wang XZ, Ron D. Stress-induced phosphorylation and activation of the transcription factor CHOP (GADD153) by P38 MAP kinase. *Science.* 1996;272(5266):1347–1349.

Wang Y, Huang S, Sah VP, et al. Cardiac muscle cell hypertrophy and apoptosis induced by distinct members of the p38 mitogen-activated protein kinase family. *J Biol Chem.* 1998;273(4):2161–2168.

Weber KT. Are myocardial fibrosis and diastolic dysfunction reversible in hypertensive heart disease? *Congest Heart Fail.* 2005;11(6):322–324.

Wettschureck N, Rutten H, Zywietz A, et al. Absence of pressure overload induced myocardial hypertrophy after conditional inactivation of Galphaq/Galpha11 in cardiomyocytes. *Nat Med.* 2001;7(11):1236–1240.

Wisneski JA, Gertz EW, Neese RA, et al. Myocardial metabolism of free fatty acids. Studies with ¹⁴C-labeled substrates in humans. *J Clin Invest.* 1987;79(2):359–366.

Wollert KC, Heineke J, Westermann J, et al. The cardiac Fas (APO-1/CD95) receptor/Fas ligand system: relation to diastolic wall stress in volume-overload hypertrophy in vivo and activation of the transcription factor AP-1 in cardiac myocytes. *Circulation.* 2000;101(10):1172–1178.

Wollnik B, Schroeder BC, Kubisch C, et al. Pathophysiological mechanisms of dominant and recessive KVLQT1 K⁺ channel mutations found in inherited cardiac arrhythmias. *Hum Mol Genet.* 1997;6(11):1943–1949.

Wyllie AH. Death from inside out: an overview. *Philos Trans R Soc Lond B Biol Sci.* 1994;345(1313):237–241.

Xu W, Liu Y, Wang S, et al. Cytoprotective role of Ca²⁺-activated K⁺ channels in the cardiac inner mitochondrial membrane. *Science.* 2002;298(5595):1029–1033.

Yamamoto C, Miyamoto A, Sakamoto M, et al. Lead perturbs the regulation of spontaneous release of tissue plasminogen activator and plasminogen activator inhibitor-1 from vascular smooth muscle cells and fibroblasts in culture. *Toxicology.* 1997;117(2–3):153–161.

Yamamoto M, Ko LJ, Leonard MW, et al. Activity and tissue-specific expression of the transcription factor NF-E1 multigene family. *Genes Dev.* 1990;4(10):1650–1662.

Yamashita K, Kajstura J, Discher DJ, et al. Reperfusion-activated Akt kinase prevents apoptosis in transgenic mouse hearts overexpressing insulin-like growth factor-1. *Circ Res.* 2001;88(6):609–614.

Yaoita H, Ogawa K, Maehara K, et al. Apoptosis in relevant clinical situations: contribution of apoptosis in myocardial infarction. *Cardiovasc Res.* 2000;45(3):630–641.

Yin T, Sandhu G, Wolfgang CD, et al. Tissue-specific pattern of stress kinase activation in ischemic/reperfused heart and kidney. *J Biol Chem.* 1997;272(32):19943–19950.

Yoon Y, Krueger EW, Oswald BJ, McNiven MA. The mitochondrial protein hFis1 regulates mitochondrial fission in mammalian cells through an interaction with the dynamin-like protein DLP1. *Mol Cell Biol.* 2003;23(15):5409–5420.

Young M, Fullerton M, Dilley R, et al. Mineralocorticoids, hypertension, and cardiac fibrosis. *J Clin Invest.* 1994;93(6):2578–2583.

Yu T, Jhun BS, Yoon Y. High-glucose stimulation increases reactive oxygen species production through the calcium and mitogen-activated protein kinase-mediated activation of mitochondrial fission. *Antioxid Redox Signal.* 2011;14(3):425–437.

Yu T, Sheu SS, Robotham JL, Yoon Y. Mitochondrial fission mediates high glucose-induced cell death through elevated production of reactive oxygen species. *Cardiovasc Res.* 2008;79(2):341–351.

Zakhari S. Cardiovascular toxicology of halogenated hydrocarbons and other solvents. In: Acosta D, ed. *Cardiovascular Toxicology.* New York: Raven Press; 1992:409–454.

Zhou S, Starkov A, Froberg MK, et al. Cumulative and irreversible cardiac mitochondrial dysfunction induced by doxorubicin. *Cancer Res.* 2001;61(2):771–777.

Zhou W, Fontenot HJ, Liu S, et al. Modulation of cardiac calcium channels by propofol. *Anesthesiology.* 1997;86(3):670–675.

Zhou W, Fontenot HJ, Wang SN, et al. Propofol-induced alterations in myocardial beta-adrenoceptor binding and responsiveness. *Anesth Analg.* 1999;89(3):604–608.

Zorzano A, Hernández-Alvarez MI, Palacín M, Mingrone G. Alterations in the mitochondrial regulatory pathways constituted by the nuclear cofactors PGC-1alpha or PGC-1beta and mitofusin 2 in skeletal muscle in type 2 diabetes. *Biochim Biophys Acta.* 2010;1797(6–7):1028–1033.

Zou Y, Hiroi Y, Uozumi H, et al. Calcineurin plays a critical role in the development of pressure overload-induced cardiac hypertrophy. *Circulation.* 2001;104(1):97–101.

chapter 19

Toxic Responses of the Skin

Robert H. Rice and Theodora M. Mauro

INTRODUCTION

As the body's first line of defense against external insult, the skin's enormous surface area (1.5-2 m²) is exposed routinely to chemicals and may inadvertently serve as a portal of entry for topical contactants. Recognizing the potential hazards of skin exposure, the National Institute of Occupational Safety and Health (NIOSH) characterized skin disease as one of the most pervasive occupational health problems in the United States. In 1982, NIOSH placed skin disease in the top 10 leading work-related diseases based on frequency, severity, and the potential for prevention. Data from the Bureau of Labor Statistics indicate that in 2004 skin disease attributed to workplace exposures accounted for nearly 16% of reported nonfatal occupational disease in private industry; incidence data indicate a rate of 4.4 cases per 10,000 or nearly 39,000 new cases per year. On that basis, the annual economic burden of dermatitis in workers in the USA has been estimated as ≈$1.2 billion (Blanciforti, 2010). Substantial reduction in the reported incidence has occurred in recent years thanks to workplace cleanup and better personal protective equipment. Nevertheless, improvements in prevention and management are needed for continued progress (Emmett, 2003). Skin conditions resulting from exposures to consumer products or occupational illnesses not resulting in lost work time are poorly recorded and tracked. Hence, the incidence of such skin diseases appears greatly underestimated.

NIOSH recently changed its skin notations to reflect more accurately the varied risks to workers after topical exposure (see DHHS(NIOSH) Publication No. 2009-147, www.cdc.gov/niosh). Previously, inhalation exposures were thought to produce the most risk to workers, with skin exposure being only a secondary exposure pathway. The new guidelines now reflect increased understanding of several pathways by which skin exposure can lead to disease: systemic toxicity via skin absorption (SYS), direct effects that damage the skin (DIR), and immune-mediated responses to chemicals that contact the skin (SEN). The new notations utilize these categories to designate hazard-specific skin notations, and have incorporated standard criteria to ensure consistency in how chemicals are designated. Determining the hazard potential of a particular chemical is based on physicochemical properties of the substance, toxicokinetic studies, epidemiological data, in vitro or in vivo laboratory testing, and in silico computational predictions. These criteria are specified in the chemical designation.

SKIN AS A BARRIER

A large and highly accessible human organ, the skin protects the body against external insults to maintain internal homeostasis. Its biological sophistication allows it to perform a myriad of functions above and beyond that of a suit of armor. Physiologically, the skin participates directly in thermal, electrolyte, hormonal, metabolic, antimicrobial and immune regulation, without which a human would perish. Rather than merely repelling noxious physical agents, the skin may react to them with a variety of defensive mechanisms that prevent internal or widespread cutaneous damage. If an insult is severe or sufficiently intense to overwhelm the protective function of the skin, acute or chronic injury becomes readily manifest in various ways. The specific presentation depends on a variety of intrinsic and extrinsic factors including body site, duration of exposure, and other environmental conditions (Table 19-1).

Skin Histology

The skin consists of two major components—the outer epidermis and the underlying dermis, which are separated by a basement membrane (Fig. 19-1). The junction ordinarily is not flat but has an

Table 19-1

Factors Influencing Cutaneous Responses

VARIABLE	COMMENT
Body site	
Palms/soles	Thick stratum corneum—good physical barrier
	Common site of contact with chemicals
	Occlusion with protective clothing
Intertriginous areas (axillae, groin, neck, finger webs, umbilicus, and genitalia)	Moist, occluded areas
	Chemical trapping
	Enhanced percutaneous absorption
Face	Exposed frequently
	Surface lipid interacts with hydrophobic substances
	Chemicals frequently transferred from hands
Eyelids	Poor barrier function—thin epidermis
	Sensitive to irritants
Postauricular region	Chemical trapping
	Occlusion
Scalp	Chemical trapping
	Hair follicles susceptible to metabolic damage
Predisposing cutaneous illnesses	
Atopic dermatitis	Increased sensitivity to irritants
	Impaired barrier function
Psoriasis	Impaired barrier function
Genetic factors	Predisposition to skin disorders
	Variation in sensitivity to irritants
	Susceptibility to contact sensitization
Temperature	Vasodilation—improved percutaneous absorption
	Increased sweating—trapping
Humidity	Increased sweating—trapping
Season	Variation in relative humidity
	Chapping and wind-related skin changes

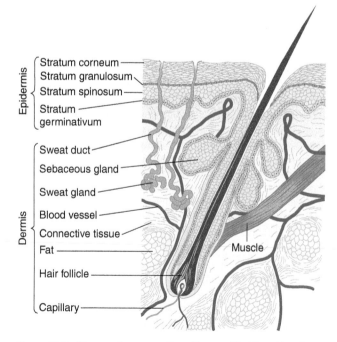

Figure 19-1. *Diagram of a cross-section of human skin.* The epidermis and pilosebaceous units are shown in pink and purple.

Labels: Epidermis: Stratum corneum, Stratum granulosum, Stratum spinosum, Stratum germinativum. Dermis: Sweat duct, Sebaceous gland, Sweat gland, Blood vessel, Connective tissue, Fat, Hair follicle, Capillary, Muscle.

undulating appearance (rete ridges). In addition, epidermal appendages (hair follicles, sebaceous glands, and eccrine glands) span the epidermis and are embedded in the dermis. In thickness, the dermis comprises approximately 90% of the skin and has largely a supportive function. It has a high content of collagen and elastin secreted by scattered fibroblasts, thus providing the skin with elastic properties. Separating the dermis from underlying tissues is a layer of adipocytes, whose accumulation of fat has a cushioning action. The blood supply to the epidermis originates in the capillaries located in the rete ridges at the dermal–epidermal junction. Capillaries also supply the bulbs of the hair follicles and the secretory cells of the eccrine (sweat) glands. The ducts from these glands carry a dilute salt solution to the surface of the skin, where its evaporation provides cooling.

The interfollicular epidermis is a stratified squamous epithelium consisting primarily of keratinocytes. These cells are tightly attached to each other by desmosomes and to the basement membrane by hemidesmosomes. Melanocytes are interspersed among the basal cells and distributed in the papilla of hair follicles. In the epidermis, these cells are stimulated by ultraviolet light to produce melanin granules. The granules are extruded and taken up by the surrounding keratinocytes, which thereby become pigmented. Migrating through the epidermis are numerous Langerhans cells, which are important participants in the immune response of skin to foreign agents.

Keratinocytes of the basal layer comprise the germinative compartment. When a basal cell divides, one of the progeny detaches from the basal lamina and migrates outward. As cells move toward the skin surface, they undergo a remarkable program of terminal differentiation. They gradually express new protein markers and accumulate keratin proteins, from which the name of this cell type is derived. The keratins form insoluble intermediate filaments accounting for nearly 40% of the total cell protein in the spinous layer. At the granular layer, the cells undergo a striking morphological transformation, becoming flattened and increasing in volume nearly 40-fold. Lipid granules fuse with the plasma membrane at the granular layer/stratum corneum interface, filling the intercellular spaces of the stratum corneum with lipid, as opposed to the aqueous intercellular solution in the viable epidermis. This lipid performs a variety of defensive functions, both in preventing diffusion of water and ions out of the body, and preventing access of toxins and bacteria into the body. It thus constitutes the major barrier to toxin entry into the skin (Elias, 2005). Meanwhile, the plasma membranes of these cells become permeable, resulting in the loss of their reducing environment and consequently in extensive disulfide bonding among keratin proteins. Cell organelles are degraded, while a protein envelope is synthesized immediately beneath the plasma membrane. The membrane is altered characteristically by the loss of phospholipid and the addition of sphingolipid.

This program of terminal differentiation, beginning as keratinocytes leave the basal layer, produces the outermost layer of the skin, the stratum corneum. No longer viable, the mature cells (called *corneocytes*) are approximately 80% keratin in content. They are gradually shed from the surface and replaced from beneath. The process typically takes two weeks for basal cells to reach the stratum corneum and another two weeks to be shed from the surface. In the skin disease psoriasis, the migration of cells to the surface is nearly 10-fold faster than normal, resulting in a stratum corneum populated by cells that are not completely mature. In instances in which the outer layer is deficient due to disease or physical or chemical trauma, the barrier to the environment that the skin provides is inferior to that provided by normal, healthy skin.

Percutaneous Absorption

Until the turn of the century, the skin was believed to provide an impervious barrier to exogenous substances. Gradually, the ability of substances to penetrate the skin, though this process generally is very slow, became appreciated. During the past 50 years, the stratum corneum has been recognized as the primary barrier (Scheuplein and Blank, 1971). Diseases (eg, psoriasis) or other conditions (eg, abrasion, wounding) in which this barrier is compromised can permit greatly increased uptake of poorly permeable substances, as does removal of the stratum corneum by tape stripping or organic solvents such as acetone. The viable layer of epidermis provides a much less effective barrier, because hydrophilic chemicals readily diffuse into the intercellular water, while hydrophobic agents can partition into cell membranes, and each can diffuse readily to the blood supply in the rete ridges of the dermis.

Probably the best-known biological membrane barrier for this purpose, the stratum corneum prevents water loss from underlying tissues by evaporation. Its hydrophobic character reflects the lipid content of the intercellular space, approximately 15% of the total volume (Elias, 1992). The lipids, a major component being sphingolipids, have a high content of long-chain ceramides, removal of which seriously compromises barrier function as measured by transepidermal water loss. The stratum corneum ordinarily is hydrated (typically 20% water), the moisture residing in corneocyte protein,

but it can take up a great deal more water upon prolonged immersion, thereby reducing the effectiveness of the barrier to chemicals with a hydrophilic character. Indeed, occlusion of the skin with plastic wrap, permitting the retention of perspiration underneath, is a commonly employed technique to enhance uptake of chemicals applied to the skin surface. Although penetration from the air is generally too low to be of concern, protection from skin uptake may be advisable for some compounds (eg, nitrobenzene) at concentrations high enough to require respirator use.

Finding the rate at which the uptake of agents through the skin occurs is important for estimating the consequences of exposure to many agents we encounter in the environment. Indeed, a regulatory strategy permitting bathing in water considered barely unfit for drinking was revised when it was realized that exposure from dermal/inhalation uptake during bathing could be comparable to that from drinking 2 L of the water (Brown *et al.*, 1984). Uptake through the skin is now incorporated in pharmacokinetic modeling to estimate potential risks from exposures. The degree of uptake depends upon the details of exposure conditions, being proportional to solute concentration (assuming it is dilute), time, and the amount of skin surface exposed. In addition, two intrinsic factors contribute to the absorption rate of a given compound: its hydrophobicity, which affects its ability to partition into epidermal lipid, and its rate of diffusion through this barrier. A measure of the first property is the commonly used octanol/water partitioning ratio (K_{ow}). This is particularly relevant for exposure to contaminated water, as occurs during bathing or swimming. However, partitioning of a chemical into the skin is greatly affected by its solubility in or adhesion to the medium in which it is applied (including soil). Similarly, very hydrophobic compounds, once in the stratum corneum, may diffuse only very slowly into less hydrophobic regions below. The second property is an inverse function of molecular weight (MW) or molecular volume. Thus, hydrophobic agents of low MW permeate the skin better than those of high MW or those that are hydrophilic. For small molecules, hydrophobicity is a dominant factor in penetration.

Although only small amounts of chemicals may penetrate the stratum corneum, those of high potency may still be very dangerous. For example, hydrophobic organophosphorus and carbamate pesticides can be neurotoxic to humans and domestic animals by skin contact. Children and adolescents harvesting tobacco are especially susceptible to poisoning by contact with nicotine, a natural pesticide present in moisture on the leaves (McKnight and Spiller, 2005). Conditions of topical treatment of livestock for pest control must take into consideration not only the tolerance of the animals but also residues in meat and milk resulting from skin penetration. High level skin exposure to chemicals considered safe at low levels can be dangerous, evident from the nervous system toxicity and deaths of babies exposed to hexachlorophene mistakenly added to talcum powder for their diapers (Martin-Bouyer *et al.*, 1982). Previous findings of *N*-nitrosamines that penetrate skin well (such as *N*-nitrosodiethanolamine) in cutting oils and cosmetics raised concern and led to their monitoring and to reduction of exposure.

Considerable empirical information has been collected on some compounds of special interest (including pharmaceuticals, pesticides, and pollutants) for use in quantifying structure–penetration relationships. From such information, relations can be obtained for skin penetration (P_{cw}) using empirically derived constants (C_1, C_2, C_3) that have the form shown below (Potts and Guy, 1992).

$$\log P_{cw} = C_1 - C_2(\text{MW}) + C_3 \log K_{ow}$$

Such relations describe steady-state conditions, in which a chemical leaves the stratum corneum at the same rate it enters. Because rates of transfer of very hydrophobic agents into the aqueous phase of the spinous layer are slow, saturation of the stratum corneum provides a depot, leading to continued penetration into the body for relatively long time periods after external exposure to a chemical stops. Recognition that such estimates overpredict uptake from short exposures has led to modeling of limited doses (Guy, 2010a).

Diffusion through the epidermis is considerably faster at some anatomical sites than others. A list in order of decreasing permeability gives the following hierarchy: foot sole > palm > forehead > abdomen (Scheuplein and Blank, 1971). Scrotal skin reportedly has the highest permeability for some topical chemicals (Fisher, 1989). Under ordinary conditions, absorption through the epidermal appendages is generally neglected, despite the ability of chemicals to bypass the stratum corneum by this route, because the combined appendageal surface area is such a small fraction of the total available for uptake. However, because loading of the stratum corneum is slow, penetration through the appendages can constitute an appreciable fraction of the total for short exposures. In some cases, the effects of appendages can even be dominant. For instance, benzo[a]pyrene penetrates the skin of haired mice several fold faster than that of hairless strains (Kao and Hall, 1987). Recent studies indicate the hair follicles serve as important routes of entry for hydrophilic agents and pharmaceuticals as well, a property that could be exploited for therapeutic purposes (Otberg et al., 2008).

Transdermal Drug Delivery The ability of the stratum corneum to serve as a reservoir for exogenously applied agents is well illustrated by the recent development of methods for the delivery of pharmaceuticals. Application of drugs to the skin can produce systemic effects, a phenomenon observed unintentionally before the ability of the skin to serve as a delivery system was appreciated. For example, topical exposure of young girls to estrogens has led to reports of pseudoprecocious puberty, while in young or adult males, such exposure has produced gynecomastia (Amin et al., 1998). Transfer of topically applied hormonal medication from a treated to an untreated individual with consequent effects on the latter is also observed (Busse and Maibach, 2011).

Specially designed patches are currently in use to deliver at least 17 different drugs (including estradiol, testosterone, nitroglycerin, scopolamine, clonidine, fentanyl, and nicotine) for therapeutic purposes (Guy, 2010b), and others are under development. The advantages of this approach over oral dosing include providing a steady infusion for extended periods (typically one-seven days), thereby avoiding large variations in plasma concentration, preventing exposure to the acidic pH of the stomach, and avoiding biotransformation in the gastrointestinal tract or from first-pass removal by the liver. The contrast in plasma concentration kinetics between different methods of delivery is particularly evident for chemicals that are rapidly metabolized, such as nitroglycerin, which has a half-life of minutes. A variety of chemicals, chosen carefully to minimize irritation or allergenicity, have been incorporated into pharmaceutical preparations to enhance absorption and penetration. In addition, encapsulating a drug in small vesicles of phospholipid or nonionic surfactant or coating nanoparticles can improve delivery through the epidermis and hair follicles (Desai et al., 2010). Finally, various microneedle systems have been studied to deliver drugs, vaccines, and gene therapy across the skin. These systems may prove especially important in delivering vaccines in areas where refrigeration for conventional vaccines is not available (Prausnitz et al., 2009).

Measurements of Penetration A pharmacokinetic approach with intact subjects has been commonly employed with experimental animals. To simplify determination of penetration kinetics,

skin flaps may be employed and the capillary blood flow monitored to measure penetration. For this purpose, pig skin has particular utility (Riviere and Brooks, 2005). Because penetration through rodent skin is usually faster than through human skin, the former can provide an overestimate for behavior of the latter. Without verification using human skin, such measurements are subject to large uncertainties due to species differences in density of epidermal appendages, stratum corneum properties (eg, thickness, lipid composition), and biotransformation rates. A promising variation minimizing species differences is to use skin grafts on experimental animals for these measurements. Human skin persists well on athymic mice and retains its normal barrier properties.

For risk assessment and pharmaceutical design, the most useful subject for experimentation is human skin. Volunteers are dosed, plasma and/or urine concentrations are quantified at suitable intervals, and amounts excreted from the body are estimated. Past measurements of penetration often used ^{14}C-labeled agents. This approach is not preferred, but use of isotopic labels now is readily feasible when coupled to ultrasensitive detection by accelerator mass spectrometry (Buchholz et al., 1999). For in vitro work, excised split-thickness skin can be employed in special diffusion chambers, though care is needed to preserve the viability of the living layer of epidermis. The chemical is removed for measurement from the underside by a fluid into which it partitions, thereby permitting continued penetration. Commonly employed is a simpler setup using cadaver skin with the lower dermis removed. This lacks biotransformation capability, but retains the barrier function of the stratum corneum. Accurate testing of percutaneous absorption of poorly soluble chemicals from environmental and pharmaceutical substrates requires attention to details of particle size, component complexes, vehicle, application rate, and skin contact. A long time goal has been to predict chemical permeability from chemical structure. Comparisons of predictive models with results from transdermal patches show good correlations, despite large discrepancies in fluxes of some compounds, and emphasize the importance of experimental details (Farahmand and Maibach, 2009).

Biotransformation

The ability of the skin to metabolize chemicals that diffuse through it contributes to its barrier function. In specific activity, phase I metabolism in the skin usually is only a small fraction ($\approx3\%$) of that in the liver (Rolsted et al., 2008), but it is capable of affecting the outcome of exposure. Biotransformation influences the biological activity of xenobiotics and topically applied drugs, leading to their degradation or their activation as skin sensitizers or carcinogens (Svensson, 2009). While overall activities are normally low, they can be induced (or suppressed). In fact, a large fraction of the pharmaceuticals used in clinical dermatology are cytochrome P450 inducers, inhibitors, or substrates (Ahmad and Mukhtar, 2004). For example, cytochromes P450 1A1 and 1B1 are inducible in the epidermis to high levels by crude coal tar (Smith et al., 2006), which is used in dermatological therapy. Well-known xenobiotic inducers of these isozymes include tetrachlorodibenzo-p-dioxin (TCDD), polycyclic aromatic hydrocarbons, and coplanar polychlorinated biphenyls. Exposure to such inducers could influence skin biotransformation and even sensitize epidermal cells to other chemicals that are not good inducers themselves, a phenomenon observable in cell culture (Walsh et al., 1995).

Biotransformation of a variety of compounds in the skin has been detected, including arachidonic acid derivatives, steroids, retinoids, amines, and polycyclic aromatic hydrocarbons, suggesting that multiple P450 activities are expressed. Using sensitive technologies, it is now evident that numerous distinct isozymes are expressed at widely varying levels. Evidence for expression of >30 CYP genes has been obtained by DNA microarray and real-time polymerase chain reaction (Hu *et al.*, 2010; Luu-The *et al.*, 2009). A recent survey of those in the CYP1-4 families indicated that half were expressed at substantially higher levels in differentiating keratinocytes (similar to spinous cells) than in basal-like cells (Du *et al.*, 2006). Species differences are apparent in the amounts of P450 activities detectable. For example, measured ethoxycoumarin-*O*-deethylase activity is 20-fold higher in mouse than human (or rat) skin. Differences of such magnitude help rationalize the observation that the rate of penetration of ethoxycoumarin is sufficient to saturate its metabolism in some species such as human but not in others such as mouse or guinea pig (Storm *et al.*, 1990). Beyond the cytochromes P450, other phase I enzymes expressed in the skin include flavin-dependent monooxygenases, aldehyde dehydrogenases, carboxylesterases, and glutathione peroxidases (Hu *et al.*, 2010). To the extent that phase I and II metabolism influences sensitization to exogenous chemicals (Svensson, 2009), they may also help rationalize species differences in allergic response.

Enzymes participating in phase II metabolism are expressed in skin. Several isozymes each of UDP glucuronosyltransferase, sulfotransferase, and glutathione *S*-transferase have been detected in human (Hu *et al.*, 2010; Luu-The *et al.*, 2009) and rodent skin (Oesch *et al.*, 2007). In general, this activity occurs at a lower rate than observed in the liver, but exceptions are evident, as in the case of quinone reductase (Khan *et al.*, 1987). Different species express different relative amounts of the various isozymes, which could alter resulting target specificities or degrees of responsiveness. Glutathione *S*-transferase, for instance, catalyzes the reaction of glutathione with exogenous electrophiles or provides intracellular transport of bound compounds in the absence of a reaction. It also facilitates the reaction of glutathione with endogenous products of arachidonate lipoxygenation (leukotrienes) to yield mediators of anaphylaxis and chemotaxis, which are elements of the inflammatory response in skin. Of the first three major transferase forms characterized in liver, the dominant form in skin of humans and rodents is the P isozyme. A comparison of human with rodent skin indicates the former has higher glutathione *S*-transferase activity but lower glutathione content, suggesting that it may be less susceptible to low doses of electrophilic substrates, whereas rodent skin could be less susceptible at higher doses when glutathione is depleted in human but not mouse skin (Jewell *et al.*, 2000).

A variety of other metabolic enzyme activities have also been detected in human epidermal cells, including sulfatases, β-glucuronidase, *N*-acetyl transferases, esterases, and reductases (Hu *et al.*, 2010; Luu-The *et al.*, 2009). In addition, the intercellular region of the stratum corneum has catabolic activities (eg, protease, lipase, glycosidase, and phosphatase) supplied by the lamellar bodies along with their characteristic lipid (Elias, 1992). The epidermis and pilosebaceous units are the most important drug targets and sites of toxic effects sites and, indeed, are the major sources of biotransformation activity in the skin. However, other cell types such as fibroblasts are known to participate in biotransformation, helping to rationalize observations that organotypic cell cultures containing underlying fibroblasts resemble natural skin in biotransformation better than those without fibroblasts (Gibbs *et al.*, 2007; Hu *et al.*, 2010; Luu-The *et al.*, 2009). Such cultures, where keratinocytes float on collagen gels at the air–liquid interface, are better skin mimics than conventional ones using established keratinocyte lines. Their development has stimulated aspirations that these in vitro models can replace much animal testing of cosmetics and potential skin toxicants.

The report that cholesterol sulfotransferase is regulated by ligands of LXR and PPAR illustrates the potential for exogenous chemicals, including pharmaceuticals, to influence such activities and thereby the barrier function of the skin (Jiang *et al.*, 2005), where penetration can be influenced by cell differentiation and biotransformation. The influence of hydroxysteroid dehydrogenases and microsomal reductase activities during percutaneous absorption is evident in studies on skin in organ culture. Biotransformation can activate prodrugs, an example being minoxidil, applied to prevent hair loss, which undergoes sulfation locally to its active form. To permit increased penetration of pharmaceuticals through the lipid barrier of the stratum corneum, prodrug design strategies have been developed that depend on epidermal esterase activity. Thus, hydrophobic esters of pharmaceuticals targeting the skin (eg, acne) could be applied to the skin surface, de-esterified during transit, and yield slow release of the active forms (Fang and Leu, 2006).

CONTACT DERMATITIS

In the occupational arena, where records are compiled on large workforces, contact dermatitis is by far the largest category (≈90%) of compensated skin disease. Using eczema of the hand as a sentinel condition, since 80% of the total reported dermatitis occurs at that location (10% on the face), reveals a prevalence of 7% to 10% among workers. Attributed to better diagnosis, more accurate identification of offending chemicals, and more effective prevention and worker education, the fraction of afflicted workers recovering without impairment has improved nearly to 80% with proper management (Belsito, 2005). However, while certain conditions carry a favorable prognosis, others (eg, chronic cumulative irritant contact dermatitis or contact allergy to nickel, chromate, formaldehyde, or rubber) frequently result in chronic disease in which changing jobs is of limited or no benefit (Belsito, 2005; Emmett, 2003). Overall, contact dermatitis falls into the two major categories of irritant and allergic forms that share important features (Watkins and Maibach, 2009). Both involve inflammatory processes and can have indistinguishable clinical characteristics of erythema (redness), induration (thickening and firmness), scaling (flaking), and vesiculation (blistering) in areas of direct contact with the chemical. Biopsies from affected sites reveal a mixed-cell inflammatory infiltrate of lymphocytes and eosinophils and spongiosis (intercellular edema), but are insufficient to distinguish the two conditions from each other or from certain other common syndromes. The two can coexist. For example, since wet cement is alkaline and often contains chromates (commonly allergenic), chronic exposure can produce a composite response.

Irritant Dermatitis

Accounting for nearly 80% of contact dermatitis cases, this condition arises from the direct action of agents on the skin. A chemical in this category is anticipated to give an adverse reaction to anyone if the concentration is high enough and the exposure time long enough. Certain chemicals at sufficient concentration produce an acute irritation, sometimes called a second-degree chemical burn, that can even result in scarring in serious cases. These include strong acids, alkalies, and powerful oxidizing and reducing agents that substantially disrupt the cornified layer, producing cytotoxicity directly. Contact with a variety of plants can also have irritant effects (Modi *et al.*, 2009). Exposure stimulates release of proinflammatory cytokines (IL1-α, IL1-β, and TNF-α) from keratinocytes. More common is chronic cumulative irritation from repeated exposures to mild irritants such as soaps, detergents, solvents and

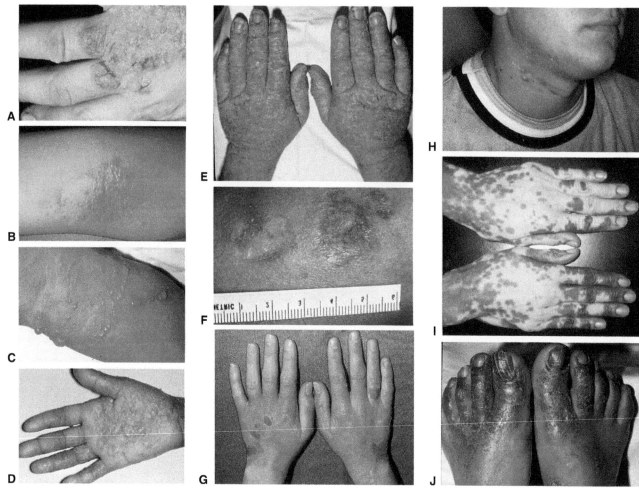

Figure 19-2. *Examples of occupational skin toxicity.* The panels, available at the NIOSH web site (http://www.cdc.gov/niosh/ocderm1.html), are a small selection from the 140-slide NIOSH program "Occupational Dermatoses—A Program for Physicians" prepared by Drs. E. Shmunes, M. M. Key, J. B. Lucas, and J. S. Taylor. (**A**) Eczema from cutting oil; (**B**) atopic irritant dermatitis; (**C**) burn from ethylene oxide; (**D**) burn from alkali exposure; (**E**) sensitization to dichromate; (**F**) beryllium granulomas; (**G**) phototoxicity from lime juice; (**H**) acne from cutting oil; (**I**) leukoderma from rubber antioxidants; and (**J**) hyperpigmentation from mercaptobenzothiazole.

cutting oils. An example of eczema from cutting oil is shown in Fig. 19-2A. The chronic friction and production of small scale trauma can wear away the lipid barrier of the stratum corneum, leading gradually to further damage (loss of cohesion, desquamation) that facilitates penetration of exogenous chemicals and may be detectable as increased transepidermal water loss. In some cases, epidermal thickening occurs without much inflammation. Chronic exposure in the occupational setting often elicits a process of "hardening," where the irritant response resolves. Of uncertain mechanism, it exhibits thicker granular layer and stratum corneum, increased permeability to irritants, altered expression of inflammatory mediators, and a parallel hardening of unexposed skin (Watkins and Maibach, 2009). In any case, increased penetrance at sites of barrier damage can facilitate exposure to chemicals that elicit subsequent toxic effects.

The skin at some anatomic sites is more sensitive than at other sites. Eyelids have a thin epidermis and are quite sensitive, for example, and the back is more sensitive than the forearm or the scalp of individuals with male pattern baldness (Zhai *et al.*, 2004). Individuals vary greatly in sensitivity to irritant dermatitis. Fig. 19-2B shows an irritant reaction on the inside of the elbow on an atopic person. The incidence of atopic dermatitis is increasing rapidly in industrialized societies, and now comprises up to 20% of the pediatric population in these societies (Elias and Schmuth,

2009). Atopic individuals are the most sensitive to irritants and exhibit a propensity to produce specific IgE antibodies to allergens and typically suffer from hay fever. These individuals usually have a poorer prognosis than nonatopics and have a higher frequency of persistent dermatitis. The best preventive measure for atopics and others is to avoid exposure to contact irritants, but in practice this strategy is difficult to implement. That atopic dermatitis has a strong genetic component led to the realization that defects in the intermediate filament aggregating protein filaggrin are strongly associated with this condition and associated development of asthma (Palmer *et al.*, 2006). That loss of filaggrin also causes ichthyosis vulgaris, a scaly skin condition with defective epidermal barrier function (Gruber *et al.*, 2011), has raised the possibility that contributions from other genetic defects in barrier function may be revealed.

Information on the irritancy of chemicals toward human skin may be obtained as part of differential diagnosis by patch testing for allergic response. The skin of laboratory animals (mice, rats, rabbits, and guinea pigs) can be used for testing, but it is thinner and more sensitive than human skin to irritants. For development of new pharmaceuticals, cosmetics, and other consumer products, a great need exists for an in vitro system to determine the potential for irritant responses. Use of human epidermal cell cultures has been increasing as reconstructed epidermal and skin models come closer to the native differentiated state. For example, a recent study compared

50 chemicals for which data on 30 are available from patch testing (Tornier *et al.*, 2006). The tests provided useful comparative data and, judging by viability (mitochondrial function), histology, and release of inflammatory mediators (IL-1α), suggested a parallel with natural skin. Such models offer advantages in convenience and cost, appear applicable to phototoxicity as well, and are more uniform in response than skin in the human population. Analyses of cellular responses by DNA microarray and proteomic methods are being explored. Although advanced, the state of maturation in such culture models is not complete, as seen by histology and barrier function, resulting in their greater sensitivity than the skin (Netzlaff *et al.*, 2005). In addition, extrapolation of the models to cumulative insult dermatitis presents a challenge.

Chemical Burns

A chemical that is extremely corrosive can produce immediate coagulative necrosis resulting in considerable tissue damage with ulceration and sloughing. Sometimes referred to as a third degree chemical burn, the damage does not have a primary inflammatory component and thus may not be classified as an irritant reaction. Examples of burns from ethylene oxide and alkali are shown in Fig. 19-2C and D. If the chemical is not quickly and completely removed, damage to the skin may continue and, with increased access to the circulation, systemic injury can occur. Table 19-2 lists some important corrosive agents giving chemical burns in the occupational arena. Certain chemical warfare agents first used in combat a century ago, such as bis-(2-chloroethyl)sulfide (sulfur mustard) or 2-chlorovinyl dichloroarsine (Lewisite), are potent vesicants upon skin contact and produce considerable damage when inhaled. Sulfur mustard was used in numerous conflicts during the last century

(Ghabili *et al.*, 2011), and the threat of use remains (Shakarjian *et al.*, 2010). A more immediate threat is chemical assault on individuals, a worldwide problem resulting in serious disfigurement and visual impairment (Milton *et al.*, 2010), especially in the developing world (Karunadasa *et al.*, 2010). Acids, typically those readily available (sulfuric, nitric, sometimes formic), are the most common agents, and the face is the most common target.

Allergic Contact Dermatitis

Allergic contact dermatitis is a delayed (T-cell mediated) hypersensitive reaction. To induce sensitization through the skin, chemical haptens generally penetrate the lipid barrier and, to be detected by the immune system, become attached to carrier proteins. The complete antigens are then processed by Langerhans cells (resident macrophages) and displayed on their surfaces with major histocompatibility complex II molecules. The Langerhans cells present the processed peptides to T helper type 1 cells in regional lymph nodes, thereby stimulating interleukin release and proliferation of the sensitive T helper cells. Over a one- to three-week period, memory T cells are thus generated and enter the circulation. Upon subsequent exposure to a specific antigen previously encountered, allergen presentation by the Langerhans cells results in a much greater response due to homing by the memory cells to the skin, their clonal proliferation and their release of cytokines chemotactic for inflammatory cells and stimulatory for their further production. Because this process takes time, the characteristic dermal infiltration and spongiosis result after a delay (latent period) of a half to several days (Mark and Slavin, 2006).

Thousands of chemicals have been reported to give rise to allergic contact dermatitis, many across a variety of occupations and

Table 19-2

Selected Chemicals Causing Skin Burns

CHEMICAL	COMMENT
Ammonia	Potent skin corrosive Contact with compressed gas can cause frostbite
Calcium oxide (CaO)	Severe chemical burns Extremely exothermic reaction—dissolving in water can cause heat burns
Chlorine	Liquid and concentrated vapors cause cell death and ulceration
Ethylene oxide	Solutions and vapors may burn Compressed gas can cause frostbite
Hydrogen chloride (HCl)	Severe burning with scar formation
Hydrogen fluoride (HF)	Severe, painful, slowly healing burns from high concentration Lower concentration causes delayed cutaneous injury Systemic absorption can lead to electrolyte abnormalities and death Calcium-containing topical medications and quaternary ammonium compounds are used to limit damage
Hydrogen peroxide	High concentration causes severe burns and blistering
Methyl bromide	Liquid exposure produces blistering and deep burns
Nitrogen oxides	Moist skin facilitates the formation of nitric acid causing severe yellow-colored burns
Phosphorus	White phosphorus continues to burn on skin in the presence of air
Phenol	Extremely corrosive even in low concentrations Systemic absorption through burn sites may result in cardiac arrhythmias, renal disease, and death
Sodium hydroxide	High concentration causes deep burns, readily denatures keratin
Toluene diisocyanate	Severe burns with contact Skin contact rarely may result in respiratory sensitization

Table 19-3

Common Contact Allergens

SOURCE	COMMON ALLERGENS	
Topical medications/ hygiene products	**Antibiotics** Bacitracin Neomycin Polymyxin Aminoglycosides Sulfonamides	**Therapeutics** Benzocaine Idoxuridine α-Tocopherol (vitamin E) Corticosteroids
	Preservatives Benzalkonium chloride Formaldehyde Formaldehyde releasers Quaternium-15 Imidazolidinyl urea Diazolidinyl urea DMDM hydantoin Methylchloroisothiazolone	**Others** Cinnamic aldehyde Ethylenediamine Lanolin p-Phenylenediamine Propylene glycol Benzophenones Fragrances Thioglycolates
Plants and trees	Abietic acid Balsam of Peru Rosin (colophony)	Pentadecylcatechols Sesquiterpene lactone Tuliposide A
Antiseptics	Chloramine Chlorhexidine Chloroxylenol Dichlorophene Dodecylaminoethyl glycine HCl	Glutaraldehyde Hexachlorophene Thimerosal (merthiolate) Mercurials Triphenylmethane dyes
Rubber products	Diphenylguanidine Hydroquinone Mercaptobenzothiazole p-Phenylenediamine	Resorcinol monobenzoate Benzothiazolesulfenamides Dithiocarbamates Thiurams
Leather	Formaldehyde Glutaraldehyde	Potassium dichromate
Paper products	Abietic acid Formaldehyde Nigrosine	Rosin (colophony) Triphenyl phosphate Dyes
Glues and bonding agents	Bisphenol A Epichlorohydrin Formaldehyde Acrylic monomers Cyanoacrylates	Epoxy resins p-(t-Butyl)formaldehyde resin Toluene sulfonamide resins Urea formaldehyde resins
Metals	Chromium Cobalt	Mercury Nickel

consumer products. Table 19-3 lists some common contact allergens, two of which among others are shown in Fig. 19-3. Because most chemicals in the chemical universe are only weakly active or infrequently encountered, much effort has focused on finding the major allergens in the population by systematic patch testing of dermatology patients. Although not measuring sensitivity in the population at large, the results are quite useful. The panel of chemicals tested can vary with geographic location to accommodate local usage, or it can be directed to specific anatomic sites such as the foot (Holden and Gawkrodger, 2005). Panels also are adapted to emerging trends as new products appear and others decline in use. Table 19-4 lists the 21 agents most commonly giving positive reactions in adult subjects (ages 19–64) in recent patch tests conducted by the North American

Contact Dermatitis Group (Warshaw et al., 2012; Yoo et al., 2010). The testing showed that individuals older than 64 exhibited rates similar to those in adults, both higher than those in children. Most such surveys reveal two-thirds of the subjects to be sensitive to at least one agent in the panel (Yoo et al., 2010). Increasing prevalence of reaction to nickel among younger subjects may reflect increasing exposure, including through body piercing (Schram et al., 2010). A number of agents (nickel, dichromate, p-phenylenediamine, and formaldehyde) have shown high prevalences of reactivity for several decades, while others, once thought innocuous, have more recently become recognized as reactive. For example, individuals exhibit sensitization to gold jewelry, dental gold, and gold coronary stents (Moller, 2010). The high prevalence of allergic contact dermatitis

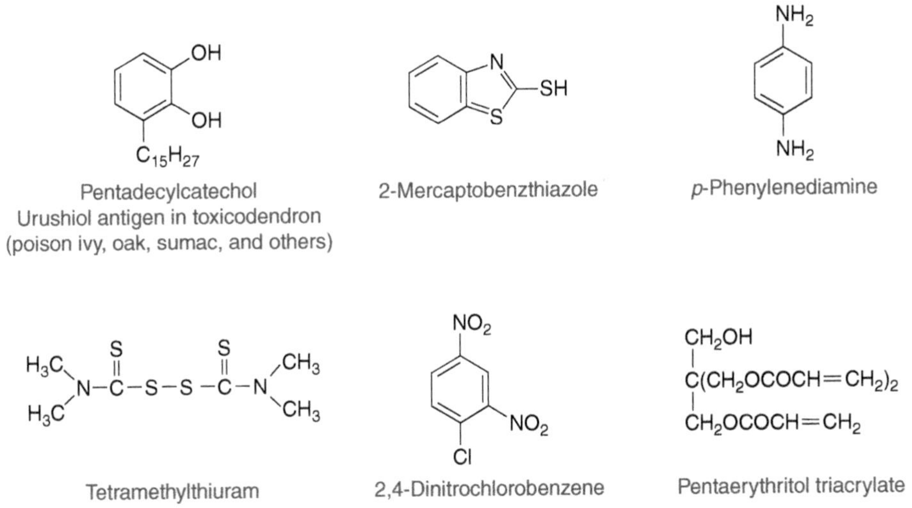

Figure 19-3. *Structural formulas of some potent contact sensitizers.*

to metals has raised concerns about possible reactions to surgical implants containing them (Basko-Plluska *et al.*, 2011), especially nickel (Schram *et al.*, 2010). An example of contact allergy to dichromate in cement is shown in Fig. 19-2E.

Table 19-4

Prevalence of Positive Reactions in Patch Test Patients

ALLERGEN	PATIENTS WITH POSITIVE PATCH TESTS (%)
Nickel sulfate	17.2
Thimerosal	10.8
Balsam of Peru	10.5
Neomycin sulfate	10.3
Sodium gold thiosulfate	10.0
Fragrance mix I	9.8
Quaternium-15	8.4
Formaldehyde	8.1
Cobalt chloride	8.1
Bacitracin	7.8
Budesonide	5.8
Methyldibromo glutaronitrile/ phenoxy ethanol	5.6
Propolis	5.4
Iodopropynyl butylcarbamate	5.4
p-Phenylenediamine	5.0
Thiuram mix	4.6
Carba mix	4.6
Benzalkonium chloride	4.3
Potassium dichromate	4.3
Fragrance mix II	3.7
Propylene glycol	3.5

SOURCE: Data from Warshaw et al. (2012).

Sensitization by ingredients in cosmetics is a common problem, and one that changes as the formulations evolve (Pascoe *et al.*, 2010). As with other consumer products, reduction in use of the most prevalent allergenic chemicals and their replacement by less allergenic substitutes are advocated. Caution in using less characterized chemicals as replacements must be exercised, however, since their allergenicity may not become evident until they reach large populations of users, as has happened in several prominent cases (Uter *et al.*, 2005). For instance, methylchloroisothiazolinone/ methylisothiazolinone, used in cosmetics, was replaced with the biocide methyldibromo glutaronitrile, which did not cause allergic contact dermatitis in initial screens. Upon widespread use, however, the latter was shown to be a potent contact allergen (Kynemund Pedersen *et al.*, 2004). Paradoxically, several chemicals that are reliably contact sensitizing are used therapeutically for papillomavirus-induced warts, skin cancer, and alopecia areata (Holzer *et al.*, 2006).

Unlike contact irritants, where the response is generally proportional to the applied dose and time, contact allergens can elicit reactions at very small doses. Nevertheless, careful analysis from human and animal testing (Arts *et al.*, 2006; Boukhman and Maibach, 2001) shows that a higher dose confers a greater likelihood of sensitization and that doses below a threshold for sensitization can have a cumulative effect. In addition, the dose required to elicit a reaction is lower after sensitization with a higher dose. Moreover, the dose dependence for sensitization displays nonlinearity, suggesting that the response of individual dendritic cells is sublinear, probably sigmoidal. Thus, more stimulation can produce a more than proportionally larger response, although at high doses saturation and sometimes even inhibition of the response become evident. This result emphasizes the importance of minimizing individual exposures. The findings also reveal a wide variation in human response to sensitization, which appears to have at least in part a genetic basis.

Diagnosis and Testing When a patient exhibits allergic contact dermatitis, finding the responsible agent is important to avoid continued exposure. For this purpose, patch testing is commonly employed by procedures refined over many years of practice since it was first employed a century ago (Mark and Slavin, 2006). On the washed backs of patients, who are not currently exhibiting contact dermatitis or using corticosteroids or other immunosuppressives, are placed patches each containing a small amount of a potential allergen. Conveniently, many of the materials are commercially available at standardized concentrations too low to produce irritant reactions.

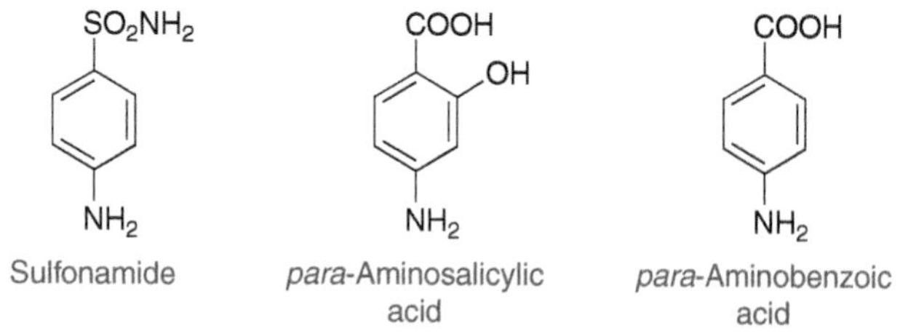

Figure 19-4. *Structural formulas of selected para-amino compounds that show cross-reactions in allergic contact sensitization.*

Certain chemicals normally are not tested because they induce too strong a response (urushiol from poison ivy) or might produce sensitization (beryllium). After two to three days, during which time a maximal reaction usually develops, the patches are removed and sites of exposure are scored for degree of response. Relevance to the patient's actual environment must be considered so that exposure in daily life can be minimized to appropriate chemicals. Interpretation of the results and environmental modification should take into account the phenomenon of cross-sensitivity, where reactivity to a compound may be evident if it shares functional groups that have provoked sensitization in another compound. Fig. 19-4 illustrates the principle with three amine compounds, and Table 19-5 lists some common cross-reacting chemicals.

Animal testing to predict allergenicity has an extended history (Ngo and Maibach, 2010). A chemical is applied to intact or abraded skin or through intradermal injection with or without adjuvant to enhance sensitization. The reaction of the skin to subsequent challenge with the chemical is then observed and graded. This approach has successfully identified some strong sensitizers relevant to human exposures, but detection of weak sensitizers on a large scale is hampered by the usual difficulties in animal testing, including small animal numbers and limited experiment time to reduce expense. In addition, extrapolation of sensitivity measurements from laboratory animals to humans presents large uncertainties. Nevertheless, the local lymph node assay performed in mice has gained attention as a way to measure the pool of sensitized T cells by their proliferation in draining lymph nodes, illustrated by a comparison of potencies of Disperse Blue 106 and 2,4-dinitrochlorobenzene (Betts *et al.*, 2005). Because sensitizers differ in potency by at least four orders of magnitude, a quantitative assay has a distinct advantage.

Increasing emphasis on reducing or eliminating animal use in toxicity testing, driven in part by regulatory initiatives, has stimulated development of integrated testing strategies, where predictions of toxic effects such as skin sensitization include physical chemical structural analysis and in vitro testing. The most important sensitization property of a chemical is its ability to form protein adducts, thus creating a complete antigen in the skin (Roberts and Aptula, 2008). Because chemicals forming protein adducts are generally electrophiles, their relative reactivity in this context likely correlates well with their ability to react with DNA and thus with their mutagenicity. Thus, information on the bacterial mutagenicity (and clastogenicity) of chemicals is valuable for estimating their sensitization potential (Mekenyan *et al.*, 2010). Protein adduct formation may be modeled well for certain chemical classes such as Michael acceptors (eg, α,β-unsaturated carbonyls), which react with protein thiols, by their reactivity with glutathione (Roberts and Natsch, 2009; Schwöbel *et al.*, 2010), which also correlates well with their toxicity toward the model organism *Tetrahymena pyriformis* (Böhme *et al.*, 2009). In such analyses, the contribution of metabolites of chemicals of interest merit consideration since, as in the case of diphenylthiourea (Samuelsson *et al.*, 2011), they may be ultimate sensitizers.

GRANULOMATOUS DISEASE

Foreign body reactions, isolating invading substances that cannot be readily removed, occur infrequently toward a variety of agents introduced into the skin through injection or after laceration or abrasion. These can produce persistent lesions with abundant inflammatory cells resembling chronic infectious conditions (eg, tuberculosis, leprosy, leishmaniasis, and syphilis) and present diagnostic challenges (Del Rosario *et al.*, 2005). In the case of silica or talc (a magnesium silicate), a resulting hard nodule may appear after a latent period of months or years as the original large particles disaggregate to assume a colloidal state. Injection of paraffin or mineral oil in the skin or contamination of wounds with starch powder cross-linked with epichlorohydrin for use in surgical gloves may also result in granulomatous reactions. Delayed allergic sensitization may occur with beryllium analogous to the reaction in the lung, and skin lesions have even been reported in individuals with life-threatening pulmonary exposure. An example of beryllium granuloma of the skin is shown in Fig. 19-2F. However, allergic sensitization may well contribute to the skin rashes that occur during acute beryllium exposure in a continuum of hypersensitivity reactions (Cummings *et al.*, 2009). Cutaneous gadolinium deposition and fibrosis are seen in the nephrogenic systemic fibrosis syndrome evidently arising from gadolinium exposure (Wilford *et al.*, 2010). Metallic mercury and zirconium compounds, formerly used in deodorants, and tattoo dyes (containing cobalt, chromium, mercury, lead, iron, cadmium, and manganese compounds) can also induce granulomatous reactions (Kaur *et al.*, 2009) that in rare cases can be induced by intense light treatment (Tourlaki *et al.*, 2010).

Table 19-5

Common Cross-Reacting Chemicals

CHEMICAL	CROSS REACTOR
Abietic acid	Pine resin (colophony)
Balsam of Peru	Pine resin, cinnamates, benzoates
Bisphenol A	Diethylstilbestrol, hydroquinone monobenzyl ether
Canaga oil	Benzyl salicylate
Chlorocresol	Chloroxylenol
Diazolidinyl urea	Imidazolidinyl urea, formaldehyde
Ethylenediamine di-HCl	Aminophylline, piperazine
Formaldehyde	Arylsulfonamide resin, chloroallyl-hexaminium chloride
Hydroquinone	Resorcinol
Methyl hydroxybenzoate	Parabens, hydroquinone monobenzyl ether
p-Aminobenzoic acid	*p*-Aminosalicylic acid, sulfonamide
Phenylenediamine	Parabens, *p*-aminobenzoic acid
Propyl hydroxybenzoate	Hydroquinone monobenzyl ether
Phenol	Resorcinol, cresols, hydroquinone
Tetramethylthiuram disulfide	Tetraethylthiuram mono- and disulfide

PHOTOTOXICOLOGY

The ultraviolet and visible spectra of solar radiation reaching the earth extend from 290 to 700 nm. Wavelengths beyond this range are either filtered by the earth's atmosphere or are insufficiently energetic to cause cutaneous pathology. Adequate doses of artificially produced UVC (<290 nm) or X-rays can produce profound physical and toxicological skin changes. The protective skin pigment melanin, synthesized in melanocytes, absorbs a broad range of radiation from UVB (290-320 nm) through the visible spectrum. Other chromophores in the skin include amino acids, primarily tryptophan and to a lesser extent tyrosine, and their breakdown products (eg, urocanic acid), which absorb light in the UVB range. Biologically, the most significant chromophore is DNA, since damage from radiation can have lasting effects on the genetic information in target cells.

Adverse Responses to Electromagnetic Radiation

The most evident acute feature of ultraviolet radiation exposure is erythema (redness or sunburn). The minimal erythema dose (MED), the smallest dose of ultraviolet light needed to induce an erythematous response, varies greatly from person to person. Vasodilation responsible for the color change is accompanied by significant alterations in a variety of inflammatory mediators from injured keratinocytes and local inflammatory cells that may be responsible for some systemic symptoms associated with sunburn such as fever, chills, and malaise. UVB (290-320 nm) is the most effective solar band to cause erythema in human skin. A substantially greater dosage of UVA (320-400) reaches the earth compared to UVB (up to 100-fold); however, its efficiency in generating erythema in humans is about 1000-fold less than that of UVB. Both UVA and UVB have been implicated in the development of melanoma and nonmelanoma skin cancers. Because of its longer wavelength and greater depth of skin penetration, UVA is likely more responsible for long-term UV effects such as wrinkling, skin atrophy, and easy bruisability. Overt pigment darkening is another typical response to ultraviolet exposure. This may be accomplished by enhanced melanin production by melanocytes or by photo-oxidation of melanin. Tanning or increased pigmentation usually occurs within three days of ultraviolet light exposure, while photo-oxidation is evident immediately. The tanning response is most readily produced by exposure to UVB and may be induced, along with erythema and DNA repair, by DNA damage. Tanning serves to augment the protective effects of melanin in the skin over the long run, but in the short run the protection afforded appears insufficient to balance the damage sustained in acquiring it, especially in fair-skinned individuals (Sheehan *et al.*, 2002).

Chronic exposure to radiation induces a variety of characteristic skin changes. For ultraviolet light, these changes accelerate or mimic aging, but the rate depends greatly on the baseline skin pigmentation of the individual. Lighter skinned people suffer from chronic skin changes with greater frequency than darker individuals, and locations such as the head, neck, hands, and upper chest are more readily involved due to their routine exposures. Pigmentary changes such as freckling and hypomelanotic areas, wrinkling, telangiectasias (fine superficial blood vessels), actinic keratoses (precancerous lesions), and malignant skin lesions such as basal and squamous cell carcinomas and malignant melanomas are all consequences of chronic exposure to ultraviolet light exposure. One significant pathophysiological response of chronic exposure to ultraviolet light is the pronounced decrease of epidermal Langerhans cells. Chronically sun exposed skin may have up to 50% fewer of these compared to photoprotected areas. This decrease may result in lessened immune surveillance of neoantigens on malignant cells and thus allow such a transformation to proceed unabated. For these reasons, gaining a tan, either naturally or through tanning salons, is not recommended (Lim *et al.*, 2011). Exposures to ionizing radiation may produce a different spectrum of disease depending upon the dose delivered. Large acute exposures will result in local redness, blistering, swelling, ulceration, and pain. After a latent period or following subacute chronic exposures, characteristic changes such as epidermal thinning, freckling, telangiectasias, and nonhealing ulcerations may occur. Also, a variety of skin malignancies have been described years after skin exposure to radiation.

Aside from the toxic nature of electromagnetic radiation, natural and environmental exposures to certain bands of light are vital for survival. Ultraviolet radiation is critical for the conversion of 7-dehydrocholesterol to previtamin D3, without which normal endogenous production of vitamin D would not take place. Blue light in the 420 to 490 nm range can be lifesaving due to its capacity to photoisomerize bilirubin (a red blood cell breakdown product) in the skin. Infants with elevated serum bilirubin, potentially neurotoxic, have difficulty clearing this by-product because of its low water solubility, but treatment with blue light renders bilirubin more water soluble and markedly augments excretion. In addition, the toxic effects of ultraviolet light have been exploited for decades through artificial light sources for treatment of hyperproliferative skin disorders such as psoriasis.

Photosensitivity

An abnormal sensitivity to ultraviolet and visible light, photosensitivity may result from endogenous or exogenous factors (Bylaite *et al.*, 2009). For instance, a variety of genetic diseases, such as xeroderma pigmentosum, impair the cell's ability to repair ultraviolet light-induced damage. The autoimmune disease lupus erythematosus also features abnormal sensitivity to ultraviolet light. In hereditary or chemically induced porphyrias, enzyme abnormalities disrupt the biosynthetic pathways producing heme, the prosthetic building block for hemoglobin, myoglobin, catalases, peroxidases, and cytochromes, leading to accumulation of porphyrin precursors or derivatives throughout the body, including the skin. These compounds in general fluoresce when exposed to light of 400 to 410 nm (Soret band), and in this excited state interact with cellular macromolecules or with molecular oxygen to generate toxic free radicals. A "constitutional" sensitivity to light (porphyria cutanea tarda) can be precipitated by alcohol, estrogens, or certain antibiotics in individuals with hereditary abnormalities in porphyrin synthesis, and an "acquired" sensitivity in general by hexachlorobenzene and mixtures of polyhalogenated aromatic hydrocarbons (Frank and Poblete-Gutiérrez, 2010) .

Phototoxicity Phototoxic reactions from exogenous chemicals may be produced by systemic or topical administration or exposure. In acute reactions, the skin can become red and blister within minutes to hours after ultraviolet light exposure. In an occupational setting, for example, exposing the skin to coal tar and sunlight can quickly produce a stinging sensation and elicit damage resembling a bad sunburn with hyperpigmentation. Phototoxic chemicals most commonly absorb ultraviolet light in the range of 320 to 400 nm (UVA), thereby assuming a higher energy excited triplet state, and either transfer an electron to other molecules or become reduced to form highly reactive free radicals (DeLeo, 2004; Moan and Peng, 2004). An oxygen-dependent photodynamic reaction commonly occurs as these excited molecules, returning to the ground state,

Table 19-6
Selected Phototoxic Chemicals
Furocoumarins
8-Methoxypsoralen
5-Methoxypsoralen
Trimethoxypsoralen
Polycyclic aromatic hydrocarbons
Anthracene
Fluoranthene
Acridine
Phenanthrene
Drugs
Tetracyclines
Sulfonamides
Sulfonylureas
Nalidixic acid
Thiazides
Phenothiazines
Nonsteroidal anti-inflammatories
Dyes
Disperse blue 35
Eosin
Acridine orange
Porphyrin derivatives
Hematoporphyrin

transfer their energy to oxygen, forming highly reactive singlet oxygen. These reactive products are capable of damaging cellular macromolecules, notably unsaturated membrane lipids, and causing cell death. The resulting damage stimulates release of a variety of immune mediators from keratinocytes and local white blood cells that recruit more inflammatory cells to the skin and thus yield the clinical signs of phototoxicity. Agents most often associated with phototoxic reactions are listed in Table 19-6.

Psoralens are good examples of agents that produce phototoxicity largely without requiring oxygen radicals. Upon entering cells, they intercalate with the DNA and then form covalent adducts and cross-links when activated by UVA. The result is to inhibit DNA synthesis and repair and cell growth or survival. Psoralens (and other phototoxins) can be encountered in a variety of food plants, including limes and celery, producing phytophotodermatitis in occupational settings where such a food is routinely handled. An example of phototoxicity from lime juice is given in Fig. 19-2G. Psoralens in combination with UVA (PUVA) are used therapeutically to inhibit growth of keratinocytes and lymphocytes in hyperproliferative conditions such as psoriasis and T-cell lymphomas. In analogous fashion, though generating reactive oxygen, photodynamic therapy is a new approach that takes advantage of the selective uptake of a photosensitizing agent, usually a porphyrin precursor, into rapidly dividing cells such as in neoplasms. The photosensitizing agent is activated by laser or continuous wave light sources ranging from 400 to 600 nm or more, resulting in selective destruction of the neoplasm (Ibbotson, 2011).

Nails often suffer toxic reactions to drugs, most commonly to systemically administered agents such as antibiotics, less commonly to topically applied agents. While various types of nail pathology may result from therapy-induced changes in cell growth or division, changes in pigmentation or detachment of the various layers of the nail plate from each other (onycholysis) often result from

photosensitive reactions, commonly phototoxic, less commonly photoallergic. Agents such as topical or systemic porphyrins, coal tar, and drugs such as the tetracycline family of antibiotics produce photodynamic toxicity, which requires generation of oxygen radicals. In contrast, topical or systemic psoralens produce onycholysis by a nonphotodynamic mechanism that does not require oxygen.

Photoallergy A photoallergen elicits an allergic response by forming a complete antigen upon absorbing ultraviolet or visible light. Light stimulates the agent either to assume an excited state that can bind directly to a carrier protein or to yield a stable photoproduct that becomes conjugated to a carrier (Andreu et al., 2010). As in the case of allergic contact dermatitis, the complete antigen formed then is processed by Langerhans cells and presented to T cells. Upon recurrent exposure to an exogenous agent and light, a delayed hypersensitivity (Type IV) reaction ensues, leading typically to eczema (erythema, vesiculation, and itching). Like phototoxins, most photoallergens respond to light in the range of 320 to 400 nm (UVA). Light sensitivity usually subsides within days but may persist for several weeks if the agent is retained in the epidermis.

Use of halogenated salicylanilides and related antimicrobial agents in widely used consumer personal care products such as soap led to many thousands of cases of photoallergy in the 1960s and 1970s. When the most active agents were removed from the market, fragrances in cosmetics and sunscreens then became conspicuous sources of photoallergy a decade later. In parallel, certain antimicrobial agents were seen to be photoallergens (Kerr and Ferguson, 2010). Currently, active ingredients in sunscreens and antimicrobial agents are the most frequently recognized causes followed by medications, fragrances, plant derivatives, and pesticides (Victor et al., 2010). Although of low risk, these agents have become widely used as the risks of extensive sun exposure have become appreciated.

Photoallergy generally is distinguishable from phototoxicity, since the former results from delayed hypersensitivity, and amounts of agent too low to give a toxic response still suffice to elicit allergy. Agents causing phototoxicity, because reactivity is generated upon light exposure, may also be photoallergenic, but the latter type of response is much less common. Among individuals with a history of photosensitivity, a recent study reported that 11% exhibited photoallergy (Victor et al., 2010). Diagnosis is best performed by patch testing with and without light exposure of the treated surface to distinguish photocontact from contact allergy. Since the offending agent may not be obvious from the patient history due to the delay between exposure to the agent and sunlight and the symptoms, a panel of test agents may include some 50 common photoallergens as well as the patient's own sunscreen and personal care products. To assist in predicting risks of photoallergy, efforts have been made to derive important chemical features among existing photoallergens that account for their reactivity toward proteins. This information, coupled with assessment of physical properties such as aqueous/lipid partitioning, is anticipated to streamline testing of new products (Barratt, 2004).

ACNE

Acne is a common affliction of the pilosebaceous units in the face, upper chest, and upper back. Found in many forms, this condition typically arises from blockage of the sebaceous duct leading from the gland to the hair follicle, resulting in retention of sebum and enlargement of the gland. In the most common form (acne vulgaris), androgen stimulation at puberty leads to high sebum production, hyperproliferation, and cornification of the ductal cells, plugging the orifice, and retention of corneocytes in the hair follicle lumen (Cunliffe *et al.*, 2004). Proliferation of resident bacteria and inflammation typically result. Long-chain fatty acids can give an acne-like response in animal models and appear to do so in sensitive individuals exposed to cosmetics. Likely acting in a similar fashion, petroleum products (oils, coal tar) in the workplace can give rise to acneiform eruptions (Ancona, 1986). Insoluble cutting oils used in machining may have this effect, as illustrated in Fig. 19-2H. Such agents, which can contain chlorinated paraffins, stimulate excessive stratification of the ductal cells, preventing their disaggregation and blocking the flow of sebum.

Chloracne

The most disfiguring form of acne in humans, chloracne, is caused by exposure to halogenated aromatic hydrocarbons. Chloracnegenic agents such as polychlorinated biphenyls (PCBs) and naphthalenes are often accompanied by the highly potent polychlorinated dibenzofuran and dioxin contaminants readily formed during synthesis of these agents or chlorinated phenolic pesticides and can arise from combustion of the latter in fires and explosions. Chloracne is a rare disease but still occurs sporadically from industrial and environmental exposures (Gawkrodger *et al.*, 2009; Passarini *et al.*, 2010). Its recalcitrant nature and its preventability make it an important occupational and environmental illness. Typically, comedones and straw-colored cysts are present behind the ears, around the eyes, shoulders, back, and genitalia. In addition to acne, hypertrichosis (increased hair in atypical locations), hyperpigmentation, brown discoloration of the nail, conjunctivitis and eye discharge may be present. Since chloracne is a marker of systemic exposure, concurrent effects in the liver and nervous system may accompany the integumentary findings. Chloracne exhibits progressive degeneration of sebaceous units, transition of sebaceous gland cells to keratinizing cells and prominent hyperkeratosis in the follicular canal. Accounting for the distinctive effects on sebaceous glands, chloracnegens have been hypothesized to shift the differentiation of stem cells in the hair follicle to an epidermal program, which may contribute to their long lasting effects (Panteleyev and Bickers, 2006).

Since the original recognition of the syndrome a century ago, effects of chloracnegens on humans have been clearly demonstrated over the last 5 decades through industrial disasters. In 1953 a chemical plant in Ludwigshafen exploded, discharging 2,4,5-trichlorophenol; in 1976 in Seveso, Italy, a reactor explosion liberated tetrachlorodibenzo-*p*-dioxin (TCDD); and in 1968 and 1979 in Japan and Taiwan, respectively, rice cooking oil was contaminated with PCBs, polychlorinated dibenzofurans and related polychlorinated aromatic hydrocarbons. Individual poisonings involving remarkably high TCDD body burdens have not been lethal despite severe chloracne (Geusau *et al.*, 2001; Sorg *et al.*, 2009). Skin toxicity can appear within months after exposure and, depending on the severity, may either be cleared quickly or remain manifest even decades after exposure ceases, reflecting the high lipid solubility, recalcitrance to metabolic clearance, and thus long half-life in humans of the responsible agents. The highly potent TCDD has a half-life in humans of ≈ 8 years (Geyer *et al.*, 2002), and highly chlorinated dibenzofurans and biphenyls are similarly persistent.

Chlorinated dioxins and dibenzofurans have substantial and reproducible effects on cellular function. TCDD is one of the most potent known inducers of CYP1A1 by virtue of its high affinity for the Ah receptor stimulating its expression. The fate of individuals afflicted with chloracne has been of particular interest in view

of the suggestion they may be more prone to other adverse health effects of exposure. So far, however, chloracne has not proven to be a sentinel biomarker for cancer (Pesatori *et al.*, 2009). Since polymorphisms in Ah receptor sequence confer differences in sensitivity to health effects in animals, analogous polymorphisms have been sought in the human population; Ah receptor polymorphisms have been identified, but as yet they have not been shown to affect responses to the receptor ligands (Okey *et al.*, 2005). In the mouse, skin symptoms analogous to chloracne in humans are dependent on the hr locus, where the (−/−) genotype is susceptible (Poland and Knutson, 1982), although subclinical acne-like symptoms have now been observed in B6C3F1 mice (Ramot *et al.*, 2009). An analogous locus has been identified in humans that governs hair loss, where mutations give a phenocopy of the generalized atrichia from loss of vitamin D receptor activity (Miller *et al.*, 2001), but a functional allele does not prevent susceptibility to chloracne.

PIGMENTARY DISTURBANCES

Melanocytes help protect the skin from harmful effects of ultraviolet light by producing the insoluble polymeric pigment melanin starting with the action of tyrosine hydroxylase. As indicated in Table 19-7, a variety of agents can interfere with normal

Table 19-7

Selected Causes of Cutaneous Pigmentary Disturbances

I. Hyperpigmentation
   Ultraviolet light exposure
   Postinflammatory changes (melanin and/or hemosiderin deposition)
   Hypoadrenalism
   Internal malignancy
   Chemical exposures
      Coal tar volatiles
      Anthracene
      Picric acid
      Mercury
      Lead
      Bismuth
      Furocoumarins (psoralens)
      Hydroquinone (paradoxical)
   Drugs
      Chloroquine
      Amiodarone
      Bleomycin
      Zidovudine (AZT)
      Minocycline

II. Hypopigmentation/depigmentation/leukoderma
   Postinflammatory pigmentary loss
   Vitiligo
   Chemical leukoderma/hypopigmentation
      Hydroquinone
      Monobenzyl, monoethyl, and monomethyl ethers of hydroquinone
      p-(*t*-Butyl)phenol
      Mercaptoamines
      Phenolic germicides
      p-(*t*-Butyl)catechols
      Butylated hydroxytoluene

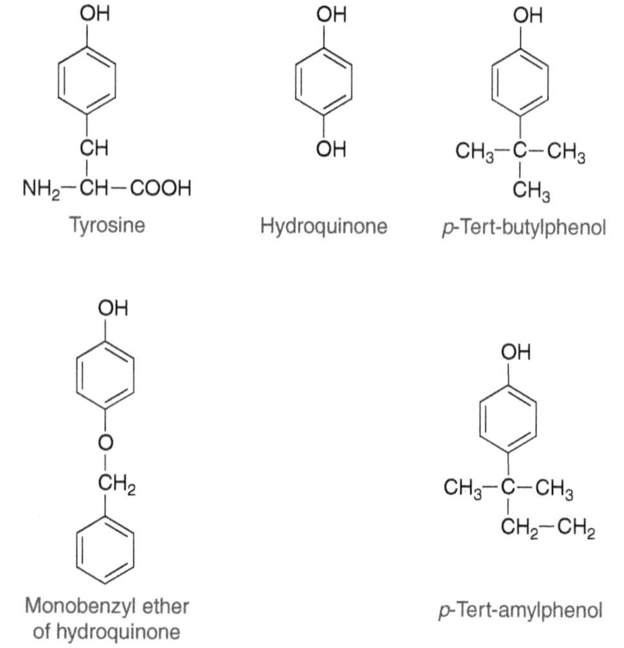

Figure 19-5. *Chemical structure of tyrosine and of selected hypo-pigmenting and depigmenting agents.*

pigmentation to yield either excessive or reduced amounts of melanin. An acquired condition of generalized pigmentation loss, leukoderma (vitiligo) has a genetic basis but is triggered by environmental influences, particularly involving generation of reactive oxygen (Guerra *et al.*, 2010). Thought likely to be of autoimmune origin, this condition is characterized by loss of melanocytes. In the occupational arena, depigmentation is well known to occur through exposure to phenols, catechols, quinones, and related compounds, several of which are shown in Fig. 19-5, that appear toxic to melanocytes. An illustration of depigmentation caused by antioxidant exposure in rubber manufacture is given in Fig. 19-2I. In case reports, the cancer chemotherapeutic imatinib mesylate has been found to give pigment loss in the epidermis, probably through its inhibition of c-Kit tyrosine kinase signaling essential for melanocyte function (Arora *et al.*, 2004), and paradoxically to give hyperpigmentation in the hard palate (Mattsson *et al.*, 2011) and repigmentation of gray hair (Etienne *et al.*, 2002). In sub-Saharan Africa and Asia, use of skin-lightening creams containing hydroquinone, corticosteroids, or mercurials is common among women. These agents produce their effects by inhibiting tyrosine hydroxylase activity or expression, but the treatments can give nonuniform effects or discoloration (ochronosis) and frequently are accompanied by undesirable cutaneous consequences including allergic contact dermatitis. Moreover, they pose risks of serious systemic effects, particularly the mercurials (nephropathy, neuropathy) and corticosteroids (adrenal suppression) (Ladizinski *et al.*, 2011). By contrast, hyperpigmentation is well known to result from exposure to phototoxic agents including coal tar, coumarin derivatives found in perfumes and certain food such as limes (shown in Fig. 19-2G) and food plants (parsley, celery), dyes in cosmetics, and elements such as lead, bismuth, and arsenic (Table 19-7). An example of excessive pigmentation from mercaptobenzothiazole is shown in Fig. 19-2J. In addition, phototoxic or photosensitive reactions commonly occur with some oral medications, most notably diuretic, antibacterial, and nonsteroidal anti-inflammatory drugs (NSAIDs) (Moore, 2002).

URTICARIA

For those allergens to which IgE antibodies have been elicited by previous or ongoing exposure, subsequent contact can lead to development of hives, typically in minutes, through an immediate type I hypersensitivity reaction. Hives are raised wheals that usually itch or sting and may appear reddish. Generally disappearing within hours and rarely lasting longer than a day or two, the symptoms result from degranulation of cutaneous mast cells by liganded IgE, leading to release of histamine and other vasoactive substances. Food allergies (Sicherer and Sampson, 2010) and pharmaceuticals (Limsuwan and Demoly, 2010) are major causes of acute urticaria, but many other causes are known (Table 19-8). Some agents (eg, opiates) can bring about direct release of histamine from mast cells without antibody mediation, while others (nonsteroidal anti-inflammatories) may do so through effects on arachidonic acid metabolism or by uncertain mechanisms. Responses lasting longer than six weeks, if not attributable to allergen exposure, frequently have an autoimmune basis such as development of autoantibodies

Table 19-8

Substances Reported to Elicit Contact Urticaria

CHEMICALS	FOODS
Anhydrides	Animal viscera
Hexahydrophthalic	Apple
Methylhexahydrophthalic	Artichoke
Maleic	Asparagus
Antibiotics	Beef
Bacitracin	Beer
Streptomycin	Carrot
Cephalosporins	Chicken
Penicillin	Deer
Rifamycin	Egg
Benzoic acid	Fish
Cobalt chloride	Lamb
Butylhydroxyanisole (BHA)	Milk
Butylhydroxytoluene (BHT)	Mustard
Carboxymethylcellulose	Paprika
Cyclopentolate hydrochloride	Peanut
Diphenyl guanidine	Potato
Diphenylmethane-4,4'-diisocyanate	Pork
Epoxy resin	Rice
2-Ethylhexyl acrylate	Sesame
Formaldehyde	Shellfish
Fragrances	Soy
Balsam of Peru	Strawberry
Cinnamic aldehyde	Tree nuts
Menthol	Turkey
Plants, woods, trees, weeds	Wheat
Latex	
Phenylmercuric acetate	
Xylene	

against the high affinity IgE receptor. Lifetime prevalence of urticaria has been estimated as 9%, of which nearly 2% occurs chronically (Zuberbier *et al.*, 2010).

Contact urticaria in an occupational setting can arise from exposure to plant or animal proteins and appears more common in atopic individuals, who are especially sensitive to irritants. Among the numerous occupations where this response occurs include hairdressers and those involving routine handling of food, plant, or animal products (Doutre, 2005). The common occupational problem of allergic contact dermatitis to rubber gloves, especially in the health care industry, reflects the variety of accelerators (carbamates, thiurams, 2-mercaptobenzothiazole, and 1,3-diphenylguanidine) and antioxidants (*p*-phenylenediamines) they contain (Cao *et al.*, 2010). The widespread use of latex rubber in medical supplies and devices, as well as gloves, has resulted in widespread sensitization to the latex proteins they contain, cross-reaction with which may even be responsible for certain food allergies (Santos and Van Ree, 2011). The latex proteins have a propensity to induce immediate type I hypersensitive reactions, where the response can range from a mild skin reaction to anaphylaxis and death (Reines and Seifert, 2005). In addition, powder used in the gloves can adsorb the allergenic proteins and distribute them through the air. Modification of the manufacturing process to produce low-protein, low-allergenic, powder free gloves has led to reappraisal of their replacement by nitrile and other gloves (Palosuo *et al.*, 2011).

A life-threatening response of anaphylactic shock, as from latex allergy, may occur from IgE-mediated massive release of histamine and other vasoactive agents from the mast cells upon systemic exposure to allergens. Certain food allergies (eg, to nuts, fish, and shellfish) are capable of producing this extreme response. Among pharmaceuticals, the best known example is penicillin, where adverse reactions must be managed carefully to avoid serious consequences (Gruchalla and Pirmohamed, 2006). Other antibiotics that can produce anaphylaxis include cephalosporins, sulfonamides, macrolides, vancomycin, tetracyclines, and fluoroquinolines; all but the last two also can produce toxic epidermal necrolysis. Insect allergens such as those in bee and wasp stings are well known to be capable of giving an anaphylactic response.

TOXIC EPIDERMAL NECROLYSIS

Toxic epidermal necrolysis is a rare life-threatening skin disease with an incidence of one to two cases per million person-years except among AIDS patients, where it is 1000-fold higher (Harr and French, 2010). At the most severe end of a spectrum of adverse cutaneous hypersensitivity reactions to drugs, this syndrome involves detachment of ≥30% of the epidermal surface from the dermis, commonly accompanied by severe erosions of mucous membranes, and has a fatality rate ≈30%. The Stevens–Johnson syndrome is a milder but still serious version of nearly the same phenomenon with up to 10% of the skin surface area affected and with a proportionally lower fatality rate. The two syndromes overlap when 10% to 30% of the skin surface is involved. Toxic epidermal necrolysis commonly resembles an upper respiratory tract infection in the first several days (fever, cough, sore throat, and malaise), but prompt diagnosis when the cutaneous lesions become evident several days later improves survival chances. Ongoing exposure to drugs first encountered during the previous month is stopped and treatment is initiated similar to that for burns, where fluid and electrolyte replacement, protection from infection, and nutritional assistance are critical. Nearly 200 drugs have been reported to cause this syndrome with major contributors being anticonvulsants, nonsteroidal

anti-inflammatories, antibacterial sulfonamides, allopurinol, and nevirapine. Mechanisms leading to this idiosyncratic drug reaction are under scrutiny to prevent its occurrence or at least to optimize treatment. Studies of genetic predisposition have revealed striking correlations between HLA genotype and susceptibility to carbamazepine, but other reports and a recent genome wide association study raise the possibility that susceptibility may depend on the agent and ethnic background (Ahmadi, 2011). A characteristic feature of the syndrome is the large-scale apoptosis of epidermal keratinocytes. Candidates for mediating apoptosis through cell surface death receptors include tumor necrosis factor and FAS ligand, which appear elevated; in addition, drug-sensitized natural killer and cytotoxic T lymphocytes, secreting granulysin, and other components of the innate immune response may participate in inducing keratinocyte death (Bellon and Blanca, 2011). Effectiveness of treatments has been difficult to evaluate, but promising approaches involve immunosuppression (cyclophosphamide, ciclosporin) or blockage of death receptors using intravenous immunoglobulin therapy (Ardern-Jones and Friedmann, 2011).

SKIN CANCER

Radiation

Radiation from ionizing wavelengths to ultraviolet wavelengths has been shown to cause skin cancer. Shortly after the discovery of radioactive elements at the turn of the 20th century, it was observed that X-rays could cause severe burns, squamous cell carcinoma, and basal cell carcinomas. X-ray-induced nonmelanoma skin cancers (NMCS) continued to be observed throughout the 20th century, as X-rays were used therapeutically until the mid-20th century for a variety of skin diseases (acne, atopic dermatitis, psoriasis, and tinea). Although NMSC from X-rays are now uncommon, dermal atrophy or sclerosis still is seen as sequelae of radiodermatitis, which sometimes develops after X-ray treatment of internal malignancies.

UV-Induced Skin Cancer

Most skin cancers in the United States now are UV-induced. The most common UV-induced skin cancers are NMSC and cutaneous malignant melanoma. NMSC are increasing in incidence and now number more than 1.2 million cases each year (Neville *et al.*, 2007). The incidence of malignant melanoma also is increasing rapidly, faster than any other malignancy (Rigel, 2008). Although melanoma occurs with much less frequency than NMSC, it accounts for most of the deaths due to skin cancer in the USA (Balk, 2011). An important new source of UV radiation is the cosmetic tanning industry (Schulman and Fisher, 2009). The American Cancer Society, The Centers for Disease Control, the American Academy of Dermatology, and the National Council on Skin Cancer Prevention all have recommended that sun tanning and tanning beds be avoided (Balk, 2011). In addition to UV exposure, particularly blistering sunburns, as a risk factor for malignant melanoma and NMSC, genetic variations in the melanocortin 1 receptor predict increased skin cancer risk, independent of hair type or skin color (Lynde and Sapra, 2010).

UVB (290-320 nm) induces pyrimidine dimers and 8-oxoguanine modifications, thereby eliciting mutations in critical genes (Melnikova and Ananthaswamy, 2005; Nishigori, 2006). The p53 tumor suppressor gene is a major target in which damage occurs early and is detectable in most resulting squamous cell carcinomas. Because the p53 protein arrests cell cycling until DNA damage is repaired and may induce apoptosis, its loss destabilizes the genome of initiated cells and gives them a growth advantage. UV light also has immunosuppressive effects that may help skin tumors survive. Nonmelanoma skin cancer incidence is highest in the tropics and is highest in pale-complexioned whites, particularly at sites on the head and neck that receive the most intense exposure. Individuals with xeroderma pigmentosum, who are deficient in repair of pyrimidine dimers, must scrupulously avoid sun exposure to prevent the occurrence of premalignant lesions that progress with continued exposure. Even when it does not cause cancer in normal individuals, sun exposure leads to premature aging of the skin. For this reason, sunbathing is discouraged and the use of sunblock lotions is encouraged, especially those that remove wavelengths up to 400 nm. Protection from solar (and other) radiation as well as chemical carcinogens is important in the occupational arena (Gawkrodger, 2004).

Polycyclic Aromatic Hydrocarbons

A landmark epidemiological investigation by Percival Pott in 1775 connected soot with the scrotal cancer prevalent among chimney sweeps in England. Since that time, substances rich in polycyclic aromatic hydrocarbons (coal tar, creosote, pitch, and soot) have become recognized as skin carcinogens in humans and animals (Voelter-Mahlknecht et al., 2007). With their variable content of polycyclic aromatic hydrocarbons and nitrosamines, mineral oils have a long history of causing skin cancer in the occupational arena among, for example, metalworkers, cotton spinners, and jute processors (Tolbert, 1997). Polycyclic aromatic compounds alone are relatively inert chemically, but they would tend to accumulate in membranes and thus perturb cell function if they were not removed. They are hydroxylated by a number of cytochrome P450 isozymes, primarily 1A1 and 1B1 in epidermal cells, and conjugated for disposal from the body. Oxidative biotransformation, however, produces electrophilic epoxides that can form DNA adducts. Phenols, produced by rearrangement of the epoxides, can be oxidized further to electrophilic quinones that generate reactive oxygen species and lead to DNA adducts, oxidized bases, and abasic sites (Park et al., 2006). Occupations at risk of skin cancer from exposure to these compounds (eg, roofing) often involve considerable sun exposure, an additional risk factor. Concern persists regarding the use of coal tar for pharmaceutical purposes (Thami and Sarkar, 2004). The combination of coal tar and UV light is useful in treating severe psoriasis, since the toxicity reduces the excessive turnover rate of keratinocytes that characterizes this disease. Repeated treatments are necessary, raising the specter of elevated risk of nonmelanoma skin cancer. However, this deleterious outcome has not been manifest clinically (Roelofzen et al., 2010). Using longer wave UVA with phototoxic psoralen derivatives (PUVA) in place of coal tar in such protocols is much less messy and avoids UVB, but produces DNA adducts and a persistent elevation of nonmelanoma skin cancer risk (Nijsten and Stern, 2003).

As a major regulator of induction of CYP1A1, and to a lesser extent CYP1B1, the aryl hydrocarbon receptor (AhR) plays a critical role in the response of epidermal cells to polycyclic aromatic hydrocarbons (Swanson, 2004). For example, mice in which the AhR gene has been functionally ablated are insensitive to skin cancer from topical application of benzo[a]pyrene (Shimizu et al., 2000). By contrast, a constitutively activated AhR expressed in mouse epidermal keratinocytes was not seen to induce neoplasia, but it did result in inflammatory skin lesions reminiscent of contact dermatitis elicited by polycyclic aromatic hydrocarbons in humans (Tauchi et al., 2005). A common AhR polymorphism reduces the sensitivity in mice by an order of magnitude to toxic effects of ligands for this receptor, while in the rat an AhR variant with more subtle transactivation properties bestows dramatic resistance to lethal effects of TCDD without altering CYP1A1 inducibility (Okey et al., 2005). Screening efforts in humans have not yet revealed AhR polymorphisms that alter human responses to receptor ligands, but polymorphisms in cytochromes P450 do exist that are regulated by the AhR and could plausibly affect skin sensitivity or function. An example is CYP2S1, which metabolizes retinoic acid (Saarikoski et al., 2005).

Mouse Skin Tumor Promotion

Through the work of numerous investigators over the past century, initially studying substances rich in polycyclic aromatic hydrocarbons, mouse skin has been developed as an important target for carcinogenicity testing (Rubin, 2001). The observed incidence of squamous cell carcinomas has been helpful in providing a biological basis for conclusions from epidemiological studies. For instance, mouse skin carcinogenicity of tobacco smoke condensate and constituents strongly supported the conclusion that tobacco smoke is carcinogenic in humans. Carcinogenicity in mouse skin is taken as evidence of a carcinogenic risk for humans generally, including for the lung (Walaszek et al., 2007). Much has been learned about the pathogenesis of squamous cell carcinomas in mouse skin that does have general applicability to human squamous cell carcinomas of the skin or other anatomic sites, a learning process now augmented with mouse strains engineered for over-expression or ablation of genes of interest (Abel et al., 2009).

Initial fractionation of coal tar showed that the carcinogenic polycyclic aromatic hydrocarbons thereby purified and identified accounted for only a small fraction of the total carcinogenicity (Rubin, 2001). This puzzling observation led to the realization that other constituents, by themselves not carcinogenic, acted as cocarcinogens. Some agents, called tumor promoters, were found effective even when applied to the mouse skin long after a single treatment with a carcinogen applied at a dose too low to give cancer alone. The latter, inducing tumors by itself at sufficiently high doses, was a "complete" carcinogen with the salient property of being genotoxic. One explanation for the commonly observed nonlinear response is that a large dose of a complete carcinogen does more than initiate cancer by damaging the DNA in cells. It is also toxic, killing some cells and thereby stimulating a regenerative response in the surviving basal cells. Tumor promoters are agents that do not cause cancer themselves, but induce tumor development in skin that has been initiated by a low dose of a carcinogen. Their promoting power generally is parallel to their ability to give sustained hyperplasia of the epidermis with continued treatment by a variety of signaling pathways (Rundhaug and Fischer, 2010). Selective stimulation of tumor growth is envisioned to occur from differential stimulation of initiated cells or due to the insensitivity of initiated cells to toxicity or to terminal differentiation induced in uninitiated cells by the promoter. Continuing efforts to understand the promotion process are envisioned to assist development of short-term tests that predict promoting potential (Curtin et al., 2006).

An advantage of the experimental model of mouse skin carcinogenesis is the ability to separate the neoplastic process into stages of initiation, promotion, and progression, and the analysis can be extended to more complicated multihit, multistage models (Owens et al., 1999). In the simplest model, the skin is treated once with a low dose of an initiator, a polycyclic aromatic hydrocarbon, for example. The skin does not develop tumors unless it is subsequently treated with a promoter, which must be applied numerous times at frequent intervals (eg, twice per week for three months). Application of the promoter need not start immediately after initiation, but if it is not continued long enough, or if it is applied before or without the initiator, tumors do not develop. A consequence of promotion then is a tendency to linearize the dose–response curve for the initiator. Although an important aspect of promotion is its epigenetic nature, papillomas arising from promotion characteristically are aneuploid. Mutations in the *c-Ha-ras* gene are commonly found in papillomas, particularly those initiated by polycyclic aromatic hydrocarbons. Eventually some of the resulting papillomas become autonomous, continuing to grow without the further addition of the promoter. Genetic damage accumulates in the small fraction of tumors that progress to malignancy.

A number of natural products are tumor promoters, many of which alter phosphorylation pathways. The best-studied example, and one of the most potent, is the active ingredient of croton oil, 12-*O*-tetradecanoylphorbol-13-acetate. This is a member of a diverse group of compounds that give transitory stimulation followed by chronic depletion of protein kinase C in mouse epidermis (Fournier and Murray, 1987). Another group of agents, an example of which is okadaic acid, consists of phosphatase inhibitors. Compounds acting by other routes are known, including thapsigargin (calcium channel modulator) and benzoyl peroxide (free radical generator). Sensitivity to tumor promotion is an important factor in the relative sensitivity to skin carcinogenesis among different mouse strains and even among other laboratory animal species. An intriguing example, TCDD is 100-fold more potent than tetradecanoylphorbol acetate in certain hairless mouse strains but virtually inactive in some nonhairless strains (Poland *et al.*, 1982). Much effort is currently focusing on the signal transduction pathways that are perturbed by treatment with such chemicals. The finding that chromate (a human lung carcinogen) in the drinking water enhances tumor yield from ultraviolet light in mouse skin suggests that generation of reactive oxygen can be effective and raises concern about the Cr(VI) drinking water standard (Davidson *et al.*, 2004).

The desire to reduce the cost and improve the effectiveness of cancer testing in animals has led to development of transgenic mice with useful properties. The Tg.AC strain, for example, exhibits a genetically initiated epidermis (Humble *et al.*, 2005). Integrated in this mouse genome is a v-Ha-ras oncogene driven by part of the ζ-globin promoter, which in this context fortuitously drives expression only in epidermis that is wounded or treated with tumor promoters. The mice display enhanced skin sensitivity to a number of nongenotoxic carcinogens and have low backgrounds of spontaneous tumors over a 26-week treatment period. They also respond to genotoxic carcinogens, which target genes that cooperate with the ras oncogene in neoplastic development (Owens *et al.*, 1995). Tg.AC mice can be employed for testing in combination with a different mouse strain that has one p53 allele inactivated, and thus displays enhanced sensitivity to genotoxic carcinogens in other tissues in addition to the skin. These genetically modified mice promise to speed up testing using fewer animals and to reduce false-positive results arising from either strain-/species-specific idiosyncrasies or high doses that could elicit secondary responses not relevant to human exposures. Although replacement of the very expensive two-year rodent carcinogenesis assay is not yet feasible, these genetically modified mice have reduced the number of such assays and assisted pharmaceutical evaluation (Jacobs, 2005).

Arsenic

An abundant element in the earth's crust that is encountered routinely in small doses in the air, water, and food, arsenic has long been known to affect human health (Hughes *et al.*, 2011). In earlier times, high exposures occurred from medications such as Fowler's solution (potassium arsenite) and from pesticides such as sodium arsenite and lead arsenate; the latter pesticides have been phased out in the USA but monomethylarsenate is still used in considerable (though decreasing) volumes in agriculture. Around the world, substantial exposures can occur as a result of mining operations to individuals who breathe the dust from ores or smelting fumes or to communities encountering leachate from tailings into waterways. Glass manufacture and food dried using coal with high arsenic content can also contribute to high exposures, and the environmental burden is increased by disposal of large volumes of wood preserved with chromated copper arsenate and of litter from poultry fed organic arsenical antibiotics. Well water derived from geological formations with high arsenic content is now recognized as a major health concern, highlighted by populations in the tens of millions at risk in Bangladesh and India (Tapio and Grosche, 2006). Previous studies of populations in southwestern Taiwan revealed an association of high arsenic exposure with altered skin pigmentation and hyperkeratosis of the palms and soles, blackfoot disease from impaired circulation reflecting endothelial cell damage, and carcinomas of the skin and several other organs (bladder, lung, and liver). More recent concentration dependence studies in Bangladesh show skin hyperpigmentation and keratoses occurring with drinking water concentrations close to 50 ppb (Argos *et al.*, 2011), the former USA drinking water standard. Synergistic effects with arsenic have now been reported with smoking, sun exposure, and fertilizer use (Melkonian *et al.*, 2011). Recognition that carcinomas of the skin and internal organs occur in humans drinking water with concentrations less than an order of magnitude higher than 50 ppb contributed to reducing the USA standard to 10 ppb as of 2006.

Due to continuing debate over the dependence of health effects on arsenic at low concentration, much effort is devoted to understanding arsenic action. Numerous mechanisms have been proposed by which arsenic serves as a carcinogen and gives other pathological effects, of which the majority could plausibly involve binding of trivalent forms to protein sulfhydryls (Kitchin and Wallace, 2008). Methylation has been considered a detoxification method, because the observed pentvalent mono- and dimethyl arsenates isolated in urine from exposed humans and animals are much less toxic than the inorganic forms. Wide species differences in methylation capability even among primates have raised the possibility that other detoxification pathways exist, and observations that the methylated forms are also found at low levels in the highly toxic trivalent state in animal tissues and in human urine have prompted re-evaluation of their roles. Exploring how the recently identified As(III)-methyltransferase influences toxic effects is anticipated to help clarify this important issue (Hughes *et al.*, 2011). For the epidermis, where little methylation has been demonstrated, effects of the inorganic forms may dominate. As shown by many labs, effects of arsenate (the most common form in drinking water) in vivo or in culture are mediated by reduction to arsenite (Patterson *et al.*, 2003).

Arsenic is a weak mutagen at best in bacteria and mammalian cells, but it does induce DNA deletions and chromosomal aberrations and acts as a comutagen, possibly by interfering with DNA repair (Rossman *et al.*, 2004). Consistent with this view, high arsenic exposure from drinking water appears to promote skin lesions in users of betel nut (McCarty *et al.*, 2006), a source of genotoxic nitrosamines known to be activated by cytochrome P450 activities in keratinocytes of the oral cavity (Miyazaki *et al.*, 2005). An important contributing factor to such phenomena, limiting DNA repair, could be arsenite inactivation of poly(ADP-ribose) polymerase-1 by binding to its zinc finger motifs (Zhou *et al.*, 2011). Similarly, in mice where the skin is irradiated with ultraviolet light, arsenic acts as a cocarcinogen (Rossman *et al.*, 2004), and in Tg.AC mice, expressing an activated ras oncogene in the epidermis, arsenic enhances phorbol ester tumor promotion (Germolec *et al.*, 1997). Among the proposed mechanisms of arsenic action, generation of reactive oxygen in target cells is a likely contributor to such carcinogenic and other pathological effects. This phenomenon has been proposed to result from activation of NADPH oxygenases (Cooper *et al.*, 2009), damage to mitochondria (Liu *et al.*, 2005), or, in the case of the methylated forms, (auto)oxidation (Kitchin and Ahmad, 2003). Pursuant to the demonstration that inorganic arsenic is a transplacental carcinogen for various tissues in mice (Waalkes *et al.*, 2004), further investigation revealed that this treatment enlarged stem cell compartments, including in the epidermis (Tokar *et al.*, 2011). Consonant with this observation, arsenite prevents differentiation and preserves stem cell character in human keratinocyte culture (Reznikova *et al.*, 2010).

REFERENCES

Abel EL, Angel JM, Kiguchi K, DiGiovanni J. Multi-stage chemical carcinogenesis in mouse skin: fundamentals and applications. *Nat Protoc.* 2009;4:1350–1362.

Ahmad N, Mukhtar H. Cytochrome P450: a target for drug development for skin diseases. *J Invest Dermatol.* 2004;123:417–425.

Ahmadi KR. Role of common genetic variants on the risk of Stevens–Johnson syndrome and toxic epidermal necrolysis. *Pharmacogenomics.* 2011;12:761–764.

Amin S, Freeman S, Maibach HI. Systemic toxicity in man secondary to percutaneous absorption. In: Roberts MS, Walters KA, eds., *Dermal Absorption and Toxicity Assessment.* New York: Marcel Dekker; 1998:103–125.

Ancona AA. Occupational acne. *Occup Med.* 1986;1:229–243.

Andreu I, Mayorga C, Miranda MA. Generation of reactive intermediates in photoallergic dermatitis. *Curr Opin Allergy Clin Immunol.* 2010;10:303–308.

Ardern-Jones MR, Friedmann PS. Skin manifestations of drug allergy. *Br J Clin Pharmacol.* 2011;71:672–683.

Argos M, Kalra T, Pierce BL, et al. A prospective study of arsenic exposure from drinking water and incidence of skin lesions in bangladesh. *Am J Epidemiol.* 2011;174:185–194.

Arora B, Kumar L, Sharma A, Wadhwa W, Kochupillai V. Pigmentary changes in chronic myeloid leukemia patients treated with imatinib mesylate. *Annals Oncol.* 2004;15:358–359.

Arts JHE, Mommers C, de Heer C. Dose–response relationships and threshold levels in skin and respiratory allergy. *Crit Rev Toxicol.* 2006;36:219–251.

Balk SJ. Ultraviolet radiation: a hazard to children and adolescents. *Pediatrics.* 2011;127:e791–e817.

Barratt MD. Structure–activity relationships and prediction of the phototoxicity and phototoxic potential of new drugs. *Altern Lab Anim.* 2004;32:511–524.

Basko-Plluska JL, Thyssen JP, Schalock PC. Cutaneous and systemic hypersensitivity reactions to metallic implants. *Dermatitis.* 2011;22:65–79.

Bellon T, Blanca M. The innate immune system in delayed cutaneous allergic reactions to medications. *Curr Opin Allergy Clin Immunol.* 2011;11:292–298.

Belsito DV. Occupatiopnal contact dermatitis: etiology, prevalence, and resultant impairment/disability. *J Am Acad Dermatol.* 2005;53:303–313.

Betts CJ, Dearman RJ, Kimber I, Maibach HI. Potency and risk assessment of a skin sensitizing disperse dye using the local lymph node assay. *Contact Dermatitis.* 2005;52:268–272.

Blanciforti LA. Economic burden of dermatitis in US workers. *J Occup Environ Med.* 2010;52:1045–1054.

Böhme A, Thaens D, Paschke A, Schüürmann G. Kinetic glutathione chemoassay to quantify thiol reactivity of organic electrophiles—application to alpha,beta-unsaturated ketones, acrylates, and propiolates. *Chem Res Toxicol.* 2009;22:742–750.

Boukhman MP, Maibach HI. Thresholds in contact sensitization: immunologic mechanisms and experimental evidence in humans—an overview. *Food Chem Toxicol.* 2001;39:1125–1134.

Brown HS, Bishop DR, Rowan CA. The role of skin absorption as a route of exposure for volatile organic compounds (VOCs) in drinking water. *Am J Public Health.* 1984;74:479–484.

Buchholz BA, Fultz E, Haack KW, et al. HPLC-accelerator MS measurement of atrazine metabolites in human urine after dermal exposure. *Analyt Chem.* 1999;71:3519–3525.

Busse KL, Maibach HI. Transdermal estradiol and testosterone transfer in man: existence, models, and strategies for prevention. *Skin Pharmacol Physiol.* 2011;24:57–66.

Bylaite M, Grigaitiene J, Lapinskaite GS. Photodermatoses: classification, evaluation and management. *Br J Dermatol.* 2009;161(suppl 3):61–68.

Cao LY, Taylor JS, Sood A, Murray D, Siegel PD. Allergic contact dermatitis to synthetic rubber gloves. *Arch Dermatol.* 2010;146:1001–1007.

Cooper KL, Liu KJ, Hudson LG. Enhanced ROS production and redox signaling with combined arsenite and UVA exposure: contribution of NADPH oxidase. *Free Radical Biol Med.* 2009;47:381–388.

Cummings KJ, Stefaniak AB, Virji MA, Kreiss K. A reconsideration of acute beryllium disease. *Environ Health Perspect.* 2009;117:1250–1256.

Cunliffe WJ, Holland DB, Jeremy A. Comedone formation: etiology, clinical presentation, and treatment. *Clin Dermatol.* 2004;22:367–374.

Curtin GM, Hanausek M, Walaszek Z, et al. Short-term biomarkers of cigarette smoke condensate tumor promoting potential in mouse skin. *Toxicol Sci.* 2006;89:66–74.

Davidson T, Kluz T, Burns FJ, et al. Exposure to chromium(VI) in the drinking water increases the susceptibility to UV-induced skin tumors in hairless mice. *Toxicol Appl Pharmacol.* 2004;196:431–437.

Del Rosario RN, Barr RJ, Graham BS, Kaneshiro S. Exogenous and endogenous cutaneous anomalies and curiosities. *Am J Dermatopathol.* 2005;27:259–267.

DeLeo VA. Photocontact dermatitis. *Dermatol Ther.* 2004;17:279–288.

Desai P, Patlolla RR, Singh M. Interaction of nanoparticles and cell-penetrating peptides with skin for transdermal drug delivery. *Molec Membrane Biol.* 2010;27:247–259.

Doutre MS. Occupational contact urticaria and protein contact dermatitis. *Eur J Dermatol.* 2005;15:419–424.

Du L, Neis MM, Ladd PA, Lanza DL, Yost GS, Keeney DS. Effects of the differentiated keratinocyte phenotype on expression levels of CYP1-4 family genes in human skin cells. *Toxicol Appl Pharmacol.* 2006;213:135–144.

Elias PM. Role of lipids in barrier function of the skin. In: Mukhtar H, ed. *Pharmacology of the Skin.* Boca Raton: CRC Press; 1992:29–38.

Elias PM. Stratum corneum defensive functions: an integrated view. *J Invest Dermatol.* 2005;125:183–200.

Elias PM, Schmuth M. Abnormal skin barrier in the etiopathogenesis of atopic dermatitis. *Curr Opin Allergy Clin Immunol.* 2009;9:437–446.

Emmett EA. Occupational contact dermatitis II: risk assessment and prognosis. *Am J Contact Dermat.* 2003;14:21–30.

Etienne G, Cony-Makhoul P, Mahon FX. Imatinib mesylate and gray hair. *N Engl J Med.* 2002;347:446.

Fang JY, Leu YL. Prodrug strategy for enhancing drug delivery via skin. *Curr Drug Discov Technol.* 2006;3:211–224.

Farahmand S, Maibach HI. Estimating skin permeability from physicochemical characteristics of drugs: a comparison between conventional models and an in vivo-based approach. *Int J Pharm.* 2009;375:41–47.

Fisher AA. Unique reactions of scrotal skin to topical agents. *Cutis.* 1989;44:445–447.

Fournier A, Murray MW. Application of phorbol ester to mouse skin causes a rapid and sustained loss of protein kinase C. *Nature.* 1987;330:767–769.

Frank J, Poblete-Gutiérrez P. Porphyria cutanea tarda—when skin meets liver. *Best Pract Res Clin Gastroenterol.* 2010;24:735–745.

Gawkrodger DJ. Occupational skin cancers. *Occupational Med.* 2004;54:458–463.

Gawkrodger DJ, Harris G, Bojar RA. Chloracne in seven organic chemists exposed to novel polycyclic halogenated chemical compounds (triazoloquinoxalines). *Br J Dermatol.* 2009;161:939–943.

Germolec DR, Spalding J, Boorman GA, et al. Arsenic can mediate skin neoplasia by chronic stimulation of keratinocyte-derived growth factors. *Mutation Res.* 1997;386:209–218.

Geusau A, Abraham K, Geissler K, Sator MO, Stingl G, Tschachler E. Severe 2,3,7,8-Tetrachlorodibenzo-p-dioxin (TCDD) intoxication: clinical and laboratory effects. *Environ Health Perspect.* 2001;109: 865–869.

Geyer HJ, Schramm K-W, Feicht EA, et al. Half lives of tetra-, penta-, hexa-, hepta- and octachlorodibenzo-p-dioxin in rats, monkeys and humans—a critical review. *Chemosphere.* 2002;48:631–644.

Ghabili K, Agutter PS, Ghanei M, Ansarin K, Panahi Y, Shoja MM. Sulfur mustard toxicity: history, chemistry, pharmacokinetics, and pharmacodynamics. *Crit Rev Toxicol.* 2011;41:384–403.

Gibbs S, van de Sandt JJM, Merk HF, Lockley DJ, Pendlington RU, Pease CK. Xenobiotic metabolism in human skin and 3D human skin reconstructs: a review. *Curr Drug Metab.* 2007;8:758–772.

Gruber R, Elias PM, Crumrine D, et al. Filaggrin genotype in ichthyosis vulgaris predicts abnormalities in epidermal structure and function. *Am J Pathol.* 2011;178:2252–2263.

Gruchalla RS, Pirmohamed M. Antibiotic allergy. *N Engl J Med.* 2006; 354:601–609.

Guerra L, Dellambra E, Brescia S, Raskovic D Vitiligo: pathogenetic hypotheses and targets for current therapies. *Curr Drug Metab.* 2010;11:451–467.

Guy RH. Predicting the rate and extent of fragrance chemical absorption into and through the skin. *Chem Res Toxicol.* 2010a;23:864–870.

Guy RH. Transdermal drug delivery. In: Schäfer-Korting M, ed. *Drug Delivery, Handbook of Experimental Pharmacology.* Vol. 197. Berlin, Germany: Springer Verlag; 2010b:399–410.

Harr T, French LE. Toxic epidermal necrolysis and Stevens–Johnson syndrome. *Orphanet J Rare Dis.* 2010;5:39.

Holden CR, Gawkrodger DJ. 10 years' experience of patch testing with a shoe series in 230 patients: which allergens are important? *Contact Dermatitis.* 2005;53:37–39.

Holzer AM, Kaplan LL, Levis WR. Haptens as drugs: contact allergens are powerful immunomodulators. *J Drugs Dermatol.* 2006;5:410–416.

Hu T, Khambatta ZS, Hayden PJ, et al. Xenobiotic metabolism gene expression in the EpiDerm™ in vitro 3D human epidermis model compared to human skin. *Toxicol In Vitro.* 2010;24:1450–1463.

Hughes MF, Beck BD, Chen Y, Lewis AS, Thomas DJ. Arsenic exposure and toxicology: a historical perspective. *Toxicol Sci.* 2011;123:305–332.

Humble MC, Trempus CS, Spalding JW, Cannon RE, Tennant RW. Biological, cellular and molecular characterisitics of an inducible transgenic skin tumor model: a review. *Oncogene* 2005;24:8217–8228.

Ibbotson SH. Adverse effects of topical photodynamic therapy. *Photodermatol Photoimmunol Photomed.* 2011;27:116–130.

Jacobs A. Prediction of 2-year carcinogenicity study results for pharmaceutical products: how are we doing? *Toxicol Sci.* 2005;88:18–23.

Jewell C, Heylings J, Clowes HM, Williams FM. Percutaneous absorption and metabolism of dinitrochlorobenzene in vitro. *Arch Toxicol.* 2000;74:356–365.

Jiang YJ, Kim P, Elias PM, Feingold KR. LXR and PPAR activators stimulate cholesterol sulfotransferase type 2 isoform 1b in human keratinocytes. *J Lipid Res.* 2005;46:2657–2666.

Kao J, Hall J. Skin absorption and cutaneous first pass metabolism of topical steroids: in vitro studies with mouse skin in organ culture. *J Pharmacol Exper Therap.* 1987;241:482–487.

Karunadasa KP, Perera C, Kanagaratnum V, Wijerathne UP, Samarasingha I, Kannangara CK. Burns due to acid assaults in Sri Lanka. *J Burn Care Res.* 2010;31:781–785.

Kaur RR, Kirby W, Maibach H. Cutaneous allergic reactions to tattoo ink. *J Cosmet Dermatol.* 2009;8:295–300.

Kerr A, Ferguson J. Photoallergic contact dermatitis. *Photodermatol Photoimmunol Photomed.* 2010;26:56–65.

Khan WA, Das M, Stick S, Javed S, Bickers DR, Mukhtar H. Induction of epidermal NAD(P)H:quinone reductase by chemical carcinogens: a possible mechanism for the detoxification. *Biochem Biophys Res Commun.* 1987;146:126–133.

Kitchin KT, Ahmad S. Oxidative stress as a possible mode of action for arsenic carcinogenesis. *Toxicol Lett.* 2003;137:3–13.

Kitchin KT, Wallace K. The role of protein binding of trivalent arsenicals in arsenic carcinogenesis and toxicity. *J Inorganic Biochem.* 2008;102:532–539.

Kynemund Pedersen L, Agner T, Held E, Johansen JD. Methyldibromo glutaronitrile in leave-on products elicits contact allergy at low concentration. *Br J Dermatol.* 2004;151:817–822.

Ladizinski B, Mistry N, Kundu RV. Widespread use of toxic skin lightening compounds: medical and psychosocial aspects. *Dermatol Clin.* 2011;29:111–123.

Lim HW, James WD, Rigel DS, Maloney ME, Spencer JM, Bhushan R. Adverse effects of ultraviolet radiation from the use of indoor tanning equipment: time to ban the tan. *J Am Acad Dermatol.* 2011;64:893–902.

Limsuwan T, Demoly P. Acute symptoms of drug hypersensitivity (urticaria, angioedema, anaphylaxis, anaphylactic shock). *Med Clin N Am.* 2010;94:691–710.

Liu SX, Davidson MM, Tang X, et al. Mitochondrial damage mediates genotoxicity of arsenic in mammalian cells. *Cancer Res.* 2005; 65:3236–3242.

Luu-The V, Duche D, Ferraris C, Meunier JR, Leclaire J, Labrie F. Expression profiles of phases 1 and 2 metabolizing enzymes in human skin and the reconstructed skin models Episkin and full thickness model from Episkin. *J Steroid Biochem Mol Biol.* 2009;116:178–186.

Lynde CW, Sapra S. Predictive testing of the melanocortin 1 receptor for skin cancer and photoaging. *Skin Therapy Lett.* 2010;15:5–7.

Mark BJ, Slavin RG. Allergic contact dermatitis. *Med Clin N Am.* 2006;90:169–185.

Martin-Bouyer G, Lebreton R, Toga M, Stolley PD, Lockhart J. Outbreak of accidental hexachlorophene poisoning in France. *Lancet.* 1982;1: 91–95.

Mattsson U, Halbritter S, Mörner Serikoff E, Christerson L, Warfvinge G. Oral pigmentation in the hard palate associated with imatinib mesylate therapy: a report of three cases. *Oral Surg Oral Med Oral Pathol Oral Radiol Endod.* 2011;111:e12–e16.

McCarty KM, Houseman EA, Quamruzzaman Q, et al. The impact of diet and betel nut use on skin lesions associated with drinking-water arsenic in Pabna, Bangladesh. *Environ Health Perspect.* 2006;114:334–340.

McKnight RH, Spiller HA. Green tobacco sickness in children and adolescents. *Pub Health Rep.* 2005;120:602–605.

Mekenyan O, Patlewicz G, Dimitrova G, et al. Use of genotoxicity information in the development of integrated testing strategies (ITS) for skin sensitization. *Chem Res Toxicol.* 2010;23:1519–1540.

Melkonian S, Argos M, Pierce BL, et al. A prospective study of the synergistic effects of arsenic exposure and smoking, sun exposure, fertilizer use, and pesticide use on risk of premalignant skin lesions in Bangladeshi men. *Am J Epidemiol.* 2011;173:183–191.

Melnikova VO, Ananthaswamy HN. Cellular and molecular events leading to the development of skin cancer. *Mutation Res.* 2005;571:91–106.

Miller J, Djabali K, Chen T, et al. Atrichia caused by mutations in the vitamin D receptor gene is a phenocopy of generalized atrichia caused by mutations in the hairless gene. *J Invest Dermatol.* 2001;117: 612–617.

Milton R, Mathieu L, Hall AH, Maibach HI. Chemical assault and skin/eye burns: two representative cases, report from the Acid Survivors Foundation, and literature review. *Burns.* 2010;36:924–932.

Miyazaki M, Sugawara ETY, Yamazaki H, Kamataki T. Mutagenic activation of betel quid-specific *N*-nitrosamines catalyzed by human cytochrome P450 coexpressed with NADH-cytochrome P450 reductase in *Salmonella typhimurium* YG7108. *Mutation Res.* 2005;581:165–171.

Moan J, Peng Q. An outline of the hundred-year history of PDT. *Anticancer Res.* 2004;23:3591–3600.

Modi GM, Doherty CB, Katta R, Orengo IF. Irritant contact dermatitis from plants. *Dermatitis.* 2009;20:63–78.

Moller H. Contact allergy to gold as a model for clinical–experimental research. *Contact Dermatitis.* 2010;62:193–200.

Moore DE. Drug-induced cutaneous photosensitivity: incidence, mechanism, prevention and management. *Drug Safety.* 2002;25:345–372.

Netzlaff F, Lehr CM, Wertz PW, Schaefer UF. The human epidermis models EpiSkin, SkinEthic and EpiDerm: an evaluation of morphology and their suitability for testing photoxicity, irritancy, corrosivity and substance transport. *Eur J Pharm Biopharm.* 2005;60:167–178.

Neville JA, Welch E, Leffell DJ. Management of nonmelanoma skin cancer in 2007. *Nat Clin Pract Oncol.* 2007;4:462–469.

Ngo MA, Maibach HI. Dermatotoxicology: historical perspective and advances. *Toxicol Appl Pharmacol.* 2010;243:225–238.

Nijsten TE, Stern RS. The increased risk of skin cancer is persistent after discontinuation of psoralen + ultraviolet A: a cohort study. *J Invest Dermatol.* 2003;121:252–258.

Nishigori C. Cellular aspects of photocarcinogenesis. *Photochem Photobiol Sci.* 2006;5:208–214.

Oesch F, Fabian E, Oesch-Bartlomowicz B, Werner C, Landsiedel R. Drug-metabolizing enzymes in the skin of man, rat, and pig. *Drug Metab Rev.* 2007;39:659–698.

Okey AB, Franc MA, Moffat ID, et al. Toxicological implications of poly-morphisms in receptors for xenobiotic chemicals: the case of the aryl hydrocarbon receptor. *Toxicol Appl Pharmacol.* 2005;207:S43–S51.

Otberg N, Patzelt A, Rasulev U, et al. The role of hair follicles in the percu-taneous absorption of caffeine. *Br J Clin Pharmacol.* 2008;65:488–492.

Owens DM, Spalding JW, Tennant RW, Smart RC. Genetic alterations cooperate with v-Ha-ras to accelerate multistage carcinogenesis in Tg.AC transgenic mouse skin. *Cancer Res.* 1995;55:3171–3178.

Owens DM, Wei SJC, Smart RC. A multihit, multistage model of chemical carcinogenesis. *Carcinogenesis.* 1999;20:1837–1844.

Palmer CN, Irvine AD, Terron-Kwiatkowski A, et al. Common loss-of-function variants of the epidermal barrier protein filaggrin are a major predisposing factor for atopic dermatitis. *Nat Genet.* 2006;38:441–446.

Palosuo T, Antoniadou I, Gottrup F, Phillips P. Latex medical gloves: time for a reappraisal. *Int Arch Allergy Immunol.* 2011;156:234–246.

Panteleyev AA, Bickers DR. Dioxin-induced chloracne—reconstructing the cellular and molecular mechanisms of a classic environmental disease. *Exp Dermatol.* 2006;15:705–730.

Park JH, Troxel AB, Harvey RG, Penning TM. Polycyclic aromatic hydro-carbon (PAH) o-quinones produced by the aldo-keto-reductases (AKRs) generate abasic sites, oxidized pyrimidines and 8-oxo-dGuo via reactive oxygen species. *Chem Res Toxicol.* 2006;19:719–728.

Pascoe D, Moreau L, Sasseville D. Emergent and unusual allergens in cos-metics. *Dermatitis.* 2010;21:127–137.

Passarini B, Infusino SD, Kasapi E. Chloracne: still cause for concern. *Dermatology.* 2010;221:63–70.

Patterson TJ, Ngo M, Aronov PA, Reznikova TV, Green PG, Rice RH. Biological activity of inorganic arsenic and antimony reflects oxidation state in cultured keratinocytes. *Chem Res Toxicol.* 2003;16:1624–1631.

Pesatori AC, Consonni D, Rubagotti M, Grillo P, Bertazzi PA. Cancer inci-dence in the population exposed to dioxin after the "Seveso accident": twenty years of follow-up. *Environ Health.* 2009;8:39.

Poland A, Knutson JC. 2,3,7,8-Tetrachlorodibeno-p-dioxin and related halogenated aromatic hydrocarbons: examination of the mechanism of toxicity. *Ann Rev Pharmacol Toxicol.* 1982;22:517–554.

Poland A, Palen D, Glover E. Tumor promotion by TCDD in skin of HRS/J hairless mice. *Nature.* 1982;300:271–273.

Potts RO, Guy RH. Predicting skin permeability. *Pharmacol Res.* 1992;9:663–669.

Prausnitz MR, Mikszta JA, Cormier M, Andrianov AK. Microneedle-based vaccines. *Curr Top Microbiol Immunol.* 2009;333:369–393.

Ramot Y, Nyska A, Lieuallen W, et al. Inflammatory and chloracne-like skin lesions in B6C3F1 mice exposed to 3,3′,4,4′-tetrachloroazobenzene for 2 years. *Toxicology.* 2009;265:1–9.

Reines HD, Seifert PC. Patient safety: latex allergy. *Surg Clin North Am.* 2005;85:1329–1340.

Reznikova TV, Phillips MA, Patterson TJ, Rice RH. Opposing actions of insulin and arsenite converge on PKCδ to alter keratinocyte proliferative potential and differentiation. *Molec Carcinog.* 2010;49:398–409.

Rigel DS. Cutaneous ultraviolet exposure and its relationship to the devel-opment of skin cancer. *J Am Acad Dermatol.* 2008;58:S129–S132.

Riviere JE, Brooks JD. Predicting skin permeability from complex chemi-cal mixtures. *Toxicol Appl Pharmacol.* 2005;208:99–110.

Roberts DW, Aptula AO. Determinants of skin sensitisation potential. *J Appl Toxicol.* 2008;28:377–387.

Roberts DW, Natsch A. High throughput kinetic profiling approach for covalent binding to peptides: application to skin sensitization potency of Michael acceptor electrophiles. *Chem Res Toxicol.* 2009;22:592–603.

Roelofzen JH, Aben KK, Oldenhof UT, et al. No increased risk of can-cer after coal tar treatment in patients with psoriasis or eczema. *J Invest Dermatol.* 2010;130:953–961.

Rolsted K, Kissmeyer AM, Rist GM, Hansen SH. Evaluation of cytochrome P450 activity in vitro, using dermal and hepatic microsomes from four species and two keratinocyte cell lines in culture. *Arch Dermatol Res.* 2008;300:11–18.

Rossman TG, Uddin AN, Burns FJ. Evidence that arsenite acts as a cocar-cinogen in skin cancer. *Toxicol Appl Pharmacol.* 2004;198:394–404.

Rubin H. Synergistic mechanisms in carcinogenesis by polycyclic aromatic hydrocarbons and by tobacco smoke: a bio-historical perspective with updates. *Carcinogenesis.* 2001;22:1903–1930.

Rundhaug JE, Fischer SM. Molecular mechanisms of mouse skin tumor promotion. *Cancers.* 2010;2:436–482.

Saarikoski ST, Rivera SP, Hankinson O, Husgafvwl-Pursianinen K. CYP2S1: a short review. *Toxicol Appl Pharmacol.* 2005;207:S62–S69.

Samuelsson K, Bergstrom MA, Jonsson CA, Westman G, Karlberg AT. Diphenylthiourea, a common rubber chemical, is bioactivated to potent skin sensitizers. *Chem Res Toxicol.* 2011;24:35–44.

Santos A, Van Ree R. Profilins: mimickers of allergy or relevant allergens? *Int Arch Allergy Immunol.* 2011;155:191–204.

Scheuplein RJ, Blank IH. Permeability of skin. *Physiol Rev.* 1971;51:702–747.

Schram SE, Warshaw EM, Laumann A. Nickel hypersensitivity: a clinical review and call to action. *Int J Dermatol.* 2010;49:115–125.

Schulman JM, Fisher DE. Indoor ultraviolet tanning and skin cancer: health risks and opportunities. *Curr Opin Oncol.* 2009;21:144–149.

Schwöbel JA, Wondrousch D, Koleva YK, Madden JC, Cronin MT, Schüürmann G. Prediction of Michael-type acceptor reactivity toward glutathione. *Chem Res Toxicol.* 2010;23:1576–1585.

Shakarjian MP, Heck DE, Gray JP, et al. Mechanisms mediating the vesi-cant actions of sulfur mustard after cutaneous exposure. *Toxicol Sci.* 2010;114:5–19.

Sheehan JM, Cragg N, Chadwick CA, Potten CS, Young AR. Repeated ultraviolet exposure affords the same protection against DNA photodam-age and erythema in human skin types II and IV but is associated with faster DNA repair in skin type IV. *J Invest Dermatol.* 2002;118:825–829.

Shimizu Y, Nakatsuru Y, Ichinose M, et al. Benzo[a]pyrene carcinogenicity is lost in mice lacking the aryl hydrocarbon receptor. *Proc Natl Acad Sci USA.* 2000;97:779–782.

Sicherer SH, Sampson HA. Food allergy. *J Allergy Clin Immunol.* 2010;125:S116–S125.

Smith G, Ibbotson SH, Comrie MM, et al. Regulation of cutaneous drug-metabolizing enzymes and cytoprotective gene expression by topical drugs in human skin in vivo. *Br J Dermatol.* 2006;155:275–281.

Sorg O, Zennegg M, Schmid P, et al. 2,3,7,8-Tetrachlorodibenzo-p-dioxin (TCDD) poisoning in Victor Yushchenko: identification and measure-ment of TCDD metabolites. *Lancet.* 2009;374:1179–1185.

Storm JE, Collier SW, Stewart RF, Bronaugh RL. Metabolism of xenobiot-ics during percutaneous penetration: Role of absorption rate and cutane-ous enzyme activity. *Fund Appl Toxicol.* 1990;15:132–141.

Svensson CK. Biotransformation of drugs in human skin. *Drug Metab Dispos.* 2009;37:247–253.

Swanson HI. Cytochrome P450 expression in human keratinocytes: an aryl hydrocarbon receptor perspective. *Chem-Biol Interact.* 2004;149:69–79.

Tapio S, Grosche B. Arsenic in the etiology of cancer. *Mutation Res.* 2006;612:215–246.

Tauchi M, Hida A, Negishi T, et al. Constitutive expression of aryl hydro-carbon receptor in keratinocytes causes inflammatory skin lesions. *Molec Cell Biol.* 2005;25:9360–9368.

Thami GP, Sarkar R. Coal tar: past, present and future. *Clin Exp Dermatol.* 2004;27:99–103.

Tokar EJ, Qu W, Waalkes MP. Arsenic, stem cells, and the developmental basis of adult cancer. *Toxicol Sci.* 2011;120:S192–S203.

Tolbert PE. Oils and cancer. *Cancer Causes Control.* 1997;8:386–405.

Tornier C, Rosdy M, Maibach HI. In vitro skin irritation testing on reconstituted human epidermis: reproducibility for 50 chemicals tested with two proptocols. *Toxicol in Vitro.* 2006;20:401–416.

Tourlaki A, Boneschi V, Tosi D, Pigatto P, Brambilla L. Granulomatous tattoo reaction induced by intense pulse light treatment. *Photodermatol Photoimmunol Photomed.* 2010;26:275–276.

Uter W, Johansen JD, Orton DI, Frosch PJ, Schnuch A. Clinical update on contact allergy. *Curr Opin Allergy Clin Immunol.* 2005;5:429–436.

Victor FC, Cohen DE, Soter NA. A 20-year analysis of previous and emerging allergens that elicit photoallergic contact dermatitis. *J Am Acad Dermatol.* 2010;62:605–610.

Voelter-Mahlknecht S, Scheriau R, Zwahr G, et al. Skin tumors among employees of a tar refinery: the current data and their implications. *Int Arch Occup Environ Health.* 2007;80:485–495.

Waalkes MP, Liu J, Ward JM, Diwan BA. Animal models for arsenic carcinogenesis: inorganic arsenic is a transplacental carcinogen in mice. *Toxicol Appl Pharmacol.* 2004;198:377–384.

Walaszek Z, Hanausek M, Slaga TJ. The role of skin painting in predicting lung cancer. *Int J Toxicol.* 2007;26:345–351.

Walsh AA, deGraffenried LA, Rice RH. 2,3,7,8-Tetrachlorodibeno-*p*-dioxin sensitization of cultured human epidermal cells to carcinogenic heterocyclic amine toxicity. *Carcinogenesis.* 1995;16:2187–2191.

Warshaw EM, Raju SI, Fowler JFJ, et al. Positive patch test reactions in older individuals: retrospective analysis from the North American Contact Dermatitis Group, 1994–2008. *J Am Acad Dermatol.* 2012;66:229–240.

Watkins SA, Maibach HI. The hardening phenomenon in irritant contact dermatitis: an interpretative update. *Contact Dermatitis.* 2009;60:123–130.

Wilford C, Fine JD, Boyd AS, Sanyal S, Abraham JL, Kantrow SM. Nephrogenic systemic fibrosis: report of an additional case with granulomatous inflammation. *Am J Dermatopathol.* 2010;32:71–75.

Yoo JY, Al Naami M, Markowitz O, Hadi SM. Allergic contact dermatitis: patch testing results at Mount Sinai Medical Center. *Skinmed.* 2010;8:257–260.

Zhai H, Fautz R, Fuchs A, Bhandarkar S, Maibach HI. Human scalp irritation compared to that of the arm and back. *Contact Dermatitis.* 2004;51:196–200.

Zhou X, Sun X, Cooper KL, Wang F, Liu KJ, Hudson LG. Arsenite interacts selectively with zinc finger proteins containing C3H1 or C4 motifs. *J Biol Chem.* 2011;286:22855–22863.

Zuberbier T, Balke M, Worm M, Edenharter G, Maurer M. Epidemiology of urticaria: a representative cross-sectional population survey. *Clin Exp Dermatol.* 2010;35:869–873.

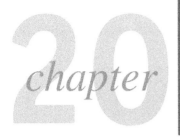

Toxic Responses of the Reproductive System

Paul M.D. Foster and L. Earl Gray Jr.

INTRODUCTION

Any evaluation of toxicity to reproduction will have as an important consideration that events may not only be on the adults having impact on their likelihood to have children, but also impact the viability and quality of life of their potential offspring and feasibly even affect later generations. That chemicals can adversely affect reproduction in males and females is not a new concept, one only has to look at the importance of drugs as contraceptives to realize how sensitive the reproductive system can be to external chemical influences to disrupt this process. Of course in these cases, the failure of normal reproduction is a desired outcome in a contraceptive, but unfortunately we have had a number of catastrophes in which such failure has been unintentional. Many of the classic examples in chemical workers, or contamination of groundwater from chemical exposure such as dibromochloropropane (DBCP) or kepone (chlordecone) have shown the sensitivity of human reproduction to these specific exposures (reviewed by Cannon et al., 1978; Faroon et al., 1995; Winker and Rudiger, 2006). There have been significant improvements in our ability to test for effects on reproduction for chemicals, agrochemicals, and drugs, but unfortunately such adverse episodes continue to occur in, for example, the more recent reports of the effects of 2-bromopropane in chemical workers (both male and female) in Korea (reviewed by Boekelheide et al., 2004).

Recent trends in human fertility, fecundity—changing social influences (age at which women have their first child), and the knowledge that populations in many western countries are no longer self-sustaining, coupled with the advent of assisted reproductive

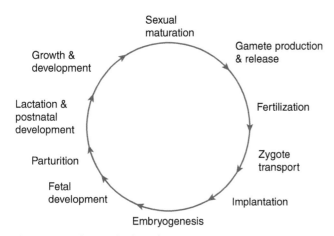

Figure 20-1. *The reproductive cycle.*

techniques (ARTs), where according to a recent paper 5.9% of all live births in Denmark used these ARTs (Andersen *et al.*, 2005), all point to the potential for declines in normal human reproduction. Underlying all these issues with human reproductive performance is the concept that exposure to environmental chemicals and drugs may be contributing to these declines.

The advent of the endocrine disruptor debate provided a major impetus to the examination of the methods used in screening and testing for reproductive (and other) toxicity, and highlighted a number of shortfalls, not least in how we should evaluate the latent effects on adults of in utero exposures. However, this chapter will not specifically address the emerging issue of the fetal origins of adult disease as proposed by Barker (see Barker *et al.*, 1989, 1993; Barker, 1995, 1999).

This chapter will take the reproductive cycle (Fig. 20-1) as the biological basis for the description of toxicity to reproduction rather than an encyclopedic approach. The basic biology of the different life stages and processes that are requisites for normal reproduction will be discussed and, where possible, the differences between experimental animals and humans highlighted (see Tables 20-1 and 20-2). These processes will then be placed into perspective by reference to a number of case studies of selected chemicals chosen to illustrate a range of modes of action and how they can perturb reproduction.

Special attention will be focused on endocrine disruption, methods proposed for screening and testing and the selection of agents with specific pharmacologies (eg, estrogen or antiandrogen) to illustrate the types of toxicities produced at different life stages.

The chapter will also provide basic information on testing methodologies for chemicals, pesticides, and drugs, but placed into the reproductive cycle framework. Thus, it will examine the life stages that are exposed and when specific evaluations are undertaken. Lastly, we have included a section on the evaluation of data and weight of evidence, specifically how one looks at concordance of end points with examples of the types of profiles observed (based on the examples used previously). We do not believe that we have seen this anywhere before, or in this context, and hopefully this will be a useful tool for students and professionals alike.

THE REPRODUCTIVE CYCLE

If one considers the purpose of the reproductive system as the production of good quality gametes, capable of fertilization, and producing a viable offspring, which in turn can successfully reproduce, then it is clear that a large number of complex processes need to be orchestrated in a precise, sequential order for optimal performance

---

Table 20-1

Examples of Reproductive Physiology Similarities Among Humans and Rats

- Steroid hormone control of reproductive function relies on testosterone, dihydrotestosterone, estradiol, and progesterone.
- CNS–hypothalamic secretion of GnRH controls pituitary release and synthesis of FSH and LH.
- FSH and LH regulate germ cell development after puberty, LH surges induce spontaneous ovulation in the female, and LH regulates testis Leydig cell testosterone production.
- Placental support of embryos. Placenta and fetal unit also produce hormones critical for pregnancy maintenance after the first week.
- Hormonal regulation of uterine function and onset of delivery.
- Androgens required to maintain male spermatogenesis and secondary sex characteristics.
- Hormone-dependent mating and other sexually dimorphic behavior. "Rough and tumble" play behavior is sexually dimorphic behavior being imprinted by early androgens.
- Lactation under complex hormonal regulation.
- Dramatic endocrine changes resulting from CNS–HPG maturation responsible for puberty in males and females. Females generally attain puberty at an earlier age than males of the same species.

CNS, Central nervous system; GnRH, gonatropin-releasing hormone; FSH, follicle-stimulating hormone; LH, luteinizing hormone; HPG, hypothalamic–pituitary–gonadal.

at different stages of the life cycle of the animals, or humans. Thus following fertilization of an egg by a sperm, the resulting zygote must be transported along the oviduct while maturing into an early embryo. This embryo is then required to implant in the uterus successfully, such that the developing conceptus can differentiate, produce a placenta, and normal embryogenesis and fetal development occur. Once the fetus has completed in utero growth and differentiation, parturition needs to occur at the correct time and the neonate be born and then proceed successfully through the lactation phase of development and be weaned.

When the male and female offspring enter puberty after infancy, they need to acquire sexual characteristics as young adults with mature reproductive systems. Acquisition of sexual maturity involves the generation of gametes by the gonads, which in turn can result in the production of the next generation. For the parental animals, once their reproductive lifespan has finished, the process of reproductive senescence then occurs. This myriad of processes all involve complex interplay between tissues and cells, the vast majority of these processes being under complex hormonal control that provides the critical signals and precise timing of these events.

Not surprisingly, it is possible to perturb this complex series of events and thus disturb the process and purpose of reproduction. Indeed, all these processes can be targets for the action of specific chemicals that can disturb these events leading to adverse effects on reproduction, such that the normal production of viable offspring cannot occur. It is thus important to consider in an evaluation of reproductive toxicity that while simple yes/no answers as to whether a particular agent can be a reproductive toxicant are possible, and indeed are used, any description of such toxicity has to be in the context of the life stage of exposure and effect. There are examples of chemicals that can have different effects on reproduction, at different life stages, via different modes of action/mechanisms. Indeed, it might be useful for this particular aspect of

Table 20-2

Examples in Which the Reproductive Strategy of the Rat Differs From That of The Human

1. The rat is a short (22.5 day) gestation species. Pregnancy in humans is 9 months.
2. The rat placenta lacks aromatase; estrogen is produced during pregnancy by the ovary. Human placental tissue expresses high levels of aromatase.
3. In the rat, sexual differentiation of the reproductive tract is perinatal, whereas central nervous system (CNS) sexual differentiation is a postnatal event, regulated to a great degree by aromatization of testosterone to estradiol (play behavior, an exception, is androgen-dependent in both rats [Hotchkiss et al., 2002, 2003] and humans [Hines, 2003]). In nonhuman primates and presumably humans, more CNS events are prenatal, and androgens are more important than in rats (Goy and Phoenix, 1972; Goy and Resko, 1972; Goy et al., 1988; Hines, 2003).
4. The rat has a 4- to 5-day estrous cycle, with no functional corporus luteum. The estrous cycle can be monitored easily by examining daily cytology. The female rat displays sexual receptivity only during estrus after "lights out" after a proestrus vaginal smear. This behavior is exquisitely dependent on estrogen followed by progesterone. Humans have a menstrual cycle approximately 28 days in duration and do not display periods of peak behavioral estrus during the cycle. Corpora luteal function is sustained for approximately 10 days by mating-induced cervical stimulatory prolactin surges in rats, whereas the human menstrual cycle has a spontaneous luteal phase of 10 to 14 days after ovulation.
5. Male rat sex behavior can be induced by estrogens and involves multiple series of ejaculations in a single mating. Mating involves approximately 10 mounts, with intromission before each ejaculation, followed by a postejaculatory interval before the onset of the next series. In nonhuman primates and presumably humans, male sex behavior is androgen mediated.
6. Both ovaries spontaneously release several ova in response to a luteinizing hormone surge into separate uterine horns, each with a separate cervix in the rat; whereas in women, a single ovum is typically ovulated during each cycle.
7. Pregnancy is easily disrupted by estrogens in rats, but not in humans. Rats, unlike humans, are a litter-bearing species. Most strains used for toxicology testing have litters of 10 to 12 pups. Spontaneous reproductive malformations are very rare in the rats, whereas in humans, some malformations such as cryptorchidism occur in 3% of newborn boys.
8. Spermatogenesis begins at approximately 5 days of age in the rat; the spermatogenic cycle is about 53 days of age, and sperm appear in the epididymis at about 55 days of age. In humans, spermatogenesis begins during puberty at 10 to 14 years of age, and the entire spermatogenic cycle is approximately 75 days in duration.
9. Puberty in the rat (as measured by the age at vaginal opening and the onset of estrous cyclicity) occurs at about 32 days of age in females and 42 days of age (as measured by preputial separation, an androgen-dependent event) in male SD and LE rat strains. In humans, puberty occurs at 9 to 12 years of age in girls, and 10 to 14 years of age in boys.
10. Fertility begins to decline in the female rat at about 6 months of age, especially if never mated and allowed to cycle continuously. Fertility begins to decline in women at about 35 years of age, and at 40 years of age, approximately 50% of women are infertile.

For a review of reproductive physiology, see Knobil and Neill (1994).

toxicity to modify the adage of Paracelsus to "It is the *timing* of the dose that makes the poison." That is the dose of the toxic chemical and its resultant effects will be dependent on when in the life stage of the organism that the chemical is administered and evaluated.

The next sections will examine some of the hormonal and other control mechanisms that have been deduced from careful physiological studies in experimental animals and humans (see Table 20-3) to provide more information as to where chemicals may

Table 20-3

Reproductive Parameters for Various Species

| SPECIES | AGE AT PUBERTY/ PERIOD | SEXUAL CYCLE DURATION (DAYS) | OVULATION | | GESTATION | |
			TIME	TYPE	IMPLANTATION (DAYS)	PARTURITION (DAYS)
Mouse	5–6 weeks	4	2–3 h	S	4–5	19 (19–21)
Rat	6–11 weeks	4–6	8–11 h	S	5–6	21–22
Rabbit	6–7 months	Indefinite	10 h	I	7–8	31 (30–35)
Hamster	5–8 weeks	4	Early estrus	S	5+	16 (15–18)
Guinea Pig	8–10 weeks	16–19	10 h	S	6	67–68
Ferret	8–12 months	Seasonal	30–36 h	I	12–13	42
Cat	6–15 months	Seasonal	24–56 h	I	13–14	63 (52–69)
Dog	6–8 months	9	1–3 days	S	13–14	61 (53–71)
Monkey	3 years	28	9–20 days	S	9	168 (146–180)
Man	12–16 years	27–28	13–15 days	S	7.5	267 (ovulation)

S, Spontaneous; I, induced.

produce their effects. Rather than provide a laundry list of chemicals that can produce effects on reproduction, one or two examples will be mentioned to illustrate the variety of processes that can be affected with referral to more detailed references. While reviewing the mammalian reproductive cycle one could start in any position, we have decided to begin with the development of the reproductive system in utero that occurs with the process of sexual differentiation of the embryo and the move forward around the cycle as depicted in Fig. 20-1.

REPRODUCTIVE DEVELOPMENT AND SEXUAL DIFFERENTIATION

During early human development, there is a short period immediately prior to sexual differentiation when the gonad is sexually indifferent and it is not until the seventh week of gestation that male and female morphological characteristics begin to develop. In rodents, the embryo remains sexually indifferent and possesses both male and female reproductive tract primordia until embryonic day 13.5 regardless of its genetic sex.

Gonadogenesis begins with proliferation of the mesodermal (coelomic) epithelium, which invades the underlying mesenchyme, resulting in a longitudinal thickening on the medial side of the mesonephros, known as the gonadal ridge (Byskov, 1986). The invading epithelium begins to form primitive sex cords in the gonadal ridge, which are surrounded by undifferentiated mesenchyme (Pelliniemi, 1975). Primordial germ cells, or primitive sex cells, are first visible in the fourth week in the caudal region of the yolk sac near the origin of the allantois and migrate along the hindgut, up the dorsal mesentery and into the gonadal ridges (Eddy *et al.*, 1981). The primordial germ cells divide mitotically during migration and continue to proliferate as they migrate under the underlying mesenchyme and are incorporated into the primary sex cords (Moore, 1982). As the primitive cords begin to form, the mesenchyme is invaded by capillaries. The indifferent gonad now consists of an outer cortex and an inner medulla. In the rodent, formation of the gonadal cords is a rapid process that occurs at gestational day 13 via transitory epithelial cell aggregates along the length of the gonadal ridge (Paranko *et al.*, 1983).

Gonadal differentiation is dependent on signals from the Y chromosome, which contains the genes necessary to induce testicular morphogenesis. One of these signals is the SRY gene, which is the sex-determining region on the short arm of the Y chromosome (Koopman *et al.*, 1990), and acts as a "switch" to initiate transcription of other genes, which contribute to testicular organogenesis. In the absence of the SRY protein, the gonad remains indifferent for a short period of time before differentiating into an ovary.

The first morphological sign of testis formation is the aggregation of primordial germ cells and somatic cells (primitive Sertoli cells). These aggregates develop from the gonadal blastema into plate-like structures, which then develop into simple arches of elongated testicular cords (Paranko *et al.*, 1983). Throughout differentiation, the testicular cords remain connected to the basal portion of the mesonephric cell mass. The cords gradually transform and extend into the medulla of the gonad, where they branch and anastomose to form a network of cords, known as the rete testis (Moore, 1982). A characteristic and diagnostic feature of testicular development is development of a thick fibrous capsule, the tunica albuginea. As this capsule develops, the connection of the prominent testicular (seminiferous) cords with the surface epithelium is disrupted. Gradually the testis separates from the regressing mesonephros, becoming suspended by its own mesentery. Concurrent

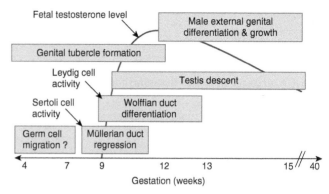

Figure 20-2. *Male sexual differentiation in humans during gestation.* (Reproduced with permission from Klonisch et al., 2004.)

with testicular cord formation, fetal Leydig cells differentiate from loosely packed, undifferentiated mesenchymal cells in the interstitium (Pelliniemi, 1975). These interstitial Leydig cells produce the male sex hormone testosterone, which induces masculine differentiation of the Wolffian duct and external genitalia. Intratesticular vasculature differentiates in the gonadal mesenchyme along with the growth of epithelial components. A testis-specific distribution of blood vessels is obvious from an early phase of testicular development (Pelliniemi, 1975). See Fig. 20-2 for a diagrammatic representation of sexual differentiation in the human male.

The fetal testis is composed of testicular cords containing supporting immature Sertoli cells and centrally placed spermatogonia, derived from the surface epithelium and primordial germ cells, respectively. These cords are surrounded by a highly vascularized interstitium containing fetal Leydig cells and mesenchyme (Pelliniemi and Niei, 1969). The testicular cords remain without a lumen throughout the fetal period. The seminiferous cords turn into tubules when the Sertoli cells undergo terminal differentiation. This occurs after birth when they finish dividing (roughly at the onset of puberty). They develop tight junctions between adjacent cells, and apical secretion of fluid begins as these cells become highly polarized. Thus, the lumen forms as Sertoli cells develop their mature phenotype.

In the rodent and human species, fetal testicular androgen production is not only necessary for proper testicular development and normal male sexual differentiation, but also differentiation of the Wolffian ducts into the epididymides, vasa deferentia, and seminal vesicles (Wilson and Lasnitzki, 1971; Veyssiere *et al.*, 1982; Imperato-McGinley *et al.*, 1992; Barker *et al.*, 1993; Berman *et al.*, 1995; Roy and Chatterjee, 1995; Silversides *et al.*, 1995; Kassim *et al.*, 1997).

Androgens derived from the Leydig interstitial cells stimulate the mesonephric (or Wolffian) ducts to form the male genital ducts, while Sertoli cells produce Müllerian inhibiting substance (MIS or Anti-Müllerian Hormone, AMH), which suppresses development of the paramesonephric (Müllerian) ducts, or female genital ducts.

There is differential maturation of the mesonephric ducts depending on location. Near the testis, some tubules persisting and are transformed into efferent ductules, which open into the mesonephric duct, forming the ductus epididymis. Distal to the epididymis, the mesonephric ducts acquire a thickening of smooth muscle to become the ductus deferens, or vas deferens (Moore, 1982).

Development of the external genitalia is similar in the two sexes. In the human, the external genitalia are indistinguishable until the ninth week of gestation, and not fully differentiated until the twelfth week of development. Development of the external genitalia coincides with gonadal differentiation. Early in the

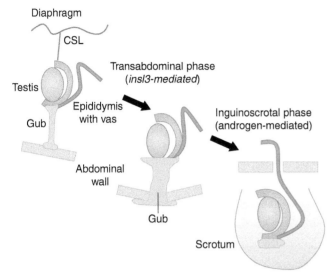

Figure 20-3. *The two distinct phases of testicular descent in mammals.* The first (transabdominal phase) mediated by insl3 from the fetal testis involving the removal of the cranial suspensory ligament (CSL) and development of the gubernaculum (gub). The second (inguinoscrotal phase) being androgen mediated. (Reproduced with permission from Klonisch *et al.*, 2004. Elsevier Science.)

fourth week of gestation, the sexually undifferentiated fetus develops a genital tubercle at the cranial end of the cloacal membrane. Labioscrotal (genital) swellings and urogenital (urethral) folds then develop on each side of the cloacal membrane. The genital tubercle then elongates forming a phallus. In response to testicular androgens, the phallus enlarges and elongates forming the penis while the labioscrotal swellings ultimately form the scrotum. At the end of the sixth week of gestation, the urorectal septum fuses with the cloacal membrane dividing the membrane into a dorsal anal and a ventral urogenital membrane. Approximately a week following, these membranes rupture forming the anus and urogenital orifice, respectively (Moore, 1982).

Fetal testicular androgens are responsible for the induction of masculinization of the indifferent external genitalia. The testis remains caudally positioned during the 10th to 15th week until entry into the inguinal canal and transabdominal descent. Testicular descent through the inguinal canal begins in the 28th week, and the testes enter the scrotum by the 32nd week. At birth, the testes reach the bottom of the scrotum (Moore, 1982). There are two critical phases of testis descent, transabdominal and inguinoscrotal, essential to move the testes into the scrotum. Although the precise mechanisms of testicular descent, and causes of cryptorchidism, remain unclear, the insulin-like peptide hormone INSL3 and fetal testicular androgens are known to play a critical role (Klonisch *et al.*, 2004; see Fig. 20-3). Cryptorchidism or undescended testes occur in about 3% of full-term and 30% of preterm males making it the most common human birth defect (Boisen *et al.*, 2004). However, in a comparative study of the prevalence of cryptorchidism in cohorts of children in Denmark and Finland a higher prevalence of cryptorchidism was observed in Denmark, with a 9% incidence rate in full-term males reported at birth (Boisen *et al.*, 2004). These data add further evidence to the concept that there is a significant geographical difference in male reproductive health in two neighboring countries, and therefore potential exposure to similar environmental effects. As the major difference was found in the milder forms of cryptorchidism, an environmental rather than a genetic basis for effect is favored. If correct, there is a need to determine the nature of the environmental agents responsible, because similar agents

may well be implicated in the trends noted in other geographically diverse countries where an increasing frequency of cryptorchidism and testicular cancer has been found (Boisen *et al.*, 2004).

Thus male, but not female, reproductive tract development is totally hormonally dependent and thus inherently more susceptible to endocrine disruption (see section "Endocrine Disruption [Including Screening and Puberty]"). It is also of note to mention that the early development and triggers of the testis are mediated by direct hormone action before the establishment of the hypothalamic–pituitary–gonadal (HPG) axis.

GAMETOGENESIS

Formation and production of gametes in mammals begin in early embryonic life with the development of primordial germ cells in the genital ridge and movement of these cells into what will become the gonads (see the "Reproductive development and sexual differentiation" section). The critical feature in the production of gametes is the process of meiosis.

The basic features of meiosis—two cell divisions with no intervening DNA replication, results in a halving of the chromosome complement—are conserved throughout evolution. Thus, it is not surprising that the general outline applies to both mammalian males and females. However, the strategies employed are remarkably different between the sexes. The mammalian oocyte begins meiosis during fetal development but arrests part-way through meiosis I and does not complete the first division until ovulation; the second division is completed only if the egg is fertilized (see Fig. 20-4). Oogenesis therefore requires several start and stop signals and, in some species (eg, the human), may last for more than 10 years. In contrast, male meiosis begins at puberty and is a continuous process, with spermatocytes progressing from prophase through the meiotic second division in little more than a week. This difference in strategy has implications for the action of toxicants and critical time periods when these cells may be vulnerable to attack (see section on male and female reproductive system). Critical to this is the understanding that the complement of oocytes available to the mammalian female is complete at birth, whereas in the male there is significant stem cell (spermatogonial) renewal to maintain the significantly higher number of germ cells available in males.

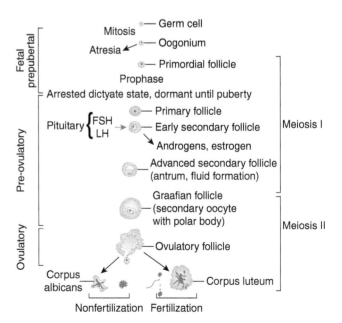

Figure 20-4. *Development of the oocyte.*

NEONATAL DEVELOPMENT

At birth, or even late in gestation, male rats display longer ano-genital distances (AGD) than do female rats with neonatal male AGD being more than twice as long as females (Gray *et al.*, 1999a). There are homologous sex differences in humans (Swan *et al.*, 2005; Longnecker *et al.*, 2007). Administration of androgen receptor (AR) antagonists or inhibitors of testosterone synthesis can demasculinize male AGD whereas androgen administration during this period lengthens female AGD (Gray *et al.*, 1994, 1999a; Wolf *et al.*, 2002; Hotchkiss *et al.*, 2007).

In addition, in many mammalian species, including humans and rats, males of the species engage in more aggressive play than do females (Hines, 2003; Hotchkiss *et al.*, 2003). In rats, play behavior is displayed for a period of a few weeks around 35 days of age and males engage in more rough and tumble aggressive play than do females. This behavior differentiates during neonatal life and exposure to antiandrogens such as flutamide or vinclozolin shortly after birth demasculinizes this behavior such that treated males engage in female-like play at about 35 days of age. In contrast, neonatal androgen treatments masculinize female rat play behavior such that they will engage in male-like levels of rough and tumble play. In humans, sexually dimorphic play behaviors are displayed fairly early in life. Congenital adrenal hyperplasia (CAH) daughters exposed to high levels of adrenal androgens in utero display male-like play (Hines and Kaufman, 1994). Normally in rats, the development of this behavior differentiates under the influence of a neonatal surge in testosterone in the first few days of pregnancy, after which fetal testis Leydig cells regress and testosterone production declines to very low levels for a few weeks until the emergence of the adult Leydig cells occurs in the testis prior to puberty (Huhtaniemi and Pelliniemi, 1992). In rodents but not humans, interestingly the first wave of spermatogenesis is initiated at about four days of age.

INFANTILE DEVELOPMENT

Later in lactation, during the infantile period of development, several key events occur in the reproductive system of rats including emergence of the nipple buds and areolae in females and maturation of the hypothalamic–pituitary axis. Emergence of the nipple buds is an event most visible around 13 days of age, which prevented in males by prenatal androgen-induced atrophy of the nipple anlagen. It is noteworthy that male rats with the shortest AGD and highest numbers of female-like nipples have a very high likelihood of displaying reproductive tract lesions such as hypospadias or epididymal agenesis (Barlow *et al.*, 2004; Hotchkiss *et al.*, 2007). Similarly, prenatally androgen-treated females with the longest AGDs and reduced infant nipple numbers are more likely to display reproductive tract malformations (retained male tissues or vaginal agenesis) than less affected females (Hotchkiss *et al.*, 2007). In addition, the effects on AGD are permanent in both sexes (Barlow *et al.*, 2004; Hotchkiss *et al.*, 2004, 2007) with nipple buds being permanent in males.

PUBERTAL DEVELOPMENT

Scientific evidence increasingly supports the concerns about environmentally induced alterations of pubertal events in girls and boys. In addition, experimental animal data are consistent with a potential role of environmental factors in inducing altered pubertal maturation in humans. Puberty is the stage of life when an individual matures from a child, through adolescence to full maturity. The process is marked by dramatic development of hormone-dependent sexual characteristics, somatic growth, and sexual and social behaviors eventually resulting in full sexual maturity and reproductive capacity. The stages of puberty in boys and girls are determined using approaches including the Tanner Stages (Marshall and Tanner, 1969; Marshall and Tanner, 1970) for breast and pubic hair development in girls and gonadal and pubic hair development in boys. Puberty in girls is also assessed using the age at menarche as a marker. Alternatively, increasing levels of estradiol or androgens in the serum prior to some of the development of some of the early physical markers can be used to determine the onset of puberty in girls and boys, respectively.

Puberty is initiated by activation of the HPG and hypothalamic–pituitary–adrenal (HPA) axes (Ojeda and Heger, 2001; Ojeda *et al.*, 2003) (see Fig. 20-5). At the onset, the HPG axis releases gonadotropin-releasing hormone (GnRH) pulses with increasing frequency and amplitude, which induces complimentary pulsatile secretions of luteinizing hormone (LH) and follicle-stimulating hormone (FSH) from the anterior pituitary (Ojeda *et al.*, 2003). In turn, LH and FSH stimulate the gonads inducing gonadarche characterized by the onset of gonadal hormone production. In the female, secretion of androgens from theca cells and estradiol from granulosa cells of maturing follicles prior to ovulation, followed by secretion of progesterone from the corpus luteum after ovulation, whereas in the male, LH stimulates testicular synthesis and secretion of androgens and insulin-like 3 peptide hormone from the Leydig cells of males. Interestingly, in most mammals including humans and rodents, puberty in the female normally precedes the age of puberty in the male.

In humans, adrenarche, the maturation of adrenal endocrine function, occurs early in pubertal development resulting in the growth of pubic hair, acne, and other secondary sex traits (Auchus and Rainey, 2004). These physical changes result from increasing adrenal synthesis and secretion of steroids including dehydroepiandrosterone (DHEA), dehydroepiandrosterone sulfate (DHEAS), and androstenedione, steroids with weak androgenic activities. Adrenarche is independent of gonadarche and typically occurs between six and eight years of age in both sexes. Adrenarche occurs only in primates and is not associated with puberty in all primate species.

Precocious puberty is defined as the onset of sexual traits before eight and nine years of age in girls and boys, respectively, whereas puberty is considered as delayed in girls if thelarche is not displayed by 13 years and at 14 years of age in boys when testicular volume of less than 4 mL (Becker and Epperson, 2006; Biro *et al.*, 2006; Den Hond and Schoeters, 2006; Himes, 2006; Muir, 2006; Ojeda *et al.*, 2006; Papathanasiou and Hadjiathanasiou, 2006; Tuvemo, 2006). Delays in boys can occur as a result of either primary hypothalamic–pituitary or gonadal failure, from head trauma or from infection. While the majority of these delays are transient, some cases are associated with gene mutations resulting in either hypogonadotropic hypogonadism or primary gonadal failure.

Of greatest concern current is the observation that in the United States and several other countries the age of onset of puberty over the past 40 years has decreased from 0.5 and 1.0 years in girls and the age at menarche has declined by about 0.2 years (Kaplowitz, 2006). Northern European countries have not reported such a trend. Similar trends in male puberty have not been observed and similar trends have not been seen in boys.

Some scientists have attributed the trends in pubertal maturation of girls to obesity rates in children. Rapid early weight gain, obesity, and early development have been associated with the development of insulin resistance and an exaggerated adrenarche

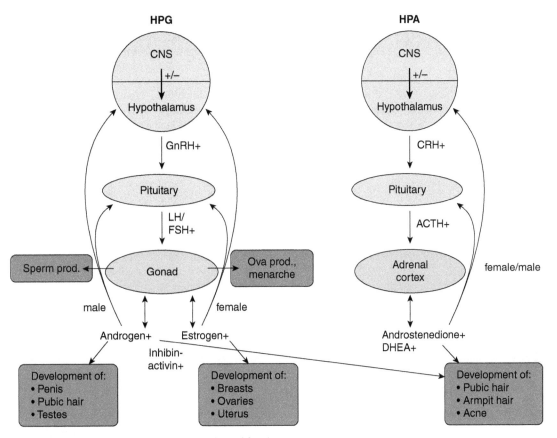

Figure 20-5. *Endocrine control of puberty in males and females.*

(Buck *et al.*, 2007). These endocrine alterations, together with elevated leptin levels and enhancement of hormonal activity by conversion of steroids to estrogens by fat cells, could affect the onset and progression of puberty in young obese girls. In addition, the role of environmental factors including endocrine disrupting chemicals (EDCs) in the etiology of this trend also is being investigated. Alterations of puberty in boys and girls can also be of genetic origin. Precocious puberty may result from early-onset of HPG function or via gonadotropin-independent alterations.

Premature thelarche and premature adrenarche are often referred to as pseudoprecocious puberty when the full spectrum of pubertal changes do not occur. Premature thelarche in girls and gynecomastia in boys are known to result from direct exposure to estrogen-containing personal care and "natural" products (Hertz, 1958; Massart *et al.*, 2006; Henley *et al.*, 2007). Although these conditions are usually resolved after termination of exposure, untoward consequences of these conditions may occur with prolonged exposure including shortened stature due to effects of estrogens, the growth plates of the long bones, and sexual–social behavior that is inappropriate for chronological age of the child (Wacharasindhu *et al.*, 2006). Concerns also have been expressed that premature thelarche may enhance the likelihood of developing diseases such as breast cancer and endometriosis.

Numerous human studies have examined the relationships between environmental factors and human puberty. Many studies have shown a positive relation between body fat and onset of the growth spurt, breast development, or menarche (Battaglia *et al.*, 2005; Dunger *et al.*, 2005; Biro *et al.*, 2006; Himes, 2006; McCartney *et al.*, 2007). Environmental exposure to persistent halogenated organic chemicals such as PCBs (Den Hond and Schoeters, 2006), DDT/DDE (Krstevska-Konstantinova *et al.*, 2001; Gladen *et al.*, 2004; Ouyang *et al.*, 2005; Charlier, 2006), brominated flame

retardants (Blanck *et al.*, 2000), dioxin (Eskenazi *et al.*, 2000; Warner *et al.*, 2004; Hauser *et al.*, 2005; Wolff *et al.*, 2005), HCB (Charlier, 2005, 2006), endosulfan (Saiyed *et al.*, 2003), and heavy metals also have been studied for associated with pubertal alterations, but a consensus about the causative role of these chemicals in altering puberty has not been achieved.

Rodent Models of Puberty

Rodents provide important animal models in the study of the genetic and environmental factors that regulate puberty. In rats, GnRH secretion is at low levels during juvenile development until GnRH release is activated by neuronal networks during puberty. During the onset of puberty, there is an increase in the excitatory amino acids and the kisspeptin peptide (Tena-Sempere, 2006) along with decreases in inhibitory neurotransmitters gamma-aminobutyric acid (GABA), and opioid peptides. In addition, several growth factors like epidermal growth factor (EGF)-like ligands and members of the EGF receptor family contribute to glia-to-neuron communication (Ojeda *et al.*, 2003, 2006). While the complete pathway triggering the onset of puberty in rodents has not yet been described, several early components have been identified including the kisspeptin-GPR-54 regulatory system. Mutations of the GPR54 receptor result in absence of puberty in humans and mice (Semple *et al.*, 2005). In addition, leptin (Vogel, 1996) and insulin-like growth factor 1 (IGF-1) (Jaruratanasirikul *et al.*, 1999) appear to be in sustaining pubertal events once the process has been initiated.

In laboratory rats, the standard landmarks of puberty in the male are the age of male preputial separation (PPS), an androgen-mediated event, and the ages of vaginal opening (VO), an estrogen-mediated event, and first estrus, with VO normally coinciding with the first estrus and the onset of estrous cycles (Goldman *et al.*, 2000). In the laboratory mouse, VO is not a useful indicator of puberty because it is not associated with the ages at first estrus and the onset of estrous cyclicity.

The ages of VO in females and PPS in male rats were included as required end points in the 1998 USEPA multigenerational test guidelines (http://www.epa.gov/opptsfrs/publications/ OPPTS_Harmonized/870_Health_Effects_Test_Guidelines/ Series/870-3800.pdf). Furthermore, it is generally agreed among risk assessors that statistically significant alterations in pubertal maturation in rats are adverse effects and these data have been used as a critical effect to establish reference doses in some cases (see the USEPA Vinclozolin Risk Assessment, 2002). Because EDCs share mechanisms of action in common with many of the drugs used to treat altered human pubertal development, it is biologically plausible that these EDCs would also alter pubertal onset in boys and girls, if children were exposed to sufficient levels of these chemicals during this critical stage of life.

Toxicants can alter puberty as a consequence of in utero, lactational, or pubertal exposures. In a multigenerational study, discerning the stage of life when exposure induced the alteration may be challenging, if possible at all, because dosing is not initiated in the parent (F_0) generation, the only generation with in utero and lactational exposure, until well after puberty. Some alternate reproductive test protocols (Gray *et al.*, 1988a) can detect pubertal alterations in the F_0 generation since they initiate exposure right after weaning. In addition, short-term studies using the pubertal male and female rat assays (EDSTAC Final Report, 1998; Gray *et al.*, 2004) can help resolve this uncertainty since exposures are initiated directly to the weanling rat and continued for 20 to 30 days for females and males, respectively. Comprehensive reviews describing the toxicology of puberty in rodents are found elsewhere (Goldman *et al.*, 2000; Stoker *et al.*, 2000; Gray *et al.*, 2004).

Studies using rats demonstrate that body weight at weaning is an important determinant of the age of VO in the female and PPS in the male. However, treatments that reduce growth by 10% or less have little effect on the attainment of the male and female pubertal landmarks. The onset of puberty can be altered in the male and female rat by disrupting the endocrine system at a variety of levels including the entire HPG axis. In addition to effects on the HPG axis, the landmarks of female rat puberty can be altered by the direct action of either estrogens or antiestrogens on VO and other components of the reproductive tract, whereas, androgens and antiandrogens can alter male rat pubertal landmarks by acting at the level of the male reproductive tract.

Because estrogen exposure in the peripubertal female rat can accelerate the onset of VO and at the age of the first estrus smear without accelerating the onset of regular estrous cycles, it is useful to monitor all three landmarks of puberty in the female in order to discriminate pseudoprecocious puberty (accelerated age at VO but not the onset of estrous cyclicity) from true precocious puberty (both the ages at VO and the onset of estrous cyclicity are accelerated).

Selected Examples of Chemicals That Alter the Onset of Pubertal Landmarks in Rats After Acute In Utero and/or Lactational Exposures

In utero exposure to 2,3,7,8-tetrachlorodibenzo-*p*-dioxin (TCDD) (a single dose of 0.001 mg/kg on gestational day [GD] 15) delays the onset of pubertal landmarks in male and female rats (Gray *et al.*, 1995, 1997b,c; Gray and Ostby, 1995). The mode of action for these effects is not known, but it likely involves permanent organizational effects of TCDD of the reproductive tract during sexual differentiation mediated via arylhydrocarbon receptor, AhR. In addition, the treated females display a persistent vaginal thread after puberty.

In utero exposure to the potent alkalating drug busulfan (at 5 and 10 mg/kg sc on GD 15) destroys fetal germ cells resulting in gonadal atrophy and delayed puberty in both male and female rats (Gray and Ostby, 1998). Some females never displayed VO, or any other pubertal landmark likely due to a total absence of primary follicles in the ovary.

Prenatal androgen administration can induce agenesis of the lower vaginal canal in females, an effect that could be missed entirely of misconstrued as just a delay in VO unless the females are retained after weaning and thoroughly examined after the normal age at puberty (Hotchkiss *et al.*, 2007). Conversely, prenatal antiandrogen treatments can result in the formation of a lower vaginal "pouch" in treated male rats (Gray *et al.*, 1994).

Administration of estrogens such as ethinyl estradiol or methoxychlor to the dam during gestation and lactation can accelerate VO in female rat offspring. In the higher dosage groups, VO can be detected as early as 10 to 15 days of age, albeit a "pin-hole" like opening (Gray *et al.*, 1989).

Peripubertal administration of EDCs can alter the onset of pubertal landmarks in male (Monosson *et al.*, 1999; Gray *et al.*, 2004) and female rats (Goldman *et al.*, 2000). Androgens play a key role in pubertal maturation in young males and antiandrogens such as vinclozolin (Monosson *et al.*, 1999), linuron (Gray *et al.*, 1999b), o,p′-DDE (Kelce *et al.*, 1995), prochloraz (Blystone *et al.*, 2007), and the phthalates (Gray *et al.*, 1999b) produce measurable delays in this process. For example, vinclozolin treatment delayed pubertal maturation, and retarded sex accessory gland and epididymal growth (at 30 and 100 mg/kg/day) (Monosson *et al.*, 1999). Serum LH (significant at all dosage levels), testosterone, and 5α-androstane,3α,17β-diol (at 100 mg/kg/day) levels were increased. Testis size and sperm production, however, were unaffected. In contrast, reproductive toxicants such as carbendazim that indirectly alter FSH levels without affecting serum testosterone fail to delay PPS even at dosage levels that cause profound alterations of testicular and hypothalamic–pituitary (FSH secretion) function (Gray *et al.*, 1990).

The ease with which a delay in PPS, a landmark of puberty in the rat, can be measured enables us to use this end point to evaluate chemicals for this form of endocrine activity. A "pubertal male assay" including an assessment of PPS is being considered by the USEPA and others (Gray *et al.*, 1997a; Gray, 1998; Stoker *et al.*, 2000) for screening chemicals for endocrine activity, as mandated by 1996 US legislation (the Food Quality Protection Act and Safe Drinking Water Act).

Selected Examples of Chemicals That Alter the Onset of Pubertal Landmarks in Rats After Peripubertal Exposures

The "pubertal female rat assay" assay has been included in the proposed EDSTAC Tier 1 Screening (T1S) battery. In this assay, weanling female rats are dosed daily by gavage for 21 days and the age at VO (puberty) is monitored and the females are necropsied at about 42 days of age (reviewed by Goldman *et al.*, 2000). Vaginal estrous cycles are also determined by daily observation by light microscopy of the cell types present in a vaginal lavage, taken from VO until necropsy. Necropsy measurements include serum thyroid hormones, and uterine and ovarian weight and histology. This assay detects alterations in thyroid hormone status, HPG function, and inhibition of steroidogenesis, estrogens, and antiestrogens. Recently, in studies from different laboratories the pubertal female assay was found to be highly reproducible and

Table 20-4

Chemicals Evaluated By the US Environmental Protection Agency (EPA) Using the Standardized Pubertal Female Rat Assay in Two Contract Laboratories or Key Studies Performed in Other Laboratories

Studies performed in Laboratory 1 for the EPA

Ethinyl estradiol: positive estrogenic control

Tamoxifen: mixed estrogen agonist–antagonist; successfully identified mixed action

Ketoconazole: inhibits steroidogenesis; caused ovarian histological changes

Methoxychlor: estrogenic pesticide; successfully detected by accelerated puberty

Phenobarbital: alters liver, hypothalamic, pituitary, and ovarian function; delays puberty

Studies performed in Laboratory 2 for the EPA

Methoxychlor: estrogenic pesticide; successfully detected by accelerated puberty

Ketoconazole: inhibits steroidogenesis; caused ovarian histological changes

Bisphenol A: weakly estrogenic plastic monomer; negative for endocrine effects

Propylthiouracil: antithyroid agent; lowered T4, increased thyroid-stimulating hormone, and caused thyroid histological changes at low doses that slightly delayed rat puberty

Fenarimol: fungicide that weakly inhibits aromatase; slight delay in puberty, but lowered T4 and retarded growth

Atrazine: herbicide that alters hypothalamic–pituitary function; delays puberty and growth

Key published studies performed in other laboratories

Methoxychlor: estrogenic pesticide; accelerates puberty (Gray *et al.*, 1989)

Polybrominated diphenyl ether: DE71; antithyroid toxicant; affected thyroid end points and delayed puberty (Stoker *et al.*, 2004)

Fadrazole: potent aromatase inhibitor; delayed puberty (Marty *et al.*, 1999)

Antarelix: gonadotropin-releasing hormone antagonist; delayed puberty (Ashby *et al.*, 2002)

Octylphenol: estrogenic surfactant; accelerates female rat puberty (Gray and Ostby, 1998)

DES: estrogenic pharmaceutical; accelerated puberty (Kim *et al.*, 2002)

Tamoxifen: a mixed agonist/antagonistic drug; accelerated puberty (Kim *et al.*, 2002)

ICI 182,780: estrogen receptor (ER) antagonist; delayed puberty (Ashby *et al.*, 2002)

ZM 189,154: ER antagonist; delayed puberty (Ashby *et al.*, 2002)

Pubertal female assay data from contract laboratories (Summary available at http://www.epa.gov/scipoly/oscpendo/assayvalidation/meetings.htm).

very sensitive to certain endocrine activities including estrogenicity, inhibition of steroidogenesis, and antithyroid activity (Gray *et al.*, 2004) (see Table 20-4).

The "pubertal male assay rat" (Gray *et al.*, 2004; Stoker *et al.*, 2000; Monosson *et al.*, 1999) detects alterations of thyroid function, HPG maturation, steroidogenesis, and altered steroid hormone function (androgen). Intact weanling males are exposed to the test substance for about 30 days, the age at puberty is determined and reproductive tissues are evaluated and serum taken for optional hormonal analyses. This assay produced reproducible responses among different labs and was sensitive to androgens, antiandrogens, inhibitors of steroidogenesis, and antithyroid activity. The chemicals studied to date in this assay are listed in Table 20-5.

When antiandrogenic chemicals are administered to juvenile male rats, these chemicals do not induce malformations of the reproductive tract, but pubertal development is delayed. Throughout puberty and into adulthood, the sex accessory glands and other androgen-dependent tissues (ie, muscles, nervous system) continue to be dependent upon testosterone (T) and 5α-dihydrotestosterone (DHT) for maturation and maintenance of function. Several androgen-dependent events occur during puberty, most notably the separation of the prepuce from the penis (PPS), followed 10 days to two weeks later by the appearance of mature sperm in the epididymis (Monosson *et al.*, 1999). During pubertal maturation, there are gradual changes in serum concentrations of testosterone (T) and of its metabolite 5α-androstanediol. In very young rats, 5α-androstanediol is present in greater quantities than T. T concentrations begin to increase, however, as 5α-reductase activity decreases in the Leydig cells,

resulting in higher serum T concentrations than androstanediol in older rats. Peak T concentrations generally occur around 50 to 60 days of age.

In addition to delaying PPS, some antiandrogens also alter serum LH and T, while others do not. In particular, peripubertal exposure to flutamide (from 23 to 38 days of age) or vinclozolin (from 23 to 55 days of age) causes reductions in prostate, seminal vesicle, and epididymis in rats whereas serum LH and testosterone are increased (Monosson *et al.*, 1999).

SEXUAL MATURITY

Hypothalamic–Pituitary–Gonadal Axis

FSH and LH are glycoproteins synthesized and released from a subpopulation of the basophilic gonadotropic cells of the pituitary gland. Hypothalamic neuroendocrine neurons secrete specific releasing or release-inhibiting factors into the hypophyseal portal system, which carries them to the adenohypophysis, where they act to stimulate or inhibit the release of anterior pituitary hormones. GnRH acts on gonadotropic cells, thereby stimulating the release of FSH and LH. Native and synthetic forms of GnRH stimulate the release of both gonadotrophic hormones.

The neuroendocrine neurons have nerve terminals containing monoamines (norepinephrine, dopamine, and serotonin) that impinge on them. Reserpine, chlorpromazine, and monoamine oxidase (MAO) inhibitors modify the content or actions of brain monoamines that affect gonadotropin production.

In the female (see Fig. 20-6 for structure of the female reproductive tract of the rat and Fig. 20-7 for basic endocrine control),

Table 20-5

Chemicals Evaluated By the US Environmental Protection Agency (EPA) Using the Standardized Pubertal Male Rat Assay in Two Contract Laboratories or Key Studies Performed in Other Laboratories

Studies performed in Laboratory 1 for the EPA
Flutamide: potent antiandrogenic drug; delayed puberty, among other effects
Ketoconazole: inhibits steroidogenesis
Methyltestosterone: androgenic drug; accelerated puberty
Phenobarbital: alters liver, hypothalamic, pituitary, and testis function; delayed puberty, among other effects
Vinclozolin: antiandrogenic fungicide; delayed puberty, among other effects
Dibutyl phthalate: plasticizer that inhibits Leydig cell testosterone function; delayed puberty, among other effects

Studies performed in Laboratory 2 for the EPA
Vinclozolin: antiandrogenic fungicide; delayed puberty, among other effects
Linuron: antiandrogenic herbicide; delayed puberty, among other effects
p,p'-DDE: antiandrogenic pesticide metabolite; delayed puberty, among other effects
Phenobarbital: alters liver, hypothalamic, pituitary, and testis function; delayed puberty, among other effects
Methoxychlor: estrogenic and antiandrogenic pesticide; reduced androgen-dependent tissues weights
Ketoconazole: inhibits steroidogenesis
Atrazine: herbicide, alters hypothalamic pituitary function; delays puberty and growth

Key published studies performed in other laboratories
Vinclozolin: androgen receptor antagonistic fungicide; delayed puberty, increase serum T and luteinizing hormone (Monosson *et al.*, 1999)
Cyproterone acetate: antiandrogenic drug; delayed puberty, among other effects
Polybrominated diphenyl ether, DE71; antithyroid toxicant; affected thyroid end points, and delayed puberty (Stoker *et al.*, 2004)
Finasteride: potent inhibitor of enzyme 5 alpha reductase required for dihydrotesterone synthesis; reduced sex gland weight (Marty *et al.*, 2001)

Pubertal female and pubertal male assay data from contract laboratories (summary available at http://www.epa.gov/scipoly/oscpendo/assayvalidation/ meetings.htm).

LH acts on thecal cells of the ovary to induce steroidogenesis, particularly the production of progesterone and androgens which are transferred to the granulosa cells which can be stimulated by FSH to produce estradiol. These steroids then feedback on the hypothalamus and pituitary to regulate gonadotropin production (see later sections on "Ovarian function").

Similarly in the male (see Fig. 20-8 for the basic structure of the male reproductive system and Fig. 20-9 for basic endocrine control), FSH acts primarily on the Sertoli cells, but it also appears to stimulate the mitotic activity of spermatogonia. LH stimulates steroidogenesis in the interstitial Leydig cells. A defect in the function of the testis (in the production of spermatozoa or testosterone) will tend to be reflected in increased levels of FSH

and LH in serum because of the lack of the "negative feedback" effect of testicular hormones.

The HPG feedback system is a very delicately modulated hormonal process. Several sites in the endocrine process can be perturbed by different chemicals.

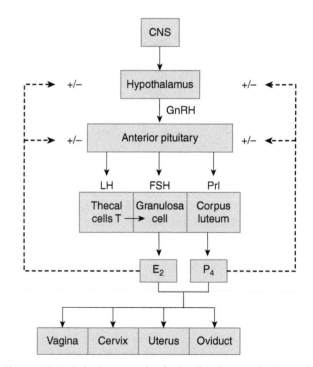

Figure 20-7. *Endocrine control of the female reproductive cycle.* CNS, central nervous system; GnRH, gonadotropin releasing hormone; LH, luteinizing hormone; FSH, follicle-stimulating hormone; Prl, Prolactin; T, testosterone; E₂, estradiol; P₄, progesterone.

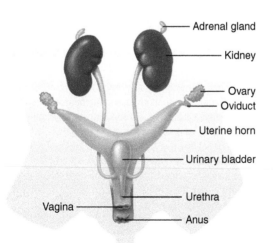

Figure 20-6. *Rat female reproductive system.*

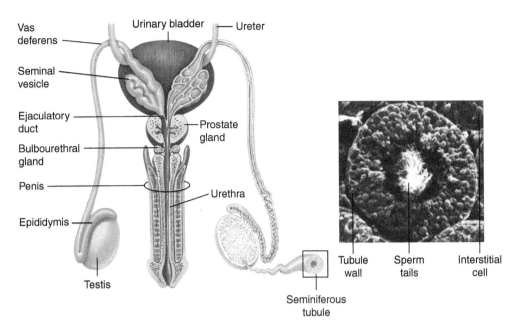

Figure 20-8. *Male reproductive system.*

Ovarian Function

Oogenesis Ovarian germ cells with their follicles have a dual origin; the theca or stromal cells arise from fetal connective tissues of the ovarian medulla, the granulosa cells from the cortical mesenchyme (Fig. 20-4). In women, about 400,000 follicles are present at birth in each human ovary. After birth, many undergo atresia, and those that survive are continuously reduced in number. Any chemical that damages the oocytes will accelerate the depletion of the pool and can lead to reduced fertility in females. About one-half of the numbers of oocytes present at birth remain at puberty; the number is reduced to about 25,000 by 30 years of age. About 400 primary follicles will yield mature ova during a woman's reproductive life span. During the approximately three decades of fecundity, follicles in various stages of growth can always be found. After menopause, follicles are no longer present in the ovary (Knobil and Neill, 1994).

Follicles remain in a primary follicle stage following birth until puberty, when a number of follicles start to grow during each ovarian cycle. However, most fail to achieve maturity. For the follicles that continue to grow, the first event is an increase in size of the primary oocytes. During this stage, fluid-filled spaces appear among the cells of the follicle, which unite to form a cavity or antrum, otherwise known as the Graafian follicle.

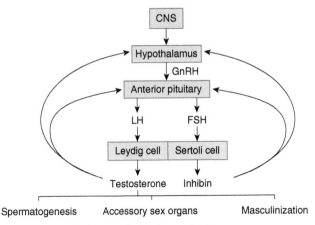

Figure 20-9. *Endocrine control of male reproduction.*

Primary oocytes undergo two specialized nuclear divisions, which result in the formation of four cells containing one-half the number of chromosomes (Fig. 20-4). The first meiotic division occurs within the ovary just before ovulation, and the second occurs just after the sperm fuses with the egg. In the first stage of meiosis, the primary oocyte is actively synthesizing DNA and protein in preparation for entering prophase. The DNA content doubles as each of the prophase chromosomes produces its mirror image. Each doubled chromosome is attracted to its homologous mate to form tetrads. The members of the tetrads synapse or come to lie side by side. Before separation, the homologous pairs of chromosomes exchange genetic material by a process known as crossing over. Thus, qualitative differences occur between the resulting gametes. Subsequent meiotic stages distribute the members of the tetrads to the daughter cells in such a way that each cell receives the haploid number of chromosomes. At telophase, one secondary oocyte and a polar body have been formed, which are no longer genetically identical.

The secondary oocyte enters the next cycle of division very rapidly; each chromosome splits longitudinally; the ovum and the three polar bodies now contain the haploid number of chromosomes and half the amount of genetic material. Although the nuclei of all four eggs are equivalent, the cytoplasm is divided unequally. The end products are one large ovum and three rudimentary ova (polar bodies), which subsequently degenerate. The ovum is released from the ovary at the secondary oocyte stage; the second stage of meiotic division is triggered in the oviduct by the entry of the sperm.

Although ovarian weight, unlike uterine weight, in the rat does not fluctuate during the estrous cycle, ovarian weight and histology can provide very useful information about the effects of toxicants on the female reproductive system. Ovarian weight can be reduced by either depletion of oocytes or disruption of the HPG axis. Toxicants affect ovarian histology inducing a variety of lesions, including polyovular follicles, oocyte depletion, interstitial cell hyperplasia, corpora albanicans, and absence of corpora lutea, for example. In addition, ovarian tissue can be cultured ex vivo after in vivo treatment or in vitro at different stages of the estrous cycle or during pregnancy to assess their steroidogenic capacity (Berman and Laskey, 1993; Gray *et al.*, 1997a; Calafat *et al.*, 2006).

Case Study—Busulfan The drug busulfan is an alkylating agent used to treat several diseases in humans including chronic myelogenous leukemia, certain myeloproliferative disorders such as severe thrombocytosis and polycythemia vera, and busulfan is also used in combination with other drugs to treat myelofibrosis. Busulfan has been used in very high doses and in combination with other drugs to destroy the bone marrow in preparation for a bone marrow transplant. Busulfan may interfere with the normal menstrual cycles in women and block sperm production in men. In addition, busulfan causes ovarian failure and prevents or delays the onset of puberty in girls (http://www.nlm.nih.gov/medlineplus/druginfo/medmaster/a682248.html).

In the rat, busulfan produces a similar profile of reproductive effects, the most dramatic occurring in utero. In rodents, endocrine function during adulthood can be altered by prenatal exposure to fetal germ cell toxicants. The ovary of the treated female offspring, lacking oocytes, developing follicles (the source of most serum estradiol), or corpora lutea (the major source of progesterone) fails to produce sex hormones. Administration of busulfan (10 mg/kg ip five–seven days before birth) specifically inhibits germ cell development (Hemsworth and Jackson, 1963) in rats. Offspring of rats dosed with 2.5 and 5 mg busulfan per kg on gestational day 14 display permanent reproductive and central nervous system (CNS) alterations (Gray and Ostby, 1998). The most severely affected females do not display estrous cycles or spontaneous sexual behavior as a consequence of this effect. Puberty was markedly delayed in females treated with 10 mg of busulfan. In male progeny, testicular (at 2.5 mg), epididymal (2.5 mg), and ejaculated sperm (5.0 mg) counts, fertility and fecundity (10 mg), measured under continuous breeding conditions, were reduced. In female progeny, fertility and fecundity (2.5 mg) and ovarian weight (5 mg) were reduced, and the incidence of constant vaginal estrus was increased (10 mg). In addition to these reproductive effects, brain weight was reduced in both sexes of all dosage groups, even though body and other nonreproductive organ weights were only affected in the high dose group (10 mg). Even though the gonads of both sexes were affected at similar dosage levels, fertility and gonadal hormone production were much more easily disrupted in female than male offspring because the steroid producing cells in the ovary fail to differentiate in the absence of the oocyte. In the male, Leydig cell numbers and steroidogenesis are not so dependent upon normal gametogenesis. Hence, the lack of oocytes in the female progeny results in a lack of estrous cyclicity and the spontaneous display of female mating behavior at proestrus. Technically, busulfan is not considered to be an EDC because the cells that it eliminates, the oocytes, do not display endocrine activity. However, this classification is of little import because in their absence, ovarian thecal and granulosa cell endocrine functions are severely impaired.

In addition to busulfan, several environmental chemicals have been shown to disrupt ovarian development and oocyte numbers in the rat or mouse. Oral administration of some of the benzidine-based dyes on days eight to 12 of pregnancy in the mouse or rat produces reproductive effects in the female offspring similar to those seen with the lower dose levels of busulfan, albeit at much higher dose levels (1 g/kg/day) (Gray and Kelce, 1996).

4-Vinylcyclohexene (VCH) is a chemical intermediate used in the production of flame retardants, flavors and fragrances, in the manufacture of polyolefins, and as a solvent and in the manufacture of its diepoxide. Low levels of occupational exposure have been measured during the production and use of 1,3-butadiene. In the mouse, VCH destroys the small preantral follicles in the ovaries (Hoyer and Sipes, 2007) and the monoepoxide metabolites, 1,2-VCH epoxide, 7,8-VCH epoxide, and the diepoxide, VCD, cause preantral follicle loss in rats as well as in mice. Mice are more susceptible to VCH than rats because they are capable of its metabolic bioactivation. Follicle destruction by VCD is selective for primordial and primary follicles and results from upregulating the rate of atresia (apoptosis) through activation of proapoptotic signaling events selectively in the small preantral follicles.

Methoxychlor (MXC) is an organochlorine pesticide and reproductive toxicant that also produces antral follicle atresia, in part by altering apoptotic regulators (Bcl-2 and Bax). MXC directly inhibits follicle growth partly by Bcl-2 and Bax pathways, and increases atresia partly through Bcl-2 pathways (Miller *et al.*, 2005) by inducing oxidative stress (Gupta *et al.*, 2006a,b). A diagrammatic representation of the sites of actions of female reproductive toxicants is presented in Fig. 20-10.

Ovarian Cycle

The cyclic release of pituitary gonadotropins involving the secretion of ovarian progesterone and estrogen is depicted in Fig. 20-11.

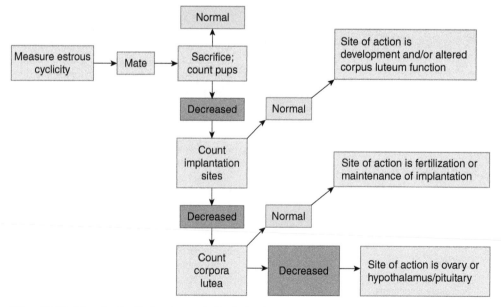

Figure 20-10. *Sites of action for female reproductive toxicants.*

Temporal comparison of menstrual versus estrous cycles

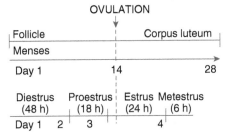

Figure 20-11. *Comparison of the human menstrual cycle with the rat estrus cycle.*

These female sex steroids determine ovulation and prepare the female accessory sex organs to receive the male sperm. Sperm, ejaculated into the vagina, must make their way through the cervix into the uterus, where they are capacitated. Sperm then migrate into the oviducts, where fertilization takes place. The conceptus then returns from the oviducts to the uterus and implants into the endometrium.

This axis can be disrupted, resulting in infertility at any level of the endocrine system. For example, chemicals that block the LH surge transiently can prevent or delay ovulation resulting in infertility or lower fecundity due to delayed fertilization of ova (Goldman *et al.*, 1993, 1994, 1997; Stoker *et al.*, 1993, 1996, 2001, 2003, 2005; Cooper *et al.*, 1994, 2000).

Postovarian Processes

Female accessory sex organs function to bring together the ovulated ovum and the ejaculated sperm. The chemical composition

and viscosity of reproductive tract fluids, as well as the epithelial morphology of these organs, are controlled by ovarian (and trophoblastic) hormones (see Fig. 20-6).

Oviducts The oviducts provide the taxis of the fimbria, which is under muscular control. The involvement of the autonomic nervous system in this process, as well as in oviductal transport of both the male and female gametes, raises the possibility that drugs known to alter the autonomic nervous system may alter function and therefore fertility. The progression of the fertilized eggs through the oviduct and uterus is under hormonal regulation and chemicals such as the estrogens can stimulate oviductal transport and interfere with uterine endometrial function, precluding implantation (Cummings and Perreault, 1990).

Uterus Uterine endometrium reflects the cyclicity of the ovary as it is prepared to receive the conceptus. The myometrium's major role is contractile. In primates, at the end of menstruation, all but the deep layers of the endometrium are sloughed. Under the influence of estrogens from the developing follicle, the endometrium increases rapidly in thickness. The uterine glands increase in length but do not secrete to any degree. These endometrial changes are called proliferative. After ovulation, the endometrium becomes slightly edematous, and the actively secreting glands become tightly coiled and folded under the influence of estrogen and progesterone from the corpus luteum. These are secretory (progestational) changes (Fig. 20-11). When fertilization fails to occur, the endometrium is shed and a new cycle begins. Only primates menstruate (Knobil and Neill, 1994).

Other mammals have estrous cycles rather than menstrual cycles, see Fig. 20-12 for a diagrammatic comparison of the human menstrual and rat estrous cycles with regard to timing and endocrine

Comparative endocrinology of menstrual and estrous cycles and early pregnancy

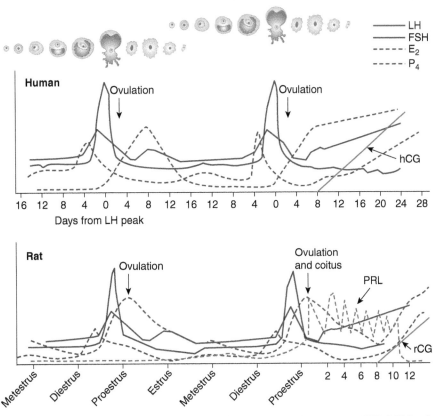

Figure 20-12. *Comparison of the timing of the human and rat cycles.* LH, luteinizing hormone; FSH, follicle-stimulating hormone; PRL, prolactin; E$_2$, estradiol; P$_4$, progesterone; hCG, human chorionic gonadotropin; rCG, rat chorionic gonadotropin.

control. In the young adult rat, the female has a four to five day estrous cycle which lacks a functional luteal phase (Knobil and Neill, 1994, Chap. 46; Cooper *et al.*, 1984). During the estrous cycle, the uterus and vagina display remarkable changes in morphology over the brief cycle. Uterine weight and fluid content increase many folds during proestrus under the influence of estrogen. The vaginal cytology also changes daily throughout the estrous cycle, and this can be monitored by examining the cytology of the cells sloughed from the vaginal epithelium into the lumen with daily vaginal lavages.

Uterine weight is a very useful index of estrogenicity in the immature or adult ovariectomized female rats. Because uterine weight and histology fluctuate greatly during the estrous cycle, studies which necropsy females at different stages of the cycle will often be too variable to detect anything but the most profound effects on these end points, but nonetheless it can still be a useful end point and should be measured. A single vaginal lavage, taken at necropsy could be used as a covariate to analyze for treatment effects. It is noteworthy that both uterine weight and ovarian histology provided useful information in a surprising number of cases in the assessment of chemicals in the Pubertal Female Rat Assay being validated by the USEPA, OSCP, and EDSP (reports available at http://www.epa.gov/scipoly/oscpendo/).

TESTICULAR STRUCTURE AND FUNCTION

Targets for Toxicity

For the adult male, the overall objective of the reproductive process is the production of gametes capable of fertilization and the production of viable offspring. In considering these processes, there are numerous potential targets for the action of chemicals upon the system (see Fig. 20-13). These would range from the action of dopamine analogs on the hypothalamus interrupting the normal secretion of GnRH, the action of estrogens on the pituitary (and hypothalamus) to interfere with gonadotropin (LH and FSH, see Fig. 20-7) production through direct effects on spermatogenesis—where the vast majority of toxicants have their site of action. However, there are specific examples of chemicals that may impair

Potential target sites

CNS   *Dopamine antagonists*

Pituitary   *estrogens*

Cd   Testicular vasculature   Pineal   *melatonin*

Spermatogenesis

Nutrition   Liver   *CCl₄*
Vit A, Zn

Epididymal maturation   *α-Chlorhydrin*

Fertilization   *Ab*

Paternal developmental toxicity   *Cyclophosphamide*

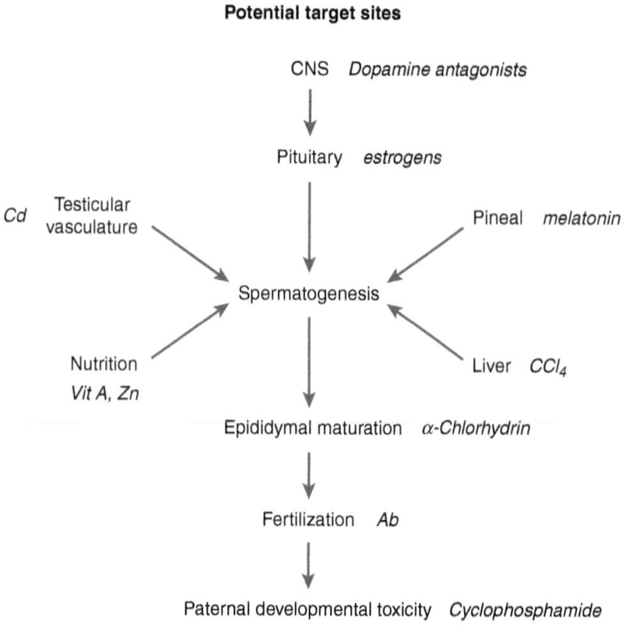

Figure 20-13. *Potential target sites for male reproductive toxicants.* Examples of agents shown in italics.

spermatogenesis via an indirect mechanism not specifically related to the HPG axis. So for example, there are a number of examples of nutritional deficits (and overexposures) of critical vitamins and minerals (eg, vitamin A and zinc) that are essential for normal reproduction. Perturbing the homeostasis of these nutrients can lead to direct effects on spermatogenesis and subsequent issues with fertility. Similarly, chemicals with direct effects on the liver (eg, CCl_4) can disturb the normal metabolism of sex steroids leading to changes in clearance (predominantly of glucuronide and sulfate conjugates of hydroxytestosterones in the male), indirectly affecting the HPG axis and exerting effects on male reproduction.

While most experimental rodents normally employed in reproductive toxicity studies do not show marked seasonality in breeding performance, there are dramatic exceptions (for example the hamster, where during the breeding season (or under lab conditions of 14 hours light and 10 hours dark) up to 10% of an adult male's body weight may be testicular tissue). In the hamster markedly changing the light:dark cycle to reduce the hours of daylight can influence melatonin levels and through a cascade of signaling responses cause regression of the testes and concurrent decreases in testicular steroids and mating behavior. This is a normal circumstance in the wild, but care should be taken in laboratory situations to ensure appropriate housing for the conduct of reproduction studies with this species.

The testis also has a finely tuned circulatory system in mammals, termed the pampiniform plexus, designed to shunt the arterial venous blood supply and aid in scrotal cooling. Some chemicals can actually target this structure and the testis circulatory system to induce ischemic shock to the testis again resulting in injury and reduced fertility, with cadmium being an example of an agent that can induce testicular damage via this "indirect" mechanism (Setchell and Waites, 1970).

Testicular Structure and Spermatogenesis

The experimenter should be cognizant of these indirect mechanisms for affecting male reproductive biology; however, the overwhelming number of chemicals known to affect the male reproductive system appears to do so by a direct effect on the testis and an interference with the process of spermatogenesis. In rodents, there is a highly efficient process for the production of sperm in large numbers. A simple cross section of the testis from a rat (see Fig. 20-14), the most common species employed in reproductive toxicity studies, indicates that not all of the seminiferous tubules have an identical morphology. The generalized structure of the rat seminiferous tubule (see Figs. 20-15 and 20-16) shows the organization of a

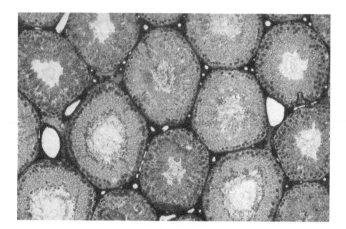

Figure 20-14. *Control testis indicating different cellular associations noted in different seminiferous tubule cross-sections.* See also Fig. 20-19.

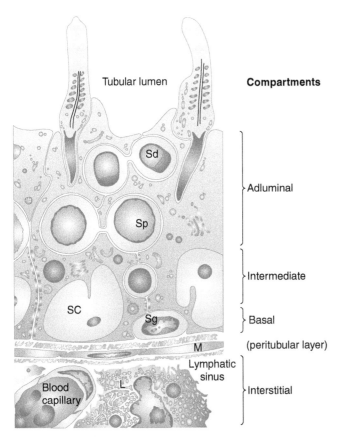

Figure 20-15. *Diagrammatic representation of a portion of a seminiferous tubule showing the cellular arrangements and testicular compartments.* Key: L, Leydig cell; M, myoepithelial peritubular cell; SC, Sertoli cell; Sd, spermatid; Sg, spermatogonium; Sp, spermatocyte (from Foster, 1988).

number of different cell types comprising germ cells at different stages of differentiation supported by a somatic cell, the Sertoli cell, that provides structure to the epithelium and numerous support functions (eg, hormonal signaling, nutrition, fluid provision, etc) and serves to maintain the haploid germ cells in a protected environment (the so-called blood–tubule barrier) since these would be recognized as foreign by the host immune system. Thus, the seminiferous tubules can be divided into a number of physiological compartments (as indicated in Fig. 20-15) that facilitate the process of spermatogenesis. The boundary of the seminiferous tubule is

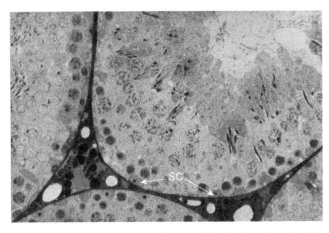

Figure 20-16. *Section of rat seminiferous tubules showing the orientation of different germ cells and Sertoli cells (SC).* Compare with Figs. 20-15 and 20-18.

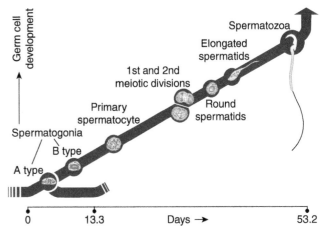

Figure 20-17. *Diagrammatic depiction of spermatogenesis in the rat.* (From Foster, 1988.)

surrounded by myoepithelial cells that aid in a peristaltic process in moving released spermatozoa present in the lumina of the tubules (at this time these sperm are both nonmotile and nonfertile) along the tubules through the rete testis (into which the seminiferous tubules open—these tubules have both ends attached to the rete) for further progression through the efferent ducts to the epididymis. It is here that a concentration of sperm and changes in their fluid environment occur as the sperm are ushered through the epididymis and acquire motility and fertilizing ability.

Spermatogenesis is an extremely ordered process in the rat (see Fig. 20-17), the spermatogonia have populations that act as the stem cells for the seminiferous tubules and a proportion of these cells then undergo a series of mitotic divisions to increase numbers, move into meiotic prophase and are then committed to becoming spermatozoa. These germ cells proceed through the various stages of prophase, preleptotene, leptotene, zygotene, and pachytene with increasingly larger cells that undertake DNA replication in preparation for the cells to enter meiosis. The germ cells enter diplotene and then diakinesis with two meiotic divisions, which eventually results in the production of the haploid spermatid population. These initially round cells then undergo an incredible metamorphosis to produce the elongated spermatozoa that mature and are then released into the seminiferous tubule lumen.

The spermatogonial stem cells undergo another round of mitotic division every approximately 13 days in the rat to produce another wave of division and differentiation (see Fig. 20-18). For the rat, the time taken for a spermatogonial stem cell to become a mature spermatozoan is approximately eight weeks (and 10 weeks for humans) with an additional 10 days to two weeks for the released sperm to mature in the epididymis and be capable for ejaculation and fertilization of the ovum. One of the consequences of these successive longitudinal waves of differentiation is the highly ordered sequence of events reflected in seminiferous tubular morphology. The most primitive germ cells, the spermatogonia, reside at the periphery of the tubule and as they mature, they move toward the tubule lumen for eventual release (in a process termed spermiation). As can be seen from Fig. 20-18, at any one time the tubule can contain cellular members from four and a half successive spermatogenic cycles, with the most primitive spermatogonia from the current cycle and the most mature, the late spermatids (about to become spermatozoa on release), generated up to 4.5 cycles earlier. Thus when we take a cross section through a seminiferous tubule, this is essentially taking a "snapshot" in time of the various spermatogenic cycles. This also explains why different tubular cross sections have different

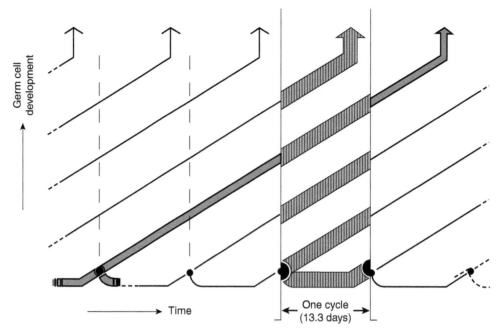

Figure 20-18. *The cyclicity of the seminiferous epithelium of the rat.* The process whereby successive spermatogenic "waves" (see Fig. 20-18) are interrelated. A transverse section of a tubule covering one cycle of the epithelium will contain cellar representatives at different stages of maturity from successive waves (from Foster, 1988).

morphologies, depending on when this "snapshot" is taken because of different cellular associations resulting from different cycles. It is possible for the various species to construct a morphological diagram of the nature of these cellular associations (Fig. 20-19 illustrates this for the rat). The most common system employed for the rat was based on that published by Leblond and Clermont (1952) and describes 14 different patterns of cellular association (or stages—usually depicted by a roman numeral). We know that different biochemical events can go on during the different stages and indeed this can provide clues as to potential mode of action of chemicals that produce stage-specific lesions. Such occurrences do occur regularly (eg, certain phthalate esters, glycol ethers, antiandrogenic agents,

etc). In the case of a phthalate ester given to an adult rat, there is a marked stage specificity in response which coincides with those stages that have the highest concentrations of FSH receptors (in the Sertoli cells of the tubule) (Creasy *et al.*, 1987). Other Sertoli cell *in vitro* data indicated that the phthalate ester metabolites responsible for *in vivo* damage could downregulate Sertoli cell responsiveness to FSH with regard to cAMP production (Lloyd and Foster, 1988), lending support to the establishment of a potential mode of action for this class of chemicals in adult rats.

At spermiation, when the step 19 spermatids are released into the seminiferous tubule lumen, the excess cytoplasm and cellular debris form a residual body that is then phagocytosed by the

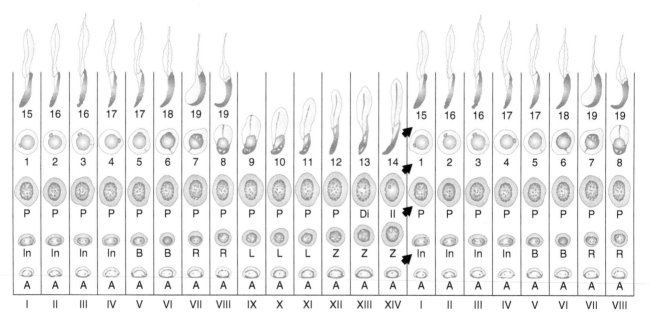

Figure 20-19. *Diagram of the 14 stages of spermatogenesis of the rat testis (after Leblond and Clermont, 1952).* Each stage (Roman numeral) contains different cellular associations of spermatogonia (A, IN or B), spermatocytes (R, resting/preleptotene; L, leptotene; Z, zygotene; P, pachytene; Di, diplotene; II, secondary), and spermatids (Arabic numerals 1–19). (Reproduced with permission from Foster, 1988.)

Sertoli cell. These bodies originate at the luminal surface of the tubule and then as they are resorbed, can be seen to move through the Sertoli cell toward the base of the tubule and eventually disappear. Delays in spermiation—that is step 19 late spermatids being retained beyond Stage VIII of the cycle are one of the more subtle, yet commonly noted testicular lesions, for example, boric acid (Gray *et al.*, 1990; Chapin and Ku, 1994); dibromoacetic acid (Linder *et al.*, 1997; Melnick *et al.*, 2007) and hormonal withdrawal (Saito *et al.*, 2000), and are sometimes accompanied by abnormal residual body formation. Having this "extra" layer of germ cells is a lesion frequently missed by pathologists without a good knowledge and appreciation of the stages of the spermatogenic cycle.

Once sperm are released into the seminiferous tubule lumen and proceed to the epididymis, they can also be the target of toxicant action. Chlorosugars and epichlorohydrin have both been shown to inhibit energy metabolism in sperm that prevents them from functioning normally. The specificity of the response was noted, at least in part, from the specific isoform of lactate dehydrogenase found in testicular germs cells (LDH-X or C4) essential for energy production. We are now learning more about the molecular events that drive fertilization, and it seems likely that here may be a potential target for the action of chemicals to disturb the process. We certainly know of the requirement for the expression of critical cell surface markers by the sperm that facilitate the normal binding of the sperm to the egg surface membrane. Lastly, there is the potential for effects in the male to induce paternally mediated developmental toxicity in the embryo/fetus. While this is not a common occurrence, it has been documented with one or two specific chemicals (eg, cyclophosphamide (Trasler *et al.*, 1985).

The number of known environmental chemicals that produce adverse responses in human males is not large. All of these have been shown to induce effects in rodents and especially the rat, although there may be differences in sensitivity based on dose. Interestingly, a number of the classic human testicular toxicants (eg, DBCP, gossypol) do not seem to produce infertility or testicular toxicity in the mouse and so the rat is more commonly employed as a model for male reproductive toxicity studies. However, this does not imply that all chemicals known to produce injury in the rats would indeed show toxicity in humans. The human does not employ a longitudinal wave for the production of sperm in the testis noted above for the rat, rather cellular associations are organized in a helical fashion that is intrinsically less efficient for sperm production (when estimated on a sperm produced per gram of tissue basis) and thus humans are usually deemed more sensitive, from the risk assessment standpoint, because there are a greater range of values for semen parameters for the human population than the rat and a lesser decrement in sperm number or function is more likely to push larger numbers of men in the population into the infertile range.

Posttesticular Processes

Following the release of mature spermatids from the seminiferous epithelium, the extraneous cytoplasm and organelles form the residual body that is phagocytosed by the Sertoli cell and moves from the periphery of the tubule to its base. These nonmotile sperm are moved along the tubules by a peristaltic-like action of the myoepithelial cells of the tubule and eventually empty into the rete testis.

In rodents, but not humans, a large blood plexus forms over the rete (which is close to the surface and near the pole of the testis) where fluid exchange can take place. Sperm are then moved into the efferent ducts that exit the testis. These ducts are rich in ER receptors (Oliveira *et al.*, 2004) and the fluid from the seminiferous tubules contains steroid hormones, but is low in overall total protein.

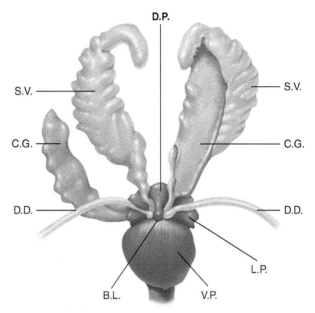

Figure 20-20. *Anatomic relation of components of rodent sex accessory glands.* D.D., ductus deferens; B.L., bladder; V.P., ventral prostate; L.P., lateral prostate; C.G., coagulating gland (also called the anterior prostate); S.V., seminal vesicle; D.P., dorsal prostate (Reproduced with permission from Hayes, 1982).

The efferent ducts then empty into the caput (head) of the epididymis which is a single highly coiled tube derived from the Wolffian duct in utero. The epididymis can be divided into three anatomical portions: the caput, corpus (body), and cauda (tail), which has a changing chemical environment and fluid composition from the efferent ducts through to the cauda. The sperm undergo maturation in the caput and corpus and begin to acquire motility, whereas the cauda is principally used for sperm storage, although expression of some critical surface markers does occur that are involved in the process of fertilization. In humans, the passage of sperm takes approximately six days and is longer in rats (~10 days). During the movement along the epididymal, tubule fluid is removed by active transport and this stage of the process is one that can be interfered with by toxicants resulting in an inappropriate environment for normal sperm development.

Most mammals possess seminal vesicles and a prostate (in experimental animals, the exception is that dogs do not have seminal vesicles) and the accessory sex organs are depicted in Fig. 20-20. The physiology and anatomy of these organs vary widely among mammalian species with the rodent having a clear lobular pattern to the prostate that is not seen in humans. These organs are predominantly glandular/secretory in nature and produce much of the seminal plasma for the ejaculation of sperm to survive within the female reproductive tract. Other contributors to the seminal plasma are the epididymis and bulbourethral (Cowper's) glands. The seminal plasma contains many nutrients for sperm motion as well as distinct proteins and ion content. Any disturbance in these components may have an effect on subsequent fertility. For example, a diminution in energy substrates can affect sperm motion characteristics. These "accessory sex organs" are androgen dependent for their function and/or development and are frequently recorded in toxicity studies as indicators of androgen action. Indeed the Hershberger assay, used as part of the EPAs screening battery for endocrine disruptors (see "Testing for Reproductive Toxicity" section), uses changes in the weights of these organs as indicators of androgen or antiandrogen action in this pharmacological screen.

Semen volume varies considerably among species ranging from relatively small (1–10 mL: like humans) to much larger (~500 mL in boars).

Erection and Ejaculation

These physiological processes are controlled by the CNS but are modulated by the autonomic nervous system. Parasympathetic nerve stimulation results in dilatation of the arterioles of the penis, which initiates an erection. Erectile tissue of the penis engorges with blood, veins are compressed to block outflow, and the turgor of the organ increases. In the human, afferent impulses from the genitalia and descending tracts, which mediate erections in response to erotic psychic stimuli, reach the integrating centers in the lumbar segments of the spinal cord. The efferent fibers are located in the pelvic splanchnic nerves (Andersson and Wagner, 1995).

Ejaculation is a two-stage spinal reflex involving emission and ejaculation. Emission is the movement of the semen into the urethra; ejaculation is the propulsion of the semen out of the urethra at the time of orgasm. Afferent pathways involve fibers from receptors in the glans penis that reach the spinal cord through the internal pudendal nerves. Emission is a sympathetic response produced by contraction of the smooth muscle of the vas deferens and seminal vesicles. Semen is ejaculated out of the urethra by contraction of the bulbocavernosus muscle. The spinal reflex centers for this portion of the reflex are in the upper sacral and lowest lumbar segments of the spinal cord; the motor pathways traverse the first to third sacral roots of the internal pudendal nerves.

Little is known concerning the effects of chemicals on erection or ejaculation (Woods, 1984). Pesticides, particularly the organophosphates, are known to affect neuroendocrine processes involved in erection and ejaculation. Many drugs act on the autonomic nervous system and affect potency (Table 20-5) (see also Buchanan and Davis, 1984; Stevenson and Umstead, 1984; Keene and Davies, 1999). Impotence, the failure to obtain or sustain an erection, is rarely of endocrine origin; more often, the cause is psychological. The occurrence of nocturnal or early-morning erections implies that the neurological and circulatory pathways involved in attaining an erection are intact and suggests the possibility of a psychological cause.

Normal penile erection depends upon the relaxation of smooth muscles in the corpora cavernosa. In response to sexual stimuli, cavernous nerves and endothelial cells release nitric oxide, which stimulates the formation of cyclic guanosine monophosphate (GMP) by guanylate cyclase. The drug sildenafil (Viagra) is used to treat erectile dysfunction; its mechanism of action resides in its ability to selectively inhibit cGMP-specific phosphodiesterase type 5. By selectively inhibiting cGMP catabolism in cavernosal smooth muscle cells, sildenafil restores the natural erectile response (cf. Goldstein *et al.*, 1998; Uckert *et al.*, 2006). In the rat, prenatal exposure to the antiandrogenic fungicide, vinclozolin, induces a significant reduction of erections at all dose levels during the ex copula penile reflex tests in male offspring (Colbert *et al.*, 2005).

Case Studies for Effects on the Male

m-Dinitrobenzene   *m*-Dinitrobenzene (*m*-DNB) has been extensively studied for its ability to produce rapid deleterious effects on the rat testis since the mid-1980s. The earliest studies using a 10 week dosing regimen (five day/week by gavage in corn oil) reported effects at 6 mg/kg/day (Linder *et al.*, 1986), while others have reported testicular injury after a single gavage oral dose of 25 to 50 mg/kg (Blackburn *et al.*, 1988). This paper also showed that the other isomers of DNB (*o*- and *p*-) were without testicular effects when given using the same dosing regime. Rehenberg *et al.*, (1988)

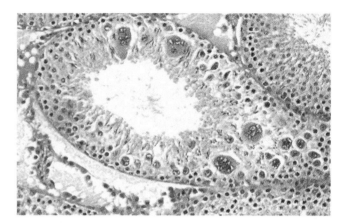

Figure 20-21. *Seminiferous tubules 24 hours after m-dinitrobenzene exposure (25 mg/kg).* Note that multinucleate giant cells and germ cell debris sloughed into the tubular lumen.

showed that the activity was via a direct mechanism not secondary to changes in the HPG axis. Foster (1989) showed that five-day dosing with 5 mg/kg/day produced a minimal to moderate testicular lesion within two weeks and with 10 mg/kg/day a moderate to severe lesion. Testicular weight remained reduced for many weeks after the treatment period with significant dose-related effects on fertility (measured by pregnancy rate and implantation success). Similar studies have shown abnormal sperm function and failure of fertilization in rat in vitro fertilization (IVF) studies (Holloway *et al.*, 1990). Detailed electron microscopic evaluation has shown initial lesions to be present in the Sertoli cells of the testis, which results rapidly in germ cell apoptosis and death. The primary testicular effects on Sertoli cells (see Fig. 20-21) are consistent with the period of infertility noted in the breeding study (see Fig. 20-22) and could also be modeled in Sertoli-germ cell cultures where the *o*- and *p*-isomers were also without effect. A futile redox cycle has been proposed to explain the difference in isomer toxicity in which only *m*-DNB is metabolized to its nitroso-metabolite and further to the hydroxylamine which is recycled back to the nitroso intermediate to reduce cellular reducing equivalents, such as reduced glutathione GSH (Foster *et al.*, 1987; Cave and Foster, 1990; Ellis and Foster, 1992; Reeve *et al.*, 2002)

Ethylene Glycol Monomethyl Ether   Since first published in 1979 (Nagano *et al.*, 1979) that ethylene glycol monomethyl ether (EGME) can elicit testicular toxicity in the mouse, there has been significant effort expended on trying to understand the mode of

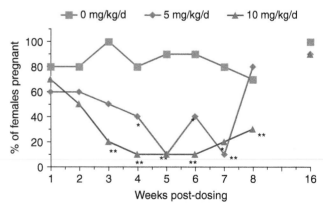

Figure 20-22. *Effect of m-dinitrobenzene on percentage of females pregnant in a serial mating study design.* Note that the range of germ cell types affected consequent to the Sertoli cell injury produced by the compound and the reversibility of the effects after 16 weeks (two spermatogenic waves—see Fig. 20-17). (Reproduced with permission from Foster, 1988.)

action for the induction of these effects. Thus far EGME has been shown to produce testicular toxicity in a wide variety of species, including nonmammals, the major toxicologically used species (rat, mouse, rabbit, and dog) with reasonable evidence that it is likely to have effects in humans should exposure be high enough. A number of studies have described the pathogenesis of the EGME lesion (predominantly in the rat), which seems to be common for the species thus far examined. The earliest features of these studies after a single dose (250 or 500 mg/kg/day) were that there are Sertoli cell vacuoles and swollen germ cell mitochondria, followed by (or concurrent with) a breakdown of the membrane between the Sertoli cell and the pachytene spermatocyte in a spermatogenic stage-specific manner. This is followed quickly (within hours) by the death of (probably those) pachytene spermatocytes (Foster *et al.*, 1983; Creasy and Foster, 1984; Creasy *et al.*, 1986). See Fig. 20-23.

EGME is metabolized to active intermediates; these are methoxyacetaldehyde and methoxyacetic acid (MAA). MAA has a longer half-life and is generally considered the more important of the two. Treating animals with MAA produces identical testicular lesions as that of the parent compound.

The spermatogenic stage-specific effects are on the pachytene spermatocytes immediately before and during meiotic division (so, in stages XII–XIV of the cycle in the rat (see Fig. 20-24), and also the early pachytene spermatocytes, at stages I–IV of the cycle). Dead germ cells can be seen as soon as 12 hours after an effective dose. Continued treatment at a low effective dose seems to affect just the vulnerable cell types, so that a window of missing cells appears downstream from the stage of damage as time progresses (see Fig. 20-24). As with other testis toxicants, higher dose levels produce a more widespread lesion involving other cell types (Foster *et al.*, 1987), producing immediate (<24 hour) and widespread damage and destruction within the tubules. The Sertoli cell

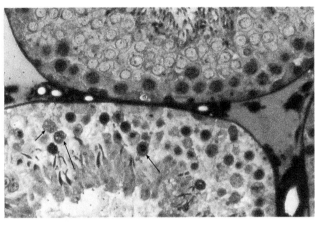

Figure 20-23. *Effect of ethylene glycol monomethyl ether (or its metabolite methoxyacetic acid) 24 hours after a single oral dose (100 mg/kg/d).* Note the damaged spermatocytes (*arrows*) in lower tubule compared to the upper normal tubule.

vacuolization regresses after about 12 hours and is not a prominent feature of this lesion as it is with other agents like hexanedione, or some of the phthalate esters. Some weak evidence of involvement of this cell type also comes from some in vitro data with isolated seminiferous tubules. In this system, molecules that inhibit transcellular calcium movement block the germ cell death from occurring, supporting a change in Sertoli cell communication to germ cells resulting in the rapid cell death after MAA treatment. Leydig cells do not seem to be pivotally involved in the pathogenesis. The lesion is not characteristic of a low-androgen testicular lesion, and reduced accessory sex organ weights are not a prominent feature associated with the early testicular pathology.

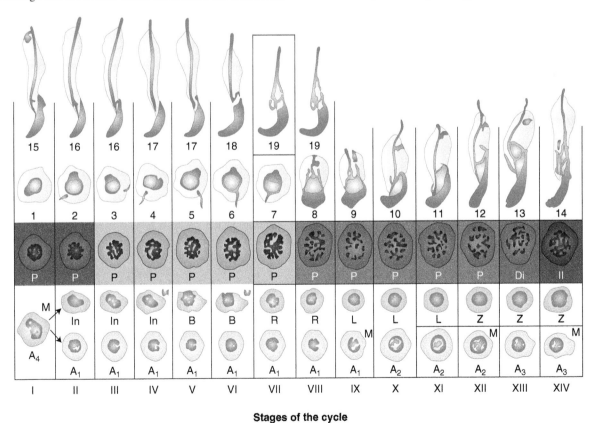

Stages of the cycle

Figure 20-24. *Stage-specific lesions induced by methoxyacetic acid.* Intensity of shading indicates magnitude of effect on spermatocytes (after Foster *et al.*, 1987).

Decrements in fertility in the rat after acute treatment with EGME are entirely consistent with the primary effect on pachytene spermatocyte germ cells, the prominent period of infertility being approximately five to six weeks after dosing when the pachytene spermatocytes should have matured to become mature sperm capable of fertilization based on the known kinetics of the process (Chapin *et al.*, 1985).

MATING BEHAVIOR IN THE RAT

Female rats are only sexually receptive on the day of proestrus, which is characterized by round nucleated and cornified epithelial cells in the vaginal lavage (Knobil and Neill, 1994, Chap. 35). The period of receptivity begins at the onset of the dark phase of their light cycle, terminating later in the evening before the next stage of the cycle, defined as estrus which is typically characterized by the display of a vaginal lavage of mostly cornified epithelial cells. Serum estradiol rises during proestrus and this is followed by initiation of an LH surge shortly after the onset of the dark phase of the light cycle, which in turn induces ovulation and a brief increase in progesterone. This is normally the only time during which the female is receptive to the male and the display of this behavior can be induced in ovariectomized female rats by a sequence of injections of estradiol for a couple of days prior to mating followed by progesterone administration a few hours before the mating trial is conducted, which must occur during the evening of the rat's diurnal cycle. Male and female rat mating behavior is sufficiently stereotyped that it can be easily quantified to assess the effects of toxicants on these behaviors (Gray *et al.*, 1988b; Gray and Ostby, 1998).

During mating, the female rat displays proceptive behaviors like ear wiggling and darting to induce the male to mount, and when mounted the female is "receptive" displaying a lordosis posture characterized by a raised head and tail and fully arched back. The female maintains this posture for several seconds. In experienced male rats, the latency to the first mount is usually on a few seconds, but inexperienced males may take much longer. When the male rat mounts the lordosing female, he will display a single pelvic thrust that may or may not result in intromission of the penis into the vagina. In rats, there is a rapid dismount after this single pelvic thrust. Within a few seconds, the male mounts again and this series continues until the male ejaculates. Ejaculation is usually identifiable by a slow dismount, after which the male retires for several minutes; a period termed the postejaculatory interval (PIE). During this period, the male produces a 22 kHz vocalization, during which the female does not display proceptive behaviors (Porter *et al.*, 2005). Following the PIE, the series repeats itself several times throughout the evening. At the beginning of the second series, the male dislodges the copulatory plug, formed from the seminal secretions. The copulatory plug normally fits close to the cervix, and it is necessary to facilitate sperm entry into the uterus. It is not unusual to find seven to eight copulatory plugs in the breeding cage the day after mating (Gray *et al.*, 1989). If mating does not occur, then the brief rise in serum progesterone declines by the next day.

In spontaneously ovulating species (eg, rodents), the endocrine events are comparable with those in the menstrual cycle. In the rabbit, the LH surge and ovulation is a neural reflex produced by copulation (Knobil and Neill, 1994).

Cervix

The mucosa of the uterine cervix does not undergo cyclic desquamation, but there are regular changes in the cervical mucus. Estrogen, which makes the mucus thinner and more alkaline, promotes the survival and transport of sperm. Progesterone makes the mucus thick, tenacious, and cellular. The mucus is thinnest at the time of ovulation and dries in an arborizing, fernlike pattern on a slide. After ovulation and during pregnancy, it becomes thick and fails to form the fern pattern. Disruptions of the cervix may be expressed as disorders of differentiation (including neoplasia), disturbed secretion, and incompetence. Exfoliative cytological (Papanicolaou's stain) and histological techniques are currently used to assess disorders of differentiation. Various synthetic steroids (eg, oral contraceptives) can affect the extent and pattern of cervical mucus.

Vagina

Estrogen produces a growth and proliferation of vaginal epithelium. The layers of cells become cornified and can be readily identified in vaginal smears. Vaginal cornification has been used as an index for estrogens. Progesterone stimulation produces a thick mucus and the epithelium proliferates, becoming infiltrated with leukocytes. The cyclic changes in the vaginal smear in rats are easily recognized. The changes in humans and other species are similar, but less apparent. Analysis of vaginal fluid or cytological studies of desquamated vaginal cells (quantitative cytochemistry) normally reflects ovarian function. However, administration of estrogenic toxicants can induce persistent vaginal cornification in both immature and adult ovariectomized females by acting directly on the cellular dynamics and cell cycling of the vaginal epithelium (Gray *et al.*, 1988b, 1989). Vaginal sampling of cells and fluid might offer a reliable and easily available external monitor of internal function and dysfunction.

FERTILIZATION

Fertilization is the process whereby the genome from one generation is passed to the next to begin the development of a new organism. In mammals, the oocyte is surrounded by two layers: an outer layer of cumulus cells and an inner layer of extracellular matrix termed the zona pellucida (see the review by Hoodbhoy and Dean, 2004). To reach the oocyte, the sperm must penetrate both layers that require high motility, the release of sperm enzymes and the presence of proteins that will facilitate binding of the sperm to the oocyte. Moreover, once fertilization has occurred, mechanisms must be in place to prevent the binding of further sperm to the fertilized oocyte (the zygote). To facilitate these activities, sperm must be capacitated (Hunter and Rodriguez-Martinez, 2004) and the secretion of enzymes (hyaluronidases) allows the sperm to penetrate through the cumulus cells to the zona pellucida. This special extracellular matrix is composed of three glycoproteins and cell surface factors then cause the sperm to release the secretory enzymes present in the acrosome via binding to the specific carbohydrates present in this matrix. The release of these enzymes enables the sperm to penetrate through the zona pellucida to then bind and fuse with the oocyte plasma membrane through specialized proteins to release the genetic material into the oocyte as the male pronucleus, which eventually combines with the genetic material from the female to form the zygote. Once sperm fusion has occurred, a "zona block" is initiated to prevent any further sperm entering through the zona pellucida and fusing with the oocyte membrane. The precise mechanisms of how this occurs have not been fully elucidated (Hoodbhoy and Dean, 2004).

IMPLANTATION

Implantation is an intricately timed event that allows mammals to nourish and protect their young during early development and results from an intimate relationship between the developing embryo and the differentiating uterus (see the diagram

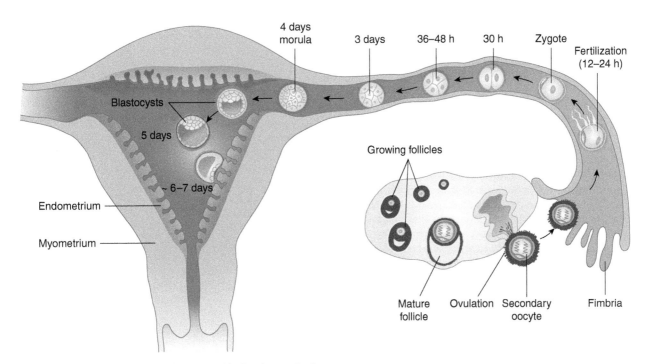

Figure 20-25. *Fertilization and implantation in the female reproductive tract.*

in Fig. 20-25). Implantation can only occur when the embryo reaches the blastocyst stage and gains implantation competency and the uterus, through steroid hormone-dependent changes, attains a receptive state. This reciprocal interaction must occur between the blastocyst and uterus together with an increase in uterine vascular permeability at the site of blastocyst attachment. There are four stages that comprise early implantation in mammals, (1) apposition and adhesion of the blastocyst to the uterine lumen, (2) penetration of the epithelium, (3) decidualization of the stromal cells, and (4) trophoblastic invasion into the stromal vasculature. These four stages can vary in length and in precise order depending on the specific species studied and is further reviewed by Schäfer-Somi (2003), Aplin and Kimber (2004), Lee and DeMayo (2004), and Tranguch *et al.* (2005). The molecular understanding of these physiological events is far from complete, with data being generated mainly from studies in the mouse that have indicated through gene ablation in the uterus, a number of critical factors and cytokines involved in implantation; however, a number of these critical gene products (eg, VEGF, BMP-2, and wnt-4) have also been shown to produce early embryonic lethality when knocked out. Another important aspect of the implantation process common to many species (and offering an experimental tool to study implantation) is the embryonic diapause (or delayed implantation) evolved as a strategy to ensure proper implantation timing depending on environmental conditions (see review by Lopes *et al.*, 2004). The regulation of this phenomenon varies widely between species ranging from photoperiod through hormonal or nutritional influences.

PLACENTA

The placenta plays a key role in pregnancy, mediating exchanges between the mother and fetus and maternal tolerance of antigens produced by the fetus. There are a huge number of different placental types exhibited by eutherian mammals that exhibit differences in both structure and endocrinology including significant difference between the major experimental animal species and humans (see

reviews by Malassine *et al.*, 2003; Enders and Carter, 2004 and Fig. 20-26). Humans and monkeys possess a hemochorial placenta. Pigs, horses, and donkeys have an epitheliochorial type of placenta, whereas sheep, goats, and cows have a syndesmochorial type of placenta. In laboratory animals (eg, rat, rabbit, and guinea pig), the placenta is termed a hemoendothelial type. Among the various species, the number of maternal and fetal cell layers ranges from six (eg, pig, horse) to a single one (eg, rat, rabbit). Primates, including humans, have three layers of cells in the placenta that a substance must pass across.

Early in implantation the blastocyst comes in contact with the endometrium, and becomes surrounded by an outer layer or syncytiotrophoblast, a multinucleated mass of cells with no discernible boundaries, and an inner layer of individual cells, the cytotrophoblast. The syncytiotrophoblast erodes the endometrium, and the blastocyst implants. Placental circulation is then established and trophoblastic function continues. The blastocysts of most mammalian species implant about day six or seven following fertilization. At this stage, the differentiation of the embryonic and extraembryonic (trophoblastic) tissues is apparent.

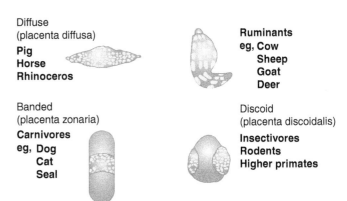

Figure 20-26. *Types of mammalian placentae.*

Trophoblastic tissue differentiates into cytotrophoblast and syncytiotrophoblast cells. The syncytiotrophoblast cells produce chorionic gonadotropin, chorionic growth hormones, placental lactogen, estrogen, and progesterone, which are needed to achieve independence from the ovary in maintaining the pregnancy. Rapid proliferation of the cytotrophoblast serves to anchor the growing placenta to the maternal tissue.

The developing placenta consists of proliferating trophoblasts, which expand rapidly and infiltrate the maternal vascular channels. Shortly after implantation, the syncytiotrophoblast is bathed by maternal venous blood, which supplies nutrients and permits an exchange of gases. Histotrophic nutrition involves yolk sac circulation; hemotrophic nutrition involves the placenta. Placental circulation is established quite early in women and primates and relatively much later in rodents and rabbits. One of the major differences in endocrine placental function between humans and rodents is in the production and regulation of progesterone necessary for the maintenance of pregnancy. In the rodent, the corpus luteum in the ovary has to produce progesterone throughout gestation and is regulated initially by pituitary prolactin secretion and then around midway through gestation by placental lactogens produced by the trophoblast. Thus, hypophysectomy (to remove pituitary influences) in a mouse does not terminate pregnancy after GD 11. In humans, the pituitary gland is not required for the initiation and maintenance of pregnancy, with maintenance of the corpus luteum to produce progesterone dependent on the secretion of human chorionic gonadotropin (hCG) by the trophoblast. There is sufficient progesterone produced by the trophoblast after eight weeks of gestation in humans to maintain pregnancy even in cases of ovariectomy.

Generally, the placenta is quite impermeable to chemicals/drugs with molecular weights of 1000 Da or more. Because most medications and xenobiotics have molecular weights of 500 Da or less, molecular size is rarely a factor in denying a drug's entrance across the placenta and into the embryo/fetus. Placental permeability to a chemical is affected by placental characteristics including thickness, surface area, carrier systems, and lipid-protein concentration of the membranes. The inherent characteristics of the chemical itself, such as its degree of ionization, lipid solubility, protein binding, and molecular size also affect its transport across the placenta.

PREGNANCY

In the female rat, during mating repeated cervical stimulation by the penis induces a surge of prolactin from the posterior pituitary within 20 minutes followed by the onset of twice-daily prolactin surges, which persist for an eight- to 13-day period. During this period, prolactin "rescues" the corpora lutea preventing regression. If sperm transport, fertilization, or implantation are blocked, then the mated female is "pseudopregnant" for about 10 to 13 days (Swingle *et al.*, 1951). During days six to 10 of pregnancy, sustained ovarian luteal function also requires pituitary LH. Pregnancy loss, that is full-litter resorption, can be induced at this stage of pregnancy by inhibition of pituitary LH secretion, which in turn causes a reduction in serum progesterone levels (Bielmeier *et al.*, 2004).

Midpregnancy of the rat is characterized by hypertrophic development of the corpus luteum, which is dependent upon transition from the early LH and prolactin-dependent phase of pregnancy to one that involves the secretion of hormones by the feto-placental unit (rCG and rPL) that induce rapid growth and differentiation of the corpora lutea, an increase in progesterone synthesis and a doubling in serum progesterone. Doody *et al.* (1991) examined the levels of expression of mRNA species encoding cholesterol side-chain cleavage cytochrome P-450 (P-450scc), 17α-hydroxylase cytochrome P-450 (P-450 17α), aromatase cytochrome P-450 (P-450AROM), and 3β-hydroxysteroid dehydrogenase (3 β-HSD) in rat ovaries during pregnancy. Expression of P-450scc mRNA is at low, but detectable levels until day 14, thereafter expression increased to high levels (day 14–21 of gestation). Levels of P-450 17α mRNA on day 10 of gestation were low and decreased further on days 14 and 17. Expression of 3β-HSD was decreased on day 10, but on days 14, 17, and 21 of gestation high mRNA levels were detectable. Ovarian expression of the three P-450AROM species is also dramatically increased between days 14 and 17 of pregnancy, but declines by day 21.

Because the transition from early to midpregnancy in the rat requires hormones from the feto-placental unit, if implantation or uterine decidualization is blocked by a chemical, then the female would resume her estrous cycles and the corpora lutea would regress (Knobil and Neill, 1994, Chap. 7). Chemicals that induce whole-litter loss at mid-to-late pregnancy may cause abortions in some of the females, whereas others fail to deliver and appear pregnant for an unusually long period of time. Effects on female fertility due to disruption of hormones during pregnancy may be difficult to detect in standard testing studies if females are mated to similarly treated males or if the chemical affects the reproductive system of both sexes. For example, with chronic di-*n*-butyl phthalate (DBP) administration at high dose levels induces whole litter loss at mid-pregnancy through reductions in ovarian progesterone production on GD 13. However, ovarian weight is not altered at GD 13 and the onset of female puberty, estrous cyclicity, and mating also were unaffected. This is in contrast to the robust reductions in testis size and histology, sex accessory gland size, and sperm counts in pubertal males treated with DBP at 500 or 1000 mg/kg/day, treated F0 females only display gross morphological reproductive alterations and reductions in uterine weights during mid-pregnancy. Hence, when female-mediated infertility is affected in this manner, it may only be apparent when treated females are mated to untreated males. Chemicals that reduce serum progesterone production during pregnancy by inhibiting progesterone synthesis also may not alter the estrous cycles in the rat since the rat estrous cycle does not have a functional luteal phase, unlike humans.

Many abortifacients induce pregnancy loss by reducing progesterone levels in the rat. Generally, reducing midpregnancy progesterone levels by half or more is sufficient to terminate pregnancy (Carnathan *et al.*, 1987). For example, treating pregnant rats with a prostaglandin F2alpha analogue ICI 81008, which reduces serum progesterone levels during pregnancy, induces full-litter loss in 40% of 300 dams, while 25% had reduced litter sizes and 35% had normal litters (Warnock and Csapo, 1975). In comparison with the 107 control dams, all treated rats with full-litter loss had a drastic reduction in mid-pregnancy plasma progesterone levels. In contrast, those animals with only a partly resorbed litters only had a moderate reduction in progesterone until day 16. In contrast to progesterone, there was no correlation between plasma estradiol-17β levels and the consequences of treatment on pregnancy.

Corpora lutea function during pregnancy also may involve androgens and insulin-like 3 peptide hormone, in concert with lactogenic hormones. Whereas some of the androgenic actions are mediated by conversion of androgens to estrogens, pure androgenic effects also have been implicated (Goyeneche *et al.*, 2002). Goyeneche *et al.* (2002) reported that AR mRNA and protein were expressed throughout gestation in the rat corpus luteum. In addition, they found that androstenedione, the main circulating androgen in pregnant rats, opposed luteal regression, reduced the number of cells undergoing apoptosis, and enhanced the levels of circulating progesterone.

PARTURITION

Parturition is a complex process involving fetal, placental, and maternal signals, and the precise molecular events controlling this physiological process are not clear. Parturition is best to be thought of as a release from the inhibitory effects of pregnancy on the myometrium of the uterus rather than an active process, although the timing and order of the precise events is an active process. For most mammals, the uterus is held in a quiescent state by high levels of progesterone and it is the decrease of progesterone that provides the trigger for parturition. In humans, this does not seem to be the case (ie, levels of progesterone do not drop). Some authors have postulated that progesterone receptor inactivity does appear to be related to onset of labor and that local metabolism of progesterone in the cervix and uterus produces a localized decrease in progesterone that initiates labor. The fetus also directly contributes to the onset of parturition by activation of its HPA axis producing increased levels of cortisol. This in turn directly upregulates steroidogenic enzymes (especially CYP 17) in the fetus and placenta, which in turn leads to changes in prostaglandin (particularly PGF2α) and oxytocin production to induce uterine contractions together with the increased activity of cytokines (including NF-κB and IL-1β). In humans, there is no CYP 17 in the placenta, which may be related to the lack of change of progesterone (see reviews by Challis et al., 2005; Mendelson and Condon, 2005; Snegovskikh et al., 2006).

LACTATION

The endocrine control of lactation is one of the most complex physiological mechanisms of human parturition. Mammogenesis, lactogenesis, galactopoiesis, and galactokinesis are all essential to assure proper lactation. Prolactin is the key hormone of lactation and seems to be the single most important galactopoietic (milk synthesis) hormone. Oxytocin, serotonin, opioids, histamine, substance P, and arginine–leucine modulate prolactin release by means of an autocrine/paracrine mechanism, whereas estrogen and progesterone hormones can act at the hypothalamic and adenohypophysial levels. Human placental lactogen and growth factors play an essential role to assure successful lactation during pregnancy with oxytocin being the most powerful galactokinetic (milk ejection) hormone (Buhimschi, 2004).

SENESCENCE

Reproductive senescence is usually preceded by a dysregulation of the HPG axis. This dysregulation leads to alterations in serum HPG hormones, accompanied an upregulation in GnRH, LH, and activin activities and a decrease in steroids in the brain. Receptors for these hormones in the brain are intimately involved in cell proliferation and differentiation in growth and development. In females, reproductive senescence is associated with a transition from regular to irregular estrus (menstrual) cycles leading to acyclicity and ultimately a loss of fertility. GnRH neurons in the brain are affected morphologically and there are changes in GnRH neurosecretion with changes in pulsatility and preovulatory release that are causal in producing acyclicity. Perinatal exposure to toxicants with estrogenic activity can defeminize the HPG axis such that the females are acyclic and infertile while less affected females display the "delayed anovulatory syndrome" and become anovulatory and acyclic at an early age (Gray et al., 1989).

In males, a decrease in androgen is noted in around 20% of fit 60-year old men, but the value of androgen supplementation is not clear with regard to reproductive senescence. Dysregulation of the HPG axis is also found in aged male rats, with elevations in FSH and LH and decreased testosterone normally found. For reviews on reproductive senescence and possible associations with cognitive function, see the studies of Atwood et al. (2005), Keefe et al. (2006), and Yin and Gore (2006).

ENDOCRINE DISRUPTION (INCLUDING SCREENING AND PUBERTY)

Currently, the potential effects of "endocrine disrupting chemicals" (EDCs) on human health and the proven effects of EDCs on wildlife are a major focus among the scientific community. In 1996, the USEPA was given a mandate under the Food Quality Protection Act and Safe Drinking Water Act to develop test protocols to screen for endocrine effects. The initial impetus for these actions arose from a work session in 1991 on "Chemically Induced Alterations in Sexual Development: The Wildlife/Human Connection" (Colborn, 1994). Recent findings have contributed to these concerns; for example, it has been suggested that in utero exposure to environmental estrogens, antiandrogens or chemicals like phthalates, or 2,3,7,8-TCDD could be responsible for the reported 50% decline in sperm counts in some areas and the apparent increase in cryptorchid testes (Toppari et al., 2001), testicular cancer (Skakkebaek, 2002), and hypospadias (Paulozzi et al., 1997; Canning, 1999; Aho et al., 2000; Toppari et al., 2001; Pierik et al., 2002; Porter et al., 2005; Nassar et al., 2007). The differences in sperm counts between regions are so large that they cannot be explained by methodological biases and "environmental effects are entirely plausible" (Jorgensen et al., 2001, 2002; Giwercman et al., 2006). Indeed, it has been proposed (Skakkebaek, 2002) that the secular deficits in these human reproductive endpoints could be plausibly linked and have an origin in fetal life as the testes are developing. These authors proposed the term testicular dysgenesis syndrome (see Fig. 20-27) to explain the interrelationship of these findings.

Phthalate exposures have been associated with reduced AGD in boys and lower testosterone levels in men. In females, exposure to EDCs during development could contribute to earlier age at puberty and to increased incidences of endometriosis and breast cancer, for example. The original focus for the discussion of "endocrine disrupters" was research on toxicants reported to possess estrogenic activity, with little consideration given to other mechanisms of endocrine toxicity; mechanisms that, in fact, may be of equal or greater concern. In addition, there has been a great deal of misinformation communicated on issues concerning endocrine disrupters; for example, nonestrogenic chemicals (ie, phthalates and p,p'-DDE) are repeatedly reported to be estrogenic. There is a lack of appreciation for the fact that many endocrine disrupters (ie, TCDD, EE) are very potent reproductive toxicants. In addition, there has been a tendency to dismiss the wildlife data as correlative, ignoring examples of clear, cause and effect relationships between chemical exposure and reproductive alterations (eg, DDT metabolite effects on birds, PCB effects on fish, and environmental estrogen effects on domestic animals). There is a lack of recognition that subtle, low dose reproductive effects seen in laboratory studies with endocrine disrupters will be difficult, if not impossible, to detect in typical epidemiological studies because of high variability normally

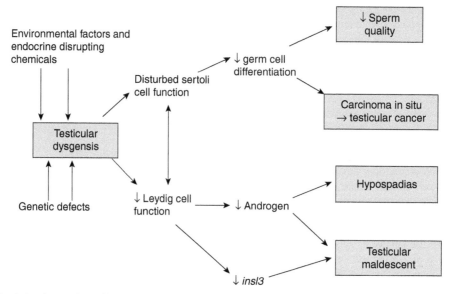

Figure 20-27. *Testicular dysgenesis syndrome.* The hypothesis that events occurring during the development of the testis in fetal life can be related to the secular increases in a number of human reproductive disorders (Data from Skakkebaek *et al.*, 2002).

seen in human reproductive function (eg, time to fertility, fecundity, and sperm measures), the delayed appearance of the reproductive lesions and a lack of high quality exposure data. There is also a lack of appreciation for the complexity of the multiple mechanisms by which a single chemical can alter the endocrine milieu, to say nothing of the complex endocrine alterations induced by mixtures of chemicals.

We are now not only concerned about pesticides and other toxic substances in the environment, but the issue has broadened considerably due to the growing awareness that the list of EDCs present in the environment from human activities includes potent pharmaceutical products and phytosterols. Among these drugs are estrogens, antibiotics, β-blockers, antiepileptics, and lipid-regulating agents. One study reported that the pharmaceuticals found as contaminants of aquatic systems included 36 of 55 pharmaceuticals and five of nine metabolites measured including antiepileptic drugs (Kolpin *et al.*, 1998, 2002, 2004).

In the area of wildlife toxicology and ecosystem health, it is apparent that clear-cut cause and effect relationships exist between exposure to EDCs and adverse effects in several vertebrate classes from fish to mammals. One challenge in interspecies extrapolation is to link laboratory mechanistic studies with EDCs to both individual and population effects in the field.

Reports of U-shaped (nonmonotonic), ultra-low dose effects and nonthreshold effects for EDCs are challenging some of the basic assumptions of risk assessment for noncancer end points. While the focus of this debate has centered on the low dose effects of bisphenol A (Nagel *et al.*, 1997; vom Saal *et al.*, 1998, 2005; Ashby *et al.*, 1999; Owens and Chaney, 2005; Welshons *et al.*, 2006), well-documented U-shaped dose response curves are known from many other in vitro and some in vivo studies. For example, administration of testosterone produces a well-characterized and reproducible U-shaped dose response for spermatogenesis (Ewing *et al.*, 1977, 1979, 1981; Robaire *et al.*, 1979) in the intact adult male rat. In vitro studies show that such responses do not always involve multiple mechanisms of action. Several AR ligands, antagonists at low-to-moderate concentrations, became AR agonists at high concentrations. Furthermore, the basic tenet of toxicology from Paracelceus (1564) that "dose alone determines the poison" is too limited for some EDCs because the timing of exposure dictates not only the

effect, but also whether the effects are adverse or beneficial. Even when administered during adult life, drugs with EDC-activity can simultaneously have a beneficial effect on one tissue and an adverse effect on another.

Known Effects of EDCs in Humans and Animals

The list of chemicals that are known to affect humans, domestic animals, and/or wildlife via functional developmental toxicity or endocrine mechanisms includes 2,3,7,8-TCDD, PCBs and polychlorinated dibenzofurans (PCDFs), methylmercury, EE, alkylphenols, plant sterols, fungal estrogens, androgens, chlordecone, DBCP, *o,p'*-DDD (Mitotane), *o,p'*-DDT, and *p,p'*-DDE (Gray *et al.*, 2001; Gray, 2002). In addition to these xenobiotics, over 30 different drugs taken during pregnancy have been found to alter human development as a consequence of endocrine disruption. These drugs are not limited to estrogens like diethylstilbestrol (DES). EDCs are known to alter human development via several mechanisms besides the estrogen receptor (ER): this includes binding to the AR, or retinoic acid (RAR, RXR) receptors, and by inhibition of steroidogenic enzymes or the synthesis of thyroid hormones. Findings on the effects of background levels of PCBs on the neurobehavioral development of the child have contributed to the concerns about the effects of EDCs on human health via alteration of hormone function including the thyroid (Brouwer *et al.*, 1999; Tan and Zoeller, 2007). In summary, there are several hundred epidemiology studies showing associations among EDCs and adverse human health effects, however, none of these has been sufficiently studied to claim that "cause and effect" exists.

Effects of Drugs on Human Sexual Differentiation

In humans (Herbst, 1973; Bardin and Catterall, 1981; Ohyama, 2004; Carmichael *et al.*, 2005) and laboratory rodents (Foster *et al.*, 2001; Fisher, 2004; Gray *et al.*, 2006), exposure to hormonally active chemicals during sex differentiation can produce pseudohermaphroditism. Androgenic drugs such as danazol and methyltestosterone can masculinize human females (ie, "female pseudohermaphroditism") (Rosa, 1984; Kingsbury, 1985; Schardein, 2000). Laboratory studies demonstrate that these chemicals alter sex differentiation in rodents as well (Duck and Katayama, 1981). The drug amino-glutethimide, which alters steroid hormone synthesis in a manner identical to many fungicides, also masculinizes human females following in utero exposure (LeMaire *et al.*, 1972; Schardein, 2000).

DES provides an unfortunate example of how in utero exposure to a potent endocrine disrupter with estrogenic activity can alter reproductive development in humans (Herbst, 1987; Shaffer, 2000; Veurink *et al.*, 2005). Although a few cases of masculinized females were noted in the late 1950s, most of the effects of DES were not apparent until after the children attained puberty. Transplacental exposure of the developing fetus to DES causes clear cell adeno-carcinoma of the vagina, as well as gross structural abnormalities of the cervix, uterus, and fallopian tube. These women are more likely to have an adverse pregnancy outcome, including spontaneous abortions, ectopic pregnancies, and premature delivery (DeCherney *et al.*, 1981). Some of the pathological effects that develop in males following fetal DES exposure appear to result from an inhibition of androgen action or synthesis (underdevelopment or absence of the vas deferens, epididymis, and seminal vesicles) and anti-Müllerian duct factor (persistence of the Müllerian ducts) (Niculescu, 1985). DES may also have caused epididymal cysts, hypotrophic testes, and infertility in males.

Effects of Plant and Fungal Products in Animals and Humans

The phytoestrogens and fungal mycotoxins are naturally occurring and widespread in nature. Farnsworth *et al.* (1975) listed over 400 species of plants that contain potentially estrogenic isoflavonoids or coumestans or were suspected of being estrogenic based on biological grounds (Farnsworth, 1990). Plants contain many other compounds in addition to estrogens that can affect reproductive performance, such as the purported antiandrogenic activity in the oil from saw palmetto (Gordon and Shaughnessy, 2003).

Although most naturally occurring environmental estrogens are relatively inactive, when compared to steroidal estrogens or DES, the phytoestrogen miroestrol is almost as potent as estradiol in vitro and even more potent than estradiol when administered orally (Cain, 1960; Matsumura *et al.*, 2005). In addition, many plant estrogens occur in such high concentrations that they induce reproductive alterations in domestic animals (Adams, 1990; Adams and Sanders, 1988). "Clover disease," which is characterized by dystocia, prolapse of the uterus, and infertility, is observed in sheep grazed on highly estrogenic clover pastures. Permanent infertility (defeminization) can be produced in ewes by much lower amounts of estrogen over a longer time period than are needed to produce "clover disease." In domestic animals, feeds contaminated with the zearalenone-producing fungus (*Fusarium* spp.) induce adverse reproductive effects in a wide variety of domestic animals, including impaired fertility in cows and hyperestrogenism in swine and turkeys (Kuiper-Goodman *et al.*, 1987).

Effects of Organochlorine Compounds in Humans

In addition to drugs and plant substances, several pesticides and toxic substances have been shown to alter human reproductive function (listed above). An accidental high dose in utero exposure to PCBs and PCDFs has been associated with reproductive alterations in boys, increased stillbirths, low birth weight, malformations, and IQ and behavioral deficits (Jacobson and Jacobson, 1997). In addition to the effects associated with this inadvertent exposure, relatively subtle adverse effects were seen in infants and children exposed to relatively low levels of PCBs and PCDFs. The authors reported that the lowest observed adverse effect levels (LOAELs) for developmental neurobehavioral and reproductive end points are currently within the range of current human body burdens based on toxicity equivalency factors.

One metabolite of DDT was found to alter adrenal function with sufficient potency to be used as a drug to reduce adrenal androgen production (Knappe *et al.*, 1997). o,p′-DDD (mitotane) is used to treat adrenal steroid hypersecretion associated with adrenal tumors. In addition to this usage, lower doses of mitotane restored menstruation in women with spanomenorrhea associated with hypertrichosis.

Occupational Exposures Occupational exposure to pesticides and other toxic substances (ie, chlordecone and DBCP) in the workplace have been associated with reduced fertility, lowered sperm counts, and/or endocrine alterations in male workers. Workers in Hopewell, VA, exposed to high levels of chlordecone, an estrogenic (Hammond *et al.*, 1979) and neurotoxic (Landrigan *et al.*, 1980) organochlorine pesticide, displayed obvious signs of intoxication, which included severe neurotoxicity and abnormal testicular function (Epstein, 1978; Reich and Spong, 1983). As this cohort was not followed, it is not known if the effects of chlordecone were completely reversible.

It is surprising to learn that occupational exposures to potential EDCs at effective concentrations apparently have not been entirely eliminated from the workplace. A series of publications from about 1990 to 1996 presented documentation of sexual impotence in chemical factory workers exposed to a DES-like stilbene derivative. National Institute of Occupational Safety and Health conducted two studies in response to complaints of impotence and decreased libido among male workers involved in the manufacture of 4,4′-diaminostilbene-2,2′-disulfonic acid (DAS), a key ingredient in the synthesis of dyes and fluorescent whitening agents (Grajewski *et al.*, 1996; Hammond *et al.*, 1987; Quinn *et al.*, 1990; Smith and Quinn, 1992; Whelan *et al.*, 1996). Both current and former workers had lower serum testosterone levels (Grajewski *et al.*, 1996) and reduced libido (Whelan *et al.*, 1996) as compared to control workers. In addition, duration of employment was negatively correlated with testosterone levels. These studies replicated the observations reported by Quinn *et al.* (1990) who reported low levels of serum testosterone and problems with impotence in male workers. In a uterotrophic assay, while DAS was only weakly to negligibly estrogenic (Smith and Quinn, 1992), a single sc 30 mg/kg dose of 4-nitrotoluene, a precursor of DAS, increased uterine weights without producing overt toxicity. Samples of DAS from the workplace displayed estrogenic activity.

Environmental Androgens

Androgenic activity has been detected in several complex environmental mixtures. There are Pulp and paper mill effluents (PME) from Florida, the Baltic Sea, the Great Lakes, and New Zealand (Ellis *et al.*, 2003; Larsson and Forlin, 2002; Parks *et al.*, 2001). PME effluents from sites on the Fenholloway River in Florida include a chemical mixture that binds AR and induces androgen-dependent gene expression in vitro. This mode of action is consistent with the masculinized female mosquitofish (*Gambusia holbrooki*) collected from contaminated sites on the river. Male-biased sex ratios of fish embryos have been reported near a pulp mill in broods of eelpout (*Zoarces viviparus*) in the vicinity of a large kraft pulp mill on the Swedish Baltic coast, suggesting that masculinizing compounds in the effluent were affecting gonadal differentiation and promoting skewed sex ratios. Efforts to date have not conclusively identified chemicals in PME responsible for androgenic activity (Durhan *et al.*, 2002).

Effluents from beef cattle concentrated animal feeding operations (CAFO) from Nebraska and Ohio have been shown to display androgenicity. Orlando *et al.* (2004) found that CAFO discharge at a site in Nebraska exhibited androgenic activity and found that fish (fathead minnow; *Pimephales promelas*) collected at the site displayed small gonads as compared to fish from a reference site. Durhan *et al.* (2006) detected the synthetic androgens 17α- and 17β-trenbolone in several water samples from a beef CAFO in Ohio, where trenbolone acetate implants were used to stimulate weight gain and the samples collected from a direct discharge from the feedlot displayed significant androgenic activity in vitro. Complementary laboratory studies revealed that both trenbolone isomers were androgenic in fathead minnows (Ankley *et al.*, 2003) and rats (Wilson *et al.*, 2002). When administered in utero, 17β-trenbolone (TB) masculinized female rat offspring, increased AGD and caused vaginal agenesis and induced male sex accessory tissues in females (Wolf *et al.*, 2002). TB binds to AR with high affinity and induces androgen-dependent gene expression in vitro at concentrations similar to those for DHT (Wilson *et al.*, 2004).

In vivo androgenicity testing using the Hershberger assay shows that TB is as potent as testosterone propionate (TP) in inducing growth of the androgen-dependent levator ani–bulbocavernosus muscles (Wilson *et al.*, 2002) being about 70 times more potent when administered sc versus orally.

Environmental Antiandrogens

Fungicides Vinclozolin and procymidone are two members of the dicarboximide fungicide class that act as AR antagonists (Kelce *et al.*, 1994; Ostby *et al.*, 1999). These pesticides, or their metabolites, competitively inhibit the binding of androgens to AR that leads to an inhibition of androgen-dependent gene expression in vitro and in vivo (Kelce *et al.*, 1997). Peripubertal administration of antiandrogens can alter the onset of pubertal landmarks in the male rat (Monosson *et al.*, 1999). Vinclozolin delays pubertal maturation, and reduces sex accessory gland and epididymal growth and increases serum LH, and testosterone and 5-androstane, 3,17-diol levels. In a Hershberger assay using castrated immature testosterone-treated male rats, vinclozolin and procymidone alone or in combination inhibited testosterone-induced growth of androgen-dependent tissues (ventral prostate, seminal vesicles, and levator ani–bulbocavernosus muscles) in a dose-additive fashion (Gray *et al.*, 2001).

Administration of vinclozolin during sexual differentiation demasculinizes and feminizes the male rat offspring such that treated males display female-like AGD at birth, retained nipples, hypospadias, suprainguinal ectopic testes, a blind vaginal pouch, and small to absent sex accessory glands (Gray *et al.*, 1994). In contrast to the phthalates and linuron (see below), even at high dosages (200 mg/kg/day), epididymal hypoplasia was rare and no cases of gubernacular agenesis were noted. At low doses, vinclozolin reduces neonatal AGD and increases the incidence of retained nipples/areolae in infant male rats. In adult life, ventral prostate weight is permanently reduced and male offspring display permanent female-like nipples (Gray *et al.*, 1999a). Treatment at 50 and 100 mg/kg/day induces hypospadias and other reproductive tract malformations. The most sensitive period of development to the disruptive effects of vinclozolin is GD 16–17 with less severe effects seen in males exposed to vinclozolin on GD 14–15 and GD 18–19. In addition, Hotchkiss *et al.* (2003) demonstrated that neonatal injection of vinclozolin at 200 mg/kg/day demasculinized aggressive play behavior in male rats at 35 days of age, indicating that CNS sexual differentiation was altered in an antiandrogenic manner.

When procymidone is administered from day 14 of pregnancy to day three after birth, AGD is shortened in male pups,

and the males display retained nipples, hypospadias, cryptorchidism, cleft phallus, a vaginal pouch, and reduced sex accessory gland size (Ostby *et al.*, 1999). Procymidone also induces fibrosis, cellular infiltration, and epithelial hyperplasia in the dorsolateral and ventral prostatic and seminal vesicular tissues in the offspring when examined as adults.

Prochloraz is a fungicide that disrupts reproductive development and function by several modes of action (Noriega *et al.*, 2005; Vinggaard *et al.*, 2000, 2002). Prochloraz inhibits the steroidogenic enzymes 17,20-lyase and aromatase and it is an AR antagonist. Wilson *et al.* (2004) found that prenatal prochloraz reduces fetal testis testosterone and increases progesterone production 10-fold on GD 18 without affecting Leydig cell insl3 mRNA levels. Prenatal prochloraz treatment delayed parturition and altered reproductive development in the male offspring in a dose-related manner (Noriega *et al.*, 2005). Treated males displayed reduced AGD and female-like areolas and high dose males displayed hypospadias, but the epididymides and gubernacular ligaments were relatively unaffected.

Linuron (Herbicide) The herbicide linuron is an AR antagonist. It binds rat and human AR and inhibits DHT-hAR induced gene expression in vitro (Lambright *et al.*, 2000; McIntyre *et al.*, 2000, 2002). In vivo treatment with linuron elicits a positive response in the Hershberger assay for antiandrogens (Lambright *et al.*, 2000). In utero linuron exposure produces dramatic effects in male rat offspring. More than half of the males exposed to 100 mg linuron/kg/day (GD14-18) display epididymal and testicular abnormalities (Gray *et al.*, 1999b) with effects seen at dosage as low as 12.5 mg/kg/day (exposed from GD 10–22) (McIntyre *et al.*, 2000). In contrast to the effects of vinclozolin and procymidone, malformed external genitalia and undescended testes were rarely displayed by linuron-exposed males. Interestingly, the syndrome of effects for linuron is atypical of an AR antagonist and more closely resembles those seen with in utero to phthalates, which inhibit fetal Leydig cell insl3 hormone levels. Wilson *et al.* (2004) found that fetal testosterone production is significantly reduced in linuron-treated fetal males demonstrating that linuron is antiandrogenic via dual mechanisms of action.

p,p′-DDE (Pesticide Metabolite) Kelce *et al.* (1995, 1997) found that p,p′-DDE displayed AR antagonism both in vivo and in vitro. In vitro, p,p′-DDE binds to the AR and inhibits androgen-dependent gene expression. In vivo, p,p′-DDE delays pubertal development in male rats by about five days at 100 mg/kg/day and inhibits androgen-stimulated tissue growth in the Hershberger assay, which uses castrated immature androgen-treated male rats (Table 20-1). p,p′-DDE administered to Long-Evans Hooded and Sprague–Dawley male rats in utero reduces AGD, induces nipples, and permanently reduces androgen-dependent organ weights (Gray *et al.*, 1999b).

Phthalates (Plasticizers) The phthalates represent a class of high production volume chemicals that alter reproductive development. While a few in vitro studies suggested that some of the phthalates are estrogenic, DBP injections do not induce an uterotrophic response or estrogen-dependent sex behavior (lordosis) in the ovariectomized adult female rats (Gray, 1998). Likewise, oral DBP or diethylhexyl phthalate (DEHP) treatments fail to accelerate VO or induce constant estrus in the intact female rats. In addition, neither the phthalate diesters nor their monoester metabolites appear to compete significantly with androgens for binding to AR at environmentally relevant concentrations (Foster *et al.*, 2001; Parks *et al.*, 2000; Stroheker *et al.*, 2005). In utero, some phthalate esters alter the development of the male rat reproductive tract at relatively low dosages. Prenatal exposure to DBP, benzyl butyl phthalate (BBP), di-isononyl phthalate (DINP), and DEHP treatment cause a syndrome of effects, including underdevelopment and agenesis of the epididymis and other androgen-dependent tissues and testicular abnormalities (Foster *et al.*, 2001; Gray *et al.*, 2000). Among the antiandrogenic EDCs, the phthalates are unique in their ability to induce agenesis of the gubernacular cords, a tissue whose development is dependent upon the peptide hormone insulin-like peptide-3. Wilson *et al.* (2004) found that the phthalates reduced both insl3 mRNA and testosterone levels during sexual differentiation of the male rat.

When pregnant SD rats are dosed by gavage with DEHP from GD 8 to day 17 of lactation with 0, 11, 33, 100, or 300 mg/kg/day, in utero exposure induces a low incidence of abnormalities consistent with the "phthalate syndrome" in the 11, 33, and 100 mg/kg/day dose groups along with subtle reductions in reproductive organ weights. In the high dose group, more than 25% of the males display testicular and/or epididymal abnormalities. Pubertal DEHP treatment alone is sufficient to delay puberty in Long Evans (LE) and SD rats due to lowered testosterone levels.

Prenatal exposure to DBP from day 10 to 22 of gestation produces effects nearly identical to those seen with DEHP, with effects occurring at dosage levels of 50 to 100 mg/kg/day (Mylchreest *et al.*, 1999, 2000). When administered in four-day periods of gestation (GD 8–11, 12–15, or 16–19), DBP at 500 mg/kg/day was most effective in altering sexual differentiation at GD 16–19 (Gray *et al.*, 1999b). When Carruthers and Foster (2005) exposed SD rats to DBP at 500 mg/kg/day for two-day periods (GD 14 and 15, 15 and 16, 16 and 17, 17 and 18, 18 and 19, or 19 and 20), they also found that the critical window for abnormal development is GD 16–18.

DBP also disrupts reproductive function in the rabbit. In rabbits exposed to 400 mg DBP/kg/day in utero (GD 15–29), male offspring exhibit reduced numbers of ejaculated sperm, testis weight, and accessory sex gland weight (Higuchi *et al.*, 2003). Additionally, DBP caused a slight increase in histological alterations of the testis, a doubling of abnormal sperm and hypospadias, hypoplastic prostate, and cryptorchid testes with carcinoma in situ-like cells were present in 1/17 DBP-treated male rabbits.

Environmental Estrogens

Methoxychlor (M) is an estrogenic pesticide that produces a variety of estrogen-like effects on the male and female rats. This pesticide requires metabolic activation in order to display full endocrine activity in vitro. The active metabolites of M bind ER and activate estrogen-dependent gene expression in vitro (Wilson *et al.*, 2005) and in vivo in the female rat, M stimulates a uterotrophic response, accelerates VO and induces constant estrus, reduces ovarian weight lacking corpora lutea and infertility in the female rat (Gray *et al.*, 1989; Chapin, 1997). Ovarian function also is altered by M exposure. In the ovariectomized female rat, M also induces estrogen-dependent reproductive and nonreproductive behaviors (Gray *et al.*, 1988b) including female sex behaviors, running wheel activity, and food consumption. Unlike estradiol, M is as effective, or is more effective, when administered orally than when it is injected.

When given to the dam during pregnancy and lactation both male and female offspring are affected, with females being the more sensitive gender with effects ranging from VO at 5 mg/kg/day and above and infertility at 100 mg/kg/day and above. At 50 mg/kg/day F_1 females display irregular estrous cycles and reduced fecundity.

F_1 male fertility is unaffected at dose levels up to 200 mg/kg/day, even though they do display permanent reductions in testis and other reproductive organ weights at 50 mg/kg/day and above.

EE is a synthetic derivative of estradiol that is very bioactive orally. This estrogen is in almost all modern formulations of combined oral contraceptive pills. Over time, formulations have decreased the EE dose from as high as 100 μg/day to as low as 20 μg/day. EE is found in many aquatic systems contaminated by sewage effluents, originating principally from human excretion. Along with natural steroidal estrogens, EE plays a major role in causing widespread endocrine disruption in wild populations of fish species and other lower vertebrate species (Jobling and Tyler, 2006).

In the immature SD and Wistar female rats, 0.3 μg/kg/day of EE is effective in inducing uterine weight when given sc, whereas orally 1.0 μg EE/kg/day stimulates uterine weight (Kanno *et al.*, 2001).

Administration of 0.5 mg EE/kg/day accelerates VO by five to seven days and induces vaginal cornification in LE and SD weanling rats. When administered to the dam during gestation and lactation over a broad dose response (0.05-50 μg/kg/day) range, F1 female LE rats display a variety of reproductive tract lesions including cleft phallus, accelerated VO, and infertility at 5 and 50 μg/kg/day whereas F1 males are less severely affected. F1 males did not display any reproductive tract malformations and seminal vesicle, ventral prostate and other androgen-dependent organ weights were not affected at any dose whereas testis and epididymal weights were reduced at 50 μg EE/kg/day. In a similar study with the SD rat, EE was only affected F1 females at 50 μg/kg/day and it was reported that they were not infertile and no effects were noted in the male offspring (Sawaki *et al.*, 2003).

EDC Screening Programs

In response to the 1996 legislative mandate for an endocrine screening and testing program, the EPA formed the Endocrine Disruptor Screening and Testing Advisory Committee (EDSTAC), which proposed a tiered screening and testing strategy for EDCs in its final report in 1998 (http://www.epa.gov/scipoly/oscpendo/history/finalrpt.htm). The EDSTAC proposal included the following: (1) a process to prioritize chemicals for evaluation and recommendations, for (2) screening (Tier 1), and for (3) testing (Tier 2) batteries. The recommended screening battery was designed to detect alterations of HPG function; estrogen, androgen, and thyroid hormone synthesis; and androgen receptor (AR) and estrogen receptor (ER)-mediated effects on mammals and other taxa. Based on a "weight-of-evidence" analysis, chemicals positive in Tier 1 would be considered as potential EDCs and subjected to testing (Tier 2). Equivocal effects in Tier 1 could be replicated or evaluated further in additional short-term assays before more extensive Tier 2 testing was initiated. Tier 1 should include assays sensitive enough to detect EDCs, whereas issues of "dose-response, relevance of the route of exposure, sensitive life stages, and adversity" would be resolved in the Tier 2 testing phase.

In Vivo Mammalian Assays EDSTAC recommended the laboratory rat as the species of choice for the endocrine screening and testing assays. In vitro assays can produce false-positive responses at high concentrations due to a lack of specificity as assay conditions deteriorate. Although such false-positives can be eliminated by experimental measurement of Ki values, few in vitro screening strategies include Ki determinations to insure that the effects seen on binding and gene expression assays are the result of competitive inhibition of ER or AR. As a result, a high

Table 20-6

Chemicals Examined in Protocols of the Organisation for Economic Cooperation and Development (OECD) and the US Environmental Protection Agency (EPA), Using Standardized Assays With Oral or Subcutaneous Dosing

OECD uterotrophic assay (four protocols—all successfully identified each chemical)
Ethinyl estradiol: positive estrogenic control
Genistein: phytoestrogen
Methoychlor: estrogenic and antiandrogenic pesticide
Nonylphenol: estrogenic "inert" ingredient and surfactant
o,p'-DDT: estrogenic pesticide
Bisphenol A: estrogenic plastic monomer
ZM 189,154: antiestrogenic pharmaceutical
Dibutyl phthalate: negative control; plasticizer that inhibits testis Leydig cells

OECD Hershberger assay (each chemical successfully identified)
Testosterone propionate: androgenic positive control
Trenbolone: androgenic veterinary pharmaceutical
Methyltestosterone: potent androgenic pharmaceutical
Linuron: antiandrogenic herbicide
p,p'-DDE: antiandrogenic pesticide metabolite
Flutamide: potent antiandrogenic pharmaceutical
Finasteride: potent inhibitor of enzyme 5α reductase required for DHT synthesis and full androgen-dependent growth of some sex accessory tissues
Vinclozolin: antiandrogenic fungicide
Procymidone: antiandrogenic fungicide

EPA in utero–lactational protocol (partially successful in identifying estrogenicity)
Methoxychlor: estrogenic and antiandrogenic pesticide

EPA execution of adult intact male assay (did not successfully identify endocrine activity of either chemical)
Linuron: antiandrogenic herbicide
Methoxychlor: estrogenic and antiandrogenic pesticide

percentage of screened chemicals that are determined to be "positives" in vitro may not be true receptor ligands. Finally, because in vitro screening assays are unable to integrate the endocrine responses seen in the whole organism, the relationships between endocrine toxicity and other systemic effects cannot be simulated in vitro. To avoid the limitations described above, the EDSTAC proposed three short-term in vivo mammalian assays for the Tier 1 Screening Battery: the uterotrophic, Hershberger, and pubertal female rat assays (Gray *et al.*, 1997a, 2002; Gray, 1998). Table 20-6 indicates the range of EDCs tested in validating these assays for use in the screening program

Uterotrophic Assay Estrogen agonists and antagonists are detected in a three-day uterotrophic assay using subcutaneous administration of the test compound. Based on the evaluation of four variations of the uterotrophic assay protocol in the OECD interlaboratory studies, all of the protocols have produced acceptable responses without regard to rat strain, diet, or housing conditions (Owens and Ashby, 2002; Kanno *et al.*, 2003a,b; Owens *et al.*, 2003, 2006; Owens and Koeter, 2003). The selected uterotrophic assays for estrogens and antiestrogens use either the intact juvenile or the castrated ovariectomized adult/juvenile female rat.

Hershberger Assay The second in vivo assay in T1S, the Hershberger assay, detects antiandrogenic activity simply by weighing androgen-dependent tissues in the castrated male rat (Gray *et al.*, 1997a, 2002; Gray, 1998; Hershberger *et al.*, 1953). In this assay, weights of the ventral prostate, Cowper's glands, seminal vesicle (with coagulating glands and fluids), glans penis, and levator ani/bulbocavernosus muscles are measured in castrated, testosterone-treated (or untreated) male rats after 10 days

of oral treatment with the test compound. This assay is very sensitive for detection of androgens and antiandrogens. Other useful end points that help reveal the mechanism of action and specificity of the response include weights of the adrenal, liver, and kidney, and measurements of serum (collected by cardiac puncture) levels of testosterone and LH. The Hershberger assay shows high sensitivity and specificity to chemicals with AR-mediated activity. Weakly antiandrogenic pesticides such as *p,p*'-DDE and linuron are easily detected in the Hershberger assay (Lambright *et al.*, 2000; Yamasaki *et al.*, 2003). Chemicals such as finasteride, which inhibit 5α-reductase activity, also are active in this assay. They dramatically reduce male accessory sex gland weight with less effect on the levator ani/bulbocavernosus muscle, which has low levels of this enzyme. Chemicals that are positive in the Hershberger assay often produce adverse effects during puberty and after in utero exposure.

Pubertal Female Rat Assay The third in vivo mammalian/rat assay included in the screening battery is the pubertal female rat assay, which has been in use for nearly two decades (Gray *et al.*, 1988a, 1989). In this assay, weanling female rats are dosed daily by gavage for 21 days while the age at VO (puberty) is monitored. The females are necropsied at about 42 days of age (reviewed by Goldman *et al.*, 2000). Measurements include serum thyroid hormones, uterine and ovarian weight, and histology. This assay detects alterations in thyroid hormone status, HPG function, inhibition of steroidogenesis, estrogens, and antiestrogens, and has been found to be highly reproducible and very sensitive to certain endocrine activities including estrogenicity, inhibition of steroidogenesis, and antithyroid activity.

Alternative Screening Assays Alternative in vivo assays were also discussed by EDSTAC and are being evaluated by the EPA. If they are of sufficient sensitivity, specificity, and relevance, they might replace or augment current T1S assays. However, whether they meet such criteria remains to be determined.

Pubertal Male Rat Assay One promising alternative assay is the pubertal male rat assay (Stoker *et al.*, 2000), which detects alterations of thyroid function, HPG maturation, steroidogenesis, and altered steroid hormone function (androgen). Intact weanling males are exposed to the test substance for approximately 30 days. The age at puberty is determined by measuring the age at PPS, and reproductive tissues are evaluated and serum taken for optional hormonal analyses. The studies conducted on contract for EPA using the pubertal male assay are also presented on the EPA EDSP web site. This assay produced reproducible responses among different laboratories and was sensitive to androgens and antiandrogens.

In Utero–Lactational Assay The EDSTAC recommended that the EPA develop and evaluate an in utero–lactational assay due to the unique sensitivity of the fetal reproductive system to disruption by some toxicants. For example, 2,3,7,8-TCDD (dioxin) alters sexual differentiation of male and female rats and hamsters at dosage levels approximately two orders of magnitude below those required to produce adverse effects in pubertal or adult rats (Gray *et al.*, 1997b,c; Stoker *et al.*, 2000). One version of the proposed in utero–lactational assay now being evaluated by the EPA takes about 80 days and uses approximately 10 litters per group (120–150 pups). In this protocol, androgens and antiandrogens can be detected in approximately two to three weeks, and EDCs with antithyroid activity can be detected in infant or weanling offspring after four to five weeks of maternal treatment.

It is important to retain flexibility in the selection of new assays and end points for the screening and testing program so that new methods can be used as replacements or to augment the assays if they offer distinct advantages over the current battery of assays. Enhancements to current life cycle and multigenerational tests are also being considered in an effort to improve the quality of the data on EDCs that will be used for risk assessments. Scientists are attempting to minimize animal use by using as few animals as possible in the most precise and sensitive assays, by incorporating sensitive in vitro assays in T1S, and by using quantitative structure activity relationships (QSAR) models or high throughput prescreening assays in the prioritization of chemicals for use in vivo. It is also possible to avoid unwarranted animal use because chemicals negative in T1S are not subject to T2T. In addition, testing statistical "false positives" can be almost entirely eliminated by ensuring that T1S assay results are replicated in T1.5 before moving to T2T. Attempts to enhance T2T by adding more sensitive end points and a more thorough assessment of the animals already on study may also lead to additional reductions in animal use.

TESTING FOR REPRODUCTIVE TOXICITY

Screens and Multigeneration Studies

The testing of materials for reproductive toxicity has been refined over many decades to provide more comprehensive assessments of a test material's ability to affect the reproductive cycle in laboratory animal models and provide appropriate information to estimate potential risk of exposure to humans. The history and evolution of reproductive toxicity guidelines for pharmaceuticals have recently been reviewed (Collins, 2006). The types of protocols and guidelines employed depend on the type of chemical being tested and its intended use(s). For example, this would involve extensive and comprehensive testing of a food use pesticide, where all the population may be exposed, while much more limited information would be required for a specific drug (eg, used to treat women for menopausal symptoms). In the specific drug case, the experimentation required would be directed at the "target" life stage(s).

It should also be noted that comprehensive testing for reproductive toxicity normally involves the simultaneous exposures of both males and females. Only with specific protocol amendments will the affected sex(es) be determined (eg, exposure of one sex, or a cross-over mating study design in which treated males and females are mated with the corresponding control animals). The details below apply to the rat, the most common species employed in reproductive toxicity studies. Suitable amendments can be made for other species (the mouse is sometimes used) and nonhuman primates occasionally employed—particularly for testing drugs.

A significant amount of attention has also been focused on the development of "screens" for reproductive toxicity as opposed to the more definitive protocols usually found in testing guidelines. Such a need has arisen primarily for the evaluation of the 80,000 chemicals used in commerce, which have no reproductive toxicity testing information. Thus, the screens currently employed (and particularly the OECD 421 and 422 guidelines) have been developed to prioritize chemicals for more comprehensive testing. Whereas such screening approaches can identify chemicals that have adverse effects on reproductive function, the dosing regimes, endpoints employed, number of dose levels used, etc serve only to provide a signal, albeit that the basic information is of a quality to set dose levels, or highlight potential areas of issue in more detailed studies. More problematic is what to do with negative data from these screens as these *do not* imply that the chemical tested is without reproductive toxicity, and may still present a risk to humans. Thus, the outcomes from such screens can be summarized as "*a positive response is a positive, but a negative response is a maybe.*" More detailed information on the proposed screening battery for EDCs is provided in section "Endocrine Disruption (Including Screening and Puberty)."

The most comprehensive assessment of reproductive toxicity would be provided by a protocol that exposes the animal model throughout the reproductive cycle (see Fig. 20-1) and involves the assessment of multiple end points at different life stages during this continuous exposure. The protocol and guideline coming closest to this ideal is the multigeneration reproduction study used for the assessment of chemicals, pesticides, and some food additives (OECD 416, EPA OPPTS 870.3800, FDA "redbook" and the NTP Reproductive Assessment by Continuous Breeding [RACB]). These all represent variations on the general theme noted in Figs. 20-28 and 20-29, and the reader is pointed to the specific guidelines for more detailed explanation of the differences. In general, parental (F_0) animals are exposed for approximately 10 weeks prior to mating (based on the duration of the spermatogenic wave of eight weeks and the passage of sperm through the epididymis and the availability of mature sperm for fertilization; see Fig. 20-16). Exposure continues through mating (and after the mating pairs are separated) continues through gestation, birth, and lactation. Litters maybe "standardized" to ensure equal lactational demand on the dams and normalize the growth of pups (litters are usually reduced to four males and four females per litter on PND 4). At weaning, F_1 litters are usually culled to one male and one female that are raised and exposed until adulthood and the exposure continues through the same processes in the second breeding generation, which usually halts at weaning of the F_2 pups. These studies normally have at least three dose levels (with the highest dose level designed to induce some toxicity) and at least 20 litters produced per dose

Multigeneration reproduction study

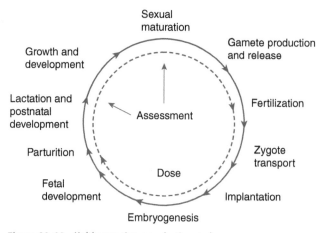

Figure 20-28. *Multigeneration reproduction study.*

group. The RACB study is unusual in that two to three litters are produced in each generation and in its latest form, four males and females are retained from the last F_1 and F_2 litters to adulthood. These multigeneration studies normally encompass detailed measurements of reproductive performance (number of pregnant females from number of pairs mated, number of females producing a litter, litter size, number of live pups with their birth weights, and sex). Measurement of growth and analysis of the reproductive

organs in the F_0 parental generation is conducted (including specific evaluations of ovarian follicles, estrous cyclicity, and sperm parameters). Similar measurements to those undertaken for the F_0 are made on the F_1 parents, but in addition offspring are normally carefully examined at birth (and sexually dimorphic end points may be collected such as AGD), at weaning, and at puberty (particularly the assessment of VO and time of first estrus in females and balanopreputial separation in males) in addition to the adult measurements of reproductive performance, organ weights, histology, etc. In the EPA multigeneration study design, only 10 adult animals per sex, per group, and per generation are required to have their tissues evaluated histologically. For the OECD 416 design, this number is increased to 20 per sex per group (ie, each male and female selected for breeding in the F_1 generation).

Generally, only one mating is performed per generation, but in the presence of equivocal data, or clear indications that effects are becoming more adverse in succeeding generations, then extra litters or generations may be added to the standard designs to clarify potential reproductive toxicity.

Testing for Endocrine Disrupting Chemicals

In a tiered screening and testing approach, only chemicals that display positive reproducible responses in Tier 1 screening (T1S—see the "Endocrine Disruption (Including Screening and Puberty)" section) or T1.5 would be evaluated further in full life cycle or multigenerational tests. In Tier 2 testing (T2T), not T1S, issues of

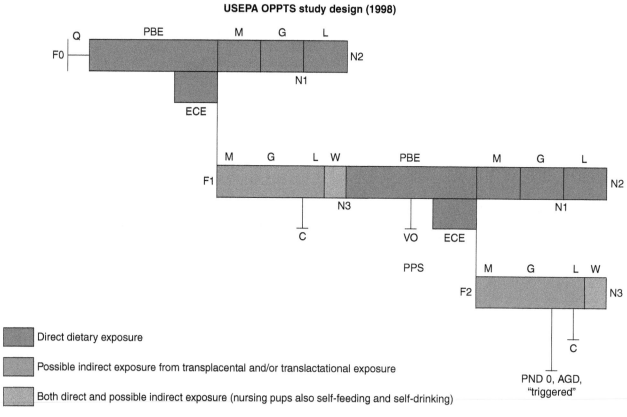

Figure 20-29. *Multigeneration reproduction study as recommended by EPA.* Key for the rat: Q, Quarantine (one week); PBE, prebreed exposure (10 weeks); M, mating (two weeks); G, gestation (three weeks); L, lactation (three weeks); VO, vaginal opening (evaluated in F1 females on postnatal day 22 to acquisition); PPS, preputial separation (evaluated in F1 males on postnatal day 35 to acquisition); W, weaning (postnatal day 21); N1, necropsy of all paternal animals (organ weights, histology, and andrological assessments); N2, necropsy of all maternal animals (organ weights, histology, and ovarian follicle assessments); N3, necropsy of selected weanlings, three/sex/litter, if possible (organ weights); ECE, estrous cyclicity evaluation (three weeks); C, Cull litters to ten pups (with equal sex ratio) on postnatal day 4; AGD, anogenital distance measured in F2 pups on postnatal day 0 if triggered by effects on F1 reproductive development; N, necropsy.

dose-response, relevance of the route of exposure, sensitive life stages, and adversity are resolved. For some endocrine activities, the number of sensitive end points and F_1 offspring examined in these assays should be expanded on a case-by-case basis.

AGD at birth and nipple/areola retention in infant female and male rats should be included in testing of androgens and antiandrogens, respectively, because they are sensitive, potentially permanent effects that are highly correlated with malformations and reproductive organ weight changes later in life (McIntyre et al., 2001). These early alterations constitute part of the antiandrogen-induced developmental syndromes. The syndrome induced by the AR antagonists differs to some degree from that induced by the phthalates, which inhibit the synthesis of fetal testosterone and insulin-like 3 peptide (insl-31) hormones.

Developmental Syndromes and Tailored Testing A careful evaluation of the male rat offspring allows one to distinguish the "phthalate syndrome," in which effects on reproductive development involve a decrease in fetal testicular testosterone and insl-3 peptide hormone biosynthesis (Gray et al., 2002; Mylchreest and Foster, 2000; Mylchreest et al., 1999; Parks et al., 2001; Wilson et al., 2004) from the "AR antagonist syndrome," induced by vinclozolin (Gray et al., 1994, 1999b; Lim et al., 2001) or flutamide (McIntyre et al., 2001). The main distinction between the two syndromes is that the phthalate syndrome includes agenesis of the testis, epididymis, and gubernacular cord. These lesions are rarely seen in the AR antagonist syndrome, even when all of the males display hypospadias. In addition, of all chemicals that interfere with the androgen-signaling pathway in the fetal male rat, only the phthalates affect Leydig cell insl-3 hormone synthesis and cause undescended testes due to gubernacular agenesis (Wine et al., 1997).

In contrast to the antiandrogens, which primarily affect the male offspring (see Table 20-7), in utero exposure to androgenic chemicals has more severe consequences for the female offspring (see Table 20-8). It is important to consider this information when tailoring T2T based on T1S results. For example, when the female rat fetus is exposed to testosterone (Hotchkiss et al., 2007) or the veterinary pharmaceutical trenbolone, agenesis of the vagina and nipples is seen at a low rate in the lower dosage groups. In fact, most of the low-dose effects of androgens in the female offspring (retained prostatic and vesicular tissues and nipple agenesis; Wolf et al., 2002; Hotchkiss et al., 2007) are effects that are likely to be missed in a standard necropsy.

When conducting a multigenerational study, it is important to summarize the data in a manner that clearly delineates the proportion of animals that are affected, indicating that they display any lesion (histological or gross pathology) consistent with the syndrome. In teratology studies, data are typically presented and analyzed in this manner, indicating the number of malformed/number observed on an individual and litter basis, whereas multigenerational studies are frequently presented and analyzed differently, even when clear teratogenic and other developmental responses are noted after birth. Multigenerational protocols are used in T2T because only these protocols expose the animals during all critical stages of development and examine reproductive function of offspring after they mature.

Although the new EPA multigenerational test provides for a comprehensive evaluation of the F_0 or parental generation, too few F_1 animals (offspring with developmental exposure) are examined after maturity to detect anything but the most profound reproductive teratogens (Gray and Foster, 2004). F_0 animals within a dose group typically respond in a similar fashion to the chemical exposure;

however, the response to toxicants in utero can vary greatly even within a litter with only a few animals displaying severe reproductive malformations in the lower dosage groups. For example, dose-related adverse reproductive effects are seen in less than 10% of the F_1 offspring treated in utero with the phthalate DINP (male reproductive malformations, Gray et al., 2000); 2,3,7,8-TCDD (permanent vaginal threads and ovarian atrophy, Gray et al., 1997c); in utero busulfan (ovarian atrophy and delayed puberty, Gray and Ostby, 1998); DEHP (epididymal and testicular lesions), and linuron (McIntyre et al., 2000), epididymal and testicular hypoplasia, and androgens (vaginal and nipple agenesis, Wolf et al., 2002). Thus, a standard multigenerational protocol that examines only one F_1 animal per sex, per litter after maturity from 20 litters per dosage group, can detect statistically significant alterations only when they are displayed by 25% or more of the offspring. Histopathological alterations must be displayed by 50% or more of the offspring because a histological examination of the reproductive tract is required only in 10 F_1 animals per sex, per dose—far too few to detect anything but the most profound effects on reproductive development. Such an approach would also create uncertainty associated with lowest observed adverse effect levels ("LOAELs") and no observed adverse effect levels ("NOAELs") identified in multigenerational studies for chemicals that do not include either a complete assessment of all of the end points that constitute the syndrome, or those included in the EPA new Multigenerational Test Guidelines.

In "transgenerational" protocols (Gray, 1998; Gray and Ostby, 1995; Gray et al., 1994, 1997c, 1999a,b, 2002; McIntyre et al., 2000, 2001; Mylchreest et al., 1998, 2000), we typically use fewer litters (7–10 per dose group), but examine all of the animals in each litter. These protocols actually use fewer animals, but provide enhanced statistical power to detect reproductive effects in the F_1 generation. Additional factors, besides detection of adverse effects at necropsy or during data analysis and interpretation, limit interpretation of data from the standard multigenerational reproduction test. The lifelong exposure of both males and females in the F_1 generation, which allows one to detect effects induced in utero, during lactation, or from direct exposure after puberty, can confound the identification of when the effect was induced (ie, during adulthood vs. development) or even the affected sex. In studies, where the dosing period normally is terminated near birth or at weaning, precludes misinterpretation of the developmental origin of reproductive effects. Nevertheless, it is clear that transgenerational protocols would not be appropriate for EDCs that induce low-dose alterations in the pubertal or adult animal in the F_0 generation.

Test Design and Numbers of F_1 Animals It is important to reiterate that the end points described above, which are sensitive to antiandrogens or androgens in utero (listed in detail in Gray and Foster, 2004), are not sensitive to xenoestrogens or some other EDCs. Thus not all EDCs should be tested similarly to the androgens or antiandrogens. Testing should be tailored based on the pharmacological activity demonstrated in T1S. In addition, the developing fetus is not always the most sensitive life stage. Some EDCs disrupt pregnancy by altering maternal ovarian hormone production in F_0 dams at dosage levels that appear to be without direct effect on the offspring (Gray et al., 1999b). In such cases, the standard EPA multigenerational protocol with minor enhancements would be recommended, or a transgenerational protocol with exposure continued after weaning. The transgenerational or in utero–lactational protocols (see Fig. 20-30) fill a gap in the testing program for EDCs that should be used only on a case-by-case basis, as indicated by the results of T1S and any Tier 1 repeat study.

Table 20-7

Detecting Developmental Reproductive Syndromes in Male Rat Offspring

Neonatal-infantile data
1. Anogenital distance at birth (1–3 days of age)
2. Areola/nipple retention in infant male rats at 13–14 days of age

External necropsy end points on all male rat offspring at maturity
1. Body weight any unusual malformations or anomalies, euthanize
2. Shave ventral surface from inguinal region to neck and count nipples and areolas (observer blind to treatment), record position of areolas and nipples.
3. Check animals for hypospadias, epispadias, cleft phallus, and measure AGD
4. Note if testes obviously undescended
5. Note if inguinal region soiled with urine
6. Note if prepuce partially or entirely detached from glans penis, especially if a persistent thread of tissue is present along frenulum.

Internal end points on all male rat offspring at maturity
1. Location of each testis (scrotal, abdominal, and gubernaclum attached to abdominal wall)
2. Gubernacular cords, present or absent, and length in mm if abnormal
3. Note if present, cranial suspensory ligaments
4. Note if testes are small, absent, fluid filled, enlarged, appear infected or other
5. Note if epididymides are small, absent, or infected (record region of effects)
6. Note if ventral prostate is small, absent, or infected
7. Note if dorsolateral prostate is small, absent, or infected
8. Note if seminal vesicles are small, absent, infected, or one side larger than the other
9. Note if coagulating glands are small absent, infected, one side larger than the other or detached from seminal vesicles.
10. Note if kidneys display hydronephrosis, calcium deposits
11. Note the presence of hydroureter
12. Note the presence of bladder stones or bloody in bladder

Weigh the following organs on all male rat offspring at maturity
1. Each testis individually (examine histology of each testis)
2. Each corpus plus caput epididymis (examine histology of each segment)
3. Each cauda epididymis (examine histology of each segment)
4. Entire seminal vesicle, plus coagulating glands with fluid as a unit, if possible
5. Entire ventral prostate, if possible
6. Each kidney
7. Paired adrenals
8. Liver
9. Levator ani plus bulbocavernosus
10. Cowper's glands as a pair, if possible
11. Glans penis
12. Pituitary
13. Brain

Histology on all male F_1 offspring at maturity
1. Both testes
2. Both epididymides
3. Prostate glands
4. Any grossly abnormal reproductive tissues

Multitude of effects of antiandrogens in male rat offspring that should be evaluated in Tier 2 testing studies displaying this activity in Tier 1 screening or other assays.

Testing Pharmaceuticals

In the case of pharmaceuticals, it is rare for multigeneration studies to be conducted, because it is not common for all the population to use a specific drug and that exposure to the drug is not necessarily chronic and over many different life stages. Typically, three specific studies are undertaken based on the recommendations of the International Conference on Harmonization of Guidelines S5A: Detection of toxicity to reproduction for medicinal products (see Collins, 2006 for specific study descriptions) although any permutation or specific design is open to the investigator to explore

specific toxicity based on the pharmacology of the drug tested. The three "most likely" studies are as follows:

1. *A study of fertility and early embryonic development* (see Fig. 20-31). Parental adults are exposed to the test chemical for two weeks (females) or four weeks (males) prior to breeding and then during breeding. Females then continue their exposure through to implantation. Males can be necropsied for the end points noted above for the multigeneration studies after pregnancy has been confirmed, and for the pregnant females, necropsy takes place any time after mid-gestation.

Table 20-8

Detecting Developmental Reproductive Syndromes in Female Rat Offspring

Neonatal-infantile data in female rat offspring
1. Anogenital distance at birth (1–3 days of age)
2. Areola/nipple agenesis (complete or faint) in infant female rats at 13–14 days of age

External necropsy end points on all female rat offspring at maturity
1. Body weight any unusual malformations or anomalies, euthanize
2. Shave ventral surface from inguinal region to neck and count nipples and areolas (observer blind to treatment), record position of areolas and nipples
3. Check animals for cleft phallus and measure AGD and position of vaginal opening
4. Note if inguinal region soiled with urine

Internal end points on all female rat offspring at maturity
1. Location of ovaries in relationship to kidneys
2. Note if absent, cranial suspensory ligaments
3. Note if ovaries are small, cystic-fluid filled, enlarged, appear infected, or other
4. Note if oviducts, uterus, or upper or lower vagina are small, absent, or infected (record region of effects) or fluid-filled
5. Note if ventral prostate tissue is present
6. Note if seminal vesicle tissue is present
7. Note if levator ani/bulbocavernosus muscle tissues are present
8. Note if other male tissues are present
9. Note if kidneys display hydronephrosis, calcium deposits
10. Note presence of hydroureter
11. Note presence of bladder stones or blood in bladder

Weigh the following organs in all female offspring at maturity
1. Paired ovaries (histology)
2. Uterus with fluid (histology)
3. Vagina
4. Each kidney
5. Paired adrenals
6. Liver
7. Pituitary
8. Brain

Histology on all female rat offspring at maturity
1. Both ovaries
2. Uterus
3. Vagina
4. Any suspected male reproductive tissues
5. Any grossly abnormal reproductive tissues

Multitude of effects of androgens in female rat offspring that should be evaluated in Tier 2 testing studies.

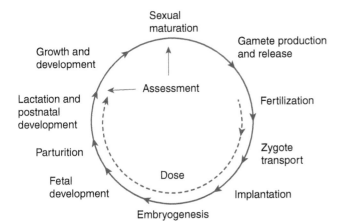

Figure 20-30. *The in utero–lactational study design under review by EPA for the assessment of endocrine active agents.*

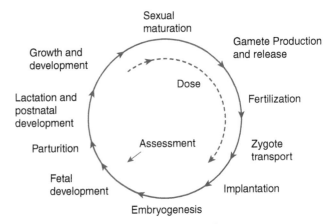

Figure 20-31. *Fertility and early embryonic study.*

Pre-and postnatal development study

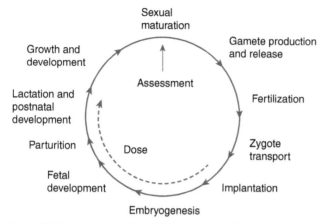

Figure 20-32. *Pre- and postnatal developmental toxicity study.* Dosing is from implantation until the litters are weaned.

Embryo-fetal development study

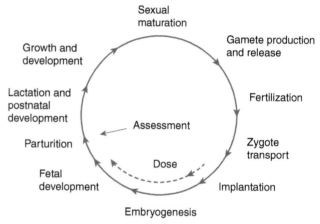

Figure 20-33. *Embryo-fetal developmental toxicity study as used by FDA guidelines.* Dosing starts at implantations and continues to closure of the hard palate with an assessment of fetuses just prior to parturition.

As with the multigeneration study, reproductive and target organs are weighed and examined histologically, sperm parameters are assessed in males and in females, the uterine implantation sites and ovarian *corpora lutea* are counted, as well as live and dead embryos.

In this study design, the selection of the dosing regimen for males has been based on pragmatism in attempting to shorten the study, rather than the biology of spermatogenesis in the test species (as employed in the multigeneration study). It is thought that the majority of chemicals that might affect the male should be detectable (by histology) after four weeks exposure; however, there are a number of exceptions to this notion. One of the significant advantages of the pharmaceutical guideline approach is that the investigator is encouraged to tailor their testing protocols to reflect the best science and available knowledge. One potential disadvantage is that the basic approach does represent a theoretical "gap" as some chemicals may not manifest a testis histological lesion in four weeks and also there is a potential disassociation of structure (testis histology and sperm parameters) from function (male breeding performance).

2. *A study of effects on pre- and post-natal development including maternal function* (see Fig. 20-32). In this study, pregnant females are exposed from implantation until weaning of their offspring (usually PND 21 in the rat). After cessation of exposure, selected offspring (one male and one female per litter) are raised to adulthood and then mated to assess reproductive competence. These animals are observed for maturation and growth (but are not exposed). Puberty indices, as employed in the multigeneration study, are measured. In addition, sensory function, reflexes, motor activity, learning, and memory are also evaluated.

3. *A study of embryo–fetal development* (see Fig. 20-33). This study tests for enhanced toxicity relative to that noted in pregnant females and unlike the previous two studies, is normally conducted in two species (typically the rat and rabbit). Exposure occurs between implantation and closure of the hard palate, and females are killed just prior to parturition. At necropsy, dams are observed for any affected organs and *corpora lutea* are counted. Live and dead fetuses counted and examined for external, visceral, and skeletal abnormalities. In the evaluation of prenatal developmental toxicity for a pesticide or other chemical (eg, OPPTS 870.3700, OECD 414), exposure of the pregnant dams is usually longer and can be continuous

throughout pregnancy or, more normally, from implantation until just prior to birth (see Fig. 20-34). Other end points measured in the dam and fetuses are identical between the pharmaceutical embryo-fetal toxicity study and that employed for evaluation of an industrial chemical or pesticide.

The FDA Center for Drug Evaluation and Research produced a draft guidance document in 2001 that explored how data should be passed through an integrative process to assess a drug for reproductive toxicity. The tool is used in a tiered manner consisting of three sections: (1) methods applicable to all datasets, (2) approaches applicable only to datasets without evidence of reproductive and developmental toxicity, and (3) approaches applicable to datasets with positive indications of reproductive and/or developmental toxicity. This integration would provide one of three summary risk conclusions that would be applied to the drug label namely—(1) not anticipated to produce reproductive and/or developmental effects above the background incidence for humans when used in accordance with the dosing information on the product label; (2) the drug may increase the incidence of adverse reproductive and/or developmental events, or (3) that the drug is expected to increase the incidence of adverse reproductive and/or developmental effects in humans when used according to the product label.

EPA prenatal developmental toxicity study

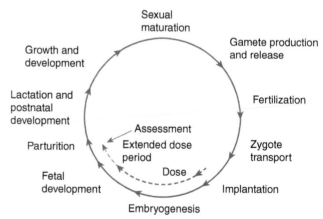

Figure 20-34. *Prenatal developmental toxicity study as used by EPA and OECD.* Note the extended dose period compared with that used in Fig. 20-33.

Single generation reproduction study

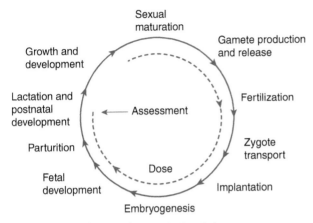

Figure 20-35. *Single generation reproduction study.*

An examination of the reproductive cycle in a comparison of these three most likely options for FDA studies indicates an obvious gap in the exposure regime for the complete reproductive cycle, namely exposure of weanlings through puberty to adulthood. However, there has been significant interest in the safe use of pharmaceuticals in pediatric populations, and unlike the more standard reproductive and developmental studies, specific studies on juvenile animals are usually performed on a case-by-case basis. The number of these types of studies has also been increasing and whether these could be combined with more standard approaches in a targeted fashion to, for example, evaluate behavioral testing after extended exposure postweaning (as would be conducted in a standard, pre- and postnatal study) or have cohabitation for assessment of fertility and fecundity of the offspring (see reviews by Hurtt *et al.*, 2004; Cappon *et al.*, 2009).

The single generation reproduction study (OECD 415) is used more frequently in Europe where specific testing guidelines for reproductive toxicity may be triggered by the tonnage production of a specific chemical. This design (see Fig. 20-35) has a common F_0 parental exposure period to that used in the multigeneration guideline (OECD multigeneration study—416). Estimates are made of the standard litter parameters and reproductive performance of the F_0 parents, but in this design the study halts at the weaning of the F_1 offspring and no estimate is made of effects on adult F_1 offspring,

nor on the ability of this generation to reproduce. This study design provides critical information on parental reproductive effects, but has very limited information on the offspring aside from pup number, growth, and survival to weaning, and thus has limited utility in the estimation of transgenerational effects, or postnatal reproductive consequences.

Newer Guidelines and Approaches

The International Life Sciences Institute sponsored a new endeavor looking at how agricultural chemicals might be assessed for toxicity, including reproductive toxicity in a proposed life stage approach (Cooper *et al.*, 2006) using an extended one-generation study (see Fig. 20-36) in the rat. This approach incorporated many of the changes made more recently to testing guidelines (including extra endocrine-related end points) and attempted to streamline the testing of agrochemicals for toxicity. The life stages protocol was one of a tiered set of proposed studies, such that all data available could be incorporated into the study design and interpretation of the data. The approach was very laudable in that it proposed (unfortunately only as an option) incorporation of toxicokinetic data generated during pregnancy and lactation into the study design, as has long been required in drug testing, to aid study design and data interpretation. In addition, end points evaluating (at least to some degree) developmental neurotoxicity and developmental immunotoxicity would be measured as a standard, rather than as a triggered option. Its major aim was to reduce the number of animals required and increase the information available on young animals. However, these compromises were not without some flaws compared to the current multigeneration study used for pesticides by EPA or OECD. The study would seek to be a substitute for the current multigeneration study in most instances. The proposal does offer the opportunity to undertake a classical multigeneration study in a second tier, but only if an adverse event was found in the Tier 1 study. Thus, a negative in the extended one-generation study could mean a halt to testing for reproductive toxicity. In particular, the paper recommends the use of the shortened exposure period before breeding the parental animals, similar to that implied in the International Conference on Harmonization of Guidelines (ICH) for fertility and early embryonic development, but it is much harder to justify that pesticides and other agricultural agents, unlike drugs, will not have human exposure at least subchronically and moreover

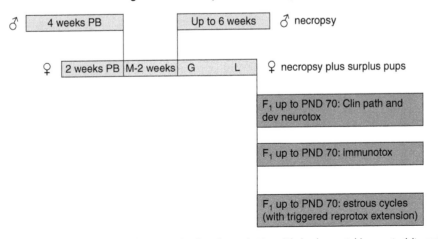

Figure 20-36. *The ILSI/ACSA life stages study for the evaluation of reproduction with developmental immunotoxicity and neurotoxicity.*

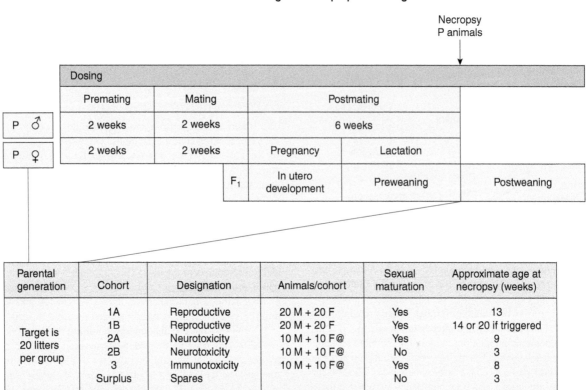

Figure 20-37. *Diagrammatic representation of the draft OECD extended one generation reproduction study.* OECD (2010), OECD Guideline for the testing of chemicals http://www.oecd.org/chemicalsafety/testingofchemicals/46466062.pdf.

the divorce of reproductive structure (eg, histopathology of the reproductive organs) from function (eg, litter parameters) could have serious implications for classification and labeling in some parts of the world.

In Europe, the advent of REACH (Registration, Evaluation, Authorization and Restriction of Chemical substances) was likely to require increased toxicity testing of chemicals at the same time that other efforts were seeking to reduce experimental animal usage. Significant attention was therefore focused on those assays that required (or produced) the largest number of experimental animals—the multigeneration reproduction study and the prenatal developmental toxicity study (usually conducted in two species). The OECD took up the challenge of finding a study that would provide adequate information for the evaluation of reproductive toxicity, but would also reduce animal numbers and has proposed a study (the extended one-generation reproduction study, based on the Cooper *et al.*'s design) for adoption (see Fig. 20-37; the final draft is available on line at http://www.oecd.org/dataoecd/23/10/46466062.pdf). It is proposed to be used for all chemicals (not just pesticides), where a much reduced toxicity database is likely to be available.

As our knowledge of critical windows of exposure has increased, particularly with the increased focus on chemicals that may have endocrine-like activity, the last 15 years has shown the need for a study where there has been a larger focus on the evaluation of potential postnatal adverse outcomes. Thus, there have been updates to standard designs to incorporate more functional end points (eg, sperm and oocyte analysis, vaginal cytology, indices of puberty, and sexual differentiation) to improve the detection of chemicals affecting reproduction and the endocrine status of animals. In particular, in current study designs, the ability to evaluate

(both detection and analysis of dose response) abnormalities of the reproductive tract routinely following in utero exposure to chemicals with endocrine activity was determined to be underpowered by several research groups (McIntyre *et al.*, 2002; Hotchkiss *et al.*, 2008; Blystone *et al.*, 2010). For example, in an evaluation of prenatal developmental toxicity, every fetus is examined for potential abnormalities (typically ~250 fetuses per group) whereas in the multigeneration study, only one male and female pup per litter from a minimum of 20 litters is examined at adulthood for adverse pathological events (ie, only 40 of the potential 250 animals/group produced). Some recent studies have shown the added value and increased statistical power of evaluating more offspring per litter by retaining them to adulthood, rather than discarding animals already produced, or performing only a gross examination at weaning, when the reproductive organs are not fully differentiated or developed (see Fig. 20-38; Blystone *et al.*, 2010). The NTP has already adopted the improved use of these animals, in its (RACB) study design, by carrying more animals through adulthood for examination, rather than removing them at weaning.

Following a workshop held by the NTP on the evaluation of tumors of the endocrine system in rodent models (Thayer and Foster, 2007), the program adopted a new default paradigm for its rat cancer bioassays that incorporates exposure during the perinatal period (ie, gestation and lactation). Before embarking on such a study, it would be customary to undertake a preliminary study that evaluated target organ toxicity (for a conventional cancer study, this would be the 90-day toxicity study) and enabled suitable dose levels to be selected for the cancer bioassay. Thus, for a long-term cancer study involving exposure during pregnancy and lactation, a shorter duration study that involved exposure during these critical developmental windows would be required. The NTP has previously used

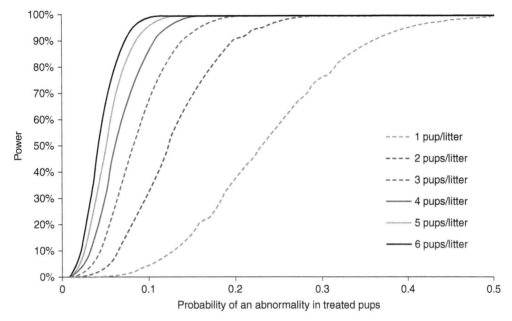

10% incidence detected 4.7% of time with 1 pup; 66.4% 3 pups; 86.5% 4 pups

Figure 20-38. *Power curves for the detection of offspring abnormalities with low background incidence (20 litters, 0% background).* Curves are presented for the probability of detecting an adverse response with increasing numbers of pups retained per litter. Note that with only one pup retained (typically the approach on most reproduction studies) the probability of detecting a 10% response (shown by the *vertical dotted line*) will be only 4.7% for one pup per litter, but 66.4% for three pups per litter and 86.5 for four pups per litter. From Blystone *et al.* (2010).

a study that has exposure for 90 days after the pups are weaned. It became apparent that this basic design could easily be adapted to provide more detailed information on reproduction and development, as well as all the necessary information to select dose levels for the cancer study. Thus, there would be a gain in information on a greater array of toxicity end points and maximize the utility of the animals that had already been produced and raised to weaning, such that the other, "stand alone" reproduction and developmental toxicity studies would not be required.

This new NTP design (see Fig. 20-39) employs pregnant animals with dosing commencing at implantation (gestation day six in the rat) and continually exposes the dams throughout gestation and lactation. At weaning (usually postnatal day 21 in the rat), the offspring would be continued to be administered the test article at the same dose level as their respective dam and are subsequently assigned to a number of different cohorts that can be considered as interchangeable "cassettes" that can be included, or not, based on the objectives of the study, or other available information. These cassettes are essentially protocols used on other standard studies and would normally include:

- An evaluation of target organ toxicity, pathology, clinical pathology, etc, similar to a current 90-day toxicity protocol—*a subchronic toxicity cohort*. This would normally require 10 animals to be evaluated per sex, per dose group.
- An evaluation of prenatal developmental toxicity—*a teratology cohort*. One male and female offspring from each litter would be selected and nonsibling matings would be performed in each group on reaching sexual maturity (~PND 110). Just prior to expected delivery, a Cesarean section would be performed on the pregnant dams for a standard evaluation of external, visceral, and skeletal abnormalities of the fetuses.
- An evaluation of breeding performance—*a littering cohort*. One male and female offspring from each litter would be selected and nonsibling matings would be performed in each

group on reaching sexual maturity (~PND 110). The pregnant dams would be allowed to deliver their litters and raise them to weaning.

On a specific case basis, other cassettes could be added, or substituted, in the protocol, including an assessment of developmental immunotoxicity and/or developmental neurotoxicity, using other standard guideline protocols.

The study would normally be conducted in the rat with a sufficient number of time-mated animals would be acquired to ensure a minimum of 20 litters per dose group with normally three dose levels, plus a vehicle control. The normal route of exposure employed on such studies would be oral (eg, dosed feed, drinking water, or gavage) and treatment would be continuous throughout the study (for gavage, direct dosing of pups may be required at least from PND 12, or as appropriate from toxicokinetic [TK] information). If no other toxicity information is available, a pilot study with a small number of pregnant dams would be required to set dose levels and potentially acquire preliminary TK data in pregnancy and lactation.

This design emphasizes a full evaluation of the F_1 animals in the study. The design uses significantly fewer animals than a RACB or a multigeneration reproduction study and generates important information on both reproduction and postnatal development, together with a pathological evaluation of all the offspring (after PND 4) when they reach adulthood to improve the ability to detect postnatal effects. A major addition will be the information achieved on prenatal developmental toxicity. The teratology and littering cohorts of animals allow the evaluation of fertility and fecundity and importantly, to maintain the relationship between structural changes in the reproductive organs and functional outcomes in the same animals. In addition, the design will be able to maintain a 10-week exposure period prior to mating of the F_1 animals to ensure that any potential male germ cell effects could be reflected in a functional outcome.

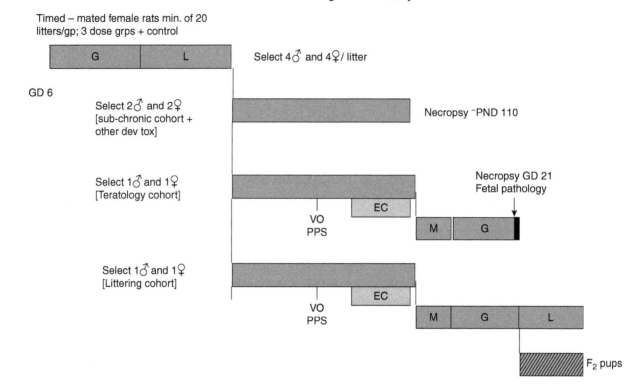

Figure 20-39. *Diagrammatic representation of the NTP modified one generation reproduction study.* Only 10 pups per sex (on reaching adulthood) are required for the subchronic cohort and thus sufficient numbers of animals would be available for evaluations of other developmental toxicity that may include effects on the developing immune or nervous systems. Key: G, Gestation; L, lactation; PND, postnatal day; GD, gestation day; M, mating; VO, vaginal opening; PPS, balanopreputial separation; EC, estrous cyclicity evaluation.

The OECD extended one generation study (Fig. 20-37), while using fewer animals than a typical multigeneration study, does have a number of significant design flaws that have been highlighted at various recent scientific meetings (eg, the Teratology Society/European Teratology Society exchange lectures in 2010; Foster, 2010a,b). Some of these issues include: (1) a truncated exposure period before breeding the F_0 animals that will only produce functional effects in males if the chemical under investigation affects epididymal sperm; (2) a failure to routinely breed F_1 animals and so not provide a full characterization of this unique exposure group; (3) the employment of internal triggers to make decisions on when breeding of the F_1 generation, or utilization of specific cohorts of animals, will occur. In particular, the triggers to be employed do not take into account the timing for the production of data from the various components of the study, to make informed decisions on whether to apply triggers, or not; (4) the adverse structural changes will not be related to functional outcomes in the same animals if the triggers are not applied correctly; and (5) the developmental neurotoxicity cohort is underpowered with only 10 animals/sex/group evaluated. Using this proposed OECD design, one could conduct a reproduction study that does not adequately evaluate fertility and fecundity in any generation.

EVALUATION OF TOXICITY TO REPRODUCTION

Concordance of End Points

As noted in the "Testing For Reproductive Toxicity", our standard testing protocols do not allow for discrimination between male and female effects except by some method modification. However, there is built-in redundancy in the number and type of end points evaluated in these studies that could indicate male, female, or effects on both sexes during testing. The following examples give an outline of the types of end points evaluated typically in rat multigeneration studies (the species most commonly used for reproductive toxicity evaluations).

There are a number of general points that the investigator should note in any estimation of potential reproductive toxicity:

- Adequacy of experimental design and conduct. Was there sufficient statistical power in the evaluation(s)?
- Occurrence of common versus rare reproductive deficits. Biological versus statistical significance.
- Use of historical control data to place concurrent control data into perspective and to estimate population background incidence of various reproductive parameters and deficits.
- Known structure–activity relationships for inducing reproductive toxicity.
- Concordance of reproductive end points (eg, did a decrease in litter size, relate to ovarian histology and changes in vaginal cytology?).
- Did the reproductive deficits become more severe with increases in dose. For example, did histological changes at one dose level become decrements in litter size and then reductions in fertility at higher dose levels in any generation?
- Did the reproductive deficits increase in prevalence (more individuals and/or more litters) with dose level in any generation?
- Special care should be taken for decrements in reproductive parameters noted in the F_1 generation (and potentially later generations) that were not seen in the F_0 generation, which may suggest developmental, as well as reproductive, toxicity.

Likewise, findings in an F_1 generation animal may (or may not) be reproduced in F_2 offspring. For example, effects in the F_1 generation on reproductive parameters may have resulted in the selection out of sensitive animals in the population, thus not producing F_2 offspring for subsequent evaluation.

The first primary indication of a decrement in reproduction is obtained from the inspection of litter parameters from a breeding and determination of any functional effects. Thus, it is normal to inspect for various treatment groups versus the control, the number of fertile pairings, the mean litter size, pup weight at birth (small litters tend to have higher pup weights), and the sex ratio (to determine if there is a selective effect on any one sex).

In the parental females, there should also be an evaluation of potential maternal toxicity that may or may not impact on the reproductive performance of these animals; these measures are crude and usually restricted to body weight, food consumption, and clinical signs. Gestation length is normally recorded (and this may be shortened or lengthened) together with any signs of dystocia. Chemicals with progestin-like activity may also produce midgestational bleeding observable on the fur/or in the cage. At weaning of the litter (usually PND 21 in the rat), the parental females are usually necropsied (if no further pairings are required) and the uteri examined for implantation sites (which can be compared to the number of offspring produced) and the ovaries examined for corpora lutea and corpora albicans. These data are not as definitive for pre- versus postimplantation loss as in the developmental toxicity study because the female will begin to cycle around postnatal day 15 and have representative corpora lutea from both the pregnancy and the new ovarian cycle(s).

In immature females after weaning, measurements can be made of the onset of puberty (which may be accelerated or delayed) through estimates of the date of VO and first estrus from vaginal smears. Some care needs to be used in the impact of other toxicity on these pubertal parameters, and it is usual to normalize based on bodyweight. However, timing of puberty should not be normalized by body weight at acquisition of puberty (since a delay will invariably mean that the females are larger compared to controls and vice versa for acceleration). Instead, it is more likely that the investigator would employ weight at weaning as a covariate in the analysis of these pubertal end points.

As the female matures estimates will be made of estrous cyclicity particularly if they are normal or abnormal (a rat normally has a four–five day cycle) and the duration of the cycles (for example, was persistent estrus or diestrus noted). Vaginal smears are also noted during mating, and the presence of a sperm positive smear would indicate a successful mating that provides at least some surrogate of normal reproductive behavior from the breeding pair.

At necropsy of the adult F_1 female, weights and histopathology would be undertaken on critical organs (eg, ovaries, uterus, pituitary and perhaps adrenal as another steroidogenic organ). Histopathology of the ovary is not straightforward and some guidelines require the evaluation of primordial follicle counts in step sections of the ovary. However, such an examination provides only limited information on one type of follicle and it is essential that the pathologists make their evaluation with regard to the normal expected patterns of the different follicular types (from primordial to antral) and when necessary undertake quantitative analysis to confirm an effect on ovarian follicular development.

In the parental males, similar types of evaluation are available to the investigator with regard to potential parental toxicity. Decreases in fertile pairings and litter size may be equally applicable for the detection of a male effect. The presence of a sperm positive smear in the female is indicative that the male has successfully mounted and mated with the female (note the presence of a copulatory plug is not the same because these may be formed from accessory sex organ fluids in the absence of sperm).

Males going through puberty can be estimated using the date of balanopreputial separation of the penis as an index. This androgen-dependent end point in the male is also corrected for growth, but the same caveats used in the female around normalization of data would apply to this male measurement. Decrements of ~10% body weight are normally without significant effect on male or female puberty indices (Carney et al., 2004). As the male matures and is bred with a female, observation of the precoital interval (the time between pairing and evidence of mating) can indicate treatment related effects on mating performance or behavior. However, it should be noted that if the female is at a random stage of estrus when introduced to the male, she may not allow mating until estrus is attained. Thus, delays of more than four to five days in precoital interval should be carefully examined.

Once a pregnancy has been achieved and there is no requirement for further matings, the parental male is necropsied and organ weights and histological examination conducted usually of the testis, epididymis, prostate, seminal vesicles, and pituitary (and perhaps adrenal as for the female as another steroidogenic organ). Some studies also include other androgen-dependent organ weights such as the Levator ani-bulbocavernosus muscle, Cowper's gland, and penis. As with the ovary, histopathological examination of the testis requires some experience and the pathologist must be familiar with the different stages of the spermatogenic cycle. Although quantitative analysis of stage frequency is rarely required (and not useful in longer term studies), the noting of specific stages that may show a predilection for injury is most helpful, as is an appreciation of the different cellular associations within the seminiferous tubule which is essential in the detection of more subtle testicular effects.

At necropsy, a number of quantitative estimates can be made of sperm production and function. These can include testicular spermatid counts following homogenization (this end point entails destruction of one testis and has to be balanced with the information obtained from histopathology). A sperm sample is also taken from the vas or cauda epididymis for examination of sperm concentration, motility, and morphology, which can be examined using manual methods. More often, computer-assisted sperm analysis is used to evaluate these sperm end points and in addition further parameters can be collected, such as forward progressive motility, which is believed more closely related to fertility. Frequently, whole cauda epididymal sperm counts are also evaluated and normalized by weight.

Evaluation of male and female offspring follows the schema outline above for adults and for animals going through puberty. In addition other useful end points may be included before weaning such as AGD, the presence of nipples and areolae (usually at postnatal day 13 before the pup fur has started to grow excessively to prevent examination), and the presence of certain reproductive tract malformations (see Tables 20-7 and 20-8). AGD and nipple retention are sexually dimorphic in the rat and under androgen control. Thus, normally AGD is twice the distance in males than females (this also seems to hold true for humans) and is dependent on levels of circulating DHT. In the normal male rat fetus, the presence of androgen around gestation day 17 causes the anlagen for the nipples to undergo apoptosis and thus males are born without nipples whereas females have the full complement of 12. The presence of an antiandrogen in males or an androgen in females would upset this balance to produce nipple retention in the males and a reduced number in the females reflective of the androgen status of these animals at critical periods of development. Some assessment must also be made of general growth of the offspring (usually bodyweight).

Consistency Across Generations

The F_0 reproductive parameters can differ markedly from those noted in the F_1 and similarly from the F_2 generation in a multigeneration study. Because exposure in a multigeneration study typically starts with the F_0 generation as young adults, critical periods of reproductive development have already taken place. The phthalates (eg, DBP; Wine *et al.*, 1997) represent a classic example of weak effects noted in the F_0 generation (all the pairs were fertile, but there was a small but significant effect on litter size and pup growth). In the F_1 generation where exposure is from conception to adulthood when these animals were bred at the same dose only 19/20 pairings resulted in a litter and thus the effects on reproduction were significantly enhanced in the F_1 generation and illustrate the importance of breeding the F_1 animals to detect functional effects on the offspring due to in utero exposure.

Differences between F_1 and F_2 generations can also arise. Here the exposure duration and critical windows of development are the same. However, since one normally only takes one male and female from each litter to generate the F_1 and F_2 parents, it is distinctly possible that a selection bias can exist (eg, if sensitive animals did not produce a litter, or the sensitive pups within a litter did not survive, then a pup from this pairing cannot be selected for further generations) and therefore potential effects may decrease in incidence or severity across generations. Other specific effects may increase severity in the F_2 versus the F_1. For example, a selective effect during in utero exposure of F_1 on the mammary gland would show the F_1 population as being normal with regard to reproduction, but when the F_1 animal becomes a parent, it cannot raise the F_2 adequately because of a mammary effect. In this instance, there would be a more profound influence on the F_2 than the F_1 litters.

Graded Effects

In a similar fashion to developmental toxicity, it is important to keep in mind the ability of changes in dose to alter the outcome of reproductive toxicity studies such that it is not just an increase in severity of a reproductive deficit that may be noted with increased dose, but potentially an increased prevalence of a specific effect (on either an individual or litter basis). There may also be an increase in the severity of the type of lesion with the full constellation of the effects only noted at the highest dose level. Thus, for example, a single compound may produce a subtle effect on testis histology at low dose levels. As the dose level increases, this lesion may become more severe, with pathology noted in the epididymis, this in turn may affect semen parameters, that result in a decrease in litter size and as the dose increases further, to a reduction in the number of fertile pairs—thus there is a continuum of effects, that may be shown by a chemical producing reproductive toxicity that are interrelated and become important in selecting appropriate effect dose levels and therefore those exposures that maybe without effect.

REFERENCES

Adams NR. Permanent infertility in ewes exposed to plant oestrogens. *Aust Vet J.* 1990;67:197–201.

Adams NR, Sanders MR. Persistent infertility in ewes after prolonged exposure to oestradiol-17 beta. *J Reprod Fertil.* 1988;84:373–378.

Aho M, Koivisto AM, Tammela TL, Auvinen A. Is the incidence of hypospadias increasing? Analysis of Finnish hospital discharge data 1970–1994. *Environ Health Perspect.* 2000;108:463–465.

Andersen AN, Gianaroli L, Felberbaum R, de Mouzon J, Nygren KG. Assisted reproductive technology in Europe, 2001. Results generated from European registers by ESHRE. *Hum Reprod.* 2005;20:1158–1176.

Andersson KE, Wagner G. Physiology of penile erection. *Physiol Rev.* 1995;75:191–236.

Ankley GT, Jensen KM, Makynen EA, et al. Effects of the androgenic growth promoter 17-beta-trenbolone on fecundity and reproductive endocrinology of the fathead minnow. *Environ Toxicol Chem.* 2003;22(6):1350–1360.

Aplin JD, Kimber SJ. Trophoblast–uterine interactions at implantation. *Reprod Biol Endocrinol.* 2004;2:48.

Ashby J, Owens W, Deghenghi R, Odum J. Concept evaluation: an assay for receptor-mediated and biochemical antiestrogens using pubertal rats. *Regul Toxicol Pharmacol.* 2002;35(3):393–397.

Ashby J, Tinwell H, Haseman J. Lack of effects for low dose levels of bisphenol A and diethylstilbestrol on the prostate gland of CF1 mice exposed in utero. *Regul Toxicol Pharmacol.* 1999;30:156–166.

Atwood CS, Meethal SV, Liu T, et al. Dysregulation of the hypothalamic–pituitary–gonadal axis with menopause and andropause promotes neurodegenerative senescence. *J Neuropathol Exp Neurol.* 2005;64:93–103.

Auchus RJ, Rainey WE. Adrenarche—physiology, biochemistry and human disease. *Clin Endocrinol.* 2004;60:288–296.

Bardin CW, Catterall JF. Testosterone: a major determinant of extragenital sexual dimorphism. *Science (New York, N.Y.)* 1981;211:1285–1294.

Barker DJ. Fetal origins of coronary heart disease. *BMJ.* 1995;311:171–174.

Barker DJ. Fetal origins of cardiovascular disease. *Ann Med.* 1999;31 (suppl 1):3–6.

Barker DJ, Hales CN, Fall CH, Osmond C, Phipps K, Clark PM. Type 2 (non-insulin-dependent) diabetes mellitus, hypertension and hyperlipidaemia (syndrome X): relation to reduced fetal growth. *Diabetologia.* 1993;36:62–67.

Barker DJ, Winter PD, Osmond C, Margetts B, Simmonds SJ. Weight in infancy and death from ischaemic heart disease. *Lancet.* 1989;2:577–580.

Barlow NJ, McIntyre BS, Foster PM. Male reproductive tract lesions at 6, 12, and 18 months of age following in utero exposure to di(*n*-butyl) phthalate. *Toxicol Pathol.* 2004;32:79–90.

Battaglia C, De Iaco P, Iughetti L, et al. Female precocious puberty, obesity and polycystic-like ovaries. *Ultrasound Obstet Gynecol.* 2005;26:651–657.

Becker AL, Epperson CN. Female puberty: clinical implications for the use of prolactin-modulating psychotropics. *Child Adolesc Psychiatr Clin N Am.* 2006;15:207–220.

Berman DM, Tian H, Russell DW. Expression and regulation of steroid 5α-reductase in the urogenital tract of the fetal rat. *Mol Endocrinol.* 1995;9:1561–1570.

Berman E, Laskey JW. Altered steroidogenesis in whole-ovary and adrenal culture in cycling rats. *Reprod Toxicol.* 1993;7:349–358.

Bielmeier SR, Best DS, Narotsky MG. Serum hormone characterization and exogenous hormone rescue of bromodichloromethane-induced pregnancy loss in the F344 rat. *Toxicol Sci.* 2004;77:101–108.

Biro FM, Khoury P, Morrison JA. Influence of obesity on timing of puberty. *Int J Androl.* 2006;29:272–277; discussion 286–290.

Blackburn DM, Gray AJ, Lloyd SC, Sheard CM, Foster PMD. A comparison of the effects of the three isomers of dinitrobenzene on the testis in the rat. *Toxicol. Appl. Pharmacol.* 92:54–64.

Blanck HM, Marcus M, Tolbert PE, et al. Age at menarche and tanner stage in girls exposed in utero and postnatally to polybrominated biphenyl. *Epidemiology (Cambridge, Mass).* 2000;11:641–647.

Blystone CR, Kissling GE, Bishop JB, Chapin RE, Wolfe GW, Foster PM. Determination of the di-(2-ethylhexyl) phthalate (DEHP) NOAEL for reproductive development in the rat: importance of the retention of extra animals to adulthood. *Toxicol Sci.* 2010;116:640–646.

Blystone CR, Lambright CS, Howdeshell KL, et al. Sensitivity of fetal rat testicular steroidogenesis to maternal prochloraz exposure and the underlying mechanism of inhibition: prochloraz reduced fetal testis testosterone. *Toxicol Sci.* 2007;97:512–519.

Boekelheide K, Darney SP, Daston GP, et al. NTP-CERHR Expert Panel Report on the reproductive and developmental toxicity of 2-bromopropane. *Reprod Toxicol.* 2004;18:189–217.

Boisen KA, Kaleva M, Main KM, et al. Difference in prevalence of congenital cryptorchidism in infants between two Nordic countries. *Lancet.* 2004;363:1264–1269.

Brouwer A, Longnecker MP, Birnbaum LS, et al. Characterization of potential endocrine-related health effects at low-dose levels of exposure to PCBs. *Environ Health Perspect.* 1999;107(suppl 4):639–649.

Buchanan JF, Davis LJ. Drug-induced infertility. *Drug Intell Clin Pharm.* 1984;18:122–132.

Buck Louis GM, Gray LE Jr, Marcus M, et al. Environmental factors and puberty timing: expert panel research needs. *Pediatrics.* 2008;121 (suppl 3):S192–S207.

Buhimschi CS. Endocrinology of lactation. *Obstet Gynecol Clin North Am.* 2004;31:963–979, xii.

Byskov AG. Differentiation of mammalian embryonic gonad. *Physiol Rev.* 1986;66:71–117.

Cain JC. Miroestrol: an oestrogen from the plant Pueraria mirifica. *Nature.* 1960;188:774–777.

Calafat AM, Brock JW, Silva MJ, et al. Urinary and amniotic fluid levels of phthalate monoesters in rats after the oral administration of di(2-ethylhexyl) phthalate and di-*n*-butyl phthalate. *Toxicology.* 2006; 217:22–30.

Canning DA. Hypospadias trends in two US surveillance systems. Rise in prevalence of hypospadias. *J Urol.* 1999;161:366.

Cannon SSB, Veazey JJM, Jackson RRS, et al. Epidemic kepone poisoning in chemical workers. *Am J Epidemiol.* 1978;107:529–537.

Cappon GD, Bailey GP, Buschmann J, et al. Juvenile animal toxicity study designs to support pediatric drug development. *Birth Defects Res B Dev Reprod Toxicol.* 2009;86:463–469.

Carmichael SL, Shaw GM, Laurent C, Croughan MS, Olney RS, Lammer EJ. Maternal progestin intake and risk of hypospadias. *Arch Pediatr Adolesc Med.* 2005;159:957–962.

Carnathan GW, Metcalf LE, Cochrane RL, Nutting EF, Black DL. Relationship between progesterone suppression and pregnancy in rats. *J Pharm Pharmacol.* 1987;39:401–404.

Carney EW, Zablotny CL, Marty MS, et al. The effects of feed restriction during in utero and postnatal development in rats. *Toxicol Sci.* 2004;82:237–249.

Carruthers CM, Foster PM. Critical window of male reproductive tract development in rats following gestational exposure to di-n-butyl phthalate. *Birth Defects Res B Dev Reprod Toxicol.* 2005;74:277–285.

Cave DA, Foster PMD. Modulation of *m*-dinitrobenzene and *m*-nitrosonitrobenzene toxicity in rat Sertoli—germ cell co-cultures. *Fund Appl Toxicol.* 1990;14:199–207.

Challis JR, Bloomfield FH, Bocking AD, et al. Fetal signals and parturition. *J Obstet Gynaecol Res.* 2005;31:492–499.

Chapin R, Dutton S, Ross M, Lamb J. Effects of ethylene glycol monomethyl ether (EGME) on mating performance and epididymal sperm parameters in F344 rats. *Fundam Appl Toxicol.* 1985;5: 182–189.

Chapin RE, Harris MW, Davis BJ, et al. The effects of perinatal/juvenile methoxychlor exposure on adult rat nervous, immune, and reproductive system function. *Fundam Appl Toxicol.* 1997;40:138–157.

Chapin RE, Ku WW. The reproductive toxicity of boric acid. *Environ Health Perspect.* 1994;102(suppl 7):87–91.

Charlier C. Endocrine effects of environmental pollutants. *Bull Mem Acad R Med Belg.* 2005;160:301–310.

Charlier C. Effects of environmental pollutants on hormone disturbances. *Bull Mem Acad R Med Belg.* 2006;161:116–124; discussion 124–116.

Colbert NK, Pelletier NC, Cote JM, et al. Perinatal exposure to low levels of the environmental antiandrogen vinclozolin alters sex-differentiated social play and sexual behaviors in the rat. *Environ Health Perspect.* 2005;113:700–707.

Colborn T. The wildlife/human connection: modernizing risk decisions. *Environ Health Perspect.* 1994;102(suppl 12):55–59.

Collins TF. History and evolution of reproductive and developmental toxicology guidelines. *Curr Pharm Des.* 2006;12(12):1449–1465.

Cooper RL, Barrett MA, Goldman JM, Rehnberg GR, McElroy WK, Stoker TE. Pregnancy alterations following xenobiotic-induced delays in ovulation in the female rat. *Fundam Appl Toxicol.* 1994;22:474–480.

Cooper RL, Lamb JC, Barlow SM, et al. A tiered approach to life stages testing for agricultural chemical safety assessment. *Crit Rev Toxicol.* 2006;36:69–98.

Cooper RL, Roberts B, Rogers DC, Seay SG, Conn PM. Endocrine status versus chronologic age as predictors of altered luteinizing hormone secretion in the "aging" rat. *Endocrinology.* 1984;114:391–396.

Cooper RL, Stoker TE, Tyrey L, Goldman JM, McElroy WK. Atrazine disrupts the hypothalamic control of pituitary-ovarian function. *Toxicol Sci.* 2000;53:297–307.

Creasy DM, Beech LM, Gray TJ, Butler WH. An ultrastructural study of ethylene glycol monomethyl ether-induced spermatocyte injury in the rat. *Exp Mol Pathol.* 1986;45:311–322.

Creasy DM, Beech LM, Gray TJB, Butler WH. The ultrastructural effects of di-*n*-pentyl phthalate on the testis of the mature rat. *Exp Mol Pathol.* 1987;46:357–371.

Creasy DM, Foster PMD. The morphological development of glycol ether-induced testicular atrophy in the rat. *Exp Mol Path.* 1984;40:169–176.

Cummings AM, Perreault SD. Methoxychlor accelerates embryo transport through the rat reproductive tract. *Toxicol Appl Pharmacol.* 1990;102:110–116.

DeCherney AH, Cholst I, Naftolin F. Structure and function of the fallopian tubes following exposure to diethylstilbestrol (DES) during gestation. *Fertil Steril.* 1981;36:741–745.

Den Hond E, Schoeters G. Endocrine disrupters and human puberty. *Int J Androl.* 2006;29:264–271; discussion 286–290.

Doody KJ, Lephart ED, Stirling D, et al. Expression of mRNA species encoding steroidogenic enzymes in the rat ovary. *J Mol Endocrinol.* 1991;6:153–162.

Duck SC, Katayama KP. Danazol may cause female pseudohermaphroditism. *Fertil Steril.* 1981;35:230–231.

Dunger DB, Ahmed ML, Ong KK. Effects of obesity on growth and puberty. *Best Pract Res Clin Endocrinol Metab.* 2005;19:375–390.

Durhan EJ, Lambright C, Wilson V, et al. Evaluation of androstenedione as an androgenic component of river water downstream of a pulp and paper mill effluent. *Environ Toxicol Chem.* 2002;21(9):1973–1976.

Durhan EJ, Lambright CS, Makynen EA, et al. Identification of metabolites of trenbolone acetate in androgenic runoff from a beef feedlot. *Environ Health Perspect.* 2006;114(suppl 1):65–68.

Eddy E, Gong D, Fenderson A. Origin and migration of primoridal germ cells in mammals. *Gamete Res.* 1981;4:333–336.

EDSTAC Final Report. 1998. Available at: http://www.epa.gov/endo/pubs/edspoverview/finalrpt.htm.

Ellis MK, Foster PMD. The metabolism of 1,3-dinitrobenzene by rat testicular subcellular fractions. *Toxicol Lett.* 1992;62:201–208.

Ellis RJ, van den Heuvel MR, Bandelj E, Smith MA, McCarthy LH, Stuthridge TR, Dietrich DR. In vivo and in vitro assessment of the androgenic potential of a pulp and paper mill effluent. *Environ Toxicol Chem.* 2003;22(7):1448–1456.

Enders AC, Carter AM. What can comparative studies of placental structure tell us?—a review. *Placenta.* 2004;25:S3–S9.

Epstein SS. Kepone—hazard evaluation. *Science Total Environ.* 1978;9:1–62.

Eskenazi B, Mocarelli P, Warner M, et al. Seveso Women's Health Study: a study of the effects of 2,3,7,8-tetrachlorodibenzo-*p*-dioxin on reproductive health. *Chemosphere.* 2000;40:1247–1253.

Ewing LL, Desjardins C, Irby DC, Robaire B. Synergistic interaction of testosterone and oestradiol inhibits spermatogenesis in rats. *Nature.* 1977;269:409–411.

Ewing LL, Gorski RA, Sbordone RJ, Tyler JV, Desjardins C, Robaire B. Testosterone–estradiol filled polydimethylsiloxane subdermal implants: effect on fertility and masculine sexual and aggressive behavior of male rats. *Biol Reprod.* 1979;21:765–772.

Ewing LL, Zirkin BR, Chubb C. Assessment of testicular testosterone production and Leydig cell structure. *Environ Health Perspect.* 1981;38:19–27.

Farnsworth NR. The role of ethnopharmacology in drug development. *Ciba Foundation Symp.* 1990;154:2–11; discussion 11–21.

Farnsworth NR, Bingel AS, Cordell GA, Crane FA, Fong HS. Potential value of plants as sources of new antifertility agents II. *J Pharm Sci.* 1975;64(5):717–754.

Faroon O, Kueberuwa S, Smith L, DeRosa C. ATSDR evaluation of health effects of chemicals. II. Mirex and chlordecone: health effects, toxicokinetics, human exposure, and environmental fate. *Toxicol Ind Health.* 1995;11:1–203.

Fisher JS. Environmental anti-androgens and male reproductive health: focus on phthalates and testicular dysgenesis syndrome. *Reproduction.* 2004;127:305–315.

Foster PM, Cook MW, Thomas LV, Walters DG, Gangolli SD. Differences in urinary metabolic profile from di-*n*-butyl phthalate-treated rats and hamsters. A possible explanation for species differences in susceptibility to testicular atrophy. *Drug Metab Dispos.* 1983;11:59–61.

Foster PM, Mylchreest E, Gaido KW, Sar M. Effects of phthalate esters on the developing reproductive tract of male rats. *Hum Reprod Update.* 2001;7:231–235.

Foster PMD. Testicular organization and biochemical function. In: Lamb JC, Foster PMD, eds. *The Physiology and Toxicology of Male Reproduction.* New York: Academic Press; 1988:7–34.

Foster PMD. Studies on the toxicity of *m*-dinitrobenzene to the testicular Sertoli cell. *Arch Toxicol Suppl.* 1989;13:3–17.

Foster PMD. The cons of the extended 1-generation study protocol: how to get better hazard information and avoid the tyranny of triggers? *Reproduct Toxicol.* 2010a;30:224–224.

Foster PMD. The cons of the extended one—generation study protocol. *Birth Defect Res A Clin Mol Teratol.* 2010b;88:325.

Foster PMD, Lloyd SC, Blackburn DM. Comparison of the in vivo and in vitro testicular effects produced by methoxy-, ethoxy- and *n*-butoxy acetic acids in the rat. *Toxicology.* 1987;43:17–30.

Giwercman A, Rylander L, Hagmar L, Giwercman YL. Ethnic differences in occurrence of TDS—genetics and/or environment? *Int J Androl.* 2006;29:291–297; discussion 304–296.

Gladen BC, Klebanoff MA, Hediger ML, et al. Prenatal DDT exposure in relation to anthropometric and pubertal measures in adolescent males. *Environ Health Perspect.* 2004;112:1761–1767.

Goldman JM, Laws SC, Balchak SK, Cooper RL, Kavlock RJ. Endocrine-disrupting chemicals: prepubertal exposures and effects on sexual maturation and thyroid activity in the female rat. A focus on the EDSTAC recommendations. *Crit Rev Toxicol.* 2000;30:135–196.

Goldman JM, Parrish MB, Cooper RL, McElroy WK. Blockade of ovulation in the rat by systemic and ovarian intrabursal administration of the fungicide sodium dimethyldithiocarbamate. *Reprod Toxicol.* 1997;11:185–190.

Goldman JM, Stoker TE, Cooper RL, McElroy WK, Hein JF. Blockade of ovulation in the rat by the fungicide sodium *N*-methyldithiocarbamate: relationship between effects on the luteinizing hormone surge and alterations in hypothalamic catecholamines. *Neurotoxicol Teratol.* 1994;16:257–268.

Goldman JM, Stoker TE, Perreault SD, Cooper RL, Crider MA. Influence of the formamidine pesticide chlordimeform on ovulation in the female hamster: dissociable shifts in the luteinizing hormone surge and oocyte release. *Toxicol Appl Pharmacol.* 1993;121:279–290.

Goldstein I, Lue TF, Padma-Nathan H, Rosen RC, Steers WD, Wicker PA. Oral sildenafil in the treatment of erectile dysfunction. Sildenafil Study Group. *N Engl J Med.* 1998;338:1397–1404.

Gordon AE, Shaughnessy AF. Saw palmetto for prostate disorders. *Am Fam Phys.* 2003;67:1281–1283.

Goyeneche AA, Calvo V, Gibori G, Telleria CM. Androstenedione interferes in luteal regression by inhibiting apoptosis and stimulating progesterone production. *Biol Reprod.* 2002;66:1540–1547.

Goy RW, Bercovitch FB, McBrair MC. Behavioral masculinization is independent of genital masculinization in prenatally androgenized female rhesus macaques. *Horm Behav.* 1988;22(4):552–571.

Goy RW, Phoenix CH. The effects of testosterone propionate administered before birth on the development of behavior in genetic female rhesus monkeys. *UCLA Forum Med Sci.* 1972;15:193–201.

Goy RW, Resko JA. Gonadal hormones and behavior of normal and pseudohermaphroditic nonhuman female primates. *Recent Prog Horm Res.* 1972;28:707–733.

Grajewski B, Whelan EA, Schnorr TM, Mouradian R, Alderfer R, Wild DK. Evaluation of reproductive function among men occupationally exposed to a stilbene derivative: I. Hormonal and physical status. *Am J Ind Med.* 1996;29:49–57.

Gray LE. Emerging issues related to endocrine disrupting chemicals and environmental androgens and antiandrogens. In: Hutzinger O. ed. *The Handbook of Environmental Chemistry.* Heidelberg: Springer-Verlag; 2002:209–248.

Gray LE Jr. Tiered screening and testing strategy for xenoestrogens and antiandrogens. *Toxicol Lett.* 1998;102–103:677–680.

Gray LE Jr, Foster PM. Significance of experimental studies for assessing adverse effects of endocrine disrupting chemicals. *Pure Appl Chem.* 2004;75:2125–2141.

Gray LE Jr, Kelce WR. Latent effects of pesticides and toxic substances on sexual differentiation of rodents. *Toxicol Ind Health.* 1996;12:515–531.

Gray LE Jr, Kelce WR, Monosson E, Ostby JS, Birnbaum LS. Exposure to TCDD during development permanently alters reproductive function in male Long Evans rats and hamsters: reduced ejaculated and epididymal sperm numbers and sex accessory gland weights in offspring with normal androgenic status. *Toxicol Appl Pharmacol.* 1995;131:108–118.

Gray LE Jr, Kelce WR, Wiese T, et al. Endocrine screening methods workshop report: detection of estrogenic and androgenic hormonal and antihormonal activity for chemicals that act via receptor or steroidogenic enzyme mechanisms. *Reprod Toxicol.* 1997a;11:719–750.

Gray LE Jr, Ostby J. Effects of pesticides and toxic substances on behavioral and morphological reproductive development: endocrine versus nonendocrine mechanisms. *Toxicol Ind Health.* 1998;14:159–184.

Gray LE Jr, Ostby J, Ferrell J, et al. A dose–response analysis of methoxychlor-induced alterations of reproductive development and function in the rat. *Fundam Appl Toxicol.* 1989;12:92–108.

Gray LE Jr, Ostby J, Furr J, Price M, Veeramachaneni DN, Parks L. Perinatal exposure to the phthalates DEHP, BBP, and DINP, but not DEP, DMP, or DOTP, alters sexual differentiation of the male Rat. *Toxicol Sci.* 2000;58:350–365.

Gray LE, Ostby J, Furr J, et al. Effects of environmental antiandrogens on reproductive development in experimental animals. *Hum Reprod Update.* 2001;7:248–264.

Gray LE Jr, Ostby J, Linder R, Goldman J, Rehnberg G, Cooper R. Carbendazim-induced alterations of reproductive development and function in the rat and hamster. *Fundam Appl Toxicol.* 1990;15:281–297.

Gray LE Jr, Ostby J, Monosson E, Kelce WR. Environmental antiandrogens: low doses of the fungicide vinclozolin alter sexual differentiation of the male rat. *Toxicol Ind Health.* 1999a;15(1–2):48–64.

Gray LE Jr, Ostby J, Sigmon R, et al. The development of a protocol to assess reproductive effects of toxicants in the rat. *Reprod Toxicol.* 1988a;2:281–287.

Gray LE Jr, Ostby J, Wilson V, et al. Xenoendocrine disrupters-tiered screening and testing: filling key data gaps. *Toxicology.* 2002;181–182, 371–382.

Gray LE Jr, Ostby JS. In utero 2,3,7,8-tetrachlorodibenzo-*p*-dioxin (TCDD) alters reproductive morphology and function in female rat offspring. *Toxicol Appl Pharmacol.* 1995;133:285–294.

Gray LE Jr, Ostby JS, Ferrell JM, Sigmon ER, Goldman JM. Methoxychlor induces estrogen-like alterations of behavior and the reproductive tract in the female rat and hamster: effects on sex behavior, running wheel activity, and uterine morphology. *Toxicol Appl Pharmacol.* 1988b;96:525–540.

Gray LE Jr, Ostby JS, Kelce WR. Developmental effects of an environmental antiandrogen: the fungicide vinclozolin alters sex differentiation of the male rat. *Toxicol Appl Pharmacol.* 1994;129:46–52.

Gray LE, Ostby JS, Kelce WR. A dose–response analysis of the reproductive effects of a single gestational dose of 2,3,7,8-tetrachlorodibenzo-*p*-dioxin in male Long Evans Hooded rat offspring. *Toxicol Appl Pharmacol.* 1997b;146:11–20.

Gray LE Jr, Wilson V, Noriega N, et al. Use of the laboratory rat as a model in endocrine disruptor screening and testing. *ILAR J.* 2004;45:425–437.

Gray LE Jr, Wilson VS, Stoker T, et al. Adverse effects of environmental antiandrogens and androgens on reproductive development in mammals. *Int J Androl.* 2006;29:96–104; discussion 105–108.

Gray LE Jr, Wolf C, Lambright C, et al. Administration of potentially anti-androgenic pesticides (procymidone, linuron, iprodione, chlozolinate, p,p'-DDE, and ketoconazole) and toxic substances (dibutyl- and diethylhexyl phthalate, PCB 169, and ethane dimethane sulphonate) during sexual differentiation produces diverse profiles of reproductive malformations in the male rat. *Toxicol Ind Health.* 1999b;15:94–118.

Gray LE, Wolf C, Mann P, Ostby JS. In utero exposure to low doses of 2,3,7,8-tetrachlorodibenzo-*p*-dioxin alters reproductive development of female Long Evans hooded rat offspring. *Toxicol Appl Pharmacol.* 1997c;146:237–244.

Gupta RK, Miller KP, Babus JK, Flaws JA. Methoxychlor inhibits growth and induces atresia of antral follicles through an oxidative stress pathway. *Toxicol Sci.* 2006a;93:382–389.

Gupta RK, Schuh RA, Fiskum G, Flaws JA. Methoxychlor causes mitochondrial dysfunction and oxidative damage in the mouse ovary. *Toxicol Appl Pharmacol.* 2006b;216:436–445.

Hammond B, Katzenellenbogen BS, Krauthammer N, McConnell J. Estrogenic activity of the insecticide chlordecone (Kepone) and interaction with uterine estrogen receptors. *Proc Natl Acad Sci USA.* 1979;76:6641–6645.

Hammond SK, Smith TJ, Ellenbecker MJ. Determination of occupational exposure to fabric brightener chemicals by HPLC. *Am Ind Hygiene Assoc J.* 1987;48:117–121.

Hauser R, Williams P, Altshul L, et al. Predictors of serum dioxin levels among adolescent boys in Chapaevsk, Russia: a cross-sectional pilot study. *Environ Health.* 2005;4:8.

Hayes AW: *Principles and Methods of Toxicology.* New York: Raven Press; 1982; from previous edition of C&D.

Hemsworth BN, Jackson H. Effect of busulphan on the developing ovary in the rat. *J Reprod Fertil.* 1963;6:229–233.

Henley DV, Lipson N, Korach KS, Bloch CA. Prepubertal gynecomastia linked to lavender and tea tree oils. *N Engl J Med.* 2007;356:479–485.

Herbst AL. Exogenous hormones in pregnancy. *Clin Obstet Gynecol.* 1973; 16:37–50.

Herbst AL. The effects in the human of diethylstilbestrol (DES) use during pregnancy. *Princess Takamatsu symposia.* 1987;18:67–75.

Hershberger LG, Shipley EG, Meyer RK. Myotrophic activity of 19-nortestosterone and other steroids determined by modified levator ani muscle method. *Proc Soc Exp Biol Med.* 1953;83:175–180.

Hertz R. Accidental ingestion of estrogens by children. *Pediatrics.* 1958;21:203–206.

Higuchi TT, Palmer JS, Gray LE Jr, Veeramachaneni DN. Effects of Dibutyl Phthalate in Male Rabbits following in Utero, Adolescent, or Postpubertal Exposure. *Toxicol Sci.* 2003;72:301–313.

Himes JH. Examining the evidence for recent secular changes in the timing of puberty in US children in light of increases in the prevalence of obesity. *Mol Cell Endocrinol.* 2006;254–255;13–21.

Hines M. Sex steroids and human behavior: prenatal androgen exposure and sex-typical play behavior in children. *Ann N Y Acad Sci.* 2003;1007:272–282.

Hines M, Kaufman FR. Androgen and the development of human sex-typical behavior: rough-and-tumble play and sex of preferred playmates in children with congenital adrenal hyperplasia (CAH). *Child Dev.* 1994;65:1042–1053.

Holloway AJ, Moore HDM, Foster PMD. The use of in vitro fertilization to detect reductions in fertility of male rats exposed to 1,3-dinitrobenzene. *Fund Appl Toxicol.* 1990;14:113–122.

Hoodbhoy T, Dean J. Insights into the molecular basis of sperm–egg recognition in mammals. *Reproduction.* 2004;127:417–422.

Hotchkiss AK, Lambright CS, Ostby JS, Parks-Saldutti L, Vandenbergh JG, Gray LE Jr. Prenatal testosterone exposure permanently masculinizes anogenital distance, nipple development, and reproductive tract morphology in female Sprague–Dawley rats. *Toxicol Sci.* 2007;96:335–345.

Hotchkiss AK, Ostby JS, Vandenbergh JG, Gray LE Jr. An environmental antiandrogen, vinclozolin, alters the organization of play behavior. *Physiol Behav.* 2003;79:151–156.

Hotchkiss AK, Parks-Saldutti LG, Ostby JS, et al. A mixture of the "antiandrogens" linuron and butyl benzyl phthalate alters sexual differentiation of the male rat in a cumulative fashion. *Biol Reprod.* 2004;71:1852–1861.

Hotchkiss AK, Rider CV, Blystone CR, et al. Fifteen years after "Wingspread"—environmental endocrine disrupters and human and wildlife health: where we are today and where we need to go. *Toxicol Sci.* 2008; 105:235–259.

Hotchkiss AK, Ostby JS, Vandenburgh JG, Gray LE Jr. Androgens and environmental antiandrogens affect reproductive development and play behavior in the Sprague-Dawley rat. *Environ Health Perspect.* 2002;110(suppl 3):435–439.

Hoyer PB, Sipes IG. Development of an animal model for ovotoxicity using 4-vinylcyclohexene: a case study. *Birth Defects Res B Dev Reprod Toxicol.* 2007;80:113–125.

Huhtaniemi I, Pelliniemi LJ. Fetal Leydig cells: cellular origin, morphology, life span, and special functional features. *Proc Soc Exp Biol Med.* 1992;201:125–140.

Hunter RH, Rodriguez-Martinez H. Capacitation of mammalian spermatozoa in vivo, with a specific focus on events in the Fallopian tubes. *Mol Reprod Dev.* 2004;67:243–250.

Hurtt ME, Daston G, Davis-Bruno K, et al. Juvenile animal studies: testing strategies and design. *Birth Defects Res B Dev Reprod Toxicol.* 2004; 71:281–288.

Imperato-McGinley J, Sanchez RS, Spencer JR, Yee B, Vaughan ED. Comparison of the effects of the 5 alpha-reductase inhibitor finasteride and the antiandrogen flutamide on prostate and genital differentiation: dose–response studies. *Endocrinology.* 1992;131:1149–1156.

Jacobson JL, Jacobson SW. Evidence for PCBs as neurodevelopmental toxicants in humans. *Neurotoxicology.* 1997;18:415–424.

Jaruratanasirikul S, Leethanaporn K, Pradutkanchana S, Sriplung H. Serum insulin-like growth factor-1 (IGF-1) and insulin-like growth factor binding protein-3 (IGFBP-3) in healthy Thai children and adolescents: relation to age, sex, and stage of puberty. *J Med Assoc Thai.* 1999;82:275–283.

Jobling S, Tyler CR. Introduction: the ecological relevance of chemically induced endocrine disruption in wildlife. *Environ Health Perspect.* 2006;114(suppl 1):7–8.

Jorgensen N, Andersen AG, Eustache F, et al. Regional differences in semen quality in Europe. *Human Reprod.* 2001;16:1012–1019.

Jorgensen N, Carlsen E, Nermoen I, et al. East-West gradient in semen quality in the Nordic-Baltic area: a study of men from the general population in Denmark, Norway, Estonia and Finland. *Human Reprod.* 2002;17:2199–2208.

Kanno J, Onyon L, Haseman J, Fenner-Crisp P, Ashby J, Owens W. The OECD program to validate the rat uterotrophic bioassay to screen compounds for in vivo estrogenic responses: phase 1. *Environ Health Perspect.* 2001;109:785–794.

Kanno J, Onyon L, Peddada S, Ashby J, Jacob E, Owens W. The OECD program to validate the rat uterotrophic bioassay. Phase 2: coded single-dose studies. *Environ Health Perspect.* 2003a;111:1550–1558.

Kanno J, Onyon L, Peddada S, Ashby J, Jacob E, Owens W. The OECD program to validate the rat uterotrophic bioassay. Phase 2: dose–response studies. *Environ Health Perspect.* 2003b;111:1530–1549.

Kaplowitz P. Pubertal development in girls: secular trends. *Curr Opin obstet Gynecol.* 2006;18:487–491.

Kassim NM, McDonald SW, Reid O, Bennett NK, Gilmore DP, Payne AP. The effects of pre- and postnatal exposure to the nonsteroidal antiandrogen flutamide on testis descent and morphology in the Albino Swiss rat. *J Anat.* 1997;190:577–588.

Keefe DL, Marquard K, Liu L. The telomere theory of reproductive senescence in women. *Curr Opin obstet Gynecol.* 2006;18:280–285.

Keene LC, Davies PH. Drug-related erectile dysfunction. *Adverse Drug React Toxicol Rev.* 1999;18:5–24.

Kelce WR, Monosson E, Gamcsik MP, Laws SC, Gray LE Jr. Environmental hormone disruptors: evidence that vinclozolin developmental toxicity is mediated by antiandrogenic metabolites. *Toxicol Appl Pharmacol.* 1994;126(2):276–285.

Kelce WR, Monosson E, Gray LE Jr. An environmental antiandrogen. *Recent Prog Horm Res.* 1995;50:449–453.

Kelce WR, Lambright CR, Gray LE, Roberts KP. Vinclozlin and p,p'-DDE alter androgen-dependent gene expression: In vivo confirmation of an androgen receptor-mediated mechanism. *Toxicol Appl Pharmacol.* 1997;142:192–200.

Kim HS, Shin JH, Moon HJ, et al. Evaluation of the 20-day pubertal female assay in Sprague-Dawley rats treated with DES, tamoxifen, testosterone, and flutamide. *Toxicol Sci.* 2002;67(1):52–62.

Kingsbury AC. Danazol and fetal masculinization: a warning. *Med J Aust.* 1985;143:410–411.

Klonisch T, Fowler PA, Hombach-Klonisch S. Molecular and genetic regulation of testis descent and external genitalia development. *Dev Biol.* 2004;270:1–18.

Knappe G, Gerl H, Ventz M, Rohde, W. The long-term therapy of hypothalamic-hypophyseal Cushing's syndrome with mitotane (o,p'-DDD)]. *Deutsche Medizinische Wochenschrift.* 1997;(1946)122:882–886. First published on Langzeit-Therapie des hypothalamisch-hypophysaren Cushing-Syndroms mit Mitotan (o,p'-DDD).

Knobil E, Neill J. *The Physiology of Reproduction.* New York: Raven Press; 1994.

Kolpin DW, Furlong ET, Meyer MT, et al. Pharmaceuticals, hormones, and other organic wastewater contaminants in U.S. streams, 1999–2000: a national reconnaissance. *Environ Sci Technol.* 2002;36:1202–1211.

Kolpin DW, Skopec M, Meyer MT, Furlong ET, Zaugg SD. Urban contribution of pharmaceuticals and other organic wastewater contaminants to streams during differing flow conditions. *Sci Total Environ.* 2004;328:119–130.

Kolpin DW, Thurman EM, Linhart SM. The environmental occurrence of herbicides: the importance of degradates in ground water. *Arch Environ Contam Toxicol.* 1998;35:385–390.

Koopman P, Munsterberg A, Capel B, Vivian N, Lovell-Badge R. Expression of a candidate sex-determining gene during mouse testis differentiation. *Nature.* 1990;348:450–452.

Krstevska-Konstantinova M, Charlier C, Craen M, et al. Sexual precocity after immigration from developing countries to Belgium: evidence of previous exposure to organochlorine pesticides. *Human Reprod.* 2001;16:1020–1026.

Kuiper-Goodman T, Scott PM, Watanabe H. Risk assessment of the mycotoxin zearalenone. *Regul Toxicol Pharmacol.* 1987;7:253–306.

Lambright C, Ostby J, Bobseine K, et al. Cellular and molecular mechanisms of action of linuron: an antiandrogenic herbicide that produces reproductive malformations in male rats. *Toxicol Sci.* 2000;56:389–399.

Landrigan PJ, Kreiss K, Xintaras C, Feldman RG, Heath CW Jr. Clinical epidemiology of occupational neurotoxic disease. *Neurobehav Toxicol.* 1980;2:43–48.

Larsson DG, Förlin L. Male-biased sex ratios of fish embryos near a pulp mill: temporary recovery after a short-term shutdown. *Environ Health Perspect.* 2002;110(8):739–742. Erratum in: *Environ Health Perspect.* 110(9):A505.

Leblond CP, Clermont Y. Definition of the stages of the seminiferous epithelium in the rat. *Ann N Y Acad Sci.* 1952;55:548–573.

Lee KY, DeMayo FJ. Animal models of implantation. *Reproduction.* 2004;128:679–695.

LeMaire WJ, Cleveland WW, Bejar RL, Marsh JM, Fishman L. Aminoglutethimide: a possible cause of pseudohermaphroiditism in females. *Amj Dis Child.* 1972;124:421–423.

Lim HN, Raipert-de Meyts E, Skakkebaek NE, Hawkins JR, Hughes IA. Genetic analysis of the INSL3 gene in patients with maldescent of the testis. *Eur J Endocrinol.* 2001;144:129–137.

Linder RE, Hess RA, Strader LF. Testicular toxicity and infertility in male rats treated with 1,3-dinitrobenzene. *J Toxicol Environ Health.* 1986;19:477–489.

Linder RE, Klinefelter GR, Strader LF, Veeramachaneni DN, Roberts NL, Suarez JD. Histopathologic changes in the testes of rats exposed to dibromoacetic acid. *Reprod Toxicol.* 1997;11:47–56.

Lloyd SC, Foster PM. Effect of mono-(2-ethylhexyl)phthalate on follicle-stimulating hormone responsiveness of cultured rat Sertoli cells. *Toxicol Appl Pharmacol.* 1988;95:484–489.

Longnecker MP, Gladen BC, Cupul-Uicab LA, et al. In utero exposure to the antiandrogen 1,1-dichloro-2,2-bis(*p*-chlorophenyl)ethylene (DDE) in relation to anogenital distance in male newborns from Chiapas, Mexico. *Am J Epidemiol.* 2007;165:1015–1022.

Lopes FL, Desmarais JA, Murphy BD. Embryonic diapause and its regulation. *Reproduction.* 2004;128:669–678.

Malassine A, Frendo JL, Evain-Brion D. A comparison of placental development and endocrine functions between the human and mouse model. *Hum Reprod Update.* 2003;9:531–539.

Marty MS, Crissman JW, Carney EW. Evaluation of the EDSTAC female pubertal assay in CD rats using 17beta-estradiol, steroid biosynthesis inhibitors, and a thyroid inhibitor. *Toxicol Sci.* 1999;52(2):269–277.

Marty MS, Crissman JW, Carney EW. Evaluation of the male pubertal onset assay to detect testosterone and steroid biosynthesis inhibitors in CD rats. *Toxicol Sci.* 2001;60:285–295.

Marshall WA, Tanner JM. Variations in pattern of pubertal changes in girls. *Arch Dis Child.* 1969;44:291–303.

Marshall WA, Tanner JM. Variations in the pattern of pubertal changes in boys. *Arch Dis Child.* 1970;45:13–23.

Massart F, Parrino R, Seppia P, Federico G, Saggese G. How do environmental estrogen disruptors induce precocious puberty? *Minerva Pediatr.* 2006;58:247–254.

Matsumura A, Ghosh A, Pope GS, Darbre PD. Comparative study of oestrogenic properties of eight phytoestrogens in MCF7 human breast cancer cells. *J Steroid Biochem Mol Biol.* 2005;94:431–443.

McCartney CR, Blank SK, Prendergast KA, et al. Obesity and sex steroid changes across puberty: evidence for marked hyperandrogenemia in pre- and early pubertal obese girls. *J Clin Endocrinol Metab.* 2007;92:430–436.

McIntyre BS, Barlow NJ, Foster PM. Androgen-mediated development in male rat offspring exposed to flutamide in utero: permanence and correlation of early postnatal changes in anogenital distance and nipple retention with malformations in androgen-dependent tissues. *Toxicol Sci.* 2001;62:236–249.

McIntyre BS, Barlow NJ, Foster PMD. Male rats exposed to linuron in utero exhibit permanent changes in anogenital distance, nipple retention, and epididymal malformations that result in subsequent testicular atrophy. *Toxicol Sci.* 2002;65:62–70.

McIntyre BS, Barlow NJ, Wallace DG, Maness SC, Gaido KW, Foster PM. Effects of in utero exposure to linuron on androgen-dependent reproductive development in the male Crl:CD(SD)BR rat. *Toxicol Appl Pharmacol.* 2000;167:87–99.

Melnick RL, Nyska A, Foster PM, Roycroft JH, Kissling GE. Toxicity and carcinogenicity of the water disinfection byproduct, dibromoacetic acid, in rats and mice. *Toxicology.* 2007;230:126–136.

Mendelson CR, Condon JC. New insights into the molecular endocrinology of parturition. *J Steroid Biochem Mol Biol.* 2005;93:113–119.

Miller KP, Gupta RK, Greenfeld CR, Babus JK, Flaws JA. Methoxychlor directly affects ovarian antral follicle growth and atresia through Bcl-2 and Bax-mediated pathways. *Toxicol Sci.* 2005;88:213–221.

Monosson E, Kelce WR, Lambright C, Ostby J, Gray LE Jr. Peripubertal exposure to the antiandrogenic fungicide, vinclozolin, delays puberty, inhibits the development of androgen-dependent tissues, and alters androgen receptor function in the male rat. *Toxicol Ind Health.* 1999;15:65–79.

Moore KL. *The Developing Human: Clinically Oriented Embryology.* Philadelphia: W. B. Saunders Company; 1982.

Mylchreest E, Cattley RC, Foster PM. Male reproductive tract malformations in rats following gestational and lactational exposure to Di(n-butyl) phthalate: an antiandrogenic mechanism? *Toxicol Sci.* 1998;43:47–60.

Mylchreest E, Foster PM. DBP exerts its antiandrogenic activity by indirectly interfering with androgen signaling pathways. *Toxicol Appl Pharmacol.* 2000;168:174–175.

Mylchreest E, Sar M, Cattley RC, Foster PMD. Disruption of Androgen-Regulated Male Reproductive Development by Di(n- Butyl) Phthalate during Late Gestation in Rats Is Different from Flutamide. *Toxicol Appl Pharmacol.* 1999;156:81–95.

Mylchreest E, Wallace DG, Cattley RC, Foster PM. Dose-dependent alterations in androgen-regulated male reproductive development in rats exposed to Di(n-butyl) phthalate during late gestation. *Toxicol Sci.* 2000; 55:143–151.

Muir A. Precocious puberty. *Pediatr Rev.* 27:373–381.

Nagano K, Nakayama E, Koyano M, Oobayashi H, Adachi H, Yamada T. Testicular atrophy of mice induced by ethylene glycol mono alkyl ethers (author's transl). *Sangyo Igaku.* 1979;21:29–35.

Nagel SC, vom Saal FS, Thayer KA, Dhar MG, Boechler M, Welshons WV. Relative binding affinity-serum modified access (RBA-SMA) assay predicts the relative in vivo bioactivity of the xenoestrogens bisphenol A and octylphenol. *Environ Health Perspect.* 1997;105:70–76.

Nassar N, Bower C, Barker A. Increasing prevalence of hypospadias in Western Australia, 1980–2000. *Arch Dis Child.* 2007;92(7):580–584.

Niculescu AM. Effects of in utero exposure to DES on male progeny. *J Obstet Gynecol Neonatal Nurs.* 1985;14:468–470.

Noriega NC, Ostby J, Lambright C, Wilson VS, Gray LE Jr. Late gestational exposure to the fungicide prochloraz delays the onset of parturition and causes reproductive malformations in male but not female rat offspring. *Biol Reprod.* 2005;72:1324–1335.

Ohyama K. Disorders of sex differentiation caused by exogenous hormones. *Nippon Rinsho.* 2004;62:379–384.

Ojeda SR, Heger S. New thoughts on female precocious puberty. *J Pediatr Endocrinol Metab.* 2001;14:245–256.

Ojeda SR, Lomniczi A, Mastronardi C, et al. Minireview: the neuroendocrine regulation of puberty: is the time ripe for a systems biology approach? *Endocrinology.* 2006;147:1166–1174.

Ojeda SR, Prevot V, Heger S, Lomniczi A, Dziedzic B, Mungenast A. The neurobiology of female puberty. *Horm Res.* 2003;60(suppl 3):15–20.

Oliveira CA, Mahecha GA, Carnes K, et al. Differential hormonal regulation of estrogen receptors ERalpha and ERbeta and androgen receptor expression in rat efferent ductules. *Reproduction.* 2004;128:73–86.

Ostby J, Kelce WR, Lambright C, Wolf CJ, Mann P, Gray LE Jr. The fungicide procymidone alters sexual differentiation in the male rat by acting as an androgen-receptor antagonist in vivo and in vitro. *Toxicol Ind Health.* 1999;15:80–93.

Ouyang F, Perry MJ, Venners SA, et al. Serum DDT, age at menarche, and abnormal menstrual cycle length. *Occup Environ Med.* 2005;62:878–884.

Owens JW, Ashby J. Critical review and evaluation of the uterotrophic bioassay for the identification of possible estrogen agonists and antagonists: in support of the validation of the OECD uterotrophic protocols for the laboratory rodent. Organisation for Economic Co-operation and Development. *Crit Rev Toxicol.* 2002;32:445–520.

Owens JW, Chaney JG. Weighing the results of differing "low dose" studies of the mouse prostate by Nagel, Cagen, and Ashby: quantification of experimental power and statistical results. *Regul Toxicol Pharmacol.* 2005;43:194–202.

Owens W, Ashby J, Odum J, Onyon L. The OECD program to validate the rat uterotrophic bioassay. Phase 2: dietary phytoestrogen analyses. *Environ Health Perspect.* 2003;111:1559–1567.

Owens W, Koeter HB. The OECD program to validate the rat uterotrophic bioassay: an overview. *Environ Health Perspect.* 2003;111:1527–1529.

Owens W, Zeiger E, Walker M, Ashby J, Onyon L, Gray LE Jr. The OECD program to validate the rat Hershberger bioassay to screen compounds for in vivo androgen and antiandrogen responses. Phase 1: use of a potent agonist and a potent antagonist to test the standardized protocol. *Environ Health Perspect.* 2006;114:1259–1265.

Papathanasiou A, Hadjiathanasiou C. Precocious puberty. *Pediatr Endocrinol Rev.* 2006;3(suppl 1):182–187.

Paranko J, Pelliniemi LJ, Vaheri A, Foidart JM, Lakkala-Paranko T. Morphogenesis and fibronectin in sexual differentiation of rat embryonic gonads. *Differentiation.* 1983;23(suppl):S72–S81.

Parks LG, Lambright CS, Orlando EF, Guillette LJ Jr, Ankley GT, Gray LE Jr. Masculinization of female mosquitofish in Kraft mill effluent-contaminated Fenholloway River water is associated with androgen receptor agonist activity. *Toxicol Sci.* 2001;62(2):257–267.

Parks LG, Ostby JS, Lambright CR, et al. The plasticizer diethylhexyl phthalate induces malformations by decreasing fetal testosterone synthesis during sexual differentiation in the male rat. *Toxicol Sci.* 2000;58(2):339–349.

Paulozzi LJ, Erickson JD, Jackson RJ. Hypospadias trends in two US surveillance systems. *Pediatrics.* 1997;100:831–834.

Pelliniemi LJ. Ultrastructure of the early ovary and testis in pig embryos. *Am J Anat.* 1975;144:89–111.

Pelliniemi LJ, Niei M. Fine structure of the human foetal testis. I. The interstitial tissue. *Z Zellforsch Mikrosk Anat.* 1969;99:507–522.

Pierik FH, Burdorf A, Nijman JM, de Muinck Keizer-Schrama SM, Juttmann RE, Weber RF. A high hypospadias rate in The Netherlands. *Human Reprod.* 2002;17:1112–1115.

Porter MP, Faizan MK, Grady RW, Mueller BA. Hypospadias in Washington State: maternal risk factors and prevalence trends. *Pediatrics.* 2005;115:e495–e499.

Quinn MM, Wegman DH, Greaves IA, et al. Investigation of reports of sexual dysfunction among male chemical workers manufacturing stilbene derivatives. *Am J Ind Med.* 1990;18:55–68.

Reeve IT, Voss JC, Miller MG. 1,3-Dinitrobenzene metabolism and GSH depletion. *Chem Res Toxicol.* 2002;15:361–366.

Rehnberg GL, Linder RE, Goldman JM, Hein JF, McElroy WK, Cooper RL. Changes in testicular and serum hormone concentrations in the male rat following treatment with m-dinitrobenzene. *Toxicol Appl Pharmacol.* 1988;95(2):255–264.

Reich MR, Spong JK. Kepone: a chemical disaster in Hopewell, Virginia. *Int J Health Serv.* 1983;13:227–246.

Robaire B, Ewing LL, Irby DC, Desjardins C. Interactions of testosterone and estradiol-17 beta on the reproductive tract of the male rat. *Biol. Reprod.* 1979;21:455–463.

Rosa FW. Virilization of the female fetus with maternal danazol exposure. *Am J Obstet Gynecol.* 1984;149:99–100.

Roy AK, Chatterjee B. Androgen action. *Crit Rev Eukaryot Gene Expr.* 1995;5:157–176.

Saito K, O'Donnell L, McLachlan RI, Robertson DM. Spermiation failure is a major contributor to early spermatogenic suppression caused by hormone withdrawal in adult rats. *Endocrinology.* 2000;141:2779–2785.

Saiyed H, Dewan A, Bhatnagar V, et al. Effect of endosulfan on male reproductive development. *Environ Health Perspect.* 2003;111:1958–1962.

Sawaki M, Noda S, Muroi T, et al. In utero through lactational exposure to ethinyl estradiol induces cleft phallus and delayed ovarian dysfunction in the offspring. *Toxicol Sci.* 2003;75(2):402–411.

Schäfer-Somi S. Cytokines during early pregnancy of mammals: a review. *Anim Reprod Sci.* 2003;75:73–94.

Schardein J. *Chemically Induced Birth Defects.* New York: Marcel Dekker Inc; 2000.

Semple RK, Achermann JC, Ellery J, et al. Two novel missense mutations in g protein-coupled receptor 54 in a patient with hypogonadotropic hypogonadism. *J Clin Endocrinol Metab.* 2005;90:1849–1855.

Setchell BP, Waites GM. Changes in the permeability of the testicular capillaries and of the 'blood-testis barrier' after injection of cadmium chloride in the rat. *J Endocrinol.* 1970;47:81–86.

Shaffer NG. DES: a continuing health concern. *Pa Med.* 2000;103:17.

Silversides DW, Price CA, Cooke GM. Effects of short-term exposure to hydroxyflutamide in utero on the development of the reproductive tract in male mice. *Can J Physiol Pharmacol.* 1995;73:1582–1588.

Skakkebaek NE. Endocrine disrupters and testicular dysgenesis syndrome. *Horm Res.* 2002;57(suppl S2):43.

Smith ER, Quinn MM. Uterotropic action in rats of amsonic acid and three of its synthetic precursors. *J Toxico Environ Health.* 1992;36:13–25.

Snegovskikh V, Park JS, Norwitz ER. Endocrinology of parturition. *Endocrinol Metab Clin North Am.* 2006;35:173–191, viii.

Stevenson JG, Umstead GS. Sexual dysfunction due to antihypertensive agents. *Drug Intell Clin Pharm.* 1984;18:113–121.

Stoker TE, Cooper RL, Goldman JM, Andrews JE. Characterization of pregnancy outcome following thiram-induced ovulatory delay in the female rat. *Neurotoxicol Teratol.* 1996;18:277–282.

Stoker TE, Goldman JM, Cooper RL. The dithiocarbamate fungicide thiram disrupts the hormonal control of ovulation in the female rat. *Reprod Toxicol.* 1993;7:211–218.

Stoker TE, Goldman JM, Cooper RL. Delayed ovulation and pregnancy outcome: effect of environmental toxicants on the neuroendocrine control of the ovary(1). *Environ Toxicol Pharmacol.* 2001;9:117–129.

Stoker TE, Jeffay SC, Zucker RM, Cooper RL, Perreault SD. Abnormal fertilization is responsible for reduced fecundity following thiram-induced ovulatory delay in the rat. *Biol Reprod.* 2003;68:2142–2149.

Stoker TE, Laws SC, Crofton KM, Hedge JM, Ferrell JM, Cooper RL. Assessment of DE-71, a commercial polybrominated diphenyl ether (PBDE) mixture, in the EDSP male and female pubertal protocols. *Toxicol Sci.* 2004;78(1):144–155.

Stoker TE, Parks LG, Gray LE, Cooper RL. Endocrine-disrupting chemicals: prepubertal exposures and effects on sexual maturation and thyroid function in the male rat. A focus on the EDSTAC recommendations. Endocrine Disrupter Screening and Testing Advisory Committee. *Crit Rev Toxicol.* 2000;30(2):197–252.

Stoker TE, Perreault SD, Bremser K, Marshall RS, Murr A, Cooper RL. Acute exposure to molinate alters neuroendocrine control of ovulation in the rat. *Toxicol Sci.* 2005;84:38–48.

Stroheker T, Cabaton N, Nourdin G, Regnier JF, Lhuguent JC, Chagnon MC. Evaluation of anti-androgenic activity of di-(2-ethylhexyl)phthalate. *Toxicology.* 2005;208:115–121.

Swan SH, Main KM, Liu F, et al. Decrease in anogenital distance among male infants with prenatal phthalate exposure. *Environ Health Perspect.* 2005;113:1056–1061.

Swingle WW, Seay P, Perlmutt J, Collins EJ, Barlow G Jr, Fedor EJ. An experimental study of pseudopregnancy in rat. *Am J Physiol.* 1951;167:586–592.

Tan SW, Zoeller RT. Integrating basic research on thyroid hormone action into screening and testing programs for thyroid disruptors. *Crit Rev Toxicol.* 2007;37:5–10.

Tena-Sempere M. KiSS-1 and reproduction: focus on its role in the metabolic regulation of fertility. *Neuroendocrinology.* 2006;83:275–281.

Thayer KA, Foster PM. Workgroup report: National Toxicology Program Workshop on hormonally induced reproductive tumors—relevance of rodent bioassays. *Environ Health Perspect.* 2007;115:1351–1356.

Toppari J, Kaleva M, Virtanen HE. Trends in the incidence of cryptorchidism and hypospadias, and methodological limitations of registry-based data. *Hum Reprod Update.* 2001;7:282–286.

Tranguch S, Daikoku T, Guo Y, Wang H, Dey SK. Molecular complexity in establishing uterine receptivity and implantation. *Cell Mol Life Sci.* 2005;62:1964–1973.

Trasler JM, Hales BF, Robaire B. Paternal cyclophosphamide treatment of rats causes fetal loss and malformations without affecting male fertility. *Nature.* 1985;316:144–146.

Tuvemo T. Treatment of central precocious puberty. *Expert Opin Investig Drugs.* 2006;15:495–505.

Uckert S, Hedlund P, Andersson KE, Truss MC, Jonas U, Stief CG. Update on phosphodiesterase (PDE) isoenzymes as pharmacologic targets in urology: present and future. *Eur Urol.* 2006;50:1194–1207; discussion 1207.

Veurink M, KosterM, Berg LT. The history of DES, lessons to be learned. *Pharm World Sci.* 2005;27:139–43.

Veyssiere G, Berger M, Jean-Faucher C, de Turckheim M, Jean C. Testosterone and dihydrotestosterone in sexual ducts and genital tubercle of rabbit fetuses during sexual organogenesis: effects of fetal decapitation. *J Steroid Biochem.* 1982;17:149–154.

Vinggaard AM, Hnida C, Breinholt V, Larsen JC. Screening of selected pesticides for inhibition of CYP19 aromatase activity in vitro. *Toxicol In Vitro.* 2000;14:227–234.

Vinggaard AM, Nellemann C, Dalgaard M, Jorgensen EB, Andersen HR. Antiandrogenic Effects in Vitro and in Vivo of the Fungicide Prochloraz. *Toxicol Sci.* 2002;69:344–353.

Vogel G. Leptin: a trigger for puberty? *Science.* 1996;274:1466–1467.

vom Saal FS, Cooke PS, Buchanan DL, et al. A physiologically based approach to the study of bisphenol A and other estrogenic chemicals on the size of reproductive organs, daily sperm production, and behavior. *Toxicol Ind Health.* 1998;14:239–260.

vom Saal FS, Nagel SC, Timms BG, Welshons WV. Implications for human health of the extensive bisphenol A literature showing adverse effects at low doses: a response to attempts to mislead the public. *Toxicology.* 2005;212:244–252, author reply 253–244.

Wacharasindhu S, Petwijit T, Aroonparkmongkol S, Srivuthana S, Kingpetch K. Bone mineral density and body composition in Thai Precocious Puberty girls treated with GnRH agonist. *J Med Assoc Thai.* 2006;89:1194–1198.

Warner M, Samuels S, Mocarelli P, et al. Serum dioxin concentrations and age at menarche. *Environ Health Perspect.* 2004;112:1289–1292.

Warnock DH, Csapo AI. Progesterone withdrawal induced by ICI 81008 in pregnant rats. *Prostaglandins.* 1975;10:715–724.

Welshons WV, Nagel SC, vom Saal FS. Large effects from small exposures. III. Endocrine mechanisms mediating effects of bisphenol A at levels of human exposure. *Endocrinology.* 2006;147:S56–S69.

Whelan EA, Grajewski B, Wild DK, Schnorr TM, Alderfer R. Evaluation of reproductive function among men occupationally exposed to a stilbene derivative: II. Perceived libido and potency. *Am J Ind Med.* 1996; 29:59–65.

Wilson JD, Lasnitzki I. Dihydrotestosterone formation in fetal tissues of the rabbit and rat. *Endocrinology.* 1971;89:659–668.

Wilson VS, Bobseine K, Gray LE Jr. Development and characterization of a cell line that stably expresses an estrogen-responsive luciferase reporter for the detection of estrogen receptor agonist and antagonists. *Toxicol Sci.* 2004;81(1):69–77.

Wilson VS, Lambright C, Furr J, et al. Phthalate ester-induced gubernacular lesions are associated with reduced insl3 gene expression in the fetal rat testis. *Toxicol Lett.* 2005;146:207–215.

Wilson VS, Lambright C, Ostby J, Gray LE Jr. In vitro and in vivo effects of 17beta-trenbolone: a feedlot effluent contaminant. *Toxicol Sci.* 2002; 70:202–211.

Wine RN, Li LH, Barnes LH, Gulati DK, Chapin RE. Reproductive toxicity of di-*n*-butylphthalate in a continuous breeding protocol in Sprague–Dawley rats. *Environ Health Perspect.* 1997;105:102–107.

Winker R, Rudiger HW. Reproductive toxicology in occupational settings: an update. *Int Arch Occup Environ Health.* 2006;79:1–10.

Wolf CJ, Hotchkiss A, Ostby JS, LeBlanc GA, Gray LE Jr. Effects of prenatal testosterone propionate on the sexual development of male and female rats: a dose–response study. *Toxicol Sci.* 2002;65:71–86.

Wolff MS, Britton JA, Russo JC. TCDD and puberty in girls. *Environ Health Perspect.* 2005;113:A17; author reply A18.

Woods JS. Drug effects on human sexual behavior. In: Woods NF, ed. *HumanSexuality in Health and Illness.* 3d ed. St. Louis: Mosby; 1984.

Yamasaki K, Sawaki M, Ohta R, et al. OECD validation of the Hershberger assay in Japan: phase 2 dose response of methyltestosterone, vinclozolin, and *p,p'*-DDE. *Environ Health Perspect.* 2003;111: 1912–1919.

Yin W, Gore AC. Neuroendocrine control of reproductive aging: roles of GnRH neurons. *Reproduction.* 2006;131:403–414.

chapter 21

Toxic Responses of the Endocrine System

Patricia B. Hoyer and Jodi A. Flaws

INTRODUCTION

Higher animals, including humans, have developed the ability to regulate their internal environment, independent of wide fluctuations in external factors, in the form of endocrine systems. An endocrine system consists of (1) an endocrine gland that secretes a hormone, (2) the hormone itself, and (3) a target tissue that responds to the hormone. The classical definition of a hormone is a chemical substance produced by a ductless endocrine gland and secreted into the blood, which carries it to a specific target organ to produce an effect (Porterfield, 2001). In addition to the humoral communication regulated by endocrine systems, the nervous system also regulates overall bodily functions (Hedge *et al.*, 1987). The two systems are intimately interconnected and normally work in close concert. One direct point at which the two systems interface involves "neuroendocrine" cells, which are special types of neurons capable of secreting humoral substances (hormones) in response to synaptic input (neurotransmitters).

The hormone-producing glands of humans include the pituitary (hypophysis), the thyroid and parathyroids, the adrenals, the gonads, and the pancreas. The mechanisms by which endocrine glands synthesize, store, and secrete hormones depend on the chemical properties of the hormone. There are primarily three chemical classes of hormones: amino acid derivatives, peptides and proteins, and steroids. The amino acid derivatives include the catecholamines, epinephrine, and norepinephrine (produced in the adrenal medulla); and the thyroid hormones, triiodothyronine (T_3) and thyroxine (T_4). A large number of hormones are peptides or proteins, such as the neurohormones of the posterior pituitary, tropic hormones of the anterior pituitary, and pancreatic hormones. Steroids are produced by the adrenal cortex, the testes, the ovaries, and in pregnancy, the placenta. These hormones are derivatives of cholesterol. In general, designation of a hormone as hydrophilic (peptides and proteins, catecholamines) or hydrophobic (thyroid hormones, vitamin D, and steroids) provides information useful in understanding the synthesis, secretion, transport, and target cell mechanism of action of that particular hormone (Table 21-1).

Circulating hormone levels are influenced by the rate of secretion from the endocrine gland, rate of metabolism, and method by

Table 21-1

Groups of Hormones

	HYDROPHILIC	HYDROPHOBIC (LIPOPHILIC)
Endocrine gland cellular storage	Yes	No
Secretion	Secretory vesicles	Passive diffusion
Transport in blood	Free*	Protein bound
Target organ receptors	Plasma membrane	Nuclear

*Catecholamines are transported on albumin.

which hormone is transported in the blood. The rate of secretion is regulated in the endocrine gland by a variety of physiological factors. The rate of hormonal metabolism or degradation in the bloodstream determines its half-life ($t_{1/2}$) in blood. The cells of the endocrine gland typically contain only a small store of synthesized hormone, although one noted exception is the thyroid that stores hormone for several months. Therefore, in response to a specific stimulus, the cells synthesize and secrete hormone directly into the bloodstream where they are normally found in very low concentrations (10^{-8} to 10^{-12} M). Although most hormones are carried by the blood, they are not all transported in the same way. Hydrophilic hormones (peptides and proteins) are freely dissolved in the plasma and do not require a specialized transport system. In contrast, given the limited aqueous solubilities of hydrophobic hormones (steroids, thyroid hormones), it is not possible for them to exist in free solution in the aqueous environment of the blood so they circulate bound to specialized serum binding proteins or to albumin. The two major functions of serum binding proteins are to (1) solubilize the hormone for transport in the blood, and (2) extend the life of the hormone in circulation ($t_{1/2}$) by protecting the small molecules from enzymatic degradation in the blood stream. The extent to which a hydrophobic hormone is protein bound varies from one hormone to another. However, in all cases, the total hormone pool is predominantly in the bound form. This is important because it is generally accepted that only the pool of free hormone is biologically active. Therefore, binding proteins also provide a large hormone reserve that can be called upon to replenish the free pool. It is the magnitude of the free pool rather than the total pool of hormone that is monitored and adjusted to maintain normal endocrine function.

Hormones elicit a wide variety of biological responses. For virtually all hormones, the initial step in this process is binding of the hormone to a receptor in its target tissue. Those receptors can be located on the plasma membrane (peptide, protein, and catecholamine hormones) or have their action in the cellular nucleus (steroids, thyroid, and vitamin D hormones). The interaction of the hormone with its receptor initiates a chain of intracellular events leading to the physiological response specific to that hormone. For each endocrine system in this chapter, the sections first briefly describe the anatomy and physiology of the normal endocrine gland because such a background is important for understanding the effects of xenobiotics on that gland. This is followed by a description of some effects of environmental chemicals on various aspects of the system's function. Mechanistic information is included whenever possible to aid in the interpretation of findings and to assess their potential for human risk.

PITUITARY GLAND

Anatomy and Physiology

The pituitary may be divided into four major subdivisions. The pars distalis (adenohypophysis or anterior pituitary) forms the largest subdivision. The pars intermedia forms the thin cellular zone between the adenohypophysis and neurohypophysis. The pars tuberalis (stalk) is a very small subdivision, highly vascularized, and is not known to secrete hormones. Finally, the pars nervosa (neurohypophysis or posterior pituitary) forms the second largest subdivision of the pituitary. There are two basic types of communication between the hypothalamus and pituitary (Fig. 21-1). (1) The adenohypophysis receives vascular supply from the median eminence. The communication between the two is endocrine in that peptide hormones are released in nerve endings of tuberoinfundibular neurons, which are neuroendocrine cells located in the median eminence. Once secreted, the peptides are transported in the blood via the pars tuberalis to the anterior pituitary. (2) The neurohypophysis receives neuronal communication from the supraoptic nucleus (SON) and paraventricular nucleus (PVN). The type of communication is neuroendocrine, the cell bodies are located in the SON and PVN, and their axons stretch through the median eminence of the hypothalamus, span the infundibular stalk, and terminate in the posterior lobe (Porterfield, 2001). These cells are called magnocellular neurons and are neuroendocrine cells. Therefore, functionally and anatomically, the posterior pituitary is an extension of the hypothalamus. In fact, the hormones produced in the posterior pituitary are actually synthesized in the neuroendocrine cell bodies located in the hypothalamus (SON and PVN).

There are a variety of mechanisms that regulate the rate of release of hormones in the neuroendocrine pathway. Superimposed on endogenous rhythms of hormone release are a number of feedback mechanisms. To maintain appropriate homeostasis, the endocrine organ must constantly monitor systemic hormone concentrations, or some function of it. This awareness is provided in

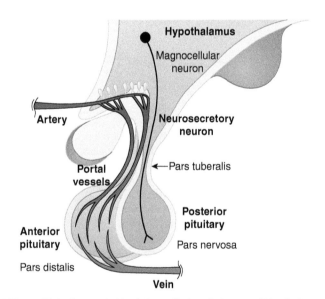

Figure 21-1. *Communication between the hypothalamus and the pituitary.* The anterior pituitary receives endocrine input from the hypothalamus in the form of peptide releasing hormones, which are transported in portal vessels to stimulate release of hormones in the anterior pituitary cells. The posterior pituitary is innervated by axons extending from magnocellular neurons with their cell bodies located in the hypothalamus. Stimulation of these cell bodies results in hormonal secretion in the posterior pituitary (Modified from Hedge *et al.*, 1987).

Table 21-2

Pituitary Cell Distribution

CELL TYPE	% CELLS IN PITUITARY	HORMONE SECRETED
Somatotrophs	50	Growth hormone (GH)
Lactotrophs	10–20	Prolactin (PRL)
Corticotrophs	15–20	Adrenocorticotropic hormone (ACTH)
Thyrotrophs	5	Thyroid stimulating
Gonadotrophs	5–15	Luteinizing hormone (LH) Follicle stimulating hormone(FSH)

the form of negative feedback loops. By this mechanism, hormones produced in the target organ feedback to reduce hypothalamic peptide and/or anterior pituitary hormone release (Hedge *et al.*, 1987). For example, high circulating levels of cortisol produced in the adrenal cortex will inhibit corticotrophin releasing hormone (CRH) release from the hypothalamus, and adrenocorticotropic hormone (ACTH) release from the pituitary.

Most of the blood supply from the hypothalamus to the pars distalis (adenohypophysis, anterior pituitary) is derived from a portal system (hypothalamo-hypophyseal vessels), which arises from a capillary network in the median eminence, transports down the pituitary stalk, then terminates in the anterior lobe. Blood flowing from the hypothalamus to the pituitary delivers hypothalamic peptides that regulate anterior pituitary hormone secretion. There are six major protein hormones secreted by five distinctive cell types in the anterior pituitary. Table 21-2 provides a summary of some of the characteristics of these five cell types.

Each type of endocrine cell in the adenohypophysis is under the control of a specific releasing hormone from the hypothalamus (Fig. 21-2). These releasing hormones are small peptides synthesized and secreted by tuberoinfundibular neurons of the hypothalamus. They are transported by short axonal processes to the median eminence, where they are released into capillaries and conveyed by the hypophyseal portal system to specific trophic hormone-secreting cells in the adenohypophysis. Each hormone stimulates the rapid release of preformed secretory granules containing a specific trophic hormone. Specific releasing hormones have been identified for thyroid-stimulating hormone (TSH), follicle-stimulating hormone (FSH) and luteinizing hormone (LH), adrenocorticotropic hormone (ACTH), and growth hormone (GH). Prolactin (PRL) secretion is stimulated by a number of factors, the most important of which appears to be thyrotropin-releasing hormone (TRH). Dopamine serves as the major prolactin-inhibitory factor to suppress PRL secretion. Another hypothalamic release-inhibitory factor is somatostatin, which inhibits secretion of growth hormone (Hadley and Levine, 2007). Regulation of the thyroid gland by TSH and the adrenal cortex by ACTH will be discussed in this chapter. Regulation of the gonads by LH and FSH is discussed in Chap. 20.

The pars nervosa (neurohypophysis; posterior pituitary) in the human secretes two important hormones. These are vasopressin, VP (or antidiuretic hormone, ADH) and oxytocin. They are nonapeptides that share a strong structural homology. ADH plays an important regulatory role in water conservation and maintenance of body fluid osmolality, blood volume, and pressure. ADH (VP) has two major effects corresponding to its two names; (1) it enhances reabsorption of water by the distal tubule and collecting ducts of the kidney producing an antidiuretic effect, which decreases osmotic pressure of the blood, and (2) it causes contraction of vascular smooth muscle producing a generalized pressor effect (Porterfield, 2001). Oxytocin stimulates contraction of smooth muscles located in the uterine myometrium to regulate fetal parturition, and in breast alveoli to regulate milk let-down during lactation.

Pituitary Toxicity

Few studies have focused on the effects of xenobiotics on the pituitary gland (Stefaneanu and Kovacs, 1991; Capen, 2001). However, studies consistently show that heavy metals may target pituitary gland structure or function (Caride *et al.*, 2010a; Lafuente and Esquifino, 1999). Cadmium affects many different cell types in the pituitary gland (Caride *et al.*, 2010a; Lafuente and Esquifino, 1999). It affects the lactotrophs by inhibiting prolactin secretion after long-term or acute exposure (Lafuente and Esquifino, 1999). The ability of cadmium to inhibit prolactin secretion may depend on the route of administration and age of the animals. In adult rats, oral and subcutaneous administrations of cadmium inhibit prolactin secretion, whereas only oral administration inhibits prolactin in pubertal animals (Lafuente and Esquifino, 1999). Cadmium also affects the gonadotrophs by inhibiting LH and FSH secretion in male and female rats (Lafuente and Esquifino, 1999). This effect of cadmium on the gonadotrophs may depend on the route of exposure because oral, but not subcutaneous administration of cadmium inhibits gonadotropin levels (Lafuente and Esquifino, 1999). Further, the ability of cadmium to affect gonadotrophs may differ with age. Studies indicate that the degree of cadmium-induced inhibition of LH and FSH is higher in older rats compared to younger rats (Lafuente and Esquifino, 1999). Similarly, cadmium affects the corticotrophs by altering ACTH levels in a manner that differs with age (Lafuente and Esquifino, 1999). Cadmium exposure increases ACTH levels in rodents exposed during puberty and decreases ACTH levels in animals exposed during adulthood. Further, cadmium may also affect the somatotrophs (Lafuente and Esquifino, 1999). Studies indicate that acute exposure to cadmium

Hypothalamic releasing hormones

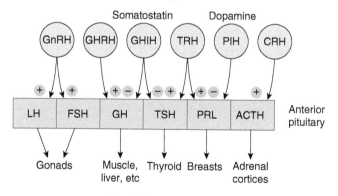

Target tissues

Figure 21-2. *Regulation of anterior pituitary hormone release (rectangles) by hypothalamic releasing hormones (circles).* Major target tissues for the anterior pituitary hormones are indicated. GnRH, gonadotropin releasing hormone; LH, luteinizing hormone; FSH, follicle-stimulating hormone; GHRH, growth hormone releasing hormone; GHIH, growth hormone inhibiting hormone (somatostatin); GH, growth hormone; TRH, thyrotropin releasing hormone; TSH, thyroid stimulating hormone; PIH, prolactin inhibiting hormone (dopamine); CRH, corticotropin releasing hormone; ACTH, adrenocorticotropic hormone. +, stimulatory; –, inhibitory (Modified from Hedge *et al.*, 1987).

decreases circulating GH levels, while treatment for a longer period (14 days) increases circulating GH levels (Lafuente and Esquifino, 1999). One study evaluated the effect of chronic exposure (30 days in drinking water) to cadmium in male Sprague–Dawley rats on circadian release of ACTH, GH, and TSH (Caride et al., 2010b). Compared with controls, cadmium delayed the 24-hour peak of ACTH release and eliminated that of GH. Interestingly, mean daily circulating levels of ACTH and TSH were increased by the metal. These findings supported that cadmium has chronotoxic effects at the level of the pituitary.

Cadmium is not the only heavy metal that affects the pituitary. Lead and mercury inhibit secretion of LH and FSH from the gonadotropes (Sikka and Wang, 2008). Further, high lead levels have been associated with increases in ADH secretion in case reports (Suarez et al., 1992).

Environmental contaminants such as polychlorinated biphenyls (PCBs) and polybrominated diphenyl ethers (PBDEs) also affect the pituitary gland (Sikka and Wang, 2008). PCBs inhibit release of LH and FSH from gonadotrophs (Sikka and Wang, 2008). They also affect the thyrotrophs by inhibiting TSH secretion (Patrick, 2009; Zoeller, 2010).

Several pesticides cause adverse effects on the pituitary (Lafuente et al., 2000; Reuber, 1984; Sikka and Wang, 2008; Wozniak et al., 2005). The insecticide dimethoate causes pituitary tumors in male and female rats (Reuber, 1984). The organochlorine pesticide methoxychlor increases prolactin levels as well as LH levels (Lafuente et al., 2000). Both dieldrin and endosulfan stimulate prolactin secretion from the pituitary cell line GH3 via a mechanism that involves increasing calcium, which stimulates the release of prolactin (Wozniak et al., 2005). Measurements were made in pubertal male Sprague–Dawley rats following prenatal and lactational exposure to endosulfan. Expression of mRNA encoding prolactin, LH, GH, and TSH was downregulated, whereas secretion of LH and GH was stimulated and prolactin and TSH were inhibited (Caride et al., 2010c). The herbicide atrazine has been demonstrated in vitro to also have direct pituitary effects by binding to the growth hormone releasing hormone receptor and inhibiting GH expression at the mRNA and protein levels (Fakhouri et al., 2010).

Several phytoestrogens affect pituitary cells (Wozniak et al., 2005). Coumestrol reduces pulsatile LH secretion and suppresses the pituitary response to exogenous gonadotropin releasing hormone (GnRH) in female rats (Dickerson and Gore, 2007; Gore, 2011). Acute genistein exposure suppresses pulsatile LH release in ovariectomized ewes (Dickerson and Gore, 2007). Chronic genistein exposure increases the pituitary size in rodents (Dickerson and Gore, 2007). Bisphenol A (BPA) increases LH secretion in adult male rats and GH content and receptors in juvenile rainbow trout (Aluru et al., 2010; Tohei et al., 2001).

A variety of chemicals used in industrial processes alter pituitary structure or function (Verma and Rana, 2009). Flame retardants (tetrabromobisphenol A and tetrachlorobisphenol A) increase proliferation in GH3 cells, a pituitary cell line (Kitamura et al., 2002). The plasticizer BPA increases GH content in rainbow trout (Aluru et al., 2010). 2-Mercaptobenzothiazole, which is used in rubber products and can come into contact with drinking water, causes pituitary tumors in chronically exposed rats and mice (Whittaker et al., 2004).

Finally, a few pharmaceutical agents have been linked to changes in the pituitary. Cyanamide, a chemical used in the treatment of alcoholics, increases pro-opiomelancortin mRNA in the anterior pituitary when coadministered with ethanol (Kinoshita et al., 2001). A safety evaluation of RO2910, a drug for treatment of HIV infection, has shown that RO2910 causes hypertrophy in the thyrotrophs (Zabka et al., 2011). The neuroleptic agent sulpiride causes the release of prolactin from the anterior pituitary in the rat and stimulates DNA replication (Capen, 2001). The administration of clomiphene prevents the stimulation of DNA synthesis produced by sulpiride, but does not affect prolactin release from the gland (Capen, 2001). These findings suggest that the intracellular prolactin content of the pituitary plays a role in the regulation of DNA synthesis through a mechanism mediated by estrogens (Capen, 2001).

ADRENAL GLANDS

The adrenals are two small glands situated on the superior poles of the kidneys (Fig. 21-3). The major physiological role of the adrenals is management of stress. Each adrenal gland is divided into two morphologically and functionally distinct regions. The adrenal cortex is the more exterior region, and the interior region is the medulla. The cortex synthesizes and secretes steroid hormones that function to regulate salt and fluid balance, glucose homeostasis, and a long-term response to stress. The medulla can be likened to a large postganglionic neuron, and secretes the catecholamines, epinephrine and norepinephrine, upon stimulation by preganglionic cholinergic sympathetic fibers. The medullary catecholamines combine with norepinephrine from sympathetic nerve endings to mediate a very rapid time frame of response to stress (Hadley and Levine, 2007). Because of the anatomic proximity of the two regions of the adrenal glands, blood from the cortex perfuses the medulla. This provides a functional association because cortisol secreted by the cortex stimulates expression of phenylethanolamine-N-methyltransferase (PNMT), the enzyme that converts norepinephrine to epinephrine in the medulla.

The adrenals have not been as widely studied in toxicology as other endocrine glands, even though it has been documented to be the most common toxicological target of all (Ribelin, 1984). In fact, the relative frequency of effects on endocrine systems reported from in vivo toxicology studies has been adrenal > testes > thyroid > ovary > pancreas > pituitary > parathyroid, with the adrenal cortex most frequently targeted (Harvey et al., 2007). This relative lack of attention in toxicology is surprising considering the critical role of the adrenals in mediating endocrine homeostasis throughout the body.

ADRENAL CORTEX

As seen in Fig. 21-3, the adrenal cortex can be divided at the cellular level into three separate zones, the zona glomerulosa (outermost), the zona fasciculata (intermediate), and the zona reticularis (innermost). The zona glomerulosa is responsible for production of the mineralocorticoid hormone, aldosterone. The glucocorticoid hormones, cortisol and corticosterone, are both secreted by the zona fasciculata and, to some extent the zona reticularis. The zona reticularis also secretes the androgens, dehydroepiandrosterone, and androstenedione (Porterfield, 2001). These adrenal androgens are thought to be involved in the onset of puberty and serve a function in postmenopausal women; however, they are of relatively little biological significance under normal circumstances.

The adrenal cortex regulates many physiological functions such as the immune system, inflammation, water and electrolyte balance, carbohydrate and protein metabolism involving such target organs as the liver, kidney, heart, bone, and nervous system (Harvey, 2010). The adrenal cortex is predisposed to the toxic

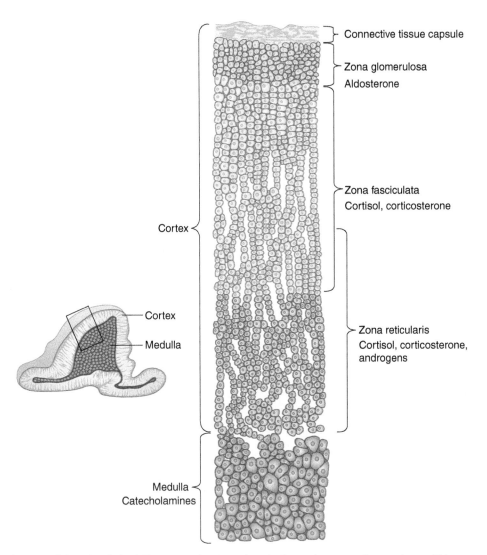

Figure 21-3. *Anatomy of the adrenal gland.* The outer region (cortex) synthesizes and secretes adrenocorticosteroid hormones. The cortex consists of three zones. The zona glomerulosa produces the mineralocorticoid aldosterone. The inner zones, fasciculata and reticularis, produce glucocorticoids, corticosterone and cortisol, as well as adrenal androgens. The inner region, medulla, synthesizes and secretes catecholamines, epinephrine, and norepinephrine (Modified from Hadley and Levine, 2007).

effects of xenobiotic chemicals for two apparent reasons. First, the adrenal cortical cells of most animal species contain large stores of lipids used primarily as substrate for steroidogenesis. Many adrenal cortical toxic compounds are lipophilic and, therefore, can accumulate in these lipid-rich cells. Second, adrenal cortical cells express enzymes involved in steroidogenesis, including those of the cytochrome P450 family, which are capable of metabolizing xenobiotic chemicals. A number of toxic xenobiotic chemicals serve as pseudosubstrates for these enzymes and can be metabolized to reactive toxic species. These reactive compounds can cause direct toxicity by covalent interactions with cellular macromolecules, or through lipid peroxidation or the generation of free radicals (Hinson and Raven, 2006).

Steroidogenesis

Adrenal steroids are synthesized from cholesterol by specific enzyme-catalyzed reactions that involve a complex shuttling of steroid intermediates between the mitochondria and endoplasmic reticulum. Histologically, adrenal cortical cells are characterized by an abundance of lipid droplets, mitochondria, and smooth endoplasmic reticulum. Lipid droplets contain cholesterol, the precursor

substrate for steroid production. The specificity of mitochondrial hydroxylation reactions in terms of precursor acted upon and the position of the substrate that is hydroxylated is confined to a specific cytochrome P450. The common biosynthetic pathway from cholesterol is the formation of pregnenolone, the basic precursor for the three major classes of adrenal steroids (Fig. 21-4).

In the zonae fasciculata and reticularis, pregnenolone is first converted to progesterone by two microsomal enzymes. Three subsequent hydroxylation reactions involve carbon atoms at the 17, 21, and 11 positions. The resulting steroid is cortisol, which is the major glucocorticoid in teleosts, hamsters, dogs, and nonhuman and human primates. Corticosterone is the major glucocorticoid produced in amphibians, reptiles, birds, rats, mice, and rabbits. It is produced in a manner similar to the production of cortisol, except that progesterone does not undergo 17α-hydroxylation and proceeds directly to 21-hydroxylation and 11β-hydroxylation.

In the zona glomerulosa, pregnenolone is converted to aldosterone by a series of enzyme-catalyzed reactions similar to those involved in cortisol formation; however, the cells of this zone lack the 17α-hydroxyprogesterone that is required to produce cortisol. Therefore, the initial hydroxylation product is corticosterone. Some of

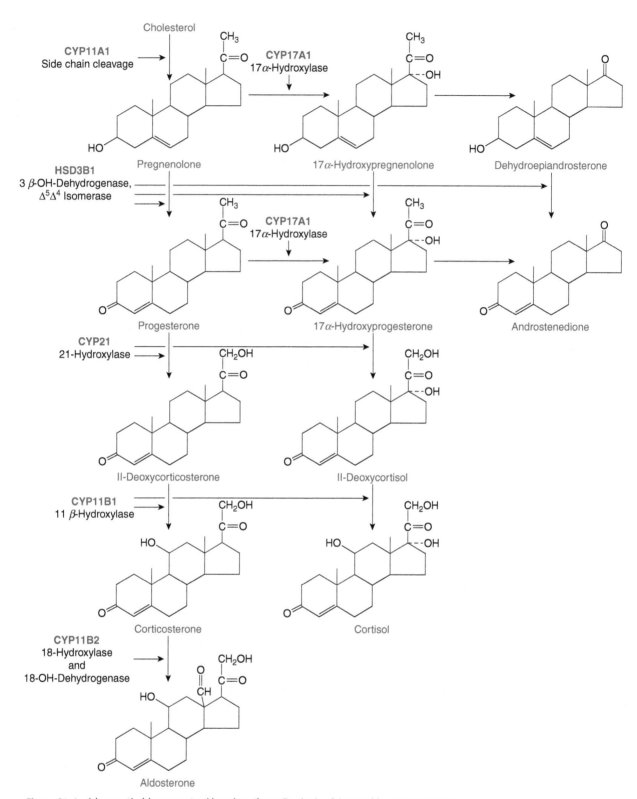

Figure 21-4. *Adrenocortical hormone steroidogenic pathway.* Synthesis of the steroids uses cholesterol as a substrate. A series of cytochrome P450 (CYP) enzymes participate in synthesis of aldosterone (zona glomerulosa) or cortisol and adrenal androgens (zonae fasciculata and reticularis). The zona glomerulosa does not express the enzyme 17α-OH (CYP17A1), whereas the zonae fasciculata and reticularis do not express the enzyme 18OH (CYP11B2) (Modified from Hadley and Levine, 2007.)

the corticosterone is acted on by 18-hydroxylase to form 18-hydroxy-corticosterone, which in turn interacts with 18-hydroxysteroid dehydrogenase to form aldosterone. Since 18-hydroxysteroid dehydrogenase is expressed only in the zona glomerulosa, it is not surprising that only this zone has the capacity to produce aldosterone.

Glucocorticoids

To better appreciate the wide-ranging effects of glucocorticoids, the effects of the hormone can be divided into normal physiological and pharmacological effects, since cortisol is therapeutically quite effective and widely prescribed. The physiological effects include (a) hepatic glucose production, gluconeogenesis (liver), (b) protein catabolism (skeletal muscle), (c) fat catabolism (adipose tissue), (d) increased bone resorption, (e) altered mood (CNS), (f) increased gastric acidity (g.i. tract), and (g) PNMT synthesis (adrenal medulla). Therapeutically, at pharmacological levels the effects of cortisol include (a) preventing vascular collapse during overwhelming stress, (b) providing an anti-inflammatory effect, and (c) invoking immunosuppression.

Adrenocortical Toxicity

The zonae fasciculata and reticularis appear to be the principal targets of xenobiotic chemicals in the adrenal cortex. Classes of chemicals known to be toxic for the adrenal cortex include short chain (three or four carbons) aliphatic compounds, lipidosis-inducers, and amphiphilic compounds (Yarrington *et al.*, 1981, 1985). In general, compounds seen to frequently produce necrosis, particularly in the zonae fasciculate and reticularis, include 7,12-dimethyl benz[*a*]anthracene (DMBA), acrylonitrile, hexadimethrine bromide, polyanethosulfonate (along with amino-caprionic acid), thioacetamide, and basic polyglutamic acid (Szabo and Lippe, 1989; Colby *et al.*, 1994). By comparison, lipidosis inducers can cause accumulations, often coalescing, of neutral fats, which may be of sufficient quantity to cause a reduction or loss of organellar function and eventual cell destruction. Examples of chemicals that directly target glucocorticoid secretion in the adrenal cortex include dimethoate, ketoconazole, spironolactone, efonidipine, mibefradil, 1-aminobenzotriazole, and various PCBs (Colby *et al.*, 1995; Harvey, 2010). Lesions that are caused may be classified as follows: endothelial damage (eg, acrylonitrile), mitochondrial damage (eg, DMNM, *o,p'*-DDD, amphenone), endoplasmic reticulum disruption (eg, triparanol), lipid aggregation (eg, aniline), lysosomal phospholipid aggregation (eg, chlorophentermine), and secondary effects due to embolization by medullary cells (eg, acrylonitrile). Tricresyl phosphate (TCP) and other triaryl phosphates cause a defect in cholesterol metabolism by blocking both uptake from serum and storage pathways. An inhibition of cytosolic neutral cholesteryl ester hydroxylase (nCEH) by triaryl phosphate results in the progressive accumulation of cholesteryl ester in the form of lipid droplets in the cytoplasm of adrenal cortical cells.

Biologically active cationic amphiphilic compounds produce a generalized phospholipidosis that involves primarily the zonae fasciculate and reticularis and produce microscopic phospholipid-rich inclusions. These compounds affect the functional integrity of lysosomes, which appear ultrastructurally to be enlarged and filled with membranous lamellae of myelin figures. Examples of compounds known to induce phospholipidosis include chloroquine, triparanol, and chlorophentermine.

In addition, there is a miscellaneous group of chemicals that affects hydroxylation and other functions of mitochondrial and microsomal fractions (eg, smooth endoplasmic reticulum) in the adrenal cortex. Examples of these compounds include *o,p'*-DDD and α-(1,4-dioxido-3-methylquinoxalin-2-yl)-*N*-methylnitrone (DMNM). Other compounds in this miscellaneous category cause their effects by means of cytochrome P450 metabolism and the production of toxic metabolites. A classic example is the activation of carbon tetrachloride, resulting in lipid peroxidation and covalent binding to cellular macromolecules of the adrenal cortex (Colby, 1988).

Adrenocortical toxicity can also involve increased secretion of endogenous glucocorticoids. Compounds that have been shown to cause this include ethanol, chlordecone, carbon disulfide, cannabinoids, cocaine, amitriptyline, and cytotoxic anticancer drugs (Harvey, 2010). Furthermore, pharmacological treatment with glucocorticoid agonists that have been widely used as anti-inflammatory agents can produce symptoms that resemble Cushing's syndrome (Harvey, 2010).

There have been documented cases of iatrogenically (physician-caused) induced adrenocortical toxicity. For example, the anesthetic etomidate and the anticonvulsant aminoglutethimide have been demonstrated to produce significant morbidity and mortality because of their potency as steroidogenic enzyme inhibitors. Aminoglutethimide inhibits CYP11A (side chain cleavage enzyme; Johansson *et al.*, 2002), whereas etomidate blocks CYP11B1 (CYPβ/18; Hinson and Raven, 2006). This iatrogenic suppression of steroidogenesis in the adrenal cortex can result in Addisonian crisis (which can be associated with fatigue, cardiovascular collapse, and death).

In Vitro Toxicity

In addition to in vivo testing for effects of xenobiotics on the adrenal cortex, much recent work has used an in vitro approach to identify the molecular targets of adrenocortical toxicity. Of particular usefulness has been the human adrenocortical carcinoma-derived NCI-H295R cell line. This cell line expresses all key enzymes necessary for steroidogenesis, and it produces all of the major steroids including progesterone, androgens, estrogens, glucocorticoids, and aldosterone (Harvey *et al.*, 2007). These cells express functional ACTH receptors as well as functional receptors for CRH, angiotensin II, vasoactive intestinal peptide, atrial natriuretic peptide, LH, human chorionic gonadotropin (hCG), tumor necrosis factor, and activin A. They respond to forskolin and isobutylmethylxanthine (cAMP induction) as well as dibutyryl cyclic AMP with stimulated corticosterone synthesis. This cell line has proven useful for identification of specific steroidogenic enzymes that are targeted by xenobiotics. A recent review article provides a useful table listing over 60 compounds that have been shown to induce functional adrenocortical and steroidogenic toxicity along with the specific enzymes targeted (Harvey *et al.*, 2007). Therefore, the H295R cell line is a versatile tool for assessment of adrenocortical function and steroidogenesis in general. Because the cell line is derived from a human source, it is also very worthwhile for hazard risk assessment.

Serum Binding Proteins

Cortisol and corticosterone are transported in blood by corticosteroid binding globulin (CBG), also called transcortin (Hedge *et al.*, 1987). When bound to CBG, the steroid is biologically inactive and cannot have its effects on target tissues, or provide negative feedback to the hypothalamic–pituitary–adrenal (HPA) axis. Thus, a chemical affecting CBG could alter the balance between free and bound hormone, and impact its availability in target tissues. Nonsteroidal anti-inflammatory drugs (NSAIDS) have been reported to decrease the binding capacity of CBG by a mechanism other than simple displacement of bound glucocorticoid (Harvey, 2010).

Target Tissue Receptors

In addition to direct effects on steroidogenesis, chemically induced changes in adrenal function can result from blockage of the action of adrenocorticoids at peripheral sites. Adrenocortical steroids and HPA axis hormones exert their effects through receptors located in target tissues throughout the body. These receptors can be upregulated or downregulated by the action of xenobiotic compounds. For example, hexachlorobenzene reduces hepatic glucocorticoid receptors in rats (Lelli *et al.*, 2007), and aminoglutethimide downregulates adrenocortical cell ACTH receptors (Fassnacht *et al.*, 1998). Other chemicals can increase adrenocortical cell ACTH receptors (Li and

Hypothalamic-pituitary-adrenal axis

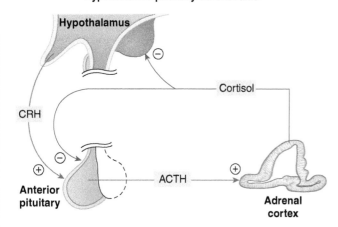

Figure 21-5. *Hypothalamic–pituitary–adrenal axis of regulation.* CRH from the hypothalamus stimulates release of ACTH from the anterior pituitary. ACTH stimulates synthesis and secretion of cortisol from the adrenal cortex. Cortisol provides inhibitory (negative) feedback on the hypothalamus and pituitary. Stress, the major stimulator of the axis, can override the feedback regulatory loop. +, Stimulatory, –, inhibitory (Modified from Hedge *et al.*, 1987).

Wang, 2005). In the first mechanism, many antisteroidal compounds (antagonists) act by competing with or binding to steroid hormone receptor sites; thereby, either reducing the number of available receptor sites or by altering their binding affinity. Spironolactone, an antimineralocorticoid, is an example of a peripherally acting adrenal cortical hormone antagonist (Los and Colby, 1994).

Neuroendocrine Regulation

The zonae fasciculata and reticularis of the adrenal cortex are under tropic control by the pituitary hormone, ACTH, which stimulates them to produce cortisol. The level of output of cortisol by the adrenal is almost entirely determined by the intensity of the ACTH stimulus. Increased cortisol produced then provides long-loop negative feedback on the hypothalamus and anterior pituitary and decreases CRH and ACTH secretion, respectively (Fig. 21-5). Stress is a major factor that can override the negative feedback control system and stimulate cortisol secretion (Hedge *et al.*, 1987). Persistent exposure of the adrenal cortex to high levels of ACTH during chronic stress can result in adrenocortical hypertrophy. Adrenal androgens are also produced in ACTH-sensitive cells; therefore, abnormal conditions of stimulation of these cells by ACTH, such as Cushings' disease, can also raise androgen secretion by the cortex. Conversely, conditions of reduced exposure of the cortex to its tropic hormone, ACTH, can result in adrenal atrophy.

Drugs that affect neuroendocrine function can indirectly affect adrenal function. For example, synthetic glucocorticoids, valproic acid, bromocriptine, cyproheptadine, ketanserin, ritanserin, somatostatin analogs, 4′-thio-beta-D-arabinofuranosylcytosine, hexachlorobenzene, alcohol, and caffeine have been shown to suppress ACTH or CRH secretion (Harvey, 2010). ACTH secretion can also be pharmacologically stimulated by, for example, caffeine, methylxanthines, adenosine analogs, 3,4-methylenedioxymethamphetamine, and di-2-ethylhexyl phthalate (Harvey, 2010). Exogenous steroids can disrupt normal function and structure of the adrenal cortex. Agonists will cause negative feedback inhibition of ACTH secretion in the pituitary and will result in atrophy of the zonae fasciculata and reticularis. On the other hand, antagonists of steroids will block hormone action in target tissues and on negative feedback, which will lead to increased ACTH secretion, and differential hyperplasia of the cortex. Generally, testing of compounds that

have a neuroendocrine site of action is only likely to be detected by in vivo studies. Because of the tropic effects of ACTH, adrenal enlargement (hypertrophy) usually results from stimulation of the HPA axis (stress or direct ACTH stimulation), or loss of feedback inhibition. Thus, adrenal hypertrophy can distinguish a neuroendocrine site of action from direct adrenocortical inhibition/suppression. Other physiological endpoints can be evaluated during testing for HPA axis stimulation. A one-month toxicology study of corticosterone administration in rats at high but physiologically relevant levels (approximating stress) observed reduced body weight gain, and lower thymus, adrenal, prostate, and seminal vesicle weights (Harvey *et al.*, 1992). The body and thymus weight effects were attributed directly to high corticosterone, and reduced prostate and seminal vesicle weights to the inhibition of LH and testosterone by corticosterone. These effects in combination with enlarged adrenals (resulting from ACTH stimulation) could be useful as indicators to rule out primary adrenocortical insufficiency (Harvey *et al.*, 2007).

Animal Testing

Special considerations for animal testing in adrenal toxicity were outlined in a recent review (Harvey *et al.*, 2007). A number of things should to be taken into account. To avoid increased glucocorticoid levels resulting from the stress of handling, sham dosing should be conducted seven to 10 days prior to the onset of dosing. If females are used, their stage of estrous cycle needs to be coordinated. Blood samples should be taken at the same time of day and should be completed within three minutes of cage disturbance to ensure nonstressed control values. Animal dosing should be via oral gavage (or the route of human exposure) to provide adequate translational relevance. A particularly useful method of testing of chemicals for effects on adrenocortical competence is the ACTH stimulation test in which ACTH is administered subcutaneously following a predetermined period of exposure of test animals to the compound of interest. Blood samples can be collected within one to three hours for assessment of glucocorticoid levels. A direct impact of the compound on the adrenal gland will be assumed if ACTH fails to elevate corticosterone levels to those seen in controls.

Mineralocorticoids

The adrenals are essential to life, mainly because of the salt-retaining function of the z. glomerulosa, but to a lesser extent, because of the stress management role of the adrenal cortex. Loss of mineralocorticoid production by the cortex results in a life-threatening retention of potassium and hypovolemic shock associated with the excessive urinary loss of sodium, chloride, and water. Aldosterone, the most important mineralocorticoid, participates in the regulation of renal sodium and potassium balance, thereby affecting blood pressure homeostasis (Hadley and Levine, 2007). Aldosterone promotes sodium reabsorption and increases the excretion of potassium and hydrogen ions by the kidney (Fig. 21-6). The ratio of the concentrations in the urine of Na^+/K^+ decreases when blood levels of aldosterone increase, and vice versa. All routes of loss of sodium and potassium from the body are controlled by aldosterone. Thus, an increase in the concentration of aldosterone in blood also decreases the Na^+/K^+ ratio of saliva, sweat, and feces.

In theory, chemicals that target steroidogenic enzymes in the pathway to aldosterone secretion could affect both aldosterone and glucocorticoid (StAR, CYP11A1, and CYP21) or only aldosterone synthesis and secretion (CYP11B1; see Harvey *et al.*, 2007).

The aldosterone-producing cells of the zona glomerulosa are controlled separately by other tropic substances, but may require permissive concentrations of ACTH. Unlike the cells of the zonae

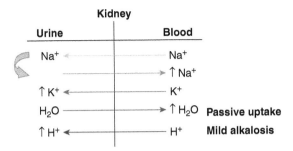

Kidney

Urine		Blood
Na⁺ ←		Na⁺
	→ ↑Na⁺
↑K⁺ ←		K⁺
H_2O →	↑H_2O	**Passive uptake**
↑H⁺ ←		H⁺	**Mild alkalosis**

Figure 21-6. Aldosterone effects on the kidney. Aldosterone stimulates reuptake of Na^+ from the filtrate while promoting K^+ excretion into the urine. Water (H_2O) is reabsorbed by passive uptake, whereas protons (H^+) are excreted along with K^+.

fasciculata and reticularis, regulation of release from the zona glomerulosa is not primarily via ACTH. The renin–angiotensin system is the primary regulator of aldosterone secretion in the adrenal cortex (Porterfield, 2001). Renin is a proteolytic enzyme synthesized and secreted in the renal juxtaglomerular apparatus (JGA). Release of renin from the JGA is stimulated by decreases in blood pressure or volume, or reduced plasma sodium. Once released, the enzyme (renin) encounters renin substrate (angiotensinogen) of hepatic origin, which is already in circulation and serves as a prohormone reservoir for angiotensin. In the blood stream, renin cleaves angiotensinogen to become angiotensin I (AgI, a decapeptide), and angiotensin converting enzyme (ACE) further cleaves AgI to produce angiotensin II (AgII). This octapeptide (AgII) is one of the most potent known physiological vasoconstrictors. However, it also acts as a tropic hormone for the zona glomerulosa cells of the adrenal cortex to stimulate synthesis and secretion of aldosterone. Because AgII constricts resistance vessels in the body to increase blood pressure, and decrease vascular capacity, this contributes to a feedback mechanism to decrease secretion of renin by JGA cells. Further, by stimulating aldosterone secretion (long loop feedback), the resulting increase in Na^+ and water retention returns blood volume and osmolality to normal. This further inhibits release of renin, providing a physiological feedback loop of regulation.

Fetal Adrenal

The adrenal cortex in the human fetus differs both structurally and functionally from that in the adult. A specialized fetal adrenal cortex exists in primates during late gestation (Mesiano and Jaffe, 1997). The cortex is composed of large polyhedral cells that produce abundant cortisol and estrogen precursors. The hormones secreted by the cortex are important for normal development of the fetus, and the steroid precursor dehydroepiandrostreone is converted to estriol by the placenta. The cells of the fetal cortex are produced in the outer cortex and migrate medially, where they undergo hypertrophy and eventually apoptosis. After birth, there is a rapid regression, apoptosis, and lysis of the fetal cortex with dilation of cortical capillaries and replacement by the typical three cortical zones. The fetal adrenal cortex is proportionately much larger than the adult gland because of the large size of the fetal zone. It is important not to misinterpret this as a lesion in neonatal primates since it represents physiological replacement of the fetal cortex with the definitive postnatal adrenal cortex.

X-Zone

Similar to the fetal cortex in primates, the X-zone in the mouse adrenal cortex is also a unique physiological phenomenon. In contrast to the fetal cortex of primates, the X-zone develops postnatally

in the inner cortex of mice and is fully formed at weaning. Its function is unknown, but it may be similar to the fetal zone in primates. After weaning, the X-zone degenerates at variable rates, depending on the sex of the mouse. In male mice, the X-zone undergoes degeneration at puberty with accumulation of intracellular fat globules. In females, the zone undergoes slow regression and degeneration during the first pregnancy. As with the fetal zone in primates, it is important not to misinterpret the degeneration associated with regression of the X-zone in mice as a lesion.

ADRENAL MEDULLA

Because it is classified as a specialized postganglionic (sympathetic) neuron, the adrenal medulla is a functional extension of the nervous system and is also called the sympathoadrenal system. Thus, the adrenal medulla comprises a branch of the sympathetic division of the autonomic nervous system. Located in the center of the adrenal gland, the physiological role of the medulla is to help maintain the constant internal environment of the body. The medulla is composed of cells called pheochromoblasts (specialized sympathetic ganglia), also known as chromaffin cells, which are the site of catecholamine synthesis and secretion. Chromaffin cells derive their name from the chromaffin reaction, the formation of a brown color due to oxidation of catecholamine stores (Tischler *et al.*, 2010). These cells are true neuroendocrine cells, which provide a direct interface between the nervous and endocrine systems. That is, sympathetic, cholinergic stimulation of the cell bodies results in secretion of catecholamines, which behave as hormones by entering the circulation and producing true endocrine effects throughout the body. Secretory granules in the chromaffin cells are the site of storage for the catecholamines, which are rapidly released upon receipt of neuronal input from a preganglionic neuron along the splanchnic nerve pathway. As a result of this stimulation, the catecholamines, epinephrine, and norepinephrine are released into the circulation. Peptides are also reported to reside in chromaffin cells. These include chromogranins and the neuropeptides enkephalin (Schultzberg *et al.*, 1978), neuropeptide Y (NPY, Varndell *et al.*, 1984), substance P (Kuramoto *et al.*, 1985), vasopressin and oxytocin (Hawthorn *et al.*, 1987), galanin (Holgert *et al.*, 1994), and neurotensin (NT, Holgert *et al.*, 1994).

Sympathetic Response

The general functions of the sympathetic division of the autonomic nervous system can be summarized as follows: (a) ensuring reciprocity to counteract and balance the tonic effects of parasympathetic stimulation to visceral structures, (b) assisting in the maintenance of the steady state functions of the body (digestion, secretion, vasomotor tone, etc), and (c) assisting in the mobilization of body reserves to meet unusual or emergency situations (fear, fright, injury, etc). Dr. Walter Cannon in 1929 was the first to suggest that activation of the sympathetic nervous system prepares an animal for "fright, fight, or flight."

Catecholamines

The sites of catecholamine synthesis in the body are the CNS, postganglionic sympathetic neurons, and the adrenal medulla. It is the adrenal medulla that is the major site of epinephrine production. In fact, 80% of the medullary output of catecholamines in humans is epinephrine. In the catecholamine biosynthetic pathway, tyrosine is acted on by tyrosine hydroxylase to produce dopa, which is converted to dopamine by dopa decarboxylase. Dopamine in turn is acted on by dopamine β-hydroxylase to form norepinephrine, which is converted to epinephrine by PNMT (Hedge *et al.*, 1987). Tyrosine hydroxylase is the principal rate-limiting step in catecholamine synthesis. The conversion of tyrosine to dopa and dopamine occurs within the cytosol of chromaffin cells. Dopamine then enters the chromaffin granule, where it is converted to norepinephrine. Norepinephrine leaves the granule and is converted to epinephrine in the cytosol, and epinephrine, reenters and is stored in the chromaffin granule. In contrast to the synthesis of catecholamines which occurs in the cytosol, neuropeptides and chromogranin-A proteins are synthesized in the granular endoplasmic reticulum and are packaged into granules in the Golgi apparatus. Release of the catecholamines is stimulated by acetylcholine from cholinergic preganglionic neurons. Catecholamine release is stimulated by acetylcholine deriving from preganglionic neurons along the splanchnic nerve. Acetylcholine activates nicotinic and muscarinic cholinergic receptors, which cooperatively stimulate the secretory response by increasing a Ca^{++} flux and activating protein kinase C. This flux involves Ca^{++} from both extracellular influx and intracellular stores. Physiological activators of release include decreased blood pressure, decreased blood glucose, decreased oxygen availability, stress or anxiety, cold, exercise, and postural hypotension. Rather than staining for the chromaffin reaction to identify catecholamine-producing cells, more recently, immunostaining for catecholamine-synthesizing enzymes tyrosine hydroxylase (TH), dopamine-β-hydroxylase (DBH), and PNMT is used to identify individual cells that produce catecholamines, and whether they synthesize epinephrine (Tischler *et al.*, 2010).

Catecholamines generally affect all tissues. However, the most pronounced effects are on the (a) heart, (b) liver, (c) skeletal muscle, (d) adipocytes, (e) vascular smooth muscle, and (f) bronchial smooth muscle.

Adrenergic Receptors

Catecholamine actions are mediated through interactions with specific classes of adrenergic receptors on target cell membranes. There are two major types of these receptors, known as α and β adrenergic receptors. The α and β classification is further divided into at least two subtypes of each, α_1 and α_2, and β_1 and β_2 (Table 21-3). Each type of receptor has its own unique pattern of distribution throughout the body (Porterfield, 2001). The relative number of each receptor type in each target organ determines, in part, the nature of the response of the organ to the catecholamines. For example, α_2 receptors predominate on insulin-secreting pancreatic B cells, whereas β receptors predominate on glucagon-secreting pancreatic A cells. The net effect is that catecholamines inhibit insulin (decreased cAMP production) and stimulate glucagon (increased cAMP production) release so that glucagon can facilitate an anti-insulin effect by increasing blood glucose. Epinephrine and norepinephrine display similar affinities for the different receptor types, with the exception of β_2 receptors that bind epinephrine 10 times greater than norepinephrine. As a result, epinephrine participates more than norepinephrine in mediating its metabolic effects. Therefore, receptor type variation on target tissues contributes to the diversity with which the sympathetic response exerts its specific effects.

General Toxicity

Examples of specific chemicals that target chromaffin cells include toxins that block voltage-gated ion channels (Alvarez *et al.*, 2008), and bacterial toxins, which block exocytosis of secretory granules, thereby, preventing catecholamine release (Gasman *et al.*, 1999). The effects of these toxins on whole animal physiology are

Table 21-3

Different Classes of Adrenergic Receptors

RECEPTOR TYPE	SIGNALING PATHWAY	RELATIVE AFFINITY	PHYSIOLOGICAL RESPONSES
α_1	↑ IP$_3$, DAG	E=NE	Vasoconstriction, uterine contraction, pupil dilation
α_2	↓cAMP	E=NE	Sphincter muscle constriction (g.i., bladder), ↓lipolysis, ↓insulin secretion
β_1	↑ cAMP	E=NE	↑heart rate, ↑cardiac output, ↑renin secretion
β_2	↑ cAMP	E>>>NE (10X)	Bronchodilation, vasodilation, uterine relaxation, ↑glycogenolysis, ↑lipolysis, smooth muscle relaxation (g.i., bladder), ↑insulin secretion

relatively unimportant due to their more global and lethal effects on the nervous system. Furthermore, the relevance of the adrenal medulla as a target organ in toxicology is highly dependent on the species, strain, and sex of the animals studied (Tischler *et al.*, 2010). The most common pathological changes seen in the adrenal medulla in toxicological studies involve proliferative lesions classified as nodular hyperplasia, although degenerative changes can also occasionally be observed.

Pheochromocytoma

The adrenal medulla can undergo a series of proliferative changes ranging from diffuse hyperplasia to benign and malignant neoplasms. The latter neoplasms have the capacity to invade locally and metastasize to distant sites. Larger benign adrenal medullary proliferative lesions are designated pheochromocytomas.

Pheochromocytomas are relatively rare in humans (Greim *et al.*, 2009). The incidence is about 1/100,000, and both sexes are affected equally. The peak incidence is ages 40 to 50, and the tumors occur bilaterally in only 10% of the cases. About 10% are malignant, 10% occur outside of the adrenal gland, and 10% are considered to be hereditary (Gimm, 2005). Pheochromocytomas in humans and rats are both composed of chromaffin cells with variable numbers of hormone-containing secretory granules. There appears to be a striking species difference in the response of medullary chromaffin cells to mitogenic stimuli, with rats being very sensitive compared to humans. In humans, pheochromocytomas are uncommon except in patients with inherited clinical syndromes of multiple endocrine neoplasia (MEN). These tumors in rats usually do not secrete excess amounts of catecholamines, whereas human pheochromocytomas episodically secrete increased amounts of catecholamines, leading to hypertension and other clinical disturbances. Further, no data are available to suggest that pheochromocytomas may be inducible in humans. In general, they are usually indolent tumors in humans and mice. These observations have increasingly led regulatory agencies to diminish the need of investigating rat pheochromocytomas for purposes of risk assessment (Tischler *et al.*, 2010).

Proliferative lesions occur in the adrenal medulla with high frequency in many strains of laboratory rats. The incidence of these lesions varies with strain, age, sex, diet, and exposure to drugs and a variety of environmental agents. Studies from the NTP historical database of two-year-old F344 rats have reported that the incidence of pheochromocytomas was 17.0% and 3.1% for males and females, respectively. Malignant pheochromocytomas were detected in 1% of males and 0.5% of females. In addition to F344 rats, other strains with a high incidence of pheochromocytomas include Wistar, NEGH (New England Deaconess Hospital), Long-Evans, and Sprague–Dawley. Pheochromocytomas are considerably less common in Osborne–Mendel, Charles River, Holtzman, and WAG/Rij rats. Most studies have revealed a higher incidence in males than in females. Crossbreeding of animals with high and low frequencies of adrenal medullary proliferative lesions results in F1 animals with an intermediate tumor frequency. For reasons not well understood, spontaneous pheochromocytomas are largely observed in aging male laboratory rats, but are relatively rare in mice (Greim et al., 2009). The differences between rats and mice have led to the suggestion that the mouse is a more suitable model for humans as regards adrenal medullary risk assessment. These medullary lesions, more frequently observed in males, can be induced by a variety of xenobiotic agents (Tischler et al., 2010).

Pheochromocytomas in rats differ from those in all other species in that they are common, often bilateral, and can be induced by many chemicals. An extensive listing of chemicals that are effective at producing proliferative lesions in rats and mice has been provided in reviews by Greim et al. (2009) and Tischler et al. (2010). Warren et al. (1966) studied over 700 pairs of rats and found that more than 50% of irradiated male rats developed adrenal medullary tumors. Substances that have been shown in NTP studies to induce pheochromocytoma in rats include metal compounds, halogenated and nonhalogenated aliphatic or aromatic hydrocarbon, aromatics, aromatic amines as well as other dyestuff, pesticides, and pharmaceuticals (Greim et al., 2009). Vitamin D is the most powerful mitogenic stimulus to cause chromaffin cell proliferation in the adrenal medulla in rats (Greim et al., 2009). Because the vitamin D effect has been seen in vivo, but not in vitro, it is thought to result from impaired calcium homeostasis, resulting in hypercalcemia.

In animals, there is no indication as yet that pheochromocytomas are induced by chemicals working through genotoxic mechanisms (Ozaki et al., 2002). Proliferation of chromaffin cells in male rats occurred following exposure to aromatic amines such as p-chloroaniline (Chhabra et al., 1991). Rather, proliferation of chromaffin cells in rats can be stimulated by chemicals that induce uncoupling of mitochondrial respiration, hypoxia, disturbances in calcium homeostasis, acute stress, and overfeeding (Greim et al., 2009). Many of the chemicals that induce pheochromocytoma in animals are uncouplers of oxidative phosphorylation, for example, acrylamide (Howland and Alli, 1986) or furan (Mugford et al., 1997).

Unlike in humans, in which they secrete high levels of epinephrine, rat pheochromocytomas are usually characterized by predominant or exclusive production of norepinephrine. Chemicals that induce pheochromocytomas in rats are pharmacologically diverse, and usually stimulate chromaffin cell proliferation by neutrally derived signals, or agents that regulate catecholamine synthesis and release. An important class of compounds that affects the rat adrenal medulla includes sugars and sugar alcohols, such as lactitol, xylitol, and sorbitol (Lynch et al., 1996).

Both nicotine and reserpine have been implicated in the development of adrenal medullary proliferative lesions in rats. Both chemicals act by a shared mechanism, because nicotine directly stimulates nicotinic acetylcholine receptors whereas reserpine causes a reflex increase in the activity of cholinergic nerve endings in the adrenal. A short dosing regimen of reserpine administration in vivo stimulates proliferation of chromaffin cells in the adult rat, and the mechanism may involve a reflex increase in neurogenic stimulation via the splanchnic nerve.

Roe and Bar (1985) have suggested that environmental and dietary factors may be more important than genetic factors as determinants of the incidence of adrenal medullary proliferative lesions in rats because the incidence of adrenal medullary lesions can be reduced by lowering the carbohydrate content of the diet. Several of the chemicals that increase the incidence of adrenal medullary lesions, such as sugar alcohols, increase absorption of calcium from the gut. Calcium ions as well as cyclic nucleotides and prostaglandins may act as mediators capable of stimulating both hormonal secretion and cellular proliferation. In summary, three dietary factors have been suggested to lead to an increased incidence of adrenal medullary proliferative lesions in chronic toxicity studies in rats (Roe and Bar, 1985). These are excessive intake of (1) food associated with feeding ad libitum; (2) calcium and phosphorus; and (3) other food components (eg, vitamin D and poorly absorbable carbohydrates), which increase calcium absorption.

Tischler et al. (1995) reported that adult rat chromaffin cells had a marked increase in bromodeoxyuridine (BrdU)-labeled nuclei in vitro following the addition of forskolin (activator of adenylate cyclase) and phorbol myristate (PMA, activator of protein kinase C), whereas mouse chromaffin cells had a minimal response to the same mitogens. This striking difference in sensitivity to mitogenic stimuli may explain the lower frequency of adrenal medullary proliferative lesions in mice compared to many rat strains. The human adrenal medulla, as in mice, has a low spontaneous incidence of proliferative lesions of chromaffin cells. Human chromaffin cells also failed to respond to a variety of mitogenic stimuli in culture (Tischler and Riseberg, 1993). These findings and others suggest that chromaffin cells of the rat represent an inappropriate model to assess the potential effects of xenobiotic chemicals on chromaffin cells of the human adrenal medulla.

A relationship exists between adenohypophyseal (anterior pituitary) hormones and the development of adrenal medullary proliferative lesions. For example, the long-term administration of growth hormone is associated with an increased incidence of pheochromocytomas as well as the development of tumors at other sites. Prolactin-secreting pituitary tumors, which occur commonly in many rat strains, also play a role in the development of proliferative medullary lesions. In addition, several neuroleptic compounds that increase prolactin secretion by inhibiting dopamine production have been associated with an increased incidence of proliferative lesions of medullary cells in chronic toxicity studies in rats.

In long-term animal studies, pheochromocytomas often are accompanied by tumors or toxic effects in other organs. They often are seen in cases involving renal, lung, and hepatic toxicity, in addition to endocrine disturbances (Greim et al., 2009). They are associated with the following conditions: hypoxia, uncoupling of oxidative phosphorylation, disturbances of calcium homeostasis, or disturbances of the hypothalamic endocrine axis (Greim et al., 2009). Additionally, pheochromocytomas often develop following treatment with substances that target enzymes in catecholamine synthesis, receptor tyrosine kinase (RET), hypoxia-inducible factor (HIF), succinate dehydrogenase, or fumarate hydratase. As with humans, pheochromocytomas can also occur in mice and rats in conjunction with MEN. This was seen in male rats after administration of propyl gallate (NTP, 1982).

In Vitro Testing

A commonly employed cell line used in neurobiology is the PC12 pheochromocytoma line derived from a rat adrenal medullary tumor (Greene and Tischler, 1976). These cells respond to nerve growth factor (NGF) by ceasing replication, extending neurites, and increasing a number of neuronal markers. This cell line is widely used in neurotoxicological studies. However, in using them, it must be considered that rat PC12 cells are representative only of a subset of chromaffin cells, and may differ in some ways from normal and neoplastic chromaffin cells of other species. At this time, there are no human chromaffin cell lines, despite numerous efforts to establish such a cell line (Tischler *et al.*, 2010).

The PC12 cell line has been useful in determining intracellular mechanisms at the molecular level that are involved in chromaffin cell signaling and proliferation. Studies with PC12 cells have shown that substances which inhibit mitochondrial function (cyanide, rotenone) or uncouple oxidative phosphorylation (dinitrophenol, *p*-trifluoromethoxyphenyl hydrazone) stimulate catecholamine secretion in the same way as occurs under hypoxic conditions. This is thought to be dependent upon Ca++ influx through voltage-gated channels (Taylor *et al.*, 2000). Proliferation of chromaffin cells can also be induced in vitro by activators of adenylate cyclase that stimulates neuropeptide receptors, as well as stimulators of protein kinase C, which stimulates muscarinic cholinergic receptors.

THYROID GLAND

General Anatomy

The thyroid gland consists of two lobes of endocrine tissue located just below the larynx on each side of the trachea with an isthmus connecting the two lobes (Fig. 21-7; Capen and Martin, 1989; Capen, 2001). A second cell type is also present, the C-cells, or parafollicular cells composing the intrafollicular spaces (Capen and Martin, 1989; Capen, 2001). The C-cells synthesize and secrete calcitonin (CT), a hormone involved in calcium homeostasis (see "Parathyroid gland" section for more details).

The thyroid secretes two hormones known as thyroxine (T_4) and triiodothyronine (T_3) (Capen and Martin, 1989; Capen, 2001; Hedge *et al.*, 1987). Both of these hormones are produced in epithelial cells in the basic functional unit of the thyroid known as the follicle (Fig. 21-8). Each follicle consists of a sphere of epithelial cells surrounding a colloidal core. The colloid material is composed of the glycoprotein thyroglobulin (TGB), which acts as a storage

Thyroid and parathyroid glands

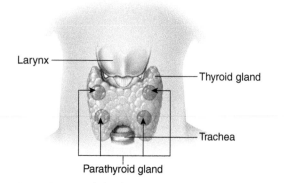

Figure 21-7. *Anatomy of the thyroid and parathyroid glands.* The schematic shows the thyroid gland in humans, which consists of two lobes of endocrine tissue, located just below the larynx on each side of the trachea with an isthmus connecting the two lobes (Modified from Porterfield, 2007).

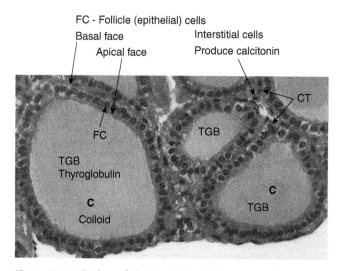

Figure 21-8. *Histology of the thyroid gland.* The micrograph shows thyroid follicles (FC) composed of epithelial cells, the site of thyroid hormone synthesis, with colloid (C), the site of thyroid hormone storage, contained in the follicular lumen. The epithelial cell contains a basal and apical face. The interstitial compartment is composed of C cells, the site of synthesis, and secretion of calcitonin (Modified from Porterfield, 2007).

depot for T_4 and T_3 (Capen and Martin, 1989; Capen, 2001). In humans, about three months of thyroid hormone is stored as TGB in the colloid (Hedge *et al.*, 1987). This represents the largest reserve of any stored hormone in the body. Generally, the level of secretory activity of follicular cells can be estimated as a direct function of their height. Cells involved in synthesizing thyroid hormone are columnar in shape, whereas quiescent cells are cuboidal (Capen and Martin, 1989; Capen, 2001).

T_4 and T_3 are important regulators of overall metabolism, and their effects are regulated within a long time frame (Capen, 2001; Hedge *et al.*, 1987). Essentially all tissues are to some degree targets for thyroid hormone. However, the primary target tissues for thyroid hormone include the liver, kidney, heart, brain, pituitary, gonads, and spleen (Capen and Martin, 1989; Capen, 2001; Zoeller *et al.*, 2007).

Some studies indicate that xenobiotics directly affect the structure of the thyroid gland (Capen, 2001). For example, some environmental chemicals such as heavy metals and red dye #3 are known to decrease the size of the colloid space (Bronnikov *et al.*, 2005; Capen and Martin, 1989; Capen, 2001). This is thought to reduce the space required for storing hormones, leading to an impaired ability of the thyroid gland to synthesize and store thyroid hormones. Chemicals such as PCBs are known to alter the appearance of the epithelial cells so that they are hypertrophic or hyperplastic in nature (Capen, 2001; Langer, 2010). This is thought to lead to excessive thyroid hormone production.

Thyroid Hormone Structure and Synthesis

Thyroid hormones are composed of two modified, covalently linked tyrosine amino acids (Fig. 21-9, Capen, 2001; Hedge *et al.*, 1987). Each of the aromatic rings of the tyrosines contains one or two iodides. T_4 contains two iodides on each aromatic ring for a total of four, while T_3 contains two iodides on the tyrosine closest to the amino acid moiety (amino and carboxy groups), and one iodide on the outer aromatic ring (Capen, 2001; Hedge *et al.*, 1987). The iodide is derived from dietary intake and is required for biologic activity. While the thyroid gland synthesizes and secretes both T_4, and T_3, it primarily releases T_4. In fact, about 90% of thyroid hormone secreted by the thyroid gland is in the form of T_4 in humans (Hedge *et al.*, 1987).

Figure 21-9. *Structure of thyroid hormone (T_3 and T_4).* The schematic shows the structures required to make T_3, T_4, and reverse T_3 (rT_3). At the apical membrane of the follicular cells, I_2 combines with tyrosine residues on thyroglobulin (TGB) to form monoiodotyrosine (MIT) and diiodotyrosine (DIT). Coupling between MIT and DIT occurs such that combined MIT and DIT forms T_3, whereas combined DIT and DIT forms T_4. T_4 from the thyroid gland can be peripherally converted to T_3 (active hormone) or rT_3 (inactive metabolite), then successively deiodinated by the monodeiodinases (Modified from Hedge *et al.*, 1987).

TGB, a glycoprotein containing large numbers of tyrosine amino acid residues, is synthesized in the epithelial cell and serves as the backbone for thyroid hormone synthesis (Capen, 2001; Hedge *et al.*, 1987). Iodine in the form of iodide (I^-) is actively transported into the epithelial cell, where it is oxidized to I_2 by thyroid peroxidase. At the apical membrane, I_2 combines with tyrosine residues on TGB to form monoiodotyrosine (MIT) and diiodotyrosine (DIT), which remain attached to TGB (Capen, 2001; Hedge *et al.*, 1987). Coupling between MIT and DIT occurs such that a combined MIT and DIT forms T_3; whereas a combined DIT and DIT forms T_4 (Hedge *et al.*, 1987; Capen, 2001).

The iodinated TGB is stored in the follicular lumen as colloid until the thyroid gland is stimulated to secrete hormone (Capen, 2001; Hedge *et al.*, 1987). Upon stimulation, iodinated TGB is endocytosed into the epithelial cell and transported in the direction of the basal membrane where lysosomal enzymes hydrolyze peptide bonds to release T_3 and T_4 for passive diffusion into the circulation (Capen, 2001; Hedge *et al.*, 1987). Remaining MIT and DIT are recycled in the epithelial cell for synthesis of new TGB (Capen, 2001; Hedge *et al.*, 1987).

T_4 from the thyroid gland can be peripherally converted to T_3 (active hormone) or reverse T_3 (rT_3, the inactive metabolite) then successively deiodinated by the monodeiodinases (Capen, 2001; Hedge *et al.*, 1987). About 40% of circulating T_4 is metabolized to T_3 by 5'-monodeiodinase, and 40% is converted to rT_3 by 5-monodeiodinase (Capen, 2001; Hedge *et al.*, 1987; Zoeller *et al.*, 2007). Additionally, about two-thirds of T_3 and all rT_3 in circulation are produced from T_4 by peripheral conversion (Capen, 2001; Hedge *et al.*, 1987). As a result, the ratio of circulating T_4 and T_3 does not reflect the ratio of these two substances when they were released from the thyroid gland. Based on a variety of observations, it appears that circulating T_4 levels provide a "sink" of prohormone that can serve as a ready supply for peripheral conversion to T_3 (the active form; Hedge *et al.*, 1987).

Several studies indicate that xenobiotics can interfere with thyroid gland function by adversely affecting the process of thyroid hormone synthesis (Jugan *et al.*, 2010; Kortenkamp, 2008; Lynch *et al.*, 2002; Mastorakos *et al.*, 2007; Sauvage *et al.*, 1998). For example, environmental chemicals such as perchlorate, chlorate, and bromate inhibit uptake of iodide and thus, decrease thyroid hormone synthesis (Crofton, 2008). Some chemicals such as genistein and daidzein in soy products, thionamides, and substituted phenols can inhibit thyroid peroxidase, blocking incorporation of iodide into TGB (Delclos and Newbold, 2007; Doerge and Chang, 2002). Further, some chemicals may interfere with monodeiodinases, leading to decreased levels of thyroid hormones. Specifically, studies have shown that red dye #3 and propylthiouracil inhibit 5'-monodeiodinase, leading to reduced serum levels of T_3 (Capen, 2001; Crofton, 2008).

Thyroid Hormone Binding Proteins

Once released into the blood, thyroid hormones are rapidly bound to high affinity serum binding proteins (Capen, 2001; Hedge et al., 1987). The result is that less than 1% of the T_3 (99.7% bound) and less than 0.1% of the T_4 (99.97% bound) are free in circulation (Hedge et al., 1987). Only the small unbound fraction of the total hormone pool has access to receptors in target cells, and thus only the unbound fraction can exert biological activity.

There are three types of thyroid hormone binding proteins: thyroid binding globulin (TBG), thyroxine-binding prealbumin (TBPA), and albumin (Hedge et al., 1987; Capen, 2001). TBG binds about 80% of the thyroid hormones, whereas TBPA and albumin each bind about 10% of the thyroid hormones (Hedge et al., 1987). Environmental chemicals such as the PCBs and PBDEs are known to displace thyroid hormones from serum binding proteins (Jugan et al., 2010; Patrick 2009; Yamauchi and Ishihara, 2006). The displacement of thyroid hormones from the binding proteins often leads to a rapid decline in serum thyroid hormone levels.

Thyroid Hormone Receptors

Thyroid hormones act by binding to thyroid hormone receptors (TRs) (Zoeller, 2005). TRs are members of the nuclear receptor superfamily of ligand-inducible transcription factors. TRs can form homodimers or heterodimers with other nuclear hormone receptors such as the retinoid X receptor (Zoeller, 2005). The homodimers and heterodimers bind to thyroid hormone response elements located in target genes and interact with coactivators and corepressors to regulate transcription. In humans, thyroid hormone receptors are the products of two genes that encode three thyroid hormone receptor isoforms known as TRα, TRβ1, and TRβ2 (Zoeller, 2005). While all three isoforms are present in most tissues, their expression differs spatially and temporally during development (Zoeller, 2005). TRα is abundant in the brain, heart, and immune system, whereas TRβ1 is particularly expressed in the brain, liver, and kidney (Zoeller, 2005).

Environmental chemicals can interfere with thyroid hormone binding to TRs and thyroid-hormone related transcription at multiple levels (Jugan et al., 2010; Kitamura et al., 2002; Patrick, 2009; Zoeller, 2005). First, some chemicals such as PBDEs can bind directly to TRs and induce either agonistic or antagonist effects (Zoeller, 2005). Interestingly, some PBDE congeners have different affinities for TRα and TRβ, whereas some congeners can bind to more than one isoform. Second, some environmental chemicals interfere with thyroid hormone binding to receptors via indirect mechanisms (Zoeller, 2005). In such cases, it is thought that the chemicals exert their effects by promoting coactivators or inhibiting corepressors. For example, BPA impairs thyroid hormone action by inhibiting T_3 binding to TR and by recruiting the nuclear corepressor N-CoR to the TR, resulting in repression of transcription (Patrick, 2009; Zoeller, 2005). Similarly, some PCBs are able to suppress TR/coactivator (SRC-1) complex-mediated transactivation, leading to suppression of TR-mediated transcription (Crofton, 2008). Third, some xenobiotics can interfere with cross talk between TRs and

other nuclear receptors. For example, hydroxyl-PCBs can partially dissociate the heterodimer TR/retinoic acid receptor from the T_3-response element (Crofton, 2008). Finally, some chemicals such as BPA and phthalates can inhibit expression of TRs (Patrick, 2009).

Thyroid Hormone Clearance

The main pathway for clearance of thyroid hormones from the serum is via conjugation to glucuronic acid or sulfate by phase II enzymes such as glucuronyl transferases (UDPGTs) and sulfo transferases (SULTs), respectively (Patrick, 2009; Zoeller, 2010). The metabolites then are transported across plasma membranes for elimination by phase III transporters, including the multidrug resistance protein 1 and the multidrug resistance-associated protein 2 (MRP2).

Some studies indicate that some xenobiotics may increase the clearance of thyroid hormones from the serum, limiting the availability of thyroid hormones to act on tissues and often resulting in symptoms of hypothyroidism (Brouwer et al., 1998; Yamauchi and Ishihara, 2006). For example, coplanar and noncoplanar PCB congeners have been shown to induce UDPGTs and SULTs, resulting in low serum T_4 levels (Crofton, 2008; Patrick, 2009). In contrast, a few studies have shown that xenobiotics such as pentachlorophenol or triclosan may inhibit SULTs, increasing the availability of thyroid hormones to act on tissues (Crofton, 2008; Jekat et al., 1994; Patrick, 2009). Studies have also shown that xenobiotics such as dioxin, rifampicin, and phenobarbital may decrease the transport of thyroid hormones into the brain and liver by inhibiting phase III transporters (Crofton, 2008).

Regulation of Thyroid Hormone Release

Thyroid hormone secretion is regulated by thyroid-stimulating hormone (TSH, thyrotropin) from the anterior pituitary gland (Capen, 2001; Hedge et al., 1987). The rate of release of TSH is under a hypothalamic–pituitary–thyroid regulatory axis involving negative feedback (Fig. 21-10). Specifically, a hypothalamic releasing hormone known as TRH directly stimulates release of TSH from the anterior pituitary gland (Hedge et al., 1987). TSH then increases secretion of T_4 and T_3 from the thyroid gland. In turn, T_4 and T_3 can feedback to the anterior pituitary to inhibit TSH release and they can

Hypothalamic-pituitary-thyroid axis

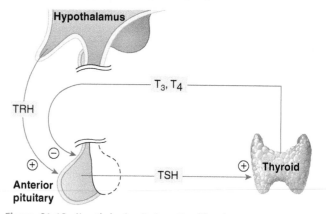

Figure 21-10. *Hypothalamic–pituitary–thyroid axis.* The hypothalamus synthesizes and secretes thyroid-releasing hormone (TRH). TRH travels to the anterior pituitary via the portal plexus and stimulates the thyrotropes to synthesize and secrete TSH. TSH acts on the thyroid gland to stimulate production and/or release of T_3 and T_4. T_3 and T_4 can then exert negative feedback control at the level of the anterior pituitary to inhibit further release of TSH (Modified from Hedge et al., 1987).

feedback to the hypothalamus to inhibit TRH release. Interestingly, most inhibition by thyroid hormones is by T_4, although T_3 can also provide some degree of inhibition (Hedge *et al.*, 1987). Further, the feedback effect is mediated primarily at the level of the anterior pituitary, although some degree of negative feedback occurs at the level of the hypothalamus (Hedge *et al.*, 1987).

In addition to these methods of regulating thyroid hormone secretion, there is a circadian rhythm of TRH and TSH release, with a decrease following the onset of sleep (Hedge *et al.*, 1987). Overall, the thyroid axis responds rapidly at the hypothalamo-pituitary unit, but beyond this level, the system is governed by processes that have extremely long time constants. Therefore, the long half-lives of thyroid hormones in circulation dampen the diurnal rhythm that is obvious in TSH levels. As a result, this rhythm is not reflected in circulating thyroid hormone concentrations. This contributes to the "sluggishness" of the system.

Xenobiotics have been shown to alter the ability of the hypothalamic–pituitary–thyroid regulatory axis to control thyroid hormone levels (Patrick, 2009; Zoeller, 2005). For example, chemicals such as PBDEs may increase TSH levels, leading to increased levels of T_4 and T_3 (Darnerud *et al.*, 2001). Alternatively, xenobiotics may inhibit TRH or TSH levels, leading to decreased levels of T_4 and T_3 (Patrick, 2009).

Physiological Effects

Thyroid hormones influence nearly every tissue in the body, in a variety of ways (Capen, 2001; Hedge *et al.*, 1987; Patrick, 2009). In spite of complexities of hormone action on target tissues, it is reasonably accurate to simply view thyroid hormone as the primary determinant of the overall metabolic rate of the body. The effects are exaggerated in states of thyroid excess (hyperthyroidism) or deficiency (hypothyroidism) and produce the clinical and biochemical manifestations of these disorders. In general, thyroid hormone stimulates both anabolic and catabolic biochemical pathways; however, its over-riding effect is catabolism (energy mobilization).

Thyroid hormone also produces significant effects on growth and development (Capen, 2001; Hedge *et al.*, 1987; Zoeller *et al.*, 2002; Zoeller, 2005). It is essential for normal development of the CNS and for maturation of the skeleton (Dickerson and Gore, 2007; Gore, 2011; Zoeller *et al.*, 2002). A deficiency of thyroid hormone in early life leads to a delay in development of the brain in animal models and humans (Dickerson and Gore, 2007; Gore, 2011; Zoeller *et al.*, 2002). Brain development is especially dependent on thyroid hormone during the first several months after birth in humans (Zoeller, 2005). If thyroid hormone levels are inadequate during this period, severe irreversible mental retardation in the form of cretinism occurs. Early diagnosis and immediate replacement with thyroid hormones can prevent these effects, and are; therefore, essential.

Thyroid Toxicity

Given the influence of thyroid hormones on numerous tissues in the body, it is not surprising that xenobiotics that affect thyroid hormone levels often cause symptoms of hypothyroidism, hyperthyroidism, or lead to significant impairment in brain development and function. Below are some specific examples of environmental chemicals that have been shown to affect thyroid hormone levels through a variety of mechanisms, resulting in adverse physiological outcomes.

PCBs PCBs are some of the best characterized thyroid disrupting chemicals (Boas *et al.*, 2009; Dickerson and Gore, 2007; Gore,

2011; Jugan *et al.*, 2010; Patrick, 2009; Zoeller, 2010). PCBs are industrial chemicals that were widely used in capacitors and transformers. They are made of two phenyl rings with varying degrees of chlorination, resulting in 209 different congeners. The production of PCBs was banned in the 1970s, but unfortunately, PCBs are persistent chemicals and thus, they are still routinely found in humans and wildlife blood samples and tissues.

PCBs are known to interfere with the thyroid system in a manner that leads to serious neurocognitive effects (Gore, 2011; Porterfield, 2000; Zoeller *et al.*, 2002). Several human studies indicate that PCB exposure in prenatal life is associated with lower full-scale and verbal IQ scores and less short-term and long-term memory and attention in postnatal life (Porterfield, 2000; Zoeller *et al.*, 2002). Rodent studies indicate that prenatal PCB exposure increases hyperactivity (Porterfield, 2000; Zoeller *et al.*, 2002). Further, rodent studies indicate that PCB exposure causes hearing disorders because the developing auditory system is sensitive to thyroid hormones (Porterfield, 2000; Zoeller *et al.*, 2002).

While PCBs may exert negative effects on animals and humans via several mechanisms, the most common pathway is thought to include PCB inhibition of thyroid hormone levels or activity (Gore, 2011; Patrick, 2009). Several studies indicate that PCBs decrease the levels of thyroid hormone by inhibiting thyroid hormone synthesis and/or increasing the metabolism of thyroid hormones by increasing phase II enzymes (Zoeller, 2010). Further, some studies indicate that PCBs interfere with thyroid hormone action by inhibiting the binding of thyroid hormones to binding proteins or blocking the ability of thyroid hormones to bind to TRs (Zoeller, 2010).

PBDEs PBDEs are also well-known thyroid disrupting chemicals (Boas *et al.*, 2009; Jugan *et al.*, 2010; Zoeller, 2010). These chemicals are flame retardants that are used in a variety of products, including electric equipment, clothing, furniture, carpeting, plastics, and paints. PBDEs are not chemically bound to products in which they are used; thus, they can leach from the products into human and wildlife tissues and into the environment over time.

The structure of PBDEs often resembles that of PCBs. Thus, it is not surprising that many of the toxic effects of PBDEs are similar to those elicited by PCBs. Like PCBs, PBDEs have been shown to inhibit thyroid hormone levels and/action, leading to serious neurocognitive deficits. PBDEs inhibit thyroid hormone levels by inducing hepatic phase II enzymes, resulting in increased metabolism of circulating thyroid hormones (Zoeller, 2010). They also can downregulate proteins required for transporting thyroid hormone into target cells and they can bind to TRs, blocking the ability of thyroid hormones to bind to TRs (Zoeller, 2010).

Perchlorate Perchlorate is another thyroid disrupting chemical (Crofton, 2008; Jugan *et al.*, 2010; Patrick, 2009; Zoeller, 2010). This chemical is widely used as a rocket propellant as well as a chemical in fireworks and airbag deployment systems. Perchlorate is also used in pharmaceutical industries. It is a highly stable and water-soluble compound and thus, it is known to persist in the environment, particularly in the water and food supply. While less is known about the effects of perchlorate on the thyroid system than about PCBs and PDBEs, a few studies indicate that perchlorate exposure inhibits thyroid hormone levels, possibly leading to hypothyroid-like outcomes (Crofton, 2008; Patrick, 2009). The mechanism of action of perchlorate is thought to be primarily by reducing iodide uptake, which ultimately reduces thyroid hormone synthesis (Patrick, 2009). It is important to note, however, that the effects of perchlorate on the thyroid gland have not been well studied and the results to date in humans are equivocal.

Pesticides Pesticides such as dichlorodiphenyltrichloroethane (DDT) and hexachlorobenzene (HCB) are known thyroid disrupting chemicals (Boas *et al.*, 2009). While both DDT and HCB have been banned in many countries, they persist in the environment due to their long environmental half-lives and thus, they may place humans and wildlife at risk for thyroid disorders. Pesticide mixtures containing DDT have been shown to increase thyroid volume and to induce antibodies that attack the thyroid gland, resulting in autoimmune thyroid disease (Boas *et al.*, 2009; Crofton, 2008; Patrick, 2009). Further, DDT has been shown to inhibit TSH receptors, blocking the ability of TSH to induce secretion of T_4 and T_3 and in turn, resulting in low circulating T_4 and T_3 levels (Boas *et al.*, 2009; Patrick, 2009). HCB has been shown to interfere with thyroid function by blocking the ability of thyroid hormones to bind to TR (Boas *et al.*, 2009; Crofton, 2008; Patrick 2009).

Perfluorinated Chemicals Perfluorinated chemicals (PFCs) are a family of chemicals used in many products due to their surface protection properties. Such products include stains and oil-resistant coatings, floor polishes, and insecticides. Some studies have shown that a PFC known as perfluorooctane sulfonate (PFOS) decreases T_4 levels in pregnant dams as well as their pups (Boas *et al.*, 2009). The PFC known as perfluorooctanic acid (PFOA) has been shown to decrease T_3 levels. While the mechanisms by which PFOS and PFOA decrease thyroid hormone levels are not completely clear, studies suggest that they upregulate phase II metabolic enzymes in the liver and increase deiodinases in the thyroid gland (Boas *et al.*, 2009).

Bisphenol A BPA is a suspected possible thyroid hormone disrupting chemical (Boas *et al.*, 2009; Zoeller, 2010). It is primarily used in the manufacture of polycarbonate plastics such as those used in baby bottles, toys, and food containers. It is also a component of dental sealants and the linings of food cans. BPA can leach out of products and enter the blood and organs. In fact, recent studies indicate that over 95% of human urine samples contain BPA, indicating continuous and widespread exposure to this chemical. Given the vast exposure of humans to BPA, it is important to consider its potential effects on the thyroid gland. Some laboratory studies have shown that BPA blocks T_3 action by antagonizing the binding of T_3 to its receptor (Zoeller, 2010). Further, some studies have shown that BPA inhibits T_3-mediated gene expression in cell lines (Zoeller, 2010). While the effects of BPA-induced inhibition of thyroid hormone action in humans are unclear, several studies suggest that BPA leads to symptoms of hypothyroidism or thyroid resistance syndrome in animal models. Further, prenatal BPA exposure has been shown to cause attention deficit hyperactivity disorder like symptoms in rodents in postnatal life (Zoeller, 2010). This effect is thought to be due to the BPA-induced inhibition of normal thyroid function, which in turn affects normal development of the neurological system (Zoeller, 2010).

Phthalates A few recent studies suggest that phthalates may act as thyroid disrupting agents; however, they are not thought to do so to the same degree as PCBs and PBDEs (Boas *et al.*, 2009; Jugan *et al.*, 2010). Phthalates are used to improve the flexibility of plastics used in a variety of products, including toys, medical tubing, plastic bottles, and cosmetics. To date, a few small human studies have shown that phthalate exposures may alter the levels of T_4 and T_3 levels in adult men and pregnant women (Jugan *et al.*, 2010). Interestingly, a by-product of phthalates produced by gram-negative bacteria has been shown to inhibit thyroperoxidase, an enzyme required for thyroid hormone synthesis (Jugan *et al.*, 2010). This results in low thyroid hormone levels and to symptoms

of hypothyroidism in humans. A few rodent studies have shown that a phthalate known as di-*n*-butyl phthalate decreases T_3 and T_4 in a dose-dependent manner (Boas *et al.*, 2009; Jugan *et al.*, 2010). The consequences of phthalate-induced changes in thyroid hormone levels in humans or rodents are unclear at this time and should be investigated in future studies.

PARATHYROID GLAND

General Anatomy

The parathyroid glands are embedded in the surface of the thyroid gland (Fig. 21-7) (Capen and Rosol, 1989; Hedge *et al.*, 1987). Humans have four parathyroid glands, which are located on the back of side of the thyroid gland (Hedge *et al.*, 1987). The parathyroid glands are composed of chief cells and oxyphil cells (Capen and Rosol, 1989; Hedge *et al.*, 1987). The main function of chief cells is to produce parathyroid hormone (PTH), whereas the function of the oxyphil cells is unknown (Capen and Rosol, 1989; Hedge *et al.*, 1987). In humans, oxyphil cells are absent at birth, appear around puberty, and increase in number with age. Thus, it is thought that they may represent structurally and functionally modified chief cells.

The parathyroid glands are critical for life (Capen and Rosol, 1989). This is largely because PTH helps maintain normal plasma calcium levels (Fig. 21-11) (Capen and Rosol, 1989; Hedge *et al.*, 1987). Calcium is required in optimal concentrations for many of life's fundamental processes: fertilization, vision, locomotion-muscle contraction, nerve conduction, blood clotting, exocytosis, cell division, and the activity of a number of enzymes and hormones (Hedge *et al.*, 1987). Therefore, the concentrations of calcium in the cellular and extracellular fluids must be maintained at a constant value. When the parathyroid glands are removed or damaged,

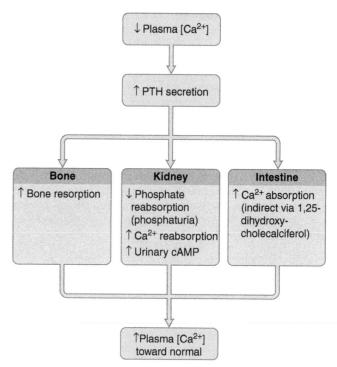

Figure 21-11. *Effects of calcium on target tissues.* Low levels of circulating Ca^{2+} stimulate and increase in secretion of parathyroid hormone (PTH). PTH helps restore normal plasma Ca^{2+} levels by acting on bone, the kidney, and the intestine (Reproduced with permission from Boron and Boulpaep, 2005).

PTH levels drop, causing a major drop in circulating calcium levels. In turn, this can lead to tetanic convulsions and death (Capen and Rosol, 1989; Hedge *et al.*, 1987).

Parathyroid Toxicity

Xenobiotic exposures may alter the structure of the parathyroid gland (Capen and Rosol, 1989). In some cases, chemicals such as the anticancer drug L-asparaginase cause death of parathyroid cells (Capen and Rosol, 1989; Capen, 2001). Specifically, studies have shown that L-asparaginase selectively destroys chief cells in rabbits. This results in a reduced size and capacity of the parathyroid to release PTH, which eventually leads to tetany and death. Studies have also shown that sublethal doses of heroin cause degenerative changes in the rat parathyroid gland (Barai *et al.*, 2009). These changes are characterized by cytoplasmic vacuolization, pyknotic nuclei in the chief cells, and dying Golgi complexes and mitochondria.

Many xenobiotic exposures have been shown to increase the size of the parathyroid gland. Lead exposure has been shown to significantly increase parathyroid gland weight (Szabo *et al.*, 1991). Some pesticides such as rotenone, malathion, and malaoxin increase proliferation of the chief cells and thus, increase the size of the parathyroid gland (Abdo *et al.*, 1988; Reuber, 1985). This scenario often results in parathyroid gland cancer. Further, fungicides such as hexachlorobenzene and bis(tri-*n*-butyltin)oxide, the antifreeze ethylene glycol, the broad-spectrum germicide *o*-benzyl-*p*-chlorophenol, and the diuretic drug hydrochlorothiazide have been shown to induce proliferation and/or adenomas in rat parathyroid glands (Andrews *et al.*, 1989; Arnold *et al.*, 1986; Bucher *et al.*, 1990; DePass *et al.*, 1986; Lijinsky and Reuber, 1987; National Toxicology Program, 1994; Wester *et al.*, 1990). Similarly, irradiation and coumarin exposure induce parathyroid gland adenomas in rodents (National Toxicology Program, 1993). It is unclear whether all of the effects of xenobiotics are due to a primary effect of the chemical on the parathyroid gland or due to effects on the kidney or bones, which in turn alter the parathyroid gland (secondary effects).

PTH Structure and Synthesis

PTH is a polypeptide hormone that is derived from a precursor molecule called preproparathyroid hormone (Fig. 21-12; Potts, 2005). In humans, preproparathyroid hormone is composed of 115 amino acid residues. The preproparathyroid hormone is cleaved by trypsin-like proteases in the Golgi zone of the chief cells to become proparathyroid hormone, which is 90 amino acids in size. Six amino acid residues are then removed from the proparathyroid hormone by proteases in the Golgi to make PTH (Capen, 2001). PTH is then packaged into secretory vesicles that migrate to the periphery of the cell, where the hormone is secreted via vesicular exocytosis (Capen, 2001; Potts, 2005). Interestingly, the structure of this hormone is highly conserved among many species, including humans, cows, pigs, dogs, rats, and chickens (Potts, 2005).

A few studies indicate that xenobiotics may interfere with the normal synthesis of PTH. Metals such as aluminum and cadmium have been shown to inhibit PTH secretion in a variety of species, including humans (Cannata *et al.*, 1983; Jeffery *et al.*, 1996; Kido *et al.*, 1991; Rignell-Hydbom *et al.*, 2009). Similarly, alcohol consumption has been shown to decrease PTH levels in pregnant rats (Keiver and Weinberg, 2003). Lithium, a drug widely used to manage manic-depressive illnesses, has been associated with a rise in PTH levels as well as abnormally high calcium levels (Matsis *et al.*, 1989). Interestingly, a longitudinal study on Gulf War I veterans showed that depleted uranium exposure was associated with significant decreases in serum levels of PTH as well as significant increases in urinary calcium (McDiarmid *et al.*, 2011; Tissandie *et al.*, 2006).

PTH Receptors

The PTH receptor is a single G-protein-coupled receptor called the PTH/PTHrP receptor (PTHR1) (Potts, 2005). This receptor is the primary receptor that mediates the traditional actions of PTH. However, it is thought other receptors exist that bind to portions of PTH or proparathyroid hormone. In humans, the gene for the PTHR1 is located on chromosome 3 and consists of 14 exons. PTHR1 has been extensively localized in bone and kidney cells (Potts, 2005).

Limited information is available about whether xenobiotics bind PTHR1 and exert agonistic or antagonistic actions. However, one study shows that xenobiotics may alter the expression of PTHR1. Specifically, studies have shown that binge alcohol drinking significantly decreases expression of PTHR1 in male rats (Callaci *et al.*, 2009).

PTH Clearance

PTH is primarily metabolized by the liver and the kidney (Capen and Rosol, 1989). It is thought that the hormone is cleaved into two major fragments (N-terminal and C-terminal) quite quickly by

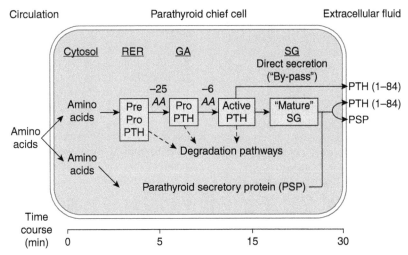

Figure 21-12. *Biosynthesis of PTH.* Active PTH is synthesized as a larger biosynthetic precursor molecule (preproPTH) that undergoes rapid posttranslational processing to proPTH prior to secretion as active PTH (amino acids 1–84) from chief cells in the parathyroid glands.

metabolic enzymes. In cows, for example, the half-life of PTH is estimated to be between three and four minutes. In dogs, the half-life of PTH is between five and six minutes, with about 60% of PTH metabolism occurring in the liver.

It is possible that xenobiotics increase the metabolism of PTH and that this leads to abnormally low levels of PTH. Alternatively, it is possible that xenobiotics decrease the metabolism of PTH and that this leads to high levels of PTH. Unfortunately, these issues have not been examined in detail and it is unclear which xenobiotics, if any, directly affect PTH metabolism.

Physiological Effects

The main physiological role of the parathyroid gland is to control circulating calcium levels (Capen and Rosol, 1989; Capen, 2001; Hedge *et al.*, 1987). Given the importance of maintaining normal levels of circulating calcium, multicellular organisms have evolved a complex system of controls to insure this constancy. Thus, PTH works in concert with CT and vitamin D (Capen, 2001; Hedge *et al.*, 1987). CT is secreted from the C cells of the thyroid gland (Capen, 2001; Hedge *et al.*, 1987). Vitamin D is produced from precursors in the skin, and it is obtained from the diet (Capen, 2001; Hedge *et al.*, 1987).

PTH serves to increase circulating calcium levels by increasing the release of calcium from bone (Capen, 2001; Hedge *et al.*, 1987). Bone is remodeled continuously during adulthood by the resorption of old bone by osteoclasts and the subsequent formation of new bone by osteoblasts (Hedge *et al.*, 1987). These two events are responsible for renewing the skeleton, while maintaining its anatomical and structural integrity. Under normal conditions, bone remodeling proceeds in cycles in which osteoclasts adhere to bone and subsequently remove it by acidification and proteolytic digestion. Shortly after the osteoclasts have left the resorption site, osteoblasts invade the area and begin the process of forming new bone by secreting osteoid (a matrix of collagen and other proteins), which is eventually mineralized (Capen, 2001; Hedge *et al.*, 1987). In regulating bone remodeling, PTH binds to osteoblasts and increases IL-6 which, along with other cytokines, causes osteoclast differentiation. In turn, this demineralizes bone and releases calcium from the bone into circulation (Capen, 2001; Hedge *et al.*, 1987).

PTH also serves to increase calcium levels by increasing the tubular reabsorption of calcium by the kidney (Capen and Rosol, 1989). Further, it inhibits the renal reabsorption of phosphate, which aids in increasing the solubility of calcium (Capen, 2001; Hedge *et al.*, 1987). PTH also enhances magnesium reabsorption, inhibits bicarbonate ion reabsorption, and blocks exchange of sodium ions by the tubules (Capen, 2001; Hedge *et al.*, 1987). These actions of PTH result in metabolic acidosis, which favors removal of calcium from plasma proteins and bones (Capen, 2001; Hedge *et al.*, 1987). In turn, this increases circulating levels of ionized calcium (Capen, 2001; Hedge *et al.*, 1987).

CT reduces circulating calcium levels by reversing the action of PTH on bone resorption (Capen and Rosol, 1989). When circulating calcium levels become high, CT is secreted by the C cells of the thyroid (Capen, 2001; Hedge *et al.*, 1987). CT serves to prevent hypercalcemia by shutting down efflux of calcium from bone. It also negatively regulates PTH to prevent kidney calcification (Capen, 2001; Hedge *et al.*, 1987).

Vitamin D_3 (cholecalciferol) is a steroid-like compound that is essential for calcium absorption in the gastrointestinal tract (Capen, 2001; Hedge *et al.*, 1987). It is derived from cholesterol, and the active form is produced from a precursor, 7-dehydrocholesterol. Exposure of the skin to ultraviolet light causes formation of vitamin D, which is biologically inert and must be activated by two sequential hydroxylations (Capen, 2001; Hedge *et al.*, 1987). The first hydroxylation occurs in the liver, and the second occurs in the kidney (Capen, 2001; Hedge *et al.*, 1987). The second conversion is stimulated by PTH activation of 1-hydroxylase enzyme activity. Vitamin D also serves to inhibit PTH actions and build bone (Capen, 2001; Hedge *et al.*, 1987).

Some xenobiotics such as pesticides and fungicides can cause excessive PTH secretion by the parathyroid gland and lead to hyperparathyroidism (Capen, 2001). However, it is important to note that most excessive PTH secretion is due to a parathyroid adenoma that is no longer under the negative feedback control of calcium. The traditional symptoms of PTH excess have been characterized as "stones, bones, and groans" for several reasons (Hedge *et al.*, 1987). First, excessive PTH levels lead to hypercalcemia, hypercalciuria, and hypophosphatemia, which often lead to the formation of renal stones. The constant supply of calcium released via unchecked bone resorption must eventually be excreted, and even though PTH normally elicits calcium reabsorption from the kidney, the consistently elevated calcium exceeds the renal threshold for reabsorption such that calcium leaks into the urine. The hallmark of this disease is abnormally increased bone resorption, leading to severe bone pain.

Xenobiotic exposures such as those to heavy metals may cause low PTH secretion and lead to hypoparathyroidism (Long *et al.*, 1992; Pounds, 1984). This condition leads to a very densely calcified skeleton, hypocalcemia, and hyperphosphatemia. Of great concern is that hypoparathyroidism often leads to tetany and death (Capen, 2001).

Regulation of PTH Release

PTH release is controlled by circulating calcium levels (Capen and Rosol, 1989). The cells in the parathyroid gland, kidney, and other cells that respond to calcium possess recognition sites for circulating calcium levels known as calcium sensors or receptors (Hedge *et al.*, 1987). Recently, the calcium sensor or calcium receptor on the parathyroid cell was cloned and determined to belong to the 7-transmembrane class of G-protein-coupled receptors linked to phospholipase C.

When the calcium receptors in the parathyroid gland sense low calcium levels, they stimulate the parathyroid gland to release PTH (Hedge *et al.*, 1987). PTH then functions to raise plasma calcium primarily by stimulating bone resorption and secondarily by enhancing renal calcium reabsorption. Further, PTH stimulates the metabolism in the kidney of vitamin D to its active hormonal form, 1,25-dihydroxyvitamin D_3 (1,25$(OH)_2D_3$) or 1,25-dihydroxycholecalciferol (Hedge *et al.*, 1987). This last effect of PTH shifts calcium recovery from the skeletal reserve and the kidney in the acute situation to intestinal absorption mediated by 1,25$(OH)_2D_3$ in the chronic situation, thereby sparing mineralized bone (Hedge *et al.*, 1987).

In general, xenobiotic exposures that interfere with the regulation of PTH could cause problems in controlling calcium levels. As mentioned above, lithium has been shown to increase PTH levels and in turn, increase circulating levels of calcium. Depleted uranium exposure has been associated with low PTH and consequently, abnormal levels of calcium in the urine (McDiarmid *et al.*, 2011).

ENDOCRINE PANCREAS

The pancreas is an organ that has both endocrine and nonendocrine functions. The acinar or exocrine portion of the pancreas is concerned primarily with the regulation of gastrointestinal function. Scattered among the pancreatic acini are the endocrine units of the pancreas, the Islets of Langerhans (Porterfield, 2001). The Islets of Langerhans comprise only 1% to 2% of the weight of the pancreas. The major physiological function of the endocrine pancreas is to serve as the primary homeostatic regulator of fuel metabolism, particularly circulating glucose. Islet cells are sensors of glucose homeostasis (maintaining balance by regulation and counterregulation) that respond to changes in their nutrient and hormonal environment. The hormones secreted by islets have major effects directly on the liver. Three major cell types within the endocrine pancreas are known to produce the hormones involved in this regulation. The most abundant cell type is the beta cell (β), the site of synthesis and secretion of insulin. Glucagon is produced by the alpha cell (α) and the delta cell (δ) is the site of somatostatin synthesis (Hadley and Levine, 2007). It is likely that a functional relationship exists between the various cell types of the islets because it is known that both glucagon and somatostatin affect insulin secretion, and that somatostatin also influences glucagon secretion.

Role of the Liver in Glucose Production

Energy for cellular metabolism can be derived from fatty acids (β oxidation) or glucose (glycolysis, TCA cycle) in the blood. The liver is the primary contributor to increasing blood glucose levels. Fig. 21-13 summarizes physiological sources of energy for cellular metabolism.

Pancreatic Hormones

Insulin The overall effects of insulin are to stimulate anabolic processes (energy storage). Specifically, insulin functions to lower blood levels of glucose, fatty acids, and amino acids and to promote their conversion to the storage form of each: glycogen, triglycerides, and protein, respectively. A number of factors affect the rate of secretion of insulin (Hedge *et al.*, 1987). The most powerful physiological stimulus is increased circulating blood glucose. In addition, an increase in the concentration of amino acids (especially arginine and leucine) and ketone bodies in blood also increase the

Hepatic glucose production

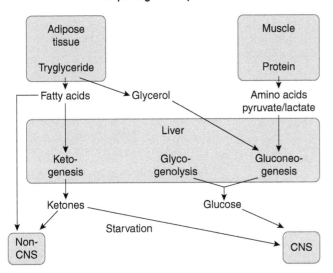

Figure 21-13. *Hepatic production of glucose.* The liver provides most of the circulating glucose in the fasting state by glycogen breakdown (glycogenolysis) and de novo synthesis (gluconeogenesis). Substrates for gluconeogenesis are provided by adipose tissue (glycerol from triglyceride breakdown) and muscle (amino acids from protein breakdown). Fatty acids from triglyceride breakdown are used to produce ketones, which can be used by the CNS for energy as an alternate to glucose during starvation.

rate of secretion of insulin. Glucagon and the gastrointestinal peptides gastrin, secretin, gastric inhibitory polypeptide also stimulate release of insulin. Conversely, insulin secretion is inhibited by hypoglycemia, epinephrine, and norepinephrine via α_2-adrenergic receptors (inhibition of cAMP production) and somatostatin.

The variety of physiological responses to insulin include (a) increased cellular glucose uptake (in most tissues), (b) lower blood glucose levels, (c) stimulated glycogen synthesis (liver, muscle), (d) stimulated glycerol production (adipose tissue), (e) increased amino acid uptake (liver, muscle), (f) inhibited lipolysis (adipose tissue), and (g) stimulated protein synthesis (replication, transcription, and translation), a mitogenic response. As regards the pathophysiology of insulin, hypersecretion produces hypoglycemia and hyposecretion produces diabetes mellitus.

Glucagon Glucagon is the primary hormone with action counterregulatory to insulin, because it stimulates catabolic processes (energy mobilization) to prevent hypoglycemia (Hedge *et al.*, 1987). The most powerful physiological stimulus of secretion of glucagon is reduced circulating blood glucose. Thus, as blood glucose levels fall (hypoglycemia), glucagon secretion increases in an attempt to restore normal homeostasis. Conversely, an increase in blood glucose levels inhibits glucagon secretion. In addition to circulating levels of glucose, glucagon secretion is regulated by other factors. The release of glucagon is stimulated by epinephrine and norepinephrine (via β-adrenergic receptors; stimulation of cAMP production), and by the amino acids, arginine, leucine, and alanine (unless accompanied by glucose ingestion). Conversely, glucagon secretion is inhibited by insulin, and somatostatin.

The physiological responses to glucagon occur mostly in the *liver* with a stimulation of glycogenolysis, gluconeogenesis (conversion of amino acids and glycerol to glucose), lipolysis, and ketogenesis (over a long time). Additionally, glucagon stimulates the secretion of insulin in pancreatic β cells. Due to the ability of other counterregulatory hormones (epinephrine, growth hormone, and cortisol) to compensate for a deficiency of glucagon, there are no significant pathological conditions associated with abnormal glucagon secretion.

Somatostatin Somatostatin was first isolated from the hypothalamus; its role in regulation of neuroendocrine function is to inhibit secretion of growth hormone in the anterior pituitary. After its identification in hypothalamic tissue, somatostatin was found in other cells of the brain, in various parts of the gastrointestinal tract, and in the δ cells of the pancreas. The generalized function of somatostatin appears to be as a hormone release inhibitor. Its physiological role within the pancreas is unknown; however, it inhibits secretion of insulin and glucagon (paracrine effect), and inhibits its own secretion (autocrine effect).

Interactions of Release

In addition to individual regulation of secretion of insulin and glucagon, the interactions of their release as relates to overall nutrient homeostasis of the individual must be considered. Although glucagon and insulin exert opposing effects on carbohydrate metabolism, they act in concert to preserve normoglycemia in the face of any perturbations that might tend to elevate or lower blood glucose (Hedge *et al.*, 1987). Many substances that influence insulin secretion also affect glucagon secretion but usually in the opposite direction. Fig. 21-14 shows how insulin and glucagon interact to maintain glucose homeostasis (normoglycemia).

Insulin and glucagon exert opposing effects on various metabolic processes (Table 21-4). Therefore, many investigators like

Insulin–glucagon interactions

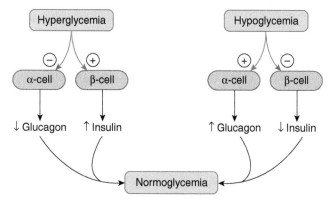

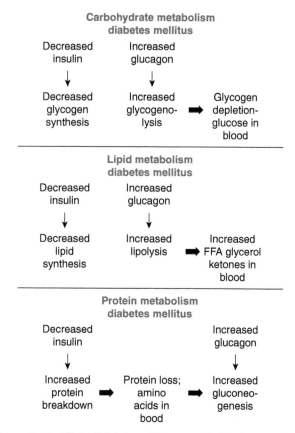

Figure 21-14. *Interactions between insulin and glucagon secretion as regulated by circulating glucose levels.* Hyperglycemia stimulates insulin and inhibits glucagon secretion. Insulin lowers blood glucose to restore normoglycemia. Hypoglycemia inhibits insulin and stimulates glucagon secretion. Glucagon mobilizes glucose from the liver to restore normoglycemia (Modified from Hedge *et al.*, 1987).

to think of the insulin-to-glucagon ratio in blood as an important determinant of the overall metabolic status. Thus, when there is a high ratio of insulin to glucagon, the effects of insulin dominate, producing a relatively anabolic state. When the ratio of insulin to glucagon is low, a catabolic state exists.

Metabolic Responses in Diabetes

Diabetes mellitus is the result of inadequate insulin action. It is usually manifest in one of two forms. Type 1 (insulin-dependent) results from autoimmune-based destruction of pancreatic β cells. Type 2 involves end organ insensitivity or resistance to insulin (non-insulin-dependent). In type 2 diabetes, insulin levels also eventually drop due to extended stress placed on pancreatic β cells. As a result of the insufficient physiological insulin action, reduced glucose removal from plasma causes hyperglycemia and a variety of metabolic alterations result. The net effect is that of increased counter-regulatory hormone dominance. These effects are summarized in Fig. 21-15. The major clinical effects in poorly controlled diabetes usually relate to progressive deterioration of function in a variety of tissues. Morbidity and mortality resulting from this disease make diabetes among the most costly of chronic diseases (Fischer, 2010). There is a genetic component associated with diabetes; however, studies in identical twins have suggested there is also most likely an environmental component to the disease. Diet,

Figure 21-15. *Effects of diabetes mellitus on metabolism.* Decreased insulin (type 1) or insulin action (type 2) inhibits glycogen, lipid, and protein synthesis. Increased glucagon stimulates glycogenolysis, lipolysis, and protein breakdown. Glycogenolysis increases circulating glucose. Increased glycerol and amino acids serve as substrates for gluconeogenesis to further increase circulating glucose.

viral disease, and exogenous chemical substances are thought to trigger a genetic predisposition to its development (Fischer, 2010).

Fig. 21-16 summarizes the clinical consequences of diabetes mellitus in which the liver becomes an overproducer of glucose resulting in glucose excretion from the kidneys. This results not only from lack of insulin action, but increased glucagon secretion (which is insulin-dependent in pancreatic α cells).

Pancreatic Toxicity

The insulin-secreting β cells are particularly sensitive to chemical attack, compared with the glucagon-secreting α and somatostatin-secreting δ cells (Malaisse *et al.*, 1982). Further, the clinical

Table 21-4

Physiological Effects of Insulin and Glucagon

	INSULIN	GLUCAGON
1. Glucose metabolism	Incr. glucose uptake	Incr. blood glucose
	Decr. blood glucose	
	Incr. glycogen synthesis	Incr. glycogenolysis
	Decr. gluconeogenesis	Incr. gluconeogenesis
2. Fat	Incr. lipogenesis	
	Decr. lipolysis	Incr. lipolysis
3. Protein	Incr. protein synthesis	–

incr., increased; decr., decreased; –, no effect.

Diabetes mellitus summary

- ♦ Liver = overproducer of glucose
  - • Increased glycogenolysis
  - • Increased gluconeogenesis
    - * ↑ a.a., glycerol, lactate/pyruvate
- ♦ Glucose spills into urine
  - • Polyurea
  - • Polydypsia (thirst)

Figure 21-16. *Physiological responses during diabetes mellitus.* Because of increased glycogenolysis and gluconeogenesis stimulated by increased glucagon, the liver becomes an overproducer of glucose. High circulating glucose levels exceed the renal threshold and glucose spills into the urine. This results in polyuria and polydipsia (thirst). a.a., amino acid.

consequences of insulin deficiency are physiologically more severe than those that would result from glucagon deficiency because the other counterregulatory hormones that oppose insulin action can compensate for reduced glucagon regulation. For those reasons, there is relatively little information about chemicals that affect α or δ cells, thus, this section will focus mainly on β-cell effects. Two chemicals that have been widely used to generate animal models of diabetes are alloxan and streptozotocin (STZ). Both of these selectively destroy pancreatic β cells, thereby causing insulin insufficiency (Scarpelli, 1989; Pisarev et al., 2009; Fischer, 2010; Adeghate, 2010). The structures of these chemicals are very different. Alloxan is a cyclic urea derivative, whereas STZ is an N-methylnitrosourea containing a deoxyglucose moiety. Each of these, however, can produce β cell destruction following a single intraperitoneal injection.

The mechanism by which alloxan is thought to have cytotoxic effects involves the generation of reactive species of oxygen, particularly the hydroxyl free radical (OH•). Isolated intact pancreatic islets synthesize and secrete insulin in response to high glucose (Fischer, 2010). A short exposure of isolated pancreatic islets to alloxan eliminates glucose-stimulated insulin secretion. There is support for this mechanism because this effect can be completely inhibited by pretreatment of islets with superoxide dismutase (SOD), catalase, diethylenetriaminepentaacetic acid, or dimethyl-urea (Fischer and Hamburger, 1980a, b). Furthermore, pancreatic islets have been shown to be deficient in the important protective factor, glutathione peroxidase (Malaisse et al., 1982). This probably contributes to the selectivity of alloxan for pancreatic β cells.

Two separate mechanisms are thought to be involved in the effects of STZ on β cells (Fischer, 2010). A single high dose of STZ causes generalized cytotoxicity and cell death, whereas low, multiple doses cause nonlethal cell damage, which results in an immune-based inflammatory response leading to cell death. High dose exposure to STZ causes alkylation of proteins and toxicity in β cells, where it decomposes to release nitric oxide. Thus, alkylation and nitric oxide-mediated injury could play a role in STZ-induced injury. Additionally, high-dose exposure to STZ causes a decrease in cellular levels of nicotinamide adenine dinucleotide (NAD). Part of the selectivity of STZ for pancreatic β cells is thought to be due to its glucose moiety, which is taken up via the glucose transporter GLUT-2 (Schnedl et al., 1994).

A common target of alloxan and STZ in pancreatic β cells is DNA (Uchigata et al., 1982). There are data to support that DNA damage occurs, poly(ADP-ribose) synthetase is activated, polyadenylation increases, and NAD declines. Pretreatment of rat pancreatic islets with the poly(adenosine diphosphate ribose) inhibitor nicotinamide prior to incubation with alloxan or STZ protects them against inhibition of proinsulin synthesis. However, in rats given these combined treatments, several months later the animals exhibit islet cell tumors (Yamagami et al., 1985).

Multiple exposure of animals to low doses of STZ demonstrates evidence of an immune system component (Fischer, 2010). There is a progressive series of changes involving infiltrating lymphocytes and macrophages in the islets, which produce inflammatory destruction of β cells 10 to 15 days after the initiation of treatment (Like et al., 1978).

Daily oral administration of the antihistamine–antiserotonin drug cyproheptadine (CPH) to rats causes progressive ultrastructural changes in the endoplasmic reticulum of β cells within two to three days of treatment (Fischer, 2010). This is accompanied by loss of insulin secretory granules. This is followed by swelling and vesiculation of the ER. The loss of pancreatic insulin appears to be due to a direct effect of CPH on insulin biosynthesis (Miller et al., 1993).

However, CPH also inhibits insulin secretion from β cells. This has been attributed to an effect of CPH on calcium influx into β cells.

CPH can be converted in rats to an epoxide metabolite desmethylcyproheptadine-10,11 (DMCPH)-epoxide. This is a major metabolite of CPH found in urine and pancreatic tissue (Fischer, 2010). Decreasing the production of this metabolite using inhibitors of drug metabolism reduces pancreatic insulin depletion caused by CPH (Chow et al., 1988). Thus, DMCPH is likely the most toxic form of the chemical.

There appear to be big species differences in β-cell toxicity. Human β-cell destruction has been demonstrated with the rodenticide Vacor (Prosser and Karam, 1978) and during treatment with the drug pentamidine (Bouchard et al., 1982). Whereas humans develop Vacor-induced diabetes, no sensitive animal has been found. Conversely, unlike in rats, STZ, when used as chemotherapy, has not caused diabetes in humans (Fischer 2010).

Insulin Resistance

Insulin resistance and defective function of pancreatic β cells usually occur sometime before the development of type 2 diabetes. Glucocorticoid treatment induces insulin resistance and enhances insulin secretion in rodents and humans (Rafacho et al., 2010). In that study, dexamethasone treatment of rats for five days resulted in hyperinsulinemia at the end of dosing, whereas 10 days following cessation of dexamethasone treatment hyperinsulinemia and insulin resistance had resolved. This provides important information as regards the therapeutic use of glucocorticoids in humans.

In a study investigating nondiabetic residents living near a deserted pentachlorophenol and chloralkali factory in Taiwan, insulin resistance was associated with increased circulating levels of dioxins and mercury (Chang et al., 2011). Furthermore, increased levels of dioxins and mercury combined were associated with even greater insulin resistance. Thus, simultaneous exposure to dioxins and mercury appears to enhance the risk of insulin resistance.

BPA, an endocrine-disruptor, is a chemical compound in the manufacture of polycarbonate plastics that is widespread in the environment. BPA exposure of pregnant mice resulted in increased insulin, leptin, triglyceride, and glycerol levels and greater insulin resistance in mothers four months postpartum (Alonso-Magdalena et al., 2010). Further, male offspring of the exposed mothers, at six months of age, demonstrated reduced glucose tolerance and increased insulin resistance. Thus, BPA may represent a risk factor for diabetes in exposed humans.

In Vitro Testing

Several cell lines are available for testing of insulin secretion. Pancreatic β-cell-derived RINm5F cells were exposed to a combination of the cytokines, IL-1β, TNF-α, and IFNγ to simulate type 1 diabetes mellitus conditions (Gurgul-Convey et al., 2011). This study showed that hydrogen peroxide produced by these cytokines reacted in the presence of trace metal Fe^{++} with nitric oxide to form highly toxic hydroxyl radicals. The authors concluded that proinflammatory cytokine-mediated β-cell death is due to nitro-oxidative stress-mediated hydroxyl radical formation in the mitochondria.

RINm5F cells were also used to investigate the role of oxidative stress in inorganic arsenic (iAs) exposure (Lu et al., 2011). A number of proapoptotic mitochondrial and cytosolic markers were investigated and found to be elevated during β-cell toxicity. The iAs-induced apoptosis and its cellular signaling events could be reversed by the antioxidant N-acetylcysteine. Therefore, it was concluded that iAs-induced oxidative stress causes apoptosis in β cells, by the mitochondria-dependent and ER stress-triggered signaling pathways. Rat-derived INS-1(832/13) cells that secrete insulin in response to glucose were also studied for the effects of exposure to iAs (Fu *et al.*, 2010). Reactive oxygen species derived from glucose metabolism provide a metabolic signal for glucose-stimulated insulin secretion from pancreatic β cells. Exposure of these cells to low levels of iAs increased an antioxidant-mediated response, and dampened glucose-stimulated insulin secretion. These findings support that low levels of arsenic can induce a cellular adaptive oxidative stress response, and disrupt β-cell function. The apoptotic as opposed to oxidative stress effects of iAs between these two studies seem to be disparate. However, two different cell lines were used, and the former study incubated the cells with higher levels of iAs (2, 5 μM), compared with the latter (0.05–0.5 μM). It is possible that oxidative stress induced at the higher levels of iAs exposure (causing cell death) is sufficient to overwhelm that which, at lower levels, plays a regulatory role in insulin secretion (inhibition). This observation suggests that the nature of the cellular response depends on the level of exposure.

REFERENCES

Abdo KM, Eustis SL, Haseman J, Huff JE, Peters A, Persing R. Toxicity and carcinogenicity of rotenone given in the feed to F344/N rats and B6C3F1 mice for up to two years. *Drug Chem Toxicol.* 1988;11(3):225–235.

Adeghate, E, Hameed, RS, Ponery, AS, et al. Streptozotocin causes pancreatic beta cell failure via early and sustained biochemical and cellular alterations. *Exp Clin Endocrinol Diabetes.* 118:699–707.

Alonso-Magdalena P, Vieira E, Soriano S, et al. Bisphenol A exposure during pregnancy disrupts glucose homeostasis in mothers and adult male offspring. *Environ Health Perspect.* 2010;118:1243–1250.

Aluru N, Leatherland JF, Vijayan MM. Bisphenol A in oocytes leads to growth suppression and altered stress performance in juvenile rainbow trout. *PLoS One.* 2010;5(5):e10741.

Alvarez YD, Ibanez LI, Uchitel OD, et al. P/Q Ca^{2+} channels are functionally coupled to exocytosis of the immediately releasable pool in mouse chromaffin cells. *Cell Calcium.* 2008;43:154–164.

Andrews JE, Courtney KD, Stead AG, Donaldson WE. Hexachlorobenzene-induced hyperparathyroidism and osteosclerosis in rats. *Fundam Appl Toxicol.* 1989;12(2):242–251.

Arnold DL, Moodie CA, Collins BT, Zawidzka ZZ, Krewski DR. Two-generation chronic toxicity study with hexachlorobenzene in the rat. *IARC Sci Publ.* 1986;77:405–410.

Barai SR, Suryawanshi SA, Pandey AK. Responses of parathyroid gland, C cells, and plasma calcium and inorganic phosphate levels in rat to sub-lethal heroin administration. *J Environ Biol.* 2009;30(5 suppl):917–922.

Boas M, Main KM, Feldt-Rasmussen U. Environmental chemicals and thyroid function: an update. *Curr Opin Endocrinol Diabetes Obes.* 2009;16:385–391.

Boron WF, Boulpaep EL, eds. *Medical Physiology.* Philadelphia PA: Elsevier; 2005).

Bouchard P, Sai P, Reach G, et al. Diabetes mellitus following pentamidine-induced hypoglycemia in humans. *Diabetes.* 1982;31:40–45.

Bronnikov VI, Goldyreva TP, Tereshchenko IV. Influence of anthropogenic pollution on thyroid structure in Perm population. *Arkh Patol.* 2005;67(6):18–21.

Brouwer A, Morse DC, Lans MC, et al. Interactions of persistent environmental organohalogens with the thyroid hormone system: mechanisms and possible consequences for animal and human health. *Toxicol Ind Health.* 1998;14(1–2):59–84.

Bucher JR, Huff J, Haseman JK, et al. Toxicology and carcinogenicity studies of diuretics in F344 rats and B6C3F1 mice. 1. Hydrochlorothiazide. *J Appl Toxicol.* 1990;10(5):359–367.

Callaci JJ, Himes R, Lauing K, Wezeman FH, Brownson K. Binge alcohol-induced bone damage is accompanied by differential expression of bone remodeling-related genes in rat vertebral bone. *Calcif Tissue Int.* 2009;84(6):474–484.

Cannata JB, Briggs JD, Junor BJ, Fell GS, Beastall G. Effect of acute aluminum overload on calcium and parathyroid-hormone metabolism. *Lancet.* 1983;1(8323):501–503.

Capen CC. Toxic responses of the endocrine system. In: Klaassen CD, ed. *Casarett & Doull's Toxicology: The Basic Science of Poisons.* New York: McGraw-Hill; 2001:711–759.

Capen CC, Martin SL. The effects of xenobiotics on the structure and function of thyroid follicular and c-cells. *Toxicol Pathol.* 1989;17(2):266–293.

Capen CC, Rosol TJ. Recent advances in the structure and function of the parathyroid gland in animals and the effects of xenobiotics. *Toxicol Pathol.* 1989;17(2):333–345.

Caride A, Fernandez-Perez B, Cabaleiro T, Lafuente A. Daily pattern of pituitary glutamine, glutamate, and aspartate content disrupted by cadmium exposure. *Amino Acids.* 2010a;38(4):1165–1172.

Caride A, Fernandez-Perez B, Cabaleiro T, et al. Cadmium chronotoxicity at pituitary level: effects on plasma ACTH, GH and TSH daily pattern. *J Physiol Biochem.* 2010b;66:213–220.

Caride A, Lafuente A, Cabaleiro T. Endosulfan effects on pituitary hormone and both nitrosative and oxidative stress in pubertal male rats. *Toxicol Lett.* 2010c;197:106–112.

Chang JW, Chen HL, Su HJ, et al. Simultaneous exposure of non-diabetics to high levels of dioxins and mercury increases their risk of insulin resistance. *J Hazard Mater.* 2011;185:749–755.

Chhabra RS, Huff JE, Haseman JK, et al. Carcinogenicity of *p*-chloroaniline in rats and mice. *Food Chem Toxicol.* 1991;29:119–124.

Chow SA, Rickert DE, Fischer LJ. Evidence that drug metabolites are involved in cyproheptadine-induced loss of pancreatic insulin. *J Pharmcol Exp Ther.* 1988;246:143–149.

Colby HD, Purcell H, Kominami, et al. Adrenal activation of carbon tetrachloride: role of microsomal P450 isozymes. *Toxicology.* 1994;94:31–40.

Colby HD, Abbott B, Cachovic, et al. Inactivation of adrenal cytochromes P450 by 1-aminobenzotriazole. Divergence of *in vivo* and *in vitro* actions. *Biochem Pharmacol.* 1995;18:1057–1062.

Colby HD. Adrenal gland toxicity: chemically induced dysfunction. *J Coll Toxicol.* 1988;7:45–69.

Crofton KM. Thyroid disrupting chemicals: mechanisms and mixtures. *Int J Androl.* 2008;31:209–223.

Darnerud PO, Erikson GS, Johannesson T, Larsen PB, Viluksela M. Polybrominated diphenyl ethers: occurrence, dietary exposure, and toxicology. *Environ Health Perspect.* 2001;109(suppl 1):49–68.

Delclos KB, Newbold R. NTP toxicity report of reproduction dose range-finding study of genistein (CAS No. 466-72-0) administered in feed to Sprague–Dawley rats. *Toxic Rep Ser.* 2007;79:C1–C2.

Depass LR, Garman RH, Woodside MD, Giddens WE, Maronpot RR, Weil CS. Chronic toxicity and oncogenicity studies of ethylene glycol in rats and mice. *Fundam Appl Toxicol.* 1986;7(4):547–565.

Dickerson SM, Gore AC. Estrogenic environmental endocrine-disrupting chemical effects on reproductive neuroendocrine function and dysfunction across the life cycle. *Rev Endocr Metab Disord.* 2007;8:143–159.

Doerge DR, Chang HC. Inactivation of thyroid peroxidase by soy isoflavones, in vitro and in vivo. *J Chromatogr B.* 2002;777:269–279.

Fakhouri WD, Nunez JL, Trail F. Atrazine binds to the growth hormone-releasing hormone receptor and affects growth hormone gene expression. *Environ Health Perspec.* 2010;118:1400–1405.

Fassnacht M, Beuschlein F, Vay S, et al. Aminoglutethimide suppresses adrenocorticotropin receptor expression in NCI-h295 adrenocortical tumor cell line. *J Endocrinol.* 1998;159:35–42.

Fischer LJ. Toxicity to the insulin secreting β-cell. In: McQueen CA, ed. *Comprehensive Toxicology*, Richburg J, Hoyer PB, eds. *Reproductive and Endocrine Toxicology.* Vol. 11. 2nd ed. Oxford, UK: Elsevier; 2010:313–337.

Fischer LJ, Hamburger SA. Inhibition of alloxan action in isolated pancreatic islets by superoxide dismutase, catalase, and metal chelator. *Diabetes.* 1980a;29:213–216.

Fischer LJ, Hamburger SA. Dimethyl urea: a radical scavenger that protects isolated pancreatic islets from the effects of alloxan and dihydroxy-fumarate exposure. *Life Sci.* 1980b;26:1405–1409.

Fu J, Woods CG, Yehuda-Shinaidman E, et al. Low-level arsenic impairs glucose-stimulated insulin secretion in pancreatic beta cells: involvement of cellular adaptive response to oxidative stress. *Environ Health Perspect.* 2010;118:864–870.

Gasman S, Chasserot-Golaz S, Vitale N, et al. Bacterial toxins: useful for studying G-proteins implicated in the mechanism of exocytosis in neurnendocrine cells. *Soc Biol.* 1999;193:451–456.

Gimm O. Pheochromocytoma-associated syndromes: genes proteins and functions of RET, VHL and SDHx. *Fam Cancer.* 2005;4:17–23.

Gore AC. Neuroendocrine targets of endocrine disruptors. *Hormones.* 2011;9(1):16–27.

Greene LA, Tischler AS. Establishment of a noradrenergic clonal line of rat adrenal pheochromocytoma cells which respond to nerve growth factor. *Proc Natl Acad Sci USA.* 1976;73:2424–2428.

Greim H, Hartwig A, Reuter U, et al. Chemically induced pheochromocytomas in rats: mechanisms and relevance for human risk assessment. *Crit Rev Toxicol.* 2009;39:695–718.

Gurgul-Convey E, Mehmeti I, Lortz S, et al. Cytokine toxicity in insulin-producing cells is mediated by nitro-oxidative stress-induced hydroxyl radical formation in mitochondria. *J. Mol. Med.* 2011;89:785–798.

Hadley ME, Levine JE, eds. *Endocrinology.* 6th ed. Upper Saddle River NJ: Pearson/Prentice Hall; 2007.

Harvey PW, Er J, Fernandes C, et al. Corticosterone does not cause testicopathology in the rat: relevance to methylxanthines, ACTH and stress. *Hum Exp Toxicol.* 1992;11:505–509.

Harvey PW, Everett DJ, Springall CJ. Adrenal toxicology: a strategy for assessment of functional toxicity to the adrenal cortex and steroidogenesis. *J Appl Toxicol.* 2007;27:103–115.

Harvey PW. Toxic responses of the adrenal cortex. In: McQueen CA, ed. *Comprehensive Toxicology,* Richburg J, Hoyer PB, eds. *Reproductive and Endocrine Toxicology.* Vol. 11. 2nd ed. Oxford, UK: Elsevier; 2010: 265–289.

Hawthorn J, Nussey SS, Henderson JR, et al. Immunohistochemical localization of oxytocin and vasopressin in the adrenal glands of rat, cow, hamster and guinea pig. *Cell Tissue Res.* 1987;250:1–6.

Hedge GA, Colby HD, Goodman RL, eds. *Clinical Endocrine Physiology.* Philadelphia PA: W.B. Saunders Company; 1987.

Hinson JP, Raven PW. Effects of endocrine-disrupting chemicals on adrenal function. *Best Pract Res Clin Endocrinol Metab.* 2006;20:111–120.

Holgert H, Dagerlind A, Hokfelt T, et al. Neural markers, peptides and enzymes in nerves and chromaffin cells in the rat adrenal medulla during postnatal development. *Brain Res Dev Brain Res.* 1994;83:35–52.

Howland RD, Alli P. Altered phosphorylation of rat neuronal cytoskeletal proteins in acrylamide induced neuorpathy. *Brain Res.* 1986;363:333–339.

Jeffery EH, Abreo K, Burgess E, Cannata J, Greger JL. Systemic aluminum toxicity: effects on bone, hematopoietic tissue and kidney. *J Toxicol Environ Health.* 1996;48(6):649–665.

Jekat FW, Meisel ML, Eckard R, Winterhoff H. Effects of pentachlorophenol (PCP) on the pituitary and thyroidal hormone regulation in the rat. *Toxicol Lett.* 1994;71(1):9–25.

Johansson MK, Sanderson JT, Lund BO. Effects of 3-MeSO$_2$-DDE and some CYP inhibitors on glucocorticoid steroidogenesis in the H295R human adrenocortical carcinoma cell line. *Toxicol In Vitro.* 2002;16:131–121.

Jugan ML, Levi Y, Blondeau JP. Endocrine disruptors and thyroid hormone physiology. *Biochem Pharmacol.* 2010;79:939–947.

Keiver K, Weinberg J. Effect of duration of alcohol consumption on calcium and bone metabolism during pregnancy in the rat. *Alcohol Clin Exp Res.* 2003;27(9):1507–1519.

Kido T, Honda R, Tsuritani I, et al. Assessment of cadmium-induced osteopenia by measurement of serum bone Gla protein, parathyroid hormone, and 1-alpha, 25-dihydroxyvitamin D. *J Appl Toxicol.* 1991;11(3):161–166.

Kinoshita H, Jessop DS, Finn DP, et al. Acetaldehyde, a metabolite of ethanol, activates the hypothalamic–pituitary–adrenal axis in the rat. *Alcohol Alcohol.* 2001;36(1):59–64.

Kitamura S, Jinno N, Ohta S, Kuroki H, Fujimoto N. Thyroid hormonal activity of the flame retardants tetrabromobisphenol A and tetrachlorobisphenol A. *Biochem Biophys Res Commun.* 2002;293(1):554–559.

Kortenkamp A. Low dose mixture effects of endocrine disrupters: implications for risk assessment and epidemiology. *Int J Androl.* 2008;31:233–240.

Kuramoto H, Kondo H, Fujita T. Substance P-like immunoreactivity in adrenal chromaffin cells and intra-adrenal nerve fibers in rats. *Histochemistry.* 1985;82:507–512.

Lafuente A, Esquifino AI. Cadmium effects on hypothalamic activity and pituitary hormone secretion in the male. *Toxicol Lett.* 1999;110: 209–218.

Lafuente A, Marquez N, Pousada Y, Pazo D, Esquifino AI. Possible estrogenic and/or antiandrogenic effects of methoxychlor on prolactin release in male rats. *Arch Toxicol.* 2000;74(4–5):270–275.

Langer P. The impacts of organochlorines and other persistent pollutants on thyroid and metabolic health. *Front Neuroendocrinol.* 2010;31(4):497–518.

Lelli SM, Caballos NR, Mazzetti MB, et al. Hexachlorobenzene as hormonal disruptor—studies about glucocorticoids: their hepatic receptors, adrenal synthesis and plasma levels on relation to impaired gluconeogenesis. *Biochem Pharmacol.* 2007;73:873–879.

Li LA, Wang PW. PCB 126 induces differential changes in androgen, cortisol and aldosterone biosynthesis in human adrenocortical H295R cells. *Toxicol Sci.* 2005;85:530–540.

Lijinsky W, Reuber MD. Pathologic effects of chronic administration of hydrochlorothiazide, with and without sodium nitrite, to F344 rats. *Toxicol Ind Health.* 1987;3(3):413–422.

Like AA, Appel MC, Williams RM, et al. Streptozotocin-induced pancreatic insulitis in mice. Morphologic and physiologic studies. *Lab Invest.* 1978;38:470–486.

Long GJ, Rounds JG, Rosen JF. Lead intoxication alters basal and parathyroid hormone-regulated cellular calcium homeostasis in rat osteosarcoma (ROS 17/2.8) cells. *Calcif Tissue Int.* 1992;50(5):451–458.

Los LE, Colby HD. Binding of spironolactone metabolites *in vivo* to renal mineralocorticoid receptors in guinea pigs. *Pharmacology.* 1994; 48:86–92.

Lu TH, Su CC, Chen YW, et al. Arsenic induces pancreatic β-cell apoptosis via the oxidative stress-regulated mitochondria-dependent and endoplasmic reticulum stress-triggered signaling pathways. *Toxicol Lett.* 2011;201:15–26.

Lynch BS, Delzell ES, Bechtel DH. Toxicology review and risk assessment of resorcinol: thyroid effects. *Regul Toxicol Pharmacol.* 2002;36(2):198–210.

Lynch BS, Tischler AS, Capen C, et al. Low digestible carbohydrates (polyols and lactose): significance of adrenal medullary proliferative lesions in the rat. *Regul Toxicol Pharmacol.* 1996;23:256–297.

Malaisse WJ, Malaisse-Lagae F, Sener A. Determinants of the selective toxicity of alloxan to the pancreatic B cell. *Proc Natl Acad Sci USA.* 1982;79:927–930.

Mastorakos G, Karoutsou EI, Mizamtsidi M, Creatsas G. The menace of endocrine disruptors on thyroid hormone physiology and their impact on intrauterine development. *Endocrine.* 2007;31(3):219–237.

Matsis PP, Fisher RA, Tasman-Jones C. Acute lithium toxicity—chorea, hypercalcemia, and hyperamylasemia. *Aust N Z J Med.* 1989;19(6): 718–720.

McDiarmid MA, Engelhardt SM, Dorsey CD, et al. Longitudinal health surveillance in a cohort of Gulf War veterans 18 years after first exposure to depleted uranium. *J Toxicol Environ Health A.* 2011;74(10):678–691.

Mesiano S, Jaffe RB. Developmental and functional biology of the primate fetal adrenal cortex. *Endocr. Rev.* 1997;18:378–403.

Miller CP, Reape TJ, Fischer LJ. Inhibition of insulin production by cyproheptadine in RINm5F rat insulinoma cells. *J Biochem Toxicol.* 1993;8:127–134.

Mugford CA, Carfagna MA, Kedderis GL. Furan-mediated uncoupling of hepatic oxidative phosphorylation in Fischer-344 rats—an early event in cell death. *Toxicol Appl Pharmacol.* 1997;144:1–11.

National Toxicology Program. NTP toxicology and carcinogenesis studies of *o*-benzyl-*p*-chlorophenol (CAS No. 120-32-1) in F344/N rats and B6C3F1 mice (gavage studies). *Natl Toxicol Program Tech Rep Ser.* 1994;424:1–304.

National Toxicology Program. NTP toxicology and carcinogenesis studies of coumarin (CAS No. 91-64-5) in F344/N rats and B6C3F1 mice (gavage studies). *Natl Toxicol Program Tech Rep Ser.* 1993;422:1–340.

NTP (National Toxicology Program). Carcinogenesis bioassay of propyl gallate (CAS No 121-79-9 in F344/N rats and B6C3F1 mice (feed study). *Technical Report Series No. 240.* Bethesda, MD: National Institutes of Health; 1982.

Ozaki K, Haseman JK, Hailey JR, et al. Association of adrenal pheochromocytoma and lung pathology in inhalation studies with particulate compounds in the male F344 rat-The National Toxicology Program experience. *Toxicol Pathol.* 2002;30:263–270.

Patrick L. Thyroid disruption: mechanisms and clinical implication in human health. *Altern Med Rev.* 2009;14:326–346.

Pisarev VB, Snigur GL, Spasov AA, et al. Mechanisms of toxic effect of streptozotocin on β-cells in the islets of Langerhans. *Bull Exp Biol Med.* 2009;148:937–939.

Porterfield SP. Thyroidal dysfunction and environmental chemicals-potential impact on brain development. *Environ Health Perspect.* 2000;108(suppl 3):433–438.

Porterfield SP. *Endocrine Physiology.* 2nd ed. St. Louis, MO: Mosby; 2001.

Potts JT. Parathyroid hormone: past and present. *J Endocrinol.* 2005; 187:311–325.

Pounds JG. Effect of lead intoxication on calcium homestasis and calcium-mediated cell function: a review. *Neurotoxicology.* 1984;5(3):295–331.

Prosser PR, Karam JH. Diabetes mellitus following rodenticide ingestion in man. *J Am Med Assoc.* 1978;239:1148–1150.

Rafacho A, Quallio S, Ribeiro DL, et al. The adaptive compensations in endocrine pancreas from glucocorticoid-treated rats are reversible after the interruption of treatment. *Acta Physiol.* 2010;200:223–235.

Reuber MD. Carcinogenicity and toxicity of malathion and malaoxon. *Environ Res* 1985;37(1):119–153.

Reuber MD. Carcinogenicity of dimethoate. *Environ Res.* 1984;34(2): 193–211.

Ribelin WE. The effects of drugs and chemicals upon the structure of the adrenal gland. *Fund Appl Toxicol.* 1984;4:105–119.

Rignell-Hydbom A, Skerfving A, Lundh T, et al. Exposure to cadmium and persistent organochlorine pollutants and its association with bone mineral density and markers of bone metabolism on postmenopausal women. *Environ Res.* 2009;109(8):991–996.

Roe FJC, Bar A. Enzootic and epizootic adrenal medullary proliferative disease of rats: influence of dietary factors which affect calcium absorption. *Hum Toxicol.* 1985;4:27–52.

Sauvage MF, Marquet P, Rousseau A, Raby C, Buxeraud J, Lachatre G. Relationship between psychotropic drugs and thyroid function: a review. *Toxicol Appl Pharmacol.* 1998;149(2):127–135.

Scarpelli DG. Toxicology of the pancreas. *Toxciol Appl Pharmacol.* 1989;101:543–554.

Schnedl WJ, Ferber S, Johnson JH, et al. STZ transport and cytotoxicity. Specific enhancement in GLUT-2 expressing cells. *Diabetes.* 1994;43:1326–1333.

Schultzberg M, Lundberg JM, Hokfelt T, et al. Enkephalin-like immunoreactivity in gland cells and nerve terminals of the adrenal medulla. *Neuroscience.* 1978;3:1169–1186.

Sikka SC, Wang, R. Endocrine disruptors and estrogenic effects on male reproductive axis. *Asian J Androl.* 2008;10(1):134–145.

Stefaneanu L, Kovacs K. Effects of drugs on pituitary fine structure in laboratory animals. *J Electron Microsc Tech.* 1991;19(1):80–89.

Suarez CR, Black LE 3rd, Hurley RM. Elevated lead levels in a patient with sickle cell disease and inappropriate secretion of antidiuretic hormone. *Pediatr Emerg Care.* 1992;8(2):88–90.

Szabo A, Merke J, Hugel U, Mall G, Stoeppler M, Ritz E. Hyperparathyroidism and abnormal 1,25(OH)$_2$ vitamin D3 metabolism in experimental lead intoxication. *Eur J Clin Invest.* 1991;21(5):512–520.

Szabo S, Lippe IT. Adrenal gland: chemically induced structural and functional changes in the cortex. *Toxicol Pathol.* 1989;17:317–329.

Taylor SC, Shaw SM, Peers C. Mitochondrial inhibitors evoke catecholamine release from pheochromocytoma cells. *Biochem Biophys Res Commun.* 2000;273:17–21.

Tischler AS, Riseberg J. Different responses to mitogenic agents by adult rat and human chromaffin cells in vitro. *Endocrine Pathol.* 1993;4: 15–19.

Tischler AS, Nyska A, Elmore SA. Toxic responses of the adrenal medulla. In: McQueen CA, ed. *Comprehensive Toxicology*, Richurg J, Hoyer PB, eds. *Reproductive and Endocrine Toxicology.* Vol. 11, 2nd ed. Oxford, UK: Elsevier; 2010:291–311.

Tischler AS, Riseberg JC, Gray R. Mitogenic and antimitogenic effects of pituitary adenylate cyclase-activating polypeptide (PACAP) in adult rat chromaffin cell cultures. *Neurosci Lett.* 1995;189:135–138.

Tissandie E, Gueguen Y, Lobaccaro JM, Paquet F, Aigueperse J, Souidi M. Effects of depleted uranium after short-term exposure on vitamin D metabolism in rat. *Arch Toxicol.* 2006;80(8):473–480.

Tohei A, Suda S, Taya K, Hashimoto T, Kogo H. Bisphenol A inhibits testicular functions and increases luteinizing hormone secretion in adult male rats. *Exp Biol Med (Maywood).* 2001;226(3):216–221.

Uchigata Y, Yamamoto H, Kawamura A, et al. Protection by superoxide dismutase, catalase, and poly(ADP-ribose) synthetase inhibitors against alloxan- and streptozotocin-induced islet DNA strand breaks and against the inhibition of proinsulin synthesis. *J Biol Chem.* 1982;257: 6084–6088.

Varndell IM, Polak JM, Allen JM, et al. Nueropeptide tyrosine (NPY) immunoreactivity in norepinephrine-containing cells and nerves of the mammalian adrenal gland. *Endocrinology.* 1984;114:1460–1462.

Verma Y, Rana SV. Endocrinal toxicity of industrial solvents—a mini review. *Indian J Exp Biol.* 2009;47(7):537–549.

Warren S, Gruzdev L, Gates O, et al. Radiation induced adrenal medullary tumors in the rat. *Arch Pathol.* 1966;82:115–118.

Wester PW, Krajinc EI, van Leeuwen FX, et al. Chronic toxicity and carcinogenicity of bis(tri-*n*-butyltin)oxide (TBTO) in the rat. *Food Chem Toxicol.* 1990;28(3):179–196.

Whittaker MH, Gebhart AM, Miller TC, Hammer F. Human health risk assessment of 2-mercaptobenzothiazole in drinking water. *Toxicol Ind Health.* 2004;20(6–10):149–163.

Wozniak AL, Bulayeva NN, Watson CS. Xenoestrogens at picomolar to nanomolar concentrations trigger membrane estrogen receptor-alpha-mediated Ca^{2+} fluxes and prolactin release in GH3/B6 pituitary tumor cells. *Environ Health Perspect.* 2005;113(4):431–439.

Yamagami T, Miwa A, Takasawa S, et al. Induction of rat pancreatic B-cell tumors by the combined administration of streptozotocin or alloxan and poly(adenosine diphosphate ribose) synthesis inhibitors. *Cancer Res.* 1985;45:1845–1849.

Yamauchi K, Ishihara A. Thyroid system-disrupting chemicals: interference with thyroid hormone binding to plasma proteins and the cellular thyroid hormone signaling pathway. *Rev Environ Health.* 2006;21(4): 229–251.

Yarrington JT, Huffman KW, Gibson JP. Adrenocortical degeneration in dogs, monkeys, and rats treated with α-(1,4-dioxido-3-methylquinoxalin-2-yl)-*N*-methylnitrone. *Toxicol Lett.* 1981;8:229–234.

Yarrington JT, Loudy DE, Sprinkel DJ, et al. Degeneration of the rat and canine adrenal cortex caused by α-(1,4-dioxido-3-methylquinoxalin-2-yl)-*N*-methylnitrone (DMNM). *Fundam Appl Toxicol.* 1985;5: 370–381.

Zabka TS, Fielden MR, Garrido R, et al. Characterization of xenobiotic-induced hepatocellular enzyme induction in rats: anticipated thyroid effects and unique pituitary gland findings. *Toxicol Pathol.* 2011;39(4):664–677.

Zoeller TR. Environmental chemicals as thyroid hormone analogues: new studies indicate that thyroid hormone receptors are targets of industrial chemicals? *MolCell Endocrinol.* 2005;242:10–15.

Zoeller TR. Environmental chemicals targeting thyroid. *Hormones.* 2010;9(1):28–40.

Zoeller RT, Dowling ALS, Herzig CTA, Iannacone EA, Gauger KJ, Bansal R. Thyroid hormone, brain development, and the environment. *Environ Health Perspect.* 2002;110(suppl 3):355–361.

Zoeller RT, Tan SW, Tyl RW. General background on the hypothalamic–pituitary–thyroid (HPT) axis. *Crit Rev Toxicol.* 2007;37(1–2): 11–53.

Toxic Agents

Toxic Effects of Pesticides

Lucio G. Costa

INTRODUCTION

Pesticides can be defined as any substance or mixture of substances intended for preventing, destroying, repelling, or mitigating pests. Pests can be insects, rodents, weeds, and a host of other unwanted organisms (Ecobichon, 2001a). Thus, pesticides occupy a rather unique position among the many chemicals that we encounter daily, in that they are deliberately added to the environment for the purpose of killing or injuring some form of life. Ideally, their injurious action would be highly specific for undesirable targets; in fact, however, most pesticides are not highly selective, but are generally toxic to many nontarget species, including humans. Thus, the use of pesticides must minimize the possibility of exposure of nontarget organisms to injurious quantities of these chemicals (Murphy, 1986).

It is not uncommon for people to refer to pesticides as a single unitary class of chemicals, while in fact the term pesticide should be equated to that of pharmaceutical drugs. As there are dozens of drugs with different therapeutic indications and different mechanisms of action, several different classes of pesticides exist, with different uses, mechanisms, and, hence, toxic effects in nontarget organisms. The most common classification of pesticides relies on the target species they act on. The four major classes (and their target pests) are those of insecticides (insects), herbicides (weeds), fungicides (fungi, molds), and rodenticides (rodents), but there are also acaricides (mites), molluscides (snails, other mollusks), miticides (mites), larvicides (larvae), and pediculicides (lice). In addition, for regulatory purposes, plant growth regulators, repellants, and attractants (pheromones) often also fall in this broad classification of chemicals. Furthermore, within each class, several subclasses exist, with substantially different chemical and toxicological characteristics. For example, among insecticides, one can find organophosphorus compounds, carbamates, organochlorines, pyrethroids, and many other chemicals. Even within each of these subclasses, significant differences can exist, as is the case, for example, of organochlorine compounds such as dichlorodiphenyltrichloroethane (DDT), aldrin, or chlordecone. Thus, detailed knowledge of the toxicological characteristics of each chemical is needed to properly evaluate its potential risks for nontarget species.

The literature pertaining to the chemistry, development, nomenclature, biotransformation and degradation, environmental effects, toxicity in target and nontarget species, and mode of action of pesticides over the past 60 years is very extensive, and the reader is referred to the monographs of O'Brien (1967), Ecobichon and Joy (1982), Hayes (1982), Wagner (1983), Matsumura (1985), Costa *et al.* (1987), Baker and Wilkinson (1990), Dikshith (1991), Hayes and Laws (1991), Chambers and Levi (1992), Satoh and Gupta (2010), and Krieger (2001, 2010), for more in-depth discussions.

HISTORICAL DEVELOPMENTS

Pesticides have been used to a limited degree since ancient times. The Ebers Papyrus, written about 1500 BC, lists preparations to expel fleas from the house. The oldest available record is Homer's mention (about 1000 BC) that Odysseus burned sulfur "…to purge the hall and the house and the court" (*Odyssey XXII*, 493–494). Pliny the Elder (AD 23–79) collected in his *Natural History* many anecdotes on the use of pesticides in the previous three to four centuries (Shepard, 1939). Dioscorides, a Greek physician (AD 40–90), knew of toxic properties of sulfur and arsenic. There are records showing that by AD 900 the Chinese were using arsenic sulfides to control garden insects. *Veratrum album* and *V. nigrum*, two species of false hellebore, were used by the Romans as rodenticides (Shepard, 1939). In 1669, the earliest known record of arsenic as an insecticide in the Western world mentioned its use with honey as an ant bait. Use of tobacco as contact insecticide for plant lice was mentioned later in the same century. Copper compounds were known since the early 1800s to have fungicidal value, and the Bordeaux mixture (hydrated lime and copper sulfate) was first used in France in 1883. Hydrocyanic acid, known to the Egyptians and the Romans as a poison, was used as a fumigant in 1877 to kill museum pests in insect collections, and carbon disulfide has been used as a fumigant since 1854 (Costa, 1987). Even in this century, until the 1930s, pesticides were mainly of natural origins or inorganic compounds. Arsenicals have played a major role in pest control, first as insecticides, and then as herbicides. Sulfur has been widely used as a fumigant since the early 1800s, and remains one of the most widely used fungicides as of today. Nicotine has been widely used as an insecticide all over the world, as has been rotenone, used as a fish poison in South America since 1725 (Costa, 1987). Mercuric chloride was used as a fungicide since 1891, slowly replaced by phenylmercury and alkylmercury. Outbreaks of poisoning with the latter compounds (Bakir *et al.*, 1973) have led to a ban of these chemicals.

The period between 1935 and 1950 was characterized by the development of major classes of pesticides, particularly insecticides. In 1939 Paul Mueller found that DDT, which had been first synthesized in 1874, acted as a poison on flies, mosquitoes, and other insects. DDT was commercialized in 1942 and was used extensively and successfully for the control of typhus epidemics, and particularly of malaria. Together with DDT, other chlorinated hydrocarbon insecticides were developed. In the early 1940s, scientists in England and France recognized the gamma isomer of hexachlorocyclohexane, commonly known as lindane, which had been first synthesized in 1825 by Faraday, as a highly potent insecticide (Ecobichon and Joy, 1982). Starting in the mid 1940s several other chlorinated insecticides were commercialized, including chlordane, heptachlor,

aldrin, and dieldrin. The organophosphorus insecticides were first synthesized in Germany in the late 1930s. Gerhard Schrader, a chemist at the I. G. FarbenIndustrie in Germany, is considered the "father" of organophosphorus insecticides. The first one, tetraethylpyrophosphate (TEEP), was brought to the market in 1944, but had little success because of its instability in aqueous solution. Several thousand molecules were synthesized by Schrader, and one (code name E605) was eventually introduced into the agricultural market under the trade name parathion, to become one of the most widely employed insecticides in this class. During those years, compounds of much greater toxicity than parathion, such as sarin, soman, and tabun, were also synthesized as potential chemical warfare agents. The mechanism of action of organophosphates, that is, inhibition of acetylcholinesterase (AChE), was soon discovered, primarily by knowledge of the effects and mechanism of action of physostigmine. This alkaloid had been isolated in 1864 from Calabar beans, the seeds of *Physostigma venenosum*, a perennial plant in tropical West Africa, and its mode of action as a cholinesterase inhibitor was identified in 1926 (Casida, 1964). Despite the early studies on physostigmine, the carbamates were introduced as insecticides only in the early 1950s. Although pyrethrum flower and extracts had been used for several centuries, pyrethrins were characterized only between 1910 and 1924 (Casida, 1980). This led then to the development of synthetic pyrethroids, the first of which, allethrin, was followed by several others in the early 1970, particularly because of the work of Michael Elliott in England and of scientists at Sumitomo Chemical Company in Japan (Casida, 2010). Several other classes of insecticides (eg, avermectins, neonicotinoids, *N*-phenylpyrazoles, diamides) have also been developed in the past few decades.

The past 60 years have also seen the development of hundreds of other chemicals used as herbicides, fungicides, and rodenticides. The development of thioureas, such as α-naphthyl thiourea (ANTU), and of anticoagulants such as warfarin, as rodenticides, dates back to the mid to late 1940s. A few years later, two important fumigants were introduced, 1,2-dichloropropene and methyl bromide. In the 1950s, phenylureas and chlorophenoxy compounds were developed as herbicides, together with the fungicides captan and folpet. Triazines, chloroacetanilides, and paraquat all widely used herbicides, came to the market in the 1960s, and so did the important class of dithiocarbamate fungicides, while the herbicide glyphosate was introduced in the mid 1970s.

ECONOMICS AND PUBLIC HEALTH

As with all chemicals, including therapeutic drugs, the use of pesticides must take into consideration the balance of the benefits that may be expected versus the possible risks of injury to human health or degradation of environmental quality. Pesticides play a major role in the control of vector-borne diseases, which represent a major threat to the health of large human populations. Pesticides of various types are used in the control of insects, rodents, and other pests that are involved in the life cycle of vector-borne diseases such as malaria, filariasis, yellow fever, viral encephalitis, typhus, and many others (Novak and Lampman, 2001). The case of DDT exemplifies the difficulty in striving a balance between benefits of its use and risks, in this case mainly to the environment. When introduced in 1942, DDT appeared to hold immense promise of benefit to agricultural economics and protection of public health against vector-borne diseases. For example, in the Italian province of Latina there were 175 new cases of malaria in 1944, but after a DDT spray control program was initiated, no new cases of malaria appeared by 1949 (Murphy, 1986). Indeed, at the time, the public health benefits of DDT were viewed so great that Mueller was awarded the Nobel

Prize in medicine in 1948. However, because of its bioaccumulation in the environment and its effects on bird reproduction, DDT was eventually banned in most countries by the mid 1970s. In South Africa, DDT was only banned in 1996, and at the time <10,000 cases of malaria were registered in that country. By the year 2000, cases of malaria had increased to 62,000, but with the reintroduction of DDT at the end of that year, cases were down to 12,500 (Maharaj *et al.*, 2005). There are still hundreds of millions of people in the world who are at risk from schistosomiasis, filariasis, and intestinal worm infestations, particularly in Africa and some Asian countries, and these major health problems require a continuous judicious use of pesticides (Novak and Lampman, 2001).

In many parts of the world, excessive loss of food crops to insects or other pests may contribute to possible starvation, and use of pesticides seems to have a favorable cost–benefit relationship (Murphy, 1986). In developed countries, pesticides allow production of abundant, inexpensive, and attractive fruits and vegetables, as well as grains. In this case, cost–benefit considerations are based on economic considerations, particularly with regard to labor costs. Along with insecticides, herbicides and fungicides play a major role in this endeavor. Loss of harvested crops by postharvest infestation by insects, fungi, and rodents is also a major problem (Ecobichon, 2001a), which is dealt with by the use of fumigants and other pesticides. Pesticides, particularly herbicides, also find useful application in forestry, during reforestation, as well as the clearing of roadways, train tracks, and utilities' rights of way. In the urban setting, pesticides find multiple uses in the home and garden area, to control insects, weeds, and other pests (Rust, 2001; Marsh, 2001). It is estimated that 75% of households in the United States utilize some form of pesticides (Table 22-1). These could include, for example, chemicals to control termite, cockroach, or rodent infestations, herbicides to control weeds in the garden, or insect repellents.

Use of Pesticides

It is commonly believed that there has been a continuous increase in the use of pesticides. While this is certainly true for the period 1950s–1980s, in the past 20 years or so, use of pesticides (as amount of active ingredient) has actually reached a plateau (Table 22-2). This is due in part to the utilization of more efficacious compounds, which require less active ingredient to be applied to obtain the same degree of pest control, and in part to the introduction of integrated pest management approaches and organic farming, at least in the developed countries. Expenditures on pesticides, however, have

Table 22-1

Number of US Households Using Pesticides (2000)

PESTICIDE TYPE	US HOUSEHOLDS (MILLIONS)	TOTAL HOUSEHOLDS (%)*
Insecticides	59	56
Herbicides	41	39
Fungicides	14	13
Repellents	53	50
Disinfectants	59	56
Any pesticide	78	74

Based on 105.5 million households and a population of 281.4 million (US Census Bureau, 2000).
SOURCE: Data from Kiely et al. (2004).

Table 22-2

Use and Expenditure on Pesticides in the United States in all Market Sectors: 1985–2000

YEAR	USE*	EXPENDITURE†
1985	1,304	6,706
1990	1,201	7,727
1995	1,210	10,781
2000	1,234	11,165

Millions of pounds of active ingredients. Excludes preservatives, specialty biocides, and chlorine/hypochlorites.
†*Millions of dollars.*
SOURCE: Data from Kiely et al. (2004).

increased (Table 22-2), as new chemicals are more expensive than older ones. In the United States, almost half of the pesticides used are herbicides, while in other countries, particularly Africa, Asia, and Central America, there is also a substantial use of insecticides (Table 22-3). Because the latter compounds are generally more acutely toxic, they contribute to the still large number of yearly pesticide poisonings (see below). Table 22-4 shows the most commonly used pesticides in the agricultural sector in the United States, while Table 22-5 indicates pesticide use by crop and by state.

Pesticides are often, if not always, used as multiagent formulations, in which the active ingredient is present together with other ingredients to allow mixing, dilution, application, and stability. These other ingredients are lumped under the term "inert" or "other" (Tominack, 2000). Although they do not have pesticidal action, such inert ingredients may not always be devoid of toxicity; thus, an ongoing task of manufactures and regulatory agencies is to assure that inert ingredients do not pose any unreasonable risk of adverse health effects (Tominack, 2000).

Exposure

Exposure to pesticides can occur via the oral or dermal routes or by inhalation. From a quantitative perspective, oral exposure lies on the extremes of a hypothetical dose–response curve. High oral doses, leading to severe poisoning and death, are achieved as a

Table 22-3

US and World Use of Pesticides: 2001

PESTICIDE	UNITED STATES MILLIONS OF POUNDS OF a.i.	%	WORLD MILLIONS OF POUNDS OF a.i.	%
Herbicides*	553	46	1870	37
Insecticides	105	9	1232	24
Fungicides	73	6	475	9
Other†	472	39	1469	29
Total	1203	100	5046	100

a.i., active ingredient.
Includes herbicides and plant growth regulators.
†*Other: rodenticides, fumigants, nematocides, molluscicides, and other chemicals.*
SOURCE: Data from Kiely et al. (2004).

Table 22-4

Most Commonly Used Conventional Pesticide Active Ingredients in the US Agricultural Market Sector in 2002

PESTICIDE TYPE	PESTICIDE	MILLIONS OF POUNDS
Insecticides	Oil	91.6
	Chlorpyrifos	8.5
	Malathion	5.1
	Aldicarb	3.4
	Terbufos	3.4
Herbicides	Glyphosate	102.3
	Atrazine	76.9
	2,4-D	40.1
	Acetochlor	36.2
	S-Metolachlor	24.8
Fungicides	Sulfur	70.9
	Copper sulfate	12.5
	Chlorothalonil	8.7
	Mancozeb	8.2
	Captan	3.1
Other pesticides	Metam-sodium	54.9
	Sulfuric acid	49.8
	1,3-Dichloropropene	29.6
	Methyl bromide*	20.6
	Chloropicrin	15.0

*Discontinued in the United States as of 2005.
SOURCE: Data from Gianessi and Reigner (2006a,b).

result of pesticide ingestion for suicidal intents, or of accidental ingestion, commonly due to storage of pesticides in improper containers. Chronic low doses, on the other hand, are consumed by the general population as pesticide residues in food, or as contaminants in drinking water. Regulations exist to ensure that pesticide residues are maintained at levels below those that would cause

Table 22-5

Pesticide Active Ingredient Use (Million of Pounds) by Crop and by State in the US Agricultural Sector: 2002

	I	H	F	O	TOTAL
Crop					
Corn	9.6	158.5			168.1
Potatoes	2.2	7.2		94.2	103.6
Soybean		91.1			91.1
Citrus	64.2	5.6	7.0		76.8
Cotton	12.7	21.7		13.8	48.2
Grapes	3.3		44.8		48.1
State					
California	29.2		65.8	30.9	125.9
Florida	58.5		9.5	15.5	83.5
Washington	11.2		7.7	25.3	44.2
Illinois		39.8			39.8
Iowa		37.3			37.3
Idaho			2.5	33.8	36.3

I, insecticide; H, herbicide; F, fungicide; O, other.
SOURCE: Data from Gianessi and Reigner (2006a,b).

any adverse effect (see below). Workers involved in the production, transport, mixing and loading, and application of pesticides, as well as in harvesting of pesticide-sprayed crops, are at highest risk for pesticide exposure. The dermal route is believed in this case to offer the greatest potential for exposure, with a minor contribution of the respiratory route when aerosols or aerial sprayings are used. In the latter cases, bystanders or individual living in proximity of the spraying may also be exposed because of off-target drifts. In the occupational setting, dermal exposure during normal handling or application of pesticides, or in case of accidental spillings, occurs in body areas not covered by protective clothing, such as the face or the hands. Furthermore, deposition of pesticides on clothing may lead to slow penetration through the tissue and/or to potential exposure of others, if clothes are not changed and washed on termination of exposure. Several methodologies exist to assess exposure by passive dosimetry, such as the use of absorbent cloth or paper patches, of biosensors, or of tracers followed by video imaging (USEPA, 1999; Fenske et al., 1986; Chester, 2010). Biological monitoring is also used, to measure the absorbed dose of pesticides. Analysis of body fluids and excreta, usually urine, for parent compound or metabolites, can provide both a quantitative and a qualitative measurement of absorbed dose. The advantage of such approach over passive dosimetry is that it evaluates actual, rather than potential, absorption, and integrates absorption from all routes of exposure (Sobus et al., 2010). In some cases, modifications of biochemical parameters or a consequence of exposure can be measured as an indication of both exposure and of a biological effect. This is the case, for example, of measurements of plasma or erythrocyte cholinesterases on exposure to organophosphorus insecticides (Storm et al., 2000).

Human Poisoning

Pesticides are not always selective for their intended target species, and adverse health effects can occur in nontarget species, including humans (Calvert et al., 2010). In the general population and in occupationally exposed workers, recurring concerns relate to a possible association between pesticide exposure and increased risk of cancer (Pearce and McLean, 2005; Jaga and Dharmani, 2005; Weichenthal et al., 2010), or neurodegenerative diseases such as Parkinson disease (Hatcher et al., 2008; Moretto and Colosio, 2011). More recently, the acknowledgment that pesticide standards are based on healthy adults, and thus may not be sufficiently protective of susceptible populations, such as children, has led to new concerns, research, and regulations (NRC, 1993; Colborn, 2006). Evidence that some pesticides may act as endocrine disruptors, possibly contributing to various adverse effects in humans, including cancer and reproductive and developmental toxicity, has also prompted additional concerns and initiatives (Porterfield, 2000; Safe, 2005; Stoker and Kavlock, 2010). Yet, from a global perspective, the major problem with pesticides remains that of acute human poisoning. The World Health Organization (WHO) estimated that there are around three million hospital admissions for pesticide poisoning each year, which result in around 220,000 deaths (WHO, 1990; Colosio et al., 2010). Most occur in developing countries, particularly in Southeast Asia, and a large percentage is due to intentional ingestion for suicide purposes (Gunnell and Eddleston, 2003). New estimates indicate that there are about 300,000 deaths due to pesticide self-poisoning each year, accounting for one third of all suicides globally (Bertolote et al., 2006; Gunnell et al., 2007). In some countries in Central and South America (eg, El Salvador, Peru), or in Asia (eg, Korea, Taiwan), pesticide self-poisoning accounts for 50% to 90% of suicides (Ajdacic-Gross et al., 2008; Chen et al., 2009).

Table 22-6

WHO-Recommended Classification of Pesticides by Hazard

| CLASS | | LD$_{50}$ IN RAT (mg/kg BODY WEIGHT) | | | |
| | | ORAL | | DERMAL | |
		SOLIDS	LIQUIDS	SOLIDS	LIQUIDS
Ia	Extremely hazardous	5 or less	20 or less	10 or less	40 or less
Ib	Highly hazardous	5–50	20–200	10–100	40–400
II	Moderately hazardous	50–500	200–2000	100–1000	400–4000
III	Slightly hazardous	Over 500	Over 2000	Over 1000	Over 4000
IV+	Unlikely to present hazard in normal use	Over 2000	Over 3000	Over 4000	Over 6000

SOURCE: Data from IPCS (2005).

The WHO has recommended a classification of pesticides by hazard, where acute oral or dermal toxicities in rats were considered (Table 22-6; IPCS, 2005). An analysis of commercially available pesticides indicates that, as a class, insecticides are the most acutely toxic. Indeed, among the 74 active ingredients listed in Class IA (extremely hazardous) and Class IB (highly hazardous), 48 (65%) are insecticides, in particular organophosphates (IPCS, 2005). Rodenticides are also highly toxic to rats, but do not present the same hazard to humans. Indeed, warfarin, one of the most widely used rodenticides, is the same chemical used as an effective "blood thinner" (anticoagulant) for prevention of stroke and other blood clot–related conditions. Herbicides, again as a class, have generally moderate to low acute toxicity, one exception being paraquat (which has a low dermal toxicity but causes fatal effects when ingested). Fungicides vary in their acute toxicity, but this is usually low. While this classification has served public health well over the years, it has been recently challenged. In a prospective cohort study in Sri Lanka, Dawson et al. (2010) have pointed out that category II (moderately hazardous; Table 22-6) comprises compounds associated with very different outcomes in humans on acute exposure for suicidal purposes. For example, the organophosphorus insecticides dimethoate, fenthion, or chlorpyrifos, the pyrethroid insecticide deltamethrin, the phenylpyrazole insecticide fipronil, and the herbicide paraquat are all listed in WHO category II; yet, the mortality rate in this study was significantly variable: 21%, 15%, 8%, 0%, 0%, and 43%, for each indicated pesticide, respectively (Dawson et al., 2010).

Reports of human poisonings worldwide underline the severe acute toxicity of certain anticholinesterase compounds and of paraquat. In Costa Rica between 1980 and 1986, 3330 individuals were hospitalized for pesticide poisoning, and 429 died. Cholinesterase inhibitors (organophosphates and carbamates) caused 63% of hospitalizations and 36% of deaths, while paraquat accounted for 24% of hospitalizations and 60% of deaths. Cholinesterase inhibitors also caused more than 70% of occupational accidents (Wesseling et al., 1993). Of 335 poisoning deaths in Manipal, India, in the 1990s, 70% were due to cholinesterase inhibitors (Mohanty et al., 2004), and similar findings were also reported in Brazil (Caldas et al., 2008).

In Sri Lanka between 1986 and 2000, hospital admissions for pesticide poisoning were 12,000 to 20,000 per year, with a 10% fatality rate (Roberts et al., 2003). Organophosphates and the organochlorine insecticide endosulfan (which was banned in 1998) were the compounds most commonly involved. In Malaysia, in the period 1999–2001, pesticide poisonings accounted for 17% of all poisoning-related admissions, but 78% of fatalities (Rajasuriar et al., 2007). Similarly, in Korea, during the period 1996–2005, deaths due to pesticide poisoning showed a gradual increase, and accounted for 58% of the total poisoning fatalities (Lee et al., 2009a). The same pattern of poisoning can be also seen in developed countries. For example, in Greece, the number of poisonings ranged between 1200 and 1700 per year during the periods 1988–1999. Of these, 40% were due to occupational exposure and 45% to accidental exposure. Organophosphates, carbamates, and paraquat were again involved in the majority of cases (Bertsias et al., 2004). In a four-year period in Japan, 346 cases of pesticide poisoning were reported; in this case 70% were due to suicide attempts. Again, cholinesterase inhibitors and paraquat were involved in more than 60% of poisonings. Death rate from poisoning with paraquat was over 70%, while it was <10% with the herbicides glyphosate or glufosinate (Nagami et al., 2005). In the state of Louisiana, >40% of all pesticide-related hospitalizations in the period 1998–2007 involved insecticides (Badakhsh et al., 2010). However, from 1995 to 2004, the overall number of pesticide poisoning in the United States has been declining, particularly for anticholinesterase insecticides (−70%), and for paraquat (−79%) (Blondell, 2007). It should also be pointed out that self-poisoning with pesticides for suicidal purposes, while very common in some countries, is the least utilized method in the United States (Ajdacic-Gross et al., 2008; Chen et al., 2009).

Regulatory Mandate

The awareness that the misuse of pesticides may pose potential health hazards has led to a realm of regulatory measures to ensure their safe use and the protection of the population. In the United States, the primary authority for pesticide regulation resides with the US Environmental Protection Agency (EPA), under the Federal Insecticide, Fungicide and Rodenticide Act (FIFRA) and the Federal Food, Drug and Cosmetic Act (FFDCA). Under FIFRA, EPA registers pesticides for use, while under FFDCA, EPA establishes maximum allowable levels of pesticide residues (tolerances) in foods and animal feeds, which are enforced by other federal agencies (Fenner-Crisp, 2001).

The first legislation passed in the United States was the Federal Insecticide Act of 1910, which only prohibited the manufacture of any insecticide or fungicide that was adulterated or misbranded. FIFRA was originally passed by Congress in 1947, adding the requirement of registration by the Secretary of Agriculture before sale of insecticides, rodenticides, fungicides, and herbicides. Amendments in subsequent years added other pesticides to FIFRA jurisdiction, and provided the US Department of Agriculture (USDA) with the authority to deny, suspend, or cancel registrations of products. In 1954, Congress amended the FFDCA to require the Food and Drug Administration (FDA) to establish tolerances for pesticides in raw agricultural commodities. This was extended four years later to processed foods. In 1970, the primary federal authority for the regulation of pesticides was transferred from USDA and FDA to the newly formed EPA. Between 1970 and 1990, FIFRA was amended several other times, to address various issues related to pesticide safety and registration processes.

In 1996, the Food Quality and Protection Act (FQPA) brought important changes to pesticide regulations in the United States that affected both FIFRA and FFDCA. For example, FQPA provided the statutory mandate, under FIFRA, for continuing the expedited consideration of applications for pesticides that may provide reduced risks for human health, nontarget species, and the environment (Fenner-Crisp, 2001). Perhaps more significant were the changes to the FFDCA mandate. In 1958, an amendment of the FFDCA, the Delaney clause (Section 409), stated that ". . . no additive shall be deemed safe if it is found to induce cancer when ingested by man or animal or if it is found, after tests which are appropriate for the evaluation of the safety of food additives, to induce cancer in man or animal. . . ." Pesticides were included in this "additive" legislation. Under FQPA, however, pesticide residues are excluded from the definition of food additive, and the Delaney clause no longer applies to residues in food. Thus, tolerances can be set also for carcinogens. FQPA also directs EPA to consider aggregate exposure in the risk assessment process, that is, exposure which occurs from all food uses for a pesticide, as well as from exposures that occur from nonoccupational sources (eg, drinking water, indoor residential or school use). Additionally, EPA must consider whether certain pesticides, as well as other substances, may have the same mechanism of toxicity, and, if so, carry out a cumulative risk assessment.

Another change introduced by FQPA gives EPA the mandate to assess special risks of pesticides to infants and children. The Agency must assess aggregate risks based on dietary consumption patterns of children, possible susceptibility of infants and children to pesticides, and cumulative effects of compounds that share the same mechanism of toxicity. In the absence of adequate data, an additional default 10-fold safety factor should be applied to ensure children's safety. Finally, provisions are included for EPA to determine whether certain substances may have endocrine-disrupting effects in humans. Additional regulations concerning pesticides are present in other laws, such as the Safe Drinking Water Act or the Clean Air Act.

Under FIFRA, all pesticides sold or distributed in the United States must be registered by the EPA. Older products, registered before 1984, must undergo a re-registration process. To register a pesticide or a formulated product, a large number of studies (over 140) are required, a process that takes several years and anywhere between $50 and $100 million. The database should include information on product and residue chemistry, environmental fate, toxicology, biotransformation/degradation, occupational exposure and reentry protection, spray drift, environmental impact on nontarget species (birds, mammals, aquatic organisms, plant, soils), environmental persistence and bioaccumulation, as well as product performance and efficacy. Table 22-7 lists the basic requirements regarding toxicology data needed for new pesticide registration (see also Chap. 2). New tiered approaches to toxicity testing for agricultural chemicals, which would reduce the use of animals and improve the risk assessment process, have been recently proposed (Doe *et al.*, 2006; Cooper *et al.*, 2006).

Other nations, such as Canada, Japan, and most European countries, have promulgated legislation similar to that of the United States for registration of pesticides. In the European Union a number of directives regulate pesticide registration; the active substance must be approved at the EU level, and the formulated products must be authorized at the Member State level. The European Commission Standard Committee on the Food Chain and Animal Health (SCFCAH) authorizes registration of new active substances, based on the initial Draft Assessment Report from a Member State, and a review by the European Food Safety Agency (EFSA). Some developing nations, with a shortage of trained technical, scientific, and legal professionals to develop their own legislation, have adopted the regulatory framework of one or another industrialized

Table 22-7

Basic Toxicology Testing Requirements for Pesticide Registration

TEST	ANIMAL SPECIES*
Acute lethality (oral, dermal, inhalation)	Rat, mouse, guinea pig, rabbit
Dermal irritation	Rabbit, rat, guinea pig
Dermal sensitization	Guinea pig
Eye irritation	Rabbit
Acute delayed neurotoxicity	Hen
Genotoxicity studies (in vitro, in vivo)	Bacteria, mammalian cells, mouse, rat, drosophila
Teratogenicity	Rabbit, rodent (mouse, rat, hamster)
Two- to four-week toxicity study (oral, dermal, inhalation)	Rat, mouse
90-Day toxicity study (oral)	Rat
Chronic toxicity study (oral; six months to two years)	Rat, dog
Oncogenicity study	Rat, mouse
Reproductive/fertility study	Rat
Developmental neurotoxicity study	Rat

Substantial efforts are being devoted to develop alternative nonanimal test systems. Nevertheless, only limited in vitro tests (for primary skin irritation) have been validated and accepted by regulatory bodies.

nation. The WHO provides guidance, particularly with the setting of acceptably daily intake (ADI) values for pesticides, through its Joint FAO/WHO Meeting on Pesticide Residues (JMPR). In a few countries, still no legislation has been introduced to curb adverse effects of pesticides on the environment and human health.

INSECTICIDES

Insecticides play a most relevant role in the control of insect pests, particularly in developing countries. All of the chemical insecticides in use today are neurotoxicants, and act by poisoning the nervous systems of the target organisms (Table 22-8) (Casida, 2009). The central nervous system of insects is highly developed and not unlike that of mammals, and the peripheral nervous system, though less complex, also presents striking similarities (Ecobichon, 1992; 2001a). Thus, insecticides are mostly not species-selective with regard to targets of toxicity, and mammals, including humans, are highly sensitive to their toxicity. When selectivity exists, this is often due to differences in detoxication pathways between insects and mammals, or due to differential interactions with their target. As a class, insecticides have higher acute toxicity toward nontarget species compared with other pesticides. Some of them, most notably the organophosphates, are involved in a great number of human poisonings and deaths each year. The literature pertaining to the chemistry, development, biotransformation, environmental effects, and toxicity in target and nontarget species of insecticides is extensive, and the reader should refer to the monographs of O'Brien (1967), Brooks (1974), Hayes (1982), Ecobichon and Joy (1982),

Table 22-8

Molecular Targets of the Major Classes of Insecticides

TARGET	INSECTICIDE	EFFECT
Acetylcholinesterase	Organophosphates	Inhibition
	Carbamates	Inhibition
Sodium channels	Pyrethroids (types I and II)	Activation
	DDT	Activation
	Dihydropyrazoles	Inhibition
Nicotinic acetylcholine receptors	Nicotine	Activation
	Neonicotinoids	Activation
GABA receptor-gated chloride channels	Cyclodienes	Inhibition
	Phenylpyrazoles	Inhibition
	Pyrethroids (type II)	Inhibition
Glutamate-gated chloride channels[*]	Avermectins	Activation
Octopamine receptors[†]	Formamidines	Activation
Mitochondrial complex I	Rotenoids	Inhibition
Ryanodine receptors	Diamides	Activation

[*]*Found only in insects. In mammals avermectins activate GABA_A receptors.*

[†]*In mammals, formamidines activate α_2-adrenoceptors.*

Matsumura (1985), Ford *et al.* (1986), Clark and Matsumura (1986), Costa *et al.* (1987), Hayes and Laws (1991), Chambers and Levi (1992), Krieger (2001, 2010), Gupta (2006), and Satoh and Gupta (2010).

Organophosphorus Compounds

Although a number of organic phosphorus (OP) compounds were synthesized in the 1800s, their development as insecticides only occurred in the late 1930s and early 1940s (Gallo and Lawryk, 1991; Costa, 1988). The German chemist Gerhard Schroeder is credited for the discovery of the general chemical structure of anticholinesterase OP compounds, and for the synthesis of the first commercialized OP insecticide (Bladan, containing tetraethyl pyrophosphate [TEPP] as the active ingredient), and for one of the most known, parathion, in 1944. Since then, hundreds of OP compounds have been made and commercialized worldwide in a variety of formulations. More than half of the insecticides used (excluding oil; Table 22-4) are OPs.

The chemistry of OPs has been thoroughly investigated (Chambers *et al.*, 2010a). The general structure of OP insecticides can be represented as follows:

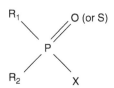

where X is the so-called leaving group, which is displaced when the OP phosphorylates AChE, and is the most sensitive to hydrolysis; R_1 and R_2 are most commonly alkoxy groups (ie, OCH_3 or OC_2H_5), although other chemical substitutes are also possible; either an oxygen or a sulfur (in this case the compound should be defined

as a phosphorothioate) is also attached to the phosphorus with a double bond. Based on chemical differences, OPs can be divided into several subclasses, which include phosphates, phosphorothioates, phosphoramidates, phosphonates, and others (Chambers *et al.*, 2010a). Fig. 22-1 shows the chemical structures of some commonly used OPs. Most are phosphorothioates, and need to be bioactivated in vivo to their oxygen analogs to exert their toxic action, but some (eg, dichlorvos, methamidophos, or the nerve agent sarin) have P=O bonds. Most OPs used as insecticides have two methoxy or ethoxy side chains (Fig. 22-1).

Biotransformation The complex array of reactions involved in the biotransformation of OPs in target and nontarget species has been the subject of extensive investigations (Tang *et al.*, 2006; Chambers *et al.*, 2010b). For all compounds that contain a sulfur bound to the phosphorus, a metabolic bioactivation is necessary for their biological activity to be manifest, as only compounds with a P=O moiety are effective inhibitors of AChE. This bioactivation consists of an oxidative desulfuration, mediated, mostly but not exclusively in the liver, by cytochrome P450 enzymes (CYPs), and leading to the formation of an "oxon," or oxygen analog of the parent insecticide (reaction 1 in Fig. 22-2). This bioactivation reaction has been known for several decades, and recent evidence has revealed a complex picture with regard to the CYP isoforms involved. Indeed, multiple CYPs have been shown to activate organophosphorothioates to their oxons, with different substrate specificities. For example, diazinon is activated by human hepatic CYP2C19, while parathion is activated primarily by CYP3A4/5 and CYP2C8, and chlorpyrifos by CYP2B6 (Kappers *et al.*, 2001; Tang *et al.*, 2001; Mutch *et al.*, 2003). In addition to oxidative desulfuration, other reactions can activate OPs (Costa, 1988). Of relevance to insecticidal OPs is thioether oxidation (formation of a sulfoxide, S=O, followed by the formation of a sulfone, O=S=O) that occurs in the leaving group moiety, and is also catalyzed by CYPs. For example, in case of the OP disulfoton, the sulfoxide and the sulfone are more potent inhibitors of AChE than the parent compound. Many other biochemical reactions are detoxication reactions, as they lead to metabolites of lesser or no toxicity (reactions 2-5 in Fig. 22-2). Some, for example, oxidative dearylation or *O*-dealkylation, are mediated by CYPs, and differences between CYPs exist also in the detoxication process. For example, dearylation of chlorpyrifos is catalyzed primarily by CYP2C19, while that of parathion by CYP2B6 (Tang *et al.*, 2001; Hodgson, 2003). Catalytic hydrolysis by phosphotriesterases, known as A-esterases (which are not inhibited by OPs), also plays an important role in the detoxication of certain OPs (reaction 5 in Fig. 22-2). One example is the enzyme paraoxonase (PON1) that hydrolyzes the oxons of chlorpyrifos and diazinon, and, at least in vitro, also of parathion (Li *et al.*, 2000; Costa *et al.*, 2002; Costa and Furlong, 2010). Noncatalytic hydrolysis of OPs also occurs when these compounds phosphorylate serine esterases classified as B-esterases, which are inhibited by OPs but cannot catalytically hydrolyze them. Examples are the carboxylesterases (CarE) and butyrylcholinesterase (BuChE), in addition to the OP target, AChE. CarE also performs a catalytic hydrolysis of the carboxylic esters of malathion, and is believed to be a major determinant of its low toxicity in mammals. Indeed, insects have low CarE activity, and inhibition of CarE by other OPs greatly potentiates the toxicity of malathion in mammals (Murphy, 1986). Glutathione *S*-transferases may also contribute to the detoxication of OPs, particularly the methoxy compounds (Abel *et al.*, 2004).

Signs and Symptoms of Toxicity and Mechanism of Action OP insecticides have high acute toxicity, with oral LD_{50} values in rat often below 50 mg/kg, although for some widely

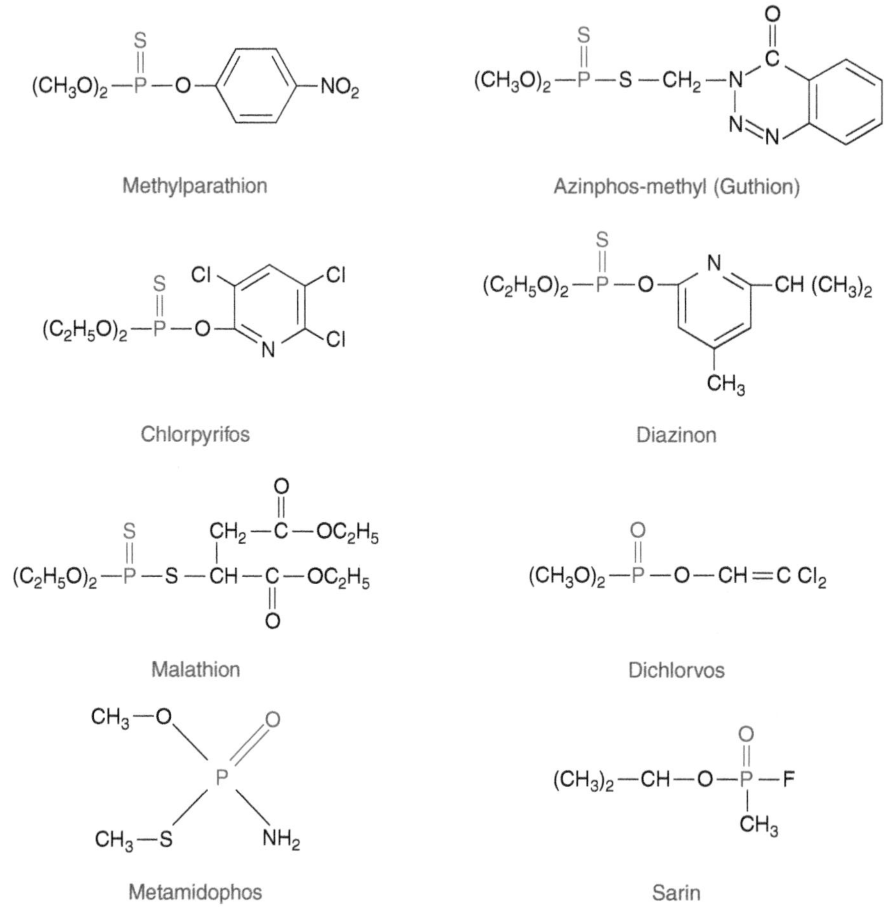

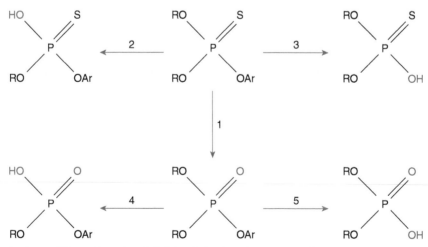

Figure 22-1. *Structures of some organophosphorus insecticides and of the nerve agent sarin.* Note that most commonly used compounds are organophosphorothioates (ie, have a P=S bond) but some, including sarin, have a P=O bond and do not require metabolic activation.

used compounds (eg, chlorpyrifos, diazinon) toxicity is somewhat lower, due to effective detoxication. One exception is malathion, which has an oral LD_{50} in rat of >1 g/kg, due, as said, to rapid detoxication by CarE. For several OPs acute dermal toxicity is also high, with some exceptions being azinphos-methyl and malathion (Murphy, 1986). The primary target for OPs is AChE, a B-esterase whose physiological role is that of hydrolyzing acetylcholine, a major neurotransmitter in the central and peripheral (autonomic and motor-somatic) nervous systems. Acetylcholine released from cholinergic nerve terminals is disposed of solely through hydrolysis by AChE. In fact, in contrast to other neurotransmitters (eg, norepinephrine or dopamine), it is choline, the product of acetylcholine hydrolysis by AChE, that is taken up by the presynaptic terminal. Hence, inhibition of AChE by OPs causes accumulation

Figure 22-2. *General scheme of biotransformation of dialkyl aryl phosphorothioate insecticides.* Reaction 1 is the bioactivation by oxidative desulfuration of the parent compound to the active metabolite, the oxon. The other reactions are enzymatic detoxication reactions that yield products that do not inhibit acetylcholinesterase. Reactions 2 and 4 are dealkylation reactions, while reaction 3 is a dearylation. All are mediated by various cytochromes P450. Reaction 5 is a hydrolytic reaction, catalyzed by paraoxonase (PON1). Note that not all reactions occur with every organophosphorus insecticide.

Table 22-9

Signs and Symptoms of Acute Poisoning with Anticholinesterase Compounds

SITE AND RECEPTOR AFFECTED	MANIFESTATIONS
Exocrine glands (M)	Increased salivation, lacrimation, perspiration
Eyes (M)	Miosis, blurred vision
Gastrointestinal tract (M)	Abdominal cramps, vomiting, diarrhea
Respiratory tract (M)	Increased bronchial secretion, bronchoconstriction
Bladder (M)	Urinary frequency, incontinence
Cardiovascular system (M)	Bradycardia, hypotension
Cardiovascular system (N)	Tachycardia, transient hypertension
Skeletal muscles (N)	Muscle fasciculations, twitching, cramps, generalized weakness, flaccid paralysis
Central nervous system (M, N)	Dizziness, lethargy, fatigue, headache, mental confusion, depression of respiratory centers, convulsions, coma

M, muscarinic receptors; N, nicotinic receptors.

of acetylcholine at cholinergic synapses, with overstimulation of cholinergic receptors of the muscarinic and nicotinic type. As these receptors are localized in most organs of the body, a "cholinergic syndrome" ensues, which includes increased sweating and salivation, profound bronchial secretion, bronchoconstriction, miosis, increased gastrointestinal motility, diarrhea, tremors, muscular twitching, and various central nervous system effects (Table 22-9). When death occurs, this is believed to be due to respiratory failure as a result of inhibition of respiratory centers in the brainstem, bronchoconstriction and increased bronchial secretion, and flaccid paralysis of respiratory muscles (Gallo and Lawryk, 1991; Lotti, 2000, 2010). The time interval between exposure and onset of symptoms varies with the route and degree of exposure, and the chemical nature of the OP. The first signs to appear are usually muscarinic, which may or may not be in combination with nicotinic signs. While respiratory failure is a hallmark of severe OP poisoning, mild poisoning and/or early stages of an otherwise severe poisoning may display no clear-cut signs and symptoms (Lotti, 2010). Therefore, diagnosis is made through symptom recognition; miosis is observed most often, followed by gastrointestinal symptoms (nausea, vomiting, abdominal pain, vomiting) and hypersalivation.

The interaction of OPs with AChE has been studied in much detail. OPs with a P=O moiety phosphorylate a hydroxyl group on serine in the active (esteratic) site of the enzyme, thus impeding its action on the physiological substrate (Fig. 22-3). The first reaction leads to the formation of a Michaelis complex, while a subsequent reaction leads to phosphorylated AChE (Table 22-10). Rates of these two reactions, which are usually very rapid, indicate the affinity of the enzyme for a given OP. The bond between the phosphorus atom and the esteratic site of the enzyme is much more stable than the bond between the carbonyl carbon of acetate (in acetylcholine) at

the same enzyme site. While breaking of the carbon–enzyme bond is complete in a few microseconds, breaking of the phosphorus–enzyme bond can take from a few hours to several days, depending on the chemical structure of the OP. Phosphorylated AChE is hydrolyzed by water at a very slow rate (Fig. 22-3; Table 22-10), and the rate of "spontaneous reactivation" depends on the chemical nature of the R substituents. Reactivation decreases in the order demethoxy > diethoxy >> diisopropoxy (Gallo and Lawryk, 1991). While water is a weak nucleophilic agent, certain hydroxylamine derivatives, known as oximes, can facilitate dephosphorylation of AChE, and are utilized in the therapy of OP poisoning (see below). Reactivation of phosphorylated AChE does not occur once the enzyme–inhibitor complex has "aged" (Fig. 22-3). Aging consists of the loss (by nonenzymatic hydrolysis) of one of the two alkyl (R) groups, and the rate of aging depends on the nature of the alkyl group. When phosphorylated AChE has aged, the enzyme can be considered to be irreversibly inhibited, and the only means of replacing its activity is through synthesis of new enzyme, a process that may take days.

Treatment of Poisoning On OP poisoning, prompt treatment is essential. Procedures aimed at decontamination and/or at minimizing absorption depend on the route of exposure. In case of dermal exposure, contaminated clothing should be removed, and the skin washed with alkaline soap (Lotti, 2010). Special attention should be exercised by medical personnel, because passive contamination may occur. In case of ingestion, procedures to reduce absorption from the gastrointestinal tract do not appear to be very effective (Lotti, 2010). Atropine represents the cornerstone of the treatment for OP poisoning; it is a muscarinic receptor antagonist, and thus prevents the action of accumulating acetylcholine on these receptors. Atropine is preferably given intravenously, although the intramuscular route is also effective. The best clinical approach is to administer doses of atropine large enough to achieve evidence of atropinization, that is, flushing, dry mouth, changes in pupil size, bronchodilation, and increased heart rate; atropinization should be maintained for at least 48 hours (Lotti, 2010). Indicative doses of atropine are 1 or 2 to 5 mg in case of mild or moderate poisoning, respectively. Higher doses by continuous infusion may be required in severe cases. Overdosage with atropine is rarely serious in OP-poisoned patients (Lotti, 2010).

Oximes, such as pralidoxime (2-PAM), are also used in the therapy of OP poisoning. 2-PAM contains a positively charged atom capable of attaching to the anionic site of AChE, and facilitates dephosphorylation of the enzyme (Fig. 22-4), thus restoring the catalytic site of AChE to its function. However, this chemical reaction occurs only when the phosphorylated AChE has not undergone aging. Dosing regimens for various oximes depend on the specific compound and the severity of OP poisoning. For example, for pralidoxime chloride, an initial 1 g dose given intravenously is recommended, followed after 15 to 30 minutes by another 1 g, if no improvement is seen. If still no improvement is seen, an infusion of 0.5 g/h can be started (Lotti, 2010). The recommended dosage schedule is aimed at achieving a plasma oxime concentration of 4 mg/L, which was shown to be effective for pralidoxime methanesulfonate in cats poisoned with a quaternary analog of sarin (Sundwall, 1961). While animal data consistently show a marked positive effect of oximes, several authors reported limited or no efficacy of oximes in the treatment of OP poisoning (Bismuth *et al.*, 1992; Singh *et al.*, 1995; Buckley *et al.*, 2005). A recent meta-analysis of several studies of OP-poisoned patients concluded that use of oximes was associated "with either a null effect or possible harm" (Peter *et al.*, 2006). On the other hand, inadequate dosing has been held as a

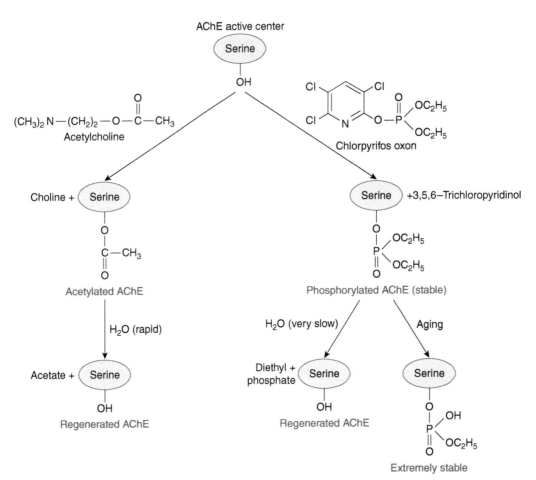

AChE active center

Figure 22-3. *Scheme of hydrolysis of acetylcholine by acetylcholinesterase (AChE) and reaction of chlorpyrifos oxon with AChE.* See text for details.

major factor for lack of response to oxime therapy (Johnson *et al.*, 2000; Eddleston *et al.*, 2002). Furthermore, poisoning by OPs bearing two methoxy groups (malathion, methyl parathion, dimethoate) is considered to be rather resistant to oxime therapy (Worek *et al.*, 1999a). Additionally, time of oxime administration following OP poisoning is crucial, as their therapeutic window is determined by the rate of aging. For example, one day after intoxication with a dimethyl phosphoryl compound, virtually all phosphorylated AChE

would be expected to be in the aged form, so that oxime therapy will be useless by that time (Johnson *et al.*, 2000). Oximes have also the potential to form stable phosphoryl oximes that have themselves anticholinesterase activity; for this reason, and because of rapid reactivation of carbamylated AChE, oximes are not indicated in case of poisoning with carbamate insecticides.

In addition to oximes, diazepam (10–20 mg) is also used in the treatment of acute OP poisoning to relieve anxiety in mild cases, and to reduce muscle fasciculations and antagonize convulsions in the more severe cases (Lotti, 2010).

Biochemical Measurements In addition to synapses, AChE is also present in red blood cells (RBC). Additionally, BuChE, also known as pseudocholinesterase, is found in plasma. The physiological functions of these enzymes in blood are yet to be discovered. Nevertheless, because activity of both enzymes is usually inhibited on exposure to OPs, their measurement is widely used as an indication of exposure, and/or biological effect of OPs. The specificity and usefulness of measurements of RBC AChE and of plasma BuChE in case of OP exposure have been debated for some time (Lotti, 1995). The main issues can be summarized as follows (Costa *et al.*, 2005): (1) different OPs may inhibit AChE or BuChE to a different degree. For example, the oxygen analogs of malathion, diazinon and chlorpyrifos, and dichlorvos, are stronger inhibitors of plasma BuChE than of RBC AChE. (2) There is a high degree of variability of enzyme activity (particularly of BuChE) among individuals, in part due to genetic differences (see below). This requires establishment of a baseline value for each individual, or, in case this is not available, of repeated postexposure measurements to determine

Table 22-10

Rates of Cholinesterase Inhibition by Carbamate and Organophosphorus Esters

$$EH + AB \underset{k_{-1}}{\overset{k_1}{\rightleftharpoons}} EHAB \xrightarrow{k_2} EA + BH \xrightarrow{k_3} EH + AOH$$

		REACTION RATES	
PARAMETER	KINETIC CONSTANT	CARBAMATE	ORGANOPHOSPHORUS
Complex formation	k_{-1}/k_1	Rapid	Rapid
Inhibition rate	k_2	Variable	Rapid to moderately rapid
Reactivation rate	k_3	Relatively rapid	Slow to extremely slow

Data from Ecobichon (2001a,b).

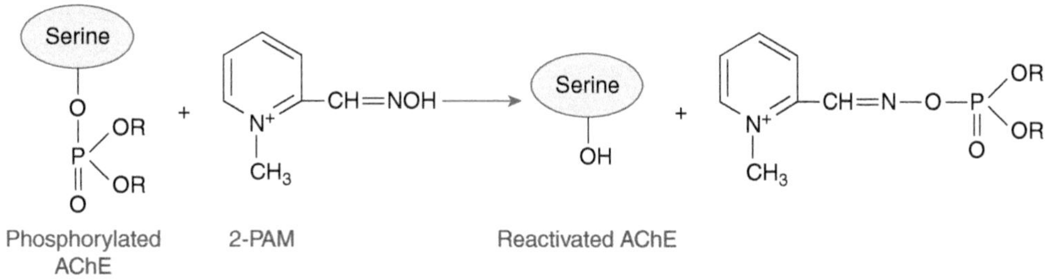

Figure 22-4. *Reactivation of phosphorylated acetylcholinesterase by pralidoxime (2-PAM).* Note that 2-PAM is only effective before the phosphorylated enzyme has undergone the aging reaction.

possible changes back toward baseline values. (3) RBC AChE activity is better correlated with target tissue (eg, brain, diaphragm) AChE than is plasma BuChE activity, as indicated by animal studies (Padilla *et al.*, 1994). There is also a good correlation between the severity of signs and symptoms of poisoning and the degree of inhibition of RBC AChE (Lotti, 2010). (4) Neither measurement is specific for a certain OP, and, indeed, other insecticides, such as carbamates, also inhibit AChE and BuChE. (5) A 30% or greater decrease of plasma BuChE from preexposure baseline raises a red flag, and requires health and workplace surveillance, and removal of the worker from the exposure; however, the toxicological significance of such decrease is still much debated (Carlock *et al.*, 1999; USEPA, 2000). Despite these caveats, measurements of plasma BuChE, and particularly of RBC AChE, remain a very valid way to determine exposure to OPs, and early biological effects of OP exposure, to be used as confirmation of diagnosis of OP poisoning, or to monitor occupationally exposed workers. Several methods exist to measure activity of these two enzymes (Reiner and Simeon-Rudolf, 2006; Wilson and Henderson, 2007). Whole blood AChE may also be measured, considering that only about 10% of the activity is due to the plasma enzyme (Worek *et al.*, 1999b).

Several analytical methods are available to measure OPs and their metabolites in body fluids; the parent compound is measured in blood, while metabolites are measured in urine (Lotti, 2010). These measurements are rarely carried out in the clinical setting, but are extensively utilized in epidemiological studies; indeed, determination of metabolite levels in urine is the most practical method to estimate exposure to OPs (Maroni *et al.*, 2000). Such metabolites include alkylphosphate derivatives, as well as chemical residues (the "leaving group") specific for each compound. The alkylphosphates or alkyl-(di)-thiophosphates are the result of metabolism of parent compounds or their oxygen analogs by CYPs or esterases. They are not specific for a certain OP, but are useful to assess exposure to (or internal dose of) several OPs. Some alkylphosphate metabolites of commonly used OPs are shown in Table 22-11. Other metabolites

Table 22-11

Examples of Alkylphosphates in Urine

METABOLITE	ORGANOPHOSPHATE
Dimethylphosphate (DMP)	Methyl parathion, methylchlorpyrifos, dichlorvos, trichlorfon
Diethylphosphate (DEP)	Parathion, diazinon, chlorpyrifos
Dimethylthiophosphate (DMTP)	Azinphos-methyl (Guthion), fenitrothion
Diethylthiophosphate (DETP)	Diazinon, parathion, chlorpyrifos

Data from Maroni et al. (2000).

are specific for certain OP compounds; for example, *p*-nitrophenol in urine is an indicator of exposure to parathion or methyl parathion, while 3,5,6-trichloropyridinol is useful to assess exposure to chlorpyrifos or methyl chlorpyrifos (Barr *et al.*, 2005). While measurements of urinary metabolites of OPs have been widely used to assess exposure to OP from occupational, environmental, and dietary sources, caution should be exercised when interpreting results, as dialkylphosphates, and also leaving groups, can be found in the environment, including food and drinks, as a result of OP degradation. This would lead to an overestimate of OP exposure (Lu *et al.*, 2005).

The Intermediate Syndrome A second distinct manifestation of exposure to OPs is the so-called intermediate syndrome, which was first conceptualized by clinicians in Sri Lanka involved in the treatment of suicide attempts (Senanayake and Karalliedde, 1987). The intermediate syndrome is seen in 20% to 50% of acute OP poisoning cases, and has been observed following exposure to a large variety of OPs (de Bleecker, 2006). The syndrome develops one to several days after the poisoning, during recovery from cholinergic manifestations, or, in some cases, when patients are completely recovered from the initial cholinergic crisis. Prominent features of the intermediate syndrome are a marked weakness of respiratory, neck, and proximal limb muscles. Mortality due to respiratory paralysis and complications ranges from 15% to 40%, and recovery in surviving patients usually takes up to 30 days. The intermediate syndrome is not a direct effect of AChE inhibition, and its precise underlying mechanisms are still unknown. The hypothesis that muscle weakness may result from nicotinic receptor desensitization due to prolonged cholinergic stimulation remains the most valid (Lotti, 2010). There is no specific treatment for the intermediate syndrome and intervention is exclusively supportive.

Organophosphate-Induced Delayed Polyneuropathy A few OPs may also cause another type of toxicity, known as organophosphate-induced delayed polyneuropathy (OPIDP). Signs and symptoms include tingling of the hands and feet, followed by sensory loss, progressive muscle weakness and flaccidity of the distal skeletal muscles of the lower and upper extremities, and ataxia (Lotti, 1992; Lotti and Moretto, 2005; Ehrich and Jortner, 2010). These may occur two to three weeks after a single exposure, when signs of both the acute cholinergic and the intermediate syndromes have subsided. OPIDP can be classified as a distal sensorimotor axonopathy. Neuropathological studies in experimental OPIDP have evidenced that the primary lesion is a bilateral degenerative change in distal levels of axons and their terminals, primarily affecting larger/longer myelinated central and peripheral nerve fibers, leading to breakdown of neuritic segments and the myelin sheaths (Ehrich and Jortner, 2010). OPIDP is not related to AChE inhibition. Indeed, one of the compounds involved in several epidemics of this neuropathy, including the so-called Ginger-Jake paralysis in the 1930s in the United States, is tri-*ortho*-cresyl phosphate (TOCP), which is a very poor AChE inhibitor. Extensive studies carried out in the past 30 years (Johnson, 1982; Johnson and Glynn, 2001; Lotti, 1992) have identified the target for OPIDP as an esterase, present in nerve tissues as well as other tissues (eg, lymphocytes), named neuropathy target esterase (NTE). Several OPs, depending on their chemical structure, can inhibit NTE, as do some non-OPs, such as certain carbamates and sulfonyl fluorides. Phosphorylation of NTE by OPs is similar to that observed for AChE. However, only OPs whose chemical structure leads to aging of phosphorylated NTE (by a process analogous to that described for AChE) can cause OPIDP. Other compounds that inhibit NTE but cannot undergo the aging reaction are not neuropathic, indicating that inhibition of NTE catalytic activity is not the mechanism of axonal degeneration. Direct evidence of the importance of the aging reaction in the initiation of OPIDP was provided by studies with stereoisomers of *O*-ethyl *O*-4-nitrophenyl phenylphosphonate (EPN); while both stereoisomers inhibit NTE, only the one that undergoes aging produces OPIDP, while the other is non-neuropathic and protective (see below; Johnson and Read, 1987). For OPIDP to be initiated, phosphorylation and subsequent aging of at least 70% of NTE is necessary, and this two-step process occurs within hours of poisoning. When the first clinical signs of OPIDP are evident some weeks later, NTE activity has recovered. Lymphocyte NTE activity has been used in animals and in humans as a marker of NTE in nervous tissue (Lotti and Moretto, 2005; Richardson *et al.*, 2009).

The physiological functions(s) of NTE are still unknown. Enzymatically NTE behaves as a B-esterase, that is, it is inhibited by OPs rather than capable of hydrolyzing them (Wijeyesakere and Richardson, 2010). NTE may be a phospholipase, as shown by its ability to hydrolyze phosphatidylcholine to glycerophosphocholine, and may thus play a role in lipid metabolism, in intraneuronal membrane trafficking, and in lipid homeostasis (Zaccheo *et al.*, 2004; Glynn, 2006; Wijeyesakere and Richardson, 2010). NTE has a 41% identity with the Swiss Cheese protein (SWS) in neurons of *Drosophila*, whose mutation leads to glial and neuronal cell death with subsequent vacuolation (Kretzschmar *et al.*, 1997). Studies in genetically modified mice have indicated that NTE is required for normal blood vessel and placental development, and that absence of brain NTE results in neuronal degeneration and loss

of endoplasmic reticulum in various brain areas (Moser *et al.*, 2004; Akossoglou *et al.*, 2004). Hypotheses to explain the consequences of OP–NTE interactions include a loss of non-esterase functions of NTE (eg, in phospholipid metabolism) that would be essential for the axon, or a gain of toxic function of phosphorylated/aged NTE (Lotti and Moretto, 2005; Wijeyesakere and Richardson, 2010). Although reductions in axonal transport have been found to precede overt clinical signs, the exact chain of events occurring between phosphorylation and aging of NTE and axonal degeneration is still unknown. Thus, the most crucial issues in the mechanisms of OPIDP development and progression remain obscure.

Although several epidemics of OPIDP have occurred in the past, its occurrence in humans is now rare. Before commercialization, OPs must undergo specific neurotoxicity testing in the hen (one of the most sensitive species) to determine whether OPIDP is produced (Moretto, 1999). High doses of OPs are used, and animals are protected from acute cholinergic toxicity with atropine, and clinical, morphological, and biochemical measurements are carried out. In vitro tests can provide the ratio of relative inhibitory potency toward AChE and NTE, but these have not been yet accepted by regulatory agencies (Ehrich *et al.*, 1997). Despite these tests, a few commercialized OPs (methamidophos, trichlorfon, chlorpyrifos) have caused OPIDP in humans, mostly as a result of extremely high exposures in suicide attempts (Lotti and Moretto, 2005). The possibility that repeated, low-level exposure to OPs may cause OPIDP is negligible, as the threshold (~70%) for NTE inhibition and aging would not be reached under these exposure conditions (Wijeyesakere and Richardson, 2010). Although it was once thought that some animal species (eg, rodents) were insensitive to OPIDP, only mice appear to be somewhat resistant (Veronesi *et al.*, 1991). On the other hand, age is an important determinant of susceptibility, with young animals displaying more resistance; in young chicks the threshold for NTE inhibition and aging is >90% versus 70% in adult hens (Peraica *et al.*, 1993). Children are also more resistant to OPIDP.

As noted earlier, compounds that inhibit NTE but do not age do not cause OPIDP. When given to experimental animals *before* a neuropathic OP, these compounds exert a protective role, by occupying the NTE active site. However, when given after a neuropathic OP, these compounds have been shown to promote OPIDP (Fig. 22-5;

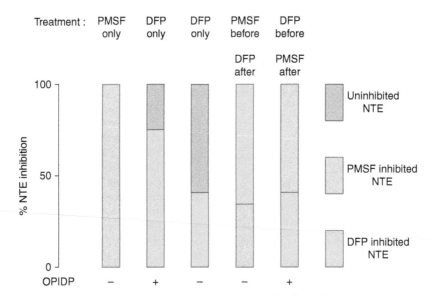

Figure 22-5. *A summary of initiation, protection, and promotion of OPIDP, showing the relationships among dosing, NTE inhibition, and clinical response, when diisopropylfluorophosphate (DFP) and phenylmethanesulfonyl fluoride (PMSF) are given alone or in combination.* (From Lotti *et al.*, 1991, with permission.)

Lotti *et al.*, 1991; Lotti, 2002a). By borrowing a terminology used for carcinogenic compounds, agents that phosphorylate NTE and age have been named initiators, while NTE inhibitors that do not initiate OPIDP but can promote it have been named promoters (Lotti, 2002a,b). It is easy to understand why the latter compounds would be protective when given before an OP initiator; however, why and how they are able to promote OPIDP is still unknown. Promoters can also potentiate axonal degeneration caused by means other than OPs, such as traumatic nerve lesion, or 2,5-hexanedione (Moretto, 2000). Furthermore, promotion has also been shown to occur, in some cases, even when the promoter is given at doses that do not inhibit NTE, suggesting that another protein, rather than NTE, may be the target for the promoting effect. Since promotion is less efficient in chicks, where the compensation/repair mechanisms are thought to be more efficient, a hypothesis is that promotion may directly affect compensation/repair mechanism(s) of the nervous system (Lotti, 2002a). Although still mechanistically mysterious, the issue of promotion may have a bearing on risk assessment of potential insecticide mixtures. Indeed, exposure to an initiator at a dose lower than that required to cause OPIDP would nevertheless result in OPIDP if followed by exposure to a promoter.

Genetic Susceptibility Genetically determined variations in biotransformation enzymes or target molecules can modify the response to OPs (Costa, 2001). As discussed earlier, CYPs are important for the activation and detoxication of OPs. Variant forms of several CYPs have been identified, and these polymorphisms confer differences in catalytic activity or levels of expression that may result in varying rates of oxidation of OPs. Limited in vitro studies have indeed shown that polymorphic forms of some CYPs (eg, CYP2C19 or CYP3A4) cause differential desulfuration and dearylation of chlorpyrifos (Hodgson, 2003), but their overall influence on OP toxicity in vivo has not been investigated. The liver and plasma A-esterase paraoxonase (PON1), which detoxifies chlorpyrifos oxon and diazoxon, also presents several polymorphisms in the coding and promoter regions, which affect the catalytic efficiency of the enzyme toward different substrates (the Q192R polymorphism), and its level of expression (eg, the C-108T polymorphism) (Costa *et al.*, 2002, 2003; Costa and Furlong, 2010). Studies in transgenic animal models have clearly indicated that PON1 "status," encompassing both the Q192R polymorphism and the level of PON1 activity, plays a most relevant role in modulating the acute toxicity of some OPs (Fig. 22-6; Li *et al.*, 2000; Cole *et al.*, 2005). Evidence that PON1 status may play a role in susceptibility to OPs in humans is also emerging (Furlong *et al.*, 2006; Hoffman *et al.*, 2009). Genetically engineered PON1s with higher catalytic efficiencies toward different OPs are also being considered as catalytic scavengers to be eventually utilized in case of OP poisoning (Stevens *et al.*, 2008; Costa and Furlong, 2010).

High levels of BuChE are present in plasma, and OPs can inhibit its activity. Although its physiological function is unclear, BuChE, by scavenging OPs, can guard against their toxicity, as the OP would be unavailable for reaction with its primary target AChE (Costa, 2001). At least 39 genetic variants of BuChE have been identified, with nucleotide alterations in the coding region. Several of these variants are silent, but they are rare; most common variants have a reduced activity and are far less efficient scavengers of cholinesterase inhibitors (Lockridge and Masson, 2000; Goodal, 2006; Lockridge *et al.*, 2010). Individuals with such BuChE variants would be predicted to be more susceptible to OP toxicity, as suggested by a study in Brazilian farmers (Fontoura-da-Silva and Chautard-Friere-Maira, 1996). To date, only a few genetic variants of human AChE have been described (Goodal, 2006). One resulted

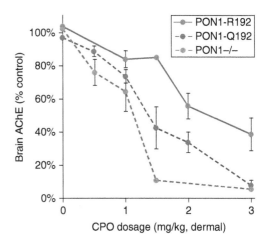

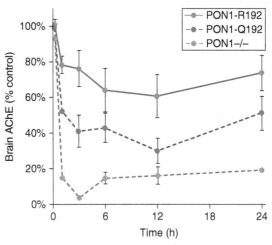

Figure 22-6. *Dose–response (top panel) and timecourse (bottom panel) of brain acetylcholinesterase (AChE) inhibition by chlorpyrifos oxon (CPO) in PON1 knockout mice (PON1–/–) or in mice expressing either of the two human PON1$_{R192}$ or PON1$_{Q192}$ transgenes in place of endogenous mouse PON1.* Note that mice lacking PON1 are most sensitive to CPO toxicity, while those expressing human PON1$_{R192}$ are most resistant. Mice expressing human PON1$_{Q192}$ show intermediate sensitivity, despite expressing similar levels of PON1. The experiments indicate the role of PON1 "status" in modulating the toxicity of CPO. (Modified with permission from Cole *et al.*, 2005.)

in an amino acid change but had no effect on the catalytic properties of the enzyme (Masson *et al.*, 1994), while a polymorphism in the distal promoter region was associated with an enhanced response to pyridostigmine (Shapira *et al.*, 2000). A third study identified several polymorphisms in the coding region that also did not appear to alter the catalytic action of AChE (Hasin *et al.*, 2004). Transgenic mice carrying one deficient AChE allele (AChE$^{+/-}$) are healthy, and display supersensitivity to OPs (Lockridge *et al.*, 2005). Genetic polymorphisms of AChE in humans that would cause partial AChE deficiency have been hypothesized, but not yet demonstrated; such individuals would be expected to display increased susceptibility to OP toxicity.

Long-Term Toxicity While the effects of acute exposure to OPs have been clearly identified and characterized by thousands of animal studies and cases of human poisonings, there is still controversy on possible long-term effects of OPs. The fact that acute exposure to high doses of OPs may result, in some cases, in long-lasting adverse health effects (particularly in the CNS) has been shown in animals, as well as humans (Sanchez-Santed *et al.*, 2004;

Rosenstock *et al.*, 1991). More controversial is the possibility that low exposure to OPs, at doses that produce no cholinergic signs, may lead to long-term adverse health effects, particularly in the central and peripheral nervous systems. Chronic exposure of animals to OPs, at doses that significantly inhibit AChE, but may not be associated with clinical signs, results in the development of tolerance to their cholinergic effects (which is mediated, at least in part, by downregulation of cholinergic receptors), and has been associated with neurobehavioral abnormalities, particularly at the cognitive level (Costa *et al.*, 1982; Prendergast *et al.*, 1998). Evidence describing long-term neuropsychological or neuropsychiatric alterations in humans on low chronic exposure is contradictory (Daniell *et al.*, 1992; Jamal and Julu, 2002), and most recent expert reviews tend to conclude that the balance of evidence does not support the existence of clinically significant neuropsychological effects, neuropsychiatric abnormalities, or peripheral nerve dysfunction in humans chronically exposed to low levels of OPs (Ray, 1998; Lotti, 2002b; Colosio *et al.*, 2003; IOM, 2000; Moretto *et al.*, 2010). Yet, research in this area, and the ensuing debate, will undoubtedly continue.

OPs as a class are not considered to be mutagenic, and there is little evidence that they may be carcinogenic. Immunotoxicity of OPs has been suggested from in vitro or high-dose animal studies, but evidence in humans is lacking. Some OPs have also endocrine-disrupting activities in vitro (Tamura *et al.*, 2003; Kitamura *et al.*, 2003), but in vivo studies, even at dose levels that inhibit brain AChE activity, have not substantiated these findings (Okahashi *et al.*, 2005).

Developmental Toxicity and Neurotoxicity A report from the National Academy of Sciences highlighted the potential higher exposure of children to pesticides (NRC, 1993), and FQPA indicates that in the risk assessment process, an additional safety factor should be included to ensure protection of children who are presumed to be more sensitive to the effects of toxicants (FQPA, 1996). Experimental data indicate that young animals are more sensitive to the acute toxicity of OPs (Costa, 2006; Pope, 2010). This increased sensitivity does not appear to be due to intrinsic differences in AChE, but rather due to lower detoxication abilities of young animals. For example, low detoxication by CYPs or PON1 accounts for the age-dependent susceptibility of parathion and chlorpyrifos, respectively (Benke and Murphy, 1975; Mortensen *et al.*, 1996; Costa and Furlong, 2010). On the other hand, as discussed earlier, the young appear to be more resistant to OPIDP. In recent years, accumulating evidence suggests that perinatal exposure to OPs may cause developmental neurotoxicity. Studies in rodents indicate that OPs can affect various cellular processes (eg, DNA replication, neuronal survival, neurite outgrowth) and noncholinergic pathways (eg, serotoninergic synaptic functions, the adenylate cylase system), and cause various behavioral abnormalities (Song *et al.*, 1997; Dam *et al.*, 1998; Jett *et al.*, 2001; Aldridge *et al.*, 2003; Ricceri *et al.*, 2003; Garcia *et al.*, 2005). Such effects are also seen at dose levels that produced no cholinergic signs of toxicity (Timofeeva and Levin, 2010). These findings, together with results of biomonitoring studies that indicate exposure of children, particularly in inner cities and farming communities, to OPs, have led to regulatory restrictions on the use of certain OPs, and to concern for their potential neurotoxic effects in children (Eskenazi *et al.*, 1999; Weiss *et al.*, 2004; Eaton *et al.*, 2008). Furthermore, specific guidelines for developmental neurotoxicity have been implemented (Tilson, 2000).

Carbamates

Carbamate insecticides have a variety of chemical structures (Fig. 22-7), but all derive from carbamic acid, the majority being

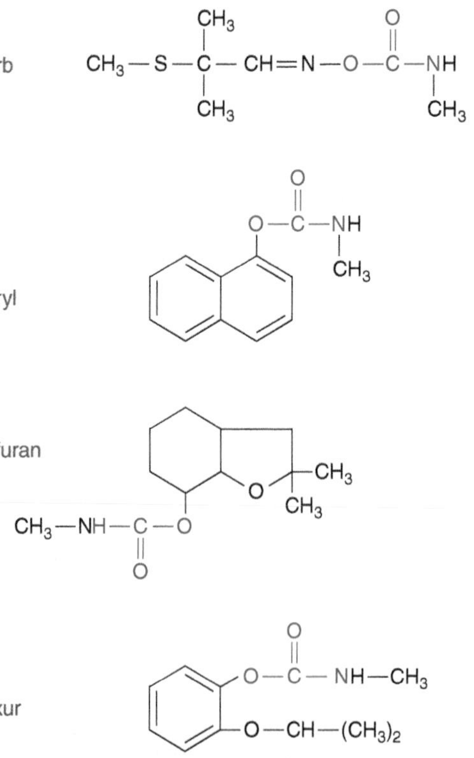

	LD$_{50}$ in rats (mg/kg)		Water solubility (g/L)
	Oral	Dermal	
Aldicarb	0.8	3.2	6.0
Carbaryl	400	>5000	0.7
Carbofuran	10	>1000	0.7
Propoxur	85	~1500	2.0

Figure 22-7. *Structures of some carbamate insecticides, with indication of acute oral and dermal toxicity in the rat, and of water solubility.*

N-methylcarbamates. They present different degrees of acute oral toxicity, ranging from moderate to low toxicity such as carbaryl, to extremely high toxicity, such as aldicarb (Fig. 22-7). Dermal toxicity is lower, but skin penetration is increased by organic solvents and emulsifiers present in most formulations (Ecobichon, 2001b). Carbamates are susceptible to a variety of enzyme-catalyzed biotransformation reactions, and the principal pathways involve oxidation and hydrolysis (Fukuto, 1972; Tang *et al.*, 2006). They do not require metabolic bioactivation, and the metabolites are for the most part devoid of biological activity, although this is not always the case. For example, two metabolites of aldicarb, the sulfoxide and the sulfone, are more potent anticholinesterases than the parent compound (Risher *et al.*, 1987). The mechanism of toxicity of carbamates is analogous to that of OPs, in that they inhibit AChE. However, inhibition is transient and rapidly reversible, since there is rapid reactivation of the carbamylated enzyme in the presence of water (Table 22-10). Additionally, carbamylated AChE does not undergo the aging reaction. The signs and symptoms of carbamate poisoning are the same observed following intoxication with OPs, and include miosis, urination, diarrhea, salivation, muscle fasciculation, and CNS effects (Table 22-9). However, differently from OPs, acute intoxication by carbamates is generally resolved within a few hours. Fig. 22-8 shows experimental data on AChE inhibition by propoxur in mice; maximal inhibition is achieved very rapidly, as carbamates are direct AChE inhibitors and do not require metabolic bioactivation, and enzyme activity returns to control levels within two hours. Carbamates also inhibit BuChE; the degree of such inhibition varies depending on the specific compound, but is generally modest after moderate exposure (when, however, inhibition of RBC and nervous tissue AChE can be substantial), and equivalent to that of AChE after severe exposure (Ecobichon, 2001b).

The transient nature of AChE inhibition following carbamate exposure poses several problems in measurements of its activity. First, measurements should be made shortly (a few hours at most) following exposure; otherwise, even if severe inhibition and symptoms of toxicity were present, the latter would be resolved, and no enzyme inhibition would be detected. Second, particular care should be taken even if blood samples are drawn shortly after exposure, as temperature and time elapsed before the assay would cause reversal of inhibition. The treatment of carbamate intoxication relies on the use of the muscarinic antagonist atropine. Use of oximes is generally not recommended, as 2-PAM has been shown to aggravate the

toxicity of carbaryl (Murphy, 1986). Yet, oximes may have beneficial effects in case of other carbamates such as aldicarb (Ecobichon, 2001b), and a current view is that concern over use of oximes in case of carbamate poisoning is unwarranted (Rossman *et al.*, 2009). There are several cases of human poisoning associated with exposure to various carbamates, in particular carbaryl (Cranmer, 1986) and propoxur (Hayes, 1982). Most cases, however, involved aldicarb. This compound, which has a very high acute toxicity, is also highly water soluble (Fig. 22-7). Although, because of this characteristic, it is not registered for use on any fruit or vegetable having high water content, its illegal uses in hydroponically grown cucumbers and in watermelons have led to outbreaks of poisoning (Goes *et al.*, 1980; Goldman *et al.*, 1990). Contamination of drinking water has also been reported (Zaki *et al.*, 1982). Carbamates can inhibit NTE, but since carbamylated NTE cannot age, they are thought to be unable to initiate OPIDP. Additionally, when given before a neuropathic organophosphate, carbamates offer protection against OPIDP (Johnson and Lawerys, 1969), but when given after, they can promote OPIDP (Lotti, 2002a). A few case reports indicate that exposure to very high dosages of methylcarbamates (eg, carbaryl, carbofuran) may result in a peripheral polyneuropathy similar to OPIDP (Dickoff *et al.*, 1987; Yang *et al.*, 2000). This would imply that aging is not required for OPIDP to develop, or, alternatively, that in these cases, carbamates may have amplified a preexisting subclinical neuropathy. Carefully conducted animal studies would be needed to substantiate this hypothesis.

Subchronic and chronic toxicity studies on carbamate insecticides have been carried out mostly for registration purposes, and their main findings (inhibition of cholinesterases, effects on organ weight and hematological parameters, histopathological changes) are described in detail by Baron (1991). Development of tolerance to some carbamates (propoxur, carbaryl) on repeated exposure has been observed, and this appears to be due to an induction of microsomal enzymes (Costa *et al.*, 1981). As a class, methylcarbamates are not mutagenic, and there is also no evidence of carcinogenicity. Embryotoxicity or fetotoxicity is observed only at maternally toxic doses (Baron, 1991). Limited evidence suggests that carbamates (eg, aldicarb) may be more acutely toxic to young animals than to adults (Moser, 1999), possibly because of lower detoxication, but this aspect has not been investigated in the same detail as for OPs.

Pyrethroids

Pyrethrins were first developed as insecticides from extracts of the flower heads of *Chrisanthenum cinerariaefolium*, whose insecticidal potential was appreciated in ancient China and Persia. However, because pyrethrins were decomposed rapidly by light, synthetic analogs, the pyrethroids, were developed (Casida, 2010). Because of their high insecticidal potency, generally low mammalian toxicity, relatively low tendency to induce insect resistance, and lack of environmental persistence, pyrethroids have encountered much success in the past 30 years, and now account for about 15% to 20% of the global insecticide market (Soderlund *et al.*, 2002). Pyrethroids are used widely as insecticides both in the house and in agriculture, in medicine for the topical treatment of scabies and head lice, and in tropical countries for malaria control, both in soaked bed nets to prevent mosquito bites and in indoor residual spraying. They are known to alter the normal function of insect nerves by modifying the kinetics of voltage-sensitive sodium channels, which mediate the transient increase in the sodium permeability of the nerve membrane that underlies the nerve action potential (Soderlund *et al.*, 2002). All pyrethroid insecticides contain an acid moiety, a central ester bond, and an alcohol moiety (Fig. 22-9). The

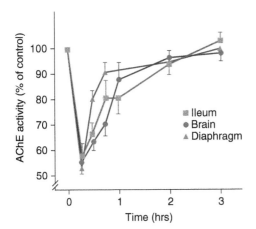

Figure 22-8. *Timecourse of acetylcholinesterase (AChE) inhibition in different tissues of mice following administration of a single dose of the carbamate insecticide propoxur (10 mg/kg, i.p.).* Note the near complete recovery of AChE activity two hours after propoxur administration. (With permission from Costa *et al.*, 1981.)

acid moiety contains two chiral carbons; thus, pyrethroids typically exist as stereoisomeric compounds (*trans* and *cis*). Additionally, some pyrethroids also have a chiral carbon on the alcohol moiety, allowing for a total of eight different stereoenantiomers. These chemical considerations are relevant, as pyrethroids' effects on sodium channels, their insecticidal activity, and their mammalian toxicity are stereospecific. The *cis* isomers are generally more toxic than the corresponding *trans* isomers (Casida *et al.*, 1983). The acute oral mammalian toxicity of pyrethroids is generally low. Values of LD_{50} range, for example, from 100 mg/kg (deltamethrin) to 10,000 mg/kg (phenothrin). To underline the relevance of stereospecificity, the LD_{50} for 1R,*trans*-resmethrin is 8000 mg/kg, but that of 1R,*cis*-resmethrin is 100 mg/kg (Casida *et al.*, 1983). The low mammalian toxicity of pyrethroids is confirmed by the fact that despite their extensive worldwide use, there are relatively few reports of human poisonings, and only a dozen deaths (Bradberry *et al.*, 2005). Most deaths occurred following accidental or intentional exposure to pyrethroids. For example, a 45-year-old man died three hours after eating beans and cheese prepared using a 10% cypermethrin solution instead of oil (Poulos *et al.*, 1982). The dermal toxicity of pyrethroids is even lower, because of limited absorption through the skin.

On absorption, pyrethroids are very rapidly metabolized through two major biotransformation routes: hydrolysis of the ester linkage, which is catalyzed by hepatic and plasma CarE, and oxidation of the alcohol moiety by cytochromes P450 (Miyamoto, 1976; Soderlund and Casida, 1977; Kaneko, 2010). These initial reactions are followed by further oxidations, hydrolysis, and conjugation with sulfate or glucuronide. The relative importance of the hydrolytic or oxidative biotransformation varies from compound to compound, and from isomer to isomer for each pyrethroid. For example, the *trans* isomer of permethrin is more susceptible to hydrolysis by CarE than the *cis* isomer (Soderlund and Casida, 1977; Ross *et al.*,

2006). Type II pyrethroids (see below) are less sensitive to hydrolysis. For instance, deltamethrin, a type II pyrethroid containing a cyano group (Fig. 22-9), and present solely as the *cis* isomer, is more extensive metabolized by hepatic cytochromes P450, particularly CYP1A2 and CYP1A1 (Vmax/Km = 34.9), than by liver CarE (Vmax/Km = 11.5) (Anand *et al.*, 2006a). Although it has been suggested that oxidative metabolism may lead in some cases to bioactivation of certain pyrethroids (Dayal *et al.*, 2003; Ray and Fry, 2006), the current line of evidence would suggest that hydrolytic and oxidative metabolism achieve detoxication of the parent, active compound (Soderlund *et al.*, 2002). Inhibition of cytochromes P450 by piperonyl butoxide indeed increases pyrethroid toxicity, and so does inhibition of CarE (Casida *et al.*, 1983). Piperonyl butoxide is added to most pyrethroid formulations as a synergist. Inhibition of CarE may be of significance if unauthorized pyrethroid/organophosphate mixtures are utilized (Ray and Forshaw, 2000). In fact, several organophosphates inhibit CarE activity, and may thus be expected to potentiate pyrethroid toxicity (Choi *et al.*, 2004). Biotransformation of pyrethroids in humans is similar to rats, with ester hydrolysis and oxidation as the predominant metabolic reactions; the latter are mostly carried out by CYP2C9 and CYP3A4 (Kaneko, 2010).

Signs and Symptoms of Toxicity and Mechanism of Action The acute mammalian toxicity of pyrethroids is well characterized (Soderlund, 2010). Based on toxic signs in rats, pyrethroids have been divided into two types (Table 22-12; Verschoyle and Aldridge, 1980). Type I compounds produce a syndrome consisting of marked behavioral arousal, aggressive sparring, increased startle response, and fine body tremor progressing to whole-body tremor and prostration (Type I or T syndrome). Type II compounds produce profuse salivation, coarse tremor progressing to choreoatetosis, and clonic seizures (Type II or CS syndrome) (Soderlund *et al.*, 2002; Ray and Fry, 2006; Soderlund, 2010). A key structural

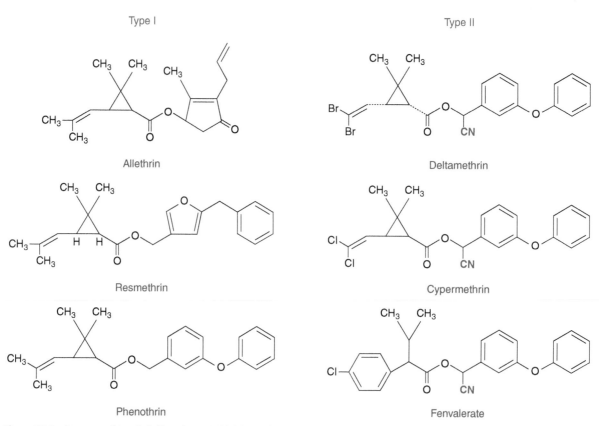

Figure 22-9. *Structures of type I (left) and type II (right) pyrethroid insecticides.* Note that all type II pyrethroids display a cyano (CN) group.

Table 22-12

Classification of Pyrethroid Insecticides Based on Toxic Signs in Rats

SYNDROME	SIGNS AND SYMPTOMS	EXAMPLES
Type I (T syndrome)	Aggressive sparring Increased sensitivity to external stimuli Whole-body tremors Prostration	Allethrin Bioallethrin Resmethrin Phenothrin
Type 2 (CS syndrome)	Pawing and burrowing Profuse salivation Coarse tremor Choreoatetosis Clonic seizures	Deltamethrin Fenvalerate Cypermethrin Cyhalothrin

difference between type I and type II pyrethroids is the presence only in the latter of a cyano group at the α carbon of the alcohol moiety of the compound (Fig. 22-9). However, certain pyrethroids (eg, cyphenothrin, flucythrinate) elude such classification, as they produce a combination of the two syndromes (Soderlund et al., 2002; Ray and Fry, 2006).

The mode of action of pyrethroids in mammals is the same as in insects, disruption of the voltage-gated sodium channels (Narahashi, 1996; Soderlund, 2010). Pyrethroids bind to the α subunit of the sodium channel and slow the activation (opening), as well as the rate of inactivation (closing), of the sodium channel, leading to a stable hyperexcitable state. Sodium channels then open at more hyperpolarized potentials, and are held open longer, allowing more sodium ions to cross and depolarize the neuronal membrane (Shafer et al., 2005). In general, type II compounds

delay the inactivation of sodium channels substantially longer (>10 milliseconds) than do type I compounds (<10 milliseconds) (Ray and Fry, 2006). Type I compounds prolong channel opening only long enough to cause repetitive firing of action potential (repetitive discharge), analogously to DDT (Vijverberg et al., 1982); type II compounds hold the channels open for such long periods that the membrane potential ultimately becomes depolarized to the point at which generation of action potential is not possible (depolarization-dependent block) (Fig. 22-10; Shafer et al., 2005). These differences in the time of opening of sodium channels are believed to be at the basis of the differences observed between the T and CS syndromes (Ray and Fry, 2006). The higher sensitivity of insects to pyrethroid toxicity, compared with mammals, is believed to result from a combination of higher sensitivity of insect sodium channels, lower body temperature (as pyrethroids show a negative temperature coefficient of action), and slower biotransformation (Ray and Fry, 2006). For example, there is a 1000-fold difference in sensitivity to allethrin between the sodium channel in cockroach and rat neurons (Narahashi et al., 2007). Type II pyrethroids, but not type I compounds, also bind to, and inhibit, GABA$_A$-gated chloride channels (Lawrence and Casida, 1983), albeit at higher concentrations than those sufficient to affect sodium channels (10^{-7} M vs 10^{-10} M). This effect is believed to contribute to the seizures that accompany severe type II pyrethroid poisoning. However, drugs that enhance GABAergic transmission (eg, diazepam) have modest effects toward deltamethrin-induced choreoatetosis or seizures (Soderlund, 2010). Type II pyrethroids, such as deltamethrin, also inhibit at low concentration (10^{-10} M) voltage-dependent chloride channels (Forshaw et al., 1993). Since agents that open these chloride channels, such as ivermectin and pentobarbital, antagonize pyrethroid-induced choreoatetosis and salivation, inhibition of maxi voltage-dependent chloride channels by pyrethroid may contribute to some of the signs associated with the type II poisoning

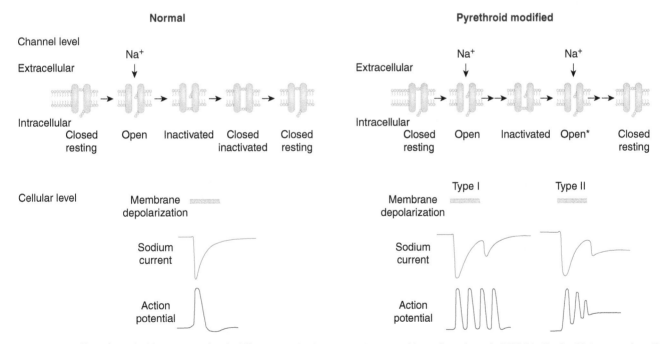

Figure 22-10. *Effect of pyrethroids on neuronal excitability.* Depolarization opens voltage-sensitive sodium channels (VSSCs) allowing Na$^+$ to enter the cell. To limit Na$^+$ entry and depolarization length, VSSCs inactivate and return to a "resting" state before reopening (top left). Pyrethroids delay inactivation (double arrows between states) of the channel and allow continued Na$^+$ flux (Open*) (top right). Under normal circumstances, depolarization leads to a rapidly inactivating current, and generates a single action potential (bottom left). Pyrethroid-modified VSSCs remain open when depolarization ends, resulting in a "tail" current. Type I compounds depolarize the cell membrane above the threshold for action potential generation, resulting in a series of action potential (repetitive firing). Type II compounds cause greater membrane depolarization, diminishing the Na$^+$ electrochemical gradient and subsequent action potential amplitude, eventually leading to depolarization-dependent block (bottom right). (From Shafer et al., 2005, with permission.)

syndrome (Forshaw *et al.*, 2000; Soderlund, 2010). Other reported targets for pyrethroids include calcium ATPase and voltage-gated calcium channels, which are, however, affected at higher concentrations (10^{-5} and 10^{-6} M, respectively). The latter interaction may be of interest, as pyrethroids have been shown to increase calcium-dependent neurotransmitter release (Soderlund, 2010). Also of note is the observation that several pyrethroids could stimulate protein kinase C–dependent protein phosphorylation at very low concentrations (10^{-13} M) (Enan and Matsumura, 1993), but whether this interaction is involved in the modulation of sodium and/or chloride channels remains to be determined.

Young animals are more sensitive to the acute toxicity of certain pyrethroids, such as deltamethrin and cypermethrin (Sheets, 2000), most likely because of a lesser capacity for metabolic detoxification (Anand *et al.*, 2006b); however, only minor age-related differences were found for other compounds (Sheets, 2000). Some studies have suggested that certain pyrethroids may cause developmental neurotoxicity, but current evidence has been judged inadequate (Shafer *et al.*, 2005). Furthermore, levels of background pyrethroid exposure (presumably through residues in the diet) in children have been found to be orders of magnitude lower than the corresponding acceptable daily intake (Heudorf *et al.*, 2004). Also, the use of deltamethrin-impregnated bed nets does not appear to pose any health risk in children and neonates (Barlow *et al.*, 2001), while substantially reducing infant mortality from malaria (Alonso *et al.*, 1991).

On occupational exposure, the primary adverse effect resulting from dermal contact with pyrethroids is paresthesia (Flannigan *et al.*, 1985; He *et al.*, 1989). Symptoms include continuous tingling or prickling or, when more severe, burning. The condition reverses in about 24 hours, and topical application of vitamin E has been shown to be an effective treatment. Paresthesia is presumably due to abnormal pyrethroid-induced repetitive activity in skin nerve terminals (Ray and Fry, 2006). Given their widespread use, reports on incidents due to pyrethroid exposure have been increasing over the past decade, although such exposures resulted in minor or no symptoms in most cases (Power and Sudakin, 2007). In a study in the US Pacific Northwest, 407 incidents involving pyrethroids were reported; effects were mainly respiratory (as exposure was predominantly by inhalation), and of low severity (Walters *et al.*, 2009).

Chronic studies with pyrethroids indicate that at high dose levels they cause slight liver enlargement often accompanied by some histopathological changes. There is little or no evidence of teratogenicity and mutagenicity (Miyamoto, 1976; Ray, 1991). An increased rate of lymphoma incidence in rodents has been reported for deltamethrin, but the effect was not dose-dependent (Cabral *et al.*, 1990). Liver tumors were found in rats on chronic exposure to permethrin, but as the mode of action appears to be due to enzyme induction and increased cell proliferation, it was judged not to be relevant to humans (Osimitz and Lake, 2009). There is no compelling evidence that pyrethroids may act as endocrine disruptors (Kim *et al.*, 2004). Pyrethroids are particularly toxic to fish, but not to birds (Miyamoto, 1976).

Organochlorine Compounds

The organochlorine insecticides include the chlorinated ethane derivatives, such as DDT and its analogs; the cyclodienes, such as chlordane, aldrin, dieldrin, heptachlor, endrin, and toxaphene; the hexachlorocyclohexanes, such as lindane; and the caged structures mirex and chlordecone (Figs. 22-11 and 22-12). From the 1940s to the 1970s–1980s, the organochlorine insecticides enjoyed wide use in agriculture, structure insect control, and malaria

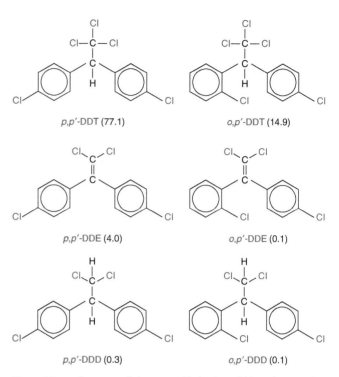

Figure 22-11. *Structures of the organochlorine insecticide p,p'-DDT and its isomers.* The percentage of each isomer present in technical grade DDT is indicated in parenthesis. DDE and DDD also result from biotransformation of DDT.

control programs. Their acute toxicity is moderate (less than that of organophosphates), but chronic exposure may be associated with adverse health effects particularly in the liver and the reproductive system. Primarily because of ecological considerations, these compounds have been banned in most countries in the past 30 years. Yet, because of their environmental persistence and high lipophilicity, exposure to these compounds continues, most notably through the diet. Furthermore, some, such as DDT, are being reintroduced in part of the world for malaria control; hence, a discussion of their toxicity has more than historical value.

DDT and Its Analogs 1,1,1-Trichloro-2,2-bis(4-chlorophenyl) ethane (DDT) was first synthesized by O. Zeidler in 1874, but its insecticidal activity was discovered only in 1939 by Paul Mueller in Switzerland. Early experiments showed that DDT was effective against a wide variety of agricultural pests, as well as against insects that transmit some of the world's most serious diseases, such as typhus, malaria, and yellow fever. In the United States, annual use of DDT rose until 1959 to about 36,000 tons, after which it declined gradually until its ban in 1972 (Rogan and Chen, 2005). However, as said, because of its high persistence, global redistribution, and its current use in many parts of the world, a discussion of the toxicology of DDT is still of relevance (Longnecker, 2005). While DDT is the universally accepted common name of the insecticide, technical trade DDT is a mixture of several isomers (Fig. 22-11), with *p,p'*-DDT being responsible for the insecticidal activity.

DDT has a moderate acute toxicity when given by the oral route, with an LD_{50} of about 250 mg/kg; *p,p'*-DDT is at least 10-fold more toxic than *o,p'*-DDT (Smith, 2010). Dermal absorption of DDT is very limited, resulting in dermal LD_{50} values of >1000 mg/kg. In humans, oral doses of 10 to 20 mg/kg produce illness, but doses as high as 285 mg/kg have been ingested accidentally without fatal results. Toxicity from dermal exposure in humans is also low, as evidenced by the lack of significant adverse health effects when

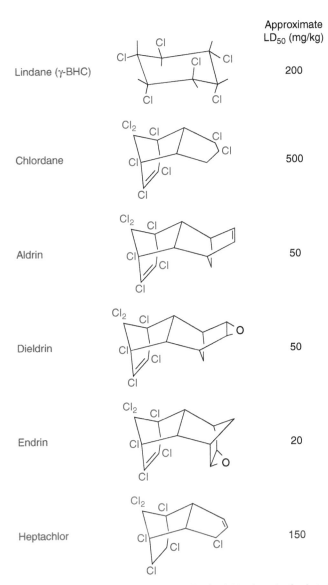

	Approximate LD$_{50}$ (mg/kg)
Lindane (γ-BHC)	200
Chlordane	500
Aldrin	50
Dieldrin	50
Endrin	20
Heptachlor	150

Figure 22-12. *Structure and acute toxicity (oral LD$_{50}$ in rat) of selected organochlorine insecticides of different chemical classes (see text for details).*

thousands of people were liberally dusted with this compound. On absorption, DDT distributes in all tissues, and the highest concentrations are found in adipose tissue. DDT is also extensively but slowly metabolized, with DDE, DDD, and DDA (in each case both the *p,p'* and the *o,p'* isomers) being the primary metabolites in humans (Smith, 2010). DDE is also stored in adipose tissue. Excretion is through the bile, urine, and the milk.

Acute exposure to high doses of DDT causes motor unrest, increased frequency of spontaneous movements, abnormal susceptibility to fear, and hypersusceptibility to external stimuli (light, touch, sound). This is followed by the development of fine tremors, progressing to coarse tremors, and eventually tonic–clonic convulsions. Symptoms usually appear several hours after exposure, and death, usually due to respiratory failure, may follow after 24 to 72 hours (Ecobichon and Joy, 1982). Signs and symptoms of poisoning are similar in most animal species, with dogs displaying prominent convulsions. There is no evidence that young animals may be more sensitive than adults to the acute toxicity of DDT, and they may actually be less sensitive (Smith, 2010). In humans, the earliest symptom of poisoning by DDT is hyperesthesia of the mouth and lower part of the face, followed by paresthesia of the same area and of the tongue.

Dizziness, tremor of the extremities, confusion, and vomiting follow, while convulsions occur only in severe poisoning.

Signs and symptoms of acute poisoning clearly point at the nervous system as the primary target for DDT toxicity (Woolley, 1982). Both in insects and in mammals, DDT interferes with the sodium channels in the axonal membrane by a mechanism similar to that of type I pyrethroids (Vijverberg *et al.*, 1982). DDT has little or no effect on the resting potential or the rising phase and peak amplitude of the action potential. However, it greatly prolongs the depolarizing (negative) afterpotential of the action potential, and this produces a period of increased neuronal excitability immediately after the spike phase. This, in turn, enhances the probability of repetitive firing, and the insurgence of a "train" of action potentials (Fig. 22-13). Voltage clamp studies have shown that the principal effect of DDT is to slow down the closing of sodium channels once they have opened, while having little or no effect on closed gates. In addition to this effect on sodium channels, DDT also affects ATPases. Although DDT inhibits Na$^+$,K$^+$-ATPase, this action would not contribute to its neurotoxic effect (Matsumura and Patil, 1969). Rather, inhibition of a Ca^{2+}-ATPase (an ecto-ATPase, located on the outside of the cell membrane) may be involved in the effects of DDT. As the function of this Ca^{2+}-ATPase is believed to be that of maintaining high external calcium concentrations, its inhibition would lower external calcium and contribute to membrane instability and repetitive firing (Matsumura and Ghiasuddin, 1979). Several neurochemical studies have also shown that DDT exposure alters the levels of some neurotransmitters such as acetylcholine, norepinephrine, and serotonin, as well as of cyclic GMP, but these effects appear to be the results, rather than the cause, of DDT-induced neurotoxicity (Woolley, 1982). Treatment for DDT poisoning focuses on the nervous system. In animals, phenytoin and calcium gluconate have been found to reduce DDT-induced tremors and mortality, respectively. In humans, in addition to decontamination and supportive treatment, diazepam or phenobarbital may be beneficial to control convulsions, if present.

While acute exposure to DDT is a rare event, chronic exposure has been, and still is, a primary concern. In this regard, an important target for DDT is the liver. DDT and DDE increase liver weight and cause hepatic cell hypertrophy and necrosis, and are potent inducers of cytochromes P450, particularly CYP2B and CYP3A (Smith, 1991, 2010). DDT has been shown to be hepatocarcinogenic in mice and rats, but results in other species are inconclusive. DDT also increased incidence of lung tumors and adenomas in mice. Both DDE and DDD were also shown to be carcinogenic, causing primarily an increase in liver tumors. DDT is not genotoxic in in vitro and in vivo tests. Based on animal data, DDT is classified as a possible human carcinogen by IARC; however, evidence of human carcinogenicity is still inconclusive. Along with many negative studies, there is some, albeit contradictory, evidence of increased risks for pancreatic cancer, liver cancer, and multiple myeloma, associated with exposure to DDT (Turosov *et al.*, 2002; Beard, 2006). Given the endocrine-disrupting actions of DDT and DDE (see below), particular attention has been devoted to possible associations between exposure to these compounds and hormonally sensitive cancers, such as those of the breast, the endometrium, and the prostate, but the results have been inconclusive (Safe, 2005; Beard, 2006).

Methoxychlor (2,2-bis(*p*-methoxyphenyl)-1,1,1-trichloroethane) is the *p,p'*-dimethoxy analog of *p,p'*-DDT. Because of its low acute toxicity (LD$_{50}$ in rat = 5000 mg/kg) and short biological half-life, its use greatly expanded following the ban of DDT. Furthermore, methoxychlor is rapidly metabolized, and does not accumulate in tissues. Although convulsions have been reported in dogs after high doses, in the rat depression of the central nervous

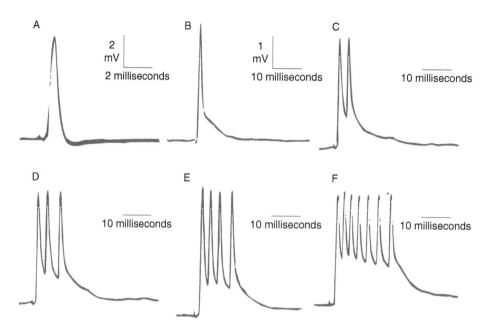

Figure 22-13. *Action potential of a single nerve fiber from the sciatic nerve of the toad Xenopus laevis, before (**A**), and 65, 85, 90, 105, and 135 minutes (**B-F**) after in vitro exposure to 10^{-4} M DDT.* Note the difference in timescale between A and B. The first observable effect is the development of a negative afterpotential (B). With time of exposure, repetitive spike discharge is initiated and increased in proportion to the amplitude of the negative afterpotential (C-F). (With permission from Van den Bercken, 1972.)

system, mild tremors, diarrhea, and anorexia were observed (Smith, 2010). On chronic exposure, methoxychlor has been found to be a modest inducer of liver microsomal enzymes, and to cause chronic nephritis, and hypertrophy of kidneys, mammary glands, and uterus. Testicular atrophy and decreased spermatogenesis were also observed. Evidences of mutagenicity and carcinogenicity are inconclusive. Methoxychlor is metabolized by CYP2C19 and CYP1A2 to demethylated compounds, which have estrogenic activity (Smith, 2010); these are likely responsible for the effects caused by methoxychlor on the reproductive system in both male and female animals.

Hexachlorocyclohexanes and Cyclodienes These two families of organochlorine insecticides comprise a large number of compounds that share a similar mechanism of neurotoxic action (Brooks, 2010). Lindane is the γ isomer of benzene hexachloride (BHC; 1,2,3,4,5,6-hexachlorocyclohexane) (Fig. 22-12). BHC is composed of eight stereoisomers, and the γ isomer is the one with insecticidal activity (Smith, 1991). Cyclodiene compounds include chlordane, dieldrin, aldrin (which is rapidly metabolized to dieldrin), heptachlor, and endrin (Fig. 22-12). Toxaphene, a complex mixture of chlorinated bornanes and camphenes, is also classified as an organochlorine insecticide. All of these compounds were introduced in the late 1940s to early 1950s, and have experienced wide use before being banned in most countries due to their persistence and environmental and human health effects. Lindane's use as an insecticide in agriculture has been banned, although it remains available as a scabicide and pediculicide in lotions and shampoos. The primary use of chlordane has been for termite control, while other compounds were primarily used in agriculture. Endrin was registered for use as a rodenticide to control voles in orchards, a testament to its rather high acute toxicity, compared with most other organochlorines (Fig. 22-12).

Lindane and cyclodienes have moderate to high acute oral toxicity (Fig. 22-12). However, in contrast to DDT, these compounds are readily absorbed through the skin. The primary target for their toxicity is the central nervous system. Unlike DDT, tremor is essentially absent, but convulsions are a prominent aspect of poisoning. These are due to the ability of these compounds to interfere with

γ-aminobutyric acid (GABA)–mediated neurotransmission. GABA is an important neurotransmitter in the mammalian and insect CNS and in the insect neuromuscular junction. GABA receptors are members of the superfamily of ligand-gated ion channels that contain a chloride ionophore; by binding to these receptors, endogenous GABA causes the opening of chloride channels resulting in hyperpolarization of the membrane. Lindane and cyclodienes bind to a specific site (the picrotoxin site) on the chloride channel, thereby blocking its opening and thus antagonizing the "inhibitory" action of GABA (Cole and Casida, 1986; Eldelfrawi and Eldefrawi, 1987; Narahashi, 1996). Treatment of acute poisoning is symptomatic; phenobarbital and diazepam can be used as anticonvulsants. Additional reported neurochemical effects of organochlorine insecticides include inhibition of Na^+,K^+-, Ca^{2+}-, and Mg^{2+}-ATPases, and changes in neurotransmitter levels.

As with DDT, these compounds are slowly metabolized, and have a tendency to bioaccumulate in adipose tissue; they are also excreted in milk. Cyclodienes are inducers of microsomal biotransformation enzymes and cause liver enlargement on chronic exposure (Smith, 1991). They are not genotoxic, but have been shown to act as tumor promoters and cause liver tumors in mice. As with DDT, they are extremely persistent in the environment, and some have endocrine-disrupting properties. Cyclodienes, and in particular dieldrin, have also been suggested as potential pesticide candidates that may contribute to the etiology of Parkinson disease, given their ability to disrupt dopaminergic neurotransmission (Hatcher *et al.*, 2008).

Mirex and Chlordecone These two organochlorine insecticides have a cage-like structure and were introduced in the late 1950s for use against fire ants and leaf-eating insects, respectively. Chlordecone (Kepone) has been the most studied because of one episode that involved 148 workers in a chlordecone-producing factory in Hopewell, Virginia, between 1973 and 1975 (Taylor *et al.*, 1978). The primary manifestation of chlordecone toxicity is the presence of tremors, which are observed in animals as well as in humans (Guzelian, 1982). The exact mechanism of chlordecone neurotoxicity has not been elucidated, but it is believed to involve inhibition of ATPases (both Na^+,K^+- and Mg^{2+}-ATPases), and

Table 22-13

Concentration of DDT in a Lake Michigan Food Chain

	DDT (ppm)
Water	0.000002
Bottom mud	0.014
Fairy shrimp	0.410
Coho salmon, lake trout	3–6
Herring gull	99

Data from Harrison et al. (1970).

ensuing inhibition of the uptake of catecholamines (Desaiah, 1982). In contrast to cyclodienes, chlordecone does not cause seizures.

Chlordecone induces hepatic drug-metabolizing enzymes, and causes hepatosplenomegaly in rats and humans. It is not mutagenic, but can induce liver tumors in rodents (Smith, 1991). Chlordecone also causes reproductive toxicity in animals, likely by mimicking the effects of excessive estrogens. Low or absent sperm count was found in chlordecone-exposed workers (Taylor *et al.*, 1978; Guzelian, 1982). Cholestyramine, an anion-exchange resin, has been shown effective in both animals and humans as a means to increase fecal excretion of chlordecone, probably by sequestering unmetabolized compound that is secreted into the intestinal lumen via biliary excretion; this interrupts enterohepatic circulation and shortens the biological half-life (Guzelian, 1982).

Environmental Ubiquity and Persistence The properties (low volatility, chemical stability, lipid solubility, slow rate of biotransformation, and degradation) that made organochlorine compounds such effective insecticides also brought about their demise because of their persistence in the environment, bioconcentration and biomagnification in food chains, and the acquisition of biologically active body burdens at higher trophic levels (Ecobichon, 2001a). Sweden banned DDT in 1970, the United States in 1972, and the United Kingdom in 1986. Most other organochlorine insecticides were also banned in the United States during this period, for example, aldrin and dieldrin in 1975, toxaphene in 1982, and chlordane in 1988. These bans occurred largely on the basis of ecological considerations. Their extensive use and their environmental persistence made them widespread pollutants. Studies

carried out in the Great Lakes region in the United States exemplify the nature and the extent of the problem. Table 22-13 shows the tendency of DDT to bioaccumulate in the food chain. Adverse effects on bird reproduction (eg, eggshell thinning) were among the first ecological effects to be identified and denounced (Carson, 1962; Peakall, 1970), and played an important role in the decision to ban DDT (USEPA, 1975). Monitoring of organochlorine insecticides in fish in the Great Lakes shows extreme high levels in 1970 (eg, 20,000 ng/g of total DDT, which also includes DDE and DDD), and a progressive decline after the use of these compounds was restricted or banned (Hickey *et al.*, 2006).

Because of their stability and high lipophilicity, organochlorines are present in adipose tissues of most individuals. For example, DDE, the breakdown product of DDT in the environment and the result of its biotransformation, is an extremely stable compound ($t_{1/2}$ = 7–11 years), which accumulates in fat, and is usually found in human tissue at the highest concentration. Studies in populations from different countries in the 1960s showed that all adipose tissue samples contained DDT at concentrations ranging from 5 to 20 mg/kg (ppm), with DDE accounting for about 60% of total DDT (WHO, 1979). Although concentrations of DDT in humans show a decreasing trend, those of DDE, which is ingested with food, particularly meat and fish, remain more constant or decrease only slightly. Organochlorine insecticides are also excreted in the milk. Although levels have decreased in most countries in the last decades (Smith, 2010), elevated levels remain in several developing countries (Table 22-14; Chao *et al.*, 2006). Data presented in Table 22-14 also indicate a differential DDE/DDT ratio among milk samples from different populations; a higher ratio is an indication of high environmental persistence and continuous bioaccumulation, while a low DDE/DDT ratio indicates recent exposure to DDT, as the biological half-life of DDT is shorter than that of DDE (Jaga and Dharmani, 2003).

Endocrine Disruption An endocrine, or hormone, disruptor can be defined as an exogenous agent that interferes with the synthesis, secretion, transport, binding, action, or elimination of natural hormones in the body that are responsible for the maintenance of homeostasis, reproduction, development, and behavior (Crisp *et al.*, 1998; Stoker and Kavlock, 2010). Several pesticides may fall into this category, and, among these, a large number are organochlorine insecticides. The *o,p'*-isomer of DDT, which comprises approximately 15% of the technical grade product (Fig. 22-11),

Table 22-14

Levels of *p,p'*-DDT and *p,p'*-DDE (ng/g Lipid) in Human Milk from Selected Countries

COUNTRY	SAMPLING YEAR	N	*p,p'*-DDT	*p,p'*-DDE	DDE/DDT	REFERENCE
Sweden	1997	40	14	129	9.2	Noren and Meironyte (2000)
Japan	1998	49	18	270	15.0	Konishi *et al.* (2001)
New Zealand	1998	53	26	626	24.1	Bate *et al.* (2002)
United Kingdom	2001–2003	54	6.2	150	24.2	Kalantzi *et al.* (2004)
Taiwan	2000–2001	30	22	301	13.7	Chao *et al.* (2006)
Mexico	1997–1998	60	651	3997	6.1	Waliszewski *et al.* (1999)
Thailand	1998	25	2600	8210	3.2	Stuetz *et al.* (2001)
China (Guangzhou)	2000	54	700	2850	4.1	Wong *et al.* (2002)
Vietnam	2000–2001	96	223	1956	8.8	Minh *et al.* (2004)
Turkey	2003	37	65	1522	28.0	Erdogrul *et al.* (2004)

Table 22-15		
Potency of DDT and Its Metabolites, and of Chlordecone, at Androgen and Estrogen Receptors		
	IC_{50} (μM)	
COMPOUND	ANDROGEN RECEPTOR	ESTROGEN RECEPTOR
p,p'-DDT	75	>1000
p,p'-DDE	5	>1000
o,p'-DDT	95	5
p,p'-DDD	90	>1000
Chlordecone	125	3
17β-Estradiol	0.5	0.002

Data from Kelce et al. (1995).

has estrogenic properties, in that it can act as an agonist at estrogen receptors (ER) α and β (Table 22-15). A metabolite of DDT, p,p'-DDE, on the other hand, inhibits androgen binding to androgen receptor (Table 22-15; Kelce *et al.*, 1995). Metabolites of the DDT analog, methoxychlor, are active as ERα agonists and ERβ antagonists and are antiandrogenic. Chlordecone also has estrogenic properties (Table 22-15; Guzelian, 1982). Other organochlorine compounds with weak estrogenic activity are dieldrin, endosulfan, toxaphene, lindane, and the β isomer of hexachlorocyclohexane (β-BHC). In all cases, the potency of the insecticides or their metabolites is several orders of magnitude less than those of the hormones. Experimental studies have shown that administration of these compounds to animals can cause hormonally mediated adverse health effects. For example, p,p'-DDE had clear antiandrogenic effect when given to fetal, pubertal, and adult male rats (Kelce *et al.*, 1995). Several studies have shown that chlordecone and methoxychlor affect the male reproductive system (Guzelian, 1982; Kavlock, 2001). Of possible relevance is the recent finding that exposure to methoxychlor during gestation (E8-E15) induced transgenerational defects in spermatogenic capacity and sperm viability, that is, these abnormalities were also observed in F2 generation animals (Anway *et al.*, 2005). All these findings, though provocative, were obtained at dosage levels that far exceed anticipated environmental exposure. It has been suggested that estrogen equivalents from phytoestrogens present in foods and beverages are several orders of magnitude higher than estrogen equivalents resulting from estrogenic organochlorine insecticide contaminants in food (Safe, 2000). The association between exposure to organochlorine compounds and possible related diseases in humans appeared to be weak (Golden *et al.*, 1998; Safe, 2005). However, the Pine River Statement recently reviewed 494 studies published between 2003 and 2008 and found that "...DDT and its breakdown product DDE may be associated with adverse health outcomes such as breast cancer, diabetes, decreased semen quality, spontaneous abortion, and impaired development in childhood..." (Eskenazi *et al.*, 2009). Early life exposure to p,p'-DDT was shown to be associated with an increased risk of breast cancer in young women (Cohn *et al.*, 2007), and of decreased triiodothyronine (T3) levels in preschool children (Alvarez-Pedrerol *et al.*, 2008). Furthermore, of 21 epidemiological studies published in 2009, nine showed no significant correlations between effects and DDT and/or DDE exposure, while 12 showed significant associations between DDT and DDE with type 2 diabetes, hormonal levels, birth mass, pancreatic duct carcinoma, and sperm parameters (Bouwman *et al.*, 2011).

DDT and Public Health: Risk–Benefit Considerations The Stockholm Convention on Persistent Organic Pollutants, ratified in 2004 by 50 states, outlawed the use of 12 industrial chemicals (the "Dirty Dozen"), including DDT. Yet, an exemption clause allows malaria-endemic nations to continue utilizing DDT for indoor residual wall spraying. The United Nations Environment Program estimates that about 25 countries would use DDT under this exemption from its ban. This situation is keeping the debate on the risks and benefits of DDT usage very much alive (Rogan and Chen, 2005; van Den Berg, 2009; Bouwman *et al.*, 2011). On one hand, the environmental and human health effects of DDT are evident; on the other hand, one has to come to grips with the burden of mortality from malaria worldwide. Indeed, there are an estimated 250 million clinical cases of malaria, causing almost one million deaths each year, mostly in children less than five years of age, and mostly in sub-Saharan Africa (van den Berg, 2009; WHO, 2010).

Thus, use of DDT might reduce mortality from malaria and overall infant mortality if spraying were carried out according to planned schedule, which is not always the case, and if malaria-transmitting mosquitoes do not become resistant to DDT, a problem that in the past has forced switching to other insecticides. The successful results obtained in South Africa in recent years (see the section "Economics and Public Health") would support a continuous use of DDT. However, although indoor residual spraying might not cause the ecological effects that caused the ban of DDT, it would expose humans to amounts of DDT that may cause adverse health effects. In this regard, reproductive outcomes are of most concern. In particular, preterm births and early weaning (decreased duration of lactation), which can lead to increased infant mortality, have been associated with DDT exposure (Chen and Rogan, 2003; Rogan and Chen, 2005), although findings are controversial (Roberts *et al.*, 2004). Nevertheless, reported DDT levels in breast milk often exceed the tolerable daily intake and would cause great concern in any developed country (Okankwo *et al.*, 2008). High serum levels of DDT have also been found in applicators when proper personal protective equipment is not utilized (Bouwman *et al.*, 2011). DDT remains a public health intervention that is cheap, long-lasting, and effective. Its judicious use should be combined with that of insecticide-treated bed nets, to prevent mosquito biting, and with a better availability of therapeutic interventions in affected populations.

Other Old and New Insecticides

Rotenoids The roots of the East Asian Derris plants, particularly *D. elliptica*, and those of *Lonchocarpus utilis* and *L. urucu* in South America contain at least six rotenoid esters, among which the most abundant is rotenone. Rotenone is used as an agricultural insecticide/acaricide, particularly in organic farming (Isman, 2006). It is rather persistent in food crops after treatment, as indicated by half-life of four days in olives (Cabras *et al.*, 2002). Rotenone is very toxic to fish; root extracts were used to paralyze fish for capture and consumption, and rotenone is still used in fishery management. Toxicity of rotenone in target and nontarget species is due to its ability to inhibit, at nanomolar concentrations, the mitochondrial respiratory chain, by blocking electron transport at NADH-ubiquinone reductase, the energy-conserving enzyme complex commonly known as complex I. Insect and fish mitochondria are particularly sensitive to complex I inhibition (Degli Esposti, 1998). Purified rotenone has a high acute toxicity in rodents and dogs, and is less toxic to rabbits and birds (Ujvary, 2010). Poisoning symptoms include initial increased respiratory and cardiac rates, clonic and tonic spasms, and muscular depression, followed by respiratory depression. Acute intoxication in humans is rare; a case report describes a fatal case in a 3.5-year-old girl who ingested an estimated 40 mg/kg of rotenone. Of note is that the label on the insecticide, which was manufactured in France and recommended for external use on animals, had stated "Natural Product–Non Toxic" (De Wilde *et al.*, 1986). An additional case report describes a fatal case in a middle aged woman after deliberate ingestion of rotenone, at a dosage estimated at 25 mg/kg (Wood *et al.*, 2005).

In recent years, rotenone has received much attention because of its potential role in the etiology of Parkinson disease. An earlier study by Heikkila *et al.* (1985) showed that stereotaxic administration to rats of rotenone damaged the dopaminergic nigrostriatal pathway, similarly to what observed with 1-methyl-4-phenylpyridinium (MPP$^+$, the active metabolite of 1-methyl-4-phenyl-1,2,3,6-tetrahydropyridine [MPTP]), a known parkinsonism-causing chemical, which is also a complex I inhibitor (Degli Esposti, 1998). More recent studies have shown that administration of rotenone to rats (2–3 mg/kg per day for one to five weeks) caused selective nigrostriatal degeneration, although inhibition of complex I was observed uniformly in brain (Betarbet *et al.*, 2000; Sherer *et al.*, 2003). The finding that rotenone also produced protein inclusions, similar to Lewy bodies, which stained positively for ubiquitin and α-synuclein, suggests that the rotenone model for Parkinson disease would be even better than the MPTP model (Betarbet *et al.*, 2002). However, the severe systemic toxicity of rotenone, the high variability across and within strains, and reports on nonspecific CNS effects (Lapointe *et al.*, 2004) have also pointed out the limitations of the rotenone model (Li *et al.*, 2005). There is no evidence of Parkinson disease–like clinical signs or neurodegenerative pathology in chronic dietary studies (Hollingworth, 2001), suggesting that although rotenone may represent a useful experimental model, its primary role in the etiology of Parkinson disease in the general population is still unproven (Hollingworth, 2001; Li *et al.*, 2005). Most recently, however, an association between use of rotenone and increased risk of Parkinson disease has been reported (Tanner *et al.*, 2011).

Nicotine The tobacco plant (*Nicotiana tabacum, N. rustica*) was introduced in Europe in 1559 from the Americas where it had long been cultivated primarily for smoking. Tobacco extracts have been used to repel and kill insects since 1690, and tobacco smoke was also used for fumigation (Ujvary, 2010). Nicotine is an alkaloid extracted from the leaves of tobacco plants, and is used as a free base or as the sulfate salt. The most notorious commercial preparation, Black Leaf 40, has been discontinued. Very little nicotine is used currently in the United States, but nicotine is still used as a minor insecticide in some Asian countries. It is a systemic insecticide effective toward a wide range of insects, including aphids, thrips, and whiteflies (Ujvary, 1999). As the primary component of tobacco used for smoking or chewing, nicotine's pharmacology and toxicology have been thoroughly investigated (Benowitz, 1996; Taylor, 1996). Nicotine exerts its pharmacological and toxic effects in mammals and insects by activating nicotinic acetylcholine receptors (nAChRs). In vertebrates, nAChRs are expressed at neuromuscular junctions, in the PNS and in the CNS; in insects, nAChRs are confined to the nervous system (Eldelfrawi and Eldefrawi, 1997). Interaction of nicotine with nAChRs produces initial stimulation followed by protracted depolarization, which results in receptor paralysis. The overall effect is the summation of stimulatory and inhibitory effects of nicotine at all sites expressing nAChRs. At high doses, parasympathetic stimulation and ganglionic and neuromuscular blockade predominate (Matyunas and Rodgers, 2001). Nicotine has a high acute toxicity in vertebrates, with LD_{50}s usually below 50 mg/kg (Ujvary, 2010). Signs and symptoms of

poisoning include nausea, vomiting, muscle weakness, respiratory effects, headache, lethargy, and tachycardia. Most cases of poisoning with nicotine occur after exposure to tobacco products, or gum or patches. Workers who cultivate, harvest, or handle tobacco may experience green tobacco sickness, caused by dermal absorption of nicotine.

Neonicotinoids Starting in the late 1970s, by various chemical modifications of nicotine and other nAChRs agonists, new classes of insecticides have been developed that contain a nitromethylene, nitroimine, or cyanoimine group, and are referred to as neonicotinoids. One of the first compounds synthesized was nithiazine, a nitromethylenyl heterocyclic compound highly toxic toward insects and with low mammalian toxicity. Nithiazine was not developed commercially because of its photo-instability. Further structure–activity studies led to the development of imidacloprid, nitenpyram, acetamiprid, and other neonicotinoid compounds (Fig. 22-14; Matsuda *et al.*, 2001). The insecticidal activity of neonicotinoids is attributed to activation of postsynaptic nAChRs, which in insects are located exclusively in the central nervous system. They are used primarily for crop protection as systemic insecticides, but are also effective against fleas in cats and dogs (Schenker *et al.*, 2003). The mammalian toxicity of neonicotinoids is similar to that of nicotine, and correlates with agonist action and binding affinity at the nAChRs. Acute oral toxicity (LD_{50}) in rats ranges from 180 to >2000 mg/kg (Fig. 22-14), while dermal toxicity is much lower (2000–5000 mg/kg), likely because of their low lipophilicity (Tomizawa and Casida, 2005). Signs and symptoms of toxicity in mammals are attributable to stimulation of nAChRs particularly in the peripheral nervous system, given their poor penetration of the blood–brain barrier (Sheets, 2010). Some neonicotinoids (imidocloprid, thiacloprid) are particularly toxic to birds, others (thiacloprid) to fish. Most neonicotinoids are not mutagenic, carcinogenic, or teratogenic. Neonicotinoids undergo limited biotransformation in mammals, involving mostly cytochrome P450–mediated oxidative reactions (Sheets, 2010; Tomizawa and Casida, 2005).

Neonicotinoids account for 10% to 15% of the total insecticide market, and their use is increasing faster than other insecticides (Matsuda *et al.*, 2001; Tomizawa and Casida, 2005). The main reason for their success lies in their selectivity profile, which is largely attributable to their specificity toward insect versus mammalian nAChRs. The nAChR consists of diverse subtypes assembled in combination from 10 α and 4 β, γ, δ, and ε subunits. The most abundant subtypes in the vertebrate nervous system are α4β2 and α7, which are insensitive and sensitive, respectively, to α-bungarotoxin. In insects, neonicotinoids have been shown to bind to at least three pharmacologically distinct nAChRs (Matsuda *et al.*, 2001; Sheets, 2010). Table 22-16 shows the in vitro effects of some neonicotinoids toward insect nAChRs and mammalian α4β2 nAChRs, and compares them with nicotine. Structural features of neonicotinoids that contribute to their selective actions at insect nAChRs have been described (Nakayama and Sukekawa, 1998; Matsuda *et al.*, 2001; Tomizawa and Casida, 2005). Given their wider availability, there is an increasing number of acute neonicotinoid poisonings, primarily due to suicidal attempts; mortality is however low (~3%), because of their receptor selectivity and low lipophilicity (Phua *et al.*, 2009).

Formamidines Formamidines, such as chlordimeform ((*N'*-(4-chloro-*o*-tolyl)-*N*,*N*-dimethylformamidine) or amitraz (*N'*-2,4-(dimethyl-phenyl)-*N*-*N*((2,4-dimethylphenyl)imino)methyl-*N*-methanimidamide), are used in agriculture and in veterinary medicine as insecticides/acaricides (Hollingworth, 1976). Their structures are closely related to the neurotransmitter norepinephrine (Fig. 22-15). In invertebrates, these compounds exert their

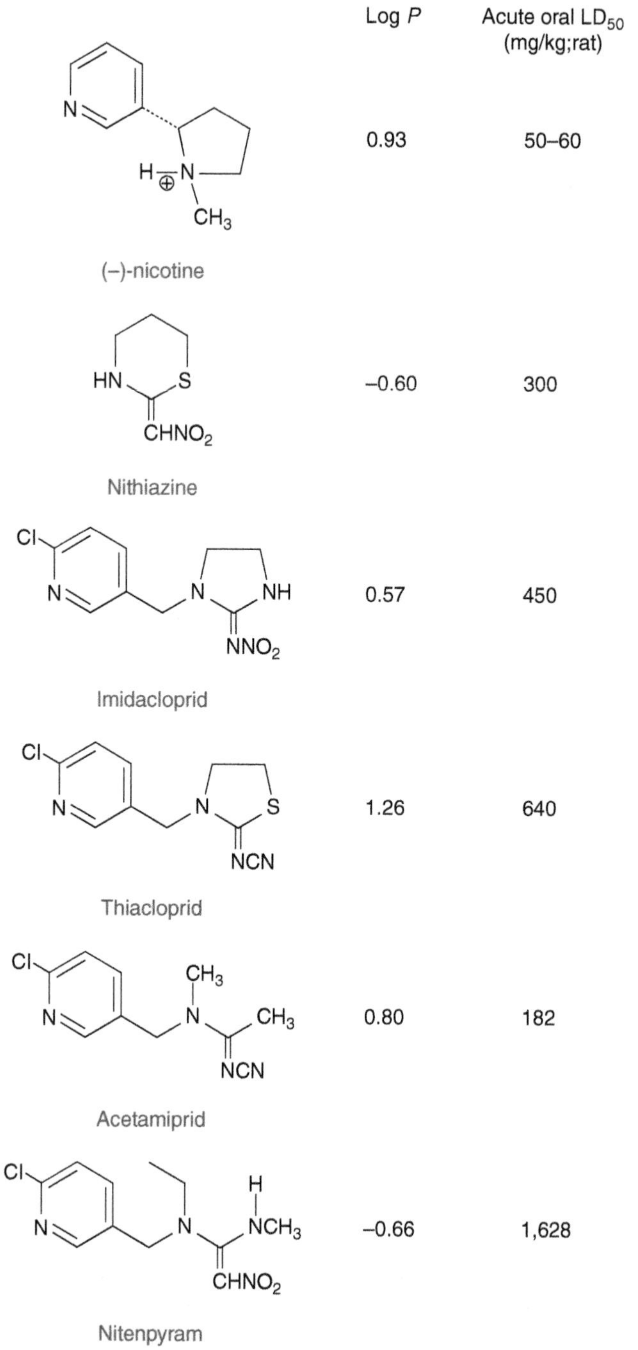

	Log P	Acute oral LD$_{50}$ (mg/kg;rat)

(−)-nicotine — 0.93 — 50–60

Nithiazine — −0.60 — 300

Imidacloprid — 0.57 — 450

Thiacloprid — 1.26 — 640

Acetamiprid — 0.80 — 182

Nitenpyram — −0.66 — 1,628

Figure 22-14. Structures of nicotine and of neonicotinoid insecticides with indication of their acute oral toxicity in rat and their octanol/water partition (P). (Data are derived from Tomizawa and Casida, 2005.)

toxicity by activating an octopamine-dependent adenylate cyclase (Nathanson, 1985). In mammals, symptoms of formamidine poisoning are sympathomimetic in nature (Beeman and Matsumura, 1973). The similarity between insect octopamine receptors and mammalian α_2-adrenergic receptors had suggested the latter as a possible target for formamidines. In vivo and in vitro studies have indeed shown that formamidines act as rather selective agonists at α_2-adrenergic receptors (Hsu and Lu, 1984; Hsu and Kakuk, 1984; Costa *et al.*, 1988; Altobelli *et al.*, 2001). Chlordimeform's metabolism plays a most relevant role in its toxicity. The *N*-demethylated metabolite (desmethylchlordimeform) is more acutely toxic than chlordimeform, and displays a >400-fold higher potency toward α_2-adrenoceptors (Ghali and Hollingsworth, 1985; Costa and Murphy,

Table 22-16

Specificity of Neonicotinoids for Insect and Vertebrate nAChRs

		IC$_{50}$ (nM)	
INSECTICIDE	INSECT	VERTEBRATE $\alpha4\beta2$	SELECTIVITY RATIO
Imidacloprid	4.6	2600	565
Acetamiprid	8.3	700	84
Thiacloprid	2.7	860	319
Nitenpyram	14.0	49,000	3500
(−)Nicotine	4000	7	0.002

SOURCE: Data from Tomizawa and Casida (2005).

1987). Two other metabolites of chlordimeform, 4-chloro-toluidine and *N*-formyl-4-chloro-*o*-toluidine, are thought to be responsible for the observed hemangioendotheliomas in mice observed in carcinogenicity studies (IPCS, 1998). Chlordimeform was classified as a probable human carcinogen (Group 2A) by IARC in 1990. Given the increasing evidence of an association between exposure to chlordimeform and 4-chloro-*o*-toluidine and bladder cancer (Popp *et al.*, 1992), chlordimeform was withdrawn from the market in 1992. Amitraz, on the other hand, remains on the market and is still used worldwide for the control of ectoparasites in farm animals and crops. In recent years several cases of acute amitraz poisoning have been reported, particularly in Turkey, and most involved children (Yaramis *et al.*, 2000; Caksen *et al.*, 2003; Elinav *et al.*, 2005; Proudfoot, 2003). Signs and symptoms of poisoning mimicked those of α_2-adrenergic receptor agonists such as clonidine, and

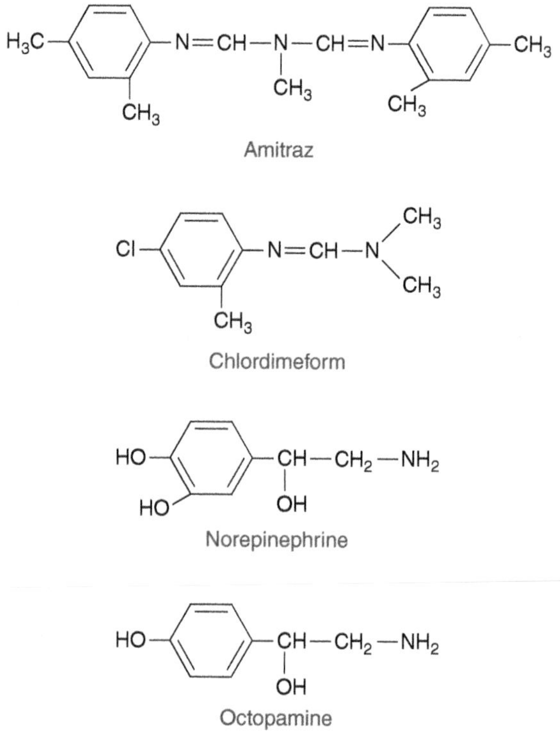

Amitraz

Chlordimeform

Norepinephrine

Octopamine

Figure 22-15. Structures of the formamidine insecticides/acaricides amitraz and chlordimeform. Structures of the mammalian neurotransmitter norepinephrine and of the insect neurotransmitter octopamine are also shown.

included nausea, hypotension, hyperglycemia, bradycardia, and miosis. No deaths occurred. A series of acute amitraz poisonings has been recently reported in South Africa, with CNS depression as the most common clinical sign (Veale *et al.*, 2011). Although α_2-adrenoceptor antagonists such as yohimbine have proven useful as antidotes in animals (Andrade and Sakate, 2003), their usefulness in managing amitraz poisoning in humans has not been evaluated.

Avermectins The avermectins are macrocyclic lactones, first isolated in 1975 from the fermentation broth of the actinomycete *Streptomyces avermitilis*, which originated from a Japanese soil sample (Campbell, 1989; Fisher and Mrozik, 1992). This fungus synthesizes eight individual avermectins, of which avermectin B_{1a} displays the highest antiparasitic activity. Currently, abamectin (a mixture of 80% avermectin B_{1a} and 20% avermectin B_{1b}) is used as an insecticide, while the semisynthetic derivatives of avermectin B_{1a}, emamectin benzoate and ivermectin, are used as insecticides, and for parasite control in human and veterinary medicine, respectively (Stevens and Breckenridge, 2001). Abamectin is used primarily to control mites, while emamectin benzoate is effective at controlling lepidopterian species in various crops. Ivermectin is used as an antihelmintic and antiparasitic agent in veterinary medicine, and in humans it has proven to be an effective treatment for infection of intestinal threadworms, onchocerciasis (river blindness), and lymphatic filariasis (Stevens and Breckenridge, 2001). In insects and nematodes, avermectins exert their toxic effects by binding to, and activating, glutamate-dependent chloride channels (Arena *et al.*, 1995). Avermectins have a high acute toxicity, with oral LD_{50}s in rats of 11 mg/kg (abamectin) to 80 mg/kg (emamectin). Toxicity is higher in neonate animals, possibly because of a deficient blood–brain barrier (Stevens and Breckenridge, 2001). Signs and symptoms of intoxication include hyperexcitability, tremors, and incoordination, followed by ataxia and coma-like sedation. These effects are due to the ability of avermectins to activate $GABA_A$ receptor-gated chloride channels in the vertebrate CNS (Pong *et al.*, 1982; Fisher and Mrozik, 1992). Activity at $GABA_A$ receptors also mediates the anticonvulsant effects of avermectins, but since the same target seems to mediate both pharmacological and toxic effects, the potential of avermectins as anticonvulsants is limited (Dawson *et al.*, 2000).

Avermectins interact with P-glycoprotein, a plasma membrane protein of the ATP-binding cassette (ABC) transporters superfamily, whose main function is the ATPase-dependent transport of foreign substances from the cell (Didier and Loor, 1996). As such, avermectins are being investigated for their potential ability to inhibit multidrug resistance of tumor cells (Korystov *et al.*, 2004). In this respect, the complete sequencing of the *S. avermitilis* genome would allow the definition of the precise biosynthetic pathways and regulatory mechanisms for avermectins, which in turn may lead to engineering of this fungus to produce pharmacological compounds of interest (Yoon *et al.*, 2004). The P-glycoprotein-mediated efflux plays an important role in attenuating the neurotoxicity and developmental neurotoxicity of avermectins (Stevens *et al.*, 2010), and P-glycoprotein polymorphisms, which may affect its function, may increase avermectin neurotoxicity in humans (MacDonald and Gladhill, 2007). Nevertheless, given the wide use of avermectins, and particularly of ivermectin in Africa, there is little evidence of adverse health effects in humans. The major effect following administration of active doses of ivermectin (0.1–0.2 mg/kg) is a severe inflammatory response (the Mazzotti reaction), characterized by pruritus, erythema, and vesicle and papulae formation, and attributable to the killing of microfilariae that dislodge from their site of infestation and are transported in the blood and body fluids (Ackerman *et al.*, 1990).

Phenylpyrazoles A relatively recent class of insecticides is that of phenylpyrazole derivatives, of which fipronil, commercialized in the mid 1990s, was the first one brought to market. Fipronil is a broad-spectrum insecticide with moderate mammalian toxicity (LD_{50} in rat: oral, 97 mg/kg; dermal, >2000 mg/kg), and a high selectivity for target species. It acts as a blocker of the $GABA_A$-gated chloride channel, but binds to a site different from the picrotoxin binding site used by organochlorine insecticides. It also has a much higher specificity for insect receptors over mammalian receptors (Hainzl *et al.*, 1998; Narahashi *et al.*, 2007). Furthermore, fipronil also potently blocks glutamate-activated chloride channels in insects; these channels are not present in mammals (Narahashi *et al.*, 2007). There is no evidence that fipronil is an eye or skin irritant, or has any mutagenic, carcinogenic, or teratogenic effects. A number of human poisonings with fipronil have been reported that resulted from accidental or intentional ingestion. Less than 20% of the patients developed seizures, and all recovered (Mohamed *et al.*, 2004; Lee *et al.*, 2010).

Diamides These compounds represent a recent class of insecticides, with a novel mechanism of action, activation of the ryanodine receptors; fubendiamide, a phthalic diamide, chlorantraniliprole, and anthranilic diamide were introduced in 2008. Ryanodine receptors are a family of calcium channels. Under normal conditions, input from the nervous system activates voltage-gated calcium channels, leading to an increase in intracellular calcium; in turn, this triggers activation of ryanodine receptors located in the muscle sarcoplasmic reticulum, resulting in the release of stored pools of calcium and initiating muscle contraction. Ryanodine, a natural alkaloid present in the shrub *Ryania speciosa*, binds to and blocks these calcium channels, thus inhibiting muscle contraction. Ryanodine itself had been utilized as an insecticide, but its mammalian toxicity precluded its further use (Satelle *et al.*, 2008). In contrast, diamides bind to a site different from ryanodine, and cause receptor activation in insects (Satelle *et al.*, 2008; Bentley *et al.*, 2010). Both flubediamide and chlorantraniliprole have an extremely favorable toxicological profile (USEPA, 2008; Bentley *et al.*, 2010), likely due to the difference between insect and mammalian ryanodine receptors, and the ability of these compounds to selectively activate insect ryanodine receptors. Acute toxicity is low (oral LD_{50} = 2000–5000 mg/kg), and there is no evidence of genotoxicity, carcinogenicity, neurotoxicity, and reproductive and developmental toxicity.

Bacillus Thuringiensis The past decade has seen increasing research and development in the area of biopesticides, that is, pesticides derived from natural materials such as plants, bacteria, and fungi. As of 2001, there were 195 registered biopesticide active ingredients in the United States, and 780 products. Biopesticides fall into three major classes: (1) microbial pesticides, which consist of a microorganism (eg, a bacterium, fungus, or protozoan) as the active ingredient. The most widely used microbial pesticides are subspecies and strains of *Bacillus thuringiensis* (Bt) that act as insecticides. Other microbial pesticides can control different kinds of pests; for example, there are fungi that can control certain weeds, and others that can kill specific insects. (2) Plant-incorporated protectants, which are pesticidal substances that plants produce from genetic material that has been added to the plant. For example, a plant can be genetically manipulated to produce the Bt pesticidal protein. (3) Biochemical pesticides, which are naturally occurring substances that control pests by nontoxic mechanisms. Examples are sex pheromones that interfere with mating of insects, or various scented plant extracts that attract insect pests to traps (Sudakin, 2003). Biopesticides represent somewhat more than 1% to 2% of the world pesticide market, and Bt products represent 80% of all biopesticides sold (Whalon and Wingend, 2003). Bt is a soil microorganism, closely related to *Bacillus cereus*, which produces proteins that are selectively toxic to certain insects. Its name comes from the German region of Thuringia, where this strain was found in 1915. Bt-based microbial insecticides were commercialized in France in 1938 and in the United States in 1961. During the stationary phase of its growth cycle, Bt forms spores that contain crystals predominantly comprising one or more Cry and/or Cyt proteins; over 150 of such proteins have been identified in Bt (Schnepf *et al.*, 1998; van Frankenhuyzen, 2009; Sanahuja *et al.*, 2011). After ingestion of Bt by an insect, the crystal proteins are solubilized, and proteolytically processed to active toxins (δ-endotoxin) in the insect's midgut. Here they bind to specific receptors in the epithelial cells and insert into the cellular membrane. Next, aggregation of inserted crystal protein occurs, resulting in the formation of pores, which lead to changes in K^+ fluxes across the epithelial cells, and to changes in pH. Ultimately, cells of the midgut epithelium are destroyed by the high pH and by osmotic lysis. Insects eventually die as a result of gut paralysis and feeding inhibition, and subsequent starvation and septicemia (Gringorten, 2001; Bravo *et al.*, 2007). Bt targets primarily leaf-feeding lepidoptera, breaks down rapidly in UV light, and exhibits low mammalian toxicity. The basis for the selective toxicity of Bt is attributed to the fact that crystalline Bt endotoxins require activation by alkalis and/or digestion, conditions absent in the mammalian stomach (Ujvary, 2010). A summary of the toxicology studies in mammals of Bt-based insecticides is provided by McClintock *et al.* (1995). Adverse health effects in humans are infrequent and include allergic reactions and infections (Ujvary, 2010). Bt genes are also expressed in a variety of crop plants, most notably cotton and corn (Sanahuja *et al.*, 2011). Thus, the plant, instead of the Bt bacterium, produces the crystal toxins that affect the insect on feeding. Resistance can develop to Bt toxins that involves alterations in the processing of Cry toxin in the insect's gut or in its binding to receptors (Whalon and Wingerd, 2003; Bravo *et al.*, 2011).

INSECT REPELLENTS

Insect-transmitted diseases remain a major source of illness and death worldwide, as mosquitoes alone transmit disease to more than 700 million persons annually (Fradin and Day, 2002). Although insect-borne diseases represent a greater health problem in tropical and subtropical climates, no part of the world is immune to their risks. For example, in 1999, the West Nile virus, transmitted by mosquitoes, was detected for the first time in the western hemisphere. In the New York City area, 62 persons infected with the West Nile virus were hospitalized and seven died (Nash *et al.*, 2001). Other arthropod-borne viral diseases (eg, equine encephalitis) and tick-borne diseases (eg, Lyme disease) are also of concern; additionally, other insect bites can be associated with variable adverse health effects, from mild irritation and discomfort to possible allergic reactions. Insect repellents are thus widely used to provide protection toward insect bites (Katz *et al.*, 2008). The best known and most widely used insect repellent is DEET, and a newer compound, picaridin, is encountering increasing success. Botanical insect repellents based on citronella or oil of eucalyptus, and a biopesticide structurally similar to the amino acid alanine are also commercialized in Europe and the United States (Fradin and Day, 2002).

DEET

DEET (*N*,*N*-diethyl-*m*-toluamide or *N*,*N*-diethyl-3-methylbenzamide) was first developed by the USDA in 1946 for use in the military, and was registered as an insect repellent for the general public

in 1957. The USEPA estimates that 30% of the US population uses DEET every year. More than 200 formulations exist with varying concentrations of DEET (commonly 4.75–40%), which are applied directly to the skin or on clothing. DEET is very effective at repelling insects, flies, fleas, and ticks, and protection time increases with increasing concentrations (Fradin and Day, 2002). The repellent mechanisms of DEET are still unknown; a recent study suggests that its efficacy is a result of direct detection and avoidance of DEET in the vapor phase by mosquitoes (Syed and Leal, 2008; Sudakin and Osimitz, 2010). Percutaneous absorption of DEET varies from 7.9% to 59%, depending on the species tested and the conditions of the study (Osimitz and Murphy, 1997). DEET undergoes oxidative biotransformation catalyzed by various cytochromes P450, and is excreted mostly in the urine (Sudakin and Trevathan, 2003). It has low acute toxicity, with LD_{50} values in the rat of 1892 mg/kg (oral) and >5000 mg/kg (dermal) (Schoenig and Osimitz, 2001). From 1961 to 2002, eight deaths were reported related to DEET: three resulted from deliberate ingestion, while two were reported following dermal exposure (Tenenbein, 1987; Bell *et al.*, 2002). The remaining three cases were children, age 17 months to six years (Zadikoff, 1979). Subchronic toxicity studies in various species did not reveal major toxic effects, with the exception of renal lesions in male rats; these were considered to be reflective of α_{2u}-globulin-induced nephropathy, a condition unique to male rats and not occurring in humans (Schoenig and Osimitz, 2001). No significant effects of DEET were seen in mutagenicity, reproductive toxicity, and carcinogenicity studies. Acute and chronic neurotoxicity studies also provided negative results (Schoenig *et al.*, 1993; Sudakin and Osimitz, 2010). Yet, several case reports over the past 40 years have indicated neurologic effects of DEET, and most of these were in children (Gryboski *et al.*, 1961; MMWR, 1989; Osimitz and Murphy, 1997; Hampers *et al.*, 1999; Petrucci and Sardini, 2000; Briassoulis *et al.*, 2001; Sudakin and Trevathan, 2003). The most common symptoms reported were seizures. Given that seizure disorders occur in 3% to 5% of children, and almost 30% of children in the United States are utilizing DEET, an association just by chance is certainly possible. Possible mechanism(s) responsible for neurotoxic effects of DEET are unknown, although it has been suggested that DEET's structure is similar to that of nikethamide, a convulsant (Briassoulis *et al.*, 2001). It has also been suggested that DEET may disrupt the permeability of the blood–brain barrier, but results are inconclusive (Abdel-Rahman *et al.*, 2002). Overall, given its long-standing and widespread use, DEET appears to be relatively safe when used as recommended (Osimitz and Murphy, 1997; Koren *et al.*, 2003). A risk assessment by the Canadian Pest Management Regulatory Agency has recommended, however, that toddlers and children, up to 12 years old, should only be exposed to products with up to 10% DEET (Sudakin and Trevathan, 2003). For all other individuals, products with up to 30% DEET can be used, as they appear safe and effective (Fradin and Day, 2002; Antwi *et al.*, 2008).

Picaridin

Picaridin (1-piperidinecarboxylic acid, 2-(hydroxyethyl),1-methyl propyl ester) was developed as an alternative to DEET. Insect repellent formulations (cream, aerosol, wipe) containing 5% to 20% picaridin are highly effective against a variety of arthropod pests, especially mosquitoes, ticks, and flies (Sangha, 2010). Its action in insects is believed to be due to the interaction with specific olfactory receptors of the arthropod (Boeckh *et al.*, 1996). In humans it is absorbed through the skin to a limited degree (90% less than in the rat), and is metabolized via hydroxylation and glucuronidation, before excretion in the urine. The toxicological profile of picaridin is unremarkable. Acute dermal toxicity is low (~5 g/kg), and NOEL values are ~200 mg/kg per day in dermal subchronic and chronic toxicity studies. There is no evidence of genotoxicity, carcinogenicity, teratogenicity, reproductive toxicity, or neurotoxicity (Sangha, 2010). When used as directed, picaridin-containing formulations are deemed to be safe and effective (Antwi et al., 2008).

HERBICIDES

Herbicides are chemicals that are capable of either killing or severely injuring plants. They represent a very broad array of chemical classes and act at a large number of sites of metabolic functions and energy transfer in plant cells (Duke, 1990; Casida, 2009). Some of the various mechanisms by which herbicides exert their biological effects are shown in Table 22-17, together with examples for each class. Another method of classification pertains to how and when herbicides are applied. Thus, *preplanting* herbicides are applied to the soil before a crop is seeded; *preemergent* herbicides are applied to the soil before the time of appearance of unwanted vegetation; and *postemergent* herbicides are applied to the soil or foliage after the germination of the crop and/or weeds (Ecobichon, 2001a). Herbicides are also divided according to the manner they are applied to plants. *Contact* herbicides are those that affect the plant that was treated, while *translocated* herbicides are applied to the soil or to above-ground parts of the plant, and are absorbed and circulated to distant tissues. Nonselective herbicides will kill all vegetation, while selective compounds are those used to kill weeds without harming the crops. In the past decade, the development of herbicide-resistant crops through transgenic technology has allowed the use of nonselective compounds as selective herbicides (Duke, 2005). A final classification, of relevance to adverse health effects in nontarget species, relies, on the other hand, on chemical structures, as indicated below.

For the past several decades, herbicides have represented the most rapidly growing sector of the agrochemical market, and these compounds now represent almost half of the pesticides used in the United States, and more than one-third of those utilized worldwide (Table 22-3). This can be ascribed in part to movement to monocultural practices, where the risk of weed infestation has increased, and to mechanization of agricultural practices because of increased labor costs. In addition to agriculture and home and garden uses, herbicides are also widely utilized in forestry management and to clear roadsides, utilities' rights of way, and industrial areas.

In terms of general toxicity, herbicides, as a class, display relatively low acute toxicity, compared, for example, with most insecticides. There are exceptions, however, such as paraquat. A number of herbicides can cause dermal irritation and contact dermatitis, particularly in individuals prone to allergic reactions. Other compounds have generated much debate for their suspected carcinogenicity or neurotoxicity. The principal classes of herbicides associated with reported adverse health effects in humans are discussed below.

Chlorophenoxy Compounds

Chlorophenoxy herbicides are characterized by an aliphatic carboxylic acid moiety attached to a chlorine- or-methyl-substituted aromatic ring. The most commonly used compound of this class is 2,4-dichlorophenoxyacetic acid (2,4-D), while others are 2,4,5-trichlorophenoxyacetic acid (2,4,5-T) and 4-chloro-2-methylphenoxyacetic acid (MCPA) (Fig. 22-16). Chlorophenoxy herbicides are chemical analogs of auxin, a plant growth hormone, and produce uncontrolled and lethal growth in target plants (Casida, 2009). Because the auxin hormone is critical to the growth of many broad-leaf plants, but is not used by grasses, chlorophenoxy compounds can suppress the growth of weeds (eg, dandelions) without affecting the grass. Once absorbed, they selectively eliminate broad-leaf plants, due to their larger leaf area and greater absorption. 2,4-D is one of the most widely used herbicides throughout the world, and is primarily used in agriculture to control weeds in corn and grain (Table 22-4), in forestry, and in lawn care practices, with over 120 commercialized formulations (Kennepohl et al., 2010). 2,4,5-T has been largely withdrawn from use because of concerns that arose from contamination of some formulations with 2,3,7,8-tetrachlorodibenzo-p-dioxin (TCDD), which can

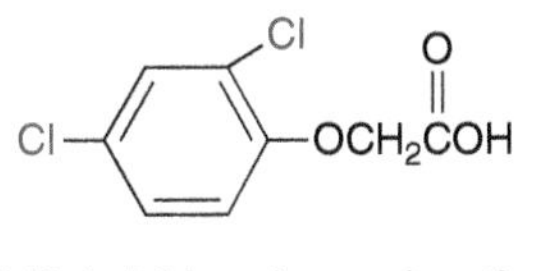

Figure 22-16. *Structures of three chlorophenoxy acid herbicides.*

Table 22-17

Some Mechanisms of Action of Herbicides

MECHANISM	CHEMICAL CLASSES (EXAMPLE)
Inhibition of photosynthesis	Triazines (atrazine), substituted ureas (diuron), uracils (bromacil)
Inhibition of respiration	Dinitrophenols
Auxin growth regulators	Phenoxy acids (2,4-D), benzoic acids (dicamba), pyridine acids (picloram)
Inhibition of protein synthesis	Dinitroanilines
Inhibition of lipid synthesis	Aryloxyphenoxyproprionates (diclofop)
Inhibition of specific enzymes • Glutamine synthetase • Enolpyruvylshikimate-3-phosphate synthetase • Acetalase synthase	 Glufosinate Glyphosate Sulfonylureas
Cell membrane disruptors	Bipyridyl derivatives (paraquat)

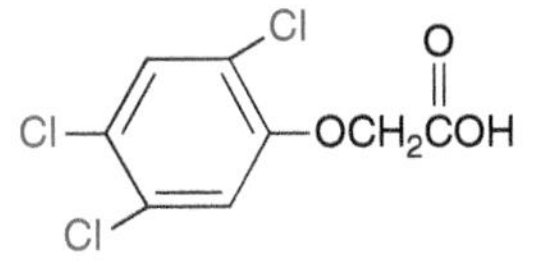

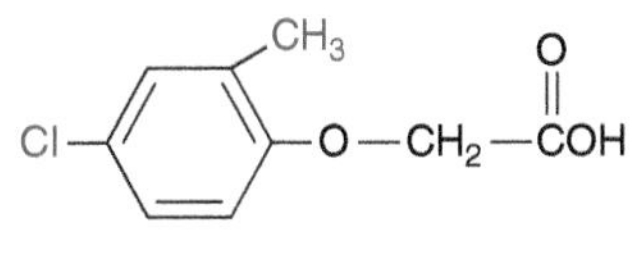

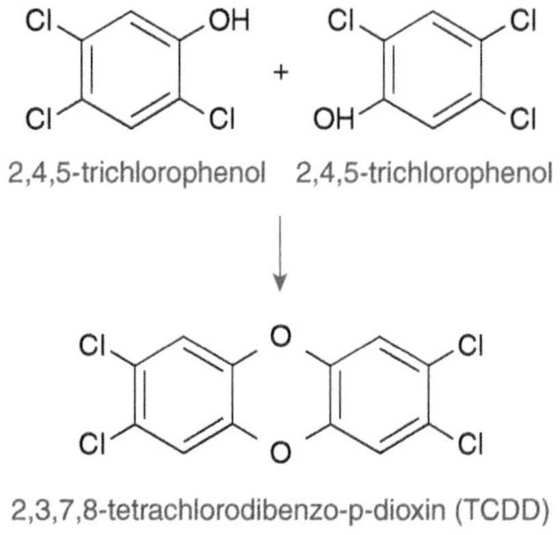

2,4,5-trichlorophenol   2,4,5-trichlorophenol

2,3,7,8-tetrachlorodibenzo-p-dioxin (TCDD)

Figure 22-17. *Formation of 2,3,7,8-tetrachlorodibenzodioxin (TCDD) during the synthesis of 2,4,5-T because of reaction between two molecules of 2,4,5-trichlorophenol.*

Table 22-18

Effect of Urine Alkalinization on Renal Clearance and Plasma Half-Life of 2,4-D

URINE pH	RENAL CLEARANCE (mL/min)	HALF-LIFE (h)
5.10–6.5	0.28	219
6.55–7.5	1.14	42
7.55–8.8	9.60	4.7

Data from Park et al. (1977).

derive from the reaction of two molecules of 2,4,5-trichlorophenol (Fig. 22-17). A 50:50 mixture of the *n*-butyl esters of 2,4,-D and 2,3,5-T, known as Agent Orange (from the color of the barrels that contained it), was extensively used as a defoliant during the Vietnam War, and was found to be contaminated with TCDD to a maximum of 47 μg/g. Exposure of military personnel and of Vietnamese population to Agent Orange has raised concerns on possible long-term health effects, particularly carcinogenicity and reproductive toxicity (IOM, 1996), which are ascribed to the presence of TCDD. Formulations of 2,4-D contain extremely low levels of polychlorinated dibenzo-*p*-dioxins (PCDDs), usually below the limit of detection of 10 ppb (Kennepohl *et al.*, 2010).

2,4-D is a compound of low to moderate acute toxicity, with oral LD_{50}s in rodents of 300 to 2000 mg/kg. The dog is more sensitive, possibly because of its less ability to eliminate organic acids via the kidney. On oral exposure, 2,4-D is rapidly absorbed, and its salts and esters rapidly dissociate or hydrolyze in vivo, so that toxicity depends primarily on the acid form. It binds extensively to serum albumin, but does not accumulate in tissues, and is excreted almost exclusively through the urine. Ingestion of 2,4-D has caused several cases of acute poisoning in humans, usually at doses above 300 mg/kg, although lower doses have been reported to elicit symptoms. Vomiting, burning of the mouth, abdominal pain, hypotension, myotonia, and CNS involvement including coma are among the clinical signs observed (Bradberry *et al.*, 2000, 2004a). Management of 2,4-D poisoning appears to be aided by urine alkalinization, through intravenous administration of bicarbonate (Proudfoot *et al.*, 2004; Bradberry *et al.*, 2004a). The rationale is that ionization of an acid, such as 2,4-D, is increased in an alkaline environment; although, at pH 5.0, practically all 2,4-D would already be ionized, further alkalinization of urine, to pH 7.5 or above, would reduce the nonionized fraction from approximately 0.53% to 0.0017%. As a result, the fraction prone to reabsorption would be >300 times lower (Bradberry *et al.*, 2004a), thus diminishing reabsorption and increasing 2,4-D elimination. Nevertheless, it has been recently recommended that additional studies be conducted to fully validate this approach in case of 2,4-D poisoning (Roberts and Buckley, 2007). Table 22-18 shows an example of the effect of urine alkalinization on 2,4-D renal clearance and plasma half-life.

Dermal exposure is by far the major route of unintentional exposure to 2,4-D in humans. Dermal absorption studies in rats, mice, and rabbit indicate an absorption of 12% to 36%; the absorption in humans, however, is lower (2%–10%), and is usually less than 6% (Ross *et al.*, 2005). Acute poisoning by 2,4-D via the dermal route is thus uncommon; no reports of systemic toxicity

following dermal exposure have been reported for over 20 years, and no fatalities have ever occurred (Bradberry *et al.*, 2004a).

The precise mechanisms of toxicity of chlorophenoxy herbicides have not been completely elucidated, but experimental studies indicate the possible involvement of three actions: (1) cell membrane damage; (2) interference with metabolic pathways involving acetyl-coenzyme A; (3) uncoupling of oxidative phosphorylation (Bradberry *et al.*, 2000). The toxicity of chlorophenoxy herbicides has been summarized in several reviews (Sterling and Arundel, 1986; Munro *et al.*, 1992; Garabrandt and Philbert, 2002; Kennepohl *et al.*, 2010). 2,4-D and its salts and esters are not teratogenic in mice, rats, or rabbits, unless the ability of the dam to excrete the chemical is exceeded. There is also no convincing evidence that 2,4-D is associated with human reproductive toxicity (Garabrandt and Philbert, 2002). Subchronic and chronic toxicity studies have not provided evidence of immunotoxicity, and there is very limited evidence that 2,4-D may affect the nervous system (Mattsson *et al.*, 1997). There are, however, several case reports suggesting an association between exposure to 2,4-D and neurologic effects such as peripheral neuropathy, demyelination and ganglion degeneration in the CNS, reduced nerve conduction velocity, myotonia, and behavioral alterations (Garabrandt and Philbert, 2002). 2,4-D-induced hypomyelination on developmental exposure has also been recently described (Konjuh *et al.*, 2008).

Numerous in vitro and in vivo studies with 2,4-D indicate that it has very little genotoxic potential (Munro *et al.*, 1992). Long-term bioassays in rats, mice, and dogs provided no evidence to suggest that 2,4-D is a carcinogen in any of these species. An earlier study in rats reported an increase in the incidence of brain astrocytomas in male animals, only at the highest dose tested (45 mg/kg per day) (Serota, 1986). However, a review of this study concluded that the observed tumors were not treatment-related (Munro *et al.*, 1992), and more recent studies did not replicate this finding (Charles *et al.*, 1996). Nevertheless, the chlorophenoxy herbicides have attracted much attention because of the association between exposure and non-Hodgkin lymphoma or soft tissue sarcoma, found in a small number of epidemiological studies (Hoar *et al.*, 1986; Hardell *et al.*, 1994). In a recent review that follows several previous ones discussing this topic (Wood *et al.*, 1987; Munro *et al.*, 1992; USEPA, 1994), Garabrandt and Philbert (2002) evaluated all cohort and case–control studies available to date, and concluded that there was no adequate evidence from epidemiological studies to conclude that exposure to 2,4-D is associated with soft tissue sarcoma, non-Hodgkinlymphoma, or Hodgkin disease. 2,4-D is classified as a Group D agent (not classifiable as to human carcinogenicity) (USEPA, 1997). It should also be noted that biomonitoring data in the United States and Canada indicate that exposure to 2,4-D in both the general and agricultural populations is well below the noncancer reference dose (Aylward *et al.*, 2010).

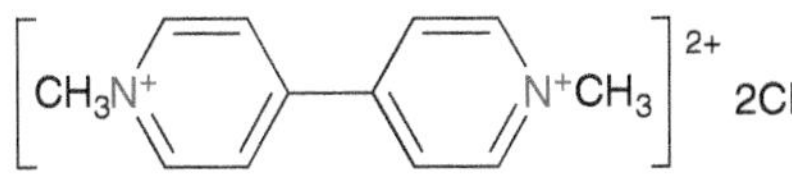

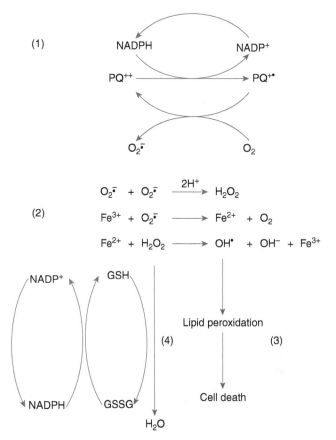

Figure 22-18. *Structures of the bipyridyl herbicides paraquat and diquat, marketed as the dichloride and dibromide salts, respectively.*

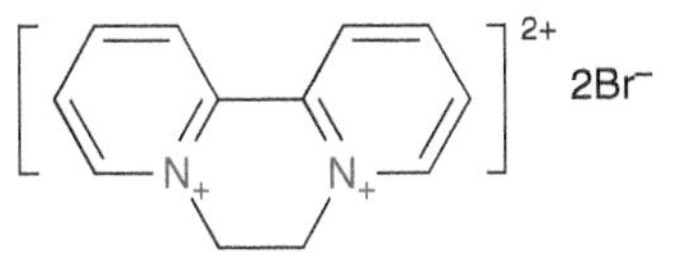

Bipyridyl Compounds

This class of herbicides comprises paraquat and diquat (Fig. 22-18). Of these, paraquat (1,1′-dimethyl-4,4′-bipyridylium dichloride) is of most toxicological concern, and will be discussed in more detail. First described in 1882, paraquat's redox properties were discovered in 1933, when the compound was called methyl viologen. Paraquat was introduced as a herbicide in 1962, and is formulated as an aqueous solution or as a granular formulation. It is a very effective, fast-acting, nonselective contact herbicide, used to control broad-leaved weeds and grasses in plantations and fruit orchards, and for general weed control (Dinis-Oliveira *et al.*, 2008; Lock and Wilks, 2010). Its redox potential (see below) explains its herbicidal activity, as well as its mammalian toxicity.

Paraquat has one of the highest acute toxicities among herbicides; its oral LD_{50} in rat is approximately 100 mg/kg, while guinea pigs, rabbits, and monkeys are more sensitive. Paraquat is more toxic when given by the i.p. route (LD_{50} in rats = 10–20 mg/kg), suggesting that it is not efficiently absorbed from the gastrointestinal tract. Absorption through intact skin is minimal, and inhalation exposure does not occur, as paraquat has no appreciable vapor pressure. On absorption, independently of the route of exposure, paraquat accumulates in the lung and the kidney, and these two organs are the most susceptible to paraquat-induced injury. Only a small fraction of paraquat is metabolized, and the greater part is excreted unchanged in the urine. Paraquat has minimal to no genotoxic activity, is not carcinogenic in rodents, has no effect on fertility, is not teratogenic, and only produces fetotoxicity at maternally toxic doses (Lock and Wilks, 2010). Thus, the major toxicological concerns for paraquat are related to its acute systemic effects, particularly in the lung, and, secondarily, the kidney. Rose *et al.* (1974) first described an energy-dependent accumulation of paraquat in lung tissue, particularly, but not exclusively, in type II alveolar epithelial cells. The loss of paraquat from lung tissue following in vivo administration is slow. Thus, the basis for the selective toxicity of paraquat to the lung resides in its ability to concentrate in alveolar type II and I cells and Clara cells. Pulmonary concentrations of paraquat can be six- to 10-fold higher than in plasma (Dinis-Oliveira *et al.*, 2008).

The mechanism(s) by which paraquat is toxic to living cells have been extensively investigated (Autor, 1974; Bus and Gibson, 1984; Smith, 1987). Paraquat can be reduced to form a free radical, which, in the presence of oxygen, rapidly reoxidizes to the cation, with a concomitant production of superoxide anion ($O_2^{\cdot-}$)

Figure 22-19. *Mechanism of toxicity of paraquat.* (1) Redox cycling of paraquat utilizing NADPH; (2) formation of hydroxy radicals leading to lipid peroxidation (3); (4) detoxication of H_2O_2 via glutathione reductase/peroxidase couple, utilizing NADPH. (Modified from Smith, 1987, with permission from Palgrave Macmillan.)

(Fig. 22-19). Thus, once paraquat enters a cell, it undergoes alternate reduction followed by reoxidation, a process known as redox cycling (Adam *et al.*, 1990). Superoxide dismutases (SOD) are a family of metalloenzymes that can dismutate superoxide anions to hydrogen peroxide and oxygen. The finding that transgenic mice lacking copper/zinc SOD show marked increased sensitivity to paraquat (Ho *et al.*, 1998) supports a role for superoxide anions in paraquat's cellular toxicity. Nevertheless, superoxide anion itself is unlikely to be the ultimate toxic species. Three hypotheses have been proposed to account for the ensuing cytotoxicity, which are not mutually exclusive (Lock and Wilks, 2010). The generation of superoxide anion and subsequently of hydroxy radicals would initiate lipid peroxidation, ultimately leading to cell death (Bus and Gibson, 1984). Intracellular redox cycling of paraquat would also result in the oxidation of NADPH, leading to its cellular depletion, which is augmented by the detoxification of hydrogen peroxide formed in the glutathione peroxidase/reductase enzyme system to regenerate GSH (Fig. 22-19). A third hypothesis is that paraquat toxicity is due to mitochondrial damage; however, paraquat does not affect complex I in isolated brain mitochondria (Richardson *et al.*, 2005).

On acute exposure to lethal doses of paraquat, mortality may occur two to five days after dosing, although death can also occur after longer periods (Clark *et al.*, 1966). Damage to alveolar epithelial cells is seen within 24 hours after exposure. Damage progresses in the following two to four days with large areas of the alveolar epithelium completely lost. This is followed by alveolar edema, extensive infiltration of inflammatory cells into the alveolar interstitium, and finally death due to severe anoxia (Smith and Heath, 1976). Survivors of this first phase, called the destructive phase, show extensive proliferation of the fibroblast in the lung. The second phase, called the proliferative phase, is characterized by attempts by the alveolar epithelium to regenerate and restore normal architecture, and presents itself as an intensive fibrosis (Smith and Heath, 1976). Some individuals who survive the first phase may still die from the progressive loss of lung function several weeks after exposure.

Attempts to develop treatments for paraquat poisoning have focused on prevention of absorption from the gastrointestinal tract, removal from the bloodstream, prevention of its accumulation in the lung, use of free radical scavengers, and prevention of lung fibrosis (Dinis-Oliveira et al., 2008; Lock and Wilks, 2010). Although some approaches have shown promises in vitro or in isolated lung tissue preparations, only the first one, removal of the ingested material by emesis or purgation of the gastrointestinal tract, has been shown to be effective in vivo in animals. Administration of dexamethasone, with induction of P-glycoprotein in several tissues including the lung, and of sodium salicylate, because of its anti-inflammatory properties, has also been shown, in animal studies, to be effective treatments for paraquat poisoning (Dinis-Oliveira et al., 2008).

Since its introduction as a herbicide, there have been thousands of episodes of acute poisoning with paraquat in humans, a large percentage of which are fatal (Malone et al., 1971; Casey and Vale, 1994; Wesseling et al., 2001; Lock and Wilks, 2010). Most cases involved ingestion of a 20% paraquat concentrate solution for suicidal purposes, or resulted from accidental poisoning due to decanting in unlabeled drink bottles or containers. To avoid the latter, in the 1980s, the manufacturers added a blue pigment, a stenching compound, and an emetic substance to the formulation, to make severe unintentional poisoning due to oral intake virtually impossible (Sabapathy, 1995). As said, absorption of paraquat across the human skin is very low (but is increased by damage to skin, and paraquat is a skin irritant), and few cases of paraquat poisoning have been reported following dermal exposure. Signs and symptoms of paraquat poisoning in humans reflect those previously described. A dose of 20 to 30 mg/kg can cause mild poisoning, while 30 to 50 mg/kg can cause delayed development of pulmonary fibrosis, which can be lethal. Higher doses usually cause death within a few days due to pulmonary edema, and renal and hepatic failure (Smith and Heath, 1976). No single therapeutic intervention, among those outlined earlier, has proven efficacious in case of severe acute paraquat poisoning (Bismuth et al., 1982). In rare instances, heart/lung transplant has been used to treat severely paraquat-poisoned patients.

Chronic exposure of experimental animals to paraquat affects the same target organs of acute toxicity, that is, the lung and the kidney, and no-effect levels have been established. Under normal use conditions, exposure to paraquat is very low and can be monitored by measuring paraquat levels in urine, as the compound is mostly excreted unchanged (Lee et al., 2009b). In the late 1970s concern was raised about possible exposure of marijuana smokers to paraquat by inhalation. Paraquat was indeed used to destroy marijuana fields, and residues were still present in the final products (Landrigan et al., 1983). However, no clinical cases were identified.

Chronic paraquat exposure has also been suggested as a possible etiological factor in the development of Parkinson disease. The first suggestion came from a study in the Canadian province of Quebec (Barbeau et al., 1986), and the hypothesis arose from the structural similarity of paraquat to MPP$^+$ ion, the toxic metabolite of MPTP. MPP$^+$ itself was initially developed as a possible herbicide, but was never commercialized. It has been argued that paraquat, being positively charged, cannot easily pass the blood–brain barrier. Yet, animal studies have shown that paraquat can cause CNS effects, most notably a neurodegeneration of dopaminergic neurons (McCormack et al., 2002). Paraquat may be transported into the brain by a neutral amino acid transporter, such as the system L carrier (LAT-1) (Shimizu et al., 2001). The ability of paraquat to cause oxidative damage through a free radical mechanism may explain the selective vulnerability of dopaminergic neurons, which are per se more susceptible to oxidative damage (McCormack et al., 2005). Paraquat neurotoxicity is, however, distinct from that of MPTP or rotenone (Richardson et al., 2005). Nevertheless, while animal studies convincingly show that paraquat can cause dopaminergic toxicity, particularly in mice, there is still no solid evidence that paraquat may be associated with Parkinson disease in humans (Li et al., 2005; Berry et al., 2010; Moretto and Colosio, 2011). Furthermore, a five- to 10-year follow-up of individuals who survived paraquat poisoning did not provide any evidence of parkinsonism (Zilker et al., 1988). However, the debate on whether exposure to paraquat may contribute to the etiology of Parkinson disease continues (Miller, 2007; Tanner et al., 2011).

Despite the chemical similarity to paraquat (Fig. 22-18), the herbicide diquat presents a different toxicological profile. Acute toxicity is somewhat lower, with oral LD$_{50}$ in rats of approximately 200 mg/kg (Lock and Wilks, 2001). Diquat is not a skin sensitizer, has minimal or no genotoxic activity, is not carcinogenic in rodents, has no effect on fertility, and is not teratogenic. In contrast to paraquat, it does not accumulate in the lung, and no lung toxicity is seen on acute or chronic exposure. On chronic exposure, target organs for toxicity are the gastrointestinal tract, the kidney, and particularly the eye. Diquat indeed causes a dose- and time-dependent appearance of cataracts in both rats and dogs (Lock and Wilks, 2001). Like paraquat, diquat can be reduced to form a free radical and then reoxidized in the presence of oxygen, with the concomitant production of superoxide anion. This process of redox cycling occurs in the eye and is believed to be the likely mechanism of cataract formation (Lock and Wilks, 2001). A limited number of cases of human poisoning with diquat have occurred. Clinical symptoms include nausea, vomiting, diarrhea, ulceration of mouth and esophagus, decline of renal functions, and neurologic effects, but no pulmonary fibrosis. As for paraquat, therapy for intoxication is directed at preventing absorption and enhancing elimination (Vanholder et al., 1981; Lock and Wilks, 2001).

Chloroacetanilides

Representative compounds of this class of herbicides are alachlor, acetochlor, and metolachlor (shown in Fig. 22-20), and butachlor and propachlor, all registered in the United States between 1967 and 1997. They are used to control herbal grasses and broad-leaf weeds in a number of crops, primarily on corn. The herbicidal action of chloroacetanilides is not fully understood, although they have been shown to inhibit the synthesis of lipids, alcohols, fatty acids, and terpenoids. Chloroacetanilides display moderate to low acute toxicity, with oral LD$_{50}$ in rat ranging from about 600 mg/kg (propachlor) to 2800 mg/kg (metolachlor). Dermal LD$_{50}$ values are usually much higher, indicating a poor absorption of these compounds across the skin (Heydens et al., 2010). Most are nonirritant, or only slightly irritant to the eye and skin, with the exception of propachlor, which causes severe irritation to the eye (Heydens et al., 2010). Subchronic and chronic toxicity studies, carried out in multiple species (mice, rats, dogs, rabbits), have identified the liver and kidney as principal target organs, and no observed adverse effect level (NOAEL) values have been established (Heydens et al., 2010). Alachlor was found to produce an ocular lesion, termed "progressive uveal degeneration syndrome," in Long–Evans rats

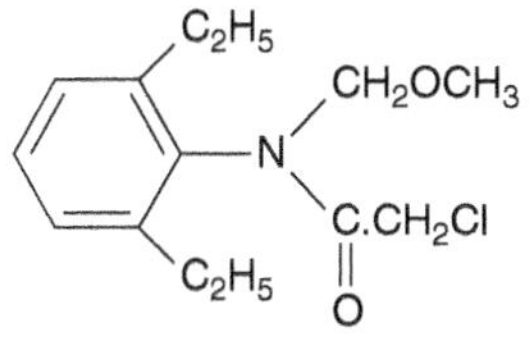

Alachlor
2-chloro-2′,6′-diethyl-N-
(methoxymethyl) acetanilide

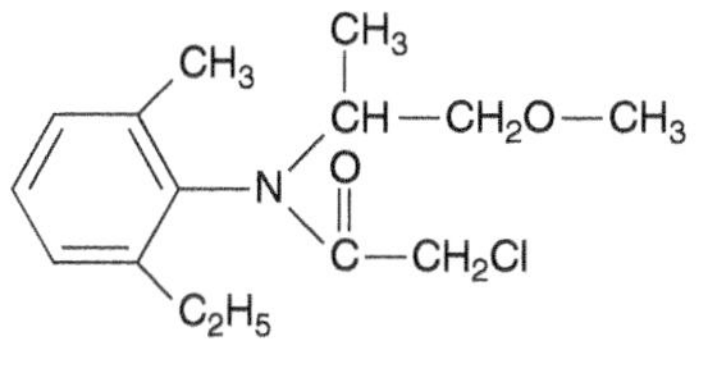

Metolachlor
2-chloro-N-(2-ethyl-6-methylpheynyl-N-
(2-methoxy-1-methylethyl)-acetamide

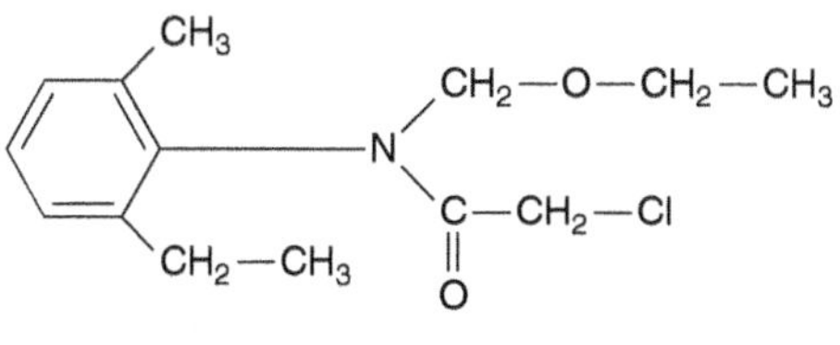

Acetochlor
2-chloro-N-(ethoxymethyl)-N-
2-ethyl-6-methylphenyl)-acetamide

Figure 22-20. *Structures of chloroacetanilide herbicides.*

(Heydens, 1998). This ocular lesion was not observed in mice, dogs, or other strains of rats. Furthermore, an investigation of similar eye abnormalities in alachlor production workers considered to have the highest alachlor exposure, far exceeding that of farmers or herbicide applicators, provided no evidence of ocular disease (Ireland *et al.*, 1994). Most of the chloroacetanilides do not appear to be teratogenic or to cause reproductive or developmental toxicity; for propachlor, slight effects on the offspring were observed in some studies at the highest dose tested (Heydens *et al.*, 2010).

Chloroacetanilides have been extensively tested for genotoxicity in vitro, in bacterial and mammalian systems, and in vivo, and these studies indicate, on the basis of a weight-of-evidence approach, that these compounds are not genotoxic (Ashby *et al.*, 1996; Heydens *et al.*, 1999, 2010). Yet, these compounds have shown to induce tumors at various sites in rats. Tumors in female mice (lung adenomas), found with alachlor and acetochlor, were considered not to be treatment-related (Ashby *et al.*, 1996; Heydens *et al.*, 1999, 2010). In rats, nasal epithelial (olfactory) tumors and thyroid follicular tumors were observed in carcinogenicity studies with alachlor, acetochlor, and butachlor, while glandular stomach tumors were found with alachlor and butachlor. These findings led to the initial classification of these compounds as probable human carcinogens (Group B2). The discovery of alachlor in well water led to cancellation of its registration in some countries, and to its restriction in others. A series of mechanistic studies in the past two decades has provided evidence that tumors observed in rats may be species-specific, show a threshold, and are not due to genotoxic mechanisms, and hence may not be relevant to humans

(Ashby *et al.*, 1996; Heydens *et al.*, 1999, 2010). Alachlor and other chloroacetanilides are extensively metabolized in rat, and more than 30 metabolites have been identified in this species, with equal quantities appearing in urine and feces; in mice, alachlor's metabolism is qualitatively similar, but significant quantitative differences are observed between these two species. In contrast, in primates alachlor is metabolized to a limited number of glutathione and glucuronide conjugates, excreted primarily in the kidney, with >90% of the dose being excreted in the urine within 48 hours. Furthermore, in rats, alachlor metabolites of intermediate molecular weight undergo biliary excretion and enterohepatic recirculation, while this phenomenon is not observed in primates. Alachlor and other chloroacetanilides undergo demethylation with the release of formaldehyde (Jacobsen *et al.*, 1991), and this compound, known to produce rat nasal tumors on inhalation exposure, was initially thought to be involved in the nasal carcinogenicity of these herbicides. However, the different nature and distribution of tumors, and additional metabolic considerations, argue against this hypothesis (Heydens *et al.*, 2010). In rats, alachlor and butachlor are initially metabolized in the liver via the cytochrome P450 pathway and by glutathione conjugation, and the metabolites undergo enterohepatic circulation and further metabolism in liver and nasal tissue, to form the putative carcinogenic metabolite diethyl quinoneimine (DEIQ) (Feng *et al.*, 1990). In the case of acetochlor, the carcinogenic metabolite is EMIQ, an acetochlor quinoneimine compound analogous to DEIQ. Quinone imines are electrophilic, deplete glutathione, and exert cellular toxicity by binding to cellular proteins, which is followed by regenerative cell proliferation. Whole-body autoradiography studies have shown that alachlor-derived protein adducts specifically localize in the nasal mucosa of rats, but not in nasal tissue from mice or monkeys. Furthermore, the ability of rat nasal tissue to form DEIQ is much higher (751-fold) than that of human nasal tissue (Wilson *et al.*, 1995). With regard to rat stomach and thyroid tumors, it is suggested that these result from tissue-specific toxicity leading to compensatory cell proliferation in the fundic mucosa, and to alterations of thyroid-stimulating hormone (TSH) homeostasis, respectively. Both are believed to be threshold-sensitive phenomena, not expected to be relevant to humans (Heydens *et al.*, 2010). Epidemiological investigations in workers involved in the manufacturing of alachlor have not demonstrated any evidence of increased mortality or cancer incidence (Leet *et al.*, 1996). As a result of these studies, alachlor has been reclassified as "likely" at high doses, but "not likely" at low doses, to be a human carcinogen, and a downgrading for acetochlor has also been suggested (Heydens *et al.*, 2010).

Triazines

The family of triazine herbicides comprises several compounds (eg, atrazine, simazine, propazine; Fig. 22-21), which have been extensively used for the preemergent and postemergent control of broadleaf weeds and certain grasses for over 30 years (Breckenridge *et al.*, 2010). Their herbicidal action is due to inhibition of photosynthesis (Casida, 2009; Brenckenridge *et al.*, 2010). Triazines have low acute oral and dermal toxicity ($LD_{50}s = 1$–2 g/kg), and chronic toxicity studies indicate primarily a decreased body weight gain as the basis for setting NOAEL values; however, in dogs, cardiotoxicity is seen with atrazine, and is used to derive the NOAEL for this compound (Gammon *et al.*, 2005). There is no evidence that triazines are teratogenic, or developmental or reproductive toxicants. The weight of evidence from in vitro and in vivo studies indicates that triazines are not genotoxic (Brusick, 1994), although a possible clastogenic effect of atrazine has been

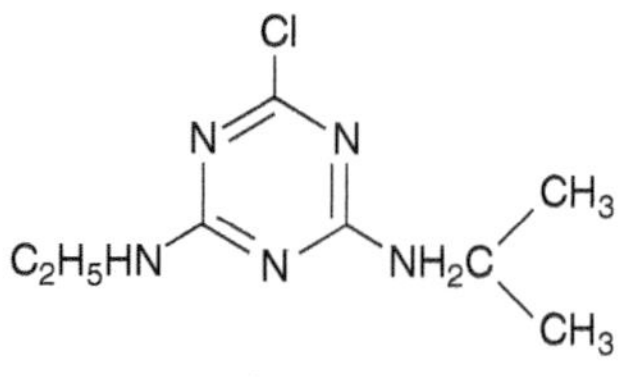

Atrazine
2-chloro-4(ethylamino)-6-
(isopropylamino)-s-triazine

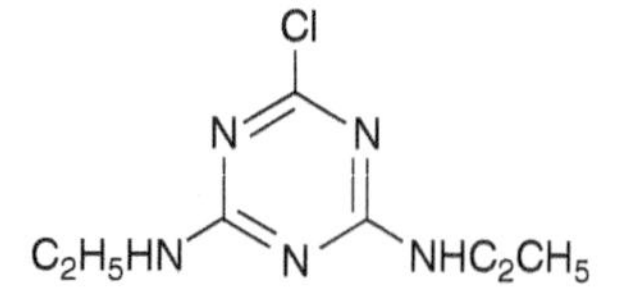

Simazine
2-chloro-4,6(ethylamino)-s-triazine

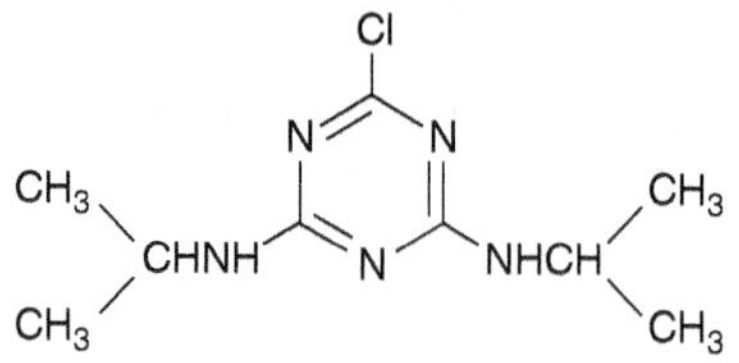

Propazine
2-chloro-4,6 bis(isopropylamino)-s-triazine

Figure 22-21. *Structures of triazine herbicides.*

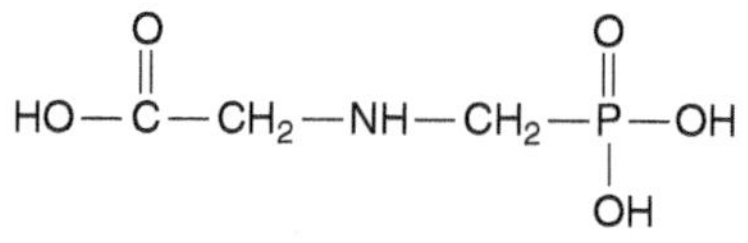

Glyphosate

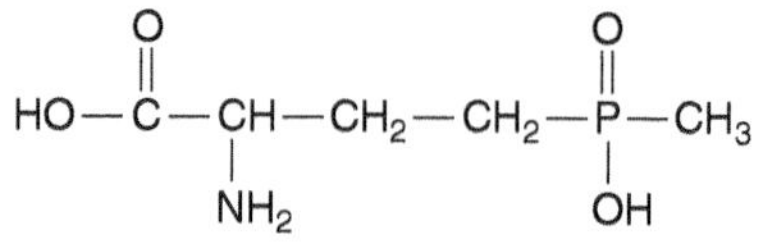

Glufosinate

Figure 22-22. *Structures of the phosphomethyl amino acids glyphosate and glufosinate.* Note that although having a P=O moiety such as organophosphates, these compounds are not acetylcholinesterase inhibitors.

suggested (Taets *et al.*, 1998). Oncogenicity studies found that triazines cause an increased incidence of mammary carcinomas in female Sprague–Dawley rats (Stevens *et al.*, 1999; Gammon *et al.*, 2005; Breckenridge *et al.*, 2010). Such tumors were not observed in male Sprague–Dawley rats, or in Fischer 344 rats or CD-1 mice of either sex (IARC, 1999; Stevens *et al.*, 1999; Breckenridge *et al.*, 2010). It is believed that such mammary tumors arise from an endocrine effect that might be expected to show a threshold. In contrast to most rodent species, female Sprague–Dawley rats have a high degree of spontaneous mammary tumors, due to their reproductive aging; they display prolonged or persistent estrus associated with high estrogen levels (Eldridge *et al.*, 1996). This is supported by the finding that ovariectomy eliminates mammary tumors in Sprague–Dawley rat that arise both spontaneously and as a result of atrazine administration (Stevens *et al.*, 1999). The possible mechanisms for the effect of atrazine involve an action on pituitary luteinizing hormone, regulated by hypothalamic gonadotropin-releasing hormone, in turn controlled by hypothalamic norepinephrine (Cooper *et al.*, 2000, 2007). Such effect was seen only at high doses of atrazine, but not at low doses, suggesting a threshold response (Breckenridge *et al.*, 2010). Most regulatory agencies have concluded that mammary tumors in female Sprague–Dawley rats are formed via a secondary, hormone-mediated mechanism, of little or no toxicological relevance to humans. Epidemiological studies of triazine herbicides and cancer have provided inconclusive results (Sathiakumar and Delzell, 1997; Rusiecki *et al.*, 2004). More recent studies have suggested an increased risk of prostate cancer associated with triazine herbicides (Mills and Yang, 2003), but this has not been substantiated by others (Alavanja *et al.*, 2003). Both atrazine and simazine are classified as Group 3 carcinogens (not classifiable as to its carcinogenicity to humans) by IARC.

Although exposure to atrazine through residues in food commodities is very low, contamination of ground water and drinking water is common. The European Union has banned the use

of atrazine in 2004, mainly because it was often detected at levels exceeding the 0.1 mg/L standard for drinking water. Recent publications have reported a possible feminization of frogs, measured in laboratory and field studies, by ppb levels of atrazine (Hayes *et al.*, 2002, 2010). However, other investigators failed to reproduce these findings (Carr *et al.*, 2003; Kloas *et al.*, 2009), and it has been argued that the conflicting results do not allow any firm conclusion in this regard (USEPA, 2003; Solomon *et al.*, 2008). In 2006, the USEPA issued a cumulative risk assessment of triazine herbicides, concluding that they posed no harm that would result to the general US population, infants, children, or other consumers (USEPA, 2006). Nevertheless, atrazine is still being investigated for its potential effects on amphibian species (Rohr *et al.*, 2008; Rohr and McCoy, 2010). Furthermore, the known hormonal effects of atrazine and other triazines call for careful evaluation of endocrine-disrupting effects of these herbicides, which may contribute to developmental, reproductive, and metabolic disorders (Villanueva *et al.*, 2005; Lim *et al.*, 2009).

Phosphonomethyl Amino Acids

The two compounds of this class are glyphosate (*N*-phosphonomethyl glycine) and glufosinate (*N*-phosphonomethyl homoalanine). Both are broad-spectrum nonselective systemic herbicides used for postemergent control of annual and perennial plants, and are marketed primarily as the isopropylamine salt (glyphosate) or ammonium salt (glufosinate). Although both compounds contain a P=O moiety (Fig. 22-22), they are not organophosphates, but rather organophosphonates, and do not inhibit AChE (Farmer, 2010).

Glyphosate Glyphosate exerts its herbicidal action by inhibiting the enzyme 5-enolpyruvylshikimate-3-phosphate synthase, responsible for the synthesis of an intermediate in the biosynthesis of various amino acids (Casida, 2009). Although important in plant growth, this metabolic pathway is not present in mammals, providing a high selectivity to this compound. The toxicity profile of technical grade glyphosate is unremarkable (Williams *et al.*, 2000; Farmer, 2010). Oral and dermal LD_{50} are >5000 mg/kg, and chronic toxicity studies show only nonspecific effects, such as failure to gain weight. It has no teratogenic, developmental, or reproductive effects. Genotoxicity and carcinogenicity studies in animals were negative; on the basis of all available evidence glyphosate has been classified as a Group E compound (evidence of noncarcinogenicity in humans) by the USEPA (Farmer, 2010).

Glyphosate is one of the most widely used herbicides in the United States (Table 22-4) and worldwide, and the development of transgenic crops that can tolerate glyphosate treatment has expanded its utilization. Given its widespread use, including the home and garden market, accidental or intentional exposure to glyphosate is inevitable. For example, in the period 2001–2003, there were over 13,000 reports to the American Association of Poisons Control Centers Toxic Exposure Surveillance System relating to glyphosate exposure (Bradberry et al., 2004b). There was a major adverse outcome in 18 patients, and five died. Several other cases of glyphosate ingestions have been published, with a 10% to 15% mortality rate (Sawada et al., 1988; Talbot et al., 1998; Lee et al., 2000; Stella and Ryan, 2004; Bradberry et al., 2004b). Given the low acute toxicity of glyphosate itself, the attention has focused on its formulation, which contains surfactants to aid its penetration. The most widely used glyphosate product is Roundup®, which is formulated as a concentrate containing water, 41% glyphosate (as isopropylamine salt), and 15% polyoxyethyleneamine (POEA). Animal studies suggest that the acute toxicity of this glyphosate formulation is due to the surfactant POEA, which has an oral LD in rat of 1200 mg/kg (Bradberry et al., 2004b). It has been recently suggested that POEA may increase cell permeability to glyphosate (Benachour and Seralini, 2009). Mild intoxication results mainly in transient gastrointestinal symptoms, while moderate or severe poisoning presents with gastrointestinal bleeding, hypotension, pulmonary dysfunction, and renal damage (Talbot et al., 1998). Dietary exposure of the general population has been estimated to be very low, only 1% to 3% of the reference dose (Farmer, 2010).

Glufosinate Glufosinate is a nonselective contact herbicide that acts by irreversibly inhibiting glutamine synthetase (Ebert et al., 1990; Casida, 2009). Plants die as a consequence of the increased levels of ammonia and deficiency of glutamine, leading to inhibition of photorespiration and photosynthetic processes (Ujvary, 2010). Mammals have other metabolizing systems that can cope with the effects on glutamine synthetase activity to a certain limit. In brain, however, inhibition of >10% of this enzyme activity is considered an adverse effect (EFSA, 2005). Glufosinate undergoes very limited metabolism and 80% to 90% is excreted unchanged in the feces (Ujvary, 2010). It has relatively low acute toxicity (oral LD_{50} in rat is 1.5 g/kg), and chronic toxicity studies provided a NOAEL of 4.5 mg/kg per day, based on decreased glutamine synthetase activity. There is no evidence of genotoxicity or carcinogenicity, or direct effects on reproductive performance and fertility. Developmental toxic effects were found in rat and rabbit, but were considered not to be relevant to humans under normal handling or use (Schulte-Hermann et al., 2006). The most commonly used form of glufosinate is as ammonium salt, which is formulated with an anionic surfactant. Several cases of acute human poisoning from glufosinate ammonium-containing products have been reported, particularly in Japan, due to suicidal intent or accidental misuse. Symptoms include gastrointestinal effects, impaired respiration, neurologic disturbance, and cardiovascular effects (Koyama et al., 1994; Watanabe and Sano, 1998; Ujvary, 2010). Although glufosinate does not inhibit cholinesterase, a reduction of RBC and plasma cholinesterase was found in poisoned patients. As is the case for glyphosate, a role for the surfactant in the acute toxicity has been proposed, particularly with regard to the cardiovascular effects (Ujvary, 2010).

FUNGICIDES

Fungal diseases are virtually impossible to control without chemical application. Fungicidal chemicals are derived from a variety of structures, from simple inorganic compounds, such as copper sulfate, to complex organic compounds. The majority of fungicides are surface or plant protectants, and are applied prior to potential infection by fungal spores, either to plants or to postharvest crops.

Other fungicides can be used therapeutically, to cure plants when an infestation has already begun. Still others are used as systemic fungicides, which are absorbed and distributed throughout the plant.

With few exceptions, fungicides have low acute toxicity in mammals. However, several produce positive results in genotoxicity tests and some have carcinogenic potentials. The effects are often associated with the mechanisms by which these compounds act on their targets, the fungi. A 1987 evaluation by the National Research Council concluded that fungicides, although accounting for only 7% of all pesticide sales, and less than 10% of all pounds of pesticides applied, accounted for about 60% of estimated dietary oncogenic risk (NRC, 1987). Some fungicides have been associated with severe epidemics of poisoning, and have thus been banned. Methylmercury was associated with poisoning in Iraq when treated grains were consumed (Bakir et al., 1973). Hexachlorobenzene (HCB), used in the 1940s–1950s to treat seed grains, was associated with an epidemic of poisoning in Turkey from 1955 to 1959 (Cam and Nigogosyan, 1963). HCB has a high cumulative toxicity and caused a syndrome called black sore, characterized by blistering and epidermolysis of the skin, pigmentation, and scarring. It also causes porphyria as well as hepatomegaly and immunosuppression (Ecobichon, 2001a). The main classes of fungicides currently in use are discussed below; additional discussions of fungicide use and toxicity can be found in Hayes (1982) and in Edwards et al. (1991).

Captan and Folpet

Captan and folpet are broad-spectrum protectant fungicides; together with captafol, which was taken off the market in 1988, they are called chloroalkylthio fungicides, due to the presence of side chains containing chlorine, carbon, and sulfur (Fig. 22-23). Captan was first registered in the United States in 1949, and folpet followed a few years later. As for most fungicides, captan and folpet have low acute oral and dermal toxicity ($LD_{50} \cong 5g/kg$), while they are very toxic by the i.p. route ($LD_{50} = 40$–50 mg/kg). They are potent eye irritants, but only mild skin irritants. Dermal absorption is low. Both are extensively and rapidly metabolized in mammals, through hydrolysis and thiol interactions, with thiophosgene being a common metabolite (Gordon, 2010). Captan and folpet, as well as thiophosgene, are mutagenic in in vitro tests; however, in vivo mutagenicity tests are mostly negative, possibly because of the rapid degradation of these compounds (Arce et al., 2010). Both fungicides induce the development of duodenal tumors in mice, and on this basis, they were classified by the USEPA as probable human carcinogens (Category B2). However, the mode of action for these tumors is thought to be not related to mutagenicity, but instead to be dependent on irritation and cell loss in the intestinal villi, followed by a compensatory increase in proliferation in the crypt compartment (Gordon, 2010). For this reason the USEPA changed the classification of captan to "not likely to be a human carcinogen when used according to label directions" (Gordon, 2007). Additionally, tumors observed in rats (renal adenomas and uterine sarcomas) are considered not to be treatment-related (Gordon, 2007, 2010). Captan and folpet share a common mechanism of toxicity with regard to the development of duodenal tumors in mice, as well as other toxicity end points, and are considered for cumulative risk assessment under the FQPA (Bernand and Gordon, 2000). The margin of exposure (MOE) for both captan and folpet is ~1,000,000, suggesting that neither should pose a cancer risk for humans. Reentry intervals for farm workers are now based on the potential for eye irritation (Gordon, 2010). Because of their structural similarity to the potent teratogen thalidomide (Fig. 22-23), chloroalkylthio fungicides have been extensively tested in reproductive/developmental studies in

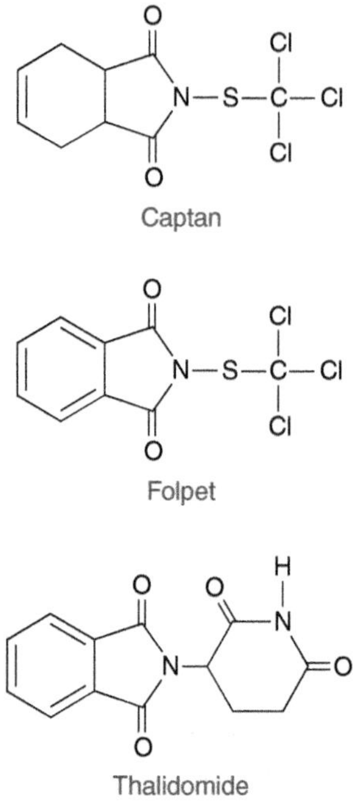

Captan

Folpet

Thalidomide

Figure 22-23. *Structures of the phthalimide fungicides captan and folpet. The structure of thalidomide is also shown, although phthalimides have been shown not to be teratogenic, despite structural similarities.*

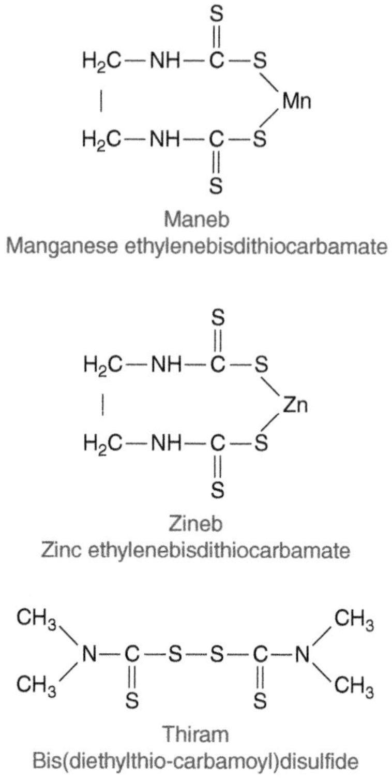

multiple species, but no evidence of teratogenicity has been found (McLaughlin *et al.*, 1969).

Dithiocarbamates

Dithiocarbamates are a group of fungicides that have been widely used since the 1940s to control about 400 fungal pathogens in a variety of crops. The nomenclature of many of these compounds arises from the metal cations with which they are associated; thus, there are, for example, maneb (Mn), ziram and zineb (Zn), and mancozeb (Mn and Zn) (Fig. 22-24). Thiram is an example of dithiocarbamate without a metal moiety (Fig. 22-24). The dithiocarbamates have low acute toxicity by the oral, dermal, and respiratory route; for example, the oral LD_{50}s in rat are >5 g/kg (Hurt *et al.*, 2010). However, chronic exposure is associated with adverse effects that may be due to the dithiocarbamate acid or the metal moiety. These compounds are metabolized to a common metabolite, ethylenethiourea (ETU); on average, 5% to 7.5% of the administered dose is converted to ETU on a weight basis (Hurt *et al.*, 2010). Formation of ETU is responsible for the effects of dithiocarbamates on the thyroid. This compound causes thyroid tumors in rats and mice, which result from the inhibition of the synthesis of the thyroid hormones thyroxine (T4) and T3. This leads to elevated serum levels of TSH, via feedback stimulation of the hypothalamus and the pituitary, and subsequent hypertrophy and hyperplasia of thyroid follicular cells, which progresses to adenomas and carcinomas (Chhabra *et al.*, 1992). Similarly, dithiocarbamates alter thyroid hormone levels, and cause thyroid hypertrophy. The hormonal mechanism of thyroid tumors implies a threshold model for hazard assessment. In addition, humans are expected to exhibit a lesser degree of sensitivity to thyroid inhibitors (Hurt *et al.*, 2010). ETU also causes liver tumors in mice, by yet unknown mechanisms, although levels of ETU resulting from fungicide metabolism at maximum tolerated doses are believed to be insufficient to produce hepatic tumors (Hurt *et al.*, 2010). Neither dithiocarbamates nor ETU are genotoxic in in vitro and in vivo tests.

Maneb
Manganese ethylenebisdithiocarbamate

Zineb
Zinc ethylenebisdithiocarbamate

Thiram
Bis(diethylthio-carbamoyl)disulfide

Figure 22-24. *Structures of three dithiocarbamate fungicides.*

Developmental toxicity and teratogenicity are observed with dithiocarbamates and ETU at maternally toxic doses, particularly in rats. These effects are ascribed to an effect of ETU on the thyroid. A key concern with chemicals affecting thyroid functions is their potential developmental neurotoxicity, given the essential role of thyroid hormones in brain development (Chan and Kilby, 2000), and this deserves further investigation. There is also some evidence that dithiocarbamates may cause neurotoxicity by mechanisms not involving ETU. High doses of several of these compounds cause hind limb paralysis, which is possibly related to the release of the carbon disulfide moiety from a common metabolite, ethylene bisisothiocyanate-sulfide (EBIS) (Johnson *et al.*, 1998; Hurt *et al.*, 2010). Chronic exposure to maneb has been associated with parkinsonism, which is likely ascribed to exposure to the manganese moiety, rather than the dithiocarbamate (Ferraz *et al.*, 1988; Meco *et al.*, 1994), particularly when there is coexposure with paraquat (Costello *et al.*, 2009). Maneb has also been shown to produce nigrostriatal degeneration when given in combination with paraquat (Thiruchelvam *et al.*, 2000), and to potentiate the neurotoxicity of MPTP (McGrew *et al.*, 2000). It has been shown that maneb affects dopaminergic neurons by inhibiting mitochondrial functions (Zhang *et al.*, 2003). This fungicide has been recently withdrawn from the US market (Keigwin, 2010).

The structure of dithiocarbamate fungicides resembles that of disulfiram, a compound used therapeutically to produce intolerance to alcohol, by virtue of its ability to inhibit aldehyde dehydrogenase. Interactions of dithiocarbamates with alcohol, leading to elevation in acetaldehyde levels, have been reported (Edwards *et al.*, 1991).

Chlorothalonil

Chlorothalonil is a halogenated benzonitrile fungicide (Fig. 22-25), first registered in the United States in 1966, and widely used to treat vegetable, ornamental, and orchard diseases (Table 22-4).

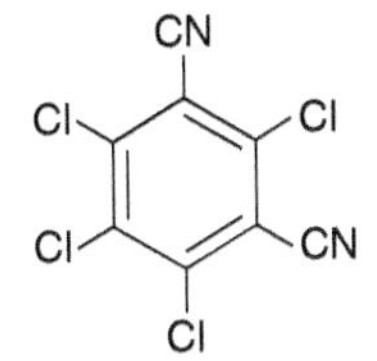

Figure 22-25. *Structures of the fungicides chlorothalonil and benomyl.*

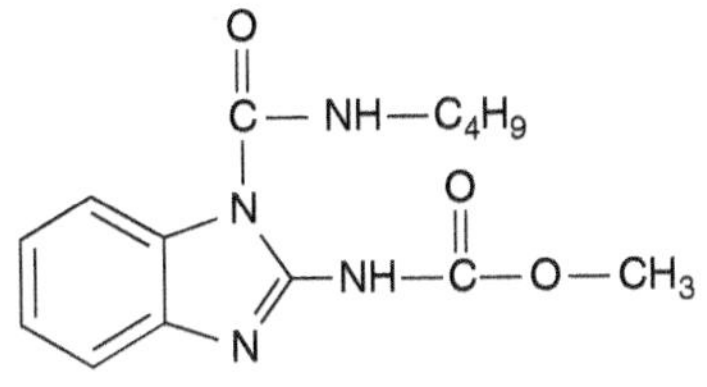

While oral and dermal toxicities are low (LD$_{50}$s = 5–10 g/kg), it is highly toxic by the intraperitoneal and inhalation routes. It also causes severe irreversible eye lesions in the rabbit, because of its irritant properties, but causes skin irritation only after repeated dermal applications. Dermal absorption is low, but following oral administration, chlorothalonil is rapidly absorbed and metabolized through glutathione conjugation, with excretion occurring primarily through the feces. Chlorathalonil is not mutagenic in in vitro and in vivo tests; however, tumors in the forestomach and the kidney have been found in chronic toxicity studies in both rats and mice, but not in dogs (Parsons, 2010). Such tumors are believed to be due to regenerative hyperplasia, and it is assumed that a threshold can be established for carcinogenicity (Parsons, 2010). Chlorothalonil is not a reproductive or developmental toxicant. Known adverse effects in humans are limited to its irritant effects on the eye and the skin.

Benzimidazoles

Benomyl is the main representative of this class of fungicides (Fig. 22-25). It inhibits fungal growth by inhibiting microtubule assembly in fungi, with minor effects in plants or mammals. Acute toxicity is low, while chronic studies have found effects in the liver, testes, bone marrow, and gastrointestinal tract (Mull and Hershberger, 2001). Allergic contact dermatitis caused by foliar benomyl residues has been reported (O'Malley, 2010). Because of its ability to disrupt microtubule assembly during cell division, benomyl causes chromosomal aberrations (aneuploidy) both in vitro and in vivo, but does not interact directly with DNA. Liver tumors have been observed in chronic oncogenicity studies in mice. The action on dividing cells has also raised concern for benomyl's potential teratogenicity and developmental toxicity. Teratogenic effects were observed following administration of high doses of benomyl and carbendazim (a metabolite of benomyl, which is commercialized as a fungicide, but not in the United States) to rats and zebrafish (Mull and Hershberger, 2001; Kim *et al.*, 2009). However, such effects were not seen in feeding studies in rats or rabbits. Anecdotal evidence suggests that maternal exposure to benomyl may result in anophthalmia in humans, but epidemiological studies did not demonstrate any convincing association (Spagnolo *et al.*, 1994). Benomyl has been shown in animals to affect the male reproductive system (decreased testicular and epididymal weight and reduced sperm count), but the mechanisms underlying these effects remain unclear (Kim *et al.*, 2009).

Inorganic and Organometal Fungicides

Several inorganic and organic metal compounds are, or have been, used as fungicides (Clarkson, 2001). The fungicidal activity of soluble copper salts was discovered as early as 1807, and by 1890 copper sulfate found extensive use, particularly in the formulation known as Bordeaux mixture (copper sulfate and calcium hydroxide). Copper sulfate has overall low toxicity and remains one of the most widely used fungicides (Table 22-4). Among organotin compounds, triphenyltin acetate is used as a fungicide, while tributyltin has long been utilized as an antifouling agent. However, because of its adverse ecological effects, particularly on oysters, its use has been banned as of 2008. It has been replaced in antifouling paints by copper, often in combination with "booster" biocides, such as the fungicides chlorothalonil or zineb, or the herbicide diuron (Dafforn *et al.*, 2011). Triphenyltin has moderate to high acute toxicity, but may cause reproductive toxicity and endocrine disruption (Golub and Doherty, 2004). Organic mercury compounds, such as methylmercury, were used extensively as fungicides in the past for the prevention of seed-borne diseases in grains and cereals. Given their high toxicity, particularly neurotoxicity, and large episodes of human poisoning (Bakir *et al.*, 1973), their use has since been banned. A discussion of organometal compounds is found in Chap. 23.

RODENTICIDES

Rats and mice can cause health and economic damages to humans. Rodents are vectors for several human diseases, including plague, endemic rickettsiosis, spirochetosis, and several others; they can occasionally bite people; they can consume large quantities of postharvest stored foods, and can contaminate foodstuffs with urine, feces, and hair, which may cause diseases. Hence, there is a need to control rodent populations. Limiting their access to feed and harborage, and trapping are two approaches; however, rodenticides still play, and will likely continue to play, an important role in rodent control. To be effective, yet safe, a rodenticide must satisfy several criteria: (a) the poison must be very effective in the target species once incorporated into bait in small quantity; (b) baits containing the poison must not excite bait shyness, so that the animal will continue to eat it; (c) the manner of death must be such that survivors do not become suspicious of its cause; and (d) it should be species-specific, with considerable lower toxicity to other animals (Murphy, 1986; Ecobichon, 2001a; Pelfrene, 2010).

The compounds used as rodenticides comprise a diverse range of chemical structures having a variety of mechanisms of action. The ultimate goal is to obtain the highest species selectivity; in some cases (eg, norbormide) advantage has been taken of the physiology and biochemistry unique to rodents. With other rodenticides, the sites of action are common to most mammals, but advantage is taken of the habits of the pest animal and/or the usage, thereby minimizing toxicity for nontarget species. Because rodenticides are used in baits that are often placed in inaccessible places, widespread exposures or contaminations are unlikely. However, toxicological problems can arise from acute accidental ingestions or from suicidal/homicidal attempts. In particular, poison centers receive thousands of calls every year related to accidental ingestions of rodenticide baits by children, most of which resolve without serious consequences.

Fluoroacetic Acid and Its Derivatives

Sodium fluoroacetate (Compound 1080) and fluoroacetamide are the main representatives of this class of rodenticides. They are white in color and odorless, and due to their high mammalian toxicity, their use is restricted to trained personnel. Both compounds have indeed high acute toxicity (oral LD_{50}s in the rat ≤ 2 and 13 mg/kg, respectively). The main targets of toxicity are the central nervous system and the heart. Fluoroacetate is incorporated into fluoracetyl-coenzyme A, which condenses with oxaloacetate to form fluorocitrate, which inhibits mitochondrial aconitase. This results in inhibition of the Krebs cycle, leading to lowered energy production, reduced oxygen consumption, and reduced cellular concentration of ATP. Blockage of energy metabolism is believed to account for most signs of toxicity, although some may be due to accumulation of citrate, which is a potent chelator of calcium ions (Pelfrene, 2010). Since 1946, when sodium fluoroacetate was introduced in the United States, several cases of human poisoning have been reported. Initial gastrointestinal symptoms are followed by severe cardiovascular effects (ventricular tachycardia, fibrillation, hypotension), as well as CNS effects (agitation, convulsions, coma). The estimated lethal dose in humans ranges from 2 to 10 mg/kg. There is no specific antidote for sodium fluoroacetate. Monacetin (60% glycerol monoacetate) has proved beneficial in the treatment of poisoned primates. Use of procainamide (for cardiac arrhythmia) and barbiturates (to control seizures) is also indicated. Use of Compound 1080 in the United States is severely restricted primarily because of toxicity to nontarget animals, such as dogs.

Thioureas

The discovery of ANTU occurred fortuitously in the mid 1940s in the Psychobiological Laboratory of Curt Richter in Baltimore. While studying thioureas, favored by geneticists for taste tests because they are so bitter to some people and tasteless to others, Richter discovered that ANTU was lethal yet tasteless to rodents, while being of low toxicity to humans (Keiner, 2005). A wide range of acute oral LD_{50} values has been reported for different species, the rat being the most sensitive at 6 mg/kg, and the monkey the least susceptible at 4 g/kg. The main target of toxicity is the lung, where ANTU causes marked edema of the subepithelial spaces of the alveolar walls. ANTU is believed to be biotransformed to a reactive intermediate that binds to lung macromolecules; however, the exact mechanism of its toxicity is unknown. Young rats are resistant to the chemical, whereas older rats become tolerant to it; both situations have been ascribed to developmentally low, or to ANTU-induced inhibition of, microsomal enzymes involved in its bioactivation (Boyd and Neal, 1976). There are no reports of human poisonings with ANTU. However, several cases involving a combination of chloralose and ANTU were reported in France; symptoms included motor agitation and coma, both characteristic of chloralose poisonings, and pulmonary effects, due to ANTU, but all patients recovered (Pelfrene, 2010). Suggestions that the presence of an impurity in ANTU, β-naphthylamine, may increase risk of bladder cancer remain unsubstantiated (Case, 1966; Pelfrene, 2010).

Anticoagulants

Following the report of a hemorrhagic disorder in cattle that resulted from the ingestion of spoiled sweet clover silage, the hemorrhagic agent was identified by University of Wisconsin biochemistry professor Karl Paul Link in 1939 as bishydroxycoumarin (dicoumarol). In 1948, a more potent synthetic congener was introduced as an extremely effective rodenticide; the compound was named warfarin, as an acronym derived from the name of the patent holder, the Wisconsin Alumni Research Foundation (Majerus and Tollefsen, 2006). In addition to their use as rodenticides, coumarin derivatives, including warfarin itself, are used as anticoagulant drugs and

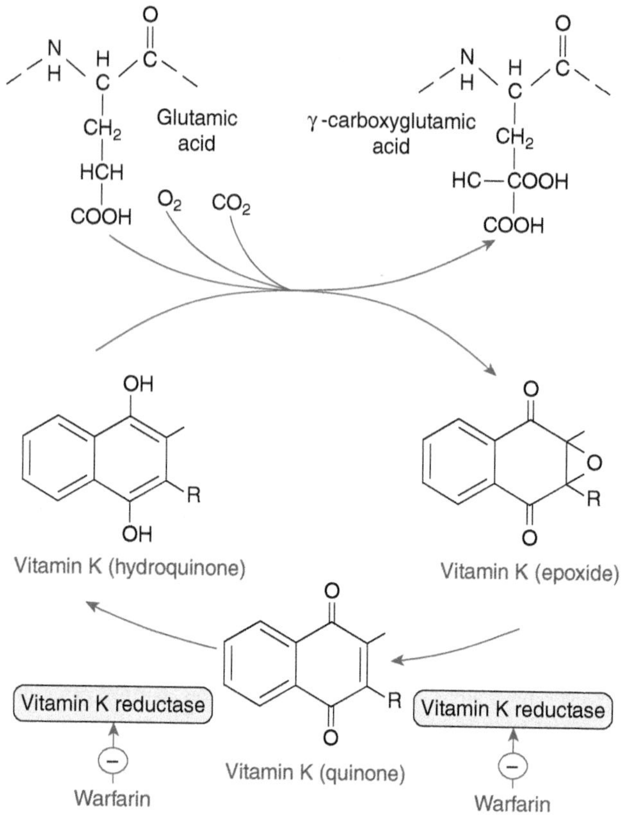

Figure 22-26. *Site of action of the anticoagulant rodenticide warfarin.* Reduced vitamin K (hydroquinone) serves as cofactor for the conversion of glutamic acid to γ-carboxyglutamic acid in the peptide chains of coagulation factors II, VII, IX, and X. During this reaction, vitamin K is oxidized to an epoxide that is then reduced to quinone and hydroquinone by vitamin K reductase, which is inhibited by warfarin.

have become a mainstay for prevention of thromboembolic disease (Majerus and Tollefsen, 2006). Coumarins antagonize the action of vitamin K in the synthesis of clotting factors (factors II, VII, IX, and X). Their specific mechanism involves inhibition of the enzyme vitamin K epoxide reductase, which regenerates reduced vitamin K necessary for sustained carboxylation and synthesis of relevant clotting factors (Fig. 22-26). The acute oral toxicity of warfarin in rats is approximately 50 to 100 mg/kg, while the 90-day dose LD_{50} has been reported as 0.077 mg/kg, indicating that multiple doses are required before toxicity develops.

Human poisonings by these agents are rare because they are dispersed in grain-based baits. However, there is a significant number of suicide or homicide attempts or of accidental consumption of warfarin. One often reported case involved a Korean family that consumed a diet of corn containing warfarin over a two-week period. Symptoms (massive bruises, hematomata, gum and nasal hemorrhage) appeared about 10 days after the beginning of the warfarin consumption. Consumption of warfarin in this episode was estimated to be in the order of 1 to 2 mg/kg per day (Lange and Terveer, 1954). Monitoring of anticoagulant therapy is done by measuring prothrombin time (PT) in comparison to normal pooled plasma. Values of international normalized ratio (INR) are then derived, with a target value of two to three. In case of poisoning, PT is significantly longer, and leads to severe internal bleeding. When INR is above five, vitamin K can be given as an antidote (Burkhart, 2001).

The appearance of rats resistant to warfarin and to other early anticoagulant rodenticides led to the development of "second-generation" anticoagulants. Some are coumarins, such as the "superwarfarins" brodifacoum or difenacoum, while others are indane-1,3-dione derivatives (diphacinone, chlorophacinone). These compounds essentially act like warfarin, but have prolonged half-lives (eg, brodifacoum 156 hours vs warfarin 37 hours), and cause very long-lasting inhibition of coagulation. Some are extremely toxic to most mammalian species; for example, the oral LD_{50} of brodifacoum is about 0.3 mg/kg in rat, rabbit, and dog (Pelfrene, 2010). During the period 2000–2003, Poison Centers in the United States reported a total of 65,891 exposures to these long-lasting anticoagulant rodenticides; of these 89% involved children under the age of six, and 96% were unintentional. Of the latter only 0.2% developed a moderate or major effect (Caravati *et al.*, 2007).

Other Compounds

Norbormide This compound was introduced in 1964 as a selective rodenticide, lethal to rats but not to other rodent species (Pelfrene, 2010). Norbormide shows a remarkable selectivity in toxicity; oral LD_{50} in rat is about 5 to 10 mg/kg, while it is >2000 mg/kg in mice. In other species, 1000 mg/kg produces no effects. Such species difference in toxicity seems to be accounted for by differences in response of the peripheral blood vessels to norbormide-induced vasoconstriction; however, the exact mechanisms of this effect and of the species specificity are not known. No cases of human intoxication with norbormide have been reported (Pelfrene, 2010).

Zinc Phosphide The toxicity of this agent can be accounted for by the phosphine gas (PH_3) formed on ingestion following a hydrolytic reaction with water in the stomach. Phosphine causes widespread cellular toxicity with necrosis of the gastrointestinal tract and injury to liver and kidney. The exact mechanism of toxicity has not been elucidated, but may involve generation of oxidative stress rather than inhibition of cytochrome *c* oxidase as initially suggested (Proudfoot, 2009). Aluminum phosphide and magnesium phosphide, which also generate phosphine, are mainly used as fumigants (Lyubimov and Garry, 2010). Several cases of human poisoning have been reported with gastrointestinal, cardiovascular, hepatic, and electrolytic balance effects (Ecobichon, 2001a; Proudfoot, 2009). Additional inorganic compounds that have been used as rodenticides include thallium sulfate and arsenic salts. Thallium sulfate has the unusual feature of causing extensive alopecia (hair loss); because of its high acute toxicity in nontarget species, it was banned in the United States in 1972 (Clarkson, 2001).

Other Some rodenticides used in the past that have become obsolete include strychnine, an extremely poisonous alkaloid derived from the seeds of *nux vomica*. Strychnine antagonizes the effect of the inhibitory neurotransmitter glycine, and is a potent convulsant. Red squill (sea onion) and its bioactive principle, scilliroside, affect the cardiovascular and central nervous systems and cause emesis; the inability of rodents to vomit explains the rather selective action in these species (Ujvary, 2010). Pyriminil is a substituted urea, introduced as a rodenticide in 1975, but withdrawn in the United States a few years later. This compound targets complex I in the mitochondria, and there are many reports of human poisoning in the short period of its use (Pelfrene, 2010). As many other ureas, it has diabetogenic properties.

FUMIGANTS

A large number of compounds are used for soil or structural fumigation, or for fumigating postharvest commodities. They are active toward insects, mites, nematodes, weed seeds, fungi, or rodents, and have in common the property of being in the gaseous form at the time they exert their pesticidal action. They can be liquids that readily vaporize (eg, ethylene dibromide), solids that can release a toxic gas on reaction with water (eg, phosphine released by aluminum phosphide), or gases (eg, methyl bromide). For soil fumigation, the compound is injected directly into the soil, which is then covered with plastic sheeting or other tarping materials, which are then sealed and kept in place for several days. By eliminating unwanted pests, this treatment enhances the quality of the crops and increases yield. For structural fumigation, the commercial or residential structure is covered by a tent, fumigated, and then aerated. Fumigation of postharvest commodities, such as wheat, cereals, and fruits, to eradicate pest infestations, typically occurs where the commodities are stored (eg, warehouses, grain elevators, ship holds). After treatment, mechanical ventilation aerates the commodity until concentration of the fumigant decreases to safe levels.

Compounds used as fumigants are usually nonselective, highly reactive, and cytotoxic. They provide a potential hazard, primarily for applicators, from the standpoint of inhalation exposure, and to a minor degree for dermal exposure or ingestion, in case of solids or liquids. Fumigant residues in food commodities are usually extremely low. Several fumigants used in the past are no longer marketed because of toxicological concerns. These include, for example, carbon disulfide, which is neurotoxic; carbon tetrachloride, a potent hepatotoxicant; 1,2-dibromo-3-chloropropane, a male reproductive toxicant; and ethylene dibromide, a carcinogen. Their toxicity is discussed in other sections of the book. Some of the most commonly used fumigants are discussed below.

Methyl Bromide

Methyl bromide (CH_3Br) is a broad-spectrum pesticide, used for soil fumigation, commodity treatment, and structural fumigation. It has been used as a fumigant for over 50 years, and its use is strictly controlled, and restricted to certified applicators wearing appropriate personal protection equipment. Since the mid 1990s, global use of methyl bromide has substantially decreased, because of environmental and toxicological concerns (Ruzo, 2006). Methyl bromide is thought to contribute to ozone depletion in the stratosphere. In 1987, with the signing of the Montreal Protocol on Substances that Deplete the Ozone Layer, the international community initiated a series of steps to reduce emissions of ozone-depleting products, including methyl bromide. As of January 2005, methyl bromide was officially phased out in the United States, while developing countries have until 2015 to phase out methyl bromide production (Ajwa *et al.*, 2010). Concerns on certain toxicological aspects of methyl bromide have also contributed to its decreasing use, and to the search of viable alternatives (Ruzo, 2006; Schneider *et al.*, 2003). Yet, as of 2002, this compound remained one of the most extensively used pesticides in the United States (Table 22-4), likely for convenience and economic reasons (Norman, 2005; McCook, 2006).

The acute toxicity of methyl bromide relates to both its concentration and the duration of exposure. For example, LC_{50} values in rats were 2833 ppm for a 30-minute exposure, and 302 ppm for an eight-hour exposure (Piccirillo and Piccirillo, 2010). Between 1953 and 1981, 301 cases of systemic poisoning and 60 fatalities resulted from use of methyl bromide as a fumigant (Alexeef and Kilgore, 1983). Additional cases of human intoxication have since been reported (Hertzstein and Cullen, 1990). Acute exposure results in respiratory, gastrointestinal, and neurologic symptoms; the latter include lethargy, headache, seizures, paresthesias, peripheral neuropathy, and ataxia, and are considered to be more relevant than other toxic effects for human risk assessment (Alexeef and Kilgore, 1983; Lifshitz and Gavrilov, 2000; Piccirillo and Piccirillo, 2010).

Acute and chronic neurotoxicity studies in rats have demonstrated behavioral effects and morphological lesions, which were concentration- and time-dependent (Piccirillo and Piccirillo, 2010). Long-lasting behavioral and neuropsychiatric effects are also seen in humans (De Haro *et al.*, 1997; Lifshitz and Gavrilov, 2000; Magnavita, 2009). The mechanism(s) underlying methyl bromide neurotoxicity are not known. Depletion of GSH in brain areas was observed following exposure of rats to methyl bromide (140 ppm for six hours per day, for five days) (Davenport *et al.*, 1992). This may be due to conjugation of methyl bromide with GSH. The role of GSH and the possible ensuing increase in oxidative stress in methyl bromide neurotoxicity remains, however, uncertain. In various subchronic toxicity studies, the NOELs for neurotoxicity range between 18 and 200 ppm, slightly higher than the overall NOEL (Piccirillo and Piccirillo, 2010). In chronic inhalation studies in rat, a primary effect was also degeneration of the nasal olfactory epithelium, which appears to be reversible (Piccirillo and Piccirillo, 2010).

Methyl bromide is positive in several genotoxicity tests in vitro and in vivo. Carcinogenicity studies produced carcinomas in the forestomach of rats following oral ingestion, and increased incidence of adenomas of the pituitary gland in male rats in an inhalation study. Other studies in rats and mice, however, provided no evidence of carcinogenicity. Methyl bromide is classified by IARC in Group 3 (not classifiable as to its carcinogenicity to humans), given the limited evidence in animals and the inadequate evidence in humans. As methyl bromide is an odorless and colorless gas, another fumigant, chloropicrin, which has a pungent odor and causes irritation of the eyes, is often used in conjunction with methyl bromide and other fumigant mixtures, to warn against potentially harmful exposures.

1,3-Dichloropropene

1,3-Dichloropropene ($C_3H_4Cl_2$), first introduced in 1945, is a soil fumigant, extensively utilized (see Table 22-4) for its ability to control soil nematodes. It has a moderate to high acute toxicity in animals (oral LD_{50} in rats: 130–713 mg/kg; dermal LD_{50}: >1200 mg/kg; inhalation LD_{50}: ~1000 ppm) (Stott *et al.*, 2001). Human fatalities following oral exposure have been reported (Hernandez *et al.*, 1994). 1,3-Dichloropropene is an irritant, and can cause redness and necrosis of the skin. It is extensively metabolized, with the mercapturic acid conjugate being the major urinary metabolite. Data on genotoxicity are contradictory, with positive in vitro, and mostly negative in vivo, results. However, some short-term genotoxicity assays may have been confused by the presence of a mutagen, epichlorohydrin, which was historically added as a stabilizing agent (Stott and Gallipudi, 2010). Carcinogenicity studies in rodents have found an increase in benign liver tumors in rats but not in mice, after oral administration (Stebbins *et al.*, 2000), and of benign lung adenomas in mice following inhalation exposure (Lomax *et al.*, 1989). The toxicology of 1,3-dichloropropene has been recently reviewed (Stott and Gallipudi, 2010). Because of its relatively favorable toxicological and environmental profiles, 1,3-dichloropropene is considered as one of the best alternatives to methyl bromide for use as a soil nematocide (Sanchez-Moreno *et al.*, 2009). However, it lacks herbicidal properties, and is often formulated with chloropicrin, which is a better fungicide (Ajwa *et al.*, 2010).

Metam-Sodium

Metam-sodium ($C_2H_4NNaS_2$) is a widely used soil fumigant (Table 22-4), whose toxic actions toward soil nematodes, fungi, and weed seeds are due to its hydrolysis product, methyl isothiocyanate

(MITC). In mammals, metam-sodium is metabolized in vivo to carbon disulfide and MITC (Pruett *et al.*, 2001). Acute toxicity is low, while on chronic exposure in various species, toxic effects in bladder, kidney, and liver have been reported. Metam-sodium is not genotoxic, and does not appear to be carcinogenic in rats, although results in mice are equivocal (Carlock and Dotson, 2010). Developmental and reproductive toxicities are seen only at maternally toxic doses. No neurotoxicity has been observed in acute and subchronic studies. In humans, metam-sodium can act as a contact sensitizer, inducing allergic dermatitis, possibly due to MITC. Main effects of acute exposure to MITC in the vapor state are irritated or burning eyes, nasal and throat irritation, nausea, coughing, and shortness of breath (Dourson *et al.*, 2010). In 1991, because of the derailment of a train car, approximately 19,000 gallons of metam-sodium was spilled into the Sacramento River in California, causing a large kill of aquatic organisms. Symptoms reported by exposed individuals included headache, eye irritation, nausea, shortness of breath, and dermatitis (Pruett *et al.*, 2001). Metam-sodium is increasingly being used as an alternative to methyl bromide (Ruzo, 2006), as it is effective against nematodes, weeds, and fungi (Ajwa *et al.*, 2010).

Sulfur Compounds

Elemental sulfur is considered the oldest of all pesticides, and its pesticidal properties were known to the ancient Greeks as early as 1000 BC (Tweedy, 1981). It is very effective for the control of many plant diseases, particularly fungal diseases, and still represents one of the most heavily used crop protection chemicals in the United States (Table 22-4). Sulfur finds its major use in grapes and tomatoes, and can be used in organic farming (Gammon *et al.*, 2010). Although generally considered an environmentally and toxicologically safe compound, elemental sulfur used as a fungicide can make the soil too acidic for the continuous optimal growth of a particular crop (Gammon *et al.*, 2010). The primary health effect in humans associated with the agricultural use of elemental sulfur is dermatitis (Gammon *et al.*, 2010). In ruminants, excessive sulfur ingestion can cause cerebrocortical necrosis (polioencephalomalacia), possibly due to its conversion by microorganisms in the rumen to hydrogen sulfide (Gammon *et al.*, 2010).

Sulfur dioxide (SO_2) is used as a fumigant, because of its antimicrobial properties, particularly in the treatment of grapes held in cold storage. It is a colorless gas with high water solubility, and is also used as a food additive (a preservative) (Gammon *et al.*, 2010).

Sulfuryl fluoride (SO_2F_2) is also used as a fumigant, particularly for structural fumigation and for postharvest fumigation of stored commodities. There is no evidence of developmental toxicity, mutagenicity, or carcinogenicity. On chronic exposure, the primary effect in multiple species is neurotoxicity, evidenced by microvacuolation in various brain areas. The mechanism is unknown (Eisenbrandt and Hotchkiss, 2010).

REFERENCES

Abdel-Rahman A, Shetty AK, Abou-Donia MB. Disruption of the blood–brain barrier and neuronal cell death in cingulate cortex, dentate gyrus, thalamus, and hypothalamus in a rat model of Gulf War syndrome. *Neurobiol Dis.* 2002;10:306–326.

Abel EL, Bammler TK, Eaton DL. Biotransformation of methyl parathion by glutathione *S*-transferases. *Toxicol Sci.* 2004;79:224–232.

Ackerman SJ, Kephart GM, Francis H, et al. Eosinophil degranulation: an immunologic determinant in the pathogenesis of the Mazzotti reaction in human onchocerciasis. *J Immunol.* 1990;144:3961–3969.

Adam A, Smith LL, Cohen GM. An evaluation of the redox cycling potencies of paraquat and nitrofurantoin in microsomal and lung slice systems. *Biochem Pharmacol.* 1990;40:1533–1539.

Ajdacic-Gross V, Weiss MG, Ring M, et al. Method of suicide: international suicide patterns derived from the WHO mortality data base. *Bull World Health Org.* 2008;86:726–732.

Ajwa H, Ntow WJ, Qin R, et al. Properties of soil fumigants and their fate in the environment. In: Krieger R, ed. *Hayes' Handbook of Pesticide Toxicology.* San Diego: Academic Press; 2010:315–330.

Akossoglou K, Malester B, Xu J, et al. Brain-specific deletion of neuropathy target esterase/Swiss Cheese results in neurodegeneration. *Proc Natl Acad Sci U S A.* 2004;101:5075–5080.

Alavanja MCR, Samanic C, Dosemeci M, et al. Use of agricultural pesticides and prostate cancer risk in the Agricultural Health Study cohort. *Am J Epidemiol.* 2003;157:800–814.

Aldridge JE, Seidler FJ, Meyer A, et al. Serotoninergic systems targeted by developmental exposure to chlorpyrifos: effects during different critical periods. *Environ Health Perspect.* 2003;111:1736–1743.

Alexeef GV, Kilgore WW. Methyl bromide. *Residue Rev.* 1983;88:101–153.

Alonso L, Lindsay SW, Armstrong JRM, et al. The effect of insecticide-treated bed nets on mortality of Gambian children. *Lancet.* 1991;337:1499–1502.

Altobelli D, Martire M, Maurizi S, et al. Interaction of formamidine pesticides with the presynaptic α_2-adrenoceptor regulating [^{3}H] noradrenaline release from rat hypothalamic synaptosomes. *Toxicol Appl Pharmacol.* 2001;172:179–185.

Alvarez-Pedrerol M, Ribas-Fito N, Torrent M, et al. Effects of PCBs, *p,p'*-DDT, *p,p'*-DDE, HCB, and β-HCH on thyroid function in preschool children. *Occup Environ Med.* 2008;65:452–457.

Anand SS, Bim KB, Padilla S, et al. Ontogeny of hepatic and plasma metabolism of deltamethrin in vitro: role in age-dependent acute neurotoxicity. *Drug Metab Dispos.* 2006b;34:389–397.

Anand SS, Bruckner JV, Haines WT, et al. Characterization of deltamethrin metabolism by rat plasma and liver microsomes. *Toxicol Appl Pharmacol.* 2006a;212:156–166.

Andrade SF, Sakate M. The comparative efficacy of yohimbine and atipamezole to treat amitraz intoxication in dogs. *Vet Hum Toxicol.* 2003;45:124–127.

Antwi FB, Shama LM, Peterson RK. Risk assessment for the insect repellents DEET and picaridin. *Regul Toxicol Pharmacol.* 2008;51:31–36.

Anway MD, Cupp AS, Uzumcu M, et al. Epigenetic transgenerational actions of endocrine disruptors and male fertility. *Science.* 2005;306:1466–1468.

Arce GT, Gordon EB, Cohen SM, et al. Genetic toxicology of folpet and captan. *Crit Rev Toxicol.* 2010;40:546–574.

Arena JP, Liu KK, Paress PS, et al. The mechanism of action of avermectins in *Caenorhabditis elegans*: correlation between activation of glutamate-sensitive chloride current, membrane binding and biological activity. *J Parasitol.* 1995;81:286–294.

Ashby J, Kier L, Wilson AGE. Evaluation of the potential carcinogenicity and genetic toxicity to humans of the herbicide acetochlor. *Hum Exp Toxicol.* 1996;15:702–735.

Autor AP. *Biochemical Mechanisms of Paraquat Toxicity.* New York: Academic Press; 1974.

Aylward LL, Morgan MM, Arbuckle TE, et al. Biomonitoring data for 2,4-dichlorophenoxyacetic acid in the United States and Canada: interpretation in a public health risk assessment context using biomonitoring equivalents. *Environ Health Perspect.* 2010;118:177–181.

Badakhsh R, Lackovic M, Ratard R. Characteristics of pesticide-related hospitalizations, Louisiana, 1998-2007. *Public Health Rep.* 2010;125:457–467.

Baker SR, Wilkinson DF, eds. *The Effects of Pesticides on Human Health.* Princeton: Princeton Scientific Publishing; 1990:438.

Bakir F, Damluji SF, Amin-Zaki L, et al. Methylmercury poisoning in Iraq. *Science.* 1973;181:230–241.

Barbeau A, Roy M, Clourier L, et al. Environmental and genetic factors in the etiology of Parkinson's disease. *Adv Neurol.* 1986;45:299–306.

Barlow SM, Sullivan FM, Lines J. Risk assessment of the use of deltamethrin on bed nets for the prevention of malaria. *Food Chem Toxicol.* 2001;39:407–422.

Baron RL. Carbamate insecticides. In: Hayes WJ, Laws ER, eds. *Handbook of Pesticide Toxicology.* San Diego: Academic Press; 1991:1125–1189.

Barr DB, Allen R, Olsson AO, et al. Considerations of selective metabolites of organophosphorus pesticides in the United States population. *Environ Res.* 2005;99:314–326.

Bate MN, Thomson B, Garrett N. Reduction in organochlorine levels in the milk of New Zealand. *Arch Environ Health.* 2002;57:591–597.

Beard J. DDT and human health. *Sci Total Environ.* 2006;355:78–89.

Beeman RW, Matsumura F. Chlordimeform: a pesticide acting upon amine regulatory mechanisms. *Nature.* 1973;242:273–274.

Bell JW, Veltri JC, Page BC. Human exposures to *N,N*-diethyl-*m*-toluamide insect repellents reported to the American Association of Poison Control Centers 1993-1997. *Int J Toxicol.* 2002;21:341–352.

Benachour N, Seralini GE. Glyphosate formulations induce apoptosis and necrosis in human umbilical, embryonic, and placental cells. *Chem Res Toxicol.* 2009;22:97–105.

Benke G, Murphy SD. The influence of age on the toxicity and metabolism of methylparathion and parathion in male and female rats. *Toxicol Appl Pharmacol.* 1975;31:254–269.

Benowitz NL. Pharmacology of nicotine: addiction and therapeutics. *Annu Rev Pharmacol Toxicol.* 1996;36:597–613.

Bentley KS, Fletcher JL, Woodward MD. Chlorantraniliprole: an insecticide of the anthranilic diamide class. In: Krieger R, ed. *Hayes' Handbook of Pesticide Toxicology.* San Diego: Academic Press; 2010:2231–2242.

Bernand BK, Gordon EB. An evaluation of the common mechanism approach to the Food Quality Protection Act: captan and four related fungicides, a practical example. *Int J Toxicol.* 2000;19:43–61.

Berry C, LaVecchia C, Nicotera P. Paraquat and Parkinson's disease. *Cell Death Differ.* 2010;17:1115–1125.

Bertolote JM, Fleischmann A, Eddleston M, et al. Deaths from pesticide poisoning: a global response. *Br J Psychiatry.* 2006;189:201–203.

Bertsias GJ, Katonis P, Tzanakakis G, et al. Review of clinical and toxicological features of acute pesticide poisoning in Crete (Greece) during the period 1991-2001. *Med Sci Monit.* 2004;10:CR622–CR627.

Betarbet R, Sherer TB, Greenamyre JT. Animal models of Parkinson's disease. *Bioessays.* 2002;24:308–318.

Betarbet R, Sherer TB, MacKenzie G, et al. Chronic systemic pesticide exposure reproduces features of Parkinson's disease. *Nat Neurosci.* 2000;3:1301–1306.

Bismuth C, Garnier R, Dolly S, et al. Prognosis and treatment of paraquat poisoning: a review of 28 cases. *Clin Toxicol.* 1982;19:461–474.

Bismuth C, Inns RH, Marrs TC. Efficacy, toxicity and clinical use of oximes in anticholinesterases poisoning. In: Ballantyne B, Marrs TC, eds. *Clinical and Experimental Toxicology of Organophosphates and Carbamates.* Oxford: Butterworth-Heinemann; 1992:555–577.

Blondell JM. Decline in pesticide poisonings in the United States from 1995 to 2004. *Clin Toxicol.* 2007;45:589–592.

Boeckh J, Breer H, Geier M, et al. Acylated 1,3-aminopropanols as repellents against bloodsucking arthropods. *Pest Sci.* 1996;48:359–373.

Bouwman H, van de Berg H, Kylin H. DDT and malaria prevention: addressing the paradox. *Environ Health Perspect.* 2011;119:744–747.

Boyd MR, Neal RA. Studies on the mechanism of toxicity and of development of tolerance to the pulmonary toxic α-naphthylthiourea (ANTU). *Drub Metab Dispos.* 1976;4:314–322.

Bradberry SM, Cage SA, Proudfoot AT, et al. Poisoning due to pyrethroids. *Toxicol Rev.* 2005;24:93–106.

Bradberry SM, Proudfoot AT, Vale JA. Poisoning due to chlorophenoxy herbicides. *Toxicol Rev.* 2004a;23:65–73.

Bradberry SM, Proudfoot AT, Vale JA. Glyphosate poisoning. *Toxicol Rev.* 2004b;23:159–167.

Bradberry SM, Watt BE, Proudfoot AT, et al. Mechanisms of toxicity, clinical features, and management of acute chlorophenoxy herbicide poisoning: a review. *Clin Toxicol.* 2000;39:111–122.

Bravo A, Gill SS, Soberon M. Mode of action of *Bacillus thuringiensis* Cry and Cyt toxins and their potential for insect control. *Toxicon.* 2007;49:423–435.

Bravo A, Likitvatanavong S, Gill SS, Soberón M. *Bacillus thuringiensis*: a story of a successful bioinsecticide. *Insect Biochem Mol Biol.* 2011;41:423–431. doi:10.1016/j.jbmb.2011.02.006.

Breckenridge CB, Elridge JC, Stevens JJ, et al. Symmetrical triazine herbicides: a review of regulatory toxicity endpoints. In: Krieger R, ed. *Hayes' Handbook of Pesticide Toxicology.* San Diego: Academic Press; 2010:1711–1723.

Briassoulis G, Niarloglou M, Hatzis T. Toxic encephalopathy associated with use of DEET insect repellents: a case analysis of its toxicity in children. *Hum Exp Toxicol.* 2001;20:8–14.

Brooks GT. *Chlorinated Insecticides. Vol I. Technology and Application; and Vol. II. Biological and Environmental Aspects.* Cleveland: CRC Press; 1974:197,249.

Brooks GT. Interactions with the gamma-aminobutyric acid A-receptor: polychlorocycloalkanes and recent congeners and other ligands. In: Krieger R, ed. *Hayes' Handbook of Pesticide Toxicology.* San Diego: Academic Press; 2010:2065–2092.

Brusick DJ. An assessment of the genetic toxicity of atrazine: relevance to human health and environmental effects. *Mutat Res.* 1994;317:133–144.

Buckley NA, Eddleston M, Szinicz L. Oximes for acute organophosphate pesticide poisoning. *Cochrane Database Syst Rev.* 2005;(1):CD005085.

Burkhart KK. Anticoagulant rodenticides. In: Ford MD, Delaney KA, Ling LJ, Erickson T, eds. *Clinical Toxicology.* Philadelphia: WB Saunders Co; 2001:848–853.

Bus JS, Gibson JE. Paraquat: model for oxidant-initiated toxicity. *Environ Health Perspect.* 1984;55:37–46.

Cabral JR, Galendo D, Laval M, et al. Carcinogenicity studies with deltamethrin in mice and rats. *Cancer Lett.* 1990;49:147–152.

Cabras P, Caboni P, Cabras M, et al. Rotenone residues in olives and in olive oil. *J Agric Food Chem.* 2002;50:2576–2580.

Caksen H, Odabas D, Arslan S, et al. Report of eight children with amitraz intoxication. *Hum Exp Toxicol.* 2003;22:95–97.

Caldas ED, Rebelo FM, Heliodoro VO, et al. Poisonings with pesticides in the Federal District of Brazil. *Clin Toxicol.* 2008;46:1058–1063.

Calvert GM, Mehler LN, Alsop J, et al. Surveillance of pesticide-related illness and injury in humans. In: Krieger R, ed. *Hayes' Handbook of Pesticide Toxicology.* San Diego: Academic Press; 2010:1313–1369.

Cam C, Nigogosyan G. Acquired toxic porphyria cutanea tarda due to hexachlorobenzene. *JAMA.* 1963;183:88–91.

Campbell WC, ed. *Ivermectin and Abamectin.* New York: Springer Verlag; 1989:363.

Caravati EM, Erdman AR, Scharman EJ, et al. Long-lasting anticoagulant rodenticide poisoning: an evidence-based consensus guideline for out-of-hospital management. *Clin Toxicol.* 2007;45:1–22.

Carlock LL, Chen WL, Gordon EB, et al. Regulating and assessing risks of cholinesterase-inhibiting pesticides: divergent approaches and interpretations. *J Toxicol Environ Health B Crit Rev.* 1999;2:105–160.

Carlock LL, Dotson TA. Metam-sodium. In: Krieger R, ed. *Hayes' Handbook of Pesticide Toxicology.* San Diego: Academic Press; 2010:2293–2306.

Carr JA, Gentles A, Smith EE, et al. Response of larval *Xenopus laevis* to atrazine: assessment of growth, metamorphosis, and gonadal and laryngeal morphology. *Environ Toxicol Chem.* 2003;22:396–405.

Carson R. *Silent Spring.* Boston: Houghton Mifflin; 1962.

Case RAM. Tumours of the urinary tract as an occupational disease in several industries. *Ann R Coll Surg Engl.* 1966;39:213–235.

Casey P, Vale JA. Deaths from pesticide poisoning in England and Wales: 1945-1989. *Hum Exp Toxicol.* 1994;13:95–101.

Casida JE. Esterase inhibitors as pesticides. *Science.* 1964;146:1011–1017.

Casida JE. Pyrethrum flowers and pyrethroid insecticides. *Environ Health Perspect.* 1980;34:189–202.

Casida JE. Pest toxicology: the primary mechanisms of pesticide actions. *Chem Res Toxicol.* 2009;22:609–619.

Casida JE. Michael Elliot's billion dollar crystals and other discoveries in insecticide chemistry. *Pest Manag Sci.* 2010;66:1163–1170.

Casida JE, Gammon DW, Glickman AH, et al. Mechanisms of selective action of pyrethroid insecticides. *Annu Rev Pharmacol Toxicol.* 1983;23:413–438.

Chambers HW, Meek EC, Chambers JE. Chemistry of organophosphorus insecticides. In: Krieger R, ed. *Hayes' Handbook of Pesticide Toxicology.* San Diego: Academic Press; 2010a:1395–1398.

Chambers JE, Levi PE, eds. *Organophosphates: Chemistry, Fate and Effects.* San Diego: Academic Press; 1992:443.

Chambers JE, Meek EC, Chambers HW. The metabolism of organophosphorus insecticides. In: Krieger R, ed. *Hayes' Handbook of Pesticide Toxicology.* San Diego: Academic Press; 2010b:1399–1407.

Chan S, Kilby MD. Thyroid hormone and fetal central nervous system development. *J Endocrinol.* 2000;165:1–8.

Chao HR, Wang SL, Lin TC, et al. Levels of organochlorine pesticides in human milk from central Taiwan. *Chemosphere.* 2006;62:1776–1785.

Charles JM, Bond DM, Jeffries TK, et al. Chronic dietary toxicity/oncogenicity studies on 2,4-dichlorophenoxyacetic acid in rodents. *Fundam Appl Toxicol.* 1996;33:166–172.

Chen A, Rogan WJ. Nonmalarial infant deaths and DDT use for malaria control. *Emerg Infect Dis.* 2003;9:960–964.

Chen YY, Park NS, Lu TS. Suicide methods used by women in Korea, Sweden, Taiwan and the United States. *J Formos Med Assoc.* 2009;108:452–459.

Chester G. Worker exposure: methods and techniques. In: Krieger R, ed. *Hayes' Handbook of Pesticide Toxicology.* San Diego: Academic Press; 2010:1127–1138.

Chhabra RS, Eustis S, Haseman JK, et al. Comparative carcinogenicity of ethylene thiourea with or without perinatal exposure in rats and mice. *Fundam Appl Toxicol.* 1992;18:405–417.

Choi J, Hodgson E, Rose RL. Inhibitions of *trans*-permethrin hydrolysis in human liver fractions by chlorpyrifos oxon and carbaryl. *Drug Metab Drug Interact.* 2004;20:233–246.

Clark DG, McElligott TF, Hurst EW. The toxicity of paraquat. *Br J Ind Med.* 1966;23:126–132.

Clark JM, Matsumura F, eds. *Membrane Receptors and Enzymes as Targets of Insecticidal Action.* New York: Plenum Press; 1986:256.

Clarkson TW. Inorganic and organometal pesticides. In: Krieger R, ed. *Handbook of Pesticide Toxicology.* San Diego: Academic Press; 2001:1357–1428.

Cohn BA, Wolff MS, Cirillo PM, et al. DDT and breast cancer in young women: new data on the significance of age of exposure. *Environ Health Perspect.* 2007;115:1406–1414.

Colborn T. A case for revisiting the safety of pesticides: a closer look at neurodevelopment. *Environ Health Perspect.* 2006;114:10–17.

Cole LM, Casida JE. Polychlorocycloalkane insecticide-induced convulsions in mice in relation to disruption of the GABA-regulated chloride ionophore. *Life Sci.* 1986;39:1855–1862.

Cole TB, Walter BJ, Shih DM, et al. Toxicity of chlorpyrifos and chlorpyrifos oxon in a transgenic mouse model of the human paraoxonase (PON1) Q192R polymorphism. *Pharmacogenet Genomics.* 2005;15:589–598.

Colosio C, Tiramani M, Maroni M. Neurobehavioral effects of pesticides: state of the art. *Neurotoxicology.* 2003;24:577–591.

Colosio C, Vellere F, Moretto A. Epidemiological studies of anticholinesterase pesticide poisoning: global impact. In: Satoh T, Gupta RC, eds. *Anticholinesterase Pesticides: Metabolism, Neurotoxicity and Epidemiology.* Hoboken, NJ: Wiley & Sons; 2010:343–355.

Cooper RL, Lamb JC, Barlow SM, et al. A tiered approach to life testing for agricultural risk assessment. *Crit Rev Toxicol.* 2006;36:69–98.

Cooper RL, Laws SC, Das PC, et al. Atrazine and reproductive function: mode and mechanism of action studies. *Birth Defects Res (Pt B).* 2007;80:98–112.

Cooper RL, Stoker TE, Tyrey L, et al. Atrazine disrupts the hypothalamic control of pituitary-ovarian function. *Toxicol Sci.* 2000;53:297–307.

Costa LG. Toxicology of pesticides: a brief history. In: Costa LG, Galli CL, Murphy SD, eds. *Toxicology of Pesticides: Experimental, Clinical and Regulatory Perspectives.* Heidelberg: Springer Verlag; 1987:1–10.

Costa LG. Organophosphorus compounds. In: Galli CL, Manzo L, Spencer PS, eds. *Recent Advances in Nervous System Toxicology.* New York: Plenum Publishing Corp; 1988:203–246.

Costa LG. Pesticide exposure. Differential risk for neurotoxic outcomes due to enzyme polymorphisms. *Clin Occup Environ Med.* 2001;1:511–523.

Costa LG. Current issues in organophosphate toxicology. *Clin Chim Acta.* 2006;366:1–13.

Costa LG, Cole TB, Jarvik GP, et al. Functional genomics of the paraoxonase (PON1) polymorphisms: effect on pesticide sensitivity, cardiovascular disease and drug metabolism. *Annu Rev Med.* 2003;54:371–392.

Costa LG, Cole TB, Vitalone A, et al. Measurement of paraoxonase (PON1) status as a potential biomarker of susceptibility to organophosphate toxicity. *Clin Chim Acta*. 2005;352:37–47.

Costa LG, Furlong CE. Paraoxonase 1: structure, function and polymorphisms. In: Satoh T, Gupta RC, eds. *Anticholinesterase Pesticides: Metabolism, Neurotoxicity, and Epidemiology*. Hoboken, NJ: John Wiley & Sons; 2010:85–95.

Costa LG, Galli CL, Murphy SD, eds. *Toxicology of Pesticides: Experimental, Clinical and Regulatory Perspectives*. Heidelberg: Springer Verlag; 1987:320.

Costa LG, Hand H, Schwab BW, et al. Tolerance to the carbamate insecticide propoxur. *Toxicology*. 1981;21:267–278.

Costa LG, Li WF, Richter RJ, et al. PON1 and organophosphate toxicity. In: Costa LG, Furlong CE, eds. *Paraoxonase (PON1) in Health and Disease: Basic and Clinical Aspects*. Norwell, MA: Kluwer Academic Publishers; 2002:165–183.

Costa LG, Murphy SD. Interaction of the pesticide chlordimeform with adrenergic receptors in mouse brain: an in vitro study. *Arch Toxicol*. 1987;59:323–327.

Costa LG, Olibet G, Murphy SD. Alpha$_2$-adrenoceptors as a target for formamidine pesticides: in vitro and in vivo studies in mice. *Toxicol Appl Pharmacol*. 1988;93:319–328.

Costa LG, Schwab BW, Murphy SD. Tolerance to anticholinesterase compounds in mammals. *Toxicology*. 1982;25:79–97.

Costello S, Cockburn M, Bronstein J, et al. Parkinson's disease and residential exposure to maneb and paraquat from agricultural applications in the Central Valley in California. *Am J Epidemiol*. 2009;169:919–926.

Cranmer MF. Carbaryl. A toxicological review and risk analysis. *Neurotoxicology*. 1986;7:247–332.

Crisp TM, Clegg ED, Cooper RL, et al. Environmental endocrine disruption: an effects assessment and analysis. *Environ Health Perspect*. 1998;106(suppl 1):11–56.

Dafforn KA, Lewis JA, Johnston EL. Antifouling strategies: history and regulation, ecological impact and mitigation. *Marine Pollut Bull*. 2011;62:453–465.

Dam K, Seidler FJ, Slotkin TA. Developmental neurotoxicity of chlorpyrifos: delayed targeting of DNA synthesis after repeated administration. *Dev Brain Res*. 1998;108:39–45.

Daniell WE, Barnhart S, Demers P, et al. Neuropsychological performance among pesticide applicators. *Environ Res*. 1992;59:217–228.

Davenport CJ, Ali SF, Miller FJ, et al. Effect of methylbromide on regional brain glutathione, glutathione *S*-transferases, monoamines, and amino acids in F344 rats. *Toxicol Appl Pharmacol*. 1992;112:120–127.

Dawson AH, Eddleston M, Senarathna L, et al. Acute human lethal toxicity of agricultural pesticides: a prospective cohort study. *PLoS Med*. 2010;7(10):e1000357.

Dawson GR, Wafford KA, Smith A, et al. Anticonvulsant and adverse effects of avermectin analogs in mice are mediated through the γ-aminobutyric acid$_A$ receptor. *J Pharmacol Exp Ther*. 2000;295:1051–1060.

Dayal M, Parmar D, Dhawan A, Ali M, Dwivedi UN, Seth PK. Effect of pretreatment of cytochrome P450 (P450) modifiers on neurobehavioral toxicity induced by deltamethrin. *Food Chem Toxicol*. 2003;41:431–437.

de Bleecker JL. Intermediate syndrome in organophosphate poisoning. In: Gupta RC, ed. *Toxicology of Organophosphate and Carbamate Compounds*. Amsterdam: Elsevier; 2006:371–380.

De Haro L, Gastaut JL, Jouglard J, et al. Central and peripheral neurotoxic effects of chronic methyl bromide intoxication. *J Toxicol Clin Toxicol*. 1997;35:29–34.

De Wilde AR, Heyndrickx A, Carton D. A case of fatal rotenone poisoning in a child. *J Forensic Sci*. 1986;31:1492–1498.

Degli Esposti M. Inhibitors of NADH-ubiquinone reductase: an overview. *Biochim Biophys Acta*. 1998;1364:222–235.

Desaiah D. Biochemical mechanisms of chlordecone neurotoxicity: a review. *Neurotoxicology*. 1982;3:103–110.

Dickoff DJ, Gerber O, Turovsky Z. Delayed neurotoxicity after ingestion of carbamate pesticide. *Neurology*. 1987;37:1229–1231.

Didier A, Loor F. The abamectin derivative invermectin is a potent P-glycoprotein inhibitor. *Anticancer Drugs*. 1996;7:745–757.

Dikshith TSS, ed. *Toxicology of Pesticide in Animals*. Boca Raton: CRC Press; 1991:255.

Dinis-Oliveira RJ, Duarte JA, Sanchez-Navarro A, et al. Paraquat poisoning: mechanisms of lung toxicity, clinical features, and treatment. *Crit Rev Toxicol*. 2008;38:13–71.

Doe JE, Boobis AR, Blacker A, et al. A tiered approach to systemic toxicity testing for agricultural risk assessment. *Crit Rev Toxicol*. 2006;36:37–68.

Dourson ML, Kahrman-Vincent MJ, Allen BC. Dose response assessment for effects of acute exposure to methyl isocyanate (MITC). *Regul Toxicol Pharmacol*. 2010;58:181–188.

Duke SO. Overview of herbicide mechanisms of action. *Environ Health Perspect*. 1990;87:263–271.

Duke SO. Taking stock of herbicide-resistant crops ten years after introduction. *Pest Manag Sci*. 2005;61:211–218.

Eaton DL, Daroff RB, Autrup H, et al. Review of the toxicology of chlorpyrifos with an emphasis on human exposure and neurodevelopment. *Crit Rev Toxicol*. 2008;38(suppl 2):1–125.

Ebert E, Leist KH, Mayer D. Summary of safety evaluation of toxicity studies of glufosinate ammonium. *Food Chem Toxicol*. 1990;28:339–349.

Ecobichon DJ. Introduction. In: Ecobichon DJ, Roy RM, eds. *Pesticides and Neurological Diseases*. Boca Raton: CRC Press; 1992:1–14.

Ecobichon DJ. Toxic effect of pesticides. In: Klaassen CD, ed. *Casarett and Doull's Toxicology. The Basic Science of Poisons*. New York: McGraw-Hill; 2001a:763–810.

Ecobichon DJ. Carbamate insecticides. In: Krieger R, ed. *Handbook of Pesticide Toxicology*. San Diego: Academic Press; 2001b:1087–1106.

Ecobichon DJ, Joy RM. *Pesticides and Neurological Diseases*. Boca Raton: CRC Press; 1982:281.

Eddleston M, Szinicz L, Eyer P, Buckley N. Oximes in acute organophosphorus pesticide poisoning: a systematic review of clinical trials. *QJM*. 2002;95:275–283.

Edwards IR, Ferry DG, Temple WA. Fungicides and related compounds. In: Hayes WJ, Laws ER, eds. *Handbook of Pesticide Toxicology*. Vol. 3. San Diego: Academic Press; 1991:1409–1470.

EFSA (European Food Safety Agency). Conclusion regarding the peer-review of the pesticide risk assessment of the active substance glufosinate. *EFSA Sci Rep*. 2005;27:1–81.

Ehrich M, Correll L, Veronesi B. Acetylcholinesterase and neuropathy target esterase inhibitions in neuroblastoma cells to distinguish organophosphorus compounds causing acute and delayed neurotoxicity. *Fundam Appl Toxicol*. 1997;38:55–63.

Ehrich M, Jortner BS. Organophosphorus-induced delayed neuropathy. In: Krieger R, ed. *Hayes' Handbook of Pesticide Toxicology*. San Diego: Academic Press; 2010:1479–1504.

Eisenbrandt DL, Hotchkiss JA. Sulfuryl fluoride. In: Krieger R, ed. *Hayes' Handbook of Pesticide Toxicology*. San Diego: Academic Press; 2010:2245–2258.

Eldelfrawi AT, Eldefrawi ME. Receptors for γ-aminobutyric acid and voltage-dependent chloride channels as targets for toxicants. *FASEB J*. 1987;1:262–271.

Eldefrawi ME, Eldefrawi AT. Comparative molecular and pharmacological properties of cholinergic receptors in insects and mammals. In: Hedin PA, Hollingworth RM, Masler, EP, Miyamoto J, Thompson DG, eds. *Phytochemicals in Pest Control*. Washington, DC: American Chemical Society; 1997:327–338.

Eldridge JC, Stevens JT, Wetzel LT, et al. Atrazine: mechanisms of hormonal imbalance in female SD rats. *Fundam Appl Toxicol*. 1996;42:2–5.

Elinav E, Shapira Y, Ofran Y, et al. Near-fatal amitraz intoxication: the overlooked pesticide. *Basic Clin Pharmacol Toxicol*. 2005;97:185–187.

Enan E, Matsumura F. Activation of phosphoinositide protein kinase C pathway in rat brain tissue by pyrethroids. *Biochem Pharmacol*. 1993;45:703–710.

Erdogrul O, Covaci A, Kurtul N, et al. Levels of organohalogenated persistent pollutants in human milk from Kahramanmaras region, Turkey. *Environ Int*. 2004;30:659–666.

Eskenazi B, Bradman A, Castorina R. Exposures to children to organophosphate pesticides and their potential health effects. *Environ Health Perspect*. 1999;107(suppl 3):409–419.

Eskenazi B, Chevrier J, Rosas LG, et al. The Pine River Statement: human health consequences of DDT use. *Environ Health Perspect.* 2009;117:1359–1367.

Farmer D. Inhibitors of aromatic acid biosynthesis. In: Krieger R, ed. *Hayes' Handbook of Pesticide Toxicology.* San Diego: Academic Press; 2010:1967–1972.

Feng P, Wilson AGE, McClanahan R, et al. Metabolism of alachlor by rat and mouse liver and nasal turbinate tissues. *Drug Metab Dispos.* 1990;18:373–377.

Fenner-Crisp PA. Risk assessment and risk management: the regulatory process. In: Krieger R, ed. *Handbook of Pesticide Toxicology.* San Diego: Academic Press; 2001:681–689.

Fenske RA, Wong SM, Leffingwell JT, et al. A video imaging technique for assessing dermal exposure. II. Fluorescent tracer testing. *Am Ind Hyg Assoc.* 1986;47:771–775.

Ferraz HB, Bertolucci PH, Pereira JS, et al. Chronic exposure to the fungicide maneb may produce symptoms and signs of CNS manganese intoxication. *Neurology.* 1988;38:550–553.

Fisher MH, Mrozik H. The chemistry and pharmacology of avermectins. *Annu Rev Pharmacol Toxicol.* 1992;32:537–553.

Flannigan SA, Tucker SB, Key MM, et al. Synthetic pyrethroid insecticides: a dermatological evaluation. *Br J Ind Med.* 1985;42:363–372.

Fontoura-da-Silva SE, Chautard-Friere-Maira EA. Butyrylcholinesterase variants (BChE and ChE1 loci) associated with erythrocyte acetylcholinesterase inhibition in farmers exposed to pesticides. *Hum Hered.* 1996;46:142–147.

Ford MG, Lunt GG, Reay RC, et al., eds. *Neuropharmacology and Pesticide Action.* Chichester: Ellis Norwood; 1986:512.

Forshaw PJ, Lister T, Ray DE. Inhibition of a neuronal voltage-dependent chloride channel by the type II pyrethroid, deltamethrin. *Neuropharmacology.* 1993;32:105–111.

Forshaw PJ, Lister T, Ray DE. The role of voltage-gated chloride channels in type II pyrethroid insecticide poisoning. *Toxicol Appl Pharmacol.* 2000;163:1–8.

FQPA (Food Quality Protection Act). Public Law 104-170; 1996.

Fradin MS, Day JF. Comparative efficacy of insect repellents against mosquito bites. *N Engl J Med.* 2002;347:13–18.

Fukuto TR. Metabolism of carbamate insecticides. *Drug Metab Rev.* 1972;1:117–152.

Furlong CE, Holland N, Richter RJ, et al. PON1 status of farm worker mother and children as a predictor of organophosphate sensitivity. *Pharmacogenet Genom.* 2006;16:183–190.

Gallo MA, Lawryk NJ. Organic phosphorus pesticides. In: Hayes WJ, Laws ER, eds. *Handbook of Pesticide Toxicology.* San Diego: Academic Press; 1991:917–1123.

Gammon DW, Aldous CN, Carr WC, et al. A risk assessment of atrazine use in California: human health and ecological aspects. *Pest Manag Sci.* 2005;61:331–355.

Gammon DW, Moore TB, O'Malley MA. A toxicological assessment of sulfur as a pesticide. In: Krieger R, ed. *Hayes' Handbook of Pesticide Toxicology.* San Diego: Academic Press; 2010:1889–1901.

Garabrandt DH, Philbert MA. Review of 2,4-dichlorophenoxyacetic acid (2,4-D) epidemiology and toxicology. *Crit Rev Toxicol.* 2002;34:233–257.

Garcia SJ, Seidler FJ, Slotkin TA. Developmental neurotoxicity of chlorpyrifos: targeting glial cells. *Environ Toxicol Pharmacol.* 2005;19:455–461.

Ghali TG, Hollingworth RM. Influence of mixed function oxygenase metabolism on the acute neurotoxicity of the pesticide chlordimeform in mice. *Neurotoxicology.* 1985;6:215–238.

Gianessi L, Reigner N. *Pesticide Use in U.S. Crop Production: 2002. Fungicides and Herbicides.* Washington, DC: CropLife Foundation; 2006a:40.

Gianessi L, Reigner N. *Pesticide Use in U.S. Crop Production: 2002. Insecticides and Other Pesticides.* Washington, DC: CropLife Foundation; 2006b:36.

Glynn P. A mechanism for organophosphate-induced delayed neuropathy. *Toxicol Lett.* 2006;162:94–97.

Goes AE, Savage EP, Gibbons G, Aaronson M, Ford SA, Wheeler HW. Suspected foodborne carbamate pesticide intoxications with the ingestion of hydroponic cucumbers. *Am J Epidemiol.* 1980;111:254–259.

Golden RJ, Noller KL, Titus-Enrstoff L, et al. Environmental endocrine modulators and human health: an assessment of biological evidence. *Crit Rev Toxicol.* 1998;28:109–227.

Goldman LR, Smith DF, Neutra RR, et al. Pesticide food poisoning from contaminated watermelons in California, 1985. *Arch Environ Health.* 1990;45:229–236.

Golub M, Doherty J. Triphenyltin as a potential human endocrine disruptor. *J Toxicol Environ Health B Crit Rev.* 2004;7:281–295.

Goodal R. Cholinesterase pharmacogenetics. In: Gupta RC, ed. *Toxicology of Organophosphate and Carbamate Compounds.* Amsterdam: Elsevier; 2006:187–198.

Gordon EB. Captan: transition from "B2" to "not likely". How pesticide registrants affected the EPA cancer classification update. *J Appl Toxicol.* 2007;27:519–526.

Gordon EB. Captan and folpet. In: Krieger R, ed. *Hayes' Handbook of Pesticide Toxicology.* San Diego: Academic Press; 2010:1915–1949.

Gringorten JL. Ion balance in the Lepidopteran midgut and insecticidal action of *Bacillus thuringiensis.* In: Isheaya I, ed. *Biochemical Sites of Insecticide Action and Resistance.* Heidelberg: Springer Verlag; 2001:167–207.

Gryboski J, Weinstein D, Ordway NK. Toxic encephalopathy apparently related to the use of an insect repellent. *N Engl J Med.* 1961;264:289–290.

Gunnell D, Eddleston M. Suicide by intentional ingestion of pesticides: a continuing tragedy in developing countries. *Int J Epidemiol.* 2003;32:902–909.

Gunnell D, Eddleston M, Phillips MR, Konradsen F. The global distribution of fatal pesticide self-poisoning: systematic review. *BMC Public Health.* 2007;7:357.

Gupta RC, ed. *Toxicology of Organophosphate and Carbamate Compounds.* Amsterdam: Elsevier; 2006:763.

Guzelian PS. Comparative toxicology of chlordecone (Kepone) in humans and experimental animals. *Annu Rev Pharmacol Toxicol.* 1982;22: 89–113.

Hainzl D, Cole LM, Casida JE. Mechanisms for selective toxicity of fipronil insecticide and its sulfone metabolite and desulfinyl photoproduct. *Chem Res Toxicol.* 1998;11:1529–1535.

Hampers LC, Oker E, Leikin JB. Topical use of DEET insect repellent as a cause of severe encephalopathy in a healthy adult male. *Acad Emerg Med.* 1999;6:1295–1297.

Hardell L, Eriksson M, Degerman A. Exposure to phenoxyacetic acids, chlorophenols or organic solvents in relation to histopathology, stage, and anatomical localization of non-Hodgkin's lymphoma. *Cancer Res.* 1994;54:2386–2389.

Harrison ML, Loucks OL, Mitchell JW, et al. Systems studies of DDT transport. *Science.* 1970;170:503–508.

Hasin Y, Avidan N, Bercovich D, et al. A paradigm for single nucleotide polymorphism analysis: the case of the acetylcholinesterase gene. *Hum Mutat.* 2004;24:408–416.

Hatcher TM, Pennell KD, Miller GW. Parkinson's disease and pesticides: a toxicological perspective. *Trends Pharmacol Sci.* 2008;29:322–329.

Hayes TB, Collins A, Lee M, et al. Hermaphroditic, demasculinized frogs after exposure to the herbicide atrazine at low ecologically relevant doses. *Proc Natl Acad Sci U S A.* 2002;99:5476–5480.

Hayes TB, Khourry V, Narayan A, et al. Atrazine induces complete feminization and chemical castration in male African clawed frogs (*Xenopus laevis*). *Proc Natl Acad Sci U S A.* 2010;107:4612–4617.

Hayes WJ. *Pesticides Studied in Man.* Baltimore: Williams & Wilkins; 1982:672.

Hayes WJ, Laws ER, eds. *Handbook of Pesticide Toxicology.* San Diego: Academic Press; 1991:1576.

He F, Wang S, Liu L, et al. Clinical manifestations and diagnosis of acute pyrethroid poisoning. *Arch Toxicol.* 1989;63:54–58.

Heikkila RE, Nicklas WJ, Vyas I, Duvoisin RC. Dopaminergic toxicity of rotenone and the 1-methyl-4-phenylpyridinium ion after their stereotaxic administration to rats: implication for the mechanism of 1-methyl-4-phenyl-1,2,3,6-tetrahydropyridine toxicity. *Neurosci Lett.* 1985;62:389–394.

Hernandez AF, Martin-Rubi JC, Ballesteros JL, et al. Clinical and pathological findings in fatal 1,3-dichloropropene intoxication. *Hum Exp Toxicol.* 1994;13:303–306.

Hertzstein J, Cullen MR. Methyl bromide intoxication in four field workers during removal of soil fumigation sheets. *Am J Ind Med.* 1990;17:321–326.

Heudorf U, Angerer J, Drexler H. Current internal exposure to pesticides in children and adolescents in Germany: urinary levels of metabolites of pyrethroid and organophosphorus insecticides. *Int Arch Occup Environ Health.* 2004;77:67–72.

Heydens WF. Summary of toxicology studies with alachlor. *J Pest Sci.* 1998;24:75–82.

Heydens WF, Lamb IC, Wilson AGE. Chloroacetanilides. In: Krieger R, ed. *Hayes' Handbook of Pesticide Toxicology.* San Diego: Academic Press; 2010:1753–1769.

Heydens WF, Wilson AGE, Kier LD, et al. An evaluation of the carcinogenic potential of the herbicide alachlor to man. *Hum Exp Toxicol.* 1999;18:363–391.

Hickey JP, Batterman SA, Chernyak SM. Trends of chlorinated organic contaminants in Great Lakes trout and walleye from 1970 to 1998. *Arch Environ Contam Toxicol.* 2006;50:97–110.

Ho YS, Magnenat JL, Gargano M, et al. The nature of antioxidant defense mechanisms: a lesson from transgenic mice. *Environ Health Perspect.* 1998;106:1219–1228.

Hoar SK, Blair A, Holmes FF, et al. Agricultural herbicide use and risk of lymphoma and soft-tissue sarcoma. *JAMA.* 1986;256:1141–1147.

Hodgson E. In vitro human phase I metabolism of xenobiotics I: pesticides and related compounds used in agriculture and public health, May 2003. *J Biochem Mol Toxicol.* 2003;17:201–206.

Hoffman JN, Keifer MC, Furlong CE, et al. Serum cholinesterase inhibition in relation to paraoxonase 1 (PON1) status among organophosphate-exposed agricultural pesticide handlers. *Environ Health Perspect.* 2009;117:1402–1408.

Hollingworth RM. Chemistry, biological activity and uses of formamidine pesticides. *Environ Health Perspect.* 1976;14:57–69.

Hollingworth RM. Inhibitors and uncouplers of mitochondrial oxidative phosphorylation. In: Krieger R, ed. *Handbook of Pesticide Toxicology.* San Diego: Academic Press; 2001:1169–1261.

Hsu WH, Kakuk TJ. Effects of amitraz and chlordimeform on heart rate and pupil diameter in rats: mediated by alpha$_2$-adrenoceptors. *Toxicol Appl Pharmacol.* 1984;73:411–415.

Hsu WH, Lu ZH. Amitraz-induced delay of gastrointestinal transit in mice: mediated by alpha$_2$-adrenergic receptors. *Drug Dev Res.* 1984;4:655–660.

Hurt S, Ollinger J, Arce G, et al. Dialkyldithiocarbamates (EBDCs). In: Krieger R, ed. *Hayes' Handbook of Pesticide Toxicology.* San Diego: Academic Press; 2010:1689–1710.

IARC (International Agency for Research on Cancer). Atrazine. *IARC Monogr Eval Carcinog Risks Hum.* 1999;73:59–113.

IOM (Institute of Medicine). *Veterans and Agent Orange. Update 1996.* Washington, DC: National Academy Press; 1996:365.

IOM (Institute of Medicine). *Gulf War and Health.* Vol. I. Washington, DC: National Academy Press; 2000:408.

IPCS (International Programme on Chemical Safety). *Chlordimeform.* Environmental Health Criteria 1999. Geneva: World Health Organization; 1998:159.

IPCS (International Programme on Chemical Safety). *The WHO Recommended Classification of Pesticides by Hazard and Guidelines to Classification: 2004.* Geneva: World Health Organization; 2005:58.

Ireland B, Acquarella, J, Farrell T, et al. Evaluation of ocular health among alachlor manufacturing workers. *J Occup Med.* 1994;36:738–742.

Isman MB. Botanical insecticides, deterrents and repellents in modern agriculture and an increasingly regulated world. *Annu Rev Entomol.* 2006;51:45–66.

Jacobsen NE, Sanders M, Toia RP, et al. Alachlor and its analogues as metabolic progenitors of formaldehyde: fate of *N*-methoxymethyl and other *N*-alkoxyalkyl substituents. *J Agric Food Chem.* 1991;39:1342–1350.

Jaga K, Dharmani C. Global surveillance of DDT and DDE levels in human tissues. *Int J Occup Med Environ Health.* 2003;16:7–20.

Jaga K, Dharmani C. The epidemiology of pesticide exposure and cancer: a review. *Rev Environ Health.* 2005;20:15–38.

Jamal GA, Julu POO. Low level exposure to organophosphate esters may cause neurotoxicity. *Toxicology.* 2002;181:22–33.

Jett DA, Navoa RV, Beckles RA, et al. Cognitive function and cholinergic neurochemistry in weanling rats exposed to chlorpyrifos. *Toxicol Appl Pharmacol.* 2001;174:89–98.

Johnson DJ, Graham DG, Amarnath V, et al. Release of carbon disulfide is a contributing mechanism in the axonopathy produced by *N,N*-diethyldithiocarbamate. *Toxicol Appl Pharmacol.* 1998;148:288–296.

Johnson MK. The target for initiation of delayed neurotoxicity by organophosphorus esters: biochemical studies and toxicological applications. *Rev Biochem Toxicol.* 1982;4:141–212.

Johnson MK, Glynn P. Neuropathy target esterase. In: Krieger R, ed. *Handbook of Pesticide Toxicology.* San Diego: Academic Press; 2001:953–965.

Johnson MK, Jacobsen D, Meredith TJ, et al. Evaluation of antidotes for poisoning by organophosphorus pesticides. *Emerg Med.* 2000;12:22–37.

Johnson MK, Lauwerys R. Protection by some carbamates against the delayed neurotoxic effects of diisopropyl phosphorofluoridate. *Nature.* 1969;222:1066–1067.

Johnson MK, Read DJ. The influence of chirality on the delayed neuropathic potential of some organophosphorus esters: neuropathic and prophylactic effects of streoisomers of ethyl phenylphosphonic acid (EPN oxon and EPN) correlate with quantities of aged and unaged neuropathy target esterase in vivo. *Toxicol Appl Pharmacol.* 1987;90:103–115.

Kalantzi OI, Martin FL, Thomas GO, et al. Different levels of polybrominated diphenyl ethers (PBDEs) and chlorinated compounds in breast milk from two UK regions. *Environ Health Perspect.* 2004;112:1086–1091.

Kaneko H. Pyrethroid chemistry and metabolism. In: Krieger R, ed. *Hayes' Handbook of Pesticide Toxicology.* San Diego: Academic Press; 2010:1635–1663.

Kappers WA, Edwards RJ, Murray S, et al. Diazinon is activated by CYP2C19 in human liver. *Toxicol Appl Pharmacol.* 2001;177:68–76.

Katz TM, Miller JH, Hebert AA. Insect repellents: historical perspectives and new developments. *J Am Acad Dermatol.* 2008;58:865–871.

Kavlock RJ. Pesticides as endocrine-disrupting chemicals. In: Krieger R, ed. *Handbook of Pesticide Toxicology.* San Diego: Academic Press; 2001:727–746.

Keigwin RP. Maneb; cancellation order for a certain pesticide registration. *Fed Reg.* 2010;75(73):19967–19968.

Keiner C. Wartime rat control, rodent ecology, and the rise and fall of chemical rodenticides. *Endeavour.* 2005;29:119–125.

Kelce WR, Stone CR, Laws SC, et al. Persistent DDT metabolite *p,p'*-DDE is a potent androgen receptor antagonist. *Nature.* 1995;375:581–585.

Kennepohl E, Munro IC, Bus JS. Phenoxy herbicides (2,4-D). In: Krieger R, ed. *Hayes' Handbook of Pesticide Toxicology.* San Diego: Academic Press; 2010:1829–1847.

Kiely T, Donaldson D, Grube A. *Pesticide Industry Sales and Usage. 2000 and 2001 Market Estimates.* Washington, DC: USEPA; 2004:33.

Kim DJ, Seok SH, Baek MW, et al. Benomyl induction of brain aromatase and toxic effects in the zebrafish embryo. *J Appl Toxicol.* 2009;29:289–294.

Kim IY, Shin JH, Kim HS, et al. Assessing estrogenic activity of pyrethroid insecticides using in vitro combination assays. *J Reprod Dev.* 2004;50:245–255.

Kitamura S, Suzuki T, Ohta S, Fujimoto N. Antiandrogenic activity and metabolism of the organophosphorus pesticide fenthion and related compounds. *Environ Health Perspect.* 2003;111(4):503–508.

Kloas W, Lutz I, Urbatzka R, et al. Does atrazine affect larval development and sexual differentiation of South African clawed frogs? *Ann N Y Acad Sci.* 2009;1163:437–440.

Konishi Y, Kuwabara K, Hori S. Continuous surveillance of organochlorine compounds in human breast milk from 1972 to 1998 in Osaka, Japan. *Arch Environ Contam Toxicol.* 2001;40:571–578.

Konjuh C, Garcia G, Lopez L, et al. Neonatal hypomyelination by the herbicide 2,4-dichlorophenoxyacetic acid. Chemical and ultrastructural studies in rats. *Toxicol Sci.* 2008;104:332–340.

Koren G. Matsui D, Bailey B. DEET-based insect repellents: safety implications for children and pregnant and lactating women. *CMAJ.* 2003;169:209–212.

Korystov YN, Ermakova NV, Kublik LN, et al. Avermectins inhibit multidrug resistance of tumor cells. *Eur J Pharmacol.* 2004;493:57–64.

Koyama K, Andou Y, Saruki K, et al. Delayed and severe toxicity of a herbicide containing glufosinate and a surfactant. *Vet Hum Toxicol.* 1994;36:17–18.

Kretzschmar D, Mason G, Sharma S, Heisenberg M, Benzer S. The Swiss Cheese mutant causes glial hyperwrapping and brain degeneration in Drosophila. *J Neurosci.* 1997;17:7425–7432.

Krieger R, ed. *Handbook of Pesticide Toxicology.* San Diego: Academic Press; 2001:1908.

Krieger R, ed. *Hayes' Handbook of Pesticide Toxicology.* San Diego: Academic Press; 2010:2342.

Landrigan PJ, Powell KE, James LE, Taylor PR. Paraquat and marijuana: epidemiologic risk assessment. *Am J Public Health.* 1983;73:784–788.

Lange PF, Terveer J. Warfarin poisoning; report of fourteen cases. *US Armed Forces J.* 1954;5:872–877.

Lapointe N, St-Hilaire M, Martinoli MG, et al. Rotenone induces non-specific central nervous system and systemic toxicity. *FASEB J.* 2004;18:717–719.

Lawrence LJ, Casida JE. Stereospecific action of pyrethroid insecticides on the γ-aminobutyric acid receptor–ionophore complex. *Science.* 1983;221:1399–1401.

Lee HL, Chen KW, Chi CH, et al. Clinical presentations and prognostic factors of a glyphosate-surfactant herbicide intoxication: a review of 131 cases. *Acad Emerg Med.* 2000;7:906–910.

Lee K, Park EK, Stoecklin-Marois M, et al. Occupational paraquat exposure of agricultural workers in large Costa Rican farms. *Int Arch Occup Environ Health.* 2009b;82:455–462.

Lee SJ, Mulay P, Diebolt-Brown B, et al. Acute illnesses associated with exposure to fipronil—surveillance data from 11 states in the United States, 2001-2007. *Clin Toxicol (Phila).* 2010;48:737–744.

Lee WJ, Cha ES, Park ES, et al. Deaths from pesticide poisoning in South Korea: trends over 10 years. *Int Arch Occup Environ Health.* 2009a;82:365–371.

Leet T, Acquavella J, Lynch C, et al. Cancer incidence among alachlor manufacturing workers. *Am J Ind Med.* 1996;30:300–306.

Li AA, Mink PJ, McIntosh LJ, et al. Evaluation of epidemiologic and animal data associating pesticides with Parkinson's disease. *J Occup Environ Med.* 2005;47:1059–1087.

Li WF, Costa LG, Richter RJ, et al. Catalytic efficiency determines the in vivo efficacy of PON1 for detoxifying organophosphates. *Pharmacogenetics.* 2000;10:767–779.

Lifshitz M, Gavrilov V. Central nervous system toxicity and early peripheral neuropathy following dermal exposure to methyl bromide. *Clin Toxicol.* 2000;38:799–801.

Lim S, Ahn SY, Song IC, et al. Chronic exposure to the herbicide atrazine causes mitochondrial dysfunction and insulin resistance. *PLoS One.* 2009;4:e5186.

Lock EA, Wilks MF. Diquat. In: Krieger R, ed. *Handbook of Pesticide Toxicology.* San Diego: Academic Press; 2001:1605–1621.

Lock EA, Wilks MF. Paraquat. In: Krieger R, ed. *Hayes' Handbook of Pesticide Toxicology.* San Diego: Academic Press; 2010:1771–1827.

Lockridge O, Duysen EG, Masson P. Butyrylcholinesterase: overview, structure and function. In: Satoh T, Gupta RC, eds. *Anticholinesterase Pesticides: Metabolism, Neurotoxicity and Epidemiology.* Hoboken, NJ: John Wiley & Sons; 2010:25–41.

Lockridge O, Duysen EG, Voelker T, Thompson CM, Schopfer LM. Life without acetylcholinesterase: the implications of cholinesterase inhibition toxicity in AChE-knockout mice. *Environ Toxicol Pharmacol.* 2005;19:463–469.

Lockridge O, Masson P. Pesticides and susceptible populations: people with butyrylcholinesterase genetic variants may be at risk. *Neurotoxicology.* 2000;21:113–126.

Lomax LG, Stott WT, Johnson KA, et al. The chronic toxicity and oncogenicity of inhaled technical grade 1,3-dichloropropene in rats and mice. *Fundam Appl Toxicol.* 1989;12:418–431.

Longnecker MP. Invited commentary: why DDT matters now. *Am J Epidemiol.* 2005;162:726–728.

Lotti M. The pathogenesis of organophosphate neuropathy. *Crit Rev Toxicol.* 1992;21:465–487.

Lotti M. Cholinesterase inhibition: complexities in interpretation. *Clin Chem.* 1995;41:1814–1818.

Lotti M. Organophosphorus compounds. In: Spencer PS, Schaumburg HH, Ludolph AC, eds. *Experimental and Clinical Neurotoxicology.* Oxford: Oxford University Press; 2000:898–925.

Lotti M. Promotion of organophosphate-induced delayed polyneuropathy by certain esterase inhibitors. *Toxicology.* 2002a;181–182:245–248.

Lotti M. Low level exposures to organophosphorus esters and peripheral nerve functions. *Muscle Nerve.* 2002b;25:492–504.

Lotti M. Clinical toxicology of anticholinesterases in humans. In: Krieger R, ed. *Hayes' Handbook of Pesticide Toxicology.* San Diego: Academic Press; 2010:1543–1589.

Lotti M, Caroldi S, Capodicasa E, et al. Promotion of organophosphate-induced delayed polyneuropathy by phenylmethanesulfonyl fluoride. *Toxicol Appl Pharmacol.* 1991;108:234–241.

Lotti M, Moretto A. Organophosphate-induced delayed polyneuropathy. *Toxicol Rev.* 2005;24:37–49.

Lu C, Bravo R, Caltabiano LM, et al. The presence of dialkylphosphates in fresh fruit juices: implications for organophosphorus pesticide exposure and risk assessments. *J Toxicol Environ Health Part A.* 2005;68: 209–227.

Lyubimov AV, Garry VF. Phosphine. In: Krieger R, ed. *Hayes' Handbook of Pesticide Toxicology.* San Diego: Academic Press; 2010:2259–2266.

Macdonald N, Gladhill A. Potential impact of ABCB1 (P-glycoprotein) polymorphisms on avermectin toxicity in humans. *Arch Toxicol.* 2007;81:553–563.

Magnavita N. A cluster of neurological signs and symptoms in soil fumigators. *J Occup Health.* 2009;51:159–163.

Maharaj R, Mthembu DJ, Sharp BL. Impact of DDT re-introduction on malaria transmission in KwaZulu-Natal. *S Afr Med J.* 2005;95:871–874.

Majerus PW, Tollefsen DM. Blood coagulation and anticoagulants, thrombolytic, and antiplatelet drugs. In: Brunton LL, ed. *Goodman and Gilman's The Pharmacological Basis of Therapeutics.* New York: McGraw-Hill; 2006:1467–1488.

Malone JDG, Carmody M, Keogh B, et al. Paraquat poisoning—a review of nineteen cases. *J Ir Med Assoc.* 1971;64:59–68.

Maroni M, Colosio C, Ferioli A, et al. Biological monitoring of pesticide exposure: a review. *Toxicology.* 2000;143:5–118.

Marsh RE. Vertebrate pest control chemicals and their use in urban and rural environments. In: Keirger R, ed. *Handbook of Pesticide Toxicology.* San Diego: Academic Press; 2001:251–262.

Masson P, Froment MT, Sorenson RC, et al. Mutation His322Asn in human acetylcholinesterase does not alter electrophoretic and catalytic properties of the erythrocyte enzyme. *Blood.* 1994;83:3003–3005.

Matsuda K, Buckingam SD, Kleier D, et al. Neonicotinoids: insecticides acting on insect nicotinic acetylcholine receptors. *Trends Pharmacol Sci.* 2001;22:573–580.

Matsumura F. *Toxicology of Insecticides.* New York: Plenum Press; 1985:598.

Matsumura F, Ghiasuddin SM. Characteristics of DDT-sensitive Ca-ATPase in the axonic membrane. In: Narahashi T, ed. *Neurotoxicology of Insecticides and Pheromones.* New York: Plenum Press; 1979:245–257.

Matsumura F, Patil KC. Adenosin triphosphatase sensitive to DDT in synapses of rat brain. *Science.* 1969;166:121–122.

Mattsson JL, Charles JM, Yano BL, et al. Single-dose and chronic dietary neurotoxicity screening studies on 2,4-dichlorophenoxyacetic acid in rats. *Fundam Appl Toxicol.* 1997;40:111–119.

Matyunas NG, Rodgers GC. Nicotine poisoning. In: Ford MD, Delaney KA, Ling LJ, Erickson T, eds. *Clinical Toxicology.* Philadelphia: WB Saunders Co; 2001:985–989.

McClintock JT, Schaffer CR, Sjobald RD. A comparative review of the mammalian toxicity of *Bacillus thuringiensis*–based pesticides. *Pestic Sci.* 1995;45:95–106.

McCook A. The banned pesticide in our soil. *Scientist.* 2006;20:40–45.

McCormack AL, Atienza JG, Johnston LC, et al. Role of oxidative stress in paraquat-induced dopaminergic cell degeneration. *J Neurochem.* 2005;93:1030–1037.

McCormack AL, Thiruchelvam M, Manning-Bog AB, et al. Environmental risk factors and Parkinson's disease: selective degeneration of nigral dopaminergic neurons caused by the herbicide paraquat. *Neurobiol Dis.* 2002;10:119–127.

McGrew DM, Irwin I, Langston JW. Ehtylene-bisdithiocarbamate enhances MPTP-induced striatal dopamine depletion in mice. *Neurotoxicology.* 2000;21:309–312.

McLaughlin J, Reynaldo EF, Lamar JK, et al. Teratology studies in rabbits with captan, folpet and thalidomide. *Toxicol Appl Pharmacol.* 1969;14:641.

Meco G, Bonifati V, Vanacore N, et al. Parkinsonism after chronic exposure to the fungicide maneb (manganese ethylene-bis-dithiocarbamate). *Scand J Work Environ Health.* 1994;20:301–305.

Miller GW. Paraquat: the red herring of Parkinson's disease research. *Toxicol Sci.* 2007;100:1–2.

Mills PK, Yang R. Prostate cancer risk in California farm workers. *J Occup Environ Med.* 2003;45:249–258.

Minh NH, Somaya M, Minh TB, et al. Persistent organochlorine residue in human breast milk from Hanoi and Hochiminh City, Vietnam: contamination, accumulation kinetics and risk assessment for infants. *Environ Pollut.* 2004;129:431–441.

Miyamoto J. Degradation, metabolism and toxicity of synthetic pyrethroids. *Environ Health Perspect.* 1976;14:15–28.

MMWR (Morbidity and Mortality Weekly Reports). Seizures temporarily associated with use of DEET insect repellents—New York and Connecticut. *MMWR.* 1989;38:678–680.

Mohamed F, Senarathna L, Percy A, et al. Acute human self-poisoning with the *N*-phenylpyrazole insecticide fipronil—a GABA$_A$-gated chloride channel blocker. *J Toxicol Clin Toxicol.* 2004;42:955–963.

Mohanty MK, Kumar V, Pastia BK, et al. An analysis of poisoning deaths in Manipal, India. *Vet Hum Toxicol.* 2004;46:208–209.

Moretto A. Testing for organophosphate delayed neuropathy. In: Maines MD, Costa LG, Reed DJ, et al., eds. *Current Protocols in Toxicology.* New York: John Wiley & Sons; 1999:11.5.1–11.5.14.

Moretto A. Promoters and promotion of axonopathies. *Toxicol Lett.* 2000;112–113:17–21.

Moretto A, Colosio C. Biochemical and toxicological evidence of neurological effects of pesticides: the example of Parkinson's disease. *Neurotoxicology.* 2011;32:383–391.

Moretto A, Tiramani M, Colosio C. Long-term neurotoxicological effects of anticholinesterases after acute or chronic exposure. In: Satoh T, Gupta RC, eds. *Anticholinesterase Pesticides: Metabolism, Neurotoxicity and Epidemiology.* Hoboken, NJ: John Wiley & Sons; 2010:97–108.

Mortensen S, Chandra S, Hooper M, et al. Maturational differences in chlorpyrifos-oxonase activity may contribute to age-related sensitivity to chlorpyrifos. *J Biochem Toxicol.* 1996;1:279–287.

Moser M, Li Y, Varpel K, et al. Placental failure and impaired vasculogenesis result in embryonic lethality for neuropathy target esterase-deficient mice. *Mol Cell Biol.* 2004;24:1667–1679.

Moser V. Companion of aldicarb and metamidophos neurotoxicity at different ages in the rat: behavioral and biochemical parameters. *Toxicol Appl Pharmacol.* 1999;157:94–106.

Mull RL, Hershberger LW. Inhibitors of DNA biosynthesis—mitosis: benzimidazoles. The benzimidazole fungicides benomyl and carbendazim. In: Krieger R, ed. *Handbook of Pesticide Toxicology.* San Diego: Academic Press; 2001:1673–1699.

Munro IC, Carlo GL, Orr JC, et al. A comprehensive, integrated review and evaluation of the scientific evidence relating to the safety of the herbicide 2,4-D. *J Am Coll Toxicol.* 1992;11:559–664.

Murphy SD. Toxic effects of pesticides. In: Klaassen CD, Amdur MO, Doull J, eds. *Casarett and Doull's Toxicology. The Basic Science of Poisons.* New York: Macmillan Publishing Co; 1986:519–581.

Mutch E, Daly AK, Leathart JBS, et al. Do multiple cytochrome P450 isoforms contribute to parathion metabolism in man? *Arch Toxicol.* 2003;77:313–320.

Nagami H, Nishigaki Y, Matsushima S, et al. Hospital-based survey of pesticide poisoning in Japan, 1998-2002. *Int J Occup Environ Health.* 2005;11:180–184.

Nakayama A, Sukekawa M. Quantitative correlation between molecular similarity and receptor-binding activity of neonicotinoid insecticides. *Pestic Sci.* 1998;52:104–110.

Narahashi T. Neuronal ion channels as the target sites of insecticides. *Pharmacol Toxicol.* 1996;78:1–14.

Narahashi T, Zhao X, Ikeda T, et al. Differential actions of insecticides on target sites: basis for selective toxicity. *Hum Exp Toxicol.* 2007;26:361–366.

Nash D, Mostashari F, Fine A, et al. The outbreak of West Nile virus infection in the New York City area in 1999. *N Engl J Med.* 2001;344:1807–1814.

Nathanson JA. Characterization of octopamine-sensitive adenylate cyclase: elucidation of a class of potent and selective octopamine-2 receptor agonists with toxic effects in insects. *Proc Natl Acad Sci U S A.* 1985;82:599–603.

Noren K, Meironyte D. Certain organochlorine and organobromine contaminants in Swedish human milk in perspective of past 20-30 years. *Chemosphere.* 2000;40:1111–1123.

Norman CS. Potential impact of imposing methylbromide phaseout on US strawberry growers: a case study of nomination for a critical use exemption under the Montreal Protocol. *J Environ Manag.* 2005;75:167–176.

Novak RJ, Lampman RL. Public health pesticides. In: Krieger R, ed. *Handbook of Pesticide Toxicology.* San Diego: Academic Press; 2001:181–201.

NRC (National Research Council). *Regulating Pesticides in Food: The Delaney Paradox.* Washington, DC: National Academy Press; 1987:288.

NRC (National Research Council). *Pesticides in the Diets of Infants and Children.* Washington, DC: National Academy Press; 1993:386.

O'Brien RD. *Insecticides: Action and Metabolism.* New York: Academic Press; 1967:332.

Okahashi N, Sano M, Miyata K, et al. Lack of evidence for endocrine disrupting effects in rats exposed to fenitrothion in utero and from weaning to maturation. *Toxicology.* 2005;206:17–31.

Okankwo JO, Mutshatsi TN, Botha B, et al. DDT, DDE and DDD in human milk from South Africa. *Bull Environ Contam Toxicol.* 2008;81:348–354.

O'Malley M. The regulatory evaluation of the skin effects of pesticides. In: Krieger R, ed. *Hayes' Handbook of Pesticide Toxicology.* San Diego: Academic Press; 2010:701–787.

Osimitz TG, Lake BG. Mode of action analysis for induction of rat liver tumors by pyrethrins: relevance to human cancer risk. *Crit Rev Toxicol.* 2009;39:501–511.

Osimitz TG, Murphy JV. Neurological effects associated with use of the insect repellent N, N-diethyl-m-toluamide (DEET). *Clin Toxicol.* 1997;35:435–441.

Padilla S, Wilson VA, Bushnell PJ. Studies on the correlation between blood cholinesterase inhibition and target tissue inhibition in pesticide-treated rats. *Toxicology.* 1994;92:11–25.

Park J, Darrien I, Prescott LF. Pharmacokinetic studies in severe intoxication with 2,4-D and mecoprop. *Proc Eur Soc Toxicol.* 1977;18:154–155.

Parsons PP. Mammalian toxicokinetics and toxicity of chlorothalonil. In: Krieger R, ed. *Hayes' Handbook of Pesticide Toxicology.* San Diego: Academic Press; 2010:1951–1966.

Peakall DB. Pesticides and the reproduction of birds. *Sci Am.* 1970;222:72–78.

Pearce N, McLean D. Agricultural exposures and non-Hodgkin's lymphoma. *Scand J Work Environ Health.* 2005;31(suppl 1):18–25.

Pelfrene AF. Rodenticides. In: Krieger R, ed. *Hayes' Handbook of Pesticide Toxicology.* San Diego: Academic Press; 2010:2153–2217.

Peraica M, Capodicasa E, Moretto A, et al. Organophosphate polyneuropathy in chicks. *Biochem Pharmacol.* 1993;45:131–135.

Peter JV, Moran JL, Graham P. Oxime therapy and outcomes in human organophosphate poisoning: an evaluation using meta-analytic techniques. *Crit Care Med.* 2006;34:502–510.

Petrucci N, Sardini S. Severe neurotoxic reaction associated with oral ingestion of low-dose diethyltoluamide-containing insect repellent in a child. *Pediatr Emerg Care.* 2000;16:341–342.

Phua DH, Lin CC, Wu ML, Deng JF, Yang CC. Neonicotinoid insecticides: an emerging cause of acute pesticide poisoning. *Clin Toxicol.* 2009;47:336–341.

Piccirillo VJ, Piccirillo AL. Methyl bromide. In: Krieger R, ed. *Hayes' Handbook of Pesticide Toxicology.* San Diego: Academic Press; 2010:2267–2279.

Pong SS, DeHaven R, Wang CC. A comparative study of avermectin B$_{1A}$ and other modulators of the γ-aminobutyric acid receptor-chloride ion channel complex. *J Neurosci.* 1982;2:966–971.

Pope C. The influence of age on pesticide toxicity. In: Krieger R, ed. *Hayes' Handbook of Pesticide Toxicology.* San Diego: Academic Press; 2010:819–835.

Popp W, Schmieding W, Speck M, et al. Incidence of bladder cancer is a cohort of workers exposed to 4-chloro-*o*-toluidine while synthesizing chlordimeform. *Br J Ind Med.* 1992;49:529–531.

Porterfield SP. Thyroidal dysfunction and environmental chemicals. Potential impact on brain development. *Environ Health Perspect.* 2000;108(suppl 3):433–438.

Poulos L, Athanaselis S, Coutselinis A. Acute intoxication with cypermethrin (NRDC 149). *J Toxicol Clin Toxicol.* 1982;19:519–520.

Power LE, Sudakin DL. Pyrethrin and pyrethroid exposure in the United States: a longitudinal analysis of incidents reported to poison centers. *J Med Toxicol.* 2007;3:94–99.

Prendergast MA, Terry AV, Buccafusco JJ. Effects of chronic, low-level organophosphate exposure on delayed recall, discrimination, and spatial learning in monkeys and rats. *Neurotoxicol Teratol.* 1998;20:115–122.

Proudfoot AT. Poisoning with amitraz. *Toxicol Rev.* 2003;22:71–74.

Proudfoot AT. Aluminum and zinc phosphide poisoning. *Clin Toxicol.* 2009;47:89–100.

Proudfoot AT, Krenzelak EP, Vale JA. Position paper on urine alkalinization. *J Toxicol Clin Toxicol.* 2004;42:1–26.

Pruett SB, Myers LP, Keil DE. Toxicology of metam sodium. *J Toxicol Environ Health Part B.* 2001;4:207–222.

Rajasuriar R, Awang R, Hashim SBH, et al. Profile of poisoning admissions in Malaysia. *Hum Exp Toxicol.* 2007;26:73–81.

Ray DE. Pesticides derived from plants and other organisms. In: Hayes WJ, Lawd ER, eds. *Handbook of Pesticide Toxicology.* San Diego: Academic Press; 1991:585–636.

Ray DE. Chronic effects of low level exposure to anticholinesterases—a mechanistic review. *Toxicol Lett.* 1998;103:527–533.

Ray DE, Forshaw PJ. Pyrethroid insecticides: poisoning, syndromes, synergies and therapy. *Clin Toxicol.* 2000;38:95–101.

Ray DE, Fry JR. A reassessment of the neurotoxicity of pyrethroid insecticides. *Pharmacol Ther.* 2006;111:174–193.

Reiner E, Simeon-Rudolf V. Methods for measuring cholinesterase activities in human blood. In: Gupta RC, ed. *Toxicology of Organophosphate and Carbamate Compounds.* Amsterdam: Elsevier; 2006:199–208.

Ricceri L, Markina N, Valanzano A, et al. Developmental exposure to chlorpyrifos alters reactivity to environmental and social cues in adolescent mice. *Toxicol Appl Pharmacol.* 2003;191:189–201.

Richardson JR, Quan Y, Sherer TB, et al. Paraquat neurotoxicity is distinct from that of MPTP and rotenone. *Toxicol Sci.* 2005;88:193–201.

Richardson RJ, Worden RM, Makhaeva GF. Biomarkers and biosensors of delayed neuropathic agents. In: Gupta RC, ed. *Handbook of Toxicology of Chemical Warfare Agents.* Amsterdam: Elsevier; 2009:859–876.

Risher JF, Miuk FL, Stara JF. The toxicologic effects of the carbamate insecticide aldicarb in mammals: a review. *Environ Health Perspect.* 1987;72:267–281.

Roberts D, Curtis C, Tren R, et al. Malaria control and public health. *Emerg Infect Dis.* 2004;10:1170–1171.

Roberts DM, Buckley N. Urinary alkalinization for acute achlorophenoxy herbicide poisoning. *Cochrane Database Syst Rev.* 2007;(1):CD005488.

Roberts DM, Karunarathna A, Buckley NA, et al. Influence of pesticide regulation on acute poisoning deaths in Sri Lanka. *Bull World Health Organ.* 2003;81:789–798.

Rogan WJ, Chen A. Health risks and benefits of bis (4-chlorophenyl)-1,1,1-trichloroethane (DDT). *Lancet.* 2005;366:763–773.

Rohr JR, McCoy K. A qualitative meta-analysis reveals consistent effects of atrazine on freshwater fish and amphibians. *Environ Health Perspect.* 2010;118:20–32.

Rohr JR, Schotthoefer AM, Raffael TR, et al. Agrochemicals increase trematode infections in declining amphibian species. *Nature.* 2008;455:1235–1239.

Rose MS, Smith LL, Wyatt I. Evidence for the energy-dependant accumulation of paraquat into rat lung. *Nature.* 1974;252:314–315.

Rosenstock L, Keifer M, Daniell WE, et al. Chronic central nervous system effects of acute organophosphate pesticide intoxication. *Lancet.* 1991;338:223–227.

Ross JH, Driver JH, Harris SA, et al. Dermal absorption of 2,4-D: a review of species differences. *Regul Toxicol Pharmacol.* 2005;41:82–91.

Ross MK, Borazjani A, Edward CC, et al. Hydrolytic metabolism of pyrethroids by human and other mammalian carboxylesterase. *Biochem Pharmacol.* 2006;71:657–669.

Rossman Y, Maharovski I, Bentur Y, et al. Carbamate poisoning: treatment recommendations in the setting of a mass casualties event. *Am J Emerg Med.* 2009;27:1117–1124.

Rusiecki JA, de Roos A, Lee WJ, et al. Cancer incidence among pesticide applicators exposed to atrazine in the Agricultural Health Study. *J Natl Cancer Inst.* 2004;96:1375–1382.

Rust MK. Insecticides and their use in urban structural pest control. In: Krieger R, ed. *Handbook of Pesticide Toxicology.* San Diego: Academic Press; 2001:243–250.

Ruzo LO. Physical, chemical and environmental properties of selected chemical alternatives for the pre-plant use of methyl bromide as soil fumigant. *Pest Manag Sci.* 2006;62:99–113.

Sabapathy NN. Paraquat formulation and safety management. In: Bismuth C, Hall AH, eds. *Paraquat Poisoning.* New York: Dekker; 1995:335–347.

Safe S. Endocrine disruptors and human health—is there a problem? An update. *Environ Health Perspect.* 2000;108:487–493.

Safe S. Clinical correlates of environmental endocrine disruptors. *Trends Endocrinol Metab.* 2005;16:139–144.

Sanahuja G, Banakar R, Twyman RM, et al. *Bacillus thuringiensis*: a century of research, development and commercial applications. *Plant Biotechnol J.* 2011;9:283–300.

Sanchez-Moreno S, Alonso-Prados E, Alonso-Prados JL, et al. Multivariate analysis of toxicological and environmental properties of soil nematocides. *Pest Manag Sci.* 2009;65:82–92.

Sanchez-Santed F, Canadas F, Flores P, et al. Long-term functional neurotoxicity of paraoxon and chlorpyrifos oxon: behavioral and pharmacological evidence. *Neurotoxicol Teratol.* 2004;26:304–317.

Sangha GK. Toxicology and safety evaluation of the new insect repellent picaridin (Saltidin). In: Krieger R, ed. *Hayes' Handbook of Pesticide Toxicology.* San Diego: Academic Press; 2010:2219–2230.

Satelle DB, Cordova D, Cheek TR. Insect ryanodine receptors: molecular targets for novel pest control chemicals. *Invert Neurosci.* 2008;8:107–119.

Sathiakumar N, Delzell E. A review of epidemiologic studies of triazine herbicides and cancer. *Crit Rev Toxicol.* 1997;27:599–612.

Satoh T, Gupta RC, eds. *Anticholinesterase Pesticides: Metabolism, Neurotoxicity and Epidemiology.* Hoboken, NJ: John Wiley & Sons; 2010:625.

Sawada Y, Nagai Y, Ueyama M, Yamamoto I. Probable toxicity of surface-active agent in commercial herbicide containing glyphosate. *Lancet.* 1988;1:299.

Schenker R, Tinembart O, Humbert-Droz E, et al. Comparative speed of kill between nitenpyram, fipronil, imidacloprid, selamectin and cythioate against adult *Ctenocephalides felis* (Bouché) on cats and dogs. *Vet Parasitol.* 2003;112:249–254.

Schneider SM, Rosskopf EN, Leesch JG, et al. United States Department of Agriculture—Agricultural Research Service research on alternatives to methyl bromide: pre-plant and post-harvest. *Pestic Manag Sci.* 2003;59:814–826.

Schnepf E, Crickmore N, Van Rie J, et al. *Bacillus thuringiensis* and its pesticidal crystal proteins. *Microbiol Mol Biol Rev.* 1998;62:775–806.

Schoenig GP, Hartnagel RE, Schardein JL, et al. Neurotoxicity evaluation of *N, N*-diethyl-*m*-toluamide (DEET) in rats. *Fundam Appl Toxicol.* 1993;21:355–365.

Schoenig GP, Osimitz TH. DEET. In: Krieger R, ed. *Handbook of Pesticide Toxicology.* San Diego: Academic Press; 2001:1439–1459.

Schulte-Hermann R, Wogan GN, Berry C, et al. Analysis of reproductive toxicity and classification of glufosinate-ammonium. *Regul Toxicol Pharmacol.* 2006;44:S1–S76.

Senanayake N, Karalliedde L. Neurotoxic effects of organophosphate insecticides. An intermediate syndrome. *N Engl J Med.* 1987;316:761–763.

Serota DG. *Combined Chronic Toxicity and Oncogenicity Study in Rats with 2,4-D Acid.* Unpublished Report 2184-102. Vienna, VA: Hazleton Laboratories Inc; 1986.

Shafer TJ, Meyer DA, Crofton KM. Developmental neurotoxicity of pyrethroid insecticides: critical review and future research needs. *Environ Health Perspect.* 2005;113:123–136.

Shapira M, Tur-Kaspa I, Bosgraaf L, et al. A transcription-activating polymorphism in the AChE promoter associated with acute sensitivity to anti-acetylcholinesterases. *Hum Mol Genet.* 2000;9:1273–1281.

Sheets LP. A consideration of age dependent differences in susceptibility to organophosphorus and pyrethroid insecticides. *Neurotoxicology.* 2000;21:57–64.

Sheets LP. Imidacloprid: a neonicotinoid insecticide. In: Krieger R, ed. *Hayes' Handbook of Pesticide Toxicology.* San Diego: Academic Press; 2010:2055–2064.

Shepard HH. *The Chemistry and Toxicology of Insecticides.* Minneapolis: Burgess Publishing Co; 1939:383.

Sherer TB, Kim JH, Betarbet R, et al. Subcutaneous rotenone exposure causes highly selective dopaminergic degeneration and α-synuclein aggregation. *Exp Neurol.* 2003;179:6–16.

Shimizu K, Ohtaki K, Matsubara K, et al. Carrier-mediated processes in blood–brain barrier penetration and neural uptake of paraquat. *Brain Res.* 2001;906:135–142.

Singh S, Batra YK, Singh SM, Wig N, Sharma BK. Is atropine alone sufficient in acute severe organophosphorus poisoning? Experience of a North West Indian hospital. *Int J Clin Pharmacol Ther.* 1995;33:628–630.

Smith AG. Chlorinated hydrocarbon insecticides. In: Hayes WJ, Laws ER, eds. *Handbook of Pesticide Toxicology.* San Diego: Academic Press; 1991:731–915.

Smith AG. Toxicology of DDT and some analogues. In: Krieger R, ed. *Hayes's Handbook of Pesticide Toxicology.* San Diego: Academic Press; 2010:1975–2032.

Smith LL. Mechanism of paraquat toxicity in the lung and its relevance to treatment. *Hum Toxicol.* 1987;6:31–36.

Smith LL, Heath D. Paraquat. *CRC Crit Rev Toxicol.* 1976;4:411–445.

Sobus JR, Morgan MK, Pleil JD, et al. Biomonitoring: uses and considerations for assessing nonoccupational human exposures to pesticides. In: Krieger R, ed. *Hayes' Handbook of Pesticide Toxicology.* San Diego: Academic Press; 2010:1021–1036.

Soderlund DM. Toxicology and mode of action of pyrethroid insecticides. In: Krieger R, ed. *Hayes' Handbook of Pesticide Toxicology.* San Diego: Academic Press; 2010:1665–1686.

Soderlund DM, Casida JE. Effects of pyrethroid structure on rates of hydrolysis and oxidation by mouse liver microsomal enzymes. *Pestic Biochem Physiol.* 1977;7:391–401.

Soderlund DM, Clark JM, Sheets LP, et al. Mechanisms of pyrethroid neurotoxicity: implications for cumulative risk assessment. *Toxicology.* 2002;171:3–59.

Solomon KR, Can JA, Du Preez LH, et al. Effects of atrazine on fish, amphibians and aquatic reptiles: a critical review. *Crit Rev Toxicol.* 2008;38:721–772.

Song X, Seidler FJ, Saleh JL, et al. Cellular mechanisms for developmental toxicity of chlorpyrifos: targeting the adenylate cyclase signaling cascade. *Toxicol Appl Pharmacol.* 1997;145:158–174.

Spagnolo A, Bianchi F, Calabro A, et al. Anophthalmia and benomyl in Italy: a multicenter study based on 940,615 newborns. *Reprod Toxicol.* 1994;8:397–403.

Stebbins KE, Johnson KA, Jeffries TK, et al. Chronic toxicity and oncogenicity studies of ingested 1, 3-dichloropropene in rats and mice. *Regul Toxicol Pharmacol.* 2000;32:1–13.

Stella J, Ryan M. Glyphosate herbicide formulation: a potentially lethal ingestion. *Emerg Med Aust.* 2004;16:235–239.

Sterling TD, Arundel AV. Health effects of phenoxy herbicides. *Scand J Work Environ Health.* 1986;12:161–173.

Stevens J, Breckenrideg CB, Wright J. The role of P-glycoprotein in preventing developmental and neurotoxicity: avermectins—a case study. In: Krieger R, ed. *Hayes' Handbook of Pesticide Toxicology.* San Diego: Academic Press; 2010:2093–2110.

Stevens JT, Breckenridge CB. The avermectins: insecticidal and antiparasitic agents. In: Krieger R, ed. *Handbook of Pesticide Toxicology.* San Diego: Academic Press; 2001:1157–1167.

Stevens JT, Breckenridge CB, Wetzel LT, et al. A risk characterization for atrazine: oncogenicity profile. *J Toxicol Environ Health.* 1999;56:69–109.

Stevens RC, Suzuki SM, Cole TB, et al. Engineered recombinant human paraoxonase 1 (rHuPON1) purified from *Escherichia coli* protects against organophosphate poisoning. *Proc Natl Acad Sci U S A.* 2008;105:12780–12784.

Stoker TE, Kavlock RJ. Pesticides as endocrine-disrupting chemicals. In: Krieger R, ed. *Hayes' Handbook of Pesticide Toxicology.* San Diego: Academic Press; 2010:551–569.

Storm E, Rozman KK, Doull J. Occupational exposure limits for organophosphate pesticides based on inhibition of red blood cell acetylcholinesterase. *Toxicology.* 2000;150:1–29.

Stott WT, Gollapudi BB. 1,3-Dichloropropene. In: Krieger R, ed. *Hayes' Handbook of Pesticide Toxicology.* San Diego: Academic Press; 2010:2281–2292.

Stott WT, Gollapudi BB, Rao KS. Mammalian toxicity of 1,3-dichloropropene. *Rev Environ Contam Toxicol.* 2001;168:1–42.

Stuetz W, Propamontol T, Erhardt JG, Classen HG. Organochlorine pesticide residues in human milk of a Hmong hill tribe living in Northern Thailand. *Sci Total Environ.* 2001;273:53–60.

Sudakin DK. Biopesticides. *Toxicol Rev.* 2003;22:83–90.

Sudakin DK, Osimitz T. DEET. In: Krieger R, ed. *Hayes' Handbook of Pesticide Toxicology.* San Diego: Academic Press; 2010:2111–2125.

Sudakin DL, Trevathan WR. DEET: a review and update of safety and risk in the general population. *J Toxicol Clin Toxicol.* 2003;41:831–839.

Sundwall A. Minimum concentrations of *N*-methylpyridinium-2-aldoxime methane sulphonate (P2S) which reverse neuromuscular block. *Biochem Pharmacol.* 1961;8:413–417.

Syed Z, Leal WS. From the cover: mosquitoes smell and avoid the insect repellent DEET. *Proc Natl Acad Sci U S A.* 2008;105:13598–13603.

Taets C, Aref S, Rayburn AL. The clastogenic potential of triazine herbicide combinations found in potable water supplies. *Environ Health Perspect.* 1998;106:197–201.

Talbot AR, Shiaw MH, Huang JS, et al. Acute poisoning with a glyphosate surfactant herbicide (Roundup): a review of 93 cases. *Hum Exp Toxicol.* 1998;10:1–8.

Tamura H, Yoshikawa H, Gaido KW, et al. Interaction of organophosphate pesticides and related compounds with the androgen receptor. *Environ Health Perspect.* 2003;111:545–552.

Tang J, Cao Y, Rose RL, et al. Metabolism of chlorpyrifos by human cytochrome P450 isoforms and human, mouse and rat liver microsomes. *Drug Metab Dispos.* 2001;29:1201–1204.

Tang J, Rose RL, Chambers JE. Metabolism of organophosphorus and carbamate pesticides. In: Gupta RC, ed. *Toxicology of Organophosphate and Carbamate Compounds.* Amsterdam: Elsevier; 2006:127–143.

Tanner CM, Kamel F, Ross GW, et al. Rotenone, paraquat and Parkinson's disease. *Environ Health Perspect.* 2011;119:866–872.

Taylor JR, Selhorst JB, Houff SA, et al. Chlordecone intoxication in man. I. Clinical observations. *Neurology.* 1978;28:626–630.

Taylor P. Agents acting at the neuromuscular junction and autonomic ganglia. In: Hardman JG, Limbird LE, eds. *Goodman & Gilman's The Pharmacological Basis of Therapeutics.* New York: McGraw-Hill; 1996:177–197.

Tenenbein M. Severe toxic reactions and death following the ingestion of diethyltoluamide-containing insect repellents. *JAMA.* 1987;258:1509–1511.

Thiruchelvam M, Richfield EK, Baggs RB, et al. The nigrostriatal dopaminergic system as a preferential target of repeated exposures to combined paraquat and maneb: implications for Parkinson's disease. *J Neurosci.* 2000;20:9207–9214.

Tilson HA. Neurotoxicology risk assessment guidelines: developmental neurotoxicology. *Neurotoxicology.* 2000;21:189–194.

Timofeeva OA, Levin ED. Lasting behavioral consequences of organophosphate pesticide exposure during development. In: Krieger R, ed. *Hayes' Handbook of Pesticide Toxicology.* San Diego: Academic Press; 2010:837–846.

Tominack RL. Herbicide formulations. *Clin Toxicol.* 2000;38:129–135.

Tomizawa M, Casida JE. Neonicotinoid insecticide toxicology: mechanisms of selective action. *Annu Rev Pharmacol Toxicol.* 2005;45:247–268.

980

Turosov V, Rakitsky V, Tomatis L. Dichlorodiphenyltrichloroethane (DDT): ubiquity, persistence, and risks. *Environ Health Perspect.* 2002;110: 125–128.

Tweedy BW. Inorganic sulfur as a fungicide. *Residue Rev.* 1981;78:43–68.

Ujvary I. Nicotine and other insecticidal alkaloids. In: Yamamoto I, Casida JE, eds. *Nicotinoid Insecticides and the Nicotinic Acetylcholine Receptor.* Tokyo: Springer Verlag; 1999:29–69.

Ujvary I. Pest control agents from natural products. In: Krieger R, ed. *Hayes' Handbook of Pesticide Toxicology.* San Diego: Academic Press; 2010:119–229.

USEPA (U.S. Environmental Protection Agency). *DDT: A Review of Scientific and Economic Aspects of the Decision to Ban Its Use as a Pesticide.* Washington, DC: USEPA; 1975:300.

USEPA (U.S. Environmental Protection Agency). *A SAB Report: Assessment of Potential 2,4-D Carcinogenicity. Review of Epidemiological and Other Data on Potential Carcinogenicity of 2,4-D.* Washington, DC: U.S. Environmental Protection Agency, Science Advisory Board; 1994.

USEPA (U.S. Environmental Protection Agency). *Carcinogenicity Peer Review (4th) of 2,4-Dichlorophenoxyacetic Acid (2,4-D).* Washington, DC: USEPA; January 29, 1997.

USEPA (U.S. Environmental Protection Agency). *Exposure Factors Handbook.* EPA/600/C-99/001. Washington, DC: US EPA, Office of Research and Development; February 1999.

USEPA (U.S. Environmental Protection Agency). *The Use of Data on Cholinesterase Inhibition for Risk Assessments of Organophosphorus and Carbamate Pesticides.* Washington, DC: USEPA: 2000:50. Available at: http://www.epa.gov/pesticides/trac/science/cholin.pdf.

USEPA (U.S. Environmental Protection Agency). *Potential Developmental Effects of Atrazine in Amphibians.* 2003. Available at: www.epa.gov/oscpmont/sap/2003/june/junemeetingreport.pdf.

USEPA (U.S. Environmental Protection Agency). *Triazine Cumulative Risk Assessment and Atrazine, Simazine and Propazine Decisions.* Washington, DC: USEPA; June 22, 2006.

USEPA (U.S. Environmental Protection Agency). *Pesticide Fact Sheet: Flubendiamide.* Washington, DC: USEPA; 2008:65.

Van den Bercken J. The effect of DDT and dieldrin on myelinated nerve fibers. *Eur J Pharmacol.* 1972;20:205–214.

van den Berg H. Global status of DDT and its alternatives for use in vector control to prevent disease. *Environ Health Perspect.* 2009;117:1656–1663.

van Frankenhuyzen K. Insecticidal activity of *Bacillus thuringiensis* crystal proteins. *J Invert Pathol.* 2009;101:1–16.

Vanholder R, Colardyn F, De Reuck J, et al. Diquat intoxication—report of two cases and review of the literature. *Am J Med.* 1981;70:1267–1271.

Veale DJ, Wium CA, Muller GJ. Amitraz poisoning in South Africa: a two year survey (2008-2009). *Clin Toxicol (Phila).* 2011;49:40–44.

Veronesi B, Padilla S, Blackmon K, et al. Murine susceptibility to organophosphorus-induced delayed neuropathy (OPIDN). *Toxicol Appl Pharmacol.* 1991;107:311–324.

Verschoyle RD, Aldridge WN. Structure–activity relationships of some pyrethroids in rats. *Arch Toxicol.* 1980;45:325–329.

Vijverberg HPM, van der Zalm JM, van den Bercken J. Similar mode of action of pyrethroids and DDT on sodium channel gating in myelinated nerves. *Nature.* 1982;295:601–603.

Villanueva CM, Durand G, Coutté MB, et al. Atrazine in municipal drinking water and risk of low birth weight, pre-term delivery, and small-for-gestational-age status. *Occup Environ Med.* 2005;62:400–405.

Wagner SL. *Clinical Toxicology of Agricultural Chemicals.* Park Ridge, NJ: Noyes Data Corporation; 1983:306.

Waliszewski SM, Aguirre AA, Infanzon RM, et al. Comparison of organochlorine pesticide levels in adipose tissue and human milk of mothers living in Veracruz, Mexico. *Bull Environ Contam Toxicol.* 1999;62:685–690.

Walters JK, Boswell LE, Green MK, et al. Pyrethrin and pyrethroid illnesses in the Pacific Northwest: a five-year review. *Public Health Rep.* 2009;124;149–159.

Watanabe T, Sano T. Neurological effects of glufosinate poisoning with a brief review. *Hum Exp Toxicol.* 1998;17:35–39.

Weichenthal S, Moase C, Chan P. A review of pesticide exposure and cancer incidence in the Agricultural Health Study cohort. *Environ Health Perspect.* 2010;118:1117–1125.

Weiss B, Amler S, Amler SW. Pesticides. *Pediatrics.* 2004;113:1030–1036.

Wesseling C, Castillo L, Elinder CG. Pesticide poisonings in Costa Rica. *Scand J Work Environ Health.* 1993;19:227–235.

Wesseling C, van Wendel De Joode B, Ruepert C, et al. Paraquat in developing countries. *Int J Occup Environ Health.* 2001;7:275–286.

Whalon ME, Wingend BA. Bt: mode of action and use. *Arch Insect Biochem Physiol.* 2003;54:200–211.

WHO (World Health Organization). *DDT and Its Derivatives. Environmental Health Criteria 9.* Geneva: WHO; 1979:194.

WHO (World Health Organization). *Public Health Impact of Pesticides Used in Agriculture.* Geneva: WHO; 1990.

WHO (World Health Organization). *World Malaria Report 2010.* Geneva: WHO; 2010:238.

Wijeyesakere SJ, Richardson RJ. Neuropathy target esterase. In: Krieger R, ed. *Hayes' Handbook of Pesticide Toxicology.* San Diego: Academic Press; 2010:1435–1455.

Williams GM, Kroes R, Munro IC. Safety evaluation and risk assessment of the herbicide Roundup and its active ingredient, glyphosate, for humans. *Regul Toxicol Pharmacol.* 2000;31:117–165.

Wilson AGE, Lau H, Asbury KJ, et al. Metabolism of alachlor by human nasal tissue. *Fundam Appl Toxicol.* 1995;15:1398.

Wilson BW, Henderson JD. Determination of cholinesterase in blood and tissue. *Curr Protoc Toxicol.* 2007;34:12.13.1–12.13.16.

Wong CK, Leung KM, Poon BH, et al. Organochlorine hydrocarbons in human breast milk collected in Hong Kong and Guangzhou. *Arch Environ Contam Toxicol.* 2002;43:364–372.

Wood DM, Alsahaf H, Streete P, et al. Fatality after deliberate ingestion of the pesticide rotenone: a case report. *Crit Care.* 2005;9:R280–R284.

Woods JS, Polissar L, Severson RK, et al. Soft tissue sarcoma and non-Hodgkin's lymphoma in relation to phenoxyherbicide and chlorinated phenol exposure in western Washington. *J Natl Cancer Inst.* 1987;78:899–910.

Woolley DE. Neurotoxicity of DDT and possible mechanisms of action. In: Prasad KN, Vernadakis A, eds. *Mechanisms of Action of Neurotoxic Substances.* New York: Raven Press; 1982:95–141.

Worek F, Diebold C, Eyer P. Dimethylphosphoryl-inhibited human cholinesterases: inhibition, reactivation and aging kinetics. *Arch Toxicol.* 1999a;73:7–14.

Worek F, Mast U, Kiderlen D, et al. Improved determination of acetylcholinesterase activity in human whole blood. *Clin Chim Acta.* 1999b;288:73–90.

Yang PY, Taso TC, Lin JL, et al. Carbofuran-induced delayed neuropathy. *J Toxicol Clin Toxicol.* 2000;38:43–46.

Yaramis A, Soker M, Bilici M. Amitraz poisoning in children. *Hum Exp Toxicol.* 2000;19:1–3.

Yoon YJ, Kim ES, Hwang YS, et al. Avermectin: biochemical and molecular basis of its synthesis and regulation. *Appl Microbiol Biotechnol.* 2004;63:626–634.

Zaccheo O, Dinsdale D, Meacock PA, et al. Neuropathy target esterase and its yeast homologue degrade phosphatidylcholine to glycerophosphocholine in living cells. *J Biol Chem.* 2004;279:24024–24033.

Zadikoff CM. Toxic encephalopathy associated with use of insect repellents. *J Pediatr.* 1979;95:140–142.

Zaki MM, Moran D, Harris D. Pesticide in ground-water: the aldicarb story in Suffolk County, New York. *Am J Public Health.* 1982;72:1391–1395.

Zhang J, Fitsanakis VA, Gu G, et al. Manganese ethylene-bis-dithiocarbamate and selective dopaminergic neurodegeneration in rat: a link through mitochondrial dysfunction. *J Neurochem.* 2003;84:336–346.

Zilker T, Fogt F, von Clarmann M. Kein Parkinsonsyndrom nach akuter paraquat intoxikation. *Klin Wochenschr.* 1988;66:1138–1141.

chapter 23

Toxic Effects of Metals

Erik J. Tokar, Windy A. Boyd,
Jonathan H. Freedman, and Michael P. Waalkes

INTRODUCTION

What is a Metal?

What defines a "metal" is not always obvious and the differences between metallic and nonmetallic elements may be subtle (Vouk, 1986). Metals are typically defined by physical properties of the element in the solid state, but can vary widely with the metallic element. General metal properties include high reflectivity (luster), high electrical conductivity, high thermal conductivity, and mechanical ductility and strength. A characteristic of metals of toxicological importance is that they may often react in biological systems by losing one or more electrons to form cations (Vouk, 1986). In the periodic table, within a group there is often a gradual transition from nonmetallic to metallic properties going from lighter to heavier atoms (eg, Group IVa transitions from carbon to lead). Metals often exhibit variable oxidation states. Various names are applied to subsets of metallic elements including alkali metals (eg, lithium and sodium), the alkaline earth metals (eg, beryllium and magnesium), the transition (or "heavy") metals (eg, cadmium), and the metalloids (eg, arsenic and antimony), the latter of which show characteristics of metals and nonmetals.

Over 75% of the elements in the periodic table are regarded as metals and several are considered metalloids. This chapter discusses metals, and certain metal complexes or molecules, that have been reported to produce significant toxicity in humans. The discussion includes major toxic metals (eg, lead, cadmium), essential metals (eg, zinc, copper), medicinal metals (eg, platinum, bismuth), and minor toxic metals including metals of technological significance (eg, indium, uranium). This chapter will also discuss toxic metalloids (eg, arsenic, antimony) and certain nonmetallic elemental toxicants (eg, selenium, fluoride). An overview of *toxic effects of metals* is shown in Fig. 23-1.

Metals as Toxicants

It cannot be stressed enough that the use of metals has been critical to the progress and success of human civilization. It is difficult to imagine an advanced civilization without extensive use of metals and metal compounds. However, metals are unique among pollutant toxicants in that they are all naturally occurring and, in many cases, are already ubiquitous to some level within the human environment. Thus, regardless of how safely metals are used in industrial processes or consumer endpoint products, some level of human exposure is inevitable. Furthermore, life evolved in the presence of metals and organisms have been forced to deal with these potentially toxic, yet omnipresent, elements. Perhaps in response

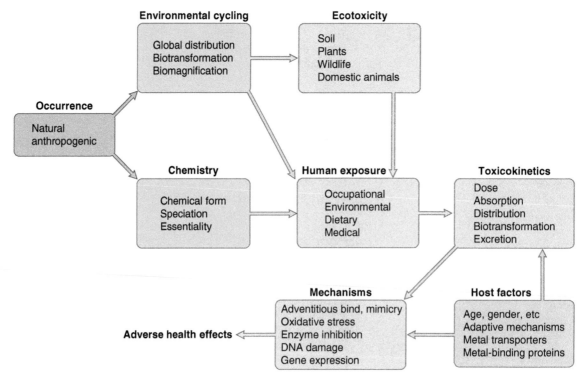

Figure 23-1. *Overview of metal toxicology.*

to, or at the very least fortuitously, many metals have become essential to various biological processes. With essentiality there is intentional bioaccumulation that involves safe transport and storage. Nonetheless, even essential metals can be toxic with increasing exposure, as they overwhelm biological systems and bind to unwanted sites. It is repeatedly seen that the nonessential toxicant metals mimic essential metals and thereby gain access to, and potentially disrupt, key cellular functions. This can also account for bioaccumulation of toxic metals without known biological function.

Metals differ from other toxic substances because, as elements, they are neither created nor destroyed by human endeavors. What human industry and civilization generally do accomplish is to concentrate metals in the biosphere. The anthropogenic contribution to the levels of metals in air, water, soil, and food is well recognized (Beijer and Jernelov, 1986). Human use of metals can also alter the chemical form or speciation of an element and thereby impact toxic potential. With a few very notable exceptions, most metals are only sparingly recycled once used. These factors combine together and tend to make metals persistent in the human environment, often resulting in protracted exposures.

Due to their very early use, metals are one of the oldest toxicants known to humans. For instance, human use of lead probably started prior to 2000 BC, when abundant supplies were obtained from ores as a by-product of smelting silver. The first description of abdominal colic in a man who extracted metals is credited to Hippocrates in 370 BC. Arsenic and mercury are discussed by Theophrastus of Erebus (370–287 BC), and Pliny the Elder (AD 23–79). Arsenic was used early on for decoration in Egyptian tombs and as a "secret poison," whereas mercury assumed almost a mystical stature in early science and was a large focus of alchemy. However, most of the use of the metals has occurred since the onset of the industrial revolution. In this regard, many of the metals of toxicological concern today were only relatively recently discovered. For instance, cadmium was first recognized in the early 1800s, and it was much later before the metal was widely used. The toxicological importance of some of the rarer or lesser used metals has increased with new applications, such as chemotherapy and microelectronics, or other emerging technologies.

Historically, metal toxicology usually concerned acute or overt, high-dose effects, such as abdominal colic from lead or the bloody diarrhea and uropenia after mercury exposures. Due to advances in our understanding of toxic potential of metals, and the accompanying improvements in industrial hygiene and stricter environmental standards, acute high-dose effects of metals are now very uncommon in the Western world. Metal toxicology has shifted focus to more subtle, chronic, low-dose effects, in which cause-and-effect relationships may not be immediately clear. These might include a level of effect that causes a change in an important, but highly complex index of an affected individual's performance, such as lower than expected IQs due to childhood lead exposure. Other important chronic toxic effects include carcinogenesis, and several metals have emerged as human carcinogens (Straif et al., 2009). In humans, defining the responsible agent for such toxicological effects can often be difficult, particularly when the endpoint disease may have a complex etiology caused by a number of different chemicals or even combinations of chemicals. In addition, humans are never exposed to only a single metal, but rather to complex mixtures. Rodent or cellular/molecular models are helpful but the metals as a class of toxicants clearly present many challenges in toxicological research.

The elemental nature of metals impacts their biotransformation and toxicity, as detoxication by destructive metabolism to subcomponents of lesser toxicity cannot occur with these atomic species. In essence, beyond elemental species metals are nonbiodegradable. This level of indestructibility combined with the bioaccumulation that can often occur contributes to the high concern for metals as toxicants. Most elemental metals tend to form ionic bonds. However, biological conjugation to form organometallic compounds can occur for various metals (Dopp et al., 2004; Drobna et al., 2010), particularly with metalloids, such as arsenic, that show mixed carbonaceous and metallic qualities. The redox capacity of a given metal or metallic compound should also be considered as part of its metabolism. The metabolism of metals is intricate and subtle but directly impacts toxic potential.

Movement of Metals in the Environment

Metals are redistributed naturally in the environment by both geologic and biological cycles. Rainwater dissolves rocks and ores and transports materials, including metals, to rivers and underground water (eg, arsenic), depositing and stripping materials from adjacent soil and eventually transporting these substances to the ocean to be precipitated as sediment or taken up into forming rainwater to be relocated elsewhere. Biological cycles moving metals include biomagnification by plants and animals resulting in incorporation into food cycles. In comparison, human activity often intentionally shortens the residence time of metals in ore deposits, and can result in the formation of new, non-naturally occurring metallic compounds. For instance, cadmium distribution mainly comes from human activities. Human industry greatly enhances metal distribution in the global environment by discharge to soil, water, and air, as exemplified by the 200-fold increase in lead content of Greenland ice since the onset of the industrial revolution. Mercury undergoes global cycling with elevated levels being found far from points of discharge, as, for example, with mercury in the Arctic Ocean. Mercury also undergoes biomethylation and biomagnification by aquatic organisms (see Fig. 23-5).

Increased distribution of metals and metal compounds in the environment, especially through anthropogenic activities, raises increasing concern for ecotoxicological effects. Reports of metal intoxication are common in plants, aquatic organisms, invertebrates, fish, sea mammals, birds, and domestic animals. The ecotoxicity of various metals is discussed under each individual section. Mercury poisoning from consumption of fish containing high levels of methylmercury and cadmium poisoning from consumption of rice grown in soils contaminated with cadmium from industrial discharges are examples of human consequences from environmental pollution.

Not all human toxicity occurs from metals deposited in the biosphere by human activity. For example, chronic arsenic poisoning from high levels of naturally occurring inorganic arsenic in drinking water is a major health issue in many parts of the world. Endemic intoxication from excess fluoride, selenium, or thallium can all occur from natural high environmental levels.

Chemical Mechanisms of Metal Toxicology

The precise chemical basis of metal toxicology is inadequately understood but a uniform mechanism for all toxic metals is implausible because of the great variation in chemical properties and toxic end points. Chemically, metals in their ionic form can be very reactive and can interact with biological systems in a large variety of ways. In this regard, a cell presents numerous potential metal-binding ligands. For instance, metals such as cadmium and mercury readily attach to sulfur in proteins as a preferred bioligand. Such adventitious binding is an important chemical mechanism by which exogenous metals exert toxic effects that can result in steric rearrangement that impairs the function of biomolecules (Kasprzak, 2002). An example would be the inhibition of enzyme activity by metal interaction at sites other than the active center, such as the inhibition of heme synthesis enzymes by lead. The inhibition of biologically critical enzymes is an important molecular mechanism of metal toxicology.

The metals can show more specific forms of chemical attack through mimicry. In this regard the toxic metals may act as mimics of essential metals, binding to physiological sites that normally are reserved for an essential element. Owing to their rich chemistry, essential metals control, or are involved in, a variety of key metabolic and signaling functions (Kasprzak, 2002; Cousins et al., 2006). Through mimicry, the toxic metals may gain access to, and potentially disrupt, a variety of important or even critical metal-mediated cellular functions. For example, mimicry for, and replacement of, zinc is a mechanism of toxicity for cadmium, copper, and nickel. Thallium mimics potassium and manganese mimics iron as a critical factor in their toxicity. Mimicry of arsenate and vanadate for phosphate allows for cellular transport of these toxic elements, whereas selenate, molybdate, and chromate mimic sulfate and can compete for sulfate carriers and in chemical sulfation reactions (Bridges and Zalpus, 2005). Organometallic compounds can also act as mimics of biological chemicals, as, for example, with methylmercury, which is transported by amino acid or organic anion transporters (Bridges and Zalpus, 2005). Indeed, molecular or ionic mimicry at the level of transport is often a key event in metal toxicity.

Another key chemical reaction in metal toxicology is metal-mediated oxidative damage. Many metals can directly act as catalytic centers for redox reactions with molecular oxygen or other endogenous oxidants, producing oxidative modification of biomolecules such as proteins or DNA. This may be a key step in the carcinogenicity of certain metals (Kasprzak, 2002). Besides oxygen-based radicals, carbon- and sulfur-based radicals may also occur. Nickel and chromium are two examples of metals that act, at least in part, by generation of reactive oxygen species (ROS) or other reactive intermediates (Kasprzak, 2002). Alternatively, metals may displace redox active essential elements from their normal cellular ligands, which, in turn, may result in oxidative cellular damage. For instance, cadmium, which is not redox active, may well cause oxidative stress through the release of endogenous iron, an element with high redox activity (Valko et al., 2006).

Metals in their ionic form can be very reactive and form DNA and protein adducts in biological systems. For example, once hexavalent chromium enters the cell it is reduced by various intracellular reductants to give reactive trivalent chromium species that form DNA adducts or DNA–protein cross-links, events likely to be important in chromium genotoxicity (Zhitkovich, 2005). Metals can also induce an array of aberrant gene expression, which, in turn, produces adverse effects. For example, nickel can induce the expression of Cap43/NDRG1, under the control of the hypoxia-inducible transcription factor (HIF-1), which is thought to play a key role in nickel carcinogenesis (Costa et al., 2005). An array of aberrant hepatic gene expressions occurs in adult mice after in utero arsenic exposure, which could be an important molecular event in arsenic hepatocarcinogenesis (Liu et al., 2006).

Factors Impacting Metal Toxicity

The standard factors that impact the toxic potential of all chemicals apply to the metals as well. Exposure-related factors include dose, route of exposure, duration, and frequency of exposure. Because metals can be quite reactive, the portal of entry is often initially the organ most affected, as with the lung after inhalation.

Host-based factors that can impact metal toxicity include age at exposure, gender, and capacity for biotransformation. For instance, it is quite clear that younger subjects are often more sensitive to metal intoxication, as, for example, with the neurotoxicity of lead in children. The major pathway of exposure to many toxic metals in children is food, and children consume more calories per pound of body weight than adults. Moreover, children have higher gastrointestinal absorption of metals, particularly lead. The rapid growth and proliferation in the perinate represent opportunities for toxic effects, including potentially carcinogenesis, of metallic agents, and several metals (eg, arsenic, nickel, lead, and chromium) are transplacental carcinogens in rodents. Fetal-stage toxicity of metals is well documented, as with methylmercury, and many metals are teratogenic. For many inorganics there is no impediment to transplacental transport, as with lead or arsenic, and human fetal blood lead levels (BLL) are similar to maternal levels. Elderly persons are also believed to be generally more susceptible to metal toxicity than younger adults. Recognition of factors that influence toxicity of a metal is important in determining risk, particularly in susceptible subpopulations.

Chemical-related factors directly impact the toxic potential of metals. This would include the precise metal compound and its valence state or speciation. For instance, methylmercury is a potent neurotoxin, whereas the inorganic mercurials primarily attack the kidney. Similarly, the oxidation state of chromium can differentiate the essential (naturally occurring trivalent chromium) from toxic species (hexavalent chromium).

Lifestyle factors such as smoking or alcohol ingestion may have direct or indirect impacts on the level of metal intoxication. For instance, cigarette smoke by itself contains many toxic metals, such as cadmium, and it is thought that smoking will double the lifetime burden of cadmium in nonoccupationally exposed individuals. Other components of cigarette smoke may also influence pulmonary effects, as, for instance, with metals that are lung carcinogens. Alcohol ingestion may influence toxicity by altering diet, reducing essential mineral intake, and altering hepatic iron deposition. The composition of the diet can significantly alter gastrointestinal absorption of various dietary metals.

The essentiality of metals has direct bearing on the toxic potential of a metal. Any "free" ionic metal would be potentially toxic due to reactive potential. The need to accumulate essential metals dictates the evolution of systems for the safe transport, storage, and utilization as well as, within limits, elimination of excess. For example, metallothionein (MT) is a metal-binding protein that may function in the homeostatic control of zinc (Cousins et al., 2006), and may represent a storage or transport form of this metal. Such factors imply that a threshold would exist for toxicity due to essential metal exposure. In this regard, the essential metallic elements would be expected to show a "U"-shaped dose–response curve in that, at very low exposure levels, toxic adverse effects would occur from deficiency, but at high exposure levels toxicity also occurs. The nonessential toxic metals can mimic essential elements and disrupt homeostasis, as with cadmium which will potentially displace zinc to bind to zinc-dependent transcription factors and enzymes (Waalkes, 2003).

Adaptive mechanisms can be critical to the toxic effects of metals, and organisms have a variety of ways in which they can adapt to otherwise toxic metal insults. Typically, adaptation is acquired after the first few exposures and can be long-lasting or transient after exposure ceases. Adaptation can be at the level of uptake or excretion, or, with some metals, through long-term storage in a toxicologically inert form. For instance, it appears enhanced arsenic efflux is involved in acquired tolerance to the metalloid on the cellular level (Liu *et al.*, 2001). Conversely, intentional sequestration of toxic metals is another adaptive tactic and examples of such long-term storage include lead inclusion bodies, which form in various organs and contain protein-immobilized lead in a distinct cellular aggresome. These bodies are thought to be protective by limiting the level of free, and therefore toxic, lead within the cell, and the inability to form such bodies clearly increases the chronic toxic effects of lead, including carcinogenesis (Waalkes *et al.*, 2004). Similarly, cadmium exposure causes the overexpression of MT that will sequester cadmium and reduce its toxicity as an adaptive mechanism (Klaassen and Liu, 1998). Metal exposure can also induce a cascade of molecular/genetic responses that may, in turn, reduce toxicity, such as with metal-induced oxidative stress responses (Valko *et al.*, 2006). It is clear that acquired metal adaptation, although allowing immediate cellular survival, may in fact be a potential contributing factor in long-term toxicity (Waalkes *et al.*, 2000). For instance, acquired self-tolerance to cadmium- or arsenic-induced apoptosis may actually contribute to eventual carcinogenesis by allowing survival of damaged cells that would otherwise have been eliminated (Hart *et al.*, 2001; Pi *et al.*, 2005).

Biomarkers of Metal Exposure

Biomarkers of exposure, toxicity, and susceptibility are important in assessing the level of concern with metal intoxication. Exposure biomarkers, such as concentrations in blood or urine, have long been used with metals. Techniques in molecular toxicology have greatly expanded the possibilities for biomarkers. Thus, in the case of chromium, DNA–protein complexes may serve as a biomarker of both exposure and carcinogenic potential. The capacity for expression of genes that potentially play protective roles against metal toxicity, as, for example, with MT and heme oxygenase, shows promise as markers of both effect and susceptibility. The use of such biomarkers may well allow identification of particularly sensitive subpopulations.

Estimates of the relationship of exposure level to toxic effects for a particular metal are in many ways a measure of the dose–response relationships discussed in great detail earlier in this book. The dose of a metal is a multidimensional concept and is a function of time as well as concentration. The most toxicologically relevant definition of dose is the amount of active metal within cells of target organs. The active form is often presumed to be the free metal, but it is technically difficult or impossible to precisely determine.

A critical indicator of retention of a metal is its biological half-life, or the time it takes for the body or organ to excrete half of an accumulated amount. The biological half-life varies according to the metal as well as the organ or tissue. For example, the biological half-lives of cadmium in kidney and lead in bone are 20 to 30 years, whereas for some metals, such as arsenic or lithium, they are only a few hours to days. For many metals, more than one half-life is needed to fully describe the retention. The half-life of lead in blood is only a few weeks, as compared with the much longer half-life in bone. After inhalation of mercury vapor, at least two half-lives describe the retention in brain, one on the order of a few weeks and the other measured in years. Continued metal exposure clearly complicates retention kinetics.

Blood, urine, and hair are the most accessible tissues for measuring metal exposure. Results from single measurements may reflect recent exposure or long-term or past exposure, depending on retention time in the particular tissue. Blood and urine concentrations usually, but not always, are reflective of more recent exposures and correlate with acute adverse effects. An exception is urinary cadmium, which may reflect kidney damage related to a renal cadmium accumulation over several decades. Hair can be useful in assessing variations in exposure to metals over the period of its growth. Analyses can be performed on segments of the hair, so that metal content of the newest growth can be compared with past exposures. Hair levels of mercury have been found to be a reliable measure of exposure to methylmercury. For most other metals, however, hair is not a reliable tissue for measuring exposure because of metal deposits from external contamination that complicate analysis.

Molecular Responses to Metal Exposure

Exposure to elevated levels of nonessential and essential metals can induce intracellular damage. This damage includes oxidative stress, which can lead to lipid peroxidation, protein denaturation, DNA damage, and organelle dysfunction. In addition, metals can disrupt the biological function/activity of proteins by either directly binding to the protein or displacing metals within metalloproteins. The ability of metals to affect gene expression is well documented. However, the role of metal-induced changes in gene expression in the etiology of human disease has only recently begun to be elucidated. Modern genomic technologies have identified hundreds to thousands of genes whose levels of expression are affected following exposure to essential and nonessential metals. Gene expression can change as a direct response to metal exposure, or to metal-induced intracellular stress, such as oxidative stress, DNA damage, or protein denaturation. The intended consequence of metal activation of gene expression is to protect the organism from metal-induced damage. Metal exposure is associated with increased expression of genes that encode proteins that: (1) remove the metal from the cell via chelation or increased export; (2) reduce the level of oxidative stress; and (3) repair the metal-induced intracellular damage. However, the inappropriate activation of gene expression following metal exposure can be a contributing factor to a variety of human pathologies (Waisberg *et al.*, 2003).

Bioinformatic analyses of the genomic data have identified dozens of transcription factors and cognate intracellular signal transduction pathways that are activated in response to a variety of metals. Several of the more frequently identified transcription factors and signaling pathways include mitogen-activated protein kinase (MAPK), nuclear factor kappa-light-chain-enhancer of activated B cells (NF-κB), heat shock factor protein 1 (HFS-1), hypoxia-inducible factor-1α and -2α (HIF-1α, -2α), phosphoinositide 3′-kinase (PI3K)/Akt signaling cascade, and metal regulatory transcription factor 1 (MTF-1). Although these transcription factors and signaling pathways affect the expression of proteins that protect the cell from metal toxicity, they do not exclusively control the expression of defense and repair proteins. For example, MAPKs phosphorylate and activate a collection of transcription factors to regulate gene expression. The MAPKs are part of a regulatory network that controls multiple cellular processes including cell growth, differentiation, cell survival, and the stress response (Pearson *et al.*, 2001). Thus, any metal that activates the MAPK signaling cascade can produce unintentional effects on these basic cellular processes. It has been proposed that the activation of MAPK pathways by metals contributes to metal-induced apoptosis (Waisberg *et al.*, 2003).

Many metal-responsive signaling pathways and the cognate transcription factors have been identified. However, the mechanisms by which metals initially activate these pathways have not been completely resolved. Metals can affect the steady-state levels of intracellular second messengers such as calcium, cAMP, cGMP, nitric oxide, and phospholipids. Cadmium and zinc affect cAMP and cGMP levels by inhibiting the cyclic nucleotide phosphodiesterase responsible for the degradation of the cyclic nucleotide (Merali *et al.*, 1975; Watjen *et al.*, 2001). ROS can activate redox-sensitive transcription factors such as NF-κB, AP-1, and p53 (Valko *et al.*, 2005). It should be noted that a single metal can affect multiple signaling pathways, transcription factors, and second messengers. Likewise, the activity of a single transcription factor can be influenced by a variety of metals. For example the activity of NF-κB is affected by copper, arsenic, vanadium, chromium, cadmium, mercury, lead, or any other metal that can induce intracellular oxidative stress (Chen and Shi, 2002; Korashy and El-Kadi, 2008; Thevenod, 2009).

In addition to affecting gene expression via transcription factors, metals can induce epigenetic changes. Epigenetic changes include posttranslational modification of histones and methylation of DNA to convert cytosine to 5-methylcytosine (Esteller, 2009). The ability of nickel, cadmium, arsenic, and chromium to induce cancer has been linked to metal-inducible epigenetic changes (Arita and Costa, 2009).

Metal-Binding Proteins and Metal Transporters

Protein binding of metals is a critical aspect of essential and toxic metal metabolism (Zalpus and Koropatnick, 2000). Many different types of proteins play roles in the disposition of metals in the body. Nonspecific binding to proteins such as serum albumin or hemoglobin acts in metal transport and tissue distribution. Metals vary in their preferred site of proteinaceous binding, and can attack a variety of amino acid residues. For instance, cysteine sulfurs are preferred by cadmium and mercury, and these residues are commonly involved with overall protein structure, while copper and nickel prefer histidine imidazole. In addition, proteins with specific metal-binding properties play special roles in the trafficking of specific essential metals, and toxic metals may interact with these proteins through mimicry. Metal-binding proteins are an important emerging issue in the physiology and toxicology of metals and only a few examples are highlighted here.

The *MTs* are an important class of intracellular metal-binding proteins that function in essential metal homeostasis and metal detoxication (Carpene *et al.*, 2007). They are small (6000 Da), soluble, and rich in internally oriented thiol ligands. These thiol ligands provide the basis for high-affinity binding of several essential and toxic metals including zinc, cadmium, copper, and mercury. The MTs are highly inducible by a variety of metals or other stimulants including oxidative stress, heat shock, and exposure to chemotherapeutic agents. MTs clearly play an important role in metal toxicity, as illustrated in the discussion of cadmium below.

Transferrin is a glycoprotein that binds most of the ferric iron in plasma and helps transport iron across cell membranes. The protein also transports aluminum and manganese. *Ferritin* is primarily a storage protein for iron. It has been suggested that transferrin may serve as a general metal detoxicant protein, since it binds a variety of toxic metals including cadmium, zinc, beryllium, and aluminum.

Ceruloplasmin is a copper-containing glycoprotein oxidase in plasma that converts ferrous iron to ferric iron, which then binds to transferrin. This protein also stimulates iron uptake by a transferrin-independent mechanism.

In all cells there are mechanisms for metal ion homeostasis that frequently involve a balance between uptake and efflux systems. A large number of membrane-bound metal transport proteins have been discovered that transport metals across cell membranes and organelles inside the cells. Metal transporters are important for cellular resistance to metals or metalloids (Rosen, 2002). For instance, enhanced efflux via multidrug resistance protein pumps is involved in acquired tolerance to arsenic (Liu *et al.*, 2001), while decreased influx via reduced calcium G-type channels is involved in acquired tolerance to cadmium (Leslie *et al.*, 2006). Over 10 zinc transporters and four Zip family proteins are involved in cellular zinc transport, trafficking, and signaling (Cousins *et al.*, 2006). The importance of metal transporters in human diseases is well illustrated by Menkes disease and Wilson disease, which are caused by genetic mutations in the copper-transport protein gene *ATP7A*, resulting in copper deficiency (Menkes), or *ATP7B*, resulting in copper overload (Wilson) (see Fig. 23-7).

Metal chaperones are a class of proteins and small molecules that move metals within cells. These molecules prevent the metal ions from roaming freely in a reactive form within the cytoplasm. They are also responsible for delivering metals into metalloproteins. Copper and manganese chaperones have been extensively studied; however, chaperones of other metals (iron, zinc, molybdenum) have been reported in microbial systems and may exist in humans (Culotta, 2006).

Pharmacology of Metals

Metals and metal compounds have a long and rich history of pharmacological use. Metallic agents, largely because of their potential toxicity, have been often used in chemotherapeutic settings. For instance, mercury was used in the treatment of syphilis as early as the 16th century. Similarly, Ehrlich's *magic bullet* (arsphenamine) was an organoarsenical. Today, many metallic chemicals remain valuable pharmacological tools in the treatment of human disease, as exemplified by the highly effective use of platinum compounds in cancer chemotherapy. In addition, inorganic arsenic has returned as a very effective chemotherapeutic and agent of choice against certain hematologic cancers. Other examples of medicinal metals used today include aluminum (antacids and buffered analgesics), bismuth (peptic ulcer), lithium (mania and bipolar disorders), and gold (arthritis). Metallic compounds find their way into a variety of pharmacological preparations as active or inactive ingredients. Traditional Chinese medicines, usually complex mixtures, can be made with toxic metals, such as mercury, as intentional ingredients (Liu *et al.*, 2008).

Treatment of metal poisoning is sometimes used to prevent, or even attempt to reverse, toxicity. The therapeutic strategy is to give metal chelators that will complex the metal and enhance its excretion (Klaassen, 2006). Most chelators are not specific and will interact with a number of metals, eliminating more than the metal of concern. In addition, the vast array of biological metal ligands is a formidable barrier to chelator efficacy as is the chelator's water/fat solubility (Klaassen, 2006). Metal chelation therapy should be considered a secondary alternative to toxic metal exposure reduction or even prevention. Chelator therapy can be used for many different metals including lead, mercury, iron, and arsenic. For detailed discussion on the pharmacology of chelation therapy, see Klaassen (2006).

MAJOR TOXIC METALS

Arsenic

Arsenic (As) is a toxic and carcinogenic metalloid. The word *arsenic* is from the Persian word *Zarnikh*, as translated to the Greek *arsenikon*, meaning "yellow orpiment." Arsenic has been known and used since ancient times as the *poison of kings and the king of poisons*. The element was first isolated in about 1250. Arsenicals

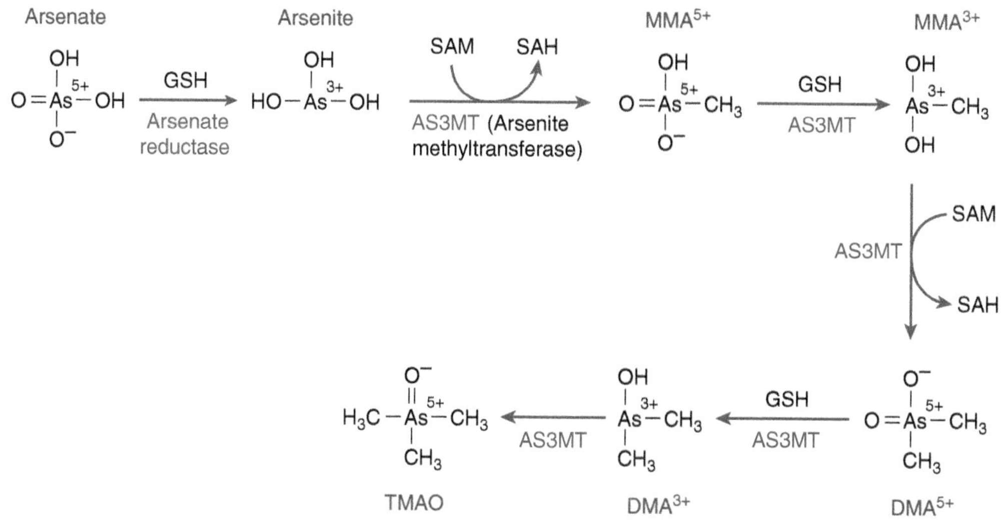

Figure 23-2. *Arsenic metabolism*. GSH, reduced glutathione; SAM, *S*-adenosylmethionine; SAH, *S*-adenosylhomocysteine; AS3MT, arsenic methyltransferase (Cyt19); MMA^{5+}, monomethylarsonic acid; MMA^{3+}, monomethylarsonous acid; DMA^{5+}, dimethylarsinic acid; DMA^{3+}, dimethylarsinous acid; TMAO, trimethylarsenic oxide.

have been used since ancient times as drugs and even today are very effective against acute promyelocytic leukemia (Sanz and Lo-Coco, 2011). Arsenic exists in the trivalent and pentavalent forms and is widely distributed in nature. The most common inorganic trivalent arsenic compounds are arsenic trioxide and sodium arsenite, while common pentavalent inorganic compounds are sodium arsenate, arsenic pentoxide, and arsenic acid. Important organoarsenicals include arsanilic acid, arsenosugars, and several methylated forms produced as a consequence of inorganic arsenic biotransformation in various organisms, including humans. Arsine (AsH$_3$) is an important gaseous arsenical.

Occupational exposure to arsenic occurs in the manufacture of pesticides, herbicides, and other agricultural products. Exposure to arsenic fumes and dusts may occur in smelting industries (ATSDR, 2005a; IARC, 2011a). Environmental arsenic exposure mainly occurs from arsenic-contaminated drinking water, which can be very high depending on the subsurface geology (IARC, 2011a). Arsenic in drinking water is generally from natural sources. Although most US drinking water contains arsenic at levels lower than 5 μg/L (ppb), it has been estimated that about 25 million people in Bangladesh alone drink water with arsenic levels above 50 ppb (IARC, 2004). Food, especially seafood, may contribute significantly to daily arsenic intake. Arsenic in seafood is largely in an organic form called arsenobetaine that is much less toxic than the inorganic forms (ATSDR, 2005a).

Toxicokinetics Inorganic arsenic is well absorbed (80%–90%) from the gastrointestinal tract, distributed throughout the body, often metabolized by methylation, and then excreted primarily in urine (NRC, 2001; IARC, 2011a; Drobna *et al.*, 2010). Arsenic compounds of low solubility (eg, arsenic trioxide, arsenic selenide, lead arsenide, and gallium arsenide) are absorbed less efficiently after oral exposure. Skin is a potential route of exposure to arsenic, and systemic toxicity has been reported in persons having dermal contact with solutions of inorganic arsenic (Hostynek *et al.*, 1993), but the relevance of this to today's exposure paradigms is limited. Airborne arsenic is largely trivalent arsenic oxide. Deposition in airways and absorption of arsenicals from lungs is dependent on particle size and chemical form. Excretion of absorbed arsenic is mainly via the urine. The whole-body biological half-life of ingested arsenic is about 10 hours, and 50% to 80% is excreted

over three days. The biological half-life of methylated arsenicals is in the range of 30 hours. Arsenic has a predilection for skin and is excreted by desquamation of skin and in sweat, particularly during periods of profuse sweating. It also concentrates in forming fingernails and hair. Arsenic exposure produces characteristic transverse white bands across fingernails (Mees' line), which appear about six weeks after the onset of symptoms of arsenic toxicity. Arsenic in the fingernails and hair has been used as a biomarker for exposure, including both current and past exposures, while urinary arsenic is a good indicator for current exposure.

Methylation of inorganic arsenic species is no longer considered as a detoxication process, as recent work has identified the highly toxic trivalent methylated arsenicals (Drobna *et al.*, 2010). Some animal species even lack arsenic methylation capacity, perhaps as an adaptation mechanism. Fig. 23-2 illustrates the biotransformation of arsenic. Arsenate (As^{5+}) is rapidly reduced to arsenite (As^{3+}) by arsenate reductase (presumably purine nucleoside phosphorylase). Arsenite is then sequentially methylated to form monomethylarsonic acid and dimethylarsinic acid (DMA^{5+}) by arsenic methyltransferase (AS3MT) or arsenite methyltransferase using *S*-adenosylmethionine (SAM) as a methyl group donor. The intermediate metabolites, monomethylarsonous acid and dimethylarsinous acid (DMA^{3+}), are generated during this process, and these trivalent methylated arsenicals are now thought to be more toxic than even the inorganic arsenic species (Aposhian and Aposhian, 2006; Thomas *et al.*, 2007; Drobna *et al.*, 2010). In humans, urinary arsenicals are composed of 10% to 30% inorganic arsenicals, 10% to 20% MMA, and 55% to 76% DMA (NRC, 2001; IARC, 2011a). However, large variations in arsenic methylation occur due to factors such as age and sex. Genetic polymorphisms impacting arsenic metabolism do exist (eg, Engström *et al.*, 2011) and the role of these in disease states is now being defined. Arsenic metabolism also changes through the course of pregnancy, reflected in higher urinary excretion of DMA and lower urinary levels of inorganic arsenic and MMA, which may have toxicological impact on the developing fetus (Hopenhayn *et al.*, 2003).

Toxicity

Acute Poisoning Ingestion of large doses (70–180 mg) of inorganic arsenic can be fatal. Symptoms of acute intoxication include fever, anorexia, hepatomegaly, melanosis, cardiac arrhythmia, and, in fatal cases, terminal cardiac failure. Acute arsenic ingestion can damage mucous membranes of the gastrointestinal tract, causing irritation, vesicle formation, and even sloughing. Sensory loss in the peripheral nervous system is the most common neurological effect, appearing at one to two weeks after large doses and consisting of Wallerian degeneration of axons, a condition that is reversible if exposure is stopped. Anemia and leucopenia, particularly granulocytopenia, occur a few days following high-dose arsenic exposure and are reversible. Intravenous arsenic infusion at clinical doses in the treatment of acute promyelocytic leukemia may be significantly or even fatally toxic in susceptible patients, and a few sudden deaths have been reported (Westervelt *et al.*, 2001). Acute exposure to a single high dose can produce encephalopathy, with signs and symptoms of headache, lethargy, mental confusion, hallucination, seizures, and even coma (ATSDR, 2005a).

Arsine gas, generated by electrolytic or metallic reduction of arsenic in nonferrous metal production, is a potent hemolytic agent, producing acute symptoms of nausea, vomiting, shortness of breath, and headache accompanying the hemolytic reaction. Exposure to arsine is fatal in up to 25% of the reported human cases and may be accompanied by hemoglobinuria, renal failure, jaundice, and anemia in nonfatal cases when exposure persists (ATSDR, 2005a).

Chronic Toxicity The skin is a major target organ in chronic inorganic arsenic exposure. In humans, chronic exposure to arsenic induces a series of characteristic changes in skin epithelium. Diffuse or spotted hyperpigmentation and, alternatively, hypopigmentation can first appear between six months and three years with chronic exposure to inorganic arsenic. Palmar-plantar hyperkeratosis usually follows the initial appearance of arsenic-induced pigmentation changes within a period of years (NRC, 2001; IARC, 2011a). Skin cancer is common with protracted high-level arsenical exposure (see below).

Liver injury, characteristic of long-term or chronic arsenic exposure, manifests itself initially as jaundice, abdominal pain, and hepatomegaly (NRC, 2001; Mazumder, 2005). Liver injury may progress to cirrhosis and ascites, even to hepatocellular carcinoma (Liu and Waalkes, 2008; Straif *et al.*, 2009; IARC, 2011a).

Repeated exposure to low levels of inorganic arsenic can produce peripheral neuropathy. This neuropathy usually begins with sensory changes, such as numbness in the hands and feet, but later may develop into a painful "pins and needles" sensation. Both sensory and motor nerves can be affected, and muscle tenderness often develops, followed by weakness, progressing from proximal to distal muscle groups. Histological examination reveals a dying-back axonopathy with demyelination, and effects are dose-related (ATSDR, 2005a).

An association between ingestion of inorganic arsenic in drinking water and cardiovascular disease has been shown (NRC, 2001; Chen *et al.*, 2005; Navas-Acien *et al.*, 2005). Peripheral vascular disease has been observed in persons with chronic exposure to inorganic arsenic in the drinking water in Taiwan. It is manifested by acrocyanosis and Raynaud's phenomenon and may progress to endarteritis and gangrene of the lower extremities (black foot disease). Arsenic-induced vascular effects have been reported in Chile, Mexico, India, and China, but these effects do not compare in magnitude or severity with black foot disease in Taiwanese populations, indicating other environmental or dietary factors may be involved (Yu *et al.*, 2002). Atherosclerotic models have been developed in mice with arsenic exposure (Srivastava *et al.*, 2009). Studies have shown an association between high arsenic exposure in Taiwan and Bangladesh and an increased risk of diabetes mellitus (Navas-Acien *et al.*, 2006; Tseng, 2008).

Immunotoxic effects of arsenic have been suggested (ATSDR, 2005a). The hematologic consequences of chronic exposure to arsenic may include interference with heme synthesis, with an increase in urinary porphyrin excretion, which has been proposed as a biomarker for arsenic exposure (Ng *et al.*, 2005).

Mechanisms of Toxicity The trivalent compounds of arsenic are thiol-reactive, and thereby inhibit enzymes or alter proteins by reacting with proteinaceous thiol groups. Pentavalent arsenate is an uncoupler of mitochondrial oxidative phosphorylation, by a mechanism likely related to competitive substitution (mimicry) of arsenate for inorganic phosphate in the formation of adenosine triphosphate. Arsine gas is formed by the reaction of hydrogen with arsenic, and is a potent hemolytic agent (NRC, 2001).

In addition to these basic modes of action, several mechanisms have been proposed for arsenic toxicity and carcinogenicity. Arsenic and its metabolites have been shown to produce oxidants and oxidative DNA damage, alteration in DNA methylation status and genomic instability, impaired DNA damage repair, and enhanced cell proliferation (NRC, 2001; Rossman, 2003). It appears that arsenic methylation is required for oxidative DNA damage by inorganic arsenic, but cells can still acquire a malignant phenotype without such metabolism (Kojima *et al.*, 2009). This indicates multiple mechanisms may be at play in carcinogenesis. Unlike many carcinogens, arsenic is not a mutagen in bacteria and acts weakly in mammalian cells, but can induce chromosomal abnormalities, aneuploidy, and micronuclei formation. Arsenic can also act as a comutagen and/or cocarcinogen (Rossman, 2003; Chen *et al.*, 2005). These mechanisms are not mutually exclusive and multiple mechanisms likely account for arsenic toxicity and carcinogenesis (Kojima *et al.*, 2009). Some mechanisms, however, may be organ specific. There is emerging evidence that arsenic can impact target tissue stem cells in various ways to facilitate oncogenic change (Tokar *et al.*, 2011).

Carcinogenicity The carcinogenic potential of arsenic was recognized over 110 years ago by Hutchinson (see IARC, 2011a), who observed an unusual number of skin cancers occurring in patients treated for various diseases with medicinal arsenicals. IARC (2011a) and NTP (2011a) have long classified arsenic as a known human carcinogen, most associated with various tumors including those of the skin, lung, and urinary bladder, and possibly kidney, liver, and prostate (Straif *et al.*, 2009; IARC, 2011a).

Arsenic-induced skin cancers include basal cell carcinomas and squamous cell carcinomas, both arising in areas of arsenic-induced hyperkeratosis. The basal cell cancers are usually only locally invasive, but squamous cell carcinomas may have distant metastases. In humans, the skin cancers often, but not exclusively, occur on areas of the body not exposed to sunlight (eg, on palms of hands and soles of feet). They also often occur as multiple primary malignant lesions. Animal models have shown that arsenic acts as a rodent skin tumor copromoter with 12-*O*-teradecanoyl phorbol-13-acetate in v-Ha-*ras* mutant Tg.AC mice (Germolec *et al.*, 1998) or as a cocarcinogen with UV irradiation in hairless mice (Rossman *et al.*, 2004).

The association of internal tumors in humans with arsenic exposure is well recognized (NRC, 2001; Straif *et al.*, 2009; IARC, 2011a; NTP, 2011a). This includes arsenic-induced tumors of the human urinary bladder, and lung, and potentially the liver, kidney, and prostate (Straif *et al.*, 2009; IARC, 2011a). In rats, the methylated arsenic species, DMA^{5+}, is a urinary bladder tumor carcinogen and promoter and produces urothelial cytotoxicity and proliferative regeneration with continuous exposure (see Tokar *et al.*, 2010a for review). It has been suggested that the relevance of this finding to inorganic arsenic carcinogenesis must be extrapolated cautiously, because it requires a high dose of DMA to produce these regenerative changes in rats (NRC, 2001).

In contrast to most other human carcinogens, it has been difficult to confirm the carcinogenicity of inorganic arsenic in experimental animals (Tokar *et al.*, 2010a). Recently, a transplacental arsenic carcinogenesis model has been established in mice. Short-term exposure of the pregnant rodents from gestation days eight to 18, a period of general sensitivity to chemical carcinogenesis, produces tumors in various tissues in the offspring as adults (Tokar *et al.*, 2010a, 2011), including sites identified in humans, such as liver and lung (Straif *et al.*, 2009; IARC, 2011a). Prenatal exposure to arsenic in mice can also enhance the sensitivity to tumor development induced by exposure to other agents after birth, and can enhance skin and bladder cancer formation (Tokar *et al.*, 2010a, 2011), again important human target sites of arsenic carcinogenesis (Straif *et al.*, 2009; IARC, 2011a). Data are emerging indicating that humans exposed during early developmental periods to inorganic arsenic show a predilection toward cancer development in later life (Smith *et al.*, 2006; Tokar *et al.*, 2011), indicating that the developmental life stage appears to be hypersensitive to arsenic carcinogenesis in rodents and humans (Tokar *et al.*, 2011).

Treatment For acute arsenic poisoning, treatment is symptomatic, with particular attention to fluid volume replacement and support of blood pressure. The oral chelator penicillamine or succimer (2,3-dimercaptosuccinic acid [DMSA]) is effective in removing arsenic from the body. Dimercaptopropanesulfonic acid (DMPS) has also been used for acute arsenic poisoning with fewer side effects (Aposhian and Aposhian, 2006). However, for chronic poisoning, chelator therapy has not proven effective in relieving symptoms (Rahman *et al.*, 2001; Liu *et al.*, 2002) except for a limited preliminary trial with DMPS (Mazumder, 2005). The best strategy for preventing chronic arsenic poisoning is by reducing exposure.

Beryllium

Beryllium (Be), an alkaline earth metal, was discovered in 1798. The name beryllium comes from the Greek *beryllos*, a term used for the mineral beryl. Beryllium compounds are divalent. Beryllium alloys are used in automobiles, computers, sports equipment, and dental bridges. Pure beryllium metal is used in nuclear weapons, aircraft, x-ray machines, and mirrors. Human exposure to beryllium and its compounds occurs primarily in beryllium manufacturing, fabricating, or reclaiming industries. Individuals may also be exposed to beryllium from implanted dental prostheses. The general population is exposed to trace amounts of beryllium through the air, food, and water, as well as from cigarette smoke (WHO, 1990a,b; ATSDR, 2002).

Toxicokinetics The primary route of exposure to beryllium compounds is through the lungs. After being deposited in the lung, beryllium is slowly absorbed into the blood. In patients accidentally exposed to beryllium dust, serum beryllium levels peak about 10 days after exposure with a biological half-life of two to eight weeks (ATSDR, 2002). Gastrointestinal and dermal absorption of beryllium is low (<1%), but incidental oral exposure to soluble beryllium compounds or exposure through damaged skin may significantly contribute to total body burden (Deubner *et al.*, 2001). Most of the beryllium circulating in the blood is bound to serum proteins, such as prealbumins and globulins. A significant part of the inhaled beryllium is stored in the bone and lungs. More soluble beryllium compounds are distributed to the liver, lymph nodes, spleen, heart, muscle, skin, and kidney. Elimination of absorbed

beryllium occurs mainly in the urine and only to a minor degree in the feces. Because of the long residence time of beryllium in the skeleton and lungs, its biological half-life is over one year (ATSDR, 2002; WHO, 1990a,b).

Toxicity

Skin Effects Exposure to soluble beryllium compounds may result in conjunctivitis and papulovesicular dermatitis of the skin, which is likely an inflammatory response to the beryllium. Beryllium exposure may also cause a delayed-type hypersensitivity reaction in the skin, which is a cell-mediated immune response. If insoluble beryllium-containing materials become embedded under the skin, a chronic granulomatous lesion develops, which may be necrotizing and ulcerative. Skin is a route of beryllium exposure and sensitization, and the beryllium sulfate skin test and the beryllium lymphocyte proliferation test have been used to identify beryllium-sensitive individuals (Fontenot *et al.*, 2002; Tinkle *et al.*, 2003). Beryllium fluoride patch test may in itself be sensitizing, which has been replaced by the use of 1% beryllium sulfate (ATSDR, 2002; Fontenot *et al.*, 2002).

Acute Chemical Pneumonitis Inhalation of beryllium can cause a fulminating inflammatory reaction of the entire respiratory tract, involving the nasal passages, pharynx, tracheobronchial airways, and the alveoli. In the most severe cases, it produces acute fulminating pneumonitis. This occurs almost immediately following inhalation of aerosols of soluble beryllium compounds, particularly the fluoride, during the ore extraction process. Fatalities have occurred, although recovery is generally complete after a period of several weeks or even months.

Chronic Granulomatous Disease Berylliosis, or chronic beryllium disease (CBD), was first described among fluorescent lamp workers exposed to insoluble beryllium compounds, particularly beryllium oxide. Granulomatous inflammation of the lung, along with dyspnea on exertion, cough, chest pain, weight loss, fatigue, and general weakness, is the most typical feature. Impaired lung function and hypertrophy of the right heart are also common. Chest x-rays show miliary mottling. Histologically, the alveoli contain small interstitial granulomas resembling those seen in sarcoidosis. In severe cases CBD may be accompanied by cyanosis and hypertrophic osteoarthropathy (WHO, 1990a,b; ATSDR, 2002). Beryllium sensitization following initial exposure can progress to CBD (Newman *et al.*, 2005). As the lesions progress, interstitial fibrosis increases, with loss of functioning alveoli, impairment of effective air-capillary gas exchange, and increasing respiratory dysfunction. CBD involves an antigen-stimulated, cell-mediated immune response. Human leukocyte antigen, T cells, and proinflammatory cytokines (TNF-α and IL-6) are believed to be involved in the pathogenesis of CBD (Fontenot *et al.*, 2002; Day *et al.*, 2006).

Carcinogenicity A number of epidemiology studies in US beryllium workers found that death due to lung cancer was increased, along with increased incidence of respiratory diseases. The increase in lung cancers is linked to high exposure levels that occurred prior to stricter exposure regulations introduced in the 1950s. The likelihood of lung cancer was greater in workers with acute beryllium disease than in those with CBD (ATSDR, 2002; Gordon and Bowser, 2003). Beryllium has been classified as a human carcinogen (IARC, 1993; NTP, 2011b).

Experimental studies confirmed carcinogenic potential of beryllium compounds by inhalation. For example, a single, short (<48-minute) exposure to 410 to 980 mg/m³ beryllium metal aerosol induced lung tumors in rats 14 months after exposure. Chronic beryllium sulfate inhalation (13 months, 0.034 mg Be/m³) resulted in 100% lung tumor incidence in rats (Gordon and Bowser, 2003). Injection of beryllium compounds also induced osteosarcomas in rabbits (WHO, 1990a,b). Beryllium compounds are negative in bacterial mutation assays. In mammalian cells, soluble beryllium compounds show weak mutagenic potential, but can induce malignant transformation. The ability of beryllium compounds to produce chromosomal aberrations is controversial, and appears to depend on the compound, dose, and experimental conditions (Gordon and Bowser, 2003). The carcinogenic mechanism of beryllium is not yet clear. Several molecular events can occur including oncogene activation (K-*ras*, c-*myc*, c-*fos*, c-*jun*, and c-*sis*), and tumor suppressor gene dysregulation (p53, p16), but mutations in *p53* or K-*ras* are not evident. Beryllium-induced lung tumors show hypermethylation of p16 leading to loss of expression, and have decreased expression of genes associated with DNA repair (Gordon and Bowser, 2003).

Cadmium

Cadmium (Cd) is a toxic transition metal that was discovered in 1817 as an impurity of "calamine" (zinc carbonate) for which it is named (from the Latin *cadmia*). Until recently the industrial use of cadmium was quite limited, but now it has become an important metal with many uses. About 75% of cadmium produced is used in batteries, especially nickel–cadmium batteries. Because of its noncorrosive properties, cadmium has been used in electroplating or galvanizing alloys for corrosion resistance. It is also used as a color pigment for paints and plastics, in solders, as a barrier to control nuclear fission, as a plastic stabilizer, and in some special application alloys. This metal is typically found in ores with other metals, and is commercially produced as a by-product of zinc and lead smelting, which are sources of environmental cadmium. Cadmium ranks close to lead and mercury as one of the top toxic substances (Nordberg *et al.*, 2007; ATSDR, 2008).

Exposure Food is the major source of cadmium for the general population. Many plants readily accumulate cadmium from soil. Both natural and anthropogenic sources of cadmium contamination occur for soil, including fallout of industrial emissions, some fertilizers, soil amendments, and use of cadmium-containing water for irrigation, all resulting in a slow but steady increase in the cadmium content in vegetables over the years (Järup *et al.*, 1998). Shellfish accumulate relatively high levels of cadmium (1–2 mg/kg), and animal liver and kidney can have levels higher than 50 µg Cd/kg. Cereal grains such as rice and wheat, and tobacco concentrate cadmium to levels of 10 to 150 µg Cd/kg. With nearby industrial emission, air can be a significant source of direct exposure or environmental contamination. Total daily cadmium intake from all sources in North America and Europe ranges from 10 to 30 µg Cd per day. Of this about 10% or less is retained (Järup *et al.*, 1998). Cigarette smoking is a major nonoccupational source of cadmium exposure, because of cadmium in the tobacco. Smoking is thought to roughly double the lifetime body burden of cadmium (Satarug and Moore, 2004).

Historically, levels of cadmium in the workplace have dramatically improved with the appreciation of its potential toxicity in humans, development of safety restrictions, and improved industrial hygiene. Inhalation is the dominant route of exposure in occupational settings. Airborne cadmium in the present-day workplace environment is generally 5 µg/m³ or less and occupational standards range from 2 to 50 µg/m³. Occupations potentially at risk from cadmium exposure include those involved with refining zinc and lead ores, iron production, cement manufacture, and industries involving fossil fuel combustion, all of which can release airborne cadmium. Other occupations include the manufacture of paint pigments, cadmium–nickel batteries, and electroplating (WHO, 1990a,b; ATSDR, 2008).

Toxicokinetics Gastrointestinal absorption of cadmium is limited to 5% to 10% of a given dose. Cadmium absorption can be increased by dietary deficiencies of calcium or iron and by diets low in protein. In the general population, women have higher blood cadmium levels than men, possibly due to increased oral cadmium absorption because of relatively low iron stores in women of childbearing age. Indeed, women showing low serum ferritin levels have twice the normal rate of oral cadmium absorption (Nordberg *et al.*, 2007). It has recently been shown that rats on an iron-deficient diet have an increased absorption of cadmium, which correlated with the upregulation of the iron transporter, DMT, which transports both iron and cadmium (Ryu *et al.*, 2004). Absorption of cadmium after inhalation is generally greater, ranging from 10% to 60%, depending on the specific compound, site of deposition, and particle size (Nordberg *et al.*, 2007; Prozialeck and Edwards, 2010). For instance, 50% of cadmium fumes, as generated in cigarette smoke, may be absorbed. It is thought that as much as 100% of cadmium eventually reaching the alveoli can be transferred to blood (Satarug and Moore, 2004).

Once absorbed, cadmium is very poorly excreted and only about 0.001% of the body burden is excreted per day. Both urinary and fecal excretory routes are operative (Satarug and Moore, 2004; ATSDR, 2008). Cadmium transport into cells is mediated through calcium channels (Leslie *et al.*, 2006) and through molecular mimicry (Zalpus and Ahmad, 2003). Gastrointestinal excretion occurs through the bile as a glutathione complex. Cadmium excretion in urine increases relative to body burden (Nordberg *et al.*, 2007; ATSDR, 2008). Cadmium is nephrotoxic, and when renal pathology is present the urinary excretion of cadmium is increased due to decreased renal absorption of filtered cadmium (Zalpus and Ahmad, 2003).

The relationship of cadmium metabolism and toxicity is shown in Fig. 23-3. Cadmium is transported in blood by binding to albumin and other higher-molecular-weight proteins. It is rapidly taken up by tissues and is primarily deposited in the liver and to a lesser extent in the kidney. In the liver, kidney, and other tissues, cadmium induces the synthesis of MT, a low-molecular-weight, high-affinity metal-binding protein (Klaassen *et al.*, 1999). Cadmium is stored in the liver primarily as cadmium–MT. Cadmium–MT may be released from the liver and transported via blood to the kidney, where it is reabsorbed and degraded in the lysosomes of the renal tubules. This releases cadmium to induce more cadmium–MT complex or cause renal toxicity.

Blood cadmium levels in nonoccupationally exposed, nonsmokers are usually less than 1 µg/L. Cadmium does not readily cross the placenta. Breast milk is not a major source of early life exposure. About 50% to 75% of the retained cadmium is found in the liver and kidneys. The biological half-life of cadmium in humans is not known exactly, but is probably in the range of 10 to 30 years (Nordberg *et al.*, 2007).

Toxicity Acute, high-dose cadmium toxicity in humans is now a rare event. Acute cadmium toxicity from the ingestion of high concentrations of cadmium in the form of heavily contaminated beverages or food causes severe irritation to the gastrointestinal epithelium. Symptoms include nausea, vomiting, and abdominal pain. Inhalation of cadmium fumes or other heated cadmium-containing materials may produce acute pneumonitis with pulmonary edema. Inhalation of large doses of cadmium can be lethal for humans (ATSDR, 2008). Acute cadmium toxicity depends on

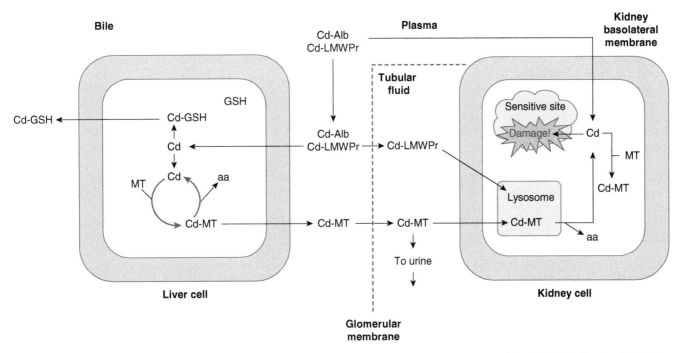

Figure 23-3. *Cadmium transport, protein binding, and toxicity.* GSH, glutathione; MT, metallothionein; aa, amino acids; Cd-Alb, Cd–albumin; Cd-LMWPr, Cd associated with low-molecular-weight proteins.

solubility of cadmium compounds (ATSDR, 2008). For instance, with acute inhalation exposures, the more soluble cadmium chloride, oxide fume, and carbonate are more toxic than the relatively less soluble sulfide (Klimisch, 1993). The major long-term toxic effects of low-level cadmium exposure are renal injury, obstructive pulmonary disease, osteoporosis, and cardiovascular disease. Cancer is primarily a concern in occupationally exposed groups. The chronic toxic effects of cadmium are clearly a much greater concern than the rare acute toxic exposures.

Nephrotoxicity Cadmium is toxic to tubular cells and glomeruli, markedly impairing renal function. Pathologically, these lesions consist of initial tubular cell necrosis and degeneration, progressing to an interstitial inflammation and fibrosis. There appears to be a critical concentration of cadmium in the renal cortex that, once exceeded, is associated with tubular dysfunction. This concentration depends on the individual, and chronic cadmium nephropathy is seen in about 10% of the population at renal concentrations of ~200 µg/g and in about 50% of the population at about 300 µg/g. Because of the potential for renal toxicity, there is considerable concern about the levels of dietary cadmium intake for the general population. In fact, it is thought that upwards of 7% of the general population may have significant cadmium-induced kidney alterations due to chronic exposure with kidney cadmium levels as low as 50 µg/g (Järup *et al.*, 1998).

Cadmium-induced renal toxicity is reflected by proteinuria as a result of renal tubular dysfunction. The predominant proteins include β2-microglobulin, *N*-acetyl-β-D-glucosaminidase (NAG), and MT, as well as retinol-binding protein, lysozyme, ribonuclease, α1-microglobulin, and immunoglobulin light chains (Chen *et al.*, 2006; Prozialeck and Edwards, 2010). The presence of larger proteins, such as albumin and transferrin, in the urine after occupational cadmium exposure suggests a glomerular effect as well. The pathogenesis of the glomerular lesion in cadmium nephropathy is not well understood (Prozialeck and Edwards, 2010). Urinary excretions of proteins and cadmium have been used as biomarkers for cadmium exposure.

The induction of MT by cadmium and the subsequent sequestration of cadmium as the cadmium–MT complex likely protect tissues from cadmium toxicity. However, if cadmium–MT complex is injected, it is acutely nephrotoxic (Nordberg, 2004). This led to the hypothesis that the cadmium–MT complex was responsible for chronic cadmium nephropathy. In this scenario, cadmium–MT released from the liver would be filtered by the kidney and reabsorbed in proximal tubule cells, where it is degraded releasing locally high levels of "free" cadmium (Fig. 23-3). Nephrotoxicity in normal rats following liver transplantation from cadmium-exposed rats supported this hypothesis (Chan *et al.*, 1993). However, MT-null mice, which are unable to produce the major forms of MT, are hypersensitive to chronic cadmium nephropathy (Liu *et al.*, 1998a), suggesting that cadmium nephropathy is not necessarily mediated through the cadmium–MT complex. Kidney pathology from a single injection of cadmium–MT also differs greatly from that induced by chronic oral inorganic cadmium exposure (Liu *et al.*, 1998b). Inorganic cadmium can be taken into the kidney from the basolateral membrane, and is more toxic than cadmium–MT to cultured renal cells (Prozialeck *et al.*, 1993; Liu *et al.*, 1994; Zalpus and Ahmad, 2003). It is likely that inorganic cadmium can bind to other low-molecular-weight proteins or other complexes for renal uptake, and these complexes can contribute to chronic cadmium nephropathy (Zalpus and Ahmad, 2003).

Chronic Pulmonary Disease Cadmium inhalation is toxic to the respiratory system in a fashion related to the dose and duration of exposure. Cadmium-induced obstructive lung disease in humans can be slow in onset, and results from chronic bronchitis, progressive fibrosis of the lower airways, and accompanying alveolar damage leading to emphysema. Pulmonary function is reduced with dyspnea, reduced vital capacity, and increased residual volume. The pathogenesis of these lung lesions is not completely understood, but can be duplicated in rodents (WHO, 1990a,b; ATSDR, 2008). The chronic effects of cadmium on the lung clearly increased the mortality of cadmium workers with high exposure.

Skeletal Effects Occupational cadmium exposure is a well-recognized cause for renal tubular dysfunction associated with hypercalciuria, renal stone formation, osteomalacia, and osteoporosis (Kazantzis, 2004). The long-term consumption of cadmium-contaminated rice caused *Itai-Itai* disease, which occurred mostly in multiparous elderly women and was characterized by severe osteomalacia and osteoporosis, resulting in bone deformities and concomitant renal dysfunction. Vitamin D deficiency and perhaps other nutritional deficiencies are thought to be cofactors in *Itai-Itai* disease. Issues with loss of bone density, height loss, and increased bone fractures have now been reported in populations exposed to far lower levels of environmental cadmium than *Itai-Itai* victims (Kazantzis, 2004). Cadmium affects calcium metabolism, at least partially through renal dysfunction, and excess excretion of calcium often occurs in the urine. The skeletal changes are possibly related to a loss or decrease of calcium absorption, and interference with the actions of parathyroid hormone, disruption of collagen metabolism, and impairment of vitamin D activity (Nordberg *et al.*, 2007), although the effects on vitamin D activity are debated (Engstrom *et al.*, 2009). Cadmium may also act directly on bone and animal studies have shown the metal stimulates osteoclast activity, resulting in the breakdown of bone matrix. Cadmium in bone interferes with calcification and bone remodeling (Wang and Bhattacharyya, 1993). In accord with human victims of *Itai-Itai*, multiparity in mice enhances the osteotoxicity of cadmium (Bhattacharyya *et al.*, 1988).

Cardiovascular Effects Some epidemiological evidence suggests cadmium may be an etiologic agent for cardiovascular disease including hypertension, although these associations are not observed in all studies (Järup *et al.*, 1998; Messner and Bernhard, 2010). The population-based US National Health and Nutrition Examination Survey (NHANES II) and studies in Belgium (Staessen *et al.*, 1996) have not supported a role for cadmium in the etiology of hypertension or cardiovascular disease in humans. Animal studies indicate that cadmium may be toxic to myocardium (Kopp *et al.*, 1982), although the relevance of these results to humans is not clear.

Neurotoxicity There are only limited data from animals and humans that cadmium can be neurotoxic (Järup *et al.*, 1998; ATSDR, 2008). Studies in humans have suggested a relationship between abnormal behavior and decreased intelligence in children and adults exposed to cadmium, but are typically complicated by exposure to other toxic metals. Furthermore, the blood–brain barrier severely limits cadmium access to the central nervous system, and a direct toxic effect appears to occur only with cadmium exposure prior to blood–brain barrier formation (young children), or with blood–brain barrier dysfunction under certain pathological conditions. Additionally, the choroid plexus epithelium may accumulate high levels of cadmium reducing access to other areas (Zheng, 2001). Although a special form of MT (MT-3) occurs in the brain, the role of MT in cadmium neurotoxicity is incompletely defined (Klaassen *et al.*, 1999).

Carcinogenicity Cadmium compounds are considered to be human carcinogens (IARC, 2011b; NTP, 2011c). In humans, occupational respiratory exposure to cadmium has been most clearly associated with lung cancer (IARC, 2011b; NTP, 2011c). Early human studies also indicated a possible link to cancer of the prostate, which has not been confirmed by more recent work (Sahmoun *et al.*, 2005), despite evidence that the prostate can be a target of cadmium carcinogenesis in rats (Waalkes, 2003). Both the kidney and pancreas accumulate high concentrations of cadmium and exposure to cadmium may also be associated with human renal

(Il'yasova and Schwartz, 2005) and pancreatic cancer (Schwartz and Reis, 2000; Kriegel *et al.*, 2006).

Multiple rodent studies have confirmed that inhalation of various cadmium compounds will lead to lung cancer (Waalkes, 2003; IARC, 2011b; NTP, 2011c). Lung tumors can also be produced by systemic cadmium exposure in mice (Waalkes, 2003). Beyond the lung, in rodents cadmium can produce a variety of tumors, including malignant tumors at the site of repository injection (subcutaneous, etc). Compounds such as cadmium chloride, oxide, sulfate, sulfide, and cadmium powder produce local sarcomas in rodents after subcutaneous or intramuscular injections. A single injection can be effective, but multiple injections of cadmium at the same site cause more aggressive sarcomas that show a higher rate of local invasion and distant metastasis. The relevance of injection site sarcoma production to human cancer is unclear. Cadmium also induces tumors of the testes, specifically benign Leydig cell tumors, but this is likely due to a high-dose mechanism involving acute testicular necrosis, degenerative testicular atrophy, and subsequent overstimulation by luteinizing hormone, factors very likely of limited relevance in humans (Waalkes, 2003). Other studies have found that cadmium exposure can induce tumors of the pancreas, adrenals, liver, kidney, pituitary, and hematopoietic system in mice, rats, or hamsters. Cadmium can be carcinogenic in animals after inhalation or oral administration or by various injection routes (Waalkes, 2003). Emerging evidence indicates that cadmium exposure significantly increases the risk of breast and endometrial cancers (McElroy *et al.*, 2006; Akesson *et al.*, 2008; Gallagher *et al.*, 2010). Various studies indicate zinc administration will generally block cadmium carcinogenesis, whereas dietary zinc deficiency can enhance the response (Waalkes, 2003; IARC, 2011b; NTP, 2011c). The mechanisms of cadmium carcinogenesis are poorly understood (Waalkes, 2003) and are generally categorized into four groups, aberrant gene expression, inhibition of DNA damage repair, inhibition of apoptosis, and induction of oxidative stress (Joseph, 2009). Cadmium appears to also work through estrogenic and non-estrogenic mechanisms in hormone-related cancers (Akesson *et al.*, 2008; Benbrahim-Tallaa *et al.*, 2009).

Treatment At the present time, there is no effective clinical treatment for cadmium intoxication. In certain cases (Itai-Itai disease, osteomalacia) vitamin D is prescribed, although its effects have not been satisfactory (Nordberg *et al.*, 2007). In experimental systems some chelators can reduce acute cadmium-induced mortality (Klaassen *et al.*, 1984), but chelation therapy for cadmium generally results in significant adverse effects.

Chromium

Chromium (Cr) was named from the Greek word "*chroma*" meaning color, because of the many colorful compounds made from it. It is part of the mineral crocoite (lead chromate), and the element was first isolated in 1798. Most naturally occurring chromium is found in the trivalent state in chromite ores, which are generally refined to ferrochromium or metallic chromium for use in industrial processes. Because trivalent chromium (Cr^{3+}) is an essential trace nutrient important for glucose metabolism, it will be discussed separately in the section "Essential Metals with Potential for Toxicity."

Hexavalent chromium (Cr^{6+}) is rarely found in nature and is formed as a by-product of various industrial processes. Most chromite ores are processed to sodium dichromate, a hexavalent chromium compound, which is used as an oxidizing agent in stainless steel production and welding, chromium plating, ferrochrome alloys and chrome pigment production, and tanning industries (Ashley *et al.*, 2003). Hexavalent chromium is a human carcinogen and produces a variety of toxic effects (ATSDR, 2008). Chromium in ambient air originates primarily from industrial sources, particularly ferrochrome production, ore refining, and chemical processing. Chromium fallout is deposited on land and water, and, eventually, in sediments. Widespread industrial uses have increased chromium levels in the environment. The hexavalent chromium compounds are also toxic to ecosystems, and microbial and plant variants occur that adapt to high chromium levels in eco-environment (Cervantes *et al.*, 2001). Up to 38% of drinking water supplies in California have detectable levels of hexavalent chromium, but little is known about the health effects from environmental exposures (Costa and Klein, 2006; Sedman *et al.*, 2006). Cobalt–chromium alloy hip replacement can increase blood levels of chromium (Bhamra and Case, 2006).

Toxicokinetics Absorption of hexavalent chromium compounds is higher (2%–10%) than that of trivalent chromium compounds (0.5%–2%). Inhaled chromium compounds are absorbed in the lung via transfer across alveolar cell membranes. Dermal absorption depends on the chemical form, vehicle, and integrity of the skin. Concentrated potassium chromate may cause chemical burns to the skin and facilitate absorption. Hexavalent chromium readily crosses cell membranes via sulfate and phosphate transporters, while trivalent chromium compounds form octahedral complexes making entry into cells difficult (ATSDR, 2008). Once in the blood, hexavalent chromium is taken up by erythrocytes, while trivalent chromium is only loosely associated with erythrocytes. Chromium compounds are distributed to all organs of the body, with high levels in liver, spleen, and kidney. Particles containing chromium can be retained in the lungs for years. Absorbed chromium is excreted primarily in urine. The half-life for excretion of potassium chromium is about 35 to 40 hours (Sedman *et al.*, 2006; ATSDR, 2008).

Once hexavalent chromium enters cells, it is reduced intracellularly by ascorbic acid, glutathione, and/or cysteine, ultimately to trivalent chromium. It is thought that the toxicity of hexavalent chromium compounds results from damage to cellular components during this process, including the generation of free radicals and the formation of DNA adducts (Zhitkovich, 2005).

Toxicity Toxic effects have been attributed primarily to airborne hexavalent chromium compounds in industrial settings. Hexavalent chromium is corrosive and may cause chronic ulceration and perforation of the nasal septum, as well as chronic ulceration of other skin surfaces (ATSDR, 2008). It elicits allergic contact dermatitis among previously sensitized individuals, which is a type IV allergic reaction inducing skin erythema, pruritus, edema, papule, and scars. The prevalence of chromium sensitivity is less than 1% among the general population (Proctor *et al.*, 1998). Occupational exposure to chromium may be a cause of asthma (Bright *et al.*, 1997). Accidental ingestion of high doses of hexavalent chromium compounds may cause acute renal failure characterized by proteinuria, hematuria, and anuria, but kidney damage from lower-level chronic exposure is equivocal (ATSDR, 2008).

Carcinogenicity Hexavalent chromium compounds are classified as *known to be human carcinogens* by the National Toxicology Program (NTP, 2011d). Occupational exposure to hexavalent chromium compounds, particularly in the chrome production and pigment industries, is associated with increased risk of lung cancer and hexavalent chromium–containing compounds are considered to be human carcinogens (IARC, 1990). Hexavalent chromium compounds are genotoxic; a review of more than 700 sets of short-term genotoxicity test results with 32 chromium compounds revealed 88% of hexavalent chromium compounds were positive, as a

function of solubility and bioavailability to target cells (De Flora, 2000). Trivalent chromium compounds were generally nongenotoxic, probably because trivalent chromium is not readily taken up by cells. Once hexavalent chromium enters cells, it is reduced by various intracellular reductants to create reactive chromium species. During the reduction process, various genetic lesions can be generated, including chromium–DNA adducts, DNA–protein cross-links, DNA–chromium intrastrand cross-links, DNA strand breaks, and oxidized DNA bases (O'Brien *et al.*, 2003; Zhitkovich, 2005). Hexavalent chromium compounds are mutagenic, causing base substitutions, deletions, and transversions in bacterial systems, and hypoxanthine guanine phosphoribosyltransferase, *supF* mutations, etc, in mammalian mutagenesis systems (Cohen *et al.*, 1993; O'Brien *et al.*, 2003).

Hexavalent chromium compounds also react with other cellular constituents during the intracellular reduction process. They can cause the generation of reactive oxygen radicals, inhibit protein synthesis, and arrest DNA replication. Hexavalent chromium can also cause disturbances of the p53 signaling pathway, cell cycle arrest, apoptosis, interference of DNA damage repair, and neoplastic transformation. All these effects could well play an integrated role in chromium carcinogenesis (O'Brien *et al.*, 2003; Costa and Klein, 2006).

Inhaled chromium compounds can penetrate many tissues in the body, and thus have the potential to cause cancer at sites other than the lung. Accumulating evidence indicates an association between cancers of the bone, prostate, hematopoietic system, stomach, kidney, and urinary bladder and hexachromium chromium exposure (Costa, 1997). Furthermore, exposure of hexavalent chromium compounds through the drinking water enhances UV-induced skin cancer in hairless mouse model (Costa and Klein, 2006). An association of hexavalent chromium in the drinking water with stomach cancer has also been reported (Sedman *et al.*, 2006).

Lead

Lead (Pb) has been used by humans for at least 7000 years, because it is easy to extract and work with and widespread. It is highly malleable and ductile as well as easy to smelt. In the early Bronze Age, lead was used with antimony and arsenic. Lead's elemental symbol, Pb, is an abbreviation of its Latin name *plumbum*. Lead in lead compounds primarily exists in the divalent form. Metallic lead (Pb^0) is resistant to corrosion and can combine other metals to form various alloys. Organolead compounds are dominated by Pb^{4+}. Inorganic lead compounds are used as pigments in paints, dyes, and ceramic glazes. Organolead compounds were once widely used as gasoline additives. Lead alloys are used in batteries, shields from radiation, water pipes, and ammunition. Environmental lead comes mainly from human activity and is listed as a top toxic substance (ATSDR, 2005b). The phasing out of leaded gasoline and the removal of lead from paint, solder, and water supply pipes have significantly lowered BLL in the general population. Lead exposure in children remains a major health concern. Lead is not biodegradable and ecotoxicity of lead remains a concern. For instance, the leaded fish sinkers or pellets lost in the bottom of lakes and river banks can be mistaken for stone and ingested by birds causing adverse effects including death (De Francisco *et al.*, 2003).

Exposure Lead-containing paint in older housing is a primary source of lead exposure in children (Levin *et al.*, 2008). Major environmental sources of lead for infants and toddlers up to four years of age is hand-to-mouth transfer of lead-containing paint chips or dust from floors of older housing (Manton *et al.*, 2000; Levin *et al.*, 2008). Lead in household dust can also come from outside of the home and may be related to lead in neighborhood soil (von Lindren *et al.*, 2003). A major route of exposure for the general population is from food and water. Dietary intake of lead has decreased dramatically in recent years, and for infants, toddlers, and young children is <5 µg per day (Manton *et al.*, 2005). A review by the EPA in 2004 found lead levels in 71% of the water systems in the United States showed <5 µg Pb/L (ppb). Only 3.6% exceeded the action level of 15 ppb. Lead in urban air is generally higher than that in rural air. Air lead in rural areas of eastern United States is typically 6 to 10 ng/m^3 (ATSDR, 2005b).

Other potential sources of lead exposure are recreational shooting, hand-loading ammunition, soldering, jewelry making, pottery making, gunsmithing, glass polishing, painting, and stained glass crafting. Workplace exposure is gradually being reduced. Herbal medicines could be potential sources of lead exposure (Levin *et al.*, 2008). Certain Ayurvedic herbal products were found to be contaminated with lead ranging up to 37 mg/g and over 55 cases of lead poisoning have been related to the ingestion of herbal medicines (Patrick, 2006).

BLL are commonly used for monitoring human exposure to lead. The uses of other biomarkers for lead exposure have been critically reviewed (Barbosa *et al.*, 2005).

Toxicokinetics Adults absorb 5% to 15% of ingested lead and usually retain less than 5% of what is absorbed. Children absorb 42% of ingested lead with 32% retention (Ziegler *et al.*, 1978). Lead absorption can be enhanced by low dietary zinc, manganese, iron, and calcium (Mahaffey, 1985; Wu *et al.*, 2011), especially in children (Mahaffey, 1985). Airborne lead is a minor component of exposure. Lead absorption by the lungs depends on the form (vapor vs particle), particle size, and concentration. About 90% of lead particles in ambient air that are inhaled are small enough to be retained. Absorption of retained lead through alveoli is relatively efficient.

Lead in blood is primarily (~99%) in erythrocytes bound to hemoglobin; only 1% of circulating lead in serum is available for tissue distribution (ATSDR, 2005b). Lead is initially distributed to soft tissues such as kidney and liver, and then redistributed to skeleton and hair. The half-life of lead in blood is about 30 days. The fraction of lead in bone increases with age from 70% of body burden in childhood to as much as 95% in adulthood, with a half-life of about 20 years. Lead released from bones may contribute up to 50% of the lead in blood, and can be a significant source of endogenous exposure. Bone lead release may be important in adults with accumulated exposure and in women due to bone resorption during pregnancy, lactation, and menopause, and from osteoporosis (Silbergeld *et al.*, 1993; Gulson *et al.*, 2003). Lead crosses the placenta, so that cord blood generally correlates with maternal BLL but is often slightly lower. Lead accumulation in fetal tissues, including brain, is proportional to maternal BLL (Goyer, 1996).

The major route of excretion of absorbed lead is the kidney. Renal excretion of lead is usually through glomerular filtrate with some renal tubular resorption. Fecal excretion via biliary tract accounts for one-third of total excretion of absorbed lead (ATSDR, 2005b).

Physiological-based pharmacokinetic (PBPK) models have been developed for lead risk assessment. The O'Flaherty model is a model for children and adults. The integrated exposure uptake (IEUBK) model was developed by EPA for predicting BLL in children. The Leggett model allows simulation of lifetime exposures and can be used to predict blood lead in both children and adults (ATSDR, 2005b).

Toxicity Lead can induce a wide range of adverse effects in humans depending on the dose and duration of exposure. The toxic effects range from inhibition of enzymes to the production of severe pathology or death (Goyer, 1990). Children are most sensitive to effects in the central nervous system, while in adults, peripheral neuropathy, chronic nephropathy, and hypertension are concerns. Other target tissues include the gastrointestinal, immune, skeletal, and reproductive systems. Effects on heme biosynthesis provide a sensitive biochemical indicator even in the absence of other detectable effects.

Neurological, Neurobehavioral, and Developmental Effects in Children Clinically overt lead encephalopathy may occur in children with high exposure to lead, probably at BLL of 70 µg/dL or higher. Symptoms of lead encephalopathy begin with lethargy, vomiting, irritability, loss of appetite, and dizziness, progressing to obvious ataxia, and a reduced level of consciousness, which may progress to coma and death. The pathological findings at autopsy are severe edema of the brain due to extravasations of fluid from capillaries in the brain. This is accompanied by the loss of neuronal cells and an increase in glial cells. Recovery is often accompanied by sequelae including epilepsy, mental retardation, and, in some cases, optic neuropathy and blindness (Goyer, 1990; Bellinger, 2005; ATSDR, 2005b; Laraque and Trasande, 2005).

The most sensitive indicators of adverse neurological outcomes are psychomotor tests or mental development indices, and broad measures of IQ. Most studies report a 2- to 4-point IQ deficit for each µg/dL increase in BLL within the range of 5 to 35 µg/dL. The Centers for Disease Control and Prevention set the goal of eliminating ≥10 µg/dL BLL in children by 2010 (CDC, 2005). However, effects of lead on IQ may occur below this level (Bellinger, 2005; Murata *et al.*, 2009). Recent studies found that deficits in cognitive and academic skills could occur with BLL <5.0 µg/dL (Lamphear *et al.*, 2000). A study of a cohort of children from pregnancy to 10 years of age found that lead exposure around 28 weeks of gestation is a critical period for later child intellectual development, and lead's effect on IQ occurs with first few micrograms of BLL (Schnaas *et al.*, 2006). Some now consider no level of lead exposure to be "safe" in childhood with regard to neurodevelopment (Bellinger, 2008).

Lead can affect the brain by multiple mechanisms (Goyer, 1996; ATSDR, 2005b). It may act as a surrogate for calcium and/or disrupt calcium homeostasis. The stimulation of protein kinase C may result in alteration of blood–brain barrier and inhibition of cholinergic modulation of glutamate-related synaptic transmissions. Lead affects virtually every neurotransmitter system in the brain, including glutamatergic, dopaminergic, and cholinergic systems. All these systems play a critical role in synaptic plasticity and cellular mechanisms for cognitive function, learning, and memory.

Neurotoxic Effects in Adults Adults with occupational exposure may demonstrate abnormalities in a number of measures in neurobehavior with cumulative exposures resulting from BLL > 40 µg/dL (Lindgren *et al.*, 1996). Peripheral neuropathy is a classic manifestation of lead toxicity in adults. More than a half-century ago, foot drop and wrist-drop characterized the house painter and other workers with excessive occupational exposure to lead but are rare today. Peripheral neuropathy is characterized by segmental demyelination and possibly axonal degeneration. Motor nerve dysfunction, assessed clinically by electrophysiological measurement of nerve conduction velocities, occurred with BLL as low as 40 µg/dL (Goyer, 1990).

Hematologic Effects Lead has multiple hematologic effects, ranging from increased urinary porphyrins, coproporphyrins, δ-aminolevulinic acid (ALA), and zinc protoporphyrin to anemia. The heme biosynthesis pathway and the sites of lead interference

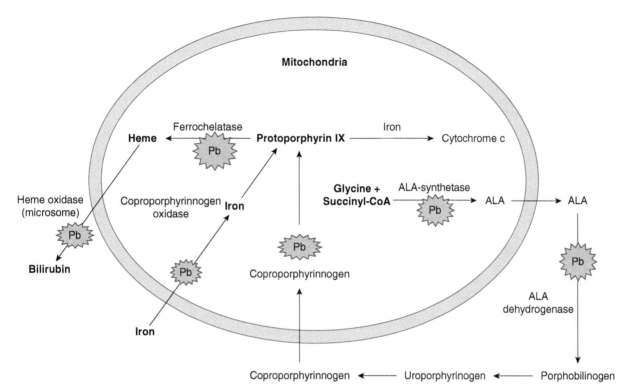

Figure 23-4. *Lead interruption of heme biosynthesis.* ALA, δ-aminolevulinate; Pb, sites for lead effects. The major lead inhibition sites are ALA dehydrogenase and ferrochelatase.

are shown in Fig. 23-4. The most sensitive effects of lead are the inhibition of δ-aminolevulinic acid dehydratase (ALAD) and ferrochelatase. ALAD catalyzes the condensation of two units of ALA to form phorphobilinogen (PBG). Inhibition of ALAD results in accumulation of ALA. Ferrochelatase catalyzes the insertion of iron into the protoporphyrin ring to form heme. Inhibition of ferrochelatase results in accumulation of protophorphyrin IX, which takes the place of heme in the hemoglobin molecule and, as the erythrocytes containing protoporphyrin IX circulate, zinc is chelated at the site usually occupied by iron. Erythrocytes containing zinc protoporphyrin are intensely fluorescent and may be used to diagnose lead exposure. Feeding lead to experimental animals also raises heme oxygenase activity, resulting in increases in bilirubin formation. Anemia only occurs in very marked cases of lead toxicity, and is microcytic and hypochromic, as in iron deficiency. The changes in ALAD in peripheral blood and excretion of ALA in urine correlate with BLL and serve as early biochemical indices of lead exposure (ATSDR, 2005b).

Genetic polymorphisms have been identified for alleles of the *ALAD* gene that may affect the toxicokinetics of lead. However, no firm evidence exists for an association between *ALAD* genotype and susceptibility to lead toxicity at background exposures, and, thus, population testing for *ALAD* polymorphism is not justified (Kelada *et al.*, 2001).

Renal Toxicity Acute lead nephrotoxicity consists of proximal tubular dysfunction and can be reversed by treatment with chelating agents. Chronic lead nephrotoxicity consists of interstitial fibrosis and progressive nephron loss, azotemia, and renal failure (Goyer, 1989). A characteristic microscopic change is the presence of intranuclear inclusion bodies. By light microscopy the inclusions are dense, homogeneous, and eosinophilic with hematoxylin and eosin staining. The bodies are composed of a lead–protein complex. The protein is acidic and contains large amounts of aspartic and

glutamic acids with little cystine. The inclusion bodies are a form of aggresome accumulating large amounts of lead in a relatively inert, nontoxic state. MT-null mice cannot form inclusion bodies following lead treatment and are hypersensitive to lead-induced nephropathy and carcinogenesis, suggesting that lead inclusion body formation requires MT as a participant (Qu *et al.*, 2002; Waalkes *et al.*, 2004). In fact, MT is found on the outer surface of lead inclusion bodies, indicating that it may transport the metal to the forming inclusion (Waalkes *et al.*, 2004). Lead nephrotoxicity impairs the renal synthesis of heme-containing enzymes in the kidney, such as heme-containing hydroxylase involved in vitamin D metabolism causing bone effects (ATSDR, 2005b). Hyperuricemia with gout occurs more frequently in the presence of lead nephropathy (Batuman, 1993). Lead nephropathy can be a cause of hypertension (Gonick and Behari, 2002).

Effects on Cardiovascular System There is evidence of a causal relationship between lead exposure and hypertension (Gonick and Behari, 2002; ATSDR, 2005b; Navas-Acien *et al.*, 2007). Analysis of data from the NHANES II for the US population, including BLL and blood pressure measurements in a general population (5803 people aged 12–74), found a correlation between BLL at relatively low levels and blood pressure (Harlan, 1988). An epidemiology reappraisal using meta-analysis of 58,518 subjects from both the general population and occupationally exposed groups from 1980 to 2001 suggested a weak, but significant association between BLL and blood pressure (Nawrot *et al.*, 2002). Elevated blood pressure is more pronounced in middle age than at young age (ATSDR, 2005b). A systematic review of human data indicates a causal relationship between lead and hypertension (Navas-Acien *et al.*, 2007).

A review of chronic lead exposure on blood pressure in experimental animals indicated that at lower doses, lead consistently produced hypertension effects, whereas at higher doses results are inconsistent (Victery, 1988). The pathogenesis of lead-induced hypertension is multifactorial including: (1) inactivation of endogenous nitric oxide and cGMP, possibly through lead-induced ROS; (2) changes in the rennin–angiotensin–aldosterone system, and increases in sympathetic activity, important humoral components of hypertension; (3) alterations in calcium-activated functions of vascular smooth muscle cells including contractility by decreasing Na$^+$/K$^+$-ATPase activity and stimulation of the Na$^+$/Ca^{2+} exchange pump; and (4) a possible rise in endothelin and thromboxane (Gonick and Behari, 2002; Vaziri and Sica, 2004).

Immunotoxicity The developing immune system is sensitive to toxic effects of lead (Dietert *et al.*, 2004). A hallmark of lead-induced immunotoxicity is a pronounced shift in the balance in T helper cell function toward Th2 responses at the expense of Th1 functions, resulting in elevated IgE levels. Increased IgE levels and inflammatory cytokines were found in lead-exposed neonatal rodents, and there is an association between BLL and elevated IgE levels in children (Karmaus *et al.*, 2005; Luebke *et al.*, 2006). Thus, lead immunotoxicity might be a risk factor for childhood asthma (Dietert *et al.*, 2004). In experimental animals, lead has been shown to target macrophages and T cells, especially CD4$^+$ T cells. In occupational exposure, lead-associated changes include altered T-cell subpopulations, reduced immunoglobulin levels, and reduced polymorphonuclear leukocyte chemotactic activity (Dietert *et al.*, 2004; Luebke *et al.*, 2006).

Bone Effects Lead has an extremely long half-life in bone, accounting for over 90% of the body lead in adults. It can affect bone by interfering with metabolic and homeostatic mechanisms including parathyroid hormone, calcitonin, vitamin D, and other hormones that influence calcium metabolism. Lead substitutes for calcium in bone (Pounds *et al.*, 1991). It is known to affect osteoblasts, osteoclasts, and chondrocytes and has been associated with osteoporosis and delays in fracture repair (Carmouche *et al.*, 2005). In children exposed to lead, a higher bone mineral density (BMD) was observed. This may be due to accelerated bone maturation through inhibition of parathyroid hormone–related peptide, may ultimately result in lower peak BMD in young adulthood, and might predispose subjects to osteoporosis later in life (Campbell *et al.*, 2004). A positive association between lead exposure and dental caries in children has been shown in a number of studies. Lead is deposited in teeth, inhibits mineralization of enamel and dentine, and affects metabolism of the cells in the dental pulp (ATSDR, 2005b). Lead in bone is recognized as a potential source for exposure to other tissues when bone is mobilized, as during pregnancy (Silbergeld, 1991).

Other Effects Lead colic is a major gastrointestinal symptom of severe lead poisoning, and is characterized by abdominal pain, nausea, vomiting, constipation, and cramps (ATSDR, 2005b). It is rarely seen today.

Lead-induced gametotoxic effects have been demonstrated in both male and female animals (Goyer, 1990). There is also evidence that lead may disrupt the hypothalamic–pituitary–gonadal axis. An increase in the maternal BLL may also contribute to premature birth and reduced birth weight (ATSDR, 2005b).

Carcinogenicity The association of lead exposure with increased human cancer risk was strengthened by recent studies (ATSDR, 2005c), and inorganic lead compounds were recently reclassified as probably carcinogenic to humans while organic lead compounds were considered not classifiable as to human carcinogenicity (IARC, 2006). A study of a cohort of 20,700 workers coexposed to lead and engine exhaust found a 1.4-fold increase in the overall cancer incidence and a 1.8-fold increase in lung cancer among those who ever had elevated BLL (Anttila *et al.*, 1995).

Another epidemiological study of 27,060 brain cancer cases and 108,240 controls who died of nonmalignant disease in the United States from 1984 to 1992 provides evidence for a potential link between occupational exposure to lead and brain cancer (Cocco *et al.*, 1998). A meta-analysis of published data on cancer incidence among workers in various industries with lead exposure indicates a significant excess of cancer deaths from stomach cancer, lung cancer, and bladder cancer (Fu and Boffetta, 1995). Analysis of eight principal studies with well-documented lead exposures suggests associations of lead exposure with increased lung and stomach cancers (Steenland and Boffetta, 2000). However, workers were not exposed to lead alone, and exposures to other potential carcinogens such as arsenic, cadmium, and engine exhausts could confound these interpretations. Lead does not appear to be directly genotoxic in vivo or in vitro, and lead may interact with other toxicants to facilitate chemical carcinogenesis (Silbergeld, 2003).

Lead is a nephrocarcinogen in adult rodents (Waalkes *et al.*, 1995, 2004; IARC, 2006). Lead-induced renal tumors also occur after perinatal exposure in the absence of the extensive chronic nephropathy (Waalkes *et al.*, 1995). MT-null mice, which do not form lead inclusion bodies, are hypersensitive to lead-induced proliferative lesions of the kidney (Waalkes *et al.*, 2004) and develop testicular teratomas (Tokar *et al.*, 2010b) compared with similarly exposed wild-type mice.

Several mechanisms have been proposed for lead-induced carcinogenesis, including regenerative repair, inhibition of DNA synthesis or repair, generation of ROS with oxidative damage to DNA, substitution of lead for zinc in transcriptional regulators, interaction with DNA-binding proteins, and aberrant gene expression (Silbergeld *et al.*, 2000; Qu *et al.*, 2002; Silbergeld, 2003).

Treatment Chelation therapy is warranted in workmen with BLL >60 μg/dL. For children, criteria have been established (Laraque and Trasande, 2005) that may serve as guidelines to assist in evaluating the individual case with potential health effects. The oral chelating agent DMSA (also called succimer) has advantages over EDTA in that it can be given orally and is effective in temporarily reducing BLL. However, DMSA neither improves long-term BLL in children nor reduces brain lead levels beyond the cessation of lead exposure alone (Cremin *et al.*, 1999; O'Connor and Rich, 1999). A recent study shows that DMSA lowered BLL in children, but had no detectable benefit on learning and behavior (Dietert *et al.*, 2004). Chelation therapy is nonetheless still recommended for children (Warniment *et al.*, 2010). Treatment of organic lead poisoning is symptomatic.

Mercury

Mercury (Hg) was named after the Greco-Roman god known for swift flight. Also called quicksilver, metallic mercury is in liquid state at room temperature. The symbol Hg was derived from the Latinized Greek *hydrargyrum*, meaning "water" and "silver." Mercury was known in ancient times from approximately 1500 BC. By 500 BC mercury was used to make amalgams with other metals. Mercury vapor (Hg^0) is much more hazardous than the liquid form. Mercury binds to other elements (such as chlorine, sulfur, or oxygen) to form inorganic mercurous (Hg^{1+}) or mercuric (Hg^{2+}) salts. This metal can form a number of stable organometallic compounds by attaching to one or two carbon atoms. Methylmercury (CH$_3$Hg$^+$, or MeHg) is the toxicologically most important organic form (ATSDR, 1999a,b). Mercurial compounds have characteristic toxicokinetics and health effects that depend on oxidation state and associated organic species.

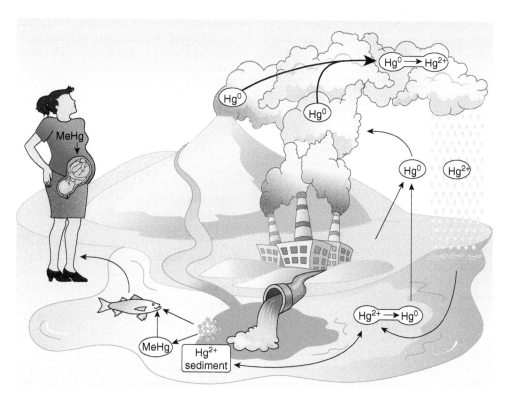

Figure 23-5. *The movement of mercury in the environment.* In nature, mercury vapor (Hg^0), a stable monoatomic gas, evaporates from the earth's surface (both soil and water) and is emitted by volcanoes. Anthropogenic sources include emissions from coal-burning power stations and municipal incinerators. After approximately one year, mercury vapor is converted to soluble form (Hg^{2+}) and returned to the earth by rainwater. It may be converted back to the vapor by microorganisms and reemitted into the atmosphere. Thus, mercury may recirculate for long periods. Mercury attached to aquatic sediments is subjected to microbial conversion to methylmercury, starting with plankton, then herbivorous fish, and finally ascending to carnivorous fish and sea mammals. This biomethylation and biomagnification result in human exposure to methylmercury through consumption of fish, and pose the health risk to humans, especially the developing fetus.

Global Cycling and Ecotoxicology Mercury exemplifies movement of metals in the environment (Fig. 23-5). Atmospheric mercury, in the form of mercury vapor (Hg^0), is derived from natural degassing of the earth's crust and through volcanic eruptions as well as from evaporation from oceans and soils. Anthropogenic sources are estimated to contribute two-thirds of the total atmospheric mercury (Lindberg *et al.*, 2007). These contributions include emissions from metal mining and smelting (mercury, gold, copper, and zinc), coal combustion, municipal incinerators, and chloralkali industries. Mercury vapor is a chemically stable monatomic gas and its residence time in atmosphere is about one year. Thus, mercury is globally distributed even from point resources. Eventually it is oxidized to a water-soluble inorganic form (Hg^{2+}), and returned to the earth's surface in rainwater. The metal may then be reduced back to mercury vapor and returned to the atmosphere, or it may be methylated by microorganisms present in sediments of bodies of fresh and ocean water. This natural biomethylation reaction produces methylmercury (MeHg). Methylmercury enters the aquatic food chain starting with plankton, then herbivorous fish, and finally ascending to carnivorous fish and sea mammals. On the top of the food chain, tissue mercury can rise to levels 1800 to 80,000 times higher than levels in the surrounding water. This biomethylation and bioconcentration result in human exposure to methylmercury through consumption of fish (Clarkson, 2002; Risher *et al.*, 2002). Organomercurial compounds are generally more toxic than inorganic mercury to aquatic organisms, aquatic invertebrates, fish, plants, and birds. Organisms in the larval stages are generally more sensitive to toxic effects of mercury (Boening, 2000).

Exposure

Dietary Exposure Consumption of fish is the major route of exposure to methylmercury. Unlike the case of polychlorinated biphenyls, which are also deposited in fat, cooking the fish does not lower the methylmercury content. Inorganic mercury compounds are also found in food. The source of inorganic mercurial is unknown but the amounts ingested are far below known toxic levels. Mercury in the atmosphere and in drinking water is generally so low that they do not constitute an important source of exposure to the general population (ATSDR, 1999a,b; Clarkson, 2002).

Occupational Exposure Inhalation of mercury vapor can occur from the working environment, as in the chloralkali industry, where mercury is used as a cathode in the electrolysis of brine. Occupational exposure may also occur during manufacture of a variety of scientific instruments and electrical control devices, and in dentistry where mercury amalgams are used in tooth restoration. In the processing of and extraction of gold, especially in developing countries, large quantities of metallic mercury are used to form an amalgam with gold. The amalgam is then heated to drive off the mercury, resulting in a substantial atmospheric release (ATSDR, 1999a,b; Eisler, 2003).

Medicinal Exposure Mercury was an important constituent of drugs for centuries and was used as an ingredient in diuretics, antiseptics, skin ointments, and laxatives. These uses have largely been replaced by safer drugs. Thimerosal contains the ethylmercury radical attached to the sulfur group of thiosalicylate (49.6% mercury by weight as ethylmercury), and has been used as a preservative in many vaccines since 1930s, although its use in children's vaccines was discontinued in 2001 over concerns that children may be exposed to excessive levels of mercury. The use of mercury amalgam in dental restoration releases mercury vapor in the oral cavity and can result in increased mercury body burden. Although the potential health effects of amalgams have been fiercely debated (Clarkson and Magos, 2006; Mutter *et al.*, 2007), the amounts are low compared with occupational exposure (Clarkson *et al.*, 2003).

Accidental Exposure Fatal mercury poisonings come mainly from accidental exposure. Elemental mercury spills can occur in many ways, such as from broken elemental mercury containers, medicinal devices, barometers, and melting tooth amalgam fillings to recover silver. Inhalation of large amount of mercury vapor can be deadly (Baughman, 2006). Oral ingestion of large amounts of inorganic mercury chloride has also been lethal in suicide cases (ATSDR, 1999a,b). A well-known organomercurial poisoning episode was from consumption of fish contaminated with methylmercury from industrial waste in Minamata, Japan. Consumption of grains and rice treated with methylmercury or ethylmercury as fungicides to prevent plant root diseases in Iraq and China also led to a significant number of poisonings (Clarkson, 2002; Risher *et al.*, 2002). Contact with even a small amount of dimethylmercury (CH_3CH_3Hg) can penetrate laboratory gloves resulting in rapid transdermal absorption, delayed cerebella damage, and death (Nierenberg *et al.*, 1998).

Toxicokinetics

Mercury Vapor Mercury vapor is readily absorbed (about 80%) in the lungs, rapidly diffuses across alveolar membranes into the blood, and distributes to all tissues in the body due to its high lipid solubility. Once the vapor has entered cells, it is oxidized to divalent inorganic mercury by tissue and erythrocyte catalase. A significant portion of mercury vapor crosses the blood–brain barrier and placenta before it is oxidized by erythrocytes, and thus shows more neurotoxicity and developmental toxicity compared with administration of inorganic mercury salts that cross membranes less rapidly. After mercury vapor undergoes oxidation, its deposition resembles inorganic mercury. Approximately 10% of mercury vapor is exhaled within a week of exposure, and that converted to inorganic mercury is excreted mainly in urine and feces, with a half-life of one to two months (Clarkson *et al.*, 2003; ATSDR, 1999a,b). Liquid metallic mercury, such as that swallowed from a broken thermometer, is only poorly absorbed by the gastrointestinal tract (0.01%), is not biologically reactive, and is generally thought to be of little or no toxicological consequence.

Inorganic Mercury Inorganic mercury is poorly absorbed from the gastrointestinal tract. Absorption ranges 7% to 15% of ingested dose, depending on the inorganic compound. A small portion of absorbed inorganic mercury is formed by reduction in tissues and exhaled as mercury vapor. The highest concentration of inorganic mercury is found in kidney, a major target. Renal uptake of mercury salts occurs through two routes: from luminal membranes in renal proximal tubule in the form of the cysteine *S*-conjugates (Cys-*S*-Hg-*S*-Cys) or from the basolateral membrane through organic anion transporters (Bridges and Zalpus, 2005). Inorganic mercury salts do not readily pass blood–brain barrier or placenta and are mainly excreted in urine and feces, with a half-life of about two months.

Methylmercury Methylmercury is well absorbed from the gastrointestinal tract. About 95% of methylmercury ingested from fish is absorbed. It is distributed to all tissues in about 30 hours. About 10% of absorbed methylmercury is distributed to the brain and 5% remains in blood. The concentration in erythrocytes is 20 times that in plasma. Methylmercury is bound to thiol-containing molecules such as cysteine (CH_3Hg-*S*-Cys), which mimic methionine to cross the blood–brain barrier and placenta through the neutral amino acid carrier. Methylmercury readily accumulates in hair, and although concentrations are proportional to that in blood, they are about 250-fold higher. Thus, hair mercury is often used as an indicator of exposure. Methylmercury undergoes extensive enterohepatic recycling, which can be interrupted to enhance fecal excretion. Methylmercury is slowly metabolized to inorganic mercury by microflora in intestine (about 1% of the body burden per day). In contrast to inorganic mercury, 90% of the methylmercury is eliminated from the body in the feces, and less than 10% is in the urine, with a half-life of 45 to 70 days (Clarkson, 2002; Risher *et al.*, 2002; Bridges and Zalpus, 2005).

The disposition of ethylmercury is similar to methylmercury. The major differences include that the conversion to inorganic mercury in body is much faster for ethylmercury, which can result in renal injury. The mercury levels in brain are lower for ethylmercury than those for methylmercury. The half-life for ethylmercury is only 15% to 20% of that for methylmercury (Clarkson *et al.*, 2003).

Toxicity

Mercury Vapor Inhalation of mercury vapor at extremely high concentrations may produce an acute, corrosive bronchitis and interstitial pneumonitis and, if not fatal, may be associated with central nervous system effects such as tremor or increased excitability. With chronic exposure to mercury vapor, the major effects are on the central nervous system. Early signs are nonspecific, and this condition has been termed the *asthenic-vegetative syndrome* or *micromercurialism*. Identification of the syndrome requires neurasthenic symptoms and three or more of the following clinical findings: tremor, enlargement of the thyroid, increased uptake of radioiodine in the thyroid, labile pulse, tachycardia, dermographism, gingivitis, hematologic changes, or increased excretion of mercury in urine. The triad of tremors, gingivitis, and erethism (memory loss, increased excitability, insomnia, depression, and shyness) has been recognized historically as the major manifestation of mercury poisoning from inhalation of mercury vapor. Sporadic instances of proteinuria and even nephrotic syndrome may occur in persons with exposure to mercury vapor, particularly with chronic occupational exposure. The pathogenesis is probably immunologically similar to that occurring after exposure to inorganic mercury (Clarkson, 2002; ATSDR, 1999a,b). Mercury vapor release from amalgam is in general too low to cause significant toxicity (Clarkson *et al.*, 2003; Factor-Litvak *et al.*, 2003; Horsted-Bindslev, 2004).

Inorganic Mercury Kidney is the major target organ for inorganic mercury (ATSDR, 1999a,b). Although a high dose of mercuric chloride is directly toxic to renal tubular cells, chronic low-dose exposure to mercury salts may induce an immunologic glomerular disease (Bigazzi, 1999). Exposed persons may develop proteinuria that is reversible after they are removed from exposure. Experimental studies have shown that the pathogenesis has two phases including an early phase characterized by an anti–basement membrane glomerulonephritis, followed by a superimposed immune complex glomerulonephritis with transiently raised concentrations of circulating immune complexes (Henry *et al.*, 1988). The pathogenesis of the nephropathy in humans appears similar, although antigens have not been characterized. In humans, the early glomerular nephritis may progress to interstitial immune complex nephritis (Pelletier and Druet, 1995; Bigazzi, 1999).

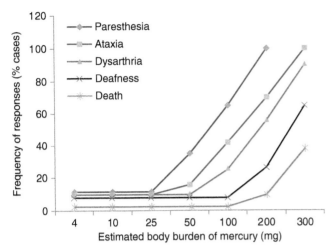

Figure 23-6. *A dose–response simulation of estimated methylmercury body burden and the onset and frequency of symptoms from Iraq epidemic poisoning in 1970s.*

Methylmercury The major human health effect from exposure to methylmercury is neurotoxicity. Clinical manifestations of neurotoxicity include paresthesia (a numbness and tingling sensation around the mouth, lips) and ataxia, manifested as a clumsy, stumbling gait, and difficulty in swallowing and articulating words. Other signs include neurasthenia (a generalized sensation of weakness), vision and hearing loss, and spasticity and tremor. These may finally progress to coma and death. Neuropathological observations have shown that the cortex of the cerebrum and cerebellum are selectively involved with focal necrosis of neurons, lysis and phagocytosis, and replacement by glial cells. These changes are most prominent in the deeper fissures (sulci), as in the visual cortex and insula. The overall acute effect is cerebral edema, but with prolonged destruction of gray matter and subsequent gliosis, cerebral atrophy results (Takeuchi, 1977). A study of the Iraq epidemic of methylmercury exposure (Bakir *et al.*, 1973) has provided dose–response estimates of the body burden of mercury required for the onset and frequency of symptoms (Fig. 23-6).

Mechanism of Toxicity High-affinity binding of divalent mercury to sulfhydryl groups of proteins in the cells is an important mechanism for producing nonspecific cell injury or even cell death. A number of general mechanisms of toxicity have been observed after mercury exposures. Although mercury does not participate in Fenton-like reactions, oxidative stress plays a significant role in mercury toxicity. Reduced glutathione levels and antioxidant enzymes have been reported in mice exposed to methylmercury (Stringari *et al.*, 2008; Franco *et al.*, 2009). Genes associated with oxidative stress have been found to be upregulated by inorganic mercury exposure using microarray studies in yeast and human cells (Kawata *et al.*, 2007; Jin *et al.*, 2008). In vitro exposures to inorganic or methylmercury also affected the MAPK signaling pathway (Kim *et al.*, 2002; Hao *et al.*, 2009). Methylmercury has also been shown to disrupt microtubules in neurites and in neonatal mice (Ferraro *et al.*, 2009; Fukushima *et al.*, 2009). Both inorganic and methylmercury damage mitochondria and disrupt intracellular calcium homeostasis (Freitas *et al.*, 1996; Konigsberg *et al.*, 2001; Cambier *et al.*, 2009).

Sensitive Subpopulations Early life stages are particularly vulnerable to mercury intoxication (Counter and Buchanan, 2004). In Minamata, Japan, pregnant women who consumed fish contaminated with methylmercury manifested mild or minimal symptoms,

but gave birth to infants with severe developmental disabilities, raising initial concerns for mercury as a developmental toxicant. Methylmercury crosses the placenta and reaches the fetus, and is concentrated to a level in fetal brain at least five to seven times that of maternal blood (Clarkson, 2002). Prenatal methylmercury exposure at high levels can induce widespread damage to the fetal brain. However, the observed effects from low-level exposures are inconsistent (Counter and Buchanan, 2004; Davidson *et al.*, 2004). In the Seychelles Children Development Study, a group with significant methylmercury exposure from a diet predominantly of fish was studied for adverse developmental effects. These children were examined six times over 11 years using extensive batteries of age-appropriate developmental end points, but no convincing associations were found except for delayed walking (Davidson *et al.*, 2006). The National Research Council reviewed the epidemiological studies relating in utero methylmercury exposure and fetal neurological development. It concluded that the current EPA reference dose (RfD) for methylmercury of 0.1 μg/kg per day or 5.8 μg/L cord blood is scientifically justifiable for protection of human health (NRC, 2000). The RfD is equivalent to 12 ppm methylmercury in maternal hair.

The safety of thimerosal (ethylmercury) used in childhood vaccines has also received extensive attention. A recent review indicates that thimerosal is safe at the doses used in vaccines, except for a potential for local hypersensitivity (Clarkson *et al.*, 2003). However, some infants may be exposed to cumulative levels of mercury during the first six months of life that may exceed EPA recommendations (Ball *et al.*, 2001). Steps have been rapidly taken to remove thimerosal from vaccines in the United States by switching to single-dose vials that do not require preservatives. Nonetheless, the World Health Organization concluded that it is safe to continue using thimerosal in vaccines, which is important for developing countries where it is essential to use multidose vials (Clarkson *et al.*, 2003).

Although the use of mercury amalgam in children can contribute to mercury exposure, the level of exposure is too low to cause significant toxicological effects (DeRouen *et al.*, 2006).

Acrodynia has occurred in children chronically exposed to inorganic mercury compounds in teething powder and diaper disinfectants, as well as to organomercurials. It is characterized by pink hands and feet (also called pink disease). These subjects are photophobic and suffer from joint pains (Clarkson, 2002).

Treatment Therapy for mercury poisoning should be directed toward lowering the concentration of mercury at the critical organ or site of injury. For the most severe cases, particularly with acute renal failure, hemodialysis may be the first measure, along with administration of chelating agents for mercury, such as cysteine, EDTA, BAL, or penicillamine. Caution should be taken to avoid inappropriate use of chelating agents in putative mercury poisoning patients (Risher and Amler, 2005).

Chelation therapy is not very helpful for alkyl mercury exposure. Biliary excretion and reabsorption by the intestine can be interrupted by oral administration of a nonabsorbable thiol resin, which can bind mercury and enhance fecal excretion (Clarkson, 2002).

Nickel

Nickel (Ni) has been in use since ancient times. However, because the ores of nickel were easily mistaken for ores of silver, a more complete understanding of nickel and its specific use came with more contemporary times. In 1751, nickel was first isolated from the ore kupfernickel (niccolite) from which it derives its name. Nickel is used in various metal alloys, including stainless steels, in electroplating, batteries, pigments, catalysts, and ceramics. Major properties of nickel alloys include strength, corrosion resistance, and good thermal and electrical conductivity. Occupational exposure to nickel occurs by inhalation of nickel-containing aerosols, dusts, or fumes, or dermal contact in workers engaged in nickel production (mining, milling, refinery, etc) and nickel-using operations (melting, electroplating, welding, nickel–cadmium batteries, etc) (ATSDR, 2005c; NTP, 2011e). Nickel, like many other metals, is ubiquitous in nature, and the general population is exposed to low levels of nickel in air, cigarette smoke, water, and food. These exposures are generally too low to be of real toxicological concern (Kasprzak *et al.*, 2003). Nickel has various oxidation states but the 2+ oxidation state is the most prevalent form in biosystems. The major soluble nickel compounds are nickel acetate, nickel chloride, nickel sulfate, and nickel nitrate. The important water-insoluble nickel compounds include nickel sulfide, nickel subsulfide, nickel oxide, nickel carbonyl, and nickel carbonate (ATSDR, 2005c).

Toxicokinetics Inhalation of nickel is the most important route toxicologically. Inhaled nickel particles are deposited in the respiratory tract and, as with all inhaled particles, the site of deposition depends on the particle size. Large particles (5–30 μm) deposit in the nasopharyngeal area via impaction, smaller particles (1–5 μm) enter the trachea and bronchiolar region by sedimentation, and particles smaller than 1 μm enter the alveolar space. About 25% to 35% of the inhaled nickel that is retained in the lungs is absorbed into the blood. The insoluble nickel particles can be taken up into cells by phagocytosis. When applied or in contact with skin, the rate of absorption depends on the rate of penetration into the epidermis, which differs for different chemical forms of nickel. In humans, about 27% of a single oral dose of nickel in drinking water is absorbed, depending on the compound, whereas only about 1% is absorbed when nickel is given with food. Intestinal nickel absorption occurs through calcium or iron channels, or by the divalent metal transport protein-1 (ATSDR, 2005c).

The main transport proteins of nickel in blood are albumin, histidine, and α_2-microglobulin. Nickelplasmin and MT also can bind and transport nickel. Following inhalation exposure, nickel is distributed to the lungs, skin, kidneys, liver, pituitary, and adrenals. The half-life of nickel is one to three days for nickel sulfate, five days for nickel subsulfide, and more than 100 days for nickel oxide (ATSDR, 2005c). Absorbed nickel is excreted into urine. Urinary nickel correlates closely with exposure to airborne levels of insoluble nickel compounds. Thus, urinary nickel may serve as a suitable measure of current nickel exposure.

The marked differences in carcinogenic activities of various nickel compounds may be due to differences in delivery of nickel ion to specific cells and subcellular target molecules. For example, injection of animals with crystalline nickel subsulfide or crystalline nickel sulfide results in a high incidence of tumors at the site of injection sites, although tumors are generally not observed in animals similarly injected with soluble nickel sulfate (IARC, 1990). The crystalline nickel particles can be actively phagocytized and apparently deliver larger quantities of nickel ions into the nucleus of local cells compared with water-soluble nickel compounds that diffuse away from the site (Kasprzak *et al.*, 2003; Costa *et al.*, 2005). Several water-soluble nickel compounds can, however, produce local malignant tumors when repeatedly injected into the peritoneal cavity of rats, suggesting repeated exposures to the target cells may be required (IARC, 1990).

Essentiality of nickel in higher organisms is questionable, although nickel may be nutritionally essential for some plants, bacteria, and invertebrates. Nickel deficiency syndromes have not been reported in humans and nickel-dependent enzymes or cofactors are unknown (Denkhaus and Salnikow, 2002).

Toxicity

Contact Dermatitis Nickel-induced contact dermatitis is the most common adverse health effect from nickel exposure and is found in 10% to 20% of the general population. It can result from exposure to airborne nickel, liquid nickel solutions, or prolonged skin contact with metal items containing nickel, such as coins and jewelry. Nickel sensitization usually arises from prolonged contact with nickel or exposure to a large dose of nickel. The resulting dermatitis is an inflammatory reaction mediated by type IV delayed hypersensitivity (ATSDR, 2005c).

Nickel Carbonyl Poisoning Metallic nickel combines with carbon monoxide to form nickel carbonyl ($Ni[CO]_4$), which decomposes to nickel and carbon monoxide on heating to 200°C (the Mond process). This reaction provides a convenient and efficient method for nickel refining. However, nickel carbonyl is extremely toxic, and can cause acute toxicity. Intoxication begins with headache, nausea, vomiting, and epigastric or chest pain, followed by cough, hyperpnea, cyanosis, gastrointestinal symptoms, and weakness. The symptoms may be accompanied by fever and leukocytosis. The more severe cases can progress to pneumonia, respiratory failure, and eventually to cerebral edema and death.

Carcinogenicity Nickel is a respiratory tract carcinogen in nickel-refining industry workers (IARC, 1990; Straif *et al.*, 2009; NTP, 2011e). Risks are highest for lung and nasal cancers among workers heavily exposed to nickel. Because the refining of nickel in some plants that were studied involved the formation of nickel carbonyl, it was believed for a time that nickel carbonyl was the principal carcinogen. However, multiple additional epidemiological studies of workers in other refineries suggest that the source of the increased risk is the mixture of nickel compounds (IARC, 1990; Straif *et al.*, 2009; NTP, 2011e). Studies often involve a complex mixture of the metal and several of its compounds making separate carcinogenic assessment challenging (Straif *et al.*, 2009; NTP, 2011e). Nickel sulfate and combinations of nickel sulfides and oxides encountered in nickel refining are considered to cause human cancer (IARC, 1990; NTP, 2011e). Human studies have also shown a strong association between primary exposure to water-soluble nickel compounds in the nickel-refinery industry and elevated cancer risk (Grimsrud and Andersen, 2010; NTP, 2011e). Nonetheless, controversy remains about the role of soluble nickel compounds in human cancer causation based on a biokinetic hypothesis that they are unable to deliver sufficient nickel to critical local targets because they are soluble (Goodman *et al.*, 2011). Metallic nickel is considered *reasonably anticipated to be a human carcinogen* based on multiple positive rodent studies (NTP, 2011e).

Studies with rats and some with mice have shown that inhaled or intratracheal instilled nickel subsulfide or nickel oxide produces lung tumors, including carcinoma, in a dose-related fashion and causes adrenal gland tumors (IARC, 1990; NTP, 2011e). Injection of various nickel compounds (generally water insoluble) at various sites (subcutaneous, intramuscular, intrarenal, etc) causes local tumors (primarily sarcomas) in laboratory animals often in a dose-related fashion (IARC, 1990; NTP, 2011e). The relevance of routes to human exposure situations is debatable, but such data are used to assess carcinogenic potential. Nickel monoxides, hydroxides, and crystalline sulfides are also considered to be carcinogenic in animals based on studies finding injection site tumors and/or lung tumors after intratracheal instillations (IARC, 1990; NTP, 2011e). Metallic nickel produces injection site tumors and lung tumors after intratracheal instillation (IARC, 1990; NTP, 2011e). Rodent carcinogenesis studies of soluble nickel compounds have also yielded positive results in rodents (Kasprzak *et al.*, 2003). For instance, water-soluble nickel acetate is a complete transplacental carcinogen for the rat pituitary and initiator of kidney tumors in the rat (Diwan *et al.*, 1992). The water-soluble nickel compounds, nickel chloride, nickel sulfate, and nickel acetate, produced local mesotheliomas or sarcomas when given by repeated intraperitoneal injection to rats (IARC, 1990), suggesting repeated exposure to soluble salts is required (IARC, 1990). In two strain A mouse studies, multiple intraperitoneal injections of nickel acetate increased lung adenocarcinoma incidence (one study) and lung tumor multiplicity (both studies; IARC, 1990). However, many rodent studies using soluble nickel compounds have been negative (Sivulka, 2005).

Mechanism for Nickel Carcinogenesis The carcinogenicity of nickel is thought to be due to the generation of ionic nickel in target cells at sites that are key for carcinogenesis (NTP, 2011e). This has allowed consideration of these compounds as a single group (Straif *et al.*, 2009; NTP, 2011e). Ionic nickel is thought to be the active and genotoxic form of the metal, and there is no reason to suspect that the mechanisms by which nickel causes cancer in experimental animals would differ from humans (NTP, 2011e).

Carcinogenic nickel particles that are phagocytized and deliver large quantities of nickel ions into the nucleus are generally not mutagenic but are clastogenic (Costa *et al.*, 2005). In this way insoluble nickel compounds can produce specific chromosomal damage, notable in the heterochromatic long arm of the X chromosome that suffers regional decondensation, frequent deletions, and other aberrations (Costa *et al.*, 2005). Nickel compounds also produce chromosomal abnormalities such as sister chromatid exchange, especially in hetrochromatin, micronuclei formation in human lymphocytes, microsatellite mutations in human lung cancer cells, and mutations in renal cells (Kasprzak *et al.*, 2003). Many studies in vitro and in vivo indicate a variety of soluble and insoluble forms of nickel cause genetic damage, including DNA damage, cell transformation, and DNA repair disruption (NTP, 2011e). The redox activity of nickel may produce ROS that could attack DNA directly (NTP, 2011e).

Epigenetic Effects A broad spectrum of epigenetic effects occurs with nickel and includes alterations in gene expression resulting from perturbed DNA methylation and posttranslational histone modification (Arita and Costa, 2009). A notable nickel-inducible gene is Cap43/NDRG1, under the control of the HIF-1. During tumor development, HIF-1 facilitates angiogenesis and regulates numerous genes including glucose transport and glycolysis, which are essential for tumor growth. A correlation of overexpression of Cap43 with the neoplastic state of the cells was noted (Costa *et al.*, 2005). Another nickel-induced gene amplification is the Ect2 gene. The Ect2 protein is overexpressed in nickel-transformed cells, which can cause microtubule disassembly and cytokinesis, and may contribute to morphological changes in cells (Clemens *et al.*, 2005). Nickel produces low, but measurable ROS in cells and depletes cellular glutathione. Oxidative DNA damage, oxidative protein damage, and lipid peroxidation, as well as inhibition of DNA repair enzymes, can be observed following nickel exposure (Kasprzak *et al.*, 2003; Valko *et al.*, 2005).

Treatment of Nickel Toxicity Sodium diethylcarbodithioate (DDTC) is the preferred drug for nickel treatment. Disulfiram, another nickel-chelating agent, has been used in nickel dermatitis and in nickel carbonyl poisoning. Other chelating agents, such as D-penicillamine and DMPS, provide some degree of protection from clinical effects (Blanusa *et al.*, 2005).

Cobalt

Cobalt (Co) is a relatively rare, ferromagnetic transition metal first isolated in the 1730s. The name cobalt comes from the German word *kobalt*, which is derived from *kobold* meaning "goblin," a name applied by miners of the time to cobalt ore, which was thought to be worthless and poisonous. Cobalt is usually not mined alone and tends to be produced primarily as a by-product of copper and nickel mining. It is useful in various alloys, where it provides corrosion and wear resistance, and in cemented carbides ("hard" metals). It is used in permanent magnets, as a paint or varnish dryer, in catalysts, and in production of pigments (ATSDR, 2004a).

Toxicokinetics The toxicokinetics and possible adverse health effects of inorganic cobalt compounds have been reviewed (De Boeck *et al.*, 2003; ATSDR, 2004a; Lison, 2007). Cobalt absorption depends on the compound. Less than 5% of an oral dose of cobalt oxide is absorbed, whereas about 30% of an oral dose of cobalt chloride is absorbed in rodents. Oral absorption of cobalt varies widely in humans, and it is estimated to be between 5% and 45%. Increasing doses of cobalt results in a decreasing proportional absorption, so increased cobalt levels tend not to cause significant accumulation. Absorption of inhaled cobalt compounds appears to be relatively effective in humans and animals. About 80% of absorbed cobalt is excreted in urine, and about 15% is excreted in feces. The liver, kidneys, adrenals, and thyroid have relatively high concentrations. The normal levels in human urine and blood are <2.0 and 0.2 to 0.5 µg/L, respectively. Cobalt in blood is largely associated with red blood cells.

Essentiality Cobalt is an essential nutrient, in small amounts, to mammals, including humans. The essential form of cobalt is cobalamin, a cobalt-containing tetrapyrrolic ring and critical component of vitamin B_{12}. Vitamin B_{12} is required for the production of red blood cells and in the prevention of pernicious anemia. Insufficient natural levels of cobalt in the diet of sheep and cattle result in cobalt deficiency disease, characterized by anemia and loss of weight or retarded growth. If other requirements for cobalt exist, they are not well defined (Herbert, 1996).

Toxicity Occupational inhalation of cobalt-containing dust in industrial settings may cause respiratory irritation at air concentrations between 0.002 and 0.01 mg/m³. Higher concentrations may be a cause of "hard metal" pneumoconiosis, a progressive form of pulmonary interstitial fibrosis. This disease is observed in workers exposed to cobalt–tungsten carbide but not observed with exposure to cobalt alone (ATSDR, 2004a; NTP, 2011f). Occupational dermal exposure is sometimes associated with an allergic dermatitis.

Cobalt can be erythropoietic when excessive amounts are ingested by most mammals, including humans. Chronic oral administration of high levels of cobalt for the treatment of anemia can cause goiter, and epidemiological studies suggest that the incidence of goiter is higher in regions containing increased levels of cobalt in water and soil. The goitrogenic effect has been elicited by the oral administration of 3 to 4 mg/kg to children in the course of treatment of sickle cell anemia. Intravenous exposure to cobalt can cause increased blood pressure, slowed respiration, tinnitus, and deafness due to nerve damage. Cardiomyopathy with signs of congestive heart failure has been associated with excessive cobalt intake (>10 mg per day), particularly from drinking beer to which cobalt was added as a foaming agent. Autopsy findings in such cases have found a 10-fold increase in the cardiac levels of cobalt. In animals, myocardial degeneration can be produced by cobalt injection. In rats cobalt injection will produce hyperglycemia due to pancreatic β-cell damage (Lison, 2007).

Based on experimental studies in animals, cobalt sulfate has been classified as *reasonably anticipated to be carcinogenic in humans* (NTP, 2011f). In rodents, inhalation of cobalt sulfate induces lung tumors, including carcinoma, in rats and mice (Bucher *et al.*, 1999). Repository injections or implantation of various cobalt compounds can produce local sarcomas in rodents (IARC, 1991). Incidence of adrenal gland tumors was also increased in female rats expose to cobalt sulfate (NTP, 2011f). The mechanisms by which cobalt produces cancer are not fully defined but potentially include inhibition of DNA repair and formation of DNA-damaging ROS, and through alterations of important cellular functions by replacing other essential metal ions (ATSDR, 2004a; NTP, 2011f).

Cobalt–tungsten carbide powders and hard metals are *reasonably anticipated to be human carcinogens* based on limited evidence of carcinogenicity from human studies and supporting evidence from studies on mechanisms of carcinogenesis (NTP, 2011f). No studies examining the carcinogenicity of cobalt–tungsten carbide powders or hard metals in animals have been identified. Potential carcinogenic mechanisms include the release of cobalt ions, increased production of ROS with resultant oxidative stress response, and by causing cytotoxicity, genotoxicity, inflammation, and apoptosis (NTP, 2011f).

Copper

Copper (Cu) has been used for many centuries. By 2000 BC, "bronze" or copper–tin alloys were in wide use in Europe. In Roman times, copper became known as *cerium* because so much of it was mined in Cyprus, and eventually Anglicized into *copper*. Copper is an essential element widely distributed in nature. Food, beverages, and drinking water are major sources of exposure in the general population. The Recommended Dietary Allowance (RDA) of copper varies according to age, and pregnancy and lactation. Daily intake of copper in adults is 0.9 mg per day, in children between 0.2 and 0.9 mg per day, and in pregnant or lactating women 1.0 to 1.3 mg per day (IOM and Food and Nutrition Board, 2001). The average daily intake of copper from food is ~1.2 to 1.7 mg per day (Chambers *et al.*, 2010).

Copper exposure in industry is primarily from inhaled particulates in mining or metal fumes in smelting operations, welding, or related activities. In the general population, exposure to elevated levels of copper can occur via metal leaching from copper plumbing or copper lined cookware (ATSDR, 2004b). Excess copper in the water represents a significant risk factor to the aquatic environment, producing endocrine disruption and other toxic effects in fish (Handy, 2003).

Toxicokinetics Approximately 55% to 75% of an oral dose of copper is absorbed from the gastrointestinal tract, primarily in the duodenum. Intestinal copper absorption can be reduced by zinc, iron, molybdate, and fructose (IOM and Food and Nutrition Board, 2001). Following intestinal absorption, copper is transported into the serum where it binds to a series of copper-binding proteins and small peptides, such as albumin, and amino acids. Although all tissues and cells contain copper, the primary sites for copper storage include the liver, which accounts for >80% of the stored copper, and brain. Within the cell, a majority of copper is complexed by glutathione, MT, and cytosolic copper chaperons, which work in conjunction with copper-ATPases to maintain copper homeostasis (Harris, 2000; Mercer, 2001). The remainder of copper is complexed

by copper-containing proteins, where the metal serves as a cofactor in enzymatic reactions (Stern, 2010). The amount of copper in the body is maintained at homeostatic levels mainly through control of excretion, although copper binding to hepatic MT may act as a form of intracellular storage. In mammals, the major route of excretion for excess copper is via the feces, with very little copper excreted into the urine. The bile is the major route of excretion from the liver. Bile secretion, enterohepatic recirculation, and intestinal reabsorption all help to maintain copper homeostasis.

Essentiality Copper is an essential component of several metalloenzymes, including type A oxidases and type B monoamine oxidases. Of the type B oxidases, cytochrome *c* oxidase is probably the most important because it catalyzes a key reaction in energy metabolism, and inherited mutational defects can result in severe pathology in humans (Hamza and Gitlin, 2002). Of the type A oxidases, lysyl oxidase plays a major role in the formation and repair of extracellular matrix by oxidizing lysine residues in elastin and collagen, thereby initiating the covalent cross-linkage (Kagan and Li, 2003). Copper/zinc superoxide dismutase (SOD) is present in most cells, particularly of the brain, thyroid, liver, lung, and blood, and helps protect from oxygen toxicity by reducing superoxide radicals to hydrogen peroxide (Valko *et al.*, 2005).

Copper deficiency is uncommon in humans, but can occur as a result of malnutrition, overdose of molybdenum, or excessive consumption of zinc (Maret and Standstead, 2006). Copper deficiency manifests clinically by hypochromic, microcytic anemia that is refractory to iron supplementation and predisposes to infection. More recently, a series of case reports has implicated acquired copper deficiency in the etiology of adult-onset progressive myeloneuropathy and in the development of severe blood disorders including myelodysplastic syndrome (Kumar *et al.*, 2005; Goodman *et al.*, 2009). This deficiency is sometimes accompanied by bone abnormalities. Less frequent manifestations are hypopigmentation of the hair and hypotonia. Biomarkers of copper deficiency include low serum and urine copper levels, ceruloplasmin concentration, and copper-dependent enzyme activities (IOM and Food and Nutrition Board, 2001).

Toxicity The upper safe limit for daily copper consumption is estimated to be 10 mg Cu per day. The most commonly reported adverse health effects of excess oral copper intake are gastrointestinal distress. Nausea, vomiting, and abdominal pain have been reported shortly after drinking solutions of copper sulfate or beverages stored in containers that readily release copper (Pizarro *et al.*, 1999). Ingestion of drinking water with >3 mg Cu/L will produce gastrointestinal symptoms. Ingestion of large amounts of copper salts, most frequently copper sulfate, may produce hepatic necrosis and death. Animal and human epidemiological studies have not found any relation between copper exposure and cancer (ATSDR, 2004b).

Hereditary Disease of Copper Metabolism

Menkes Disease This is a rare sex-linked genetic defect in copper metabolism resulting in copper deficiency in male infants. It is characterized by peculiar hair, failure to thrive, severe mental retardation, neurological impairment, connective tissue dysfunction, and death usually by three to five years of age. The majority of the pathologies associated with Menkes disease can be linked to deficiencies in copper-containing proteins (Tümer and Møller, 2010). Bones are osteoporotic with flared metaphases of the long bones and bones of the skull. There is extensive degeneration of the cerebral cortex and of white matter. The gene responsible for Menkes disease, *ATP7A*, belongs to the family of ATPases and is

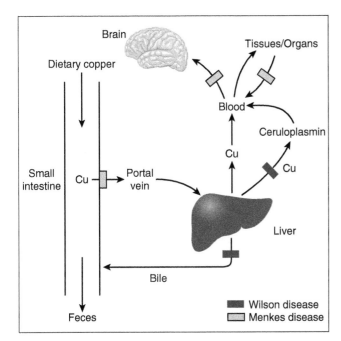

Figure 23-7. *Pathways of copper in the body and defects in Menkes and Wilson diseases.* Copper is absorbed by the enterocytes of the small intestine and transported across the basolateral membrane of enterocytes into the portal circulation. The latter process is defective in Menkes disease patients and results in accumulation of copper in the enterocytes and overall copper deficiency in the body. Most of the newly absorbed copper is normally taken up by the liver. In cases of copper overload, excess copper is excreted in the bile and this process is blocked in Wilson disease, as is the delivery of copper to ceruloplasmin, the principal copper carrier in the blood. Other low-molecular-weight proteins such as Cu–metallothionein and Cu-histidine are also proposed to be important sources of copper to tissues. The transport of copper to the brain is blocked in patients with Menkes disease, leading to the severe neurological abnormalities. (Adapted from Mercer, 2001, with permission from Elsevier.)

a copper transporter (Fig. 23-7). Deficiency in this copper transporter in Menkes disease blocks copper transportation across the basolateral membrane of intestinal cells into the portal circulation, resulting in accumulation of copper in the enterocytes and systemic copper deficiency in the body. The transport of copper to the brain is also blocked, causing severe neurological abnormalities. Animal models for copper deficiency support the importance of adequate copper intake during embryogenesis and early development (Shim and Harris, 2003). Supplementation with copper-histidine has been shown to delay disease progression of the disease and successfully increase life span (Kodama *et al.*, 2011).

Wilson Disease This is an autosomal recessive genetic disorder of copper metabolism characterized by the excessive accumulation of copper in liver, brain, kidneys, and cornea (Huster, 2010). Serum ceruloplasmin is low and serum copper not bound to ceruloplasmin is elevated. Urinary excretion of copper is high. Clinical abnormalities of the nervous system, liver, kidneys, and cornea are related to copper accumulation. Patients with Wilson disease have impaired biliary excretion of copper, which is believed to be the fundamental cause of the hepatic copper overload. Wilson disease is associated with hepatic diseases ranging from mild hepatitis to acute liver failure. There is also an increased incidence of hepatocarcinoma in patents with Wilson disease (Wang *et al.*, 2002). Neurological symptoms associated with Wilson disease include dystonia, tremor, dysarthria, and psychiatric disturbances. Genetic studies have identified the defect in copper transport as mutations

of the Wilson disease locus (WND) on chromosome 13, encoding P-type ATPase (*ATP7B*) (Huster, 2010). There appear to be several polymorphisms of the defect, which may explain the clinical variability in the disorder. Diagnosis may be suspected with elevated serum copper but must be confirmed by liver biopsy and elevated liver copper (normally 15-55 µg/g vs >250 µg/g in Wilson disease).

Hereditary Aceruloplasminemia This is the autosomal recessive genetic disorder of copper-binding protein ceruloplasmin, associated with the iron overload syndrome. Clinical signs and symptoms, which result from iron overload in the brain, include mental confusion, memory loss, dementia, cerebellar ataxia, altered motor function, retinal degeneration, and diabetes (Xu *et al.*, 2004). Ceruloplasmin-null mice accumulate iron predominantly in organs of reticuloendothelial system. In these mice, hematologic indices and serum iron are abnormal by 10 weeks of age, with profound iron overload in the spleen and liver. Hepatic copper deposition is also approximately doubled in these mice. However, neurodegeneration and diabetes are not observed in these mice (Shim and Harris, 2003).

Indian Childhood Cirrhosis (ICC) This is a disorder occurring in young children characterized by jaundice due to an insidious and progressive liver disease. Two distinguishing features are a widespread brown orcein staining (indicating copper) and intralobular hepatic fibrosis progressing to portal cirrhosis and chronic inflammation. The etiology is not known but it is suspected that bottle feeding of milk contaminated with copper from storage in brass vessels may be important. However, epidemiological studies also suggest an autosomal recessive genetic component because of strong familial occurrence and high consanguinity among affected children (WHO, 1998a,b).

Idiopathic Copper Toxicosis or Non-Indian Childhood Cirrhosis This is a rare disorder in children similar to ICC occurring in some Western countries. The largest series of cases are reported from the Tyrol region of Austria. This population also used copper vessels to store milk, and the incidence of the disorder has declined since replacement of the copper vessels. A number of other cases have been reported from other parts of the world, some from increased amounts of copper in the drinking water (WHO, 1998a,b).

Treatment Treatment for Wilson disease and other diseases of copper overload includes copper chelators and supplementation with zinc salts. Clinical improvement can be achieved by chelation of copper with D-penicillamine, Trien (triethylenetetramine 2HCl), zinc acetate, and tetrathiomolybdate. The combination of tetrathiomolybdate and zinc acetate is more effective (Brewer, 2005). *N*-Acetylcysteine amide can cross the blood–brain barrier and was developed to help prevent neurodegenerative disorders (Cai *et al.*, 2005).

Iron

Iron (Fe) is a highly abundant transition metal that came into use around 4000 BC. An early source of iron was from fallen meteorites and the name may derive from the Ethruscan word *aisar* that means "the gods." Iron is an essential metal for erythropoiesis and a key component of hemoglobin, myoglobin, heme enzymes, metalloflavoprotein enzymes, and mitochondrial enzymes. Physiologically, iron mainly exists as the ferrous (2+) and ferric (3+) forms. Toxicological considerations are important in terms of iron deficiency, accidental acute exposures, and chronic iron overload due to idiopathic hemochromatosis or as a consequence of excess dietary iron or frequent blood transfusions (Papanikolaou and Pantopoulos, 2005; Weinberg, 2010).

Toxicokinetics Iron metabolism is regulated by a complex series of events that maintain homeostasis, mainly involving absorption, storage, and excretion (Wang and Pantopoulos, 2011; Theil, 2011). Heme iron from meat, poultry, and fish is highly bioavailable. Nonheme iron absorption is influenced by its solubility and by other dietary factors, such as ascorbic acid which enhances uptake. Absorption involves movement of ferrous ions from the intestinal lumen into the mucosal cells via the divalent metal transporter protein 1 (DMT1) among several other transporters (Theil, 2011). The metal is then transferred from the mucosal cell to the plasma, where iron is bound to transferrin for transport and distribution. A β_1-globulin produced in the liver, transferrin, delivers iron to tissues by binding to transferrin receptor-1 on the cell membrane, followed by endocytosis. Intracellular iron homeostasis is regulated by a complex coordination of iron trafficking and iron storage involving an iron response element/iron regulatory protein system and antioxidant response elements (Wang and Pantopoulos, 2011; Theil, 2011). The human body contains ~3 to 5 g of iron. About two-thirds of body iron is in hemoglobin, 10% is in myoglobin and iron-containing enzymes, and the remainder is bound to iron storage proteins such as ferritin and hemosiderin, stored in liver and reticuloendothelial cells in the spleen and bone marrow. Iron stores serve as a reservoir to supply cellular iron needs, mainly for hemoglobin production. Erythrocyte destruction and production are responsible for most iron turnover. Hepcidin, a small peptide of liver origin, modulates iron absorption in response to erythropoiesis (Papanikolaou and Pantopoulos, 2005). The major route of excretion of iron is into the gastrointestinal tract and eventually the feces.

Essentiality and Deficiency Iron deficiency is the most common nutritional deficiency worldwide, affecting infants, young children, and women of childbearing age and is considered a major public health issue (Theil, 2011). The critical period for iron deficiency in children is between the ages of six months and two years. The major manifestation of iron deficiency is anemia with microcytic hypochromic red blood cells. Other effects of iron deficiency include impaired psychomotor development and intellectual performance, decreased resistance to infection, adverse pregnancy outcomes, and possibly increased susceptibility to lead and cadmium toxicity. Oral ferrous sulfate is the treatment of choice for iron deficiency.

Toxicity Acute iron poisoning from accidental ingestion of iron-containing dietary supplements is the most common cause of acute toxicity. It most often occurs in children. This type of poisoning decreased following the introduction of childproof lids on prescription medicines and vitamin supplements. Severe toxicity occurs after the ingestion of more than 0.5 g of iron or 2.5 g of ferrous sulfate. Toxicity occurs about one to six hours after ingestion. Symptoms include abdominal pain, diarrhea, and vomiting. Of particular concern are pallor or cyanosis, metabolic acidosis, liver damage, and cardiac collapse. Death may occur in severely poisoned children within 24 hours. Supportive therapy and iron chelation with deferoxamine (also known as desferrioxamine) should be used as soon as possible. Inhalation of iron oxide fumes or dust may cause pneumoconiosis in occupational settings (Doherty *et al.*, 2004).

Chronic iron toxicity from iron overload in adults is a relatively common problem. There are three basic ways in which excessive amounts of iron can accumulate in the body. The first is hereditary hemochromatosis due to abnormal absorption of iron from the intestinal tract. Hereditary hemochromatosis is an autosomal recessive

disorder attributed to mutation in the hemochromatosis gene. The second possible cause of iron overload is excess intake via the diet or from oral iron preparations. The third circumstance in which iron overload can occur is repeated blood transfusions for some form of refractory anemia and is referred to as *transfusional siderosis*. The pathological consequences of iron overload are similar regardless of the basis. *Hemosiderosis* refers to increased iron stores in the form of hemosiderin. The body iron content can increase 20 to 40 g, up to 10 times higher than normal levels. *Hemochromatosis* refers to excessive deposition of iron that causes organ damage, often resulting in fibrosis. Inhalation of iron oxide fumes or dust by workers in hematic mines (mainly Fe_2O_3), steel workers, and welders may produce siderosis (nonfibrotic), and in some cases silicosis (fibrotic) in the lung, with increases in total body iron (Doherty *et al.*, 2006). Liver iron overload from hereditary hemochromatosis appears to be associated with an increased risk for hepatocellular carcinoma, as well as with other malignancies (Papanikolaou and Pantopoulos, 2005). Oxidant stress would be a presumable carcinogenic mode of action.

Increased body iron may play a role in the development of cardiovascular disease, including cardiomyopathy (Gujja *et al.*, 2010). It is suspected that iron may produce free radical damage resulting in artherosclerosis and ischemic heart disease (Alpert, 2004). It is clear that mortality from cardiovascular disease is correlated with liver iron overload (Yuan and Li, 2003; Gujja *et al.*, 2010). Several neurodegenerative disorders are associated with aberrant iron metabolism in the brain, such as neuroferritinopathy, aceruloplasminemia, and manganism (Aschner *et al.*, 2005; Papanikolaou and Pantopoulos, 2005).

Treatment Desferrioxamine is the chelator of choice for the treatment of acute iron intoxication and chronic iron overload. Iron chelators have also been proposed for the treatment of cancers with iron overload (Buss *et al.*, 2004).

Magnesium

Magnesium (Mg) was recognized as an element in 1755. The name originates from the Greek word for a district in Thessaly called *Magnesia*. Magnesium is a nutritionally essential metal that plays a key role in a wide range of important fundamental cellular reactions (Herroeder *et al.*, 2011). Nuts, cereals, seafood, and meats are good dietary sources of magnesium. The drinking water content of magnesium increases with hardness of the water. Magnesium citrate, oxide, sulfate, hydroxide, and carbonate are widely taken as antacids or cathartics. Magnesium hydroxide, or milk of magnesia, is one of the universal antidotes for poisoning. Topically, the sulfate is also used to relieve inflammation. Parenteral administration of magnesium sulfate has been used in the treatment of seizures associated with eclampsia of pregnancy and acute nephritis.

Toxicokinetics Oral magnesium is absorbed mainly in the small intestine. The colon also absorbs some magnesium. Calcium and magnesium are competitive with respect to absorption, and excess calcium will partially inhibit magnesium absorption. Serum magnesium levels are remarkably constant. Magnesium is excreted into the digestive tract by the bile and in pancreatic and intestinal juices. Approximately 60% to 65% of the total body magnesium is in the bone, 27% in muscle, 6% to 7% in other organs, and only 1% is in extracellular fluid. Of the magnesium filtered by the glomeruli, about 95% is reabsorbed, an important factor in maintaining homeostasis.

Essentiality and Deficiency Magnesium is a cofactor of many enzymes. In the glycolytic cycle, there are seven key enzymes that require divalent magnesium. Magnesium-containing enzymes are also involved in the citric acid cycle and in β-oxidation of fatty acids. Deficiency may occur as a complication of various disease states such as malabsorption syndromes, renal dysfunction, and endocrine disorders. Magnesium deficiency in humans causes neuromuscular irritability, frank tetany, and even convulsions. Magnesium deficiency induces an inflammatory syndrome (Mazur et al., 2007), and is a risk factor for diabetes mellitus, hypertension, hyperlipidemia, and ischemic heart diseases (Ueshima, 2005). Supplementation of magnesium, by either intravenous or oral administration, is beneficial.

Toxicity In industrial exposures, no ill effects are produced with a twofold increase in serum magnesium, although concurrent increases occur in serum calcium. Inhaled freshly generated magnesium oxide can cause metal fume fever, similar to that caused by zinc oxide. In nonoccupationally exposed individuals, toxicity can occur when magnesium-containing drugs, usually antacids, are ingested chronically by persons with serious renal failure. The toxic effects may progress from nausea and vomiting to hypotension, electrocardiograph abnormalities, central nervous system effects, coma, and systolic cardiac arrest (Herroeder et al., 2011). Magnesium toxicity can sometimes be counteracted with calcium infusion.

Manganese

Manganese (Mn) was in use in prehistoric times. Paints that were pigmented with manganese dioxide can be traced back 17,000 years. The pure element was isolated in 1774 and named after the Latin *magnes*, meaning "magnet." Manganese is an essential metal required for many metabolic and cellular functions. Manganese metalloenzymes include arginase, glutamine synthetase, phosphoenolpyruvate decarboxylase, and manganese SOD (Aschner and Aschner, 2005). Manganese is also a cofactor for a number of enzymatic reactions. It exists in many valences but the divalent cation is by far the predominant species within cells. Divalent manganese may be oxidized to the more reactive and toxic trivalent form. The major source of manganese intake is from food. Vegetables, grains, fruits, nuts, and tea are rich in manganese. Daily manganese intake ranges from 2 to 9 mg (ATSDR, 2008). The adequate intake is 2.3 and 1.8 mg per day for adult men and women, respectively (IOM, 2002).

Occupational exposures to high concentrations of manganese can occur in a number of settings, including manganese dioxide mines and smelters. Significant exposure can also occur in factories making manganese steel alloys, electrical coils, batteries, glass, and welding rods, and during production of potassium permanganate ($KMnO_4$). The industrial use of manganese has expanded in recent years as a ferroalloy in the iron industry and as a component of alloys used in welding (Crossgrove and Zheng, 2004).

Environmental exposures are often associated with manganese-based organometallic pesticides, maneb and mancozeb. Manganese intoxication has also been reported after ingestion of contaminated water (Crossgrove and Zheng, 2004; ATSDR, 2008). There is current interest in the toxicology of manganese-containing fuel additive methylcyclopentadienyl manganese tricarbonyl (MMT). In addition, manganese compounds, such as mangafodipir, are increasingly used as MRI enhancers in clinical imaging techniques.

Toxicokinetics Approximately 1% to 5% of ingested manganese is normally absorbed. Interactions between manganese and iron, as well as other divalent elements, occur and impact the toxicokinetics of manganese especially following oral exposure (Roth

and Garrick, 2003). Iron and manganese can compete for the same binding protein in serum (transferrin) and the same transport systems (DMT1). Inhalation of particulate manganese may result in direct transfer to brain tissue via the olfactory system (Tjalve and Henriksson, 1999). Within the plasma, manganese is largely bound to γ-globulin and albumin, with a small fraction bound to transferrin. Manganese concentrates in mitochondria, so that tissues rich in these organelles, such as pancreas, liver, kidneys, and intestines, have the highest concentrations of manganese. It readily crosses the blood–brain barrier and accumulates in specific brain regions (Crossgrove and Zheng, 2004). Manganese is eliminated in the bile and reabsorbed in the intestine. The principal route of manganese excretion is with the feces. Biliary excretion is poorly developed in neonates and exposure during this period may result in increased delivery of manganese to the brain and other tissues (Aschner and Aschner, 2005).

Essentiality and Deficiency Manganese deficiency has been produced in many species of animals, but questions remain about whether deficiency has actually been demonstrated in humans (WHO, 1996). Deficiency in animals results in impaired growth, skeletal abnormalities, and disturbed reproductive function.

Toxicity Chronic manganese-induced neurotoxicity (manganism) is of great concern and the brain is considered the most sensitive organ to manganese. Manganism affects the release of dopamine from dopaminergic neurons, the same neurons affected by Parkinson disease. While both conditions lead to some similar neurological effects, effects on dopaminergic neurons are not the same, also causing distinct behavioral effects (Guilarte, 2010). Neurotoxicity due to inhalation of airborne manganese ranging from 0.027 to 1 mg Mn/m³ has been reported in a number of occupational settings. Overt manganism occurs in workers exposed to aerosols containing extremely high levels of manganese (>1–5 mg Mn/m³). Neurotoxicity also occurs following ingestion of manganese-contaminated water (1.8–14 ppm; Aschner et al., 2005). Manganism is associated with elevated brain levels of manganese, primarily in those areas known to contain high concentrations of nonheme iron, such as the substantia nigra, basal ganglia, caudate–putamen, globus pallidus, and subthalamic nuclei (Aschner et al., 2007). Early manifestations of manganese neurotoxicity include headache, insomnia, memory loss, muscle cramps, and emotional instability. Initial outward symptoms progress gradually and are mainly psychiatric. As exposure continues and the disease progresses, patients may develop prolonged muscle contractions (dystonia), decreased muscle movement (hypokinesia), rigidity, hand tremor, speech disturbances, and festinating "cock-walk" gait. These signs are associated with damage to dopaminergic neurons that control muscle movement (Crossgrove and Zheng, 2004; Aschner et al., 2005). Specialized T1-weighted magnetic resonance brain imaging of manganism patients indicates high levels in the basal ganglia and especially in the globus pallidus.

Inhalation of manganese-containing dust in certain occupational settings can lead to an inflammatory response in the lung. Symptoms of lung irritation and injury may include cough, bronchitis, pneumonitis, and, occasionally, pneumonia (ATSDR, 2008). Men working in plants with high concentrations of manganese dust show an incidence of respiratory disease that is 30 times greater than normal. Manganese exposure also alters cardiovascular function in animals and humans, as evidenced by abnormal electrocardiogram and the inhibition of myocardial contraction. Manganese dilates blood vessels and induces hypotension (Jiang and Zheng, 2005). When manganese is combined with bilirubin, it produces intrahepatic cholestasis by acting on the synthesis and degradation of cholesterol and the inhibition of the transport pump Mrp2 (Akoume *et al.*, 2004). Liver cirrhosis is a major contributing factor for hepatic encephalopathy, often associated with increased manganese levels in the brain (Mas, 2006).

Interactions between manganese and iron play a role in manganese toxicity. The coaccumulation of iron with manganese in the globus pallidus raises the concern that iron may be a contributing factor facilitating neuronal cell loss during manganese intoxication. Chronic exposure to manganese alters iron concentrations in blood and cerebrospinal fluid, presumably due to manganese–iron interaction at certain iron–sulfur-containing proteins, which regulate iron homeostasis. Manganese intoxication in monkeys causes elevated iron deposition in the globus pallidus and substantia nigra. The excess iron may produce oxidative stress via the Fenton reaction, leading to neuronal damage. Dysfunctional iron metabolism has also been seen in manganism patients. Serum parameters associated with iron metabolism, such as ferritin, transferrin, and total-iron-binding capacity, are significantly altered (Roth and Garrick, 2003; Crossgrove and Zheng, 2004). High levels of total iron and iron-associated oxidative stress, decreased ferritin, and abnormal mitochondrial complex-1 have been repeatedly reported in postmortem samples of substantia nigra from manganism patients.

Available data indicate that inorganic manganese is not carcinogenic in humans or rodents, and negative in the Ames test, but may cause DNA damage and chromosome aberrations in vitro in mammalian cells (Gerber *et al.*, 2002).

Molybdenum

Molybdenum (Mo) was first separated from lead and graphite in 1778. The name "molybdenum" was derived from Greek *molybdos* meaning "lead-like." As an essential element, molybdenum acts as a cofactor for four enzymes in humans: sulfite oxidase, xanthine oxidase, aldehyde oxidase, and mitochondrial amidoxime reductase (Mendel and Bittner, 2006). Molybdenum exists in five oxidation states but the predominant species are Mo^{4+} and Mo^{6+}. Molybdenum concentration in food varies considerably depending on the local environment. Molybdenum is added in trace amounts to fertilizers to stimulate plant growth. The human requirement for molybdenum is low and easily provided by a common US diet. The RDA for molybdenum is 45 µg per day (IOM and Food and Nutrition Board, 2001).

The most important mineral source of molybdenum is molybdenite (MoS_2). The industrial uses of this metal include the manufacture of high-temperature-resistant steel alloys for gas turbines and jet aircraft engines and in the production of catalysts, lubricants, and dyes. Ammonium tetrathiomolybdate is used as a molybdenum-donating copper chelator in treatment of Wilson disease (Brewer, 2003).

Toxicokinetics Water-soluble molybdenum compounds are readily absorbed when ingested. In animals, gastrointestinal absorption varies between 75% and 95%. In humans, absorption of molybdenum after oral intake varies from 28% to 77% (Vyskocil and Viau, 1999). Once absorbed, molybdenum rapidly appears in blood and most tissues. The highest molybdenum concentrations are found in kidneys, liver, and bones. Very little molybdenum appears to cross the placenta. When elevated exposure is ceased, tissue concentrations quickly return to normal levels. Molybdenum metabolism is related to copper and sulfur. Exposure to molybdenum decreases intestinal absorption of copper and sulfate, and impairs the sulfation of chemicals (Boles and Klaassen, 2000). Excretion, primarily via the urine, is rapid and 36% to 90% of a dose of molybdenum is excreted in urine in experimental animals.

In humans, the urinary excretion ranges from 17% to 80% of the total dose. Very little (<1%) of molybdenum excretion is via bile (Vyskocil and Viau, 1999). When consuming a low-molybdenum diet, the intestinal molybdenum absorption and tissue uptake are increased, while urinary excretion is decreased to reduce the molybdenum loss. With high dietary intake, urinary excretion can be dramatically increased to help eliminate excess molybdenum (Novotny and Turnlund, 2006).

Essentiality and Deficiency Molybdenum deficiency has been described in various animal species and consists of disturbances in uric acid metabolism and sulfite metabolism. Molybdenum cofactor (Moco) deficiency is a pleiotropic genetic disorder characterized by the loss of the molybdenum-dependent enzymes sulfite oxidase, xanthine oxidoreductase, and aldehyde oxidase, due to mutations in the genes involved with Moco biosynthesis. This rare human genetic metabolic disorder is characterized by severe neurodegeneration resulting in early childhood death (Schwarz, 2005).

Toxicity Molybdenum is of low toxicity. Chronic exposure to excess molybdenum in humans is characterized by high uric acid levels in serum and urine. A gout-like syndrome has been observed in inhabitants exposed to high levels of environmental molybdenum or among workers exposed to molybdenum in a copper–molybdenum plant (Vyskocil and Viau, 1999). When inhaled, both metallic molybdenum and sparingly soluble molybdenum trioxide have been reported to cause pneumoconiosis. Recent work in animal models suggests that combinations of molybdenum and copper can significantly affect male reproduction (Wirth and Mijal, 2010). Molybdenosis (teart) is a form of molybdenum poisoning that produces a disease in ruminants similar to copper deficiency (Barceloux, 1999a,b). Generally, soluble molybdenum compounds are more toxic than insoluble compounds. In many ways molybdenum toxicity resembles copper deficiency. Treatment with supplemental copper can often reverse the adverse effects of excess molybdenum (Vyskocil and Viau, 1999). Conversely, treatment of Wilson disease with molybdenum compounds is used to reduce copper burden. Molybdenum treatment may also be beneficial for angiogenesis, inflammation, and other disorders associated with excess copper (Brewer, 2003).

Selenium

Selenium (Se) was discovered in 1817, and named after the Greek word *selene* meaning moon. Although technically a nonmetal, certain forms have metal-like properties. Selenium is an essential element found in selenoproteins and deficiency is recognized in humans and animals (Högberg and Alexander, 2007). It is also toxic and high doses cause overt selenium poisoning (*selenosis*). The availability and the toxic potential of selenium compounds are related to their chemical forms and, most importantly, to solubility. Selenium occurs in nature and biological systems as selenate (Se^{6+}), selenite (Se^{4+}), selenide (Se^{2+}), and elemental selenium (Se^0) (Fairweather-Tait *et al.*, 2010).

Foods are a good source of selenium. Seafood (especially shrimp), meat, milk products, and grains provide the largest amounts in the diet. Levels of selenium in river water vary depending on environmental and geologic factors. Combustion of coal and other fossil fuels are the primary sources of airborne selenium compounds. Occupational exposure comes from selenium refining operations, metal smelting, and milling operations, incineration of rubber tires, and municipal waste. Rocks and soil, plants, and tobacco are other sources of selenium exposure (Högberg and Alexander, 2007; Fairweather-Tait *et al.*, 2010).

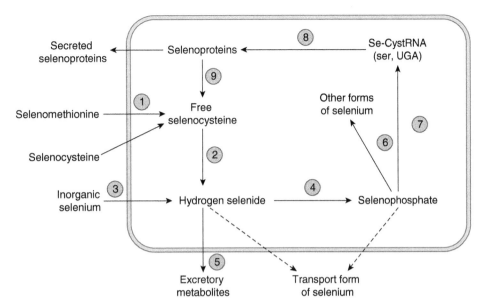

Figure 23-8. *Selenium metabolism pathways.* (1) The transsulfuration pathway; (2) selenocysteine β-lyase; (3) reduction by glutathione; (4) selenophosphate synthetase; (5) methylation; (6) replacement of sulfur in tRNA by selenium; (7) replacement of oxygen in serine to produce selenocysteine; (8) decoding of UGA in mRNA with insertion of selenocysteine into primary structure of protein; and (9) proteolytic breakdown of proteins. The origin and identity of the transport form for selenium is unknown, as indicated by the broken lines.

Toxicokinetics Orally administered selenite, selenate, and selenomethione are readily absorbed, often greater than 80%, whereas elemental selenium and selenides are virtually insoluble and poorly absorbed. Because of their insolubility, these forms may be regarded as an inert selenium sink. Monogastric animals have higher intestinal absorption than ruminants, probably because selenite is reduced to an insoluble form in rumen. Selenium accumulates in many tissues, with the highest accumulation in the liver and kidney. It is transferred through the placenta to the fetus, and it also appears in milk. Levels in milk are dependent on dietary intake. Selenium in red blood cells is associated with glutathione peroxidase and is about three times more concentrated than in plasma. Selenium is primarily eliminated in urine and feces. In cases of acute exposure to toxic concentrations of selenium, significant amounts are eliminated in expired air, causing the characteristic "garlic breath" (Högberg and Alexander, 2007; Fairweather-Tait *et al.*, 2010).

Selenium metabolism is well regulated in order to meet several metabolic needs (Fig. 23-8). Inorganic selenium and selenocysteine undergo stepwise reduction to the key intermediate hydrogen selenide, which is either transformed to selenophosphate for selenoprotein synthesis or excreted into breath or urine after being transformed into methylated metabolites of selenide (Högberg and Alexander, 2007; Fairweather-Tait *et al.*, 2010). Selenophosphate is involved in the synthesis of selenocystein tRNA according to the UGA code for the selenocysteine residue. The translation of selenoprotein mRNA requires *cis*-acting sequences in the mRNA and transacting factors dedicated to selenocysteine incorporation (Högberg and Alexander, 2007). Selenoprotein synthesis is highly dependent on selenium availability.

Essentiality and Deficiency Selenium is notable for its actions in antioxidant systems through involvement in over 20 selenoproteins (Högberg and Alexander, 2007; Fairweather-Tait *et al.*, 2010). For instance, glutathione peroxidase is the selenium-dependent enzyme that reduces peroxides using glutathione, and thereby protects membrane lipids, proteins, and nucleic acids from damage by oxidants or free radicals. The enzyme thioredoxin reductase is another selenium-dependent enzyme that has an important role in body's defense against oxidative damage. Selenoprotein P is the major plasma selenoprotein, and serves as an antioxidant in the extracellular space and transports selenium from the liver to other tissues. Selenium W is a low-molecular-weight selenoprotein and may have redox functions. Iodothreonine deiodinases are selenoproteins contributing to systemic or local thyroid hormone homeostasis. Selenium content in endocrine tissues (thyroid, adrenals, pituitary, testes, and ovary) is higher than that in many other organs. Hormones and growth factors also regulate expression of selenoproteins (Kohrle *et al.*, 2005).

The most extensively documented deficiency of selenium in humans is Keshan disease. This is an endemic cardiomyopathy first discovered in Keshan County in China where there are very low concentrations of selenium in the soil and food. Keshan disease patients show very low plasma selenium levels. This deficiency occurs most frequently in children under 15 years of age and in women of childbearing age and is characterized by various degrees of cardiomegaly and cardiac decompensation. Deficiency of selenium also occurs in domestic animals and rodents. Selenium supplementation reduces these adverse effects (Fairweather-Tait *et al.*, 2010).

Kashin–Beck disease is an osteoarthropathy found in areas where combined deficiency of selenium and iodine occurs with elevated exposure to mycotoxin and fulvic acids (Fairweather-Tait *et al.*, 2010). Selenium deficiency is a major contributing factor in this disease. Other potential effects of selenium deficiency include immune dysfunction, and susceptibility to cancer or infectious/ inflammatory diseases (Högberg and Alexander, 2007; Fairweather-Tait *et al.*, 2010). Established tolerable upper intake limits of selenium in adults are 200 to 300 μg per day (Duffield-Lillico *et al.*, 2002; Högberg and Alexander, 2007). Metabolic balance studies in adults indicate about 50 to 70 μg per day is required to maintain selenium balance and presumably to satisfy selenium requirement (Högberg and Alexander, 2007). Data indicate that daily intake less than 20 μg can cause Keshan disease.

Toxicity Acute selenium toxicity in humans is rare. Intentional or accidental ingestion of a large dose of sodium selenate or sodium selenite can be life-threatening. Symptoms of fatal selenium intoxication include nausea and vomiting, followed by pulmonary edema and rapid cardiovascular collapse (Fairweather-Tait *et al.*, 2010).

Chronic selenium toxicity (*selenosis*) can occur with environmental exposure when the intake exceeds the excretory capacity. Effects are mainly dermal and neurological including hair and fingernail loss, tooth discoloration, numbness, paralysis, and occasional hemiplegia. Selenosis occurred in several villages in China where people were exposed to very high selenium in food (Fairweather-Tait *et al.*, 2010). Intoxication from environmental selenium has also been noted in people residing in Venezuela and South Dakota. Selenium toxicity in animals was recognized in South Dakota when the livestock that had been grazed in areas with high soil selenium developed *alkali disease* and *blind staggers*. In a study of people living in this area, poor dentition, a yellowish discoloration of the skin, skin eruptions, and diseased fingernails and toenails were found (Fairweather-Tait *et al.*, 2010).

Plants vary in their ability to accumulate selenium. Grasses, grains, and most weeds do not accumulate selenium even when grown in high selenium areas, so that these plants add little to the selenium content of livestock feed. But there are several plant species that are classified as "selenium accumulators" and they may contain selenium at very high concentrations (100–10,000 mg/kg). These plants usually grow in nonagricultural areas and when consumed by livestock may cause selenium intoxication. Selenium has produced loss of fertility and congenital defects and is considered embryotoxic and teratogenic in animals (ATSDR, 2003a,b; Högberg and Alexander, 2007).

Selenium has various bioinorganic interactions, which may affect the toxicity of selenium or other metals. It forms insoluble complexes with various metals, as, for example, with arsenic. Selenium complexation can increase the biliary excretion of various metals. Selenium forms complexes with copper, and toxicity of either selenium or copper is influenced by the intake of the other elements. The methylation of selenium can influence other methylation reactions, and can alter arsenic metabolism and toxicity (Zeng *et al.*, 2005). Selenium prevents the toxic effects of cadmium and can reduce the toxic effects of methylmercury. The mechanisms for these interactions are only partially understood, but their occurrence influences the determination of safe and toxic levels of selenium for the general population (WHO, 1996).

Some epidemiological data have linked low blood selenium levels and increased cancer risk in various populations (ATSDR, 2003a,b). Selenium supplementations appear to decrease human cancer rates, especially for prostate cancer (Duffield-Lillico *et al.*, 2002; Fairweather-Tait *et al.*, 2010). Increasing selenium content of forage crops has been shown to be beneficial in reducing cancer risk. Some experimental evidence supports a role for selenium in reduction of spontaneous tumors or tumors formed by organic carcinogens in rats and mice. On the other hand, selenium sulfide is considered *reasonably anticipated to be a human carcinogen* based on multiple positive rodent studies where tumors of the lung or liver were produced after exposure via stomach tube (NTP, 2011g).

Trivalent Chromium

Essentiality Trivalent chromium (Cr^{3+}) is a naturally occurring essential trace nutrient serving an important role in glucose metabolism by enhancing insulin signaling (IOM and Food and Nutrition Board, 2001). The glucose tolerance factor is a complex of trivalent chromium, nicotinic acid, and amino acids, and physiologically potentiates the action of insulin in glucose, lipid, and protein metabolism (IOM and Food and Nutrition Board, 2001). Other effects of trivalent chromium include the beneficial roles in growth,

immune response, and stress. The tissue levels of chromium are reduced among diabetic individuals, but the effects of chromium supplementation in type 2 diabetes are still controversial (Cefalu and Hu, 2004). The adequate intake of chromium is now proposed as 35 and 25 μg/kg per day for men and women, respectively, which is lower than previous 50 to 200 μg per day. Chromium picolinate contains Cr^{3+} and is a top-selling nutritional supplement. It was thought to have adverse effects and perhaps the potential to cause cancer (Vincent, 2004), but an in-depth study of chronic chromium picolinate feeding has now shown no evidence of carcinogenesis in male or female mice or female rats only and equivocal evidence of a response (preputial gland tumors) in male rats (Stout *et al.*, 2010).

Zinc

Zinc (Zn) was named from German *zink* meaning tin. It has been used since ancient times in alloys and medicines. An essential metal, zinc deficiency results in severe health consequences. In contrast, zinc toxicity is relatively uncommon and occurs only at very high exposure levels. Zinc is ubiquitous in the environment and is present in most foodstuffs, water, and air. The major route of zinc intake is through the diet, the contents of which vary from 5.2 to 16.2 mg Zn per day (ATSDR, 2005d). RDA for zinc in children less than three years old is 3 mg per day; this value increases to 8 mg per day for children between four and 13 years old. For men >14 years old the RDA is 11 mg per day, while for women it is 8 to 9 mg per day, which increases to 12 to 13 mg per day during pregnancy (Yates *et al.*, 2001).

Occupational exposure to dusts and fumes of metallic zinc occurs in zinc mining and smelting. The zinc content of substances in contact with galvanized copper or plastic pipes may be high. Many countries regulate workplace levels of zinc oxide fume and dust at levels between 5 and 10 mg/m^3 (WHO, 1998a,b).

Toxicokinetics The absorption of zinc from the gastrointestinal tract is homeostatistically regulated. About 20% to 30% of ingested zinc is absorbed. Zinc uptake from the intestinal lumen involves passive diffusion and a carrier-mediated process through zinc-specific transmembrane transporters such as ZnT-1. Intestinal absorption of zinc can be reduced by dietary fiber, phytates, calcium, and phosphorus, while amino acids, picolinic acid, and prostaglandin E2 can enhance zinc absorption. Once absorbed, zinc is widely distributed throughout the body. The total zinc content of the human body is in the range of 1.5 to 3 g, most of which is found in muscle (60%), bone (30%), skin/hair (8%), liver (5%), and pancreas (3%). The highest concentrations of zinc are found in prostate, pancreas, liver, and kidney. In plasma, zinc concentration is about 1 mg/L, and is bound to albumin (60%–80%), which represents the metabolically active pool of zinc. The remainder is bound to α_2-macroglobulin and transferrin. Zinc is excreted in both urine and feces. The concentration of zinc in the plasma is not a sensitive indicator of zinc status and does not reflect the dose–response relationship between zinc levels in the body and effects at various target sites. Zinc ions are involved as intercellular and intracellular messengers, and the homeostasis of zinc has to be tightly controlled. The most reliable index of zinc status is the determination of zinc balance, using a U-shaped homeostatic model to analyze the relationship between intake and excretion (WHO, 1998a,b).

Zinc is an effective inducer of MT synthesis and, when MT is saturated in intestinal cells, zinc absorption is decreased. MT is also an important storage depot for cellular zinc. Liver MT concentration is influenced by hormonal factors, including adrenocorticotropic hormone and parathyroid hormone, and various stimuli that impact zinc metabolism. The high concentration of zinc in the prostate is probably related to the rich content of zinc-containing enzyme acid phosphatase.

Essentiality and Deficiency More than 300 catalytically active zinc metalloenzymes and 2000 zinc-dependent transcription factors exist (Ziegler and Filer, 1996; Cai *et al.*, 2005). Zinc participates in a wide variety of metabolic processes, supports a healthy immune system, and is essential for normal growth and development during pregnancy, childhood, and adolescence. Zinc deficiency is related to poor dietary zinc intake, dietary phytate (inositol hexakisphosphate) intake, chronic illness, or over supplementation with iron or copper (Prasad, 2004). Symptoms of zinc deficiency include growth retardation, appetite loss, alopecia, diarrhea, impaired immune function, cognitive impairments, dermatitis, delayed healing of wounds, taste abnormalities, and impaired sexual function (Prasad, 2004; Cai *et al.*, 2005; Cousins *et al.*, 2006). *Acrodermatitis enteropathica* is a rare autosomal recessive disorder involving zinc deficiency that can begin to appear after weaning from breast or formula feeding. The deficiency is due to mutations in a zinc-specific transporter that is highly expressed in the intestine. The disease is characterized by periorificial and acral dermatitis, alopecia, and diarrhea (Maverakis *et al.*, 2007). Zinc supplementation, alone or with other micronutrients, is recommended for zinc-deficient children, especially in developing countries.

Therapeutic uses of zinc include the treatment of acute diarrhea in infants with severe zinc deficiency, the treatment of common cold by its antiviral and immunomodulatory effects, therapy for Wilson disease to help reduce copper burden and to induce MT, and in the prevention of blindness in age-related macular degeneration (Prasad, 2004).

Toxicity Acute zinc toxicity from excessive ingestion is uncommon, but gastrointestinal distress and diarrhea have been reported following ingestion of beverages standing in galvanized cans. Following inhalation of zinc oxide, and to a lesser extent other zinc compounds, the most common effect is "metal fume fever" characterized by fever, chest pain, chills, cough, dyspnea, nausea, muscle soreness, fatigue, and leukocytosis. Acute inhalation of high levels of zinc chloride as in the military use of "smoke bombs" results in more pronounced damage to the mucous membrane including interstitial edema, fibrosis, pneumonitis, bronchial mucosal edema, and ulceration. Chronic intakes of zinc (150–450 mg per day) have been associated with low copper status, altered iron function, and reduced immune function. Recently, excessive use of denture adhesive cream has been recognized as a potential source for zinc toxicity. These individuals ingest 350 to 1200 mg of zinc per day (Hedera *et al.*, 2009). Following long-term exposure to lower doses of zinc (60 mg per day), symptoms generally result from a decreased dietary copper absorption, leading to early symptoms of copper deficiency, such as decreased erythrocyte number or decreased hematocrit (Yates *et al.*, 2001).

Neuronal Toxicity Zinc has dual effects in the brain. As an essential cofactor for numerous enzymes and proteins, zinc deficiency may alter activity of the antioxidant enzyme Cu–Zn SOD, resulting in excess free radicals that are damaging to cell membranes (Valko *et al.*, 2005). A genetic abnormality of Cu–Zn SOD may be the basis of a familial form of amyotrophic lateral sclerosis (Selverstone Valentine *et al.*, 2005). Zinc can also act as a neurotransmitter for normal brain functions (Frederickson *et al.*, 2005; Cousins *et al.*, 2006). It modulates the solubility of β-amyloid in the brain and protects against β-amyloid toxicity, but excess zinc may trigger neuronal death that is independent or synergistic with the toxic effect of β-amyloid (Valko *et al.*, 2005). In contrast, excess zinc released by oxidants can act as a potent neurotoxin (Frederickson *et al.*, 2005). Synaptically released zinc might contribute to excitotoxic brain injury, and the release of excess, toxic free zinc into the brain that occurs during excitotoxic brain injury could be a factor that sets the stage for the later development of Alzheimer disease.

Pancreatic Toxicity Because large amounts of zinc accumulate in secretory granules of pancreatic islet β-cells, zinc released under certain conditions can affect the function or survival of islet cells and cause β-cell death. Excess dietary zinc is associated with damage to exocrine pancreas. A single, high-dose injection of zinc increases plasma α-amylase activity and can produce fibrosis and necrosis of pancreatic exocrine cells, but does not affect the islets of Langerhans cells (Cai *et al.*, 2005).

Zinc and Carcinogenicity Epidemiological studies of workers in electrolytic zinc and copper refining industries have not found an increased incidence of cancer associated with occupational zinc inhalation. Oral zinc supplementation does not appear to have a significant effect on cancer incidence (ATSDR, 2005d). In contrast, zinc deficiency may be associated with increased risk of cancer in humans (Prasad and Kucuk, 2002). Zinc supplementation could decrease oxidative stress and improve immune function, which may be a possible mechanism for its cancer preventive activity (Prasad and Kucuk, 2002). In experimental animals, zinc prevents cadmium-induced testicular cancer, but facilitates cadmium-induced prostate tumors (Waalkes, 2003).

METALS RELATED TO MEDICAL THERAPY

Aluminum

Aluminum (Al) is the third most abundant element in the earth's crust after oxygen and silicon. Elemental aluminum was first identified in 1827. Due to its high reactivity, aluminum is not found in the free state in nature. Chemical compounds of aluminum occur typically in the trivalent state (Al^{3+}). As a hard trivalent ion, aluminum binds strongly to oxygen donor ligands such as citrate and phosphate. The chemistry of aluminum compounds is complicated by a tendency to hydrolyze and form polynuclear species, many of which are sparingly soluble (Harris *et al.*, 1996).

Aluminum has many uses, mainly in the form of alloys, and finds use in packing, construction, transportation, electrical applications, and beverage cans. Aluminum compounds are also used as food additives. Human exposure to aluminum comes primarily from food and secondarily from drinking water. The amount of aluminum in the food supply is small compared with pharmaceutical use of aluminum in antacids and buffered analgesics (Soni *et al.*, 2001). Occupational exposures to aluminum occur during mining and processing, as well as in aluminum welding. The levels of exposure can vary greatly according to the type of industry and hygiene conditions. Inhalation of aluminum-containing dust particles is of health concern (Sjögren *et al.*, 2007).

Aluminum exists predominantly in forms that are innocuous to humans and most species. However, acidic conditions, such as acid rain or dry acid deposition, can dramatically increase the amount of aluminum in ecosystems, resulting in well-described destructive effects on plants, fish, and other wildlife. However, aluminum is not bioaccumulated to any significant extent except in the tea plant (Sparling and Lowe, 1996).

Toxicokinetics Aluminum is poorly absorbed following either oral or inhalation exposure and is essentially not absorbed dermally. Inhalation of particulate aluminum may result in direct transfer to brain tissue via the olfactory system (Tjalve and Henriksson, 1999).

Less than 1% of aluminum in the diet is absorbed. Absorption from the gut depends largely on pH and the presence of complexing ligands, particularly carboxylic acids, through which aluminum becomes absorbable. For example, intestinal absorption is enhanced in the presence of citrate. Biological speciation is also of major importance in distribution and excretion of aluminum in mammals (Sjögren *et al.*, 2007). In plasma, 80% to 90% of aluminum binds to transferrin, an iron transport protein with receptors in many tissues. The transferrin pathway is also considered a mechanism for aluminum transport across the blood–brain barrier (Yokel, 2006). Lung, liver, and bone have the highest concentrations of aluminum (Sjögren *et al.*, 2007). Aluminum is removed from blood by the kidneys and excreted in urine. In patients with impaired renal function, tissue aluminum concentrations can increase and are associated with encephalopathy and osteomalacia.

Aluminum compounds can alter absorption of other elements in the gastrointestinal tract. For instance, aluminum inhibits fluoride absorption and may decrease the absorption of calcium and iron compounds and salicylic acid, which, in turn, may affect the absorption of aluminum (Exley *et al.*, 1996). The binding of phosphorus by aluminum in the intestinal tract can lead to phosphate depletion and, potentially, osteomalacia. Aluminum interacts with calcium in bone and kidney, resulting in aluminum osteodystrophy (Goyer, 1997). Aluminum may also alter gastrointestinal tract motility by inhibition of acetylcholine-induced contractions, which is probably why aluminum-containing antacids often cause constipation.

Toxicity Acute aluminum toxicity is rare. Most cases of aluminum toxicity in humans are observed in patients with chronic renal failure, or in persons exposed to aluminum in the workplace, with the lung, bone, and central nervous system as major target organs. Aluminum affects similar target organs in animals and can produce developmental effects.

Lung and Bone Toxicity Occupational exposure to aluminum dust can produce lung fibrosis in humans, but this effect is probably due to lung overload caused by excessive deposition of dust (Sjögren *et al.*, 2007). Osteomalacia has been associated with excessive intake of aluminum-containing antacids in otherwise healthy individuals. This is assumed to be due to interference with intestinal phosphate absorption. Osteomalacia also can occur in uremic patients exposed to aluminum in the dialysis fluid. In these patients, osteomalacia may be a direct effect of aluminum on bone mineralization as bone levels are high (Soni *et al.*, 2001).

Neurotoxicity Aluminum is neurotoxic to experimental animals, with wide species and age variations. In susceptible animals, such as rabbits and cats, aluminum toxicity is characterized by progressive neurological impairment resulting in death associated with status epilepticus (WHO, 1997). The most prominent early pathological change is the accumulation of neurofibrillary tangles (NFTs) in large neurons, proximal axons, and dentrites of neurons of many brain regions. This is associated with loss of synapses and atrophy of the dendritic tree. Not all species show this reaction to aluminum. For instance, rats fail to develop NFTs or encephalopathy and monkeys develop NFTs only after more than a year of aluminum infusion. Impairment of cognitive and motor function and behavioral abnormalities are often observed. Whereas studies in animals have provided some insights into the mechanisms of the neurotoxicity of aluminum in experimental models, the relationship to any human disease is still uncertain.

Dialysis Dementia This is a progressive, neurological syndrome reported in patients on long-term intermittent hemodialysis for chronic renal failure (Sjögren *et al.*, 2007). The first symptom in these patients is a speech disorder followed by dementia, convulsions, and myoclonus. The disorder, which typically arises after three to seven years of dialysis treatment, may be due to aluminum intoxication. The aluminum content of brain, muscle, and bone increases in these patients. Sources of the excess aluminum may be from oral aluminum hydroxide commonly given to these patients or from aluminum in dialysis fluid derived from the tap water used to prepare the dialysate fluid. The high serum aluminum concentrations may be related to increased parathyroid hormone levels that are due to low blood calcium and osteodystrophy common in patients with chronic renal disease. The syndrome may be prevented by avoiding the use of aluminum-containing oral phosphate binders and by monitoring of aluminum in the dialysate.

The Chamorro people of the Marina Islands in the Western Pacific Ocean, particularly Guam and Rota, have an unusually high incidence of neurodegeneration of the Alzheimer type. Garruto *et al.* (1984, 1985) noted that the volcanic soils of the regions of Guam with a high incidence of amyotrophic lateral sclerosis and parkinsonism–dementia syndromes (ALS-PD) contained high concentrations of aluminum and manganese and were low in calcium and magnesium. They postulated that a low intake of calcium and magnesium induced secondary hyperparathyroidism, resulting in an increase in the deposition of calcium, aluminum, and other toxic metals, and eventually in neuronal injury and death. How and why aluminum enters the brain of these people is unclear. The incidence of these disorders dramatically decreased or disappeared during the past 60 years, possibly as the result of radical socioeconomic, ethnographic, and ecological changes brought about by the rapid westernization of Guam, rather than genetic factors (Garruto *et al.*, 1985; Plato *et al.*, 2003).

Alzheimer Disease A possible relationship between aluminum and Alzheimer disease has been a matter of speculation for decades (Sjögren *et al.*, 2007; Bondy, 2010). The basis for this relationship is the finding of increased aluminum levels in Alzheimer brains and neurofibrillary lesions in experimental animals, and the fact that aluminum is associated with various components of the pathological lesions in Alzheimer brain tissue. However, elevated aluminum levels in Alzheimer brains may be a consequence and not a cause of the disease. The reduced effectiveness of the blood–brain barrier in Alzheimer might allow more aluminum into the brain. Also, recent studies have raised the possibility that the staining methods in earlier studies may have led to aluminum contamination (Makjanic *et al.*, 1998; Bondy, 2010). Furthermore, the NFTs seen in aluminum encephalopathy differ structurally and chemically from those in Alzheimer (WHO, 1997). Epidemiological studies examining the role of aluminum exposure in Alzheimer disease arrive at conflicting conclusions. An examination of 20 epidemiological studies concluded that there is not enough evidence to support a primary causative role of aluminum in Alzheimer disease, and aluminum does not induce Alzheimer pathology in vivo in any species, including humans (WHO, 1997). However, there is increasing evidence suggesting a link between aluminum in the brain and other neurodegenerative diseases (Kawahara, 2005; Bondy, 2010).

Treatment Chelation therapy for aluminum, mostly in dialyzed and/or uremic patients, resembles that for iron overload, with deferoxamine and deferiprone (Blanusa *et al.*, 2005).

Bismuth

Bismuth (Bi) is a metal with a stable valence of 3+. The name *bisemutum* is from German *Wismuth*, perhaps from the term *weiße Masse*, for "white mass." It was confused in early times with tin and lead due to its resemblance to those elements. Bismuth was shown to be distinct from lead in 1753. The solubility of most bismuth salts is low but can be affected by pH and the presence of sulfhydryl or hydroxy-containing ligands. The significance of environmental and occupational bismuth exposure is unclear. Human exposure to bismuth generally is due to medicinal use.

Trivalent insoluble bismuth salts such as bismuth subnitrate, subcarbonate, and subgallate are used for various gastrointestinal disorders including diarrhea, flatulence, constipation, cramps, and dyspepsia. Colloidal bismuth subcitrate, bismuth subsalicylate, and ranitidine bismuth citrate are widely used to treat peptic ulcer and *Helicobacter pylori*–associated gastritis. Outdated medicinal applications include the use of bismuth salts for treatment of syphilis, malaria, warts, stomatitis, and infections of the upper respiratory tract (Slikkerveer and de Wolff, 1996). A potential application includes the use of bismuth subnitrate to prevent cisplatin nephrotoxicity, probably due to a specific induction of renal MT (Kondo *et al.*, 2004), although this does not appear to have been applied in practice. The use of α-particle-emitting bismuth compounds as radiotherapeutic agents and as antitumor agents shows some promise (Wild *et al.*, 2011).

Toxicokinetics Most bismuth compounds are insoluble and poorly absorbed from the gastrointestinal tract or when applied to the skin. The three widely used compounds, colloidal tripotassium dicitrato bismuthate, bismuth subsalicylate, and ranitidine bismuth citrate, are all poorly absorbed (<1%) (Tillman *et al.*, 1996). The highest concentrations of bismuth are found in kidneys, and to a lesser extent in the brain, liver, and bone (Slikkerveer and de Wolff, 1996; Larsen *et al.*, 2005). Passage of bismuth into the amniotic fluid and fetus has been demonstrated. Bismuth is cleared from the body through urine and feces (Gregus and Klaassen, 1986). Traces of bismuth can be found in milk and saliva. The elimination half-life is reported to be about 21 days, depending on bismuth compounds.

Toxicity Bismuth-containing medications are consumed worldwide and the risk of bismuth-related toxicity in the general population is relatively low. The main target organs for bismuth toxicity are kidney, brain, and bone (Slikkerveer and de Wolff, 1996; Tillman *et al.*, 1996; Larsen *et al.*, 2005). Acute renal injury is related to very high doses of bismuth, or to oral intake of organic bismuth compounds such as bismuth sodium triglycocollamate or thioglycollate, particularly in children. The tubular epithelium is the primary site of toxicity, where bismuth produces degeneration of renal tubular cells and nuclear inclusion bodies composed of bismuth–protein complex analogous to those found with lead exposure (Fowler and Goyer, 1975). A large single oral dose of colloidal bismuth subcitrate damages the proximal tubes, but the damage is reversible in both humans and animals (Leussink *et al.*, 2001).

An episode of bismuth-associated encephalopathy in France in the 1970s revealed a potential neurotoxic effect of bismuth, although it cannot be exclusively attributed to bismuth alone (Slikkerveer and de Wolff, 1996). High amounts of bismuth were found in the reticular and hypothalamic nuclei, in the oculomotor and hypoglossal nuclei, and in Purkinje cells after an eight-month exposure to bismuth. Axonal transport seems to influence the distribution of bismuth. Ultrastructurally, accumulation of bismuth was seen in lysosomes (Larsen *et al.*, 2005).

Treatment The most effective treatment of bismuth toxicity is to discontinue bismuth intake. Chelation therapy using dimercaprol (BAL), DMSA, and DMPS reduces the bismuth concentration in most organs (especially kidney and liver) and increase elimination of bismuth in urine. BAL was the only chelator effective in

lowering brain bismuth concentrations (Slikkerveer and de Wolff, 1996).

Gallium

Gallium (Ga) has a very low melting point with the main valence state of 3+ (gallic), although the 2+ (gallous) form can also form stable gallium compounds. Gallium, stemming from *Gallia* meaning Gaul or France, was predicted to exist prior to being discovered in 1875 by its characteristic spectrum. Gallium is of interest because of the use of radiogallium as a diagnostic tool for the localization of bone lesions. Nonradioactive gallium nitrate has been used as an antitumor agent and in the treatment of hypercalcemia. Gallium is obtained as a by-product of copper, zinc, lead, and aluminum refining and is used in high-temperature thermometers, as a substitute for mercury in arc lamps, as a component of metal alloys, and as a seal for vacuum equipment. Gallium arsenide is a widely used semiconductor material. Gallium is the only metal other than mercury that is liquid at or near room temperature.

Toxicokinetics Gallium salts are sparingly absorbed from the gastrointestinal tract, but accumulation in tissues can be observed after repeated administrations. The oral bioavailability is improved with gallium complexes such as gallium maltolate. Gallium accumulates mainly in bone, inflammatory lesions, and tumors, as well as in the liver, spleen, and kidney. It binds to plasma transferrin and enters cells by iron transport mechanisms. Urine is the major route of gallium excretion with lesser amounts in the feces (Fowler and Sexton, 2007; Chitambar, 2010).

Toxicity The trivalent gallium cation biologically resembles ferric iron. It affects cellular acquisition of iron by binding to transferrin and interacts with the iron-dependent enzyme ribonucleotide reductase, resulting in decreased dNTP pools and inhibition of DNA synthesis (Chitambar, 2010). The abundance of transferrin receptors and ribonucleotide reductase renders tumor cells susceptible to the cytotoxicity of gallium. Use of bolus intravenous injection of gallium nitrate in the treatment of lymphoma and bladder cancer is limited by potential nephrotoxicity, which can be reduced by slow continuous infusion over several days (Chitambar, 2010). Gallium nitrate is an effective treatment for cancer-related hypercalcemia and diseases associated with accelerated bone loss including myeloma, bone metastasis, Paget disease, and osteoporosis. It accumulates in metabolically active regions of bone and favorably alters the mineral properties to enhance hydroxyapatite crystallization and reduce mineral solubility. Gallium inhibits osteoclastic bone resorption without poisoning the osteoclast cells, yielding a skeletal system with increased calcium and phosphate content and improved strength (Chitambar, 2010). Adverse effects may include nausea, vomiting, and anemia. Less frequent are gallium-induced neurological, pulmonary, and dermatologic effects.

Acute and chronic toxicity to lung (including alveolar and bronchioalveolar tumors), testes, and kidney is associated with exposures of gallium arsenide in animals, although the role of the individual metals in this response is unclear (Tanaka, 2004; Chitambar, 2010). There is little information regarding adverse effects of gallium compounds following occupational exposure, but renal toxicity was the primary side effect of gallium nitrate treatment in human clinical trials (Fowler and Sexton, 2007).

Gold

Gold (Au) was well known and highly valued since prehistoric times. It is widely distributed but usually in small quantities. The metal has a number of industrial uses because of its electrical and thermal conductivity. Monovalent organogold salts (eg, auranofin, aurothioglucose, gold sodium thiomalate) are used for the treatment of rheumatoid arthritis. Monovalent and trivalent coordinated gold complexes have antitumor potential (Kostova, 2006). Colloidal gold or gold nanoparticles are used to label subcellular structures for electron microscopy, carriers for drugs, and photothermal agents (Khlebtsov and Dykman, 2011).

Toxicokinetics Gold salts are poorly absorbed from the gastrointestinal tract. The more water-soluble, therapeutic gold compounds are absorbed after intramuscular injection, and peak concentration in blood is reached in two to six hours. Gold is initially bound to serum albumin, and then distributes to various tissues. With continued therapy, the concentration of gold in synovium of affected joints is 10 times that of muscle, bone, or fat. Gold deposits are also found in macrophages, kidney, liver, testes, and skin. About 60% to 90% of gold is excreted via the kidney while 10% to 40% occurs via biliary excretion into feces. Chelators such as dimercaprol may increase the excretion of gold. Gold has a long biological half-life, and elevated tissue and blood levels can be demonstrated for months after cessation of treatment.

Toxicity Contact dermatitis is the most frequently reported toxic reaction to gold and is sometimes accompanied by stomatitis, probably involving an allergic mechanism. Gold-induced allergic responses include delayed hypersensitivity, formation of intracutaneous nodules and immunogenic granuloma, as well as the occurrence of eczema (Hostynek, 1997).

The use of gold in the form of organic salts to treat rheumatoid arthritis may be complicated by the development of proteinuria and the nephrotic syndrome, which morphologically consists of immune complex glomerulonephritis, with granular deposits along the glomerular basement membrane and in the mesangium (Bigazzi, 1999; Hostynek, 1997). The pathogenesis of the immune complex disease is not certain, but gold may behave as a hapten and generate the production of antibody complexes for the glomerular deposits (Viol *et al.*, 1977).

The health risks associated with gold mining, especially miners who used elemental mercury to amalgamate and extract gold, have been reviewed (Eisler, 2003). Gold miners have increased frequency of pulmonary diseases, including tumors, and increased prevalence of infectious diseases. Mercury intoxication associated with gold mining activities is well documented (Eisler, 2003).

There are limited data on the human toxicity associated with exposure to gold nanoparticles. In vivo and in vitro studies suggest that toxicity is related to the shape of the nanomaterial (Tarantola *et al.*, 2011). Intravenous injection of gold nanoparticles is associated with inflammatory responses (Khlebtsov and Dykman, 2011).

Lithium

Lithium (Li) is one of the lightest metallic elements. It was discovered in 1817, and the name was derived from the Greek *lithos* for stone. On the periodic table of the elements, lithium shares its group with sodium and potassium, and is widely distributed in nature. Lithium is used in batteries, alloys, catalysts, photographic materials, and the aerospace industry. Lithium hydride produces hydrogen on contact with water and is used in manufacturing electronic tubes, in ceramics, and in chemical analysis. Groundwater contamination from man-made waste disposal could be a risk factor for the aquatic environment (Kszos and Stewart, 2003). Lithium carbonate and lithium citrate are widely used for mania and bipolar disorders. In this regard, lithium is active possibly through its effects on signal transduction, such as phosphoinositide hydrolysis,

glycogen synthase kinase-3, and neurotropic cascades (Lenox and Hahn, 2000; Quiroz *et al.*, 2004). Topical applications of lithium succinate are still used in the treatment of seborrheic dermatitis (Sparsa and Bonnetblanc, 2004).

Toxicokinetics Lithium is readily absorbed from the gastrointestinal tract, with peak therapeutic levels at 30 minutes to three hours postingestion. It is not bound to plasma proteins, but associates with red blood cells. Lithium is distributed to total body water with higher levels in kidney, thyroid, and bone, as compared with other tissues. Excretion is chiefly through the kidneys with 80% of the filtered lithium reabsorbed. The usual elimination half-life is 12 to 27 hours, but it may rise to nearly 60 hours if renal function is compromised. Lithium can substitute for sodium or potassium on several membrane-bound transport proteins. It enters cells via the amiloride-sensitive sodium channel or the Na/H^+ exchanger. The greater part of lithium is retained in the cells, perhaps at the expense of potassium. In general, it may be competing with sodium at certain sites, such as in renal tubular reabsorption (Timmer and Sands, 1999).

Toxicity From the industrial point of view, except for lithium hydride, neither are the other salts considered hazardous nor is the metal very toxic itself. Lithium hydride is intensely corrosive and may produce burns on the skin because of the formation of hydroxides (Cox and Singer, 1981). Intoxications related to lithium exposure are mainly related to its medicinal uses (Timmer and Sands, 1999), as the therapeutic index of lithium is very narrow. In this regard, 0.7 to 1.2 mmol/L is considered an adequate therapeutic blood level, while blood levels only threefold higher commonly result in severe symptoms such as seizures and coma. The toxic responses to lithium include neuromuscular changes (tremor, muscle hyperirritability, and ataxia), central nervous system disorders (blackout spells, epileptic seizures, slurred speech, coma, psychosomatic retardation, and increased thirst), cardiovascular disturbances (cardiac arrhythmia, hypertension, and circulatory collapse), gastrointestinal symptoms (anorexia, nausea, and vomiting), and renal damage (albuminuria and glycosuria). The renal lesions are believed to be due to temporary hypokalemic nephritis. Long-term sequelae from acute lithium poisoning include cognitive losses such as impaired memory, attention and executive functions, and visuospatial deficits (Brumm *et al.*, 1998).

Chronic lithium nephrotoxicity and interstitial nephritis may occur with long-term exposure even when lithium levels remain within the therapeutic range. Lithium nephrotoxicity primarily targets distal and collecting tubes, with a higher incidence of proteinuria and associated glomerular pathology (Markowitz *et al.*, 2000). Chronic lithium-induced neurotoxicity, nephritis, and thyroid dysfunction may occur, especially in susceptible patients with identifiable clinical risk factors such as nephrogenic diabetes insipidus, older age, abnormal thyroid function, and impaired renal function (Oakley *et al.*, 2001).

Acute lithium overdose produces neurological sequelae and cardiac toxicity, which can be fatal (Offerman *et al.*, 2010). The toxicity may be treated by the administration of diuretics (amiloride) and lowering of blood levels via hemodialysis. Treatment with diuretics must be accompanied by replacement of water and electrolytes (Timmer and Sands, 1999).

Platinum

Platinum (Pt) is a malleable, ductile, silvery-white noble metal. Naturally occurring platinum and platinum-rich alloys have been known for a long time. The first European reference to platinum appeared in 1557 and the element was isolated in 1741. In platinum compounds, the maximum oxidation state is 6+, while the 2+ and 4+ valences are most stable. Platinum is found in nature either in the metallic form or in a number of mineral forms in various ores. Environmental platinum levels are very low. Platinum compounds are used as automobile catalysts, in jewelry, in electronics, and in dental alloys. Platinum coordination complexes are very important antitumor agents. Occupational exposure can be higher than the exposure limit of 2 $\mu g/m^3$ in some settings (WHO, 1991).

Toxicokinetics Following a single inhalation exposure, most of the inhaled platinum is rapidly cleared from the lungs by mucociliary action, swallowed, and excreted in the feces, with half-life of about 24 hours. A small portion is detected in the urine, indicating very little platinum is absorbed. After intravenous administration of clinical doses, the drug has an initial elimination half-life in plasma of 25 to 50 minutes. More than 90% of the platinum in the blood is covalently bound to plasma proteins. After administration of the main metallochemotherapeutic form, *cis*-dichlorodiammine platinum(II) (cisplatin), high concentrations are found in the kidney, liver, intestine, spleen, and testes, but there is poor penetration into the brain. Only a small portion of the drug is excreted by the kidney during the first six hours. By 24 hours up to 25% is excreted, while by five days up to 43% of the administered dose is recovered in the urine (WHO, 1991; Hardman *et al.*, 2001).

Toxicity Platinum can produce profound hypersensitivity reactions in susceptible individuals (WHO, 1991). The signs of hypersensitivity include urticaria, contact dermatitis of skin, and respiratory distress, ranging from irritation to an asthmatic syndrome, following exposure to platinum dust. The skin and respiratory changes are termed *platinosis*. They are mainly confined to persons with a history of industrial exposure to soluble compounds such as sodium chloroplatinate, although cases resulting from the wearing of platinum jewelry have been reported (WHO, 1991). The complex salts of platinum may act as powerful allergens, particularly ammonium hexachloroplatinate and hexachloroplatinic acid. Platinum salt sensitization may persist for years after cessation of exposure (Brooks *et al.*, 1990). Halogeno complex salts of platinum are potent allergens provoking Type I allergic symptoms in platinum refining workers. Skin prick tests can detect sensitization at an early stage and are the mainstay of surveillance programs (WHO, 1991; Linnett, 2005).

Antitumor Effects of Platinum Complexes The platinum-coordinated complexes are important antitumor agents, including cisplatin, carboplatin, and oxaliplatin (Hardman *et al.*, 2001; Wang, 2010). They are routinely administered, often in combination with other anticancer drugs, in the treatment of a wide spectrum of malignancies, especially epithelial cancers. Platinum complexes are neutral and have a pair of *cis*-leaving groups. Low intracellular chloride concentrations favor hydrolysis of chloride-leaving groups in cisplatin to yield a positively charged molecule, which then reacts with DNA and proteins, forming both intrastrand and interstrand DNA cross-links with guanine and/or adenine. In tumor cells, the replication of DNA is impaired due to cisplatin-induced DNA cross-links, while in normal cells, guanine is repaired before replication. The formation of DNA adducts with platinum is also responsible for cytotoxicity (WHO, 1991; Hardman *et al.*, 2001; Wang, 2010).

Carcinogenic Effects of Platinum Complexes Although cisplatin has antitumor activity in humans, it is considered *reasonably anticipated to be a human carcinogen* (NTP, 2011h) or a *probable human carcinogen* (IARC, 1987). Cisplatin is clearly carcinogenic

in rodents (NTP, 2011h). In fact, in mice deficient in MT, cisplatin can induce liver carcinoma at clinically relevant doses (Waalkes *et al.*, 2006). There are several other positive rodent studies with cancer end points after treatment with the metallochemotherapeutic (NTP, 2011h). Cisplatin is a strong mutagen in bacterial systems and causes chromosomal aberrations in cultured hamster cells and a dose-dependent increase in sister chromatid exchanges.

Toxicities of Platinum Antitumor Complexes Cisplatin is a nephrotoxin, which often compromises its usefulness as a therapeutic agent. Platinum compounds with antitumor activity produce proximal and distal tubular cell injury, mainly in the corticomedullary region, where the concentration of platinum is highest. Associated with cisplatin nephrotoxicity is the risk for electrolyte abnormalities. In comparison, carboplatinum and oxaliplatinum, given at standard chemotherapeutic doses, are not considered as highly nephrotoxic (Markman, 2003).

Neurotoxicity is another dose-limiting factor, particular when platinum complexes are combined with other potential neurotoxic drugs such as paclitaxel. Hearing loss can occur and can be unilateral or bilateral but tends to be more frequent and severe with repeated doses. Marked nausea and vomiting occur in most patients receiving the platinum complexes but can be controlled with ondansetron or high dose of corticosteroids. Bone marrow suppression, manifested as anemia, neutropenia, and thrombocytopenia, is relatively common during treatment with platinum complexes, especially when given in combination with fluorouracil. Carboplatin treatment has a higher myelotoxic risk than cisplatin and oxaliplatin (Hardman *et al.*, 2001; Markman, 2003).

MINOR TOXIC METALS

Antimony

Antimony (Sb) is a metalloid that belongs to the same periodic group as arsenic. It was recognized in antiquity (3000 BC or earlier) in various compounds for its fine casting qualities, and the description of its isolation appeared in 1540. The name antimony may have come from the Greek words "anti" and "monos," which means "opposed to solitude" as it was thought never to exist in its pure form. Most antimony compounds are of trivalent and pentavalent states. Antimony has many uses including in alloys, and in production of fireproofing chemicals, ceramics, glassware, and pigments. It is used medically in the treatment of the parasitic diseases, schistosomiasis and leishmaniasis (De Boeck *et al.*, 2003; Sundar and Chakravarty, 2010). Occupational antimony exposure comes from industrial emissions. Food is the major route for environmental exposure, but the exposure levels are generally low. The average daily intake from food and water is estimated at about 5 μg (ATSDR, 1992; Sundar and Chakravarty, 2010).

The disposition of antimony in the body resembles that of arsenic. Most antimony compounds are absorbed from the lung and the gastrointestinal tract. The major sites of antimony accumulation are the liver, kidney, lung, spleen, and blood. The accumulation of antimony in blood may be due to high affinity of trivalent antimony for erythrocytes (ATSDR, 1992). In humans and rodents, pentavalent antimony is only sparingly reduced to the trivalent form, and evidence of antimony methylation in mammals is low (Ogra, 2009). The pentavalent form is predominantly excreted in urine, whereas trivalent antimony is conjugated to GSH and is excreted via the bile and found mainly in feces.

Toxicity Most information about antimony toxicity has been obtained from industrial experiences (Sundar and Chakravarty, 2010).

Occupational exposures are usually by inhalation of dust containing antimony compounds, such as the pentachloride, trichloride, trioxide, and trisulfide (Sundar and Chakravarty, 2010). Acute toxicity from the pentachloride and trichloride exposures includes rhinitis and, in severe exposures, even acute pulmonary edema. Chronic exposure by inhalation of other antimony compounds results in rhinitis, pharyngitis, trachitis, and, over the longer term, bronchitis and eventually pneumoconiosis with obstructive lung disease and emphysema. Transient skin eruptions (antimony spots) may occur in workers with chronic exposure (Sundar and Chakravarty, 2010). Trivalent forms of antimony appear more toxic and may produce cardiotoxicity involving arrhythmias and myocardial damage, although the evidence of heart disease from industrial exposure to antimony is not strong (Sundar and Chakravarty, 2010). In rodent subchronic/chronic studies with antimony potassium tartrate, relatively low toxicity was reported (Lynch et al., 1999).

The chemicotoxicological similarity between arsenic and antimony has prompted research on mutagenic and carcinogenic potential of antimony compounds. Antimony trioxide is considered an animal carcinogen (IARC, 1987; Sundar and Chakravarty, 2010), but human data on antimony are difficult to evaluate with the frequent coexposure to arsenic (Leonard and Gerber, 1996; De Boeck et al., 2003). Antimony compounds are generally negative in nonmammalian genotoxicity tests, whereas mammalian tests usually give positive results for trivalent but negative results for pentavalent antimony compounds. The in vivo potential of antimony to induce chromosome aberrations appears inconsistent (Leonard and Gerber, 1996; De Boeck et al., 2003).

The metal hydride of antimony, stibine (SbH_3), is a highly toxic gas that can be generated when antimony is exposed to reducing acids or when certain batteries are overcharged. High-purity stibine is also used in the production of semiconductors and, like arsine (AsH_3), causes hemolysis.

Barium

Barium (Ba) is an alkaline earth metal found in the environment in the 2+ oxidation state. It was first identified in 1774, and named from the Greek word barys meaning "heavy." Barium and barium compounds (barium carbonate, sulfate, chloride, and hydroxide) are used in ceramics, electronics, insecticides, rodenticides, pigments, and as x-ray contrast media. Barium is relatively abundant in nature and is found in plants and animal tissue. Some foods, such as Brazil nuts, pecans, and seafood, may contain high amounts of barium. Barium from natural sources may exceed Federal government standards in some freshwater, although the amount found in food and water usually is not high enough to be a health concern. Occupational exposure to barium primarily occurs in workers who inhale barium sulfate from working with the ore, barite, and barium carbonate dust during mining and manufacturing (ATSDR, 2007).

Insoluble barium sulfate is not absorbed from the gastrointestinal tract, and is nontoxic to humans. Ingested soluble compounds are absorbed, but vary greatly and are affected by many factors such as age, duration, dose, and amounts of other elements in the intestine. Aerosols of soluble barium compounds are well absorbed in the lung. Bone and teeth are the major sites of barium deposition, containing up to 90% of the body burden. The remainder of barium in the body is found in soft tissues, such as the lung, aorta, brain, heart, spleen, liver, and pancreas (Dallas and Williams, 2001). Once filtered by the glomeruli, barium is reabsorbed by the renal tubules with only small amounts appearing in the urine. The major route of barium excretion is the feces. The elimination half-life is about one to two weeks.

Toxicity Occupational poisoning by barium is uncommon, but a benign pneumoconiosis (baritosis) may result from inhalation of barium sulfate (barite) dust or barium carbonate. This is not incapacitating and is usually reversible with cessation of exposure. Intentional or accidental poisoning from ingestion of an acute toxic dose (over 200 mg) of soluble barium salt results in intractable vomiting, severe diarrhea, and gastrointestinal hemorrhage. Cardiac arrest is often the cause of death (ATSDR, 2007). Profound hypokalemia and muscle weakness progressing to flaccid paralysis are the hallmarks of barium poisoning (Johnson and VanTassell, 1991). The mechanism of toxicity probably involves the blocking of calcium-activated potassium channels responsible for cellular efflux of potassium. As a result, intracellular potassium rises and extracellular levels fall leading to hypokalemia. The progressive muscle weakness seen in barium intoxication in humans could be due to barium-induced hypokalemia rather than a direct effect on muscles, which is not observed in experimental animals. Treatment with intravenous potassium appears beneficial.

Following long-term exposure to barium, nephrotoxicity has been observed in rats and mice. Animal studies designed to assess cardiovascular function have not found significant alterations. Barium compounds are not considered carcinogenic in rodents and there is no evidence in humans (Dallas and Williams, 2001; ATSDR, 2007).

Cesium

Cesium (Cs) is a soft silvery-gold alkali metal discovered in 1860, and named from the Latin word caesius meaning "sky blue." Similar to mercury and gallium, metallic cesium exists in the liquid state at slightly above room temperature, and is used in vacuum tubes and in atomic clocks. Cesium compounds only have the 1+ oxidation state, and are used as catalysts in inorganic chemistry, in pharmaceuticals, as well as in scintillation counters. [137]Cesium is a by-product of nuclear reactions and is used in radiation therapy (ATSDR, 2004c).

The Chernobyl nuclear plant accident in 1986 resulted in a large release of cesium into the atmosphere, which then spread as radioactive fallout into the soil, rivers, and lakes, causing serious ecological problems in Northern Europe. The transfer of radiocesium into the food chain and into sheep and reindeer may contribute to human cesium exposure (Howard and Howard, 1997). These ecological issues remain in some areas even decades after the original accident (Bell and Shaw, 2005).

Most cesium compounds are water soluble and are well absorbed through inhalation, ingestion, or skin contact. Once in the blood, cesium is rapidly distributed throughout the body, with higher concentrations in kidneys, skeletal muscle, liver, and red blood cells (Leggett et al., 2003). Cesium can cross the placenta and appears in milk. It mimics potassium for cellular transport. Urinary excretion is the primary route of elimination of cesium from the body. The biological half-life of cesium is variable, ranging from 50 to 150 days (ATSDR, 2004c). A physiologically based kinetic model has been developed to describe the distribution and retention of cesium in humans (Leggett et al., 2003).

Toxicity

Radioactive Cesium Exposure to radioactive cesium ([134]Cs and ^{137}Cs) is of much greater human health concern than exposure to nonradioactive cesium. The initial symptoms following radioactive cesium exposure include nausea, vomiting, and diarrhea. Local skin blistering is common when there is significant dermal contact. With continued exposure to radioactive cesium, adverse neurological and developmental effects can be observed. Symptoms can eventually progress to bone morrow suppression, infection, hemorrhage, and even death (ATSDR, 2004c).

Nonradioactive Cesium Compounds Stable cesium (^{133}Cs) compounds are relatively less toxic. High-dose exposure can cause irritation to the gastrointestinal tract and to the eye (ATSDR, 2004c). Cardiac arrhythmia and QT wave prolongation have been observed in several case reports following ingestion of cesium salts as homeopathic remedies for cancer treatment (ATSDR, 2004c; Dalal *et al.*, 2004). Adverse developmental effects of cesium chloride have been observed in rodents (Messiha, 1994). Prussian blue has been approved in the treatment of cesium poisoning (Thompson and Callen, 2004).

Fluorine

Fluorine (F) was isolated in 1886 by Henri Moissan for which he was awarded the 1906 Nobel Prize in chemistry. Fluorides are organic and inorganic compounds containing the nonmetallic element fluorine. Fluoride is an essential component for normal mineralization of bones and dental enamel, and it has been widely used to reduce the prevalence and severity of dental caries in children and adults. Flurosilicic acid and sodium fluorosilicate have been used in water fluoridation since 1940s. Adequate intake level is about 0.05 mg/kg per day in adults but is much lower for infants (ATSDR, 2003a,b). Toxicologically important fluoride compounds include hydrogen fluoride and sodium fluoride. The major sources of fluoride intake in the general population are water, food, and fluoride-containing dental products. However, excessive intake of fluorides has been observed from environmental sources, including from drinking water with naturally high fluoride (Meenakshi and Maheshwari, 2006), or from exposure to indoor fluoride air pollution from the use of high fluoride-containing coal (Liu *et al.*, 2002).

Fluorides are readily absorbed (75%–90%) from the gastrointestinal tract. Once absorbed, fluorides are rapidly distributed throughout the body. Approximately 99% of the fluoride in the body is found in bones and teeth. Fluoride is incorporated into bone by replacing the hydroxyl ion in hydroxyapatite to form hydroxyfluoapatite. Fluoride in bone can be remobilized slowly as a result of the ongoing process of bone remodeling, especially in the young children. Fluoride is readily transferred across the placenta but poorly transferred to breast milk. Fluorides are mainly excreted in urine. Plasma and urine fluoride levels are related to fluoride intake and are a biomarker for excess exposure, while hair, fingernails, and tooth enamel are indicators of long-term response (ATSDR, 2003a,b).

Toxicity

Dental Fluorosis Excessive fluoride intake from water during the period of enamel formation in children can cause dental fluorosis. In its mild form, dental fluorosis is characterized by white, opaque areas on the tooth surface. In its severe form, it is manifested as yellowish brown to black stains and severe pitting of the teeth. Dental fluorosis incidence and severity in some instances can be decreased by the cessation of water fluoridation (Clark *et al.*, 2006). Inappropriate use of fluoride toothpaste and fluoride supplements in young children is a risk factor for dental fluorosis (Browne *et al.*, 2005). Dental fluorosis is more common and severe in areas of endemic environmental fluorosis (Meenakshi and Maheshwari, 2006).

Skeletal Fluorosis Long-term exposure to very high oral doses of fluoride or occupational exposure to cryolite dusts can result in skeletal fluorosis. Cases of skeletal fluorosis are predominantly found in developing countries and are associated with high fluoride intake coupled with malnutrition (ATSDR, 2003a,b; Meenakshi and Maheshwari, 2006). Skeletal fluorosis does not usually manifest symptomatically until the disease attains an advanced stage. Fluoride is mainly deposited in the neck, knee, pelvic, and shoulder joints and/or bones, which makes it difficult to move or walk. The symptoms of skeletal fluorosis are similar to arthritis, and early on include sporadic pain, back stiffness, burning-like sensation, pricking and tingling in the limbs, muscle weakness, and chronic fatigue. These symptoms are associated with abnormal calcium deposits in bones and ligaments. In the advanced stage, symptoms include osteoporosis in long bones, and bone outgrowth. The vertebrae may fuse together and eventually the victim may be crippled (crippling skeletal fluorosis), a disability often accompanied by kyphosis (humpbacked) or lordosis (arched back).

There are conflicting data regarding the association between fluoride exposure and the incidence of osteosarcoma, a rare bone tumor (ATSDR, 2003a,b). A case–control study in the United States found an association between fluoride exposure in drinking water during childhood and the incidence of osteosarcoma among males but not among females (Bassin *et al.*, 2006). The National Toxicology Program in a rodent study found no evidence of carcinogenic activity in male or female mice or female rats exposed to sodium fluoride in the drinking water (NTP, 1990), although equivocal evidence of a response was observed in male rats based on a few osteosarcomas that occurred with a weak dose–response trend (NTP, 1990). Caution should be taken before any conclusions are made from such data and more studies are needed (Douglass and Joshipura, 2006).

Other health effects include respiratory tract, skin, and eye irritation following inhalation exposure to hydrogen fluoride or fluorine gas. Gastrointestinal symptoms occur with excess ingestion of fluoride (ATSDR, 2003a,b). Chronic endemic fluorosis may also lead to muscle fiber degeneration, low hemoglobin levels, skin rashes, neurological manifestations, compromised immunity, and endocrine effects (Meenakshi and Maheshwari, 2006). Endemic fluorosis from coal burning in China often occurs concurrently with arsenicosis (Liu *et al.*, 2002).

Germanium

Germanium (Ge) is considered a metalloid such as antimony and arsenic, and was named in honor of the discoverers' homeland Germany. The discovery of germanium as a predicted analog of silicon in the 1880s was a key confirmation of the developing theory of elemental periodicity. Chemically similar to tin, germanium can form a large number of organometallic compounds such as dimethyl germanium and germanium tetrahydride. Stable oxidation states include divalent and tetravalent germanium. In the semiconductor industry, germanium transistors found countless uses in solid state electronics up to the mid 1970s, but then were largely replaced by silicon. Currently it is used in infrared night vision systems, in fiber optics, in electronics, in solar cells, as a polymerization catalyst, and in alloys with other metals. Silicon germanide (SiGe) is rapidly becoming an important semiconductor metal for use in high-speed integrated circuits. Germanium is commercially derived from zinc ore processing or as a combustion by-product of certain coals. Ultrapure germanium can be obtained from other metals by fractional distillation of the volatile germanium tetrachloride.

The diet is the dominant source of germanium exposure in the general population while occupational exposure is predominantly by inhalation. Germanium concentrations in most foods are similar to the natural abundance level of about 0.6 to 1.3 ppm in soils, although higher levels have been reported in some canned foods (Faroon *et al.*, 2007). Daily germanium intake from food in humans is reported to be about 1.5 mg, of which 96% is absorbed (Faroon *et al.*, 2007). Intake of germanium from drinking water appears negligible. Considerable amounts of germanium are emitted into the air by coal combustion, although exposure from air is limited in the general population. There is no evidence of any essential function of germanium.

Inorganic germanium compounds are rapidly and effectively absorbed after oral exposure. Elemental germanium particles are likewise rapidly cleared from the lung and soon appear in distant tissues (Faroon *et al.*, 2007). Absorbed germanium is widely distributed throughout the body with the highest concentrations occurring in many tissues including the liver, kidney, and spleen. Absorption and distribution appears to be largely independent of the germanium compound, as both sodium germanate and tetraethylgermanium are widely distributed without evidence of selective retention or storage after oral exposure in mice. In both humans and laboratory animals, germanium is excreted mainly via the kidneys with whole-body half-life of one to four days. Hair and nails may be useful media for biological monitoring (Faroon *et al.*, 2007).

There appear to be no reports on systemic toxicity of germanium after occupational exposure. There are, however, at least 31 case reports of renal failure in humans after ingestion of inorganic or organometallic germanium compounds mainly through consumption of germanium-containing dietary supplements or elixirs for various diseases (Takeuchi *et al.*, 1992; Tao and Bolger, 1997). Among these cases nine deaths were reported (Tao and Bolger, 1997). Levels of germanium consumed were ~15 to 300 g and were ingested over a period of two to 36 months (Tao and Bolger, 1997). Excessive germanium consumption from such sources induces various symptoms including renal dysfunction involving tubular degeneration, anemia, muscle weakness, and peripheral neuropathy. Recovery of renal function is slow and incomplete (Tao and Bolger, 1997). Although reports on the efficacy of germanium supplementation against diseases such as cancer and AIDS persist, germanium supplementation has not been clearly shown to be of value and the USFDA considers such germanium products to present a potential human health risk (Tao and Bolger, 1997).

Spirogermanium (2-aza-8-germanspiro[4,5] decane-2-propamine-8,8-diethyl-*N*,*N*-dimethyl dichloride) was neurotoxic to humans after intravenous injection for the treatment of cancer. The effects were reversible and included ataxia and seizures. Neurotoxic effects are also observed in dogs (Faroon *et al.*, 2007).

There is no evidence of germanium carcinogenicity in humans. In rodents, limited testing indicates germanium is not carcinogenic in rats and it has no mutagenic activity (Faroon *et al.*, 2007). Dimethyl germanium oxide can produce embryonic resorption and fetal malformations in animals (Faroon *et al.*, 2007).

Indium

Indium (In) is a posttransitional metal, named after the indigo line in its atomic spectrum, which was discovered and isolated in the 1860s. It is a rare metal with a principal valence state of 3+ and is recovered as a by-product of zinc smelting. In its metallic forms, indium is used in liquid displays, semiconductors, alloys, solders, and as a hardening agent for bearings. Indium arsenide and indium phosphide are chemical forms commonly used in semiconductors (Tanaka, 2004). The most common isotope of indium is slightly radioactive, a characteristic exploited in medical imaging and nuclear medicine. Indium is considered to be a nonessential metal.

The human daily intake of indium has been estimated in the range of 8 to 10 µg. The most common routes of exposure for the general population are inhalation and ingestion while in occupational exposure inhalation predominates and dermal absorption is possible with the use of indium for nanotechnology. Indium compounds are poorly absorbed when ingested or after intratracheal instillation but may show moderate absorption after inhalation (Zheng *et al.*, 1994; Fowler, 2007). Indium derived from oral or intratracheal instillation of indium phosphide is uniformly distributed between major organs and is excreted in the urine and feces (Zheng *et al.*, 1994). Ionic indium is transported bound to transferrin and is cleared from the blood within three days of an intravenous injection in mice (Fowler, 2007).

Toxicity There appear to be no meaningful reports of local or systemic indium toxicity in humans after oral or inhalation exposure. Animal data on indium indicate that toxicity is related to the chemical form and route of exposure (NTP, 2001). Acute toxicity in animals is generally greatest after inhalation or intravenous injection, and limited after oral exposure (NTP, 2001). In this regard, intravenous injection of indium chloride in mice or rats produces extensive renal and liver necrosis (Fowler, 2007). Intratracheal instillation of indium chloride produces severe inflammation and pulmonary damage with fibrosis in mice (Blazka *et al.*, 1994). Lung instillation of indium phosphide can produce alveolar or bronchiolar cell hyperplasia in hamsters (Tanaka *et al.*, 1996). The intratracheal instillation of indium phosphide produces little systemic toxicity (Oda, 1997). Inhalation of indium tin oxide is a potential risk for lung diseases in humans (Nagano *et al.*, 2011). The developmental toxicity of indium has been recently reviewed by Nakajima *et al.* (2008). Indium trichloride showed no evidence of reproductive toxicity in mice, although it did adversely affect fetal survival. Teratogenic effects have been observed with intravenously injected indium compounds in rats and hamsters, but not in mice. Oral indium is teratogenic only at doses that induce maternal toxicity. Inhalation of indium phosphide or oral exposure to indium chloride by pregnant rats results in fetal indium concentrations that are similar to maternal blood levels (NTP, 2001; Nakajima *et al.*, 2008) indicating the placenta does not perturb indium.

Because of its use in the microelectronics industry, indium phosphide was tested recently by the National Toxicology Program (NTP, 2001). After inhalation of indium phosphide for up to two years there was clear evidence of pulmonary carcinogenic activity in both male and female rats and mice. This included production of lung adenoma and carcinoma after inhalation of indium phosphide. Concurrent genetic toxicity testing, specifically micronucleated erythrocytes in peripheral mouse blood, was negative (NTP, 2001). Further study indicated inhaled indium phosphide particles likely acted through chronic inflammation in conjunction with production of ROS and epithelial cell proliferation (Gottschling *et al.*, 2001). Inhalation of indium tin oxide aerosol for two years increased the incidence of malignant lung tumors in male and female rats, but had no carcinogenic effect in mice (Nagano *et al.*, 2011).

Palladium

Palladium (Pd) belongs to the platinum group metals. It was discovered in 1803, and named after the asteroid Pallas. Palladium occurs together with other platinum group metals (platinum, rhodium, ruthenium, iridium, and osmium) at a very low concentration in earth crust, and is recovered as a by-product of refining nickel, platinum, and other base metals. Palladium compounds commonly exhibit oxidation state of 2+, although compounds with oxidation state 4+ are observed. Organopalladium compounds also exist. Palladium is used in automobile catalysts, in dentistry (for crowns and bridges), in electrical appliances, and in jewelry and coinage.

Environmental palladium levels are increasing, but exposure in the general population is low. Dental alloys and work in metal refining or catalyst manufacture can be major sources of palladium exposure (WHO, 2002; Satoh, 2007).

Palladium chloride is poorly absorbed from the gastrointestinal tract or from subcutaneous injection sites. After intravenous administration of palladium compounds, palladium is distributed to kidney, liver, spleen, lung, and bone. In cells, palladium compounds likely complex with amino acids, proteins, DNA, and other macromolecules. Orally administered palladium is poorly absorbed and eliminated in feces, whereas intravenous palladium is mainly eliminated in the urine. Half-lives range from five to 12 days (WHO, 2002; Satoh, 2007).

Toxicity Palladium sensitization is a health concern, as very low doses are sufficient to cause allergic reactions in susceptible individuals (Satoh, 2007). Persons with known nickel allergy may be especially susceptible. Contact dermatitis is a main manifestation of palladium sensitivity, unlike that with platinum. Immediate hypersensitivity (type I) reactions to palladium have been reported in refinery workers sensitized to platinum (Ravindra et al., 2004). Palladium sensitization is often from dental alloys or jewelry. Occupational exposure to palladium salts may cause skin and eye irritation, and occasionally asthma (WHO, 2002; Satoh, 2007).

There is limited evidence that palladium chloride is carcinogenic after oral exposure in rodents, but the validity of this study has been questioned based on increased longevity of the treated group and lack of a specific target site (Ravindra et al., 2004; Satoh, 2007). Palladium compounds are negative in bacterial mutagenicity tests and in micronucleus test in human peripheral lymphocytes. Tetraammine palladium hydrogen carbonate induced a clastogenic response to lymphocytes in vitro but did not produce positive results in the micronucleus test (WHO, 2002). Some organopalladium complexes have been shown to have antitumor potential similar to that of cisplatin (WHO, 2002; Abu-Surrah and Kettunen, 2006).

Silver

Sliver (Ag) is a rare, naturally occurring element found as a soft, "silver"-colored metal. It was known since ancient times and was separated from lead as early as 4000 BC. The chemical symbol for silver, Ag, is from its Latin name *argentum*. Metallic silver and 1+ oxidation forms are common. Silver metal is used for jewelry, silverware, electronic equipment, and dental filling. Soluble silver salts (eg, silver nitrate, silver sulfide) have been used to treat bacterial infection. Silver halide is used in the manufacture of photographic plates, while silver sulfadiazine is used in the treatment of burns. Occupational exposure occurs mainly from inhalation of silver fumes and dusts in a number of settings (ATSDR, 1990; Drake and Hazelwood, 2005). Dietary intake is in the range of 70 to 90 μg per day, which is much less than the silver intake from medicinal uses. For drinking water disinfection, WHO permissible level is 0.1 mg silver/L (Pelkonen et al., 2003).

One of the recent uses of silver is in silver nanoparticles (AgNP), materials with sizes ranging from 1 to 100 nm, containing 20 to 15,000 atoms of silver. Because of their antimicrobial activity, AgNP are used in a variety of consumer products including medical devices, disinfectants, appliances, textiles, and water treatment. The primary routes of exposure for AgNP include lung skin and gastrointestinal tract (Chen and Schluesener, 2008; Ahamed et al., 2010). It has been reported that levels of AgNP >20 mg/kg iv is toxic (Shoults-Wilson et al., 2011).

Sliver compounds can be absorbed orally, by inhalation, and through damaged skin. Ingested silver compounds are absorbed

at a level of less than 10%, and only 2% to 4% is retained in tissues. Metallic silver and insoluble silver compounds are not readily taken up by the body, and pose minimal health risk (Drake and Hazelwood, 2005). In mice given drinking water containing silver nitrate (0.03 mg/L for two weeks), silver was widely distributed to most tissues including muscle, cerebellum, spleen, duodenum, heart, lung, liver, and kidney (Pelkonen et al., 2003). Silver can cross the blood–brain barrier and produce long-lasting deposits in many structures of the nervous system (Rungby, 1990) and is located almost exclusively in lysosomes of neuronal cells (Stoltenberg et al., 1994). Uptake of silver into lysosomes probably occurs through a carrier-mediated process (Havelaar et al., 1998). Autopsy findings after silver treatment of burn victims indicate the highest levels occur in skin, gingiva, cornea, liver, and kidneys. Urine silver analysis as a biomarker is useful only following a high degree of exposure because little silver is excreted in urine.

Toxicity The most common health effects associated with prolonged exposure to silver compounds are the development of a characteristic, irreversible pigmentation of the skin (argyria) and/or the eyes (argyrosis). The affected area becomes bluish-gray or ash gray. This is most prominent in the areas of the body exposed to sunlight, as light acts as a catalyst by triggering the photoreduction of these compounds to form metallic silver, similar to the process of developing a photographic negative. Metallic silver is subsequently oxidized by tissue and is bound as silver sulfide. Black silver sulfide and silver selenide complexes bound to tissue are identified as silver particle deposits. Argyria has two forms, local and general. Localized argyria is caused by direct, local contact with silver such as through jewelry, and involves the formation of gray-blue patches on the skin or may manifest itself in the conjunctiva of the eye. In generalized argyria, the skin shows widespread pigmentation, often spreading from the face to most uncovered parts of the body.

Chelating therapy and dermal abrasion are ineffective in removing silver deposits from the body and there is no effective treatment for argyria. Argyria can be considered a mechanism for detoxication of silver by sequestering it in the tissues as nontoxic silver–protein complexes or silver sulfide (ATSDR, 1990; Drake and Hazelwood, 2005).

The respiratory tract may be affected in severe cases of silver intoxication. Chronic bronchitis has also been reported to result from medicinal use of colloidal silver (ATSDR, 1990). Large oral doses of silver nitrate may cause severe gastrointestinal irritation due to its caustic action. Lesions of the kidneys and lungs and arteriosclerosis have been attributed to both industrial and medicinal exposures. Animal experiments indicate that silver may disturb copper metabolism (Hirasawa et al., 1994) and that MT may protect against the toxic action of silver (Shinogi and Maezumi, 1993).

Relatively little is known concerning the human toxicity of AgNP. Prolonged exposure to high levels of AgNP in rodents is associated with alveolar inflammation and slight liver damage (Ahamed et al., 2010, Table 1). In addition, AgNP produced damage to the blood–brain barrier, astrocyte swelling, and caused neuronal degeneration in rodents (Tang et al., 2009).

Tellurium

Tellurium (Te) is a metalloid chemically related to selenium and sulfur. Discovered in the 1780s, tellurium is named after the Latin word for earth (*tellus*). It is naturally found as the telluride of gold or combined with various other metals. Produced most often as a by-product of electrolytic copper refining, tellurium is used as an additive to improve metallurgic characteristics of copper, steel, and lead alloys (Gerhardsson, 2007). Tellurium vapor is used in "daylight" lamps and as a semiconductor in combination with other metals. It is also used in explosives, specialized glass, and thermo-electric and electronic devices.

Tellurium in food is probably in the form of tellurates. The estimated human daily intake is about 100 µg. Condiments, dairy products, nuts, and fish have relatively high concentrations of tel-lurium. Some plants, such as cactus, accumulate tellurium from the soil. The average body burden in humans is about 600 mg, mainly in bone.

The biochemistry and toxicity of inorganic and organometallic tellurium compounds have been reviewed (Taylor, 1996; Nogueira *et al.*, 2004). Soluble tetravalent tellurates, absorbed into the body after oral administration, are reduced to tellurides, partly methyl-ated, and then exhaled as dimethyl telluride. The dimethylated form is responsible for the characteristic garlic odor in persons intoxi-cated by tellurium compounds. Food is the main source of tellurium for the general population, while in industrial exposure inhalation would predominate. Some organometallic tellurium compounds are absorbed through the skin. Respiratory absorption data are limited, but inhaled tellurium compounds are likely well absorbed. After oral exposure of tellurides, 10% to 20% of the ingested dose is absorbed (Gerhardsson, 2007). The kidney, bone, and liver accu-mulate tellurium and it is estimated that bone stores may have a half-life of up to two years or more (Gerhardsson, 2007). The urine and bile are the principal routes of excretion. Tellurium crosses the blood–brain barrier and the placenta.

Toxicity Of toxicological importance are elemental tellurium, the gases hydrogen telluride and tellurium hexafluoride, and the water-soluble sodium or potassium tellurites and tellurates (Gerhardsson, 2007). Many organometallic forms of tellurium exist. Tellurates and tellurium are of generally low toxicity, but tellurites are typi-cally more toxic. Acute intoxication by inhalation results in sweat-ing, nausea, a metallic taste, and garlic smelling breath. In fact, garlic breath is an indicator of exposure to tellurium by dermal, inhalation, or oral routes. The cases of tellurium intoxication reported from industrial exposure do not appear to have been life-threatening. Two deaths occurred within six hours of accidental poisoning by mistaken injection of sodium tellurite (instead of sodium iodine) into the ureters during retrograde pyelography (Gerhardsson, 2007). The victims had garlic breath, renal pain, cyanosis, vomiting, stupor, and loss of consciousness. The amount of sodium telluride injected was about 2 g.

In rats, chronic exposure to high doses of tellurium diox-ide produces renal and hepatic injury (Gerhardsson, 2007). Rats fed metallic tellurium at 1% of the diet develop demyelination of peripheral nerves (Goodrum, 1998), probably due to the inhibition of cholesterol biosynthesis (Laden and Porter, 2001). Remyelination occurs after cessation of tellurium exposure (Morell *et al.*, 1994). Tellurium compounds are genotoxic and/or mutagenic in hamster fibroblasts, fungus and bacteria (Degrandi *et al.*, 2010), rat astro-cytes (Roy and Hardej, 2011), human blood cells (Santos *et al.*, 2009), and human promyelocytic cells (Sailer *et al.*, 2004). In most cases, exposure to these compounds led to oxidative stress and DNA damage, and apoptosis was the predominant mechanism of cell death.

There are no data on human or animal carcinogenicity of tel-lurium; however, there are studies indicating an anticarcinogenic effect of tellurium (Gerhardsson, 2007). Lifetime exposure to sodium tellurite at 2 mg Te/L drinking water had no effect on tumor incidence in rats. Some tellurium compounds show mutagenic

potential (Gerhardsson, 2007). Tellurium compounds produce hydrocephalus in rats after gestational exposure between days nine and 15.

Thallium

Thallium (Tl) is one of the most toxic metals. Thallium (from the Greek *thallos* meaning "a green shoot or twig") was discovered in 1861. The thallium ion has a similar charge and ion radius as the potassium ion, and its toxic effects may result from interference with the biological functions of potassium. In addition, thallium disrupts mitochondrial function leading to increases in intracellu-lar oxidative stress and apoptosis (Hanzel and Verstraeten, 2006, 2009).

Thallium is obtained as a by-product of the refining of iron, cadmium, and zinc, and is used as a catalyst in alloys, and in opti-cal lenses, jewelry, low-temperature thermometers, semiconduc-tors, dyes, pigments, and scintillation counters. It has been used medicinally as a depilatory. Thallium compounds, chiefly thallous sulfate, were used as rat poisons and insecticides. Once the com-monest sources of human thallium poisoning, the use of thallium as rodenticides or insecticides is now banned (WHO, 1996; Peter and Viraraghavan, 2005). Industrial poisoning is a special risk in the manufacture of fused halides for the production of lenses and win-dows. Naturally high thallium concentration in soils and consequent uptake into edible plants in Southwest Guizhou, China, caused locally endemic chronic thallium poisoning (Xiao *et al.*, 2004).

Thallium is absorbed through the skin and gastrointestinal tract. The highest concentrations after thallium poisoning are in the kidney. Following the initial exposure, large amounts are excreted in urine during the first 24 hours, but after that urinary excretion becomes slow and the feces become an important route of excre-tion. The half-life of thallium in humans has been reported to range from one to 30 days and depends on the initial dose. Thallium undergoes enterohepatic recirculation. Prussian blue, the most commonly used antidote, is given orally to break the enterohepatic recycling by trapping thallium secreted into bile and carrying it into the feces (WHO, 1996). Thallium can transfer across the placenta and is found in breast milk, and may cause toxicity in the offspring (Hoffman, 2000).

Toxicity The triad of gastroenteritis, polyneuropathy, and alo-pecia is regarded as the classic syndrome of thallium poisoning (WHO, 1996). Other signs and symptoms also occur depending on the dose and duration of exposure. The estimated acute lethal dose in humans is 10 to 15 mg/kg. Death is due mainly to renal, cen-tral nervous system, and cardiac failure within a few days to two weeks (WHO, 1996; Galvan-Arzate and Santamaria, 1998; Peter and Viraraghavan, 2005).

Alopecia is the best known effect of thallium poisoning. Depilation begins about 10 days after ingestion and complete hair loss can occur in about one month. Other dermal signs may include palmar erythema, acne, anhydrosis, and dry scaly skin due to toxic effects of thallium on sweat and sebaceous glands. After oral inges-tion of thallium, gastrointestinal symptoms occur, including nausea, vomiting, gastroenteritis, abdominal pain, and gastrointestinal hem-orrhage. Neurological symptoms usually appear two to five days after acute exposure, depending on age and the level of exposure. A consistent and characteristic feature of thallium intoxication in humans is the extreme sensitivity of the legs, followed by the "burn-ing feet syndrome" and paresthesia. Central nervous system toxic-ity is manifest by hallucinations, lethargy, delirium, convulsions, and coma. The acute cardiovascular effects of thallium are initially manifested by hypotension and bradycardia due to direct effects of thallium on sinus node and cardiac muscle. This is followed by hypertension and tachycardia due to vagal nerve degeneration. In severe cases, cardiac failure occurs (Mulkey and Oehme, 1993).

Major symptoms of chronic thallium poisoning include anorexia, headache, and abnormal pain. Other toxic effects of thallium include fatty infiltration and necrosis of the liver, nephritis, pulmonary edema, degenerative changes in the adrenals, and degeneration of the peripheral and central nervous system. In severe cases, alopecia, blindness, and even death have been reported as a result of long-term systemic thallium intake.

A recent review on thallium poisoning during pregnancy in humans gives a range of fetal effects from severe toxicity to normal development. The only consistent effect identified is a trend toward prematurity and low birth weight in children exposed to thallium during early gestation (Hoffman, 2000). Evidence that thallium is mutagenic or carcinogenic is scanty (Leonard and Gerber, 1997). In contrast, it may be teratogenic, especially with regard to cartilage and bone formation, but most of the evidence comes from birds and not mammals.

Treatment Therapy for thallium intoxication combines forced diuresis, use of activated charcoal, prevention of reabsorption by administration of Prussian blue, and administration of potassium ferric hexacyanoferrate (WHO, 1996). Prussian blue is the recommended drug of choice in acute thallium poisoning (Hoffman, 2003). Desferrioxamine has also been tested and shown to remove thallium from the body (Fatemi *et al.*, 2007).

Tin

Tin (Sn) is a silver-white metal. The name tin derives from the Anglo-Saxon, *tin*, through the Latin, *stannum*. Tin is one of the earliest metals known and was used as a component of bronze from antiquity. Because of its hardening effect on copper, tin was used in bronze implements as early as 3500 BC. However, the pure metal was not used until 600 BC. Metallic tin can combine with chloride, sulfur, or oxygen to form inorganic tin compounds (stannous, Sn^{2+}; and stannic, Sn^{4+}). Tin can also bind with carbon to form a number of toxicologically important organotin compounds including dimethyltin, dibutyltin, dioctyltin, triphenyltin, and tricyclohexyltin (ATSDR, 2005e). Currently, tin is used in the manufacture of various alloys, such as bronze and brass, for fabricating window glass and in solders, but was previously widely used in food packaging. Stannic chlorides are used in dyeing textiles. Organic tin compounds have been used in fungicides, bactericides, and slimicides, as well as in plastics as stabilizers. The average daily intake of tin from all sources is about 4.0 mg, considerably lower than the 17 mg estimated in previous decades, thanks to better food packaging technology (Winship, 1988; Blunden and Wallace, 2003). Organotin compounds are ubiquitous contaminants in the environment. Bioconcentration in aquatic organisms and ecotoxicity are dependent on the bioavailability of the particular compounds. Some tin compounds, especially organotins, show high bioavailability and may pose adverse effects toward aquatic ecosystems (Fent, 1996; Ostrakhovitch and Cherian, 2007).

Inorganic tin compounds are poorly absorbed after oral, inhalation, or dermal exposures. For example, only 3% of stannous and <1% of stannic compounds are absorbed from the gastrointestinal tract (Rudel, 2003). The majority of an oral dose of inorganic tin is excreted in the feces, while only a small portion of absorbed tin is eliminated via urine (Rudel, 2003; Ostrakhovitch and Cherian, 2007). Studies on animals reveal that administration of inorganic tin compounds reduces copper absorption (Yu and Beynen, 1995). The organotin compounds, particularly trimethyltin and triethyltin

compounds, are better absorbed than inorganic tins (Ostrakhovitch and Cherian, 2007). The tissue distribution of tin from these organometallic compounds shows the highest concentration in the bone, liver, kidney, and lung, with smaller amounts in the muscle, spleen, heart, or brain. Tetraethyltin, triethyltin, and diethyltin undergo dealkylation to ethyltin compounds, whereas tributyltin is dealkylated to di- and mono-butyltin compounds. Phenyltin compounds undergo dearylation, mainly by microsome monooxygenase and P450 enzymes (Winship, 1988; ATSDR, 2005e).

Toxicity Metallic tin and inorganic tin compounds are relatively nontoxic. Ingestion of food items contaminated with high levels of inorganic tins may cause acute gastroenteritis, while chronic inhalation of inorganic tins (eg, stannic oxide dust or fumes) may lead to benign nonfibrotic pneumoconiosis called *stannosis* (ATSDR, 2005e; Ostrakhovitch and Cherian, 2007).

Some organic tin compounds are highly neurotoxic, particularly triethyltin and trimethyltin, and cause encephalopathy and cerebral edema (Ostrakhovitch and Cherian, 2007). Toxicity declines as the number of carbon atoms in the chain increases. An outbreak of neurotoxicity of almost epidemic nature took place in France in the 1950s due to the oral ingestion of a preparation (Stalinon) containing diethyltin diiodide for the treatment of skin disorders (WHO, 1980). Trimethyltin produces degenerative lesions in the hippocampus and associated structure of the limbic system in primates and rodents. The lesions are characterized by neuron cell apoptosis with astrocyte swelling and gliosis. Microglia and astrocyte activation with the production of proinflammatory cytokines may well contribute to the lesion. Triethyltin produces cerebral edema in experimental animals (Rohl and Sievers, 2005; ATSDR, 2005e).

Triphenyltin, tributyltin, dibutyltin, and dioctyltin compounds produce immunotoxicity in experimental animals, characterized by thymic atrophy, and suppression of T-cell-mediated immune response (ATSDR, 2005e; Ostrakhovitch and Cherian, 2007). Acute burns or subacute dermal irritation has been reported among workers as a result of dermal tributyltin exposure (Ostrakhovitch and Cherian, 2007). Exposure of pregnant animals to organotin compounds such as tributyltin and triethyltin may induce developmental and endocrine-disrupting effects (Adeeko *et al.*, 2003; ATSDR, 2005e; Ostrakhovitch and Cherian, 2007).

Experimental studies have failed to find convincing evidence of carcinogenicity, mutagenicity, or teratogenicity of inorganic tin compounds (Winship, 1988). There is inadequate information to assess carcinogenic potential of organotin compounds in animals, and they are considered not classifiable as to human carcinogenicity (ATSDR, 2005e). Inhalation of indium tin oxide increased the incidence of malignant lung tumors in male and female rats (Nagano *et al.*, 2011), but these effects may be due to exposure to the indium (see the section "Indium"). Studies of genotoxicity of organotin compounds have given mixed results depending on the specific compound and test system. Triphenyltin compounds are potential chromosome mutagens, inducing production of micronuclei and sister chromatid exchange in Chinese hamster cells (Ostrakhovitch and Cherian, 2007).

Titanium

Discovered in 1791, titanium is named for the *Titans* of Greek mythology. Most titanium compounds are in the 4+ oxidation state (titanic), but the 3+ oxidation state (titanous) and 2+ compounds can occur. Titanium can form organometallic compounds. Because of its resistance to corrosion, inertness, and tensile strength, titanium has many metallurgic applications, and finds use in aircraft, armor plating, naval ships, missiles, and as a component of surgical implants and prostheses. Titanium dioxide (TiO_2), the most widely used titanium compound, is used as a white pigment in paints, paper, toothpaste, and plastics, as a food additive to whiten flour, in dietary products and confections, and as a whitener in cosmetics (Lomer *et al.*, 2004). Titanium complexes (such as titanium diketonate and budotitane) and titanocene complexes (such as titanocene dichloride) have undergone clinical trials as cancer chemotherapeutics (Caruso and Rossi, 2004; Kostova, 2009). Titanium tetrachloride ($TiCl_4$) is used to make titanium metal and other titanium-containing compounds. Occupational exposures to $TiCl_4$ can be of toxicological concern (ATSDR, 1997).

Approximately 3% of an oral dose of inorganic titanium is absorbed. The majority of the absorbed dose is excreted in the urine while unabsorbed titanium is excreted in the feces. The normal urinary concentration of titanium has been estimated at 10 μg/L (Kazantzis, 1981), and the estimated total body burden of titanium is about 15 mg. As a result of inhalation exposure, titanium accumulates in the lungs where it remains for long periods of time. Lung burdens increase with age and vary according to geographic location. Concentrations of titanium in liver (8 μg/g) and kidney (6 μg/g) are similar. Titanium may circulate in plasma bound to transferrin (Messori *et al.*, 1999), which is thought to be a mediator for delivery of titanium to tumor cells (Desoize, 2004).

Toxicity   Occupational inhalation exposure to $TiCl_4$ can produce mild to severe pulmonary injury because it undergoes rapid hydrolysis on contact with water to form hydrochloric acid, titanium oxychloride, and TiO_2. Occupational exposure to titanium dioxide occurs during production. TiO_2 is classified as a nuisance particulate with a threshold limit value of 10 mg/m³ (ACGIH, 2005). Inhalation and instillation of titanium particles coated with alumina and/or amorphous silica produce mild and reversible pulmonary effects. The base pigment-grade and/or nanoscale TiO_2 particles produce minimal pulmonary toxicity, regardless of particle size and surface area (Warheit *et al.*, 2005, 2006). In general, TiO_2 has been considered toxicologically inert regardless of route of exposure.

Epidemiological studies in humans have not found the association of titanium exposure with increased risk of lung cancer and chronic respiratory diseases (Fayerweather *et al.*, 1992; Fryzek *et al.*, 2003; IARC, 2010). Exposure of rats to TiO_2 via inhalation or intratracheal instillations caused malignant lung tumors (Jin and Berlin, 2007; IARC, 2010). The titanium compound, titanocene, when suspended in trioctanoin and injected intramuscularly, is carcinogenic in rats and mice (Jin and Berlin, 2007). According to IARC, there is inadequate evidence in humans and sufficient evidence in animals for the carcinogenicity of TiO_2 (IARC, 2010).

Titanium compounds and related metallocenes have recently shown chemotherapeutic activity toward gastrointestinal, breast, lung, and skin cancer (Desoize, 2004; Kostova, 2009; Olszewski and Hamilton, 2010). The mechanism of action of titanium compounds appears different from platinum compounds, and nephrotoxicity and myelotoxicity are not prominent. TiO_2 nanoparticles have photocatalytic activity raising concerns over their use in sunscreens. While some studies show TiO_2 particles cause oxidative damage to DNA (IARC, 2010), much about the safety or toxicity of these nanoparticles is still unknown making their use in sunscreens somewhat controversial (Burnett and Wang, 2011; Wiesenthal *et al.*, 2011).

Uranium

Uranium (U) is an actinide metal with a long history of human use. It was discovered by the German chemist Martin Kloproth in 1789 in a mineral called pitchblende, and was named after Uranus, the planet, which had been discovered eight years earlier. Uranium naturally occurs in three radioisotopes: [234]U, [235]U, and [238]U. The isotope [235]U is of particular interest in nuclear weapons and nuclear reactions. Thus, uranium ore is chemically enriched to increase [235]U content from 0.72% to 2% to 4%. The by-product of this process is called depleted uranium, which has decreased [235]U and has 40% less radioactivity than natural uranium (ATSDR, 1999a,b). Depleted uranium has been used in military applications as warheads and tank armor. Nonmilitary uses include counterweights in airplanes and shields against radiation in hospitals (Craft *et al.*, 2004). The chemical toxicity of uranium compounds is a health concern, rather than their radiation. Depleted uranium has the same chemical toxicity potential as natural uranium (ATSDR, 1999a,b; Craft *et al.*, 2004).

Uranium has five oxidation states but only the 4+ and 6+ forms are stable enough to be of practical importance. The 6+ oxidation state forms the uranyl ion (UO^{2+}), which further forms water-soluble compounds and is an important species of uranium in body fluids. The uranyl ion is also the most prevalent form in the environment (Sheppard *et al.*, 2005). The ecotoxicity of uranium and uranyl carbonate complexes to plants, aquatic life, and birds has been recently reviewed (Sheppard *et al.*, 2005).

Absorption of uranium compounds is low by all exposure routes. Absorption of inhaled uranium compounds occurs in respiratory tract via transfer across cell membranes, and is dependent on the particle size and solubility. Absorption from the gastrointestinal tract can vary from 0.1% to 6%, depending on the specific uranium compound. Once in the blood, uranium is distributed to the organs of the body. Uranium in body fluids generally exists as uranyl ion complexed with citrate and bicarbonate. Uranium preferentially distributes to bone (66%), liver (16%), kidney (8%), and then other tissues (10%). Two-thirds of the uranium in the blood is excreted in urine over the first 24 hours, but bone deposits of uranium last for about 1.5 years (ATSDR, 1999a,b; Craft *et al.*, 2004).

Toxicity   The kidney is the most sensitive organ for uranium toxicity. The primary target is the renal proximal tubule, but the glomeruli may also be affected. Biomarkers of tubular effects include enzymuria, and increased excretion of low-molecular-weight proteins, amino acids, and glucose. Glucosuria is the most persistent biomarker for uranium-induced tubular dysfunction. Biomarkers for glomerular toxicity include urinary albuminuria, and elevated blood creatinine and urea nitrogen. Pathological and functional changes occur within days following acute exposure and are manifested by injury to renal tubular epithelial cells. Renal effects from acute exposure to uranium appear to have some relationship to peak kidney concentrations regardless of chemical form and route of exposure and are usually transient or reversible (Diamond and Zalpus, 2005). Overt renal effects are observed with peak kidney uranium concentrations above 2 μg U/g, but mild renal tubular dysfunction from chronic exposure may occur at even lower renal concentrations. There appears to be a trend toward increase in severity of renal toxicity with increase in length exposure and urinary uranium levels (Thun *et al.*, 1985; Squibb *et al.*, 2005).

Challenges remain for establishing any causal relationship between human uranium exposure and birth defects and/or gonadal endocrine dysfunction, because these studies are confounded by coexposure to other toxicants and inadequate exposure assessments (Craft *et al.*, 2004; Hindin *et al.*, 2005). However, uranium and depleted uranium can be developmental toxicants when given orally or subcutaneously to mice. Decreased fertility, embryo/fetal toxicity, teratogenicity, and reduced growth of the offspring have been observed in rodents following uranium exposure during different periods of gestation. Bone is a major site of uranium accumulation, and chronic uranium intoxication may result in diminished bone growth and osteoporosis. There is also increasing concern of potential neurotoxicity of uranium (Craft *et al.*, 2004; Jiang and Aschner, 2006).

A higher incidence of lung cancer has been found in uranium miners and is probably due to radon and its daughter products, but not to uranium itself (ATSDR, 1999a,b). Gulf war veterans who were wounded subsequent to the explosion of armor-piercing shells containing depleted uranium often retain small fragments of the metal. This has created concern for the potential long-term effects of such embedded uranium fragments. Although there are no human data, a study in rats indicates that embedded depleted uranium fragments can cause localized proliferative reactions and sarcomas in rats (Hahn *et al.*, 2002). However, many types of implanted pellets will cause local sarcomas in rats (Hahn *et al.*, 2002).

Vanadium

Vanadium (V) is a transition metal discovered in the early 1800s and is named after the goddess of beauty in Scandinavian mythology, *Vanadis*, because of its beautiful multicolored chemical compounds. It is an essential trace element for microorganisms and bacteria, but definitive evidence for essentiality in mammals is lacking and no specific biochemical function for vanadium has been defined in humans (Lagerkvist and Oskarsson, 2007). Vanadium has several oxidation states, the most common being 3+, 4+, and 5+. The metal can be found as halides, such as the tetrachloride, and oxides, such as vanadium pentoxide. Organometallic vanadium compounds are generally unstable. Vanadium is recovered from vanadium-containing ores and from fossil fuels. Vanadium compounds are used in the production of special steels and alloys, in the manufacture of pigments, in photography, and as catalysts.

Food is the major source of human exposure in the general population (Lagerkvist and Oskarsson, 2007). Significant amounts of vanadium are found in seafood, mushrooms, dill seed, milk, meat, cereals, and vegetables. Concentrations in the drinking water largely depend on geographic location. Concentrations in rural air are much lower than in urban air, largely due to fossil fuel combustion. The dietary daily intake is estimated in the range from 10 to 60 μg (Lagerkvist and Oskarsson, 2007).

The lungs absorb about 25% of soluble vanadium compounds, but the absorption of vanadium salts from the gastrointestinal tract is generally poor (Lagerkvist and Oskarsson, 2007). Some dermal absorption of soluble compounds is possible but probably represents a minor route for humans. Once absorbed, extracellular vanadium will be in the form of vanadate (5+) and most likely in the vanadyl (4+) form after entering cells. After experimental exposure by various routes in rodents, the highest amounts of vanadium are found in the bone, kidney, liver, and spleen (Lagerkvist and Oskarsson, 2007). Brain levels are considerably lower than other tissues indicating limited transport across the blood–brain barrier. After oral exposure, vanadium shows a multicompartmental pattern with potential for accumulation and retention particularly in the bone (Lagerkvist and Oskarsson, 2007).

Toxicity The toxicity of vanadium compounds usually increases as the valence increases, the pentavalent compounds being the most toxic. After occupational exposure to airborne vanadium, its toxic actions are largely confined to irritation of the respiratory tract, eyes, and skin (Lagerkvist and Oskarsson, 2007). Interestingly, there is usually a latent period of one to six days before the adverse effects of vanadium appear, although the effects are usually reversible. Bronchitis and bronchopneumonia are more frequent in workers exposed to vanadium compounds. In industrial exposures to vanadium pentoxide dust, a characteristic greenish-black discoloration of the tongue occurs due to deposition of vanadium. There is some evidence that a sensitization reaction may occur with repeated exposures (Lagerkvist and Oskarsson, 2007). Gastrointestinal distress, nausea, vomiting, abdominal pain, cardiac palpitation, tremor, nervous depression, and kidney damage have also been linked with industrial vanadium exposure (Barceloux, 1999a,b).

There is clear evidence that inhaled vanadium pentoxide is carcinogenic in mice and rats producing benign and malignant lung tumors in a large NTP study (Ress *et al.*, 2003). Vanadium can act as a tumor promoter in the mouse lung (Rondini *et al.*, 2010). There are no data indicating a carcinogenic potential for vanadium compounds in humans, although vanadium pentoxide inhalation causes a variety of DNA damage in exposed workers (Ehrlich *et al.*, 2008). Vanadium compounds can be mutagenic in some systems (Lagerkvist and Oskarsson, 2007). Further work is required on vanadium carcinogenicity. Reproductive toxicology data are sparse and inconsistent, but there is some evidence of teratogenic potential in hamsters or mice (Lagerkvist and Oskarsson, 2007).

There are a variety of proposed pharmacological uses for vanadium compounds, including lowering cholesterol, triglycerides, and glucose levels, and some evidence indicates it can prevent tumor growth or formation in rodents (Lagerkvist and Oskarsson, 2007).

ACKNOWLEDGMENTS

This work was supported by the Division of the National Toxicology Program, National Institute of Environmental Health Sciences (NIEHS). This chapter may be the work product of an employee or group of employees of the NIEHS, National Institutes of Health (NIH); however, the statements contained herein do not necessarily represent the statements, opinions, or conclusions of the NIEHS, NIH or the US government. Neither the content of this publication necessarily reflect the views or the policies of the Department of Health and Human Services, nor does mention of trade names, commercial products, or organizations imply endorsement by the US government.

REFERENCES

Abu-Surrah AS, Kettunen M. Platinum group antitumor chemistry: design and development of new anticancer drugs complementary to cisplatin. *Curr Med Chem.* 2006;13:1337–1357.

ACGIH. TLVs and BEIs for chemical substances and physical agents. In: American Conference of Governmental Industrial Hygienists; 2005; Cincinnati, OH.

Adeeko A, Li D, Forsyth DS. Effects of in utero tributyltin chloride exposure in the rat on pregnancy outcome. *Toxicol Sci.* 2003;74:407–415.

Ahamed M, Alsalhi MS, Siddiqui MK. Silver nanoparticle applications and human health. *Clin Chim Acta.* 2010;411:1841–1848.

Akesson A, Julin B, Wolk A. Long-term dietary cadmium intake and postmenopausal endometrial cancer incidence: a population-based prospective cohort study. *Cancer Res.* 2008;68:6435–6441.

Akoume MY, Tuchweber B, Plaa GL, Yousef IM. The role of mdr2 in manganese-bilirubin induced cholestasis in mice. *Toxicol Lett.* 2004;148:41–51.

Alpert PT. New and emerging theories of cardiovascular disease: infection and elevated iron. *Biol Res Nurs.* 2004;6:3–10.

Anttila A, Heikkila P, Pukkala E, et al. Excess lung cancer among workers exposed to lead. *Scand J Work Environ Health.* 1995;21:460–469.

Aposhian HV, Aposhian MM. Arsenic toxicology: five questions. *Chem Res Toxicol.* 2006;19:1–15.

Arita A, Costa M. Epigenetics in metal carcinogenesis: nickel, arsenic, chromium and cadmium. *Metallomics.* 2009;1:222–228.

Aschner JL, Aschner M. Nutritional aspects of manganese homeostasis. *Mol Aspects Med*. 2005;26:353–362.

Aschner M, Erikson KM, Dorman DC. Manganese dosimetry: species differences and implications for neurotoxicity. *Crit Rev Toxicol*. 2005;35:1–32.

Aschner M, Guilarte TR, Schneider JS, et al. Manganese: recent advances in understanding its transport and neurotoxicity. *Toxicol Appl Pharmacol*. 2007;221:131–147.

Ashley K, Howe AM, Demange M, et al. Sampling and analysis considerations for the determination of hexavalent chromium in workplace air. *J Environ Monit*. 2003;5:707–716.

ATSDR. *Toxicological Profile for Silver*. Atlanta, GA: Agency for Toxic Substances and Disease Registry; 1990:1–145.

ATSDR. *Toxicological Profile for Antimony*. Atlanta, GA: Agency for Toxic Substances and Disease Registry; 1992:1–207.

ATSDR. *Toxicological Profile for Titanium Tetrachloride*. Atlanta, GA: Agency for Toxic Substances and Disease Registry; 1997:1–109.

ATSDR. *Toxicological Profile for Mercury (Update)*. Atlanta, GA: Agency for Toxic Substances and Disease Registry; 1999a:1–485.

ATSDR. *Toxicological Profile for Uranium (Update)*. Atlanta, GA: Agency for Toxic Substances and Disease Registry; 1999b:1–398.

ATSDR. *Toxicological Profile for Beryllium (Update)*. Atlanta, GA: Agency for Toxic Substances and Disease Registry; 2002:1–247.

ATSDR. *Toxicological Profile for Fluorides, Hydrogen Fluoride, and Fluorine (Update)*. Atlanta, GA: Agency for Toxic Substances and Disease Registry; 2003a:1–356.

ATSDR. *Toxicological Profile for Selenium (Update)*. Atlanta, GA: Agency for Toxic Substances and Disease Registry; 2003b:1–418.

ATSDR. *Toxicological Profile for Cobalt*. Atlanta, GA: Agency for Toxic Substances and Disease Registry; 2004a:1–486.

ATSDR. *Toxicological Profile for Copper (Update)*. Atlanta, GA: Agency for Toxic Substances and Disease Registry; 2004b:1–272.

ATSDR. *Toxicological Profile for Cesium*. Atlanta, GA: Agency for Toxic Substances and Disease Registry; 2004c:1–244.

ATSDR. *Toxicological Profile for Arsenic (Update)*. Atlanta, GA: Agency for Toxic Substances and Disease Registry; 2005a:1–357.

ATSDR. *Toxicological Profile for Lead (Update)*. Atlanta, GA: Agency for Toxic Substances and Disease Registry; 2005b:1–577.

ATSDR. *Toxicological Profile for Nickel (Update)*. Atlanta, GA: Agency for Toxic Substances and Disease Registry; 2005c:1–351.

ATSDR. *Toxicological Profile for Zinc (Update)*. Atlanta, GA: Agency for Toxic Substances and Disease Registry; 2005d:1–307.

ATSDR. *Toxicological Profile for Tin (Update)*. Atlanta, GA: Agency for Toxic Substances and Disease Registry; 2005e:1–376.

ATSDR. *Toxicological Profile for Barium*. Atlanta, GA: Agency for Toxic Substances and Disease Registry; 2007:1–143.

ATSDR. *Toxicological Profile for Cadmium (Update)*. Atlanta, GA: Agency for Toxic Substance and Disease Registry; 2008:1–512.

Bakir F, Damluji SF, Amin-Zaki L, et al. Methylmercury poisoning in Iraq. *Science*. 1973;181:230–241.

Ball LK, Ball R, Pratt RD. An assessment of thimerosal use in childhood vaccines. *Pediatrics*. 2001;107:1147–1154.

Barbosa F Jr, Tanus-Santos JE, Gerlach RF, et al. A critical review of biomarkers used for monitoring human exposure to lead: advantages, limitations, and future needs. *Environ Health Perspect*. 2005;113:1669–1674.

Barceloux DG. Molybdenum. *J Toxicol Clin Toxicol*. 1999a;37:231–237.

Barceloux DG. Vanadium. *J Toxicol Clin Toxicol*. 1999b;37:265–278.

Bassin EB, Wypij D, Davis RB, et al. Age-specific fluoride exposure in drinking water and osteosarcoma (United States). *Cancer Causes Control*. 2006;17:421–428.

Batuman V. Lead nephropathy, gout, and hypertension. *Am J Med Sci*. 1993;305:241–247.

Baughman TA. Elemental mercury spills. *Environ Health Perspect*. 2006;114:147–152.

Beijer K, Jernelov A. General chemistry of metals. In: Friberg L, Nordberg GF, Voul VB, eds. *Handbook on the Toxicology of Metals*. New York: Elsevier; 1986:68–84.

Bell JN, Shaw G. Ecological lessons from the Chernobyl accident. *Environ Int*. 2005;31:771–777.

Bellinger DC. Lead. *Pediatrics*. 2005;113:1016–1022.

Bellinger DC. Very low lead exposures and children's neurodevelopment. *Curr Opin Pediatr*. 2008;20:172–177.

Benbrahim-Tallaa L, Tokar EJ, Diwan BA, et al. Cadmium malignantly transforms normal human breast epithelial cells into a basal-like phenotype. *Environ Health Perspect*. 2009;117:1847–1852.

Bhamra MS, Case CP. Biological effects of metal-on-metal hip replacements. *Proc Inst Mech Eng*. 2006;220:379–384.

Bhattacharyya MH, Whelton BD, Peterson DP, et al. Skeletal changes in multiparous mice fed a nutrient-sufficient diet containing cadmium. *Toxicology*. 1988;50:193–204.

Bigazzi PE. Metals and kidney autoimmunity. *Environ Health Perspect*. 1999;107(suppl 5):753–765.

Blanusa M, Varnai VM, Piasek M, et al. Chelators as antidotes of metal toxicity: therapeutic and experimental aspects. *Curr Med Chem*. 2005;12:2771–2294.

Blazka ME, Tepper JS, Dixon D, et al. Pulmonary response of Fischer 344 rats to acute nose only inhalation of indium trichloride. *Environ Res*. 1994;67:68–83.

Blunden S, Wallace T. Tin in canned food: a review and understanding of occurrence and effect. *Food Chem Toxicol*. 2003;41:1651–1662.

Boening DW. Ecological effects, transport, and fate of mercury: a general review. *Chemosphere*. 2000;40:1335–1351.

Boles JW, Klaassen CD. Effects of molybdate and pentachlorophenol on the sulfation of acetaminophen. *Toxicology*. 2000;146:23–35.

Bondy SC. The neurotoxicity of environmental aluminum is still an issue. *Neurotoxicology*. 2010;31:575–581.

Brewer GJ. Tetrathiomolybdate anticopper therapy for Wilson's disease inhibits angiogenesis, fibrosis and inflammation. *J Cell Mol Med*. 2003;7:11–20.

Brewer GJ. Neurologically presenting Wilson's disease: epidemiology, pathophysiology and treatment. *CNS Drugs*. 2005;19:185–192.

Bridges CC, Zalpus RK. Molecular and ionic mimicry and the transport of toxic metals. *Toxicol Appl Pharmacol*. 2005;204:274–308.

Bright P, Burge PS, O'Hickey SP. Occupational asthma due to chrome and nickel electroplating. *Thorax*. 1997;52:28–32.

Brooks SM, Baker DB, Gann PH, et al. Cold air challenge and platinum skin reactivity in platinum refinery workers. Bronchial reactivity precedes skin prick response. *Chest*. 1990;97:1401–1407.

Browne D, Whelton H, O'Mullane D. Fluoride metabolism and fluorosis. *J Dent*. 2005;33:177–186.

Brumm VL, van Gorp WG, Wirshing W. Chronic neuropsychological sequelae in a case of severe lithium intoxication. *Neuropsychiatr Neuropsychol Behav Neurol*. 1998;11:245–249.

Bucher JR, Hailey JR, Roycroft JR, et al. Inhalation toxicity and carcinogenicity studies of cobalt sulfate. *Toxicol Sci*. 1999;49:56–67.

Burnett ME, Wang SQ. Current sunscreen controversies: a critical review. *Photodermatol Photoimmunol Photomed*. 2011;27:58–67.

Buss JL, Greene BT, Turner J, et al. Iron chelators in cancer chemotherapy. *Curr Top Med Chem*. 2004;4:1623–1635.

Cai L, Li XK, Song Y, et al. Essentiality, toxicology and chelation therapy of zinc and copper. *Curr Med Chem*. 2005;12:2753–2763.

Cambier S, Bénard G, Mesmer-Dudons N, et al. At environmental doses, dietary methylmercury inhibits mitochondrial energy metabolism in skeletal muscles of the zebra fish (*Danio rerio*). *Int J Biochem Cell Biol*. 2009;41:791–799.

Campbell JR, Rosier RN, Novotny L, et al. The association between environmental lead exposure and bone density in children. *Environ Health Perspect*. 2004;112:1200–1203.

Carmouche JJ, Puzas JE, Zhang X, et al. Lead exposure inhibits fracture healing and is associated with increased chondrogenesis, delay in cartilage mineralization, and a decrease in osteoprogenitor frequency. *Environ Health Perspect*. 2005;113:749–755.

Carpene E, Andreani G, Isani G. Metallothionein functions and structural characteristics. *J Trace Elem Med Biol*. 2007;21(suppl 1):35–39.

Caruso F, Rossi M. Antitumor titanium compounds. *Mini Rev Med Chem*. 2004;4:49–60.

CDC. Blood lead levels—United States, 1999–2002. *Morb Mortal Wkly Rep (MMWR)*. 2005;54:513–516.

Cefalu WT, Hu FB. Role of chromium in human health and in diabetes. *Diabetes Care.* 2004;27:2741–2751.

Cervantes C, Campos-Garcia J, Devars S, et al. Interactions of chromium with microorganisms and plants. *FEMS Microbiol Rev.* 2001;25:335–347.

Chambers A, Krewski D, Birkett N, et al. An exposure–response curve for copper excess and deficiency. *J Toxicol Environ Health B Crit Rev.* 2010;13:546–578.

Chan HM, Zhu LF, Zhong R, et al. Nephrotoxicity in rats following liver transplantation from cadmium-exposed rats. *Toxicol Appl Pharmacol.* 1993;123:89–96.

Chen CJ, Hsu LI, Wang CH, et al. Biomarkers of exposure, effect, and susceptibility of arsenic induced health hazards in Taiwan. *Toxicol Appl Pharmacol.* 2005;206:198–206.

Chen F, Shi X. Intracellular signal transduction of cells in response to carcinogenic metals. *Crit Rev Oncol Hematol.* 2002;42:105–121.

Chen L, Jin T, Huang B, et al. Critical exposure level of cadmium for elevated urinary metallothionein—an occupational population study in China. *Toxicol Appl Pharmacol.* 2006;215:93–99.

Chen X, Schluesener HJ. Nanosilver: a nanoproduct in medical application. *Toxicol Lett.* 2008;176:1–12.

Chitambar CR. Medical applications and toxicities of gallium compounds. *Int J Environ Res Public Health.* 2010;7:2337–2361.

Clark DC, Shulman JD, Maupome G, et al. Changes in dental fluorosis following the cessation of water fluoridation. *Community Dent Oral Epidemiol.* 2006;34:197–204.

Clarkson TW. The three modern faces of mercury. *Environ Health Perspect.* 2002;110(suppl 1):11–23.

Clarkson TW, Magos L. The toxicology of mercury and its chemical compounds. *Crit Rev Toxicol.* 2006;36:609–662.

Clarkson TW, Magos L, Myers GJ. The toxicology of mercury—current exposures and clinical manifestations. *N Engl J Med.* 2003;349:1731–1737.

Clemens F, Verma R, Ramnath J, et al. Amplification of the Ect2 protooncogene and over expression of Ect2 mRNA and protein in nickel compound and methylcholanthrene-transformed 10T1/2 mouse fibroblast cell lines. *Toxicol Appl Pharmacol.* 2005;206:138–149.

Cocco P, Dosemeci M, Heineman EF. Brain cancer and occupational exposure to lead. *J Occup Environ Med.* 1998;40:937–942.

Cohen MD, Kargacin B, Klein CB, et al. Mechanisms of chromium carcinogenicity and toxicity. *Crit Rev Toxicol.* 1993;23:255–281.

Costa M. Toxicity and carcinogenicity of Cr(VI) in animal models and humans. *Crit Rev Toxicol.* 1997;27:431–442.

Costa M, Davidson TL, Chen H, et al. Nickel carcinogenesis: epigenetics and hypoxia signaling. *Mutat Res.* 2005;592:79–88.

Costa M, Klein CB. Toxicity and carcinogenicity of chromium compounds in humans. *Crit Rev Toxicol.* 2006;36:155–163.

Counter SA, Buchanan LH. Mercury exposure in children: a review. *Toxicol Appl Pharmacol.* 2004;198:209–230.

Cousins RJ, Liuzzi JP, Lichten L. Mammalian zinc transport, trafficking, and signals. *J Biol Chem.* 2006;281:24085–24089.

Cox M, Singer I. Lithium. In: Bronner F, Coburn JW, eds. *Disorders of Mineral Metabolism.* New York: Academic Press; 1981:369–438.

Craft E, Abu-Qare A, Flaherty M, et al. Depleted and natural uranium: chemistry and toxicological effects. *J Toxicol Environ Health B Crit Rev.* 2004;7:297–317.

Cremin JD Jr, Luck ML, Laughlin NK, et al. Efficacy of succimer chelation for reducing brain lead in a primate model of human lead exposure. *Toxicol Appl Pharmacol.* 1999;161:283–293.

Crossgrove J, Zheng W. Manganese toxicity upon overexposure. *NMR Biomed.* 2004;17:544–553.

Culotta VC. Metallochaperones and metal ion homeostasis. In: *Encyclopedia of Inorganic Chemistry.* Wiley Online Library; 2006.

Dalal AK, Harding JD, Verdino RJ. Acquired long QT syndrome and monomorphic ventricular tachycardia after alternative treatment with cesium chloride for brain cancer. *Mayo Clin Proc.* 2004;79:1065–1069.

Dallas CE, Williams PL. Barium: rationale for a new oral reference dose. *J Toxicol Environ Health B Crit Rev.* 2001;4:395–429.

Davidson PW, Myers GJ, Weiss B. Mercury exposure and child development outcomes. *Pediatrics.* 2004;113(4 suppl):1023–1029.

Davidson PW, Myers GJ, Weiss B, et al. Prenatal methyl mercury exposure from fish consumption and child development: a review of evidence and perspectives from the Seychelles Child Development Study. *Neurotoxicology.* 2006;27:1106–1109.

Day GA, Stefaniak AB, Weston A, et al. Beryllium exposure: dermal and immunological considerations. *Int Arch Occup Environ Health.* 2006;79:161–164.

De Boeck M, Kirsch-Volders M, Lison D. Cobalt and antimony: genotoxicity and carcinogenicity. *Mutat Res.* 2003;533:135–152.

De Flora S. Threshold mechanisms and site specificity in chromium(VI) carcinogenesis. *Carcinogenesis.* 2000;21:533–541.

De Francisco N, Ruiz Troya JD, Aguera EI. Lead and lead toxicity in domestic and free living birds. *Avian Pathol.* 2003;32:3–13.

Degrandi TH, de Oliveira IM, d'Almeida GS, et al. Evaluation of the cytotoxicity, genotoxicity and mutagenicity of diphenyl ditelluride in several biological models. *Mutagenesis.* 2010;25:257–269.

Denkhaus E, Salnikow K. Nickel essentiality, toxicity, and carcinogenicity. *Crit Rev Oncol Hematol.* 2002;42:35–56.

DeRouen TA, Martin MD, Leroux BG, et al. Neurobehavioral effects of dental amalgam in children: a randomized clinical trial. *JAMA.* 2006;295:1784–1792.

Desoize B. Metals and metal compounds in cancer treatment. *Anticancer Res.* 2004;24:1529–1544.

Deubner DC, Lowney YW, Paustenbach DJ, et al. Contribution of incidental exposure pathways o total beryllium exposures. *Appl Occup Environ Hyg.* 2001;16:568–578.

Diamond GL, Zalpus R. Nephrotoxicity of metals. In: Tarloff JB, Lash LH, eds. *Toxicology of the Kidney.* 3rd ed. Boca Raton: CRC Press; 2005:971–979:chap 22.

Dietert RR, Lee JE, Hussain I, et al. Developmental immunotoxicology of lead. *Toxicol Appl Pharmacol.* 2004;198:86–94.

Diwan BA, Kasprzak KS, Rice JM. Transplacental carcinogenic effects of nickel(II) acetate in the renal cortex, renal pelvis and adenohypophysis in F344/NCr rats. *Carcinogenesis.* 1992;13:1351–1377.

Doherty MJ, Healy M, Richardson SG, et al. Total body iron overload in welder's siderosis. *Occup Environ Med.* 2004;61:82–85.

Doherty MJ, Healy M, Richardson SG, et al. Total body iron overload in welder's siderosis. *Occup Environ Med.* 2006;61:82–85.

Dopp E, Hartmann LM, Florea AM, et al. Environmental distribution, analysis, and toxicity of organometal(loid) compounds. *Crit Rev Toxicol.* 2004;34:301–333.

Douglass CW, Joshipura K. Caution needed in fluoride and osteosarcoma study. *Cancer Causes Control.* 2006;17:481–482.

Drake PL, Hazelwood KJ. Exposure-related health effects of silver and silver compounds: a review. *Ann Occup Hyg.* 2005;49:575–585.

Drobna Z, Walton FS, Harmon AW, Thomas DJ, Styblo M. Interspecies differences in metabolism of arsenic by cultured primary hepatocytes. *Toxicol Appl Pharmacol.* 2010;245:47–56.

Duffield-Lillico AJ, Reid ME, Turnbull BW, et al. Baseline characteristics and the effect of selenium supplementation on cancer incidence in a randomized clinical trial: a summary report of the Nutritional Prevention of Cancer Trial. *Cancer Epidemiol Biomarkers Prev.* 2002;11:630–639.

Ehrlich VA, Nersesyan AK, Atefie K, et al. Inhalative exposure to vanadium pentoxide causes DNA damage in workers: results of a multiple end point study. *Environ Health Perspect.* 2008;116:1689–1693 [erratum in *Environ Health Perspect.* 2009;117(1):A15].

Eisler R. Health risks of gold miners: a synoptic review. *Environ Geochem Health.* 2003;25:325–345.

Engström A, Skerving S, Lidfeldt J, et al. Cadmium-induced bone effect is not mediated via low serum 1,25-dihydroxy vitamin D. *Environ Res.* 2009;109:188–192.

Engström K, Vahter M, Mlakar SJ, et al. Polymorphisms in arsenic (+III oxidation state) methyltransferase (AS3MT) predict gene expression of AS3MT as well as arsenic metabolism. *Environ Health Perspect.* 2011;119:182–188.

Esteller M. *Epigenetics in Biology and Medicine.* Boca Raton: CRC Press; 2009.

Exley C, Burgess E, Day JP, et al. Aluminum toxicokinetics. *J Toxicol Environ Health.* 1996;48:569–584.

Factor-Litvak P, Hasselgren G, Jacobs D, et al. Mercury derived from dental amalgams and neuropsychologic function. *Environ Health Perspect.* 2003;111:719–723.

Fairweather-Tait SJ, Bao Y, Broadley MR, et al. Selenium in human health and disease. *Antioxid Redox Signal.* 2010;14:1337–1383.

Faroon OM, Keith LS, Hansen H, et al. Germanium. In: Nordberg GF, Fowler BA, Nordberg M, eds. *Handbook of the Toxicology of Metals.* 3rd ed. New York: Elsevier; 2007:557–567.

Fatemi SJ, Amiri A, Bazargan MH, et al. Clinical evaluation of desferrioxamine (DFO) for removal of thallium ions in rat. *Int J Artif Organs.* 2007;30:902–905.

Fayerweather WE, Karns ME, Gilby PG, et al. Epidemiologic study of lung cancer mortality in workers exposed to titanium tetrachloride. *J Occup Med.* 1992;34:164–169.

Fent K. Ecotoxicology of organotin compounds. *Crit Rev Toxicol.* 1996;26:1–117.

Ferraro L, Tomasini MC, Tanganelli S, et al. Developmental exposure to methylmercury elicits early cell death in the cerebral cortex and long-term memory deficits in the rat. *Int J Dev Neurosci.* 2009;27:165–174.

Fontenot AP, Maier LA, Canavera SJ, et al. Beryllium skin patch testing to analyze T cell stimulation and granulomatous inflammation in the lung. *J Immunol.* 2002;168:3627–3634.

Fowler BA. Indium. In: Nordberg GF, Fowler BA, Nordberg M, Friberg LT, eds. *Handbook on the Toxicology of Metals.* New York: Elsevier; 2007:569–576.

Fowler BA, Goyer RA. Bismuth localization within nuclear inclusions by x-ray microanalysis. Effects of accelerating voltage. *J Histochem Cytochem.* 1975;23:722–726.

Fowler BA, Sexton MJ. Gallium and semiconductor compounds. In: Nordberg GF, Fowler BA, Nordberg M, Friberg LT, eds. *Handbook on the Toxicology of Metals.* New York: Elsevier; 2007:547–555.

Franco JL, Posser T, Dunkley PR, et al. Methylmercury neurotoxicity is associated with inhibition of the antioxidant enzyme glutathione peroxidase. *Free Radic Biol Med.* 2009;47:449–457.

Frederickson CJ, Koh JY, Bush AI. The neurobiology of zinc in health and disease. *Nat Rev Neurosci.* 2005;6:449–462.

Freitas AJ, Rocha JB, Wolosker H, et al. Effects of Hg2+ and CH3Hg+ on Ca2+ fluxes in rat brain microsomes. *Brain Res.* 1996;738:257–264.

Fryzek JP, Chadda B, Marano D, et al. A cohort mortality study among titanium dioxide manufacturing workers in the United States. *J Occup Environ Med.* 2003;45:400–409.

Fu H, Boffetta P. Cancer and occupational exposure to inorganic lead compounds: a meta-analysis of published data. *Occup Environ Med.* 1995;52:73–81.

Fukushima N, Furuta D, Hidaka Y, Moriyama R, Tsujiuchi T. Post-translational modifications of tubulin in the nervous system. *J Neurochem.* 2009;109:683–693.

Gallagher CM, Chen JJ, Kovach JS. Environmental cadmium and breast cancer risk. *Aging.* 2010;2:804–814.

Galvan-Arzate S, Santamaria A. Thallium toxicity. *Toxicol Lett.* 1998;99:1–13.

Garruto RM, Fukatsu R, Yanagihara R, et al. Imaging of calcium and aluminum in neurofibrillary tangle-bearing neurons in parkinsonism dementia of Guam. *Proc Natl Acad Sci U S A.* 1984;81:1875–1879.

Garruto RM, Yanagihara R, Gajdusek DC. Disappearance of high-incidence amyotrophic lateral sclerosis and parkinsonism–dementia on Guam. *Neurology.* 1985;35:193–198.

Gerber GB, Leonard A, Hantson P. Carcinogenicity, mutagenicity and teratogenicity of manganese compounds. *Crit Rev Oncol Hematol.* 2002;42:25–34.

Gerhardsson L. Tellurium. In: Nordberg GF, Fowler BA, Nordberg M, Friberg LT, eds. *Handbook on the Toxicology of Metals.* New York: Elsevier; 2007:815–825.

Germolec DR, Spalding J, Yu HS, et al. Arsenic enhancement of skin neoplasia by chronic stimulation of growth factors. *Am J Pathol.* 1998;153:1775–1785.

Gonick HC, Behari JR. Is lead exposure the principal cause of essential hypertension? *Med Hypotheses.* 2002;59:239–246.

Goodman BP, Bosch EP, Ross MA, et al. Clinical and electrodiagnostic findings in copper deficiency myeloneuropathy. *J Neurol Neurosurg Psychiatry.* 2009;80:524–527.

Goodman JE, Prueitt RL, Thakali S, et al. The nickel ion bioavailability model of the carcinogenic potential of nickel-containing substances in the lung. *Crit Rev Toxicol.* 2011;41:142–174.

Goodrum JF. Role of organotellurium species in tellurium neuropathy. *Neurochem Res.* 1998;23:1313–1319.

Gordon T, Bowser D. Beryllium: genotoxicity and carcinogenicity. *Mutat Res.* 2003;533:99–105.

Gottschling BC, Maronpot RR, Hailey JR, et al. The role of oxidative stress in indium phosphide-induced lung carcinogenesis in rats. *Toxicol Sci.* 2001;64:28–40.

Goyer RA. Mechanisms of lead and cadmium nephrotoxicity. *Toxicol Lett.* 1989;46:153–162.

Goyer RA. Lead toxicity: from overt to subclinical to subtle health effects. *Environ Health Perspect.* 1990;86:177–181.

Goyer RA. Results of lead research: prenatal exposure and neurological consequences. *Environ Health Perspect.* 1996;104:1050–1054.

Goyer RA. Toxic and essential metal interactions. *Annu Rev Nutr.* 1997;17:37–50.

Gregus Z, Klaassen CD. Disposition of metals in rats: a comparative study of fecal, urinary, and biliary excretion and tissue distribution of eighteen metals. *Toxicol Appl Pharmacol.* 1986;85:24–38.

Grimsrud TK, Andersen A. Evidence of carcinogenicity in humans of water-soluble nickel salts. *J Occup Med Toxicol.* 2010;5:7.

Guilarte TR. Manganese and Parkinson's disease: a critical review and new findings. *Environ Health Perspect.* 2010;118:1071–1080.

Gujja P, Rosing DR, Tripodi DJ, Shizukuda Y. Iron overload cardiomyopathy: better understanding of an increasing disorder. *J Am Coll Cardiol.* 2010;21;56:1001–1012.

Gulson BL, Mizon KJ, Korsch MJ, et al. Mobilization of lead from human bone tissue during pregnancy and lactation—a summary of long-term research. *Sci Total Environ.* 2003;303:79–104.

Hahn FF, Guilmette RA, Hoover MD. Implanted depleted uranium fragments cause soft tissue sarcomas in the muscles of rats. *Environ Health Perspect.* 2002;110:51–59.

Hamza I, Gitlin JD. Copper chaperones for cytochrome *c* oxidase and human disease. *J Bioenerg Biomembr.* 2002;34:381–388.

Handy RD. Chronic effects of copper exposure versus endocrine toxicity: two sides of the same toxicological process? *Comp Biochem Physiol Part A.* 2003;135:25–38.

Hanzel CE, Verstraeten SV. Thallium induces hydrogen peroxide generation by impairing mitochondrial function. *Toxicol Appl Pharmacol.* 2006;216:485–492.

Hanzel CE, Verstraeten SV. Tl(I) and Tl(III) activate both mitochondrial and extrinsic pathways of apoptosis in rat pheochromocytoma (PC12) cells. *Toxicol Appl Pharmacol.* 2009;236:59–70.

Hao C, Hao W, Wei X, et al. The role of MAPK in the biphasic dose–response phenomenon induced by cadmium and mercury in HEK293 cells. *Toxicol In Vitro.* 2009;23:660–666.

Hardman JG, Limbird LE, Gilman AG, eds. The *Pharmacological Basis of Therapeutics.* New York: McGraw-Hill; 2001:1432–1435.

Harlan WR. The relationship of blood lead levels to blood pressure in the US population. *Environ Health Perspect.* 1988;78:9–13.

Harris ED. Cellular copper transport and metabolism. *Annu Rev Nutr.* 2000;20:291–310.

Harris WR, Berthon G, Day JP, et al. Speciation of aluminum in biological systems. *J Toxicol Environ Health.* 1996;48:543–568.

Hart BA, Potts RJ, Watkin RD. Cadmium adaptation in the lung—a double-edged sword? *Toxicology.* 2001;160:65–70.

Havelaar AC, de Gast IL, Snijders S. Characterization of a heavy metal ion transporter in the lysosomal membrane. *FEBS Lett.* 1998;436:223–227.

Hedera P, Peltier A, Fink JK, et al. Myelopolyneuropathy and pancytopenia due to copper deficiency and high zinc levels of unknown origin II. The denture cream is a primary source of excessive zinc. *Neurotoxicology.* 2009;30:996–999.

Henry GA, Jarnot BM, Steinhoff MM, et al. Mercury-induced renal autoimmunity in the MAXX rat. *Clin Immunol Immunopathol.* 1988;49:187–203.

Herbert V. Vitamin B-12. In: Ziegler EE, Filer LJ eds. *Present Knowledge in Nutrition*. Washington, DC: ILSI; 1996:191–205.

Herroeder S, Schönherr ME, De Hert SG, et al. Magnesium—essentials for anesthesiologists. *Anesthesiology*. 2011;114:971–993.

Hindin R, Brugge D, Panikkar B. Teratogenicity of depleted uranium aerosols: a review from an epidemiological perspective. *Environ Health*. 2005;26:4–17.

Hirasawa F, Sato M, Takizawa Y. Organ distribution of silver and the effect of silver on copper status in rats. *Toxicol Lett*. 1994;70:193–201.

Hoffman RS. Thallium poisoning during pregnancy: a case report and comprehensive literature review. *J Toxicol Clin Toxicol*. 2000;38:767–775.

Hoffman RS. Thallium toxicity and the role of Prussian blue in therapy. *Toxicol Rev*. 2003;22:29–40.

Högberg J, Alexander J. Selenium. In: Nordberg GF, Fowler BA, Nordberg M, Friberg LT, eds. *Handbook on the Toxicology of Metals*. New York: Elsevier; 2007:783–807.

Hopenhayn C, Huang B, Christian J, et al. Profile of urinary arsenic metabolites during pregnancy. *Environ Health Perspect*. 2003;111:1888–1891.

Horsted-Bindslev P. Amalgam toxicity—environmental and occupational hazards. *J Dent*. 2004;32:359–365.

Hostynek JJ. Gold: an allergen of growing significance. *Food Chem Toxicol*. 1997;35:839–844.

Hostynek JJ, Hinz RS, Lorence CR, et al. Metals and the skin. *Crit Rev Toxicol*. 1993;23:171–235.

Howard BJ, Howard DC. Health impacts of large releases of radionuclides. The radioecological significance of semi-natural ecosystems. *Ciba Found Symp*. 1997;203:21–45.

Huster D. Wilson disease. *Best Pract Res Clin Gastroenterol*. 2010;24:531–539.

IARC. *IARC Monographs on the Evaluation of Carcinogenic Risks to Humans. Overall Evaluations of Carcinogenicity: An Updating of IARC Monographs*. Vols. 1-42. Lyon, France: IARC; 1987.

IARC. *IARC Monographs on the Evaluation of Carcinogenic Risks to Humans. Chromium, Nickel and Welding*. Vol. 49. Lyon, France: IARC; 1990:1–677.

IARC. *IARC Monographs on the Evaluation of Carcinogenic Risks to Humans. Chlorinated Drinking Water Chlorination By-Products, Some Other Halogenated Compounds Cobalt and Cobalt Compounds*. Vol. 52. Lyon, France: IARC; 1991:1–544.

IARC. *IARC Monographs on the Evaluation of Carcinogenic Risks to Humans. Beryllium, Cadmium, Mercury and Exposures in the Glass Manufacturing Industry*. Vol. 58. Lyon, France: IARC; 1993:41–117.

IARC. *IARC Monographs on the Evaluation of Carcinogenic Risks to Humans. Arsenic in Drinking Water: Some Drinking Water Disinfectants and Contaminants, Including Arsenic*. Vol. 84. Lyon, France: IARC; 2004:269–477.

IARC. *IARC Monographs on the Evaluation of Carcinogenic Risks to Humans. Inorganic Lead and Organic Lead Compounds*. Vol. 87. Lyon, France: IARC; 2006.

IARC. *IARC Monographs on the Evaluation of Carcinogenic Risks to Humans. Carbon Black, Titanium Dioxide, and Talc*. Vol. 93. Lyon, France: IARC; 2010:193–276.

IARC. *IARC Monographs on the Evaluation of Carcinogenic Risks to Humans. Arsenic and Arsenic Compounds*. Vol. 100c. Lyon, France: IARC; 2011a.

IARC. *IARC Monographs on the Evaluation of Carcinogenic Risks to Humans. Cadmium and Cadmium Compounds*. Vol. 100c. Lyon, France: IARC; 2011b.

Il'yasova D, Schwartz GG. Cadmium and renal cancer. *Toxicol Appl Pharmacol*. 2005;207:179–186.

IOM (Institute of Medicine), Food and Nutrition Board. *Dietary Reference Intakes for Vitamin A, Vitamin K, Arsenic, Boron, Chromium, Copper, Iodine, Iron, Manganese, Molybdenum, Nickel, Silicon, Vanadium, and Zinc*. Washington, DC: National Academic Press; 2001:1–769.

Järup L, Berglund M, Elinder CG, et al. Health effects of cadmium exposure—a review of the literature and a risk estimate. *Scand J Work Environ Health*. 1998;24(suppl 1):1–51.

Jiang GC, Aschner M. Neurotoxicity of depleted uranium: reasons for increased concern. *Biol Trace Elem Res*. 2006;110:1–18.

Jiang Y, Zheng W. Cardiovascular toxicities upon manganese exposure. *Cardiovasc Toxicol*. 2005;5:345–354.

Jin T, Berlin M. Titanium. In: Nordberg GF, Fowler BA, Nordberg M, Friberg LT, eds. *Handbook on the Toxicology of Metals*. New York: Elsevier; 2007:861–870.

Jin YH, Dunlap PE, McBride SJ, et al. Global transcriptome and deletome profiles of yeast exposed to transition metals. *PLoS Genet*. 2008;4:e1000053.

Johnson CH, VanTassell VJ. Acute barium poisoning with respiratory failure and rhabdomyolysis. *Ann Emerg Med*. 1991;20:1138–1142.

Joseph P. Mechanisms of cadmium carcinogenesis. *Toxicol Appl Pharmacol*. 2009;238:272–279.

Kagan HM, Li W. Lysyl oxidase: properties, specificity, and biological roles inside and outside of the cell. *J Cell Biochem*. 2003;88:660–672.

Karmaus W, Brooks KR, Nebe T, et al. Immune function biomarkers in children exposed to lead and organochlorine compounds: a cross-sectional study. *Environ Health*. 2005;4:1–10.

Kasprzak KS. Oxidative DNA and protein damage in metal-induced toxicity and carcinogenesis. *Free Radic Biol Med*. 2002;32:958–967.

Kasprzak KS, Sunderman FW Jr, Salnikow K. Nickel carcinogenesis. *Mutat Res*. 2003;533:67–97.

Kawahara M. Effects of aluminum on the nervous system and its possible link with neurodegenerative diseases. *J Alzheimers Dis*. 2005;8:171–182 [discussion 209–215].

Kawata K, Yokoo H, Shimazaki R, et al. Classification of heavy-metal toxicity by human DNA microarray analysis. *Environ Sci Technol*. 2007;41:3769–3774.

Kazantzis G. Role of cobalt, iron, lead, manganese, mercury, platinum, selenium, and titanium in carcinogenesis. *Environ Health Perspect*. 1981;40:143–161.

Kazantzis G. Cadmium, osteoporosis and calcium metabolism. *Biometals*. 2004;17:493–498.

Kelada SN, Shelton E, Kaufmann RB, et al. Delta-aminolevulinic acid dehydratase and lead toxicity, a HuGE review. *Am J Epidemiol*. 2001;154:1–13.

Khlebtsov N, Dykman L. Biodistribution and toxicity of engineered gold nanoparticles: a review of in vitro and in vivo studies. *Chem Soc Rev*. 2011;40:1647–1671.

Kim SH, Johnson VJ, Sharma RP. Mercury inhibits nitric oxide production but activates proinflammatory cytokine expression in murine macrophage: differential modulation of NF-kappaB and p38 MAPK signaling pathways. *Nitric Oxide*. 2002;7:67–74.

Klaassen CD. Heavy metals and heavy-metal antagonists. In: Brunton LL, Lazo JS, Parker KL, eds. The *Pharmacological Basis of Therapeutics*. New York: McGraw-Hill; 2006:1753–1775.

Klaassen CD, Liu J. Induction of metallothionein as an adaptive mechanism affecting the magnitude and progression of toxicological injury. *Environ Health Perspect*. 1998;106(suppl 1):297–300.

Klaassen CD, Liu J, Choudhuri S. Metallothionein: an intracellular protein to protect against cadmium toxicity. *Annu Rev Pharmacol Toxicol*. 1999;39:267–294.

Klaassen CD, Waalkes MP, Cantilena LR Jr. Alteration of tissue disposition of cadmium by chelating agents. *Environ Health Perspect*. 1984;54:233–242.

Klimisch HJ. Lung deposition, lung clearance and renal accumulation of inhaled cadmium chloride and cadmium sulphide in rats. *Toxicology*. 1993;84:103–124.

Kodama H, Fujisawa C, Bhadhprasit W. Pathology, clinical features and treatments of congenital copper metabolic disorders—focus on neurologic aspects. *Brain Dev*. 2011;33:243–251.

Kohrle J, Jakob F, Contempre B, et al. Selenium, the thyroid, and the endocrine system. *Endocr Rev*. 2005;26:944–984.

Kojima C, Ramirez DC, Tokar EJ, et al. Requirement of arsenic biomethylation for oxidative DNA damage. *J Natl Cancer Inst*. 2009;101:1670–1680.

Kondo Y, Himeno S, Satoh M, et al. Citrate enhances the protective effect of orally administered bismuth subnitrate against the nephrotoxicity of *cis*-diamminedichloroplatinum. *Cancer Chemother Pharmacol*. 2004;53:33–38.

Königsberg M, López-Díazguerrero NE, Bucio L, et al. Uncoupling effect of mercuric chloride on mitochondria isolated from an hepatic cell line. *J Appl Toxicol.* 2001;21:323–329.

Kopp SJ, Glonek T, Perry HM Jr, et al. Cardiovascular actions of cadmium at environmental exposure levels. *Science.* 1982;217:837–839.

Korashy HM, El-Kadi AO. The role of redox-sensitive transcription factors NF-kappaB and AP-1 in the modulation of the Cyp1a1 gene by mercury, lead, and copper. *Free Radic Biol Med.* 2008;44:795–806.

Kostova I. Gold coordination complexes as anticancer agents. *Anticancer Agents Med Chem.* 2006;6:19–32.

Kostova I. Titanium and vanadium complexes as anticancer agents. *Anticancer Agents Med Chem.* 2009;9:827–842.

Kriegel AM, Soliman AS, Zhang Q, et al. Serum cadmium levels in pancreatic cancer patients from the East Nile Delta region of Egypt. *Environ Health Perspect.* 2006;114:113–119.

Kszos LA, Stewart AJ. Review of lithium in the aquatic environment: distribution in the United States, toxicity and case example of groundwater contamination. *Ecotoxicology.* 2003;12:439–447.

Kumar N, Elliott MA, Hoyer JD, et al. "Myelodysplasia," myeloneuropathy, and copper deficiency. *Mayo Clin Proc.* 2005;80:943–946.

Laden BP, Porter TD. Inhibition of human squalene monooxygenase by tellurium compounds: evidence of interaction with vicinal sulfhydryls. *J Lipid Res.* 2001;42:235–240.

Lagerkvist BJ, Oskarsson A. Vanadium. In: Nordberg GF, Fowler BA, Nordberg M, eds. *Handbook on the Toxicology of Metals.* 3rd ed. New York: Elsevier; 2007:905–923.

Lamphear BP, Dietrich K, Auinger P, et al. Cognitive deficits associated with blood lead concentrations <10 µg/dL in US children and adolescents. *Public Health Rep.* 2000;115:521–529.

Laraque D, Trasande L. Lead poisoning: successes and 21st century challenges. *Pediatr Rev.* 2005;26:435–443.

Larsen A, Stoltenberg M, Sondergaard C, et al. In vivo distribution of bismuth in the mouse brain: influence of long-term survival and intracranial placement on the uptake and transport of bismuth in neuronal tissue. *Basic Clin Pharmacol Toxicol.* 2005;97:188–196.

Leggett RW, Williams LR, Melo DR, et al. A physiologically based biokinetic model for cesium in the human body. *Sci Total Environ.* 2003;317:235–255.

Lenox RH, Hahn CG. Overview of the mechanism of action of lithium in the brain: fifty-year update. *J Clin Psychiatry.* 2000;61(suppl 9):5–15.

Leonard A, Gerber GB. Mutagenicity, carcinogenicity and teratogenicity of antimony compounds. *Mutat Res.* 1996;366:1–8.

Leonard A, Gerber GB. Mutagenicity, carcinogenicity and teratogenicity of thallium compounds. *Mutat Res.* 1997;387:47–53.

Leslie EM, Liu J, Klaassen CD, et al. Acquired cadmium resistance in metallothionein-I/II(−/−) knockout cells: role of the T-type calcium channel Cacnalpha1G in cadmium uptake. *Mol Pharmacol.* 2006;69:629–639.

Leussink BT, Slikkerveer A, Engelbrecht MR, et al. Bismuth overdosing-induced reversible nephropathy in rats. *Arch Toxicol.* 2001;74:745–754.

Levin R, Brown MJ, Kashtock ME, et al. Lead exposures in U.S. children, 2008: implications for prevention. *Environ Health Perspect.* 2008;116:1285–1293.

Lindberg S, Bullock R, Ebinghaus R, et al. A synthesis of progress and uncertainties in attributing the sources of mercury in deposition. *Ambio.* 2007;36:19–32.

Lindgren KN, Masten VL, Ford DP. Relation of cumulative exposure to inorganic and neuropsychological test performance. *Occup Environ Med.* 1996;53:472–477.

Linnett PJ. Concerns for asthma at pre-placement assessment and health surveillance in platinum refining—a personal approach. *Occup Med (Lond).* 2005;55:595–599.

Lison D. Cobalt. In: Nordberg GF, Fowler BA, Nordberg M, Friberg LT, eds. *Handbook on the Toxicology of Metals.* New York: Elsevier; 2007:511–528.

Liu J, Chen H, Miller DS, et al. Overexpression of glutathione *S*-transferase pi and multidrug resistance transport proteins is associated with acquired tolerance to inorganic arsenic. *Mol Pharmacol.* 2001;60:302–309.

Liu J, Habeebu SS, Liu Y, et al. Acute CdMT injection is not a good model to study chronic Cd nephropathy: comparison of chronic CdCl2 and CdMT exposure with acute CdMT injection in rats. *Toxicol Appl Pharmacol.* 1998b;153:48–58.

Liu J, Liu Y, Habeebu SS, et al. Susceptibility of MT-null mice to chronic CdCl2-induced nephrotoxicity indicates that renal injury is not mediated by the CdMT complex. *Toxicol Sci.* 1998a;46:197–203.

Liu J, Liu Y, Klaassen CD. Nephrotoxicity of CdCl2 and Cd-metallothionein in cultured rat kidney proximal tubules and LLC-PK1 cells. *Toxicol Appl Pharmacol.* 1994;128:264–270.

Liu J, Shi JZ, Yu LM, et al. Mercury in traditional medicines: is cinnabar toxicologically similar to common mercurials? *Exp Biol Med.* 2008;233:810–817.

Liu J, Waalkes MP. Liver is a target of arsenic carcinogenesis. *Toxicol Sci.* 2008;105:24–32.

Liu J, Xie Y, Ducharme DM, et al. Global gene expression associated with hepatocarcinogenesis in adult male mice induced by in utero arsenic exposure. *Environ Health Perspect.* 2006;114:404–411.

Liu J, Zheng B, Aposhian HV, et al. Chronic arsenic poisoning from burning high-arsenic-containing coal in Guizhou, China. *Environ Health Perspect.* 2002;110:119–122.

Lomer MCE, Hutchinson C, Volkert S, et al. Dietary sources of inorganic microparticles and their intake in healthy subjects and patients with Crohn's disease. *Br J Nutr.* 2004;92:947–955.

Luebke RW, Chen DH, Dietert R. The comparative immunotoxicity of five selected compounds following developmental or adult exposure. *J Toxicol Environ Health B Crit Rev.* 2006;9:1–26.

Lynch BS, Capen CC, Nestmann ER, et al. Review of subchronic/chronic toxicity of antimony potassium tartrate. *Regul Toxicol Pharmacol.* 1999;30:9–17.

Mahaffey KR. Factors modifying susceptibility to lead toxicity. In: Mahaffey KR, ed. *Dietary and Environmental Lead: Human Health Effects.* New York: Elsevier; 1985:373–420.

Makjanic J, McDonald B, Chen LHCP, et al. Absence of aluminium in neurofibrillary tangles in Alzheimer's disease. *Neurosci Lett.* 1998;240: 123–126.

Manton WI, Angle CR, Krogstrand KL. Origin of lead in the United States diet. *Environ Sci Technol.* 2005;15:8995–9000.

Manton WI, Angle CR, Stanek KL, et al. Acquisition and retention of lead by young children. *Environ Res.* 2000;82:60–80.

Maret W, Standstead HH. Zinc requirements and the risks and benefits of zinc supplementation. *J Trace Elem Med Biol.* 2006;20:3–18.

Markman M. Toxicities of the platinum antineoplastic agents. *Expert Opin Drug Saf.* 2003;2:597–607.

Markowitz GS, Radhakrishnan J, Kambham N, et al. Lithium nephrotoxicity: a progressive combined glomerular and tubulointerstitial nephropathy. *J Am Soc Nephrol.* 2000;11:1439–1448.

Mas A. Hepatic encephalopathy: from pathophysiology to treatment. *Digestion.* 2006;73(suppl 1):86–93.

Maverakis E, Fung MA, Lynch PJ, et al. Acrodermatitis enteropathica and an overview of zinc metabolism. *J Am Acad Dermatol.* 2007;56: 116–124.

Mazumder DN. Effect of chronic intake of arsenic-contaminated water on liver. *Toxicol Appl Pharmacol.* 2005;206:169–175.

Mazur A, Maier JA, Rock E. Magnesium and the inflammatory response: potential physiopathological implications. *Arch Biochem Biophys.* 2007;458:48–56.

McElroy JA, Shafer MM, Trentham-Dietz A, et al. Cadmium exposure and breast cancer risk. *J Natl Cancer Inst.* 2006;98:869–873.

Meenakshi RC, Maheshwari SK. Fluoride in drinking water and its removal. *J Hazard Mater.* 2006;137:456–463.

Mendel RR, Bittner F. Cell biology of molybdenum. *Biochim Biophys Acta.* 2006;1763:621–635.

Merali Z, Kacew S, Singhal RL. Response of hepatic carbohydrate and cyclic AMP metabolism to cadmium treatment in rats. *Can J Physiol Pharmacol.* 1975;53:174–184.

Mercer JF. The molecular basis of copper-transport diseases. *Trends Mol Med.* 2001;7:64–69.

Messiha FS. Developmental toxicity of cesium in the mouse. *Gen Pharmacol.* 1994;25:395–400.

Messner B, Bernhard D. Cadmium and cardiovascular diseases: cell biology, pathophysiology, and epidemiological relevance. *Biometals.* 2010;23:811–822.

Messori L, Orioli P, Banholzer V, et al. Formation of titanium(IV) transferrin by reaction of human serum apotransferrin with titanium complexes. *FEBS Lett.* 1999;442:157–161.

Morell P, Toews AD, Wagner M, et al. Gene expression during tellurium-induced primary demyelination. *Neurotoxicology.* 1994;15:171–180.

Mulkey JP, Oehme FW. A review of thallium toxicity. *Vet Hum Toxicol.* 1993;35:445–453.

Murata K, Iwata T, Dakeishi M, et al. Lead toxicity: does the critical level of lead resulting in adverse effects differ between adults and children? *J Occup Health.* 2009;51:1–12.

Mutter J, Naumann J, Guethlin C. Comments on the article "The toxicology of mercury and its chemical compounds" by Clarkson and Magos (2006). *Crit Rev Toxicol.* 2007;37:537–549.

Nagano N, Nishizawa T, Umeda Y, et al. Inhalation carcinogenicity and chronic toxicity of indium-tin-oxide in rats and mice. *J Occup Health.* 2011;53:175–187.

Nakajima M, Usami M, Nakazawa K, et al. Developmental toxicity of indium: embryotoxicity and teratogenicity in experimental animals. *Congenit Anom Kyoto.* 2008;48:145–150.

Navas-Acien A, Guallar E, Silbergeld EK, et al. Lead exposure and cardiovascular disease—a systematic review. *Environ Health Perspect.* 2007;115:472–482.

Navas-Acien A, Sharrett AR, Silbergeld EK, et al. Arsenic exposure and cardiovascular disease: a systematic review of the epidemiologic evidence. *Am J Epidemiol.* 2005;162:1037–1049.

Navas-Acien A, Silbergeld EK, Streeter RA, et al. Arsenic exposure and type 2 diabetes: a systematic review of the experimental and epidemiological evidence. *Environ Health Perspect.* 2006;114:641–648.

Nawrot TS, Thijs L, Den Hond EM, et al. An epidemiological re-appraisal of the association between blood pressure and blood lead: a meta-analysis. *J Hum Hypertens.* 2002;16:123–131.

Newman LS, Mroz MM, Balkissoon R, et al. Beryllium sensitization progresses to chronic beryllium disease: a longitudinal study of disease risk. *Am J Respir Crit Care Med.* 2005;171:54–60.

Ng JC, Wang JP, Zheng B, et al. Urinary porphyrins as biomarkers for arsenic exposure among susceptible populations in Guizhou province, China. *Toxicol Appl Pharmacol.* 2005;206:176–184.

Nierenberg DW, Nordgren RE, Chang MB, et al. Delayed cerebellar disease and death after accidental exposure to dimethylmercury. *N Engl J Med.* 1998;338:1672–1676.

Nogueira CW, Zeni G, Rocha JB. Organoselenium and organotellurium compounds: toxicology and pharmacology. *Chem Rev.* 2004;104:6255–6285.

Nordberg GF. Cadmium and health in the 21st century—historical remarks and trends for the future. *Biometals.* 2004;17:485–489.

Nordberg GF, Nogawa K, Nordberg M, *et al.* Cadmium. In: Nordberg GF, Fowler BA, Nordberg M, Friberg LT, eds. *Handbook on the Toxicology of Metals.* New York: Elsevier; 2007:445–486.

Novotny JA, Turnlund JR. Molybdenum kinetics in men differ during molybdenum depletion and repletion. *J Nutr.* 2006;136:953–977.

NRC. *Toxicological Effects of Methylmercury.* Committee on the Toxicological Effects of Methylmercury, Board on Environmental Studies and Toxicology, Commission on Life Sciences. Washington, DC: National Research Council, National Academy Press; 2000:1–344.

NRC. *Arsenic in the Drinking Water (Update).* Washington, DC: National Research Council, National Academy Press; 2001:1–225.

NTP. NTP toxicology and carcinogenesis studies of sodium fluoride (CAS no. 7681-49-4) in F344/N rats and B6C3F1 mice (drinking water studies). *Natl Toxicol Program Tech Rep Ser.* 1990;393:1–448.

NTP. Toxicology and carcinogenesis studies of indium phosphide (CAS no. 22398-90-7) in F344/N rats and B6C3F1 mice (inhalation studies). *Natl Toxicol Program Tech Ser.* 2001;499:7–340.

NTP. *Arsenic and Inorganic Arsenic Compounds.* National Toxicology Program Report on Carcinogens. 12th ed. Research Triangle Park, NC: NTP; 2011a:50–53.

NTP. *Beryllium and Beryllium Compounds.* National Toxicology Program Report on Carcinogens. 12th ed. Research Triangle Park, NC: NTP; 2011b:67–70.

NTP. *Cadmium and Cadmium Compounds.* National Toxicology Program Report on Carcinogenes. 12th ed. Research Triangle Park, NC: NTP; 2011c:80–83.

NTP. *Chromium Hexavalent Compounds.* National Toxicology Program Report on Carcinogens. 12th ed. Research Triangle Park, NC: NTP; 2011d:106–109.

NTP. *Nickel Compounds and Metallic Nickel.* National Toxicology Program Report on Carcinogens. 12th ed. Research Triangle Park, NC: NTP; 2011e:280–283.

NTP. *Cobalt Sulfate and Cobalt–Tungsten Carbide: Powders and Hard Metals.* National Toxicology Program Report on Carcinogens. 12th ed. Research Triangle Park, NC: NTP; 2011f:113–118.

NTP. *Selenium Sulfide.* National Toxicology Program Report on Carcinogens. 12th ed. Research Triangle Park, NC: NTP; 2011g:376–377.

NTP. *Cisplatin.* National Toxicology Program Report on Carcinogens. 12th ed. Research Triangle Park, NC: NTP; 2011h:110–111.

Oakley PW, Whyte IM, Carter GL. Lithium toxicity: an iatrogenic problem in susceptible individuals. *Aust N Z J Psychiatry.* 2001;35:833–840.

O'Brien TJ, Ceryak S, Patierno SR. Complexities of chromium carcinogenesis: role of cellular response, repair and recovery mechanisms. *Mutat Res.* 2003;533:3–36.

O'Connor ME, Rich D. Children with moderately elevated lead levels: is chelation with DMSA helpful? *Clin Pediatr (Phila).* 1999;38:325–331.

Oda K. Toxicity of a low level of indium phosphide (InP) in rats after intra-tracheal instillation. *Ind Health.* 1997;35:61–68.

Offerman SR, Alsop JA, Lee J, Holmes JF. Hospitalized lithium overdose cases reported to the California Poison Control System. *Clin Toxicol.* 2010;48:443–448.

Ogra Y. Toxicometallomics for research on the toxicology of exotic metalloids based on speciation studies. *Anal Sci.* 2009;25:1189–1195.

Olszewski U, Hamilton G. Mechanisms of cytotoxicity of anticancer agents. *Anticancer Agents Med Chem.* 2010;10:302–311.

Ostrakhovitch EA, Cherian MG. Tin. In: Nordberg GF, Fowler BA, Nordberg M, Friberg LT, eds. *Handbook on the Toxicology of Metals.* New York: Elsevier; 2007:839–859.

Papanikolaou G, Pantopoulos K. Iron metabolism and toxicity. *Toxicol Appl Pharmacol.* 2005;202:199–211.

Patrick L. Lead toxicity, a review of the literature. Part 1: exposure, evaluation, and treatment. *Altern Med Rev.* 2006;11:2–22.

Pearson G, Robinson F, Beers Gibson T, et al. Mitogen-activated protein (MAP) kinase pathways: regulation and physiological functions. *Endocr Rev.* 2001;22:153–183.

Pelkonen KH, Heinonen-Tanski H, Hanninen OO. Accumulation of silver from drinking water into cerebellum and musculus soleus in mice. *Toxicology.* 2003;186:151–157.

Pelletier L, Druet P. Immunotoxicology of metals. In: Goyer RA, Cherian MG. eds. *Handbook of Experimental Pharmacology.* Vol. 115. Heidelberg, Germany: Springer-Verlag; 1995:77–92.

Peter AL, Viraraghavan T. Thallium: a review of public health and environmental concerns. *Environ Int.* 2005;31:493–501.

Pi J, He Y, Bortner C, et al. Low level, long-term inorganic arsenite exposure causes generalized resistance to apoptosis in cultured human keratinocytes: potential role in skin co-carcinogenesis. *Int J Cancer.* 2005;116:20–26.

Pizarro F, Olivares M, Gidi V, Araya M. The gastrointestinal tract and acute effects of copper in drinking water and beverages. *Rev Environ Health.* 1999;14:231–238.

Plato CC, Garruto RM, Galasko D, et al. Amyotrophic lateral sclerosis and parkinsonism dementia complex of Guam: changing incidence rates during the past 60 years. *Am J Epidemiol.* 2003;157:149–157.

Pounds JG, Long GJ, Rosen JF. Cellular and molecular toxicity of lead in bone. *Environ Health Perspect.* 1991;91:17–32.

Prasad AS. Zinc deficiency: its characterization and treatment. *Met Ions Biol Syst.* 2004;41:103–137.

Prasad AS, Kucuk O. Zinc in cancer prevention. *Cancer Metastasis Rev.* 2002;21:291–295.

Proctor DM, Fredrick MM, Scott PK, et al. The prevalence of chromium allergy in the United States and its implications for setting soil cleanup: a cost-effectiveness case study. *Regul Toxicol Pharmacol.* 1998;28:27–37.

Prozialeck WC, Edwards JR. Early biomarkers of cadmium exposure and nephrotoxicity. *Biometals*. 2010;23:793–809.

Prozialeck WC, Wellington DR, Lamar PC. Comparison of the cytotoxic effects of cadmium chloride and cadmium–metallothionein in LLC-PK1 cells. *Life Sci*. 1993;53:PL337–PL342.

Qu W, Diwan BA, Liu J, et al. The metallothionein-null phenotype is associated with heightened sensitivity to lead toxicity and an inability to form inclusion bodies. *Am J Pathol*. 2002;160:1047–1056.

Quiroz JA, Gould TD, Manji HK. Molecular effects of lithium. *Mol Interv*. 2004;4:259–272.

Rahman MM, Chowdhury UK, Mukherjee SC, et al. Chronic arsenic toxicity in Bangladesh and West Bengal, India—a review and commentary. *J Toxicol Clin Toxicol*. 2001;39:683–700.

Ravindra K, Bencs L, Van Grieken R. Platinum group elements in the environment and their health risk. *Sci Total Environ*. 2004;318:1–43.

Ress NB, Chou BJ, Renne RA, et al. Carcinogenicity of inhaled vanadium pentoxide in F344/N rats and B6C3F1 mice. *Toxicol Sci*. 2003;74:287–296.

Risher JF, Amler SN. Mercury exposure: evaluation and intervention the inappropriate use of chelating agents in the diagnosis and treatment of putative mercury poisoning. *Neurotoxicology*. 2005;26:691–699.

Risher JF, Murray HE, Prince GR. Organic mercury compounds: human exposure and its relevance to public health. *Toxicol Ind Health*. 2002;18:109–160.

Rohl C, Sievers J. Microglia is activated by astrocytes in trimethyltin intoxication. *Toxicol Appl Pharmacol*. 2005;204:36–45.

Rondini EA, Walters DM, Bauer AK. Vanadium pentoxide induces pulmonary inflammation and tumor promotion in a strain-dependent manner. *Part Fibre Toxicol*. 2010;7:9.

Rosen BP. Transport and detoxification systems for transition metals, heavy metals and metalloids in eukaryotic and prokaryotic microbes. *Comp Biochem Physiol A Mol Integr Physiol*. 2002;133:689–693.

Rossman TG. Mechanism of arsenic carcinogenesis: an integrated approach. *Mutat Res*. 2003;533:37–65.

Rossman TG, Uddin AN, Burns FJ. Evidence that arsenite acts as a cocarcinogen in skin cancer. *Toxicol Appl Pharmacol*. 2004;198:394–404.

Roth JA, Garrick MD. Iron interactions and other biological reactions mediating the physiological and toxic actions of manganese. *Biochem Pharmacol*. 2003;66:1–13.

Roy S, Hardej D. Tellurium tetrachloride and diphenyl ditelluride cause cytotoxicity in rat hippocampal astrocytes. *Food Chem Toxicol*. 2011;49:2564–2574.

Rudel H. Case study: bioavailability of tin and tin compounds. *Ecotoxicol Environ Saf*. 2003;56:180–189.

Rungby J. An experimental study on silver in the nervous system and on aspects of its general cellular toxicity. *Dan Med Bull*. 1990;37:442–449.

Ryu DY, Lee S-J, Park DW, et al. Dietary iron regulates intestinal cadmium absorption through iron transporters in rats. *Toxicol Lett*. 2004;152:19–25.

Sahmoun AE, Case LD, Jackson SA, et al. Cadmium and prostate cancer: a critical epidemiologic analysis. *Cancer Invest*. 2005;23:256–263.

Sailer BL, Liles N, Dickerson S, et al. Organotellurium compound toxicity in a promyelocytic cell line compared to non-tellurium-containing organic analog. *Toxicol In Vitro*. 2004;18:475–482.

Santos DB, Schiar VPP, Paixão MW, et al. Hemolytic and genotoxic evaluation of organochalogens in human blood cells *in vitro*. *Toxicol In Vitro*. 2009;23:1195–1204.

Sanz MA, Lo-Coco F. Modern approaches to treating acute promyelocytic leukemia. *J Clin Oncol*. 2011;29:495–503.

Satarug S, Moore MR. Adverse health effects of chronic exposure to low-level cadmium in foodstuffs and cigarette smoke. *Environ Health Perspect*. 2004;112:1099–1103.

Satoh H. Palladium. In: Nordberg GF, Fowler BA, Nordberg M, eds. *Handbook on the Toxicology of Metals*. 3rd ed. New York: Elsevier; 2007:759–768.

Schnaas L, Rothenberg SJ, Flores M-F, et al. Reduced intellectual development I children with prenatal lead exposure. *Environ Health Perspect*. 2006;114:791–797.

Schwartz GG, Reis IM. Is cadmium a cause of human pancreatic cancer? *Cancer Epidemiol Biomarkers Prev*. 2000;9:139–145.

Schwarz G. Molybdenum cofactor biosynthesis and deficiency. *Cell Mol Life Sci*. 2005;62:2792–2810.

Sedman RM, Beaumont J, McDonald TA, et al. Review of the evidence regarding the carcinogenicity of hexavalent chromium in drinking water. *J Environ Sci Health C Environ Carcinog Ecotoxicol Rev*. 2006;24:155–182.

Selverstone Valentine J, Doucette PA, Zittin Potter S. Copper–zinc superoxide dismutase and amyotrophic lateral sclerosis. *Annu Rev Biochem*. 2005;74:563–593.

Sheppard SC, Sheppard MI, Gallerand MO, et al. Derivation of ecotoxicity thresholds for uranium. *J Environ Radioact*. 2005;79:55–83.

Shim H, Harris ZL. Genetic defects in copper metabolism. *J Nutr*. 2003;133(5 suppl 1):1527S–1531S.

Shinogi M, Maeizumi S. Effect of preinduction of metallothionein on tissue distribution of silver and hepatic lipid peroxidation. *Biol Pharm Bull*. 1993;16:372–374.

Shoults-Wilson WA, Zhurbich OI, McNear DH, et al. Evidence for avoidance of Ag nanoparticles by earthworms (*Eisenia fetida*). *Ecotoxicology*. 2011;20:385–396.

Silbergeld EK. Lead in bone: implications for toxicology during pregnancy and lactation. *Environ Health Perspect*. 1991;91:63–70.

Silbergeld EK. Facilitative mechanisms of lead as a carcinogen. *Mutat Res*. 2003;533:121–133.

Silbergeld EK, Sauk J, Somerman M, et al. Lead in bone: storage site, exposure source, and target organ. *Neurotoxicology*. 1993;14:225–236.

Silbergeld EK, Waalkes M, Rice JM. Lead as a carcinogen: experimental evidence and mechanisms of action. *Am J Ind Med*. 2000;38:316–323.

Sivulka DJ. Assessment of respiratory carcinogenicity associated with exposure to metallic nickel: a review. *Regul Toxicol Pharmacol*. 2005;43:117–133.

Sjögren B, Iregren A, Elinder CG, et al. Aluminum. In: Nordberg GF, Fowler BA, Nordberg M, Friberg LT, eds. *Handbook on the Toxicology of Metals*. New York: Elsevier; 2007:339–352.

Slikkerveer A, de Wolff FA. Toxicity of bismuth and its compounds. In: Chang LW, Magos L, Suzuki T, eds. *Toxicology of Metals*. New York: CRC Press; 1996:439–454.

Smith AH, Marshall G, Yuan Y, et al. Increased mortality from lung cancer and bronchiectasis in young adults after exposure to arsenic in utero and in early childhood. *Environ Health Perspect*. 2006;114:1293–1296.

Soni MG, White SM, Flamm WG, et al. Safety evaluation of dietary aluminum. *Regul Toxicol Pharmacol*. 2001;33:66–79.

Sparling DW, Lowe TP. Environmental hazards of aluminum to plants, invertebrates, fish, and wildlife. *Rev Environ Contam Toxicol*. 1996;145:1–127.

Sparsa A, Bonnetblanc JM. Lithium. *Ann Dermatol Venereol*. 2004;131:255–261.

Squibb KS, Leggett RW, McDiarmid MA. Prediction of renal concentrations of depleted uranium and radiation dose in Gulf War veterans with embedded shrapnel. *Health Phys*. 2005;89:267–273.

Srivastava S, Vladykovskaya EN, Haberzettl P, et al. Arsenic exacerbates atherosclerotic lesion formation and inflammation in ApoE–/– mice. *Toxicol Appl Pharmacol*. 2009;241:90–100.

Staessen JA, Buchet JP, Ginucchio G, et al. Public health implications of environmental exposure to cadmium and lead: an overview of epidemiological studies in Belgium. Working Groups. *J Cardiovasc Risk*. 1996;3:26–41.

Steenland K, Boffetta P. Lead and cancer in humans: where are we now? *Am J Ind Med*. 2000;38:295–299.

Stern BR. Essentiality and toxicity in copper health risk assessment: overview, update and regulatory considerations. *J Toxicol Environ Health A*. 2010;73:114–127.

Stoltenberg M, Juhl S, Poulsen EH. Autometallographic detection of silver in hypothalamic neurons of rats exposed to silver nitrate. *J Appl Toxicol*. 1994;14:275–280.

Stout MD, Nyska A, Bishop JB, et al. NTP toxicology and carcinogenesis studies of chromium picolinate monohydrate (CAS No. 27882-76-4) in F344/N rats and B6C3F1 mice (feed studies). *Natl Toxicol Program Tech Rep Ser*. 2010;556:1–194.

Straif K, Benbrahim-Tallaa L, Baan R, et al. A review of human carcinogens—part C: metals, arsenic, dusts, and fibres. *Lancet Oncol*. 2009;10:453–454.

Stringari J, Nunes AKC, Franco JL, et al. Prenatal methylmercury exposure hampers glutathione antioxidant system ontogenesis and causes long-lasting oxidative stress in the mouse brain. *Toxicol Appl Pharmacol.* 2008;227:147–154.

Sundar S, Chakravarty J. Antimony toxicity. *Int J Environ Res Public Health.* 2010;7:4267–4277.

Takeuchi A, Yoshizawa N, Oshima S, et al. Nephrotoxicity of germanium compounds: report of a case and review of the literature. *Nephron.* 1992;60:436–442.

Takeuchi T. Neuropathology of Minamata disease in Kumamoto: especially at the chronic stage. In: Roisin L, Shiaki H, Greevic N, eds. *Neurotoxicology.* New York: Raven Press; 1977:235–246.

Tanaka A. Toxicity of indium arsenide, gallium arsenide, and aluminium gallium arsenide. *Toxicol Appl Pharmacol.* 2004;198:405–411.

Tanaka A, Hisanaga A, Hirata M, et al. Chronic toxicity of indium arsenide and indium phosphide to the lungs of hamsters. *Fukuoka Igaku Zasshi.* 1996;87:108–115.

Tang J, Xiong L, Wang S, et al. Distribution, translocation and accumulation of silver nanoparticles in rats. *J Nanosci Nanotechnol.* 2009;9:4924–4932.

Tao SH, Bolger PM. Hazard assessment of germanium supplements. *Regul Toxicol Pharmacol.* 1997;25:211–219.

Tarantola M, Pietuch A, Schneider D, et al. Toxicity of gold-nanoparticles: synergistic effects of shape and surface functionalization on micromotility of epithelial cells. *Nanotoxicology.* 2011;5:254–268.

Taylor A. Biochemistry of tellurium. *Biol Trace Elem Res.* 1996;55:231–239.

Theil EC. Iron homeostasis and nutritional iron deficiency. *J Nutr.* 2011;141:724S–728S.

Thevenod F. Cadmium and cellular signaling cascades: to be or not to be? *Toxicol Appl Pharmacol.* 2009;238:221–239.

Thomas DJ, Li J, Waters SB, et al. Arsenic (+3 oxidation state) methyltransferase and the methylation of arsenicals. *Exp Biol Med.* 2007;232:3–13.

Thompson DF, Callen ED. Soluble or insoluble Prussian blue for radiocesium and thallium poisoning? *Ann Pharmacother.* 2004;38:1509–1514.

Thun MJ, Baker DB, Steenland K, et al. Renal toxicity in uranium mill workers. *Scand J Work Environ Health.* 1985;11:83–90.

Tillman LA, Drake FM, Dixon JS, et al. Review article: safety of bismuth in the treatment of gastrointestinal diseases. *Aliment Pharmacol Ther.* 1996;10:459–467.

Timmer RT, Sands JM. Lithium intoxication. *J Am Soc Nephrol.* 1999;10:666–674.

Tinkle SS, Antonini JM, Rich BA. Skin as a route of exposure and sensitization in chronic beryllium disease. *Environ Health Perspect.* 2003;111:1202–1208.

Tjalve H, Henriksson J. Uptake of metals in the brain via olfactory pathways. *Neurotoxicology.* 1999;20:181–195.

Tokar EJ, Benbrahim-Tallaa L, Ward JM, et al. Cancer in experimental animals exposed to arsenic and arsenic compounds. *Crit Rev Toxicol.* 2010a;40:912–927.

Tokar EJ, Diwan BA, Waalkes MP. Early life inorganic lead exposure induces testicular teratoma and renal and urinary bladder preneoplasia in adult metallothionein-knockout mice but not in wild type mice. *Toxicology.* 2010b;276:5–10.

Tokar EJ, Qu W, Waalkes MP. Arsenic, stem cells, and the developmental basis of adult cancer. *Toxicol Sci.* 2011;120(suppl 1):S192–S203.

Tseng CH. Cardiovascular disease in arsenic-exposed subjects living in the arseniasis hyperendemic areas in Taiwan. *Atherosclerosis.* 2008;199:12–18.

Tümer Z, Møller LB. Menkes disease. *Eur J Hum Genet.* 2010;18:511–518.

Ueshima K. Magnesium and ischemic heart disease: a review of epidemiological, experimental, and clinical evidences. *Magnes Res.* 2005;18:275–284.

Valko M, Morris H, Cronin MT. Metals, toxicity and oxidative stress. *Curr Med Chem.* 2005;12:1161–1208.

Valko M, Rhodes CJ, Moncol J, et al. Free radicals, metals and antioxidants in oxidative stress induced cancer. *Chem Biol Interact.* 2006;160:1–40.

Vaziri ND, Sica DA. Lead-induced hypertension: role of oxidative stress. *Curr Hypertens Rep.* 2004;6:314–320.

Victery W. Evidence for effects of chronic lead exposure on blood pressure in experimental animals: an overview. *Environ Health Perspect.* 1988;78:71–76.

Vincent JB. Recent developments in the biochemistry of chromium(III). *Biol Trace Elem Res.* 2004;99:1–16.

Viol GW, Minielly JA, Bistricki T. Gold nephropathy: tissue analysis by X-ray fluorescent spectroscopy. *Arch Pathol Lab Med.* 1977;101:635–640.

von Lindren IH, Spalinger SM, Bero BN, et al. The influence of soil remediation on lead in house dust. *Sci Total Environ.* 2003;303:59–78.

Vouk VB. General chemistry of metals. In: Friberg L, Nordberg GF, Vouk VB, eds. *Handbook on the Toxicology of Metals.* New York: Elsevier; 1986:14–35.

Vyskocil A, Viau C. Assessment of molybdenum toxicity in humans. *J Appl Toxicol.* 1999;19:185–192.

Waalkes M. Cadmium carcinogenesis. *Mutat Res.* 2003;533:107–120.

Waalkes MP, Diwan BA, Ward JM, et al. Renal tubular tumors and atypical hyperplasias in B6C3F1 mice exposed to lead acetate during gestation and lactation occur with minimal chronic nephropathy. *Cancer Res.* 1995;55:5265–5271.

Waalkes MP, Fox DA, States JC, et al. Metals and disorders of cell accumulation: modulation of apoptosis and cell proliferation. *Toxicol Sci.* 2000;56:255–261.

Waalkes MP, Liu J, Goyer RA, Diwan BA. Metallothionein-I/II double knockout mice are hypersensitive to lead-induced kidney carcinogenesis: role of inclusion body formation. *Cancer Res.* 2004;64:7766–7772.

Waalkes MP, Liu J, Kasprzak KS, et al. Hypersusceptibility to cisplatin carcinogenicity in metallothionein-I/II double knockout mice: production of hepatocellular carcinoma at clinically relevant doses. *Int J Cancer.* 2006;119:28–32.

Waisberg M, Joseph P, Hale B, Beyersmann D. Molecular and cellular mechanisms of cadmium carcinogenesis. *Toxicology.* 2003;192:95–117.

Wang C, Bhattacharyya MH. Effect of cadmium on bone calcium and 45Ca in nonpregnant mice on a calcium-deficient diet: evidence of direct effect of cadmium on bone. *Toxicol Appl Pharmacol.* 1993;120:228–239.

Wang J, Pantopoulos K. Regulation of cellular iron metabolism. *Biochem J.* 2011;434:365–381.

Wang X. Fresh platinum complexes with promising antitumor activity. *Anticancer Agents Med Chem.* 2010;10:396–411.

Wang XW, Hussain SP, Huo TI, et al. Molecular pathogenesis of human hepatocellular carcinoma. *Toxicology.* 2002;181–182:43–47.

Warheit DB, Brock WJ, Lee KP, et al. Comparative pulmonary toxicity inhalation and instillation studies with different TiO2 particle formulations: impact of surface treatments on particle toxicity. *Toxicol Sci.* 2005;88:514–524.

Warheit DB, Webb TR, Sayes CM, et al. Pulmonary instillation studies with nanoscale TiO2 rods and dots in rats: toxicity is not dependent upon particle size and surface area. *Toxicol Sci.* 2006;91:227–236.

Warniment C, Tsang K, Galazka SS. Lead poisoning in children. *Am Fam Physician.* 2010;81:751–757.

Watjen W, Benters J, Haase H, et al. Zn2+ and Cd2+ increase the cyclic GMP level in PC12 cells by inhibition of the cyclic nucleotide phosphodiesterase. *Toxicology.* 2001;157:167–175.

Weinberg ED. The hazards of iron loading. *Metallomics.* 2010;2:732–740.

Westervelt P, Brown RA, Adkins DR, et al. Sudden death among patients with acute promyelocytic leukemia treated with arsenic trioxide. *Blood.* 2001;98:266–271.

WHO. *IPCS Environmental Health Criteria. Tin and Organotin Compounds: A Preliminary Review.* Vol. 15. Geneva: World Health Organization; 1980.

WHO. *IPCS Environmental Health Criteria. Beryllium.* Vol. 106. Geneva: World Health Organization; 1990a:1–210.

WHO. *IPCS Environmental Health Criteria. Cadmium.* Vol. 134. Geneva: World Health Organization; 1990b:1–220.

WHO. *IPCS Environmental Health Criteria. Platinum.* Vol. 125. Geneva: World Health Organization; 1991:1–167.

WHO. *IPCS Environmental Health Criteria. Thallium.* Vol. 182. Geneva: World Health Organization; 1996.

WHO. *IPCS Environmental Health Criteria. Aluminum.* Vol. 194. Geneva: World Health Organization; 1997:1–282.

WHO. *IPCS Environmental Health Criteria. Copper.* Vol. 200. Geneva: World Health Organization; 1998a:1–360.

WHO. *IPCS Environmental Health Criteria. Zinc.* Vol. 221. Geneva: World Health Organization; 1998b:1–360.

WHO. *IPCS Environmental Health Criteria. Palladium.* Vol. 226. Geneva: World Health Organization; 2002:1–201.

Wiesenthal A, Hunter L, Wang S, et al. Nanoparticles: small and mighty. *Int J Dermatol.* 2011;50:247–254.

Wild D, Frischknecht M, Zhang H, et al. Alpha- versus beta-particle radiopeptide therapy in a human prostate cancer model (213Bi-DOTA-PESIN and 213Bi-AMBA versus 177Lu-DOTA-PESIN). *Cancer Res.* 2011;71:1009–1018.

Winship KA. Toxicity of tin and its compounds. *Adverse Drug React Acute Poisoning Rev.* 1988;7:19–38.

Wirth JJ, Mijal RS. Adverse effects of low level heavy metal exposure on male reproductive function. *Syst Biol Reprod Med.* 2010;56:147–167.

Wu Y, Yang X, Ge J, et al. Blood lead level and its relationship to certain essential elements in the children aged 0 to 14 years from Beijing, China. *Sci Total Environ.* 2011;409:3016–3020.

Xiao T, Guha J, Boyle D, et al. Environmental concerns related to high thallium levels in soils and thallium uptake by plants in southwest Guizhou, China. *Sci Total Environ.* 2004;318:223–244.

Xu X, Pin S, Gathinji M, et al. Aceruloplasminemia: an inherited neurodegenerative disease with impairment of iron homeostasis. *Ann N Y Acad Sci.* 2004;1012:299–305.

Yates AA, Trumbo P, Schlicker S, et al. Dietary reference intakes: vitamin A, vitamin K, arsenic, boron, chromium, copper, iodine, iron, manganese, molybdenum, nickel, silicon, vanadium, and zinc. *J Am Diet Assoc.* 2001;101:294–301.

Yokel RA. Blood–brain barrier flux of aluminum, manganese, iron and other metals suspected to contribute to metal-induced neurodegeneration. *J Alzheimers Dis.* 2006;10:223–253.

Yu HS, Lee CH, Chen GS. Peripheral vascular diseases resulting from chronic arsenical poisoning. *J Dermatol.* 2002;29:123–130.

Yu S, Beynen AC. High tin intake reduces copper status in rats through inhibition of copper absorption. *Br J Nutr.* 1995;73:863–869.

Yuan XM, Li W. The iron hypothesis of atherosclerosis and its clinical impact. *Ann Med.* 2003;35:578–591.

Zalpus RK, Ahmad S. Molecular handling of cadmium in transporting epithelia. *Toxicol Appl Pharmacol.* 2003;186:163–188.

Zalpus RK, Koropatnick J. *Molecular Biology and Toxicology of Metals.* New York: Taylor & Francis; 2000.

Zeng H, Uthus EO, Combs GF Jr. Mechanistic aspects of the interaction between selenium and arsenic. *J Inorg Biochem.* 2005;99:1269–1274.

Zheng W. Toxicology of choroid plexus: special reference to metal-induced neurotoxicities. *Microsc Res Tech.* 2001;52:89–103.

Zheng W, Winter SM, Kattnig MJ, et al. Tissue distribution and elimination of indium in male Fischer 344 rats following oral and intratracheal administration of indium phosphide. *J Toxicol Environ Health.* 1994;43:483–494.

Zhitkovich A. Importance of chromium–DNA adducts in mutagenicity and toxicity of chromium(VI). *Chem Res Toxicol.* 2005;18:3–11.

Ziegler EE, Edwards BB, Jensen RL, et al. Absorption and retention of lead by infants. *Pediatr Res.* 1978;12:29–34.

Ziegler EE, Filer LJ, eds. *Present Knowledge in Nutrition.* Washington, DC: ILSI; 1996:1–684.

chapter 24

Toxic Effects of Solvents and Vapors

James V. Bruckner, S. Satheesh Anand,
and D. Alan Warren

INTRODUCTION

The term *solvent* refers to a class of organic chemicals of variable lipophilicity and volatility. These properties, coupled with small molecular size and lack of charge, make inhalation the major route of exposure and provide for ready absorption across membranes of the lung, gastrointestinal (GI) tract, and skin. In general, the lipophilicity of solvents increases with increasing numbers of carbon and/or halogen atoms, while volatility decreases. Organic solvents are frequently used to dissolve, dilute, or disperse materials that are insoluble in water. As such they are widely employed as degreasers and as constituents of paints, varnishes, lacquers, inks, aerosol spray products, dyes, and adhesives. Other uses are as intermediates in chemical synthesis, and as fuels and fuel additives. Most organic solvents are refined from petroleum. Many such as naphthas and

gasoline are complex mixtures, often consisting of hundreds of compounds. Early in the 20th century, there were perhaps a dozen or so known and commonly used solvents. By 1981, this number had climbed to approximately 350 (OSHA, 2006).

Solvents are classified largely according to molecular structure or functional group. Classes of solvents include aliphatic hydrocarbons, many of which are halogenated (ie, halocarbons), aromatic hydrocarbons, alcohols, ethers, esters/acetates, amides/amines, aldehydes, ketones, and complex mixtures that defy classification. The main determinants of a solvent's inherent toxicity are: (1) its number of carbon atoms; (2) whether it is saturated or has double or triple bonds between adjacent carbon atoms; (3) its configuration (ie, straight chain, branched chain, or cyclic); (4) whether it is halogenated; and (5) the presence of functional groups. Some

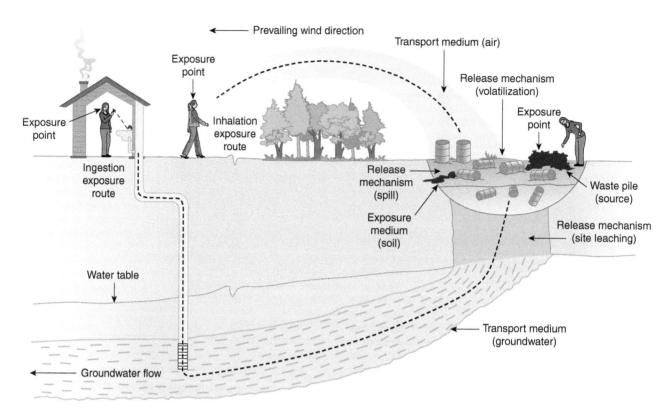

Figure 24-1. *Solvent exposure pathways and media.* (Adapted from EPA, 1989.)

class-wide generalizations regarding toxicity can be made. For example, the more lipophilic a hydrocarbon, the more potent a central nervous system (CNS) depressant it is; amides/amines tend to be potent sensitizers; aldehydes are particularly irritating; hydrocarbons that are extensively metabolized tend to be more cytotoxic/mutagenic; and many unsaturated, short-chain halocarbons are animal carcinogens. The toxicity of solvents within the same class can vary dramatically. For example, both 1,1,1-trichloroethane (TRI) and 1,1,2-trichloroethylene (TCE) are halocarbons with three chlorine atoms, yet unsaturated TCE is carcinogenic in the rat and mouse, but TRI is not. Similar results have been reported for 2,4- and 2,6-diaminotoluene in rodents, as only the 2,4-isomer is capable of inducing significant hepatocyte proliferation and liver tumors. Slight structural differences in solvent metabolites are also of toxicological consequence. The peripheral neuropathy induced by *n*-hexane and 2-hexanone is dependent on the production of the γ-diketone metabolite 2,5-hexanedione. Diketones lacking the gamma structure are not neurotoxic. Thus, subtle differences in chemical structure can translate into dramatic differences in toxicity.

Nearly everyone is exposed to solvents during their normal activities. Consider, for example, a person who works in an aircraft factory as a metal degreaser (TCE exposure), drives to the neighborhood bar after work and has a few drinks (ethanol exposure) and cigarettes (benzene and styrene exposure), stops on the way home at a self-service filling station for gasoline (benzene, toluene, 1,3-butadiene, etc, exposure) and the dry cleaner's for laundry (tetrachloroethylene [PERC] exposure), and after dinner enjoys his hobby of model shipbuilding that requires the use of glue (toluene exposure). While everyone may not identify with the above scenario, detailed surveys of indoor and outdoor air, such as the Environmental Protection Agency's (EPA's) Total Exposure Assessment Methodology (TEAM) and National Human Exposure Assessment Survey (NHEXAS) studies, indicate that airborne solvent exposure is unavoidable (Wallace, 1990; Clayton *et al.*, 1999). Drinking water is also a common source

of solvent exposure due to discharge of solvents into surface and groundwaters and the presence of disinfection by-products, including the animal carcinogen chloroform ($CHCl_3$). Trichloroacetic acid (TCA) and dichloroacetic acid (DCA), metabolites of TCE and PERC, are also common drinking water disinfection by-products.

Environmental exposures to solvents in air and groundwater are frequent subjects of toxic tort litigation, despite concentrations that are typically in the low parts per billion (ppb) or parts per trillion (ppt) ranges. Multiple exposure pathways frequently exist (Fig. 24-1). Although not represented in Fig. 24-1, household use of solvent-contaminated water may result in solvent intake from inhalation and dermal absorption as well as ingestion (Weisel and Jo, 1996; Nuckols *et al.*, 2005). In many cases, risk assessment guidelines stipulate that risks be determined for physiologically diverse individuals who are exposed to several solvents by multiple exposure pathways. As an aid to the risk assessment process, the US EPA has derived toxicity factors for many of the most common solvents. These toxicity factors are referred to as reference concentrations (RfCs), reference doses (RfDs), and cancer slope factors (CSFs). Values for a number of these are available from the EPA's online Integrated Risk Information System (IRIS). Additional sources of exposure guidelines for non-cancer end points are found in the *Toxicological Profiles* of the US Agency for Toxic Substances and Disease Registry (ATSDR). These profiles often contain minimal risk levels (MRLs) that are derived in a similar manner to EPA's RfCs and RfDs, but are frequently based on different critical studies or derived with different uncertainty factors.

Occupational solvent exposures involve situations ranging from a secretary using typewriter correction fluid to the loading and off-loading of tanker trucks with thousands of gallons of gasoline. The greatest industrial use of solvents is as metal degreasers. This work environment is typically where the highest exposures occur, mainly via inhalation and secondarily via dermal contact. An estimated 10 million people are potentially exposed to organic solvents in the workplace (OSHA, 2006). Many of the most severe exposures to solvents have occurred as a result of their use in confined spaces with inadequate ventilation. While the US Occupational Safety and Health Administration (OSHA) has established legally enforceable permissible exposure limits (PELs) for over 100 solvents, most PELs are outdated. The majority of existing PELs were adopted from a list of threshold limit values (TLVs) previously published by the American Conference of Governmental Industrial Hygienists (ACGIH). Many current TLVs are more stringent than PELs but do not carry the weight of law. Whereas the ACGIH's TLVs for an eight-hour workday, 40-hour workweek are designed to be protective for a working lifetime, its short-term exposure limits (STELs) and ceiling values are designed to protect against the acute effects of high-level, short-term solvent exposure. If warranted, ACGIH will assign a skin notation to a solvent, indicating that a significant contribution to overall exposure is possible by the dermal route, by either contact with vapors or direct skin contact with the liquid. ACGIH also categorizes chemicals for carcinogenicity in animals and humans. Biological monitoring in the workplace should find increasing use as technologic advances are made, because it often provides a better measure of exposure than classic industrial hygiene monitoring. The ACGIH has published over 50 Biological Exposure Indices (BEIs), on which basis the safety of internal measures of exposure can be judged (ACGIH, 2012).

Most solvent exposures involve a mixture of chemicals, rather than a single compound (see the section "Solvent Mixtures"). Our knowledge of the toxicity of solvent mixtures is rudimentary relative to the toxicology of individual solvents. While the assumption is frequently made that the toxic effects of solvents are additive, the chemicals may also interact synergistically or antagonistically. For example, repetitive alcohol consumption induces certain cytochrome P450s (CYPs), and may therefore enhance the metabolic activation of other solvents to cytotoxic metabolites. Ethanol intake near the time of exposure to such solvents, in contrast, may competitively inhibit their metabolism and be protective. Another well-characterized example of solvent antagonism is the competitive metabolic interaction between benzene and toluene (Medinsky et al., 1994). Coexposure to these chemicals results in diminished benzene metabolism, genotoxicity, and erythropoietic toxicity relative to that which follows benzene exposure alone. It is now recognized that significant data gaps exist in the area of mixtures toxicology, and that these can be significant sources of uncertainty in risk assessments. Physiologically based toxicokinetic (PBTK) models are being developed by different research groups to predict the impact of metabolic induction and inhibition on the kinetics of individual components of specific mixtures (see the section "Physiological Modeling").

Although some solvents are much less hazardous than others, virtually all can cause adverse effects. Provided that the dose or concentration is sufficient, most have the potential to induce some level of narcosis and cause respiratory and mucous membrane irritation. A number of solvents are animal carcinogens, but only a handful have been classified as known human carcinogens. Herein lies a major challenge for toxicology—determining the human relevance of tumors observed in chronic, high-dose rodent studies. As with other chemicals, whether adverse health effects occur from solvent exposure is dependent on several factors: (1) toxicity/carcinogenicity of the solvent; (2) exposure route; (3) amount or rate of exposure; (4) duration of exposure; (5) individual susceptibility; and (6) interactions with other chemicals. Adverse health effects may occur acutely and be readily discernible, or they may result from chronic exposure and have insidious onset. Numerous epidemiological studies of environmentally and occupationally exposed populations have been conducted for some solvents, but most human risk assessments remain heavily reliant on extrapolation from high-dose animal studies. One must bear in mind that the toxic effects and their underlying mechanisms discussed herein may be operative only in certain animal species or strains and under certain exposure conditions. Care must therefore be taken in generalizing beyond the experimental conditions under which data are collected. While a relatively small number of commercially available solvents is discussed in this chapter, those selected for discussion are thought to best demonstrate principles of solvent toxicology, are of particular commercial importance, and/or are currently garnering significant attention from the toxicological and regulatory communities. A book chapter that examines solvents from an organ systems standpoint, in contrast to discussion of individual solvents, is that of Gerr and Letz (1998).

IS THERE A SOLVENT-INDUCED CHRONIC ENCEPHALOPATHY?

The CNS depressant effects of acute, high-level exposures and the potential for permanent neurologic damage in chronic solvent abusers are not a matter of debate. It is also clear that chronic, moderate-to-high-level exposure to a few solvents such as n-hexane and carbon disulfide (CS_2) can cause specific degenerative changes in the CNS or the peripheral nervous system (PNS). Far less clear is whether chronic, low-level exposure to virtually any solvent or solvent mixture can produce a pattern of neurologic dysfunction referred to as *painters' syndrome, organic solvent syndrome, psychoorganic syndrome, and chronic solvent encephalopathy* (CSE). CSE is characterized by nonspecific symptoms (eg, headache, fatigue, mood disturbances, and sleep disorders) with or without changes in neuropsychological function. There is a reversible form of CSE referred to as *neuroasthenic syndrome* that consists of symptoms only, and both "mild" and "severe" forms accompanied by objective signs of neuropsychological dysfunction that may or may not be fully reversible. This syndrome was first described in the Scandinavian occupational literature in the late 1970s, in solvent-exposed painters (Axelson et al., 1976; Arlien-Soborg et al., 1979). Since that time, numerous studies from Scandinavia have been published purporting that solvents as a class have chronic neurotoxic properties. These countries, as well as a few others in Europe (ie, Germany, Austria, and Belgium), have passed legislation recognizing CSE as a compensable occupational disability (Triebig and Hallermann, 2001). Scientists outside of Scandinavia, including many in the United States, have generally been less willing to recognize CSE as a legitimate disease state and have published studies to the contrary (Triebig et al., 1988; Bleecker et al., 1991; Spurgeon et al., 1994).

In response to the numerous reports of CSE, two conferences were convened in 1985. The first was held in Copenhagen by the Nordic Council of the World Health Organization (WHO, 1985). The second, in Raleigh, North Carolina, was attended by an international group of scientists from academia, industry, and government (Cranmer, 1986). The categorization scheme that resulted from the Raleigh meeting is presented in Table 24-1. The WHO scheme is similar. Among those who utilize the categorization scheme, it is generally believed that the most severe CSE category, type 3, results from repeated, severe intoxications like those experienced by solvent abusers. CSE types 1 and 2, on the other hand, are thought to be associated with prolonged, low-to-moderate-level exposure common to work environments. A major criticism of the categorization scheme is the lack of consideration of inhaled solvent concentration and exposure duration. While no consensus exists, even most CSE proponents believe that solvent exposure must occur for approximately 10 years before clinical symptoms are manifest. Citing growing acceptance of CSE outside of Scandinavia, some scientists and

Table 24-1

Proposed Categories of Solvent-Induced Encephalopathy

CATEGORY	CLINICAL MANIFESTATIONS
Type 1	*Symptoms only*: The patient complains of nonspecific symptoms such as fatigability, memory impairment, difficulty in concentration, and loss of initiative. These symptoms are reversible if exposure is discontinued, and there is no objective evidence of neuropsychiatric dysfunction
Type 2A	*Sustained personality or mood change*: There is a marked and sustained change in personality involving fatigue, emotional lability, impulse control, and general mood and motivation
Type 2B	*Impairment in intellectual function*: There is difficulty in concentration, impairment of memory, and a decrease in learning capacity. These symptoms are accompanied by objective evidence of impairment. There may also be minor neurologic signs. The complete reversibility of type 2B is questionable
Type 3	*Dementia*: In this condition, marked global deterioration in intellect and memory is often accompanied by neurologic signs and/or neuroradiologic findings. This condition is, at best, poorly reversible, but is generally nonprogressive once exposure has ceased

SOURCE: Reproduced from Cranmer (1986), with permission from Elsevier.

physicians advocate for refinement of existing diagnostic criteria and a unified categorization scheme (van der Hoek *et al.*, 2000, 2001).

CSE researchers typically rely on self-reported symptoms and a clinical neuropsychological evaluation (Table 24-2), and to a much lesser extent on diagnostic tests such as electroencephalography and computerized brain tomography. It has been argued that the neuropsychological tests are of questionable validity, sensitivity, specificity, and predictive value. It has also been noted that many investigations of CSE are fraught with methodological flaws. For example, CSE investigators frequently fail to measure premorbid function

Table 24-2

Functions that may be Assessed in a Neuropsychological Evaluation

Psychomotor functions
    Reaction time
    Motor speed and dexterity
    Eye–hand coordination
Sustained attention/concentration and perceptual speed
Verbal and nonverbal memory
    Immediate memory
    Delayed memory
Learning
Visual constructive ability
Conceptual ability
Evaluation of personality and affect

SOURCE: Reproduced from Cranmer (1986), with permission from Elsevier.

or intellect; employ a reference population; control adequately for the potential confounders of age, alcohol use, other CNS diseases, and other chemicals; corroborate functional deficits with objective evidence of brain disease; and/or examine exposure–response relationships. The importance of doing so is best exemplified by the reanalysis of individuals originally reported in the seminal study by Arlien-Soborg *et al.* (1979) to have "painters' syndrome." When the influences of age, education, and intelligence were considered, the previously reported reduction in neuropsychological test scores disappeared (Gade *et al.*, 1988). Another example is that of Cherry *et al.* (1985), who demonstrated the importance of matching solvent-exposed and control groups for preexposure intellect before making a diagnosis of CSE. More recently, Albers *et al.* (2000) reportedly found no objective evidence of toxic encephalopathy among 52 railroad workers with long-term solvent exposure and diagnosis of CSE.

It is evident that resolution of the controversial issue of CSE will come only through the conduct of well-designed and controlled epidemiological studies, especially considering the absence of an appropriate animal model. Brief, but insightful reviews of CSE by Rosenberg (1995) and Schaumburg and Spencer (2000) have been published. These reviews conclude that the current literature, including the "landmark" North American study of 187 paint-manufacturing workers (Bleecker *et al.*, 1991), does not support chronic low-level solvent exposure as a cause of *symptomatic* CNS or PNS dysfunction. This does not preclude, however, the possibility that such exposure can be associated with *subclinical* cognitive dysfunction in the form of slight psychomotor and attentional deficit disorders. For the viewpoint of CSE proponents, readers are directed to texts by Arlien-Soborg (1992) and Kilburn (1998).

SOLVENT ABUSE

Inhalants are volatile substances that can be inhaled to induce a psychoactive or mind-altering effect. Their abuse has become a major drug problem worldwide, particularly in disadvantaged populations and among adolescents (Williams and Storck, 2007). The epidemiology of inhalant abuse in the United States is receiving considerable attention (Spiller, 2004; Wu *et al.*, 2004), with almost 13.1% 8th graders claiming to have used inhalants according to a recent National Institute on Drug Abuse (NIDA)–sponsored survey (Johnston *et al.*, 2008). Solvents are among the most popular classes of drugs of abuse, given their presence in a multitude of inexpensive, readily available products that are legal to buy and possess. These products are used for common household and industrial purposes and include paint thinners and removers, dry-cleaning fluids, degreasers, gasoline, glues, typewriter fluid, nail polish remover, felt-tip marker fluids, and aerosols such as fabric protector sprays and spray paints. Solvents are often among the first drugs used by children and adolescents. Early use of inhalants is often a precursor to abuse of multiple illegal substances (Wu *et al.*, 2004). Research suggests that adverse socioeconomic conditions, a history of child abuse, poor grades, and dropping out of school are all factors contributing to inhalant abuse (NIDA, 2012).

Solvent abuse is a unique exposure situation in that participants repeatedly subject themselves to vapor concentrations high enough to produce effects that resemble alcohol intoxication. Solvents can be breathed in through the nose or the mouth by "sniffing" or "snorting" vapors from containers, spraying aerosols directly into the nose or mouth, "bagging" by inhaling vapors from a plastic or paper bag, or "huffing" from a solvent-soaked rag stuffed into the mouth (NIDA, 2012). Although dependent on the pattern of inhalation, blood levels of solvents typically peak a few minutes after inhalation begins, and the abuser can begin to experience effects after a matter of seconds. While intoxication may last only a few minutes, abusers frequently seek to prolong the "high" by inhaling repeatedly over the course of several hours. In extreme circumstances, death may be a consequence of cardiac arrhythmias, asphyxiation, and/or cachexia.

Relatively little is known about the neuropharmacology of abused solvents, although they appear to have much in common with the classical CNS depressant drugs such as ethanol and barbiturates, including the potential for tolerance and dependence (Balster, 1998). Commonly used solvents have been shown to alter the function of a variety of ligand-gated ion channels, including those activated by glycine, gamma-aminobutyric acid (GABA), and N-methyl-D-aspartate (NMDA) (Beckstead et al., 2000; Cruz et al., 2000). Recent evidence links high-level toluene exposure in rats to increased dopaminergic neurotransmission within the mesolimbic reward pathway, an effect thought to underlie the abuse potential of numerous drugs (Reigel and French, 2002; Reigel et al., 2004). Toluene, as well as TCE and TRI, has been shown to enhance serotonin-3 receptor function, which has also been implicated in the reinforcing properties of abused drugs (Lopreato et al., 2003).

Whereas the intoxicating effects achieved through acute solvent abuse are reversible, abuse may be continued for years and result in residual organ damage. For example, chronic abuse of products containing n-hexane and methyl-n-butyl ketone can cause peripheral neuropathies. Blood dyscrasias, liver damage, kidney injury, and hearing impairment are seen in patients who have abused solvents injurious to these organs. It has been known for some time that the brain is not spared residual damage, with long-term neurologic and psychological sequelae (Caldemeyer et al., 1996; Lubman et al., 2008). Rosenberg et al. (2002) reported increased incidences of neurologic and neuropsychological effects in chronic solvent abusers compared with a control group of chronic drug abusers. Solvent abusers did significantly worse on tests of working memory and executive cognitive function, and a much higher percentage of the patients (44.0% vs 25.5%) had structural abnormalities in subcortical regions of the brain (ie, basal ganglia, cerebellum, pons, and thalamus) as visualized by MRI (Fig. 24-2). Solvent abusers also showed moderate to severe diffuse abnormality of the

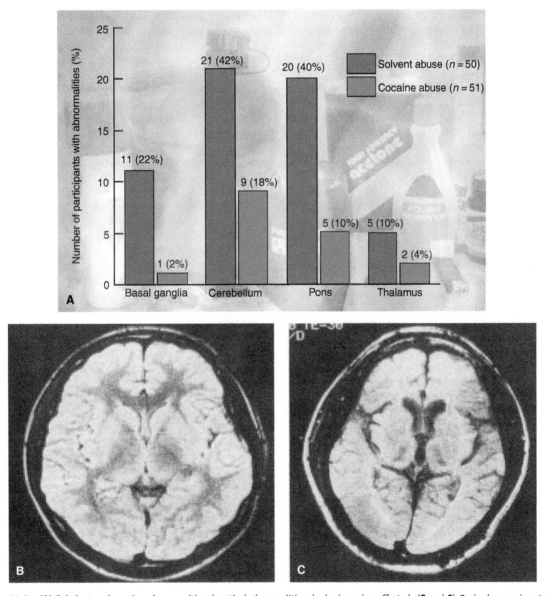

Figure 24-2. *(A) Inhalant and cocaine abusers with subcortical abnormalities, by brain region affected. (B and C) Brain damage in a toluene abuser.* (A) Magnetic resonance imaging (MRI) scans of chronic inhalant abusers and chronic cocaine abusers showed more frequent occurrence of abnormalities in the basal ganglia, cerebellum, pons, and thalamus for those who abused solvents. (Methias, 2002.) MRI shows marked atrophy (shrinkage) of brain tissue in a toluene abuser (C) compared with a nonabusing individual (B). Note the smaller size and the larger empty (dark) space within the toluene abuser's brain. The white outer circle in each image is the skull. (Available electronically at http://www.drugabuse.gov/PDF/RRInhalants.pdf.) (Courtesy of Neil Rosenberg, MD, as published in NIDA *Research Report Series*, March 2012.)

cerebral white matter, consistent with that seen in earlier studies of neuropsychologically impaired toluene abusers (Rosenberg *et al.*, 1988a,b). This condition was termed "white matter dementia," as myelinated neurons are white in appearance. It was characterized primarily by diffuse cerebral, cerebellar, and brainstem atrophy, and ventricular enlargement (Fig. 24-2). Dementia in toluene abusers has been referred to as "toluene leukoencephalopathy" (Filley *et al.*, 2004). Leukoencephalopathy, also known as multifocal demyelinating disease, involves structural alteration of cerebral white matter, in which the myelin sheaths that cover nerve fibers are destroyed but axons are largely spared. Thus, toluene is among a long list of white matter toxins identified to date.

ENVIRONMENTAL CONTAMINATION

Widespread use of solvents has resulted in their dissemination throughout the environment (Fig. 24-1). Everyone is exposed daily to solvents, as reflected by their common occurrence in blood of nonoccupationally exposed populations (Churchill *et al.*, 2001; Sexton *et al.*, 2005; Blount *et al.*, 2006). Because solvents as a chemical class are volatile, the preponderance of solvents entering the environment does so by evaporation. The majority of the more volatile organic chemicals (VOCs) volatilize when products containing them (eg, aerosol propellants, paint thinners, cleaners, and soil fumigants) are used as intended. Solvent loss into the atmosphere also occurs during production, processing, storage, and transport activities, resulting in elevated concentrations in air in the proximity of point sources. Winds dilute and disperse solvent vapors across the world. Atmospheric concentrations of most VOCs are usually extremely low (ie, nondetectable to nanograms or a few micrograms per cubic meter of air). Relatively high atmospheric concentrations of certain solvents (eg, 10–520 $\mu g/m^3$, or 3–163 ppb of benzene) have been measured in urban areas, around petrochemical plants, and in the immediate vicinity of hazardous waste sites. Motor vehicle exhaust is a major contributor to hydrocarbon emissions (Mohamed *et al.*, 2002). Fraser *et al.* (1998) measured very high levels of benzene, toluene, ethylbenzene, and xylenes in a Los Angeles roadway tunnel.

Solvent contamination of drinking water supplies is a major health concern. Although the majority of a solvent spilled onto the ground evaporates, some may permeate the soil and migrate through it until reaching groundwater or an impermeable material. In years past, the more lipophilic solvents were generally regarded as water insoluble. It is now recognized that all solvents are soluble in water to some extent. Some (eg, alcohols, ketones, glycols, and glycol ethers) are freely water soluble. Maximum solubilities of some common hydrocarbon solvents range from 10 mg/L (ppm) for *n*-hexane to 24,000 ppm for bromochloromethane. High concentrations of VOCs are sometimes found in the effluent of facilities of rubber producers, chemical companies, petrochemical plants, and paper mills. Concentrations diminish rapidly after VOCs enter bodies of water, primarily due to dilution and evaporation. VOCs in waters rise to the surface or sink to the bottom, according to their density. VOCs on the surface will largely evaporate. VOCs on the bottom must depend on solubilization in the water or mixing by current or wave action to reach the surface. VOCs in groundwater tend to remain trapped until the water reaches the surface, although some are subject to microbial modification. Concentrations in well water are rarely high enough for acute or subacute toxicity to be of concern. The very low levels of some solvents typically found in water have, however, caused a great deal of concern and debate about their toxic and carcinogenic potential (NTP, 1993a).

Potential health effects of solvent contaminants of water have received considerable attention over the past >40 years. A report by Mason and McKay (1975), of an increased incidence of cancer in persons who drank water from the Mississippi River, prompted the EPA to analyze the water supply of New Orleans. The finding of approximately 76 synthetic organic chemicals, many of which were solvents, prompted passage of the Safe Drinking Water Act in 1974. $CHCl_3$ is the most frequently found VOC in finished drinking water supplies in the United States (ATSDR, 1997a). It and certain other trihalomethanes are formed by reaction of the chlorine added as a disinfectant with natural organic compounds present in the water. Levels of solvents found in drinking water in the United States are typically in the nanogram per liter (ppt) to microgram per liter (ppb) range, although concentrations in the low milligram per liter (ppm) range are found in water from wells situated in solvent plumes from hazardous waste sites and other point discharges. Of the thousands of chemicals found at hazardous waste sites, six of the 10 most commonly present in groundwater are solvents (Pohl *et al.*, 2008).

People are subjected to solvents in environmental media by inhalation, ingestion, and skin contact. Considerable effort was devoted by the EPA, from 1979 to 1985, to assess personal exposure to solvents in different locales of the United States. TRI, PERC, benzene, xylenes, and ethylbenzene were most frequently found in highest concentrations (~1–32 $\mu g/m^3$) in air (Wallace *et al.*, 1987). Exhaled breath levels of some chemicals (eg, $CHCl_3$, ethylbenzene) corresponded to indoor air levels. Personal activities (eg, smoking, visiting a dry cleaner or service station) and occupational exposures were thought to be largely responsible for exposures to other VOCs (eg, benzene, toluene, xylenes, and PERC) (Ashley *et al.*, 1994). Subsequent studies, accounting for all pertinent exposure pathways, were conducted by the EPA in the mid-1990s (Gordon *et al.*, 1999). Elliott *et al.* (2006) more recently reported indoor exposures to VOCs did not have adverse effects on the respiratory function of 953 adults surveyed, with the exception of 1,4-dichlorobenzene, a component of air fresheners, toilet bowl deodorants, and mothballs. It should be recognized that $CHCl_3$ and other VOCs volatilize to some degree during home water usage, particularly when the water is heated. Thus, a significant proportion of one's total exposure to VOCs in tap water can occur via inhalation (Weisel and Jo, 1996), although the contribution of dermal exposure is relatively modest (Thrall *et al.*, 2002).

TOXICOKINETICS

Toxicokinetic (TK) studies are playing an increasingly important role in reducing uncertainties in risk assessments of solvents (Andersen, 2003; Dixit *et al.*, 2003; Clewell *et al.*, 2004). The fundamental goal of TK studies is to delineate the uptake and disposition of chemicals and certain of their metabolites in the body. It is now recognized that toxicity is a dynamic process, in which the degree and duration of injury of a target tissue are dependent on the net effect of toxicodynamic (TD) and TK processes including systemic absorption, tissue deposition, metabolism, interaction with cellular components, elimination, and tissue repair. Estimation of risk of toxicity from TK data is based on the fundamental concept that the intensity of response from an administered dose is dependent on the amount(s) of biologically active chemical moiety(ies) present in a target tissue (ie, the tissue dose). A related concept is that the tissue dose in a given target organ in one species will have the same degree of effect as an equivalent target organ dose in a second species. This concept of tissue dose equivalence appears to be applicable in many cases to solvents (Andersen, 1987), although TD differences are possible. Gaining an understanding of how the processes that govern solvent kinetics vary with dose, route of exposure, species, and even different individuals greatly reduces the number of assumptions that have to be made in assessment of health risks from exposure and effect data.

Volatility and lipophilicity are two of the most important properties of solvents that govern their absorption and deposition in the body. Most solvents are volatile under normal usage conditions, although volatility varies from compound to compound. Lipophilicity can also vary substantially, from quite water soluble (eg, glycols, esters, and alcohols) to quite lipid soluble (eg, halocarbons and aromatic hydrocarbons). Many solvents of particular concern at present are relatively lipid soluble and volatile, hence their designation as VOCs. These compounds have relatively low molecular weight and are uncharged. Thus, they pass freely through membranes from areas of high to low concentration by passive diffusion.

Absorption

The majority of systemic absorption of inhaled VOCs occurs in the alveoli, although limited absorption has been demonstrated to occur in the upper respiratory tract (Stott and McKenna, 1984). Gases in the alveoli are thought to equilibrate almost instantaneously with blood in the pulmonary capillaries. Blood:air partition coefficients (PCs) of VOCs are important determinants of the extent of their uptake. A PC is defined by Gargas *et al.* (1989) as the ratio of concentration of VOC achieved between two different media at equilibrium. As blood is largely aqueous, the more hydrophilic solvents have relatively high blood:air PCs, which favor extensive uptake. Gargas *et al.* (1989) determined in vitro PCs for 55 VOCs in F344 rats. Human blood:air values were measured for 36 of the compounds. Because VOCs diffuse from areas of high concentration to those of low concentration, increases in respiratory rate (to maintain a high alveolar concentration) and in cardiac output/pulmonary blood flow (to maintain a large concentration gradient by removing capillary blood containing the VOC) enhance systemic absorption.

Systemic uptake of solvents during ongoing inhalation exposures is dependent on tissue loading and metabolism, in addition to the factors noted above. Percent uptake is initially high, but progressively declines as the chemical accumulates in tissues, and the level of chemical in venous blood returning in the pulmonary circulation increases. A near steady state, or equilibrium, will be reached on inhalation of a fixed concentration of lipophilic solvents. The approach to equilibrium is asymptotic. Despite continued inhalation of lipophilic solvents, concentrations in the blood and tissues (other than fat) generally only increase modestly. Percent uptake remains relatively constant for the duration of exposure, with metabolism and accumulation in adipose tissue largely responsible for the continuing absorption. Hydrophilic solvents take considerably longer to reach steady state, due to the extended time required for equilibration of chemical in inspired air with that in total body water.

Solvents are well absorbed from the GI tract. Peak blood concentrations are observed within a few minutes of dosing fasted subjects, although the presence of fatty food in the GI tract can significantly delay absorption of lipophilic solvents. It is now usually assumed that 100% of an oral dose of most solvents is absorbed systemically. The vehicle or diluent in which a solvent is ingested can affect its absorption and TK. Kim *et al.* (1990a,b), for example, found that a corn oil vehicle served as a reservoir in the gut to delay GI absorption of carbon tetrachloride (CCl_4) in rats. Although bioavailability of CCl_4 given in corn oil and in an aqueous emulsion was the same, peak blood CCl_4 levels and acute hepatotoxicity were much lower in the corn oil group. Other factors that can influence the oral absorption of certain classes of chemicals have relatively little influence on most lipophilic solvents, due to their rapid passive diffusion in the entire GI tract.

Dermal absorption of solvents can result in both local and systemic effects. Skin contact with vapors and concentrated solutions of solvents is a common occurrence in the workplace. Dermal contact with solvent contaminants of water can also occur in the home and in recreational settings (Weisel and Jo, 1996; Gordon *et al.*, 2006). Lipophilic solvents penetrate the stratum corneum, the skin's barrier to absorption, by passive diffusion. Important determinants of the rate of dermal absorption of solvents include the chemical concentration, surface area exposed, exposure duration, integrity and thickness of the stratum corneum, and lipophilicity and molecular weight of the solvent (EPA, 1998a). Skin penetration can be quantified in laboratory animals and humans by a variety of in vitro and in vivo techniques (Morgan *et al.*, 1991; Nakai *et al.*, 1999). Although absorption rates measured by these methods may vary numerically, there is often good agreement in their relative ranking of chemicals' ability to penetrate the skin. Dermal permeability constants are typically two to four times lower for human than for rodent skin (McDougal *et al.*, 1990). The extent of dermal absorption in occupational and environmental exposure settings should be taken into account when conducting risk assessments of solvents.

Transport and Distribution

Chemicals and nutrients absorbed into portal venous blood from the GI tract can be removed from the bloodstream by first-pass, or presystemic elimination. As VOCs are rapidly absorbed and human intestinal epithelium apparently does not contain cytochrome P450 2E1 (CYP2E1) (Paine *et al.*, 2006), the primary CYP isoform that metabolizes low doses of many VOCs, their first-pass GI metabolism should be negligible. Blood in the portal venous circulation passes through the liver before entering the arterial circulation. Solvents are also subject to exhalation by the lungs during their first pass through the pulmonary circulation. Therefore, solvents that are well metabolized and quite volatile are most efficiently eliminated before they reach the arterial blood. The efficiency of the hepatic first-pass elimination is thus dependent on the chemical, as well as the rate at which it arrives in the liver. Pulmonary first-pass elimination, in contrast, is believed to be a zero-order process, as a fixed percentage of the chemical is thought to exit the pulmonary blood at each pass through the pulmonary circulation. Indeed, Lee *et al.* (1996) demonstrated in rats that pulmonary first-pass elimination of TCE was relatively constant over a range of doses, but that hepatic elimination was inversely related to dose. Thirty years ago Andersen (1981) theorized that the liver was capable of removing "virtually all" of an orally administered VOC, if the amount in the portal blood was not great enough to saturate metabolism. Liu *et al.* (2009) could not detect TCE (limit of quantitation = 25 pg/ml) in the arterial blood of rats gavaged with 0.1 μg TCE/kg in an aqueous emulsion, but did find TCE at bolus doses ≥1 μg/kg. Interestingly, bioavailability was consistently ~12% in the dosage range of 100 to 5000 μg TCE/kg. These findings indicate that first-pass elimination affords extrahepatic organs substantial, if not complete protection from environmentally encountered levels of well-metabolized VOCs.

Solvents are transported by the arterial blood and taken up by tissues according to their blood flow and mass and tissue:blood PCs (Astrand, 1983). Relatively hydrophilic solvents solubilize in plasma. Nevertheless, as much as 50% of such chemicals may still be carried by erythrocytes (Lam *et al.*, 1990). These researchers found that lipophilic solvents do not bind appreciably to plasma proteins or hemoglobin, but partition into hydrophobic sites in these molecules. Lipophilic solvents also partition into phospholipids, lipoproteins, and cholesterol present in the blood. The brain is an example of a rapidly perfused tissue with a relatively high lipid content. Lipophilic solvents therefore quickly accumulate in the brain after the initiation of exposures (Warren *et al.*, 2000). Inhalation of halothane, TCE, and $CHCl_3$ can produce CNS effects as profound as surgical anesthesia within as little as one to two minutes. Redistribution to poorly perfused, lipoidal tissues will subsequently occur. Adipose tissue gradually accumulates relatively large amounts of VOCs, and then slowly releases them back into the blood, due to high fat:blood PCs and low blood perfusion rates.

Route of exposure can significantly influence target organ deposition and toxicity of solvents. Much of the pre-1980s toxicology database for solvents comprised results of inhalation studies. Inhalation is the major route of occupational exposure to these chemicals. Since then, much attention has been focused on potential health effects of VOC contaminants of drinking water. Due to the initial paucity of oral data, regulatory agencies sometimes extrapolated directly from inhalation data to predict risks of ingested VOCs. Such a practice is obviously not scientifically valid, when physiological differences in the absorption pathways are taken into account. All the cardiac output passes through the pulmonary circulation versus ~20% for the GI tract. Also, the alveolar surface area for absorption is approximately 20 times that of the entire GI tract in humans. VOCs absorbed in the lungs directly enter the arterial circulation and are transported throughout the body. In contrast, VOCs absorbed from the GI tract largely enter the portal circulation and are subject to first-pass elimination by both the liver and the lungs. The GI epithelium contains certain monooxygenases, notably CYP3A in rats (Mitschke *et al.*, 2008) and CYP3A4 in humans (Ding and Kaminsky, 2003), although these isozymes do not participate to a significant extent in metabolism of most solvents. The liver, however, takes up and metabolizes a portion of many VOCs following ingestion (Sanzgiri *et al.*, 1997). It is not surprising then that extrahepatic organs receive a relatively high dose on inhalation of VOCs.

The pattern of ingestion of solvents can significantly influence their TK and health effects. For convenience, test chemicals are typically given daily to animals as a single bolus by gavage in short- and long-term oral toxicity and carcinogenicity studies. Actual human exposures to solvents in drinking water are quite different, in that people typically ingest water in divided doses. High, daily gavage doses of $CHCl_3$ and other halocarbons have produced hepatocellular carcinoma in B6C3F1 mice. No evidence of hepatic tumorigenesis was seen, however, when these mice were given the same doses of the chemical in their drinking water (Jorgenson *et al.*, 1985; Klaunig *et al.*, 1986). Female B6C3F1 mice exhibited hepatocellular necrosis and regenerative hyperplasia when gavaged with $CHCl_3$. Consumptions of the same doses in water were without ill effect (Larson *et al.*, 1994). Similarly, the maximum blood level of CCl_4 was found to be much higher and hepatotoxicity more severe in rats dosed with CCl_4 by gavage, than in those given the same dose over two hours by gastric infusion (Sanzgiri *et al.*, 1995). Oral bolus doses of solvents can cause damage of extrahepatic organs by exceeding the capacity of hepatic and pulmonary first-pass elimination, as well as protection and repair processes of hepatocytes.

Elimination

The rate of systemic elimination of different solvents varies considerably. The two major routes of systemic elimination of VOCs are metabolism and exhalation. The rate and extent of metabolic clearance are dose- and compound-dependent. Exhalation is determined largely by the rate of pulmonary blood flow, the chemical's

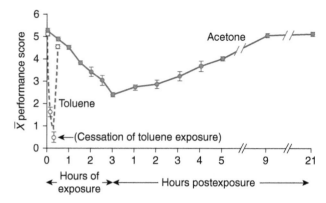

Figure 24-3. *Comparison of the induction of and recovery from toluene and acetone narcosis.* Rats inhaled 45 mg/L of toluene or acetone for 20 minutes or three hours, respectively. Animal performance/reflexes were monitored periodically as measures of the degree of CNS depression. (Reproduced from Bruckner and Peterson, 1981, with permission from Elsevier.)

blood:air PC, and the alveolar ventilation rate. The more volatile, lipophilic VOCs are exhaled the most readily, because they have the lower blood:air PCs (Gargas *et al.*, 1989). A good "case in point" is the comparison of toluene with acetone. The extent of CNS depression caused by each chemical is dependent on the concentration of the parent compound present in the brain (Bruckner and Peterson, 1981). As can be seen in Fig. 24-3, recovery of rats from toluene anesthesia occurs within minutes of exposure cessation. This can be attributed to redistribution of toluene from the brain to body fat and other tissues, as well as to relatively rapid metabolism and exhalation. In contrast, recovery from acetone narcosis does not occur for at least nine hours postexposure. As acetone is water soluble, limited amounts are deposited in the brain. It is instead distributed in the considerable volume of the blood and other body water. Clearance of acetone is slow due to its large volume of distribution and its relatively slow metabolism and exhalation. Acetone's water solubility is responsible for its relatively high blood:air PC and retention in the blood. Thus, acetone is available for diffusion into the brain and induction of a modest degree of CNS depression for a prolonged time.

Body fat plays an important role in the elimination of lipophilic solvents. Blood concentrations of such solvents drop very rapidly during the initial elimination phase following cessation of exposure. This so-called redistribution phase is characterized by rapid diffusion of solvents from the blood into tissues. Equilibration of adipose tissue is prolonged due to the small fraction of cardiac output (~3%) supplying fat depots. Body fat increases the volume of distribution and total body burden of lipophilic solvents. De-equilibration from adipose tissue during the terminal elimination phase is prolonged, due to low blood flow and high fat:blood PCs. Sato *et al.* (1975) demonstrated slower elimination of benzene from female than from male rats and humans, due to the females' higher body fat content. Rats with excess body fat experienced leukopenia during chronic benzene exposure, whereas their thinner counterparts did not.

Metabolism

Biotransformation plays a key role in modulating the toxicities of many solvents. Organic solvents are poorly soluble in water. Certain cellular enzymes can convert them to relatively water-soluble derivatives, which may be more readily eliminated in the largely aqueous urine and/or bile. Conversion of a bioactive parent compound to a less bioactive or inactive metabolite(s) that is(are) efficiently eliminated is termed *metabolic inactivation*, or *detoxification*. Toluene, for example, accumulates in neuronal membranes and inhibits their functions. It is metabolized to hydroxyl and carboxyl metabolites, which are too polar to accumulate or remain in substantial quantities in neuronal membranes. Thus, metabolism serves to detoxify and to accelerate the elimination of toluene. Metabolism of other solvents can produce reactive metabolites that are cytotoxic and/or mutagenic. This phenomenon is known as *metabolic activation*, or *bioactivation*. Benzene, for example, is oxidized to a variety of epoxides, quinones, and semiquinones that can produce hematopoietic toxicities and leukemia (Snyder, 2004). Benzene and many other VOCs are converted via multiple metabolic pathways to products of varying toxicity. Some of these competing pathways are considered bioactivation, others detoxification pathways. A variety of factors can influence the prominence of the different pathways and hence alter toxicity outcomes.

The initial step in biotransformation of relatively lipophilic solvents is catalyzed primarily by microsomal CYPs. They are a "superfamily" of hemoproteins that act as terminal oxidases of the mixed-function oxidase (MFO) system. Their mode of action is described in Chap. 6. CYPs can catalyze a number of oxidative reactions, as well as certain reductive reactions (Omiecinski *et al.*, 1999). Fifty seven different human CYP isoforms have been identified, but six (CYPs 2D6, 2C9, 3A4, 1A2, 2C19, and 2E1) account for the majority of xenobiotic metabolism (Rendic, 2002; Guengerich, 2006). CYPs are generally thought to have broad, overlapping substrate specificities, as demonstrated by Kobayashi *et al.* (2002) in rats. Xenobiotic metabolism under physiological conditions may favor one or two isoforms as the primary catalysts for a given chemical. Different isoforms can predominate at different concentrations of a chemical.

The outcome of exposure to a potentially toxic solvent can depend on the relative abundance of CYP isoforms. Expression of CYPs can differ considerably as a result of genetic polymorphisms and exposure to chemicals that induce or inhibit specific isoforms. A number of factors have been found to be sources of individual variability in CYP induction (Tang *et al.*, 2005). Inheritable gene alterations, such as base changes and deletions, can result not only in functionally deficient enzymes but also in the absence of certain P450s (Ma *et al.*, 2004). As CYPs have different modes of regulatory control, their expression in response to various inducers and inhibitors varies. It should also be recognized that frequently there are interspecies differences in the presence, regulation, and catalytic activities of CYPs (Lewis *et al.*, 1998; Guengerich, 2006).

There has been a focus on identification of CYPs that participate in the metabolism of individual solvents. Nakajima *et al.* (1992a) found that low concentrations of TCE in rat liver were metabolized primarily by CYP2E1, a constitutive high-affinity, low-capacity isoform. CYP2B1/2, a low-affinity, high-capacity form, predominated under high-dose (substrate) conditions. CYP2E1 was observed to be a major contributor to the metabolism of TCE and benzene, but not toluene. CYP1A1 catalyzed the formation of *o*-cresol, but not benzyl alcohol from toluene. CYP1A1 oxidized TCE in mice but not in rats. Thus, CYP isoforms exhibit species selectivity, substrate selectivity, and regioselectivity for solvents (Nakajima, 1997).

CYP2E1 is a major catalyst of the oxidation of a variety of low-molecular-weight xenobiotics, including many solvents. It is found predominantly in liver, with lower levels present in kidneys, lungs, brain, testes, and other extrahepatic tissues of rodents and humans. Guengerich *et al.* (1991) reported that human CYP2E1 is primarily responsible for oxidation of some 16 halogenated and aromatic hydrocarbons, including benzene, styrene, $CHCl_3$, TCE, and vinyl chloride. These compounds are oxidized to electrophilic metabolites, capable of causing cytotoxicity and/or mutagenicity (Raucy *et al.*, 1993). The isozyme is also responsible for reduction of CCl_4 to free radicals (see the discussion of CCl_4 in this chapter). CYP2E1 activity is associated with the pathogenesis of alcoholic cirrhosis, through formation of highly reactive oxygen radicals and acetaldehyde from ethanol (Caro and Cederbaum, 2004; Gonzalez, 2005; Lu and Cederbaum, 2008). CYP2E1 is inducible by ethanol, acetone, pyridazine, chlorzoxazone, isoniazid, and other of its substrates. Activity of the isoform varies from species to species and from human to human (Snawder and Lipscomb, 2000). Overnight fasting is widely recognized to induce CYP2E1, due in part to release of acetone during lipolysis (Bruckner *et al.*, 2002). Starving rats, however, apparently must engage in coprophagy for induction to occur (Chung *et al.*, 2001). Such differences in CYP2E1 activity/levels may play a major role in susceptibility to the toxicity and carcinogenicity of ethanol and a number of other solvents.

A variety of environmental factors can predispose people to harmful effects of solvents by altering P450s (Lof and Johanson, 1998). Ethanol is an effective CYP2E1 inducer when ingested repeatedly in substantial amounts (see the section "Exogenous Factors"). The person who drinks in such a manner may be subject to potentiation of solvent toxicity, due to increased solvent metabolic activation (Manno *et al.*, 1996). Conversely, ethanol consumed at about the same time as a solvent exposure can be protective by competitively inhibiting metabolic activation of the solvent. Thus, the timing of exposures is important. Folland *et al.* (1976) reported severe CCl_4-induced hepatorenal injury in workers at an isopropyl alcohol bottling plant. These subjects' preexposure to the alcohol, which is metabolized to acetone, had markedly induced CYP2E1. Their induced condition resulted in a substantial increase in the metabolic activation and cytotoxicity of CCl_4, on inhalation of normally nontoxic concentrations of the halocarbon.

The metabolic basis of solvent interactions receives considerable attention. The consequence of CYP2E1 induction by one solvent or drug depends on the nature of the second solvent. Kaneko *et al.* (1994) reported that ethanol pretreatment of rats has a more profound effect on the TK of TRI (poorly metabolized) than of TCE (well metabolized). Similarly, ethanol pretreatment of rats results in a greater increase in metabolism and hepatotoxicity of CCl_4 (relatively poorly metabolized) than of $CHCl_3$ (well metabolized) (Wang *et al.*, 1997). As capacity-limited (ie, metabolic capacity of the liver) metabolism prevails for poorly metabolized solvents, irrespective of dose, induction of their metabolism could be toxicologically significant in high (occupational) or low (environmental) exposure settings. In contrast, alterations of the bioactivation of low doses of well-metabolized solvents should be of little consequence, as their biotransformation is perfusion (ie, hepatic blood flow) limited. Lipscomb *et al.* (2003), for example, utilized a PBTK model to calculate that a sixfold interindividual difference in TCE metabolism resulted in <2% change in the total amount of TCE oxidized by persons inhaling only 50 ppm for eight hours or drinking 2 L of water containing 5 ppb TCE. Under such circumstances, interindividual metabolic differences should have little influence on cancer risks posed by trace levels of such solvents.

Physiological Modeling

PBTK models have been developed to provide predictions of chemical concentrations in blood and tissues as a function of time. They are thus used to relate the administered, or external, dose to the blood and/or tissue (internal) dose of parent compound and/or bioactive moiety. If there is sufficient knowledge of the physiology of the test animal/tissue and interactions of the bioactive moiety with cellular components and ensuing responses, physiologically based toxicodynamic (PBTD) models can be developed (Conolly, 2002). Relatively few PBTD models have been published to date for solvents. Tan *et al.* (2003) linked an existing PBTK model for $CHCl_3$ with data for hepatocellular death and regenerative hyperplasia to predict liver tumor response in mice. Luke *et al.* (2010) expanded upon the work of Tan *et al.* (2003) by developing biologically based dose–response (BBDR) models for $CHCl_3$ and CCl_4, based on key events of cytotoxicity and proliferation, to forecast liver tumor incidence in female B6C3F1 mice. The BBDR models consisted of a chemical-specific PBPK model for each chemical linked to a PBPD model of cytotoxicity and cellular proliferation, linked in turn to a clonal growth model to predict tumor incidence. Tan *et al.* (2011) have recently utilized models to evaluate the likelihood of TK and TD interactions of different chemical mixtures.

Development of PBTK models for anesthetic gases was initially undertaken in the 1920s and 1930s. Modeling was used in the design of experiments and dosage regimens for drugs, but the practice was not extended to industrial chemicals until the 1970s and 1980s. A "benchmark" paper by Ramsey and Andersen (1984) described the development of a PBTK model for styrene. By 1995, PBTK models had been developed for ~50 chemical environmental contaminants (Leung and Paustenbach, 1995). Approximately 28 of these 50 chemicals were solvents. Andersen (2003) more recently identified approximately 700 papers that dealt with PBTK models and/or their applications to toxicology and risk assessment. Thus, physiological models are being developed and used with increasing frequency to incorporate dosimetry and mechanistic data into noncancer and cancer risk assessments (Krishnan and Johanson, 2005).

Physiological modeling accounts for species- and dose-dependent shifts from linear to nonlinear kinetics, which impact tissue doses of bioactive moiety or moieties. The models are well suited for species-to-species extrapolations, because human physiological and metabolic parameter values can be inserted into animal models, and simulations of target tissue doses and effects in humans generated. Thus, solvent exposures necessary to produce the same target organ dose in humans, as those found experimentally to cause unacceptable cancer or noncancer risks in test animals, can be determined for some chemicals with reasonable certainty. In the limited number of cases where there may be species differences in tissue sensitivity, PBTD models must be used to forecast toxicologically effective target organ doses.

The influence of interindividual variability in model parameters has been receiving considerable attention (Price *et al.*, 2003). Jonsson and Johanson have performed model fitting in a Bayesian framework using Markov chain Monte Carlo (MCMC) simulation to reduce parameter uncertainty for methylene chloride (MC) (2001) and styrene (2002). A Bayesian analysis of a PBPK model for TCE yielded improved agreement of simulated and empirical TK data (Hack *et al.*, 2006). Covington *et al.* (2007) utilized this methodology to estimate that only ~2% of low inhaled doses of PERC are metabolized by humans to TCA. Qui *et al.* (2010) subsequently reported a similar finding when they used the approach in an expanded and more detailed assessment of PERC kinetics and TCA production. The percentage is far lower than has been assumed by regulatory agencies in the absence of data. Hierarchial analyses are proving quite useful in characterization of model parameter uncertainty and variability, and thereby in providing improved predictions of internal dosimetry for risk assessments.

PBTK modeling is finding increasing use in estimating exposure levels that result in concentrations of solvents measured in blood, exhaled breath, or urine (ie, biomarkers) in humans. Bois (2001) pointed out the need to apply PBTK models to large and poorly characterized human populations that have highly variable exposures, activity, physiology, and kinetics. A procedure termed *reverse dosimetry* has been employed to reconstruct population exposures from limited biomarker data (Clewell *et al.*, 2008). Reverse dosimetry, integrating PBPK modeling with exposure pattern characterization, Monte Carlo analysis, and other statistical tools, has been successfully employed to estimate distributions of exposures consistent with concentrations of TCE (Sohn *et al.*, 2004), $CHCl_3$ (Tan *et al.*, 2006), and other trihalomethanes (Tan *et al.*, 2007) quantified in human blood or exhaled breath. These exposure distributions can be compared with occupational and environmental exposure guidelines, in order to evaluate potential health risks in different situations.

POTENTIALLY SENSITIVE SUBPOPULATIONS

There is considerable variability in responses of humans to solvents and other xenobiotics. Although information on interindividual differences in the kinetics and toxicity of solvents is usually limited, some significant differences are reported and should be taken into account in risk assessments (Grassman *et al.*, 1998; Hattis *et al.*, 1999). Children within specific age groups appear to be even more variable than adults (Hattis *et al.*, 2003). Current EPA cancer and noncancer risk assessment practices are generally considered to be quite protective of potentially vulnerable subgroups, due to the use of multiple uncertainty factors and conservative default assumptions.

Endogenous Factors

Children Currently, there is considerable interest in regulatory and scientific issues related to protection of children's health (Landrigan and Goldman, 2011). The potential sensitivity of infants and children to pesticides and other chemicals was brought to the public's attention by a National Academy of Sciences' report (NAS, 1993). Ensuing Presidential Executive Order 13045 in 1997 directed all federal agencies to make protection of children a high priority and to consider risks to children when making policies and setting standards. The resulting Food Quality Protection Act of 1996 dictated that an additional 10-fold safety/uncertainty factor be used in pesticide risk assessments when pediatric toxicity and TK data are unavailable. This is almost always the case for insecticides, solvents, and other chemicals. Application of the 10-fold children's safety factor to nonpesticides has been considered. The Pediatric Research Equity Act of 2003 requires pharmaceutical companies seeking FDA's approval of new drugs to assess a compound's safety and efficacy at different doses in pediatric patients or surrogates.

Very little information is available on the toxic potential of solvents and most other chemicals in infants and children. There are several well-known examples of compounds (eg, lead, thalidomide, chloromycetin, and diazepam) to which fetuses or neonates are particularly susceptible. Results of experiments with chlorpyrifos (CPF) in immature rats raised enough concern about possible neurodevelopmental disorders in children that use of a number of organophosphates was severely restricted, and they have largely been removed from the home-use market (Colborn, 2006). Compilations of maximally tolerated doses (MTDs) of chemotherapeutic drugs are among our most definitive data on age-dependent toxicity in humans. Clinical trials of diverse groups of antineoplastic drugs have revealed that their toxic effects are often similar qualitatively, and usually differ quantitatively by a factor of ≤ 2 (NAS, 1993). MTDs for anticancer drugs in children are frequently higher than those for adults (Bruckner, 2000). Ginsberg *et al.* (2002) assembled a database with which TK parameters for adults and children can be compared for 45 drugs. These developmental metabolic profiles are relevant to some solvents and other environmental chemicals.

Increasing numbers of toxicology studies are being carried out in immature laboratory animals. Some of the most comprehensive data sets available are compilations of LD_{50} values from experiments with immature rodents (Goldenthal, 1971). These and other data reveal that immature rodents are more sensitive to most but not to all chemicals (Hasegawa *et al.*, 2007). Variances are usually no more than two to threefold, but can be as much as 10-fold. The younger and more immature a subject, the more different its response from that of the adult. The newborn mouse and rat more nearly resemble the human fetus during the third trimester than during the human neonate's initial weeks and months of life. Thus, it is not surprising that newborn rodents would be much more sensitive to many toxicants than adult rodents and human newborns. Growth and maturation are, of course, much more rapid in rodents. A few days' growth of mice and rats can result in substantial changes in metabolism, disposition, and toxicity (Ginsberg *et al.*, 2004a,b). It is generally accepted that there are *windows of vulnerability*, or periods during the development of the nervous, audiovisual, immune, reproductive, endocrine, and other organ systems when the intricate, fragile maturational processes may be particularly sensitive to xenobiotics (Dorman *et al.*, 2001; Scheuplein *et al.*, 2002). These windows occur at different ages and last for different periods of time in different species. This makes the choice of an appropriate animal model for children complex and cross-species comparisons more difficult than usual with adult risk assessments (Ginsberg *et al.*, 2004a,b; Morford *et al.*, 2004).

Despite a paucity of data, some logical assumptions can be made about age-dependent changes in the TK and toxicity of solvents. GI absorption of solvents would not be expected to vary with age, as most solvents are absorbed rapidly and completely by passive diffusion from the entire GI tract. Systemic absorption of inhaled solvents may be greater in infants and children. Their cardiac output and respiratory rates are relatively high, although their alveolar surface area is lower than that of adults (Sarangapani *et al.*, 2003). Reduced plasma protein binding in neonates and infants may be of consequence for certain solvent metabolites. Low-binding capacity for TCA, for example, could result in more of the mouse hepatocarcinogen being available for hepatic uptake, as well as for renal clearance. Extracellular water, expressed as percent of body weight, is highest in newborns and diminishes through childhood. The larger volume of distribution for water-soluble solvents results in their slower clearance and longer duration of action. Body fat is high from approximately six months to three years of age, and then steadily decreases until adolescence, when it increases again in females. As lipophilic solvents accumulate in adipose tissue, more body fat would result in higher body burdens, slower clearance, and longer duration of action.

Changes in xenobiotic biotransformation during maturation may have the greatest impact on susceptibility to chemical toxicity and carcinogenicity. Poisonings of premature and term human newborns by benzyl alcohol, hexachlorophene, diazepam, chloramphenicol, and certain other compounds are primarily attributable to deficits in hepatic Phase II metabolic (ie, conjugative) capacity. Maturational studies of human liver reveal that CYP isoforms are expressed asynchronously (Cresteil, 1998). There have been comprehensive efforts to characterize the ontogeny of human hepatic Phase I (Hines and McCarver, 2002; Stevens *et al.*, 2003; Johnsrud *et al.*, 2003) and Phase II (McCarver and Hines, 2002) enzymes from gestation to adolescence. Levels of CYP2E1, the

primary catalyst of oxidation of a variety of solvents, are very low in fetal liver, increase steadily for the first year, and remain relatively constant through adolescence (Cresteil, 1998; Johnsrud *et al.*, 2003). Blanco *et al.* (2000) failed to find an age-related difference in the maximal in vitro activity of CYP2E1 or other CYP isoforms in liver microsomes from donors from infancy to 93 years old. More rapid systemic clearance of many compounds by young children than by adults (Ginsberg *et al.*, 2002) is generally believed to result from the child's liver's larger volume and more rapid perfusion rate (Murry *et al.*, 1995; Sarangapani *et al.*, 2002). Glomerular filtration and renal tubular secretion are quite low at birth, but increase substantially during the first six months to one year (Scheuplein *et al.*, 2002). The half-life of creatinine, a substance eliminated entirely by glomerular filtration, is about half the adult value at one year. The net result of multiple age-related TK changes, some with offsetting effects, is difficult to predict.

A number of authorities have advocated the use of PBTK/TD models to collectively account for the unique and changing characteristics of children (Clewell *et al.*, 2004; Daston *et al.*, 2004). A few PBTK models have been published for predicting the internal dosimetry of chemicals in immature rats. Timchalk *et al.* (2007) developed a BBDR model for chloropyrifos (CPF), a widely used organophosphate insecticide. More pronounced depression of erythrocyte and brain cholinesterase activities, apparently resulting from higher CPF-oxon blood and brain levels, was forecast in preweanling than in adult rats. Rodriguez *et al.* (2007) used PBTK modeling to forecast the TK of six inhaled VOCs (TCE, PERC, benzene, $CHCl_3$, MC, and methyl ethyl ketone) in 10-day-old and adult rats. VOC blood levels were forecast to be up to 3.8-fold higher in the preweanlings, due primarily to their lower metabolism and faster respiration. Many of the input parameters were estimated or scaled, however, rather than measured. Empirical data were not provided to assess the accuracy of the simulations. Tornero-Velez *et al.* (2010) developed a PBTK model that clarified why preweanling rats are more susceptible than adults to the acute toxicity of deltamethrin (DLM), a pyrethroid insecticide. These researchers were among the first to rely primarily on age-specific input parameters and to demonstrate concordance between measured and simulated timecourses of a bioactive moiety (ie, the neurotoxic parent compound). Blood and brain levels of DLM were inversely related to age in 10-, 21-, 40-, and 90-day-old rats. Sensitivity analyses showed V_{maxs} (Anand *et al.*, 2006a) for CYP- and carboxylesterase (hydrolytic)–mediated clearance pathways significantly influenced both blood and brain dosimetry. Inefficient metabolic detoxification was thus a major contributor to preweanling rats' susceptibility to DLM, although immaturities in other kinetic processes may also be factors. Age-specific CYP levels and CPF bioactivation and inactivation in liver microsomes and plasma are currently being measured and used to model organophosphate TK and cholinesterase inhibition in humans (Foxenberg *et al.*, 2011; Smith *et al.*, 2011). Determination and utilization of age-specific input parameters will continue to improve the accuracy of immature human PBTK–TD predictions.

Effort is being devoted to development of PBTK models for VOCs in human infants and children. Clewell *et al.* (2004) constructed what they termed a life-stage model to simulate blood levels of four solvents (isopropanol, vinyl chloride, MC, and PERC) and their primary metabolites in different life stages. This was intended to be a preliminary model, in view of the lack of validated models for the younger groups and the required number of simplifying assumptions in the face of uncertainties about many age-specific parameters. In general, dose metrics for the chemicals across life stages were within a factor of two, except during the early postnatal period when the largest TK differences occurred. Gentry *et al.*

(2003) took a similar approach to forecast internal dosimetry of vinyl chloride, isopropanol, MC, and PERC in human offspring during pregnancy and lactation. In general, blood concentrations of the VOCs were lower in neonates during lactation than in the fetus during gestation. Fetal/neonatal VOC exposures were generally several orders of magnitude lower than maternal exposures. Sarangapani *et al.* (2002) developed a PBTK model that integrated key age-specific respiratory tract parameters, such that the disposition of four VOCs (styrene, vinyl chloride, isopropanol, and PERC) could be forecast in children and adults. Differences in blood levels of parent compounds in infants and adults were comparable or varied <2-fold during the first year of life. Nong *et al.* (2006) incorporated measured age-specific liver volumes and CYP2E1 content into a PBPK model for toluene to predict internal doses (blood levels) of the parent compound in adults and in children of different age groups. CYP2E1 content was the key model input parameter for neonates, whereas liver blood flow rate was predominant after a few months of age. Combined interindividual and interage variability in the areas under blood level versus time curves (AUCs) was within a factor of 2, except for the neonates, who had somewhat higher AUCs.

The aforementioned findings suggest that differences in dosimetry of parent solvents across life stages are usually well within the 3.3 TK component of the classical 10-fold intraspecies uncertainty factor. Relative little work has been done, however, to model solvent metabolite dosimetry in different age groups. Potential PD differences should also be taken into account in children's risk assessments.

Elderly Age-related changes in effects of xenobiotics have primarily been of interest in the field of drug therapy (Bressler and Bahl, 2003; McLean and LeCouteur, 2004). More attention is now being paid to exposures and vulnerabilities of the elderly to other chemicals (Geller and Zenick, 2005). The EPA encourages evaluation of toxicity across the entire lifespan, with a focus on life stages with their own unique sensitivity (Brown *et al.*, 2008). Data are sorely lacking, however, on the relative susceptibility of geriatric populations to solvents and many other industrial chemicals. The aging CNS undergoes changes (eg, neuronal loss, altered neurotransmitter and receptor levels, and reduced adaptability to effects of toxicants) (Ginsberg *et al.*, 2005), which may predispose to more pronounced neurologic effects by solvents. Older people do appear to be more sensitive to the CNS depressant effects of ethanol, due in part to lower gastric alcohol dehydrogenase (ADH) activity (Seitz *et al.*, 1993). Kiesswetter *et al.* (1997) observed the most pronounced neurobehavorial effects in older workers with the highest single or mixed organic solvent exposures. Memory, attention, visual perception, and motor skills diminish with aging, even in the absence of chemical exposure. Thus, these findings could be interpreted as merely additive (ie, aging + solvents effects), or as exacerbation during a vulnerable life stage. Paradoxically, a subsequent investigation by Kiesswetter *et al.* (2000), this time of toluene-exposed rotogravure printers, revealed fewer symptoms and better psychometric performance in older workers with higher exposure levels. A limited number of studies of this phenomenon by other investigators are no more definitive.

Investigations of adverse effects of solvents on old animals have been quite limited. Attention has been primarily focused on age-related susceptibility of rodents to liver damage. Susceptibility varies dramatically from one chemical to another. Rikans and Hornbrook (1997) reviewed studies showing increased susceptibility of geriatric F344 rats to allyl alcohol, but there was no apparent age dependency with bromobenzene. Results varied with species, strain, and gender. CCl_4 hepatotoxicity was less severe in 28-month-old female F344 rats than in young adults. Wauthier *et al.* (2004) saw no changes in CYP2E1 protein or mRNA in 18-month-old male Wistar rats, but did observe decreased CYP2E1 activity. The investigators attributed this phenomenon to oxidative stress on the isoform. More severe CCl_4-induced DNA damage in hepatocytes from older mice was shown to be due to preexisting oxidative DNA damage and a higher incidence of DNA strand breaks in the older animals (Lopez-Diazguerrero *et al.*, 2005). Thus, it appears normal aging processes may be accentuated by chemical stressors.

There are few pertinent geriatric animal or human toxicology studies, but age-specific factors that govern the TK of solvents have received considerable attention. Clewell *et al.* (2002) and Sarangapani *et al.* (2003) compiled comprehensive reviews and evaluations of age-specific TK parameters, although data for many age groups are inadequate. Splanchnic blood flow decreases with age more rapidly than cardiac output. This is unlikely to significantly affect the GI absorption of solvents, as they are readily absorbed by passive diffusion. Dermal absorption could be influenced by loss of integrity of the stratum corneum, reduction in skin surface lipids, and atrophy of the dermal capillary network (Roskos *et al.*, 1989). Total lung capacity does not change with age, but vital capacity (mobile volume) diminishes progressively due to loss of lung elasticity and strength of the respiratory muscles. Residual capacity (fixed volume) increases with progressive narrowing and closure of small airways (Ritschel, 1988). Other alterations that may contribute to lower pulmonary absorption include decreases in alveolar surface area, membrane permeability and capillary blood volume, and thicker alveolar cell membranes (Clewell *et al.*, 2002). Nevertheless, inhalation PBTK model predictions of steady-state blood concentrations of isopropanol, styrene, vinyl chloride, and PERC differed very little among 10-, 15-, 25-, 50-, and 75-year-old humans (Sarangapani *et al.*, 2003).

Age influences the distribution of xenobiotics in the body, as well as their metabolism and elimination (Mangoni and Jackson, 2003). With aging, body fat content usually increases substantially at the expense of the lean mass (ie, skeletal muscle) and body water. Thus, polar solvents tend to reach higher blood levels during exposures. Relatively lipid-soluble solvents accumulate in adipose tissue and are released slowly to sites of action, metabolism, and elimination. Ginsberg *et al.* (2005) assembled clearance and half-life data for 46 drugs in 4500 subjects. Clearance was typically slower and half-life longer after the age of 60 years, particularly in those 80 to 84 years old. Cardiac output diminishes 30% to 40% between the ages of 25 and 65 years, as do renal and hepatic blood flows (McLean and Le Couteur, 2004). This research group and Clewell *et al.* (2002) concluded that reduced hepatic clearance of flow- and capacity-limited xenobiotics in the elderly was due primarily to reductions in liver blood flow and liver size. McLean and Le Couteur (2004) presented evidence that aging of the sinusoidal endothelium reduced oxygen delivery and drug transfer from blood to hepatocytes. Schmucker (2005) and Herrlinger and Klotz (2001) did not find significant relationships between aging and CYP activities in human liver. Cotreau *et al.* (2005) did describe some reports of age-related decreases in CYP3A4, an isoform important in metabolism of a number of drugs in humans, but of limited relevance to solvent metabolism.

Recent findings indicate that toxic compounds, both xenobiotics and certain products of intermediary metabolism, are major contributors to macromolecular damage and dysregulation involved in aging (Zimniak, 2008). Important endogenous toxicants include reactive carbonyl compounds and electrophiles formed by peroxidation of polyunsaturated lipids. Enzymes capable of reducing carbonyl groups and glutathione S-transferases (GSTs) are key protection mechanisms. Lee *et al.* (2008) characterized age-related changes in the expression of a substantial number of xenobiotic-metabolizing enzymes in the liver of aged male F344 and Brown Norway rats. GST expression diminished with age. Most data, however, indicate that Phase II (conjugation) pathways in humans are not altered by aging (Mitchell *et al.*, 2011). Maurya and Rizvi (2010) reported an increase in plasma GST activity and antioxidant potential in a study of 80 healthy male and female human subjects 18 to 85 years old. It was hypothesized that this was in response to increased production of reactive oxygen moieties with advancing age.

Information is available on certain age-related aspects of xenobiotic clearance other than metabolism. Plasma protein binding of drugs generally remains unaltered or diminishes modestly with age (Grandison and Boudinot, 2000). Hepatic and/or renal dysfunction more often account for altered protein binding. Little information apparently exists on effects of aging on most transporters (Kinirons and O'Mahony, 2004), although Lee *et al.* (2008) did see diminished expression of efflux transporters in the livers of aging male rats. Renal clearance diminishes with advancing age, due to parallel annual decreases of ~0.65% in glomerular filtration and maximal tubular secretory capacity beyond the age of 30 years. The foregoing TK factors may significantly influence the internal dosimetry of polar solvent metabolites, and in turn certain responses of geriatric populations.

PBTK models should be useful for integrating age-related physiological and metabolic changes into a quantitative framework to forecast their net effect on blood and tissue timecourses of parent compounds and metabolites. Very few such "geriatric" models, however, have been published. McMahon *et al.* (1994) employed a PBTK model to demonstrate that reduced urinary elimination of benzene metabolites by geriatric mice was due to decreased renal blood flow rather than altered formation of metabolites. Corley *et al.* (2005c) incorporated a number of age-, gender-, and species-specific physiological and biochemical parameters into a preexisting PBTK model for 2-butoxyethanol (BE), in order to predict the kinetics of BE and butoxyacetic acid (BAA), BE's major metabolite, in male and female mice and rats of different ages. The life-stage PBTK model of Clewell and colleagues was used to simulate human blood concentrations of several VOCs and their major metabolite (or metabolic rate) from infancy to the age of 75 years (Sarangapani *et al.*, 2003). Blood levels of the parent compounds remained relatively constant during adulthood, but metabolite levels or amounts metabolized frequently varied during the pediatric and geriatric years. In a subsequent publication, blood levels of PERC and its major metabolite, TCA, were predicted to progressively rise during adulthood and old age by a PBTK model. Clewell *et al.*, (2004) attributed this phenomenon to relatively low pulmonary and metabolic clearance, coupled with accumulation of the lipophilic solvent in ample amounts of adipose tissue. Much work remains to be done to refine these generic PBTK models and to integrate them with significant geriatric PD changes (Burton *et al.*, 2005).

Gender Some of the physiological and biochemical differences between men and women have the potential to alter tissue dosimetry and health effects of certain solvents (Vahter *et al.*, 2007). Clewell *et al.* (2002) have provided one of the most comprehensive reviews of the potential impact of gender differences on chemicals' TK. There was no convincing evidence of sex differences in GI absorption rate constants. The investigators located few data on gender-dependent dermal or pulmonary absorption of solvents or other chemicals. Sarangapani *et al.* (2003) published tables of a number of factors (eg, cardiac output, pulmonary ventilation rate, and pulmonary surface area) that dictate pulmonary absorption of

VOCs. These rates and values were generally higher for males, but a PBPK model's predictions of steady-state blood concentrations for inhaled isopropanol, styrene, vinyl chloride, and PERC were largely sex-independent (Sarangapani *et al.*, 2003).

Distribution of water- and lipid-soluble solvents can vary substantially between men and women (Schwartz, 2003). Most men have more lean body mass and larger body size. Women typically have smaller volumes of distribution for polar solvents, but larger volumes of distribution for lipophilic solvents (Gandhi *et al.*, 2004). Lean body mass decreases from 76% to 52%, and body fat increases from 33% to 49% in females between the ages of 25 and 65 to 70 years. Nomiyama and Nomiyama (1974) found that women retain less inhaled acetone and ethyl acetate than similarly exposed men. Levels of toluene and TCE in expired air of females were lower, reflecting greater fat deposition and retention of these lipophilic chemicals. Similarly, women exhibited significantly higher respiratory uptake of 1,3-butadiene, another lipophilic VOC (Lin *et al.*, 2001b). Clewell and Andersen (2004) utilized their life-stage PBTK model to predict blood levels of PERC and TCA, its major metabolite, in men and women over a lifetime of daily ingestion of 1 µg PERC/kg. The women were predicted to attain significantly higher blood PERC and TCA concentrations, ostensibly due to PERC's greater storage in fat and its relatively low pulmonary and metabolic clearance.

The major sex differences in P450-mediated hepatic metabolism in rats are not seen in humans or most other mammals. Rinn *et al.* (2004) did see significant differences in gene expression in the liver, kidney, and reproductive tissues of male and female mice. Some of the differentially expressed genes involve drug and steroid metabolism, but the biological significance of these variances is unknown. No marked gender differences in P450-catalyzed oxidation reactions have been identified in humans (Mugford and Kedderis, 1998). Other investigators have described modestly higher levels and activities of certain liver P450s in males, including CYP2E1, CYP1A2, and CYP2D6 (Schwartz, 2003). Many CYP3A substrates do not exhibit sex-dependent differences in clearance, although some researchers report differences for certain substrates (Cotreau *et al.*, 2005). Gender-specific metabolism data for most hydrocarbon solvents are lacking. Men exhibit somewhat lower blood ethanol levels than women on ingestion of equal doses, due in part to more extensive ADH-catalyzed metabolism of the alcohol by the male gastric mucosa (Frezza *et al.*, 1990). UDP-glucuronyl transferase activity appears to be somewhat higher in males. Women seem to have modestly lower glomerular filtration rates, although information on gender-dependent renal tubular secretion and reabsorption processes is lacking.

A gender-specific PBTK model was developed to assess the relative risks of benzene exposures (Brown *et al.*, 1998). Women were found to have a higher blood:air PC, a higher percent of body fat, and higher maximum rate of benzene metabolism than men. They exhibited higher blood benzene levels and a 23% to 26% increase in benzene metabolism, potentially placing them at greater risk than men with equivalent exposures.

Relatively little is known about potential influences of contraceptives, hormone replacement therapy, or pregnancy on the metabolism and disposition of xenobiotics (Gleiter and Gundert-Remy, 1996). The menstrual cycle with its hormone changes may influence the metabolism of some xenobiotics (Fletcher *et al.*, 1994). Watanabe *et al.* (1997) found that estradiol changes during the estrous cycle of rats affected both UDP-glucuronyl transferase and NADPH-cytochrome *c* reductase activities. Experiments by Nakajima *et al.* (1992b) demonstrated that pregnancy of rats resulted in significant reductions in hepatic CYP content, as well as the metabolism of both toluene and TCE. Pregnancy results in a 40% increase in tidal volume, which may increase the absorption of inhaled VOCs. Plasma volume increases ~50% in pregnant women, resulting in a decrease in albumin concentration and plasma protein binding of many drugs (Fletcher *et al.*, 1994). Cardiac output increases ~50%, due to increases in stroke volume and heart rate (Silvaggio and Mattison, 1994). Uterine blood flow, renal plasma flow, and glomerular filtration rise substantially, although no information on hepatic blood flow is apparently available. These TK factors need to be considered when assessing risks and setting occupational exposure limits for these subpopulations.

The effects of pregnancy on peroxisome proliferator–activated receptors (PPARs) are being investigated. PPARs are transcription factors that belong to the nuclear hormone receptor superfamily. They regulate genes involved in cell differentiation, development, and metabolism. The three identified and described PPAR isoforms are peroxisome proliferator–activated receptor alpha (PPARα), PPARβ/δ, and PPARγ. Among the isoforms, PPARγ has the greatest influence on cellular homeostasis and carcinogenicity. However, all three PPAR isoforms play essential roles in physiological change and development in the fetoplacental unit. Abnormalities in PPAR-regulated pathways may be implicated in reproductive and gestational disease (Toth *et al.*, 2007; Borel *et al.*, 2008). Two TCE and PERC metabolites, TCA and DCA, can induce modest PPARα activation in humans. The combined effects of pregnancy and low-level PPAR activation, if any, are unknown.

Gentry *et al.* (2003) described an approach for use of PBTK modeling to compare maternal and fetal/neonatal blood and tissue dosimetry during pregnancy and lactation. In general, blood levels of isopropanol, vinyl chloride, MC, and PERC were predicted to be lower in the human neonate during lactation than in the fetus during gestation. Simulated vinyl chloride levels, for example, were four orders of magnitude lower in the neonates. Fetal/neonatal isopropanol levels were forecast to be orders of magnitude lower than maternal levels. Corley *et al.* (2003) reviewed PBTK/TD modeling of the developing embryo, fetus, and neonate.

Genetics A variety of genetic polymorphisms for biotransformation have been found to occur at different frequencies in different ethnic groups. Polymorphisms for xenobiotic-metabolizing enzymes may affect the quantity and quality of enzymes and the outcomes of exposures to solvents and other chemicals (Wormhoudt *et al.*, 1999). It is important to note that culturally linked environmental factors also contribute to ethnic differences in metabolism and disposition of solvents and other chemicals. It is often difficult to disentangle the influences of genetic traits from those of different lifestyles, socioeconomic status, and geographic settings.

Ethnic differences in regulating the expression of CYP isozymes and other enzymes are associated with some variations in xenobiotic metabolism and susceptibility to certain cancers (Raunio *et al.*, 1995; Weber, 1999). Shimada *et al.* (1994) found that Caucasians had higher total hepatic CYP levels than Japanese. Caucasians exhibited higher CYP2E1 activities, as reflected by aniline *p*-hydroxylation and 7-ethoxycoumarin *O*-deethylation. Individuals with two linked polymorphisms in the transcription regulatory region of the CYP2E1 gene exhibited greater expression of the isoform. Reported frequencies of these rare alleles were 2% in Caucasians, 2% to 5% in African Americans, and 24% to 27% in Japanese (Kato *et al.*, 1992). Kawamoto *et al.* (1995) found that a CYP2E1 polymorphism in Japanese workers did not affect metabolism of toluene to benzoic acid, but that CYP1A1 and aldehyde dehydrogenase (ALDH2) polymorphisms did. ALDH2 deficiency can result in elevated CNS levels of toluene and benzaldehyde

(Wilkins-Haug, 1997) in toluene-exposed individuals. About half of the Japanese population lacks ALDH2, due to a structural point mutation in the ALDH2 gene. Pronounced interethnic differences in rates of ethanol metabolism have been associated with a number of ADH and aldehyde dehydrogenase (ALDH) polymorphisms (Pastino *et al.*, 2000). Results of investigations of relationships between occurrence of defective alleles for CYP2E1 and cancer incidence have been contradictory. Studies with more statistical power of selected ethnic groups are needed. Molecular markers clearly indicate variances in CYP genes, but biologically plausible mechanisms linking specific genotypes with specific outcomes need to be established.

Ethnic differences have been demonstrated for some Phase II biotransformation reactions. GSTs are a family of enzymes, some of which promote the detoxification of electrophilic metabolites by catalyzing their conjugation with reduced glutathione (GSH). In contrast, GST theta–mediated conjugation with GSH is the first step in metabolic activation of MC to formaldehyde, a putative carcinogen (see the section "Methylene Chloride"). Individuals with a null/null genotype for GST theta are thus at a lower risk of developing cancer from MC (El-Masri *et al.*, 1999; Haber *et al.*, 2002). The prevalence of this genotype ranges from 10% in Mexican Americans to 60% to 65% in Chinese and Koreans (Nelson *et al.*, 1995). GST theta also catalyzes dehalogenation of DCA to glyoxylic acid. DCA, a minor product of TCE and PERC oxidation, is a hepatocarcinogen in high doses in mice and rats. It is cleared more slowly from the systemic circulation of persons with a GST theta polymorphism, possibly resulting in increased risk of liver cancer on TCE or PERC exposure (Shroads *et al.*, 2011). GSTs participate in conjugating relatively small percentages of doses of TCE and PERC, but these pathways can lead to production of cytotoxic, mutagenic metabolites in the kidney. Contrary to findings in a more limited study, Wiesenhutter *et al.* (2007) saw no association between deletion polymorphisms of GST-T1 and GST-M1 and incidence of renal cell cancer (RCC) in 134 RCC cases (20 with TCE exposure) and 401 matched controls. More recently Moore *et al.* (2010) studied gene variants in 1097 RCC cases and 1476 controls. A significant association was found between TCE exposure and RCC in individuals with at least one intact GST-T1 allele, but not in individuals with two deleted alleles.

Genetic polymorphisms, variable transporter activities, genetic variants of receptors and regulatory proteins, and environmental factors can play roles in individual variability in CYP induction (Tang *et al.*, 2005). Lipscomb *et al.* (1997) described substantial differences in activity and/or content of CYP2E1 within the US population. Lipscomb (2004) incorporated extremes in CYP2E1-mediated metabolism into a PBTK model for TCE and found there was very little impact on TCA dosimetry. Intersubject differences in hepatic blood flow did have a pronounced effect on TCE biotransformation, as TCE is an extensively metabolized (blood flow limited) compound. Wenker *et al.* (2001) similarly reported that interindividual genetic polymorphisms in CYP2E1 and several other CYPs did not affect the metabolism of styrene, another flow-limited compound. Kedderis (1997) utilized a PBTK modeling approach to confirm this phenomenon, and found the opposite to be true for poorly metabolized (capacity limited) VOCs such as PERC and CCl_4.

Exogenous Factors

P450 Inducers Considerable effort has been devoted to investigation of effects of different enzyme inducers on xenobiotic metabolism and toxicity. Preexposure to drugs and other compounds, which induce CYP isoforms that metabolically activate chemicals, can markedly potentiate the chemicals' toxicity/carcinogenicity (Gut *et al.*, 1993; Ioannides and Lewis, 2004; Dekant, 2009). As described in the subsection "Metabolism" in the section "Toxicokinetics," CYP2E1 is a high-affinity, low-capacity isoform responsible for activation of a wide variety of low-molecular-weight hydrocarbon and halocarbon solvents to cytotoxins and mutagens (Guengerich *et al.*, 1991). A number of CYP2E1 substrates (eg, ethanol and other alcohols, acetone and other ketones, pyridine and pyridazine, isoniazid, acetaminophen, chlorzoxazone) can act as inducers of the isoform. The minimal hepatocytotoxicity caused by a low dose of CCl_4 alone (Panel B, Fig. 24-4) can be contrasted with the centrilobular necrosis (Panel C, Fig. 24-4) in rats pretreated with 2-butanol before the same CCl_4 dose (Traiger and Bruckner, 1976). CYP2E1 is present in many tissues, as are other CYPs that metabolize solvents. Although levels/activities are highest in liver, induction in extrahepatic tissues can result in increased metabolic activation in situ that may be toxicologically significant. It is worthy of note that many chemicals that induce CYPs also induce detoxifying enzymes (eg, epoxide hydrolase, glucuronyltransferases, and sulfotransferases). Thus, the net outcome of preexposure to an inducing agent on solvent toxicity should be addressed on a case by case basis. A number of naturally occurring organosulfur compounds in allium vegetables have been demonstrated to induce Phase II enzymes in the liver, kidney, intestines, and lungs of Wistar rats (Guyonnet *et al.*, 1999).

It should be recognized that timing of exposures to ≥2 CYP substrates is important. Sato *et al.* (1991) demonstrated that ethanol competitively inhibited the biotransformation of TCE when the exposures were concurrent. Alternatively, preexposure to the alcohol induced TCE metabolism. As described previously in the subsection "Metabolism" in the section "Toxicokinetics," increased metabolic capacity in an individual is of little consequence for environmentally encountered levels of blood flow–limited (ie, extensively metabolized) solvents (eg, TCE, vinyl chloride, MC, and $CHCl_3$). Thus, genetically predisposed or induced individuals should be at no greater cancer risk from oxidative metabolites of low doses of these solvents than the average person.

P450 Inhibitors An increasing number of drugs and other chemicals, dietary supplements, fruit juices, and vegetable constituents are being identified as inhibitors and/or inducers of CYPs, Phase II enzymes, and efflux transporters (Lin and Lu, 2001; Huang and Lesko, 2004). It should be recalled that mechanisms of P450 inhibition can be categorized as reversible, quasireversible, and irreversible. Reversible inhibition is transient, with the normal function of the CYP continuing after elimination of the inhibitor. Both quasireversible and irreversible inhibitions result from the enzyme's formation of a reactive metabolite. With quasireversible inhibition, the metabolite and enzyme form a complex that is so stable that the intact enzyme may or may not be available for further metabolism. With mechanism-based or suicide inhibition, the reactive metabolite irreversibly inhibits the enzyme by binding to its active site. Experiments by Lilly *et al.* (1998) indicate that this is the mechanism by which epoxide metabolites of *trans-* and *cis-*1,2-dichloroethylene inhibit CYP2E1. Fisher *et al.* (2004) subsequently reported that metabolites generated from a single oral dose of CCl_4 as low as 1 mg/kg are suicide inhibitors of CYP2E1 and CYP2B2 in B6C3F1 mice. The net result of this action by CCl_4 was reduced formation of TCA from coadministered PERC. Blobaum (2006) described reversible inactivation of CYP2E and CYP2B isoforms during their mechanism-based inactivation by small *tert*-butyl terminal alkynes.

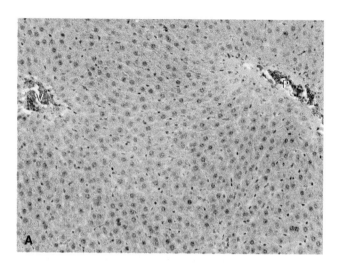

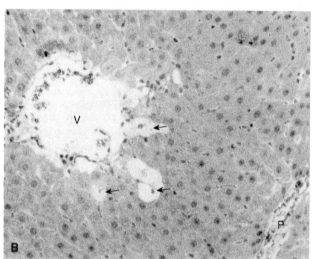

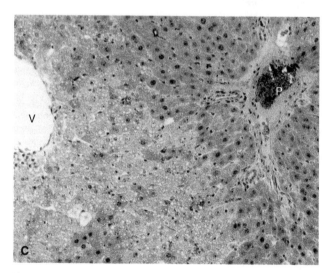

Figure 24-4. *Potentiation of CCl_4 hepatotoxicity by 2-butanol.* Rats were (**A**) untreated; (**B**) given 0.1 mL CCl_4/kg IP; or (**C**) pretreated with 2-butanol (2.2 mL/kg PO) 16 hours before 0.1 mL/kg CCl_4 IP. Central veins and portal triads are designated V and P, respectively. Occasional hepatocytes (arrows) adjacent to the central vein are vacuolated in "B." Note the demarcation between vacuolated/necrotic centrilobular and midzonal cells, and normally appearing periportal cells in "C." Hematoxylin and eosin stain. (A and C) ×315; (B) ×480. (Reproduced from Traiger and Bruckner, 1976, with permission from ASPET.)

Flavanoids in grapefruit juice were one of the first classes of naturally occurring compounds to be documented to produce clinically significant increases in internal levels of therapeutic agents metabolized by CYP3A4 (Chan *et al.*, 1998). Flavanoids in red wine exerted a similar effect on intestinal CYP3A4, but white wine had little influence. Bergamottin, a furanocoumarin in grapefruit and lime juice, was subsequently found to inhibit human CYP3A4 activity (Bailey *et al.*, 2003) as well as intestinal P-glycoprotein efflux transporters (Dresser and Bailey, 2003). St. John's wort, a top-selling dietary supplement taken for depression, selectively induced CYP3A4 in the small intestine (Huang and Lesko, 2004). *Echinacea* inhibited human intestinal CYP3A, but induced hepatic CYP3A. Ginsenosides exhibited no or weak inhibition of several human CYPs, but some of the compounds' major intestinal metabolites inhibited a wide range of CYPs (Liu *et al.*, 2006). Certain components of *Ginkgo biloba*, frequently used for memory impairment, were potent inhibitors of human recombinant CYP1B1, CYP1A1, and CYP1A2 (Chang *et al.*, 2006). Identification of isoform-selective, nontoxic inhibitors may eventually lead to modulation of human xenobiotic metabolism for therapeutic purposes. There are large interindividual responses to CYP enzyme inducers and inhibitors (Lin and Lu, 2001).

Lifestyle Exercise can significantly affect the kinetics of xenobiotics, but is often not considered in occupational risk assessments of solvents. It increases two of the major determinants of VOC uptake, alveolar ventilation rate and cardiac output/pulmonary blood flow. Polar solvents with relatively high blood:air PCs (eg, acetone, ethanol, and ethylene glycol [EG]) are very rapidly absorbed into the pulmonary circulation. Alveolar ventilation is rate limiting for these chemicals. In contrast, pulmonary blood flow and metabolism are rate limiting for uptake of the more lipophilic solvents (Johanson and Filser, 1992). Heavy exercise can increase pulmonary uptake of relatively polar solvents as much as fivefold in human subjects (Astrand, 1983). Light exercise doubles uptake of relatively lipid-soluble solvents, but no further increases occur at higher workloads. Blood flow to the liver and kidneys diminishes with exercise, so biotransformation of well-metabolized solvents and urinary elimination of polar metabolites may be diminished (Lof and Johanson, 1998). Dankovic and Bailer (1994) modified the human PBTK model of Reitz *et al.* (1989) for MC to reflect light work conditions. The modified model predicted that light exercise would result in a twofold increase in hepatic MC deposition and in metabolite formation via CYP- and GSH-dependent pathways. Jonsson *et al.* (2001) developed a population PBTK model for humans inhaling MC during moderate to heavy exercise. Increased workload was predicted by PBTK modeling to produce an 87% increase in internal exposure to components of a mixture of toluene, ethylbenzene, and xylene (Dennison *et al.*, 2005).

Dietary habits can influence the absorption, metabolism, and toxicity of solvents in several ways. Factors that influence gastric emptying would not be expected to influence systemic absorption of VOCs, as VOCs are very rapidly absorbed by passive diffusion throughout the GI tract. The mere presense of food in the GI lumen, however, can inhibit absorption by reducing contact of the chemical with the GI epithelium. VOCs in the GI tract partition into dietary lipids, largely remaining there until the lipids are emulsified and absorbed. This serves to substantially delay uptake of lipophilic solvents such as CCl4, resulting in lower, but prolonged blood CCl4 levels and diminished hepatotoxicity in rats (Kim *et al.*, 1990a). Food intake increases splanchnic blood flow, which favors GI absorption. The elevation in liver blood flow would be expected to enhance the biotransformation of low doses of well-metabolized

solvents, but to have relatively little effect on metabolism of relatively high (ie, saturating) doses. Consumption of a high-fat diet results in a selective increase in hepatic CYP2E1 activity and protein levels in male Sprague–Dawley (S-D) rats (Raucy *et al.*, 1991). Elevation of plasma ketone bodies appears to be implicated in this process, because acetone is a potent CYP2E1 inducer. Carbohydrate deficiency has been recognized for many years to enhance the metabolism of a series of VOCs in rats, but not to alter their conjugation (Sato and Nakajima, 1985). Psoralens (found in parsley, parsnip, and celery) reduce CYP1A2 activity, whereas food cooked over charcoal enhances it. Effects of other foods, fruit juices, and food supplements are addressed in the sections "P450 Inducers" and "P450 Inhibitors."

Fasting for one to three days can significantly alter the hepatotoxicity of medium to high doses of VOCs that undergo metabolic activation. Fasting results in decreased hepatic concentrations of reduced GSH, due to cessation of intake of amino acids required for its synthesis. GSH plays a key role in detoxifying electrophilic metabolites of a number of VOCs, such as 1,1-dichloroethylene (DCE) (Jaeger *et al.*, 1974). Conversely, conjugation of GSH with TCE or PERC can lead to formation of limited quantities of cytotoxic, mutagenic metabolites (see the sections "Trichloroethylene" and "Tetrachloroethylene"). Fasting (~8–24 hours) results in induction of liver CYP2E1 and increase in metabolism of a number of aromatic hydrocarbons and halocarbons (Nakajima *et al.*, 1982). The hepatotoxicity of DCE and CCl4, which require CYP2E1-catalyzed metabolic activation, is more severe in fasted animals. In contrast, long-term food deprivation (ie, starvation) results in decreased synthesis and activity of CYPs.

Many physiological and biochemical processes that impact solvent TK exhibit circadian, or diurnal, rhythms. A series of investigations has been conducted to delineate molecular control mechanisms of diurnal oscillation in mammals. The phenomenon appears to be controlled by a "master pacemaker" in the suprachiasmatic nuclei (SCN) of the hypothalamus of mice (Teboul *et al.*, 2009). Genetic and genomic analyses of the SCN and liver indicate that a relatively small number of output genes are directly regulated by core oscillator components. Rate-limiting steps in major cellular pathways/processes are being identified as key sites of circadian regulation. Experiments reveal that transcriptional feedback is required for maintenance of circadian rhythmicity (Sato *et al.*, 2006).

Several research groups have discovered circadian rhythms in susceptibility of rats to liver damage by various VOCs, including CCl4, CHCl3, DCE, ethanol, and styrene (Labrecque and Belanger, 1991). In each instance, the chemicals were most toxic when given during the initial part of the rodents' dark/active cycle. Low hepatic GSH levels at this time were an important contributing factor to the increased liver injury by DCE and CHCl3. Restricted food intake during sleep resulted in lipolysis and formation of acetone, which contributed to the diurnal induction of CYP2E1 and the ensuing increases in hepatic metabolic activation and cytotoxicity of CCl4 in male rats during the early part of the animals' active cycle (Bruckner *et al.*, 2002). Skrzypinska-Gawrysiak *et al.* (2000) also observed that male mice were most susceptible to CCl4 hepatotoxicity when dosed at a similar time. Clearance rates for a number of well-metabolized compounds, including ethanol (Sturtevant *et al.*, 1978) and nicotine (Gries *et al.*, 1996), are maximal in human subjects during the first part of their active/wake cycle. Hepatic blood flow and acetone levels in expired air of humans peak before breakfast. Thus, humans may also be more susceptible during this time to the toxicity of solvents that undergo metabolic activation.

Ethanol is an effective CYP2E1 inducer when ingested repeatedly in substantial amounts. There are numerous reports of marked potentiation of hepatic or renal damage by ethanol or other alcohols in persons occupationally exposed to potent hepatorenal toxicants, such as CCl_4 (Folland *et al.*, 1976; Manno *et al.*, 1996). CCl_4 is not extensively metabolized, but its free radical metabolites are extremely cytotoxic.

A group of moderate drinkers exposed to TRI vapor at 175 ppm showed a significant increase in metabolism and metabolic clearance of the chemical (Johns *et al.*, 2006). TRI is a relatively nontoxic, poorly metabolized solvent. Kaneko *et al.* (1994) exposed ethanol-pretreated rats by inhalation of TCE or TRI at 50 to 1000 ppm. TRI metabolism was enhanced at all vapor concentrations, but TCE metabolism was enhanced by ethanol only at the highest vapor concentration (1000 ppm), as its biotransformation is perfusion-limited (limited by hepatic blood flow). Low levels of TCE entering the liver are extensively metabolized, even in nondrinkers who still have substantial CYP2E1 activity. Kedderis (1997) predicted that a 10-fold increase in CYP2E1 activity in humans inhaling TCE at 10 ppm would result in only a 2% increase in TCE metabolism by the liver. Thus, increased bioactivation capacity due to ethanol or other factors should not increase risks of toxicity or cancer from low-level exposures to TCE, DCE, MC, vinyl chloride, benzene, or other extensively metabolized VOCs. In contrast, Kedderis (1997) predicted a 10-fold increase in CYP2E1 activity would result in a 3.8-fold increase in PERC metabolites in the liver of persons inhaling 10 ppm PERC. Increased bioactivation of less extensively metabolized VOCs could thus enhance risks of low-level exposures to such chemicals.

Timing of ethanol consumption and VOC exposure is important. Prior repeated exposure to ethanol is necessary for substantial CYP2E1 synthesis to occur. Concurrent exposure to ethanol and a VOC, however, may often be protective from both well-metabolized and poorly metabolized solvents. If both a VOC and ethanol are metabolized by CYP2E1, the xenobiotics compete for available isozyme. Muller *et al.* (1975) observed that concurrent intake of ethanol and inhalation of TCE at 50 ppm by human subjects resulted in a marked decrease in urinary excretion of TCE's major metabolites, TCA and trichloroethanol (TCOH). In this instance, ethanol would afford protection against these oxidative metabolites. Metabolism of ethanol produces an excess of NAD, a cofactor that favors formation of TCOH from chloral hydrate (CH), at the expense of TCA. Reduced formation of TCA would be protective against TCA-induced hepatic tumors. Larson and Bull (1989), however, observed this interaction in rats only with very high doses of TCE and ethanol.

Medications and drugs of abuse that induce or inhibit CYP2E1 and other enzymes involved in the metabolism of VOCs can potentially alter the chemicals' toxicity or carcinogenicity. Nakajima *et al.* (1992a) showed that pretreatment of rats with phenobarbital, ethanol, or 3-methylcholanthrene significantly increased TCE oxidation. The same would be expected to occur in humans at high TCE doses. Some drugs (such as cycloheximide, disulfiram, and chloramphenicol) and the aforementioned natural constituents of plants inhibit CYP2E1. Those compounds, in sufficient doses, would be protective against high doses of TCE and other VOCs that are bioactivated by CYP2E1.

Tobacco smoke contains a number of compounds that are strong CYP inducers. Polycyclic hydrocarbons, such as 3-methylcholanthrene, are potent inducing agents. The polycyclic hydrocarbons primarily stimulate synthesis of CYP1A1 and CYP1A2, isozymes that play a modest role in catalyzing the biotransformation of TCE (Nakajima *et al.*, 1992a). Nicotine, however, is a strong CYP2E1 inducer in rats (Micu *et al.*, 2003). Cigarette smoke is known to induce CYP2E1 in both rodents and humans.

Yue *et al.* (2009) recently observed that chronic nicotine treatment also increased voluntary ethanol intake by rats, thereby further enhancing hepatic CYP2E1 and CYP2B1/2 levels.

Solvent Mixtures Many occupational and environmental exposures to VOCs involve multiple chemicals. That is particularly true of contaminated environmental media, in that widespread use of solvents leads to their volatilization and entry into surface waters and groundwater. VOCs spilled onto the ground evaporate, although some often leaches through porous soils into groundwater and remains trapped there. The groundwater at about 90% of 1608 hazardous waste sites on the US National Priorities List contains VOCs. TCE is the most frequently found of all chemicals, followed by lead, PCE, and benzene (Pohl *et al.*, 2008). The most common four-component VOC mixture is TCE, PCE, TRI, and 1,1-dichloroethane. ATSDR (2004) published a toxicological profile addressing potential health risks posed by this four-component mixture. Many US cities' drinking water supplies also contain complex mixtures of VOCs. Total concentrations generally range from ppt to ppb (Moran *et al.*, 2007; Rowe *et al.*, 2007). Trace amounts of a variety of VOCs are also present in the blood of many nonoccupationally exposed members of the general population (Churchill *et al.*, 2001; Blount *et al.*, 2006).

Most studies have involved experiments with binary or ternary mixtures. One chemical may have no effect on, potentiate (enhance), or antagonize (inhibit) adverse actions of a second or third chemical (Tan *et al.*, 2011). Knowledge of mechanisms of VOC interactions involves largely the influence of one VOC on the metabolic activation or inactivation of another. Koizumi *et al.* (1982) published the results of one of the first such studies. They found that coexposure of rats to PERC and TRI resulted in significant suppression of TRI metabolism. Workers exposed to TCE and PERC were found to have lower urinary concentrations of TCE metabolites than workers exposed to TCE alone (Seiji *et al.*, 1989). The interaction resulted from competitive metabolic inhibition, wherein the amounts of the combined chemicals exceeded the metabolic capacity of the study subjects. Such an interaction is protective against cytotoxicity and carcinogenicity, in that the bioactivation of both TCE and PERC is reduced. Conversely, systemic concentrations of parent VOCs would be increased, and this might enhance neurologic effects of sufficiently high doses (Pohl and Scinicariello, 2011).

PBTK modeling has been used by several research groups to predict the metabolic and toxicological consequences of exposure to VOC mixtures. Competitive metabolic inhibition was evident in a PBTK modeling approach to studying TCE and 1,1-DCE (El-Masri *et al.*, 1996) and TCE and vinyl chloride (Barton *et al.*, 1995). Later PBTK modeling efforts predicted interaction thresholds below which competitive metabolic inhibition would not occur. Dobrev *et al.* (2001), for example, reported that the thresholds for interaction of TCE with PERC and TRI vapor in rats were 25 and 135 ppm, respectively, when the TCE concentration was 50 ppm. Those findings imply that protection from adverse effects caused by oxidative metabolites would occur in occupational settings when vapor concentrations were relatively high. An increase in blood TCE concentrations under these exposure conditions, however, was predicted to result in a disproportionate increase in formation of nephrotoxic GSH conjugation products in humans (Dobrev *et al.*, 2002). Competitive metabolic inhibition, with potentiation or protection from adverse effects of VOCs, would not occur on exposure to environmentally relevant concentrations.

Additivity of toxic effects of chemicals that act by similar mechanisms is typically assumed in the absence of experimental evidence to the contrary. Stacey (1989) studied the joint action of

TCE and PERC on the liver and kidneys of rats. Combined administration of near-toxic-threshold doses of the two solvents produced modest hepatorenal toxicity. Jonker *et al.* (1996) provided evidence that TCE and PERC in combination with two other similarly acting solvents affected kidney weight in rats given subtoxic doses of each chemical by gavage for 32 days. Competitive metabolic inhibition, as described above, would result in less than additive adverse effects when metabolites are the bioactive moieties (Pohl and Scinicariello, 2011). Goldsworthy and Popp (1987) found that the joint effect of TCE and PERC on peroxisome proliferation in the liver and kidneys of mice and rats was less than additive. Competitive metabolic inhibition at relatively high exposure levels of toluene, ethylbenzene, and xylene has been predicted by PBTK modeling to result in higher internal exposures (and CNS depressant effects) than would occur with simple additivity (Dennison *et al.*, 2005).

Few toxicity or carcinogenicity studies of complex chemical mixtures including VOCs have been conducted. The National Toxicology Program (NTP, 1993a) supplied F344 rats and B6C3F1 mice with drinking water containing 24 contaminants for up to 26 weeks. The mixture contained TCE, PERC, MC, TRI, DCE, 1,1-dichloroacetic acid, other solvents, heavy metals, polychlorinated biphenyls, and a phthalate. The total no-observed-adverse-effect level (NOAEL) for histological changes in the liver was 11 ppm in rats. Suppression of immune function occurred in female mice that consumed 756 ppm of the mixture for two weeks or 378 ppm for 13 weeks. A follow-up study in chemically tumor-initiated rats showed that the contaminant mixture did not promote preneoplastic foci in the liver (Benjamin *et al.*, 1999). Wang *et al.* (2002a) supplied ICR mice with water containing $CHCl_3$, 1,1-dichloroacetic acid, DCE, TRI, TCE, and PERC for 16 and 18 months. There was a trend of increasing frequency of hepatocellular neoplasms in the male mice and an increasing incidence of mammary adenocarcinomas in the high-dose female mice. The total concentration of VOCs in the drinking water of females was about 1555 ppb. Most of the mixture was TCE (471 ppb) and PERC (606 ppb). These concentrations are far lower than have previously been reported to produce tumors. The results must be regarded as preliminary, in that the study design had a number of limitations, and the results have not been replicated. In addition, male B6C3F1 mice are particularly susceptible to hepatic tumors (Haseman *et al.*, 1998) and mice metabolically activate a substantially greater proportion of VOC doses than do humans.

Diseases Illness can be a major source of variability in response to solvents. Impaired drug metabolism and clearance are commonly seen in patients with cirrhosis and hepatitis (Welling and Pool, 1996). Reduced metabolism of solvents may result from decrease in hepatic parenchymal mass, diminished enzymatic activity, and/or decreased portal blood flow (Morgan and McLean, 1995). Lower levels of CYP2E1, CYP1A2, and GSH are seen in livers of patients with cirrhosis (Murray, 1992). Reduced P450-catalyzed metabolic activation of certain solvents can be protective, but diminished capacity to conjugate electrophilic metabolites with GSH would have the opposite effect. Plasma levels of albumin and α_1-acid glycoprotein fall in cirrhotic patients. Thus, plasma protein binding of many xenobiotic metabolites decreases and their rate of elimination increases (Morgan and McLean, 1995). Definitive information is lacking, however, on the net effect of common liver diseases on solvents.

Chronic kidney disease is becoming increasingly prevalent in the United States over the past decade (Coresh *et al.*, 2007). Progressive loss of kidney function leads to impaired renal excretion of numerous chemicals and metabolites that may be toxic or pharmacologically active. Kidney disease can affect uptake and efflux transporters and metabolic enzymes in the liver and the GI tract (Nolin *et al.*, 2008). Chronic renal failure can result in downregulation of the expression of some liver CYPs, but have no effect on others (Leblond *et al.*, 2001). Effects on hepatic clearance of therapeutic chemicals can thus vary widely. The mechanisms of these effects on gene expression are unclear, as is their applicability to solvents. The plasma protein binding of many xenobiotics is reduced in patients with compromised renal function, apparently due to retention of substances that compete for protein-binding sites, as well as reduced albumin synthesis. Clearance of highly metabolized xenobiotics thus appears to depend on potentially offsetting influences of altered metabolism, decreased plasma protein binding, and decreased renal excretion (Yuan and Venitz, 2000). Impairment of renal metabolic activation via oxidation or β-lyase-mediated conversion of GSH metabolic intermediates of TCE and PERC (see the sections "Trichloroethylene" and "Tetrachloroethylene" for details) to reactive, mutagenic metabolites would be protective.

Diabetes mellitus is a metabolic disease characterized by hyperglycemia as a result of insulin deficiency (Type I) or insulin resistance (Type II). Type II accounts for 90% of cases. Approximately 21 million people suffer from diabetes in the United States. A prominent effect of chemically induced Type I diabetes in rats is induction of CYP2E1. Elevation of acetone, but apparently not the other ketone bodies, is responsible for the CYP2E1 increase. Hypoinsulinemia may play a role, in that insulin downregulates CYP2E1 mRNA in rat hepatoma cells and primary cultures of rat hepatocytes (Cheng and Morgan, 2001). In contrast, CYP2E1 is not affected in Type II diabetic animals (Sawant *et al.*, 2004). Neither Type I nor Type II diabetes influences CYP2E1 activity in humans (Lucas *et al.*, 1998; Cheng and Morgan, 2001). Nevertheless, animal studies show that Type II diabetes increases susceptibility to hepatotoxicants including allyl alcohol and CCl_4 (Sawant *et al.*, 2004), apparently due to inhibition of tissue repair. Devi and Mehendale (2005, 2006) subsequently demonstrated inhibition of expression of genes involved in cell division and protease inhibitors, as well as enhanced gene expression of proteases in Type I diabetic rats. These events may be important in delayed tissue repair following chemical cytotoxicity in diabetics.

Persons with bacterial infections may be more sensitive to cytotoxic actions of solvents. Endotoxin, which includes a lipopolysaccharide (LPS), is released from the cell wall of gram-negative organisms. The LPS causes the release of inflammatory mediators, which alter cell membranes, intercellular signaling, and gene expression (Roth *et al.*, 1997). These effects may render cells more susceptible to damage by solvents and other chemicals. Exposure of animals to small amounts of endotoxin potentiates liver injury by CCl_4, halothane, allyl alcohol, ethanol, and other solvents (Roth *et al.*, 1997). Endotoxin apparently activates Kupffer cells to release inflammatory mediators and cytotoxic moieties to hepatocytes (Thurman, 1998).

CHLORINATED HYDROCARBONS

Trichloroethylene

TCE was widely used as a solvent and metal degreasing chemical in the United States from the early 1900s to 1980s (Bakke *et al.*, 2007). Workers were initially subjected routinely to quite high exposures. NIOSH (1989) estimated that 401,000 persons at 23,225 plants in the United States were potentially exposed to TCE. TCE has been identified at over one half of the nearly 1300 hazardous waste sites that make up the EPA's National Priorities List (ATSDR, 2006a; Pohl *et al.*, 2008). It is released into the atmosphere from

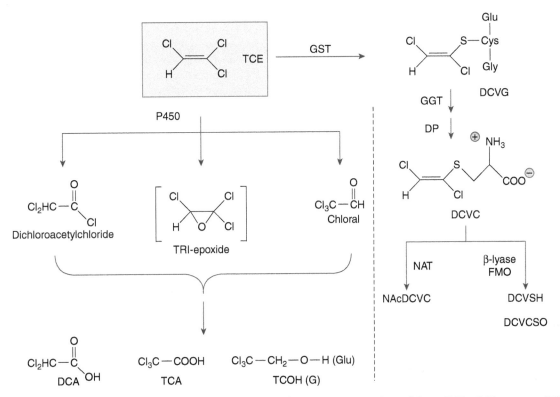

Figure 24-5. *General scheme of metabolism for TCE. Abbreviations*: β-Lyase, cysteine conjugate β-lyase; DCA, dichloroacetate; DCVC, *S*-(1,2-dichlorovinyl)-L-cysteine; DCVSH, 1,2-dichlorovinylthiol; DCVCSO, DCVC sulfoxide; DCVG, *S*-(1,2-dichlorovinyl)glutathione; DP, dipeptidase; FMO, flavin-containing monooxygenase; GGT, γ-glutamyltransferase; GST, GSH *S*-transferase; P450, cytochrome P450; TCA, trichloroacetate; TCOH, trichloroethanol; TCOG, TCOH glucuronide. (Reproduced from Lash *et al.*, 2005, with permission from Elsevier.)

vapor degreasing operations; however, direct discharges to surface waters and groundwater from disposal operations have been frequent occurrences. As a result, TCE can be released to indoor air by vapor intrusion through underground walls and floors and by volatilization from the water supply. TCE has recently received a great deal of attention from the scientific and regulatory communities, due in large part to the EPA's effort to update the chemical's two-decade-old risk assessment (EPA, 2009).

Moderate to high doses of TCE, as with other halocarbons, are associated with a number of noncancer toxicities (ATSDR, 1997d; Barton and Das, 1996). TCE has been implicated in the development of autoimmune disorders and immune system dysfunction (Blossom and Gilbert, 2006; Cooper *et al.*, 2009; Lan *et al.*, 2010), and has been investigated for its potential as a male reproductive toxicant (Forkert *et al.*, 2003; Xu *et al.*, 2004). The effect of gestational exposure to TCE or its oxidative metabolites on cardiac development is a subject that has invoked considerable debate, as conflicting results have been published (Fisher *et al.*, 2001; Johnson *et al.*, 2003; Watson *et al.*, 2006). The issue of TCE's potential effect on ocular development has also recently reemerged (Warren *et al.*, 2006). Nevertheless, cancer remains the dominant issue for TCE. TCE and its potential health risks have recently been reviewed by the NAS (2006, 2009), Jollow *et al.* (2009), and the EPA (2009).

Metabolism The adverse effects of TCE, other than CNS depression, are generally believed to be associated with TCE's metabolites. CNS depression is due to the parent compound and a major metabolite, TCOH. Knowledge of TCE's metabolism in different species and under different exposure conditions is thus a prerequisite to understanding its mechanisms of action and assessing human health risks. A great deal of experimentation at many biological levels has been conducted over the last five decades to these ends.

TCE is rapidly and extensively absorbed into the systemic circulation via the oral and inhalation routes. Dermal absorption is considerably slower and less extensive. The majority of TCE is oxidized in the liver, while a small amount is conjugated in the liver with GSH by GSTs. The oxidative pathway is shown on the left of Fig. 24-5, while the GSH pathway is shown on the right. This diagram is a simplification of a more complex metabolic scheme described in detail by Lash *et al.* (2000a).

The initial step in the oxidative pathway is catalyzed by microsomal CYPs. CYP2E1, as described previously in the subsection "Metabolism" in the section "Toxicokinetics," is the primary isozyme responsible for oxidation of low concentrations of TCE (Lipscomb *et al.*, 1997; Ramdhan *et al.*, 2008; Kim and Ghanayem, 2006). CYP-catalyzed oxidation of TCE in rodents and humans, in decreasing order of magnitude, is as follows: mice >> rats > humans (Lash *et al.*, 2000a). Whether or not TCE is initially converted to TCE oxide is controversial. Cai and Guengerich (2001) were able to detect formation of trace amounts of the epoxide by phenobarbital-induced rat liver CYPs, but not by human liver CYPs. The majority of TCE is apparently converted to an oxygenated TCE–CYP intermediate, which rearranges to form chloral, a major metabolic intermediate. Chloral is oxidized to chloral hydrate (CH), a sedative and hypnotic still widely used in medical and dental procedures for infants and children (Buck, 2005; Heistein *et al.*, 2006). CH is both oxidized to TCA and reduced to TCOH. Much TCOH is conjugated with glucuronic acid (GLU) and excreted in the urine. TCOH–GLU that is excreted in the bile is extensively hydrolyzed in the gut, reabsorbed, and oxidized in part to TCA (Stenner *et al.*, 1997). Chiu *et al.* (2007) observed that concentrations of TCA were significantly lower than TCOH and TCOH–GLU concentrations in the blood of humans who inhaled TCE at 1 ppm for six hours. Modest amounts of DCA apparently are produced from TCA and TCOH in mice, but relatively little DCA is formed in rats or humans. Trace amounts of DCA were detected in one study of TCE-exposed humans (Fisher *et al.*, 1998) but not in other studies (Lash *et al.*, 2000b; Bloemen *et al.*, 2001). Very high doses of both TCA and DCA have been shown to be hepatic carcinogens in mice (Bull, 2000). It is generally accepted that TCA is a nongenotoxic liver carcinogen in B6C3F1 mice, although its ability to cause liver cancer in humans has been discounted by findings in numerous laboratory investigations (Bull, 2000). The possible role of DCA in human liver cancer is even more controversial (Walgren *et al.*, 2005; Caldwell and Keshava, 2006; Klaunig *et al.*, 2007).

The GSH conjugation pathway is quite similar qualitatively, but not quantitatively, in rats and humans. The initial step in this second, minor pathway involves conjugation of TCE with GSH to form *S*-(1,2-dichlorovinyl)GSH (DCVG). DCVG formation occurs primarily in the liver at a rate about 10 times greater in rats than in humans (Green *et al.*, 1997). Much of the DCVG is excreted via the bile into the intestines and converted to *S*-(1,2-dichlorovinyl)-L-cysteine (DCVC). That metabolite is reabsorbed and taken up by the liver, where a portion is detoxified by *N*-acetylation. Bernauer *et al.* (1996) exposed rats and humans to TCE vapor at up to 160 ppm for six hours. The rats excreted eight times more *N*-acetyl-DCVC in their urine than did the human volunteers at each exposure level. Some DCVC is taken up by the kidneys and further metabolized by the enzyme β-lyase to *S*-(1,2-dichlorovinyl)thiol (DCVSH). DCVSH is then converted to highly reactive products, including DCVC sulfoxide (DCVCS), chlorothioketene, and thionoacylchloride (Lash *et al.*, 2000a). Metabolic activation of DCVC to chlorothioketene was shown to occur 11 times more rapidly in rats than in humans (Green *et al.*, 1997). Lash *et al.* (2001) also demonstrated that cultured rat renal cells were more sensitive to DCVC than human renal cells. Chlorothioketene and similarly unstable congeners are capable of covalently binding to renal cellular proteins and DNA. This results in genotoxicity and cytotoxicity, with ensuing regenerative hyperplasia and potentially renal cell cancer (RCC).

Modes of Carcinogenic Action in Target Tissues Both metabolic pathways are implicated in the carcinogenicity of TCE: reactive metabolite(s) of the GSH pathway in kidney tumors in rats and oxidative metabolites in liver and lung tumors in mice. That tumor formation in many cases is species-, strain-, sex-, and route of exposure–dependent has provided clues as to TCE's modes of carcinogenic action. Whereas substantial progress has been made on the mechanistic front, the reader should not infer from the text that follows that all modes of action are known with absolute certainty.

Liver Cancer It is well established that TCE, when given chronically in very high doses by gavage, can produce an increased incidence of hepatocellular carcinoma in B6C3F1 mice, but not in other strains of mice or in rats. This differential susceptibility can be explained in part by the greater capacity of the mouse to bioactivate relatively large quantities of TCE via the oxidative pathway. The B6C3F1 mouse produces a substantially larger amount of TCA after TCE exposures than do unresponsive strains of mouse, rats, or humans. The susceptibility of the B6C3F1 mouse is also likely related to the high (42.2%) incidence of liver adenoma/carcinoma in male controls (Haseman *et al.*, 1998). This phenomenon may be due to an abnormally high population of spontaneously initiated cells in these animals' liver. Mice express very low levels of epoxide hydrolase (Lorenz *et al.*, 1984), the enzyme that catalyzes the hydrolytic degradation/detoxification of reactive epoxide metabolites of TCE and other VOCs.

CH induces hepatic tumors in male B6C3F1 mice, but not in F344 rats (Leaky *et al.*, 2003). Female B6C3F1 mice gavaged with

up to 100 mg CH/kg per day for 104 weeks showed no increase in liver tumors, but the male mice did exhibit increased incidences of hepatoma and/or hepatocellular carcinoma. CH is rapidly converted to TCA and TCOH in rodents and humans. Merdink *et al.* (2008) detected only trace amounts of DCA in blood and urine of male human subjects dosed with 500 or 1500 mg of CH. An epidemiology study of the possible association of short-term clinical administration of CH as a sedative–hypnotic and cancer risk in 2290 patients was conducted by Haselkorn *et al.* (2006). The authors concluded there was no persuasive evidence of a causal relationship between CH and cancer in humans.

TCA and DCA are the most likely candidates for proximate hepatocarcinogens produced by TCE's oxidative pathway. TCA is a species-specific carcinogen that induces peroxisome proliferation and hepatocellular carcinoma in male and female B6C3F1 mice when administered in very high doses in drinking water or by gavage. It does not produce liver tumors in any strain of rats tested under these conditions (NAS, 2006, 2009). Very high doses of DCA, however, produce hepatic tumors in both B6C3F1 mice and F344 rats. Large, repeated doses of DCA and TCA initially stimulate, and then depress the growth of normal hepatocytes (Bull, 2000). This may confer a growth advantage to initiated cells, and is referred to as *negative selection*. At high tumorigenic doses, DCA (but not TCA) is thought to stimulate cell replication within liver tumors. If indeed both DCA and TCA contribute to tumorigenesis, findings by Bull *et al.* (2002) indicate they do so by distinct mechanisms. DCA-promoted liver tumors differed phenotypically from those promoted by TCA. DCA- and TCA-induced tumors also differ as to whether their depression of cytosine methylation is reversible on cessation of treatment (Tao *et al.*, 1998). This is particularly important as DNA hypomethylation, including that of the proto-oncogenes c-jun and c-myc, may be an epigenetic mechanism for the tumorigenicity of DCA and TCA (Tao *et al.*, 2004). It appears that hypomethylation due to TCA and DCA induces DNA replication and prevents the methylation of newly synthesized strands of DNA (Ge *et al.*, 2001). Tao *et al.* (2000) have reported that DCA and TCA do so by virtue of their depletion of *S*-adenosylmethionine, which normally supplies the methyl group for the methylation process. It should be recognized that these are not genotoxic mechanisms. The effects disappear as soon as these metabolites are eliminated.

A primary mode of action of TCA and to a smaller extent DCA is activation of PPARα. As peroxisomes contain a variety of oxidative enzymes, PPARα activation produces oxidative stress, which can be manifest as lipid peroxidation, oxidative DNA damage, and transcription factor activation (O'Brien *et al.*, 2005). Stimulation of PPARα can enhance DNA replication, resulting in expansion of some clones of hepatocytes and suppression of apoptosis, so initiated and precancerous cells will be spared. Male wild-type mice dosed orally with TCE exhibit hepatocyte proliferation and changes in expression of genes involved in cell growth (Laughter *et al.*, 2004). PPARα-null mice are refractory to those effects, which are associated with carcinogenesis. Mice expressing human PPARα fail to show increases in markers of cell proliferation and are resistant to liver cancer if treated with PPARα agonists (Morimura *et al.*, 2006; Yang *et al.*, 2008). The concentration of PPARα in human cells is about 10% of that in the livers of rodents (Palmer *et al.*, 1998; Klaunig *et al.*, 2003). Many toxicologists have judged that the mode of action for hepatic carcinogenesis observed in mice after administration of peroxisome proliferation–inducing drugs and other chemicals, such as TCA, makes it unlikely that such chemicals pose a hepatic cancer risk in humans (Cattley *et al.*, 1998; Clewell and Andersen, 2004; Klaunig *et al.*, 2007; Gonzalez and Shah, 2008). It was concluded by an expert review panel that the PPARα mode of action for liver cancer in mice is not relevant to humans (NAS, 2006). However, others have raised questions about the interpretation of PPARα actions and whether it is the only relevant mode of action for such chemicals (Keshava and Caldwell, 2006). This continues to be a subject of active debate (NAS, 2008).

It is important to recognize that stimulation or inhibition of cell growth through PPARα activation ceases when the metabolites are eliminated (Miller *et al.*, 2000). Thus, such alteration of cell signaling is not a genotoxic mechanism of action. Very high concentrations of DCA and CH have a weak genotoxic action in vitro. Bull (2000) and Moore and Harrington-Brock (2000), however, conclude that it is unlikely that those metabolites would cause tumors in any organ through genotoxicity or mutagenicity at exposure concentrations relevant to humans.

Lung Cancer As discussed in the review paper by Green (2000), inhaled TCE is carcinogenic to the mouse lung but not to that of the rat. Oral TCE is not carcinogenic to the lung, probably due to first-pass hepatic metabolism that limits the amount of TCE reaching the lungs. The primary target of TCE in the mouse lung is the nonciliated Clara cell. Cytotoxicity is characterized by vacuolization and increased replication of these cells in the bronchiolar epithelium. A dose-dependent reduction in the CYP activity in Clara cells is observed as well. This loss of metabolic activation capacity can be thought of as an adaptive response. Clara cells recover morphologically during repeated daily inhalation exposures to TCE.

Chloral is the putative toxicant responsible for pulmonary tumor formation. Clara cells of the mouse efficiently metabolize TCE to chloral. Chloral accumulates, due to its efficient production and low activity of ADH, the enzyme responsible for its reduction to TCOH. The Clara cells' lack of glucuronosyltransferase, the enzyme that normally catalyzes the formation of TCOH–GLU, has also been implicated in chloral accumulation. Species differences in susceptibility of the lung to TCE are due in part to mouse lung Clara cells having a much higher level of CYP2E1 than those of the rat, and thus a much higher capacity to metabolize TCE to chloral. Also, Clara cells in mice are much more numerous than in rats. Clara cells are rare in human lungs. A critical role for chloral is supported by the findings that its administration to mice, but not TCA or TCOH, causes Clara cell toxicity identical to that of TCE. Chloral does appear to have some genotoxic potential, especially in regard to inducing aneuploidy. However, the fact that tumors are not seen in species where cytotoxicity does not occur strongly implicates cytotoxicity and reparative proliferation in tumor formation. In an effort to test the hypothesis that bronchiolar damage by TCE is associated with bioactivation within Clara cells, Forkert *et al.* (2006) administered TCE i.p. to CD-1 mice. The result was dose-dependent production of dichloroacetyl lysine adducts in Clara cells (used as an in vivo marker of TCE metabolism) that correlated with bronchiolar damage. The work also suggested that CYP2F2 may play a more important role than CYP2E1 in TCE metabolism and cytotoxicity within the mouse lung (Forkert *et al.*, 2005).

Kidney Cancer TCE was given in corn oil to F344/N rats and B6C3F1 mice of both sexes by gavage five times weekly at doses up to 1000 mg/kg in rats and 6000 mg/kg in mice in a 13-week study, as well as up to 1000 mg/kg to both species and sexes in a 103-week study (NTP, 1990). A low, but statistically significant increase in renal tumor incidence was observed only in the male rats given TCE at 1000 mg/kg for two years. Two-year gavage studies of TCE, in four additional rat strains, were also conducted (NTP, 1988). In all strains of rats tested, cytomegaly and karyomegaly of tubular cells in the renal corticomedullary region were seen. Frank toxic nephropathy was observed with higher frequency in male rats

beginning at 52 weeks of exposure. Renal adenomas or adenocarcinomas were occasionally seen in male rats of different strains after two years of the repetitive, high-dose oral exposure regimen.

Adverse effects of TCE on the kidneys are due largely to metabolites formed via the GSH conjugation pathway (Lash *et al.*, 2000b). As described previously, conjugation of TCE with GSH to form DCVG occurs primarily in the liver. DCVG is secreted into bile and blood. That in the bile is converted in the gut to DCVC, which is reabsorbed into the bloodstream. Humans have a lower capacity than rats to metabolize TCE by the GSH pathway. Lash *et al.* (1999) were able to detect DCVG in the blood of humans who inhaled TCE at 50 or 100 ppm for four hours, but Bloeman *et al.* (2001) could not find DCVG or DCVC in the urine of similarly exposed subjects. DCVG in the blood is taken up by the kidneys and metabolized to DCVC by γ-glutamyltransferase and a dipeptidase. Lash *et al.* (2001) observed the following decreasing order of toxic potency in freshly isolated rat cortical cells: DCVC > DCVG >> TCE. DCVC can be detoxified by acetylation or activated further by two pathways: (1) cleavage by renal cytosolic and mitochondrial β-lyases to dichlorothioketene, which in turn can lose a chloride ion to yield chlorothioketene or tautomerize to form chlorothionacyl chloride (the latter two moieties are very reactive and acylate proteins and DNA); and (2) oxidation by renal CYPs or flavin-containing monooxygenases to DCVCS, a reactive epoxide. Lash *et al.* (1994) reported that DCVCS was a more potent nephrotoxicant than DCVC in vitro and in vivo in rats. Apoptosis was observed after as little as one hour of incubation of cultured human renal proximal tubular (RPT) cells with DCVC and DCVCS (Lash *et al.*, 2003, 2005). Cellular proliferation, accompanied by increased expression of proteins associated with cellular growth, differentiation, stress and apoptosis, was also an early response to low doses. Necrosis, however, was a late, high-dose phenomenon. Exposure of human RPT cells to DCVC at lower concentrations for 10 days also resulted in expression of genes associated with cell proliferation, apoptosis, and stress (Lash *et al.*, 2005), as well as repair and DCVC metabolism (Lash *et al.*, 2006).

Animal studies typically provide insight into mode of action, but in the case of TCE-induced RCC, human studies have been of significant value. Bruning *et al.* (1997a) analyzed tumor tissues from 23 RCC patients with occupational histories of long-term, high-level TCE exposure. Tumor cell DNA was isolated and analyzed for somatic mutations of the von Hippel–Lindau (VHL) tumor suppressor gene. Compared with VHL gene mutation rates of 33% to 55% in unexposed RCC patients, all 23 TCE-exposed RCC patients exhibited aberrations of the VHL gene. In a follow-up study, Brauch *et al.* (1999) sought to determine whether TCE produced a specific mutation of the VHL gene. These investigators analyzed VHL gene sequences in DNA isolated from RCC tissues from patients exposed to high levels of TCE in metal-processing factories. Renal cell tumors of TCE-exposed patients showed somatic VHL mutations in 33 of 44 cases (75%). Of the 33 cases with VHL mutations, a specific mutational hot spot at VHL nucleotide 454 was observed in 13 cases. The nucleotide 454 mutation was not found in any of the 107 RCC patients without TCE exposure or among 97 healthy subjects, 47 of whom had a history of TCE exposure. These data suggest that the VHL gene may be a specific and susceptible target of reactive GSH pathway metabolites, a concept strengthened by a more recent study reporting VHL nucleotide 454 mutation among TCE-exposed but not in nonexposed RCC patients (Brauch *et al.*, 2004). More recently, however, Charbotel *et al.* (2007) found no associations between the number and type of VHL mutations in TCE-exposed and unexposed RCC patients. The subject awaits further clarification (Chow and Devesa, 2008).

The aforementioned reactive products of DCVC are both cytotoxic and mutagenic. Adverse effects on proximal tubule cells include alkylation of cytosolic and mitochondrial structural and enzymatic proteins, oxidative stress, marked ATP depletion, and perturbations of calcium homeostasis. Tubular necrosis ensues, with subsequent proliferation that can alter gene expression, which may modify cell growth and differentiation. Genes associated with stress, apoptosis, repair, and proliferation were upregulated almost twofold in cultured human renal tubular cells exposed to subtoxic doses of DCVC for 10 days (Lock et al., 2006). Mechanisms of noncarcinogenic and carcinogenic action are discussed in detail by Lash et al. (2000b) and Lock and Reed (2006).

Bruning and Bolt (2000) opine that reactive metabolite(s) of the GSH pathway may have a genotoxic effect on the proximal tubule of the human kidney, but that full development of a malignant tumor requires a promotional effect such as cell proliferation in response to tubular damage. If this is true, RCC secondary to TCE exposure would be a threshold response. The question of whether chronic tubular damage is a prerequisite to renal tumor formation is quite important. Evidence has come from the use of electrophoresis to examine protein excretion patterns in the urine of RCC patients with and without a history of chronic, high-level TCE exposure (Bruning et al., 1996). Protein excretion patterns indicative of tubular damage were identified in all their 17 TCE-exposed cases, but in only about one half of 35 controls. Bruning et al. (1999) subsequently published the results of a larger study supportive of this concept. Approximately 93% of 41 RCC patients with high TCE exposure exhibited elevated urinary α_1-microglobulin excretion versus 46% of 50 RCC patients without a history of TCE exposure. Similar findings were reported in an updated study by Bolt et al. (2004), and in an investigation by Green et al. (2004) of 70 electronics workers who inhaled an average of 32 ppm TCE for four years.

Results of an investigation by Mally et al. (2006) provide additional insight into the TCE renal carcinogenesis threshold premise. A strain of rats (Eker) uniquely susceptible to renal carcinogens was administered 100, 250, 500, and 1000 mg TCE/kg by gavage five days per week for 13 weeks. The Eker rat is a unique animal model for RCC, carrying a germ-line alteration of the Tsc-2 tumor suppressor gene. Results showed a significant increase in cell proliferation in renal tubular cells but no increase in preneoplastic renal lesions or tumor incidence. In vitro studies were conducted on primary Eker rat renal epithelial cells by exposing them to the TCE metabolite DCVC dissolved in water at 10 to 50 µM for eight, 24, and 72 hours. Concentrations of DCVC that reduced rat renal cell survival to 50% also resulted in cell transformation. No carcinogen-specific mutations were identified in the VHL or Tsc-2 tumor suppressor genes in the transformed cells. RCCs in the Eker rat have substantial similarities to human RCC. It is not entirely clear that this or any contemporary experimental animal model adequately mirrors humans with regard to the effects of TCE-induced mutations in the VHL gene, but the authors firmly suggest that TCE-mediated renal carcinogenicity may occur only secondarily to nephrotoxicity and sustained regenerative cell proliferation.

Metabolism of TCE by the GSH pathway is similar qualitatively, but not quantitatively in rats and humans. N-Acetyl-DCVC, the major detoxification product of DCVC, was found in the urine of humans and rats after six hours of inhalation of up to 160 ppm TCE (Bernauer et al., 1996). Cumulative excretion of the N-acetyl derivative was seven- to eight-fold higher in the rats. Bruning et al. (1997b) originally reported an increased likelihood of RCC patients with high TCE exposure having a functional GST isozyme GSTT1 or GSTM1 genotype. This isozyme GSTT1 is thought to be primarily involved in TCE metabolism, while GSTM1 is thought to

detoxify epoxides. A reassessment by the investigators of a larger population, however, revealed no such relationships (Wiesenhutter et al., 2007). Moore et al. (2010), recently completed an assessment of an even larger population. There was an increased risk of RCC in workers with at least one intact GSTT1 allele, but not in persons with two deleted alleles (ie, null genotype).

It is also worthy of note that male rats and humans are apparently at greater risk of TCE-induced kidney cancer than their female counterparts. Blood DCVG concentrations were 3.4-fold higher in male than in female volunteers inhaling 50 or 100 ppm TCE (Lash et al., 1999). Male rats display higher GSH conjugation, γ-glutamyl transpeptidase activity, and cysteine conjugate β-lyase activity than female rats. Taken together, results of the cited studies indicate that both male humans and male rats possess GSH conjugation capacity and can produce the critical TCE metabolite DCVC. Renal carcinoma has been observed in male rats and male workers when both have been exposed to very high TCE concentrations for prolonged periods of time. These observations show data congruence, indicating that the conjugation pathway plays a central role in induction of renal carcinoma in males of both species. As described previously, rats have a significantly greater capacity to metabolically activate TCE to DCVC by this pathway than do humans. Rat renal cortical cells, in turn, are more susceptible to injury by DCVC than their human counterparts.

Cancer Epidemiology Studies There have been many published studies of cancer incidence and mortality in TCE-exposed populations. Most of the epidemiology studies in the United States prior to 2000 involved workers in the aircraft maintenance and manufacturing industries. There were also investigations of Swedish, Finnish, German, and Danish worker cohorts. Results of these assessments have been mixed, ranging from no association to limited evidence. The major studies with some exposure data constituted what the Wartenberg et al. (2000) meta analysis referred to as Tier I studies, which received a greater weighting when making causal inferences than lower tier cohort, case–control, and community-based investigations. Among the Tier I studies, evidence for an excess incidence of cancer was strongest for kidney (rate ratios [RR] = 1.7, 95% confidence interval [CI] = 1.1–2.7), liver (RR = 1.9, CI = 1.0–3.4), and non-Hodgkin lymphoma (NHL) (RR = 1.5, CI = 0.9–2.3) (Wartenberg et al., 2000).

The report of Henschler et al. (1995) was the first in a series of German studies that have provided some of the strongest evidence to date for an association between TCE and RCC. These authors described a cohort of male cardboard factory workers who were exposed to moderate to extremely high concentrations of TCE vapor. By the closing date of the study, five of the 169 exposed workers had been diagnosed with kidney cancer versus none of the 190 controls. This resulted in standardized incidence ratios (SIRs) of 7.97 (CI = 2.59–18.59) and 9.66 (CI = 3.14–22.55), using Danish and German Cancer Registry data for comparison, respectively. German researchers also conducted a hospital-based case–control study with 58 RCC patients and 84 patients from accident wards who served as controls. Of the 58 RCC patients, 19 had histories of occupational TCE exposure of at least two years, compared with only 5 of the controls. After adjustment for potential confounders, an association between RCC and long-term exposure to TCE was reported (odds ratio [OR] = 10.80, CI = 3.36–34.75) (Vamvakas et al., 1998). In an expanded German case–control study of 134 RCC cases and 401 controls, excess risks for those working longest with TCE (OR = 1.8, CI = 1.01–3.20) and those experiencing narcotic symptoms (OR = 3.71, CI = 1.80–7.54) were reported (Bruning et al., 2003). Narcosis was thought to be associated with peak exposures. These workers reported frequent dizziness, requiring them to seek fresh air several times daily. More recent investigations have generally involved surveys of populations with lower exposures. The results of these investigations have been suggestive of an association between TCE and RCC, although some findings were negative or did not reach statistical significance (Alexander *et al.*, 2006; Boice *et al.*, 2006; Chang *et al.*, 2005; Mandel *et al.*, 2006; Raaschou-Nielsen *et al.*, 2003; Wong, 2004). A number of these assessments involved a limited number of subjects. Charbotel *et al.* (2006) studied 86 RCC patients and 316 matched controls from an area in France with high TCE exposures in local industries. There was a 64% increase in RCC risk with TCE exposure, with the risk doubling in persons with a high cumulative dose, increasing more when peak exposures were also taken into account (OR = 2.74, CI = 1.06–7.07). The OR was still high, but not statistically significant after adjusting for exposure to cutting fluids, because of the study's lack of power. Chow and Devesa (2008) reviewed recent epidemiological evidence of a rising incidence of RCC in the United States. Cohort studies showed associations with smoking, obesity, diminished physical activity, hypertension, and certain chemical exposures.

Epidemiological evidence of NHL or cancer of the liver, lung, or other organs has been weaker than that for the kidney. There appeared to be a dose-dependent increase in the SIR for NHL with increased duration of TCE exposure in Danish workers (Raaschou-Nielsen *et al.*, 2003). These researchers also reported a SIR of 1.7 for esophageal adenocarcinoma. Seidler *et al.* (2007) described the association between TCE exposure of >35 ppm per year and malignant lymphoma (OR = 2.1, CI = 1.0–4.8) as being of borderline statistical significance. Lan *et al.* (2010) recently observed a dose-dependent decline in major types of lymphocytes in TCE-exposed workers in China. Little or no association with NHL incidence was seen by Boice *et al.* (2006) or Zhao *et al.* (2005) in aerospace employees. Evidence of lung cancer in persons occupationally exposed to TCE is limited to nonexistent (Boice *et al.*, 2006; Hansen *et al.*, 2001; Zhao *et al.*, 2005; Raaschou-Nielsen *et al.*, 2003). The latter group of scientists' estimates of SIRs for lung cancer, for example, were 1.4 for men and 1.9 for women. Most estimates of liver cancer risk in TCE-exposed workers have also been low. SIRs of 2.6 (Hansen *et al.*, 2001) and 2.8 (Raaschou-Nielsen *et al.*, 2003), resulting from a small number of cases, were among the highest reported.

Risk Assessment Attempts to understand the mechanistic underpinnings of TCE's carcinogenicity in rodent models and their relevance to humans have resulted in a *massive* body of published data. TCE provides a stellar example of how experimental data from laboratory and epidemiological studies may or may not impact cancer risk assessment in a regulatory context. The EPA began in the 1990s to revise its guidelines for cancer risk assessment. The final EPA *Guidelines for Carcinogen Risk Assessment* were released in March 2005. TCE was utilized as a pilot chemical for evaluation and implementation of this guidance document. The guidelines emphasize a scientific "weight of evidence" approach that includes characterization of dose–response relationships, modes of action, and metabolic/TK processes. Where adequate data are available to support reversible binding of the carcinogenic moiety to biological molecules as the initiating event, a nonlinear (ie, threshold) risk assessment/approach is to be used. Otherwise, the default assumption of a linear (ie, no-threshold) model/approach is to be used to estimate cancer risk. As described above, there is considerable evidence that TCE's oxidative metabolites act via nongenotoxic modes of action. PPARα activation and induction of mouse liver tumors

were judged to be irrelevant to humans (NAS, 2006). The EPA, in its 2001a draft *TCE Risk Assessment*, concluded it was difficult to establish with sufficient certainty the important TCE metabolites, the key events they cause, and their relevance to humans. Despite a substantial increase in information in the last decade, EPA scientists (Caldwell and Kesheva, 2006) contend that knowledge of mechanisms and human relevance is still insufficient to depart from the default assumption. This is exemplified by the critical response of EPA scientists (Caldwell *et al.*, 2006) to the attempt of Clewell and Andersen (2004, 2006) to apply a margin of exposure approach (nonlinear dose–response extrapolation) in their TCE risk assessment. In contrast to liver cancer, kidney cancer is widely accepted to be qualitatively similar in rats and humans, although rats form greater quantities of reactive metabolites via the GSH pathway. Despite genotoxic events, kidney tumor formation in humans is generally believed to require promotion resulting from frank cytotoxicity. Caldwell and Kesheva (2006), however, opine that there may be other modes of action of multiple metabolites operative at low doses. This logic has been retained in the EPA's most recent *IRIS Toxicological Review of TCE* (2009).

The EPA (2001a) draft *TCE Risk Assessment* elicited considerable debate, which prompted the EPA and other federal agencies to request a scientific review of the document by a NAS expert panel. Their report was released in 2006. It concluded there was concordance between rat and human studies of renal carcinogenicity. The preponderance of evidence indicated that humans would be much less susceptible than mice to liver and lung carcinogenesis. It was recommended, among other things, that a new meta-analysis of epidemiological data be conducted. Kelsh and his coworkers recently completed meta-analyses of occupational study data. Studies were classified as group I or II, depending on the quality of their design and exposure assessment. The summary relative risk estimate (SRRE) across all such studies was 1.42 (CI = 1.17–1.77) for kidney cancer (Kelsh *et al.*, 2010). The same research group performed meta-analyses for occupational TCE exposures and liver cancer (Alexander *et al.*, 2007) and NHL (Mandel *et al.*, 2006). The highest SSREs calculated for liver cancer and NHL in any study groupings were 1.30 and 1.59, respectively. The authors noted the results of many studies were inconsistent, information on TCE exposure was often quite limited, and recognized confounding factors were not always taken into account. NAS (2009) recently evaluated published occupational epidemiology studies, and concluded there was limited/suggestive evidence of associations between chronic TCE exposure and kidney cancer. Evidence was deemed inadequate/insufficient to determine whether there was an association with NHL or cancer of the liver, lung, or any other organ. In contrast, Scott and Chiu (2006) opined that modest RR elevations (1.5–2.0) typically reported in positive epidemiology studies provided support for the kidney, liver, and lymphatic systems as target organs. The EPA (2009), in its *IRIS* document released in September 2011, concluded there was convincing evidence of a causal association between TCE exposure and kidney cancer. Epidemiological evidence was said to be less compelling for NHL, and even more limited for liver cancer. Nevertheless, TCE was characterized by the EPA as "carcinogenic in humans by all routes of exposure." This is a departure from previous national and international classifications.

Tetrachloroethylene

Tetrachloroethylene (perchloroethylene, PERC) is commonly used as a dry cleaner, fabric finisher, degreaser, rug and upholstery cleaner, paint and stain remover, solvent, and chemical intermediate. The highest exposures usually occur in occupational settings via inhalation. Much attention is being focused on adverse health effects that may be experienced by dry cleaners and other persons living in the proximity of such facilities (Garetano and Gochfeld, 2000). Echeverria *et al.* (1995), for example, reported adverse effects on visuospatial functions in dry cleaners. PERC is frequently detected in the low ppt range in the breath and blood of the general populace (Ashley *et al.*, 1994; Churchill *et al.*, 2001; Blount *et al.*, 2006). Although releases are primarily to the atmosphere, PERC enters surface and groundwaters by accidental and intentional discharges (ATSDR, 1997c). Levels in the ppb range were reported in municipal water in areas of New England, where PERC was used in a process to treat plastic water pipe (Paulu *et al.*, 1999). Pohl *et al.* (2008) reported that PERC was the third most frequently found chemical contaminant in groundwater at hazardous waste sites in the United States. A dry cleaner adjacent to Camp Lejeune, in North Carolina, was the source of PERC contamination of some wells that supplied drinking water to the marine base. This contamination prompted a recent study of potential health effects in employees and persons stationed at the base (NAS, 2009).

Metabolism The systemic disposition and metabolism of PERC and TCE are similar in many respects, although PERC is much less extensively metabolized (ATSDR, 1997c; Chiu *et al.*, 2007). Both chemicals are well absorbed from the lungs and GI tract, distributed to tissues according to their blood flow and lipid content, partially exhaled unchanged, and metabolized. PERC, like TCE, is metabolized by CYP-catalyzed oxidation and GSH conjugation. CYP2E1, however, is not thought to play a major role, in that PERC is considered to be oxidized primarily by the CYP2B family in the rat (Hanioka *et al.*, 1995). In humans, CYP2B6 is the primary isoform responsible for PERC metabolism, and there are minor contributions by CYP1A1 and CYP2C8 (White *et al.*, 2001). The initial metabolite is the epoxide PERC oxide. This metabolic intermediate can be biotransformed to several products (Lash and Parker, 2001). The primary one is trichloroacetyl chloride, which reacts with water to form TCA, the predominant PERC metabolite found in the urine of rodents and humans (Birner *et al.*, 1996; Volkel *et al.*, 1998). Some TCA is converted to DCA.

A small proportion of absorbed PERC undergoes conjugation with GSH to form *S*-(1,2,2-trichlorovinyl)GSH (TCVG). That initial metabolic step is catalyzed by GSTs and occurs primarily in the liver. TCVG is converted to *S*-(1,2,2-trichlorovinyl)-L-cysteine (TCVC). TCVC, like the DCVC formed from TCE, is both detoxified in the liver by *N*-acetylation and metabolically activated by β-lyases in the kidneys. 2,2-Dichlorothioketene can decompose to DCA. Hence, DCA is derived from both GSH- and CYP-dependent biotransformation of PERC. PERC is conjugated with GSH more extensively by rats (1%–2%) (Dekant *et al.*, 1986) than is TCE (<0.005%) (Green *et al.*, 1997). The extent of GSH conjugation of PERC increases when the oxidative pathway begins to become saturated at high exposure levels. Metabolic products of GSH conjugates of TCE and PERC are primary contributors to these halocarbons' nephrotoxicity (Lash *et al.*, 2007).

Modes of Cytotoxicity/Carcinogenicity PERC-induced hepatic injury is believed to be a consequence of its oxidative metabolism (Lash and Parker, 2001). Although PERC is more poorly metabolized by CYPs than TCE, two additional intermediate metabolites of PERC contribute to its hepatocytotoxicity: the initial oxidation product, PERC oxide, and one of its convertants, trichloroacetyl chloride. TCA is primarily responsible for activation of the nuclear receptor PPARα, which stimulates peroxisomal enzymes and selected CYPs involved in lipid metabolism. This results in peroxisome proliferation, which generates reactive oxygen moieties that can cause lipid peroxidation, cellular injury, and altered expression of cell-signaling proteins (Bull, 2000). Lash *et al.* (2007) more recently demonstrated that CYP inhibition resulted in reduced injury of hepatocytes isolated from male F344 rats and exposed to PERC. GSH depletion increased cellular injury, apparently because of a shift from the GSH to the oxidative pathway.

The metabolism and mode of nephrotoxicity of PERC and TCE appear to be quite similar, although PERC and its metabolites are somewhat more potent. Renal effects of both halocarbons are due primarily to metabolites formed via the GSH pathway (Lash and Parker, 2001). The sites, enzymes, and products associated with PERC biotransformation are almost identical to those associated with TCE. The primary difference is that TCVG and TCVC are produced from PERC, and DCVG and DCVC are formed from TCE. TCVC can be detoxified by acetylation or cleaved by renal cytosolic and mitochondrial β-lyases to trichlorothioketene, which loses a chloride ion to form dichlorothioketene. The latter is a very reactive moiety that binds to cellular proteins and DNA. TCVC, as noted above, can be enzymatically oxidized to form the very reactive TCVC sulfoxide (TCVCS) (Krause *et al.*, 2003). TCVCS was shown to be more nephrotoxic than TCVC in male rats after i.p. injection (Elfarra and Krause, 2007). TCVC caused more pronounced necrosis of RPT cells in male rats than did DCVC after i.v. injection (Birner *et al.*, 1997). Lash *et al.* (2002) similarly found that PERC and TCVG were more toxic than TCE and DCVG in vivo to renal cortical cells of F344 rats. Cells from male rats were more sensitive than cells from females to PERC- and TCVG-induced mitochondrial state 3 respiratory inhibition and cytotoxicity. Isolated rat hepatocytes and their mitochondria, however, were unaffected by PERC and TCVC. Elevated GSH levels enhanced TCE-induced and PERC-induced cytotoxicity in suspensions of rat renal cortical cells but not hepatocytes (Lash *et al.*, 2007). Thus, PERC's GSH metabolites are both sex- and organ-specific.

Hepatorenal Toxicity PERC, like TCE, has a limited ability to adversely affect the liver or kidneys of rodents. Near-lethal i.p. doses of PERC were required to cause acute liver injury in mice (Klaassen and Plaa, 1966). Buben and O'Flaherty (1985) saw manifestations of modest hepatocellular damage in male mice given 500 to 2000 mg PERC/kg daily for six weeks by corn oil gavage. A lack of dose dependence reflected saturation of metabolic activation in this dosage range. Philip *et al.* (2007) reported that male mice given 150 to 1000 mg PERC/kg by aqueous gavage initially exhibited a dose-dependent increase in serum alanine aminotransferase (ALT) activity, but levels of the enzyme regressed substantially over a 30-day dosing period. Hayes *et al.* (1986) found no consistent dose-related changes in any clinical chemistry parameter in male or female rats that consumed up to 1440 mg PERC/kg in their drinking water for 90 days. Liver injury was not seen in B6C3F1 mice or Osborne–Mendel rats gavaged with up to ~1000 mg/kg daily for 78 weeks (NCI, 1977a,b). Dose-dependent karyomegaly was observed in the renal proximal tubule (RPT) epithelium of mice and rats inhaling PERC for 103 weeks (NTP, 1986). This change was most prominent in the male rats. Tinston (1995) reported mild, progressive glomerulonehropathy and increased pleomorphism of renal tubular nuclei in male but not female rats that inhaled 1000 ppm PERC for up to 19 weeks. Green *et al.* (1990) found increases in protein droplets and cell proliferation in the proximal tubular epithelium of male F344 rats gavaged with 1500 mg PERC/kg daily for up to 42 days. These alterations were accompanied by an increase in α_{2u}-globulin, a male rat-specific protein (Fig. 24-6). Goldsworthy *et al.* (1988) reported similar findings in male but not female F344 rats gavaged for 10 days with 1000 mg PERC/kg per

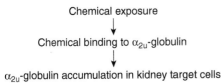

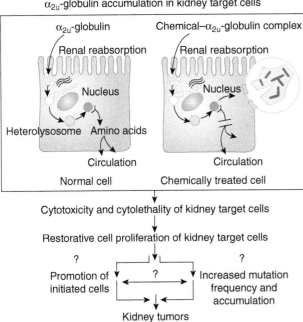

Figure 24-6. *Proposed mechanism of solvent-induced kidney cancer in male rats involving α_{2u}-globulin.* (Used with permission from Borghoff *et al.*, 1996a.)

day. The accumulation of α_{2u}-globulin is cytotoxic, causing cellular necrosis and compensatory cellular proliferation in the P2 segment of renal proximal tubules (Borghoff *et al.*, 1990).

Humans should be less susceptible to hepatorenal injury by PERC than rodents, due to lower target organ doses of the parent compound and its bioactive metabolites. Rats achieve a substantially higher internal dose of VOCs than do humans on inhalation exposures. Volkel *et al.* (1998) subjected rats and people to identical PERC inhalation regimens. Blood TCA concentrations were 3 to 10 times higher in the rats. DCA was not detectable in human urine, but substantial amounts were found in rat urine. A study of the urinary excretion of total trichloro-metabolites by PERC-exposed workers led Ohtsuki *et al.* (1983) to conclude that the capacity of humans to metabolize PERC was rather low. Lash and Parker (2001) noted that saturation of PERC metabolism occurred at lower doses in humans than in rodents. This indicates that humans have lower capacity to form biologically active metabolites from moderate to high PERC doses. The difference is reflected in the finding of much lower concentrations of protein adducts in the blood of humans than in the blood of rats subjected to equivalent PERC inhalation exposures (Pahler *et al.*, 1999).

PERC has limited ability to damage the liver of humans. Stewart *et al.* (1977) found no evidence of hepatotoxicity in six male and six female volunteers exposed randomly to PERC at 0, 25, or 100 ppm 5.5 hours per day, five days per week for 11 weeks. Serum ALT activity was not increased in 22 dry cleaners examined by Lauwerys *et al.* (1983). A research group in Italy studied 141 employees exposed to PCE in small laundries and dry-cleaning shops (Gennari *et al.*, 1992). No worker exhibited clinical signs of hepatic dysfunction or abnormal serum enzyme concentrations, although there did appear to be an increase in one isozyme of

γ-glutamyltransferse, which was said to be associated with hepatobiliary impairment. Another investigation of dry cleaners failed to reveal increases in serum enzymes, but did show mild to moderate changes in hepatic parenchyma revealed by ultrasonography (Brodkin *et al.*, 1995). Thus, considerable experience in occupational settings demonstrates that humans may develop mild but reversible liver injury on chronic exposure to high concentrations of PERC (ATSDR, 1997c).

Occupational exposures to PERC vapor have led to several reports of mild renal tubular damage (ATSDR, 1997c). Employees of dry-cleaning shops have been the subjects of a number of studies of potential kidney effects. Increased concentrations of urinary lysosomal or β-glucuronidase activity were described in dry cleaners exposed to 10 ppm (Franchini *et al.*, 1983) and 23 ppm PERC (Vyskocil *et al.*, 1990) for 9 to 14 years. In a more comprehensive study, a number of urinary indices indicative of early glomerular and tubular changes were increased in 50 dry cleaners who inhaled ~15 ppm PERC for 10 years (Mutti *et al.*, 1992). Verplanke *et al.* (1999) monitored several indices of tubular and glomerular function in Dutch dry-cleaning workers, but found an increase only in retinol-binding protein in their urine. Other investigators have failed to find evidence of renal effects in such populations. A laboratory study of 10 male and 10 female adults, who inhaled PERC at up to 150 ppm for as long as 7.5 hours per day for five days, did not show changes from preexposure baseline BUN levels (Stewart *et al.*, 1981). Hake and Stewart (1977) described a dry cleaner who was found unconscious in a pool of PERC, where he had been for an estimated 12 hours. Laboratory tests revealed hematuria and proteinuria that lasted for 10 and 20 days, respectively. Mild hepatic damage was revealed by transient increases in serum enzymes. On the basis of the foregoing occupational experiences, PERC has shown limited ability to cause diffuse changes along the nephron, although extremely high exposures can lead to pronounced changes in humans.

Cancer Bioassays in Rodents High, chronic doses of PERC have been demonstrated to produce species-specific and in certain cases strain- and gender-specific tumors in some organs of mice and rats. Male and female B6C3F1 mice, gavaged with very high doses of PERC (stabilized with epichlorohydrin) for up to 78 weeks, exhibited an increase in hepatocellular carcinoma (NCI, 1977a). No increase in tumor incidence was seen in Osborne–Mendel rats. A significant increase in hepatocellular neoplasms (adenomas and carcinomas combined) was seen in B6C3F1 mice inhaling 100 or 200 ppm PERC for two years (NTP, 1986). There was also a low incidence of renal adenomas and carcinomas in male but not female F344 rats exposed for two years to 200 or 400 ppm PERC vapor. The incidence of renal neoplasms in the males was 1 of 49 controls, 3 of 49 exposed at 200 ppm, and 4 of 49 exposed at 400 ppm (NTP, 1986). Even though the changes were not statistically significant, it was noted that these particular tumors are *rare* in F344/N male rats, so they were believed to have been caused by PERC exposure. There was also a significant increase over controls in mononuclear-cell leukemia (MNL) in the male and female rats, but it was not clearly dose-dependent. The incidence of this form of leukemia can exceed 70% in F344 controls (Caldwell, 1999; Ishmael and Dugard, 2006). MNL in this rat strain apparently arises from large granular lymphocytes. This lukemic origin is very uncommon in humans (Caldwell, 1999). Gliomas were found in two female and four male F344/N rats exposed to PERC at 400 ppm and in one control male (NTP, 1986). The increase in incidence of this tumor was not statistically significant. Thus, the brain tumors were not considered by NTP (1986) to have been induced by exposure to PERC. The overall incidence of Leydig cell (testicular) tumors was

70%, 80%, and 82% in the 0-, 200-, and 400-ppm groups, respectively. Haseman *et al.* (1998) reported that NTP control F344 rats have an extremely high spontaneous incidence (89.1%) of Leydig cell tumors. Therefore, these tumors are believed to be irrelevant to men (Ishmael and Dugard, 2006). No increases in lung proliferative lesions seen in B6C3F1 mice of either sex after inhalation of PERC at 100 or 200 ppm for 103 weeks, nor were lung neoplasms seen in male or female F344/N rats exposed at 200 or 400 ppm for 103 weeks (NTP, 1986).

Cancer Epidemiology Studies There have been many epidemiology studies of cancer incidence and mortality in groups of dry cleaners and other persons occupationally exposed to PERC (ATSDR, 1997c; NAS, 2009; EPA, 2008). Some researchers have reported findings of excess incidences of different cancers, while others have not. Frequently, there was not a determination of the degree or duration of PERC exposure, or consideration of major confounding factors (eg, exposure to other solvents/ chemicals, smoking, alcohol consumption, socioeconomic status). Nevertheless, there was sufficient information for Weiss (1995) to conclude that cigarette smoking and alcohol consumption could only partially account for an increased rate of esophageal cancer in dry cleaners. In this instance kidney cancer incidence did not appear to be elevated. Blair *et al.* (2003) conducted and updated a mortality assessment of a cohort of dry cleaners and found an increased risk of death from esophageal cancer (standardized mortality ratio [SMR] = 2.2, 95% CI = 1.5-3.3). No exposure–response pattern was seen. Chang *et al.* (2005) did not find any cases of esophageal cancer in a Taiwanese cohort of electronics workers, while Lynge *et al.* (2006) observed a decreased incidence in dry cleaners in Nordic countries. Nevertheless, NAS (2009) concluded there was limited/suggestive evidence of an association between chronic PERC exposure and esophageal cancer.

There has been little evidence of an association between occupational PERC exposure and liver cancer. Increased incidences or mortality were not seen in cohort studies (Blair *et al.*, 2003; Chang *et al.*, 2005) or in a case–control study (Lynge *et al.*, 2006). A RR of just 0.76 (CI = 0.38–1.52) was estimated in the latter investigation of Nordic dry-cleaning workers. A mortality odds ratio (MOR) of 2.57 (CI = 1.21–5.46) was reported by Lee *et al.* (2003) in another case–control study, but the exposure assessment was weak. The NAS (2009) recently concluded there was insufficient/inadequate evidence to determine whether an association exists between chronic PERC exposure and hepatobiliary cancer.

Epidemiology studies of populations exposed to PERC generally have shown no increase in risk of lung cancer. Blair *et al.* (2003), however, in an updated mortality analysis of dry cleaners, reported a SMR of 1.5 (CI = 1.2–1.9) for workers with medium to high exposures. This study adequately characterized exposures and included a relatively large number of subjects. Thus, the NAS (2009) concluded there is limited/suggestive evidence of an association between chronic PERC exposure and lung cancer.

Investigations of kidney cancer risk in PERC-exposed populations have yielded mixed results. A number of studies have not revealed an increased risk (Blair *et al.*, 2003; Boice *et al.*, 1999; Lynge *et al.*, 2006; Mundt *et al.*, 2003; Ruder *et al.*, 2001). However, some of the assessments lacked power due to a limited number of study subjects. Although Blair *et al.* (2003) reported a very low SMR for kidney cancer deaths in dry cleaners with little or no PERC exposures, the SMR was 1.5 for those with medium or high exposure. Increased incidences have also been reported by Mandel *et al.* (1995), Pesch *et al.* (2000), and McCredie and

Stewart (1993). The NAS (2009) concluded there is limited/suggestive evidence of an association between chronic PERC exposure and kidney cancer in humans.

Risk Assessment A great deal of research has been conducted to characterize PERC's dose–response relationships, modes of action, and metabolism/TK in rodents and humans. It is apparent from the previous discussion there is a considerable body of information available from human experience/exposures to PERC, as well as extensive data sets from studies in different species of laboratory animals. Both types of data are important in assessing risks to human health. Knowledge of the relevance of the animal data to humans is essential in order to meaningfully extrapolate from one species to another.

Humans appear to be less susceptible than rodents to the toxic or carcinogenic actions of PERC, as they are to those of TCE. Humans absorb less inhaled PERC and TCE, attain lower target organ doses of the parent compounds, have lower oxidative and GSH conjugation capacity, and inactivate epoxide intermediates more efficiently. On equivalent inhalation exposures of Wistar rats and humans to PERC, the rats excreted substantially larger amounts of TCA, DCA, and acetylated TCVC (Volkel *et al.*, 1998). These observations were consistent with in vitro findings of greater conversion of PERC to TCVC by rat liver cytosol and of 10-fold higher β-lyase-mediated metabolism of TCVC by rat than by human kidney (Green *et al.*, 1990). These data indicate that the human kidney has limited capacity to generate reactive metabolites from PERC by the GSH and β-lyase pathways. Biotransformation of PERC by the GSH conjugation pathway appears to be quite similar qualitatively, but not quantitatively in male rats and humans.

PERC-induced accumulation of $\alpha_{2\mu}$-globulin in the P2 segment of renal proximal tubules and the accompanying cytotoxic and regenerative changes are *unique* to the male rat (Borghoff *et al.*, 1990). $\alpha_{2\mu}$-Globulin is synthesized under androgenic control in the liver of male rats, reabsorbed by the P2 segment, and undergoes hydrolytic digestion. Accumulation of $\alpha_{2\mu}$-globulin in cytoplasmic droplets elicits tubular cell necrosis and compensatory cell proliferation (Goldsworthy *et al.*, 1988). Sustained cell proliferation can promote clonal expansion of spontaneously or chemically initiated cells in proximal tubules to form preneoplastic and neoplastic lesions (Swenberg, 1993). The increase in cell proliferation is reversible, as is the binding of halocarbon metabolites to $\alpha_{2\mu}$-globulin. Thus, this mode of action is not genotoxic and is considered by International Agency for Research on Cancer (IARC) and the EPA to be irrelevant to humans. Melnick and Kohn (1999), however, argue that some data are inconsistent with this conclusion, and that alternative mechanisms may exist. Doi *et al.* (2007) find some contribution of $\alpha_{2\mu}$-globulin nephropathy to renal tumors produced by several structurally diverse chemicals in rats, but conclude that other critical processes are probably involved.

Several comprehensive reviews of PERC's toxicity and carcinogenicity have been published. Lash and Parker (2001) compiled an excellent review of the metabolism, toxicity, and modes of toxicity of the chemical in laboratory animals and humans. The NAS (2009) recently published an evaluation of risks of use of TCE- and PERC-contaminated drinking water. It contained an extensive review of the metabolism, toxicity, and carcinogenicity of the two VOCs. The EPA (2008) released a draft document in support of its IRIS risk assessment, entitled *Toxicological Review of Tetrachloroethylene (Perchloroethylene)*. Quite recently, the NAS (2010) published a review of the EPA document. Questions were raised that called into question the soundness and reliability of EPA's proposed toxicity and cancer risk estimates. Stated weaknesses included a lack of critical analysis of data, preference given to studies (eg, genotoxicity, epidemiological) showing positive results, and lack of an integrated consideration of the weight of evidence. It is anticipated this review will result in EPA's publication of a revised PERC risk assessment document.

1,1,1-Trichloroethane

TRI (methyl chloroform) is a widely used organic solvent. Its popularity as a metal degreaser, general purpose solvent, spot cleaner, and component of aerosols and a variety of household products increased substantially with the decline in manufacture of other halocarbons found to be high-dose rodent carcinogens and potential human carcinogens (ATSDR, 2006b). Utilization of TRI diminished during the 1990s, however, due to its ozone-depleting properties (Doherty, 2000). The VOC was to be phased out under the Montreal Protocol by 2002, but is still manufactured in the United States and utilized as a precursor for hydrofluoro-carbons. TRI is also still present in some cleaning products. It was found in groundwater at 21% of hazardous waste sites surveyed in the United States (Pohl et al., 2008). TRI and other VOCs in groundwater can remain trapped for years and serve as a source of low-level exposure. The highest exposures to TRI occur via inhalation in occupational settings, but many persons encounter the VOC at home by use of commercial products and tap water containing it. Ashley et al. (1994) reported TRI and other VOCs in the blood of 75% of >600 non-occupationally exposed individuals. TRI and TCE were also frequently detected in a subset of 982 adults examined in the NHANES III survey (Churchill et al., 2001), and in 951 members of the general population (Blount et al., 2006).

Toxicokinetics and Metabolism The TK of TRI has been characterized in rodents and in humans. TRI is rapidly and extensively absorbed from the lungs (Schumann et al., 1982) and GI tract (White et al., 2013). Systemic uptake and blood levels are elevated in humans inhaling TRI and other VOCs when they exercise (Astrand et al., 1973). Dallas et al. (1989) observed that uptake of inhaled TRI by rats diminished from >80% to 50% to 60% during two hours of exposure, due to its systemic accumulation as a result of slow metabolism. Monster et al. (1979) similarly noted in humans that the capacity of the body to absorb TRI vapor was less than for TCE, due to TRI's relatively poor metabolism. White et al. (2013) reported the bioavailability of comparable oral doses of TRI and TCE in rats to be ~85% and 45%, respectively. TRI, like other VOCs, is distributed throughout the body, with fat achieving the highest concentrations (Schumann et al., 1982). As TRI biotransformation is quite limited, the VOC is cleared primarily by exhalation by rodents (Reitz et al., 1988; Schumann et al., 1982) and humans (Nolan et al., 1984).

A number of PBTK models for TRI in rodents and in humans have been published. Lu et al. (2008) recently evaluated the suitability of each of these for use in the EPA IRIS database. The model of Reitz et al. (1988) proved the most satisfactory, in that it accurately predicted the time-course of TRI in mouse, rat, and human blood for different inhalation scenarios. No empirical data were available for assessing the accuracy of simulations of brain TRI levels. Warren et al. (1998), however, demonstrated a high degree of correlation between brain and blood levels in TRI-exposed mice and rats, as well as reasonable correlation between brain levels and CNS effects of the VOC. TK data from human and rodent studies were used by Lu et al. (2008) to simulate internal dose metrics for appropriate human exposure scenarios for derivation of IRIS reference values.

Toxicity The primary pharmacological manifestation of acute or chronic inhalation of TRI is CNS depression, ranging in severity from slight headache or dizziness to anesthesia and death (ATSDR, 2006b). The current TLV of 350 ppm was established to prevent decrements in workers' mental and physical functions. Volunteers who inhaled 450 ppm TRI for four hours showed no effects on psychophysiological functions (Salvini et al., 1971). Two of 11 other subjects inhaling 500 ppm TRI 6.5 to 7.0 hours daily for five days exhibited difficulty balancing on one foot (Stewart et al., 1969). Muttray et al. (2000) found no psychophysiological effects in volunteers breathing 200 ppm TRI for four hours, but did report EEG changes and slight tiredness in their subjects. Warren et al. (2000) observed rapid, parallel increases in blood and brain TRI concentrations in mice inhaling the VOC. Mice breathing high vapor levels initially exhibited increased locomotor activity, followed by decreased activity. Mattsson et al. (1993) saw large evoked potential and EEG changes in F344 rats during inhalation of 2000 ppm TRI, but no evidence of neurotoxicity (eg, residual neurologic functional or morphological changes) after 13 weeks of exposure of ≤2000 ppm six hours daily, five days per week. Most studies of long-term occupational exposures have not revealed residual neurologic effects, although one assessment of workers subject to near-anesthetic vapor levels did reveal deficits in memory and balance (ATSDR, 2006b). It is worthy of note that very high inhaled concentrations of TRI, particularly when accompanied by hypoxia and stress, can sensitize the myocardium to catecholamines, producing cardiac arrhythmias (Reinhardt et al., 1973).

TRI has a very limited cytotoxic potential, ostensibly due to its limited biotransformation to relatively nontoxic metabolites. A near-lethal acute i.p. dose (3350 mg TRI/kg) was required to significantly enhance serum ALT activity in mice (Klaassen and Plaa, 1966). Male rats given a single oral dose of ~2500 mg/kg exhibited a transient increase in serum aspartate aminotransferase activity, but no ALT increase (Tyson et al., 1983). These enzymes are released from damaged or necrotic hepatocytes into the bloodstream. Male rats gavaged five times weekly for as long as 12 days with up to 5 g TRI/kg died from effects of repeated, protracted CNS depression, but exhibited only slight hepatotoxicity (Bruckner et al., 2001). Quast et al. (1988) saw only minimal histological changes in the liver of F344 rats inhaling 1500 ppm TRI six hours daily, five times per week for up to two years. Rats gavaged daily for 21 days with a high dose of TRI showed increased urinary N-acetyl-β-D-glucosaminidase (NAG) activity, but no microscopic evidence of injury indicative of renal toxicity (NTP, 1996). Liver and/or kidney injury are usually absent or quite modest in occupationally exposed populations, even in fatal cases (ATSDR, 2006b). A report by Hodgson et al. (1989) is an exception. They described four TRI-exposed workers who exhibited elevated serum ALT activity and fatty vacuolation of hepatocytes. In addition, Brogen et al. (1986) reported that 10% of a group of metal workers exposed to TRI, TCE, and Freon 113 had elevated NAG activity in their urine.

Potential Carcinogenicity The NCI (1977b) conducted a 78-week study in which B6C3F1 mice and F344 rats of both sexes received high doses of TRI daily by gavage. There was no increase in cancers attributable to TRI. In a screening study, Maltoni et al. (1986) observed an apparent increase in leukemias in male and female S-D rats gavaged with 500 mg TRI/kg per day for 104 weeks. Statistical analyses were not presented, and the authors stated that definite conclusions could not be drawn from their work due to limitations in the design and number of animals. A two-year inhalation study in B6C3F1 mice and F344 rats of both sexes revealed no evidence of tumorigenicity due to TRI (Quast et al., 1988). Few

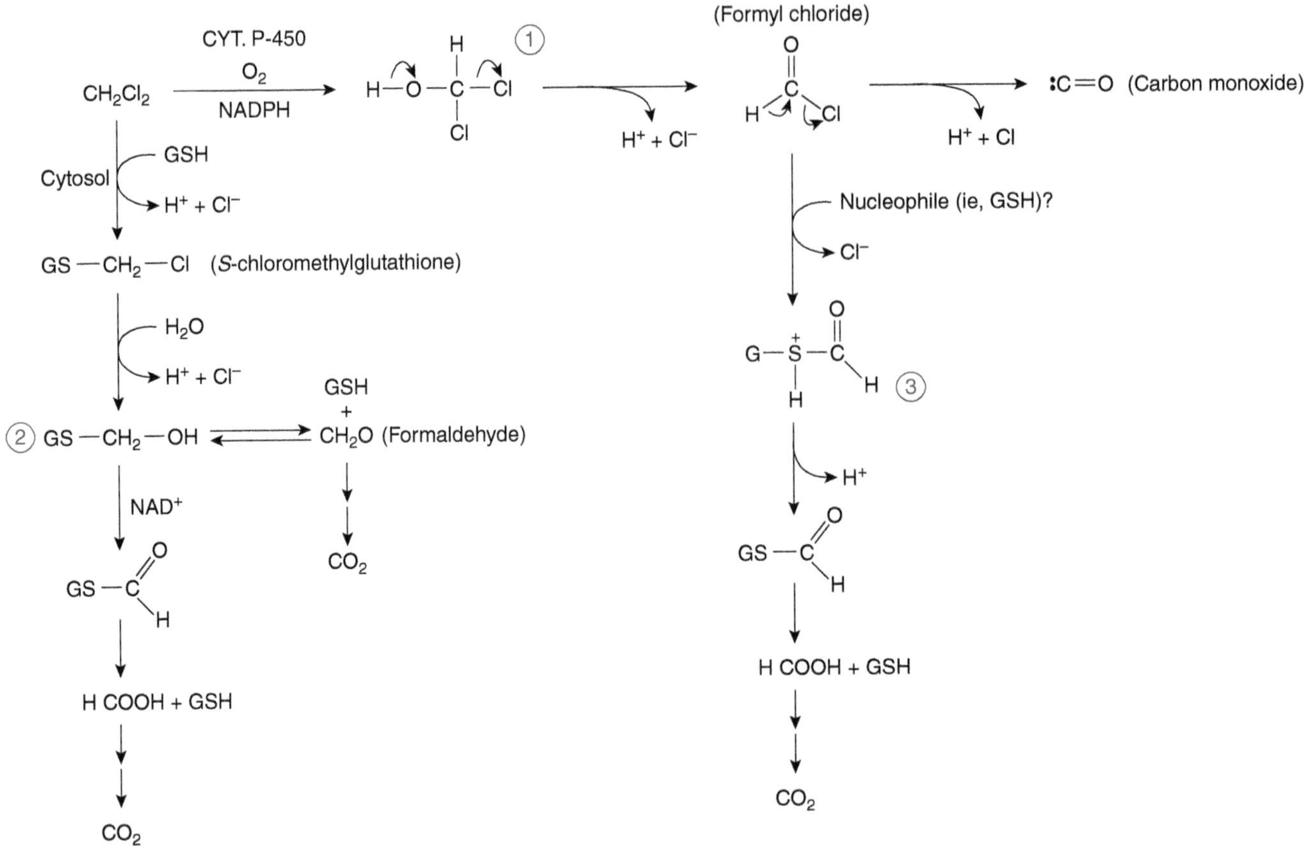

Figure 24-7. *Proposed pathways for methylene chloride (CH₂Cl₂) metabolism.* (1) Mixed-function oxidase pathway; (2) glutathione transferase pathway; and (3) nucleotide pathway. (Modified from Andersen *et al.*, 1987, with permission from Elsevier.)

epidemiological studies of TRI-exposed populations have been conducted. Infante-Rivard *et al.* (2005) did report a high risk (OR = 7.55, 95% CI = 0.92–61.97) of childhood leukemia in offspring of women exposed to TRI from two years before pregnancy up to birth. Recently, Gold *et al.* (2011) reported an OR of 1.8 (1.1–2.9) for multiple myeloma in persons exposed to TRI. It should be recognized that workers are commonly exposed to multiple solvents in the workplace. TRI is currently assigned the classification of D (not classifiable as to carcinogenicity in humans) by the EPA (1998b).

Methylene Chloride

MC (dichloromethane) has enjoyed widespread use as a solvent in industrial processes, manufacture of drugs, degreasing agents, aerosol propellants, agriculture, and food preparation. It was commonly used to decaffeinate coffee and tea. Thus, large numbers of people have been exposed occupationally and in the home. The primary route of exposure to this very volatile solvent is inhalation. The preponderance of MC escaping into the environment does so by volatilization (ATSDR, 2000a). The VOC is also frequently found in wastewater discharges and in air and water at hazardous waste sites (Pohl *et al.*, 2008).

Metabolism The TK of MC has been well characterized in humans and rodents. MC is rapidly absorbed and distributed throughout the body (Angelo *et al.*, 1986). Inhaled MC reached a near steady state in the blood of human subjects with one to two hours of continuous exposure (DiVincenzo and Kaplan, 1981). Less than 5% of the absorbed dose was exhaled unchanged. Approximately 25% to 34% was exhaled as carbon monoxide (CO), the major end metabolite of MC. Exposure of the volunteers

to 50, 100, 150, and 200 ppm for 7.5 hours produced peak blood carboxyhemoglobin saturations of 1.9%, 3.4%, 5.3%, and 6.8%, respectively. MC was very rapidly eliminated from the body and did not accumulate over a five-day exposure regimen. As shown in Fig. 24-7, metabolism of MC in humans and rodents is believed to occur via three pathways (Andersen *et al.*, 1987). One entails CYP2E1-catalyzed oxidation to CO via formyl chloride, a reactive intermediate. The second, a GSH-mediated pathway, involves the theta-class GST, GST-T1. Oxidation is a high-affinity, low-capacity pathway that predominates at the relatively low MC concentrations present in occupational and environmental settings. The GST conjugation is a low-affinity, high-capacity pathway operative at the high exposure levels used in cancer bioassays (Green, 1997). With the third and minor pathway, it is postulated that CO_2 is also formed via the oxidative pathway by reaction of formyl chloride with a nucleophile such as GSH (Watanabe and Guengerich, 2006). The abilities of different species to metabolize MC in the liver by the GST pathway are as follows: mouse >> rat > human high conjugators > hamster > human nonconjugators (Reitz *et al.*, 1989; Thier *et al.*, 1998). Interindividual variation in the ability to biotransform MC via GST-T1 is associated with genetic polymorphisms in humans (Haber *et al.*, 2002).

PBTK models for MC have been developed to assess the relative importance of the oxidative and GST pathways in MC's toxicity and carcinogenicity. A PBTK model by Andersen *et al.* (1987) was validated by comparing simulations of blood MC time-course data with data from experiments with mice, rats, and humans. Tumor incidences in mice in chronic bioassays by NTP (Mennear *et al.*, 1988) and Serota *et al.* (1986a,b) were consistent with model predictions of liver and lung doses of GSH metabolites, but not oxidative metabolites. After extensive review, the EPA adopted this model as a reasonable means of extrapolating NTP bioassay results in mice to humans. This was the first use of PBTK modeling by EPA in a cancer risk assessment. Other investigators such as Reitz *et al.* (1988, 1989) published deterministic models for MC, which also provided internal dosimetry point estimates of GST pathway metabolites. Forecasts of relatively low tissue doses of GST metabolites in humans resulted in part from the need to saturate the oxidative pathway before appreciable GSH metabolites could be formed.

Recently, probabilistic PBTK models for MC have been developed, which allow for inclusion of intraspecies and interspecies variability in model predictions, as well as quantitative assessment of model uncertainty. Values for model input parameters and TK data from rodent studies from a variety of sources were subjected to MCMC analysis, a Bayesian optimization technique. With this approach, the prior input information can be combined to obtain posterior distributions of key model parameters. El-Masri *et al.* (1999) and Jonsson and Johanson (2001) used Bayesian analysis solely to evaluate the influence of GST-T1 polymorphism on human cancer risk. Marino *et al.* (2006) used MCMC analysis to develop a probabilistic PBTK model for MC in mice. The resulting dose metrics (mg MC metabolized by GST/L tissue per day) were three- to four-fold higher than contemporary EPA estimates. David *et al.* (2006) applied this modeling approach to humans. Inclusion of GSH nonconjugators resulted in a unit cancer risk estimation 500-fold lower than the EPA unit risk at that time. The EPA (2010a) recently concluded in an extensive assessment that this was the best available PBTK model, despite some uncertainties.

Modes of Toxicity/Carcinogenicity

MC has a quite limited cytotoxicity potential. Male and female B6C3F1 mice consuming up to ~2000 mg MC/kg per day in their drinking water for 90 days showed no adverse effects (Kirschmann *et al.*, 1986). Similarly dosed male and female F344 rats exhibited mild to moderate hepatocellular lipid vacuolation and elevated serum enzyme activities at daily dosage levels as low as 166 to 209 mg/kg per day (Kirschmann *et al.*, 1986). Hepatic centrilobular vacuolation and focal necrosis occurred in the liver of rats inhaling 500 to 4000 ppm MC six hours per day, five days per week for two years (Burek *et al.*, 1984; Mennear *et al.*, 1988). Manifestations of kidney damage have been rare in laboratory animals, but have occasionally been reported in persons subjected to high vapor levels (ATSDR, 2000a; EPA, 2010a). There is little information on the identity of MC metabolites that adversely affect the liver or kidney. As described previously, the CO formed by oxidation of MC binds to hemoglobin to produce dose-dependent increases in carboxyhemoglobin. Offspring of pregnant rats inhaling low concentrations of CO have been reported to exhibit permanent learning and memory impairment (De Salvia *et al.*, 1995). It is generally accepted that tissue hypoxia can contribute to CNS depressant effects of MC. There are few reports of residual neurologic dysfunction in MC-exposed workers (Lash *et al.*, 1991; ATSDR, 2000a).

There has been a great deal of research to define mechanisms of MC carcinogenicity, in order to more clearly understand the relevance of the murine tumors to humans (Green, 1997). Liver and lung tumors in mice do not seem to be associated with overt cytotoxicity or increased replicative DNA synthesis (Maronpot *et al.*, 1995). Induction of the tumors in mice is generally believed to be due to a reactive intermediate generated via the GST pathway (Andersen *et al.*, 1987). GST-T1 in liver and lung catalyzes conversion of MC to *S*-(chloromethyl)glutathione (GSCH$_2$Cl), which apparently breaks down rapidly to GSH and formaldehyde. Both

GSCH$_2$Cl and formaldehyde are reactive with DNA. MC is usually mutagenic in bacterial assays containing GSH/GST activity. MC produces DNA single-strand breaks (SSBs) in vitro in mouse hepatocytes and lung Clara cells, in which GST is localized in the nucleus (Mainwaring *et al.*, 1996). DNA SSBs were induced in mouse hepatocytes by a 60-fold lower MC concentration than in rat hepatocytes. Rat liver does not show preferential nuclear localization of GST-T1. Some human hepatocytes apparently exhibit nuclear localization, others cytoplasmic (Sherratt *et al.*, 2002). Negative results have been seen in a variety of genotoxicity assays with rat or hamster cell lines with little or no GST activity (EPA, 2010a). Positive results for sister chromatid exchanges, chromosomal aberrations, and the micronucleus test have been obtained in experiments with human cell lines and isolated cells. Negative results were seen in unscheduled DNA synthesis, DNA SSBs, and DNA–protein cross-links (DPX). There is limited evidence of formation of GSCH$_2$Cl DNA adducts in some hybrid in vitro systems, but the adducts' instability presents considerable technical challenges to their study. They have yet to be isolated in vivo. Formaldehyde produces both DPX and SSBs, indicative of its prominent role in MC's carcinogenicity (Graves and Green, 1996).

Cancer Bioassays in Rodents

High, chronic exposures to MC have been found to produce species- and gender-specific tumors in some organs of mice and rats. Serota *et al.* (1986a,b) administered a series of doses of MC to F344 rats and B6C3F1 mice in their drinking water for two years. The male mice showed a trend for an increase in hepatocellular adenomas and carcinomas, but the modest response was not dose-dependent. There was a statistically significant increase in neoplastic nodules or hepatocellular carcinoma in some groups of female F344 rats. Burek *et al.* (1984) saw a significant increase in salivary gland sarcomas in male S-D rats that inhaled 3500 ppm six hours per day, five days per week for two years. The number of benign mammary tumors per tumor-bearing female S-D rat increased with increasing concentration of exposure, although the number of tumor-bearing rats was not significantly elevated over controls. Similarly exposed hamsters were unaffected. In a two-year follow-up study (Nitschke *et al.*, 1988), female S-D rats inhaling 500 ppm MC also only exhibited an increased number of benign mammary tumors per tumor-bearing rat. No increase in malignant tumors was manifest in male rats. NTP conducted an inhalation study, in which F344/N rats and B6C3F1 mice inhaled up to 4000 ppm MC six hours daily, five times weekly for two years (Mennear *et al.*, 1988). There were weak trends for neoplastic nodules and hepatocellular carcinoma, as well as benign mammary tumors in female rats. Male and female mice inhaling 2000 or 4000 ppm MC exhibited statistically significant, dose-dependent increases in hepatocellular adenoma and carcinoma, as well as bronchoalveolar adenoma and carcinoma. There were similar findings in a follow-up study of female B6C3F1 mice inhaling 2000 ppm MC for two years (Maronpot *et al.*, 1995). The incidences of these hepatic and lung tumors in control B6C3F1 mice are quite high (Haseman *et al.*, 1998).

Cancer Epidemiology Studies

Despite a substantial number of epidemiology studies of MC-exposed workers, evidence of associations between MC and specific tumors is not strong. There have been four cohort mortality studies of employees at facilities where MC was used as a solvent for cellulose acetate. There were no increased risks of cancer mortality for all tissues or for lung or breast. In just one assessment was there an elevated risk (SMR = 2.98 [95% CI = 0.81–7.63]) of death from liver and biliary tract cancer (Lanes *et al.*, 1993). This was apparently the sole report of increased hepatic cancer mortality in an occupational population.

No investigations provide evidence of an association between MC and lung or kidney cancer (ATSDR, 2000a; EPA, 2010a). Cantor *et al.* (1995) conducted a case–control study of 33,509 occupationally exposed women, but found little association between MC exposure probability and breast cancer mortality. Blair *et al.* (1998), however, reported a RR of 3.0 (1.0–8.8) for breast cancer in 3605 women employed at Hill Air Force Base. Blair *et al.* (1998) also estimated RRs of 3.0 (0.9–10.0) and 3.4 (0.9–13.2) for NHL and multiple myeloma, respectively, in MC-exposed aircraft maintenance employees of both sexes. Occasionally, excess risks of other cancers have been found in highly exposed groups. Gibbs *et al.* (1996), for example, computed a statistically significant SMR of 2.08 for prostate cancer death of cellulose acetate workers with a latency period of at least 20 years since their first exposure to 350 to 700 ppm MC. In a study of association between MC and astrocytic brain cancer, Heineman *et al.* (1994) calculated an OR of 2.4 for males with a high probability of MC exposure and for intense exposure versus unexposed controls. Lastly, Infante-Rivard *et al.* (2005) reported an increased risk of childhood leukemia (OR = 3.22 [0.88–11.7]) in offspring of mothers with probable or definite occupational MC exposure. Nevertheless, most investigations have revealed weak or no apparent associations between relatively high MC inhalation exposures in industry and cancers (Dell *et al.*, 1999; Starr *et al.*, 2006).

Risk Assessment A considerable body of scientific information supports the following conclusion: should MC be a carcinogen in humans, it is much less potent than in rodents, notably mice. DPX were detected in hepatocytes that had been isolated from B6C3F1 mice and incubated for two hours with MC. They were not found in hepatocytes of F344 rats, Syrian golden hamsters, or three human subjects (Casanova *et al.*, 1996, 1997). RNA–formaldehyde cross-links, however, were found in hepatocytes of all species. These links were four-, seven-, and 14-fold higher in cells from mice than in cells from rats, humans, and hamsters, respectively. Metabolism of MC via the GSH pathway is an order of magnitude greater in mouse than in rat liver. Metabolic rates in hamster and human liver are even lower (Reitz *et al.*, 1989; Thier *et al.*, 1998; Sherratt *et al.*, 2002). High GST-T1 activity was measured in the nuclei of mouse centrilobular hepatocytes. Mice may be unique in that the extensive metabolic activation of MC to an unstable intermediate occurs in the proximity of the DNA. It would be useful in future PBTK models to include subcompartments for cytosolic and nuclear GST activities (Starr *et al.*, 2006). GST-T1 was also detected in relatively high levels in mouse lung Clara cells and ciliated cells at alveolar/bronchiolar junctions (Mainwaring *et al.*, 1996). Clara cells are present in much lower numbers in rats, and are rare in human lungs. GSCH$_2$Cl apparently causes SSB in vivo and in vitro in DNA of mouse liver and lung (Graves *et al.*, 1995). No DNA breaks were detected in hamster or human hepatocytes in vitro.

The EPA (2010a,b) has recently concluded that MC is likely to be carcinogenic in humans and appears to act via a mutagenic mode of action. The designation of "likely to be carcinogenic in humans" was based largely on the NTP (Mennear *et al.*, 1988) findings of cancer at two sites (liver and lung) in male and female B6C3F1 mice. More limited findings of certain tumors in MC-exposed rats were considered to be supporting evidence. Epidemiological studies were said to provide some evidence of an association between occupational MC exposure and brain and liver cancer. As described in the previous paragraph, bioactivation of MC is qualitatively, but not quantitatively similar in mice and humans. Due to the similarity, the EPA (2010a) reasons that the apparent mode of action (mutagenicity of GST pathway metabolites) is biologically plausible

in humans. The currently recommended inhalation risk value is ~47-fold lower than the previous IRIS value. EPA classifies MC as likely to be carcinogenic in humans.

Carbon Tetrachloride

CCl$_4$ previously enjoyed widespread use as a solvent, cleaning agent, fire extinguisher, synthetic intermediate, grain fumigant, and human anthelmintic. Its use has steadily declined since the 1970s, due to its hepatorenal toxicity, carcinogenicity, and contribution to atmospheric ozone depletion (ATSDR, 2005). Nevertheless, CCl$_4$ appears to be ubiquitous in ambient air in the United States, and it is still found in some water wells and waste sites. CCl$_4$ is a classic hepatotoxin, but kidney injury is often more severe in humans.

The timecourse of CCl$_4$-induced acute liver injury has been well characterized (ATSDR, 2005). Early signs of hepatocellular injury in rats include dissociation of polysomes and ribosomes from rough endoplasmic reticulum, disarray of smooth endoplasmic reticulum, inhibition of protein synthesis, and triglyceride accumulation. Hypomethylation of RNA is thought to contribute to inhibition of lipoprotein synthesis, thereby playing a role in steatosis (Clawson *et al.*, 1987). Ingested CCl$_4$ reaches the liver, undergoes metabolic activation, produces lipid peroxidation, covalently binds, and inhibits microsomal ATPase activity within minutes in rats. Single cell necrosis, evident five to six hours postdosing, progresses to maximal centrilobular necrosis within 24 to 48 hours. Most microsomal enzyme activities are significantly depressed (Recknagel *et al.*, 1989). A variety of cytoplasmic enzymes are released from dead and dying hepatocytes into the bloodstream. The activity of these enzymes in serum generally parallels the extent of necrosis in the liver. Cellular regeneration, manifest by increased DNA synthesis and cell cycle progression, is maximal 36 to 48 hours postdosing (Rao *et al.*, 1997).

The metabolism of CCl$_4$ is required for its conversion to a variety of cytotoxic agents. It is widely recognized that CCl$_4$ is bioactivated by cytochromes P450 via reductive dehalogenation to the trichloromethyl radical (CCl$_3$•), which can react in turn with oxygen to form trichloromethyl peroxy free radicals (CCl$_3$OO•). Both unstable radicals bind covalently to a variety of cellular components including enzymatic and structural proteins and polyunsaturated fatty acids in membranes. This results in lipoperoxidation, loss of intracellular and cellular membrane integrity, and leakage of enzymes (Plaa, 2000; Weber *et al.*, 2003). By-products of lipid peroxidation include reactive aldehydes, which can form adducts with proteins and DNA, contributing to cytotoxicity and carcinogenicity, respectively (Manibusan *et al.*, 2007). Liu *et al.* (1995) have proposed that CCl$_4$ oxidative stress in the liver enhances nuclear factor kappa B activity, which in turn promotes expression of proinflammatory cytotoxic cytokines. Shi *et al.* (1998) proposed apoptosis as an additional/alternate mechanism of CCl$_4$-induced cell death.

Perturbation of intracellular calcium (Ca^{2+}) homeostasis appears to be an integral part of CCl$_4$ cytotoxicity (Stoyanovsky and Cederbaum, 1996). Increased cytosolic Ca^{2+} levels may result from influx of extracellular Ca^{2+} due to plasma membrane damage and from decreased intracellular Ca^{2+} sequestration. Elevation of intracellular Ca^{2+} in hepatocytes can cause activation of phospholipase A$_2$ and exacerbation of membrane damage (Glende and Recknagel, 1992). Elevated Ca^{2+} may also be involved in alterations in calmodulin and phosphorylase activity, as well as changes in nuclear protein kinase C activity (Omura *et al.*, 1999). High intracellular Ca^{2+} levels activate a number of catabolic enzymes including proteases, endonucleases, and phospholipases, which kill cells via apoptosis or necrosis (Weber *et al.*, 2003). The hydrolytic enzyme calpain mediates progression of acute CCl$_4$-induced liver injury by leaking from dying hepatocytes and attacking neighboring cells (Limaye *et al.*, 2003). Ca^{2+} may stimulate the release of cytokines and eicosanoids from Kupffer cells. Edwards *et al.* (1993) demonstrated that destruction of Kupffer cells prior to CCl_4 dosing of rats resulted in significant reductions in neutrophil infiltration and hepatocellular injury. Macrophages are known to release a number of inflammatory mediators, such as tumor necrosis factor alpha (TNF-α), that are cytotoxic (Morio *et al.*, 2001).

Development of cellular resistance and tissue repair are important in limiting CCl_4 hepatotoxicity, and in recovery (Mehendale, 2005). Alterations in transmembrane carrier proteins have been discovered in hepatocytes of CCl_4-treated mice. CCl_4 results in reduced expression of genes associated with extraction of bile acids and organic ions from sinusoidal blood, as well as upregulation of certain detoxification genes (Aleksunes *et al.*, 2005). It also produces differential upregulation of multidrug resistance proteins that are involved in export of oxidative stress products and metabolites. Hepatocellular regeneration has been shown to begin within six hours of a small dose of CCl_4, just as centrilobular necrosis is becoming evident (Lockard *et al.*, 1983). This early phase regeneration (arrested G_2 hepatocytes activated to proceed through mitosis) is followed at ~24 hours by the secondary phase of regeneration (hepatocytes mobilized from G_0/G_1 to proceed through mitosis) (Bell *et al.*, 1988). CCl_4 hepatotoxicity is obviously a complex, multifactorial process that is likely to continue to receive considerable attention.

CCl_4 has frequently been used as a model hepatotoxic compound with which to examine the influence of various factors that alter P450s. CYP2E1 is primarily responsible for catalyzing the bioactivation of low doses of CCl_4 in humans. CYP3A contributes to the metabolism of higher doses (Zangar *et al.*, 2000). The preeminent role of CYP2E1 in animals is clearly demonstrated by the protection afforded to CCl_4-treated rodents by CYP2E1 antibody (Castillo *et al.*, 1992), the CYP2E1 inhibitor 3-amino-1,2,4-triazole (Padron *et al.*, 1996), and the absence of CYP2E1 expression (Wong *et al.*, 1998). As discussed previously in the subsection "P450 Inducers," a variety of conditions that induce CYP2E1 potentiate CCl_4 hepatotoxicity in test animals and humans. Sufficient doses of CYP2E1 inhibitors, including natural constituents of foods (described in the subsection "P450 Inhibitors"), can inhibit CCl_4 toxicity (Lieber, 1997). Taieb *et al.* (2005) discovered protein 8, a transcription factor that regulates the expression of genes that protect cells from stress, rapidly triggering CYP2E1 downregulation in CCl_4-dosed mice, thereby minimizing CCl_4 bioactivation.

CCl_4 has been found to be a hepatocarcinogen in rodents, but there is relatively little experimental evidence on whether it is genotoxic or carcinogenic in humans (ATSDR, 2005; EPA, 2010b). There have been extensive studies of its potential genotoxic and mutagenic effects, but the results are largely negative in bacterial and in mammalian systems. Araki *et al.* (2004) did report that CCl_4 was mutagenic in a strain of *E. coli* that is particularly sensitive to oxidative damage. As early as the 1940s, the National Cancer Institute conducted a series of chronic bioassays in which very high oral bolus doses of CCl_4 were given to mice and rats. Large increases over controls in incidences of liver tumors were found in male and female mice (ATSDR, 2005). Relatively little was seen in rats, but hamsters were susceptible to CCl_4-induced liver cancer. Recently, Nagano *et al.* (2007) published the results of a study in which F344 rats and BDF1 mice of both sexes were exposed six hours daily, five times weekly for 104 weeks to 0, 5, 25, or 125 ppm CCl_4 vapor. There was a significant increase in hepatocellular adenomas and carcinomas in the male and female rats at the highest exposure level. Significant increases in these tumors and in adrenal pheochromocytomas were manifest in the 25- and 125-ppm male and female mice. There was

a statistically significant, but more modest elevation in hepatocellular adenomas, but not carcinomas, in the 5-ppm female mice. Degenerative and necrotic hepatic changes were seen in livers of all groups of animals with liver tumors except the 5-ppm female mice. There has been limited evidence of associations between occupational CCl_4 exposure and certain cancers described in some epidemiology studies, but the data were not conclusive. Exposures to CCl_4 were poorly characterized and confounded by the concurrent exposures of most subjects to other chemicals in workplaces. There were no reported associations with liver cancer.

The weight of scientific evidence indicates that CCl_4 is more likely an indirect than a direct acting mutagen/carcinogen (EPA, 2010b). Manibusan *et al.* (2007) concluded that sustained cell death, regeneration, and proliferation enhance the likelihood of unrepaired spontaneous lipid peroxidation and endonuclease-induced mutations that may lead to hepatocarcinogenesis. Jiang *et al.* (2004) observed changes in expression of genes involved in cell death, proliferation, DNA damage, and fibrogenesis in livers of mice given a high CCl_4 dose daily for four weeks. Four weeks after cessation of this treatment, most gene expression profiles returned to control levels, except fibrogenesis. Bioactivated CCl_4 can apparently exert modest genotoxic effects, such as DNA breakage and related sequelae only under highly cytotoxic conditions. ACGIH (2012) assigned CCl_4 the designation of A2 (suspected human carcinogen), in light of its threshold mode of action and its very weak or absent genotoxicity. Germany placed CCl_4 into its category 4, indicating that genotoxicity plays no, or at most a minor, role in its mode of action (MAK, 2011). The EPA (2010b), however, recently categorized the chemical as "likely to be carcinogenic to humans." Despite acknowledging the correlation between hepatocellular cytotoxicity, regenerative hyperplasia, and induction of liver tumors in rodents, concern about the reactivity of direct and indirect products of CCl_4 metabolism and about limited knowledge of key events led the agency to conclude that "the mode of action was unknown." This led to use of a linear model to estimate human cancer risks from oral and inhalation exposures. PBPK models were used to estimate mouse internal doses and human equivalent doses as part of this risk assessment.

Chloroform

The primary use of $CHCl_3$ (trichloromethane) is in the production of the refrigerant chlorodifluoromethane (Freon 22), but this use is diminishing as chlorine-containing fluorocarbons are phased out under the Montreal Protocol. $CHCl_3$ was among the first inhalation anesthetics, but it was replaced by safer compounds after about 1940. It is a by-product of drinking water chlorination and has been measured in municipal drinking water supplies in concentrations as high as several hundred ppb, although levels are usually <25 ppb (ATSDR, 1997a). $CHCl_3$ has also been found in ppb concentrations in swimming pool water and surrounding air (Aggazzotti *et al.*, 1995). Like many other halocarbons, $CHCl_3$ can invoke CNS symptoms at subanesthetic concentrations similar to those of alcohol intoxication and can sensitize the myocardium to catecholamines, possibly resulting in cardiac arrhythmias.

The reproductive and developmental toxicities of $CHCl_3$ are rather unremarkable. Schwetz *et al.* (1974) found that inhalation of 100 to 300 ppm $CHCl_3$ by pregnant rats caused a high incidence of fetal resorption, retardation of fetal development, and a low incidence of fetal anomalies. Murray *et al.* (1979) reported that gestational exposure to 100 ppm $CHCl_3$ resulted in the decreased ability of mice to maintain pregnancy, as well as cleft palate, decreased fetal weight and length, and decreased ossification in pups. Very high CHCl$_3$ concentrations retarded development and induced diffuse cell death in cultured rat embryos (Brown-Woodman *et al.*, 1998). These studies support CHCl$_3$ as a weak teratogen, but negative studies employing maternally toxic doses argue against this characterization (Thompson *et al.*, 1974; NTP, 1997a). The EPA's 2001 IRIS profile for CHCl$_3$ notes that in reproductive/developmental studies, maternal toxicity and fetal effects occurred at doses higher than those that produced liver toxicity.

Hepatotoxicity serves as the basis for EPA's benchmark dose–based RfD (EPA, 2001b). Under certain conditions CHCl$_3$ is hepatotoxic and nephrotoxic. These toxicities are potentiated by aliphatic alcohols, ketones, DCA, and TCA (Davis, 1992). Albeit at low doses, numerous disinfection by-products such as the rodent carcinogens TCA and DCA are routinely consumed with CHCl$_3$ in finished drinking water. For this reason, mixture studies are particularly relevant. Consider, for example, the studies of Pereira *et al.* (2001) in which *N*-methyl-*N*-nitrosourea-initiated B6C3F1 mice were exposed to DCA with or without CHCl$_3$. CHCl$_3$ prevented hypomethylation, which would have resulted in increased mRNA expression of the proto-oncogene c-myc and promotion of liver tumors by DCA. Conversely, CHCl$_3$ increased DCA-induced DNA hypomethylation and enhanced the DCA promotion of kidney tumors. Thus, concurrent exposure to two rodent carcinogens, CHCl$_3$ and DCA, resulted in less than additive activity in one organ and synergism in another (Pereira *et al.*, 2001; Tao *et al.*, 2005). This exemplifies the difficulty in assessing the risks posed by solvent mixtures.

Tolerance or adaptation to CHCl$_3$'s hepatorenal toxicity and carcinogenicity has been observed in some mouse strains after repeated exposure. This phenomenon was first investigated by Pereira and Grothaus (1997), who reported pre-exposure of mice to low doses of CHCl$_3$ in drinking water–induced resistance to hepatotoxicity and cell proliferation following a higher gavage dose. This was presumed at the time to result from suicidal inhibition of the CYPs responsible for CHCl$_3$'s activation. More recently, mice exposed daily for 7, 14, and 30 days were found to have a robust regenerative response in target tissues, which prevented the progression of injury (Anand *et al.*, 2005). Blood and tissue levels of CHCl$_3$ after repeated exposure were substantially lower than those following a single exposure, owing to increased elimination of CHCl$_3$ via exhalation (Anand *et al.*, 2006b). These same researchers also reported that priming mice with CHCl$_3$ prior to a lethal dose stimulated compensatory hepatogenic and nephrogenic repair, limiting the progression of injury and resulting in 100% survival. Relative to unprimed mice, there was no difference in hepatic or renal CYP2E1 activity, although GSH and GSH reductase activity were upregulated in the kidney (but not in the liver), with a consequent decrease in renal covalent binding. The area under the blood level versus time curve (AUC) was 40% lower in primed versus unprimed mice, but increased elimination via exhalation was not responsible for the reduction in internal exposure in this particular case (Philip *et al.*, 2006). Taken together, these studies suggest that TK and TD factors contribute to the tolerance observed to CHCl$_3$ toxicity. Mehendele and colleagues have conducted a series of other studies with CHCl$_3$, alone or in combination with other hepatotoxicants, to further discern the role of tissue repair in toxicant-induced injury. These studies have provided valuable insight into the importance of both the timing of the tissue repair response and its magnitude as pivotal determinants of the outcome of toxicant-induced injury, emphasizing the need to consider repair processes in predictive toxicology (Anand *et al.*, 2003, 2005; Mehendale, 2005).

The status of CHCl$_3$ as a rodent carcinogen is indisputable. It causes liver and kidney tumors that are species-, strain-, sex-, and route of exposure–dependent. CHCl$_3$-induced liver tumors in mice and their dependence on ongoing liver necrosis were reported near the end of World War II (Eschenbrenner and Miller, 1945). These same authors observed that male but not female mice suffered kidney necrosis. This observation was supported by the report of Roe *et al.* (1979) that CHCl$_3$ ingested in a toothpaste base resulted in renal tumors in male but not female mice. This sex difference is thought to be attributable to testosterone-mediated differences in renal CYP activity (Smith *et al.*, 1984). The NCI (1976) cancer bioassay demonstrated renal tumors in male rats and an extremely high incidence of liver tumors in both sexes of B6C3F1 mice gavaged with CHCl$_3$ in corn oil. In 1985, Jorgenson and colleagues reported that daily doses of CHCl$_3$ in drinking water comparable to those in the NCI gavage assay also produced renal tumors in rats, but failed to cause liver tumors in B6C3F1 mice. This finding provided evidence that the dose rate of CHCl$_3$ was a determinant of liver tumor formation, supporting the existence of a threshold mechanism. Hard *et al.* (2000) have reevaluated the kidneys from the Jorgenson *et al.* (1985) study and have confirmed the presence of chronic renal tubule injury, indicative of renal tumor formation via an epigenetic mechanism. In what may be a landmark study, Larson *et al.* (1994) compared cytotoxicity and cell proliferation in female B6C3F1 mice given CHCl$_3$ by gavage in corn oil versus ad libitum ingestion in drinking water. As seen in Fig. 24-8, the hepatocyte labeling index, a measure of the proliferative response, differed between the two exposure regimens at comparable doses. Pereira (1994) reported essentially the same observation. This suggests that ingestion of CHCl$_3$ in small increments, similar to drinking water patterns of humans, fails to produce a sufficient amount of cytotoxic metabolite(s) per unit time to overwhelm detoxification and other protective mechanisms.

Potentiation of CHCl$_3$'s toxicity by CYP inducers and protection by GSH and P450 inhibitors suggest that a metabolite, presumably phosgene, is responsible for CHCl$_3$'s hepatorenal toxicity. Both target organs metabolize CHCl$_3$ to phosgene. There is evidence that CYP2E1 and CYP2B1/2 metabolically activate CHCl$_3$. The former isoform is thought to catalyze CHCl$_3$ metabolism at a lower substrate concentration than the latter (Nakajima *et al.*, 1995). By using an irreversible CYP2E1 inhibitor and CYP2E1 knockout mice, Constan *et al.* (1999) have demonstrated that metabolism of CHCl$_3$ by CYP2E1 is required for liver and kidney necrosis and cell proliferation. The electrophilic intermediate generated by CHCl$_3$'s metabolism (ie, phosgene) is initially detoxified by covalently binding to cytosolic GSH. Once GSH is depleted, phosgene is free to covalently bind to hepatic and renal proteins and lipids. Such binding damages membranes and other intracellular structures, leading to necrosis and subsequent reparative cellular proliferation. Sustained proliferation with repeated exposures promotes tumor formation in rodents by irreversibly "fixing" spontaneously altered DNA and clonally expanding initiated cells. The expression of certain genes, including *myc* and *fos*, is altered during regenerative cell proliferation in response to CHCl$_3$-induced cytotoxicity (Sprankle *et al.*, 1996; Kegelmeyer *et al.*, 1997). While the identity of phosgene's intracellular targets is largely unknown, Guastadisegni *et al.* (1999) have reported that phosgene reacts with phosphatidylethanolamine (PE). The adduct formed appears to consist of two PE moieties cross-linked at the amino head groups by the carbonyl moiety of phosgene. CHCl$_3$-modified PE preferentially accumulates on inner mitochondrial membranes, inducing ultrastructural modifications and inhibiting functions of the organelle. These researchers observed the induction of hepatic apoptosis and necrosis in CHCl$_3$-treated rats and pointed out that apoptosis may be initiated by the release of regulatory factors normally sequestered in mitochondria, in particular Ca^{2+}. Evidence that Ca^{2+} perturbation plays

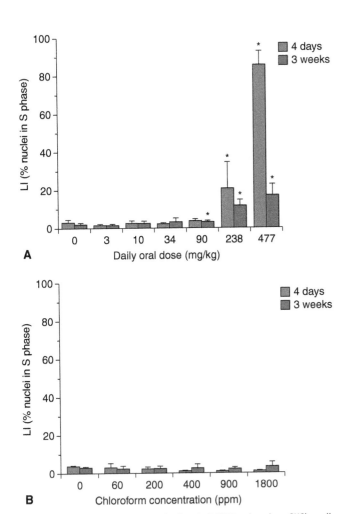

Figure 24-8. *Hepatocyte liver LI in female B6C3F1 mice given CHCl₃ orally in corn oil (**A**) or drinking water (**B**) for four days or three weeks.* The LI is defined as the percent of hepatocyte nuclei positive for 5-bromo-2'-deoxyuridine immunohistochemical staining (ie, percent of cells in the S phase, the period of DNA synthesis during the cell cycle). Values represent the mean ± SD for five mice. Asterisks (*) denote a significant difference from similarly treated control mice (<0.05). Note that 1800 ppm CHCl₃ in water corresponds to a cumulative uptake of 329 mg/kg per day. (Reproduced with permission from Larson *et al.*, 1994.)

a role in CHCl₃ toxicity comes from a report of Ca^{2+} mobilization in Madin–Darby canine kidney cells using Fura-2 as a Ca^{2+} probe. CHCl₃, albeit in millimolar concentrations, increased the cytosolic Ca^{2+} levels by releasing Ca^{2+} from multiple sites within the cell (Jan *et al.*, 2000).

There is no evidence of covalent binding of CHCl₃ metabolites to nucleic acids. There is binding to nuclear histone, which plays a key role in controlling DNA expression and might be a mechanism of CHCl₃'s carcinogenicity (Diaz and Castro, 1980; Fabrizi *et al.*, 2003). It has been hypothesized that the induction of oxidative stress and depletion of GSH by CHCl₃ may lead to indirect genotoxicity that could contribute to carcinogenicity. This hypothesis is supported by the small dose-dependent increase in M(1) dG adducts (malondialdehyde reacts with DNA to form adducts to deoxyguanosine), DNA strand breakage, and lipid peroxidation in CHCl₃-treated rat hepatocytes in the absence of any increase in DNA oxidation (Beddowes *et al.*, 2003). Such a mechanism would still be threshold dependent, given its reliance on the initial depletion of antioxidants.

The EPA (2001b) classifies CHCl₃ as a probable human carcinogen (group B2), meaning there is sufficient evidence

for carcinogenicity in animals and inadequate or no evidence in humans. Experimental evidence and the prevailing opinion that CHCl₃ is nongenotoxic indicates that the relationship between CHCl₃ dose and tumor formation is nonlinear. The EPA has, as is called for in its *Guidelines for Carcinogen Risk Assessment* (EPA, 2005), considered mode of action in the determination of CHCl₃'s cancer risk and relied on a nonlinear dose–response approach and the use of margin of exposure analysis. In doing so, the Agency concluded that the RfD for noncancer effects, based on the dog study of Heywood *et al.* (1979), was adequately protective for cancer by the oral route on the basis of cancer and noncancer effects having a common link through cytotoxicity. The wealth of mechanistic data available continues to inform the risk assessment for CHCl₃. For example, Constan *et al.* (2002) exercised a PBTK dosimetry model to compare hepatic responses in mice and humans with inhaled CHCl₃. They concluded that no safety factor was needed to account for interspecies differences in inhalation cancer risk. Additionally, Tan *et al.* (2003) have published a PBTK/TD model for CHCl₃ to describe the plausible mechanism linking the hepatic metabolism of CHCl₃ to hepatocellular killing and regenerative proliferation, thereby creating a predictive model that most accurately reflects the current science.

AROMATIC HYDROCARBONS

Benzene

Benzene produced commercially in the United States is derived primarily from petroleum. It has been utilized as a general purpose solvent, but it is now used principally in the synthesis of other chemicals (ATSDR, 2006c). The percentage by volume of benzene in gasoline is 1% to 2%. Benzene plays an important role in unleaded gasoline (UG) due to its antiknock properties. Inhalation is the primary route of exposure in industrial and in everyday settings. Benzene is present in the atmosphere both from natural sources such as forest fires and oil seeps and from industrial uses including automobile exhaust and gasoline vapor emission. Cigarette smoke is the major source of benzene in the home (Wallace, 1996). Smokers have benzene body burdens that are six to 10 times greater than those of nonsmokers. Passive smoke can be a significant source of benzene exposure to nonsmokers. Because of the health risks of benzene exposure, the use and environmental release of this chemical has significantly diminished in the last two decades.

There is strong evidence from epidemiological studies that high-level benzene exposures result in an increased risk of acute myelogenous leukemia (AML) in humans (Bergsagel *et al.*, 1999; ATSDR, 2006a). Evidence of increased risks of other cancers in such populations is less compelling. Only AML incidence was significantly elevated in the largest cohort study to date, in which ~75,000 benzene-exposed workers in 12 cities in China were evaluated (Yin *et al.*, 1996). Types of cancer other than AML have been tentatively attributed to benzene. Marginal, nonsignificant increases were seen for lung cancer and chronic myelogenous leukemia. Some investigations of persons exposed to engine exhausts have reported a significant association with multiple myeloma. Bezabeth *et al.* (1996) and Bergsagel *et al.* (1999) have concluded, however, that there is no scientific evidence to support a causal relationship between benzene exposure and multiple myeloma or NHL. Increased incidences of malignant lymphomas and a variety of solid tumors were found in male and female B6C3F1 mice dosed orally with high doses of benzene for up to 103 weeks (Huff *et al.*, 1989). Male and female F344 rats in this bioassay exhibited excesses of

Zymbal gland, skin, and oral cavity carcinomas. Benzene exposure via inhalation, dermal, and i.p. routes also produced a variety of tumors in rodents. Thus, benzene is clearly an animal and human carcinogen, but major species differences exist.

The most important adverse effect of benzene is hematopoietic toxicity, which precedes leukemia. Chronic, high benzene exposure can lead to bone marrow damage, which may be manifest initially as anemia, leukopenia, thrombocytopenia, or a combination of these. Bone marrow depression appears to be dose-dependent in both laboratory animals and humans. Continued exposure may result in marrow aplasia and pancytopenia, an often fatal outcome. Survivors of aplastic anemia frequently exhibit a preneoplastic state, termed myelodysplasia, which may progress to myelogenous leukemia (Snyder, 2002; Bird *et al.*, 2005). Decreased lymphocyte counts are shown to be the early and consistent finding in animals and humans following benzene exposure (Goldstein, 1988). Hematologic effects in workers with prolonged benzene exposure in the range of one to 30 ppm and above have been well documented (Ward *et al.*, 1996). However, there is conflicting evidence for effects at levels <1 ppm, the permissible exposure level (PEL) recommended by US OSHA. Three large epidemiological studies (two in the United States and one in the Netherlands) have not revealed any difference in blood

parameters between exposed (<1 ppm) and nonexposed workers (Collins *et al.*, 1997; Tsai *et al.*, 2004; Swaen *et al.*, 2010). However, Lan *et al.* (2004) have reported dose-dependent hematotoxicity in approximately 250 Chinese shoe workers who inhaled low (≤1 to ≥10 ppm) levels of benzene. Exposures of 100 of these employees to ≤1 ppm reduced mature white cell and platelet counts, as well as myeloid progenitor cell colony formation. The progenitors were more sensitive to benzene than mature white cells. Polymorphisms in myeloperoxidase (an enzyme that metabolizes benzene to toxic quinones and free radicals) and NAD(P)H:quinone oxidoreductase (an enzyme that protects against these moieties) conferred increased susceptibility to white cell decreases. Turtletaub and Mani (2003) found that formation of DNA and protein adducts in mouse liver and bone marrow was dose-dependent over a range of benzene doses, the lowest of which was 5 μg/kg.

Adverse health outcomes of chronic benzene exposure have been known for a long time, but the mechanisms by which benzene causes effects remain incompletely understood. The toxicity of benzene is dependent on its metabolites. Thus, it is essential to understand the metabolism of benzene in order to address its mechanisms of toxicity. The initial metabolic step (Fig. 24-9), oxidation of benzene to an epoxide (ie, benzene oxide), is catalyzed

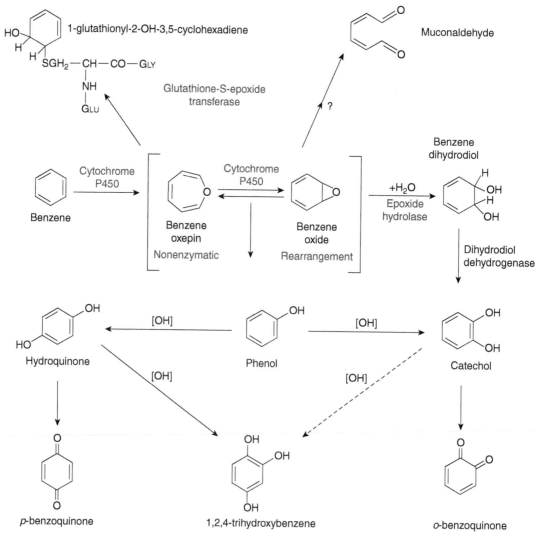

Figure 24-9. *Biotransformation of benzene.* A question mark leads from the oxepin-oxide compartment to muconaldehyde because the substrate for the ring opening has yet to be identified. The dotted line leading to 1,2,4-trihydroxybenzene (1,2,4-T) indicates that it is not clear what the relative contributions of hydroquinone and catechol are to 1,2,4-T. (Modified and used with permission from Rangan and Snyder, 1997.)

primarily by hepatic CYP2E1. Valentine *et al.* (1996) demonstrated that benzene-treated transgenic CYP2E1 knockout mice had relatively low levels of all benzene metabolites in their urine. A five-day, 200-ppm benzene inhalation regimen produced severe genotoxicity and cytotoxicity in wild-type B6C3F1 mice, but no adverse effects in the knockout mice. Benzene oxide, which is in equilibrium with its oxepin form, is further metabolized by three pathways: (1) conjugation with GSH to form a premercapturic acid, which is converted to phenylmercapturic acid; (2) rearrangement nonenzymatically to form phenol; and (3) hydration by epoxide hydrolase to benzene dihydrodiol, which in turn can be oxidized by dihydrodiol dehydrogenase to catechol. If phenol is hydroxylated in the *ortho* position, more catechol will be formed. Catechol can be converted to *o*-benzoquinone. If benzene is hydroxylated in the *para* position, *p*-hydroquinone is formed. It can be oxidized to *p*-benzoquinone. The *o*- and *p*-benzoquinones are considered to be among the ultimate toxic metabolites of benzene. Another potentially toxic metabolite, muconaldehyde, may arise from ring opening of oxepin. Muconaldehyde undergoes a series of reactions that ultimately lead to *t,t*-muconic acid, an end metabolite found in the urine (Golding and Watson, 1999; Snyder, 2004).

Liver is the primary metabolic organ, while bone marrow is the target organ for benzene. Transport of primary metabolites and further metabolism in bone marrow is believed by many authorities to play the key role in myelotoxicity. Levels of DNA and protein adducts were significantly higher in bone marrow than in liver of benzene-dosed mice (Turtletaub and Mani, 2003). Bernauer *et al.* (1999) measured activity and levels of CYP2E1 in liver and bone marrow of five strains of mice of varying sensitivity to benzene. CYP2E1 amounts and activities were considerably greater in liver than in marrow, but no interstrain differences were seen in either tissue. It is likely that non-CYP enzymes (eg, peroxidase, myeloperoxidase, and cyclooxygenase) play an important role in generation of semiquinones and quinones in bone marrow (Ross *et al.*, 1996). Lindstrom *et al.* (1997) have reported that benzene oxide has an estimated half-life of 7.9 minutes in rat blood, and thus may be able to travel from liver to bone marrow. The quinones are thought to be too reactive to be transported in the bloodstream. Reactivity of muconaldehyde in the presence of GSH suggests that this metabolite would not reach bone marrow; however, metabolites of muconaldehyde, which are less reactive, could be transported to bone marrow and reoxidized. It has been generally accepted that phenolic conjugates are formed in the liver and transported via the blood to the bone marrow, where they are hydrolyzed and oxidized to quinones. Researchers have been unable to reproduce benzene toxicity by giving individual phenolic metabolites to animals, but co-administration of its metabolites, phenol and muconaldehyde with hydroquinone, reproduced the myelotoxic effects of benzene (Witz *et al.*, 1996; Monks *et al.*, 2010). Snyder (2004) concluded that benzene hematopoietic toxicity and leukemogenesis are primarily a function of the bone marrow, a site remote from the liver where substantial benzene metabolism occurs.

Benzene's metabolic pathways appear to be qualitatively, though not quantitatively, similar in species studied to date (Henderson, 1996). Mice have a greater overall capacity to metabolize benzene than do rats or primates. Mani *et al.* (1999) reported good correlation between protein–DNA adduct levels in bone marrow and susceptibility to benzene genotoxicity and carcinogenesis in F344 rats and three strains of mice. The B6C3F1 mouse shows the highest adduct levels and is the most sensitive of the animals tested. Powley and Carlson (1999) reported similar findings on measurement of benzene metabolism in mouse, rat, rabbit, and human lung and liver microsomes. A paucity of information is available on the ability of human bone marrow to metabolically activate benzene and/or its metabolites. Rappaport *et al.* (2009) suggested that humans metabolize benzene to phenol and muconic acid by two enzymes, a high-affinity enzyme which is active primarily below 1 ppm, leading to muconic acid, and a low-affinity enzyme active primarily above 1 ppm, leading to phenol. The authors also suggested that CYP2E1 was active primarily at higher concentrations and CYP2E1 and CYP2A13 could be contributing at lower concentrations.

Factors that alter the metabolism of benzene have the potential to influence the hematopoietic toxicity and carcinogenicity of the VOC. Pretreatment of rats with ethanol, a CYP2E1 inducer, enhanced metabolism of benzene and potentiated its acute and subacute myelotoxicity in rats (Nakajima *et al.*, 1985) and mice (Marrubini *et al.*, 2003). Phenobarbital had a negligible effect. Pretreatment of male B6C3F1 mice with acetone, another CYP2E1 inducer, increased benzene oxidation by about fivefold (Kenyon *et al.*, 1996). Pretreatment with diethyldithiocarbamate, a CYP2E1 inhibitor, completely abolished benzene oxidation. Coexposure of F344 rats to gasoline and benzene resulted in competitive metabolic inhibition (Travis *et al.*, 1992). Metabolism of benzene by hepatic microsomes from 10 human donors was directly proportional to CYP2E1 activity in the samples (Seaton *et al.*, 1994). Thus, it would be anticipated that CYP2E1 polymorphisms may influence susceptibility to benzene toxicity. Male mice have consistently been found to be more sensitive than females to genotoxic effects of benzene. PBTK analysis of data from gas uptake experiments with B6C3F1 mice of both sexes revealed that the optimized maximum rate of benzene metabolism was twice as high in males (Kenyon *et al.*, 1996). It is not known whether there is a sex-dependent difference in benzene metabolism in humans. Sato *et al.* (1975) saw a more rapid rate of pulmonary elimination of benzene in men than in women following inhalation of 25 ppm for two hours. Benzene was retained longer in the females due to their higher body fat content. Unfortunately, most epidemiology studies of benzene-exposed workers have not provided a gender comparison. Li *et al.* (1994) did not see a statistically significant difference in cancer mortality between male and female workers exposed to benzene, although risks tended to be somewhat higher for males. Polymorphisms in enzymes involved in benzene metabolism such as CYP2E1, epoxide hydrolase, myeloperoxidase, GSTs, and quinone reductases will also influence the toxicity of benzene.

There are a number of cell populations in the bone marrow that may serve as targets for benzene metabolites. Benzene exposure in vivo results in inhibited growth and development of pluripotential bone marrow stem cells. More mature precursors, such as stromal cells and erythroid and myeloid colony-forming units, are also affected. Trush *et al.* (1996) point out that hydroquinone-induced inhibition of interleukin (IL)-1 synthesis by stromal macrophages results in altered differentiation of myeloid and lymphoid cells that are normally active in immune responses. These investigators also note that killing of stromal macrophages and fibroblasts could result in such a pronounced reduction of cytokines and growth factors that immature and committed hematopoietic progenitors would die from apoptosis. The erythroid series is more susceptible than the myeloid series to benzene-induced cytotoxicity. Immature myeloid cells can proliferate when the development of erythroid cells is restricted and acquire neoplastic characteristics on dedifferentiation. The end result is AML (Golding and Watson, 1999).

Investigations of benzene toxicity/leukemogenesis have uncovered a variety of potential mechanisms (Golding and Watson, 1999; Snyder, 2002; Bird *et al.*, 2005). As mentioned before, experimental evidence indicates that the complementary actions of benzene and several of its metabolites are required for myelotoxicity. It has been recognized for 20 years that a number of benzene metabolites can bind covalently to GSH, proteins, DNA, and RNA. This can result in disruption of the functional hematopoietic microenvironment by inhibition of enzymes, destruction of certain cell populations, and alteration of the growth of other cell types. Covalent binding of hydroquinones to spindle fiber proteins will inhibit cell replication (Smith, 1996). In vitro studies have established that reactive benzene metabolites bind covalently to DNA of several tissues of different species. Through the use of accelerator mass spectrophotometry, Creek et al. (1997) have demonstrated DNA binding in mice exposed to extremely low ^{14}C-benzene levels. The binding was dose-dependent over a wide range of doses. DNA adduct levels were so low, however, that this mechanism alone may be insufficient to fully account for leukemogenic effects. The role of the aryl hydrocarbon receptor (AhR) in benzene-induced hematoxicity is emerging. AhR-knockout mice were completely resistant to hematotoxicity of benzene, suggesting a central role of AhR in benzene toxicity (Yoon et al., 2002), but the mechanisms for this receptor are still under investigation. A recent review of literature by Gasiewicz et al. (2010) indicated that AhR regulates the expression of enzymes involved in benzene toxicity and plays a major role in the regulation of hematopoietic stem cells. In order to identify critical data gaps and prioritize research, Meek and Klaunig (2010) proposed five key events in the mode of action for benzene-induced leukemia: (1) benzene metabolism via CYP; (2) interaction of benzene metabolites with target cells in the bone marrow; (3) formation of initiated, mutated target cells; (4) selective proliferation of the mutated cells; and (5) production of leukemia.

It appears likely that oxidative stress contributes to benzene toxicity. As the bone marrow is rich in peroxidase activity, phenolic metabolites of benzene can be activated there to reactive quinone derivatives. Ross et al. (1996) discovered that myeloperoxidase present in murine and human progenitor cells could bioactivate hydroquinone to p-benzoquinone. Electron spin resonance experiments by Hiraku and Kawanishi (1996) revealed the formation of a semiquinone radical in p-benzoquinone-treated HL-60 cells (a human myeloid cell line). This suggested that reactive oxygen moieties (eg, O_2^- and H_2O_2) are produced via the formation of the semiquinone radicals. These active oxygen species can cause DNA strand breaks or fragmentation, leading to cell mutation or apoptosis, respectively. Ross et al. (1996), however, pointed out that quinones can also inhibit proteases involved in induction of apoptosis. These authors noted that modulation of apoptosis may lead to aberrant hematopoiesis and neoplastic progression. Badham et al. (2010) recently demonstrated that in utero exposure to benzene in mice increased oxidative stress in fetal tissue. The increase in oxidative stress was also associated with changes in redox-sensitive signaling pathways involved in normal hematopoiesis.

A number of biomarkers of exposure to benzene have been developed and carefully evaluated. Concentrations of the parent compound in exhaled breath parallel blood concentrations. Clayton et al. (1999) reported a high correlation between the extent of smoking-related activities and levels of benzene in exhaled breath of humans. Urinary excretion of a variety of benzene metabolites (ie, phenol, catechol, hydroquinone, 1,2,4-trihydroxybenzene, S-phenylmercapturic acid, and t,t-muconic acid) has been shown to be correlated with benzene exposure in occupational settings. Phenol, catechol, and hydroquinone, however, are neither sensitive nor specific biomarkers, because relatively high levels are found in nonexposed individuals (Medeiros et al., 1997). Similarly, t,t-muconic acid is not specific, because it is a metabolite of sorbic acid, a common food additive. Boogaard and van Sittert (1996) conclude that S-phenylmercapturic acid, an end product of the conjugation of benzene oxide and GSH, is a suitable urinary biomarker for low-level benzene exposure because of its specificity and relatively long half-life. Adducts to hemoglobin and cysteine groups of proteins have been demonstrated in rodents, but not in humans. DNA damage has been detected in benzene-exposed workers (Liu et al., 1996; Andreoli et al., 1997), although such measures have not yet found widespread acceptance as biomarkers of effect.

A number of PBTK models have been developed to aid in predicting risks of myelotoxicity and leukemia posed to humans by benzene. Medinsky et al. (1989) published one of the first such models for benzene. They assumed that benzene metabolism followed Michaelis–Menten kinetics and occurred via benzene oxide. B6C3F1 mice, which are more sensitive than F344 rats to benzene myelotoxicity, were predicted to metabolize two to three times more inhaled benzene. This and other PBTK models do not accurately simulate some laboratory data sets. Modeling benzene metabolism and disposition is difficult because of its inherent complexity and variability. In light of intricate dose–response relationships, Medinsky et al. (1996) emphasized the importance of considering competitive metabolic interactions between benzene and its metabolites, as well as the balance between enzymatic activation and inactivation processes. Cole et al. (2001) employed in vitro metabolic parameters for several pathways to construct a PBTK model that simulated most tissue dosimetry data sets for benzene-exposed mice quite well. Yokley et al. (2006) described a PBTK model that simulated tissue doses of benzene, benzene oxide, phenol, and hydroquinone in humans exposed orally and by inhalation. A MCMC statistical technique was used to assess dissimilarities in population distributions of key model parameters. Variability in metabolic parameters and certain physiological parameters (eg, organ weight) had to be inputed to accurately predict the range of human values.

Benzene is concluded to be a known human carcinogen by regulatory agencies around the world. The IARC classifies benzene as a Group 1 carcinogen (carcinogenic to humans). Benzene is characterized as a known human carcinogen for all routes of exposures based on strong evidence in human and laboratory animals (EPA, 2007). Maximum contaminant levels (MCLs) of 0.005 and 0.01 mg/L have been established for benzene in drinking water (EPA, 2002; WHO, 2004). For the protection of workers, OSHA (2005) has established a TLV of 0.5 ppm as an eight-hour time-weighted average (TWA). ACGIH has also established a BEI for benzene of 25 µg of S-phenylmercapturic acid and 500 µg of t,t-muconic acid/g of creatinine for a urine sample collected at the end of a workshift. Readers are encouraged to review the recent NTP's 12th Report on Carcinogens and ATSDR's Toxicological Profile for Benzene (2006c) for other regulatory levels for benzene exposure.

Toluene

Toluene is present in paints, lacquers, thinners, cleaning agents, glues, and many other products. It is also used in the production of other chemicals. Gasoline, which contains 5% to 7% toluene by weight, is the largest source of atmospheric emissions and exposure of the general populace (ATSDR, 2000b). Inhalation is the primary route of exposure, although skin contact occurs frequently. Toluene is a favorite of solvent abusers, who intentionally inhale high concentrations to achieve a euphoric effect (Filley et al., 2004). Large amounts of toluene enter the environment each year by volatilization. Relatively small amounts are released in industrial wastewater. Toluene is frequently found in water, soil, and air at hazardous waste sites (Pohl et al., 2008).

Toluene TK has been thoroughly characterized in humans and laboratory animals. Toluene is well absorbed from the lungs and

GI tract. It rapidly accumulates in and can affect the brain, due to that organ's high rate of blood perfusion and relatively high lipid content. Toluene subsequently is deposited in other tissues according to their lipid content, with adipose tissue attaining the highest levels.

Toluene is well metabolized, but a portion is exhaled unchanged. CYPs catalyze metabolism of toluene primarily to benzyl alcohol and lesser amounts of cresols. Benzyl alcohol is converted by ADH and ALDH to benzoic acid, which is primarily conjugated with glycine and eliminated in the urine as hippuric acid. Nakajima et al. (1992a) reported that CYP2E1 and CYP2C11 are primarily responsible for catalyzing the initial hydroxylation step in rat liver at low and high toluene levels, respectively. CYP2E1 is most active at low doses in humans (Nakajima et al., 1997). Benignus et al. (1998) attempted to use a PBTK model to relate toluene blood concentrations to behavioral effects in rats and humans. It appeared that humans were more sensitive to increases in blood levels, but more rat data and much more human data are needed for model validation.

The CNS is the primary target organ of toluene and other alkylbenzenes. Cardiac, renal, and hepatic toxicities as well as fetal alcohol-like syndrome have occasionally been reported. Increased incidence of spontaneous abortion was linked to toluene exposure at workplaces, but has not been supported by the results of animal testing. Manifestations of acute exposure range from slight dizziness and headache to unconsciousness, respiratory depression, and death. Occupational inhalation exposure guidelines are established to prevent significant decrements in psychomotor functions. Acute encephalopathic effects are rapidly reversible on cessation of exposure (Fig. 24-3), and are not associated with neuroimaging changes (Filley et al., 2004). Subtle neurologic effects have been described in some groups of occupationally exposed individuals. Exposure to ~100 ppm toluene for years may result in subclinical effects, as evidenced by altered brainstem auditory-evoked potentials (Abbate et al., 1993) and changes in visual-evoked potentials (Vrca et al., 1995). Foo et al. (1990) reported a good correlation between toluene exposure and poor scores on neurobehavioral tests of 30 female rotogravure workers. In contrast, severe neurotoxicity is often diagnosed in persons who have abused toluene for a prolonged period. A relatively specific neurobehavioral profile is manifest including inattention, apathy, memory dysfunction, diminished visuospatial skills, frontal lobe dysfunction, and psychiatric symptoms (Filley et al., 2004). Magnetic resonance imaging reveals ventricular enlargement, cerebral atrophy, and white matter hyperintensity, a characteristic profile termed toluene leukoencephalopathy. Such changes represent severe, chronic myelin toxicity. More advanced neuroimaging techniques may be able to reveal mild, subtle changes associated with early alterations in myelin of workers as well as toluene abusers (Caldemeyer et al., 1996; Filley et al., 2004). Rat pups subjected to high doses of toluene on days six to 19 of gestation exhibited a significant reduction in myelination per forebrain cell when they were 21 days old (Gospe and Zhou, 1998).

There is limited information on mechanisms by which toluene and similar solvents produce acute or residual CNS effects (Balster, 1998). The Meyer–Overton theory of partitioning of the lipophilic parent compounds into membrane lipids has been widely accepted for a century. It has been proposed that the presence of solvent molecules in cholesterol-filled interstices between phospholipids and sphingolipids changes membrane fluidity, thereby altering intercellular communication and normal ion movements (Engelke et al., 1996). Such a process is reversible. An alternate hypothesis is that toluene partitions into hydrophobic regions of proteins and interacts with them, thereby altering membrane-bound enzyme activity and/

or receptor specificity in a reversible manner (Balster, 1998). Other evidence suggests that toluene and other VOCs may act acutely by enhancing $GABA_A$ receptor function (Mihic et al., 1994), attenuating NMDA receptor-stimulated calcium flux (Cruz et al., 1998), attenuating nicotinic acetylcholine receptors (Bale et al., 2002), enhancing glycine receptors (Bale et al., 2005), and/or activating dopaminergic systems (von Euler, 1994). Using an in vivo microdialysis study and a schedule-controlled operant behavioral task, it was shown that glutamate levels were decreased in mice after acute toluene exposure (Win-Shwe et al., 2009). In addition to neurotransmitter systems, immune and hypothalamic neurohormonal systems also are proposed to play a role in toluene-induced neurotoxicity (Win-Shwe and Fujimaki, 2010). Hester et al. (2011) demonstrated altered expression of genes associated with synaptic transmission and plasticity following acute toluene exposure. The mechanism of chronic toluene neurotoxicity is unknown. Toluene is known to be deposited in brain areas with the highest myelin content. Astrocytosis frequently accompanies myelin disruption (Gotohda et al., 2000; Filley et al., 2004).

As toluene is metabolized by CYPs, ADH, and ALDH, the chemical can interact with other xenobiotics metabolized by these enzymes. Concurrent exposure to solvents metabolized by the same CYP isoforms can result in competitive metabolic inhibition. Inoue et al. (1988) observed that benzene and toluene suppressed one another's metabolism in humans. Thus, the risk of leukopenia in workers exposed to benzene and toluene should be less than that in workers exposed to benzene alone. Pryor and Rebert (1992) found that toluene greatly reduced manifestations of peripheral neuropathy caused by n-hexane in rats. Although no interaction between toluene and xylenes was seen in humans inhaling low levels of each, simultaneous exposure to higher levels results in mutual metabolic suppression (Tardif et al., 1991). Prior exposure to P450 inducers can result in increased rates of toluene metabolism/elimination and more rapid recovery from toluene-induced CNS depression. Nakajima and Wang (1994) observed that high concentrations of inhaled toluene moderately induced four of the six CYP isoforms that metabolize it, but inhibited the other two in rat liver.

High-level prenatal toluene exposures have produced growth and skeletal retardations in offspring of rodents and humans. The term "fetal solvent syndrome" was used to describe toluene-abusing women's children who exhibit microcephaly and cranial facial features similar to those with fetal alcohol syndrome (FAS) (Wilkins-Haug, 1997). Exposure to a pattern of binge toluene abuse caused growth retardation, gross morphological anomalies, skeletal abnormalities, and soft tissue anomalies in a dose-related fashion (Bowen et al., 2009). Growth and skeletal retardation were the common findings in the developmental toxicity studies in animals. The reproductive and developmental toxic potential of toluene was evaluated in a two-generation study of S-D rats (Roberts et al., 2003). Both sexes of each generation were exposed to 0, 100, 500, or 2000 ppm toluene vapor six hours per day, seven days per week for 80 days premating and for 15 days of mating. Pregnant animals were also exposed from gestation days one to 20 and lactation days five to 21. No adverse effects were seen at any dose on fertility, reproductive performance, or maternal or pup behavior. Reduced fetal body weight and skeletal anomalies associated with growth retardation were manifest in the offspring of both generations subjected to 2000 ppm, but not to lower vapor levels (Roberts et al., 2003).

Existing studies suggest that toluene is not carcinogenic or mutagenic. IARC classified toluene as not classifiable as a human carcinogen. ACGIH (2012) has established a TLV of 20 ppm as an eight-hour TWA to protect workers from subclinical changes in blue-yellow color vision and the potential for spontaneous abortion.

The current ACGIH BEI for toluene is 0.02 mg of toluene/L blood, 0.03 mg toluene/L urine, and 0.3 mg *o*-cresol/g of creatinine for urine collected at the end of a workshift.

Xylenes and Ethylbenzene

Large numbers of people are exposed to xylenes and ethylbenzene occupationally and environmentally (Wallace *et al.*, 1987). Xylenes (ATSDR, 2006d) and ethylbenzene (ATSDR, 2010a), like benzene and toluene, are major components of gasoline and fuel oil. The primary uses of xylenes and ethylbenzene industrially are as solvents and synthetic intermediates. Most of these aromatics that are released into the environment evaporate into the atmosphere. They may also enter groundwater from oil and gasoline spills, leakage of storage tanks, and migration from waste sites.

The TK and acute toxicity of toluene, xylenes, and other aromatic solvents are quite similar. Xylenes and the others are well absorbed from the lungs and GI tract, distributed to well-perfused and lipophilic tissues such as liver, fat, brain, and skin, exhaled unchanged to some extent, well metabolized by hepatic P450s, and largely excreted as urinary metabolites (Lof and Johanson, 1998). Nielsen and Alarie (1982) state that the potency of benzene and a series of alkylbenzenes, as sensory irritants of the upper respiratory tract of mice, increases with increasing lipophilicity. Acute lethality of hydrocarbons (ie, CNS depressant potency) also varies directly with lipophilicity (Swann *et al.*, 1974). Some of the alkylbenzenes including xylenes and ethylbenzene are shown to be ototoxic in rats. There is limited evidence that chronic occupational exposure to xylenes is associated with residual neurologic effects (ATSDR, 2006d). Limited human data suggest that systemic effects associated with ethylbenzene exposure are respiratory tract and ocular irritation, possible ototoxicity, and hematologic alterations (ATSDR, 2010a). Exposure conditions, including the presence of other solvents, have usually not been characterized in such reports. Uchida *et al.* (1993), for example, reported increased subjective CNS symptoms in workers exposed for approximately seven years to a mean of 21 ppm xylenes. Neither was the prevalence of symptoms dose-dependent nor were other solvent exposures characterized. This vapor concentration is significantly lower than current occupational exposure standards in the United States, which are established on the basis of acute irritancy or CNS effects. Savolainen *et al.* (1981) observed improved performance on a series of psychophysiological tests by humans inhaling 200 ppm *m*-xylene for four hours. An excitatory stage is often initially manifest in subjects, followed by functional inhibition with higher vapor concentrations and/or longer exposure periods. The current PEL in the United States for xylenes and ethylbenzene is 100 ppm.

Xylenes and ethylbenzene appear to have very limited capacity to adversely affect organs other than the CNS. Mild, transient liver and/or kidney toxicity have/has occasionally been reported in humans exposed to high vapor concentrations of xylenes. Little evidence of hepatorenal injury is typically manifest in laboratory animals (ATSDR, 2006c). Xylenes and ethylbenzene increase liver weight and moderately induce liver CYPs in laboratory animals (ATSDR, 2006c, 2010a). The *o*, *p*, and *m* isomers of xylene vary somewhat in their capacity to induce various CYP isoforms in different organs of rats (Backes *et al.*, 1993). Concurrent exposure to an alkylbenzene and another compound metabolized by P450s generally results in their competitive metabolic inhibition. Competitive metabolic interaction between xylene and ethylbenzene following inhalation exposure has been reported (Campbell and Fisher, 2007). Preexposure to an alkylbenzene, conversely, can result in increased metabolism of the other chemical.

The majority of alkylbenzenes do not appear to be genotoxic or carcinogenic. Ethylbenzene and styrene are two exceptions. Kidney injury and an increased incidence of renal adenoma and carcinoma (combined) were found in male F344 rats exposed to 750 ppm ethylbenzene for up to two years (NTP, 1997b). However, no association has been found between the occurrence of tumors and exposure to ethylbenzene in humans. A battery of in vivo and in vitro genetic toxicity assays has shown that ethylbenzene is not genotoxic. IARC classified ethylbenzene as a possible human carcinogen.

Styrene

Styrene is primarily used in the manufacture of polystyrene items and in copolymers with acrylonitrile or 1,3-butadiene to produce synthetic rubber, latex, and reinforced plastics (Gibbs and Mulligan, 1997). Worker exposures in the rubber industry are of greatest concern toxicologically. Styrene is also often detected in the blood of nonoccupationally exposed populations (Churchill *et al.*, 2001; Blount *et al.*, 2006). Sources include tobacco smoke, auto exhaust, and emissions from building materials. Discharges from industry are the major source of environmental pollution (ATSDR, 2010b).

CNS effects and mucous membrane and respiratory irritation are the most commonly reported effects in humans following styrene exposure. Workers exposed to ~25 ppm exhibit signs of mild hepatic injury and cholestasis (Brodkin *et al.*, 2001). Styrene is damaging to the nasal epithelium of rats and mice, and hepatotoxic and pneumotoxic in mice. Species differences in styrene toxicity can be explained by metabolic differences. Styrene is metabolized principally by CYP2E1 in liver and CYP2F2 in lung to styrene-7,8-oxide (SO) (Linhart *et al.*, 2000; Carlson, 2003). SO, the ultimate toxicant, can bind covalently to proteins and nucleic acids. This epoxide is detoxified by the actions of epoxide hydrolase and GST (Carlson, 2010; Chung *et al.*, 2006). SO is detoxified much more efficiently by epoxide hydrolase in rats and humans than in mice. Among the three species, mouse liver and lungs have the highest capacity to form SO from styrene (ATSDR, 2010b).

There is considerable debate as to whether styrene is a human carcinogen. It is carcinogenic to the forestomach of orally dosed mice and rats (Roe, 1994). Results of in vitro and in vivo mutagenicity and genotoxicity studies of styrene have been mixed (ATSDR, 2010b). Chromosomal aberrations, micronuclei, and/or sister chromatid exchange have been reported in employees in some high-exposure occupational settings, but not in others. Increased rates of different cancers have been reported in workers exposed to 1,3-butadiene and styrene in the synthetic rubber industry. The excesses of cancers have largely been attributed to 1,3-butadiene, although styrene may modify the actions of 1,3-butadiene and/or be implicated itself (Matonoski *et al.*, 1997). Occasional findings of small increases in incidences of lymphatic and hematopoietic neoplasms in epidemiological studies of workers exposed primarily to styrene are not very robust (IARC, 2002; ATSDR, 2010b). No increases in any tumors were seen in male or female S-D rats exposed six hours daily, five days weekly for 104 weeks to as high as 1000 ppm styrene vapor (Cruzan *et al.*, 1998). A similar inhalation cancer bioassay, however, revealed increases in pulmonary adenomas and/or carcinomas in male and female CD-1 mice (Cruzan *et al.*, 2001). Gavage studies have yielded variable results (ATSDR, 2010b). In a NCI (1979) study, dose-related increases in the combined incidence of benign and malignant lung tumors were noted in mice following chronic gavage dosing. In an oral study in which pregnant dams were given a single dose of styrene on gestation day 17, and offspring were exposed to high oral doses once weekly for 16 weeks after weaning, a significant increase in lung tumors was observed in these offspring following a 100-week exposure period (Ponomarkov and Tomatis, 1978). The same authors reported no significant tumor incidences in a second study in which a different strain of mice was exposed to much lower doses of styrene on gestation day 17 followed by once a week exposure of offspring for 120 weeks. Lung tumor response observed in mice is most likely due to cytotoxicity caused by the in situ formation of SO, followed by cell proliferation (ATSDR, 2010b). The relevance of mouse lung tumors to humans has been questioned due to species differences in lung metabolism of styrene (Carlson, 2008).

Workers in the reinforced plastics industry are exposed to styrene and SO. Tornero-Velez and Rappaport (2001) used a modified PBTK model to predict the relative contributions of inhaled styrene and SO to systemic levels of SO in humans. Inhaled SO was forecast to present the greater cytogenetic hazard. Sarangapani et al. (2002) created a PBTK model with a multicompartment representation of the respiratory tract that included species-specific quantitative information on physiology, cellular composition, and metabolic capacity. The model-based analysis indicated that humans would be 100-fold less susceptible than mice to pulmonary tumors, based on predictions of SO concentrations in terminal bronchioles. Wenker et al. (2001) attempted to correlate key CYP metabolic capacities of 20 male volunteers with styrene clearance. Lack of correlation was attributed to the low inhaled vapor concentrations and styrene's blood flow–limited metabolism.

Based on the limited evidence in humans and evidence in mice, NTP (2011) recently classified styrene as "reasonably anticipated to be a human carcinogen," and IARC classified it as "possibly carcinogenic to humans." For workers' protection, OSHA (2006) has established a PEL of 100 ppm, and ACGIH has established a TLV of 20 ppm as an eight-hour TWA (ACGIH, 2012).

ALCOHOLS

Ethanol

Many humans experience greater exposure to ethanol (ethyl alcohol, alcohol) than to any other solvent. Not only is ethyl alcohol used as an additive in gasoline, as a solvent in industry, in many household products, and in pharmaceuticals, but it is also heavily consumed in intoxicating beverages. Frank toxic effects are less important occupationally than injuries resulting from psychomotor impairment. Driving under the influence of alcohol is, of course, the major cause of fatal auto accidents. In many states in the United States, a blood alcohol level of 80 mg/100 mL blood (80 mg%) is prima facie evidence of "driving while intoxicated." One's blood alcohol level and the time necessary to achieve it are controlled largely by the rapidity and extent of consumption of the chemical. Ethanol is distributed in body water and to some degree in adipose tissue. Alcohol is eliminated by urinary excretion, exhalation, and metabolism. The blood level in an average adult decreases by $\approx$ 16 mg% per hour. Thus, a person with a blood alcohol level of 120 mg% would require $\approx$ eight hours to reach negligible levels.

Ethanol is metabolized to acetaldehyde by three enzymes: the major pathway involves ADH-catalyzed oxidation to acetaldehyde. ADHs are present in various tissues including stomach, lung, eye, and liver, but the highest concentrations are found in the cytoplasm of hepatocytes (Yin et al., 1999). While hepatic ADH largely contributes to ethanol oxidation in humans (Lee et al., 2006), a PBTK model indicates both hepatic and gastric ADH contribute to first-pass metabolism of ethanol in rats, with gastric ADH playing a greater role at lower ethanol doses (Pastino and Conolly, 2000).

The oxidation ADH catalyzes is reversible, but the acetaldehyde that is formed is rapidly oxidized by aldehyde dehydrogenase (ALDH) to acetate. Liver mitochondrial ALDH is the major enzyme responsible for acetaldehyde clearance. However, a recent PBTK model predicted the reversible conversion of acetaldehyde to alcohol by ADH to be an essential step in the systemic clearance of acetaldehyde (Umulis et al., 2005). A second enzyme, catalase, utilizes H_2O_2 supplied by the actions of NADPH oxidase and xanthine oxidase. There is usually little H_2O_2 available in hepatocytes to support the reaction, so it is unlikely that catalase will normally account for more than 10% of ethyl alcohol metabolism. The third enzyme, CYP2E1, is the principal isoform of the hepatic microsomal ethanol oxidizing system.

Ethanol interacts with other solvents that are also metabolized by ADH and CYP2E1. It can be an effective antidote for poisoning by methanol, ethylene glycol (EG), and diethylene glycol (DEG). As ethyl alcohol has a relatively high affinity for ADH, it competitively inhibits the metabolic activation of other alcohols and glycols. Preexposure to a single high dose or multiple doses of ethanol can induce CYP2E1, thereby enhancing the metabolic activation and potentiating the toxicity of a considerable number of other solvents and drugs such as acetaminophen (Lieber, 1997; Klotz and Ammon, 1998). Manno et al. (1996), for example, describe heavy drinkers who developed severe hepatorenal toxicity from CCl_4 exposures, which caused no ill effects in nondrinkers. Other alcohols, such as 2-butanol (Fig. 24-4), can have analogous effects (Traiger and Bruckner, 1976). Chronic heavy drinkers may develop more severe hepatotoxicity associated with acetaminophen overdosing than nonalcoholics, due to increased formation and reduced detoxification of toxic metabolites (Riordan and Williams, 2002; Rumack, 2004). Such interactions are also described in the sections "Metabolism" and "Exogenous Factors."

A variety of factors that modulate ADH, CYP2E1, and ALDH can influence adverse effects experienced by drinkers. Relatively low ADH and CYP2E1 activities increase systemic alcohol levels and prolong its effects, while low ALDH results in elevated acetaldehyde levels. Long-term ingestion of high alcohol doses can lead to alcohol dependency and cirrhosis, whereas high acetaldehyde levels may result in acute toxicity due to covalent binding to proteins and other macromolecules (Niemela, 1999). Ethanol-metabolizing enzymes exist in multiple molecular forms that are genetically controlled. Genetic polymorphisms of these enzymes contribute to different disease outcomes in different ethnic and racial populations (Crabb et al., 2004; Russo et al., 2004). Asians have higher frequencies of an ADH1*2 variant, which encodes for a rapidly metabolizing form of ADH, preventing alcoholism. White and black populations in the United States predominantly have an ADH1*1 allele (Russo et al., 2004), which encodes for a relatively inactive ADH (Lee et al., 2006), leading to increased risk of alcohol dependency. As for ALDH, approximately 50% of Asians have high levels of the inactive allele, ALDH2*2. Hence, this population experiences acetaldehyde-induced flushing, tachycardia, nausea, vomiting, and hyperventilation on alcohol consumption. Whereas this syndrome offers protection against developing alcoholism, it increases the risk of acetaldehyde-related cancers, including esophageal, stomach, colon, lung, head, and neck tumors (Vasiliou et al., 2004). The proposed mechanism for these cancers is that constant interaction of acetaldehyde with DNA leads to mutations in procarcinogenic or antiapoptotic genes (Israel et al., 2011). While higher frequencies of ADH1*2 and ALDH*2 result in increased internal exposure of acetaldehyde, the incidences of esophageal, stomach, colon, lung, head, and neck tumors in individuals who carry ADH1*2 is markedly less. A possible explanation for this difference is that the increase in acetaldehyde levels in ADH1*2 individuals is brief due to further metabolism of acetaldehyde by ALDH, whereas ALDH2*2 individuals have sustained exposure to acetaldehyde. Hispanics, on the other hand, have very low levels of ADH1*2 and ALDH2*2, predisposing them to alcoholism and their offspring to fetal alcohol syndrome (FAS). Disulfiram, an ALDH inhibitor, is used to treat alcoholism, by enhancing acetaldehyde levels when alcohol is consumed. Whereas CYP2E1 polymorphism is reported in humans (Zintzaras *et al.*, 2006), its role in the pathogenicity of alcoholism is still unclear.

Gender differences in responses to ethanol are well recognized. Women are more sensitive to alcohol, and exhibit higher mortality at lower levels of consumption than men (Sato *et al.*, 2001; Brienza and Stein, 2002). They exhibit somewhat higher blood levels than men following ingestion of equivalent doses of ethanol (Pikaar *et al.*, 1988). This phenomenon appears to be due in part to more extensive ADH-catalyzed metabolism of ethanol by the male gastric mucosa (Frezza *et al.*, 1990; Seitz *et al.*, 1993). Kinetic data indicate that hepatic ADH does not play a role in the sex difference in first-pass elimination of ethanol, although Chrostek *et al.* (2003) did report higher activities of ADH isoforms that efficiently oxidize ethanol in the liver of male subjects. Sex differences in ethanol metabolism in the remainder of the body appear to be small or nonexistent. A second factor contributing to the higher blood ethanol levels and greater CNS effects in women is their smaller volume of distribution for relatively polar solvents such as alcohols. It is well known that women are more susceptible to alcohol-induced hepatitis and cirrhosis (Thurman, 2000). A postulated mechanism for this sex difference is described below.

Alcohol now is recognized as the leading preventable cause of birth defects and developmental disorders (review in Warren *et al.*, 2011). The severity of birth defects resulting from exposure of the developing embryo or fetus to alcohol is determined by multiple factors, including genetic background, timing and level of alcohol exposure, pattern of drinking, and nutritional status. Peak maternal blood alcohol concentration is apparently the most important determinant of the likelihood of alcohol-related developmental effects. Overconsumption during all three trimesters of pregnancy can result in certain manifestations, dependent on the period of gestation during which ingestion occurs. The most serious adverse consequence of prenatal alcohol exposure is FAS, which has an estimated prevalence that ranges from 0.5 to 7.0 cases per 1000 births in the United States. Diagnostic criteria for FAS include: (1) heavy maternal alcohol consumption during gestation; (2) prenatal and postnatal growth retardation; (3) craniofacial malformations including microcephaly; and (4) mental retardation. However, there are other alcohol-related brain and behavioral abnormalities that are not diagnosed as FAS because of the lack of abnormal facial features. This range of deficits now is referred to as fetal alcohol spectrum disorders (FASD) and is estimated to occur in 1% of births.

Despite an intensive research effort for three decades, the mechanisms underlying FAS remain unclear. Exposure of embryonic tissue to ethanol adversely affects many cellular functions critical to development, including protein and DNA synthesis, uptake of critical nutrients such as glucose and amino acids, and changes in several kinase-mediated signal transduction pathways (Shibley and Pennington, 1997). Alcohol may also harm the fetus indirectly as a result of the mother's malnutrition. Numerous mechanisms have been suggested as contributing to alcohol-induced fetal damage, although none has been established with certainty (Goodlett and Horn, 2001). Some studies have suggested that oxidative stress on fetal tissues is responsible (Henderson *et al.*, 1999), while others have implicated ethanol's effects on neurotransmitter-gated ion channels, particularly the NMDA receptor (Costa *et al.*, 2000), and its ability to trigger cell death via necrosis and apoptosis (Ikonomidou *et al.*, 2000; Goodlett and Horn, 2001). Others have reported that ethanol produces a long-lasting reduction in synaptic efficacy (Bellinger *et al.*, 1999) and alters the fetal expression of developmentally important genes such as msx2 and insulin-like growth factors (Singh *et al.*, 1996; Rifas *et al.*, 1997). Recent studies suggest that ethanol-induced NMDA receptor antagonism and GABA receptor agonist activity-mediated apoptosis play critical roles in learning impairment (Ikonomidou *et al.*, 2000; Olney *et al.*, 2002; Toso *et al.*, 2006). Acetaldehyde may also contribute to the development of FAS, as it is shown to accumulate in the fetal brain after prenatal alcohol exposure (Hamby-Mason *et al.*, 1997) and to be cytotoxic to cultured embryonic brain cells (Lee *et al.*, 2005). Other potential mechanisms of FASD include: (1) alterations in the regulation of gene expression (eg, reduced retinoic acid signaling, altered DNA methylation), (2) interference with mitogenic and growth factor responses involved in neural stem cell proliferation, migration, and differentiation; (3) disturbances in molecules that mediate cell–cell interactions (L1, NCAM, loss of trophic support); and (4) derangements of glial proliferation, differentiation, and function (Guerri *et al.*, 2009; Ramsay, 2010).

Genetic variability in metabolic enzymes is another proposed mechanism for FAS. A role for CYP2E1 in the induction of FAS has been hypothesized, given its expression in human cephalic tissues during embryogenesis (Boutelet-Bochan *et al.*, 1997). Results of in vitro experiments indicate that human CYP2E1 is effective in production of reactive oxygen intermediates (eg, hydroxy radicals, superoxide anion, and H_2O_2) and in causation of lipid peroxidation (Dai *et al.*, 1993). Membrane lipids and a variety of enzymes are targets for free radical attack. Albano *et al.* (1999) have demonstrated a marked increase in covalent binding of hydroxyethyl radicals to hepatic microsomal proteins from rats following chronic ethanol administration. There is not yet direct evidence that hydroxyethyl radicals contribute to lipid peroxidation, but they do readily react with α-tocopherol, GSH, and ascorbic acid, thereby potentially lowering liver antioxidant levels in vivo. Albano *et al.* (1999) also describe evidence that hydroxyethyl radical–protein adducts in hepatocytes induce immune responses, which may contribute to chronic ethanol hepatotoxicity (ie, alcoholic liver disease [ALD]).

ALD is one of the most prevalent and fatal conditions of alcohol abuse. It is the 12th leading cause of death in the United States. The progression of ALD follows a characteristic pattern marked by appearance of fatty liver, hepatocyte necrosis, inflammation, regeneration nodules, fibrosis, and cirrhosis. Despite extensive research, the mechanisms underlying ALD are still unclear. It is postulated that chronic alcohol consumption increases the gut permeability to lipopolysaccharide (LPS), an endotoxin that is a major constituent of the outer membrane of gram-negative bacteria. LPS binds to receptors in Kupffer cells to produce reactive oxygen species (ROS), which activate nuclear regulatory factor kappa beta (NF-κB), leading to TNF-α and other inflammatory mediators that are cytotoxic to hepatocytes and chemoattractants for neutrophils (Bautista, 2000; Diehl, 2000). These mediators include ILs, prostaglandins, free radicals, and eicosanoids. TNF-α signaling also increases mitochondrial ROS, which trigger apoptotic cell death in the liver. Apoptotic cells in turn result in an increased inflammatory response. Proinflammatory cytokines and oxidative stress stimulate collagen synthesis by hepatic stellate cells, leading to alcoholic fibrosis (Lieber, 2004). Chronic alcohol consumption also inhibits components of innate immunity, such as natural killer (NK) cells. The inhibition of NK cells decreases NK cell-mediated killing of stellate cells, contributing to fibrosis (Miller *et al.*, 2011; Mandrekar and Szabo, 2009).

Alcohol-induced oxidative stress is thought to cause liver injury by promoting the development of both humoral and cellular immune responses (Vidali *et al.*, 2008). CYP2E1 can generate ROS during its catalytic cycle. Because CYP2E1 metabolizes ethanol and increases during ethanol exposure, it is suggested to play a significant role in ethanol-induced liver toxicity. Lu *et al.* (2010) recently reported that wild-type mice and humanized CYP2E1 (knock-in) mice had significant ethanol-induced oxidative stress and fatty liver, but CYP2E1 knockout mice did not have these changes.

Acetaldehyde is capable of upregulating collagen synthesis either directly or indirectly by inducing TGF-β1. Hence, polymorphisms of ALDH can increase the risk of fibrosis (Purohit and Brenner, 2006). Kupffer cells of female rats are more sensitive to endotoxin than those of males. Estrogen increases the sensitivity of Kupffer cells of rats to endotoxin, leading to increased production of TNF-α and death of hepatocytes (Thurman, 2000; Yin *et al.*, 2000; Colantoni *et al.*, 2003). This phenomenon is thought to account in part for the more severe hepatitis and cirrhosis commonly seen in female alcoholics (Thurman, 2000).

Alcohol-induced damage of the liver and other tissues is thought to result in part from nutritional disturbances, as well as toxic effects (Lieber, 2004; DiCecco and Francisco-Ziller, 2006). Lack of money, poor judgment, prolonged inebriation, and appetite loss contribute to poor nutrition and weight loss in alcoholics. A high percentage of calories in the alcoholic's diet is furnished by alcohol. Malabsorption of thiamine, diminished enterohepatic circulation of folate, degradation of pyridoxal phosphate, and disturbances in the metabolism of vitamins A and D can occur (Mezey, 1985). Prostaglandins released from endotoxin-activated Kupffer cells may be responsible for a hypermetabolic state in the liver. With the increase in oxygen demand, the viability of centrilobular hepatocytes would be most compromised, due to their relatively poor oxygen supply (Thurman, 1998). Metabolism of ethanol via ADH and ALDH results in a shift in the redox state of the cell. The metabolites and the more reduced state can result in hyperlactacidemia, hyperlipidemia, hyperuricemia, and hyperglycemia, leading to increased steatosis and collagen synthesis (Lieber, 2004).

Alcoholism can result in damage of extrahepatic tissues. Alcoholic myopathy is one of the more common consequences, occurring in 50% of alcohol abusers. The condition is characterized by reductions in skeletal muscle mass and strength (Adachi *et al.*, 2003; Preedy *et al.*, 2003). Alcoholic cardiomyopathy is a complex process that occurs in 20% to 25% of alcoholics. It results from decreased synthesis of cardiac contractile proteins, attack of oxygen radicals, increases in endoplasmic reticulum Ca²⁺-ATPase, and an antibody response to acetaldehyde–protein adducts (Richardson *et al.*, 1998; Preedy *et al.*, 2003). Interestingly, light to moderate drinking is reported to protect against atherosclerosis in the carotid artery, a major cause of ischemic stroke (Hillbom, 1999). Alcohol increases high-density lipoprotein (HDL) cholesterol by inducing the constituents, apo I and II, by increasing catabolism of very low-density lipoproteins and chylomicrons, and by delaying HDL catabolism (Kolovou *et al.*, 2006). It is also hypothesized that ethanol metabolism in the vascular wall may inhibit oxidation of low-density lipoproteins (LDL), a requisite for atherogenesis. Phenolic antioxidants in wines may also inhibit LDL oxidation as well as reduce platelet aggregation. Conversely, heavy drinking appears to deplete antioxidants and have the opposite effects (Hillbom, 1999; Kolovou *et al.*, 2006). Recent heavy drinking increases the risk of both hemorrhagic and ischemic strokes. Other organ systems can be adversely affected in alcoholics including the brain and GI tract (Kril *et al.*, 1997; Rajendram and Preedy, 2005).

Table 24-3

Possible Mechanisms of Ethanol Carcinogenicity

Congeners: additives and contaminants in alcoholic beverages influence carcinogenicity

CYP2E1 induction by ethanol increases metabolic activation of procarcinogens

Ethanol acts as a solvent for carcinogens, enhancing their absorption into tissues of the upper GI tract. Ethanol affects the actions of certain hormones on hormone-sensitive tissues

Immune function is suppressed by alcohol

Absorption and bioavailability of nutrients are reduced by alcohol

SOURCE: Adapted with permission from Ahmed (1995).

There is concern about the role of ethyl alcohol in carcinogenesis, due to the frequent consumption of alcoholic beverages by millions of people. IARC (1988) concluded that there was "sufficient evidence" for causation of tumors of the oral cavity, pharynx and larynx, esophagus, and liver of humans. In a 2007 meeting, IARC added breast and colorectal cancers to the list of cancers causally linked with alcohol consumption (Baan *et al.*, 2007). Genotoxic effects by acetaldehyde and elevated estrogen levels are likely mechanisms for breast cancer (Boffeta and Hashibe, 2006). According to the World Health Organization Global Burden of Disease Project, drinking accounts for ~3.2% of all deaths and 3.6% of all cancers (Rehm *et al.*, 2004). The original associations between alcohol and cancers came primarily from epidemiological case–control and cohort studies. One such cohort study of 276,000 American men showed an increase in total cancer risk with increasing ethanol consumption (Boffeta and Garfinkel, 1990). In support of epidemiological studies, a rat study showed that ethanol induces tumors in various organs including oral cavity, tongue, and lips (Soffritti *et al.*, 2002). While mechanisms for alcohol-related carcinogenesis are not fully understood, metabolism plays a major role (Seitz and Stickel, 2007). Ethanol is shown to induce CYP2E1, which is known to generate ROS that damage DNA, lipids, and proteins. Additionally, acetaldehyde, which is carcinogenic to humans, reacts with DNA, forming adducts. Evidence suggests that the risk of alcohol-induced cancer in humans is modulated by genetic polymorphisms in enzymes responsible for alcohol metabolism, folate metabolism, and DNA repair (Boffeta and Hashibe, 2006). Ethanol may also stimulate carcinogenesis by inhibiting DNA methylation and interfering with retinoic acid metabolism. Ethanol and smoking act synergistically to cause oral, pharyngeal, and laryngeal cancers. Age, sex, and ethnicity have also been reported to be factors. It is generally accepted that alcohol induces liver cancer by causing cirrhosis or other chronic liver damage and/or by enhancing the bioactivation of other carcinogens (Table 24-3).

An international symposium (Purohit *et al.*, 2005), sponsored by the National Institute on Alcohol Abuse and Alcoholism in 2004, concluded that chronic ethanol consumption may promote carcinogenesis by: (1) production of acetaldehyde, a weak mutagen and carcinogen; (2) induction of CYP2E1 and its associated oxidative stressors and conversion of procarcinogens to carcinogens; (3) depletion of *S*-adenosylmethionine (SAM) and, consequently, induction of global DNA hypomethylation; (4) increased production of inhibitory guanine nucleotide regulatory proteins and components of extracellular signal-regulated kinase-mitogen-activated protein kinase signaling; (5) accumulation of iron and associated oxidative stress; (6) inactivation of the tumor suppressor gene *BRCA1* and increased estrogen responsiveness (primarily in the breast); and (7) impairment of retinoic acid metabolism. Jeannot *et al.* (2011) recently reported that ethanol may act by promoting spontaneously initiated cells, especially *H-ras* mutated cells.

Methanol

Methanol (methyl alcohol, wood alcohol, and CH_3OH) is primarily used as a starting material for the synthesis of chemicals such as formaldehyde, acetic acid, methacrylates, ethylene glycol (EG), and methyl *tertiary*-butyl ether (MTBE). CH_3OH is found in windshield washer fluid, carburetor cleaners, antifreeze, and copy machine toner, and serves as fuel for Sterno™ heaters, and model airplanes. It also functions as a denaturant for some ethyl and iso-propyl alcohols, rendering them unfit for consumption. It is used to a limited extent as an alternative fuel for fleet vehicles (usually in a mixture of 85% CH_3OH and 15% gasoline) and is being explored as a gasoline additive and hydrogen source for fuel cell vehicles. Exposure of the general population also occurs via the consumption of fruits, fruit juices, vegetables, and alcoholic beverages that contain free CH_3OH or CH_3OH precursors. Indirect exposure occurs via the hydrolysis of the artificial sweetener, aspartame, and subsequent CH_3OH absorption from the gut. Very low-level exposures may occur via ambient air and drinking water. Of all chemicals reported, CH_3OH was ranked No. 1 for fugitive air emissions, No. 3 for point source air emissions, and No. 2 for surface water discharges according to the 2004 Toxic Release Inventory (EPA, 2006a). Nevertheless, persistence and bioaccumulation in the environment are not expected. The consumption of adulterated "bootleg" whiskey is a major cause of CH_3OH poisoning.

Serious CH_3OH toxicity is most commonly associated with ingestion. Left untreated, acute CH_3OH poisoning in humans is characterized by an asymptomatic latent period of 12 to 24 hours followed by formic acidemia, ocular toxicity, coma, and in extreme cases death (Lanigan, 2001). Visual disturbances generally develop between 18 and 48 hours after ingestion and range from mild pho-tophobia and misty or blurred vision to markedly reduced visual acuity and complete blindness (Eells *et al.*, 1996). Although there is considerable variability among individuals in susceptibility to CH_3OH, a frequently cited lethal oral dosage is 1 mL/kg. Blindness and death have been reported with dosages as low as 0.1 mL/kg (ATSDR, 1993). CH_3OH's target within the eye is the retina, specifically the optic disk and optic nerve. Optic disk edema and hyperemia are seen, along with morphological alterations in the optic nerve head and the intraorbital portion of the optic nerve. Both axons and glial cells exhibit altered morphologies (Kavet and Nauss, 1990). Rods and cones, the photoreceptors of the retina, are also altered functionally and structurally (Seme *et al.*, 1999). Evidence is accumulating that Müller cells, neuroglia that function in the maintenance of retinal structure and in intracellular and intercellular transport, are early targets of CH_3OH (Garner *et al.*, 1995a). There are indications of mitochondrial disruption in Müller and photoreceptor cells, which is consistent with the long-held view that formate inhibits the energy-generating mitochondrial enzyme, cytochrome *c* oxidase, which is critical for the proper functioning of highly oxidative organs such as the retina. This mechanism might explain, at least in part, CH_3OH's selective toxicity to photoreceptors and other highly metabolically active cells (Eells *et al.*, 1996). Interestingly, exposure of rats to monochromatic red radiation from light-emitting diode arrays can aid in the recovery of rod and cone function in CH_3OH-treated rats and protect the retina from histopathological changes characteristic of formate toxicity (Eells *et al.*, 2003). This "photobiomodulation" is thought to be mediated by the ability of monochromatic red to near-IR light to improve mitochondrial respiratory chain function (ie, increase cytochrome *c* oxidase activity), thereby initiating a signaling cascade that promotes cellular proliferation and cytoprotection.

Significant species differences exist in the susceptibility of CH_3OH toxicity. Acute ocular toxicity, metabolic acidosis, CNS depression, and death noted in humans are not seen with rodents. Conversely, rodents can be susceptible to delayed adverse effects of methanol such as developmental toxicity. Therefore, elucidation of the mechanism of CH_3OH's acute toxicity was hampered for years by the lack of appropriate animal models. Largely based on the work of Gilger and Potts (1955), it became apparent that only nonhuman primates respond to CH_3OH similarly to humans. Humans and non-human primates metabolize CH_3OH to formaldehyde (HCOH) by ADH, whereas rodents utilize catalase. In all mammalian species, HCOH is very rapidly converted via formaldehyde dehydrogenase (FLDH) to formate, which is further metabolized to CO_2. The conversion of formate to CO_2 occurs via a two-step, tetrahydrofolate (THF)-dependent pathway. First, formate is converted to 10-formyl-THF by formyl-THF synthetase, after which 10-formyl-THF is oxidized to CO_2 by formyl-THF dehydrogenase (F-THF-DH). Because rodents have much higher hepatic THF levels than primates, formate does not accumulate as it does in humans and monkeys (Medinsky and Dorman, 1995; Martinasevic *et al.*, 1996). Another possible explanation is the lower F-THF-DH activity in primate liver (Johlin *et al.*, 1989). It is further speculated that primates are more susceptible to CH_3OH and formate toxicity due to their relative inability to excrete excess formate via the kidneys (Smith and Taylor, 1982). Irregardless, susceptibility to CH_3OH-induced ocular toxicity is dependent on the relative rate of formate clearance. Dietary and chemical depletion of endogenous folate cofactors in rats has been shown to increase formate accumulation following CH_3OH, resulting in the development of metabolic acidosis and ocular toxicity similar to that observed in humans (Eells *et al.*, 1996, 2000). Sweeting *et al.* (2011) reported that rabbits, similar to humans and monkeys, metabolize CH_3OH by ADH and exhibit slower CH_3OH clearance and increased formate accumulation, suggesting that rabbits resemble primates and humans more closely than rodents. A simplified scheme of CH_3OH metabolism is presented in Fig. 24-10.

For years there was considerable debate whether HCOH or formate was responsible for CH_3OH's ocular toxicity. The finding

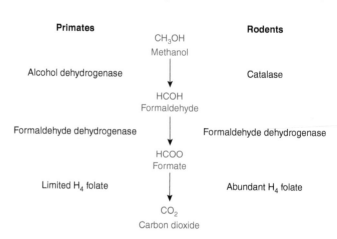

Figure 24-10. *Scheme for the metabolism of methanol.* Major enzymes are listed for primates (left) and rodents (right). Conversion of formate to CO_2 is rapid in rodents, but relatively slow in primates. (Used with permission from Dorman and Welsch, 1996.)

that HCOH does not accumulate following CH_3OH treatment, even in folate-deficient monkeys that are profoundly sensitive to CH_3OH, argues against a role for HCOH. Also, species of differing susceptibility exhibit comparable blood HCOH half-lives. In contrast, formate has been shown to accumulate in the human and monkey following CH_3OH treatment. CH_3OH-derived formate has also been quantified in the vitreous humor, retina, and to a lesser extent the optic nerve (Eells *et al.*, 1996). Moreover, CH_3OH-induced retinal dysfunction, as indicated by diminution of the amplitude of electroretinogram (ERG) *a* and *b* waves, is negatively correlated in a linear fashion with blood formate concentrations (Eells *et al.*, 1996). Others have reported similar relationships between blood formate and ERG responses indicative of photoreceptor dysfunction (Seme *et al.*, 1999). Formate has also been shown to induce ocular toxicity in monkeys and formate oxidation-inhibited rats in the absence of metabolic acidosis or a reduction in blood pH (Martin-Amat *et al.*, 1978; Eells *et al.*, 1996). Direct incubation of formate with cultured ocular cells caused ATP depletion and cytotoxicity (Treichel *et al.*, 2003). Thus, formate appears to act as a direct ocular toxin and not indirectly through the induction of an acidotic state, although acidosis may potentiate formate toxicity (since the inhibition of cytochrome oxidase increases as pH decreases and acidosis allows for greater diffusion of formic acid into cells).

The question has been raised whether ocular toxicity is simply a function of circulating formate reaching the visual tract, or whether metabolism in retinal or optic nerve tissues generates toxic metabolites locally. This is a legitimate question considering that metabolism of CH_3OH to HCOH via peroxisomal enzymes (catalase) has been demonstrated in rat retina in vitro (Garner *et al.*, 1995a), and the presence of cytoplasmic formaldehyde dehydrogenase (FLDH) activity has been demonstrated in several regions of the rat and mouse eye, including the retina (Messiha and Price, 1983; McCaffery *et al.*, 1991). By use of a folate-deficient rat model, Garner *et al.* (1995b) showed that a level of blood formate generated by i.v. infusion of pH-buffered formate did not diminish the ERG *b*-wave amplitude generated by Müller cells of the retina, as did a comparable blood level of formate derived from CH_3OH. This suggests that the intraretinal metabolism of CH_3OH is necessary for the initiation of retinal toxicity by formate. Not only are the enzymes necessary to produce formate present in the retina, but so too are folate and F-THF-DH. The latter was found to be localized in the mitochondria of Müller cells, prompting the suggestion that F-THF-DH may serve a dual role, one protective of the Müller cell and the other toxic. Protection would come in the form of formate oxidation, and toxicity from the over-consumption or depletion of ATP required for formate metabolism via the folate pathway (Martinasevic *et al.*, 1996).

The aforementioned findings raise concerns about the safety of CH_3OH exposure. Chamber studies of human volunteers exposed to 200 ppm CH_3OH for four or six hours showed no blood formate accumulation above background (Lee *et al.*, 1992; d'Alessandro *et al.*, 1994). Whereas this might be considered evidence that exposure at the 2012 ACGIH TLV and OSHA PEL of 200 ppm poses no risk of ocular toxicity, such an interpretation may not be valid, given that ocular toxicity may be a function of intraretinal CH_3OH metabolism rather than circulating formate levels.

The effects of acute, high CH_3OH exposures are well characterized compared with those of chronic, low-level exposures. Few reproductive/developmental studies and even fewer cancer bioassays have been conducted, due to the fact that rodents are not an ideal animal model for CH_3OH. Nonetheless, Soffritti *et al.* (2002) conducted a bioassay in which S-D rats received CH_3OH in their drinking water (0, 500, 5000, or 20,000 ppm ad libitum) for 104 weeks.

The investigators concluded that CH_3OH was a multipotent carcinogen. However, they referenced two Japanese bioassays that found no evidence of carcinogenicity in B6C3F1 mice or F344 rats exposed 20 hours per day to 10, 100, or 1000 ppm CH_3OH by inhalation for 18 and 24 months, respectively (NEDO, 1987; Katoh, 1989). A recent review of carcinogenicity and genetic toxicity studies concluded that CH_3OH is not likely to be carcinogenic in humans (Cruzan, 2009).

The NTP Center for the Evaluation of Risks to Human Reproduction released a monograph on CH_3OH's reproductive/developmental toxicity, largely based on an expert panel report (NTP, 2003, 2004b). Among the conclusions was that CH_3OH is a potential developmental toxicant in humans, provided a high enough blood concentration of the parent compound (assumed to be the proximate teratogen) is achieved. As this conclusion was largely based on data in rodents that metabolize CH_3OH much differently than humans, its validity has been called into question (Clary, 2003). As such, the few reproductive/developmental studies in nonhuman primates are particularly informative. These studies reported that maternal exposure of monkeys to inhaled CH_3OH (200, 600, or 1800 ppm, 2.5 hours per day, seven days per week prior to breeding and throughout pregnancy) was not associated with maternal toxicity, reproductive loss, or congenital malformations in offspring, but was associated with a six- to eight-day reduction in the mean length of pregnancy (Burbacher *et al.*, 2004a,b). Studies in rodents and rodent whole embryo cultures have implicated dysregulated cell death in the pathogenesis of CH_3OH-induced malformations, examined GSH status in the developing conceptus as it relates to vulnerability, and explored the basis for the increased sensitivity of the mouse embryo compared with that of the rat (Harris *et al.*, 2003, 2004; Degitz *et al.*, 2004; Hansen *et al.*, 2005). Because the disposition of CH_3OH and formic acid in rabbits was similar to humans, Sweeting *et al.* (2010) considered rabbits as an appropriate model for assessing the risk of human developmental toxicity. Three strains of mice and New Zealand rabbits were given a single dose of CH_3OH during gestation. Two strains of mice were susceptible to CH_3OH teratogenicity; one strain of mice and the rabbits were resistant. Despite similar CH_3OH and formic acid disposition in three strains of mice, the finding that one strain did not exhibit teratogenic effects suggests mechanisms other than pharmacokinetics could be involved. A role for ROS is suspected. The study also raised concerns about using rodents as a surrogate to predict human developmental toxicity of CH_3OH.

Whereas there is still much to be learned about the mechanisms of CH_3OH toxicity, what is known allows for effective therapies, if they are applied in a timely manner. The American Academy of Clinical Toxicology has published practice guidelines for the treatment of CH_3OH poisoning (Barceloux *et al.*, 2002). In cases of severe CH_3OH poisoning, there is a direct correlation between the formic acid concentration and increased morbidity and mortality. Sodium bicarbonate is usually given i.v. to correct severe acidosis, and case reports suggest that it may enhance renal formate excretion. Metabolic blockade is usually achieved with ethanol or 4-methylpyrazole (fomepizole), both acting as effective competitive inhibitors of ADH. Folate or folinic acid (activated folate) therapy is also indicated to increase the efficiency of formate oxidation. Hemodialysis is generally indicated when acidemia, high CH_3OH concentrations, or visual symptoms are present, although there are conflicting data on whether it appreciably shortens the elimination half-life of formate (Kerns *et al.*, 2002; Hantson *et al.*, 2005). Lastly, the treatment threshold of 20 mg CH_3OH/dL of blood in a nonacidotic patient arriving early for care has been questioned as being overly conservative. This stems from a comprehensive review of worldwide CH_3OH poisonings that identified 126 mg/dL as the lowest early blood CH_3OH level ever clearly associated with acidosis (Kostic and Dart, 2003). CH$_3$OH exemplifies the benefits of knowing a chemical's mode of action when treating the poisoned patient. This knowledge also aids in identifying potentially sensitive subpopulations, such as those suffering from dietary folate deficiency. Research suggests, however, that even in a state of folate deficiency, the body probably contains sufficient folate stores to effectively detoxify small doses of CH$_3$OH-derived formate from exogenous sources (Medinsky *et al.*, 1997).

GLYCOLS

Ethylene Glycol

EG (1,2-dihydroxyethane) is a constituent of antifreeze, deicers, hydraulic fluids, drying agents, and inks, and is used to make plastics and polyester fibers. Workers may be exposed dermally or by inhalation when solutions containing EG are heated or sprayed. The most important exposure route is ingestion, as EG may be accidentally swallowed, taken deliberately in suicide attempts, or used as a cheap substitute for ethanol. "Antifreeze" poisoning occurs frequently in cats and dogs that find its taste appealing. In 2004, there were 5562 human cases of EG exposure reported by the American Association of Poison Control Centers (23 fatal), nearly 40% of which were treated in a health care facility (Watson *et al.*, 2005). EG enters the environment as a result of disposal of industrial and consumer products containing the chemical. It partitions into surface water and groundwater, but does not persist in any environmental medium and is practically nontoxic to aquatic organisms (Staples *et al.*, 2001).

The TK profile of EG is well characterized. All laboratory mammals and humans metabolize EG similarly. A series of papers has been published describing the TK of EG in S-D rats and CD-1 mice after administration of a single dose by the i.v., oral, or percutaneous routes (Frantz *et al.*, 1996a-c). Absorption from the GI tract of rodents and humans is very rapid and virtually complete, whereas cutaneous and pulmonary absorption is relatively slow and less extensive. Once absorbed, EG is distributed throughout the total body water. As illustrated in Fig. 24-11, EG is metabolized by NAD$^+$-dependent ADH to glycolaldehyde and on to glycolic acid (GA). GA is oxidized to glyoxylic acid by GA oxidase and lactic dehydrogenase. Glyoxylic acid may be converted to formate and CO$_2$, or oxidized by glyoxylic acid oxidase to oxalic acid (OA) (Wiener and Richardson, 1988; Frantz *et al.*, 1996b). The rate-limiting step in the metabolism of EG is the conversion of GA to glyoxylic acid. EG has a half-life in humans of three to 8.6 hours (Leth and Gregersen, 2005). Under conditions of repetitive, low-dose exposure, EG is not expected to bioaccumulate, given its rapid metabolism and elimination. Pregnancy status has no bearing on the TK of EG, GA, or OA, as demonstrated by comparisons of pregnant and nonpregnant S-D rats (Pottenger *et al.*, 2001).

The minimum acute lethal dose of EG in humans is estimated at ~1.4 mL/kg, which equates to 100 mL for a 70-kg adult (LaKind *et al.*, 1999; Hess *et al.*, 2004). Acute poisoning entails three clinical stages after an asymptomatic period, during which EG is metabolized: (1) a period of inebriation, the duration and degree depending on dose; (2) the cardiopulmonary stage 12 to 24 hours after exposure, characterized by tachycardia and tachypnea, which may progress to cardiac failure and pulmonary edema; and (3) the renal toxicity stage 24 to 72 hours postexposure. Metabolic acidosis, due largely to GA accumulation, can develop and become progressively more severe during stages 2 and 3 (Jacobsen *et al.*, 1984; Moreau *et al.*, 1998; Egbert and Abraham, 1999). Hypocalcemia can result from Ca^{2+} chelation by OA to form Ca^{2+} oxalate monohydrate (COM) crystals. Deposition of these crystals in kidney tubules is associated with organ damage and potentially with acute renal failure. Nephrotoxicity

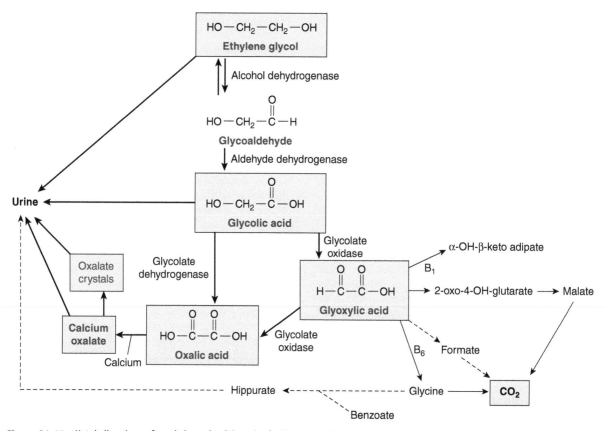

Figure 24-11. *Metabolic scheme for ethylene glycol in animals.* Key metabolites that have been observed in vivo are highlighted in boxes. Dashed lines are theoretical pathways that have not been verified in vivo or in vitro. (Used with permission from Corley *et al.*, 2005a.)

appears to be an acute, high-dose phenomenon, as no demonstrable kidney damage has been reported in occupational studies of groups such as airport deicing workers or Finnish auto mechanics (Laitinen *et al.*, 1995; Gerin *et al.*, 1997). COM crystal deposition has been reported in the walls of CNS blood vessels, with associated inflammation, edema, and sometimes neuropathy (Froberg *et al.*, 2006).

Based on high-dose rodent studies, including two lifetime dietary studies, EG has very limited chronic toxicity potential, exhibits no evidence of carcinogenicity, and does not appear to be a reproductive toxicant (DePass *et al.*, 1986; NTP, 1993b). However, it can cause adverse developmental effects such as skeletal and soft tissue malformations and delayed ossification when administered during gestation at high doses (≥500 mg/kg per day) (ATSDR, 1997b). GA appears to be the proximate developmental toxicant, with metabolic acidosis playing an exacerbating, but not obligatory role (Carney *et al.*, 1996, 1999). Pottenger *et al.* (2001) have demonstrated that at teratogenic doses of EG, blood levels of GA are disproportionately high relative to the EG dose, further supporting GA as the proximate teratogen and implying a role for metabolic saturation. Corley *et al.* (2005d) have detailed the key events in EG-induced developmental toxicity and suggest the disruption of *hox* gene expression, fluid imbalance, and dysregulation of cell death in the embryo as mechanistic possibilities. The mechanism of GA's teratogenic action remains largely unknown, however, as does the relevance of defects in rodents given the absence of reported developmental effects in humans. The NTP Center for the Evaluation of Risks to Human Reproduction has released a monograph on EG's reproductive/developmental toxicity largely based on an expert panel report (NTP, 2004d,f). The overall conclusion was that EG exposures below the level of metabolic saturation should not result in developmental toxicity in humans. Further, because environmental and occupational exposures to humans are two to three orders of magnitude lower than those expected to result in metabolic saturation, such exposures are of negligible concern. Corley *et al.* (2005a) have developed a PBTK model of EG and GA and compared internal dose surrogates in rats and humans. Based on the comparisons, they also concluded that occupationally or environmentally exposed humans are unlikely to achieve blood levels of GA that have been associated with developmental toxicity in rats.

The chief concern about EG is renal toxicity after high-dose, acute exposure. Although EG must be metabolized to toxic intermediates to induce kidney damage, the specific metabolite(s) and underlying mechanism(s) responsible remain to be fully elucidated. There is agreement, however, that the process involves a toxicant-induced proximal tubular necrosis leading to loss of renal function. Poldelski *et al.* (2001) exposed isolated mouse proximal tubule segments and human proximal tubular epithelial cells (HK-2) to GA, glycoaldehyde, glyoxylate, or OA for 15 to 60 minutes, on which basis they concluded glycoaldehyde and glyoxylate are the principal metabolites responsible for EG nephrotoxicity. This is contrary to the prevailing opinion that renal toxicity is due to the terminal metabolite, OA, which precipitates in the kidney in the form of COM crystals (Guo and McMartin, 2005). Corley *et al.* (2005d) have listed the key mechanistic events in the renal toxicity of EG: (1) metabolism of EG to OA via GA; (2) concentration of OA in tubular urine → precipitation of OA with Ca^{2+} → buildup of COM crystals in renal tubular epithelium → adherence of COM crystals to the plasma membrane of proximal tubular cells → subsequent intracellular uptake of COM crystals by endocytosis; and (3) physical trauma by COM crystals and/or production of free radicals and lipid peroxidation leading to cell necrosis, apoptosis, and renal tubular degeneration. Clearly, the weight of evidence implicates OA is critical in the induction of renal damage, but a possible role for less frequently observed hippuric acid crystals and direct cytotoxicity by

other metabolites cannot be ruled out. In vitro assays have indicated that both oxalate and COM crystals are injurious to renal epithelial cells (Thamilselvan and Khan, 1998). Also, renal damage has been observed occasionally following exposure to EG, without documentation of crystals in the kidney.

The intracellular target(s) of COM crystals is(are) not known with certainty, but it is well established that mitochondrial damage is a major mechanism for chemically mediated renal tubular necrosis. As such, COM crystals in the cytoplasm could directly affect mitochondria or be metabolized to release the oxalate ion that could do so. McMartin and Wallace (2005) hypothesized as much and demonstrated that COM produced a dose-dependent decrease in state 3 respiration in isolated rat kidney mitochondria, which they believe may be responsible for induction of mitochondrial permeability transition (MPT). MPT is characterized by an otherwise inpenetrant inner mitochondrial membrane undergoing transformation, whereby it becomes penetrable to solutes or large molecules. As a result of MPT, mitochondria undergo a rapid and progressive osmotic swelling, depolarization of mitochondrial membrane potential, and inhibition of oxidative phosphorylation/ATP synthesis, all of which can lead to either oncotic/ischemic cell death or apoptotic cell death. Additional insight into the pathogenesis of EG-induced renal damage has been provided by Chen *et al.* (2004), who provided male rats with 0.75% EG in their drinking water for two, four, and eight weeks, after which the kidneys were processed for RNA isolation and microarray analysis using a rat-based chip. Changes in the expression of genes associated with tubular structure and function, oxidative damage, and inflammation were common. Increased expression of mitochondrial uncoupling protein was also observed, providing additional evidence of a mitochondrial target. EG has also been used as a model crystal-forming renal toxicant to determine the basis for COM crystal retention in the kidney. Studies with EG suggest that crystal retention in the kidney may depend on the expression of the proteins hyaluronan, osteopontin, and their mutual cell surface receptor CD44, all of which are upregulated in response to renal injury/inflammation, and under normal circumstances play a role in reestablishment of epithelial barrier integrity and restoration of renal function. However, their upregulation could turn a noncrystal-binding epithelium into a crystal-binding one, thereby setting the stage for crystal retention and renal injury (Asselman *et al.*, 2003; Verhulst *et al.*, 2003).

In cases of severe EG poisoning, early diagnosis and aggressive therapeutic intervention are essential for a favorable clinical outcome. A plasma EG level of 20 mg/dL is considered the threshold for kidney toxicity, if therapeutic strategy is based on EG concentration alone (Hess *et al.*, 2004). However, no signs of renal injury have developed in patients at initial plasma GA concentrations of up to 10.1 mM or 76.7 mg/dL (Brent *et al.*, 1999; Hess *et al.*, 2004). In any case, treatment of EG poisoning involves three primary goals: (1) correction of the patient's metabolic acidosis; (2) inhibition of EG metabolism to its toxic metabolites; and (3) removal of EG and its toxic metabolites by hemodialysis, if necessary. As Guo and McMartin (2005) demonstrated that the renal cytotoxicity of COM crystals is potentiated by severe acidosis, its correction with bicarbonate should help ameliorate the development of renal toxicity. As with CH_3OH, ethanol and 4-methylpyrazole (fomepizole) are frequently given as antidotes for EG poisoning and can prevent renal injury if given early in the course of intoxication. These ADH inhibitors block EG's metabolic bioactivation, thus minimizing the formation of toxic metabolites and allowing EG to be eliminated unchanged by the kidneys. There is increasing evidence that i.v. fomepizole may be more efficacious than ethanol as an antidote and obviate the need for hemodialysis in most EG-poisoned patients with normal renal function (Moreau *et al.*, 1998; Brent *et al.*, 1999;

Sivilotti *et al.*, 2000; Scalley *et al.*, 2002). Watson (2000) has even stated that the results of fomepizole therapy support the recommendation that ethanol's use should be limited to settings where fomepizole is not available or contraindicated. The same editorial by Watson also supports the use of hemodialysis for renal insufficiency or metabolic acidosis rather than the traditional criterion of serum EG concentrations >50 mg/dL. Interestingly, Corley and McMartin (2005) have refined a previously published PBTK model for EG and its GA metabolite in rats and humans to include hemodialysis, ethanol, and fomepizole as therapeutic interventions. This enabled the model to describe data from several human case reports of EG poisoning and demonstrated that fomepizole, if administered early enough, can indeed be more effective than ethanol or hemodialysis in inhibiting EG metabolism.

From a regulatory standpoint, EPA has established a RfD of 2 mg/kg per day based on kidney toxicity in the chronic rat feeding study by DePass *et al.* (1986) (EPA, 2006b). Palmer and Brent (2005) have recently derived a toxicity value of 43.7 mg/kg per day based on a NOAEL for acute renal toxicity in humans using international programme for chemical safety guidelines. Although considerably higher than EPA's RfD, it is comparable to the benchmark dose 0.5 ($BMD_{0.5}$) for EG-induced nephrotoxicity of 49 mg/kg per day derived by Health Canada (2000).

Diethylene Glycol

DEG is similar in physicochemical properties to EG, but has a higher boiling point, viscosity, and specific gravity. It serves as a chemical intermediate in the production of polyester resins and polyurethanes, and as a solvent for shellacs and printing ink. It is hygroscopic, which leads to applications as a drying agent for natural and industrial gases, a humectant for cork and paper, and an additive in cosmetics.

DEG's use as an excipient in a liquid sulfanilamide preparation resulted in 105 deaths in the United States in 1937. This incident prompted passage of the Food, Drug and Cosmetic Act of 1938 (Wax, 1995). Use of DEG-contaminated propylene glycol (PG) or glycerin in various pharmaceuticals has caused multiple fatalities from renal failure in Nigeria, Bangladesh, India, and Haiti. In the Haitian incident, 109 cases of acute renal failure (with 88 deaths) were identified in children who received a locally manufactured acetaminophen syrup containing DEG-contaminated glycerin (O'Brien *et al.*, 1998). The median lethal dose of DEG was estimated at 1.34 mL/kg. Renal failure was the "hallmark" finding in these cases, but hepatitis, pancreatitis, and severe neurologic manifestations (eg, encephalopathy, optic neuritis with retinal edema, and unilateral facial paralysis) were frequently seen. Alfred *et al.* (2005) have presented seven cases of DEG poisoning characterized by metabolic acidosis, renal failure, and, in three patients, neurotoxicity.

Compared with EG, toxicological data for DEG in animals are quite limited. Consistent with observations in human poisonings, Fitzhugh and Nelson (1946) reported dose-dependent hepatorenal injury in rats that consumed diets containing DEG. Kraul *et al.* (1991) reported oliguria or polyuria, proteinuria, and other manifestations indicative of renal tubule injury in rats given a single i.p. dose of DEG. Similar to EG, renal tubular necrosis and COM crystal deposition in tubules have been observed following acute exposure of male rats (Hebert *et al.*, 1978). As for reproductive/developmental effects, high-dose gavage and dietary studies during gestation in mice, rats, and rabbits have largely been negative for embryotoxicity and teratogenicity (Ballantyne and Snellings, 2005). One study in mice employing a continuous breeding protocol has revealed diminished reproductive performance and fertility, as well as limited data

on craniofacial malformations in live-born and dead pups at drinking water exposures equivalent to 6.1 g/kg per day (Williams *et al.*, 1990). Citing this lone positive result and the developmental toxicity profile of EG, Ballantyne and Snellings (2005) gavaged CD-1 mice and CD rats with a range of DEG doses (559-11,180 mg/kg per day) on gestation days six to 15. They reported no embryotoxic or teratogenic effects at any dose in either species, except for delayed ossification consistent with reduced fetal body weight in rats.

Like EG, DEG is well absorbed from the GI tract, distributed throughout total body water and organs on the basis of blood flow, and initially metabolized by ADH and subsequently by ALDH (Heilmair *et al.*, 1993). The ether linkage of DEG is not cleaved and no appreciable amounts of EG or EG metabolites are formed from DEG, although small amounts of OA have occasionally been reported (Hebert *et al.*, 1978; Winek *et al.*, 1978). Based on studies in rats and dogs, unchanged DEG recovered in urine constitutes the majority of oral doses, with a single urinary metabolite, (2-hydroxyethoxy)acetic acid, accounting for most of the remainder (Lenk *et al.*, 1989; Wiener and Richardson, 1989; Mathews *et al.*, 1991). Differences in the toxicity/potency of DEG and EG can thus be explained by differences in their TK profiles. DEG's nephrotoxic moiety(ies) has(have) not been positively identified. As with EG, ADH inhibitors can be effective antidotes for DEG, as demonstrated by the use of fomepizole and hemodialysis to successfully treat a 17-month-old girl who ingested DEG (Brophy *et al.*, 2000).

Propylene Glycol

PG is used as an intermediate in the synthesis of polyester fibers and resins, as a component of automotive antifreeze/coolants, and as a deicing fluid for aircraft. As PG is "generally recognized as safe" by the FDA, it is a constituent of many cosmetics, processed foods, and tobacco products, and serves as a diluent for oral, dermal, and i.v. drug preparations (ATSDR, 1997b). The most important routes of exposure in the general population are ingestion and dermal contact with products containing the compound. The use and disposal of deicing solutions is the major means by which PG is released to the environment. PG has a high mobility in soil and the potential to leach into groundwater, but is neither persistent nor bioaccumulative. Its soil and water half-lives are a few days under aerobic or anaerobic conditions. Workers in industries involved in manufacturing or use of products containing PG may be exposed to concentrations higher than the general population, particularly when these materials are heated or sprayed.

PG has a very low order of acute and chronic toxicity (ATSDR, 1997b; LaKind *et al.*, 1999). No organ system has been identified as a target for acute or chronic injury by PG, and there have been no accounts of human fatalities. Glover and Reed (1996) reported a typical clinical case in which a two-year-old child experienced CNS depression and anion gap acidosis after ingesting a hair gel containing PG. Clinical studies and case reports speak of individuals with reactions to PG-containing drug preparations where preexisting conditions exist. For example, a patient with renal insufficiency secondary to chronic cocaine use developed metabolic acidosis after receiving lorazepam for sedation in which PG was a component of the i.v. formulation (Cawley, 2001). Wilson *et al.* (2000) reported a case of nearly fatal PG toxicity after i.v. diazepam in high doses for alcohol withdrawal. These same authors report on a case series detailing the risk of PG toxicity from i.v. benzodiazepine therapy (Wilson *et al.*, 2005).

Toxicity studies of PG in laboratory animals can be found in the literature, but findings of adverse effects are rare. Christopher *et al.* (1990) noted increases in anion gap acidosis, CNS depression, and ataxia in cats ingesting high doses of PG, consistent with progressively elevated plasma lactate levels. PG has not been shown to be mutagenic and was negative for carcinogenicity in a chronic feeding study of male and female rats (Gaunt *et al.*, 1972). As for PG's reproductive/developmental toxicity, the NTP Center for the Evaluation of Risks to Human Reproduction released a monograph on the subject largely based on an expert panel report (NTP, 2004e,g). The overall conclusion was that there is negligible concern for adverse developmental/reproductive toxicity from PG exposures in humans, because animal studies have shown no such effect even at the highest doses tested.

PG's TK profile explains its relative lack of toxicity. As with other glycols, PG is readily absorbed from the GI tract and distributed throughout total body water and to organs on the basis of blood flow. Approximately 55% of PG is metabolized by ADH to lactaldehyde, while a significant percentage (~45%) is excreted unchanged by the kidneys (Morshed *et al.*, 1988). PG has a mean serum half-life in humans of two to four hours. Whereas excessive lactic acid from lactaldehyde metabolism is primarily responsible for metabolic acidosis observed in extreme exposures, lactate is a good substrate for gluconeogenesis, an efficient detoxification mechanism (NTP, 2004e,g). This detoxification mechanism typically does not allow lactic acid to accumulate to toxic levels, even under saturable metabolic conditions. The rate-limiting step in PG metabolism is its conversion to lactaldehyde. Saturation of this metabolic step in humans occurs at doses eight- to 10-fold lower than observed in laboratory animals. This is protective, because PG has a lower general toxicity than its metabolites (NTP, 2004e,g). As for EG and DEG, ADH inhibitors may competitively inhibit PG metabolism and thus be beneficial in the PG-poisoned patient. This is exemplified by a case of coingestion of ethanol and PG-containing antifreeze by a 61-year-old man absent of significant acid–base disturbance and minimal lactate elevation (Brooks and Wallace, 2002).

Two structural analogues of PG also have low hazard profiles. Both dipropylene glycol (DPG) and tripropylene glycol (TPG) are widely used in personal care products such as perfumes, facial makeup, stick deodorants, and shaving and skin-care preparations. Their low hazard profiles are predictable, given that DPG is rapidly converted to PG, and TPG is rapidly hydrolyzed to DPG, which is further hydrolyzed to PG. The toxicity of these compounds has been summarized (UNEP, 1994, 2001). A negative DPG cancer bioassay was conducted in F344 rats and B6C3F1 mice receiving the chemical via drinking water (Hooth *et al.*, 2004; NTP, 2004c).

GLYCOL ETHERS

If one alcohol residue of EG ($HO–CH_2–CH_2–OH$) is replaced by an ether, the resulting compound is a monoalkyl glycol ether such as EG monomethyl ether, also called 2-methoxyethanol (2-ME; $CH_3–O–CH_2–CH_2–OH$). If both alcohols are replaced by ethers, the result is a dialkyl glycol ether such as EG dimethyl ether ($CH_3–O–CH_2–CH_2–O–CH_3$). The alkyl group at the end of the ether linkage may be a straight or branched short-chain moiety (eg, methyl, ethyl, *n*-propyl, isopropyl, or butyl). The butyl moiety results in one of the most widely used glycol ethers, 2-butoxyethanol (2-BE) ($CH_3–CH_2–CH_2–CH_2–O–CH_2–CH_2–OH$). Acetates of monoalkyl ethers such as 2-methoxyethanol (2-ME) acetate ($CH_3–CO–O–CH_2–CH_2–O–CH_3$) are also common solvents that undergo rapid ester hydrolysis to their parent glycol ethers in vivo, and thus tend to exhibit the same toxicity profiles as unesterified glycols. Glycol ethers exhibit properties of both alcohols and ethers and are thus soluble in water and most organic solvents. This dual solubility and a favorable evaporation rate make glycol ethers very popular solvents for surface coatings such as varnishes and latex paints. Glycol ethers also find use as solvents in paint thinners and strippers, inks, metal cleaning products, liquid soaps, and household cleaners, and are used as jet fuel anti-icing additives and in semiconductor fabrication. Human exposure occurs mainly via inhalation, but also by dermal absorption.

Although glycol ether metabolism varies with chemical structure, some generalizations are possible (Fig. 24-12). For EG monoalkyl ethers, the major metabolic pathway is oxidation via

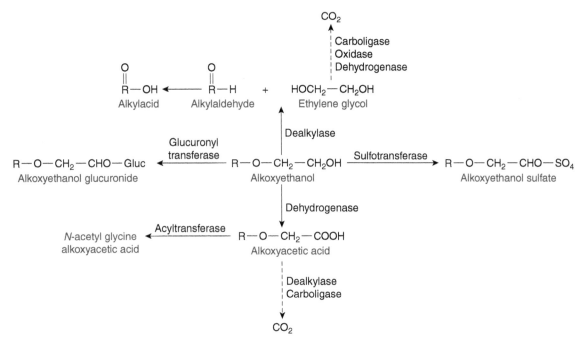

Figure 24-12. *Metabolism of glycol ethers.* R denotes alkyl group of $–CH_3$, $–CH_2–CH_3$, or $–CH_2–CH_2–CH_2–CH_3$ for methoxyethanol, ethoxyethanol, or butoxyethanol, respectively. The formation of alkoxy glucuronide or sulfate conjugates has been identified only for butoxyethanol. (Reproduced from Medinsky *et al.*, 1990, with permission from Elsevier.)

ADH and ALDH to alkoxyacetic acids. For example, 2-ME and 2-BE are metabolized to methoxyacetic acid (MAA; CH_3–CO–O–CH_2–O–CH_3) and BAA (CH_3–CO–O–CH_2–O–CH_2–CH_2–CH_2–CH_3), respectively. The competing O-dealkylase pathway results in the cleavage of the ether linkage to form EG and an alkyl aldehyde. Medinsky *et al.* (1990) reported that the relative contribution of the oxidative pathway to metabolism of EG ethers increases with increasing alkyl chain length, whereas that of the O-dealkylase pathway decreases. In contrast, the propylene series of glycol ethers (eg, propylene glycol monomethyl ether [PGME]) is predominantly biotransformed to PG via O-dealkylation. Glycol ethers may also be conjugated with glucuronide or sulfate, but this is thought to occur mainly after saturation of other metabolic pathways.

In vitro and in vivo toxicity studies demonstrate that some glycol ethers and their oxidative metabolites are reproductive, developmental, hematologic, and immunologic toxicants by all exposure routes. A few have also tested positive in rodent cancer bioassays. The metabolism of glycol ethers is considered a prerequisite to their toxicity, as the alkoxyacetic acids are usually regarded as the ultimate toxicants. Their acetaldehyde precursors have also been implicated on occasion. A critical role for metabolism is supported by the differential toxicities of glycol ethers metabolized via the oxidative and O-dealkylase pathways (Miller *et al.*, 1984; Ghanayem *et al.*, 1987). This differential toxicity has resulted in a dramatic shift away from the production and use of certain low-molecular-weight EG ethers and their acetate esters (eg, 2-ME and 2-ethylene glycol monoethyl ether or 2-EE) toward those with more favorable toxicity profiles such as EG, DEG, and triethylene glycol butyl ethers and those in the low-molecular-weight propylene series such as PGME (de Ketttenis, 2005; Spencer, 2005). Like several glycol ethers of the ethylene series, PBTK models have been developed for PGME and its acetate in rats and humans and exercised for risk assessment, including derivation of a RfC and a RfD (Corley *et al.*, 2005b; Kirman *et al.*, 2005; Lemazurier *et al.*, 2005). Structure–activity relationships have been discerned in studies of glycol ethers with various chemical substitution patterns (Hardin *et al.*, 1984; Rawlings *et al.*, 1985; Hardin and Eisenmann, 1987; Ghanayem *et al.*, 1989). The reproductive and developmental toxicities of the monoalkyl glycol ethers, for example, tend to decrease with increasing alkyl chain length, whereas hematotoxicity increases. Thus, structure–activity relationships may not be universally applicable across multiple toxicological end points.

Reproductive Toxicity

Epidemiological studies have reported associations between glycol ether exposure and increased risk for spontaneous abortion, menstrual disturbances, and subfertility among women employed in the semiconductor industry (Schenker *et al.*, 1995; Correa *et al.*, 1996; Chen *et al.*, 2002; Hsieh *et al.*, 2005). These associations appear biologically plausible, given the reproductive toxicity of 2-ME and its active metabolite, MAA, is manifested as ovarian luteal cell hypertrophy and increased progesterone production in the female rat. Furthermore, MAA increased progesterone production in cultured human luteal cells at the same concentration it did in rat luteal cells, implying that it has the potential to alter ovarian luteal function in women (Almekinder *et al.*, 1997; Davis *et al.*, 1997). Reproductive effects, primarily reversible spermatotoxicity, have also been described for men exposed to glycol ethers, in some cases at concentrations well below current OSHA PELs for 2-ME (25 ppm) and 2-EE (200 ppm). For instance, Welch *et al.* (1988) found that painters exhibited oligospermia and azoospermia following average exposure to 2-EE and 2-ME at 2.7 and 0.8 ppm,

respectively. In addition, men exposed to a mean level of 6.6-ppm 2-EE in a foundry had decreased numbers of sperm per ejaculate (Ratcliffe *et al.*, 1989). Lastly, a large case–control study of male fertility clinic patients revealed a highly significant association between a diagnosis of impaired fertility and the detection of ethoxyacetic acid in urine (Veulemans *et al.*, 1993).

Testicular effects in men are supported by experimental observations in animals including seminiferous tubule atrophy, abnormal sperm head morphology, necrotic spermatocytes, decreased sperm motility and count, and infertility (Lamb *et al.*, 1984; Foote *et al.*, 1995; Watanabe *et al.*, 2000). Spermatocytes are among the first cells to be visibly affected following glycol ether exposure and their death involves apoptosis (Chapin *et al.*, 1984; Brinkworth *et al.*, 1995; Ku *et al.*, 1995). Creasy and Foster (1984) noted a consistent order of spermatocyte susceptibility following oral administration of 2-ME or 2-EE to rats: dividing spermatocytes > early pachytene spermatocytes > late pachytene spermatocytes > mid-pachytene spermatocytes. Spermatocytes in the leptotene/zygotene stages of cell division, late-stage spermatids, and spermatogonia can be affected if the dose is increased and exposure prolonged.

As for mechanism of action, studies suggest several possibilities. Beattie *et al.* (1984) reported that rates of lactate accumulation in cultured rat Sertoli cells were significantly decreased by MAA. Lactate is the preferred metabolic substrate of spermatocytes. Also, 2-EE has been shown to increase oxygen consumption and decrease ATP levels in pachytene spermatocytes in a manner consistent with an uncoupled oxidative state (Oudiz and Zenick, 1986). Mebus *et al.* (1989) have, in addition, demonstrated that serine, acetate, sarcosine, and glycine attenuated the spermatotoxicity of 2-ME in the rat, suggesting MAA may interfere with the availability of one-carbon units for incorporation into purine and pyrimidine bases necessary for nucleic acid synthesis in pachytene spermatocytes. A mechanistic role for Ca^{2+} has been hypothesized and investigated in a series of studies by Chapin and colleagues. Ghanayem and Chapin (1990) observed that a Ca^{2+} channel blocker afforded protection against 2-ME-induced pachytene spermatocyte cell death. These authors reasoned that 2-ME perturbed Ca^{2+} homeostasis, which is consistent with observations of spermatocyte mitochondrial disruption. Involvement of Ca^{2+} was further suggested by observations that 2-ME activates a Ca^{2+}-dependent nuclease, cyclophilin A, found in pachytene spermatocytes and associated with spermatocyte apoptosis (Wine *et al.*, 1997). Whereas an increase in intracellular Ca^{2+} is thought to trigger endonuclease activation, the protection afforded by Ca^{2+} channel blockers against MAA-induced spermatocyte apoptosis is apparently not mediated by preventing a rise in intracellular free Ca^{2+} (Li *et al.*, 1997). Rather, because an intact relationship between Sertoli and germ cells is necessary for the morphological expression of MAA-induced spermatocyte apoptosis, it was reasoned that spermatocyte apoptosis is mediated by Sertoli cell–generated factor(s). This hypothesis proposes that transfer of this factor(s) from Sertoli cells into germ cells (or initiation of spermatocyte apoptosis by 2-ME-damaged Sertoli cells through direct Sertoli cell to germ cell communication) can be inhibited by Ca^{2+} channel blockers through their membrane-stabilizing effects and/or interaction with protein kinase C and/or calmodulin, both of which have demonstrated roles in apoptosis. The inhibition of protein kinase C and calmodulin has been shown to block MAA-induced spermatocyte cell death (Li *et al.*, 1997).

Jindo *et al.* (2001) advanced the research of their predecessors by using cultured seminiferous tubules of juvenile rats to demonstrate that MAA-induced spermatocyte apoptosis could be blocked with protein kinase inhibitors. Several kinases (eg, Src) increased immediately *around* dying spermatocytes in the immediate proximity of Sertoli cells. An increase was also noted in the phosphorylation of the endoplasmic reticulum chaperone glucose-regulated protein 94, known also as endoplasmin, which was located *inside* dying spermatocytes. This work implicates a role for kinase activity in the pathogenesis of MAA-induced spermatocyte apoptosis and suggests the involvement of Sertoli cells. Yet another investigation examined the role of tyrosine kinase pp60 (rat testicular Src), a tyrosine kinase encoded by the Src gene and involved in an array of cell signaling pathways, for its involvement in 2-ME-induced spermatocyte apoptosis. Sertoli cell cytoplasm was observed to be the principal site of Src immunoreactivity in control testis, while 2-ME treatment significantly induced Src expression in dying spermatocytes. In addition, MAA-induced apoptosis was blocked using Src inhibitors, further supporting a role for rat testicular Src in Sertoli–germ cell communication and spermatocyte toxicity of 2-ME (Wang *et al.*, 2000). Furthermore, a suppression subtractive hybridization technique using whole testes from 2-ME-treated mice was employed to create mouse testis cDNA libraries enriched for gene populations either upregulated or downregulated by 2-ME (Wang and Chapin, 2000). A total of 70 clones was screened, and 6 of them were shown to be differentially expressed in the 2-ME lesion, three with increased expression, and three were suppressed. Interestingly, predicted peptide sequences of the six genes revealed several conserved motifs such as phosphorylation sites for protein kinase C and tyrosine kinase. Importantly, these gene changes were apparent at multiple germ cell stages and were localized in multiple germ cell types (Sertoli, interstitial, and peritubular cells). This further suggests the involvement of cell types other than the dying spermatocyte in the pathogenesis of 2-ME-induced spermatocyte death and helps explain the requirement for *intact* seminiferous tubules for in vitro replication of the pathology observed in vivo.

Developmental Toxicity

Exposure to certain glycol ethers during organogenesis (eg, 2-ME and 2-EE) is toxic to the developing embryo, with effects seen in several animal models including nonhuman primates (Hardin *et al.*, 1986; Scott *et al.*, 1989). Others such as EG butyl, propyl, and monohexyl ethers, and most PG ethers either have not induced fetal malformations or have a lower potential for developmental toxicity (Tyl *et al.*, 1989; Spencer, 2005). Structural anomalies in rodents have included a variety of minor skeletal variations, hydrocephalus, exencephaly, cardiovascular malformations, dilatation of the renal pelvis, craniofacial anomalies, and digit malformations. In the absence of structural defects, electrocardiograms of fetal rats from dams treated with 2-ME during gestation showed persistent, aberrant QRS waves, suggestive of an intraventricular conduction delay (Toraason and Breitenstein, 1988). Neurobehavioral changes and regional brain alterations of several neurotransmitters in offspring of rats treated with 2-ME or 2-EE have been reported (Nelson and Brightwell, 1984).

Little is known about the mechanism by which glycol ethers exert their developmental effects. 2-ME has served as a model toxicant to investigate the disposition of weak acids in the maternal–fetal unit and the hypothesis that weak acids such as MAA exert their effects by altering embryonic pH at critical stages of organogenesis (Nelson *et al.*, 1989; Clarke *et al.*, 1992; O'Flaherty *et al.*, 1995; Terry *et al.*, 1995). Ambroso *et al.* (1998) have applied confocal laser scanning microscopy, classical histopathology, and in situ immunohistochemistry to demonstrate that 2-ME caused a dose-dependent increase and expansion of apoptosis in gestation day eight mouse embryos that could underlie 2-ME-induced neural tube defects. Such a mechanism has also been hypothesized for malformations induced by several prototypical teratogens such as retinoic acid and ethanol.

Few epidemiological studies have addressed developmental effects of glycol ethers. Saavedra *et al.* (1997) described facial malformations and varying degrees of mental retardation in 44 offspring of mothers who were exposed occupationally to 2-ME and EG at a factory producing capacitors in Mexico. There are a few reports published from a multicenter case–control study in Europe designed to investigate the role of maternal exposures at work and congenital malformations (Ha *et al.*, 1996; Cordier *et al.*, 1997; Lorente *et al.*, 2000). Preliminary results (Ha *et al.*, 1996) of evaluation of offspring of mothers who were exposed to glycol ethers at work during pregnancy found excesses of oral clefts (OR = 2.0; 95% CI = 1.1–4.1) and CNS malformations (OR = 1.8; 95% CI = 1.1–3.3). In a study of 984 cases of major congenital malformations, Cordier *et al.* (1997) reported an overall OR of congenital malformations associated with glycol ether exposure of 1.44 (95% CI = 1.10–1.90), with significant associations for glycol ether exposure with cleft lip, multiple anomalies, and neural tube defects. Lorente *et al.* (2000) studied 100 mothers of babies with oral clefts and 751 mothers of healthy babies and reported a nonsignificant OR of 1.7 (95% CI = 0.9–3.3) for maternal occupational exposure to glycol ethers and cleft lip, with or without cleft palate. Maldonado *et al.* (2003) have reviewed the epidemiological evidence and determined that it is insufficient to determine whether occupational exposure to glycol ethers causes human congenital malformations.

Out of concern for the potential of EG monoalkyl ethers as developmental toxicants, several PBTK models have been developed. Hays *et al.* (2000) developed a PBTK model for 2-ME and MAA in the pregnant rat that was capable of predicting embryonic concentrations. Gargas *et al.* (2000a,b) applied a PBTK model to estimate inhaled concentrations of 2-EE, its acetate ester, and 2-ME in humans that would result in blood levels equivalent to those observed at the rat NOAELs and LOAELs for developmental effects. Sweeney *et al.* (2001) applied Monte Carlo simulations to the models of Gargas and coworkers to account for the variability in TK and TD factors among humans and animals and derived occupational exposure limits to protect workers from developmental effects of 2-ME and 2-EE that were one to two orders of magnitude lower than current OSHA PELs. It is worthy of note that 2-ME has been largely removed from commerce due to its teratogenic potency.

Hematotoxicity

Some glycol ethers are hemolytic to red blood cells (RBCs). Typically, the osmotic balance of cells is disrupted, they imbibe water and swell, their ATP concentration decreases, and hemolysis occurs (Ghanayem, 1989). Nyska *et al.* (1999) reported that subchronic exposure to 2-BE causes disseminated thrombosis and bone infarctions in female, but not male rats, likely due to impedance of blood flow by intravascular hemolysis. It is thought that females might be susceptible, because they are less efficient in eliminating BAA, the hemolytic metabolite of 2-BE, and exhibit higher peak blood BAA levels. Young adult rats are more resistant to the hematologic effects of 2-BE than older rats, an observation attributed to depressed degradation and renal clearance of BAA in the older rats.

Species differ dramatically in their sensitivities to glycol ether–induced RBC deformity and hemolysis. Humans are less susceptible than rodents. This lower susceptibility even applies to RBCs from potentially sensitive subpopulations, such as the elderly and persons with hereditary blood disorders (Udden, 1994; Udden and Patton, 1994). A good example of using PBTK models in human risk assessment has been published by Corley et al. (1994). Based on comparisons of model output with data collected by Udden and colleagues on levels of 2-BE required to affect osmotic fragility of human RBCs, Corley and coworkers concluded that humans are unlikely to achieve hemolytic blood levels of BAA unless very large volumes of 2-BE are intentionally ingested. Udden (2005) has recently reported on the hemolytic effects of diethylene glycol butyl ether (DGBE) and its principal metabolite, butoxyethoxyacetic acid (BEAA), using rat and human RBCs in vitro. BEAA had weak hemolytic activity on rat erythrocytes, which is consistent with the finding of mild hemolysis when DGBE is administered to rats by gavage. However, such effects were absent in human RBCs exposed to DGBE or BEAA, indicating that it is unlikely hemolysis will occur in humans exposed to DGBE. Johnson et al. (2005) recently confirmed DGBE's low order of hematotoxicity in a 13-week drinking water study in F344 rats that identified a NOAEL of 250 mg/kg per day, with minimal but statistically significant decreases in RBC count, hemoglobin, and hematocrit at 1000 mg/kg per day.

Hoflack et al. (1997) have shown 2-BE capable of inducing apoptosis in a human leukemia cell line and have hypothesized that the hematopoietic toxicity of 2-BE may be the result of its ability to induce apoptotic cell death. However, once inside the cell it is not entirely clear how hemolysis is accomplished, although the RBC membrane has long been the suspected target. Udden and Patton (2005) have utilized BAA to examine the mechanism of glycol ether hemolysis in rat RBCs in vitro. They concluded that the mode of action of BAA is to cause a colloid osmotic lysis of the RBC and speculated the following scenario: BAA causes Na^+ and Ca^{2+} to enter the cell → Ca^{2+} initially has a protective effect via the Ca^{2+}-activated potassium channel, which facilitates the loss of potassium, thereby compensating for the osmotic effect of increased cell Na^+ → Ca^{2+} subsequently has deleterious effects through activation of proteases and the loss of the normal asymmetric distribution of phospholipids (eg, phosphatidylserine) in the membrane bilayer. These authors noted that preliminary studies in their laboratory have shown the movement of phosphatidylserine from the inner to the outer leaflet of the lipid bilayer of rat RBCs incubated with BAA. This "externalization" of phosphatidylserine is associated with adhesion of RBCs to endothelial cells and the generation of thrombin, which is most interesting given reports of disseminated thrombosis and infarction in 2-BE-treated rats (Nyska et al., 1999; Ghanayem et al., 2001).

Immunotoxicity/Carcinogenicity

Based on changes in thymus and splenic weights/cellularities and a variety of in vitro and in vivo immune function assays, the immune system is a potential target for the oxidative metabolites of some glycol ethers. 2-ME and MAA have been employed almost exclusively in immunotoxicity investigations of glycol ethers. Not only have adult animals proven susceptible, but also 2-ME exposure of pregnant mice induces fetal thymic atrophy/hypocellularity and a reduction in fetal liver prolymphocytes with potential implications for fetal immunity (Holladay et al., 1994). Using B6C3F1 mice and gavage exposure, House et al. (1985) were among the first to report that 2-ME and MAA reduced thymus weight. Kayama et al. (1991) subsequently reported that 2-ME selectively depleted immature thymocytes in mice. Exon et al. (1991) reported not only thymic atrophy in rats exposed to 2-ME in drinking water but also decreased antibody production, decreased splenocyte production of interferon-γ, and a reduction in spleen cellularity. Around the

same time, the first in a lengthy series of studies by Smialowicz and colleagues was published (Smialowicz et al., 1991a,b, 1992, 1994; Williams et al., 1995; Kim and Smialowicz, 1997). This series has reported decreased thymus weights, reduced lymphoproliferative responses to mitogens, and reduced IL-2 production in splenocytes of F344 rats exposed to 2-ME by gavage. It has also generated data indicating that not all glycol ethers are immunosuppressive, that mice are relatively insensitive to glycol ether immunosuppression compared with rats, and that rats of various strains show differential sensitivities. The Smialowicz series has further demonstrated that the relative insensitivity of mice is not a function of their more rapid clearance of MAA; that 2-ME is immunotoxic when applied dermally to F344 rats; and that questions remain as to 2-ME's proximate immunotoxicant, as 2-methoxyacetaldehyde is more immunotoxic than MAA based on the ability to suppress IgM and IgG production by lymphocytes in F344 rats.

As for cancer, only a few chronic bioassays have been conducted with glycol ethers. Two-year inhalation bioassays of 2-BE in F344 rats and B6C3F1 mice revealed some evidence of carcinogenicity in male mice, based on increased incidences of hemangiosarcoma of the liver, as well as some evidence of carcinogenic activity in female mice, based on increased incidences of forestomach squamous cell papilloma or carcinoma (mainly papilloma) (NTP, 2000). In June 2004, an IARC working group evaluated the cancer risk of 2-BE and concluded that it is not likely to be carcinogenic to humans at environmental concentrations at or below the RfD and RfC (Cogliano et al., 2005). Likewise, EPA's IRIS profile for 2-BE currently indicates that the human carcinogenic potential of 2-BE cannot be determined at this time (EPA, 2012). Since NTP's bioassays were completed, numerous studies have shed light on 2-BE's possible modes of action related to liver hemangiosarcomas and forestomach tumors and their implications for risk assessment (Park et al., 2002; Siesky et al., 2002; Poet et al., 2003; Boatman et al., 2004; Klaunig and Kamendulis, 2005; Corthals et al., 2006). As discussed by Gift (2005), these studies suggest the following scenario: 2-BE consumed while grooming is metabolized to irritant metabolites in the forestomach and/or irritant metabolites are formed in the upper respiratory tract and swallowed → chronic irritation → inflammation → hyperplastic effects → forestomach tumors. As for liver hemangiosarcomas, the following is suggested: 2-BE is metabolized to BAA → BAA causes hemolysis of RBCs → hemosiderin (iron) derived from released hemoglobin is taken up by and stored in phagocytic cells (eg, Kupffer cells) of the spleen and liver → oxidative damage and increased synthesis of endothelial DNA are initiated by ROS from excess iron or Kupffer cells, producing cytokines/growth factors that suppress apoptosis and promote cell proliferation → endothelial DNA mutations → potentiation and promotion of hepatic neoplastic cell populations. As further discussed by Gift (2005), the evidence suggests nonlinear modes of action in both cases and questionable human relevance of both tumor types. Several PBTK models have been developed and subsequently refined for 2-BE and BAA to aid in risk assessments (Corley et al., 1994, 2005c; Lee et al., 1998; Franks et al., 2006).

Spencer et al. (2002) have reported a two-year inhalation bioassay of PGME in F344 rats and B6C3F1 mice that did not result in increases in neoplasia in either species except for kidney adenomas in male rats related to α_{2u}-globulin nephropathy. In contrast, a two-year inhalation bioassay with propylene glycol mono-t-butyl ether (PGMBE) in F344 rats and B6C3F1 mice also resulted in α_{2u}-globulin nephropathy in male rats, as well as liver tumors in male and female B6C3F1 mice at the highest concentration tested (1200 ppm) (NTP, 2004a; Doi et al., 2004). Dill et al. (2004) have published information on PGMBE TK in rats and mice that demonstrate saturation of PGMBE metabolism/elimination at this tumor-producing concentration. The genotoxicity of some glycol ethers and their metabolites has been evaluated, with most exhibiting a lack of genotoxic potential and others yielding weakly positive responses in certain tests. Therefore, the role of genetic toxicology in the toxicities discussed above cannot be summarily dismissed, but is of unknown significance (Elliot and Ashby, 1997; NTP, 2000; Ballantyne and Vergnes, 2001).

FUELS AND FUEL ADDITIVES

Automotive Gasoline

Automotive gasoline is a complex mixture of hundreds of hydrocarbons predominantly in the C_4 to C_{12} range. The sheer number of people exposed in the manufacture, distribution, and use of gasoline makes characterization of its acute and chronic toxicities important. Generalizations regarding gasoline toxicity must be made with care, because its composition varies with the crude oil from which it is refined, the refining process, and the use of specific additives. Experiments conducted with fully vaporized gasoline may not be predictive of actual risk, because humans are exposed primarily to the more volatile components in the range of C_4 and C_5. These hydrocarbons are generally regarded as less toxic than their higher-molecular-weight counterparts. Concern about gasoline exposure is fueled in part by the toxicities of certain components, some of which are classified by EPA as known or probable human carcinogens (eg, benzene and 1,3-butadiene). The ACGIH has established a TLV for gasoline of 300 ppm to prevent ocular and upper respiratory tract irritation and a STEL of 500 ppm to avoid acute CNS depression.

Inhalation exposure to gasoline has been measured for service station attendants, self-service customers, truck drivers, distribution workers, and workmen removing leaking underground storage tanks (Kearney and Dunham, 1986; Shamsky and Samimi, 1987). In one survey, short-term exposures of self-service customers averaged about 6 ppm. The TLV is rarely exceeded in occupationally exposed individuals, due in part to the use of vapor scavenging systems. Brief exposures in excess of the STEL have, however, been documented for workers engaged in bulk handling operations (Phillips and Jones, 1978). The most extreme exposures occur to those intentionally sniffing gasoline for its euphoric effects. Several case reports of acute and chronic encephalopathies are testament to the dangers of this habit (Valpey et al., 1978; Fortenberry, 1985). In these cases, the identity of the offending agent(s) is often unclear. Gasoline is one of the most popular and lethal inhalants (Spiller, 2004; Wu et al., 2004), with deaths reported even among Aboriginal people in South Australia (Byard et al., 2003). An all too common occurrence is the ingestion of gasoline during siphoning events. This is typically followed by a burning sensation in the mouth and pharynx, as well as nausea, vomiting, and diarrhea resulting from GI irritation. If aspirated into the lungs, gasoline may produce pulmonary epithelial damage, edema, and pneumonitis. Thus, emetic therapy for gasoline ingestion is usually contraindicated.

Between 1986 and 2004, EPA identified 447,233 releases from underground petroleum storage tanks, many of which threaten groundwater that serves as the primary drinking water source for nearly one half of the US population. Despite the number of releases, few community health studies have been conducted, and those that have are typically driven by concerns over leukemia risk owing to gasoline's benzene content. Consider, for example, the retrospective cohort study of the "Tranguch Gasoline Spill" in

northeastern Pennsylvania (Patel et al., 2004). The standard incidence ratio for leukemia of all types was significantly elevated (4.40; 95% CI = 1.09–10.24), consistent with that reported by the Pennsylvania Department of Health. However, the excess was based on only four cases, two of which had a history of smoking, a potential confounder. In addition, exposure was not well characterized, and only two of the subjects had AML, the leukemia type most strongly associated with benzene. Such a study exemplifies the problem with inferring causation for environmentally exposed populations based on limited data.

Reese and Kimbrough (1993) and Caprino and Togna (1998) have reviewed the acute toxicity of gasoline and its additives. Like some other solvents, gasoline can sensitize the heart to catecholamines, defat the skin on repeated contact, and induce hepatic CYPs and UDP-glucuronyltransferase activities (Poon et al., 1995). The question of whether there is a "fetal gasoline syndrome" has been raised, although case reports are confounded by tetraethyl lead, alcohol abuse, and the possibility that an aberrant gene is distributed within the small Amerindian population where the cases reside (Hunter et al., 1979). There is a paucity of data on the reproductive toxicity of gasoline, but reports of enhanced estrogen metabolism and uterine atrophy among unleaded gasoline (UG)-treated mice suggest that this end point warrants investigation (Standeven et al., 1994a). Although dated, the study of Lykke and Stewart (1978) is of interest, because rats exposed to leaded gasoline at one-third the ACGIH TLV (ie, 100 ppm) for 40 hours per week for six to 12 weeks were observed to have a progressive interstitial fibrosis of the lungs associated with irregular alveolar collapse.

Prior to the identification of α_{2u}-globulin as the principal accumulating protein in the syndrome referred to as α_{2u}-globulin nephropathy, Kuna and Ulrich (1984) reported regenerative epithelium and dilated tubules in the kidneys of male rats exposed to 1552 ppm UG for 90 days. At about the same time, a chronic inhalation study revealed not only nephropathy but also increased renal tumors in male rats (MacFarland et al., 1984). Subsequent studies by Halder et al. (1986) and Aranyi et al. (1986) showed that such nephropathy could not be produced by exposure of rats to a mixture of the butane and pentane components of gasoline or the 0°F to 145°F gasoline distillation fraction. These are thought to be more representative of human occupational exposures than wholly vaporized gasoline. In addition, the authors of a gavage screening study of 15 pure hydrocarbons and gasoline fractions concluded that branched aliphatic alkane components were primarily responsible for the nephropathy (Halder et al., 1985).

Investigations of mechanisms of the nephropathy and renal tumors included an assessment of unscheduled (a measure of genotoxicity) and replicative DNA synthesis (a measure of cell proliferation) in rat kidney cells exposed in vitro and in vivo to UG. No unscheduled DNA synthesis occurred, even at a tumorigenic dose, while a five- to eightfold increase in cell proliferation was observed (Loury et al., 1987). In a publication the same year by Olson et al. (1987), UG was reported to result in an increase in hyaline droplets harboring large accumulations of α_{2u}-globulin within proximal convoluted tubule epithelial cells. It was hypothesized that α_{2u}-globulin accumulated secondary to a defect in renal lysosomal degradation of the protein (Fig. 24-6). Supportive evidence for this hypothesis came from the demonstration that inhibition of the lysosomal peptidase, cathepsin B, caused a rapid accumulation of phagolysosomes and α_{2u}-globulin in the kidney similar to that of UG (Olson et al., 1988).

Further progress in elucidating the mechanism of α_{2u}-globulin nephropathy came from the demonstration that the UG component, 2,2,4-trimethylpentane (TMP), itself an inducer of α_{2u}-globulin nephropathy, was metabolized to 2,4,4-trimethyl-2-pentanol (TMPOH), which was selectively retained by the kidney of male rats. Subsequently, it was demonstrated that the sex-specific retention of TMPOH in the kidney was due to reversible binding with α_{2u}-globulin. This binding rendered the protein less digestible by lysosomal enzymes, which accounted for its accumulation (Charbonneau and Swenberg, 1988). This accumulation, in turn, led to cellular degeneration and necrosis, primarily in the P_2 segment of the proximal tubule. In response, regenerative proliferation occurs and promotes formation of renal cell tumors by irreversibly "fixing" spontaneously altered DNA and clonally expanding initiated cells. The promotional effects of gasoline and TMP on atypical cell foci and renal cell tumors have been demonstrated in male rats following initiation with N-ethyl-N-hydroxyethylnitrosamine (Short et al., 1989). NCI–Black–Reiter male rats, the only rat strain not to synthesize α_{2u}-globulin, are resistant to gasoline- and TMP-induced nephropathy (Dietrich and Swenberg, 1991). Thus, gasoline and TMP have been of great value in elucidating the mechanism of α_{2u}-globulin nephropathy and shedding light on its implications for renal tumorigenesis. Most toxicologists, and indeed the EPA, have concluded that renal tumors secondary to α_{2u}-globulin nephropathy are of little relevance, because humans do not synthesize α_{2u}-globulin.

Chronic inhalation of gasoline at high concentrations has also resulted in increased hepatocellular adenomas and carcinomas in female B6C3F1 mice, possibly due to the promotion of spontaneously initiated cells that occur with unusually high frequency in this mouse strain (MacFarland et al., 1984). This possibility is supported by reports that UG is a CYP inducer, mitogen, and liver tumor promoter in N-nitrosodiethylamine (DEN)-initiated female B6C3F1 mice (Standeven and Goldsworthy, 1993; Standeven et al., 1995; Moser et al., 1996a). CYP induction by UG has been attributed to "heavy UG" (components with boiling points >100°C), whereas mitogenic activity is highly concentrated in UG components boiling from 100°C to 132°C, for which the 2,2,3-, 2,2,4-, and 2,3,4-trimethylpentane isomers appear at least partially responsible (Standeven and Goldsworthy, 1994). It has been hypothesized that the liver tumor-promoting activity of UG is secondary to its estrogen antagonism, given that (1) UG is not a hepatocarcinogen in male mice; (2) estrogen inhibits liver tumor development initiated in mice but potentiates liver tumor promotion by UG; and (3) UG induces hepatic estrogen metabolism (Standeven et al., 1994b). The hypothesis that liver tumor promotion by UG depends on its interaction with estrogen is supported by the demonstration that tumor-promoting activity of UG was greatly attenuated in ovariectomized mice relative to intact mice (Moser et al., 1997). Further, the addition of estrogen to DEN-treated mice substantially reduces the percentage of hepatic foci with decreased levels of TGF-β1 compared with DEN-treated control mice or DEN + UG-treated mice, suggesting a promotional mechanism involving estrogen and the dysregulation of tumor growth factor(s) (Moser et al., 1996c). Whereas much attention has been given to its promotional potential, UG may also damage DNA, as it reportedly induces unscheduled DNA synthesis in hepatocytes from male and female mice treated in vivo and in cultured mouse, rat, and human hepatocytes (IARC, 1989b). The epidemiological evidence for an association between gasoline exposure and cancer in humans is inconclusive. Raabe (1993) has reviewed the carcinogenic potential of gasoline. IARC (1989b) classifies it as possibly carcinogenic to humans (Group 2B) primarily due to its benzene content. A comprehensive review of gasoline toxicity is provided in ATSDR's (1995) Toxicological Profile for Gasoline.

Vehicle emissions from gasoline combustion are a major contributor to urban air pollution, which is at unhealthy levels in numerous cities. In response, the Clean Air Act Amendments of 1990 require the use of oxygenated gasoline in such areas. Oxygenated gasoline contains additives that add oxygen to gasoline, thereby boosting its octane quality, enhancing combustion, and reducing exhaust emissions. MTBE and ethanol are the two most common oxygenates, although use of the former is being rapidly phased out due to widespread groundwater contamination and health concerns. As a result, the demand for ethanol–gasoline blends is increasing dramatically, raising concerns about how the two components might interact toxicologically. There is a dearth of information on this issue, but a four-week inhalation study of an ethanol–gasoline mixture (6130-ppm ethanol and 500-ppm gasoline) in rats concluded that coexposure showed additive and possibly some synergistic effects on growth, neurochemistry, and histopathology of the adrenal gland and respiratory tract. Effects were described as generally mild and adaptive in nature, and returned to normal after exposure cessation (Chu et al., 2005). The risks and benefits of ethanol as an oxygenate are discussed in detail by Williams et al. (2003), who point out several reasons why ethanol in gasoline can increase groundwater plume lengths and persistence of gasoline constituents in groundwater if ethanol blends are released into the environment. The most obvious concern is that longer or more persistent gasoline plumes could lead to a higher probability of gasoline constituents affecting public water wells. Meanwhile, another fuel additive, methylcyclopentadienyl manganese tricarbonyl (MMT), is receiving attention due to concerns that it could increase manganese inhalation exposures and pose a risk for neurotoxicity. The combustion of MMT gasoline results in the emission of fine Mn particulates mainly as Mn sulfate and Mn phosphate and smaller amounts of oxides. Several studies characterizing vehicular exhaust using MMT gasoline and describing the TK and neurobehavioral toxicity of Mn have been recently published, some of which were mandated by EPA (Normandin et al., 2004; Dorman et al., 2009; Reaney et al., 2006; Tapin et al., 2006). Gasoline engine exhaust has been classified as possibly carcinogenic to humans (Group 2B), based largely on sufficient evidence in animals when condensates and exhaust extracts are tested (IARC, 1989a).

Methyl *tertiary*-Butyl Ether

MTBE's high octane rating made it a logical replacement for tetraethyl lead as an octane booster for gasoline, and later as a gasoline oxygenator. As an oxygenator, MTBE makes fuel combustion more complete, thereby reducing pollutant emissions from automobile exhaust. MTBE may be added to gasoline at levels up to 15% by volume in order to comply with the 1990 Amendments to the Clean Air Act. By 1997, it was being used at the rate of 10 million gal per day, with more than one-third of the usage in California (Williams et al., 2000a). While routine, low-level exposure of customers occurs at self-service stations, heightened concern about MTBE has resulted primarily from its contamination of groundwater by leaking underground gasoline tanks. It is highly water soluble, travels faster and farther in water than other gasoline components, and is resistant to degradation.

MTBE is well absorbed following oral, inhalation, and dermal exposure of humans and rats (Dekant et al., 2001; Prah et al., 2004; McGregor, 2006). The majority of absorbed MTBE is exhaled unchanged. Some MTBE is oxidized to *tert*-butyl alcohol (TBA) and HCOH. Whereas this oxidation is primarily CYP2A6-mediated in humans (Hong et al., 1999), it is largely CYP2B1-mediated in rats (Turini et al., 1998). TBA is relatively water soluble, so it tends to remain in the blood and extracellular fluid, and is slowly exhaled. It is further metabolized, first to 2-methyl-1,2-propanediol and then to 2-hydroxyisobutyrate, the major urinary metabolites of MTBE. In addition, glucuronide and sulfate conjugates of TBA are found in trace amounts in urine. Although HCOH is one of the oxidative metabolites of MTBE, it is undetectable after MTBE exposure in humans and rats, presumably due to its rapid metabolism. PBTK models have been developed to describe the dosimetry of MTBE and TBA following inhalation and oral exposures in rats and humans (Borghoff *et al.*, 1996b; Licata *et al.*, 2001).

Concern about MTBE has led to numerous toxicity studies in humans and rodents, and a number of reviews of MTBE's toxicity are available (ATSDR, 1996b; EPA, 1997; Borak *et al.*, 1998; McGregor, 2006; WHO, 1998). The review of Borak *et al.* (1998) focuses on the acute human health effects of MTBE. It concludes, based on 19 reports of inhalation exposure to MTBE alone or in gasoline and 12 reports of parenteral MTBE administration to dissolve cholesterol gallstones, that no significant association exists between MTBE exposure and the acute symptoms commonly attributed to it. These symptoms include headache, eye, nose and throat irritation, cough, nausea, dizziness, and disorientation. The more recent review of McGregor (2006) is supportive of this conclusion.

In 1988, the EPA and industry developed a Testing Consent Order for MTBE under the Toxic Substances Control Act that precipitated investigations of MTBE's potential two-generation reproductive toxicity, developmental toxicity, in vivo mutagenicity, subchronic inhalation toxicity, oncogenicity, and neurotoxicity. Results of these studies are a major addition to the toxicity literature on MTBE and define several NOAELs (Bevan *et al.*, 1997a,b; Bird *et al.*, 1997; Daughtrey *et al.*, 1997; Lington *et al.*, 1997; McKee *et al.*, 1997). The publication of Bird and colleagues is actually a recapitulation of reports by Chun *et al.* (1992) and Burleigh-Flayer *et al.* (1992), both of which are of particular value, as they represent two of only three MTBE cancer bioassays. In the study by Chun *et al.*, male and female F344 rats were exposed to 0, 400, 3000, or 8000 ppm MTBE vapor six hours per day, five days per week for 24 months. In the other inhalation study, Burleigh-Flayer *et al.* (1992) subjected male and female CD-1 mice to the same exposure regimen for 18 months. The only oral chronic bioassay is that by Belpoggi *et al.* (1995, 1997), who subjected male and female S-D rats by olive oil gavage to 0, 250, or 1000 mg/kg MTBE four days per week for two years. The results of the three MTBE animal cancer bioassays are presented in Table 24-4. In addition, Cirvello *et al.* (1995) and NTP (1995) have reported some evidence for the carcinogenicity of TBA in the kidney and thyroid after long-term drinking water exposure.

Taken at face value, one might interpret these cancer bioassay findings as ample evidence of carcinogenicity in animals and suggestive of a cancer risk for humans. The relevance of these findings to humans, however, has been a source of debate among toxicologists. Critics have questioned these studies on the basis of (1) the appropriateness of a combined incidence category for leukemias and lymphomas; (2) the possibility that renal tumors were secondary to male rat-specific α_{2u}-globulin nephropathy; (3) the possibility that Leydig cell tumors were a function of abnormally low testicular tumor rates in control animals or increased survival time of treated rats; (4) the questionable relevance of testicular tumors in rats to humans, given the species' differential responses of Leydig cells to proliferative stimuli; (5) the possibility that liver and kidney tumors are the result of high-dose-induced chronic cytotoxicity, cell death, and reparative cell proliferation; (6) the questionable relevance of inhalation bioassays to prediction of drinking water risks; and (7) the use of an oil rather than a water-dosing vehicle, which could unduly influence MTBE's oral TK. Mennear (1997) and McGregor (2006) have discussed a number of these issues.

As an outgrowth of the uncertainties surrounding MTBE's human carcinogenicity risk, several mechanistic studies have been published. For example, after only 10 days of MTBE inhalation exposure, a strong positive linear relationship between renal α_{2u}-globulin concentration and cell proliferation was seen in the male F344 rat (Prescott-Matthews *et al.*, 1997). This study, unlike the chronic bioassay of Chun *et al.* (1992), definitively identified the accumulating protein as α_{2u}-globulin. Williams and Borghoff (2001) have shown that TBA interacts with α_{2u}-globulin, which explains its accumulation in the male rat kidney following MTBE or TBA exposure. MTBE has been shown to be a hepatic mitogen in the female mouse, but not a promoter of tumor formation in DEN-initiated female mouse liver (Moser *et al.*, 1996b). It has been suggested in light of these findings that MTBE may promote the growth of spontaneously initiated cell populations having genetic lesions different from those produced by DEN. Casanova and Heck (1997) have reported a lack of concentration, species, and sex dependence in the formation of HCOH-induced DPX and RNA–HCOH adducts in isolated female CD-1 mouse hepatocytes incubated with MTBE. As the cancer bioassay data suggest that hepatocarcinogenicity varies with all of these factors, these results do not support a role for HCOH in MTBE-induced liver tumor formation. Studies also indicate that MTBE causes endocrine dysregulation in rodents at high doses, suggesting the possibility that MTBE-induced tumor formation is hormonally mediated (Moser *et al.*, 1998; Williams *et al.*, 2000b). Changes in triiodothyronine, luteinizing hormone, testosterone, and estradiol levels have been discussed as possible mechanisms of MTBE-induced Leydig cell cancer (Williams and Borghoff, 2000; Williams *et al.*, 2000b; de Peyster *et al.*, 2003). Although it is generally accepted that MTBE induces certain tumors in animals through nongenotoxic mechanisms, experiments indicate that MTBE is mutagenic in a few in vitro test systems (Williams-Hill *et al.*, 1999; Zhou *et al.*, 2000).

Several mechanistic issues surrounding MTBE's toxicity, particularly its carcinogenicity, have yet to be resolved. Nonetheless, citing widespread groundwater contamination and health concerns, numerous states have instituted phased-in partial or complete bans of MTBE. This is in keeping with the opinion of EPA's *Blue Ribbon Panel on Oxygenates in Gasoline* that, in 1999, agreed that with

Table 24-4

Summary Results of MTBE Cancer Bioassays

AUTHORS	ANIMAL STRAIN/SPECIES	EXPOSURE ROUTE	POSITIVE RESULTS
Chun *et al.* (1992)	Fischer 344 rats	Inhalation	Kidney and testicular tumors (males)
Burleigh-Flayer *et al.* (1992)	CD-1 mice	Inhalation	Liver adenomas (females)
Belpoggi *et al.* (1995)	Sprague–Dawley rats	Oral	Testicular tumors (males) Leukemia + lymphoma (females)

the use of MTBE and other gasoline additives threats to drinking water supplies should be substantially reduced. To date, independent expert review groups who have assessed MTBE inhalation health risks (eg, "Interagency Assessment of Oxygenated Fuels") have not concluded that the use of MTBE-oxygenated gasoline poses an imminent threat to public health. EPA's Office of Water has concluded that available data are not adequate to estimate potential health risks of MTBE at low exposure levels in drinking water, but that the data support the conclusion that MTBE is a potential human carcinogen at high doses. Fortunately, water containing MTBE has an unpleasant taste and odor, which may alert consumers to the fact that their water is contaminated. Based on the results of studies of taste and odor thresholds for humans, an advisory guidance range of 20 to 40 µg/L has been set by the EPA to assure consumer acceptance and provide a large margin of safety from toxicity and carcinogenicity. California has both derived a cancer potency estimate and adopted a Public Health Goal of 13 ppb for MTBE in drinking water. While many advocate the suspension of MTBE's use in reformulated gasoline, such a decision should weigh the benefits against the risks associated with increased auto emissions of carcinogenic VOCs and the public health impact of increased CO_2 emissions and ozone formation. Two articles that discuss this subject in considerable detail are by Spitzer (1997) and Erdal et al. (1997).

Jet Fuel

Jet A, jet propellant-8 (JP-8), and JP-8+100 are the predominant jet fuels in use today. All are kerosene-like mixtures of hundreds of aliphatic and aromatic hydrocarbons. Jet A is commercial aviation fuel, whereas JP-8 and JP-8+100 are military fuels. JP-8 is a mixture of Jet A plus three additives, whereas JP-8+100 contains JP-8 and an additional additive package. JP-8 is now the recognized battlefield fuel for all NATO forces and is used not only for aircraft but also for ground vehicles and other equipment such as generators, cooking stoves, and tent heaters (NAS, 2003). Owing to slight differences in hydrocarbon composition and additives, JP-8 differs from its predecessor fuels (eg, JP-4 and JP-5) in ways that impart added safety, enhance combat aircraft survivability, simplify battlefield logistics, and promote standardization with commercial jet fuel.

Civilian and military personnel are exposed to jet fuel by inhalation and dermal contact. Exposure can occur to liquid, vapor, or aerosol, each phase having a distinct composition and toxicity profile. Exposure is prevalent in aircraft refueling and maintenance operations and ground crews positioned behind jet aircraft during "cold starts" can become "drenched" in aerosol emissions. Jet fuel can be released into the environment by in-flight jettisoning and spills or leaks to soil or water during use, storage, or transportation. In many cases, the US Department of Defense (DoD) is responsible for the cost of remediating contaminated military sites and contractor facilities, not to mention its responsibility to safeguard the health of military personnel. It is thus in DoD's interest to accurately characterize the toxicity of jet fuel. Much of the research conducted to date has been funded by the military. The Navy's Occupational Safety and Health Standards Board has proposed an eight-hour TWA PEL of 350 mg/m³ and a 15-minute STEL of 1800 mg/m³ for jet fuel vapors, but notes that exposure to aerosols that are much more toxic may necessitate reevaluation. The NAS Subcommittee on Jet Propulsion Fuel 8 recommended that the eight-hour TWA be considered interim until further research is completed, and that the STEL be lowered to 1000 mg/m³ to avoid acute CNS effects (NAS, 2003).

The complexity of jet fuel mixtures presents multiple challenges to toxicologists and risk assessors alike. One such challenge is to generate experimental exposures to jet fuel that accurately reflect those occurring in humans. The NAS Subcommittee on JP8 has reviewed the methods used to generate exposure atmospheres in several published studies using aerosol/vapor mixtures and suspects that the JP-8 concentrations may have been underreported, particularly in studies by Witten and colleagues (NAS, 2003). Therefore, it seems prudent at this time to discuss aerosol/vapor exposures in qualitative terms only. Because of concerns surrounding the quantitative accuracy of the exposure atmospheres, the NAS Subcommittee recommended an examination of the methods used for their characterization. To this end, Dietzel et al. (2005) have developed and validated a GC/MS method for JP-8, which was subsequently used to characterize the aerosol and vapor fractions of aerosolized fuel in one of the University of Arizona-based inhalation chambers previously utilized by Witten and colleagues.

Jet A, JP-8, and JP-8+100 have similar toxicity profiles, which suggests their toxicities are largely a function of hydrocarbon content rather than additives. Toxicity data on jet fuels have been well summarized (ATSDR, 1998; NAS, 2003; Ritchie et al., 2003), but there remain several data gaps including genotoxicity. Most toxicity studies of jet fuels have focused on the two main portals of entry (ie, lung and skin) and the immune system. In subchronic and chronic rodent inhalation studies of jet fuel vapor, the chief findings have been renal toxicity and neoplasia in male rats consistent with α_{2u}-globulin nephropathy (Mattie et al., 1991; Bruner et al., 1993). Whereas the liver, kidneys, and testes in humans are not considered particularly sensitive targets of jet fuels, proteomic analyses of these tissues have been conducted in male rats subchronically exposed to JP-8 vapor (Witzmann et al., 2000a,b, 2003). Similarly, gene expression in the whole brain of rats repeatedly exposed to JP-8 vapor has been examined (Lin et al., 2001a, 2004), driven largely by reports of cognitive and motor deficits and neurochemical changes in jet fuel–exposed workers and experimental animals (Baldwin et al., 2001; Ritchie et al., 2001; Rossi et al., 2001; Bell et al., 2005).

Pulmonary Effects The pulmonary effects of an aerosol/vapor mixture of JP-8 were initially investigated in rats with nose-only exposures designed to simulate military flightline exposures (Hays et al., 1995; Pfaff et al., 1995, 1996). Functional changes in the form of increases in pulmonary resistance and alveolar permeability were accompanied by a decrease in the concentration of the tachykinin substance P (SP) in bronchoalveolar lavage fluid. Pathological changes were observed in lower pulmonary structures including inflammation of the terminal bronchioles, degeneration of alveolar type II epithelial (AIIE) cells, and disruption of terminal bronchial airway epithelium. Most interestingly, the activity of neutral endopeptidase (NEP), an enzyme responsible for the metabolism of SP in the lung, was increased by exposure and a significant inverse relationship between SP and NEP activity demonstrated. Thus, JP-8 appears to exhibit a rather novel mechanism of lung injury that involves the reduction or depletion of SP due to its enhanced metabolism by NEP.

Because SP participates in the maintenance of airway epithelial cell competency, the effect of JP-8 and n-tetradecane (C_{14}), a primary constituent of JP-8, on epithelial barrier integrity was examined in vitro using paracellular mannitol flux in BEAS-2B human bronchial epithelial cells (Robledo et al., 1999). Noncytotoxic concentrations of JP-8 and C_{14} produced dose-dependent increases in transepithelial mannitol flux that spontaneously reversed to control values over a 48-hour recovery period. This suggests that JP-8 and C_{14} compromise the integrity of intercellular tight junctions that may precede and initiate the pathological alterations observed in

whole animal studies. Evidence was also collected that SP's protective effect on the lung is largely mediated through the plasma membrane–bound neurokinin receptor, NK_1, present on airway epithelium from the trachea to the respiratory bronchioles (Robledo and Witten, 1999).

Among the most affected alveolar cells in rodent studies are AIIE cells. In support of the hypothesis that apoptotic cell death is responsible at least partially for JP-8's cytotoxicity in the lung, Stoica et al. (2001) reported that JP-8 results in morphological and biochemical changes characteristic of apoptosis in the rat AIIE cell line, RLE-6TN. Further, Boulares et al. (2002) have collected data that strongly suggest JP-8 triggers apoptosis in rat lung epithelial cells by inducing the generation of ROS, depleting/reducing intracellular GSH, and markedly decreasing mitochondrial membrane potential, thereby initiating the apoptotic cascade (ie, caspase-3 activation and DNA fragmentation).

A characteristic feature of the lung inflammatory response to JP-8 in rodents is vacuolization of AIIE cells and accumulation of pulmonary alveolar macrophages (PAM). The findings of Wang et al. (2002b) suggest that JP-8 causes proinflammatory cytokine secretion by not only PAM but also AIIE cells. The prolonged production of proinflammatory cytokines, together with the proteases produced by activated macrophages and neutrophils, is capable of producing a sustained immune response with increased risk for lung damage. Moreover, cocultures of AIIE cells and primary PAM indicate that the balance of cytokines released in response to JP-8 could possibly be regulated in vivo by cross-communication between the two cell types. Espinoza et al. (2005) showed that the JP-8-induced expression of proinflammatory cytokine genes in AEII cells was mediated by the activation of PARP-1 (an enzyme coactivator of NF-κB) and NF-κB (a transcription factor that controls the expression of a variety of genes involved in inflammatory responses). The release of cytokines in the lung in response to JP-8 is similar to cytokine release from epidermal cells, which is thought to mediate, at least in part, the dermal and immune toxicities of JP-8 (see below). Further insight into the pulmonary effects of jet fuel has come from examinations of aerosolized JP-8's effect on gene and protein expression in lung cytosol and lung tissue of rats and mice (Witzmann et al., 1999; Drake et al., 2003; Espinoza et al., 2005).

Immune Effects The immune system appears to be as susceptible to jet fuel as the lung, if not more so. Detrimental effects on the immune system of mice have been reported for aerosolized Jet A, JP-8, and JP-8+100 (Harris et al., 2001a). Some effects were apparent just one hour after a single inhalation exposure with continued deterioration with each successive exposure (Harris et al., 2002). As first reported by Harris et al. (1997a), mice exposed nose-only to a JP-8 aerosol/vapor mix exhibited decreased spleen and thymus weights and cellularities and an altered number of viable immune cells in lymph nodes, bone marrow, and peripheral blood. Depending on the immune tissue examined, different immune cell subpopulations were lost, including T and B cells and macrophages. In addition, JP-8 affected immune function as demonstrated by a concentration-dependent suppression of T-cell proliferation on stimulation with the mitogen concanavalin A. In a short-term exposure study, Harris et al. (1997b) determined that JP-8-induced immunotoxicity persisted for at least one month after insult. These same authors later expanded the number of immune parameters examined and reported that aerosolized JP-8 exposure of mice nearly completely ablated NK cell function, suppressed the generation of lymphokine-activated killer cell activity, suppressed the generation of cytotoxic T lymphocytes from precursor T cells, and inhibited helper T-cell activity (Harris et al., 2000).

Ullrich (1999) has demonstrated that dermal application of JP-8 to mice can induce immune suppression. Ullrich found IL-10, a cytokine with potent immunosuppressive activity, in the serum of JP-8 dermally treated mice. He interpreted this as suggestive of an immune-suppressive mechanism involving the upregulation of cytokine release. In a follow-up study, Ullrich and Lyons (2000) demonstrated that the immunosuppressive effect of dermally applied JP-8 appears to be specific to cell-mediated immune reactions (ie, T-helper cell-driven cell-mediated immunity), as JP-8 had no effect on antibody production in immunized mice. Further, their study again implicated the release of cytokines from epidermal cells in immunosuppression, particularly prostaglandin E2 (PGE2) and IL-10. Ramos et al. (2004) have subsequently used platelet-activating factor (PAF) receptor antagonists to show that the PAF receptor, a signaling phospholipid which upregulates PGE2 synthesis by keratinocytes, plays a critical role in jet fuel–induced immune suppression. Ramos et al. (2002) have also demonstrated that the dermal application of JP-8 and Jet A suppresses delayed-type hypersensitivity and immunologic memory on rechallenge with a fungal pathogen, suggesting that jet fuel exposure may depress the protective effect of prior vaccination. Similar to that seen for pulmonary toxicity, aerosolized SP can both prevent and reverse some facets of JP-8-induced immunotoxicity, suggesting a key mechanistic role for the neuropeptide (Harris et al., 1997c, 2001b). As reported for AIIE cells, JP-8 also induces apoptosis in primary mouse thymocytes (Stoica et al., 2001). Exposure of mice to JP-8 in utero reportedly has implications for the immune system (Keil et al., 2003).

Dermal Effects Owing to reports of severe contact dermatitis among military personnel, the dermal toxicity of jet fuel has been the subject of intensive investigation. A recent examination of dermal exposure in 124 US Air Force fuel cell maintenance workers, using a noninvasive tape-strip technique and naphthalene as a surrogate, confirmed that the skin provides a significant exposure route for JP-8 (Chao et al., 2005). Dermal absorption and penetration of JP-8 and its component hydrocarbons have been examined in vitro using dermatomed rat skin and static diffusion cells and in vivo in weanling pigs (McDougal et al., 2000; Singh et al., 2003). Their cutaneous toxicity has been explored in pigs, rats, rabbits, and in vitro using human epidermal keratinocytes (HEK) (Kabbur et al., 2001; Monteiro-Riviere et al., 2001; Chou et al., 2003; Singh and Singh, 2004). Dermal exposure to jet fuel can lead to skin irritation and sensitization and the disruption of skin barrier function. Research implicates cytokine release, oxidative stress, and DNA damage/fragmentation as mechanistic underpinnings (Allen et al., 2000; Rogers et al., 2001; Gallucci et al., 2004). Chronic dermal application of middle distillate fuels such as jet fuel can be weakly carcinogenic, although it has been effectively argued that such tumorigenicity is secondary to chronic irritation (Nessel, 1999; Nessel et al., 1999).

The ultrastructural analysis of pig skin exposed to cotton fabric saturated with jet fuel suggests that the primary effect of exposure is damage of the stratum corneum barrier (Monteiro-Riviere et al., 2004). This same publication reported that IL-8 release from HEK after JP-8 exposure was decreased by SP, which is an agonist for the NK_1 receptor present in keratinocytes and mechanistically linked to IL release. The attenuation of IL release in keratinocytes by SP and the protection SP affords against pulmonary and immunotoxicity suggests that there may be a common mechanistic linkage to these toxicities. However, studies suggest that jet fuel–induced cell death in skin is via necrosis, not apoptosis as observed in some other cell types such as AIIE cells and T lymphocytes (Stoica et al.,

2001). This was also demonstrated by Rosenthal *et al.* (2001), who observed JP-8-induced necrotic rather than apoptotic cell death in mouse skin fibroblasts and HEK in culture or grafted onto nude mice. These authors used immunoblot analysis to determine that necrosis of HEK appeared to be associated with the perturbation of the ratio between antisurvival and prosurvival members of the Bcl-2 family of proteins (ie, the toxic, higher level of JP-8 decreased levels of the prosurvival proteins Bcl-2 and Bcl-x$_L$, while simultaneously elevating levels of the antisurvival proteins Bad and Bak). This has led to the suggestion that high intrinsic levels of Bcl-2 and Bcl-x$_L$ may prevent apoptotic death of keratinocytes at low concentrations of JP-8, whereas modulation of Bcl-2 family members by high doses may lead to necrotic cell death.

As the skin allows for the selective absorption and penetration of various jet fuel components, one cannot assume that the internal or target tissue dose of chemical is qualitatively or quantitatively the same as that of the external dose (McDougal and Robinson, 2002). This has led to efforts to identify the offending components of jet fuel mixtures. Using static diffusion cells, McDougal *et al.* (2000) identified 12 components of JP-8 that fully penetrated rat skin and six components, all aliphatic hydrocarbons, which were partially absorbed or retained by the skin. This led these researchers to speculate that the aliphatic components of jet fuel may be the cause of skin irritation. Allen *et al.* (2001) exposed HEK to micromolar concentrations of four aliphatic hydrocarbon components of jet fuel and found that they all induced IL-8 release at subtoxic doses, further implicating aliphatic components. However, Chou *et al.* (2002) exposed HEK to 10 aliphatic jet fuel hydrocarbons (C6-C16) and found that the higher cytotoxicity of the shorter chain aliphatics did not correlate with their ability to induce IL-8 release, which peaked at midchain lengths (ie, C9-C13). The toxicological interactions of jet fuel's aromatic and aliphatic components on HEK cells have also been explored (Yang *et al.*, 2006). The cytotoxicity and IL-8 release from these "mixed" hydrocarbon exposures were not always predictable based on the cytotoxic and IL-8 profiles of individual components. Muhammad *et al.* (2005) have exposed pigs topically to cotton fabric soaked with one of eight aliphatic hydrocarbons or one of six aromatic hydrocarbons and monitored skin irritation. Based on these data, coupled with data on IL-8 release, in vitro absorption, and cytotoxicity, they postulate that tridecane and tetradecane may be the two most important hydrocarbons responsible for jet fuel–induced skin irritation. Jet fuel exemplifies the difficulty in accurately predicting the dermal risk posed by a complex mixture based on limited knowledge of a few individual components. Progress toward this end has recently been made, as Kim *et al.* (2006) have published a dermatotoxicokinetic model of the skin that quantitatively characterizes the TK of three aromatic and three aliphatic jet fuel components following application of a single dose of JP-8 to the forearm of human volunteers. As in lung tissue and lung cytosol of rodents, the capacity of JP-8 to alter gene or protein expression in HEK has been thoroughly examined (Espinoza *et al.*, 2004; Witzmann *et al.*, 2005; Chou *et al.*, 2006).

CARBON DISULFIDE

The toxicity of CS$_2$ was first recognized during the 19th century, when it was widely employed as a solvent to soften rubber. CS$_2$ is listed as a Clean Air Act Chemical because of reported high emissions and the potential for human exposure. The major uses of CS$_2$ are in the production of rayon fiber, cellophane, and CCl$_4$ and as a solubilizer for waxes and oils (ATSDR, 1996a). Historically, exposures were particularly high during the early period of rayon production, and studies of these workers have been very informative as

to CS$_2$'s toxicity. Human exposure is predominantly occupational, although CS$_2$ has been identified in at least 200 current or former EPA National Priority List hazardous waste sites (ATSDR, 1996a). Most industrial releases are to the atmosphere. The general public may be subjected to low vapor levels as demonstrated by detection of CS$_2$ in samples of breath and indoor and outdoor air surveyed in and around New York City (Phillips, 1992). Exposure to dithiocarbamate pesticides and drugs (eg, the alcohol aversion drug, disulfiram) can result in indirect exposure to CS$_2$, as it is a product of their metabolism. However, there is evidence that the metabolic production of CS$_2$ is not a unifying explanation for the neuropathies frequently associated with dithiocarbamate exposure (Tonkin *et al.*, 2000; Mulkey, 2001).

The relative contributions of parent compound and metabolites to most CS$_2$-induced toxicities are unknown. Two distinct metabolic pathways for CS$_2$ exist: (1) the direct interaction of CS$_2$ with free amine and sulfhydryl groups of amino acids and polypeptides to form dithiocarbamates and trithiocarbonates; and (2) microsomal metabolism of CS$_2$ to reactive sulfur intermediates capable of covalently binding tissue macromolecules (Graham *et al.*, 1995) (Fig. 24-13). The conjugation of CS$_2$ with sulfhydryls of cysteine or GSH results in the formation of 2-thiothiazolidine-4-carboxylic acid (TTCA), which is excreted in urine and has been frequently used as a biomarker of CS$_2$ exposure, especially among viscose rayon workers (Riihimaki *et al.*, 1992; Lee *et al.*, 1995). Several limitations of TTCA as a biomarker have been noted, and covalently cross-linked erythrocyte spectrin and hemoglobin have been discussed as potential alternatives (Valentine *et al.*, 1993, 1998). Nonetheless, the current ACGIH BEI for CS$_2$ is 0.5 mg of TTCA/g of creatinine for a urine sample collected at the end of a workshift (ACGIH, 2012).

A few comprehensive reviews of CS$_2$'s toxicity have been published (Beauchamp *et al.*, 1983; ATSDR, 1996a; WHO, 2002; Gelbke *et al.*, 2009). CS$_2$ is capable of targeting multiple organ systems including the cardiovascular system, CNS and PNS, male and female fertility, and eyes (retinal angiopathy and impairment of color vision). CS$_2$ toxicity requires frequent and prolonged exposures in occupational settings. The nervous and cardiovascular systems have garnered the most attention. The most common neurotoxic effect is a distal sensorimotor neuropathy that preferentially affects long axons in the PNS and CNS (particularly the ascending and descending tracks of the spinal cord and the visual pathways). Encephalopathy with motor and cognitive impairment has also been reported following chronic, low-level exposure to CS$_2$ (Graham *et al.*, 1995). Several MRI studies report diffuse white matter lesions in chronically exposed workers similar to that described for "toluene leukoencephalopathy" among solvent abusers (Cho *et al.*, 2002; Ku *et al.*, 2003). For those particularly interested in the nervous system, the classic paper by Richter (1945) detailing his observations of chronic CS$_2$ poisoning in monkeys is recommended. Rosenberg (1995) described the following clinical syndromes associated with CS$_2$: (1) acute and chronic encephalopathy (often with prominent psychiatric manifestations); (2) polyneuropathy (both peripheral and cranial); (3) Parkinsonism; and (4) asymptomatic CNS and PNS dysfunction. Pathological changes occur in both the CNS and PNS. CNS pathology consists of neuronal degeneration throughout the cerebral hemispheres, with maximal diffuse involvement in the frontal regions. Cell loss is also noted in the globus pallidus, putamen, and cerebellar cortex, with loss of Purkinje cells. Vascular abnormalities with endothelial proliferation of arterioles may be seen, sometimes associated with focal necrosis or demyelination. PNS changes consist primarily of myelin swelling and fragmentation and large focal axonal swellings, characteristic of distal axonopathy.

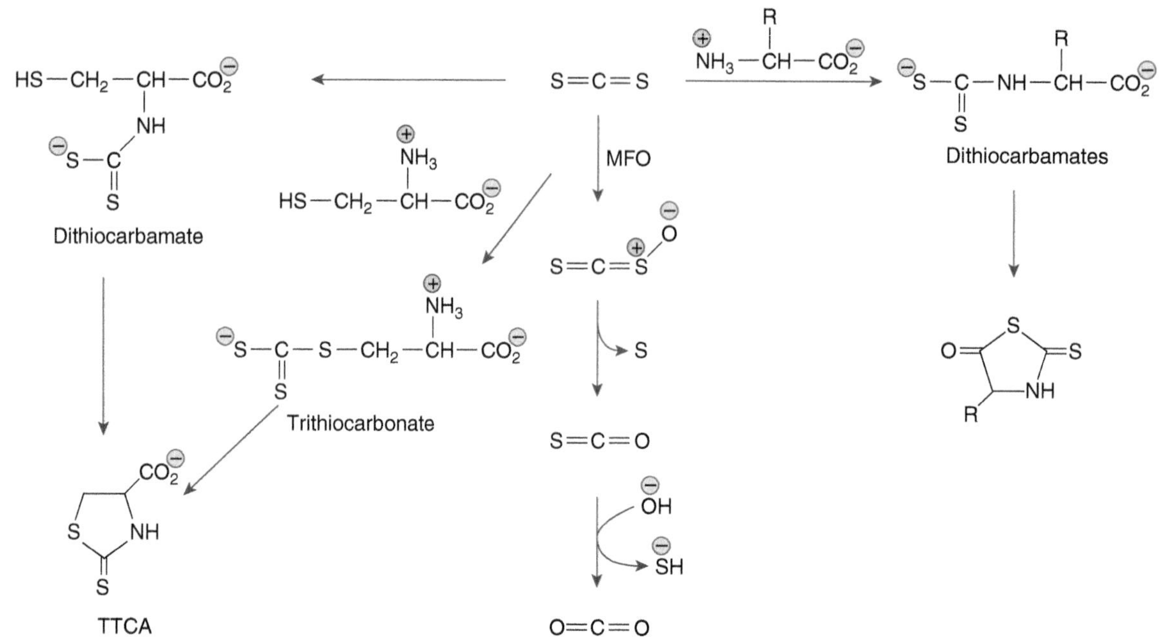

Figure 24-13. *Metabolism of carbon disulfide (CS₂).* CS₂ is metabolized by the mixed-function oxidase (MFO) system to carbonyl sulfide, atomic sulfur, and HS⁻. Reaction of CS₂ with sulfhydryls of cysteine or GSH yields trithiocarbonates, which can cyclize to form thiazolidine-2-thione-4-carboxylic acid (TTCA). Reaction of CS₂ with amino groups of amino acids results in dithiocarbamate derivatives, which can cyclize to yield 2-thio-5-thiazolidinones; reaction of cysteine amine could also produce TTCA. CS₂ is also metabolized in the liver by P450s to an unstable oxygen intermediate, which spontaneously generates atomic sulfur, carbonyl sulfide (COS), and CO₂. (Reproduced with permission from Graham *et al.*, 1995.)

Significant contributions to the understanding of CS₂'s neurotoxicity have come from collaborative research by the NIEHS, EPA, and several universities (Harry *et al.*, 1998; Sills *et al.*, 2005). Studies were conducted with F344 rats subchronically exposed to a range of CS₂ concentrations, in order to define the onset and temporal progression of neurotoxicity as manifest by multiple end points. These specific end points included TK changes in blood CS₂ levels and urinary TTCA, covalent cross-linking of blood and spinal cord proteins, alterations in axon/Schwann cell interactions as indicated by nerve growth factor mRNA expression, morphology of distal axonopathy, nerve conduction velocity and action potential, and behavioral assessment using a functional observational battery. This research showed sensitive end points at the cellular level that progressed to alterations in hindlimb and forelimb function, followed by electrophysiological and morphological changes. The TK data provided useful information about internal exposure to CS₂, but their use in the prediction of biological effects was limited (Moorman *et al.*, 1998). The collaborative efforts support the theory that the axonal degeneration that underlies CS₂'s central–peripheral neuropathy results from the reaction of CS₂ (and perhaps carbonyl sulfide [COS]) with protein amino groups to yield initial adducts (dithiocarbamate derivatives). The adducts decompose to an electrophile (isothiocyanate for CS₂ and isocyanate for COS), which in turn reacts with protein nucleophiles on neurofilaments to cause covalent protein cross-linking. Progressive cross-linking of neurofilaments occurs during neurofilament transport along the axon, and covalently cross-linked masses of neurofilaments are thought to occlude axonal transport at the nodes of Ranvier, ultimately resulting in axonal swelling and degeneration (similar to that seen with 2,5-hexanedione). It should be noted that several other mechanisms for the disruption of neurofilament transport that underlie CS₂'s axonopathy have been proposed including impaired energy metabolism, metal ion chelation by CS₂'s dithiocarbamate derivatives, induction of vitamin deficiency, and disruption of cytoskeletal

protein association by the increased phosphorylation of neurofilaments (Wilmarth *et al.*, 1993; Graham *et al.*, 1995).

One of the potentially more important outcomes of the collaborative research effort described above was the identification of thiourea cross-linking structures on erythrocyte spectrin and hemoglobin. This cross-linking exhibited a linear dose–response over the range of inhaled CS₂ concentrations examined, was detectable at subneurotoxic exposure levels, preceded axonal structural damage, and was positively correlated with neurofilament cross-linking (ie, spectrin and hemoglobin cross-linking reflects neurofilament cross-linking). These findings suggest the utility of spectrin and hemoglobin cross-linking as sensitive biomarkers of exposure and effect, and potential alternatives or supplements to TTCA, which was found to lack dose proportionality in the same studies (Valentine *et al.*, 1997, 1998; Moorman *et al.*, 1998).

Numerous worker studies support an association between CS₂ exposure and cardiovascular disease and related mortality. Elevated mortality from cardiovascular disease has been reported among viscose rayon workers in Finland, the United Kingdom, the United States, Scandinavia, and Poland (WHO, 2002). Viscose rayon worker studies reporting excess cardiovascular morbidity expand the range to Germany (Drexler *et al.*, 1996) and Japan (Takebayashi *et al.*, 2004). Further support for a CS₂–cardiovascular disease link comes from examination of cardiovascular disease risk factors in workers, and to a lesser extent experimental rodent studies. In workers, CS₂ exposure has been associated with elevations in blood pressure, total and LDL cholesterol, triglycerides, apolipoproteins, and lipid peroxidation in plasma, as well as reductions in HDL and antioxidant status (Vanhoorne *et al.*, 1992; Wronska-Nofer *et al.*, 2002; Luo *et al.*, 2003). Wronska-Nofer (1979) conducted studies in rats supporting a role for CS₂ in the elevation of blood cholesterol, whereas Lewis *et al.* (1999) found that exposure to as little as 50 ppm CS₂ significantly enhanced the rate of arterial fat deposition in mice placed on a Western style, high-fat diet. Sulsky *et al.*

(2002) have reviewed 37 studies addressing the CS_2–cardiovascular disease association and concluded that epidemiological evidence for an association was "mixed," with an effect on total and/or LDL cholesterol being the most consistent finding but of limited magnitude and uncertain clinical significance. Tan *et al.* (2002) conducted a meta-analysis of 11 cohort studies on CS_2's cardiovascular effects, which showed a small but significant correlation between CS_2 exposure and cardiovascular disease prevalence (pooled RR = 1.56; 95% CI = 1.12–2.1). Taken together, studies suggest that CS_2 has the ability to accelerate atherosclerosis. Further, some have speculated that like neurotoxicity, protein cross-linking may also be involved in CS_2's promotion of the atherosclerotic process (Lewis *et al.*, 1999).

Price *et al.* (1997) pointed out that the cardiovascular mortality excesses seen in most published studies were among workers chronically exposed to high concentrations that no longer are observed in the workplace. These authors reviewed historical exposure and mortality data in the viscose rayon industry and estimated that chronic exposures of 15 to 20 ppm would not be associated with an increased risk of mortality due to ischemic heart disease. They were also instrumental in applying the benchmark dose method toward the establishment of EPA's RfC for CS_2 of 0.7 mg/m^3 (~0.22 ppm), which is based on reduced maximum motor conduction velocity in the peroneal nerves of the NIOSH cohort of viscose rayon workers reported by Johnson *et al.* (1983) (Price *et al.*, 1996; EPA, 2006c). For the protection of workers, OSHA has established a PEL of 20 ppm as an eight-hour TWA with an acceptable ceiling concentration of 30 ppm. The NIOSH recommended exposure limit (REL) of 1 ppm with a STEL of 10 ppm. The ACGIH TLV was reduced from 10 to 1 ppm in 2006, as an eight-hour TWA based on neurologic end points. As a result, the ACGIH has also reduced CS_2's BEI from 5 to 0.5 mg TTCA/g creatinine in 2009. Gelbke *et al.* (2009) reviewed the health effects of CS_2 in viscose industry and concluded that while some uncertainties exist, available data generally support a REL of 10 ppm.

REFERENCES

Abbate C, Giorgianni C, Munao F, Brecciaroli R. Neurotoxicity induced by exposure to toluene. An electropyhysiologic study. *Int Arch Occup Environ Health*. 1993;64:389–392.

ACGIH (American Conference of Governmental Industrial Hygienists). *Threshold Limit Values (TLVs) and Biological Exposure Indices (BEIs)*. Cincinnati, OH: ACGIH; 2012. Available at: www.acgih.org.

Adachi J, Asano M, Ueno Y, et al. Alcoholic muscle disease and biomembrane perturbations. *Nutr Biochem*. 2003;14:616–625.

Aggazzotti G, Fantuzzi G, Righi E, Predieri G. Environmental and biological monitoring of chloroform in indoor swimming pools. *J Chromatogr A*. 1995;710:181–190.

Ahmed FE. Toxicological effects of ethanol or human health. *Crit Rev Toxicol*. 1995;25:347–367.

Albano E, French SW, Ingelman-Sundberg M. Hydroxyethyl radicals in ethanol hepatotoxicity. *Front Biosci*. 1999;4:533–540.

Albers JW, Wald JJ, Garabrant DH, et al. Neurologic evaluation of workers previously diagnosed with solvent-induced toxic encephalopathy. *J Occup Environ Med*. 2000;42:410–423.

Aleksunes LM, Slitt AM, Cherrington NJ, et al. Differential expression of mouse hepatic transporter genes in response to acetaminophen and carbon tetrachloride. *Toxicol Sci*. 2005;83:44–52.

Alexander DD, Kelsh MA, Mink PJ. A meta-analysis of occupational trichloroethylene exposure and liver cancer. *Int Arch Occup Environ Health*. 2007;81:127–143.

Alexander DD, Mink PJ, Mandel JH, Kelsh MA. A meta-analysis of occupational trichloroethylene exposure and multiple myeloma or leukemia. *Occup Med*. 2006;56:485–493.

Alfred S, Coleman P, Harris D, et al. Delayed neurologic sequelae resulting from epidemic diethylene glycol poisoning. *Clin Toxicol*. 2005;43:155–159.

Allen DG, Riviere JE, Monteiro-Riviere NA. Identification of early biomarkers of inflammation produced by keratinocytes exposed to jet fuels jet A, JP-8, and JP-8 (100). *J Biochem Mol Toxicol*. 2000;14:231–237.

Allen DG, Riviere JE, Monteiro-Riviere NA. Analysis of interleukin-8 release from normal human epidermal keratinocytes exposed to aliphatic hydrocarbons: delivery of hydrocarbons to cell cultures via complexation with α-cyclodextrin. *Toxicol In Vitro*. 2001;15:663–669.

Almekinder JL, Lennard DE, Walmer DK, et al. Toxicity of methoxyacetic acid in cultured human luteal cells. *Fundam Appl Toxicol*. 1997;38:191–194.

Ambroso JL, Stedman DB, Elswick BA, Welsch F. Characterization of cell death induced by 2-methoxyethanol in CD-1 mouse embryos on gestation day 8. *Teratology*. 1998;58:231–240.

Anand SS, Kim K-B, Padilla S, et al. Ontogeny of hepatic and plasma metabolism of deltamethrin in vitro: role in age-dependent acute neurotoxicity. *Drug Metab Dispos*. 2006a;34:389–397.

Anand SS, Mumtaz MM, Mehendale HM. Dose-dependent liver regeneration in chloroform, trichloroethylene and allyl alcohol ternary mixture hepatotoxicity in rats. *Arch Toxicol*. 2005;79:671–682.

Anand SS, Philip BK, Palkar PS, et al. Adaptive tolerance in mice upon subchronic exposure to chloroform: increased exhalation and target tissue regeneration. *Toxicol Appl Pharmacol*. 2006b;213:267–281.

Anand SS, Soni MG, Vaidya VS, et al. Extent and timeliness of tissue repair determines the dose-related hepatotoxicity of chloroform. *Int J Toxicol*. 2003;22:25–33.

Andersen ME. A physiologically based toxicokinetic description of the metabolism of inhaled gases and vapors: analysis at steady state. *Toxicol Appl Pharmacol*. 1981;60:509–526.

Andersen ME. Tissue dosimetry in risk assessment, or what's the problem here anyway? In: Gillette JR, Jollow P, Chairs. *Drinking Water and Health*. Vol. 8. Washington, DC: National Academy Press; 1987:8–26.

Andersen ME. Toxicokinetic modeling and its applications in chemical risk assessment. *Toxicol Lett*. 2003;138:9–27.

Andersen ME, Clewell HJ III, Gargas ML, et al. Physiologically based pharmacokinetics and the risk assessment process for methylene chloride. *Toxicol Appl Pharmacol*. 1987;87:185–205.

Andreoli C, Leopardi P, Crebelli R. Detection of DNA damage in human lymphocytes by alkaline single cell gel electrophoresis after exposure to benzene or benzene metabolites. *Mutat Res*. 1997;377:95–104.

Angelo MJ, Pritchard AB, Hawkins DR, et al. The pharmacokinetics of dichloromethane. II. Disposition in Fischer 344 rats following intravenous and oral administration. *Food Chem Toxicol*. 1986;24:975–980.

Araki A, Kamigaito N, Sasaki T, Matsushima T. Mutagenicity of carbon tetrachloride and chloroform in *Salmonella typhimurium* TA 98, TA 100, TA 1535, and TA 1537, and *Escherichia coli* WP2uvrA/pKM101 and WP2/pKM101, using a gas exposure method. *Environ Mol Mutagen*. 2004;43:128–133.

Aranyi C, O'Shea WJ, Halder CA, et al. Absence of hydrocarbon-induced nephropathy in rats exposed subchronically to volatile hydrocarbon mixtures pertinent to gasoline. *Toxicol Ind Health*. 1986;2:85–98.

Arlien-Soborg P. *Solvent Neurotoxicity*. Boca Raton, FL: CRC Press; 1992.

Arlien-Soborg P, Bruhn P, Gyldensted P, Melgaard B. Chronic painters' syndrome: chronic toxic encephalopathy in house painters. *Acta Neurol Scand*. 1979;60:149–156.

Ashley DL, Bonin MA, Cardinali FL, et al. Blood concentrations of volatile organic compounds in a nonoccupationally exposed US population and in groups with suspected exposure. *Clin Chem*. 1994;40:1401–1404.

Asselman M, Verhulst A, de Broe ME, Verkoelen CF. Calcium oxalate crystal adherence to hyaluronan-, osteopontin-, and CD44-expressing injured/regenerating tubular epithelial cells in rat kidneys. *J Am Soc Nephrol*. 2003;14:3155–3166.

Astrand I. Effect of physical exercise on uptake, distribution and elimination of vapors in man. In: Fiserova-Bergerova V, ed. *Modeling of Inhalation Exposure to Vapors: Uptake, Distribution, and Elimination*. Vol. 2. Boca Raton, FL: CRC Press; 1983:107–130.

Astrand I, Kilbom A, Wahlberg I, Ovrum P. Methyl chloroform exposure. I. Concentration in alveolar air and blood at rest and during exercise. *Work Environ Health.* 1973;10:69–81.

ATSDR (Agency for Toxic Substances and Disease Registry). Methanol toxicity. *Am Fam Physician.* 1993;47:163–171.

ATSDR (Agency for Toxic Substances and Disease Registry). *Toxicological Profile for Gasoline.* Atlanta, GA: Public Health Service; 1995.

ATSDR (Agency for Toxic Substances and Disease Registry). *Toxicological Profile for Carbon Disulfide.* Atlanta, GA: Public Health Service; 1996a.

ATSDR (Agency for Toxic Substances and Disease Registry). *Toxicological Profile for Methyl t-Butyl Ether.* Atlanta, GA: Public Health Service; 1996b.

ATSDR (Agency for Toxic Substances and Disease Registry). *Toxicological Profile for Chloroform.* Atlanta, GA: Public Health Service; 1997a.

ATSDR (Agency for Toxic Substances and Disease Registry). *Toxicological Profile for Ethylene Glycol and Propylene Glycol.* Atlanta, GA: Public Health Service; 1997b.

ATSDR (Agency for Toxic Substances and Disease Registry). *Toxicological Profile for Tetrachloroethylene.* Atlanta, GA: Public Health Service; 1997c.

ATSDR (Agency for Toxic Substances and Disease Registry). *Toxicological Profile for Trichloroethylene.* Atlanta, GA: Public Health Service; 1997d.

ATSDR (Agency for Toxic Substances and Disease Registry). *Toxicological Profile for Jet Fuels (JP-5 and JP-8).* Atlanta, GA: Public Health Service; 1998.

ATSDR (Agency for Toxic Substances and Disease Registry). *Toxicological Profile for Methylene Chloride.* Atlanta, GA: Public Health Service; 2000a.

ATSDR (Agency for Toxic Substances and Disease Registry). *Toxicological Profile for Toluene.* Atlanta, GA: Public Health Service; 2000b.

ATSDR (Agency for Toxic Substances and Disease Registry). *Interaction Profile for 1,1,1-Trichloroethane, 1,1-Dichloroethane, Trichloroethylene and Tetrachloroethylene.* Atlanta, GA: Public Health Service; 2004.

ATSDR (Agency for Toxic Substances and Disease Registry). *Toxicological Profile for Carbon Tetrachloride.* Atlanta, GA: Public Health Service; 2005.

ATSDR (Agency for Toxic Substances and Disease Registry). *ToxFAQs for Trichloroethylene (TCE).* Atlanta, GA: Public Health Service; 2006a. Available at: http://www.atsdr.ege.gov/tfacts19.html.

ATSDR (Agency for Toxic Substances and Disease Registry). *Toxicological Profile for 1,1,1-Trichloroethane (Update).* Atlanta, GA: Public Health Service; 2006b.

ATSDR (Agency for Toxic Substances and Disease Registry). *Toxicological Profile for Benzene.* Atlanta, GA: Public Health Service; 2006c.

ATSDR (Agency for Toxic Substances and Disease Registry). *Toxicological Profile for Xylenes.* Atlanta, GA: Public Health Service; 2006d.

ATSDR (Agency for Toxic Substances and Disease Registry). *Toxicological Profile for Ethylbenzene.* Atlanta, GA: Public Health Service; 2010a.

ATSDR (Agency for Toxic Substances and Disease Registry). *Toxicological Profile for Styrene.* Atlanta, GA: Public Health Service; 2010b.

Axelson O, Hane M, Hogstedt C. A case-referent study of neuropsychiatric disorders among workers exposed to solvents. *Scand J Work Environ Health.* 1976;2:14–20.

Baan R, Straif K, Grosse Y, et al. Carcinogenicity of alcoholic beverages. WHO International Agency for Research on Cancer Monograph Working Group. *Lancet Oncol.* 2007;8:292–293.

Backes WL, Sequeira DJ, Cawley GF, Eyer CS. Relationship between hydrocarbon structure and induction of P450: effects on protein levels and enzyme activities. *Xenobiotica.* 1993;23:1353–1366.

Badham HJ, Renaud SJ, Wan J, Linn LM. Benzene-induced oxidative stress: effects on embryonic signaling pathways. *Chem Biol Interact.* 2010;184:218–221.

Bailey DG, Dresser GK, Bend JR. Bergamottin, lime juice, and red wine as inhibitors of cytochrome P450 3A4 activity: comparison with grapefruit juice. *Clin Pharmacol Ther.* 2003;73:529–537.

Bakke B, Stewart PA, Waters MA. Use of and exposure to trichloroethylene in U.S. industry: a systematic literature review. *J Occup Environ Hyg.* 2007;4:375–390.

Baldwin CM, Houston FP, Podgornik MN, et al. Effects of aerosol-vapor JP-8 jet fuel on the functional observational battery, and learning and memory in the rat. *Arch Environ Health.* 2001;56:216–226.

Bale AS, Smothers CT, Woodward JJ. Inhibition of neuronal nicotine acetylcholine receptors by the abused solvent, toluene. *Br J Pharmacol.* 2002;137:375–383.

Bale AS, Tu Y, Carpenter-Hyland EP, et al. Alterations in glutamatergic and gabaergic ion channel activity in hippocampal neurons following exposure to the abused solvent toluene. *Neuroscience.* 2005;30:197–206.

Ballantyne B, Snellings WM. Developmental toxicity study with diethylene glycol dosed by gavage to CD rats and CD-1 mice. *Food Chem Toxicol.* 2005;43:1637–1646.

Ballantyne B, Vergnes JS. In vitro and in vivo genetic toxicology studies with diethylene glycol monohexyl ether. *J Appl Toxicol.* 2001;21:449–460.

Balster RL. Neural basis of inhalant abuse. *Drug Alcohol Depend.* 1998;512:207–214.

Barceloux DG, Bond GR, Krenzelok EP, et al. American Academy of Clinical Toxicology practice guidelines on the treatment of methanol poisoning. *J Toxicol Clin Toxicol.* 2002;40:415–446.

Barton HA, Creech JR, Godin CS, et al. Chloroethylene mixtures: pharmacokinetic modeling and in vitro metabolism of vinyl chloride, trichloroethylene, and *trans*-1,2-dichloroethylene in rat. *Toxicol Appl Pharmacol.* 1995;130:237–247.

Barton HA, Das S. Alternative for a risk assessment on chronic noncancer effects from oral exposure to trichloroethylene. *Regul Toxicol Pharmacol.* 1996;24:269–285.

Bautista AP. Impact of alcohol on the ability of Kupffer cells to produce chemokines and its role in alcoholic liver disease. *J Gastroenterol Hepatol.* 2000;15:349–356.

Beattie PJ, Welsh MJ, Brabec MJ. The effect of 2-methoxyethanol and methoxyacetic acid on Sertoli cell lactate production and protein synthesis in vitro. *Toxicol Appl Pharmacol.* 1984;76:56–61.

Beauchamp RO, Bus JS, Popp JA, et al. A critical review of the literature on carbon disulfide toxicity. *Crit Rev Toxicol.* 1983;11:169–278.

Beckstead MJ, Weiner JL, Eger EI, et al. Glycine and gamma-aminobutyric acid (A) receptor function is enhanced by inhaled drugs of abuse. *Mol Pharmacol.* 2000;57:1199–1205.

Beddowes EJ, Faux SP, Chipman JK. Chloroform, carbon tetrachloride and glutathione depletion induce secondary genotoxicity in liver cells via oxidative stress. *Toxicology.* 2003;187:101–115.

Bell AN, Young RA, Lockard VG, Mehendale HM. Protection of chlordecone-potentiated carbon tetrachloride hepatotoxicity and lethality by partial hepatectomy. *Arch Toxicol.* 1988;61:392–405.

Bell IR, Brooks AJ, Baldwin CM, et al. JP-8 jet fuel exposure and divided attention test performance in 1991 Gulf War veterans. *Aviat Space Environ Med.* 2005;76:1136–1144.

Belliger FP, Bedi KS, Wilson P, Wilce PA. Ethanol exposure during the third trimester equivalent results in long-lasting decreased synaptic efficacy but not plasticity in the CA1 region of the rat hippocampus. *Synapse.* 1999;31:51–58.

Belpoggi F, Soffritti M, Filippini F, Maltoni C. Results of long-term experimental studies on the carcinogenicity of methyl *tert*-butyl ether. *Ann N Y Acad Sci.* 1997;837:77–95.

Belpoggi F, Soffritti M, Maltoni C. Methyl-*tertiary*-butyl ether (MTBE)—a gasoline additive—causes testicular and lymphohaematopoietic cancers in rats. *Toxicol Ind Health.* 1995;11:119–149.

Benignus VA, Boyes WK, Bushnell PG. A dosimetric analysis of behavioral effects of acute toluene exposure in rats and humans. *Toxicol Sci.* 1998;43:186–195.

Benjamin SA, Yang RS, Tessari JD, et al. Lack of promotional effects of groundwater contaminant mixtures on the induction of preneoplastic foci in rat liver. *Toxicology.* 1999;137:137–149.

Bergsagel DE, Wong O, Bergsagel PL, et al. Benzene and multiple myeloma: appraisal of the scientific evidence. *Blood.* 1999;94:1174–1182.

Bernauer U, Birner G, Dekant W, Henschler D. Biotransformation of trichloroethene: dose-dependent excretion of 2,2,2-trichloro-metabolites and mercapturic acids in rats and humans after inhalation. *Arch Toxicol.* 1996;70:338–346.

Bernauer U, Vieth B, Ellrich R, et al. CYP2E1-dependent benzene toxicity: the role of extrahepatic benzene metabolism. *Arch Toxicol.* 1999;73:189–196.

Bevan C, Neeper-Bradley TL, Tyl RW, et al. Two-generation reproductive toxicity study of methyl *tertiary*-butyl ether (MTBE) in rats. *J Appl Toxicol.* 1997a;17(S1):S13–S19.

Bevan C, Tyl RW, Neeper-Bradley TL, et al. Developmental toxicity evaluation of methyl *tertiary*-butyl ether (MTBE) by inhalation in mice and rabbits. *J Appl Toxicol.* 1997b;17(S1):S21–S29.

Bezabeth S, Engel A, Morris CB, Lamm SH. Does benzene cause multiple myeloma? An analysis of the published case–control literature. *Environ Health Perspect.* 1996;104(suppl 6):1393–1398.

Bird MG, Burleigh-Flayer HD, Chun JS, et al. Oncogenicity studies of inhaled methyl *tertiary*-butyl ether (MTBE) in CD-1 mice and F-344 rats. *J Appl Toxicol.* 1997;17:S45–S55.

Bird MG, Greim H, Snyder R, Rice JM. International symposium: recent advances in benzene toxicity. *Chem Biol Interact.* 2005;153–154:1–5.

Birner G, Bernauer U, Werner M, Dekant W. Biotransformation, excretion, and nephrotoxicity of haloalkane-derived cysteine S-conjugates. *Arch Toxicol.* 1997;72:1–8.

Birner G, Rutkowska A, Dekant W. N-Acetyl-S-(1,2,2-trichlorovinyl)-L-cysteine and 2,2,2-trichloroethanol: two novel metabolites of tetrachloroethylene in humans after occupational exposure. *Drug Metab Dispos.* 1996;14:41–48.

Blair A, Hartge P, Stewart PA, et al. Mortality and cancer incidence of aircraft maintenance workers exposed to trichloroethylene and other organic solvents and chemicals: extended follow-up. *Occup Environ Med.* 1998;55:161–171.

Blair A, Petralia SA, Stewart PA. Extended mortality following a cohort of dry cleaners. *Ann Epidemiol.* 2003;13:50–56.

Blanco JG, Harrison PL, Evans WE, Relling MV. Human cytochrome P450 maximal activities in pediatric versus adult liver. *Drug Metab Dispos.* 2000;28:379–382.

Bleecker ML, Bolla KI, Agnew J, et al. Dose-related subclinical neurobehavioral effects of chronic exposure to low levels of organic solvents. *Am J Ind Med.* 1991;19:715–728.

Blobaum AL. Mechanism-based inactivation and reversibility: is there a new trend in the inactivation of cytochrome P450 enzymes? *Drug Metab Dispos.* 2006;34:1–7.

Bloemen LJ, Monster AC, Kezic S, et al. Study on the cytochrome P-450- and glutathione-dependent biotransformation of trichloroethylene in humans. *Int Arch Occup Environ Health.* 2001;74:102–108.

Blossom SJ, Gilbert KM. Exposure to a metabolite of the environmental toxicant, trichloroethylene, attenuates CD4+ T cell activation-induced cell death by metalloproteinase-dependent FasL shedding. *Toxicol Sci.* 2006;92:103–114.

Blount BC, Kobelski RJ, McElprang DO, et al. Quantification of 31 volatile organic compounds in whole blood using solid-phase microextraction and gas chromatography–mass spectrometry. *J Chromatogr B.* 2006;832:292–301.

Boatman R, Corley R, Green T, et al. Review of studies concerning the tumorigenicity of 2-butoxyethanol in B6C3F1 mice and its relevance for human risk assessment. *J Toxicol Environ Health B Crit Rev.* 2004;7:385–398.

Boffeta P, Garfinkel L. Alcohol drinking and mortality among men enrolled in an American Cancer Society prospective study. *Epidemiology.* 1990;1:342–348.

Boffeta P, Hashibe M. Alcohol and cancer. *Lancet Oncol.* 2006;7:149–156.

Boice JD, Marano DE, Cohen SS, et al. Mortality among Rocketdyne workers who tested rocket engines, 1948-1999. *J Occup Environ Med.* 2006;48:1070–1092.

Boice JD Jr, Marano DE, Fryzek JP, et al. Mortality among aircraft manufacturing workers. *Occup Environ Med.* 1999;56:581–597.

Bois FY. Applications of population approaches in toxicology. *Toxicol Lett.* 2001;120:385–394.

Bolt HM, Lammert M, Selinski S, Bruning T. Urinary alpha 1-microglobulin excretion as a biomarker of renal toxicity in trichloroethylene-exposed persons. *Int Arch Occup Environ Health.* 2004;77:186–190.

Boogaard PJ, van Sittert NJ. Suitability of S-phenylmercapturic acid and *trans-trans*-muconic acid as biomarkers for exposure to low concentrations of benzene. *Environ Health Perspect.* 1996;104(suppl 6):1151–1157.

Borak J, Pastides H, Van Ert M, et al. Exposure to MTBE and acute human health effects: a critical literature review. *Hum Ecol Assess.* 1998;4:177–200.

Borel V, Gallot D, Marceau G, et al. Placental implications of peroxisome proliferator-activated receptors in gestation and parturition. *PPAR Res.* 2008;2008:758562.

Borghoff SJ, et al. *CIIT Activities.* 1996a;16:1–8.

Borghoff SJ, Murphy JE, Medinsky MA. Development of physiologically based pharmacokinetic model for methyl *tertiary*-butyl ether and *tertiary*-butanol in male Fischer-344 rats. *Fundam Appl Toxicol.* 1996b;30:264–275.

Borghoff SJ, Short BG, Swenberg JA. Biochemical mechanisms and pathobiology of α_{2u}-globulin nephropathy. *Annu Rev Pharmacol Toxicol.* 1990;30:349–367.

Boulares AH, Contreras FJ, Espinoza LA, Smulson ME. Roles of oxidative stress and glutathione depletion in JP-8 jet fuel-induced apoptosis in rat lung epithelial cells. *Toxicol Appl Pharmacol.* 2002;180:92–99.

Boutelet-Bochan H, Huang Y, Juchau MR. Expression of CYP2E1 during embryogenesis and fetogenesis in human cephalic tissues: implications for the fetal alcohol syndrome. *Biochem Biophys Res Commun.* 1997;238:443–447.

Bowen SE, Irtenkauf S, Hannigan JH, Stefanski AL. Alterations in rat fetal morphology following abuse patterns of toluene exposure. *Reprod Toxicol.* 2009;27:161–169.

Brauch H, Weirich G, Hornauer MA, et al. Trichloroethylene exposure and specific somatic mutations in patients with renal cell carcinoma. *J Natl Cancer Inst.* 1999;91:854–861.

Brauch H, Weirich G, Klein B, et al. VHL mutations in renal cell cancer: does occupational exposure to trichloroethylene make a difference? *Toxicol Lett.* 2004;151:301–310.

Brent J, McMartin K, Phillips S, et al. Fomepizole for the treatment of ethylene glycol poisoning. Methylpyrazole for Toxic Alcohols Study Group. *N Engl J Med.* 1999;340:832–838.

Bressler R, Bahl JJ. Principles of drug therapy for the elderly patient. *Mayo Clin Proc.* 2003;78:1564–1577.

Brienza RS, Stein MD. Alcohol use disorders in primary care: do gender-specific differences exist? *J Gen Intern Med.* 2002;17:387–397.

Brinkworth MH, Weinbauer GF, Schlatt S, Nieschlag E. Identification of male germ cells undergoing apoptosis in adult rats. *J Reprod Fertil.* 1995;105:25–33.

Brodkin CA, Daniell W, Checkoway H, et al. Hepatic ultrasonic changes in workers exposed to perchloroethylene. *Occup Environ Med.* 1995;52:679–685.

Brodkin CA, Moon J-D, Camp J, et al. Serum hepatic biochemical activity in two populations of workers exposed to styrene. *Occup Environ Med.* 2001;58:95–102.

Brogen C-H, Christensen JM, Rasmussen K. Occupational exposure to chlorinated organic solvents and its effect on renal excretion of N-acetyl-beta-D-glucosaminidase. *Arch Toxicol.* 1986;9(suppl):460–464.

Brooks DE, Wallace KL. Acute propylene glycol ingestion. *J Toxicol Clin Toxicol.* 2002;40:513–516.

Brophy PD, Tenebein M, Gardner J, et al. Childhood diethylene glycol poisoning treated with alcohol dehydrogenase inhibitor fomepizole and hemodialysis. *Am J Kidney Dis.* 2000;35:958–962.

Brown EA, Shelley ML, Fisher JW. A pharmacokinetic study of occupational and environmental exposure with regard to gender. *Risk Anal.* 1998;18:205–213.

Brown RC, Barone S, Kimmel CA. Children's health risk assessment: incorporating a lifestage approach into the risk assessment process. *Birth Defects Res.* 2008;83:511–521.

Brown-Woodman PDC, Hayes LC, Huq F, et al. In vitro assessment of the effect of halogenated hydrocarbons: chloroform, dichloromethane, and dibromomethane on embryonic development of the rat. *Teratology.* 1998;57:321–333.

Bruckner JV. Differences in sensitivity of children and adults to chemical toxicity: the NAS panel report. *Regul Toxicol Pharmacol.* 2000;31:280–285.

Bruckner JV, Kyle GM, Luthra R, et al. Acute, short-term and subchronic oral toxicity of 1,1,1-trichloroethane in rats. *Toxicol Sci.* 2001;60:363–372.

Bruckner JV, Peterson RG. Evaluation of toluene and acetone inhalant abuse. I. Pharmacology and pharmacodynamics. *Toxicol Appl Pharmacol.* 1981;61:27–38.

Bruckner JV, Ramanathan R, Lee KM, Muralidhara S. Mechanisms of circadian rhythmicity of carbon tetrachloride hepatotoxicity. *J Pharmacol Exp Ther.* 2002;300:273–281.

Bruner RH, Kinkead ER, O'Neill TP, et al. The toxicologic and oncogenic potential of JP-4 jet fuel vapors in rats and mice: 12-month intermittent inhalation exposures. *Fundam Appl Toxicol.* 1993;20:97–110.

Bruning T, Bolt HM. Renal toxicity and carcinogenicity of trichloroethylene: key results, mechanisms, and controversies. *Crit Rev Toxicol.* 2000;30:253–285.

Bruning T, Golka K, Makropoulos V, Bolt HM. Preexistence of chronic tubular damage in cases of renal cell cancer after long and high exposure to trichloroethylene. *Arch Toxicol.* 1996;70:259–260.

Bruning T, Lammert M, Kempkes M, et al. Influence of polymorphisms of GSTM1 and GSTT1 for risk of renal cell cancer in workers with long-term high occupational exposure to trichloroethene. *Arch Toxicol.* 1997b;71:596–599.

Bruning T, Mann H, Melzer H, et al. Pathological excretion patterns of urinary proteins in renal cell cancer patients exposed to trichloroethylene. *Occup Med.* 1999;49:299–305.

Bruning T, Pesch B, Wisenhutter B, et al. Renal cell cancer risk and occupational exposure to trichloroethylene: results of a consecutive case–control study in Arnsberg, Germany. *Am J Ind Med.* 2003;43:274–285.

Bruning T, Weirich G, Hornauer MA, et al. Renal cell carcinomas in trichloroethene (TRI) exposed persons are associated with somatic mutations in the von Hippel–Lindau (VHL) tumour suppressor gene. *Arch Toxicol.* 1997a;71:332–335.

Buben JA, O'Flaherty EJ. Delineation of the role of metabolism in the hepatotoxicity of trichloroethylene and perchloroethylene. A dose–effect study. *Toxicol Appl Pharmacol.* 1985;78:105–122.

Buck ML. The use of chloral hydrate in infants and children. *Pediatr Pharmacother.* 2005;11:1–4.

Bull RJ. Mode of action of liver tumor induction by trichloroethylene and its metabolites, trichloroacetate and dichloroacetate. *Environ Health Perspect.* 2000;108(suppl 2):241–259.

Bull RJ, Orner GA, Cheng RS, et al. Contribution of dichloroacetate and trichloroacetate to liver tumor induction in mice by trichloroethylene. *Toxicol Appl Pharmacol.* 2002;182:55–65.

Burbacher TM, Grant KS, Shen DD, et al. Chronic maternal methanol inhalation in nonhuman primates (*Macaca fascicularis*): reproductive performance and birth outcome. *Neurotoxicol Teratol.* 2004a;26:639–650.

Burbacher TM, Shen DD, Lalovic B, et al. Chronic maternal methanol inhalation in nonhuman primates (*Macaca fascicularis*): exposure and toxicokinetics prior to and during pregnancy. *Neurotoxicol Teratol.* 2004b;26:201–221.

Burek JD, Nitschke KD, Bell TJ, et al. Methylene chloride: a two-year inhalation toxicity and oncogenicity study in rats and hamsters. *Fundam Appl Toxicol.* 1984;4:30–47.

Burleigh-Flayer HD, Chun JS, Kintigh WJ. *Methyl tertiary Butyl Ether: Vapor Inhalation Oncogenicity Study in CD Mice.* Export, PA: Bushy Run Research Center; 1992.

Burton DA, Allen MC, Bird JL, Faragher RA. Bridging the gap: ageing, pharmacokinetics and pharmacodynamics. *J Pharm Pharmacol.* 2005;57:671–679.

Byard RW, Chivell WC, Gilbert JD. Unusual facial markings and lethal mechanisms in a series of gasoline inhalation deaths. *Am J Forensic Med Pathol.* 2003;24:298–302.

Cai H, Guengerich FP. Reaction of trichloroethylene and trichloroethylene oxide with cytochrome P450 enzymes: inactivation and sites of modification. *Chem Res Toxicol.* 2001;14:451–458.

Caldemeyer KS, Armstrong SW, George KK, et al. The spectrum of neuroimaging abnormalities in solvent abuse and their clinical correlation. *J Neuroimag.* 1996;6:167–173.

Caldwell DJ. Review of mononuclear cell leukemia in F-344 rat bioassays and its significance to human cancer risk: a case study using alkyl phthalates. *Regul Toxicol Pharmacol.* 1999;30:40–53.

Caldwell JC, Evans MV, Marcus AH, et al. Comments on article "Applying mode-of-action and pharmacokinetic considerations in contemporary cancer risk assessments: an example with trichloroethylene" by Clewell and Andersen. *Crit Rev Toxicol.* 2006;36:291–294.

Caldwell JC, Keshava N. Key issues in the modes of action and effects of trichloroethylene metabolites for liver and kidney tumorigenesis. *Environ Health Perspect.* 2006;114:1457–1463.

Campbell JL Jr, Fisher JW. A PBPK modeling assessment of the competitive metabolic interactions of JP-8 vapor with two constituents, *m*-xylene and ethylbenzene. *Inhal Toxicol.* 2007;19:265–273.

Cantor KP, Stewart PA, Brinton LA, Dosemaci M. Occupational exposures and female breast cancer mortality in the United States. *J Occup Environ Med.* 1995;37:336–348.

Caprino L, Togna GI. Potential health effects of gasoline and its constituents: a review of current literature (1990–1997) on toxicological data. *Environ Health Perspect.* 1998;106:115–125.

Carlson GP. In vitro metabolism of styrene to styrene oxide in liver and lung of CYP2E1 knockout mice. *J Toxicol Environ Health A.* 2003;66:861–869.

Carlson GP. Critical appraisal of the expression of cytochrome P450 enzymes in human lung and evaluation of the possibility that such expression provides evidence of potential styrene tumorigenicity in humans. *Toxicology.* 2008;254:1–10.

Carlson GP. Metabolism and toxicity of styrene in microsomal epoxide hydrolase-deficient mice. *J Toxicol Environ Health A.* 2010;74:1689–1699.

Carney EW, Freshour NL, Dittenber DA, Dryzga MD. Ethylene glycol developmental toxicity: unraveling the roles of glycolic acid and metabolic acidosis. *Toxicol Sci.* 1999;50:117–126.

Carney EW, Liberacki AB, Bartels MJ, Breslin WJ. Identification of proximate toxicant for ethylene glycol developmental toxicity using rat whole embryo culture. *Teratology.* 1996;53:38–46.

Caro AA, Cederbaum AI. Oxidative stress, toxicology, and pharmacology of CYP2E1. *Annu Rev Pharmacol Toxicol.* 2004;44:27–42.

Casanova M, Bell DA, Heck H d'A. Dichloromethane metabolism to formaldehyde and reaction of formaldehyde with nucleic acids in hepatocytes of rodents and humans with and without glutathione *S*-transferase T1 and M1 genes. *Fundam Appl Toxicol.* 1997;37:168–180.

Casanova M, Conolly RB, Heck H d'A. DNA–protein cross-links (DPX) and cell proliferation in B6C3F1 mice but not Syrian golden hamsters exposed to dichloromethane: pharmacokinetics and risk assessment with DPX as dosimeter. *Fundam Appl Toxicol.* 1996;31:103–116.

Casanova M, Heck H d'A. Lack of evidence for the involvement of formaldehyde in the hepatocarcinogenicity of methyl *tertiary*-butyl ether in CD-1 mice. *Chem Biol Interact.* 1997;105:131–143.

Castillo T, Koop DR, Kamimura S, et al. Role of cytochrome P-450 2E1 in ethanol-, carbon tetrachloride- and iron-dependent microsomal lipid peroxidation. *Hepatology.* 1992;16:992–996.

Cattley RC, DeLuca J, Elcombe C, et al. Do peroxisome proliferating compounds pose a hepatocarcinogenic hazard to humans? *Regul Toxicol Pharmacol.* 1998;27:47–60.

Cawley MJ. Short-term lorazepam infusion and concern for propylene glycol toxicity: case report and review. *Pharmacotherapy.* 2001;21:1140–1144.

Chan WK, Nguyen LT, Miller VP, Harris RZ. Mechanism-based inactivation of human cytochrome P450 3A4 by grapefruit juice and red wine. *Life Sci.* 1998;62:135–142.

Chang TKH, Chen J, Yeung EYH. Effect of *Ginkgo biloba* extract on procarcinogen-bioactivating human CYP enzymes: identification of isorhamnetin, kaempferol, and quercetin as potent inhibitors of CYP1B1. *Toxicol Appl Pharmacol.* 2006;213:18–26.

Chang YM, Tai CF, Yang SC, et al. Cancer incidence among workers potentially exposed to chlorinated solvents in an electronics factory. *J Occup Health.* 2005;47:171–180.

Chao YC, Gibson RL, Nylander-French LA. Dermal exposure to jet fuel (JP-8) in US Air Force personnel. *Ann Occup Hyg.* 2005;49:639–648.

Chapin RE, Dutton SD, Ross MD, et al. The effects of ethylene glycol monomethyl ether on testicular histology in F344 rats. *J Androl.* 1984;5:369–380.

Charbonneau M, Swenberg JA. Studies on the biochemical mechanism of α_u-globulin nephropathy in rats. *CIIT Activities.* 1988;8:1–5.

Charbotel B, Fevotte J, Hours M, et al. Case–control study on renal cell cancer and occupational exposure to trichloroethylene. Part II: epidemiological aspects. *Ann Occup Hyg.* 2006;50:777–787.

Charbotel B, Gad S, Caiola D, et al. Trichloroethylene exposure and somatic mutations of the VHL gene in patients with renal cell carcinoma. *J Occup Med Toxicol.* 2007;2:13–20.

Chen DH, Kaung HL, Miller CM, et al. Microarray analysis of changes in renal phenotype in the ethylene glycol rat model of urolithiasis: potential and pitfalls. *BJU Int.* 2004;94:637–650.

Chen PC, Hsieh GY, Wang JD, Cheng TJ. Prolonged time to pregnancy in female workers exposed to ethylene glycol ethers in semiconductor manufacturing. *Epidemiology.* 2002;13:191–196.

Cheng P-Y, Morgan ET. Hepatic cytochrome P450 regulation in disease states. *Curr Drug Metab.* 2001;2:165–183.

Cherry NH, Hutchins H, Pace T, Waldron JA. Neurobehavioral effects of repeated occupational exposure to toluene and paint solvents. *Br J Ind Med.* 1985;42:291–300.

Chiu WA, Micallef S, Monster AC, Bois FY. Toxicokinetics of inhaled trichloroethylene and tetrachloroethylene in humans at 1 ppm: empirical results and comparisons with previous studies. *Toxicol Sci.* 2007;95:23–26.

Cho SK, Kim RH, Yim SH, et al. Long-term neuropsychological effects and MRI findings in patients with CS_2 poisoning. *Acta Neurol Scand.* 2002;106:269–275.

Chou CC, Riviere JE, Monteiro-Riviere NA. Differential relationship between the carbon chain length of jet fuel aliphatic hydrocarbons and their ability to induce cytotoxicity vs. interleukin-8 release in human epidermal keratinocytes. *Toxicol Sci.* 2002;69:226–233.

Chou CC, Riviere JE, Monteiro-Riviere NA. The cytotoxicity of jet fuel aromatic hydrocarbons and dose-related interleukin-8 release from human epidermal keratinocytes. *Arch Toxicol.* 2003;77:384–391.

Chou CC, Yang JH, Chen SD, et al. Expression profiling of human epidermal keratinocyte response following 1-minute JP-8 exposure. *Cutan Ocul Toxicol.* 2006;25:141–153.

Chow W-H, Devesa SS. Contemporary renal cell epidemiology. *Cancer J.* 2008;14:288–301.

Christopher MM, Eckfeldt JH, Eaton JW. Propylene glycol ingestion causes D-lactic acidosis. *Lab Invest.* 1990;62:114–118.

Chrostek L, Jelski W, Szmitkowski M, Puchalski Z. Gender-related differences in hepatic activity of alcohol dehydrogenase isoenzymes and aldehyde dehydrogenase in humans. *J Clin Lab Anal.* 2003;17:93–96.

Chu I, Poon R, Valli V, et al. Effects of an ethanol–gasoline mixture: results of a 4-week inhalation study in rats. *J Appl Toxicol.* 2005;25:193–199.

Chun JS, Burleigh-Flayer HD, Kintigh WJ. *Methyl tertiary Butyl Ether: Vapor Inhalation Oncogenicity Study in Fisher 344 Rats.* Export, PA: Bushy Run Research Center; 1992.

Chung HC, Sung SH, Kim JS, et al. Lack of cytochrome P450 2E1 (CYP2E1) induction in the rat liver by starvation without coprophagy. *Drug Metab Dispos.* 2001;29:213–216.

Chung J-K, Yuan W, Liu G, Zheng J. Investigation of bioactivation and toxicity of styrene in CYP2E1 transgenic cells. *Toxicology.* 2006;226:99–106.

Churchill JE, Ashley DL, Kaye WE. Recent chemical exposures and blood volatile organic compound levels in a large population-based sample. *Arch Environ Health.* 2001;56:157–166.

Cirvello JD, Radovsky A, Heath JE, et al. Toxicity and carcinogenicity of *t*-butyl alcohol in rats and mice following chronic exposure in drinking water. *Toxicol Ind Health.* 1995;11:151–165.

Clarke DO, Duignan JM, Welsch F. 2-Methoxyacetic acid dosimetry–teratogenicity relationships in CD-1 mice exposed to 2-methoxyethanol. *Toxicol Appl Pharmacol.* 1992;114:77–87.

Clary JJ. Methanol, is it a developmental risk to humans? *Regul Toxicol Pharmacol.* 2003;37:83–91.

Clawson GA, MacDonald J, Woo C. Early hypomethylation of 2-0-ribose moieties in hepatocytes cytoplasmic ribosomal RNA underlies the protein synthesis defect produced by CCl_4. *J Cell Biol.* 1987;105:705–711.

Clayton CA, Pellizzari ED, Whitmore RW, et al. National Human Exposure Assessment Survey (NHEXAS): distributions and associations of lead, arsenic and volatile organic compounds in EPA Region 5. *J Expos Anal Environ Epidemiol.* 1999;9:381–392.

Clewell HJ, Andersen ME. Applying mode-of-action and pharmacokinetic considerations in contemporary cancer risk assessments: an example with trichloroethylene. *Crit Rev Toxicol.* 2004;34:385–445.

Clewell HJ, Andersen ME. Response to comments by Caldwell *et al.* on article "Applying mode-of-action and pharmacokinetic considerations in contemporary cancer risk assessments: an example with trichloroethylene." *Crit Rev Toxicol.* 2006;36:295–298.

Clewell HJ, Gentry PR, Covington TR, et al. Evaluation of the potential impact of age- and gender-specific pharmacokinetic differences on tissue dosimetry. *Toxicol Sci.* 2004;79:381–393.

Clewell HJ, Tan YM, Campbell JL, Andersen ME. Quantitative interpretation of human biomonitoring data. *Toxicol Appl Pharmacol.* 2008;231:122–133.

Clewell HJ, Teeguarden J, McDonald T, et al. Review and evaluation of the potential impact of age- and gender-specific pharmacokinetic differences on tissue dosimetry. *Crit Rev Toxicol.* 2002;32(5):329–389.

Cogliano VJ, Grosse Y, Baan RA, et al. Meeting report: summary of IARC monographs on formaldehyde, 2-butoxyethanol, and 1-*tert*-butoxy-2-propanol. *Environ Health Perspect.* 2005;113:1205–1208.

Colantoni A, Idilman R, De Maria N, et al. Hepatic apoptosis and proliferation in male and female rats fed alcohol: role of cytokines. *Alcohol Clin Exp Res.* 2003;27:1184–1189.

Colborn T. A case for revisiting the safety of pesticides: a closer look at neurodevelopment. *Environ Health Perspect.* 2006;114:10–17.

Cole CE, Tran HT, Schlosser PM. Physiologically based pharmacokinetic modeling of benzene metabolism in mice through extrapolation from in vitro to in vivo. *J Toxicol Environ Health A.* 2001;62:439–465.

Collins JJ, Ireland BK, Easterday PA, et al. Evaluation of lymphopenia among workers with low-level benzene exposure and the utility of routine data collection. *J Occup Environ Med.* 1997;39:232–237.

Conolly R. The use of biologically based modeling in risk assessment. *Toxicology.* 2002;181–182:275–279.

Constan AA, Sprankle CS, Peters JM, et al. Metabolism of chloroform by cytochrome P4502E1 is required for induction of toxicity in the liver, kidney, and nose of male mice. *Toxicol Appl Pharmacol.* 1999;160:120–126.

Constan AA, Wong BA, Everitt JI, Butterworth BE. Chloroform inhalation exposure conditions necessary to initiate liver toxicity in female B6C3F1 mice. *Toxicol Sci.* 2002;66:201–208.

Cooper GS, Markris SL, Nietert PG, Jinot J. Evidence of autoimmune-related effects of trichloroethylene exposure from studies in mice and humans. *Environ Health Perspect.* 2009;117:696–702.

Cordier S, Bergeret A, Goujard J, et al. Congenital malformations and maternal occupational exposure to glycol ethers. *Epidemiology.* 1997;8:355–363.

Coresh J, Selvin E, Stevens LA, et al. Prevalence of chronic kidney disease in the United States. *JAMA.* 2007;398:2038–2047.

Corley RA, Bartels MJ, Carney EW, et al. Development of a physiologically based pharmacokinetic model for ethylene glycol and its metabolite, glycolic acid, in rats and humans. *Toxicol Sci.* 2005a;85:476–490.

Corley RA, Bormett GA, Ghanayem BI. Physiologically based pharmacokinetics of 2-butoxyethanol and its major metabolite, 2-butoxyacetic acid, in rats and humans. *Toxicol Appl Pharmacol.* 1994;129:61–79.

Corley RA, Gies RA, Wu H, Weitz KK. Development of a physiologically based pharmacokinetic model for propylene glycol monomethyl ether and its acetate in rats and humans. *Toxicol Lett.* 2005b;156:193–213.

Corley RA, Grant DM, Farris E, et al. Determination of age and gender differences in biochemical processes affecting the disposition of 2-butoxyethanol and its metabolites in mice and rats to improve PBPK modeling. *Toxicol Lett.* 2005c;156:127–161.

Corley RA, Mast TJ, Carney EW, et al. Evaluation of physiologically based models of pregnancy and lactation for their application in children's health risk assessments. *Crit Rev Toxicol.* 2003;33:137–211.

Corley RA, McMartin KE. Incorporation of therapeutic interventions in physiologically based pharmacokinetic modeling of human clinical case reports of accidental or intentional overdosing with ethylene glycol. *Toxicol Sci.* 2005;85:491–501.

Corley RA, Meek ME, Carney EW. Mode of action: oxalate crystal-induced renal tubule degeneration and glycolic acid-induced dysmorphogenesis—renal and developmental effects of ethylene glycol. *Crit Rev Toxicol.* 2005d;35:691–702.

Correa A, Gray R, Cohen R, et al. Ethylene glycol ethers and risks of spontaneous abortion and subfertility. *Am J Epidemiol.* 1996;143:707–717.

Corthals SM, Kamendulis LM, Klaunig JE. Mechanism of 2-butoxyethanol-induced hemangiosarcomas. *Toxicol Sci.* 2006;92:378–386.

Costa ET, Savage DD, Valenzuela CF. A review of the effects of prenatal or early postnatal ethanol exposure on brain ligand-gated ion channels. *Alcohol Clin Exp Res.* 2000;24:706–715.

Cotreau MM, von Moltke LL, Greenblatt DJ. The influence of age and sex on the clearance of cytochrome P450 3A substrates. *Clin Pharmacokinet.* 2005;44:33–60.

Covington TR, Gentry PR, Van Landingham CB, et al. The use of Markov chain Monte Carlo uncertainty analysis to support a public health goal for perchloroethylene. *Regul Toxicol Pharmacol.* 2007;47:1–18.

Crabb DW, Matsumoto M, Chang D, You M. Overview of the role of alcohol dehydrogenase and aldehyde dehydrogenase and their variants in the genesis of alcohol-related pathology. *Proc Nutr Soc.* 2004;63:49–63.

Cranmer JM. Proceedings of the workshop on neurobehavioral effects of solvents. *Neurotoxicology.* 1986;7:1–95.

Creasy DM, Foster PMD. The morphological development of glycol ether-induced testicular atrophy in the rat. *Exp Mol Pathol.* 1984;40:169–176.

Creek MR, Mani C, Vogel JS, Turteltaub KW. Tissue distribution and macro-molecular binding of extremely low doses of [^{14}C]-benzene in B6C3F1 mice. *Carcinogenesis.* 1997;18:2421–2427.

Cresteil T. Onset of xenobiotic metabolism in children: toxicological implications. *Food Add Contam.* 1998;15(suppl):45–51.

Cruz SL, Balster RL, Woodward JJ. Effects of volatile solvents on recombinant *N*-methyl-D-aspartate receptors expressed in *Xenopus* oocytes. *Br J Pharmacol.* 2000;131:1303–1308.

Cruz SL, Mirshahi T, Thomas B, et al. Effects of the abused solvent toluene on recombinant *N*-methyl-D-aspartate and non-*N*-methyl-D-aspartate receptors expressed in *Xenopus* oocytes. *J Pharmacol Exp Ther.* 1998;286:334–340.

Cruzan G. Assessment of the cancer potential of methanol. *Crit Rev Toxicol.* 2009;39:347–363.

Cruzan G, Cushman JR, Andrews LS, et al. Chronic toxicity/oncogenicity study of styrene in CD rats by inhalation exposure for 104 weeks. *Toxicol Sci.* 1998;46:266–281.

Cruzan G, Cushman JR, Andrews LS, et al. Chronic toxicity/oncogenicity study of styrene in CD-1 mice by inhalation exposure for 104 weeks. *J Appl Toxicol.* 2001;21:185–198.

d'Alessandro A, Osterloh JD, Chuwers P, et al. Formate in serum and urine after controlled methanol exposure at the threshold limit value. *Environ Health Perspect.* 1994;102:178–181.

Dai Y, Rashba-Step J, Cederbaum AI. Stable expression of human cytochrome P4502E1 in HepG2 cells: characterization of catalytic activities and production of reactive oxygen intermediates. *Biochemistry.* 1993;32:6928–6937.

Dallas CE, Ramanathan R, Muralidhara S, et al. The uptake and elimination of 1,1,1-trichloroethane during and following inhalation exposures in rats. *Toxicol Appl Pharmacol.* 1989;98:385–397.

Dankovic DA, Bailer AJ. The impact of exercise and intersubject variability on dose estimates for dichloromethane derived from a physiologically based pharmacokinetic model. *Fundam Appl Toxicol.* 1994;22:20–25.

Daston G, Faustman E, Ginsberg G, et al. A framework for assessing risks to children from exposure to environmental agents. *Environ Health Perspect.* 2004;112:238–256.

Daughtrey WC, Gill MW, Pritts IM, et al. Neurotoxicological evaluation of methyl *tertiary*-butyl ether in rats. *J Appl Toxicol.* 1997;17(S1):S57–S64.

David RM, Clewell HJ, Gentry PR, et al. Revised assessment of cancer risk to dichloromethane. II. Application of probabilistic methods to cancer risk determinations. *Regul Toxicol Pharmacol.* 2006;45:55–65.

Davis BJ, Almekinder JL, Flagler N, et al. Ovarian luteal cell toxicity of ethylene glycol monomethyl ether and methoxy acetic acid in vivo and in vitro. *Toxicol Appl Pharmacol.* 1997;142:328–337.

Davis ME. Dichloroacetic acid and trichloroacetic acid increase chloroform toxicity. *J Toxicol Environ Health.* 1992;37:139–148.

de Ketttenis P. The historic and current use of glycol ethers: a picture of change. *Toxicol Lett.* 2005;156:5–11.

de Peyster A, MacLean KJ, Stephens BA, et al. Subchronic studies in Sprague–Dawley rats to investigate mechanisms of MTBE-induced Leydig cell cancer. *Toxicol Sci.* 2003;72:31–42.

De Salvia MA, Cagiano R, Carratu MR, et al. Irreversible impairment of active avoidance behavior in rats prenatally exposed to mild concentrations of carbon monoxide. *Psychopharmacology.* 1995;122:66–71.

Degitz SJ, Rogers JM, Zucker RM, Hunter ES III. Developmental toxicity of methanol: pathogenesis in CD-1 and C57BL/6J mice exposed in whole embryo culture. *Birth Defects Res A Clin Mol Teratol.* 2004;70:179–184.

Dekant W. The role of biotransformation and bioactivation in toxicity. In: Luch A, ed. *Molecular Clinical and Environmental Toxicology.* Vol. 1. Switzerland: Birkhauser Verlag; 2009:57–86.

Dekant W, Bernauer U, Rosner E, Amberg A. Biotransformation of MTBE, ETBE, and TAME after inhalation or ingestion in rats and humans. *Res Rep Health Eff Inst.* 2001;102:29–71.

Dekant W, Metzler M, Henschler D. Identification of S-(1,2,2-trichlorovinyl)-*N*-acetylcysteine as a urinary metabolite of tetrachloroethylene: bioactivation through glutathione conjugation as a possible explanation for its nephrocarcinogenicity. *J Biochem Toxicol.* 1986;1:57–71.

Dell LD, Mundt KA, McDonald M, et al. Critical review of the epidemiology literature on the potential cancer risks of methylene chloride. *Int Arch Occup Environ Health.* 1999;72:429–442.

Dennison JE, Bigelow PL, Mumtaz, MM, et al. Evaluation of potential toxicity from co-exposure to three CNS depressants (toluene, ethylbenzene, and xylene) under resting and working conditions using PBPK modeling. *J Occup Environ Hyg.* 2005;2:127–135.

DePass LR, Garman RH, Woodside MD, et al. Chronic toxicity and oncogenicity studies of ethylene glycol in rats and mice. *Fundam Appl Toxicol.* 1986;7:547–565.

Devi SS, Mehendale HM. Disrupted G1 to S phase clearance via cyclin signaling impairs liver tissue repair in thioacetamide-treated type I diabetic rats. *Toxicol Appl Pharmacol.* 2005;207:89–102.

Devi SS, Mehendale HM. Microarray analysis of thioacetamide-treated type I diabetic rats. *Toxicol Appl Pharmacol.* 2006;212:69–78.

DeVincenzo GD, Kaplan CJ. Effect of exercise or smoking on the uptake, metabolism and excretion of methylene chloride vapor. *Toxicol Appl Pharmacol.* 1981;59:141–148.

Diaz G, Castro JA. Covalent binding of chloroform metabolites to nuclear proteins—no evidence for binding to nucleic acids. *Cancer Lett.* 1980;9:213–218.

DiCecco SR, Francisco-Ziller N. Nutrition in alcoholic liver disease. *Nutr Clin Pract.* 2006;21:245–254.

Diehl AM. Cytokine regulation of liver injury and repair. *Immunol Rev.* 2000;174:160–171.

Dietrich DR, Swenberg JA. NCI–Black–Reiter (NBR) male rats fail to develop renal disease following exposure to agents that induce α-2u-globulin (α2u) nephropathy. *Fundam Appl Toxicol.* 1991;16:749–762.

Dietzel KD, Campbell JL, Bartlett MG, et al. Validation of a gas chromatography/mass spectrometry method for quantification of aerosolized Jet Propellant 8. *J Chromatogr A.* 2005;1093:11–20.

Dill J, Fuciarelli A, Lee K, et al. Toxicokinetics of propylene glycol mono-*t*-butyl ether following intravenous or inhalation exposure in rats and mice. *Inhal Toxicol.* 2004;16:271–290.

Ding X, Kaminsky LS. Human extrahepatic cytochromes P450: function in xenobiotic metabolism and tissue-selective chemical toxicity in the respiratory and gastrointestinal tracts. *Annu Rev Pharmacol Toxicol.* 2003;43:149–173.

DiVincenzo GD, Kaplan CJ. Uptake, metabolism, and elimination of methylene chloride vapor by humans. *Toxicol Appl Pharmacol.* 1981;59:130–140.

Dixit R, Riviere J, Krishnan K, Andersen ME. Toxicokinetics and physiologically based toxicokinetics in toxicology and risk assessment. *J Toxicol Environ Health B.* 2003;6:1–40.

Dobrev ID, Andersen ME, Yang RS. In silico toxicology: stimulating inter-action thresholds for human exposure to mixtures of trichloroethylene, tetrachloroethylene, and 1,1,1-trichloroethane. *Environ Health Perspect.* 2002;110:1031–1039.

Dobrev ID, Andersen ME, Yang RSH. Assessing interaction thresholds for trichloroethylene in combination with tetrachloroethylene and 1,1,1-tri-chloroethane using gas uptake studies and PBPK modeling. *Arch Toxicol.* 2001;75:134–144.

Doherty RE. A history of the production and use of carbon tetrachloride, tetrachloroethylene, trichloroethylene and 1,1,1-trichloroethane in the United States: part 2—trichloroethylene and 1,1,1-trichloroethane. *J Environ Forensics.* 2000;1:83–93.

Doi AM, Hill G, Seely J, et al. $\alpha_{2\mu}$-Globulin in nephropathy and renal tumors in National Toxicology Program studies. *Toxicol Pathol.* 2007;35: 533–540.

Doi AM, Roycroft JH, Herbert RA, et al. Inhalation toxicology and carcino-genesis studies of propylene glycol mono-*t*-butyl ether in rats and mice. *Toxicology.* 2004;199:1–22.

Dorman DC, Allen SL, Byczkowski JZ, et al. Methods to identify and char-acterize developmental neurotoxicity for human health risk assessment. III. Pharmacokinetics and pharmacodynamic considerations. *Environ Health Perspect.* 2001;109(suppl 1):101–111.

Dorman DC, Struve MF, Clewell HJ III, Andersen ME. Application of phar-macokinetic data to the risk assessment of inhaled manganese. *Toxicol Sci.* 2009;108:22–34.

Dorman DC, Welsch F. *CIIT Activities.* 1996;16:1–7.

Drake MG, Witzmann FA, Hyde J, Witten ML. JP-8 jet fuel exposure alters protein expression in the lung. *Toxicology.* 2003;191:199–210.

Dresser GK, Bailey DG. The effects of fruit juices on drug disposition: a new model for drug interactions. *Eur J Clin Invest.* 2003;33(suppl 2):10–16.

Drexler H, Ulm K, Hardt R, et al. Carbon disulphide: IV. Cardiovascular function in workers in the viscose industry. *Int Arch Occup Environ Health.* 1996;69:27–32.

Echeverria D, White RF, Sampaio C. A behavioral evaluation of PCE expo-sure in patients and dry cleaners: a possible relationship between clinical and preclinical effects. *J Occup Environ Med.* 1995;37:667–680.

Edwards MJ, Keller BJ, Kauffman FC, Thurman RG. The involvement of Kupffer cells in carbon tetrachloride toxicity. *Toxicol Appl Pharmacol.* 1993;119:275–279.

Eells JT, Henry MM, Lewandowski MF, et al. Development and character-ization of a rodent model of methanol-induced retinal and optic nerve toxicity. *Neurotoxicology.* 2000;21:321–330.

Eells JT, Henry MM, Summerfelt P. Therapeutic photobiomodulation for methanol-induced retinal toxicity. *Proc Natl Acad Sci U S A.* 2003;100: 3439–3444.

Eells JT, Salzman MM, Lewandowski MR, Murray TG. Formate-induced alterations in retinal function in methanol-intoxicated rats. *Toxicol Appl Pharmacol.* 1996;140:58–69.

Egbert PA, Abraham K. Ethylene glycol intoxication: pathophysiology, diagnosis, and emergency management. *ANNA J.* 1999;26:295–302.

Elfarra AA, Krause RJ. *S*-(1,2,2-Trichlorovinyl)-L-cysteine sulfoxide, a reactive metabolite of *S*-(1,2,2-trichlorovinyl)-L-cysteine formed in rat liver and kidney microsomes, is a potent nephrotoxicant. *J Pharmacol Exp Ther.* 2007;321:1095–1101.

Elliot BM, Ashby J. Review of the genotoxicity of 2-butoxyethanol. *Mutat Res.* 1997;387:89–96.

Elliott L, Longnecker MP, Kissling GE, London SJ. Volatile organic com-pounds and pulmonary function in the Third National Examination Survey. *Environ Health Perspect.* 2006;114:1210–1214.

El-Masri HA, Bell DA, Portier CJ. Effects of glutathione transferase theta polymorphism on the risk estimates of dichloromethane to humans. *Toxicol Appl Pharmacol.* 1999;158:221–230.

El-Masri HA, Tessari JD, Yang RS. Extrapolation of an interaction threshold for the joint toxicity of trichloroethylene and 1,1-dichloro-ethylene: utilization of a PBPK model. *Arch Toxicol.* 1996;70: 527–539.

Engelke M, Tahti H, Vaalavirta L. Perturbation of artificial and biological membranes by organic compounds of aliphatic, alicyclic and aromatic structure. *Toxicol In Vitro.* 1996;10:111–115.

EPA. *Risk Assessment Guidance for Superfund. Human Health Evaluation Manual Part A, Interim Final.* Washington, DC: Office of Emergency and Remedial Response; 1989.

EPA (U.S. Environmental Protection Agency). *Drinking Water Advisory: Consumer Acceptability Advice and Health Effects Analysis on Methyl tertiary-Butyl Ether (MtBE).* Washington, DC: Office of Water; December 1997.

EPA (U.S. Environmental Protection Agency). *Risk Assessment Guidance for Superfund. Human Health Evaluation Manual Supplemental Guidance, Dermal Risk Assessment, Interim Guidance.* Vol. I. Washington, DC: Office of Emergency and Remedial Response; 1998a.

EPA (Environmental Protection Agency). *On-Line Integrated Risk Information System (IRIS) Substance File—1,1,1-Trichloroethane.* Washington, DC: EPA; 1998b. Available at: http://www.epa.gov/iris/subst/0020.htm.

EPA (U.S. Environmental Protection Agency). *Trichloroethylene Health Risk Assessment: Synthesis and Characterization.* External review draft. EPA/600/P-01/002A. Washington, DC: National Center for Environmental Assessment; 2001a.

EPA (U.S. Environmental Protection Agency). *On-Line Integrated Risk Information System (IRIS) Substance File—Chloroform.* Washington, DC: EPA; 2001b. Available at: http://www.epa.gov/iris/subst/0025.htm.

EPA (U.S. Environmental Protection Agency). *National Primary Drinking Water Regulations.* EPA/816/F-02/013. Washington, DC: Office of Ground Water and Drinking Water; 2002. Available at; http://www.epa.gov/safewater/mcl.html.

EPA (U.S. Environmental Protection Agency). *Guidelines for Carcinogen Risk Assessment.* Risk Assessment Forum, EPA/630/P-03/001F. Washington, DC: EPA; 2005.

EPA (U.S. Environmental Protection Agency). *EPA Toxics Release Inventory.* 2006a. Available at: http://semanticcommunity.info/EPA/Web.

EPA (U.S. Environmental Protection Agency). *On-Line Integrated Risk Information System (IRIS) Substance File—Ethylene Glycol.* Washington, DC: EPA; July 30, 2006b. Available at: http://www.epa.gov/iris/subst/0238.htm.

EPA (U.S. Environmental Protection Agency). *On-Line Integrated Risk Information System (IRIS) Substance File—Carbon Disulfide.* Washington, DC: EPA; July 17, 2006c. Available at: http://www.epa.gov/iris/subst/0217.htm.

EPA (U.S. Environmental Protection Agency). *On-Line Integrated Risk Information System (IRIS) Substance File—Benzene.* Washington, DC: EPA; 2007. Available at: http://www.epa.gov/iris/subst/index.html.

EPA (U.S. Environmental Protection Agency). *Toxicological Review of Tetrachloroethylene (Perchloroethylene).* In support of IRIS. External review draft, EPA/635/R-08/011A. Washington, DC: EPA; 2008.

EPA (U.S. Environmental Protection Agency). *Toxicological Review of Trichloroethylene.* In support of IRIS. External review draft, EPA/635/R-09/011A. Washington, DC: EPA; 2009.

EPA (U.S. Environmental Protection Agency). *Toxicological Review of Dichloromethane (Methylene Chloride). In Support of IRIS.* External review draft, EPA/635/R-10/003A. Washington, DC: EPA; 2010a.

EPA (U.S. Environmental Protection Agency). *On-Line Integrated Risk Information System (IRIS) Substance File—Carbon Tetrachloride.* Washington, DC: EPA; 2010b. Available at: http://www.epa.gov/iris/subst/0020.htm.

EPA (U.S. Environmental Protection Agency). *On-Line Integrated Risk Information System (IRIS) Substance File—Ethylene Glycol Monobutyl Ether (EGBE) (2-Butoxyethanol).* Washington, DC: EPA; August 1, 2012. Available at: http://www.epa.gov/iris/subst/0500.htm.

Erdal S, Gong H Jr, Linn WS, Rykowski R. Projection of health benefits from ambient ozone reduction related to the use of methyl *tertiary* butyl ether (MTBE) in the reformulated gasoline program. *Risk Anal.* 1997;17:693–704.

Eschenbrenner AB, Miller E. Induction of hepatomas in mice by repeated oral administration of chloroform, with observations on sex differences. *J Natl Cancer Inst.* 1945;5:251–255.

Espinoza LA, Li P, Lee RY, et al. Evaluation of gene expression profile of keratinocytes in response to JP-8 jet fuel. *Toxicol Appl Pharmacol.* 2004;200:93–102.

Espinoza LA, Valikhani M, Cossio MJ, et al. Altered expression of γ-synuclein and detoxification-related genes in lungs of rats exposed to JP-8. *Am J Resp Cell Mol.* 2005;32:192–200.

Exon JH, Mather GG, Bussiere JL. Effects of subchronic exposure of rats to 2-methoxyethanol or 2-butoxyethanol: thymic atrophy and immunotoxicity. *Fundam Appl Toxicol.* 1991;16:830–840.

Fabrizi L, Taylor GW, Canas B, et al. Adduction of the chloroform metabolite phosgene to lysine residues of human histone H2B. *Chem Res Toxicol.* 2003;16:266–275.

Filley CM, Halliday W, Kleinschmidt-DeMasters BK. The effects of toluene on the central nervous system. *J Neuropathol Exp Neurol.* 2004;63:1–12.

Fisher J, Lumpkin M, Boyd J, et al. PBPK modeling of the interaction between carbon tetrachloride and tetrachloroethylene in mice. *Environ Toxicol Pharmacol.* 2004;16:93–105.

Fisher JW, Channel SR, Eggers JS, et al. Trichloroethylene, trichloroacetic acid, and dichloroacetic acid: do they affect fetal rat heart development? *Int J Toxicol.* 2001;20:257–67.

Fisher JW, Mahle D, Abbas R. A human physiologically based pharmacokinetic model for trichloroethylene and its metabolites, trichloroacetic acid and free trichloroethanol. *Toxicol Appl Pharmacol.* 1998;152:339–359.

Fitzhugh OG, Nelson AA. Comparison of the chronic toxicity of triethylene glycol with that of diethylene glycol. *J Ind Hyg Toxicol.* 1946;28:40–43.

Fletcher CV, Acosta CP, Strykowski JM. Gender differences in human pharmacokinetics and pharmacodynamics. *J Adolesc Health.* 1994;15:619–629.

Folland DS, Schaffner W, Ginn EH, et al. Carbon tetrachloride toxicity potentiated by isopropyl alcohol. *JAMA.* 1976;236:1853–1856.

Foo SC, Jeyaratnam J, Koh D. Chronic neurobehavioral effects of toluene. *Br J Ind Med.* 1990;47:480–484.

Foote RH, Farrell PB, Schlafer DH, et al. Ethylene glycol monomethyl ether effects on health and reproduction in male rabbits. *Reprod Toxicol.* 1995;9:527–539.

Forkert P-G, Baldwin RM, Millen B, et al. Pulmonary bioactivation of trichloroethylene to chloral hydrate: relative contributions of CYP2E1, CYP2F, and CYP2B1. *Drug Metab Dispos.* 2005;33:1429–1437.

Forkert P-G, Lash L, Tardif R, et al. Identification of trichloroethylene and its metabolites in human seminal fluid of workers exposed to trichloroethylene. *Drug Metab Dispos.* 2003;31:306–311.

Forkert P-G, Millen B, Lash LH, et al. Pulmonary bronchiolar cytotoxicity and formation of dichloroacetyl lysine protein adducts in mice treated with trichloroethylene. *J Pharmacol Exp Ther.* 2006;316:520–529.

Fortenberry JD. Gasoline sniffing. *Am J Med.* 1985;79:740–744.

Foxenberg RJ, Ellison CA, Knaak JB, et al. Cytochrome P450-specific human PBPK/PD models for the organophosphorus pesticides: chlorpyrifos and parathion. *Toxicology.* 2011;285:57–66.

Franchini I, Cavtorta A, Falzoi M, et al. Early indicators of renal damage in workers exposed to organic solvents. *Int Arch Occup Environ Health.* 1983;52:1–9.

Franks SJ, Spendiff MK, Cocker J, Loizou GD. Physiologically based pharmacokinetic modeling of human exposure to 2-butoxyethanol. *Toxicol Lett.* 2006;162:164–173.

Frantz SW, Beskitt JL, Grosse CM, et al. Pharmacokinetics of ethylene glycol. I. Plasma disposition after single intravenous, peroral, or percutaneous doses in female Sprague–Dawley rats and CD-1 mice. *Drug Metab Dispos.* 1996a;24:911–921.

Frantz SW, Beskitt JL, Grosse CM, et al. Pharmacokinetics of ethylene glycol. II. Tissue distribution, dose-dependent elimination, and identification of urinary metabolites following single intravenous, peroral or percutaneous doses in female Sprague–Dawley rats and CD-1 mice. *Xenobiotica.* 1996b;26:1195–1220.

Frantz SW, Beskitt JL, Tallant MJ, et al. Pharmacokinetics of ethylene glycol. III. Plasma disposition and metabolic fate after single increasing intravenous, peroral, or percutaneous doses in the male Sprague–Dawley rat. *Xenobiotica.* 1996c;26:515–539.

Fraser MP, Cass GR, Simoneit BRT. Gas-phase and particle-phase organic compounds emitted from motor vehicle traffic in a Los Angeles roadway tunnel. *Environ Sci Technol.* 1998;32:2051–2060.

Frezza M, di Padova C, Pozzato G, et al. High blood alcohol levels in women. The role of decreased gastric alcohol dehydrogenase activity and first-pass metabolism. *N Engl J Med.* 1990;322:95–99.

Froberg K, Dorion RP, McMartin KE. The role of calcium oxalate crystal deposition in cerebral vessels during ethylene glycol poisoning. *Clin Toxicol.* 2006;44:315–318.

Gade A, Mortensen EL, Bruhn P. "Chronic painter's syndrome." A reanalysis of psychological test data in a group of diagnosed cases, based on comparisons with matched controls. *Acta Neurol Scand.* 1988;77:293–306.

Gallucci RM, O'Dell SK, Rabe D, Fechter LD. JP-8 jet fuel exposure induces inflammatory cytokines in rat skin. *Int Immunopharmacol.* 2004;4:1159–1169.

Gandhi M, Aweeka F, Greenblatt RM, Blaschke TF. Sex differences in pharmacokinetics and pharmacodynamics. *Annu Rev Pharmacol Toxicol.* 2004;44:499–523.

Garetano G, Gochfeld M. Factors affecting tetrachloroethylene concentrations in residences above dry cleaning establishments. *Arch Environ Health.* 2000;55:59–68.

Gargas ML, Burgess RJ, Voisard DE, et al. Partition coefficients of low-molecular-weight volatile chemicals in various liquids and tissues. *Toxicol Appl Pharmacol.* 1989;98:87–99.

Gargas ML, Tyler TR, Sweeney LM, et al. A toxicokinetic study of inhaled ethylene glycol monomethyl ether (2-ME) and validation of a physiologically based pharmacokinetic model for the pregnant rat and human. *Toxicol Appl Pharmacol.* 2000a;165:53–62.

Gargas ML, Tyler TR, Sweeney LM, et al. A toxicokinetic study of inhaled ethylene glycol ethyl ether acetate and validation of a physiologically based pharmacokinetic model for rat and human. *Toxicol Appl Pharmacol.* 2000b;165:63–73.

Garner CD, Lee EW, Louis-Ferdinand RT. Muller cell involvement in methanol-induced retinal toxicity. *Toxicol Appl Pharmacol.* 1995a;130:101–107.

Garner CD, Lee EW, Terzo TS, Louis-Ferdinand RT. Role of retinal metabolism in methanol-induced retinal toxicity. *J Toxicol Environ Health.* 1995b;44:43–56.

Gasiewicz TA, Singh KP, Casado FL. The aryl hydrocarbon receptor has an important role in the regulation of hematopoiesis: implications for benzene-induced hematopoietic toxicity. *Chem Biol Interact.* 2010;184:246–251.

Gaunt IF, Carpanini FM, Grasso P, Lansdown AB. Long-term toxicity of propylene glycol in rats. *Food Cosmet Toxicol.* 1972;10:151–162.

Ge R, Yang S, Kramer PM, et al. The effect of dichloroacetic acid and trichloroacetic acid on DNA hypomethylation and cell proliferation in B6C3F1 mice. *J Biochem Mol Toxicol.* 2001;15:100–106.

Gelbke HP, Goen T, Maurer M, Sulsky SI. A review of health effects of carbon disulfide in viscose industry and a proposal for an occupational exposure limit. *Crit Rev. Toxicol.* 2009;39(suppl 2):1–126.

Geller AM, Zenick H. Aging and the environment: a research framework. *Environ Health Perspect.* 2005;113:1257–1262.

Gennari P, Naldi M, Motta R, et al. Gamma-glutamyltransferase isozymes pattern in workers exposed to tetrachloroethylene. *Am J Ind Med.* 1992;21:661–671.

Gentry PR, Covington TR, Clewell HJ III. Evaluation of the potential impact of pharmacokinetic differences on tissue dosimetry in offspring during pregnancy and lactation. *Regul Toxicol Pharmacol.* 2003;38:1–16.

Gerin M, Patrice S, Begin D, et al. A study of ethylene glycol exposure and kidney function of aircraft de-icing workers. *Int Arch Occup Environ Health.* 1997;69:255–265.

Gerr F, Letz R. Organic solvents. In: Rom WD, ed. *Environmental and Occupational Medicine.* 3rd ed. Philadelphia: Lippincott-Raven; 1998:1091–1108.

Ghanayem BI. Metabolic and cellular basis of 2-butoxyethanol-induced hemolytic anemia in rats and assessment of human risk in vitro. *Biochem Pharmacol.* 1989;38:1679–1684.

Ghanayem BI, Burka LT, Matthews HB. Metabolic basis of ethylene glycol monobutyl ether (2-butoxyethanol) toxicity: role of alcohol and aldehyde dehydrogenases. *J Pharmacol Exp Ther.* 1987;242:222–231.

Ghanayem BI, Burka LT, Matthews HB. Structure–activity relationships for the in vitro hematotoxicity of n-alkoxyacetic acids, toxic metabolites of glycol ethers. *Chem Biol Interact.* 1989;70:339–352.

Ghanayem BI, Chapin RE. Calcium channel blockers protect against ethylene glycol monomethyl ether (2-methoxyethanol)-induced testicular toxicity. *Exp Mol Pathol.* 1990;52:279–290.

Ghanayem BI, Long PH, Ward SM, et al. Hemolytic anemia, thrombosis, and infarction in male and female F344 rats following gavage exposure to 2-butoxyethanol. *Exp Toxicol Pathol.* 2001;53:97–105.

Gibbs BF, Mulligan CN. Styrene toxicity: an ecotoxicological assessment. *Ecotoxicol Environ Saf.* 1997;38:181–194.

Gibbs GW, Amsel J, Soden K. A cohort mortality study of cellulose triacetate-fiber workers exposed to methylene chloride. *J Occup Environ Med.* 1996;38:693–697.

Gift JS. U.S. EPA's IRIS assessment of 2-butoxyethanol: the relationship of noncancer to cancer effects. *Toxicol Lett.* 2005;156:163–178.

Gilger AP, Potts AM. Studies on the visual toxicity of methanol: V. The role of acidosis in experimental methanol poisoning. *Am J Ophthalmol.* 1955;39:63–86.

Ginsberg G, Hattis D, Miller R, Sonawane B. Pediatric pharmacokinetic data: implications for environmental risk assessment for children. *Pediatrics.* 2004a;113:973–983.

Ginsberg G, Hattis D, Russ A, Sonawane B. Pharmacokinetic and pharmacodynamic factors that can affect sensitivity to neurotoxic sequelae in elderly individuals. *Environ Health Perspect.* 2005;113: 1243–1249.

Ginsberg G, Hattis D, Sonawane B, et al. Evaluation of child/adult pharmacokinetic differences from a database derived from the therapeutic drug literature. *Toxicol Sci.* 2002;66:185–200.

Ginsberg G, Slikker W Jr, Bruckner JV, Sonawane B. Incorporating children's toxicokinetics into a risk framework. *Environ Health Perspect.* 2004b;112:272–283.

Gleiter CH, Gundert-Remy U. Gender differences in pharmacokinetics. *Eur J Drug Metab Pharmacokinet.* 1996;21:123–128.

Glende EA Jr, Recknagel RO. Phospholipase A2 activation and cell injury in isolated rat hepatocytes exposed to bromotrichloromethane, chloroform and 1,1-dichloroethylene as compared to effects of carbon tetrachloride. *Toxicol Appl Pharmacol.* 1992;113:159–162.

Glover ML, Reed MD. Propylene glycol: the safe diluent that continues to cause harm. *Pharmacotherapy.* 1996;16:690–693.

Gold LS, Stewart PA, Milliken, K, et al. The relationship between multiple myeloma and occupational exposure to six chlorinated solvents. *Occup Environ Med.* 2011;68:391–399.

Goldenthal EI. A compilation of LD50 values in newborn and adult animals. *Toxicol Appl Pharmacol.* 1971;18:185–207.

Golding BT, Watson WP. Possible mechanisms of carcinogenesis after exposure to benzene. In: Singer B, Bartsch H, eds. *Exocyclic DNA Adducts in Mutagenesis and Carcinogenesis.* Lyons, France: ARC; 1999:75–88. IARC Publication No. 150.

Goldstein BD. Benzene toxicity. *Occup Med.* 1988;33:541–554.

Goldsworthy TL, Lyght O, Bumett VL, Popp JA. Potential role of α-2μ-globulin, protein droplet accumulation, and cell replication in the renal carcinogenicity of rats exposed to trichloroethylene, perchloroethylene and pentachloroethane. *Toxicol Appl Pharmacol.* 1988;96:367–379.

Goldsworthy TL, Popp JA. Chlorinated hydrocarbon-induced paroxisomal enzyme activity in relation to species and organ carcinogenicity. *Toxicol Appl Pharmacol.* 1987;88:225–233.

Gonzalez FJ. Role of cytochromes P450 in chemical toxicity and oxidative stress: studies with CYP2E1. *Mutat Res.* 2005;569:101–110.

Gonzalez FJ, Shah YM. PPARα: mechanism of species differences and hepatocarcinogenesis of peroxisome proliferators. *Toxicology.* 2008;246: 2–8.

Goodlett CR, Horn KH. Mechanisms of alcohol-induced damage to the developing nervous system. *Alcohol Res Health.* 2001;25:175–184.

Gordon SM, Brinkman MC, Ashley DL, et al. Changes in breath trihalomethane levels resulting from household water-use activities. *Environ Health Perspect.* 2006;114:514–521.

Gordon SM, Callahan PJ, Nishioka MG, et al. Residential environmental measurements in the National Human Exposure Assessment Survey (NHEXAS) pilot study in Arizona: preliminary results for pesticides and VOCs. *J Expos Anal Environ Epidemiol.* 1999;9:456–470.

Gospe SM Jr, Zhou SS. Toluene abuse embryopathy: longitudinal neurodevelopmental effects of prenatal exposure to toluene in rats. *Reprod Toxicol.* 1998;12:119–126.

Gotohda T, Takunaga I, Kubo S, et al. Effect of toluene inhalation on astrocytes and neutrotrophic factor in rat brain. *Forensic Sci Int.* 2000;113: 233–238.

Graham DG, Amarnath V, Valentine WM, et al. Pathogenetic studies of hexane and carbon disulfide neurotoxicity. *Crit Rev Toxicol.* 1995;25: 91–112.

Grandison MK, Boudinot FD. Age-related changes in protein binding of drugs: implications for therapy. *Clin Pharmacokinet.* 2000;38:271–290.

Grassman JA, Kimmel CA, Neumann DA. Accounting for variability in responsiveness in human risk assessment. In: Neumann DA, Kimmel CA, eds. *Human Variability in Response to Chemical Exposures.* Washington, DC: International Life Sciences Institute; 1998:1–26.

Graves RJ, Coutts C, Green T. Methylene chloride-induced DNA damage: an interspecies comparison. *Carcinogenesis.* 1995;16:1919–1926.

Graves RJ, Green T. Mouse liver glutathione S-transferase mediated metabolism of methylene chloride to a mutagen in the CHO/HRPT assay. *Mutat Res.* 1996;367:143–150.

Green T. Methylene chloride induced mouse liver and lung tumors: an overview of the role of mechanistic studies in human safety assessment. *Hum Exp Toxicol.* 1997;16:3–13.

Green T. Pulmonary toxicity and carcinogenicity of trichloroethylene: species differences and modes of action. *Environ Health Perspect.* 2000;108(suppl 2):261–264.

Green T, Dow J, Ellis MK, et al. The role of glutathione conjugation in the development of kidney tumors in rats exposed to trichloroethylene. *Chem Biol Interact.* 1997;105:99–117.

Green T, Dow J, Ong CN, et al. Biological monitoring of kidney function among workers occupationally-exposed to trichloroethylene. *Occup Environ Med.* 2004;61:312–317.

Green T, Odum J, Nash JA, et al. Perchloroethylene-induced rat kidney tumors: an investigation of the mechanisms involved and their relevance to humans. *Toxicol Appl Pharmacol.* 1990;103:77–89.

Gries J-M, Benowitz N, Verotta D. Chronopharmacokinetics of nicotine. *Clin Pharmacol Ther.* 1996;60:385–395.

Guastadisegni C, Balduzzi M, Mancuso MT, Di Consiglio E. Liver mitochondria alterations in chloroform-treated Sprague–Dawley rats. *J Toxicol Environ Health.* 1999;57:415–429.

Guengerich FP. Cytochrome P450s and other enzymes in drug metabolism and toxicity. *AAPS J.* 2006;8:E101–E111.

Guengerich FP, Kim DH, Iwasaki M. Role of human cytochrome P-450 IIE1 in the oxidation of many low molecular weight cancer suspects. *Chem Res Toxicol.* 1991;4:168–179.

Guerri C, Bazinet A, Riley EP. Foetal alcohol spectrum disorders and alterations in brain and behavior. *Alcohol Alcohol.* 2009;44:108–114.

Guo C, McMartin KE. The cytotoxicity of oxalate, metabolite of ethylene glycol, is due to calcium oxalate monohydrate formation. *Toxicology.* 2005;208:347–355.

Gut I, Terelius Y, Frantik E, et al. Exposure to various benzene derivatives differently induces cytochromes P450 2B1 and P450 2E1 in rat liver. *Arch Toxicol.* 1993;67:237–243.

Guyonnet D, Siess M-H, Le Bon A-M, Suschetet M. Modulation of phase II enzymes by organosulfur compounds from allium vegetables in rat tissues. *Toxicol Appl Pharmacol.* 1999;154:50–58.

Ha M-C, Cordier S, Dananche B, et al. Congenital malformations and occupational exposure to glycol ethers: a European collaborative case–control study. *Occup Hyg.* 1996;2:417–421.

Haber LT, Maier A, Gentry PR, et al. Genetic polymorphisms in assessing interindividual variability in delivered dose. *Regul Toxicol Pharmacol.* 2002;35:177–197.

Hack CE, Chiu WA, Zhao QJ, Clewell HJ. Bayesian population analysis of a harmonized physiologically based pharmacokinetic model of trichloroethylene and its metabolites. *Regul Toxicol Pharmacol.* 2006;46:63–83.

Hake CL, Stewart RD. Human exposure to tetrachloroethylene: inhalation and skin contact. *Environ Health Perspect.* 1977;21:231–238.

Halder CA, Holdsworth CE, Cockrell BY, Piccirillo VJ. Hydrocarbon nephropathy in male rats: identification of the nephrotoxic components of unleaded gasoline. *Toxicol Ind Health.* 1985;1:67–87.

Halder CA, Van Gorp GS, Hatoum NS, Warne TM. Gasoline vapor exposures. Part II. Evaluation of the nephrotoxicity of the major C4/C5 hydrocarbon components. *Am Ind Hyg Assoc J.* 1986;47:173–175.

Hamby-Mason R, Chen JJ, Schenker S, et al. Catalase mediates acetaldehyde formation from ethanol in fetal and neonatal rat brain. *Alcohol Clin Exp Res.* 1997;21:1063–1072.

Hanioka N, Jinno H, Toyo'oka T, et al. Induction of rat liver drug metabolizing enzymes by tetrachloroethylene. *Arch Environ Contam Toxicol.* 1995;28:273–280.

Hansen J, Raaschou-Nielson O, Christensen JM, et al. Cancer incidence among Danish workers exposed to trichloroethylene. *J Occup Environ Med.* 2001;43:133–139.

Hansen JM, Contreras KM, Harris C. Methanol, formaldehyde, and sodium formate exposure in rat and mouse conceptuses: a potential role of the visceral yolk sac in embryotoxicity. *Birth Defects Res A Clin Mol Teratol.* 2005;73:72–82.

Hantson P, Haufroid V, Wallemacq P. Formate kinetics in methanol poisoning. *Hum Exp Toxicol.* 2005;24:55–59.

Hard GC, Boorman GA, Wolf DC. Re-evaluation of the 2-year chloroform drinking water carcinogenicity bioassay in Osborne–Mendel rats supports chronic renal tubule injury as the mode of action underlying the renal tumor response. *Toxicol Sci.* 2000;53:237–244.

Hardin BD, Eisenmann CJ. Relative potency of four ethylene glycol ethers for induction of paw malformations in the CD-1 mouse. *Teratology.* 1987;35:321–328.

Hardin BD, Goad PT, Burg JR. Developmental toxicity of four glycol ethers applied cutaneously to rats. *Environ Health Perspect.* 1984;57:69–74.

Hardin BD, Goad PT, Burg JR. Developmental toxicity of diethylene glycol monomethyl ether (diEGME). *Fundam Appl Toxicol.* 1986;6:430–439.

Harris C, Dixon M, Hansen JM. Glutathione depletion modulates methanol, formaldehyde and formate toxicity in cultured rat conceptuses. *Cell Biol Toxicol.* 2004;20:133–145.

Harris C, Wang SW, Lauchu JJ, Hansen JM. Methanol metabolism and embryotoxicity in rat and mouse conceptuses: comparisons of alcohol dehydrogenase (ADH1), formaldehyde dehydrogenase (ADH3), and catalase. *Reprod Toxicol.* 2003;17:349–357.

Harris DT, Sakiestewa D, Robledo RF, Witten M. Immunotoxicological effects of JP-8 jet fuel exposure. *Toxicol Ind Health.* 1997a;13:43–55.

Harris DT, Sakiestewa D, Robledo RF, Witten M. Short-term exposure to JP-8 jet fuel results in long-term immunotoxicity. *Toxicol Ind Health.* 1997b;13:559–570.

Harris DT, Sakiestewa D, Robledo RF, Witten M. Protection from JP-8 jet fuel induced immunotoxicity by administration of aerosolized substance P. *Toxicol Ind Health.* 1997c;13:571–588.

Harris DT, Sakiestewa D, Robledo RF, et al. Effects of short-term JP-8 jet fuel exposure on cell-mediated immunity. *Toxicol Ind Health.* 2000;16:78–84.

Harris DT, Sakiestewa D, Titone D, et al. Jet fuel-induced immunotoxicity. *Toxicol Ind Health.* 2001a;16:261–265.

Harris DT, Sakiestewa D, Titone D, et al. Substance P as prophylaxis for JP-8 jet fuel-induced immunotoxicity. *Toxicol Ind Health.* 2001b;16:253–259.

Harris DT, Sakiestewa D, Titone D, et al. JP-8 jet fuel exposure results in immediate immunotoxicity, which is cumulative over time. *Toxicol Ind Health.* 2002;18:77–83.

Harry GJ, Graham DG, Valentine WM, et al. Carbon disulfide neurotoxicity in rats: VIII. Summary. *Neurotoxicology.* 1998;19:159–162.

Hasegawa R, Hirata-Koizumi M, Dourson M, et al. Pediatric susceptibility to 18 industrial chemicals: a comparative analysis of newborn with young animals. *Regul Toxicol Pharmacol.* 2007;47:296–307.

Haselkorn T, Whittemore AS, Udaltsova N, Friedman GD. Short-term chloral hydrate administration and cancer in humans. *Drug Saf.* 2006;29:67–77.

Haseman JK, Hailey JR, Morris RW. Spontaneous neoplasm incidences in Fischer 344 rats and B6C3F1 mice in two-year carcinogenicity studies: a National Toxicology Program update. *Toxicol Pathol.* 1998;26:428–441.

Hattis D, Banati P, Goble R, Burmaster DE. Human interindividual variability in parameters related to health risks. *Risk Anal.* 1999;19:711–726.

Hattis D, Ginsberg G, Sonawane B, et al. Differences in pharmacokinetics between children and adults—II. Children's variability in drug elimination half-lives and in some parameters needed for physiologically-based pharmacokinetic modeling. *Risk Anal.* 2003;23:117–142.

Hayes JR, Condie LW Jr, Borzelleca JF. The subchronic toxicity of tetrachloroethylene (perchloroethylene) administered in the drinking water of rats. *Fundam Appl Toxicol.* 1986;7:119–125.

Hays AM, Parliman G, Pfaff JK, et al. Changes in lung permeability correlate with lung histology in a chronic exposure model. *Toxicol Ind Health.* 1995;11(3):325–336.

Hays SM, Elswick BA, Blumenthal GM, et al. Development of a physiologically based pharmacokinetic model of 2-methoxyethanol and 2-methoxyacetic acid disposition in pregnant rats. *Toxicol Appl Pharmacol.* 2000;163:67–74.

Health Canada. *Priority Substances List. State-of-the-Science Report for Ethylene Glycol.* Ontario: Health Canada and Environment Canada; 2000. Available at: http://www.ec.gc.ca/substances/ese/eng/psap/final/ethyleneglycol.cfm.

Hebert JL, Fabre M, Auzepy P, Paillas J. Acute experimental poisoning by diethylene glycol: acid base balance and histological data in male rats. *Toxicol Eur Res.* 1978;1:2890–2894.

Heilmair R, Lenk W, Lohr D. Toxicokinetics of diethylene glycol (DEG) in the rat. *Arch Toxicol.* 1993;67:655–666.

Heineman EF, Cocco P, Gomez MR, et al. Occupational exposure to chlorinated aliphatic hydrocarbons and risk of astrocytic brain cancer. *Am J Ind Med.* 1994;26:155–169.

Heistein LC, Ramaciotti C, Scott WA, et al. Chloral hydrate sedation for pediatric echocardiography: physiologic responses, adverse events, and risk factors. *Pediatrics.* 2006;117:e434–e441.

Henderson GI, Chen JJ, Schenker S. Ethanol, oxidative stress, reactive aldehydes, and the fetus. *Front Biosci.* 1999;4:D541–D550.

Henderson RF. Species differences in the metabolism of benzene. *Environ Health Perspect.* 1996;104(suppl 6):1173–1175.

Henschler D, Vamvakas S, Lammert M, et al. Increased incidence of renal cell tumors in a cohort of cardboard workers exposed to trichloroethene. *Arch Toxicol.* 1995;69:291–299.

Herrlinger C, Klotz U. Drug metabolism and drug interactions in the elderly. *Best Pract Res Clin Gastroenterol.* 2001;15:897–918.

Hess R, Bartels MJ, Pottenger LH. Ethylene glycol: an estimate of tolerable levels of exposure based on a review of animal and human data. *Arch Toxicol.* 2004;78:671–680.

Hester SD, Johnstone AF, Boyes WK, et al. Acute toluene exposure alters expression of genes in the central nervous system associated with synaptic structure and function. *Neurotoxicol Terotol.* 2011;33:521–529.

Heywood R, Sortwell RJ, Noel PRB, et al. Safety evaluation of toothpaste containing chloroform. III Long-term study in beagle dogs. *J Environ Pathol Toxicol.* 1979;2:835–881.

Hillbom M. Oxidants, antioxidants, alcohol and stroke. *Front Biosci.* 1999;4:67–71.

Hines RN, McCarver DG. The ontogeny of human drug-metabolizing enzymes: phase I oxidative enzymes. *J Pharmacol Exp Ther.* 2002;300:355–360.

Hiraku Y, Kawanishi S. Oxidative DNA damage and apoptosis induced by benzene metabolites. *Cancer Res.* 1996;56:5172–5178.

Hodgson MJ, Heyl AE, Van Thiel DH. Liver disease associated with exposure to 1,1,1-trichloroethane. *Arch Intern Med.* 1989;149:1793–1798.

Hoflack J-C, Vasseur P, Poirier GG. Glycol ethers induce death and necrosis in human leukemia cells. *Biochem Cell Biol.* 1997;75:415–425.

Holladay SD, Comment CE, Kwon J, Luster MI. Fetal hematopoietic alterations after maternal exposure to ethylene glycol monomethyl ether: prolymphoid cell targeting. *Toxicol Appl Pharmacol.* 1994;129:53–60.

Hong J-Y, Wang Y-Y, Bondoc FY, et al. Metabolism of methyl *tert*-butyl ether and other gasoline ethers by human liver microsomes and heterologously expressed human cytochromes P450: identification of CYP2A6 as a major catalyst. *Toxicol Appl Pharmacol.* 1999;160:43–48.

Hooth MJ, Herbert RA, Haseman JK, et al. Toxicology and carcinogenesis studies of dipropylene glycol in rats and mice. *Toxicology*. 2004;204: 123–140.

House RV, Lauer LD, Murray MJ, et al. Immunological studies in B6C3F1 mice following exposure to ethylene glycol monomethyl ether and its principal metabolite methoxyacetic acid. *Toxicol Appl Pharmacol*. 1985;77: 358–362.

Hsieh GY, Wang JD, Cheng TJ, Chen PC. Prolonged menstrual cycles in female workers exposed to ethylene glycol ethers in the semiconductor manufacturing industry. *Occup Environ Med*. 2005;62:510–516.

Huang S-M, Lesko LJL. Drug–drug, drug–dietary supplement, and drug–citrus fruit and other food interactions: what have we learned? *J Clin Pharmacol*. 2004;44:559–569.

Huff JE, Haseman JK, DeMarini DM, et al. Multiple-site carcinogenicity of benzene in Fischer 344 rats and B6C3F1 mice. *Environ Health Perspect*. 1989;82:125–163.

Hunter AGW, Thompson D, Evans JA. Is there a fetal gasoline syndrome? *Teratology*. 1979;20:75–80.

IARC (International Agency for Research on Cancer). *IARC Monographs on the Evaluation of Carcinogenic Risks to Humans: Alcohol Drinking*. Vol. 44. Lyons, France: World Health Organization; 1988:251–259.

IARC (International Agency for Research on Cancer). *IARC Monographs on the Evaluation of Carcinogenic Risks to Humans. Diesel and Gasoline Engine Exhausts and Some Nitroarenes*. Vol. 46. Lyons, France: World Health Organization; 1989a.

IARC (International Agency for Research on Cancer). *IARC Monographs on the Evaluation of Carcinogenic Risks to Humans. Occupational Exposures in Petroleum Refining: Crude Oil and Major Petroleum Fuels*. Vol. 45. Lyons, France: World Health Organization; 1989b.

IARC (International Agency for Research on Cancer). *Summaries and Evaluations—Styrene (Group 2B)*. Vol. 82. Lyons, France: World Health Organization; 2002:437.

Ikonomidou C, Bittigau P, Ishimaru MJ, et al. Ethanol-induced apoptotic neurodegeneration and fetal alcohol syndrome. *Science*. 2000;287:1056–1060.

Infante-Rivard C, Siemiatycki R, Nadon L. Maternal exposure to occupational solvents and childhood leukemia. *Environ Health Perspect*. 2005; 113:787–792.

Inoue O, Seiji K, Watanabe T, et al. Mutual metabolic suppression between benzene and toluene in man. *Int Arch Occup Environ Health*. 1988;60: 15–20.

Ioannides C, Lewis DFV. Cytochrome P450 in the bioactivation of chemicals. *Curr Top Med Chem*. 2004;5:1767–1788.

Ishmael J, Dugard PH. A review of perchloroethylene and rat mononuclear cell leukemia. *Regul Toxicol Pharmacol*. 2006;45:178–184.

Israel Y, Rivera-Meza M, Quintanilla ME, et al. Acetaldehyde burst protection of ADH1B*2 against alcoholism: an additional hormesis protection against esophageal cancers following alcohol consumption? *Alcohol Clin Exp Res*. 2011;35:306–810.

Jacobsen D, Ovrebo S, Ostborg J, Sejersted OM. Glycolate causes the acidosis in ethylene glycol poisoning and is effectively removed by hemodialysis. *Acta Med Scand*. 1984;216:409–416.

Jaeger RJ, Conolly R, Murphy SD. Effect of 18 hr fast and glutathione depletion on 1,1-dichloroethylene-induced hepatotoxicity and lethality in rats. *Exp Mol Pathol*. 1974;20:187–198.

Jan CR, Chen LW, Lin MW. Ca^{2+} mobilization evoked by chloroform in Madin–Darby canine kidney cells. *J Pharmacol Exp Ther*. 2000;292: 995–1001.

Jeannot E, Pogribny IP, Breland FA, Rusyn I. Chronic administration of ethanol leads to an increased incidence of hepatocellular adenoma by promoting H-ras-mutated cells. *Cancer Lett*. 2011;301:161–167.

Jiang Y, Liu J, Waalkes M, Kang YJ. Changes in gene expression associated with carbon tetrachloride-induced liver fibrosis persist after cessation of dosing in mice. *Toxicol Sci*. 2004;79:404–410.

Jindo T, Wine RN, Li L-H, Chapin RE. Protein kinase activity is central to rat germ cell apoptosis induced by methoxyacetic acid. *Toxicol Pathol*. 2001;29:607–616.

Johanson G, Filser JG. Experimental data from closed chamber gas uptake studies in rodents suggest lower uptake rate of chemical than calculated from literature values on alveolar ventilation. *Arch Toxicol*. 1992;66:291–295.

Johlin FC, Swain E, Smith C, Tephly TR. Studies on the mechanism of methanol poisoning: purification and comparison of rat and human liver 10-formyltetrahydrofolate dehydrogenase. *Mol Pharmacol*. 1989;35:745–750.

Johns DO, Daniell WE, Shen DD, et al. Ethanol induced increase in the metabolic clearance of 1,1,1-trichloroethane in human volunteers. *Toxicol Sci*. 2006;92:61–70.

Johnson BL, Boyd J, Burg JR, et al. Effects on the peripheral nervous system of workers' exposure to carbon disulfide. *Neurotoxicology*. 1983;4:53–65.

Johnson KA, Baker PC, Kan HL, et al. Diethylene glycol monobutyl ether (DGBE): two- and thirteen-week oral toxicity studies in Fischer 344 rats. *Food Chem Toxicol*. 2005;43:467–481.

Johnson PD, Goldberg SJ, Mays MZ, Dawson BV, et al. Threshold of trichloroethylene contamination in maternal drinking waters affecting fetal heart development in the rat. *Environ Health Perspect*. 2003;111: 289–292.

Johnsrud EK, Koukouritaki SB, Divakaran K, et al. Human hepatic CYP2E1 expression during development. *J Pharmacol Exp Ther*. 2003;307:402–407.

Johnston LD, O'Malley PM, Bachman JG, Schulenberg JE. *Monitoring the Future National Results on Adolescent Drug Use: Overview of Key Findings*. Bethesda, MD: National Institute on Drug Abuse, 2008;1–67. NIH Publication No. 09-7401.

Jollow DJ, Bruckner JV, McMillan DC, et al. Trichloroethylene risk assessment: a review and commentary. *Crit Rev Toxicol*. 2009;39:782–797.

Jonker D, Woutersen RA, Fernon VJ. Toxicity of mixtures of nephrotoxicants with similar or dissimilar mode of action. *Food Chem Toxicol*. 1996;34:1075–1082.

Jonsson F, Bois F, Johanson G. Physiologically based pharmacokinetic modeling of inhalation exposure of humans to dichloromethane during moderate to heavy exercise. *Toxicol Sci*. 2001;89:209–218.

Jonsson F, Johanson G. A Bayesian analysis of the influence of GSTT1 polymorphism on the cancer risk estimate for dichloromethane. *Toxicol Appl Pharmacol*. 2001;174:99–112.

Jonsson F, Johanson G. Physiologically based modeling of the inhalation kinetics of styrene in humans using a Bayesian population approach. *Toxicol Appl Pharmacol*. 2002;179:35–49.

Jorgenson TA, Meierhenry EF, Rushbrook CJ, et al. Carcinogenicity of chloroform in drinking water to male Osborne–Mendel rats and female B6C3F1 mice. *Fundam Appl Toxicol*. 1985;5:760–769.

Kabbur MB, Rogers JV, Gunasekar PG, et al. Effect of JP-8 jet fuel on molecular and histological parameters related to acute skin irritation. *Toxicol Appl Pharmacol*. 2001;175:83–88.

Kaneko T, Wang P-Y, Sato A. Enzymes induced by ethanol differently affect the pharmacokinetics of trichloroethylene and 1,1,1-trichloroethane. *Occup Environ Med*. 1994;51:113–119.

Kato S, Shields PG, Caparoso NE, et al. Cytochrome P450IIE1 genetic polymorphisms, racial variation, and lung cancer risk. *Cancer Res*. 1992;52:6712–6715.

Katoh M. New Energy Development Organization data. Presented at: The Methanol Vapors and Health Effects Workshop: What We Know and What We Need to Know—Summary Report. Washington, DC: ILSI Risk Science Institute/U.S. Environmental Protection Agency/Health Effects Institute/American Petroleum Institute, A-7; 1989.

Kavet R, Nauss KM. The toxicity of inhaled methanol vapors. *Crit Rev Toxicol*. 1990;21:21–50.

Kawamoto T, Koga M, Murata K, et al. Effects of ALDH2, CYP1A1, and CYP2E1 genetic polymorphisms and smoking and drinking habits on toluene metabolism in humans. *Toxicol Appl Pharmacol*. 1995;133: 295–304.

Kayama F, Yamashita U, Kawamoto T, Kodama Y. Selective depletion of immature thymocytes by oral administration of ethylene glycol monomethyl ether. *Int J Immunopharmacol*. 1991;13:531–540.

Kearney CA, Dunham DB. Gasoline vapor exposures at a high volume service station. *Am Ind Hyg Assoc J*. 1986;47:535–539.

Kedderis GL. Extrapolation of in vitro enzyme induction data to humans in vivo. *Chem Biol Interact*. 1997;107:109–121.

Kegelmeyer AE, Sprankle CS, Horesovsky GJ, Butterworth BE. Differential display identified changes in mRNA levels in regenerating livers from chloroform-treated mice. *Mol Carcinogen*. 1997;20: 288–297.

Keil DE, Warren DA, Jenny MJ, et al. Immunological function in mice exposed to JP-8 jet fuel in utero. *Toxicol Sci.* 2003;76:347–356.

Kelsh MA, Alexander DD, Mink PJ, Mandel JH. Occupational trichloro-ethylene exposure and kidney cancer: a meta-analysis. *Epidemiology.* 2010;21:95–102.

Kenyon EM, Kraichely RE, Hudson KT, Medinsky MA. Differences in rates of benzene metabolism correlate with observed genotoxicity. *Toxicol Appl Pharmacol.* 1996;136:49–56.

Kerns W, Tomaszewski C, McMartin K, et al. Formate kinetics in methanol poisoning. *Clin Toxicol.* 2002;40:137–143.

Keshava N, Caldwell JC. Key issues in the role of peroxisome proliferator-activated receptor agonism and cell signaling in trichloroethylene toxic-ity. *Environ Health Perspect.* 2006;114:1464–1470.

Kiesswetter E, Sietmann B, Seeber A. Standardization of a questionnaire for neurotoxic symptoms. *Environ Res.* 1997;73:73–80.

Kiesswetter E, Sietmann B, Zupanic M, Seeber A. Neurobehavioral study on the interactive effects of age and solvent exposure. *Neurotoxicology.* 2000;21:685–696.

Kilburn KH. *Chemical Brain Injury.* New York: Van Nostrand Reinhold; 1998.

Kim B-S, Smialowicz RJ. The role of metabolism in 2-methoxyethanol induced suppression of in vitro polyclonal antibody responses by rat and mouse lymphocytes. *Toxicology.* 1997;123:227–239.

Kim D, Andersen ME, Nylander-French LA. A dermatotoxicokinetic model of human exposures to jet fuel. *Toxicol Sci.* 2006;93:22–33.

Kim D, Ghanayem BI. Comparative metabolism and disposition of tri-chloroethylene in CYP2E1–/– and wild-type mice. *Drug Metab Dispos.* 2006;34:2020–2027.

Kim HJ, Bruckner JV, Dallas CE, Gallo JM. Effect of dosing vehicles on the pharmacokinetics of orally administered carbon tetrachloride in rats. *Toxicol Appl Pharmacol.* 1990a;102:50–60.

Kim HJ, Oden'hal S, Bruckner JV. Effect of oral dosing vehicles on the acute hepatotoxicity of carbon tetrachloride in rats. *Toxicol Appl Pharmacol.* 1990b;102:34–49.

Kinirons MT, O'Mahony MS. Drug metabolism and aging. *Br J Clin Pharmacol.* 2004;57:540–544.

Kirman CR, Sweeney LM, Corley R, Gargas ML. Using physiologically-based pharmacokinetic modeling to address nonlinear kinetics and changes in rodent physiology and metabolism due to aging and adapta-tion in deriving reference values for propylene glycol methyl ether and propylene glycol methyl ether acetate. *Risk Anal.* 2005;25:271–284.

Kirschmann JC, Brown NM, Coots RH, et al. Review of investigations of dichloromethane metabolism and subchronic oral toxicity as the basis for the design of chronic oral studies in rats and mice. *Food Chem Toxicol.* 1986;24:943–949.

Klaassen CD, Plaa GL. Relative effects of various chlorinated hydrocar-bons on liver and kidney function in mice. *Toxicol Appl Pharmacol.* 1966;9:139–151.

Klaunig JE, Babich MA, Baetcke KP, et al. PPARalpha agonist-induced rodent tumors: modes of action and human relevance. *Crit Rev Toxicol.* 2003;33:655–780.

Klaunig JE, Babich MA, Cook JC, et al. PPARα and effects of TCE. *Environ Health Perspect.* 2007;115:A14–A15.

Klaunig JE, Kamendulis LM. Mode of action of butoxyethanol-induced mouse liver hemangiosarcomas and hepatocellular carcinomas. *Toxicol Lett.* 2005;156:107–115.

Klaunig JE, Ruch RJ, Pereira MA. Carcinogenicity of chlorinated methane and ethane compounds administered in drinking water to mice. *Environ Health Perspect.* 1986;69:89–95.

Klotz U, Ammon E. Clinical and toxicological consequences of the induc-tive potential of ethanol. *Eur J Clin Pharmacol.* 1998;54:7–12.

Kobayashi K, Urashima K, Shimada N, Chiba K. Substrate specificity for rat cytochrome P450 (CYP) isoforms: screening with cDNA-expressed systems in rats. *Biochem Pharmacol.* 2002;63:889–896.

Koizumi A, Kumai M, Ikeda M. In vivo suppression of 1,1,1-trichloroethane metabolism by co-administered tetrachloroethylene: an inhalation study. *Bull Environ Contam Toxicol.* 1982;29:196–199.

Kolovou GD, Salpea KD, Anagnostopoulou KK, Mikhailidis DP. Alcohol use, vascular disease, and lipid-lowering drugs. *J Pharmacol Exp Ther.* 2006;318:1–7.

Kostic MA, Dart RC. Rethinking the toxic methanol level. *J Toxicol Clin Toxicol.* 2003;41:793–800.

Kraul H, Jahn F, Braunlich H. Nephrotoxic effects of diethylene glycol (DEG) in rats. *Exp Pathol.* 1991;42:27–32.

Krause RJ, Lash LH, Elfarra AA. Human kidney flavin-containing monoxy-genases and their potential roles in cysteine S-conjugate metabolism and nephrotoxicity. *J Pharmacol Exp Ther.* 2003;304:185–191.

Kril JJ, Halliday GM, Svoboda MD, Cartwright H. The cerebral cortex is damaged in chronic alcoholics. *Neuroscience.* 1997;79:983–998.

Krishnan K, Johanson G. Physiologically-based pharmacokinetic and toxicokinetic models in cancer risk assessment. *J Environ Sci Health.* 2005;23:31–53.

Ku MC, Huang CC, Kuo HC, et al. Diffuse white matter lesions in carbon disulfide intoxication: microangiopathy or demyelination. *Eur Neurol.* 2003;50:220–224.

Ku WW, Wine RN, Chae BY, et al. Spermatocyte toxicity of 2-methoxy-ethanol (ME) in rats and guinea pigs: evidence for the induction of apop-tosis. *Toxicol Appl Pharmacol.* 1995;134:100–110.

Kuna RA, Ulrich CE. Subchronic inhalation toxicity of two motor fuels. *J Am Coll Toxicol.* 1984;3:217–229.

Labrecque G, Belanger PM. Biological rhythms in the absorption, distri-bution, metabolism and excretion of drugs. *Pharmacol Ther.* 1991;52: 95–107.

Laitinen J, Liesivuori J, Savolainen H. Exposure to glycols and their renal effects in motor servicing workers. *Occup Med.* 1995;45:259–262.

LaKind JS, McKenna EA, Hubner RP, Tardiff RG. A review of the com-parative mammalian toxicity of ethylene glycol and propylene glycol. *Crit Rev Toxicol.* 1999;29:331–365.

Lam C-W, Galen TJ, Boyd JF, Pierson DL. Mechanism of transport and distribution of organic solvents in blood. *Toxicol Appl Pharmacol.* 1990;104:117–129.

Lamb JC IV, Gulati DK, Russell VS, et al. Reproductive toxicity of ethyl-ene glycol monoethyl ether tested by continuous breeding of CD-1 mice. *Environ Health Perspect.* 1984;57:85–90.

Lan O, Zhang L, Li G, et al. Hematotoxicity in workers exposed to low levels of benzene. *Science.* 2004;306:1774–1776.

Lan Q, Zyang L, Tang X, et al. Occupational exposure to trichloroethylene is associated with a decline in lymphocyte subsets and soluble CD27 and CD30 markers. *Carcinogenesis.* 2010;31:1592–1596.

Landrigan PJ, Goldman LR. Children's vulnerability to toxic chemicals: a challenge and opportunity to strengthen health and environmental policy. *Health Affairs.* 2011;30:842–850.

Lanes SF, Rothman KJ, Dreyer NA, et al. Mortality update of cellulose fiber production workers. *Scand J Work Environ Health.* 1993;19:426–428.

Lanigan S. Final report on the safety assessment of methyl alcohol. *Int J Toxicol.* 2001;20(suppl 1):57–85.

Larson JL, Bull RJ. Effect of ethanol on the metabolism of trichloroethyl-ene. *J Toxicol Environ Health.* 1989;28:395–406.

Larson JL, Wolf DC, Butterworth BE. Induced cytotoxicity and cell pro-liferation in the hepatocarcinogenicity of chloroform in female B6C3F1 mice: comparison of administration by gavage in corn oil vs ad libitum in drinking water. *Fundam Appl Toxicol.* 1994;22:90–102.

Lash AA, Becker CE, So Y, Shore M. Neurotoxic effects of methylene chloride: are they long lasting in humans? *Br J Ind Med.* 1991;48: 418–426.

Lash LH, Fisher JW, Lipscomb JC, Parker JC. Metabolism of trichloroeth-ylene. *Environ Health Perspect.* 2000a;108(suppl 2):177–200.

Lash LH, Parker JC. Hepatic and renal toxicities associated with perchloro-ethylene. *Pharmacol Rev.* 2001;53:177–208.

Lash LH, Parker JC, Scott CS. Modes of action of trichloroethylene for kidney tumorigenesis. *Environ Health Perspect.* 2000b;108(suppl 2):225–240.

Lash LH, Putt DA, Brashear WT, et al. Identification of S-(1,2-dichlorovinyl) glutathione in the blood of human volunteers exposed to trichloroethyl-ene. *J Toxicol Environ Health A.* 1999;56:1–21.

Lash LH, Putt DA, Huang P, et al. Modulation of hepatic and renal metabolism and toxicity of trichloroethylene and perchloroethylene by alterations in status of cytochrome P450 and glutathione. *Toxicology.* 2007;235:11–26.

Lash LH, Putt DA, Hueni SE, et al. Roles of necrosis, apoptosis, and mitochondrial dysfunction in *S*-(1,2-dichlorovinyl)-L-cysteine sulfoxide-induced cytotoxicity in primary cultures of human renal proximal tubular cells. *J Pharmacol Exp Ther.* 2003;305:1163–1172.

Lash LH, Putt DA, Hueni SE, Horwitz BP. Molecular markers of trichloroethylene-induced toxicity in human kidney cells. *Toxicol Appl Pharmacol.* 2005;206:157–168.

Lash LH, Putt DA, Parker JC. Metabolism and tissue distribution of orally administered trichloroethylene in male and female rats: identification of glutathione- and cytochrome P-450-derived metabolites in liver, kidney, blood, and urine. *J Toxicol Environ Health A.* 2006;69: 1285–1309.

Lash LH, Qian W, Putt DA, et al. Renal and hepatic toxicity of trichloroethylene and its glutathione-derived metabolites in rats and mice: sex-, species- and tissue-dependent differences. *J Pharmacol Exp Ther.* 2001;297:155–164.

Lash LH, Qian W, Putt DA, et al. Renal toxicity of perchloroethylene and *S*-(1,2,2-trichlorovinyl)glutathione in rats and mice: sex- and species-dependent differences. *Toxicol Appl Pharmacol.* 2002;179: 163–171.

Lash LH, Sausen PJ, Duescher RJ. Roles of cysteine β-lyase and S-oxidase in nephrotoxicity: studies with *S*-(1,2-dichlorovinyl)-4-cysteine and *S*-(1,2-dichlorovinyl)-L-cysteine sulfoxide. *J Pharmacol Exp Ther.* 1994;269:374–383.

Laughter AR, Dunn CS, Swanson CL, et al. Role of the peroxisome proliferators-activated receptor alpha (PPARalpha) in responses to trichloroethylene and metabolites, trichloroacetate and dichloroacetate in mouse liver. *Toxicology.* 2004;203:83–98.

Lauwerys R, Herbrand J, Buchet JP, et al. Health surveillance of workers exposed to tetrachloroethylene in dry cleaning shops. *Int Arch Occup Environ Health.* 1983;52:69–77.

Leaky JEA, Seng JE, Latendresse JR, et al. Dietary controlled carcinogenicity study of chloral hydrate in male B6C3F1 mice. *Toxicol Appl Pharmacol.* 2003;193:266–280.

Leblond F, Guevin C, Demers C, et al. Downregulation of hepatic cytochrome P450 in chronic renal failure. *J Am Soc Nephrol.* 2001;12:326–332.

Lee BL, Yang XF, New AL, Ong CN. Liquid chromatographic determination of urinary 2-thiothiazlidine-4-carboxylic acid, a biomarker of carbon disulphide exposure. *J Chromatogr B.* 1995;668:265–272.

Lee EW, Terzo TS, D'Arcy JB, et al. Lack of blood formate accumulation in humans following exposure to methanol vapor at the current permissible exposure limit of 200 ppm. *Am Ind Hyg Assoc J.* 1992;53:99–104.

Lee JS, Ward WO, Wolf DC, et al. Coordinated changes in xenobiotic metabolizing enzyme gene expression in aging male rats. *Toxicol Sci.* 2008;106:263–283.

Lee KM, Bruckner JV, Muralidhara S, Gallo JM. Characterization of presystemic elimination of trichloroethylene and its nonlinear kinetics in rats. *Toxicol Appl Pharmacol.* 1996;139:262–271.

Lee KM, Dill JA, Chou BJ, Roycroft JH. Physiologically based pharmacokinetic model for chronic inhalation of 2-butoxyethanol. *Toxicol Appl Pharmacol.* 1998;153:211–226.

Lee LJ, Chung CW, Ma YC, et al. Increased mortality odds ratio of male liver cancer in a community contaminated by chlorinated hydrocarbons in groundwater. *Occup Environ Med.* 2003;60:364–369.

Lee RD, An SM, Kim SS, et al. Neurotoxic effects of alcohol and acetaldehyde during embryonic development. *J Toxicol Environ Health A.* 2005;68:2147–2162.

Lee SL, Chau GY, Yao CT, et al. Functional assessment of human alcohol dehydrogenase family in ethanol metabolism: significance of first-pass metabolism. *Alcohol Clin Exp Res.* 2006;30:1132–1142.

Lemazurier E, Lecomte A, Robidel F, Bois FY. Propylene glycol monomethyl ether. A three-generation study of isomer beta effects on reproduction and developmental parameters in rats. *Toxicol Ind Health.* 2005;21:33–40.

Lenk W, Lohr D, Sonnenbichler J. Pharmacokinetics and biotransformation of diethylene glycol and ethylene glycol in the rat. *Xenobiotica.* 1989;19:961–979.

Leth PM, Gregersen M. Ethylene glycol poisoning. *Forensic Sci Int.* 2005;155:179–184.

Leung H-W, Paustenbach DJ. Physiologically based pharmacokinetic and pharmacodynamic modeling in health risk assessment and characterization of hazardous substances. *Toxicol Lett.* 1995;79:55–65.

Lewis DFV, Ioannides C, Parke DV. Cytochrome P450 and species differences in xenobiotic metabolism and activation of carcinogen. *Environ Health Perspect.* 1998;106:633–641.

Lewis JG, Graham DG, Valentine WM, et al. Exposure of C57BL/6 mice to carbon disulfide induces early lesions of atherosclerosis and enhances arterial fatty deposits induced by a high fat diet. *Toxicol Sci.* 1999;49: 124–132.

Li G-L, Linet MS, Hayes RB, et al. Gender differences in hematopoietic and lymphoproliferative disorders and other cancer risks by major occupational group among workers exposed to benzene in China. *J Occup Med.* 1994;36:875–881.

Li L-H, Wine RN, Miller DS, et al. Protection against methoxyacetic-acid-induced spermatocyte apoptosis with calcium channel blockers in cultured rat seminiferous tubules: possible mechanisms. *Toxicol Appl Pharmacol.* 1997;144:105–119.

Licata AC, Dekant W, Smith CE, Borghoff SJ. A physiologically based pharmacokinetic model for methyl *tert*-butyl ether in humans: implementing sensitivity and variability analyses. *Toxicol Sci.* 2001;62: 191–204.

Lieber CS. Cytochrome P4502E1: its physiological and pathological role. *Physiol Rev.* 1997;77:517–544.

Lieber CS. Alcoholic fatty liver: its pathogenesis and mechanism of progression to inflammation and fibrosis. *Alcohol.* 2004;34:9–19.

Lilly PD, Thorton-Manning JR, Gargas ML, et al. Kinetic characterization of CYP2E1 inhibition in vivo and in vitro by the chloroethylenes. *Arch Toxicol.* 1998;72:609–621.

Limaye PB, Apte UM, Shankar K, et al. Calpain release from dying hepatocytes mediates progression of acute liver injury induced by model hepatotoxicants. *Toxicol Appl Pharmacol.* 2003;191:211–226.

Lin B, Ritchie GD, Rossi J III, Pancrazio JJ. Identification of target genes responsive to JP-8 exposure in the rat central nervous system. *Toxicol Ind Health.* 2001a;17:262–269.

Lin B, Ritchie GD, Rossi J III, Pancrazio JJ. Gene expression profiles in the rat central nervous system induced by JP-8 jet fuel vapor exposure. *Neurosci Lett.* 2004;363:233–238.

Lin JH, Lu AYH. Interindividual variability in inhibition and induction of cytochrome P450 enzymes. *Annu Rev Pharmacol Toxicol.* 2001;41:535–567.

Lin Y-S, Smith TJ, Kelsey KT, Wypij D. Human physiological factors in respiratory uptake of 1,3-butadiene. *Environ Health Perspect.* 2001b; 109:921–926.

Lindstrom AB, Yeowell-O'Connell K, Waidyanatha S, et al. Measurement of benzene oxide in the blood of rats following administration of benzene. *Carcinogenesis.* 1997;18:1637–1641.

Lington AW, Dodd DE, Ridlon SA, et al. Evaluation of 13-week inhalation toxicity study on methyl *t*-butyl ether (MTBE) in Fischer 344 rats. *J Appl Toxicol.* 1997;17(S1):S37–S44.

Linhart I, Gut I, Smejkal J, Novak J. Biotransformation of styrene in mice. Stereochemical aspects. *Chem Res Toxicol.* 2000;13:36–44.

Lipscomb JC. Evaluating the relationship between variance in enzyme expression and toxicant concentration in health risk assessment. *Hum Ecol Risk Assess.* 2004;10:39–55.

Lipscomb JC, Garrett CM, Snawder JE. Cytochrome P450-dependent metabolism of trichloroethylene: interindividual differences in humans. *Toxicol Appl Pharmacol.* 1997;142:311–318.

Lipscomb JC, Teuschler LK, Swartout J, et al. The impact of cytochrome P450 2E1-dependent metabolic variance on a risk-relevant pharmacokinetic outcome in humans. *Risk Anal.* 2003;23:1221–1238.

Liu L, Zhang Q, Feng J, et al. The study of DNA oxidative damage in benzene-exposed workers. *Mutat Res.* 1996;370:145–150.

Liu S-L, Esposti SD, Yao T, et al. Vitamin E therapy of acute CCl₄-induced hepatic injury in mice is associated with inhibition of nuclear factor kappa B binding. *Hepatology.* 1995;22:1474–1481.

Liu Y, Bartlett MG, White CA, et al. Presystemic elimination of trichloroethylene in rats following environmentally relevant oral exposures. *Drug Metab Dispos.* 2009;37:1994–1998.

Liu Y, Zhang J-W, Li W, et al. Ginsenoside metabolites, rather than naturally occurring ginsenosides, lead to inhibition of human cytochrome P450 enzymes. *Toxicol Sci*. 2006;91:356–364.

Lock EA, Barth JL, Argraves SW, Schnellmann RG. Changes in gene expression in human renal proximal tubule cells exposed to low concentrations of *S*-(1,2-dichlorovinyl)-L-cysteine, a metabolite of trichloroethylene. *Toxicol Appl Pharmacol*. 2006;216:319–330.

Lock EA, Reed CJ. Trichloroethylene: mechanisms of renal toxicity and renal cancer and relevance to risk assessment. *Toxicol Sci*. 2006;91:313–331.

Lockard VG, Mehendale HM, O'Neal RM. Chlordecone-induced potentiation of carbon tetrachloride hepatotoxicity: a morphometric and biochemical study. *Exp Mol Pathol*. 1983;39:246–256.

Lof A, Johanson G. Toxicokinetics of organic solvents: a review of modifying factors. *Crit Rev Toxicol*. 1998;28:571–650.

Lopez-Diazguerrero NE, Luna-Lopez A, Gutierrez-Ruiz MC, et al. Susceptibility of DNA to oxidative stressors in young and aging mice. *Life Sci*. 2005;77:2840–2854.

Lopreato GF, Phelan R, Borghese CM, et al. Inhaled drugs of abuse enhance serotonin-3 receptor function. *Drug Alcohol Depend*. 2003;70:11–15.

Lorente C, Cordier S, Bergeret A, et al. Maternal occupational risk factors for oral clefts. Occupational exposure and congenital malformation working group. *Scand J Work Environ Health*. 2000;26:137–145.

Lorenz J, Glatt HR, Fleishmann R, et al. Drug metabolism in man and its relationship to that in three rodent species: monooxygenase, epoxide hydrolase, and glutathione *S*-transferase activities in subcellular fractions of lung and liver. *Biochem Med*. 1984;32:43–56.

Loury DJ, Smith-Oliver T, Butterworth BE. Assessment of unscheduled DNA and replicative DNA synthesis in rat kidney cells exposed in vitro or in vivo to unleaded gasoline. *Toxicol Appl Pharmacol*. 1987;87:127–140.

Lu Y, Cederbaum AI. CYP2E1 and oxidative liver injury by alcohol. *Free Radic Biol Med*. 2008;44:723–738.

Lu Y, Rieth S, Lohitnavy M, et al. Application of PBPK modeling in support of the derivation of toxicity reference values for 1,1,1-trichloroethane. *Regul Toxicol Pharmacol*. 2008;50:249–260.

Lu Y, Wu D, Wang X, et al. Chronic alcohol-induced liver injury and oxidant stress are decreased in cytochrome P4502E1 knockout mice and restored in humanized cytochrome P4502E1 knock-in mice. *Free Radic Biol Med*. 2010;49:1406–1416.

Lubman DI, Yucel M, Lawrence AJ. Inhalant abuse among adolescents: neurobiological considerations: *Br J Pharmacol*. 2008;154:316–326.

Lucas D, Farez C, Bardou LG, et al. Cytochrome P450 2E1 activity in diabetic and obese patients as assessed by chlorzoxazone hydroxylation. *Fundam Clin Pharmacol*. 1998;12:553–558.

Luke NS, Sams R, DeVito MJ, et al. Development of a quantitative model incorporating key events in a hepatotoxic mode of action to predict tumor incidence. *Toxicol Sci*. 2010;115:253–266.

Luo JC, Chang HY, Chang SJ, et al. Elevated triglyceride and decreased high density lipoprotein level in carbon disulfide workers in Taiwan. *J Occup Environ Med*. 2003;45:73–78.

Lykke AWJ, Stewart BW. Fibrosing alveolitis (pulmonary interstitial fibrosis) evoked by experimental inhalation of gasoline vapours. *Experientia*. 1978;34:498.

Lynge E, Andersen A, Rylander L, et al. Cancer in persons working in dry cleaning in the Nordic countries. *Environ Health Perspect*. 2006;114:213–219.

Ma JD, Nafziger AN, Bertino JS Jr. Genetic polymorphisms of cytochrome P450 enzymes and the effect on interindividual, pharmacokinetic variability in extensive metabolizers. *J Clin Pharmacol*. 2004;44:447–456.

MacFarland HN, Ulrich CE, Holdsworth CE, et al. A chronic inhalation study with unleaded gasoline vapor. *J Am Coll Toxicol*. 1984;3:231–248.

Mainwaring GW, Williams SM, Foster JR, et al. The distribution of theta-class glutathione *S*-transferase in the liver and lung of mouse, rat and human. *Biochem J*. 1996;318:297–303.

MAK. *List of MAK and BAT Values*. Report No. 48. Deutsche Forschungsgemeinschaft. Germany: Commission for the Investigation of Health Hazards of Chemical Compounds in the Work Area; 2011. Available at: http://www.dfg.de.

Maldonado G, Delzell E, Tyl RW, Sever LE. Occupational exposure to glycol ethers and human congenital malformations. *Int Arch Occup Environ Health*. 2003;76:405–423.

Mally A, Walker CL, Everitt JI, et al. Analysis of renal cell transformation following exposure to trichloroethene in vivo and its metabolite *S*-(dichlorovinyl)-L-cysteine in vitro. *Toxicology*. 2006;224:108–118.

Maltoni C, Cotti G, Patella V. Results of long-term carcinogenicity bioassays on Sprague-Dawley rats of methyl chloroform, administered by ingestion. *Acta Oncol*. 1986;7:101–107.

Mandel JH, Kelsh MA, Mink PJ. Occupational trichloroethylene exposure and non-Hodgkin's lymphoma: a meta-analysis and review. *Occup Environ Med*. 2006;63:597–607.

Mandel JS, McLaughlin JK, Schlehofer B, et al. International renal-cell cancer study. IV. Occupation. *Int J Cancer*. 1995;61:601–605.

Mandrekar P, Szabo G. Signaling pathways in alcohol-induced liver inflammation. *J Hepatol*. 2009;50:1258–1266.

Mangoni AA, Jackson SHD. Age-related changes in pharmacokinetics and pharmacodynamics: basic principles and practical applications. *Br J Clin Pharmacol*. 2003;57:6–14.

Mani C, Freeman S, Nelson DO, et al. Species and strain comparisons in the macromolecular binding of extremely low doses of [^{14}C] benzene in rodents using accelerator mass spectrophotometry. *Toxicol Appl Pharmacol*. 1999;159:83–90.

Manibusan MK, Odin M, Eastmond DA. Postulated carbon tetrachloride mode of action: a review. *J Environ Sci Health C*. 2007;25:185–209.

Manno M, Rezzadore M, Grossi M, Sbrana C. Potentiation of occupational carbon tetrachloride toxicity by ethanol abuse. *Hum Exp Toxicol*. 1996;15:294–300.

Marino DJ, Clewell HJ, Gentry PR, et al. Revised assessment of cancer risk to dichloromethane. I. Bayesian PBPK and dose–response modeling in mice. *Regul Toxicol Pharmacol*. 2006;45:44–54.

Maronpot RR, Devereux TR, Hegi M, et al. Hepatic and pulmonary carcinogenicity of methylene chloride in mice: a search for mechanisms. *Toxicology*. 1995;102:73–81.

Marrubini G, Castoldi AF, Coccini T, Manzo L. Prolonged ethanol ingestion enhances benzene myelotoxicity and lowers urinary concentrations of benzene metabolite levels in CD-1 mice. *Toxicol Sci*. 2003;75:16–24.

Martin-Amat G, McMartin KE, Hayreh SS, et al. Methanol poisoning: ocular toxicity produced by formate. *Toxicol Appl Pharmacol*. 1978;45:201–208.

Martinasevic K, Green MD, Baron J, Tephly TR. Folate and 10-formyltetrahydrofolate dehydrogenase in human and rat retina: relation to methanol toxicity. *Toxicol Appl Pharmacol*. 1996;141:373–381.

Mason TJ, McKay FW. *U.S. Cancer Mortality by County: 1950–1969*. NIH Publication No. 74-615. Bethesda, MD: National Cancer Institute; 1975.

Mathews JM, Parker MK, Matthews HB. Metabolism and disposition of diethylene glycol in rat and dog. *Drug Metab Dispos*. 1991;19:1066–1070.

Matonoski G, Elliott E, Tao X, et al. Lymphohematopoietic cancers and butadiene and styrene exposure in synthetic rubber manufacture. *Ann N Y Acad Sci*. 1997;837:157–169.

Mattie DR, Alden CL, Newell TK, et al. A 90-day continuous vapor inhalation toxicity study of JP-8 jet fuel followed by 20–21 months of recovery in Fischer 344 rats and C57BL/6 mice. *Toxicol Pathol*. 1991;19:77–87.

Mattsson JL, Albee RR, Lomax LG, et al. Neutoxicologic examination of rats exposed to 1,1,1-trichloroethane vapor for 13 weeks. *Neurotoxicol Teratol*. 1993;15:313–326.

Maurya PK, Rizvi SI. Age-dependent changes in glutathione-*S*-transferase: correlation with total plasma antioxidant potential and red cell intracellular glutathione. *Ind J Clin Biochem*. 2010;25:398–400.

McCaffery P, Tempst P, Lara G, Drager U. Aldehyde dehydrogenase as a positional marker in the retina. *Development*. 1991;112:693–702.

McCarver DG, Hines RH. The ontogeny of human drug-metabolizing enzymes: phase II conjugative enzymes and regulatory mechanisms. *J Pharmacol Exp Ther*. 2002;300:361–366.

McCredie M, Stewart JH. Risk factors for kidney cancer in New South Wales, IV. Occupation. *Br J Ind Med*. 1993;50:349–354.

McDougal JN, Jepson GW, Clewell HJ III, et al. Dermal absorption of organic chemical vapors in rats and humans. *Fundam Appl Toxicol.* 1990;14:299–308.

McDougal JN, Pollard DL, Weisman W, et al. Assessment of skin absorption and penetration of JP-8 jet fuel and its components. *Toxicol Sci.* 2000;55:247–255.

McDougal JN, Robinson PJ. Assessment of dermal absorption and penetration of components of a fuel mixture (JP-8). *Sci Total Environ.* 2002;288:23–30.

McGregor D. Methyl *tertiary*-butyl ether: studies for potential human health hazards. *Crit Rev Toxicol.* 2006;36:319–358.

McKee RH, Vergnes JS, Galvin JB, et al. Assessment of the in vivo mutagenic potential of methyl *tertiary*-butyl ether. *J Appl Toxicol.* 1997;17(S1):S31–S36.

McLean AJ, Le Couteur DG. Aging biology and geriatric clinical pharmacology. *Pharmacol Rev.* 2004;56:163–184.

McMahon TF, Medinsky MA, Birnbaum LS. Age-related changes in benzene disposition in male C57BL/6N mice described by a physiologically based model. *Toxicol Lett.* 1994;74:241–253.

McMartin KE, Wallace KB. Calcium oxalate monohydrate, a metabolite of ethylene glycol, is toxic for rat renal mitochondrial function. *Toxicol Sci.* 2005;84:195–200.

Mebus CA, Welsch F, Working PK. Attenuation of 2-methoxyethanol induced testicular toxicity in the rat by simple physiological compounds. *Toxicol Appl Pharmacol.* 1989;99:110–121.

Medeiros AM, Bird MG, Witz G. Potential biomarkers of benzene exposure. *J Toxicol Environ Health.* 1997;51:519–539.

Medinsky MA, Dorman DC. Recent developments in methanol toxicity. *Toxicol Lett.* 1995;82/83:707–711.

Medinsky MA, Dorman DC, Bond JA, et al. Pharmacokinetics of methanol and formate in female cynomolgus monkeys exposed to methanol vapors. *Res Rep Health Eff Inst.* 1997;77:1–38.

Medinsky MA, Kenyon EM, Seaton MJ, Schlosser PM. Mechanistic considerations in benzene physiological model development. *Environ Health Perspect.* 1996;104(suppl 6):1399–1404.

Medinsky MA, Sabourin PJ, Lucier G, et al. A physiological model for simulation of benzene metabolism by rats and mice. *Toxicol Appl Pharmacol.* 1989;99:193–206.

Medinsky MA, Schlosser PM, Bond JA. Critical issues in benzene toxicity and metabolism: the effect of interactions with other organic chemicals on risk assessment. *Environ Health Perspect.* 1994;102(suppl 9):119–124.

Medinsky MA, Singh G, Bechtold WE, et al. Disposition of three glycol ethers administered in drinking water to male F344/N rats. *Toxicol Appl Pharmacol.* 1990;102:443–455.

Meek ME, Klaunig JE. Proposed mode of action of benzene-induced leukemia: interpreting available data and identifying critical data gaps for risk assessment. *Chem Biol Interact.* 2010;184:279–285.

Mehendale HM. Tissue repair: an important determinant of final outcome of toxicant-induced injury. *Toxicol Pathol.* 2005;33:41–51.

Melnick RL, Kohn MC. Possible mechanisms of induction of renal tubule cell neoplasms in rats associated with α2u-globulin: role of protein accumulation versus ligand delivery to the kidney. In: Cappen CC, Dybing E, Rice JM, Wilbourn JD, eds. *Species Differences in Thyroid, Kidney and Urinary Bladder Carcinogenesis.* Lyons, France: IARC; 1999:119–137. IARC Publication No. 147.

Mennear JH. Carcinogenicity studies on MTBE: critical review and interpretation. *Risk Anal.* 1997;17:673–681.

Mennear JH, McConnell EE, Huff JE, et al. Inhalation and carcinogenesis studies of methylene chloride (dichloromethane) in F344/N rats and B6C3F1 mice. *Ann N Y Acad Sci.* 1988;534:343–351.

Merdink JL, Robison LM, Stevens DK, et al. Kinetics of chloral hydrate and its metabolites in male human volunteers. *Toxicology.* 2008;245:130–140.

Messiha FS, Price J. Properties and regional distribution of ocular aldehyde dehydrogenase in the rat. *Neurobehav Toxicol Teratol.* 1983;5:251–254.

Methias R. Chronic solvent abusers have more brain abnormalities and cognitive impairment than cocaine abusers. *NIDA Notes.* 2002;17(4).

Mezey E. Metabolic effects of ethanol. *Fed Proc.* 1985;44:134–138.

Micu AL, Miksys S, Sellers DL, et al. Rat hepatic CYP2E1 is induced by very low nicotine doses: an investigation of induction, time course, dose response and mechanism. *J Pharmacol Exp Ther.* 2003;306:941–947.

Mihic SJ, McQuilkin SJ, Eger EI, et al. Potentiation of γ-aminobutyric acid type A receptor-mediated chloride currents by novel halogenated compounds correlated with their abilities to induce general anesthesia. *Mol Pharmacol.* 1994;46:851–857.

Miller AM, Horiguchi N, Jeong W-I, et al. Molecular mechanisms of alcoholic liver disease: innate immunity and cytokines. *Alcohol Clin Exp Res.* 2011;35:787–793.

Miller JH, Minard KR, Wind RA, et al. In vivo MRI measurements of tumor growth induced by dichloroacetate: implications for mode of action. *Toxicology.* 2000;145:115–125.

Miller RR, Hermann EA, Young JT, et al. Ethylene glycol monomethyl ether and propylene glycol monomethyl ether: metabolism, disposition, and subchronic inhalation toxicity studies. *Environ Health Perspect.* 1984;57:233–239.

Mitchell SJ, Kane AE, Hilmer SN. Age-related changed in the hepatic pharmacology and toxicology of paracetamol. *Curr Gerontol Geriatr Res.* 2011;2011:1–14.

Mitschke D, Reichel A, Fricker G, Moenning U. Characterization of cytochrome P450 expression along the entire length of the intestine of male and female rats. *Drug Metab Dispos.* 2008;36:1039–1045.

Mohamed MF, Kang D, Aneja VP. Volatile organic compounds in some urban locations in United States. *Chemosphere.* 2002;47:863–882.

Monks TJ, Butterworth M, Lau SS. The fate of benzene-oxide. *Chem Biol Interact.* 2010;184:201–206.

Monster AC. Difference in uptake, elimination, and metabolism in exposure to trichloroethylene, 1,1,1-trichloroethane and tetrachloroethylene. *Int Arch Occup Environ Health.* 1979;42:311–317.

Monteiro-Riviere N, Inman A, Riviere J. Effects of short-term high-dose and low-dose exposure to Jet A, JP-8 and JP-8 + 100 jet fuels. *J Appl Toxicol.* 2001;21:485–494.

Monteiro-Riviere NA, Inman AO, Riviere JE. Skin toxicity of jet fuels: ultra-structural studies and the effects of substance P. *Toxicol Appl Pharmacol.* 2004;195:339–347.

Moore LE, Boffetta P, Karami S, et al. Occupational trichloroethylene exposure and renal carcinoma risk: evidence of genetic susceptibility by reductive metabolism gene variants. *Cancer Res.* 2010;70:6527–6536.

Moore MM, Harrington-Brock K. Mutagenicity of trichloroethylene and its metabolites: implications for the risk assessment of trichloroethylene. *Environ Health Perspect.* 2000;108(suppl 2):215–223.

Moorman MP, Sills RC, Collins BJ, Morgan DL. Carbon disulfide neurotoxicity in rats: II. Toxicokinetics. *Neurotoxicology.* 1998;19:89–97.

Moran MJ, Zogorski JS, Squillace PJ. Chlorinated solvents in groundwater of the United States. *Environ Sci Technol.* 2007;41:74–81.

Moreau CL, Kerns W II, Tomaszewski CA, et al. Glycolate kinetics and hemodialysis clearance in ethylene glycol poisoning. META Study Group. *J Toxicol Clin Toxicol.* 1998;36:659–666.

Morford LL, Henck JW, Breslin WJ, DeSesso JM. Hazard identification and predictability of children's health risk from animal data. *Environ Health Perspect.* 2004;112:266–271.

Morgan DJ, McLean AJ. Clinical pharmacokinetic and pharmacodynamics considerations in patients with liver disease. An update. *Clin Pharmacokinet.* 1995;29:370–391.

Morgan DL, Cooper SW, Carlock DL, et al. Dermal absorption of neat and aqueous volatile organic chemicals in the Fischer 344 rat. *Environ Res.* 1991;55:51–63.

Morimura K, Cheung C, Ward JM, et al. Differential susceptibility of mice humanized for peroxisome proliferator-activated receptor (alpha) to Wy-14,643-induced liver carcinogenesis. *Carcinogenesis.* 2006;27:1074–1080.

Morio LA, Chiu H, Sprowles KA, et al. Distinct roles of tumor necrosis factor-α and nitric oxide in acute liver injury induced by carbon tetrachloride in mice. *Toxicol Appl Pharmacol.* 2001;172:44–51.

Morshed KM, Nagpaul JP, Majumdar S, et al. Kinetics of propylene glycol elimination and metabolism in the rat. *Biochem Med Metab Biol.* 1988;39:90–97.

Moser GJ, Wolf DC, Harden R, et al. Cell proliferation and regulation of negative growth factors in mouse liver foci. *Carcinogenesis*. 1996c;17:1835–1840.

Moser GJ, Wolf DC, Sar M, et al. Methyl *tertiary* butyl ether-induced endocrine alterations in mice are not mediated through the estrogen receptor. *Toxicol Sci*. 1998;41:77–87.

Moser GJ, Wolf DC, Wong BA, Goldsworthy TL. Loss of tumor-promoting activity of unleaded gasoline in *N*-nitrosodiethylamine-initiated ovariectomized B6C3F1 mouse liver. *Carcinogenesis*. 1997;18:1075–1083.

Moser GJ, Wong BA, Wolf DC, et al. Comparative short-term effects of methyl *tertiary* butyl ether and unleaded gasoline vapor in B6C3F1 mice. *Fundam Appl Toxicol*. 1996a;31:173–183.

Moser GJ, Wong BA, Wolf DC, et al. Methyl *tertiary* butyl ether lacks tumor-promoting activity in *N*-nitrosodiethylamine-initiated B6C3F1 female mouse liver. *Carcinogenesis*. 1996b;17:2753–2761.

Mugford CA, Kedderis GL. Sex-dependent metabolism of xenobiotics. *Drug Metab Rev*. 1998;30:441–498.

Muhammad F, Monteiro-Riviere NA, Riviere JE. Comparative in vivo toxicity of topical JP-8 jet fuel and its individual hydrocarbon components: identification of tridecane and tetradecane as key constituents responsible for dermal irritation. *Toxicol Pathol*. 2005;33:258–266.

Mulkey ME. *The Determination of Whether Dithiocarbamate Pesticides Share a Common Mechanism of Toxicity*. Internal memorandum. Washington, DC: U.S. EPA Office of Pesticide Programs; December 19, 2001:1–38. Available at: http://www.epa.gov/oppsrrdl/cumulative/dithiocarb.pdf.

Muller G, Spassowski M, Henschler D. Metabolism of trichloroethylene in man. III. Interaction of trichloroethylene and ethanol. *Arch Toxicol*. 1975;33:173–189.

Mundt KA, Birk T, Burch MT. Critical review of the epidemiological literature on occupational exposure to perchloroethylene and cancer. *Int Arch Occup Environ Health*. 2003;76:473–491.

Murray FJ, Schwetz BA, McBride JG, Staples RE. Toxicity of inhaled chloroform in pregnant mice and their offspring. *Toxicol Appl Pharmacol*. 1979;50:515–522.

Murray M. P450 enzymes. Inhibition mechanisms, genetic regulation and effects of liver disease. *Clin Pharmacokinet*. 1992;23:132–146.

Murry DJ, Crom WR, Reddick WE, et al. Liver volume as a determinant of drug clearance in children and adolescents. *Drug Metab Dispos*. 1995;23:1110–1116.

Mutti A, Alinovi R, Bergamaschi E, et al. Nephropathies and exposures to perchloroethylene in dry-cleaners. *Lancet*. 1992;340:189–193.

Muttray A, Kurten R, Jung D, et al. Acute effects of 200 ppm 1,1,1-trichloroethane on the human EEG. *Eur J Med Res*. 2000;5:375–384.

Nagano K, Sasaki T, Umeda Y, et al. Inhalation carcinogenicity and chronic toxicity of carbon tetrachloride in rats and mice. *Inhal Toxicol*. 2007;19:1089–1103.

Nakai JS, Stathopulos PB, Campbell GL, et al. Penetration of chloroform, trichloroethylene, and tetrachloroethylene through human skin. *J Toxicol Environ Health*. 1999;58:157–170.

Nakajima T. Cytochrome P450 isoforms and the metabolism of volatile hydrocarbons of low relative molecular mass. *J Occup Health*. 1997;39:83–91.

Nakajima T, Elovaara E, Okino T, et al. Different contributions of cytochrome P450 2E1 and P450 2B1/2 to chloroform hepatotoxicity in rat. *Toxicol Appl Pharmacol*. 1995;133:215–222.

Nakajima T, Koyama Y, Sato A. Dietary modification of metabolism and toxicity of chemical substances—with special reference to carbohydrate. *Biochem Pharmacol*. 1982;31:1005–1011.

Nakajima T, Okuyama S, Yonekura I, Sato A. Effects of ethanol and phenobarbital administration on the metabolism and toxicity of benzene. *Chem Biol Interact*. 1985;55:23–38.

Nakajima T, Wang R-S. Induction of cytochrome P450 by toluene. *Int J Biochem*. 1994;26:1333–1340.

Nakajima T, Wang R-S, Elovaara E, et al. A comparative study on the contribution of cytochrome P450 isozymes to metabolism of benzene, toluene and trichloroethylene in rat liver. *Biochem Pharmacol*. 1992a;43:251–257.

Nakajima T, Wang R-S, Elovaara E, et al. Toluene metabolism by cDNA-expressed human hepatic cytochrome P450. *Biochem Pharmacol*. 1997;53:271–277.

Nakajima T, Wang R-S, Katakura Y, et al. Sex-, age- and pregnancy-induced changes in the metabolism of toluene and trichloroethylene in rat liver in relation to the regulation of cytochrome P450IIE1 and P450IIC11 content. *J Pharmacol Exp Ther*. 1992b;261:869–874.

NAS (National Academy of Sciences). *Pesticides in the Diets of Infants and Children*. National Research Council. Washington, DC: National Academy Press; 1993:1–12.

NAS (National Academy of Sciences). *Toxicologic Assessment of Jet-Propulsion Fuel 8*. Washington, DC: National Academies Press; 2003.

NAS (National Academy of Sciences). *Assessing the Human Health Risks of Trichloroethylene: Key Scientific Issues*. Washington, DC: National Academy Press; 2006.

NAS (National Academy of Sciences). *Mouse Liver Tumors: Benefits and Constraints on Use in Human Health Risk Assessment, Qualitative and Quantitative Aspects*. Risk Analysis Issues and Reviews Newsletter No. 2. Washington, DC: National Academy Press; 2008.

NAS (National Academy of Sciences). *Contaminated Water Supplies at Camp Lejeune: Assessing Potential Health Effects*. Washington, DC: National Academy Press; 2009.

NAS (National Academy of Sciences). *Review of the Environmental Protection Agency's Draft IRIS Risk Assessment of Tetrachloroethylene*. Washington, DC: National Academy Press; 2010.

NCI (National Cancer Institute). *Carcinogenesis Bioassay of Chloroform*. National Technical Information Service No. PB264018/AS. Bethesda, MD: NCI; 1976.

NCI (National Cancer Institute). *Bioassay of Tetrachloroethylene for Possible Carcinogenicity*. DHEW Publication No. NIH 77-813. Bethesda, MD: NCI; 1977a.

NCI (National Cancer Institute). *Bioassay of 1,1,1-Trichloroethane for Possible Carcinogenicity*. DHEW Publication No. NIH 77-803, NCI-CG-TR-3. Bethesda, MD: NCI; 1977b.

NCI (National Cancer Institute). Bioassay of Styrene for Possible Carcinogenicity. Technical Report Series No. 185. NIH 79–1741, NCI-CG-TR-185. Bethesda, MD, 1979.

NEDO (New Energy Development Organization). *Toxicological Research of Methanol as a Fuel for Power Station: Summary Report on Test with Monkeys, Rats and Mice*. Tokyo: New Energy Development Organization; 1987:1–296.

Nelson BK, Brightwell WS. Behavioral teratology of ethylene glycol monomethyl and monoethyl ethers. *Environ Health Perspect*. 1984;57:43–46.

Nelson BK, Vorhees CV, Scott WJ, Hastings L. Effects of 2-methoxyethanol on fetal development, postnatal behavior, and embryonic intracellular pH of rats. *Neurotoxicol Teratol*. 1989;11:273–284.

Nelson HH, Wiencke JK, Christiani DC, et al. Ethnic differences in the prevalence of the homozygous deleted genotype of glutathione *S*-transferase theta. *Carcinogenesis*. 1995;16:1243–1245.

Nessel CS. A comprehensive evaluation of the carcinogenic potential of middle distillate fuels. *Drug Chem Toxicol*. 1999;22:165–180.

Nessel CS, Freeman JJ, Forgash RC, McKee RH. The role of dermal irritation in the skin tumor promoting activity of petroleum middle distillates. *Toxicol Sci*. 1999;49:48–55.

NIDA (National Institute on Drug Abuse). *Research Report Series: Inhalant Abuse*. NIH Publication No. 12-3818. Bethesda, MD: National Institute on Drug Abuse; 2012:1–8.

Nielsen GD, Alarie Y. Sensory irritation, pulmonary irritation, and respiratory stimulation by airborne benzene and alkylbenzenes: prediction of safe industrial exposure levels and correlation with their thermodynamic properties. *Toxicol Appl Pharmacol*. 1982;65:459–477.

Niemela O. Aldehyde–protein adducts in the liver as a result of ethanol-induced oxidative stress. *Front Biosci*. 1999;4:506–513.

NIOSH (National Institute of Occupational Safety and Health). *1981-83 National Occupational Exposure Survey (NOAES)*. Atlanta, GA: National Institute of Occupational Safety and Health; 1989.

Nitschke KD, Burek JD, Bell TJ, et al. Methylene chloride: a 2-year inhalation toxicity and oncogenicity study in rats. *Fundam Appl Toxicol*. 1988;11:48–59.

Nolan RJ, Freshour NL, Rick DL, et al. Kinetics and metabolism of inhaled methyl chloroform (1,1,1-trichloroethane) in male volunteers. *Fundam Appl Toxicol*. 1984;4:654–662.

Nolin TD, Naud J, Leblond FA, Pichette V. Emerging evidence of the impact of kidney disease on drug metabolism and transport. *Clin Pharmacol Ther*. 2008;83:898–903.

Nomiyama K, Nomiyama H. Respiratory retention, uptake and excretion of organic solvents in man. *Int Arch Arbeitsmed*. 1974;32:75–83.

Nong A, McCarver DG, Hines RN, Krishnan K. Modeling interchild differences in pharmacokinetics on the basis of subject-specific data on physiology and hepatic CYP2E1 levels: a case study with toluene. *Toxicol Appl Pharmacol*. 2006;214:78–87.

Normandin L, Ann Beaupre L, Salehi F, et al. Manganese distribution in the brain and neurobehavioral changes following inhalation exposure of rats to three chemical forms of manganese. *Neurotoxicology*. 2004;25:433–441.

NTP (National Toxicology Program). *Toxicology and Carcinogenesis Studies of Tetrachloroethylene (Perchloroethylene) in F344/N Rats and B6C3F1 Mice*. Research Triangle Park, NC: National Toxicology Program; 1986.

NTP (National Toxicology Program). *Toxicology and Carcinogenesis Studies of Trichloroethylene in Four Strains of Rats (ACI, August, Marshall, Osborne–Mendel) (Gavage Studies)*. NIH Publication No. 88-2529. Research Triangle Park, NC: National Toxicology Program; 1988.

NTP (National Toxicology Program). *Carcinogenesis Studies of Trichloroethylene (Without Epichlorohydrin) in F344/N Rats and B6C3F1 Mice (Gavage Studies)*. NIH Publication No. 90-1779. Research Triangle Park, NC: National Toxicology Program; 1990.

NTP (National Toxicology Program). *Toxicity Studies of a Chemical Mixture of 25 Groundwater Contaminants Administered in Drinking Water to F344/N Rats and B6C3F1 Mice*. Technical Report Series No. 35; NIH Publication No. 93-3384. Research Triangle Park, NC: National Toxicology Program; 1993a.

NTP (National Toxicology Program). *Toxicology and Carcinogenesis Studies of Ethylene Glycol in B6C3F1 Mice (Feed Studies)*. NIH Publication No. 93-3144. Research Triangle Park, NC: National Toxicology Program; 1993b.

NTP (National Toxicology Program). *Toxicology and Carcinogenesis Studies of t-Butyl Alcohol in F344/N Rats and B6C3F1 Mice*. Technical Report Series No. 436; NIH Publication No. 95-3167. Research Triangle Park, NC: National Toxicology Program; 1995.

NTP (National Toxicology Program). *NTP Technical Report on Renal Toxicity Studies of Selected Halogenated Ethanes Administered by Gavage to F344/N Rats*. Toxicity Report Series 45, NIH Publication No. 96-3935. Research Triangle Park, NC: National Toxicology Program; 1996.

NTP (National Toxicology Program). Chloroform. NTP reproductive assessment by continuous breeding study. *Environ Health Perspect*. 1997a;105(suppl 1):285–286.

NTP (National Toxicology Program). *Toxicology and Carcinogenesis Studies of Ethylbenzene in F344/N Rats and B6C3F1 Mice (Inhalation Studies)*. Research Triangle Park, NC: National Toxicology Program; 1997b.

NTP (National Toxicology Program). NTP toxicology and carcinogenesis studies 2-butoxyethanol (CAS no. 111-76-2) in F344/N rats and B6C3F1 mice (inhalation studies). *Natl Toxicol Program Tech Rep Ser*. 2000;484:1–290.

NTP (National Toxicology Program). *NTP-CERHR Monograph on the Potential Human and Reproductive and Developmental Effects of Methanol*. NIH Publication No. 03-4478. Research Triangle Park, NC: NTP-Center for the Evaluation of Risks to Human Reproduction, U.S. DHHS; September 2003.

NTP (National Toxicology Program). NTP technical report on the toxicology and carcinogenesis studies of propylene glycol mono-t-butyl ether (CAS no. 57018-52-7) in F344/N rats and B6C3F1 mice and a toxicology study of propylene glycol mono-t-butyl ether in male NBR rats (inhalation studies). *Natl Toxicol Program Tech Rep Ser*. 2004a;515:1–306.

NTP (National Toxicology Program). NTP-CERHR expert panel on the reproductive and developmental toxicity of methanol. *Reprod Toxicol*. 2004b;18:303–390.

NTP (National Toxicology Program). NTP toxicology and carcinogenesis studies of dipropylene glycol (CAS no. 25265-71-8) in F344/N rats and B6C3F1 mice (drinking water studies). *Natl Toxicol Program Tech Rep Ser*. 2004c;511:6–260.

NTP (National Toxicology Program). NTP-CERHR expert panel report on the reproductive and developmental toxicity of ethylene glycol. *Reprod Toxicol*. 2004d;18:457–532.

NTP (National Toxicology Program). NTP-CERHR expert panel report on the reproductive and developmental toxicity of propylene glycol. *Reprod Toxicol*. 2004e;18:533–579.

NTP (National Toxicology Program). *NTP-CERHR Monograph on the Potential Human Reproductive and Developmental Effects of Ethylene Glycol*. NTP CERHR MON 11:1-III36. Research Triangle Park, NC: National Toxicology Program; 2004f.

NTP (National Toxicology Program). *NTP-CERHR Monograph on the Potential Human Reproductive and Developmental Effects of Propylene Glycol (PG)*. NTP CERHR MON 12:i-III6. Research Triangle Park, NC: National Toxicology Program; 2004g.

NTP (National Toxicology Program). *12th Report on Carcinogens (ROC)*. Public Health Service. 2011. Available at: http://niehs.nih.gov/go/roc12.

Nuckols JR, Ashley DL, Lyu C, et al. Influence of tap water quality and household water use activities on indoor air and internal dose levels of trihalomethanes. *Environ Health Perspect*. 2005;113:863–870.

Nyska A, Maronpot RR, Long PH, et al. Disseminated thrombosis and bone infarction in female rats following inhalation exposure to 2-butoxyethanol. *Toxicol Pathol*. 1999;27:287–294.

O'Brien KL, Selanikio JD, Hecdivert C, et al. Epidemic of pediatric deaths from acute renal failure caused by diethylene glycol poisoning. *JAMA*. 1998;279:1175–1180.

O'Brien ML, Spear BT, Glauert HP. Role of oxidative stress in peroxisome proliferator mediated carcinogenesis. *Crit Rev Toxicol*. 2005;35:61–88.

O'Flaherty EJ, Nau H, McCandless D, et al. Physiologically based pharmacokinetics of methoxyacetic acid: dose–effect considerations in C57BL/6 mice. *Teratology*. 1995;52:78–89.

Ohtsuki T, Sato K, Koizumi A, et al. Limited capacity of humans to metabolize tetrachloroethylene. *Int Arch Occup Environ Health*. 1983;51:381–390.

Olney JW, Wozniak DF, Farber NB, et al. The enigma of fetal alcohol neurotoxicity. *Ann Med*. 2002;34:109–119.

Olson MJ, Garg BD, Murty CVR, Roy AK. Accumulation of α2u-globulin in the renal proximal tubules of male rats exposed to unleaded gasoline. *Toxicol Appl Pharmacol*. 1987;90:43–51.

Olson MJ, Mancini MA, Garg BD, Roy AK. Leupeptin-mediated alteration of renal phagolysosomes: similarity to hyaline droplet nephropathy of male rats exposed to unleaded gasoline. *Toxicol Lett*. 1988;41:245–254.

Omiecinski CJ, Remmel RP, Hosagrahara VP. Concise review of the cytochrome P450s and their roles in toxicology. *Toxicol Sci*. 1999;4:151–156.

Omura M, Katsumata T, Misawa H, Yamaguchi M. Decreases in protein kinase and phosphatase activities in the liver nuclei of rats exposed to carbon tetrachloride. *Toxicol Appl Pharmacol*. 1999;160:192–197.

OSHA (Occupational Safety and Health Administration). *Benzene. Limits for Air Contaminants. Occupational Safety and Health Standards*. Code of Federal Regulations. 29 CFR 1910.1028. Washington, DC: U.S. Department of Labor; 2005. Available at: http://www.osha.gov/comp-links.html.

OSHA (Occupational Safety and Health Administration). *Solvents*. July 3, 2006. Available at: http://www.osha.gov/archive/oshinfo/priorities/solvents.html.

Oudiz D, Zenick H. In vivo and in vitro evaluations of spermatotoxicity induced by 2-ethoxyethanol treatment. *Toxicol Appl Pharmacol*. 1986;84:576–583.

Padron AG, de Toranzo EGD, Castro JA. Depression of liver microsomal glucose 6-phosphatase activity in carbon tetrachloride-poisoned rats. Potential synergistic effects of lipid peroxidation and of covalent binding of haloalkane-derived free radicals to cellular components in the process. *Free Radic Biol Med*. 1996;21:81–87.

Pahler A, Parker J, Dekant W. Dose-dependent protein adduct formation in liver, kidney, and blood of rats and in human blood after perchloroethylene inhalation. *Toxicol Sci*. 1999;48:5–13.

Paine MF, Hart HL, Ludington SS, et al. The human intestinal cytochrome P450 "pie". *Drug Metab Dispos*. 2006;34:880–886.

Palmer CN, Hsu MH, Griffin KJ, et al. Peroxisome proliferator activated receptor α expression in human liver. *Mol Pharmacol.* 1998;53: 14–22.

Palmer RB, Brent J. Derivation of a chemical-specific adjustment factor (CSAF) for use in the assessment of risk from chronic exposure to ethylene glycol: application of international programme for chemical safety guidelines. *Toxicol Appl Pharmacol.* 2005;207:576–584.

Park J, Kamendulis LM, Klaunig JE. Effects of 2-butoxyethanol on hepatic oxidative damage. *Toxicol Lett.* 2002;126:19–29.

Pastino GM, Conolly RB. Application of a physiologically based pharmacokinetic model to estimate the bioavailability of ethanol in male rats: distinction between gastric and hepatic pathways of metabolic clearance. *Toxicol Sci.* 2000;55:256–265.

Pastino GM, Flynn EJ, Sultatos LG. Genetic polymorphisms in ethanol metabolism: issues and goals for physiologically based pharmacokinetic modeling. *Drug Chem Toxicol.* 2000;23:179–201.

Patel AS, Talbott EO, Zborowski JV, et al. Risk of cancer as a result of community exposure to gasoline vapors. *Arch Environ Health.* 2004;59:497–503.

Paulu C, Aschengrau A, Ozonoff D. Tetrachloroethylene-contaminated drinking water in Massachusetts and the risk of colon-rectum, lung, and other cancers. *Environ Health Perspect.* 1999;107:265–271.

Pereira MA. Route of administration determines whether chloroform enhances or inhibits cell proliferation in the liver of B6C3F1 mice. *Fund Appl Toxicol.* 1994;23:87–92.

Pereira MA, Grothaus M. Chloroform in drinking water prevents hepatic cell proliferation induced by chloroform administered by gavage in corn oil to mice. *Fundam Appl Toxicol.* 1997;37:82–87.

Pereira MA, Kramer PM, Conran PB, Tao L. Effect of chloroform on dichloroacetic acid and trichloroacetic acid-induced hypomethylation and expression of c-myc gene and on their promotion of liver and kidney tumors in mice. *Carcinogenesis.* 2001;22:1511–1519.

Pesch B, Haerting J, Ranft U, et al. Occupational risk factors for renal cell carcinoma: agent-specific results from a case–control study in Germany. *Int J Epidemiol.* 2000;29:1014–1024.

Pfaff J, Parton K, Lantz RC, et al. Inhalation exposure to JP-8 jet fuel alters pulmonary function and substance P levels in Fischer 344 rats. *J Appl Toxicol.* 1995;15:249–256.

Pfaff JK, Tollinger BJ, Lantz RC, et al. Neutral endopeptidase (NEP) and its role in pathological pulmonary change with inhalation exposure to JP-8 jet fuel. *Toxicol Ind Health.* 1996;12:93–103.

Philip BK, Anand SS, Palkar PS, et al. Subchronic chloroform priming protects mice from a subsequently administered lethal dose of chloroform. *Toxicol Appl Pharmacol.* 2006;216:108–121.

Philip BK, Mumtaz MM, Latendresse JR, Mehendale HM. Impact of repeated exposure on toxicity of perchloroethylene in Swiss Webster mice. *Toxicology.* 2007;232:1–14.

Phillips CF, Jones RK. Gasoline vapor exposures during bulk handling operations. *Am Ind Hyg Assoc J.* 1978;39:118–128.

Phillips M. Detection of carbon disulfide in breath and air: a possible new risk factor for coronary artery disease. *Int Arch Occup Environ Health.* 1992;64:119–123.

Pikaar NA, Wedel M, Hermus RJJ. Influence of several factors on blood alcohol concentrations after drinking alcohol. *Alcohol Alcohol.* 1988;23: 289–297.

Plaa GL. Chlorinated methanes and liver injury: highlights of the past 50 years. *Annu Rev Pharmacol Toxicol.* 2000;40:43–65.

Poet TS, Soelberg JJ, Weitz KK, et al. Mode of action and pharmacokinetic studies of 2-butoxyethanol in the mouse with an emphasis on forestomach dosimetry. *Toxicol Sci.* 2003;71:176–189.

Pohl HR, Scinicariello F. The impact of CYP2E1 genetic variability on risk assessment of VOC mixtures. *Regul Toxicol Pharmacol.* 2011;59: 364–374.

Pohl HR, Tarkowski S, Buczynska A, et al. Chemical exposures at hazardous waste sites: experiences from the United States and Poland. *Environ Toxicol Pharmacol.* 2008;25:283–291.

Poldelski V, Johnson A, Wright S, et al. Ethylene glycol-mediated tubular injury: identification of critical metabolites and injury pathways. *Am J Kidney Dis.* 2001;38:339–348.

Ponomarkov V, Tomatis L. Effects of long-term oral administration of styrene to mice and rats. *Scand J Work Environ Health.* 1978;4(suppl 2): 127–135.

Poon R, Chu IH, Bjarnason S, et al. Short-term inhalation toxicity of methanol, gasoline, and methanol/gasoline in the rat. *Toxicol Ind Health.* 1995;11:343–361.

Pottenger LH, Carney EW, Bartels MJ. Dose-dependent nonlinear pharmacokinetics of ethylene glycol metabolites in pregnant (GD 10) and nonpregnant Sprague–Dawley rats following oral administration of ethylene glycol. *Toxicol Sci.* 2001;62:10–19.

Powley MW, Carlson GP. Species comparison of hepatic and pulmonary metabolism of benzene. *Toxicology.* 1999;139:207–217.

Prah J, Ashley D, Blount B, et al. Dermal, oral, and inhalation pharmacokinetics of methyl *tertiary* butyl ether (MTBE) in human volunteers. *Toxicol Sci.* 2004;77:195–205.

Preedy VR, Ohlendieck K, Adachi J, et al. The importance of alcohol-induced muscle disease. *Clin Sci.* 2003;104:287–294.

Prescott-Matthews JS, Wolf DC, Wong BA, Borghoff SJ. Methyl *tert*-butyl ether causes α2u-globulin nephropathy and enhanced renal cell proliferation in male Fischer-344 rats. *Toxicol Appl Pharmacol.* 1997;143:301–314.

Price B, Bergman TS, Rodriguez M, et al. A review of carbon disulphide exposure data and the association between carbon disulfide exposure and ischemic heart disease mortality. *Regul Toxicol Pharmacol.* 1997;26:119–128.

Price B, Berner T, Henrich RT, et al. A benchmark concentration for carbon disulfide: analysis of the NIOSH carbon disulfide exposure database. *Regul Toxicol Pharmacol.* 1996;24:171–176.

Price PS, Conolly RB, Chaisson CF, et al. Modeling interindividual variation in physiological factors used in PBPK models in humans. *Crit Rev Toxicol.* 2003;33:469–503.

Pryor GT, Rebert CS. Interactive effects of toluene and hexane on behavior and neurophysiologic responses in Fischer-344 rats. *Neurotoxicology.* 1992;13:225–234.

Purohit V, Brenner DA. Mechanisms of alcohol-induced hepatic fibrosis: a summary of the Ron Thurman Symposium. *Hepatology.* 2006;43: 872–878.

Purohit V, Khalsa J, Serrano J. Mechanisms of alcohol-associated cancers: introduction and summary of the symposium. *Alcohol.* 2005;35: 155–160.

Quast JF, Calhoun LL, Frauson LE. 1,1,1-Trichloroethane formulation: a chronic inhalation toxicity and oncogenicity study in Fischer 344 rats and B6C3F1 mice. *Fundam Appl Toxicol.* 1988;11:611–625.

Qui J, Chien Y-C, Bruckner JV, Fisher JW. Bayesian analysis of a physiologically based model for perchloroethylene in humans. *J Toxicol Environ Health A.* 2010;73:74–91.

Raabe GK. Review of the carcinogenic potential of gasoline. *Environ Health Perspect.* 1993;101:35–38.

Raaschou-Nielsen O, Hansen J, McLaughlin JK, et al. Cancer risk among workers at Danish companies using trichloroethylene: a cohort study. *Am J Epidemiol.* 2003;158:1182–1192.

Rajendram R, Preedy VR. Effect of alcohol consumption on the gut. *Dig Dis.* 2005;23:214–221.

Ramdhan DH, Kamijima M, Yamada N, et al. Molecular mechanism of trichloroethylene-induced hepatotoxicity mediated by CYP2E1. *Toxicol Appl Pharmacol.* 2008;231:300–307.

Ramos G, Kazimi N, Nghiem DX, et al. Platelet activating factor receptor binding plays a critical role in jet fuel-induced immune suppression. *Toxicol Appl Pharmacol.* 2004;195:331–338.

Ramos G, Nghiem DX, Walterscheid JP, Ullrich SE. Dermal application of jet fuel suppresses secondary immune reactions. *Toxicol Appl Pharmacol.* 2002;180:136–144.

Ramsay M. Genetic epigenetic insights into fetal alcohol spectrum disorders. *Genome Med.* 2010;2:27–35.

Ramsey JC, Andersen ME. A physiologically based description of the inhalation pharmacokinetics of styrene in rats and humans. *Toxicol Appl Pharmacol.* 1984;73:159–175.

Rangan U, Snyder R. Scientific update on benzene. *Ann NY Acad Sci.* 1997;837:105–112.

Rao PS, Mangipudy RS, Mehendale HM. Tissue injury and repair as parallel and opposing responses to CCl4 hepatotoxicity: a novel dose–response. *Toxicology.* 1997;118:181–193.

Rappaport SM, Kim S, Lan Q, et al. Evidence that humans metabolize benzene via two pathways. *Environ Health Perspect.* 2009;117:946–952.

Ratcliffe JM, Schrader SM, Clapp DE, et al. Semen quality in workers exposed to 2-ethoxyethanol. *Br J Ind Med.* 1989;46:399–406.

Raucy JL, Kraner JC, Lasker JM. Bioactivation of halogenated hydrocarbons by cytochrome P4502E1. *Crit Rev Toxicol.* 1993;23:1–20.

Raucy JL, Lasker JM, Kraner JC, et al. Induction of cytochrome P450IIE1 in the obese overfed rat. *Mol Pharmacol.* 1991;39:275–280.

Raunio H, Husgafvel-Pursianinen K, Anttila S, et al. Diagnosis of polymorphisms in carcinogen-activating and inactivating enzymes and cancer susceptibility: a review. *Gene.* 1995;159:113–121.

Rawlings SJ, Shuker DE, Webb M, Brown NA. The teratogenic potential of alkoxy acids in post-implantation rat embryo culture: structure–activity relationships. *Toxicol Lett.* 1985;28:49–58.

Reaney SH, Bench G, Smith DR. Brain accumulation and toxicity of Mn(II) and Mn(III) exposures. *Toxicol Sci.* 2006;93:114–124.

Recknagel RO, Glende EA Jr, Dolak JA, Waller RL. Mechanisms of carbon tetrachloride toxicity. *Pharmacol Ther.* 1989;43:139–154.

Reese E, Kimbrough RD. Acute toxicity of gasoline and some additives. *Environ Health Perspect.* 1993;101(suppl 6):115–131.

Rehm J, Room R, Monteiro M, et al. Alcohol use. In: Ezzati M, Lopez A, Rodgers A, Murray C, eds. *Comparative Quantification of Health Risks. Global and Regional Burden of Disease Attributable to Selected Major Risk Factors.* Geneva: WHO; 2004:960–1108.

Reigel AC, Ali SF, Torinese S, French ED. Repeated exposure to the abused inhalant toluene alters levels of neurotransmitters and generates peroxynitrite in nigrostriatal and mesolimbic nuclei in rat. *Ann N Y Acad Sci.* 2004;1025:543–551.

Reigel AC, French ED. Abused inhalants and central reward pathways: electrophysiological and behavioral studies in the rat. *Ann N Y Acad Sci.* 2002;965:281–291.

Reinhardt CT, Mulllin LS, Maxfield ME. Epinephrine-induced cardiac arrhythmia potential of some common industrial solvents. *J Occup Med.* 1973;15:953–955.

Reitz RH, McDougal JN, Himmelstein MW, et al. Physiologically-based pharmacokinetic modeling with methylchloroform: implications for interspecies, high dose/low dose, and dose route extrapolations. *Toxicol Appl Pharmacol.* 1988;95:185–199.

Reitz RH, Mendrala AL, Guengerich FP. In vitro metabolism of methylene chloride in human and animal tissues: use in physiologically based pharmacokinetic models. *Toxicol Appl Pharmacol.* 1989;97:220–246.

Rendic S. Summary of information on human CYP enzymes: human P450 metabolism data. *Drug Metab Rev.* 2002;34:83–448.

Richardson PJ, Patel VB, Preedy VR. Alcohol and the myocardium. *Novartis Found Symp.* 1998;216:35–45.

Richter R. Degeneration of the basal ganglia in monkeys from chronic carbon disulfide poisoning. *J Neuropathol Exp Neurol.* 1945;4:324–353.

Rifas L, Towler DA, Avioli LV. Gestational exposure to ethanol suppresses msx2 expression in developing mouse embryos. *Proc Natl Acad Sci U S A.* 1997;94:7549–7554.

Riihimaki V, Kivisto H, Peltonen K, et al. Assessment of exposure to carbon disulfide in viscose production workers from urinary 2-thiothiazolidine-4-carboxylic acid determinations. *Am J Ind Med.* 1992;22:85–97.

Rikans LE, Hornbrook KR. Age-related susceptibility to hepatotoxicants. *Environ Toxicol Pharmacol.* 1997;4:339–344.

Rinn JL, Rozowsky JS, Laurenzi IJ, et al. Major molecular differences between mammalian sexes are involved in drug metabolism and renal function. *Dev Cell.* 2004;6:791–800.

Riordan SM, Williams R. Alcohol exposure and paracetamol-induced hepatotoxicity. *Addict Biol.* 2002;7:191–206.

Ritchie GD, Rossi J III, Nordholm AF, et al. Effects of repeated exposure to JP-8 jet fuel vapor on learning of simple and difficult operant tasks by rats. *J Toxicol Environ Health.* 2001;64:385–415.

Ritchie GD, Still KR, Rossi J, et al. Biological and health effects of exposure to kerosene-based jet fuels and performance additives. *J Toxicol Environ Health B.* 2003;6:357–451.

Ritschel WA. Physiology of the aged respiratory system. In: Ritschel WA, ed. *Gerontokinetics: The Pharmacokinetics of Drugs in the Elderly.* Caldwell, NJ: The Telford Press; 1988:7.

Roberts LG, Bevans AC, Schreiner CA. Development and reproductive toxicity evaluation of toluene vapor in the rat. I. Reproductivity toxicity. *Reprod Toxicol.* 2003;17:649–658.

Robledo RF, Barber DS, Witten ML. Modulation of bronchial epithelial cell barrier function by in vitro jet propulsion fuel 8 exposure. *Toxicol Sci.* 1999;51:119–125.

Robledo RF, Witten ML. NK1-receptor activation prevents hydrocarbon-induced lung injury in mice. *Am J Physiol.* 1999;276:L229–L238.

Rodriguez CE, Mahle DA, Gearhart JM, et al. Predicting age-appropriate pharmacokinetics of six volatile organic compounds in the rat utilizing physiologically based pharmacokinetic modeling. *Toxicol Sci.* 2007;98:43–56.

Roe FJ. Styrene: toxicity studies—what do they show? *Crit Rev Toxicol.* 1994;24(suppl 1):S117–S125.

Roe FJC, Palmer AK, Worden AN, Van Abbe NJ. Safety evaluation of toothpaste containing chloroform. I. Long-term studies in mice. *J Environ Pathol Toxicol.* 1979;2:799–819.

Rogers JV, Gunasekar PG, Garrett CM, et al. Detection of oxidative species and low-molecular weight DNA in skin following dermal exposure with JP-8 jet fuel. *J Appl Toxicol.* 2001;21:521–525.

Rosenberg NL. Neurotoxicity of organic solvents. In: Rosenberg NL, ed. *Occupational and Environmental Neurology.* Newton, MA: Butterworth-Heinemann; 1995:71–113.

Rosenberg NL, Grigsby J, Dreisbach J, et al. Neuropsychologic and MRI abnormalities associated with chronic solvent abuse. *J Toxicol Clin Toxicol.* 2002;40:21–34.

Rosenberg NL, Kleinschmidt-DeMasters BK, Davis KA, et al. Toluene abuse causes central nervous system white matter changes. *Ann Neurol.* 1988a;23:611–614.

Rosenberg NL, Spitz MC, Filley CM, et al. Central nervous system effects of chronic toluene abuse—clinical, brainstem evoked response and magnetic resonance imaging studies. *Neurotoxicol Teratol.* 1988b;10:489–495.

Rosenthal DS, Simbulan-Rosenthal CMG, Liu WF, et al. Mechanisms of JP-8 jet fuel cell toxicity. II. Induction of necrosis in skin fibroblasts and keratinocytes and modulation of levels of Bcl-2 family members. *Toxicol Appl Pharmacol.* 2001;171:107–116.

Roskos KV, Maibach HI, Guy RH. The effect of aging on percutaneous absorption in man. *J Pharmacokinet Biopharm.* 1989;17:617–630.

Ross D, Siegel D, Schattenberg DG, et al. Cell-specific activation and detoxification of benzene metabolites in mouse and human bone marrow: identification of target cells and potential role for modulation of apoptosis in benzene toxicity. *Environ Health Perspect.* 1996;104(suppl 6):1177–1182.

Rossi J III, Nordholm AF, Carpenter RL, et al. Effects of repeated exposure of rats to JP-5 or JP-8 jet fuel vapor on neurobehavioral capacity and neurotransmitter levels. *J Toxicol Environ Health A.* 2001;63:397–428.

Roth RA, Harkema JR, Pestka JP, Ganey PE. Is exposure to bacterial endotoxin a determinant of susceptibility to intoxication from xenobiotic agents? *Toxicol Appl Pharmacol.* 1997;147:300–311.

Rowe BL, Toccalino PL, Moran MJ, et al. Occurrence and potential human-health relevance of volatile organic compounds in drinking water from domestic wells. *Environ Health Perspect.* 2007;115:1539–1546.

Ruder AM, Ward EM, Brown DP. Mortality in dry-cleaning workers: an update. *Am J Ind Med.* 2001;39:121–132.

Rumack BH. Acetaminophen misconceptions. *Hepatology.* 2004;40:10–15.

Russo D, Purohit V, Foudin L, Salin M. Workshop on alcohol use and health disparities 2002: a call to arms. *Alcohol.* 2004;32:37–43.

Saavedra D, Arteaga M, Tena M. Industrial contamination with glycol ethers resulting in teratogenic damage. *Ann N Y Acad Sci.* 1997;837:126–137.

Salvini M, Binaschi S, Riva M. Evaluation of the psychological functions in humans exposed to the threshold limit value of 1,1,1-trichloroethane. *Br J Ind Med.* 1971;28:286–292.

Sanzgiri UY, Kim HJ, Muralidhara S, et al. Effect of route and pattern of exposure on the pharmacokinetics and acute hepatotoxicity of carbon tetrachloride. *Toxicol Appl Pharmacol.* 1995;134:148–154.

Sanzgiri UY, Srivatsan V, Muralidhara S, et al. Uptake, distribution, and elimination of carbon tetrachloride in rat tissues following inhalation and ingestion exposures. *Toxicol Appl Pharmacol.* 1997;143:120–129.

Sarangapani R, Gentry PR, Covington TR, et al. Evaluation of the potential impact of age- and gender-specific lung morphology and ventilation rate on the dosimetry of vapors. *Inhal Toxicol.* 2003;15:987–1016.

Sarangapani R, Teeguarden JG, Cruzan G, et al. Physiologically based pharmacokinetic modeling of styrene and styrene oxide respiratory-tract dosimetry in rodents and humans. *Inhal Toxicol.* 2002;14:789–834.

Sato A, Endoh K, Kaneko T, Johanson G. Effects of consumption of ethanol on the biological monitoring of exposure to organic solvent vapors: a simulation study with trichloroethylene. *Br J Ind Med.* 1991;48:548–556.

Sato A, Nakajima T. Enhanced metabolism of volatile hydrocarbons in rat liver following food deprivation, restricted carbohydrate intake, and administration of ethanol, phenobarbital, polychlorinated biphenyl and 3-methylcholanthrene: a comparative study. *Xenobiotica.* 1985;15:67–75.

Sato A, Nakajima T, Fujiwara Y, Murayama N. Kinetic studies on sex difference in susceptibility to chronic benzene intoxication with special reference to body fat content. *Br J Ind Med.* 1975;32:321–328.

Sato N, Lindros KO, Baraona E, et al. Sex difference in alcohol-related organ injury. *Alcohol Clin Exp Res.* 2001;25:40S–45S.

Sato TK, Yamada RG, Ukai H, et al. Feedback repression is required for mammalian clock function. *Nat Genet.* 2006;38:312–319.

Savolainen K, Riihimaki V, Laine R, Kekoni J. Short-term exposure of human subjects to *m*-xylene and 1,1,1-trichloroethane. *Int Arch Occup Environ Health.* 1981;49:89–98.

Sawant SP, Dnyanmote AV, Shankar K, et al. Potentiation of carbon tetrachloride hepatotoxicity and lethality in type 2 diabetic rats. *J Pharmacol Exp Ther.* 2004;308:694–704.

Scalley RD, Ferguson DR, Piccaro JC, et al. Treatment of ethylene glycol poisoning. *Am Fam Physician.* 2002;66:807–812.

Schaumburg HH, Spencer PS. Organic solvent mixtures. In: Spencer PS, Schaumburg HH, eds. *Experimental and Clinical Neurotoxicology.* 2nd ed. New York: Oxford University Press; 2000:894–897.

Schenker MB, Gold EB, Beaumont JJ, et al. Association of spontaneous abortion and other reproductive effects with work in the semiconductor industry. *Am J Ind Med.* 1995;28:639–659.

Scheuplein R, Charnley G, Dourson M. Differential sensitivity of children and adults to chemical toxicity. I. Biological basis. *Regul Toxicol Pharmacol.* 2002;35:429–447.

Schmucker DL. Age-related changes in liver structure and function: implications for disease? *Exp Gerontol.* 2005;40:650–659.

Schumann AM, Fox TR, Watanabe PG. [14C] methyl chloroform (1,1,1-trichloroethane): pharmacokinetics in rats and mice following inhalation exposure. *Toxicol Appl Pharmacol.* 1982;62:390–401.

Schwartz JB. The influence of sex on pharmacokinetics. *Clin Pharmacokinet.* 2003;42:107–121.

Schwetz BA, Leong BK, Gehring PJ. Embryo- and fetotoxicity of inhaled chloroform in rats. *Toxicol Appl Pharmacol.* 1974;28:442–451.

Scott CS, Chiu WA. Trichloroethylene cancer epidemiology: a consideration of selected issues. *Environ Health Perspect.* 2006;114:1471–1478.

Scott WJ, Fradkin R, Wittfoht W, Nau H. Teratologic potential of 2-methoxyethanol and transplacental distribution of its metabolite, 2-methoxyacetic acid, in non-human primates. *Teratology.* 1989;39:363–373.

Seaton MJ, Schlosser PM, Bond JA, Medinsky MA. Benzene metabolism by human liver microsomes in relation to cytochrome P450 2E1 activity. *Carcinogenesis.* 1994;15:1799–1806.

Seidler A, Mohner M, Berger J, et al. Solvent exposure and malignant lymphoma: a population-based case–control study in Germany. *J Occup Med Toxicol.* 2007;2:2–12. Available at: http://www.occup-med.com/content/2/1/2.

Seiji K, Inoue O, Jin C, et al. Dose excretion relationship in tetrachloroethylene-exposed workers and the effect of tetrachloroethylene co-exposure on trichloroethylene exposure. *Am J Ind Med.* 1989;16:675–684.

Seitz HK, Egerer G, Simanowski UA, et al. Human gastric alcohol dehydrogenase activity: effect of age, sex, and alcoholism. *Gut.* 1993;34:1433–1437.

Seitz HK, Stickel F. Molecular mechanisms of alcohol-mediated carcinogenesis. *Natl Rev Cancer.* 2007;7:599–612.

Seme MT, Summerfelt P, Henry MM, et al. Formate-induced inhibition of photoreceptor function in methanol intoxication. *J Pharmacol Exp Ther.* 1999;289:361–370.

Serota DG, Thakur AK, Ulland BM, et al. A two-year drinking-water study of dichloromethane in rodents. I. Rats. *Food Chem Toxicol.* 1986a;24:951–958.

Serota DG, Thakur AK, Ulland BM, et al. A two-year drinking-water study of dichloromethane in rodents. II. Mice. *Food Chem Toxicol.* 1986b;24:959–963.

Sexton K, Adgate JL, Church TR, et al. Children's exposure to volatile organic compounds as determined by longitudinal measurements in blood. *Environ Health Perspect.* 2005;113:342–349.

Shamsky S, Samimi B. Organic vapors at underground gasoline tank removal sites. *Appl Ind Hyg.* 1987;2:242–245.

Sherratt PJ, Williams S, Foster J, et al. Direct comparison of the nature of mouse and human GST T1-1 and the implications on dichloromethane carcinogenicity. *Toxicol Appl Pharmacol.* 2002;179:89–97.

Shi J, Aisaki K, Ikawa Y, Wake K. Evidence of hepatocyte apoptosis in rat liver after the administration of carbon tetrachloride. *Am J Pathol.* 1998;153:515–525.

Shibley IA, Pennington SN. Metabolic and mitotic changes associated with the fetal alcohol syndrome. *Alcohol Alcohol.* 1997;32:423–434.

Shimada T, Yamazaki H, Mimura M, et al. Interindividual variations in human liver P-450 enzymes involved in the oxidation of drugs, carcinogens and toxic chemicals: studies with liver microsomes of 30 Japanese and 30 Caucasians. *J Pharmacol Exp Ther.* 1994;270:414–423.

Short BG, Steinhagen WH, Swenberg JA. Promoting effects of unleaded gasoline and 2,2,4-trimethylpentane on the development of atypical cell foci and renal tubular cell tumors in rats exposed to *N*-ethyl-*N* hydroxyethylnitrosamine. *Cancer Res.* 1989;49:369–378.

Shroads AL, Langaee T, Coats BS, et al. Human polymorphisms in the glutathione transferase zeta 1/maleylacetoacetate isomerase gene influence the toxicokinetics of dichloroacetate. *J Clin Pharmacol.* 2012;52:837–849 [online]. Available at: http://jcp.sagepub.com/content/early/2011/06/01/0091700114056664.

Siesky AM, Kamendulis LM, Klaunig JE. Hepatic effects of 2-butoxyethanol in rodents. *Toxicol Sci.* 2002;70:252–260.

Sills RC, Harry GJ, Valentine WM, Morgan DL. Interdisciplinary neurotoxicity inhalation studies: carbon disulfide and carbonyl sulfide research in F344 rats. *Toxicol Appl Pharmacol.* 2005;207:S245–S250.

Silvaggio T, Mattison D. Setting occupational health standards: toxicokinetic differences among and between men and women. *J Occup Med.* 1994;36:849–854.

Singh S, Singh J. Dermal toxicity and microscopic alteration by JP-8 jet fuel components in vivo in rabbit. *Environ Toxicol Pharm.* 2004;16:153–161.

Singh S, Zhao K, Singh J. In vivo percutaneous absorption, skin barrier perturbation, and irritation from JP-8 jet fuel components. *Drug Chem Toxicol.* 2003;26:135–146.

Singh SP, Ehmann S, Snyder AK. Ethanol-induced changes in insulin-like growth factors and IGF gene expression in the fetal brain. *Proc Soc Exp Biol Med.* 1996;212:349–354.

Sivilotti ML, Burns MJ, McMartin KE, Brent J. Toxicokinetics of ethylene glycol during fomepizole therapy: implications for management. For the Methylpyrazole for Toxic Alcohols Study Group. *Ann Emerg Med.* 2000;36:114–125.

Skrzypinska-Gawrysiak M, Piotrowski JK, Sporny S. Circadian variations in hepatotoxicity of carbon tetrachloride in mice. *Int J Occup Med Environ Health.* 2000;13:165–173.

Smialowicz RJ, Riddle MM, Luebke RW, et al. Immunotoxicity of 2-methoxyethanol following oral administration in Fischer 344 rats. *Toxicol Appl Pharmacol.* 1991a;109:494–506.

Smialowicz RJ, Riddle MM, Rogers RR, et al. Evaluation of the immunotoxicity of orally administered 2-methoxyacetic acid in Fischer 344 rats. *Fundam Appl Toxicol.* 1991b;17:771–781.

Smialowicz RJ, Riddle MM, Williams WC, et al. Species and strain comparisons of immunosuppression by 2-methoxyethanol and 2-methoxyacetic acid. *Int J Immunopharmacol.* 1994;16:695–702.

Smialowicz RJ, Williams WC, Riddle MM, et al. Comparative immunosuppression of various glycol ethers orally administered to Fischer 344 rats. *Fundam Appl Toxicol.* 1992;18:621–627.

Smith EN, Taylor RT. Acute toxicity of methanol in the folate-deficient acatalasemic mouse. *Toxicology.* 1982;25:271–287.

Smith JH, Maita K, Sleight SD, Hook JB. Effect of sex hormone status on chloroform nephrotoxicity and renal mixed function oxidases in mice. *Toxicology.* 1984;30:305–316.

Smith JN, Timchalk C, Bartels MJ, Poet TS. In vitro age-dependent enzymatic metabolism of chlorpyrifos and chlorpyrifos-oxon in human hepatic microsomes as well as chloropyrifos oxon in plasma. *Drug Metab Dispos.* 2011;39:1353–1362.

Smith MT. The mechanism of benzene-induced leukemia: a hypothesis and speculations on the causes of leukemia. *Environ Health Perspect.* 1996;104(suppl 6):1219–1225.

Snawder JE, Lipscomb JC. Individual variance of cytochrome P450 forms in human hepatic microsomes: correlation of individual forms with xenobiotic metabolism and implications in risk assessment. *Regul Toxicol Pharmacol.* 2000;32:200–209.

Snyder R. Benzene and leukemia. *Crit Rev Toxicol.* 2002;32:155–210.

Snyder R. Xenobiotic metabolism and the mechanism(s) of benzene toxicity. *Drug Metab Rev.* 2004;36:531–547.

Soffritti M, Belpoggi F, Cevolani D, et al. Results of long-term experimental studies on the carcinogenicity of methyl alcohol and ethyl alcohol in rats. *Ann N Y Acad Sci.* 2002;982:46–69.

Sohn MD, McKone TE, Blancato JN. Reconstructing population exposure from dose biomarkers: inhalation of trichloroethylene (TCE) as a case study. *J Expos Sci Environ Epidemiol.* 2004;14:204–213.

Spencer PJ. New toxicity data for the propylene glycol ethers—a commitment to public health and safety. *Toxicol Lett.* 2005;156:181–188.

Spencer PJ, Crissman JW, Stott WT, et al. Propylene glycol monomethyl ether (PGME): inhalation toxicity and carcinogenicity in Fischer 344 rats and B6C3F1 mice. *Toxicol Pathol.* 2002;30:570–579.

Spiller HA. Epidemiology of volatile substance abuse (VSA) cases reported to US poison control centers. *Am J Drug Alcohol Abuse.* 2004;30: 155–165.

Spitzer HL. An analysis of the health benefits associated with the use of MTBE reformulated gasoline oxygenated fuels in reducing atmospheric concentrations of selected volatile organic compounds. *Risk Anal.* 1997;17:683–691.

Sprankle CS, Larson JL, Goldsworthy SM, Butterworth BE. Levels of *myc, fos*, Ha-*ras*, *met* and hepatocyte growth factor mRNA during regenerative cell proliferation in female mouse liver and male rat kidney after a cytotoxic dose of chloroform. *Cancer Lett.* 1996;101: 97–106.

Spurgeon A, Glass DC, Calvert IA, et al. Investigation of dose related neurobehavioral effects in paintmakers exposed to low levels of solvents. *Occup Environ Med.* 1994;51:626–630.

Stacey NH. Toxicity of mixtures of trichloroethylene, tetrachloroethylene and 1,1,1-trichloroethane: similarity of in vitro to in vivo responses. *Toxicol Ind Health.* 1989;5:441–450.

Standeven AM, Blazer DG, Goldsworthy TL. Investigation of antiestrogenic properties of unleaded gasoline in female mice. *Toxicol Appl Pharmacol.* 1994a;127:233–240.

Standeven AM, Goldsworthy TL. Promotion of preneoplastic lesions and induction of CYP2B by unleaded gasoline vapor in female B6C3F1 mouse liver. *Carcinogenesis.* 1993;14:2137–2141.

Standeven AM, Goldsworthy TL. Identification of hepatic mitogenic and cytochrome P-450-inducing fractions of unleaded gasoline in B6C3F1 mice. *J Toxicol Environ Health.* 1994;43:213–224.

Standeven AM, Wolf DC, Goldsworthy TL. Interactive effects of unleaded gasoline and estrogen on liver tumor promotion in female B6C3F1 mice. *Cancer Res.* 1994b;54:1198–1204.

Standeven AM, Wolf DC, Goldsworthy TL. Promotion of hepatic preneoplastic lesions in male B6C3F1 mice by unleaded gasoline. *Environ Health Perspect.* 1995;103:696–700.

Staples CA, Williams JB, Craig GR, Roberts KM. Fate, effects and potential environmental risks of ethylene glycol: a review. *Chemosphere.* 2001;43:377–383.

Starr TB, Matanoski G, Anders MW, Andersen ME. Workshop overview: reassessment of the cancer risk of dichloromethane in humans. *Toxicol Sci.* 2006;91:20–28.

Stenner RD, Merdink JL, Stevens DK, et al. Enterohepatic recirculation of trichloroethanol glucuronide as a significant source of trichloroacetic acid. *Drug Metab Dispos.* 1997;25:529–535.

Stevens JC, Hines RN, Gu C, et al. Developmental expression of the major human hepatic CYP3A enzymes. *J Pharmacol Exp Ther.* 2003;307: 573–582.

Stewart RD, Gay HH, Schaffer AW, et al. Experimental human exposure to methyl chloroform vapor. *Arch Environ Health.* 1969;19:467–472.

Stewart RD, Hake CL, Forster HV, et al. *Tetrachloroethylene: Development of a Biologic Standard for the Industry Worker by Breath Analysis.* Contract No. HSM 99-72-83. NIOSH-MCOW-ENVM-PCE-74-6. NTIS No. PB82-152166. Cincinnati, OH: National Institute of Occupational Safety and Health; 1981.

Stewart RD, Hake CL, Wu A, et al. *Effects of Perchloroethylene/Drug Interaction on Behavior and Neurological Function.* Final Report PB-83-17460. Washington, DC: National Institute of Occupational Safety and Health; 1977.

Stoica BA, Boulares AH, Rosenthal DS, et al. Mechanisms of JP-8 jet fuel toxicity. I. Induction of apoptosis in rat lung epithelial cells. *Toxicol Appl Pharmacol.* 2001;171:94–106.

Stott WT, McKenna MJ. The comparative absorption and excretion of chemical vapors by the upper, lower and intact respiratory tract of rats. *Fundam Appl Toxicol.* 1984;4:594–602.

Stoyanovsky DA, Cederbaum AI. Thiol oxidation and cytochrome P450-dependent metabolism of CCl_4 triggers Ca^{2+} release from liver microsomes. *Biochemistry.* 1996;35:15839–15845.

Sturtevant RP, Sturtevant FM, Pauly JE, Scheving LE. Chronopharmacokinetics of ethanol. *Int J Clin Pharmacol.* 1978;16:594–599.

Sulsky SI, Hooven FH, Burch MT, Mundt KA. Critical review of the epidemiological literature on the potential cardiovascular effects of occupational carbon disulfide exposure. *Int Arch Occup Environ Health.* 2002;75:365–380.

Swaen GM, van Amelsvoort L, Twisk JJ, et al. Low level occupational benzene exposure and hematological parameters. *Chem Biol Interact.* 2010;184:94–100.

Swann HE Jr, Kwon BK, Hogan GK, Snellings WM. Acute inhalation toxicology of volatile hydrocarbons. *Am Ind Hyg Assoc J.* 1974;35: 511–518.

Sweeney LM, Tyler TR, Kirman CR, et al. Proposed occupational exposure limits for select ethylene glycol ethers using PBPK models and Monte Carlo simulations. *Toxicol Sci.* 2001;62:124–139.

Sweeting JN, Siu M, McCallum GP, et al. Species differences in methanol and formic acid pharmacokinetics in mice, rabbits and primates. *Toxicol Appl Pharmacol.* 2010;247:28–35.

Sweeting JN, Siu M, Wiley MJ, Wells PG. Species- and strain-dependent teratogenicity of methanol in rabbits and mice. *Reprod Toxicol.* 2011;31:50–58.

Swenberg JA. $\alpha_{2\mu}$-Globulin nephropathy: review of the cellular and molecular mechanisms involved and their implications for human risk assessment. *Environ Health Perspect.* 1993;101:39–44.

Taieb D, Malicet C, Garcia S, et al. Inactivation of stress protein 8 increases murine carbon tetrachloride hepatotoxicity via preserved CYP2E1 activity. *Hepatology.* 2005;42:176–182.

Takebayashi T, Nishiwaki Y, Uemura T, et al. A six year follow up study of the subclinical effects of carbon disulphide exposure on the cardiovascular system. *Occup Environ Med.* 2004;61:127–134.

Tan X, Peng X, Wang F, et al. Cardiovascular effects of carbon disulfide: meta-analysis of cohort studies. *Int J Hyg Environ Health.* 2002;205:473–477.

Tan Y-M, Butterworth BE, Gargas ML, Conolly RB. Biologically motivated modeling of chloroform cytolethality and regenerative cellular proliferation. *Toxicol Sci.* 2003;75:192–200.

Tan Y-M, Clewell H, Campbell J, Andersen M. Evaluating pharmacokinetic and pharmacodynamic interactions with computational models in supporting cumulative risk assessment. *Int J Environ Res Public Health.* 2011;8:1613–1630.

Tan Y-M, Liao KH, Clewell HJ. Reverse dosimetry: interpreting trihalomethanes biomonitoring data using physiologically based pharmacokinetic data. *J Expos Sci Environ Epidemiol.* 2007;17:591–603.

Tan Y-M, Liao KH, Conolly RB, et al. Use of a physiologically based pharmacokinetic model to identify exposures consistent with human biomonitoring data for chloroform. *J Toxicol Environ Health A.* 2006;69:1727–1756.

Tang C, Lin JH, Lu AYH. Metabolism-based drug–drug interactions: what determines individual variability in cytochrome P450 induction? *Drug Metab Dispos.* 2005;33:603–613.

Tao L, Kramer PM, Ge R, Pereira MA. Effect of dichloroacetic acid and trichloroacetic acid on DNA methylation in liver and tumors of female B6C3F1 mice. *Toxicol Sci.* 1998;43:139–144.

Tao L, Li Y, Kramer PM, et al. Hypomethylation of DNA and the insulin-like growth factor-II gene in dichloroacetic and trichloroacetic acid-promoted mouse liver tumors. *Toxicology.* 2004;196:127–136.

Tao L, Wang W, Li L, et al. DNA hypomethylation induced by drinking water disinfection by-products in mouse and rat kidney. *Toxicol Sci.* 2005;87:344–352.

Tao L, Yang S, Xie M, et al. Effect of trichloroethylene and its metabolites, dichloroacetic acid and trichloroacetic acid, on the methylation and expression of c-Jun and c-Myc protooncogenes in mouse liver: prevention by methionine. *Toxicol Sci.* 2000;54:399–407.

Tapin D, Kennedy G, Lambert J, Zayed J. Bioaccumulation and locomotor effects of manganese sulfate in Sprague–Dawley rats following subchronic (90 days) inhalation exposure. *Toxicol Appl Pharmacol.* 2006;211:166–174.

Tardif R, Lapare S, Plaa GL, Brodeur J. Effect of simultaneous exposure to toluene and xylene on their respective biological exposure indices in humans. *Int Arch Occup Environ Health.* 1991;63:279–284.

Teboul M, Grechez-Cassiau A, Guillaumond F, Delaunnay F. How nuclear receptors tell time. *J Appl Physiol.* 2009;107:1965–1971.

Terry KK, Elswick BA, Welsch F, Conolly RB. Development of a physiologically based pharmacokinetic model describing 2-methoxyacetic acid disposition in the pregnant mouse. *Toxicol Appl Pharmacol.* 1995;132:103–114.

Thamilselvan S, Khan SR. Oxalate and calcium oxalate crystals are injurious to renal epithelial cells: results of in vivo and in vitro studies. *J Nephrol.* 1998;11:66–69.

Thier R, Wiebel FA, Hinkel A, et al. Species differences in the glutathione transferase GSTT1-1 activity towards the model substrates methyl chloride and dichloromethane in liver and kidney. *Arch Toxicol.* 1998;72:622–629.

Thompson DJ, Warner SD, Robinson VB. Teratology studies on orally administered chloroform in the rat and rabbit. *Toxicol Appl Pharmacol.* 1974;29:348–357.

Thrall KD, Weitz KK, Woodstock AD. Use of real-time breath analysis and physiologically based pharmacokinetic modeling to evaluate dermal absorption of aqueous toluene in human volunteers. *Toxicol Sci.* 2002;68:280–287.

Thurman RG. Mechanisms of hepatic toxicity II. Alcoholic liver injury involves activation of Kupffer cells by endotoxin. *Am J Physiol.* 1998;275:G605–G611.

Thurman RG. Sex-related liver injury due to alcohol involves activation of Kupffer cells by endotoxin. *Can J Gastroenterol.* 2000;14:129D–135D.

Timchalk C, Kousba AA, Poet TS. An age-dependent physiologically based pharmacokinetic/pharmacodynamic model for the organophosphorus insecticide in the preweanling rat. *Toxicol Sci.* 2007;98:348–365.

Tinston DJ. *Perchloroethylene: Multigeneration Inhalation Study in the Rat.* Report No. CTL/P/4907. Alderley Park, Cheshire, UK: Zenca Central Laboratory; 1995.

Tonkin EG, Erve JC, Valentine WM. Disulfiram produces a non-carbon disulfide-dependent schwannopathy in the rat. *J Neuropathol Exp Neurol.* 2000;59:786–797.

Toraason M, Breitenstein M. Prenatal ethylene glycol ether (EGME) exposure produces electrocardiographic changes in the rat. *Toxicol Appl Pharmacol.* 1988;95:321–327.

Tornero-Velez R, Mirfazaelian A, Kim K-B, et al. Evaluation of deltamethrin kinetics and dosimetry in the maturing rat using a PBPK model. *Toxicol Appl Pharmacol.* 2010;244:208–217.

Tornero-Velez R, Rappaport SM. Physiological modeling of the relative contributions of SO derived from direct inhalation and from styrene metabolism to the systemic dose in humans. *Toxicol Sci.* 2001;64:151–161.

Toso L, Roberson R, Woodard J, et al. Prenatal alcohol exposure alters GABA(A)alpha(5) expression: a mechanism of alcohol-induced learning dysfunction. *Am J Obstet Gynecol.* 2006;195:1038–1044.

Toth B, Hornung D, Scholz S, et al. Peroxisome proliferator-activated receptors: new players in the field of reproduction. *Am J Reprod Immunol.* 2007;58:289–310.

Traiger GJ, Bruckner JV. The participation of 2-butanone in 2-butanol-induced potentiation of carbon tetrachloride hepatotoxicity. *J Pharmacol Exp Ther.* 1976;196:493–500.

Travis CC, Fox MT, Simmons WM, Lyon BF. Co-exposure to gasoline vapor decreases benzene metabolism in Fischer-344 rats. *Toxicol Lett.* 1992;62:231–240.

Treichel JL, Henry MM, Skumatz CM, Eells JT, Burke JM. Formate, the toxic metabolite of methanol, in cultured ocular cells. *Neurotoxicology.* 2003;24:825–834.

Triebig G, Claus D, Csuzda I, et al. Cross-sectional epidemiological study on neurotoxicity of solvents in paints and lacquers. *Int Arch Occup Environ Health.* 1988;60:233–241.

Triebig G, Hallermann J. Survey of solvent related chronic encephalopathy as an occupational disease in European countries. *Occup Environ Med.* 2001;58:575–581.

Trush MA, Twerdok LE, Rembish SJ, et al. Analysis of target cell susceptibility as a basis for the development of a chemoprotective strategy against benzene-induced hematotoxicities. *Environ Health Perspect.* 1996;104(suppl 6):1227–1234.

Tsai SP, Fox EE, Ransdell JD, et al. A hematology surveillance study of petrochemical workers exposure to benzene. *Regul Toxicol Pharmacol.* 2004;40:67–73.

Turini A, Amato G, Longo V, Gervasi PG. Oxidation of methyl- and ethyl-*tertiary*-butyl ethers in rat liver microsomes: role of the cytochrome P450 isoforms. *Arch Toxicol.* 1998;72:207–214.

Turtletaub KW, Mani C. Benzene metabolism in rodents at doses relevant to human exposure from urban air. *Res Rep Health Eff Inst.* 2003;113:1–26.

Tyl RW, Ballantyne B, France KA, et al. Evaluation of the developmental toxicity of ethylene glycol monohexyl ether vapor in Fischer 344 rats and New Zealand white rabbits. *Fundam Appl Toxicol.* 1989;12:269–280.

Tyson CA, Hawk-Prather K, Story DL, et al. Correlations of *in vitro* and *in vivo* hepatotoxicity for five haloalkanes. *Toxicol Appl Pharmacol.* 1983;70:289–302.

Uchida Y, Nakatsuka H, Ukai H, et al. Symptoms and signs in workers exposed predominantly to xylenes. *Int Arch Occup Environ Health.* 1993;64:597–605.

Udden MM. Hemolysis and deformability of erythrocytes exposed to butoxyacetic acid, a metabolite of 2-butoxyethanol: II. Resistance in red blood cells from humans with potential susceptibility. *J Appl Toxicol.* 1994;14:97–102.

Udden MM. Effects of diethylene glycol butyl ether and butoxyethoxyacetic acid on rat and human erythrocytes. *Toxicol Lett.* 2005;156:95–101.

Udden MM, Patton CS. Hemolysis and deformability of erythrocytes exposed to butoxyacetic acid, a metabolite of 2-butoxyethanol: I. Sensitivity in rats and resistance in normal humans. *J Appl Toxicol.* 1994;14:91–96.

Udden MM, Patton CS. Butoxyacetic acid-induced hemolysis of rat red blood cells: effect of external osmolarity and cations. *Toxicol Lett.* 2005;156:81–93.

Ullrich SE. Dermal application of JP-8 jet fuel induces immune suppression. *Toxicol Sci.* 1999;52:61–67.

Ullrich SE, Lyons HJ. Mechanisms involved in the immunotoxicity induced by dermal application of JP-8 jet fuel. *Toxicol Sci.* 2000;58:290–298.

Umulis DM, Gurmen NM, Singh P, Fogler HS. A physiologically based model for ethanol and acetaldehyde metabolism in human beings. *Alcohol.* 2005;35:3–12.

UNEP (United Nations Environment Programme). *SIDS Initial Assessment Report for SIAM 2—Tripropylene Glycol.* July 1994. Available at: http://www.inchem.org/documents/sids/sids/24800-44-0.pdf.

UNEP (United Nations Environment Programme). *SIDS Initial Assessment Report for 11th SIAM—Dipropylene Glycol (Mixed Isomers and*

Dominant Isomer). January 2001. Available at: http://www.inchem.org/documents/sids/sids/25265-71-8.pdf.

Vahter M, Gochfeld M, Casati B, et al. Implications of gender differences for human health risk assessment and toxicology. *Environ Res.* 2007;104:70–84.

Valentine JL, Lee SS-T, Seaton MJ, et al. Reduction of benzene metabolism and toxicity in mice that lack CYP2E1 expression. *Toxicol Appl Pharmacol.* 1996;141:205–213.

Valentine WM, Amarnath V, Amarnath K, et al. Covalent modification of hemoglobin by carbon disulfide: III. A potential biomarker of effect. *Neurotoxicology.* 1998;19:99–108.

Valentine WM, Amarnath V, Graham DG, et al. CS2-mediated cross-linking of erythrocyte spectrin and neurofilament protein: dose response and temporal relationship to the formation of axonal swellings. *Toxicol Appl Pharmacol.* 1997;142:95–105.

Valentine WM, Graham DG, Anthony DC. Covalent cross-linking of erythrocyte spectrin by carbon disulfide in vivo. *Toxicol Appl Pharmacol.* 1993;121:71–77.

Valpey R, Sumi SM, Copass MK, Goble GJ. Acute and chronic progressive encephalopathy due to gasoline sniffing. *Neurology.* 1978;28:507–510.

Vamvakas S, Bruning T, Thomasson B, et al. Renal cell cancer correlated with occupational exposure to trichloroethene. *J Cancer Res Clin Oncol.* 1998;124:374–382.

van der Hoek JAF, Verberk MM, Hageman G. Criteria for solvent-induced chronic toxic encephalopathy: a systematic review. *Int Arch Occup Environ Health.* 2000;73:362–368.

van der Hoek JAF, Verberk MM, van der Laan G, Hageman G. Routine diagnostic procedures for chronic encephalopathy induced by solvents: survey of experts. *Occup Environ Med.* 2001;58:382–385.

Vanhoorne MH, De Bacquer D, De Backer G. Epidemiological study of the cardiovascular effects of carbon disulphide. *Int J Epidemiol.* 1992;21:745–752.

Vasiliou V, Pappa A, Estey T. Role of human aldehyde dehydrogenases in endobiotic and xenobiotic metabolism. *Drug Metab Rev.* 2004;36:279–299.

Verhulst A, Asselman M, Persy VP, et al. Crystal retention capacity of cells in the human nephron: involvement of CD44 and its ligands hyaluronic acid and osteopontin in the transition of a crystal binding—into a non-adherent epithelium. *J Am Soc Nephrol.* 2003;14:107–115.

Verplanke AJ, Leummens MH, Herber RF. Occupational exposure to tetrachloroethylene and its effects on the kidneys. *J Occup Environ Med.* 1999;41:11–16.

Veulemans H, Steeno O, Maschelein R, Groeseneken D. Exposure to ethylene glycol ethers and spermatogenic disorders in man: a case–control study. *Br J Ind Med.* 1993;50:71–78.

Vidali M, Stewart SF, Albano E. Interplay between oxidative stress and immunity in the progression of alcohol-mediated liver injury. *Trends Mol Med.* 2008;14:63–71.

Volkel W, Friedewald M, Lederer E, et al. Biotransformation of perchloroethene: dose-dependent excretion of trichloroacetic acid, dichloroacetic acid, and N-acetyl-S-(trichlorovinyl)-l-cysteine in rats and humans after inhalation. *Toxicol Appl Pharmacol.* 1998;153:20–27.

von Euler G. Toluene and dopaminergic transmission. In: Isaacon RL, Jensen KF, eds. *The Vulnerable Brain and Environmental Risk. Toxins in Air and Water.* Vol. 3. New York: Plenum Press; 1994:301–321.

Vrca A, Bozicevic D, Karacic V, et al. Visual evoked potentials in individuals exposed to long-term low concentrations of toluene. *Arch Toxicol.* 1995;69:337–340.

Vyskocil A, Emminger S, Tejral J, et al. Study on kidney function in female workers exposed to perchloroethylene. *Hum Exp Toxicol.* 1990;9:377–380.

Walgren JL, Kurtz DT, McMillan JM. Lack of direct mitogenic activity of dichloroacetate and trichloroacetate in cultured rat hepatocytes. *Toxicology.* 2005;211:220–230.

Wallace L. Major sources of exposure to benzene and other volatile organic chemicals. *Risk Anal.* 1990;10:59–64.

Wallace L. Environmental exposure to benzene: an update. *Environ Health Perspect.* 1996;104(suppl 6):1129–1136.

Wallace LA, Pellizzari ED, Hartwell TD, et al. A TEAM study: personal exposures to toxic substances in air, drinking water, and breath of 400 residents of New Jersey, North Carolina, and North Dakota. *Environ Res.* 1987;43:290–307.

Wang FI, Kuo ML, Shun CT, et al. Chronic toxicity of a mixture of chlorinated alkanes and alkenes in 1CR mice. *J Toxicol Environ Health.* 2002a;65:279–291.

Wang PY, Kaneko T, Tsukada H, et al. Dose- and route-dependent alterations in metabolism and toxicity of chemical compounds in ethanol-treated rats: difference between highly (chloroform) and poorly (carbon tetrachloride) metabolized hepatotoxic compounds. *Toxicol Appl Pharmacol.* 1997;142:13–21.

Wang S, Young RS, Sun NN, Witten ML. In vitro cytokine release from rat type II pneumocytes and alveolar macrophages following exposure to JP-8 jet fuel in co-culture. *Toxicology.* 2002b;173:211–219.

Wang W, Chapin RE. Differential gene expression detected by suppression subtractive hybridization in the ethylene glycol monomethyl ether-induced testicular lesion. *Toxicol Sci.* 2000;56:165–174.

Wang W, Wine RN, Chapin RE. Rat testicular Src: normal distribution and involvement in ethylene glycol monomethyl ether-induced apoptosis. *Toxicol Appl Pharmacol.* 2000;163:125–134.

Ward E, Hornung R, Morris J, et al. Risk of low red or white blood cell count related to estimated benzene exposure in a rubberworker cohort. *Am J Ind Med.* 1996;29:247–257.

Warren DA, Bowen SE, Jennings WB, et al. Biphasic effects of 1,1,1-trichloroethane on the locomotor activity of mice: relationship to blood and brain solvent concentrations. *Toxicol Sci.* 2000;56:365–373.

Warren DA, Graeter LJ, Channel SR, et al. Trichloroethylene, trichloroacetic acid, and dichloroacetic acid: do they affect eye development in the Sprague–Dawley rat? *Int J Toxicol.* 2006;25:279–284.

Warren DA, Reigle TG, Muralidhara S, Dallas CE. Schedule-controlled operant behavior of rats during 1,1,1-trichloroethane inhalation: relationship to blood and brain solvent concentrations. *Neurotoxicol Teratol.* 1998;20:143–153.

Warren KR, Hewitt BG, Thomas JD. Fetal alcohol spectrum disorders: research challenges and opportunities. *Alcohol Res Health.* 2011;34:4–14.

Wartenberg D, Reyner D, Scott CS. Trichloroethylene and cancer: epidemiologic evidence. *Environ Health Perspect.* 2000;108(suppl 2):161–176.

Watanabe A, Nakano Y, Endo T, et al. Collaborative work to evaluate toxicity on male reproductive organs by repeated dose studies in rats 27. Repeated toxicity study on ethylene glycol monomethyl ether for 2 and 4 weeks to detect effects on male reproductive organs in rats. *J Toxicol Sci.* 2000;25:259–266.

Watanabe K, Guengerich FP. Limited reactivity of formyl chloride with glutathione and relevance to metabolism and toxicity of dichloromethane. *Chem Res Toxicol.* 2006;19:1091–1096.

Watanabe M, Tanaka M, Tateishi T, et al. Effects of the estrous cycle and the gender differences on hepatic drug metabolizing enzyme activities. *Pharmacol Res.* 1997;35:477–480.

Watson RE, Jacobson CF, Williams AL, et al. Trichloroethylene-contaminated drinking water and congenital heart defects: a critical analysis of the literature. *Reprod Toxicol.* 2006;21:117–147.

Watson WA. Ethylene glycol toxicity: closing in on rational, evidence-based treatment. *Ann Emerg Med.* 2000;36:139–141.

Watson WA, Litovitz TL, Rodgers GC Jr, et al. 2004 annual report of the American Association of Poison Control Centers Toxic Exposure Surveillance System. *Am J Emerg Med.* 2005;23:589–666.

Wauthier V, Verbeeck RK, Calderan PB. Age-related changes in the protein and mRNA levels of CYP2E1 and CYP3A isoforms as well as in their hepatic activities in Wistar rats. What role for oxidative stress? *Arch Toxicol.* 2004;78:131–138.

Wax PM. Elixirs, diluents, and the passage of the 1938 Federal Food, Drug and Cosmetic Act. *Ann Intern Med.* 1995;122:456–461.

Weber LWD, Boll M, Stampfl A. Hepatoxicity and mechanisms of action of haloalkanes: carbon tetrachloride as a toxicological model. *Crit Rev Toxicol.* 2003;33:105–136.

Weber WW. Populations and genetic polymorphisms. *Mol Diagn.* 1999;4:299–307.

Weisel CP, Jo WK. Ingestion, inhalation, and dermal exposures to chloroform and trichloroethene from tap water. *Environ Health Perspect.* 1996;104:48–51.

Weiss NS. Cancer in relation to occupational exposure to perchloroethylene. *Cancer Causes Control.* 1995;6:257–266.

Welch LS, Schrader SM, Turner TW, Cullen MR. Effects of exposure to ethylene glycol ethers on shipyard painters: II. Male reproduction. *Am J Ind Med.* 1988;14:509–526.

Welling PG, Pool WF. Effect of liver disease on drug metabolism and pharmacokinetics. In: Cameron RG, Feuer G, De la Iglesia FA, eds. *Drug Induced Hepatotoxicity.* Berlin: Springer-Verlag; 1996:367–394.

Wenker MAM, Kerzic S, Monster AC, de Wolff FA. Metabolic capacity and interindividual variation in toxicokinetics of styrene in volunteers. *Hum Exp Toxicol.* 2001;20:221–228.

White CA, Muralidhara S, Hines C, et al. Effects of oral dosage regimen and rate on first-pass elimination and toxicokinetics of 1,1,1-trichloroethane and trichloroethylene. *Toxicol Appl Pharmacol.* 2013.

White INH, Razvi N, Gibbs AH, et al. Neoantigen formation and clastogenic action of HCFC-123 and perchloroethylene in human MCL-5 cells. *Toxicol Lett.* 2001;124:129–138.

WHO (World Health Organization)/Nordic Council of Ministers. *Chronic Effects of Organic Solvents on the Central Nervous System and Diagnostic Criteria.* Copenhagen: WHO; 1985.

WHO (World Health Organization of the United Nations). *Environmental Health Criteria 206: Methyl tertiary-Butyl Ether.* Geneva: WHO; 1998.

WHO (World Health Organization). *Concise International Chemical Assessment Document 46—Carbon Disulfide.* Geneva: WHO; 2002:1–64. Available at: http://www.inchem.org/documents/cicads/cicads/cicad46.htm.

WHO (World Health Organization). *Guidelines for Drinking Water Quality.* 3rd ed. Geneva: WHO; 2004. Available at: http://www.who.int/water_sanitation_health/drug/gdwq3/en/.

Wiener HL, Richardson KE. The metabolism and toxicity of ethylene glycol. *Res Commun Subst Abuse.* 1988;9:77–87.

Wiener HL, Richardson KE. Metabolism of diethylene glycol in male rats. *Biochem Pharmacol.* 1989;38:539–541.

Wiesenhutter B, Selinski S, Golka K, et al. Re-assessment of the influence of polymorphisms of phase-II metabolic enzymes on renal cell cancer risk of trichloroethylene-exposed workers. *Int Arch Occup Environ Health.* 2007;81:247–251.

Wilkins-Haug L. Teratogen update: toluene. *Teratology.* 1997;55:145–151.

Williams J, Reel JR, George JD, Lamb JC IV. Reproductive effects of diethylene glycol and diethylene glycol monoethyl ether in Swiss CD-1 mice assessed by a continuous breeding protocol. *Fundam Appl Toxicol.* 1990;14:622–635.

Williams JF, Storck M. Inhalant abuse. *Pediatrics.* 2007;119:1009–1017.

Williams PR, Cushing CA, Sheehan PJ. Data available for evaluating the risks and benefits of MTBE and ethanol as alternative fuel oxygenates. *Risk Anal.* 2003;23:1085–1115.

Williams PRD, Scott PK, Sheehan PJ, Paustenbach DJ. A probabilistic assessment of household exposures to MTBE in California drinking water. *Hum Ecol Risk Assess.* 2000a;6:827–849.

Williams TM, Borghoff SJ. Induction of testosterone biotransformation enzymes following oral administration of methyl *tert*-butyl ether to male Sprague–Dawley rats. *Toxicol Sci.* 2000;57:147–155.

Williams TM, Borghoff SJ. Characterization of *tert*-butyl alcohol binding to alpha2u-globulin in F-344 rats. *Toxicol Sci.* 2001;62:228–235.

Williams TM, Cattley RC, Borghoff SJ. Alterations in endocrine responses in male Sprague–Dawley rats following oral administration of methyl *tert*-butyl ether. *Toxicol Sci.* 2000b;54:168–176.

Williams WC, Riddle MM, Copeland CB, et al. Immunological effects of 2-methoxyethanol administered dermally or orally to Fischer 344 rats. *Toxicology.* 1995;98:215–223.

Williams-Hill D, Spears CP, Prakash S, et al. Mutagenicity studies of methyl-*tert*-butylether using the Ames tester strain TA102. *Mutat Res.* 1999;446:15–21.

Wilmarth KR, Viana ME, Abou-Donia MB. Carbon disulfide inhalation increases Ca²⁺/calmodulin-dependent kinase phosphorylation of cytoskeletal proteins in the rat central nervous system. *Brain Res.* 1993;628:293–300.

Wilson KC, Reardon C, Farber HW. Propylene glycol toxicity in a patient receiving intravenous diazepam. *N Engl J Med.* 2000;343:815.

Wilson KC, Reardon C, Theodore AC, Farber HW. Propylene glycol toxicity: a severe iatrogenic illness in ICU patients receiving IV benzodiazepines: a case series and prospective, observational pilot study. *Chest.* 2005;128:1674–1681.

Wine RN, Ku WW, Li LH, Chapin RE. Cyclophilin A is present in rat germ cells and is associated with spermatocyte apoptosis. Reproductive Toxicology Group. *Biol Reprod.* 1997;56:439–446.

Winek CL, Shingleton DP, Shanor SP. Ethylene and diethylene glycol toxicity. *Clin Toxicol.* 1978;13:297–324.

Win-Shwe TT, Fujimaki H. Neurotoxicity of toluene. *Toxicol Lett.* 2010;198:93–99.

Win-Shwe TT, Hojo R, Mitsushima D, et al. Establishment of mouse model to assess brain neurotransmitter level and learning performance simultaneously following toxic chemical exposure: using in vivo microdialysis and schedule-controlled operant behavior. *J UOEH.* 2009;31:1–11.

Witz G, Zhang Z, Goldstein BD. Reactive ring-opened aldehyde metabolites in benzene hematotoxicity. *Environ Health Perspect.* 1996;104(suppl 6): 1195–1199.

Witzmann FA, Bauer MD, Fieno AM, et al. Proteomic analysis of simulated jet fuel exposure in the lung. *Electrophoresis.* 1999;20:3659–3669.

Witzmann FA, Bauer MD, Fieno AM, et al. Proteomic analysis of the renal effects of simulated occupational jet fuel exposure. *Electrophoresis.* 2000a;21:976–984.

Witzmann FA, Bobb A, Briggs GB, et al. Analysis of rat testicular protein expression following 91-day exposure to JP-8 jet fuel vapor. *Proteomics.* 2003;3:1016–1027.

Witzmann FA, Carpenter RL, Ritchie GD, et al. Toxicity of chemical mixtures: proteomic analysis of persisting liver and kidney protein alterations induced by repeated exposure of rats to JP-8 jet fuel vapor. *Electrophoresis.* 2000b;21:2138–2147.

Witzmann FA, Monteiro-Riviere NA, Inman AO, et al. Effect of JP-8 jet fuel exposure on protein expression in human keratinocyte cells in culture. *Toxicol Lett.* 2005;160:8–21.

Wong FW-Y, Chan W-Y, Lee SS-T. Resistance to carbon tetrachloride-induced hepatotoxicity in mice which lack CYP2E1 expression. *Toxicol Appl Pharmacol.* 1998;153:109–118.

Wong O. Carcinogenicity of trichloroethylene: an epidemiologic assessment. *Clin Occup Environ Med.* 2004;4:557–589.

Wormhoudt LW, Commandeur JNM, Vermeulen NPE. Genetic polymorphisms of human *N*-acetyltransferase, cytochrome P450, glutathione-*S*-transferase, and epoxide hydrolase enzymes: relevance to xenobiotic metabolism and toxicity. *Crit Rev Toxicol.* 1999;29:59–124.

Wronska-Nofer T. Various disorders of cholesterol metabolism and their effect on the development of experimental arteriosclerosis in rats exposed to carbon disulfide. *Med Proc.* 1979;30:121–134.

Wronska-Nofer T, Chojnowska-Jezierska J, Nofer JR, et al. Increased oxidative stress in subjects exposed to carbon disulfide (CS₂)—an occupational coronary risk factor. *Arch Toxicol.* 2002;76:152–157.

Wu L-T, Pilowsky DJ, Schlenger WE. Inhalant abuse and dependence among adolescents in the United States. *J Am Acad Child Adolesc Psychol.* 2004;43:1206–1214.

Xu H, Tanphaichitr N, Forkert PG, et al. Exposure to trichloroethylene and its metabolites causes impairment of sperm fertilizing ability in mice. *Toxicol Sci.* 2004;82:590–597.

Yang JH, Lee CH, Monteiro-Riviere NA, et al. Toxicity of jet fuel aliphatic and aromatic hydrocarbon mixtures on human epidermal keratinocytes: evaluation based on in vitro cytotoxicity and interleukin-8 release. *Arch Toxicol.* 2006;80:508–523.

Yang Q, Nagano T, Shah R, et al. The PPARα-humanized mouse: a model to investigate species differences in liver toxicity mediated by PPARα. *Toxicol Sci.* 2008;101:132–139.

Yin M, Ikejima K, Wheeler MD, et al. Estrogen is involved in early alcohol-induced liver injury in a rat enteral feeding model. *Hepatology.* 2000;31:117–123.

Yin SJ, Han CL, Lee AI, Wu CW. Human alcohol dehydrogenase family. Functional classification, ethanol/retinol metabolism, and medical implications. *Adv Exp Med Biol.* 1999;463:265–274.

1112

Yin S-N, Hayes RB, Linet MS, et al. A cohort study of cancer among benzene-exposed workers in China: overall results. *Am J Ind Med.* 1996;29:227–235.

Yokley K, Tran HT, Pekari K, et al. Physiologically based pharmacokinetic (PBPK) modeling of benzene in humans: a Bayesian approach. *Risk Anal.* 2006;26:925–942.

Yoon BI, Hirabayashi Y, Kawasaki Y, et al. Aryl hydrocarbon receptor mediates benzene-induced hematotoxicity. *Toxicol Sci.* 2002;70:150–156.

Yuan R, Venitz J. Effect of chronic renal failure on the disposition of highly hepatically metabolized drugs. *Int J Clin Pharmacol Ther.* 2000;38:245–253.

Yue J, Khokhar J, Miksys S, Tyndale RF. Differential induction of ethanol-metabolizing CYP2E1 and nicotine-metabolizing CYP2B1/2 in rat liver by chronic nicotine treatment and voluntary ethanol intake. *Eur J Pharmacol.* 2009;609:88–95.

Zangar RC, Benson JM, Burnett VL, Springer DL. Cytochrome P450 2E1 is the primary enzyme responsible for low-dose carbon tetrachloride metabolism in human liver microsomes. *Chem Biol Interact.* 2000;125:233–243.

Zhao Y, Krishnadasan A, Kennedy N, et al. Estimated effects of solvents and mineral oils on cancer incidence and mortality in a cohort of aerospace workers. *Am J Ind Med.* 2005;48:249–258.

Zhou W, Yuan D, Huang G, et al. Mutagenicity of methyl *tertiary* butyl ether. *J Environ Pathol Toxicol Oncol.* 2000;19:35–39.

Zimniak P. Detoxification reactions: relevance to aging. *Ageing Res Rev.* 2008;7:281–300.

Zintzaras E, Stefanidis I, Santos M, Vidal F. Do alcohol-metabolizing enzyme gene polymorphisms increase the risk of alcoholism and alcoholic liver disease? *Hepatology.* 2006;43:352–361.

Toxic Effects of Radiation and Radioactive Materials

David G. Hoel

INTRODUCTION

Ionizing radiations such as γ-rays and x-rays are radiations that have sufficient energy to displace electrons from molecules. These freed electrons then have the capability of damaging other molecules and, in particular, DNA. Thus, the potential health effects of low levels of radiation are important to understand in order to be able to quantify their effects. For example, it has been estimated that 10% of lung cancers are attributable to radon exposures. In recent years the amount of radiation that the public receives has greatly increased due to medical applications, especially the higher doses associated with computed tomography (CT) scans. Currently 50% of radiation exposures are from medical, 48% from environmental (primarily radon), and 2% from consumer products. The average yearly total effective exposure to individuals is 6.2 mSv. For an extensive analysis, the reader is referred to National Council on Radiation Protection (NCRP) Report 160. Fig. 25-1 taken from the report gives a summary breakdown of exposure sources.

Biological effects of radiation are primarily damage to the DNA. Atoms of the DNA target may be directly ionized or indirectly affected by the creation of a free radical that can interact with the DNA molecule. In particular, the hydroxyl radical is predominant in DNA damage. For radiation particles such as neutrons and α particles the damage is primarily direct, whereas for photons such as x-rays, about two-third of the DNA damage in mammalian cells is due to hydroxy radicals. The study of health effects of ionizing radiation is complicated by the fact that there are various types of radiation, from x-ray photons to heavy charged particles encountered in space. Within any type of radiation the potential damage also depends on the energy level of the photons or particles.

Cancer has been the major adverse health effect of ionizing radiation. It has been well studied epidemiologically, as well as in the laboratory and in animal toxicological studies. More recently, there has been a concern with possible cardiovascular effects, cataractogenesis, and possibly immunosceneses. At one time there was considerable concern about the possible heritable effects, but the risks now appear to be small. The issues with chemicals are the risks at low doses, and with radiation the effects of acute versus chronic exposures. Most radiation risk analyses depend on epidemiological studies. There have been many that have large populations and varied exposures. There is, however, a need for better radiobiological understanding of potential health effects in order to estimate low-dose effects, sensitive subgroups, and radiation types and energies that have not been adequately studied.

RADIATION BACKGROUND

Types of Ionizing Radiation

When ionizing radiation passes through matter, it has the energy to ionize atoms so that one or more of its electrons can be dislodged and chemical bonds broken. Ionizing radiation is of two types: particulate and electromagnetic waves. Particulate radiation may either be electrically charged (α, β, proton) or have no charge (neutron). Ionizing electromagnetic radiation (photons) in the form of x-rays or γ-rays has considerably more energy than nonionizing radiation, such as ultraviolet and visible light. Radionuclides (ie, radioactive atoms), being unstable, release both electromagnetic and particulate radiation during their radioactive decay. The radionuclides

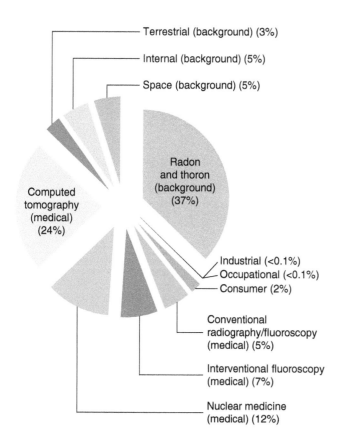

Figure 25-1. *Percent contribution of total effective dose to individuals (NCRP Report 160).*

decay into either stable elements or through a decay chain of successive radionuclides called decay daughters. The types of radiation emitted, its rate of decay, and the energies of the released radiation are unique to each type of radionuclide. The charged particles are directly ionizing because they ionize molecules by direct collisions with the molecules' electrons. Photons can travel relatively long distances, and after interacting with an electron in a material, the photon transfers some or all of its energy to the electron. The energetic electrons (ie, photoelectrons or Compton electrons) are released, producing an indirect ionization. There are three basic radionuclide decay series: thorium, neptunium, and uranium series. The uranium decay series is illustrated in Fig. 25-2, and Table 25-1 gives the details.

The rate of energy dissipation by a single event is referred to as linear energy transfer (LET). The LET of a charged particle is the average energy lost due to interactions per unit length of its trajectory given as kiloelectron volts per micrometer (keV/μm). x-Rays, γ-rays, and β particles of similar energies produce sparse ionization tracks and are classified as low-LET radiation. Particulate radiation (eg, neutrons and α particles) causes interactions with large amounts of energy being dissipated within short distances. α Particles (helium nucleus), which are released from the nucleus of some radionuclides, are slow-moving with a positive charge. Although they cannot penetrate a piece of paper or skin, they are of concern if ingested or inhaled. The most recognized example is the lung cancer risk from the inhalation of radon (Rn222) and its daughter products. LET depends on the energy of the particle; for example, the LET of a 5-MeV α particle would be 100 keV/μm. Neutrons released during nuclear chain reactions have a greater range and lower LET (20 for a 2.5-MeV neutron). A 250-keV x-ray has an LET of 2 to 3 and a Cobalt 60 γ-ray 0.2 to 0.3. A β particle is a simple electron that is released from the nucleus when a neutron

converts into a proton, and it has similar low-LET values depending again on its energy.

The rate of decay of a radionuclide is exponential with a decay rate constant λ that is then simply $Ae^{-\lambda t}$ for time t and initial quantity of the radionuclide A. The radiological half-life is the time required for the radionuclide to lose 50% of its activity by decay. Each radionuclide has its own unique half-life as illustrated in Table 25-1. For example, the half-life of iodine 131 is eight days while for cesium 137 it is 20 years. If a radionuclide is internally deposited in an individual, the actual half-life is obtained by taking the reciprocal of the sum of the reciprocals of the radiological half-life and the biological half-life; that is, $1/T = 1/T_r + 1/T_b$ where T is the half-life, T_r is the radiological half-life, and T_b is the biological half-life. For more extensive and detailed information the reader is referred to Biological Effects of Ionizing Radiation (BEIR) VII and the text by Turner (2007).

Relative Biological Effectiveness and Quality Factors

The various types of ionizing radiation have similar biological effects that occur because of the ionization of molecules. However, without knowing the type of radiation, one cannot specify how much radiation is needed to produce a specific biological effect. This is because a given absorbed dose (energy per unit mass) of x-rays does not have the same biological effect as an identical dose of neutrons. The relative effectiveness of different types of radiation in producing biological changes depends on deposition of energy, that is, LET. In order to deal with this problem the International Council of Radiation Protection (ICRP) developed the concept of relative biological effectiveness (RBE). It is defined in BEIR V as

"Biological potency of one radiation as compared with another to produce the same biological endpoint. It is numerically equal to the inverse of the ratio of absorbed doses of the two radiations required to produce equal biological effects. The reference radiation is often 200-kV x-rays."

The difficulty is that the RBE may differ depending on the biological endpoint and it may also be dose-dependent. When dose is not specified, it is assumed that the RBE is at the low-dose limit (see BEIR VII). The RBE increases as a function of LET, reaching a maximum at about 100 keV/μm. Interestingly, it was pointed out by Hall and Giaccia (2005) that at the density of ionization of 100 keV/μm, the average separation between ionization events, just coincides with the diameter of the DNA double helix. Thus, radiation with this density has the highest probability of causing a double-stranded break by the passage of a single charged particle.

For regulatory purposes, the ICRP introduced the related concept of "quality factor" (Q) or weighting factor w_R. It is defined as an LET-dependent factor by which doses are multiplied to obtain a quantity that corresponds to the degree of biological effect produced by x-rays and low-energy γ-rays. Table 25-2 gives the current weighting factors, whereas Fig. 25-3 plots the values for various neutron energy levels (taken from ICRP 103).

The "equivalent dose" to an organ or tissue is then defined as $H_T = \Sigma_R w_R D_{TR}$ where D_{TR} is the dose to the organ from radiation type R. For public health purposes, ICRP further defines "effective dose" as $E = \Sigma_T w_T H_T$ where w_T are tissue-weighting factors (Table 25-3). It should be noted that these are the currently recommended ICRP values although the Nuclear Regulatory Agency is using previous values (eg, 0.25 instead of 0.08 for gonads possibly because of previous concerns about genetic effects). For the radionuclides there are also the terms "committed equivalent dose" and "committed effective dose," which simply means the total accumulative dose for 50 years after the exposure. Finally "total

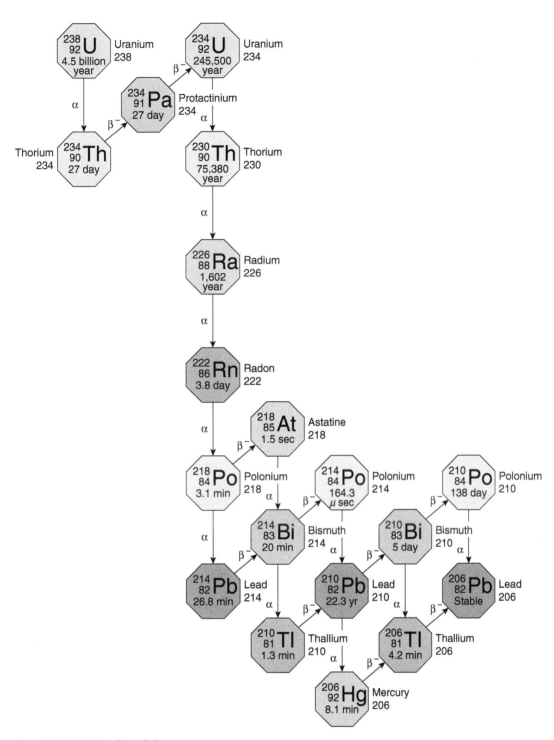

Figure 25-2. *Uranium decay chain.*

effective dose equivalent" (TEDE) means the sum of the effective dose equivalent (for external exposures) and the committed effective dose equivalent (for internal exposures).

Units of Radiation Activity and Dose

The basic unit of radiation activity is the Becquerel (Bq), which is nuclear disintegrations per second. The older unit of activity is the Curie (Ci), which corresponds to the number of disintegrations in one second from 1 g of radium 226 or 1 Ci = 3.7×10^{10} decays per second; thus, 1 Bq = 2.7×10^{-11} Ci. The EPA continues to use the old unit of activity with regard to radon. For example, the EPA's

level of concern for radon in the home currently is 4 pCi/L, which is equivalent to 148 Bq/m^3.

The basic unit of dose is the Gray (Gy), which is the amount of energy released in a given mass of tissue. One Gray is defined as 1 joule of energy released in 1 kg of tissue. The older dose unit of rad (100 erg/g) is 1/100 of a Gray. The other common measure is the Sievert (Sv), which is a dose equivalent; that is, the dose in Gray multiplied by the appropriate quality factor. The dose equivalent rem is rad multiplied by the quality factor. Because ^{60}Co γ-rays and 240 keV x-rays have a quality factor of one, we see Sv and Gy are used interchangeably in studies. Less common is the roentgen (R) that quantifies exposure, and is the number of ionizations in a cubic

Table 25-1

Radioisotopes in the Uranium Decay Series

NUCLIDE	DECAY MODE	HALF-LIFE (a = YEAR)	ENERGY RELEASED, MeV	PRODUCT OF DECAY
^{238}U	α	4.468×10^9 a	4.270	^{234}Th
^{234}Th	β$^-$	24.10 days	0.273	^{234m}Pa
^{234m}Pa	β$^-$ 99.84 % IT 0.16 %	1.16 min	2.271 0.074	^{234}U ^{234}Pa
^{234}Pa	β$^-$	6.70 h	2.197	^{234}U
^{234}U	α	245,500 a	4.859	^{230}Th
^{230}Th	α	75,380 a	4.770	^{226}Ra
^{226}Ra	α	1602 a	4.871	^{222}Rn
^{222}Rn	α	3.8235 days	5.590	^{218}Po
^{218}Po	α 99.98 % β$^-$ 0.02 %	3.10 min	6.115 0.265	^{214}Pb ^{218}At
^{218}At	α 99.90 % β$^-$ 0.10 %	1.5 s	6.874 2.883	^{214}Bi ^{218}Rn
^{218}Rn	α	35 ms	7.263	^{214}Po
^{214}Pb	β$^-$	26.8 min	1.024	^{214}Bi
^{214}Bi	β$^-$ 99.98 % α 0.02 %	19.9 min	3.272 5.617	^{214}Po ^{210}Tl
^{214}Po	α	0.1643 ms	7.883	^{210}Pb
^{210}Tl	β$^-$	1.30 min	5.484	^{210}Pb
^{210}Pb	β$^-$	22.3 a	0.064	^{210}Bi
^{210}Bi	β$^-$ 99.99987% α 0.00013%	5.013 days	1.426 5.982	^{210}Po ^{206}Tl
^{210}Po	α	138.376 days	5.407	^{206}Pb
^{206}Tl	β$^-$	4.199 min	1.533	^{206}Pb
^{206}Pb	–	Stable	–	–

Table 25-2

Recommended Radiation Weighting Factors

RADIATION TYPE	RADIATION WEIGHTING FACTOR, w_R
Photons	1
Electrons and muons	1
Protons and pions	2
Alpha particles, fission fragments, heavy ions	20
Neutrons	See Fig. 25-3

The "equivalent dose" to an organ or tissue is then defined as $H_T = \Sigma_R w_R D_{TR}$, where D_{TR} is the dose to the organ from radiation type R. For public health purposes.

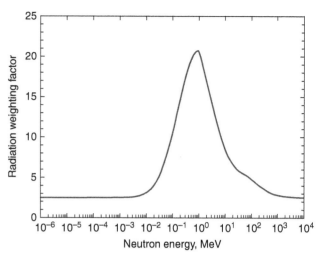

Figure 25-3. *Neutron weighting factor by energy level.*

meter of air produced by x-rays or γ radiation. Because 1 roentgen of γ- and x-ray gives an absorbed dose to tissue of about 1 rad (10 mSv), they are nearly equivalent. For radon and its daughters, a different exposure system is used. Considering the uranium miner studies, exposure is expressed as a working level (WL), which is defined by BEIR VI as follows:

"Any combination of the short-lived progeny of radon in 1 L of air, under ambient temperature and pressure, that results in the ultimate emission of 1.3×10^5 MeV of α particle energy. This is approximately the total amount of energy released over a long period of time by the short-lived progeny in equilibrium with 100 pCi of radon. 1 WL = 2.08×10^{-5} Jm^{-3}."

For cumulative exposure, a working level month (WLM) is used, which is the exposure to one WL for one working month of 170 hours.

RADIOBIOLOGY

Radiation biology has made significant progress in our understanding of radiation effects at low doses. BEIR VII and, more recently, Dauer *et al.* (2010) go into great detail describing our current knowledge as it pertains to radiation-induced cancer. Currently radiation cancer risk extrapolations make two assumptions: namely that the basic mode of action is linearly related to dose and that the individual cell is the unit of risk. However, effects occurring in nontargeted cells such as with induced genomic instability and

Table 25-3

Recommended Tissue Weighting Factors

TISSUE	w_T	$\Sigma_T w_T$
Bone-marrow, colon, lung, stomach, breast, remainder tissues*	0.12	0.72
Gonads	0.08	0.08
Bladder, esophagus, liver, thyroid	0.04	0.16
Bone surface, brain, salivary glands, skin	0.01	0.04
	Total	1.00

* Remainder tissues: adrenals, extrathoracic (ET) region, gall bladder, heart, kidneys, lymphatic nodes, muscle, oral mucosa, pancreas, prostate, small intestine, spleen, thymus, uterus/cervix.

bystander effects, suggest that responses can occur nonuniformly over time at the tissue level. How cells in tissues react to radiation effects is not well understood. There are many complexities in the cancer process that are not explained by the "single-cell biophysical hit" model of radiation-induced cancer, which is the basis for the linear no-threshold (LNT) model used for low-dose cancer risk assessments. Damage from ionizing radiation appears to increase linearly with dose, but recent data suggest that the processing and repair of induced damage could be nonlinear. The understanding of these processes is necessary for low-dose risk estimation. Following irradiation, various protective cellular processes occur that depend on the degree of damage and the tissue type. These mechanisms include DNA repair, intracellular metabolic oxidation/reduction reactions, cell cycle checkpoint controls, cellular signaling, senescence, and apoptosis (see Dauer *et al.*, 2010).

The BEIR VII report reviewed in detail the effects of DNA damage after exposure to low doses of ionizing radiation. After an exposure to 5 mGy of low-LET radiation (average background per year), each cell nucleus is on average hit by one electron, resulting in 5 to 10 damaged bases, 2.5 to 5 single-strand breaks and 0.25 double-strand breaks.

Nontargeted Radiation Effects

Exposure to ionizing radiation can result in direct damage to the irradiated cells as well as producing effects in cells that were not irradiated (bystander effects). These nontargeted effects can occur in the nonirradiated neighbors of irradiated cells and at sites distant from the irradiated cells. Effects can also be observed in the progeny of an irradiated cell (genomic instability). Both targeted and nontargeted effects can result in DNA mutations, gene amplifications, chromosomal rearrangements, carcinogenesis, and cell death.

Bystander Effects Radiation-induced bystander effects are those in which cells that have not been directly exposed to ionizing radiation react as though they have been exposed by receiving a biochemical signal from a radiation-exposed cell. That is, they show chromosomal instability and other abnormalities, or die. BEIR VII concluded that for high-LET radiation a bystander effect has been shown for inducing cell lethality, chromosome aberrations, sister-chromatid exchanges, mutations, genomic instability, signal transduction pathways, and in vitro transformation. For low-LET radiation, the bystander effect has been limited to cell lethality and lethal mutations.

These bystander cells can be either adjacent or at some distance from the radiation-exposed cell. Not all cells can produce bystander signals or react to them. The important issue from a risk assessment view is whether bystander effects are beneficial (eg, adaptive response and apoptosis [removal of damaged cells]) or detrimental to the nonexposed cells, and what impact they may have on dose response at low doses. It should be noted that most observed effects are detrimental, but beneficial effects are more difficult to measure. However, bystander effects demonstrate that the organism and tissues communicate and are responding as an organized structure to radiation insult. Large DNA deletions are the major type of radiation-induced mutations. In bystander cells, however, the types of mutations are similar to those that occur spontaneously, with the majority being point mutations. These differences are important in understanding risk at low doses (Dauer *et al.*, 2010).

BEIR VII quotes Sawant *et al.* (2001) on high-LET bystander in vitro studies that "These results, if applicable in vivo, would have significant consequences in terms of radiation risk extrapolation to low doses, implying that the relevant target for radiation oncogenesis

is larger than an individual cell, and that the risk of carcinogenesis would increase more slowly, if at all, at higher doses—an effect seen in vivo, as well as epidemiologically. Thus, a simple linear extrapolation of radiation risk from high doses (where they can be measured) to lower doses (where they must be inferred) would be of questionable validity." In other words, it is speculated that there could be a convex, downward-curving dose–response relationship at low doses, and that extrapolation of data from high doses could lead to an underestimate of the effect at low doses of high-LET radiation. Finally, BEIR VII concludes that "until molecular mechanisms of the bystander effect are elucidated, especially as related to an intact organism, and until reproducible bystander effects are observed for low-LET radiation in the dose range of 1–5 mGy, where an average of about one electron track traverses the nucleus, a bystander effect of low dose, low-LET radiation that might result in a dose-response curving either upward or downward should not be assumed." For an in-depth review of bystander effects both in vitro and in vivo see the papers by Morgan (2003a,b) as well as Mothersill (2004, 2005) and Liu *et al.* (2006).

Genomic Instability Genomic instability has been defined as the increase in rate of acquiring genetic change, and induced genomic instability can be observed in the progeny of irradiated cells and can persist for many generations (Morgan, 2003a,b). When a cell is saturated in repairing radiation damage it may change its gene-product profile without any specific genetic damage. This has been suggested as a cause of genomic instability, which is an anti-inflammatory response, and is a risk for malignancy (Barcellos-Hoff, 2005). There is a need for the understanding of the molecular targets and processes responsible for genomic instability in order to understand the dose response and why the frequency saturates at 10% to 30% of the surviving cells. This may be due to the fact that only a fraction of cells in a particular part of the cell cycle are susceptible. It is believed that genomic instability could be linked to the loss of telomere maintenance and too short telomeres as a mechanism in cancer development. Chromosome instability can also be initiated by double-strand breaks that result in the loss of a telomere that protects the chromosome end and prevents chromosome fusion. The induction of chromosomal aberrations plays an important role in genomic instability. There is also some evidence that reactive oxygen species (ROS) may play a role. BEIR VII concludes "However, until the molecular mechanisms responsible for genomic instability and its relationship to carcinogenesis are understood, extrapolation of the limited dose-response data for genomic instability to radiation-induced cancers in the low-dose range <100 mGy is not warranted."

Adaptive Response Cells that are exposed to a low priming dose of radiation (eg, 10–20 mGy) followed in a short time interval with a larger challenge dose (eg, 1 Gy), the frequency of chromosomal aberrations induced by the challenge dose was found to be less than that from the challenge dose given alone. This effect is referred to as "adaptive response" (Tapio and Jacob, 2007). Studies have also shown that low doses of radiation may reduce the biological background effect. This has been shown for cell transformation and chromosomal damage. It has also been observed that the normal rate of cell transformation (Redpath *et al.*, 2006) and chromosome damage can be decreased to below the normal background level after an initial low-dose radiation exposure. Adaptive responses have been observed both in vitro and in vivo for both cancer and genetic effects, which suggests that low doses may decrease radiation risk. These adaptive responses suggest that enhancing normal repair or protective processes make it possible to decrease the risk for low-dose radiation-induced cancer (Dauer *et al.*, 2010).

In BEIR VII's assessment of adaptive response, they state that data are needed when both the priming and challenging doses are low (<100 mGy) and when doses are delivered over several weeks or months at low dose rates or with fractionated exposures. They also suggest that the adaptive response studies using malignant transformation assays using immortalized cell lines may not be relevant to normal nonimmortalized cells. Finally BEIR VII states "Thus, it is concluded that any useful extrapolations for dose-response relationships in humans cannot be made from the adaptive responses observed in human lymphocytes or other mammalian cellular systems. Therefore, at present, the assumption that any stimulatory effects of low doses of ionizing radiation substantially reduce long-term deleterious radiation effects in humans is unwarranted."

Hormesis

The BEIR VII committee defined hormesis as "the stimulating effect of small doses of substances which in larger doses are inhibitory" (see Calabrese *et al.*, 2007 for a review). They concluded that the preponderance of available experimental data does not support the idea that low levels of ionizing radiation have a beneficial effect, and the possible mechanisms remain obscure. Further, they state "At this time, the assumption that any stimulatory hormetic effects from low doses of ionizing radiation will have a significant health benefit to humans that exceeds potential detrimental effects from radiation exposure at the same dose is unwarranted." Research actively continues in this area and the BEIR committee recommends the need for research on the possible mechanisms for hormesis at low radiation doses.

Gene Expression

Gene expression profiling for monitoring ionizing radiation exposure has become an active area of research. It has been shown that dose, dose rate, radiation quality, and time since exposure result in variations in the response of genes, so that gene expression signatures may be markers of radiation exposure. Changes in gene expression in human cell lines occur after as little as 0.02 Gy γ-rays (Amundson and Fornace, 2001; Amundson *et al.*, 2003). Using gene expression methods, Ory *et al.* (2011) and Ugolin *et al.* (2011), were able to distinguish a number of post-Chernobyl thyroid tumors and postradiotherapy thyroid tumors from their sporadic counterparts. These techniques, if applicable to low-dose radiation exposures, could be very useful in radiation epidemiological studies (see Maenhaut *et al.*, 2011).

SUMMARY

Cancer being the primary health concern from exposure to ionizing radiation, there is a focus on mechanisms and dose response as they relate to the induction of chromosomal aberrations and gene mutations because cancer is believed to be associated with these cellular responses. Experimental data indicate that the dose–response relationship over a range of 20 to 100 mGy is most likely to be linear, and not significantly affected by either an adaptive or a bystander effect. Data in this dose range for genomic instability are generally not available. The question of the shape of the dose–response relationship up to 20 mGy remains uncertain. The future of understanding low-dose radiation cancer risks will depend on the continued advancement of molecular biology, gene expression analysis, and computational biology.

CANCER EPIDEMIOLOGY

Epidemiological studies have been extensive and provide the basis for our understanding of radiation-induced cancer effects. These studies provide a wide range of exposures including populations at high natural background exposures, occupational studies, populations exposed to nuclear testing and reactor accidents, A-bomb survivor studies, and the follow-up of patients having had high-dose medical radiation therapies. Radiation cancer studies are no different from other types of occupational and environmental cancer studies in that radiation-induced cancers are not distinguishable pathologically, and there are usual issues of exposure confounding, long latencies (eg, 10–20 years for solid tumors), levels of exposure, and study size. Generally for acute exposures only epidemiological studies with exposures to relatively high doses of radiation (greater than 0.15 Sv) have shown such an excess of cancer. Because of these difficulties, the most informative studies are those that involve a large number of individuals with large radiation doses and follow-up of several decades.

Epidemiological assessment of cancer in populations exposed to radiation has been the principal source of information used by regulatory groups. The National Academies series of BEIR reports provides this information through expert committee analyses. The most recent report BEIR VII is restricted to the health effects of low-LET radiation (eg, γ-ray, x-ray). The BEIR VI report is solely devoted to radon, whereas BEIR IV is focused on radionuclides. BEIR V is a previous version of BEIR VII. The BEIR reports, besides reviewing the scientific literature on radiation health effects, develop quantitative cancer risk models for low-LET exposures, as well as radon exposures. The United Nations Scientific Committee on the Effects of Atomic Radiation (UNSCEAR) reports also review the literature on cancer and noncancer effects of radiation exposures. They developed quantitative cancer risk models and applied them to various populations. More recently, the International Agency for Research on Cancer (IARC), in their monograph series, evaluated cancer effects for various types of radiation exposures (IARC report 100D). This qualitative analysis determined for each radiation type which cancer sites are considered to be causal. A brief summary was published after the meeting and the findings are reproduced here in Table 25-4 (El Ghissassi *et al.*, 2009). We see from Table 25-4 that there are numerous Class 1 cancer sites for γ-ray and x-ray, while only lung cancer is associated with radon exposures.

A-bomb Survivor Studies

The Radiation Effects Research Foundation (RERF), and its predecessor the Atomic Bomb Casualty Commission (ABCC), have reported a series of mortality studies on a fixed population (Life Span Study [LSS] cohort) of 120,321 individuals. These included A-bomb survivors and residents who were not present at the time of the bombing (NIC, not in city, 26,529). The most recent report is the 14th in the series and covers the years 1950–2003, and includes both cancer and noncancer mortality (Ozasa *et al.*, 2012). There are also studies on cancer incidence, with the most recent for solid cancers during the period 1958–1998 and for hematopoietic tumors during 1950–2001 (Preston *et al.*, 2007; Hsu *et al.*, 2012). RERF also publishes analyses of individuals in the Adult Health Study (AHS), which is a subcohort of LSS with 22,400 individuals and an additional 1000 *in utero* exposed. This subcohort is oversampled with more individuals who were exposed to the higher doses. Members of the AHS are given physical examinations every two years, and this provides much clinical data as well as biological samples. Details of the RERF study cohorts, publications, and databases can be accessed at the RERF web site.

The LSS cohort's exposures are a whole-body exposure, which then allows for comparisons between specific cancer sites and their relative risks. The cohort is not likely to have many confounding issues because the basis of the dose estimation is the distance from the hypocenter. Finally the AHS subcohort allows for clinical,

Table 25-4

IARC: Tumors Sites With Sufficient Evidence of Human Carcinogenicity

RADIATION TYPE	MAJOR STUDY POPULATIONS	TUMOR SITES (AND TYPES) ON WHICH SUFFICIENT EVIDENCE IS BASED
α-particle and β-particle emitters		
Radon-222 and decay products	General population (residential exposure), underground miners	Lung
Radium-224 and decay products	Medical patients	Bone
Radium-226, radium-228, and decay products	Radium-dial painters	Bone, paranasal sinus, and mastoid process (radium-226 only)
Thorium-232 and decay products	Medical patients	Liver, extrahepatic bile ducts, gall bladder, leukemia (excluding CLL)
Plutonium	Plutonium-production workers	Lung, liver, bone
Phosphorus-32	Medical patients	Acute leukemia
Fission products, including strontium-90	General population, following nuclear reactor accident	Solid cancers, leukemia
Radioiodines, including iodine-131	Children and adolescents, following nuclear reactor accident	Thyroid
X-radiation or γ-radiation	Atomic-bomb survivors, medical patients; in utero exposure (offspring of pregnant medical patients and of atomic-bomb survivors)	Salivary gland, esophagus, stomach, colon, lung, bone, skin (BCC), female breast, urinary bladder, brain and CNS, leukemia (excluding CLL), thyroid, kidney (atomic-bomb survivors, medical patients); multiple sites (in utero exposure)
Solar radiation	General population	Skin (BCC, SCC, melanoma)
UV-emitting tanning devices	General population	Skin (melanoma), eye (melanoma, particularly choroid and ciliary body)

BCC, basal cell carcinoma; CLL, chronic lymphocytic leukemia; CNS, central nervous system; SCC, squamous cell carcinoma.

lifestyle, and biological measurements, which help to assure the lack of confounding and effect modifiers in the dose calculations. The problem with the cohort is that the results are extrapolated from a group of Japanese who survived the bombing and have different background cancer rates than other populations (eg, Pierce, 2007).

The number of individuals in the LSS cohort is shown by city and colon dose (Gy) in Table 25-5 (adapted from Ozasa et al., 2012). Although most individuals have low estimated doses, there is a good range of doses, with sufficient numbers at the higher doses for analysis and risk modeling. The individual dose reconstructions have evolved over the years with the current system completed in 2002 and referred to as DS02 (dosimetry system 2002). The uncertainty in the dosimetry is estimated to be about 30% and has been modeled for risk assessment purposes (see Pierce et al., 1990 and Little et al., 2008).

The results of the mortality data show that for total solid cancers, the excess relative risk decreases with attained age and age at exposure. The modeled data are illustrated in Fig. 25-4, which is extracted from Ozasa et al. (2012). The excess relative risks for individual cancer sites and other causes of mortality are shown in Fig. 25-5, again from the Ozasa et al. (2012) analysis.

Recently there have been sufficient incidence data so that both BEIR VII and UNSCEAR (2006) can model cancer incidence risk by cancer site. BEIR V previously used mortality data for their risk analyses. The most recent cancer incidence data for solid tumors, used by BEIR VII in their risk modeling, included the years 1958–1998, given in the publication by Preston et al. (2007). Each individual cancer site is analyzed and discussed in detail in the article by Preston. For total solid tumor incidence the estimated excess relative risk per Gy is 0.47 (0.40–0.54).

Table 25-5

Number of LSS Cohort Members by Colon Dose (Gy)

	TOTAL*	<0.005	0.005–	0.1–	0.2–	0.5–	1.0–	2.0–	UNKNOWN[†]	NIC[‡]	TOTAL[§]
Hiroshima	58,494	21,697	22,733	5037	5067	2373	1152	435	3442	20,179	82,214
Nagasaki	28,117	16,812	7228	937	1289	1051	611	189	3616	6350	38,107
Total	86,611	38,509	29,961	5974	6356	3424	1763	624	7058	26,529	120,321

*Total number of subjects with a reconstructed dose.
[†]Those subjects with an unknown dose.
[‡]Not in the cities of Hiroshima or Nagasaki at the time of the bombing.
[§]Total of those with either a reconstructed dose, an unknown dose, or were NIC.

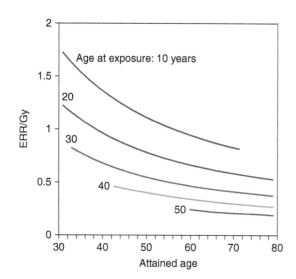

Figure 25-4. *LSS solid tumor mortality excess relative risk.*

Coincidently it is also 0.47 for solid tumor mortality study as shown in Fig. 25-5.

Occupational Studies

Nuclear Worker Studies There have been numerous worker studies over the years among nuclear workers, primarily at governmental facilities. In most of these studies, mortality rates were compared with those in the general population. In most cases, the cancer mortality rates were less than those for the general public, which may be due to the healthy worker effect and differences between nuclear workers and the public. For those studies with external radiation dose estimates solid cancer risk estimates either increased or decreased with dose and had large confidence intervals (CIs; see BEIR VII for details). As an example in a nested case–control study of workers at the Portsmouth Naval Shipyard (PNS), 1097 lung cancer deaths were age-matched with 3291 controls among the cohort of 37,853 civilian workers (Yiin *et al.*, 2007). After adjusting for confounders such as asbestos and welding fumes, lung cancer risk was associated with radiation exposure. However when work-related medical x-rays, which occur more frequently among radiation monitored workers, were included, lung cancer was no longer associated with radiation dose. The medical x-rays were of the same magnitude as the work exposures of the monitored workers. Because the individual covariates were associated with lung cancer risk, this study shows the importance of incorporating potential confounders in occupational radiation studies.

To address the problem of varied results, IARC carried out a joint analysis of seven nuclear facilities in Canada, the UK, and the USA, and is referred to as the three-country study (Cardis *et al.*, 1995). This analysis involved a total of 95,673 workers and 3830 cancer deaths. The study estimated a slightly negative ERR per Sv of –0.9 (90% CI –0.4, 0.3) for total solid cancers, but observed a significant increase in mortality of both acute and chronic myelogenous leukemia. Also, multiple myeloma was significantly increased with increasing dose in the study. Although negative for total solid cancers this result was not inconsistent with the risk estimates derived from the A-bomb studies.

The three-country study was followed by the 15-country study that involved a joint analysis of over 400,000 nuclear workers from 154 facilities (Cardis, 2007). As seen in Table 25-6 the number of workers and person-years at risk (pyr) are much greater in the 15-country study. However, the numbers of workers at the higher cumulative exposures is much lower. This is due to the elimination of workers in the 15-country cohorts who were monitored for internal exposures and also those who may have received an acute exposure of some significance. The study reported significant increases in smoking-related solid cancer mortality but not for leukemias, which was essentially the opposite of the three-country findings. There are a number of issues with the 15-country study as discussed in Dauer (2010), namely, questions about the exclusion of workers included in the previous (three-country) study, such as the Idaho National Engineering Laboratory cohort, and exclusion of workers who were considered to have had potential for high internal dose. Also of concern is the inability to deal with smoking and the undue influence given to the results for one country, namely Canada, where risk estimates are very high and error-prone (Ashmore *et al.*, 2010). The increase in overall solid cancer incidence would no longer be significant if the Canadian cohort were excluded; however, it would be consistent with risk estimates projected from the A-bomb studies.

A series of analyses of workers at the Russian nuclear facility at Mayak have been published. The Mayak workers generally experienced very high doses from both internal (plutonium, α particles) and external radiation exposures. Plutonium body burdens were based on urine analyses. Worker exposures of Pu239 and 240 and external exposures have been reassessed by Vasilenko *et al.* (2007). High levels of body burdens of plutonium greater than 7.4 kBq (mean 76 kBq) were found to have a relative risk of liver cancer of 17 (Gilbert *et al.*, 2000) and 7.9 for bone cancer (Koshurnikova *et al.*, 2000). Small nonsignificant increases were seen at low doses. These studies were based on the mortality experience of 11,000 workers. In a larger group of 21,000 workers 655 lung cancer deaths were evaluated (Gilbert *et al.*, 2004). In contrast to the high-dose effects on the liver and bone, the effects of plutonium on lung cancer were found to be consistent with a linear dose response. Plutonium exposures to workers in the USA and the UK were much lower, and cancer increase was not observed except possibly for a nonsignificant increase in lung cancer (Omar *et al.*, 1998; Wiggs *et al.*, 1994; Wilkinson *et al.*, 1987). Also, experimental studies of plutonium administered to beagle dogs have predicted these high-dose effects in workers (eg, Wilson *et al.*, 2010). The dogs overpredicted the bone and liver cancers risks but the lung cancers were similar.

Medical Radiation Workers It is estimated that there are 2.3 million medical radiation workers worldwide. Radiologists and radiological technologists have been studied epidemiologically for many years. These workers were some of the earliest exposed to radiation with the first finding in 1902 that radiation can cause skin cancer. It was recognized in the 1940s that radiologists had increased rates of leukemia (eg, Ulrich, 1946). More recently Yoshinaga and others at the NCI reviewed cancer mortality from eight international cohorts involving 270,000 subjects (Yoshinaga *et al.*, 2004). By far the greatest number of workers were from the study of 146,000 US technologists (Mohan *et al.*, 2003). In this study there were increases in breast cancer and non-chronic lymphocytic leukemias (CLLs), based on years worked for those employed before 1950 when exposures were much higher than today. The cohorts consistently show increases in leukemias for the early years with less consistency for skin cancer and breast cancer (Yoshinaga *et al.*, 2004).

The US Radiologic Technologists (USRT) health study is a large study (90,000 subjects with about 75% females), first contacted in 1983–1998, and is representative of the population of technologists with good employment history information and data on other risk factors such as smoking. Radiation monitoring (badges)

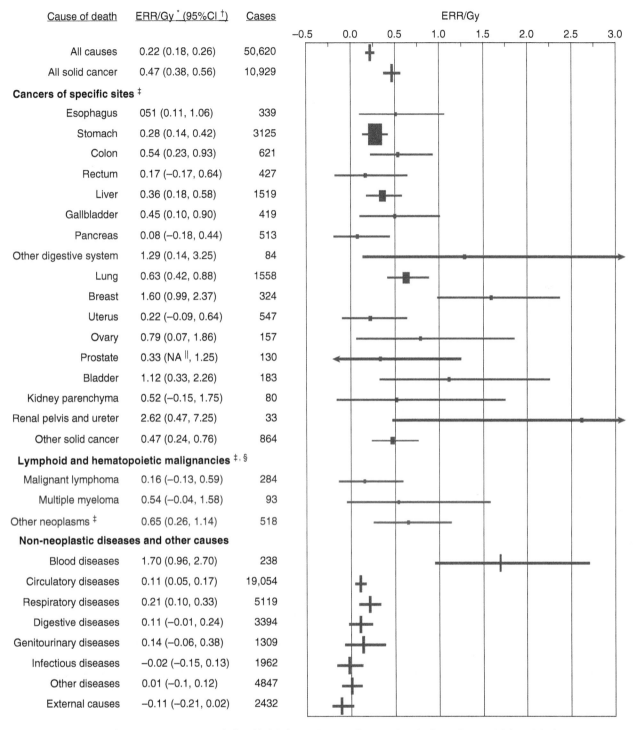

Cause of death	ERR/Gy* (95%CI†)	Cases
All causes	0.22 (0.18, 0.26)	50,620
All solid cancer	0.47 (0.38, 0.56)	10,929
Cancers of specific sites ‡		
Esophagus	051 (0.11, 1.06)	339
Stomach	0.28 (0.14, 0.42)	3125
Colon	0.54 (0.23, 0.93)	621
Rectum	0.17 (−0.17, 0.64)	427
Liver	0.36 (0.18, 0.58)	1519
Gallbladder	0.45 (0.10, 0.90)	419
Pancreas	0.08 (−0.18, 0.44)	513
Other digestive system	1.29 (0.14, 3.25)	84
Lung	0.63 (0.42, 0.88)	1558
Breast	1.60 (0.99, 2.37)	324
Uterus	0.22 (−0.09, 0.64)	547
Ovary	0.79 (0.07, 1.86)	157
Prostate	0.33 (NA‖, 1.25)	130
Bladder	1.12 (0.33, 2.26)	183
Kidney parenchyma	0.52 (−0.15, 1.75)	80
Renal pelvis and ureter	2.62 (0.47, 7.25)	33
Other solid cancer	0.47 (0.24, 0.76)	864
Lymphoid and hematopoietic malignancies ‡, §		
Malignant lymphoma	0.16 (−0.13, 0.59)	284
Multiple myeloma	0.54 (−0.04, 1.58)	93
Other neoplasms ‡	0.65 (0.26, 1.14)	518
Non-neoplastic diseases and other causes		
Blood diseases	1.70 (0.96, 2.70)	238
Circulatory diseases	0.11 (0.05, 0.17)	19,054
Respiratory diseases	0.21 (0.10, 0.33)	5119
Digestive diseases	0.11 (−0.01, 0.24)	3394
Genitourinary diseases	0.14 (−0.06, 0.38)	1309
Infectious diseases	−0.02 (−0.15, 0.13)	1962
Other diseases	0.01 (−0.1, 0.12)	4847
External causes	−0.11 (−0.21, 0.02)	2432

Figure 25-5. *LSS mortality 1950–2003: excess relative risk (ERR).* *ERR was estimated using the linear dose model, in which city, sex, age at exposure, and attained age were included in the background rates, but not allowing radiation effect modification by those factors. †Confidence interval. Horizontal bars show 95% confidence intervals. ‡The size of plots for site-specific cancers was proportional to the number of cases. §ERR (95% CI) of leukemia was 3.1 (1.8, 4.3) at 1 Gy and 0.15 (−0.01, 0.31) at 0.1 Gy based on a linear quadratic model with 318 cases (not displayed in the figure). ‖The lower limit of 95% CI was lower than zero, but not specified by calculation.

was introduced in the 1950s and is beginning to be used in the analyses (Simon *et al.*, 2006). Recently Rajaraman *et al.* (2006) analyzed lung cancer in the cohort and did not find increases after adjustments for smoking. The USRT health study will continue with improved dosimetry and longer follow-up times. These studies will continue to be important because they involve low doses of continuous exposure in contrast to the acute exposure of the A-bomb survivors.

Chernobyl Cleanup Workers The Chernobyl cleanup workers are of interest because of their higher exposures compared with other nuclear workers. It has been estimated that there were 600,000 workers, with 240,000 of the workers exposed during 1986–1987 and having an average exposure of 100 mSv (Cardis *et al.*, 2006). Ivanov *et al.* (2006) reported an analysis of 55,718 workers who had yearly physical examinations. The analysis covered two five-year periods 1991–1995 and 1996–2001, with a total of 1370

Table 25-6

IARC Nuclear Worker Studies

	STUDY	SUBJECT	pyr	DEATHS			
	3-country	95,673	2.1 million	18,993			
	15-country	407,291	5.2 million	15,825			
	DEATHS PER mSv INTERVAL						
	0–10	10–50	50–100	100–200	200–400	400+	
3-country	9582	3728	989	702	586	238	
15-country	13608	3728	855	492	268	42	

pyr-person years at risk.

cancer cases. The average dose for these workers during 1985–1986 was 130 mSv. Although there was an increase in the incidence of solid tumors, it was not significant. Cancer mortality was evaluated in a smaller cohort of workers (29,003 with 651 cancer deaths). The excess relative risk for solid tumors was significant (ERR = 1.52 per Gy) and the increase was observed in the highest dose interval (mean 200 mSv) with no increase in the lower-dose interval (mean 100 mSv). Besides solid tumors, a significant increase in leukemia incidence was observed for those with exposures greater than 0.15 Gy, compared with workers with lower exposures (Ivanov, 2007). Also, increases in the incidence of cardiovascular disease were observed among those at higher exposures.

A smaller cohort (10,332) of Chernobyl cleanup workers from the Baltic States was reported by Rahu *et al.* (2006). The mean exposure was 109 mGy, and 155 incidental cancer cases were observed. Although there were increases in thyroid (seven cases) and brain cancer (eleven cases), they were not dose-related and were likely the result of close surveillance and multiple comparisons.

Other than for leukemias, the follow-up period has been relatively short and it is thus too soon to conclude much about solid cancer risks. The relatively high reconstructed doses make it important to continue the follow-up of the cohorts and to evaluate the exposures and their uncertainties.

Nuclear Worker Registries The National Dose Registry of Canada includes 206,620 workers for the period 1951–1987. Ashmore *et al.* (1998) analyzed 5426 deaths and reported an increase in total cancer mortality among males (ERR = 3% per 10 mSv), which was marginally significant but not for any particular cancer, including leukemia. There was not a significant increase among females who comprised about half of the workers, but generally had much lower recorded doses. Sont *et al.* (2001) analyzed the Registry for cancer incidence of 191,333 workers for the period 1951–1988. Using national rates, the standardized incidence ratio (SIR) for all cancer was significantly less than 1 (SIR = 0.88 [90% CI 0.85, 0.92]). Leukemia was also significantly less than 1. When doses were used, the ERR for all cancer was 2.5 (90% CI 1.2, 4.0) and 5.4 (90% CI 0.2, 20.0) for leukemia. One difficulty with these analyses is that the cohort includes dental (0.3 mSv mean accumulative dose), medical (3.95 mSv), industrial (4.78 mSv), and nuclear workers (31.98 mSv), whose lifestyles may well differ as do their radiation exposures.

Muirhead *et al.* (2009) analyzed both mortality and incidence of the UK National Registry of Radiation Workers (124,723 workers). Total solid tumors were increased, ERR = 0.28 per Sv among 23,326 deaths and ERR = 0.27 among 11,165 malignant incident cases. Leukemias were also increased with ERR = 1.7 for mortality

and 1.8 for incidence. Other than leukemia, individual cancer sites were not significantly increased. The increases for solid tumors and leukemias were significant using a 90% CI but not for a 95% CI.

Nonoccupationally Exposed Groups

Studies of the Techa River Exposures A joint US and Russian program has been evaluating the health effects of those living near the Techa River. During the early 1950s radioactive waste from the Mayak nuclear production facility was released into the river. A dose reconstruction system has been developed (Degteva *et al.*, 2000, 2007) and applied to a cohort of 30,000 people. Exposures were 55% internal from food and water, primarily of Cs 137 and Sr 89, 90. A mortality analysis based on 1842 solid cancer deaths estimated an ERR = 0.92 (0.2, 1.7) per Gy and 6.5 (1.8, 24) for 61 leukemia deaths (Krestinina *et al.*, 2007). Cancer incidence for a subcohort of 17,000 individuals with 1836 cases reported an ERR = 1.0 per Gy with a mean cumulative exposure of 40 mGy stomach dose and mean bone marrow dose of 30 mGy. There are some uncertainties about the exposures in the early years, which may have been underestimated and, if increased, would reduce the risk estimates (Cardis, 2007).

High Natural Background Radiation Areas In 2000, a series of articles were published in a supplement issue of the *Journal of Radiation Research* that described the results of a joint China–Japan collaborative research program, which studied the population living in the high background radiation areas in Yangjiang, China. Cancer mortality was analyzed for the period 1979–1995 for 125,000 individuals, which accumulated 1.7 million person-years with 10,415 deaths including 1003 cancer deaths and a population average annual effective exposure of 6.4 mSv (Tao *et al.*, 2000). Comparing individuals in the high background area to those in a control area, the relative risk was 0.99 (0.87, 1.14) for total cancer mortality. Dividing the high background area into low, medium, and high radiation exposures, the relative risks for nonleukemia cancer mortality actually decreased with dose (1.07, 0.98, and 0.91, respectively).

In an additional analysis, Sun *et al.* (2000) modeled the cancer risk using Poisson regression. The cumulative dose groups were in five 100-mSv intervals with the largest being 400+ mSv. The modeled solid tumor mortality risk did not increase with dose and was estimated to be negative but not significantly different from zero.

Recently Tao *et al.* (2012) analyzed cancer mortality (956 cases) among 31,604 people in the Yangjiang area between 1979 and 1998. The mean cumulative radiation dose was 84.8 mGy, with 21.6 mGy for those in the control area. The excess relative risk for solid cancers was ERR = –1.01 per Gy (95% –2.93, 0.95). Liver cancer is a major cancer site and was negatively correlated with dose but is difficult to correctly diagnose. If liver cancer is removed from the analysis then the ERR for solid cancers became 0.19 (–1.87, 3.04).

To evaluate the dose reconstruction, Jiang *et al.* (2000) calculated the correlation between estimated radiation exposure and frequency of dicentric and ring chromosomes, which are recognized as a good biomarker of radiation exposure. They observed that for those in the high radiation background area, the incidence of these markers agrees with what has been observed in other studies of radiation exposures and chromosome aberrations. This result provides some evidence in support of the program's exposure estimates. In conclusion, the high background Chinese studies have not shown an increase in cancer incidence at low dose and dose rate exposures.

The coastal area of Kerala, India, is a region of high natural radiation background that has been well studied. Nair *et al.* (2009) published an analysis of cancer incidence and individually determined γ exposures in the region. A cohort of 70,000 individuals (age 30–84 years) were followed for 10.5 years, which resulted in 1379 cancer cases including 30 leukemias. The researchers also obtained individual data on smoking, education, occupation, and other possible cancer risk factors for their analysis. Cumulative dose intervals ranged from 0–49 mGy to 500+ mGy. For total cancers and for leukemia there were no increases observed among any of the dose intervals compared to the lowest dose interval. Excluding leukemia, the overall excess relative risk for cancer was estimated to be –0.13 per Gy (95% CI –0.58, 0.46). Leukemia was not increased. The analysis included tobacco use and other risk factors that usually are not available in most other radiation epidemiological studies.

Although not a high background study, Kendall *et al.* (2012) studied childhood cancers in relation to natural background radiation in Great Britain. Using the National Registry of Childhood Tumours, the study involved over 27,000 cancer cases and matched controls with radiation exposures estimated on the basis of the mother's residence at time of birth. The mean cumulative dose from birth until diagnosis was 4 mSv. The study found a significant increase in leukemias with an estimated ERR of 12% (95% CI 3, 22) per mSv of γ exposure to the red marrow. Other cancers were not significantly increased and radon was not a significant risk factor.

Semipalatinsk Fallout-Related Exposures The Semipalatinsk area of Kazakhstan has been studied for possible cancer effects resulting from radiation exposures from local fallout of the Soviet atomic nuclear weapons testing program. Bauer *et al.* (2005) studied six rural districts that had measurable levels of exposure and compared the individuals in the districts with six villages that were several hundred kilometers east of the nuclear test site. Follow-up of the populations began five to ten years after the nuclear testing. Using soil samples taken in 1963 of strontium and cesium as well as information on the types of weapons, a dose reconstruction was developed for external and internal exposures. This dose reconstruction was based on the eight most dose-contributing nuclear tests.

For the purpose of analysis the approximate 10,000 individuals in the exposed area were matched with a group of 10,000 in the distant comparison area.

Cancer rates were considerably higher in the exposed groups of individuals, which resulted in significant dose–response relationships for most solid tumors. There appeared, however, to be an undefined bias in the distant control group since the rate ratios increased relatively little among the exposure categories. The authors' estimate for total solid tumors was ERR/Sv = 0.81 (0.46; 1.33), which

is similar to the A-bomb cancer risk estimates. The CIs are fairly narrow but the uncertainty in the dose reconstruction was not included in the analysis. The lack of a dose response is possibly explained by the fact that the study was ecological in nature.

Other Nonoccupational Studies

Buildings With Cobalt 60 A group of 7271 individuals who resided in buildings with high levels of Cobalt 60 contaminated steel in Taiwan have been studied by Hwang *et al.* (2006). The average cumulative exposure was about 50 mSv, and after a follow-up period of 16 years, a total of 141 cancer cases were identified. For total solid cancers (82 cases) compared to the national rates, the total cancers were less than expected, but thyroid cancer (seven cases) and non-Hodgkin lymphoma (five cases) were significantly increased. This is a small study that shows little effect of continuous exposure. It is also difficult to interpret because the exposed population was likely of a higher social economic status (SES) than the general comparison population.

More recently Hwang *et al.* (2008) reported significant increases in leukemia excluding CLL, and marginally significant increases in breast cancer. This was based on a dose–response analysis using an exposure assessment system developed to reconstruct the doses to the individuals. The average cumulative dose was 48 mGy.

Populations Residing Near Nuclear Facilities Ecological cancer studies have been carried out in the vicinity of nuclear power plants in many countries. There has often been reported an unexplained increase in childhood leukemia (Laurier *et al.*, 2002; Baker and Hoel, 2007). Spix *et al.* (2008) and Kaatsch *et al.* (2008) conducted a childhood cancer case–control study in the areas in the vicinity of 16 German nuclear power plants. They observed 1592 cancer cases with 593 cases of leukemia among children under the age of five during the period 1983–2003. Children within 5 km of a nuclear facility had a significant increase in leukemias, but not for other cancers (37 leukemia cases and 54 controls). It was not possible to measure for possible confounders. The authors stated that radiation exposures near these German nuclear power plants are less than the natural background radiation by a factor of 1000 to 100,000.

In France a study of childhood leukemia among children living in the vicinity of the 29 French nuclear sites reported 670 cases, with 729 cases expected from national rates (White-Koning *et al.*, 2004). They observed no trend in leukemia rates with respect to distance. For those within 5 km of a facility, there were 65 leukemia cases, with 75 expected, and for children less than five years of age, there were 39 leukemia cases with 40 cases expected.

Evrard *et al.* (2006) analyzed childhood leukemia, which included three additional years of follow-up from the White-Koning study. Instead of the usual distance surrogate for dose, the researchers estimated doses to the bone marrow based upon the nuclear plants' radioactive discharges. The Institute for Radiation Protection and Nuclear Safety combined the radionuclide discharge data and the local climate data to model the environmental exposure levels. Estimated doses to the red marrow for those in the vicinity of the nuclear sites ranged from 0.06 to 1.33 μSv per year. There were a total of 750 leukemia cases (age <15 years) with 795 expected and 394 among those less than five years of age (415 expected). There was no trend of leukemia incidence based on yearly exposure rates. The authors concurred with the authors of the German study by estimating that the doses due to releases in the vicinity of the nuclear facilities are approximately 1000 to 100,000 times lower than the average dose due to natural radiation sources.

Table 25-7

WHO's Estimated Proportion of Lung Cancer Attributable to Radon

COUNTRY	MEAN INDOOR RADON, Bq/m³	RISK ESTIMATE USED IN CALCULATION	PERCENTAGE OF LUNG CANCER ATTRIBUTED TO RADON, %	ESTIMATED NO. OF DEATHS DUE TO RADON-INDUCED LUNG CANCER EACH YEAR
Canada (Brand *et al.*, 2005)	28	BEIR VI	7.8	1400
Germany (Menzler *et al.*, 2008)	49	European pooling study*	5	1896
Switzerland (Menzler *et al.*, 2008)	78	European pooling study*	8.3	231
United Kingdom (AGIR, 2009)	21	European pooling study* BEIR IV	3.3 6	1089 2005
France (Catelinois *et al.*, 2006)	89	European pooling study BEIR VI	5 12	1234 2913
United States (BEIR VI, 1999)	46	BEIR VI	10–14	15,400–21,800

with adjustment for year-to-year variation in indoor radon concentrations.

The recent COMARE report (2011), focused on leukemias in children around nuclear power plants. The report discusses in detail the German studies as well as studies in other countries. Importantly Kinlen (1988, 2011) describes the concept of population mixing, which basically is the idea that workers arriving in a typically rural area bring foreign infectious agents that in turn will affect local childhood leukemias. In his article Kinlen (2011) focuses on the nuclear power plant studies and the German results in particular. The Kinlen hypothesis of population mixing has been discussed by some authors to explain increased leukemia effects in children when there is no evidence of radiation exposures from the nuclear plants.

The National Research Council (2012) released a review of studies around nuclear facilities with recommendations on how a study could be carried out in the United States using cancer registry data. Previously the NCI (Jablon *et al.*, 1991) analyzed cancer mortality rates in those counties with nuclear power reactors compared with control counties. Basically no differences were found; however, the use of counties as the analysis unit is likely to be too great a geographical area to detect any possible small effects.

Radionuclides

Radon There have been some human studies involving exposures to radionuclides but the data are limited other than for radon, that has been extensively studied. Radon is a natural radioactive gas produced by the decay of uranium and thorium. Originally, exposures to radon and its daughter radionuclides among uranium miners and some other groups of miners established that high exposures were a clear risk for lung cancer. Cancer causation has been restricted to lung cancer but there are also some suggestions that leukemia risk may also be an issue (see the BEIR VI and IARC 100D reports). More recently there have been many case–control studies in the United States and Europe of lung cancer and radon exposure in the home. These studies have been brought together for joint analyses of those studies carried out in Europe (13 studies Darby *et al.*, 2006) and for those studies from North America (seven studies Krewski *et al.*, 2006). The analysis by Darby, as well as Krewski, observed

the data to be best fit by a linear function in dose, with Darby estimating the excess relative risk of lung cancer to be 0.08 per 100 Bq/m³ and 0.10 in the Krewski analysis. The lung cancer risk was also significantly increased when the cases were restricted to exposures less than 200 Bq/m³. The lung cancer effects were also consistent, with the risks projected downward from the higher exposed uranium miners, that is, 0.12 per 100 Bq/m³. When Darby adjusted the data for uncertainties in the radon exposure estimates, the excess relative risk increased to 0.16. BEIR IV, which also includes chapters on radionuclides other than radon, provides tables giving the excess lifetime relative risk for various ages at first exposure, exposure level, and period of exposure. This is done for both males and females and for smokers and never smokers. These tables were not included in the newer BEIR VI report on radon; however, Chen (2005) published similar tables using the newer BEIR VI risk models. Currently (eg, Darby *et al.*, 2006) the risk analyses find that the relative risk for lung cancer and radon exposure is independent of smoking status. Average radon levels in the home for various countries is given in the *WHO Handbook on Indoor Radon 2009* and estimates that 3% to 16% of lung cancer is attributable to radon in the home depending on the risk model used. From Table 25-7 we see that for the United States, with an average level of 46 Bq/m³, and using BEIR VI risk models, the attributable lung cancer risk is 10% to 14%.

Radium There are 25 isotopes of radium of which four occur naturally (Radium 223, 224, 226, and 228); the others are man-made or decay products of man-made radionuclides. Radium 226 with a half-life of 1601 years is by far the common natural form, followed by 228 with a half-life of 5.75 years. Radium 223 and 224 have half-lives of only a few days. Except for radium 228, which is a β emitter, the other three are all α emitters. The different isotopes have been used both occupationally as luminescent paint on watches and instruments (Radium 226 and 228) and in medical applications (Radium 223 and 224). These uses, as well as radium found environmentally in drinking water, have provided material for many epidemiological studies. Beginning in the 1920s, young women worked painting the dials of watches with paint containing radium 226 and 228. Many of them "pointed" the tips of their paintbrushes by mouth resulting in ingestion of relatively large amounts of radium for some of the women. A cohort of 1476 of these dial painters has been established with careful exposure reconstruction (Rowland et al., 1978). Radium as a bone seeker resulted in increases in bone cancer as well as paranasal sinus cancers. Although about one-half of the cohort had cumulative exposures less than 1 Gy, there were no bone cancers for those who were exposed to less than 10 Gy, which using a quality factor of 20 for α irradiation gives 200 Sv. In a statistical modeling of the bone cancers, it was estimated that 5 Gy was a threshold level (Hoel and Carnes, 2004). During the 1940's instrument dials were painted in Britain without the tipping of brushes by mouth (Baverstock and Papworth, 1989). In a follow-up of this cohort, cancers and bone cancers in particular were not increased.

Bone sarcomas were also the major cancer effect among patients with tuberculosis and ankylosing spondylitis who were treated with high doses of Radium 224 (mean bone surface dose of 30 Gy) in two cohort studies in Germany (Nekolla et al., 2010; Wick et al., 1999). There were increases in bone cancer in both studies, but there were also some increases in other cancer sites (Nekolla et al., 2010).

Plutonium Plutonium is used for nuclear weapons production, and in the production of mixed oxide fuels. Most of the exposure to plutonium is to workers involved in the processing of plutonium in nuclear weapons (Pu 239) and in nuclear power generation (Pu 238). Several groups of workers exposed to plutonium have been studied in the USA, United Kingdom, and Russian. The major exposure to plutonium is by inhalation and is retained primarily in the lung, liver, and bone, and has been studied in the USA, United Kingdom, and the Russian Federation. The most informative studies are those of workers employed at the Russian Mayak plant where exposures to plutonium were substantial. Dose–response relationships have been shown for cancers of the lung, liver, and bone over a wide range of doses (see Gilbert et al., 2000, 2004; Koshurnikova et al., 2000; Sokolnikov et al., 2008). Internal estimated plutonium doses were very high: up to 5+ Gy for lung, 23 Gy for liver, and 144 Gy for bone surface.

Radioiodine Releases from nuclear facilities of fission-product radionuclides deposited in the environment as well as internal doses from the ingestion of foods containing fission products have been the result of the Chernobyl and Fukushima accidents. Cesium 134 and 137 as well as Iodine 131 were the most important radionuclides exposures that potentially are health risks. Besides nuclear accidents, there are studies of the health effects from exposures to nuclear testing fallout from the Nevada test site and the testing in the South Pacific. The major observable health effect has been childhood thyroid cancer resulting from the β emitter Iodine 131, which has a half-life of only eight days. From studies of external radiation exposures in the A-bomb survivor studies as well as the children who were treated by radiation for tinea capitis (ring worm present on the scalp), it is clear that radiation is a risk for thyroid cancer for exposures to adolescents. Ron et al. (1995), in a pooled analysis of the studies of external exposures, observed for childhood exposures that the excess relative risk per Gy was 7.7 (95% CI 2.1, 28.7). Iodine 131 is of particular concern because it is taken up by the thyroid gland. Cardis et al. (2005) studied 276 case patients with thyroid cancer and 1300 controls, ages less than 15 years at the time of the Chernobyl accident. Individual doses were estimated for each subject based on their location and diets at the time of the accident. A dose–response relationship was observed between Iodine 131 dose to the thyroid received in childhood and thyroid

cancer risk. For a dose of 1 Gy, the estimated odds ratio (OR) of thyroid cancer ranged from 5.5 to 8.4 depending on the risk model. The risk of radiation-related thyroid cancer was three times higher in iodine-deficient areas and the use of potassium iodide as a supplement reduced this risk of radiation-related thyroid cancer by a factor of 3. Cardis et al. (2006) further predict that within Europe by 2065 about 16,000 cases of thyroid cancer and 25,000 cases of other cancers may be expected due to radiation from the accident, whereas several hundred million cancer cases are expected from other causes. Ron (2007) estimated that 90% of the thyroid cancer was due to the ingestion of iodine 131.

NONCANCER EPIDEMIOLOGY

Cardiovascular Disease

Fig. 25-5 shows that there are mortality effects of radiation exposure in the A-bomb studies besides cancer. What is of particular interest is cardiovascular disease (CVD) mortality, because although it may have a lower relative risk from radiation exposure than solid tumors, it accounts for more total background deaths. Atherosclerosis is an inflammatory disease of the arteries, which can lead to ischemia of the heart. In a study of inflammatory biomarkers (TNF-α, IL-10, IgM, IgA, and IFN-γ) as well as erythrocyte sedimentations rates among A-bomb survivors, it was shown that these markers were associated with radiation exposure. It has been estimated that an exposure of 1 Sv was equivalent to an increase in immunological age of nine to 10 years (see Hoel, 2006 for a discussion). The LSS data show a linear dose response for heart disease mortality but curvilinear for stroke mortality (Shimizu et al., 2010). It is not clear whether there are effects at acute exposures below 0.5 Gy. A current review of what we scientifically understand about CVD and radiation can be found in Darby et al. (2010), and a meta-analysis of the epidemiological studies in Little et al. (2012).

Cataracts

Cataracts were one of the earliest radiation-associated effects found after the discovery of x-rays. It has long been believed that it results from only high doses of radiation to the lens of the eye. For example, the ICRP estimates that acute exposures of 0.5 to 2 Sv are required to cause detectable lens opacities and 5 Sv for vision-impairing cataracts. For protracted exposures, they estimate the dose thresholds as 5 and 8 Sv. There are basically three types of cataracts that are described by Asbell et al. (2005). These types are nuclear or nuclear sclerosis, cortical, and posterior-subcapsular (PS) cataracts. Each of these clinical types has its known risk factors such as cigarette smoking for nuclear and possibly PS cataracts, while UV-B is a risk factor for cortical cataracts. Ionizing radiation is a risk factor for both cortical and PS cataracts but not nuclear sclerotic cataracts (Rafnsson et al., 2005; Worgul et al., 2007). Recent studies have, however, suggested that radiation exposures to the lens confer the risk of opacities at doses well under 1 Sv. The most carefully studied population for relating ionizing radiation and cataracts is the A-bomb survivors. In an ophthalmological screen of members of the adult heath study, the researchers found a statistically significant dose response for PS opacities OR = 1.41 (threshold 0.7 Gy) and for cortical opacities OR = 1.29 (threshold 0.6 Gy). A greater risk for PSC opacities was observed for those exposed at a younger age. In a subsequent study of survivors who had lens removal surgery the radiation risk was estimated to be OR = 1.39 with a low estimated threshold of 0.1 Gy (10 rem). There was no evidence of an association of nuclear cataracts with radiation exposure.

Shore *et al.* (2010) has shown that among Japanese A-bomb survivors, the risks for cataracts requiring lens surgery are at doses under 1 Gy. The CI on the dose threshold for cataract surgery indicated that the data are consistent with a dose threshold ranging from 0 to 0.8 Gy. What is not known is what are the risks at continuous or protracted exposures. Also there is limited evidence that those exposed at a younger age are at greater risk. The question of thresholds of effect continues to be undecided, with no consensus at this point in time. Classically, PSC opacities were considered to be the risk of ionizing radiation exposure to the lens. Several studies have also found that radiation affects cortical opacities. As far as the degree of risk is concerned, the typical estimate from the studies suggests that 1 Gy of exposure to the lens would correspond to a relative risk of about 1.4 for PSC and somewhat less for cortical opacities. For a general discussion of the scientific issues see Blakley *et al.* (2010).

Mental Effects

In the A-bomb survivor analyses, significant effects on the developing brain were observed among those exposed during the period of the eighth week through 25th week of gestation. During the most sensitive period of eight to 15 weeks, there was an increased frequency of severe mental retardation, a diminution in IQ scores and school performances, as well as an increase in the occurrence of seizures. During this sensitive period there is a rapid increase in the number of neurons; they migrate to the cerebral cortex where they lose their capacity to divide, becoming perennial cells. Of the 30 cases of severe retardation, 60% had small head sizes and of those with small head sizes about 10% were retarded. Also the highest IQ score among the 30 cases was 64. For retardation, the dose–response appears linear with an estimated threshold at about 0.2 Gy. At about 1 Gy the statistical regression estimates about 50% retardation. The data also suggest that at 1 Gy there is a loss of 25 to 31 IQ points with no observed effect below 0.1 Gy (Otake *et al.*, 1990, 1991 also see COMARE, 2004).

DISCUSSION

The major issue in radiation health effects is the causation of cancer. We now see noncancer effects such as CVD at low-dose and also low dose-rate exposures that occur at environmental levels and in diagnostic medical screening. Currently the LNT model is used to estimate these effects well below what can be observed in epidemiological studies. The simple defense of the LNT model is that the physical energy deposition of ionizing radiation increases cancer risk linearly with increasing dose, and the carcinogenic effectiveness is constant independent of dose. The French National Academy of Sciences and the French National Academy of Medicine (Tubiana *et al.*, 2005) has taken an opposing view on the appropriateness of the use of the LNT model. It is generally agreed that epidemiological studies have been unable to detect increases in cancer below exposures of 100 mSv. The French Academy's reason for believing that thresholds may be present and that the LNT overestimates risk is based on radiobiology. It is recognized that a cell is not passively affected by the accumulation of lesions induced by ionizing radiation. The cell reacts through at least three main mechanisms: first by reacting against radiation-induced ROS; secondly by eliminating damaged cells by either apoptosis or through cell death during mitosis of unrepaired cells; and thirdly by immunosurveillance systems that eliminate clones of transformed cells. The Academy states that experimental data strongly suggest that a practical threshold exists, but the current data do not indicate at what dose or dose rate of radiation it becomes trivial, probably somewhere between 10 and 50 mGy (Tubiana, 2005). For a recent debate see Brenner (2009) and Averbeck (2009). The BEIR VII committee concluded

"The committee judged that the linear no-threshold model (LNT) provided the most reasonable description of the relation between low-dose exposure to ionizing radiation and the incidence of solid cancers that are induced by ionizing radiation."

The answer awaits further progress in radiobiology.

A second question is whether there is a dose and dose rate effectiveness factor (DDREF) greater than one. In other words, are chronic exposures less of a cancer risk than an acute exposure such as from the A-bomb studies that provide the quantitative risk estimates? Previously a value of two had been used until BEIR VII concluded that it should be 1.5. Recently it has been argued that it should probably be equal to one (Jacob *et al.*, 2009). Animal studies have generally suggested that a DDREF is appropriately between 2 and 10 (BEIR V); however, these studies were generally conducted at relatively high doses.

For a much more in-depth reading of health effects of ionizing radiation the reader is referred to two outstanding text books (Hall and Giacca, 2005; and Mettler and Upton, 1995). For an understanding of radiation exposures there are several available health physics texts (eg, Cember and Johnson, 2009). Finally BEIR VII is a very good source of the current scientific understanding of biology, toxicology, and epidemiology of radiation exposures. Further committee conclusions about health effects can be found in IARC volume 100D and UNSCEAR (2006).

REFERENCES

Advisory Group on Ionising Radiation AGIR. Radon and public health radiation, Chemicals and environmental hazards. Health Protection Authority. 2009. http://www.hpa.org.uk/web/HPAwebFile/HPAweb_C/1243838496865.

Amundson SA, Fornace AJ Jr. Gene expression profiles for monitoring radiation exposure. *Radiat Prot Dosim.* 2001;97(1):11–16.

Amundson SA, Lee RA, Koch-Paiz CA, et al. Differential responses of stress genes to low dose-rate gamma irradiation. *Mol Cancer Res.* 2003;1(6):445–452.

Asbell PA, Dualan I, Mindel J, Brocks D, Ahmad M and S Epstein. Age-related cataracts. *Lancet.* 2005;365:599–609.

Ashmore JP, Gentner NE, Osborne RV. Incomplete data on the Canadian cohort may have affected the results of the study by the International Agency for Research on Cancer on the radiogenic cancer risk among nuclear industry workers in 15 countries. *J Radiol Prot.* 2010;30(2):121–129.

Ashmore JP, Krewski D, Zielinski JM, Jiang H, Semenciw R, Band PR. First analysis of mortality and occupational radiation exposure based on the National Dose Registry of Canada. *Am J Epidemiol.* 1998;148:564–574.

Averbeck D. Does scientific evidence support a change from the LNT model for low-dose radiation risk extrapolation? *Health Phys.* 2009;97(5):493–504.

Baker PJ, Hoel DG. Meta-analysis of standardized incidence and mortality rates of childhood leukaemia in proximity to nuclear facilities. *Eur J Cancer Care (Engl).* 2007;16(4):355–363.

Barcellos-Hoff MH. Integrative radiation carcinogenesis: interactions between cell and tissue responses to DNA damage. *Semin Cancer Biol.* 2005;15(2):138–148.

Bauer S, Gusev BI, Pivina LM, Apsalikov KN, Grosche B. Radiation exposure due to local fallout from Soviet atmospheric nuclear weapons testing in Kazakhstan: solid cancer mortality in the Semipalatinsk historical cohort, 1960–1999. *Radiat Res.* 2005;164(4 pt 1):409–419.

Baverstock KF, Papworth DG. The UK radium luminizer survey. *BIR report.* 1989;21:72–79.

BEIR. Health effects of Radon and other internally deposited alpha-emitters. Advisory Committee on the Biological Effects of Ionizing Radiation. BEIR IV. National Academy of Sciences; 1988.

BEIR. Health effects of exposure to low levels of ionizing radiation. *National Research Council Advisory Committee on the Biological Effects of Ionizing Radiation. BEIR V.* Washington, DC: National Academy of Sciences; 1990.

BEIR. Health effects of exposure to radon. *National Research Council Advisory Committee on the Biological Effects of Ionizing Radiation. BEIR VI.* Washington, DC: National Academy of Sciences; 1999.

BEIR. Health risks from exposure to low levels of ionizing radiation. *National Research Council Advisory Committee on the Biological Effects of Ionizing Radiation. BEIR VII phase 2.* Washington, DC: National Academy of Sciences; 2006.

Blakely EA, Kleiman NJ, Neriishi K, et al. Radiation cataractogenesis: epidemiology and biology. *Rad Res.* 2010;173(5):709–717.

Brand K, Zielinski J, Krewski D. Residential radon in Canada: an uncertainty analysis of population and individual lung cancer risk. *Risk Anal.* 2005;25:253–269.

Brenner DJ. Extrapolating radiation-induced cancer risks from low doses to very low doses. *Health Phys.* 2009;97(5):505–509.

Calabrese EJ, Bachmann KA, Bailer AJ, et al. Biological stress response terminology: integrating the concepts of adaptive response and preconditioning stress within a hormetic dose-response framework. *Toxicol Appl Pharmacol.* 2007;222(1):122–128.

Cardis E. Commentary: low dose-rate exposures to ionizing radiation. *Int J Epidemiol.* 2007;36(5):1046–1047.

Cardis E, Gilbert ES, Carpenter L, et al. Effects of low doses and low dose rates of external ionizing radiation: cancer mortality among nuclear industry workers in three countries. *Radiat Res.* 1995;142(2):117–132.

Cardis E, Howe G, Ron E, et al. Cancer consequences of the Chernobyl accident: 20 years on. *J Radio Prot.* 2006;26:127–140.

Cardis E, Kesminiene A, Ivanov V, et al. Risk of thyroid cancer after exposure to ^{131}I in childhood. *J Natl Cancer Inst.* 2005;97:724–732.

Cardis E, Vrijheid M, Blettner M, et al. The 15-Country Collaborative Study of Cancer Risk among radiation workers in the nuclear industry: estimates of radiation-related cancer risks. *Radiat Res.* 2007;167(4):396–416.

Catelinois O, Rogel A, Laurier D, et al. Lung cancer attributable to indoor radon exposure in France: impact of the risk models and uncertainty analysis. *Environ Health Perspect.* 2006;114(9):1361–1366.

Cember H, Johnson TE. *Introduction to Health Physics.* 4th ed. New York: McGraw Hill Medical; 2009.

Chen J. Estimated risks of radon-induced lung cancer for different exposure profiles based on the new EPA model. *Health Phys.* 2005;88:323–333.

COMARE, Committee on Medical Aspects of Radiation in Environment (COMARE). Eighth report. *Review of Pregnancy Outcomes Following Preconceptional Exposure to Radiation.* Chilton: National Radiological Protection Board; 2004.

COMARE, Committee on Medical Aspects of Radiation in the Environment (COMARE). Fourteenth report. *Further Consideration of the Incidence of Childhood Leukaemia Around Nuclear Power Plants in Great Britain.* London: Health Protection Agency for the Committee on Medical Aspects of Radiation in the Environment; 2011.

Darby SC, Cutter DJ, Boerma M, et al. Radiation-related heart disease: current knowledge and future prospects. *Int J Radiat Oncol Biol Phys.* 2010;76(3):656–665.

Darby S, Hill D, Deo H, et al. Residential radon and lung cancer: detailed results of a collaborative analysis of individual data on 7148 subjects with lung cancer and14208 subjects without lung cancer from 13 epidemiologic studies in Europe. *Scand J Work Environ Health.* 2006;32(suppl 1):1–83.

Dauer LT, Brooks AL, Hoel DG, Morgan WF, Stram D, Tran P. Review and evaluation of updated research on the health effects associated with low-dose ionising radiation. *Radiat Prot Dosim.* 2010:140:103–136.

Degteva MO, Kozheurov VP, Tolstykh EI, et al. Dose reconstruction system for the exposed population living along the Techa River. *Health Phys.* 2000;78(5):542–554.

Degteva MO, Shagina NB, Tolstykh EI, et al. An approach to reduction of uncertainties in internal doses reconstructed for the Techa River population. *Radiat Prot Dosim.* 2007;127(1–4):480–485.

El Ghissassi F, Baan R, Straif K, et al. Special report: policy a review of human carcinogens—Part D: radiation. *Lancet Oncol.* 2009;10:751–752.

Evrard AS, Hemon D, Morin A, et al. Childhood leukaemia incidence around French nuclear installations using geographic zoning based on gaseous discharge dose estimates. *Br J Cancer.* 2006;94(9):1342–1347.

Gilbert ES, Koshurnikova NA, Sokolnikov M, et al. Liver cancers in Mayak workers. *Radiat Res.* 2000;154, 246–252.

Gilbert ES, Koshurnikova NA, Sokolnikov ME, et al. Lung cancer in Mayak workers. *Radiat Res.* 2004;162(5):505–516.

Hall E, Giaccia A. *Radiobiology for the Radiologist.* 6th ed. Lippincott Williams & Wilkins; 2005.

Hoel DG. Ionizing radiation and cardiovascular disease. *Ann NY Acad Sci.* 2006;1076:309–317.

Hoel DG, Carnes B. Cancer dose-response analysis of the radium dial workers. *Proceedings from HEIR 2004 9th International Conference on Health Effects Incorporated Radionuclides*; 2004:169–173.

Hsu W, Preston D, Soda M, et al. The incidence of leukemia, lymphoma, and multiple myeloma among atomic bomb survivors: 1950-2001. *Radiat Res.* 2012 (to appear).

Hwang SL, Guo HR, Hsieh WA, et al. Cancer risks in a population with prolonged low dose-rate gamma-radiation exposure in radiocontaminated buildings, 1983-2002. *Int J Radiat Biol.* 2006;82(12):849–858.

Hwang SL, Hwang JS, Yang YT, et al. Estimates of relative risks for cancers in a population after prolonged low-dose-rate radiation exposure: a follow-up assessment from 1983 to 2005. *Radiat Res.* 2008;170:143–148.

International Commission on Radiological Protection. The 2007 Recommendations of the International Commission on Radiological Protection. ICRP publication 103. *Ann ICRP.* 2007;37(2–4):1–332.

IARC. A review of human carcinogens: Part D radiation. *IARC Monogr Eval Carcinog Risks Hum.* 2009;100D:1–362.

Ivanov VK, Late cancer and noncancer risks among Chernobyl emergency workers of Russia. *Health Phys.* 2007;93(5):470–479.

Ivanov VK, Tsyb AF, Vasilenko EK, et al. Cancer morbidity and mortality among the liquidators of the Chernobyl accident: estimation of radiation risks. *Radiats Biol Radioecol.* 2006;46(2):159–166.

Jablon S, Hrubec Z, Boice JD Jr. Cancer in populations living near nuclear facilities. A survey of mortality nationwide and incidence in two states. *JAMA.* 1991;265(11):1403–1408.

Jacob P, Ruhm W, Walsh L, Blettner M, Hammer G, Zeeb H. Is cancer risk of radiation workers larger than expected? *Occup Environ Med.* 2009;66:789–796.

Jiang T, Hayata I, Wang C, et al. Dose-effect relationship of dicentric and ring chromosomes in lymphocytes of individuals living in the high background radiation areas in China. *J Radiat Res (Tokyo).* 2000;41(suppl):63–68.

Kaatsch P, Spix C, Schulze-Rath R, Schmiedel S, Blettner M. Leukaemia in young children living in the vicinity of German nuclear power plants. *Int J Cancer.* 2008;122(4):721–726.

Kendall GM, Little MP, Wakeford R, et al. A record-based case–control study of natural background radiation and the incidence of childhood leukaemia and other cancers in Great Britain during 1980–2006. *Leukemia.* 2012;1–7.

Kinlen L. Evidence for an infective cause of childhood leukaemia: comparison of a Scottish new town with nuclear reprocessing sites in Britain. *Lancet.* 1988;2(8624):1323–1327.

Kinlen L. Childhood leukemia, nuclear sites, and population mixing. *Br J Cancer.* 2011;104:12–18.

Koshurnikova NA, Gilbert ES, Sokolnikov M, et al. Bone cancers in Mayak workers. *Radiat Res.* 2000;154:237–245.

Krestinina LY, Davis F, Ostroumova EV, et al. Solid cancer incidence and low-dose-rate radiation exposures in the Techa River cohort: 1956-2002. *Int J Epidemiol.* 2007;36(5):1038–1046.

Krewski D, Lubin JH, Zielinski JM, et al. A combined analysis of North American case-control studies of residential radon and lung cancer. *J Toxicol Environ Health A.* 2006;69:533–597.

Laurier D, Grosche B, Hall P. Risk of childhood leukaemia in the vicinity of nuclear installations--findings and recent controversies. *Acta Oncol.* 2002;41(1):14–24.

Little MP, Azizova TV, Bazyka D, et al. Systematic review and meta-analysis of circulatory disease from exposure to low-level ionizing radiation and estimates of potential population mortality risks. *Environ Health Perspect.* 2012 (to appear).

Little MP, Hoel DG, Molitor J, Boice JD, Wakeford R, Muirhead CR. New models for evaluation of radiation-induced lifetime cancer risk and its uncertainty employed in the UNSCEAR 2006 report. *Radiat Res.* 2008;169(6):660–676.

Liu Z, Mothersill CE, McNeill FE, et al. A dose threshold for a medium transfer bystander effect for a human skin cell line. *Radiat Res.* 2006;166:19–23.

Maenhaut C, Detours V, Dom G, Handkiewicz-Junaky D, Oczko-Wojciechowska M, Jarzab B. Gene expression profiles for radiation-induced thyroid cancer. *Clin Oncol.* 2011;23:282–288.

Menzler S, Piller G, Gruson M, Rosario AS, Wichmann H, Kreienbrock L. Population attributable fraction for lung cancer due to residential radon in Switzerland and Germany. *Health Phys.* 2008;95:179–189.

Mettler F, Upton AC. *Medical Effects of Ionizing Radiation.* 3rd ed. WB Saunders Co; 2008.

Mohan AK, Hauptmann M, Freedman DM, et al. Cancer and other causes of mortality among radiologic technologists in the United States. *Int J Cancer.* 2003;103:259–267.

Morgan WF. Non-targeted and delayed effects of exposure to ionizing radiation: I. Radiation-induced genomic instability and bystander effects in vitro. *Radiat Res.* 2003a;159(5):567–580.

Morgan WF. Non-targeted and delayed effects of exposure to ionizing radiation: II. Radiation-induced genomic instability and bystander effects in vivo, clastogenic factors and transgenerational effects. *Radiat Res.* 2003b;159(5):581–596.

Mothersill C, Seymour CB. Radiation-induced bystander effects—implications for cancer. *Nat rev Cancer.* 2004;4(2):158–164.

Mothersill C, Seymour C. Radiation-induced bystander effects: are they good, bad or both? *Med Confl Surviv.* 2005;21(2):101–110.

Muirhead CR, O'Hagan JA, Haylock RGE, et al. Mortality and cancer incidence following occupational radiation exposure: third analysis of the National Registry for Radiation Workers. *Br J Cancer.* 2009;100:206–212.

Nair RRK, Rajan B, Akiba S, et al. Background radiation and cancer incidence in Kerala, India-Karanagappally cohort study. *Health Phys.* 2009;96(1):55–66.

NCRP Report No. 160. *Ionizing Radiation Exposure of the Population of the United States.* Bethesda, MD: National Council on Radiation Protection and Measurements; 2009.

National Research Council. *Analysis of Cancer Risks in Populations Near Nuclear Facilities: Phase 1.* Washington, DC: National Academy Press; 2012.

Nekolla EA, Walsh L, Spiess H. Incidence of malignant diseases in humans injected with radium-224. *Radiat Res.* 2010;174:377–386.

Omar RZ, Barber JA, Smith PJ. Cancer mortality and morbidity among plutonium workers at the Sellafield plant of British Nuclear Fuels. *Br J Cancer.* 1998;79:1288–1301.

Ory C, Ugolin N, Levalois C, et al. Gene expression signature discriminates sporadic from post-radiotherapy-induced thyroid tumors. *Endocr Relat Cancer.* 2011;18:193–206.

Otake M, Schull WJ, Neel JV. Congenital malformations, stillbirths, and early mortality among the children of atomic bomb survivors: a reanalysis. *Radiat Res.* 1990;122:1–11.

Otake M, Schull WJ, Yoshimaru T. Brain damage among the prenatally exposed. *J Radiat Res.* 1991;32(suppl):249–264.

Ozasa K, Shimizu Y, Suyama A, et al. Studies of the mortality of atomic bomb survivors, report 14, 1950–2003: an overview of cancer and non-cancer diseases. *Radiat Res.* 2012;177(3):229–243.

Pierce DA, Stram DO, Vaeth M. Allowing for random errors in radiation dose estimates for the atomic bomb survivor data. *Radiat Res.* 1990;123(3):275–284.

Pierce DA, Vaeth M, Shimizu Y. Selection bias in cancer risk estimation from A-bomb survivors. *Radiat Res.* 2007;167(6):735–741.

Preston DL, Ron E, Tokuoka S, et al. Solid cancer incidence in atomic bomb survivors: 1958–1998. *Radiat Res.* 2007;168:1–64.

Rafnsson V, Olafsdottir E, Hrafnkelsson J, et al. Cosmic radiation increases the risk of nuclear cataract in airline pilots: a population based case-control study. *Arch Ophthalmol.* 2005;123:1102–1105.

Rahu M, Rahu K, Auvinen A, et al. Cancer risk among Chernobyl cleanup workers in Estonia and Latvia, 1986-1998. *Int J Cancer.* 2006;119(1):162–168.

Rajaraman P, Sigurdson AJ, Doody MM, et al. Lung cancer risk among US Radiologic Technologists, 1983-1998. *Int J Cancer.* 2006;119(10):2481–2486.

Redpath JL. Suppression of neoplastic transformation in vitro by low doses of low let radiation. *Dose Response.* 2006;4(3):302–308.

Ron E. Thyroid cancer incidence among people living in areas contaminated by radiation from the Chernobyl accident. *Health Phys.* 2007;93(5):502–511.

Ron E, Lubin JH, Shore RE, et al. Thyroid cancer after exposure to external radiation: a pooled analysis of seven studies. *Radiat Res.* 1995;141:259–277.

Rowland RE, Sterhney AF, HF Lucas. Dose-response relationships for female radium dial workers. *Radiat Res.* 1978;76:368–383.

Sawant SG, Randers-Pehrson G, Geard CR, Brenner DJ, Hall EJ. The bystander effect in radiation oncogenesis: I. Transformation in C3H 10T1/2 cells in vitro can be initiated in the unirradiated neighbors of irradiated cells. *Radiat Res.* 2001;155:397–401.

Shimizu Y, Kodama K, Nishi N, et al. Radiation exposure and circulatory disease risk: Hiroshima and Nagasaki atomic bomb survivor data, 1950–2003. *BMJ.* 2010;340:193.

Shore RE, Neriishi J, Nakashima E. Epidemiological studies of cataract risk at low to moderate radiation doses: (not) seeing is believing. *Radiat Res.* 2010;174:889–894.

Simon SL, Weinstock RM, Doody MM, et al. Estimating historical radiation doses to a cohort of U.S. radiologic technologists. *Radiat Res.* 2006;166(1 pt 2):174–192.

Sokolnikov ME, Gilbert ES, Preston DL, et al. Lung, liver and bone cancer mortality in Mayak workers. *Int J Cancer.* 2008;123:905–911.

Sont WN, Zielinski JM, Ashmore JP, et al. First analysis of cancer incidence and occupational radiation exposure based on the National Dose Registry of Canada. *Am J Epidemiol.* 2001;153(4):309–318.

Spix C, Schmiedel S, Kaatsch P, Schulze-Rath R, Blettner M. Case-control study on childhood cancer in the vicinity of nuclear power plants in Germany 1980-2003. *Eur J Cancer.* 2008;44(2):275–284.

Sun Q, Akiba S, Tao Z, et al. Excess relative risk of solid cancer mortality after prolonged exposure to naturally occurring high background radiation in Yangjiang, China. *J Radiat Res (Tokyo).* 2000;41(suppl):43–52.

Tao Z, Akiba S, Zha Y, et al. Cancer and non-cancer mortality among inhabitants in the high background radiation area of Yangjiang, China (1979-1998). *Health Phys.* 2012;102(2):173–181.

Tao ZF, Zha YR, Akiba, et al. Cancer mortality in the high background radiation areas of Yangjiang, China during the period between 1979 and 1995. *J Radiat Res (Tokyo).* 2000;41(suppl):31–41.

Tapio S, Jacob V. Radioadaptive response revisited. *Radiat Environ Biophys.* 2007;46(1):1–12.

Tubiana M. Dose-effect relationship and estimation of the carcinogenic effects of low doses of ionizing radiation: the Joint Report of the Académie Des Sciences (Paris) and of the Académie Nationale de Medicine. *Int J Radiat Oncol Biol Phys.* 2005;63:317–319.

Tubiana M, Aurengo A, Averbeck D, et al. *Dose-effect Relationships and Estimation of the Carcinogenic Effects of Low Doses of Ionizing Radiation.* Académie des Sciences Report March 30, 2005, Nat Acad Med (France). Académie Nationale de Médicine Report; 2005.

Turner JE. *Atoms, Radiation, and Radiation Protection.* 3rd ed. John Wiley & Sons; 2007.

Ugolin N, Ory C, Lefevre E, et al. Strategy to find molecular signatures in a small series of rare cancers: validation for radiation-induced breast and thyroid tumors. *PLoS ONE.* 2011;6(8):e23581.

Ulrich H. The incidence of leukemia in radiologists. *N Engl J Med.* 1946;234:45–46.

United Nations Effects of Ionizing Radiation. *Volume 1: Report to the General Assembly, Scientific Annexes A and B; Volume II UNSCEAR.* New York: United Nations; 2006.

Vasilenko EK, Khokhryakov VF, Miller SC, et al. Mayak workers dosimetry study: an overview. *Health Phys.* 2007;93(3):190–206.

Wick RR, Nekolla EA, Gossner W, Kellerer AM. Late effects in ankylosing spondylitis patients treated with 224Ra. *Radiat Res.* 1999;152(suppl): S8–S11.

White-Koning ML, Hemon D, Laurier D, et al. Incidence of childhood leukaemia in the vicinity of nuclear sites in France, 1990-1998. *Br J Cancer.* 2004;91(5):916–922.

Wiggs LD, Johnson ER, Cox-DeVore CA, Voelz GL. Mortality through 1990 among white male workers at the Los Alamos National Laboratory: considering exposures to plutonium and external ionizing radiation. *Health Phys.* 1994;67:577–588.

Wilkinson GS, Tietjen GL, Wiggs LD, et al. Mortality among plutonium and other radiation workers at a plutonium weapons facility. *Am J Epidemiol.* 1987;125:231–250.

Wilson DA, Mohr L, Frey GD, Lackland D, Hoel DG. Lung, liver and bone cancer mortality after plutonium exposure in beagle dogs and nuclear workers. *Health Phys.* 2010;98:42–52.

Worgul BV, Kundiyev YI, Sergiyenko NM, et al. Cataracts among Chernobyl clean-up workers: implications regarding permissible eye exposures. *Radiat Res.* 2007;167:233–243.

Yiin JH, Silver SR, Daniels RD, Zaebst DD, Seel EA, Kubale TL. A nested case-control study of lung cancer risk and ionizing radiation exposure at the Portsmouth Naval Shipyard. *Radiat Res.* 2007;168(3):341–348.

Yoshinaga S, Mabuchi K, Sigurdson AJ, Doody MM, Ron E. Cancer risks among radiologists and radiology technologists: review of epidemiology studies. *Radiology.* 2004;233(2):313–321.

chapter 26

Toxic Effects of Plants and Animals

John B. Watkins, III

INTRODUCTION

History is replete with stories of the earliest humans using plant extracts and animal venoms for hunting, war, assassination, and political intrigue for millennia. Even the Ebers Papyrus, which dates to around 1550 BC, describes concoctions using plant substances as primary ingredients. The toxic properties of plants and animals often enhance their ability to survive. These toxic adaptations reflect how the organism interacts with its surroundings and with its predators. Some toxic compounds are used primarily to aid an animal in obtaining food while plants have developed toxic properties to specifically ward off being used as food. These toxic compounds are invaluable in the insight that they provide into the systems that they disrupt and poison. One major complication to the study of plant and animal poisons arises from their complexity as mixtures. Studies readily separate and evaluate individual components, but it is very difficult to use purified components to make the original toxin or venom. Nevertheless, extensive study of many toxins has contributed to a greater understanding of their biology and chemistry. Toxins

Table 26-1

Poisoning Syndromes Caused by Plants

SYNDROME	GENERA	MECHANISM(S)
Antimuscarinic	*Atropa, Datura, Hyoscyanmus, Solanum*	Blockade of muscarinic cholinoceptors
Cardiotoxic	*Adenium, Digitalis, Convallaria, Nerium*	Inhibition of cellular Na$^+$,K$^+$-ATPase increases contractility, enhanced vagal effect
Convulsants	*Anemone, Conium, Labrunum, Nicotinia, Ranunculus*	Blockade of gamma-aminobutyric acid (GABA) receptor on the neuronal chloride channel, alteration of acetylcholine homeostasis, mimic excitatory amino acids, sodium channel alteration, hypoglycemia
Cyanogenic	*Eriobotrya, Hydrangea, Prunus*	Gastric acid hydrolysis of cyanogenic glycosides releases cyanide
Dysrhythmia	*Acotinum, Rhododendron, Veratrum*	Sodium channel activation
Nicotinic	*Conium, Laburnum, Lobelia, Nicotinia*	Stimulation of nicotinic cholinoceptors
Pyrrolizidine	*Crotalaria, Heliotropium, Senecia*	Pyrroles injure endothelium of hepatic or pulmonary vasculature leading to veno-occlusive disease and hepatic necrosis
Toxalbumin	*Abrus, Ricinus*	Protein synthesis inhibitors leading to multiple organ system failure

have been utilized as tools to study human biochemistry and physiology in order to pave the way for new pharmaceuticals. In fact, some components are in active development for clinical use. Clinical evaluation of human poisoning is complicated by questionable identification of plant or animal species and the inability to quantify the level of exposure. In this chapter, an overview of specific plant and animal toxins and their effects will precede a short discussion of the considerable effort to harness natural pharmacopeia for clinical use.

INTRODUCTION TO PLANT TOXICITIES

The plant kingdom contains potentially 300,000 species, and the toxic effects of plants serve primarily as defense mechanisms against natural predators. Toxicity in humans can result from simply touching as well as ingesting plants to cause a truly wide array of deleterious effects. Toxic effects on humans can range from simple hay fever caused by exposure to plant pollen all the way to serious systemic reactions caused by ingestion of specific plants. Table 26-1 lists some of the poisoning syndromes that plants can produce (Nelson *et al.*, 2007).

There are many variables that can affect the concentration of a plant's toxin and that can be a major factor in the severity of

reaction one will experience on exposure. These factors include what part of the plant exposure is from, the age of the plant, amount of sunlight and soil quality that the plant has grown in, and genetic differences within a species. Also, plant toxins fall under a number of different chemical structures, which is useful in understanding related toxins. Table 26-2 lists some of the common classifications.

The number and variety of plants that have some level of toxicity are far too many to be discussed here. Criteria for inclusion for discussion are based on how frequently human exposure occurs, the seriousness of these exposures, and also how well the toxic agent is scientifically understood. Excellent source material can be found in the comprehensive texts by Dart (2004), Cameron *et al.* (2009), Leikin and Paloucek (2008), and Nelson *et al.* (2007).

TOXIC EFFECTS BY ORGAN

Skin

Irritant Contact Dermatitis Plants that cause irritation of the skin on contact are rather common (Nelson *et al.*, 2007). A list of such plants containing their family, genus, and common names can be found in Table 26-3. The trichomes, or barb-like hairs (Fig. 26-1),

Table 26-2

Chemical Classification of Plant Toxins

CHEMICAL CATEGORY	GENERA	EXAMPLES
Alkaloids	*Atropa, Senecio, Nicotinia, Coffea, Papaver, Solanum, Acotinum*	Tropines, pyrrolizidines, pyridines, purines, isoquinolines, steroids, diterpines
Glycosides	*Digitalis, Aesculus*	Steroids, coumarins
Proteinaceous compounds	*Abrus, Amanitin, Lathyrus*	Toxalbumins (abrin, ricin), polypeptides (amatoxins, phallotoxins, phalloidin), amines (aminopropionitrile)
Organic acids	*Caladium, Dieffenbachia, Rheum*	Oxalates
Alcohols	*Cicuta, Eupatorium*	Cicutoxin, tremetol
Resins and resinoids	*Cannabis, Rhus*	Tetrahydrocannabinol, urushiol

Table 26-3

Selective Plants Producing Contact Dermatitis

BOTANICAL FAMILY	GENUS SPECIES	COMMON NAME
Amaryllidaceae	*Narcissus*	Narcissus
Apocynaceae	*Nerium oleander*	Oleander
Bromeliaceae	*Ananas comosus*	Pineapple
Asteraceae	*Ambrosia, Aster, Chrysanthemum, Rudbeckia hirta, Tagetes minuta*	Ragweed, aster, chrysanthemum, Blackeyed Susan, Mexican marigold
Euphorbiaceae	*Ricinus communis*	Castor bean
Fumariaceae	*Dicentra spectabilis*	Bleeding heart
Ginkgoaceae	*Ginkgo biloba*	Ginkgo
Liliaceae	*Allium cepa*	Onion
Myrtaceae	*Eucalyptus globulus*	Eucalyptus
Pinaceae	*Abies balsamea*	Balsam fir
Saxifragaceae	*Hydrangea*	Hydrangea
Solanaceae	*Lycopersicon esculentum, Solanum carolinense, S. turerosum*	Tomato, horse nettle, potato
Umbelliferae	*Daucus carota, Heracleum lanatum*	Carrot, cow parsnip
Urticaceae	*Urtica dioica, U. urens*	Stinging nettle

found on stinging nettles (*Urtica* species, Urticaceae) puncture skin on contact and release an irritating sap containing a mixture of formic acid, histamine, acetylcholine, and serotonin (Kavalali, 2003). Various species of *Urtica* can be found all over the world; however,

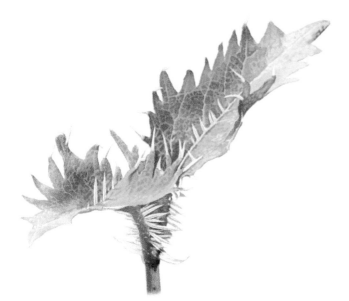

Figure 26-1. *Stinging hairs of Urtica ferox (nettles).*

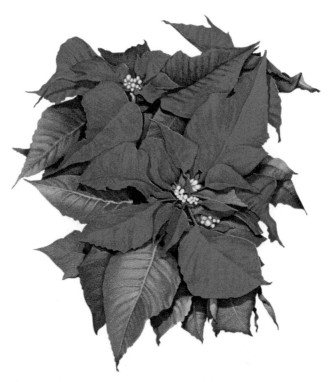

Figure 26-2. *Euphorbia pulcherrima (poinsettia).*

the most dangerous is *U. ferox* (poisonous tree nettle), which is most common in New Zealand. Exposure has been reported to cause death in humans and animals. *Mucuna pruriens* (cowhage), which also deploys its toxin via barbed trichomes on contact, may cause pain, itching, erythema, and vesication. Mucinain, contained in the toxin, is the proteinase responsible for causing the pruritus (Southcott and Haegi, 1992).

Certain species of *Ranunculus* (buttercup) contain a compound known as ranunculin, which is enzymatically broken down into the toxin protoanemonin. On contact with skin, protoanemonin found in *Anemone* (buttercup) is converted to anemonin, which is the irritant directly responsible for the resulting dermatitis. If ingested, protoanemonin may cause severe irritation of the gastrointestinal tract (Kelch *et al.*, 1992).

Damage to the stems or leaves of the genus *Euphorbia* (Euphorbiaceae, spurge family) causes exudation of a milky latex that contains diterpene esters that are irritating to the skin. *Euphorbia marginata* (snow-on-the-mountain) is a common plant in the United States that is used in flower arrangements by florists. Dermal contact with its latex can cause skin irritation (Urushibata and Kase, 1991). Also, serious eye irritation has been reported (Frohn *et al.*, 1993). The poinsettia (*Euphorbia pulcherrima*, Fig. 26-2), which is ubiquitous at holiday times, may cause contact dermatitis (Massermanian, 1998).

Allergic Contact Dermatitis Many people have experienced allergic dermatitis, most frequently from contact with poison ivy. Allergic dermatitis is an actual allergic reaction occurring within the skin as opposed to just a response to the presence of an irritant (Johnson *et al.*, 1972). Due to this immunological component, the severity of the reaction can range widely.

Philodendron scandens (Araceae, arum family) and the toxicodendron group of plants, which contains *Rhus radicans* (poison ivy, Fig. 26-3), *Rhus diversiloba* (poison oak), and *Rhus vernix* (poison sumac), are all known to cause allergic dermatitis. *P. scandens* is a common houseplant that produces allergenic resorcinols, especially

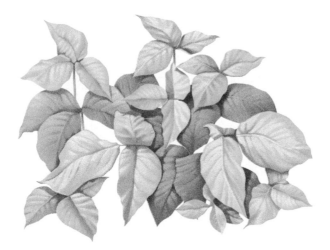

Figure 26-3. *Toxicodendron radicans (poison ivy).*

5-*n*-heptadecatrienyl resorcinol (Knight, 1991). In the *Rhus* species the allergen is a fat-soluble substance called urushiol that can penetrate the stratum corneum where it then binds to Langerhans cells in the epidermis. These haptenated cells then migrate to lymph nodes, where T cells are activated resulting in the allergic response (Kalish and Johnson, 1990). Ingestion of *Rhus* species has been reported to cause generalized dermatitis (Oh *et al.*, 2003). Sap of the mango fruit (*Magnifera indica*, Anacardiaceae) can also cause allergic dermatitis due to the presence of oleoresins that, with repeated exposure, will cross-react with allergens of poison ivy (Tucker and Swan, 1998).

Alkaloids present in the sap of daffodils, hyacinths, and tulips can sometimes cause irritation. Irritation can also be caused by contact with needle-like crystals of calcium oxalate, also known as raphides, which are present on these plants' bulbs (Gude *et al.*, 1988). The major culprit is the compound tulipalin-A, which causes "tulip fingers" from handling tulip bulbs (Christensen and Kristiansen, 1999). Tulipalin-A can be found in concentrations up to 2%. A safe threshold for this allergen is considered to be 0.01% (Hausen *et al.*, 1983). Table 26-4 contains more plants that cause irritation due to oxalates.

"Latex-fruit syndrome" is the result of cross-sensitivity to latex in rubber gloves and some fruits. *Hevea brasiliensis* (the latex tree) produces prohevein, a chitin-binding polypeptide that is also found in several plants. Hevein, a 43–amino acid N-terminal fragment of prohevein, is the major binding component (Kolarich *et al.*, 2005). Individuals who are allergic to rubber latex may become sensitized to fruits containing a chitinase with a hevein-like domain, such as banana, kiwi, tomato, and avocado (Blanco *et al.*, 1999).

Lichens, such as species of *Usnea* and *Cladonia*, are known to cause dermatitis due to the production of usnic acid (a benzofuran) and related acids (Aalto-Korte *et al.*, 2005). Usnic acid has also been implicated in hepatotoxicity following use of certain nonprescription weight loss supplements (Han *et al.*, 2004).

Photosensitivity Dermatitis does not necessarily have to be caused by skin contact. Consumption of *Hypericum perforatum* (St. John's wort) by animals can lead to serious dermatitis and even may be life threatening. The toxic agent is hypericin (a bianthraquinone) that, once ingested and dispersed systemically, causes photosensitization of the animal's skin. On exposure to sunlight, edematous lesions form on areas of skin that are not protected by hair such as the nose and ears (Sako *et al.*, 1993). Photosensitization caused by St. John's wort in humans is a rare occurrence; however, an increased response to therapeutic exposure to ultraviolet therapy has been reported (Beattie *et al.*, 2005).

Table 26-4

Selective Plants Causing Gastrointestinal Irritation Due to Release of Raphides of Oxalates

BOTANICAL FAMILY	SCIENTIFIC NAME	COMMON NAME
Amaranthaceae	*Halogeton glomeratus*	Saltlover, halogeton
Araceae	*Alocasia macrorrhiza*	Giant taro
	Anthurium andreanum	Flamingo Lily
	Caladium bicolor	Caladium
	Dieffenbachia sp.	Dumbcane
	Epipremnum sp.	Pothos, Devil's Ivy
	Monstera sp.	Shingle plant, Swiss Cheese plant
	Philodendron scandens	Philodendron
	Scindapsus aureus, Pothosaureus	Marble queen
	Spathiphyllum sp.	Peace Lily
	Syngonium podophyllum	Arrowhead plant
Chenopodiaceae	*Spinacia oleracea*	Spinach
Commelinaceae	*Tradescantieae* sp.	Spiderworts
Onagraceae	*Fushsia* sp.	Fuchsia
Oxalidaceae	*Oxalis* sp.	Wood sorrel
Palmae	*Caryotamitis*	Fishtail palm
Polygonaceae	*Rheum rhaponticum*	Rhubarb
Portulacaceae	*Portulaca* sp.	Purslane
Vitaceae	*Parthenocissus quinquefolia*	Virginia creeper
	Parthenocissus triscupidata	Boston ivy, Japanese creeper

Respiratory Tract

Allergic Rhinitis "Hay fever" or rhinitis from inhalation of plant pollens is a seasonal problem for many individuals. A chromosomal association in these individuals is under investigation (Blumenthal *et al.*, 2006). Trees, grasses, and weeds are all responsible to contributing to airborne pollen. Grass species *Poa* and *Festuca* are major contributors along with pollen from several weed genera in the Asteraceae (eg, mugwort, *Artemisia vulgaris*, in Europe, and ragweed, *Ambrosia* sp., in North America, Fig. 26-4). The common denominator in the various pollen allergens is the conserved binding domain known as profiling, which is also found in birch pollen (Hirschwehr *et al.*, 1998). Asthma and rhinitis have been linked to individuals who are exposed to cascara sagrada (*Rhamnus purshiana*) (Giavina-Bianchi *et al.*, 1997), or workers in greenhouses in which bell peppers are growing (Groenewoud *et al.*, 2006).

Cough Reflex Workers who process peppers have a significantly increased incidence of coughing when specifically handling *Capsicum annuum* (sweet pepper) and *Capsicum frutescens* (red pepper). These two types of peppers produce the major irritants

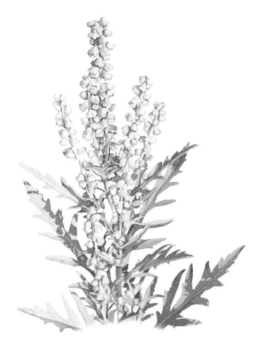

Figure 26-4. *Ambrosia psilostachya (western ragweed).*

capsaicin (*trans*-8-methyl-*N*-vanillyl-6-nonenamide) and dihydrocapsaicin (Surh *et al.*, 1998). Specific nerves in the airway have been found to be capsaicin-sensitive, which leads to the irritation and cough (Blanc *et al.*, 1991).

Toxin-Associated Pneumonia The pneumotoxin, 4-ipomeanol, is produced in sweet potato roots (*Ipomea batatas*, Convolvulaceae) by the mold *Fusarium solani*. 4-Ipomeanol is activated by human cytochrome P450s to an intermediate that binds to DNA (Alvarez-Diez and Zheng, 2004). In cattle and rabbits, the major P450 activator is CYP4B1 found in the lung that results in pneumonia. In the mouse, CYP4B1 is most abundant in the kidneys that results in renal toxicity and in humans multiple subsets of liver P450 enzymes are responsible for activating 4-ipomeanol (Baer *et al.*, 2005).

Gastrointestinal System

Direct Irritant Effects Ingestion of a toxic plant can cause irritation of the gastrointestinal tract often resulting in nausea, vomiting, and diarrhea. Many different compounds produced by plants can cause mild to severe versions of these effects. A list of plants known to cause these effects is provided in Table 26-5. Ingestion of ripe tung nuts (*Aleurites fordii*) causes abdominal pain, vomiting, and diarrhea. Outbreaks of poisoning are most likely to occur in children (Lin *et al.*, 1996).

Toxic quinolizidine alkaloids are found in buffalo beans, also known as buffalo peas (*Thermopsis rhombifolia*), which grow naturally in the western United States. Ingestion by children causes nausea, vomiting, dizziness, and abdominal discomfort (McGrath-Hill and Vicas, 1997). Also, consumption by livestock of the mature plant with seeds has been reported to be fatal.

Nuts from *Aesculus hippocastanum* (horse chestnut, Fig. 26-5) and *Aesculus glabra* (Ohio buckeye) contain a glucoside called esculin. Ingestion by humans causes gastroenteritis, which increases in severity with the number of nuts consumed.

Table 26-5

Selective Plants Causing Gastrointestinal Irritation

COMMON NAME	SCIENTIFIC NAME	TOXIC PART	TOXIN
Amaryllis	*Hippeastrum equestre*	Bulb	Lycorine
Barberry	*Berberis vulgaris*	Root	Protoberberine and other isoquinoline alkaloids
Boxwood	*Buxus* sp.	Leaves, stems	Steroidal alkaloids
Buttercup	*Ranunculus* sp.	All parts	Ranunculin, protoanemonin
Crown of thorns	*Euphorbia milii*	All parts	Resiniferatoxin
Daffodil	*Narcissus*	All, especially bulb	Lycorine, narcissin, phenanthridine alkaloids
English Ivy	*Hedera helix*	All parts	Hederin from hederagenin
Euonymus	*Euonymus* sp.	All parts	Alkaloids
Hyacinth	*Hyacinthus orientalis*	Bulb	Calcium oxalate, lycorine
Iris	*Iris*	Bulb	Irritant resin
Mayapple	*Podophyllum peltatum*	Green fruit, roots	Podophyllotoxin
Mistletoe	*Phoradendron flavescens*	Berries, other parts	Phoratoxin
Pokeweed	*Phytolacca americana*	All parts	Phytolaccatoxin, related triterpines
Purging nut	*Jatropha curcas*	Seeds	Jatrophin (curcin) (toxalbumin)
Tung nut	*Aleurites fordii*	Nut	Derivative of phorbol, saponins, toxalbumins
Wiseria	*Wisteria sinensis*	Pods	Wistarine (glycoside)

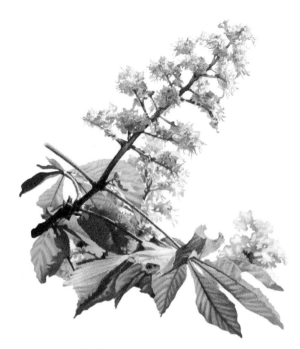

Figure 26-5. *Aesculus hippocastanum.*

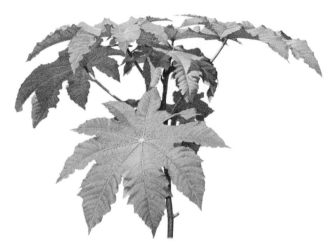

Figure 26-6. *Ricinus communis (castor bean plant).*

Fortunately, esculin is poorly absorbed by the gastrointestinal tract of humans and its systemic effects are usually limited. However, in cattle, esculin may be hydrolyzed in the rumen resulting in release of the aglycone to cause systemic effects. This can lead to nervous system stimulation—marked by a stiff-legged gait and, in severe poisoning, tonic seizures with opisthotonus (Casteel *et al.*, 1992). The triperpene saponin β-aescin in horse chestnut seed extract may have value in treatment of venous insufficiency in humans (Siebert *et al.*, 2002).

Antimitotic Effects Podophyllotoxin is found in *Podophyllum peltatum* (May apple, Berberidaceae) especially in its foliage and roots. In low doses, mild purgation occurs; however, overdose results in nausea and severe paroxysmal vomiting (Frasca *et al.*, 1997). By binding microtubules, podophyllotoxin blocks mitosis from proceeding. This has made podophyllotoxin of interest for treatment of cancer (Schacter, 1996).

Found in the bulbs of *Colchicum autumnale* (autumn crocus, Liliaceae), colchicine blocks the formation of microtubules ultimately preventing successful mitosis. Ingestion of these bulbs causes severe gastroenteritis (nausea, vomiting, diarrhea, and dehydration). Severe poisoning can result in confusion, hematuria, neuropathy, renal failure and cardiotoxicity (Mendis, 1989).

Protein Synthesis Inhibition The family Euphorbiaceae contains several genera that are known to be very toxic. The castor bean (*Ricinus communis*, Fig. 26-6) is an ornamental plant that produces seeds that, if eaten by children or adults, causes no symptoms of poisoning for several days after ingestion. Gradually, gastroenteritis develops resulting in some loss of appetite, with nausea, vomiting, and diarrhea. If a fatal dose is ingested, the gastroenteritis becomes extremely severe and is marked by persistent vomiting, bloody diarrhea, and icterus followed by death within six to eight days. A fatal dose for a child can be as few as five seeds and may be as low as 20 seeds for an adult. However, fatality occurs in less than 10% of ingestions when a "fatal" dose is consumed owing to the fact that the toxic protein is largely destroyed during digestion. The toxic agents are two lectins found in the beans: ricin I and ricin II of which ricin II is more toxic. Ricin II is made up of an A-chain

and a B-chain. The B-chain is responsible for helping the A-chain get inside the cell. It binds to a terminal galactose residue on the cell membrane that then allows for the A-chain to be endocytosed (Wu *et al.*, 2006). Once inside, the A-chain inactivates the 60s ribosomal subunit of cells by catalytic depurination of an adenosine residue within the 28s rRNA (Bantel *et al.*, 1999), thereby blocking protein synthesis.

The seeds of *Abrus precatorius* (jequirity bean, Leguminosae) contain lectins known as abrins. Abrin-a, one of four isoabrins produced by the plant, has the highest inhibitory effect on protein synthesis and consists of an A-chain and a B-chain (Tahirov *et al.*, 1994). Similar to ricin, the A-chain directly inhibits protein synthesis while the B-chain is responsible for getting the A-chain inside the cell (Ohba *et al.*, 2004). The LD_{50} of abrin when injected in mice is less than 0.1 μg/kg making abrin one of the most toxic substances known.

Plants that produce only A-chains are not nearly as toxic as those that pair them with a B-chain. Young shoots of pokeweed (*Phytolacca americana*, Phytolaccaceae, Fig. 26-7) can be ingested without toxicity; however, consumption of mature leaves and berries may cause nausea and diarrhea. The plant produces three isozymes of single-chain lectins that are capable of inhibiting protein synthesis in cells. However, these do not readily pass through a

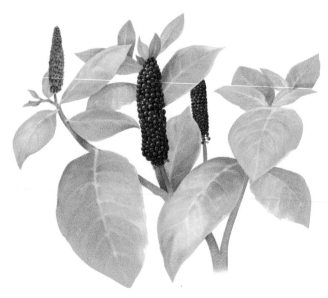

Figure 26-7. *Phytolacca americana (pokeweed).*

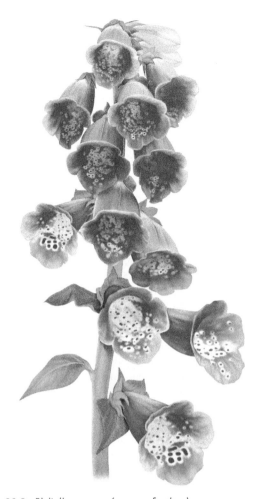

Figure 26-8. *Digitalis purpurea (common foxglove).*

cells membrane but are capable of doing so with the help of a virus (Monzingo *et al.*, 1993).

Wisteria floribunda (Leguminosae) is a common ornamental climbing vine that develops seeds in the fall. Ingestion of these seeds can cause severe gastroenteritis. Just a few seeds can produce headache, nausea, and diarrhea within hours, followed by dizziness, confusion, and hematemesis (Rondeau, 1993). The toxic agent is a lectin that binds *N*-acetylglucosamine on mammalian neurons.

Cardiovascular System

Cardioactive Glycosides The best known cardioactive glycoside is *Digitalis purpurea* (foxglove, Scrophulariaceae, Fig. 26-8). However, others exist in the lily family, such as squill (*Scilla maritima*), which contains scillaren, and lily of the valley (*Convallaria majalis*), which contains convallatoxin in the bulbs, that have actions similar to digitalis. Also, milkweeds (*Asclepias* species, Asclepiadaceae) contain glycosides (Roy *et al.*, 2005). Other cardiotoxic plants can be found in Table 26-6. The cardiac glycoside desglucouzarin in *Asclepias asperula*, like digitalis, inhibits Na$^+$,K$^+$-ATPase (Abbott *et al.*, 1998). Two plants in the Apocynaceae (oleander family) also contain cardioactive glycosides. *Thevetia peruviana* (yellow oleander) is a common ornamental plant in the United States whose seeds contain the highest concentration of cardiac glycosides. The fatal dose to an adult is eight to 10 seeds (Prabhasankar *et al.*, 1993). Clinical aspects of oleander toxicosis in sheep have been described (Aslani *et al.*, 2004). Also, oleander poisoning may not be fatal (Pietsch *et al.*, 2005).

Table 26-6

Selective Plants Causing Cardiotoxicity

COMMON NAME	SCIENTIFIC NAME	TOXIC PART	TOXIN
Azalea	*Rhodendron* sp.	All	Grayanotoxins
Death camus	*Zigadenus*	All	Zygadenine, veratrine
Foxglove	*Digitalis* sp.	Leaves, seeds	Digitalis glycosides
Larkspur	*Delphenium ambiguum*	All	Delphinine
Lily of the valley	*Convallaria majalis*	All	Convallarin, convallamarin
Milkweed	*Asclepias* sp.		(Hydroxycinnamoyl) desglucouzarin
Monkshood	*Aconitum* sp.	Leaves, roots, seeds	Aconitine, aconine
Oleander	*Nerium oleander*	All	Oleandrin, oleandrosine

Actions on Cardiac Nerves Toxic alkaloids found in *Veratrum viride* (American hellebore, Liliaceae, Fig. 26-9), *Veratrum album* (European hellebore), and *Veratrum californicum* cause nausea, emesis, hypotension, and bradycardia on ingestion. *Veratrum album* has been used for centuries to "slow and soften the pulse." The mixture of alkaloids includes protoveratrine, veratramine, and jervine that affects the heart by causing a repetitive response to a single stimulus resulting from prolongation of the sodium current (Jaffe *et al.*, 1990). The bulbs of the wild camas (Zigadenus paniculatus and other species of Zigadenus, Liliaceae) contain Veratrum-like alkaloids (Peterson and Rasmussen, 2003).

Aconitum species, which have been used in western and eastern medicine for centuries, produce the toxic alkaloids aconitine, mesaconitine, and hypoaconitine. Poisoning may occur on

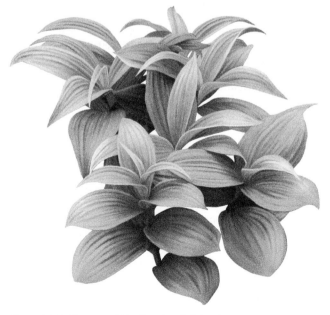

Figure 26-9. *Veratrum viride (American hellebore).*

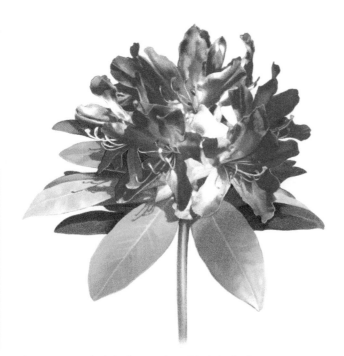

Figure 26-10. *Rhododendron ponticum (rhododendron).*

ingestion but severity varies with the concentration of the alkaloids, which depends on species, place of origin, time of harvest, and processing procedures (Chan *et al.*, 1994). Along with cardiac arrhythmias and hypotension, ingestion causes gastrointestinal upset and neurological symptoms. The alkaloids work by causing a prolonged sodium current with slowed repolarization in cardiac muscle (Peper and Trautwein, 1967) and in nerve fibers (Murai *et al.*, 1990).

Grayanotoxins are produced exclusively by several genera of Ericaceae (heath family) and in particular they are found in *Rhododendron ponticum* (Fig. 26-10; Onat *et al.*, 1991) *R. macrophyllum* (Casteel and Wagstaff, 1989), and *Kalmia angustifolia* (Burke and Doskotch, 1990). Ingestion of honey contaminated with grayanotoxins, brought there by bees, can produce a severe reaction called "mad honey poisoning." The poisoning resembles aconitine poisoning in that there is bradycardia, hypotension, oral parasthesia, and gastrointestinal upset. Severe poisoning can result in respiratory depression and eventually loss of consciousness. Grayanotoxins bind to sodium channels in cardiac and muscle cells resulting in increased sodium conductance (Maejima *et al.*, 2002).

Vasoactive Chemicals American mistletoe (*Phoradendron flavescens*) and European mistletoe (*Viscum album*, Loranthaceae) are members of the same family and both produce a toxin that is marked for its effect on the cardiovascular system. Both phoratoxin (produced by American mistletoe) and viscotoxin (produced by European mistletoe) cause hypotension, vasoconstriction of the vessels in skin and skeletal muscle, and bradycardia resulting from negative inotropic actions on heart muscle. Phoratoxin is only one-fifth as active as the viscotoxins (Rosell and Samuelsson, 1988). Although serious poisoning from the plants is rare, it is possible to induce anaphylaxis with repeated injections of mistletoe extract (Bauer *et al.*, 2005).

Ingestion of the fungus *Claviceps purpurea* (ergot), which grows on grains that are used for food, causes vasoconstriction. The "ergot gene cluster" is required for production of ergot alkaloids (Coyle and Panaccione, 2005; Haarmann *et al.*, 2005). Ergot poisoning was called "St. Anthony's fire" due to the blackened appearance of the limbs of some victims. In extreme cases, the

vasoconstriction was severe enough that gangrene would develop in the extremities. Abortion in pregnant women is also common after ingestion of ergot-contaminated grains. *Acremonium coenophialum*, a fungus which grows on the grass tall fescue (*Festuca arundinacea*), produces some ergot alkaloids. Grazing cattle that ingest the contaminated grass develop "fescue toxicosis" (Blodgett, 2001; Hill *et al.*, 1994). This condition results in decreased weight gain, decreased reproductive performance, and increased peripheral vasoconstriction. Pulmonary infection from *Acremonium strictum* has been noted in a horse (Pusterla *et al.*, 2005).

Liver

Hepatocyte Damage Pyrrolizidine alkaloids can be found in *Senecio* (groundsel, Asteraceae) and within four genera of Boraginaceae, *Echium* (bugloss), *Cynoglossum* (hound's tongue), *Heliotropium* (heliotrope), and *Symphytum* (comfrey) Altamirano *et al.*, 2005; Mei *et al.*, 2005. Ingestion of significant concentrations of these alkaloids causes liver damage in the form of hepatic veno-occlusive disease associated with lipid peroxidation (Bondan *et al.*, 2005). Cattle that graze on grass contaminated with *Senecio* have been found to develop hepatitis that can progress to death if allowed to continue grazing. Human deaths have also been reported in several countries and in Afghanistan, an epidemic of hepatic veno-occlusive disease arose from consumption of a wheat crop contaminated by *Heliotropium* (Tandon *et al.*, 1978). The liver damage caused by ingestion clinically appears to be similar to cirrhosis and some hepatic tumors that can easily be mistaken to be the source of the disease (McDermott and Ridker, 1990). Consumption of these plants leads to a form of the Budd–Chiari syndrome, which is hallmarked by portal hypertension and obliteration of the small hepatic veins. Human consumption can occur from drinking "comfrey tea" that contains *Symphytum* (Rode, 2002). There are species differences in metabolism of the pyrrolizidine alkaloids (Huan *et al.*, 1998).

Lantana camara (Verbenaceae), a shrub native to Jamaica, has been shown to poison livestock, particularly in India. Cattle grazing on the plant develop bile-related disorders including cholestasis and hyperbilirubinemia. Several triterpenoids have been isolated from the plant and in particular lantadene A (22-β-angeloyloxy-3-oxo-olean-12-en-28-oic acid) has been shown to be hepatotoxic (Sharma *et al.*, 1991).

Mushroom Toxins Most nonedible mushrooms may cause mild discomfort and are not life threatening; however, repeated ingestion of the false morel, *Gyromitra esculenta*, has been found to cause hepatitis (Michelot and Toth, 1991). The toxin gyromitrin is generally inactivated by boiling. Most fatal poisonings related to wild mushrooms are from ingestion of different species within *Amanita*, *Galerina*, and *Lepiota* (Karlson-Stiber and Persson, 2003). The dangerousness of *Amanita phalloides* (Fig. 26-11) and *Amanita ocreata* is why they are named "death cap" and "death angel," respectively. Two types of toxins, phalloidin and amatoxins, can be found within *A. phalloides*. Phalloidin is capable of binding actin in muscle cells; however, it is not readily absorbed during digestion, which limits its harmful effects (Cappell and Hassan, 1992). Unfortunately, α-, β-, and γ-amanitins are readily absorbed due to being molecularly much smaller than phalloidin. Of the amatoxins, α-amanitin is the most toxic as it inhibits protein synthesis in hepatocytes by binding to RNA polymerase II (Jaeger *et al.*, 1993). In addition to liver, intestinal mucosa and kidneys are also affected and serious clinical signs develop about three days after ingestion. In cases of severe poisoning, a liver transplant may be required. Amatoxin-α irreversibly inhibits acetylcholinesterase (Hyde and Carmichael, 1991).

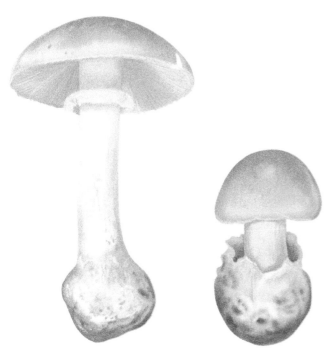

Figure 26-11. *Amanita phalloides (death cap).*

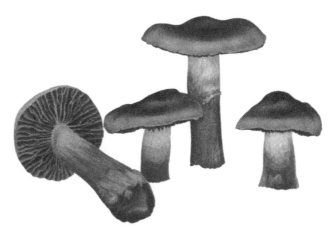

Figure 26-12. *Cortinarius rubellus (deadly webcap).*

Mycotoxins Fumonisin toxins are produced by the fungus *Fusarium* that is known to grow on corn. Consumption of contaminated corn by horses leads to equine leukoencephalomalacia that is marked by lethargy, ataxia, convulsions, and ultimately death (Norred, 1993). The liver is the most affected organ in many species including horses, pigs, chickens, and rats (Riley *et al.*, 1994). Ingestion in humans has been suggested to be associated with esophageal cancer (Yoshizawa *et al.*, 1994). Fumonisins are diesters of propane-1,2,3-tricarboxylic acid and a pentahydroxyicosane containing a primary amino acid (Gurung *et al.*, 1999) that is similar to sphingosine. This similarity is responsible for their toxicity as they block the enzymes involved in sphingolipid biosynthesis (Norred, 1993). In contrast, mycoestrogenic zearalenone induces CYP3A enzymes (Ding *et al.*, 2006). Aflatoxin B1 has been shown to form guanine adducts and induce apoptosis in human hepatocytes (Reddy *et al.*, 2006).

Kidney and Bladder

Carcinogens The bracken fern (*P. aquilinum*), which is extremely common worldwide, is the only higher plant known to be carcinogenic in animals under natural feeding conditions. The commonest bladder tumors in cattle are epithelial and mesenchymal neoplasms (Kim and Lee, 1998). Ptaquiloside, a norsesquiterpene glucoside, is the known carcinogen present in the fern and it has been found to alkylate adenines and guanines of DNA (Rasmussen *et al.*, 2003; Shakin *et al.*, 1999). Bovine consumption of bracken fern has been shown to significantly increase chromosomal aberrations (Lioi *et al.*, 2004). Also, evidence has been found that consumption of young bracken fern shoots by humans is associated with cancers of the mouth and throat (Alonso-Amelot and Avendano, 2002).

Kidney Tubular Degeneration Species of *Xanthium* (cocklebur, Asteraceae) have been found to contain the toxin carboxyatractyloside, which causes microvascular hemorrhages in multiple organs (Turgut *et al.*, 2005). Livestock poisoning has been noted to cause the outward signs of depression and dyspnea; however, internally the toxin causes tubular degeneration and necrosis in the kidney and centrilobular necrosis in the liver (del Carmen Mendez *et al.*, 1998).

Consumption of the mushroom species *Cortinarius* has been found to cause acute renal failure but different species vary widely in toxicity and, therefore, edibility. In an investigation of a series of 135 poisonings related to *Cortinarius* ingestion, where death occurred in almost 15% of the cases, renal biopsy showed acute degenerative tubular lesions with inflammatory interstitial fibrosis (Bouget *et al.*, 1990). *Cortinarius orellanus* and *C. rubellus* (Fig. 26-12) contain the deadly toxin orellanin, which triggers renal failure. Table 26-7 lists the common and scientific names and toxins for selective plants that are capable of inducing nephrotoxicity.

Blood and Bone Marrow

Anticoagulants Fungal infections in sweet clover (*Melilotus alba*) have been found to produce dicumarol, a coumarin derivative that is a potent anticoagulant. Deaths in cattle have been reported and are caused by hemorrhages (Puschner *et al.*, 1998).

Bone Marrow Genotoxicity *Argemone* (Papaveraceae), a species of poppy, produces sanguinarine, a benzophenanthridine alkaloid that is known to intercalate DNA and have carcinogenic potential (Das *et al.*, 2005). Studies in mice have shown that a single low dose of argemone oil increases chromosomal aberrations in bone marrow cells (Ansari *et al.*, 2004).

Table 26-7

Selective Plants Producing Nephrotoxicity

COMMON NAME	SCIENTIFIC NAME	PART	TOXIN
Autumn crocus	*Colchicum autumnale*	Bulb	Colchicine
Castor bean	*Ricinus communis*	All	Ricin, recinine
Daphne	*Daphne mezereum*	Leaves, fruits	Daphnin, mezerein (diterpenoid)
Impila	*Callilepis laureola*	Tubers	Atractyloside
Mushrooms	*Amanita phalloides*	All	Amatoxin
	Cortinarius sp.	All	Orellanine
Water hemlock	*Cicuta maculata*	Roots	Cicutoxin

Table 26-8

Selective Plants Producing Neurotoxicity

COMMON NAME	SCIENTIFIC NAME	PART	TOXIN	MECHANISM
Acacia tree	*Acacia willardiana*	Seeds	Willardiine	Glutamate receptor agonist
Alga	*Digenea simplex* *Chondria armata*	All	Kainic acid Domoic acid	Depolarization of glutamate-gated channels
Betel nut	*Areca catechu*	Nut	Guvacine Arecoline	GABA uptake inhibitor, anticonvulsant Stimulates muscarinic cholinoceptors; CNS stimulation
Buckthorn; Coyotillo	*Karwinskia humboldtiana*	Seeds, leaves	Tullidinol	Demyelination of motor neurons leading to paralysis
Chrysanthemum	*Chrysanthemum cinerarifolium*	Seeds	Pyrethrins	Stimulate sodium efflux from neurons in insects
Deadly nightshade	*Atropa belladonna*	Berries	Tropine alkaloid	Blockade of muscarinic cholinoceptors
Fly agaric mushroom	*Amanita muscaria*	All	Muscarine Muscimol	Stimulates muscarinic cholinoceptors; CNS stimulation GABA receptor agonist
Rhododendron	*Rhododendron* sp.	Leaves	Grayanotoxins	Stimulate sodium channel and membrane depolarization
Ryania	*Ryania speciosa*	Stems	Ryanodine	Stimulates calcium channels and muscle contraction
Poison nut tree	*Strychnos nux vomica*	All, especially seeds	Strychnine	Glycine receptor antagonist that produces convulsions
Tobacco	*Nicotiana tabacum*	Leaves	Nicotine	Nicotinic cholinoceptor agonist (low doses) or antagonist (high doses); CNS stimulation

Cyanogens Cyanogens are found in a wide variety of plants including the kernels of apples, cherries, and peaches. The highest concentrations are found in the seeds of the bitter almond, *Prunus amygdalus* var *amara*. However, small children are susceptible to amygdalin poisoning if they consume enough peach (*Prunus persica*) kernels. Fortunately, the concentration present in seeds of apples is low enough that they are unlikely to cause a problem. Metabolism of amygdalin releases hydrocyanic acid that binds to the ferric ion in methemoglobin, which, if severe enough, results in cyanide poisoning with death from asphyxiation (Bromley *et al.*, 2005; Jorgensen *et al.*, 2005; Rosling, 1993). Severe cyanide poisoning can occur with so-called vitamin supplements (O'Brien *et al.*, 2005).

Cassava produced from *Manihot esculenta* (Euphorbiaceae) is a major food source for some regions of Africa. The raw root contains a cyanogenic glucoside linamarin that is removed during processing of the root for human consumption. Unfortunately, local processing may be inadequate and that can lead to ingestion of linamarin. Chronic ingestion has been suggested to be the cause of epidemics of konzo, a form of tropical myelopathy with sudden onset of spastic paralysis (Tylleskar *et al.*, 1992).

Nervous System

Epileptiform Seizures The common and scientific names for selective plants that produce neurotoxins can be found in Table 26-8. Within the family Apiaceae, which contains carrots, the fleshy tubers of *Cicuta maculata* (water hemlock, Fig. 26-13) produce neurotoxic cicutoxin (a C17-polyacetylene). Consumption of a single tuber can result in fatal poisoning, characterized by tonic–clonic convulsions, owing to the cicutoxin binding to GABA-gated chloride channels (Uwai *et al.*, 2000).

Members of the mint family (Labiatae) such as pennyroyal (*Hedeoma*), sage (*Salvia*), and hyssop (*Hyssopus*) are well known for their essential oils containing monoterpenes. Ingestion of these

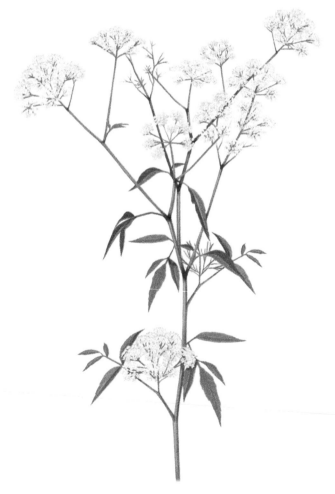

Figure 26-13. *Cicuta maculate (water hemlock)*.

monoterpenes in concentrations much higher than those used for flavoring can cause tonic–clonic convulsions. In particular, menthol is a selective modulator of inhibitory ligand-gated channels (Hall *et al.*, 2004).

Certain species within *Strychnos* (Loganiaceae) produce strychnine and brucine, which are known to cause increased CNS stimulation by blocking glycine-gated chloride channels. *Strychnos nux vomixa*, a small tree native to India, produces seeds that have been implicated in cases of unintentional poisoning (Wang *et al.*, 2004).

Excitatory Amino Acids Red algae (*Digenia simplex*) under certain conditions can proliferate rapidly leading to the notorious beach vacating "red tide" and producing kainic acid. Kainic acid may be ingested by humans who eat filter-feeding mussels that have eaten red algae. Acute symptoms are most notably gastrointestinal distress, headache, hemiparesis, confusion, and seizures. Severe exposure can result in severe memory deficits and sensorimotor neuropathy (Teitelbaum *et al.*, 1990). Isodomoic acid from *Nitzschia* sp. has seizure-inducing properties (Kotaki *et al.*, 2005).

The fungi *Amanita muscaria* (fly agaric, Fig. 26-14) and *Amanita pantherian* (panther agaric) produce the excitatory amino acid ibotenic acid (isoxazole amino acid) and its derivative muscimol that is neurotoxic (Li and Oberlies, 2005). Poisoning produces central nervous system depression, ataxia, hysteria, and hallucinations. Myoclonic twitching and seizures sometimes develop (Benjamin, 1992). Other genera of fungi have been marked for their hallucinogenic actions, notably *Psilocybe*, which contains psilocin and psilocybin (Tsujikawa *et al.*, 2003).

Willardiine, an agonist on glutamate receptors, has been isolated from *Acacia willardiana*, *Acacia lemmoni*, *Acacia millefolia*, and *Mimosa asperata* (Gmelin, 1961) and causes excitation of the nervous system. Seeds from the legume *Lathyrus sativus* (grass pea) also contain an excitatory amino acid known as β-*N*-oxalyl-L-α,β-diaminopropionic acid (Warren *et al.*, 2004). Consumption of seeds over long periods can cause lathyrism to develop. Affected individuals have corticospinal motor neuron degeneration with severe spastic muscle weakness and atrophy but little sensory involvement (Spencer *et al.*, 1986). Thiocyanate from linamarin can stimulate neuronal glutamate receptors, leading to degeneration of corticospinal motor pathways (Spencer, 1999).

Motor Neuron Demyelination *Karwinskia humboldtiana* is a shrub found in the southwestern United States, Mexico, and Central

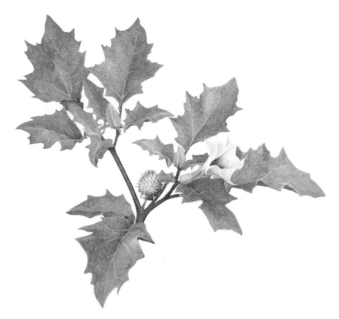

Figure 26-15. *Datura stramonium (jimson weed)*.

America that produces anthracenones in its seeds. Both human and livestock poisonings have been known to occur (Bermundez *et al.*, 1986). Several days following ingestion, ascending flaccid paralysis develops with demyelination of large motor neurons in the legs and eventually leads to bulbar paralysis in fatal cases (Martinez *et al.*, 1998). In addition to neurotoxicity, the anthracenones in *Karwinskia*, especially peroxisomicine A$_2$, cause lung atelectasis, emphysema, and massive liver necrosis. Inhibition of catalase in peroxisomes has been proposed as the mechanism of cell toxicity (Martinez *et al.*, 1997).

Cerebellar Neurons The legumes *Swainsonia cansescens*, *Astragalus lentiginosus* (spotted locoweed), and *Oxytropis sericea* (locoweed) produce a toxic indolizidine alkaloid called swainsonine. These weeds can be accidentally consumed by grazing cattle causing aberrant behavior with hyperexcitability and locomotor difficulty (James *et al.*, 1991). In fatal cases there is cytoplasmic foamy vacuolation of cerebellar neurons. Swainsonine causes marked inhibition of liver lysosomal and cytosomal α-mannosidase and Golgi mannosidase II resulting in abnormal accumulation of brain glycoproteins and mannose-rich oligosaccharides that ultimately causes cell death (Tulsiani *et al.*, 1988). *Embellisia* fungi from locoweed produce a locoweed-like toxicosis (McLain-Romero *et al.*, 2004).

Parasympathetic Stimulation Certain mushrooms of the genera *Inocybe*, *Clitocybe*, and *Omphalatus* contain significant amounts of muscarine, the principal neurotransmitter in the parasympathetic nervous system. Consumption of one these species results in extreme parasympathetic activation resulting in diarrhea, sweating, salivation, and lacrimation (de Haro *et al.*, 1999).

Parasympathetic Block Atropine, L-hyoscyamine, and scopolamine are belladonna alkaloids that can be found in varying concentrations in several genera of Solanaceae such as *Datura stramonium* (jimson weed, Fig. 26-15), *Hyoscyamus niger* (henbane), *Atropa belladonna* (deadly nightshade, Fig. 26-16), and *Duboisia myoporoides* (pituri). These alkaloids all effectively block the muscarinic receptor, essentially turning off the parasympathetic drive at the target organ. This explains why tachycardia, dry mouth, dilated pupils, and decreased gastrointestinal motility all occur

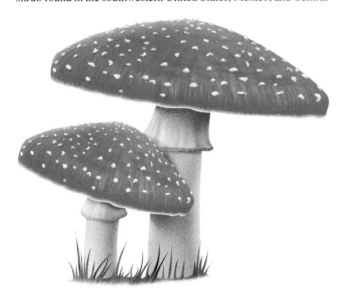

Figure 26-14. *Amanita muscaria (fly agaric)*.

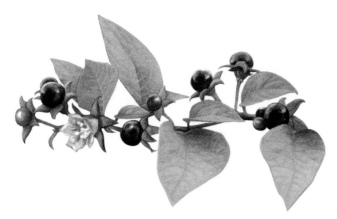

Figure 26-16. *Atropa belladonna (deadly nightshade).*

on ingestion of these toxins (Smith *et al.*, 1991). Consumption of grains contaminated with seeds from Datura sp produce poisoning typical of belladonna alkaloids (van Muers *et al.*, 1992). Of the three alkaloids, scopolamine is the most potent; however, sizable doses of L-hyoscyamine or atropine can produce similar effects. Large doses can cause confusion, bizarre behavior, hallucinations, and subsequent amnesia and in severe intoxication, tachycardia may be completely absent (Caksen *et al.*, 2003).

The seeds of *Solanum dulcamara* (bittersweet), which are used in flower arrangements, contain the glycoalkaloid solanine that on ingestion causes tachycardia, dilated pupils, and hot and dry skin—symptoms similar to atropine poisoning (Ceha *et al.*, 1997).

Sensory Neuron Block Capsaicin found in *C. annuum* (sweet pepper) and *C. frutescens* (red pepper) causes a burning sensation on vanilloid-type (VR1) sensory receptors. It also desensitizes the transient potential vanilloid 1 receptor (TRPV1) of sensory endings of C-fiber nociceptors to stimuli, a property which has therapeutic use in treating chronic pain (Szalcsany, 2002). Capsaisin also can relax ileal smooth muscle (Fujimoto *et al.*, 2006). Fortunately, desensitization produced by capsaicin is not due to cell death (Dedov *et al.*, 2001). Polygodial, a sesquiterpene found in *Polygonum hydropiper*, also desensitizes the TRPV1 (Andre *et al.*, 2006), whereas resiniferatoxin activates TRVP1 (Raisinghani *et al.*, 2005). Pyrethum from chrysanthemum flowers blocks sodium channels in the insect nervous system (McGovern and Bakley, 1999).

Skeletal Muscle and Neuromuscular Junction

Neuromuscular Junction Anabasine, an isomer of nicotine, is present in *Nicotiana glauca* (tree tobacco, Solanaceae) and produces prolonged depolarization of the junction after a period of excessive stimulation. Consumption of *N. glauca* leaves can result in flexor muscle spasm and gastrointestinal irritation, followed by severe, generalized weakness, and respiratory compromise (Mellick *et al.*, 1999). Curare, which is used as a poison placed on the tips of arrows, is also a potent neuromuscular blocking agent and is obtained from tropical species of *Strychnos toxifera* and *Chondrodendron tomentosum. Anabaena flosaquae*, a species of alga, can produce under the right conditions a neurotoxin anatoxin A that is known to be fatal. Anatoxin A, ingested by animals that drink pond water with the alga present, depolarizes and blocks the animal's nicotinic and muscarinic acetylcholine receptors, which can cause death from respiratory arrest within minutes to hours (Short and Edwards, 1990).

Delphinium barbeyi (tall larkspur, Ranunculaceae), which grows naturally in the western United States, contains

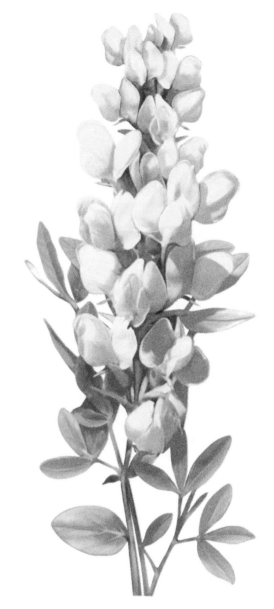

Figure 26-17. *Thermopsis montana (mountain goldenbanner).*

methyllycaconitine. Ingestion of the toxin by cattle results in muscle tremors and ataxia followed by prostration and can ultimately lead to respiratory arrest in fatal cases. Methyllycaconitine is similar to curare in that it has a high affinity for the acetylcholine receptor at the neuromuscular junction. Physostigmine has been used successfully as an antagonist to treat some cases of methyllycaconitine poisoning (Pfister *et al.*, 1994).

Skeletal Muscle Damage Certain species of *Thermopsis* produce seeds that contain quinolizidine alkaloids. Human poisoning from eating the seeds is rare, but cases have been reported in young children who experienced abdominal cramps, nausea, vomiting, and headache lasting up to 24 hours (Spoerke *et al.*, 1988). Livestock grazing on *Thermopsis montana* (false lupine, mountain goldenbanner, Fig. 26-17) develop locomotor depression and recumbency due to areas of necrosis in skeletal muscle that have been found on autopsy (Keeler and Baker, 1990).

Consumption of *Cassia obtusifolia* (sicklepod, Leguminosae) seeds by livestock causes a degenerative myopathy in cardiac and skeletal muscle. Extracts of *C. obtusifolia* have been found to

Foliage and seeds of *Leucaena leucocephala*, *Leucaena glauca*, and *Mimosa pudica* contain a toxic amino acid, mimosine, which on ingestion by cattle leads to uncoordinated gait, goiter, and reproductive disturbances including infertility and fetal death (Kulp *et al.*, 1996). Mimosine has been found to arrest the cell cycle in late G1 phase that helps explain its toxic effects (Perry *et al.*, 2005).

Lectins present in bitter melon seeds (*Momordica charantia*, Curcurbitaceae) have antifertility, abortifacient, and embryotoxic actions on ingestion. Components of the lectins known as momorcharins are known to induce midterm abortion in humans (Wang and Ng, 1998).

Caulophyllum thalictroides (blue cohosh, Berberidaceae) contains a toxin known as caulophylline that is teratogenic in rats (Kennelly *et al.*, 1999) and herbal preparations of blue cohosh have been used to terminate pregnancy (Jones and Lawson, 1998). In fact, nicotine toxicity may result from blue cohosh use as an abortifacient (Rao and Hofman, 2002).

Teratogens Ingestion of *V. californicum* (California false hellebore, Liliaceae, Fig. 26-19) by pregnant sheep is known to cause malformations in its offspring that can include cyclopia,

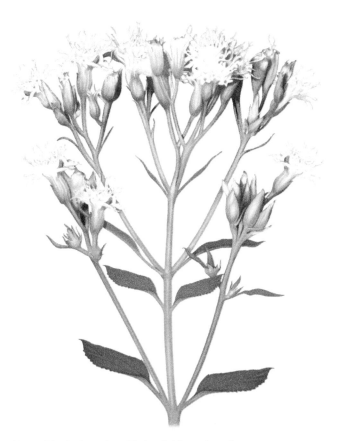

Figure 26-18. *Ageratina altissima (white snakeroot).*

inhibit NADH-oxidoreductase in bovine and swine mitochondria in vitro (Lewis and Shibamoto, 1989).

White snakeroot (*Ageratina altissima*, Asteraceae, Fig. 26-18), a common plant in the central and western United States, can be accidentally eaten by grazing cattle. On ingestion, the cattle exhibits tremors and humans who drink the milk of an affected cow can get "milk sickness" (Beier *et al.*, 1993). The toxic effects are attributed to tremetone, a benzofuran, which blocks gluconeogenesis from lactate, resulting in acidosis, tremor, and ultimately death (Polya, 2003).

Bone and Tissue Calcification

Bone and Soft Tissue Consumption of *Solanum malacoxylon* (Solanaceae) by sheep and cows can cause a marked decrease in bone calcium and calcification of the entire vascular system due to the presence of a water-soluble vitamin D–like substance. In severe cases other organs can also be affected such as the lungs, joint cartilage, and kidney.

Consumption of *Cestrum diurnum* (day-blooming jasmine, Solanaceae) and *Cestrum laevigatum* has been found to cause hypercalcemia and soft tissue calcification in grazing cattle (Durand *et al.*, 1999) and chickens (Mello and Habermehl, 1992), which is due to the presence of a dihydroxyvitamin D_3 glycoside in the leaves (Durand *et al.*, 1999). Hay that has been contaminated with *C. laevigatum* caused a marked centrilobular and midzonal hepatic necrosis in goats (Peixato *et al.*, 2000).

Reproduction and Teratogenesis

Abortifacients Besides its actions on the nervous system, swainsonine, the active alkaloid in the legumes *Astragalus* and *Oxytropus*, also causes abortions in pregnant livestock that accidentally ingest locoweeds (Bunch *et al.*, 1992).

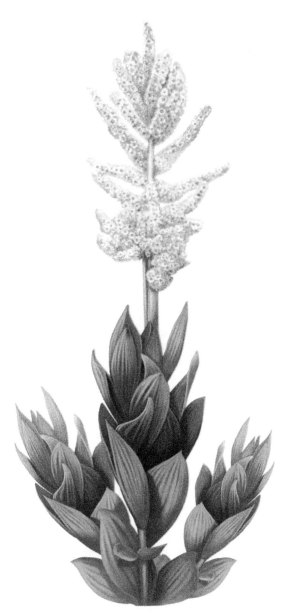

Figure 26-19. *Veratrum californicum (California false hellebore).*

exencephaly, and microphthalmia. As with most teratogens, the severity of malformations depends on what developmental stage the fetus is in at the time of exposure. Limb defects are common with exposure during the fourth to fifth week of gestation; fetal stenosis of the trachea will occur with ingestion on days 31 to 33 (Omnell *et al.*, 1990). Many other species of animals are susceptible to *V. californicum* poisoning including cows, goats, chickens, rabbits, rats, and mice (Omnell *et al.*, 1990), hamsters (Gaffield and Keeler, 1993), lambs (Keeler, 1990), and rainbow trout embryos (Crawford and Kocan, 1993). The toxic alkaloid called jervine causes teratogenesis by blocking cholesterol synthesis that, among other things, prevents a proper response of fetal target tissue to the sonic hedgehog gene (Shh). Shh has an important role in proper developmental patterning of head and brain, and blocking cholesterol synthesis has been shown experimentally to cause a loss of midline facial structures (Cooper *et al.*, 1998).

Pregnant cattle grazing on *Lupinus caudatus* and *Lupinus formosus* (lupines, Leguminosae), *N. glauca* (tree tobacco, Solanaceae), and *Conium maculatum* (poison hemlock, Solanaceae) have been found to experience a myriad of fetal deformations if ingestion occurs during a sensitive gestational period. The toxic alkaloids in these plants are anagyrine (*L. caudatus*), ammodendrine (*L. formosus*), anabasine (*N. glauca*), and coniine (*C. maculatum*, Forsyth *et al.*, 1996). It is thought that these alkaloids depress fetal movements that can lead to malformations (Lopez *et al.*, 1999).

CLINICAL STUDY OF PLANT POISONS

Recent research concerning the use of plant toxins in a clinical setting has blossomed (Ball and Kowdley, 2005). A number of factors make plant toxins of particular interest including their diverse effects, availability, and cost. With a growing group of people who wish to return to a more "natural" way of life, a medicine that is derived straight from a plant is much more marketable than one that is completely chemically synthesized. For example, root extract of the African Uzara plant has been used as an antidiarrheal remedy for centuries; however, its mechanism of action was only speculative. Recent research has shown that Uzara root extract reduced chloride secretion by the gut specifically by inhibiting Na⁺,K⁺-ATPase. This effect was seen even in the presence of cholera toxin that causes potent diarrhea by increasing chloride secretion in the gut (Schulzke *et al.*, 2011). Interestingly, anemonin, which is the active skin irritant produced by species of *Ranunculus* (buttercup), has been found to show potent anti-inflammation effects under certain conditions. The compound was found to reduce nitric oxide production that resulted in a lessened inflammatory response to inflammatory stimuli (Lee *et al.*, 2008). This mechanism could provide a new anti-inflammatory treatment modality and is being tested for possible medical use. Silymarin and usuic acid may have promise as anticancer agents (Mayer *et al.*, 2005a,b). Finally, seed extract from *M. pruriens* is used by native Nigerians as a pretreatment for snakebites from *Naja sputatrix* (Javan spitting cobra). When this was tested in rats, the seed extract helped protect against the cardiorespiratory and neuromuscular depressant effects of the snake venom (Fung *et al.*, 2011). Thus, old herbal remedies are a ripe field of study for many of their effects can be beneficial yet toxic at high enough concentrations. A goal for new research is to elucidate the mechanism of action so that treatments can be tailored to the individual needs and toxic effects can be avoided or interactions with conventional drugs can be minimized (Izzo and Ernst, 2001). As our knowledge of plant toxins and their mechanisms of action expands, the number of new and clinically useful plant remedies and medical products is bound to increase. Technological advances

in chemical purification and identification will permit better toxic characterization as well (Arilla *et al.*, 2006).

SUMMARY OF PLANT TOXICITIES

Toxic chemicals produced by plants can cause something as innocuous as a mild rash on the skin all the way to death by respiratory arrest. It is important to remember that these toxins are first and foremost defense mechanisms against natural predators. However, we benefit greatly from plants as many have produced potent antibiotics and pharmacologic therapies for myriad diseases that afflict humans.

INTRODUCTION TO ANIMAL VENOMS

The animal kingdom consists of more than 100,000 species spread through major phyla including arthropods, mollusks, chordates, etc (Mebs, 2002). Venomous animals are capable of producing a poison in a highly developed exocrine gland or group of cells and can deliver their toxin during a biting or stinging act. The venom is the sum of all natural venomous substances produced in the animal (Ménez *et al.*, 2006). Conversely, poisonous animals have no specific mechanism or structure for the delivery of their poisons, and poisoning usually takes place through ingestion. Venomous or poisonous animals are widely distributed throughout the animal kingdom, from the unicellular protistan *Alexandrium* (*Gonyaulax*) to certain mammals, including the platypus and the short-tailed shrew. At least 400 species of snakes are considered dangerous to humans. Myriad venomous and poisonous arthropods exist, and toxic marine animals are found in almost every sea and ocean (Russell and Nagabhushanam, 1996; Mackessy, 2010; Mebs, 2002).

Animal venom may play a role in offense (as in the capture and digestion of food), in the animal's defense (as in protection against predators or aggressors), or in both functions. Venoms used in an offensive posture are generally associated with the oral pole, as in the snakes and spiders, while those used in a defensive function are usually associated with the aboral pole or with spines, as in the stingrays and scorpion fishes. In the snake, the venom provides a food-getting mechanism. Its secondary function is its defensive status. In contrast, in venomous spiders, toxin is used to paralyze the prey before the extraction of hemolymph and body fluids. The venom is not primarily designed to kill the prey, but it is only to immobilize the organism for feeding. The same can be said for scorpions, although they do use their venom in defense. In fishes, such as the scorpion fishes and stone fishes, and in elasmobranches, such as the stingray, the venom apparatus is generally used in the animal's defense. Poisonous animals, on the other hand, usually derive their toxins through the food chain. As such, poison is often a metabolite produced by microorganisms, plants, or animals. Poisons are sometimes concentrated as they pass through the food chain from one animal to another. It is also worth noting that animal and plant toxins tend to differ significantly in their chemical complexity, yet both are capable of causing massive harm. Plant toxins tend to be smaller compounds or proteins and often times a single offending substance can be pinpointed. Conversely, animal toxins must be studied in the context of the entire venom or poison that typically is very complex and contains many individual toxic compounds and very large proteins that essentially work together to cause their effects. Just the same as the preceding section on plant toxins, certain criteria were employed to effectively narrow down the animal toxins discussed. Specifically considered were how often does human exposure occur, how significant is an exposure, and in general how much is known about the animal's toxic properties.

PROPERTIES OF ANIMAL TOXINS

Venoms are very complex, containing polypeptides, high- and low-molecular-weight proteins, amines, lipids, steroids, aminopolysaccharides, quinones, glucosides, and free amino acids, as well as serotonin, histamine, and other substances. Some venoms are known to consist of more than a hundred proteins. The venom is a source of peptides and proteins that act on myriad exogenous targets such as ion channels, receptors, and enzymes within cells and on cell membranes (Ménez *et al.*, 2006). Studying venom is important for several reasons. First, venoms offer valuable insight into the systems they act on such as the cardiovascular system, nervous system, coagulation, and homeostasis. Second, venoms are useful as a source of potential new drugs, with at least five agents already on the market and dozens undergoing preclinical or clinical trials (Menez *et al.*, 2005). Third, a greater understanding of venoms favors development of improved protection against envenomation (Ménez *et al.*, 2006).

Novel instrument developments have permitted the greater application of mass spectrometry, coupled with various separation technologies, to tease out the complexity of natural venoms, thereby identifying the peptide and protein components of venoms (Escoubas, 2006). The technology allows considerable resolution of extremely small amounts of venom. Fig. 26-20 demonstrates the application of gel filtration and high-pressure liquid chromatography (HPLC), as cone snail venom was fractionated into numerous peptides with varying activities (Olivera *et al.*, 1990). Similar fractionations have been performed on many other types of venom to identify the individual components. Unfortunately, studying the chemistry, pharmacology, and toxicology of venoms requires isolating and dismantling the venoms and losing the synergy among multiple components. Nevertheless, advanced technology will permit peptide sequencing, and the characterization of posttranslational modifications, such as glycosylation, and the discovery of new pharmacophores. Most venoms probably exert their effects on almost every cell and tissue, and their principal pharmacologic properties are usually determined by the amount of a fraction that accumulates at an activity site. Table 26-9 reveals the extremely large range in the LD_{50} of different toxic compounds and venoms injected intravenously into mice.

The bioavailability of a venom is determined by its composition, molecular size, amount or concentration gradient, solubility, degree of ionization, and the rate of blood flow into that tissue, as well as the properties of the engulfing surface itself. The venom can be absorbed by active or passive transport, facilitated diffusion, or pinocytosis, among other physiologic mechanisms. Besides the bloodstream, the lymph circulation not only carries surplus interstitial fluid produced by the venom but also transports larger molecular components and other particulates back to the bloodstream. Thus, the larger toxins of snake venoms, particularly those of Viperidae, probably enter the lymphatic network preferentially and then are transported to the central venous system in the neck (Russell, 2001). Because lymphatic capillaries, unlike blood capillaries, lack a basement membrane and have fibroelastic "anchoring filaments," they can readily adjust their shape and size, facilitating absorption of excess interstitial fluid along with macromolecules contained in a venom.

The site of action and metabolism of venom is dependent on its diffusion and partitioning along the gradient between the plasma and the tissues where the components are deposited. Once the toxin reaches a particular site, its entry to that site is dependent on the rate of blood flow into that tissue, the mass of the structure, and the partition characteristics of the toxin between the blood and the particular

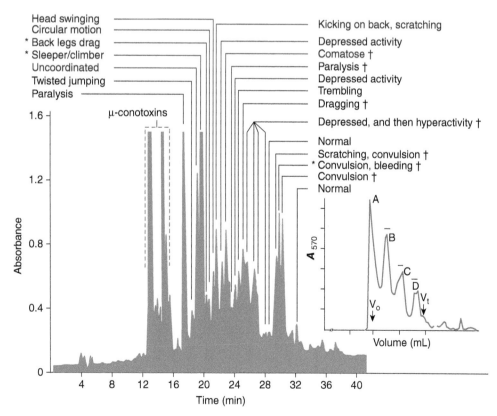

Figure 26-20. *Multiple biologically active components were obtained from Conus geographus venom by first subjecting the venom to gel filtration on Sephadex G-25 into four fractions and then separation of fraction B (which contains the α-conotoxins) by high-pressure liquid chromatography on a VYDAC C18 column using a trifluoroacetic acid–acetonitrile gradient.* Various peak fractions were then injected intracerebrally into mice and different responses were noted. (†) The fraction was lethal in at least one injected animal. (Reprinted with permission from Olivera *et al.*, 1990.)

Table 26-9

Intravenous LD$_{50}$ Values of Selected Toxins Determined in Mice

TOXIN SOURCE	COMMON NAME	LD$_{50}$ (μg/kg)
Clostridium botulinum	Botulinum toxin	0.0003
Crotalus viridis helleri	Southern pacific rattlesnake	1.3
Crotalus adamanteus	Eastern diamondback	1.5
Oxyuranus scutellatus	Australian taipan	2
Crotalus atrox	Western diamondback	2.2
Agkistrodon piscivorus	Eastern cottonmouth	4
Agkistrodon contortrix	Copperhead	11
Androctonus australis	North African scorpion	17
Notechis scutatus	Australian tiger snake	25
Naja siamensis	Indochinese spitting cobra	75

SOURCES: Data from Mebs (2002) and Russell (2001).

tissue. Receptor sites appear to have highly variable degrees of sensitivity. In the case of complex venoms, there may be several, if not many, receptor sites. There is also considerable variability in the sensitivity of those sites for the different components of a venom.

A venom may also be metabolized in several or many different tissues before undergoing excretion. Some venom components are metabolized distant to the receptor site(s) and may never reach the primary receptor in a quantity sufficient to affect that site. The amount of a toxin that tissues can metabolize without endangering the organisms may also vary. Organs or tissues may contain enzymes that catalyze a host of reactions, including deleterious ones. Once a venom component is metabolically altered, the end substance is excreted primarily through the kidneys. The intestines play a minor role, and the contributions by the lungs and biliary system have not been determined. Excretion may be complicated by the direct action of the venom on the kidneys themselves.

ARTHROPODS

There are more than one million species of arthropods, generally divided into 25 orders, of which only about 10 orders are of significant venomous or poisonous importance. These include the arachnids (scorpions, spiders, whip scorpions, solpugids, mites, and ticks), the myriapods (centipedes and millipedes), the insects (water bugs, assassin bugs, and wheel bugs), beetles (blister beetles), Lepidoptera (butterflies, moths, and caterpillars), and Hymenoptera (ants, bees, and wasps). Several texts and papers that deal with venomous and poisonous arthropods are available (Bettini, 1978; Pick, 1986; Cohen and Quistad, 1998; Russell, 2001; Kuhn-Nentwig, 2003; Isbister *et al.*, 2004).

The number of deaths from arthropod stings and bites is unknown. In Mexico, parts of Central and South America, North Africa, and India, deaths from scorpion stings, for instance, exceed several thousand a year. Spider bites probably do not account for more than 200 deaths a year worldwide. A common problem faced by physicians in suspected spider bites relates to the differential diagnosis. The arthropods most frequently involved in the

misdiagnoses were ticks (including their embedded mouthparts), mites, bedbugs, fleas (infected flea bites), Lepidoptera insects, flies, vesicating beetles, water bugs, and various stinging Hymenoptera. Among the disease states that were confused with spider or arthropod bites or stings were erythema chronicum migrans, erythema nodosum, periarteritis nodosum, pyroderma gangrenosum, kerion cell-mediated response to a fungus, Stevens–Johnson syndrome, toxic epidermal necrolysis, herpes simplex, and purpura fulminans. Any arthropod may bite or sting and not eject venom. Finally, some arthropod venom poisonings accentuate the symptoms and signs of an existing undiagnosed subclinical disease that further complicates diagnosis.

ARACHNIDA

Scorpions

Of the more than 1000 species of scorpions, the stings of more than 75 can be considered of sufficient importance to warrant medical attention (Keegan, 1980; Polis, 1990; Russell, 2001). Some of the more important scorpions are noted along with their location in Table 26-10. In addition, members of the genera *Pandinus*, *Hadrurus*, *Vejovis*, *Nebo*, and some of the others are capable of inflicting painful and often erythematous lesions.

Many scorpion venoms contain low-molecular-weight proteins, peptides, amino acids, nucleotides, and salts, among other components (Possani *et al.*, 2000; Goldin, 2001; Rodriguez de la Vega and Possani, 2004, 2005). The neurotoxic fractions are generally classified on the basis of their molecular size; the short-chain toxins are composed of 20 to 40 amino acid residues with three or four disulfide bonds and appear to affect potassium or chloride channels, while the long-chain toxins have 58 to 76 amino acid residues (6500–8500 Da) with four disulfide bonds and affect mainly the sodium channels (Mouhat *et al.*, 2004). These particular toxins may have an effect on both voltage-dependent channels. The amino acid content is known for more than 90 species, and there appears to be a high number of cysteine residues in most of these venoms. The toxins can selectively bind to a specific channel of excitable cells, thus impairing the initial depolarization of the action potential in the nerve and muscle that results in their neurotoxicity. It appears that the way some scorpion venoms differently affect mammalian, as opposed to insect tissues, is related to the structural basis of the gates in the two organisms. Not all scorpions, however,

Table 26-10

Location of Some Medically Important Scorpions

GENUS	DISTRIBUTION
Androctonus species	North Africa, Middle East, Turkey
Buthus species	France and Spain to Middle East and north Africa, Mongolia, China
Buthotus species	Africa, Middle East, central Asia
Centruroides species	North, Central, South America
Heterometrus species	Central and southeast Asia
Leiurus species	North Africa, Middle East, Turkey
Mesobuthus species	Turkey, India
Parabuthus species	Southern Africa
Tityus species	Central and South America

have fractions that affect neuromuscular transmission. Recently, Rodriguez de la Vega and Possani (2005) constructed a phylogenetic tree using 191 different amino acid sequences from long-chain peptides and discussed their functional divergence and extant biodiversity. The effects of scorpion venom on various potassium channels have been reviewed (Rodriguez de la Vega and Possani, 2004).

The symptoms and signs of scorpion envenomation differ considerably depending on the species (Russell, 2001). Common offenders are members of the family Vejovidae, generally found in the southwestern and western United States, Central America, and South America. Their sting gives rise to localized pain, swelling, tenderness, and mild parasthesia. Systemic reactions are rare, although weakness, fever, and muscle fasciculations have been reported.

Envenomations by some members of the genus *Centruroides* are clinically the most important, particularly in the western United States. The bark scorpion, *C. exilicauda*, is often found hiding under the loose bark of trees or in dead trees or logs, and may frequent human dwellings. Straw to yellowish-brown or reddish-brown in color, it is often easily distinguishable from other scorpions in the same habitat by its long, thin telson, or tail, and its thin pedipalps, or pincer-like claws. In children, their sting may produce initial pain, although some children do not complain of pain and are unaware of the injury. The area becomes sensitive to touch, and merely pressing lightly over the injury will elicit an immediate retraction. Usually there is little or no local swelling and only mild erythema. The child becomes tense and restless and shows abnormal and random head and neck movements. Often the child will display roving eye movements. *Centruroides vittatus*, the striped bark scorpion (Fig. 26-21), is commonly involved in envenomation but fatalities are rare. In their review of *Centruroides sculpturatus* stings, Rimsza *et al.* (1980) noted visual signs, including nystagmus roving eye and oculogyric movements, in 12 of 24 patients stung by this scorpion. Tachycardia is usually evident within 45 minutes as well as some hypertension. Although this is not seen in children as early or as severely as in adults, it is often present within an hour following the sting. Respiratory and heart rates are increased, and by 90 minutes the child may appear quite ill. Fasciculations may be seen over the face or large muscle masses, and the child may complain of generalized weakness

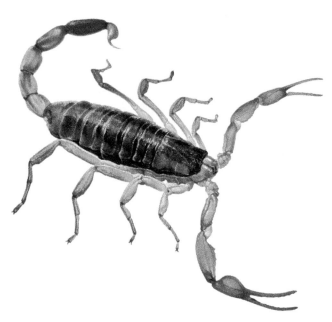

Figure 26-21. *Centruroides vittatus (striped bark scorpion).*

and display some ataxia or motor weakness. Opisthotonos is not uncommon. The respiratory distress may proceed to respiratory paralysis. Excessive salivation is often present and may further impair respiratory function. Slurring of speech may be present, and convulsions may occur. If death does not occur, the child usually becomes asymptomatic within 36 to 48 hours.

In adults the clinical picture is somewhat similar, but there are some differences (Russell, 2001). Almost all adults complain of immediate pain after the sting, regardless of the *Centruroides* species involved. Adults do not show the restlessness that is seen in children. Instead, they are tense and anxious. They develop tachycardia and hypertension, and respirations are increased. They may complain of difficulties in focusing and swallowing. In some cases, there is some general weakness and pain on moving the injured extremity. Convulsions are very rare, but ataxia and muscle incoordination may occur. Most adults are asymptomatic within 12 hours, but may complain of generalized weakness for 24 hours or more.

Spiders

Of the 30,000 or so species, at least 200 have been implicated in significant bites on humans. Spiders are predaceous, polyphagous arachnids that generally feed on insects or other arthropods. Additional information on spider bites can be found elsewhere (Gertsch, 1979; Maretiê and Lebez, 1979; Russell, 2001). Table 26-11 provides a short list of spiders with their associated toxins and the targets of their toxins.

All spiders except the Uloboridae family possess a venom apparatus that produces neurotoxins designed to paralyze or kill prey. Spider venoms are complex mixtures of low-molecular-weight components, including inorganic ions and salts, free acids,

Table 26-11

Some Significant Spiders, Their Toxins, and the Targets of the Toxins

SPIDER	PEPTIDE	TARGET*
Acanthoscurria gomesiana	Gomesin	PLM
Agelenopsis aperta	ω-AfaI-IVA	Ca^{2+}
	μ-Afatoxin 1-6	Na^+
Grammostola spatula	HaTx1,2	K^+
	GsMTx2,4	MS
	GSTxSIA	Ca^{2+}
Hadronyche versuta	ω-ACTX-Hv1a	Ca^{2+}
	ω-ACTX-Hv2a	Ca^{2+}
	δ-ACTX-Hv1a	Na^+
Heteroscodra maculate	HmTx1,2	K^+
Ornithoctonus huwena	Huwentoxin I	Ca^{2+}
	Huwentoxin IV	Na^+
Psalmopoeus cambridgei	PcTx1	ASIC
Phrixotrichus auratus	PaTx1,2	K^+
Thrixopelma pruriens	ProTxI,II	Na^+

Additional species, their toxins, and their targets may be obtained in the article by Corzo and Escoubas (2003).
*PLM, phospholipid membranes; Ca^{2+}, K^+, and Na^+, calcium, potassium, and sodium ion channels; MS, mechanosensitive ion channels; ASIC, acid-sensing ion channels.

glucose-free amino acids, biogenic amines and neurotransmitters, and polypeptide toxins. The acylpolyamines, composed of a hydrophobic aromatic carboxylic acid linked to a lateral chain of one to nine aminopropyl, aminobutyl, or aminopentyl units, are voltage-dependent open-channel blockers (sodium, calcium, and potassium channels) and/or blockers of the ion channel associated with glutamate receptors. They also act on nicotinic acetylcholine receptors. The acylpolyamines possess insecticidal activity and induce fast insect paralysis via a reversible block of the insect neuromuscular junction. Polypeptide toxins include the ion channel blockers, pore-forming peptides, and enzymes. In particular, hanatoxins 1 and 2 have allowed characterization of voltage-dependent potassium channels (Swartz and MacKinnon, 1995; Yellen, 2002). The ω-agatoxins have been demonstrated to block voltage-sensitive vertebrate calcium channels (Corzo and Escoubas, 2003). The ω-atracotoxins have greater selectivity on insect voltage-sensitive calcium channels (Wang *et al.*, 2001). Many more spiders and the spider peptide toxins have been studied to date (Fatehi *et al.*, 1997; Liu *et al.*, 1997; Corzo and Escoubas, 2003; Adams, 2004; Kuhn-Nentwig *et al.*, 2004; Rodriguez de la Vega and Possani, 2004; Ushkaryov *et al.*, 2004; Wilson and Alewood, 2006). The small spider peptide toxins are relatively easy to produce by chemical synthesis or by recombinant means. Peptide toxins from spiders have proved useful in discriminating between different cellular components of native ion channel currents and for the molecular isolation and designation of cellular receptors (Escoubas *et al.*, 2000; Corzo and Escoubas, 2003; Adams, 2004).

Poor case definition and spider identification contribute to the controversy regarding the clinical consequences and inappropriate diagnosis of spider bites worldwide. Many patients never see the spider, yet many skin lesions or areas of necrosis are attributed to spider bites. The medically important spiders include the *Agelenopsis* sp., *Latrodectus* sp., *Loxosceles* sp., *Atrax* sp., *Hadronyche* sp., and *Phoneutria* sp. Table 26-12, summarized from Isbister and White (2004), lists local and systemic effects for known cases of major spider groups in Australia.

Agelenopsis Species (American Funnel Web Spiders) The American funnel web spider (*Agelenopsis aperta*) contains three classes of agatoxins that target ion channels (Adams, 2004). The α-agatoxins appear to be use-dependent, noncompetitive antagonists of the glutamate receptor channels. These are low-molecular-weight acylpolyamines that are devoid of amino acids. Mass spectrometry analysis has identified more than 33 α-agatoxins in *A. aperta* venom (Chesnov *et al.*, 2001). The μ-agatoxins are 36 to 37 amino acid, C-terminal amidated, peptides with four internal disulfide bridges (Skinner *et al.*, 1989). These μ-agatoxins cause increased spontaneous release of neurotransmitter from presynaptic terminals and repetitive action potentials in motor neurons. In addition, the μ-agatoxins are specific for insect sodium channels. The ω-amatoxins are a structurally diverse group of peptides that are selective for voltage-activated calcium channels. There are four types of ω-amatoxins that can be distinguished by sequence similarity and their spectrum of action against insect and vertebrate calcium channels. The action of the α-agatoxins is synergized by the μ-agatoxins causing channels to open at the normal resting potentials. It is interesting to note that the agatoxins are used as selective pharmacologic probes to characterize ion channels in organs such as brain and heart, and have been evaluated as candidate biopesticides.

Latrodectus Species (Widow Spiders) Found throughout the world in all continents with temperate or tropical climates, these spiders are commonly known as the black widow, brown widow, or red-legged spider. They, however, have many other common names in English: hourglass, poison lady, deadly spider, red-bottom spider, T-spider, gray lady spider, and shoe-button spider. Although both male and female widow spiders are venomous, only the female has fangs that are large and strong enough to penetrate the human skin. Mature *Latrodectus mactans* females range in body length from 10 to 18 mm, whereas males range from 3 to 5 mm (Fig. 26-22). These spiders have a globose abdomen varying in color from gray to brown to black, depending on the species. In the black widow, the abdomen is shiny black with a red hourglass or red spots and sometimes with white spots on the venter (Russell, 2001).

The latrotoxins, a family of high-molecular-weight proteins that are found in *Latrodectus* venoms, target different classes of animals including vertebrates, insects, and crustaceans (Grishin, 1998, 1999; Ushkaryov *et al.*, 2004). The toxins are synthesized as large precursors containing around 1000 amino acid residues (around 132–156 kDa) that undergo proteolytic processing to 110 to 130 kDa and activation in the lumen of the venom gland. Mature latrotoxins are structurally conserved and contain multiple ankyrin

Table 26-12

Comparison of Clinical Effects of Bites by Some Spiders of Australia

CLINICAL EFFECTS	*LACTRODECTUS* REDBACK SPIDERS	*STEATODA* CUPBOARD SPIDERS	LAMPONIDAE WHITE-TAIL SPIDERS	MYGALOMORPHAEFWS, MOUSE SPIDERS, TRAPDOOR SPIDERS
Severe pain (%)	62	26	27	49
Duration of pain	36 h	6 h	5 min	60 min
Fang marks (%)	6	17	17	58
Initial erythema	74	96	83	36
Swelling (%)	7	9	8	13
Itchiness (%)	38	48	44	0
Nausea, vomiting, headache, malaise (%)	35	30	9	36
Distal limb bite (%)	46	52	82	91

SOURCE: Data from Isbister and White (2004).

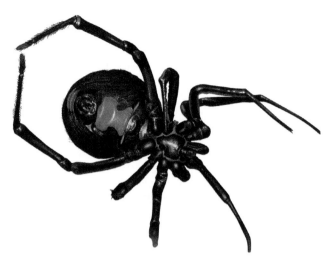

Figure 26-22. *Latrodectus mactans (female black widow spider).*

repeats. At least seven different latrotoxins have been isolated and all are large acidic proteins (pI ~5.0–6.0). Some are called latroinsectotoxins because they affect insects but not vertebrates, and one protein called α-latrocrustatoxin is active only in crayfish. All latrotoxins stimulate massive release of neurotransmitters after binding to specific neuronal receptors.

α-Latrotoxin is the most studied protein that is toxic only to vertebrates and not to insects or crustaceans (Ushkaryov *et al.*, 2004). It is a presynaptic toxin that is said to exert its toxic effects on the vertebrate central nervous system depolarizing neurons by increasing intracellular [Ca^{2+}] and by stimulating exocytosis of neurotransmitters from nerve terminals (Holz and Habener, 1998). The purported three-dimensional structure of α-latrotoxin consists of tetrameric complexes with a central channel that inserts into the lipid bilayer. A G-protein-coupled receptor latrophilin and a single-transmembrane receptor neurenin are high-affinity binding sites for α-latrotoxin (Ushkaryov *et al.*, 2004). The latrotoxins act by both calcium-dependent and calcium-independent mechanisms. In fact, a mutant recombinant α-latrotoxin that does not form pores has been invaluable in furthering our understanding of the multiple actions of the toxin (Volynski *et al.*, 2003). α-Latrotoxin and its mutants are versatile tools for the study of exocytosis. In particular, studies with this toxin have helped confirm the vesicular hypothesis of transmitter release (Hurlbut *et al.*, 1990), establish the requirement of calcium ion for endocytosis (Ceccarelli and Hurlbut, 1980), characterize individual neurotransmitter sites in the central nervous system (Auger and Marty, 1997), and identify two families of important neuronal cell surface receptors (Krasnoperov *et al.*, 1997).

Bites by the black widow are described as sharp and pinprick-like, followed by a dull, occasionally numbing pain in the affected extremity and by pain and cramps in one or several of the large muscle masses (Russell, 2001). Rarely is there any local skin reaction except during the first 60 minutes following the bite. Muscle fasciculations frequently can be seen within 30 minutes of the bite. Sweating is common, and the patient may complain of weakness and pain in the regional lymph nodes, which are often tender on palpation and occasionally are enlarged; lymphadenitis is frequently observed. Pain in the low back, thighs, or abdomen is a common complaint, and rigidity of the abdominal muscles is seen in most cases in which envenomation has been severe. Severe paroxysmal muscle cramps may occur, and arthralgia has been reported. Hypertension is a common finding, particularly in the elderly after moderate to severe envenomations. Blood studies are usually normal.

Loxosceles **Species (Brown or Violin Spiders)** These primitive spiders are variously known in North America as the fiddleback spider or the brown recluse (Fig. 26-23). There are over 100 species of *Loxosceles*. The abdomen of these spiders varies in color from grayish to orange and reddish-brown to blackish and is distinct from the pale yellow to reddish-brown background of the cephalothorax. This spider has six eyes grouped in three dyads. Females average 8 to 12 mm in body length, whereas males average 6 to 10 mm. Both males and females are venomous (Russell, 2001).

The venom of *Loxosceles* spiders appears to contain phospholipase, protease, esterase, collagenase, hyaluronidase, deoxyribonuclease, ribonuclease, dipeptides, dermonecrosis factors, and sphingomyelinase D. The venom has coagulation and vasoconstriction properties and it causes selective vascular endothelial damage. There are adhesions of neutrophils to the capillary wall with sequestration and activation of passing neutrophils by the perturbed endothelial cells (Patel *et al.*, 1994). In *Loxosceles intermedia*, the toxic effects appear to be associated with a 35-kDa protein that demonstrates a complement-dependent hemolytic activity and a dermonecrotic-inducing factor. ^{31}P-Nuclear magnetic resonance assay of the four bands representing proteins, measuring 34 kDa in the venom, produced three proteins with sphingomyelinase D activity (Merchant *et al.*, 1998). An endotoxemic-like shock, showing eosinophilic material in the proximal and distal tubules and tubular necrosis, was the most common histopathological finding, preceded in mice by prostration, acute cachexia, hypothermia, neurological changes, and hemoglobinuria (Tambourgi *et al.*, 1998).

The bite of this spider produces about the same degree of pain as does the sting of an ant, but sometimes the patient may be unaware of the bite. In most cases, a local burning sensation, which may last for 30 to 60 minutes, develops around the injury. Pruritus over the area often occurs, and the area becomes red, with a small blanched area surrounding the reddened bite site. Skin temperature usually is elevated over the lesion area. With significant envenomations, the reddened area enlarges and becomes purplish during the subsequent one to eight hours. It often becomes irregular in shape, and as time passes, hemorrhages may develop throughout the area. A small bleb or vesicle may form at the bite site, increase in size, and rupture with subsequent pustule formation. The red hemorrhagic area continues to enlarge, as does the pustule. The whole area may become swollen and painful, and lymphadenopathy is common. During the early stages, the lesion often takes on a bull's-eye appearance, with a central white vesicle surrounded by the reddened area and ringed by a whitish or bluish border. The central

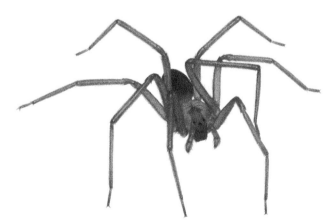

Figure 26-23. *Loxosceles reclusa (male brown recluse spider) with the violin pattern on the dorsal cephalothorax.*

UNIT V

TOXIC AGENTS

pustule ruptures, and necrosis to various depths can be visualized (Russell, 2001).

In serious bites, the lesion can measure 8×10 cm^2 with severe necrosis invading muscle tissue. On the face, large lesions resulting in extensive tissue destruction and requiring subsequent plastic surgery sometimes are seen after bites by *Loxosceles laeta* in South America. Systemic symptoms and signs include fever, malaise, stomach cramps, nausea and vomiting, jaundice, spleen enlargement, hemolysis, hematuria, and thrombocytopenia. Fatal cases, while rare, usually are preceded by intravascular hemolysis, hemolytic anemia, thrombocytopenia, hemoglobinuria, and renal failure (Russell, 2001).

Steatoda **Species** These spiders are variously known as the false black widow, combfooted, cobweb, or cupboard spiders. The female of *Steatoda grossa* differs from *L. mactans* and *Latrodectus hesperus* in having a purplish-brown abdomen rather than a black one. It is less shiny, and its abdomen is more oval than round. It may have pale yellow or whitish markings on the dorsum of the abdomen, and no markings on the venter. The abdomen of some species is orange, brown, or chestnut in color, and often bears a light band across the anterior dorsum (Russell, 2001).

The venom of *Steatoda paykulliana* stimulates the release of transmitter substances similar to *Latrodectus* venom (Cavalieri *et al.*, 1987). The venom is said to form ionic channels permeable for bivalent and monovalent cations, and the duration of time in the open state depends on the membrane potential (Sokolov *et al.*, 1984). *S. paykulliana* venom induces strong motor unrest, clonic cramps, exhaustion, ataxia, and then paralysis in guinea pigs. Bites by *S. grossa* or *Steatoda fulva* in the United States have been followed by local pain, often severe; induration; pruritus; and the occasional breakdown of tissue at the bite site (Russell, 2001).

Cheiracanthium **Species (Running Spiders)** The 160 species of this genus have an almost circumglobal distribution, although only four or five species have been implicated in bites on humans (Russell, 2001). *Cheiracanthium punctorium*, *Cheiracanthium inclusum*, *Cheiracanthium mildei*, *Cheiracanthium diversum*, and *Cheiracanthium japonicum* are often implicated in envenomations. The abdomen is convex and egg shaped and varies in color from yellow, green, or greenish-white to reddish-brown; the cephalothorax is usually slightly darker than the abdomen. The chelicerae are strong, and the legs are long, hairy, and delicate. The spider ranges in length from 7 to 16 mm. Like *Phidippus* jumping spiders but even more so, *Cheiracanthium* tends to be tenacious and sometimes must be removed from the bite area. For that reason there is a high degree of identification following the bite of these spiders. The most toxic venom fraction is said to be a protein of 60 kDa, and the venom is high in norepinephrine and serotonin.

The patient usually describes the bite by *C. inclusum* as sharp and painful, with the pain increasing during the first 30 to 45 hours. The patient complains of dull pain over the injured part. A reddened wheal with a hyperemic border develops. Small petechiae may appear near the center of the wheal. Skin temperature over the lesion is often elevated, but body temperature is usually normal. Lymphadenitis and lymphadenopathy may develop. *C. japonicum* produces more severe manifestations, including severe local pain, nausea and vomiting, headache, chest discomfort, severe pruritus, and shock (Russell, 2001).

Theraphosidae **Species (Tarantulas)** True tarantulas are members of the family Theraphosidae and there are around 800 species that are distributed worldwide, but especially in tropical or semitropical regions. Tarantulas are predators and they feed on various vertebrate and invertebrate preys that are captured after envenomation with venoms that act rapidly and irreversibly on the central and peripheral nervous systems. In humans, reported bites elicit mild to severe local pain, strong itching, and tenderness that may last for several hours. Edema, erythema, joint stiffness, swollen limbs, burning feelings, and cramps are common. In more severe cases, strong cramps and muscular spasms lasting up to several hours may be observed. *Poecilotheria* and *Stromatopelma* sp. appear to be most toxic to humans, although no fatalities have been reported (Escoubas and Rash, 2004).

Tarantula venoms have been extensively studied, and modern purification often uses orthogonal HPLC separations that combine reversed-phase and ion-exchange chromatography. Most spider peptide toxins appear to have basic pI in the nine to 11 range (Escoubas *et al.*, 2000). At least 33 peptide toxins have been described from various tarantula venoms. These have a molecular weight of 3000 to 5700 Da, and targets include voltage-gated potassium, sodium, and calcium channels, tetrodotoxin-sensitive channels, and acid-sensing ion channels, which are sensitive to extracellular pH (reviewed by Escoubas and Rash, 2004). At least two distinct structural motifs have been characterized: the inhibitory cystine knot (ICK) with a consensus sequence of $C_IX_{3-7}-C_{II}X_{3-8}-C_{III}X_{0-7}-C_{IV}X_{1-4}-C_VX_{4-13}-C_{VI}$ and disulfide bond pairing of C_I-C_{IV}, $C_{II}-C_V$, and $C_{III}-C_{VI}$ (Craik *et al.*, 2001), and the disulfide-directed β-hairpin (DDH) motif that comprises an antiparallel β-hairpin stabilized by two disulfide bridges (Wang *et al.*, 2000). Tarantula toxins have been classified as long-loop ICK, short-loop ICK, or DDH toxins (Escoubas and Rash, 2004).

Theraphosid spiders contain several toxins that are being evaluated for development as antiarrhythmic or as antinociceptive drugs. In particular, *Grammostola* mechanotoxin 4 from *Grammostola spatulata* has considerable promise as an antiarrhythmic. Protoxin I and II from *Thrixopelma pruriens* have promise as analgesics because they inhibit the tetrodotoxin-resistant sodium channels (Middleton *et al.*, 2002).

Future work on the toxins of tarantulas will encompass genomic and proteomic approaches. Expanding knowledge suggests trends in the association of primary and three-dimensional structures with pharmacologic activity. Continued improvement in isolation and purification technologies plus the combination of cDNA library screening with mass spectrometry will prove invaluable in characterization of toxin function and definition of toxin targets.

Ticks

Many of the approximately 900 species of ticks are associated with disease in humans and wild and domesticated animals (Rash and Hodgson, 2002; Barker and Murrell, 2004; Steen *et al.*, 2006). Tick paralysis is caused by the saliva of certain ticks of the families Ixodidae, Argasidae, and Nuttalliellidae. The tick bite involves insertion of cutting, tube-like mouthparts through the host's skin with anchoring so that the tick can feed for hours, days, or weeks. Saliva from the salivarium flows outward initially and the blood meal flows inward afterward. Ticks are known to transmit the organisms causing Lyme disease, Rocky Mountain spotted fever, babesiosis, leptospirosis, Q fever, ehrlichiosis, typhus, tick-borne encephalitis, and others. In fact, the import of immunosuppression by tick saliva in the transmission of flaviviruses has been discussed (Nuttall and Labuda, 2003).

Tick saliva contains a number of active constituents (Steen *et al.*, 2006). For example, saliva from *Ixodes scapularis* contains apyrase (ATP-diphosphohydrolase), which hydrolyzes ADP that is released at the bite site thereby inhibiting ADP-induced platelet aggregation (Mans *et al.*, 1998); kininase (ACE-like protein or angiotensin-converting enzyme-like protein), which hydrolyzes circulating kinins and reduces the host inflammatory response (Franciscchetti *et al.*, 2003); glutathione peroxidase (Das *et al.*, 2001); serine protease inhibitors, which inhibit coagulation enzymes (Valenzuela, 2004); an anticomplement protein that inhibits an enzyme in the alternative pathway for complement (Valenzuela *et al.*, 2000); an amine-binding protein that binds serotonin, histamine, and other biogenic amines (Sangamnetdej *et al.*, 2002); and prostanoids (PGE_2 and $PGF_2\alpha$) (Inokuma *et al.*, 1994). A discussion of toxins from other species may be found elsewhere (Cavassani *et al.*, 2005; Steen *et al.*, 2006).

Potentially 50 species of ticks are associated with clinical paralysis (Russell, 2001). As tick bites are often not felt, the first evidence of envenomation may not appear until several days later, when small macules 3 to 4 mm in diameter develop that are surrounded by erythema and swelling, often displaying a hyperemic halo. The patient often complains of difficulty with gait, followed by paresis and eventually locomotor paresis and paralysis. Problems in speech and respiration may ensue and lead to respiratory paralysis if the tick is not removed. The saliva of *Ixodes holocyclus* has yielded a peptide holocyclotoxin-1 that may cause paralysis (Masina and Broady, 1999). Peak paralytic activity was found between 60 and 100 kDa, and was a trimer of a neurotoxic protein subunit of 23 kDa (Crause *et al.*, 1993). Symptoms resolve rapidly on removal of the tick (Russell, 2001).

CHILOPODA (CENTIPEDES)

These elongated, many-segmented brownish-yellow arthropods have a pair of walking legs on most segments, and they are fast moving, secretive, and nocturnal and are found worldwide. They feed on other arthropods and even small vertebrates and birds. The first pair of legs behind the head is modified into poison jaws. Centipedes range in length from 3 to almost 300 mm. In the United States, the prevalent biting genus is a *Scolopendra* species. The venom is concentrated within the intracellular granules, discharged into vacuoles of the cytoplasm of the secretory cells, and moved by exocytosis into the lumen of the gland; from thence ducts carry the venom to the jaws (Ménez *et al.*, 1990).

Centipede venoms contain high-molecular-weight proteins, proteinases, esterases, 5-hydroxytryptamine, histamine, lipids, and polysaccharides (Mebs, 2002). Such venom contains a heat-labile cardiotoxic protein of 60 kDa that produces, in humans, changes associated with acetylcholine release (Gomes *et al.*, 1983). The bite produces two tiny punctures, sharp pain, immediate bleeding, redness, and swelling often lasting for 24 hours. Localized tissue changes and necrosis have been reported, and severe envenomations may cause nausea and vomiting, changes in heart rate, vertigo, and headache. In the most severe cases, there can be mental disturbances (Bush *et al.*, 2001; Russell, 2001; Mebs, 2002).

DIPLOPODA (MILLIPEDES)

Ranging in length from 20 to 300 mm, these arthropods are cylindrical, worm-like creatures, mahogany to dark brown or black in color, and bearing two pairs of jointed legs per segment. In Australia and New Guinea particularly, the repellent secretions expelled from the sides of their bodies contain a toxin of benzoquinone derivatives plus a variety of complex substances such as iodine and hydrocyanic acid, which the animal makes use of to produce hydrogen cyanide (Kuwahara *et al.*, 2002). Some species can spray these defensive secretions, and eye injuries are not uncommon. The lesions produced by millipedes consist of a burning or prickling sensation and development of a yellowish or brown-purple lesion; subsequently, a blister containing serosanguinous fluid forms, which may rupture. Eye contact can cause acute conjunctivitis, periorbital edema, keratosis, and much pain; such an injury must be treated immediately (Russell, 2001).

INSECTA

Heteroptera (True Bugs)

The clinically most important of the true bugs are the Reduviidae (the reduviids): the kissing bug, assassin bug, wheel bug, or conenose bug of the genus *Triatoma* (Russell, 2001). Generally, they are parasites of rodents and common in the nests of wood rat or in wood piles. These are elongated bugs with freely movable, cone-shaped heads, and straight beaks. The most commonly involved species appear to be *Triatoma protracta*, *Triatoma rubida*, *Triatoma magista*, *Reduvius personatus*, and *Arilus cristatus*. The average length of these bugs is 19 mm. The venom of these bugs appears to have apyrase activity and to lack 5-nucleotidase, inorganic pyrophosphatase, phosphatase, and adenylate kinase activities, but it is fairly rich in protease properties. It inhibits collagen-induced platelet aggregation. Three peptides isolated from the saliva of predatory reduviids are 34 to 36 amino acid residues in size, are calcium channel blockers similar to ω-conotoxins, and belong to the four-loop disulfide bridge scaffold structural class (Corzo *et al.*, 2001). The bites of *Triatoma* species are painful and give rise to erythema, pruritus, increased temperature in the bitten part, localized swelling, and—in those allergic to the saliva—systemic reactions such as nausea and vomiting and angioedema. With some bites the wound area will slough, leaving a depression.

The water-dwelling true bugs are of at least three families, Naucoridae, Belostomatidae, and Notonectidae, which are capable of biting and envenomating humans (Russell, 2001). They are found in lakes, ponds, marshes, quiet fresh water, and swimming pools. *Lethocerus americanus*, a Belostomatidae, ranges in length from 12 to 70 mm, but some water bugs may reach 150 mm. The dorsal side is usually tan or brown, but it may be brightly colored, while the ventral side is brown. They are very strong insects and can immobilize snails, tadpoles, salamanders, and even small fish and water snakes. Water bug saliva is said to contain digestive enzymes, neurotoxic components, and hemolytic fractions. ApoLp-III isolated from the hemolymph of *Lathocerus medius* is about 19 kDa and has an amino acid composition high in methionine. If molested, water bugs will bite, and their bites give rise to immediate pain, some localized swelling, and possibly induration and formation of a small papule.

Hymenoptera (Ants, Bees, Wasps, and Hornets)

Formicidae (Ants) Most ant species sink their powerful mandibles into the flesh, providing leverage, and then drive their stings into the victim. Most ants have stings, but those that lack them can spray a defensive secretion from the tip of the gaster, which is often placed in the wound of the bite. Ants of the different species vary considerably in length, ranging from less than 1.5 to over 35 mm. Clinically important stinging ants are the harvesting ants (*Pagonomyrmex*), fire ants (*Solenopsis*), and little fire ants (*Ochetomyrmex*). The harvester ants are large red, dark brown, or black ranging in size from 6 to 10 mm and having fringes of long hairs on the posterior of their heads (Russell, 2001).

The venoms of the ants vary considerably. The venoms of the Ponerinae, Ecitoninae, and *Pseudomyrmex* are proteinaceous in character. The Myrmicinae venoms are a mixture of amines, enzymes, and proteinaceous materials, histamine, hyaluronidase, phospholipase A, and hemolysins, which hemolyze erythrocytes and mast cells. Formicinae ant venom contains about 60% formic acid. Fire ant venoms are poor in polypeptides and proteins, but are rich in alkaloids such as solenopsine (Russell, 2001; Mebs, 2002). The sting of the fire ant gives rise to a painful burning sensation, after which a wheal and localized erythema develop, leading in a few hours to a clear vesicle. Within 12 to 24 hours, the fluid becomes purulent and the lesion turns into a pustule. It may break down or become a crust or fibrotic nodule. In multiple stings there may be nausea, vomiting, vertigo, increased perspiration, respiratory difficulties, cyanosis, coma, and even death. Cross-exposure to the venom of other species of ants is possible. Allergic reactions and fatal anaphylactic shock are seen in sensitized victims (Hoffman, 2006). Treatment of ant stings is dependent on their number, whether an allergic reaction is involved, and whether there are possible complications.

Apidae (Bees)

This family includes the bumble bees, honeybees, carpenter bees, and yellow jackets. The commonest stinging bees are *Apis mellifera* and the Africanized bee, *Apis mellifera adansonii*, and the incidence of Hymenoptera poisonings is increasing. The venom of the Africanized bee is not remarkably different from that of the European bee, *A. m. mellifer* (Fig. 26-24). The former bee is smaller and gives less venom, but its aggressiveness is such that attacks of 50 to hundreds of bees are not unusual (Russell, 2001).

The venom contains biologically active peptides, such as melittin, apamine, mast cell–degranulating peptide, and others, as well as phospholipases A$_2$ and B, hyaluronidase, histamine, dopamine, monosaccharides, and lipids (Mebs, 2002). Melittin, which is secreted as the 70 amino acid prepromelittin, consists of 26 amino acids with no cysteines that have natural detergent-like properties and causes erythrocyte lysis. Melittin also forms tetramers with pores, thereby facilitating ion transport through membranes. In particular, melittin tetramers cause a breakdown of the resting potential and rapid depolarization of nociceptors, which induces pain (Demsey, 1990; Bechinger, 1997). The compound apamine contains 18 amino acids cross-linked by two disulfide bridges. Apamine is a blocker of calcium-dependent potassium

channels and is thought to be the "lethal factor" (Habermann, 1984). In addition to apamine, mast cell–degranulating peptide is also a basic peptide containing 22 amino acids with two disulfide bonds. Besides stimulating release of histamine, this peptide specifically inhibits voltage-dependent potassium channels (Dreyer, 1990; Baku, 1999).

Bee stings typically produce immediate, sharp or burning pain, slight local erythema, and edema followed by itching. The edema may vary depending on location of the sting. It is said that 50 stings can be serious and lead to respiratory dysfunction, intravascular hemolysis, hypertension, myocardial damage, hepatic changes, shock, and renal failure. With 100 or more stings, death can occur. In patients who are allergic to bee stings, immediate allergic reaction with the risk of anaphylactic shock requires urgent medical treatment (Mebs, 2002; Hoffman, 2006).

Vespidae (Wasps)

This family includes wasps and hornets. These venoms contain a high content of peptides, which include mastoparan in wasps and hornets and crabolin from hornet venom. These peptides release histamine from mast cells and consist of 13 to 17 amino acids with no disulfide bridges. Other peptides named wasp kinins cause immediate pain, vasodilation, and increased vascular permeability leading to edema. These venoms also contain phospholipases and hyaluronidases, which contribute to the breakdown of membranes and connective tissue to facilitate diffusion of the venom. These proteins also contribute to the allergenicity of the venoms (Mebs, 2002; Hoffman, 2006).

Lepidoptera (Caterpillars, Moths, and Butterflies)

The urticating hairs, or setae, of caterpillars are effective defensive weapons that protect some species from predators. The setae are attached to unicellular poison glands at the base of each hair. Both the larvae and the adults are capable of stinging, either by direct contact with the setae or indirectly when the creature becomes irritated. It appears that contraction of the caterpillar's abdominal muscles is sufficient to release the barbs from their sockets, allowing them to become airborne. The toxic material found in the venom glands contains aristolochic acids, cardenolides, kallikrein, and histamine among other substances. Fibrinolytic activity has been found in 16 and 18 kDa components (isoelectric point of 8.5); coagulation defects such as prolonged prothrombin and partial thromboplastin times have been detected, and decreases in fibrinogen and plasminogen have been noted. It is thought that the hemorrhagic syndrome cannot be classified as being either totally fibrinolytic or a syndrome such as disseminated intravascular coagulopathy. The spicules of *Thaumetopoea pityocampa* contain a 28-kDa toxin called thaumetopoein, which is a strong dermal irritant and highly allergenic peptide (Kawamoto and Kumada, 1984; Russell, 2001; Mebs, 2002).

In some parts of the world the stings of several species of Lepidoptera give rise to a bleeding diathesis, often severe and sometimes fatal. Envenomation by members of the family Saturniidae, the buck moths, the grapeleaf skeletonizer (family Zygaenidae), the puss moth (family Megalopygidae), and the brown-tailed moth (*Euproctis* species) generally gives rise to little more than immediate localized itching and pain, usually described as burning, followed in some cases by urticaria, edema, and occasionally fever. The hemolymph and spicules contain highly active clotting enzymes, a protease with fibrinolytic activity and an enzyme that activates prothrombin. In the more severe cases—often due to *Megalopyge*, Dioptidae, *Automeris*, and *Hemileuca* species—there is localized

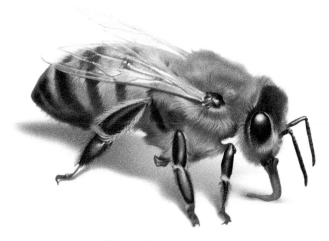

Figure 26-24. *Apis mellifera mellifera (honey bee).*

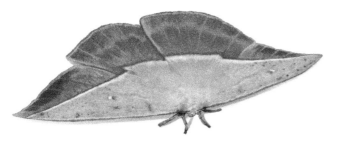

Figure 26-25. *Lonomia oblique (giant silkworm moth).*

pain as well as papules (sometimes hemorrhagic) and hematomas; on occasions there may also be headache, nausea, vomiting, hematuria, lymphadenitis, and lymphadenopathy. Contacts with larvae of the saturnid moths in South America (*Lonomia acheolus* and *Lonomia oblique*, Fig. 26-25) can cause severe coagulopathy, due to inhibition of clotting factor XIII by a venom component called lonomine V. Severe envenomation can cause cerebral hemorrhage and death (Guerrero *et al.*, 1999).

MOLLUSCA (CONE SNAILS)

Human interest in this group of mollusks has been due to the beautiful patterns on their shells. Cone snails were known to Roman scholars and natural history collectors, as the shells were often made into jewelry. The first record of fatality from cone snail sting may be found in the book of Rumphius from 1705. The genus *Conus* is a group of approximately 500 species of carnivorous predators found in marine habitats that use venom as a weapon for prey capture (Fig. 26-26). Cone snails have a venom duct for synthesis and storage of venom and hollow harpoon-like teeth for injection of the venom (Rockel *et al.*, 1995).

Cone snails may be divided into three groups depending on preferred prey. The largest group contains worm-hunting species

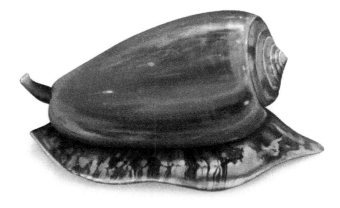

Figure 26-26. *Conus geographus (geography cone).*

that feed on polychaetes (segmented marine worms in the phylum Annelida). The second group is molluscivorous and hunts other gastropods. The final group is piscivorous and has venoms that rapidly immobilize fish (Olivera, 1997, 2002; Mebs and Kauferstein, 2005).

There are probably over 100 different venom components per species (Terlau and Olivera, 2004). Components have become known as conotoxins, which may be rich in disulfide bonds, and conopeptides. Molecular targets include G-protein-coupled receptors, neuromuscular transporters, and ligand- or voltage-gated ion channels. Some components have enzymatic activity.

Fig. 26-27 provides an overview of peptidic *Conus* venom components, indicating gene superfamilies, disulfide bond characteristics, and general targets (McIntosh *et al.*, 1999; Olivera, 2002). The two major divisions of *Conus* toxins are the disulfide-rich conotoxins and the peptides that lack multiple disulfide cross-links. The arrangement of cysteines in the primary sequence is restricted to only a few patterns, which may be diagnostic of

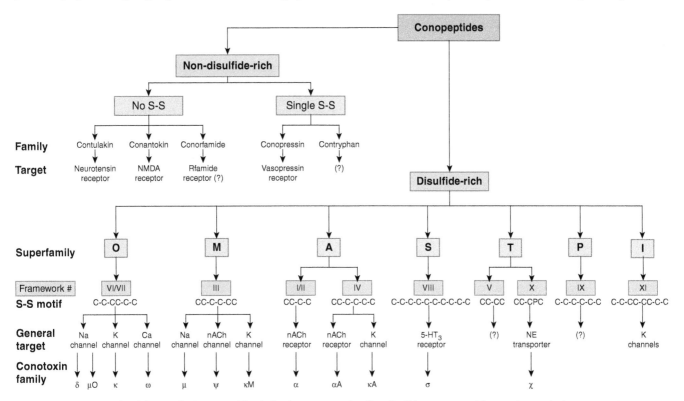

Figure 26-27. *Organizational diagram for Conus peptides, indicating gene superfamilies, disulfide patterns, and known pharmacologic targets.* Only the superfamilies of the disulfide-rich peptides are shown. (Used with permission from Terlau and Olivera, 2004.)

the gene superfamily. Most disulfide-rich conotoxins are small and consist of 12 to 30 amino acids. These toxins contain an unusually diverse complement of posttranslationally modified amino acids, including hydroxyproline, *O*-glycosylated serine or threonine, γ-carboxyl-glutamate, sulfated tyrosine, and D-amino acids (Craig *et al.*, 1999). Apparently, the posttranslational modification enzyme γ-carboxylase is present in their venom ducts (Bandyopadhyay *et al.*, 2002). The enzyme has a recognition signal in the pro region of the precursor that instructs the enzyme to modify specific amino acid residues in the mature toxin region. Thus, the pro region of conopeptide precursors provides potential anchor-binding sites for posttranslational modification enzymes (Hooper *et al.*, 2000).

Cone snails could be called sophisticated practitioners of combination drug therapy. After injection, multiple conopeptides act synergistically to affect the targeted prey. The term toxin cabal has been applied to this coordinated action of the conopeptide mixture. The fish-hunting species *Conus purpurascens* apparently has two distinct cabals whose effects differ in time and space. The "lightning-strike cabal" causes immediate immobilization of the injected prey because various venom components inhibit voltage-gated sodium channel inactivation and block potassium channels, resulting in massive depolarization of axons in the vicinity of the injection site and a tetanic state. The second physiologic cabal, the "motor cabal," acts more slowly as conotoxins must be distributed throughout the body of the prey. The overall result is total inhibition of neuromuscular transmission. Various conopeptides inhibit presynaptic calcium channels that control neurotransmitter release, the postsynaptic neuromuscular nicotinic receptors, and the sodium channels involved in the muscle action potential (Terlau *et al.*, 1996).

Conopeptides can affect many ion channels (Olivera *et al.*, 1994; Terlau and Olivera, 2004). For example, μ-conotoxins are peptides with 22 to 25 amino acids and six cysteine residues that block sodium currents by acting at a site that overlaps the tetrodotoxin-sensitive site of sodium channels. The main effect of the unusually hydrophobic δ-conotoxins, which are peptides with an inhibitory cysteine knot motif pattern of disulfide bridges, is the inhibition of the fast inactivation of sodium currents, which affects the shape and duration of the action potential. This can lead to a massive electrical hyperexcitation of the complete organism. The κ-, κA-, and κM-conotoxins target potassium channels. The ω-conotoxins are peptides that target calcium channels, and these toxins have been widely used in neuroscience research. A characteristic feature of the ω-conotoxins is their high content of basic amino acids. One peptide, ω-conotoxin MVIIA from *Conus magus*, has been developed as ziconotide (Prialt®) for the treatment of intractable pain (Olivera, 2000). Other conotoxins are being studied as potential antinociceptive agents.

Conopeptides also target ligand-gated ion channels that mediate fast synaptic transmission (Kandel *et al.*, 2000). One major group of ligand-gated ion channels is activated by acetylcholine, serotonin, γ-aminobutyric acid, or glycine. These proteins differ in ligand specificity and selectivity for the permeant ion. The second family activates the glutamate receptors, *N*-methyl-D-aspartate and kainate/AMPA receptors. A third group activates synaptic transmission at certain synapses via the ATP receptors. It is evident from Fig. 26-27 that there are conopeptides that target these three different families of ligand-gated ion channels. It is clear that our understanding of the structure and function of conopeptides is rapidly expanding and additional information regarding these toxins is available in an excellent review (Terlau and Olivera, 2004).

REPTILES

Lizards

The Gila monster (*Heloderma suspectum*, Fig. 26-28) and the beaded lizards (*Heloderma horridum*) are divided into five subspecies. These large, corpulent, relatively slow moving, and largely nocturnal reptiles have few enemies other than humans. They are far less dangerous than is generally believed. Their venom is transferred from venom glands in the lower jaw through ducts that discharge their contents near the base of the larger teeth of the lower jaw. The venom is then drawn up along grooves in the teeth by capillary action (Brown and Carmony, 1991). The venom of this lizard has serotonin, amine oxidase, phospholipase A, a bradykinin-releasing substance, helodermin, gilatoxin, and low-proteolytic as well as high-hyaluronidase activities, but lacks phosphomonoesterase and phosphodiesterase, acetylcholinesterase, nucleotidase, ATPase, deoxyribonuclease, ribonuclease, amino acid oxidase, and fibrinogenocoagulase activities. The clinical presentation of a helodermatid bite can include pain, edema, hypotension, nausea, vomiting, weakness, and diaphoresis. No antivenin is commercially available. Treatment is supportive (Strimple *et al.*, 1997).

The venom has been shown to contain a 25-kDa protein, helothermine, containing 223 amino acids and four pairs of disulfide bonds, which appears to inhibit Ca²⁺ flux from the sarcoplasmic reticulum (Morrissette *et al.*, 1995; Nobile *et al.*, 1996). A fraction causing hemorrhage in internal organs and the eye, a glycoprotein of 210 amino acid residues with plasma kallikrein-like properties, has also been described (Datta and Tu, 1997). A 35 amino acid residue, helodermin produces hypotension that is partially attributed to activation of glibenclamide-sensitive K⁺ channels (Horikawa *et al.*, 1998). In fact, helospectin I and II and helodermin are nonamidated, vasoactive intestinal peptide-like peptides, isolated from the salivary gland venom of the lizards *H. suspectum* and *H. horridum*, which have strong and potent vasodilator effects (Uddman *et al.*, 1999).

Snakes

General Information and Classification Snakes have a three-chambered heart and rely almost exclusively on an enlarged right lung (which spans approximately half of the body length) for respiration. Of the approximately 2700 known species of snakes, about 20% are considered to be venomous (Mebs, 2002; Mackessy, 2010). Venomous snakes primarily belong to the following families: Viperidae (vipers), Elapidae, Atractaspididae, and Colubridae.

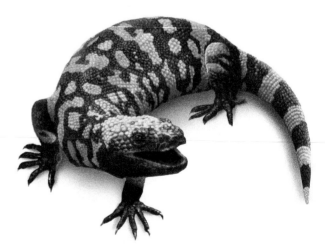

Figure 26-28. *Heloderma suspectum (Gila monster).*

The vipers are further divided into subfamilies, an example of which is the Crotalinae, or pit vipers, which possess a pit between the eyes and nostrils that serves as a heat sensor to detect warm-blooded animals. Some of the subfamilies are regarded as separate families altogether depending on the classification scheme. Overall the Colubridae are considered the largest venomous family, and are composed of nearly 60% of all snakes. The Atractaspididae family is known for burrowing into the ground and possessing the ability to expose their fangs without opening their mouth.

Another characteristic that is often used for self-defense or hunting prey is mimicry (O'Shea, 2005). Scale pattern and coloration provide distinct boundaries in the wild and often carry unspoken warnings based on a reputation for snake venom toxicity for a given species. If a relatively harmless species is able to mimic the physical characteristics, especially color patterns, of a well-known highly toxic counterpart, then other potential predators may recognize both snakes as toxic and not pursue either.

Fang anatomy and dentition are good indicators of such factors as snake habitat and feeding habits (O'Shea, 2005). In general, the anatomical structure of fangs makes it nearly impossible for snakes to chew their prey. The distinct curvature of the fangs is engineered not only for puncturing skin and delivering venom but also for swallowing whole prey as well. The teeth and jaw structure are relatively mobile and effectively facilitate the positioning of whole prey for swallowing. The skull and jaw possess an extremely high degree of responsiveness to stimuli. The jaw does not actually dislocate; however, it is able to rapidly reposition itself to capture, contain, and swallow prey. In addition to the capabilities of the teeth, fangs, and jaws, the classic fork-shaped tongue is another tool for identifying prey (O'Shea, 2005).

The Viperidae fang structure is regarded as the most developed and efficient means of venom, or toxin, delivery to prey. The venom gland is positioned at the base of a long (~30 mm) hollow retractable fang (Mebs, 2002; Weinstein *et al.*, 2010). Muscle pressure on the gland determines the amount of venom released. Another highly developed venom delivery apparatus is characteristic of the spitting cobras, aptly named for their ability to project venom via glands that protrude from the base of the fang opening (Mebs, 2002). Venom is carried toward the prey, or target, via forceful exhalation that is accompanied by a hissing sound. Toxin delivery via venom exposure is the primary mechanism by which snakes immobilize and kill their prey. Toxin type and specificity is dependent on the species; however, most venom consists of complex networks of toxins that affect variable organ systems and interact with one another increasing the overall potency.

It is estimated that there are over 2.5 million snakebites annually, and that over 100,000 victims will die (Mackessy, 2010; White, 2005). Information resources available to physicians on management of snakebite victims may be found at the Clinical Toxinology Resources Web site—www.toxinology.com—or other appropriate references (Dart, 2004; Tintinalli *et al.*, 2004).

Snake Venoms These venoms are complex mixtures: proteins and peptides, consisting of both enzymatic and nonenzymatic compounds, make up over 90% of the dry weight of the venom (Phui Yee *et al.*, 2004). Snake venoms also contain inorganic cations such as sodium, calcium, potassium, magnesium, and small amounts of zinc, iron, cobalt, manganese, and nickel. The metals in snake venoms are likely catalysts for metal-based enzymatic reactions. For example, in the case of some elapid venoms, zinc ions appear to be necessary for anticholinesterase activity, and calcium may play a role in the activation of phospholipase A and the direct lytic factor. Some proteases appear to be metalloproteins. Some snake venoms also contain

carbohydrates (glycoproteins), lipids, and biogenic amines, such as histamine, serotonin, and neurotransmitters (catecholamines and acetylcholine) in addition to positively charged metal ions (Russell, 2001; Mebs, 2002; Menez, 2003; Ramos and Selistre-de-Araujo, 2006). The complexity of snake venom components is illustrated nicely in Fig. 26-29 (Ramos and Selistre-de-Araujo, 2006).

Actions of snake venoms can be said to be broad ranging in several areas (O'Shea, 2005). A simplistic approach would group toxin components as neurotoxins, coagulants, hemorrhagins, hemolytics, myotoxins, cytotoxins, and nephrotoxins. Neurotoxins produce neuromuscular paralysis ranging from dizziness to ptosis; to ophthalmoplegia, flaccid facial muscle paralysis, and inability to swallow; to paralysis of larger muscle groups; and finally to paralysis of respiratory muscles and death by asphyxiation. Coagulants may have initial procoagulant action that uses up clotting factors leading to bleeding. Coagulants may directly inhibit normal clotting at several places in the clotting cascade or via inhibition of platelet aggregation. In addition, some venom components may damage the endothelial lining of blood vessels leading to hemorrhage. Bite victims may show bleeding from nose or gums, from the bite site, and in saliva, urine, and stools. Myotoxins can directly impact muscle contraction leading to paralysis or cause rhabdomyolysis or the breakdown of skeletal muscle. Myoglobinuria, or a dark brown urine, and hyperkalemia may be noted. Cytotoxic agents have proteolytic or necrotic properties leading to the breakdown of tissue. Typical signs include massive swelling, pain, discoloration, blistering, bruising, and wound weeping. Sarafotoxins, which are found only in burrowing asps of Afro-Arabia, cause coronary artery constriction that can lead to reduced coronary blood flow, angina, and myocardial infarction. Finally, nephrotoxins can cause direct damage to kidney structures leading to bleeding, damage to several parts of the nephron, tissue oxygen deprivation, and renal failure.

Enzymes At least 26 different enzymes have been isolated from snake venoms, which can be a sequence of 150 to 1500 amino acids (Menez, 2003). No single snake venom contains all 26 enzymes and some important snake venom enzymes are shown in Fig. 26-29.

Proteolytic enzymes that catalyze the breakdown of tissue proteins and peptides include peptide hydrolases, proteases, endopeptidases, peptidases, and proteinases. Several proteolytic enzymes may be in a single venom. The proteolytic enzymes have molecular weights between 20,000 and 95,000. Some are inactivated by ethylenediaminetetraacetic acid (EDTA) and certain reducing agents. Metals appear to be intrinsically involved in the activity of certain venom proteases and phospholipases. The crotalid venoms examined so far appear to be rich in proteolytic enzyme activity. Viperid venoms have lesser amounts, whereas elapid and sea snake venoms have minimal, if any, proteolytic activity. Venoms that are rich in proteinase activity are associated with marked tissue destruction (Russell, 2001).

Collagenase is a specific kind of proteinase that digests collagen. This activity has been demonstrated in the venoms of a number of species of crotalids and viperids. The venom of *Crotalus atrox* (Fig. 26-30) digests mesenteric collagen fibers but no other proteins. EDTA inhibits the collagenolytic effect, but not the argine esterase effect.

Hyaluronidase cleaves internal glycoside bonds in certain acid mucopolysaccharides resulting in a decrease in the viscosity of connective tissues. The breakdown in the hyaluronic barrier allows other fractions of venom to penetrate the tissues, causing hyaluronidase to be called "spreading factor." The degree to which hyaluronidase contributes to the extent of edema produced by the whole venom is not known (Kemparaju *et al.*, 2010).

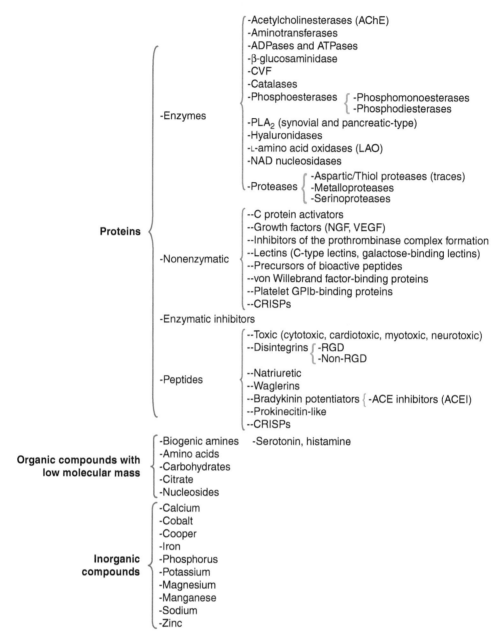

Figure 26-29. *Components of snake venoms.* ACE, angiotensin-converting enzyme; CRISP, cysteine-rich secretory protein; CVF, cobra venom factor–like proteins; LAO, L-amino acid oxidase; PLA$_2$, phospholipase A2; RGD, arginine–glycine–aspartate. (Used with permission from Ramos and Selistre-de-Araujo, 2006.)

Phospholipase A$_2$ (PLA$_2$) enzymes are widely distributed throughout the tissues of animals, plants, and bacteria, and have been well studied in snake venoms (Doley *et al.*, 2010; Ohno *et al.*, 2003; Soares and Giglio, 2003). Mammalian PLA$_2$ enzymes are involved in fertilization and cell proliferation, and have been implicated in respiratory ailments such as asthma, as well as skin conditions such as psoriasis (Kini, 2003; Soares and Giglio, 2003). PLA$_2$ catalyzes the Ca^{2+}-dependent hydrolysis of the 2-acyl ester bond, producing free fatty acids and lysophospholipids. However, liberation of pharmacologically active products and effects independent of enzymatic action may contribute to their overall action. In general, mammalian PLA$_2$s are considered to be nontoxic and do not elicit the same pharmacologic effects as similar enzymes in snake venoms.

As of 2003, over 280 PLA$_2$ enzymes had been classified, sharing at least 40% identity in their amino acid sequences (Kini, 2003; Soares and Giglio, 2003). Many PLA$_2$s have been sequenced.

They have approximately 120 amino acids and 14 cysteine residues forming seven disulfide bonds. Surface residue recognition and covalent/noncovalent bonds stabilize complexes for receptor binding. Specific amino acid residues play an important role in the diversification and overall function of the PLA$_2$s. Of note, histidine, lysine, cysteine, and methionine have been well studied for their contribution to enzyme structure and function (Soares and Giglio, 2003). For example, alkylation of His48 diminishes the hydrolytic capabilities of certain toxins. Alkylation of amino acids has proven to effectively mitigate PLA$_2$ toxicity and has been proposed as an antivenom treatment (Soares and Giglio, 2003). PLA$_2$s interact with other toxins in the venom as well, often resulting in synergistic reactions. Similarly, snake venom PLA$_2$ enzymes can be separated into three major groupings depending on their pharmacologic activities: low-toxicity enzymes (LD$_{50}$ >1 mg/kg), high-toxicity enzymes (1 mg/kg > LD$_{50}$ > 0.1 mg/kg),

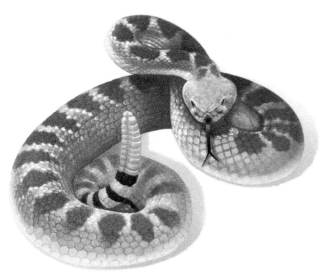

Figure 26-30. *Crotalus atrox (western diamondback rattlesnake)*.

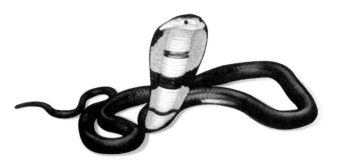

Figure 26-32. *Naja nigricollis (black necked spitting cobra)*.

and presynaptically acting toxins (LD$_{50}$ <0.1 mg/kg) (Rosenberg, 1990). Although the sequences of these enzymes are homologous and their enzymatically active sites are identical, they differ widely in their pharmacologic properties. For example, taipoxin, a PLA$_2$ enzyme from the venom of the Australian elapid *Oxyuranus scutellatus* (Fig. 26-31), has an intravenous LD$_{50}$ in mice of 2 µg/kg, whereas the neutral PLA$_2$ from *Naja nigricollis* (Fig. 26-32) has an LD$_{50}$ of 10,200 µg/kg, even though *N. nigricollis* PLA$_2$ is enzymatically more active (Russell, 2001).

Arginine ester hydrolase is one of a number of noncholinesterases found in snake venoms. The substrate specificities are directed to the hydrolysis of the ester or peptide linkage, to which an argine residue contributes the carboxyl group. This activity is found in many crotalid and viperid venoms and some sea snake venoms but is lacking in elapid venoms with the possible exception of *Ophiophagus hannah*. Some crotalid venoms contain at least three chromatographically separable arginine ester hydrolases. The bradykinin-releasing and perhaps bradykinin-clotting activities of some crotalid venoms may be related to esterase activity.

Two distinct classes of fibrin(ogen)olytic enzymes, the metalloproteinases and the serine proteinases, have been isolated from venom of Viperidae, Elapidae, and Crotalidae snake families (Swenson and Markland, 2005). These two classes of proteinases differ in mechanism of action and their target in fibrin(ogen), but ultimately they break down fibrin-rich clots and help to prevent further clot formation. The properties of fibrolase, an α-chain fibrinolytic metalloproteinase from *Agkistrodon contortrix contortrix* (Fig. 26-33) venom, and β-fibrinogenase, a β-chain fibrinogenase from *Vipera lebetina*, are provided in Table 26-13. Properties of some additionally characterized fibrin(ogen)ases are listed in Table 26-14. It is apparent that there are major differences in the properties of these enzymes from different snakes even though they have similar catalytic properties. An exciting development from the research on these enzymes is that one specific recombinant fibrinolytic enzyme derived from fibrolase called alfimeprase is progressing through clinical trials for the treatment of peripheral arterial occlusions.

The snake venom hemorrhagic metalloproteinases (SVMP) are enzymes that disrupt the hemostatic system and they are characterized by their domain structure into four primary classes, PI to PIV (Fox and Serrano, 2010). SVMPs are synthesized in vivo as multimodular proteins that comprise a signal peptide, a prodomain, and a metalloprotease domain (SVMP PI). SVMP potency tends to increase by class and those within the PIV class are larger and comprise additional disulfide bonds (Calvette *et al.*, 2003, 2005). Class PII proteins exhibit a C-terminal disintegrin domain. The PII metalloproteases block the function of integrin receptors, a function that could alleviate a variety of pathological conditions such

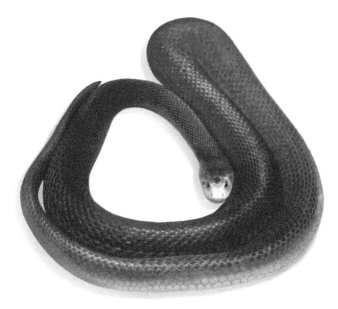

Figure 26-31. *Oxyuranus scutellatus (Australian costal taipan)*.

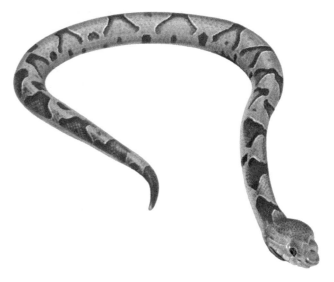

Figure 26-33. *Agkistrodon contortrix contortrix (copperhead)*.

Table 26-13

Miscellaneous Properties of Some α-Chain and β-Chain Fibrin(ogen)ases

PROPERTIES	α-CHAIN FIBRINOGENASE	β-CHAIN FIBRINOGENASE
Common name	Fibrolase	β-Fibrinogenase
Class of enzyme	Metalloproteinase	Serine protease
Chain length	203 amino acids	232 amino acids
Molecular weight	~22.7 kDa	~26 kDa
pI	6.8	~3
Carbohydrate content	None	>30%
pH optimum	7.1–7.4	8.5–9.5

SOURCE: Data from Swenson and Markland (2005).

as inflammation, tumor angiogenesis and metastasis, and thrombosis. The integrin-blocking specificity of this class of metalloproteins is highly dependent on the conformation of the inhibitory loop, and thus the placement and bonding of cysteine residues. More specifically, within the inhibitory loops, RGD-containing disintegrins are specific to the class PII metalloproteases (Calvette et al., 2003, 2005). Class PIII SVMPs exhibit the disintegrin-like domain and the C-type lectin-like domain is present in PIV SVMPs. The metalloproteinase domain or catalytic domain is composed of about 215 amino acids and has metal-dependent endopeptidase activity (Calvette et al., 2005). SVMPs degrade proteins such as laminin, fibronectin, type IV collagen, and proteoglycans from the endothelial basal membrane; degrade fibrinogen and von Willebrand factor enhancing the hemorrhagic action; and inhibit platelet aggregation and stimulate release of cytokines (Ramos and Selistre-de-Araujo, 2006).

The proteolytic action of thrombin and thrombin-like snake venom enzymes is shown in Table 26-15. This table compares ancrod (from *Calloselasma rhodostoma*), batroxobin (from *Bothrops moojeni*), crotalase (from *Crotalus adamanteus*), gabonase

Table 26-14

Miscellaneous Properties of Some α-Chain and β-Chain Fibrin(ogen)ases

PROPERTIES	α-CHAIN FIBRINOGENASE	α-CHAIN FIBRINOGENASE	α-CHAIN FIBRINOGENASE	β-CHAIN FIBRINOGENASE
Genus species	*Bothops neuwiedi*	*Agkistrodon halys*	*Lachesis stenophrys*	*Agkistrodon blomhoffi brevicadus*
Common name	Neuwiedase	Brevilysin L6	LSF	Brevinase
Chain length	198 amino acids	203 amino acids	>200 amino acids	233 amino acids
Molecular weight	22.5 kDa	22.7 kDa	24 kDa	25.7 kDa
pI	5.9	4.8	ND	5.5
Carbohydrate content	<1%	None	Glycosylated	ND
pH optimum	7.4–8.0	8.5–9.5	ND	5.5–8.5

ND, not determined.
SOURCE: Data from Swenson and Markland (2005).

Table 26-15

Comparison of Thrombin and Thrombin-like Snake Venom Enzyme Actions

ENZYMES	FIBRINOPEPTIDES RELEASED	ACTION ON HUMAN FIBRINOGEN			
		CHAIN DEGRADATION	ACTIVATION OF FACTOR XIII	PROTHROMBIN FRAGMENT CLEAVAGE	PLATELET AGGREGATION AND RELEASE
Thrombin	A – B	α(A)	Yes	Yes	Yes
Thrombin-like enzymes	A[*]	α(A)[†] or β(B)[‡]	No	Yes or no[§]	No
Agkistrodon c. contortrix venom	B	ND	Incomplete	ND	No
Bitis gabonica venom	A + B	ND	Yes	ND	ND

ND, not determined.
[*]Includes ancrod, batroxobin, crotalase, and the enzyme from T. okinavensis.
[†]Ancrod (batroxobin degrades α(A) chain of bovine but not human fibrinogen).
[‡]Crotalase.
[§]Fragment I released by crotalase and Agkistrodon contortrix venom, but not by ancrod or batroxobin.
SOURCE: Data from Russell (2001).

Table 26-16

Comparison of Snake Venom Thrombin-Like Enzymes

VENOM ENZYME	MOLECULAR WEIGHT	CARBOHYDRATE CONTENT (%)	ACTIVE SITE SERINE
Agkistrodon contortrix contortrix	100,000	ND	+
Bitis gabonica	32,500	ND	ND
Bothrops marajoensis	31,400	High	+
Bothrops moojeni	36,000	5.8	+
Calloselasma rhodostoma	59,000	36.0	+
Crotalus adamantus	32,700	8.3	+
Crotalus horridus horridus	19,400	Very low	ND
Deinagkistrodon acutus	33,500	13.0	+
Trimeresurus gramineus	27,000	25.0	+
Trimeresurus okinavensis	34,000	6.0	+

ND, not determined.
SOURCE: Data from Russell (2001).

Table 26-17

Snake Venom Proteins Active on the Hemostatic System

GENERAL FUNCTIONAL ACTIVITY	SPECIFIC BIOLOGICAL ACTIVITY
Procoagulant	Activates factors II, V, IX, X, and protein C Fibrinogen clotting
Anticoagulant	Factor IX/factor X–binding protein Thrombin inhibitor Phospholipase A
Fibrinolytic	Fibrin(ogen) degradation Plasminogen activation
Vessel wall interactive	Hemorrhagic

SOURCES: Data from Markland (1998) and Russell (2001).

(from *Bitis gabonica*), and venzyme (from *A. contortrix*). Table 26-16 shows the molecular size of some thrombin-like enzymes. A recent contribution on snake toxins, using mass spectrometric immunoassay and bioactive probe techniques, has been published by Ramirez *et al*. (1999a,b). Considerable study has been given to the hemostatic properties of venoms (Markland, 1998; Phillips *et al*., 2010). The hemostatically active components are summarized in Table 26-17.

Phosphomonoesterase (phosphatase) is widely distributed in the venoms of all families of snakes except the colubrids (Dhananjaya *et al*., 2010). It has the properties of an orthophosphoric monoester phosphohydrolase. There are two nonspecific phosphomonoesterases, and they have optimal pH at 5.0 and 8.5. Many types of venom contain both acid and alkaline phosphatases, whereas others contain one or the other.

Phosphodiesterase has been found in the venoms of all families of poisonous snakes. It is an orthophosphoric diester phosphohydrolase that releases 5-mononucleotide from the polynucleotide chain and thus acts as an exonucleotidase, attacking DNA and RNA. More recently, it has been found that it also attacks derivatives of arabinose.

Acetylcholinesterase was first demonstrated in cobra venom and is widely distributed throughout the elapid venoms (Ahmed *et al*., 2010). It is also found in sea snake venoms but is totally lacking in viperid and crotalid venoms. It catalyzes the hydrolysis of acetylcholine to choline and acetic acid. The role of the enzyme in snake venoms is not clear, but may function to catalyze the hydrolysis of acetylcholine thereby facilitating tetanic paralysis and capture of prey.

RNase is present in some snake venoms in small amounts as the endopolynucleotidase RNase. It appears to have specificity toward pyrimidine-containing pyrimidyladenyl bonds in DNA. The optimum pH is 7 to 9 when ribosomal RNA is used as the substrate. This enzyme in *Naja oxiana* venom has a molecular weight of 15,900.

DNase acts on DNA to produce predominantly trinucleotides or higher oligonucleotides that terminate in 3′-monoesterified phosphate. *C. adamanteus* venom contains two DNases, with optimum pH at 5 and 9.

5′-Nucleotidase is a common constituent of all snake venoms; in most instances it is the most active phosphatase in snake venoms. It specifically hydrolyzes phosphate monoesters, which link with a 5′ position of DNA and RNA. It is found in greater amounts in crotalid and viperid venoms than in elapid venoms. The molecular weight as determined from amino acid composition and gel filtration with *Naja naja atra* venom has been estimated at 10,000. The enzyme from *N. naja* venom is enhanced by Mg^{2+}, is inhibited by Zn^{2+}, is inactivated at 75°C at pH 7.0 or 8.4, and has an isoelectric point of about 8.6. That from *Agkistrodon halys blomhoffi* shows a pH optimum of 6.8 to 6.9, with activity being enhanced by Mg^{2+} and Mn^{2+} and inhibited by Zn^{2+}. The enzyme has a low order of lethality (Russell, 2001).

Nicotinamide adenine dinucleotide (NAD) nucleotidase has been found in a number of snake venoms. This enzyme catalyzes the hydrolysis of the nicotinamide *N*-ribosidic linkage of NAD, yielding nicotinamide and adenosine diphosphate riboside. Its optimum pH is 6.5 to 8.5; it is heat labile, losing activity at 60°C. Nucleotidases function as ADP scavengers thereby acting as potent inhibitors of platelet aggregation.

L-Amino acid oxidase has been found in all snake venoms examined so far and it is what gives the characteristic yellow color to the venom. This enzyme catalyzes the oxidation of L-α-amino and α-hydroxy acids. This activity results from a group of homologous enzymes with molecular weights ranging from 85,000 to 150,000. The mouse intravenous LD_{50} of the enzyme from *C. adamanteus* venom was 9.13 mg/kg body weight, approximately four times less than the lethal value of the crude venom, and this enzyme had no effect on nerve, muscle, or neuromuscular transmission (Russell, 2001; Tan and Fung, 2010).

Polypeptides Snake venom polypeptides are low-molecular-weight proteins that do not have enzymatic activity. More than

80 polypeptides with pharmacologic activity have been isolated from snake venoms. Interested readers will find definitive reviews on these peptides in the works of Lee (1979), Eaker and Wadström (1980), and Gopalakrishnakone and Tan (1992). Most of the lethal activity of the poison of the sea snake *Laticauda semifasciata* was recovered as two toxins, erabutoxin-a and erabutoxin-b, using carboxymethylcellulose chromatography; 30% of the proteins were erabutoxins. More recently, erabutoxin-a, a short-chain curamimetic, has been crystallized in monomeric and dimeric forms (Nastopoulos *et al.*, 1998). Erabutoxin-b is said to be relatively ineffective at the mammalian neuromuscular junction (Vincent *et al.*, 1998). Another curamimetic, a long-chain polypeptide, is α-cobratoxin, while a novel "neurotoxin" from *N. naja atra*, having 61 amino acid residues and eight cystine residues, has been isolated by Chang *et al.* (1997).

Disintegrins are a family of short cysteine-rich polypeptides and are divided into five subgroups based on the combination of length and number of disulfide bonds of polypeptides. In general, the disintegrins comprise 40 to 100 amino acids. Their small size coupled with a relatively dense network of disulfide bonds contributes to the tertiary structure of these compounds and high potency of such small compounds. Disintegrins are released in venoms via proteolytic processes of PII metalloproteinases, whereas structures similar in form and function to disintegrins, or disintegrin-like, are subject to PIII processes (Calvette *et al.*, 2005). Monomeric disintegrins can vary from about 50 residues and four disulfide bonds as in echistatin and obtustatin to around 70 amino acid residues and six disulfide bridges as in albolabrin, barbourin, and halysin, to over 84 amino acids and seven disulfide bonds for bitistatin and salmosin-3. Dimeric disintegrins are about 67 amino acids long and contain four intrachain disulfide linkages and two between-chain bonds. Examples include contortrostatin and acostatin. The monomeric disintegrin-like chemicals contain around 100 amino acids and eight disulfide bonds, and include trimelysin-I, bothropasin, and jararhagin (Calvette *et al.*, 2003; Ramos and Selistre-de-Araujo, 2006).

RGD (argine–glycine–asparagine) and non-RGD-containing disintegrins coexist in certain venoms and exhibit affinities for variable ligand receptors. In such cases, one copy of the gene encodes for the more conserved RGD function of platelet aggregation, whereas the duplicated genes have drifted toward facilitating other biological functions. Modeling and structure analysis of cyclic RGD peptides has implicated the importance of amino acid sequences on the C-terminal of the RGD sequence; furthermore, the physical features such as size of the integrin-binding loop contribute to the receptor-binding capabilities (Calvette *et al.*, 2005). In general, the amino acid residues of this region of the RGD sequence are not well conserved and are thought to play a key role in determining integrin receptor-binding specificity. There are additional mechanisms within the C-terminal region, which include conformational epitopes that are utilized to alter receptor-binding capabilities.

The small basic polypeptide myotoxins are widely distributed in *Crotalus* snake venoms. The specific agent crotamine from *Crotalus durissus terrificus* venom induces skeletal muscle spasms and paralysis by changing the inactivation process of sodium channels, which are inhibited by tetrodotoxin and potentiated by veratridine and grayanotoxin, leading to depolarization of the neuromuscular junction. Crotamine is composed of 42 amino acid residues and three disulfide bonds. The crotamine gene contains 1.8 kbp and has three exons that are separated by a long phase-1 and a short phase-2 intron and mapped to chromosome 2. In addition, the three-dimensional structure has been published, and the structural topology is similar to that of other three disulfide bridge containing peptides such as human β-defensins and scorpion sodium

channel toxin. These structural properties enable crotamine to have a unique cell penetrating ability allowing the toxin to concentrate in the nucleus by means of a probable receptor-independent mechanism. It is interesting to note that topology and diversification of functional folds are common themes in animal venom peptides acting on ion channels and other targets (Menez, 1998; Mouhat *et al.*, 2004; Oguiura *et al.*, 2006).

Toxicology In general, the venoms of rattlesnakes and other New World crotalids produce alterations in the resistances and often in the integrity of blood vessels, changes in blood cells and blood coagulation mechanisms, direct or indirect changes in cardiac and pulmonary dynamics, and—with crotalids such as *C. durrissus terrificus* and *C. scutulatus*—serious alterations in the nervous system and changes in respiration. In humans, the course of the poisoning is determined by the kind and amount of venom injected; the site where it is deposited; the general health, size, and age of the patient; the kind of treatment; and those pharmacodynamic principles noted earlier in this chapter. Death in humans may occur within less than one hour or after several days, with most deaths occurring between 18 and 32 hours. Hypotension or shock is the major therapeutic problem in North American crotalid bites (Russell, 2001).

Snakebite Treatment The treatment of bites by venomous snakes is now so highly specialized that almost every envenomation requires specific recommendations. However, three general principles for every bite should be kept in mind: (1) snake venom poisoning is a medical emergency requiring immediate attention and the exercise of considerable judgment; (2) the venom is a complex mixture of substances of which the proteins contribute the major deleterious properties, and the only adequate antidote is the use of specific or polyspecific antivenom; and (3) not every bite by a venomous snake ends in an envenomation. Venom may not be injected. In almost 1000 cases of crotalid bites, 24% did not end in a poisoning. The incidence with the bites of cobras and perhaps other elapids is probably higher. The reader is referred to other appropriate texts for appropriate treatment of snakebites (Russell, 2001; Dart, 2004; Sholl *et al.*, 2004; Tintinalli *et al.*, 2004; Singletary and Holstege, 2006; Smith and Bush, 2010; see also www.toxinology.com).

Snake Venom Evolution Considerable efforts are being expended to examine the complex process by which snake venom components are thought to have changed over the years. This evaluation involves tracing the ancestral roots of toxins, which is made even more cumbersome due to the distinct differences in the speed at which individual components of a venom evolve. The current assemblage of snake venoms with regard to functionality and ancestral protein activity is outlined in Table 26-18 (Fry, 2005). In general, the toxins from ancestral proteins that were constructed of dense networks of cysteine cross-linkages are considered among the most diverse today in terms of toxicological insult.

The evolution of the PLA$_2$s appears to be directed toward modifying the molecular surface in order to maximize the diversity of the pharmacologic properties of each isozyme component (Kini and Chan, 1999; Li *et al.*, 2005). As PLA$_2$s are not crucial for snake survival, mutations in some PLA$_2$ isozymes may be ignored and allowed to progress, thereby expediting the evolution in comparison to other more critical enzymes in which mutations are monitored more closely and not allowed to progress. The functionality of PLA$_2$ isozymes can be significantly hindered by increased rates of mutations within highly conserved regions of the amino acid sequence, which could in turn displace cysteine residues and alter the tertiary protein structure. However, increased mutation of a

Table 26-18

Basal Bioactivities of Some Toxin Types

TOXIN	ACTIVITY
3FTx	α-Neurotoxicity, blocks nicotinic acetylcholine receptor
ADAM	In Viperidae venoms, proteolytic cleavage of C-terminal domains results in direct fibrinolytic activity, liberation of disintegrins, which inhibit platelet aggregation
Cobra venom factor	Causes unregulated activation of complement cascade, hemolysis, cytolysis
Crotamine	Myonecrosis, modifies voltage-gated sodium channels
Factor V	In taipan and brown snake venom, combines with toxic form of factor X to convert prothrombin to thrombin
Kallikrein	Increases vascular permeability, stimulates inflammation, and reduces blood pressure
Kunitz	Inhibits plasmin and thrombin and other serine proteases, blocks L-type calcium channels
L-Amino oxidase	Induces apoptosis, decreases platelet aggregation, inhibits blood factor IX
PLA$_2$	Releases arachidonic acid from phospholipids, resulting in inflammation and tissue destruction
VEGF	Increases permeability of vascular bed causing hypotension and shock
Whey acidic proteins	Inhibit leukoproteinases

SOURCE: Data from Fry (2005).

particular subset of enzymes, such as the PLA$_2$s, may be a result of a shift in ecological niche. A recent study (Li *et al.*, 2005) reports a shift in the diet composition of the marbled sea snake as the root cause of decelerated evolution of the PLA$_2$ enzymes. The diet change from live prey to fish eggs essentially negated the need for PLA$_2$ enzymes to immobilize live prey for swallowing and digestion. Future research could focus on the declining need for PLA$_2$s, and on the altered digestive enzyme composition that has likely occurred as a result of diet shift.

ANTIVENOM

Antivenoms have been produced against most medically important snake, spider, scorpion, and marine toxins. Animals immunized with venom develop a variety of antibodies to the many antigens in the venom. Antivenom consists of venom-specific antisera or antibodies concentrated from immune serum to the venom. Antisera contain neutralizing antibodies: one antigen (monospecific) or several antigens (polyspecific). Monovalent antivenoms have a high neutralization capacity, which is desirable against the venom of a specific animal. Polyvalent antisera are typically used to cover several venoms, such as snakes from a geographic region. Polyvalent preparations usually required higher doses or volumes than monovalent antivenoms. Neutralization capacity of antivenom is highly variable as there are no enforced international standards. Antivenom may cross-react with venoms from distantly related species and may not react with venom from the intended species. Nevertheless, in general, the antibodies bind to the venom molecules, rendering them ineffective.

Antivenoms are available in several forms: intact IgG antibodies or fragments of IgG such as F(ab)$_2$ and Fab. The molecular weight of the intact IgG is about 150,000, whereas that of Fab is approximately 50,000. The molecular size of IgG prevents its renal excretion and produces a volume of distribution much smaller than that of Fab. The elimination half-life of IgG in the blood is approximately 50 hours. Its ultimate fate is not known, but most IgG is probably taken up by the reticuloendothelial system and degraded with the antigen attached. Fab fragments have an elimination half-life of about 17 hours, and are small enough to permit renal excretion.

All antivenom products may produce hypersensitivity reactions. Type I (immediate) hypersensitivity reactions are caused by antigen cross-linking of endogenous IgE bound to mast cells and basophils. Binding of antigen by a mast cell may cause the release of histamine and other mediators, producing an anaphylactic reaction. Once initiated, anaphylaxis may continue despite discontinuation of antivenom administration. Type III hypersensitivity (serum sickness) may develop several days after antivenom administration. In these cases, antigen–antibody complexes are deposited in different areas of the body, often producing inflammatory responses in the skin, joints, kidneys, and other tissues. Fortunately, these reactions are rarely serious. The risks of anaphylaxis should always be considered when one is deciding whether to administer antivenom, and thus antivenom should be given only by intravenous infusion under medical supervision (Heard *et al.*, 1999; Russell, 2001; Mebs, 2002; Dart, 2004; Tintinalli *et al.*, 2004; www.toxinology.com).

POTENTIAL CLINICAL APPLICATION OF VENOMS

Animal venoms are being used as research and clinical tools based on their high affinity for specific targets and well-studied pharmacologic properties (Cherniack, 2010, 2011; Mayer *et al.*, 2010; Menez, 1998, 2003; Dimarcq and Hunneyball, 2003; Escoubas and Rash, 2004). Toxin specificities for receptors and channels that facilitate the interface and coordination of neuromuscular activity are utilized and manipulated to study, model, diagnose, and sometimes treat acute and degenerative conditions. On closer examination of α-bungarotoxin and candoxin nicotinic acetylcholine receptor specificity, plans are under way to utilize the reversible and irreversible receptor binding in muscular and neuronal tissues, respectively, in Alzheimer patients (Phui Yee *et al.*, 2004). In addition to treating neurological diseases, specific α-toxins (longer chained) are also studied for their antiangiogenic capabilities in treating malignant tumor growth in patients suffering from small cell lung carcinoma (Tsetlin and Hucho, 2004). In cases such as this, there is an inherent trade-off between promoting some degree of neurological deficit in light of combating tumor growth. Toxins such as the snake venom thrombin-like enzymes are valuable tools in both research and therapeutic applications. Similarly, fibrin(ogen)olytic enzymes that break down fibrin-rich clots preventing further clot formation may be useful as controls in blood clotting research or to treat heart attacks and strokes (Castro *et al.*, 2004; Marsh and Williams, 2005; Swenson and Markland, 2005). To facilitate research, the complement-activating cobra venom factor has been produced by recombinant techniques (Vogel *et al.*, 2004). These pharmazooticals include reptilase-R, bothrocethin, stypven, ecarin, and protac.

Active research efforts have noted that animal venoms contain components that can reduce pain, can selectively kill specific cancers, may reduce the incidence of stroke via effects on blood coagulability, and function as antibiotics. Numerous compounds have been isolated from marine animals (Bingham *et al.*, 2010; Newman *et al.*, 2009), including the anticancer agents plinabulin, tasidotin, bryostatin 1, hemiasterlin, and salinosporamide A (also known as marizomib). The compound epibatidin comes from the skin of the South American frog, *Epipedobates tricolor*, and a synthetic derivative ABT-594 appears to be more effective than morphine without being addictive. TM 601 is derived from the Israeli yellow scorpion and attacks malignant brain tumors called glioma tumors responsible for two-thirds of the cases of brain cancer, without harming healthy cells. ET 743, which comes from sea squirts, is being tested for treatment of ovarian cancer and soft tissue sarcoma. Ancrod is an anticoagulant with potential to prevent cell damage and death when someone suffers a stroke. The active ingredient comes from the venom of the Malaysian pit viper. In Germany, where Ancrod has been marketed for a number of years, a specially built facility houses about 3000 snakes. Several other sources of anticoagulants are being examined. A substance called magainin 2, which comes from the skin of frogs, is an effective antibiotic to which bacteria do not appear to develop resistance. The clotting enzyme batroxobin is an ingredient in reptilase and has been used in the development of fibrin glue, which is used in surgery to stop diffuse bleeding from liver or lung by covering the surface with a thin layer of fibrin.

Another major area of investigation and success involves the venom components that act as enzyme inhibitors. In particular, venom peptides from *Bothrops jararaca* were initially called bradykinin-potentiating peptides and lowered blood pressure. After further research, it became clear that these peptides were inhibitors of angiotensin I–converting enzyme, and chemical modification leads to orally active agents such as captopril.

Venom toxins can also be used as a component of the toxin–receptor–antibody complex for diagnosis of autoimmune disorders (Menez, 2003). In addition to providing a promising means for researching and treating muscular and neurological diseases and cancer, work is being conducted on designing methods by which to consistently reconstruct and conform the overall toxin structure to bind to a specific protein, such as HIV (Menez, 2003).

It has been shown that leeches, earthworms, helminths, snails, centipedes, spiders, and ticks all produce substances with potential clinical applications, such as osteoarthritis, deep vein thrombosis, antimicrobial action, inflammatory bowel disease, analgesia, and hyperlipidemia (Cherniack, 2011). In particular, approximately 14 anticoagulant chemicals have been isolated from the leech, including hirudin and lepirudin, apyrase, collagenase, hyaluronidase, and eglin (Lubenow and Greinacher, 2002; Massart *et al.*, 2009). Tick saliva contains proteins that inhibit human kallikrein and factors XIa and XIIa (Mazzuca *et al.*, 2007). Earthworms contain proteins with anticoagulant, antimicrobial, and anti-inflammatory bowel disease properties (Joo *et al.*, 2009; Reddy and Fried, 2009; Ruyssers *et al.*, 2010). Bees can provide honey, royal jelly, and propolis, which all have antimicrobial properties, and the venom contains apamin and mellitin, which have anti-inflammatory properties. Additional details of the clinical applications of animal saliva and venom may be found in Cherniack (2010, 2011).

Additional work is being conducted on animals such as the mongoose, hedgehog, and opossum, which all embody a high level of resistance to snakebites. Blood from these animals contains proteins between 400 and 700 amino acids long that inhibit hemorrhagins. The exact mechanism of the many components in animal venoms that produce toxicity or resistance to certain toxins has yet to be determined. Further research will require a multidisciplinary approach involving techniques from parasitology, chemistry, molecular biology, genomics, proteomics, physiology, pharmacology, and toxicology.

CONCLUSION

The myriad toxins produced by plants and animals range from the relative simplicity of small chemical agents to the exceedingly complex proteinaceous toxins. The effects of these compounds are amazingly diverse and can range from local irritation to systemic destruction and death. The interplay between toxin and organism is often hard to study due to difficulty involved in recreating the interaction in the laboratory. One must also not forget the interactions that arise between toxins and substances already present in the organism. These interactions can act to worsen or reduce the poisonous outcome. As laboratory techniques become more sophisticated and new methods are developed, research concerning toxins and their effects will continue to grow.

ACKNOWLEDGMENT

The author gratefully acknowledges the assistance of Peter Joseph Massa in the preparation of this chapter.

REFERENCES

Aalto-Korte K, Lauerma A, Alanko K. Occupational allergic contact dermatitis from lichens in present-day Finland. *Contact Dermatitis.* 2005;52:36–38.

Abbott AJ, Holoubek CG, Martin RA. Inhibition of Na+, K+-ATPase by the cardenolide 6′-O-(E-4-hydroxycinnamoyl) desglucouzarin. *Biochem Biophys Res Commun.* 1998;251:256–259.

Adams ME. Agatoxins: ion channel specific toxins from the American funnel web spider, *Agelenopsis aperta. Toxicon.* 2004;43:509–525.

Ahmed M, Rocha JBT, Morsch VM, Schetinger MRC. Snake venom acetylcholinesterase. In: Mackessy SP, ed. *Handbook of Venoms and Toxins of Reptiles.* Boca Raton: CRC Press/Taylor & Francis; 2010:207.

Alonso-Amelot ME, Avendano M. Human carcinogenesis and bracken fern: a review of the evidence. *Curr Med Chem.* 2002;9:675–686.

Altamirano JC, Gratz SR, Wolnik KA. Investigation of pyrrolizidine alkaloids and their N-oxides in commercial comfrey-containing products and botanical materials by liquid chromatography electrospray ionization mass spectrometry. *JAOAC Int.* 2005;88:406–412.

Alvarez-Diez TM, Zheng J. Mechanism-based inactivation of cytochrome P450 3A4 by 4-ipomeanol. *Chem Res Toxicol.* 2004;17:150–157.

Andre E, Campi B, Trevisani M, et al. Pharmacological characterisation of the plant sesquiterpenes polygodial and drimanial as vanilloid receptor agonists. *Biochem Pharmacol.* 2006;71:1248–1254.

Ansari KM, Chauhan LK, Dhawan A, et al. Unequivocal evidence of genotoxic potential of argemone oil in mice. *Int J Cancer.* 2004;112: 890–895.

Arilla MC, Gonzalez-Rioja R, Ibarrola I, et al. A sensitive monoclonal antibody-based enzyme-linked immunosorbent assay to quantify *Parietaria judaica* major allergens, Par j1 and Par j2. *Clin Exp Allergy.* 2006;36:87–93.

Aslani MR, Movassaghi AR, Mhori M, et al. Clinical and pathological aspects of experimental oleander (*Nerium oleander*) toxicosis in sheep. *Vet Res Commun.* 2004;28:609–616.

Auger C, Marty A. Heterogeneity of functional synaptic parameters among single release sites. *Neuron.* 1997;19:139–150.

Baer BR, Rettie AE, Henne KR. Bioactivation of 4-ipomeanol by CYP4B1: adduct characterization and evidence for an enedial intermediate. *Chem Res Toxicol.* 2005;18:855–864.

Baku A. Mast cell degranulating (MCD) peptide: a prototypic peptide in allergy and inflammation. *Peptides.* 1999;20:415–420.

Ball KR, Kowdley KV. A review of *Silybum marianum* (milk thistle) as a treatment for alcoholic liver disease. *J Clin Gastroenterol.* 2005;39:520–528.

Bandyopadhyay PK, Garrett JE, Shetty RP, et al. γ-Carboxylation: an extra-cellular post-translational modification that antedates the divergence of molluscs, arthropods and chordates. *Proc Natl Acad Sci U S A.* 2002;99:1264–1269.

Bantel H, Engels IH, Voelter W, et al. Mistletoe lectin activates caspase-8/FLICE independently of death receptor signaling and enhances anti-cancer drug-induced apoptosis. *Cancer Res.* 1999;59:2038–2090.

Barker SC, Murrell A. Systematics and evolution of ticks with a list of valid genus and species names. *Parasitology.* 2004;129:S15–S36.

Bauer C, Oppel T, Rueff F, et al. Anaphylaxis to viscotoxins of mistletoe (*Viscum album*) extracts. *Ann Allergy Asthma Immunol.* 2005;94:86–89.

Beattie PE, Dawe RS, Traynor NJ, et al. Can St. John's wort (*Hypericin*) ingestion enhance the erythremal response during high-dose ultraviolet A1 therapy? *Br J Dermatol.* 2005;153:1187–1191.

Bechinger B. Structure and functions of channel-forming peptides: magainins, cecropins, melittin and alamethicin. *J Membr Biol.* 1997;156:197–211.

Beier RC, Norman JO, Reagor JC, et al. Isolation of the major component in white snakeroot that is toxic after microsomal activation: possible explanation of sporadic toxicity of white snakeroot plants and extracts. *Nat Toxins.* 1993;1:286–293.

Benjamin DR. Mushroom poisoning in infants and children. *J Toxicol Clin Toxicol.* 1992;30:13–22.

Bermudez MV, Gonzalez-Spencer D, Guerrero M, et al. Experimental intoxication with fruit and purified toxins of buckthorn (*Karwinskia humboldtiana*). *Toxicon.* 1986;24:1091–1097.

Bettini S, ed. *Arthropod Venoms.* Heidelberg: Springer; 1978.

Bingham J-P, Mitsunaga E, Bergeron ZL. Drugs from slugs—past, present and future perspectives of ώ-conotoxin research. *Chem Biol Interact.* 2010;183:1–18.

Blanc P, Liu D, Juarez C, et al. Cough in hot pepper workers. *Chest.* 1991;99:27–32.

Blanco C, Diaz-Perales A, Collada C, et al. Class I chitinases as potential panallergens involved in the latex-fruit syndrome. *J Allergy Clin Immunol.* 1999;103(pt 1):507–513.

Blodgett DJ. Fescue toxicosis. *Vet Clin North Am Equine Pract.* 2001;17:567–577.

Blumenthal MN, Langefeld CD, Barnes KC, et al. A genome-wide search for quantitative trait loci contributing to variations in seasonal pollen reactivity. *J Allergy Clin Immunol.* 2006;117:79–85.

Bondan C, Soares JC, Cecim M, et al. Oxidative stress in the erythrocytes of cattle intoxicated with *Senecio* sp. *Vet Clin Pathol.* 2005;34:353–357.

Bouget J, Bousser J, Pats B, et al. Acute renal failure following collective intoxication by *Cortinarius orellanus. Intensive Care Med.* 1990;16:506–510.

Bromley J, Hughes BG, Leong DC, et al. Life-threatening interaction between complementary medicines: cyanide toxicity following ingestion of amygdalin and vitamin C. *Ann Pharmacother.* 2005;39:1566–1569.

Brown DE, Carmony NB. *Gila Monster.* Silver City, NM: High Lonesome Books; 1991.

Bunch TD, Panter KD, James LK. Ultrasound studies of the effects of certain poisonous plants on uterine function and fetal development in livestock. *J Anim Sci.* 1992;70:1639–1643.

Burke JW, Doskotch RW. High field I H- and 13 C-NMR assignments of grayanotoxins I, IV and XIV isolated from *Kalmia angustifolia. J Nat Prod.* 1990;53:131–137.

Bush SP, King BO, Norris RL, et al. Centipede envenomation. *Wilderness Environ Med.* 2001;12:93–99.

Caksen H, Odabas D, Akabayram S, et al. Deadly nightshade (*Atropa belladonna*) intoxication: an analysis of 49 children. *Hum Exp Toxicol.* 2003;22:665–668.

Calvette JJ, Marcinkiewicz C, Monleon D, et al. Snake venom disintegrins: evolution of structure and function. *Toxicon.* 2005;45:1063–1074.

Calvette JJ, Moreno-Murciano MP, Theakston RDG, et al. Snake venom disintegrins: novel dimeric disintegrins and structural diversification by disulfide bond engineering. *Biochem J.* 2003;372:725–734.

Cameron P, Jelinek G, Kelly A-M, Murray L, Brown AFT, Heyworth J. *Textbook of Adult Emergency Medicine.* 3rd ed. New York: Churchill Livingstone/Elsevier; 2009.

Cappell MS, Hassan T. Gastrointestinal and hepatic effects of *Amanita phalloides* ingestion. *J Clin Gastroenterol.* 1992;15:225–228.

Casteel SW, Johnson GC, Wagstaff DJ. *Aesculus glabra* intoxication in cattle. *Vet Hum Toxicol.* 1992;34:55.

Casteel SW, Wagstaff DJ. Rhododendron macrophyllum poisoning in a group of sheep and goats. *Vet Hum Toxicol.* 1989;31:176–177.

Castro HC, Zingali RB, Albuquerque MG, et al. Snake venom thrombin-like enzymes: from retilase to now. *Cell Mol Life Sci.* 2004;61:843–856.

Cavalieri M, D'Urso D, Lassa A, et al. Characterization and some properties of the venom gland extract of a theridiid spider (*Steatoda paykulliana*) frequently mistaken for black widow spider (*Latrodectus tredecimguttatus*). *Toxicon.* 1987;25:965–974.

Cavassani KA, Aliberti JC, Dias ARV, et al. Tick saliva inhibits differentiation, maturation and function of murine bone-marrow derived dendritic cells. *Immunology.* 2005;114:235–245.

Ceccarelli B, Hurlbut WP. Ca2+-dependent recycling of synaptic vesicles at the frog neuromuscular junction. *J Cell Biol.* 1980;87:297–303.

Ceha LJ, Presperin C, Young E, et al. Anticholinergic toxicity from nightshade berry poisoning responsive to physostigmine. *J Emerg Med.* 1997;15:65–69.

Chan TYF, Tomlinson B, Crichley JAJH, et al. Herb-induced aconitine poisoning presenting as tetraplegia. *Vet Hum Toxicol.* 1994;36:133–134.

Chang LS, Chou YC, Lin SR, et al. A novel neurotoxin, cobrotoxin b, from *Naja naja atra* venom: purification, characterization and gene organization. *J Biochem.* 1997;122:1252–1259.

Cherniack EP. Bugs as drugs, part 1: insects. The "new" alternative medicine for the 21st century? *Altern Med Rev.* 2010;15:124–135.

Cherniack EP. Bugs as drugs, part two: worms, leeches, scorpions, snails, ticks, centipedes and spiders. *Altern Med Rev.* 2011;16:50–58.

Chesnov S, Bigler L, Hesse M. The acylpolyamines from the venom of the spider *Agelenopsis aperta. Helv Chim Acta.* 2001;84:2178–2197.

Christensen LP, Kristiansen K. Isolation and quantification of tuliposides and tulipalins in tulips (*Tulipa*) by high-performance liquid chromatography. *Contact Dermatitis.* 1999;40:300–309.

Cohen E, Quistad GB. Cytotoxic effects of arthropod venoms on various cultured cells. *Toxicon.* 1998;36:353–358.

Cooper MK, Porter JA, Young RE, et al. Teratogen-mediated inhibition of target tissue response to Shh signalling. *Science.* 1998;280:1603–1610.

Corzo G, Adachi-Akahane S, Nagao T, et al. Novel peptides from assassin bugs (Hemiptera: Reduviidae): isolation, chemical and biological characterization. *FEBS Lett.* 2001;499:256–261.

Corzo G, Escoubas P. Pharmacologically active spider peptide toxins. *Cell Mol Life Sci.* 2003;60:2409–2426.

Coyle CM, Panaccione DG. An ergot alkaloid biosynthesis gene and clustered hypothetical genes from *Aspergillus fumigatus. Appl Environ Microbiol.* 2005;71:3112–3118.

Craig AG, Bandyopadhyay P, Olivera BM. Post-translationally modified peptides from *Conus* venoms. *Eur J Biochem.* 1999;264:271–275.

Craik DJ, Daly NL, Waine C. The cysteine knot motif in toxins and implications for drug design. *Toxicon.* 2001;39:43–60.

Crause JC, Vershoor JA, Coetzee J, et al. The localization of paralysis toxin in granules and nuclei of prefed female *Rhipicephalus evertsi evertsi* tick salivary gland cells. *Exp Appl Acarol.* 1993;17:357–363.

Crawford L, Kocan RM. Steroidal alkaloid toxicity to fish embryos. *Toxicol Lett.* 1993;66:175–181.

Dart RC, ed. *Medical Toxicology.* 3rd ed. Philadelphia: Lippincott; 2004.

Das M, Ansari KM, Dhawan A, et al. Correlation of DNA damage in epidemic dropsy patients to carcinogenic potential of argemone oil and isolated sanguinarine alkaloid in mice. *Int J Cancer.* 2005;117: 709–717.

Das S, Bannerjee G, DePonte K, et al. Salp25D, an *Ixodes scapularis* antioxidant, is 1 of 14 immunodominant antigens in engorged tick salivary glands. *J Infect Dis.* 2001;184:1056–1064.

Datta G, Tu AT. Structure and other chemical characterizations of gila toxin, a lethal toxin from lizard venom. *J Pept Res.* 1997;50:443–450.

de Haro L, Prost N, David JM, et al. Syndrome sudorien ou muscarinien. *Presse Med.* 1999;28:1069–1070.

Dedov VN, Mondadi S, Armati PJ, et al. Capsaicin-induced depolarisation of mitochondria in dorsal root ganglion neurons is enhanced by vanilloid receptors. *Neuroscience.* 2001;103:219–226.

del Carmen Mendez M, dos Santos RS, Riet-Correa F. Intoxication by *Xanthium cavanillesii* in cattle and sheep in southern Brazil. *Vet Hum Toxicol.* 1998;40:144–147.

Demsey CE. The actions of melittin on membranes. *Biochim Biophys Acta.* 1990;1031:143–161.

Dhananjaya BL, Vishwanath BS, D'Souza CJM. Snake venom nucleases, nucleotidases and phosphomonoesterases. In: Mackessy SP, ed. *Handbook of Venoms and Toxins of Reptiles.* Boca Raton: CRC Press/ Taylor & Francis; 2010:155.

Dimarcq J-L, Hunneyball I. Pharma-entomology: when bugs become drugs. *Drug Discov Today.* 2003;8:107–110.

Ding X, Lichti K, Staudinger JL. The mycoestrogen zearalenone induces CYP3A through activation of the pregnane X receptor. *Toxicol Sci.* 2006;91:448–455.

Doley R, Zhou X, Kini RM. Snake venom phospholipase A_2 enzymes. In: Mackessy SP, ed. *Handbook of Venoms and Toxins of Reptiles.* Boca Raton: CRC Press/Taylor & Francis; 2010:173.

Dreyer F. Peptide toxins and potassium channels. *Rev Physiol Biochem Pharmacol.* 1990;115:93–116.

Durand R, Figueredo JM, Mendoza E. Intoxication in cattle from *Cestrum diurnum. Vet Hum Toxicol.* 1999;41:26–27.

Eaker D, Wadström T, eds. *Natural Toxins.* Elmsford, NY: Pergamon Press; 1980.

Escoubas P. Mass spectrometry in toxinology: a 21st-century technology for the study of biopolymers from venoms. *Toxicon.* 2006;47:609–613.

Escoubas P, Diochot S, Corzo G. Structure and pharmacology of spider venom neurotoxins. *Biochimie.* 2000;82:893–907.

Escoubas P, Rash L. Tarantulas: eight-legged pharmacists and combinatorial chemists. *Toxicon.* 2004;43:555–574.

Fatehi M, Rowan EG, Harvey AL, et al. Polyamine FTX-3.3 and polyamine amide sFTX-3.3 inhibit presynaptic calcium currents and acetylcholine release at mouse motor nerve terminals. *Neuropharmacology.* 1997;36:185–194.

Forsyth CS, Speth RC, Wecker L, et al. Comparison of nicotinic receptor binding and biotransformation of coniine in the rat and chick. *Toxicol Lett.* 1996;89:175–183.

Fox JW, Serrano SMT. Snake venom metalloproteinases. In: Mackessy SP. ed. *Handbook of Venoms and Toxins of Reptiles.* Boca Raton: CRC Press/Taylor & Francis; 2010:95.

Francischetti IBM, Mather TN, Ribeiro JMC. Cloning of a salivary gland metalloprotease and characterization of gelatinase and fibrino(gen)lytic activities in the saliva of the lyme disease tick vector *Ixodes scapularis. Biochem Biophys Res Commun.* 2003;305:869–875.

Frasca T, Brett AS, Yoo SD. Mandrake toxicity. *Arch Intern Med.* 1997;157:2007–2009.

Frohn A, Frohn C, Steuhl KP, et al. Wolfsmilchveratzung. *Ophthalmology.* 1993;90:58–61.

Fry BG. From genome to "venome": molecular origin and evolution of the snake venom proteome inferred from phylogenetic analysis of toxin sequences and related body proteins. *Genome Res.* 2005;15:403–420.

Fujimoto S, Mori M, Tsushima H, et al. Capsaicin-induced, capsazepine-insensitive relaxation of the guinea-pig ileum. *Eur J Pharmacol.* 2006;530:144–151.

Fung SY, Tan NH, Sim SM, et al. *Mucuna pruriens* seed extract pretreatment protects against cardiorespiratory and neuromuscular depressant effects of *Naja sputatrix* (Javan spitting cobra) venom in rats. *Indian J Exp Biol.* 2011;49:254–259.

Gaffield W, Keeler RF. Implications of C-5, C-6 unsaturation as a key structural factor in steroidal alkaloid-induced mammalian teratogenesis. *Experientia.* 1993;49:922–924.

Gertsch WJ. *American Spiders.* 2nd ed. New York: Van Nostrand Reinhold; 1979.

Giavina-Bianchi PF Jr, Castro FF, Machado ML, et al. Occupational respiratory allergic disease induced by *Passiflora alata* and *Rhamnus purshiana. Ann Allergy Asthma Immunol.* 1997;79:449–454.

Gmelin R. Isolierung von Willardiin [3-(1-uracyl)-L-alanin] aus den samen von *Acacia millefolia, Acacia lemmoni* und *Mimosa asperata. Acta Chem Scand.* 1961;15:1188–1189.

Goldin AL. Resurgence of sodium channel research. *Annu Rev Physiol.* 2001;63:871–894.

Gomes A, Datta A, Sarangi B, et al. Isolation, purification and pharmacodynamics of a toxin from the venom of centipede, *Scolopendra subspinipes dehaani* Brandt. *Ind J Exp Biol.* 1983;21:203–207.

Gopalakrishnakone P, Tan CK, eds. *Recent Advances in Toxinology Research.* Singapore: National University of Singapore; 1992.

Grishin E. Polypeptide neurotoxins from spider venoms. *Eur J Biochem.* 1999;264:276–280.

Grishin EV. Black widow spider toxins: the present and the future. *Toxicon.* 1998;36:1693–1701.

Groenewoud GC, de Groot H, van Wijk RG. Impact of occupational and inhalant allergy on rhinitis-specific quality of life in employees of bell pepper greenhouses in the Netherlands. *Ann Allergy Asthma Immunol.* 2006;96:92–97.

Gude M, Hausen MD, Heitsch H, et al. An investigation of the irritant and allergenic properties of daffodils (*Narcissus pseudonarcissus,* Amaryllidaceae): a review of daffodil dermatitis. *Contact Dermatitis.* 1988;19:1–10.

Guerrero B, Perales J, Gil San Juan A, Arocha-Pinango CL. Effect on platelet FXIII and partial characterization of Lonomin V, a proteolytic enzyme from *Lonomia achelous* caterpillars. *Thromb Res.* 1999;93:243–252.

Gurung NK, Rankens DL, Shelby RA. In vitro ruminal disappearance of fumonisin B1 and its effects on in vitro dry matter disappearance. *Vet Hum Toxicol.* 1999;41:196–199.

Haarmann T, Machado C, Lubbe Y, et al. The ergot alkaloid gene cluster in *Claviceps purpurea*: extension of the cluster sequence and intra species evolution. *Phytochemistry.* 2005;66:1312–1320.

Habermann E. Apamin. *Pharmacol Ther.* 1984;25:255–270.

Hall AC, Turcotte CM, Betts BA, et al. Modulation of human GABAA and glycine receptor currents by menthol and related monoterpenoids. *Eur J Pharmacol.* 2004;506:9–16.

Han D, Matsumaru K, Rettori D, et al. Usnic acid-induced necrosis of cultured mouse hepatocytes: inhibition of mitochondrial function and oxidative stress. *Biochem Pharmacol.* 2004;67:439–451.

Hausen BM, Prater E, Shubert H. The sensitizing capacity of *Alstroemeria* cultivars in man and guinea pig. *Contact Dermatitis.* 1983;9:46–54.

Heard K, O'Malley GF, Dart RC. Antivenom therapy in the Americas [review]. *Drugs.* 1999;58:5–15.

Hill NS, Thompson FN, Dawe DL, et al. Antibody binding by circulating ergot alkaloids in cattle grazing tall fescue. *Am J Vet Res.* 1994;55:419–424.

Hirschwehr R, Heppner C, Spitzauer S, et al. Allergens, IgE mediators, inflammatory mechanisms. *J Allergy Clin Immunol.* 1998;101: 196–206.

Hoffman DR. Hymenoptera venom allergens. *Clin Rev Allergy Immunol.* 2006;30:109–128.

Holz GG, Habener JF. Black widow spider alpha-latrotoxin: a presynaptic neurotoxin that shares structural homology with the glycogen-like peptide-1 family of insulin secretagogic hormones. *Comp Biochem Physiol B Biochem Mol Biol.* 1998;121:177–184.

Hooper D, Lirazon MB, Schoenfeld R, et al. Post-translational modification: a two dimensional strategy for molecular diversity of *Conus* peptides. In: Fields GB, Tam JP, Barany G, eds. *Peptides for the New Millennium: Proceedings of the Sixteenth American Peptide Symposium.* Dordrecht, The Netherlands: Kluwer; 2000.

Horikawa N, Kataha K, Watanabe N, et al. Glibenclamide-sensitive hypotension produced by heolodermin assessed in the rat. *Biol Pharm Bull.* 1998;21:1290–1293.

Huan J-Y, Mironda CL, Buhler DR, et al. Species differences in the hepatic microsomal enzyme metabolism of the pyrrolizidine alkaloids. *Toxicol Lett.* 1998;99:127–137.

Hurlbut WP, Iezzi N, Fesce R, et al. Correlation between quantal secretion and vesicle loss at the frog neuromuscular junction. *J Physiol.* 1990;425:501–526.

Hyde EG, Carmichael WW. Amatoxin-a(s), a naturally occurring organophosphate, is an irreversible active site-directed inhibitor of acetylcholinesterase (E.C.3.1.1.7). *J Biochem Toxicol.* 1991;6:195–201.

Inokuma H, Kemp DH, Willadsen P. Comparison prostaglandin E2 in salivary gland of *Boophilus microplus*, *Haemaphysalis longicornis* and *Ixodes holocyclus* and quantification of PGE2 in saliva, hemolymph, ovary and gut of B. microplus. *J Vet Med Sci.* 1994;56:1217–1218.

Isbister GK, Volschenk ES, Seymour JE. Scorpion stings in Australia: five definite stings and a review. *Int Med J.* 2004;34:427–430.

Isbister GK, White J. Clinical consequences of spider bites: recent advances in our understanding. *Toxicon.* 2004;43:477–492.

Izzo AA, Ernst E. Interactions between herbal medicines and prescribed drugs: a systematic review. *Drugs.* 2001;61:2163–2175.

Jaeger A, Fehl F, Flesch F, et al. Kinetics of amatoxins in human poisoning: therapeutic implications. *Clin Toxicol.* 1993;31:63–80.

Jaffe AM, Gephardt D, Courtemanche L. Poisoning due to ingestion of *Veratrum viride* (false hellebore). *J Emerg Med.* 1990;8:161–167.

James LF, Panter KE, Broquist HP, et al. Swainsonine-induced high mountain disease in calves. *Vet Hum Toxicol.* 1991;33:217–219.

Johnson RA, Baer H, Kirkpatrick CH, et al. Comparison of the contact allergenicity of the four pentadecylcatechols derived from poison ivy urushiol in human subjects. *J Allergy Clin Dermatol.* 1972;49:27–35.

Jones TK, Lawson BM. Profound neonatal congestive heart failure caused by maternal consumption of blue cohosh herbal medication. *J Pediatr.* 1998;132:550–552.

Joo SS, Won TJ, Kim JS, et al. Inhibition of coagulation activation and inflammation by a novel factor Xa inhibitor synthesized from the earthworm *Eisenia andrei*. *Biol Pharm Bull.* 2009;32:253–258.

Jorgensen K, Bak S, Busk PK, et al. Cassava plants with a depleted cyanogenic glucoside content in leaves and tubers. *Plant Physiol.* 2005;139:363–374.

Kalish RS, Johnson KL. Enrichment and function of urushiol (poison ivy)-specific T lymphocytes in lesions of allergic contact dermatitis to urushiol. *J Immunol.* 1990;145:3706–3713.

Kandel ER, Schwartz JH, Jessel TM. *Principles of Neural Sciences.* 4th ed. New York: McGraw-Hill; 2000.

Karlson-Stiber C, Persson H. Cytotoxic fungi—an overview. *Toxicon.* 2003;42:339–349.

Kavalali G. The chemical and pharmacological aspects of *Urtica*. In: Kavalali GM, ed. *Urtica*. New York: Taylor & Francis; 2003:25–39.

Kawamoto F, Kumada N. Biology and venoms of Lepidoptera. In: Tu A, ed. *Insect Poisons, Allergens, and Other Invertebrate Venoms.* Vol. 2. New York: Marcel Dekker; 1984:292.

Keegan HL. *Scorpions of Medical Importance.* Jackson, MI: University Press of Mississippi; 1980.

Keeler RF. Early embryonic death in lambs induced by *Veratrum californicum*. *Cornell Vet.* 1990;80:203–207.

Keeler RF, Baker DC. Myopathy in cattle induced by alkaloid extracts from *Thermopsis montana*, *Laburnum anagyroides* and a *Lupinus* sp. *J Comp Pathol.* 1990;103:169–182.

Kelch WJ, Kerr LA, Adair HS, et al. Suspected buttercup (*Ranunculus bulbosus*) toxicosis with secondary photosensitization in a Charolais heifer. *Vet Hum Toxicol.* 1992;34:238–239.

Kemparaju K, Girish KS, Nagaraju S. Hyaluronidases, a neglected class of glycosidases from snake venom: beyond a spreading factor. In: Mackessy SP, ed. *Handbook of Venoms and Toxins of Reptiles.* Boca Raton: CRC Press/Taylor & Francis; 2010:237.

Kennelly EJ, Flynn TJ, Mazzola EP, et al. Detecting potential teratogenic alkaloids from blue cohosh rhizomes using an in vitro rat embryo culture. *J Nat Prod.* 1999;62:1385–1389.

Kim D-Y, Lee Y-S. Ovine copper poisoning and *Pteridium aquilinum*-associated bovine urinary bladder tumor in Korea. *J Toxicol Soc.* 1998;23(suppl 4):645–646.

Kini RM. Excitement ahead: structure, function and mechanism of snake venom phospholipase A2 enzymes. *Toxicon.* 2003;42:827–840.

Kini RM, Chan YM. Accelerated evolution and molecular surface of venom phospholipases A2 enzymes. *J Mol Evol.* 1999;48:125–132.

Knight TE. Philodendron-induced dermatitis: report of cases and review of the literature. *Cutis.* 1991;48:375–378.

Kolarich D, Altmann F, Sunderasan E. Structural analysis of the glycoprotein allergen Hev b 4 from natural rubber latex by mass spectrometry. *Biochim Biophys Acta.* 2005;46:946–953.

Kotaki Y, Furio EF, Satake M, et al. Production of isodomoic acids A and B as major toxin components of a pennate diatom *Nitzschia navis-varingica*. *Toxicon.* 2005;46:946–953.

Krasnoperov VG, Bittner MA, Beavis R, et al. α-Latrotoxin stimulates exocytosis by the interaction with a neuronal G-protein-coupled receptor. *Neuron.* 1997;18:925–937.

Kuhn-Nentwig L. Antimicrobial and cytolytic peptides of venomous arthropods. *Cell Mol Life Sci.* 2003;60:2651–2668.

Kuhn-Nentwig L, Schaller J, Nentwig W. Biochemistry, toxicology and ecology of the venom of the spider *Cupiennius salei* (Ctenidae). *Toxicon.* 2004;43:534–553.

Kulp KS, Valliet PR, Richard P. Mimosine blocks cell cycle progression by chelating iron in asynchronous human breast cancer cells. *Toxicol Appl Pharmacol.* 1996;139:356–364.

Kuwahara Y, Omura H, Tanabe T. 2-Nitroethenylbenzenes as natural products in millipede defense secretions. *Naturwissenschaften.* 2002;89:308–310.

Lee C-Y, ed. *Snake Venoms*. New York, Springer Verlag; 1979.

Lee TH, Huang NK, Lai TC, et al. Anemonin, from *Clematis crassifolia*, potent and selective inducible nitric oxide synthase inhibitor. *J Ethnopharmacol.* 2008;116:518–527.

Leikin JB, Paloucek FP. Poisoning and Toxicology Handbook. New York: Informa Healthcare; 2008.

Lewis DC, Shibamoto T. Effects of *Cassia obtusifolia* (sicklepod) extracts and anthraquinones on muscle mitochondrial function. *Toxicon.* 1989;27:519–529.

Li C, Oberlies NH. The most widely recognized mushroom: chemistry of the genus *Amanita*. *Life Sci.* 2005;78:532–538.

Li M, Fry BG, Kini RM. Putting the brakes on snake venom evolution: the unique molecular evolutionary patterns of *Aipysurus eydouxii* (marbled sea snake) phospholipase A2 toxins. *Mol Biol Evol.* 2005;22:934–941.

Lin TJ, Hsu CI, Lee KH, et al. Two outbreaks of acute tung nut (*Aleurites fordii*) poisoning. *J Toxicol Clin Toxicol.* 1996;34:87–92.

Lioi MB, Barbieri R, Borzacchiello G, et al. Chromosome aberrations in cattle with chronic enzootic haematuria. *J Comp Pathol.* 2004;131:233–236.

Liu M, Nakazawa K, Inoue K, et al. Potent and voltage-dependent block by philanthotoxin-343 of neuronal nicotinic receptor/channels in PC12 cells. *Br J Pharmacol.* 1997;122:379–385.

Lopez TA, Cid MS, Bianchini ML. Biochemistry of hemlock (*Conium maculatum*) alkaloids and their acute and chronic toxicity in livestock: a review. *Toxicon.* 1999;37:841–865.

Lubenow N, Greinacher A. Hirudin in heparin-induced thrombocytopenia. *Semin Thromb Hemost.* 2002;28:431–438.

Mackessy SP. *Handbook of Venoms and Toxins of Reptiles.* Boca Raton: CRC Press/Taylor & Francis; 2010.

Maejima H, Kinoshita E, Yuki T, et al. Structural determinants for the action of grayanotoxin in D1 S4-S5 and D4 S4-S5 intracellular linkers of sodium channel alpha-subunits. *Biochem Biophys Res Commun.* 2002;295:452–457.

Mans BJ, Gaspar ARMD, Louw AI, et al. Purification and characterization of apyrase from the tick, *Ornithodoros savignyi*. *Comp Biochem Physiol B Biochem Mol Biol.* 1998;120:617–624.

Maretiĉ Z, Lebez D. *Araneism.* Belgrade, Yugoslavia: Nolit Belgrade; 1979.

Markland FS. Snake venoms and their hemostatic system. *Toxicon.* 1998;36:1749–1800.

Marsh N, Williams V. Practical applications of snake venom toxins in haemostasis. *Toxicon.* 2005;45:1171–1181.

Martinez FJ, Duron RR, de Torres NW, et al. Experimental evidence for toxic damage induced by a dimeric anthracenon: diast T-514 (peroxisome A2). *Toxicol Lett.* 1997;90:155–162.

Martinez HR, Bermudez MV, Rangel-Guerra RA, et al. Clinical diagnosis in *Karwinskia humboldtiana* polyneuropathy. *J Neurol Sci.* 1998;154:49–54.

Masina S, Broady KW. Tick paralysis: development of a vaccine. *Int J Parasitol.* 1999;29:535–541.

Massart D, Sohawon S, Noordally O. Medicinal leeches. *Rev Med Brux.* 2009;30:533–536.

Massermanian A. Contact dermatitis due to *Euphorbia pulcherrima* Willd, simulating a phototoxic reaction. *Contact Dermatitis.* 1998;38:113–114.

Mayer AMS, Glaser KB, Cuevas C, et al. The odyssey of marine pharmaceuticals: a current pipeline perspective. *Trends Pharmacol Sci.* 2010;31:255–265.

Mayer KE, Myers RP, Lee SS. Silymarin treatment of viral hepatitis. *J Viral Hepat.* 2005a;12:559–567.

Mayer M, O'Neill MA, Murray KE, et al. Usnic acid: a non-genotoxic compound with anti-cancer properties. *Anticancer Drugs.* 2005b;16:805–809.

Mazzuca M, Heurteaux C, Alloui A, et al. A tarantula peptide against pain via ASIC1a channels and opioid mechanisms. *Nat Neurosci.* 2007;10:943–945.

McDermott WV, Ridker PM. The Budd–Chiari syndrome and hepatic venoocclusive disease. *Arch Surg.* 1990;125:525–527.

McGovern TW, Barkley TM. Botanical briefs: chrysanthemum—*Dendranthema* spp. *Cutis.* 1999;63:319–320.

McGrath-Hill CA, Vicas IM. Case series of *Thermopsis* exposures. *J Toxicol Clin Toxicol.* 1997;35:659–665.

McIntosh JM, Santos AD, Olivera BM. *Conus* peptides targeted to specific nicotinic acetylcholine receptor subtypes. *Annu Rev Biochem.* 1999;68:59–88.

McLain-Romero J, Creamer R, Zepeda H, et al. The toxicosis of *Embellisia* fungi from locoweed (*Oxytropis lambertii*) is similar to locoweed toxicosis in rats. *J Anim Sci.* 2004;82:2169–2174.

Mebs D. *Venomous and Poisonous Animals.* Stuttgart: Medpharm; 2002.

Mebs D, Kauferstein S. Ichthyotoxicity caused by marine cone snail venoms? *Toxicon.* 2005;46:355–356.

Mei N, Guo L, Fu PP, et al. Mutagenicity of comfrey (*Symphytum officinale*) in rat liver. *Br J Cancer.* 2005;92:873–875.

Mellick LB, Makowski T, Mellick GA, et al. Neuromuscular blockade after ingestion of tree tobacco (*Nicotiana glauca*). *Ann Emerg Med.* 1999;34:101–104.

Mello JR, Habermehl GG. Calcinogenic plants and the incubation effect of rumen fluid. *Dtsch Tierarztl Wochenschr.* 1992;99:371–376.

Mendis S. Colchicine cardiotoxicity following ingestion of *Gloriosa superba* tubers. *Postgrad Med J.* 1989;65:752–755.

Menez A. Functional architectures of animal toxins: a clue to drug design? *Toxicon.* 1998;36:1557–1572.

Menez A. *The Subtle Beast: Snakes, from Myth to Medicine.* New York: Taylor & Francis; 2003.

Menez A, Gillet D, Grishin E. In: Gillet D, Johannes L, eds. *Recent Research Developments on Toxins from Bacteria and Other Organisms.* Trivandrum, India: Research Signpost; 2005.

Ménez A, Stocklin R, Mebs D. "Venomics" or: the venomous systems genome project. *Toxicon.* 2006;47:255–259.

Ménez A, Zimmerman K, Zimmerman S, et al. Venom apparatus and toxicity of the centipede *Ethmostigmus rubripes* (Chilopoda, Scolopendridae). *J Morphol.* 1990;206:303–312.

Merchant ML, Hinton JF, Geren CR. Sphingomyelinase D activity of brown recluse spider (*Loxosceles reclusa*) venom as studied by 31 P-NMR: effects on the time-course of sphingomyelin hydrolysis. *Toxicon.* 1998;36:537–545.

Michelot D, Toth B. Poisoning by *Gyromitra esculenta*—a review. *J Appl Toxicol.* 1991;11:235–243.

Middleton RE, Warren VA, Kraus RL, et al. Two tarantula peptides inhibit activation of multiple sodium channels. *Biochemistry.* 2002;41:14734–14747.

Monzingo AF, Collins EJ, Ernst SR, et al. The 2.5 A structure of pokeweed antiviral protein. *J Mol Biol.* 1993;233:705–715.

Morrissette J, Kratezschmar J, Haendler B, et al. Primary structure and properties of helothermine, a peptide toxin that blocks ryanodine receptors. *Biophys J.* 1995;68:2280–2288.

Mouhat S, Jouirou B, Mosbah A, et al. Diversity of folds in animal toxins acting on ion channels. *Biochem J.* 2004;378:717–726.

Murai M, Kimura I, Kimura M. Blocking effects of hypoaconitine and aconitine on nerve action potentials in phrenic nerve–diaphragm muscles of mice. *Neuropharmacology.* 1990;29:567–572.

Nastopoulos D, Kanellopoulos PN, Tsernoglov D. Structure of dimeric and monomeric erabutoxin a refined at 1.5 A resolution. *Acta Crystallogr D Biol Crystallogr.* 1998;54:964–974.

Nelson LS, Shih RD, Balik MJ. *Handbook of Poisonous and Injurious Plants.* New York: Springer; 2007.

Newman DJ, Cragg GM, Battershill CN. Therapeutic agents from the sea: biodiversity, chemo-evolutionary insight and advances to the end of Darwin's 200th year. *Diving Hyperbaric Med.* 2009;39:216–225.

Nobile M, Noceti F, Prestipino G, et al. Helothermine, a lizard venom toxin, inhibits calcium current in cerebellar granules. *Exp Brain Res.* 1996;110:15–20.

Norred WP. Fumonisins—mycotoxins produced by *Fusarium moniliforme.* *J Toxicol Environ Health.* 1993;38:309–328.

Nuttall PA, Labuda M. Dynamics of infection in tick vectors and at the tick–host interface. *Adv Virus Res.* 2003;60:233–272.

O'Brien B, Quigg C, Leong T. Severe cyanide toxicity from "vitamin supplements." *Eur J Emerg Med.* 2005;12:257–258.

Oguiura N, Boni-Mitake M, Radis-Baptista G. New view on crotamine, a small basic polypeptide myotoxin from South American rattlesnake venom. *Toxicon.* 2006;46:363–370.

Oh SH, Haw CR, Lee MH. Clinical and immunologic features of systemic contact dermatitis from ingestion of *Rhus* (Toxicodendron). *Contact Dermatitis.* 2003;48:251–254.

Ohba H, Moriwaki S, Bakalova R, et al. Plant-derived abrin-a induces apoptosis in cultured leukemic cell lines by different mechanisms. *Toxicol Appl Pharmacol.* 2004;195:182–193.

Ohno M, Chijiwa T, Oda-Ueda N, et al. Molecular evolution of myotoxic phospholipases A2 from snake venom. *Toxicon.* 2003;42:841–854.

Olivera BM. *Conus* venom peptides, receptor and ion channel targets and drug design: 50 million years of neuropharmacology. *Mol Biol Cell.* 1997;8:2101–2109.

Olivera BM. ω-Conotoxin MVIIA: from marine snail venom to analgesic drug. In: Fusetani N, ed. *Drugs from the Sea.* Basel: Karger; 2000.

Olivera BM. *Conus* venom peptides: reflections from the biology of clades and species. *Annu Rev Ecol Syst.* 2002;33:25–42.

Olivera BM, Miljanich G, Ramachandran J, et al. Calcium channel diversity and neurotransmitter release: the ω-conotoxins and ω-agatoxins. *Annu Rev Biochem.* 1994;63:823–867.

Olivera BM, Rivier J, Clark C, et al. Diversity of *Conus* neuropeptides. *Science.* 1990;249:257–263.

Omnell ML, Sun FRP, Keeler RF, et al. Expression of *Veratrum* alkaloid teratogenicity in the mouse. *Teratology.* 1990;42:105–119.

Onat FY, Yegen BC, Lawrence R, et al. Mad honey poisoning in man and rat. *Rev Environ Health.* 1991;9:3–9.

O'Shea M. *Venomous Snakes of the World.* Princeton: Princeton University Press; 2005.

Patel KA, Modur V, Zimmerman GA. The necrotic venom of the brown recluse spider induces dysregulated endothelial cell-dependent neutrophil activation. Differential induction of GM-CSF, IL-8, and E-selectin expression. *J Clin Invest.* 1994;94:631–642.

Peixato PV, Brust LC, Duarte MD, et al. *Cestrum laevigatum* poisoning in goats in southeastern Brazil. *Vet Hum Toxicol.* 2000;42:13–14.

Peper K, Trautwein W. The effect of aconitine on the membrane current in cardiac muscle. *Pflugers Arch.* 1967;296:328–336.

Perry C, Sastry R, Nasrallah IM, et al. Mimosine attenuates serine hydroxymethyltransferase transcription by chelating zinc. Implications for inhibition of DNA replication. *J Biol Chem.* 2005;280:396–400.

Peterson MC, Rasmussen GJ. Intoxication with foothill camas (*Zigadenus paniculatus*). *J Toxicol Clin Toxicol*. 2003;41:63–65.

Pfister JA, Panter KE, Manners GD. Effective dose in cattle of toxic alkaloids from tall larkspur (*Delphinium barberi*). *Vet Hum Toxicol*. 1994;36:10–11.

Phillips DJ, Swernson SD, Markland FS. Thrombin-like snake venom serine proteinases. In: Mackessy SP, ed. *Handbook of Venoms and Toxins of Reptiles*. Boca Raton: CRC Press/Taylor & Francis; 2010:139.

Phui Yee JS, Nanling G, Afifiyan F, et al. Snake postsynaptic neurotoxins: gene structure, phylogeny and applications in research and therapy. *Biochimie*. 2004;86:137–149.

Pick T, ed. *Venoms of the Hymenoptera*. London: Academic Press; 1986.

Pietsch J, Oertel R, Trautmann S, et al. A non-fatal oleander poisoning. *Int J Legal Med*. 2005;119:236–240.

Polis GA, ed. *The Biology of Scorpions*. Stanford, CA: Stanford University Press; 1990:482.

Polya G. *Biochemical Targets of Plant Bioactive Compounds*. London: Taylor & Francis; 2003:583.

Possani LD, Merino E, Corona M, et al. Peptides and genes encoding for scorpion toxins that affect ion-channels. *Biochimie*. 2000;82:861–868.

Prabhasankar P, Raguputhi G, Sundaravadivel B, et al. Enzyme-linked immunosorbent assay for the phytotoxin thevetin. *J Immunoassay*. 1993;14:279–296.

Puschner B, Galey FD, Holstege DM, et al. Sweet clover poisoning in California. *J Am Vet Med Assoc*. 1998;212:857–859.

Pusterla N, Holmberg TA, Lorenzo-Figueras M, et al. *Acremonium strictum* pulmonary infection in a horse. *Vet Clin Pathol*. 2005;34:413–416.

Raisinghani M, Pabbidi RM, Premkumar LS. Activation of transient receptor potential vanilloid 1 (TRPV1) by resiniferatoxin. *J Physiol*. 2005;567(pt 3):771–786.

Ramirez M, Rivera E, Ereu C. Fifteen cases of atropine poisoning after honey ingestion. *Vet Hum Toxicol*. 1999a;41:19–20.

Ramirez MS, Sanchez EE, Garcia-Prieto C, et al. Screening for fibrinolytic activity in 8 viperid venoms. *Comp Biochem Physiol C Pharmacol Toxicol Endocrinol*. 1999b;124:91–98.

Ramos OHP, Selistre-de-Araujo HS. Snake venom metalloproteases—structure and function of catalytic and disintegrin domains. *Comp Biochem Physiol C Toxicol Pharmacol*. 2006;142:328–346.

Rao RB, Hoffman RS. Nicotinic toxicity from tincture of blue cohosh (*Caulophyllum thalictroides*) used as an abortifacient. *Vet Hum Toxicol*. 2002;44:221–222.

Rash LD, Hodgson WC. Pharmacology and biochemistry of spider venoms. *Toxicon*. 2002;40:225–254.

Rasmussen LH, Jensen LS, Hansen HC. Distribution of the carcinogenic terpene ptaquiloside in bracken fronds, rhizomes (*Pteridium aquilinum*), and litter in Denmark. *J Chem Ecol*. 2003;29:771–778.

Reddy A, Fried B. An update on the use of helminths to treat Crohn's and other autoimmunune diseases. *Parasitol Res*. 2009;104:217–221.

Reddy L, Odhav B, Bhoola K. Aflatoxin B1-induced toxicity in HepG2 cells inhibited by carotenoids: morphology, apoptosis and DNA damage. *Biol Chem*. 2006;387:87–93.

Riley RT, Hinton DM, Chamberlain WJ, et al. Dietary fumonisin B1 induces disruption of sphingolipid metabolism in Sprague–Dawley rat: a new mechanism of nephrotoxicity. *J Nutr*. 1994;124:594–603.

Rimsza ME, Zimmerman DR, Bergeson PS. Scorpion envenomation. *Pediatrics*. 1980;66:298–302.

Rockel D, Korn W, Kohn AJ. *Manual of the Living Conidae*. Weisbaden, Germany: Verlag Christa Hemmen; 1995.

Rode D. Comfrey toxicity revisited. *Trends Pharmacol Sci*. 2002;23:497–499.

Rodriguez de la Vega RC, Possani LD. Current views on scorpion toxins specific for K+–channels. *Toxicon*. 2004;43:865–875.

Rodriguez de la Vega RC, Possani LD. Overview of scorpion toxins specific for Na+ channels and related peptides: biodiversity, structure–function relationships and evolution. *Toxicon*. 2005;46:831–844.

Rondeau ES. Wisteria toxicity. *J Toxicol*. 1993;31:107–112.

Rosell S, Samuelsson B. Effect of mistletoe viscotoxin and phoratoxin on blood circulation. *Toxicon*. 1988;26:975–987.

Rosenberg P. Phospholipases. In: Shier WT, Mebs D, eds. *Handbook of Toxinology*. New York: Marcel Dekker; 1990:67.

Rosling R. Cyanide exposure from linseed. *Lancet*. 1993;341:177.

Roy MC, Chang FR, Huang HC, et al. Cytotoxic principles from the formosan milkweed, *Asclepias curassavica*. *J Nat Prod*. 2005;68:1494–1499.

Russell FE. Toxic effects of animal venoms. In: Klaassen CD, ed. *Casarett and Doull's Toxicology: The Basic Science of Poisons*. 6th ed. New York: McGraw-Hill; 2001:945.

Russell FE, Nagabhushanam R. *The Venomous and Poisonous Marine Invertebrates of the Indian Ocean*. Enfield, NH: Science Publications; 1996:271.

Ruyssers NE, De Winter BY, De Man JG, et al. *Schistosoma mansoni* proteins attenuate gastrointestinal motility disturbances during experimental colitis in mice. *World J Gastroenterol*. 2010;16:703–712.

Sako MDN, Al-Sultan II, Saleem AN. Studies on sheep experimentally poisoned with *Hypericum perforatum*. *Vet Hum Toxicol*. 1993;35:298–300.

Sangamnetdej S, Paesen GC, Slovak M, et al. A high affinity serotonin- and histamine-binding lipocalin from tick saliva. *Insect Mol Biol*. 2002;11:79–86.

Schacter L. Etopside phosphate: what, why, where and how? *Semin Oncol*. 1996;23(suppl 13):1–7.

Schulzke JD, Andres S, Amasheh M, Fromm A, Günzel D. Anti-diarrheal mechanism of the traditional remedy Uzara via reduction of active chloride secretion. *PLoS One*. 2011;6(3):e18107.

Shakin M, Smith BL, Prakash AS. Bracken carcinogens in the human diet. *Mutat Res*. 1999;443:69–79.

Sharma OP, Dawra RK, Pattabhi V. Molecular structure, polymorphism, and toxicity of lantadene A, the pentacyclic triterpenoid from the hepatotoxic plant *Latana camara*. *J Biochem Toxicol*. 1991;6:57–63.

Sholl JM, Rathlev NK, Olshaker JS. *Wilderness Medicine*. Philadelphia: WB Saunders; 2004.

Short SO, Edwards WC. Blue green algae toxicosis in Oklahoma. *Vet Hum Toxicol*. 1990;32:558–560.

Siebert U, Brach M, Sroczynski G, et al. Efficacy, routine effectiveness, and safety of horse chestnut seed extract in the treatment of chronic venous insufficiency. A meta-analysis of randomized controlled trials and large observational studies. *Int Angiol*. 2002;21:305–315.

Singletary EM, Holstege CP. Bites and stings: insects, marine, mammals and reptiles. In: Aghababian RV, ed. *Essentials of Emergency Medicine*. Sudbury, MA: Jones and Bartlett; 2006.

Skinner WS, Adams ME, Quistad GB, et al. Purification and characterization of two classes of neurotoxins from the funnel web spider *Agelenopsis aperta*. *J Biol Chem*. 1989;264:2150–2155.

Smith EA, Meloan CE, Pickell JA, et al. Scopolamine poisoning from homemade "moon flower" wine. *J Anal Toxicol*. 1991;15:216–219.

Smith J, Bush S. Envenomations by reptiles in the United States. In: Mackessy SP, ed. *Handbook of Venoms and Toxins of Reptiles*. Boca Raton: CRC Press/Taylor & Francis; 2010:475.

Soares AM, Giglio JR. Chemical modifications of phospholipases A2 from snake venoms: effects on catalytic and pharmacological properties. *Toxicon*. 2003;42:855–868.

Sokolov IuV, Chanturiia AN, Lishko VK. Channel-forming properties of *Steatoda paykulliana* spider venom [Russian]. *Biofizika*. 1984;29:620–623.

Southcott RV, Haegi LAR. Plant hair dermatitis. *Med J Aust*. 1992;156:623–628.

Spencer PS. Food toxins, AMPA receptors and motor neuron diseases. *Drug Metab Rev*. 1999;31:561–587.

Spencer PS, Roy DN, Ludolph A, et al. Lathyrism: evidence for the role of the neuroexcitatory amino acid, BOAA. *Lancet*. 1986;2:1066–1067.

Spoerke DG, Murphy MM, Wruk KM, et al. Five cases of *Thermopsis* poisoning. *J Toxicol Clin Toxicol*. 1988;26:397–406.

Steen NA, Barker SC, Alewood PF. Proteins in the saliva of the *Ixodida* (ticks): pharmacological features and biological significance. *Toxicon*. 2006;47:1–20.

Strimple PD, Tomassoni AJ, Otten EJ, et al. Report on envenomation by a Gila monster (*Heloderma suspectum*) with a discussion of venom apparatus, clinical findings, and treatment. *Wilderness Environ Med*. 1997;8:111–116.

Surh Y-J, Lee E, Lee JM. Chemoprotective properties of some pungent ingredients present in red pepper and ginger. *Mutat Res.* 1998;404:259–267.

Swartz KJ, MacKinnon R. An inhibitor of the Kv2.1 potassium channel isolated from the venom of a Chilean tarantula. *Neuron.* 1995;15:35–42.

Swenson S, Markland FS Jr. Snake venom fibrin(ogen)olytic enzymes. *Toxicon.* 2005;45:1021–1039.

Szalcsany J. Capsaicin receptors as target molecules on nociceptors for development of novel analgesic agents. In: Keri G, Toth I, eds. *Molecular Pathomechanisms and New Trends in Drug Research.* London: Taylor & Francis; 2002:319–333.

Tahirov THO, Lu T-H, Liaw Y-C, et al. A new crystal form of abrina from the seeds of *Abrus precatorius. J Mol Biol.* 1994;235:1152–1153.

Tambourgi DV, Petricevich VL, Magnoli FC, et al. Endotoxemic-like shock induced by *Loxosceles* spider venoms: pathological changes and putative cytokine mediators. *Toxicon.* 1998;36:391–403.

Tan N-H, Fung S-Y. Snake venom L-amino acid oxidases. In: Mackessy SP, ed. *Handbook of Venoms and Toxins of Reptiles.* Boca Raton: CRC Press/Taylor & Francis; 2010:221.

Tandon HD, Tandon BN, Mattocks AR. An epidemic of veno-occlusive disease of the liver in Afghanistan. *Am J Gastroenterol.* 1978;70:607–613.

Teitelbaum JS, Zatorre RJ, Carpenter S, et al. Neurologic sequelae of domoic acid intoxication due to the ingestion of contaminated mussels. *N Engl J Med.* 1990;322:1781–1787.

Terlau H, Olivera BM. *Conus* venoms: a rich source of novel ion channel-targeted peptides. *Physiol Rev.* 2004;84:41–68.

Terlau H, Shon K, Grilley M, et al. Strategy for rapid immobilization of prey by a fish-hunting cone snail. *Nature.* 1996;381:148–151.

Tintinalli JE, Kelen GD, Stapczynski JS, eds. *Emergency Medicine: A Comprehensive Study Guide.* 6th ed. New York: McGraw-Hill; 2004.

Tsetlin VI, Hucho F. Snake and snail toxins acting on nicotinic acetylcholine receptors: fundamental aspects and medical applications. *FEBS Lett.* 2004;557:9–13.

Tsujikawa K, Kanamori T, Iwata Y, et al. Morphological and chemical analysis of magic mushrooms in Japan. *Forensic Sci Int.* 2003;138:85–90.

Tucker MO, Swan CR. The mango–poison ivy connection. *N Engl J Med.* 1998;339:235.

Tulsiani DR, Broquest HP, James LF, et al. Production of hybrid glycoprotein and accumulation of oligosaccharides in the brain of sheep and pigs administered swainsonine or locoweed. *Arch Biochem Biophys.* 1988;264:607–617.

Turgut M, Alhan CC, Gurgoze M, et al. Carboxyatractyloside poisoning in humans. *Ann Trop Paediatr.* 2005;25:125–134.

Tylleskar T, Banca M, Bikongi N, et al. Cassava cyanogens and konzo, an upper motoneuron disease found in Africa. *Lancet.* 1992;339:208–211.

Uddman R, Goadsby PJ, Jansen-Olesen I, et al. Helospectin-like peptides: immunochemical localization and effects on isolated cerebral arteries and on local cerebral blood flow in the cat. *J Cerebral Blood Flow Metab.* 1999;19:61–67.

Urushibata O, Kase K. Irritant contact dermatitis from *Euphorbia marginata. Contact Dermatitis.* 1991;24:155–157.

Ushkaryov YA, Volnski KE, Ashton AC. The multiple actions of black widow spider toxins and their selective use in neurosecretion studies. *Toxicon.* 2004;43:527–542.

Uwai K, Ohashi K, Takaya Y, et al. Exploring the structural basis of neurotoxicity in C(17)-polyacetylenes isolated from water hemlock. *J Med Chem.* 2000;43:4508–4515.

Valenzuela JG. Blood-feeding arthropod salivary glands and saliva. In: Marquardt WC, ed. *Biology of Disease Vectors.* Amsterdam: Elsevier; 2004:chap 28.

Valenzuela JG, Charlab R, Mather TN, et al. Purification, cloning and expression of a novel salivary anticomplement protein from the tick *Ixodes scapularis. J Biol Chem.* 2000;275:18717–18723.

van Meurs A, Cohen A, Edelbroek P. Atropine poisoning after eating chapattis contaminated with *Datura stramonium* (thorn apple). *Trans R Soc Trop Med Hyg.* 1992;86:221.

Vincent A, Jacobson L, Curran L. Alpha-bungarotoxin binding to human muscle acetylcholine receptor. *Neurochem Int.* 1998;332:427–433.

Vogel C-W, Fritsinger DC, Hew BE. Recombinant cobra venom factor. *Mol Immunol.* 2004;41:191–199.

Volynski KE, Capogna M, Ashton AC, et al. Mutant α-latrotoxin (LTXN4C) does not form pores and causes secretion by receptor stimulation. This action does not require neurexins. *J Biol Chem.* 2003;278:31058–31066.

Wang H, Ng TB. Ribosome inactivating protein and lectin from bitter melon (*Momordica charantia*) seeds: sequence comparison with related proteins. *Biochem Biophys Res Commun.* 1998;253:143–146.

Wang X, Connor M, Smith R, et al. Discovery and characterization of a family of insecticidal neurotoxins with a rare vicinal disulfide bridge. *Nat Struct Biol.* 2000;7:505–513.

Wang X, Connor M, Wilson D, et al. Discovery and structure of a potent and highly specific blocker of insect calcium channels. *J Biol Chem.* 2001;276:40306–40312.

Wang Z, Zhao J, Xing J, et al. Analysis of strychnine and brucine in postmortem specimens by RP-HPLC: a case report of fatal intoxication. *J Anal Toxicol.* 2004;28:141–144.

Warren BA, Patel SA, Nunn PB, et al. The *Lathyrus* excitotoxin beta-N-oxalyl-L-alpha, beta diaminopropionic acid is a substrate of the L-cystine/L-glutamate exchanger system xc-. *Toxicol Appl Pharmacol.* 2004;200:83–92.

Weinstein SA, Smith TL, Kardong KV. Reptile venom glands: form, function and future. In: Mackessy SP, ed. *Handbook of Venoms and Toxins of Reptiles.* Boca Raton: CRC Press/Taylor & Francis; 2010:65.

White J. Snake venoms and coagulopathy. *Toxicon.* 2005;45:951–967.

Wilson D, Alewood PF. Taxonomy of Australian funnel-web spiders using rp-HPLC/ESI-MS profiling techniques. *Toxicon.* 2006;47:614–627.

Wu JH, Singh T, Herp A, et al. Carbohydrate recognition factors of the lectin domains present in the *Ricinus communis* toxic protein (ricin). *Biochemie.* 2006;88:201–217.

Yellen G. The voltage-gated potassium channels and their relatives. *Nature.* 2002;419:35–42.

Yoshizawa T, Yamashita A, Luo Y. Fumonisin occurrence in corn from high- and low-risk areas for human esophageal cancer in China. *Appl Environ Microbiol.* 1994;60:1626–1629.

27 chapter

Toxic Effects of Calories

Martin J. Ronis, Kartik Shankar,
and Thomas M. Badger

BIOLOGY OF EATING AND DIGESTION

All biotic organisms derive energy from food to sustain life and this energy "drives" various cellular functions, including digestion, metabolism, pumping blood, and muscle contractions. Nutrients can broadly be defined as chemical substances found in food that are necessary for proper growth and development, reproduction, and repair following injury. Based on their chemical nature, nutrients can be grouped into organic (carbon-containing) and inorganic classifications. Carbohydrates, proteins, fats, and vitamins comprise the former, while minerals and water are inorganic nutrients essential for life (Stipanuk, 2006). Inorganic nutrients such as minerals can be absorbed into the body through food and are generally incorporated into the food chain through environmental sources (soil, water). Minerals comprise ~4% of the body weight in humans and in combination with water furnish a major part of the obligatory milieu necessary for cellular functioning (pH, osmolarity). Macrominerals are those whose abundance is generally 0.01% of body weight or daily required amounts exceed 100 mg per day. Calcium, phosphorous, sodium, and magnesium fall in this group. Other minerals that are not as abundant can be equally important for an organism. Trace minerals are defined as minerals whose concentration is <0.01% of total body weight. Other alternative definitions include nutrients whose requirements are below 1 ppm. Iron, zinc, copper, iodine, selenium, and molybdenum are six essential trace elements with established recommended dietary allowances. Overall, trace nutrients perform a variety of important functions, including transport of oxygen (iron as a part of hemoglobin), catalysis of biological reactions as component of enzymes (iron, zinc), and as part of other organic molecules (selenocysteine). While inorganic compounds serve important roles in physiology, the energy in food is derived from metabolism of organic substances. Organic compounds are generally synthesized by living cells from simpler molecules. For example, green plants and marine phytoplankton utilize photosynthesis to convert the very simple molecule carbon dioxide into more complex, energy-rich compounds such as carbohydrates using the energy from the sunlight. Because most bacteria and higher organisms cannot carry out photosynthesis, they derive their energy by metabolism of preformed organic molecules, such as carbohydrates. In general, bacteria utilize simpler organic molecules and animals and humans require more complex macronutrients (proteins, fats, and carbohydrates) to meet their needs.

Digestion of Foods

Common foods are a complex matrix and before the nutrients in food can be utilized they invariably need to undergo digestion. The process of digestion is a remarkable orchestration of many complex biochemical and physiological events, which occurs throughout the gastrointestinal (GI) tract, involving mechanical and chemical breakdown of food into simpler nutrients that are amenable for absorption. The upper GI tract consists of oral cavity, esophagus, and stomach. Breakdown of food begins in the mouth via the actions of enzymes in saliva. Movement of food between sections of the GI tract is restricted via sphincters or valves. In the stomach, food is acted upon by gastric juices, which are secretions from the cardiac, oxyntic, and pyloric glands in the stomach. Gastric juice contains high amounts of hydrochloric acid that is secreted from gastric parietal cells. This along with the enzymes pepsin and α-amylase acts upon proteins and carbohydrates, respectively, to generate polypeptides and simpler sugars (such as dextrins from starch). Digestion in the small intestine is aided by numerous enzymes supplied by the pancreas, liver, and gall bladder, which drain into the proximal part called the duodenum. Bile made in the liver and secreted from the gall bladder aids in the absorption of fats from the diet. Pancreatic juice contains digestive enzymes including carboxypeptidases, lipases, amylases, and nucleases. Pancreatic secretions also contain bicarbonate and divalent cations (mostly sodium and potassium) that help neutralize the acidic composition of the partially digested food from the stomach. Almost half of ingested carbohydrates and proteins, and 90% of ingested fat are digested by pancreatic enzymes. In addition to the enzymes, the small intestine itself secretes numerous enzymes including aminopeptidases, lipases, and disaccharidases.

The latter parts of the small intestine, the jejunum and ileum, are primary sites of absorption of nutrients. The surface of the small intestine is uniquely adapted to facilitate the absorption of digested nutrients. The surface area of the intestinal mucosa available for absorption is greatly increased due to a combination of folds called valvulae conniventes (folds of Kerckring) and finger-like projections (villi) that are lined with enterocytes. The luminal surface of the enterocytes is further lined by microvilli that give the mucosal surface brush-border-like appearance. The luminal and basolateral surfaces of the enterocytes are rich in transporters that mediate uptake of nutrients into the enterocytes. Absorption of nutrients into enterocytes may be accomplished by diffusion, facilitated diffusion, or active transport. Luminal digestion of complex carbohydrates involves breakdown via salivary and pancreatic amylases into dextrins that undergo further digestion to simple monosaccharides in the membrane. These are transported into the enterocytes by active transport (glucose, galactose) or via facilitated diffusion (fructose). Digestion of proteins begins in the stomach and continues in the lumen of the small intestine. The jejunum is the site of absorption of amino acids and dipeptides and tripeptides by amino acid and peptide carriers in the enterocyte brush border. Lipids in the diet such as triacylglycerols are hydrolyzed by pancreatic and intestinal lipases to free fatty acids or monoacylglycerol. Bile salts along with phospholipids facilitate the absorption of lipids by forming emulsified complexes called micelles. After uptake into the enterocyte fatty acids are reesterified and packaged into chylomicrons that exit the enterocyte into the lymphatic system. Macronutrient molecules (amino acids, sugars, and fatty acids) that end up in the circulation undergo metabolism in various tissues to be either oxidized to extract energy or stored for future utilization.

Integrated Fuel Metabolism

The requirement for energy to fuel cellular functions in all organisms is continuous. However, food consumption is intermittent. Hence, most organisms have developed processes to store energy from a meal to be utilized until the next meal. Energy in the body is derived from three main nutrient classes: carbohydrates, protein, and fat, which in turn are made up of sugars, amino acids, and free fatty acids, respectively. The principal circulating fuels in the body, glucose and free fatty acids, are stored as glycogen and triglycerides, respectively. Highest concentrations of glycogen are present in the liver and skeletal muscle, which is a macromolecule consisting of branching chains of glucose held together by α-1,4 and 1,6 linkages. Triglycerides are stored in adipose depots in specialized cells (adipocytes) within large lipid droplets. While total body protein constitutes a large percentage of the energy, unlike fats and carbohydrate, protein is not normally utilized as storage form of energy. Proteins are critical in maintaining structure and function and are catabolized for energy only as a last-ditch effort, under extreme conditions. The energetic value of macromolecules per gram of tissue is influenced based on their hydration. While the theoretical energy content of glycogen is ~4 cal/g, due to its highly hydrophilic nature, each gram of glycogen is associated with two to three times its weight of water. Hence, in reality glycogen provides approximately 1 kcal/g of actual energy. This makes storage of energy predominantly in the form of glycogen quite inefficient. In contrast, because triglycerides are stored in a mostly nonaqueous milieu, fat tissue is energy dense, yielding close to the theoretical 9.4 cal/g of triglyceride. Hence, most animals have developed systems to convert glucose into lipids (lipogenesis) and adipose depots to store de novo synthesized lipids.

The interconversion of fuel sources and release in the time of need is designed to address three priorities of fuel utilization (Shulman *et al.*, 2003). Maintaining a stable supply of substrate for utilization by the brain is the first priority. Because the brain has little to no stored energy in the form of glycogen or triglycerides, it exclusively depends on the liver for maintaining a continuous supply of glucose. Blood glucose concentrations are maintained within a narrow range (55–140 mg/dL) via a number of interrelated mechanisms that are highly conserved. Unlike the brain, the heart and to some degree the liver and skeletal muscles derive most of their energy needs through the oxidation of fatty acids. Maintenance of protein reserves and replenishment of proteins (enzymes, cytoskeletal proteins, contractile proteins) following feeding is the next important function of fuel metabolism. Finally, conversion of existing nutrients into their storage forms (glycogen and triglycerides) is carried via anabolic biological pathways (glycogenesis and lipogenesis).

Hormonal messages generated by the endocrine cells of the pancreas, adipose tissue (adipokines), and GI tract (gut neuropeptides) are critical to orchestrating the multiple processes associated with fuel flux and metabolism. Insulin is the principal hormone required to manage nutrient fuels in both fed and fasted states. The presence and subsequent absorption of food in the GI tract and rise in blood glucose stimulates insulin secretion from the pancreas. Through its actions on various signaling pathways, insulin promotes glucose uptake in peripheral tissues, glycogen synthesis in the liver and muscle, lipid synthesis in adipocytes, and amino acid and protein synthesis in most cells. Insulin also acts to restrain catabolic processes such as lipolysis, gluconeogenesis, and protein degradation, which classically occur under states of low insulin (such as fasting). Following the immediate disposal of absorbed nutrients, the body enters a postabsorptive (early fasting) state, during which energy can no longer be derived from glucose directly from the meal (Ruderman *et al.*, 2005). In this state, serum levels of insulin start to decrease, and the liver begins catabolic processes, first glycogenolysis and then de novo synthesis of glucose (from gluconeogenic precursors, lactate and fatty acids, and glycerol). The substrates for gluconeogenesis arrive from anaerobic metabolism of glucose in red blood cells or metabolism of triglycerides and fatty acids (in adipose tissues). If food remains unavailable for a further protracted period of time, glycogen levels are almost completely depleted in both the muscle and liver and amino acids (released from breakdown of proteins) become the primary source for glucose production. A rise in glucagon and glucocorticoids (such as cortisol) also characterizes this state. These hormones promote lipolysis and breakdown of glycogen.

Set-Point Theory and Neural Control of Energy Balance

A number of redundant feedback mechanisms operate to maintain the homeostasis of energy in living systems. These mechanisms eventually regulate the balance between food intake and energy expenditure to maintain fuel reserves at preset levels. Under steady-state conditions, energy consumed is normally metabolized and utilized to maintain basic metabolic rate and thermogenesis, and carry out cellular processes, organ-specific functions, and movement (muscle contractions). Excess fuels are converted to triglycerides and stored in adipose tissues. Because adipose tissue is the major depot of preserving energy, signals derived from the periphery signal to regions in the brain that coordinate energy balance. When total energy consumed equals the total energy required to meet basal metabolic needs, growth, thermogenesis, and physical activity, the individual is in energy balance, and maintaining this balance will result in relatively stable weight and healthy body composition. When energy intake exceeds the actual energy expenditure, weight gain ensues and body composition can become problematic. The existence of a precise energy balance system is illustrated by considering normal variations in weight among groups of individuals over time. Over the course of a year, the average adult male consumes about one million cal, yet body weight of most weight-stable individuals does not fluctuate more than 1 lb. Even a small (~5%) error in matching intake and expenditure would result in a net change of approximately 6 kg of body weight. Therefore, it is obvious that mechanisms operating within the body can regulate energy balance with exquisite precision.

One theory called the "set-point" hypothesis proposes that food intake and energy expenditure are coordinately regulated by defined regions in the central nervous system that signal to maintain a relatively constant level of energy reserve and body weight (Keesey and Hirvonen, 1997). It is posited that the status of energy stores is sensed by the central nervous system and changes in the afferent signal result in adjustments in food intake and/or energy expenditure. Implicitly, the model requires the existence of four major components of an energy homeostasis system: afferent signals relaying the levels of energy stores, efferent processes regulating energy storage and expenditure, efferent mechanisms controlling ingestive behavior, and integrative centers in the brain to coordinate these processes. Studies have shown that the hypothalamus plays a central role in the control of energy balance, especially food intake. The hormone leptin, secreted in proportion to body fat stores from the adipose tissue, was the first signal to be identified to be a homeostatic regulator of energy balance. Leptin acts on metabolic-sensing neurons in the brain receptor-mediated actions, regulating signaling pathways that in effect decrease food intake (Friedman and Leibel, 1992). Leptin also has potent neurotrophic actions in the brain.

Two populations of neurons are seat of appetite control machinery in the brain, both of which are sensitive to leptin's actions (among other neuropeptides), one expressing orexigenic peptides neuropeptide-Y (NPY) and agouti-related peptide (AGRP) and the other expressing anorexigenic peptides proopiomelanocortin (POMC) and cocaine- and amphetamine-regulated transcript (CART). These are located in the arcuate nucleus of the hypothalamus. Downstream projections from these neurons interact with the melanocortin receptor neurons and the neurons in the paraventricular nucleus of the hypothalamus. In addition to the hypothalamic control of appetite per se, reward and hedonic processes of "liking" and "wanting" food occur in the ventral striatum of the midbrain in conjunction with the mesolimbic dopamine system. In addition, the corticolimbic system of reward is controlled by areas in the prefrontal cortex, which integrates sensory, emotional, and cognitive information to coordinate behavioral responses (Lenard and Berthoud, 2008). Hence, the homeostatic control of energy balance fits into the larger decision scheme of choice behavior via a complex neural system.

METHODS TO ASSESS ENERGY BALANCE

Assessing Caloric Intake

In animal studies, caloric intake can be quantitatively monitored by measuring the amount of food consumed by animals in metabolic cages. Caloric intake can be derived by multiplying the quantity (g per day) of diets consumed with the caloric density of the diet. Knowledge of caloric intake is important in many experimental designs where pair-feeding a parallel cohort of animals is necessary. In clinical studies, assessing caloric intake can be performed in a number of ways, each with its strengths and limitations. A prospective method to collect information about current intake is maintenance of *food records*. These are usually carried out for a specific duration of time (three to seven days, generally including both week and weekend days) during which a written record of all food and beverages consumed is maintained. Quantification is performed by estimation of weights or actual weighing of foodstuff, and hence food records provide both qualitative and quantitative data. Advantages include high reliability as records do not rely on memory and can provide detailed records of diet and nutrient intake. However, weighed records are both labor and cost intensive and place higher burden on participants. Habitual eating habits can be influenced by the process of recording and the reliability of the method decreases over long periods of data collection. Collected data are analyzed using a nutritional database such as the Nutrition Data System for Research (University of Minnesota). Several methods of dietary assessment rely on retrospective collection of food intake. The *diet history* and *food recall* are commonly used methods in clinical research, where a trained individual obtains details of participant's habitual dietary intake in-person or over the phone. Details may include portion sizes, cooking methods, and patterns of eating. The techniques allow a large amount of descriptive data to be collected. Most usually, the interviewer incorporates a 24-hour or three-day window in which detailed recall is obtained. Burden on the participant is low; however, the technique involves considerable training and time on the part of the researcher. Recall interviews can sometimes be time-consuming and several recalls may be necessary to obtain useful information. Again, analysis of the collected data using a nutritional database is necessary to get quantitative measures of nutrient and caloric intakes. *Food frequency questionnaires* (FFQ) are tools that can be self-administered or provided in an interview setting to participants. FFQ collect information about consumption of each food from a list of foods over a specified period of time (eg last six months). They are devoid of specific data regarding the portion sizes and cooking method and are not an appropriate method for quantifying intakes. However, FFQ are useful in gathering information on long-term food patterns, in a low-burden and inexpensive method. Both of these methods are merely estimations and can have significant errors.

Assessing Caloric Content of Foods

Accurate assessment of the caloric value of foods is essential for effective nutritional management in clinical and public policy arenas. Classical investigations by Professor Atwater and his colleagues providing the general calorie factors of 4, 9, and 4 for the major sources of energy—carbohydrate, fat, and protein—have been widely used. Both fats and carbohydrates can be completely oxidized to water and carbon dioxide, while protein is incompletely oxidized and partly excreted from the body as urea. The heat released by combustion of a food in a bomb calorimeter is a measure of its gross energy. However, not all the ingested energy will be available for metabolism and digestible energy refers to the fraction following losses of energy as fecal energy and gases from microbial fermentation. The truly metabolizable energy can be derived by accounting for lost energy in urine (mainly from nitrogen) and on the body surface. Analytical methods to determine the macronutrients in food, protein, fat, and carbohydrates in addition to alcohol and other organic acids, have been described widely (Tontisirin *et al.*, 2003). Protein content is mainly determined via estimating nitrogen content by either the Kjeldahl method or hydrolysis of proteins into amino acids and then measuring concentrations using gas or high-pressure liquid chromatography. Fat content can be assessed by measuring the sum of methanol–chloroform extractable total fatty acids that can be expressed as triglyceride equivalents. Total fat can also be assessed by gravimetric methods. Carbohydrate content is generally measured by difference as the remaining energy after accounting for protein, fat, alcohol, and ash. This measure of carbohydrate included energy from fiber as well as some components that may strictly not be carbohydrates (organic acids).

Assessing Energy Expenditure

The process of oxidative phosphorylation couples the oxidation of nutrients with the synthesis of high-energy molecules (viz, adenosine triphosphate [ATP]), the main energy currency of the cell. The energy stored with these molecules is utilized to power all the biochemical processes in cells, which encompass metabolism, growth, and cell division. The total energy expenditure (TEE) or metabolic cost for an average adult ranges from 1500 to 3000 kcal per day. A calorie is defined as a unit of energy that is required to raise the temperature of 1 g of water by 1°C. TEE is primarily composed of three components: (1) basal energy expenditure, (2) thermic effect of food (TEF), (3) energy expenditure associated with physical activity (EEPA). While most of the variance in daily TEE is accounted for by the three aforementioned components, a small fraction of energy expenditure is accounted for by adaptive thermogenesis (energetic cost of cold adaptation). Basal energy expenditure, also called as resting energy expenditure (REE), is the energy expended when the individual is lying down and at complete rest, generally after sleep in the postabsorptive state. REE accounts for almost 60% of TEE (Gropper *et al.*, 2005). A close surrogate of REE is the resting metabolic rate (RMR). TEF, which accounts for 10% to 15% of TEE, is the energy expenditure associated with the digestion, absorption, and storage of food. EEPA consists of (1) expenditure related to planned exercise and (2) nonexercise activity thermogenesis (NEAT). The former refers to purposeful physical activity, which varies in most individuals and is negligible in individuals who do not participate in exercise. However, even in individuals who do undertake regular exercise, NEAT contributes the greater proportion to EEPA. NEAT includes all energy expenditure from occupational and leisure activities (sitting, climbing stairs, walking, fidgeting, etc).

Components of energy expenditure can be measured using either (1) direct or (2) indirect calorimetry. The basic principle in direct calorimetry is to measure the actual heat produced by the organism in a highly controlled environment as an estimate of energy expenditure. In large organisms (such as human subjects) this is generally impractical due to the large inherent capacity to store heat. Further, due to limitations in the design, complexity, and cost of carrying out direct calorimetry, it is seldom utilized. The most commonly used methods to estimate energy expenditure, therefore, involve indirect calorimetry. Since most aerobic organisms derive energy from oxidation reactions, consumption of oxygen can serve as reliable surrogate for heat production. Using experimentally derived estimates for energy yields per mole of oxygen for the main fuel substrates, heat production can be calculated based on the quantity of oxygen consumed. Indirect calorimetry can be coupled with specific tracer techniques to examine the utilization and metabolism of specific substrates in both whole body and tissue-specific compartments. The ratio of carbon dioxide expired and oxygen consumed is called the respiratory quotient (RQ). RQ estimates can be useful in understanding both energy expenditure and overall substrate oxidation. An RQ value of 1.0 suggests that carbohydrate is being oxidized, because under these conditions the amount of oxygen required for oxidation of glucose is equal to the amount of carbon dioxide produced. The representative average RQ values for carbohydrate, fat, and protein are 1.0, 0.7, and 0.8, respectively. Indirect calorimetry can be assessed in animals by placing them in closed chambers in which airflow is controlled at specified flow rates. Oxygen and carbon dioxide concentrations are assessed using gas analyzers to calculate RQ values. Specialized chambers that are commercially available integrate measurement of body weights, food and water intake, activity, and oxygen consumption in a single chamber. In human subjects, the same principle is utilized to assess oxygen consumption in a variety of designs. A simple metabolic cart can be utilized to assess basal metabolic rate (BMR) in individuals over a short 30-minute period while the individual is in the supine position, but not asleep. Estimates of 24-hour RMR can be calculated by extrapolation. Metabolic carts can be adapted to estimate energy expenditure during physical activity such as treadmill running to estimate maximal oxygen consumption (VO_2 max). However, these measurements only estimate the REE component of TEE. Room calorimeters allow estimating the true TEE by measuring oxygen consumption during all aspects of free living, including postmeal thermic expenditure and during physical activity. These studies require the participant to be isolated in a room calorimeter and are expensive to undertake and maintain. Another method to estimate TEE in free-living subjects utilizes measurement of stable isotopes $^2H_2$ (deuterium) and ^{18}O. In this technique referred to as "doubly labeled water," a stable isotope of water is given to individuals ($H_2^{18}O$ and ^2H_2O) and the disappearance of the labeled tracer in blood and urine is assessed over three- to six-week time period. The labeled water incorporates into the body water pool and estimates either the water turnover alone (^2H label) or the turnover of water and production of CO_2 (^{18}O label). The difference between the two rates of loss of the two labels corresponds to the rate of production of CO_2. The amount of oxygen consumed is indirectly calculated via food records (food quotient) over the assessment period. RQ and energy expenditure can then be calculated using the volumes of oxygen and carbon dioxide. RMR estimates can also be calculated nonexperimentally based on derived equations. Equations such as the Harris–Benedict equation and the Mifflin and St. Jeor equation utilize the person's body weight, body surface area, age, gender, and height.

Assessing Body Composition

Body composition assessments are aimed at describing the overall mass of an individual organism in terms of its molecular or nutrient components: water, fat mass, lean mass, protein, and minerals. In a simple two-compartment model of body composition assessment, total body mass is divided into fat mass (essential and nonessential fat) and fat-free mass (including lean mass and water). Lean mass in this scenario includes protein, carbohydrate, and minerals. A number of techniques have been developed to indirectly assess either specific components or all measures of body composition.

Anthropometric Analysis Body mass is an obvious, but poor surrogate to relative fat mass. While individuals with greater body weight (mass) per height tend to have greater fat mass, total body weight may also be determined by increased muscle mass. Taller people on average have greater weight and weight and/or body composition also changes more dynamically with age. Hence, the simplest indirect measure of body fatness is the relative proportion of weight to height, more commonly referred to as body mass index (BMI). BMI is derived by ratio of mass (in kilograms) and square of height (in meters). The advantage of BMI is that it is easy to compute and large worldwide reference datasets exist. BMI, however, is only an estimate and because BMI does not always reflect fat mass, care must be taken when using BMI as a fat index. Other anthropometric estimates of body composition include measurement of skin folds and circumference at various sites (abdomen, waist, hip). The general assumption is that total body fat is proportional to the fat deposited beneath the skin. Measurements can be analyzed by utilizing several regression models that predict percent body fat. Five commonly employed sites include triceps, subscapula, suprailiac, abdomen, and thigh. While the technique is inexpensive to perform, sites chosen for analysis and skill of the anthropometrist influence the accuracy of the results.

Hydrodensitometry The principle used to calculate body density using hydrostatic weighing has been known since antiquity when the Greek mathematician Archimedes showed that the density of an object is the ratio of its weight in air to its loss of weight in water. Using the density of the whole body and correcting for residual air in the lungs and GI tract, the relative body fat can be estimated using derived equations by Siri or Brozek. This procedure is also known as underwater weighing.

Air Displacement Plesmography This procedure employs the same principles as underwater weighing described above, except rather than the body displacing water, it displaces air. This allows the body volume to be calculated and then body fat can be calculated. This is probably the most accurate, precise, and cost-effective measure of total body fat, and is employed widely in clinical research in the United States.

Absorptiometry This is one of the most widely used tools in assessing body composition. In this technique imaging is performed throughout the entire body by a photon beam. Most investigations using this technique use either a dual-photon source (gadolinium) or x-ray at two different energy levels (dual-energy x-ray

absorptiometry [DXA]). Hence, this allows imaging of both soft tissues and bone. The attenuation of the x-ray signal received on the detector is proportional to the density of the tissue. Percentage of body fat, lean tissue, and bone mineral density can be computed for the whole body or specific sites based on the analysis of images.

Computerized Tomography While utilizing similar principles of differential x-ray attenuation through body, computerized tomography is used to produce three-dimensional "slices" or cross-sectional images of the subject. This is made possible by positioning the x-ray source and detectors on opposite poles of a circular tube within which the subject is imaged. The ability to generate 3D images allows regional localization of adipose tissues, muscles, and organs (liver). Using the image data, percent body fat and lean mass can be calculated.

Nuclear Magnetic Resonance (NMR) NMR works by interpreting radio-frequency signals of excited nuclei in an external magnetic field. The physical characteristics of the hydrogen atom differ when the hydrogen is located on protein, fat, or water and this can be detected and quantitated to determine body composition. Magnetic resonance imaging (MRI) is an extremely powerful imaging technique with high-resolution capacity and employed widely as a clinical diagnostic tool. Images acquired are three-dimensional allowing detailed analysis of body composition and regional fat and lean mass distribution with depots and ectopic deposition within tissues. While MRI has several advantages in terms of assessing the distribution of body fat, its expense relative to NMR makes it less used, and other considerations such as the requirement for the participant to lay still during the scanning period and the extreme noise make MRI less applicable than NMR for children.

Electrical Impedance Bioelectrical impedance analysis (BIA) and total body electrical conductivity (TOBEC) measure total body composition based on measuring electrical impedance (the inverse of conductance) of an electric current passed through the body. The conductance of a weak painless current through the body (which serves as an electrolytic medium) is utilized to infer lean body mass and fat mass. Lean mass has more water and greater conductivity than fat mass and predictive equations are employed to derive fat and lean body mass.

Total Body Water Body fat and lean mass can be calculated by estimating total body water using stable isotopes. Dilution of water containing specific concentrations of labeled isotope (either deuterium or ^{18}O) is usually assessed. Concentrations of isotopes are measured in blood or urine over a timecourse following a two- to six-hour equilibration period. Since body water occupies 73.2% of lean mass, fat-free mass can be computed based on total body water. Using a three-compartment model fat mass can be calculated. The method is significantly influenced by hydration status and assumptions are confounded by water present in fat tissue. While the cost of chemicals and collection of samples is not high, analysis of stable isotopes can be expensive.

Assessing Physical Activity

Accurate quantification of physical activity in free-living subjects is challenging. Methods utilizing self-reported diaries and questionnaires tend to overestimate physical activity. Devices such as accelerometers and pedometers can be utilized to empirically estimate activity. Accelerometers are versatile and cost-effective and can measure activity with little subject burden. Existing accelerometers come in varying degrees of sophistication from simple pedometers that count steps to models that can assess motion in three dimensions. An important challenge in utilizing accelerometers is to convert the count data into energy expenditure, which is done using different regression models.

BIOLOGY OF OBESITY

Obesity Risk: Genes, Epigenetics, and Fetal Environment

Access to plentiful food has been unpredictable throughout most of human (and animal) developmental history, marked by periods of feast or famine. In evolutionary terms, fitness and survival of an individual were likely to be closely related to the ability to maximally seek, acquire, consume, and store energy (as fat) when food was available, and to select for mechanisms that reduce energy expenditure during times when food is scarce. Thus, selection favored so-called thrifty genes that orchestrate anabolic processes over energy-consuming ones and provide selective advantage to those who possessed them during periods of food deprivation (Neel, 1962). However, the advent of agrarian lifestyle and recent industrialization has meant that much of the developed and emerging world now has a drastically altered environment. Food is generally available for most people and our lifestyles require less physical activity and exertion. Hence, the genetic legacy of once beneficial thrifty genes placed in an environment of caloric abundance acts as a powerful engine for weight gain, obesity, and its associated metabolic dysfunction. Recently questions have been raised whether the selection of thrifty genes occurred because of a true advantage contributing to survival. Speakman has proposed that natural variation and random mutation (genetic drift) in genes controlling hypothalamic energy balance set-points occurred in human evolution as human beings developed fire and social behaviors, and were released from risk of predation. This theory referred to as the "drifty gene" hypothesis better explains why even in societies where obesity is high, not everyone becomes obese (Speakman, 2008). Obesity is a highly heritable trait and studies comparing monozygotic with dizygotic twins indicate that 40% to 75% of the interindividual difference in trait is accounted for by genetic variability. Several genes whose disruption causes severe monogenic forms of familial obesity have been described. Remarkably, most of these genes impair central control of food intake. However, the genetic basis of nonsyndromic (common) obesity has remained elusive.

Recent genome-wide association studies (GWAS) have been highly effective in identifying common genetic variants that impact adiposity and other aspects of the metabolic syndrome (MetS). To date 50 such obesity-associated loci have been identified with high confidence (O'Rahilly and Farooqi, 2008). Of these the FTO (fat mass and obesity associated) is unequivocally associated with increased risk of obesity. Individuals who are homozygous for the high-risk (AA) allele weigh on average 3 kg more than individuals who do not carry any risk allele. New meta-analysis of GWAS studies including ~250,000 subjects has revealed 18 novel loci associated with BMI. Overall, the presently identified loci in combination still explain only a small proportion of obesity. Epigenetic regulation of gene expression is another area that might explain the underlying differences in susceptibility to obesity.

Epigenetics is loosely defined as heritable changes in modifications to the DNA that do not alter the DNA sequence. DNA methylation and covalent modification of histone tails are examples of epigenetic regulation. It is clear that epigenetic mechanisms are involved in basic cell functions including proliferation, differentiation, and growth. Because DNA methylation patterns can also be affected by environmental influences (in utero environment,

exposure to xenobiotics, stress), it is plausible that interaction of certain risk alleles and epigenetic mechanisms are responsible for susceptibility to obesity.

The incidence of obesity continues to rise and prevalence even among infants is rapidly rising. As for many chronic diseases, it is now widely accepted that increased susceptibility to obesity can be programmed in utero and early postnatal life. This hypothesis referred to as the "fetal origin of adult disease" is derived from the findings by Professor David Barker and colleagues at the University of Southampton, who discovered an inverse relationship between birth weight and risk of mortality due to coronary heart disease (Barker et al., 1989). Over the last two decades, epidemiological studies have extended the initial associations between birth weight and later cardiovascular disease to include associations between early growth patterns and risk for hypertension, insulin resistance, type 2 diabetes, and obesity in later life. Experimentally manipulating birth weights in a variety of animal models (rats, mice, sheep, pigs) also recapitulates the developmental programming phenotype (McMillen and Robenson, 2005). Another important influence on risk of obesity in later life is maternal body composition (fat mass) at conception and gestational weight gain. Studies in women and experimental models clearly indicate that maternal diet and body composition during pregnancy influence aspects of metabolism and appetite regulation in the offspring (Shankar et al., 2008). The mechanisms of such programming presumably involve epigenetic mechanisms.

TOXICITY RELATED TO EXCESS CALORIC INTAKE/OBESITY

Many of the adaptive, physiological responses to a positive energy balance produced as a result of overeating and inadequate physical activity result in toxicity over the long term. Short-term coordinated changes in metabolic pathways in white adipose tissue in response to overfeeding result in excess energy storage in the form of triglycerides and increased size of preexisting adipocytes (hypertrophy), and this also leads to formation of new adipocytes through hyperplasia (Virtue and Vidal-Puig, 2010). However, management of excess ingested energy over the long term can be complex. Under such conditions, the efficiency of energy storage in adipose tissue is decreased and the body has to resort to several different options to store energy in addition to fat, such as in ectopic sites, which may in fact be detrimental. As plasma concentrations of nonesterified fatty acids (NEFA) increase as a result of ingestion of high-fat diets and as a result of hydrolysis of triglycerides in the fat, triglycerides begin to accumulate in nonadipose tissues such as liver, skeletal muscle, and the pancreas as lipid droplets. The presence of excess NEFA and lipid metabolites in these tissues results in direct and indirect toxic actions leading to insulin resistance, inflammation, and tissue damage.

In addition, adipose tissue from obese individuals releases chemokines and cytokines, the so-called adipokines, which contribute to a state of "metabolic inflammation" (Gustafson, 2010; Dulloo et al., 2010). Fat is also an endocrine organ and the pattern of adipokines produced by adipose tissue in obesity differs substantially from that seen in lean individuals (Cornier et al., 2008).

NEFA and the other factors released from adipose tissue contribute to the development of the Metabolic Syndrome "MetS" in some overweight and obese individuals. This is a cluster of components including insulin resistance, disruptions in lipid homeostasis (dyslipidemia), and elevated blood pressure that substantially increase the risk for development of cardiovascular disease and type 2 diabetes. MetS is also associated with other comorbidities including nonalcoholic fatty liver disease (NAFLD) and reproductive dysfunction and elevated serum insulin in response to insulin resistance contributes to increased cancer risk associated with obesity. As a consequence, overall mortality is increased and life span is shortened with increasing caloric intake, body weight, and adiposity, whereas caloric restriction (CR), at least in animal models, has been shown to substantially increase life span.

Adaptation of Liver and Adipose Tissue to Excess Calories

Triglycerides and glycogen are used by the body to store excess caloric energy. This is a homeostatic mechanism that maintains energy sources such as blood glucose levels between meals. Dietary fats are transported in blood from the gut to the liver and adipose tissue by lipoprotein particles called chylomicrons. In both tissues, local hydrolysis of triglycerides in the capillary bed by the enzyme lipoprotein lipase results in the release of free fatty acids that are subsequently taken up into hepatocytes and adipocytes via fatty acid transport proteins (FATPs) and the scavenger receptor CD36. As they enter the cell, free fatty acids that are toxic are immediately conjugated with acetyl CoA and are bound to intracellular fatty acid–binding proteins before reesterification with glycerol to form triglyceride lipid droplets in the cytosol. Such droplets are highly dynamic and are coated with PAT proteins (named after *p*erilipin, *a*dipophilin, and the *t*ail-interacting protein). Adipophilin and perilipin have important roles in droplet stabilization and regulation of triglyceride turnover. The hepatocyte cytosol contains many small droplets that vary in size depending on the length of time after a meal, dietary fat to carbohydrate ratio, type of dietary fat, and overall caloric intake relative to metabolic requirements. The small hepatic lipid droplets function as a temporary energy storage site, whereas in adipocytes the small lipid droplets fuse to form a single large storage droplet and can serve as a longer-term storage site. In the hours after a meal, triglycerides from the hepatic droplets are incorporated into the lipoprotein VLDL, which is secreted into the plasma and which transports hepatic triglycerides to the adipose tissue for storage. Removal of triglycerides from VLDL by lipoprotein lipase in adipose and other peripheral tissues results in generation of the more dense lipoprotein LDL, which is subsequently recycled by the liver as the result of endocytosis on binding to the LDL receptor (Olson, 1998).

Although obesity is often associated with overconsumption of high-fat diets, it can develop from excessive caloric intake of any food energy source, including carbohydrates and proteins. Although overall consumption of dietary fat has declined in the United States over the past two decades, the proportion of obesity has increased to epidemic levels. In part this is due to excessive intake of simple carbohydrates that have increased as dietary fat consumption has decreased. Dietary carbohydrates are converted to monosaccharides, mainly glucose and fructose, which are further metabolized in the liver and peripheral tissues. Excess glucose can be stored in the liver in the form of the glucose polymer glycogen that accumulates as cytosolic granules and can make up as much as 7% of liver weight. However, the majority of excess hepatic glucose is metabolized via glycolysis and the citric acid cycle to acetyl CoA and is shunted into de novo fatty acid and triglyceride synthesis.

Recent DNA microarray analysis of gene expression in human adipose tissue biopsies suggests that coordinated upregulation of lipogenesis occurs in fat rapidly and directly as a result of increased caloric intake independent of changes in body weight (Franck *et al.*, 2011). Evidence for increases in adipose tissue glucose transport, and fatty acid and triglyceride biosynthesis has also been obtained from microarray analysis of fat from rats overfed a mixture of

simple carbohydrates and fat (Shankar *et al.*, 2010). The increase in triglyceride synthesis in both liver and fat after consumption of excess calories appears to be driven by activation of two important diet-sensitive transcription factors: sterol regulatory element-binding protein (SREBP-1c) and carbohydrate response element-binding protein (ChREBP) (Postic and Girard, 2008), and this process in fat ultimately drives adipose tissue hypertrophy. In addition to fat cells getting larger, excess calories also trigger proliferation and differentiation of preadipocytes in adipose tissue depots into new adipocytes, a process known as hyperplasia. However, the degree to which hyperplasia contributes to the ability of fat stores to expand in response to the need to store excess energy relative to hypertrophy remains unclear. What is clear is that in some individuals, there is a limit to which adipose tissue can expand safely without damage to adipocytes and that when this limit is reached toxicity results.

Recent studies have shown that when fat mass increases excessively, adipose tissue undergoes extensive structural remodeling. An extracellular matrix (ECM) with high concentrations of collagen fibrils and fibronectin appears to be essential for maintenance of the structural integrity of adipocytes and for preadipocyte differentiation (Divoux and Clement, 2011). However, at the point when adipocytes reach a certain size limit within a particular fat pad, hypoxia appears to develop possibly as a result of restricted blood flow. This triggers expression of the transcription factor hypoxia-inducible factor 1 (HIF-1α). Evidence from HIF-1α transgenic and knockout mice suggests that HIF-1α regulates inappropriate ECM remodeling and development of fibrosis in adipose tissue in response to hypoxia and obesity (Halberg *et al.*, 2009). Fibrosis has been reported to be increased in subcutaneous adipose tissue from obese subjects compared with lean subjects both by staining of collagen fibrils and by analysis of col6a3 gene expression and the percentage of fibrosis in white adipose tissue has been shown to correlate with inflammation in morbidly obese subjects (Divoux and Clement, 2011). Further evidence linking adipose tissue ECM with limitations in the ability of fat pads to expand to store excess caloric energy and for limited adipocyte hypertrophy to precede the development of obesity-linked pathologies such as inflammation and MetS comes from studies with mice in which genes involved in ECM formation have been knocked out. The protein SPARC is required for appropriate collagen synthesis during ECM remodeling. Both SPARC–/– mice and obesity-prone ob/ob mice where the collagen VI gene has been deleted display increased adipocyte and fat pad size, loose ECM structure, and reduced inflammation and metabolic disturbances after high-fat feeding. It is thought that complex interactions between enlarging adipocytes and a fibrotic ECM trigger activation of MAP kinase pathways such as c-Jun N-terminal kinase (JNK) resulting in development of adipocyte insulin resistance, apoptosis, and necrosis, which in turn results in activation of resident macrophages in the fat and an inflammatory response (Divoux and Clement, 2011) (see Fig. 27-1).

Ectopic Fat Deposition

In general, there is a positive correlation between increased BMI and inappropriate accumulation of lipids in tissues other than fat. The major sites for this ectopic fat deposition are liver and skeletal muscle. However, lipid accumulation in other tissues such as small intestine, pancreas, and uterus has also been reported to be associated with chronic consumption of high-fat diets and development of obesity. Correlation between central (visceral) adiposity, waist circumference, and ectopic fat deposition is better than for BMI and is also highly correlated with progressive insulin resistance. However, the relationship between adiposity, ectopic fat

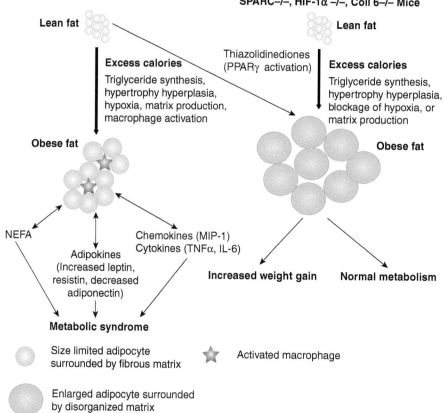

Figure 27-1. *Effects of excess calories (energy) on fat morphology under conditions leading to metabolic syndrome (left) or following stimulation of adipocyte differentiation and hyperplasia by thiazolidinedione treatment/in knockout mice incapable of normal responses to hypoxia (HIF-1α −/−)/in knockout mice incapable of normal extracellular matrix production (SPARC−/−, Coll 6−/−) (right).*

accumulation in liver and muscle, and insulin resistance is highly complex and is strongly affected by diet composition, exercise, and race (Lara-Castro and Garvey, 2008).

In the liver, intrahepatocellular lipid accumulation, also known as fatty liver, or steatosis, is defined as an increase in hepatic lipid content above 5% by weight and is characterized in paraffin-stained sections by the appearance of multiple round empty vacuoles in hepatocytes displacing the nucleus to the periphery of the cell. To confirm that steatosis is actually present, additional staining of frozen sections for triglycerides using stains such as Oil Red O is required. Abnormal lipid accumulation in the liver in the absence of heavy alcohol usage is referred to as non-alcoholic fatty liver disease (NAFLD) and is associated with a wide spectrum of hepatic dysfunction. The incidence of NAFLD in the general population including children has increased in line with increasing incidence of obesity and is observed in >50% of adult obese patients (Browning *et al.*, 2004). Simple steatosis is generally reversible with weight loss and/or lifestyle modification (diet and exercise). However, a small proportion of patients progress to more severe liver pathologies (see below). Hepatic lipid accumulation can occur as the result of one or more of the following: (1) increased fatty acid supply to the liver and increased fatty acid transporter expression; (2) increased de novo fatty acid and triglyceride synthesis; (3) decreased fatty acid oxidation; and (4) decreased synthesis and/or secretion of VLDL. Which of these processes predominates depends on the degree of obesity, total caloric intake, and diet composition. As the capacity of adipose tissue to expand is compromised with increasing BMI and insulin resistance develops in adipocytes, there is an increase in plasma non-esterified free fatty acids (NEFA) as the result of increased hydrolysis of triglycerides in fat by two enzymes—hormone-sensitive

lipase and adipose triglyceride lipase. Increased hepatic exposure to NEFA derived from adipose tissue or from dietary fats has been reported to increase fatty acid transporter expression in hepatocytes (Baumgardner *et al.*, 2008a; Marecki *et al.*, 2011). In contrast, excess calories in the form of simple carbohydrates results in increased de novo hepatic fatty acid synthesis (Shankar *et al.*, 2010). The type of dietary fat can also influence the development of steatosis. For example, it has been shown that saturated and polyunsaturated fatty acids can interfere with VLDL secretion relative to monounsaturated fatty acids via different mechanisms; whereas polyunsaturated fatty acids provoke oxidative stress and degradation of ApoB100 in hepatocytes, saturated fatty acids appear to block VLDL secretion via stimulation of an unfolded protein response and endoplasmic reticulum (ER) stress (Pan *et al.*, 2004; Caviglia *et al.*, 2011). In addition to increased NEFA, adipose tissue inflammation also appears to significantly contribute to development of NAFLD. Positive correlations have been reported between expression of macrophage markers in adipose tissue and liver fat content independent of total fat mass (Lara-Castro and Garvey, 2008).

Moreover, disrupted adipokine secretion also plays a role. The adipokine adiponectin acts on the liver to inhibit fatty acid synthesis and increase fatty acid degradation through activation of the AMP kinase cascade, downstream inhibition of SREBP-1c, and activation of the transcription factor peroxisome proliferator–activated receptor (PPAR)α. Reduced serum concentrations of adipokine adiponectin that accompany development of obesity will result in increased hepatic fatty acid synthesis and reduced fatty acid degradation and thus contribute to development of steatosis (Shankar *et al.*, 2010).

The other major site of ectopic fat deposition in obesity is skeletal muscle in the form of intramyocellular lipid (IMCL). Skeletal muscle contains an intracellular pool of stored triglyceride that exchanges with circulating free fatty acids. Although older methods such as biochemical extraction and computer tomography scans could quantitate muscle tissue triglycerides, more recent approaches such as Oil Red O staining of frozen sections and proton NMR spectroscopy are capable of quantifying IMCL distinct from extramyocellular fat in muscle tissue. Using these methods, IMCL has been shown to positively correlate with visceral adiposity. Various mechanisms have been proposed to underlie accumulation of IMCL in obesity. In adults it has been suggested that changes in intracellular distribution of the fatty acid transporter CD36 from soluble to membrane-associated pools are responsible for increased import of NEFA and triglyceride accumulation (Nickerson *et al.*, 2007). In contrast, data from a pediatric model of obesity demonstrated increased CD36 mRNA and protein expression in skeletal muscle associated with appearance of IMCL (Marecki *et al.*, 2011).

Metabolic Syndrome

The development of central obesity as a result of overnutrition and a sedentary lifestyle leads to a clustering of metabolic and physiological components in some individuals that is associated with a doubling of cardiovascular disease risk and a fivefold increase in incidence of type 2 diabetes originally described as "syndrome X" by Reaven (1988) or "insulin resistance syndrome" and more recently as MetS (Cornier *et al.*, 2008). Although the definition of MetS differs by health agency, all tend to agree that the core components include central obesity (waist circumference), insulin resistance (increased fasting glucose above 100 mg/dL and increased fasting insulin, as a result of impaired glucose uptake into skeletal muscle/fat and increased glucose output by the liver, resulting from end-organ insensitivity to insulin), dyslipidemia (decreased serum HDL below 40 mg/dL in men and 50 mg/dL in women, and increased serum triglycerides above 150 mg/dL), and hypertension (blood pressure higher than 130/85). The worldwide incidence of MetS is increasing rapidly with the obesity epidemic and is influenced by sex, age, and ethnicity. In the United States, prevalence of MetS is around 30% with higher rates in Mexican Americans than in white non-Hispanics and African Americans and increases with age into the sixth decade. Although there are no established criteria

for MetS in children and adolescents and prevalence values depend on age, population studied, and definition, among adolescents, overall incidence has been estimated to be 4.2% rising to 28.7% in those classified as obese (Cook *et al.*, 2008).

Although there does not appear to be a common unifying pathophysiological cause for all components of MetS, central obesity and insulin resistance appear to be the major drivers of this condition. The majority of obese individuals are insulin resistant but the correlation between obesity and insulin resistance is better for abdominal obesity/waist circumference than it is for overall BMI and better for whites than for African Americans. Moreover, weight loss following the feeding of low-calorie diets or following bariatric surgery rapidly leads to marked improvements in insulin sensitivity. However, the relationship between obesity and whole-body insulin resistance is not direct but appears to be mediated through increased circulating fatty acids and ectopic fat deposition particularly in IMCL in skeletal muscle (Fig. 27-2). Consumption of a very low-calorie diet in obese subjects for as little as five days has been shown to produce marked decreases in IMCL and enhanced insulin sensitivity without significant changes in body fat mass (Lara-Castro *et al.*, 2008). It has been suggested that reductions in glucose import into skeletal muscle with IMCL result from inhibition of translocation of the glucose transporter GLUT-4 from cytosolic- to membrane-associated compartments through the action of IMCL metabolites such as diacylglycerol, long-chain fatty acid CoAs, ceramides, and oxidized lipids (Pan *et al.*, 1997). Insulin resistance in muscle is accompanied by evidence of impaired mitochondrial function. However, it is unclear if this is a consequence of or contributor to IMCL (Lara-Castro and Garvey, 2008). Reduced glucose transport also occurs in insulin-resistant adipose tissue itself and the negative effects of obesity are exacerbated because reduced insulin signaling in adipocytes also enhances expression of hormone-sensitive and adipose triglyceride lipases to further increase the release of NEFA (Cornier *et al.*, 2008). The relationship between liver steatosis and hepatic insulin resistance is less clear and the question of whether NAFLD is a cause or a consequence of hepatic insulin resistance remains unresolved (Cohen *et al.*, 2011). Insulin resistance in liver leads to excess glucose production as the result of a reduced ability of insulin to suppress the gluconeogenic enzyme phosphoenolpyruvate

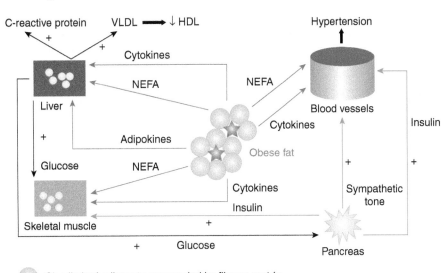

Figure 27-2. *Pathogenesis of metabolic syndrome.*

carboxykinase (PEPCK). This contributes to systemic hyperglycemia and increased pancreatic insulin production. Insulin resistance and steatosis are strongly correlated and interventions that lead to lower plasma insulin levels also decrease liver triglyceride content. Moreover, patients producing hepatic insulin as a result of metastatic insulin-secreting tumors develop steatosis in the surrounding hepatocytes. However, the suggestion that steatosis causes hepatic insulin resistance is contradicted by data from genetically manipulated mouse models where reduced fatty acid mobilization, reduced fatty acid oxidation, and defective choline synthesis are all associated with development of steatosis, but where hepatic insulin sensitivity is maintained (Cohen *et al.*, 2011).

The dyslipidemia associated with MetS is believed to be a direct consequence of increased VLDL secretion by the liver. Increased serum triglycerides are generally associated with a change in HDL size and lipid composition, and reduction of serum HDL concentration as a result of increased clearance via the kidney. Several different mechanisms have been proposed to explain the rise in blood pressure associated with MetS. Insulin acts both directly as a vasodilator and secondarily to increase sodium resorption from the kidney. Evidence suggests that under conditions of insulin resistance, the vasodilatory effects of insulin are lost while the renal effect on sodium resorption is maintained. In addition, fatty acids can act directly to mediate vasoconstriction and both fatty acids and insulin can increase the activity of the sympathetic nervous system. Adipokines, such as leptin and resistin, have also been implicated in the pathogenesis of obesity-associated hypertension (Cornier *et al.*, 2008).

Therapeutic Options for Managing Metabolic Syndrome

Since it is unclear that there is a unifying mechanism underlying the constellation of metabolic and physiological abnormalities that make up MetS, management can be problematic. Lifestyle modifications in the obese, including diets producing stable weight loss and long-term increased physical activity or bariatric surgery (discussed below), are of benefit in treating all the components of MetS, but suffer from limited compliance and significant risk of complications in the case of surgery. Therefore, routine clinical management of MetS has focused on pharmaceutical therapies for insulin resistance/hyperglycemia, dyslipidemia, and hypertension to reduce the risks of cardiovascular disease and type 2 diabetes.

Several classes of drugs are used to target insulin resistance. Metformin acts on the liver to reduce hepatic glucose production as a result of activation of the AMP kinase pathway (Boyle *et al.*, 2010). Moreover, metformin is relatively nontoxic and has been shown to reduce progression from hyperglycemia to type 2 diabetes and the incidence of cardiovascular disease (Knowler *et al.*, 2002; Ratner *et al.*, 2005). Thiazolidinediones such as pioglitazone and rosiglitazone also improve insulin sensitivity and slow progression of diabetes in about 50% of patients as a result of activation of the transcription factor PPARγ in extrahepatic tissues and increasing circulating levels of adiponectin (Gerstein *et al.*, 2006; Cho and Momose, 2008). However, increased insulin sensitivity is associated with an expansion of adipose tissue and significantly increased body weight because PPARγ regulates adipocyte differentiation. Moreover, a recently discovered adverse effect of thiazolidinediones is increased bone loss and an increased risk of osteoporosis, since PPARγ activation in bone inhibits osteoblastogenesis and stimulates accumulation of fat cells in bone marrow (Lecka-Czernik, 2010). Additional concerns have been raised regarding

potential for increased cardiovascular problems in patients taking rosiglitazone (Palee *et al.*, 2011).

Dyslipidemia associated with MetS is a major modifiable risk factor for cardiovascular disease. Increased triglycerides and low HDL levels are often accompanied by increased total and LDL cholesterol and LDL is a primary target for cholesterol-lowering therapy. Standard first-line therapy is statin inhibitors of 3-hydroxy-3-methyl glutaryl coenzyme A (HMG-CoA), the rate-limiting step in cholesterol biosynthesis, such as atorvastatin (Lipitor®). These compounds improve overall lipid profiles by decreasing LDL concentrations 20% to 40%, increasing HDL 5% to 10%, and decreasing triglycerides 7% to 30% (McFarlane *et al.*, 2002). Although generally well tolerated, atorvastatin results in muscle or joint pain in 5% of patients. Muscle pain can be an indication of rhabdomyolysis (muscle breakdown). In addition, liver injury as indicated by elevated serum values of liver enzymes such as alanine aminotransferase (ALT) has been reported in some users (Bakker-Arkema *et al.*, 1996). Statins are often used in combination with bile acid sequestrants such as ezetimibe or niacin to further reduce LDL and triglycerides and raise HDL levels. In addition to statins, high doses of 2 to 4 g of fish oil omega-3 fatty acids such as eicosapentaenoic acid (EPA) and docosahexaenoic acid (DHA) have been shown to reduce serum triglycerides by 20% to 40% (Cornier *et al.*, 2008).

Control of hypertension is also the key to prevention of cardiovascular events. Many antihypertensive drugs are available and are taken chronically. The most commonly prescribed are adrenergic β-blockers, which inhibit sympathetic inputs to reduce cardiovascular output and slow heart rate. Despite substantial decreases in systolic and diastolic blood pressure, long-term prospective studies suggest that treated hypertensive men continue to have a much greater risk of stroke and coronary heart disease than normotensive men of the same age in the second decade of treatment (Deshmukh *et al.*, 2008). This may be due to metabolic side effects, particularly increased serum triglycerides and lowering of HDL. In addition, diuretics are often given in combination with β-blockers. This can result in reductions of serum potassium and increased occurrence of gout in patients with marginal uric acid concentrations. Other front-line antihypertensive drugs are the angiotensin-converting enzyme (ACE) inhibitors. ACE inhibitors work on the renin–angiotensin system by preventing the conversion of angiotensin I to angiotensin II and reducing production of the hormone aldosterone. Aldosterone acts to reduce sodium and water excretion and is a direct vasoconstrictor. ACE inhibitors reduce arteriolar resistance, increase venous capacity, and increase cardiac output while increasing sodium excretion. ACE inhibitors in general have favorable effects on lipid profile.

Nonalcoholic Steatohepatitis (NASH)

As described above, ectopic fat deposition in the liver is strongly correlated with obesity and insulin resistance. Although NAFLD is not considered a core symptom of MetS, it is often a comorbidity. Fatty liver is very common being found in 30% of autopsies and in >80% of the obese. However, for reasons that remain unclear, in the majority of cases, steatosis is reversible and relatively asymptomatic. The disease progression of NAFLD is first to NASH, which is characterized by cell death, inflammation, and fibrosis, then to cirrhosis in which liver function is significantly impaired, and ultimately to hepatocellular carcinoma (Fig. 27-3) (Cohen *et al.*, 2011). Only about 30% of individuals with NAFLD show evidence of progression of pathology to NASH and of these, only 20% to 30% progress further to cirrhosis

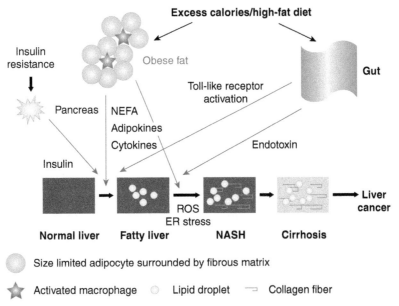

Figure 27-3. *Progression of nonalcoholic fatty liver disease (NAFLD).* ROS, Reactive oxygen species; ER stress, Endoplasmic reticulum stress.

within 10 years. Of those with NASH-induced cirrhosis, 4% to 27% ultimately develop liver cancer. NASH was first described by Ludwig *et al.* in 1980 in a group of obese adults without a history of alcohol abuse and has increased in prevalence with the obesity epidemic to about 2% to 3% of the US population. It is also increasingly observed in the pediatric population including cases in children as young as two years of age (Loomba *et al.*, 2009). Although steatosis can be diagnosed noninvasively using ultrasound or imaging, improved methods for early detection of NASH are urgently required. Although elevated serum ALT values increase the likelihood of NASH, up to 59% of NASH patients had normal ALTs and at present, only liver biopsy can provide accurate diagnosis.

Our understanding of the molecular mechanisms whereby NAFLD pathology progresses is hampered by lack of an animal model that recapitulates all aspects of the human disease (Hebbard and George, 2011). Until recently, a widely held "two-hit" hypothesis held that progression of NAFLD to NASH requires initial development of steatosis followed by several possible second hits. These include oxidative stress resulting from lipid peroxidation and mitochondrial dysfunction and ER stress triggered by protein misfolding resulting from direct lipotoxicity of saturated fatty acids. In addition, bacterial overgrowth and increased gut permeability resulting from chronic consumption of high-fat diets can increase plasma endotoxin levels resulting in Kuppfer cell activation and inflammation. An initiating role for steatosis in NASH progression is supported by human studies of NAFLD heritability. NAFLD, NASH, and cirrhosis cluster in families and one genetic variant consistently associated with appearance of NAFLD is a missense mutation in the PNPLA3 (adiponutrin) gene. PNPLA3 has triglyceride hydrolase activity that is lost on mutation, consistent with the accumulation of liver fat. In addition, treatment with insulin sensitizers, bariatric surgery, and lifestyle modification (diet and exercise) resulting in weight loss and reduction of hepatic fat content improve NASH liver pathology (Cohen *et al.*, 2011). More recently the two-hit hypothesis has been modified into a multiple interrelated hit theory as evidence has accumulated that factors derived from obese adipose tissue such as adipokines and the proinflammatory cytokine tumor necrosis factor (TNFα), activation of the endogenous immune system through Toll-like receptors, and

ER stress can all increase hepatic fat accumulation in addition to producing inflammation (Hebbard and George, 2011; Tilg and Moschen, 2010). The development of necroinflammatory injury in NASH livers appears to depend on oxidative stress and TNF. Treatment with dietary antioxidants such as the glutathione precursor *N*-acetylcysteine and vitamin E has recently been shown to prevent increases in serum ALT, suppress hepatic production of TNF, and improve NASH pathology (Baumgardner *et al.*, 2008a,b; Sanyal *et al.*, 2010). Development of fibrosis subsequent to NASH appears to involve activation of hepatic stellate cells by the cytokine transforming growth factor β (TGFβ) and inappropriate secretion of matrix components, particularly collagen, as a result of regenerative wound-healing responses to chronic liver injury and proliferative regenerative responses also ultimately promote development of hepatocellular carcinomas (Dooley *et al.*, 2009; Matsuzaki, 2009; Nejak-Gowen and Monga, 2011).

Alteration in Drug Pharmacokinetics and Metabolism in Obesity and NAFLD

Obesity and fatty liver disease can have significant effects on drug pharmacokinetics, metabolism, and therapeutic efficacy with the potential to result in adverse drug reactions (Hanley *et al.*, 2010; Merrell and Cherrington, 2011).

The most significant change in drug pharmacokinetics associated with obesity is likely to be in volume of distribution (Vd), and this determines loading dose selection. Vd estimates the extent to which a drug distributes into extravascular tissues and this in turn will depend on the drug's physiochemical properties, binding to plasma proteins, and tissue blood flow. The Vd of lipid-soluble drugs that partition readily into adipose tissue is likely to be significantly increased in obesity because obese individuals have a larger fat compartment into which the drug can distribute. In contrast, Vd for hydrophilic drugs that do not readily partition into fat may be relatively unaffected (Hanley *et al.*, 2010). For example, whereas the Vd for the highly lipophilic drug docetaxel is increased by more than 400 L in the obese, the Vd for the water-soluble drug daptomycin is increased by only 2 to 4 L. There are little data to suggest that obesity significantly alters drug binding to albumin or other plasma proteins. However, reductions in tissue blood flow and altered cardiovascular function have been observed in obesity and may further alter Vd. Increases in Vd in obesity may significantly alter drug efficacy. For example, the disposition of lipid-soluble oral contraceptives such as ethinyl estradiol have been shown to be altered in obesity and increased weight may be associated with increased risk of failure of contraception. In such circumstances drug loading dose should be adjusted by total body weight or BMI.

The major influence determining the steady-state plasma concentration of a drug in a maintenance dose regimen is clearance (CL). This in turn depends on rate of metabolism and expression of drug transporters. Obesity and NAFLD appear to have variable effects on hepatic phase I and II drug metabolism and on transporters. However, significant species differences in regulation of these enzymes and transporters and lack of appropriate animal models for NAFLD/NASH make extrapolation of much of the experimental data to the clinic problematic (Merrell and Cherrington, 2011). Obesity and NAFLD have been shown to increase expression of the cytochrome P450 enzyme CYP2E1 in both animal models and human clinical studies. CYP2E1 is involved in the metabolism of ethanol, solvents, and volatile anesthetics such as halothane and enflurane. In contrast, hepatic expression of CYP1A2 that metabolizes approximately 15% of therapeutic drugs including anticoagulants, antidepressants, antihypertensive drugs, and cyclooxygenase-2 inhibitors appears to be consistently suppressed. The effects of NAFLD/NASH on expression of other cytochrome P450 enzymes are inconsistent. However, increases have been observed in expression of other phase I enzymes including NAD(P)H quinone oxidoreductase, the mitochondrial form of epoxide hydrolase, and several aldehyde dehydrogenases in animal models of NAFLD. Less is known about the effects of NAFLD/NASH on drug conjugation and transport. Decreased expression of sulfotransferases has been reported in NASH patients, but effects on drug glucuronidation are inconsistent and glutathione conjugation appears mixed despite observations of GSH depletion in human NAFLD patients. Recent studies in experimental rat models of NAFLD suggest decreased expression of hepatic uptake transporters such as NTCP and the OATPs and increased expression of efflux transporters, such as the multidrug resistance-associated proteins Mrp2, Mrp3, and Mrp4 (Fischer *et al.*, 2009; Lickteig *et al.*, 2007). This was accompanied by a proportional shift in elimination of acetaminophen metabolites from bile to urine.

Drug elimination as measured by half-life is affected by both Vd and CL and thus may also be altered in obesity. Half-life is calculated using the following formula: $t_{1/2} = (\ln 2 \times Vd)/CL$, and thus changes in both Vd and CL can influence drug half-life. For example, the $t_{1/2}$ of the antidepressant diazepam is markedly increased in obese subjects as a result of increased Vd even though CL is unchanged.

Endocrine Dysfunction in Obesity, Metabolic Syndrome, and NAFLD

A wide spectrum of endocrine disruption is associated with obesity and MetS. Obesity in pregnancy can result in many complications including gestational diabetes, pregnancy-associated hypertension, preeclampsia, and fetal abnormalities including neural tube defects, spina bifida, heart defects, and cleft palate (Kulie *et al.*, 2011). In addition, delays in milk production and decreased duration of breast-feeding have been associated with obesity in women as a result of hormonal and metabolic effects on mammary gland development during pregnancy.

As discussed above, hyperglycemia resulting from systemic insulin resistance provokes a compensatory increase in insulin

secretion from the pancreas in obese individuals. Hyperinsulinemia then appears to have secondary effects on other endocrine systems. For example, growth hormone (GH) secretion is dramatically suppressed by obesity in both adults and children, but can be reversed by weight loss (Kreitschmann-Andermahr *et al.*, 2010). Mechanisms appear to involve direct feedback effects of insulin on the pituitary and a reduction in secretion of the endogenous GH-releasing peptide ghrelin that is produced by the stomach and hypothalamic centers. In addition, although reductions in GH lead to a decrease in hepatic synthesis and serum concentrations of total insulin-like growth factor (IGF-1) in the obese, paradoxically obesity results in a suppression of IGF-binding proteins and thus an increase in free IGF-1. Free IGF-1 can also exert a negative feedback on GH secretion. In addition to effects on the GH–IGF axis, hyperinsulinemia also appears to increase adrenal androgen production and reduce plasma concentrations of sex hormone–binding globulin (SHBG) in obese prepubertal girls (Burt Solorzano and McCartney, 2010). Increased serum concentrations of free androgens appear to explain, in part, why childhood obesity is associated with earlier pubertal development. Rodent studies of high-fat feeding have demonstrated accelerated vaginal opening that was reversed by both androgen receptor blockade and normalization of glucose homeostasis with metformin. Hyperandrogenization also appears to explain the increased incidence of polycystic ovary syndrome (PCOS) in obese adolescent girls with MetS, anovulatory cycles, and subfertility in obese women of childbearing age. Increased adipose tissue mass also results in increased estrogen production as a result of androgen aromatization in fat tissues. This may also contribute to accelerated puberty in girls. Surprisingly, in obese boys, data suggest that puberty may be delayed. This may also be related to increased aromatization of androgens in adipose tissue because negative feedback of estrogens at the level of the hypothalamic–pituitary axis may result in reduced luteinizing hormone secretion and reduced testosterone production (hypogonadotropic hypogonadism). In addition to suppression in GH and gonadotropin secretion, hypothyroidism is common in individuals with MetS. Reduced thyroid hormone concentrations may exacerbate NASH progression in the liver by increasing triglyceride synthesis, reducing fatty acid oxidation, and increasing hepatic cholesterol concentrations by reducing conversion to bile acids (Loria *et al.*, 2009).

Obesity and Cancer Risk

Increased BMI is well known to be associated with significantly increased risk of a number of cancers. These include sex-steroid-dependent endometrial, breast, and prostate cancer, GI tract cancers such as esophageal adenocarcinoma, and colon cancer and renal cancer (Table 27-1). Several mechanisms have been proposed related to endocrine and metabolic disturbances associated with obesity (Roberts *et al.*, 2010). As described above, systemic insulin resistance results in hyperinsulinemia and reduces plasma IGF-1-binding protein levels to increase free IGF-1 concentrations. Insulin and IGF-1 cross-talk through each other's receptors to stimulate cell proliferation via activation of MAP-kinase cascades resulting in increased phosphorylation of ERK and via activation of Wnt-β-catenin pathways. In addition, they exert antiapoptotic effects through PI-3 kinase pathways. Increased sex steroid concentrations in obesity promote growth of tumors in the mammary gland, endometrium, and prostate. Adipokines may also play a role in promotion of obesity-associated cancers. Leptin that is increased as fat mass increases is proproliferative, antiapoptotic, and proinflammatory and promotes new blood vessel formation (angiogenesis). In contrast, adiponectin that is suppressed in obesity has the opposite

Table 27-1		
Estimated Risk Ratios* for Cancer in Relation to BMI		
CANCER TYPE	MEN	WOMEN
Colon cancer	1.24	1.09
Gallbladder cancer	—	1.59
Leukemia	1.08	1.17
Malignant melanoma	1.17	—
Multiple myeloma	1.11	1.11
Esophageal adenocarcinoma	1.52	1.51
Renal cancer	1.24	1.34
Thyroid cancer	1.33	1.14
Prostate cancer	1.03	—
Postmenopausal breast cancer	—	1.12
Endometrial cancer[†]	—	1.73

Per increase in BMI by 5 kg/m^2 (Roberts et al., 2010).
[†]*For BMIs above 27 kg/m^2.*

properties and is inversely associated with the presence of cancer. Additional potential associations between obesity and cancer may involve depletion of cellular antioxidant systems as a result of the low-grade chronic systemic inflammation that accompanies morbid obesity and the possibility that mesenchymal stromal cells arising from expanding white adipose tissue may be recruited to tumors to promote angiogenesis and drive tumor progression (Roberts et al., 2010).

HEALTH BENEFITS AND LIFE EXTENSION ASSOCIATED WITH CALORIC RESTRICTION

The opposite of overfeeding is CR (also known as dietary restriction). Over the past two decades, CR has been repeatedly shown to increase life span and reduce age-related disease in comparison with ad libitum feeding in a wide variety of organisms including yeast, nematodes, fruit flies, fish, many rodent species, and dogs (Smith et al., 2010). Recently, Colman et al. (2009) have reported similar findings in rhesus monkeys and a multisite human randomized clinical research study is currently in progress funded by the National Institute on Aging (NIA): Comprehensive Assessment of Long-Term Effects of Reducing Intake of Energy (the CALERIE study, http://calerie.dcri.duke.edu/index.html). Preliminary data suggest reproduction of many of the results from animal studies including reduced fat and lean mass, reduced insulin, reduced energy expenditure, lower core body temperature, and improved lipid profiles. It has been suggested that the increased health and longevity associated with CR is related to reduced energy flow, increased insulin sensitivity, and reduced inflammation (Ye and Keller, 2010). Studies in yeast, C. elegans, and Drosophila have suggested that the life span–enhancing effects of CR are mediated through activation of a family of histone deacetylases known as the sirtuins (Sir), which act as sensors of nutrient flux (Smith et al., 2010). Intensive studies are underway to identify CR mimetics that might have the same benefits as CR on long-term health and longevity without the necessity for imposed food restriction. Most work has focused on the grape polyphenol resveritol that has been shown to activate Sir2 and to mimic CR effects to increase life span

in yeast, C. elegans, Drosophila, and fish in the absence of nutrient alteration. A second CR mimetic receiving significant attention is rapamycin, an inhibitor of the nutrient signaling mediator target of rapamycin (TOR).

TREATMENT OF OBESITY

Lifestyle Modification: Dieting and Exercise

As applied to body composition, dieting involves a plan or regimen to improve body composition. Trimming excess body fat generally requires reductions in total caloric intake, increases in the TEE (exercise or physical activity), and modifications in diet composition. This combined strategy is intended to reduce energy intake to a level low enough to drive the body to utilize stored fat as an energy source, thereby burning body fat.

Almost any commercially available diet plan on the market can achieve body weight loss and reduction of total fat mass. For example, people who use the Atkins diet, which is a diet high in protein and fat and very low in carbohydrates, definitely lose weight. The major problem is sustaining a healthy body composition. Most dieters return to their predieting weight and body composition (or worse) because they never achieve a true lifestyle change that meets their expectations. Comprehensive lifestyle changes that promote sustainability include two major and closely linked components: (1) learning to consume only the amount of calories from high-quality foods necessary to support basal body energy needs plus energy needs to maintain physical activity; and (2) selecting a reasonable physical activity plan that fits into the dieters' overall lifestyle patterns. Sustaining healthy body composition after significant weight loss seems to occur only in those individuals who can find a way to limit their intake of a healthy diet that they find acceptable in terms of taste, costs, and ease (food availability and ease and speed of preparation), plus an exercise regime that is acceptable in terms of access (eg, equipment, facilities, walking trails), appropriateness (eg, age-related, intensity levels), and time (eg, duration required, timing within a workday). Thus, losing weight and getting a healthy body composition comes down to energy balance, that is, consuming less energy than needed to maintain a given body composition. Maintaining a health body composition requires that energy intake equals energy expenditure. Promoting health in the context of a healthy body composition can be best achieved by including a physical activity plan, and this usually leads to healthier muscle, improved insulin sensitivity, normalization of blood lipid profiles, and improved cardiovascular measures.

Determining the energy needs is the easiest part of a plan, whereas limiting caloric intake, increasing physical activity, and sustaining these components of a plan are more difficult. In terms of energy, 3500 cal is stored in 1 lb of fat. So to lose or take off that pound of fat, the body needs to be forced to "burn" 3500 cal from adipose tissue. That pound of fat was formed over time and under conditions in which calorie intake exceeded caloric output. The energy in food eaten can be "cost accounted" roughly as follows: (1) energy required to digest and absorb food; (2) energy utilized to support basal functions such as pumping blood and breathing; (3) energy for body functions other than basal functions such as walking and playing golf; and (4) nonutilized food calories such as food components not fully digested or absorbed. Most generally healthy people have similar energy expenditure needs as described in points 1, 2, and 4 above, although there clearly are individual differences. The energy expenditure of a body at rest is termed the BMR and it can be estimated by the Harris–Benedict equations. Energy expenditures also differ by age, gender, and body

size (height and weight). For example, according to the Harris–Benedict equations, a man and a woman (each healthy and normal body composition) of age 66 years, weighing 160 lb, and 70 in tall would have a BMR of 1528 and 1372 cal, respectively. However, if they were each of age 18 years, their BMR would be 1854 and 1598 cal, respectively. No matter what a person's excess weight might be, there will always be the need for energy to meet the BMR. The energy needs of BMR could be met by diet or, in the case of overweight individuals, body energy stores such as fat. Because there are other nutrient needs besides energy (eg, nitrogen, amino acids, essential fatty acids, vitamins, minerals, and trace elements), an overweight individual will always have needs for a healthy diet, even for the short term, so fasting is usually not a long-term option to burn all excess stored body fat. Thus, to burn excess body fat, daily energy expenditure needs to exceed the energy expenditure of BMR and this comes mainly from physical activity.

The general public tends to overestimate the energy expenditure for various physical activities. It also finds it difficult to practically translate the often-recommended amount of physical activity (30 minutes of activity per day) into a daily regimen. Part of this is due to the difficultly in determining the energy expenditure amount, because the energy expended by an individual on 30 minutes of physical activity differs according to body weight, body composition, health, physical conditioning, and the activity itself (eg, walking, jogging at 4 miles/h, running a four-minute mile, or swimming a mile). In addition, overweight people are usually not accustomed to physical activity at the intensity level and duration needed to induce the body to burn body fat stores that lead to significant body fat reduction. This, when combined with the necessary changes in the diet composition and reductions in caloric intake, makes it difficult to lose body fat and more difficult to maintain a healthy body composition. The most common physical activity used in weight loss programs is walking. Walking 30 minutes at a rate of 4 miles/h for the 160-lb man or woman described above will burn approximately 180 cal. So if an overweight individual were to maintain the same caloric intake (and same diet) and just increase his or her activity level to 30 minutes of walking at 4 miles/h (a total of 2 miles per day), the calculated fat loss would be 1 lb every 20 days. If he or she also reduced the caloric intake by 180 cal a day and has the same walk schedule, he or she would reduce the time to lose 1 lb of weight to about 10 days. Thus, the way to reduce body fat (adipose tissue) is to consume less calories than expended (energy deficit) and the rate of fat loss is directly related to the level of the energy deficit (ie, caloric intake vs caloric expenditure).

Complicit in any plan to burn body fat stores is that some portion of the TEE must be met by fat stores. This requires a diet intake situation that: (1) provides fewer calories than required to meet BMR + any physical activity expenditure; (2) reduces or prevents lipogenesis; and (3) promotes lipolysis. There are several ways and several commercially available diet systems in which this can be accomplished. One of the most widely used diet systems, the Atkins diet, claims to accomplish this by increasing protein (and consequently fat) and limiting carbohydrates. Below the theory of this diet is presented as an illustration.

Following a meal containing an abundance of simple carbohydrates, blood glucose levels rise and glucose gets converted into glycogen by the liver and stored there for future energy use. Maximal glycogen storage is between about eight and 14 hours, depending on factors such as an individual's metabolism. As glucose enters cells, blood glucose concentrations would fall if not for the liver converting the glycogen back to glucose and releasing it back into the blood. This is a mechanism for maintaining glucose in the normal range between meals. Glucose is the body's energy source of choice.

Use of glucose as the primary energy source seems to be prioritized by cell and organ type, with nerve cells having the highest priority. This means that if body glucose stores become scarce, the brain will be the last organ able to use glucose as its primary source. In this case, if another carbohydrate-containing meal is not consumed and blood glucose levels dropped to very low levels, lower priority organs (such as muscle) would need another source of energy and this source is fatty acids released from fat stores (lipolysis). Just like glycogen is the storage form for glucose, fat is the storage source for fatty acids and tissues can easily burn fatty acids when glucose is absent. As liver glycogen stores become minimal, amino acids are converted to glucose (gluconeogenesis). This can support nerve cell metabolism for a while, but eventually the brain will switch from burning pure glucose and start to utilize ketone bodies produced in the liver from fatty acids as an additional energy source. High ketone levels in the blood and tissues are known as ketosis.

Insulin has a major influence on carbohydrate, fat, and protein metabolism. Under conditions of adequate carbohydrate intake, insulin causes excess sugar not utilized as fuel to be stored as fat and prevents utilization of fat as an energy source. Thus, a high-carbohydrate diet tends to induce insulin secretion, which promotes carbohydrate energy storage as fat and tends to reduce the utilization of fat as an energy source. In theory, the low carbohydrate, high protein intake promoted in the Atkins diet forces the body to burn more fat. This would call for the body to switch from using pure carbohydrates for fuel to using more fat for fuel and the source of this fat is the adipose tissue. Thus, when insulin levels are normal, the body will begin to burn its own fat as fuel, thereby resulting in body weight loss.

Toxic Effects of Dieting

There are potential toxic effects associated with some diet plans. Dieting as described in this chapter is based on the use of a healthy diet that meets the daily nutrient needs of the body, but at a reduced caloric intake and with increased moderate physical activity. The overarching premise is to provide adequate nutrients for normal cellular function, while reducing caloric intake to a level that forces the use of fat stores as an energy source to meet the energy expenditure above the caloric intake. If the diet does not include all the required nutrients (an imbalanced diet), metabolism will suffer and with time this can result in health problems. This is true whether in the case of deficiency of specific nutrients (deficiency disorders such as anemia or osteoporosis) or toxicity caused by excesses of a particular nutrient (such as thyroid impairment, vitamin deficiencies, mental confusion). Some popular diet plans call for excess intake of a particular food and these can not only alter metabolism but also interfere with medications. For example, the popular grapefruit diet can lead to inhibition of drug-metabolizing enzymes such as the cytochrome P450 CYP3As that metabolize 60% of all therapeutic medications. This may increase drug concentrations to toxic levels, increase drug–drug interactions, and result in potential health problems (Ameer and Weintraub, 1997; Kiani and Imam, 2007).

Another potential adverse effect of dieting is known as the yo-yo effect or weight cycling. This occurs with repeated dieting interspersed with periods of no dieting. This is caused when a dieter starts one diet and loses a significant amount of body weight and body fat, but cannot maintain the diet and stops to return to the prediet routine. The fat and body weight are regained, often times to an even greater body fat. In fact, the yo-yo experience may actually result in a condition in which the dieter is more efficient in gaining weight. This results in the dieter selecting another

diet plan, loss of weight, failure to maintain the diet, and return to overweight or obese conditions. There are often periods of depression and fatigue associated with this cycling behavior and the end results are extreme emotional and physical ramifications. Whether the yo-yo dieter has other health issues remains ill-defined and controversial.

Drug Therapy for Weight Loss

In addition to the diet plans described above, many overweight individuals turn to drug therapy to help lose body weight. Appetite suppressants, for example, sympathomimetics such as diethylpropion, attempt to lessen the psychological motivation for food, usually by acting on central nervous system appetite control centers, such as those in the hypothalamus (Guaraldi *et al.*, 2011). Although sympathomimetics can be used for long periods of time, their appetite-reducing effects tend to decrease after a few weeks in many people. Thus, appetite suppressants are often used in the early stages of a weight loss program. People are likely to lose weight while taking sympathomimetics, but the weight loss is generally temporary without modifications in diet composition, eating behavior, and physical activity. Short-term use is usually accompanied by minor side effects such as thirst, irritability, constipation, stomach pain, dizziness, dryness of mouth, heightened sense of well-being, headache, irritability, nausea, nervousness or restlessness, trembling or shaking, and trouble sleeping. However, long-term use of appetite suppressants often times leads to more serious side effects: intracerebral hemorrhage, acute dystonia, myocardial injury, psychosis, cerebral arteritis, cardiac arrhythmias, heart valve damage, and even fatal pulmonary hypertension. These side effects have led to the withdrawal of several such products from the market. Drug interactions are also known to occur, especially with high blood pressure medicine, stimulants, MAO inhibitors (eg, furazolidone, linezolid, phenelzine, selegiline, tranylcypromine), any other weight loss medicine, and decongestants such as are commonly found in over-the-counter cough and cold medicines.

Surgical Interventions

Surgery is another avenue to improve body composition in obesity. One of the most radical surgical treatments is the class operations known as bariatric surgeries. The end goal is to limit food intake by reducing the capacity of the stomach, but also having patients feel satiated. Bariatric surgery is actually a term that includes several surgical procedures (such as sleeve gastrectomy, gastric plication, gastric banding, gastric bypass surgery); all are aimed at helping obese patients lose weight. Weight loss is achieved by resecting and linking the small intestines to a small stomach pouch (gastric bypass surgery), removal of a portion of the stomach (sleeve gastrectomy), or reducing the size of the stomach with an implanted medical device (gastric banding) or sutures (gastric plication). These procedures are generally credited with significant long-term loss of body fat and body weight, which leads to improvement of secondary conditions caused by obesity, including type 2 diabetes, risk of cardiovascular disease, and the rate of mortality (Robinson, 2009).

These operations are most commonly used to treat morbid obesity and the comorbidities associated with it. Thus, bariatric surgery may be recommended for people with a BMI >40. These procedures have also been used successfully with obese individuals with BMI 30 to 40, especially when there are serious coexisting medical conditions such as hypertension, impaired glucose tolerance, diabetes mellitus, hyperlipidemia, and obstructive sleep apnea. Most bariatric procedures result in rapid weight loss, which is also associated with gallstones, and many surgeons prefer to remove the gallbladder at the time of bariatric surgery. Malabsorption and nutritional deficiency can occur because of reduced absorptive area. This can reduce calcium and vitamin absorption. Poor calcium absorption can occur because calcium transporters are located in areas of the intestine (duodenum) that may be removed with bariatric surgery. This can cause metabolic bone disease (osteopenia) and secondary hyperparathyroidism that increase in bone turnover. Combined, these conditions decrease bone mass and increase risk of fracture. Other deficiencies including iron and micronutrients such as vitamin B_{12}, fat-soluble vitamins, thiamine, and folate are common. Many patients will need to take a daily multivitamin pill for life to compensate for reduced absorption of essential nutrients. Because patients cannot eat a large quantity of food, physicians typically recommend a diet that is relatively high in protein and low in fats and alcohol.

Liposuction is another surgical procedure widely used to improve body composition by physically and surgically removing body fat. It is the most common "plastic surgical procedure" in the United States. However, there are significant risks with this procedure and these are mainly associated with: (1) the aggressiveness with which the procedure is performed, especially the amount of tissue sucked from the body; (2) the venues in which the procedures are performed; and (3) the amount of anesthesia used to sedate patients during increasingly lengthy procedures. The mortality rate of the late 1990s was approximately 20 per 100,000 or 1 per 5000 cases (de Jong and Grazer, 2001).

ECONOMIC, SOCIOLOGICAL, AND LEGAL ASPECTS OF THE OBESITY EPIDEMIC

Health Insurance and Obesity

Obesity is not considered an illness for most insurance purposes. However, obesity can affect the cost of health insurance because as a group, obese people have a significantly greater risk of cardiovascular disease, hypertension, type 2 diabetes, and other health issues than lean people. Thus, insurance companies factor obesity into the cost of first-time insurance purchasers. Furthermore, people who are already insured may unknowingly not have sufficient insurance to cover health problems associated with obesity. Several health insurance companies use BMI as a measure of obesity and use BMI to compute disease risk and health insurance premiums. Obesity can result in high premiums and in the case of morbidly obese individuals, insurers may decline their application. Obesity is also regarded by insurance companies as a substantial risk for both life and disability policies.

Mortality statistics for life insurance were the earliest indicator that the cost of obesity to the individual was decreased life span and increased illness, particularly diseases affecting the cardiovascular and musculoskeletal systems. The prevalence of coronary heart disease rises with increases in the BMI in both men and women. Hypertension and diabetes in the obese add further to the risks of vascular disease. Cigarette smoking also greatly augments the health risks of obesity in both sexes.

The risk of death and medical problems increase with the degree or severity of obesity (as indicated by fat mass or BMI). The type of obesity (as indicated by body shape or fat distribution) is another aspect of obesity considered by insurance companies. Abdominal obesity has been positively correlated with the risk of heart disease and stroke. Thus, some insurance companies set rates in part on fat distribution. Disability insurance rates are also affected by body composition, as cardiovascular disease or musculoskeletal

illness associated with obesity greatly increases the chances of disabilities. All of these factors are used in decision making as to whether to insure an individual and the cost of premiums. Clearly, costs increase proportionally with the degree of obesity.

Changing the Environment: Family and Community Approaches to Healthy Eating and Physical Activity

The development of obesity within an individual, a community, or a country is complex and the central cause(s) or reason(s) underlying the rapid rise in obesity in the United States and the world is not well understood. The end results in terms of body composition and secondary medical problems associated with obesity are better understood than the root causes of the obesity epidemic. One factor, however, that has received much attention relates to basic practices that were common in past decades when the general population was leaner, but are lacking now when obesity is so prevalent.

Prior to 1970, the average BMI was 25.1 for men and 24.9 for women in the United States. Physical education (PE) classes were a regular feature of school curriculums; most meals were prepared at home using fresh produce, meats, and dairy products. School lunches were prepared at schools. It was common for children to walk or ride bicycles to school and to participate in games requiring physical activity during school recess and after school and on weekends. There were no computer games and fast food restaurants did not supply such a large proportion of the daily total calories. In the 1990s and 2000s, there are few schools with PE classes and fewer meals cooked from fresh components consumed at home and the lifestyle of today's children and adults is far more sedentary than that prior to 1970. As a consequence, by 2002, average BMI for US men had risen to 27.8 and average BMI for US women to 28.1.

One approach to fighting the obesity issue is to bring back many of those practices used in the past. There are initiatives to establish community gardens, build community walking and riding trails, and teach people cooking and shopping skills that lead to healthier meal preparation. School systems are starting to return to PE classes on a regular basis and remove high-density foods and drinks from vending machines. Although these efforts have been increasing in effort throughout the United States, it is still too early to confirm their effectiveness in reversing the obesity trend.

Food security and access to quality foods is an important issue throughout the United States, regardless of whether in rural America or in the inner city. In many areas there is ready access only to convenience food stores where there is a lack of fresh vegetable and meats and the prices are higher than in a conventional supermarket. The type of food available is poor quality and energy dense, which leads to obesity. These areas have been termed "food deserts." Providing access to higher-quality fresh food to people living in these areas will improve nutrition and when combined with education on how to select and prepare the food and linked to some form of physical activity, it is hoped that body composition and health will improve in these areas.

Food Labels

The Food and Drug Administration (FDA) is responsible for assuring that foods sold in the United States are properly labeled. This applies to foods produced domestically, as well as foods from foreign countries. The Federal Food, Drug, and Cosmetic Act (FD&C Act) and the Fair Packaging and Labeling Act are the federal laws governing food products under FDA's jurisdiction. The Nutrition Labeling and Education Act (NLEA), which amended the FD&C Act, requires most foods to bear nutrition labeling. The FDA requires food labels that bear nutrient content claims and certain health messages to comply with specific requirements.

Food labeling is required for most prepared foods, such as breads, cereals, canned and frozen foods, snacks, desserts, drinks, etc. Nutrition labeling for raw produce (fruits and vegetables) and fish is voluntary. Dietary supplements are a special category of products under the general umbrella of foods, but which has separate labeling requirements. "Functional foods" or "nutraceuticals" are regulated by FDA under the authority of the FD&C Act, but they are not specifically defined by law.

Food labels can be an important factor to help consumers in their food choices that can help prevent obesity and other diseases. Federal law requires that a minimal amount of information be listed on food packaging, including ingredients and nutrition data. The FDA monitors labeling language for such issues as fat, protein, carbohydrate, and other nutrient contents and the purported ability of a particular food to prevent medical problems. Suspicious or doubtful claims or misleading statements about nutrition and health benefits on food packages can be challenged by the FDA and companies that receive warning letters have 15 days to inform the agency of corrective action. Although there has been a formal process by which a health claim can be made, foods generally are not permitted to make disease-fighting claim. The types of claims often challenged by the FDA include warding off maladies such as arthritis, cancer, and heart disease.

The Patient Protection and Affordable Care Act of 2010 establishes requirements for nutrition labeling of standard menu items for chain restaurants, similar retail food establishments, and chain vending machine operators. The most important information that must be provided for standard menu items is the number of calories in each standard menu item and a statement on the menu that puts the calorie information in the context of a recommended total daily caloric intake. In addition to restaurant menus, food sold from vending machines operated by persons who own or operate 20 or more vending machines must disclose the amount of calories in a clear and conspicuous manner.

Governmental and Corporate Issues

There has been increasing pressures from local, state, and federal governments to regulate various aspects of food as a means of promoting health and reducing obesity and the secondary consequences of obesity. Food labeling is just one example of government intervention, whereby food processors and restaurants must provide a measure of nutrient and/or caloric content. New York City was the first to pass a law requiring calorie counts to be posted next to prices on menus in some restaurants so consumers would also know the "caloric cost" of each food selection, with the hope that they will make healthy food choices. California became the first state to prohibit restaurants from using "artery-clogging trans fats" in preparing their food. Airlines and the FAA are dealing with complaints from passengers being "infringed on" by overlapping obese passengers and obese passengers complaining about abuse taken from leaner passengers. In an effort to reduce insurance costs and improve work performance, there is also a trend for the business community to set standards associated for overweight and obese workers in a manner similar to that employed for smokers. Civil rights advocates and others are concerned that there is a growing impetus for government intervention and one wonders if the time will come when "big brother" mandates what and how much one can eat.

REFERENCES

Ameer B, Weintraub RA. Drug interactions with grapefruit juice. *Clin Pharmacokinet.* 1997;33:103–121.

Bakker-Arkema RG, Davidson MH, Goldstein RJ, et al. Efficacy and safety of a new HMG-CoA reductase inhibitor atorvastatin, in patients with hypertriglyceridemia. *JAMA.* 1996;275:128–133.

Barker DJ, Winter PD, Osmond C, et al. Weight in infancy and death from ischemic heart disease. *Lancet.* 1989;2:577–580.

Baumgardner JN, Shankar K, Hennings L, et al. A new rat model for nonalcoholic steatohepatitis utilizing overfeeding of diets high in polyunsaturated fat by total enteral nutrition. *Am J Physiol.* 2008a;294:G27–G38.

Baumgardner JN, Shankar K, Hennings L, et al. *N*-Acetylcysteine attenuates progression of liver pathology in a rat model of non-alcoholic steatohepatitis. *J Nutr.* 2008b;138:1872–1879.

Boyle JG, Salt IP, McKay GA. Metformin action on AMP-activated protein kinase: a translational research approach to understanding a potential new therapeutic target. *Diabet Med.* 2010;27:1097–1106.

Browning JD, Szczepaniak LS, Dobbins R, et al. Prevalence of hepatic steatosis in an urban population in the United States: impact of ethnicity. *Hepatology.* 2004;40:1387–1395.

Burt Solorzano CM, McCartney CR. Obesity and the pubertal transition in girls and boys. *Reproduction.* 2010;140:399–410.

Caviglia JM, Gayet C, Ota T, et al. Different fatty acids inhibit apolipoprotein B100 secretion by different pathways: unique roles for endoplasmic reticulum stress, ceramide and autophagy. *J Lipid Res.* 2011;52:1636–1651.

Cho N, Momose Y. Peroxisome proliferator-activated receptor gamma agonists as insulin sensitizers: from the discovery to recent progress. *Curr Top Med Chem.* 2008;8:1483–1507.

Cohen JC, Horton JD, Hobbs HH. Human fatty liver disease: old questions and new insights. *Science.* 2011;332:1519–1523.

Colman RJ, Anderson RM, Johnson SC, et al. Caloric restriction delays disease onset and mortality in rhesus monkeys. *Science.* 2009;325(5937):201–204.

Cook S, Weitzman M, Auinger P, et al. Prevalence of a metabolic syndrome phenotype in adolescents: findings from the third National Health and Nutrition Examination Survey 1999-2002. *J Pediatr.* 2008;152:160–164.

Cornier MA, Dabelea D, Hernandez TL, et al. The metabolic syndrome. *Endocr Rev.* 2008;29:777–822.

de Jong RH, Grazer FM. Perioperative management of cosmetic liposuction. *Plast Reconstructr Surg.* 2001;107:1039–1044.

Deshmukh M, Lee HW, McFarlane SI, et al. Antihypertensive medications and their effects on lipid metabolism. *Curr Diab Rep.* 2008;8:214–220.

Divoux A, Clement K. Architecture and the extracellular matrix: the still unappreciated components of adipose tissue. *Obes Rev.* 2011;12:e494–e503.

Dooley S, Weng H, Mertens PR. Hypotheses on the role of TGF beta in the onset and progression of hepatocellular carcinoma. *Dig Dis.* 2009;27:93–101.

Dulloo AG, Jacquet J, Solinas G, et al. Body composition phenotypes in pathways to obesity and the metabolic syndrome. *Int J Obes.* 2010;34:S4–S17.

Fischer CD, Lickteig AJ, Augustine LM, et al. Experimental non-alcoholic fatty liver disease results in decreased hepatic uptake transporter expression and function in rats. *Eur J Pharmacol.* 2009;613:119–127.

Franck N, Gummesson A, Jernas M, et al. Identification of adipocyte genes regulated by caloric intake. *J Clin Endocrinol Metab.* 2011;96:E413–E418.

Friedman JM, Leibel RL. Tackling a weighty problem. *Cell.* 1992;69:217–220.

Gerstein HC, Yusuf S, Bosch J, et al. Effect of rosiglitazone on the frequency of diabetes in patients with impaired glucose tolerance or impaired fasting glucose: a randomized controlled trial. *Lancet.* 2006;368:1096–1105.

Gropper SS, Smith JL, Groff JL. Body composition and energy expenditure. In: Gropper SS, Smith JL, Groff JL, eds. *Advanced Nutrition and Human Metabolism.* Belmont, CA: Thomson Wadsworth; 2005:519–550.

Guaraldi F, Pagotto U, Pasquali R. Predictors of weight loss and maintenance in patients treated with antiobesity drugs. *Diabetes Metab Syndr Obes.* 2011;4:229–243.

Gustafson B. Adipose tissue, inflammation and atherosclerosis. *J Atheroscler Thromb.* 2010;17:332–341.

Halberg N, Khan T, Trujillo ME, et al. Hypoxia-inducible factor 1 alpha induces fibrosis and insulin resistance in white adipose tissue. *Mol Cell Biol.* 2009;29:4467–4483.

Hanley MJ, Abernethy DR, Greenblatt DJ. Effect of obesity on the pharmacokinetics of drugs in humans. *Clin Pharmacokinet.* 2010;49:71–87.

Hebbard L, George J. Animal models of nonalcoholic fatty liver disease. *Nat Rev Gastroenterol Hepatol.* 2011;8:35–44.

Keesey RE, Hirvonen MD. Body weight set-points: determination and adjustment. *J Nutr.* 1997;127:1875S–1883S.

Kiani J, Imam SZ. Medicinal importance of grapefruit juice and its interaction with various drugs. *Nutr J.* 2007;6:33.

Knowler WC, Barrett-Connor E, Fowler SE, et al. Reduction in the incidence of type 2 diabetes with lifestyle intervention or metformin. *N Engl J Med.* 2002;346:393–403.

Kreitschmann-Andermahr I, Suarez P, Jennings R, et al. GH/IGF-1 regulation in obesity—mechanisms and practical consequences in children and adults. *Horm Res Pediatr.* 2010;73:153–160.

Kulie T, Slattengren A, Redmer J, et al. Obesity and women's health. An evidence-based review. *J Am Board Fam Med.* 2011;24:75–85.

Lara-Castro C, Garvey T. Intracellular lipid accumulation in liver and muscle and the insulin resistance syndrome. *Endocrinol Metab Clin North Am.* 2008;37:841–856.

Lara-Castro C, Newcomer BR, Rowell J, et al. Effects of short term very low-calorie diet on intramyocellular lipid and insulin sensitivity in nondiabetic and diabetic subjects. *Metabolism.* 2008;57:1–8.

Lecka-Czernik B. Bone loss in diabetes: use of antidiabetic thiazolidinediones and secondary osteoporosis. *Curr Osteoporosis Res.* 2010;8:178–184.

Lenard NR, Berthoud HR. Central and peripheral regulation of food intake and physical activity: pathways and genes. *Obesity.* 2008;16:S11–S22.

Lickteig AJ, Fischer CD, Augustine LM, et al. Efflux transporter expression and acetaminophen metabolite excretion are altered in rodent models of non-alcoholic fatty liver disease. *Drug Metab Dispos.* 2007;25:1970–1978.

Loomba R, Sirlin CB, Schwimmer JB, et al. Advances in pediatric nonalcoholic fatty liver disease. *Hepatology.* 2009;50:1282–1293.

Loria P, Carulli L, Bertolotti M, Lonardo A. Endocrine and liver interaction: the role of endocrine pathways in NASH. *Nat Rev Gastroenterol Hepatol.* 2009;6:236–247.

Ludwig J, Viggiano TR, McGill DB, et al. Nonalcoholic steatohepatitis: Mayo Clinic experiences with a hitherto unnamed disease. *Mayo Clin Proc.* 1980;55:434–438.

Marecki JC, Ronis MJJ, Badger TM. Ectopic fat disposition and insulin resistance develop after overfeeding of a high fat diet to prepubertal rats despite increased adiponectin signaling, *J Nutr Biochem.* 2011;22:142–152.

Matsuzaki K. Modulation of TGF beta signaling during progression of chronic liver diseases. *Front Biosci.* 2009;14:2923–2934.

McFarlane SI, Muniyappa R, Francisco R, et al. Clinical review 145: pleiotropic effects of statins: lipid reduction and beyond. *J Clin Endocrinol Metab.* 2002;87:1451–1458.

McMillen IC, Robenson JS. Developmental origins of the metabolic syndrome: prediction, plasticity and programming. *Physiol Rev.* 2005;85:571–633.

Merrell M, Cherrington NJ. Drug metabolism alterations in nonalcoholic steatohepatitis. *Drug Metab Rev.* 2011;43:317–334.

Neel JV. Diabetes mellitus a 'thrifty' genotype rendered detrimental by 'progress'? *Am J Hum Genet.* 1962;14:352–362.

Nejak-Gowen KN, Monga SP. Beta catenin signaling, liver regeneration and hepatocellular cancer: sorting the good from the bad. *Semin Cancer Biol.* 2011;21:44–58.

Nickerson JG, Momken I, Benton CR, et al. Protein-mediated fatty acid uptake: regulation by contraction, AMP-activated protein kinase and endocrine signals. *Appl Physiol Nutr Metab.* 2007;32:865–873.

Olson RE. Discovery of the lipoproteins, their role in fat transport and their significance as risk factors. *J Nutr.* 1998;128:439S–443S.

O'Rahilly S, Farooqi IS. Human obesity: a heritable neurobehavioral disorder that is highly sensitive to environmental conditions. *Diabetes.* 2008;57:2905–2910.

Palee S, Chattipakorn S, Phromminitikul A, et al. PPAR gamma activator, rosiglitazone: is it beneficial or harmful to the cardiovascular system? *World J Cardiol.* 2011;26:144–152.

Pan DA, Lilloja S, Kriketos AD, et al. Skeletal muscle triglyceride levels are inversely related to insulin action. *Diabetes.* 1997;46:983–988.

Pan M, Cederbaum AI, Zhang YL, et al. Lipid peroxidation and oxidant stress regulate hepatic apolipoprotein B degradation and VLDL production. *J Clin Invest.* 2004;113:1277–1287.

Postic C, Girard J. Contribution of de novo fatty acid synthesis to hepatic steatosis and insulin resistance: lessons from genetically engineered mice. *J Clin Invest.* 2008;118:829–838.

Ratner R, Goldberg R, Haffner S, et al. Impact of intensive lifestyle and metformin therapy on cardiovascular disease risk factors in the diabetes prevention program. *Diabetes Care.* 2005;26:977–980.

Reaven GM. Banting lecture 1988, role of insulin resistance in human disease. *Diabetes.* 1988;37:1595–1607.

Roberts DL, Dive C, Renehan AG. Biological mechanisms linking obesity and cancer risk: new perspectives. *Annu Rev Med.* 2010;61:301–316.

Robinson MK. Editorial, surgical treatment of obesity—weighing the facts. *N Engl J Med.* 2009;361:520.

Ruderman NB, Myers MG, Chipkin SR, Tornheim K. Hormone–fuel interrelationships: fed state, starvation and diabetes mellitus. In: Kahn CR, Weir GC, King GL, Jacobson AM, Moses AC, Smith RJ, eds. *Joslin's Diabetes Mellitus.* Boston, MA: Lippincott Williams and Wilkins; 2005:127–144.

Sanyal AJ, Chalasani N, Kowdley KV, et al. Pioglitazone, vitamin E, or placebo for nonalcoholic steatohepatitis. *N Engl J Med.* 2010;362:1675–1685.

Shankar K, Harrell A, Kang P, et al. Carbohydrate-responsive gene expression in the adipose tissue of rats. *Endocrinology.* 2010;151: 153–164.

Shankar K, Harrell A, Liu X, et al. Maternal obesity at conception programs obesity in the offspring. *Am J Physiol Regul Integr Comp Physiol.* 2008;294:R528–R538.

Shulman GI, Barrett EJ, Sherwin RS. Integrated fuel metabolism. In: Porte D, Sherwin RS, Baron A, Ellenberg M, Rifkin H, eds. *Ellenberg and Rifkin's Diabetes Mellitus.* New York, NY: McGraw-Hill; 2003:1–14.

Smith DL, Nagy T, Allison DB. Calorie restriction: what recent results suggest for the future of aging research. *Eur J Clin Invest.* 2010;40:440–450.

Speakman JR. Thrifty genes for obesity, an attractive, but flawed idea and an alternative perspective: the 'drifty gene' hypothesis. *Int J Obes.* 2008;32:1611–1617.

Stipanuk M. Nutrients: history and definitions. In: Stipanuk M, ed. *Biochemical, Physiological, Molecular Aspects of Human Nutrition.* St. Louis: Saunders Elsevier; 2006:3–12.

Tilg H, Moschen AR. Evolution of inflammation in nonalcoholic fatty liver disease: the multiple parallel hits hypothesis. *Hepatology.* 2010;52:1836–1846.

Tontisirin K, Maclean WC, Warwick P. Food Energy: Methods of Analysis and Conversion Factors: Report of a Technical Workshop, Vol. 77 of FAO Food and Nutrition Paper, Issue 77 of Food Energy, Rome, 3–6 December 2002, 2003.

Virtue S, Vidal-Puig A. Adipose tissue expandability, lipotoxicity and the metabolic syndrome—an allostatic perspective. *Biochem Biophys Acta.* 2010;1801:338–349.

Ye J, Keller JN. Regulation of energy metabolism by inflammation: a feedback response in obesity and calorie restriction. *Aging.* 2010; 2:361–368.

Unit VI

Environmental Toxicology

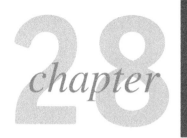

chapter 28

Nanotoxicology

Gunter Oberdörster, Agnes B. Kane,
Rebecca D. Klaper, and Robert H. Hurt

INTRODUCTION

Since the classic talk by Richard Feynman (1959) entitled "There Is Plenty of Room at the Bottom," nanotechnology has grown to a multibillion dollar industry worldwide, with 1300 nanotechnology-enabled products in commercial use by 2010 (Woodrow Wilson Center, 2012). The potential of adverse effects from exposure to "nanophase materials" was already pointed out earlier (Oberdörster and Ferin, 1992; Oberdörster *et al.*, 1992), and concerns about human and environmental health and safety of engineered nanomaterials (ENMs) were initially raised in 2003 (Colvin, 2003). Since then, toxicity of high volume, commercial nanomaterials including nanosilver, fullerenes, quantum dots, carbon nanotubes (CNTs), and metal oxide nanoparticles (NPs) have been summarized in several reviews (Borm *et al.*, 2006; Nel *et al.*, 2006; Donaldson *et al.*, 2004; Boczkowski and Hoet, 2009; Krug and Wick, 2011; Kunzmann *et al.*, 2011). New ENMs and composites are continually emerging with potential for significant commercial applications in energy generation, environmental sensing and remediation, aerospace and defense, and medical diagnosis and therapy. Examples of nanoscale materials of different shapes and sizes are depicted in Fig. 28-1. Investigation of

the magnitude of release of manufactured nanomaterials and their subsequent fate, transport, transformation, and potential for human and environmental exposure and toxicity (Fig. 28-2) is an urgent priority (Mueller and Nowack, 2008).

The National Nanotechnology Initiative (NNI, http://www.nano.gov/) defines nanotechnology as the understanding and control of matter at the nanoscale at dimensions between approximately 1 and 100 nm, where unique phenomena enable novel applications. Roco (2005) defined the sizes as ranging from the intermediate length scale between a single atom or molecule and about 100 molecular diameters or about 100 nm, and emphasizes the ability to measure and transform at this nanoscale and exploiting the properties and functions specific for the nanoscale.

The European Union (EU Commission, 2011) defined nanomaterial as a natural incidental or material containing particles as free, aggregates, or agglomerates, with 50% or more (by number) of them in the number size distribution in the range 1 to 100 nm of one or more of the external dimension, and expressed specific concerns for environment, health, safety, and also competitiveness. Because some nanoscale materials are less than 1 nm, it was clarified that fullerenes, graphene flakes, and single-walled carbon nanotubes (SWCNTs) below 1 nm are considered nanomaterials.

Nanoscale materials

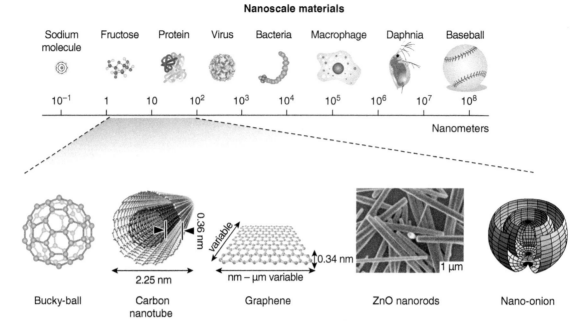

Figure 28-1. *Length scales for natural and synthetic structures (above) and some examples of engineered nanomaterials of varying size and shape (below).*

The continuing introduction of nanoscale materials into consumer products, such as TiO_2 in sunscreen creams, antibacterial Ag in textiles, multiwalled carbon nanotubes (MWCNTs) in sport equipment together with increasing numbers of publications reporting toxic responses mostly observed in in vitro studies, has led to increasing concern and more public awareness about potential adverse health effects, fostered particularly also by alarmist headlines in the popular press. Unrealistic high doses as well as questionable study designs are most often to blame. Thus, questions have to be raised about real versus perceived risk of nanotechnology applications, what is hype, what is reality? To provide

answers to these questions is one of the goals of the subdiscipline of nanotoxicology.

Nanotoxicology can be defined as the study of adverse effects of nanomaterials on living organisms and the environment. As illustrated in Fig. 28-2, there are multiple occasions for exposures to nanomaterials of humans and the environment and there is a serious need for investigation of the potential to cause adverse effects. The need of more toxicological research with the goal of characterizing risks associated with nanotechnology becomes even more urgent when considering the many beneficial and promising applications of nanotechnology for the betterment of human life, in particular

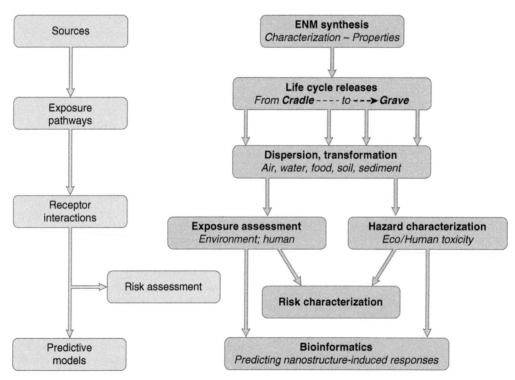

Figure 28-2. *Research phases for assessing human and environmental safety of engineered nanomaterials.*

Table 28-1

Ultrafine/Nanoparticles (<100 nm): Natural and Anthropogenic Sources

NATURAL	ANTHROPOGENIC	
	UNINTENTIONAL	*INTENTIONAL*
gas to particle conversions	internal combustion engines	engineered nanoparticles:
forest fires	power plants	*(controlled size and shape, designed for*
volcanoes *(hot lava)*	incinerators	*functionality)*
viruses	airplane jets	*metals, semiconductors, metal oxides*
biogenic magnetite:	metal fumes	*carbon, polymers*
magnetotactic bacteria;	*(smelting, welding, etc)*	*nanospheres, -wires, -needles, -tubes,*
protoctists, mollusks, arthropods,	polymer fumes	*-shells, -rings, -platelets;*
fish, birds, human brain, meteorite?	other fumes	*untreated, coated*
ferritin (12.5 nm)	heated surfaces	*(nanotechnology applied to many products:*
microparticles *(<100 nm)*	frying, broiling, grilling	*cosmetics, medical, fabrics, electronics, optics,*
(activated cells)	electric motors	*displays, etc)*

From: Oberdörster et al., 2007a,b

also for prophylactic, therapeutic, and diagnostic medical applications. The applications of nanotechnology for human health defines the new field of *nanomedicine*, and the development of new nano-enabled medical technologies must be accompanied by nanotoxicity studies to characterize undesirable effects and ensure the safety of new therapies and medical devices.

The field of nanotoxicology evolved from research of ambient airborne ultrafine particles (UFPs), particles up to about 100 nm from diverse anthropogenic and natural emission sources, including tailpipe emissions, power plants, volcanic eruptions, forest fires, and others, as summarized in Table 28-1, which gives examples of three classes: natural NPs, unintentional anthropogenic NPs, and intentional or engineered anthropogenic NPs. The same toxicological concerns and problems need to be addressed for UFPs and ENMs, they require similar research strategies with respect to study design and characterizing effects and underlying mechanisms at the primary portal of entry and in remote secondary organs. However, not only well-established respiratory tract and air pollution toxicology (see Chaps. 15 and 29) form the basis for nanotoxicology, but findings and knowledge accumulated in other traditional fields of research

provide useful complementary information and foundations for nanotoxicology. For example, virology (nanosized structures–cell interactions), metal and polymer-fume toxicology (small particle size and systemic effects), silica toxicology (particle surface reactivity), fiber toxicology (particle shape and biopersistence), radionuclide toxicology (chemistry and biokinetics), and lung deposition studies/modeling (respiratory tract dosimetry) (Oberdörster *et al.*, 2007a,b). Input from these research areas will help in the design of studies and interpretation of results of nanotoxicological research. For example, a major challenge is to correlate the distinct physicochemical characteristics of engineered nanostructures with their toxicological behavior, as will be discussed later.

Of utmost importance for nanotoxicology, as for toxicology in general, are dose-related issues. In particular, administered doses are mostly extraordinarily high when compared to doses achieved in vivo under realistic exposure scenarios. Slikker *et al.* (2004) stressed that the dose-dependent mechanisms are due to saturation processes underlying toxic responses between typical high acute experimental doses and lower human doses from realistic exposures (Fig. 28-3). Although high doses are justifiable for hazard characterization,

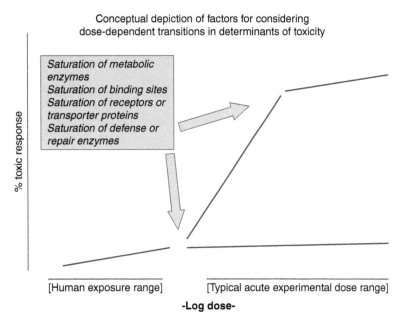

Conceptual depiction of factors for considering
dose-dependent transitions in determinants of toxicity

Saturation of metabolic enzymes
Saturation of binding sites
Saturation of receptors or transporter proteins
Saturation of defense or repair enzymes

% toxic response

[Human exposure range]   [Typical acute experimental dose range]

-Log dose-

Figure 28-3. *Conceptual depiction of factors for considering dose-dependent transitions in determinants of toxicity.* (From: Slikker Jr., *et al.*, 2004.)

ignoring real-world exposure situations may lead to erroneous conclusions about associated risks and causative mechanisms. Thus, consideration of the impact of dose, dose rate (influenced by dosing method in vitro and in vivo), and dosimetry should always be given highest priority when assessing nanomaterial toxicity. Dosimetry involves quantifying by measuring or calculating the amount of nanomaterials per body, per organ, per cell (microdosimetry), tissue or airway generation (inhalation route of exposure). Dosimetry should not be confused with "dosemetric," which is defining a dose in terms of an inherent property (physical, chemical, reactivity) of nanostructures. Neither should dosimetry or dosemetric be mixed up with "exposure." These issues will be discussed in more detail later.

The goals of nanotoxicology are to identify and characterize a hazard of ENMs for purposes of risk assessment for humans and the environment require a highly multidisciplinary team approach, covering expertise in toxicology, biology, chemistry, physics, material science, geology, exposure assessment, physiological-based pharmacokinetic (PBPK), and fate and transport modeling, and medicine is necessary to develop testing strategies, establish toxicity ranking, determine "safe" exposure levels, and derive preventive exposure guidelines. As depicted in Fig. 28-2, exposures throughout the lifecycle of ENMs, from their source to their disposal have to be considered. Dispersion and intermediate transformations in air, water, food, and soil are important modifiers of ENM—receptor interactions. Identifying underlying mechanisms of such interactions will aid in assessing risk and establishing preventive measures. Developing predictive models is a distant goal for both human and eco-nanotoxicology.

NANOMATERIAL BASICS

Perspectives: Engineered Nanoparticles Versus Ambient Particulate Matter

A large body of publications on the toxicology of airborne ambient particulate matter (PM) has shown that they can elicit adverse effects not only in the respiratory tract but also in secondary organs and systemically (see Chap. 29 on Air Pollution). An extensive critical review of the health effects of fine particulate air pollution (Pope and Dockery, 2006) pointed out that exposure to the smallest fraction of PM, referred to as UFPs or $PM_{0.1}$, particles smaller than 0.1 μm or 100 nm, has been associated with effects in the cardiovascular and central nervous system as a consequence of their translocation to and distribution via blood circulation and neurons. It is noteworthy that the definition of UFPs is based on the same maximum dimension (100 nm) as the US federal definition of nanotechnology. As will be discussed later, translocation of UFP and engineered nanoparticles (ENPs) has been clearly demonstrated, but only small amounts are translocating, and thus direct interaction of the translocated particles with organs beyond the lung may not be the sole explanation for their effects. Epidemiological studies have demonstrated that a major factor for inducing adverse effects from ambient particulate air pollution—including UFP—is susceptibility such as pre-existing disease (asthma, cardiovascular disease, diabetes), age (very young, elderly), or genetic background (polymorphism).

Table 28-2

What is Different: Nanoparticles Versus Larger Particles (*respiratory tract as portal-of-entry*)

	NANOPARTICLES (<100 nm)	LARGER PARTICLES (>500 nm)
General characteristics:		
Ratio: number or surface area/volume or mass	high	low
Agglomeration in air, liquids	likely (dependent on medium and surface)	less likely
Deposition mechanism in respiratory tract	diffusion; throughout resp. tract	sedimentation, impaction, interception; throughout resp. tract
Protein/lipid adsorption in vitro	very effective and important	less effective
Protein/lipid adsorption in vivo	yes	some
Translocation to secondary target organs:	yes	generally not (to liver under "overload")
Clearance		
• mucociliary	probably yes	efficient
• by alveolar macrophages	poor	efficient
• into or across lung epithelium	yes	mainly under overload
• lymphatic	yes	under overload
• blood circulation	yes	under overload
• sensory neurons (uptake + transport)	yes	not likely
Cell entry/uptake	yes (caveolae; clathrin; lipid rafts; diffusion)	yes (primarily phagocytic cells)
• mitochondria	yes	no
• nucleus	yes (<40 nm)	no
Effects (*caveat: dose!*):		
at secondary target organs	yes	(no)
at portal of entry (resp. tract)	yes	yes
• inflammation	yes	yes
• oxidative stress	yes	yes
• activation of signaling pathways	yes	yes
• genotoxicity, carcinogenicity	probably yes	some

Data from: Oberdörster et al., 2009

Properties and Behaviors of ENPs Versus Larger Particles

Table 28-2 contrasts differences between NPs (<100 nm) and larger particles (>500 nm) in terms of some general characteristics, translocation propensity, interactions with cells and effects, assuming inhalation exposure, and the respiratory tract as the portal of entry. Biological systems do not perceive a precise boundary at the 100 nm size threshold, but rather a gradual transition between nano- and larger-sized particles, and therefore, the 100 to 500 nm size is shown but not covered in the table.

Marked differences—which will be discussed in the following sections—between the two size classes are as follows: The high number and surface area per unit volume, which makes them chemically more reactive (eg, as catalysts) and similarly increases their biological/toxicological activity toward cells and tissues; the underlying mechanisms for deposition of inhaled particles in the respiratory tract, which is governed by diffusion or Brownian motion for NP, and by sedimentation, impaction, and interception for larger particles; and there is a difference with regard to the extent and impact of adsorption of proteins and lipids (corona formation) at the primary portal of entry and secondary target sites.

Efficient mucociliary and alveolar macrophage-mediated elimination following deposition in the respiratory tract is efficient for both nano- and larger particles once they are internalized by macrophages. NPs inhaled and deposited as singlets, however, are too small to be efficiently recognized and phagocytized by alveolar macrophages (Oberdörster *et al.*, 2005; Semmler-Behneke *et al.*, 2007; Geiser *et al.*, 2008)—unless they are aggregated or agglomerated to form larger particles—and thus overall alveolar macrophage-mediated clearance in the lung is poor. In contrast, uptake by epithelial cells and translocation into blood and lymphatic circulation occurs regularly for NPs, and only under heavy overload conditions for larger particles. Uptake of nanosized particles into sensory nerve endings of the tracheobronchial tree has also been described (Hunter and Undem, 1999), which is unlikely to occur for large particles.

Differences in cell entry mechanisms between NPs and larger particles and intracellular distribution to mitochondria and the nucleus are discussed in subsequent sections. With regard to the type of effects induced at the primary site of entry there does not seem to be a fundamental difference. However, effects in secondary organs are more likely to develop, possibly aided by a direct effect of translocated NP.

Manufactured NPs show a range of other size-dependent properties and behaviors. Among these are depressed melting points, size-dependent electronic band gaps, a quantum mechanical effect that gives rise to size-tunable fluorescence in quantum dots (semiconductor NPs), and confined plasmon resonance, which shifts the light absorption and scattering in a way that alters the colors of nanoscale materials from their larger-sized counterparts giving—for example—rise to nanosilver particles that are yellow and gold NPs that appear red. Unique size-dependent properties of NPs form the basis for many of their technological uses, but their significance for biological effect still needs to be evaluated.

Classes of ENMs

Manufactured nanomaterials have an enormous range of chemical composition, geometry, and complexity ranging from simple isometric forms (NPs), one-dimensional (1D) forms (fibers or tubes), and two-dimensional (2D) forms (plate-like or disk-like materials).

A large fraction of the stable elements in the periodic table have now been cast into NPs, or incorporated as part of a nanocomposite structure. Nanomaterials can be manufactured from metals, metal oxides, sulfides or selenides, carbon, polymers, or from biological molecules including lipids, carbohydrates, peptides, proteins, and nucleic acid oligomers. Fig. 28-4 presents a nanomaterial classification system based on a matrix involving geometry (particles, 1D forms, 2D forms) and chemistry (metals, semiconductors, ceramics, carbons, polymers; Tran and Nguyen, 2011; Rosenthal *et al.*, 2011; Cassee *et al.*, 2011; Feng and Liu, 2011; Duncan, 2011). The combination of geometry and materials chemistry gives rise to vast number of potential nanomaterials. Not all will be commercially significant, but many are being synthesized and characterized in R&D laboratories around the world. Nanomaterials may be applied to surfaces such as biomedical implants to enhance their function and biocompatibility, incorporated into nanostructured solids or composites to improve strength, conductivity, and durability, and fabricated into complex, active structures for chemical or biological sensors or other devices.

There are many approaches for synthesizing and manufacturing nanomaterials. Some methods use high-temperature processing in the vapor phase, such as inert gas condensation, flame synthesis, or "floating catalyst" chemical vapor deposition (Zhang *et al.*, 2011). These processes produce dry powders that can lead to occupational exposures when reactors are open or the powdered materials are handled or transferred. Other methods such as physical or chemical vapor deposition grow nanostructures on substrates. Substrate-bound nanostructures are less likely to cause exposures of concern, but can become detached during processing or use. A large class of methods uses solution processing, also known as "colloidal synthesis" (Tran and Nguyen, 2011). These methods involve reagent addition to liquid solvents to nucleate NPs that remain suspended in the liquid. This class of methods is less likely to lead to inhalation exposures, but they can occur if the liquid is subjected to ultrasonication, which can produce mists, or if the NPs are dried into powders or transferred onto substrates and dried for further processing (Hallock *et al.*, 2009).

Finally, most nanotoxicology research has focused on a limited set of nanomaterials with high manufacturing volume or the potential for high manufacturing volume in the near term (including ZnO, TiO$_2$, fullerenes, CNTs, nanosilver, quantum dots). Increasingly, the nanotoxicology field will have to focus on the other materials under development, especially as technological applications for those materials approach commercialization. It will be a major challenge for the nanotoxicology field to acquire the data necessary for risk assessment on the many new nanoproducts that are anticipated over the coming decades. Finally, as nanoscience progresses, there will be less emphasis on simple geometries and chemistries (see Fig. 28-4) and more emphasis on complex material structures that combine nanoelements into active or smart structures (Dvir *et al.*, 2011). Early examples of this are the synthesis of two-component or "dumbbell-shaped" NPs composed of gold and iron oxide (Xu *et al.*, 2007) or iron-platinum nanowires (Wang *et al.*, 2007). Understanding the toxicological profile of complex nanoassemblies will also present a major challenge to the field in the future.

Physicochemical Properties of Nanomaterials Relevant for Toxicity

Table 28-3 summarizes the nanomaterial properties known or thought to be relevant to biological responses. These properties are discussed in more detail in the section below, or in some cases in later sections on mammalian toxicity and ecotoxicity.

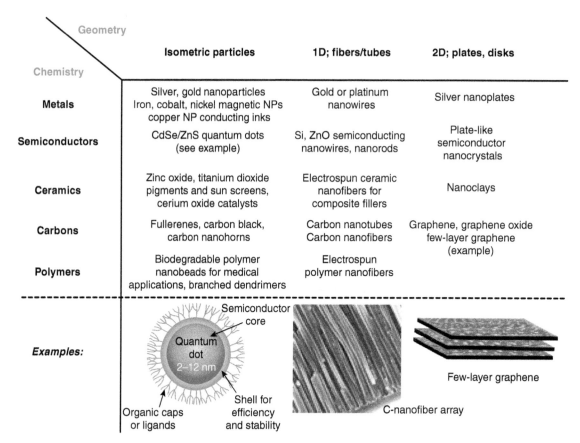

	Isometric particles	1D; fibers/tubes	2D; plates, disks
Metals	Silver, gold nanoparticles Iron, cobalt, nickel magnetic NPs copper NP conducting inks	Gold or platinum nanowires	Silver nanoplates
Semiconductors	CdSe/ZnS quantum dots (see example)	Si, ZnO semiconducting nanowires, nanorods	Plate-like semiconductor nanocrystals
Ceramics	Zinc oxide, titanium dioxide pigments and sun screens, cerium oxide catalysts	Electrospun ceramic nanofibers for composite fillers	Nanoclays
Carbons	Fullerenes, carbon black, carbon nanohorns	Carbon nanotubes Carbon nanofibers	Graphene, graphene oxide few-layer graphene (example)
Polymers	Biodegradable polymer nanobeads for medical applications, branched dendrimers	Electrospun polymer nanofibers	

Geometry

Chemistry

Examples:

Semiconductor core

Quantum dot 2–12 nm

Organic caps or ligands

Shell for efficiency and stability

C-nanofiber array

Few-layer graphene

Figure 28-4. *Classification of nanomaterials by geometry and chemistry.* The examples in this matrix illustrate the diversity in engineered nanomaterials, a diversity that continues to increase as new nanomaterials are synthesized.

Surface Area and Reactivity Nanomaterials display unique chemical and physical properties that can be exploited for novel consumer, industrial, defense, and medical applications, but these properties may also contribute to adverse environmental and health effects. At the nanoscale, chemical and physical forces govern the assembly of atoms or molecules resulting in nanostructures with a high surface-to-volume or surface-to-mass ratio. For example, 5 nm NPs have 1000 times the surface area of 5 μm particles of the same chemical composition and at the same airborne mass concentration. This high surface area of suspended NPs is responsible for increased surface reactivity, increased adsorption of chemicals, and strong catalytic activity. As particle diameter decreases below ~100 nm, the number of exposed surface molecules increases sharply (Fig. 28-5; Oberdörster *et al.*, 2005). High surface reactivity is a desirable property for catalysis; however, the large number of exposed surface molecules or atoms exposes surface defects, vacant sites, and dangling chemical bonds that enhance chemical and redox reactivity. Thus, the NP surface has high surface area, high surface energy, and high surface reactivity relative to micron-sized particles of the same chemical composition (Fenoglio *et al.*, 2011).

Table 28-3

Physicochemical NP Properties Relevant to Toxicology

Size *(aerodynamic, hydrodynamic)* **Size distribution** **Shape** **Agglomeration/aggregation state** **Density** *(material, bulk)* **Chemical composition and phase** • crystallinity • dissolution and toxicant (ion) release • coatings and bioavailable contaminants • biopersistence **Surface properties** • surface area (external, internal) • electrical charge (zeta potential) • redox activity • hydrophobicity/hydrophilicity • adsorptive capacity for biomolecules **Nanoscale quantum and magnetic properties (?)**	**Properties can change** • with method of production, preparation process, storage • when introduced into physiol. media, organism

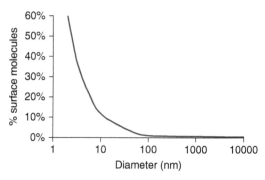

Figure 28-5. *Fraction of molecules in a particle that lie on its surface as a function of particle size.* (From: Fissan, 2008.)

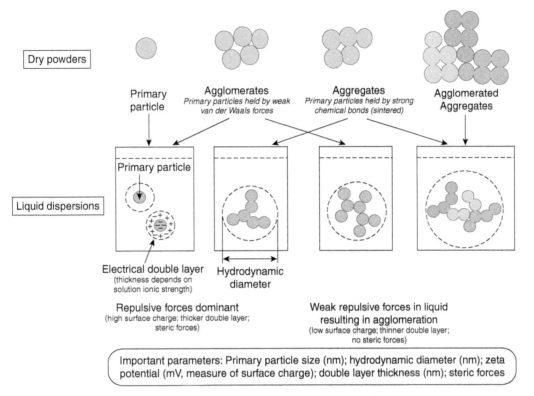

Important parameters: Primary particle size (nm); hydrodynamic diameter (nm); zeta potential (mV, measure of surface charge); double layer thickness (nm); steric forces

Figure 28-6. *Agglomeration and aggregation of nanoparticles in liquids and as dry powders.* (Modified from Jiang *et al.*, 2009.)

Surface Charge NPs have a strong tendency to form aggregates or agglomerates in the dry state, and in many cases also in liquid suspension (Fig. 28-6). This tendency is a natural consequence of small size, which leads to intermolecular attractive forces that are strong relative to gravity or to other forces that disrupt aggregates. Attractive forces between particles are determined by size, density, chemistry, and surface charge. In water, hydrophobic forces drive the agglomeration of many NP types. To obtain stable dispersions of unagglomerated nanomaterials, it is typically necessary to add macromolecular coatings that prevent particle–particle attachment through steric hindrance, or to impart an electrical charge on the NP surfaces that lead to particle–particle repulsion. A common indicator of surface charge is the "zeta potential," which is the electrical potential at the outer surface of a sphere that includes the particle and adjacent water molecules that travel with the particle during its motion. A common rule of thumb is that the zeta potential must be >30 mV or <−30 mV for repulsion to be sufficiently strong to avoid agglomeration. In physiological fluids or seawater, sodium chloride, and other ions "screen" the particle surface charge and lower the zeta potential, often causing aggregation. This property is a complicating factor in nanotoxicology assays (discussed below) and is a challenge for some biomedical applications. NPs may also adsorb molecules from their environment that *increase* stability (Nel *et al.*, 2009). Following injection or inhalation, NPs become coated with biomolecules such as serum albumin, an amphiphilic protein that carries poorly soluble molecules in the blood, or phospholipids in lung surfactant lining the alveoli as discussed in detail subsequently. For drug delivery applications (De Jong and Borm, 2008), NPs may be coated with biocompatible surfactants such as sodium cholate, or by biocompatible polymers such as phospholipid-polyethylene glycol (PEG) that stabilize colloidal suspensions of NPs through steric hindrance—a mechanism separate from electrostatic repulsion as indicated by zeta potential.

Surface Chemistry The unique physicochemical properties of nanomaterials responsible for their enhanced surface reactivity in biological systems are summarized in Fig. 28-7. Small size, high surface reactivity, and surface chemistry of NPs govern different types of interactions with biological molecules. High surface area and exposed surface atoms or molecules promote increased dissolution and release of ions from metallic or metal oxide NPs relative to bulk particles of the same chemical composition. For example, Ag^+ ions can be slowly released from nanosilver particles in aqueous environments by oxidation (Liu and Hurt, 2010). This property accounts for much of the bactericidal properties of clothes, toys, and medical devices coated or impregnated with nanosilver particles. Metal ions are toxic to bacteria and aquatic organisms by inhibition of enzymes and transport proteins. Silver ions have been shown to induce swelling of the lamellae of trout gills due to inhibition of carbonic anhydrase and Na^+/K^+ ATPase activity (Scown *et al.*, 2010). ZnO NPs are incorporated into sunscreens where they absorb ultraviolet (UV) light; however, in water, Zn^{+2} ions are rapidly released and cause acute toxicity (Xia *et al.*, 2008a). Surface hydrophilicity of charged NPs increases their ability to be suspended in water, whereas surface hydrophobicity of fullerenes or graphene repels water and enables these hydrophobic nanomaterials to partition into lipid membranes and gain entry into target cell (Sayes *et al.*, 2005; Titov *et al.*, 2010). TiO_2 NPs are used in sunscreens because they absorb UV radiation, but are too small to scatter visible light and appear transparent to the human eye. UV absorption can also lead to formation of electron/hole pairs that react on the particle surface to generate reactive oxygen species (ROS) such as superoxide anion ($O_2^{\cdot-}$) from molecular oxygen (O_2) (Schilling *et al.*, 2010). Surface defects, especially on crystalline NPs, expose electron donor/acceptor active groups that donate an electron to molecular oxygen also generating superoxide anion. Spontaneous or photoactivated generation of electrons accounts for the semiconductor properties of fullerenes and some metal oxide NPs (Xia *et al.*, 2006).

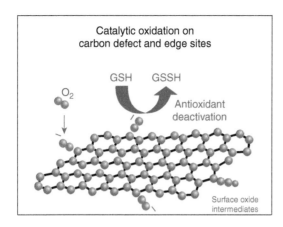

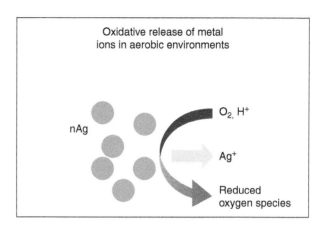

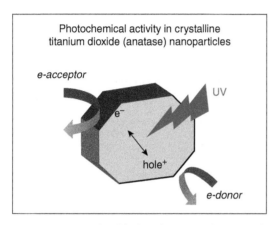

Figure 28-7. *Examples of biological reactivity of nanoparticles.*

CNTs are synthesized in the presence of metal catalysts, usually iron, nickel, or cobalt, and may contain redox-active metal residues that can undergo redox cycling and iron-catalyzed generation of highly reactive hydroxyl radical (OH•) via Fenton chemistry (Kagan *et al.*, 2006; Guo *et al.*, 2007). Nanomaterials with high surface area can adsorb organic molecules such as polycyclic aromatic hydrocarbons that are potentially carcinogenic (Yang *et al.*, 2006) and quinones that also participate in redox cycling and generation of free radicals (Nel *et al.*, 2006). Cationic NPs that have surface amide groups and cationic dendrimers are especially cytotoxic because they induce membrane damage, especially in lysosomes where the "proton sponge effect" leads to accumulation of water and chloride ions and osmotic rupture (Xia *et al.*, 2008b).

In summary, surface properties are major determinants of biological reactivity due to (1) high surface area, (2) surface charge, (3) hydrophobicity and partitioning into lipid membranes, (4) dissolution and release of metal ions, and (5) redox activity leading to generation of ROS (Nel *et al.*, 2006; 2009; Xia *et al.*, 2008b; Stone *et al.*, 2009).

Unique Quantum and Magnetic Properties NPs also display unique quantum and magnetic properties relative to micronsized particles. For example, noble metal NPs show preferred wavelengths for absorption and scattering of light due to resonant electron oscillations. This "confined plasmon resonance" phenomenon is shown by 40 to 100 nm diameter gold or silver NPs and leads to color shifts that impart a yellow color to nanosilver and a red color to some types of nanogold (Tran and Nguyen, 2011). Ferromagnetic NPs (eg, iron, nickel, cobalt, and some oxides)

less than about 10 nm in diameter exhibit the property of superparamagnetism. These particles respond strongly to an external magnetic field but have no permanent magnetic moment in the absence of the field because thermal energy is sufficient to cause fluctuations in the small magnetic dipole associated with each particle (Cole *et al.*, 2011). This property is exploited for contrast enhancement in diagnostic MRI and for hyperthermia induced by an external magnetic field to kill tumors targeted by magnetic NPs (Fortin *et al.*, 2007).

Geometry and Dimensions The geometry and dimensions of nanomaterials are also important in cellular uptake, systemic translocation, and potential toxicity as described in detail (Section III). Nanomaterials can enter target cells by passive diffusion, direct physical penetration, or active, receptor-mediated uptake by endocytosis or phagocytosis depending on their size and extent of agglomeration. For example, small NPs up to 50 nm in diameter appear to enter cells and subcellular organelles, including mitochondria and the nucleus, by passive diffusion (Geiser *et al.*, 2005; Chithrani, 2010). SWCNTs have been shown to directly puncture bacterial cells leading to osmotic lysis and death (Kang *et al.*, 2007; Akhavan and Ghaderi, 2010). SWCNTs have been reported to translocate from the alveoli into the interstitium of the lung where they promote collagen deposition and interstitial fibrosis (Wang *et al.*, 2011a). Rigid, long, high aspect ratio nanomaterials, similar to amphibole asbestos fibers (Palomaki *et al.*, 2011), are recognized by macrophages; however, they undergo incomplete uptake or frustrated phagocytosis (Shi *et al.*, 2011) resulting in impaired clearance from the lungs, lysosomal disruption, and activation of the inflammasome resulting in release of proinflammatory cytokines (Hamilton *et al.*, 2009; Donaldson *et al.*, 2010).

Biopersistence Finally, biopersistence of ENMs is an important factor in their environmental and biological toxicity. Biopersistence is related to dissolution, which not only produces biologically active ionic species (as discussed above), but can also degrade the particle and eventually clear it from biological tissue or the natural environment. ZnO NPs are an excellent example of an ENM that can exhibit acute cellular toxicity due to rapid release of Zn^{2+} ions. The rate of dissolution of metal oxides is increased by natural organic matter in the aequous environment (Xia *et al.*, 2008b); therefore, these NPs have low biodurability and it is predicted that they would not bioaccumulate in the environment. Following uptake by macrophages at the site of entry, metallic and metal oxide NPs reach the acidic endolysosomal compartment where release of metal ions is accelerated. Intracellular release of Zn^{2+} or Ni^{2+} ions, for example, is linked with significant acute toxicity to target cells in the lungs (Xia *et al.*, 2008b; Liu *et al.*, 2007; Pietruska *et al.*, 2011). ZnO NP dissolution is very rapid and is considered unlikely to be biopersistent in the lungs and induce chronic lung disease. In contrast, poorly soluble metallic nickel NPs appear to induce sustained intracellular release of Ni^{2+} ions resulting in persistent inflammation (Lu *et al.*, 2009) and activation of the HIF1-α signaling pathway in human lung epithelial cells (Pietruska *et al.*, 2011) that has been linked to nickel carcinogenicity (Costa *et al.*, 2005). Jakubek *et al.* (2009) reported that release of yttrium ions in trace levels from CNTs displaces Ca^{2+} from voltage-gated calcium channels with implications for neuronal activity. So far, no chronic rodent carcinogenicity assays have been conducted to assess whether inhalation of metal or metal oxide NPs can induce lung cancer or neurological disease.

In contrast, carbon nanomaterials are potentially biodurable raising concern that they could bioaccumulate in the environment or be biopersistent in the lungs and other organs following inhalation during occupational exposure or direct injection or implantation in biomedical applications (Bianco *et al.*, 2011). Some commercial types of long, rigid, high aspect ratio CNTs have been shown to induce toxicological endpoints similar to carcinogenic asbestos fibers (Sanchez *et al.*, 2009) as discussed in detail below. Biopersistence in the lungs and pleural or peritoneal spaces is an important physicochemical characteristic of asbestos and man-made mineral fibers associated with carcinogenicity (Bernstein *et al.*, 2005). Several recent studies have shown that carboxylated SWCNTs do undergo oxidative degradation in the presence of the plant enzyme, horseradish peroxidase and H_2O_2 (Allen *et al.*, 2008; 2009) or following exposure to phagolysosomal simulant fluid containing H_2O_2 to mimic the lysosomal compartment of macrophages (Liu *et al.*, 2010c). Oxidized or nitrogen-doped MWCNTs also showed both exfoliation of the concentric tubes and shortening in the presence of horseradish peroxidase and H_2O_2 (Zhao *et al.*, 2011). Oxidatively degraded SWCNTs did not induce lung inflammation or toxicity following pharyngeal aspiration in mice (Kagan *et al.*, 2010) providing proof-of-principle for deliberate design of engineered CNTs that are biodegradable and less likely to induce acute or chronic disease following inhalation or injection for tumor imaging or drug delivery (Bianco *et al.*, 2011). Graphene oxide nanosheets have also been shown to be degraded in the presence of horseradish peroxidase and H_2O_2 (Kotchey *et al.*, 2011) or by *Shewanella* bacteria that chemically reduce graphene oxide to graphene (Salas *et al.*, 2010).

These studies provide novel approaches for biodegradation of ENMs and prevention of long-term adverse environmental and health impacts.

THE NANOMATERIAL BIOLOGICAL INTERFACE

The high surface area of NPs provides a platform for adsorption of a variety of biological molecules including proteins, lipids, and nucleic acids. Dawson and his coworkers described in detail rapid binding of proteins in biological fluids to the surface of NPs that they defined as the "protein corona" (Lynch *et al.*, 2007). The protein corona is a dynamic interface between the NP and its local environment that governs its initial interaction with target cells (Dutta *et al.*, 2007; Walczyk *et al.*, 2010). The interaction of nanomaterials with blood plasma proteins has been investigated in most detail due to its importance in drug delivery, circulation time, organ distribution, and clearance (Karmali and Simberg, 2011). Protein adsorption is related to surface charge, hydrophobicity, and radius of curvature; however, NPs of diverse chemical composition and structure (eg, iron oxide NPs, polymeric NPs, and CNTs) avidly adsorb albumin, complement, fibrinogen, immunoglobulins, and apolipoproteins (Nel *et al.*, 2009). Protein adsorption and dissociation is a complex, dynamic phenomenon (Cedervall *et al.*, 2007a,b). Quantitative techniques to predict and characterize protein adsorption have been developed (Xia *et al.*, 2010). The consequences of protein adsorption to NPs are less clear; although, depending on the NP surface, proteins may denature resulting in loss of normal structure and function, or altered enzyme activity, or unfolding that exposes new antigenic determinants. NPs of diverse chemical composition also induce protein fibrillation or aggregation to form amyloid fibrils in an acellular system (Linse *et al.*, 2007). An important potential pathological consequence of serum protein adsorption to NPs is binding of fibrinogen leading to formation of blood clots (Khandoga *et al.*, 2010).

NPs that are inhaled into the respiratory tract or ingested into the gastrointestinal tract encounter a mucus layer that provides a natural barrier to penetration of particulates and microorganisms. Mucus is a complex glycoprotein composed of hydrophilic, dispersed regions and hydrophobic, globular domains. NPs may adhere to mucins causing enlargement of the pore size with increased susceptibility to penetration of microorganisms (Wang *et al.*, 2011b; Shvedova *et al.*, 2007). Smaller, charged NPs may be repelled by the hydrophilic domains and will not be able to penetrate the mucus layer (Lai *et al.*, 2009; Cone *et al.*, 2009; Wang *et al.*, 2011b). Aquatic organisms (Klaine *et al.*, 2008) and bacterial biofilms (Rodrigues and Elimelech, 2010) are surrounded by similar extracellular barriers that may prevent NP penetration. If inhaled NPs penetrate into the alveoli of the lungs, they encounter the lung lining fluid covering a thin film of surfactant lipids. Natural or synthetic lung lining fluid, which is a mixture of serum albumin and dipalmitoylphosphatidylcholine binds readily to a range of NPs and enhances their dispersion for use in toxicological assays (Sager *et al.*, 2007; Porter *et al.*, 2008).

ENPs also bind nucleic acids and have been proposed as gene delivery devices (Chou *et al.*, 2011). Depending on their chirality, SWCNTs may show sequence-specific DNA binding (Tu *et al.*, 2009). Graphene oxide nanosheets preferentially bind single-stranded RNA or DNA and protect it from enzymatic degradation (Lu *et al.*, 2010). Small graphene oxide nanosheets can also intercalate into double-stranded DNA and induce DNA breaks in the presence of Cu^{2+} ions (Ren *et al.*, 2010). Size-dependent binding of gold NPs into the major groove of DNA has also been reported (Schmid, 2008).

TOXICITY MECHANISMS

The emerging nanotechnology industry has generated fear and distrust among the public about unpredictable toxicity and unintended consequences of human exposure to ENMs (Bainbridge, 2002; Cobb and Macoubrie, 2004). Despite these concerns, there has not yet been an outbreak of human disease associated with exposure to ENMs, although potentially long latency periods between exposure and manifestation of effects require continued vigilance to prevent future problems. The mechanistic pathways associated with toxicity that have been discovered using various in vitro and in vivo assays are predictable based on the physicochemical properties of ENMs (Nel et al., 2009; Meng et al., 2009). Some of these toxicity pathways were identified by studying UFPs associated with ambient air pollution (Xia et al., 2006), whereas others are the consequence of intracellular release of toxic metal ions (Xia et al., 2008b). Oxidative stress due to direct generation of ROS at the surface of NPs or indirectly by target cells following internalization of NPs (Unfried et al., 2007) is a common mechanism responsible for toxicity of ENMs. The most vulnerable subcellular organelles and physiological functions that can be perturbed by exposure to ENPs are summarized in Table 28-4. Depending on the dose, duration of exposure, type of NP, and the target cell, the cellular responses may be minimal and reversible, involve activation of adaptive responses, or severe, leading to significant changes in cell structure and function that may culminate in cell death (Meng et al., 2009). Specific examples of toxicity endpoints induced by exposure to ENMs will be used to summarize our current understanding of mechanisms relevant for nanotoxicology. Most of the mechanistic studies use a variety of in vitro cellular toxicity assays and relatively high concentrations for 24 to 48 hours of exposure. As discussed in detail below, extrapolation from these short-term, high-concentration exposures in vitro to chronic, low-dose exposures in vivo is problematic. Given the wide range of ENMs currently in commercial production or in the early development stages, understanding toxicity pathways is essential for developing a rationale strategy for in vitro screening and prioritization for chronic animal testing based on new principles for toxicity testing in the 21st century (Simmons et al., 2009; Walker and Bucher, 2009; Silbergeld et al., 2011).

The cell wall of bacteria and the plasma membrane of eukaryotic cells are the initial barriers to penetration of NPs into target cells. Both gram-negative and gram-positive bacteria have thick cell walls composed of complex lipids and peptidoglycans, respectively. Bacteria do not actively take up particulates; however, several investigators have shown direct physical penetration of bacterial cell walls especially by SWCNTs (Kang et al., 2007, 2008; Liu et al., 2009), graphene and graphene oxide nanowalls (Akhavan and Ghaderi, 2010), and zinc oxide NPs (Liu et al., 2009). Carbon nanomaterials are proposed to act as "nanodarts" creating holes in the plasma membrane resulting in extracellular release of cytoplasmic contents as assessed by efflux of ribosomal RNA and decreased survival (Liu et al., 2009).

A wide range of NPs have been designed to facilitate delivery of imaging agents, genes, proteins, and drugs into mammalian cells: metallic and iron oxide NPs, silica NPs, quantum dots, biocompatible polymers, liposomes, micelles, and dendrimers (Chou et al., 2011). Target cells may recognize untargeted NPs that bind to surface scavenger receptors (Kanno et al., 2007; Hirano et al., 2008), lectin receptors (Zhang and Monteiro-Riviere, 2010), and Toll-like receptors that recognize hydrophobic domains (Seong and Matzinger, 2004). NPs can also be designed to target specific cell surface receptors triggering internalization by phagocytosis, macropinocytosis, or endocytosis mediated by clathrin, caveolae, or lipid rafts (Nel et al., 2009; Lajoie and Nabi, 2010). In order to facilitate gene, protein or drug delivery, NPs can be engineered to escape from endosomes or lysosomes by coating with pH-sensitive polymers, viral capsids, cations, or biodegradable carriers (Chou et al., 2011).

Eukaryotic cells can actively internalize a variety of ENPs using energy-dependent, receptor-mediated endocytosis or phagocytosis (Zhao et al., 2011). Following endocytosis or phagocytosis, NPs follow a well-defined intracellular pathway usually leading to fusion with lysosomes (Oh and Swanson, 1996). The kinetics and mechanisms of cell uptake vary depending on the target cell, size, shape, and surface modifications (Chithrani, 2010). Most NPs and microparticles are stored in membrane-bound vesicles, endosomes, or phagosomes; however, a subset of NPs including mesoporous silica NPs and superparamagnetic iron oxide NPs coated with chitosan undergo exocytosis or release from endothelial cells (Slowing et al., 2011) and macrophages (Serda et al., 2010). Exosomes are derived from sorting endosomes and multivesicular bodies; smaller NPs show greater exocytosis than particles in the range of 30 to 50 nm (Chithrani, 2010; Serda et al., 2010). Selective coating of NPs to favor delivery to exosomes can be exploited for drug delivery to vascularized tumors or to promote cell–cell transfer of genes and proteins (Slowing et al., 2011).

NPs that are recognized by surface receptors may activate cell-type-specific signaling pathways leading to cell proliferation or death by apoptosis, stress-related signaling, or calcium-mediated signal transduction events (Unfried et al., 2007). Dysregulated intracellular calcium ion homeostasis may be the consequence of influx across a damaged plasma membrane permeability barrier or release of calcium ions from the major intracellular storage sites, mitochondria, and endoplasmic reticulum. Sustained elevation in intracellular calcium can cause cell death by necrosis (Xia et al., 2006).

In addition, small polystyrene NPs and metallic NPs and dendrimers have been shown to enter a variety of target cells by passive diffusion in an energy-independent process (Lesniak et al., 2005; Geiser et al., 2005). Following uptake by diffusion, these small NPs are not compartmentalized into membrane-bound vesicles or lysosomes but are found free in the cytoplasm where they may secondarily enter the mitochondria or even the nucleus.

Mitochondria are the site of aerobic respiration and generation of adenosine triphosphate (ATP). Small NPs have been observed inside mitochondria (Li et al., 2003; Xia et al., 2006) where they may disrupt electron transport in the inner mitochondrial membrane and generate excess endogenous ROS. Direct or indirect generation of ROS in target cells exposed to a variety of

Table 28-4

In Vitro Mechanisms of Nanoparticle Toxicity

1. Damage to cell wall and plasma membrane
2. Interference with electron transport and aerobic respiration
3. Induction of oxidant stress
4. Activation of cell signaling pathways
5. Perturbed ion homeostasis
6. Release of toxic metal ions from internalized nanoparticles
7. Disruption of lysosomal membrane integrity
8. Incomplete uptake or frustrated phagocytosis
9. Interference with cytoskeletal function
10. DNA and chromosomal damage

engineered or ambient NPs is a major mechanism leading to cell toxicity and cell death (Nel *et al.*, 2006; Unfried *et al.*, 2007). Excess ROS that are not detoxified by endogenous antioxidant defenses can damage cellular membranes via lipid peroxidation, inactivate structural proteins, enzymes, and ion pumps, and damage nuclear DNA. A "hierarchical stress response" to oxidant-induced injury has been proposed by Nel *et al.* (2006). Low levels of ROS can activate transcription factors leading to upregulated expression of antioxidant defense-related genes. The second tier of response to ROS is activation of redox-sensitive transcription factors that upregulate genes involved in inflammation, proinflammatory cytokines and chemokines (Albrecht *et al.*, 2004). Finally, high or sustained production of ROS can lead to irreversible mitochondrial injury and cell death by apoptosis or necrosis (Nel *et al.*, 2006).

Endocytosis and phagocytosis of NPs by target cells usually results in fusion with and sequestration in membrane-bound lysosomes (Russell *et al.*, 2009; Chitharani, 2010). Uptake of quantum dots, CNTs containing metal catalyst residues, or metallic and metal oxide NPs provides a pathway for intracellular delivery of toxic metal ions by a "Trojan horse mechanism" (Limbach *et al.*, 2005). In the acidic environment of lysosomes, cadmium ions can be released from quantum dots, redox-active iron from iron oxide NPs, and other toxic metal ions including nickel from CNTs or metallic and metal oxide NPs (Liu *et al.*, 2008; Pietruska *et al.*, 2011). This mechanism may also be exploited to release drug cargoes into the cytoplasm following NP-mediated delivery (De Jong and Borm, 2008).

Cellular uptake of long, rigid, high aspect ratio nanomaterials including CNTs, metallic nanowires, and nanorods is especially hazardous for target cells in the lungs (Donaldson *et al.*, 2010). Macrophages are the initial cells to phagocytize inhaled particulates deposited in the airways or alveoli (Geiser, 2010). Rigid, high aspect ratio ENMs show similar interactions with macrophages as amphibole asbestos fibers. If they are longer than the diameter of macrophages (~10 µm), rigid elongated nanostructures show incomplete uptake or phagocytosis with prolonged generation of ROS by the respiratory burst mechanism of phagocytes and extracellular release of damaging lysosomal enzymes. Rigid, high aspect ratio nanomaterials also cause permeabilization of the lysosomal membrane resulting in release of cathepsins into the cytoplasm and activation of the inflammasome (Hamilton *et al.*, 2009). Cathepsins are proteases active at neutral pH and can cleave precursors of proinflammatory cytokines that can initiate inflammatory reactions in the lungs (Biswas *et al.*, 2011) as well as activate procaspases leading to death by apoptosis (Boya and Kroemer, 2008). Activation of the inflammasome, the cytoplasmic protein complex where this proteolytic cleavage and activation occurs, is also triggered by uptake of crystalline minerals including silica and asbestos fibers (Dostert *et al.*, 2008).

Incomplete sequestration of long, rigid, high aspect ratio NPs in lysosomes may also promote their release into the cytoplasm resulting in physical interference with cytoskeletal function. Cytoskeletal disruption can cause impaired cell motility, for example, macrophage-mediated clearance of asbestos fibers and high aspect ratio NPs is impaired resulting in sustained lung injury, inflammation, and fibrosis (Donaldson *et al.*, 2010) as discussed below. In other organs, NP-mediated interference with cytoskeletal-mediated transport may occur, for example, impaired bile transport and secretion by hepatocytes (Johnston *et al.*, 2010a). In dividing cells, high aspect ratio NPs may physically interfere with the mitotic apparatus resulting in chromosomal missegregation and polyploidy (Sargent *et al.*, 2010).

Finally, NPs may translocate into the nucleus by diffusion through nuclear pores or via nucleocytoplasmic transport (Unfried *et al.*, 2007). Quantum dots (Hoshino *et al.*, 2004), silicon dioxide NPs (Chen and von Mikecz, 2005), and gold NPs (Pante and Kunn, 2002) have been detected in the nucleus. Small gold NPs may intercalate into DNA (Schmid, 2008) and generate ROS that may induce oxidative DNA damage (Kang *et al.*, 2010). Silicon dioxide NPs have been shown to induce intranuclear protein aggregates of histones, topoisomerase I, and fibrillarin, although the functional consequences of this intranuclear protein aggregation are unknown (Unfried *et al.*, 2007).

CAVEATS IN NANOTOXICOLOGY ASSAYS

The unique physical and chemical properties of solid materials at the nanoscale contribute to serious technical limitations and potentially misleading results using conventional toxicology assays. Due to their high surface area and hydrophobicity, NPs can adsorb vital dyes, cell culture micronutrients, or released cytokines (Monteiro-Riviere and Inman, 2006; Casey *et al.*, 2007,2008; Guo *et al.*, 2008; Stone *et al.*, 2009). High surface area carbon nanomaterials such as SWCNTs and graphene have the greatest potential to adsorb aromatic amino acids and vitamins by π–π interactions with their hydrophobic graphenic surfaces (Guo *et al.*, 2008). Adsorption of bacterial lipopolysaccharide or endotoxin (a component of the cell wall of gram-negative bacteria) is a major concern because even low levels of endotoxin can activate macrophages and dendritic cells (Vallhov *et al.*, 2006). Genotoxicity endpoints are especially sensitive to NP-induced artifacts, for example, particle agglomerates interfere with the comet assay, used to detect DNA breaks and cytochalasin B used in the cytokinesis-arrested micronucleus assay, can interfere with NP uptake (Doak *et al.*, 2009; Stone *et al.*, 2009). NP agglomerates in physiological saline may also induce greater cytotoxicity than well-dispersed NPs; however, controls must be included to rule out toxicity of the dispersant (Wick *et al.*, 2007). In all toxicological studies, well-characterized positive and negative reference samples should be included over a range of doses and exposure times.

ENMs are highly complex and have unique chemical and physical properties relative to bulk materials of the same chemical composition. Complete materials characterization is required for adequate interpretation of toxicological studies (Warheit, 2008; Stone *et al.*, 2009). Nanotoxicologists must collaborate with chemists, engineers, and materials scientists in an interdisciplinary research team in order to understand the chemical, physical, and structural properties responsible for biological interactions and potential toxicity of nanomaterials. The relevance of in vivo extrapolation from high-dose, short-term, in vitro toxicity assays is discussed in more detail below.

SAFETY CONSIDERATIONS IN NANOMATERIAL DESIGN

In principle, it should be possible to engineer NPs with desirable surface properties for commercial or biomedical applications, for example, to control their size and geometry in order to prevent indiscriminate entry into cells and frustrated phagocytosis. Capping or coating of NPs using antioxidants such as tocopheryl-polyethylene-glycol-succinate (Yan *et al.*, 2007) may decrease toxicity. Release of toxic metal ions from quantum dots and iron oxide NPs can be minimized using inorganic shells or biocompatible polymers such as chitosan or alginate (De Jong and Borm, 2008). CNTs, fullerenes, and graphene are easily surface functionalized; for example, covalent functionalization with carboxyl groups has been reported to decrease toxicity of these pristine carbon nanomaterials (Sayes *et al.*, 2005, 2006; Sasidharan *et al.*, 2011). There is some evidence that CNTs are less pathogenic if short in length, or if entangled to hide their fibrous nature (Poland *et al.*, 2008). A long-term goal of mechanistic nanotoxicology is to reveal structure-activity relations that may allow the design of safe nanomaterials through re-engineering or reformulation (Hutchison *et al.*, 2008).

CASE STUDY: DESIGNING SAFER SUNSCREENS

Zinc oxide and TiO_2 NPs are widely used in sunscreens because they show less scattering of visible light and appear transparent, while effectively absorbing UV light in both the UVB and UVA wavelengths (Wang and Tooley, 2011). Due to its rapid dissolution in water releasing toxic Zn^{2+} ions, zinc oxide NPs are considered as potential environmental toxicants (Kahru and Dubourguier, 2010). Xia *et al.* (2011) deliberately doped zinc oxide NPs with iron (1%–10% by weight) that significantly retarded release of Zn^{2+} ions in water and physiological saline solutions. Zn^{2+} ions inhibit hatching of zebrafish embryos. Pristine zinc oxide NPs also inhibited hatching; however, iron-doped NPs were less inhibitory in this assay. Similarly, iron-doped zinc NPs induced significantly less lung injury and inflammation than pristine zinc oxide NPs following intratracheal instillation in rodents. This study provides proof-of-principle for safe design of ENPs to minimize potential environmental toxicity and adverse health effects.

TiO_2 NPs are used commercially in foods (candy, chewing gum), personal care products (shampoos, shaving creams, toothpastes), sunscreens, and paints and photocatalytic coatings for buildings and windows (Weir *et al.*, 2012). In 2010, 5000 metric tons of TiO_2 NPs were produced (Landsiedel *et al.*, 2010) and have been detected in effluents from waste water treatment plants where they may enter surface water (Westerhoff *et al.*, 2011).

The potential of zinc oxide and TiO_2 NPs to induce phototoxicity and penetrate into the dermis has been a major concern for human safety of sunscreens (Wang and Tooley, 2011). These mineral-based sunscreens cause less skin irritation and produce fewer allergic reactions than chemical-based sunscreens. The pristine NPs used in sunscreens form aggregates 30 to 150 nm in diameter; in this size range, these NPs are photoreactive and may generate ROS. Although uncoated TiO_2 NPs exhibit phototoxicity, following coating with hydrophobic stabilizers used in sunscreen formulations, no phototoxicity was detected in a cell culture assay system (Schilling *et al.*, 2010). A series of skin penetration studies using both ex vivo and in vivo models also showed that these NPs do not penetrate deeper than the outer most layer or stratum corneum of intact skin (Schilling *et al.*, 2010). However, TiO_2 NPs suspended in cyclopentasiloxane fluid used in cosmetics did penetrate into hair follicles of shaved skin of micropigs (Senzui *et al.*, 2010). Finally, young pigs were exposed to UVB light producing sunburn and an in vitro skin perfusion system was used to assess penetration of sunscreens containing zinc oxide or TiO_2 NPs. Only superficial penetration into the upper layers of the epidermis was observed and no zinc or titanium above untreated control levels was observed in the perfusate (Monteiro-Riviere *et al.*, 2011). Collectively, these in vitro and in vivo toxicology assays suggest that the benefits of protection against carcinogenic UV light radiation provided by sunscreens formulated with zinc oxide or TiO_2 NPs outweigh the minimal risks associated with phototoxicity, DNA damage, and skin penetration into shaved or sunburned skin.

MAMMALIAN TOXICOLOGY

Introduction

Nanotoxicology, the science of effects of ENMs on living organisms, is a rapidly growing discipline aimed at identifying and characterizing nanomaterial toxicity that will serve—in combination with exposure data—the ultimate goal of performing a meaningful risk assessment (National Academy of Sciences, 1983). Many ENMs exhibit unique and desirable catalytic, optical, structural, or electronic properties that make them attractive in diverse technological areas, including multiple manufacturing industries and environmental and medical applications. At the same time, concerns have been raised regarding potential acute and chronic adverse effects due to their physicochemical properties in combination with nanostructures, for example, an elongated fiber-like shape of CNTs (Johnston *et al.*, 2010b).

CNTs are a prime example of the two opposing faces of nanomaterials: Many highly desirable properties that are suitable for numerous beneficial applications contrast with reports of serious adverse effects in experimental animals. For example, the excitement about future uses of CNTs in biomedical applications for delivery of drugs, genes, and biosensors or as tissue engineering scaffolds (Liu *et al.*, 2008; Li *et al.*, 2010; Liang and Chen, 2010) is dampened by reports of inflammatory fibrogenic and even mesotheliogenic effects in laboratory rodents (Shvedova *et al.*, 2005; Takagi *et al.*, 2008; Jacobsen *et al.*, 2008; Poland *et al.*, 2008; Sakamoto *et al.*, 2009). Results of a number of in vitro studies in different cell systems also revealed an oxidative stress-inducing proinflammatory potential of CNTs (Hirano *et al.*, 2010; Vankoningsloo *et al.*, 2010; Pacurari *et al.*, 2008; Sanchez *et al.*, 2011; Monteiro-Riviere *et al.*, 2005); however, other in vitro studies did not confirm such effects (De Nicola *et al.*, 2007; Fenoglio *et al.*, 2006; Flahaut *et al.*, 2006; Pulskamp *et al.*, 2007).

As will be discussed later, a common problem with in vitro studies is that very high doses/concentrations in culture media are used that have no relevance for realistic in vivo conditions. Moreover, results of in vitro assays can be misleading due to interference of the nanomaterials to be tested with the testing reagents, adsorption of induced mediators (Worle-Knirsch *et al.*, 2006; Han *et al.*, 2011), or interference with optical measurements (Pfaller *et al.*, 2009); general problems related to sensitivity and reliability of in vitro systems have also been discussed (Jones and Grainger, 2009). A most recent example of reliability problems of in vitro assays in evaluating the toxicity of CNTs is described by Haniu *et al.* (2011) reporting contradictory results of increased as well as decreased cell viability as well as either no or high cytokine release when the same CNT and the same cell type were dosed using different dispersants for pretreatment.

Concepts of Nanotoxicology

The previous section discussed the importance of physicochemical properties of ENM. Table 28-3 summarizes several of these properties that are known to affect biological/toxicological effects. The size and size distribution are important determinants—thermodynamic and aerodynamic—for the deposition efficiency of inhaled materials throughout the respiratory tract. (See Fig. 28-6.) The quality of dispersion in liquid media can be determined by measuring the hydrodynamic diameter, which is important information for in vitro studies and the ENM behavior in blood and lymph circulation. The shape of ENM (tubes, fibers, planes) influences their aerodynamic and hydrodynamic behavior and is of special significance for cellular uptake, for example, a fiber shape of straight nanotubes with a length exceeding the diameter of alveolar macrophages so

Table 28-5

Time for Number Concentration to Halve and Particle Size to Double by Simple Monodisperse Coagulation

STARTING AIRBORNE CONCENTRATION (number/cm³)	TIME TO REACH HALF THE CONC. (½ N_S)	TIME TO DOUBLE PARTICLE SIZE ($N_D = 0.125\ N_S$)
10^{14}	20 µs	140 µs
10^{12}	2 ms	14 ms
10^{10}	0.2 s	1.4 s
10^{8}	20 s	140 s
10^{6}	33 min	4 h
10^{4}	55 h	16 days
10^{2}	231 days	4 year

Data from: Hinds, 1982

that they cannot be completely phagocytosed (frustrated or incomplete phagocytosis) resulting in potent activation and release of inflammatory mediators (Kane and Hurt, 2008). Individual NPs tend to agglomerate (held together by relatively weak forces, eg, Van der Waals forces) or they are aggregated when produced (sintered together or firmly bundled in the case of fibers) (Teleki *et al.*, 2008; ISO/TS 27687, 2008; Taurozzi *et al.*, 2011). Oftentimes, larger structures in the form of agglomerated aggregates are formed (Fig. 28-6), both in the airborne state and as liquid suspensions.

The terms "agglomeration" and "aggregation" are often used interchangeably, yet ISO/DIS (2011) defines them as based on the forces that keep the primary particles together (agglomerates: weakly bound with external surface area similar to the sum of surface areas of individual components; aggregates: strongly bonded or fused with the external surface significantly smaller than the sum of calculated surface areas of individual components). Both agglomerates and aggregates are also termed "secondary particles" (ISO/DIS, 2011).

The formation of agglomerates of aerosols (coagulation) depends on their number concentration in the airborne state and is a function of time (Hinds, 1982). The effect of such time-dependent agglomeration on decreasing the number of airborne particle concentration and on increasing the overall particle size is illustrated in Table 28-5 assuming simple monodisperse coagulation in still, undisturbed air. For example, it takes only 20 µs for a very high number concentration of 10^{14} particles/cm³ to decrease by half, whereas it takes 231 days if the initial concentration is only 100 particles/cm³. Similarly, in order to double the initial particle size because of a resulting increase in the agglomerate particle size, it takes 140 µs for the initially very high concentration, but four years for the low concentration. This dramatic shift in particle size distribution needs to be considered when high concentrations of airborne NPs are measured close to their source.

The agglomeration and the aggregation state of ENM will significantly influence their bulk and apparent density. For example, the specific density of TiO_2 is ~4 g/cm³, whereas the bulk density (density of a powdered material including interparticle spaces) of nano-TiO_2 depending on primary particle size ranges from 0.13 to 0.54 g/cm³. Bulk density—interchangeably also described as apparent or packing density—can be measured by pouring the ENM powder into a fixed volume of a graduated cylinder (freely settled). The volume of the measured mass/cm³ includes the particle volume, the interparticle void volume, and any internal pore

volume. Using MWCNTs as an example, the specific density of the base material, carbon, is ~2 g/cm³, but the bulk density of MWCNT was reported as ranging between 0.043 and 0.31 g/cm³ (Ma-Hock *et al.*, 2009; Pauluhn, 2010). The density achieved by packing of individual agglomerate structures of different MWCNT obviously plays an important role for differences of the bulk or packing density, as do the dimensions of length and diameter, the straightness of the tubes and the form and size of tangled structures. Knowledge of bulk density is important for understanding the aerodynamic behavior of ENM and their deposition in the respiratory tract. In simple general terms, the aerodynamic diameter (D_{ae}) of an aerosol is correlated with the physical geometric particle diameter (D_{geom}) as $D_{ae} = D_{geom} \times \sqrt{rho}$ (rho = material density in g/cm³). For particles below 1 µm, a slip-correction factor needs to be added. For highly agglomerated ENM, it may be preferred to replace the true material density with the value of bulk or apparent density in order to more accurately estimate the aerodynamic diameter.

A low bulk density obviously increases the volume of ENM after uptake into cells relative to the volume occupied by the same mass of nonagglomerated material. A volumetric overload concept for alveolar macrophages has been proposed by Morrow (1988), who suggested that when a phagocytized volume of 60% of the normal macrophage volume is reached, movement and clearance function is completely abolished, and that a retardation of the clearance function of macrophages starts when ~6% of the cell's volume is exceeded by phagocytized particles. Pauluhn (2010) applied this concept of volumetric overload to results of his subchronic inhalation study with MWCNT in rats for estimating an occupational exposure level.

Surface characteristics of ENM are a critical determinant for interpreting dose–response relationships (surface area as dosemetric), and for nanomaterial cell interactions. Uptake into cells is influenced by their surface charge, surface reactivity, the chemistry of surface coatings [functional groups, polymeric coatings] and also surface defects to the material as-synthesized, or introduced during surface functionalization or processing such as acid purification or ultrasonication for dispersion).

Solubility and solubilization rate are of interest because the shortened biopersistence of NP in the organism terminates any NP-size-related effects. Zinc oxide is an example of an NP that undergoes rapid dissolution, thereby giving rise to high ionic zinc concentrations and induction of inflammation and oxidative stress (Xia *et al.*, 2008b) in contrast to poorly soluble CeO_2 or TiO_2 NPs. Many ENPs are insoluble in the as-produced form (eg, metallic Ag^+ and Ni^{2+} metallic NPs), and do not undergo simple dissolution, but can undergo chemical oxidation, a kind of nano-corrosion, in solution, in tissue, or in the environment to produce soluble species (eg, Ag^+ and Ni^{2+}) in a process that gradually degrades and eliminates the particle state (Liu and Hurt, 2010; Liu *et al.*, 2010a; Pietruska *et al.*, 2011). Such NPs can act via a "Trojan Horse" mechanism in that they are taken up into cells and subsequently dissolve, thereby creating a very high intracellular ionic metal concentration that is cytotoxic (Limbach *et al*, 2007). The same ionic concentration outside the cell will elicit no or only a modest response because of selective cell barriers preventing metal ions from entering the cell. The results by Xia *et al.* (2008b) and Limbach *et al.* (2007) are based on in vitro studies. Donaldson *et al.* (2009) have cautioned that great care should be taken in interpreting that oxidative stress induction by particles observed in vitro will also occur in vivo. This is not to say that the "Trojan Horse" effect does not occur in vivo, it has been described and is being used in designing drug delivery via NP for therapeutic applications (Iezzi *et al.*, 2012; Kreuter, 2004). The cautionary note is more generally directed toward the extrapolation of in vitro-based oxidative stress results to in vivo conditions.

It is a major challenge for nanotoxicological studies that many of these properties, once they have been determined for a given ENM, are not stable but can change when prepared for toxicological testing or during storage or testing. Alterations can occur through oxidation or dissolution (above), or through adsorption of proteins and lipids once they have been taken up into different compartments of the organism, has become an important area of research (Cederval *et al.,* 2007a,b; Lundqvist *et al.,* 2008; Monopoli *et al.,* 2011), yet methods to study these changes on the surface of ENMs in vivo still need to be developed.

Dosemetrics

Given the importance of physicochemical properties of ENM as determinants of their biological/toxicological properties, the question of the proper dosemetrics has been raised. Toxicologists are used to thinking in units of mass or molarity when characterizing a dose or concentration. However, several in vitro and in vivo studies with NP have shown that expressing dose–response relationships on a convenient mass basis may not be as informative as the surface area of the NP (Oberdörster *et al.,* 1992; Donaldson *et al.,* 1996; Tran *et al.,* 2000). Fig. 28-8 shows the pulmonary inflammatory dose–response relationships of two sizes of TiO$_2$ particles induced by intratracheal instillation in rats. A significantly greater influx of inflammatory neutrophils into the lung was induced by 25 nm TiO$_2$ per unit mass than by 250 nm TiO$_2$. The result is a very steep dose–response for the nanosized TiO$_2$ and a flatter dose–response for the larger TiO$_2$. Likewise, there was a clear separation of the dose–response when based on the number as dosemetric; however, when the same data were expressed based on particle surface area, a common dose–response relationship emerged (Fig. 28-8).

Although the concept of particle surface area as dosemetric is biologically plausible because it is the surface of particles that interacts with cell structures, the total surface area may only be a surrogate of the actual biologically relevant surface. As was discussed above, there are a number of surface properties (Table 28-3) that affect interaction with cells. Thus, identifying a biologically available surface area will be of great value for defining a proper dosemetric. At present, the specific surface area of ENMs (m^2/g) is most commonly measured by vapor adsorption, in which the number of vapor molecules (usually nitrogen) adsorbed on solid surfaces is measured over a range of standard conditions and the surface area estimated by application of the BET theory (Brunauer *et al.,* 1938). Both the external and existing inner surface (porosity) in pores larger than the nitrogen molecule are determined by this technique. There is a need for standardization of the method with regard to the use of nitrogen or other gases (Kr; Ar) because different molecule sizes will "see" and report different surface areas in molecular-sized pores (<0.4 nm). Measurements of BET surface area can also contribute to differentiation between agglomerated and aggregated structures, for example, agglomerated NPs have essentially the same specific surface area as the same mass of individual primary particles, whereas aggregated particles have a somewhat lower specific surface area than the same mass of primary particles (ISO/TS 27687, 2008). The measured surface area can then be converted to a BET equivalent particle size for nonporous spherical particles (Teleki *et al.,* 2008).

In addition to mass, number and surface area as dimensions for a dosemetric, the volume of NPs has been suggested as another dosemetric. This suggestion is based on the interpretation of earlier long-term inhalation studies in rats in which very high concentrations of different poorly soluble particles of low cytotoxicity had resulted in highly overloaded alveolar macrophages so that their

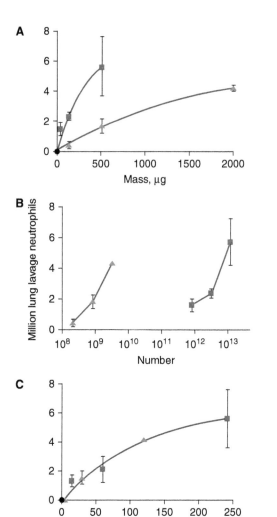

▲ Fine TiO$_2$ (250 nm)   ■ Ultrafine (25 nm) TiO$_2$ ● Saline

Figure 28-8. *Inflammatory cell response (neutrophil number in lung lavage of rats 24 hours after intratracheal instillation of two sizes of TiO$_2$ particles expressed by different dosemetrics.* Particle-mass (**A**); -number (**B**); -surface area (**C**). (Reproduced with permission from Oberdörster *et al.,* 2007a.)

normal clearance function was severely impaired or had come to a standstill. Based on the results of these studies, Morrow (1988) formulated a "particle overload" hypothesis: When the volume of phagocytized particles in alveolar macrophages exceeds 6% of the normal macrophage volume, their physiological clearance function becomes impaired; if the phagocytized volume reaches 60%, the clearance function ceases completely. For certain ENMs the volume that they occupy can be very high, for example, larger agglomerates of MWCNT, forming a loosely packed (low specific density) structure that takes up a large volume when taken up by alveolar macrophages in the lung. Pauluhn (2010) has applied this volumetric overload concept to results of a well-performed subchronic rat inhalation study for estimation of a human occupational exposure limit.

Follow-up studies to the mechanistic basis of lung particle overload point to particle surface area of agglomerated phagocytized nanosized and larger particles as dosemetric, which appears to correlate better with the impaired clearance function of alveolar macrophages rather than the phagocytized volume (Oberdörster *et al.,* 1994; Tran *et al.,* 2000). Whether particle volume or particle surface area are the more appropriate dosemetric to use in

Table 28-6

Mass/Number/Surface Area Correlations for Selected NPs

PARTICLE TYPE	DIAMETER nm	DENSITY g/cm³	SPC. SRF. AREA m²/g	SPC. NUMBER #/g	AIRBORNE CONC. OF 100 µg/m³	
					SURFACE cm²/m³	NUMBER #/m³
Pt	50	21.09	5.69	7.24×10^{14}	5.69	7.24×10^{10}
Gold	50	19.3	6.22	7.91×10^{14}	6.22	7.92×10^{10}
Ag	50	10.5	11.43	1.46×10^{15}	11.43	1.46×10^{11}
Cu	50	8.9	13.48	1.72×10^{15}	13.48	1.72×10^{11}
Al	50	2.7	44.44	5.65×10^{15}	44.44	5.65×10^{11}
TiO_2(R)	50	4.23	28.37	3.61×10^{15}	28.37	3.61×10^{11}
TiO_2(A)	50	3.9	30.77	3.92×10^{15}	30.77	3.92×10^{11}
C	50	2.26	53.10	6.76×10^{15}	53.10	6.76×10^{11}
Polystyrene	50	1.05	114.3	1.46×10^{16}	114.3	1.46×10^{12}
	5		1143.0	1.46×10^{19}	1143.0	1.46×10^{15}
	10		571.4	1.82×10^{18}	571.4	1.82×10^{14}
	100		57.14	1.82×10^{15}	57.14	1.82×10^{11}
	1000		5.71	1.82×10^{12}	5.71	1.82×10^{8}

CHAPTER 28 NANOTOXICOLOGY

situations of particle overload of the lung is still to be determined, yet—as pointed out before—it is important to remember that not only physical –volume, surface area—but also chemical—surface associated—properties of NPs are critical determinants of effects resulting from NP–cell interactions (Table 28-3).

Among the different dosemetrics discussed in this section, particle number is of particular importance with respect to characterizing exposure. Exposure concentrations in the air are expected to be very low, which makes it difficult to determine the precise concentration based on measuring mass. However, a low mass of NP consists of a huge number of particles that can reliably be measured in the airborne state using scanning mobility particle sizers or concentration particle counters. Thus, NP number as an exposure-metric for mainly isometric type NP is a valuable component for exposure characterization.

Table 28-6 shows the correlation among the different dosemet-rics of different 50 nm-sized isometric NPs, with specific material densities ranging from 21 to 1 g/cm³. Volume is not listed in this table because it depends on the bulk or packing density, which is different from the material density because of additional void spaces between the packed NP. Surface area and number per unit mass and per 100 µg/m³ air volume vary greatly. The table also shows that a 200-fold change of particle size from 5 nm to 1000 nm results in a more than six orders of magnitude change in number concentration with only a 20-fold change in surface area for all NP (shown for polystyrene in Table 28-6). However, although these correlations can readily be established for dry powders, even when they consist of polydisperse particle sizes, these correlations will change upon inhalation and disposition in the body because of different deposition and biodistribution efficiencies in the lungs and other organs.

Portals of Entry

The respiratory tract, the gastrointestinal (GI) tract, and skin are the main organs of direct exposure to ENM. For medical application, injection (intravenous, intramuscular, subcutaneous, and other) will also be an important entry route into the organism. Intake via the respiratory tract is a most prevalent exposure route for occupational exposures; additives of ENM to food (TiO_2; SiO_2) and potential contamination of food from nano-enabled packaging materials result in exposure via GI tract (Jani et al., 1990; 1994; Hoet et al., 2004; FAO/WHO, 2009; Loeschner et al., 2011). Based on available data, translocation of nanomaterials in vivo across GI-tract epithelial cells seems to be limited; Trouiller et al. (2009), however, described DNA damage in bone marrow cells following very high gavage dosing of rats. Skin exposure via cosmetics and skin-care products occurs, although penetration of healthy skin by NP has not been demonstrated (Monteiro-Riviere et al., 2011; Prow et al., 2011; Schneider et al., 2009). Some penetration of quantum dots (~30 nm) applied to the skin of mice after UV radiation-induced sunburn was found (Mortensen et al., 2008). Because the respiratory tract is a major route for humans to exposure of nanomaterials, the following sections will focus on this portal of entry to discuss biokinetics, effects, and concepts for in vivo and in vitro toxicity testing.

Dosing of the Respiratory Tract

The following sections focus on the respiratory tract as portal-of-entry of airborne ENM.

Dosing of the respiratory tract of laboratory rodents as the portal-of-entry for airborne ENMs is mostly and conveniently done by intratracheal instillation (rats) or oropharyngeal aspiration and intranasal instillation (mice), which administer materials as a bolus in a second or less. However, inhalation is the only physiological method and should be considered the gold standard for exposure to airborne materials. Obvious major differences between bolus-type and inhalation exposures relate to the dose rate (see discussion later), use of anesthesia, the distribution of administered material within the respiratory tract, and the need for special expertise and equipment required for inhalation but not bolus-type exposures. Although most of the differences between inhalation- and instillation-type delivery are well known and have been discussed in a Society of Toxicology (SOT)-sponsored White Paper (Driscoll et al., 2000), the limitations of using and interpreting results from bolus-type dosing are most often not considered (Table 28-7). Driscoll et al. concluded with several recommendations when intratracheal instillation can be applied. These included evaluation

Table 28-7

Instillation Versus Inhalation

ADVANTAGES	DISADVANTAGES
• Low cost	• non-physiological
• simple technique	• invasive delivery
• less material needed	• very high dose rate
• delivered dose is known	• usually also high dose, overwhelming lung defenses
• ranking of toxicities	• bypassing upper respiratory tract
• avoiding fur contamination (*handling hazard*)	• different distribution in lower resp. tract:
• lower risk to investigators	more central, more heterogeneous, less uniform
• nonrodent-respirable aerosol can be delivered (*human health*	• focal high lung burdens
relevant)	• potential impact of vehicle on distribution, effects,
• specific areas of lung can be dozed (*larger animals*)	material to be tested
• screening for deciding concentr. for inhalation	• potential confounder of anesthesia
• identifying toxic components of mixture	• multiple instillations to reduce heterogeneity

Note: Qualitatively, both methods yield similar results for variety of biologic endpoints—(pulmonary inflammation; fibrosis; susceptibility to infection, allergic sensitization, PSP lung tumors).
But: Requires thorough understanding of differences between both methods to avoid misinterpretation of instillation results.
SOURCE: Data from Driscoll et al., 2000.

of comparative toxicity: screening, ranking, range of doses, comparing to reference material; evaluation of material not respirable by rodents; to minimize interference of clumping and localized inflammation, only <~100 μg/rat should be used. The authors also mention situations when instillation should not be considered: For determining deposition pattern in lung to mimic inhalation; toxic effects in the upper respiratory tract; not to use for materials that react with vehicle; they also cautioned that short-term clearance (mucociliary) is not reflected accurately.

Of special importance is the tremendous difference in the delivered dose rate: Bolus-type delivery occurs within a fraction of a second, whereas inhalation at realistic concentrations takes hours to months of exposure in order to deposit the same dose in the lung. Treating a dose delivered by bolus to be the same as a dose that has accumulated in the lung over a life-long exposure is scientifically not justifiable and needs to be discouraged (Oberdörster, 2012). Inundating cells abruptly with an extraordinarily high dose does overwhelm the cell's defense mechanisms and leaves no time for developing adaptive responses. Consequently, underlying mechanisms of effects induced by such unrealistic high doses are different from those induced by relevant doses and dose rates (Slikker *et al.*, 2004, see Fig. 28-3). With respect to the administered dose rate, Fig. 28-9 illustrates a tremendous difference of inducing a pulmonary inflammation by either intratracheally instilling (~0.5 second duration) 200 μg of TiO_2 NP versus depositing the same dose by inhalation over a period of four hours or four days (4 × 4 hours). The difference in dose rate is four to five orders of magnitude, with a strong inflammatory response at the highest dose rate (instillation) and no response at the lowest dose rate (inhalation).

Evidence that extremely high doses acutely administered within a very short time overwhelm the organism's or the cell's defenses so an adaptive response cannot be mounted was presented in a rat inhalation study with nanosized particles using exposure to UFPs (~18 nm count median diameter) of polytetrafluoroethylene (PTFE) fumes (Johnston *et al.*, 2000). PTFE fumes, similar to metal fumes, when freshly generated consist of nanosized particles, which are highly reactive and are known to give rise to polymer fume and metal fume fever in occupationally exposed workers (Drinker *et al.*, 1927a,b; Drinker and Drinker,1928; Seidel *et al.*, 1991; Lee and Seidel, 1991). When groups of rats were exposed for five minutes on each of three days to either filtered air or to a

concentration (~50 μm³) of these PTFE fumes, followed on day four by a 15-minute exposure of both groups to the same concentration of PTFE fumes, the pre-exposed rats survived without any significant adverse pulmonary responses (not significantly different from rats that were sham exposed on all days), whereas the filtered air pre-exposed rats died within three hours after the 15-minute PTFE exposure (Fig. 28-10a). Estimated deposited dose of PTFE in the lung was only ~60 ng. Further lung tissue analyses revealed that the PTFE pre-exposed rats had mounted a strong "adaptive" response (increased antioxidant and chemokine mRNA), whereas nonadapted rats were unable to induce such response (Fig. 28-10b). Evidence for such adaptation following inhalation exposure to nanosized particles in humans was already reported eight decades ago when Drinker *et al.* (1927b) described that repeat exposure to zinc oxide fumes induced "resistance" in

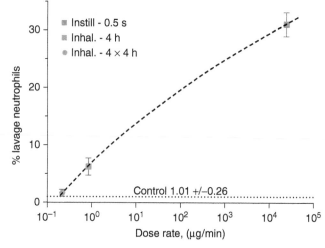

Figure 28-9. *Dose-rate—response correlation: Deposition of 200 μg nano-TiO_2 in the lungs of rats either by instillation(high dose rate) or by inhalation (low dose rate) induces widely differing pulmonary inflammatory responses as determined by the appearance of inflammatory neutrophils in lung lavage (Figure provided by G. Oberdörster).*

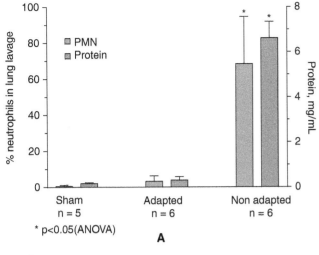

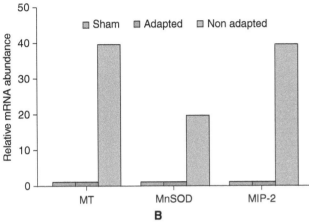

Figure 28-10. *Preventing acute pulmonary injury in rats from inhalation of polymer fume (PTFE, nanosized particles, ~18 nm count median diameter by inducing adaptation with repeated five minute. PTFE pre-exposures on each of three days prior to 15 minutes to exposure on day four.* **A.** Adapted rats show no inflammatory response assessed by neutrophil cells in lung lavage, nonadapted rats develop severe lung injury after 15 minute. PTFE exposure. Control rats were sham-exposed on all four days. **B.** Change in relative abundance of lung mRNA in PTFE adapted and nonadapted and sham-exposed control rats (Johnston *et al.*, 2000).

human subjects. Adaptive responses are important physiological protective mechanisms, which need to be considered when interpreting results of nanomaterial toxicity testing. However, the organism's capacity to adapt may not only be compromised by sudden very high acute exposures of short duration (high dose and high dose rate) but may also be impaired in susceptible parts of the population.

Despite the limitations of bolus-type delivery, they may be viewed as "proof of principle" or "hypothesis-forming studies," with the findings to be confirmed by subsequent inhalation studies. Although results from bolus-type studies are useful for toxicity ranking against known positive or negative control ENMs, they cannot be used for quantitative risk assessment. Other in vivo bolus-type deliveries involve intravenous, intraperitoneal, or intrapleural injections. If used for safety assessment of medicinal applications of ENMs, including CNTs, an appropriate range of doses should be applied. If, on the other hand, intravenous or intracavitary injections are used to simulate doses resulting from translocation of inhaled CNTs after deposition in the lung, results have to be viewed with caution. The amount of NPs translocating from the lung to the blood circulation and subsequently to secondary organs are very low, on the order of 1% to 3% (Kreyling *et al.*, 2002; 2009). Furthermore,

the translocation rate from the lung is very low, it occurs over hours and days, which contrasts with the immediate very high dose rate of injection. Bolus-associated problems have been discussed above, and confirmation of results from such "proof of principle" studies by follow-up inhalation studies is desirable.

The pretreatment of ENMs in preparation of bolus-delivery dosing is an additional difference compared to inhalation and may raise some concern: The recommendation to use dispersants in order to administer the materials in a well-dispersed mode (Fubini *et al.*, 2010; Taurozzi *et al.*, 2011) results in the coating of the treated nanomaterials that changes their surface properties and renders them different relative to their pristine state when inhaled under real-world exposure conditions. Although inhaled ENMs will also be coated by lipids and proteins of the lung lining fluid once deposited, such protein corona is likely to change upon translocation to interstitial and blood compartments based on the "concept of differential adsorption" (Müller and Heinemann, 1989). This concept states that the physicochemical properties of nanomaterials, such as size, surface properties, shape, dissolution, and others when in contact with media in the different body compartments determine protein and lipid adsorption and desorption patterns and thereby influence biodistribution across barriers and in target tissues and cells (Fig. 28-11). This concept has been further developed more recently by Dawson's group (Cederval *et al.*, 2007a; Lundqvist *et al.*, 2008; Walcyzk *et al.*, 2010) who describe the formation of hard and soft protein coronas around NPs upon incubation with blood plasma. Future studies have to show how pretreatment of ENMs for bolus-type in vivo administration will affect both biodistribution and effects. In vitro experiments with different cell types have already demonstrated that the use of different dispersants with MWCNTs resulted in contradictory results (Haniu *et al.*, 2011).

The three different methods of bolus-type dosing of the respiratory tract—intranasal instillation; intratacheal instillation; oropharyngeal aspiration—represent a convenient way to obtain first or preliminary data about effects in the respiratory tract. The limitations and caveats of using these modes of administration—as pointed out in the preceding paragraphs—should be taken into account when interpreting the results. Immediate short-term inflammatory responses will be induced, and these early bolus-associated effects are likely to also influence long-term effects. For example, when Li *et al.* (2007) compared pulmonary responses to inhaled and

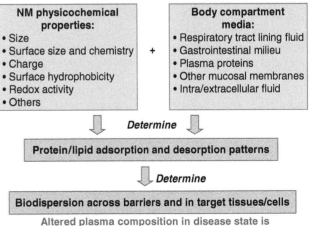

Figure 28-11. *Physicochemical properties of nanomaterials influence the adsorption of proteins and lipids from different organs, which affect the biodistribution of nanomaterials.* (Modified from Müller and Heinemann, 1989.)

intratracheally instilled MWCNTs in rats, they observed a much lower response in terms of pulmonary pathology after inhalation despite a higher lung burden from inhalation compared to instillation. It is of interest though, that in another study similar inflammatory, granulomatous and fibrotic responses were observed in mice following inhalation and oropharyngeal aspiration of SWCNTs. In fact, inhalation exposure was more potent than aspiration of an equivalent mass (estimated) of SWCNTs one to 28 days after inhalation exposure to a high concentration (5 mg/m³, four days @ 5 h/day) or oropharyngeal aspiration of 5 and 10 µg (Shvedova et al., 2008). The authors suggested that the similarity of responses between inhalation and aspiration exposure to SWCNTs in mice may be due to smaller SWCNT structures by inhalation of a dry aerosol versus aspiration of a suspension containing micrometer-sized agglomerates. However, both the Li et al. (2007) and Shvedova et al. (2008) studies only estimated the doses deposited in the lung upon inhalation based on inhaled concentration and size distribution and retained doses were not confirmed by actual measurements. In addition, the inhalation exposure by Li et al. was carried out with a static system, that is, MWCNTs were introduced into the exposure chamber as an aerosol and kept there for 90 minutes to slowly settle down while the rats were exposed. This makes it very difficult to determine the actual exposure concentration because it continually decreased, and changes in particle size due to rapid settling of the aerodynamically larger particles will occur. A dynamic exposure system with continuously generated aerosol is the standard and preferred method for inhalation exposures.

Respiratory Tract Deposition

Inhalation by humans of airborne ENM at the workplace or when handling powders of ENM results in significant deposition in the three compartments of the respiratory tract: the nasopharyngeal region from nose/mouth to the larynx; the tracheobronchial region from larynx to terminal bronchioles; and the alveolar region from the first generation of respiratory bronchioles (bronchioles with some alveoli) to the last generation of alveolar ducts. The deposition efficiency of inhaled particles depends on several particle characteristics, the anatomical structure of the airways, and breathing parameters. Particle size, size distribution, density, and shape are most important for their aerodynamic and thermodynamic diameter, which govern deposition in the respiratory tract by inertial impact, gravitational settling, and displacement by diffusion. In addition, interception (in particular for elongated structures or fibers) and electrostatic image forces (positive charge on particles attracted by negative epithelial surface) play a role in certain conditions (see Chap. 15).

Because in vivo toxicological studies are mostly performed in experimental animals, and because of anatomical and some physiological differences in the respiratory system, knowledge about variations in the behavior of inhaled particles is essential for interpreting results of animal inhalation studies with respect to dosimetric *extrapolation* to humans. Several particle deposition models have been developed based on mathematical modeling and supported by results of numerous human studies using inhalation of benign particles of different sizes. The two most frequently used models are the extensive international commission on radiation protection (ICRP) (1994) model for humans, and a user-friendly (computer) Multiple Path Particle Dosimetry (MPPD) model for rats and humans (Asgharian et al., 1999). Each of these models is based on results of an extensive database of particle deposition studies in humans (ICR Panel MPPD) and in rats (MPPD). These data have been incorporated into mathematical equations describing airborne particle behavior due to impaction, sedimentation,

and diffusion for different airway geometries in humans and rats. There is good general agreement between results of the two models, although some quantitative differences exist. It should be kept in mind that these are still models to estimate the deposition in the respiratory tract depending on particle parameters, airway geometrics, and breathing modes. Interindividual time values can be very different from the averages that are calculated by the models.

Fig. 28-12 compares the deposition fractions for monodispersed particles of sizes from about 1 nm to 20 µm diameter between humans and rats based on the MPPD model, assuming unit density material. For both species nasal breathing is assumed, which is the obligatory mode for rats. For NPs below 100 nm (in the thermodynamic size range, less than ~0.5 µm), there is only a small difference in deposition between nasal- and oral-breathing mode, whereas these differences become more pronounced for larger particles in the aerodynamic size range (starting at ~0.5 µm). The mechanisms by which inhaled particles are depositing changes from diffusion (due to bombardment of particles by air molecules) as exclusive mechanism for airborne single NPs to gravitational sedimentation and inertial impaction for the larger particles. Comparing deposition efficiencies between rats and humans, similarities but also differences become obvious: Qualitatively, size-dependent deposition fractions are similar; for example, there is a lowest point of deposition for inhaled particles in both species around the size of

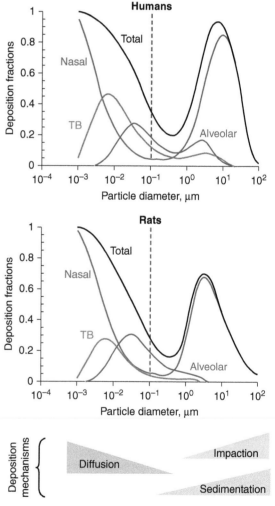

Figure 28-12. *Model predictions of deposition fractions for different particle sizes in humans and rats.* Nanosized particles are left of dashed line (<100 nm); their deposition is governed by diffusion (Brownian motion of air molecules) (Figure provided by B. Asgharian).

0.5 μm, which is due to the fact that at this size the combined impact of diffusional displacement and gravitational settling is minimal, so they are most persistent in the air. Of interest is that—contrary to a general misconception—the smallest inhaled particles (<5 nm) are not depositing in the most distal areas of the lung, but in the upper extrathoracic region. Thus, the nasal filtering capacity is effective for both the smallest and largest particles.

Obvious differences between rats and humans are the maximum size of particles that are respirable, that is, will reach the alveolar region. In rats, this is about 5 μm aerodynamic size, in humans about 15 μm. Although these sizes are outside the range of single NP, airborne NP occur for the most part as agglomerates, which can reach μm size equivalent aerodynamic diameters. The concept of rat versus human respirability also applies to smaller μm size particles. Even for submicron-sized particles rat/human deposition fractions are not necessarily the same. Thus, if a rat inhalation study is designed to simulate a human exposure scenario with an aerodynamic median particle size of 5 μm, not much of the aerosol will reach the rat's alveolar region. Instead, attempts should be made to streamline the particle size for the rat study such that the deposited dose in the alveolar region is similar between the two species relative to alveolar surface area.

The deposition curves in Fig. 28-12 imply that inhaled particles of ~20 nm have similar deposition efficiencies in all three regions of the respiratory tract. However, a more judicious analysis reveals that the alveolar region actually receives the least amount of these NPs when the deposited dose is expressed per unit surface area (Fig. 28-13). The data in this figure are derived from the MPPD model, assuming an eight-hour exposure to 20 nm monodispersed TiO_2 NPs under nasal-breathing conditions for rats and humans. As can be seen, the deposited dose normalized for surface area is less than 1 ng/cm² in the alveolar region, and is highest for the extrathoracic nasopharyngeal region. This result should also serve as a reminder that realistic in vivo doses to cells of the respiratory tract are mostly orders of magnitude lower than doses that are typically applied in vitro to lung epithelial cell cultures. Moreover, the deposited dose in Fig. 28-13 had accumulated over an eight-hour exposure, which is different from a high in vitro dose

Distribution of deposition enhancement factors of 5 μm-diameter unit density particles for a 60 L/min minute ventilation   **1207**

CHAPTER 28 NANOTOXICOLOGY

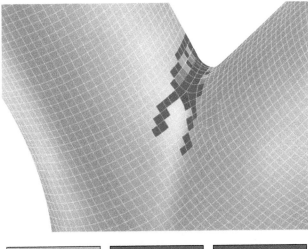

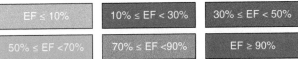

| EF ≤ 10% | 10% ≤ EF < 30% | 30% ≤ EF < 50% |
| 50% ≤ EF <70% | 70% ≤ EF <90% | EF ≥ 90% |

Figure 28-14. *Distribution of hotspots of deposition on carinal ridges of the bronchial region in the human respiratory tract.* The enhancement factor is largest for aerodynamically large particles, but is very low for airborne nanosized particles. (From: Balásházy *et al.*, 2003.)

rate, similar to dose rate differences between in vivo instillation and inhalation (see Fig. 28-8).

The development of deposition hotspots in the respiratory tract during particle inhalation is often cited as justification for using high doses in vitro studies (Phalen *et al.*, 2006). These hotspots occur at the bifurcations (carinal ridges) of the upper generations of the tracheobronchial region where due to impaction more particles per unit surface will deposit compared to the average deposition per unit surface over the length of the airways (Fig. 28-14). Concentrations up to several 100-fold higher than on average in the airway may be accumulated for larger particles. However, as Balásházy *et al.* (2003) pointed out using computer modeling, the size of the area receiving the highest concentration is the size of square (patch) with a sidelength of only 0.1 nm, and airborne NPs are contributing to these hotspots to a lesser degree only: for a patch size of 1 mm the enhancement factor is about 30-fold for 1 to 100 nm particles. In the alveolar region where the airflow is very low, no deposition hotspots for NPs exist (Balásházy *et al.*, 2008). This non-homogeneous depositoin and formation of hotspots seems to correlate with predilection sites for bronchial carcinoma (Schlesinger and Lippmann, 1978; Balásházy *et al.*, 2003), which is further enhanced by less effective mucociliary clearance at carinal ridges.

Respiratory Tract Clearance and Disposition of NP: Nanomaterials

Once NP are deposited in the respiratory tract they will encounter physiological clearance mechanisms in the nasal–oropharyngeal, tracheobronchial, and alveolar region as described under *Particle Clearance* in Chap. 15. However, there are several differences that separate NP from larger particles as indicated in Table 28-2. Alveolar macrophages generally are attracted to deposited particles by chemotactic signals generated at the site of deposition, for example C5 via activation of complement by particles (Warheit *et al.*, 1988a,b).

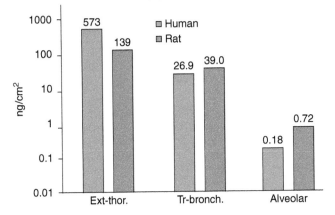

Deposition per unit surface area (cm²) over eight-hour exposure at 100 μg/m³ (nasal breathing, resting conditions)
Nanoparticle size: CMD = 20 nm; GSD = 1.0
Density: ρ = 1 g/cm³

Figure 28-13. *Deposited amount of inhaled nanoparticles of 20 nm diameter (density 1 g/cm³) in the three regions of the respiratory tract of humans and rats, calculated with the Multiple Path Particle Dosimetry model (see text).* Assumed is an inhaled concentration of 100 μg/m³ over an eight-hour exposure with nasal breathing under resting conditions. Deposition is normalized per cm² of surface area of a specific airway region.

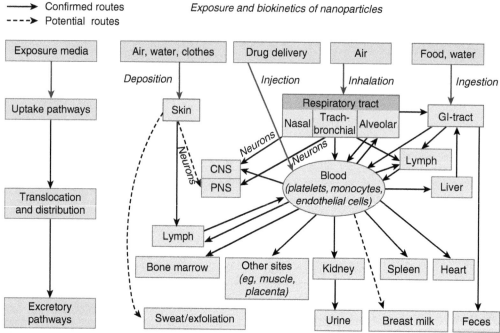

Figure 28-15. *Exposure and biokinetics of nanoparticles routes of exposure and biokinetics (uptake, distribution, elimination) of nanomaterials.* Translocation rates in general are very low (see text). (Modified from Oberdörster *et al.*, 2005.)

Nanosized particles may be too small to generate such signal; studies in rodents with inhaled particles ranging from nano- to micro-size have shown that in vivo macrophage surveillance in terms of phagocytosis and clearance of nanosized particles is rather poor (Oberdörster *et al.*, 2005; Semmler-Behneke *et al.*, 2007; Geiser *et al.*, 2008), so that deposited NP will interact with epithelial cells. Uptake into the pulmonary interstitium occurs, and there is evidence that some of the interstitialized NP reenter the airways, possibly the smaller conducting airways, from where they are cleared via the mucociliary escalator (Semmler-Behneke *et al.*, 2007).

Translocation into the interstitium and subsequently into blood and lymph circulation distinguishes nanoparticles from microparticles. Fig. 28-15 depicts the blood compartment as a plenum from which any tissue/organ can be reached by circulating NP. However, the amount of NP translocating from the lung to the blood circulation and accumulation in secondary organs is very low, as results from rat inhalation studies with NP have shown, about 1% to 2% of the lung deposit (Kreyling *et al.*, 2002, 2009; Semmler-Behneke, 2007). Long-term retention studies with radioactive iridium NPs (15–20 nm) have shown that clearance of NP in extrapulmonary organs following the initial accumulation is very efficient so that after six months, with the exception of liver and spleen, only minor amounts—below level of detection—were still present. Liver and spleen also had decreased sharply to levels of less than 0.05% of the initial lung burden. In general, the overall pattern of long-term clearance from the lungs of rats was similar to that of microparticles with retention halftimes of 70 to 90 days. Elimination of NP from the body occurred via feces (Semmler *et al.*, 2004) and via urine for smaller NPs (see below). Despite the low translocation rates of NP from the portal of entry to secondary organs and efficient clearance, it has to be considered that a continuous exposure may result in significant accumulation in some secondary organs. Significant efforts should, therefore, be made to design studies to assess the biokinetic behavior of ENM following relevant exposures.

Biokinetic studies have shown that organs with major reticuloendothelial system (RES) functions, such as liver and spleen, take up most circulating NP. Coating NP with PEG prevents this uptake by phagocytes and thereby the circulation time is increased, which may be desirable for medical diagnostic or therapeutic applications (Ballou *et al.*, 2004). Other RES organs for accumulation of nanomaterials include the bone marrow and the developing organism in utero. Like the liver and spleen, the bone marrow can receive similarly high or even higher doses of blood-borne NPs (Rinderknecht *et al.*, 2007). As a major RES organ, studies need to be designed to determine responses of stem cells in bone marrow upon interaction with ENM in vivo. A recent study in mice after administration of very high doses in drinking water of TiO_2 NP (~25 nm) for five days reported induction of DNA double strand breaks in bone marrow cells (Trouiller *et al.*, 2009). The authors interpreted this finding as secondary to a systemic inflammatory response, multiple other organs also showed oxidative stress responses and genotoxicity. The authors did not attempt to determine the amount of TiO_2 in different organs, which would have strengthened the study.

Organs with tight endothelial junctions, in particular the central nervous system, will not likely accumulate blood-borne NPs, unless the tight blood–brain barrier is damaged or NP surface has been specially modified (Kreuter, 2004). For example, coating NP with the surfactant polysorbate 80 made it possible to deliver a drug loaded into NP across the blood–brain barrier (BBB), to the brain. Translocation across the BBB was facilitated via the endothelial low-density lipoprotein (LDL), receptor, and coating of the NP with ApoE-lipoprotein achieved the same result. The drug was either released to diffuse into the brain after NP uptake into the endothelial cells or via NP transport into the brain (Kreuter, 2004). In either case, the mechanism for drug delivery may be based on a "Trojan Horse" effect in that the coated NP mimic lipoprotein particles. This underlines again the importance of protein adsorption (corona formation) for the biodistribution of NP following uptake into the organism.

Nanomaterials and the Brain

Fig. 28-16 depicts four basic translocation pathways of inhaled NP from the upper and lower respiratory tract into the CNS. In addition to the blood circulation—which does not efficiently contribute to

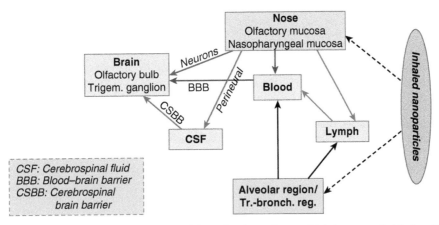

From respiratory tract to brain:
Potential translocation pathways of nanoparticles

Figure 28-16. *From the respiratory tract to the brain: Potential translocation pathways of inhales nanomaterials from the upper and lower respiratory tract.* Note that the BBB is very tight and that neuronal pathway circumvent this barrier. (From: Oberdörster *et al.*, 2009.)

CNS translocation because of the very tight blood–brain barrier—there is uptake into the lymphatic system—again feeding back into the blood circulation—and transport in or next to sensory neurons from the upper respiratory tract. Perineural translocation along the olfactory nerve will deliver NP into the cerebrospinal fluid (CSF), as reported by Czerniawska (1970) and Zhang *et al.* (2006). To what degree transport into brain tissue may be inhibited due to a cerebrospinal brain barrier needs to be assessed in further studies. The most efficient pathway of NP translocation to the CNS appears to be via olfactory sensory neurons from the nasal olfactory mucosa directly to the olfactory bulb (Oberdörster *et al.*, 2009). The discovery of this nose to brain connection as a NP passageway goes back to early studies demonstrating this pathway for polio virus ~30 nm transport from the nose to the brain in nonhuman primates following intranasal instillation (Brodie and Elridge, 1934; Bodian and Howe, 1941), and subsequently visualized by transmission electron microscopy (TEM), with silver-coated gold NP (50 nm) instilled intranasally into squirrel monkeys (De Lorenzo, 1970). More recent inhalation studies with insoluble carbon NP (~36 nm) and poorly soluble Mn-oxide NP (~30 nm) confirmed the olfactory nerve system as an efficient mechanism for airborne NP to reach the CNS (Oberdörster *et al.*, 2004; Elder *et al.*, 2006). Inflammatory responses in the olfactory bulb and several brain regions were induced by 12 days of manganese oxide exposure at concentrations that are lower than those experienced by arc welders after exposure to a mixture of nanosized particles—including manganese oxides. Other nasal instillation studies in mice, applying enormous high doses, reported oxidative stress and inflammatory responses (Wang *et al.*, 2008a,b). Results of epidemiological studies of impaired cognitive function and of neurodegenerative brain pathology associated with exposure to traffic-related particles raised the question as to whether ambient UFPs as constituents of urban air pollution may be etiologically involved (Calderon-Garciduenas *et al.*, 2011; Weuve *et al.*, 2012). Whether such etiological link exists is still to be investigated. The plausibility of a respective hypothesis is supported by findings that loss of olfactory function has been described as a common characteristic of neurodegenerative diseases, that is, Parkinson, Alzheimer, and Huntington disease (Barrios *et al.*, 2007; Doty, 2008; Kovács, 2004; Moberg and Doty, 1997).

In the same study by Trouiller *et al.* (2009) mentioned before, the authors had also exposed pregnant mice to TiO$_2$ NP in drinking water for 10 days. The offspring had a higher frequency of DNA deletions in the retina when examined at 20 days of age. Due to the extraordinarily high dose of 500 mg/kg and the lack of verifying TiO$_2$ in fetal tissues, these results have to be interpreted with caution. Other studies evaluating exposure of the fetus to NP size-dependent translocation across the placenta in mice, with smaller quantum dots transferring more readily than larger ones (Chu *et al.*, 2010). Takeda *et al.* (2009) injected TiO$_2$ NP subcutaneously in pregnant mice (100 µg/mouse on each of four days). They identified TiO$_2$ NP in testis and brain of the six-week-old male offspring. The authors also observed reduced daily sperm production and apoptotic cells in the olfactory bulb of these offspring. Results of this bolus-type injection study maybe viewed as a proof-of-principle study for demonstrating placenta penetration because of the unphysiological mode of delivery of a high dose and high dose rate; however, the same group had reported in a mouse inhalation study with diesel exhaust the presence of UFPs in the brain of offspring and increased apoptosis of Purkinje cells in the cerebellum (Sugamata *et al.*, 2006).

Elimination of Nanomaterials

Elimination pathways for ENM from the body (Fig. 28-15) include mainly feces and urine. Urinary excretion is restricted to nanostructures <5.5 nm in size for metal-based NP (Choi *et al.*, 2007), limited by the hydrodynamic diameter of the particle that may change in circulation due to protein adsorption. This general principle appears to be different for circulating fibrous structures of ENM. Singh *et al.* (2006) and Lacerda *et al.* (2008) reported that even 20 to 30 nm diameter MWCNT with length between 0.5 and 2 µm were collected in urine of rats following intravenous application. They explain this phenomenon by a hydrodynamic lining up of nanotubes so they will pass through glomerular pores. The fecal excretory clearance pathways consist of several inputs: One is mucociliary clearance of deposited particles from the airways into the GI tract; another is via hepatobiliary clearance of blood-borne ENM via liver and bile into the small intestine. This elimination pathway is suggested by results from Semmler-Behnke *et al.* (2007), and it is also a well-known excretory path for heavy metals in the blood (Clarkson *et al.*, 1988).

With regard to the CNS, no data on ENM elimination are available yet. It is conceivable that the CSF via its connections to the nasal lymphatic system (Czerniawska, 1970) and to the blood circulation could be an excretory pathway for the brain, which needs to be investigated in future studies. Indeed, Segal (2000) concluded from their review on CSF barriers that the CSF may both act as a compartment for distribution of substances to many brain regions, but also can act as an elimination route for waste products into the blood circulation because the brain has no lymphatics.

Another clearance pathway of deposited ENM in the lung involves translocation via interstitium or lymph to the pleura and subsequent elimination via lymphatic openings (stomata) on the parietal pleura to mediastinal lymph nodes from where NP may enter the blood circulation via the right and left thoracic ducts. This pathway is of particular importance for fiber-shaped ENM because the size of the parietal stomata prevents efficient clearance of structures >10 μm in length. Indeed, collection of lymph from the right thoracic duct of dogs that had been dosed intrabronchially with amosite asbestos showed only fibers <9 μm in length appearing in the collected lymph (Oberdörster et al., 1988). As a consequence, the interaction of the retained longer fibers in the pleural cavity with mesothelial cells induce inflammatory and granulomatous responses and in long-term potentially mesothelioma (Donaldson et al., 2010). The following section discusses experimental in vivo data from bolus-type and inhalation studies of the toxicology of CNT that confirm the possibility of a mesotheliogenic response, but also caution to extrapolate directly to realistic inhalation exposures without further verification. A critical appraisal of the available in vivo study concludes this section.

CASE STUDY: MWCNTs

Bolus-type Exposures

As described in the previous paragraphs, bolus-type delivery has been the preferred method of dosing to identify as a first step of the potential hazard of ENM. The advantages and disadvantages need to be considered when interpreting the results, in particular the rationale for the administered dose levels causing potential bolus associated responses should be critically considered. Several doses covering a reasonable range, also including a positive or negative control material for ranking purposes, should be part of a well-designed study. Knowledge about actual—if available—or anticipated exposure levels should be used to justify a selected dose range. Key is a careful physicochemical characterization of CNTs with respect to their original specification (pristine state) as well as any modification due to treatment (dispersants, sonification) prior to administration. Specifically, the presence of impurities (eg, metals, organics, amorphous carbon) needs to be considered.

Early intratracheal instillation studies in rats and mice with SWCNTs were performed with very high doses (up to 1.25 mg/rat and 0.5 mg/mouse), causing severe lung injury with rapid persistent granuloma formation including mortality (Warheit et al., 2004; Lam et al., 2004). Doses were so high to induce even physical blockage of conducting airways. Pharyngeal aspiration of lower doses with purified SWCNTs in mice at lower doses caused interstitial fibrosis and granulomatous lesions, possibly due to the existence of large agglomerates in the administered suspension (Shvedova et al., 2005). Subsequent aspiration studies in mice confirmed these findings in mice, showing also that the responses were not affected by the metal content; however, the degree of dispersion influenced responses such that administration of the same mass dose of well-dispersed SWCNTs caused greater and more persistent responses than poorly dispersed SWCNTs (Shvedova et al., 2008; Mercer et al., 2008).

MWCNTs delivered to rats by intratracheal instillation (0.5–5 mg/rat) also induced inflammatory, granulomatous, and fibrotic responses; these responses were lower when the material was ground such that the length of the MWCNTs was reduced from 6 to 0.7 μm (Muller et al., 2005). Another study compared pulmonary responses to purified MWCNTs in mice when given either by instillation (50 μg/mouse) or inhalation (32.6 mg/m³, 6 h/day, up to 15 days, estimated to result in 70–210 μg in the lung) (Li et al., 2007). Despite the higher lung dose following inhalation, only moderate effects were induced, whereas instillation resulted in severe inflammation and alveolar wall destruction, demonstrating a stark difference between responses induced by the two modes of dosing with the physiological inhalation exposure avoiding the high bolus-related response. As already mentioned before, the results of both the Li et al. and Shvedova et al. studies have to be interpreted with caution because of the uncertainty of the deposited doses in the lung following inhalation.

Other studies with instilled high doses (up to 1.75 mg/rat) of MWCNTs in rats reported transient inflammatory responses with persistent alveolar wall thickening (Liu et al., 2008). Transient inflammation and granulomatous responses in rats were also reported by Kobayashi et al. (2010) at lower instilled MWCNT doses, whereas Porter et al. (2010) observed a rapid and persistent fibrotic response in mice following aspiration of purified MWCNTs in mice (10–80 μg/mouse) which was confirmed by morphometric (lung tissue) analysis by Mercer et al. (2011). Additional evaluations of MWCNT responses in rats and mice confirmed inflammatory, granulomatous, and fibrotic responses following instillation or aspiration dosing (Porter et al., 2010; Aiso et al., 2011; Han et al., 2010).

Translocation of aspirated MWCNT to the pleura following aspiration in mice was also reported (Porter et al., 2010) including penetration into the intrapleural space of mice following aspiration (Mercer et al., 2010). A six-hour inhalation exposure of mice to a very high concentration of 30 mg/m³ confirmed that inhaled MWCNT can reach the subpleural wall (space between peripheral alveoli and visceral pleura) are localized within subpleural macrophages (Ryman-Rasmussen et al., 2009a). In summary, bolus-type delivery of CNTs to the respiratory tract of rats and mice revealed induction of dose-dependent significant inflammatory, granulomatous, and fibrogenic responses; they showed also that MWCNTs can reach subpleural and intrapleural sites.

Other bolus-type studies delivered MWCNTs into the peritoneal cavity (intraperitoneal injection, or i.p.)—as a surrogate for the mesothelial lining of the pleural cavity—in order to expose mesothelial cells directly for assessing a mesotheliogenic response. Takagi et al. (2008) found, indeed, mesothelioma induction one year following very high i.p. doses in p53 heterozygous mice, which was similar to the positive crocidolite asbestos control. A follow-up study with lower i.p. injection of 50 μg/mouse confirmed this finding (Kanno et al., 2010). Similarly, Sakamoto et al. (2009) induced peritoneal mesothelioma in rats, following high-dose MWCNT injection intrascrotally. Poland et al. (2008) also suggested an asbestos-like response after inducing mesothelial granuloma with amosite asbestos and with long straight but not with short MWCNT two weeks after i.p. injection in mice. Follow-up i.p. studies showed the importance of lymphatic (Fig. 28-17) clearance of fiber structures from the pleural cavity (Murphy et al., 2011): Lymphatic stomata (Wang et al., 1975) in the parietal pleura with diameters of 3 to 10 μm in rodents (Shinohara et al., 1997) act as an effective clearance pathway for shorter fibers, whereas longer ones will be retained and induce inflammatory, oxidative stress responses progressing to mesothelioma. Such length-dependent plural retention and lymphatic clearance was demonstrated by Murphy et al. (2011)

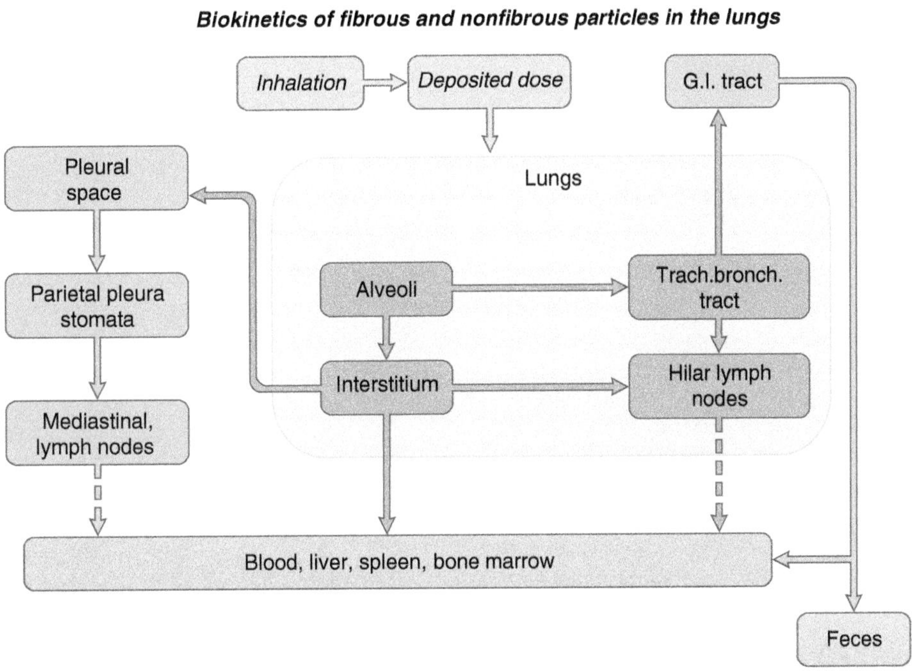

Figure 28-17. *Important translocation pathways of deposited particles in the lung that reach the interstitium are via lymphatic channels to hilar lymph nodes; or migration toward the pleura with subsequent uptake into lymphatic openings (stomata) and clearance toward mediastinal lymph nodes.* Both hilar and mediastinal lymph nodes drain into the right lymphatic duct to reach the jugular vein in the neck area.

after using i.p. injection of different types of MWCNTs and other nanotubes. Only long but not short or entangled MWCNTs caused significant mesothelial cell proliferation and granuloma formation and fibrosis. These i.p. injection studies in rodents clearly show the potential of CNTs, specifically MWCNTs, to induce severe adverse length-dependent effects at mesothelial sites once they reach the pleural cavity. Appropriate inhalation studies in rodents need to be designed to determine the translocation of inhaled, generally highly agglomerated airborne CNTs from deposition sites in the lung to the pleura and to confirm the findings from bolus aspiration studies with well-dispersed CNTs.

Inhalation Studies

Relatively few inhalation studies with CNTs in rodents have been reported (Table 28-8). Most of these were of short duration (hours to a few days), and only two were designed as subchronic 13-week inhalation studies (Ma-Hock *et al.*, 2009; Pauluhn, 2010) and two as four-week inhalation studies (Oyabu *et al.*, 2011; Morimoto *et al.*, 2012a). The value of short-term inhalation studies for risk characterization can be questioned because such exposures to CNTs at realistic low concentrations are not likely to reveal certain chronic effects if long latency periods are involved. Although unreasonable, very high concentrations with short exposures maybe helpful for purposes of hazard identification and toxicity ranking—which could be achieved at less cost and effort by bolus-type studies—they are not useful for deriving a no observed adverse effect level (NOAEL) or for quantitative risk assessment. Thus, most meaningful and best justified for the risk assessment process would be a subchronic multiconcentration (minimum three concentrations) study with sufficient postexposure observation. However, short-term, even one-term, exposure to a relevant concentration is very useful for dosimetric purposes when determining the biodistribution from deposition sites in the lung to secondary organs. Of course, a prerequisite is the availability of sensitive detection methods, such as radioactive labeling (Kreyling

et al., 2009) or use of a nonleachable catalyst firmly attached to or imbedded within the CNTs.

The choice of the mode of inhalation exposure—whole-body or nose-only—is up to the investigator. Generally, for long-term chronic exposures, whole-body is preferred because the tight confinement of rodents during nose-only exposures induces additional stress, despite careful adaptation prior to starting exposures (Rothenberg *et al.*, 2000; Fawcett *et al.*, 1994; Pare and Glavin, 1986; Udelsman *et al.*, 1993; Sistonen *et al.*, 1992). The disadvantage of whole-body exposure is the contamination of the animals' fur with aerosolized CNTs, which may lead to additional oral intake due to preening. However, the additional dose is very low, and GI-tract exposure is part of any inhalation exposure due to bronchial clearance of the deposited material.

Most of the CNT inhalation studies were performed with MWCNTs; only two used SWCNTs. Exposure concentrations ranged from 0.1 to 32.6 mg/m^3 either one concentration only up to four concentrations in a study, and duration from six hours to 13 weeks. Outcomes (Table 28-8) range from no significant effects to severe pulmonary inflammation/oxidative stress responses; one study reported systemic effects including cytokine and oxidative stress responses in the spleen (Mitchell *et al.*, 2007). Given the diversity of the used CNTs and the different exposure methods, aerosol preparation, the airborne CNT characteristics, and different endpoints, the wide range of responses should come as no surprise. Although these studies show the potential of inhaled SWCNT and inhaled MWCNT to cause lung injury, transiently or more persistently, the two subchronic multiconcentration 13-week studies allow a more complete assessment of the toxicity of MWCNTs that could be used for deriving occupational exposure limits (Pauluhn, 2010).

Although bolus-type delivery did result in pleural effects and translocation of MWCNT toward pleural sites as discussed before, no pleural effects were seen in the 13-week inhalation studies, except pleural thickening at the two highest exposure concentrations (Pauluhn, 2010). Movement of inhaled MWCNT to subpleural sites was observed by Ryman-Rasmussen *et al.* (2009a) when

Table 28-8

Carbon Nanotube Inhalation Studies in Rodents

AUTHOR AND YEAR	CNT	SPECIES (EXPOSURE)	AEROSOL	CONCENTRATION mg/m³	DURATION	FINDINGS
Li *et al.*, 2007; 2009	MWCNT	mouse (whole-body)	powder; no info. static system	32.6 (average) decreasing from 80 mg/m³ to 1 mg/m³ in 90 min.	6 h/day (4 × 90 min) 8; 16; 24 day (once every other day)	moderate proliferation and thickening of alveolar wall lung lavage increase of protein, lactate dehydrogenase (LDH), alkaline phosphatase (ALP) and acid phosphatase (ACP)
Mitchell *et al.*, 2007	MWCNT	mouse (whole-body)	powder; mass median aerodynamic diameter (MMAD) 0.7–1 μm and 1.8 μm	0.3; 1; 5	6/day 7; 14 days	no lung inflammation or tissue damage; transient systemic immunosuppression; cytokine upregulation and oxidative stress in spleen
Shvedova *et al.*, 2008	SWCNT	mouse (whole-body)	powder; mass mode aerodynamic diameter 4.2 μm	5.5	5 h/day 4 days	multifocal granulomatous pneumonia, interst. fibrosis; oxidative stress; K-ras mutation lung
Ryman-Rasmussen *et al.*, 2009	MWCNT	mouse (whole-body)	Collison jet nebulizer from suspension with pluronic F-68, MMAD ~0.16–0.21 μm	1; 30	6 h	CNT embedded in subpleural wall and in subpleural macrophages; subpleural fibrosis; no pleural fibrosis or granuloma up to 154 weeks postinhalation
Ryman-Rasmussen *et al.*, 2009b	MWCNT	mouse, OVA allergic model (whole-body)	Collison jet nebulizer from suspension with pluronic F-68; MMAD 0.714 μm	100	6 h	MWCNT throughout lung in macrophages and epithelial cells; fibrosis in OVA sensitized mice, but not in normal mice; elevated platelet derived growth factor (PDG) in nonsensitized mice; OVA and MWCNT act synergistically
Ma-Hock *et al.*, 2009	MWCNT	rat (nose-only)	powder MMAD 0.7–2.0 geometric standard deviation (GSD) 2.1–3.6	0.1; 0.5; 2.5	6 h/day 5 day/week 13 weeks	increased lung weights granulomatous inflammation fibrotic changes no lung lavage data LOAEL 0.1 mg/m³
Pauluhn *et al.*, 2010	MWCNT	rat (nose-only)	powder MMAD 2.74–3.41 GSD 1.98–2.14	0.1; 0.4; 1.5; 6.0	6 h/day 5 day/week 13 weeks	increased lung weights pre-manufacturing notice (PMN), increased in lung lavage; granulomatous inflammation fibrosis pleural thickening (high concs.) NOAEL 0.1 mg/m³
Oyabu *et al.*, 2011; and Morimoto *et al.*, 2012(a)	MWCNT (short)	rat (whole-body)	jet nebulizer, aqueous suspension with Triton-X: GMD 63 nm GSD = 1.5 geometric mean length (GML) = 1.1 μm GSD = 2.7 70% single fibers	0.37	6 h/day 5 day/week 4 weeks	~70 μg lung deposition measured; retention T½ = 54 days; slight increase in lung weight; increase of chemokines and myeloperoxidase in lung lavage
Morimoto *et al.*, 2012(b)	SWCNT	rat (whole-body)	jet nebulizer, aqueous suspension, Tween 80 pretreated; bundles: (ropes): 0.2 × 0.7 μm 90% well dispersed	0.03; 0.13	6 h/day 5 day/week 4 weeks	calculated lung burden: 1.8 and 8.8 μg; no significant changes in lung lavage neutrophils or protein, (ALP), chemokines, (CINCs), HO-1 level; no lung pathology

individual fibers and very fine agglomerates (160–210 nm) were generated from a liquid suspension following a single six-hour very high concentration exposure of 30 mg/m³. However, pleural fibrosis or granuloma did not develop up to 22 weeks postexposure. The small size of the aerosol as well as an extremely high dose may have been a factor in a deeper peripheral lung deposition. A follow-up six-hour study by Ryman-Rasmussen et al., (2009b) with inhaled MWCNT in an ovalbumin (OVA), allergic mouse model found a synergistic effect; MWCNT alone did not induce fibrosis in non-sensitized mice. This result is in contrast to their earlier study where a six-hour exposure to a three-fold lower concentration did induce subpleural fibrosis in mice (Ryman-Rasmussen et al., 2009a). The larger aerosol size in the second study may have prevented significant deposition in the peripheral lung.

Regarding a comparison between MWCNT- and SWCNT-induced pulmonary or secondary organ effects, the only medium-term (four weeks) SWCNT inhalation study in rats (Morimoto et al., 2012a) did not observe any effect; however, estimated lung burdens were just 1.8 and 8.8 µg, about the same as the lowest concentration in the Pauluhn (2010) study with MWCNTs that also did not show any effect (NOAEL).

Critical Appraisal of CNT In Vivo Studies

Several intrapleural injection studies with MWCNTs in mice have indicated that CNTs have a mesotheliogenic potential, discussed in the previous section. In addition, intratracheal instillation studies in rats and oropharyngeal aspiration studies with MWCNTs and SWCNTs have confirmed a pulmonary inflammatory and oxidative stress inducing potential. These results have raised concern that CNTs may represent and give rise to another case of asbestos toxicity and pathology, in particular insidious because of the decades-long latency period from exposure to manifestation of mesothelioma. Controversy exists regarding the applicability of results of intracavitary injection studies for regulatory purposes. European regulations for synthetic mineral fibers exonerate those from being classified as a carcinogen if it can be shown that the material fulfills one of the following conditions (EC Directive 97/69/EC, Nota Q, 1997):

- a short-term biopersistence test by inhalation has shown that the fibers longer than 20 µm have a weighted half-time less than 20 days, or
- a short-term biopersistence test by intratracheal instillation has shown that the fibers longer than 20 µm have a weighted half-time less than 40 days, or
- an appropriate intraperitoneal test has shown no evidence of excess carcinogenicity, or
- absence of relevant pathogenicity or neoplastic changes in a suitable long-term inhalation test.

This regulation is based on a number of experimental studies going back to Stanton et al. (1981) and Pott et al. (1987) that showed induction of tumors when different types of asbestos and persistent synthetic mineral fibers were directly injected into the pleural or peritoneal cavity. However, use of this test for regulatory purposes has not been established in the United States; the test has been criticized because of the massive doses being used leading to fibrotic reactions thereby interfering with and overwhelming physiological defense mechanisms. As to whether present European regulations will be applied to CNTs is questionable because they have been issued for man-made vitreous (silicate) fibers and the high bolus doses and associated caveats should be considered.

Still, results of CNT intracavitary injection studies summarized in this section have defined the potential of CNTs to induce

mesothelioma, depending on their dimension (>10 µm) and their agglomeration state. Longer-term inhalation studies need to confirm these findings; presently, two subchronic inhalation studies with agglomerated MWCNTs did not confirm a mesotheliogenic response, although high concentrations in the mg/m³ range showed some pleural thickening. Additionally, acute short-term inhalation studies using relevant exposure concentrations of long (>10 µm) and short (<5 µm) MWCNTs are also needed in order to determine the biodistribution of physiologically administered CNTs (inhalation) to secondary organs. Biodistribution based on bolus-type delivery using pretreatment with dispersants and lengthy sonication may be different quantitatively and qualitatively.

Longer-term inhalation studies with intentionally well-dispersed CNTs are not available, although two four-week studies using aerosolization from an aqueous suspension of short MWCNTs and short SWCNTs in rats with use of dispersants and two acute six-hour studies with short MWCNTs in mice using dispersant suspension resulting in smaller aerodynamic diameters reported more peripheral, even subpleural, deposition, but no pleural effects. This appears to be in agreement with results from intraperitoneal injection studies, which did not show an adverse effect of short, straight MWCNTs because of effective removal by lymphatic clearance.

Obviously, given the importance of the physicochemical properties of CNTs for inducing adverse effects, it is of utmost importance to determine these properties, in particular as they appear in the airborne state at sites of human exposures, at occupational sites, or for the consumer. Adding dispersants for testing purposes will change surface properties; conceptually, inhalation studies in experimental animals for purposes of hazard identification should mimic human exposure conditions with regard to airborne size distribution. Of course, differences in respirability between humans and rats/mice have to be considered, and—if necessary—adjustments be made without use of surface altering dispersants or harsh physical treatment.

Appropriately designed multiconcentration subchronic inhalation studies, including a longer recovery period, are essential for deriving NOAELs; results can be used as basis for deriving occupational exposure levels (OELs) by applying rodent/human dosimetric adjustments (Fig. 28-18). Using results from bolus-type studies is difficult and raises questions, although national institute for occupational safety and health (NIOSH) (2011) has combined results of fibrotic responses from diverse bolus-type and inhalation studies to derive a provisional recommended exposure level (REL) of 7 µg/m³. This REL is based on dose–response data from the available studies with bolus-type and short-term inhalation exposures and a subchronic inhalation study. Differences in lengths, use of dispersants, impact of hugely different dose rates between the studies were not considered. NIOSH (2011) suggested, though, that the mass-based REL may not be sufficiently sensitive for detecting CNTs by air sampling and calls for research to determine the most sensitive dosemetrics.

Collectively, the available in vivo toxicological database of CNTs have identified a fibrogenic and mesotheliogenic effect (hazard identification). No pulmonary tumorigenic effect has been reported so far, in contrast to studies with biopersistent asbestos. An asbestos-like mesothelioma response has only been observed following direct i.p. injection of MWCNTs; confirmation following inhalation is still lacking although it is conceivable that the old paradigm of dose–dimension–durability for fiber carcinogenicity applies also to CNTs: they are quite durable (though some studies have now reported degradation of carboxylated SWCNT by peroxidases in vitro, see below), and their dimensions in terms of length and agglomeration/entanglement appear to be important for pleural effects. Of course, other properties (chemistry, surface reactivity) may play a role as well. Thus, as long as no conclusive data regarding carcinogenic effects of realistic exposure to CNTs are available,

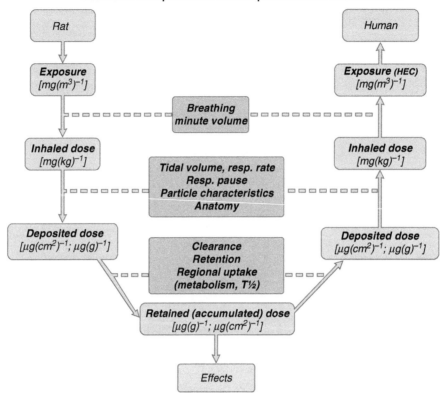

Figure 28-18. *Dosimetric extrapolation of deposition and retention in the respiratory tract from rats to humans: The concept is to achieve the same retained dose in the lungs of humans as has been found at the end of a long-term chronic inhalation study in rats.* According to the scheme above, use of a dosimetric extrapolation model for rats and humans (see text) allows to estimate the respective Human Equivalent Concentration (HEC). (Oberdörster, 1989.)

exposure should be avoided with appropriate measures (ventilation, filtration, personal protective equipment). There is an obvious and urgent need to perform additional long-term (subchronic to chronic) inhalation studies to assess the carcinogenic potential of CNTs and derive protective OELs.

Biological Degradation of Carbon Nanomaterials CNTs have been generally regarded as stable nondegradable materials, which has important implications for long-term health effects following inhalation into the lungs (Donaldson *et al.*, 2006). Recently, however, SWCNT degradation has been observed in acellular assays that simulate the phagolysosome of macrophages, but only if the tubes have been surface carboxylated, which introduces collateral defects in the side walls (Liu *et al.*, 2010c). Carboxylated tubes are also susceptible to biodegradation by exposure to hydrogen peroxide and horseradish peroxidase (Allen *et al.*, 2008, 2009; Kagan *et al.*, 2010) or hypochlorite and the mammalian enzyme myeloperoxidase (Kagan *et al.*, 2010). Kotchey *et al.* (2011) also reported that graphene oxide, but not reduced graphene oxide, is susceptible to oxidative attack by hydrogen peroxide and horseradish peroxidase. These observations may enable design of safer carbon materials (Yan *et al.*, 2011) that are potentially biodegradable in order to minimize adverse environmental and human health impacts. However, degradation of CNTs in vivo is still to be confirmed.

TOXICITY TESTING

Although numerous in vitro and in vivo studies have reported toxic effects of different ENMs, results are often conflicting and hazards are overstated due to poor understanding and knowledge about the

appropriateness of applied doses and concentrations and their relevance to realistic exposures. This issue will be further discussed later. A conceptual testing paradigm is shown in Fig. 28-19. In order to perform risk assessment or to derive OELs, exposure and hazard data are required. To identify and characterize a hazard, in vitro and in vivo studies will be useful, and results should be derived via well-designed dose–response relationships. Key considerations for designing such studies include careful physicochemical characterization of the ENM to be tested, justification of the method(s) of dosing, selection of target cells, tissues or animal species, and appropriate endpoints. Reference materials may also be included in order to rank unknown ENMs against a known positive and/or negative control. Whereas in vitro data alone permit toxicity ranking, appropriately performed in vivo studies (using inhalation when dealing with airborne materials) will allow a full risk assessment because exposure and dosimetric extrapolation to humans can be performed. In the long-term, in silico studies may be developed to assess a hazard, and in even a more distant future to predict human risk. Ideally, knowledge about anticipated human exposure would be necessary to inform both animal exposure studies as well as in vitro dosing.

In vivo animal studies obviously are not generally predicting human exposures: the lower loops in Fig. 28-19 are referring to dosimetric correlations between in vitro/in vivo and in vivo animals/in vivo humans, going in both directions with the goal to (a) inform the design of in vivo animal studies using available human exposure data, (b) use exposure–dose–response information from animal studies to compare with human data. The upper one directional animal to human loop is referring to extrapolating effects and mechanisms from relevant (based on dosimetric relevancy) animal studies to humans, with the goal to be predictive for deriving

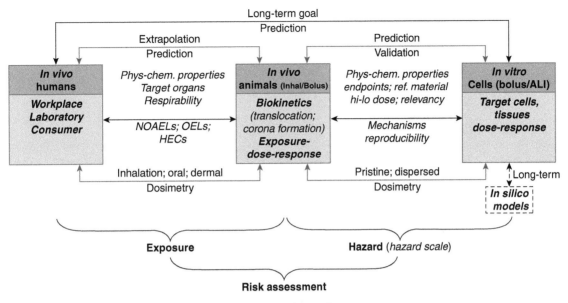

Figure 28-19. *Concepts and goals of nanomaterial toxicity testing (see text).*

"safe" exposure levels or OELs; thus, an animal study can be used to predict human equivalent exposure concentrations or OELs. An example for this approach is the recent subchronic rat inhalation study with MWCNT by Pauluhn (2010).

The following paragraphs focus on concepts and results of in vivo experiments as basis for use in the risk assessment process using as example CNTs. However, a need for in vitro studies should be stressed as far as uncovering underlying mechanisms of effects are concerned, provided that the caveats pointed out above are considered. In addition, despite these limitations, in vitro studies are useful for toxicity ranking of nanomaterials for the purpose of hazard identification (Rushton *et al.*, 2010). In contrast, the design of in vivo studies allows the full evaluation of exposure–dose–response relationships, which is necessary for the process of risk assessment (Fig. 28-19).

Some important points should be considered when designing exposure–dose–response studies with CNTs in experimental animals. The major exposure route for CNTs to be expected is via inhalation at manufacturing sites and during distribution and usage (handling, refilling, disposal), although ingestion and dermal exposures also occur but have not received as much attention (Fig. 28-15). For medicinal applications, injection is an important route of exposure requiring specific awareness with respect to assuring desired beneficial (pharmacological) outcomes yet avoiding undesirable (toxicological) responses (Kolosnaj *et al.*, 2010). For example, Yang *et al.* (2010) concluded from their studies with SWCNT that the desired pharmacological target organelle for drug delivery by SWCNT are the cell lysosomes, whereas the mitochondria are the target organelles for SWCNT toxicity. These aspects will not be discussed further.

In Vitro Dosimetry

The importance of dose rate for bolus-type delivery of ENM in vivo vis-à-vis inhalation has been stressed in previous sections. As most ENM toxicity studies are performed using in vitro assays, which are generally short-term, dosing-related questions are highly relevant. Teeguarden *et al.* (2007) pointed out that the dose received by the cell is a function of colloidal dynamics or "particokinetics"

in the culture medium governed by diffusion and settling phenomena, which in turn is governed by particle and media properties that include particle size, agglomeration/aggregation state, shape, density, and charge. This is very different from chemicals dissolved in culture medium and requires a thorough evaluation of particle dosimetry in vivo. At equal mass concentrations in the medium, the magnitude of the cellular dose of ENM will differ significantly from those implied by the media concentration. This can give rise to significant misinterpretation of responses and is likely to contribute to differences in results between different laboratories. For example, particles of the same material but of different sizes will settle onto cells in culture at different rates; and particles of the same size but different densities will also settle differently so that the time for particles to reach the cell layer at the bottom of a dish can vary widely. Similar to the aerodynamic behavior of airborne particles, the hydrodynamic behavior in culture medium expressed as their transport velocity shows a minimum of movement for intermediate sizes where the combination of gravitational settling and diffusional movement is lowest.

Fig. 28-20 illustrates the different mechanisms that determine the in vitro particle kinetics for particle sizes from 1 nm to 1000 nm (Hinderliter *et al.*, 2010). A typical U-shaped form depicting faster transport at both ends of the range of sizes and a slowest transport for particles around 20 to 60 nm is the result of the competing forces and particle and media characteristics. Temperature, mixing, and advection also add to the complexity of particle movement in the media. Teeguarden's group developed an In Vitro Sedimentation Diffusion and Dosimetry (ISDD) model for predicting the in vitro behavior and cell doses of particles. Fig. 28-21 shows the results of example calculations from this model. It indicates that for large TiO_2 particles (500 nm) the dose received by the cells in a dish with 3.1 mm media height is very fast. In contrast, 30 and 50 nm particles have a long deposition rate; only 50% of the media dose has reached the cells by 24 hours. TiO_2 NP sizes in between still have not reached the full dose by 24 hours, whereas 200 nm TiO_2 NP are fully settled by 10 hours.

Results of the ISDD prediction shown in Fig. 28-21 have to be verified by experiments. The value of this model lies in the clear separation between exposure (concentration in the

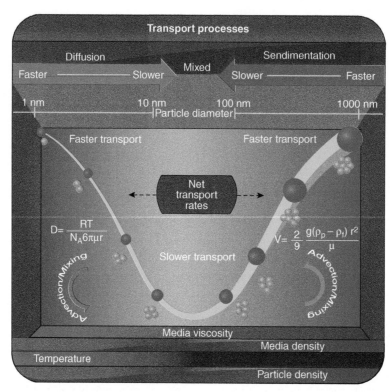

Figure 28-20. *In vitro sedimentation, diffusion and dosimetry (ISDD) model: particle transport/deposition processes for in vitro systems.* (See text). (Reproduced with permission from Hinderliter *et al.*, 2010.)

cell medium), the deposited dose on the cell surface, and—depending on cellular uptake—the cellular dose. These doses can be expressed by different metrics: mass, number, or surface area of the nanomaterial. Knowledge about the time to deposit a certain dose allows to consider dose rate as a determinant for responses, as was discussed for in vivo exposures (Fig. 28-8). In vitro dosing is often perceived as a bolus-type delivery, similar to in vivo instillation or aspiration studies. However, as the results in Fig. 28-21 show, in vitro dosing with NP is not necessarily equivalent to an instantaneous bolus. The ISDD model allows to express the deposited dose per unit cell surface area of cultured epithelial cells of the respiratory tract and thereby (*i*) compare

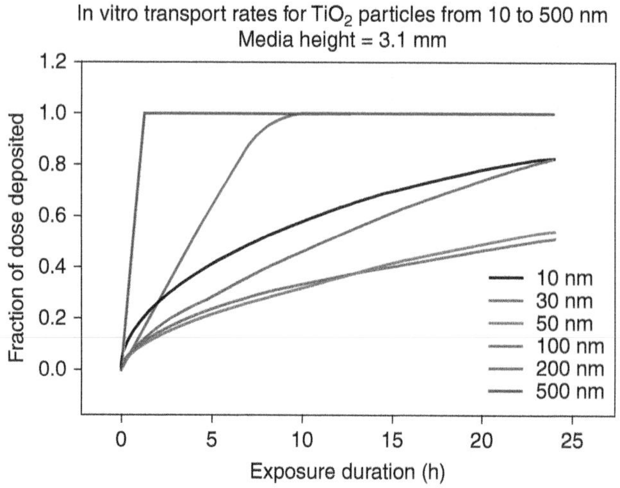

responses to the same in vivo dose per unit cell surface (based on MPPD model, Fig. 28-13), (*ii*) use in vivo-derived doses from a given exposure concentration to design in vitro studies that include realistic doses, and (*iii*) use in vitro dosimetry results and response to verify in vivo. Likewise, doses applied in vitro to cells from secondary organs (eg, CNS, bone marrow) can be estimated by the ISDD model and better justified by results from in vivo biokinetic studies with respect to doses distributed to these secondary organs. An important difference, however, between in vivo inhalation and in vitro cell exposure is the pristine state of inhaled nanomaterials, whereas for in vitro exposures nanomaterials are either treated with dispersants to separate the particles and achieve spatially uniform dosing, or else culture media constituents (serum proteins) will adsorb to the NP surface to aid in their dispersion. Surface modification is known to affect responses of ENM (Haniu *et al.*, 2011), and this possibility needs to be considered when designing and interpreting in vitro results.

An alternative in vitro methodology that avoids pretreatment of NP with surfactants or proteins prior to testing is exposure via an air liquid interface (ALI) system (Savi *et al.*, 2008; Holder *et al.*, 2008; Lenz *et al.*, 2009; de Bruijne *et al.*, 2009; Volckens *et al.*, 2009; Tang *et al.*, 2011; Xie *et al.*, 2012). Respiratory tract epithelial cells are grown on porous culture cell inserts and exposed to NP generated the same way as done for in vivo inhalation studies. Before exposure, culture medium is withdrawn so that only the basal cell surface is in contact with the medium and deposition of the aerosolized NP on the apical cell surface simulates realistic in vivo inhalation exposure. Comparative results between conventional in vitro and ALI exposure seems to confirm the apparent advantage and greater sensitivity of the ALI system (Holder *et al.*, 2008; Volckens *et al.*, 2009). However, transition of cell cultures from growing in suspension to the ALI system for exposure is likely to cause changes in gene expression, which needs to be considered using appropriate control groups (Ross *et al.*, 2007).

Figure 28-21. *In vitro sedimentation, diffusion and dosimetry (ISDD) model: prediction for in vitro transport rates for TiO₂ particles from 10 to 500 nm, assuming a media height in the culture dish of 3.1 mm.* (Reproduced with permission from Hinderliter *et al.*, 2010.)

Predictive Toxicology

The NNI developed a comprehensive Environmental, Health, and Safety Research Strategy (NanoEHS research, NNI, 2011) in which urgent research needs for nanomaterial measurements, human exposure assessment, human health, environmental health, risk assessment and risk management methods, and for the input of informatics and modeling for NanoEHS research are discussed. This initiative of the US Government's interagency program for coordinating research and development and for enhancing communication and collaborative activities in nanoscale science, engineering, and technology emphasizes the NAS risk assessment paradigm (1983) as the basis for NanoEHS research. As illustrated in Fig. 28-19, data about hazard and exposure are key for the risk assessment process. Critical elements for hazard identification based on toxicity testing of ENM are detailed information about their physicochemical properties prior to any experiments, the selection of appropriate target cells, validation of in vitro assays in terms of correlation and relevancy to in vivo results, the inclusion of biokinetics in the design of in vivo studies, and the inclusion of realistic doses in the design of dose–response in vitro and in vivo studies. Biokinetic information is crucial to identify potential secondary target organs based on significant accumulation of ENM. In order to determine relevant doses, information about exposures occurring at anticipated real-world exposure scenarios, either measured or estimated, is essential. With this information, exposure–dose–response (in vivo, rodents) and dose–response (in vitro, target cells) relationships can be established to both characterize a hazard and assess a risk (see below). In terms of toxicity ranking, it is desirable to include reference materials in the study design so that a hazard can be expressed relative to a positive (high hazard) or negative (low hazard) control ENM. Mechanistic information discovered through in vitro assays will further aid in the characterization of hazard, provided that the mechanism is operative at relevant doses/concentrations. High-dose and high dose rate-induced mechanisms may not be considered relevant and may give rise to improper classification. An awareness of dosimetry-related aspects is of highest importance (Fig. 28-19) for the risk assessment process, which often gets lost or is ignored because of a misconception of risk being analogous to hazard. Risk is a function of hazard and exposure, and neither aspect alone can determine risk.

The immediate goal of ENM toxicity testing is hazard characterization and the establishment of respective predictive tests. These should ideally be based on validated in vitro studies, for example high throughput in vitro assays, so that ethically controversial animal studies can be replaced if they only serve the purpose of hazard identification. A distant goal is the use eventually of in silico models. However, at present, animal studies are still indispensable for obtaining crucial information about long-term effects of ENM and to obtain results for risk assessment. For example, available data from subchronic (three months) inhalation studies (Ma-Hock *et al.*, 2009; Pauluhn, 2010) provide crucial information for deriving a NOAEL or lowest observed adverse effect level (LOAEL) that can be used for dosimetric extrapolation of OELs for humans.

Fig. 28-18 depicts a conceptual approach for deriving a human equivalent concentration (HEC) from results of a long-term rat inhalation study. The HEC is based solely on the equivalency of the retained dose, expressed per unit mass, or epithelial surface area of the lung. The retained dose can be expressed by different metrics, for example, rather than using the mass of ENM, as is conventional, the surface area or even number of particles might be

Individual organism measure	Population measure	Community measure	Ecosystem measure
Development Behavior Stress Growth Tumor incidence Egg production Survival	Reproduction LD50, LC50 Genetic diversity Mutation rate Change in recruitment	Bacterial diversity Presence of sensitive species	Nutrient cycling Degradation of habitat Missing food chain links Presence/ absence of functional groups

Figure 28-22. *Measures of ecological effect at the different levels.*

used. Pauluhn (2010) used the metric of particle volume retained in alveolar macrophages to estimate an OEL from the experimentally found NOAEL in a three-month rat inhalation study with MWCNT. As was done in that study, it is highly desirable that the design of a rat study includes the measurement of the retained lung burden; if this is not available, the retained dose can be estimated using a particle deposition and retention model with inputs of rat-specific breathing and airway parameters and the aerosol characteristics of the ENM used in the rat study. The same aerosol characteristics and human-specific airway and breathing parameters then as inputs to a human model are then used to determine the HEC. It should be noted that this dosimetric extrapolation should not necessarily imply that the response in humans is the same as in rats. Differences in species sensitivity may require the use of an additional safety factor. The advantage of using the retained dose as the basis is that other particle size distributions specific to human exposures at a workplace can be used instead of the rat aerosol. (Oller and Oberdörster, 2010).

Transition, Human—Eco-nanotoxicology

The goals of nanotoxicology are to identify and characterize a hazard of ENMs for purposes of risk assessment for humans and the environment require a highly multidisciplinary team approach, covering expertise in toxicology, biology, chemistry, physics, material science, geology, exposure assessment, PBPK and fate and transport modeling, and medicine is necessary to develop testing strategies, establish toxicity ranking, determine "safe" exposure levels and derive preventive exposure guidelines. As depicted in Fig. 28-2, exposures throughout the lifecycle of ENMs, from their source to their disposal, have to be considered. Dispersion and intermediate transformations in air, water, food, and soil are important modifiers of ENM-receptor interactions. Identifying underlying mechanisms of such interactions will aid in assessing risk and establishing preventive measures. Developing predictive models is a distant goal for both human and eco-nanotoxicology.

ECOTOXICOLOGY OF ENMS

Environmental Uses and Exposures to Nanomaterials

As with many chemicals in the marketplace, it is estimated that a portion of the nanomaterials used in industry and consumer products will enter the greater environment during some part of their life cycle, either through waste during production or through product use. The exponential increase in use of ENMs in a multitude of industries and consumer products has been documented by the Woodrow Wilson Center's project on Emerging Technologies, which as of March 2011 estimated that self-identified nanomaterial products had grown from 54 to over 1300 in five years. This list likely underestimates the number of uses of nanomaterials as it only includes products easily identified as containing nanomaterials and does not include other known uses of nanomaterials including industrial catalysts, wastewater treatment, in addition to environmental cleanup technologies and pesticides, which would directly place nanomaterials into the environment. Most of the uses identified are in cosmetics, clothing (where nanomaterials are often added for antimicrobial and antiodor functions), personal care products and sporting goods. The most common nanomaterials included in these products are silver and carbon nanomaterials. Other chemicals used in personal care products, cosmetics, and clothing have been found to wash into the wastewater treatment system and end up in the aquatic environment either directly from the treatment facilities or through land applications of biosolids from wastewater treatment plants. It is anticipated that some of the nanomaterial components may have the same fate, and indeed a few documented cases indicate this may be possible (Wang *et al.*, 2012) but a majority of the estimates of potential environmental release of these chemicals is from modeling based on data from other compounds without regard to specific properties of nanomaterials compared to their bulk counterparts (Mueller and Nowack, 2008, Gottschalk *et al.*, 2009, 2010). These studies estimate that concentrations in the environment can range from ng/L to ug/L with many agglomerating into larger than nanosized units and much of the NP mass binding to solids and removed into biosolid waste. However, despite these removal potentials, it has been shown that NPs can be emitted through the wastewater process in the NP size range in significant quantities (Westerhoff *et al.*, 2011).

Nanomaterials directly applied to a particular ecosystem, such as those for cleanup of environmental toxicants or as part of a pesticide formulation may also lead to exposures. Nanoscale zero-valent iron and titanium dioxide are currently being evaluated as a removal technology to treat groundwater systems and some surface water or soil systems for metals, arsenic, organic chemicals such as chlorinated solvents, polychlorinated biphenyl's (PCB's), and benzenes (Elliot and Zhang, 2001; Chen and von Mikecz, 2005; Quinn *et al.*, 2005). Poly(ethylene) glycol-modified urethane has been proposed for the sequestration and enhanced bioavailability for degradation of organic contaminants (Tungittiplakorn, 2005). Pesticide formulations containing carbon-based nanomaterials and others have been sent to the US environmental protection agency (EPA), for evaluation and are assumed to be in development.

Ecological Risk Assessment of Manufactured Nanomaterials

One of the unusual aspects of the field of nanotechnology is the way in which the science of the risk of these materials to the environment has been instigated relatively early in the adoption of the technology. For most other contaminants, the risk assessment has largely been retrospective often decades after the chemical has been in the marketplace and is now distributed across the globe into many environmental compartments. The goal of this science to date has been to determine how a particulate form of a chemical in a nanosize range influences its toxicity versus its larger bulk counterparts. A further goal is to determine how small changes in surface chemistries, size, shape, and structure affect the interaction with organisms in the environment with the goal of informing industry on safe development. However, there are issues in assessing the risk of nanomaterials that are unique to this class of

potential contaminant, and therefore the process of assessing risk also has unique considerations (some that have been mentioned in dealing with human health considerations). The assessment of ecological risk is also complicated that human health assessments as there are more species involved and higher level impacts on populations, communities of organisms and ecosystem function need to be considered. The methods to evaluate the potential impacts of nanomaterials at higher levels of organization (community, ecosystem) have not been developed as is the case with many other chemicals.

The basic framework used for ecological risk assessment (Fig. 28-23) (EPA EPA/630/R-95/002F) involves problem formulation, analysis, and risk characterization. Problem formulation involves selecting endpoints of concern and developing a plan for determining impacts on important endpoints (such as a species decline, ecosystem changes). Analysis involves evaluating the potential for exposure to stressors and potential effects at those exposure levels. Risk characterization involves taking the information on important endpoints and the analysis of exposure and effects data to determine the importance of a stressor. For nanomaterials most of the ecological risk assessment research has been conducted as the analysis of effects of a limited number of commercially available materials, using traditional acute single-organism mortality endpoints of a few select species and with little information regarding sublethal types of effects or other endpoints of concern at the community or ecosystem level. In addition, the concentrations of exposures are much higher than what is considered to be a probable environmental level. As such it is difficult to draw conclusions of the actual risk of many of even the most common materials and the conclusion is often that these particles may not cause any impact as no acute toxicity is seen. Nanomaterials may also be transformed within the environment, and therefore the toxicity of the initial nanomaterial may not provide a complete idea of the toxicity over the lifetime of the material (Nowack *et al.*, 2012). Part of this is due to the relative newness of this field, the particulate nature of the potential toxicants, and other challenges surrounding the methods for determining toxicity, methods for measuring potential exposures, and uncertainty in estimates of how the materials will be used in the future marketplace. Agencies involved in protecting public and environmental health in individual countries as well as international agencies are grappling with methods to develop a structure to assess risk for all nanomaterials and make predictions regarding new ones as they come on the marketplace. This assessment may take time as methods development needs to progress with the field of nanotechnology as new materials are being developed. The current state of the field is represented below, but the reader should keep in mind that it is rapidly changing.

Toxicity of Manufactured Nanomaterials

Complications of Assays Traditionally, ecotoxicology assays follow standard protocols and involve a group of species that has been selected to be representative of various organisms in the environment including Daphnia, bacteria, fish, birds, and insects. The most standard assays involve 24- to 48-hour exposures and mortality endpoints such as LD50. Other standard assays for these species include month-long trials assessing growth and reproduction, tumor development, and other endpoints. Some issues arise in conducting these assays for nanomaterials, which is one of the reasons the current toxicological information regarding nanomaterials is variable. Some of the major issues in toxicology assays include delivery of nanomaterials in media and approximating environmental conditions, characterizing exposures, maintaining

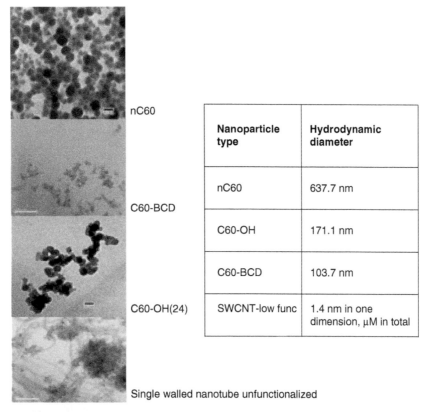

Nanoparticle type	Hydrodynamic diameter
nC60	637.7 nm
C60-OH	171.1 nm
C60-BCD	103.7 nm
SWCNT-low func	1.4 nm in one dimension, µM in total

nC60

C60-BCD

C60-OH(24)

Single walled nanotube unfunctionalized

Figure 28-23. *Example of the differences in larger particle agglomerates with nanomaterial.* All three of these are fullerene particle; however, the unfunctionalized particles are two to six times larger agglomerates in a pure water suspension compared with the functionalized counterparts. The stability in suspension also differs with functionalization (represented by the zeta potential).

exposures throughout an assay, and determining the state of exposure throughout an assay. For example, many nanomaterials are not easily dispersible and aggregate substantially when introduced into common exposure media. A hydrophobic particle will aggregate with other particles in water and to an even greater extent when salts are introduced into the media as is the case with many aquatic systems. This causes several issues when determining toxicity. First, the nanomaterial aggregate may no longer be in the nanosize range (hydrodynamic diameter >100 nm). In some cases this larger aggregate is nevertheless more toxic than its bulk chemical counterpart. This has not been shown with all nanomaterials, however, and is controversial. Second, the nanomaterials as they aggregate settle out of suspension, so depending on the organism involved the actual exposure may change over time as particles are effectively removed from suspension, or they may increase as some organisms (Daphnia) collect particles not only from the water column but from the bottom of the vessel. Some researchers have attempted to suspend the nanomaterials using solvents or detergents for better distribution. Studies have shown the solvent or detergent when not removed from the nanomaterials sufficiently can cause toxicity (Lovern and Klaper 2006; Henry *et al.*, 2007; Kovochich *et al.*, 2009) and in others the data indicates that this smaller aggregate size created by the additive changes the toxicity (eg, Lovern and Klaper 2006). Researchers have attempted to circumvent this issue by either changing the surface chemistry of the nanomaterial to make it more readily suspendable by adding a hydrophilic functional group or by altering the exposure conditions to include organic material that assists in suspension. Each of these approaches raises its own issues for toxicology. Changing the surface chemistry of a nanomaterial can also change its toxicity (Klaper *et al.*, 2010). The relationship between surface chemistry

and toxicity is important to understand because surface functionalization is an important aspect of nanomaterial formulation for industrial applications. So determining the impact of different surface chemistry changes is a necessary part of not only ecotoxicology but nanotoxicology in general. A bigger issue is that many coatings can cause toxicity on their own regardless of whether it is attached to the nanomaterial, and has also shown to be removed in certain cases by the organisms in the test media, or the environment the organism inhabits, which dramatically changes the properties of the nanomaterial through the experiment (Roberts *et al.*, 2007). Is the toxicity then due to the original particle or now to the altered form of the nanomaterial?

As part of determining the dose an organism actually encounters is determining how much of any nanomaterial actually reaches the organism and is taken up into the organism and its tissues. There are several difficulties in measuring uptake including identifying the nanomaterial within the matrix of the organism versus inside the organism, for some nanomaterials the issue is distinguishing the nanomaterial from the matrix of the organism or environment either due to their small size relative to other aggregates in a sample, or because of the chemical similarity of the nanomaterial with the matrix (carbon-based nanomaterials in tissue, for example). Bulk extractions of these materials have provided some indication of potential concentrations (Westerhoff, Furgeson refs) but missing is the finer detail regarding location and structure of nanomaterials within a matrix, which is necessary to determine that the nanomaterial itself is causing an effect and not its byproduct or a secondary physiological response. Another issue in conducting a normal ecotoxicological assay using nanomaterials is the issue of calculating the dose as a mass versus surface area as reported above. Most nanomaterials when reaching the environment are not in a spherical uniform form, which complicates any calculations of dose based on surface area.

The real adverse impacts of nanomaterials may not be due to ambient environmental concentrations that arise but may be due to some subset of materials that are persistent and biomagnify in the environment. Research indicates that various nanomaterials are taken up by organisms in the environment and much is excreted by the organism within hours (Lovern et al., 2008; Petersen et al., 2009). In addition, gold nanomaterials and cadmium selenide quantum dots have been shown to accumulate in tissues of organisms and are able pass from one level to another in simple food chain experiments (Judy et al., 2011; Werlin et al., 2011). These include microbial food chains and those involving consumption of algae or bacteria into protozoa, herbivores, or detritivores. However, nanomaterials passing from one level to the next do not guarantee biomagnification up the entire food chain as seen in quantum dot studies using transfers from Daphnia to zebrafish or where protozoa take up quantum dots and accumulate them to a greater extent than the media concentration but rotifers feeding on the protozoa do not show further increases in concentrations of nanomaterials (Holbrook et al., 2008; Lewinski et al., 2011).

Ecotoxicity of Nanomaterials

The studies on the toxicity of ENMs to date have largely focused on simple structures of fullerenes, CNTs, metal oxides, and gold and silver particles with a few examples of the impacts of nanomaterials with varying surface chemistries or functional groups. The major conclusion from these data is that toxicity varies with the type of nanomaterial and is not universal across materials. There are varying degrees of toxicity depending on the type of nanomaterial, organism studied, and the co-occurrence of other environmental factors such as UV light, organic carbon, or low pH. The most common endpoints monitored in nanoecotoxicology are acute mortality measures with traditional toxicological models species such as Daphnia, zebrafish, trout, and Arabidopsis. Most studies find some degree of toxicity but the concentrations of most nanomaterials that are needed to kill half of the sample population are in the mg/L range, which is far above the estimates of potential exposures to any nanomaterial. Nanomaterials may enter other organisms just as they do humans and other mammals, through external contact with outer tissues and breathing structures (gill, skin), and through ingestion. Nanomaterials have been shown to be ingested with and without food present in most situations thus leading to contact with internal structures. The greatest damage measured has been to gill structures in fish and in digestive tissues in other species (Zhu et al., 2008; Bilberg et al., 2010). In terrestrial studies, plants have been shown to accumulate nanomaterials in root tissues and it is assumed that inhalation is possible in certain terrestrial situations but impacts on birds and mammals other than rats has not been demonstrated.

Fullerenes and CNTs were some of the first nanomaterials investigated for their potential environmental impact. Fullerenes have been shown to be lethal to Daphnia and microbial organisms (eg, Lovern and Klaper 2006; Zhu et al., 2006). However, ecotoxicity studies have indicated that the damaging impacts of these nanomaterials can be dramatically impacted by the method of introduction into exposure media. This includes introduction by solvent carriers or by altering the materials with surface chemistries that make them more water soluble. Unmodified fullerene nanomaterials may only be toxic at very high doses mg/L and mg/kg soil (Zhu et al., 2006; Li and Alvarez 2011; Mouchet et al., 2011) and have been shown to have little impact on bacterial communities and protozoa (Johansen et al., 2008). However, increasing their solubility through either solvent or detergent introduction or by changing surface chemistry can also increase their toxicity to aquatic species (Klaper et al., 2010).

Silver nanomaterials are some of the most widely used materials and appear to demonstrate the greatest toxicity of materials investigated in the literature. Silver in particular is toxic at ug/L doses to a variety of organisms (George et al., 2011; Bilberg et al., 2012). However, silver and other metal nanomaterials are subject to dissolution even with various coatings and their entire toxicity may be due to the ionic component of an exposure rather than the nanomaterial form (Kennedy et al., 2010). These metal ions may accumulate in the body of organisms after ingestion of nanomaterials and contribute to toxicity (Asharani et al., 2008, Li et al., 2011). Rather than creating a free radical in media the impacts of metal nanomaterials may be due to metal imbalance in cells after uptake and accumulation leading to apoptosis and cellular disregulation (Kao et al., 2012). However, it has been suggested that the dissolution and ionic form of the metals is not the sole reason for nanometal toxicities (Griffit et al., 2007). Nanosilver and possibly other nanomaterials based on soft metals may also react with environmental sulfides to produce silver sulfide nanomaterials, in which the silver bioavailability and toxicity is much reduced (Kim et al., 2010; Liu and Hurt 2010).

Mechanisms of Toxicity

As in mammalian toxicology studies, oxidative stress has been implicated as a major way in which nanomaterials exert toxicity either by generating free radicals within the suspension media or by changing the chemistry of the cells in which they come in contact. Metal oxide nanomaterials in particular have been found to generate oxidative stress. Hydroxyl radicals and oxidative stress have been found to increase over time in the presence of metal oxides and UV light (Yu et al., 2011). As in human tissues the stimulation of oxidative stress pathways alone are not an indication of harm and may be countered by adaptation by the organism to exposure. Mortimer et al. (2010) found that despite oxidative stress in initial assays, toxicity decreased over time in protozoa after exposure to metal oxide nanomaterials. However, Klaper et al. (2009) found that acute assays of oxidative stress do provide an early indicator of mortality of Daphnia in chronic assays for a variety of nanomaterial types. Metal oxide nanomaterials appear to have greater toxicity than their bulk counterparts. Titanium dioxide nanomaterials generate more ROS per gram than similar macroparticulates (Xiong et al., 2011). However, they do not differ from larger aggregates in their toxicity to developing fish (Zhu et al., 2008). Most studies have found a greater difference among nanomaterials composed of different metal oxides than the difference between the bulk and nanomaterial form of these compounds.

Metal nanomaterials have been found to cause a suite of effects, which in fish include negative impacts on respiration, oxidative stress, and development (Zhu et al., 2008; Shaw and Handy, 2011), in Caenorhabditis elegans increased mortality and decreased reproduction (Wang et al., 2012) and inhibit algal growth (Peng et al., 2011). Differences among metal oxides may be a result of differential solubilities in media.

The toxicity of nanomaterials to aquatic organisms can be greatly dependent upon the interaction of nanomaterials with the media to which they are introduced (Figs. 28-24 to 28-26). For example, dissolution of metal oxides and metal nanomaterials is greatly impacted by the characteristics of the media such as pH and salt content. Li et al. (2011) found that zinc oxide nanomaterials were most toxic in ultrapure water followed by salt, lithium borate (LB), and phosphate buffer saline (PBS), buffers. In the

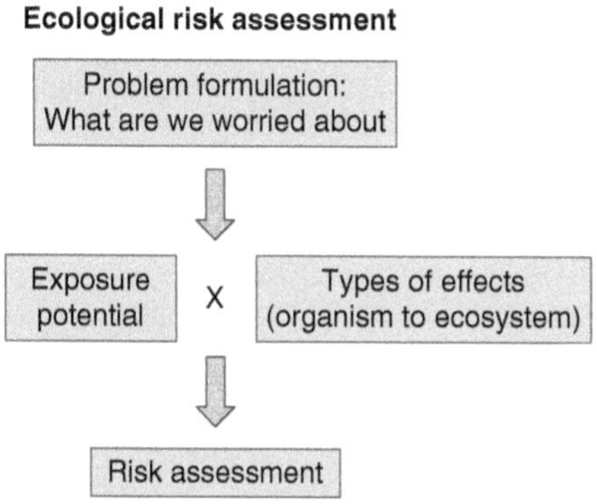

Ecological risk assessment

Problem formulation:
What are we worried about

↓

Exposure potential   X   Types of effects (organism to ecosystem)

↓

Risk assessment

Figure 28-24. *Ecological risk assessment involves determining the types of concerns we have regarding a particular stressor and its impacts, determining the potential for exposure to environmental compartments, the types of potential impacts a stressor (in this case a nanomaterial) may have at those exposures and using those two factors together to determine the risk to the environment.* With most nanomaterials we are relatively certain, environments such as freshwater systems that are receivers of wastewater will be exposed and most likely agricultural areas that receive solid wastes. The level of exposure is still in question and we have only begun to examine the types of effects. We have some information on model species such as Daphnia and trout as to the chance of mortality and some physiological effects in the acute exposure but little information is available on chronic low-level exposures. As such, it is currently premature to determine the actual risk to the environment.

environment, toxicity may differ with the presence of organic matter and the specific interaction of organic matter with a nanomaterial will differ depending on its composition. The degree of interaction of nanomaterial and organic matter has been shown to impact

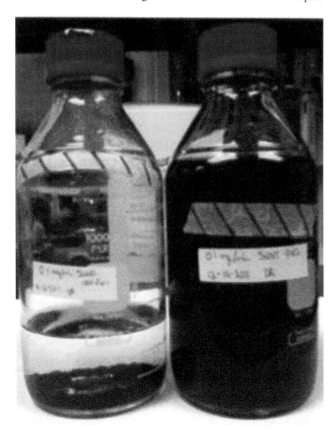

Figure 28-25. *Suspension characteristics can have a significant impact on toxicity. In this case single-walled nanotubes that have been functionalized with polyethylene glycol remain in suspension (on right) where their unfunctionalized counterparts do not (on left).*

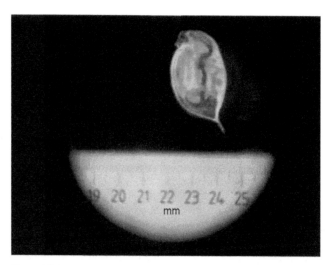

Figure 28-26. *Aquatic organisms, such as Daphnia magna, readily take up nanomaterials from the environment and their guts are rapidly filled with nanomaterials.* Some of these materials have been found to cross the gut barrier and translocate into other tissues within the organism.

toxicity (Gao *et al.*, 2009). Toxicity of particles sorbed to natural organic matter can be significantly greater (Edgington *et al.*, 2010) or diminished (Blinova *et al.*, 2010). Toxicity of nanomaterials can be significantly impacted by the surface chemistry, capping agents, and coatings of the particles. Additions of functional groups have been shown to increase toxicity in some cases (Klaper *et al.*, 2009; Klaper *et al.*, 2010) and decrease toxicity in others (Allen *et al.*, 2009). A few studies have also examined the influence of aging of nanomaterials in the environment on their toxicity.

Nanomaterials may also impact the bioavailability and toxicity of other contaminants in the environment. Fullerene and CNT particles in particular have been shown to bind to various organic contaminants with the strength of the association dependent upon the compound. Sorption to these nanomaterials can increase concentrations of bound organics by up to 60%, which if ingested could increase their toxicity (Baun *et al.*, 2008).

As many nanomaterial exposures in the environment will occur at relatively low levels (ug to ng/L exposures), it is important to use assays other than LD50 to indicate the most relevant environmental effect. Including sublethal assays of physiology, assays of impacts of chronic low-level exposures, monitoring of alternative endpoints such as reproduction, growth, and at a higher level changes in community structure and ecosystem function are essential. Nanomaterials cause a shift in overall behavior in Daphnia, which can indicate a greater susceptibility to predators and a greater energy cost leading to decreased reproduction (Lovern *et al.*, 2007; Braush *et al.*, 2011). Various nanomaterials have been shown to impact development and physiology of fish species causing greater apoptosis in tissues, stress, and other impacts including structural effects (Chen *et al.*, 2011; Shaw and Handy 2011; Truong *et al.*, 2012; Xiong *et al.*, 2011). As the immune response is the first interaction of foreign substances with an organism, it has been shown that nanomaterials are stimulatory to the immune system of fish in particular and have an effect that is equal to the response to bacterial cell components, which may indicate an eventual cost to the organism (Klaper *et al.*, 2010; Jovanovic *et al.*, 2011). Nanomaterials also have the potential to be mutagenic and in flies cause mutations that alter the phenotype significantly into the second generation (Vecchio *et al.*, 2012).

Measurements of impacts at the community and ecosystem level are uncommon for nanomaterials, as they are for chemical toxicants with a much longer toxicology history. The existing studies indicate that community structure is impacted by the same nanomaterials that show toxicity and developmental impacts such as metals and metal oxides. Cerium dioxide and silver nanomaterials have a significant impact on marine microbial communities and microbial communities in wastewater—decrease in degradation potential and productivity (Fabrega *et al.*, 2011; Garcia *et al.*, 2012). They also cause shifts in decomposition communities in freshwater streams (Pradhan *et al.*, 2011). Nanomaterials such as unfunctionalized fullerenes that have been shown to be less toxic exhibit no impact on soil community structure (Tong *et al.*, 2007), macrophyte structure (Velzeboer *et al.*, 2011), or mutagenesis across generations (Nyberg *et al.*, 2008) but do cause shifts in community composition of soil bacteria (Johansen *et al.*, 2008). The overall composition may also be altered as microbial communities on mucus secretions of carp are different in those that have been exposed to fullerenes (Letts *et al.*, 2011). The overall community impact is greatly affected by complexity in environmental samples (Kang *et al.*, 2009).

Ecosystem impacts may be impacted by these community effects as bacterial community function has a great impact on nutrient cycling. CNTs have been shown to impact microbial activity (Chung *et al.*, 2011) and fullerenes, silver and CdSe quantum dots impact sediment bacterial oxidation of organics (Gao *et al.*, 2009).

REFERENCES

Aiso S, Yamazaki K, Umeda Y, et al. Pulmonary toxicity of intratracheally instilled carbon nanotubes in male Fischer 344 rats. *Ind Health*. 2011;48(6):783–795.

Akhavan O, Ghaderi E. Toxicity of graphene and graphene oxide nanowalls against bacteria. *ACS Nano*. 2010;4:5731–5736.

Albrecht C, Borm PJ, Unfried K. Signal transduction pathways relevant for neoplastic effects of fibrous and non-fibrous particles. *Mutat Res*. 2004;553:23–35.

Allen BL, Kotchey GP, Chen Y, et al. Mechanistic investigations of horseradish peroxidase-catalyzed degradation of single-walled carbon nanotubes. *J Am Chem Soc*. 2009;131:17194–17205.

Allen BL, Kichambare PD, Gou P, et al. Biodegradation of single-walled carbon nanotubes through enzymatic catalysis. *Nano Lett*. 2008;8:3899–3903.

Asgharian B, Miller FJ, Subramaniam RP. Dosimetry software to predict particle deposition in humans and rats. *CIIT Activities*. 1999;19(3):1–6.

Asharani PV, Lian Wu Y, Gong Z, Valiyaveettil S. Toxicity of silver nanoparticles in zebrafish models. *Nanotechnology*. 2008.

Bainbridge W. Public attitudes towards nanotechnology. *J Nanopart Res*. 2002;4:461–470.

Balashazy I, Hofmann W, Helstracher T. Local particle deposition patterns may play a key role in the development of lung cancer. *J Appl Physiol*. 2003;94:1719–1725.

Balashazy IW, Hofmann W, Farkas F, Madas BG. Three-dimensional model for aerosol transport and deposition in expanding and contracting alveoli. *Inhal Toxicol*. 2008;20(6):611–621.

Ballou B, Lagerholm BC, Ernst LA, Bruchez MP, Waggoner AS. Noninvasive imagaing of quantum dots in mice. *Bioconjugate Chem*. 2004;15:79–86.

Barrios FA, Gonzalez L, Favila R, et al. Olfaction and neurodegeneration in HD. *Neuroreport*. 18:73 (2007).

Bilberg K, Hovgaard MB, Besenbacher F, Baatrup E. In vivo toxicity of silver nanoparticles and silver ions in Zebrafish (Danio rerio). *J Toxicol*. 2012;2012:293784.

Baun A, Sørensen SN, Rasmussen RF, Hartmann NB, Koch CB. Toxicity and bioaccumulation of xenobiotic organic compounds in the presence of aqueous suspensions of aggregates of nano-C(60). *Aquat Toxicol*. 2008;86(3):379–387.

Bernstein D, Castranova V, Donaldson K, et al. Testing of fibrous particles: short-term assays and strategies. *Inhalation Toxicology*. 2005;17:497–537.

Bianco A, Kostarelos K, Prato M. Making carbon nanotubes biocompatible and biodegradable. *Chem Commun (Camb)*. 2011;47:10182–10188.

Bilberg K, Malte H, Wang T, Baatrup E. Silver nanoparticles and silver nitrate cause respiratory stress in Eurasian perch (Perca fluviatilis). *Aquat Toxicol*. 2010;96(2):159–165.

Biswas R, Bunderson-Schelvan M, Holian A. Potential role of the inflammasome-derived inflammatory cytokines in pulmonary fibrosis. *Pulm Med*. 2011;2011:105707.

Blinova I, Ivask A, Heinlaan M, Mortimer M, Kahru A. Ecotoxicity of nanoparticles of CuO and ZnO in natural water. *Environ Pollut*. 2010;158(1):41–47.

Boczkowski J, Hoet P. What's new in nanotoxicology? Implications for public healthfrom a brief review of the 2008 literature. *Nanotoxicology*. 2009.

Bodian D, Howe HA. Experimental studies on intraneural spread of poliomyelitis virus. Bordley JI, (ed). Bulletin of the Johns Hopkins Hospital. Baltimore, The Johns Hopkins Press; 1941:LXVIII248–267.

Borm P J A, Robbins D, Haubold S, et al. The potential risks of nanomaterials: a review carried out for ECETOC. *Part Fibre Toxicol*. 2006;3(11).

Boya P, Kroemer G. Lysosomal membrane permeabilization in cell death. *Oncogene*. 2008;27:6434–6451.

Brausch KA, Anderson TA, Smith PN, Maul JD. The effect of fullerenes and functionalized fullerenes on Daphnia magna phototaxis and swimming behavior. *Environ Toxicol Chem*. 2011;30(4):878–884.

Brodie M, Elvidge AR. The portal of entry and transmission of the virus of poliomyelitis. *Science*. 1934;79(2045):235–236.

Brunauer S, Emmett PH, Teller E. Adsorption of gases in multimolecular layers. *J Am Chem Soc*. 1938;60:309–319.

Calderon-Garciduenas L, Engle R, Mora-Tiscareno A, et al. Exposure to severe urban air pollution influences cognitive outcomes, brain volume and systemic inflammation in clinically healthy children. *Brain Cogn*. 2011;77:345–355.

Casey A, Herzog E, Davoren M, Lyng FM, Byrne HJ, Chambers G. Spectroscopic analysis confirms the interactions between single walled carbon nanotubes and various dyes commonly used to assess cytotoxicity. *Carbon*. 2007;45:1425–1432.

Casey A, Herzog E, Lyng FM, Byrne HJ, Chambers G, Davoren M. Single walled carbon nanotubes induce indirect cytotoxicity by medium depletion in A549 lung cells. *Toxicol Lett*. 2008;179:78–84.

Cassee FR, van Balen EC, Singh C, et al. Exposure, health and ecological effects review of engineered nanoscale cerium and cerium oxide associated with its use as a fuel additive. *Crit Rev Toxicol*. 2011;41:213–229.

Cederval T, Lynch I, Foy M, et al. Detailed identification of plasma proteins adsorbed on copolymer nanoparticles. *Angew Chem Int Ed*. 2007b;46:5754–5756.

Cedervall T, Lynch I, Lindman S, et al. Understanding the nanoparticle-protein corona using methods to quantify exchange rates and affinities of proteins for nanoparticles. *Proc Natl Acad Sci U S A*. 2007a;104:2050–2055.

Chen J, Dong X, Xin Y, Zhao M. Effects of titanium dioxide nano-particles on growth and some histological parameters of zebrafish (Danio rerio) after a long-term exposure. *Aquat Toxicol*. 2011;101(3–4):493–499.

Chen M, von Mikecz A. Formation of nucleoplasmic protein aggregates impairs nuclear function in response to SiO2 nanoparticles. *Exp Cell Res*. 2005;305:51–62.

Chithrani DB. Intracellular uptake, transport, and processing of gold nanostructures. *Mol Membr Biol*. 2010;27:299–311.

Choi HS, Liu W, Misra P, et al. Renal clearance of quantum dots. *Nature Biotechnology*. 2007;25(10):1165–1170.

Chou LY, Ming K, Chan WC. Strategies for the intracellular delivery of nanoparticles. *Chem Soc Rev*. 2011;40:233–245.

Chu M, Wu Q, Yang H, et al. Transfer of quantum dots from pregnant mice to pups across the placental barrier. *Small*. 2010;6(5):670–678.

Chung H, Son Y, Yoon TK, Kim S, Kim W. The effect of multi-walled carbon nanotubes on soil microbial activity. *Ecotoxicol Environ Saf*. 2011;74(4):569–575.

Clarkson TW, Friberg L, Nordberg GF, Sager PR, eds. *Biological Monitoring of Toxic Metals*. Plenum Press;1988:686.

Cobb MD, Macoubrie J. Public perceptions about nanotechnology: risks, benefits and trust. *J Nanoparticle Res*. 2004;6(4):395–405.

Cole AJ, Yang VC, David AE. Cancer theranostics: the rise of targeted magnetic nanoparticles. *Trends Biotechnol*. 2011;29:323–332.

Colvin VL. The potential environmental impact of engineered nanomaterials. *Nat Biotechnol*. 2003;21:1166–1170.

Cone RA. Barrier properties of mucus. *Adv Drug Deliv Rev*. 2009;61:75–85.

Costa M, Davidson TL, Chen H, et al. Nickel carcinogenesis: epigenetics and hypoxia signaling. *Mutat Res*. 2005;592:79–88.

Czerniawska A. Experimental investigations on the penetration of 198Au from nasal mucous membrane into cerebrospinal fluid. *Acta Otolaryng*. 1970;70:58–61.

de Bruijne, Ebersviller S, Sexton KG, et al. Design and testing of Electrostatic Aerosol in Vitro Exposure System (EAVES): an alternative exposure system for particles. *Inhal Toxicol*. 2009;21(2):91–101.

De Jong WH, Borm PJ. Drug delivery and nanoparticles:applications and hazards. *Int J Nanomed*. 2008;3:133–149.

De Lorenzo A. The olfactory neuron and the blood-brain barrier. In: *Taste and smell in vertebrates*. Wolstenholme G, Knight J, eds. London: J. & A. Churchill; 1970:151–176.

De Nicola M, Gattia D, Bellucci S, et al. Effect of different carbon nanotubes on cell viability and proliferation. *J Phys Condens Matter*. 2007;19(39):395013.

Doak SH, Griffiths SM, Manshian B, et al. Confounding experimental considerations in nanogenotoxicology. *Mutagenesis*. 2009;24:285–293.

Donaldson K, Aitken R, Tran L, et al. Carbon nanotubes: a review of their properties in relation to pulmonary toxicology and workplace safety. *Toxicol Sci*. 2006;92:5–22.

Donaldson K, Beswick PH, Gilmour PS. Free radical activity associated with the surface of particles: a unifying factor in determining biological activity? *Toxicol Lett*. 1996;88(1–3):293–298.

Donaldson K, Murphy FA, Duffin R, Poland CA. Asbestos, carbon nanotubes and the pleural mesothelium: a review and the hypothesis regarding the role of long fibre retention in the parietal pleura, inflammation and mesothelioma. *Part Fibre Toxicol*. 2010;7(1):5.

Donaldson KP, Borm PJ, Castranova V, Gulumian M. The limits of testing particle-mediated oxidative stress *in vitro* in predicting diverse pathologies; relevance for testing of nanoparticles. *Part Fibre Toxicol*. 2009;6:13.

Donaldson K, Stone V, Tran CL, Kreyling W, Borm PJA. Nanotoxicology (editorial)—a new frontier in particle toxicology relevant to both the workplace and general environment and to consumer safety. *Occup Environ Med*. 2004;61:727–728.

Dostert C, Petrilli V, Van Bruggen R, Steele C, Mossman BT, Tschopp J. Innate immune activation through Nalp3 inflammasome sensing of asbestos and silica. *Science*. 2008;320:674–677.

Doty RL. The olfactory vector hypothesis of neurodegenerative disease: is it viable? *Ann Neurol*. 2008;63:7.

Drinker K, Drinker PRM. Metal fume fever: V. results of the inhalation by animals of zinc and magnesium oxide fumes. *J Ind Hyg*. 1928;10:56–71.

Drinker P, Finn JL, Thomson RM. Metal fume fever II: resistance acquired by inhalation of zinc oxide on two successive days. *J Ind Hyg*. 1927a;9:98–105.

Drinker P, Thomson RM, Finn JL. Metal fume fever IV: threshold doses of zinc oxide preventive measures and the chronic effects of repeated exposures. *J Ind Hyg*. 1927b;9:331–345.

Driscoll K, Costa DL, Hatch G, et al. Intratracheal instillation as an exposure technique for the evaluation of respiratory tract toxicity: uses and limitations. *Toxicol Sci*. 2000;55:24–35.

Duncan R. Polymer therapeutics as nanomedicines: new perspectives. *Curr Opin Biotechnol*. 2011;22:492–501.

Dutta D, Sundaram SK, Teeguarden JG, et al. Adsorbed proteins influence the biological activity and molecular targeting of nanomaterials. *Toxicol Sci*. 2007;100(1):303–315.

Dvir T, Timko BP, Kohane DS, Langer R. Nanotechnological strategies for engineering complex tissues. *Nat Nanotechnol*. 2011;6:13–22.

EC Directive 97/69/EC, Nota Q: EU Commission, directive dated 5 December 1997. (http://eur-lex.europa.eu/LexUriServ/LexUriServ.do?uri=CELEX:31997L0069:EN:HTML).

Edgington AJ, Roberts AP, Taylor LM, et al. The influence of natural organic matter on the toxicity of multiwalled carbon nanotubes. *Environ Toxicol Chem*. 2010;29(11):2511–2518.

Elder A, Gelein R, Silva V, et al. Translocation of inhaled ultrafine manganese oxide particles to the central nervous system. *Environ Health Perspect*. 2006;114:1172–1178.

Elliott D, Zhang W. Field assessment of nanoparticles for groundwater treatment. *Environ Sci Technol*. 2001;35:4922–4926.

European Commission. Commission Recommendation of.... on the definition of the term "nanomaterial". Brussels: European Commission; 2011.

(EU), E.C. Commission Recommendation on the definition of nanomaterial. *Official J European Union*. 2011/696/EU. 2011 (adopted).

Fabrega J, Luoma SN, Tyler CR, Galloway TS, Lead JR. Silver nanoparticles: behaviour and effects in the aquatic environment. *Environ Int*. 2011;37(2):517–531.

Fissan H. Nachhaltige nanotechnologie. In: *Nordrhein-Westfälische Akademie der Wissenschaften*. Germany, Herstellung: Ferdinand Schöningh, Paderborn; 2008; ISBN: 978-3-506-76565-9.

Food and Agriculture Organization of the United Nations/World Health Organization. FAO/WHO Expert Meeting on the Application of Nanotechnologies in the Food and Agriculture Sectors: Potential Food Safety Implications. Meeting Report. Rome; 2009:104.

Fawcett TW, Sylvester SL, Sarge KD, Morimoto RI, Holbrook NJ. Effects of neurohormonal stress and aging on the activation of mammalian heat shock factor 1. *J Biol Chem*. 1994;269(51):32272–32278.

Feng L, Liu Z. Graphene in biomedicine: opportunities and challenges. *Nanomedicine (Lond)*. 2011;6:317–324.

Fenoglio I, Fubini B, Ghibaudi EM, Turci F. Multiple aspects of the interaction of biomacromolecules with inorganic surfaces. *Adv Drug Deliv Rev*. 2011;63:1186–1209.

Fenoglio I, Tomatis M, Lison D, et al. Reactivity of carbon nanotubes: free radical generation or scavenging activity? *Free Radic Biol Med*. 2006;40:1227–1233.

Feynman R. *There's Plenty of Room at the Bottom*. Classic talk given on 12/29/59 at the American Physical Society at Caltech. First published in Caltech Engineering and Science, Volume 23:5, February 1960, pp 22–36.

Flahaut E, Durrieu MC, Remy-Zolghadri M, Bareille R, Baquey CH. Investigation of the cytotoxicity of CCVD carbon nanotubes towards human umbilical vein endothelial cells. *Carbon*. 2006;44(6):1093–1099.

Fortin JP, Wilhelm C, Christin JS. Size-sorted anionic iron oxide nanomagnets as colloidal mediators for magnetic hyperthermia. *J Am Chem Soc*. 2007;129:2628–2635.

Fubini B, Ghiazza M, Fenoglio I. Physico-chemical features of engineered nanoparticles relevant to their toxicity. *Nanotoxicology*. 2010;4(4):347–363.

García A, Delgado L, Torà JA, et al. Effect of cerium dioxide, titanium dioxide, silver, and gold nanoparticles on the activity of microbial communities intended in wastewater treatment. *J Hazard Mater*. 2012;199–200:64–72.

Gao J, Youn S, Hovsepyan A, et al. Dispersion and toxicity of selected manufactured nanomaterials in natural river water samples: effects of water chemical composition. *Environ Sci Technol*. 2009;43(9):3322–3328.

Geiser M, Casaulta M, Kupferschmid B, Schulz H, Semmler-Behnke M, Kreyling W. The role of macrophages in the clearance of inhaled ultrafine titanium dioxide particles. *Am J Respir Cell Mol Biol*. 2008;38: 371–376.

Geiser M, Kreyling WG. Deposition and biokinetics of inhaled nanoparticles. *Part Fibre Toxicol*. 2010;7:2.

Geiser M, Rothen-Rutishauser B, Kapp N, et al. Ultrafine particles cross cellular membranes by nonphagocytic mechanisms in lungs and in cultured cells. *Environ Health Perspect*. 2005;113:1555–1560.

George S, Xia T, Rallo R, et al. Use of a high-throughput screening approach coupled with in vivo zebrafish embryo screening to develop hazard ranking for engineered nanomaterials. *ACS Nano*. 2011;5(3):1805–1817.

Gottschalk F, Sonderer T, Scholz RW, Nowack B. Modeled environmental concentrations of engineered nanomaterials (TiO(2), ZnO, Ag, CNT, Fullerenes) for different regions. *Environ Sci Technol*. 2009;43(24):9216–9222.

Gottschalk F, Sonderer T, Scholz RW, Nowack B. Possibilities and limitations of modeling environmental exposure to engineered nanomaterials by probabilistic material flow analysis. *Environ Toxicol Chem.* 2010;29(5):1036–1048.

Griffitt RJ, Weil R, Hyndman KA, et al. Exposure to copper nanoparticles causes gill injury and acute lethality in zebrafish (Danio rerio). *Environ Sci Technol.* 2007;41(23):8178–8186.

Guo L, Liu X, Vaslet C, Hurt RH, Kane AB. Iron bioavailability and redox activity in diverse carbon nanotube samples. *Chem Mater.* 2007;19:3472–3478.

Guo L, Von Dem Bussche A, Buechner M, Yan A, Kane AB, Hurt RH. Adsorption of essential micronutrients by carbon nanotubes and the implications for nanotoxicity testing. *Small.* 2008;4:721–727.

Hallock MF, Greenlay P, DiBerardinis L, Kallin D. Potential risks of nanomaterials and how to safely handle materials of uncertain toxicity. *J Chem Health Saf.* 2009;16:16–23.

Hamilton RF, Wu N, Porter D, Buford M, Wolfarth M, Holian A. Particle length-dependent titanium dioxide nanomaterials toxicity and bioactivity. *Part Fibre Toxicol.* 2009;6:35.

Han GH, Andrews R, Gairola CG. Acute pulmonary response of mice to multi-wall carbon nanotubes. *Inhal Toxicol.* 2010;22:340–347.

Han X, Gelein R, Corson N. Validation of an LDH assay for assessing nanoparticle toxicity. *Toxicology.* 2011;287:99–104.

Haniu H, Saito N, Matsuda Y, et al. Effect of dispersants of multi-walled carbon nanotubes on cellular uptake and biological responses. *Intl J Nanomed.* 2011;6:3295–3307.

Henry TB, Menn FM, Fleming JT, Wilgus J, Compton RN, Sayler GS. Attributing effects of aqueous C60 nano-aggregates to tetrahydrofuran decomposition products in larval zebrafish by assessment of gene expression. *Environ Health Perspect.* 2007;115(7):1059–1065.

Hinderliter PM, Minard KR, Orr G, Chrisler WB et al. ISDD: a computational model of particle sedimentation, diffusion and target cell dosimetry for in vitro toxicity studies. *Part Fibre Toxicol.* 2010;7:36.

Hinds WC. Time for number concentration to halve and particle size to double by simple monodisperse coagulation. In: *Aerosol Technology.* John-Wiley, New York; 1982:235–239.

Hirano S, Fujitani Y, Furuyama A, Kanno S. Uptake and cytotoxic effects of multi-walled carbon nanotubes in human bronchial epithelial cells. *Toxicol Appl Pharmacol.* 2010;249(1):8–15.

Hirano S, Kanno S, Furuyama A. Multi-walled carbon nanotubes injure the plasma membrane of macrophages. *Toxicol Appl Pharmacol.* 2008; 232(2):244–251.

Hoet PHM, Bruske-Hohlfeld I, Salata OV. Nanoparticles - known and unknown health risks. *J Nanobiotechnol.* 2004;2(12):12–27.

Holbrook RD, Murphy KE, Morrow JB, Cole KD. Trophic transfer of nanoparticles in a simplified invertebrate food web. *Nat Nanotechnol.* 2008;3(6):352–355.

Holder AL, Lucas D, Goth-Goldstein R, Koshland CP. Cellular response to diesel exhaust particles strongly depends on the exposure method. *Toxicol Sci.* 2004;103(1):108–115.

Hoshino A, Fujioka K, Oku T, et al. Physicochemical properties and cellular toxicity of nanocrystal quantum dots depend on their surface modification. *Nano Letters.* 2004;4(11):2163–2169.

Hunter DD, Undem BJ. Identification and substance P content of vagal afferent neurons innervating the epithelium of the guinea pig trachea. *Am J Respir Crit Care Med.* 1999;159:1943–1948.

Hutchison JE. Greener nanoscience: a proactive approach to advancing applications and reducing implications of nanotechnology. *ACS Nano.* 2008;2:395–402.

ICRP. *Annals of the ICRP, Human Respiratory Tract Model for Radiological Protection.* Vol. 24 (1–3). ICRP Publication 66, Pergamon; 1994.

Iezzi R, Guru B, Glybina IV, et al. Dendrimer-based targeted intravitreal therapy for sustained attenuation of neuroinflammation in retinal degeneration. *Biomaterials.* 2012;33:979–988.

ISO/DIS 26824. *Particle characterization of particulate systems—Vocabulary.* ISO/TS; 2011.

ISO/TS 27687. *Nanotechnologies—Terminology and Definitions for Nano-objects—Nanoparticle, Nanofibre and Nanoplate.* ISO/TS; 2008.

Jacobsen NR, Pojana G, White P, et al. Genotoxicity, cytotoxicity, and reactive oxygen species induced by single-walled carbon nanotubes and C(60) fullerenes in the FE1-Mutatrade mark-Mouse lung epithelial cells. *Environ Mol Mutagen.* 2008;49(6):476–487.

Jakubek LM, Marangoudakis S, Raingo J, Liu X, Lipscombe D, Hurt RH. The inhibition of neuronal calcium ion channels by trace levels of yttrium released from carbon nanotubes. *Biomaterials.* 2009;30:6351–6357.

Jani PU, Halbert GW, Langridge J, Florence AT. Nanoparticle uptake by the rat gastrointestinal mucosa: quantitation and particle size dependency. *J Pharm Pharmacol.* 1990;42:821–826.

Jani PU, McCarthy DE, Florence AT. Titanium dioxide (rutile) particle uptake from the rat GI tract and translocation to systemic organs after oral administration. *Int J Pharm.* 1994;105:157–168.

Jiang J, Oberdörster G, Biswas P. Characterization of size surface charge, and agglomeration state of nanoparticle dispersons for toxicological studies. *J Nanopart Res.* 2009;11:77–89.

Judy JD, Unrine JM, Bertsch PM. Evidence for biomagnification of gold nanoparticles within a terrestrial food chain. *Environ Sci Technol.* 2011;45(2):776–781. Epub 2010 Dec 3.

Johansen A, Pedersen AL, Jensen KA, et al. Effects of C60 fullerene nanoparticles on soil bacteria and protozoans. *Environ Toxicol Chem.* 2008;27(9):1895–1903.

Johnston CJ, Finkelstein, JN, Mercer P, et al. Pulmonary effects induced by ultrafine PTFE particles. *Toxicol Appl Pharmacol.* 2000;168:208–215.

Johnston HJ, Hutchison GR, Christensen FM, et al. A critical review of the biological mechanisms underlying the *in vivo* and *in vitro* toxicity of carbon nanotubes: the contribution of physico-chemical characteristics. *Nanotoxicology.* 2010a;4(2):207–246.

Johnston HJ, Semmler-Behnke M, Brown DM, Kreyling W, Tran L, Stone V. Evaluating the uptake and intracellular fate of polystyrene nanoparticles by primary and hepatocyte cell lines in vitro. *Toxicol Appl Pharmacol.* 2010b;242:66–78.

Jones CF, Grainger DW. *In vitro* assessments of nanomaterial toxicity. *Adv Drug Deliv Rev.* 2009;61(6):438–456.

Jovanović B, Anastasova L, Rowe EW, Zhang Y, Clapp AR, Palić D. Effects of nanosized titanium dioxide on innate immune system of fathead minnow (Pimephales promelas Rafinesque, 1820). *Ecotoxicol Environ Saf.* 2011;74(4):675–683.

Kagan VE, Konduru NV, Feng W. Carbon nanotubes degraded by neutrophil myeloperoxidase induce less pulmonary inflammation. *Nat Nanotechnol.* 2010;5:354–359.

Kagan VE, Tyurina YY, Tyurin VA, et al. Direct and indirect effects of single walled carbon nanotubes on RAW 264.7 macrophages: role of iron. *Toxicol Lett.* 2006;165:88–100.

Kahru A, Dubourguier HC. From ecotoxicology to nanoecotoxicology. *Toxicology.* 2010;269:105–119.

Kane AB, Hurt RH. Nanotoxicology: the asbestos analogy revisited. *Nat Nanotechnol.* 2008;3(7):378–379.

Kang B, Mackey MA, El-Sayed MA. Nuclear targeting of gold nanoparticles in cancer cells induces DNA damage, causing cytokinesis arrest and apoptosis. *J Am Chem Soc.* 2010;132(5):1517–1519.

Kang S, Herzberg M, Rodrigues DF, Elimelech M. Antibacterial effects of carbon nanotubes: size does matter! *Langmuir.* 2008;24:6409–6413.

Kang S, Pinault M, Pfefferle LD, Elimelech M. Single-walled carbon nanotubes exhibit strong antimicrobial activity. *Langmuir.* 2007;23:8670–8673.

Kang S, Mauter MS, Elimelech M. Microbial cytotoxicity of carbon-based nanomaterials: implications for river water and wastewater effluent. *Environ Sci Technol.* 2009;43(7):2648–2653.

Kanno J, Takagi A, Nishimura T, Hirose A. Mesothelioma induction by micrometer-sized multi-walled carbon nanotube intraperitoneally injected to p53 heterozygous mice. *Toxicologist.* 2010;114:A1397.

Kanno S, Furuyama A, Hirano S. A murine scavenger receptor MARCO recognizes polystyrene nanoparticles. *Toxicol Sci.* 2007;97:398–406.

Kao YY, Chen YC, Cheng TJ, Chiung YM, Liu PS. Zinc oxide nanoparticles interfere with zinc ion homeostasis to cause cytotoxicity. *Toxicol Sci.* 2012;125(2):462–472.

Karmali PP, Simberg D. Interactions of nanoparticles with plasma proteins: implication on clearance and toxicity of drug delivery systems. *Expert Opin Drug Deliv.* 2011;8:343–357.

Kennedy AJ, Hull MS, Bednar AJ, et al. Fractionating nanosilver: importance for determining toxicity to aquatic test organisms. *Environ Sci Technol*. 2010;44(24):9571–9577.

Khandoga A, Stoeger T, Khandoga AG, et al. Platelet adhesion and fibrinogen deposition in murine microvessels upon inhalation of nanosized carbon particles. *J Thromb Haemost*. 2010;8:1632–1640.

Kim BY, Rutka JT, Chan WC. Nanomedicine. *N Engl J Med*. 2010; 363:2434–2443.

Klaine SJ, Alvarez PJ, Batley GE, et al. Nanomaterials in the environment: behavior, fate, bioavailability, and effects. *Environ Toxicol Chem*. 2008;27:1825–1851.

Klaper R, Arndt D, Setyowati K, Chen J, Goetz F. Functionalization impacts the effects of carbon nanotubes on the immune system of rainbow trout, Oncorhynchus mykiss. *Aquat Toxicol*. 2010;100(2):211–217.

Klaper R, Crago J, Barr J, Arndt D, Setyowati K, Chen J. Toxicity biomarker expression in daphnids exposed to manufactured nanoparticles: changes in toxicity with functionalization. *Environ Pollut*. 2009;157(4):1152–1156.

Kobayashi N, Naya M, Ema M, et al. Biological response and morphological assessment of individually dispersed multi-wall carbon nanotubes in the lung after intratracheal instillation in rats. *Toxicology*. 2010;276(3):143–153.

Kolosnjaj-Tabi J, Hartman KB, Boudjemaa S, et al. *In vivo* behavior of large doses of ultrashort and full-length single-walled carbon nanotubes after oral and intraperitoneal administration to Swiss mice. *ACS Nano*. 2010;4(3):1481–1492.

Kotchey GP, Allen BL, Vedala H, et al. The enzymatic oxidation of graphene oxide. *ACS Nano*. 2011;5:2098–2108.

Kovács T. Mechanisms of olfactory dysfunction in aging and neurodegenerative disorders. *Ageing Res Rev*. 2004;3:215.

Kovochich M, Espinasse B, Auffan M, et al. Comparative toxicity of C60 aggregates toward mammalian cells: role of tetrahydrofuran (THF) decomposition. *Environ Sci Technol*. 2009;43(16):6378–6384.

Kreuter J. Influence of the surface properties on nanoparticle-mediated transport of drugs to the brain. *J. Nanosci Nanotechnol*. 2004;4:484–488.

Kreyling W, Semmler M, Erbe F, et al. Translocation of ultrafine insoluble iridium particles from lung epithelium to extrapulmonary organs is size dependent but very low. *J Toxicol Environ Health A*. 2002;65(20): 1513–1530.

Kreyling WG, Semmler-Behnke M, Seitz J, et al. Size dependence of the translocation of the inhaled iridium and carbon nanoparticle aggregates from the lung of rats to the blood and secondary target organs. *Inhalation Toxicol*. 2009;21(S1):55–60.

Krug HF, Wick P. Nanotoxicology: an interdisciplinary challenge. *Angew Chem Int Ed*. 2011;50:1260–1278.

Kunzmann A, Andersson B, Thurnherr T, et al. Toxicology of engineered nanomaterials: focus on biocompatibility, biodistribution and biodegradation. *Biochimica et Biophysica Acta*. 2011;1810:361–373.

Lacerda L, Soundararajan A, Singh R, et al. Dynamic imaging of functionalized multi-walled carbon nanotube systemic circulation and urinary excretion. *Adv Mater*. 2008;20:225–230.

Lai SK, Wang YY, Hanes J. Mucus-penetrating nanoparticles for drug and gene delivery to mucosal tissues. *Adv Drug Deliv Rev*. 2009;61:158–171.

Lajoie P, Nabi IR. Lipid rafts, caveolae, and their endocytosis. *Int Rev Cell Mol Biol*. 2010;282:135–163.

Lam GW, James JT, McCluskey R, Hunter RL. Pulmonary toxicity of single-wall carbon nanotubes in mice 7 and 90 days after intratracheal instillation. *Toxicol Sci*. 2004;77:125–134.

Landsiedel R, Ma-Hock L, Kroll A, et al. Testing metal-oxide nanomaterials for human safety. *Adv Mater*. 2010;22:2601–2627.

Lee KP, Seidel WC. Pulmonary response of rats exposed to polytetrafluoroethylene and tetrafluoroethylene hexafluoropropylene copolymer fume and isolated particles. *Inhal Toxicol*. 1991;3:237–264.

Lenz AG, Karg E, Lentner B, et al. A dose-controlled system for air-liquid interface cell exposure and application to zinc oxide nanoparticles. *Part Fibre Toxicol*. 2009;6:32.

Lesniak W, Bielinska AU, Sun K, et al. Silver/dendrimer nanocomposites as biomarkers: fabrication, characterization, in vitro toxicity, and intracellular detection. *Nano Lett*. 2005;5:2123–2130.

Letts RE, Pereira TC, Bogo MR, Monserrat JM. Biologic responses of bacteria communities living at the mucus secretion of common carp (Cyprinus carpio) after exposure to the carbon nanomaterial fullerene (C60). *Arch Environ Contam Toxicol*. 2011;61(2):311–317.

Lewinski NA, Zhu H, Ouyang CR, et al. Trophic transfer of amphiphilic polymer coated CdSe/ZnS quantum dots to Danio rerio. *Nanoscale*. 2011;3(8):3080–3083.

Li D, Alvarez PJ. Avoidance, weight loss, and cocoon production assessment for Eisenia fetida exposed to C_{60} in soil. *Environ Toxicol Chem*. 2011;30(11):2542–2545.

Li JG, Li QN, Xu JY, et al. The pulmonary toxicity of multi-wall carbon nanotubes in mice 30 and 60 days after inhalation exposure. *J Nanosci Nanotechnol*. 2009;9:1384–1387.

Li JG, Li WX, Xu JY, et al. Comparative study of pathological lesions induced by multiwalled carbon nanotubes in lungs of mice by intratracheal instillation and inhalation. *Environ Toxicol*. 2007;22:415–421.

Li M, Zhu L, Lin D. Toxicity of ZnO nanoparticles to Escherichia coli: mechanism and the influence of medium components. *Environ Sci Technol*. 2011;45(5):1977–1983.

Li N, Sioutas C, Cho A, et al. Ultrafine particulate pollutants induce oxidative stress and mitochondrial damage. *Environ Health Perspect*. 2003;111:455–460.

Li X, Fan Y, Watari F. Current investigations into carbon nanotubes for biomedical application. *Biomed Mater*. 2010;5(2):22001.

Liang F, Chen B. A review of biomedical applications of single-walled carbon nanotubes. *Curr Med Chem*. 2010;17:10–24.

Limbach LK, Li Y, Grass RN, et al. Oxide nanoparticle uptake in human lung fibroblasts: effects of particle size, agglomeration, and diffusion at low concentrations. *Environ Sci Technol*. 2005;39:9370–9376.

Limbach LK, Wick P, Manser P, et al. Exposure of engineered nanoparticles to human lung epithelial cells: influence of chemical composition and catalytic activity on oxidative stress. *Environ Sci Technol*. 2007;41(11):4158–4163.

Linse S, Cabaleiro-Lago C, Xue WF, et al. Nucleation of protein fibrillation by nanoparticles. *Proc Natl Acad Sci U S A*. 2007;104:8691–8696.

Liu J, Hurt RH. Ion release kinetics and particle persistence in aqueous nano-silver colloids. *Env Sci Tech*. 2010;44:6:2169–2175.

Liu J, Sonshine D, Shervani S, Hurt RH. Controlled release of biologically active silver from nanosilver surfaces. *ACS Nano*. 2010a; 4(11):6903–6913.

Liu S, Ng AK, Xu R, et al. Antibacterial action of dispersed single-walled carbon nanotubes on Escherichia coli and Bacillus subtilis investigated by atomic force microscopy. *Nanoscale*. 2010b;2: 2744–2750.

Liu S, Wei L, Hao L, et al. Sharper and faster "nano darts" kill more bacteria: a study of antibacterial activity of individually dispersed pristine single-walled carbon nanotube. *ACS Nano*. 2009;3:3891–3902.

Liu X, Guo L, Morris D, Kane AB, Hurt RH. Targeted removal of bioavailable metal as a detoxification strategy for carbon nanotubes. *Carbon*. 2008;46:489–500.

Liu X, Hurt RH, Kane AB. Biodurability of single-walled carbon nanotubes depends on surface functionalization. *Carbon*. 2010c;48:1961–1969.

Liu Y, He L, Mustapha A, Li H, Hu ZQ, Lin M. Antibacterial activities of zinc oxide nanoparticles against Escherichia coli O157:H7. *J Appl Microbiol*. 2009;107:1193–1201.

Liu Z, Chen K, Davis C, et al. Drug delivery with carbon nanotubes for *in vivo* cancer treatment. *Cancer Res*. 2008;68(16):6652–6660.

Liu Z, Sun X, Nakayama-Ratchford N, Dai H. Supramolecular chemistry on water-soluble carbon nanotubes for drug loading and delivery. *ACS Nano*. 2007;1:50–56.

Loeschner K, Hadrup N, Ovortrup K, et al. Distribution of silver in rats following 28 days of repeated oral exposure to silver nanoparticles or silver acetate. *Part Fibre Toxicol*. 2011;8:18.

Lovern SB, Owen H, Klaper R. Electron microscopy of gold nanoparticle intake in the gut of Daphnia magna. *Nanotoxicology*. 2008;2(1):43–48.

Lovern SB, Strickler JR, Klaper R. Behavioral and physiological changes in Daphnia magna when exposed to nanoparticle suspensions (titanium dioxide, nano-C_{60}, and $C_{60}HxC_{70}Hx$). *Environ Sci Technol*. 2007; 41(12):4465–4470.

Lovern S, Klaper R. Daphnia magna mortality when exposed to titanium dioxide and fullerene nanoparticles. *Environ Toxicol Chem.* 2006; 25(4):1132–1137.

Lu CH, Zhu CL, Li J, Liu JJ, Chen X, Yang HH. Using graphene to protect DNA from cleavage during cellular delivery. *Chem Commun (Camb).* 2010;46:3116–3118.

Lu S, Duffin R, Poland C, et al. Efficacy of simple short-term in vitro assays for predicting the potential of metal oxide nanoparticles to cause pulmonary inflammation. *Environ Health Persp*ect. 2009;117:241–247.

Lundqvist M, Stigler J, Elia G, et al. Nanoparticle size and surface properties determine the protein corona with possible implications for biological impacts. *Proc Natl Acad Sci USA.* 2008;105(38):14265–14270.

Lynch I, Cedervall T, Lundqvist M, Cabaleiro-Lago C, Linse S, Dawson KA. The nanoparticle-protein complex as a biological entity; a complex fluids and surface science challenge for the 21st century. *Adv Colloid Interface Sci.* 2007;134–135:167–174.

Ma-Hock L, Trenmann S, Strauss V, et al. Inhalation toxicity of multi-wall carbon nanotubes in rats exposed for 3 months. *Toxicol Sci.* 2009; 112:468–481.

McNeil SE. Nanotechnology for the biologist. *J Leukocyte Biol.* 2005; 78:585–594.

Meng H, Xia T, George S, Nel AE. A predictive toxicological paradigm for the safety assessment of nanomaterials. *ACS Nano.* 2009;3:1620–1627.

Mercer RR, Hubbs AF, Scabilloni JF, et al. Distribution and persistence of pleural penetrations by multi-walled carbon nanotubes. *Particle Fibre Toxicol.* 2010;7:28.

Mercer RR, Hubbs AF, Scabilloni JF, et al. Pulmonary fibrotic response to aspiration of multi-walled carbon nanotubes. *Particle Fibre Toxicol.* 2011;8:21.

Mercer RR, Scabilloni J, Wang L, et al. Alteration of deposition pattern and pulmonary response as a result of improved dispersion of aspirated single walled carbon nanotubes in a mouse model. *Am J Physiol Lung Cell Mol Physiol.* 2008;294:L87–L97.

Mitchell LA, Gao J, Wal RV, et al. Pulmonary and systemic immune response to inhaled multiwalled carbon nanotubes. *Toxicol Sci.* 2007;100(1): 203–214.

Moberg PJ, Doty RL. Olfactory function in Huntington's disease patients and at-risk offspring. *Int J Neurosci.* 1997;89:133.

Monopoli MP, Bombelli FB, Dawson KA. Nanobiotechnology: nanoparticle coronas take shape. *Nat Nanotechnol.* 2011;6(1):11–12.

Monteiro-Riviere NA, Inman AO. Challenges for assessing carbon nanomaterial toxicity to the skin. *Carbon.* 2006;44:1070–1078.

Monteiro-Riviere NA, Nemanich RJ, Inman AO, Wang YY, Riviere JE. Multi-walled carbon nanotube interactions with human epidermal keratinocytes. *Toxicol Lett.* 2005;155(3):377–384.

Monteiro-Riviere NA, Wiench K, Landsiedel R, Schulte S, Inman AO, Riviere JE. Safety evaluation of sunscreen formulations containing titanium dioxide and zinc oxide nanoparticles in UVB sunburned skin: an in vitro and in vivo study. *Toxicol Sci.* 2011;123:264–280.

Morimoto Y, Hirohashi M, Ogami A, et al. Pulmonary toxicity of well-dispersed multi-call carbon nanotubes following inhalation and intratracheal instillation. *Nanotoxicology.* 2012a;6(6):587–599.

Morimoto Y, Hirohashi M, Kobayashi N, et al. Pulmonary toxicity of well-dispersed multi-call carbon nanotubes after inhalation. *Nanotoxicology.* 2012b. In press.

Morrow PE. Possible mechanisms to explain dust overloading of the lungs. *Fund Appl Tox.* 1988;10:369–384.

Mortensen LJ, Oberdörster G, Pentland AP, DeLouise LA. In vivo skin penetration of quantum dot nanoparticles in the murine model: the effect of UVR. *Nano Lett.* 2008. http://pubs.acs.org/journals/nalefd/index.html.

Mortimer M, Kasemets K, Kahru A. Toxicity of ZnO and CuO nanoparticles to ciliated protozoa Tetrahymena thermophila. *Toxicology.* 2010; 269(2–3):182–189.

Mouchet F, Landois P, Datsyuk V, et al. International amphibian micronucleus standardized procedure (ISO 21427-1) for in vivo evaluation of double-walled carbon nanotubes toxicity and genotoxicity in water. *Environ Toxicol.* 2011;26(2):136–145.

Mueller NC, Nowack B. Exposure modeling of engineered nanoparticles in the environment. *Environ Sci Technol.* 2008;42:4447–4453.

Muller J, Huaux F, Moreau N. Respiratory toxicity of multi-wall carbon nanotubes. *Toxicol Appl Pharmacol.* 2005;207:221–231.

Müller RH, Heinemann S. In: Gurny R, Junginger HE, eds. Bioadhesion–Possibilities and Future trends. Stuttgart: Wissenschaftliche Verlagsgesellschaft; 1989:202–214.

Murphy FA, Poland CA, Duffin R, et al. Length-dependent retention of carbon nanotubes in the pleural space of mice initiates sustained inflammation and progressive fibrosis on the parietal pleura. *Am J Pathol.* 2011;178:2587–2600.

National Academy of Sciences. *Risk assessment in the Federal Government: Managing the process.* 1983.

National Nanotechnology Initiative. *NNI Environmental, Health, and Safety Research Strategy.* National Science and Technology Council Committee on Technology, Subcommittee on Nanoscale Science, Engineering and Technology; 2011.

Nel A, Xia T, Madler L, Li N. Toxic potential of materials at the nanolevel. *Science.* 2006;311:622–627.

Nel AE, Madler L, Velegol D, et al. Understanding biophysicochemical interactions at the nano-bio interface. *Nat Mater.* 2009;8:543–557.

NIOSH. Current Intelligence Bulletin. *Occupational Exposure To Carbon Nanotubes.* 2011. www.cdc.gov/niosh/docket/review/docket161A/.

Nowack B, Ranville JF, Diamond S, et al. Potential scenarios for nanomaterial release and subsequent alteration in the environment. *Environ Toxicol Chem.* 2012;31(1):50–59.

Nyberg L, Turco RF, Nies L. Assessing the impact of nanomaterials on anaerobic microbial communities. *Environ Sci Technol.* 2008; 42(6):1938–1943.

Oberdörster G. Dosimetric principles for extrapolating results of rat inhalation studies to humans, using nickel as an example. *Health Phys.* 1989;57(suppl 1):213–220.

Oberdörster G. Nanotoxicology: in vitro–in vivo dosimetry [letter to editor]. *Environ Health Perspect.* 2012;120:a13–a13. http://dx.doi.org/10.1289/ehp.1104320.

Oberdörster G, Elder A, Rinderknecht A. Nanoparticles and the brain: cause for concern? *J Nanosci Nanotechnol.* 2009;9:4996–5007.

Oberdörster G, Ferin J, Gelein R, et al. Role of the alveolar macrophage in lung injury: studies with ultrafine particles. *Environ Health Perspect.* 1992;97:193–197.

Oberdörster G, Ferin J. Metal compounds used in new technologies: metal oxides of ultrafine particles have increased pulmonary toxicity. In: Merian E, Haerdi W, eds. *Metal Compounds in Environment & Life.* Northwood, UR: Science & Technology Ltrs. and Science Reviews, Inc; 1992:443–450.

Oberdörster G, Ferin J, Lehnert BE. Correlation between particle size, in vivo particle persistence, and lung injury. *Environ Health Perspect.* 1994;102(suppl 5):173–179.

Oberdörster G, Morrow PE, Spurny K. Size dependent lymphatic short term clearance of amosite fi bers in the lung. *Ann Occup Hyg.* 1988;32 (suppl, inhaled particles VI):149–156.

Oberdörster G, Oberdörster E, Oberdörster J. Nanotoxicology: an emerging discipline evolving from studies of ultrafine particles. *Environ Health Perspect.* 2005;113:823–839.

Oberdörster G, Oberdörster E, Oberdörster J. Correspondence: concepts of nanoparticle dose metric and response metric. *Environ Health Perspect.* 2007a;115(6):A290.

Oberdörster G, Stone V, Donaldson K. Toxicology of nanoparticles: a historical perspective. *Nanotoxicology.* 2007b;1(1):2–25.

Oberdörster G, Sharp Z, Atudorei V, et al. Translocation of inhaled ultrafine particles to the brain. *Inhalation Toxicol.* 2004;16(6–7):437–445.

Oh YK, Swanson JA. Different fates of phagocytosed particles after delivery into macrophage lysosomes. *J Cell Biol.* 1996;132:585–593.

Oller A, Oberdörster G. Incorporation of particle size differences between animal studies and human workplace aerosols for deriving exposure limit values. *Regul Toxicol Pharmacol.* 2010;57:181–194.

Oyabu T, Myojo T, Morimoto Y, et al. Biopersistence of inhaled MWCNT in rat lungs in a 4-week well-characterized exposure. *Inhal Toxicol.* 2011; 23(13):784–791.

Pacurari M, Yin XJ, Ding M, et al. Oxidative and molecular interactions of multi-wall carbon nanotubes (MWCNT) in normal and malignant human mesothelial cells. *Nanotoxicology.* 2008;2(3):155–170.

Palomaki J, Valimaki E, Sund J, et al. Long, needle-like carbon nanotubes and asbestos activate the NLRP3 inflammasome through a similar mechanism. *ACS Nano*. 2011;5:6861–6870.

Pante N, Kann M. Nuclear pore complex is able to transport macromolecules with diameters of about 39 nm. *Mol Biol Cell*. 2002;13:425–434.

Pare WP, Glavin GB. Restraint stress in biomedical research: a review. *Neurosci Biobehav Rev*. 1986;10:339–370.

Pauluhn J. Subchronic 13—week inhalation exposure of rats to multiwalled carbon nanotubes: toxic effects are determined by density of agglomerate structures, not fibrillar structure. *Toxicol Sci*. 2010;113:226–242.

Peng X, Palma S, Fisher NS, Wong SS. Effect of morphology of ZnO nanostructures on their toxicity to marine algae. *Aquat Toxicol*. 2011; 102(3–4):186–196.

Petersen EJ, Akkanen J, Kukkonen JVK, Weber WJ Jr. Biological uptake and depuration of carbon nanotubes by Daphnia magna. *Environ Sci Technol*. 2009;43(8):2969–2975.

Pfaller TR, Colognato R, Nelissen I, et al. The suitability of different cellular in vitro immunotoxicity and genotoxicity methods for the analysis of nanoparticle-induced events. *Nanotoxicology*. 2009:21. [epub ahead of print]

Phalen RF, Oldham MJ, Nel AE. Tracheobronchial particle dose considerations for in vitro toxicology studies. *Toxicol Sci*. 2006;92(1):126–132.

Pietruska JR, Liu X, Smith A, et al. Bioavailability, intracellular mobilization of nickel, and HIF-1α activation in human lung epithelial cells exposed to metallic nickel and nickel oxide nanoparticles. *Toxicol Sci*. 2011;124(1):138–148.

Poland C, Duffin R, Kinloch I, et al. Carbon nanotubes introduced into the abdominal cavity of ICR show asbestos-like pathogenicity in a pilot study. *Nat Nanotechnol*. 2008:423–428.

Pope CAI, Dockery DW. Health effects of fine particulate air polluton: lines that connect. *J Air Waste Manage Assoc*. 2006;56:709–742.

Porter D, Sriram I, Wolfarth M, et al. A biocompatible medium for nanoparticle dispersion. *Nanotoxicology*. 2008;2:144–154.

Porter DW, Hubbs AF, Mercer RR, et al. Mouse pulmonary dose- and time course-responses induced by exposure to multi-walled carbon nanotubes. *Toxicology*. 2010;269(2–3):136–147.

Pott F, Ziem U, Reiffer F-J, et al. Carcinogenicity studies on fibres, metal compounds and some other dusts in rats. *Exp Pathol*. 1987;32: 129–152.

Pradhan A, Seena S, Pascoal C, Cássio F. Can metal nanoparticles be a threat to microbial decomposers of plant litter in streams? *Microb Ecol*. 2011;62(1):58–68.

Prow TW, Grice JE, Lin LL, et al. Nanoparticles and microparticles for skin drug delivery. *Adv Drug Deliv Rev*. 2011;63(6):470–491.

Pulskamp K, Diabaté S, Krug HF. Carbon nanotubes show no sign of acute toxicity but induce intracellular reactive oxygen species in dependence on contaminants. *Toxicol Lett*. 2007;168(1):58–74.

Quinn J, Geiger C, Clausen C, et al. Field demonstration of DNAPL dehalogenation using emulsified zero-valent iron. *Environ Sci Technol*. 2005; 39(5):1309–1318.

Ren H, Wang C, Zhang J, et al. DNA cleavage system of nanosized graphene oxide sheets and copper ions. *ACS Nano*. 2010;4:7169–7174.

Rinderknecht A, Elder A, Prud'homme R, Gindy M, Harkema J, Oberdörster G. Surface functionalization affects the role of nanoparticle disposition. *Am J Respir Crit Care Med*. 2007;175:A246.

Roberts AP, Mount AS, Seda B, et al. In vivo biomodification of lipid-coated carbon nanotubes by Daphnia magna. *Environ Sci Technol*. 2007;41(8):3025–3029.

Roco MC. Environmentally responsible development of nanotechnology. *Environ Sci Technol*. 2005;39:106A–112A.

Rodrigues DF, Elimelech M. Toxic effects of single-walled carbon nanotubes in the development of E. coli biofilm. *Environ Sci Technol*. 2010;44:4583–4589.

Rosenthal SJ, Chang JC, Kovtun O, McBride JR, Tomlinson ID. Biocompatible quantum dots for biological applications. *Chem Biol*. 2011;18:10–24.

Ross AJ, Dailey LA, Brighton LE, Devlin RB. Transcriptional Profiling of Mucociliary Differentiation in Human Airway Epithelial Cells. *Am J Respir Cell Mol Biol*. 2007;37:169–185.

Rothenberg SJ, Parker RM, York RG, et al. Lack of effects of nose-only inhalation exposure on testicular toxicity in male rats. *Toxicol Sci*. 2000;53:127–134.

Rushton EK, Jiang J, Leonard SS, et al. Concept of assessing nanoparticle hazards considering nanoparticle dosemetric and chemical/biological response metrics. *J Toxicol Environ Health A*. 2010;73(5): 445–461.

Russell DG, Vanderven BC, Glennie S, Mwandumba H, Heyderman RS. The macrophage marches on its phagosome: dynamic assays of phagosome function. *Nat Rev Immunol*. 2009;9:594–600.

Ryman-Rasmussen JP, Cesta MF, Brody AR, et al. Inhaled carbon nanotubes reach the subpleural tissue in mice. *Nat Nanotechnol*. 2009a;4: 747–751.

Ryman-Rasmussen JP, Tewksbury EW, Moss OR, et al. Inhaled multiwalled carbon nanotubes potentiate airway fibrosis in murine allergic asthma. *Am J Respir Cell Mol Biol*. 2009b;40(3):349–358.

Sager TM, Porter DW, Robinson VA, Lindsley WG, Schwegler-Berry DE, Castranova V. Improved method to disperse nanoparticles for in vitro and in vivo investigation of toxicity. *Nanotoxicol*. 2007;1:118–129.

Sakamoto Y, Nakae D, Fukumori N, et al. Induction of mesothelioma by a single intrascrotal administration of multi-wall carbon nanotube in intact male Fischer 344 rats. *J Toxicol Sci*. 2009;34(1):65–76.

Salas EC, Sun Z, Luttge A, Tour JM. Reduction of graphene oxide via bacterial respiration. *ACS Nano*. 2010;4:4852–4856.

Sanchez VC, Pietruska JR, Miselis NR, Hurt RH, Kane AB. Biopersistence and potential adverse health impacts of fibrous nanomaterials: what have we learned from asbestos? *Wiley Interdiscip Rev Nanomed Nanobiotechnol*. 2009;1:511–529.

Sanchez VC, Weston P, Yan A, Hurt RH, Kane AB. A 3-dimensional in vitro model of epithelioid granulomas induced by high aspect ratio nanomaterials. *Part Fibre Toxicol*. 2011;8(1):17.

Sargent LM, Reynolds SH, Castranova V. Potential pulmonary effects of engineered carbon nanotubes: in vitro genotoxic effects. *Nanotoxicology*. 2010;4:396–408.

Sasidharan A, Panchakarla LS, Chandran P, et al. Differential nano-bio interactions and toxicity effects of pristine versus functionalized graphene. *Nanoscale*. 2011;3:2461–2464.

Savi M, Kalberer M, Lang D, et al. A novel exposure system for the efficient and controlled deposition of aerosol particles onto cell cultures. *Environ Sci Technol*. 2008;42(15):5667–5674.

Sayes CM, Gobin AM, Ausman KD, Mendez J, West JL, Colvin VL. Nano-C60 cytotoxicity is due to lipid peroxidation. *Biomaterials*. 2005;26:7587–7595.

Sayes CM, Liang F, Hudson JL, et al. Functionalization density dependence of single-walled carbon nanotubes cytotoxicity in vitro. *Toxicol Lett*. 2006;161:135–142.

Schilling K, Bradford B, Castelli D, et al. Human safety review of "nano" titanium dioxide and zinc oxide. *Photochemical & photobiological sciences*. *Photochem Photobiol Sci*. 2010;9:495–509.

Schlesinger RB, Lippmann M. Selective particle deposition and bronchogenic carcinoma. *Environmental Res*. 1978;15:424–431.

Schmid G. The relevance of shape and size of Au55 clusters. *Chem Soc Rev*. 2008;37:1909–1930.

Schneider M, Stracke F, Hansen S, Schaefer UF. Nanoparticles and their interactions with the dermal barrier. *Dermato-Endocrinology*. 2009;1(4):197–206.

Scown TM, van Aerle R, Tyler CR. Review: do engineered nanoparticles pose a significant threat to the aquatic environment? *Crit Rev Toxicol*. 2010;40:653–670.

Segal MB. The choroid plexuses and the barriers between the blood and the cerebrospinal fluid. *Cell and Mol Neurobiol*. 2000;20:183.

Seidel WC, Scherer KV Jr, Cline D Jr, et al. Chemical, physical, and toxicological characterization of fumes produced by heating tetrafluoroethene homopolymer and its copolymers with hexafluoropropene and perfluoro(propyl vinyl ether). *Chem Res Toxicol*. 1991;4:229–236.

Semmler-Behnke M, Takenaka S, Fertsch S, et al. Efficient elimination of inhaled nanoparticles from the alveolar region: evidence for interstitial uptake and subsequent re-entrainment onto airways epithelia. *Environ Health Perspect*. 2007;115(5):728–733.

Semmler M, Seitz J, Erbe F, et al. Long-term clearance kinetics of inhaled ultrafine insoluble iridium particles from the rat lung, including transient translocation into secondary organs. *Inhal Toxicol.* 2004;16(6/7):453–459.

Senzui M, Tamura T, Miura K, Ikarashi Y, Watanabe Y, Fujii M. Study on penetration of titanium dioxide (TiO(2)) nanoparticles into intact and damaged skin in vitro. *J Toxicol Sci.* 2010;35:107–113.

Seong SY, Matzinger P. Hydrophobicity: an ancient damage-associated molecular pattern that initiates innate immune responses. *Nat Rev Immunol.* 2004;4:469–478.

Serda RE, Mack A, van de Ven AL, et al. Logic-embedded vectors for intracellular partitioning, endosomal escape, and exocytosis of nanoparticles. *Small.* 2010;6:2691–2700.

Shaw BJ, Handy RD. Physiological effects of nanoparticles on fish: a comparison of nanometals versus metal ions. *Environ Int.* 2011; 37(6):1083–1097.

Shi X, von dem Bussche A, Hurt RH, Kane AB, Gao H. Cell entry of one-dimensional nanomaterials occurs by tip recognition and rotation. *Nat Nanotechnol.* 2011;6:714–719.

Shinohara H. Distribution of lymphatic stomata on the pleural surface of the thoracic cavity and the surface topography of the pleural mesothelium in the golden hamster. *Anat Rec.* 1997;249:16–23.

Shvedova AA, Kisin ER, Mercer R, et al. Unusual inflammatory and fibrogenic pulmonary responses to single walled carbon nanotubes in mice. *Am J Physiol Lung Cell Mol. Physiol.* 2005;289:698–708.

Shvedova AA, Kisin E, Murray AR, et al. Inhalation vs. aspiration of single-walled carbon nanotubes in C57BL/6 mice: inflammation, fibrosis, oxidative stress, and mutagenesis. *Am J Physiol Lung Cell Mol Physiol.* 2008;295(4):L552–L565.

Shvedova AA, Sager T, Murray AR, et al. Critical issues in the evaluation of possible adverse pulmonary effects from airborne nanoparticles. *Nanotoxicology, Characterization, Dosing and Health Effects.* New York, London: Informa Healthcare, USA Inc; 2007.

Silbergeld EK, Contreras EQ, Hartung T, et al. Nanotoxicology: "the end of the beginning"—signs on the roadmap to a strategy for assuring the safe application and use of nanomaterials. *Altex.* 2011;28:236–241.

Simmons SO, Fan CY, Ramabhadran R. Cellular stress response pathway system as a sentinel ensemble in toxicological screening. *Toxicol Sci.* 2009;111:202–225.

Singh R, Pantarotto D, Lacerda L, et al. Tissue biodistribution and blood clearance rates of intravenously administered carbon nanotube radiotracers. *Proc Natl Acad Sci U S A.* 2006;103(9):3357–3362.

Sistonen L, Sarge KD, Phillips B, et al. *Mol Cell Biol.* 1992;12: 4104–4111.

Slikker W Jr, Andersen ME, Bogdanffy MS, et al. Dose-dependent transitions in mechanisms of toxicity. *Toxicol Appl Pharmacol.* 2004; 201(3):203–225.

Slowing II, Vivero-Escoto JL, Zhao Y, et al. Exocytosis of mesoporous silica nanoparticles from mammalian cells: from asymmetric cell-to-cell transfer to protein harvesting. *Small.* 2011;7:1526–1532.

Stanton MF, Layard M, Tegeris A, et al. Relation of particle dimension to carcinogenicity in Amphibole asbestoses and other fibrous minerals. *JNCL.* 1981;67:965–975.

Stone V, Johnston H, Schins RP. Development of in vitro systems for nanotoxicology: methodological considerations. *Crit Rev Toxicol.* 2009;39:613–626.

Sugamata M, Uhara T, Takano H, Oshio S, Takeda K. Maternal diesel exhaust exposure damages newborn murine brains. *J Health Science.* 2006;52(1):82–84.

Takagi A, Hirose A, Nishimura T, et al. Induction of mesothelioma in p53+/- mouse by intraperitoneal application of multi-wall carbon nanotube. *J Toxicol Sci.* 2008;33(1):105–116.

Takeda K, Suzuki K-i, Ishihra A, et al. Nanoparticles transferred from pregnant mice to their offspring can damage the genital and cranial nerve systems. *J Health Sci.* 2009;55(1):95–102.

Tang T, Gminski R, Könczöl M, Modest C, Armbruster B, Mersch-Sundermann V. Investigations on cytotoxic and genotoxic effects of laser printer emissions in human epithelial A549 lung cells using an air/liquid exposure system. *Environ Mol Mutagen.* 2011.

Taurozzi JS, Hackley VA, Wiesner MR. Ultrasonic dispersion of nanoparticles for environmental, health and safety assessment—issues and recommendations. *Nanotoxicology.* 2011;5:711–729.

Teeguarden JG, Hinderliter PM, Orr G, Thrall BD, Pounds JG. Particokinetics in vitro: dosimetry considerations for in vitro nanoparticle toxicity assessments. *Toxicol Sci.* 2007;95(2):300–312.

Teleki A, Wengeler R, Wengeler L, Nirschl H, Pratsinis SE. Distinguishing between aggregates and agglomerates of flame-made TiO$_2$ by high-pressure dispersion. *Powder Technol.* 2008;181: 292–300.

Titov AV, Kral P, Pearson R. Sandwiched graphene—membrane superstructures. *ACS Nano.* 2010;4:229–234.

Tong Z, Bischoff M, Nies L, Applegate B, Turco RF. Impact of fullerene (C60) on a soil microbial community. *Environ Sci Technol.* 2007; 41(8):2985–2991.

Tran CL, Buchanan D, Cullen RT, Searl A, Jones AD, Donaldson K. Inhalation of poorly soluble particles. II. Influence of particle surface area on inflammation and clearance. *Inhal Toxicol.* 2000;12:1113–1126.

Tran TH, Nguyen TD. Controlled growth of uniform noble metal nanocrystals: aqueous-based synthesis and some applications in biomedicine. *Colloids Surf B, Biointerfaces.* 2011;88:1–22.

Trouiller B, Reliene R, Westbrook A, Solaimani P, Schiestl RH. Titanium dioxide nanoparticles induce DNA damage and genetic instability in vivo in mice. *Cancer Res.* 2009;69(22):8784–8789.

Truong L, Saili KS, Miller JM, Hutchison JE, Tanguay RL. Persistent adult zebrafish behavioral deficits results from acute embryonic exposure to gold nanoparticles. *Comp Biochem Physiol C Toxicol Pharmacol.* 2012;155(2):269–274.

Tu X, Manohar S, Jagota A, Zheng M. DNA sequence motifs for structure-specific recognition and separation of carbon nanotubes. *Nature.* 2009;460:250–253.

Tungittiplakorn W, Cohen C, Lion LW. Engineered polymeric nanoparticles for bioremediation of hydrophobic contaminants. *Environ Sci Technol.* 2005;39(5):1354–1358.

Udelsman R, Blake MJ, Stagg CA, et al. Vascular heat shock protein expression in response to stress. *J Clin Invest.* 1993;91:465–473.

Unfried K, Albrecht C, et al. Cellular responses to nanoparticles: target structures and mechanisms. *Nanotoxicology.* 2007;1:52–71.

Vallhov H, Qin J, Johansson SM, et al. The importance of an endotoxin-free environment during the production of nanoparticles used in medical applications. *Nano Lett.* 2006;6:1682–1686.

Vankoningsloo S, Piret J-P, Saout C, et al. Cytotoxicity of multi-walled carbon nanotubes in three skin cellular models: effects of sonication, dispersive agents and corneous layer of reconstructed epidermis. *Nanotoxicology.* 2010;4(1):84–97.

Vecchio G, Galeone A, Brunetti V, et al. Mutagenic effects of gold nanoparticles induce aberrant phenotypes in Drosophila melanogaster. Nanomedicine. 2012;8(1):1–7.

Velzeboer I, Kupryianchyk D, Peeters ET, Koelmans AA. Community effects of carbon nanotubes in aquatic sediments. *Environ Int.* 2011; 37(6):1126–1130.

Volckens J, Dailey L, Walters G, Devlin RB. Direct particle-to-cell deposition of coarse ambient particulate matter increases the production of inflammatory mediators from cultured human airway epithelial cells. *Environ Sci Technol.* 2009;43(12):4595–4599.

Walczyk D, Bombelli FB, Monopoli MP, et al. What the cell "sees" in bionanoscience. *J Am Chem Soc.* 2010;132:5761–5768.

Walker NJ, Bucher JR. A 21st century paradigm for evaluating the health hazards of nanoscale materials? *Toxicol Sci.* 2009;110:251–254.

Wang C, Hou Y, Kim J, Sun S. A general strategy for synthesizing FePt nanowires and nanorods. *Angew Chem Int Ed Engl.* 2007;46: 6333–6335.

Wang J, Chen, C, Liu Y, et al. Potential neurological lesion after nasal instillation of TiO(2) nanoparticles in the anatase and rutile crystal phases. *Toxicol Lett.* 2008a;183(1–3):72–80.

Wang J, Liu Y, Jiao F, et al. Time-dependent translocation and potential impairment on central nervous system by intranasally instilled TiO(2) nanoparticles. *Toxicology.* 2008b;254(1–2):82–90.

Wang NS. The preformed stomatas connecting the pleural cavity and the lymphatics in the parietal pleura. *Amer Rev Resp Dis.* 1975;111:12–20.

Wang SQ, Tooley IR. Photoprotection in the era of nanotechnology. Semin Cutan Med Surg. 2011;30:210–213.

Wang X, Xia T, Ntim SA, et al. Dispersal state of multiwalled carbon nanotubes elicits profibrogenic cellular responses that correlate with fibrogenesis biomarkers and fibrosis in the murine lung. ACS Nano. 2011a;5:9772–9787.

Wang YY, Lai SK, So C, Schneider C, Cone R, Hanes J. Mucoadhesive nanoparticles may disrupt the protective human mucus barrier by altering its microstructure. PloS One. 2011b;6:e21547.

Wang Y, Westerhoff P, Hristovski KD. Fate and biological effects of silver, titanium dioxide, and C_{60} (fullerene) nanomaterials during simulated wastewater treatment processes. J Hazard Mater. 2012;201–202:16–22. Epub 2011 Nov 7. PubMed PMID: 22154869.

Warheit DB. How meaningful are the results of nanotoxicity studies in the absence of adequate material characterization? Toxicol Sci. 2008; 101:183–185.

Warheit DB, Hartsky MA, Stefaniak MS. Comparative physiology of rodent pulmonary macrophages: in vitro functional responses. J Appl Physiol. 1988a;64(5):1953–1959.

Warheit DB, Laurence BR, Reed KL, Rouch DH, Reynolds GAM, Webb TR. Comparative pulmonary toxicity assessment of single-wall carbon nanotubes in rats. Toxicol Sci. 2004;77:117–125.

Warheit DB, Overby LH, George G, Brody AR. Pulmonary macrophages are attracted to inhaled particles on alveolar surfaces. Exp Lung Res. 1988b;14:51–66.

Weir A, Westerhoff P, Fabricius L, Hristovski K, von Goetz N. Titanium dioxide nanoparticles in food and personal care products. Environ Sci Technol. 2012;46(4):2242–2250.

Werlin R, Priester JH, Mielke RE, et al. Biomagnification of cadmium selenide quantumdots in a simple experimental microbial food chain. Nat Nanotechnol. 2011;6(1):65–71.

Westerhoff P, Song G, Hristovski K, Kiser MA. Occurrence and removal of titanium at full scale wastewater treatment plants: implications for TiO_2 nanomaterials. J Environ Monit. 2011;13:1195–1203.

Weuve J, Puett RC, Schwartz J, et al. Exposure to particulate air pollution and cognitive decline in older women. Arch Intern Med. 2012; 172(3):219–227.

Wick P, Manser P, Limbach LK, et al. The degree and kind of agglomeration affect carbon nanotube cytotoxicity. Toxicol Lett. 2007;168:121–131.

Woodrow Wilson Center. 2012: http://www.nanotechproject.org/inventories/consumer/analysis_draft/

Worle-Knirsch JM, Pulskamp K, Krug HF. Oops they did it again! Carbon nanotubes hoax scientists in viability assays. Nano Lett. 2006;6(6): 1261–1268.

Xia T, Kovochich M, Brant J, et al. Comparison of the abilities of ambient and manufactured nanoparticles to induce cellular toxicity according to an oxidative stress paradigm. Nano Lett. 2006;6:1794–1807.

Xia T, Kovochich M, Liong M, et al. Comparison of the mechanism of toxicity of zinc oxide and cerium oxide nanoparticles based on dissolution and oxidative stress properties. ACS Nano. 2008a;2:2121–2134.

Xia T, Kovochich M, Liong M, Zink JI, Nel AE. Cationic polystyrene nanosphere toxicity depends on cell-specific endocytic and mitochondrial injury pathways. ACS Nano. 2008b;2:85–96.

Xia T, Zhao Y, Sager T, et al. Decreased dissolution of ZnO by iron doping yields nanoparticles with reduced toxicity in the rodent lung and zebrafish embryos. ACS Nano. 2011;5:1223–1235.

Xia XR, Monteiro-Riviere NA, Riviere JE. An index for characterization of nanomaterials in biological systems. Nat Nanotechnol. 2010;5: 671–675.

Xie Y, Williams NG, Tolic A, et al. Aerosolized ZnO nanoparticles induce toxicity in alveolar type ii epithelial cells at the air-liquid interface. Toxicol Sci. 2012;125(2):450–461.

Xiong D, Fang T, Yu L, Sima X, Zhu W. Effects of nano-scale TiO_2, ZnO and their bulk counterparts on zebrafish: acute toxicity, oxidative stress and oxidative damage. Sci Total Environ. 2011;409(8): 1444–1452.

Xu C, Xie J, Ho D, et al. Au-Fe3O4 dumbbell nanoparticles as dual-functional probes. Angew Chem Int Ed Engl. 2008;47:173–176.

Yan A, Von Dem Bussche A, Kane AB, Hurt RH. Tocopheryl polyethylene glycol succinate as a safe, antioxidant surfactant for processing carbon nanotubes and fullerenes. Carbon. 2007;45:2463–2470.

Yan L, Zhao F, Li S, Hu Z, Zhao Y. Low-toxic and safe nanomaterials by surface-chemical design, carbon nanotubes, fullerenes, metallofullerenes, and graphenes. Nanoscale. 2011;3:362–382.

Yang K, Zhu L, Xing B. Adsorption of polycyclic aromatic hydrocarbons by carbon nanomaterials. Environ Sci Technol. 2006;40: 1855–1861.

Yang Z, Zhang Y, Yang Y, et al. Pharmacological and toxicological target organelles and safe use of single-walled carbon nanotubes as drug carriers in treating Alzheimer disease. Nanomedicine. 2010;6(3): 427–441.

Yu LP, Fang T, Xiong DW, Zhu WT, Sima XF. Comparative toxicity of nano-ZnO and bulk ZnO suspensions to zebrafish and the effects of sedimentation, ·OH production and particle dissolution in distilled water. J Environ Monit. 2011;13(7):1975–1982.

Zhang LW, Monteiro-Riviere NA. Lectins modulate multi-walled carbon nanotubes cellular uptake in human epidermal keratinocytes. Toxicol In Vitro. 2010;24:546–551.

Zhang Q, Huang JQ, Zhao MQ, Qian WZ, Wei F. Carbon nanotube mass production: principles and processes. ChemSusChem. 2011;4: 864–889.

Zhang QZ, Zha L-S, Zhang Y, et al. The brain targeting efficiency following nasally applied MPEG-PLA nanoparticles in rats. J Drug Target. 2006; 14(5):281–290.

Zhao F, Zhao Y, Liu Y, Chang X, Chen C, Zhao Y. Cellular uptake, intracellular trafficking, and cytotoxicity of nanomaterials. Small. 2011;7: 1322–1337.

Zhao Y, Allen BL, Star A. Enzymatic degradation of multiwalled carbon nanotubes. J Phys Chem A. 2011;115:9536–9544.

Zhu S, Oberdörster E, Haasch ML. Toxicity of an engineered nanoparticle (fullerene, C60) in two aquatic species, Daphnia and fathead minnow. Mar Environ Res. 2006;62(suppl):S5–S9.

Zhu X, Zhu L, Lang Y, Chen Y. Oxidative stress and growth inhibition in the freshwater fish Carassius auratus induced by chronic exposure to sublethal fullerene aggregates. Environ Toxicol Chem. 2008; 27(9):1979–1985.

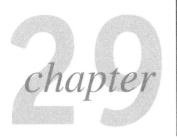

chapter 29

Air Pollution*

Daniel L. Costa and Terry Gordon

AIR POLLUTION IN PERSPECTIVE

The second half of the 20th century was marked by remarkable changes in how the public viewed its relationship to the environment. Until that time, national pride and prosperity were often depicted as an expanse of urban factories with smokestacks belching opaque dark clouds of industrial effluent into a neutral blue sky. But the price of that unchecked human progress through the first half of the century led to several air pollution catastrophes highlighting the profoundly detrimental impact that reckless prosperity could have on the environment. These images of "modern" life gradually gave rise to public outcry for governmental action to protect air quality and public health—a challenge to industry that had been focused on economic growth alone. The ensuing 50 years of regulatory legislation in the United States and Western Europe along with cost-efficient innovations by the private sector have remade this industrial image in most technologically developed nations.

Ironically, as regulatory control measures began to reduce emissions from stationary industrial sources of air pollution, highways to "open spaces" and urban flight took many people to the suburbs with its cleaner air and safe, comfortable lifestyle. Meanwhile,

the developing world saw little of this growth and what has grown is frequently cast-off old technology and variants of exploitation by the Western corporations attracted by abundant resources, a cheap workforce, and few regulations of constraints. This situation has persisted into the 21st century but is evolving with broader globalization of improved technology and communication.

The change in land use and demography in the United States in the 1950s and 1960s altered the national character and distribution of air pollution. The commute from suburban home to city workplace back to suburban home led increasingly to congested thoroughfares, whose emissions contributed to a photochemical cauldron of oxidant air pollution around expanding metro–suburban areas. Moreover, postwar population growth and rising expectations for a better (peace-time) standard of living led to unrestrained consumption, including inexpensive gasoline for commuting and recreation.

Today, the search is worldwide for cheap oil to fuel transportation and goods movement as easily accessible North American oil resources have been greatly diminished. International sources are increasingly prominent. For nontransportation sectors of industry and electricity generation, low cost and domestic availability have brought coal to the top of the energy pyramid. Other energy sources, natural gas and biomass in its varied forms, are being intensively explored to meet the energy demands of modern life. Most notable as a potential major resource is natural gas, which is being recovered through less conventional methods (eg, fracking) which in 2012 is thought by some to be the next revolution in energy

*This chapter has been reviewed by the US Environmental Protection Agency, and approved for publication. Approval does not signify that the contents necessarily reflect the views and the policies of the Agency.

Counties designated "nonattainment"
for Clean Air Act's National Ambient Air Quality Standards (NAAQS)*

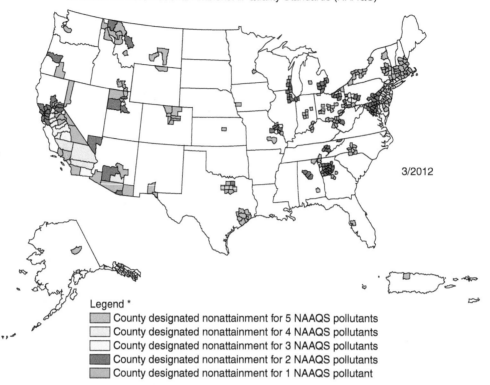

3/2012

Legend *

□ County designated nonattainment for 5 NAAQS pollutants
□ County designated nonattainment for 4 NAAQS pollutants
□ County designated nonattainment for 3 NAAQS pollutants
■ County designated nonattainment for 2 NAAQS pollutants
■ County designated nonattainment for 1 NAAQS pollutant

Figure 29-1. *Areas in the United States not in attainment (as of September 2012) for the NAAQS criteria pollutants: O_3, PM_{10} or $PM_{2.5}$, SO_2, and Pb.* There were no nonattainment areas for NO_2 and CO (http://www.epa.gov/oaqps001/greenbk/mapnpoll.html).

resources. Decades to come will see an evolution in our energy portfolio driven by cost and access, environmental impacts including climate change, and technological innovation. Nevertheless, so long as organically derived fuel is combusted to derive energy, its potential for impact on air quality and on public health and the environment will remain.

While great strides have been made in balancing regulation and technology to reduce emissions from stationary and mobile sources, unsatisfactory air quality continues to impose a risk to public and environmental health even in highly developed countries throughout the world. More than half the US population resides in counties that are not in compliance with current National Ambient Air Quality Standards (NAAQS) (Fig. 29-1). These noncompliant areas correspond well with where people live and work and reflect the redistribution of population growth from major urban and industrial centers. Air pollutants can also be transported across many miles such that previously pristine, rural areas have measurable pollution above their historic background levels. Indeed, as the developing world grows industrially, air pollution now is intercontinental with transport through the atmosphere via pathways close to the earth's surface as well as upper atmosphere. Emissions of precursors of ozone can come from hundreds of miles away and contribute to local pollution levels; likewise other emissions such as mercury from coal-fired power plants in Asia can account for the majority of US deposition on land and in streams many thousands of miles from the original sources (Hemispheric Transport of Air Pollution, 2010).

While episodes of extreme air pollution are rare in the Western world today, occasionally, unusual meteorological stagnations exaggerate typical air pollution patterns in both the levels of pollutants and their expanse (eg, 1995 in the United Kingdom and Western Europe). Likewise, in specific locales prone to stagnations due to

topography (eg, Utah Valley through the 1980s–1990s) or where there exists a single dominant source (eg, port areas, transport terminals, or smelters), repeated episodic or even patterned poor air quality can impact public health. From a broader public community perspective, typical exposures are characterized by prolonged periods of relatively low, cyclic levels of complex mixtures of photochemically transformed industrial and mobile emissions with occasional moderate excursions due to weather patterns. As pollution now extends even into remote and wilderness areas, significant damage to flora and crops can also occur.

The situation in many developing countries experiencing rapid population growth, industrialization, and economic expansion is reminiscent of the urban, industrial pollution in the United States and Europe more than half a century ago. The lessons of Western industrial nations and the consequences of inadequate air pollution control in some countries have not necessarily outweighed economic drivers or public health concerns. For example, despite being a modern economic center, two marathoners died in Hong Kong in February 2006 while running on a weekend during a protracted period of severe air pollution. Just as in US history, the urban air in rapidly industrialized nations simply reflects poor air quality management and the desire to prosper economically. Air pollutant levels in some of the developing urban centers can run 10 or more times those of the United States today, and their expanding worldwide distribution contributes substantially to the global burden of many air pollutants such as mercury, particulate matter (PM), sulfate/SO_2, and major global warming pollutants such as black carbon, CO_2, and methane. A willingness to balance worldwide economic growth and industrialization using lessons learned from the misadventures of the Second Industrial Revolution and the Age of the Automobile will determine the impact of the "new" global economy on the health of both the earth and its inhabitants.

Other issues facing many parts of the developing world tie closely to domestic culture and economy, as well as to the level of technological sophistication. Prime among these problems is exposure to carbon and soot from combustion of biomass in cooking and heating in domestic stoves. Approximately three billion people worldwide use biomass for home cooking in households with little ventilation. The World Health Organization (WHO) estimates two million deaths per year result from these exposures, especially women who are exposed day in and day out over many years, often with their infant children by their sides. Understanding the intersection of technological as well as socioeconomic and political challenges will be at the core of any resolution to these issues.

The gathering of scientific information regarding the impacts of air pollution on human health began with general indices of haziness or the darkness of a spot on a filter. The interest in learning causation drove science to focus more on individual pollutants to better understand the linkages with health and to aid in mitigation of risk. In turn, this knowledge was used both to develop public health standards and to establish regulatory controls. Despite the obvious complexities of urban air pollution, it was felt that single pollutant regulations were the best path to success, and, indeed, great strides have been made in that regard. However, research agendas are evolving to include the study of multipollutant interaction and transformation of individual pollutant components within atmospheric systems—a truer reflection of real-world exposure complexities. These multipollutant approaches entail sophisticated statistical models and empirical study designs, all with the goal of a more complete systems-based understanding of air pollution and risk to maximize benefits while minimizing costs and unintended consequences.

This chapter will present an overview of the current state of knowledge regarding air pollution and its ensuing impacts on human health, and the role of toxicology and translational biology in unraveling the complexities to allow for informed assessment of risk. As such, the contextual complexities of regulatory decisions and risk assessment will also be addressed. The intent is to provide the reader with both a fundamental knowledge and appreciation of the nature of the problem, how traditional and modern-day approaches aid in this understanding, as well as a sense of the uncertainties in need of future investigation to resolve issues even before they arise.

A Brief History of Air Pollution and Its Regulation

For most of history, air pollution has been a problem of microenvironments and domestic congestion. The smoky fires of early cave and hut dwellers choked the air inside their homes, and even when the emissions were vented outdoors, they simply combined with those of the neighbors to settle around the village on damp cold nights. With urbanization and a concomitant decrease in forest wood as a source of fuel to heat and cook, the need for energy led to the burning of easily accessible, dirty coal and the ambient release of sulfurous, sooty smoke. Industrialization brought kilns to make quicklime for construction and metal smelters needed for the development of progressive "modern" cities, only to push smoke and chemical emissions into the air. Unfortunately, the city dwellers who worked near these industries had to endure the bad air, while those of wealth frequently had country homes to which they could escape. The poor quality of urban air has been captured historically by many writers including Charles Dickens, who noted London's fogs in his writings, all the way back to the ancients such as Seneca, the Roman philosopher, who in AD 61 wrote: "As soon as I had

gotten out of the *heavy air* of Rome, and from the *stink* of the chimneys thereof, which being stirred, poured forth whatever *pestilential vapors and soot* they had enclosed in them, I felt an *alteration to my disposition*" (emphasis added: Miller and Miller, 1993).

Historically, efforts to regulate air pollution have, like today, competed with national, regional, and industrial economies, and, as a result, they have evolved slowly. Early on, in the time of Greece and Rome, individual civil suits could be levied against local polluters, although these were of marginal success. Beginning in the 13th century, community-based outcries received some recognition by governing officials; one example was the banning of "sea coal" from lime kilns and domestic heaters in London by Edward I. Enforcement, however, was not effective and the populace largely resigned itself to polluted air as part of urban life. By the 17th century, England, in the middle of several decades that some refer to as "the little ice age," depleted its forest wood resources, which only increased reliance on sea coal for domestic heating. Meanwhile, Percival Pott's discovery that chimney soot was related to the incidence of scrotal cancer in chimney sweeps led to some in the health community to recommend: "Fly the city, shun its turbid air; breathe not the chaos of eternal smoke…" (Brimblecombe, 1999)—essentially the same advice advanced by Seneca 1600 years earlier. In the late 18th century, the industrial revolution, which was powered by the burning of "cleaner" mined coal, added a second dimension to urban air pollution. These emissions were more acidic and hung in the air longer than the fluffy soot of the cheaper sea coal. Continued soiling of buildings and damage to nearby crops brought community boards to address sanitary reforms to cut the worse of the pollution peaks and episodes, but any gains were soon offset by growth. By the end of the 19th century and into the early 20th century, power plants were being built to provide energy for factories and eventually to light homes in the Western world. Steel mills and other industries proliferated along riverbanks and lakeshores, oil refineries rose in port cities, and near oil fields smelters roasted and refined metals in areas near large mineral deposits.

By 1925, air pollution was common to all industrialized nations. However, people slowly grew less tolerant of the nuisance of acidic-soot corrosion of all exposed surfaces and the general discomfort that came with smoky air—this acidic, sooty form of air pollution was termed *reducing* air pollution because of its reducing chemical nature. Public surveys were initiated—in Salt Lake City in 1926, New York City in 1937, and Leicester, Great Britain, in 1939—to bring political attention to the problem and promote the implementation of controls (Miller and Miller, 1993). However, it was the cumulative impact of the great air pollution disasters in the Meuse Valley, Belgium, in 1930; Donora, Pennsylvania, in 1948; and the great London fog of 1952 that indicted air pollution as a health risk. In the United States, California was already leading the way with passage of the Air Pollution Control Act of 1947 to regulate the discharge of opaque smokes. Visibility problems in Pittsburgh during the 1940s had also prompted efforts to control smoke from local industries. At the national level, however, it was the initiative of President Truman that provided the federal impetus to deal with air pollution. His early efforts culminated in congressional passage of a series of acts starting with the Air Pollution Control Act of 1955 under the Eisenhower administration.

The prosperity of the late 1950s and the accompanying suburban sprawl introduced the third and perhaps most chemically complex dimension of air pollution. The term *smog*, though originally coined to describe the mixture of smoke and fog that hung over large cities such as London, was curiously adopted for the eye-irritating photochemical reaction products of auto exhaust that blanketed cities such as Los Angeles and Mexico City. Early federal legislation addressing stationary sources was soon expanded to include automobile-derived pollutants in the United States (the Clean Air Act [CAA] of 1963, amended in 1967, and the Motor Vehicle Air Pollution Control Act of 1965). The landmark CAA Amendments of 1970 evolved from the early legislation, and, despite being only an amendment, it was revolutionary. It recognized the problem of air pollution as a national issue and set forth a plan to control it. The Act charged the newly instituted US Environmental Protection Agency (USEPA) with the responsibility to protect the public from the hazards of polluted outdoor air. Seven "criteria" air pollutants (ozone [O_3], sulfur dioxide [SO_2], PM, nitrogen dioxide [NO_2], carbon monoxide [CO], lead [Pb], and total hydrocarbons—the last now dropped from the list, leaving six criteria pollutants) were specified as significant health hazards in need of *individual* NAAQS. These NAAQS were mandated for review every five years as to the adequacy of the existent standard to protect human health (Table 29-1), although adherence to this schedule has generally not been achieved. The explosion in the literature databases for the criteria pollutants and the extensive review and commentary process has typically led to delays in completing the process on schedule. In 2006, however, this process was streamlined through the creation of an Integrated Science Assessment (ISA) to replace each Criteria Document where the findings since the last assessment could be integrated with older studies (summarized with the foundation literature confined to tables and an appendix). This ISA is combined with a Risk and Exposure Assessment into a Policy Assessment to develop a range of proposed standards based on risk analyses. The US EPA Administrator considers proposals from both "evidence"- and "risk"-based assessments to establish policy and set the NAAQS (*www.epa.gov/ttn/naaqs/naaqs_process_report_march2006.pdf*). With regard to the Primary NAAQS, only health criteria can be considered in the development of the standard, including safety considerations for potentially susceptible groups. The Secondary NAAQS consider agricultural

and structural welfare. Economic impacts are not to be involved in the standard setting process itself—only in assessing the cost of the implementation procedures. Other hazardous air pollutants (HAPs), of which there were eight listed in 1970, were to undergo health assessments to establish emission controls—today there are 189 (see below). The CAA of 1970 was by far the most far-reaching legislation to control air pollution to date.

The accidental release of 30 tons of methyl isocyanate vapor into the air of the shanty village of Bhopal, India, on December 3, 1984, killed an estimated 3000 people within hours of the release, with several thousand delayed deaths and 200,000 injured or permanently impaired. The tragedy shocked the world, and raised the issue of HAPs in the United States to a new level of concern. While such a disaster has never struck the United States, accidental industrial releases or spills of toxic chemicals are surprisingly common, with 4375 cases recorded between 1980 and 1987, inflicting 11,341 injuries and 309 deaths (Waxman, 1994). The Toxic Release Inventory (TRI) of 650 chemicals reported annually by industry is required by EPA and suggests a decrease in releases (~9% in 10 years across land, water, and air), but these data are self-reported and do not include most of the 80,000 low-volume chemicals in use today.

The HAPs, which had been the stepsister of the criteria pollutants for more than a decade after the passage of the 1970 CAA, have since garnered more public and policy attention. There is concern not only for the acute effects of accidental releases of fugitive or secondary chemicals—such as phosgene, benzene, butadiene, and dioxin, into the air of populated industrial centers—but also for potential chronic health effects, with cancer often being the focus of attention. The slow progress of regulatory decisions on HAPs (only eight between 1970 and 1990) led to a mandated acceleration of the process under the CAA amendment of 1990. Section 112(b) currently lists 189 chemicals or classes of chemicals for which special standards and risk assessments are required. The chemicals listed are those of greatest concern on the basis of toxicity (including cancer) and estimated release volumes. Currently, there is a list of 33 HAPs from the list of 189 that are deemed to be of greatest concern, so-called list of the "dirty 30." Emissions of HAPs are mandated for control to the maximal achievable control technology (MACT), and any residual health risk after MACT is to be considered in a separate quantitative risk assessment. The database for this process utilizes existing knowledge or, if necessary, mandates further research by the emitter. While many of these chemicals are now better controlled than in the past, residual risk estimates are yet to be completed for many HAPs. The database from which these assessments are made is called the Integrated Risk Information System (IRIS, www.epa.gov/iris/index.html) and currently contains 550 chemicals that have health data.

Emissions from motor vehicles include a number of HAPs (eg, benzene, butadiene) as well as NAAQS pollutants (eg, CO, NO_x, PM), but are addressed primarily under the CAA Title II, Emission Standards for Mobile Sources. The reduction of emissions from mobile sources is complex and involves both fuel formulation and engine/vehicle reengineering. Refinements in combustion engineering are ongoing making use of advanced computerized ignition and timing, but fuel properties have drawn most recent attention for improvement. For example, to reduce wintertime CO, several oxygenates (including ethers and alcohols) have been formulated into fuels to both reduce cold-start emissions and enhance overall combustion. Perhaps the most prominent of the ethers is methyl *tertiary*-butyl ether (MTBE), which became a controversial additive in the early 1990s, arising in part from odor and reports of asthma-like reactions by some individuals during auto refueling. However,

Table 29-1

US National (Primary) Ambient Air Quality Standards*

POLLUTANT	PRIMARY/ SECONDARY	AVERAGING TIME	LEVEL
Sulfur dioxide	Primary	1 h	75 ppb
	Secondary	3 h	0.5 ppm
Carbon monoxide	Primary	1 h	35 ppm
		8 h	9 ppm
Ozone	Primary and secondary	8 h	0.075 ppm
Nitrogen dioxide	Primary	1 h	100 ppb
		Annual	53 ppb
Particulates: PM_{10}	Primary and secondary	24 h	150 μg/m³
$PM_{2.5}$	Primary and secondary	24 h	35 μg/m³
		Annual	15 μg/m³
Lead	Primary and secondary	Rolling three-month average	0.15 μg/m³

*For detailed information regarding policy and precise statistical and time-based computations to achieve attainment, contact EPA Web site: http://www.epa.gov/air/criteria.html.

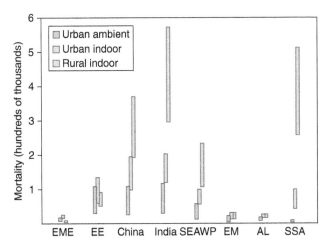

Figure 29-2. *Excess mortality due to outdoor and indoor particulate matter in various international economic groupings.* Bottom and top of each bar represent the lower and upper estimates of mortality, respectively, computed using the methodology of Schwela (2000): established market economies (EME), Eastern Europe (EE), China, India, Southeast Asia/Western Pacific (SEAWP), Eastern Mediterranean (EM), Latin America (AL), and Sub-Saharan Africa (SSA). (Modified from Fig. 2.6 by D. Schwela, *Air Pollution in the Megacities of Asia—Seoul Workshop Report: Urban Air Pollution Management and Practice in Major and Megacities of Asia.*)

the controversy took an unexpected twist; MTBE has been removed from fuel, not because of health concerns associated with airborne exposure but rather due to leakage from service-station storage tanks into groundwater. Ironically, this prescribed remedy for an air problem evolved into an unexpected problem: groundwater contamination. This example illustrates the broad complexity of all pollution control measures in that unappreciated factors can transcend engineering or other targeted features if a broader systematic assessment is not undertaken. Nevertheless, fuel additives have been developed to boost octane ratings of fuels and/or improve engine performance and combustion (eg, organic oxygenates, methylcyclopentadienyl manganese tricarbonyl [MMT], platinum compounds for diesel). These additives are reviewed under Title II because of concerns regarding the potential changes in combustion product reactivity or the introduction of metals into the environment, reminiscent of use of lead in fuels from the 1930s to the 1970s, when lead fuel additives were banned in the United States.

Internationally, the magnitude and control of air pollution sources vary considerably, especially among developing nations, which often forgo concerns for health and welfare because of cost and the desire to achieve prosperity. Fig. 29-2 illustrates the international variation in air pollution–related mortality (outdoor and indoor) based on economic groupings. It is clear that there are wide differences reflecting economic imbalances—particularly prominent are the indoor particulate levels in developing nations where biomass combustion is used for heating and cooking. These regions also contain many of the megacities of the world with major air pollution problems. The political upheaval in Eastern Europe since 1990 has revealed the consequences of decades of uncontrolled industrial air pollution. While vast improvements are now evident in this area, as industries are being modernized and emissions controlled, many Asian, African, and South American cities have virtually unchecked air pollution. Some nations as well as the WHO have adopted air quality standards as a rational basis for guiding control measures, but the lack of binding regulations and/or economic fortune impedes significant controls and improvements (Lipfert, 1994). In addition to local socioeconomic and political concerns, emissions of air pollutants have spawned problems

of "international pollution." Long-range transport of polluted air masses from one country to another has been anticipated as a global issue for several years (Reuther, 2000). This issue was the subject of some controversy between Canada and the United States in the late 1980s and into the 1990s as a result of the air mass transport of acid sulfates from industrial centers of the Midwestern United States to southern Ontario. However, reduction in SO_2 emissions has somewhat relieved the tension over the last several years (Fig. 29-3). Improvement in NO_x, also a product of stationary source fossil fuel burning, is also apparent. Importantly, growing prosperity in China has led to enormous growth in its power sector and coal combustion resulting in transoceanic transport of airborne mercury such that transported mercury now accounts for the majority of mercury deposition in the waters and land in the United States (Seigneur *et al.*, 2004).

TOOLS TO ASSESS RISKS ASSOCIATED WITH AIR POLLUTION

Risk assessment is a formalized process, originally described in the landmark 1983 National Research Council report, whereby toxicity, exposure, and dose-dependent outcome data can be systematically integrated to estimate risk to a population. Fig. 29-4 provides a modified version of the paradigm of the NAS (NRC, 1983), incorporating recent interest in providing evidence of "accountability" that the regulations indeed do have impacts. The health database for any air pollutant may comprise data from animal toxicology, controlled human studies, and/or epidemiology. But, because each of these research approaches has inherent strengths and limitations, an appropriate assessment of an air pollutant requires the careful integration and interpretation of data from all three methodologies. Thus, one should be aware of the attributes of each (Table 29-2).

Epidemiological studies reveal associations between exposure to a pollutant(s) and the health effect(s) in the *community* or *population* of interest. Because data are garnered directly under real-world exposure conditions and often involve large numbers of people, the data are of direct utility to regulators assessing pollutant impacts. With proper design and analysis, studies can explore either acute or long-term exposures and theoretically can examine patterns in mortality and morbidity, both acute and chronic, especially if these responses appear disproportionately in population subsets (ie, sensitive groups). Why, then, is this approach to the study of air pollution not the exclusive choice of regulators in decision making? The problem is that it is difficult to control confounding personal variables in the population. Factors such as genetic diversity and lifestyle differences among individuals, and population mobility are difficult to control. Perhaps most problematic is the lack of adequate exposure data—especially on a personal basis. Exposure assessment is often one of the major weaknesses of an epidemiological study, not only because of the difficulties of assessing exposure (as a measure of dose) to the pollutant of interest but also because it is difficult to segregate a single pollutant from correlated copollutants and other environmental influences, such as meteorology. Thus, only associations, and not causality, can be drawn between the broad-based exposure data and effects observed in epidemiology studies. Causal relationships are sometimes inferred in the presence of strong statistical significance, but such determinations are likely to be criticized. However, recent advances in exposure estimation and study design and analysis (eg, time series) have allowed epidemiologists to examine relationships with greater confidence and specificity. These models limit the impact of covariates and longer time-based influences and thus allow epidemiologists to tease out effects of short-term pollution not accessible formerly

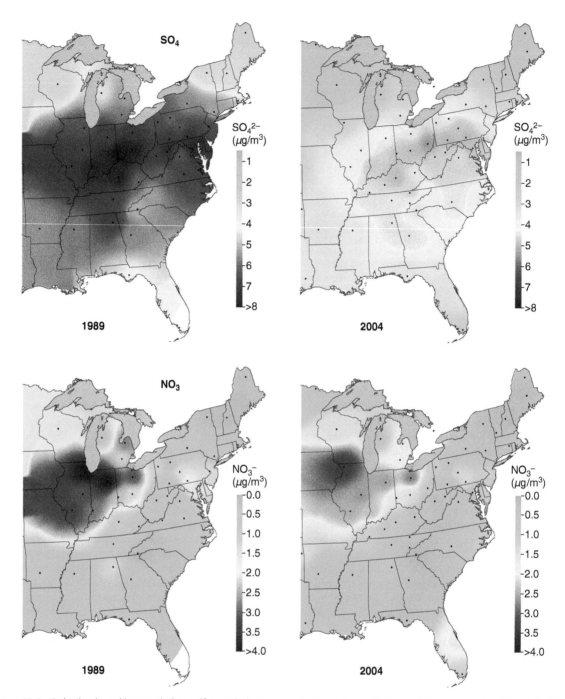

Figure 29-3. *Reduction in ambient particulate sulfate and nitrate concentrations between 1989 and 2004 in the eastern half of the United States (from CASTNet monitoring data).* Sulfates and nitrates arising from industrial centers of the Midwest contribute to acid rain deposition (see Fig. 29-13). Sulfates are readily dispersed toward the eastern half of the country. Nitrates arise from the industrial centers as well as metropolitan areas and show both a local and dispersed pattern. (Adapted with permission from Clean Air Status and Trends Network—http://www.epa.gov/castnet/mapconc_e.html.)

(Schwartz, 1991). Similarly, newer approaches that employ field studies—sometimes called *panel studies*—incorporate time-series design and multiple regression analyses of more focused and complete exposure data (ideally personal) and targeted clinical end points in the exposed population under study. The end points often derive from empirical human and animal studies and therefore have a priori conceptual ties. The advent of new genetic approaches for characterizing polymorphisms of potentially influential traits (eg, glutathione *S*-transferase M1 [GSTM1]; Tujague *et al.*, 2006) opens the genomic door for assessing gene–environment interactions. These factors may well underlie a significant portion of the human

susceptibility to air pollution. Novel approaches such as this are evident in the most recent studies of PM air pollution (see below).

Studies that involve *controlled human exposures* have been used extensively to evaluate the criteria air pollutants regulated by the USEPA. Because most people are exposed to these pollutants in their daily lives, human volunteers can be ethically exposed to them in a highly controlled fashion (with the exception of Pb, which has cumulative and irreversible effects). Exposures are conducted in a controlled environment (usually in a chamber or with a mask) and are generally of short or limited repeat durations, given assurances that all responses are reversible. Clearly, data of this type are very

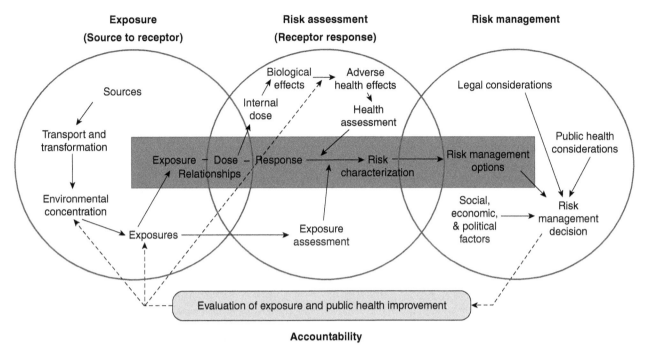

Figure 29-4. *NRC risk assessment paradigm.* Components of *risk assessment* within the left circle provide data to development of *risk management* as depicted in the right circle, modified to include an "accountability" component as a means to address air quality management impacts on the process risk reduction (National Research Council, 1983).

valuable in assessing potential human risk, since they are derived from the species of concern and are rooted in well-established clinical knowledge and experience.

Suspected "susceptible or sensitive" individuals (see below) representing potential higher-risk groups can also be studied to better understand the breadth of response in the exposed public. However, clinical studies have several practical limitations. Ethical issues are involved in every aspect of a clinical test; potentially irreversible effects and carcinogenicity are also always of concern,

along with the definition of an acceptable level of hyperresponsiveness in so-called sensitive individuals who volunteered to participate in the study. Likewise for any test subject, there are obvious restrictions on the invasiveness of biological procedures, although sophistication in medical technology has made accessible a large array of molecular biomarkers from peripheral blood and nasal, bronchial, and alveolar lavage fluids as well as biopsied cells from airway segments (Devlin *et al.*, 1991; Salvi *et al.*, 1999). With the advent of cutting-edge genomic and proteomic high-throughput

Table 29-2

Strengths and Weaknesses of Disciplinary Approaches for Obtaining Health Information

DISCIPLINE	POPULATION	STRENGTHS	WEAKNESSES
Epidemiology	Communities	Natural exposure	Difficult to quantify exposure
			Many covariates
	Diseased groups	No extrapolation	
		Isolates susceptibility trait	Minimal dose–response data
		Long-term, low-level effects	Association versus causation
	Field/panel groups	Good exposure data	Usually short-term
		Fewer covariates	Volunteers
		Focus on host traits	Expensive
		Utilizes clinical evaluations	
Clinical studies	Experimental	Controlled exposures	Artificial exposures
	Diseased subjects	Few covariates	Acute effects only
		Isolates susceptibility trait	Hazards
		Cause–effect	Volunteers
Toxicology	Animals	Maximum control	Human extrapolation
		Dose–response data	Realistic models of human disease?
		Cause–effect	
	In vitro systems	Rapid data acquisition	In vivo extrapolation
		Mechanisms	

SOURCE: Data from Boubel et al. (1994), with permission.

technologies, new tools are emerging to identify responses in humans and the relationships to innate susceptibility. Obviously, the issue of cost, the limited numbers of subjects that can be practically evaluated, and the inability to address chronic exposure issues remain constraints on human testing. Where partnerships with animal toxicology studies have been established, studies in laboratory animal species can sometimes provide ethical justification for at least limited direct human exposure for addressing critical questions. Analogously, in vitro studies in both human and animal cell and tissue systems, often augmented with similar genomic tools, allow the elucidation of mechanisms of toxicity. These basic biological responses inform extrapolation models that link animal data to humans, and they support the feasibility and preclude risks that may reside in human studies with some toxic air pollutants (see below).

Animal toxicology is used to predict or corroborate, through plausible mechanisms, suspected effects in humans. In the absence of human data, animal toxicology constitutes the essential first step of risk assessment: *hazard identification*. Animal toxicology is often required before any controlled human exposure can be conducted. It is particularly useful in elucidating pathogenic mechanisms involved in toxic injury or disease, providing basic knowledge that is critical to extrapolating databases across species, estimating uncertainties, and determining the relevance of information to humans. Knowledge of the toxic mechanism(s) provides the underpinnings to the "plausibility" of findings in the human context and, under carefully defined and highly controlled circumstances, may allow *quantitative* estimates of risk to human populations. Animal toxicology studies have been used to investigate all of the criteria air pollutants and many of the HAPs as well. The strength of this discipline is that it can involve methods that are not practical in human studies and can provide more rapid turnaround of essential toxicity data under diverse exposure concentrations and durations. The minimization of uncontrolled variables (eg, genetic and environmental) may be the greatest strength of the animal bioassay.

The clear limitation of animal studies in human risk assessment lies in the unknowns that weaken the extrapolation of findings in animals to the day-to-day human life scenario. Ideally, a test animal is selected with knowledge that it responds in a manner similar to that of the human (*homology*). *Qualitative* extrapolation of homologous effects is not unusual with many toxic inhalants, but *quantitative* extrapolation is frequently clouded by uncertainties of the relative *sensitivity* of the animal or specific target tissue compared with that of the human. Uncertainties about the target tissue dose also loom large, constituting the first obstacle to quantitative extrapolation (see below). With respect to the target tissue dose, however, most animal toxicologists make every effort to keep exposure concentrations at 5- to 10-fold that of the anticipated human exposure until appropriate dosimetric data can be ascertained. An often overlooked issue is that the dose to the target (lung region) for the test animal is frequently less than that of the human under similar exposure conditions—especially when exposures are conducted during dormancy for the animals (Wichers *et al.*, 2006). Most human inhalation studies involve exercise exposure paradigms where increased ventilation augments dose. Thus, in the absence of exercise, higher doses may be needed to achieve a group response among a limited pool of genetically similar animals (maybe 6–10) to represent a large population effect. However, it must be appreciated that mechanisms may well differ at different dose levels and some responses may be misleading if assessed only at the higher dose levels. Despite these limitations, however, animal studies have provided the largest database on a wide range of air toxicants and have proven utility in predicting human adverse responses to chemicals. New high-throughput technologies offer great promise

in shortening the toxicity assessment process and reducing costs of both the test process and the consumption of animals, but it remains to be seen how this new technology aids in the quantitative assessment of toxic inhalants.

To be effective, any health assessment should consider the strengths and weaknesses of the approaches selected to estimate actual toxic risk. In the larger picture, other scientific disciplines can be highly valuable to a more accurate assessment of the impact of air pollution on society. The atmospheric sciences, particularly the chemical and physical sciences, provide insights into exposure by better characterizing what is in the air. Better pollutant characterization, linked to exposure assessment, can only strengthen epidemiological outcome associations. Similarly, better air characterization and dose estimates support toxicity evaluations based on biological test systems. In the latter case, the uncertainties of dose relevancy can be reduced and linkages to defined pollutant physicochemical attributes and interactions can be pursued. Recreating realistic exposure environments to the extent possible is invaluable to developing models to estimate human risk.

Lastly, studies of botanical responses to air pollutants are now appreciated more than ever. Not only are commercial and native vegetation affected by pollution but also some plant species are being exploited as sensitive "sentinels," warning of the impacts of pollution on both human and environmental receptors. When considered collectively, economists can inform regulators and the public at large of the cumulative impact and adversity of pollution on our quality and standard of living (Maddison and Pierce, 1999). Interestingly, some basic mechanisms (eg, the involvement of antioxidants) between plants and animals have remarkable parallels.

Animal-to-Human Extrapolation: Issues and Mitigating Factors

The value of animal toxicology in inhalation studies is highly dependent on the ability to extrapolate or relate empirical findings to real-world human scenarios. Several factors of study design play into the process of extrapolation (eg, exposure concentration, duration, and patterns), but most important is the selection of the animal species that will serve as the toxicological model. Therefore, this selection should involve more than considerations of cost and convenience. Whenever possible, effects that are homologous and involve the same mode of action between the study species and the human should guide the decision of the most appropriate test species. For example, if upper airway irritant responses such as bronchoconstriction are anticipated (eg, SO_2 or formaldehyde), then the guinea pig, with its human-like reactive airway reflexes, should be selected over the rat, which is not particularly responsive in this regard. However, if the underlying molecular events in tissue remodeling are of interest, then rat or mouse might better serve as a model because of cellular mechanistic parallels with human tissue responses. In part, the availability of probes to aid in such studies could factor into the selection of the rodent strain as well. Additionally, as inbred strains of rats and mice differ in their neutrophilic responsiveness to deep lung inhalants (eg, O_3), contrasting responsiveness or the mode of action may be more revealing and support one strain over another in its selection for study (Costa *et al.*, 1985). Other innate differences in sensitivity among species may also relate to differences in lung structure, regional distribution of cell types having varied metabolism, genetic polymorphisms, or antioxidant defenses. Genetic control of responses such as inflammation have been identified in mice where a specific quantitative trait locus (*Inf2*) on chromosome 17 exhibits a more robust neutrophilic response to O_3 (Bauer and Kleeberger, 2010). Thus, when a test animal strain is selected where such nuances are unclear or unknown, the replication of responses in multiple species builds confidence in the finding as being homologous or having species-conserved modes of action that are relevant to the human and bear careful consideration in a risk assessment.

An essential, but often overlooked, part of response extrapolation from species to species is knowledge of the relative dosimetry of the pollutant along the respiratory tract. Significant advances in studies of the distribution of gaseous and particulate pollutants have been made through the use of empirical and mathematical models, the latter of which incorporate parameters of respiratory anatomy and physiology, fluid dynamics, and physical chemistry into predictions of deposition and retention. Empirical models combined with theoretical models aid in relating animal toxicity data to humans and help refine the study of injury mechanisms due to better estimates of the target dose. Fig. 29-5 illustrates the application of such an approach to the reactive gas O_3 and insoluble 0.6-μm spherical particles, respectively, as each is distributed along the respiratory tract of humans and rats. Anatomic differences between the species clearly affect the deposition of both gases and particles, but the relative distributions are quite similar. This is not surprising if one argues teleologically that the lungs of each species evolved with similar functional drivers (ie, O_2–CO_2 exchange, blood acid/base balance), mechanical impediments, and environmental stresses. One needs only a cursory review of the comparative lung physiology literature to appreciate the allometric

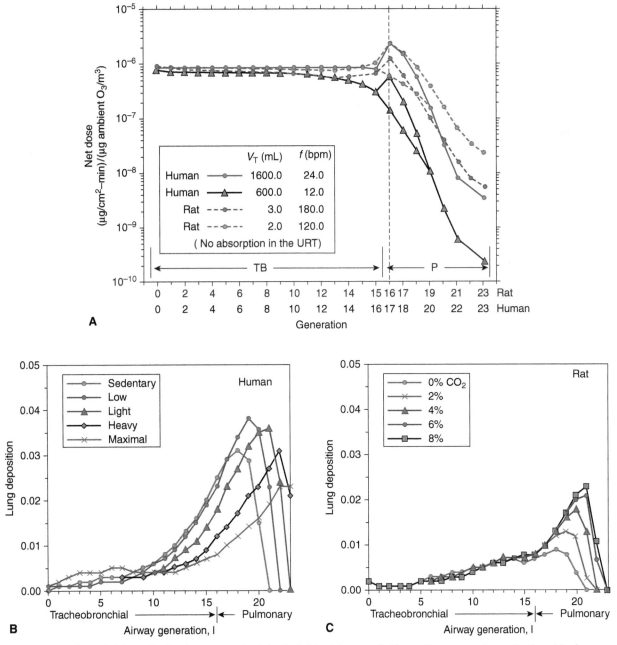

Figure 29-5. *Theoretical (normalized to the concentration in inspired air) uptake curves for the reactive gas ozone in a resting/exercising human and a rat (A).* Likewise, the percent deposition in the airways of a 0.6 μm insoluble particle in the respiratory tracts of a resting/exercising human (**B**) and rat (**C**). Eight percent inspired CO_2 in the rat augments ventilation up to threefold. Airway generation refers to that airway branch numbered from the trachea (0). (Panel A is from Overton and Miller, 1987, and panels B and C are from Martonen *et al.*, 1992. Reproduced with permission.)

consistency of the mammalian respiratory tract to meet the challenge of breathing air. This design coherency has provided the fundamental rationale for the use of animal models for the study of air pollutants. With knowledge of ventilation parameters, one should be able to compute nominal tissue doses based on lung surface area using available published data.

OVERARCHING CONCEPTS

What is an Adverse Health Effect?

Establishing criteria to define an "adverse effect" of air pollution is difficult. When relating a health effect to an air pollutant, a response must be appreciated at two levels—that of the individual and that of the population. Clearly, an effect on an individual can be beyond an acceptable limit potentially putting that person's overall health in jeopardy, but this response may be lost in an index reflecting a population-based response. The risk to a population reflects the averaging of individual responses or risks and may be measured as a shift in the normal distribution of some index of response for that population. Hence, on average, the entire population may be judged to be at some enhanced risk. These two forms of risk are clearly related, but most often in practice, the population risk is considered most appropriate from a public health perspective. It is also generally most credibly quantifiable. However, subpopulations that carry some related risk factor may represent a more limited group with unusual risk that too may be quantifiable. Such a group is often called a susceptible subpopulation.

Defining an air pollutant effect as "adverse" within the range of effects that may result from exposure is not always straightforward. Clearly, in humans, some effects would pass uncontested as adverse, for example, death, acute life-threatening dysfunction or disease, irreversible impairments, and pain. In animal models, pathology has traditionally been the hallmark of an adverse effect. In either humans or animals, however, other effects that reflect minor and temporary dysfunctions or discomfort could be argued as not warranting significant or costly concern, especially if the effects are minor and transient with no long-term untoward outcomes. This vein of thought would simply attribute these effects to be within normal physiologic ranges and are readily compensated within functional or biochemical reserve. Thus, if one is to try to assess the impacts of air pollution on health, it is desirable that there exist some objective criteria to define what is indeed adverse based on the nature and the magnitude of the effect under evaluation. Moreover, distinguishing an air pollution effect from other adverse stimuli or disease processes can be complex and fraught with confounding factors, such as smoking and negative lifestyle factors.

Not surprisingly, air pollution impacts have long been focused on the lung as the primary target organ. With regard to acute effects in humans, the American Thoracic Society in 1985 issued a position paper that attempted to define an adverse effect related to air pollution in terms of its impact on lung function (where, eg, a 10% or more drop in forced vital capacity [FVC] was deemed adverse); at that time, lung function was the primary human health effect that could be studied under controlled inhalation conditions. The definition of "adverse" was revised in 2000, because of the many advances in clinical medicine and empirical health sciences, to include seven broad areas: biomarkers, quality of life, physiologic impacts, symptoms, clinical outcomes, mortality, and population health versus individual risk (American Thoracic Society, 2000). The summary conclusion states that caution should be exercised in evaluating the many new biomarkers

of effect (especially cell and molecular markers), as there is need for validation that *small* changes in these markers represent a progression along a course to disease or permanent impairment. Since that time, further advances in molecular markers and systems assessment of toxic pathways have opened a new dimension of evaluation of health outcomes where their detailed pathogenesis can be examined. Of course, many of the same questions arise as to the criteria to define when a pathogenic process is qualitatively or quantitatively adverse, but clearly the ability to measure effects and understand their nature and relationship to chronic disease is advancing rapidly.

Susceptibility

A common thread through all of these subject areas is the influential role of susceptibility, which can take the form of hyperresponsiveness or loss of reserve. What is a minor reversible effect in the majority of individuals may be a dysfunction that cannot be reversed or compensated in certain individuals (Fig. 29-6). Obvious examples would be cardiopulmonary-compromised individuals who function with little or no reserve. In the end, however, the 2000 ATS statement acknowledges the limits of definitions and the importance of value judgment in the final assessment. Implied in this position is that a loss in quality of life due to air pollution as well as enduring its associated effects may also be designated as adverse. As science continues to advance, especially in the realm of molecular biology where small signals can be detected that may forecast an adverse effect or otherwise may identify individuals or groups at risk, the definition of adverse will certainly need reexamination. That same sensitivity in measurement that serves to predict an adverse effect must be separated from signals that are essential for homeostasis and the maintenance of life. Clearly, dissecting and defining these phenomena will have implications not only for assessing clinical adversity but also for predictive toxicology.

In actuality, there is no widely accepted definition for a "susceptible" individual and quite frequently the term is used interchangeably with "vulnerable." The USEPA, however, separates

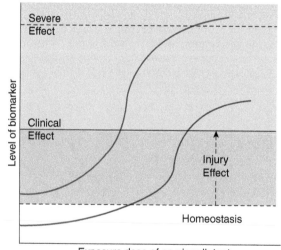

Figure 29-6. *Schematic illustration of the elements of the dose response to an air pollutant(s) of a susceptible versus a healthy individual.* The hypothetical susceptible individual may be more sensitive or may have a *loss of reserve*, either of which results in an *inability to maintain homeostasis*. The *leftward shift or increased slope* in the dose–response curve suggests an increase in responsiveness. Either situation may contribute to sensitivity and the likelihood of enhanced progression from subtle to severe outcomes.

Table 29-3

Factors that Influence the Response of Individuals or Subpopulations to Ambient Air Pollutants

SUSCEPTIBILITY FACTORS	VULNERABILITY/ EXPOSURE FACTORS
Preexisting cardiopulmonary disease	Proximity to point source
Genetic factors	Proximity to high-traffic-volume roadway
Age	Occupation
Gender	Activity level
Race/ethnicity	Use of air conditioning/building leakiness
Obesity	In utero exposure
Pregnancy	Geographic location (eg, East vs West coast of the United States)
Diabetes	Lower social economic status

Adapted from Table 4-1 of SO$_2$ Integrated Science Assessment, 2010 (http://cfpub.epa.gov/ncea/cfm/recordisplay.cfm?deid=198843).

the two terms and utilizes "vulnerability" to refer to extrinsic (ie, nonbiological) factors (eg, an increased exposure to ambient air pollutants because one's school is located adjacent to a high-traffic-volume roadway), whereas "susceptibility" refers to intrinsic biological factors such as genetics, age, or preexisting disease. Regardless of the precise definition, a susceptible subpopulation encompasses both intrinsic and extrinsic factors that increase the response to air pollution. As demonstrated in both toxicological and epidemiological studies, a combination of factors influences the incidence and magnitude of adverse responses of susceptible subpopulations to inhaled pollutants (Table 29-3). For example, over the last 20 years, hundreds of publications have documented association between ambient PM levels and increases in cardiopulmonary morbidity and mortality. Age has been consistently shown to influence health outcomes, and the association between ambient air pollution and increases in hospital admissions for asthma is driven by the response seen in children. Conversely, the association between episodic exposure to PM and cardiac mortality is strongest in those over 65 years of age.

Susceptible subpopulations that show exaggerated responsiveness to pollutants merit special mention. The existence of sensitive individuals and groups is well accepted among those who conduct air pollution health assessments, but relatively little is actually known about the host traits that render certain individuals sensitive to inhaled particles and gases. This appreciation for sensitive populations is specifically noted in the CAA, where protection of these groups is mandated in the setting of the NAAQS in the United States. There are some definable subgroups that are considered inherently more susceptible, including children, the elderly, and those with a preexisting disease (eg, asthma, cardiovascular disease, lung disease). The importance of susceptibility in air pollutant responses is gaining more and more attention as test subject responses that were once considered "outliers" in a controlled chamber study may well be evidence of unusual responsiveness.

In some cases, susceptibility may simply reflect differences in dosimetry. Children spend more time outdoors than adults, are more active, and have basal ventilation rates that exceed adults on a volume to body weight ratio, and therefore may experience overall greater dose to the lungs. Certainly, rapidly growing tissues may also factor in and may have contributed, perhaps with dosimetry factors, to epidemiology findings that polluted urban air retards lung growth (Gauderman *et al.*, 2004). Similarly, adult humans and animals with obstructive airway disease, for example, may have "hotspots" of particle deposition in the airways that exceed normal local tissue doses many-fold (Kim and Kang, 1997; Sweeney *et al.*, 1995). Another often underappreciated aspect of susceptibility relates to the loss of functional reserve or compensation due to age or disease, perhaps altering a response threshold or impairing recovery and the reestablishment of homeostasis. Air pollution–induced changes in physiologic measurements such as blood pressure or heart rate may be easily restored in a young healthy individual but not in a more fragile older person with cardiovascular disease.

As already noted, there is also growing interest in gene–environment interactions where genetic differences can influence responsiveness. For example, because the variability in response to ozone was much greater among human subjects than within subjects exposed to ozone in a controlled clinical exposure setting, research in the 1990s suggested that genetic factors influence the response to ozone (McDonnell, 1991). This observation was preceded by an animal study in which significant interstrain differences were found in inbred mice exposed to high levels of ozone (Goldstein *et al.*, 1973). Since these early studies, human (controlled exposure and epidemiology studies) and animal studies have clearly shown that the response to an inhaled pollutant is dependent on genetics. In humans, GSTM1 polymorphisms affect ~50% of the population and, thus, any defect in gene function may undermine antioxidant defenses in those individuals (McCunney, 2005). A number of studies have shown that the null (deletion) GSTM1 genotype, in comparison to the normal wild-type allele, is associated with a greater response to ozone and that the observed pulmonary function changes are even larger if other gene variants involved in oxidative stress are present. Unfortunately, the majority of human studies have examined the contribution of only a handful of gene variants at a time. Current state-of-the-art techniques, however, will now permit the study of the individual and interactive role of numerous (and someday all) gene polymorphisms in the response to inhaled pollutants. Animal studies have advanced from classical quantitative linkage analysis studies of single sensitive and resistant inbred mouse strains to haplotype mapping studies that take advantage of the complete sequencing or deep SNP analysis of multiple inbred mouse strains. Similarly, in human studies, we now have the capability to perform genome-wide association (GWA) studies that link up to one million SNPs or haplotypes with a given phenotype/disease in large (ie, tens of thousands) population studies. Not surprisingly, these GWA studies have determined that individual gene polymorphisms contribute to only a small fraction of the variability in response or disease. Thus, at present, genetic susceptibility, as well as overall susceptibility, to inhaled pollutants is a complex concept that bears significantly on any response. Individual variations in response to ambient air pollution may reflect differences in dose, sensitivity, and/or compensation. As a result, outcomes among individuals may be similar, but the balance of contributing factors that underlie the individual response may be multifactorial.

The study of adverse effects in human volunteers undergoing controlled exposure to air pollutants is ethically limited, but it is even more so for compromised human subjects. Such studies of susceptibility are confined to subjects of only modest suspected risk such as mild asthmatics, healthy older adults, and asymptomatic cardiopulmonary subjects. Inroads have nevertheless been made in recent years because of more thorough prestudy assessments of potential risk factors, allowing researchers to design studies that need not carry undue risk of serious complications. New molecular methods also allow more sensitive assessment of putative biomarkers of response. Additionally, the development of more appropriate animal models of disease or dysfunction (eg, obese or diabetic mouse models) provides a useful adjunct to explore susceptibility factors more extensively prior to study in humans. Hence, coordinated studies in animals and human subjects are proving to be useful to investigate specific questions such as the roles of preexisting disease, diet (eg, antioxidant content), exercise (as it relates to dosimetry), age, gender, and race. The goal of such susceptibility studies is to elucidate patterns, common factors, or pathways that may inform potential intervention or mitigation strategies as well as basic information to reduce the uncertainties regarding risk factors (Kodavanti *et al.*, 1998).

To augment genome studies in humans, recent advances in molecular biology allow the assessment of phenotypic traits in animal models tied to identifiable genes that are homologous to humans. Natural variants in mouse genetics and specially bioengineered transgenic and knockout strains (and in some cases rats) are now widely used to explore the mechanistic basis of phenotypic responses to air pollutants. These new biological tools hold great promise in better understanding responses and establishing gene–environment interactions that may underlie variation in human responsiveness. Transgenic strains can be devised to express desired gene-linked traits using genes inserted from humans as well as other animal models, while knockout models with specific genes removed or silenced can be made devoid of specific traits to isolate responsiveness mechanisms to a toxic challenge. These engineered animal models add to the availability of natural mutants that have been inbred historically to "fix" a desired genotype with a specific phenotype expression (Glasser and Nogee, 2006; Shapiro, 2007). Current technology can also target specific genes for isolated expression in the lung (eg, if linked to surfactant protein C), and in some cases controlled by genes that an investigator can switch on or off using a pharmacologic or chemical prechallenge. These advances allow the dissection of underlying mechanisms under very controlled scenarios and avoid the problems of having a gene be inappropriately active or inactive through all life stages or throughout all body tissues.

To date, the emphasis of studies using these genetically modified animal models has been on mechanisms associated with disease pathogenesis (Suga *et al.*, 2000; Yoshida and Whitsett, 2006). Among the most popular uses of knockout and transgenic mice has been in the study of inflammatory cytokines and associated products in asthma, where the expression of specific mediators is thought to be under the control of single genes. Analogous models derived to exhibit a desired pathology or disease stemming from a genetic defect—for example, involving lung structure or growth (eg, cystic fibrosis or emphysema)—may serve as a surrogate of the human condition (eg, O'Donnell *et al.*, 1999). These models are not limited to the lung but include other risk factors to study such provocative associations between air pollution and atherosclerosis and cardiac disease (eg, ApoE$^{-/-}$; Sun *et al.*, 2005; Chen *et al.*, 2010).

The use of genetically modified animal models in air pollution research has generally lagged behind that of basic science and toxicology in general. The reasons for this are likely many, including practicality and expenses, but may relate to the difficulties in incorporating such data into conventional risk assessment paradigms. However, with recent interest in susceptible groups,

there has been a definitive upswing in the use of pharmacologically or naturally altered, as well as bioengineered, animal models to more closely link mechanistic profiles to basic human biology. Ozone has been a common test pollutant in these new studies, since more is known about O_3 and its effects in humans than about any other air pollutant. Frequently, these studies address aspects of inflammation and antioxidant capacity relative to challenge by O_3 and other oxidants (Kleeberger *et al.*, 2000; Shore *et al.*, 2009). But with the current interest in PM health effects, these and other models are being redirected. Examples include strain differences and acid-coated PM (Ohtsuka *et al.*, 2000), and hypertransferrinemic mice and metal-rich PM (Ghio *et al.*, 2000). Among rats, the spontaneously hypertensive rat (SHR) and its variants have gained considerable popularity since hypertension is thought to be a human risk factor and because this rat model resembles human hypertension with serum oxidant imbalances, heart disease, as well as its sensitivity to lung injury from inhalants (Kodavanti *et al.*, 2005). The curious are directed to the rapidly evolving literature in this area of research.

EXPOSURE

Air Pollution: Sources and Personal Exposure

Six major air pollutants (PM, O_3, NO_x, SO_2, CO, and Pb) are considered ubiquitous to industrialized communities and are thought to carry the greatest risk to human and environmental health. With the exception of O_3, these pollutants are emitted by anthropogenic combustion processes along with the myriad of special chemical compounds (mostly volatile organic compounds [VOCs]) considered under the category of HAPs. There are many natural sources of air pollutants as well (eg, volcanoes, wildfires, windblown dust, natural biogenic vapors) but it is the anthropogenic sources that emit pollutants that concentrate where people live that raise concerns about their potential health impacts. These factors do not dismiss the significance of potential risks posed by the natural emissions but put focus on the potential for human exposure and risk.

Great strides have been made in reducing the emissions of some pollutants. Airborne Pb is down >98% in the United States since it was removed from motor vehicle gasoline in 1973. Similar measures were taken throughout Europe in the 1970s and 1980s. The United Nations Environment Program has been actively advising all countries in the world to use only unleaded gasoline and currently only a small number of countries have not restricted the use of Pb in gasoline. What remains in ambient air emanates from a few isolated stationary sources and re-entrained Pb in road dust. Of the other five criteria pollutants, overall emissions have been cut 63% since 1970, while at the same time the US Gross National Product (GNP) has increased 204%. Energy consumption has increased 25%, and vehicle miles driven have increased 168% (National Emissions Inventory [NEI] Air Pollutant Emissions Trends, 2011 {http://www.epa.gov/ttnchie1/trends/}]). The changing profile of pollutant emissions since 1900 is reflected in Fig. 29-7. Since 2001, air quality has continued to improve with reductions in ambient SO_2 being largest (−50%) (http://epa.gov/airtrends/2011/report/ozone.pdf). O_3, which is formed in the air from emitted precursors of both natural and man-made sources, has changed the least (∼−13%). Obviously, for any specific locality, air quality can vary depending on the emission profiles of local sources, geographic topography, and meteorology. In the vicinity of a smelter, for example, SO_2, metals, and/or PM may dominate the pollutant profile, while a refinery air shed might be dominated by VOCs and other

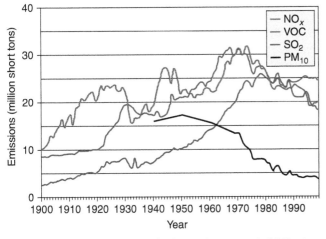

Figure 29-7. *Emission trend for volatile organic compounds (VOC), nitrogen oxides (NO$_x$), sulfur dioxide (SO$_2$), and particulate matter (PM <10 μm) from 1900 (or when records began) to 1998.* Note that since the passage of the Clean Air Act of 1970, most emissions have decreased or, in the case of nitrogen oxides, have leveled off. (Reproduced with permission from U.S. EPA, 2000a.)

carbonaceous products. In suburban areas, where the automobile is the main source of pollution, CO, VOCs, and NO_2 would prevail along with their primary photochemical product, O_3. NO_x releases (including NO_2) by stationary sources also contribute to the local O_3 levels along with that derived secondarily from auto emissions. In all, in 2010 about 124 million people in the United States lived in counties that have violations of the NAAQS designed to minimize risks to the criteria pollutants. However, it is clear that with continued population growth and demands on energy and transportation, efficiencies continue to reduce pollutant emissions substantially—with CO_2 reductions being the next great challenge (Fig. 29-8).

Assessing exposure to an air pollutant has long rested on observational measures of what is in the air. Indeed, much of epidemiology as will be discussed below rests on the principle that what

is in the air reflects what an individual is actually exposed to and ultimately inhales. Exposure science is advancing rapidly and now utilizes approaches that range from novel statistical treatments of traditional exposure metrics to sophisticated models that systematically involve aerodynamic and microenvironmental characteristics to estimate or predict exposures to individuals or populations. The treatment of this subject is well beyond the scope of this chapter (Zou *et al.*, 2009), but the concept is critical to any toxicological evaluation of air pollutants. It also bears heavily on the appropriate approach to conducting inhalation studies in animal models to study air pollutants. Typically, inhalation studies of animals involve square-wave exposure patterns, although it is well appreciated that human exposures vary spatially and temporally. Moreover, animal studies are generally done during the workday (daytime), which is the nocturnal sleep time of most rodent models. In the latter case, one might expect different ventilation patterns in sleeping rodents as compared with those in humans in their daytime activities and perhaps inverted diurnal biochemical activities associated with feeding cycles. Such differences may not have significant impacts on animal toxicological results but the potential for differences needs to be appreciated and respected in translational or interpretational activities.

Indoor versus Outdoor People in the United States (and in most industrialized nations) spend in excess of 80% of their time indoors while at work, school, and home or between these places in an automobile (Robinson and Nelson, 1998). Generally, the time spent indoors is disproportionately higher for adults, who have relatively less time to participate in outdoor activities, especially during the day, when outdoor pollutants are usually at their highest levels. The increased outdoor activity pattern for children is changing and potentially has consequences such as the increased risk of obesity and other health/growth parameters. Perhaps the most significant risk factor in indoor air for children is the presence of asthma. With nearly 10% of children with asthma, the risk of exposure to pollutants and allergens in concentrated form is particularly great.

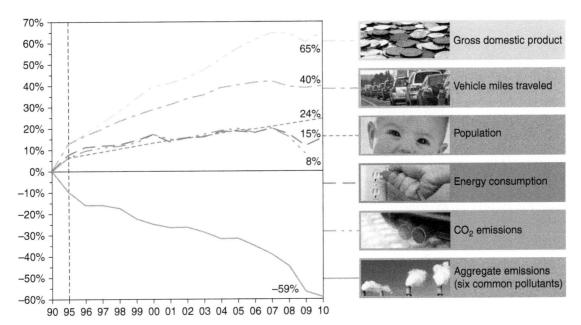

Figure 29-8. *Comparison of growth measures and emissions from 1990 to 2010.* During this period the US population, energy consumption, and CO_2 production grew in parallel (the latter affected after 2007 by the economy), while miles traveled and the economy grew substantially more over this time. Meanwhile, the six common air pollutants fell by more than half, indicative of great advances in industrial and motor vehicle efficiencies. (Figure used with permission. *Our Nation's Air—Status and Trends through 2010*—http://www.epa.gov/airtrends/2011/.)

As to the issue of total exposure, children and outdoor workers are thought to be more likely to encounter outdoor air pollution at its worst; in fact, the relatively high physical activity levels of these subgroups leads to larger doses of any given pollutant being delivered to the lungs. Thus, while it is important to characterize and track pollution levels in outdoor air, a realistic exposure estimate is perhaps best achieved when some indoor/outdoor proportionality can be included as well as some indicator of physical activity. From these data, it would be possible to estimate lung dose, although uncertainties can increase with each increment of personal detail. Defining personal exposure can be extremely difficult, as personal monitoring is tedious and expensive, and can sometimes be confounded by other contributions to the indicator being monitored. Hence, exposure measures are typically drawn from ambient measurements or derived from models developed from studies of groups of people carefully characterized across personal exposure modifiers—exercise, personal lifestyles, etc.

The indoor environment has gained appreciation as a major contributor to total personal exposure. The energy crisis of the 1970s spurred efforts to increase home and building insulation, reduce infiltration of outside air, and minimize energy consumption. At the same time, indoor sources of air contaminants have been on the rise from household products and furnishings, which—when combined with poorly ventilated heating systems and overall reductions in air exchange rates—give rise to potentially unhealthy indoor air environments. As people begin to notice patterns of odors, microbiological growth, and even ill health, measures of indoor air become a significant part of environmental risk assessment. Personal exposure has, therefore, come to include the myriad of potential sources, both outdoors and indoors.

It is clear now that indoor air can at times be more complex than outdoor air, a point often raised in challenging the legitimacy of studies that rely solely on outdoor monitoring data. Nevertheless, the national monitoring network for the criteria pollutants has been shown to reflect human exposure reasonably well for some pollutants, especially those that are nonreactive. Indeed, outdoor air permeates the indoor environment in spite of the reduced air exchange in most buildings. However, many variables determine how well components of the outdoor air infiltrate. The current evidence suggests that the average insulated home has about one air change per hour, resulting in indoor concentrations of pollutants that range from 30% to 80% of those outdoors. For nonreactive gases (eg, CO), there could likely be nearly a 1:1 indoor/outdoor ratio in the absence of a "sink" for that gas; the ratio for fine PM (<2.5 μm) could also be fairly high (~0.4–0.7), since these particles can easily penetrate through cracks and open spaces. In contrast, the indoor/outdoor ratio of O_3 would likely be low (<0.3) because of its reactivity. Obviously, household differences in the use of window ventilation and air conditioning can also be important variables. Not to be overlooked, of course, are independent indoor sources of contamination where the ratio of an indoor pollutant to that outdoors can even exceed 1 (eg, NO_2). Particles and gases from tobacco smoke, unvented space heaters, and poorly vented fireplaces and wood stoves as well as fresh paint and cleaning agents can be significant indoor sources. Attention is also being directed toward the many and varied insidious sources of indoor contaminants: certain soils and construction masonry emit radon, gas cooking appliances emit NO_x, sidestream tobacco smoke emits PM, CO, and a host of carcinogenic polyaromatics, and carpets, furnishings, dry-cleaned clothes, and household air fresheners can emit a wide range of VOCs. Responses appear also to be affected by ambient comfort factors such as temperature and humidity. Additionally, some of these chemicals can even interact with one another as has been found to occur with O_3 diffused indoors reacting with VOCs emitted from household cleaners to form small particles. The complexity of these multiple sources underscores the importance of appreciating the total exposure scenario if we are to understand the nature of air pollution and its potential effects on human health (Fig. 29-9).

There remain two broadly defined illnesses that were identified in the 1980s that are largely unique to the indoor building environment (Brooks and Davis, 1992). The first is "sick building syndrome" (SBS), which is a collection of ailments defined by a set of persistent symptoms enduring at least two weeks (Table 29-4) and appears to occur in at least 20% of those exposed. The pattern is complaints by the building inhabitants, typically of unknown specific etiology sometimes even with ambient measurements, but is relieved sometime after an affected individual leaves the offending building (Hayes et al., 1995). Frequently but not always, this syndrome occurs in new, poorly ventilated, or recently refurbished office buildings. The suspected causes include combustion products, cleaning chemicals, biological emissions from mold, and vapor emissions from furnishings frequently exacerbated by discomfort. The perception of irritancy to the eyes, nose, and throat ranks among the predominant symptoms that can become intolerable with repeated exposures. Controlled clinical studies have shown concentration- and duration-dependent worsening of sensory discomfort after exposure to a complex mixture of 22 VOCs commonly found in the indoor environment (Molhave et al., 1986). The many factors contributing to such responses are poorly understood but include various host susceptibility factors such as personal stress and fatigue, diet, and alcohol use. Current biomarkers of response used in the laboratory include sensory irritancy to the eyes in volunteer test subjects and sometimes in animals. However, in general, animal studies using standard measures of sensory irritation or other corporal end points have had limited success in assessing SBS and related syndromes. Human perception factors are believed to be critical to the response patterns.

The second syndrome (building-related illnesses) is a group of illnesses that, in contrast to the SBS, consists of well-documented conditions with defined diagnostic criteria and generally recognizable etiology. These illnesses typically call for conventional medical treatment strategies, because simply exiting the building where the illness was contracted may not readily reverse the symptoms. Several biocontaminant-related illnesses (eg, legionnaires' disease, hypersensitivity pneumonitis, humidifier fever) fall into this group, as do allergies to animal dander, dust mites, and cockroaches. Medical treatment and mitigation of exposure (source elimination or personal protection) are generally needed to abate symptoms. Some typical outdoor pollutants can also be problematic indoors—most notably, CO from poorly vented heaters. Indoor exposures to NO_2 can pose problems as well, especially in people who may be sensitive—such as asthmatics. At times, however, when the concentrations of CO, NO_2, and many VOCs (passively emitted from new furniture or rugs, or from molds in the ventilation system) result in less discernible or definable signs and symptoms, the responses may be misdiagnosed as SBS, which can complicate assessment of the situation.

Many inhalants, such as NO_2 and trichloroethylene (a VOC common to the indoor air arising from chlorinated water or dry-cleaned clothes), have been shown in animal toxicology studies to suppress immune defenses and allow opportunistic pathogens to proliferate in the lung. The involvement of immunologic suppression is a particularly controversial, yet important attribute of indoor pollution because of its insidious nature and its implications for all building-related illnesses. This problem is further complicated

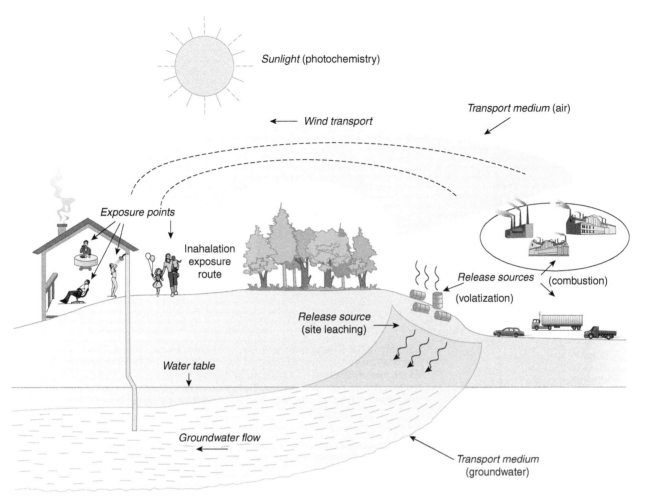

Figure 29-9. *Illustration of contributors to the total personal exposure paradigm showing how these indoor and outdoor factors interact.*

in that complex indoor environments comprising of chemicals and biologicals (dust mites, fungi, molds, etc) may also lead to unexpected interactions that remain virtually unstudied and thus are underappreciated in the assessment of indoor pollution.

Recently, there have been incidents that highlight indoor air pollution. Post Hurricane Katrina (2005) deployment of trailers where people lived for extended periods resulted in exposure to formaldehyde from urea foam insulation with a myriad of effects on inhabitants—notably children. And more recently, wallboard of Chinese origin, which had sulfate and other chemical components on the sealant surface paper that vaporized into the air, resulted in a wide array of symptoms among inhabitants as well as corrosion of some materials. Clearly, the indoor environment is not to be underestimated as to its potential for impact on human health.

Indoor Air in the Developing World Pollution of the indoor environment in the developing world is a major issue; in some parts of the world this issue actually overrides outdoor air pollution. In the more urbanized environments, there is indoor infiltration of outdoor pollutants unhampered due to poor housing stock. Superimposed on the infiltration of ambient air pollutants are indoor emissions from cooking practices, the cultural use of incense, tobacco, and various other substances, such as perfumes. In less developed communities, unvented or poorly vented cookstoves that burn biomass are used much as they have been for centuries. The emissions from these cookstoves accumulate indoors exposing families, and especially women and children, to soot and account for two million deaths around the world (Fig. 29-10). Chronic lung diseases, such as bronchitis, emphysema, and cancer, are major killers of exposed women while children suffer from bronchitis and various other infectious lung diseases. The cookstove issue is the focus of a UN Foundation called the Global Alliance for Clean Cookstoves (http://www.unfoundation.org/assets/pdf/global-alliance-for-clean-cookstoves-factsheet.pdf), which is a multinational effort to replace existing dirty stoves with clean culturally practical alternative cooking stoves and devices. The black carbon (soot) emitted from the dirty stoves is also believed to be a major contributor to global climate change.

Table 29-4

Symptoms Commonly Associated with the Sick Building Syndromes

Eyes, nose, and throat irritation
Headaches
Fatigue
Reduced attention span
Irritability
Nasal congestion
Difficulty breathing
Nosebleeds
Dry skin
Nausea

SOURCE: Data from Brooks and Davis (1992), with permission.

1246

Deaths from indoor smoke from solid fuels

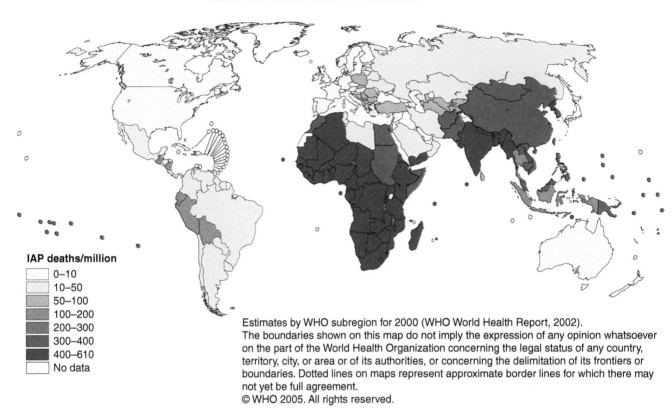

Estimates by WHO subregion for 2000 (WHO World Health Report, 2002).
The boundaries shown on this map do not imply the expression of any opinion whatsoever on the part of the World Health Organization concerning the legal status of any country, territory, city, or area or of its authorities, or concerning the delimitation of its frontiers or boundaries. Dotted lines on maps represent approximate border lines for which there may not yet be full agreement.
© WHO 2005. All rights reserved.

IAP deaths/million
- 0–10
- 10–50
- 50–100
- 100–200
- 200–300
- 300–400
- 400–610
- No data

Figure 29-10. *Illustration of contribution of burning solid fuels to global mortality.* The map shows considerable country-by-country differences in total deaths per million inhabitants that can be attributed to combustion of solid fossil fuels such as wood and other biomass materials.

The Evolving Profile of Outdoor Air Pollution Classically, ambient air pollution was distinguished on the basis of the chemical redox nature of its primary components. Dickens's 18th-century "London's particular" referred to a chilled, acrid fog resulting from the accumulation of SO_2 and smoke from incomplete combustion during frequent meteorological inversions. This acidic mix reacts with surfaces, corroding metal and eroding masonry, characteristic of reductive chemistry. These reducing-type atmospheres have long been associated with smelting and related combustion-based industries (as along the Meuse River in 1930 and Donora, Pennsylvania, in 1948) as well as with large, urban centers (eg, London in 1952, New York in 1962) burning coal or other dirty fossil fuels for energy. In contrast, Los Angeles has always had a characteristically "oxidant-type" pollution consisting of NO_x and other secondary photochemical oxidants, such as O_3, aldehydes, and electron-hungry hydrocarbon radicals. By virtue of its regional topography and summer meteorology, Los Angeles is particularly prone to trap traffic emissions, while other areas, such as Atlanta, are simply plagued by stagnant, humid summer air.

The classical types of air pollution were implicitly seasonal. Reducing-type air pollution occurred during winter periods of oil and coal combustion for heating and power coupled with meteorological inversions, while the oxidant atmospheres occurred during the warmer months of spring and summer, when sunlight is most intense and can catalyze reactions among the constituents of auto exhaust. Today the urban distinctions between reducing and oxidant smogs have become largely an academic or historic exercise. Most US urban areas have virtually eliminated smoky, sulfurous emissions (through regulation and a changing national industrial profile) and now with suburban sprawl have a proliferation of automobiles that contribute tons of oxidant precursors into the ambient air. However, in the Midwest there remains still relatively heavy industrial activity that continues to emit SO_2, albeit much less than decades ago, but whose emissions are targeted for further reduction. These emissions continue to have important regional implications as they undergo complex cloud chemistry to form sulfate and impact visibility (regional haze) as well as contribute significantly to PM mass, the primary metric linked to human health effects (Zeger *et al.*, 2008). The air above metropolitan areas in the eastern half of the United States is currently composed of regional reducing pollutants that distribute and blanket a large segment of the country as well as temporally and spatially varied local source pollutants (HAPs) and secondary oxidant pollutants. Increasingly, oxidants and sulfates formed high in the atmosphere are transported across regions to other locales. In the East, sulfates may still predominate over nitrates in the air, in contrast to the Southwest United States, but nitrates occupy a higher ratio of the pollutant mix than ever due in large part to the growth in traffic. No longer is the Northeastern air pollution simply a sulfur-based problem. Adding further to the complexity of the ambient air profile is that not only has the composition of the urban haze changed but also the ambient chemistry has affected its temporal patterns. Long extended periods of O_3 (8–12 hours) now prevail over wide areas such as southern California and the US Southeast and even along the Northeast corridor. The prototypic spike pattern of an hour or two depicted for Los Angeles in the 1970s, and assumed to be the norm for photochemical processes, has changed. In part, the chemical mixes are different as is the distribution of the sources (motor vehicle traffic). As climate change progresses, there is expectation that the underlying chemistry will change further altering these patterns because the assumptions and data that led to current O_3 control measures will be undermined.

UNIT VI

ENVIRONMENTAL TOXICOLOGY

Outside the United States, many international megacities remain plagued by the classic reducing and oxidant forms of air pollution. For example, uncontrolled industrial and coal-fired power plant emissions surrounding cities such as Beijing and the northern sectors of Mexico City are dominated by sulfurous, particulate emissions, whereas southern Mexico City, Santiago, and Tokyo have substantially (although not exclusively) automobile-associated oxidant smogs. Impacts on health, visibility, and general welfare are clear and are bringing ever increasing public concern in an all too familiar scenario played out in the United States in the mid-20th century. Urban air pollution is a worldwide problem, where the estimate of people exposed to O_3 at potentially harmful levels exceeds 480 million (Schwela, 1996), with a recent estimate of attributable yearly mortality at 700,000 (Anenberg et al., 2010). The WHO estimates of PM-related mortality are at 1.3 million per year (WHO, 2009).

EPIDEMIOLOGICAL EVIDENCE OF HEALTH EFFECTS

Outdoor Air Pollution

Acute and Episodic Exposures A number of air pollution incidents have been documented where pollutant concentrations rose to levels that are clearly hazardous to human health. Where a single chemical has been accidentally released (eg, methyl isocyanate in Bhopal, India), establishing the relationship between cause and ill effect is straightforward. However, most air pollution situations involve complex atmospheres, and establishing a specific cause other than the air pollution incident itself can be difficult. Three acute episodes of community air pollution are considered classic (Meuse Valley, Belgium—1930; Donora, Pennsylvania—1948; and London, United Kingdom—1952). In each event, community inhabitants were clearly affected adversely; hospitalizations were concomitant with an elevated mortality rate. Likewise, each involved a meteorological inversion (cold air capped above by a blanket of warm air, with little or no vertical air mixing) that prevailed for three to five days, during which time the concentration of an array of combustion pollutants rose well above the normal levels for these already heavily polluted areas. No actual measurements of pollution were made in the Meuse Valley and Donora, but crude daily averages of smoke and SO_2 of the London smog incident were recorded—estimated at 4.5 mg/m^3 and 1.34 ppm, respectively, on the worst day. Brief (on the order of hours) peaks of these pollutants certainly were much higher. During the Meuse Valley episode, 65 people died, while in Donora the number was 20. These deaths are considered "excess" deaths when compared with normal mortality rates for that time of year that were likely already affected by the background air pollution.

The "London smog" of 1952 was a true disaster with an estimated 4000 excess deaths during the event itself with perhaps thousands more in the weeks to follow. Hospital admissions increased dramatically, mainly among the elderly and those with preexisting cardiac and/or respiratory disease. Even otherwise healthy pedestrians, their visibility limited to as little as 3 ft, covered their noses and mouths in an attempt to minimize their exposure to the acrid air. Many reports of sudden death were reported among workers commuting on bicycle or on foot with symptoms described as "choking." People with preexisting cardiac and lung problems were particularly affected. It is ironic that 16 years earlier, shortly after the Meuse Valley episode, Firkert (1936) predicted that 3200 deaths would occur should a Meuse-like smog strike London. Although the London incident brought the issue of air pollution to the public consciousness, additional episodes occurred with the 1956 and 1962 incidents being among the most notable. But none were of the magnitude seen in 1952. Interestingly, in December 1991, London experienced a winter inversion smog alert, but one with a very different modern pollutant profile: NO_2 at 423 ppb, black smoke at 148 μg/m^3, and SO_2 at 72 ppb (five, four times, and twice the seasonal average, respectively). The differences between this episode and previous episodes were that the air pollution was neither of the magnitude of earlier events nor completely dominated by coal emissions as traffic was at this point a major source of oxidant emissions (Anderson, 1999). Overall increases in mortality and hospital admissions were not so apparent, but regional comparisons suggested impacts among the elderly and cardiopulmonary-impaired (mortality: ↑ 14% cardiovascular and ↑ 22% respiratory; ↑ 43% for respiratory admissions). Susceptible individuals are always the first to respond to these pollution episodes, but the impacts eventually are widespread.

During the latter half of the 20th century, other cities experienced notable air pollution events; among these were New York City, Steubenville, Ohio; Pittsburgh, Pennsylvania; Athens, Greece; and major regions of Western Europe from the Netherlands to the Ruhr Valley of Germany. Major episodes of anthropogenic air pollution continue to decrease in the developed world, in both frequency and intensity, but "natural" events such as the vegetation/forest fires of Indonesia of 1997 and 1998, greater Moscow in 2009, and northern California in 2009 and 2010 all saw significant impacts on regional air quality and public health. The impacts of these fires, like that of the US Northwest in 2003, were tracked as their plumes dispersed across the country.

So much had the air cleared in much of the United States from the late 1960s into the 1970s that many thought that the problem of industrial pollution was on its way to full resolution. Smoke from factory chimneys was less visible and the air epidemiology of the times showed little health impact. However, in the 1980s, it was realized that smoky skies were largely due to carbonaceous material and that more efficient burning had eliminated much of what could be seen in the air. But the sulfur in fuel emitted as sulfur dioxide reacted in clouds to form acidic sulfate and traveled great distances depositing and acidifying lakes and streams and at the same time painting the leaves and the ground resulting in defoliation of forests (Calvert et al., 1985). There were also new studies showing that acid haze with O_3 was associated with emergency room visits among susceptible populations—for example, asthmatics (Bates and Sizto, 1987). A series of studies showed acute effects of regional summer haze in areas of central and Northeastern North America. These two- to three-day episodes of haze were typified by increases in O_3 and acid and neutralized (ammonium) sulfates, characteristic of the new generation of pollution in many US urban areas. Interestingly, the apparent combined temporal or sequential patterns of O_3 and sulfate were associated with the health effects, and neither constituent seemed to be acting alone. Similar results were reported for the upstate New York area as well (Thurston et al., 1992), but it seemed the acidity as [H$^+$] of the haze was the active toxicant. Studies of children at summer camps, where children are active and outdoors most of the day, had reported decrements in daily measured pulmonary function on days of haze when both O_3 and acidity levels were elevated. The responses appeared to exceed those predicted by chamber studies of O_3 alone, suggesting dose differences or interactions between haze components (Lippmann, 1989). Clinical studies in adolescent asthmatics and animal studies lent further support to the belief that H$^+$ can affect airway function, particularly in the presence of O_3. Studies in the South and Southwest similarly found effects in young asthmatics and diminished performance in athletes, but these appeared to relate more specifically to O_3, since sulfate was less prominent in the ambient air of these regions. Yet these epidemiological and field studies showing associations with "acid" haze could not be replicated in the laboratory with either animal or human exposure studies. There could be any number of reasons for this lack of coherence but the exposure concentrations were often orders of magnitude more than in the ambient air. When refined acid measurements in ambient air were used, the consistency of the findings could not be reliably replicated. With no *apparent* impact on mortality in epidemiological studies, the focus of air pollution toxicology focused more and more on O_3 where clinical and animal exposure studies easily could measure impacts on lung function. It was felt that O_3 was the likely culprit and its ubiquity in urban air argued for greater and greater attention. Indeed, many health effects could be ascribed to oxidant/irritant properties of O_3.

Of the many air pollution studies over the last 25 years, none have had more impact on the perception of pollutant risk and the direction of research today than a series of epidemiological studies that showed an association between PM mass concentration (as measured by the regulatory monitoring network in the United States) and daily mortality. These studies departed from conventional epidemiological methods used for air pollution studies in the United States and utilized novel time-series analyses that could more easily blunt the impact of weather, smoking, and other variables that might obscure patterns in health variables linked to the air monitoring data. These studies showed significant and consistent associations between health outcomes of ambient PM at levels previously thought to be safe. Prior to this period, measurable effects of PM and SO_2 were not easily detected below the 24-hour means for smoke and SO_2—250 $\mu g/m^3$ and 0.19 ppm, respectively. In fact, the new findings showed effects, as evidenced by increases in mortality and morbidity rates at or below contemporaneous NAAQS levels (1987: 50 $\mu g/m^3$, annual mean; 150 $\mu g/m^3$ daily maximum for PM of diameter <10 μm [PM_{10}]). Time-series analyses are based on Poisson regression modeling to distinguish changes in daily death counts (or hospital admissions) associated with short-term changes in air pollution. The studies initially found effects with cruder measures of PM—total suspended particulate material (TSP), which includes virtually all particles <100 μm in mass median aerodynamic diameter (MMAD—a median particle size normalizing the particle to unit density and spherical shape for aerodynamic comparison). These studies were followed with stronger associations with particles considered inhalable—PM_{10} (an MMAD at which PM is aerodynamically separated at an initial 50% efficiency at 10 μm and increasingly at smaller sizes). Beginning in the mid-1990s, even stronger associations have been found with an analogous but fully and deeply respirable particle—$PM_{2.5}$. As the PM diameter gets smaller, it better represents anthropogenic sources of pollution. The statistical methodology applied in these time-series studies had an advantage over conventional regression analyses in that it could detect short-term trends and minimized the effects of other pollutants and potential confounders with longer time constants (Schwartz, 1991; reviewed by Pope and Dockery, 2006).

In contrast to the three epidemiological studies used by the US EPA to develop the 1987 PM_{10} NAAQS, there were more than 30 such studies for the 1997 revision and the promulgation of the new index, $PM_{2.5}$ NAAQS ([15 $\mu g/m^3$, annual mean; 65 $\mu g/m^3$ daily maximum for PM of diameter <2.5 μm [$PM_{2.5}$]). These studies showed a significant health impact of PM, linked to mass and not necessarily sulfate or any other constituent. In 2006, the PM NAAQS was revised keeping the annual $PM_{2.5}$ NAAQS at 15 $\mu g/m^3$, with a tightening of the daily maximum to 35 $\mu g/m^3$. The NAAQS for PM is reviewed about every five years depending on legal or procedural issues as data accrue; an update on the primary (human)

standards for $PM_{2.5}$ (fine PM) and $PM_{2.5-10}$ (coarse PM) is expected in the 2012 time frame. The PM NAAQS is specifically noted since of all the NAAQS, it has the greatest impact on human health of any US regulation in terms of both cost and benefit. As a result, the health science (epidemiology, clinical human exposure and animal toxicology studies) is scrutinized more than any other US regulatory decision.

PM stands as the preeminent air pollutant because of its health impact as well as the pollutant that opened the door to unsuspected targets of injury. The major health outcome revealed in the study of PM has been the involvement of the cardiovascular system as a prime target for adverse impact, and not the lung as historically assumed. While the heart, as part of the cardiopulmonary system, has always held an indirect role in health impacts or disease from air pollution, both epidemiological and toxicological studies now point to major cardiac involvement in PM-associated mortality. Current thinking is that cardiac-mediated effects are more germane to the PM-associated mortality findings than pulmonary effects (Brook *et al.*, 2010). Not surprisingly, effects are most apparent in subpopulations already compromised by cardiopulmonary and perhaps vascular diseases (eg, diabetes). There exists no one generally accepted mechanism or mode of action to account for these findings (Costa, 2000; Brook *et al.*, 2010). However, several pathways have been proposed that attempt to link exposure and cardiac effects that may or may not include pulmonary mediation. These potential mechanisms are illustrated in Fig. 29-11.

From a toxicological perspective, it has been difficult to accept that the association between PM and health outcomes is not somehow linked to particle composition rather than mass alone. The linkage to mass and not composition is counterintuitive, especially in light of the fact that all PM is not constitutively identical. The actual "biochemical lesion" caused by PM is generally thought to involve oxidant mechanisms (generation of reactive oxygen and perhaps nitrogen species) by constituents or attributes (eg, reactive surface area) of the particles at the cell or molecular level. Initially, there was a credibility hurdle ("biologically plausibility") that day-to-day fluctuations in the mass concentration of ~10 $\mu g/m^3$ airborne PM would result in an increase of about 0.6% to 1% (excess) mortality. However, there now exist several plausible hypotheses that have some degree of empirical support: metals, organics, nanosize with reactive surfaces, and constitutive oxidants to name those most prominent.

The experience with PM has expanded the thinking of the possible extrapulmonary effects of other air pollutants. Potential links to cardiovascular toxicity of several of the NAAQS pollutants have been demonstrated, although not with the consistency of PM. Moreover, there are new data showing pollutant-related impacts on birth outcomes, postnatal development, and neurologic health. In the latter case, it is unclear if these effects are related to vascular impacts such as those caused by PM or to other systemic oxidant intermediates.

Long-Term Exposures Epidemiological studies of the chronic effects of air pollution are difficult to conduct by the very nature of the goal: outcomes associated with long-term exposures. Looking back in time with retrospective, cross-sectional studies was the common approach, but those studies frequently were confounded with unknown variables and inadequate historical exposure data. A good example of the problem of confounding is cigarette smoking. Without extensive information on both active and passive smoking, the ability to discern the impact of an air pollution disease outcome such as chronic bronchitis and emphysema would be greatly impaired. Prospective studies, on the other hand, have the advantage of more precise control of confounding variables, such

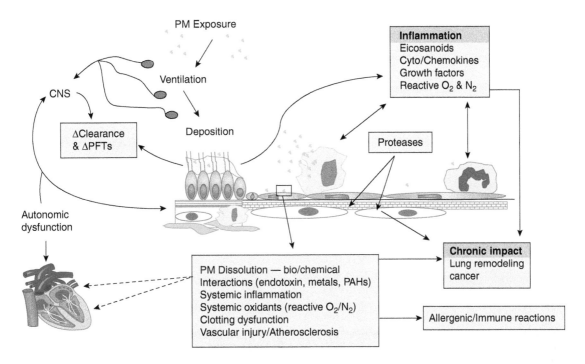

Figure 29-11. *Schematic of the multiple mechanisms thought to function in cardiopulmonary response(s) to air pollutants—derived from current hypothesized mechanisms for particulate matter.*

as the tracking of urinary cotinine as an index of tobacco smoke exposure, but they can be very expensive and require substantial time and dedication on the part of both the investigators and the study population. Depending on the study size and design, exposure assessments can be complex, and the loss of subjects due to dropout is sometimes unpredictable.

Despite these deficiencies and problems, there are both retrospective and prospective epidemiology studies that have tackled the issue of long-term air pollution health effects. In general, these studies have suggested a positive association between urban pollution and progressive pulmonary impairments. On the one hand, cross-sectional studies in the Los Angeles Air Basin have found evidence of accelerated "aging-like" loss of lung function in people living for extended periods in regions of high oxidant pollution, when compared with that in people living in areas where sea air circulation lowers overall pollutant concentrations (Detels *et al.*, 1991). Similarly, exposure to SO$_2$ and PM in the Netherlands over a 12-year period was shown prospectively to gradually impair lung function (Van De Lende *et al.*, 1981). And even rural areas in western Pennsylvania, which are swept by reducing-type pollutants transported from Midwestern industrial centers, have been shown to have a higher incidence of respiratory symptoms as determined from a questionnaire-based design (Schenker *et al.*, 1983). While a negative impact of any specific pollutant followed in these studies is difficult to dissect, the message that long-term exposure to air pollution contributes to deterioration of lung health seems clear.

Among the most detailed prospective epidemiological studies of chronic health effects across a range of levels of air pollution has been the so-called Harvard Six Cities Study begun in the early 1970s. The cities were chosen to represent a range of air quality based on SO$_2$ and PM—it was designed as a study of "acid" air pollution. Early on in the study, there was great dependence on routine regional air monitoring data, but over time the investigators themselves conducted the air analyses of exposure microenvironments (local and indoor). The initial design of these studies included the gathering of parental questionnaire data (including approximately 20,000 people) about the prevalence of respiratory problems in school children and has continued over 30 years along with periodic assessments of pulmonary function. When compared across cities, [H$^+$] (measured in four of the six cities) was correlated (Fig. 29-12D) better than was sulfate with the prevalence of bronchitis in children aged 10 to 12 (Speizer, 1989). However, as the assessment program evolved, more detailed study revealed mortality associations with PM as represented in Fig. 29-12A-C. The role of [H$^+$] in relation with acute mortality was less convincing than that associated with the sulfate or PM$_{2.5}$ (sulfates co-associate with fine PM in the atmosphere) (Dockery *et al.*, 1993). More importantly with regard to long-term health, this study showed very significant effects of PM on the life spans of people living in Steubenville, Ohio—the dirtiest of the industrial centers. Over a 15-year period, the average human life span was reduced by about two years due to PM exposure. These findings were corroborated by a prospective cohort-based mortality study using a database collected on over 500,000 people by the American Cancer Society (ACS) across 151 cities from 1982 to 1989 (Pope *et al.*, 1995). The study showed a 15% to 17% increased mortality risk over seven years due to PM, about equivalent to the risk of smoking over that period. Subsequently, Pope *et al.* (2002) reported results of a 10-year and again an 18-year follow-up study of the ACS cohort (Pope *et al.*, 2011). These updated analyses, which included gaseous copollutant and new fine particle measurements, and more comprehensive personal information on the enrollees, confirmed the linkage of health effects, including an increased risk of lung cancer, with PM$_{2.5}$ exposures. These findings reinforce the concerns for potential chronic health impacts of PM and the heightened risk of premature death from lifelong air pollution exposure. There is currently a 10-year study (results expected ~2015) to assess the impact of air pollution, with emphasis on PM, on atherosclerosis in humans as part of the Multi-Ethnic Study of Atherosclerosis Air Pollution (MESA AIR; http://depts.washington.edu/mesaair/).

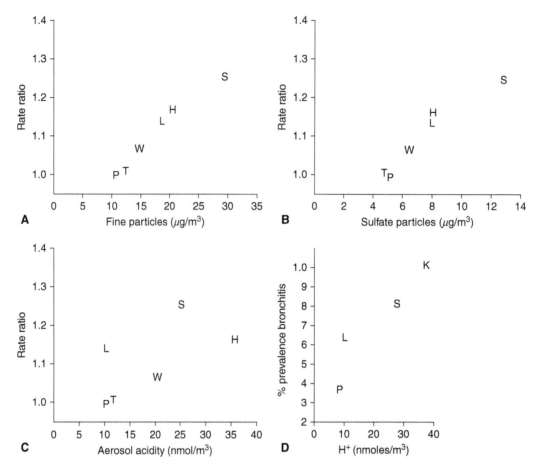

Figure 29-12. *Data from the Harvard Six Cities Studies indicating the superior relationship of PM$_{10}$ and sulfate to mortality rates (**A-C**) in contrast to acidity (**D**), which correlates better with the prevalence of bronchitis in children.* Reproduced with permission from Speizer (1989) (D) and Dockery *et al.* (1993) (A-C).

POLLUTANTS OF OUTDOOR AMBIENT AIR

Classic Reducing-Type Air Pollution

The acute air pollution episodes of the 20th century showed that high concentrations of the reducing-type air pollution, characterized by SO$_2$ and smoke, are capable of producing dramatic human health effects. Empirical studies in human subjects and animals have long stressed the irritancy of SO$_2$ and its role in these incidents, while the full potential for interactions among the copollutants in the smoky, sulfurous mix has a mixed record of replication in the human exposure laboratory. Because of its history, SO$_2$ is often thought of as the prototypic air pollutant of the industrial age, and as such it has a detailed historical literature base. It is an irritant gas that has a toxicology of its own and, through atmospheric reactions, can transform photochemically into sulfites or sulfates within a secondarily irritant particle. The impact of SO$_2$ emissions on irritancy, the formation of secondary particles that affect visibility, and its damaging acidification of the environment have been the focus of much regulation for coal-fired power plants since 1970. Levels are greatly reduced (>60%) in the United States and continue to fall under new cross-state regulations.

Sulfur Dioxide

General Toxicology Sulfur dioxide is a water-soluble irritant gas. As such, it is absorbed predominantly in the upper airways. It is a sensory irritant and can stimulate bronchoconstriction and mucus secretion in a number of species, including humans. Early studies with relatively high exposure concentrations of SO$_2$ showed airway cellular injury and subsequent proliferation of mucus-secreting

goblet cells. This attribute of SO$_2$ has led to its use (>250 ppm) in the production of laboratory animal models of bronchitis and airway injury (Kodavanti *et al.*, 2000). At much lower concentrations (<1 ppm), such as might be encountered in the polluted ambient air of industrialized areas, long-term residents experience a higher incidence of bronchitis. In fact, prior to the breakup of the Soviet block, many eastern European cities were renowned for widespread public affliction with bronchitis; 20 years later, the prevalence of bronchitis was greatly reduced (von Mutius *et al.*, 1994). While other factors (diet, access to health care, other pollutants) may well have been involved in this reversal, reductions in ambient smoke and SO$_2$ are generally thought to be the most important.

The concentrations of SO$_2$ likely to be encountered in the United States are lower still—on average, considerably less than 0.01 ppm. Rats exposed for 70 to 170 hours to 0.1, 1.0, and 20 ppm exhibited reduced clearance of inert particles, while dogs exposed to 1 ppm for a year had slowed tracheal mucociliary transport. Analogously, mouse models show that mice exposed to 0.1 ppm were more susceptible to bacterial infections. The fact that the low-concentration exposures showed marked effects when extended over longer periods is consistent with the epidemiological associations between SO$_2$ exposure and bronchitis. The evidence is not clear, however, as some studies show no overt long-term pulmonary pathology. Guinea pigs and monkeys, for example, showed no effect on lung function or pathology after a year of continuous exposure to concentrations of 0.1 to 5 ppm SO$_2$ (Alarie *et al.*, 1970, 1972).

The penetration of SO$_2$ into the lungs is greater during mouth as opposed to nose breathing. An increase in the airflow during deep rapid breathing augments penetration of the gas into the deeper lung.

As a result, persons exercising would inhale more SO_2 and, as noted with asthmatics, are likely to experience greater irritation. Once deposited along the airway, SO_2 dissolves into surface lining fluid as sulfite or bisulfite and is readily distributed throughout the body. It is thought that the sulfite interacts with sensory receptors in the airways to initiate local and centrally mediated bronchoconstriction.

Pulmonary Function Effects The basic pulmonary response to inhaled SO_2 is mild bronchoconstriction, which is reflected as a measurable increase in airflow resistance due to narrowing of the airways. Concentration-related increases in resistance have been observed in guinea pigs, dogs, and cats as well as humans. Exposure of isolated segments of the nose or airways of dogs and guinea pigs appeared to alter resistance in a manner consistent with receptor-mediated sensory stimulation. Airflow resistance increased more when the gas was introduced through a tracheal cannula than via the nose, since nasal scrubbing of the water-soluble gas was bypassed. Isolated nasal exposures increased airflow resistance through the nose largely as a result of mucosal swelling, but the irritant effect appeared to signal the more distal airways as well. Direct exposure of the trachea had a more dramatic effect on airflow resistance. Exposure of the intact nose also induced some response, consistent with the existence of a nasal neural network being involved in bronchoconstriction (Frank and Speizer, 1965; Nadel *et al.*, 1965). Intravenous injection of atropine (a parasympathetic receptor blocker) or cooling of the cervical vagal nerves abolishes bronchoconstriction in the cat model; rewarming of the nerve reestablishes the response. The rapidity of the response and its reversal emphasize the parasympathetic tonal change in airway smooth muscle. Studies in human subjects have confirmed the predominance of parasympathetic mediation, but histamine from inflammatory cells may play a secondary role in the bronchoconstrictive responses of asthmatics.

Human subjects exposed to 1, 5, or 13 ppm SO_2 for just 10 minutes exhibit a rapid bronchoconstrictive response, with 1 to 3 ppm being a threshold for most if exercise is involved. Exposures to 0.25 to 1 ppm for a few hours can induce bronchoconstriction in adult and adolescent subjects with clinically defined mild asthma (Sheppard *et al.*, 1981; Koenig *et al.*, 1981). Findings such as these (responses <0.5 ppm) have raised concerns about potential adverse effects in this sensitive subpopulation when it is exposed to peaks of SO_2 that are known to occur near point sources.

Chronic Effects Only a few long-term studies have been conducted with SO_2 at levels approaching those found in ambient air. Alarie *et al.* (1970) exposed guinea pigs to 0.1, 1.0, or 5.7 ppm SO_2 continuously for a year without adverse impact on lung mechanics. Similarly, monkeys exhibited no alteration in pulmonary function when exposed continuously for 78 weeks to 0.1, 0.6, and 1.3 ppm SO_2 (Alarie *et al.*, 1972). Even in the presence of 0.1 mg/m^3 sulfuric acid, dogs exposed 16 hours a day for 18 months to 0.5 ppm SO_2 showed no impairment in pulmonary function (Vaughan *et al.*, 1969). Higher levels of SO_2 for protracted periods of time (dogs to 5 ppm for 225 days [Lewis *et al.*, 1969]; rats to 350 ppm for 30 days [Reid, 1963]) have been shown to alter airway mucus secretion, goblet cell topography, or lung function, but these results are of little relevance to typical SO_2 levels in ambient air.

Sulfuric Acid and Related Sulfates The conversion of SO_2 to sulfate is favored in the environment with subsequent ammonia neutralization to ammonium sulfate [$(NH_4)_2SO_4$] or ammonium bisulfate [NH_4HSO_4]. During oil and coal combustion or the smelting of metal ores, sulfuric acid condenses downstream of the combustion processes with available metal ions and water vapor to form submicrometer sulfuric acid fume and sulfated fly ash. Sulfur dioxide continues to oxidize to sulfate within dispersing smokestack plumes, which can be augmented by the presence of free soluble or partially coordinated transition metals such as iron, manganese, and vanadium within the effluent ash. When coal is burned, the acid may adsorb to the surface or solubilize in ultrafine (<0.1 μm) metal oxide particles during emission. Photochemical reactions also promote acid sulfate formation via both metal-dependent and independent mechanisms, but studies have shown that most of the oxidation of SO_2 occurs within plumes as they disperse in the atmosphere. Stack emissions may undergo long-range transport to areas distant from the emission source, allowing considerable time for sunlight-driven chemistry. Although the fine particle sulfates may exist as fine sulfuric acid (the primary source of free H$^+$), partially or fully neutralized forms of sulfate predominate due to the abundance of natural atmospheric ammonia. As fine PM sulfates are transported long distances, they may contribute to regional summer haze and pose a health hazard to certain groups such as asthmatics (Koenig *et al.*, 1989), and may also stress the general environment as acid rain (Calvert *et al.*, 1985) (Fig. 29-13). The CAA and

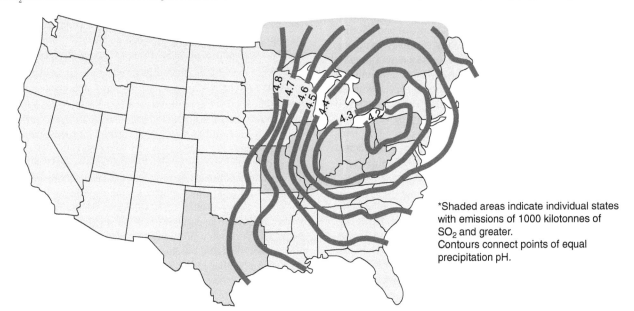

*Shaded areas indicate individual states with emissions of 1000 kilotonnes of SO_2 and greater.
Contours connect points of equal precipitation pH.

Figure 29-13. *Areas in 1988 where precipitation in the East fell below pH 5: acid rain.* The acidity of the air in the east is thought to result from air mass transport of fine sulfated particulate matter from the industrial centers of the Midwest (U.S. EPA, 2000a).

subsequent regulations for the reduction of sulfur emissions (eg, the 1990 Acid Rain Program and the 2012 Cross State Air Pollution Rule) continue to reduce the environmental acidification and visibility problems associated with transport and deposition of acidic products formed from stack emissions in North America.

General Toxicology Sulfuric acid irritates by virtue of its ability to protonate (H^+) receptor ligands and other biomolecules. This action can either directly damage membranes or activate sensory reflexes that initiate inflammation. Ammonia, which exists in free air at about 25 ppb and in much higher concentrations within the mammalian naso-oropharynx (in the human up to 350 ppm), is capable of neutralizing most of the irritant acidic sulfates (Utell *et al.*, 1989). Neutralization can also be quite efficient in standard whole-body animal exposure studies, in which excreta and bacteria in the chambers interact, giving rise to in-chamber ammonia concentrations up to 1100 ppb—more than enough to fully neutralize neat sulfuric acid up to several mg/m^3 (Higuchi and Davies, 1993).

Interestingly, there is considerable species variability in sensitivity to sulfuric acid, with guinea pigs being quite responsive to acid sulfates, in contrast to rats, which seem generally resistant. The reasons for this difference relate to sensory fiber network density in the airways, and probably not on differences in neutralization by ammonia in the airway. The sensitivity of healthy humans appears to fall somewhere in between, with asthmatic humans being perhaps best modeled by the guinea pig. Overall, however, the collective data involving animals and humans are remarkably coherent (Amdur, 1989).

Unlike other irritants, such as O_3 (see below), inhaled sulfuric acid does not appear to stimulate a classic neutrophilic lung inflammation. Rather, eicosanoid homeostasis appears to be disturbed resulting in macrophage dysfunction and altered host defense.

Pulmonary Function Effects Sulfuric acid produces an increase in flow resistance in guinea pigs due to reflex airway narrowing, or bronchoconstriction, which impedes the flow of air into and out of the lungs. This response might be thought of as a defensive measure to limit the inhalation of air containing noxious gases, but this explanation may be more teleological than fact. The magnitude of the response is related to both acid concentration and particle size (Amdur *et al.*, 1978). Early studies indicated that as particle size was reduced from 7 μm to the submicrometer range, the concentration of sulfuric acid necessary to induce a response and the time to the onset of the response fell significantly. With large particles, even the sensitive guinea pig was able to withstand an exceedingly high (30 mg/m^3) challenge with little change in pulmonary resistance, in contrast to the <1 mg/m^3 challenge needed with the 0.3-μm particles (Amdur *et al.*, 1978). Human asthmatics exposed to 2 mg/m^3 of acid fog (10 μm) for one hour, a very high concentration for an asthmatic, experienced variable respiratory symptoms suggesting irritation, but no changes in spirometry were elicited (Hackney *et al.*, 1989). The apparent reason for this PM size–based differential is probably the scrubbing of large particles in the nose, while small particles are able to penetrate deep into the lung. The thicker mucus blanket of the nose may also blunt (by dilution or neutralization by mucus buffers) much of the irritancy of the deposited acid. In contrast, the less shielded distal airway tissues, with higher receptor density, would be expected to be more sensitive to the acid particles reaching that area (Costa and Schlegele, 1998). Regional sensitivity and the longer residence times of a deposited particle relative to SO_2 gas are reflected in the relatively protracted recovery times observed in acid-exposed guinea pigs compared with those in animals exposed to SO_2 alone.

Asthmatics appear to be somewhat more sensitive to the bronchoconstrictive effects of sulfuric acid than are healthy individuals, but published studies have been inconsistent in this finding (Koenig *et al.*, 1989; Utell *et al.*, 1984). Asthma generally is characterized by hyperresponsive airways, so their tendency to constrict at low acid concentrations would be expected, just as asthmatic airways are sensitive to nonspecific airway smooth muscle agonists (eg, carbachol, histamine, exercise). The variability may well relate to differences in the degree of impairment or underlying inflammation in the subjects, but this hypothesis remains to be confirmed. Airway hyperreactivity has been observed as an acute response in guinea pigs two hours after a one-hour exposure to 200 μg/m^3 sulfuric acid and appears to be associated with pulmonary inflammation. Likewise in rabbits, increased airway reactivity was associated with arachidonate metabolites, products of both epithelial and inflammatory cells. The general correlation between airway responsiveness and inflammation that appears to be important in grading asthma severity and risk of negative clinical outcomes may also be predictive of responses to environmental stimuli.

Effects on Mucociliary Clearance and Macrophage Function Sulfuric acid alters the clearance of particles from the lung. Using insoluble, radioactively labeled ferric oxide particles as a probe, as little as a single one-hour exposure in donkeys, rabbits, and human subjects can slow clearance. Mucus clearance appears to vary directly with the acidity ($[H^+]$) of the acid sulfate, with sulfuric acid having the greatest effect and ammonium sulfate the smallest (Schlesinger, 1984). Curiously, there appears to be a biphasic response to acid. In general, brief, single exposures of <250 μg/m^3 accelerate clearance, while high concentrations of >1000 μg/m^3 clearly depress clearance. With repeated daily exposures to low levels, there appears to be a cumulative (concentration times duration) dose-related depression of clearance. Longer-term exposure of rabbits to low-level acid also results in hyperplasia of airway mucosecretory cells (Gearhart and Schlesinger, 1989).

Collectively, there seems to be coherence in the data to rank sulfate irritancy: sulfuric acid > ammonium bisulfate > ammonium sulfate. Acidity $[H^+]$ appears to be the primary driver on most respiratory effects attributable to the acid sulfates even at the level of pulmonary macrophages. Lavaged rabbit macrophage phagocytosis was affected more after a single exposure to 500 μg/m^3 sulfuric acid than after exposure to 2000 μg/m^3 ammonium bisulfate (Schlesinger *et al.*, 1990). Nevertheless, in the complexity of summer haze, it remains unclear whether the bioactive form of $[H^+]$ is more appropriately assayed as free ion concentration (as pH) or as total available ion concentration (titratable H^+).

Chronic Effects Not surprisingly, sulfuric acid induces qualitatively similar effects in the airways as found at high concentrations of SO_2. As a fine aerosol, sulfuric acid deposits deeper along the respiratory tract, and its high specific acidity imparts greater effect on various cells (eg, phagocytes and epithelial cells). Thus, a primary concern with regard to chronic inhalation of acidic aerosols is the potential for bronchitis, since this has been a problem in occupational settings in which employees are exposed to sulfuric acid mists (eg, battery plants). Early studies in the donkey (later confirmed in a rabbit model) have provided fundamental data on this issue. The depression of clearance observed in donkeys exposed repeatedly (100 μg/m^3 one hour per day for six months) raises concerns that a similar response (potentially contributing to chronic bronchitis) can occur in humans. Studies with cigarette smoke showed parallel responses.

Studies conducted with sulfuric acid in the rabbit are in general agreement with the early findings in the donkey (Schlesinger,

1984). The initial early stimulation of clearance with subsequent depression has been shown to occur over 12 months with as little as two hours per day at 125 µg/m³ sulfuric acid (Schlesinger *et al.*, 1992). Related studies also have demonstrated that the airways of exposed animals become progressively more sensitive to challenge with acetylcholine, show a progressive decrease in diameter, and experience an increase in the number of secretory cells, especially in the smaller airways. These studies have expanded our knowledge of the biological response and its exposure-based relationship to sulfuric acid. It seems reasonable to postulate that chronic daily exposure of humans to ~100 µg/m³ sulfuric acid may lead to impaired clearance and mild chronic bronchitis. The possibility that chronic irritancy may elicit bronchitis-like disease in susceptible individuals (perhaps over a lifetime or in children because of dose differences) appears to be reasonable.

Particulate Matter

PM was referred to as "soot" in the "reducing-type" air pollution of the classic episodes. The major constituents of this soot consisted of incompletely burned carbonaceous materials, acid sulfates, various metals, and silicates associated with the solid nature of the fuel. Metals were abundant, with a considerable amount of zinc in the form of zinc sulfate—as reported from postepisode analyses of the Donora PM. Soot is indicative of poorly (inefficiently) combusted fuel. Over time, combustion technology and improved fuels provided gains by increasing efficiency and minimizing gross soot emissions. Improvements in combustion methods simultaneously reduced the size of emitted particles and overall less mass. A side benefit of the smaller particles was the reduction in light diffraction through the emissions and hence a less visible plume. As such, much of the early cleanup was largely achieved through technological improvements. Carbon in fuel that is not fully oxidized to CO_2 persists in elemental form or as products of incomplete combustion—organic carbon. Oxidized S becomes sulfate and many of the metals appear as oxides. As noted above, sulfate was long suspected as the culprit of most health impacts associated with stationary sources, but this relationship is less discernable in contemporary particle epidemiology and toxicology.

In the last 20 years PM has reemerged as the dominant issue in the air pollution community, overtaking O_3 as the pressing air pollution health issue. The reason for this shift was the emergence of epidemiology data consistently showing increased mortality, an adverse effect of greatest import with the major impact on the cost/benefit analyses. As already noted, the collective studies showed health impacts (both morbidity and mortality) at levels of PM thought to be "safe" with no apparent threshold (reviewed in Pope and Dockery, 2006). Over time, science advances and reanalyses have confirmed the initial mortality findings. Several hypotheses that lend "biological plausibility" to the findings have emerged along with several "ancillary" impacts of PM on health not previously realized. The impacts of PM on health appear to be ever expanding, beyond lung effects, perhaps with even greater cardiovascular effects and an ever growing body of data suggesting impacts on neurologic and reproductive health, as well as growth and development.

PM in the atmosphere can be solid, liquid, or a combination of both with a mélange of organic, inorganic, and biological compounds. The compositional matrix of PM can vary significantly depending on the emission source and secondary transformations, many of which involve gas to particle conversions. Long-range transport of emissions or transformation products can contribute significantly to the regional matrix of PM, particularly in the case of sulfate of East Coast $PM_{2.5}$. Particles of larger size tend to have more local sources, the reason being that they are formed from dispersed dust and attrition of materials. Being of larger size, they tend to "fall out" or settle from the air due to gravity (although winds can in fact carry these particles great distances—eg, Sahara desert particles have been found on the US East Coast). Particles in the range of 10 to 2.5 µm ($PM_{10-2.5}$—coarse PM) are highly inhalable by humans. In the urban setting there is considerable spatial and temporal heterogeneity of coarse PM while $PM_{2.5}$ appears more homogenous throughout a regional environment. The size designation of fine and coarse PM is based on their relative respirability—those in the range of PM_{10} are inhalable into the larger thoracic airways while the $PM_{2.5}$ is inhalable into the deeper reaches (gas exchange areas) of the lung (see Chap. 15).

The large epidemiological database contending that PM elicits both short- and long-term health effects is largely founded on data from monitoring networks used for PM regulation. As such, the PM-associated effects appear to be dependent on the gravimetric measures that these networks yield. From this, it might then be argued that the effects are not influenced by particle composition (eg, inorganic and organic components). Further, because the findings strengthen with decreasing particle size (eg, total suspended particulate mass [pre-1978 index], PM_{10}, $PM_{2.5}$), it is the mass concentration of PM, despite compositional complexity and variation, that is the index of choice. However, toxicologists argue that a mass-based relationship contradicts the basic tenets of conventional air pollution toxicology, which is rooted in the concept of chemical-specific toxicities. A number of hypotheses that draw on various physical and chemical attributes of PM have also been offered in search of a "biologically plausible" explanation for the reported epidemiological observations. However, no one constituent has been identified as singularly determinant of the spectrum of health impacts. The smallest particles, which derive from anthropogenic combustion activities, appear to drive many of the health effects of particles. Prominently included among the causative hypotheses that tie toxicity to particle characteristics are metals, organics, acidity, size distribution (focusing on the unique bioactivity of ultrafine PM—PM <0.1 µm), PM oxidant activity or reactivity, and the presence of potentially toxic or allergenic biologicals. However, at present, there remains insufficient understanding of the relative importance of these theories to choose one over another, especially if the spectrum of heath effects is included. As a result, there seems to be insufficient reason to unseat the PM mass-based correlation with health outcomes as the driver of regulatory policies. Although the laboratory animal and human toxicological database is growing rapidly with regard to the issue of causation, much remains to be learned before new regulatory indices can be considered.

From research directed initially toward potential occupational hazards, it is known that several metals and silicates that make up much of the inorganic phase of PM can be cytotoxic to lung cells. Organic constituents, as well, can induce toxicity either directly or via metabolism product—some of which are genotoxic. Other PM attributes may also come into play. Studies focusing on very small, ultrafine particles suggest that although these particles are low in mass, they are high in number and thus provide substantial reactive particle surface to interact with biological substances. Less is known about the role of biologically derived materials, such as endotoxin, glucans, plant glycoproteins, and bioallergen fragments, which may elicit rudimentary inflammatory responses in the lung. The involvement of biologicals may be greatest in agricultural and indoor exposure environments. There has been considerable interest in PM–copollutant interactions, but our knowledge in this area is somewhat limited and has spurred toxicologists to better access the experience and knowledge of atmospheric scientists as to the atmospheric interactions that are most relevant to biological outcomes.

Metals There have been many standard acute and subchronic rodent inhalation studies with specific metal compounds, often as oxides, chlorides, or sulfates. These exposure studies relate most appropriately to occupational exposures. The varied systemic toxicities of metal compounds are presented in detail elsewhere in this book; however, it should be appreciated that the effects of metals delivered by inhalation may differ from their impacts when administered by other routes. Metals may arise from natural as well as anthropogenic activities, and as a result metals are a common constituent in ambient PM. The metal profiles among regions differ appreciably in concentration and type and they also differ by the size mode of PM. Coarse PM (2.5–10 μm) arises largely from natural sources and thus has prominent earthen metals such as iron, sodium, silica, and magnesium—usually in oxide forms. Combustion-derived metals reflect the fuel source. For example, oil may have vanadium, nickel, and perhaps zinc and iron, while coal may have zinc and selenium. Their chemical forms vary from water-soluble salts to oxide and phosphate forms. Other metals are emitted from vehicles burning fuels to which metal compounds were added to alter functionality (eg, lead, manganese, platinum) or as engine wear and catalyst by-products. Similarly, metals may also derive from brake (copper, iron), tire (zinc), and dispersed road (earthen silicates) wear. Metals have many biological properties, some essential to life while others being directly toxic to cells or act indirectly in a pro-oxidant toxic fashion. Thus, metals have garnered considerable interest regarding their role in PM toxicity (Costa and Dreher, 1997).

Metal compounds can be separated nominally by physicochemical characteristics: those that are essentially water-insoluble (eg, metal oxides and hydroxides such as those that might be released from high-temperature combustion sources or derived from the geocrustal matrix) and those that are soluble or somewhat soluble in water (often chlorides or sulfates such as those that might form under acidic conditions in a smoke plume or leach from acid-hydrated silicate particles in the atmosphere). Solubility appears to play a role in the toxicity of many inhaled metals by enhancing metal bioavailability (eg, nickel from nickel chloride vs nickel oxide), but insolubility can also be a critical factor in determining toxicity by increasing pulmonary residence time within the lung (eg, insoluble cadmium oxide vs soluble cadmium chloride). Moreover, some metals, either in their soluble forms or when partially coordinated on the surface of silicate or bioorganic materials, can promote electron transfer to form reactive oxidants. Complexes with particulate organic material in a partially hydrated form (as might be promoted by the presence of sea salt) have been shown to interact with poorly soluble metals to free coordination sites that again are pro-oxidant (Kieber et al., 2005). Thus, caution is warranted in assessing inhaled PM-associated metals, as both their chemical and physical attributes and their interaction with cocontaminants in PM may influence their apparent toxicity. Simply measuring total metal mass to estimate effects in the lung can be misleading.

Perhaps the most compelling evidence for a role of soluble metals in PM toxicity derives from a series of studies on PM sampled in Utah Valley where a large open hearth steel mill went from full production to a one-year hiatus due to a strike and then resumed its open hearth operations. These studies related the metal content of PM sampled in the area to plant operation showing a reduction in total PM as well as a reduction of >90% PM metal content during the strike. Studies of hospital admissions for a variety of lung ailments and death rates showed reductions during the strike and toxicological studies where PM extractions from the operational and shutdown periods were tested in human and animal lungs, as well as on human lung epithelial cells, all correlated with plant operations, PM metal content, and the findings in parallel population studies (Pope, 1996; Dye et al., 2001; Ghio, 2004).

Gas–Particle Interactions As already noted, these gas–particle interactions can be extremely complex involving multiple components of the particles, gases/vapors, and sunlight. However, more than 40 years ago, generic binary interactions between particles and gases in the absence of light were shown to alter the toxicity of either the particle or the gas acting alone. The guinea pig bronchoconstriction model used for many years by Amdur and associates showed early on that SO_2 can interact with hydrated metal salts to potentiate particle irritancy. The mechanism(s) behind this interaction has yet to be fully discerned, but it appears to involve solubility of SO_2 in a hydrated aerosol and the ability of the metal to catalyze the oxidation of the dissolved SO_2 to sulfate. In the case of sodium chloride aerosol, potentiation appeared to be governed primarily by the solubility of SO_2 in the salt droplet and enhanced respiratory penetration. The metal salts of manganese, iron, and vanadium, on the other hand, catalyzed the formation of sulfate. Studies in humans have been less revealing about such interactions, but this database affirms the need to consider the complexity of the atmospheric challenge in estimating biological outcomes.

Complex chemistry also occurs within the effluent of the combustion source. Using a laboratory-scale furnace, the emission mix of sulfuric acid and metal oxide particles common to metal smelting and coal combustion was used to explore potential plume interactions that might impact respiratory irritancy (Amdur et al., 1986). These emitted metal oxide particles, once aged and cooled, were a mixture of singlet and agglomerated ultrafine particles that would be expected to distribute throughout the lung on inhalation. Exposures in guinea pigs of 30 to 60 μg/m³ sulfuric acid combined with ultrafine zinc oxide produced progressive decreases in DL_{CO}, total lung capacity, and vital capacity and increases in cells, protein, and a variety of enzymes in lavage fluid that were not completely resolved 96 hours after exposure (Amdur, 1989). It is unclear whether the acid was on the surface of the particles or made the metal more soluble, but the combination was clearly more toxic than acid alone. These effects greatly exceeded the changes in airway resistance found with relatively simple, binary mixture of SO_2 and water-soluble metal salts.

Combustion studies using different coals again emphasized the significance of surface-associated acidic S-compounds. Ultrafine combustion particles from Illinois No. 6 coal had a layer of sulfuric acid adsorbed on the surfaces resulting in greater effects in guinea pigs than the more alkaline Montana lignite. Despite the greater sulfur content of the Montana coal, this emission ultrafine particle had neutralized the irritating sulfate (Chen et al., 1990). Similar studies using inert carbon black appear consistent with its role as carrier for reactive gases such as O_3 and various aldehydes to enhance delivery of toxic materials to the deep lung (Jakab, 1992). The result of the latter study was enhanced infectivity when the carbon-gas preexposed test animals were subsequently exposed to pathologic bacteria.

Similar interactions may result from gaseous pollutants that impair the clearance of particles from the lung or otherwise alter their metabolism. Studies by Laskin at New York University in the 1960s showed an intriguing interaction of SO_2 and benzo(a)pyrene. It was thought that impaired clearance and greater residence time in the lung led to the enhanced probability of carcinogenic expression of the particle. Similarly, rats exposed to an urban eight-hour daily profile of O_3 for six weeks, followed by a five-hour exposure to asbestos, were found to retain three times as many fibers as did the controls 30 days postexposure. The fibers were deposited in the distal airways and penetrated more deeply into airway tissues making them less accessible to phagocytic removal (Pinkerton *et al.*, 1989). These studies, together with those focusing on irritancy and infectivity, raise the prospect that realistic exposure scenarios of gaseous and particulate pollutants can interact through either chemical or physiologic mechanisms to enhance health risks of complex polluted atmospheres.

Ultrafine Carbonaceous Matter Ultrafine carbon particles (often called black carbon) typically result from high-temperature pyrolysis or as the product of atmospheric transformation involving organic vapors and sunlight. The size of these particles allows them to slip between gas molecules moving primarily by diffusion and principles of Brownian motion. Agglomeration on surfaces or other particles in the air is their primary mode of dissipation. When concentrations exceed ~1 million/cm^3, they rapidly agglomerate with each other to form larger clumps or chains of ultrafine particles. As an air pollutant, therefore, elemental carbon particles generally do not exist as singlets except near their emission points—for example, traffic or other high-temperature sources. Fine PM consists in part of agglomerates of carbonaceous organic material that if partially oxidized may be somewhat soluble in water. Some organic materials, which exist in the vapor form, condense on the ultrafine carbon (eg diesel PM). Estimates of the carbonaceous (including organic) content of ambient fine PM vary considerably but are nominally considered to be about 10% to 60% of the total mass depending on the urban or regional area. The sources of organic carbon are varied and include the combustion products of natural smoke (eg, forest fires), engine exhaust, and stationary sources as well as transformed condensates from VOCs in the air. Elemental carbon in diesel PM frequently combines into long ultrafine chains, with variably complex organics associated with its surface depending on the combustion conditions. It has been estimated that diesel contributes about 7% of the fine urban PM emissions, which, when expressed as an annual US average, is about 2 μg/m^3 (USEPA, 1993)—but focus estimates (urban canyons) vary widely. The higher use of diesel fuel in Europe and areas of concentrated trucking in the United States has led to estimates as high as 30% of ambient fine PM mass. Elemental carbon has traditionally been associated with traffic, but it is a better marker of older vehicles as new engine technology for diesels, designed to meet new emission standards in 2007 and 2010, emits substantially (>98%) less black carbon. Automobiles release even less. The expected result over the next 20 years, with the turnover of truck fleets in particular, is a great reduction in ambient levels of elemental carbon.

Recent epidemiological and field studies with PM have been focusing on black carbon as an index of traffic and have reported strong associations between traffic (through the carbon indicator) and health effects. Most notably the observed adverse effects have been cardiovascular, thus giving some credence to hypotheses that ultrafine particles somehow find their way into the systemic circulation (see below) or trigger systemic inflammation that links to the cardiovascular effects (Peters, 2006; Tong *et al.*, 2010). The penetration of ultrafine particles into the circulation under experimental conditions appears to be composition dependent (Kreyling *et al.*, 2009).

Diesel particles vary widely in the ratio of organic and elemental carbonaceous materials, which in empirical studies has been shown to influence toxic outcomes, such as to their inflammatory and carcinogenic potential (Singh *et al.*, 2004). Some diesel particles also appear to have adjuvant activity when tested with bioallergens in both animals and humans (Diaz-Sanchez *et al.*, 1999). When reacted in vitro with O_3, there appears to be an enhancement of lung inflammation relative to the diesel or O_3 alone (Madden *et al.*, 2000). However, it is important to realize that diesel particles should not be equated with whole diesel exhaust that also contains significant amounts of gaseous pollutants: NO_x, CO, and SO_x as well as various VOCs and carbonyl irritants. Exposure to diluted diesel exhaust in humans reveals that the exhaust mix is inflammogenic and to a degree cytotoxic to airway cells (Ghio *et al.*, 2012). The use of diesel particles alone in toxicology studies does not seem to display similar toxicity, thus underscoring the potential importance of interactions among air pollutants as a critical consideration in air pollution toxicity (Mauderly and Samet, 2009).

Elemental carbon itself is generally considered to be of low toxicity, although long-term, high-concentration exposure conditions in rats can lead to lung "overload" where there is evidence of lung damage and carcinogenicity (addressed below). In the environment, carbon has the potential to act as a carrier of certain irritant gases as was noted earlier. However, carbon in the ultrafine mode (<0.1 μm) has been suggested to be more toxic than the fine mode (2.5 μm) form, perhaps due to enhanced surface reactivity or tissue penetration (Oberdorster *et al.*, 2002; Donaldson *et al.*, 1998). Size is not the only factor as it appears that composition of the ultrafine particle also contributes to its effects and behavior (Kreyling *et al.*, 2009). Ultrafine particles in the environment exist in extremely high numbers but contribute negligibly to mass. Recent commercial introduction of "engineered" nanoparticles brings many of the same concerns as ultrafines by virtue of their similar sizes. Additionally, being "engineered" particles, they may possess design features that "natural" combustion ultrafine (or nano) particles do not.

Chronic Effects and Cancer The role of air pollution in human lung cancer is difficult to assess because the vast majority of respiratory cancers result from cigarette smoking. The ACS study noted above (Pope *et al.*, 2011) showed a significant linkage between PM and lung cancer, but in general it has been difficult to show these effects for the many HAP compounds that occur as urban air pollutants and are also thought to be carcinogenic. However, most of the HAPs and even fewer (about 10%) of the more than 2800 compounds that have been identified in the air have been assayed for carcinogenic potency. Fig. 29-14 gives estimates of the relative contributions of various chemicals to the lung cancer rate that are *not* associated with cigarette smoking, which, for outdoor air, is estimated to be about 2000 cases per year (Lewtas, 1993). This compares with about 2000 cases per year for passive environmental tobacco smoke and >100,000 cases per year for smokers. VOCs and nitrogen-containing and halogenated organics account for most of the compounds that have been studied with animal and genotoxicity bioassays. Most of these compounds are derived from combustion sources ranging from tobacco to power plants to incinerators to motor vehicles. Other potential carcinogens arise from mobile sources (including diesel) as products of incomplete combustion as well as their atmospheric transformation products. Fugitive or accidental chemical releases also figure into the many chemicals in ambient air. The National Scale Air Toxics Assessment (NATA) is an assessment of the cancer and noncancer risks associated with ambient HAPs (www.epa.gov/nata2005/). The profile of outdoor carcinogens contrasts with that of indoor air, where the sources are thought to derive largely from environmental tobacco smoke and radon, with some contribution from off-gassed organics (eg, adhesives, carpet polymers, cleaning agents). Human exposure to

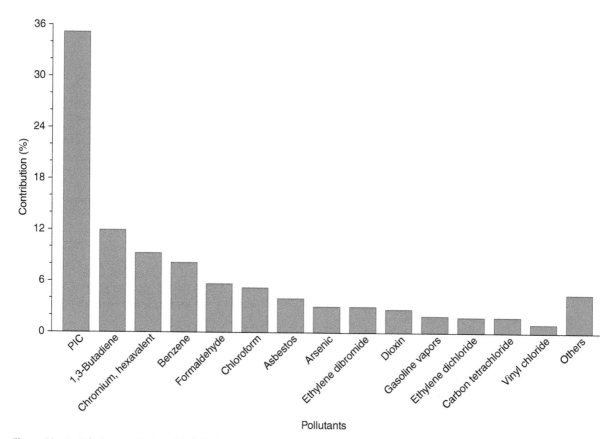

Figure 29-14. *Relative contribution of individual airborne hazardous pollutants to lung cancer rates after removal of tobacco smoke cancer.* The total number of cancers from non-tobacco-smoke sources is estimated to be about 2000 per year. PIC, products of incomplete combustion. (Reproduced with permission from Lewtas, 1993.)

airborne toxicants is highly complex compositionally as well as in its temporal and spatial heterogeneity.

The lung cancer risk of any individual is some function of the carcinogenic nature of the substance, the amount of material deposited in the lungs, which is itself a function of the concentration in the ambient air, the physical and chemical properties of the inhalant that may determine deposition efficiency, and the cumulative volume of air inhaled. Of course, the innate susceptibility of the individual (including genotype and environmental factors such as diet, etc) is also likely to be important. A significant body of data suggests that the majority of lung cancer risk from ambient air pollution lies within the PM fraction. Among the many potent chemicals are the polycyclic organic chemicals, along with a group of less-volatile organics sometimes referred to as "semivolatiles" (including nitroaromatics). These persistent organics associate with the PM matrix and thus could have a prolonged residence time at deposition sites within the respiratory tract. Genetic bioassays have revealed the potent mutagenicity, and presumably carcinogenicity, of various chemical fractions of ambient aerosols (Lewtas, 2007). Some of these compounds require metabolic transformation to activate their potency while others may be detoxified by their metabolism. Not to be forgotten, although not a feature of this chapter, are carcinogenic vapors such as benzene that are inhaled but have target tissues away from the lung—in the case of benzene, bone marrow leukemia.

The cells lining the respiratory tract turn over relatively quickly, since they interface with the ambient environment with every breath. Conceptually, their DNA would thus be vulnerable to carcinogenic or oxidant-induced replication errors that, when fixed as mutations, could give rise to tumors. Copollutants, such as irritant gases, that initiate inflammation may promote carcinogenic activity by damaging cells and further enhancing their turnover.

For example, there is experimental evidence that benzo(*a*)pyrene inhaled by rats whose respiratory tracts have been chronically exposed to SO$_2$ are prone to bronchogenic carcinomas. Likewise, epidermoid carcinomas were produced in mice that inhaled ozonized gasoline vapors, containing many reactive organic products, but only if these mice had been previously infected with influenza virus and presumably had inflamed lungs. Many believe that the so-called rural–urban gradient of lung cancer, apparent even when corrected for cigarette smoking, is a product of such complex interactions. Thus, while the phenomenon of environmental lung cancer remains poorly understood, there is general sentiment for the early opinion expressed by Kotin and Falk in 1963: "Chemical, physical and biological data unite to form a constellation that strongly implicates the atmosphere as one dominant factor in the pathogenesis of lung cancer." At the time of this statement, however, the role of tobacco smoke was not widely appreciated.

To understand the role of inhaled particles to non-cigarette-smoke-related lung cancer, chronic exposure studies have been conducted with a number of particles ranging from titanium dioxide and carbon to diesel exhaust and coal fly ash aerosol. Of these substances, diesel exhaust has been the most extensively studied (reviewed by Cohen and Nikula, 1999; Ghio *et al.*, 2012). The primary concern with diesel has been the suspicion that it can induce lung cancer (thus its IARC classification as a Group 1 human carcinogen). However, the evidence from over 40 occupational studies (primarily railway yard, truck, and bus workers) implicating diesel exhaust as a mild carcinogen continues to be debated because of a variety of confounding issues (Gamble, 2010). Taking the empirical data alone, however, carcinogenicity is suggested by several chronic exposure studies in animals and in vitro data indicating mutagenicity in *Salmonella* bacteria and enhanced sister chromatid exchange rates in Chinese hamster ovary cells. (The latter genotoxic effects have been linked to the nitroarenes associated with the diesel PM.) Rodent studies, unfortunately, have not fully resolved the question of human carcinogenic risk because of the overload needed to yield positive results, and the tumors develop only in the rat. At high concentrations of diesel PM (3.5 and 7 mg/m³), normal mucociliary clearance in the rodent models becomes overwhelmed, resulting in a progressive buildup of particles in the lungs. By 12 months in the rat, clearance irreversibly decreases to cessation with concomitant inflammation, oxidant generation, epithelial hyperplasia, and fibrosis. Rats seem to react more to this circumstance. Particle agglomerates within the alveolar lumen become the focus of inflammation, injury, and the eventual development of adenosarcomas and squamous cell carcinomas. At lower concentrations, where the particle buildup does not occur, tumors do not develop.

"Overload" is a common finding at the highest exposure concentrations of chronic particle inhalation bioassays. While this phenomenon is not likely in humans exposed to ambient PM, it is a hypothesis worthy of consideration in a discussion of particle health effects, as it relates to the interpretation of toxicological data relevant to product use and industrial exposures. Several poorly soluble particles (PSPs) have induced lung tumors in chronic rat bioassays under conditions of overload; tumors have not developed under similar conditions in mice and hamsters. Among these particles are titanium dioxide, carbon black, toner dust, talc, and diesel emission; the potential for tumors is especially marked when the particles are in the ultrafine mode. In the rat, the timecourse and pattern of accumulation, chronic inflammation, epithelial hyperplasia, and tumorigenesis are essentially the same for all of the particles. In contrast, the degree of active inflammation in the mouse and hamster under similar overload conditions appears less intense, and thus is an important distinction among the species that relates to their relative sensitivities. On one hand, such exposures do not typically demonstrate classic in vivo genotoxicity, although bulky adducts and other modifications to DNA have been described after in vivo exposure to carbon black and diesel exhaust (reviewed by Schins and Knaapen, 2007). Also, mutation of the *hprt* (hypoxanthine guanine phosphorybosyl transferase) gene was found in rat epithelial cells cultured with bronchoalveolar lavage from chronic carbon black– and titanium dioxide–treated rats (Driscoll *et al.*, 1997). Even though these few studies have demonstrated inert particle-induced modifications to DNA, generalizing this finding to overload cancers, not surprisingly, remains controversial. Typically, the pathways leading to lung cancer by relatively inert and PSPs (eg, carbon black and diesel exhaust particles) are thought to be secondary and involve pathways such as oxidative stress rather than a primary carcinogenesis mechanism such as DNA mutations (Greim *et al.*, 2001). The closest analogy in humans would be coal miners who do not appear to have an enhanced risk of lung cancer except when smoking is not involved.

The issue, then, is whether rat bioassay cancer data under conditions of overload are relevant to risk assessment. A review by an expert panel (ILSI, 2000) concluded that rats, while apparently unique in this response, may represent a sensitive subgroup, and that tumorigenesis data from the rat bioassay under conditions of overload cannot be summarily dismissed as not relevant to the consideration of cancer risk in humans. However, the data should be interpreted and weighed in the context of lower concentrations and the tumor incidence and pathology found therein.

Photochemical Air Pollution

Photochemical air pollution (notably O_3) remains the most elusive of the criteria pollutants to bring under control. It arises secondarily

from a series of complex reactions in the troposphere activated by the ultraviolet (UV) spectrum of sunlight. In addition to O_3, it comprises a mixture of nitric oxides (NO_x), aldehydes, peroxyacetyl nitrates (PAN), and a myriad of aromatics and alkenes along with analog reactive radicals. If SO_2 is present, sulfates may also be formed and, collectively, they yield "summer haze." Likewise, the complex chemistry can generate organic PM, nitric acid vapor, and various condensates. Attempts to mitigate photochemical smog (especially O_3) by controlling hydrocarbon and/or NO_x emissions have proven difficult due to the complex stoichiometry of atmospheric photochemistry. Some progress has been made in controlling peak values in the United States (regulated by the pre-1997 one-hour NAAQS), but the longer-time-frame eight-hour NAAQS has seen generally less progress. Because of a particularly strong regulatory effort in Southern California, however, the average number of high ozone days per year dropped by 33% between 2000 and 2010 (State of the Air, 2012) in the Los Angeles–Long Beach–Riverside metropolitan area, the most polluted part of the United States, in terms of ambient ozone levels.

From the point of view of the toxicology of photochemical air pollutant gases, O_3 is by far the toxicant of greatest concern. It is highly reactive and more toxic than NO_x, and because its generation is fueled through cyclic hydrocarbon radicals, it reaches greater concentrations than the hydrocarbon radical intermediates. The gaseous hydrocarbons, so integral to the chemistry, are no longer listed collectively as a criteria pollutant in the United States since they do not have a strong health-based driver. In general, the concentrations of the hydrocarbon precursors in ambient air do not reach levels high enough to produce acute toxicity, although some individual compounds fall under the HAPs rule. Rather, the importance of these hydrocarbons stems from their role in the chain of photochemical reactions.

Although O_3 is of toxicological importance in the troposphere, in the stratosphere it plays a critical protective role. About 10 to 50 km above the earth's surface, UV light directly splits molecular O_2 into atomic $O^\bullet$, which then combines with O_2 to form O_3. The O_3 also dissociates back but much more slowly. The result is an accumulation of O_3 to several ppm within a relatively thin strip of the stratosphere forming an effective "permanent" barrier by absorbing the short-wavelength UV in the chemical process. This barrier had in recent years been threatened by various anthropogenic emissions (Cl_2 gas and certain chlorofluorocarbons) that enhance O_3 degradation (creation of an "O_3 hole"), but recent restrictions on the use of these degrading chemicals seem to have been effective in reversing this process. The benefits are believed to be a reduction of excess UV light infiltration to the earth's surface and reduced skin cancer risk.

This protective issue is quite different in the troposphere, where accumulation of O_3 serves no known purpose and poses a threat to the respiratory tract. Near the earth's surface, NO_2 arising from combustion processes efficiently absorbs longer-wavelength UV light, from which a free O atom is cleaved, initiating the following simplified series of reactions:

$$NO_2 + h\nu \text{ (UV light)} \rightarrow O^\bullet + NO^\bullet \qquad (29\text{-}1)$$

$$O^\bullet + O_2 \rightarrow O_3 \qquad (29\text{-}2)$$

$$O_3 + NO^\bullet \rightarrow NO_2 \qquad (29\text{-}3)$$

This process is inherently cyclic, with NO_2 regenerated by the reaction of the $NO^\bullet$ and O_3. In the absence of unsaturated hydrocarbons (olefins and substituted aromatics) arising from fuel vaporization or combustion, as well as biogenic terpenes, this series of reactions would approach a steady state with little buildup of O_3. The free electrons of the double bonds of unsaturated hydrocarbons are attacked by free atomic $O^\bullet$, resulting in oxidized compounds and radicals that react further with $NO^\bullet$ to produce more NO_2. Thus, the balance of the reactions sequence shown in Eqs. (29-1) to (29-3) is tipped to the right, leading to buildup of O_3. This reaction is particularly favored when the sun's intensity is greatest at midday, utilizing the NO_2 provided by morning rush-hour traffic. Carbonyl compounds (especially short-chained aldehydes) are also by-products of these reactions. Formaldehyde and acrolein account for about 50% and 5%, respectively, of the total aldehyde content in urban atmospheres. Peroxyacetyl nitrate (CH_3COONO_2), often referred to as PAN, and its homologs also arise in urban air, most likely from the reaction of the peroxyacyl radicals with NO_2. In the evening when sun intensity wanes, the second rush-hour peak of NO_2 shifts the balance back by reacting with O_3 bringing the daytime peak concentration slowly down. In assessing the excess adverse effects of O_3, it is important to determine the background level of ambient O_3. Interestingly, background levels of ozone in North America are known to peak as high as 0.14 ppm (one hour), particularly in high elevation regions such as Wyoming, although the contribution of these transient one-hour levels of ozone to public health is unclear. This high altitude peak concentration is thought to be due to a combination of high VOC levels, NO_x, and the additional UV light reflected off snow cover. However, other factors such as season, thickness of boundary layers, vertical intrusions from the stratosphere, and long-range transport also play roles in determining background levels of O_3 in North America.

Short-Term Exposures to Smog

In the 1950s to 1960s, early air pollution toxicologists were challenged by the complexity of photochemical air pollution both to ascertain its potential to adversely affect human health and to determine what about these atmospheres was responsible for the effects. The focus was immediately placed on O_3 because its toxicity was found to be very high even at low ppm concentrations. Concerns that the complex atmosphere was even more hazardous led to a number of studies with actual (outdoor-derived) or synthetic (photolyzed laboratory-prepared atmospheres) smog in an attempt to assess the potency of the actual pollution mix. When human subjects were exposed to real-world photochemical air pollution (Los Angeles ambient air pumped into a laboratory exposure chamber), they experienced changes in lung function similar to those described in controlled clinical studies of O_3 alone (ie, reduction in spirometric lung volumes; see below), thus supporting the view that this oxidant was the pollutant of primary concern. Acute animal studies using synthetic atmospheres (usually irradiated auto exhaust) provided supportive evidence indicating deep lung damage, primarily within the small airway and proximal alveolar epithelium.

Thus, O_3 appeared to be the prime toxicant in many of these early studies; there was some evidence that other copollutants were involved in the effects observed with smog. When guinea pigs were exposed to irradiated auto exhaust, airway resistance increased quickly, in contrast to the pattern of O_3 alone, where less effect is seen on resistance than on breathing rate. This indicated that a more soluble irritant(s) probably was active, presumably reactive aldehydes. Thus, the array of effects of a complex atmosphere may be more diverse than would be predicted if it were assumed that O_3 alone was responsible. Interestingly, the focus over time has been almost exclusively on O_3, perhaps with the emphasis coming from the regulatory perspective tied to this single pollutant.

Chronic Exposures to Smog

Epidemiological studies in human populations as well as empirical studies in laboratory animals have attempted to link degenerative lung disease with chronic exposure to photochemical air pollution. Cross-sectional and prospective field studies have suggested an accelerated loss of lung function in people living in areas of high pollution. However, as with many studies of this type, there were problems with confounding factors (meteorology, imprecise exposure assessment, and population variables). Studies have been conducted in children living in modern-day Mexico City, which has oxidant and PM levels far in excess of any city in the United States. These studies have focused on the nasal epithelium as an exposure surrogate for pulmonary tissues, using biopsy and lavage methodologies to assess damage. Dramatic effects were found in exposed children, consisting of severe epithelial damage and metaplasia as well as permanent remodeling of the nasal epithelium. When children migrated into Mexico City from cleaner, nonurban regions, even more severe damage was observed, suggesting that the tissue remodeling in the permanent residents imparted some degree of incomplete adaptation. Because the children were of middle-class origin, these observations were less likely confounded by socioeconomic variables (Calderon-Garcidueñas et al., 1992). Changes in lung hyperinflation as estimated by x-ray tomography and impaired lung function have been reported among similarly exposed children living in Mexico City (Calderon-Garcidueñas et al., 2003) raising further concerns of long-term effects. Recently, a more mechanistic panel study demonstrated that the epithelial cell damage in the nasal cavity of Mexico City children was inversely correlated with glutathione peroxidase, a marker of oxidative stress (Hernández-Escobar et al., 2009).

A now classic synthetic smog study in animals was undertaken at the Cincinnati EPA laboratory in the mid-1960s in an attempt to address the potential for long-term lung disease. Beagle dogs were exposed on a daily basis (16 hours) for nearly six years, followed by a clean air recovery period of about three years (Lewis et al., 1974). A series of physiologic measurements were made on the dogs after the exposure, and after their three-year recovery. They were then moved to the College of Veterinary Medicine at the University of California at Davis. The lungs of the dogs then underwent extensive morphologic examination to correlate with the physiology. The dogs had been exposed to nonirradiated auto exhaust (group 1), irradiated auto exhaust (group 2), SO_2 plus sulfuric acid (group 3), the two types of exhaust plus the sulfur mixture (groups 4 and 5), and a high and a low level of NO_x (groups 6 and 7). The irradiated exhaust contained oxidant (measured as O_3) at about 0.2 ppm and NO_2 at about 0.9 ppm. The raw exhaust contained minimal concentrations of these materials and about 1.5 ppm NO. Both forms of exhaust also contained about 100 ppm CO. The control group did not show time-related lung function changes, but all the exposure groups had functional abnormalities, most of which persisted or worsened over the three-year recovery period in clean air. Enlargement of airspaces and loss of interalveolar septa in proximal acinar regions were most severe in dogs that were exposed to NO_x and SO_x with irradiated exhaust (Hyde et al., 1978). These studies described a morphologic lesion that was degenerative and progressive in nature, not unlike that of chronic obstructive pulmonary disease (COPD)—a condition most often associated with lifelong tobacco smoking.

Long-term "sentinel animal" studies in polluted cities have been attempted whereby the animals live in the same highly polluted air to which people are exposed. Such approaches have had a troubled past, but newer studies appear to be better controlled for the problems of infection, inappropriate animal care (eg, heat), and variable exposure atmospheres. One such study, conducted in rats exposed for six months to the air of São Paulo, Brazil, found considerable airway damage, lung function alterations, and altered mucus rheology (Saldiva *et al.*, 1992). The concentrations of O_3 and PM in São Paulo frequently exceed daily maximum values (in the summer months of February and March) of 0.3 ppm and 75 μg/m^3, respectively. This collage of effects is not unlike a composite of injury one might suspect from a mixed atmosphere of oxidants and acid PM in controlled laboratory animal studies. Strangely enough, however, a seven-week study in rats exposed to the polluted Mexico City air, which had induced significant lesions in children, did not reveal any nasal or lung histopathology in F-344 rats (Moss *et al.*, 2001). While there is no clear reason for the apparent differences in the findings, it is important to appreciate that all sentinel studies have elements of exposure that may be uncontrolled and hence at times can yield conflicting findings.

Ozone

General Toxicology Ozone is the primary oxidant of concern in photochemical smog because of its inherent bioreactivity and its concentration relative to other reactive species. Although it depends on the meteorological conditions of a given year, approximately 129 million Americans lived in areas not in absolute compliance with the 8-hour NAAQS in 2010. Progress has been made in reducing ambient O_3 levels and Los Angeles, for example, has not exceeded the Stage 1 smog alert (one-hour peak of 0.20 ppm or more) since 1998 and dropped the number of exceedances of the 0.075 ppm NAAQS in half from 1990 to 2011. Unlike SO_2 and the reducing-type pollution profile discussed above, current mitigation strategies for O_3 have been only marginally successful despite significant reductions in individual automobile emissions. These reductions have been offset by population growth, which brings with it additional vehicles and vehicle miles driven. With suburban sprawl and the downwind transport of air masses from populated areas to more rural environments, the geographic distribution of those exposed has also expanded, as has the temporal profile of individual exposure. In other words, ambient O_3 exposures are no longer stereotyped as brief one- to two-hour peaks. Instead, there is more typically a prolonged period of exposure of six hours or more at or near the NAAQS level. This important change in the exposure profile to O_3 has given rise to concerns that cumulative damage over an exposure of several hours may be more significant than brief pulse-like exposures, and that, as a result, many more people are at risk than was previously thought. With the 1997 revision of the US O_3 NAAQS to include an eight-hour daily average of 0.08 ppm, more cities and suburban areas find themselves in violation of the standard. If indeed the damage to the lung is cumulative over an eight-hour time period, then people in areas of compliance but with exposure levels near the standard may be affected. The American Lung Association estimates that nearly 50% of US inhabitants live in counties that are not in O_3 compliance (State of the Air, 2012). Perhaps of greater significance is that of those who might be considered susceptible due to age and/or preexistent cardiopulmonary impairments, 80% to 90% live in those areas that fail to comply with the present O_3 NAAQS.

Ozone induces a variety of effects in humans and experimental animals at concentrations that occur in many urban areas (reviewed by Lippmann, 1989; U.S. EPA, 2004). These effects include morphologic, functional, immunologic, and biochemical alterations. Because of its low water solubility, a substantial portion of inhaled O_3 penetrates deep into the lung, but its reactivity is such that about 17% and 40% is scrubbed by the nasopharynx of resting

rats and humans, respectively (Hatch *et al.*, 1994; Gerrity *et al.*, 1988). The reason for the higher degree of scrubbing in humans is unclear, but the finding is reproducible. Moreover, the mouth as well as the nose appears to scrub. Nevertheless, regardless of species, the region of the lung that is predicted to have the greatest O_3 deposition (dose per surface area) is the centriacinar region, from the terminal bronchioles to the alveolar ducts, also referred to as the proximal alveolar ductal region (Overton and Miller, 1987). Because O_3 penetration increases with increased tidal volume and flow rate, exercise increases the dose to the target area. Using $^{18}O_3$ (a nonradioactive isotope of oxygen), Hatch and coworkers have shown that the dose to the distal lung and the degree of damage to the lung as determined by leakage of plasma protein into the alveolar space (as collected by bronchoalveolar lavage) in exercising human subjects exposed to 0.4 ppm for two hours with intermittent periods of 15 minutes of exercise (threefold normal ventilation on average) are similar to those in resting rats exposed for the same length of time to 2.0 ppm. Thus, it is important to consider the role of exercise-associated dosimetry in a study of O_3 or any inhalant before making cross-study comparisons, especially if that comparison is across species.

Animal studies indicate that the acute morphologic responses to O_3 involve epithelial lining cells along the entire respiratory tract. The pattern of injury parallels the dosimetry profile, with the majority of damage occurring in the distal lung. Along the conducting airways, ciliated cells appear to be most sensitive to O_3, while Clara cells and mucus-secreting cells are the least sensitive. Studies in the rat nose indicate that O_3 also is an effective mucus secretagogue. In the alveolar region, type 1 epithelia are very sensitive to O_3 relative to type 2 cells, which have an active metabolic machinery. The more resistant type 2 cells serve as the stem cells for the replacement of type 1 cells. Ultrastructural damage to alveolar epithelia can be observed in rats after a few hours at 0.2 ppm, but sloughing of cells in the distal airway generally requires concentrations above 0.8 ppm. Recovery occurs within a few days, and there appears to be no residual pathology. Hence, from animal studies, it would appear that a single exposure to O_3 at a relatively low concentration is not likely to cause permanent damage. On a gross level, when a bronchoscope is used to peer into the human bronchus after O_3 exposure, the airways appear "sunburned" and, as with mild skin sunburn, recovery is typical. What is uncertain is the impact of repeated "sunburning" of the airways and lung.

Studies have shown particular sensitivity to O_3-induced inflammation in neonatal rats that decreased with age into adulthood. However, enhanced sensitivity to O_3 again appears in older rats as evidenced by interstitial edema that is not seen in younger adult animals. Older rats have lower ascorbate in the lung and this diminishment of antioxidant capacity may be in part responsible. Elderly humans, however, seem less responsive to the lung function impacts of high ambient O_3. The reasons for this are unclear, but caution in linking lung function and inflammation in the O_3 response is warranted.

The mechanisms by which O_3 causes injury have been studied using cellular as well as cell-free systems. As a powerful oxidant, O_3 seeks to extract electrons from other molecules. The surface fluid lining the respiratory tract and the cell membranes that underlie the lining fluid contain a significant quantity of polyunsaturated fatty acids (PUFA), either free or as part of the lipoprotein structures of the cell. The double bonds within these fatty acids have a labile, unpaired electron that is easily attacked by O_3 to form ozonides that progress through a less stable zwitterion or trioxolane (depending on the presence of water); these ultimately recombine or decompose to lipohydroperoxides, aldehydes, and hydrogen peroxide. These

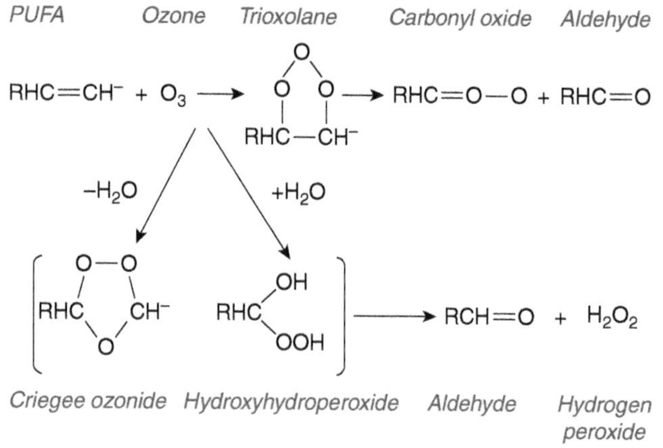

PUFA   Ozone   Trioxolane   Carbonyl oxide   Aldehyde

$$RHC{=}CH^- + O_3 \longrightarrow \underset{RHC{-}CH^-}{O{-}O{-}O} \longrightarrow RHC{=}O{-}O + RHC{=}O$$

$-H_2O$ $+H_2O$

$$\left[\underset{O}{RHC}\overset{O{-}O}{\underset{}{CH^-}} \quad RHC\overset{OH}{\underset{OOH}{}} \right] \longrightarrow RCH{=}O + H_2O_2$$

Criegee ozonide   Hydroxyhydroperoxide   Aldehyde   Hydrogen peroxide

Figure 29-15. *Major reaction pathways of O_3 with lipids in lung lining fluid and cell membranes.* (Adapted with permission from U.S. EPA, 1996.)

pathways are thought to initiate propagation of lipid radicals and auto-oxidation of cell membranes and macromolecules (Fig. 29-15).

Evidence of free radical–related damage in vivo includes detection of exhaled breath pentane and ethane and tissue measurements of diene conjugates. Damage to the air–blood interface disrupts its barrier function and promotes inflammation. Inflammatory cytokines (eg, interleukins 6, 8, and others, TNF) are released from epithelial cells and macrophages that mediate early responses and initiate repair. This inflammatory process is generally transient, but it may also interact with neural irritant responses to affect lung function acutely. The latter response may have implications for those with preexistent inflammation or disease.

Pulmonary Function Effects Exposure to O_3 produces a variety of pulmonary function changes and human subjects appear to be more sensitive than animal models. Early studies showed that exercising human subjects exposed for two to three hours to 0.12 to 0.4 ppm O_3 experience reversible concentration-related decrements in forced exhaled volumes (FVC and forced expiratory volume in one second [FEV_1]) (McDonnell *et al.*, 1983). Because of the concern that prolonged periods of exposure (six–eight hours) may lead to cumulative effects, similar protocols with lower exposure and exercise levels were extended up to 6.6 hours. In these studies, exposures to 0.12, 0.10, and 0.08 ppm induced progressive lung function impairment during the course of the exposure (Horstman *et al.*, 1989). The pattern of response was a function of exposure time such that functional changes were not detectable at 1 or 2 hours but reached significance by four to six hours. Decrements in FEV_1 after 6.6 hours at 0.12 ppm averaged 13.6% and were comparable to that observed after a two-hour exposure to 0.22 ppm with much heavier exercise. These studies were then followed up with exposures to even lower O_3 concentrations. The latter controlled human exposure studies demonstrated that multihour exposures to 0.06 and 0.08 ppm O_3 (with exercise) produced small but statistically significant mean decreases in FEV_1 (in the range of 3%–4%) as well as increases in respiratory symptoms and inflammation. It is noteworthy that in these and other controlled human exposure studies with O_3, considerable interindividual differences in response were observed, thus confirming the many animal studies showing that the response to ozone is dependent on many innate factors such as age, diet, genetics, preexisting disease, and gender.

It is not clear what mechanisms underlie the altered lung function (in terms of changes in FEV_1) produced by O_3. Although chest pain/discomfort is thought to contribute to O_3-induced decreases in an effort-dependent lung function maneuver such as FEV_1, there is also evidence that the decrements in lung function are vagally

mediated, and that the response can be abrogated by analgesics, such as ibuprofen and opiates, which also reduce pain and inflammation (see below). Thus, pain reflexes involving C-fiber networks are thought to be important in the reduction in forced expiratory volumes. On the other hand, animal studies show a prominent role for vagal reflexes in altered airway reactivity and bronchoconstriction. There is also evidence to implicate vagal reflexes in cardiac as well as thermal regulation, at least in rodents.

Airway responsiveness to specific (eg, allergen) and nonspecific (eg, cold air, inhaled methacholine) bronchoconstriction is another commonly used test of the pulmonary response to inhaled pollutants such as O_3. These types of tests are very important because airway hyperresponsiveness is a central feature of asthma and asthmatics are a sizeable subpopulation (7%–9% of the total population in the United States) that may be particularly sensitive to the adverse respiratory effects of inhaled pollutants. A number of animal models have demonstrated that O_3 induces airway hyperresponsiveness and that innate factors such as genetics, diet, and obesity can modify this effect. For the most part, many of these studies have utilized O_3 exposure concentrations that are far above ambient levels. Importantly, controlled human exposure studies have not only verified the findings of the high-dose animal studies but also demonstrated adverse effects at concentrations relevant to ambient O_3 levels. Airway hyperreactivity to nonspecific agonists in humans has been reported after acute exposure to as little as 0.08 ppm O_3. It is widely thought that hyperreactive airways may be a marker of predisposition to other pollutants such as sulfuric acid or aeroallergens, but such evidence is limited.

Inflammation of the Lung and Host Defense The mechanism by which O_3 produces decrements in pulmonary function is not fully understood and its link to airway inflammation is unclear. For example, O_3-induced lung dysfunction does not appear to be enhanced in asthmatics whose lungs are generally in a state of inflammation. Asthmatics are, however, clearly more sensitive to the bronchoconstrictive effects of both SO_2 and sulfuric acid aerosols. Other factors that play a role in the pulmonary response to O_3 include age and obesity. Animal studies have demonstrated that O_3-induced lung injury and inflammation is greater in neonatal compared with that in adult rabbits, rats, and mice (Vancza *et al.*, 2009). In addition to age as a susceptibility factor, a series of studies has shown that obesity predisposes mice to the adverse effects of O_3. Because obesity is associated with ongoing systemic inflammation, it suggests that a preexisting physiologic or disease state enhances the adverse effects of O_3.

Both human and animal studies have demonstrated that sensitivity to O_3 appears to have a genetic component as well. Studies in inbred stains of mice have shown that O_3-induced pulmonary neutrophilia, airway hyperresponsiveness, and permeability are significantly affected by SNPS in a single gene linked to the Toll-like receptor 4 (Tlr4) locus that has been associated with endotoxin sensitivity (Kleeberger *et al.*, 2000). Further research has determined that the involvement of an innate immunity factor such as Tlr4 in the multifaceted response to O_3 involves the release of hyaluronan fragments that appear to directly activate the Tlr4 cascade in mice (Li *et al.*, 2011). The role of genetic polymorphisms in the pulmonary response to O_3 is complicated, however, and many other pathways including TNF, IL-1, Nrf-2, and NF-κB can modulate the response to O_3 in animal models (Bauer and Kleeberger, 2010).

The growth of genomic and proteomic technologies has made it possible to begin studies in humans to define genetic linkages to O_3 sensitivity. These studies have typically focused on genes involved in oxidative stress pathways. For example, again using

Mexico City as a backdrop, it was found that a polymorphism in GSTM1 (as noted above with regard to PM) appears to convey O_3 sensitivity as well (Romieu *et al.*, 2004). Similarly, functional polymorphisms in the catalase and the myeloperoxidase genes have been associated with enhanced response to ambient ozone. More detailed controlled O_3 chamber exposures have confirmed that genetic polymorphisms in these and other genes, including NAD quinone oxidoreductase (NQO), GSTP1, heme oxygenase-1, and TNF, are associated with responsiveness to ozone and that gene–gene interactions are involved.

Because of the strong epidemiological evidence that O_3 can exacerbate asthma (eg, increased hospital admissions) and the inability of epidemiology studies to demonstrate causality, investigators have utilized chamber studies to test the hypothesis that O_3 enhances the immune response to allergens. The potential for O_3 to influence allergic sensitization or challenge–responses has received a significant amount of investigation in animal studies. Enhanced response to allergen challenge has been noted in a number of animal species exposed to ozone. Biochemical, cellular, and pulmonary function parameters of allergic response have all been observed to increase in sensitized animals exposed to O_3 prior to antigen challenge. Ozone's effect on allergic asthma also occurs at the sensitization stage in which repeated exposure to O_3 before or during the sensitization process exacerbates a range of allergic end points. Thus, in general, animal studies have shown the ability of O_3 to enhance the allergic process under different conditions, but evidence of this in humans is less strong. Controlled studies of heightened antigen responsiveness in allergic subjects have only been suggestive, with enhancement of allergic rhinitis after 0.5 ppm for four hours. However, diary studies of asthmatic nurses reported worsened allergy symptoms, as well as durations thereof, at concentrations of O_3 near the NAAQS (Schwartz, 1992). Similarly, eosinophils and IL-4, central components of allergic asthma, were increased in some but not all human chamber studies of O_3 exposure (U.S. EPA ISA, 2012).

Early research showed that exposure to O_3 before a challenge with aerosols of infectious agents produces a higher incidence of infection than is seen in control animals (Coffin and Blommer, 1967). Studies have demonstrated that this type of effect can be a direct result of altered phagocytosis by macrophages in O_3-exposed mice previously infected with an aerosol of *Streptococcus* (group C) bacteria (Gilmour *et al.*, 1993). The host resistance model has shown responsiveness to an exposure as low as 0.08 ppm for three hours. The susceptibility of mice and hamsters to *Klebsiella pneumoniae* aerosol is also increased by prior exposure to O_3. In the rat, altered microbe-killing may relate to membrane or receptor damage in macrophages, thus impairing the production of bactericidal agents such as superoxide anions. The rat appears less susceptible than mice because it has a more vigorous PMN response to bacteria than do mice, which seems to compensate for macrophage impairments. This is yet another example of where susceptibility lies more in the inability to compensate than in the initial responsiveness to a given challenge. It is not clear whether O_3's impairment of bacterial infections in the lung also extends to viral infections. While there is epidemiological evidence of ambient O_3 being associated with increased hospital admissions for viral and bacterial infections, animal studies have shown mixed results for O_3's effect on viral infections, although some of the contradictory findings may be a result of experimental design differences (eg, O_3 exposure occurring before or after viral infection).

Chronic Effects Morphometric studies of the centriacinar region of rats exposed for 12 hours per day for six weeks to 0.12 or 0.25 ppm O_3 have shown hyperplasia and hypertrophy of type 1 alveolar cells (smaller and thicker cells) coupled with damage and alterations in ciliated and Clara cell populations in small airways (Barry *et al.*, 1988). A collective cross-protocol analysis of type 1 cell hypertrophy was conducted; type 1 cell thickness appeared to be linearly related to the O_3 C × T (Chang *et al.*, 1991, 1992). This finding suggested that over a season, the impact of O_3 in the distal lung may be cumulative and perhaps more importantly may be without threshold. The biological significance of this change is unclear—it may be part of a compensatory response to "thicken" that part of the alveolar duct junction that receives the greatest dose and is most affected. This response may be protective since the thickened cells were also smaller, offering therefore a smaller exposure surface to the incoming O_3. This changed morphology could limit membrane damage. When returned to clean air, most of the epithelial morphologic changes regressed, but there was evidence of residual interstitial remodeling below the epithelium in the alveolar duct region. Examination of autopsied lung specimens from young smokers shows many analogous tissue lesions that come to be described as the "smoldering" precursor of emphysema. A long series of studies at the University of California, Davis, has examined the structural and functional changes produced in nonhuman primates exposed chronically to O_3. Because of the greater similarity of monkey respiratory tract to that of humans, the burden of extrapolation from rodent study results to risk assessment for humans is lessened, and these studies have proven important in establishing the causality of many of the long-term effects of O_3 observed in epidemiology studies. Episodic exposure of adult monkeys to 0.25 ppm O_3 for 18 months produced physiologic, cellular, and biochemical changes in the lung. Exposure to as little as 0.2 ppm O_3 for up to 90 days was found to produce cellular changes throughout the respiratory tract. Nasal lesions were accompanied by changes in cell populations in the respiratory bronchioles. In the second phase of these studies, infant rhesus monkeys were cyclically exposed to 0.5 ppm O_3 for eight hours per day for five days followed by several days of exposure to air. While the study design did not permit a comparison of the responsiveness of infant versus adult monkeys, the infant monkeys showed evidence of structural changes that parallel epidemiology studies linking lung growth and development with exposure to air pollution. The infant monkeys also showed a significant interaction between sensitization to house dust mite antigen and ozone. While antigen or ozone alone produced small changes in baseline airway resistance and airway responsiveness, antigen plus ozone produced more than additive effects on both parameters.

Studies involving episodic exposures of rats and monkeys using a pattern of alternating months of O_3 (0.25 ppm) for 18 months indicate that there may be carryover effects, notably thickening of interstitial fibrous matrix (Tyler *et al.*, 1988, 1991). These interstitial changes were quantitatively similar regardless of the twofold difference in the cumulative exposure dose (ie, C × T). This would imply that a pattern of exposure resembling seasonal O_3 patterns might result in more serious lesions than predicted by dose alone—indeed more than would have occurred had the exposure been continuous. Hence, the concept of "more dose = more effect" may not hold in chronic episodic scenarios for O_3, as it appears to do with uninterrupted exposures. The number of episodes experienced may well be more significant to long-term outcomes than total dose—a phenomenon not unlike that of repeated sunburning and deterioration of the skin.

Studies of lung function in rodents exposed chronically to O_3 have been conducted, but have yielded mixed results at relevant exposure concentrations. Generally, the dysfunction is reflective of stiffened or fibrotic lungs, particularly at higher concentrations.

There have been two prominent chronic O_3 studies—the EPA 18-month chronic study fashioned after a realistic urban exposure profile with a peak exposure of 0.25 ppm (Chang *et al.*, 1992; Costa *et al.*, 1995) and the National Toxicology Program (NTP)–Health Effects Institute (HEI Report, 1994/1995) study of 0.125 to 1 ppm for 20 months (square wave; six hours per day; five days per week). From an environmental relevance perspective, the $C \times T$ doses for these studies were similar, but the urban profile study produced evidence for centriacinar interstitial fibrosis suggesting a possible influence of the exposure pattern. There was no general biochemical evidence for fibrosis (Last *et al.*, 1994), as reported in monkey and rat studies that had been conducted at higher O_3 concentrations. If one attempts to compare these results with the Cincinnati beagle study, one finds that the synthetic smog atmosphere showed degenerative and not fibrotic lung lesions. However, it should be noted that the air pollutant mixture used in the beagle study both was more complex and involved considerably higher concentrations than more recent studies.

The ability of O_3 to induce tolerance to itself is a curious phenomenon that has implications for both episodic and chronic exposures. Classic O_3 tolerance takes the form of protection against a high or even lethal dose in animals that received a very low initial challenge or challenges several days before. This term, *tolerance*, is sometimes used to describe "adaptation" or acclimatization over time to near-ambient levels of O_3, and, as such, has led to some confusion. However, with regard to "adaptation" to O_3, the process begins during and immediately after the initial exposure and progresses to completion in at most two to four days. This adaptive phenomenon has been well established in humans with regard to lung function and has been correlated with several inflammatory end points (Devlin *et al.*, 1993). Lavage lactate dehydrogenase (LDH; a marker of cell injury) and elastase (enzymatically active against lung matrix material), interestingly, do not appear to adapt in humans based on the Devlin study. An analogous pattern of adaptation of functional and biochemical end points (including LDH and elastase) in rodents also takes place with repeated exposures up to a week. But to date, the linkages between acute, adaptive, and long-term process remain unclear, since over longer periods of exposure both morphologic and functional effects do appear to develop. The precise mechanism for O_3 adaptation is not known and several theories abound, including changes in cell profiles, lung surface fluids, and induced antioxidants. Few studies have tackled the problem but in rats the adaptation of the neutrophilic response appears to be related to the induction of an endogenous acute-phase response (McKinney *et al.*, 1998). On the other hand, adaptation to lung function changes in rats after chronic exposure appears linked to lung antioxidants such as ascorbic acid (Wiester *et al.*, 2000). The significance of this finding in humans is uncertain because ascorbic acid is not endogenously synthesized as it is in the rat. However, self-administration of ascorbate has been shown to reduce O_3-induced lung function decrements in adults (Mudway *et al.*, 1999), and in children, supplementation with ascorbate and α-tocopherol lessened nasal inflammatory responses to O_3 in Mexico City (Sienra-Monge *et al.*, 2004). Despite these interesting findings, it remains unclear if antioxidant supplements can protect humans from long-term O_3 effects given the many mechanisms that may be involved in the various responses. How these interplay with long-term adaptation and the likelihood of degenerative disease is unclear.

Ozone Interactions with Copollutants An approach simplifying the complexity of synthetic smog studies, yet addressing the issue of pollutant interactions involves the exposure of laboratory animals or humans to binary or more complex synthetic mixtures of pollutants that occur together in ambient air. The most frequent combination involves interactions of O_3 and NO_2 or O_3 and PM (eg, sulfuric acid or diesel particles). Not surprisingly, study design adds a level of complexity in interpretation such that evidence exists supporting either augmentation or antagonism of lung function impairments, lung pathology, and other indices of injury. This apparent conflict in the findings only emphasizes the need to carefully consider the myriad of factors that might affect studies involving multiple determinants and the nature of the exposure that is most relevant to reality.

When O_3 and NO_2 (1 and 14 ppm, respectively) were administered to rats from a premixed retention chamber, the resulting damage evident in bronchoalveolar lavage exceeded that of either toxicant alone, regardless of the temporal sequence of exposure (Gelzleichter *et al.*, 1992). Biochemical and histological indices of fibrogenesis also were increased in related studies (Last *et al.*, 1994). In retrospect, it was hypothesized that the two oxidants formed relatively stable intermediate nitrogen radicals that were more toxic than either gas alone. At lower, more realistic concentrations (0.3 ppm O_3 and 3.0 ppm NO_2), where this reaction would not be favored, the impact of these irritants on rabbits was only additive (Schlesinger *et al.*, 1991). This contrast in response serves to illustrate that the tenets of dose dependency that hold for any single-toxicant response may be of equal or more importance when two or more pollutants coexist and have the potential to interact.

Studies of O_3 mixed with acid aerosols also have shown enhanced or antagonistic responses that were time-dependent during the period of exposure. On the one hand, as noted above, field studies of children in camps and studies of asthma admissions in the Northeast and in Canada suggested an interaction of acid and O_3 underlying responses to summer haze. Yet, in an experimental setting with rabbits exposed over an extended period, there was exposure duration–specific evidence of enhanced as well as antagonized secretory cell responses with combined O_3 (0.1 ppm) and sulfuric acid (125 μg/m³) over the course of the one-year exposure (Schlesinger *et al.*, 1992). As the number of interacting variables increases, so does the difficulty in interpretation. Studies of complex atmospheres involving acid-coated carbon combined with O_3 at near-ambient levels also show varied evidence of interaction on lung function and macrophage receptor activity (Kleinman *et al.*, 1999). As such, the platform of any multicomponent study is its statistical design and the ability to either separate or determine the nature of the interacting variables. However, it is indeed the complex mixture to which people are exposed that we wish to evaluate. Creative approaches to understanding mixture responses are a likely part of the new agenda that toxicologists will need to address in the future (Mauderly, 2006).

Nitrogen Dioxide

General Toxicology Nitrogen dioxide, like O_3, is a deep lung irritant that can produce pulmonary edema if it is inhaled at high concentrations. It is a much less potent irritant and oxidant than O_3, but NO_2 can pose clear toxicological problems. Potential life-threatening exposure is a real-world problem for farmers, as near-lethal high levels of NO_2 can be liberated from fermenting fresh silage. Being heavier than air, the generated NO_2 and CO_2 displace air and oxygen at the base of silo and diffuse into closed spaces where workers can inadvertently get exposed to very high concentrations perhaps with depleted oxygen. Typically, shortness of breath rapidly ensues with exposures nearing 75 to 100 ppm NO_2, with delayed edema and symptoms of pulmonary damage. Not surprisingly, the symptoms are collectively termed "silo-filler's disease." Nitrogen dioxide is also an important indoor pollutant, especially in homes with unventilated gas stoves or kerosene heaters (Spengler and Sexton, 1983) or, in developing countries, with the unvented burning of biomass fuels (Kumie *et al.*, 2009). Under such circumstances, very young children and their mothers who spend considerable time indoors may be especially at risk. In general, indoor environments with NO_2 sources achieve concentrations far in excess of those observed outdoors at central monitoring sites. Peak levels of NO_2 near high-traffic-volume roadways can be several-fold higher than away from roadways and are thus similar to peak levels observed indoors with unvented stoves (ie, 0.2–0.5 ppm). Interestingly, protocols that simulate an urban (rush-hour) or household (cooking) patterns of two daily peaks superimposed on a low continuous background concentration have elicited effects in experimental animals that continuous exposure to NO_2 did not evoke, suggesting an important dependency on exposure profile. Among the common air pollutants, empirical studies of NO_2 have frequently shown greater effects with higher peak concentrations at equivalent $C \times T$ steady-state concentrations.

Although the distal lung lesions produced by acute NO_2 are similar among species, there exist differences in species sensitivity. Where direct comparison is possible, guinea pigs, hamsters, and monkeys appear more sensitive than rats, although comparative dosimetry information might explain some of this difference. As in the case of O_3, theoretical dosimetry studies indicate that NO_2 is deposited along the length of the respiratory tree, with preferential deposition being in the distal airways. Not surprisingly, the pattern of damage to the respiratory tract reflects this profile: damage is most apparent in the terminal bronchioles, just a bit more proximal in the airway than is seen with O_3. At high concentrations, the alveolar ducts and alveoli are also affected, with type 1 cells again showing their sensitivity to oxidant challenge. In the airways of these animals there is also damage to epithelial cells in the bronchioles, notably with loss of ciliated cells, as well as a loss of secretory granules in Clara cells. Thus, the pattern of injury of NO_2 is quite similar to that of O_3, although its potency is about an order of magnitude lower.

Pulmonary Function Effects Exposure of normal human subjects to concentrations of ≤4 ppm NO_2 for up to three hours produces no consistent effects on spirometry. However, a study has shown slightly enhanced airway reactivity with 1.5 to 2.0 ppm. Interestingly, ascorbic acid pretreatment of human subjects appeared to protect them from this hyperreactivity (Mohsenin, 1987). Whether asthmatics have a particular sensitivity to NO_2 is a controversial issue. A number of factors appear to be involved (eg, exercise, inherent sensitivity of the asthmatic subject, exposure method). Some studies have reported effects in some individuals at 0.2 ppm, which approximates an indoor level in a household with an unvented gas stove. Recent meta-analyses, which have incorporated the findings of many studies to achieve a weight-of-evidence perspective, support an effect of NO_2 on asthmatics, but it is not clear if the small but statistically significant changes in airway hyperresponsiveness in asthmatics exposed to NO_2 below 0.6 ppm are adverse. As for an appropriate animal model, only very high concentrations (10 ppm NO_2) invoke an irritancy response in guinea pigs (tachypnea); these levels are well above those a person probably would encounter in everyday life. However, NO_2 has been found to be associated with mortality in some time-series studies of air pollution attempting to tease out specific pollutant effects (focusing mainly on PM) (Gold *et al.*, 2000; Samoli *et al.*, 2006). These epidemiology studies have demonstrated that each 20 to 30 ppb increase in NO_2 results in a small but significant increase in acute cardiovascular and respiratory

mortality. Similarly, NO_2 has been associated with increased hospital admissions and emergency room visits, but these epidemiology studies are confounded by the coexposure to multiple pollutants. Thus, as stressed elsewhere, it is important that epidemiology studies results be interpreted with caution when considering causality and that controlled human exposure and animal studies be utilized, within ethical limits, to confirm the biological plausibility of the effect of NO_2, or any other pollutant, on the cardiopulmonary system. This caution obviously extends to many recent studies that have consistently linked adverse health outcomes with living near high-traffic-volume roadways. Because of the many constituents present in the exhaust of both gas and diesel combustion engines, as well as their ever changing chemistry, it is unclear from these studies whether NO_2 is acting as a marker or surrogate for vehicular traffic rather than as an indication of a specific NO_2 effect. These studies have found correlates with cardiovascular deaths, which have raised new questions of the mechanisms by which pollutants might affect health in susceptible subgroups (Rosenlund *et al.*, 2006).

Inflammation of the Lung and Host Defense Unlike O_3, NO_2 does not induce significant neutrophilic inflammation in humans at exposure concentrations encountered in the ambient outdoor environment. There is some evidence for bronchial inflammation after four to six hours at 2.0 ppm, which approximates the highest transient peak indoor levels of this oxidant. Exposures at 2.0 to 5.0 ppm have been shown to affect T lymphocytes, particularly CD8[+] cells and natural killer cells that function in host defenses against viruses. Although these concentrations may be high, epidemiological studies variably show effects of NO_2 on respiratory infection rates in children, especially in indoor environments. Animal models, by contrast, have for years shown associations between NO_2 and bacterial infection (Gardner, 1984). As noted for other effects, the incidence of infection in exposed models appears to be governed more by the peak exposure concentration than by exposure duration. The effects are ascribed to suppression of macrophage function and clearance from the lung, in the form of suppressed bactericidal and/or motility functions of macrophages from rabbits exposed to 0.3 ppm for three days (Schlesinger, 1987). Similar effects have been reported in humans exposed to 0.10 ppm for 6.6 hours (Devlin *et al.*, 1991).

Toxicological studies of the interaction of NO_2 with viruses also suggest enhanced infectivity. Squirrel monkeys infected with nonlethal levels of A/PR-8 influenza virus and then exposed continuously to 5 or 10 ppm NO_2 suffered high mortality rates; 6/6 monkeys exposed to 10 ppm died within three days, while only 1/3 exposed to 5 ppm died (Henry *et al.*, 1970). Other experiments suggest that exposure of squirrel monkeys for five months to 5 ppm NO_2 depresses the formation of protective antibodies against the A/PR-8 influenza virus. Controlled human studies with virus challenges, however, have been inconclusive, perhaps because of low subject numbers. One study showed decreased virus inactivation by alveolar macrophages recovered from four of nine subjects when cultured and exposed for 3.5 hours to 0.6 ppm NO_2 in vitro. The responsive macrophages produced interleukin-1, a known cytokine modulator of immune cell function (Frampton *et al.*, 1989). Thus, the potential for augmented risk of viral infection associated with NO_2 exposure remains unclear and suggests a role for underlying host susceptibility. This concern would be greatest for children, especially during seasonal use of unvented gas heaters, who have less mature pulmonary immune function.

Chronic Effects Concern about the chronic effects of NO_2 stems from early observations that a continuous 30-day, 30-ppm exposure produces emphysema in hamsters. Whether the result of this exposure scenario relates to cyclic human exposures at 1/100th that level is unclear. On the one hand, an 18-month study in rats exposed to an urban pattern of NO_2 in which a daily background of 0.5 ppm peaked at 1.5 ppm for 4 hours each day showed little ultrastructural damage to the distal lung (Chang et al., 1988). On the other hand, mice exposed for a year to a base level of 0.2 ppm NO_2 with a one-hour spike of 0.8 ppm twice a day, five days per week (Miller et al., 1987) displayed effects that differed between the base-only and peak-only exposure groups. The base level produced no effects, while the overlaid peaks induced slight functional impairment and augmented susceptibility to bacterial infection. Early studies (Ehrlich and Henry, 1968) showed that clearance of bacteria from the lungs is suppressed with 0.5 ppm NO_2 through 12 months of exposure. Interestingly, studies with a similar double diurnal peak design for NO_2, with NO used as a negative control, showed more pronounced effects of NO on alveolar septal remodeling than did NO_2 (Mercer et al., 1995). These and similar studies utilizing varied peak-plus-baseline NO_x exposures indicate the importance of exposure profile for at least this pollutant.

Other Oxidants

While a number of other reactive oxidants have been identified in photochemical smog, most are short-lived because of their reaction with copollutants. PAN, which is thought to be responsible for much of the eye-stinging activity of smog, is known to exist in smog situations. It is more soluble and reactive than O_3, and hence rapidly decomposes in mucous membranes before it can penetrate into the respiratory tract. The cornea is a sensitive target and is prominent in the burning/stinging discomfort often associated with oxidant smogs. A few studies with high levels of PAN have shown that it can cause lung damage and have mutagenic activity in bacteria, but it is not likely that these scenarios are relevant to ambient levels of PAN.

Aldehydes

Carbonyl compounds, notably short-chained (2-4 C) aldehydes, are common photo-oxidation products of unsaturated hydrocarbons. Two aldehydes are of major interest by virtue of their concentrations and irritancy: formaldehyde (HCHO) and acrolein (H_2C=CHCHO). They contribute to the odor as well as eye and sensory effects of smog. Formaldehyde accounts for about 50% of the estimated total aldehydes in polluted air, while acrolein, the more irritating of the two, accounts for about 5% of the total. Acetaldehyde (C_3HCHO) and many other longer-chain aldehydes make up the remainder, but they are not as intrinsically irritating, exist at low concentrations, and have less solubility in airway fluids. Formaldehyde and particularly acrolein are also found in mainstream tobacco smoke (~90 and ~8 ppm, respectively, per puff) and are likely to be found at lower levels in sidestream smoke as well. Formaldehyde is also an important indoor air pollutant and can often achieve higher concentrations indoors than outdoors due to off-gassing by new upholstery or other furnishings. In the United States, the formaldehyde off-gassing issue was highlighted in the controversy surrounding the trailer homes provided to hurricane-displaced home owners in Katrina-New Orleans-2005.

Empirical studies have shown that formaldehyde and acrolein are competitive agonists for similar irritant receptors in the airways. Thus, irritation may be related not to "total aldehyde" concentration but to specific ratios of acrolein and formaldehyde. Their relative difference in solubility, with formaldehyde being somewhat more water-soluble and thus having more nasopharyngeal uptake, may

distort this relationship under certain exposure conditions (eg, exercise). On the other hand, acrolein is very reactive and may interact easily with many tissue macromolecules and, for example, can form DNA adducts.

Formaldehyde

Formaldehyde is a primary sensory irritant. Because it is very soluble in water, it is absorbed in mucous membranes in the nose, upper respiratory tract, and eyes. The dose–response curve for formaldehyde is steep: 0.5 to 1 ppm yields a detectable odor, 2 to 3 ppm produces mild irritation, and 4 to 5 ppm is intolerable to most people. Formaldehyde is thought to act via sensory C-fibers that signal locally as well as through the trigeminal nerve to reflexively induce bronchoconstriction through the vagus nerve. In guinea pigs, a one-hour exposure to about 0.3 ppm of formaldehyde induces an increase in airflow resistance accompanied by a smaller decrease in compliance (Amdur, 1960). Respiratory frequency and minute volume also decreased, but these changes were not statistically significant until >10 ppm. The no observed effect level (NOEL) using these lung function criteria is about 0.05 ppm. The general pattern of the irritant response and its rapid recovery is similar to that produced by higher concentrations of SO_2. Like SO_2, breathing through a tracheal cannula to bypass nasal scrubbing greatly augments the irritant response, indicating that deep lung irritant receptors can also be activated by this vapor.

The irritancy of inhaled formaldehyde vapor, again like SO_2, has been shown to be potentiated by water-soluble salt aerosols. Irritancy appears to be augmented in proportion to the aerosol concentration, but the potentiation could not be accounted for by a simple aerosol "carrier" effect (Amdur, 1960). Moreover, reversal of bronchoconstriction was slower than had been observed with SO_2. Thus, it appeared that the vapor-aerosol itself constituted a new irritant species, the product of a chemical transformation of formaldehyde—perhaps methylene hydroxide. In addition to interactions with water-soluble particles, formaldehyde has been shown to interact with carbon-based particles (Jakab, 1992) to augment bacterial infectivity in a murine model. In this case, the potentiation appears to correlate with the surface carrying capacity of the inhaled particle.

Two aspects of formaldehyde toxicology have brought it from relative obscurity to the forefront of attention in recent years. One is its near ubiquitous presence in indoor atmospheres as an off-gassed product of construction materials such as plywood, furniture, or improperly polymerized urea-formaldehyde foam insulation (Spengler and Sexton, 1983). Complaints of formaldehyde irritation in industry have been reported at 50 ppb (Horvath et al., 1988). In studies relating household formaldehyde to chronic effects, children were found to have significantly lower peak expiratory flow rates (about 22% in homes with 60 ppb) than did unexposed children and asthmatic children were affected below 50 ppb. Thus, this irritant vapor can cause respiratory effects, and perhaps act as an allergen, at commonly experienced exposure levels (Krzyzanowski et al., 1990). Also, there is epidemiological evidence, sometimes inconsistent, that formaldehyde is associated with asthma (McGwin, 2010) and lower respiratory tract infections in children (Roda et al., 2011).

A longtime concern regarding formaldehyde has been its potential carcinogenicity. In 2004, IARC concluded, based on a thorough review of the published data, that formaldehyde was a probable human carcinogen; IARC deemed that there was "sufficient" epidemiological evidence that formaldehyde causes nasopharyngeal cancer, "strong but not sufficient" evidence of leukemia, and limited evidence of sinonasal cancer, along with "sufficient" evidence that formaldehyde causes nasal cancer in animals (Cogliano, 2005). Nasal cancer had been induced empirically with formaldehyde vapor in a two-year study where rats were exposed to 2, 6, or 14 ppm six hours per day, five days per week. The incidence of nasal squamous cell carcinomas was zero in the control and 2-ppm groups, 1% in the 6-ppm group, and 44% in the 14-ppm group. Mice were much less sensitive; only one carcinoma was seen at 14 ppm. The detection of DNA adducts in the two species paralleled the difference in the incidence of tumors as well as regional dosimetry. Formaldehyde, with its large and diverse database and potential public health impact, has remained the focus of considerable debate among modelers and risk assessors. The arguments behind this debate crosses both cancer and noncancer considerations and is beyond that which can be discussed in this chapter. The reader is encouraged to sample the recent literature (eg, Conolly et al., 2004; Nielsen et al., 2010).

Acrolein

Because acrolein is an unsaturated aldehyde, it is more reactive than formaldehyde. It penetrates a bit deeper into the airways and may not have the same degree of sensory irritancy but it may cause more damage. Concentrations below 1 ppm cause irritation of the eyes and the mucous membranes of the respiratory tract. Exposure of guinea pigs to ≥0.6 ppm reversibly increased pulmonary flow resistance and tidal volume and decreased respiratory frequency (Murphy et al., 1963). With irritants of this type, flow resistance is increased by concentrations below those that cause the classic decrease in frequency seen with sensory irritants. This suggests that increases in flow resistance would be produced by far lower concentrations of acrolein than were tested. The mechanism of increased resistance appears to be mediated through both a local C-fiber and centrally mediated cholinergic reflexes (Bessac and Jordt, 2010). Ablation of the C-fiber network and atropine (muscarinic blocker) block this response.

Exposures of rats to 0.4, 1.4, or 4.0 ppm for six hours per day, five days per week for 13 weeks resulted in paradoxical effects on lung function (Costa et al., 1986). The lowest concentration resulted in hyperinflation of the lung with an apparent reduction in small-airway flow resistance, while the highest concentration resulted in airway injury and peribronchial inflammation and fibrosis. The intermediate concentration was functionally not different from the control, although airway pathology was evident. It appears that the high-concentration response reflected the cumulative irritant injury and remodeling as a result of the repeated acrolein, while the low-concentration group had little overt damage and appeared to have slightly stiffened airways, perhaps a result of the protein cross-linking action of acrolein. The pathology in these rats contrasts with that found in formaldehyde studies of similar duration where more upper airway involvement was observed. Ambient exposure to acrolein probably would be about 10% to 20% of the low concentration used in the subchronic study discussed above. Because of a lack of sufficient human data, these animal data were used to perform a risk assessment analysis that showed an excess risk to humans for the adverse effect of ambient levels of acrolein on pulmonary function (Woodruff et al., 2007). However, ambient concentrations of acrolein are well below those found in mainstream tobacco smoke and the occupational exposure levels. As reviewed elsewhere (Bein and Leikauf, 2011), acrolein produces a wide range of adverse pulmonary effects including lung cancer that may be linked mechanistically to p53 (a tumor suppressor gene) DNA adducts and mutations.

Thus, as a class the aldehydes can be very irritating and may constitute a significant fraction of the discomfort and sensation experienced during an oxidant pollution episode, especially in mixed atmospheres containing particles.

Carbon Monoxide

Carbon monoxide is classed toxicologically as a chemical asphyxiant because its toxic action stems from its formation of carboxyhemoglobin, preventing oxygenation of the blood for systemic transport. The fundamental toxicology of CO and the physiologic factors that determine the level of carboxyhemoglobin attained in the blood at various atmospheric concentrations of carbon monoxide are detailed in Chap. 11.

The normal concentration of carboxyhemoglobin (COHb) in the blood of nonsmokers is about 0.5%. This is attributed to endogenous production of CO from heme catabolism. Blood COHb is a function of the concentration in air, the length of exposure, and the ventilation of the exposed individual. Uptake is said to be ventilation-limited, implying that virtually all the CO inspired in a breath is absorbed and bound to the available hemoglobin. Thus, continuous exposure of human subjects to 30 ppm CO leads to an equilibrium value of 5% COHb. The Haldane equation is used to compute the COHb equilibrium under a given exposure situation. The equilibrium values generally are reached after eight hours or more of exposure, but the time required to reach equilibrium can be shortened by physical activity.

Carbon monoxide emissions from automobiles have progressively decreased since the 1970s. Increased combustion efficiency and catalytic converters have reduced emissions at the tailpipe by more than 90%. However, motor vehicles still account for two thirds of urban CO. Depending on the location in a community, traffic density, vehicle types and age, and the urban structure, CO concentrations can vary widely. Concentrations predicted inside passenger compartments of motor vehicles in downtown traffic were almost three times those for central urban areas and five times those expected in residential areas. Occupants of vehicles traveling on expressways had CO exposures somewhere between those in central urban areas and those in downtown traffic and concentrations in underground garages, tunnels, and buildings over highways can still reach high levels. But it must be kept in mind that there are many sources of CO—anywhere combustion is ongoing. Certainly both main and sidestream tobacco smoke are a source. Home heating systems and mobile auxiliary heating sources emit CO that when used inappropriately (ie, unventilated) can create life-threatening circumstances.

No overt clinical human health effects have been demonstrated for COHb levels below 2%, while levels above 40% cause fatal asphyxiation. However, there is evidence that in some people COHb in the range of 2.0% to 2.4% can elicit acute cardiovascular effects. A 90-minute exposure to about 50 ppm CO would likely result in COHb levels of ~2.5%, with a resultant impairment of time-interval discrimination even in healthy subjects; at approximately 5% COHb, there is an impairment of other psychomotor faculties. At 5% COHb in nonsmokers (the median COHb value for smokers is about 5%), however, maximal exercise duration and maximal oxygen consumption are reduced (Aronow, 1981). Clear cardiovascular changes also may be produced by exposures sufficient to yield COHb in excess of 5%. These include increased cardiac output, arteriovenous oxygen difference, and coronary blood flow in patients without coronary disease. Decreased coronary sinus blood PO_2 occurs in patients with coronary heart disease, and this would impair oxidative metabolism of the myocardium. In the early 1990s, a series of studies in subjects with cardiovascular disease was conducted in several laboratories under the sponsorship of the Health Effects Institute (HEI) to determine the potential for angina pectoris when they exercised moderately with COHb levels in the range of 2% to 6% (Allred *et al.*, 1989). The results of these studies indicate that premature angina can occur under these conditions but that the potential for the induction of ventricular arrhythmias remains uncertain.

Carbon monoxide has been implicated as a potentially important copollutant of PM with potential human health effects at low ambient levels. Independent CO effects have been reported in some epidemiological studies of ambient air pollution, but its singular role versus indicator role (for traffic) continues to be debated. The fact that effects noted in these studies are cardiovascular and involve angina and effects on EKG patterns lends credence to a role for CO in epidemiological health outcomes. Other data from epidemiological studies have shown a linkage between CO and some general CNS indices as well as birth outcomes. The sensitivity of newer analysis methods for these population studies is revealing previously unappreciated health effects. Among these are preterm births, cardiac birth defects, and infant mortality in the postneonatal period. Moreover, toxicological studies with animals also suggest potential developmental risks.

Reducing CO emissions is a major goal because of its high hazard—a colorless and odorless nonirritant—so technical combustion engineering advances are being pursued as well as changes in fuel formulations. The introduction of gasoline oxygenates such as MTBE in the 1990s and other ether derivatives constitutes attempts to enhance fuel combustion and reduce CO emissions. The experience with MTBE (as noted earlier) has led to such formulations being approached with some caution with greater attention being placed on assessments of potential unexpected consequences.

Hazardous Air Pollutants

HAPs (so-called air toxics) represent an inclusive classification for air pollutants of anthropogenic origin that are generally of measurable quantity in the air, and are not covered in the Criteria Pollutant list. They are covered under Section 112 of the CAA. Selected regulatory issues of the HAPs were discussed above. Most exposure estimates for these pollutants are derived from emission inventories that are modeled into the National Air Toxics Assessment (www.epa.gov/ttn/atw/nata/sitemap.html). The most recent NATA assessment (2005) used 2005 data on 177 of the 188 HAPs, plus diesel PM. The diverse nature of even 33 of the 188 HAPs (the so-called dirty 30 noted above) complicates a general discussion of their toxicology because the group includes various classes of organic chemicals (by structure, eg, acrolein, benzene), minerals (eg, asbestos), polycyclic hydrocarbon particulate material (eg, benzo(a)pyrene), and various metals and metal compounds (eg, mercury, beryllium compounds) and pesticides (eg, carbaryl, parathion).

The focus to date on the HAPs has been on their potential carcinogenicity, as shown in chronic bioassays, mutagenicity tests in bacterial systems, structure–activity relationships, or—in a few special cases (eg, benzene, asbestos)—their known carcinogenicity in humans. These cancers need not be, and generally are not, pulmonary. Noncancer issues frequently relate to direct lung toxicants that, on fugitive emissions or accidental release, might risk those with preexisting diseases (eg, asthma) or might lead to chronic lung disease. The assessment of noncancer risk by air toxics to any organ system is based on the computation of long-term risk reference exposure concentrations (RfCs) to which individuals may be exposed over a lifetime without adverse, irreversible injury. This approach to HAP assessment is discussed in detail by Jarabek and Segal (1994). An analogous short-term RfC method has been developed for exposures up to 30 days. Of the noncancer risks deemed

highest in this analysis, acrolein ranks at the top based on emission inventories, the potential for exposure, and its inherent irritancy. Discussion of this topic and an approach to mixed exposures to noncancer HAPs has been reviewed (Costa, 2004).

Accidental versus "Fence-Line" Exposures

The relationship between the effects associated with an accidental release of a large quantity of a volatile chemical into the air from a point source such as a chemical plant and the effects associated with a chronic low-level exposure over many years or a lifetime is not clear. With regard to cancer, which defaults to a linearized model of dose and effect (though some alternative models can be used if there are appropriate data), the issue is fairly straightforward. Any exposure must be minimized if not eliminated if cancer risk is to be kept as close to zero as possible. With noncancer risks, the roles of nonspecific or specific host defenses, thresholds of response, and repair and recovery after exposure complicate the assessment of risk. In large part, the issue here relates to $C \times T$. Can we better relate disease or injury to *cumulative dose* or *peak* concentration for protracted exposures? Is there an exposure peak beyond which a cumulative approach fails (ie, the effect is concentration-driven), or is concentration always the dominant determinant? Many of these questions have yet to be answered, not to mention their specificity with regard to individual compounds and tissues affected.

Methyl isocyanate provides a contrast between the effects of a large accidental release and those produced by cyclic or continuous small fugitive vapor releases. The reactive nature of methyl isocyanate with aqueous environments is of such magnitude that on inspiration, almost immediate mucous tissue corrosion can be perceived. The vapor undergoes hydrolysis within the mucous lining of the airways to generate hydrocyanic acid, which destroys the airway epithelium and causes acute bronchoconstriction and edema. The damage is immediately life-threatening at concentrations above 50 ppm; at 10 ppm, it is damaging in minutes. These concentrations are in the range of the dense vapor cloud that for several hours enshrouded the village of Bhopal bordering the Union Carbide pesticide plant. Studies in guinea pigs showed the immediate irritancy of this isocyanate, which in just a few minutes also resulted in significant pathology (Alarie *et al.*, 1987). Rats exposed to 10 or 30 ppm for two hours also showed severe airway and parenchymal damage, which did not resolve in surviving rats; transient effects were seen at 3 ppm. Even six months after exposure, the airway and lung damage remained, having evolved into patchy, mostly peribronchial fibrosis with associated functional impairments (Stevens *et al.*, 1987). There was also cardiac involvement secondary to the damage to the pulmonary parenchyma and arterial bed. As a result, there was pulmonary hypertension and right-sided heart hypertrophy. This same spectrum of health effects has resulted in disability and deaths of thousands of initial survivors since the incident.

In the United States, methyl isocyanate has been measured in Katawba Valley, Texas, as a result of small but virtually continual fugitive releases of the vapor into the community air ("fence-line") from an adjoining region with several chemical plants. While these levels of methyl isocyanate are not sufficient to cause the damage seen in Bhopal, there is concern that low-level exposure over many years may have more diffuse, chronic effects. Residents complain of odors and a higher frequency of respiratory disorders, but clear evidence of injury or disease is lacking.

Phosgene is best known for its use as a war gas, but it is also a common intermediate reactant used in the chemical industry, particularly in pesticide formulation. It is also a constituent of photochemical smog. Because of its direct pulmonary reactivity, it lends itself to use as a model pulmonary toxicant for studies addressing C × T relationships. These studies suggest that there may be a threshold below which compensatory and other bodily defenses (eg, antioxidants) may be able to cope with long-term low-level exposure (tolerance). For phosgene, this appears to be at or below the current threshold limit value of 0.1 ppm for eight hours. At higher concentrations, however, concentration appears to be the primary determinant of injury or disease regardless of duration. Thus, even though there is some adaptation with time, there continues to be a concentration-driven response that exceeds that predicted by C × T. This relationship appears to be different from that of O_3 at ambient levels, which can be approximated acutely by the C × T paradigm.

THE MULTIPOLLUTANT REALITY OF AIR POLLUTION

The pollutants in the atmosphere of any community vary considerably in space and time, and are charged by the varied output from a wide range of sources, only to be transformed stoichiometrically by a patterned intensity of sunlight. These complexities have been daunting to toxicologists for decades and have prompted scientists and risk assessors to adopt a reductionist approach—nominally one pollutant at a time. While the reductionist approach has been very successful in diminishing pollutants of primary concern and improving public health, it is widely thought that there are likely chemical and physiologic interactions between and among pollutants that are of public health consequence and have not been appreciated. Indeed, interactions are more likely to be apparent as exposure concentrations decrease, and while we might expect synergistic interactions as found with some particles and SO_2, it may be that antagonisms are prevalent. As the science and the statistical methods to look at interactions have improved, there is renewed interest in multipollutant toxicology.

Recent publications are revisiting this issue (Mauderly and Samet, 2009; NRC Report on Air Quality, 2004), where scientists from all sectors are trying to determine if there are approaches to studying interactions (Dominici *et al.*, 2010; Vedal and Kaufman, 2011), synthesizing or modeling findings (Johns *et al.*, 2012), and then translating models into practical approaches to reducing the most important mixtures and components and thereby health risk (Fann *et al.*, 2011). There is yet to be any consensus on any of these aspects of multipollutant science other than this is the appropriate time to reinitiate the discussion. Early toxicology studies used complex mixtures, some of which were photochemically altered (discussed earlier), and epidemiology found that different mixtures appeared to vary in their health impacts, only to abandon the task. But the revival of the PM story, and that it is itself a mixture, and that progress has been made in understanding its toxicity and some of the key attributes that drive the PM mixture, suggest that the challenge to reengage the issue is reasonable and likely marks the next dimension of air pollution toxicology. While single pollutant approaches to air pollution research, health assessments, and ambient air quality standard setting have been successful in reducing air pollution over the past few decades, there is a clear need for parallel efforts within both the scientific and the regulatory/policy communities to advance methods for evaluating and managing the effects of air pollution in a multipollutant manner.

CONCLUSIONS

In writing this textbook chapter on air pollution toxicology, the authors' goal has been to relate empirical studies in animals to phenomena known to occur in humans through epidemiological or controlled clinical study. The breadth and complexity of the problem of air pollution—from the development of credible databases to supporting regulatory action and decision making—has been the theme throughout. The classic and still most important air pollutants provide a foundation for understanding and appreciating the nuances of the issues and strategies for air pollution control and protection of public health. The key role of the toxicologist is to develop sensitive methods to assay responses to low pollutant concentrations, apply these methods to relevant exposure scenarios and test species, and develop paradigms to relate empirical toxicological data to real life through an understanding of mechanism. Last, the toxicologist must continually integrate laboratory data with those of epidemiology and clinical study to ensure their maximum utility.

REFERENCES

Alarie Y, Ferguson JS, Stock MF, et al. Sensory and pulmonary irritation of methyl isocyanate in mice and pulmonary irritation and possible cyanide-like effects of methyl isocyanate in guinea pigs. *Environ Health Perspect.* 1987;72:159–168.

Alarie YC, Ulrich CE, Busey WM, et al. Long-term continuous exposure of guinea pigs to sulfur dioxide. *Arch Environ Health.* 1970;21:769–777.

Alarie YC, Ulrich CE, Busey WM, et al. Long-term continuous exposure to sulfur dioxide in cynomolgus monkeys. *Arch Environ Health.* 1972;24:115–128.

Allred EN, Bleeker ER, Chaitman BR, et al. Short-term effects of carbon monoxide exposure on individuals with coronary heart disease. *N Engl J Med.* 1989;321:1426–1432.

Amdur MO. The response of guinea pigs to inhalation of formaldehyde and formic acid alone and with a sodium chloride aerosol. *Int J Air Pollut.* 1960;3:201–220.

Amdur MO. Sulfuric acid: the animals tried to tell us: 1989 Herbert E. Stokinger lecture. *Appl Ind Hyg Assoc J.* 1989;4:189–197.

Amdur MO, Dubriel M, Creasia DA. Respiratory response of guinea pigs to low levels of sulfuric acid. *Environ Res.* 1978;15:418–423.

Amdur MO, Sarofim AF, Neville M, et al. Coal combustion aerosols and SO_2: an interdisciplinary analysis. *Environ Sci Technol.* 1986;20:139–145.

American Lung Association State of the Air: 2012. Available at: http://www.stateoftheair.org/.

American Thoracic Society. What constitutes an adverse health effect of air pollution? *Am J Respir Crit Care Med.* 2000;161:665–673.

Anderson HR. Health effects of air pollution episodes. In: Holgate ST, Samet JM, Koren H, Maynard RL, eds. *Air Pollution and Health.* London, Academic Press; 1999:461–484.

Anenberg SC, Horowitz LW, Tong DQ, West JJ. An estimate of the global burden of anthropogenic ozone and fine particulate matter on premature human mortality using atmospheric modeling. *Environ Health Perspect.* 2010;118:1189–1195.

Aronow WS. Aggravation of angina pectoris by two percent carboxyhemoglobin. *Am Heart J.* 1981;101:154–157.

Barry BE, Mercer RR, Miller FJ, et al. Effects of inhalation of 0.25 ppm O3 on the terminal bronchioles of juvenile and adult rats. *Exp Lung Res.* 1988;14:225–245.

Bates DV, Sizto R. Air pollution and hospital admissions in southern Ontario: the acid summer haze effect. *Environ Res.* 1987;65:172–194.

Bauer AK, Kleeberger SR. Genetic mechanisms of susceptibility to ozone-induced lung disease. *Ann N Y Acad Sci.* 2010;1203:113–119.

Bein K, Leikauf GD. Acrolein—a pulmonary hazard. *Mol Nutr Food Res.* 2011;55:1342–1360.

Bessac BF, Jordt SE. Sensory detection and responses to toxic gases: mechanisms, health effects, and countermeasures. *Proc Am Thorac Soc.* 2010;7:269–277.

Boubel RW, Fox DL, Turner DB, et al. *Fundamentals of Air Pollution.* 3rd ed. New York: Academic Press; 1994:107.

Brimblecombe P. Air pollution and health history. In: Holgate ST, Samet JM, Koren H, Maynard RL, eds. *Air Pollution and Health.* London: Academic Press; 1999:10.

Brook RD, Rajagopalan S, Pope CA 3rd, et al. Particulate matter air pollution and cardiovascular disease: an update to the scientific statement from the American Heart Association. *Circulation.* 2010;121:2331–2378.

Brooks BO, Davis WF: *Understanding Indoor Air Quality.* Boca Raton, FL: CRC Press; 1992.

Calderon-Garcidueñas L, Mora-Tiscareno A, Fordham LA, et al. Respiratory damage in children exposed to urban pollution. *Pediatr Pulmonol.* 2003;36(2):148–161.

Calderon-Garcidueñas L, Osorno-Velazquez A, Bravo-Alvarez H, et al. Histopathological changes of the nasal mucosa in southwest metropolitan Mexico City inhabitants. *Am J Pathol.* 1992;140:225–232.

Calvert JG, Lazrus A, Kok GL, et al. Chemical mechanisms of acid generation in the troposphere. *Nature.* 1985;317:27–35.

Chang L, Huang Y, Stockstill BL, et al. Epithelial injury and interstitial fibrosis in the proximal alveolar regions of rats chronically exposed to a simulated pattern of urban ambient ozone. *Toxicol Appl Pharmacol.* 1992;115:241–252.

Chang L, Miller FJ, Ultman J, et al. Alveolar epithelial cell injuries by subacute exposure to low concentrations of ozone correlate with cumulative exposure. *Toxicol Appl Pharmacol.* 1991;109:219–234.

Chang LY, Mercer RR, Stockstill BL, et al. Effects of low levels of NO_2 on terminal bronchiolar cells and its relative toxicity compared to O_3. *Toxicol Appl Pharmacol.* 1988;96:451–464.

Chen LC, Lam HF, Kim EJ, et al. Pulmonary effects of ultrafine coal fly ash inhaled by guinea pigs. *J Toxicol Environ Health.* 1990;29:169–184.

Chen LC, Quan C, Hwang JS, et al. Atherosclerosis lesion progression during inhalation exposure to environmental tobacco smoke: a comparison to concentrated ambient air fine particles exposure. *Inhal Toxicol.* 2010;22(6):449–459.

Coffin DL, Blommer EJ. Acute toxicity of irradiated auto exhaust: its indication by enhancement of mortality from streptococcal pneumonia. *Arch Environ Health.* 1967;15:36–38.

Cogliano VJ. IARC monographs, leukemia, nasopharyngeal cancer, sinonasal cancer. *Environ Health Perspect.* 2005;113:1205–1208.

Cohen AJ, Nikula KJ. The health effects of diesel exhaust: laboratory and epidemiology studies. In: Holgate ST, Samet JM, Koren HS, Maynard RL, eds. *Air Pollution and Health.* San Diego: Academic Press; 1999:707–745.

Conolly RB, Kimbel JS, Janszen D, et al. Human respiratory tract cancer risks of inhaled formaldehyde: dose–response predictions derived from biologically-motivated computational modeling of a combined rodent and human dataset. *Toxicol Sci.* 2004;82:279–296.

Costa DL. Particulate matter and cardiopulmonary health: a toxicologic perspective. *Inhal Toxicol.* 2000;12(suppl 3):35–44.

Costa DL. Issues that must be addressed for risk assessment of mixed exposures: the U.S. EPA experience with air quality. *J Toxicol Environ Health A.* 2004;67(3):195–207.

Costa DL, Dreher KL. Bioavailable transition metals in particulate matter mediate cardiopulmonary injury in healthy and compromised animal models. *Environ Health Perspect.* 1997;105(suppl 5):1053–1060.

Costa DL, Kutzman RS, Lehmann JR, et al. Altered lung function and structure in the rat after subchronic exposure to acrolein. *Am Rev Respir Dis.* 1986;133:286–291.

Costa DL, Schafrank SN, Wehner RW, et al. Alveolar permeability to protein in rats differentially susceptible to ozone. *J Appl Toxicol.* 1985;5(3):182–186.

Costa DL, Schlegele E. Irritant air pollutants. In: Swift DL, Foster WM, eds. *Air Pollutants and the Respiratory Tract.* New York: Marcel Dekker; 1998:119–145.

Costa DL, Tepper JS, Stevens MA, et al. Restrictive lung disease in rats chronically exposed to an urban profile of ozone. *Am J Respir Crit Care Med.* 1995;151:1512–1518.

Detels R, Tashkin DP, Sayre JW, et al. The UCLA population studies of CORD: X. A cohort study of changes in respiratory function associated with chronic exposure to SO_x, NO_x, and hydrocarbons. *Am J Public Health.* 1991;81:350–359.

Devlin RB, Folinsbee LJ, Biscardi F, et al. Attenuation of cellular and biochemical changes in the lungs of humans exposed to ozone for five consecutive days. *Am Rev Respir Dis.* 1993;147:A71.

Devlin RB, McDonnell WF, Mann R, et al. Exposure of humans to ambient levels of ozone for 6.6 hours causes cellular and biochemical changes in the lung. *Am J Respir Cell Mol Biol.* 1991;4:72–81.

Diaz-Sanchez D, Garcia MP, Wang M, et al. Nasal challenge with diesel exhaust particles can induce sensitization to a neoallergen in the human mucosa. *J Allergy Clin Immunol.* 1999;104(6):1183–1188.

Dockery DW, Pope CA, Xu X, et al. An association between air pollution and mortality in six U.S. cities. *N Engl J Med.* 1993;329(24):1753–1759.

Dominici F, Peng RD, Barr CD, Bell ML. Protecting human health from air pollution: shifting from a single-pollutant to a multipollutant approach. *Epidemiology.* 2010;21:187–194.

Donaldson K, Li XY, MacNee W. Ultrafine (nanometre) particle mediated lung injury. *J Aerosol Sci.* 1998;29:553–560.

Driscoll KE, Deyo LC, Carter JM, et al. Effects of particle exposure and particle-elicited inflammatory cells on mutation in rat alveolar epithelial cells. *Carcinogenesis.* 1997;18(2):423–430.

Dye JA, Lehmann JR, McGee JK, et al. Acute pulmonary toxicity of particulate matter filter extracts in rats: coherence with epidemiologic studies in Utah Valley residents. *Environ Health Perspect.* 2001;109(suppl 3):395–403.

Ehrlich R, Henry MC. Chronic toxicity of nitrogen dioxide: I. Effect on resistance to bacterial pneumonia. *Arch Environ Health.* 1968;17:860–865.

Fann N, Roman HA, Fulcher CM, et al. Maximizing health benefits and minimizing inequality: incorporating local-scale data in the design and evaluation of air quality policies. *Risk Anal.* 2011;31:908–922.

Firkert M. Fog along the Meuse Valley. *Trans Faraday Soc.* 1936;32:1192–1197.

Frampton MW, Smeglin AM, Roberts NJJ, et al. Nitrogen dioxide exposure *in vivo* and human macrophage inactivation of influenza virus *in vitro*. *Environ Res.* 1989;48:179–192.

Frank NR, Speizer FE. SO_2 effects on the respiratory system in dogs: changes in mechanical behavior at different levels of the respiratory system during acute exposure to the gas. *Arch Environ Health.* 1965;11:624–634.

Gamble J. Lung cancer and diesel exhaust: a critical review of the occupational epidemiology literature. *Crit Rev Toxicol.* 2010;40:189–244.

Gardner DE. Oxidant induced enhanced sensitivity to infection in animal models and their extrapolation to man. *J Toxicol Environ Health.* 1984;13:423–439.

Gauderman WJ, Avol E, Gilliland F, et al. The effect of air pollution on lung development from 10 to 18 years of age. *N Engl J Med.* 2004;351(11):1057–1067.

Gearhart JM, Schlesinger RB. Sulfuric acid-induced changes in the physiology and structure of the tracheobronchial airways. *Environ Health Perspect.* 1989;79:127–136.

Gelzleichter TR, Witschi H, Last JA. Synergistic interaction of nitrogen dioxide and ozone on rat lungs: acute responses. *Toxicol Appl Pharmacol.* 1992;116:1–9.

Gerrity TR, Weaver RA, Bernsten J, et al. Extrathoracic and intrathoracic removal of ozone in tidal breathing humans. *J Appl Physiol.* 1988;65:393–400.

Ghio AJ. Biological effects of Utah Valley ambient air particles in humans: a review. *J Aerosol Med.* 2004;17:157–164.

Ghio AJ, Carter JD, Richards JH, et al. Diminished injury in hypertranferrinemic mice after exposure to a metal-rich particle. *Am J Physiol Lung Cell Mol Physiol.* 2000;278(5):L1051–L1061.

Ghio AJ, Smith CB, Madden MC. Diesel exhaust particles and airway inflammation. *Curr Opin Pulm Med.* 2012;18:144–150.

Gilmour MI, Park P, Doerfler D, Selgrade MK. Ozone-enhanced pulmonary infection with *Streptococcus zooepidemicus* in mice: the role of alveolar macrophage function and capsular virulence factors. *Am Rev Respir Dis.* 1993;147:753–760.

Glasser SW, Nogee LM. Genetically engineered mice in understanding the basis of neonatal lung disease. *Semin Perinatol.* 2006;30:341–349.

Gold DR, Litonjua A, Schwartz J, et al. Ambient pollution and heart rate variability. *Circulation.* 2000;101(11):1267–1273.

Goldstein BD, Lai LY, Ross SR, Cuzzi-Spada R. Susceptibility of inbred mouse strains to ozone. *Arch Environ Health.* 1973;27:412–413.

Greim H, Borm PJA, Schins RPF, et al. Toxicity of fibers and particles. Report of the workshop held in Munich, Germany. *Inhal Toxicol.* 2001;13:101–119.

Hackney JD, Linn WS, Avol EL. Acid fog: effects on respiratory function and symptoms in healthy asthmatic volunteers. *Environ Health Perspect.* 1989;79:159–162.

Hatch GE, Slade R, Harris LP, et al. Ozone dose and effect in humans and rats: a comparison using oxygen-18 labeling and bronchoalveolar lavage. *Am J Respir Crit Care Med.* 1994;150:676–683.

Hayes SM, Gobbell RV, Ganick NR, eds. *Indoor Air Quality: Solutions and Strategies.* New York: McGraw-Hill; 1995.

Hemispheric Transport of Air Pollution. Available at: http://www.htap.org/activities/2010_Final_Report.htm.

Henry MC, Findlay J, Spengler J, Ehrlich R. Chronic toxicity of NO$_2$ in squirrel monkeys: III. Effect on resistance to bacterial and viral infection. *Am Ind Hyg Assoc J.* 1970;20:566–570.

Hernández-Escobar SA, Avila-Casado MC, Soto-Abraham V, et al. Cytological damage of nasal epithelium associated with decreased glutathione peroxidase in residents from a heavily polluted city. *Int Arch Occup Environ Health.* 2009;82:603–612.

Higuchi MA, Davies DW. An ammonia abatement system for whole-body animal inhalation exposures to acid aerosols. *Inhal Toxicol.* 1993;5:323–333.

Horstman DH, Folinsbee LJ, Ives PJ, et al. Ozone concentration and pulmonary response relationships for 6.6 hours with five hours of moderate exercise to 0.08, 0.10, and 0.12 ppm. *Am Rev Respir Dis.* 1989;142:1158–1162.

Horvath E, Anderson H, Pierce W, et al. Effects of formaldehyde on mucous membranes and lungs: a study of an industrial population. *JAMA.* 1988;259:701–707.

Hyde D, Orthoefer J, Dungworth D, et al. Morphometric and morphologic pulmonary lesions in beagle dogs chronically exposed to high ambient levels of air pollutants. *Lab Invest.* 1978;38(4):455–469.

ILSI Report. The relevance of the rat lung response to particle overload for human risk assessment: a workshop consensus report. ILSI Risk Science Institute Workshop Participants. *Inhal Toxicol.* 2000;12:101–117.

Jakab GJ. Relationship between carbon black particulate-bound formaldehyde, pulmonary antibacterial defenses and alveolar macrophage phagocytosis. *Inhal Toxicol.* 1992;4:325–342.

Jarabek AM, Segal SA. Noncancer toxicity of inhaled toxic air pollutants: available approaches for risk assessment and risk management. In: Patrick DR, ed. *Toxic Air Pollution Handbook.* New York: Van Nostrand Reinhold; 1994:100–132.

Johns DO, Stanek L, Walker K, et al. Practical advancement of multipollutant scientific and risk assessment approaches for ambient air pollution. *Environ Health Perspect.* 2012;120(9):1238–1242 [electronic].

Kieber RJ, Skrabal SA, Smith BJ, Willey JD. Organic complexation of Fe(II) and its impact on the redox cycling of iron in rain. *Environ Sci Technol.* 2005;39(6):1576–1583.

Kim CS, Kang TC. Comparative measurement of lung deposition of inhaled fine particles in normal subjects and patients with obstructive airway disease. *Am J Respir Crit Care Med.* 1997;155(3):899–905.

Kleeberger SR, Reddy S, Zhang LY, et al. Genetic susceptibility to ozone-induced lung hyperpermeability. Role of toll-like receptor 4. *Am J Respir Cell Mol Biol.* 2000;22(5):620–627.

Kleinman MT, Mautz WJ, Bjarnason S. Adaptive and non-adaptive responses in rats exposed to ozone, alone and in mixtures, with acidic aerosols. *Inhal Toxicol.* 1999;11(3):249–264.

Kodavanti UP, Costa DL, Bromberg P. Rodent models of cardiopulmonary disease: their potential applicability in studies of air pollutant susceptibility. *Environ Health Perspect.* 1998;106(suppl 1):111–130.

Kodavanti UP, Mebane R, Ledbetter A, et al. Variable pulmonary responses from exposure to concentrated ambient air particles in a rat model of bronchitis. *Toxicol Sci.* 2000;54(2):441–451.

Kodavanti UP, Schladweiler MC, Ledbetter AD, et al. Consistent pulmonary and systemic responses from inhalation of fine concentrated ambient particles: roles of rat strains used and physicochemical properties. *Environ Health Perspect.* 2005;113(11):1561–1568.

Koenig JQ, Covert DS, Pierson WE. Effects of inhalation of acidic compounds on pulmonary function in allergic adolescent subjects. *Environ Health Perspect.* 1989;79:127–137, 173–178.

Koenig JQ, Pierson WE, Horike M, Frank R. Effects of SO$_2$ plus NaCl aerosol combined with moderate exercise on pulmonary function in asthmatic adolescents. *Environ Res.* 1981;25:340–348.

Kotin P, Falk HF. Atmospheric factors in pathogenesis of lung cancer. *Cancer Res.* 1963;7:475–514.

Kreyling WG, Semmler-Behnke M, Seitz J, et al. Size dependence of the translocation of inhaled iridium and carbon nanoparticle aggregates from the lung of rats to the blood and secondary target organs. *Inhal Toxicol.* 2009;21(suppl 1):55–60.

Krzyzanowski M, Quackenboss JJ, Lebowitz MD. Chronic respiratory effects of indoor formaldehyde exposure. *Environ Res.* 1990;52:117–125.

Kumie A, Emmelin A, Wahlberg S, et al. Magnitude of indoor NO2 from biomass fuels in rural settings of Ethiopia. *Indoor Air.* 2009;19:14–21.

Last JA, Gelzleichter TR, Harkema J, Hawk S. *Consequences of Prolonged Inhalation of Ozone on Fischer-344/N Rats: Collaborative Studies. Part I: Content and Cross-Linking of Lung Collagen.* Research Report No. 65. Cambridge, MA: Health Effects Institute; April 1994.

Lewis TR, Campbell KI, Vaughan TR Jr. Effects on canine pulmonary function: via induced NO$_2$ impairment, particulate interaction, and subsequent SO$_x$. *Arch Environ Health.* 1969;18:596–601.

Lewis TR, Moorman WJ, Yang YY, Stara JF. Long-term exposure to auto exhaust and other pollutant mixtures. *Arch Environ Health.* 1974;21:102–106.

Lewtas J. Airborne carcinogens. *Pharmacol Toxicol.* 1993;72(suppl 1):55–63.

Lewtas J. Air pollution combustion emissions: characterization of causative agents and mechanisms associated with cancer, reproductive, and cardiovascular effects. *Mutat Res.* 2007;636:95–133.

Li Z, Potts-Kant EN, Garantziotis S, Foster WM, Hollingsworth JW. Hyaluronan signaling during ozone-induced lung injury requires TLR4, MyD88, and TIRAP. *PLoS One.* 2011;6(11):e27137.

Lipfert FW. *Air Pollution and Community Health: A Critical Review and Data Sourcebook.* New York: Van Nostrand Reinhold; 1994:10–57.

Lippmann M. Health effects of ozone: a critical review. *J Air Pollut Control Assoc.* 1989;39:67–96.

Madden MC, Richards J, Daily LA, et al. Effect of ozone on diesel exhaust particle toxicity in the rat lung. *Toxicol Appl Pharmacol.* 2000;168:140–148.

Maddison D, Pierce D. Costing the health effects of poor air quality. In: Holgate ST, Samet JM, Koren H, Maynard RL, eds. *Air Pollution and Health.* London: Academic Press; 1999:917–930.

Martonen TB, Zhang Z, Yang Y. Interspecies modeling of inhaled particle deposition patterns. *J Aerosol Sci.* 1992;23(4):389–406.

Mauderly JL. Health hazards of complex environmental exposures: a difficult challenge to inhalation toxicology. *Inhal Toxicol.* 2006;18:137–141.

Mauderly JL, Samet JM. Is there evidence for synergy among air pollutants in causing health effects? *Environ Health Perspect.* 2009;117:1–6.

McCunney RJ. Asthma, genes, and air pollution. *J Occup Environ Med.* 2005;47(12):1285–1291.

McDonnell WF. Intersubject variability in human acute ozone responsiveness. *Pharmacogenetics.* 1991;1:110–113.

McDonnell WF, Horstman DH, Hazucha MJ, et al. Pulmonary effects of ozone exposure during exercise: dose–response characteristics. *J Appl Physiol.* 1983;5:1345–1352.

McGwin G, Lienert J, Kennedy JI. Formaldehyde exposure and asthma in children: a systematic review. *Environ Health Perspect.* 2010;118:313–317.

McKinney WJ, Jaskot RH, Richards JH, et al. Cytokine mediation of ozone-induced pulmonary adaptation. *Am J Respir Cell Mol Biol.* 1998;18:696–705.

Mercer RR, Costa DL, Crapo JD. Effects of prolonged exposure to low doses of nitric oxide on the alveolar septa of the adult rat lung. *Lab Invest.* 1995;73(1):1–9.

Miller FJ, Graham JA, Raub JA, et al. Evaluating the toxicity of urban patterns of oxidant gases: II. Effects in mice from chronic exposure to nitrogen dioxide. *J Toxicol Environ Health.* 1987;21:99–112.

Miller FW, Miller RM. *Environmental Hazards: Air Pollution—A Reference Handbook. Contemporary World Issues.* Santa Barbara, CA: ABC-CLIO; 1993:1–18.

Mohsenin V. Effect of vitamin C on NO_2-induced airway hyperresponsiveness in normal subjects. *Am Rev Respir Dis.* 1987;136:1408–1411.

Molhave LB, Bach B, Pederson O. Human reactions to low concentrations of volatile organic compounds. *Environ Int.* 1986;12:165–167.

Moss OR, Gross EA, James RA, et al. Respiratory tract toxicity in rats exposed to Mexico City air. *Res Rep Health Effects Inst.* 2001;(100):1–24.

Mudway IS, Krishna MT, Frew AJ, et al. Compromised concentrations of ascorbate in fluid lining the respiratory tract in human subjects after exposure to ozone. *Occup Environ Med.* 1999;56(7):473–481.

Murphy SD, Klingshirn DA, Ulrich CE. Respiratory response of guinea pigs during acrolein inhalation and its modification by drugs. *J Pharmacol Exp Ther.* 1963;141:79–83.

Nadel JA, Salem H, Tamplin B, Tokiwa Y. Mechanism of bronchoconstriction during inhalation of sulfur dioxide. *J Appl Physiol.* 1965;20:164–167.

National Research Council (NRC). *Air Quality Management in the United States.* Report by the Committee on Air Quality Management in the United States, Board on Environmental Studies and Toxicology, Board on Atmospheric Sciences and Climate, Division on Earth and Life Studies. Washington, DC: The National Academy Press; 2004.

National Research Council (NRC). *Risk Assessment in the Federal Government: Managing the Means.* Committee on the Institutional Means for Assessment of Risks to Public Health. Washington, DC: National Academy Press; 1983.

Nielsen GD, Wolkoff P. Cancer effects of formaldehyde: a proposal for an indoor air guideline value. *Arch Toxicol.* 2010;84:423–446.

Oberdorster G, Sharp Z, Atudorei V, et al. Extrapulmonary translocation of ultrafine carbon particles following whole-body inhalation exposure of rats. *J Toxicol Environ Health A.* 2002;65(20):1531–1543.

O'Donnell MD, O'Conner CM, FitzGerald MX, et al. Ultrastructure of lung elastin and collagen in mouse models of spontaneous emphysema. *Matrix Biol.* 1999;18(4):357–360.

Ohtsuka Y, Clarke RW, Mitzner W, et al. Interstrain variation in murine susceptibility to inhaled acid-coated particles. *Am J Physiol Lung Cell Mol Physiol.* 2000;278(3):L469–L476.

Overton JH, Miller FJ. Modeling ozone absorption in the respiratory tract. 80th Annual Meeting of the Air Pollution Control Association; 1987; paper no. 87–99.4.

Peters A. Commentary: inflamed about ultrafine particles? *Int J Epidemiol.* 2006;35:1355–1356.

Pinkerton KE, Brody AR, Miller FJ, Crapo JD. Exposure to low levels of ozone results in enhanced pulmonary retention of inhaled asbestos fibers. *Am Rev Respir Dis.* 1989;140(4):1075–1081.

Pope CA 3rd, Thun MJ, Namboodiri MM, et al. Particulate air pollution as a predictor of mortality in a prospective study of U.S. adults. *Am J Respir Crit Care Med.* 1995;151(3 pt 1):669–674.

Pope CA 3rd. Particulate pollution and health: a review of the Utah valley experience. *J Expo Anal Environ Epidemiol.* 1996;6:23–34.

Pope CA 3rd, Burnett RT, Thun MJ, et al. Lung cancer, cardiopulmonary mortality, and long-term exposure to fine particulate air pollution. *JAMA.* 2002;287(9):1132–1141.

Pope CA 3rd, Burnett RT, Turner MC, et al. Lung cancer and cardiovascular disease mortality associated with ambient air pollution and cigarette smoke: shape of the exposure–response relationships. *Environ Health Perspect.* 2011;119:1616–1621.

Pope CA III, Dockery DW. 2006 critical review—health effects of fine particulate air pollution: lines that connect. *J Air Waste Manag Assoc.* 2006;56:709–748.

Reid L. An experimental study of hypersecretion of mucus in the bronchial tree. *Br J Exp Pathol.* 1963;44:437–440.

Reuther CG. *Focus*—winds of change: reducing transboundary air pollutants. *Environ Health Perspect.* 2000;108(4):A170–A175.

Robinson J, Nelson WC. *National Human Activity Pattern Survey Data Base.* Research Triangle Park, NC: U.S. Environmental Protection Agency; 1998.

Roda C, Kousignian I, Guihenneuc-Jouyaux C, et al. Formaldehyde exposure and lower respiratory infections in infants: findings from the PARIS cohort study. *Environ Health Perspect.* 2011;119:1653–1658.

Romieu I, Sienra-Monge JJ, Ramirez-Aguilar M, et al. Genetic polymorphism of GSTM1 and antioxidant supplementation influence lung function in relation to ozone exposure in asthmatic children in Mexico City. *Thorax.* 2004;59(1):8–10.

Rosenlund M, Berglind N, Pershagen G, et al. Long-term exposure to urban air pollution and myocardial infarction. *Epidemiology.* 2006;17(4):383–390.

Saldiva PHN, King M, Delmonte VLC, et al. Respiratory alterations due to urban air pollution: an experimental study in rats. *Environ Res.* 1992;57:19–33.

Salvi S, Blomberg A, Rudell B, et al. Acute inflammatory responses in the airways and peripheral blood after short-term exposure to diesel exhaust in healthy human volunteers. *Am J Respir Crit Care Med.* 1999;159:702–709.

Samoli E, Aga E, Touloumi G, et al. Short-term effects of nitrogen dioxide on mortality: an analysis within the APHEA project. *Eur Respir J.* 2006;27(6):1129–1138.

Schenker MB, Samet JM, Speizer FE, et al. Health effects of air pollution due to coal combustion in the Chestnut Ridge region of Pennsylvania: results of cross-sectional analysis in adults. *Arch Environ Health.* 1983;38:325–330.

Schins RP, Knaapen AM. Genotoxicity of poorly soluble particles. *Inhal Toxicol.* 2007;19(suppl 1):189–198.

Schlesinger RB. Comparative irritant potency of inhaled sulfate aerosol: effects on bronchial mucociliary clearance. *Environ Res.* 1984;34:268–279.

Schlesinger RB. Intermittent inhalation of nitrogen dioxide: effects on rabbit alveolar macrophages. *J Toxicol Environ Health.* 1987;21:127–139.

Schlesinger RB, Chen LC, Finkelstein I, Zelikoff JT. Comparative potency of inhaled acidic sulfates: speciation and the role of hydrogen ion. *Environ Res.* 1990;52:210–224.

Schlesinger RB, Gorczynski JE, Dennison J, et al. Long-term intermittent exposure to sulfuric acid aerosol, ozone, and their combination: alterations in tracheobronchial mucociliary clearance and epithelial secretory cells. *Exp Lung Res.* 1992;18:505–534.

Schlesinger RB, Weidman PA, Zelikoff JT. Effects of repeated exposures to ozone and nitrogen dioxide on respiratory tract prostanoids. *Inhal Toxicol.* 1991;3:27–36.

Schwartz J. Particulate air pollution and daily mortality in Detroit. *Environ Res.* 1991;56:204–213.

Schwartz J. Air pollution and the duration of acute respiratory symptoms. *Arch Environ Health.* 1992;47(2):116–122.

Schwela DH. Exposure to environmental chemicals relevant for respiratory hypersensitivity: global aspects. *Toxicol Lett.* 1996;86:131–142.

Schwela DH. *The World Health Organization Guidelines for Air Quality. Part 1: Exposure–Response Relationships and Air Quality Guidelines.* Geneva: WHO; 2000:29–34.

Seigneur C, Vijayaraghavan K, Lohman K, Karamchandani P, Scott C. Global source attribution for mercury deposition in the United States. *Environ Sci Technol.* 2004;38:555–569.

Shapiro SD. Transgenic and gene-targeted mice as models for chronic obstructive pulmonary disease. *Eur Respir J.* 2007;29:375–378.

Sheppard DA, Saisho A, Nadel JA, Boushey HA. Exercise increases sulfur dioxide induced bronchoconstriction in asthmatic subjects. *Am Rev Respir Dis.* 1981;123:486–491.

Shore SA, Lang JE, Kasahara DI, et al. Pulmonary responses to subacute ozone exposure in obese vs. lean mice. *J Appl Physiol.* 2009;107:1445–1452.

Sienra-Monge JJ, Ramirez-Aguilar M, Moreno-Macias H. Antioxidant supplementation and nasal inflammatory responses among young asthmatics exposed to high levels of ozone. *Clin Exp Immunol.* 2004;138(2):317–322.

Singh P, DeMarini DM, Dick CA, et al. Sample characterization of automobile and forklift diesel exhaust particles and comparative pulmonary toxicity in mice. *Environ Health Perspect.* 2004;112(8):820–825.

Speizer FE. Studies of acid aerosols in six cities and in a new multi-city investigation: design issues. *Environ Health Perspect.* 1989;79:61–68.

Spengler JD, Sexton K. Indoor air pollution: a public health perspective. *Science.* 1983;221:9–17.

Stevens MA, Fitzgerald S, Menache MG, et al. Functional evidence of persistent airway obstruction in rats following a two-hour inhalation exposure to methyl isocyanate. *Environ Health Perspect.* 1987;72: 89–94.

Suga T, Kurabayashi M, Sando Y, et al. Disruption of the klotho gene causes pulmonary emphysema in mice. *Am J Respir Cell Mol Biol.* 2000;22:26–33.

Sun Q, Wang A, Jin X, et al. Long-term air pollution exposure and acceleration of atherosclerosis and vascular inflammation in an animal model. *JAMA.* 2005;294(23):3003–3010.

Sweeney TD, Skornik WA, Brain JD, et al. Chronic bronchitis alters the pattern of aerosol deposition in the lung. *Am J Respir Crit Care Med.* 1995;151(2 pt 1):482–488.

The Collaborative Ozone Project Group. *Health Effects Report: Consequences of Prolonged Inhalation of Ozone on F344 Rats: Collaborative Studies.* Studies I–XIII, Report #65. Boston: Health Effects Institute; 1994–1995.

Thurston GD, Ito K, Kinney PL, Lippmann M. A multi-year study of air pollution and respiratory hospital admissions in three New York state metropolitan areas: results for 1988 and 1989 summers. *J Expo Anal Environ Epidemiol.* 1992;2:429–450.

Tong H, Cheng WY, Samet JM, Gilmour MI, Devlin RB. Differential cardiopulmonary effects of size-fractionated ambient particulate matter in mice. *Cardiovasc Toxicol.* 2010;10:259–267.

Tujague J, Bastaki M, Holland N, et al. Antioxidant intake, GSTM1 polymorphism and pulmonary function in healthy young adults. *Eur Respir J.* 2006;27:282–288.

Tyler WS, Tyler NK, Hinds D, et al. Influence of exposure regimen on effects of experimental ozone studies: effects of daily and episodic and seasonal cycles of exposure and post-exposure. Presented at: 84th Annual Meeting of the Air Waste Management Association; 1991; Vancouver, BC, Canada. Paper No. 91–141.5.

Tyler WS, Tyler NK, Last JA, et al. Comparison of daily and seasonal exposures of young monkeys to ozone. *Toxicology.* 1988;50:131–144.

U.S. EPA. *Air Quality Criteria Document for Ozone and Photochemical Oxidants.* 600/P-93/004cF, NCEA. Research Triangle Park, NC: U.S. EPA; 1996.

U.S. EPA. *National Air Pollutant Emission Trends Reports: 1998.* EPA 454/R-00-002. Research Triangle Park, NC: U.S. EPA, Office of Air Quality Planning and Standards; March 2000a:21.

U.S. EPA. *Air Quality Criteria for Particulate Matter (October 2004).* Washington, DC: U.S. Environmental Protection Agency; 2004. EPA 600/P-99/002aF-bF.

USEPA. *Motor Vehicle-Related Air Toxics Study.* EPA 420-R-93-005. Ann Arbor, MI: Office of Mobile Sources; 1993.

U.S. EPA ISA (Integrated Science Assessment). Available at: http://www. epa.gov/ncea/isa/ozone.htm. 2012.

Utell MJ, Mariglio JA, Morrow PE, et al. Effects of inhaled acid aerosols on respiratory function: the role of endogenous ammonia. *J Aerosol Med.* 1989;2:141–147.

Utell MJ, Morrow PE, Hyde RW. Airway reactivity to sulfate and sulfuric acid aerosols in normal and asthmatic subjects. *J Air Pollut Control Assoc.* 1984;34:931–935.

Van De Lende R, Kok TJ, Reig RP, et al. Decreases in VC and FEV_1 with time: indicators for effects of smoking and air pollution. *Bull Eur Physiopathol Respir.* 1981;17:775–792.

Vancza EM, Galdanes K, Gunnison A, Hatch G, Gordon T. Age, strain, and gender as factors for increased sensitivity of the mouse lung to inhaled ozone. *Toxicol Sci.* 2009;107:535–543.

Vaughan TR, Jennelle LF, Lewis TR. Long-term exposure to low levels of air pollutants: effects on pulmonary function in the beagle. *Arch Environ Health.* 1969;19:45–50.

Vedal S, Kaufman JD. What does multi-pollutant air pollution research mean? *Am J Respir Crit Care Med.* 2011;183:4–6.

von Mutius E, Martinez FD, Fritzsch C, et al. Prevalence of asthma and atopy in two areas of West and East Germany. *Am J Respir Crit Care Med.* 1994;149(2 pt 1):358–364.

Waxman HA. Title III of the 1990 Clean Air Act amendments. In: Patrick DR, ed. *Toxic Air Pollution Handbook.* New York: Van Nostrand Reinhold; 1994:25–32.

WHO. *Global Health Risks: Mortality and Burden of Disease Attributable to Selected Major Risks.* ISBN 978 92 4 156387 1. Geneva: World Health Organization; 2009.

Wichers LB, Rowan WH, Nolan JP, et al. Particle deposition in spontaneously hypertensive rats exposed via whole-body inhalation: measured and estimated dose. *Toxicol Sci.* 2006;93(2):400–410.

Wiester MJ, Winsett DW, Richards JE, et al. Ozone adaptation in mice and its association with ascorbic acid in the lung. *Inhal Toxicol.* 2000;12:577–590.

Woodruff TJ, Wells EM, Holt EW, Burgin DE, Axelrad DA. Estimating risk from ambient concentrations of acrolein across the United States. *Environ Health Perspect.* 2007;115:410–415.

Yoshida M, Whitsett JA. Alveolar macrophages and emphysema in surfactant protein-D-deficient mice. *Respirology.* 2006;11:S37–S40.

Zeger SL, Dominici F, McDermott A, Samet JM. Mortality in the Medicare population and chronic exposure to fine particulate matter. *Environ Health Perspect.* 2008;116:1614–1619.

Zou B, Wilson JG, Zhan FB, Zeng Y. Air pollution exposure assessment methods utilized in epidemiological studies. *J Environ Monit.* 2009;11:475–490.

Applications
of Toxicology

Ecotoxicology

Richard T. Di Giulio and Michael C. Newman

INTRODUCTION

Ecotoxicology is the science of contaminants in the biosphere and their effects on constituents of the biosphere (Newman, 2010). It follows from this definition that ecotoxicologists examine large-scale ecological phenomenon (Preston, 2002) in addition to those normally addressed in toxicology: ecotoxicology has an overarching goal of explaining and predicting effect or exposure phenomena at several levels of biological organization (Fig. 30-1). Essential explanations and models include those applied in conventional toxicology and a range of environmental sciences.

Although Truhaut's original definition of this new science encompassed effects to humans (Truhaut, 1977), most recent definitions of ecotoxicology do not. Relevant effects to nonhuman targets range from biomolecular to global. Taking on the classic toxicology vantage initially, suborganismal and organismal effects were emphasized during ecotoxicology's nascent stage; however, studies of higher level effects and interactions are becoming increasingly commonplace as the science matures. Such indirect effects[1] were initially considered problematic and reluctantly relegated to secondary importance (Fleeger *et al.*, 2003) relative to direct effects to individuals. Indirect effects are now known to be as important as direct effects to nonhuman targets (Fleeger *et al.*, 2003; Chapman, 2004). As the need to predict major effects to populations, communities, ecosystems, and other higher level entities has become increasingly apparent, more cause–effect models relevant to these higher levels

of biological organization are added to the conventional set of toxicology models applied by pioneering ecotoxicologists.

Contaminant chemical form, phase association, and movement among components of the biosphere are also central issues in ecotoxicology because they determine exposure, bioavailability, and realized dose. The context of these biogeochemical studies has expanded in the last several decades to encompass issues of larger scale such as global movement of persistent organic pollutants (POPs) (Wania and Mackay, 1996).

From a practical vantage, ecotoxicology informs decision makers about ecological risks associated with contamination. Risk to ecological entities is estimated or predicted by combining exposure and effect information. Risk might involve diminished fitness of individuals, increased risk of local population extinction, a drop in species diversity, or reduced nutrient cycling or primary productivity. Because potential ecological end points are so diverse, the ecological risk framework tends to be more flexible than that of the conventional human health risk assessment (Fig. 30-2). This important role of ecotoxicology in ecological risk assessment (ERA) will be discussed in more detail below.

SOME DISTINCT ASPECTS OF EXPOSURE

Predicting exposure and effect is difficult for all relevant ecological entities. In contrast to human toxicology in which information about a few species might be used to predict harm to one (humans), ecotoxicology commonly uses sparse information for a few species to predict effects to many species and their interactions. Exposure pathways, bioavailability, bioaccumulation, and toxicant transfer for all relevant ecological entities are also difficult issues requiring considerable effort to adequately understand.

---

[1]Indirect effects are effects of toxicants mediated by another ecosystem component (Krivtsov, 2004) such as those that might occur to a flowering plant if a pesticide were to eliminate its primary insect pollinator.

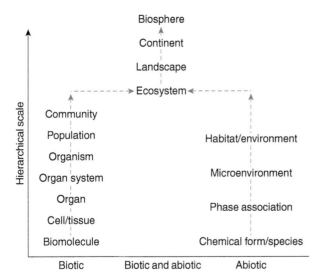

Figure 30-1. *Ecological scales relevant to ecotoxicology.* Solely biological scales relevant to ecotoxicology range from the molecular to the community levels: solely abiotic scales range from the chemical to the entire habitat. Biotic and abiotic components are usually combined at levels above the ecological community and habitat. The ecological community and physico-chemical habitat combined to form the ecosystem. Ecological systems can be considered at the landscape scale, such as the combination of marine, freshwater, and terrestrial systems at a river's mouth. Recently, the continental and biospheric scales have become relevant as in the cases of ozone depletion, acid precipitation, and global warming.

Relevant exposure routes are the conventional ingestion, inhalation, and dermal absorption. But unique features of exposure pathways must be accommodated for species that ingest a wide range of materials using distinct feeding mechanisms, breathe gaseous or liquid media using different structures, and come into dermal contact with a variety of gaseous, liquid, and solid media.

Prediction of oral exposure can be limited because species feed on different materials; however, conventional principles regarding oral bioavailability remain relevant. As an example, some birds are uniquely at high risk of lead poisoning because they ingest and then use lead shot as grit. Shot are ground together in their gizzards under acidic conditions, releasing significant amounts of dissolved lead (Kendall *et al.*, 1996). As true with humans (ie, the ionic hypothesis of Mathews, 1904), the dissolved form of lead is more available to do harm than solid lead shot. Similar high risk of lead poisoning is present for some raptors feeding on game birds whose tissues can contain lead shot (Wayland and Bollinger, 1999). Complex sorting of filtered materials on the gills of bivalve molluscs strongly influences the metal content and bioavailability of the material that eventually passes into their guts (Allison *et al.*, 1998). Some invertebrate species have elaborate feeding structures that are also involved in respiration (eg, lugworms and bivalve molluscs) or locomotion (copepods and other zooplankton species). Some zooplankton species feed and digest algal cells in such a way that only metals soluble in the algal cytosol are bioavailable (Reinfelder and Fisher, 1991). Unlike mammalian species, many invertebrate species are capable of sequestering large amounts of metals in intracellular granules (Mason and Nott, 1981). Incorporation of metals into granules by prey species reduces metal bioavailability to predators (Nott and Nicolaidou, 1993). Just as noted with 5-fluoruracil administration or chronic ethanol consumption, some pollutant exposures cause malabsorption by damaging the intestine wall. A relevant situation would be intestinal damage to otters caused by ingestion during grooming of oiled fur (Lipscomb *et al.*, 1996; Ormseth and Ben-David, 2000).

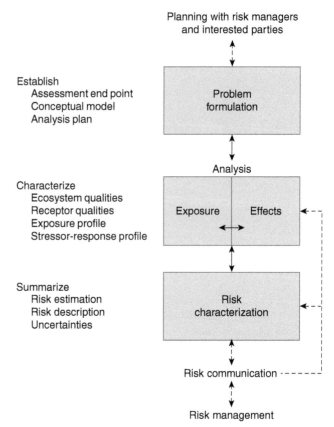

Figure 30-2. *The general form of an ecological risk assessment including problem formulation, analysis, and risk characterization stages.* Problem formulation is done in dialog with risk managers and stakeholders, and involves a clear statement of the ecological entity to be assessed, a conceptual model for the process, and a plan for conducting the assessment. The analysis stage involves exposure and effects characterizations. Using the context developed during problem formulation and information organized together in the analysis stage, a statement of risk and associated uncertainties are made in the risk characterization stage.

The principles remain the same in all of these cases but critical exposure pathway details are different.

Many techniques applied to determining human oral bioavailability are available to the ecotoxicologist; however, as just illustrated, modifications are needed for the many pathways for nonhuman species exposure. Typical are those associated with estimating contaminant bioavailability in aquatic environments. As an example, biomimetic and related extraction methods used to predict human oral bioavailability can be modified to predict sediment-bound contaminant bioavailabilities. Sediments are placed into contact with biomimetic solutions (Chen and Mayer, 1998; Leslie *et al.*, 2002) or digestive fluids taken from organisms (Mayer *et al.*, 1996; Weston and Maruya, 2002), and the amount of extracted contaminant used to estimate bioavailability.

Estimation of chemical speciation is central to predicting bioavailability of water-associated contaminants. Speciation can determine the bioavailability of dissolved metals. Movements of nonionic and ionizable organic compounds across the gut or gills are strongly influenced by lipid solubility and the pH-partition theory, respectively. Consequently, determination of a compound's lipophilicity or calculation of pH- and pK_a-dependent ionization facilitates some predictive capability for bioavailability. A common application of this approach would be estimation of water pH effects on ammonia toxicity as the consequence of the ease with which unionized ammonia passes through gills relative to ionized ammonia (Lloyd and Herbert, 1960). The free ion activity model (FIAM) states that uptake and toxicity of cationic trace metals are best predicted from their free ion activity or concentration (Campbell and Tessier, 1996), although exceptions exist to this extension of the ionic hypothesis. Consequently, dissolved metal exposure assessments often begin by estimating the amount of a metal present as the free ion. Normally, such calculations require only thermodynamic modeling based on measured concentrations of dissolved cations and anions. Lipid partitioning is often used to predict dissolved, nonionizing organic compound accumulation in and effects to aquatic biota. The propensity for an organic compound to accumulate in aquatic organisms increases with lipid solubility as often described with a simple quantitative structure activity relationship (QSAR) (Neely *et al.*, 1974; Mackay, 1982; Chiou, 1985; Connell, 1990). The log of the octanol–water partition coefficient (log K_{ow}) is used to predict measures such as the bioconcentration factor (BCF; the quotient of the concentration in the organism and that in the water from which the organic compound is being accumulated):

$$BCF = \frac{C_{Organism}}{C_{Water}}.$$

Bioavailability, bioaccumulation, or exposure concentrations for sediment-associated toxicants are also approached by considering chemical speciation and phase partitioning. Metals in sediments are either incorporated into one of many solid phases or dissolved in the interstitial waters surrounding the sediment particles. Bioavailabilities of metals in these different forms are difficult to predict (Luoma, 1989) but, nonetheless, various schemes have been applied to that end. Bioavailable metals have been estimated by normalizing sediment metal concentrations to easily extracted iron and manganese concentrations because solid iron and manganese oxides sequester metals in poorly bioavailable solid forms (Luoma and Bryan, 1978). Other chemical extraction methods have been applied with some success (Tessier *et al.*, 1984). A pragmatic method for predicting sediment metal bioavailability has emerged that is based on the assumption that the sediment metal form of most concern is the dissolved metal. Further, for many metals and sediments, the dissolved interstitial metal concentrations are determined by equilibrium between solid (iron and manganese) sulfides and the interstitial water:

$$Cd^{2+} + FeS_{Solid} \leftrightarrow CdS_{Solid} + Fe^{2+}.$$

Because the equilibrium so favors formation of metal sulfide (CdS in this case) at the expense of FeS, insignificant amounts of dissolved metal will be present in the interstitial waters if enough FeS is present. This premise has given rise to a standard technique for determining whether sediments might contain enough metal to warrant concern (Di Toro *et al.*, 1990). First, a sediment aliquot is extracted with cold hydrochloric acid. Then the amounts of sulfide (acid volatile sulfides [AVS]) and simultaneously extracted metals (SEM) are measured in that extract. The difference between the SEM and AVS suggests whether or not enough metal will be dissolved in the interstitial waters to warrant concern. This method has enjoyed wide application and was recently refined by Di Toro *et al.* (2005) by including metal partitioning to sediment organic matter. Some ecotoxicologists such as Lee *et al.* (2000) suggest that further refinement remains to be done because metal exposure of organisms that ingest sediment particulates is not fully defined by interstitial water concentrations alone.

Bioavailability and accumulation of sediment-associated organic compounds are predicted with tools similar to those described for waters. The bioavailability of ionizable organic compounds can be approximated with the pH-partition hypothesis that relates the availability of an ionizable compound to the diffusion of its unionized form through membranes as determined by pH and pK_a. Availability of nonionizing organic compounds for accumulation can often be estimated with its log K_{ow} and equilibrium partitioning theory as described already for accumulation from waters. The challenge with nonionizing organic compounds becomes adequately defining the phases between which the compound is partitioning. This might be done by estimating the partitioning of the compound between sediment solid phases and the interstitial water as done by Di Toro *et al.* (1991). Descriptions of nonionizing organic compound bioaccumulation from sediments can also entail normalization of concentrations to phases thought to be dictating partitioning:

$$\text{Biota sediment accumulation factor (BSAF)} = \frac{\mu g/kg \text{ lipid}}{\mu g/kg \text{ organic carbon}},$$

where the mass of compound in the organisms is divided by kilograms of organism-associated lipid and the mass of compound in the sediment is divided by kilograms of sediment-associated organic carbon.

Another issue of importance to the ecotoxicologist is the possibility of biomagnification, the increase in contaminant concentration as it moves through a food web. As will be described below, biomagnification can result in harmful exposures to species situated high in the food web such as birds of prey.

TOXICANT EFFECTS

While determining *exposure* comprises one half of the risk assessment paradigm, the other half, understanding chemical effects, lies at the heart of toxicology and, hence, comprises the focus of this chapter. The effects, or deleterious consequences of chemical exposures, can be enormously diverse as demonstrated by previous chapters, and investigated by numerous techniques. One approach to this complex topic of ecotoxicological effects, which we employ here, is to organize effects according to biological levels of organization. Thus, one may consider effects, in ascending order, at the subcellular (molecular and biochemical), cellular, organismal, population, community, and ecosystem levels of organization. As noted earlier, an important distinction between traditional biomedical, or human health-oriented, toxicology and ecotoxicology is the emphasis by the latter on higher levels of biological organization, specifically populations, communities, and ecosystems, while biomedical toxicology focuses on lower levels, from organismal and below. This difference arises from the focus of biomedical toxicology on one species and concerns for protecting the health of individuals of that species. Ecotoxicology, in contrast, deals with, theoretically at least, all species, and in line with other aspects of natural resource management, the primary concern is one of sustainability. That is, policies and regulations surrounding chemical effects in natural ecosystems are designed to protect ecological features such as population dynamics, community structures, and ecosystem functions. In this light, the individual organism is essentially viewed as expendable, as long as these higher level variables are protected. An exception here is that of endangered or threatened species, where the loss of an individual may have unacceptable legal or ecological consequences.

While higher levels of organization comprise the ultimate focus of those concerned with chemical pollution of natural systems, the science of ecotoxicology includes studies across the entire range. Studies at lower levels (cellular and below) provide

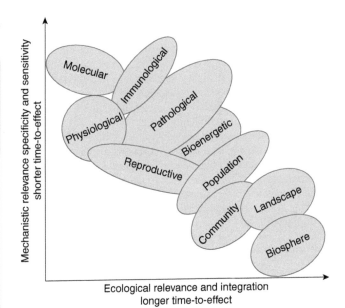

Figure 30-3. Hierarchical types of effects considered in ecotoxicology, indicating relative attributes such as mechanistic versus ecological relevance and time lags between exposure and observable effect. Based on artwork kindly provided by S. Marshall Adams, Oak Ridge National Laboratory.

insights into mechanisms of toxicity that can be valuable for making predictions among related compounds or species, and establishing cause–effect relationships in field studies, for generating useful "biomarkers" of chemical exposure and effect, and for providing insights into higher level, particularly population level, effects. Studies at the organism level have historically played a dominant role in regulatory ecotoxicology; many traditional bioassays, described later, can be viewed as organismal-level queries. Again, understanding effects at the population and higher levels can be viewed as the "gold standard" in ecotoxicology. However, because these effects can require a relatively long time beyond the initial exposure of a system to emerge, their quantification is often difficult, and they generally do not serve to identify the nature of the stressor. Thus, the elucidation of effects of chemical pollutants, as well as other stressors, in natural systems draws on multiple approaches and conclusions are generally based on the weight of evidence available. Examples of effects, or end points, that can be measured spanning levels of organization and their relative sensitivities and ecological relevancies are illustrated in Fig. 30-3. The originator of this figure, Adams (Oak Ridge National Laboratory), has discussed the importance of integrating studies across levels of organization and mathematical approaches for accomplishing this (Adams, 2000).

In the following sections, we describe important chemical effects that have been addressed at different levels of biological organization in ecotoxicological contexts, including illustrative examples. It is beyond the scope of this chapter to provide discussions of all chemicals that have received ecotoxicological attention. Other chapters in this text, particularly those in Unit V, provide detailed information for most classes of chemicals of concern as pollutants of natural systems, albeit in a primarily mammalian context. Many of the effects described are relevant to other animals, and of course mammals do occur in natural systems! Some plant-specific effects will be addressed herein. It should be noted that, while we have employed a biological level of organization approach as a meaningful way to organize and convey a complex array of information, the phenomena we have categorized into various levels are ultimately interwoven, as will become apparent.

Molecular and Biochemical Effects

This lowest level of organization includes fundamental processes associated with the regulation of gene transcription and translation, biotransformation of xenobiotics, and the deleterious biochemical effects of xenobiotics on cellular constituents including proteins, lipids, and DNA. These effects have been described elsewhere throughout this book in various contexts related to human health. Here we will highlight some aspects of subcellular effects that have received particular attention in the context of ecotoxicology. Research in this area has been performed for a variety of reasons, including the elucidation of mechanisms of adaptation and toxicity, understanding species similarities and differences (eg, to compare selected wildlife species with standard mammalian models, and to identify particularly sensitive species), and to develop useful biomarkers of chemical exposure and toxicity for environmental assessments. More in-depth discussions are provided in monographs such as Hoffman *et al.* (2003a,b), Newman (2010), Mommsen and Moon (2005), and Di Giulio and Hinton (2008).

Gene Expression and Ecotoxicogenomics

A long-standing mechanistic issue in toxicology concerns chemical effects on gene and protein expression. Xenobiotics can affect gene transcription through interactions with transcription factors and/or the promoter regions of genes that bind transcription factors in the process of activating transcription. In the context of environmental toxicology, perhaps the most studied xenobiotic effects involve ligand-activated transcription factors. These intracellular receptor proteins recognize and bind specific compounds, thus forming a complex that binds to specific promoter regions of genes, thereby activating transcription of mRNAs, and ultimately translation of the associated protein. Two examples of substantial importance in ecotoxicology that illustrate these interactions involve the estrogen receptor (ER) and the aryl hydrocarbon receptor (AHR).

Estrogen Receptor A number of chemicals have been shown to perturb various components of the endocrine system, and the identification and elucidation of "endocrine disruptors" has been a subject of much research and regulatory action in recent years, in the contexts of both human and wildlife health (see Chap. 10; Rotchell and Ostrander, 2003). Perhaps the most studied component of the vertebrate endocrine system in this context is the ER, particularly ER-α, and responses associated with it. The dominant natural ligand for this nuclear receptor is estradiol (E2); binding of E2 with ER produces a complex that can then bind to estrogen response elements (ERE) of specific genes that contain one or more EREs, thereby causing gene transcription (see Fig. 30-4). Genes regulated in this manner by E2–ER play various important roles in, for example, sexual organ development, behavior, fertility, and bone integrity (Deroo and Korach, 2006).

A number of chemicals including certain drugs and environmental pollutants can serve as ligands for ER; in most cases these "xenoestrogens" activate gene transcription, that is, similar to E2, acting as receptor agonists. The first xenoestrogen identified was diethylstilbestrol (DES), a drug used to prevent miscarriage in the 1940s to the 1970s until it was discovered to have profound developmental effects in some offspring of women receiving the treatment (Trimble, 2001). In recent years, a number of environmental pollutants with estrogenic activity have been identified, including certain chlorinated hydrocarbon insecticides (eg, DDT, methoxychlor, endosulfan), surfactants (nonylphenol), some

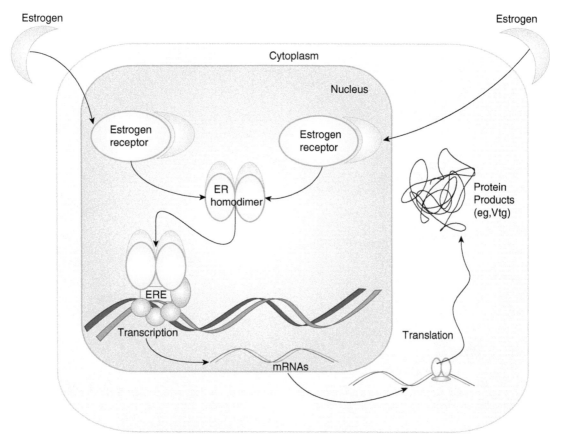

Figure 30-4. *A simplified model of estrogen receptor signaling including the estrogen receptor (ER), which on binding to native hormone ligand (estrogen) or xenoestrogen (see Fig. 30-5) forms the transcriptionally active ER homodimer complex that binds to genes containing estrogen response elements (ERE) and thereby upregulates transcription and translation of genes/proteins regulated by the system, such as vitellogenin (Vtg).* Kindly provided by Carla Rosenfeld, Duke University.

polychlorinated biphenyls (PCBs), bisphenol A (used in plastic manufacturing), and ethinyl estradiol, a synthetic estrogen used in birth control pills and observed in municipal effluents and surface waters (Shelby *et al.*, 1996; Larsson *et al.*, 1999; van der Oost *et al.*, 2003; see Fig. 30-5). With the exception of ethinyl estradiol, these pollutants exhibit relatively low binding affinities to ER, as compared with E2 or DES (Shelby *et al.*, 1996); however, environmental exposures may be sufficient to perturb reproduction or development.

Evidence for such "endocrine disruptions" by environmental xenoestrogens appears to be overall stronger for wildlife than for humans, likely due to instances of elevated exposures that are less prone to confounding factors than is typically the case for human exposures. Also, egg-laying vertebrates provide a unique biomarker of estrogen exposure that has contributed to ecotoxicological studies in this area. Vitellogenin (Vtg) is a protein that is normally produced by the liver of females and transported via the bloodstream to the ovary where, as a key component of yolk, it provides nourishment to the developing embryo. The production of Vtg is regulated by the estrogen–ER system. Interestingly, males of egg-laying vertebrate species contain the molecular machinery to produce Vtg, but production and circulating levels are normally very low, due to low titers of estrogen. However, exposures of males to estrogen and xenoestrogens upregulate Vtg production, which can be readily measured in blood samples. Consequently, elevated Vtg in males of these species is a useful biomarker of estrogenic chemical exposures (Sumpter and Jobling, 1995; see the section "Biomarkers"). Examples include rainbow trout (*Oncorhynchus mykiss*) caged in surface waters below industrial or municipal

effluent sources enriched in alkylphenolic surfactants in the United Kingdom (Harries *et al.*, 1997) or natural and synthetic estrogens in Sweden (Larsson *et al.*, 1999), and whitefish (*Coregonus lavaretus*) caged near paper mill effluents in Finland (Mellanen *et al.*, 1999). While the bulk of research related to estrogenic compounds in natural systems has focused on fish, this approach has merit for other egg-laying vertebrates (Lorenzen *et al.*, 2003; Huang *et al.*, 2005), and for some invertebrates that produce Vtg-like proteins (Porte *et al.*, 2006).

Aryl Hydrocarbon Receptor The AHR is a member of the basic helix–loop–helix Per ARNT Sim (bHLH-PAS) family of receptors/transcription factors that play roles in development, as sensors of the internal and external environment in order to maintain homeostasis, and in establishment and maintenance of circadian clocks (Denison and Nagy, 2003; Hahn *et al.*, 2005). The AHR is among the most intensively studied receptors in toxicology due to its role in regulating a number of genes coding for proteins involved in xenobiotic metabolism, and its responsiveness to a number of widespread environmental contaminants, as well as some drugs and endogenous compounds. The AHR is a ligand-activated cytosolic receptor that on binding to a ligand traverses to the nucleus where it complexes with another transcription factor, the AHR nuclear translocator (ARNT) protein (Fig. 30-6) to form a transcriptionally active dimer. This AHR–ARNT complex binds to promoter sequences of genes regulated by the AHR system; these promoters are most often referred to as "xenobiotic response elements" (XRE) or "dioxin response elements" (DRE).

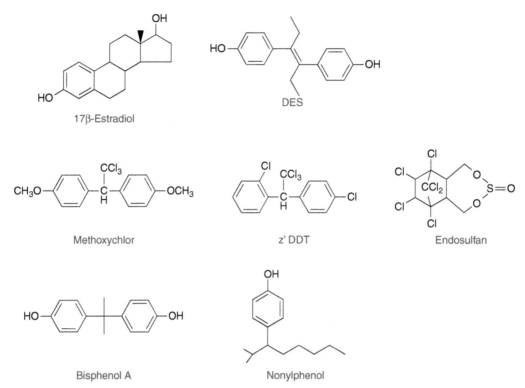

Figure 30-5. *Estrogen receptor agonists, including a native estrogen (17β-estradiol), the drug diethylstilbestrol (DES), a surfactant component (nonylphenol), an industrial intermediate (bisphenol A), and several pesticides (remainder).*

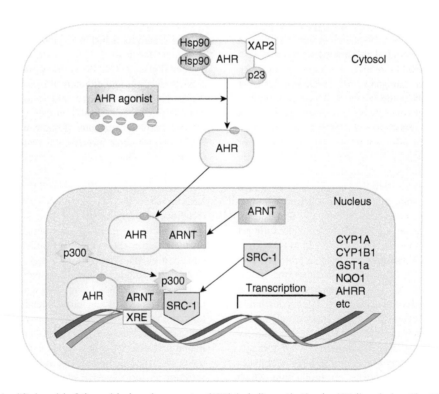

Figure 30-6. *A simplified model of the aryl hydrocarbon receptor (AHR) including activation by AHR ligands (see Fig. 30-7) that allows for dimerization with the AHR nuclear transporter (ARNT) that forms the transcriptionally active complex that binds to xenobiotic response elements (XRE) and thereby upregulates a number of genes, including several involved in biotransformation, indicated here, as well as the AHR repressor (AHRR) that provides negative feedback control of the system.* Hsp90, XAP2, and p23 are chaperone proteins; SRC-1 and p300 are examples of coregulator proteins involved in transcription. Kindly provided by Carrie Fleming and Carla Rosenfeld, Duke University.

Characterized genes that are upregulated by the AHR system in large part code for enzymes involved in the metabolism of lipophilic chemicals, including organic xenobiotics and some endogenous substrates such as steroid hormones. These enzymes include specific cytochrome P450s (mammalian CYP1A1, 1A2, and 1B1 and their counterparts in other vertebrates), a glutathione transferase (GST), a glucuronosyl transferase (UDPGT), an alcohol dehydrogenase (ALD), and a quinone oxidoreductase (NQO). In addition to these enzymes, AHR–ARNT upregulates the AHR repressor protein (AHRR), which then competes with AHR for ARNT. This results in a transcriptionally inactive complex and effectively provides a negative feedback loop for controlling AHR-mediated gene transcription (Hahn *et al.*, 2005). The biotransformation enzymes regulated by the AHR system are described in detail in Chap. 6. Briefly, they play key roles for transforming many lipophilic chemicals, including numerous common organic contaminants, into more water-soluble, and hence excretable, products. However, this biotransformation activity can result in production of highly reactive products that are more toxic than their parent compounds, that is, "activation."

Of particular relevance to the present discussion, however, is the ability of some ubiquitous pollutants to act as AHR ligands and markedly upregulate gene transcription via the AHR–ARNT signaling pathway described above (Denison and Nagy, 2003). In some cases, this can be interpreted as an adaptive response—the organism is reacting to exposure to a lipophilic xenobiotic in order to enhance its elimination. However, as noted above, biotransformation can also lead to enhanced toxicity of some substrates. The two major classes of pollutants that have members that act as ligands for the AHR and upregulate gene expression (and thereby "induce" biotransformation enzymes) and have received the greatest attention in ecotoxicology are the polycyclic aromatic hydrocarbons (PAHs) and the polyhalogenated aromatic hydrocarbons (pHAHs); examples of both are provided in Fig. 30-7. The most studied pHAHs are particular "coplanar" PCBs and chlorinated dioxins. Whereas some PAHs and pHAHs share the ability to activate the AHR, important differences between these classes exist. PAHs, whether they are ligands for the AHR or not, are overall very good substrates for the biotransformation systems upregulated via the AHR, which can act to both detoxify and enhance the toxicity of some PAHs (discussed in the section "Cancer"). In general, pHAH-type AHR ligands are more potent AHR ligands and enzyme inducers than PAHs, but due to extensive halogenation

are much poorer substrates for biotransformation. One of the most potent ligands for the AHR is the dioxin, 2,3,7,8-tetrachlorodibenzodioxin (TCDD), which is highly recalcitrant to biotransformation (Denison and Nagy, 2003).

In similarity with xenoestrogen-mediated inductions of Vtg via the ER, the inducibility of biotransformation enzymes via the AHR by xenobiotics has been used for biomonitoring. In this regard, enzymatic activities associated with the CYP1As have been the most widely used AHR-related biomarker, particularly an activity that appears highly specific for these CYPs, ethoxyresorufin O-deethylase (EROD), which is most often measured in liver tissue of vertebrates. Elevated activities of EROD in various vertebrates have been associated with exposures to PCBs, dioxins, PAHs, and complex mixtures of these associated with, for example, harbor sediments, municipal effluents, paper mill effluents, refinery effluents, and crude oil spills (Custer *et al.*, 2001; van der Oost *et al.*, 2003; Miller *et al.*, 2005). Invertebrate AHR homologues examined do not bind to ligands similarly to vertebrate AHRs and do not demonstrate protein inductions analogous to those observed in vertebrates (Butler *et al.*, 2001; Hahn, 2002; Chaty *et al.*, 2004). PAH and pHAH toxicities and the potential roles played by their interactions with the AHR will be discussed at various points in subsequent sections of this chapter, and related discussions from a human health standpoint appear in other chapters.

Genomics and Ecotoxicogenomics Recent advances in gene sequencing and associated techniques for investigating mechanism underlying gene expression have revolutionized molecular biology. These advances are rapidly permeating many areas of biological research, including toxicology and environmental science. Underlying these advances are very large projects to sequence the entire genomes of various species, such as the highly publicized Human Genome Project that was completed in 2003 (Little, 2005). Other species that have been completely or largely sequenced include the mouse, rat, cow, dog, chimpanzee, chicken, zebrafish (*Danio rerio*), puffer fish (*Fugu rubripes*), medaka (*Oryzias latipes*), fruit fly (*Drosophila melanogaster*), a sea urchin (*Strongylocentrotus purpuratus*), a soil nematode (*Caenorhabditis elegans*), a yeast (*Saccharomyces cerevisiae*), and rice (*Oryza sativa*), and the number of species sequenced is anticipated to expand rapidly (see www.genome.gov; Crollius and Weissenbach, 2005). Genome sequencing set the stage for genome-wide analysis of gene expression ("transcriptomics");

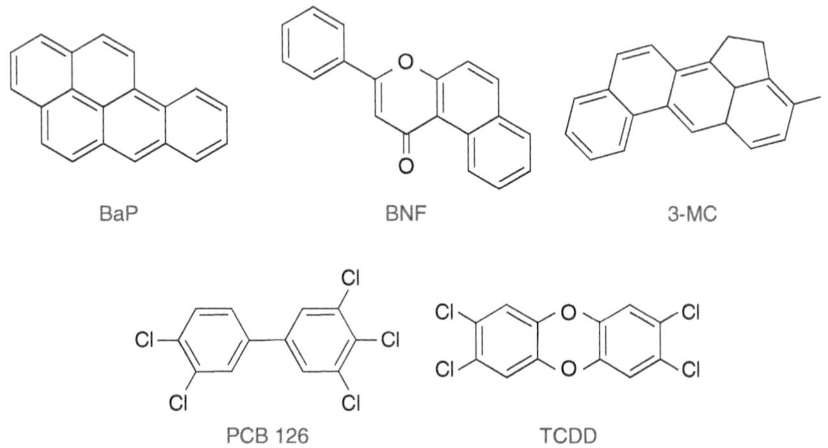

BaP   BNF   3-MC

PCB 126   TCDD

Figure 30-7. *Representative ligands of the aryl hydrocarbon receptor, including 2,3,7,8-tetrachlorodibenzodioxin (TCDD), a coplanar polychlorinated biphenyl (PCB 126), two polycyclic aromatic hydrocarbons (benzo(a)pyrene [BaP] and 3-methylcholanthrene [3-MC]), and a flavone (β-naphthoflavone [BNF]).*

cDNAs for known genes can be spotted on glass slides, or chips, resulting in "microarrays" that can be employed to quantify relative levels, that is, expression, of mRNAs for those genes in samples of interest. The study of changes in gene expression arising from chemical exposures is a key component of "toxicogenomics" (Schmidt, 2002). Microarrays for genomes or genome components of interest (such as genes associated with stress responses, carcinogenesis, and development) are commercially available for many species, and rapidly expanding. Also advancing rapidly are related analyses of global changes in proteins (the translation products of mRNAs), referred to as "proteomics," and resulting metabolite profiles (amounts of sugars, lipids, amino acids, etc, in various tissues that are controlled in part by enzyme activities), referred to as "metabolomics." A major complexity in these global analyses is the extremely large data sets that arise, for example, when one examines the responses of thousands of genes from organisms exposed to one or more concentrations of a chemical at one or more time points. This has led to the development of the field of "bioinformatics" that includes the application of sophisticated statistical and computing approaches for revealing biologically meaningful patterns of gene expression such as relationships to cellular signaling pathways. "Omics" is a term used to refer collectively to these interrelated approaches (ie, transcriptomics, proteomics, metabolomics, and bioinformatics).

Omics have spread into the science and applications of ecotoxicology, collectively termed ecotoxicogenomics. As is the case for human health-oriented toxicogenomics, ecotoxicogenomics has great potential for elucidating impacts of chemicals of ecological concern and ultimately for playing an important role in ERAs and regulatory ecotoxicology (Snape *et al.*, 2004; Ankley *et al.*, 2006; Watanabe and Iguchi, 2006). Specific areas to which this emerging field can contribute include prioritization of chemicals investigated in ERAs, identification of modes of action of pollutants, identification of particularly sensitive species, and effect prediction at higher levels of organization. As in other areas of ecotoxicology, a major complexity faced is the vast array of species of potential concern. This is a particularly problematic issue in ecotoxicogenomics that requires substantial species-specific molecular information. However, as mentioned earlier, the number of ecologically relevant species for which this information is becoming available is expanding rapidly, and is likely to accelerate as tools are refined. Moreover, as information grows, genomic approaches hold great promise for identifying appropriate surrogate species for laboratory studies used in basic ecotoxicological research and in support of regulatory ecotoxicology (Benson and Di Giulio, 2006).

Protein Damage The study of chemical effects on proteins, particularly enzymes, has a long history in toxicology. Of particular interest within ecotoxicology are the inhibitions of acetylcholinesterase (AChE) by certain pesticides and of delta-aminolevulinic acid dehydratase (ALAD) by lead. AChE degrades the neurotransmitter acetylcholine, and in so doing, controls nerve transmission in cholinergic nerve tracts. The widely used organophosphate and carbamate classes of insecticides kill by inhibiting AChE, and this mechanism is operative for "nontarget" organisms including invertebrates, wildlife, and humans. (See Chap. 22 for a detailed discussion of these pesticides and AChE inhibition.) Of particular ecological concern have been the ingestions of AChE-inhibiting insecticides with food items or granular formulations (mistaken as seed or grit) by birds and exposures to aquatic animals from agricultural runoff (Mineau, 1991; Carr *et al.*, 1997; Wilson *et al.*, 2001). In many field studies, effects of these insecticides on mortality, and relationships between AChE inhibition and mortality, have

been of primary concern. However, relationships between AChE inhibition and important sublethal impacts such as behavior have also been observed (Sandahl *et al.*, 2005).

ALAD catalyzes the rate-limiting step of heme synthesis, a key component of cytochromes, hemoglobin, and myoglobin, and ALAD activity is very sensitive to inhibition by lead (ATSDR, 1999). This sensitivity has been exploited widely as a biomarker for lead exposure in humans and wildlife. In wildlife, concerns for lead exposure have included ingestion by birds of spent lead shot used in hunting (Kendall *et al.*, 1996), accumulation of lead by wildlife living near highways (Birdsall *et al.*, 1986), and aquatic organisms inhabiting surface waters contaminated by lead from mine runoff and other industrial activities (Schmitt *et al.*, 2005). In addition to enzyme inhibition, chemicals can damage proteins in other ways, including oxidative damage as described below, and by forming stable adducts similar to those formed with DNA, also discussed below.

Oxidative Stress The classic depiction of aerobic respiration shows molecular oxygen (O_2) as the terminal electron acceptor, with its reduction resulting ultimately in water as high-energy intermediates (NADH, $FADH_2$) are oxidized and cellular energy is captured as ATP. This reduction of O_2 to H_2O requires four electrons that are sequentially added; this process is tightly coupled so that the one-, two-, and three-electron intermediates are released at low amounts (less than 0.1% of O_2 inspired; Fridovich, 2004). These intermediates are, in sequence, the superoxide anion radical ($O_2^{\bullet-}$), hydrogen peroxide (H_2O_2), and the hydroxyl radical ($^{\bullet}OH$). This tight coupling is fortunate because these intermediates, produced during aerobic respiration and other O_2-consuming or -producing processes (such as photosynthesis and CYP-mediated biotransformations), are potentially deleterious products that can indiscriminately damage cellular components; hence, they are referred to as "reactive oxygen species" (ROS). Some ROS, including $O_2^{\bullet-}$ and $^{\bullet}OH$, are free radicals, that is, they possess an unpaired electron; among ROS, $^{\bullet}OH$ is particularly reactive and toxic. In order to defend themselves from the damaging effects of ROS, all aerobic organisms have evolved complex antioxidant defense systems that include enzymatic and nonenzymatic components (Halliwell and Gutteridge, 1999). Antioxidant enzymes include superoxide dismutases that convert $O_2^{\bullet-}$ to H_2O_2, catalases and peroxidases that detoxify peroxides including H_2O_2, and enzymes involved in the production and maintenance of reduced glutathione (GSH) such as glutamate–cysteine ligase (GCL) and glutathione reductase (GR). Low-molecular-weight, nonenzymatic antioxidants include vitamins A, C, and E, and GSH.

Oxidative stress has been defined as "a disturbance in the prooxidant–antioxidant balance in favor of the former, leading to potential damage" (Sies and Cadenas, 1985)—that is, the point at which the production of ROS exceeds the capacity of antioxidants to prevent damage. Numerous environmental contaminants can act as prooxidants and enhance the production of ROS. The resulting oxidative damage can account wholly or partially for toxicity (Halliwell and Gutteridge, 1999). Mechanisms by which chemicals can enhance ROS production include redox cycling, interactions with electron transport chains (notably in mitochondria, microsomes, or chloroplasts), and photosensitization.

Redox cycling is perhaps the most common mechanism by which a diverse array of chemicals including many environmental pollutants generates intracellular ROS. Redox cycling chemicals include diphenols and quinones, nitroaromatics and azo compounds, aromatic hydroxylamines, bipyridyliums, and certain metal chelates, particularly of copper and iron (Di Giulio *et al.*, 1989; Halliwell and Gutteridge, 1999). These include compounds

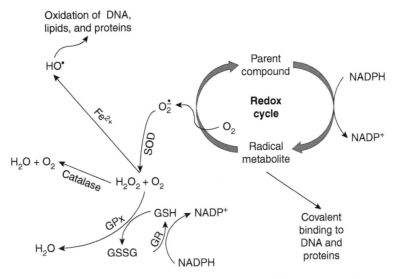

Figure 30-8. *Overview of oxidative stress, including reactive oxygen species stimulation initially by redox cycling, key antioxidant defenses, and potential deleterious biochemical effects.* "Parent compound" in redox cycle could include a number of chemicals such as quinones, nitroaromatics, azo dyes, paraquat and diquat, and transition metal chelates.

of broad industrial use, many pesticides, ubiquitous elements, and metabolic products of numerous pollutants. In the redox cycle, the parent compound accepts an electron from a reduced cofactor, such as NADH or NADPH; this reaction is typically catalyzed by a reductase such as xanthine oxidase or cytochrome P450 reductase (Kappus, 1986). In the presence of O_2, the unpaired electron of the radical metabolite is donated to O_2, yielding $O_2^{\bullet-}$ and regenerating the parent compound; importantly, the parent compound can repeat this cycle until it is cleared or metabolized to an inactive product. In the course of each redox cycle, two potentially deleterious events occur—a high-energy reducing equivalent is expended (eg, the oxidation of NADPH to $NADP^+$) and an oxygen radical is produced. A generalized redox cycle that includes associations with cellular toxicities and antioxidant defenses comprises Fig. 30-8.

Additionally, pHAH AHR ligands such as coplanar PCBs and TCDD can enhance ROS production, possibly by inducing CYP1A activity and concomitantly interfering with electron flow mediated by these enzymes (Schlezinger and Stegeman, 2001). PAHs can also upregulate CYP1A and can enhance the production of ROS-generating redox-active quinone metabolites, in contrast to uncoupling mechanisms proposed for pHAHs; Nebert *et al.* (2000) discuss potential mechanisms by which AHR agonists can produce oxidative stress. The herbicide paraquat is phytotoxic due to interference with chloroplast electron transport. Interestingly, it is a very potent lung toxicant because of its specific uptake by this tissue and subsequent redox cycling (Halliwell and Gutteridge, 1999). Another important mechanism particularly significant in aquatic systems is photosensitization. Ultraviolet (UV) radiation (specifically UVB and UVA) can penetrate surface waters to depths dependent on the wavelength of the radiation and the clarity of the water. The UV radiation generates ROS and other free radicals via excitation of photosensitizing chemicals, including common pollutants of aquatic systems (Larson and Weber, 1994). For example, due to photosensitization, many PAHs are orders of magnitude more acutely toxic to aquatic organisms in the presence of UV radiation than in its absence (Arfsten *et al.*, 1996; Ankley *et al.*, 1997). The ecological relevance of photosensitization, however, is controversial (McDonald and Chapman, 2002).

As noted, ROS are generally indiscriminant molecules and can potentially damage any cellular component. Well-characterized

biochemical impacts of ROS include oxidations of unsaturated lipid components of membranes ("lipid peroxidation"), oxidations of amino acids and proteins (resulting in, eg, the addition of carbonyl groups), and DNA oxidations resulting in products such as 8-hydroxy-guanosine and thyme glycol (Halliwell and Gutteridge, 1999). Another important impact is perturbed redox status (Schafer and Buettner, 2001). Healthy cells typically maintain high ratios of cofactors in their reduced, high-energy state relative to their oxidized state (eg, $NADH/NAD^+$, $NADPH/NADP^+$, and GSH/GSSG), as the reduced forms are those most employed for energy production, biosynthesis, and antioxidant defense, for example. The ROS can drive redox status to a more oxidized state by several direct and indirect mechanisms, potentially reducing cell viability. These ROS-mediated impacts and others have been associated with a number of human diseases including atherosclerosis, arthritis, cancer, and neurodegenerative diseases such as Alzheimer disease, Parkinson disease, and amyotrophic lateral sclerosis (Halliwell and Gutteridge, 1999). With the exception of cancer (see below), the role of ROS in specific diseases in wildlife has received little attention. However, numerous studies have documented oxidative stress-mediated biochemical and cellular effects in wildlife associated with environmental contamination (Bainy *et al.*, 1996; Livingstone, 2001; van der Oost et al., 2003; Dorval *et al.*, 2005; Winston and Di Giulio, 1991). As with humans and various animal models for human disease, it is reasonable to assume that oxidative stress comprises an important mechanism accounting in part for the toxicity of diverse pollutants to free-living organisms. Also, oxidative stress is involved in the effects of air pollutants on plants and likely plays a role in forest diebacks observed downwind of industrialized areas (Richardson *et al.*, 1989; Hippeli and Elstner, 1996).

DNA Damage The importance of DNA as a molecular target in toxicology is indicated by the devotion of Chap. 9 of this text to genetic toxicology. As indicated, perhaps the most pressing human health issue associated with xenobiotic–DNA interactions is cancer. Cancer is also an important health outcome associated with chemical exposures in wildlife, particularly for bottom-dwelling fishes, as discussed in the section "Cancer." Of greater concern in ecotoxicology versus human health are other, multigenerational effects of pollutants on genetic structures and resulting phenotypes of populations and communities, through both direct effects on DNA (mutations) and indirect effects (selection); this topic is discussed in the subsection "Population" in the section "Toxicant Effects."

Chemical contaminants can damage DNA through several mechanisms, including the formation of DNA–xenobiotic adducts, by causing strand breaks, and by oxidations of DNA bases. In the context of ecotoxicology, the most widely studied form of damage has been the formation of stable DNA adducts, particularly by PAHs. In order to form these adducts, PAHs must first be activated to reactive metabolites by enzyme systems such as the cytochrome P450s. The bulk of PAHs metabolized to various oxidized products (such as phenols, diols, and epoxides) is subsequently conjugated by phase II enzymes (such as GSH, sulfate, and glucuronosyl transferases; see Chap. 6); however, some fraction can react with DNA, mainly through covalent bonding with DNA bases. The most studied example of this is benzo(a)pyrene (BaP), which can be metabolized to the highly reactive benzo(a)pyrene diol epoxide (BPDE) that can bond to DNA. In field studies, the resulting large adducts of DNA with BPDE and other activated PAHs and related compounds can be measured with the highly sensitive ^{32}P-postlabeling assay (Phillips, 1997). This technique has been used extensively to monitor DNA adducts in benthic fish and bivalves inhabiting systems contaminated with hydrocarbons, particularly PAHs (Maccubbin, 1994; Reichert et al., 1998; Shugart, 2000; Amat et al., 2004). Other forms of DNA damage that have been investigated in ecotoxicological studies include DNA strand breaks and oxidized DNA bases (Shugart, 2000; Malins et al., 2006).

Once DNA damage has occurred, whether from chemical exposures or other causes (respiration, UV radiation, viral interactions, normal wear and tear), several subsequent outcomes can occur, including the following: the damage can be properly repaired, the damage can lead to cell death, or a resulting change in DNA structure (base sequence) can become fixed and passed on to daughter cells, that is, mutation occurs. Complex DNA repair systems have been elucidated in prokaryotic and eukaryotic organisms (see Chaps. 8 and 9), and while these systems have received relatively little attention in species of ecological relevance, it is a safe assumption that these conserved systems are qualitatively similar across diverse phyla. Overall, these systems exhibit a remarkable capacity for surveying the cellular genome, detecting damage such as oxidations, adducts, and strand breaks, and repairing the damage by, for example, removing a damaged base and replacing it with the correct base. However, misrepair does sometime occur, with the result that an incorrect base is incorporated. Depending on the gene involved and the site within the gene, this change may lead to cell death, or may result in a mutation that may have no effect (occurs at noncritical base sequence) or one that leads to functional change in the protein coded by the gene. Some chemicals cause cancer by mutating genes that play pivotal roles in cellular growth and differentiation, particularly oncogenes and tumor suppressor genes. Examples of discoveries of activated genes (in liver tumors) in field studies include the K-ras oncogene in tomcod (Microgadus tomcod) from the Hudson River, New York (Wirgin et al., 1989), and in winter flounder (Pseudopleuronectes americanus) collected from Boston Harbor (McMahon et al., 1990), and the retinoblastoma (Rb) tumor suppressor gene in the marine flatfish, dab (Limanda limanda), from the United Kingdom (du Corbier et al., 2005).

Cellular, Tissue, and Organ Effects

Cells Cellular organelles that have received attention as targets in species of ecological interest include mitochondria, lysosomes, and nuclei. Most free-living organisms routinely experience energy deficits. For example, food resources are often highly depleted during the winter for many animals, which adapt by conserving energy (by hibernating or lowering metabolism) or by storing energy beforehand (as the case for many migratory birds). Thus, effects of pollutants on mitochondrial energy metabolism can be of particular importance to wildlife. For example, Sokolova and coworkers (Sokolova, 2004; Cherkasov et al., 2006) have elegantly described the effects of cadmium on several aspects of mitochondrial function in isolated gill and hepatopancreas cells from the eastern oyster (Crassostrea virginica), and noted a marked synergy between the metal and increasing environmental temperatures. Lysosomes are involved in the degradation of damaged organelles and proteins, and also sequester a wide variety of environmental contaminants, including metals, PAHs, and nanoparticles (Moore, 2006). The accumulation of xenobiotics by lysosomes can elicit membrane damage, or "membrane instability," which has been used as an early warning measure of pathological chemical effects in both invertebrates and vertebrates (Hwang et al., 2002; Kohler et al., 2002; Moore et al., 2006).

In addition to specific damage to DNA bases described above, chemical effects on nuclei have been examined in ecological contexts with additional techniques. Micronuclei are chromosomal fragments that are not incorporated into the nucleus at cell division, and chemical exposures can markedly increase their frequency. Elevated micronuclei numbers have been observed, for example, in fish erythrocytes from polluted coastal sites in California (Hose et al., 1987) and in hemocytes in clams from a PCB-polluted harbor in Massachusetts (Dopp et al., 1996). Also, a standardized higher plant (Tradescantia) assay for micronuclei has been used for monitoring air pollution (Solenska et al., 2006). A cell-based assay that has been used widely in environmental applications is the comet assay. In this assay, cells are imbedded in agarose, lysed and subjected to gel electrophoresis, and the features of the resulting "comet's tail" on the gel used to assess DNA damage. With appropriate manipulations, the comet assay can be employed to detect and distinguish among a variety of genotoxicities including strand breaks, oxidative damage, and adducts (Moller, 2006). It has been used in a variety of field applications, particularly with bivalves (Steinert, 1999; Nigro et al., 2006), fish (Klobicar et al., 2010), and mice (Husby and McBee, 1999).

Histopathology The detailed microscopic analysis of the structure of cells and tissues can provide important links among chemical exposures, cellular targets and mechanisms, and effects at the organismal level (Hinton, 1994). Moreover, the determination that tissue damage has occurred as demonstrated by histopathological analysis is extremely useful for inferring that a significant deleterious effect has occurred. However, the substantial expertise required for proper histopathological analyses of this nature and the oftentimes time- and labor-intensive nature of these analyses has perhaps limited the application of this powerful approach in ecotoxicological contexts. Nevertheless, histopathological analysis has played an important role in confirming chemically mediated tissue damage in numerous laboratory and field studies. For example, Pacheco and Santos (2002) integrated histopathological analysis with biochemical studies of the effects of various environmental contaminants on the European eel (Anguilla anguilla), and Devlin (2006) similarly incorporated this approach in studies of the effects of methylmercury in fathead minnows (Pimephales promelas). Handy et al. (2002) relied on histopathology in a study of fish health in rivers in southern England. Wester et al. (2002) reviewed the application and potential contributions of histopathology in aquatic toxicology, particularly in the context of small fish models. In subsequent sections concerning organismal-level impacts, other examples of the use of histopathology will be provided.

Target Organs Descriptions of chemical impacts on all organ systems of the myriad species relevant to ecotoxicology are beyond the scope of this chapter. Other chapters in this volume address key target organs in the mammalian context, and much of this is relevant to other vertebrates. Target organ toxicology is also the subject of comprehensive reviews by Schlenk and Benson (2001) concerning marine and freshwater fishes, and by Gardner and Oberdorster (2005) concerning reptiles. Relevant information in marine mammals was reviewed in Vos *et al.* (2002). We are unaware of similar reviews for birds or invertebrates. The unique properties of the avian respiratory system and its utility for investigating respiratory system toxicity and air pollution were reviewed by Brown *et al.* (1997).

Another important target organ in ecotoxicology that is not covered elsewhere in this text is the respiratory organ of nonmammalian aquatic vertebrates and many invertebrates, the gill; gills of fishes have received the most attention as targets of toxicants. The gill epithelium is the major site of gas exchange, ionic regulation, acid–base balance, and nitrogenous waste excretions for fishes and other aquatic animals (Evans, 1987). Gills are immersed in a major exposure medium for these animals (surface water), so metabolically active epithelial cells are in direct contact with this medium. They also receive blood supply directly from the heart, through the ventral aorta. Thus, it is not surprising that gills comprise a very important target for many environmental pollutants, due to their critical physiological functions, central position in blood circulation pathways, and intimate relationship with the environment. The basic structure of fish gills is composed of branchial arches from which extend numerous filaments; from the filaments extend the lamellae (Wendelaar Bonga and Lock, 2008). The lamellae are covered by a layer of epithelial cells that function in gas exchange, whereas the filament epithelium is dominated by other cell types, including pavement cells, mucous cells, and chloride cells; chloride cells are the primary location for ATPase activity and ion channels involved in ion transport.

Common structural lesions in gills caused by a diverse array of chemicals include cell death (via necrosis and apoptosis), rupture of the epithelium, hyperplasia and hypertrophy of various cell populations that can lead to lamellar fusion, epithelial swelling, and lifting of the respiratory epithelium from the underlying tissue (Wendelaar Bonga and Lock, 2008). Chloride cells have received particular attention due to their key role in ionic homeostasis. For example, metals such as cadmium, copper, lead, silver, and zinc have been shown to interfere with their function in ion transport. In some cases, this may be due to inhibition of ATPase activities and/or increased membrane permeability (Spry and Wood, 1985; Wendelaar Bonga and Lock, 1992; Li *et al.*, 1998; Rogers *et al.*, 2003; Bury, 2005). The stress response, which results in elevated blood concentrations of epinephrine and cortisol, and associated responses such as increased cardiac output and elevated blood pressure, can also perturb ionic balance by promoting passive loss of ions such as Na^+ and Cl^- (Wendelaar Bonga and Lock, 2008). A variety of contaminants have been shown to evoke the stress response in fish, sometimes concomitantly with perturbations in ionic balance (Hontela, 1997; Webb and Wood, 1998; Chowdhury *et al.*, 2004). Also, gill damage appears to be the primary cause of the acute toxicity of PAH-mediated phototoxicity in fish (see the section "Oxidative Stress"). Weinstein *et al.* (1997) reported histopathological impacts of UV + fluoranthene in gills of fathead minnows including severe damage to mucosal cells, inflammation,

and apparent accumulation of lipid peroxidation products; these effects likely resulted in respiratory stress, and lethality. This study elegantly demonstrates a progression from biochemical mechanism (oxidative stress) to target organ damage (gill respiration) to an important organismal impact (death). Mortality and important sublethal organismal impacts that have received substantial attention among ecotoxicologists comprise the following section.

Organismal Effects

Mortality In similarity with impacts on human health, chemical pollution of the environment does not in most cases attain levels sufficient to outright kill wildlife. Concern in the ecotoxicological context is overall more for long-term, chronic impacts on organismal variables such as reproduction and development, behavior, and disease susceptibility, and how such impacts parlay into impacts at population and higher levels of organization. However, numerous cases of wildlife mortalities (particularly birds) due to exposures to chemical pollution have been observed, including cases associated with chronic oil discharges (Wiese and Robertson, 2004) and major oil releases from events such as the Exxon Valdez tanker wreck in Alaska (Peterson *et al.*, 2003) and the 1991 Gulf War (Evans *et al.*, 1993), lead from spent shot (Clark and Scheuhammer, 2003) and mines (Henny, 2003), and pesticide exposures (Mineau *et al.*, 1999). While not a direct toxic chemical effect, hypoxia can be an important cause of fish and invertebrate mortality in aquatic systems; anthropogenic inputs of nutrients associated with sewage or fertilizers that enhance the growth of phytoplankton can cause or exacerbate hypoxia (Paerl *et al.*, 1999; Wu, 2002). While direct mortality may not be a commonplace effect of toxic chemicals in natural systems, mortality comprises a major end point in toxicity testing, discussed later.

Reproduction and Development Impacts on reproduction and development comprise perhaps the greatest concern among potential sublethal effects of xenobiotics on animals inhabiting natural systems. This is due to sensitivities of the physiological processes involved that have been described for a number of pollutants, and the importance of reproduction and development to population dynamics, a key ecological concern. Moreover, the discovery of the effects of some organochlorine insecticides on avian reproduction (particularly eggshell thinning) and resulting population crashes of several predatory bird species, and the public's awareness through the publication of Carson's *Silent Spring* in 1962, can be associated with the birth of ecotoxicology. Concern for reproductive and developmental effects has blossomed in recent years, with the widespread detection of endocrine disruptors in the environment.

A variety of environmental contaminants have been associated with reproductive and/or developmental effects in wildlife populations, with this association supported by controlled laboratory studies. Chlorinated hydrocarbons have continued to generate concerns, although many (DDT and other insecticides, and PCBs) have had their production and use sharply curtailed. For example, DDT, its major metabolite in birds (DDE), and PCBs have been associated with reproductive and developmental impacts in bird populations in the Great Lakes, southern California, the Puget Sound, and the Arctic (Fry, 1995; Custer *et al.*, 1999; Bustnes *et al.*, 2005). Also, alligators (*Alligator mississippiensis*) inhabiting a DDT-polluted lake in Florida have exhibited reproductive and developmental perturbations (Guillette *et al.*, 2000). Evidence also indicates that PCBs impact marine mammal reproduction, including that of bottlenose dolphins (*Tursiops truncates*) (Schwacke *et al.*, 2002; Wells *et al.*, 2005).

Deleterious impacts on fish reproduction have been associated with environmental exposures to a number of contaminants. Case studies include PAHs (and other chemicals) accumulated in sediments in urban areas and harbors in the Puget Sound (Johnson *et al.*, 1993) and northeastern United States (Johnson *et al.*, 1994) or associated with oil spills such as the Exxon Valdez (Sol *et al.*, 2000). Other examples include effluents from bleached paper mills in various locations, including Canada (Munkittrick *et al.*, 1991), and selenium, for example, emanating from coal-fired power plant fly ash stored near freshwater lakes (Lemly, 2002) or in streams due to coal mine runoff (Holm *et al.*, 2005). Notably, selenium produced severe developmental effects in water birds feeding in a created wetland in central California (Kesterson National Wildlife Refuge) that concentrated naturally occurring selenium (Ohlendorf, 2002). Additionally, severe developmental anomalies have also been observed in natural populations of marine gastropods exposed to tributyltin (TBT), which has been used extensively as an antifouling paint on ship hulls (Ruiz *et al.*, 2005).

The developmental effects of dioxins (TCDD) and coplanar PCBs on vertebrate development have received substantial attention. To some extent, this work was motivated by analyses that indicated that these compounds were responsible for population crashes of Great Lakes' fisheries (particularly lake trout, *Salvelinus namaycush*, in Lake Ontario) in the 1950s and 1960s, as well as for developmental impacts on other wildlife, particularly piscivorous birds and mammals in the region (Gilbertson *et al.*, 1991; Cook *et al.*, 2003). Laboratory investigations, largely with fish and bird models, have shown that embryo development is very sensitive to these compounds, and such effects likely underlaid the population crashes (Fairbrother *et al.*, 1999; Cook *et al.*, 2003). These investigations have included elegant mechanistic studies that revealed cardiac development was particularly sensitive to these chemicals, and concluded that developmental perturbations are largely receptor mediated, that is, they are dependent on binding of the chemical (such as TCDD) with the AHR described above (Hankinson, 1995; Heid *et al.*, 2001; Tanguay *et al.*, 2003; Antkiewicz *et al.*, 2005). Much of the more recent work in this area has been done with zebrafish (*D. rerio*), a powerful model for molecular and developmental toxicology due to ease of visually examining development through a clear chorion, rapid development (approximately four days from fertilization to hatch), and abundant genetic information, including gene sequences (Carney *et al.*, 2006). For example, with a known gene sequence, one can design morpholinos to block translation of specific mRNAs; morpholinos are oligonucleotides with a modified "backbone" that renders them stable (resistant to DNA/RNAase activities) and thus able to transiently block translation of specific protein targets. Carney *et al.* (2004) employed morpholinos to knock down AHR translation in zebrafish embryos, which greatly reduced the developmental toxicity of TCDD, confirming the role of the AHR in dioxin toxicity. Morpholinos were also employed to investigate the role of CYP1A; for example, its upregulation via TCDD activation of the AHR could enhance oxidative stress. Teraoka *et al.* (2003) observed marked reductions of TCDD toxicity with either AHR or CYP1A morpholinos, while Carney *et al.* (2004) observed protection with the AHR but not the CYP1A morpholino. While the role of CYP1A in dioxin effects on development remains unclear, pathways downstream of the AHR other than CYP1A are likely involved.

Similar concerns have emerged for the developmental effects of PAHs, particularly in fish. Hydrocarbons, in large part PAHs, associated with oil spills, contaminated sediments, paper mill effluents, and creosote used for wood treatment have profound developmental effects in fish embryos (Billiard *et al.*, 1999; Carls *et al.*,

1999; Meyer *et al.*, 2002). In many cases, the effects observed visually appear similar to those observed in fish embryos exposed to dioxins and coplanar PCBs, and include malformed hearts ("tube heart"), craniofacial deformities, hemorrhaging, and edema of the pericardium and yolk sac, the latter resulting in a distended, faintly blue yolk sac and hence a name given to this syndrome—"blue sac disease" (Spitsbergen *et al.*, 1991). The mechanisms by which PAHs produce this effect are unresolved, and likely include more than a single mechanism—not surprising in light of the myriad of chemicals comprising hydrocarbon/PAH mixtures in the environment. In some cases, effects appear to be AHR-independent. Incardona *et al.* (2005) concluded in studies with zebrafish and employing morpholinos that in weathered crude oil, tricyclic PAHs (such as phenanthrene and dibenzothiophene [DBT], the latter a sulfur-substituted PAH) accounted for the bulk of cardiovascular teratogenesis, and rather than mediating toxicity, the AHR–CYP1A pathway afforded some protection. Wassenberg and Di Giulio (2004a) and Wassenberg *et al.* (2005) observed marked synergies in the developmental toxicity to killifish (*Fundulus heteroclitus*) embryos between higher molecular weight PAHs that are AHR agonists (BaP and BNF) and PAHs that inhibit CYP1A (α-naphthoflavone [ANF], fluoranthene, DBT, and carbazole—a nitrogen-substituted PAH). Also, ANF enhanced the toxicity of a water-based extract of sediments contaminated with weathered creosote (Wassenberg and Di Giulio, 2004b). In subsequent studies with zebrafish embryos investigating the synergistic toxicity of BNF and ANF, the AHR morpholino provided protection, while the CYP1A morpholino enhanced toxicity (Billiard *et al.*, 2006). Collectively, these PAH studies suggest that in the context of embryo toxicity, CYP1A plays a protective role, presumably by mediating metabolism and clearance of these metabolically labile compounds. This is in contrast to the metabolism-resistant dioxin-like compounds, where CYP1A either appears to play a role in mediating toxicity or has no effect. For some PAHs, such as lower molecular weight (tricyclic) PAHs that have little or no activity as AHR ligands, developmental toxicity appears AHR-independent, while the developmental toxicity of some higher molecular weight PAHs that are AHR agonists appears in part AHR-mediated. In addition, oxidative stress may play a role in the developmental toxicity of some PAHs to fish embryos (Bauder *et al.*, 2005). PAHs comprise a ubiquitous class of contaminants that appear to be generally increasing in the environment, reflecting urbanization, population growth, and use of fossil fuels (Van Metre and Mahler, 2005).

Contaminant effects on development are often difficult to discern in field studies, due to the small size of embryos and the fact that developmental impacts generally either are lethal or greatly reduced survival. However, early life stages of most organisms are generally more sensitive to xenobiotics than other life stages; thus, developmental impacts merit careful attention by ecotoxicologists.

Disease Susceptibility Disease plays an important role in regulating and sometimes seriously impacting populations of free-living organisms. Of great concern are interactions between disease organisms and environmental contaminants, particularly potential impacts of chemicals on immune systems that render organisms more susceptible to disease. The question is often raised about how chemical pollution elevates the role of disease in population viability and dynamics.

Both field observational and laboratory experimental studies motivate this concern. For example, forensic evidence suggested that pHAHs such as dioxins and PCBs may have played a role in mass mortalities of seals and other marine mammals in the Baltic Sea that were directly attributed to viral infections

(Ross *et al.*, 1996). Captive harbor seals (*Phoca vitulina*) fed fish from the Baltic Sea displayed a number of immune system deficits relative to seals fed fish from uncontaminated Atlantic Ocean sites, including impaired natural killer (NK) cell activity, in vitro T-lymphocyte function, antigen-specific in vitro lymphocyte proliferative responses, and in vivo delayed-type hypersensitivity and antibody responses to ovalbumin. These effects were correlated with greater concentrations of TCDD equivalents in fish from the Baltic Sea. In a case–control study using long-term data from studies of marine mammal strandings in the United Kingdom, Hall *et al.* (2006) concluded that each 1 mg/kg increase in total PCB concentrations in blubber resulted in an average increase in mortality due to infectious disease of 2% in harbor porpoises (*Phocoena phocoena*). In a study of free-ranging logger-head sea turtles (*Caretta caretta*) collected in North Carolina, Keller *et al.* (2006) observed significant correlations between selected immune responses (lysozyme activity and lymphocyte proliferation) and concentrations of PCBs and chlorinated insecticides (DDE and chlordanes); these correlations were supported by in vitro studies with these chemicals in isolated turtle leukocytes. Similarly, Auffret *et al.* (2006) observed responses associated with immunosuppression in mussels (*Mytilus galloprovincialis*) that generally tracked chemical pollution gradients in the western Mediterranean Sea. Using available laboratory and field data, Loge *et al.* (2005) developed a model to assess the effects of environmental stressors, including chemicals, on disease susceptibility in migrant juvenile salmon in the Columbia River Basin, Washington. They concluded that chemical and nonchemical stressors contributed equally to disease-induced mortalities that were predicted to range from 3% to 18% of the population, depending on residence time.

Numerous laboratory studies have demonstrated chemical impacts on immune systems in animals of ecological relevance. These include effects of pesticides on amphibians (Albert *et al.*, 2007), PCBs on channel catfish (*Ictalurus punctatus*) (Rice and Schlenk, 1995), heavy metals on rainbow trout (Sanchez-Dardon *et al.*, 1999), PAHs on bivalves (Wootton *et al.*, 2003), and flame retardants (polybrominated diphenyl ethers [PBDEs]) on American kestrels (*Falco sparverius*) (Fernie *et al.*, 2005). Fairbrother *et al.* (2004) reviewed the literature concerning effects of chemicals on immune systems of birds, emphasizing potential impacts on wildlife species, and Zelikoff *et al.* (2002) performed a similar review for fish. The potential effects of chemicals on immune function and disease susceptibility in wildlife is clearly a very important subject in ecotoxicology and one likely to see significant advances in the near future as powerful genomic tools become more available for representative species.

Behavior The impacts of chemicals on animal behavior have received significant attention among ecotoxicologists. Relatively subtle effects on behaviors associated with, for example, mating and reproduction, foraging, predator–prey interactions, preference/avoidance of contaminated areas, and migration have potentially important ramifications for population dynamics. However, difficulties in objective quantifications of behaviors and laboratory to field extrapolations appear to have limited the application of this area to ERAs, and by extension, perhaps to funds available for basic research. In some cases, however, biochemical mechanisms underlying behavioral effects have been elucidated that may assist with these issues and provide useful biomarkers for behavioral toxicants in field studies.

As noted by Rand (1985), chemicals causing behavioral effects in wildlife are often known from mammalian studies to be neurotoxicants. For example, in an early study, Grue *et al.* (1982) noted reduced nest attentiveness in female starlings dosed with the AChE-inhibiting organophosphate insecticide dicrotophos; this study took advantage of the relative ease of attracting wild starlings to artificial nest boxes that is advantageous for detailed studies, a phenomenon that has been employed in subsequent avian ecotoxicological studies (Parker and Goldstein, 2000). Grue *et al.* (1997) and Walker (2003) reviewed the behavioral effects in birds of these and other neurotoxic insecticides.

Behavioral effects of insecticides have also been observed in fish. For example, Scholz *et al.* (2000) reported adverse impacts of the organophosphate diazinon on olfactory-mediated behaviors such as the alarm response and homing in the Chinook salmon (*Oncorhynchus tshawytscha*), and Sandahl *et al.* (2005) observed similar thresholds for the effects of another organophosphate (chlorpyrifos) on swimming and feeding behaviors and on AChE inhibition in coho salmon (*O. kistich*). The effects of pollutants, including pesticides, on fish behavior were reviewed by Scott and Sloman (2004).

Mercury, particularly as methylmercury, comprises another potent neurotoxicant that has been shown to perturb behavior in wildlife. For example, golden shiners (*Notemigonus crysoleucas*) fed diets containing methylmercury that resulted in tissue mercury concentrations consistent with those observed in this species in northern US lakes exhibited perturbed predator avoidance behaviors (Webber and Haines, 2003). In a study employing fish captured in the field and brought into the laboratory for behavioral analysis, Smith and Weis (1997) observed that killifish captured from a mercury-polluted tidal creek in New Jersey exhibited reduced feeding activity and greater mortality due to predation than killifish from an uncontaminated site. Using mercury concentrations in feathers as a marker for exposure, Heath and Frederick (2005) observed a negative correlation between mercury exposure and nesting activity among White Ibises (*Eudocimus albus*) in the Florida Everglades that may be related to behavioral effects. In studies with wild mink (*Mustela vision*) collected in Canada, Basu *et al.* (2005) observed significant correlations between mercury concentrations in brains and densities of neurochemical receptors (cholinergic and dopaminergic) associated with animal behavior. The effects of mercury on wildlife, including behavioral impacts, were reviewed by Wolfe *et al.* (1998).

Environmental contaminants not generally thought of as neurotoxicants have also been shown to perturb behavior. For example, cadmium and copper have been shown to impact olfactory neurons and associated behaviors (preference/avoidance to chemicals, including pheromones) in several fish species (Saucier *et al.*, 1991; Baker and Montgomery, 2001; Baldwin *et al.*, 2003). Copper exposure in zebrafish also led to loss of neurons in the peripheral mechanosensory system ("lateral line"), which could lead to altered behaviors associated with schooling, predator avoidance, and rheotaxis (physical alignment of fish in a current) (Linbo *et al.*, 2006). Carvalho and Tillitt (2004) reported loss of retinal ganglion cells in rainbow trout exposed to TCDD; these cells link the eye with the brain, and in this study deficits in visual acuity and prey capture rates were noted in TCDD-exposed fish. Clearly, numerous mechanisms of chemical toxicity can result in behavioral impacts, including direct toxicity to neurons, alterations in hormones that modulate behaviors, and impaired energy metabolism. In some cases, impaired behavior may comprise a sublethal impact with substantive ecological consequence (Scott and Sloman, 2004).

Cancer Beginning in the 1960s, numerous cases of cancer epizootics in wildlife that are associated with chemical pollution, particularly in specific fish populations, have been reported in North America and northern Europe (Harshbarger and Clark; 1990; Vethaak, 1992). As in humans, cancer in these animals occurs largely in relatively older age classes and therefore is oftentimes considered a disease unlikely to directly impact population dynamics or other ecological parameters. However, this may not always be the case, particularly in species that require many years to attain sexual maturity and/or have low reproductive rates. In any event, the occurrence of high incidences of cancer in wildlife populations raises serious concerns for environmental quality at those locations experiencing these epizootics. For these reasons, as well as for concerns for human health in these areas, and the advantages of alternative models such as fish for understanding chemical carcinogenesis, these epizootics have motivated substantial research in several areas relevant to human health and ecotoxicology.

In field studies of cancer outbreaks in aquatic and marine systems, typically only selected species exhibit elevated cancer rates associated with chemical contamination. A major contributor to this differential cancer susceptibility in wild fish populations is clearly lifestyle; benthic (bottom-dwelling) species such as brown bullhead (*Ameriurus nebulosus*) and white sucker (*Catostomus commersoni*) in freshwater systems, and English sole (*Parophrys vetulus*) and winter flounder (*P. americanus*) in marine systems generally exhibit the highest cancer rates in polluted systems (Baumann, 1998). The bulk of chemicals in these systems associated with cancer epizootics, such as PAHs, PCBs, and other halogenated compounds, reside in sediments; benthic fish live in contact with these sediments and prey in large measure on other benthic organisms. Thus, benthic fish experience greater exposures to carcinogens than other species in these systems. Inherent biological differences may also play a role in species susceptibilities to chemical carcinogenesis; for example, laboratory studies have revealed marked differences among fish species in their abilities to activate PAH procarcinogens to DNA adduct-forming metabolite as well as to detoxify them through phase II metabolism (Collier *et al.*, 1992; Hasspieler *et al.*, 1994; Ploch *et al.*, 1998).

In their analysis of cancer epizootics in fish, Harshbarger and Clark (1990) concluded that cancers of the liver (hepatocellular neoplasms) had the strongest associations with chemical pollution, although cancers have been observed in other tissues in wild fish as well (Ostrander and Rotchell, 2005). PAHs appear to be the most implicated class of carcinogens associated with liver neoplasms in fish cancer epizootics. Studies implicating a key role for PAHs (and key PAH sources) include English sole in the Puget Sound (various urban and industrial sources; Malins *et al.*, 1987), brown bullhead in the Black River, Ohio (a coal-coking facility; Baumann and Harshbarger, 1998), and in the Potomac River watershed near Washington, DC (various point and nonpoint discharges; Pinkney *et al.*, 2001), and killifish in the Elizabeth River, Virginia (a wood treatment plant using creosote; Vogelbein *et al.*, 1990). As stated earlier, PAHs appear to comprise a class of contaminant generally increasing in the environment. The metabolism of PAHs such as BaP to reactive metabolites that form DNA adducts that initiates carcinogenesis, or conversely to excretable conjugates, was described earlier. It is noteworthy that the molecular and biochemical pathways underlying chemical carcinogenesis, such as PAH metabolism, DNA damage, and effects on oncogenes, are qualitatively similar between most fish and mammalian species examined.

This recognition of shared pathways has in part contributed to the use of various fish models for studying chemical carcinogenesis from a human health as well as from a broader environmental

standpoint. An important historical event was the identification in Italy, France, and the United States during the 1950s and 1960s of aflatoxin as a potent liver carcinogen in farm-raised rainbow trout (Sinnhuber *et al.*, 1977). Subsequently aflatoxin, a fungal toxin produced by *Aspergillus flavus* that is of concern where grains and nuts are stored in wet conditions, was found to be carcinogenic to mammals including humans. Thus, the rainbow trout observations led to the discovery of a new and important class of chemical carcinogens, and the recognition that fish can be very sensitive to chemical carcinogenesis. Since that time, other fish species have been employed for laboratory studies related to chemical carcinogenesis, particularly medaka (*O. latipes*) and platyfish/swordtails hybrids (*Xiphophorus* spp.); zebrafish also show promise as a laboratory model (Ostrander and Rotchell, 2005). Compared with rodent models, fish models have advantages of reduced costs for propagation and housing, briefer time intervals between exposures and the expression of tissue changes indicative of carcinogenesis, and greater feasibility of performing large-scale studies with many animals to quantify dose–response relationships.

It is noteworthy that the great bulk of reports of elevated cancer rates in free-living animals occur in fish, with few reports of potentially chemically related cancers to our knowledge in other vertebrates. California sea lions (*Zalophus californianus*) stranded along the central California coast were found to have elevated cancer rates (18%), and concentrations of DDT and PCBs were greater in animals with cancer versus those determined to die of other causes (Ylitalo *et al.*, 2005). Martineau *et al.* (2002) reported elevated cancer rates (also 18%) in carcasses of beluga whales (*Delphinapterus leucas*) stranded along the shores of the St. Lawrence River estuary in Quebec, a system with elevated levels of PAHs. The authors noted that beluga was the only species of marine mammal among 20 inhabiting this system that exhibited elevated cancer rates, and that cancers are rare worldwide in marine mammals. It is likely that elevated exposures play an important role in the relatively high frequency of reports of cancers in benthic fishes; relative inherent sensitivities among mammals, birds, reptiles, amphibians, and fishes are unclear.

Population

A population is a collection of individuals of the same species that occupy the same space and within which genetic information can be exchanged. The study of populations is a central theme in ecological sciences and ecotoxicology is no exception. Assessment of toxicant effects on populations has been important in ecotoxicology since its inception (Newman, 2001). A well-known, early instance is the sharp drop and then slow recovery of coastal populations of osprey (Spitzer *et al.*, 1978) and brown pelican (Anderson *et al.*, 1975) that occurred as a consequence of widespread DDT and DDE spraying and eventual banning. Another was the enhanced, genetically based tolerance of pest insect populations chronically sprayed with pesticides (Mallet, 1989). Industrial melanism, the premier example in biology textbooks of natural selection in wild populations, is another example of population ecotoxicology (Newman, 2001). Population ecotoxicology covers a wide range of topics with core research themes being (1) epidemiology of chemical-related disease, (2) effects on general population qualities including demographics and persistence, and (3) population genetics.

The level of belief warranted for possible contaminant-related effects in nonhuman populations is assessed by applying routine epidemiological methods. Many methods described in epidemiology textbooks (Anders, 1993; Woodward, 2005) are applied to

Table 30-1

A Summary of One Popular Set of Rules of Thumb (Data from Fox, 1991) for Assessing Plausibility of a Causal Association in an Ecological Epidemiology

RULE	DESCRIPTION
1. Strength of association	How strong the association is between the possible cause and the effect, for example, a very large relative risk
2. Consistency of association	How consistently is there an association between the possible cause and the effect, for example, consistent among several studies with different circumstances
3. Predictive performance	How good is the prediction of effect made from the presence/level of the possible cause
4. Monotonic trend	How consistent is the association between possible cause and effect to a monotonic trend (ie, either a consistent increase or decrease in effect level/prevalence with an increase in exposure)
5. Inconsistent temporal sequence	The effect, or elevated level of effect, occurs before exposure to the hypothesized cause
6. Factual implausibility	The hypothesized association is implausible given existing knowledge
7. Inconsistency with replication	Very poor reproducibility of association during repeated field assessments encompassing different circumstances or repeated formal laboratory testing

NOTE: *According to Fox, the first four rules are most useful in supporting a causal hypothesis if found to be true (ie, very strong, consistent, predictive, or monotonic association). The others are most useful for lessening belief in the causal hypothesis if true.*

nonhuman populations, although with a slightly different balance because much more experimental exposure data are potentially available for nonhuman populations than for human populations. Rules of thumb for gauging the level of belief warranted by evidence that emerged from human epidemiology are also applied in population ecotoxicology. Hill's nine aspects of human disease association (Hill, 1965) might be used directly or after minor modification. As an example, Fox (1991) (Table 30-1) modified such rules of thumb to accommodate slight differences in the subject matter and approaches in population ecotoxicology. Conventional epidemiological descriptors and models are also applied. For example, Horness *et al.* (1998) quantified prevalence and relative risks for neoplastic liver lesions in English sole inhabiting areas with different sediment concentrations of PAHs. Logistic regression models were also used to identify relationships between these lesions and chemical and biological risk factors (Myers *et al.*, 1994).

Defining and predicting alterations in population size, dynamics, and demographic composition due to toxicant exposure has always been central in ecotoxicology and has become increasingly so in the last 20 years as regulatory agencies such as the US Environmental Protection Agency clearly reinforced their long-standing commitment to understanding chemical exposure effects on natural population viability.

Protecting populations is an explicitly stated goal of several Congressional and Agency mandates and regulations. Thus it is important that ecological risk assessment guidelines focus upon protection and management at the population, community, and ecosystem levels....

Environmental Protection Agency (1991)

Ecological theory and research (eg, Forbes and Calow, 1999) also indicate that metrics of effect to individuals are not especially good metrics of toxicant exposure effects to populations.

Models of exposed population dynamics suggest that reductions on population densities are not the only important changes brought about by chemical exposure. Some species populations fluctuate within a range of densities. These fluctuations are characteristic of the species strategy for maintaining itself in various types of habitats and toxicant exposure could potentially change this range (Simkiss *et al.*, 1993). Combined with decreases in population densities driven by external forces such as weather events, these toxicant-induced modifications of the average population densities and dynamics can increase the risk of a population's density falling so low that local extinction occurs (Newman, 1995).

Demographic qualities can change with toxicant exposure in ways that influence the risk of local population extinction. Toxicants can change a species population's vital rates, that is, age- and sex-dependent death, birth, maturation, and migration rates, in complex ways. These changes in combination determine the population density and distribution of individuals among ages and sexes during exposure. The population's ability to resist external forces that reduce its size is determined by these demographic features (Gard, 1992; Sherratt *et al.*, 1999; Kammenga and Laskowski, 2000; Aubone, 2004). Consequently, considerable research effort is being spent on demographic methods for predicting exposed population changes and risks of extinction.

Demography explores vital rates of populations composed of individuals that differ in age and sex. Individuals in field populations can also differ in their spatial distribution and this influences the impact of toxicants (Newman, 2001). Individuals of the same species often are grouped into subpopulations within a habitat and all of these subpopulations together comprise a metapopulation (Fig. 30-9). Subpopulations in the metapopulation have different levels of exchange and different vital rates that depend on the nature of their habitat. Spatial distances and obstacles or corridors for migration influence migration among patches: habitat quality determines vital rates. An inferior habitat, such as a grossly contaminated one, can act as a sink into which individuals migrate from nearby superior (source) habitat. Migration can rescue a subpopulation or reduce its risk of local extinction. An individual migrating from the contaminated habitat to an uncontaminated one can express an adverse effect despite its present distance from the contamination, that is, the action-at-distance hypothesis of ecotoxicology (Spromberg *et al.*, 1998). The viability of the metapopulation can also be as strongly influenced by maintaining important migration corridors among subpopulations and protecting high-quality habitats (ie, keystone habitats) as by the general level of contamination within the metapopulation's habitat (Mauer and Holt, 1996; O'Connor, 1996; Spromberg *et al.*, 1998; Newman, 2001).

The genetics of exposed populations are studied to understand changes in tolerance to toxicants and to document toxicant influence on field populations. The capacity of some populations to become more tolerant of toxicants via selection is well documented. A few examples include increased tolerance of pine mice to endrin (Webb and Horsfall, 1967) and rats to warfarin (Partridge, 1979) after years

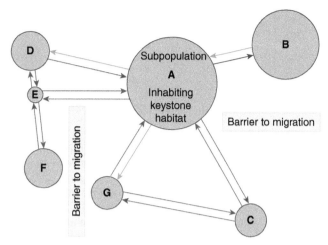

Figure 30-9. *Metapopulations are composed of subpopulations that differ in their vital rates and tendency to exchange individuals.* In this illustration, subpopulation A occupies a keystone habitat. The loss of subpopulation A would devastate the metapopulation. Also, loss of the migration corridor between subpopulations A, B, and D would devastate the metapopulation. In contrast, the loss of subpopulation F would not influence the metapopulation to the same degree.

of application of these agents for rodent control. More recently, Ownby *et al.* (2002) documented enhanced tolerance in populations of an estuarine fish chronically exposed to PAHs. Although genetically based increases in tolerance are well documented in wild populations, many exposed populations probably find themselves in situations in which they cannot adapt adequately because their genetic resources, nature of the toxicant, or spatial/temporal context within which the enhanced tolerance must evolve are inadequate. Also, in an ecotoxicological sense, all cases of increased tolerance do not fit the conventional context manifested in the examples just given. Some do not involve suborganismal changes to biochemical or anatomical features resulting in enhanced tolerance. For example, industrial melanism increases a peppered moth's fitness in the presence of soot by reducing its likelihood of being taken by a predator. The dominant light form of this moth has a lowered fitness in the presence of dark soot, and genetically based changes in color increase its fitness. The selective mechanism here is ecological, that is, fitness relative to avoiding visual predators.

Genetic qualities are also used to infer past toxicant influence in an exposed population. For example, Mulvey *et al.* (2002, 2003) showed distinct genetic qualities in estuarine fish populations exposed to high concentrations of PAHs. Another piece of evidence demonstrating past toxicant influence on populations can be a change in genetic diversity. A drop in genetic diversity in populations is thought to be an adverse effect because genetic diversity is required in populations to evolutionarily adapt to environmental changes. Toxicants can influence genetic diversity by purely stochastic means. Genes can be lost in the population if the population is so drastically reduced in size that the chance of a rare gene being lost between generations becomes very high. Also, the average rate at which the frequency of a rare gene decreases through time due to genetic drift increases as the effective population size decreases. The effective population is the number of individuals contributing genes to the next generation so toxicant-related changes in demographic qualities can also accelerate genetic drift.

Community

An ecological community is an interacting assemblage of species populations occupying a defined habitat at a particular time.

Populations in a community interact in many ways and, because these many interactions are complex, a community has properties that are not predictable from those of its component populations. Some species have such a crucial role (keystone species) or numerical dominance (dominants) that they are essential to maintaining community structure.[2] Other species contribute to the nature of the community in more subtle ways.

Ambiguity exists about the importance of all the species in a community relative to maintaining overall structure and balancing essential functions such as nutrient cycling, primary productivity, community respiration, and detritus processing. The redundant species hypothesis suggests that species function redundantly: if a species were lost, another with a similar function would increase in numbers to compensate. Only certain critical species such as dominant or keystone species are essential to the community. The rivet popper hypothesis suggests otherwise. Each species in a community is similar to one of the many rivets holding an airplane fuselage together. Each lost rivet contributes to a gradual weakening of the fuselage that will lead eventually to a failure in function. By analogy, each species disappearance diminishes a community's functioning.

Ecotoxicologists remain divided about which hypothesis is most relevant. Pratt and Cairns (1996) argue from evidence and a conservative stance that the rivet popper is the most appropriate. Ecotoxicologists and regulators who pragmatically set standards based on concentrations that will not harm more than a specified percentage of species in a community (eg, Stephan *et al.*, 1985) assume that the redundant species hypothesis is more pertinent. Although the redundant species hypothesis is assumed to be correct in many ERAs (Solomon and Sibley, 2002), recent theory (Loreau, 2004), modeling (Naeem *et al.*, 1994), and experimental evidence (Tilman, 1996; Tilman *et al.*, 1996; Salminen *et al.*, 2001) seem to support the rivet popper hypothesis. Biodiversity tends to foster community stability and function.

Communities take on characteristic structures as predicted by the Law of Frequencies: the number of individual organisms in a community is related by some function to the number of species in the community (Fig. 30-10). Ecotoxicants[3] can alter the resulting community structure in predictable ways by either directly impacting the fitness of individuals in populations that make up the community or altering population interactions. Community ecotoxicologists spend considerable effort trying to understand and predict ecotoxicant influences on community structure and essential functions.

Direct effects involve removal of a population or metapopulation from the community by reducing the Darwinian fitness of individuals enough that the population falls below some critical minimum size. Indirect effects can involve interference with

---

[2]In its most rudimentary context, community structure refers to the number of species present and the numbers of individuals present in each of these species. It can also refer to the distribution of species among different functional groups such as decomposers, detritivores, primary producers, primary consumers such as herbivores, secondary consumers such as carnivores that consume herbivores, etc.

[3]The conventional context for the term toxicant becomes difficult to retain without some qualification when dealing with populations, communities, and other higher level entities because an agent does not necessarily have to directly interact with the individual in order to harm it. As an example, an agent might eliminate a prey species, leading indirectly to the disappearance of a predator species that depended on it for sustenance. The "toxicant" did not poison the predator, yet it caused its demise nonetheless. A distinct term, ecotoxicant, is often applied to avoid confusion in such cases.

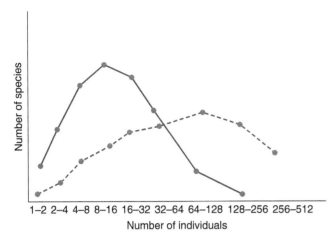

Figure 30-10. *Log-normal model of species abundance for an unexposed (solid line and red points) and toxicant-exposed community (dashed line and blue points).* Communities have distinct structure as shown here with the typical log-normal species abundance model. As first described by data from Patrick (1973), ecotoxicants tend to lower the mode of the species abundance curve and stretch the right tail outward. Ecotoxicants result in fewer intermediate abundance species and more extremely abundant species.

interspecies competition, predator–prey interactions, host–disease/parasite interactions, or symbiotic relationships such as pollination. The simplest competition model (Lotka–Volterra model) can be used to illustrate the potential for both direct and indirect effects on populations:

$$\frac{dN_1}{dt} = r_1 N_1 \left[1 - \frac{N_1}{K_1} - \frac{\alpha_{12} N_2}{K_1} \right],$$

$$\frac{dN_2}{dt} = r_2 N_2 \left[1 - \frac{N_2}{K_2} - \frac{\alpha_{21} N_1}{K_2} \right],$$

where N_1 and N_2 are the population sizes of competitors 1 and 2, K_1 and K_2 the carrying capacities of the environment for competitors 1 and 2, r_1 and r_2 the intrinsic rate of population increase (ie, birth rate – death rate) for competitors 1 and 2, α_{12} the competition coefficient quantifying the impact of the presence of competitor 2 on competitor 1, and α_{21} the impact of competitor 1 on competitor 2. Not only can exposure directly impact birth rates, death rates, and carrying capacity of each species, but it can also influence species persistence by shifting competition coefficients in favor of another species. Mathematically, it can be shown that the two competitors depicted in the Lotka–Volterra model can coexist only if two conditions are met, $K_1 < K_2/\alpha_{21}$ and $K_2 < K_1/\alpha_{12}$. So, a population can be lost from a community as readily by changing its competitive interactions as by directly changing its death and reproductive rates. Similar statements can be made about changes in predator–prey, host–disease, and various symbiotic interactions. As an example, concern expressed recently about unintended pesticide reductions in the number and diversity of pollinators in European farmlands (Newman *et al.*, 2006) could be partially responsible for the recently reported decline in insect-pollinated plant species in Britain and The Netherlands (Biesmeijer *et al.*, 2006). In another instance, reduced habitat cover and insect densities in European farmlands has had a significant impact on grey partridge populations (Rands, 1985; Chiverton, 1999). As another and final example involving predator–prey interactions, amphibian tadpole exposure to endosulfan increases the risk of predation by dragonfly larvae (Broomhall, 2002). None of these examples involves a direct

poisoning by a toxicant, but instead, involves an ecotoxicant that adversely modifies species interactions.

Structural changes to communities can be detected in species abundance plots (see Fig. 30-10) or shifts in conventional community metrics calculated from community samples taken in the proximity of contaminated sites. Common metrics for species richness, diversity, and evenness are used to express changes in biodiversity. Richness is simply the number of species in the sampled community, or if a relative number of species in different communities is all that is needed, the number of species expected in a specified sample size such as a rarefaction richness estimate of 12 species in a sample of 100 individuals from a community. Evenness is a measure of how equitably the individuals in a community are spread among the species. Finally, diversity (heterogeneity) indices combine the elements of richness and evenness into one number. Generally, but not always, ecotoxicants lower species richness, evenness, and overall diversity. The regulatory premise is that these changes reflect a diminished community.

Recently, structural and functional qualities in communities have been combined to generate multimetric indices such as the Biotic Index of Integrity (IBI) (Karr, 1991). Ecological insight is used to select and then numerically combine community qualities such as species richness, health of individual animals in a sample, and the number of individuals in a sample belonging to a particular functional group, such as number of piscivorous fish. The IBI score for a study site is calculated and compared with that expected for an unimpacted site in order to estimate its biological integrity.

Another central theme in community ecotoxicology is toxicant transfer during trophic interactions. Toxicant concentrations can decrease (biodiminution), remain constant, or increase (biomagnification) with each trophic transfer within a food web. POPs with moderately high lipid solubility ($5 < \log K_{ow} < 7$ or 8; Thomann, 1989; Connell, 1990) and minimal metabolic breakdown in an organism can biomagnify to harmful concentrations. Metals that biomagnify are mercury and the alkali metals, cesium and rubidium. Zinc, an essential metal that is actively regulated in individuals, can exhibit biomagnification or biominification depending on whether ambient levels are below or above those required by the organism to function properly. Biominification is facilitated in a marine food web after sequestration in intracellular phosphate granules of molluscan prey species (Nott and Nicolaidou, 1993) and biomagnification by active regulation in zinc-deficient terrestrial communities (Beyer, 1986). The biomagnification of mercury is enhanced by its microbial transformation to methylmercury. Biomagnification of the potassium analogs, cesium and rubidium, is facilitated by the differences in their influxes and effluxes that favor retention in organisms (Rowan and Rasmussen, 1994; Campbell *et al.*, 2005).

Quantifying the trophic position of a species in a community is essential to modeling biomagnification. Most trophic systems are not simple "food chains." Most individuals in a community can feed on different species depending on their life stage, seasons, and relative abundances of prey species. These trophic interactions are best described as occurring in a trophic web, not a trophic chain.

Conveniently, trophic position of an individual within a complex food web can be quantified with nitrogen isotopes. Generally, ^{14}N passes through biochemical pathways faster than ^{15}N, resulting in excretion of waste with a slightly higher $^{14}N/^{15}N$ ratio than in ingested food. The relative amounts of ^{14}N and ^{15}N will be slightly biased toward the heavy isotope in tissues of a species relative to those of its food source(s). This discrimination between the heavy and light N isotopes continues through food webs, allowing the trophic position of each participating species to be estimated. The metric used for this purpose, the $\delta^{15}N$, expresses the quotient of

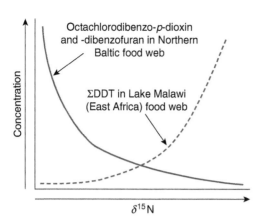

Figure 30-11. *Modeling ecotoxicant concentration versus trophic position as quantified with $\delta^{15}N$.* Power models were applied to octachlorodibenzo-*p*-dioxin/dibenzofuran concentrations in a North Baltic food chain (data from Broman *et al.*, 1992) and the ΣDDT (sum of primarily the *p,p'* isomers of DDD, DDE, and DDT) in food webs of Lake Malawi (data from Kidd *et al.*, 2001). Biomagnification and minification were evident for ΣDDT and octachlorodibenzo-*p*-dioxin/dibenzofuran, respectively.

these two isotopes in the biological tissue of interest relative to the quotient expected in the atmosphere:

$$\delta^{15}N = 1000 \left[\frac{[^{15}N_{Tissue}]/[^{14}N_{Tissue}]}{[^{15}N_{Air}][^{14}N_{Air}]} - 1 \right].$$

The change in toxicant concentrations within food webs is modeled using the $\delta^{15}N$, which quantifies trophic position of the species from which the tissue sample was taken (Fig. 30-11). Linear and exponential models are commonly applied:

$$\text{Concentration} = a + b\delta^{15}N,$$
$$\text{Concentration} = 10^{a+b\delta^{15}N} \quad \text{or} \quad e^{a+b\delta^{15}N}.$$

Ecosystem to Biosphere

Ecosystems are the functional unit of ecology composed of the ecological community and its abiotic habitat. Systems ecologists try to describe and predict energy and mass cycling in and flow from ecosystems. The ecotoxicologist's interest in ecosystems includes understanding how toxicants diminish an ecosystem's capacity to perform essential functions and to understand toxicant movement enough to assess exposure within different ecosystem components.

Many of the effects described above for exposed communities are relevant here. As an example, Allred and Giesy (1988) demonstrated that elevating cadmium concentrations in an artificial stream reduced decomposition rates of dead leaves. Odum (1985) suggested that other changes to be expected with increased ecosystem stress include an increased loss of nutrients, increased community respiration, and an imbalance of primary production and respiration.

Studies of toxicant movement within ecological systems are conducted at extremely different scales (Fig. 30-12). Conventional ecosystem studies involve descriptions of contaminant concentrations and movements in easily defined ecosystems such as lakes, forests, or fields. Some toxicants, especially those subject to wide dispersal by air or water, cannot be completely understood in this framework so a landscape scale might be chosen instead. As an example, acid precipitation might be examined in the context of an entire watershed, mountain range, or even a continental region. As another example (see Fig. 30-12, top right panel), the fish tissue concentrations of a PCB congener and other POPs were measured

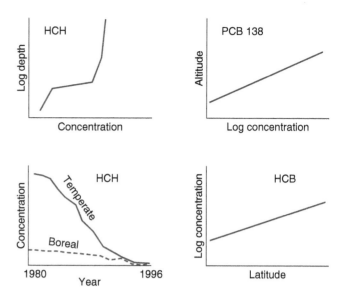

Figure 30-12. *Examples of scales relevant to assessments of ecotoxicant distributions.* The smallest scale example (top left) is the vertical distribution of α-hexachlorocyclohexane (HCH) in a stratified region of the Sea of Japan (data from Chernyak *et al.*, 1995). A slightly larger scale is reflected in the change in the polychlorinated biphenyl congener PCB 138 in tissues of fish inhabiting European lakes at different altitudes (top right panel, data from Fernandez and Grimait, 2003). Representing a subcontinental scale study is the temporal change in atmospheric α-hexachlorocyclohexane concentrations in temperate and boreal regions of central northern Europe (bottom left panel, data from Wania *et al.*, 1999). The largest scale encompasses the entire earth, showing the influence of latitude on hexachlorobenzene (HCB) concentration in tree bark (bottom right panel, data from Simonich and Hites, 1995).

in high mountain region lakes of Europe. Concentrations for several were related to the altitude at which a lake sat. The relationships between altitude and concentrations of the various POPs was interpreted based on atmospheric movement of the POPs and each POP's propensity to either volatilize or condense at a particular altitude-dependent temperature regime. Still other ecotoxicants require a global context in order to fully understand their movements and accumulation. As an example, hexachlorobenzene concentration in tree bark collected worldwide showed a clear latitudinal gradient. Its global distribution and those of other sampled POPs were a function of their relative volatilities. The volatile hexachlorobenzene moved more readily toward the poles than less volatile POPs such as endosulfan and DDT. The differential global movement of POPs due to differences in volatility and partitioning behavior was called global distillation (Wania and Mackay, 1996). The balance between a POP's tendency to condense or evaporate at different latitude-related temperatures determines its atmospheric mobility and its ultimate global deposition pattern (Wania and Mackay, 1996).

APPROACHES

Many approaches have been developed to detect and quantify contaminant effects. These span the levels of organization described above. Approaches widely applied in ecotoxicology include standardized toxicity tests deigned to meet regulatory needs and biomarkers for organismal exposure and effects. For higher levels, a range of ecological methods exists for population, community, and ecosystem effects. Other techniques such as geographic information system (GIS) analysis of impacts allow the ecotoxicologist to assess impact encompassing large spatial scales. These approaches and examples of their applications are described in this section.

Toxicity Tests

Toxicity testing encompassing representative animals and plants at different levels of organization offers a practical approach to characterize chemical effects on biological systems. While it is widely known that toxicity tests cannot mimic the complex interactions and variable conditions of natural ecosystems, they address the potential direct effects of toxic substances on individual ecosystem components in a controlled and reproducible manner. A number of testing guidelines have been put forth by regulatory bodies and organizations worldwide to meet requirements for chemical registration or authorization (OECD, 1981; MAFF, 1985; US EPA OPPTS, 1996a; ASTM International, 2006), with numerous subsequent revisions. Different sets of guidelines apply to specific countries, regions, or products, and can differ significantly in their requirements. The harmonized guidelines put forth by the US EPA Office of Prevention, Pesticides and Toxic Substances (US EPA OPPTS, 1996a) were created in an attempt to lessen variations in testing requirements, and bring together requirements from the Organisation for Economic Co-Operation and Development (OECD), the US EPA Office of Pollution Prevention and Toxics (OPPT), and the Office of Pesticide Programs (OPP).

Ecotoxicology tests feature a wide variety of aquatic (including algae, invertebrates, tadpoles, bivalves, shrimp, fish), avian (quail, duck), and terrestrial species (soil microorganisms, crops, honey bees, earthworms, wild mammals). Species are selected based on their traditional use as laboratory animals, but also on ecological relevance, which further complicates global harmonization of ecological testing. In addition, special considerations apply to testing of aquatic species due to the unmistakable differences in the way aquatic species are exposed to toxicants (US EPA OPPTS, 1996b). For instance, water quality monitoring and investigation of the solubility and stability of the test substance under the conditions of testing, along with determination of nominal versus measured concentrations, are common practices in aquatic toxicology. Testing can be conducted in aqueous systems without renewal of the test substance (static), renewal at predetermined time intervals (static-renewal), or continuous flow of test substance through the test compartment (flow-through).

Acute toxicity testing consists of single species exposed to various concentrations of the test substance. The most common end point in acute tests is death, although abnormal behavioral or other gross observations are commonly noted, and nonlethal end points occasionally apply (eg, immobilization for daphnids, shell deposition in oysters). Variations in acute toxicity studies comprise testing of different species (such as fresh vs saltwater fish, bobwhite quail vs mallard duck), life stages (embryo, larva, juvenile), environmental influences (eg, presence of organic material), or sediment exposures. Data from different test concentrations and time points are used to derive concentration–response curves and predicted values such as the LC_{50} (median lethal concentration), EC_{50} (median effective concentration), or IC_{50} (median inhibition concentration). The LC_{50} represents the concentration of test substance killing 50% of the tested animals and EC_{50} the concentration of test substance affecting 50% of the test population during a specified period of time, such as growth; the IC_{50} is the concentration causing a 50% reduction in a nonquantal measurement (such as movement) for the test population. More quantitative values derived from acute tests are the lowest observed effect concentration (LOEC), that is, the lowest concentration where an effect is observed, and the no observed effect concentration (NOEC), the highest concentration resulting in no adverse effects.

Short-term laboratory studies conducted with single species are useful for rapid screening, provide information on thresholds for effects and selective and comparative toxicity, and can be used as range finders to guide subsequent, often more involved studies. Long-term and reproductive studies evaluate the effects of substances on organisms over extended periods of time and/or sequential generations (chronic toxicity, life cycle, reproduction). End points include both quantal (such as mortality) and nonquantal (reproduction, growth) measurements, and can be used to derive additional values, other than previously mentioned in acute toxicity tests. These include the calculation of threshold values, such as the maximum acceptable toxicant concentration (MATC), which is the maximum chemical concentration not toxic to test organisms, and the BCF, which estimates the tissue concentration in relation to the average exposure concentration in the test medium (eg, water).

Unique to ecotoxicology are the more elaborate microcosm, mesocosm, and field studies. Microcosms are representative aquatic or terrestrial ecosystems created under laboratory conditions that include a number of relevant species (such as protozoa, plankton, algae, plants, invertebrates). Simulated field studies or mesocosms can be created in the laboratory or in the field (eg, artificial streams, ponds) or consist of enclosures of existing habitats, containing representative soil, water, and biota. Lastly, full-scale field studies (aquatic organisms, terrestrial wildlife, pollinators) evaluate the effects of a substance on wildlife under real-life scenarios of actual use conditions of a product (eg, pesticide field usage rate), and thus, are more complicated, subject to considerable variability, and require extensive background knowledge of the local population and community dynamics.

As a final point, plant studies are a significant component of ecological toxicity testing, particularly for pesticide registration, and involve tiered testing of both target area and nontarget terrestrial and aquatic plants. Target area plants are those that are present in the area where the substance will be routinely used (application area), but which are not anticipated to be affected. Nontarget plants are those outside of the intended use area. End points of phytotoxicity include seedling emergence and growth, vegetative vigor, and rhizobium–legume toxicity, among others, and central to the toxicity testing with plants are the substrate and environmental conditions, which greatly influence plant health.

Biomarkers

The Nuclear Regulatory Commission (NRC, 1989) defined a biomarker as "a xenobiotically induced variation in cellular or biochemical components or processes, structures, or function that is measurable in a biological system or sample." In the context of ecotoxicology, this definition has been modified slightly to refer to biochemical, physiological or histological indicators of either exposure to or effects of xenobiotic chemicals at the suborganismal or organismal level (Huggett *et al.*, 1992). The term is most often employed to refer to molecular, physiological, and organismal responses to contaminant exposure that can be quantified in organisms inhabiting or captured from natural systems. A response that is limited to laboratory studies falls outside the generally held concept of a biomarker.

By definition, biomarkers do not directly provide information concerning impacts on the higher levels of organization that ecotoxicology ultimately endeavors to discern. Nevertheless, biomarkers often provide important ancillary tools for discerning contaminant exposures and potential impacts of ecological importance. The development and use of biomarkers in ecotoxicology is motivated by several factors. These include the inherent instabilities of many contaminants (such as PAHs and many pesticides) that make measures of exposure by direct tissue residue analysis difficult, the relative biological sensitivity of many biomarkers, the chemical specificity of some biomarkers that serve to contribute to the identification of chemicals having biological effects, and relatedly, the linkage of some biomarkers to underlying mechanisms of toxic action. Additionally, while populations and higher level effects are of greatest concern, variables associated with these levels are oftentimes relatively insensitive to chemicals and other stressors, take long periods of time to become manifest, and/or have difficult or imprecise methods for their analysis. Thus, biomarkers can provide sensitive early warning signals of incipient ecological damage (van der Oost *et al.*, 2003), in essence an ecological counterpart to the "canary in the coal mine" approach for preventing harm to coal miners. However, biomarkers do not provide adequate standalone data in the context of ecological assessments of contaminant effects. At this time and for the foreseeable future, such assessments generally involve a "weight of evidence approach," coalescing information obtained from chemical analyses, toxicity tests, biomarkers, and ecological indicators (sometimes referred to as "bioindicators"; see Adams *et al.*, 1989).

In earlier discussions, a number of contaminant effects at the organismal level and below that have been utilized as biomarkers were pointed out. These include effects with some degree of chemical specificity and relationship to a mechanism of toxicity (AChE inhibition by organophosphate and carbamate insecticides, ALAD inhibition by lead, DNA–PAH adducts), responses associated with exposures to chemicals acting through a common receptor (Vtg induction by ER agonists such as natural and synthetic estrogens, some surfactants, plasticizers, and pesticides; CYP1A induction by AHR agonists such as certain pHAHs and PAHs), and broader indices of cellular stress or tissue damage, such as markers of oxidative stress, lysosomal membrane stability, and histopathology. Numerous other identified mechanisms of toxicity, indices of chemical exposure, and cellular and organismal impacts have been exploited, with varying degree of success, as biomarkers (see reviews by Huggett *et al.*, 1992; Peakall, 1992; Adams, 2000; van der Oost *et al.*, 2003). In addition, new biomarkers continue to emerge; for example, considerable attention is now being given to biomarkers arising from advances in genomic technologies, discussed above.

In considering the development or use of a selected biomarker, several issues and limitations warrant consideration. For example, while sensitivity is overall an advantage of many biomarkers, it can sometimes raise important questions surrounding interpretation. For example, some molecular and biochemical measures are very sensitive to chemical exposures, but their ramifications for organismal health are unclear. For this reason, some distinguish between biomarkers of exposure and biomarkers of effect (see reviews cited above). However, this distinction is often blurred and is subject to an individual's view of what constitutes a significant biological chemical effect; some may say the formation of DNA adduct is a significant effect, while others will argue that such adducts only indicate exposure and will require tumor formation to occur before denoting an effect. Certainly most would agree that the tumor is a clearer marker of effect than the adducts, and something more readily grasped by policy makers and the general public. On the other hand, tumors are far less sensitive as a biomarker, a key *raison d'etre*; such trade-offs merit consideration.

Chemical specificity among biomarkers is also highly variable and is imbued with trade-offs. In some cases, such as where one has a good idea of the nature of contaminants likely to occur at a site, chemical-specific biomarkers will likely be most informative. In contrast, if such information is lacking, or mixtures encompassing

several classes of chemicals likely occur, nonspecific markers may be superior. In most cases, suites of biomarkers prove to be most effective, although the larger the suite, the more time-intensive and costly the analysis will be, another trade-off. Another important consideration is the influence on the biomarker of variables other than those of concern (chemical contamination). Effects of environmental variables such as temperature, time of day or year, salinity and dissolved oxygen, and physiological variables such as sex, age, reproductive status, and nutritional status need to be controlled for or at least understood and accounted for. Many biomarkers are invasive and require sacrifice of the organism in order to obtain needed tissues. This can be problematic, particularly in cases involving rare species or charismatic species such as marine mammals. In such cases, and in others where feasible, the use of noninvasive biomarkers is either preferred or required (Fossi and Marsili, 1997). In summary, biomarkers can provide powerful tools as early warning signals of ecological damage, to assist in assessments of environmental contamination, and in determining the effectiveness of various environmental management decisions such as cleanups. However, careful case-specific thought must go into the selection of biomarkers, and they rarely are efficacious alone.

Population

Population-level effects are quantified with both field and laboratory approaches (see Newman, 2001, 2013). Population density is the most common of field population qualities measured in surveys of contaminated habitats. Quadrat, mark-recapture, and removal-based methods are applied. The density of individuals in a series of random quadrats within the area of interest is used to estimate densities in quadrat methods. The total population size can be estimated with knowledge of the total number of quadrats in the area of interest. In cases in which individuals are mobile and capable of avoiding being counted in a quadrat, a mark-recapture method might be applied instead. This involves marking a subset of individuals from the population, allowing them to randomly mix back into the population, and resampling the population. The number of marked and unmarked individuals taken, and the total number originally marked, can be used to estimate population size. Removal-based methods involve repeated sampling of the population without replacement, noting how the number collected per unit of effort declines through the sequence of samplings, and extrapolating this trend down to the point (total number caught previous to a sampling) at which no more individuals will be taken. This point is an estimate of the population size. Obviously, this approach is useful only if sampling decreases the catch noticeably between sampling episodes.

As noted earlier in discussions of metapopulations, the spatial distribution of individuals in a habitat is important to understand. Fortunately, well-established methods are available for this task. Methods vary depending on whether the sampling units are discrete or arbitrary. An arbitrary unit might be the number of razor clam per square meter of beach or number of a zooplankton species per cubic meter of water. A discrete sampling unit might be the number of mallard ducks per pond or squirrels per oak tree. Some methods associated with discrete sampling units attempt to fit the spatial pattern to a specific distribution. Methods for arbitrary sampling units include quadrat-based or distance-to-nearest-neighbor approaches as described by Krebs (1998).

Demographic surveys or experiments can be conducted for exposed populations. Some studies explore age-specific vital rates but others are designed to explore vital rates for different life ages such as nestling, fledgling, juvenile, and adult. Most result in data sets that can be analyzed profitably using either a simple life table or more involved matrix analysis. The matrix method allows one to describe the population state and also to understand the sensitivity of the population to effects occurring to vital rates for various ages or stages (Caswell, 2001). The value of such studies lies in the ability to integrate effects to several effects into a projection of population consequences. Demographic studies are becoming more common in ecotoxicology, especially with species amenable to laboratory manipulation (Jansen et al., 2001; Tanaka and Nakanishi, 2001; Chandler et al., 2004).

Conventional studies of increased tolerance after generations of exposure and molecular genetic surveys of exposed populations are the primary approaches by which genetic consequences are assessed. Increased tolerance is usually detected by subjecting individuals from the chronically exposed population and a naïve population to toxicant challenge and formally testing for tolerance differences. A recent example is the study by Ownby et al. (2002) of enhanced tolerance for a PAH-exposed population of killifish from Elizabeth River (Virginia). Alternatively, a change associated with a tolerance mechanism might be examined in chronically exposed and naïve populations. As an example, Meyer et al. (2003) found upregulated antioxidant defenses in the same populations of exposed Elizabeth River killifish studied by Ownby et al. (2002). Close examinations of population genetics associated with contaminated habitats are also used to infer consequences of multigenerational exposure. Continuing with the Elizabeth River killifish example, Mulvey et al. (2002, 2003) examined the genetic qualities of fish sampled within the Elizabeth River estuary using allozymes and mDNA. Clear evidence was found using both tools for the influence of contamination on the population genetics of killifish subpopulations within the estuary.

Community and Ecosystem

Most community and ecosystem effects studies by ecotoxicologists use modified methods developed in community and systems ecology (see Magurran, 1988, for method descriptions). Recent books such as Newman (2010) and Newman and Clements (2008) provide some details of ecotoxicological applications of these methods. Several general approaches are taken. The approach affording the most control and ability to replicate treatments involves laboratory microcosms. A microcosm is a simplified system that is thought to possess the community or ecosystem qualities of interest. The experimental control and reproducibility associated with microcosms come at the cost of losing ecological realism. Is the laboratory microcosm actually responding in a way that provides insight about how the actual community or ecosystem would respond? Microcosm studies are so common throughout the ecotoxicological literature that standard methods have been proposed for their execution (Taub, 1997). As a microcosm example, Clarke (1999) established invertebrate communities in the laboratory to determine the influence of oil drilling muds on offshore benthic communities. Relative to the issue of community redundancy discussed above, zinc-amended soil microcosms were used in another case by Salminen et al. (2001) and provided minimal evidence to support the current reliance on the redundant species theory by ecological risk assessors. Gaining back some realism by giving up some degree of tractability, outdoor mesocosms are also applied to community and ecosystem ecotoxicology. Mesocosms are larger experimental systems, usually constructed outdoors that also attempt to simulate some aspect of an ecosystem such as community species composition. Often, terrestrial ecotoxicologists apply the term enclosure instead of

mesocosm for such experimental units. Aquatic mesocosms can be artificial ponds such as those developed by Woin (1998), streams such as those used by Kreutzweiser et al. (2000), or river segments such as those used by Culp et al. (2000). Terrestrial mesocosms can be pens, enclosures, or large soil plots depending on the effects being quantified. An example of a terrestrial mesocosm study is that conducted by Korthals et al. (1996) of the effects of long-term copper exposure to soil nematode communities. Field studies are the third means of exploring effects at the community or ecosystem level. The high realism of associated findings from field studies is balanced against the difficulty of achieving true replication and sufficient control of other factors influencing the system's response. Field studies can involve manipulations such as introducing toxicant into replicate water bodies; however, the majority of field studies involve biomonitoring of an existing, notionally impacted, community or ecosystem. This might involve close examination of species composition and comparison to that expected or measured in a similar, but uncontaminated, system. Most biomonitoring efforts focus on community structure instead of function because it is generally believed that changes in community structure will be seen before those in functions. As examples, metal effects on invertebrate and plant community structure were studied by Peeters et al. (2000) and Strandberg et al. (2006), respectively. Despite the tendency to study community structure, study of functions can provide valuable insights as in the case of Day (1993), who found changes in photosynthesis in periphytic algae in response to herbicide exposure. Because mesocosm and field studies involve data generation in the presence of many uncontrolled variables and poor replication or pseudoreplication, multivariate statistical techniques for recognizing patterns among locations or through time are commonly applied, for example, Landis et al. (1997) and Kedwards et al. (1999).

Landscape to Biosphere

The creation and eventual convergence of several key technologies facilitate ecotoxicological study at the landscape to biosphere vantages. These same technologies have also allowed the emergence of large context, environmental disciplines such as landscape[4] ecology (Forman and Godron, 1986), global ecology (Rambler et al., 1989), and global biogeochemistry (Butcher et al., 1992) that contribute concepts to large-scale ecotoxicology efforts.

Technologies for acquiring, processing, and analyzing large amounts of information have been essential. Archived and new imagery from satellites and high-altitude platforms is now integrated with off-the-shelf GIS software with affordable computers. Much of this imagery is gathered with remote sensing technologies, that is, technologies that do not require physical contact with the feature being measured. However, arrays of sensors are rapidly coming together such as the network coastal observing systems that are quickly linking to form a readily accessible real-time data stream for all of our oceans. Remote sensing data from satellites or aircraft provide information for wide spatial areas and the rapidly emerging, ground- or water-based observing system networks have begun to produce extremely rich data streams. Such technologies facilitate ecotoxicological explorations at spatial scales that were impossible to consider only a few decades ago.

---

[4]A landscape is formally defined by Forman and Godron (1986) as a heterogeneous landscape that is "composed of a cluster of interacting ecosystems that is repeated in a similar form throughout." Each ecosystem is a part of a whole landscape much as a tessera is part of a mosaic or a subpopulation is part of a metapopulation.

ECOLOGICAL RISK ASSESSMENT

ERA applies ecotoxicological knowledge in support of environmental decision making. The ERA approach is an adaptation of human risk assessment methods, notably those articulated in the National Academy of Sciences paradigm (National Research Council, 1983). Adaptations are needed to accommodate differences in exposure pathways and the entities for which risk is to be estimated. Risk might be to an endangered or threatened species, or to a damaged natural resource for which remuneration might be required from a responsible party. In such cases, the ERA might estimate risk to individuals. Alternatively, as emphasized in the above EPA quote, the risk might be to a local species population or to the integrity of an ecological community. A widely dispersed ecotoxicant such as acid precipitation or widely used product such as the herbicide, atrazine, might require assessment of risk at a landscape or subcontinental scale. A recent example of such a risk assessment is that for atrazine, a herbicide used throughout North America (Solomon *et al.*, 1996). Ecotoxicants requiring a global ERA might include greenhouse gases contributing to global warming, hydrofluorocarbons depleting the ozone layer, and POPs that accumulate to harmful concentrations in polar regions far from their point of release at highly industrialized latitudes.

Adaptations are based on the context of an ERA. Some ERAs address existing situations. Considerable field information might be available for such a retroactive ERA and epidemiological methods might be applied advantageously. In contrast, predictive ERAs assess possible risk associated with a future or proposed toxicant exposure. In this case, the ERA might rely more heavily on exposure modeling and laboratory-derived effects data. A special case of predictive risk assessment is a life cycle assessment in which "cradle-to-grave" predictions are done for a product that includes all aspects of its raw material extraction, manufacture, distribution, use, and final disposal. Finally, an ERA will be structured slightly differently if it compares the ecological risk of one or more options. An example would be the comparative risk associated with a spill of bunker oil versus Orimulsion® (a bitumen-based fossil fuel). Such a comparative risk assessment might draw insight and data from existing spill sites, laboratory tests, and exposure models. Despite adaptations and differing contexts, most ERAs have the same general form (see Fig. 30-2).

Risk assessors, risk managers, and key stakeholders engage in initial planning together with the intention of formulating a clear statement of the problem. What valued ecological entity or quality is being assessed (assessment end point) is defined. A conceptual model is created that links the assessment end point and the toxicant, including descriptions of exposure pathways and possible effects. A clear statement of possible or predicted effects (risk hypothesis) is formulated. A clear formulation of the problem with concurrence of key stakeholders is critical to the ERA because of the diversity of possible assessment end points and exposure pathways.

Exposure characterization describes or predicts contact between the toxicant and the assessment end point. Depending on the ERA context, this could involve a simple calculation of average exposure, or a temporally and spatially explicit description of amounts present in relevant media. Toxicant sources, transport pathways, kinds of contact, and potential costressors are also defined.

Ecological effects characterization describes the qualities of any potential effects of concern, describes the connection between the potential effects and the assessment end point, and describes how changes in the level of exposure might influence the effects manifesting in the assessment end point. Normally, a statement about the strength of evidence associated with the descriptions is presented in the ecological effects characterization. As a common example of evidentiary uncertainty often requiring explanation is the measurement end point. It is not always desirable to derive effects information directly from an assessment end point such as an endangered species so uncertainty is introduced by gauging effects to a surrogate (measurement end point). Ecological effects characterizations must describe the justifiable confidence in extrapolating from measurement to assessment end points.

Risk characterization uses the analysis of exposure and ecological effects to address the risk question(s) posed in the problem formulation. This can involve an explicit statement of risk, that is, the probability of a specified intensity of an adverse effect occurring to the assessment end point. Often, the information needed to make such an explicit statement is absent and a qualitative statement of the likelihood of an adverse effect is made instead. Regardless of whether a quantitative or qualitative statement of risk is produced, the risk characterization must provide details surrounding the statement, including important uncertainties.

INTERCONNECTIONS BETWEEN ECOSYSTEM INTEGRITY AND HUMAN HEALTH

As noted at the beginning of this chapter, while the original definition of ecotoxicology included effects on humans, most subsequent treatments exclude discussions of humans except as a source of contaminants, with some notable exceptions (eg, Newman, 2010). This ecotoxicology chapter, imbedded in a book focused on human or biomedical toxicology, describes the younger science of elucidating chemical effects in natural systems. While ecotoxicology has features distinct from biomedical toxicology, it is important to consider parallelisms in the two fields and, more broadly, interconnections between human health and ecological integrity, or health. While obviously related, biomedical and ecological toxicology have historically exhibited relatively little coordination or collaboration among scientists across these fields. This is likely due to a number of reasons, including the different levels of biological organization considered, as well as different academic cultures populating the two fields. However, it is questionable if this gulf has been in the best interest of understanding chemical effects, and ultimately protecting both human and ecological health. This concern has prompted several broad discussions intended to bridge this divide and enhance interdisciplinary natural and social scientific research in these areas (see reviews by Costanza *et al.*, 1992; Di Giulio and Monosson, 1996; Di Giulio and Benson, 2002).

This gulf has resulted in two fields that, while largely disconnected, parallel one another and share common paradigms such as dose–response, toxicokinetics, mechanisms of action, and risk assessment frameworks. However, by generally ignoring how chemicals and other anthropogenic stressors that degrade ecosystems can ultimately impact human health and well-being, and vice versa, an opportunity to holistically understand the results of environmental contamination is lost. Miranda *et al.* (2002) developed a conceptual model for elucidating the interconnections paradigm that links natural and social systems in a circular manner with continuous feedbacks, as opposed to parallel linear models (exposure to response, in either humans or ecosystems) that dominate toxicology currently. In this conceptual model, the natural system produces both positive outputs (such as natural resources, raw materials) and negative outputs (eg, hurricanes, disease vectors) to the social system. The culture and institution of the social system in turn transforms the natural system outputs in various ways and subsequently delivers various positive outputs (consumer goods, conservation efforts) and negative outputs (pollution, deforestation) to the natural system. These outputs influence the quantity and quality of life (human and nonhuman) of the natural system, and the circular flow of resources continually creates conditions that influence the well-being of individuals, societies, and ecosystems, now and in the future.

This rather abstract model formalizes the interconnections between human and ecological health that most of us intuitively sense. Some of these connections, in the context of environmental pollution, are obvious. Chemical contamination of seafoods valued by humans is one example. Others are less clear but potentially very significant, such as human impacts on aquatic systems that foster the propagation of human disease vectors, or human impacts on global climate that may concomitantly impact humans and ecosystems in varied and complex ways. Also important to consider is the matter of human perceptions of their environment; people's sense of the health of the environment in which they live (whether their perception is correct or not) can have substantial impacts on their mental and physical health (O'Keefe and Baum, 1996). As noted by Kendall *et al.* (2001), "the indirect effects of environmental pollution may, in the end, be more important than the direct effects for human health."

There are significant indications that these fields are converging and meaningful interactions are increasing. The inclusion of an ecotoxicology chapter in this text is favorable evidence. This trend is motivated in part by the genomics revolution that provides powerful methods for evaluating fundamental biological similarities across species, including those employed in biomedical and ecotoxicological research. Research in this area has revealed genetic similarities, or conservation, in many genes and the proteins they code for that are important to organismal adaptations and impacts due to environmental stressors, including chemicals (Eaton *et al.*, 2006). Certainly many important species differences also exist that contribute to the great complexity of understanding human–ecological interconnections, but as pointed out by Winston *et al.* (2002), "in the final analysis, the biological similarities across living systems are probably more impressive than the differences." Discussions among diverse scientists of the promises, limitations, and potential applications of genomics for elucidating cross-species extrapolations are provided by Benson and Di Giulio (2006). Such cross-fertilizations among biomedical and environmental scientists, as well as social scientists and policy makers, are likely to enhance all areas, and catalyze the integrated protection of human and ecosystem health.

ACKNOWLEDGMENT

A special thanks to Dr Adriana M. Doi for her expert assistance.

REFERENCES

Adams SM. Evaluating effects of contaminants on fish health at multiple levels of biological organization: extrapolating from lower to higher levels. *Hum Ecol Risk Assess.* 2000;6:15–27.

Adams SM, Shepard KL, Greeley MS, Jimenez BD, Ryon MG, Shugart LR. The use of bioindicators for assessing the effects of pollutant stress on fish. *Mar Environ Res.* 1989;28:459–464.

Albert A, Drouillard K, Haffner GD, Dixon B. Dietary exposure to low pesticide doses causes long-term immunosuppression in the leopard frog (*Rana pipiens*). *Environ Toxicol Chem.* 2007;26:1179–1185.

Allison N, Millward GE, Jones MB. Particle processing by *Mytilus edulis*: effects on bioavailability of metals. *J Exp Mar Biol Ecol.* 1998;22:149.

Allred PM, Giesy JP. Use of in situ microcosms to study mass loss and chemical composition of leaf litter being processed in a blackwater stream. *Arch Hydrobiol.* 1988;114:231.

Amat A, Pfol-Leskowicz A, Burgeot T, Castegnaro M. DNA adducts as a biomarker of pollution: field study on the genotoxic impact evolution of the *Erika* oil spills on mussels (*Mytilus edulis*) over a period of eleven months. *Polycyclic Aromatic Compounds.* 2004;24:713–732.

Anders A. *Biostatistics for Epidemiologists.* Boca Raton, FL: CRC Press; 1993.

Anderson DW, Jehl JR, Risebrough RW, Woods LA, Deweese LR, Edgecomb WG. Brown pelicans: improved reproduction off the Southern California Coast. *Science.* 1975;190:806.

Ankley GT, Daston GP, Degitz SJ, et al. Toxicogenomics in regulatory ecotoxicology. *Environ Sci Technol.* 2006;40:4055–4065.

Ankley GT, Erickson RJ, Sheedy BR, et al. Evaluation of models for predicting the phototoxic potency of polycyclic aromatic hydrocarbons. *Aquat Toxicol.* 1997;37:37–50.

Antkiewicz DS, Burns CG, Carney SA, Peterson RE, Heideman W. Heart malformation is an early response to TCDD in embryonic zebrafish. *Toxicol Sci.* 2005;84:368–377.

Arfsten DP, Schaeffer DJ, Mulveny DC. The effects of near ultraviolet radiation on the toxic effects of polycyclic aromatic hydrocarbons in animals and plants: a review. *Ecotoxicol Environ Saf.* 1996;33:1–24.

ASTM International. *Annual Book of ASTM Standards, Volume 11.05, Pesticides; Environmental Assessment; Hazardous Substances and Oil Spill Responses.* West Conshohocken, PA: ASTM International; 2006.

ATSDR. *Toxicological Profile for Lead.* Washington, DC: U.S. Department of Health and Human Services, Agency for Toxic Substances and Disease Registry; 1999.

Aubone A. Loss of stability owing to a stable age structure skewed toward juveniles. *Ecol Model.* 2004;175:55.

Auffret M, Rousseau S, Boutet I, et al. A multiparametric approach for monitoring immunotoxic responses in mussels from contaminated sites in Western Mediterranean. *Ecotoxicol Environ Saf.* 2006;63:393–405.

Bainy ACD, Saito E, Carvalho PSM, Junqueira VBC. Oxidative stress in gill, erythrocytes, liver and kidney of Nile tilapia (*Oreochromis niloticus*) from a polluted site. *Aquat Toxicol.* 1996;34:151–162.

Baker CF, Montgomery JC. Sensory deficits induced by cadmium in banded kokopu, *Galaxias fasciatus*, juveniles. *Environ Biol Fishes.* 2001;62:455–464.

Baldwin DH, Sandahl JF, Labenia JS, Scholz NL. Sublethal effects of copper on coho salmon: impacts on nonoverlapping receptor pathways in the peripheral olfactory nervous system. *Environ Toxicol Chem.* 2003;22:2266–2274.

Basu N, Klenavic K, Gamberg M, et al. Effects of mercury on neurochemical receptor-binding characteristics in wild mink. *Environ Toxicol Chem.* 2005;24:1444–1450.

Bauder MB, Palace VP, Hodson PV. Is oxidative stress the mechanism of blue sac disease in retene-exposed trout larvae? *Environ Toxicol Chem.* 2005;24:694–702.

Baumann PC. Epizootics of cancer in fish associated with genotoxins in sediment and water. *Mutat Res Rev Mutat Res.* 1998;411:227–233.

Baumann PC, Harshbarger JC. Long term trends in liver neoplasm epizootics of brown bullhead in the Black River, Ohio. *Environ Monit Assess.* 1998;53:213–223.

Benson WH, Di Giulio RT, eds. *Emerging Molecular and Computational Approaches for Cross-Species Extrapolations.* New York: Taylor & Francis; 2006.

Beyer WN. A reexamination of biomagnifications of metals in terrestrial food chains. *Environ Toxicol Chem.* 1986;5:863–864.

Biesmeijer JC, Roberts SPM, Reemer M, et al. Parallel declines in pollinators and insect-pollinated plants in Britain and the Netherlands. *Science.* 2006;313:351.

Billiard SM, Querbach K, Hodson PV. Toxicity of retene to early life stages of two freshwater fish species. *Environ Toxicol Chem.* 1999;18:2070–2077.

Billiard SM, Timme-Laragy AR, Wassenberg DM, Cockman C, Di Giulio RT. The role of the aryl hydrocarbon receptor pathway in mediating synergistic developmental toxicity of polycyclic aromatic hydrocarbons to zebrafish. *Toxicol Sci.* 2006;92:526–536.

Birdsall CW, Grue CE, Anderson A. Lead concentrations in bullfrog (*Rana catesbeiana*) and green frog (*Rana clamitans*) tadpoles inhabiting highway drainages. *Environ Pollut.* 1986;40A:233–247.

Broman D, Naf C, Rolff C, Zebuhr Y, Fry B, Hobbie J. Using ratios of stable nitrogen isotopes to estimate bioaccumulation and flux of polychlorinated dibenzo-*p*-dioxins (PCDDs) and dibenzofurans (PCDFs) in two food chains from the Northern Baltic. *Environ Toxicol Chem.* 1992;11:331.

Broomhall S. The effects of endosulfan and variable water temperature on survivorship and subsequent vulnerability to predation in *Litoria citropa* tadpoles. *Aquat Toxicol.* 2002;61:243.

Brown RE, Brain JD, Wang N. The avian respiratory system: a unique model for studies of respiratory toxicosis and for monitoring air quality. *Environ Health Perspect.* 1997;105:188–200.

Bury NR. The changes to apical silver membrane uptake, and basolateral membrane silver export in the gills of rainbow trout (*Oncorhynchus mykiss*) on exposure to sublethal silver concentrations. *Aquat Toxicol.* 2005;72:135–145.

Bustnes JO, Miland O, Fjeld M, et al. Relationships between ecological variables and four organochlorine pollutants in an artic glaucous gull (*Larus hyperboreus*) population. *Environ Pollut.* 2005;136:175–185.

Butcher SS, Charlson RJ, Orians GH, Wolfe GV. *Global Biogeochemical Cycles.* London: Academic Press; 1992.

Butler RA, Kelley ML, Powell WH, Hahn ME, Van Beneden RJ. An aryl hydrocarbon receptor (AHR) homologue from the soft-shell clam, *Mya arenaria*: evidence that invertebrate AHR homologues lack 2,3,7,8-tetrachlorodibenzo-*p*-dioxin and beta-naphthoflavone binding. *Gene.* 2001;278:223–234.

Campbell LM, Fask AT, Wang X, Kock G, Muir DCG. Evidence for biomagnifications of rubidium in freshwater and marine food webs. *Can J Fish Aquat Sci.* 2005;62:1161–1167.

Campbell PGC, Tessier A. Ecotoxicology of metals in the aquatic environment: geochemical aspects. In: Newman MC, Jagoe CH, eds. *Ecotoxicology. A Hierarchical Treatment.* Boca Raton, FL: CRC Press; 1996:11.

Carls MG, Rice SD, Hose JE. Sensitivity of fish embryos to weathered crude oil: part I. Low-level exposure during incubation causes malformations, genetic damage, and mortality in larval Pacific herring (*Clupea pallasi*). *Environ Toxicol Chem.* 1999;18:481–493.

Carney SA, Peterson RE, Heideman W. 2,3,7,8-Tetrachlorodibenzo-*p*-dioxin activation of the aryl hydrocarbon receptor/aryl hydrocarbon receptor nuclear translocator pathway causes developmental toxicity through a CYP1A-independent mechanism in zebrafish. *Mol Pharmacol.* 2004;66:512–521.

Carney SA, Prasch AL, Heideman W, Peterson RE. Understanding dioxin developmental toxicity using the zebrafish model. *Birth Defects Res A.* 2006;76:7–18.

Carr RL, Ho LL, Chambers JE. Selective toxicity of chlorpyrifos to several species of fish during an environmental exposure: biochemical mechanisms. *Environ Toxicol Chem.* 1997;16:2369–2374.

Carson R. *Silent Spring.* Boston: Houghton Mifflin; 1962.

Carvalho PSM, Tillitt DE. 2,3,7,8-TCDD effects on visual structure and function in swim-up rainbow trout. *Environ Sci Technol.* 2004;38:6300–6306.

Caswell H. *Matrix Population Models. Construction, Analysis, and Interpretation.* Sunderland, MA: Sinauer Associates; 2001.

Chandler GT, Cary TL, Bejarano AC, Pender J, Ferry JL. Population consequences of fipronil and degradates to copepods at field concentrations: an integration of life cycle testing with Leslie matrix population modeling. *Environ Sci Technol.* 2004;38:6407.

Chapman PM. Indirect effects of contaminants. *Mar Pollut Bull.* 2004; 48:411.

Chaty S, Rodius F, Vasseur P. A comparative study of the expression of CYP1A and CYP4 genes in aquatic invertebrate (freshwater mussel, *Unio tumidus*) and vertebrate (rainbow trout, *Oncorhynchus mykiss*). *Aquat Toxicol.* 2004;69:81–93.

Chen Z, Mayer LM. Mechanisms of Cu solubilization during deposit feeding. *Environ Sci Technol.* 1998;32:770.

Cherkasov AS, Biswas PK, Ridings DM, Ringwood AH, Sokolova IM. Effects of acclimation temperature and cadmium exposure on cellular energy budgets in the marine mollusk *Crassostrea virginica*: linking cellular and mitochondrial responses. *J Exp Biol.* 2006;209:1274–1284.

Chernyak SM, McConnell LL, Rice CP. Fate of some chlorinated hydrocarbons in arctic and far eastern ecosystems in the Russian Federation. *Sci Total Environ.* 1995;75:160–161.

Chiou CT. Partition coefficients of organic compounds in lipid–water systems and correlations with fish bioconcentration factor. *Environ Sci Technol.* 1985;19:57.

Chiverton PA. The benefits of unsprayed cereal crop margins to grey partridge *Perdix perdix* and pheasants *Phasianu colchicus* in Sweden. *Wildl Biol.* 1999;5:8.

Chowdhury MJ, Pane EF, Wood CM. Physiological effects of dietary cadmium acclimation and waterborne cadmium challenge in rainbow trout: respiratory, ionoregulatory, and stress parameters. *Comp Biochem Physiol.* 2004;139C:163–173.

Clark AJ, Scheuhammer AM. Lead poisoning in upland-foraging birds of prey in Canada. *Ecotoxicology.* 2003;12:23–30.

Clarke KR. Nonmetric multivariate analysis in community-level ecotoxicology. *Env Toxicol Chem.* 1999;18:118–127.

Collier TK, Singh SV, Awasthi YC, Varanasi U. Hepatic xenobiotic metabolizing enzymes in 2 species of benthic fish showing different prevalences of contaminant-associated liver neoplasms. *Toxicol Appl Pharmacol.* 1992;113:319–324.

Connell DW. *Bioaccumulation of Xenobiotic Compounds.* Boca Raton, FL: CRC Press; 1990.

Cook PM, Robbins JA, Endicott DD, et al. Effects of aryl hydrocarbon receptor-mediated early life stage toxicity on lake trout populations in Lake Ontario during the 20th century. *Environ Sci Technol.* 2003;37: 3864–3877.

Costanza R, Norton BG, Haskell BD, eds. *Ecosystem Health. New Goals for Environmental Management.* Washington, DC: Island Press; 1992.

Crollius HR, Weissenbach J. Fish genomics and biology. *Genome Res.* 2005;15:1675–1682.

Culp JM, Lowell RB, Cash KJ. Integrating mesocosm experiments with field and laboratory studies to generate weight-of-evidence risk assessments for large rivers. *Environ Toxicol Chem.* 2000;19:1167.

Custer TW, Custer CM, Dickerson K, Allen K, Melancon MJ, Schmidt LJ. Polycyclic aromatic hydrocarbons, aliphatic hydrocarbons, trace elements, and monooxygenase activity in birds nesting on the North Platte River, Casper, Wyoming, USA. *Environ Toxicol Chem.* 2001;20:624–631.

Custer TW, Custer CM, Hines RK, et al. Organochlorine contaminants and reproductive success of double-crested cormorants from Green Bay, Wisconsin, USA. *Environ Toxicol Chem.* 1999;18:1209–1217.

Day KE. Short-term effects of herbicides on primary productivity of periphyton in lotic environments. *Ecotoxicology.* 1993;2:123.

Denison MS, Nagy SR. Activation of the aryl hydrocarbon receptor by structurally diverse exogenous and endogenous chemicals. *Annu Rev Pharmacol Toxicol.* 2003;43:309–334.

Deroo BJ, Korach KS. Estrogen receptors and human disease. *J Clin Invest.* 2006;116:561–570.

Devlin EW. Acute toxicity, uptake and histopathology of aqueous methyl mercury to fathead minnow embryos. *Ecotoxicology.* 2006;15:97–110.

Di Giulio RT, Benson WE. *Interconnections between Human Health and Ecological Integrity.* Pensacola, FL: SETAC Press; 2002.

Di Giulio RT, Hinton DE, eds. *The Toxicology of Fishes.* CRC Press. 2008.

Di Giulio RT, Monosson E, eds. *Interconnections between Human and Ecosystem Health.* London: Chapman and Hall; 1996.

Di Giulio RT, Washburn PC, Wenning RJ, Winston GW, Jewell CS. Biochemical responses in aquatic animals: a review of determinants of oxidative stress. *Environ Toxicol Chem.* 1989;8:1103–1123.

Di Toro DM, Mahony JD, Hansen DJ, et al. Toxicity of cadmium in sediments: the role of acid volatile sulfide. *Environ Toxicol Chem.* 1990;9:1487.

Di Toro DM, McGrath JA, Hansen DJ, et al. Predicting sediment metal toxicity using a sediment biotic ligand model: methodology and initial application. *Environ Toxicol Chem.* 2005;24:2410–2427.

Di Toro DM, Zarba CS, Hanson DJ, et al. Technical basis for establishing sediment quality criteria for nonionic organic chemicals using equilibrium partitioning. *Environ Toxicol Chem.* 1991;10:1541–1583.

Dopp E, Barker CM, Schiffmann D, Reinisch CL. Detection of micronuclei in hemocytes of *Mya arenaria*: association with leukemia and induction with an alkylating agent. *Aquat Toxicol.* 1996;34:31–45.

Dorval J, Leblond V, Deblois C, Hontela A. Oxidative stress and endocrine endpoints in white sucker (*Catostomus commersoni*) from a river impacted by agricultural chemicals. *Environ Toxicol Chem.* 2005;24: 1273–1280.

du Corbier FA, Lyons BP, Stentiford GA, Rotchell JM. The role of the retinoblastoma gene in liver tumor development in fish. *Environ Sci Technol.* 2005;39:9785–9790.

Eaton D, Gallagher E, Hooper M, et al. Species differences in response to toxic substances: shared pathways of toxicity—values and limitations of omic technologies to elucidate mechanism or mode of action. In: Benson WH, Di Giulio RT, eds. *Emerging Molecular and Computational Approaches for Cross-Species Extrapolations.* New York: Taylor & Francis; 2006.

Environmental Protection Agency. *Summary Report on Issues in Ecological Risk Assessment.* EPA/625/3-91/018. Springfield, VA: NTIS; 1991.

Evans DH. The fish gill: site of action and model for toxic effects of environmental pollutants. *Environ Health Perspect.* 1987;71:47–58.

Evans MI, Syemens P, Pilcher CWT. Short-term damage to coastal bird populations in Saudi-Arabia and Kuwait following the 1991 Gulf War marine pollution. *Mar Pollut Bull.* 1993;27:157–161.

Fairbrother A, Ankley GT, Birnbaum LS, et al. Reproductive and developmental toxicology of contaminants in oviparous animals. In: Di Giulio RT, Tillitt DE, eds. *Reproductive and Developmental Effects of Contaminants in Oviparous Vertebrates.* Pensacola, FL: SETAC Press; 1999:283–361.

Fairbrother A, Smits J, Grasman KA. Avian immunotoxicology. *J Toxicol Environ Health Crit Rev.* 2004;7B:105–137.

Fernandez P, Grimait JO. On the global distribution of persistent organic pollutants. *CHIMIA.* 2003;57:514.

Fernie KJ, Mayne G, Shutt JL, et al. Evidence of immunomodulation in nestling American kestrels (*Falco sparverius*) exposed to environmentally relevant PBDEs. *Environ Pollut.* 2005;138:485–493.

Fleeger JW, Carman KR, Nisbet RM. Indirect effects of contaminants in aquatic ecosystems. *Sci Total Environ.* 2003;317:207.

Forbes VE, Calow P. Is per capita rate of increase a good measure of population-level effects in ecotoxicology? *Environ Toxicol Chem.* 1999;18: 1544.

Forman RTT, Godron M. *Landscape Ecology.* New York: Wiley; 1986.

Fossi MC, Marsili L. The use of non-destructive biomarkers in the study of marine mammals. *Biomarkers.* 1997;2:205–216.

Fox G. Practical causal inference for ecoepidemiologists. *J Toxicol Environ Health.* 1991;33:359.

Fridovich I. Mitochondria: are they the seat of senescence? *Aging Cell.* 2004;3:13–16.

Fry DM. Reproductive effects in birds exposed to pesticides and industrial chemicals. *Environ Health Perspect.* 1995;103(suppl 7):165–171.

Gard TC. Stochastic models for toxicant-stressed populations. *Bull Math Biol.* 1992;54:827.

Gardner SC, Oberdorster E. *Toxicology of Reptiles.* Boca Raton, FL: Taylor and Francis; 2005.

Gilbertson M, Kubiak T, Ludwig J, et al. Great Lakes embryo mortality, edema, and deformities syndrome (GLEMEDS) in colonial fish-eating birds—similarity to chick edema disease. *J Toxicol Environ Health.* 1991;33: 455–520.

Grue CE, Gilbert PL, Seeley ME. Neurophysiological and behavioral changes in non-target wildlife exposed to organophosphate and carbamate pesticides: thermoregulation, food consumption, and reproduction. *Am Zool.* 1997;37:369–388.

Grue CE, Powell GVN, McChesney MJ. Care of nestlings by wild female starlings exposed to an organo-phosphate pesticide. *J Appl Ecol.* 1982; 19:327–335.

Guillette LJ, Crain DA, Gunderson MP, et al. Alligators and endocrine disrupting contaminants: a current perspective. *Am Zool.* 2000;40:438–452.

Hahn ME. Aryl hydrocarbon receptors: diversity and evolution. *Chem Biol Interact.* 2002;141:131–160.

Hahn ME, Merson RR, Karchner SI. Xenobiotic receptors in fish: structural and functional diversity and evolutionary insights. In: Mommsen TP, Moon TW, eds. *Environmental Toxicology, Vol 6, Biochemistry and Molecular Biology of Fishes.* Netherlands: Elsevier; 2005.

Hall AJ, Hugunin K, Deaville R, et al. The risk of infection from polychlorinated biphenyl exposure in the *harbor porpoise* (*Phocoena phocoena*): a case–control approach. *Environ Health Perspect.* 2006;114:704–711.

Halliwell B, Gutteridge JMC. *Free Radicals in Biology and Medicine.* 3rd ed. Oxford, UK: Oxford University Press; 1999.

Handy RD, Runnalls T, Russell PM. Histopathologic biomarkers in three spined sticklebacks, *Gasterosteus aculeatus*, from several rivers in Southern England that meet the freshwater fisheries directive. *Ecotoxicology.* 2002;11:467–479.

Hankinson O. The aryl hydrocarbon receptor complex. *Annu Rev Pharmacol Toxicol.* 1995;35:307–340.

Harries JE, Sheahan DA, Jobling S, et al. Estrogenic activity in five United Kingdom rivers detected by measurement of vitellogenesis in caged male trout. *Environ Toxicol Chem.* 1997;16:534–543.

Harshbarger JC, Clark JB. Epizootiology of neoplasms of bony fish of North America. *Sci Total Environ.* 1990;94:1–32.

Hasspieler BM, Behar JV, Di Giulio RT. Glutathione-dependent defense in channel catfish (*Ictalurus punctatus*) and brown bullhead (*Ameriurus nebulosus*). *Ecotoxicol Environ Saf.* 1994;28:82–90.

Heath JA, Frederick PC. Relationships among mercury concentrations, hormones, and nesting effort of White Ibises (*Eudocimus albus*) in the Florida Everglades. *Auk.* 2005;122:255–267.

Heid SE, Walker MK, Swanson HI. Correlation of cardiotoxicity mediated by halogenated aromatic hydrocarbons to aryl hydrocarbon receptor activation. *Toxicol Sci.* 2001;61:187–196.

Henny CJ. Effects of mining lead on birds: a case history at Coeur d'Alene Basin, Idaho. In: Hoffman DJ, Rattner BA, Burton GA Jr, Cairns J Jr, eds. *Handbook of Ecotoxicology.* 2nd ed. Boca Raton, FL: Lewis; 2003.

Hill AB. The environment and disease: association or causation? *Proc R Soc Med.* 1965;59:295.

Hinton DE. Cells, cellular responses, and their markers in chronic toxicity. In: Malins DC, Ostrander GK, eds. *Aquatic Toxicology: Molecular, Biochemical, and Cellular Perspectives.* Boca Raton, FL: Lewis; 1994: 207–239.

Hippeli S, Elstner EF. Mechanisms of oxygen activation during plant stress: biochemical effects of air pollutants. *J Plant Physiol.* 1996;148:249–257.

Hoffman DJ, Marn CM, Marois KC. Sublethal effects in avocet and stilt hatchlings from selenium-contaminated sites. *Environ Toxicol Chem.* 2003a;21:561–566.

Hoffman DJ, Rattner BA, Burton GA, Cairns J, eds. *Handbook of Ecotoxicology.* Boca Raton, FL: Lewis/CRC Publishers; 2003b.

Holm J, Palace V, Siwik P, et al. Developmental effects of bioaccumulated selenium in eggs and larvae of two salmonid species. *Environ Toxicol Chem.* 2005;24:2373–2381.

Hontela A. Endocrine and physiological responses to xenobiotics in fish: role of glucocorticoid hormones. *Rev Toxicol.* 1997;1:1–46.

Horness BH, Lomax DP, Johnson LL, Myers MS, Pierce SM, Collier TK. Sediment quality thresholds: estimates from hockey stick regression of liver prevalence in English sole (*Pleuronectes vetulus*). *Environ Toxicol Chem.* 1998;17:872.

Hose JE, Cross JN, Smith SG, Diehl DL. Elevated circulating erythrocyte micronuclei in fishes from contaminated sites off southern California. *Mar Environ Res.* 1987;22:167–176.

Huang YW, Matthews JB, Fertuck KC, Zacharewski TR. Use of *Xenopus laevis* as a model for investigating in vitro and in vivo endocrine disruption in amphibians. *Environ Toxicol Chem.* 2005;24:2002–2009.

Huggett RJ, Kimerle RA, Mehrle PM Jr, Bergman HL, eds. *Biomarkers. Biochemical, Physiological, and Histological Markers of Anthropogenic Stress.* Boca Raton, FL: Lewis; 1992.

Husby MP, McBee K. Nuclear DNA content variation and double-strand DNA breakage in white-footed mice (*Peromyscus leucopus*) collected from abandoned strip mines, Oklahoma, USA. *Environ Toxicol Chem.* 1999;18:926–931.

Hwang HM, Wade TL, Sericano JL. Relationship between lysosomal membrane destabilization and chemical body burden in eastern oysters (*Crassostrea virginica*) from Galveston Bay, Texas, USA. *Environ Toxicol Chem.* 2002;21:1268–1271.

Incardona JP, Carls MG, Teraoka H, et al. Aryl hydrocarbon receptor-independent toxicity of weathered crude oil during fish development. *Environ Health Perspect.* 2005;113:1755–1762.

Jansen A, Forbes VE, Parker ED Jr. Variation in cadmium uptake, feeding rate, and life-history effects in the gastropod *Potamopyrgus antipodarum*: linking toxicant effects on individuals to the population level. *Environ Toxicol Chem.* 2001;20:2503.

Johnson L, Casillas E, Sol S, Collier T, Stein J, Varanasi U. Contaminant effects on reproductive success in selected benthic fish. *Mar Environ Res.* 1993;35:165–170.

Johnson LL, Stein JE, Collier TK, Casillas E, Varanasi U. Indicators of reproductive development in prespawning female winter flounder (*Pleuronectes americanus*) from urban and nonurban estuaries in the northeast United States. *Sci Total Environ.* 1994;141:241–260.

Kammenga J, Laskowski R. *Demography in Ecotoxicology.* Chichester, UK: Wiley; 2000.

Kappus H. Overview of enzyme systems involved in bio-reduction of drugs and in redox cycling. *Biochem Pharmacol.* 1986;35:1–6.

Karr JR. Biological integrity: a long-neglected aspect of water resource management. *Ecol Appl.* 1991;1:66.

Kedwards TJ, Maund SJ, Chapman PF. Community level analysis of ecotoxicological field studies: I. Biological monitoring. *Environ Toxicol Chem.* 1999;18:149.

Keller JM, McClellan-Green PD, Kucklick JR, Keil DE, Peden-Adams MM. Effects of organochlorine contaminants on loggerhead sea turtle immunity: comparison of a correlative field study and in vitro exposure experiments. *Environ Health Perspect.* 2006;114:70–76.

Kendall RJ, Anderson TA, Baker RJ, et al. Ecotoxicology. In: Klaassen CD, ed. *Casarett and Doull's Toxicology, the Basic Science of Poisons.* 6th ed. New York: McGraw-Hill; 2001.

Kendall RJ, Lacher TE Jr, Bunck C, et al. An ecological risk assessment of lead shot exposure in non-waterfowl avian species: upland game birds and raptors. *Environ Toxicol Chem.* 1996;15:4–20.

Kidd KA, Bootsma HA, Hesslein RH, Muir DCG, Hecky RE. Biomagnification of DDT through the benthic and pelagic food webs of Lake Malawi, East Africa: importance of trophic level and carbon source. *Environ Sci Technol.* 2001;35:14–20.

Klobicar GI, Stambuk A, Pavlica M, Sertic Peric M, Kutuzovic Hackenberger B, Hylland K. Genotoxicity monitoring of freshwater environments using caged carp (*Cyprinus carpio*). *Ecotoxicology.* 2010;19:77–84.

Kohler A, Wahl E, Soffker K. Functional and morphological changes of lysosomes as prognostic biomarkers of toxic liver injury in a marine flatfish (*Platichthys flesus* (L.)). *Environ Toxicol Chem.* 2002;21:2434–2444.

Korthals GW, Alexiev AD, Lexmond TM, Kammenga JE, Bongers T. Long-term effects of copper and pH on the nematode community in an agroecosystem. *Environ Toxicol Chem.* 1996;15:979.

Krebs CJ. *Ecological Methodology.* 2nd ed. New York: Benjamin Cummings; 1998.

Kreutzweiser DP, Capell SS, Scarr TA. Community-level responses by stream insects to NEEM products containing azadirachtin. *Environ Toxicol Chem.* 2000;19:855.

Krivtsov V. Investigations of indirect relationships in ecology and environmental science: a review and the implications for comparative theoretical ecosystem analysis. *Ecol Model.* 2004;174:37.

Landis WG, Matthews RA, Matthews GB. Design and analysis of multispecies toxicity tests for pesticide registration. *Ecol Appl.* 1997;7:1111.

Larson RA, Weber EJ. *Reaction Mechanisms in Environmental Organic Chemistry.* Boca Raton, FL: Lewis Publishers; 1994.

Larsson DGJ, Adolfsson-Erici M, Parkkonen J, et al. Ethinyloestradiol—an undesired fish contraceptive? *Aquat Toxicol.* 1999;45:91–97.

Lee B-G, Griscom SB, Lee J-K, et al. Influences of dietary uptake and reactive sulfides on metal bioavailability from aquatic sediments. *Science.* 2000;287:282.

Lemly AD. Symptoms and implications of selenium toxicity in fish: the Belews Lake case example. *Aquat Toxicol.* 2002;57:39–49.

Leslie HA, Oosthoek AJP, Busser FJM, Kraak MHS, Hermens JLM. Biomimetic solid-phase microextraction to predict body residues and toxicity of chemicals that act by narcosis. *Environ Toxicol Chem.* 2002;21:229.

Li J, Quabius ES, Wendelaar Bonga SE, Flik G, Lock RAC. Effects of water-borne copper on branchial chloride cells and Na⁺/K⁺-ATPase activities in Mozambique tilapia (*Oreochromis mossambicus*). *Aquat Toxicol.* 1998;43:1–11.

Linbo TL, Stehr CM, Incardona JP, Scholz NL. Dissolved copper triggers cell death in the peripheral mechanosensory system of larval fish. *Environ Toxicol Chem.* 2006;25:597–603.

Lipscomb TP, Harris RK, Rebar AH, Ballachey BE, Haebler RJ. *Exxon Valdez Oil Spill State/Federal Natural Resource Damage Assessment, Final Report. Pathological Studies of Sea Otters (Marine Mammal Study 6–11).* Anchorage, AK: US FWS; June 1996.

Little PFR. Structure and function of the human genome. *Genome Res.* 2005;15:1759–1766.

Livingstone DR. Contaminant-stimulated reactive oxygen species production and oxidative damage in aquatic organisms. *Mar Pollut Bull.* 2001;42:656–666.

Lloyd R, Herbert DWM. The influence of carbon dioxide on the toxicity of un-ionized ammonia to rainbow trout (*Salmo gairdneri* Richardson). *Ann Appl Biol.* 1960;48:399.

Loge FJ, Arkoosh MR, Ginn TR, Johnson LL, Collier TK. Impact of environmental stressors on the dynamics of disease transmission. *Environ Sci Technol.* 2005;39:7329–7336.

Loreau M. Does functional redundancy exist? *Oikos.* 2004;104:606.

Lorenzen A, Williams KL, Moon TW. Determination of the estrogenic and antiestrogenic effects of environmental contaminants in chicken embryo hepatocyte cultures by quantitative-polymerase chain reaction. *Environ Toxicol Chem.* 2003;22:2329–2336.

Luoma SN. Can we determine the biological availability of sediment-bound trace elements? *Hydrobiologia.* 1989;379:176–177.

Luoma SN, Bryan GW. Factors controlling the availability of sediment-bound lead to the estuarine bivalve *Scrobicularia plana*. *J Mar Biol Assoc UK.* 1978;58:793.

Maccubbin AE. DNA adduct analysis in fish: laboratory and field studies. In: Malins DC, Ostrander GK, eds. *Aquatic Toxicology: Molecular, Biochemical, and Cellular Perspectives.* Boca Raton, FL: Lewis Publishers; 1994:267–294.

Mackay D. Correlation of bioconcentration factors. *Environ Sci Technol.* 1982;16:274.

MAFF (Ministry of Agriculture, Forestry and Fisheries). *Guidance on Toxicological Study Data for Application of Pesticide Registration.* No. 59-Nousan-4200. Japan: Ministry of Agriculture, Forestry and Fisheries; 1985.

Magurran AE. *Ecological Diversity and its Measurement.* Princeton, NJ: Princeton University Press; 1988.

Malins DC, Anderson KM, Stegeman JJ, et al. Biomarkers signal contaminant effects on the organs of English sole (*Parophrys vetulus*) from Puget Sound. *Environ Health Perspect.* 2006;114:823–829.

Malins DC, Krahn MM, Brown DW, et al. Toxic chemicals in marine sediment and biota from Mukilteo, Washington: relationships with hepatic neoplasms and other hepatic lesions in English sole (*Parophrys vetulus*). *J Natl Cancer Inst Monogr.* 1987;74:487–494.

Mallet J. The evolution of insecticide resistance: have the insects won? *Trends Ecol Evol.* 1989;14:336.

Martineau D, Lemberger K, Dallaire A, et al. Cancer in wildlife, a case study: beluga from the St. Lawrence estuary, Quebec, Canada. *Environ Health Perspect.* 2002;110:285–292.

Mason AZ, Nott JA. The role of intracellular biomineralized granules in the regulation and detoxification of metals in gastropods with special reference to the marine prosobranch *Littorina littorea*. *Aquat Toxicol.* 1981;1:239.

Mathews AP. The relation between solution tension, atomic volume, and the physiological action of elements. *Am J Physiol.* 1904;10:290.

Mauer BA, Holt RD. Effects of chronic pesticide stress on wildlife populations in complex landscapes: processes at multiple scales. *Environ Toxicol Chem.* 1996;15:420.

Mayer LM, Chen Z, Findlay RH, et al. Bioavailability of sedimentary contaminants subject to deposit-feeder digestion. *Environ Sci Technol.* 1996;30:2641.

McDonald BG, Chapman PM. PAH phototoxicity—an environmentally irrelevant phenomenon? *Mar Pollut Bull.* 2002;44:1321–1326.

McMahon G, Huber LJ, Moore MJ, Stegeman JJ, Wogan GN. Mutations in c-Ki-ras oncogenes in diseased livers of winter flounder from Boston Harbor. *Proc Natl Acad Sci U S A.* 1990;87:841–845.

Mellanen P, Soimasuo M, Holmbloom B, Oikari A, Santti R. Expression of the Vitellogenin gene in the liver of juvenile whitefish (*Coregonus lavaletus* L. s.l.) exposed to effluents from pulp and paper mills. *Ecotoxicol Environ Saf.* 1999;43:133–137.

Meyer JN, Nacci D, Di Giulio RT. Cytochrome P4501A (CYP1A) in killifish (*Fundulus heteroclitus*): heritability of altered expression and relationship to survival in contaminated sediments. *Toxicol Sci.* 2002;68: 69–81.

Meyer JN, Smith JD, Winston GW, Di Giulio RT. Antioxidant defenses in killifish (*Fundulus heteroclitus*) exposed to contaminated sediments and model prooxidants: short-term and heritable responses. *Aquat Toxicol.* 2003;65:377.

Miller KA, Assuncao MGL, Dangerfield NJ, Bandiera SM, Ross PS. Assessment of cytochrome P450 1A in harbour seals (*Phoca vitulina*) using a minimally-invasive biopsy approach. *Mar Environ Res.* 2005;60:153–169.

Mineau P, ed. *Cholinesterase-Inhibiting Insecticides: Their Impact on Wildlife and the Environment.* Amsterdam, The Netherlands: Elsevier; 1991.

Mineau P, Fletcher MR, Glaser LC, et al. Poisoning of raptors with organophosphorus and carbamate pesticides with emphasis on Canada, US and UK. *J Raptor Res.* 1999;33:1–37.

Miranda ML, Mohai P, Bus J, et al. Policy concepts and applications. In: Di Giulio RT, Benson WH, eds. *Interconnections between Human Health and Ecological Integrity.* Pensacola, FL: SETAC Press; 2002.

Moller P. The alkaline comet assay: towards validation in biomonitoring of DNA damaging exposures. *Basic Clin Pharmacol Toxicol.* 2006;98:336–345.

Mommsen TP, Moon TW. *Environmental Toxicology. Biochemistry and Molecular Biology of Fishes.* Vol. 6. Amsterdam, The Netherlands: Elsevier; 2005.

Moore MN. Do nanoparticles present ecotoxicological risks for the health of the aquatic environment? *Environ Int.* 2006;32:967–976.

Moore MN, Allen JI, McVeigh A. Environmental prognostics: an integrated model supporting lysosomal stress responses as predictive biomarkers of animal health status. *Mar Environ Res.* 2006;61:278–304.

Mulvey M, Newman MC, Vogelbein W, Unger MA. Genetic structure of *Fundulus heteroclitus* from PAH-contaminated and neighboring sites in the Elizabeth and York Rivers. *Aquat Toxicol.* 2002;61:195.

Mulvey M, Newman MC, Vogelbein W, Unger MA, Ownby DR. Genetic structure and mtDNA diversity of *Fundulus heteroclitus* populations from PAH-contaminated and neighboring sites. *Environ Toxicol Chem.* 2003;22:671.

Munkittrick KR, Portt CB, van der Kraak GJ, et al. Impact of bleached kraft mill effluent on population characteristics, liver MFO activity, and serum steroid levels of a Lake Superior white sucker (*Catostomus commersoni*) population. *Can J Fish Aquat Sci.* 1991;48:1371–1380.

Myers MS, Stehr CM, Olson OP, et al. Relationships between toxicopathic hepatic lesions and exposure to chemical contaminants in English sole (*Pleuronectes vetulus*), starry flounder (*Platichthys stellatus*), and white croaker (*Genyonemus lineatus*) from selected marine sites on the Pacific coast, USA. *Environ Health Perspect.* 1994;102:200.

Naeem S, Thompson LJ, Lawler SP, Lawton JH, Woodfin RM. Declining biodiversity can alter the performance of ecosystems. *Nature.* 1994;6473:734–737.

National Research Council. *Risk Assessment in the Federal Government: Managing the Process.* Washington, DC: National Academy of Sciences; 1983.

Nebert DW, Roe AL, Dieter MZ, Solis WA, Yang Y, Dalton TP. Role of the aromatic hydrocarbon receptor and [*Ah*] gene battery in the oxidative stress response, cell cycle control, and apoptosis. *Biochem Pharmacol.* 2000;59:65–85.

Neely WK, Branson DR, Blau GE. Partition coefficient to measure bioconcentration potential of organic chemicals in fish. *Environ Sci Technol.* 1974;8:1113.

Newman MC. *Population Ecotoxicology.* Chichester, UK: Wiley; 2001.

Newman MC. *Fundamentals of Ecotoxicology.* 3rd ed. Boca Raton, FL: Lewis/Taylor and Francis; 2010.

Newman MC. *Quantitative Methods.* Boca Raton, FL: CRC/Taylor and Francis; 2013.

Newman MC, Clements WH. *Ecotoxicology, A Comprehensive Treatment.* Boca Raton, FL: Taylor & Francis/CRC; 2008.

Newman MC, Crane M, Holloway G. Does pesticide risk assessment in the European Union assess long-term effects? *Rev Environ Toxicol.* 2006;187:1.

Nigro M, Falleni A, Del Barga I, et al. Cellular biomarkers for monitoring estuarine environments: transplanted versus native mussels. *Aquat Toxicol.* 2006;77:339–347.

Nott JA, Nicolaidou A. Bioreduction of zinc and manganese along a molluscan food chain. *Comp Biochem Physiol.* 1993;104A:235.

NRC (Nuclear Regulatory Commission). *Biologic Markers in Reproductive Toxicology.* Washington, DC: National Academy Press; 1989.

O'Connor RJ. Toward the incorporation of spatiotemporal dynamics into ecotoxicology. In: Rhodes OE Jr, Chesser RK, Smith MH, eds. *Population Dynamics in Ecological Space and Time.* Chicago, IL: The University of Chicago Press; 1996:281.

Odum EP. Trends expected in stressed ecosystems. *Bioscience.* 1985;35:419.

OECD (Organisation for Economic Co-Operation and Development). *OECD Guidelines for the Testing of Chemicals.* Paris, France: OECD Publishing; 1981.

Ohlendorf HM. The birds of Kesterson Reservoir: a historical perspective. *Aquat Toxicol.* 2002;57:1–10.

O'Keefe MK, Baum A. Perceptions of ecosystem health, stress and human well-being. In: Di Giulio RT, Monosson E, eds. *Interconnections between Human and Ecosystem Health.* London: Chapman and Hall; 1996.

Ormseth OA, Ben-David M. Ingestion of crude oil: effects on digesta retention times and nutrient uptake in captive river otters. *J Comp Physiol B.* 2000;170:419.

Ostrander GK, Rotchell JM. Fish models of carcinogenesis. In: Mommsen TP, Moon TW, eds. *Environmental Toxicology, Biochemistry and Molecular Biology of Fishes.* Vol. 6. Amsterdam, The Netherlands: Elsevier; 2005.

Ownby D, Newman MC, Mulvey M, Unger M, Vogelbein W. Fish (*Fundulus heteroclitus*) populations with different exposure histories differ in tolerance of creosote-contaminated sediments. *Environ Toxicol Chem.* 2002;21:1897.

Pacheco M, Santos MA. Biotransformation, genotoxic, and histopathological effects of environmental contaminants in European eel (*Anguilla anguilla* L.). *Ecotoxicol Environ Saf.* 2002;53:331–347.

Paerl HW, Pinckney JL, Fear JM, Peierls BL. Ecosystem responses to internal and watershed organic matter loading: consequences for hypoxia in the eutrophying Neuse river estuary, North Carolina, USA. *Mar Ecol Prog Ser.* 1999;166:17–25.

Parker ML, Goldstein MI. Differential toxicities of organophosphate and carbamate insecticides in the nestling European starling (*Sturnus vulgaris*). *Arch Environ Contam Toxicol.* 2000;39:233–242.

Partridge GG. Relative fitness of genotypes in a population of *Rattus norvegicus* polymorphic for warfarin resistance. *Heredity.* 1979;43:239.

Patrick R. Use of algae, especially diatoms in the assessment of water quality. *ASTM Spec Tech Bull.* 1973;528:76.

Peakall D. *Animal Biomarkers as Pollution Indicators.* New York: Chapman and Hall; 1992.

Peeters ETHM, Gardeniers JJP, Koelmans AA. Contribution of trace metals in structuring *in situ* macroinvertebrate community composition along a salinity gradient. *Environ Toxicol Chem.* 2000;19:1002.

Peterson CH, Rice SD, Short JW, Esler D, Bodkin BE, Irons DB. Long-term ecosystem response to the Exxon Valdez oil spill. *Science.* 2003;302:2082–2086.

Phillips DH. Detection of DNA modifications by the ^{32}P-postlabelling assay. *Mutat Res.* 1997;178:1–12.

Pinkney AE, Harshbarger JC, May EB, Melancon MJ. Tumor prevalence and biomarkers of exposure in brown bullheads (*Ameiurus nebulosus*) from the tidal Potomac River, USA, watershed. *Environ Toxicol Chem.* 2001;20:1196–1205.

Ploch SA, King LC, Kohan MJ, Di Giulio RT. Comparative *in vitro* and *in vivo* benzo(*a*)pyrene–DNA adduct formation and its relationship to CYP1A activity in two species of Ictalurid catfish. *Toxicol Appl Pharmacol.* 1998;149:90–98.

Porte C, Janer G, Lorusso LC, et al. Endocrine disruptors in marine organisms: approaches and perspectives. *Comp Biochem Physiol.* 2006;143C:303–315.

Pratt JR, Cairns J Jr. Ecotoxicology and the redundancy problem: understanding effects on community structure and function. In: Newman MC, Jagoe CH, eds. *Ecotoxicology. A Hierarchical Treatment.* Boca Raton, FL: CRC/Lewis; 1996:347.

Preston BL. Indirect effects in aquatic ecotoxicology: implications for ecological risk assessment. *Environ Manage.* 2002;29:311.

Rambler MB, Margulis L, Fester R. *Global Ecology. Towards a Science of the Biosphere.* Boston: Academic Press; 1989.

Rand GM. Behavior. In: Rand GM, Petrocelli AR, eds. *Fundamentals of Aquatic Toxicology.* Washington, DC: Hemisphere; 1985:221–263.

Rands MRW. Pesticide use on cereals and the survival of grey partridge *Perdix perdix* chicks in a field experiment. *J Appl Ecol.* 1985;22:49.

Reichert WL, Myers MS, Peck-Miller K, et al. Molecular epizootiology of genotoxic events in marine fish: linking contaminant exposure, DNA damage, and tissue-level alterations. *Mutat Res Rev Mutat Res.* 1998;411:215–225.

Reinfelder JR, Fisher NS. The assimilation of elements ingested by marine copepods. *Science.* 1991;251:794.

Rice CD, Schlenk D. Immune function and cytochrome P4501A activity after acute exposure to 3,3,4,4,5-pentachlorobiphenyl (PCB 126) in channel catfish. *J Aquat Anim Health.* 1995;7:195–204.

Richardson CJ, Di Giulio RT, Tandy NE. *Free Radical Mediated Processes as Markers of Air Pollution Stress in Trees. Biologic Markers of Air-Pollution Stress and Damage in Forests.* Washington, DC: National Academy Press; 1989:251–260.

Rogers JT, Richards JG, Wood CM. Ionoregulatory disruption as the acute toxic mechanism for lead in the rainbow trout (*Oncorhynchus mykiss*). *Aquat Toxicol.* 2003;64:215–234.

Ross P, De Swart R, Addison R, et al. Contaminant-induced immunotoxicity in harbour seals: wildlife at risk? *Toxicology.* 1996;112:157–169.

Rotchell JM, Ostrander GK. Molecular markers of endocrine disruption in aquatic organisms. *J Toxicol Environ Health B.* 2003;6:453–495.

Rowan DJ, Rasmussen JB. Bioaccumulation of radioceasium by fish: the influence of physicochemical factors and trophic structure. *Can J Fish Aquat Sci.* 1994;51:2388–2410.

Ruiz JM, Barreiro R, Gonzalez JJ. Biomonitoring organotin pollution with gastropods and mussels. *Mar Ecol Prog Ser.* 2005;287:169–176.

Salminen J, Van Gestel CAM, Oksanen J. Pollution-induced community tolerance and functional redundancy in a decomposer food web in metal-stressed soil. *Environ Toxicol Chem.* 2001;20:2287.

Sanchez-Dardon J, Voccia I, Hontela A, et al. Immunomodulation by heavy metals tested individually or in mixtures in rainbow trout (*Oncorhynchus mykiss*) exposed *in vivo*. *Environ Toxicol Chem.* 1999;18:1492–1497.

Sandahl JF, Baldwin DH, Jenkins JJ, Scholtz NL. Comparative thresholds for acetylcholinesterase inhibition and behavioral impairment in coho salmon exposed to chlorpyrifos. *Environ Toxicol Chem.* 2005;24:136–145.

Saucier D, Astic L, Rioux P. The effects of early chronic exposure to sublethal copper on the olfactory discrimination of rainbow trout, *Oncorhynchus mykiss*. *Environ Biol Fishes.* 1991;30:345–351.

Schafer FQ, Buettner GR. Redox environment of the cell as viewed through the redox state of the glutathione disulfide/glutathione couple. *Free Radic Biol Med.* 2001;30:1191–1212.

Schlenk D, Benson W. *Target Organ Toxicity in Marine and Freshwater Teleosts.* New York: Taylor and Francis; 2001.

Schlezinger JJ, Stegeman JJ. Induction and suppression of cytochrome P450 1A by 3,3,4,4,5-pentachlorobiphenyl and its relationship to oxidative stress in the marine fish scup (*Stenotomus chrysops*). *Aquat Toxicol.* 2001;52:101–115.

Schmidt CW. Toxicogenomics. *Environ Health Perspect.* 2002;110: A750–A755.

Schmitt CJ, Whyte JJ, Brumbaugh WG, Tillitt DE. Biochemical effects of lead, zinc, and cadmium from mining on fish in the Tri-States district of northeastern Oklahoma, USA. *Environ Toxicol Chem.* 2005;24:1483–1495.

Scholz NL, Truelove NK, French BL, et al. Diazinon disrupts antipredator and homing behaviors in Chinook salmon (*Oncorhynchus tshawytscha*). *Can J Fish Aquat Sci.* 2000;57:1911–1918.

Schwacke LH, Voit EO, Hansen LJ, et al. Probabilistic risk assessment of reproductive effects of polychlorinated biphenyls on bottlenose dolphins (*Tursiops truncatus*) from the southeast United States coast. *Environ Toxicol Chem.* 2002;21:2752–2764.

Scott GR, Sloman KA. The effects of environmental pollutants on complex fish behaviour: integrating behavioural and physiological indicators of toxicity. *Aquat Toxicol.* 2004;68:369–392.

Shelby MD, Newbold RR, Tully DB, Chae K, Davis VL. Assessing environmental chemicals for estrogenicity using a combination of in vitro and in vivo assays. *Environ Health Perspect.* 1996;104:1296–1300.

Sherratt TN, Roberts G, Williams P, et al. A life-history approach to predicting the recovery of aquatic invertebrate populations after exposure to xenobiotic chemical. *Environ Toxicol Chem.* 1999;18:2512.

Shugart L. DNA damage as a biomarker of exposure. *Ecotoxicology.* 2000;9:329–340.

Sies H, Cadenas E. Oxidative stress: damage to intact cells and organs. *Philos Trans R Soc Lond B Biol Sci.* 1985;311:617–631.

Simkiss K, Daniels S, Smith RH. Effects of population density and cadmium toxicity on growth and survival of blowflies. *Environ Pollut.* 1993;81:41.

Simonich SL, Hites RA. Global distribution of persistent organochlorine compounds. *Science.* 1995;269:1861.

Sinnhuber RO, Hendricks JD, Wales JH, Putnam GB. Neoplasms in rainbow trout, a sensitive animal model for environmental carcinogenesis. *Ann N Y Acad Sci.* 1977;298:389–408.

Smith GM, Weis JS. Predator–prey relationships in mummichogs (*Fundulus heteroclitus* (L)): effects of living in a polluted environment. *J Exp Mar Biol Ecol.* 1997;209:75–87.

Snape JR, Maund SJ, Pickford DB, Hutchinson TH. Ecotoxicogenomics: the challenge of integrating genomics into aquatic and terrestrial ecotoxicology. *Aquat Toxicol.* 2004;67:143–154.

Sokolova IM. Cadmium effects on mitochondrial function are enhanced by elevated temperatures in a marine poikilotherm, *Crassostrea virginica* Gmelin (Bivalvia: Ostreidae). *J Exp Biol.* 2004;207:2639–2684.

Sol SY, Johnson LL, Horness BH, Collier TK. Relationship between oil exposure and reproductive parameters in fish collected following the Exxon Valdez oil spill. *Mar Pollut Bull.* 2000;40:1139–1147.

Solenska M, Micieta K, Misik M. Plant bioassays for an in situ monitoring of air near an industrial area and a municipal solid waste—Zilina (Slovakia). *Environ Monit Assess.* 2006;115:499–508.

Solomon KR, Baker DB, Richards RP, et al. Ecological risk assessment of atrazine in North America surface waters. *Environ Toxicol Chem.* 1996;15:31–76.

Solomon KR, Sibley P. New concepts in ecological risk assessment: where do we go from here? *Mar Pollut Bull.* 2002;44:279.

Spitsbergen JM, Walker MK, Olson JR, Peterson RE. Pathological alterations in early life stages of lake trout, *Salvelinus namaycush*, exposed to 2,3,7,8-tetrachloro-*para*-dioxin as fertilized eggs. *Aquat Toxicol.* 1991;19:41–71.

Spitzer PR, Risebrough RW, Walker W II, et al. Productivity of ospreys in Connecticut–Long Island increases as DDE residues decline. *Science.* 1978;202:333.

Spromberg JA, John BM, Landis WG. Metapopulation dynamics: indirect effects and multiple distinct outcomes in ecological risk assessment. *Environ Toxicol Chem.* 1998;17:1640.

Spry DJ, Wood CM. Ion flux rates, acid–base status, and blood gases in rainbow trout, *Salmo gairdneri*, exposed to toxic zinc in natural soft water. *Can J Fish Aquat Sci.* 1985;42:1332–1341.

Steinert SA. DNA damage as a bivalve biomarker. *Biomarkers.* 1999;4:492–496.

Stephan CE, Mount DI, Hansen DJ, Gentile JH, Chapman GA, Brungs WA. *Guidelines for Deriving Numerical National Water Quality Criteria for the Protection of Aquatic Organisms and their Uses.* Duluth, MN: US EPA; 1985.

Strandberg B, Axelsen JA, Pedersen MB, Jensen J, Attrill MJ. Effect of a copper gradient on plant community structure. *Environ Toxicol Chem.* 2006;25:743.

Sumpter JP, Jobling S. Vitellogenesis as a biomarker for estrogenic contamination of the aquatic environment. *Environ Health Perspect.* 1995;103(suppl 7):173–178.

Tanaka Y, Nakanishi J. Life history elasticity and the population-level effect of *p*-nonylphenol on *Daphnia galeata. Ecol Res.* 2001;16:41.

Tanguay RL, Andreasen EA, Walker MK, Peterson RE. Dioxin toxicity and aryl hydrocarbon receptor signaling in fish. In: Schecter A, Gasiewicz TA, eds. *Dioxins and Health.* Hoboken, NJ: Wiley; 2003: 603–628.

Taub FB. Unique information contributed by multispecies systems: examples from the standardized aquatic microcosm. *Ecol Appl.* 1997;7: 1103–1110.

Teraoka H, Dong W, Tsujimoto Y, et al. Induction of cytochrome P450 1A is required for circulation failure and edema by 2,3,7,8-tetrachlorodibenzo-*p*-dioxin in zebrafish. *Biochem Biophys Res Commun.* 2003;304: 223–228.

Tessier A, Campbell PGC, Auclair JC, Bisson M. Relationships between partitioning of trace metals in sediments and their accumulation in the tissues of the freshwater mollusc *Elliptio complanata* in a mining area. *Can J Fish Aquat Sci.* 1984;41:1463.

Thomann RV. Bioaccumulation model of organic chemical distribution in aquatic food chains. *Environ Sci Technol.* 1989;23:699.

Tilman D. Biodiversity: population versus ecosystem stability. *Ecology.* 1996;77:350.

Tilman D, Wedin D, Knops J. Productivity and sustainability influenced by biodiversity in grassland ecosystems. *Nature.* 1996;379:718.

Trimble EL. A guest editorial: update on diethylstilbestrol. *Obstet Gynecol Surv.* 2001;56:187–189.

Truhaut R. Ecotoxicology: objectives, principles and perspectives. *Ecotoxicol Environ Saf.* 1977;1:151.

US EPA OPPTS. *OPPTS Harmonized Guidelines, Series 850—Ecological Effects Test Guidelines.* Washington, DC: Office of Prevention, Pesticides, and Toxic Substances, U.S. Environmental Protection Agency; 1996a.

US EPA OPPTS. *Ecological Effects Test Guidelines, OPPTS 850.1000. Special Considerations for Conducting Aquatic Laboratory Studies.* EPA 712–C–96–113. Washington, DC: Office of Prevention, Pesticides, and Toxic Substances, U.S. Environmental Protection Agency; 1996b.

van der Oost R, Beyer J, Vermeulen NPE. Fish bioaccumulation and biomarkers in environmental risk assessment. *Environ Toxicol Pharmacol.* 2003;13:57–149.

Van Metre PC, Mahler BJ. Trends in hydrophobic organic contaminants in urban and reference lake sediments across the United States, 1970–2001. *Environ Sci Technol.* 2005;39:5567–5574.

Vethaak ADT. Fish disease as a monitor for marine pollution: the case of the North Sea. *Rev Fish Biol Fish.* 1992;2:1–32.

Vogelbein WK, Fournie JW, Van Veld PA, Huggett RJ. Hepatic neoplasms in the mummichog *Fundulus heteroclitus* from a creosote-contaminated site. *Cancer Res.* 1990;50:5978–5986.

Vos JG, Bossart G, Fournier M, O'Shea T. *Toxicology of Marine Mammals.* New York: Taylor and Francis; 2002.

Walker CH. Neurotoxic pesticides and behavioural effects upon birds. *Ecotoxicology.* 2003;12:307–316.

Wania DM, Mackay D. Tracking the distribution of persistent organic pollutants. *Environ Sci Technol.* 1996;30:390A.

Wania DM, Mckay D, Li Y-F, Bidleman TF, Strand A. Global chemical fate of α-hexachlorocyclohexane. 1. Evaluation of a global distribution model. *Environ Toxicol Chem.* 1999;18:1390.

Wassenberg D, Nerlinger A, Battle L, Di Giulio R. Effects of the PAH heterocycles, carbazole and dibenzothiophene, on *in vivo* and *in vitro* CYP1A activity and PAH-derived embryotoxicity. *Environ Toxicol Chem.* 2005;24:2526–2532.

Wassenberg DM, Di Giulio RT. Synergistic embryotoxicity of polycyclic aromatic hydrocarbon aryl hydrocarbon receptor agonists with cytochrome P4501A inhibitors in *Fundulus heteroclitus. Environ Health Perspect.* 2004a;112:1658–1664.

Wassenberg DM, Di Giulio RT. Teratogenesis in *Fundulus heteroclitus* embryos exposed to a creosote-contaminated sediment extract and CYP1A inhibitors. *Mar Environ Res.* 2004b;58:163–168.

Watanabe H, Iguchi T. Using ecotoxicogenomics to evaluate the impact of chemicals on aquatic organisms. *Mar Biol.* 2006;149:107–115.

Wayland M, Bollinger T. Lead exposure and poisoning in bald eagles and golden eagles in the Canadian prairie provinces. *Environ Pollut.* 1999;104:341.

Webb NA, Wood CM. Physiological analysis of the stress response associated with acute silver nitrate exposure in freshwater rainbow trout (*Oncorhynchus mykiss*). *Environ Toxicol Chem.* 1998;17:579–588.

Webb RE, Horsfall F Jr. Endrin resistance in pine mouse. *Science.* 1967;156:1762.

Webber HM, Haines TA. Mercury effects on predator avoidance behavior of a forage fish, golden shiner (*Notemigonus crysoleucas*). *Environ Toxicol Chem.* 2003;22:1556–1561.

Weinstein JE, Oris JT, Taylor DH. An ultrastructural examination of the mode of UV-induced toxic action of fluoranthene in the fathead minnow, *Pimephales promelas. Aquat Toxicol.* 1997;39:1–22.

Wells RS, Tornero V, Borrell A, et al. Integrating potential life-history and reproductive success data to examine relationships with organochlorine compounds for bottlenose dolphins (*Tursiops truncatus*) in Sarasota Bay, Florida. *Sci Total Environ.* 2005;349:106–119.

Wendelaar Bonga SE, Lock RAC. Toxicants and osmoregulation in fish. *Neth J Zool.* 1992;42:478–493.

Wendelaar Bonga SE, Lock RAC. The osmoregulatory system. In: Di Giulio RT, Hinton DE, eds. *The Toxicology of Fishes.* CRC Press. 2008.

Wester PW, van der Ven LTM, Vethaak AD, Girnwis GCM, Vos JG. Aquatic toxicology: opportunities for enhancement through histopathology. *Environ Toxicol Pharmacol.* 2002;11:289–295.

Weston DP, Maruya KA. Predicting bioavailability and bioaccumulation with in vitro digestive fluid extraction. *Environ Toxicol Chem.* 2002;21:962.

Wiese FK, Robertson GJ. Assessing seabird mortality from chronic oil discharges at sea. *J Wildl Manage.* 2004;68:627–638.

Wilson L, Martin PA, Elliot JE, Mineau P, Cheng KM. Exposure of California quail to organophosphorus insecticides in apple orchards in the Okanagan Valley, British Columbia. *Ecotoxicology.* 2001;10:79–90.

Winston GW, Adams SM, Benson WH, et al. Biological bases of similarities and differences. In: Di Giulio RT, Benson WH, eds. *Interconnections between Human Health and Ecological Integrity.* Pensacola, FL: SETAC Press; 2002.

Winston GW, Di Giulio RT. Prooxidant and antioxidant mechanisms in aquatic organisms. *Aquat Toxicol.* 1991;19:137–161.

Wirgin I, Currie D, Garte SJ. Activation of the K-ras oncogene in liver tumors of Hudson River tomcod. *Carcinogenesis.* 1989;10: 2311–2315.

Woin P. Short- and long-term effects of the pyrethroid insecticide fenvalerate on an invertebrate pond community. *Ecotoxicol Environ Saf.* 1998;41:137.

Wolfe MF, Schwarzbach S, Sulaiman RA. Effects of mercury on wildlife: a comprehensive review. *Environ Toxicol Chem.* 1998;17:146–160.

Woodward M. *Epidemiology. Study Design and Data Analysis.* 2nd ed. Boca Raton, FL: Chapman & Hall/CRC; 2005.

Wootton EC, Dyrynda EA, Ratcliffe NA. Comparisons of PAH-induced immunomodulation in three bivalve mollusks. *Aquat Toxicol.* 2003;65:13–25.

Wu RSS. Hypoxia: from molecular responses to ecosystem response. *Mar Pollut Bull.* 2002;45:35–45.

Ylitalo GM, Sten JE, Hom T, et al. The role of organochlorines in cancer-associated mortality in California sea lions (*Zalophus californianus*). *Mar Pollut Bull.* 2005;50:30–39.

Zelikoff JT, Carlson E, Li Y, et al. Immunotoxicity biomarkers in fish: development, validation and application for field studies and risk assessment. *Hum Ecol Risk Assess.* 2002;8:253–263.

Food Toxicology

Frank N. Kotsonis and George A. Burdock

INTRODUCTION TO FOOD TOXICOLOGY

The typical Western diet contains hundreds of thousands of substances naturally present in food and many more, which are formed in situ when food is cooked or processed. Many of these substances affect the nutritional and esthetic qualities of food including appearance and organoleptic properties (ie, flavor, texture, or aroma) that determine whether or not we will even try the food or take a second bite. Whereas substances present in food may be nutritional and/or gratifying, they may not necessarily be "safe" in *any* amount or for *any* intended use. The Federal Food, Drug and Cosmetic (FD&C) Act gives the Federal government the authority to ensure that all foods involved in interstate commerce are safe. Congress, in writing the Act (and its subsequent amendments), understood that safety cannot be proved absolutely and indicated instead that the safety standard for substances added to food can be no more than a *reasonable certainty of no harm*. As will be pointed out in other sections of this chapter, the language of the FD&C Act effectively provides for practical and workable approaches to the assessment of safety for food, food ingredients, and food contaminants. Because food is highly complex, the legal framework provided by Congress for the regulation of food and substances in food was kept simple so that it would work.

The basic element of the framework is that food, which is defined as articles or components of articles used for food or drink for humans or animals, bears the presumption of safety (Sections 201[f] and 402[a][1] of the FD&C Act). This means that a steak or a potato is presumed to be safe unless it contains a poisonous or deleterious substance in an amount, which is shown to make it *ordinarily injurious* to health. In essence, this presumption of safety was born of necessity. If the hundreds of thousands of substances naturally present in food were subject to the same strictures and limitations that apply to added substances, virtually all food would be suspect and food shortages could easily result. To avoid such crises, Congress developed a safety standard that would not force regulatory authorities to ban common, traditional foods. In cases in which the substance is not naturally present in food but is a contaminant or added ingredient, the safety standard is quite different. This standard decrees a food to be adulterated if it contains any poisonous or deleterious substance that *may render it injurious*.

Thus, for additives and contaminants, Congress recognized that these substances are not as complex as food and should therefore meet a higher standard of safety. However, because neither the law nor Food and Drug Administration (FDA) or US Department of Agriculture (USDA) regulations explicitly define the term "safety" for substances added to food, scientists and their legal and regulatory counterparts have worked out operational definitions for the safety of such substances.

As with food, a practical and workable approach must be found for the contaminants of added ingredients, because all substances contain a myriad of contaminants at trace or even undetectable amounts with current technology. In this case, the approach involves setting specification limits on contaminants that are intended to exclude the possibility that the level present in an additive *may render* the food to which the substance is added, *unsafe*. It should be emphasized that specifications can serve their purpose of assuring suitable purity only if the manufacturing processes used are adequately controlled to assure consistency in the quality and purity of the product. The philosophy by which specifications are established for substances added to food embodies the belief that not all risks are worthy of regulatory concern and control (ie, the concept of *de minimis*).[1] Implicit in this philosophy is the important unifying concept of *threshold of regulation* in food safety assessment (Flamm *et al.*, 1994, 2002).

Food, as stated earlier, contains hundreds of thousands of substances, most of which have not been fully characterized or tested. The presumption that a food is safe is based on a history of common use and that the consumption of certain foods is deeply rooted in tradition. When the uncertainty about the risk of the added substance is small compared with the uncertainties attending food itself, the standard of "reasonable certainty of no harm" for the added substance has been satisfied. Thus, for food-like substances, the presumption is that the substance resembles food, is digested and metabolized as food, and consequently raises fewer toxicological and safety-related questions than do non-food–like substances.

Moreover, when non-food–like substances are added in only very small or trace amounts, the low levels of exposure aid in demonstrating that the intended conditions of use of these substances are safe. These broad generalizations, however, do not suffice to exempt these food ingredients from the requirements of thorough safety evaluation.

Over the past two decades, there has been increasing interest on the part of consumers regarding the health-enhancing properties of foods and the components they contain. Substances such as phytosterols from vegetable oils and isoflavones from soy have been isolated and added to other foods at elevated levels to impart cholesterol-lowering properties. Such products have raised regulatory questions about whether these substances are functioning as drugs, and should they be regulated as such, or whether they should be viewed as new nutrients and allowed in foods, as are the historically recognized nutrients, vitamin C and iron. Some experts in nutritional science have concluded that the concept of nutrients should be expanded to include a growing number of desirable food constituents that produce quantifiable health benefits related to disease prevention (Sansalone, 1999). This isolation of, and fortification with, new food components will necessitate a thorough evaluation of safety at the intended level of intake and for the population at large (Mackey and Kotsonis, 2002).

Lastly, in many parts of the world, food safety (ie, food free of microbiological, chemical, and radionuclide contamination) and food security (ie, availability of food) represent *by far* the major food concerns faced by consumers. Thus, although our vigilance in assuring the safety of substances added to food (often with safety factors of 100 to a million) is not trivial in the context of our culture, we should not lose sight of other parts of the world where availability of potable water and sustaining caloric intake, represent daily challenges.

Uniqueness of Food Toxicology

The nature of food is responsible for the uniqueness of food toxicology. Food occupies a position of central importance in virtually all cultures and, although good agricultural practice has improved the quality of unprocessed food, most food cannot be commercially produced in a definable environment under strict quality controls. Food generally cannot meet the rigorous standards of chemical identity, purity, and good manufacturing practice met by most consumer products. The fact that food is harvested from the soil, the sea, inland waters, or is derived from land animals, which are subject to the unpredictable forces of nature, makes the constancy of raw (unprocessed) food unreliable. Therefore, it is clear that meat, milk, eggs and produce are held to a different standard than the ingredients of processed food, as a practical matter dictated by necessity.

Food also acquires uniqueness from its essential nutrients, which, such as Vitamin A, may be toxic at levels only 10-fold above those required to prevent deficiencies. The evaluation of food ingredients often must rely on reasoning unique to food science in the sense that such substances may be normal constituents of food or modified constituents of food as opposed to the types of substances ordinarily addressed in the fields of occupational, environmental, and medical toxicology. Assessing the safety of such substances, which are added to food for their technical effects, often focuses on digestion and metabolism occurring in the gastrointestinal (GI) tract. The reason for this focus is that in many cases, an ingested substance is not absorbed through the GI tract; only products of its digestion are absorbed, and these products may be identical to those derived from natural food.

---

[1] *de minimis non curat praetor* or *de minimis non curat lex*, that is, the law is not interested in trivial matters. In this sense, a risk so small it is not worthy of concern.

Table 31-1

Food as a Complex Mixture

NUTRIENTS	NONNUTRIENTS
Carbohydrates	Naturally occurring substances
Proteins	Food additives
Lipids	Contaminants
Minerals	Products of food processing
Vitamins	

SOURCE: Smith RL. Does one man's meat become another man's poison? Trans Medl Soc London Nov. 1991;11:6. With permission from Medical Society of London.

Table 31-2

Nonnutrient Substances in Food

FOOD	NUMBER OF IDENTIFIED NONNUTRIENT CHEMICALS
Cheddar cheese	160
Orange juice	250
Banana	325
Tomato	350
Wine	475
Coffee	625
Beef (cooked)	625

SOURCE: Smith RL. Does one man's meat become another man's poison? Trans Medl Soc Lond Nov. 1991;11:6. With permission from Medical Society of London.

Nature and Complexity of Food

Food is an exceedingly complex mixture of nutrient and non-nutrient substances, whether it is consumed as a raw agricultural product or as highly processed ready-to-eat foods such as a "Meal Ready to Eat" military ration (Table 31-1). The Western diet consists of items of caloric and noncaloric value, that is, carbohydrates supply 47% of caloric intake, fats supply 37%, and protein supplies 16% (all three of which would be considered "macronutrients"), whereas minerals and vitamins, the "micronutrients," have no caloric value but are no less essential for life.

Nonnutrient substances are often characterized in the popular literature as being contributed by food processing, but nature provides the vast majority of nonnutrient constituents. For instance, even among "natural" (or minimally processed) foods, there are far more nonnutrient than nutrient constituents (Table 31-2). Many of these nonnutrient substances are vital for the growth and survival of the plant, including hormones and naturally occurring pesticides, estimated at approximately 10,000 by Gold et al. (1992). Some of these substances may be antinutrients such as lectins, saponins, trypsin, and/or chymotrypsin inhibitors in soybeans, phytates that may bind minerals (also present in soybeans) and antithiamines (in fish and plants), and there may also be frankly toxic constituents such as tomatine or cycasin. An idea of the large number of substances present in food is given in the database VCF Volatile Compounds in Food 12.3 (latest version) (VCF, 2010), in which approximately 7800 volatile substances are noted as occurring in one or more of the 485 different foods. However, this is only the tip of the iceberg, as the number of nonvolatile and/or yet unidentified natural chemicals in food vastly exceeds the number that has been identified to date.

Nonnutrient substances are also added to food as a result of processing, and in fact, 21 CFR 170.3(o) lists 32 categories of direct additives, of which, there are about 3000 individual substances. Approximately 2000 of these added ingredients are flavor ingredients, most of which already occur naturally in food and are non-nutritive (Burdock, 2002). Of the 2000 flavoring ingredients that may be added to food, approximately one-third are used at concentrations below 10 ppm (Hall and Oser, 1968), about the same concentration as is found naturally.

Importance of the Gastrointestinal Tract

FDA considers that humans consume approximately 1500 g of food and an equal amount of liquid per day; therefore, within a year, humans ingest on the average 548 kg of food (or about 1200 lbs). To respond to this load, it is easy to appreciate the fact that the gut is a large, complex, and dynamic organ with several layers of organization and a vast absorptive surface that has been estimated to be 250 m^2 or more (Hall, 2011). The GI transit time provides for adequate exposure of ingesta to a variety of processing conditions including, but not limited to, variable pH, digestive acids and enzymes (trypsin, chymotrypsin, etc, from the pancreas and carbohydrases, lipases, and proteases from the enterocytes), saponification agents (in bile), and a luxuriant bacterial flora (estimated to be 100 trillion organisms in adults), the latter of which provide a repertoire of metabolic capability not shared by the host (eg, fermentation of "nondigestible" sugars such as xylitol and sorbitol) (Drasar and Hill, 1974; Vickery et al., 2011). In addition, the enterocytes (intestinal epithelium) possess an extensive capacity for the metabolism of xenobiotics that may be second only to the liver, with a full complement of phase (type) I and phase (type) II reactions present. This enteric monooxygenase system is analogous to the liver, as both systems are located in the endoplasmic reticulum of cells, require NADPH and O$_2$ for maximum activity, are inhibited by many of the same substances, and are qualitatively similar in their response to enzyme induction (Hassing et al., 1989).

The constituents of food and other ingesta (eg, drugs, contaminants, inhaled pollutants dissolved in saliva and swallowed) are a physicochemically heterogeneous lot and, as a result, the intestine has evolved into a relatively impermeable membrane with specialized mechanisms of absorption that have developed, which allow only certain substances to gain access to the body from the intestinal lumen. The four primary mechanisms for absorption are passive (or simple) diffusion, facilitated diffusion/cotransport, active transport, and pinocytosis. With some exceptions, each of these mechanisms characteristically transfers a defined group of constituents from the lumen into the body, although some substances may use more than one mechanism, such as fructose (Table 31-3). As is noted in the table, xenobiotics and other substances may compete for passage into the body.

Aiding this absorption is the rich vascularization of the intestine, with a normal rate of blood flow in the portal vein of approximately 1.2 L/h/kg; however, after a meal, there is a 30% increase in blood flow through the splanchnic area (Concon, 1988). It follows then, that substances which affect blood flow, also tend to affect the rate of absorption of other materials; an example is alcohol, which tends to increase blood flow to the stomach and thus enhances its own absorption as well as other substances. Few stimuli tend to

Table 31-3

Systems Transporting Enteric Constituents

SYSTEM	ENTERIC CONSTITUENT
Passive diffusion	Water, chloride, fats (as micelles), short- and medium-chain fatty acids
Facilitated diffusion	Fructose, D-xylose, 6-deoxy-1,5-anhydro-D-glucitol, glutamic acid, aspartic acid, short-chain fatty acids, glucose, and galactose, xenobiotics with carboxy groups, sulfates, glucuronide esters, lead, cadmium, zinc
Active transport	Cations, anions, sugars, vitamins, nucleosides (pyrimidines, uracil, and thymine, which may be in competition with 5-fluorouracil and 5-bromouracil), cobalt, manganese (which competes for the iron transportation system)
Pinocytosis	Long-chain lipids, vitamin B_{12} complex, azo dyes, maternal antibodies, botulinum toxin, hemagglutinins, phalloidins, *E coli* endotoxins, virus particles

Table 31-4

Factors Affecting Intestinal Absorption and Rate of Absorption

EXAMPLE	FACTOR
Gastric emptying rate	Increased fat content
Gastric pH	Antacids, stress, H_2-receptor blockers
Intestinal motility	Diarrhea due to intercurrent disease, laxatives, dietary fiber, disaccharide intolerance, amaranth
Food content	Lectins of *Phaseolus vulgaris* (inhibition of glucose absorption and transport)
Surface area of small intestine	Short-bowel syndrome
Intestinal blood flow	Alcohol
Intestinal lymph flow	Tripalmitin
Enterohepatic circulation	Chlordecone (prevented by cholestyramine)
Permeability of mucosa	Inflammatory bowel disease, celiac disease
Inhibition of digestive processes	Catechins of tea, which inhibit sucrase and therefore glucose absorption
Concomitant drug therapy	Iron salts/tetracycline

SOURCE: Modified from Hoensch HP, Schwenk M. Intestinal absorption and metabolism of xenobiotics in humans. In: Schiller CM, ed. Intestinal Toxicology. New York: Raven Press, 1984:169–192. With permission from Lippincott Williams & Wilkins.

decrease flow to this area, with the possible exception of energetic muscular activity and hypovolemic shock.

Lymph circulation is important in the transfer of fats, large molecules (such as botulinum toxin), benzo[*a*]pyrene, 3-methylcholanthrene, and *cis*-dimethylaminostilbene (Chhabra and Eastin, 1984). Small- to medium-chain fatty acids are absorbed directly and do not require conversion to monoglycerides and do not rely on the triglyceride → micelle → chylomicron pathway (Hall, 2011). Lymph has a flow rate of about 1 to 2 mL/h/kg in humans, and a few factors are known to influence its flow including tripalmitin, which has been shown to double the flow and therefore double the absorption of materials such as *p*-aminosalicylic acid and tetracycline (Chhabra and Eastin, 1984). Another factor that lends importance to lymph is the fact that the lymph empties via the thoracic duct into the point of junction of the left internal jugular and subclavian veins, preventing "first-pass" metabolism by the liver, unlike substances transported by the blood.

Many food ingredients are modified proteins, carbohydrates, fats, or components of such substances. Thus, understanding the changes these substances undergo in the GI tract, their possible effect on the GI tract, and whether they are absorbed or affect the absorption of other substances is critical to an understanding of food toxicology and safety assessment. Some of the factors that may affect GI absorption and the rate of absorption are listed in Table 31-4.

Apart from its duties of absorption and metabolism, the GI tract is also the largest immunologic organ in the body and is constantly exposed to a large number of antigens in food (approximately 88 kg of protein annually) and commensal and ingested bacteria. One cell layer away from these antigens is the lamina propria of the GI tract, which contains the mucosal-associated lymphoid tissue, comprised of lymphocytes and antigen-presenting cells, as well as unique dendritic cells, which interact with dietary antigens and ultimately determine whether an antigen is tolerated or an immune response is launched (Brandtzaeg, 2010; Vickery *et al.*, 2011).

SAFETY STANDARDS FOR FOODS, FOOD INGREDIENTS AND CONTAMINANTS

The FD&C Act Provides for a Practicable Approach

As incredible as it may seem, there were few specifics regulating food until the Food Additives Amendment of 1958; the original Pure Food and Drug Act of 1906 only stipulated that food should not be "filthy, putrid, or unfit for consumption." In the meantime, many other facets of commerce had seen significant regulatory oversight initiated: animal feed (~1902), the Meat Inspection Act (1906) and, drugs and cosmetics (1938). The 1938 amendment superseded the 1906 Act and initiated the important concept of requiring *premarket approval* of a product, but only for drugs, not food ingredients. In practice, the 1938 amendment was found to have less benefit than expected for consumers or manufacturers and created a financial burden on FDA. That is, on one hand, the manufacturer was largely unrestricted on the addition of substances to food. On the other hand, the burden of proof was on FDA to show the lack of safety of an ingredient (requiring resource demands for testing) and once FDA declared an ingredient injurious to health, the manufacturer was forced to prove that it was "harmless *per se*" (ie, harmless at all doses) or forego the use of the substance in any amount. The "harmless *per se*" concept ignores the basic rule of toxicology that the "dose makes the poison."

By the early 1950s, it was obvious that the law in place was unworkable and a mechanism for decision making was needed to determine the safe use of foods, the hundreds of ingredients already in use in food, and finished (processed) foods derived from the ingredients. Congress understood that a requirement for premarket (regulatory) approval of all of the ingredients would create an unimaginable burden in terms of costs of testing and time to review each food additive petition and such a process made no sense, knowing that many of these substances, such as spices, had been in use for over a thousand years. At the same time, it was untenable to simply "grandfather" ingredients already in use because for some, there were no safety data or history of use upon which a decision of safety could be based. In the end, Congress decided that all ingredients added to food were food additives (which would be approved by FDA), unless they were generally recognized as safe (GRAS) (a decision left to experts inside or outside of FDA and not requiring FDA approval); this act had the effect of avoiding a log jam of food additive petitions that would likely not be resolved to this day. Congress discarded the safety *per se* concept and developed the Act, which, by itself and subsequent regulations, mitigated potential harm to the consumer through the creative use of specifications, process and manufacturing controls (Good Manufacturing Practice), action levels, tolerances, warning labels, and outright prohibitions.

The Application of Experience: Generally Recognized as Safe

The FD&C Act permits the addition of substances to food to accomplish a specific technical effect if use of the substance is determined to be GRAS. The Act does not require the FDA to make this determination, although it does not exclude the agency from making such decisions. The Act instead requires that scientific experts base a GRAS determination on the adequacy of safety, as shown through scientific procedures or through experience based on common use in food before January 1, 1958, under the intended conditions of use of the substance (FD&C Act, section 201[s]).

In addition to allowing GRAS substances to be added to food, the Act provides for a class of substances that are regulated food additives, which are defined as "any substances the intended use of which results in its becoming a component... of any food... if such substance is not generally recognized... to be safe." Hence, a legal distinction is drawn between regulated food additives and GRAS substances. Regulated food additives must be approved and regulated for their intended conditions of use by the FDA under 21 CFR 172–179 before they can be marketed. Under section 409 of the Act, the requirements for data to support the safe use of a food additive are described in general terms. The requirements or recommended methods for establishing safe conditions of use for an additive are available in the form of guidelines issued by the FDA. These guidelines, referred to as the Redbook, provide substance and definition to the safety standard applicable to regulated food additives: "reasonable certainty of no harm under conditions of intended use" (Burdock and Carabin, 2004).

Use of Tolerances

If a food contains an *unavoidable* contaminant even with the use of current good manufacturing practice (cGMP), it may be declared unfit as food if the contaminant may render the food injurious to health. Thus, for a food itself to be declared unfit, it must be ordinarily injurious, while an unavoidable contaminant in food need only pose the risk of harm for the food to be found unfit, and subject to FDA action. The reason for the dichotomy is practicality. Congress recognized that if authority were granted to ban traditional foods for reasons that go beyond clear evidence of harm to health, the agency would be subject to pressure to ban certain foods.

Foods containing unavoidable contaminants are not automatically banned because such foods are subject to the provisions of section 406 of the FD&C Act, which indicates that the quantity of unavoidable contaminants in food may be limited by regulation for the protection of public health and that any quantity of a contaminant, which exceeds the fixed limit, shall be deemed unsafe. This authority has been used by the FDA to set limits on the quantity of unavoidable contaminants in food by regulation (tolerances) or by informal action levels, which do not have the force of law. Such action levels have been set for aflatoxins, fumonisins, and patulin (Table 31-5). Action levels have the advantage of offering greater flexibility than is provided by tolerances. Whether tolerances or action levels are applied to unavoidable contaminants of food, the FDA attempts to balance the health risk posed by unavoidable contaminants against the loss of a portion of the food supply. In contrast, contaminants in food that are *avoidable* by cGMP are deemed to be unsafe under section 406 if they are considered poisonous or deleterious. Under such circumstances, the food is typically declared *adulterated* and unfit for human consumption. The extent to which consumers who are already in possession of such food must be alerted depends on the health risk posed by the contaminated food. If there is a reasonable probability that the use of or exposure to such a food will cause serious adverse health consequences or death, the FDA will seek a Class I recall, which provides the maximum public warning, the greatest depth of recall, and the most follow-up. Classes II and III represent progressively less health risk and require less public warning, less depth of recall, and less follow-up (21 CFR 7.3).

Pesticide Residues A pesticide is defined under the Federal Insecticide, Fungicide, and Rodenticide Act (FIFRA), as any substance used to control or mitigate pests (such as insects, rodents, weeds, or fungi), or intended for use as a plant growth regulator, defoliant, or desiccant. In the United States, the regulation of pesticides is the responsibility of the Environmental Protection Agency (EPA) and is accomplished under both FIFRA and the FD&C Act. FIFRA governs the registration, sale, and use of all pesticides. It is illegal to use a pesticide unless it is specifically registered and labeled for the intended use. In order to obtain registration, an applicant must supply EPA with data on pesticide composition, mammalian and ecological toxicity, environmental fate, and potential human and environmental exposures.

Table 31-5

FDA Action Levels for Mycotoxins

COMMODITY	LEVEL (ng/g)
Aflatoxins	
All products, except milk, designated for humans	20
Aflatoxins: Milk	0.5
Patulin: Apple juice	50
Deoxynivalenol (DON or vomitoxin): All finished wheat products that may be consumed by humans	1000
Fumonisins, Total ($FB_1 + FB_2 + FB_3$)	
Degermed dry milled corn product	2000
Cleaned corn intended for popcorn	3000
Cleaned corn for masa production	4000

SOURCE: *Mycotoxins in domestic foods (http://www.cfsan.fda.gov/~comm/cp07001.html)*

A major part of the registration process for most pesticides involves the establishment of tolerances. The EPA must establish tolerances, or exemptions from tolerances, for all pesticides that may come into contact with food or feed, that is, those intended for use during the production, storage, transportation, or processing of food or feed crops, on livestock, or in food-handling establishments. The tolerances are intended to represent the highest expected residue levels from legal uses of the pesticide. All pesticide tolerances are now established under Section 408 of the FD&C Act. Prior to 1996, if pesticide residues in processed foods exceeded those in raw agricultural commodities, they were considered to be intentional food additives and were required to be assigned "Food Additive Tolerances" under Section 409 of the Act. If the pesticide chemical in question had been classified by the EPA as a human or animal carcinogen, the Delaney clause would be invoked and the Section 409 food additive tolerance(s) could be denied on that basis. However, the Food Quality Protection Act (FQPA) of 1996 revised Section 201(s) of the FD&C Act to exclude pesticides from the definition of *food additive*—even in the case of concentrated residues in processed fractions. Although an additional tolerance for a processed fraction is still required if the pesticide residue in the fraction exceeds the tolerance for the raw agricultural commodity, that tolerance is now established under Section 408 rather than Section 409. Consequently, although the Delaney clause has *not* been repealed from Section 409, and continues to apply to intentional food additives *other than pesticides*, it is no longer applicable for *pesticides*.

Prior to 1996, the EPA used 100× as a default safety factor when conducting risk assessments to ensure that the necessary food and feed tolerances would be safe for human health. However, FQPA also requires that an additional 10× safety factor "shall be applied for infants and children to take into account potential pre- and postnatal toxicity and completeness of the data with respect to exposure and toxicity to infants and children." It further states, however, that "the Administrator may use a different margin of safety for the pesticide chemical residue only if, on the basis of reliable data, such margin will be safe for infants and children."

Drugs Used in Food-producing Animals The Federal Food, Drug, and Cosmetic Act (FFDCA) (section 201[g]) defines the term "drugs" as "articles intended for use in the diagnosis, cure, mitigation, treatment, or prevention of disease in man or other animals" and "articles (other than food) intended to affect the structure or any function of the body of man or other animals." An animal drug "means any drug intended for use for animals other than man" [section 201(w) of the FD&C Act]. The Center for Veterinary Medicine, the arm of the FDA responsible for regulation of animal feed and drugs, considers that any substance added to animal feed used for growth promotion and increased food production is a drug. Determination of the potential human health hazards associated with animal drug residues is complicated by the metabolism of an animal drug, which results in residues of many potential metabolites.

The primary factors that must be considered in the evaluation of animal drugs are (1) consumption and absorption by the target animal, (2) metabolism of the drug by the target food animal, (3) excretion and tissue distribution of the drug and its metabolites in food animal products and tissues, (4) consumption of food animal products and tissues by humans, (5) potential absorption of the drug and its metabolites by humans, (6) potential metabolism of the drug and its metabolites by humans, and (7) potential excretion and tissue distribution in humans of the drug, its metabolites, and the secondary human metabolites derived from the drug and

its metabolites. Thus, the pharmacokinetic and biotransformation characteristics of both the animal and the human must be considered in an assessment of the potential human health hazard of an animal drug.

For new animal drugs (ie, those not declared GRAS and effective), safety assessment is concerned primarily with residues that occur in animal food products (milk, cheese, etc) and edible tissues (muscle, liver, etc). Toxicity studies in the target species (chicken, cow, pig, etc) should provide data on metabolism and the nature of metabolites, along with data on the drug's pharmacokinetics. During this phase, the parent drug and its metabolites are evaluated both qualitatively and quantitatively in the animal products of concern (eggs, milk, meat, etc). This may involve the development of sophisticated analytic methodologies. Once these data are obtained, it is necessary to undertake an assessment to determine potential human exposure to these compounds from the diet and other sources, pursuant to the establishment of a tolerance.

To comply with the Congressional intent regarding the use of animal drugs in food-producing animals as required in the no residue provision of the Delaney clause, the FDA began to build a system for conducting risk assessment of carcinogens in the early 1970s (FDA, 1977). In the course of developing a policy and/or regulatory definition for "no residue," the FDA was compelled to address the issue of residues of metabolites of animal drugs known to induce cancer in humans or animals. As the number of metabolites may range into the hundreds, it became apparent that as a practical matter, not every metabolite could be tested with the same thoroughness as the parent animal drug. This forced the FDA to consider threshold assessment for the first time. Threshold assessment combines information on the structure and in vitro biological activity of a metabolite for the purpose of determining whether carcinogenicity testing is necessary (Flamm *et al.*, 1994, 2002). If testing is necessary and if the substance is found to induce cancer, the FDA's definition states that a lifetime risk of one in a million is equivalent to the meaning of "no residue" as intended by Congress.

Tolerance Setting Foods are regarded as such because they are edible—they cannot be unpalatable or toxic—and foods must have nutritional, hedonic, or satietal value, otherwise there would be no point in consuming them. Therefore, FD&C Act presumes that traditionally consumed foods (produce such as apples or carrots and animal products, including meat, milk, and eggs) are safe if they are free of contaminants. The fact that foods contain many natural substances, some of which are toxic at a high concentration, is in itself an insufficient basis under the Act for declaring a food as being unfit for human consumption. In practice, a food containing a poisonous or deleterious substance may be considered adulterated (unfit for consumption), the exception being that if the substance is naturally present as a constituent of that food in a quantity that is not ordinarily injurious (§409 of the Act). The implementation of the use of this concept (a) allows the presence of solanaceous glycoalkaloids (SGAs) in potatoes, as the SGAs occur naturally in potatoes, (b) but only allows the SGAs to be present at a nontoxic level (defined as "not ordinarily injurious"), and (c) effectively prohibits the addition (or presence) of SGAs in foods where SGAs would not appear naturally (such as in wheat products, where the SGAs could only be present as a contaminant). A tolerance has considerable reach—for example, a potato might have an acceptable level of SGA at the point of harvesting, but if subject to mishandling during shipping, handling, or storage, the potato may generate additional SGA to a point in excess of the prescribed tolerance.

Table 31-6

Direct Food Additives by Functionality

NUMBER	DESIGNATION	DESCRIPTION	EXAMPLES
170.3(o) (1)	Anticaking agents and free-flow agents	Substances added to finely powdered or crystalline food products to prevent caking, lumping, or agglomeration	Glucitol, sodium ferrocyanide, silicon dioxide
(3)	Antioxidants	Substances used to preserve food by retarding deterioration, rancidity, or discoloration due to oxidation	Butylated hydroxyanisole, butylated hydroxytoluene, propyl gallate
(9)	Enzymes	Enzymes used to improve food processing and the quality of the finished food	Papain, rennet, pepsin
(12)	Flavor agents and adjuvants	Substances added to impart or help impart a taste or aroma in food	Cinnamon, citral, *p*-cresol, thymol, Zingerone
(19)	Nonnutritive sweeteners	Substances having less than 2 % of the caloric value of sucrose per equivalent unit of sweetening capacity	Aspartame, neotame, sucralose, saccharin

Food and Color Additives Despite the initial successes with GRAS status following passage of the 1958 amendment, colors were designated additives in the Color Additives Amendment of 1960 and thereby not eligible for GRAS status, thus requiring a Color Additive Petition. As per the FD&C Act (§201[t]), "a color is a dye, pigment, or other substance...when added or applied to a food, drug, or cosmetic, or to the human body or any part thereof, is capable (alone or through reaction with other substance) of imparting color thereto...." Blacks, whites, and intermediate grays also are included in this definition. A provision in the Act and in the regulation (21 CFR §70.3[f]) exempts the use of a substance, which although imparting color to the final product, it is not a color *per se*. For example, food ingredients such as cherries, green or red peppers, chocolate, and orange juice, which contribute their own natural color when mixed with other foods, are not regarded as color additives (such as chocolate to produce chocolate milk); but where a food substance such as beet juice is deliberately used as a color, as in pink lemonade, it is a color additive. Although a color additive has only one function, a food additive may have any one of 32 functionalities (Table 31-6).

There are two distinct types of color additives that have been approved for food use: those requiring certification by FDA chemists and those exempt from certification. Certification, which is based on chemical analysis, is required for each batch of most organic synthesized colors because they may contain impurities that may vary from batch to batch. Most certified colors approved for food use bear the prefix FD&C. Certification involves in-depth chemical analysis of major and trace components of each individual batch of color additives by FDA chemists and is required before any batch can be released for commercial use. Such color additives consist of aromatic amines or aromatic azo structures (FD&C Blue No. 1, Blue No. 2, Green No. 3, Red No. 3, Red No. 40, Yellow No. 5, and Yellow No. 6) that cannot be synthesized without a variety of impurities. Orange B and Citrus Red No. 2 are the only certified food colors that lack the FD&C designation (21 CFR 74 Subpart A). Two additional color designations reference the range of approved use: FD&C colors, which indicate use in foods, drugs, and cosmetics; and D&C colors, which indicate their use solely in drugs and cosmetics, not foods.

The estimated daily intakes (EDI) of certified color additives for the US population and the acceptable daily intakes (ADIs) determined from toxicology studies are in Table 31-7. The calculated values of the EDIs assume an even distribution of the respective

Table 31-7

Per Capita Intakes of Certified Colors Additives for the US Population

COLOR ADDITIVE	US POPULATION PER CAPITA EDI (mg/person/day)	ADI (mg/person/day) US POPULATION (60-kg PERSON)	ADI (mg/person/day) CHILDREN (30-kg CHILD)
FD&C Blue No. 1	1.72	720	360
FD&C Blue No. 2	1.95	150	75
FD&C Green No. 3	0.038	150	75
FD&C Red No. 3	0.61	150	75
FD&C Red No. 40	17.91	420	210
FD&C Yellow No. 5	12.06	300	150
FD&C Yellow No. 6	10.74	225	113

SOURCE: FDA. Background Document for the Food Advisory Committee: Certified Color Additives in Food and Possible Association with Attention Deficit Hyperactivity Disorder in Children March 30–31, 2011.

Table 31-8

Summary of the Toxicity Tests Recommended for Different Levels of Concern[*]

	CONCERN LEVELS		
TOXICITY STUDIES[†]	I	II	III
Short term tests for genetic toxicity	X	X	X
Metabolism and pharmacokinetic studies		X	X
Short-term (28-day) toxicity studies with rodents	X[‡]		
Subchronic (90-day) toxicity studies with rodents		X[‡]	X[‡]
Subchronic (90-day) toxicity studies with nonrodents		X[‡]	
Reproduction studies with teratology phase		X[‡]	X[‡]
One-year toxicity studies with nonrodents			X
Carcinogenicity studies with rodents			X[§]
Chronic toxicity/carcinogenicity studies with rodents			X[§,‖]

[*] *The Redbook. Available at: http://www.fda.gov/Food/GuidanceComplianceRegulatoryInformation/ GuidanceDocuments/FoodIngredientsandPackaging/Redbook/default.htm. Accessed October 24, 2011.*
[†] *Not including dose range-finding studies, if appropriate.*
[‡] *Including neurotoxicity and immunotoxicity screens.*
[§] *An in utero phase is recommended for one of the two recommended carcinogenicity studies with rodents, preferably the study with rats.*
[‖] *Combined study may be performed as separate studies.*

additives for the entire population. A comparison of these levels indicates that the EDIs are well below the ADIs in both adults and children (FDA, 2011a, 2011b).

Despite the fact that aromatic amines are generally considered relatively toxic substances, the FD&C colors are notably nontoxic. The principal reason involves sulfonation of the aromatic amine or azo compound that constitutes a color additive. Such sulfonic acid groups are highly polar, which, combined with their high molecular weight, prevents them from being absorbed by the GI tract or entering cells. All the FD&C food colors have been extensively tested in all Concern Level (CL) III tests (Table 31-8) and have been found to be "remarkably" nontoxic (refer to section titled. Assignment of Concern Level and Required Testing).

Food colors that are exempt from certification typically have not been subjected to such extensive testing requirements. The exempt food colors are derived primarily from natural sources. Whereas synthetic food colors have received the majority of public, scientific, and regulatory attention, natural color agents are also an important class. Currently, 26 color additives have been given exemption from certification in 21 CFR 73. These agents consist of a variety of natural compounds generally obtained by various extraction and treatment technologies. Included in this group of colors are preparations such as dried algae meal, beet powder, grape skin extract, fruit juice, paprika, caramel, carrot oil, cochineal extract, ferrous gluconate, and iron oxide. A problem encountered in attempts to regulate these additives is the lack of a precise chemical definition of many of these preparations. With a few exceptions such as caramel, which is the most widely used color, the natural colors have not been heavily used. In part, this may be due to economic reasons, but these colors generally do not have the uniformity and intensity characteristic of the synthetic colors, therefore necessitating higher concentrations to obtain a specific color intensity. They also lack the chemical and color stability of the synthetic colors and have a tendency to fade with time.

Concerns about certified color additives (synthetic dyes) were raised in the 1970s by Dr. Benjamin Feingold, a pediatrician, who claimed that these additives were linked to behavior changes and hyperactivity in children and proposed a diet free of synthetic dyes. Recently, the FDA and FDA's Food Advisory Committee confirmed earlier findings that there is not enough evidence to conclude that certified color additives contribute to hyperactivity in children in the general population (FDA, 20lla and 2011b).

The maximal intake of food colors is estimated to be ~53.5 mg/day, whereas the average intake per day is ~15 mg (Committee on Food Protection, 1971). Only about 10% of the food consumed in the United States contains food colors. The foods that utilize food colors in order of the quantity of color utilized are (1) beverages, (2) candy and confections, (3) dessert powders, (4) bakery goods, (5) sausages (casing only), (6) cereals, (7) ice cream, (8) snack foods, and (9) gravies, jams, jellies, and so forth (Committee on Food Protection, 1971).

The Importance of Labeling The importance of labeling was first realized in its ability to protect consumers from economic fraud by requiring that the weight and exact contents of the product be stated; otherwise, the product was *mislabeled*. Later, it became obvious that labels could also serve a purpose in assuring the safety of the consumer by including safety warnings for particularly susceptible groups, including those exhibiting allergies or food intolerance.

Food allergies have a considerable impact on modern society. There is no known cure for food allergies and although accidental exposure is common, avoidance of the offending foods is the only successful noninterventional approach. Food allergy is the leading cause of anaphylaxis, a severe type of allergic reaction requiring hospitalization. It is estimated that 3% to 4% of adults and about 6% of young children in the United States suffer from food allergies, and food allergies account for 35% to 50% of all cases of anaphylaxis, the latter of which has increased from 21,000 per year in 1999 to 51,000 per year in 2008 (AAAAI, 2011). Food allergies are reported to cause approximately 150 to 200 fatalities annually (AAAAI, 2011).

Effective from January 1, 2006, as a result of the Food Allergen Labeling and Consumer Protection Act of 2004 (FALCPA), manufacturers are required to identify the presence of ingredients that contain protein derived from milk, eggs, fish, crustacean shellfish, tree nuts, peanuts, wheat, or soybeans. These eight major food allergens account for 90% of food allergic reactions. In addition, FALCPA labeling regulations require declaration of the specific type of tree nut (eg, almonds, pecans, or walnuts), the species of fish (eg, bass, flounder, or cod), and the kind of crustacean shellfish (eg, crab, lobster, or shrimp). FALCPA requires, with a few exceptions, the label on a food product (eg, conventional foods, dietary supplements, infant formula, and medical foods) that is or contains an ingredient (such as a spice, flavoring, coloring, or incidental additive) that includes a "major food allergen" (Carabin and Magnuson, 2006). Also, because the source of ingredients such as lecithin, flour, or whey may not be obvious to the consumer, the source must follow the name of the ingredient. For example, the above ingredients must be given on the labels as follows—lecithin (soy), flour (wheat) and whey (milk); alternatively, immediately after or next to the list of ingredients in a "contains" statement—for example "Contains wheat, milk and soy."[2]

Labeling requirements for nonallergens include those for intolerance (eg, lactose or gluten intolerance) or, for example, the presence of phenylalanine for phenylketonuria patients, are especially important when these substances may be present in foods where their presence may not be expected. Label warnings also include those warning of a threshold for a laxative effect (eg, polydextrose, mannitol, sorbitol). The FDA has indicated that, at this time, it is not aware of any information that foods developed through genetic engineering differ as a class in any attribute from foods developed through conventional means that would warrant a special label (Thompson, 2000). The FDA allows companies to include on the label of a product any statement as long as the statement is truthful and not misleading.

Methods Used to Evaluate the Safety of Foods, Ingredients, and Contaminants

Safety Evaluation of Direct Food and Color Additives The basic concept that forms the foundation for the safety evaluation of direct food and color additives is the recognition that the safety of any substance added to food must be established on the basis of the intended conditions of use in food. Factors that need to be taken into account include (1) the purpose for use of the substance, (2) the food to which the substance is added, (3) the concentration level used in the proposed foods, and (4) the population expected to consume the substance.

The evaluation of a new food additive is a complicated and expensive undertaking, especially when the additive will be widely used in many foods. Each additive can pose unique safety questions depending on its chemistry, stability in use, metabolism, safety study results, and estimated human exposure. Integral to a discussion of exposure is the concept of the "whole food additive." This refers to the additive, the degradation or conversion products arising from the use of the additive in foods, and the impurities found in the manufactured additive itself (Kotsonis and Hjelle, 1996).

Exposure: The Estimated Daily Intake As noted earlier, prior to 1958, the FDA held to the philosophy that food additives

(and potential contaminants) should not be harmful at any level. This is impractical, as many substances critical to life, such as vitamin A or even water, are toxic at high doses. These examples underscore the fact that exposure level is a major factor in a safety evaluation, and is reflected in the FDA's *Toxicological Principles for the Safety Assessment of Direct Food Additives and Color Additives Used in Food* (FDA, 1982a),[3] a source used to determine what testing methods should be done to determine the safe use of a substance.

In food additive safety determinations, exposure is usually referred to as EDI and is based on the daily intake (I) of the food in which the substance will be used and the concentration (C) of the substance in the food. Many food ingredients are used in several different food categories, but as an example, if an additive is used *only* in breakfast cereals at a concentration that does not exceed 20 μg/g (ppm) and the mean daily intake of breakfast cereals is 175 g/person/day, the EDI is calculated at 3500 μg/person/day. As most food additives are used in many foods, the total exposure is the sum of the exposures from each of the food categories. The formula for exposure to food additive B is $EDI_B = (C_Bf \times I_f) + (C_Bg \times I_g) + (C....)$ where C_Bf and C_Bg are the concentration of B in food category f and g, respectively. I_f and I_g are the daily intake of food category f and g, respectively. Therefore, the EDI is the sum of the individual contributions of B in each of the food categories.

The same principles may be applied to the estimation of the consumption of residue from secondary direct additives (substances not intended to remain in a food after the technical effect has been accomplished, examples include processing agents such as solvents, sanitizers, and defoaming agents) and contaminants. Additional information on the exposure to direct food additives and contaminants has been made available by the agency's Center for Food Safety and Applied Nutrition.[4]

Calculating the EDI raises several basic questions: (1) how does one determine the amount of a food additive that is added to each food category and (2) how are food categories determined? To determine the amount of food additive added to each food category, the amount or, if a range, the highest end of the range of use levels for the new substance is used. These food group maximums are not to be exceeded by a food manufacturer based on the cGMP regulation (cGMPs; 21 CFR 110), which requires a manufacturer not to add more of an additive than is reasonably required to achieve the specific technical effect of the food additive.

General food categories have been specified by the FDA (21CFR170.3(n)). A sample of the categories is presented in Table 31-9. These categories were derived from a survey of food additives conducted by the National Academy of Sciences/National Research Council and published in 1972 (NRC/NAS, 1979). This survey pioneered the use of categorizing foods, but changes in the consumption patterns of the US population, in addition to changes in the types of foods available, have necessitated the generation of additional, more current data.

---

[2]Available at: http://www.fda.gov/Food/ResourcesForYou/Consumers/ucm079311.htm. Accessed April 28, 11.

[3]The Agency is in the process of updating the Redbook and is now making Redbook 2000 chapters available electronically (http://www.cfsan.fda.gov/~redbook/red-toca.html). The Redbook 2000 chapters now substitute for or supplement, guidance available in the 1982 Redbook I and in the 1993 Draft Redbook II, which can be obtained from the Office of Food Additive Safety. As additional chapters of Redbook 2000 are completed, they will be made available electronically.

[4]US FDA, Center for Food Safety and Applied Nutrition, Office of Premarket Approval, September, 1995. Available online at http://www.cfsan.fda.gov/~dms/opa-cg8.html.

Table 31-9

Food Categories

NUMBER	DESIGNATION	DESCRIPTION	EXAMPLES
170.3(n) (1)	Baked goods and baking mixes	Includes all ready-to-eat and ready-to bake products, flours, and mixes requiring preparation before serving	Doughnuts, bread, croissants, cake mix, cookie dough
(2)	Beverages, alcoholic	Includes malt beverages, wines, distilled liquors, and cocktail mix	Beer, malt liquor, whiskey, liqueurs, wine coolers
(4)	Breakfast cereals	Includes ready-to-eat and instant and regular hot cereals	Oatmeal (both regular and instant), farina, corn flakes, wheat flakes
(42)	Sugar substitutes	Including granulated, liquid, and tablet sugar substitutes	Aspartame, neotame

More contemporary data on food intake has been calculated through the use of food consumption surveys (Table 31-10). Food consumption databases have specific characteristics and are based on particular assumptions. Methods commonly used by regulatory agencies, manufacturers, nutritionists, and general researchers for assessing food consumption by individuals include 24-hour dietary recalls, dietary records, food frequency records, and dietary history accounts (Matulka, 2005). For example, one database may be based on an individual's food intake from the past 24 hours, whereas another may utilize dietary records taken over a three-day period of time, and yet another may cover average consumption

Table 31-10

Databases for Estimating Food Intake

The Nationwide Food Consumption Survey, USDA, 1987–1988[*]
Estimates of Daily Intake (NRC/NAS), 1979 (Abrams, 1992)
The FDA Total Diet Study, Egan SK, Bolger PM, Carrington CD (2007).
Update of the US FDA's Total Diet Study Food List and Diets. JESEE 2007(17):573–582.
Foods Commonly Eaten in the United States, 1994–1996 USDA (Smiciklas-Wright, 2002)
USDA Economic Research Service Reports Continuing Survey of Food Intakes by Individuals (CSFII), USDA, 1985, 1986, 1989[*], 1990, 1991, 1994–1996, 1998[*]
NHANES I, II, III
WWEA[*,†], USDA 2001–2002, 2003–2004, 2005–2006, 2007–2008 (USDA, 2010)

NHANE, National Health and Nutrition Examination Survey; USDA, US Department of Agriculture; WWEA, What We Eat In America.
[*] *Indicates current use by FDA.*
[†] *WWEA is the dietary intake component of the NHANES. WWEIA is conducted as a partnership between the USDA and the US Department of Health and Human Services (DHHS). WWEIA represents the integration of two nationwide surveys—USDA's Continuing Survey of Food Intakes by Individuals (CSFII) and HHS' NHANES. Under the integrated framework, DHHS is responsible for the sample design and data collection. USDA is responsible for the survey's dietary data collection methodology, development, and maintenance of the food and nutrient databases used to code and process the data, and data review and processing. The two surveys were integrated in 2002.*
SOURCE: Courtesy Matulka R, personal communication.

over 14 days. Some databases may provide only general population consumption values, whereas others may provide a detailed breakout of particular subpopulations (eg, the elderly, women, teenagers).

In safety assessments, one must consider other sources of consumption for the intended use of the food additive, such as whether it is already used in food for another purpose, is used in nonfood products (eg, toothpaste, lipstick, drugs, or dietary supplements), or the additive occurs naturally in foods. In summary, to estimate human consumption of a particular food substance, it is necessary to know (1) the levels of the substance in food, (2) the daily intake of each food containing the substance, (3) the distribution of food intake within the population, and (4) the potential exposure to the substance from nonfood sources (Tennant, 2002).

Before a food additive is approved, evidence is required by regulatory agencies that indicate the additive is safe for its intended use(s) and that the EDI for the additive is less than its ADI (Butchko and Kotsonis, 1996). Regulatory agencies may impose restrictions on certain uses of food additives if the EDI exceeds the ADI, or restricts future approvals for new categories of use. Chronic, long-term rodent toxicity studies are usually used in determining the ADI. These studies are used to determine the no-observed-adverse-effect level (NOAEL) for the additive. To provide an adequate level of safety from animal to human extrapolation, a 100-fold safety factor is usually employed to account for species differences and the interindividual variation among humans, to determine the ADI for a food additive. This factor provides a reasonable certainty in estimating safe doses in humans from animal studies (Lehman and Fitzhugh, 1954).[5]

Assignment of Concern Level and Required Testing

Structure-activity relationships are now the basis for developing many therapeutic drugs, pesticides, and food additives. These relationships are put to good use in the Toxicological Principles for the Safety Assessment of Direct Food Additives and Color Additives Used in Foods (FDA, 1982a), which describes a qualitative "decision tree" that assigns categories to substances on the basis of the structural and functional groups in the molecule. Additives with functional groups with a high order of toxicity are assigned to category C, those of unknown or intermediate toxicity are assigned to category B, and those with a low potential for toxicity are assigned to category A. For example, a simple saturated hydrocarbon alcohol

---

[5]This is the original source of the 100-fold safety factor.

Table 31-11

Assignment of Concern Level*

STRUCTURE CATEGORY A	STRUCTURE CATEGORY B	STRUCTURE CATEGORY C	CONCERN LEVEL
<0.05 ppm in the total diet (<0.0012 mg/kg/day) or	<0.025 ppm in the total diet (<0.00063 mg/kg/day) or	<0.0125 ppm in the total diet (<0.00031 mg/kg/day) or	I
≥0.05 ppm in the total diet (≥0.0012 mg/kg/day) or	≥0.025 ppm in the total diet (≥0.00063 mg/kg/day) or	≥0.0125 ppm in the total diet (≥0.00031 mg/kg/day) or	II
≥1 ppm in the total diet (≥0.025 mg/kg/day)	≥0.5 ppm in the total diet (≥0.0125 mg/kg/day)	≥0.25 ppm in the total diet (≥0.0063 mg/kg/day)	III

*The Redbook. Available at: http://www.fda.gov/Food/GuidanceComplianceRegulatoryInformation/GuidanceDocuments/ FoodIngredientsandPackaging/Redbook/default.htm. Accessed October 24, 2011.

such as pentanol would be assigned to category A. Similarly, a substance containing an α,β-unsaturated carbonyl function, epoxide, thiazole, or imidazole group would be assigned to category C. Thus, based on structure assignment and calculated exposure, the CLs are assigned (Table 31-11). For example, 0.03 ppm of a substance in Structure Category B would be assigned CL II. In contrast, the same dose (ie, 0.03 ppm) of a substance in Structure Category A would be assigned to the lesser CL I.

Once the CL is established, a specific test battery is mandated (Table 31-8). The tests for CL III are the most demanding and provide the greatest breadth for the determination of adverse biological effects, including effects on reproduction. The tests are comprehensive enough to detect nearly all types of observable toxicity, including malignant and benign tumors, preneoplastic lesions, and other forms of chronic toxicity. The tests for CL II are of intermediate breadth. These tests are designed to detect the most toxic phenomena other than late-developing histopathological changes. The short-term (genotoxicity) tests are intended to identify substances for which chronic testing becomes critical. The CL I test battery is the least broad, as is appropriate for the level of hazard which substances in this category may pose. However, if untoward effects are noted, additional assessment becomes necessary. Studies of the absorption, distribution, metabolism, and elimination characteristics of a test substance are recommended before the initiation of toxicity studies longer than 90 days' duration. Of particular importance for many proposed food ingredients are data on their processing and metabolism in the GI tract.

Unique to food additive carcinogenicity testing is the controversial use of protocols that include an in utero phase. Under such protocols, parents of test animals are exposed to the test substance for four weeks before mating and throughout mating, gestation, and lactation. Most countries and international bodies do not subscribe to the combining of an in utero phase with a rat carcinogenicity study, as this presents a series of logistical and operational problems and substantially increases the cost of conducting a rat carcinogenicity study. The FDA began requesting in utero studies of the food industry in the early 1970s, when it was determined from lifetime feeding studies that the artificial sweetener saccharin produced bladder tumors in male rats when in utero exposure was included. Subsequently, the FDA required the food, drug, and cosmetic color industries to conduct lifetime carcinogenicity feeding studies of 18 color additives in rats using an in utero exposure phase.

Genetic toxicity tests are done to test chemicals for potential carcinogenicity and to assess whether a chemical may induce heritable genetic damage. Currently, genetic toxicity assays can be divided into three major groups: (1) forward and reverse mutation assays (eg, point mutations, deletions), (2) clastogenicity assays detecting structural and numerical changes in chromosomes (eg, chromosome aberrations, micronuclei), and (3) assays that identify DNA damage (eg, DNA strand breaks, unscheduled DNA synthesis).

Because the correlation between carcinogens and mutagens has proved to be less than desirable, as has been demonstrated by false-positive and false-negative findings when carcinogens and noncarcinogens have been examined in genetic toxicity tests, it is recommended that several tests be selected from a battery of tests. It should be kept in mind that as the number of tests employed increases, the possibility of false-negative results increases as well. Consequently, the National Toxicology Program (NTP) has advised that the vast majority of carcinogens are detected by both the *Salmonella* assay and rodent micronucleus tests.[6]

Safety Determination of Indirect Food Additives Indirect food additives are food additives that are not added directly to food, but enter food by migrating from surfaces that contact food. These surfaces may be from packaging material (eg, cans, paper, plastic) or the coating of packaging materials or surfaces used in processing, holding, or transporting food. As defined in the Act, a food contact substance is "any substance intended for use as a component of materials used in manufacturing, packing, packaging, transporting, or holding food if such use is not intended to have a technical effect in such food."

Essential to demonstrating the safety of an indirect additive are extraction studies with food-simulating solvents. The FDA recommends the use of three food-simulating solvents—10% ethanol, 50% ethanol, and corn oil or a synthetic triglyceride—for aqueous and acidic, alcoholic, and fatty foods, respectively (FDA, 2002a). The conditions of extraction depend in part on the intended conditions of use. Extraction studies are used to assess the level or quantity of a substance that might migrate and become a component of food, leading to consumer exposure.

To convert extraction data from packaging material into anticipated consumer exposure, the FDA has determined the fraction

[6]Available at: http://ntp.niehs.nih.gov/?objectid=12F22374-B4D0-2B5B-B021C109307FCD12. Accessed August 31, 2011.

of the US diet which comes into contact with different classes of material: glass, metal (coated and uncoated), paper (coated and uncoated), and polymers. For each class, the FDA has assigned a "consumption factor" (CF), which is the fraction of the total diet that comes into contact with an individual class of material.

The fraction of individual food types (aqueous, acidic, alcoholic, fatty) for which such packaging material is used is referred to as the food-type-distribution factor (f_T). To calculate cumulative estimated daily intake (CEDI), the following equation is used:

$$\text{CEDI} = \text{CF} \times [(f_{T\text{aqueous}} + f_{T\text{acidic}}) \times (\text{ppm of migrating substance in } 10\% \text{ ethanol}) + (f_{T\text{alcoholic}} \times \text{ppm of migrating substance in } 50\% \text{ ethanol}) + (f_{T\text{fatty}} \times \text{ppm of migrating substance in corn oil})] \times 3 \text{ kg/person/day}$$
$$= \text{mg/person/day}^7.$$

For additives with virtually no migration (<0.5 ppb), in which the CEDIs correspond to 1.5 μg/person/day, no safety studies are recommended. Migration levels, as determined by extraction studies, that are greater than 0.5 to 50 ppb (150 μg/person/day), in vitro genotoxicity tests should include bacterial mutagenicity and cytogenetic evaluation of chromosomal damage using mammalian cells or an in vitro mouse lymphoma assay. Where there is significant migration, that is, 50 ppb to 1 ppm (3 mg/person/day), genetic toxicity tests should be conducted and the substance should be further evaluated by two subchronic oral toxicity studies (one in a rodent species and one in a nonrodent species). The studies should provide an adequate basis for determining an ADI for the indirect additive or a constituent in the indicated range of CEDIs. In addition, the results of these studies will help determine whether longer-term or specialized safety tests (eg, metabolism studies, teratogenicity studies, reproductive toxicity studies, neurotoxicity studies, and immunotoxicity studies) should be conducted to assess the safety of these substances. For cumulative exposure greater than 1 ppm, FDA recommends submission of a food additive petition (FDA, 2002a).

Safety Requirements for GRAS Substances In spite of the fact that the FD&C Act and the relevant regulations scrupulously avoid defining food except in a functional sense—"food means articles used for food or drink for man or other animals...[and includes] chewing gum, and articles used for components of any such article"—it regards foods as GRAS when they are added to other food, for example, green beans in vegetable soup (Kokoski *et al.*, 1990; Burdock and Carabin, 2004). It also regards a number of food ingredients as GRAS, and these ingredients are listed under 21 CFR 182, 184, and 186. However, the language used acknowledges that there are substances the FDA considers to be GRAS, which are not listed. This accomplishes two things: (1) It leaves the door open for additional nonlisted substances to be affirmed as GRAS by the agency and (2) reinforces the concept that substances can be deemed GRAS whether or not they are listed by the FDA or on a publicly available list. A list of substances regarded as GRAS is given in Table 31-12. It is important to reemphasize that GRAS substances, though used like food additives, are not food additives. Although the distinction may seem to be one of semantics, it allows GRAS substances to be exempt from the premarket clearance requirements of a food additive petition, an opportunity to demonstrate safety through a history of safe use, and an exemption

Table 31-12

Examples of GRAS Substances and Their Functionality

CFR NUMBER	SUBSTANCE	FUNCTIONALITY
Substances GRAS 21 CFR 182		
182.2122	Aluminum calcium silicate	Anticaking agent
182.8985	Zinc chloride	Nutrient supplement
Direct food substances affirmed as GRAS 21 CFR 184		
184.1005	Acetic acid	Several
184.1355	Helium	Processing aid
Indirect food substances affirmed as GRAS 21 CFR 186		
186.1025	Caprylic acid	Antimicrobial
186.1374	Iron oxides	Ingredient of paper and paperboard
Notified GRAS substances With "No Objection"		
GRN 305	*Carnobacterium maltaromaticum* strain CB1 (viable and heat-treated)	(Antimicrobial) inhibitor of *Listeria monocytogenes*
GRN 211	Xanthan gum (with reduced pyruvate)	Stabilizer, emulsifier, thickener, suspending and bodying agent, and foam enhancer

GRAS, generally recognized as safe.

from the Delaney carcinogens clause because that clause of the Act pertains only to food additives.[8]

Although the courts have ruled that GRAS substances must be supported by the same quantity and quality of safety data that support food additives, this does not mean that the data must be identical in nature and character to that for a food additive. For uses of substances to be eligible for classification as GRAS, there must be common knowledge throughout the scientific community about the safety of substances directly or indirectly added to food (21 CFR 170.30); this is termed the "common knowledge standard" by FDA.[9] The studies relied on for concluding that a given use of a substance is GRAS must be published in the scientific literature. Such studies are unlikely to be conducted in accordance with FDA-recommended protocols, as these studies often are done for reasons unrelated to FDA approval and the data are thus not identical in nature and character to those for a food additive.

GRAS status also can be based on experience with common use in food before January 1, 1958,[10] which further distinguishes GRAS data requirements from those demanded of food additives. However,

---

[7] The 3 kg is FDA's value for daily food consumption, which, when multiplied by mg/kg (ppm) and the weighting factors, reduces to milligrams of the additive *per* day.

[8] See Assessment of Carcinogens.

[9] Available at: http://www.cfsan.fda.gov/?rdb/opa-g092.html. Accessed April 10, 2006.

[10] There are some exceptions to this rule. In at least one case, FDA has indicated that use before 1958 was not sufficient to demonstrate safety. (See GRAS Notice No. GRN 00040 on mineral oil). Available at: http://www.cfsan.fda.gov/?rdb/opa-g040.html. Accessed April 9, 2006.

in 1974, the FDA promulgated a regulation (21CFR170.3(f)) defining the term "common use in food" for purposes of section 201(s) of the FD&C Act as follows: "'[c]ommon use in food' means a substantial history of consumption of a substance by a significant number of *consumers in the United States*[11]." This requirement for use in the United States was challenged in court and held invalid on appeal.[12] In its decision, the court indicated that in the legislative history of the Act, discussion centered on a prolonged history of safe use, rather than a geographical restriction. Although the geographical limitation is no longer mentioned in the regulation, documentation of safe use in whatever domain relied upon must be clearly established. The FDA has made it clear, that although an ingredient may have an extensive history of use prior to 1958, this does not place it beyond regulatory reach, as new data generated must be taken into account—new data may trump history of use.[13]

FDA does have the last word as indicated in 21 CFR §170.38. The Commissioner, on his own initiative or on the petition of any interested person, may issue a notice in the Federal Register proposing to determine that a substance is not GRAS and is possibly an unsafe food additive subject to section §409 of the Act and subject to recall. Anyone has 60 days to respond to this notice, FDA will review the responses and act on its determination (ie, affirmation of the GRAS status or possible recall).

Lastly, because a GRAS determination does not have to be reported to FDA, the GRAS process should not be thought of as a refuge for those substances with a weak or "cherry-picked" data package that might not survive the scrutiny of a GRAS subjected to the voluntary notification procedure or those GRAS determinations approved by unqualified "experts" (FD&C §201(s); *Federal Register* 75: 81536–81543, December 28, 2010). Placing a substance in commerce that has not met the appropriate requirements can have consequences; under the Food Safety Modernization Act, signed into law January 4, 2011, new powers were conferred to FDA regarding adulterants in the food supply, including mandatory recall and substantive civil and criminal penalties.

Establishing Safe Conditions of Use for New Foods, Macroingredients and New Technologies

New and novel foods or ingredients and new technologies present new challenges and may require innovative methods for determining safety. For example, with each new additive, it has been traditional (and rooted in a regulation such as 21 CFR 170.22) to establish an ADI, which is usually based on 1/100 of the NOEL (or NOAEL) established in animal testing. This works well for additives projected to be consumed at a level of 1.5 g/day or less (which is equal to or less than 25 mg/kg), for this extrapolates at a 100-fold safety factor to consumption by a rat at a level of 2500 mg/kg/day (about 5% of the rat's diet). The problem arises when a new food or macroingredient substitute becomes a substantive part of the diet (estimated to constitute as much as 15%–20%). For example, a macroingredient substitute or food projected to be consumed at a level of just 5% of the diet (150 g/day) would require the test animal (rat) to consume 250 g/kg/day, or slightly more than the 25% of the rat's body weight. To administer test substance in the diet at such high levels is an untenable test requirement; at such high

levels in the feed, dietary (ie, nutrient) displacement occurs and the investigator would establish an effect level only for malnutrition in the test animal, not for the toxicity of the macroingredient. Further, for some essential nutrients, such as vitamins A and D and iron, doses 100 times the nutritional use level would be toxic (Kokoski *et al.*, 1990). The answer therefore lies in the careful interpretation of toxicological data and the conduct, where appropriate, of special studies to assess drug interactions, nutrient interactions changes in gut flora, changes in gut activity, and the like (Munro, 1990; Borzelleca, 1992a,b). Also, it may be appropriate to consider what effect, if any, macroingredients may have on individuals with compromised digestive tracts, those dependent on laxatives, and those on high fiber diets, etc.

The regulatory approval of a new food additive is generally based on traditional toxicology studies. The rationale is that data from such studies will adequately predict adverse effects that could occur in humans. However, such studies, especially for novel foods, may not be adequate. Therefore, although human studies are not generally required for food additives, in the case of novel foods, human studies are likely essential in evaluating their safety (Stargel *et al.*, 1996).

Another useful tool in ensuring the safety of a food additive is monitoring it after its approval, or postmarketing surveillance. With widespread use of a food additive, *monitoring for consumption* can determine whether actual consumption exceeds the EDI and *monitoring for anecdotal complaints* may identify adverse health effects that escaped detection in earlier studies. This could be especially important for novel foods when traditional toxicology studies are not done at large multiples of the EDI (Butchko *et al.*, 1994, 1996). Also, mandated reporting to the Reportable Food Registry (mandated reporting of any reasonable probability that an article of human food or animal food/feed [including pet food] will cause serious adverse health consequences or death to humans or animals), although meant to detect adulteration, may also serve to provide information of a critical nature. Thus, the combination of traditional toxicity studies, special animal and human studies, and possibly postmarketing surveillance will ensure the safety of consumers and provide evidence to justify a safety factor different from 100.

Transgenic Plant (and New Plant Varieties) Policy Crops have been genetically modified using conventional breeding methods for more than a hundred years to produce new plant varieties with improved characteristics. Methods such as wide crosses of distantly related species that normally would not interbreed and mutagenesis of developing seeds using radiation or chemical mutagens have been successfully employed to produce genetic variation for selection of improved plant varieties. Over the past 10 to 15 years, scientists have employed biotechnology to add one or more specific genes into crops like soybean, corn, cotton, and canola to improve pest and disease management, resulting in agronomic, economic, environmental, health, and social benefits for farmers (Brooker and Barfoot, 2005; James, 2006, 2011). For example, a significant portion of the corn and cotton crops planted in the United States contains genes derived from the common soil bacterium *Bacillus thuringiensis* (Bt) that produce insect control proteins. Bt insect control proteins are toxic to certain caterpillar insect pests that attack corn and cotton plants but have no apparent effect on nontarget organisms (EPA, 1988; McClintock *et al.*, 1995; Mendelsohn *et al.*, 2003; OECD, 2007). By enabling the corn and cotton plants to protect themselves from this insect pest, the use of this product can reduce the need for and use of conventional insecticides (Gianessi and Carpenter, 1999; James, 2011).

Irrespective of the breeding method used to produce a new plant variety, tests must be done to ensure that the levels of nutrients

---

[11]Emphasis added.

[12]*Fmali Herb, Inc. v Heckler*, 715 F2d 1385 [9th Cir.1983].

[13]Available at: http://www.cfsan.fda.gov/?rdb/opa-g071.html. Accessed April 10, 2006.

or toxins in the plants have not changed and that the food is still safe to consume. For food/feed from biotechnology-derived crops, compositional analyses are done to ensure that the levels of key nutrients or toxins are comparable to food from conventional varieties. This is also done for a few conventionally bred crops where levels of important toxins such as glycoalkaloids in potatoes and erucic acid in rapeseed oil have been monitored. The International Life Sciences Institutes (ILSI, 2006; Alba *et al.*, 2010) supports a large crop composition database that provides information on the natural variability in composition for conventional corn, soybean, and cotton crops. This database provides a reference for comparing the nutrient composition of new crop varieties (Drury *et al.*, 2008; Lundry *et al.*, 2008; Harrigan *et al.*, 2010; Herman *et al.*, 2010). Animal feeding studies are also done with biotechnology-derived crops fed over several weeks to months to a variety of farm animal species to ensure that the performance (feed efficiency, milk production, etc) is comparable to that of conventional controls (Flachowsky *et al.*, 2005, 2007). Food safety studies have also been done with various biotechnology-derived crops to ensure that there are no treatment-related adverse findings (EFSA, 2008). The European Food Safety Authority (EFSA, 2008) reviewed the published animal feeding studies that have been done and concluded that in the majority of the studies there was no evidence of adverse effects. Clearly, new proteins produced in plant varieties must be nontoxic and not have the characteristics of proteins known to cause allergies. Thus, the proteins produced in genetically modified crops are evaluated for toxicity and allergenicity (Sjoblad *et al.*, 1992; Betz *et al.*, 2000; Pariza and Johnson, 2001, Metcalfe *et al.*, 1996; Astwood *et al.*, 2003; Delaney *et al.*, 2008; Hammond and Cockburn, 2008; Goodman *et al.*, 2008; Thomas *et al.*, 2009; Codex, 2009; Parrott *et al.*, 2010; EFSA, 2008, 2011a). The DNA that is introduced into genetically modified plants to direct the production of such new proteins has been determined to be GRAS (FDA, 1992).

The safety of new plant varieties (transgenic plants, genetically modified plants) is regulated primarily under the FDA's postmarket authority [section 402(a)(1) of the FD&C Act]. This section, previously applied to occurrences of unsafe levels of toxicants in food, is now applied to new plant varieties whose composition has been altered by an added substance. The new policy that has been applied to plants containing substances that are GRAS [Federal Register 57(104): 22984–23005]. The *Federal Register* notice (May 29, 1992) indicates that "[i]n most cases, the substances expected to become components of food as a result of genetic modification of a plant will be the same as or substantially similar to substances commonly found in food, such as proteins, fats and oils, and carbohydrates." The notice also indicates the responsibility of the FDA to exercise the premarket review process when the "objective characteristics of the substance raise questions of safety." In regard to substances within the new variety that are not similar to substances commonly found in food, a food additive petition may have to be filed.

The *Federal Register* notice offers points of consideration for the safety assessment of new plant varieties (Table 31-13). Accompanying these points of consideration are a decision flowchart and advice that the FDA be consulted on certain findings, for example, transference of allergens from one plant to another, a change in the concentration or bioavailability of nutrients, and the introduction of a new macroingredient.

In the United States, new plant varieties are regulated not only by the FDA, but also by the EPA and USDA. The FDA is responsible for the safety and labeling of foods and feeds derived from crops, irrespective of the method used to produce the new plant variety. The EPA is responsible for assuring the safety of pesticides; thus, in the example cited above whereby a pesticide is produced in a new plant variety, this product would also fall under EPA's

Table 31-13

Points of Consideration in the Safety Assessment of New Plant Varieties

Toxicants known to be characteristic of the host and donor species

The potential that food allergens will be transferred from one food source to another

The concentration and bioavailability of important nutrients for which a food crop is ordinarily consumed

The safety and nutritional value of newly introduced proteins

The identity, composition, and nutritional value of modified carbohydrates or fats and oils

jurisdiction. The USDA's Animal and Plant Health Inspection Service has responsibility for the environmental safety of field-testing and commercial planting of new plant varieties.

The developer of a biotechnology-derived crop variety must obtain registration from not only the country of origin but from importing countries as well (OECD, 1993). A variety of European/Global Scientific authorities (WHO, 1995; FAO, 1996; OECD, 1997; Codex, 2009; EFSA 2008, 2011a) have provided guidance on the safety assessment process for food and feed derived from biotechnology-derived crops. The process considers two main categories of potential risks: those related to the properties and function of the introduced protein(s), and those related to the whole food crop since insertion of the introduced gene(s) into the plant genome theoretically could cause unintended environmental effects. As in conventional crop breeding, agronomic studies carried out under diverse environmental conditions are used to screen for varieties that exhibit unintended changes so they can be eliminated from development. A review of research projects covering a period of more than 25 years done by the European Commission conclude that "biotechnology, and in particular GMO's, are not per se more risky than for example conventional plant breeding technologies" (EU, 2010).

Food Macroingredients The safety assessment of food ingredients consumed in large amounts presents some unique issues. Such ingredients include bulking agents (such as sorbitol, xylitol, or modified starches) to provide mass to the final product. For example, if one teaspoon of sugar (~4 g) is required to sweeten a cup of coffee, it would take only about 20 mg of aspartame to have the same effect—an amount too small for the consumer to measure accurately, so the familiar blue table-top packet will include aspartame and many times that amount in bulking agent. Bulking agents can be used on a larger scale, such as modified starches, synthetic starch (polydextrose), or indigestible fiber, to provide bulk to a meal, employing non-nutritive bulk to promote satiety.

Potential issues associated with macroingredients are (1) physical—a primary mechanical effect resulting from consumption of large amounts of any, especially a nondigestible, material that may result in mechanical blockage of the GI tract (such as konjac gum) or, the reverse, as demonstrated by certain sugar alcohols or polydextrose, which, because of their inability to undergo digestion, may result in osmotic diarrhea at high doses; (2) physical—a secondary effect of preventing absorption of other substances such as calcium and zinc loss because of the presence of phytic acid in certain plant fiber resulting in the formation of insoluble phosphates or the potential for loss of fat-soluble vitamins consequent to the use of large amounts of fat mimetics; (3) primary and secondary nutritional displacement: (a) primary—frank nutritional loss resulting from prolonged use of a nutrient substitute, and (b) secondary loss—the potential loss of micronutrients present in the substituted food and/or potential secondary (possibly undefined) benefits of consuming the displaced food; (4) possibly a toxic effect, but more likely a nontoxic metabolic or physiological effect, may occur as the result of exceeding the capacity of the user to metabolize or excrete the macroingredient, whereas the system in place was adequate for the displaced ingredient at its historic level of consumption; and, (5) toxicity—the amounts consumed by humans may exceed the proportionate amounts that could be given to test animals, which may have contained toxicants whose effects were not realized in the test animals, but may be seen in humans because of the increased consumption—minor processing impurities (eg, antinutrients such as trypsin inhibitors) or contaminants (eg, metals, reaction products such as furan or acrylamide, mycotoxins) may assume greater-than-usual importance (IPCS, 1987; IOM, 1999).

Nanotechnology Nanotechnology as applied to food science is a truly transformational technology, such as genetic engineering of plants and Nicolas Appert's invention of airtight food preservation were for previous generations. What makes nanoparticles (nanoengineered materials [NEM]) so unique is that conventional-sized particles (greater than 100 nm) obey conventional Newtonian physics, in which the individual atoms of a molecule or element act as a sum of all the parts. In contrast, NEM tend to obey the laws of quantum physics because their surface-to-mass ratio is so much greater—and with individual atoms closer to the surface, these individual atoms exercise much more influence on the physicochemical properties of the substance, often conferring physical properties much different than a conventional-sized particle (EPA, 2007; NNI, 2011). Potential differences of NEM as compared to their historical-sized counterparts include particle charge, melting point, solubility, surface tension, and many other characteristics that are normally thought of as immutable. In short, at the nanodimension, many new properties and thus new applications are possible for substances whose properties were previously thought to be known and fully exploited (Burdock, 2011).

There is no universal agreement on what constitutes a NEM, although the EFSA has defined a nanomaterial as a material that meets at least one of the following criteria: (1) consists of particles with one or more external dimensions in the size range of 1 to 100 nm for more than 1% of their number within the size distribution; (2) has internal or surface structures in one or more dimensions in the size range of 1 to 100 nm; and/or (3) has a specific surface area by volume greater than 60 m²/cm³, excluding materials consisting of particles with a size lower than 1 nm (EFSA, 2011b). Although FDA has declined to specifically define nanomaterial, in some recent (June, 2011) draft guidelines, it does offer two points industry might consider (1) "[w]hether an engineered material or end product has at least one dimension in the nanoscale range (approximately 1–100 nm)," and (2) "[w]hether an engineered material or end product exhibits properties or phenomena, including physical or chemical properties or biological effects, that are attributable to its dimension(s), even if these dimensions fall outside the nanoscale range, up to 1 μm."[14]

The GI tract is a particularly formidable digestive and protective organ with the stomach at a pH approaching 1.0, vigorous pancreatic enzymes, bile salts, and the luxuriant bacterial flora. The objective of this rugged environment is primarily for destruction of ingested pathogens and reduction of foods to absorbable particles.

The GI tract is an organ for selective absorption and is the first barrier to substances that should not be absorbed (eg, large molecules or charged molecules such as aluminum lakes of colors) or those substances that serve their function best by not being absorbed (eg, fiber). In this rugged environment, nanotechnology can provide a protective barrier (encapsulation technology) to allow labile substances to sustain their integrity until absorbed in the appropriate area of the intestine. Nanotechnology can also enhance absorption; for example, under normal circumstances, less than 20% of a dose of vitamin E is absorbed; however, the resistance of the intestine may be overcome and absorption enhanced by the ability of nano-sized particles to migrate through cells (transposition) or gain entry between enterocytes or through the use of encapsulation technology (Oberdörster, et al., 2005; Kwok, 2011).

The question then arises as to what impact nanotechnology might have on this balance of selective absorption, as many of the principles of absorption (as well as distribution, metabolism, and excretion) may be affected (EPA, 2007). For example, because the intestinal barrier may act as a safety mechanism by slow absorption of a substance, what effects might be seen when the rate and extent of absorption become equivalent to that of an intravenous injection? Likewise, the absence of teratological effects of many substances may be due to their inability to cross the placental barrier, or the lack of central nervous system (CNS) toxicity the result of their inability to cross the blood–brain barrier. Further, for a nanoparticle whose design allows easy entry, as the result of, for example, its size or coating, what effect will this attribute have on the ability of the target species to eventually excrete the particle (Burdock and Williams, 2008). Lastly, a striking observation regarding effects of such particles on health is their ability to generate toxic effects at the site of initial deposition as well as significant systemic toxic responses (EPA, 2004).

The above is not to imply that nano-sized particles have never been with us, as homogenization of milk has always resulted in some nano-sized micelles and a milling or grinding process is going to produce some particles <100 nm. No specific toxicity has been reported as the result of ingestion of nano-sized particles in food, but this may be because of the low level of exposure to the incidental presence of nano-sized particles or there may be observed effects of previously unknown origin and the linkage to nanoparticles has not been made. The physicochemical characteristics of NEM distinguish themselves from the parent substance in a non-NEM format; thus, regulatory agencies are in the process of promulgating guidelines for testing.

In January of 2011, the EFSA produced draft guidelines calling for toxicity testing of NEM, with special reference to in vitro genotoxicity testing (especially if a reactive oxygen species might be generated), ADME studies (likely to be the most affected by nanoparticles and metabolism and excretion parameters are important indicators of biopersistence and bioaccumulation), and a 90-day repeated dose study in rodents. Secondary in the strategy for NEM vetting are in vitro digestion studies, reproduction/developmental studies, and possibly chronic toxicity/carcinogenicity testing. Further, even prior to hazard identification (toxicity testing) is the mandate to characterize the NEM, which includes, but is not limited to, chemical composition, particle size (at least two methods and including size range and number distribution), physical form and morphology, particle and mass concentration, surface chemistry, surface charge, redox potential, dissolution/solubility, viscosity, density, pH, chemical reactivity/catalytic activity, photocatalytic activity, and others as appropriate (EFSA, 2011b). Importantly, as emphasized in the EFSA document, "If not indicated otherwise by consideration of the data, the conventional default uncertainty factors of 10 for inter- and 10 for intraspecies differences should be

[14]"Considering Whether an FDA-regulated Product Involves the Application of Nanotechnology" (draft) Guidance for Industry. Available at: http://www.fda.gov/RegulatoryInformation/Guidances/ucm257698.htm. Accessed August 20, 2011.

applied, as currently there are no indications for a need to modify these factors" (EFSA, 2011b).

FDA has not yet promulgated specific guidelines for testing, as FDA prefers to regulate on a product-by-product basis and does not regulate a technology per se, as this would tend to stifle innovation. However, as noted in its June, 2011 "Points to Consider…," FDA emphasizes examining particle behavior and characteristics (even if outside traditional 100-nm boundaries) "…because properties and phenomena of materials at the nanoscale enable applications that can affect safety, effectiveness, performance, quality, and, where applicable, public health impact of FDA-regulated products." FDA provides several examples to illustrate the changes that may be brought about by the use of nanotechnology, "…dimension-dependent properties or phenomena may be used for functional effects such as increased bioavailability, decreased dosage, or increased potency of a drug product, decreased toxicity of a drug product, better detection of pathogens, enhanced protection offered by improved food packaging materials, or improved delivery of a functional ingredient or a nutrient in food." FDA indicates these attributes may be brought about by changes typical of NEM, that is, "[T]he properties and phenomena may be due to altered chemical, biological, or magnetic properties, altered electrical or optical activity, increased structural integrity, or other unique characteristics of nanoscale materials not normally observed in their larger counterparts." In conclusion, FDA makes it very plain that conversion of an approved product (GRAS or food additive) to the nanoscale or producing changes to the material that may elicit the type of behavior seen at the nanoscale may well render the material unsafe. That is, the FDA statement to this effect is, "these changes may raise questions about the safety, effectiveness, performance, quality, or public health impact of the products."

Functional Foods

Functional foods are those foods (or food ingredients) whose contribution to the structure and function of the body exceeds their nutritive value. Functional foods include vegetable oil sterol esters and phytostanol esters (block cholesterol absorption), olestra (a medium for frying foods, but not absorbed by the GI tract and therefore does not contribute to caloric intake), fiber (promotes growth of beneficial bacteria, which lowers colonic pH, displaces pathogens, etc), resveratrol (antioxidant), decosahexaenoic acid and eicosapentaenoic acid (DHA/EPA) (essential fatty acids that play a role in reduction of risk of cardiovascular disease), equol (ameliorates symptoms of menopause without concomitant estrogen stimulation), and dimethyl glycine (antioxidant, improves oxygen utilization). Although these foods (or food ingredients) are consumed as such or added to food, they lack a regulatory niche and have been referred to by various names including "bioactive foods" (Rulis, 2005) or more commonly, "nutraceuticals." These are foods or food ingredients, not drugs, as long as the claims for them do not indicate they are "intended for use in the diagnosis, cure, mitigation, treatment, or prevention of disease in man or other animals" (the definition of a drug, FFDCA §201(g)(1)(B)). FDA has held that claims for any beneficial effects for these ingredients (as food ingredients) must be based on their nutritive value; however, these same ingredients, when sold as a dietary supplement, may include claims for the beneficial effects, irrespective of nutritive value as long as the claim is truthful and not misleading.

Fiber Dietary fiber belongs to the broad category of carbohydrates. Fiber can be classified into soluble (eg, gums, pectins in fruits, peas, and beans), insoluble (eg, cellulose, whole grain foods, tomato skins), or mixed (eg, bran), and fermentable (eg, pectins, inulins, oligosaccharides) or nonfermentable (eg, cellulose,

lignans) (Carabin and Flamm, 1999). Fiber sources are now also divided according to those found naturally in plants (*dietary fiber*—cellulose, pectin gums, etc) and isolated or synthetic fibers (*functional fiber*—resistant starch, pectin, and commercially produced fibers such as PGX—a molecule produced from konjac, alginate, and xanthan gums) (Carabin *et al.*, 2009).

Insoluble, nonfermentable fibers are known for their bulking effect that decreases transit time and increases fecal mass. The extent of fermentation of fiber depends on its physical and chemical structure. Fermentable dietary fiber is acted upon by colonic anaerobic bacteria leading to the production of lactic acid, short-chain fatty acids (acetate, propionate, and butyrate), and gases (H_2, CO_2, and CH_4) (Roberfroid, 1993). Modulating effects of fiber considered beneficial for overall health are: (a) increased water-holding capacity of the stool, (b) increase in stool volume and decreased transit time, (c) increased vitamin and mineral absorption, (d) as the product of fermentation, an increase in the colonic bifidobacteria and lactobacilli count (lowering of pH and subsequent decrease in the pathogenic types of bacteria), (e) fermentation also gives rise to absorption of certain organic compounds (eg, short chain fatty acids that promote immune function), and (f) histological and functional changes in the intestinal epithelium (Roberfroid, 1993, 2007; Carabin and Flamm, 1999; Greger, 1999; Scholz–Ahrens and Schrezenmeir, 2007).

In general, dietary fiber has not been shown to exhibit toxicity upon repeated dosing, to be genotoxic or carcinogenic and in general, to adversely affect glycemic control, lipid metabolism, or colonic flora (Carabin and Flamm, 1999). Fiber can enhance uptake of minerals, if phytic acid (hexakisphosphate, a plant storage form of phosphate) is not present. The only potential adverse effect is the inability of the consumer to tolerate the ingested fiber (which may result in GI discomfort, including gas, or diarrhea), the extent of which is generally related to the average degree of polymerization (DP) of the fiber. DP for various fermentable products includes inulin (DP = 2–60, DP_{avg} = 12) and oligofructose (DP = 2–8, DP_{avg} = 4) (Roberfroid, 2007); in general, the lower the average DP, the quicker the fermentation time and the increased possibility of intestinal discomfort. Therefore, clinical "tolerance studies" are conducted to determine the reaction of test subjects de novo or following an acclimation period (Carabin *et al.*, 2010).

DMG Dimethylglycine (*N*,*N*-dimethylglycine or DMG) is present in a broad range of foods including meats (especially liver), grains, legumes, and other edible plants (Balch and Balch, 1997). A necessary and endogenous component of human, animal, and plant metabolism, DMG is an intermediary metabolite in cellular choline and betaine metabolism and is involved in a variety of biological roles, including a major role in the contribution of glycine for synthesis of glutathione, an endogenous antioxidant (Friesen *et al.*, 2007). Additional to and independent of its role in glutathione synthesis, the scavenging potential of orally administered DMG for free radicals has also been demonstrated in rats with ulcers; also, DMG neutralized free radicals and inhibited lipid peroxidation to reduce oxidative stress under conditions of depleted glutathione concentrations (Hariganesh and Prathiba, 2000).

Although DMG has been available since the 1970s as a dietary supplement for the improvement of athletic performance (Tonda and Hart, 1992), its efficacy as a performance enhancer in humans has not been confirmed (Harpaz *et al.*, 1985; Bishop *et al.*, 1987). DMG may, however, act to enhance the immune system (Reap and Lawson, 1990) and has been suggested to assist in the maintenance of aged mitochondria (Pak and Jeong, 2010).

In animal feed (eg, swine and poultry feeds), DMG acts as an external emulsification agent and improves the digestibility of crude fat, protein, and nitrogen-free components, which makes these fractions more available for nutritional purposes (Cools *et al.*, 2010; Kalmar *et al.*, 2010). Emulsifiers have been used for years in swine feeds to improve nutrient digestibility and, due to improved nutrient utilization, to decrease feed costs (Jones *et al.*, 1992; Dierick and Decuypere, 2004). As an added benefit for commercial broilers, the metabolic and nonenzymatic antioxidant properties of DMG also improve oxygen utilization and reduce oxidative stress. Improved oxygen utilization compensates for the inadequate cardiovascular system that makes modern broiler strains susceptible to the development of pulmonary hypertension and ascites, which in turn can result in high (>25%) mortality and financial loss (Kalmar *et al.*, 2010). The reduction of oxidative stress, a known physiological factor in the pathogenesis of ascites (Bottje and Wideman, 1995), attenuates the progression of pulmonary hypertension. DMG has also been shown to increase oxygen uptake and retard the formation of lactic acid in rats, rabbits, and horses under stressed conditions (Meduski *et al.*, 1980; Levine *et al.*, 1982) and to reduce recovery periods for equine and canine athletes (Gannon and Kendall, 1982; Rose *et al.*, 1989).

Safety Requirements for Dietary Supplements

Following a nearly 70-year history of questions concerning the regulatory classification of dietary supplements (during which time dietary supplements had been variously classified as drugs or unapproved food additives), on October 15, 1994, President Clinton signed into law the Dietary Supplement Health and Education Act. Relevant to this discussion on safety, the amendment to the Act is significant in several respects: (1) a dietary ingredient must have its origin as a constituent of food or a metabolite thereof (see FFDCA§201(ff) of the act for a complete list); (2) there is a different standard of safety for dietary supplements than for food ingredients, that is, a "reasonable *expectation* of no harm" in contrast to that for food ingredients, "a reasonable *certainty* of no harm"; (3) a genuine grandfathering provision allowing history of use to count for all or part of the determination of safety with no notification required for (a) a dietary ingredient in use before October 15, 1994, or (b) if an equivalent amount had already been approved for use in food, or (c) if an equivalent amount is present in a food that has been consumed for at least 25 years; (4) a requirement for notification of the FDA for any "new" dietary ingredient and that the notification should describe the rationale used to determine the "reasonable expectation of no harm"; and, (5) the burden of proof of lack of safety is the responsibility of FDA.

A troubling finding is that in 1994, the FDA estimated that 4000 dietary supplements were on the market. The agency now says there are more than 55,000 products on the market, but in the interval of October 1994 to July of 2011, the agency has received only 700 new dietary-ingredient notifications (filings).[15] Of those filings, approximately 70% have been rejected by FDA as being incomplete (inadequate identification of the product, errors in directions for use, inadequate evidence of safety, etc). This high rejection rate fuelled demands for guidelines from the agency on what should be included in a notification and how the safety requirements might be met. The agency ultimately responded with draft guidelines in July, 2011.[16]

Unlike the testing guidelines for food ingredients, wherein functional groups and exposure dictate the CL and resulting testing regimen, testing guidelines for dietary supplements rely heavily on proposed exposure of the material as a supplement versus historical exposure (length of exposure and quantity of exposure) of that material (Table 31-14).

Assessment of Carcinogens

Carcinogenicity as a Special Problem Congress provided the FDA with wide latitude in assessing safety and assuring a safe food supply with one exception. That exception is a provision of the FD&C Act known as the Delaney clause, which prohibits the approval of regulated food additives "found to induce cancer when ingested by man or animals" [sections 409(c)(3)(A), 706(b)(5)(B), and 512(d)(1)(H)].

The Delaney prohibition applies only to the approval of food additives, color additives, and animal drugs; it does not apply to unavoidable contaminants or GRAS substances or ingredients sanctioned by the FDA or USDA before 1958. The clause also does not apply to constituents that are present in food or color additives or animal drugs, provided that the level of such contaminants can be demonstrated to be safe and the whole additive, including its contaminants, is not found to induce cancer in humans or animals. This interpretation of the Delaney clause was set forth by the FDA in its so-called "constituent policy" published on April 2, 1982, as an Advanced Notice of Proposed Rulemaking. The policy mandates the development and use of animal carcinogenicity data and probabilistic risk assessment to establish a safe level for the contaminant in the additive under its intended conditions of use.

The constituent policy and, as will be discussed later, the implementation of the so-called diethylstilbestrol (DES) proviso for animal drugs under the Delaney clause have forced the FDA to develop a means for establishing safe levels for carcinogenic substances. The DES proviso allows the addition of carcinogenic animal drugs to animal feed if they leave no residue in edible tissue as determined by an approved analytic procedure. To do this, the FDA has turned to the use of probabilistic risk assessment in which tumor data in animals are mathematically extrapolated to an upper bound risk in humans exposed to particular use levels of the additive. The FDA takes the position that considering the many conservative assumptions inherent in the procedure, an upper bound lifetime risk of one cancer in a million individuals is the biological equivalent of zero.

Much controversy surrounds the use of risk assessment procedures, in part because estimates of risk are highly dependent on the many assumptions that must be made. The common practice of testing at a maximum tolerated dose (MTD) (Williams and Weisburger, 1991) raises the question of appropriateness to human exposure. Do high test doses cause physiological changes unlike those from human exposure? The basic assumption in quantitative risk assessment (QRA) is that the dose–response curve is linear beneath the lowest observable effect and may result in the calculation of relatively high risks even at doses that are much lower than the lowest dose that produces cancer in experimental animals. QRA is more a process than a science; many steps in the process are based on assumptions, not proven scientific facts. If only the most conservative assumptions are made throughout the process, many will represent overestimates of human risk by 10- or 100-fold, leading to a combined overestimate of perhaps a million-fold or more. Table 31-15 provides some rough estimates of potential ranges of uncertainty that might lead to large overestimates (Flamm and Lorentzen, 1988).

Historically, the FDA has employed a high threshold for establishing that a food or color additive has been found to induce cancer

---

[15]Available at: http://www.sltrib.com/sltrib/politics/52397201-90/companies-dietary-fda-guidance.html.csp. Accessed August 18, 2011.

[16]Available at: http://www.fda.gov/Food/GuidanceComplianceRegulatoryInformation/GuidanceDocuments/DietarySupplements/ucm257563.htm. Accessed August 18, 2011.

Table 31-14

Dietary Supplement Safety Testing Recommendations Matrix*

DOCUMENTED HISTORICAL USE	PROPOSED USE OF THE NEW DIETARY INGREDIENT		TWO-STUDY GENETIC TOXICITY BATTERY†	THREE-STUDY GENETIC TOXICITY BATTERY‡	14-DAY RANGE-FINDING ORAL STUDY IN ANIMALS	90-DAY SUBCHRONIC ORAL STUDY IN ANIMALS§	ONE-GENERATION RODENT REPRODUCTIVE STUDY‖	MULTIGENERATION RODENT REPRODUCTIVE STUDY‖	TERATOLOGY STUDY IN ANIMALS‖	ONE-YEAR CHRONIC TOXICITY OR TWO-YEAR CARCINOGENESIS STUDY IN ANIMALS¶	SINGLE-DOSE TOLERABILITY AND/OR ADME STUDY IN ANIMALS AND/OR HUMANS¶	REPEAT-DOSE TOLERABILITY AND/OR ADME STUDY IN ANIMALS AND/OR HUMANS¶
Daily chronic	Intermittent	< Hx use#	Documented history of use should be sufficient as evidence of safety									
		> Hx use	✓		✓	✓			✓		✓	
	Daily chronic	< Hx use	Documented history of use should be sufficient as evidence of safety									
		> Hx use	✓		✓	✓	✓		✓	✓		✓
Intermittent	Intermittent	< Hx use	Documented history of use should be sufficient as evidence of safety									
		> Hx use	✓		✓	✓					✓	
	Daily chronic	< Hx use		✓	✓	✓	✓		✓			
		> Hx use		✓	✓	✓	✓	✓	✓	✓		✓
No history	Daily chronic			✓	✓	✓	✓	✓	✓	✓		✓
	Intermittent			✓	✓	✓			✓			✓

*Draft Guidance for Industry: Dietary Supplements: New Dietary Ingredient Notifications and Related Issues (http://www.fda.gov/Food/GuidanceComplianceRegulatoryInformation/GuidanceDocuments/DietarySupplements/ucm257563.htm#table2. Accessed August 9, 2011).

†A two-study genetox battery (bacterial mutagenesis and in vitro cytogenetics) that includes a test for gene mutations in bacteria, either an in vitro mouse lymphoma thymidine kinase+/− gene mutation assay (preferred) or another suitable in vitro test with cytogenetic evaluation of chromosomal damage using mammalian cells.

‡A three-study genetic toxicity (genetox) battery includes tests cited in the two-study genetox battery, plus an in vivo test for chromosomal damage using mammalian hematopoietic cells.

§In general, if there is no history of use, two species should be used for 90-day subchronic studies. In addition, the one-year chronic toxicity study or two-year carcinogenesis study should be done in two species. However, the one-year chronic toxicity study, two-year carcinogenesis study, or second subchronic study may not be necessary in some cases based on the amount and type of historical use data or the duration of use of the NDI, if significantly shorter than lifetime daily use.

‖Reproductive and teratology testing is not needed if the product is labeled as not for use by women of childbearing age, pregnant or lactating women, and children 13 and younger.

¶Special studies such as one-year chronic toxicity studies in animals, two-year carcinogenicity studies in animals, and ADME, bioavailability, and tolerability studies in animals and/or humans should be conducted on a case-by-case basis, as appropriate, if the toxicology data or the identity of the NDI raise a special safety concern.

#Historical use.

Table 31-15

Uncertainty Parameters and Their Associated Range of Risk Factors

UNCERTAINTY PARAMETERS	ESTIMATED RANGE (FACTOR)
Extrapolation model	1–10,000
Total dose vs dose rate	30–45
Most-sensitive sex/strain vs average sensitivity	1–100
Sensitivity of human vs test animal	1–1000
Potential synergism or antagonism with other carcinogens or promoters	1–1000?
Total population vs target population, potential vs actual market penetration	1–1000
Absorptive rate (gut, skin, lung) for animals at high dose vs humans at low dose	1–10
Dose scaling: mg/kg body weight, ppm (diet, water, feed) surface area	1–15
Upper confidence on users or exposed	1–10
Specifications or tolerances	1–10
Limits of detection vs actual levels	1–1000
Additivity vs nonadditivity of multiple sites	1–3
Survival or interim sacrifice adjustments	1–2
Knowledge of only high-end plateau dose response	1–10
Error or variation in detection methods	1–10
Adjustments for less than lifetime bioassays	1–100
Adjustments for intermittent and less than lifetime human exposure	1–100
Use vs nonuse of historical data	1–2
Upper confidence and lower confidence limits vs expected values in extrapolation level of acceptable risk	1–1000
Level of acceptable risk	1–1000
Adding or not adding theoretical risks from many substances	1–100

SOURCE: Flamm WG, Lorentzen RJ. Quantitative risk assessment (qra): A special problem in the approval of new products. In Cothern CR, Mehlman MA, Marcus WL, eds. Risk Assessment and Risk Management of Industrial and Environmental Chemicals. Princeton, NJ: Princeton Scientific Publishing Co, Inc; 1988.

when ingested by humans or animals. If these additives are found to induce cancer, they cannot be approved for foods or colors, no matter how small the estimated risk. In the end, very few substances have been disapproved or banned because of the Delaney clause. Two indirect food additives (Flectol H and mercaptoimidazole) that migrate from packaging material were banned. Among direct additives, safrole, cinnamyl anthranilate, thiourea, and diethylpyrocarbonate were banned because of the Delaney clause, and diethylpyrocarbonate because it forms urethane.

A number of substances (eg, butylated hydroxyanisole [BHA], xylitol, methylene chloride, sorbitol, trichloroethylene, nitrilotriacetic acid [NTA], diethylhexyl phthalate, melamine, formaldehyde, bentonite) listed in the Code of Federal Regulation as food additives are also listed as carcinogens by NTP, the International Agency for Research on Cancer (IARC), or the state of California (under the Safe Drinking Water and Toxic Enforcement Act of 1986, also known as Proposition 65). How is this possible, and on what basis do these food additive listings continue?

Despite the fact that tests and conditions exist under which each of these substances will produce cancer in animals, the FDA has found it possible to continue listing these substances as food additives. The reasoning applied in almost every case is based on secondary carcinogenesis. The one exception is formaldehyde,

which is carcinogenic only on inhalation, and there are compelling reasons to believe that inhalation is not an appropriate test in this case (Flamm and Frankos, 1985). Therefore, formaldehyde is not treated as a carcinogen prohibited by the Delaney clause.

For BHA, which induces forestomach cancer, the concept has been advanced that its carcinogenicity is attributable primarily to a cycle of irritation and restorative hyperplasia (Clayson *et al.*, 1986). For xylitol, a sugar alcohol, an increase in bladder tumors and adrenal pheochromocytomas are considered secondary to calcium imbalance resulting from the indigestibility of sugar alcohols and their fermentation in the lower GI tract. Sorbitol, another sugar alcohol, behaves in a similar manner. For NTA, the argument is secondary carcinogenesis, and although specific explanations vary, the mechanism involving zinc imbalance has considerable scientific support.

Thus, the FDA has generally interpreted the phrase "found to induce cancer when ingested by man or animals" as excluding cancers that arise through many secondary means. Therefore, to be a carcinogen under the Delaney clause, a food or color additive must be demonstrated to induce cancer by primary means when ingested by humans or animals or to induce cancer by other routes of administration that are found to be appropriate. This is interpreted to mean that the findings of cancer must be clearly reproducible and that the cancers found are not secondary to nutritional, hormonal, or physiological imbalances. This position allows the agency to argue that changing the level of protein or fat in the diet does not induce cancer but simply modulates tumor incidence (Kritschevsky, 1994).

Biological Versus Statistical Significance Much can be learned about the proper means of assessing carcinogenicity data by studying large databases for substances that have been tested for carcinogenicity many times. The artificial sweetener cyclamate is an example. The existence of more than a dozen studies on cyclamate and the testing of multiple hypotheses at dozens of different organ and tissue sites in all these studies led to the awareness that the overall false-positive error rate could be inflated if individual findings were viewed out of context (FDA, 1984). Therefore, very careful attention must be paid to the totality of the evidence.

The possibility of false-negative error is always of concern because of the need to protect public health. However, it should be recognized that any attempt to prove absolutely that a substance is not carcinogenic is futile. Therefore, an unrelenting effort to minimize false-negative errors can produce an unacceptably high probability of a false positive. Further, demanding certainty (ie, a zero or implicitly an extremely low probability of false-negative error) has negative consequences for an accurate decision-making process. This is the case because it severely limits the ability to discriminate between carcinogens and noncarcinogens on the basis of bioassays (FDA, 1984).

In addition to the false-positive/false-negative trap, which is a statistical matter, there are many potential biological traps. The test substance, typically administered at high MTDs, may affect one or more of the many biological processes known to modulate tumor incidence at a specific organ site without causing an induction of tumors at that or any other site. Nutritional imbalances such as choline deficiency are known to lead to a high incidence of liver cancer in rats and mice. Simple milk sugar (lactose) is known to increase the incidence of Leydig cell tumors in rats. Caloric intake has been shown to be a significant modifying factor in carcinogenesis. Impairment of immune surveillance by a specific or nonspecific means (stress) affecting immune responsiveness and hormonal imbalance can result in higher incidences of tumors at specific organ sites. Hormonal imbalance, which can be caused by hormonally active agents (eg, estradiol) or by other substances that act indirectly, such as vitamin D, may result in an increased tumor incidence. Chronic cell injury and restorative hyperplasia resulting from treatment with lemon flavor (D-limonene) probably are responsible for renal tumor development in male rats by mechanisms that are of questionable relevance to humans (Flamm and Lehman–McKeeman, 1991). In these examples, the increases in tumor incidence at specific organ sites probably are secondary to significant changes in normal physiological balance and homeostasis. Moreover, the increases in tumor incidence, and hence the increases in the risk of cancer, probably would not occur except at toxic doses (Ames and Gold, 1997).

To preserve the ability of a bioassay to discriminate between carcinogens and noncarcinogens, the possibility of false-positive or false-negative results and the possibility of secondary effects must be considered. To be meaningful, evaluations must be based on the weight of evidence. Particular attention must be given to the many factors that are used in deciding whether tumor incidences are biologically as well as statistically significant. These factors include (1) the historical rate of the tumor in question (is it a rare tumor, or does it occur frequently in the controls?); (2) the survival histories of dosed and test animals (did dosed animals survive long enough to be considered "at risk" and what effect did chemical toxicity and reduced survival have in the interpretation of the data?); (3) the patterns of tumor incidence (was the response dose-related?); (4) the biological meaningfulness of the effect (was it experimentally consistent with

the evidence from related studies and did it occur in a target organ?); (5) the reproducibility of the effect with other doses, sexes, or species; (6) evidence of hyperplasia, metaplasia, or other signs of an ongoing carcinogenic process (is the effect supported by a pattern of related non-neoplastic lesions, particularly at lower doses?); (7) evidence of tumor multiplicity or progression; and (8) the strength of the evidence of an increased tumor incidence (what is the magnitude of the P value, for pairwise comparison and for trend?).

A good discussion of the use of these factors by scientists in deciding whether a substance induces cancer in animals is contained in the notice of a final rule permanently listing FD&C Yellow No. 6 (51 *Federal Register* 41765–41783, 1988). An elevation of tumor incidence in rats was identified at two organ and/or tissue sites: (1) medullary tumors of the adrenal glands in female rats only and (2) renal cortical tumors in female rats only. Scientists at the FDA concluded that the increase in medullary tumors of the adrenal glands in female rats did not suffice to establish that FD&C Yellow No. 6 is a carcinogen. The basis for the decision was (1) a lack of dose response, (2) the likelihood of false positives, (3) the lack of precancerous lesions, (4) morphological similarity of adrenal medullary lesions in treated and control rats, (5) an unaffected latency period, (6) a lack of effect in male rats, and (7) a comparison with other studies in which there was no association between exposure to FD&C Yellow No. 6 and the occurrence of adrenal medullary tumors.

A similar judgment was made with respect to the cortical renal lesions in female rats, which were not found to provide a basis for concluding that FD&C Yellow No. 6 can induce cancer of the kidneys. The main reasons leading to this conclusion were (1) the relatively common occurrence of proliferative renal lesions in aged male control rats (28 months or older), (2) the lack of renal tumors in treated males despite their usually greater sensitivity to renal carcinogens, (3) the lack of malignant tumors indicating no progression of adenomas to a malignant state, (4) the lack of a decreased latency period compared with controls, (5) the coincidence of renal proliferative lesions and chronic renal disease, (6) the lack of genotoxicity, and (7) a lack of corroborative evidence from other studies that suggests a treatment-related carcinogenic effect of FD&C Yellow No. 6 on the kidney. Both these examples emphasize the importance of considering all the evidence in attempting to decide the significance of any subset of data.

As essential elements, vitamins, sugars, and calories by themselves can increase tumor incidence in test animals; the mechanism by which tumors arise as the result of exposure to food or food ingredients is critically important to assessing the relevance of the finding to the safety of the substance under its intended conditions of use in food. In an earlier review, McClain (2002) discussed mechanistic consideration in the regulation and classification of chemical carcinogens. More recently, Cohen and Arnold (2011) reviewed chemical carcinogenesis and included discussions on mechanism and testing of carcinogens as well as on mode of action and human relevance.

Carcinogenic Contaminants The Delaney clause, which prohibits the addition of carcinogens to food, could ban many food additives and color additives if strictly interpreted to include contaminants of additives within its definition. Clearly, this was not Congress's intent, and just as clearly, the FDA needed to develop a common sense policy for addressing the problem that all substances, including food and color additives, may contain carcinogenic contaminants at some trace level.

Toward this end, the agency argued (FDA, 1982b) that banning food and color additives simply because they have been found or are known to contain a trace level of a known carcinogen does not make sense because all substances may contain carcinogenic contaminants. The agency asserted in its constituent policy that the mere fact an additive contains a contaminant known to be carcinogenic should not automatically lead the agency to ban that food additive but should instead cause the agency to consider the health risks it poses based on its level of contamination and the conditions of its use (FDA, 1977).

ADVERSE REACTIONS TO FOOD OR FOOD INGREDIENTS

Up to 25% of respondents in a survey indicated they had experienced an adverse reaction to a food at some point in their lives (Chapman *et al.*, 2006). Assuming these respondents were not exposed to a frank toxin and, that in fact, they consumed foods not reported harmful to others, these adverse reactions could be divided into allergies, idiosyncratic reactions (often confined to a specific demographic exhibiting a genetic anomaly), an anaphylactoid reaction, a food-drug interaction or, a metabolic (or normal physiological reaction) as the result of a wilful action of the consumer (such as overconsumption or inadequate processing of the food) (Table 31-16).

The categories in this section are not exhaustive, nor all inclusive, and one substance may produce a number of effects. For example, an adverse reaction to wheat can be exhibited in a variety of ways: (1) acute IgE-medicated reactions, (2) local inhalational reactions (eg, Baker asthma), (3) systemic reactions that occur when wheat is ingested following exercise and, (4) cell-mediated reactions in atopic dermatitis and celiac disease (Chapman *et al.*, 2006).

Table 31-16

Adverse Reaction to Food: Definition of Terms

TERM	DEFINITION	CHARACTERISTICS/EXAMPLES
Adverse reaction (sensitivity) to a food	General term that can be applied to a clinically abnormal response attributed to an ingested food or food additive	Any untoward pathological reaction resulting from ingestion of a food or food additive. May be immune-mediated
Food hypersensitivity (allergy)	An immunological reaction and may occur only in some patients, may occur after only a small amount of the substance is ingested, and is unrelated to any physiological effect of the food or food additive	Immune-mediated (cellular or humoral response), requires prior exposure to antigen or cross-reacting antigen. First exposure may have been asymptomatic
Food anaphylaxis	A classic allergic hypersensitivity reaction to food or food additives	A humoral immune response most often involving IgE antibody and release of chemical mediators. Mortality may result
Food intolerance	A general term describing an abnormal physiological response to an ingested food or food additive; this reaction may be an immunological, idiosyncratic, metabolic, pharmacological, or toxic response.	Any untoward pathological reaction resulting from ingestion of a food or food additive. Reaction may be immune-mediated. Examples include celiac disease (intolerance to wheat, rye, barley, oats).
Food toxicity (poisoning)	A term use to imply an adverse effect caused by the direct action of a food or food additive on the host recipient without the involvement of immune mechanisms. This type of reaction may involve nonimmune release of chemical mediators. Toxins may be contained within food or released by microorganisms or parasites contaminating food products	Not immune-mediated. May be caused by bacterial endo- or exotoxin (eg, hemorrhagic *E coli*), fungal toxin (eg, aflatoxin), tetrodotoxin from pufferfish, domoic acid from mollusks, histamine poisoning from fish (scombroid poisoning), nitrate poisoning (ie, methemoglobinuria).
Food idiosyncrasy	A quantitatively abnormal response to a food substance or additive; this reaction differs from its physiological or pharmacological effect and resembles hypersensitivity but does not involve immune mechanisms. Food idiosyncratic reactions include those which occur in specific groups of individuals who may be genetically predisposed	Not immune-mediated, favism (hemolytic anemia related to deficiency of erythrocytic glucose-6-phosphate dehydrogenase), fish odor syndrome, beeturia, lactose intolerance, fructose intolerance, asparagus urine, red wine intolerance
Anaphylactoid reaction to a food	An anaphylaxis-like reaction to a food or food additive as a result of nonimmune release of chemical mediators. This reaction mimics the symptoms of food hypersensitivity (allergy)	Not immune-mediated. Scombroid poisoning, sulfite poisoning, red wine sensitivity
Food–drug interaction	A change in the pharmacokinetic or pharmacodynamic action of a drug as the result of ingestion of a food	Not immune-mediated. Ingestion of fats, phytates or fiber to change absorption; upregulation of genes by *Brassica*, polyunsaturated fats; unregulation of polypeptide transporters by St Johns wort.
Metabolic food reaction	Toxic effects of a food when eaten in excess or improperly prepared	Cycasin, vitamin A toxicity, goiterogens, licorice

SOURCE: Adapted from Anderson JA, Sogn DD, eds. Adverse Reactions to Foods. Washington, DC: US Department of Health and Human Services; 1984.

Table 31-17

Symptoms of IgE-mediated Food Allergies

Cutaneous	Urticaria (hives), eczema, dermatitis, pruritus, rash
Gastrointestinal	Nausea, vomiting, diarrhea, abdominal cramps
Respiratory	Asthma, wheezing, rhinitis, bronchospasm
Other	Anaphylactic shock, hypotension, palatal itching, swelling including tongue and larynx, methemoglobinemia*

An unusual manifestation of allergy reported to occur in response to soy or cow milk protein intolerance in infants.

SOURCE: *Murray KF, Christie, DL. Dietary protein intolerance in infants with transient methemoglobinemia and diarrhea. J Pediatr. 1993;122:90. With permission from Elsevier.*

Adapted from Taylor SL, Scanlan RA, eds. Food Toxicology: A Perspective on the Relative Risks. New York: Marcel Dekker; 1989. With permission from Copyright Clearance Center.

Food Allergy

Food hypersensitivity (allergy) refers to a reaction involving an immune-mediated response. Such a response is generally IgE-mediated, although IgG4- and cell-mediated immunity may also play a role in some instances (Fukutomi *et al.*, 1994). What generally distinguishes food allergy from other reactions is the involvement of immunoglobulins, basophils, or mast cells (the latter being a source of mediating substances including histamine and bradykinin for immediate reactions and prostaglandins and leukotrienes for slower-developing reactions) and a need for a prior exposure to the allergen or a cross-reactive allergen. An allergic reaction may be manifested by one or more of the symptoms listed in Table 31-17. The list of foods known to provoke allergies is long and is probably limited only by what people are willing to eat, although milk, egg, peanut, tree nut, fish, and shellfish account for more than 50% of all food allergies (Schneider–Chafen *et al.*, 2010). Although cutaneous reactions and anaphylaxis (a severe allergic reaction, resulting in a drop of blood pressure, and may be fatal) are the most common symptoms associated with food allergy, the body is replete with a repertoire of responses that are rarely confined to only a few foods.

Eosinophilic esophagitis (EoE) is a newly recognized chronic disease that can be associated with food allergies. EoE is characterized by inflammation and accumulation of eosinophils in the esophagus. Symptoms include nausea, vomiting, and abdominal pain after eating and can resemble acid reflux. In severe cases, difficulty in swallowing solid food or solid food sticking in the esophagus may be manifested; in infants, this disease may be associated with a failure to thrive (NIAID, 2011).

A curious type of food allergy, the so-called exercise-induced food allergy (or exercise-induced anaphylaxis or exercise-induced asthma), is apparently provoked by exercise, which has been immediately preceded or followed by the ingestion of food. Chapman *et al.* (2006) have divided the patients into two subsets, one of which may develop a reaction in temporal proximity to any type of food and the second subset within temporal proximity to certain foods including, but not limited to, shell fish, cephalopods, peach, grapes, tomato, wheat, buckwheat, celery, dairy products, chicken, matsutake mushrooms, and "solid" food (Taylor *et al.*, 1989; Taylor and Helfe, 2002; Chapman *et al.*, 2006). The exact mechanism is unknown, but it may involve enhanced mast cell responsiveness to physical stimuli and/or diminished metabolism of histamine, similar to red wine allergy (Taylor and Scanlan, 1989).

Non-IgE–mediated immunological reactions to foods include (1) food-induced enterocolitis and colitis, (2) malabsorption syndromes (such as celiac disease), (3) cow's milk-induced syndromes, and (4) dermatitis herpetiformis (which, despite the name, has nothing to do with the herpes virus, but an immunological reaction to dietary gluten with IgA involvement (Chapman *et al.*, 2006)). Food intolerance in patients with chronic fatigue syndrome may not have much of an allergic component, but has been shown to be a somatization trait of patients with depressive symptoms and anxiety disorders (Manu *et al.*, 1993).

Chemistry of Food Allergens Food allergens are generally glycoproteins with molecular weights ranging from 10 kDa to 70 kDa (Chapman *et al.*, 2006). Although almost all foods contain one or more proteins, a few foods are associated more with allergic reactions than are others. For example, anaphylaxis to peanuts is more common than is anaphylaxis to other legumes (eg, peas, soybeans). Similarly, although allergies may occur from bony fishes, there is no basis for cross-reactivity to other types of seafood (eg, molluscs and crustaceans), although dual (and independent) sensitivities may exist. Interestingly, patients who are allergic to milk usually can tolerate beef and inhaled cattle dander, and patients allergic to eggs usually can tolerate ingestion of chicken and feather-derived particles (Anderson and Sogn, 1984), although in the "bird-egg" syndrome, patients can be allergic to bird feathers, egg yolk, egg white, or any combination of the three (DeBlay *et al.*, 1994; Szepfalusi *et al.*, 1994),

Some of the allergenic components of common food allergens are listed in Table 31-18. Although food avoidance is usually the best means of protection, it is not always possible because (1) the content of some prepared foods may be unknown (eg, the presence of eggs or cottonseed oil); (2) there is the possibility of contamination of food from unsuspected sources (eg, *Penicillium* in cheeses or meat, *Candida albicans*) (Dayan, 1993; Dorion *et al.*, 1994), and cow's milk antigens in the breast milk of mothers who have consumed cow's milk (Halken *et al.*, 1993)); (3) the presence of an allergen in a previously unknown place (the insertion of Brazil nut DNA into soybeans and subsequent appearance of the allergic 2S protein in soybean products (Nordlee *et al.*, 1996)); and (4) there is a lack of knowledge about the phylogenetic relationships between food sources (eg, legumes include peas, soybeans, and peanuts).

Cross-reactivity has not been well studied, but can have severe consequences nonetheless. The latex-fruit syndrome is an example of a sensitivity of latex, which cross-reacts with the proteins in fruit, the most commonly cited of which are banana, avocado, and kiwi. Seed storage proteins (particularly the 2S albumin family) appear to be the common denominator for allergy to sesame, mustard, sunflower, and cottonseed (Chapman *et al.*, 2006).

Demographics of Food Allergy and Intolerance Although children appear to be the most susceptible to food allergy, with adverse reactions occurring in 4% to 6% of infants, the incidence appears to taper off with maturation of the digestive tract, with only 1% to 2% of young children (4–15 years) susceptible (Fuglsang *et al.*, 1993). The increase in the number of adults exhibiting food allergy may be due in part to an expanded food universe, that is, an increased willingness to try different foods. In one study, allergies among young children were most commonly to milk and eggs, whereas allergies that developed later in life tended to be to fruit and vegetables (Kivity *et al.*, 1994).

Table 31-18

Known Allergenic Food Proteins

FOOD	ALLERGIC PROTEINS
Cow's milk	Casein (Dorion *et al.*, 1994; Stoger and Wuthrich, 1993) β-Lactoglobulin (Piastra *et al.*, 1994; Stoger and Wuthrich, 1993) α-Lactalbumin (Bernaola *et al.*, 1994; Stoger and Wuthrich, 1993)
Egg whites	Ovomucoid (Bernhisel-Broadbent *et al.*, 1994) Ovalbumin (Fukutomi *et al.*, 1994, Bernhiesel-Broadbent *et al.*, 1994)
Egg yolks	Livetin (DeBlay *et al.*, 1994; Szepfalusi *et al.*, 1994)
Peanuts	Ara h II (Dorion *et al.*, 1994) Peanut I (Sachs *et al.*, 1981)
Soybeans	β-Conglycinin (7S fraction) (Rumsey *et al.*, 1994) Glycinin (11S fraction) (Rumsey *et al.*, 1994) Gly mIA (Gonzalez *et al.*, 1992) Gly mIB (Gonzalez *et al.*, 1992) Kunitz trypsin inhibitor (Brandon *et al.*, 1986)
Codfish	Gad cI (O'Neil *et al.*, 1993)
Shrimp	Antigen II (Taylor *et al.*, 1989)
Green peas	Albumin fraction (Taylor *et al.*, 1989)
Rice	Glutelin fraction (Taylor *et al.*, 1989) Globulin fraction (Taylor *et al.*, 1989)
Cottonseed	Glycoprotein fraction (Taylor *et al.*, 1989)
Peach guava, banana, mandarin, strawberry	30 kD protein (Wadee *et al.*, 1990)
Tomato	Several glycoproteins (Taylor *et al.*, 1989)
Wheat	Gluten (Stewart-Tull and Jones, 1992) Gliadin (O'Hallaren, 1992) Globulin (O'Hallaren, 1992) Albumin (O'Hallaren, 1992)
Okra	Fraction I (Manda *et al.* 1992)

SOURCE: *Modified from Taylor SL, Scanlan RA, eds. Food Toxicology: A Perspective on the Relative Risks. New York: Marcel Dekker; 1989:265. With permission from Copyright Clearance Center.*

Familial relationships also play a role. Schrander *et al.* (1993) noted that among infants with cow's milk protein intolerance, 65% had a positive family history for atopy (first- or second-degree relatives) compared with 35% of healthy controls.

Food Idiosyncrasy

Food idiosyncrasies are generally defined as *quantitatively* abnormal responses to a food substance or additive; this reaction differs from the physiological effect, and although it may resemble hypersensitivity, it does not involve immune mechanisms. Food idiosyncratic reactions include those that occur in specific groups of individuals who may be genetically predisposed. Examples of such reactions and the foods that probably are responsible are given in Table 31-19.

Lactose Intolerance Probably the most common idiosyncratic reaction is lactose intolerance, a deficiency of the lactase enzyme needed for the metabolism of the lactose in cow's milk. A lack of this enzyme results in fermentation of lactose to lactic acid and an osmotic effect on the bowel, with resultant symptoms of malabsorption and diarrhea. Lactose intolerance is lowest in northern Europe in 3% to 8% of the population; it reaches 70% in southern Italy and Turkey and nearly 100% in Southeast Asia (Anderson and Sogn, 1984; Gudmand-Hoyer, 1994). Lactose intolerance is prominent among blacks with an incidence of 27% in black children ages 12 to 24 months, which may increase to 33% by age six years (Juambeltz *et al.*, 1993).

Favism (Glucose-6-phosphate Dehydrogenase Deficiency) Favism is the adverse reaction by certain glucose-6-phosphate dehydrogenase (G6PD)–deficient individuals to certain foods, resulting in a type of debilitating hemolytic anemia that can be fatal. There are nearly 400 different types of G6PD deficiencies (G6PDD) affecting nearly 400 million people, but classically described favism has a distinct geographical demographic (Mediterranean countries, including Italy, Greece, Spain, Portugal, and Turkey). Favism may well be the oldest enzymopathy, as it was recognized even by the early Greek mathematician Pythagoras, who is said to have warned his students against eating fava beans (Luzzatto *et al.*, 2001).

Consumption of fava beans (broad beans) results in the release of the pyrimidine aglycones divicine and isouramil, which in combination with ascorbic acid and other possible cofactors ultimately interfere with G6PD in its task to regenerate reduced glutathione.

Table 31-19

Idiosyncratic Reactions to Foods

FOOD	REACTION	MECHANISM	REFERENCE
Fava beans	Hemolysis, sometimes accompanied by jaundice and hemoglobinuria; also, pallor, fatigue, nausea, dyspnea, fever and chills, abdominal and dorsal pain.	Pyrimidine aglycones in fava bean cause irreversible oxidation of GSH in G-6-PD–deficient erythrocytes by blocking NADPH supply, resulting in oxidative stress of the erythrocyte and eventual hemolysis.	Chevion *et al.*, 1985
Chocolate	Migraine headache	Phenylethylamine-related (?)	Gibb *et al.*, 1991; Settipane, 1987
Beets	Beetanuria: passage of red urine (often mistaken for hematuria)	Excretion of beetanin in urine after consumption of beets	Smith, 1991
Asparagus	Odorous, sulfurous-smelling urine	Autosomal dominant inability to metabolize methanthiol of asparagus and consequent passage of methanthiol in urine.	Smith, 1991
Red Wine	Sneezing, flush, headache, diarrhea, skin itch, shortness of breath	Diminished histamine degradation: deficiency of diamine oxidase (?) Histamines present in wine	Wantke *et al.*, 1994
Choline- and carnitine-containing foods	Fish odor syndrome: foul odor of body secretions	Choline and carnitine metabolized to trimethylamine in gut by bacteria, followed by absorption but inability to metabolize to odorless trimethylamine *N*-oxide.	Ayesh *et al.*, 1993
Milk	Abdominal pain, bloating, diarrhea	Lactase deficiency	Mallinson, 1987
Fructose-containing foods	Abdominal pain, vomiting, diarrhea, hypoglycemia	Reduced activity of hepatic aldolase B toward fructose-1-phosphate.	Frankland, 1987; Catto-Smith and Adams, 1993

Because red blood cells are exposed to relatively high concentrations of oxidants, the lack of glutathione activity leads to oxidative cross-linking of erythrocyte membrane proteins and consequent distortion of the cell and oxygen-carrying capacity is impaired. Ca^{+2}-ATPase activity may be reduced and intracellular proteolytic enzymes may be activated, resulting in hemolysis. The end-stage process, hemolysis, often results within 2 to 24 hours following consumption of the beans. An episode may also be initiated by inhalation of pollen from the fava plant flower. Symptoms include fever, jaundice, dark red urine, headache, and increased heart rate. Affected individuals become weak and experience pain in the back and abdomen.

G6PDD is an X-linked recessive disease (mapped to Xq28 and close to the genes controlling hemophilia A and color blindness), with many variants and some unknown cofactors, such that not all individuals react the same to an identical amount of fava beans, if there is any reaction at all. Indeed, the beans themselves have variable amounts of divicine and isouramil, with the greatest amount in the springtime. In addition to this sensitivity to fava beans, individuals also may not tolerate certain drugs including, but not limited to, primaquine-type antimalarials, sulfonamides and sulfones, naldixic acid, methylene blue, and some chemicals such as naphthalene (mothballs) and trinitrotoluene. If there is an upside to G6PDD, it may be its association with resistance to malaria (Luzzattto *et al.*, 2001; Anonymous, 2002; Brunton *et al.* 2006; Beutler, 2008; Khoo, 2010).

Asian Flush Syndrome Many Asians are known to metabolize alcohol poorly and following adequate alcohol intake, exhibit facial flushing, nausea, dizziness, tachycardia, sweating, etc. The intolerance is the inability to effectively metabolize acetaldehyde to acetate (by NAD^+-dependent ALDH2), the second step in ethanol detoxification, leading to a build-up of acetaldehyde.

There is a superfamily of aldehyde dehydrogenases (ALDH) and eight are found in human DNA, but the most studied are ALDH1 (a cytosolic form) and ALDH2 (a mitochondrial form). A variant of ALDH2, found in approximately 50% of Asians, upon sequencing, was found to be a single glutamate-to-lysine substitution at position 487, and although the enzyme was active, the K_m for NAD^+ was so elevated the enzyme was functionally inactive. This acetaldehyde buildup is functionally similar to that produced chemically by disulfiram (tetraethylthiuram disulfide or Antabuse), which inhibits the enzyme, although the cytosolic form is more sensitive to disulfiram than the mitochondrial form. Asian flush syndrome has been reported in Japanese, Chinese, and Koreans and quantitative estimations in Japanese have shown 40% lack of ALDH2 activity. ALDH2 deficiency is a dominant negative trait, with homozygotes having essentially no ALDH2 activity, but heterozygotes having reduced but detectable activity. The lack of ALDH2 in a large portion of Asians may, in part, account for a comparatively low rate of alcoholism among Asians.

Alcohol dehydrogenase is also important in alcohol metabolism and σ-alcohol dehydrogenase of the stomach was missing in approximately 30% of those biopsied (Crabb *et al.*, 2004). Although this missing enzyme led to an increased level of alcohol reaching the blood stream, it is unlikely to produce a meaningful contribution to Asian flush syndrome (Steinmetz, *et al.*, 1997; Crabb *et al.*, 2004).

Table 31-20

Anaphylactoid Reactions to Food

FOOD	REACTION	MECHANISM	REFERENCE
Western Australian salmon (*Arripis truttaceus*)	Erythema and urticaria of the skin, facial flushing and sweating, palpitations, hot flushes of the body, headache, nausea, vomiting, and dizziness	Scombroid poisoning; high histamine levels demonstrated in the fish	Smart, 1992
Fish (spiked with histamine)	Facial flushing, headache	Histamine poisoning; histamine concentration in plasma correlated closely with histamine dose ingested	Van Gelderen *et al.*, 1992
Cape yellow tail (fish) (*Seriola lalandi*)	Skin rash, diarrhea, palpitations, headache, nausea and abdominal cramps, paraesthesia, unusual taste sensation, and breathing difficulties	Scombroid poisoning, treated with antihistamines	Muller *et al.*, 1992
Sulfite sensitivity	Bronchospasm, asthma	Sulfite oxidase deficiency to meta-bisulfites in foods and wine	Smith, 1991
Tuna, albacore, mackerel, bonito, mahimahi, and bluefish	Reaction resembling an acute allergic reaction	Scombroid poisoning treated with antihistamines and cimetidine	Lange, 1988
Cheese	Symptoms resembling acute allergic reaction	Responds to antihistamines; histamine poisoning?	Taylor, 1986

Anaphylactoid Reactions

Anaphylactoid reactions are historically thought of as reactions mimicking anaphylaxis through direct application of histamine, the primary mediator of anaphylactic reactions. Anaphylactoid reactions occur following ingestion of scombroid fish (eg, tuna, mackerel, bonito) that have high levels of histidine in their flesh, as well as some nonscombroid fish such as mahi mahi and bluefish. The fish flesh has been acted upon by microorganisms whose growth involves production of histidine decarboxylase to produce histamine, the essential ingredient for the anaphylactoid reaction (Table 31-20) (Clark *et al.*, 1999). Because histamine is heat-stable, cooking has relatively little effect on the outcome. Symptoms of scombroid poisoning include skin flushing, pruritus, throbbing headache, dizziness, nausea, vomiting, abdominal cramps, and diarrhea (Codori and Marinopoulos, 2009). Characteristics distinguishing scombrotoxicosis from enteric pathogens are the relatively sudden onset (10–30 minutes) and the skin flushing of the head, neck and upper torso.

Scombrotoxicosis was reported to be mimicked by the direct ingestion of 90 mg of histamine in unspoiled fish (Van Gelderen *et al.*, 1992), but according to Taylor (1986), the effect of simply ingesting histamine does not produce the equivalent effect. Instead, Taylor claims that histamine ingested with spoiled fish appears to be much more toxic than is histamine ingested in an aqueous solution as a result of the presence of histamine potentiators in fish flesh. The apparent mechanism of potentiation involves the inhibition of intestinal histamine-metabolizing enzymes (diamine oxidase), which causes increased histamine uptake. Melnik *et al.* (1997) proposed that anaphylactoid responses may be the sum of several mechanisms: (1) an increased intake of biogenic amines (including histamine) with food, (2) an increased synthesis by the intestinal flora, (3) a diminished catabolism of biogenic amines by the intestinal mucosa, and (4) an increased release of endogenous histamine from mast cells and basophils by histamine-releasing food. Scombrotoxicosis in the absence of high histamine levels (less than the FDA action level for tuna of 50 mg histamine/10-g fish) was

reported by Gessner *et al.* (1996). Ijomah *et al.* (1991) claimed that dietary histamine is not a major determinant of scombrotoxicosis because potency is not positively correlated with the dose and volunteers tend to fall into susceptible and nonsusceptible subgroups. Ijomah *et al.* (1991) suggested that endogenous histamine released by mast cells plays a significant role in the etiology of scombrotoxicosis, whereas the role of dietary histamine is minor. An exception to this endogenous histamine theory was described by Morrow *et al.* (1991), who found the expected increase in urinary histamine in scombroid-poisoned individuals but did not find an increase in urinary 9α, 11β-dihydroxy-15-oxo-2,3,18, 19-tetranorprost-5-ene-1, 20-dioic acid, the principal metabolite of prostaglandin D_2, a mast cell secretory product; thus, no mast cell involvement was indicated.

Food-Drug Interactions

Once known as pharmacological food reactions or as "false food allergies" (Moneret–Vautrin, 1987), these adverse reactions were thought to be exaggerated responses to pharmacological agents in food and possibly due to receptor sensitization. However, the majority of food and drug interactions are actually the result of food-induced changes in drug bioavailability or metabolism (ie, *pharmacokinetic* interactions), although some are the result of *pharmacodynamic* interactions. For drugs with a narrow therapeutic index and the need for dose titration, even small changes in the dose–response effects can have great consequences (Schmidt and Dalhoff, 2002). The potential to alter therapeutic effect can be great and in recognition of the role that food plays, test meals are now given to determine their effect on drug therapeutic effect (FDA, 2002b).

Pharmacokinetic effects on absorption (eg, gastric pH, gastric emptying, lymphatic flow) were described earlier. Examples of foods affecting a number of cytochromes, Phase II enzymes, and transporters are provided in Table 31-21; the effects on CYP3A4 and P-glycoprotein may be the clinically most important (Harris *et al.*, 2003). Other dietary ingredients that may produce an effect on the overall pharmacokinetics of drugs would include substances that change the pH of urine or simply the presence

Table 31-21

Food–drug Interactions (Activity may be Enhanced or Inhibited)

ENZYME OR TRANSPORTER	FOOD	DRUG
CYP1A2	Caffeine, theophylline, grapefruit juice (naringen and furanocoumarins bergamottin and dihydroxybergamotin), grape juice, cruciferous vegetables, apiaceous vegetables, cooked meat	Clozapine, fluvoxamine, imipramine
CYP2E1	Watercress and possibly other isothiocyanate-containing cruciferous vegetables; polyunsaturated fatty acids (corn oil, menhaden oil)	Ethanol, halothane, enflurane
CYP3A4	Grapefruit juice, orange juice, red wine, possibly other polyphenol-containing substances, St Johns wort, garlic	Ketoconazole, cyclosporin, erythromycin, protease inhibitors, 3-hydroxy-3-methylglutaryl-coenzyme A (HMG-CoA) reductase inhibitors
UGT and GST	Brussel sprouts, cabbage, watercress, broccoli	Acetominophen, oxazepam, morphine, ibuprofen
P-glycopeptide and OATP	Vegetables, fruit juice, St Johns wort	Digoxin, cyclosporine, pravastatin

GST, glutathione-S-transferases; OATP, organic anion–transporting polypeptides; UGT, uridine diphosphate glycuronosyltransferases.

of fiber in the intestine. Examples of pharmacodynamic interactions might include the effect of unsaturated fatty acids in the diet on anticoagulants or membrane potentials of the membranes in which they become incorporated, or high potassium intake from potassium-rich foods and the risk of hyperkalemia during therapy with angiotensin-converting enzyme inhibitors or spironolactone (Schmidt and Dalholff, 2002). Other pharmacodynamic interactions might include phytoestrogens and other estrogen-stimulating substances during treatment for hormonally sensitive cancers (eg, breast and prostate) and caffeine or other stimulatory

methylxanthines from coffee, chocolate, and soft drinks flavored with guarana, during treatment for hypertension.

Metabolic Food Reactions

Metabolic or physiologic food reactions are distinct from other categories of adverse reactions in that the foods are more or less commonly eaten and demonstrate toxic effects only when eaten to excess or improperly processed (Table 31-22). The susceptible population exists as a result of its own behavior, that is, the

Table 31-22

Metabolic Food Reactions

FOOD	REACTION	MECHANISM	REFERENCE
Lima beans, Cassava roots, millet (sorghum) sprouts, bitter almonds, apricot and peach pits	Cyanosis	Cyanogenic glycosides releasing hydrogen cyanide on contact with stomach acid	Anderson and Sogn, 1984
Cabbage family, turnips, soybeans, radishes, rapeseed and mustard	Goiter (enlarged thyroid)	Isothiocyanates, goitrin, or S-5-vinyl-thiooxazolidone interferes with utilization of iodine	Anderson and Sogn, 1984; van Etten and Tookey, 1985
Unripe fruit of the tropical tree Blighia sapida, common in Caribbean and Nigeria	Severe vomiting, coma, and acute hypoglycemia sometimes resulting in death, especially among the malnourished	Hypoglycin A, isolated from the fruit, may interfere with oxidation of fatty acids, so that glycogen stores have to be metabolized for energy, with depletion of carbohydrates, resulting in hypoglycemia	Evans, 1985
Leguminosae, Cruciferae	Lathyritic symptoms: neurological symptoms of weakness, leg paralysis, and sometimes death	L-2-4-Diaminobutyric acid inhibition of ornithine transcarbamylase of the urea cycle, inducing ammonia toxicity	Evans, 1985
Licorice (glycyrrhizic acid)	Hypertension, cardiac enlargement, sodium retention	Glycyrrhizic acid mimicking mineralocorticoids	Farese et al., 1991
Polar bear and Chicken liver	Irritability, vomiting, increased intracranial pressure, death	Vitamin A toxicity	Bryan, 1984
Cycads (cycad flour)	Amyotrophic lateral sclerosis (humans), hepatocarcino genicity (rats and nonhuman primates)	Cycasin (methylazoxymethanol); primary action is methylation, resulting in a broad range of effects from membrane destruction to inactivation of enzyme systems.	Matsumoto, 1985; Sieber et al., 1980

"voluntary" consumption of food as a result of a limited food supply or an abnormal craving for a specific food.

Excess Consumption of a Normally Nontoxic Food

Glycyrrhizism—Licorice and Hypokalemia A "pica" or abnormal craving was reported by Bannister *et al.,* (1977), who noted hypokalemia leading to cardiac arrest in a 58-year-old woman who had been eating about 1.8 kg of licorice per week. In "glycyrrhizism," or licorice intoxication, glycyrrhizic acid is the active component, with an effect resembling that of aldosterone, which suppresses the renin-angiotensin-aldosterone axis, resulting in the loss of potassium. Clinically, hypokalemia with alkalosis, cardiac arrhythmias, muscular symptoms together with sodium retention and edema, and severe hypertension are observed. The syndrome may develop at a level of 100 g licorice/day but gradually abates upon withdrawal of the licorice (Isbrucker and Burdock, 2006).

Isothiocyanates, Thiocyanates, and Goiter Isothiocyanates are present in a number of foods, especially cruciferous vegetables, including mustard and horseradish (as allyl isothiocyanate), which provide the "bite" associated with these foods, and in watercress (as methyl isothiocyanate), which confers a slight zaniness to the taste. In mustard seed, the glycoside, sinigrin, is acted upon by myrosin in the presence of water and when the seed is injured, liberating the (allyl)-isothiocyanate, a potent antimicrobial (especially antifungal). Other members of the *Brassica* family, including broccoli, kale, and cabbage, release a thiocyanate ion. Once ingested, both the iso- and thiocyanates bind iodine in the body, preventing its organification, leading to *diffuse hyperplastic (iodine-deficient) goiter*. Although the degree to which I^- is bound by the thiocyanates is not comparable to say, perchlorate anion (ClO_4^-), nevertheless, in areas of low iodine and high *Brassica* consumption, pathology could result (Capen *et al.,* 2002; Farwell and Braverman, 2006). Ermans *et al.* (1972) indicate that chronic consumption of thiocyanate may play a role in endemic cretinism. Paradoxically, excess iodine may also cause goiter (ie, *iodine-excess goiter*). Excess iodine appears primarily to block the release of T3 and T4 from thyroglobulin and interferes with peroxidation of $2I^-$ to I_2 and disrupts the conversion of monoiodothyronine to diiodothyronine (Capen *et al.,* 2002). The FDA is aware of the possibility of iodine toxicity and has placed limits on iodine in kelp, the products of which have extensive use in food (21CFR172.365).

Nutmeg, Myristicin, and Hallucinations Myristicin is a naturally occurring insecticide and acaricide that is found in nutmeg and mace (*Myristica* spp) at concentrations of 1.3% and 2.7%, respectively (Hallstrom and Thuvander, 1997). It is also present in black pepper, carrot, celery, parsley, and dill (Deshpande, 2002). It is estimated that the average total intake of myristicin from dietary sources is on the order of a few mg per person per day (Hallstrom and Thuvander, 1997). Myristicin is a weak inhibitor of monoamine oxidase and is structurally related to mescaline. At a dose level of 6 to 7 mg/kg body weight (bw), it may cause psychotropic effects in man such as increased alertness and a feeling of irresponsibility, freedom, and euphoria. Unpleasant symptoms, such as nausea, tremor, tachycardia, anxiety, and fear have also been reported in humans ingesting this dose. Although the metabolism of myristicin resembles that of safrole, there is no evidence to suggest that myristicin is carcinogenic (Hallstrom and Thuvander, 1997).

At the concentrations normally present in spices or food, the likelihood of toxicity arising from myristicin is low. However, ingestion of greater than 5 g of nutmeg (corresponding to 1–2 mg/kg bw myristicin) has produced toxicological symptoms in humans that are similar to alcohol intoxication. Because the myristicin content of nutmeg is approximately 1% to 3%, it is likely that other components of nutmeg in addition to myristicin contribute to nutmeg toxicity (Hallstrom and Thuvander, 1997; Dolan *et al.,* 2010).

Improperly Prepared Food

Cassava and Konzo Konzo is a progressive and irreversible spastic paraparesis or tetraparesis resulting from the inadequate processing of the root and leaves of cassava (*Manihot esculenta*), a hardy plant found in sub-Saharan Africa. Recent outbreaks have occurred in the Democratic Republic of Congo, Central African Republic, Tanzania, and Mozambique. For many people, cassava is a survival food and outbreaks are associated with an agricultural crisis or in periods of food insecurity. Where cassava is routinely eaten, the outbreaks are naturally associated during the cassava harvest period, when the fruit is most plentiful and would constitute a major portion of the diet. The incidence is highest in children and young women and is often associated with populations with decreased intake of sulfur-containing amino acids, and in an iodine-deficient population there is an exacerbation of cretinism. The disease is the result of the cyanogenic glucosides, primarily linamarin (α-hydroxyisobutyronitrile-β-D-glucopyranoside), which is converted to cyanohydrin, cyanide, and cyanate (OCN). Victims have increased serum and urinary thiocyanate concentrations (Cliff *et al.,* 2011; Kassa *et al.,* 2011). Although konzo is often the end product of chronic consumption, in lower and/or less frequent doses, responses include acute intoxication (dizziness, headache, nausea, vomiting, etc). In chronic doses insufficient to cause typical konzo, responses include ataxic neuropathy, loss of sensorium in hands, blindness, deafness, and weakness (Bradbury *et al.,* 2011).

Avoidance of the toxic effects of linamarin is relatively straightforward, but requires a process that takes time and the availability of potable water. The vegetable should be ground to a flour, placed in a flat pan or tray, and sufficient water added to essentially double the volume. The container is placed in the sun for two hours or the shade for five hours. This technique activates the luminase, which produces cyanohydrins, which break down to cyanide. Evaporation of the water allows the cyanide to be released harmlessly into the air and the cyanide will be reduced approximately three- to sixfold, at which time the flour may be made into the traditional porridge (Bradbury *et al.,* 2011).

Cyanogenic glycosides are present in animal feed (flax, *Trifolium repens* L, or white clover and sorghum species) and are a concern because of the large amounts animals may ingest. Poisoning in dogs has been reported following ingestion of macadamia nuts, which contain the cyanogenic glucoside, proteacin (Swenson *et al.,* 1989; Hansen *et al.,* 2000). Clinical signs include weakness, depression, vomiting, ataxia, and tremor, among others. Clinical signs were reported within 12 hours in most cases and most resolved within less than 24 hours; the average amount of macadamia nuts ingested to produce symptoms was 11.7 g/kg bw (Hansen *et al.,* 2000). Cyanogenic glycosides are also present in the pits/seeds of members of the genus, *Prunus* (cherry, peach, and apricot pits and apple seeds), but these are rarely eaten (Barceloux, 2008a).

Cycads (and Lytico-Bodig Disease) Following WW II and the occupation of Guam and neighboring islands by the US, Army physicians noted the native Chamorro people as having an especially high rate of amyotrophic lateral sclerosis (ALS or Lou Gehrig disease or specifically; in this case, *Western Pacific amyotrophic lateral sclerosis* or *lytico-bodig disease*). Lytico-bodig disease was often seen in combination with the tremorous symptoms of Parkinson's disease or, a dementia similar to Alzheimer's disease and sometimes, a combination of all three of these diseases.

A combination of the latter two diseases has been referred to as parkinsonism–dementia (PD) complex. ALS is characterized by progressive weakness of the extremities, muscle spasticity, fasiculations, and followed by atrophy. The PD complex is characterized by bradykinesia, tremor, decreased blink reflex, muscle rigidity, etc, with eventual flexion contractures and progressive dementia (Matsumoto, 1985; Barceloux, 2009a; Cox and Bradley, 2009).

The source of the disease(s) is exposure to cycad seed kernel and to a somewhat lesser extent, consumption of the flying fox (*Pteropus mariannus*), a mammal known to consume large amounts of cycad seed. The cycad responsible for intoxication is *Cycas micronesica*, not *Cycas circinalis*, as was previously thought. The cycad was a traditional food source for the Chamorro until the 1960s. What is in dispute is the actual causative agent and its origin. The cycad is known to contain the neurotoxins β-*N*-methylamino-L-alanine (BMAA) and methylazoxymethanol β-D-glucoside (cycasin). There is evidence that BMAA may be the product of symbiotic cyanobacteria, instead of the plant itself.

Among people who have used cycads for food, the method of detoxification is remarkably similar. The seeds and stems are cut into small pieces and soaked in water for several days and then are dried and ground into flour. The effectiveness of leaching the toxins from the bits of flesh is most directly dependent on the size of the pieces, the duration of soaking, and the number of water changes (Matsumoto, 1985; Barceloux, 2009a; Cox and Bradley, 2009).

The Grass Pea and Neurolathyrism Another starvation- and poverty-influenced disease is neurolathyrism, clinically indistinguishable from konzo produced by cassava, but attributed to the excessive intake of the grass pea (*Lathyrus sativus* L) and the causative agent, β-*N*-oxalyl-L-α-β-diaminopropionic acid (OADP). The grass pea is a hardy legume that is tolerant to drought, water logging, and salinity and is fairly insect-resistant. It may be among the first to blossom following a flood and silting over of fields. Its growth is now mainly confined to the Indian Subcontinent, Ethiopia and to a lesser extent in Europe, Australia, Asia, and North Africa. The grass pea is often part of a diet for people with no other choices and, despite is widespread reputation as a food with toxic consequences, it is sometimes grown as rotation crop because it fixes nitrogen and is fairly protein- and carbohydrate-rich. As a consequence of its ease of cultivation and nutrients, grass pea flour is often mixed with chickpea. Contributing factors to the toxic effects experienced by the victims, may also include low dietary sulfur amino acids and trace metal deficiencies, but clearly, the largest cohort of victims are those that have the greatest exposure, including hungry children supplementing meager meals with the wild-growing peas or those with the greatest caloric demand and, thus, often the family breadwinner. Detoxification methods include presoaking the pea seeds in cold or hot (50°C) water or cooking in boiling water (alkaline or acidic solutions), roasting at high temperature, or fermentation—all processes result in measureable (but variable) diminution of the OADP, but never total elimination of the toxin (Jiao *et al.*, 2011; Kumar *et al.*, 2011).

OADP is a nonprotein amino acid and comes in an α- and β-form (30:70 ratio at room temperature) with the former less toxic than the latter and heating can convert some β-form to the less-toxic α-form. Concentration of the toxin in the grass pea is dependent on the particular strain and a host of nutrient and environmental variables and even symbiotic relationships with the nitrogen-fixing bacteria on the roots. The toxin is subtle and hyperexcites the neuron causing spastic movements of the legs and, eventually, paralysis, with muscular rigidity and weakness, although with no loss in sensitivity. The disease is characterized by degeneration of pyramidal-tract neurons in the spinal cord and in the area of the cortex controlling the legs. The cascade of events leading to pathology involves excitotoxicty and oxidative stress involving Ca^{++} homeostasis, and may be a model for ALS (Kumar *et al.*, 2011; Van Moorhem *et al*, 2011).

Ostrich Fern Fronds (Fiddleheads) Fiddleheads (crosiers) are the unfurled fronds of the ostrich fern (*Matteuccia struthiopteris*) and are a seasonal delicacy harvested commercially in the Northeastern United States and in coastal provinces of Canada. Called fiddleheads because their spiral appearance resembles the scroll configuration of a stringed instrument or the crosier of a Bishop's staff.

The ostrich fern was a spring vegetable for American Indians of eastern North America and became part of the regular diet of settlers to New Brunswick in the late 1700s. Until recently, it was consumed primarily in the Maritime Provinces of Canada and in the Northeastern United States. The ferns are available commercially either canned or frozen, but since the early 1980s, farmers' markets and supermarket chains have sold fresh ferns in season. None of the fiddlehead ferns of eastern and central North America previously have been reported to be poisonous. Although some ferns may be carcinogenic, the ostrich fern has been considered to be safe to eat either raw or cooked. However, in May 1994, outbreaks of food poisoning were associated with eating raw or lightly cooked fiddlehead ferns in New York and eastern Canada. In one incident, approximately 60% of restaurant patrons consuming raw or minimally processed ferns (eg, light sautéing) experienced nausea, vomiting, abdominal cramps, and/or diarrhea within hours (onset can range from 30 minutes to 12 hours and the illness generally lasts two hours) (Health Canada, 2010). Those consuming ferns subjected to more rigorous processing (eg, boiling for at least six minutes) did not experience symptoms. The authors speculated the ferns contained a heat-labile toxin and recommended that ferns be boiled for 10 minutes prior to eating (MMWR, 1994).

Pre- and Postharvest Changes

Cucumbers and Cucurbitacins Members of the *Cucurbitacea* family (zucchini, cucumbers, pumpkins, squash, melons, and gourds) produce cucurbitacins (oxygenated tetracyclic terpenes) that act as movement arresters and compulsive feeding stimulants for Diabriticine beetles (corn rootworms and cucumber beetles). Because cucurbitacins act as feeding stimulants, they are added to insecticidal baits to increase efficacy (Martin *et al.*, 2002). To most nondiabrotic herbivores, such as humans, cucurbitacin is perceived as extremely bitter, even at nanogram amounts (Subbiah, 1999).

Under normal circumstances, cucurbitacins are produced at low enough concentrations the bitterness is not detectable by humans. However, in response to stresses such as high temperatures, drought, low soil fertility, and low soil pH, concentrations of cucurbitacins may increase and cause the fruits to have a bitter taste (Feather, 2010). Occasional cases of stomach cramps and diarrhea have occurred in people ingesting bitter zucchini. Twenty-two cases of human poisoning from ingestion of as little as 3 g of bitter zucchini were reported in Australia from 1981 to 1982, and in Alabama and California in 1984. The cultivar implicated in the Australia poisonings was "Blackjack" (Burfield, 2008).

Solanine and Chaconine The humble potato, *Solanum tuberosum*, may produce toxic steroidal glycoalkaloids if exposed to light in the field or during storage or otherwise stressed by mechanical damage or improper storage or sprouting. Previously known only as "solanine" or now, (total) SGAs, the major players are α-solanine and α-chaconine and are normally present in amounts of <5 mg/100 g of tuber fresh weight, although a normal toxin load in potatoes of 20 to 100 mg/kg tuber is considered safe. The toxins are not affected by normal baking, frying, or microwave cooking temperatures, but will undergo significant degradation at 210°C (410°F) for 10 minutes, where the SGA are reduced 40% (Barceloux, 2008b). SGAs inhibit cholinesterases and can alter the effects of neuromuscular blocking drugs and anesthetics (Sorensen, 2002). Low doses of these glycoalkaloids can produce GI upset with diarrhea, vomiting, and severe abdominal pain. At higher doses, neurological symptoms are evident with drowsiness and apathy, confusion, weakness, and vision disturbances, followed by loss of consciousness and sometimes, death in the absence of supportive treatment.

Rodents do not absorb solanines as well as humans and the LD_{50} is >1000 mg/kg in mice and 590 mg/kg in the rat, values that are 300 to 500 times more than the toxic dose of 2 mg/kg in humans and, in which, the estimated lethal dose may be as little as 3 to 6 mg/kg. There was thought to be an association of potato (and SGA) consumption with neural tube defects in children, although prospective studies have not borne out this hypothesis, nor has this effect been seen in animal testing (ICPS, 1993).

In the 1960s, a new variety of potato was produced from a cross of a Delta Gold with a wild type from Peru. The new variety called "Lenape" was tested as a "new potato" for roasting with meats and vegetables. Upon eating the potato, however, the grower was sickened and upon analysis, the potato was found to have high levels of SGAs. It was later determined that a product of the breeding process, the gene for glycoalkaloids, was stimulated to produce a high level of SGA. Immediately, all the seed potato growers were contacted and stocks were recalled or destroyed (Fedoroff and Brown, 2004).

Furocoumarins in Parsnips, Celery, Earl Grey Tea, and Perfume

Furocoumarins are phytoalexins (natural pesticides) produced by the plant in defense against predators including viruses, bacteria, fungi, insects, and animals and, in the latter, have been shown to be phototoxic and photomutagenic. Furocoumarins are present in cold-pressed oils (but not distilled oil) of citrus fruit (oranges [esp, bergamot], lemons, and limes) and are extensively used as fragrance ingredients and as flavor ingredients, including use in Earl Grey tea and halva (a sesame paste confection). Although concentrations of furocoumarins tend to be high in cold-pressed citrus oil, exposure to humans is fairly low (citrus flavor for soft drinks and, importantly, margarita mix, are made from the distilled oils). Concentration of furocoumarins in vegetables (the family Apiacae/Umbelliferae—carrots, parsley, celery, and parsnips) is low, but the risk of adverse effects is greater because mistreatment of the vegetables can result in increased furocoumarin levels and a relatively large amount of the vegetable could be consumed in a single day.

Postharvest treatment of parsnips can greatly influence the concentration of furocoumarins. Ceska et al. (1986) reported that older "spoiled" and diseased parsnips freely available in grocery stores may contain furocoumarin concentrations 2500% higher than fresh parsnips. Microbial infection of parsnip roots can result in a dramatic increase in furocoumarin levels. Furocoumarin concentrations (the sum of five furocoumarins: angelicin, isopimpinellin, 5-methoxypsoralen (MOP), 8-MOP, and psoralen) in freshly harvested parsnips are generally lower than 2.5 mg/kg and do not increase after storage at −18°C for up to 50 days. In contrast, storage of whole parsnips (but not cubes or homogenate) at 4°C resulted in a marked biphasic increase of furocoumarin concentrations (to approximately 40 mg/kg) after seven or 38 days of storage. A dramatic increase in furocoumarin concentrations (up to 566 mg/kg) was observed when whole parsnips were kept at room temperature over 53 days, resulting in a visible microbial (mold) presence (Ostertag et al., 2002).

In celery, infection with fungal pathogens has been shown to produce trimethylpsoralen (which is absent from plants that are not infected) and increased concentrations of 8-MOP. The resulting "pink rot" has caused repeated outbreaks of photophytodermatitis in commercial celery handlers (Zobel and Brown, 1991). Fungal infection also has been shown to stimulate a 155-fold increase in furocoumarin production in carrots (Wagstaff 1991).

Americans may well consume 1.3 mg furocoumarins/day (0.02–0.023 mg/kg/day), although consumption of 200 g of infected parsnips could result in an exposure of 100 mg. A therapeutic dose (treatment of psoriasis) is 0.5 to 0.6 mg 8-MOP/kg bw and the lowest phototoxic dose known is 0.23 mg/kg bw/day. Furocoumarins are phototoxic in combination with UVA exposure. Furocoumarins are also known to be cytotoxic and mutagenic as the result of furocoumarins intercalating between base pairs of DNA, which when exposed to UVA form covalent photoadducts. Furocoumarins have shown carcinogenicity in rats (37.4 mg/kg bw/day × 2 years) and hepatotoxicity in dogs (48 mg/kg) and induce vomiting in monkeys at 6 mg/kg bw/day (SKLM, 2006; Raquet and Schrenk, 2009; Dolan et al., 2010; Guth et al., 2011).

TOXIC SUBSTANCES IN FOOD

Heavy Metals

There are 92 natural elements; approximately 22 are known to be essential nutrients of the mammalian body and are referred to as micronutrients (Concon, 1988). Among the micronutrients are iron, zinc, copper, manganese, molybdenum, selenium, iodine, cobalt, and even aluminum and arsenic. However, among the 92 elements, lead, cadmium, and mercury are familiar as contaminants (or at least have more specifications setting their limits in food ingredients). The prevalence of these elements as contaminants is not due so much to their ubiquity in nature but rather to their use by humans.

Lead Although the toxicity of lead is well known, lead may also be an essential trace mineral. A lead deficiency induced by feeding rats <50 ppb lead (vs 1000 ppb in controls) over one or more generations produced effects on the hematopoietic system, decreased iron stores in the liver and spleen, and caused decreased growth (Kirchgessner and Reichmayer-Lais, 1981), but apparently not as a result of an effect on iron absorption. Although the toxic effects of lead are discussed elsewhere in this text, it is important to note that its effects are profound (especially in children) and appear to be long-lasting because mechanisms for excretion appear to be inadequate in comparison to those for uptake (Linder, 1991). Foods may become contaminated with lead if they are grown, stored, or processed under conditions that could introduce larger amounts of lead into the food, such as when a root crop is grown in soil that has been contaminated from the past use of leaded pesticides.

Over the years, recognition of the serious nature of lead poisoning in children has caused the World Health Organization (WHO) and FDA to adjust the recommended tolerable total lead intake from all sources of not more than 100 μg/day for infants up to six months old and not more than 150 μg/day for children from six months to two years of age to the considerably lower range of 6 to 18 μg/day as a provisional tolerable range for lead intake in a 10-kg child. The FDA is recommending that lead levels in candy products likely to be consumed frequently by small children do not exceed 0.1 ppm because such levels are achievable under good manufacturing practices and would not pose a significant risk to small children for adverse effects. This recommended maximum level is consistent with the FDA's longstanding goal of reducing lead levels in the food supply (FDA, 2005).

Initiatives to reduce the level of lead in foods, such as the move to eliminate lead-soldered seams in soldered food cans that was begun in the 1970s and efforts to eliminate leachable lead from ceramic ware glazes, have resulted in a steady decline in dietary lead intake (Shank and Carson, 1992). However, lead remains in the diet as the result of still extant lead water pipe (EPA, 2011) and has triggered recent recalls of containers (lead in stainless steel brandy flasks) and food (lead in turmeric spice and, ironically, in a bubble gum called "Toxic Waste") (FDA, 2011c, d, and e).

Cadmium Cadmium is a relatively rare commodity in nature and usually is associated with shale and sedimentary deposits. It is often found in association with zinc ores and in lesser amounts in fossil fuel. Although rare in nature, it is a nearly ubiquitous element in American society because of its industrial uses in plating, paint pigments, plastics, and textiles. Exposure to humans often occurs through secondary routes as a result of dumping at smelters and refining plants, disintegration of automobile tires (which contain cadmium-laden rubber), subsequent seepage into the soil and groundwater, and inhalation of combustion products of cadmium-containing materials. The estimated yearly release of cadmium from automobile tires alone ranges from 5.2 to 6.0 metric tons (Davis, 1970; Lagerwerff and Sprecht, 1971). However, in the absence of an overt environmental contamination, food remains the primary source for cadmium uptake for nonsmokers (EFSA, 2009).

Cadmium, like mercury, can form alkyl compounds, but unlike mercury, the alkyl derivatives are relatively unstable and consumption almost always involves the inorganic salt. Of two historical incidents of cadmium poisoning, one involved the use of cadmium-plated containers to hold acidic fruit slushes before freezing. Up to 13 to 15 ppm cadmium was found in the frozen confection, 300 ppm in lemonade, and 450 ppm in raspberry gelatin. Several deaths resulted. A more recent incident of a chronic poisoning involved the dumping of mining wastes into rice paddies in Japan. Middle-aged women who were deficient in calcium and had multiple pregnancies seemed to be the most susceptible. Symptoms included hypercalciuria; extreme bone pain from osteomalacia; lumbago; pain in the back, shoulders, and joints; a waddling gait; frequent fractures; proteinuria; and glycosuria. The disease was called *itai-itai* (ouch-ouch disease) as a result of the pain with walking. The victims had a reported intake of 1000 μg/day, approximately 200 times the normal intake of unexposed populations (Yamagata and Shigematsu, 1970). Cadmium exposure has also been associated with cancer of the breast, lung, large intestine, and urinary bladder (Newberne, 1987).

Cadmium absorption is greatest with pulmonary exposure, but it is relatively low (3%–5%) after dietary exposure to humans, although absorption is effected by several factors including nutritional status (eg, low body iron), number of pregnancies, and general health. Cadmium is retained in the kidney and liver in the body, with a very long biological half-life ranging from 10 to 30 years. Cadmium is primarily toxic to the proximal tubular cells of the kidney and tends to accumulate in the cortex of the kidney, eventually leading to renal failure. Bone demineralization occurs with prolonged exposure, as illustrated in the Japanese exposure, which may be secondary to renal dysfunction (EFSA, 2009).

JECFA (2005) investigated cadmium consumption for several countries including the United States and found that the greatest impacts of maximum (allowable) levels (ML) were seen with stem/root vegetables, other vegetables, and molluscs (41%, 68%, and 42%, respectively, when the lowest MLs were used), which represented an insignificant change over a previous intake assessment. Therefore, the current total intake of cadmium was only 40% to 60% of the Provisional Tolerable Weekly Intake (PTWI) of 7 μg/kg bw/week established several years ago, and a slight variation of 1% to 6% due to the use of the proposed new maximum limits is of no significance in terms of risk to human health (JECFA, 2005).

Mercury Exposure to elemental mercury is relatively rare, although it was once responsible for an occupational disease of hat manufacturers, as elemental mercury was used for the curing of animal pelts. Inhalation of the mercury fumes led to mental deterioration, subsequently named "mad hatter syndrome." The effects of mercury were more pronounced following the application of mercurial ointments for treatment of syphilis and gave rise to the pun "a night with Venus is followed by a lifetime with Mercury" (Waldron, 1983).

Of interest to food toxicology is the methyl derivative, methyl mercury, formed by bacterial action in an aquatic environment from anthropogenic and natural sources of elemental mercury. Anthropogenic sources include burning of coal (which contains mercury), chloralkali process, and other sources of elemental mercury discharge into aquatic environments. In the case of Minamata, Japan, there was a direct discharge of methyl mercury into the environment. Methyl mercury exposure may cause neurological paresthesias, ataxia, dysarthria, hearing defects, and death. Developmental delays have been documented in children borne of mothers exposed to methyl mercury (Carrington and Bolger, 1992). Other than direct exposure to methyl mercury, exposure usually comes about as the result of methyl mercury becoming incorporated into the food chain. Near the peak of the food chain, methyl mercury becomes concentrated in fish including, bonito (*Sarda* spp), halibut (*Hippoglossus* spp), mackerel (*Scomberomorus* spp), marlin (*Makaira* spp), shark (all species), swordfish (*Xiphias gladius*), and bluefin tuna (*Thunnus* spp). The selection of these species for monitoring and tolerance setting was based on historical data on levels of methyl mercury found in fish consumed in the United States. The selection was also based on an FDA action level of 1.0 ppm in the edible portion of fish (FDA, 2001). However, the allowable level of mercury depends on whether the mercury was "added," that is, did the presence of mercury arise from an anthropogenic source (ie, was the fish caught in an area known for mercury discharge or was it naturally present in the environment?) (Hutt *et al.*, 2007).

Halogenated Hydrocarbons (Polychlorinated and Polybrominated Hydrocarbons)

Polychlorinated Hydrocarbons Halogenated hydrocarbons have been with us for some time, and given their stability in water and resistance to oxidation, ultraviolet light, microbial degradation, and other sources of natural destruction, halogenated organics will persist in the environment for some time to come, albeit in minute amounts. However, with the introduction of chlorinated hydrocarbons as pesticides in the 1930s, diseases associated with an insect vector such as malaria were nearly eliminated. In the industrialized world, chlorinated organics brought the promise of nearly universal solvents, and their extraordinary resistance to degradation made them suitable for use as heat-transfer agents and carbonless copy paper, among other uses. As a result of their facile nature, their resulting wide-range uses, and resistance to degradation (and ease of detection), chlorinated hydrocarbons have been found in a wide variety of foods (Table 31-23).

Table 31-23

Examples of Chlorinated Hydrocarbons in British Food

FOOD	CHLORINATED HYDROCARBONS (µg/kg)								
	CHCl$_3$	CCl$_4$	TCE	TCEY	TTCE	PCE	HCB	HCBD	PerCE
Milk	5.0	0.2		0.3	—	—	1.0	0.08	0.3
Cheese	33.0	5.0		3.0	0.0	0.0	0.0	0.0	2.0
Butter	22.0	14.0		10.0	—	—	—	2.0	13.0
Chicken eggs	1.4	0.5		0.6	0.0	0.0	0.0	0.0	0.0
Beef steak	4.0	7.0	3.0	16.0	0.0	0.0	0.0	0.0	0.9
Beef fat	3.0	8.0	6.0	12.0					1.0
Pork liver	1.0	9.0	4.0	22.0	0.5	0.4			5.0
Margarine	3.0	6.0	—		0.8				7.0
Tomatoes	2.0	4.5	—	1.7	1.0		70.1	0.8	1.2
Bread (fresh)	2.0	5.0	2.0	7.0	—	—	—	—	1.0
Fruit drink (canned)	2.0	0.5	—	5.0		0.8			2.0

CHCl$_3$, chloroform; CCl$_4$, carbon tetrachloride; HCB, hexachlorobenzene; HCBD, hexachlorobutadiene; PCE, pentachloroethane; PerCE, perchloroethylene; TCE, trichloroethane; TCEY, trichloroethylene; TTCE, tetrachloroethane.

SOURCE: Modified from McConnell G, Ferguson DM, Pearson CR. Chlorinated hydrocarbons and the environment. Endeavour. 1975;34:13–18. With kind permission from Elsevier Science Ltd, The Boulevard, Langford Lane, Kidlington OX5 1GB, UK.

There have been only a few incidents of mass poisonings via food, two of which involved cooking oil contaminated with polychlorinated organics. The first became known as *yusho*, or rice oil disease, from rice oil contamination originally thought to be confined to polychlorinated biphenyls (PCBs), but has since been revised to include polychlorinated quarterphenyls and polychlorinated dibenzofurans (PCDFs) (Kanagawa *et al.*, 2008). The poisoning occurred in 1968 in Japan and affected approximately 2000 individuals. The most vulnerable were newborns of poisoned mothers. The liver and skin were the most severely affected. Symptoms included dark brown pigmentation of nails; acne-like eruptions; increased eye discharge; visual disturbances; pigmentation of the skin, lips, and gingiva; swelling of the upper eyelids; hyperemia of the conjunctiva; enlargement and elevation of hair follicles; itching; increased sweating of the palms; hyperkeratotic plaques on the soles and palms; and generalized malaise. Recovery requires several years (Anderson and Sogn, 1984; Guo *et al.*, 2003), although more recent authors claim that recovery is gradual even at the 37-year mark, as some patients exhibit symptoms specific to the disease including, but not limited to, hyperglyceridemia, pulmonary disorders, and intractable headache, which were added to the initial diagnostic criteria (Kanagawa *et al.*, 2008). The second incident occurred in 1979 in Yucheng, Taiwan, which also involved PCB-contaminated cooking oil and exposed a similar number of people as the earlier incident in Japan (Guo *et al.*, 2003). The total intakes of PCBs and PCDFs for Yusho and Yucheng victims were estimated to be 633 and 3.4 mg and 973 and 3.84 mg, respectively (Masuda, 1985).

Polychlorinated biphenyls are not formed naturally and were manufactured for use as insulators in electrical machinery, although manufacturing was banned in the United States in 1977. Despite the persistence of chlorinated hydrocarbons in our environment and their reported ubiquity, their low degree of demonstrable toxicity at ambient levels indicates a relatively low risk to humans. Ames *et al.* (1987) described a method for interpreting the differing potencies of carcinogens and human exposures: the percentage human exposure dose/rodent potency dose (HERP). Using this method, they claimed that the hazard from trichloroethylene-contaminated water in Silicon Valley or Woburn, Massachusetts, or the daily dietary intake from dichlorodiphenyltrichloroethane (DDT) (or its product, dichlorodiphenyldichloroethylene [DDE]) at a HERP of 0.0003% to 0.004% is considerably less than the hazard presented by the consumption of symphytine in a single cup of comfrey herb tea (0.03%) or the hazard presented by aflatoxin in a peanut butter sandwich (0.03%). The FDA's authority to set tolerances has been used only once in establishing levels for PCBs (21 CFR 109.15 and 109.30).

Polybrominated Hydrocarbons Polybrominated biphenyls (PBBs) and polybrominated biphenyl ethers (PDBEs) (the latter are also called brominated diphenyl oxides) were used as fire retardants in, among other things, household furniture, airplane seat upholstery, and children's pajamas, all of which had been identified as sources of preventable disfiguring burns and tragic deaths. Uses also extended to electrical equipment, paint, and plastics, and PBBs have been manufactured globally by several companies.

Appropriately, one of the names under which PPBs were sold was "FireMaster." Tragedy struck in Michigan in 1973, when FireMaster was placed in bags labeled "NutriMaster" (a magnesium oxide animal feed supplement). Several farms received feed contaminated by FireMaster and feed consumption and milk production dropped by as much as 50%, but the causative agent remained a mystery. As the result of a persistent dairy farmer and more than one serendipitous event (eg, a chromatograph left on by accident, allowing PBBs to elute after a considerable period of time), PBBs were identified as the causative agent. It was found that approximately 650 lbs of PBB had entered the food chain through milk and other dairy products, as well as beef, pork, sheep, poultry, and egg products (Fries, 1985; MDCH, 2011). Over 500 Michigan farms were quarantined, and approximately 30,000 cattle, 4500 swine,

1500 sheep, and 1.5 million chickens were destroyed, along with over 800 tons of animal feed, 18,000 pounds of cheese, 2500 pounds of butter, 5 million eggs, and 34,000 pounds of dried milk products (MDCH, 2011). The incident was eventually publicized in 1981 as a television movie entitled "Bitter Harvest." PBB-exposed Michigan residents had a variety of complaints including nausea, abdominal pain, loss of appetite, joint pain, fatigue, and weakness, and although a cause–effect relationship could not be established for these symptoms, there is a fairly strong case for development of acne from exposure to PBBs.

Like PCBs, many distinct isomers are possible of PBB and PBDE, but the three main commercial products are pentabromodiphenyl oxide or ether, octabromodiphenyl oxide or ether, and decabromodiphenyl oxide or ether. Since the Michigan incident, the production of PBBs has declined, but with a concomitant increase in demand for PBDEs. Worldwide demand for PBDEs in 2001 was estimated at 70,000 metric tons. These substances are chemically rugged entities and are very resistant to acids, bases, heat, light, reduction, and oxidation—all advantages for their intended use, but disadvantages when discharged into the environment. Interestingly, PBDEs are reported to occur naturally and are produced by *Vibrio* spp, in association with sponges of the *Dysidea* genus. Conversely, some environmental remediation may occur with two strains of *Pseudomonas* isolated from runoff areas of the Michigan manufacturer.

Absorption of PBDEs is limited with some 80% to 90% of a dose eliminated in the feces unchanged; degree of bromination is inversely proportional to absorption, but once absorbed, PBDEs are persistent and bioaccumulating. PBDEs in rat subchronic studies produced effects in liver, kidney, and thyroid in males and females. Liver enlargement, associated with increased metabolism, was reported at doses of 1 to 10 mg/kg bw. DecaBDE at 2.5% and 5% of the diet to mice and rats was carcinogenic. PBDEs are not genotoxic, but are reported to have reproductive effects in rats and rabbits. Data for humans were reported as being incomplete. Because of the limited amount of data, the JECFA committee could not allocate a Provisional Tolerable Weekly Intake (PTWI) (deBoer *et al.*, 2000; JECFA, 2005).

Nitrosmaines, Nitrosamides, and *N*-Nitroso Substances

Nitrogenous compounds such as amines, amides, guanidines, and ureas can react with oxides of nitrogen (NO_x) to form *N*-nitroso compounds (NOCs) (Hotchkiss *et al.*, 1992). The NOCs may be divided into two classes: the nitrosamines, which are *N*-nitroso derivatives of secondary amines, and nitrosamides, which are *N*-nitroso derivatives of substituted ureas, amides, carbamates, guanidines, and similar compounds (Mirvish, 1975).

Nitrosamines are stable compounds, whereas many nitrosamides have half-lives on the order of minutes, particularly at pH >>6.5. Both classes have members that are potent animal carcinogens, but by different mechanisms. In general, the biological activity of an NOC is thought to be related to alkylation of genetic macromolecules. *N*-nitrosamines are metabolically activated by hydroxylation at an α-carbon. The resulting hydroxyalkyl moiety is eliminated as an aldehyde, and an unstable primary nitrosamine is formed. The nitrosamine tautomerizes to a diazonium hydroxide and ultimately to a carbonium ion. Nitrosamides spontaneously decompose to a carbonium ion at physiological pH by a similar mechanism (Hotchkiss *et al.*, 1992). This is consistent with in vitro laboratory findings because nitrosamines require S9 for activity and nitrosamides are mutagenic de novo.

Table 31-24

Sources of Dietary NOCs

The use of nitrate and/or nitrite as intentional food additives, both of which are added to fix the color of meats, inhibit oxidation, and prevent toxigenesis.

Drying processes in which the drying air is heated by an open-flame source. NO_x is generated in small amounts through the oxidation of N_2, which nitrosates amines in the foods. This is the mechanism for contamination of malted barley products.

NOCs can migrate from food contact materials such as rubber bottle nipples.

NOCs can inhabit spices, which may be added to food

Cooking over open flames (eg, natural gas flame) can result in NOC formation in foods by the same mechanism as drying.

NOC, N-nitroso compounds.
SOURCE: Adapted with permission from Hotchkiss JH, Helser MA, Maragos CM, et al. Nitrate, nitrite, and N-nitroso compounds: food safety and biological implications. In: Finley JW, Robinson SF, Armstrong DJ, eds. Food Safety Assessment. Washington, DC: American Chemical Society; 1992:400–418.

NOCs originate from two sources: environmental formation and endogenous formation (Table 31-24). Environmental sources have declined over the last several years but still include foods (eg, nitrate-cured meats) and beverages (eg, malt beverages), cosmetics, occupational exposure, and rubber products (Hotchkiss, 1989). NOCs formed in vivo may actually constitute the greatest exposure and are formed from nitrosation of amines and amides in several areas, including the stomach, where the most favorable conditions exist (pH 2–4), although consumption of H_2-receptor blockers or antacids decreases the formation of NOCs.

Environmentally, nitrite is formed from nitrate or ammonium ions by certain microorganisms in soil, water, and sewage. In vivo, nitrite is formed from nitrate by microorganisms in the mouth and stomach, followed by nitrosation of secondary amines and amides in the diet. Sources of nitrate and nitrite in the diet are given in Table 31-25. Many sources of nitrate are also sources of vitamin C. Another possibly significant source of nitrate is well water; although the levels are generally in the range of 21 µM, levels of 1600 µM (100 mg/L) have been reported (Hotchkiss *et al.*, 1992). However, on the average, Western diets contain 1 to 2 mmol nitrate/person/day (Hotchkiss *et al.*, 1992). Nitrosation reactions can be inhibited by preferential, competitive neutralization of nitrite with naturally occurring and synthetic materials such as vitamin C, vitamin E, sulfamate, antioxidants such as butylated hydroxytoluene, BHA, and gallic acid, and even amino acids or proteins (Hotchkiss, 1989; Hotchkiss *et al.*, 1992).

N-nitrosoproline is the most common nitrosoamine present in humans and is excreted virtually unchanged in the urine. The basal rate of urinary excretion of nitrosoproline, which is claimed to be noncarcinogenic, is 2 to 7 g/day in subjects on a low-nitrate diet (Oshima and Bartsch, 1981).

Epidemiological studies have not provided compelling evidence of a causal association between nitrate exposure and human cancer nor has a causal link been shown between NOCs, preformed in the diet or endogenously synthesized, and the incidence of human cancer (Gangolli, 1999). The cancer risk of nitrite, nitrate, and processed meats is weak and inconclusive, and the risk must be weighed against the health benefits of restoring NO homeostasis via dietary nitrite and nitrate. These benefits should be considered

Table 31-25

Nitrate and Nitrite Content of Food

VEGETABLES	NITRATE (ppm)	NITRITE (ppm)	MEAT	NITRATE (ppm)	NITRITE (ppm)
Artichoke	12	0.4	Unsmoked side bacon	134	12
Asparagus	44	0.6	Unsmoked back bacon	160	8
Green beans	340	0.6	Peameal bacon	16	21
Lima beans	54	1.1	Smoked bacon	52	7
Beets	2400	4	Corned beef	141	19
Broccoli	740	1	Cured corned beef	852	9
Brussel sprouts	120	1	Corned beef brisket	90	3
Cabbage	520	0.5	Pickled beef	70	23
Carrots	200	0.8	Canned corn beef	77	24
Cauliflower	480	1.1	Ham	105	17
Celery	2300	0.5	Smoked ham	138	50
Corn	45	2	Cured ham	767	35
Radish	1900	0.2	Belitalia (garlic)	247	5
Rhubarb	2100	NR	Pepperoni (beef)	149	23
Spinach	1800	2.5	Summer sausage	135	7
Tomatoes	58	NR	Ukranian sausage (Polish)	77	15
Turnip	390	NR	German sausage	71	17
Turnip greens	6600	2.3			

NR, not reported.
SOURCE: Data from Hotchkiss JH, Helser MA, Maragos CM, et al. Nitrate, nitrite, and N-nitroso
compounds: food safety and biological implications. In: Finley JW, Robinson SF, Armstrong DJ, eds.
Food Safety Assessment. Washington, DC: American Chemical Society; 1992:400–418.

before arriving at any new regulatory or public health guidelines (Milkowski *et al.*, 2010).

Food-borne Molds and Mycotoxins

Molds have served humans for centuries in the production of foods (eg, ripening cheese) and have provided various fungal metabolites with important medicinal uses; they also may produce secondary metabolites with the potential to produce severe adverse health effects, including behavioral changes (Cousins *et al.*, 2005). It is possible that ergot mycotoxins may have exerted a major role in restricting population expansion and only the reduced dependency on rye cereal as the staple food in the sixteenth and seventeenth centuries, arising from the introduction of wheat and potatoes, allowed the steady upward movement in population growth in Europe (CAST, 2003; IFST, 2006a).

Mycotoxins are secondary fungal metabolites (ie, not essential for survival of the mold) secreted into the microenvironment around the mold. Mycotoxins represent a diverse group of chemicals that can occur in a variety of plants used as food, including commodities such as cereal grains (barley, corn, rye, wheat), coffee, dairy products, fruits, nuts, peanuts, and spices. A few mycotoxins also can occur in animal products derived from animals that consume contaminated feeds (eg, milk). However, because commodities are eaten in the greatest amounts, the mycotoxins present in these foods represent the greatest risk (Cousins *et al.*, 2005).

The current interest in mycotoxicosis was generated by a series of reports in 1960–1963 that associated the death of turkeys in England (so-called turkey X disease) and ducklings in Uganda with the consumption of peanut meal feeds containing mold products produced by *Aspergillus flavus* (Stoloff, 1977). The additional discovery of aflatoxin metabolites (eg, aflatoxin M_1 in milk) led to more intensive studies of mycotoxins and to the identification of a variety of these compounds associated with adverse human health effects, both retrospectively and prospectively.

Moldy foods are consumed throughout the world during times of famine, as a matter of taste, and through ignorance of their adverse health effects. Epidemiological studies designed to ascertain the acute or chronic effects of such consumption are few. Data from animal studies indicate that the consumption of food contaminated with mycotoxins has the potential to contribute to a variety of human diseases (Miller, 1991). Reports of acute intoxications are few; however, prolonged exposure to small quantities of mycotoxin may lead to more insidious effects including growth retardation, birth defects, impaired immunity, decreased disease resistance, and tumor formation in humans and decreased production in farm animals (CAST, 2003).

With some exceptions, molds can be divided into two main groups: "field fungi" and "storage fungi." The former group contains species that proliferate in and under field conditions and do not multiply readily once grain is in storage. Field fungi may be superseded and overrun by storage fungi if conditions of moisture and oxygen allow.

Importantly, the presence of a toxigenic mold does not guarantee the presence of a mycotoxin, which is elaborated only under certain conditions. Further, more than one mold can produce the same mycotoxin (eg, both *Aspergillus flavus* and several *Penicillium* species produce the mycotoxin cyclopiazonic acid) (El-Banna *et al.*, 1987; Truckness *et al.*, 1987). Also, more than one mycotoxin may be present in an intoxication; that is, as in the outbreak of turkey X disease, there is speculation that aflatoxin and cyclopiazonic acid both exerted an effect, but the profound effects of aflatoxin would have overshadowed those of cyclopiazonic acid (Miller, 1989). Although there are many different mycotoxins and subgroups (Table 31-26), this discussion will be confined largely to four of the more important: aflatoxins, trichothecenes, fumonisins, and ochratoxin A.

Organic foods, produced without the use of insecticides and fungicides, may be more susceptible to mycotoxin contamination than foods produced using conventional agricultural practices. For example, higher levels of ochratoxin were found in organic cereal when compared to nonorganic cereal and cereal products in Spain and Portugal (Juan *et al.*, 2008). The UK Food Standards Agency found several organic maize meal products highly contaminated with fumonisin mycotoxins, whereas conventionally produced maize meal products analyzed concurrently had levels below recommended limits (UK Food Standards Agency, 2003). Because European agriculture faces a growing demand by consumers for organic produce, the European Union has established a project called "safe organic vegetables and vegetable products by reducing risk factors and sources of fungal contaminants throughout the production chain" focusing on organic carrots and reduction of alternaria toxins (EU, 2002).

Aflatoxins Among the various mycotoxins, the aflatoxins have been the subject of the most intensive research because of the potent hepatocarcinogenicity and toxicity of aflatoxin B_1 in

Table 31-26

Selected Mycotoxins Produced by Various Molds and Some of Their Effects and Commodities Potentially Contaminated

MYCOTOXIN	SOURCE	EFFECT	COMMODITIES CONTAMINATED
Aflatoxins B_1, B_2, G_1, G_2	*Aspergillus flavus, A parasiticus*	Acute aflatoxicosis, carcinogenesis	Corn, peanuts, and others
Aflatoxin M_1	Metabolite of AFB_1	Hepatotoxicity	Milk
Fumonisins B_1, B_2. B_3, B_4, A_1, A_2	*Fusarium verticillioides*	Renal and liver carcinogenesis	Corn
Trichothecenes (for example, T-2, deoxynivalenol, diacetoxyscirpenol)	*Fusarium, Myrothecium*	Hematopoietic toxicity, meningeal hemorrhage of brain, "nervous" disorder, necrosis of skin, hemorrhage in mucosal epithelia of stomach and intestine, emesis, feed refusal, immune suppression.	Cereal grains, corn
Zearalenones	*Fusarium*	Estrogenic effect	Corn, grain
Cyclopiazonic acid	*Aspergillus, Penicillium*	Muscle, liver, and splenic toxicity	Cheese, grains, peanuts
Kojic acid	*Aspergillus*	Hepatotoxic?	Grain, animal feed
3-Nitropropionic acid	*Arthrinium sacchari, A saccharicola, A phaeospermum*	Central nervous system impairment	Sugarcane
Citreoviridin	*Penicillium citreoviride, P toxicarium*	Cardiac beriberi	Rice
Cytochalasins E, B, F, H	*Aspergillus* and *Penicillium*	Cytotoxicity	Corn, cereal grain
Sterigmatocystin	*Aspergillus versiolar*	Carcinogenesis	Corn
Penicillinic acid	*Penicillium cyclopium*	Nephrotoxicity, abortifacient	Corn, dried beans, grains
Rubratoxins A, B	*Penicillium rubrum*	Hepatotoxicity, teratogenic	Corn
Patulin	*Penicillium patulum*	Carcinogenesis, liver damage	Apple and apple products
Ochratoxin	*Aspergillus ochraceus, A carbonarius, Penicillium verrucosum*	Endemic nephropathy, carcinogenesis	Grains, peanuts, grapes, green coffee
Citrinin	*Aspergillus* and *Penicillium*	Nephrotoxicity	Cereal grains
Penitrem(s)		Tremors, incoordination, bloody diarrhea, death	Moldy cream cheese, English walnuts, hamburger bun, beer
Ergot alkaloids	*Clavicepts purpurea*	Ergotism	Grains

rats. Epidemiological studies conducted in Africa and Asia suggest that it is a human hepatocarcinogen, and various other reports have implicated the aflatoxins in incidences of human toxicity (Krishnamachari *et al.*, 1975; Peers *et al.*, 1976; Kensler *et al.*, 2011).

Generally, aflatoxins occur in susceptible crops as mixtures of aflatoxins B_1, B_2, G_1, and G_2, with only aflatoxins B_1 and G_1 demonstrating carcinogenicity. A carcinogenic hydroxylated metabolite of aflatoxin B_1 (termed aflatoxin M_1) can occur in the milk from dairy cows that consume contaminated feed. Aflatoxins may occur in a number of susceptible commodities and products derived from them, including edible nuts (peanuts, pistachios, almonds, walnuts, pecans, and Brazil nuts), oil seeds (cottonseed and copra), and grains (corn, grain sorghum, and millet) (Stoloff, 1977). In tropical regions, aflatoxin can be produced in unrefrigerated prepared foods. The two major sources of aflatoxin contamination of commodities are field contamination, especially during times of drought and other stresses, which allow insect damage that opens the plant to mold attack, and inadequate storage conditions. Since the discovery of their potential threat to human health, progress has been made in decreasing the level of aflatoxins in specific commodities in developed countries. For example, in the United States and Western European countries, control measures include ensuring adequate storage conditions and careful monitoring of susceptible commodities for aflatoxin level and the banning of lots that exceed the action level for aflatoxin B_1.

Aflatoxin B_1 is acutely toxic in all species studied, with an LD_{50} ranging from 0.5 mg/kg for the duckling to 60 mg/kg for the mouse (Wogan, 1973). Death typically results from hepatotoxicity. Aflatoxin B_1 is also highly mutagenic, hepatocarcinogenic, and possibly teratogenic. A problem in extrapolating animal data to humans is the extremely wide range of species susceptibility to aflatoxin B_1. For instance, whereas aflatoxin B_1 appears to be the most hepatocarcinogenic compound known for the rat, the adult mouse is essentially totally resistant to its hepatocarcinogenicity.

Aflatoxin B_1 is an extremely reactive compound biologically, altering a number of biochemical systems. The hepatocarcinogenicity of aflatoxin B_1 is associated with its biotransformation to a highly reactive electrophilic epoxide, which forms covalent adducts with DNA, RNA, and protein. Damage to DNA is thought to be the initial biochemical lesion resulting in the expression of the pathological tumor growth (IARC, 2002). Species differences in the response to aflatoxin may be due in part to differences in biotransformation and susceptibility to the initial biochemical lesion (Monroe and Eaton, 1987).

Trichothecenes Trichothecenes are toxic sesquiterpenoid compounds that have an epoxide functionality that is apparently crucial for their toxicity (Desjardins *et al.*, 1993). They include many different chemical entities that all contain the trichothecene nucleus (Ellison and Kotsonis, 1975) and are produced primarily by *Fusarium*, but also by a number of commonly occurring molds, including *Myrothecium*, *Trichothecium*, *Stachybotrys*, and *Cephalosporium*. The trichothecenes were first discovered during attempts to isolate antibiotics, and although some show antibiotic activity, their toxicity has precluded their use as therapeutic agents. *Fusarium* head blight, caused by trichothecene-producing *Fusarium* species, is a destructive disease of cereal grain crops that has a worldwide economic impact (Fouroud and Eudes, 2009). Consumption of contaminated grain has been associated with intestinal irritation in mammals and can lead to feed refusal in livestock and other toxic responses (Eriksen and Pettersson, 2004). There have been many reported cases of trichothecene toxicity in farm animals and a few in humans. One of the most famous cases of presumed human toxicity associated with the consumption of trichothecenes occurred in Russia during 1944 around Orenburg, Siberia. Disruption of agriculture caused by World War II resulted in millet, wheat, and barley being overwintered in the field. Consumption of these commodities resulted in vomiting, skin inflammation, diarrhea, and multiple hemorrhages, among other symptoms. About 10% of the population was affected and mortality rates were as high as 60% in some counties (Ueno, 1977; Beardall and Miller, 1994), and was subsequently identified as alimentary toxic aleukia (CAST, 2003). Trichothecenes are protein synthesis inhibitors known to bind to ribosomes. The acute LD_{50}s of the trichothecenes range from 0.5 to 70 mg/kg, and although there have been reports of possible chronic toxicity associated with certain members of this group, more research will be needed before the magnitude of their potential to produce adverse human health effects is understood (Sato and Ueno, 1977). The extent of toxicity associated with the trichothecenes in humans and farm animals is poorly understood, owing in part to the number of entities in this group and the difficulty of assaying for these compounds (JECFA, 2001).

Fumonisins Fumonisins are mycotoxins produced by *Fusarium verticillioides* (formerly known as *F moniliforme*) and several other *Fusarium* species. Corn products contaminated with *F verticilliodes* are responsible for agriculturally important diseases in horses and swine (ICPS, 2000) and are actively being evaluated to determine how great a threat they pose to public health. Initial evidence of the involvement of *F verticilliodes*–produced toxins in human disease was reported by Marasas *et al.* (1988), who found that an increased incidence of esophageal cancer was associated with the consumption of contaminated corn (maize) by humans in a region in South Africa. Fumonisins have been associated with cancer, reproductive toxicity (neural tube defects), and acute disease outbreaks where low-quality corn is consumed on a regular basis (Cousins *et al.*, 2005). Fumonisins target different organs in different species, but the underlying mechanism is a disruption of lipid metabolism by inhibition of ceramide synthetase, an enzyme integral to the formation of complex lipids for use in membranes (ICPS, 2000; IARC, 2002).

Corn borer insect pests cause damage to the developing grain, which enables spores of the toxin-producing fungi, *Fusarium*, to germinate. The fungus then proliferates, which leads to ear and kernel rot and the production of potentially hazardous levels of fumonisins. Corn varieties, which express the Bt insect control proteins, have been shown to contain significantly reduced levels of fumonisin because the Bt protein significantly reduces the corn borer–induced tissue damage in corn products (Munkvold *et al.*, 1997, 1999; Masoero *et al.*, 1999; Hammond *et al.*, 2004; Papst *et al.*, 2005; Ostry *et al.*, 2010; Folcher *et al.*, 2010).

Ochratoxin A This mycotoxin is primarily produced by *Aspergillus ochraceus*, *A carbonarius*, and *Penicillium verrucosum*, and human exposure occurs as the result of contamination of small grains (barley, wheat, and corn), coffee beans, and grapes. The effects of ochratoxin A were discovered as the result of feeding the mycotoxin to pigs, who subsequently drank copious amounts of water, urinated near continuously, and exhibited pain in the area of the kidney. Ochratoxin A is nephrotoxic and carcinogenic in mice and rats. Ochratoxin A is absorbed from the GI tract and enters the enterohepatic circulation; it is also absorbed by the proximal and distal tubules of the kidney. It binds tightly to albumin in the blood and can therefore have a very long serum half-life. Epidemiological evidence indicates nearly half the European population is exposed to ochratoxin A and there is an association of endemic nephropathy and renal tumors in humans in parts of Eastern Europe (CAST, 2003).

Ethyl Carbamate

Ethyl carbamate or urethane, the ethyl ester of carbamic acid, was used for many years as an intravenous anesthetic until its mutagenic and carcinogenic properties became known. It has since been classified by the International Agency for Research on Cancer (IARC) as "possibly carcinogenic to humans" (Group 2B) and "reasonably anticipated to be a human carcinogen" by the NTP (2004a). The primary use of urethane is as a chemical intermediate in the preparation of amino resins, with lesser uses as a solubilizer in the manufacture of pesticides, fumigants, and cosmetics and as an intermediate for pharmaceuticals and biochemical research. It is allowed in some anticonvulsant drugs at a level of 1 ppm and is still used as a veterinary anesthetic. Urethane has been found in fermented foods and beverages including liquor, wine, beer, bread, soy sauce, and yogurt. Diethylpyrocarbonate, an inhibitor of fermentation, can form ethyl carbamate.

Ethyl carbamate is easily absorbed and undergoes CYP2E1-mediated metabolic activation to vinyl carbamate epoxide, which binds covalently to nucleic acids and proteins, producing adducts. Ethyl carbamate is a multisite carcinogen with a short latency period. Single doses or short-term oral dosing at 100 to 200 mg/kg BW/day has been shown to induce tumors in mice, rats, and hamsters. Intake estimates from food and alcoholic beverages range from a mean of 0.015 μg/kg BW/day to 0.080 μg/kg BW/day for high-end users. The benchmark dose lower confidence limit as set by JECFA is 0.3 mg/kg BW/day, which yields a margin of safety of 20,000 (JECFA, 2005).

Fluoride

Fluorine, in the form of fluoride, is nearly ubiquitous in nature. Primary human exposure is via drinking water, although it is also present in some foods, notably some teas, vegetables, and marine fish. Exposure also occurs via processed food made with fluoridated water or produce washed with fluoridated water (the so-called 'halo' effect). The greatest nondietary source is fluoridated toothpaste (NRC, 2006). Fluoride taken in water has a high degree of bioavailability with an absorption of 90%, whereas fluoride taken in food is approximately 50% absorbed. Consumption of fluoride results in uptake by bone and teeth, where enamel crystallites form fluorhydroxyapatite in place of the naturally formed hydroxyapatite; the former being stronger and more acid-resistant than the latter, resisting and even reversing the initiation and progression of dental caries. Ionic fluoride rarely exists in blood, most is trapped by bone tissue, where new bone growth is stimulated and this mechanism has served as the basis of some treatments for osteoporosis (WHO, 1996).

Fluorosis occurs as the result of high fluoride intake and may be complicated by low calcium intake; it is cumulative and endemic to some areas of the world (eg, China and India). Fluorosis is dose-responsive, producing a range of effects from cosmetic (mottling of teeth) to adverse functionality (skeletal fluorosis). Enamel fluorosis occurs as the result of high fluoride consumption prior to tooth eruption (ie, in children up to the age of eight years, exposed to water with a fluoride content of ≥4 mg/L) and can range from a mild discoloration of the tooth surface to severe (brown) staining and pitting of the teeth to the point of enamel loss (NRC, 2006). In skeletal fluorosis, in the asymptomatic, preclinical stage, patients have an increased bone density. Stage 1 skeletal fluorosis is characterized

by occasional stiffness, pain in joints, or some osteosclerosis of the pelvis and vertebra. Stage 2 skeletal fluorosis is characterized by sporadic pain, stiffness of joints, and osteosclerosis of the pelvis and spine, although mobility is not severely affected. In Stage 3 (rarely seen in the United States), there may be crippling, dose-related calcification of ligaments, osteosclerosis, exotoses, osteoporosis of long bones, muscle wasting, and neurological effects due to hypercalcification of vertebrae (at this point, bone ash fluoride may be two to three times that of the bones of normal subjects). Although it is agreed that skeletal fluorosis is the result of prolonged exposure to increased amounts of fluoride, because the incidence of crippling skeletal fibrosis continues to be rare even in geographic areas of high exposure, unidentified intervening metabolic or dietary factors may have rendered skeletons more or less susceptible. Other effects attributed to excess fluoride include lower IQs and decreased thyroid function, increased calcitonin activity, increased parathyroid hormone activity, secondary hyperparathyroidism, impaired glucose tolerance, and possible effects on timing of sexual activity (NRC, 2006). The reports of possible carcinogenic effects of fluoride, including those of the bone (osteosarcoma), are tentative and mixed (NRC, 2006; Douglass and Joshipura, 2006).

Guidelines for fluoridation of the public water supply recommend addition at levels of 0.7 to 1.2 mg/L, to achieve target Adequate Intake (AI) levels based on a 2 L water/day intake by adults, with adjustments in warmer regions where water intake is high in the summer months, or where fluoride occurs naturally at high levels (eg, some areas of Colorado, 11.2 mg/L; Oklahoma, 12.0 mg/L; New Mexico, 13.0 mg/L; and Idaho, 15.9 mg/L). Although the essentiality of fluoride has not been described, an AI has been established for various age groups as a balance between caries resistance and possible fluorosis of teeth. For example, the AI for infants is 0.01 mg/day, for adult females and males is 3 and 4 mg/d, respectively, and there is a range of graduated AIs for intervening age groups (IOM, 1997).

Toxins in Fish, Shellfish, and Turtles

There are a number of marine (seafood) toxins (to be distinguished from marine venoms), many of which are not confined to a single species (over 400 species have been associated with ciguatera toxicity). Some of these toxins occur with sporadic frequency and nonpredictability, indicating an environmental influence and can often be traced to the presence of an algae (including dinoflagellates) or commensurate bacteria. However, some marine toxins appear to be specific to a single genus or species and are therefore innate to that taxonomic group.

Marine Toxins

Ciguatera Poisoning   The "cigua" in ciguatera toxin is derived from the Spanish name for the sea snail *Turbo pica* in which the symptoms were first reported. Ciguatera and related toxins (scaritoxin and maitotoxin) are ichthyosarcotoxic neurotoxins (anticholinesterase) and are found in 11 orders, 57 families, and over 400 species of fish as well as in oysters and clams. The penultimate toxin (gambiertoxin) is produced by the dinoflagellate *Gambierdiscus toxicus*, commonly isolated from microalgae growing on or near coral reefs that have ingested the dinoflagellate. The pretoxin appears to pass through the food chain and is biotransformed upon transfer to or by the ingesting fish to the active form, which is consumed by mammals. Other toxins, including palytoxin and okadaic acid, unrelated to gambiertoxin, may be present in ciguarteric fish and may contribute to toxicity. The asymptomatic period is three to five hours after consumption but may last up to 24 hours. The onset is sudden and symptoms may include abdominal pain, nausea, vomiting, and watery diarrhea; muscular aches; tingling and numbness of the lips, tongue, and throat; a metallic taste; temporary blindness; and paralysis. Deaths have occurred. Recovery usually occurs within 24 hours, but tingling may continue for a week or more. The intraperitoneal (i.p.) LD_{50} of maitotoxin in mice is 50 ng/kg (Bryan, 1984; Liston, 2000).

Palytoxin Poisoning Palytoxin is produced by the zoanthid soft coral of the genus *Palythoa*, and fish, crabs, and polychaete worms, living in close association with or eating this mass, may become contaminated with palytoxin. The toxin is not part of the stinging nematocyst of the coral, but may be produced by female polyps and mature eggs of the organism, possibly requiring the presence of symbiotic algae (possibly the dinoflagellate *Ostreopsis siamensis*). Palytoxin, in various forms, is produced by any number of species, including *P tuberculosa* in the tropical waters in the Pacific and Japan, *P mammilosa* and *P caribaeorum* in the West Indies and Puerto Rico, and in the Bahamas, *P vestitus* and other *Palythoa* spp. On occasion, the coral becomes detached from its anchorage and becomes a soft floating mass with a seaweed or moss-like appearance, a very attractive feeding ground for fish. Indigenous peoples of Hawaii knew this as *limu-make-o-Hana* (the deadly seaweed of Hana) and some are said to have smeared the moss on spear points to enhance their utility as a weapon (Onuma *et al.,* 1999; Tan and Lau, 2000; Tosteson, 2000).

The toxin has been reported in mackerel, parrotfish, and several species of crabs. Victims report a bitter, metallic taste from the meat (most often muscle, liver, ovary, and digestive tract), followed immediately by nausea, vomiting, and diarrhea. Within several hours, symptoms include myoglobinuria, a burning sensation around the mouth and extremities, muscle spasms, dyspnea, and dysphonia. Cause of death may be the result of myocardial injury, although it is known in vitro to be a powerful hemolysin.

Although there are several isoforms and possibly minor toxins associated with palytoxin (depending on the producing species), the predominant action is as a ouabain-sensitive Na^+K^+ ATPase inhibitor. Unlike ouabain, palytoxin has no effect on H^+-, Ca^{2+}-, or H^+/K^+-transporting ATPases. The toxin is quite effective with intravenous LD_{50} of 0.078, 0.45, 0.033, and 0.089 µg/kg for monkeys, mice, dogs, and rats, respectively. The standard assay is measured in mouse units (MU), the time taken to kill a mouse weighting 20 grams in four hours following intraperitoneal (i.p.) injection of 0.25 mL (Tan and Lau, 2000; Tosteson, 2000).

Abalone Poisoning (Pyropheophorbide) Abalone poisoning is caused by abalone viscera poison (located in the liver and digestive gland) of the Japanese abalone, *Haliotis discus* and *H sieboldi*, and is unusual in that it causes photosensitization; Hashimoto *et al.* (2010) report the toxin was also found in the midgut glands of cultured scallops (*Patinopecten yessoensis*) gathered in early spring in Japan. The toxin, pyropheophorbide a, is stable to boiling, freezing, and salting. The development of symptoms is contingent on exposure to sunlight. The symptoms are of sudden onset and include a burning and stinging sensation over the entire body, a prickling sensation, itching, erythema, edema, and skin ulceration on parts of the body exposed to sunlight (Bryan, 1984; Shiomi, 1999). Paralytic shellfish toxin (PST) has been detected in abalone, probably through consumption of the mossworm, a plankton feeder that also clings to seaweed and some shellfish (Takatani *et al.,* 1997).

Pheophorbide b ethyl ester has been isolated from a *Chlorella vulgaris* dietary supplement (Chee *et al.,* 2008), and pheophorbide a and phyloerythrin were putatively identified as the causative substance in photosensitization and erythematopurpuric eruptions on the skin of patients with a history of consuming chlorella dietary supplements (Jitsukawa *et al.,* 1984). Pyropheophorbide, pheophorbide, and similar phototoxic agents are breakdown products of chlorophyll.

Dinoflagellate Poisoning (Paralytic Shellfish Poisoning or PSP; Saxitoxin) The etiological agent in dinoflagellate poisoning is saxitoxin or related compounds and is found in mussels, cockles, clams or soft shell clams, butter clams, scallops, and shellfish broth. Bivalve mussels are the most common vehicles. Saxitoxin, originally isolated from toxic Alaskan butter clams (*Saxidomus giganteus*) is actually a family of neurotoxins and includes neosaxitin and gonyautoxin one through four. All block neural transmission at the neuromuscular junction by binding to the surface of the sodium channels and interrupting the flow of Na^+ ions; apical vesicles (AV) nodal conduction may be suppressed, there may be direct suppression of the respiratory center and progressive reduction of peripheral nerve excitability. Saxitoxin produces parathesia and neuromuscular weakness without hypotension and lacks the emetic and hypothermic action of tetrodotoxin. Moderate symptoms are produced by 120 to 180 µg/person and are reversible within hours or days, whereas 80 µg of purified toxin per 100 g of tissue (0.5–2 mg/person) may be lethal, due to asphyxiation, usually within 12 hours of ingestion. The toxin is an alkaloid and is relatively heat-stable. The toxin is produced by several genera of plankton (*Gonyaulax* [now known as *Alexandrium*] *catenella*, *G acatenella*, and *G tamarensis*, *Pyrodinium* spp, *Ptychodiscus brevis*, *Gymnodinium catenatum*, and others), and during red tide blooms may reach 20 to 40 million/mL. Toxic materials are stored in various parts of the body of shellfish. Digestive organs, liver, gills, and siphons contain the greatest concentrations of poison during the warmer months. Distribution is worldwide (Bryan, 1984; Clark *et al.,* 1999; Liston, 2000). The tolerance for Paralytic Shellfish Poisoning (PSP) for clams, mussels, and oysters is 80 µg/100 g meat (Compliance Policy Guideline, 540.250).

Neurotoxic Shellfish Poisoning Traditionally limited to the coast of Florida, *Gymnodinium breve* form red tide blooms containing polycyclic ether toxins called brevetoxins (based on the backbone structure of the molecule, they are generally divided into Type 1 or Type 2), with Type 2 the most often found. Brevetoxins bind to voltage-dependent sodium channels and strength of binding varies with the specific affinity of the toxin and thus the relative potency. Symptoms of Neurotoxic Shellfish Poisoning (NSP) include nausea, tingling, and numbness of the oral area, loss of motor control, and severe muscular ache, all of which resolve in a few days and no deaths have been reported, unlike PSP. An additional route of entry for mammals may result from inhalation of aerosolized toxin as the result of the relative ease of lysis of the unarmored *G breve* organism during the breaking of waves on the shore. Symptoms of this type of exposure are seen as irritation of the throat and upper respiratory tract. A "kill" of nearly 150 manatees was reported during an unprecedented large outbreak of the toxin, although the specific mode of transmission is uncertain. Human exposure is primarily via consumption of filter-feeding organisms, which may concentrate the toxin (Van Dolah, 2000). An FDA Action Level for NSP in food has been set at 0.8 ppm brevetoxin-2 equivalent (SNIC, 2007).

Amnesic Shellfish Poisoning (Domoic Acid) Consumption of mussels harvested from the area off Prince Edward Island in 1987 resulted in gastroenteritis, and many older consumers or those with underlying chronic diseases experienced neurological symptoms including memory loss. Despite treatment, three patients (71–84 years old) died within 11 to 24 days. The poisoning was attributed to domoic acid produced by the diatom *Nitzschia pungens* f *multiseries* (now called *Pseudonitzschia multiseries*), which had been ingested by the mussels during the normal course of feeding. Occurrence of domoic acid has also been reported in California shellfish and produced by *Nitzchia pseudodelicatissima* and in anchovies (resulting in pelican deaths) produced by *N pseudoseriata* (now called *Pseudonitzschia australis*). Domoic acid has been reported in shellfish in other provinces of Canada, and in the United States, in Alaska, Washington, and Oregon and may be as frequent as PSP toxins. Domoic acid has also been reported in seaweed. Domoic acid was reported in Japan in 1958 and was isolated from the red algae, *Chondria armata*.

In the Canadian outbreak, mice injected with extracts (as in the PSP assay) died within 3.5 hours. The mice exhibited a scratching syndrome uniquely characteristic of domoic acid that was followed by increasingly uncoordinated movements and seizures until the mice died. Levels of domoic acid >40 μg/g wet weight of mussel meat caused the mouse symptoms (Canadian authorities require cessation of harvesting when levels approach 20 μg/g.). Mice and rats can generally tolerate 30 to 50 mg/kg. Domoic acid is dose-responsive in humans, with no effect at 0.2 to 0.3 mg/kg, mild GI symptoms at 0.9 to 2.0 mg/kg, and the most serious symptoms at 1.9 to 4.2 mg/kg with GI effects and neurological effects, including dizziness, disorientation, lethargy, seizures, and permanent loss of short-term memory. Although rodents appear to be more tolerant, the fatalities in humans were likely associated with underlying illness. Domoic acid is an analog of glutamine, a neurotransmitter, and of kainic acid; the toxicity of all three is similar, as they are excitatory and act on three types of receptors in the CNS with the hippocampus being the most sensitive. Domoic acid may be a more potent activator of kainic acid receptors than kainic acid itself. The stimulatory action may lead to extensive damage of the hippocampus, but less severe injury to the thalamic and forebrain regions (Todd, 1993; Clark *et al*, 1999; Van Dolah, 2000). An FDA Action Level for amnesic shellfish poisoning has been set at 20-ppm domoic acid, except in the viscera of Dungeness crab, where 30 ppm is permitted (SNIC, 2007).

Innate Marine Toxins There are naturally occurring toxins in some species that do not involve marine algae or other environmental influences, but are innate to the particular marine species. The first example is Escolar (*Lepidocybium flavobrunneum*), and Oilfish or Cocco (*Ruvettus pretiosus*), a marine fish of the snake mackerel family, which are sometimes sold under the category of "butterfish," and contain a strong purgative oil, that when consumed can cause diarrhea known as gempylid fish poisoning, gempylotoxism, or keriorrhea (FDA, 2010a). The toxin consists of wax esters (C32, C34, C36, and C38 fatty acid esters), the primary component of which is $C_{34}H_{66}O_2$ (Ukishima *et al.*, 1987); these constitute a substantive portion of the lipid present in these fish (14%–25% by weight). Escolar oil contains >90% wax esters (Nichols *et al.*, 2001). Ingestion of fish containing wax esters in large amounts, coupled with their indigestibility and low melting point, results in diarrhea (Berman *et al.*, 1981). No tolerances have been established, and the FDA recommends avoidance of these fish (Dolan *et al.*, 2010; FDA, 2010a).

A second example of an innate toxin is tetramine found in the salivary glands of *Buccinum, Busycon,* or *Neptunia* spp, a type of whelk or sea snail that is distributed in temperate and tropic waters and has long been a food source for humans. These whelks are associated with a heat-stable neurotoxin, tetramine, which upon ingestion by humans causes, among other symptoms, eyeball pain, headache, dizziness, abdominal pain, ataxia, tingling in the fingers, nausea, and diarrhea (Reid *et al.*, 1988; Kim *et al.*, 2009). Power *et al.* (2002) report that the highest concentration of tetramine is in

the salivary gland (up to 6530 μg/g), but varies according to season. Reid *et al.* (1988) reported levels of 37.5 μg tetramine/g of salivary gland tissue (Reid *et al*, 1988). Because the whelk is a predator of bivalves, it is assumed the toxin is used for food procurement (Power *et al.*, 2002). Although the FDA recommends removal of the salivary gland to avoid possible intoxication (FDA, 2010b), tetramine is present in other tissues, albeit at lesser concentrations (Anthoni *et al.*, 1989; Dolan *et al.*, 2010).

The third and last example is the meat of the Greenland shark (*Somniosus microcephalus*) and the related member of the dogfish family, the pacific sleeper shark (*Somniosus pacificus*), is known to be poisonous to both man and dogs. The causative agent is trimethylamine oxide, which breaks down to trimethylamine in the gut, probably by enteric bacteria. The result is absorption of trimethylamine, which acts as a neurotoxin, producing ataxia in both humans and dogs. However, the flesh may be consumed if boiled several times with changes of water, or as the Inuit people prepare it, by burying it in the ground and allowing the meat to go through several freezing and thawing cycles (Anthoni *et al.*, 1991; Benz *et al.*, 2004; Idboro, 2008; Dolan *et al.*, 2010).

Microbiological Agents—Preformed Bacterial Toxins

Although the United States likely has the safest and cleanest food supply in the world, most food-related illnesses in the United States result from microbial contamination. Food-borne disease outbreaks are tracked by the Centers for Disease Control and Prevention (CDC) in Atlanta, Georgia. The CDC reports that there are approximately 400 outbreaks of food-borne disease per year involving 10,000 to 20,000 people. However, the actual frequency may be as much as 10 to 200 times as high because (1) an outbreak is classified as such only when the source can be identified as affecting two or more people and (2) most home poisonings are mild or have a long incubation time and are therefore not connected to the ingested food, go unreported, and are often felt to be only a "24-hour bug." Naturally, because of differences in virulence and opportunity, some species are more likely than others to cause outbreaks.

If all the microbiological food-borne health concerns could be divided into two categories—*poisonings* and *infections*—the former would include chemical poisonings and intoxications, which may have a plant, animal, or microbial origin. In the infections category, food acts as a vector for organisms that exhibit their pathogenicity once they have multiplied inside the body. Infections include the two subcategories: enterotoxigenic infections (with the release of toxins following colonization of the GI tract) and invasive infections in which the GI tract is penetrated and the body is invaded by organisms.

There are a number of food toxins of microbial origin; however, discussion in this chapter will be limited to preformed bacterial toxins—that is, those toxins elaborated by bacteria concomitant to their residence and growth in or on the food *prior* to ingestion. Importantly, the bacteria need not be present for the intoxication to take place because the bacteria may have been killed by heat while the toxin survives. Bacterial toxins may be divided on the basis of activity: *emetic toxins* (ie, *Bacillus cereus*), which produce their effect by binding to specific receptors in the duodenum, *neurotoxins* (whose action is self-explanatory), and *enterotoxins*, which are protein toxins having action on the *enteric* cells of the intestine. Enterotoxins can be subdivided into cytotoxic enterotoxins which disrupt the cell membrane or other vital functions of the cell and cytotonic enterotoxins, which enter the epithelial cell and cause diarrhea without direct membrane disruption or cell death (Granum, 2006).

Bacterial toxins may also be divided on the basis of their origin: an *endotoxin* is generally a lipopolysaccharide membrane constituent released from a dead or dying Gram-negative bacteria, and these toxins are nonspecific and stimulate inflammatory responses from macrophages including, but not limited to prostaglandins, thromboxanes, interleukins, and other mediators of immunity; *exotoxins*, which are synthesized and released (usually by Gram-positive bacteria) and are not an integral part of the organism, but may enhance its virulence. Some bacteria, such as *Shigella* spp, *Staphylococcus aureus*, or *Escherichia coli*, can elaborate both endotoxin and exotoxin.

Clostridium botulinum, C butyricum, and C baratti

Food botulism rarely causes illness because the confluence of conditions required for its occurrence—*Clostridia* in the presence of low acidity, high water activity, absence of preservatives, ambient temperature, and anaerobic environment—such a combination rarely occurs in foods, but botulinum poisoning remains important, the result of its potency (Sobel *et al.*, 2004). All *Clostridia* are Gram-positive, spore-forming anaerobes. Botulism is a product of the toxins: A (the predominant form in the United States), B (the predominant form in Europe), E (the predominant form in Northern latitudes), and F that may be produced by one or more strains of *C botulinum*, *C butyricum* (Type E only), and *C baratti*; toxins C and D cause botulism in animals. Type G has not caused any human cases. *C botulinum* toxins are categorized as Group I to IV on the basis of toxin produced; additionally, Group I is proteolytic in culture (liquefying egg white, gelatin, and other solid proteins). The toxin is elaborated in foods, wounds, and infant gut and is neurotoxic, interfering with acetylcholine at peripheral nerve endings. Botulinum neurotoxins induce blockage of voluntary motor and autonomic cholinergic neuromuscular junctions, which prevent motor fiber stimulation. Clinical illness is characterized by cranial nerve palsies, followed by descending flaccid muscle paralysis, which can involve the muscles of respiration. Although ptosis and dysarthria may be mistaken for signs of encephalopathy, patients are fully alert, and the results of a sensory examination are normal. Recovery often takes weeks to months (Sobel *et al.*, 2004). Although the spores are among the most heat-resistant, the toxins are heat-labile (the toxin may be rendered harmless at 80°C–100°C for five–10 minutes). Botulinum toxins are large zinc metalloproteins of ~150,000 Da, composed of two parts, a 50,000-Da piece, the catalytic subunit, and the 100,000-Da piece containing an *N*-terminal translocation domain and a *C*-terminal binding domain. The structural features are similar to tetanus toxin. For Types B, D, F, and G (and tetanus toxin), the target protein is vesicle-associated membrane protein (VAMP/synaptobrevin), a protein associated with the synaptic vesicle. Types A and E cleave a protein associated with the presynaptic membrane, ANAP25. Botulinum toxin C cleaves SNAP25 and syntaxin, another protein involved in exocytosis. Although intracellular mechanisms of botulinum and tetanus toxins are similar, symptoms are different because different populations of neurons are targeted. The symptoms may include respiratory distress and respiratory paralysis that may persist for six to eight months. The case fatality rate in the United States is 4% (Sobel *et al.*, 2004) and the poison is fatal in three to 10 days; a lethal dose is approximately 1 ng.

Current methods for detecting botulinum toxin include a mouse bioassay and an enzyme-linked immunosorbent assay. The mouse bioassay is the accepted standard, where the mouse is injected with a lethal dose, the signs of which should develop in eight hours and, if not, the mouse is observed for four days. The mouse bioassay can also be used to differentiate between the toxin types by mixing neutralizing antibodies with the sample, prior to injection. Determining

which mice survive following specific combinations of toxin and antisera, determines the specific toxin type. The absolute amount of toxin detected in the mouse bioassay is not well defined but is thought to be 10 to 20 pg/mL for type A (Barr *et al.*, 2005).

Sources and reservoirs for *Clostridia* include soil, mud, water, and the intestinal tracts of animals. Foods associated with botulinum toxin include improperly canned low-acid foods (green beans, corn, beets, asparagus, chili peppers, mushrooms, spinach, figs, baked potato, cheese sauce, beef stew, olives, and tuna). The toxin also may occur in smoked fish, fermented food (seal flippers, salmon eggs), and improperly home-cured hams. An increasing source of poisonings is from the use of flavored oils or oil infusion, most typically in garlic-in-oil preparations. In 1993, FDA required acidification of such preparations to prevent the growth of *Clostridia* (FDA, 2005a). Whereas a proteolytic strain of *C botulinum* (Group I) may cause the food to appear and smell "spoiled" (by-products include isobutyric acid, isovaleric acid, and phenylpropionic acid), this is not the case with nonproteolytic strains, many of which can flourish and elaborate toxin at temperatures as low as 3°C (Loving, 1998; Belitz and Grosch, 1999; Crane, 1999; Lund and Peck, 2000).

The successful use of nitrates in meat to prevent spoilage by *C botulinum* resulted in the petitioning of FDA by the USDA to have sodium and potassium nitrate approved for use by "prior sanction" (21 CFR 181.33). The mechanism of nitrates is believed to be due to an inactivation by nitric oxide of iron-sulfur proteins such as ferrodoxin and pyruvate oxidoreductase within the germinated cells. The activity is dependent on the pH and is proportional to the level of free HNO_2; 100 mg nitrate/kg of meat is necessary for the antimicrobial effect, although this effect can be enhanced with ascorbates and chelating agents. Other antibacterials that prevent *C botulinum* include nisin (used in cheese spreads), parabens, phenolic antioxidants, polyphosphates, and carbon dioxide (Belitz and Grosch, 1999; Lund and Peck, 2000).

Clostridium perfringens

Unlike *C botulinum*, the primary reservoir for *C perfringens* is the intestinal tract of warm-blooded animals (including humans). Most incidences of *C perfringens* food poisoning are associated with the consumption of roasted meat that has been contaminated with intestinal contents at slaughter, followed by roasting and inadequate storage, allowing *C perfringens* growth and enterotoxin Clostridium perfringens enterotoxin (CPE) to be elaborated (although some CPE may actually be released during a "second-sporulation" process in the stomach of the victim). Virtually all food poisoning is produced by type A strain, although a particularly severe form (a necrotic enteritis called "pig-bel" among indigenous peoples of the New Guinea highlands or in Germany known as "Darmbrand") is produced by type C strain, which has a mortality rate of 15% to 25% even with treatment. The toxin is normally trypsin-sensitive, but people with low intakes of protein or who consume trypsin-inactivating foods (eg, sweet potatoes) are more at risk than carnivorous people with normal trypsin levels (Granum and Brynestad, 1999; Granum, 2006).

CPE is enterotoxic and follows an ordered series of events, first causing cellular ion permeability, followed by macromolecular (DNA, RNA) synthesis inhibition, morphological alteration, cell lysis, and villi tip desquamation and severe fluid loss. This is manifested by abdominal cramping, and diarrhea occurs within eight to 16 hours, although symptoms are of short duration, one day or less. Foods associated with *C perfringens* poisoning include cooked meat or poultry, gravy, stew, and meat pies. *C perfringens* is also associated with the production of another 11 toxins, including those associated with gas gangrene (Hobbs *et al.*, 1953; Hauschild, 1971; Walker, 1975; Hobbs, 1976; Crane, 1999; Labbe, 2000).

Bacillus cereus *Bacillus cereus* is also a Gram-positive, spore-forming rod, but is an aerobe or facultative anaerobe. *Bacillus cereus* is a causative agent of emetic or diarrheagenic exo- and enterotoxins elaborated in food. The emetic thermostable toxin (surviving 259°F for 90 minutes) is called cerulide (a small cyclic peptide, 1.2 kDa, that acts on 5-HT_3 receptors stimulating the vagus afferent nerve) and is produced by serotypes 1, 3, and 8; it is also resistant to pH and proteolysis, but is not antigenic. The diarrheagenic thermolabile toxin (surviving 133°F for 20 minutes) is produced by serotypes 1, 2, 6, 8, 10, and 19 and may also be produced in situ in the lower intestine of the host. The diarrheal form may actually consist of three toxins, one of which is hemolytic (Granum, 2006). Reservoirs are soil and dust. Foods associated with this organism and its toxic properties include boiled and fried rice (principally the emetic form), while the diarrheal form has a wider occurrence and may be found in meats, stews, pudding, sauces, dairy products, vegetable dishes, soups, and meat loaf (Goepfert *et al.*, 1972; Gilbert, 1979; Bryan, 1984; Crane, 1999; Granum and Lund, 1997). The foods associated with the two types somewhat reflect the geographic distribution of the types, as the emetic type predominates in Japan, whereas in North America and Europe, the diarrhea type is most often seen.

Evidence is accumulating that other species of *Bacillus* may elaborate food toxins, including Bt, *B subtilis*, *B licheniformis*, and *B pumilis* (Crane, 1999; Granum and Baird-Parker, 2000; Granum, 2006). A notable exception is *B cereus* var *toyoi*, a naturally occurring, nontoxigenic, and nonpathogenic strain. *B toyoi* has been tested in a variety of systems, including conventional toxicity studies and tests for enterotoxicity and genotoxicity, and determined to be safe for its intended use in animal feed as a probiotic to promote digestive health (Williams *et al.*, 2009). *B toyoi* has been approved for addition to swine, bovine, poultry, and rabbit feed in the European Communities.

Staphylococcus aureus Staphylococcal intoxication includes staphyloenterotoxicosis and staphylococcus food poisoning. *S aureus* produces a wide variety of exoproteins, including toxic shock syndrome toxin-1 (TSST-1), the exfoliative toxins ETA and ETB, leukocidin, and the staphylococcal enterotoxins (SE) (SEA, SEB, SECn,[17] SED, SEE, SEG, SHE, and SEI). TSST-1 and the SE are also known as pyrogenic toxin superantigens on the basis of their biological characteristics. There is a relatively wide degree of molecular diversity among SE toxins and this is thought to be the result of adaptation to allow for a broad range of potential hosts (Monday and Bohach, 1999). Some, but not all, SE require Zn^{++} for superantigen activity. Although enterotoxemia only develops from ingestion of large amounts of SE, emesis is produced as the result of stimulation of the putative SE receptors in the abdominal viscera, followed by a cascade of inflammatory mediator release. All the SE toxins share a number of properties: an ability to cause emesis and gastroenteritis in primates, superantigenicity, intermediate resistance to heat and pepsin digestion, and tertiary structural similarity, including an intramolecular disulfide bond. Induction of emesis separates the SE toxins from TSST-1, but the induction of emesis is not directly correlated to superantigen activity (Granum, 2006). The exact link between superantigenicity and lethality by the SE toxins and TSST-1 is not known, but may be dependent upon cytotoxicity for certain cells, possibly in the kidneys, liver, or vascular endothelium (Monday and Bohach, 1999). Sources of *Staphylococcus* include nose and throat discharges, hands and skin,

infected cuts, wounds, burns, boils, pimples, acne, and feces. The anterior nares of humans are the primary reservoirs. Other reservoirs include mastitic udders of cows and ewes (responsible for contamination of unpasteurized milk) and arthritic and bruised tissues of poultry. Foods usually are contaminated after cooking by persons cutting, slicing, chopping, or otherwise handling them, and then keeping them at room temperature for several hours or storing them in large containers. Foods associated with staphylococcal poisoning include cooked ham; meat products, including poultry and dressing; sauces and gravy; cream-filled pastry; potatoes; ham; poultry; fish salads; milk; cheese; bread pudding; and generally high-protein leftover foods (Cohen, 1972; Bryan, 1976, 1984; Minor and Marth, 1976; Crane, 1999; Dinges *et al.*, 2000).

E coli Although *E coli* does not produce a preformed toxin, it deserves mention because of the overwhelming publicity the emergent strain O157:H7 has received (H and O refer to flagellar antigens and virulence markers). There are four categories of *E coli* associated with diarrheal disease: enteropathogenic, enterotoxigenic, enteroinvasive, and Vero cytotoxin–producing *E coli* (VTEC). The classification VTEC also includes "shiga-like toxin"–producing *E coli* and "shiga toxin"–producing *E coli* (STEC). Enterohemorrhagic *E coli* (EHEC) refers to those strains producing bloody diarrhea and are a subset of VTEC. The reference to shiga toxin is the result of the clinical similarity of the bloody diarrhea caused by EHEC to that caused by *Shigellae*. Each of the diseases presented by the four categories is also associated with one or more toxins (Willshaw *et al.*, 2000). The symptoms of STEC infections vary, but commonly include severe stomach cramps, diarrhea (often bloody), and vomiting, and about 5% to 10% of those diagnosed with STEC infections develop hemolytic uremic syndrome, a potentially life-threatening complication because the kidneys may stop working (CDC, 2010).

Cattle are a significant reservoir of *E coli*; therefore, it is logical that most outbreaks in the United States have been associated with hamburgers and other beef products, although raw vegetables (often fertilized with manure) and unpasteurized apple cider and juice have been reported as sources of outbreaks. Outbreaks in Europe are more often associated with contamination of recreational waters (swimming pools, lakes, etc). Other sources of contamination include person-to-person contact (especially in families and among institutionalized persons) and contact with farm animals especially following educational farm visits (Karch *et al.*, 1999).

The subject of organic food has increasingly captured the public interest. As a result, numerous studies have been done comparing the nutritional and health benefits of organic and conventional foods. When currently available literature was reviewed, there was no compelling evidence that there are nutrition-related health effects from the consumption of organically produced foods (Dangour *et al.*, 2010, Gueguen and Pascal, 2010).

Within this issue, there is a debate concerning the use of organic fertilizers (eg, cow manure) in organic and conventional farming, which may contain *E coli* O157:H7 (Stephenson, 1997). Data reported to the US CDC in 1996, and tabulated in a CDC document entitled "Clusters/Outbreaks of *E coli* O157:H7 reported to CDC in 1996," show that approximately 10% of all *E coli* O157:H7 infections reported that year were from organically grown lettuce, although organic foods apparently account for less than 1% of the total food supply.

At the basis of the potential problem is the use of inadequately treated manure for fertilizer. Human cases of *E coli* O157:H7 infection have been reported from consumption of contaminated lettuce, potatoes, radish sprouts, alfalfa sprouts, cantaloupe, and

---

[17]"n" indicating seven subtypes.

unpasteurized apple cider and juice (Karch *et al.*, 1999). Adequate treatment of manure requires composting the manure for a minimum of three months during which the heap must reach a temperature of 60°C and although this may be adequate to kill vegetative pathogens, it will not destroy spore-formers such as *Clostridium perfringens* or *C botulinum*. Survival of viruses and protozoa during composting is not known (Anonymous, 1999).

Bovine Spongiform Encephalopathy

Bovine spongiform encephalopathy (BSE) was first identified in Great Britain in 1986. BSE is a neurological disease classified as a transmissible spongiform encephalopathy (TSE) and is similar to TSEs in other species including scrapie (sheep and goats), transmissible mink encephalopathy (ranch-bred mink), chronic wasting disease (CWD) (mule deer and elk), exotic ungulate encephalopathy (captive exotic bovoids such as bison, orynx, kudu), and feline spongiform encephalopathy (domestic cats and zoo Felidae). TSEs among humans include kuru, Creutzfeldt–Jakob Disease (CJD) and "new variant" CJD (nvCJD), and Gerstmann–Sträussler–Scheinker syndrome (to be distinguished from CJD by an earlier onset and that it tends to run in families). There is compelling epidemiological and laboratory evidence of a causal association between the BSE outbreak in cattle in Great Britain and the new human prion disease nvCJD (CDC, 2011).

Clinically, these diseases present neurological deterioration and wasting, with the incubation period and interval from clinical onset to inexorable death determined by the dose of infective agent, its virulence, and the genetic makeup of the victim. The incubation of BSE in cattle is generally four to five years (range of 20 months–18 years) and an interval of 1 to 12 months from presentation of clinical signs to death. Characteristic histological lesions in the brain and spinal cord are vacuolation and "spongiform" changes. BSE fibrils (long strands of host glycoprotein called prion protein [PrP]) in spinal cord preparations may be seen with electron microscopy following detergent extraction and proteinase K digestion. BSE/scrapie tissues with highest infectivity are brain and spinal cord, followed by retina, spleen, tonsil lymph nodes, distal ileum, and proximal colon. The infective agent can be transferred using preparations of neural tissue from infected animals across species barriers. The most effective method of transfer is direct injection into the brain or spinal cord, but transfer has been reported with intraperitoneal injection and oral dosing. Vertical transfer (mother to offspring) has been reported among domestic cattle, and lateral transfer through biting or injury (especially among mink) has also been reported. Indirect transmission of CWD has been reported recently (Miller *et al.*, 2004); CWD of mule deer (*Odocoileus hemionus*) can be transmitted from environments contaminated by excreta 2.2 years earlier or decomposed carcasses ~1.8 years earlier.

It is generally agreed that the infective agent is likely a variant of scrapie (endemic to sheep) and was transferred to cattle from rendered sheep via inadequately processed meat and bone meal protein supplement. There is strong evidence and general agreement that the outbreak was amplified and spread throughout the UK cattle industry by feeding rendered (contaminated) bovine meat- and-bone meal to young calves. Disputes have arisen about other details of BSE and its relationship to other TSEs and effects in humans because of an expectation of conformation by BSE to historical principles of disease transmission. Recently, the human susceptibility to sheep and goat passaged-BSE prions was evaluated using transgenic mice expressing PrP and evidence was provided suggesting that humans might be equally or more susceptible to sheep or goat BSE agent compared to that of cattle (Padilla *et al.* 2011).

Responsive to concerns about transmission, new enhanced BSE-related feed bans went into effect in Canada in 2007 and in the United States in 2009. The enhanced bans prohibit most proteins, which include potentially BSE infectious tissues from all animal feeds, pet foods, and fertilizers not just from cattle feed as required by bans instituted in 1997 (CDC, 2011).

The currently most accepted theory is that the infective agent is a modified form of a normal cell surface component known as prion protein PrP^c (α-helix form), which when introduced into an organism causes a conversion of PrP^c into a likeness of itself (ie, the isoform), but then designated as the pathogenic form, PrP* or PrP^{sc} for scrapie or PrP^{res} for protease resistant (β-pleated sheet form) (Flechsig and Weissmann, 2004; Frosch *et al.*, 2005). The agent does not possess nucleic acid. The pathogenic form of the protein, PrP*, is both less soluble and more resistant to enzyme degradation than the normal form. The protein is resistant to heat, antimicrobials, ultraviolet-, or ionizing radiation, and is not consistently inactivated with alcohol, formaldehyde, glutaraldehyde, or sodium hydroxide. Phenol and sodium hypochlorite disinfection have had variable success.

Investigators have concluded that the agent in nvCJD and BSE is the same strain and may be the same agent in feline spongiform encephalopathy and exotic ungulate encephalopathy. Although this information might indicate a simple mode of transmission, workers with the highest potential incidence of exposure to BSE or TSE (sheep farmers, butchers, veterinarians, cooks, and abattoir workers) do not have an unusually high incidence of nvCJD (Prusiner, 1991; Collee, 2000). Likewise, hemophilic patients have not reflected an increased incidence of nvCJD, although CJD transmission has been documented as the result of injections of human growth hormone or gonadotrophin (derived from human pituitary gland), implantation of dura mater and corneas, and even infected electroencephalographic (EEG) electrodes and neurosurgical instruments (Prusiner, 1994; Lee *et al.*, 1998; Collee, 2000).

Substances Produced by Cooking or Processing

Heterocyclic Amines Tolerances cannot be set for contaminants that are produced as a result of an action taken by the consumer because the home is out of the jurisdiction of FDA. An example of this type of contaminant is heterocyclic amines (HCAs), which are generated during cooking. HCAs were discovered serendipitously by Japanese investigators who, while examining the mutagenicity of smoke generated by charred foods, found that the extracts of the charred surfaces of the meat and fish were quantitatively more mutagenic than could be accounted for by the presence of polycyclic aromatic hydrocarbons (Sugimura *et al.*, 1989). Collectively, there are more than 20 HCAs. They are formed as a result of high-temperature cooking of proteins (especially those containing high levels of creatinine) and carbohydrates. Normally, as a result of such heating, desirable flavor components are formed, for example, pyrazines, pyridines, and thiazoles. Intermediates in the formation of these substances are dihydropyrazines and dihydropyridines, which in the presence of oxygen form the flavor components; however, in the presence of creatinine, HCAs are formed (Table 31-27) (Chen and Chiu, 1998; Schut and Snyderwine, 1999).

These substances are rapidly absorbed by the GI tract, are distributed to all organs, and decline to undetectable levels within 72 hours. HCAs behave as electrophilic carcinogens (Table 31-28). They are metabolized first by *N*-hydroxylation

Table 31-27

Amounts of Heterocyclic Amines in Cooked Foods

SAMPLE	AMOUNT (ng/g) IN COOKED FOOD				
	IQ	MeIQx	4,8-DiMeIQx	Trp-P-1	Trp-P-2
Broiled beef	0.19	2.11		0.21	0.25
Fried ground beef	0.70	0.64	0.12	0.19	0.21
Broiled chicken		2.33	0.81	0.12	0.18
Broiled mutton		1.01	0.67		0.15
Food-grade beef extract		3.10			

4,8-DiMeIQx, 2-amino-3,4-8-trimethyl-imidazo[4,5-f]quinoxaline; IQ, 2-amino-3,4-dimethylimidazo[4,5-f]quinolone; MeIQx, 2-amino-3,8-dimethylimidazo[4,5-f]quinoxaline; Trp-P-1, 3-Amino-1,4-dimethyl-pyrido(4,3-b)indole; trp-p-2, 3-amino-1-methyl-pyrido(4,3-b)indole.

SOURCES: Sugimura T, Wakabayashi K, Nagao M, et al. Heterocyclic amines in cooked food. In: Taylor SL, Scanlan RA, eds. Food Toxicology: A Perspective on the Relative Risks. New York: Marcel Dekker; 1989:45. With permission from Copyright Clearance Center. Adamson RH. Mutagens and carcinogens formed during cooking of foods and methods to minimize their formation. Cancer Prevention. 1990:1–7. With permission from Lippincott Williams & Wilkins.

followed by further activation by *O*-acetylation or *O*-sulfonation to react with DNA. DNA adducts are formed with guanosine in various organs, including the liver, heart, kidney, colon, small intestine, forestomach, pancreas, and lung. Unreacted substances are subject to phase II detoxication reactions and are excreted via the urine and feces. In vitro, HCAs require metabolic activation, with some requiring *O*-acetyltransferase and others not. Although much of the mutagenicity testing has been carried out in TA98 and TA100, these substances are mutagenic in mammalian cells both in vitro and in vivo, *Drosophila*, and other strains of *Salmonella* (Munro *et al.*, 1993; Skog *et al.*, 1998; Sugimura and Wakabayashi, 1999).

Table 31-28

Mutagenicity and Carcinogenicity of Heterocyclic Amines

HCA	NUMBER OF REVERTANTS n/g (STRAIN TA98)	CARCINOGENICITY	
		SPECIES	STATISTICALLY SIGNIFICANT TUMORS
MeIQ	47,000,000	Mouse	Liver, forestomach
		Rat	Zymbal gland, oral cavity, colon, skin, mammary gland
IQ	898,000	Mouse	Liver, forestomach, lung
		Rat	Liver, mammary gland, Zymbal gland
		Monkey	Liver, metastasis to lungs
MeIQx	417,000	Mouse	Liver, lung, lymphoma, leukemia
		Rat	Liver, Zymbal gland, clitoral gland, skin
Glu-P-1	183,000	Mouse	Liver, blood vessels
		Rat	Liver, small and large intestine, brain, clitoral gland, Zymbal gland
Glu-P-2	930	Mouse	Liver, blood vessels
		Rat	Liver, small and large intestine, Zymbal gland, brain, clitoral gland
DiMeIQx	126,000	No data	
Trp-P-1	8990	Mouse	Liver
		Rat	Liver, metastasis to lungs
Trp-P-2	92,700	Mouse	Liver, lung
		Rat	Liver, clitoral gland
PhIP	1800	Mouse	Liver, lung, lymphoma
		Rat	Colon, mammary gland

4,8-DiMeIQx, 2-amino-3,4-8-trimethyl-imidazo[4,5-f]quinoxaline; Glu-P-1, 2-Amino-6-methyldipyrido(1,2-a:3',2'-d)imidazole; Glu-P-2, 2-Amino-dipyrido(1,2-a:3',2'-d)-imidazole; IQ, 2-amino-3,4-dimethylimidazo[4,5-f]quinolone; MeIQ, 2-Amino-3,4-dimethylimidazo(4,5-f)quinolone; MeIQx, 2-amino-3,8-dimethylimidazo[4,5-f]quinoxaline; Trp-P-1, 3-Amino-1,4-dimethyl-pyrido(4,3-b)indole; Trp-P-2, 1-Methyl-3-amino-5H-pyrido(4,3-b)indole; PhIP, 2-Amino-1-methyl-6-phenylimidazo(4,5-b)pyridine.

SOURCE: Adapted from Sugimura T, Wakabayashi K, Nagao M, et al. Heterocyclic amines in cooked food. In: Taylor SL, Scanlan RA, eds. Food Toxicology: A Perspective on the Relative Risks. New York: Marcel Dekker; 1989:36–43. With permission from Copyright Clearance Center.

Table 31-29

Representative Concentrations of Acrylamide in Several Foods (JECFA, 2005)

FOOD	MEAN CONC. (μg/kg)	REPORTED MAXIMUM (μg/kg)
Cereal-based products		
Breads and rolls	446	3436
Pastry and cookies	350	7834
Breakfast cereals	96	1346
Roots and tubers		
Baked potato	169	1270
Potato chips	752	4080
French fries	334	5312
Coffee		
Coffee, brewed, ready to drink	13	116
Coffee extracts	1100	4948
Coffee, decaffeinated	668	5399
Coffee substitutes	845	7300
Vegetables		
Raw, boiled, and canned	4.2	25
Processed (toasted, baked, fried, grilled)	59	202
Infant formula	<5	15
Baby food (biscuits)	181	1217

Acrylamide Prior to 2002, when Swedish investigators detected acrylamide in food (Table 31-29), it was of interest only to specialists in worker safety, as this chemical is an important intermediate in the manufacture of polyacrylamides. Although there are many industrial and manufacturing uses of polyacrylamides, the bulk of production are used as chemical flocculants for water treatment, oil recovery, and in construction of dam foundations, tunnels, and sewers—consumer exposure is largely incidental (NTP, 2004b). End users are exposed to polyacrylamide, which is not toxic as long as the monomer is not present. Acrylamide (the monomer) was known to be a neurotoxin, creating morphological changes in peripheral nerves at doses as low as 1 mg/kg BW/day. Much more is now known about acrylamide and its primary metabolite, glycidamide, which is produced from acrylamide by the enzyme CYP2E1; both acrylamide and glycidamide will form adducts with hemoglobin. Acrylamide is absorbed rapidly and extensively (23%–48% of the administered dose to rodents) from the GI tract. Both acrylamide and glycidamide are largely eliminated as mercapturic acid conjugates. Repeated dosing of acrylamide (in drinking water at 21 mg/kg BW/day for 40 days) produces morphological changes in the brain areas critical for learning, memory, and other cognitive functions (ie, cerebral cortex, thalamus, and hippocampus) (JECFA, 2005). Acrylamide was classified as "probably carcinogenic to humans" (IARC Group 2A) by the IARC (IARC, 1994) and "reasonably anticipated to be a human carcinogen" by the NTP (2004b).

Acrylamide is formed in foods that are high in carbohydrate, but low in protein, which are subjected to processing temperatures of at least 120°C. These high-temperature processing conditions are largely the same as required for the Maillard reaction, which imparts a toasted, or baked (ie, "crust"), flavor to breads, toast, and other baked goods, breaded meats and vegetables for sautéing or frying, and production of French fries and potato chips. Most acrylamide is formed in the final stages of baking, grilling, or frying as the moisture content of the food falls and the surface temperature rises (JECFA, 2005). The presence of ammonium bicarbonate as a leavening agent increases the formation of acrylamide.

A critical element is the presence of asparagine, and amino acids competing with asparagine in the Maillard reaction, which reduces the levels of acrylamide in the final product. Strategies for mitigation focus on reduction of asparagine through use of asparaginase, breeding and selection of low-asparagine plants, and prolonged yeast fermentation; alternatively, processing temperature could be lowered (JECFA, 2005).

Acrylamide intake estimates range from 0.3 to 2.0 μg/kg BW/day for the average population, with the 90th to 97th percentile at 0.6 to 3.5 μg/kg BW/day and the 99th percentile at up to 5.1 μg/kg BW/day. Primary sources include french fries (1%–30%), potato chips (6%–46%), coffee (13%–39%), pastry and cookies (10%–20%), and bread and rolls/toasts (10%–30%). The NOEL for morphological change in nerves and for reproductive effects is 200 and 2000 μg/kg BW/day, respectively (JECFA, 2005).

Furan Furan was once known only as an industrial chemical intermediate in the synthesis of polymers used to prepare temperature-resistant structural laminates and to prepare copolymers used in machine dishwashing products. Furan has recently been found to occur in a number of foods that undergo heat treatment, such as canned and jarred foods, including baby food. It is considered by IARC (1995) to be possibly carcinogenic to humans. According to the NTP, furan is hepatotoxic and shows clear evidence of carcinogenicity in both sexes and both species of mice and rats (NTP, 1993). Furan is produced in a variety of experimental systems, including heating of sugars (eg, glucose, lactose, fructose, xylose, rhamnose), heating sugars in the presence of amino acids or protein (eg, alanine, cysteine, casein), and thermal degradation of vitamins (ascorbic acid, dehydroascorbic acid, thiamine) (FDA, 2004).

Furan has been found in a small number of heat-treated foods, including coffee, canned meat, baked bread, cooked chicken, sodium caseinate, filberts (hazelnuts), soy protein isolate, hydrolyzed soy protein, rapeseed protein, fish protein concentrate, and caramel (FDA, 2004). Very little information has been developed on furan levels in food.

Miscellaneous Contaminants in Food

Despite normal precautions taken to protect ourselves from known toxins, some toxins have a propensity to appear unexpectedly in unfamiliar places. Cases in point here include honey poisoning, as documented by Xenophon, who when describing the "Retreat of the Ten Thousand" from Asia back to Greece, the soldiers entered an area rich in honeycombs and seized upon the food. Xenophon noted that the soldiers then "went off their heads" appearing to first be drunk, but then in a state a delirium—a description fitting what we know today about grayanotoxins from mountain laurel and other species.

Mountain laurel (*Kalima* spp), rhododendron, and azaleas (*Rhododendron* spp) all possess grayanotoxins of which there may be as many as 60, but the most potent are grayanotoxins I and III (Gunduz *et al.*, 2008). The toxins are present in the shoots, leaves, twigs, and flowers. Honey made from flowers of these plants is toxic to humans, and after an asymptomatic period of four to six hours, salivation, malaise, vomiting, diarrhea, tingling of the skin, muscular weakness, headache, visual difficulties, coma, and convulsions occur. Symptoms are proportional to dose, and atropine administration is indicted as a primary treatment modality (Gunduz *et al.*, 2008). Life-threatening bradycardia and arterial hypotension may occur. Needless to say, beekeepers maintain apiaries well away from these species of plants.

A similar poisoning can occur with oleander (*Nerium oleander* and *N indicum*), where honey made from the flowers, meat roasted on oleander sticks, or milk from a cow that eats the foliage can produce prostrating symptoms. The oleander toxin consists of a series of cardiac glycosides: thevetin, convallarin, steroidal, helleborein, ouabain, and digitoxin. Sympathetic nerves are paralyzed; the cardiotoxin stimulates the heart muscles similar to the action of digitalis, and gastric distress ensues (Anderson and Sogn, 1984; VonMalottki and Wiechmann, 1996). Although certainly as possible as the story captured by Xenophon, the stories about scouts sickened from roasting hot dogs on oleander sticks have not been documented and are likely apocryphal.

Closer to home and prevalent in the Midwest in the 18th and 19th centuries, was a mysterious scourge called "milk sickness" also known as "puking fever," "sick stomach," "the slows," and "the trembles"; thousands of people have been reported as dying, including Abraham Lincoln's mother, Nancy Hanks Lincoln. In humans, milk sickness is characterized by loss of appetite, listlessness, weakness, vague pains, muscle stiffness, vomiting, abdominal discomfort, constipation, foul breath, and finally, coma. For many years, the origin of milk sickness was unknown because there was nothing comparable in Europe (origin of most of the pioneers) and the outbreaks were sporadic. It was not recognized until the late 19th and early 20th century, that white snakeroot (*Ageratina altissima* née *Eupatorium rugosum*) and rayless goldenrod (*Bigelowia* spp, *Haplopappus heterophyllus*, and *Isocoma pluriflora*), when eaten by cattle, were the source. The sporadic nature of outbreaks became clear when it was realized that cattle would consume these plants in over-grazed pasture or in years of drought; additionally, the toxin levels in plants can vary considerably, making identification of the source of poisonings difficult. Tremetol or tremetone is the toxic agent and consists of a mixture of sterols and derivatives of methyl ketone benzofuran. The three major benzofuran ketones are tremetone, dehydrotremetone, and 3-oxyangeloyl-tremetone (Panter and James, 1990; Lee *et al.*, 2009; NPS, 2010; Dolan *et al.*, 2010).

CONCLUSION

Foods are regarded as such because they are edible. Therefore, they cannot be unpalatable or toxic, and foods must have nutritional, hedonic, or satietal value, otherwise there would be no point in consuming them. How then, could a food be toxic and still be considered a food—there are two principal means: (1) an ordinarily nontoxic food has become toxic (through some act of man or nature), if even for a small subpopulation (eg, allergy, intolerance); or (2) overconsumption of a food not ordinarily considered toxic at historic levels of use. This shift between toxic and nontoxic or toxic only for a select group would have had the potential for making the role of regulators charged with protecting the health of the public nearly impossible; however, the FD&C Act provides for some thoughtful and pragmatic solutions for achieving a balance of acceptable risk and unavoidable circumstances through the creative use of specifications, process and manufacturing controls, action levels, tolerances, warning labels, and outright prohibitions.

In the end, it is important to emphasize that the vast majority of food-borne illnesses are attributable to microbiological contamination of food and arise from the pathogenicity and/or toxicity of the contaminating organism. Thus, the overwhelming concern for food safety, in the United States and elsewhere, remains directed toward preserving the microbiological integrity of food. On a planet where for many people, food safety and food security is a daily challenge, FDA and other regulatory agencies have played a significant role in assuring a remarkably safe and available food supply in the United States.

REFERENCES

AAAAI (American Academy of Allergy, Asthma and Immunology): Allergy Statistics, 2011 (http://www.aaaai.org/media/statistics/allergy-statistics.asp#foodallergy), (site visited 28 April 2011).

Abrams IJ. Using the menu census survey to estimate dietary intake. Post-market surveillance of aspartame. In: Finley JW, Robinson, SF, Armstrong, DJ, eds. *Food Safety Assessment*. Washington DC: American Chemical Society; 1992:201–213.

Adamson RH, Snyderwine EG, Thorgeirsson UP, et al. Metabolic processing and carcinogenicity of heterocyclic amines in nonhuman primates. *Princess Takamatsu Symp*. 1990;21:289–301.

Alba R, Phillips A, Mackie S, et al. Improvements to the International Life Sciences Institute crop composition database. *J Food Compos Anal*. 2010;23:741–748.

Ames BN, Gold LS. Environmental pollution, pesticides, and the prevention of cancer: Misconceptions. *FASEB J*. 1997;11:1041.

Ames BN, Magaw R, Gold LS. Ranking possible carcinogenic hazards. *Science*. 1987;236:271.

Anderson JA, Sogn DD, eds. *Adverse Reactions to Foods*. Washington, DC: US Department of Health and Human Services; 1984.

Anonymous. *Glucose-6-Phosphate Dehydrogenase Deficiency*. Danbury, CT: National Organization for Rare Disorders; 2002:7.

Anonymous. Organic food. *Food Sci Technol Today*. 1999;13:108.

Anthoni U, Bohlin L, Larsen C, et al. The toxin tetramine from "edible" whelk *Neptunea antiqua*. *Toxicon*. 1989;27:717–723.

Anthoni U, Christophersen C, Gram L, et al. Poisonings from flesh of the Greenland shark *Somniosus microcephalus* may be due to trimethylamine. *Toxicon*. 1991;29:1205–1212.

Astwood JD, Bannon GA, Dobert RL, et al. Food biotechnology and genetic engineering. In: Metcalf DD, Sampson HA, Simon RA, eds. *Food Allergy*. 3rd ed. Maiden, MA: Blackwell Scientific Inc; 2003.

Ayesh R, Mitchell SC, Zhang A, et al. The fish odour syndrome: biochemical, familial and clinical aspects. *Br Med J*. 1993;307:655.

Balch JF, Balch PA. Elements Health. Dimethylglycine (DMG). *Prescription for Nutritional Healing*. 2nd ed. Garden City Park, New York: Avery Publishing Group; 1997:38.

Bannister B, Gibsburg G, Shneerson T. Cardiac arrest due to licorice induced hypokalemia. *BMJ*. 1977;2:738.

Barceloux DG. Cycad seeds and chronic neurologic disease (*Cycas* species). *Dis Mon*. 2009a;55:353–360.

Barceloux DG. Cyanogenic foods (cassava, fruit kernels and cycad seeds). *Medical Toxicology of Natural substances: Foods, Fungi, Medicinal Herbs, Toxic Plants and Venomous Animals*. Hoboken, NJ: John Wiley and Sons; 2008a:44–53.

Barceloux DG. Potatoes, tomatoes, and solanine toxicity (*Solanum tuberosum* L., *Solanum lycopersicum* L.). *Medical Toxicology of Natural substances: Foods, Fungi, Medicinal Herbs, Toxic Plants and Venomous Animals*. Hoboken, NJ: John Wiley and Sons; 2008b:77–83.

Barr JR, Moura H, Boyer AE, et al. Botulinum neurotoxin detection and differentiation by mass spectrometry. *Emerg Infect Dis*. 2005;11:1578–1583. Available at: http://www.cdc.gov/ncidod/EID/vol11no10/04-1279.htm. Accessed March 22, 2006.

Beardall JM, Miller JD. Diseases in humans with mycotoxins as possible causes. In: Miller JD, Trenhold HL, eds. *Mycotoxins in Grain. Compounds Other than Aflatoxin*. St. Paul, MN: JEagan Press; 1994:487.

Belitz HD, Grosch W. *Food Chemistry*. Berlin: Springer-Verlag; 1999:992.

Benz GW, Hocking R, Kowunna Sr A, et al. A second species of Arctic shark: Pacific sleeper shark *Somniosus pacificus* from Point Hope Alaska. *Polar Biol*. 2004;27:250–252.

Berman P, Harley EH, Spark AA. Keriorrhoea—the passage of oil per rectum—after ingestion of marine wax esters. *S Afr Med J*. 1981;59: 791–792.

Bernaola G, Echechipia S, Urrutia I, et al. Occupational asthma and rhinoconjunctivitis from inhalation of dried cow's milk caused by sensitization to alpha-lactalbumin. *Alergy*. 1994;49:189.

Bernhisel-Broadbent J, Dintzis HM, Dintzis RZ, et al. Allergenicity and antigenicity of chicken egg ovomucoid (Gal d III) compared with ovalbumin (Gal d I) in children with egg allergy and in mice. *J Allergy Clin Immunol*. 1994;93:1047.

Betz FS, Hammond BG, Fuchs RL. Safety and advantages of *Bacillus thuringiensis* -protected plants to control insect pests. *Regul Toxicol Pharmacol*. 2000;32(2):156.

Beutler E. Glucose-6-phosphate dehydrogenase deficiency: a historical perspective. *Blood*. 2008;111:16–24.

Bishop PA, Smith JF, Young B. Effects of *N′ N′*-dimethylglycine on physiological response and performance in trained runners. *J Sports Med Phys Fitness*. 1987;27:53.

Borzelleca JF. Macronutrient substitutes: Safety evaluation. *Regul Toxicol Pharmacol*. 1992a;16:253.

Borzelleca JF. The safety evaluation of macronutrient substitutes. *Crit Rev Food Sci Nutr*. 1992b;32:127.

Bottje WG, Wideman RF. Potential role of free radicals in the pathogenesis of pulmonary hypertension syndrome. *Poult and Avian Biol Rev*. 1995;6:211–231.

Bradbury JH, Cliff J, Denton IC. Uptake of wetting method in Africa to reduce cyanide poisoning and konzo from cassava. *Food and Chem Toxicol*. 2011;49:539–542.

Brandon DL, Haque S, Friedman M. Antigenicity of native and modified Kunitz soybean trypsin inhibitors. *Adv Exp Med Biol*. 1986;199:449.

Brandtzaeg P. Food allergy: separating the science from the mythology. *Nat Rev Gastroenterol Hepatol*. 2010;7:380–400.

Brooker G, Barfoot P. GM Crops—The global economic and environmental impact—the first nine years 1996–2004. *Ag Bio Forum*. 2005;8(2–3):187.

Brunton LL, Lazo JS, Parker K. *Goodman and Gilman's The Pharmacological Basis of Therapeutics*.11th ed. NY: McGraw-Hill Medical Publishing; 2006:2021.

Bryan FL. Diseases transmitted by foods—A classification and summary. In: Anderson JA, Sogn DN, eds. *Adverse Reactions to Foods*, Appendix. Washington, DC: US Department of Health and Human Services; 1984:1–101.

Bryan FL. *Staphylococcus aureus*. In: Defigueiredo MP, Splittstoesser DF, eds. *Food Microbiology: Public Health and Spoilage Aspects*. Westport, CT: AVI; 1976.

Burdock GA, Carabin IC. Generally recognized as safe (GRAS): History and description. *Toxicol Lett*. 2004;150(1):3.

Burdock GA. No small thing. *Nutritional Outlook*. 2011;14:56–57.

Burdock GA, Williams LD. Nanotechnology's impact on functional foods, supplements. *Natural Products Insider*. 2008:58:60. Available at: http://www.naturalproductsinsider.com/articles/2008/08/nanotechnologys-impact-on-functional-foods-suppl.aspx. Accessed April 10, 2011.

Burdock GA. Regulation of flavor ingredients. In: Kotsonis FN, Mackey M, eds. *Nutritional Toxicology*. New York: Taylor & Francis; 2002:316.

Burfield T. Coumarin: The real story. 2008. Available at: http://www.leffingwell.com/Coumarin%20-%20the%20real%20story%20update2.pdf. Accessed July 21, 2010.

Butchko H, Kotsonis F. Acceptable daily intake and estimation of consumption. In: Tschanz C, Butchko HH, Stargel WW, Kotsonis FN, eds. *The Clinical Evaluation of a Food Additive, Assessment of Aspartame*. Boca Raton, FL: CRC Press; 1996:43.

Butchko HH, Tschanz C, Kotsonis FN. Postmarketing surveillance of food additives. *Regul Toxicol Pharmacol*. 1994;20:105.

Butchko HH, Tschanz C, Kotsonis FN. Postmarketing surveillance of anecdotal medical complaints. In: Tschanz C, Butchko HH, Stargel WW, Kotsonis FN, eds. *The Clinical Evaluation of a Food Additive, Assessment of Aspartame*. Boca Raton, FL: CRC Press; 1996:183.

Capen CC, DeLellis RA, Yarrington JT. Endocrine system. In: Haschek WM, Rousseaux CG, Wallig MA, eds. *Handbook of Toxicologic Pathology*. 2nd edn. San Diego, CA: Academic Press; 2002:681.

Carabin IC, Magnuson BA. New labeling requirements for food allergens. *Nutr Outlook*. 2006;9:28.

Carabin IC, Flamm GW. Evaluation of safety of inulin and oligofructose as dietary fiber. *Regul Toxicol Pharm*. 1999;30:268–282.

Carabin IG, Gahler R, Lyon MR, et al. Correlating preclinical, clinical and post-marketing surveillance data: A case study. *NBT*. 2010;6:12–17.

Carabin IG, Lyon MR, Wood S, et al. Supplementation of the diet with the functional fiber PolyGlycoplex® is well tolerated by healthy subjects in a clinical trial. *Nutr J*. 2009;8:9.

Carrington CD, Bolger PM. An assessment of the hazards of lead in foods. *Regul Toxicol Pharm*. 1992;16:265–272.

CAST (Council for Agricultural Science and Technology). *Mycotoxins: Risks in Plant, Animal, and Human Systems*, Task Force Report No. 139. Ames, Iowa; 2003:199.

Catto-Smith AG, Adams A. A possible case of transient hereditary fructose intolerance. *J Inherit Metab Dis*. 1993;16:73.

CDC. BSE (Bovine Spongiform Encephalopathy, or Mad Cow Disease). March 17, 2011.

CDC. *Escherichia coli* O157:H7 general review (updated on July 21, 2010).

Ceska O, Chaudhary SK, Warrington PJ, et al. Naturally-occurring crystals of photocarcinogenic furocoumarins on the surface of parsnip roots sold as food. *Experentia*. 1986;42:1302–1304.

Chapman JA, Bernstein IL, Lee RE, et al. Food allergy: a practice parameter. *Ann Allergy Asthma Immunol*. 2006;96:S1–S68.

Chee CF, Rahman NA, Zain SM, et al. Pheophorbide b ethyl ester from a *Chlorella vulgaris* dietary supplement. *Acta Crystallographica Sect E Struct Rep Online*. 2008;64:1986.

Chen BH, Chiu CP. Analysis, formation and inhibition of heterocyclic amines in foods: An overview. *J Food Drug Anal*. 1998;6:625.

Chevion M, Mager J, Glaser G. Naturally occurring food toxicants: Favismproducing agents. In: Rechcigl M, Jr. ed. *CRC Handbook of Naturally Occurring Food Toxicants*. Boca Raton, FL: CRC Press; 1985:63.

Chhabra RS, Eastin WC Jr. Intestinal absorption and metabolism of xenobiotics in laboratory animals. In: Schiller CM, ed. *Intestinal Toxicology*. New York: Raven Press; 1984:145.

Clark RF, Williams SR, Nordt SP, et al. A review of selected seafood poisonings. *Undersea Hyperb Med*. 1999;26:175.

Clayson DB, Iverson F, Nera F, et al. Histopathological and radioautographical studies on the forestomach of F344 rats treated with butylated hydroxyanisole and related chemicals. *Food Chem Toxicol*. 1986;24:1171.

Cliff J, Muquingue H, Nhassico D, et al. Knozo and continuing cyanide intoxication from cassava in Mozambique. *Food Chem Toxicol*. 2011;49: 631–635.

Codex Alimentarius Commission. *Foods Derived From Modern Biotechnology*. 2nd ed. Rome: FAO/WHO; 2009:1–78.

Codori N, Marinopoulos S. Scombroid fish poisoning after eating seared tuna. *Southern Med J.* 2009;103:382–384.

Cohen JO, ed. *The Staphylococci.* New York: Wiley-Interscience; 1972.

Cohen SM, Arnold LL. Chemical Carcinogenesis. *Toxicol Sci.* 2011; 120(S1):S76–S92.

Collee JG. Transmissible spongiform encephalopathies. *The Microobiological Safety and Quality of Food.* Gaithersburg, MD: Aspen; 2000:1589.

Committee on Food Protection. *Food Colors.* Washington, DC: National Academy of Sciences; 1971.

Concon J. *Food Toxicology.* New York: Marcel Dekker; 1988.

Cools A, Maes D, Buyse J, et al. Effect of *N,N* dimethylglycine supplementation in parturition feed for sows on metabolism, nutrient digestibility and reproductive performance. *Animal.* 2010;4:2004–2011.

Cousins MA, Riley RT, Pestka JJ. Foodborne mycotoxins: Chemistry, biology, ecology, and toxicology. In: Fratamico PM, Bhunia AK, eds. *Foodborne Pathogens: Microb Molec Biol.* Norfok, UK: Horizon Scientific Press; 2005:164.

Cox PA, Bradley WG. Beyond Guam: Cyanobacteria, BMAA and sporadic amyotrophic lateral sclerosis. *ALS.* 2009;10:5–6.

Crabb DW, Matsumoto M, Chang D, et al. Overview of the role of alcohol dehydrogenase and aldehyde dehydrogenase on their variants in the genesis of alcohol-related pathology. *P Nutr Soc.* 2004;63:49–63.

Crane JK. Preformed bacterial toxins. *Clin Lab Med.* 1999;19:583.

Dangour AD, Lock K, Hayter A, et al. Nutrition-related health effect of organic foods: a systematic review. *Am J Clin Nutr.* 2010;92:203–210.

Davis WE. *National Inventory of Sources and Emissions of Cadmium, Nickel, and Asbestos. Cadmium.* Section 1. Report PB 192250. Springfield, VA: National Technical Information Service; 1970.

Dayan AD. Allergy to antimicrobial residues in food: Assessment of the risk to man. *Vet Microbiol.* 1993;35:213.

DeBlay F, Hoyet C, Candolfi E, et al. Identification of *alpha* livetin as a cross reacting allergen in bird-egg syndrome. *Allergy Proc.* 1994; 15:77.

deBoer J, deBoer K, Boon JP. Polybrominated biphenyls and diphenylethers. In: Passivirta J, ed. *The Handbook of Environmental Chemistry Vol. 3 Part K. New types of Persistent Halogenated Compounds.* Berlin: Springer-Verlag; 2000:61–94.

Delaney B, Astwood JD, Cunny H, et al. Evaluation of protein safety in the context of agricultural biotechnology. ILSI International Food Biotechnology Committee Task Force on Protein Safety. *Food Chem Toxicol.* 2008;46:S71–S97.

Deshpande SS. Food additives. *Handbook of Food Toxicology.* New York: Marcel Dekker; 2002:219–284.

Desjardins AE, Hohn TM, McCormick SP. Trichothecene biosynthesis in *Fusarium* species: chemistry, genetics, and significance. *Microbiol Rev.* 1993;57:595–604.

Dierick NA, Decuypere JA. Influence of lipase and/or emulsifier addition on the ileal and faecal nutrient digestibility in growing pigs fed diets containing 4% animal fat. *J Sci Food Agric.* 2004;84:1443–1450.

Dinges MM, Orwin PM, Schlievert PM. Exotoxins of *Staphylococcus aureus. Microbiol Rev.* 2000;13:16.

Dolan LC, Matulka RA, Burdock GA. Naturally occurring food toxins. *Toxins.* 2010;2:2289–2332.

Dorion BJ, Burks AW, Harbeck R, et al. The production of interferon-*gamma* in response to a major peanut allergy, Arh h II, correlates with serum levels of IgE anti-Ara h II. *J Allergy Clin Immunol.* 1994; 93:93.

Douglass CW, Joshipura K. Caution needed in fluoride and osteosarcoma study. *Cancer Causes Control.* 2006;17:481–482.

Drasar BS, Hill MJ. *Human Intestinal Flora.* New York: Academic Press; 1974.

Drury SM, Reynolds TL, Ridley WP, et al. Composition of forage and grain from second-generation insect-protected corn MON 89034 is equivalent to that of conventional corn (*Zea mays* L.). *J Ag Food Chem.* 2008;56:4623–4630.

Egan SK, Bolger PM, Carrington CD. Update of the US FDA's total diet study food list and diets. *JESEE.* 2007;17(9):573–582.

El-Banna AA, Pitt JI, Leistner L. Production of mycotoxins by *Penicillium* species. *Syst Appl Microbiol.* 1987;10(1):42.

Ellison RA, Kotsonis FN. C-13 NMR assignments in trichothecene mycotoxins. *J Organic Chem.* 1975;41(3):493–495.

Environmental Protection Agency. Guidance for the re-registration of pesticide products containing *Bacillus thuringiensis* as the active ingredient. *Re-registration Stand.* 1988;540:RS-89-023.

Environmental Protection Agency. *Air Quality Criteria For Particulate Matter.* Report Number EPA/600/P-99/002a,bF., Washington, DC: USEPA;2004. Available at: http://cfpub.epa.gov/ncea. Accessed April 9, 2006.

Environmental Protection Agency. *Nanotechnology White Paper*, EPA 100/B-07/001. Washington, DC: Science Policy Council, USEPA; 2007. Available at: http://www.epa.gov/nanoscience/files/epa_nano_wp_2007. pdf. Accessed October 24, 2011.

Environmental Protection Agency. *Notification of a Public Meeting of the SAB Drinking Water Committee Augmented for the Review of the Effectiveness of Partial Lead Service Line Replacements Federal Register 76.* Science Advisory Board Staff Office; 2011:13181–13182.

Eriksen GS, Pettersson H. Toxicological evaluation of trichothecenes in animal feed. *Anim Feed Sci Technol.* 2004;114:205–239.

Ermans AM, Delange F, Van der Velden M, et al. Possible role of cyanide and thiocyanate in the etiology of endemic cretinism. *Adv Exp Med Biol.* 1972;30:455.

EU Commission. A decade of GMO-funded research, 2001–2010. European Commission. Directorate-General for Research Communication Unit B-1049 Brussels, 2010. Available at: http://ec.europa.eu/research/research-eu.

EU. Safe organic vegetables. The development of strategies to ensure a safe organic food supply by minimizing mycotoxin risks: The carrot—Alternaria model, 2002. Available at: http://www.seedcentre.nl/Projects/EU SafeOrganicVegetables/safe organic vegetables.htm.

European Food Safety Authority. Safety and nutritional assessment of GE plants and derived food and feed: the role or animal feeding trials. Report of the EFSA GMO Panel Working Group on Animal Feeding Trials. *Food Chem Toxicol.* 2008;46:S2–S70.

European Food Safety Authority. Scientific opinion cadmium in food. Scientific opinion of the panel on contaminants in the food chain (Question No EFSA-Q-2007-138). *The EFSA J.* 2009;980:1–139. Available at: http://www.efsa.europa.eu/en/scdocs/doc/980.pdf. Accessed April 10, 2011.

European Food Safety Authority. Draft Scientific Opinion—Guidance on risk assessment concerning potential risks arising from applications of nanoscience and nanotechnologies to food and feed. Parma, Italy, 2011b. Available at: http://www.efsa.europa.eu/en/consultationsclosed/call/scaf110114.htm. Accessed April 10, 2011.

European Food Safety Authority. Scientific Opinion. Guidance for risk assessment of food and feed from genetically modified plants. *The EFSA J.* 2011a;9:1–37.

Evans CS. Naturally occurring food toxicants: Toxic amino acids. In: Rechcigl M, Jr., ed. *CRC Handbook of Naturally Occurring Food Toxicants.* Boca Raton, FL: CRC Press; 1985:3.

FAO. *Biotechnology and Food Safety. Report of a Joint FAO/WHO Consultation.* FAO Food and Nutrition Paper 61. Rome, Italy: FAO; 1996.

Farese RV, Biglieri EG, Shackleton CHL, et al. Licorice-induced hypermineralocorticoidism. *N Engl J Med.* 1991;325:1223.

Farwell AP, Braverman LE. Thyroid and antithyroid drugs. In: Brunton LL, Lazo JS, Parker KL, eds. *Goodman and Gilmans, The Pharmacological Basis of Therapeutics.* 11th ed. New York: McGraw-Hill; 2006:1511.

FDA. Food producing animals: criteria and procedures for evaluating assays for carcinogenic residues. *Fed Regist.* 1977;42.

FDA. *Toxicological Principles for the Safety Assessment of Direct Food Additives and Color Additives used in Food.* Washington, DC: U.S. Food and Drug Administration, Bureau of Foods; 1982a.

FDA. Policy for regulating carcinogenic chemicals in food and color additives. *Fed Regist.* 1982b;47:14464.

FDA. Scientific review of the long-term carcinogen bioassays performed on the artificial sweetener, cyclamate. *Report of the Cancer Assessment Committee for Food Safety and Applied Nutrition.* Washington, DC: Food and Drug Administration; 1984.

FDA. Statement of policy: foods derived from new plant varieties. *Fed Regist.* 1992;57:104–22984.

FDA. Methyl Mercury. *Fish and Fisheries Products Hazards and Controls Guidance*, 3rd ed. 2001:chap 10. Available at: http://www.fda.gov/Food/GuidanceComplianceRegulatoryInformation/GuidanceDocuments/Seafood/ucm092041.htm. Accessed July 21, 2010.

FDA. Guidance for industry: Preparation of food contact notifications and food additive petitions for food contact substances—Chemistry recommendations. *CFSAN/Office of Food Additive Safety.* Washington, DC: Food and Drug Administration; 2002a. Available at: http://www.cfsan.fda.gov/~dms/opa2pmnc.html. Accessed April 16, 2006.

FDA. Guidance for industry. Feed-effect bioavailablity and fed bioequivalence studies. Rockville, MD: Food and Drug Administration; 2002b. Available at: http://www.fda.gov/cder/guidance/5194fnl.pdf. Accessed April 16, 2006.

FDA. Furan in food, thermal treatment: Request for data and information. *Fed Regist.* 2004;69:25911.

FDA. Lead in candy likely to be consumed frequently by small children: recommended maximum level and enforcement policy (draft guidance). 2005. Available at: http://www.cfsan.fda.gov/~dms/pbguid2.html. Accessed April 8, 2006.

FDA. Food preservation and potentially hazardous food. *Potentially Hazardous Food: The evolving Definition of Temperature Control for Safety.* 2005a. Available at: http://www.fda.gov/Food/FoodSafety/RetailFoodProtection/FoodborneIllnessandRiskFactorReduction/RetailFoodRiskFactorStudies/ucm111305.htm. Accessed October 24, 2011.

FDA. United States Food and Drug Administration (FDA). Bad Bug Book. *Foodborne Pathogenic Microorganisms and Natural Toxins Handbook. BBB-Gemphylotoxin.* 2010a. available at: http://www.fda.gov/Food/FoodSafety/FoodborneIllness/FoodborneIllnessFoodbornePathogensNaturalToxins/BadBugBook/ucm071191.htm. Accessed July 21, 2010.

FDA. United States Food and Drug Administration (FDA). Scombrotoxin (histamine) Formation (a chemical hazard). *Fish and Fisheries Products Hazards and Controls Guidance.* 3rd ed. 2010b:chap 7. Available at: http://www.fda.gov/Food/GuidanceComplianceRegulatoryInformation/GuidanceDocuments/Seafood/FishandFisheriesProductsHazardsandControlsGuide/ucm091910.htm. Accessed August 31, 2010.

FDA. Background Document for the Food Advisory Committee. *Certified Color Additives in Food and Possible Association with Attention Deficit Hyperactivity Disorder in Children.* FDA; 2011a.

FDA. Quick Minutes. *Food Advisory Committee Meeting Minutes March 30-31, 2011 Certified Color Additives in Food and Possible Association with Attention Deficit Hyperactivity Disorder in Children.* FDA; 2011b.

FDA. E&J Brandy announces a nationwide recall of stainless steel flasks due to possible lead risk, 2011c. Available at: http://www.fda.gov/Safety/Recalls/ucm245046.htm. Accessed April 23, 2011.

FDA. B&M, Inc. conducts voluntary nationwide recall of 6 lot numbers of Archer Farms ground turmeric due to excessive lead levels, 2011d. Available at: http://www.fda.gov/Safety/Recalls/ucm251639.htm. Accessed April 23, 2011.

FDA. Candy Dynamics recalls Toxic Waste® Short Circuits™ bubble gum, 2011e. Available at: http://www.fda.gov/Safety/Recalls/ucm248548.htm. Accessed April 23, 2011.

Feather S. Growing zucchini. Why your garden zucchinis might taste bitter, 2010. Available at: http://www.donnan.com/Zucchini.htm. Accessed July 21, 2010.

Fedoroff NV, Brown NM. *Mendel in the Kitchen.* Washington, DC: Joseph Henry Press; 2004:171.

Flachowsky G, Chesson A, Aulrich K. Animal nutrition with feeds from genetically modified plants. *Arch Anim Nutr.* 2005;59(1):1.

Flachowsky G, Aulrich K, Bohme H, et al. Studies on feeds from genetically modified plants (GMP)—Contributions to nutritional and safety assessment. *Anim Feed Sci Technol.* 2007;133:2–30.

Flamm WG, Frankos V. Nitrates: Laboratory evidence In: Walk NJ, Doll R, eds. *Interpretation of Negative Epidemiological Evidence for Carcinogenicity.* Lyons, France: IARC Scientific Publications No. 65; 1985:85.

Flamm WG, Kotsonis FN, Hjelle JJ. Threshold of regulation: A unifying concept in food safety assessment. In: Kotsonis F, Mackey M, Hjelle J, eds. *Nutritional Toxicology.* New York: Raven Press; 1994:223.

Flamm WG, Kotsonis FN, Hjelle JJ. Threshold of regulation: A unifying concept in food safety assessment. In: Kotsonis F, Mackey M, Hjelle J, eds. *Nutritional Toxicology.* 2nd edn. New York: Taylor & Francis; 2002:190.

Flamm WG, Lehman-McKeeman LD. The human relevance of the renal tumor-inducing potential of *d*-limonene in male rats: Implications for risk assessment. *Regul Toxicol Pharmacol.* 1991;13:70.

Flamm WG, Lorentzen RL. Quantitative risk assessment (QRA): A special problem in approval of new products. In: Mehlman M, ed. *Risk Assessment and Risk Management.* Princeton, New Jersey: Princeton Scientific Publishing; 1988:91.

Flechsig E, Weissmann C. The role of PrP in health and disease. *Curr Mol Med.* 2004;4:337.

Folcher L, Delos M, Marengue E, et al. Lower mycotoxin levels in Bt maize. *Agron Sustain Dev.* 2010;30:711–719.

Fouroud NA, Eudes F. Trichothecene in cereal grains. *Int J Mol Sci.* 2009; 10:137–173.

Frankland AW. Anaphylaxis in relation to food allergy. In: Brostoff J, Challacombe SJ, eds. *Food Allergy and Intolerance.* Philadelphia: Bailliere and Tindall; 1987:456.

Fries GF. The PBB episode in Michigan: an overall appraisal. *CRC Crit Rev Toxicol.* 1985;16:105–156.

Friesen RW, Novak EM, Hasman D, et al. Relationship of dimethylglycine, choline, and betaine with oxoproline in plasma of pregnant women and their newborn infants. *J Nutr.* 2007;137:2641–2646.

Frosch MP, Anthony DC, DeGirolami U. The central nervous system. In: Kumar V, Abbas AK, Fausto N, eds. *Robbins and Cotran Pathologic Basis of Disease.* Philadelphia: Elsevier Saunders; 2005:1380.

Fuglsang G, Madsen C, Saval P, et al. Prevalence of intolerance to food additives among Danish school children. *Pediatr Allergy Immunol.* 1993; 4(3):123.

Fukutomi O, Kondo N, Agata H, et al. Timing of onset of allergic symptoms as a response to a double-blind, placebo-controlled food challenge in patients with food allergy combined with a radioallergosorbent test and the evaluation of proliferative lymphocyte responses. *Int Arch Allergy Immunol.* 1994;104(4):352.

Gangolli SD. Nitrate, nitrite and *n*-nitroso compounds. In: Ballantyne B, Marrs T, Turner P, eds. *General and Applied Toxicology.* New York: Stockton Press; 1999:2111.

Gannon JR, Kendall RVA. A clinical evaluation of *N,N*-Dimethylglycine (DMG) and diisopropylammonium dichloroacetate (DIPA) on the performance of racing greyhounds. *Canine.* 1982;9:7–11.

Gessner BD, Hokama Y, Isto S. Scombrotoxicosis-like illness following the ingestion of smoked salmon that demonstrated low histamine levels and high toxicity on mouse bioassay. *Clin Infect Dis.* 1996;23:1316.

Gianessi LP, Carpenter JE. *Agricultural Biotechnology: Insect Control Benefits.* National Center for Food and Agricultural Policy; 1999.

Gibb CM, Davies PT, Glover V, et al. Chocolate is a migraine-provoking agent. *Cephalalgia.* 1991;11(2):93.

Gilbert R: *Bacillus cereus* gastroenteritis. In: Reimann H, Bryan FL, eds. *Food-Borne Infections and Intoxications.* 2nd ed. New York: Academic Press; 1979.

Goepfert JM, Spira WM, Kim HU. *Bacillus cereus*: Food poisoning organism: A review. *J Milk Food Technol.* 1972;35:213.

Gold LS, Slone TH, Stern BR, et al. Rodent carcinogens: Setting priorities. *Science.* 1992;258:261.

Gonzalez R, Polo F, Zapatero L, et al. Purification and characterization of major inhalant allergens from soybean hulls. *Clin Exp Allergy.* 1992;22(8):748.

Goodman R, Vieths S, Sampson HA, et al. Allergenicity assessment of genetically modified crops—what makes sense? *Nature Biotech.* 2008;26:73–81.

Granum PE, Baird-Parker TC. *Bacillus* species. In: Lund BM, Baird-Parker TC, Gould GW, eds. *The Microbiological Safety and Quality of Food.* Gaithersburg, MD: Aspen; 2000:1029.

Granum PE, Brynestad S. Bacterial toxins as food poisons. In: Alouf JE, Freer JH, eds. *The Comprehensive Sourcebook of Bacterial Protein Toxins.* 2nd ed. New York: Academic Press; 1999:669.

Granum PE, Lund T. *Bacillus cereus* and its food poisoning toxins. *FEMS Microbiol Lett.* 1997;157:223.

Granum PE. Bacterial toxins as food poisons. In: Alouf JE, Popoff MR, eds. *The Comprehensive Sourcebook of Bacterial Protein Toxins*, 3rd ed. New York: Elsevier/Academic Press; 2006:949.

Greger JL. Nondigestible carbohydrates and mineral bioavailability. *J Nutr.* 1999;129:1434S–1435S.

Gudmand-Hoyer E. The clinical significance of disaccharide maldigestion. *Am J Clin Nutr.* 1994;59(suppl 3):735S.

Gueguen L, Pascal G. Le point sur la valeur nutritionnelle et sanitaire des aliments issus de l'agriculture biologique. *Cahiers de Nutrition et de Dietetique.* 2010;45(3):130–143.

Gunduz A, Turedi S, Russell RM, et al. Clinical review of grayanotoxin/mad honey poisoning past and present. *Clin Toxicol.* 2008;46:437–442.

Guo YL, Yu ML, Hsu CC. The Yucheng rice oil poisoning incident. *Dioxins and Health.* Hoboken, NJ: Hoboken Press; 2003:893.

Guth S, Habermeyer M, Schrenk D, et al. Update of the toxicological assessment of furanocoumarins in foodstuffs (Update of the SKLM statement of 23/24 September 2004)—Opinion of the Senate Commission on Food Safety (SKLM) of the German Research Foundation (DFG). *Mol Nutr Food Res.* 2011;55:1–4.

Halken S, Host A, Hansen LG, et al. Preventive effect of feeding high-risk infants a casein hydrolysate formula or an ultrafiltrated whey hydrolysate formula. A prospective, randomized, comparative clinical study. *Pediatr Allergy Immunol.* 1993;4(4):173.

Hall JE. *Guyton and Hall Textbook of Medical Physiology.* 12th ed. PA: Saunders; 2011:1–1091.

Hall R, Oser B. The safety of flavoring substances. *Residue Rev.* 1968;24:1.

Hallstrom H, Thuvander A. Toxicological evaluation of myristicin. *Natural Toxins.* 1997;5:186–192.

Hammond BG, Campbell KW, Pilcher CD, et al. Lower fumonisin mycotoxin levels in the grain of Bt corn grown in the United States in 2000–2002. *J Agric Food Chem.* 2004;52(5):1390.

Hammond B, Cockburn A. The safety assessment of proteins introduced into crops developed through agricultural biotechnology: a consolidated approach to meet current and future needs. In: Hammond BG, ed. *Food Safety of Proteins in Agricultural Biotechnology.* New York: CRC Press, Taylor and Francis; 2008:259–288.

Hansen SR, Buck WB, Meerdink G, et al. Weakness, tremors, and depression associated with macadamia nuts in dogs. *Vet Hum Toxicol.* 2000;42:18–21.

Hariganesh K, Prathiba J. Effect of dimethylglycine on gastric ulcers in rats. *J Pharm Pharmacol.* 2000;52:1519–1522.

Harpaz M, Otto RM, Smith TK. The effect of $N'N'$-dimethylglycine ingestion upon aerobic performance. *Med Sci Sports Exerc.* 1985;17:287.

Harrigan GG, Lundry D, Berman K, et al. Natural variation in crop composition and the impact of transgenesis. *Nature Biotech.* 2010;28(5):402–404.

Harris RZ, Jang GR, Tsunoda S. Dietary effects on drug metabolism and transport. *Clin Pharmacokinet.* 2003;42:1071.

Hashimoto S, Ueno K, Takahashi K, et al. Photosensitivity in mice caused by pyropheophorbide in the midgut gland of the scallop *Patinopecten yessoensis* observed in diarrhetic shellfish poisoning mouse bioassays. *Fisheries Sci.* 2010;76:529–536.

Hassing JM, Al-Turk WA, Stohs SJ. Induction of intestinal microsomal enzymes by polycyclic aromatic hydrocarbons. *Gen Pharmacol.* 1989;20(5):695.

Hauschild AHW. *Clostridium perfringens* enterotoxin. *J Milk Food Technol.* 1971;34:596.

Health Canada. Food safety tips for fiddleheads, 2010. Available at: http://www.hc-sc.gc.ca/fn-an/securit/kitchen-cuisine/fiddlehead-fougere-eng.php. Accessed April 8, 2011.

Herman RA, Phillips AM, Lepping MD, et al. Compositional safety of event DAS-40278-9 (AAD-1) herbicide-tolerant maize. *GM Crops.* 2010;1–5:294–311.

Hobbs BC, Smith ME, Oakley CL, et al. *Clostridium welchii* food poisoning. *J Hyg (Lond).* 1953;51:75.

Hobbs G. *Clostridium botulinum* and its importance in fishery products. *Adv Food Res.* 1976;22:135.

Hotchkiss JH. Relative exposure to nitrite, nitrate, and *N*-nitroso compounds from endogenous and exogenous sources. In: Taylor SL, Scanlan RA, eds. *Food Toxicology: A Perspective on the Relative Risks.* New York: Marcel Dekker; 1989:57.

Hotchkiss JH, Helser MA, Maragos CM, et al. Nitrate, nitrite, and *N*-nitroso compounds: Food safety and biological implications. In: Finley JW, Robinson SF, Armstrong DJ, eds. *Food Safety Assessment.* Washington, DC: American Chemical Society; 1992:400.

Hutt PB, Merrill RA, Grossman LW. *Food and Drug Law.* 3rd ed. New York, NY: Foundation Press; 2007:369.

Idboro CJ. *The Pangnirtung Inuit and the Greenland Shark* [master's thesis]. Canada: University of Manitoba; 2008. Available at: http://www.umanitoba.ca/institutes/natural_resources/canadaresearchchair/thesis/Idrobo.Masters%20Thesis.Feb%2009.pdf. Accessed July, 2010.

IFST (Institute of Food Science and Technology Trust Fund). Mycotoxins: Information statement. 2006a. Available at: http://www.ifst.org/myco.pdf. Accessed March 12, 2006.

Ijomah P, Clifford MN, Walker R, et al. The importance of endogenous histamine relative to dietary histamine in the aetiology of scombrotoxicosis. *Food Addit Contam.* 1991;8(4):531.

International Agency for Research on Cancer. Acrylamide. *Some Industrial Chemicals.* Vol. 60. Working Group on the Evaluation of Carcinogenic Risk to Humans. Lyon, France: IARC Press; 1994:389.

International Agency for Research on Cancer. Dry cleaning, some chlorinated solvents and other industrial chemicals. *IARC Monographs on the Evaluation of Carcinogenic Risks to Humans.* Vol 63. Lyon, France: IARC Press; 1995:394.

International Agency for Research on Cancer. Some traditional herbal medicines, some mycotoxins, naphthalene and styrene. *IARC Working Group on the Evaluation of Carcinogenic Risk to Humans.* Lyon, France: IARC Press, 2002, p. 171.

International Chemical Safety Programme. *Fumonisin B1, Environmental Health Criteria 219.* Geneva: United Nations Environmental Programme, the International Labour Organization and the World Health Organization International Programme on Chemical Safety; 2000:153.

International Chemical Safety Programme. *Solanine and Chaconine.* Environmental Health Criteria 764 (WHO Food Additives Series 30); 1993 Available at: http://www.inchem.org/documents/jecfa/jecmono/v30je19.htm. Accessed April 15, 2006.

International Life Sciences Institute. ILSI Crop Composition Database, version 3 (www.crop-composition.org), 2006.

Institute of Medicine. *Enhancing the Regulatory Decision-Making Approval Process for Direct Food Ingredient Technologies.* Washington, DC: National Research Council; 1999:158.

Institute of Medicine. Fluoride. *Dietary Reference Intakes for Calcium, Phosphorus, Magnesium, Vitamin D and Fluoride.* Washington, DC: National Academy Press; 1997:288:chap 8.

International Programme on Chemical Safety. Principles for the safety assessment of food additives and contaminants in food. *Environmental Health Criteria 70.* Geneva: World Health Organization; 1987:174.

Isbrucker RA, Burdock GA. Risk and safety assessment on the consumption of licorice root (*Glycyrrhiza* sp.), its extract and powder as a food ingredient, with emphasis on the pharmacology and toxicology of glycyrrhizin. *Regul Toxicol Pharmacol.* 2006;46(3):167.

James C. *Global Status of Commercialized Biotech/GM Crops—2005.* Executive summary in *ISAA Briefs* No. 34. International Service for the Acquisition of Agri-Biotech Applications, (ISAA); 2006:1.

James C. *ISAAA Briefs.* Brief 42. Global Status of Commercialized Biotech/GM Crops: 2010. Ithaca, NY: ISAAA; 2011.

Jiao CJ, Jiang JL, Ke LM, et al. Factors affecting β-ODAP content in *Lathyrus sativus* and their possible physiological mechanisms. *Food Chem Tox.* 2011;49:543–549.

Jitsukawa K, Suizu R, Hidano A. Chlorella photosensitization. New phytophotodermatosis. *Int J Dermatol.* 1984;23:263–268.

Joint Expert Committee on Food Additives. *Summary and Conclusions of the Sixty-fourth Meeting of the Joint FAO/WHO Expert Committee on Food Additives (JECFA).* 2005:47. Available at: http://www.fda.gov/downloads/Food/FoodSafety/FoodContaminantsAdulteration/ChemicalContaminants/Acrylamide/UCM194526.pdf. Accessed May 9, 2011.

Joint FAO/WHO Expert Committee on Food Additives. *Safety Evaluation of Certain Mycotoxins in Food*. WHO Food Additives Series 47. Geneva: WHO; 2001:419.

Jones DB, Hancock JD, Harmon DL, et al. Effects of exogenous emulsifiers and fat sources on nutrient digestibility, serum lipids, and growth performance in weanling pigs. *J Animal Sci*. 1992;70:3473–3482.

Juambeltz JC, Kula K, Perman J. Nursing caries and lactose intolerance. *ASDC J Dent Child*. 1993;60(4):377.

Juan C, Molto JC, Lino CM, et al. Determination of ochratoxin A in organic and non-organic cereals and cereal products from Spain and Portugal. *Food Chem*. 2008;107(1):525–530.

Kalmar ID, Cools A, Buyse J, et al. Dietary *N,N*-dimethylglycine supplementation improves nutrient digestibility and attenuates pulmonary hypertension syndrome in broilers. *J Anim Physiol Anim Nutr*. 2010;94(6):e339–e347.

Kanagawa Y, Matsumoto S, Koike S, et al. Association of clinical findings of Yusho patients with serum concentrations of polychlorinated biphenyls, polychlorinated quterphenyls and 2,3,4,7,8-pentachlorodibenz ofuran more than 30 years after the poisoning event. *Environ Health*. 2008;7:47–58.

Karch H, Bielaszewska M, Bitzan M, et al. Epidemiology and diagnosis of Shiga toxin-producing *Escherichia coli* infections. *Diagn Microbiol Infect Dis*. 1999;34:229.

Kassa RM, Kasensa NL, Monterroso VH, et al. On the biomarkers and mechanisms of konzo, a distinct upper motor neutron disease associated with food (cassava) cynogenic exposure. *Food Chem Tox*. 2011;49:571–578.

Kensler TW, Roebuck BD, Wogan GN, et al. Aflatoxin: A 50-year odyssey of mechanistic and translational toxicology. *Toxicol Sci*. 2011; 120(S1):S28–S48.

Khoo KK. Glucose-6-dehydrogenase deficiency and malaria. *Aust Med J*. 2010;3:422–425.

Kim JH, Lee KJ, Suzuki T, et al. Identification of tetramine, a toxin in whelks, as the cause of a poisoning incident in Korea and the distribution of tetramine in fresh and boiled whelk (*Neptunea intersculpta*). *J Food Prot*. 2009;72:1935–1940.

Kirchgessner M, Reichlmayer-Lais AM. *Trace Element Metabolism in Man and Animals (TEMA-4)*. Canberra: Australian Academy of Science; 1981.

Kivity S, Sunner K, Marian Y. The pattern of food hypersensitivity in patients with onset after 10 years of age. *Clin Exp Allergy*. 1994;24:1.

Kokoski CJ, Henry SH, Lin CS, et al. Methods used in safety evaluation. In: Branen AL, Davidson PM, Salminen S, eds. *Food Additives*. New York: Marcel Dekker; 1990.

Kotsonis FN, Hjelle JJ. The safety assessment of aspartame: Scientific, and regulatory considerations. In: Tschanz C, Butchko HH, Stargel W, Kotsonis FH, eds. *The Clinical Evaluation of a Food Additive. Assessment of Aspartame*. Boca Raton, FL: CRC Press; 1996:23.

Krishnamachari KAVR, Bhat RV, Nagarajan V, et al. Hepatitis due to aflatoxicosis. *Lancet*. 1975;1(7915):1061.

Kritschevsky D. The role of fat, calories and fiber in disease. In: Kotsonis F, Mackey M, Hjelle J, eds. *Nutritional Toxicology*. New York: Raven Press; 1994:67.

Kumar S, Bejiga G, Ahmed S, et al. Genetic improvement of grass pea for low neutrotoxin (β-ODAP) content. *Food Chem Toxicol*. 2011;49:589–600.

Kwok J. Dietary Supplements and Bioavailability: Looking for Some Action? *Nutritional Outlook*. 2011. Available at: http://www.nutrition-aloutlook.com/article/bioavailability-does-size-matter. Accessed April 10, 2011.

Lagerwerff JV, Sprecht AW. Occurrence of environmental cadmium and zinc and their uptake by plants. In: Hemphill DD, ed. *Proceedings of the University of Missouri 4th Annual Conference on Trace Substances in Environmental Health*. Columbia: University of Missouri; 1971:85.

Lange WR. Scombroid poisoning. *Am Fam Physician*. 1988;37:163.

Lee CA, Ironside JW, Bell JE, et al. Retrospective neuropathological review of prion disease in UK haemophilic patients. *Thromb Haemost*. 1998;80:909.

Lee ST, Davis TZ, Gardner DR, et al. Quantitative method for the measurement of three benzofuran ketones in rayless goldenrod (*Isocoma pluriflora*) and white snakeroot (*Ageratina altissima*) by high-performance liquid chromatography (HPLC). *J Agric Food Chem*. 2009;57:5639–5643.

Lehman AJ, Fitzhugh OG. 100-Fold margin of safety. *Quarterly Bulletin of the Association of Food and Drug Officials of the United States*. 1954:33.

Levine SV, Myhre GD, Smith GL, et al. Effect of a nutritional supplement containing *N,N*-dimethylglycine (DMG) on the racing standardbred. *Equine Practice Nutrition*. 1982;4:17–20.

Linder MC. *Nutritional Biochemistry and Metabolism*, 2nd ed. Norwalk, CT: Appleton and Lange; 1991.

Liston J. Fish and shellfish poisoning, in Lund BM, Baird-Parker TC, Gould GW (eds.) *The Microbiological Safety and Quality of Food*. Gaithersburg, MD: Aspen; 2000:1518.

Loving AL. Botulism in flavored oils—a review. *Dairy, Food and Environmental Sanitation*. 1998;18:438.

Lund BM, Peck MW. Clostridium botulinum. In: Lund BM, Baird-Parker TC, Gould GW, eds. *The Microbiological Safety and Quality of Food*. Gaithersburg, MD: Aspen; 2000:1057.

Lundry DR, Ridley WP, Meyer JJ, et al. Composition of grain, forage, and processed fractions from second-generation glyphosate-tolerant soybean, MON 89788, is equivalent to that of conventional soybean (*Glycine max* L.). *J Ag Food Chem*. 2008;56:4611–4622.

Luzzatto L, Mehta A, Vulliamy T. Glucose 6-phosphate dehydrogenase deficiency. In: Scriver CR, Beaudet AL, Sly WS, Valle D, eds. *The Metabolic and Molecular Bases of Inherited Disease*. Vol. 3. 8th ed. New York: McGraw-Hill Medical Publishing Division; 2001:4517–4553.

Mackey M, Kotsonis FN. Functional foods: Regulatory and scientific considerations. In: Kotsonis F, Mackey M, Hjelle J, eds. *Nutritional Toxicology*. 2nd ed. New York: Taylor & Francis; 2002:243.

Mallinson CN. Basic functions of the gut. In: Brostoff J, Challacombe SJ, eds. *Food Allergy and Intolerance*. Philadelphia: Bailtiere and Tindalf; 1987:27.

Manda F, Tadera K, Aoyama K. Skin lesions due to Okra (*Hibiscus esculenius* L.): proteolytic activity and allergenicity of okra. *Contact Dermatitis*. 1992;26(2):95.

Manu P, Matthews DA, Lane TJ. Food intolerance in patients with chronic fatigue. *Int J Eat Disord*. 1993;13:203.

Marasas WFO, Jaskiewicz K, Venter FS, et al. Fusarium moniliforme contamination of maize in oesophageal cancer areas in the transkei. *S Afr Med J*. 1988;74:110.

Martin PAW, Blackburn M, Schroder RFW, et al. Stabilization of cucurbitacin E-glycocide, a feeding stimulant for diabroticite beetles, extracted from bitter Hawkesbury watermelon. *J Insect Sci*. 2002;2:1–6.

Masoero F, Moschini M, Rossi F, et al. Nutritive value, mycotoxin contamination and *in vitro* rumen fermentation of normal and genetically modified corn (CryIA(B)) grown in northern Italy. *Maydica*. 1999; 44:205.

Masuda Y. Health status of Japanese and Taiwanese after exposure to contaminated rice oil. *Environ Health Perspect*. 1985;60:321–325.

Matsumoto H. Cycasin, in Rechcigl M Jr, ed. *CRC Handbook of Naturally Occurring Food Toxicants*. Boca Raton, FL: CRC Press; 1985:43.

Matulka RH. Understanding ingredient consumption analysis. *Nat Prod Ind Insid*. 2005;10:46.

McClain RM. Mechanistic considerations in the regulation and classification of chemical carcinogens. In: Kotsonis FN, Mackey M, Hjelle JJ, eds. *Nutritional Toxicology*. 2nd ed. New York: Taylor & Francis; 2002:387.

McClintock JT, Schaffer CR, Sjoblad RD. A comparative review of the mammalian toxicity of *Bacillus thuringiensis*-based pesticides. *Pestic Sci*. 1995;45:95.

MDCH (Michigan Department of Community Health). PBBs (Polybrominated Biphenyls) in Michigan. Frequently Asked Questions, 2011 Available at: http://www.michigan.gov/documents/mdch_PBB_FAQ_92051_7.pdf. Accessed May 7, 2011.

Meduski JW, Hyman SKR, Kim KTP, et al. Decrease of lactic acid concentration in blood of animals given *N,N*-dimethylglycine. (Presentation Abstract) Pacific Slope Biochemical Conference. July 7-9, 1980, University of California, San Diego, 1980:37.

Melnik B, Szliska C, Noehle M, et al. Food intolerance: Pseudoallergic reactions induced by biogenic amines. *Allergo J*. 1997;20:163.

Mendelsohn M, Kough J, Vaituzis Z, et al. Are Bt crops safe? *Nature Biotech*. 2003;21(9):1003–1009.

Metcalfe DD, Astwood JD, Townsend R, et al. Assessment of the allergenic potential of foods derived from genetically engineered crop plants. *Crit Rev Food Sci Nutr*. 1996;36(S):S165.

Milkowski A, Garg H, Coughlin JR, et al. Nutritional epidemiology in the context of nitric oxide biology: a risk–benefit evaluation for dietary nitrite and nitrate. *Nitric Oxide*. 2010;22:110–119.

Miller CD. *Selected Toxicological Studies of the Mycotoxin CyclopiazonicAcid in Turkeys*. (dissertation). Ann Arbor, MI: University of Michigan Dissertation Services; 1989.

Miller MW, Williams ES, Hobbs NT, et al. Environmental sources of prion transmission in mule deer. *Emerg Infect Dis*. 2004;10:1003.

Miller SA. Food additives and contaminants. In: Amdur MO, Doull J, Klaassen CD, eds. *Toxicology: The Basic Science of Poisons*. New York: Taylor & Francis; 1991:819.

Minor TE, Marth EH. *Staphylococci and their Significance in Foods*. Amsterdam: Elsevier; 1976.

Mirvish SS. Formation of *N*-nitroso compounds: Chemistry kinetics, and *in vivo* occurrence. *Toxicol Appl Pharmacol*. 1975;31:325.

MMWR. Ostrich fern poisoning—New York and Western Canada. *MMWR Morb Mortal Wkly Rep*. 1994;43:677.

Monday SR, Bohach GA. Properties of *Staphylococcus aureus* enterotoxins and toxic shock syndrome toxin-1. In: Alouf JE, Freer JH, eds. *The Comprehensive Sourcebook of Bacterial Protein Toxins*. 2nd ed. New York: Academic Press Limited; 1999:589.

Moneret-Vautrin DA. Food intolerance masquerading as food allergy: false food allergy. In: Brostoff J, Challacombe SJ, eds. *Food Allergy and Intolerance*. Philadelphia: Balliere Tindall; 1987:836.

Monroe DH, Eaton DL. Comparative effects of butylated hydroxyanisole on hepatic *in vivo* DNA binding and *in vitro* biotransformation of aflatoxin B$_1$ in the rat and mouse. *Toxicol Appl Pharmacol*. 1987; 90:401.

Morrow JD, Margiolies GR, Rowland J, et al. Evidence that histamine is the causative toxin of scombroid-fish poisoning. *N Engl J Med*. 1991; 324(11):716.

Muller GJ, Lamprechi JH, Barnes JM, et al. Scombroid poisoning: Case series of 10 incidents involving 22 patients. *S African Med J*. 1992; 81(8):427.

Munkvold GP, Hellmich RL, Rice LR. Comparison of fumonisin concentrations in kernels of transgenic Bt maize hybrids and nontransgenic hybrids. *Plant Dis*. 1999;83:130.

Munkvold GP, Hellmich RL, Showers WB. Reduced fusarium ear rot and symptomless infection in kernels of maize genetically engineered for European corn borer resistance. *Phytopathology*. 1997;87:1071.

Munro IC. Issues to be considered in the safety evaluation of fat substitutes. *Food Chem Toxicol*. 1990;28:751.

Munro IC, Kennepohl E, Erickson RE, et al. Safety assessment of ingested heterocyclic amines: Initial report. *Regul Toxicol Pharmacol*. 1993;17:S1.

National Toxicology Program. *Toxicology and Carcinogenesis Studies of Furan (CAS No. 110-00-9) in F344/N Rats and B6C3F1 Mice (gavage studies)*, NTP Technical Report No. 402. Research Triangle Park, NC: US Department of Health and Human Services, Public Health Service, National Institutes of Health; 1993.

National Toxicology Program. Acrylamide. *Report on Carcinogens*. 11th ed. Washington, DC: US Department of Health and Human Services, Public Health Service; 2004b. (http://ntp-server.niehs.nih.gov/index.cfm?objectid=32BA9724-F1F6-975E-7FCE50709CB4C932) (site visited 15 April 2006).

National Toxicology Program. Urethane. *Report on Carcinogens*. 11th ed. Washington, DC: U.S. Department of Health and Human Services, Public Health Service; 2004a. (http://ntp-server.niehs.nih.gov/index.cfm?objectid=32BA9724-F1F6-975E-7FCE50709CB4C932) (site visited 15 April 2006).

Newberne PM. Mechanisms of interaction and modulation of response. In: Vouk VB, Butler GC, Upton AC, et al., eds. *Methods for Assessing the Effects of Mixtures of Chemicals*. New York: Wiley; 1987:555.

NIAID (National Institute of Allergy and Infectious Disease). *Food Allergy: Eosinophilic Esophagitis and Food Allergy*. 2011. Available at: http://www.niaid.nih.gov/topics/foodAllergy/understanding/Pages/eoe.aspx. Accessed May 9, 2011.

Nichols, PD, Mooney, BD, Elliott, NG. Unusually high levels of non-saponifiable lipids in the fishes escolar and rudderfish: identification by gas and thin-layer chromatography. *Journal of Chromatography A*. 2001; 936:183–191.

NNI (National Nanotechnology Initiative). What's so special about the nanoscale? 2011. available at: http://www.nano.gov/nanotech-101/special. Accessed October 24, 2011.

Nordlee JA, Taylor SL, Townsend JA, et al. Transgenic soybeans containing Brazil nut 2S storage protein issues regarding allergenicity. In: Eisenbrand G, et al., eds. *Food Allergies and Intolerances*. New York: VCH Publishers; 1996:196.

NPS (National Park Service). Lincoln Boyhood National Memorial. The plant that killed Nancy Hanks Lincoln, 2010. (http://www.nps.gov/archive/libo/white_snakeroot3.htm) (site visited 21 July 2010).

NRC (National Research Council). *Fluoride in Drinking Water: A Scientific Review of EPA's Standards*. Washington, DC: National Academy Press; 2006:576.

NRC/NAS (National Research Council/National Academy of Science). *The 1977 Survey of Industry on the Use of Food Additives by the NRC/NAS*. October 1979, U.S. Department of Commerce, NTIS PB 80-113418. Volume III: *Estimates of Daily Intake*. Committee on GRAS list survey—Phase III Food and Nutrition Committee, National Research Council, 1979.

Oberdörster G, Oberdörster E, Oberdörster J. Nanotoxicology: An emerging discipline evolving from studies of ultrafine particles. *Environ Health Perspect*. 2005;113(7): 823–839.

OECD (Organization for the Economic Co-operation and Development). *Safety Evaluation of Foods Derived by Modern Biotechnology: Concepts and Principles*. Paris: OECD Press; 1993.

OECD (Organization for the Economic Co-operation and Development). *Report of the Workshop on the Toxicological and Nutritional Testing of Novel Foods*, SG/ICGB(98)1. Paris: OECD Press; 1997.

OECD (Organization for the Economic Co-operation and Development). Consensus document on safety information on transgenic plants expressing *Bacillus thuringiensis*–derived insect control proteins. In: *Joint Meeting of the Chemicals Committee and the Working Party on Chemicals, Pesticides and Biotechnology*, Paris, France; 2007.

O'Hallaren MT. Baker's asthma and reactions secondary to soybean and grain dust. In: Bardana EJ Jr, Montanaro A, O'Hallaren MT, eds. *Occupational Asthma*. Philadelphia: Hanley and Belfus; 1992:107.

O'Neil C, Helbling AA, Lehrer SB. Allergic reactions to fish. *Clin Rev Allergy*. 1993;11(2):183.

Onuma Y, Satake M, Ukena T, et al. Identification of putative palytoxin as the cause of clupeotoxism. *Toxicon*. 1999;37(1):55.

Oshima H, Bartsch H. Quantitative estimation of endogenous nitrosation in humans by monitoring *N*-nitrosoproline excreted in the urine. *Cancer Res*. 1981;41:3658.

Ostertag E, Becker T, Ammon J, et al. Effects of storage conditions on furocoumarin levels in intact, chopped or homogenized parsnips. *J Agric Food Chem*. 2002;50:2565–2570.

Ostry V, Ovesna J, Skarkova J, et al. A review of the comparative data concerning *Fusarium* mycotoxins in Bt maize and non-Bt isogenic maize. *Mycotox Res*. 2010;26:141–145.

Padilla D, Beringue V, Espinosa JC, et al. Sheep and goat BSE propagate more efficiently than cattle BSE in human PrP transgenic mice. *PLoS Pathog*. 2011;7(3):e1001319.

Pak YK, Jeong JH. Mitochondria: The secret chamber of therapeutic targets for age-associated degenerative diseases. *Biomol Ther*. 2010; 18:235–245.

Panter KE, James LF. Natural plant toxicants in milk: a review. *J Anim Sci*. 1990;68:892–904.

Papst C, Utz HF, Melchinger AE, et al. Mycotoxins produced by *Fusarium* spp. In isogenic Bt *vs*. non-Bt maize hybrids under European corn borer pressure. *Agron J*. 2005;97:219.

Pariza MW, Johnson EA. Evaluating the safety of microbial enzyme preparations used in food processing: Update for a new century. *Regul Toxicol Pharmacol*. 2001;33(2):173.

Parrott W, Chassy B, Ligon J, et al. Application of food and feed safety assessment principles to evaluate transgenic approaches to gene modulation in crops. *Food Chem Tox*. 2010;48:1773–1790.

Peers FG, Gilman GA, Linsell CA. Dietary aflatoxins and human liver cancer: a study in Swaziland. *Int J Cancer*. 1976;17:167.

Piastra M, Stabile A, Fioravanti G, et al. Cord blood mononuclear cell responsiveness to beta-lactoglobulin: T-cell activity in "atopy-prone" and "non-atopy-prone" newborns. *Int Arch Allergy Immunol*. 1994;104:358.

Power AJ, Keegan BG, Nolan K. The seasonality and role of the neurotoxin tetramine in the salivary glands of the red whelk *Neptunea antiqua* (L.). *Toxicon*. 2002;40:419–425.

Prusiner SB. *Prion Diseases of Animals and Humans*. Washington, DC: Toxicology Forum; 1991:203.

Prusiner SB. Prion diseases of humans and animals. *J R Coll Physicians*. 1994;28:1.

Raquet N, Schrenk D. Relative photomutagenicity of furocoumarins and limettin in the hypoxanthine phosphoribosyl transferase assay in V79 cells. *Chem Res Toxicol*. 2009;22:1639–1647.

Reap EA, Lawson JW. Stimulation of the immune response by dimethylglycine, a nontoxic metabolite. *J Lab Clin Med*. 1990;115(4):481–486.

Reid TMS, Gould IM, Mackie IM, et al. Food poisoning due to the consumption of red whelks (*Neptunea antiqua*). *Epidemiol Infect*. 1988;101:419–424.

Roberfroid MBL. Dietary fiber, inulin and oligofructose: a review comparing their physiological effects. *Crit Rev Food Sci Nutr*. 1993;33:103–148.

Roberfroid MB. Inulin-type fructans: functional food ingredients. *J Nutr*. 2007;137:2493S–2502S.

Rose RJ, Schlierf HA, Knight PK, et al. Effects of *N,N*-dimethylglycine on cardiorespiratory function and lactate production in thoroughbred horses performing incremental treadmill exercise. *Vet Rec*. 1989;125:268–271.

Rulis A. Food Safety and Nutritional Risk. Bioactive Food Components.In: *6th Joint CSL/JIFSAN Symposium on Food Safety and Nutrition*. July, 2005. University of Maryland, University College, Inn and Conference Center, Adelphi, MD, 2005.

Rumsey GL, Siwicki AK, Anderson DP, et al. Effect of soybean protein on serological response, non-specific defense mechnisms, growth, and protein utilization in rainbow trout. *Vet Immunol Immunopathol*. 1994;41:323.

Sachs MI, Jones RT, Yunginger JW. Isolation and partial characterization of a major peanut allergen. *J Allergy Clin Immunol*. 1981;67:27.

Sansalone W, ed. *What is a Nutrient: Defining the Food-Drug Continuum*. Washington, DC: Proceedings, Georgetown University, Center for Food and Nutritional Policy; 1999:82.

Sato N, Ueno Y. Comparative toxicities of trichothecenes. In: Rodericks JV, Hesseltine CW, Mehlman MA, eds. *Mycotoxins in Human and Animal Health*. Park Forest South, IL: Pathtox Publishers; 1977:295.

Schmidt LE, Dalhoff K. Food-drug interactions. *Drugs*. 2002;62:1481.

Schneider-Chafen JJ, Newberry SJ, Riedl MA, et al. Diagnosing and managing common food allergies: a systematic review. *JAMA*. 2010;303:1848–1856.

Schrander JJ, van den Bogart JP, Forget PP, et al. Cow's milk protein intolerance in infants under 1 year of age: a prospective epidemiological study. *Eur J Pediatr*. 1993;52(8):640.

Scholz-Ahrens K, Schrezenmeir J. Inulin and oligofructose and mineral metabolism: the evidence from animal trials. *J Nutr*. 2007;137:2513S–2523S.

Schut HAJ, Snyderwine EG. DNA adducts of heterocyclic amine food mutagens: implications for mutagenesis and carcinogenesis. *Carcinogenesis*. 1999;20:353.

Settipane GA. The restaurant syndromes. *N Engl Reg Allergy Proc*. 1987;8:39.

Shank FR, Carson KL. What is safe food? In: Finley JW, Robinson SF, Armstrong DJ, eds. *Food Safety Assessment*. Washington, DC: American Chemical Society; 1992:26.

Shiomi K. Toxins in marine animals. *J Jpn Assn Acute Med*. 1999;10:4.

Sieber SM, Correa P, Dalgard DW, et al. Carcinogenicity and hepatotoxicity of cycasin and its aglycone methylazoxymethanol acetate in nonhuman primates. *JNCI*. 1980;65:177.

Sjoblad RD, McClintock JT, Engler R. Toxicological considerations for protein components of biological pesticide products. *Regul Toxicol Pharmacol*. 1992;15(1):3.

SKLM. Toxikologische Beurteilung von Furocumarinen in Lebensmitteln [Toxicological assessment of furanocoumarins in foodstuffs];

German version from 23th/24th September 2004; in *Deutsche Forschungsgemeinschaft, Lebensmittel und Gesundheit II, Sammlung der Beschlu.sse und Stellungnahmen [German Research Foundation, Food and Health II, Collection of Decisions and Statements] (1997–2004), Communication 7*. Weinheim: Wiley-VCH Verlag GmbH & Co. KGaA; 2005. English Version 'Toxicological assessment of furanocoumarins in foodstuffs' adopted on 22 September 2006.

Skog KI, Johannsson MAE, Jagerstad MI. Carcinogenic heterocyclic amines in model systems and cooked foods: A review on formation, occurrence and intake. *Food Chem Toxicol*. 1998;36:879.

Smart DR. Scombroid poisoning: a report of seven cases involving the Western Australian salmon, *Arripis truttaceus*. *Med J Aust*. 1992;157:748.

Smiciklas-Wright H, Mitchell DC, Mickle SJ, et al. Foods Commonly Eaten in the United States, 2002 (http://www.ars.usda.gov/sp2userfiles/place/12355000/pdf/portion.pdf).

Smith RL. Does one man's meat become another man's poison? *Trans Med Soc Lond*. 1991;11:6.

SNIC (Seafood Network Information Center). Natural toxins. 2007:chap 6. Available at: http://seafood.ucdavis.edu/haccp/compendium/chapt26.htm. Accessed June 6, 2010.

Sobel J, Tucker N, Sulka A, et al. Foodborne botulism in the United States, 1990–2000. *Emerg Infect Dis*. 2004;10:1606.

Sorensen JM. Herb-drug, food-drug, nutrient-drug, and drug-drug interactions: Mechanisms involved and their medical implications. *J Altern Complement Med*. 2002;8:293.

Stargel WW, Sanders PG, Tschanz C, et al. Clinical studies with food additives. In: Tschanz C, Butchko HH, Stargel WW, Kotsonis FN, eds. *The Clinical Evaluation of a Food Additive. Assessment of Aspartame*. Boca Raton, Florida: CRC Press; 1996:11.

Steinmetz CG, Xie P, Weiner H, et al. Structure of mitochondrial aldehyde dehydrogenase: the genetic component of ethanol aversion. *Structure*. 1997;5:701–711

Stephenson J. Public health experts take aim at a moving target: foodborne infections. *JAMA*. 1997;277:97.

Stewart-Tull DE, Jones AC. Adjuvanted oral vaccines should not induce allergic responses to dietary antigens. *FEMS Microbiol Lett*. 1992; 79:489.

Stoger P, Wuthrich B. Type I allergy to cow milk proteins in adults: a retrospective study of 34 adult milk- and cheese-allergic patients. *Int Arch Allergy Immunol*. 1993;102:399.

Stoloff L. Aflatoxins – an overview. In: Rodericks JV, Hesseltine CW, Mehlman MA, eds. *Mycotoxins in Human and Animal Health*. Park Forest South, IL: Pathtox; 1977.

Subbiah V. Method of isolating cucurbitacin. 1999 (Patent). Available at: http://www.freepatentsonline.com/5925356.html. Accessed April 24, 2011.

Sugimura T, Wakabayashi K, Nagao M, et al. Heterocyclic amines in cooked food. In: Taylor SL, Scanlan RA, eds. *Food Toxicology: A Perspective on the Relative Risks*. New York: Marcel Dekker; 1989:31.

Sugimura T, Wakabayashi K. Carcinogens in foods. In Shils ME, ed. *Modern Nutrition in Health and Disease*. Baltimore: Williams and Wilkins; 1999:1255.

Swenson WK, Dunn JE, Conn EE. Cyanogenesis in the Proteaceae. *Phytochemistry*. 1989;28:821–823.

Szepfalusi Z, Ebner C, Pandjaitan R, et al. Egg yolk *alpha*-livetin (chicken serum albumin) is a cross-reactive allergen in the bird-egg syndrome. *J Allergy Clin Immunol*. 1994;93:932.

Takatani T, Akaeda H, Arakawa O, et al. Occurrence of paralytic shellfish poison (PSP) in bivalves, along with mossworm adherent to their shells, collected from Fukue Island, Nagasaki, Japan during 1995 and 1996. *J Food Hygienic Soc Jpn*. 1997;38:430.

Tan CH, Lau CO. Chemistry and detection. In: Botana LM, ed. *Seafood and Freshwater Toxins. Pharmacology, Physiology and Detection*. New York: Marcel Dekker; 2000:533.

Taylor SL. Histamine food poisoning: toxicology and clinical aspects. *Crit Rev Toxicol*. 1986;17(2):91.

Taylor SL, Hefle SL. Allergic reactions and food intolerances. In: Kotsonis F, Mackey M, Hjelle J, eds. *Nutritional Toxicology*. 2nd ed. New York: Taylor & Francis; 2002:93.

Taylor SL, Nordlee JA, Rupnow JH. Food allergies and sensitivities. In: Taylor SL, Scanlan RA, eds. *Food Toxicology: A Perspective on the Relative Risks*. New York: Marcel Dekker; 1989:255.

Tennant D. Estimation of food chemical intake. In: Kotsonis F, Mackey M, Hjelle J, eds. *Nutritional Toxicology*. 2nd ed. New York: Taylor & Francis; 2002:263.

Thomas K, MacIntosh S, Bannon G, et al. Scientific advancement of novel protein allergenicity evaluation: an overview of the HESI Protein Allergenicity Technical Committee (2000-2008). *Food Chem Toxicol*. 2009;47:1041–1050.

Thompson L. Are Bioengineered foods safe. *FDA Consum*. 2000;34:18.

Todd ECD. Domoic acid and amnesic shellfish poisoning: a review. *J Food Prot*. 1993;56:69.

Tonda ME, Hart LL. *N,N* dimethylglycine and *L*-carnitine as performance enhancers in athletes. *Ann Pharmacother*. 1992;26:935–937.

Tosteson MT. Mechanism of action, pharmacology and toxicology. In: Botana LM, ed. *Seafood and Freshwater Toxins. Pharmacology, Physiology and Detection*. New York: Marcel Dekker; 2000:549.

Truckness MW, Mislivec PB, Young K, et al. Cyclopiazonic acid production by cultures of *Aspergillus* and *Penicillium* species isolated from dried beans, corn meal, macaroni, and pecans. *J Assoc Off Anal Chem*. 1987;70:123.

Ueno Y. Trichothecenes: overview address. In: Rodericks JV, Hesseltine CW, Mehlman MA, eds. *Mycotoxins in Human and Animal Health*. Park Forest South, IL: Pathtox; 1977:189.

UK Food Standards Agency. Available at: http://www.food.gov.uk/news/newsarchive/maize. Accessed September 10, 2003.

Ukishima Y, Masui T, Masubara S, et al. Wax components of escolar (Lepidocybium flavobrunneum) and its application to base of medicine and cosmetics. *Yakugaku Zasshi*. 1987;107:883–890.

United States Department of Agriculture. What We Eat In America (NHANES), 2010. Available at: http://www.ars.usda.gov/Services/docs.htm?docid=13793.

USDA Economic Research Service Reports Continuing Survey of Food Intakes by Individuals (CSFII). USDA; 1994–1996, 1998. Available at: http://www.ars.usda.gov/Services/docs.htm?docid=14531.

Van Dolah FM. Diversity of marine and freshwater algal toxins. In: Botana LM, ed. *Seafood and Freshwater Toxins. Pharmacology, Physiology and Detection*. New York: Marcel Dekker; 2000:19.

Van Etten CH, Tookey HL. Glucosinotates. In: Rechcigl J, Jr, ed. *CRC Handbook of Naturally Occurring Food Toxicants*. Boca Raton, FL: CRC Press; 1985:15.

Van Gelderen CE, Savelkoul TJ, van Ginkel LA, et al. The effects of histamine administered in fish samples to healthy volunteers. *J Toxicol Clin Toxicol*. 1992;30(4):585.

Van Moorhem M, Lambein F, Leyhaert L. Unraveling the mechanism of β-N-oxalyl-α,β-diaminopropionic acid (β-ODAP) induced excitotoxicity and toxidative stress, relevance for neurolathyrism prevention. *Food Chem Toxicol*. 2011;49:550–555.

Vickery BP, Chin S, Burks AW. Pathophysiology of food allergy. *Pediatr Clin North Am*. 2011;58:363–376.

Volatile Compounds in Food. 2010. Available at: http://www.vcf-online.nl/VcfHome.cfm. Accessed April 25, 2011.

VonMalottki K, Wiechmann HW. Acute life threatening bradycardia: food poisoning by Turkish wild honey. *Dtsch Med Wochenschr*. 1996;121:936.

Wadee AA, Boting L2Da, Rabson AR. Fruit allergy: demonstration of IgE antibodies to a 302Dkd protein present in several fruits. *J Allergy Clin Immunol*. 1990;85:801.

Wagstaff D. Dietary exposure to furocoumarins. *Regul Toxicol Pharmacol*. 1991;14:261–272.

Waldron H. Did the Mad Hatter have mercury poisoning? *Br Med J*. 1983;287:1961.

Walker HW. Foodborne illness from *Clostridium perfringens*. *CRC Crit Rev Food Sci Nutr*. 1975;7:71.

Wantke F, Gotz M, Jarisch R. The red wine provocation test: Intolerance to histamine as a model for food intolerance. *Allergy Proc*. 1994;15(1):27.

WHO. *Application of the Principles of Substantial Equivalence to the Safety Evaluation of Foods or Food Components from Plants Derived by Modern Biotechnology*. Report WHO/FNU/FOS/95.1. Geneva: World Health Organization (WHO); 1995.

WHO. Fluoride. *Trace Elements in Human Nutrition and Health*. Geneva: World Health Organization (WHO); 1996:187:chap 15.

Williams GM, Weisburger JH. Chemical carcinogenesis. In: Amdur MO, Doull J, Klaassen CD, eds. *Toxicology: The Basic Science of Poisons*. New York: Raven Press; 1991:127.

Williams LD, Burdock GA, Jiménez G, et al. Literature review on the safety of Toyocerin® a non-toxigenic and non-pathogenic *Bacillus cereus* var. *toyoi* preparation. *Regul Toxicol Pharmacol*. 2009;55:236–246.

Willshaw GA, Cheasty T, Smith HR. *Escherichia coli*. In: Lund BM, Baird-Parker TC, Gould GW, eds. *The Microbiological Safety and Quality of Food*. Gaithersburg, MD: Aspen; 2000:1136.

Wogan GN. Aflatoxin carcinogenesis. In: Busch H, ed. *Methods in Cancer Research*. New York: Academic Press; 1973:309.

Yamagata N, Shigematsu I. Cadmium pollution in perspective. *Inst Public Health Tokyo Bull*. 1970;19:1.

Zobel AM, Brown SA. Dermatitis-inducing psoralens on the surfaces of seven medicinal plant species. *J Toxic, Cutan, and Ocular Toxic*. 1991;10:223–231.

Analytical and Forensic Toxicology

Bruce A. Goldberger and Diana G. Wilkins*

"What is there that is not poison? All things are poison and nothing without poison.
Solely the dose determines that a thing is not a poison."

                                —Paracelsus

It is impossible to consider the topic of forensic toxicology without discussing analytical toxicology in detail, as analytical toxicology has its roots in forensic applications. Therefore, it is logical to discuss these mutually dependent areas together. Analytical toxicology involves the application of the tools of analytical chemistry to the qualitative and/or quantitative estimation of chemicals that may exert effects on living organisms. Generally, the chemical that is to be measured (the analyte) is a xenobiotic that may have been altered or transformed by metabolic actions of the organism. Frequently, the specimen that is to be analyzed consists of a matrix composed of body fluids or solid tissues removed from the organism. Both the identity of the analyte and the complexity of the matrix can present formidable problems to an analytical toxicologist.

Forensic toxicology involves the use of toxicology for the purposes of the law (Cravey and Baselt, 1981). Although this broad definition includes a wide range of applications, such as regulatory toxicology and urine testing to detect drug use, by far the most common application is to identify any chemical that may serve as a causative agent in inflicting death or injury on humans, or in causing damage to property. Frequently, as a result of such unfortunate incidents, charges of liability or criminal intent are brought that must be resolved by the judicial system. At times, indirect or circumstantial evidence is presented in an attempt to prove cause and effect. However, there is no substitute for the unequivocal identification of a specific chemical substance that is demonstrated to be present in tissues from the victim at a sufficient concentration to explain the injury with a reasonable degree of scientific probability

or certainty. For this reason, forensic toxicology and analytical toxicology have long shared a mutually supportive partnership.

To aid in deciding whether adverse effects of xenobiotics contribute to death, injury, or other harm to persons or property, great efforts are made to initiate and implement analytical procedures in a forensically credible manner. Laws prescribing punishment to drug-impaired drivers are evidence of attempts to mitigate impaired driving. The measurement of ethanol in blood or breath at specific concentrations is generally required to prove impairment by this agent (Fisher *et al.*, 1968). Similarly, the decade of the 1980s saw a growing response by society to the threat of drug abuse. Identification of drug users through testing urine for the presence of drugs or their metabolites, using methods and safeguards developed by forensic toxicologists, have become required by law (Department of Health and Human Services, 1988).

The diagnosis and treatment of health problems induced by chemical substances and the closely allied field of therapeutic drug monitoring also rely greatly on analytical toxicology. Although the analytes are present in biological matrices similar to those obtained for traditional forensic toxicology, the results must be reported rapidly to be of use to clinicians in treating patients. This requirement of a rapid turnaround time often limits the number of chemicals that can be measured because analytical methods, equipment, and personnel must all be available for a swift response to toxicological emergencies. More recently, analytical toxicology methods have also been employed for the detection of drugs and other chemicals used for the purpose of performance-enhancement, which can also require rapid reporting in selected settings, including athletic events.

Occupational toxicology and regulatory toxicology also require analytical procedures for their implementation or monitoring. In occupational toxicology, the analytical methods used to monitor threshold limit values and other criteria for estimating the exposure of workers to toxic hazards may utilize simple, nonspecific, but economical screening devices. However, to determine the actual exposure of a worker, it is necessary to analyze blood, urine, breath, or another specimen by employing methods similar to those

*Drs Goldberger and Wilkins acknowledge the contribution of Alphonse Poklis, PhD, to this chapter in previous editions significant of Casarett & Doull's Toxicology.

used in clinical or forensic toxicology. For regulatory purposes, a variety of matrices (eg, food, water, air) must be examined for extremely small quantities of analytes. Frequently, this requires the use of sophisticated methodology with extreme sensitivity. Both of these applications of analytical toxicology impinge on forensic toxicology because an injury or occupational disease in a worker can result in a legal proceeding, as well as can occur with a violation of a regulatory law.

Other applications of analytical toxicology occur frequently during the course of experimental studies. Confirmation of the concentration of dosing solutions and monitoring of their stability often can be accomplished with the use of simple analytical techniques. The bioavailability of a dose may vary with the route of administration and the vehicle used. Blood concentrations can be monitored as a means of establishing this important parameter. In addition, an important feature in the study of any toxic substance is the characterization of its metabolites as well as the distribution of the parent drug, together with its metabolites, to various tissues. This requires sensitive, specific, and valid analytical procedures. Similar analytical studies can be conducted within a temporal framework to gain an understanding of the dynamics of the absorption, distribution, metabolism, and excretion of toxic chemicals.

It is evident that analytical toxicology is intimately involved in many aspects of experimental and applied toxicology. Because toxic substances include all chemical types and the measurement of toxic chemicals may require the examination of biological or nonbiological matrices, the scope of analytical toxicology is broad. Nevertheless, a systematic approach and a reliance on the practical experience of generations of forensic toxicologists can be used in conjunction with the sophisticated tools of analytical chemistry to provide the data needed to better understand the hazards of toxic substances.

ANALYTICAL TOXICOLOGY

In light of the statement by Paracelsus five centuries ago, "All substances are poisons: there is none which is not a poison," analytical toxicology potentially encompasses all chemical substances. Forensic toxicologists learned long ago that when the nature of a suspected poison is unknown, a systematic, standardized approach must be used to identify the presence of most common toxic substances. An approach that has stood the test of time was first suggested by Chapuis in 1873 in *Elements de Toxicologie*. It is based on the origin or nature of the toxic agent (Petersen *et al.*, 1923). Such a system can be characterized as follows:

1. Gases
2. Volatile substances
3. Corrosive agents
4. Metals
5. Anions and nonmetals
6. Nonvolatile organic substances
7. Miscellaneous

Closely related to this descriptive classification is the method for separating a toxic agent from the matrix in which it is embedded. The matrix is generally a biological specimen such as a body fluid or tissue. The agent of interest may exist in the matrix in a simple solution or may be bound to protein and other cellular constituents. The challenge is to separate the toxic agent in sufficient purity and quantity to permit it to be characterized and quantified. At times, the parent compound is no longer present in large enough amounts to be separated. In this case, known metabolites may indirectly provide a measure of the parent substance (Hawks and Chiang, 1986). With other substances, interaction of the poison with tissue components

may require the isolation or characterization of a protein adduct (SanGeorge and Hoberman, 1986; Stockham and Blanke, 1988). Methods for separation have long provided a great challenge to analytical toxicologists. Over the previous 20 years, improved methods have become available that permit direct measurement of some analytes without prior separation from the matrix.

Gases are most simply measured by means of gas chromatography. Some gases are extremely labile, and the specimen must be collected and preserved at temperatures as low as that of liquid nitrogen. Generally, the gas is carefully liberated by incubating the specimen at a predetermined temperature in a sealed container. The gas, freed from the matrix, collects in the empty "headspace" between the specimen and the sealed container, where it can be sampled and injected into the gas chromatograph. Other gases, such as carbon monoxide, interact with proteins. These gases can be carefully released from the protein, or the adduct can be measured independently, as in the case of carboxyhemoglobin.

Volatile substances are generally liquids of a variety of chemical types. The temperature at which they boil is sufficiently low such that older methods of separation employed microdistillation or diffusion techniques. Gas chromatography is the simplest approach for simultaneous separation and quantitation of volatile substances. The simple alcohols (eg, ethanol) can be measured by injecting a diluted body fluid directly onto the analytical column of the gas chromatograph. A more common approach is to use the headspace technique, as is done for gases, after incubating the specimen in a sealed vial at an elevated temperature.

Corrosives include mineral acids and bases. Many corrosives consist of ions that are normal tissue constituents. Clinical chemical techniques can be applied to detect these ions when they are in great excess over normal concentrations. Because these ions are endogenous constituents, the corrosive effects at the site of contact of the chemical, together with other changes in blood chemistry values, can confirm the ingestion of a corrosive substance.

Metals are encountered frequently as occupational and environmental hazards. Elegant analytical methods are available for most metals even when they are present at extremely low concentrations. Classic separation procedures involve destruction of the organic matrix by chemical or thermal oxidation. This leaves the metal to be identified and quantified in the inorganic residue. Unfortunately, this prevents the determination of the metal in the oxidation state or in combination with other elements, as it existed when the metal compound was absorbed. For example, the toxic effects of metallic mercury, mercurous ion, mercuric ion, and dimethylmercury are all different. Selected analytical methods must be capable of determining the speciation and relative amount of each form present to interpret the degree of toxicity. The analytical difficulty in doing so has resulted in the unfortunate practice of describing the toxicity of metals as if each metal existed as a single entity.

Toxic anions and nonmetals present an analytical challenge. With the exception of phosphorus, these agents are rarely encountered in an uncombined form. Some anions can be trapped in combination with a stable cation, after which the organic matrix can be destroyed, as with metals. Others can be separated from the bulk of the matrix by dialysis, after which they are detected by colorimetric or chromatographic techniques. Still others are detected and measured by ion-specific electrodes.

The *nonvolatile organic substances* constitute the largest group of substances that must be considered by analytical toxicologists. This group includes drugs, both prescribed and illicit, pesticides, natural products, pollutants, and industrial compounds. These substances are solids or liquids with high boiling points. Thus, separation procedures generally rely on differential extractions of biological fluids and tissues (Fig. 32-1). These extractions often are

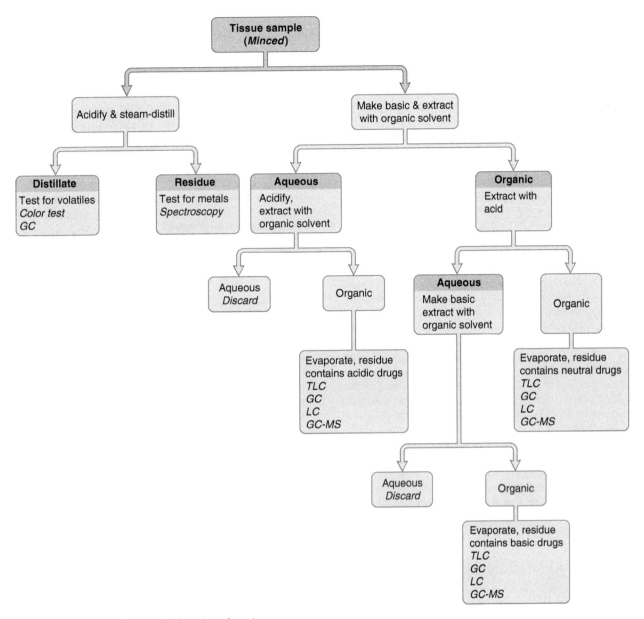

Figure 32-1. *A scheme of separation for poisons from tissues.*

inefficient, and recovery of the analyte from the matrix may be poor. When the nature of the analyte is known, immunoassay procedures, if available are useful because they allow a toxicologist to avoid using separation procedures. These compounds can be classified as follows:

1. Organic strong acids
2. Organic weak acids
3. Organic bases
4. Organic neutral compounds
5. Organic amphoteric compounds

Separation of the classes specified above is generally achieved by adjusting the acidity of the aqueous matrix and extracting with a water-immiscible solvent or a solid-phase sorbent material. Finally, a *miscellaneous* category must also be included to cover the large number of compounds that cannot be detected by the routine application of the methods described above. Venoms and other toxic mixtures of proteins, or uncharacterized constituents fall into this class. Frequently, if antibodies can be produced against the active

constituent, an immunoassay may be the most practical means of detecting and measuring these highly potent and difficult-to-isolate substances. Unfortunately, unless highly specific monoclonal antibodies are used, the analytical procedure may not be acceptable for forensic purposes. Most frequently, specific analytical procedures must be developed for each analyte of this type. At times, biological endpoints are utilized to semiquantify the concentration of the isolated product.

ROLE IN GENERAL TOXICOLOGY

In almost all experimental studies in toxicology, an agent, generally a single chemical substance is administered in known amounts to an organism. It is universally acknowledged that the chemical under study must be either pure, or the nature of any contaminant well-characterized, to enable interpretation of the experimental results with validity. However, it is a common practice to proceed with the experimental study without verifying the identity and purity of the compound. Not only does this practice lead to errors in establishing an accurate dose, but, depending on the nature of the study, other erroneous conclusions may be drawn. For example, the presence of related compounds in the dosage form of a tricyclic antidepressant led to erroneous conclusions about the metabolic products of the drug when it was administered together with the unidentified contaminants (Saady *et al.*, 1981). An even greater error may result when a small amount of a contaminant may be supertoxic. A well-publicized example of this error involved the presence of dioxin in mixtures of the defoliants 2,4-D and 2,4,5-T (Panel on Herbicides, 1971) used during the Vietnam War as Agent Orange. Some of the adverse effects of Agent Orange may have been due to the low concentration of dioxin in those mixtures. Other researchers have reported that the toxicity of mixtures of polybrominated biphenyls may be due to the high toxicity of specific components, whereas other brominated biphenyls are relatively nontoxic (Mills *et al.*, 1985).

A related application of analytical toxicology is the monitoring of dosage forms or solutions for stability throughout the course of an experimental study. Chemicals may degrade when in contact with air, by exposure to ultraviolet or other radiation, by interaction with constituents of the vehicle or dosing solution, and by other means. Developing an analytical procedure by which these changes can be recognized and corrected is essential in achieving consistent and reliable results over the course of a study (Blanke, 1987; Peters *et al.*, 2007).

Finally, analytical methods are necessary to determine the bioavailability of a compound that is under study. Some substances with low water solubility are difficult to introduce into an animal, and a variety of vehicles may be investigated. However, a comparison of the blood concentrations for the compound under study provides a simple means of comparing the effectiveness of vehicles. Introducing a compound into the stomach in an oil vehicle may not be the most effective means of enhancing the absorption of that compound (Granger *et al.*, 1987). Rather than observing dose–effect relationships, it may be more accurate to describe blood (serum) concentration–effect relationships.

ROLE IN FORENSIC TOXICOLOGY

The duties of a forensic toxicologist in postmortem investigations include the qualitative and quantitative analysis of drugs or poisons in biological specimens collected at autopsy and the interpretation of the analytical findings with respect to the physiological and behavioral effects of the detected chemicals on the deceased at the time of injury and/or death.

The complete investigation of the cause or causes of sudden death is an important civic and legal responsibility. The responsibility of establishing the cause of death rests with the medical examiner or coroner, but success in arriving at the correct conclusion often depends on the combined efforts of the pathologist and the toxicologist. The cause of death in cases of poisoning cannot be proved beyond contention without toxicological analysis that confirms the presence of the toxicant in either body fluids or tissues of the deceased.

Many drugs or poisons do not produce characteristic pathological lesions; their presence in the body can be demonstrated only by chemical methods of isolation and identification. If toxicological analyses are limited, deaths resulting from poisoning may be erroneously ascribed to an entirely different cause or poisoning may be designated as the cause of death without empirical proof. Thus, limiting analysis may have significant legal and social consequences.

Additionally, a toxicologist can furnish valuable evidence concerning the circumstances surrounding a death. Such cases commonly involve demonstrating the presence of intoxicating concentrations of ethanol in victims of automotive or industrial accidents, or measurements of concentrations of carbon monoxide in fire victims. Arson is commonly used to conceal homicide. The degree of carbon monoxide saturation of the blood may indicate whether the deceased died as a result of the fire or was dead before the fire started. Also, licit or illicit psychoactive drugs often play a significant role in the circumstances associated with sudden or violent death. The behavioral toxicity of many illicit drugs may explain the bizarre or "risk-taking" behavior of the deceased that led to his or her demise. At times, a negative toxicological finding is of particular importance in assessing the cause of death. For example, toxicology studies may demonstrate that a person with a seizure disorder was not taking the prescribed medication and that this noncompliance contributed to the fatal event.

Additionally, the results of postmortem toxicological testing provide valuable epidemiological and statistical data. Forensic toxicologists are often among the first to alert the medical community to new epidemics of substance abuse (Poklis, 1982) and the dangers of abusing over-the-counter drugs (Garriott *et al.*, 1985). Similarly, they often determine the chemical identity and toxicity of novel analogs of psychoactive agents that are subject to abuse, including "designer drugs" such as "china white" (methylfentanyl) (Henderson, 1988), "ecstasy" (methylenedioxy-methamphetamine) (Dowling *et al.*, 1987), and GHB (gamma-hydroxybutyric acid) (Andresen *et al.*, 2011). More recently, several newer groups of designer drugs, including the synthetic cathinones and derivatives such as 4-methylmethcathinone (mephedrone) and methylone (Cawrse *et al.*, 2012; Prosser and Nelson, 2012), 3,4-methylenedioxypyrovalerone and 5,6-methylenedioxy-2-aminoindane (MDAI) (Gallagher *et al.*, 2012; Coppola and Mondola, 2012; Ross *et al.*, 2012), and products containing synthetic cannabinoids, such as "K2" and "Spice" (Seely *et al.*, 2012), among others, have emerged as new trends, particularly among young age groups (Rosenbaum *et al.*, 2012).

Today, there are numerous specialized areas of study in the field of toxicology; however, it is the forensic toxicologist who is obliged to assist in the determination of the cause of death for a court of law and who has been historically recognized by the title "toxicologist."

Until the 19th century, physicians, lawyers, and law enforcement officials harbored extremely faulty notions about the signs and symptoms of poisoning (Thorwald, 1965). Unless a poisoner was literally caught in the act of the crime, there was no way to establish whether the victim died from poisoning. In the early 18th century, a Dutch physician, Hermann Boerhoave, theorized that various poisons in a hot, vaporous condition yield characteristic odors. He placed substances suspected of containing poisons on hot coals and evaluated their smells. Although Boerhoave was not successful in applying his method, he was the first to suggest a chemical method for proving the presence of poison.

White arsenic (arsenic trioxide) has been widely used with murderous intent for over a thousand years. Therefore, it is not surprising that the first milestones in the chemical isolation and identification of a poison in body tissues and fluids were described for arsenic. In 1775, Karl Wilhelm Scheele, a Swedish chemist, discovered that white arsenic is converted to arsenous acid by chlorine water. The addition of metallic zinc reduced the arsenous acid to poisonous arsine gas. If gently heated, the evolving gas would deposit metallic arsenic on the surface of a cold vessel. In 1821, Serullas utilized the decomposition of arsine for the detection of small quantities of arsenic in stomach contents and urine in poisoning cases. In 1836, James M. Marsh, a chemist at the Royal British Arsenal in Woolwich, applied Serullas' observations in developing the first reliable method to determine the presence of an absorbed poison in body tissues and fluids such as liver, kidney, and blood. After acid digestion of the tissues, Marsh generated arsine gas, which was drawn through a heated capillary tube. The arsine decomposed, leaving a dark deposit of metallic arsenic. Quantitative measures were performed by comparing the length of the deposit from known concentrations of arsenic with those of the test specimens.

The 1800s witnessed the development of forensic toxicology as a scientific discipline. In 1814, Mathieiv J. B. Orfila (1787–1853), widely considered the "father of toxicology," published *Traité des Poisons*, the first systematic approach to the study of the chemical and physiological nature of poisons (Gettler, 1977). Orfila's role as an expert witness in many famous murder trials, particularly his application of the Marsh test for arsenic in the trial of the poisoner Marie Lafarge, aroused both popular and scholarly interest in the new science. As dean of the medical faculty at the University of Paris, Orfila trained numerous students in forensic toxicology.

The first successful isolation of an alkaloidal poison was performed in 1850 by Jean Servias Stas, a Belgian chemist, using a solution of acetic acid in warm ethanol to extract nicotine from the tissues of the murdered Gustave Fougnie. As modified by the German chemist Fredrick Otto, the Stas–Otto method was quickly applied to the isolation of numerous alkaloidal poisons, including colchicine, coniine, morphine, narcotine, and strychnine. In the latter half of the 19th century, European toxicologists were in the forefront of the development and application of forensic sciences, providing valuable evidence of poisoning. A number of these trials became "causes célèbres" and the testimony of forensic toxicologists captured the imagination of the public and increased awareness of the development and application of toxicology. It was thought that murderers could no longer poison with impunity.

In the United States, Rudolph A. Witthaus, professor of chemistry at Cornell University Medical School, made many contributions to toxicology and called attention to the new science by performing analyses for the city of New York in several famous morphine poisoning cases, including the murder of Helen Potts by Carlyle Harris and that of Annie Sutherland by Dr Robert W. Buchanan. In 1911, Witthaus and Tracy C. Becker edited a four-volume work on medical jurisprudence, forensic medicine, and toxicology—the first standard forensic textbook published in the United States. In 1918, the city of New York established a medical examiner's system, and the appointment of Dr Alexander O. Gettler as toxicologist marked the beginning of modern forensic toxicology in this country. Although Dr Gettler made numerous contributions to the science, perhaps his greatest was the training and direction he gave to future leaders in forensic toxicology. Many of his associates went on to direct laboratories in medical examiner and coroner systems in major urban centers throughout the country.

In 1949, the American Academy of Forensic Sciences (AAFS) was established to support and further the practice of legal (forensic) medicine in the United States. The members of the Toxicology Section represented the vast majority of forensic toxicologists working in medical examiners' and coroner offices', as well as numerous referral laboratories. Several other international, national, and local forensic science organizations, such as the Society of Forensic Toxicologists and the California Association of Toxicologists, offer a forum for the exchange of scientific data pertaining to analytical techniques and case reports involving new or infrequently used drugs and poisons. The International Association of Forensic Toxicologists (TIAFT) founded in 1963 with over 1400 members from all regions of the world facilitates worldwide collaboration in resolving the technical problems confronting toxicology.

In 1975, the American Board of Forensic Toxicology (ABFT) was formed to examine and certify forensic toxicologists. One of the stated objectives of the board is "to make available to the judicial system, and other publics, a practical and equitable system for readily identifying those persons professing to be specialists in forensic toxicology who possess the requisite qualifications and competence." Those certified as Diplomates of the Board must have a doctor of philosophy or doctor of science degree, have at least three years of full-time professional experience, and pass a written examination. In 2000, the Board began certifying "forensic toxicology specialists." Specialists must have a master's or bachelor's degree and three years of full-time professional experience and must pass a written examination. In 2012, there are approximately 140 Diplomates and 95 Specialists certified by the Board. In 1998, the Board began an accreditation program for forensic toxicology laboratories. ABFT accredited laboratories must conform to standards of having qualified, experienced personnel and forensically sound procedures for the handling of evidence, analysis of specimens, and reporting of results. Laboratories must pass bi-annual on-site inspections, which include a review of laboratory procedures and casework.

TOXICOLOGICAL INVESTIGATION OF A POISON DEATH

The toxicological investigation of a poison death may be divided into three steps: (1) obtaining the case history and suitable specimens, (2) the toxicological analyses, and (3) the interpretation of the analytical findings.

Case History and Specimens

Today, thousands of compounds are readily available that are lethal if ingested, injected, or inhaled. Usually, a limited amount of specimen is available on which to perform analyses; therefore it is imperative that, before the analyses are initiated, as much information as possible concerning the facts of the case be collected. The age, sex, weight, medical history, and occupation of the decedent as well as any treatment administered before death, the gross autopsy findings, the drugs available to the decedent, and the interval between the onset of symptoms and death should be noted. In a typical year, a postmortem toxicology laboratory will perform analyses for such diverse poisons as over-the-counter medications (eg, analgesics, antihistamines), prescription drugs (eg, benzodiazepines, opioids), drugs of abuse (eg, cocaine, marijuana, methamphetamine), and gases (eg, inhalants, carbon monoxide). Obviously, a thorough investigation of the death scene including a tentative identification of the administered poison is helpful prior to beginning the analysis (Ernst *et al.*, 1982).

The pathologist at autopsy usually performs the collection of postmortem specimens for analysis. Specimens of many different body fluids and organs are necessary, as drugs and poisons display varying affinities for body tissues (Fig. 32-2). Therefore, detection of a poison is more likely in a tissue in which it accumulates. A large quantity of each specimen is needed for thorough toxicological analysis because a procedure that extracts and identifies one compound or class of compounds may be ineffective in extracting and identifying others (Table 32-1). Autolytic and putrefactive changes, however, may reduce specimen quality and therefore alter the selection and utility of individual specimens on a case-by-case basis. Further improvements in our knowledge regarding degradation mechanisms, as well as specimen-handling protocols to increase storage stability, may enable the forensic toxicologist to

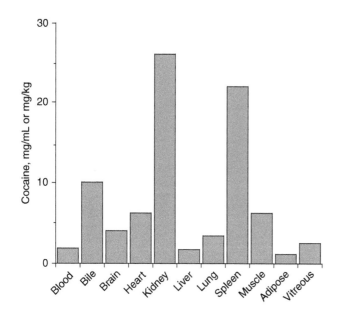

Figure 32-2. *Cocaine tissue distribution in a fatal poisoning.* (Data drawn from Poklis A, Mackell MA, Graham M. Disposition of cocaine in a fatal poisoning in man. *J Anal Toxicol.* 1985;9:227–229.)

circumvent possible analytical and interpretive difficulties (Dinis-Oliveira *et al.*, 2010).

When collecting the specimens, the pathologist labels each container with the date and time of autopsy, the name of the decedent, the identity of the sample, an appropriate case identification number, and his or her signature or initials. It is paramount that the handling of all specimens be authenticated and documented. A form developed at the collection site that identifies each specimen is submitted to the laboratory with the specimens. The form is signed and dated by the pathologist, and subsequently by any individual handling, transferring, or transporting the specimens. In legal terms, this form constitutes a "chain-of-custody" of specimens documenting all transfers. The chain-of-custody enables a toxicologist to introduce his or her results into legal proceedings, having established that the specimens analyzed were obtained from the decedent.

Fluids and tissues should be collected before embalming, as this process will dilute or chemically alter the poisons present,

Table 32-1

Suggested List of Specimens and Amounts to be Obtained at Autopsy

SPECIMEN	QUANTITY
Brain	50 g
Liver	50 g
Kidney	50 g
Heart blood	25 mL
Peripheral blood	10 mL
Vitreous humor	All available
Bile	All available
Urine	All available
Gastric contents	All available

SOURCE: Data from SOFT/AAFS Forensic Toxicology Laboratory Guidelines (2006).

rendering their detection difficult or impossible. Conversely, methyl or ethyl alcohol may be a constituent of embalming fluid, thereby affecting interpretation of the analytical findings.

Although forensic toxicology laboratories typically receive blood, urine, liver tissue, and/or stomach contents for identification of xenobiotics, they have been increasingly called upon to meet the analytical challenges of many alternative types of samples (Skopp, 2004; Flanagan *et al.*, 2005; Kronstrand and Druid, 2006; Gallardo and Queiroz, 2008). Nontraditional matrices, such as bone marrow, hair, and nails, among others, may be submitted to the laboratory. For example, on occasion, toxicological analysis is requested for cases of burned, exhumed, putrefied, and skeletal remains. In such instances, it is necessary to analyze unusual specimens such as bone marrow, hair, nails, skeletal muscle, vitreous humor, and even insects (Inoue, 1992). Numerous drugs have been successfully identified in bone marrow and bone washings from skeletal remains even after decomposition and burial (Benko, 1985; Drummer, 2010; Cartiser *et al.*, 2011). Similarly, the vitreous humor of the eye is isolated and sequestered from putrefaction, charring, and trauma; thus, it is a useful specimen for the detection of most drugs, anions, and even volatile poisons such as alcohols, ketones, and glycols (Coe, 1993; Bévalot *et al.*, 2011). Hair analysis is a rapidly growing technique in forensic toxicology and has been used to measure individual exposure to heavy metals, such as arsenic, mercury, and lead, as well as many drugs of abuse and other pharmaceuticals, pesticides, and plastics (Yamaguichi *et al.*, 1975; McKenzie, 1978; Baumgartner *et al.*, 1981; Hambidge, 1973; Puschel *et al.*, 1983; Suzuki, 1984; Marigo *et al.*, 1986; Schroeder and Nason, 1989; Strang *et al.*, 1990; Martz, 1988; Harkey and Henderson, 1989; Shen *et al.*, 2002; Boumba *et al.*, 2006). Analysis of hair for selected drugs has been utilized as an adjunct specimen in forensic settings for postmortem examinations for many years (Baumgartner *et al.*, 1979; Couper *et al.*, 1995; Gaillard and Pepin, 1997; Pragst *et al.*, 1997; Rollins *et al.*, 1997; Yegles *et al.*, 1997; Villain *et al.*, 2005; Muller *et al.*, 2000; Pragst and Balikova, 2006; Kintz, 2010; Barroso *et al.*, 2011). Nails, another keratinized matrix, have also been used to determine exposure to selected xenobiotics in both antemortem and postmortem cases (Palmeri *et al.*, 2000; Garside, 2010). Limited data are available to support a direct correlation between quantitative hair and nail values and drug doses in forensic cases; however, qualitative results have been accepted as indicators of previous drug or xenobiotic exposure.

Finally, in severely decomposed bodies, the absence of blood and/or the scarcity of solid tissues suitable for analysis have led to the collection and testing of maggots (fly larvae) feeding on the body (Pounder, 1991). The fundamental premise underlying maggot analysis is that if drugs or intoxicants are detected, they could only have originated from the decedent's tissues on which the larvae were feeding. Surprisingly, analysis of maggots is rather straightforward, requiring no special methodology beyond that routinely applied in toxicology laboratories. Case reports have documented the detection of numerous drugs and intoxicants in maggots collected from decomposed bodies. The compounds detected include barbiturates, benzodiazepines, phenothiazines, morphine, and malathion. Controlled studies in which maggots were allowed to feed on tissues to which drugs had been added have demonstrated the accumulation of propoxyphene, amitriptyline and nordiazepam, among others, in the larvae (Goff *et al.*, 1993; Gagliano-Candela and Aventaggiato, 2001; Pien *et al.*, 2004).

Toxicological Analysis

Before the analysis begins, several factors must be considered, including the amount of specimen available, the nature of the poison sought, and the possible biotransformation of the poison.

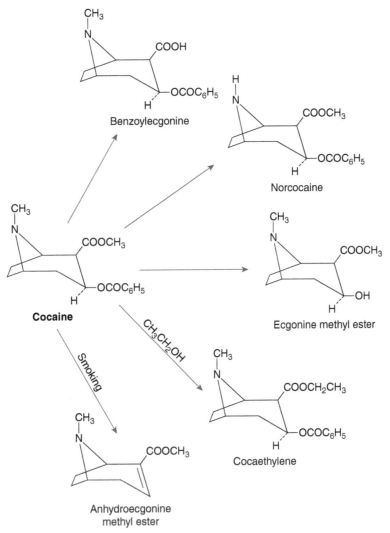

Figure 32-3. *Biotransformation and pyrolysis products of cocaine.*

In cases involving oral administration of the poison, the gastrointestinal (GI) contents are analyzed first because large amounts of residual unabsorbed poison may be present. The urine may be analyzed next, as the kidney is the major organ of excretion for most poisons and high concentrations of toxicants and/or their metabolites often are present in urine. After absorption from the GI tract, drugs or poisons are carried to the liver before entering the general systemic circulation; therefore, the first analysis of an internal organ is conducted on the liver. If a specific poison is suspected to have caused or contributed to a death, the toxicologist may first analyze the tissues and fluids in which the poison concentrates.

A thorough knowledge of drug biotransformation is often essential before an analysis is performed. The parent compound and any major pharmacologically-active metabolites should be isolated and identified. In some instances, the metabolites provide the only evidence that a drug or poison has been administered. Many screening tests, such as immunoassays, are specifically designed to detect not the parent drug but its major urinary metabolite. An example of the relationship of pharmacokinetic and analytical factors is provided by cocaine. The major metabolites of cocaine biotransformation are benzoylecgonine and ecgonine methyl ester (Fig. 32-3). The co-ingestion of alcohol with cocaine results in the hepatic transesterification of cocaine to form cocaethylene (Hime *et al.*, 1991), a psychoactive metabolite. The disposition of these compounds in various body fluids and hair is shown in Fig. 32-4. Thus, the initial testing of urine to determine cocaine use is performed with immunoassays specifically designed to detect the presence of benzoylecgonine, the major urinary metabolite. In contrast, if saliva or hair is tested, parent cocaine, as well as metabolites,

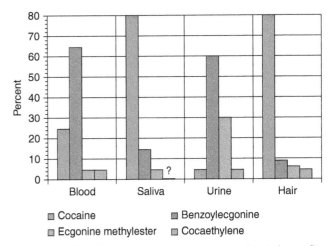

Figure 32-4. *Disposition of cocaine and cocaine metabolites in human fluids and hair.* (Data redrawn from Spiehler V. Society of Forensic Toxicology Conference on Drug Testing in Hair. Tampa, FL: October 29, 1994.)

are also sought. To determine a profile of each analyte present in a specimen, chromatographic procedures such as gas chromatography-mass spectrometry (GC-MS) are used, which facilitates the simultaneous separation and quantification of each compound.

The analysis may be complicated by the normal chemical changes that occur during the decomposition of a cadaver. The autopsy and toxicological analysis should be started as soon after death as possible. The natural enzymatic and nonenzymatic processes of decomposition and microbial metabolism may destroy a poison that was present at death or produce substances or compounds with chemical and physical properties similar to those of commonly encountered poisons. As early as the 1870s, the so-called cadaveric alkaloids isolated from the organs of putrefied bodies were known to produce color test reactions similar to those produced by morphine and other drugs. These cadaveric alkaloids resulted from the bacterial decarboxylation of the amino acids ornithine and lysine, producing putrescine and cadaverine, respectively (Evans, 1963). Similarly, during decomposition, phenylalanine is converted to phenylethylamine, which has chemical and physical properties very similar to those of amphetamine. The hydrolysis, oxidation, or reduction of proteins, nucleic acids, and lipids may generate numerous compounds, such as hydroxylated aliphatic and aromatic carboxylic acids, pyridine and piperidine derivatives, and aromatic heterocyclics such as tryptamine and norharmane (Kaempe, 1969). All these substances may interfere with the isolation, identification, and quantitation of the toxicants being sought. The concentration of cyanide and ethyl alcohol and the carbon monoxide saturation of the blood may be decreased or increased, depending on the degree of putrefaction and microbial activity. However, many poisons—such as arsenic, barbiturates, mercury, and strychnine—are extremely stable and may be detectable many years after death.

Before analysis, the purity of all chemicals used in laboratory procedures should be established. The purity of the primary reference material used to prepare calibrators and controls should be verified, and the salt form or degree of hydration should be determined (Blanke, 1989). All reagents and solvents should be of the highest grade possible and should be free of contaminants that may interfere with or distort analytical findings. For example, the chloroform contaminants phosgene and ethyl chloroformate may react with primary or secondary amine drugs to form carbamyl chloride and ethyl carbamate derivatives (Cone *et al.*, 1982). Specimen containers, lids, and stoppers should be free of contaminants such as plasticizers, which often interfere with chromatographic or GC-MS determinations. Care should be exercised to ensure a clean laboratory environment. This is of particular concern in the analysis of metals, as aluminum, arsenic, lead, and mercury are ubiquitous environmental and reagent contaminants.

Forensic toxicology laboratories analyze specimens by using a variety of analytical procedures. Initially, nonspecific tests designed to determine the presence or absence of a class or group of analytes may be performed directly on the specimens. Examples of tests used to rapidly screen urine are the FPN (ferric chloride, perchloric, and nitric acid) color test for phenothiazine drugs and immunoassays for the detection of amphetamines, benzodiazepines, and opiate derivatives, among others. Positive results obtained with these tests must be confirmed by a second analytical procedure that identifies the particular drug. The detection limit of the confirmatory test should be lower than that of the initial nonspecific test. Some analytical procedures identify specific compounds. Even in such instances, a second test should be performed to identify and confirm the presence of the analyte. The second test should be based on a chemical or physical principle different from that of the first test. Such additional testing is performed to establish an unequivocal identification of the drugs or poisons present. Whenever possible, the most specific test for the compound of interest should be performed. Today, GC-MS and liquid chromatography-mass spectrometry (LC-MS) are the most widely applied methodology in toxicology and are generally accepted as unequivocal identification for all drugs. Analyte identification is typically based on the retention time in the chromatographic system coupled with the characteristic ion fragmentation spectrum in the mass spectrometer. The analyte mass spectrum is the pattern of mass-to-charge ion fragments and their relative abundance.

Analytical methods must be of sufficient rigor to provide accurate and reliable qualitative and quantitative data. Numerous approaches for the use of quality control have been suggested, and professional organizations have developed recommendations for the implementation of quality control in forensic laboratories (Goldberger *et al.*, 1997; Ferrara *et al.*, 1998; Scientific Working Group for Forensic Toxicology). The limit of detection, the lowest concentration of analyte reliably identified by the assay, and the specificity of all qualitative methods should be well documented. The laboratory must demonstrate that the assay response of blank or negative calibrators (controls) does not overlap with the response of the lowest-positive calibrator. In certain instances, qualitative identification of a poison or drug is sufficient to resolve forensic toxicology issues. However, most cases require reliable estimates of poison concentrations for forensic interpretation. For quantitative analysis, the accuracy, precision, linearity, and specificity of the procedure must also be established. Linearity should be determined by using at least one drug-free and three drug-fortified calibrators whose concentrations bracket the anticipated concentrations in the biological specimen. Precision, which statistically demonstrates the variance in the value obtained, is determined by replicate analyses of a specimen of a known concentration. Additional assay parameters, such as analyte stability and recovery from the biological matrix, for example, can also be determined. For a variety of reasons, a quantitative result occasionally will deviate spuriously from the true value. Therefore, replicate quantitative determinations are highly recommended when sufficient specimen volume is available (Blanke, 1987).

When unusual samples such as bone marrow, fingernails, hair, and maggots are analyzed, the extraction efficiency of a procedure may vary greatly, depending on the complexity of the matrix. Therefore, all calibrators and controls should be prepared in the same matrix type as the specimens and analyzed concurrently with the specimens. Often the matrix is "unique" or impossible to match, such as decomposed or embalmed tissue. In these instances, the method of "standard additions" may be used. Known amounts of the analyte of interest are added to specimen aliquots and these are analyzed. The concentration of poison in the test specimen is determined by comparing the proportional response of the "poison fortified" specimens to that of the test specimens.

Interpretation of Analytical Results

Once the analysis of the specimens is complete, the toxicologist must interpret his or her findings with regard to the physiological or behavioral effects of the toxicants on the decedent at the concentrations found. Specific questions may be answered, such as the route of administration, the dose administered, and whether the concentration of the toxicant present was sufficient to cause death or alter the decedent's actions enough to cause his or her death. Assessing the physiological or behavioral meanings of analytical results is often the most challenging aspect confronted by the forensic toxicologist.

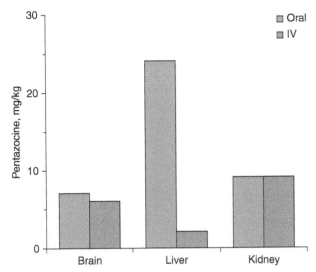

Figure 32-5. *Comparison of pentazocine distribution in fatal poisonings due to intravenous injection and oral administration.* (Data from Baselt RC. *Disposition of Toxic Drugs and Chemicals in Man.* 2nd ed. Davis, CA: Biomedical Publications; 1982:603–606, and Poklis A, MacKell MA. Toxicological findings in deaths due to pentazocine: a report of two cases. *Forensic Sci Int.* 1982;20:89–95.)

In determining the route of administration, the toxicologist notes the results of the analysis of the various specimens. As a general rule, the highest concentrations of a poison are found at the site of administration. Therefore, the presence of large amounts of drugs and/or poisons in the GI tract and liver indicates oral ingestion, while higher concentrations in the lungs than in other visceral organs can indicate inhalation or intravenous injection. The ratio or relative distribution of drugs in different tissues may also differentiate oral from parenteral administration (Fig. 32-5). Drugs may also be detected in the tissue surrounding an injection site following intramuscular or intravenous injection. Smoking is a popular route of administration for abusers of controlled substances (illicit) such as cocaine, heroin, marijuana, and phencyclidine. Pyrolysis of these drugs leads to the inhalation not only of the parent drug, but also of characteristic breakdown products of combustion. For example, a major pyrolysis product of "crack" cocaine smoking is anhydroecgonine methyl ester (Martin *et al.*, 1989) (Fig. 32-3). Thus, identification of relatively high concentrations of this compound along with cocaine or cocaine metabolites in urine or other body fluids or tissues may indicate smoking as the route of cocaine administration (Jacob *et al.*, 1990).

The presence of a toxic material in the GI tract, regardless of the quantity, does not provide sufficient evidence to establish that agent as the cause of death. It is necessary to demonstrate that absorption of the toxicant has occurred and that it has been transported by the general circulation to the target organ in order to exert its lethal effect. This is established by blood and tissue analysis. An exception to the rule is provided by strong, corrosive chemicals such as sulfuric acid, lye, and phenol, which exert their deleterious effects by directly digesting tissue, causing hemorrhage and shock. The results of urinalysis are often of little benefit in determining the physiological effects of a toxic agent. Urine results establish only that the poison was present in the body at some time before death. Correlation of urine values with physiological effects is poor because of various factors that influence the rate of excretion of specific compounds and the urine volume.

The physiological effects of most drugs and poisons are generally correlated with their concentrations in blood or blood fractions such as plasma and serum. Indeed, in living persons, this association is the basis of therapeutic drug monitoring. However, postmortem blood has been described as a fluid resembling blood that is obtained from the vasculature after death. Therefore, interpretation of postmortem blood results requires careful consideration of the case history, the site of collection, and postmortem changes. The survival time between the administration of a poison and death may be sufficiently long to permit biotransformation and excretion of the agent. Blood values may appear to be nontoxic or consistent with therapeutic administration. Death from hepatic failure after an acetaminophen overdose usually occurs at least three to four days after ingestion. Postmortem acetaminophen concentrations in blood may be consistent with the ingestion of therapeutic doses. Therefore, fatal acetaminophen overdose is determined by case history, central lobular necrosis of the liver, and, if available, analysis of serum specimens collected from the decedent when he or she was admitted to the emergency department (Price *et al.*, 1991). Furthermore, emergency medical treatment—such as the administration of fluids, plasma extenders, bicarbonate, diuretics, and blood transfusions—may dilute, remove, or enhance the elimination of toxic agents. Similarly, prolonged survival on a mechanical respirator, hemodialysis, or hemoperfusion may substantially reduce initially lethal blood concentrations of poisons.

For a long time, it was generally assumed that postmortem blood drug concentrations were more or less uniform throughout the body. However, in the 1970s, several investigators noted that postmortem concentrations of digoxin in heart blood greatly exceeded those in simultaneously collected femoral blood. They also observed that postmortem blood concentrations, particularly in heart blood, exceeded the expected values at the time of death (Vorpahl and Coe, 1978; Aderjan *et al.*, 1979). This postmortem increase in blood digoxin concentrations was apparently due to release of the drug from tissue stores, particularly the myocardium. Subsequently, other researchers demonstrated that for many drugs, blood concentrations in the same body vary greatly depending on the site from which the specimen is collected—subclavian vein, thoracic aorta, inferior vena cava, femoral vein, and so forth. For example, in a case of fatal multiple drug ingestion, analysis of postmortem blood collected from 10 different sites demonstrated imipramine concentrations that differed by as much as 760% (2.1–16.0 mg/L) (Jones and Pounder, 1987). In an extensive investigation, Prouty and Anderson (1990) demonstrated that postmortem blood drug concentrations were not only site-dependent but also increased greatly over the interval between death and specimen collection, particularly in heart blood. This increase over the postmortem interval was most pronounced for basic drugs with large apparent volumes of distribution, such as tricyclic antidepressants.

In an overt drug overdose, postmortem blood concentrations are elevated sufficiently to render an unmistakable interpretation of fatal intoxication. However, in many cases, the postmortem redistribution of drugs may significantly affect the interpretation of analytical findings. For drugs whose volume of distribution, plasma half-life, and renal clearance vary widely from person to person or that undergo postmortem redistribution, tissue concentrations readily distinguish therapeutic administration from drug overdose (Apple, 1989). Therefore, to provide a foundation of reasonable medical certainty in regard to the role of a drug in the death of an individual, it is recommended that, in addition to heart blood, a peripheral blood specimen and tissues be analyzed.

The analysis of tissue specimens is important for the estimation of a "minimal administered dose" or body burden of a drug or poison. In order to calculate a minimum body burden, it is necessary to analyze as many different body tissues and fluids as possible to determine the concentrations of the drug present. The concentration of drug in each separate specimen is then multiplied by the total weight or volume of that particular tissue or fluid. In this manner, the total amount of drug in each different tissue or fluid is determined. The amounts of drug in each separate tissue and fluid are then added together to give the total body burden or minimal administered dose. This simple approach has often proven extremely effective in resolving legal medical issues. For example, lidocaine is commonly administered in 50- to 100-mg bolus injections as an antiarrythmic agent for ventricular arrhythmia during resuscitation efforts. Because of poor circulation and tissue perfusion during arrhythmias, lidocaine is not well distributed in the body of the victim of a fatal heart attack. Postmortem bloods often exceed 50 mg/L in such cases, whereas values for effective antiarrhythmic prophylaxis do not exceed 5 mg/L. Therefore, a blood lidocaine value of 50 mg/L may be an artifact of resuscitation efforts or might represent a fatal overdose. Tissue distribution studies have resolved this issue in both accidental and homicidal poisoning with lidocaine (Poklis *et al.*, 1984).

Postmortem toxicology results are often used to corroborate investigative findings. Improved methods for determining drug exposure, with respect to longer time frames, are advantageous because drug concentrations in plasma, urine, and liver often reflect only the dosage taken within (at most) the last several days prior to sampling. Compared to traditional biological matrices, keratinized tissues such as hair and nails provide a longer window of detection for drugs and other compounds due to their slow growth and possible permanent retention of drugs. The presence of certain xenobiotics and their metabolites, have been demonstrated in human hair or nails at times when plasma and urine drug concentrations are not measurable (Rollins *et al.*, 1997; Garside, 2010), which can provide evidence of exposure to these agents weeks, months, or even years prior to death. It has been suggested that for some xenobiotics, hair also serves to characterize the drug exposure over time. For example, the analysis of sequential sections of hair provides a reliable correlation with the pattern of arsenic exposure (Smith, 1964). Significant increases in the arsenic content of the root and the first 5 mm of the hair occur within hours after the ingestion of arsenic. The germinal cells are in relatively close equilibrium with circulating arsenic; thus, as arsenic concentrations in blood rise or fall, so does arsenic deposition in growing hair. Normal arsenic content in hair varies with nutritional, environmental, and physiological factors; however, the maximum upper limit of normal deposition with a 99% confidence limit in persons not exposed to arsenic is 5 mg/kg (Shapiro, 1967). Hair grows at a rate of approximately 1.06 cm per month (LeBeau *et al*, 2011). Therefore, analysis of 1.0-cm segments provides a monthly pattern of exposure (Fig. 32-6). Such analyses can be performed in cases of homicidal poisoning to demonstrate that increases in arsenic deposition in the victim's hair correlate with times when a poisoner had an opportunity to administer the poison. Continuously elevated hair arsenic values indicate chronic rather than acute poisoning as the cause of death. A similar approach using segmental analysis of hair has been used to determine patterns of exposure for various drugs and their metabolites; however, care must be taken in order to account for the potential effects of haircuts, chemical treatments, and other environmental insults that may have occurred to the hair during the time frame of interest.

A new extension of forensic toxicology is the analysis of impurities of illicit drug synthesis in biological specimens. Many drugs of abuse, particularly methamphetamine are illicitly manufactured in clandestine laboratories. There are several popular methods of

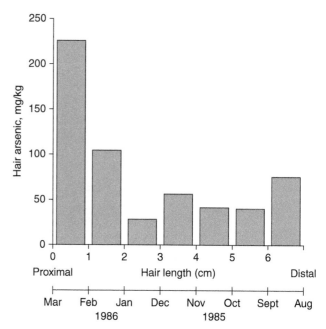

Figure 32-6. *Results of neutron activation analysis for arsenic in sequential sections of hair, demonstrating chronic arsenic poisoning.* Increased exposure in the first two sections is consistent with fatal events. Lower values in section three are consistent with two weeks of hospitalization. (Data from Poklis A, Saady JJ. Arsenic poisoning: acute or chronic? Suicide or murder? *Am J Forensic Med Pathol.* 1990;11:226–232.)

methamphetamine synthesis; when these are applied in clandestine laboratories, side reactions or incomplete conversion of the reactants yield an impure mixture of methamphetamine and synthetic impurities. These impurities can be characteristic of a particular synthetic method and their detection in biological specimens can indicate the use of an illicitly produced drug that is not a legal pharmaceutical product; suggest the synthetic method that was used to produce the drug; point to a possible common source of illicit production; and provide a link between manufacturers, dealers, and users. An example of impurity analysis was the detection of metabolites of α-benzyl-*N*-methylphenethylamine (BNMPA) in the urine of abusers of methamphetamine (Moore *et al.*, 1996b) and in a case of fatal drug overdose involving methamphetamine (Moore *et al.*, 1996a). BNMPA is an impurity arising from the synthesis of methamphetamine via the Leukart reaction using phenyl-2-propanone (P2P) synthesized from phenylacetic acid. Clandestine laboratories often must synthesize the P2P starting material, as its sale and distribution is regulated by the Federal Drug Enforcement Agency.

As discussed above, a wide range of tissues are available for the purpose of identifying xenobiotics in postmortem specimens. In contrast, for many years, traditional specimens used for the detection and quantification of substances in antemortem biological specimens have been limited to whole blood, plasma, serum, and urine, largely due to their ease of collection and accessibility in the living. More recently, the advent of improved analytical techniques with greater sensitivity and selectivity, including GC-MS/MS and LC-MS/MS, have expanded the array of biological specimens in which substances can be detected. These specimens include oral fluid (saliva), sweat, meconium, amniotic fluid, breast milk, and semen among others. In oral fluid, for example, the pharmacokinetics of many drugs and metabolites is closely aligned to that of blood pharmacokinetics, and thus can serve as an alternative matrix for illicit and therapeutic drug detection (Bosker and Huestis, 2009; Spiehler and Cooper, 2010), as well as detection of exposure to environmental toxicants and pesticides (Lanaro *et al.*, 2011; Yang *et al.*, 2011).

CRIMINAL POISONING OF THE LIVING

Over the past few decades, forensic toxicologists have become more involved in the analysis of specimens obtained from living victims of criminal poisonings. Generally, this increase in testing is a result of two types of cases: (1) administration of drugs to incapacitate victims of kidnapping, robbery, or sexual assault and (2) poisoning as a form of child abuse.

For centuries, those severely intoxicated from alcohol often became victims of kidnapping, robbery, or sexual assault. The kidnapping of drunks in seaports was a common way of obtaining sailors for long commercial voyages such as those involved in whaling. Late in the 19th century, the mixing of the powerful hypnotic chloral hydrate with alcohol produced the legendary "Mickey Finn." While alcohol is still often a primary factor in cases of alleged sexual assault, common drugs of abuse or other psychoactive drugs are often involved (Table 32-2). Of particular concern are the many potent inductive agents medically administered prior to general anesthesia. Many of these drugs, such as benzodiazepines and phenothiazines, are available today through illicit sources or legal purchase in foreign countries. When administered surreptitiously, they cause sedation and incapacitate the victim while also producing amnesia in the victim as to the events while drugged, without causing severe central nervous system depression. These cases often present a difficult analytical challenge to the toxicologist. Usually, the victim does not bring forth an allegation of assault until 24 hours to several days after the attack. Thus, the intoxicating drug may have been largely eliminated or extensively metabolized such that extremely low concentrations of drug or metabolites are present in the victim's blood, urine, and/or hair specimens. Sophisticated, highly sensitive analytical methods such as GC-MS or LC-MS may be required to accurately identify drugs in such specimens. To provide guidance in the choice of analytical approaches to such cases, recommendations for the toxicological investigation of sexual assaults have been formulated (LeBeau *et al.*, 1999; Society of Forensic Toxicologists).

Poisoning as a form of child abuse involves the deliberate administration of toxic or injurious substances to a child, usually by a parent or other caregiver. The victims of such poisonings range in age from a few months to the teens. Common agents used to intentionally poison children have included syrup of ipecac, table salt, laxatives, diuretics, antidepressants, sedative-hypnotics, and narcotics (Yin, 2010; American Association of Poison Control Centers, 2011; Oral *et al.*, 2011). The motivation for such heinous behavior is in the province of psychiatry, not toxicology. However, toxicologists must have some understanding of the nature of these poisonings to aid in the investigation of such cases. In some instances, it is a form of child battering committed by persons with low tolerance to the child's upsetting behaviors. The poison may be given to an infant to stop its crying or be force-fed to older children as a form of punishment. Such behavior is characteristic of persons with a cultural background where violence toward children is common or who have severe personality disorders or other mental illnesses. "Munchausen syndrome by proxy" is another form of child poisoning (Murray, 1997). The term *Munchausen syndrome* (MS) is used to describe patients who seek admission to hospitals with apparent illness along with plausible, dramatic, albeit fictitious medical histories. Such people seek medical treatment solely to assume the role of a patient and receive the attention derived from this deception. "MS by proxy" refers to the situation in which an individual, usually a parent, presents not himself or herself but a child with a fictitious illness often induced by physical or chemical means. The purpose of the poisoning is not to kill the child but to induce signs and symptoms of illness that will assure medical attention. Thereby, the parent as caregiver gains the craved attention. Given a fictitious case history and the obvious illness of the child, these cases are almost always and understandably misdiagnosed. Often, the child may be chronically poisoned at home and in the hospital for as long as a year before suspicion leads to the collection of specimens for extensive toxicological testing. Although the parent may not have intended such an outcome, some children have died from fatal poisoning in these situations. As in the case of sexual assault, sophisticated MS testing methods may be required to detect such agents as emetine and cephaeline, the emetic alkaloids in syrup of ipecac. Testing in these cases is best performed in a laboratory with forensic experience, as positive drug findings will usually result in some form of legal proceeding.

FORENSIC URINE DRUG TESTING

Concerns regarding the potentially adverse consequences of substance abuse for the individual, the workplace, and society have led to widespread urine analysis for controlled or illicit drugs (Gust and Walsh, 1989). Currently, such testing is conducted routinely by the military services, regulated transportation and nuclear industries, many federal and state agencies, public utilities, federal and state criminal justice systems, and numerous private businesses and industries. Significant ethical and legal ramifications are associated with such testing. Those having positive test results may not receive employment, be dismissed from a job, be court-martialed, or suffer a damaged reputation.

To assure the integrity of workplace urine testing, two certification programs currently accredit forensic urine-testing laboratories. Laboratories conducting testing of federal employees are required to be certified under the Department of Health and Human Services Mandatory Guidelines for Workplace Drug Testing as published in the April 11, 1988, *Federal Register* (Department of Health and Human Services, 1988). The College of American Pathologists (CAP) also conducts a certification program for urine drug testing laboratories. The federal program regulates the process from specimen collection through testing to the reporting of results,

Table 32-2

Distribution of Drugs of Abuse Encountered Urine Specimens in 1179 Cases of Alleged Sexual Assault*

RANK	DRUG/DRUG GROUP	INCIDENCE
1	No drugs found	468
2	Ethanol	451
3	Cannabinoids	218
4	Benzoylecgonine (cocaine metabolite)	97
5	Benzodiazepines	97
6	Amphetamines	51
7	Gamma-hydroxybutyrate (GHB)	48
8	Opiates	25
9	Propoxyphene	17
10	Barbiturates	12

*Thirty five percent of the drug-positive specimens were positive for more than one drug.
SOURCE: Data from ElSohly MA, Salamone SJ. Prevalence of drugs used in cases of alleged sexual assault. J Anal Toxicol. 1999;23(3):141–146.

Table 32-3

Forensic Urine Drug Testing Analytes and Cutoff Concentrations

ANALYTE	CONCENTRATION (ng/mL)	
	INITIAL TEST	CONFIRMATORY TEST
Marijuana metabolites	50	
Δ-9-tetrahydrocannabinol-9-carboxylic acid	–	15
Cocaine metabolites	150	
Benzoylecgonine	–	100
Opiate metabolites	2000	
Morphine	–	2000
Codeine	–	2000
6-Acetylmorphine	10	10
Phencyclidine	25	25
Amphetamines	500	
Amphetamine	–	250
Methamphetamine	–	250
MDMA	500	
MDMA	–	250
MDA	–	250
MDEA	–	250

SOURCE: *Department of Health and Human Services: Mandatory guidelines for federal workplace drug testing programs. Fed Reg. 53(69), 11983, April 11, 1988; revised: Fed Reg. 73(228), 71880, November 25, 2008. http://edocket.access.gpo.gov/2008/pdf/E8-26726.pdf.*

whereas the CAP program allows flexibility in the construction of programs servicing a broad range of clients. Both programs involve proficiency testing and periodic on-site inspection of laboratories.

Forensic urine drug testing (FUDT) differs from other areas of forensic toxicology in which urine is the only specimen analyzed and testing is performed for a limited number of drugs and metabolites. Under the federal certification program, analyses are performed for a limited number of classes or drugs of abuse (Table 32-3). While FUDT laboratories may typically analyze 100 to 1000 urine specimens daily, only a relatively small number of those specimens are positive for drugs. To handle this large workload, initial testing is performed by immunoassays on rapid, high-throughput chemistry analyzers. A confirmation analysis in FUDT-certified laboratories is performed by GC-MS and LC-MS/MS.

Proper FUDT is a challenge to good laboratory management. As with all forensic activities, every aspect of the laboratory operation must be thoroughly documented—specimen collection, chain of custody, quality control procedures, method validation, testing, qualifications of personnel, and the reporting of results. The laboratory facility must be constructed and operated to assure total security of specimens and documents. Confidentiality of all testing results is paramount; only specifically authorized persons should receive the results. The presence of a controlled or illicit drug in a single random urine specimen is generally accepted as proof of recent or past substance abuse. However, positive urine drug findings are only evidence that, at some time before the collection of the

sample, the individual was administered the drug, self-administered it, or was exposed to it. Positive urine tests do not prove impairment from drug abuse or addiction.

FUDT results are reported only as positive or negative for the drugs sought. Cutoff values are established for both the initial and confirmation assays (Table 32-3). The cutoff value is a concentration at or above which the assay is administratively considered positive. Below the cutoff value, the assay is reported to be negative for that drug or drug class. Obviously, drugs may be present below the cutoff concentration. However, the use of cutoff values allows uniformity in the drug testing and reporting of results. All test reports indicate the drug tested and its cutoff value. FUDT laboratories must be thoroughly familiar with all regulatory and analytical issues related to urine testing and devise strategies to resolve uncertainties.

Many individuals who are subject to regulated urine testing have devised techniques to mask their drug use either by physiological means such as the ingestion of diuretics or by attempting to adulterate the specimen directly with bleach, vinegar, or other products that interfere with the initial immunoassay tests (Warren, 1989; George and Braithwaite, 1996; Ferslew et al., 2003; Paul, 2004; Burrows et al., 2005). Thus, specimens are routinely tested for adulteration by checking urinary pH, creatinine, and specific gravity, nitrates, chromates, and noting any unusual color or smell. Recently, a mini-industry has developed to sell various products that are alleged to "beat the drug test." These products contain chemicals that, when added to a urine specimen, interfere with either the initial or confirmatory drug test (Dasgupta et al., 2007; Jaffee et al., 2007; Larson et al., 2008). For example, several of these products contain glutaraldehyde, which will react with the nitrogen atoms of the antibody proteins of the immunoassay screening test, thereby cross-linking the antibodies and inactivating the assay. However, this disruption of the test is so complete that the immunoassay analyzer records almost no signal, thus indicating possible adulteration of the specimen. Another adulterant, for the marijuana metabolite urine test, contains sodium nitrite. In acidic urine, the nitrite salt is converted to nitrous acid which then converts the marijuana metabolites to nitroso derivatives, rendering them undetectable by routine GC-MS analysis (Lewis et al., 1999). Often, the pH of the urine is insufficiently acidic for complete nitroso conversion of the tetrahydrocannabinol (THC) metabolite, THC-carboxylic acid. Thus, the urine will screen positive by the initial immunoassay. When urine is acidified to extract the THC acid metabolite for MS confirmation testing, the metabolite is completely oxidized and undetectable. However, the deuterated THC–carboxylic acid added to the sample as the internal standard of the confirmation test is also completely destroyed. Failure to detect the internal standard readily alerts the analyst that an oxidant adulterant had been added to the urine. In such cases, a quantitative test for nitrite is performed. Nitrite may be present in urine from numerous internal and external sources such as foods, drugs, pathological conditions, and infection from nitrate-reducing microorganisms. However, none of these sources produces urinary nitrite concentrations that even begin to approach those obtained by the addition of adulterant amounts of potassium nitrite equal to 1000 mg/L (Urey et al., 1998). Most chemical adulterants can be detected in urine by specific colorimetric tests that can be readily adapted to high-volume auto-analyzers (Table 32-4). Thus, FUDT laboratories now routinely test not only for drugs of abuse but also for a wide variety of chemical adulterants. In most instances, a positive test result for adulteration has a consequence similar to a positive drug test.

There may be valid reasons other than substance abuse for positive drug findings, such as therapeutic use of controlled substances, inadvertent intake of drugs via food, and passive inhalation. For

Table 32-4

Urine Adulterants Detected by Chemical Test

ADULTERANT	DETECTION METHOD
Acids, baking soda	pH
Bleach	Smell, color test
Detergents, diuretics, salt	Specific gravity
Diuretics	Creatinine, specific gravity
Glutaraldehyde	Color test, gas chromatography
Nitrite	Color test
Pyridinium chlorochromate	Color test, atomic absorption spectrophotometry (chromate), gas chromatography (pyridine)

example, the seed of *Papaver somniferum*, poppy seed, is a common ingredient in many pastries and breads. Depending on their botanical source, poppy seeds may contain significant amounts of morphine. Several studies have demonstrated that the ingestion of certain poppy-seed foods results in the urinary excretion of readily detectable concentrations of morphine (ElSohly and Jones, 1989). Morphine is a major urinary metabolite of heroin. Therefore, to readily differentiate heroin abuse from poppy-seed ingestion, analysis may be performed for 6-acetylmorphine, a unique heroin metabolite (Fehn and Megges, 1985).

Even over-the-counter medications may present potential problems for laboratories conducting urine drug testing. Methamphetamine may occur as a racemic mixture of D- and L-optical isomers. D-Methamphetamine, a Schedule II controlled substance, is a potent central nervous system stimulant subject to illicit drug abuse, while L-methamphetamine (L-desoxyephedrine) is an alpha-adrenergic stimulant available in over-the-counter Vicks inhalers as a nasal decongestant. Cross-reactivity of L-desoxyephedrine with the initial immunoassay screening test may occur after excessive use of the Vicks inhaler (Poklis and Moore, 1995). Additionally, the most popular conformational GC-MS products for amphetamines are achiral. Therefore, if such analyses are performed, a "false-positive" result for D-methamphetamine may be reported. This dilemma is easily resolved if confirmation testing is done with a chiral GC-MS procedure, which can readily resolve the stereoisomers of methamphetamine (Fitzgerald *et al.*, 1988).

HUMAN PERFORMANCE TESTING

Forensic toxicology activities also include the determination of the presence of ethanol and other drugs and chemicals in blood, breath, or other specimens and the evaluation of their role in modifying human performance and behavior. The most common application of human performance testing is to determine impairment while driving under the influence of ethanol (DUI) or drugs (DUID). Although operation of a motor vehicle is a common experience to most people, few appreciate the complexity of mental and physical functioning involved. A driver must simultaneously coordinate fine motor skills in tracking the road course and applying pressure to accelerator or brake—with visual attention immediately in front, to the horizon, and to the periphery of the vehicle—while continuously judging distance, speed, and appropriateness of response to signals, traffic, and unexpected events. The threshold blood alcohol concentration (BAC) for diminished driving performance of these complex functions in many individuals is as low as 0.04 g/dL,

the equivalent of ingestion of two beers within an hour's time to an average size person. The statutory definition of DUI in all 50 states is a BAC of 0.08 g/dL. These concentrations are consistent with diminished performance of complex driving skills in the vast majority of individuals. Over the past half century, an enormous amount of data has been developed correlating blood ethanol concentrations with intellectual and physiological impairment, particularly of the skills associated with the proper operation of motor vehicles. Numerous studies have demonstrated a direct relationship between an increased BAC in drivers and an increased risk of involvement in vehicular accidents (Council on Scientific Affairs, 1986). For example, alcohol impaired driving fatalities accounted for approximately one-third of all motor vehicle traffic fatalities in the United States in 2010 (National Highway Traffic Safety Administration, 2012).

During the past decade, there has been growing concern about the deleterious effects of drugs other than ethanol on driving performance. Several studies have demonstrated a relatively high occurrence of drugs in impaired or fatally injured drivers (White *et al.*, 1981; Mason and McBay, 1984). These studies tend to report that the highest drug-use accident rates are associated with the use of such illicit or controlled drugs as cocaine, benzodiazepines, marijuana, and phencyclidine. However, most studies test for only a few drugs or drug classes, and the repeated reporting of the same drugs may be a function of limited testing. Before "driving under the influence of drugs" testing is as readily accepted by the courts as ethanol testing, many legal and scientific problems concerning drug concentrations and driving impairment must be resolved (Consensus Report, 1985). The ability of analytical methodology to routinely quantify minute concentrations of drug in blood must be established. Also, drug-induced driving impairment at specific blood concentrations in controlled tests and/or actual highway experience must be demonstrated.

COURTROOM TESTIMONY

The forensic toxicologist often is called upon to testify in legal proceedings. As a general rule of evidence, a witness may testify only to facts known to him or her. The witness may offer opinions solely on the basis of what he or she has observed (Moenssens *et al.*, 1973). Such a witness is called a "lay witness." In contrast, the toxicologist is referred to as an "expert witness." A court recognizes a witness as an expert if that witness possesses knowledge or experience in a subject that is beyond the range of ordinary or common knowledge or observation. An expert witness may provide two types of testimony: objective testimony and "opinion." Objective testimony by a toxicologist usually involves a description of his or her analytical methods and findings. When a toxicologist testifies as to the interpretation of his or her analytical results or those of others, that toxicologist is offering an "opinion." Lay witnesses cannot offer such opinion testimony, as it exceeds their ordinary experience.

Before a court permits opinion testimony, the witness must be "qualified" as an expert in his or her particular field. In qualifying someone as an expert witness, the court considers the witness's education, on-the-job training, work experience, teaching or academic appointments, and professional memberships and publications as well as the acceptance of the witness as an expert by other courts. Qualification of a witness takes place in front of the jury members, who consider the expert's qualifications in determining how much weight to give his or her opinions during their deliberations.

Whether a toxicologist appears in criminal or civil court, workers' compensation, or parole hearings, the procedure for testifying is the same: direct examination, cross-examination, and redirect examination. The attorney who has summoned the witness to testify conducts direct examination. Testimony is presented in a question-and-answer format. The witness is asked a series of questions that allow him or her to present all facts or opinions relevant to the successful presentation of the attorney's case. During direct examination, an expert witness has the opportunity to explain to the jury the scientific bases of his or her opinions. Regardless of which side has called the toxicologist to court, the toxicologist should testify with scientific objectivity. Bias toward his or her client and prejudgments should be avoided. An expert witness is called to provide informed assistance to the jury. The jury, not the expert witness, determines the guilt or innocence of the defendant.

After direct testimony, the opposing attorney questions the expert. During this cross-examination, the witness is challenged as to his or her findings and/or opinions. The toxicologist will be asked to defend his or her analytical methods, results, and opinions. The opposing attorney may imply that the expert's testimony is biased because of financial compensation, association with an agency involved in the litigation, or personal feelings regarding the case. The best way to prepare for such challenges before testimony is to anticipate the questions the opposing attorney may ask.

After cross-examination, the attorney who called the witness may ask additional questions to clarify any issues raised during cross-examination. This allows the expert to explain apparent discrepancies in his or her testimony raised by the opposing attorney. Often, an expert witness is asked to answer a special type of question, the "hypothetical question." A hypothetical question contains only facts that have been presented in evidence. The expert is then asked for his or her conclusion or opinion based solely on this hypothetical situation. This type of question serves as a means by which appropriate facts leading to the expert's opinion are identified. Often, these questions are extremely long and convoluted. The witness should be sure he or she understands all the facts and implications in the question. Like all questions, this type should be answered as objectively as possible.

ROLE IN CLINICAL TOXICOLOGY

Analytical toxicology in a clinical setting plays a role very similar to its role in forensic toxicology. As an aid in the diagnosis and treatment of toxic incidents, as well as in monitoring the effectiveness of treatment regimens, it is useful to clearly identify the nature of the toxic exposure and measure the amount of the toxic substance that has been absorbed. Frequently, this information, together with the clinical state of the patient, permits a clinician to relate the signs and symptoms observed to the anticipated effects of the toxic agent. This may permit a clinical judgment as to whether the treatment must be vigorous and aggressive or whether simple observation and symptomatic treatment of the patient are sufficient.

A cardinal rule in the treatment of poisoning cases is to remove any unabsorbed material, limit the absorption of additional poison, and hasten its elimination. The clinical toxicology laboratory serves an additional purpose in this phase of the treatment by monitoring the amount of the chemical remaining in circulation or measuring what is excreted. In addition, the laboratory can provide the data needed to permit estimations of the total dosage or the effectiveness of treatment by changes in known pharmacokinetic parameters of the drug or other chemical ingested.

Although the instrumentation and the methodology used in a clinical toxicology laboratory are similar to those utilized by a

forensic toxicologist, a major difference between these two applications is responsiveness. In emergency toxicology testing, results must be communicated to the clinician within hours to be meaningful for therapy. A forensic toxicologist may carefully choose the best method for a particular test and conduct replicate procedures to assure maximum accuracy. A clinical laboratory cannot afford this luxury and may sacrifice accuracy for a rapid turnaround time. Additionally, because it is impossible to predict when toxicological emergencies will occur, a clinical laboratory must provide rapid testing 24 hours a day, every day of the year.

Primary examples of the usefulness of emergency toxicology testing are the rapid quantitative determination of acetaminophen, salicylate, alcohols, and glycol serum concentrations in instances of suspected overdose. Acetaminophen serum values related to the time after ingestion (see Chap. 33) not only indicate an overdose, but provide a prognosis for possible delayed hepatotoxicity and the need to continue administration of N-acetylcysteine antidote. In addition, continuous monitoring of serum values permits an accurate pharmacokinetic calculation of the ingested dose (Melethil et al., 1981). Similarly, salicylate serum values related to the time after ingestion may indicate an overdose, providing a prognosis for possible delayed severe metabolic acidosis and the need for lifesaving dialysis treatment. Continuous monitoring of serum salicylate values permits an accurate assessment of the efficacy of dialysis.

Ethanol is the most common chemical encountered in emergency toxicology. Although relatively few fatal intoxications occur with ethanol alone, serum values are important in the assessment of behavioral, physiologic, and neurological function, particularly in trauma cases where the patient is unable to communicate and surgery with the administration of anesthetic or analgesic drugs is indicated. Intoxications from accidental or deliberate ingestion of other alcohols or glycols—such as methanol from windshield deicer or paint thinner, isopropanol from rubbing alcohol, and ethylene glycol from antifreeze—are often encountered in emergency departments. Following ingestion of methanol or ethylene glycol, patients often present with similar neurological symptoms and severe metabolic acidosis due to the formation of toxic aldehyde and acid metabolites. A rapid quantitative serum determination for these intoxicants will indicate the severity of intoxication and the possible need for dialysis therapy. Alcohol infusion, in order to saturate the enzyme alcohol dehydrogenase, blocks the conversion of methanol and ethylene glycol to their toxic metabolites. Continuous monitoring of serum values not only permits an assessment of the clearance of the intoxicant by dialysis, but also assures a proper infusion rate of alcohol for effective antidotal concentrations (Fig. 32-7). To provide effective service to the emergency department, laboratories should have available chromatographic methods for the rapid separation and detection of alcohols and glycols (Edinboro et al., 1993).

The utilization of the analytical capabilities of a clinical toxicology laboratory has increased enormously in recent years. Typically, the laboratory performs testing not only for the emergency department but also for a wide variety of other medical departments, as drugs and toxic agents may be a consideration in diagnosis. Urine is analyzed from substance abuse treatment facilities to monitor the administration of methadone or other therapeutic agents and/or to assure that patients do not continue to abuse drugs. Similarly, psychiatrists, neurologists, and physicians treating patients for chronic pain need to know whether patients are self-administering drugs before such patients undergo psychiatric or neurological examinations. Analysis for drugs of abuse in

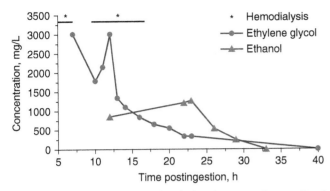

Figure 32-7. *Serum ethylene glycol and ethanol concentrations monitored during dialysis and ethanol infusion therapy.* (Data from the Toxicology Laboratory, Medical College of Virginia Hospital, Richmond, VA.)

meconium and urine obtained from neonates is used to corroborate the diagnosis of withdrawal symptoms in newborns and document fetal exposure to controlled substances. Toxic metal determinations, such as blood lead concentration, are often performed to assess possible toxic metal exposure or severity of toxicity. Analysis of heavy metals in 24-hour urine specimens is often used to rule out toxic metal exposure as a cause of symmetrical peripheral neuropathy prior to the diagnosis of neurological disorders such as Guillian–Barré syndrome. The clinical toxicology laboratory may often perform unique diagnostic tests that require sophisticated analytical capabilities such as GC-MS and LC analysis for organic acids and amino acids to detect inborn errors of metabolism in infants and children. Methods for the analysis of abnormal organic acids will also detect acidic drugs and other intoxicants such as salicylates, ethylene glycol, GHB, and valproic acid. Another such diagnostic test requiring sensitive chromatography is the timed metabolism of lidocaine to its monoethylglycinexylidide (MEGX) metabolite (O'Neal and Poklis, 1996). The rate of this conversion is a sensitive indicator of hepatic dysfunction and is often used to assess hepatic viability in donor livers prior to transplantation. MEGX formation may also be useful in monitoring the severity of the histological condition of patients with chronic hepatitis and cirrhosis (Shiffman *et al.*, 1994).

ROLE IN THERAPEUTIC MONITORING

Historically, the administration of drugs for long-term therapy was based largely on experience. A dosage amount was selected and administered at appropriate intervals based on what the clinician had learned was generally tolerated by most patients. If the drug seemed ineffective, the dose was increased; if toxicity developed, the dose was decreased or the frequency of dosing was altered. At times, a different dosage form might be substituted. Establishing an effective dosage regimen was particularly difficult in children and the elderly.

The factors responsible for individual variability in responses to drug therapy include the rate and extent of drug absorption, distribution, and binding in body tissues and fluids, rate of metabolism and excretion, pathological conditions, and interaction with other drugs (Blaschke *et al.*, 1985). Monitoring of the plasma or serum concentration at regular intervals will detect deviations from the average serum concentration, which, in turn, may suggest that one or more of these variables need to be identified and corrected.

With multiple administrations of a given drug at regular intervals, plasma drug concentrations will gradually increase and eventually reach a plateau over the course of therapy. The plateau is referred to as a steady state condition, whereas the amount of drug absorbed is in equilibrium to the amount of drug eliminated. Dosage regimes are calculated so that plasma drug concentrations during steady state conditions are within the therapeutic range, and monitoring such conditions assures that an effective concentration is present. For drugs that have a defined correlation between serum values and undesired toxic effects, the lowest serum value immediately prior to dosing (trough) and the highest expected serum concentration (peak) are monitored to assure efficacy and minimize toxicity.

Because the drug being administered is known, qualitative characterization of the analyte generally is not required. Quantitative accuracy is required, however. Frequently, the methodology applied is important, particularly in regard to its selectivity. For example, methods that measure the parent drug and its metabolites are not ideal unless the individual analytes can be quantified separately. Depending on the drug, metabolites may or may not be active to a different degree than the parent drug. The cardiac antiarrhythmic drug procainamide is acetylated during metabolism to form *N*-acetylprocainamide (NAPA). This metabolite has antiarrythmic activity of almost equal potency to that of the parent drug procainamide. There is bimodal genetic variation in the activity of the *N*-acetyltransferase for procainamide, so that, in "fast acetylators," the concentration of NAPA in the serum may exceed that of the parent drug. For optimal patient management, information should be available about the concentrations of both procainamide and NAPA in serum (Bigger and Hoffman, 1985).

Because absolute characterization of the analyte is not necessary for many drugs, immunoassay procedures are commonly used. This is particularly true of drugs with extremely low serum concentrations, such as cardiac glycosides, and drugs that are difficult to extract because of a high degree of polarity, such as the aminoglycoside antibiotics. In these cases, serum can be conveniently assayed directly by using commercially available kits for immunoassays.

The chromatographic methods in which an appropriate internal standard is added are favored when more than one analyte is to be quantified or if metabolites with structures similar to those of the parent drugs must be distinguished. Because the nature of drugs is varied, many different analytical techniques may be applied, including atomic absorption spectrophotometry for measuring lithium used to treat manic disorders. Virtually all the tools of the analyst may be used for specific applications of analytical toxicology. Drugs that are commonly monitored during therapy are presented in Table 32-5.

SUMMARY

The analytical techniques employed by forensic toxicologists have continued to expand in complexity and improve in reliability and sensitivity. Many new analytical tools have been applied to toxicological problems in almost all areas of the field, and the technology continues to open new areas of research. Forensic toxicologists continue to be concerned about conducting unequivocal identification of toxic substances in such a manner that the results can withstand a legal challenge. The issues of substance abuse, designer drugs, increased potency of therapeutic agents, and widespread concern about pollution, and the safety and health of workers present challenges to the analyst's knowledge, skills, and abilities. As these challenges are met, analytical toxicologists will continue to play a substantial role in the expansion of the discipline of toxicology.

Table 32-5

Drugs Commonly Indicated for Therapeutic Monitoring

Antiarrythmics
Digoxin
Digitoxin
Lidocaine
Procainamide and *N*-acetylprocainamide
Quinidine

Antibiotics
Amikacin
Chloramphenicol
Gentamicin
Tobramycin
Vancomycin

Anticancer
Methotrexate

Anticonvulsants
Carbamazepine
Gabapentin
Lamotrigine
Phenobarbital
Phenytoin
Primidone
Topiramate
Valproic acid
Zonisamide

Antidepressants
Amitriptyline/nortriptyline
Desipramine/imipramine
Doxepin/nordoxepin

Antipsychotics
Clozapine
Pimozide

Bronchodilators
Caffeine
Theophylline

Immunosuppressants
Azathioprine
Cyclosporine
Mycophenolic acid
Sirolimus
Tacrolimus

Mood stabilizing
Lithium

REFERENCES

Aderjan R, Bahr H, Schmidt G. Investigation of cardiac glycoside levels in human postmortem blood and tissues determined by a special RIA procedure. *Arch Toxicol.* 1979;42:107–114.

American Association of Poison Control Centers. Drugs used in child maltreatment. *Prescrire Int.* 2011;20(120):236–237.

Andresen H, Aydin BE, Mueller A, Iwersen-Bergmann S. An overview of gamma-hydroxybutyric acid: pharmacodynamics, pharmacokinetics, toxic effects, addiction, analytical method, and interpretation of results. *Drug Test Anal.* 2011;3(9):660–668.

Apple FS. Postmortem tricyclic antidepressant concentrations: assessing cause of death using parent drug to metabolite ratio. *J Anal Toxicol.* 1989;13:197–198.

Barroso M, Gallardo E, Vieira DN, López-Rivadulla M, Queiroz JA. Hair: a complementary source of bioanalytical information in forensic toxicology. *Bioanalysis.* 2011;3(1):67–79.

Baumgartner A, Jones P, Baumgartner W. Detection of phencylidine in hair. *J Forensic Sci.* 1981;26:576–581.

Baumgartner W, Jones P, Baumgartner W, Black C. Radioimmunoassay of hair for determining opiate-abuse histories. *J Nucl Med.* 1979;20:748–752.

Benko A. Toxicological analysis of amobarbital and glutethimide from bone tissue. *J Forensic Sci.* 1985;30:708–714.

Bévalot F, Gustin MP, Cartiser N, Le Meur C, Malicier D, Fanton L. Interpretation of drug concentrations in an alternative matrix: the case of meprobamate in vitreous humor. *Int J Legal Med.* 2011;25(3):463–468.

Bigger JT Jr, Hoffman BF. Antiarrhythmic drugs. In: Gilman AG, Goodman LS, Rall TW, Murad F, eds. *The Pharmacological Basis of Therapeutics.* 7th ed. New York: Macmillan; 1985:763.

Blanke RV. Quality assurance in drug-use testing. *Clin Chem.* 1987;33:41B–45B.

Blanke RV. *Validation of the Purity of Standards.* Irving, TX: Abbott Laboratories, Diagnostic Division; 1989.

Blaschke TF, Nies AS, Mamelock RD. Principles of therapeutics. In: Gilman AG, Goodman LS, Rall TW, Murad F, eds. *The Pharmacological Basis of Therapeutics.* 7th ed. New York: Macmillan; 1985:52.

Bosker WM, Huestis MA. Oral fluid testing for drugs of abuse. *Clin Chem.* 2009;55(11):1910–1931.

Boumba VA, Ziavrou KS, Vougiouklakis T. Hair as a biological indicator of drug use, drug abuse or chronic exposure to environmental toxicants. *Int J Toxicol.* 2006;25(3):143–163.

Burrows DL, Nicolaides A, Rice PJ, Dufforc M, Johnson DA, Ferslew KE. Papain: a novel urine adulterant. *J Anal Toxicol.* 2005;29(5):275–295.

Cartiser N, Bévalot F, Fanton L, Gaillard Y, Guitton J. State-of-the-art of bone marrow analysis in forensic toxicology: a review. *Int J Legal Med.* 2011;125(2):181–198.

Cawrse BM, Levine B, Jufer RA, et al. Distribution of methylone in four postmortem cases. *J Anal Toxicol.* 2012;36(6):434–439.

Chapuis E. *Elements de Toxicologie,* 1873, cited in Peterson F, Haines WS, Webster RW. *Legal Medicine and Toxicology.* 2nd ed. Vol 2. Philadelphia, PA: WB Saunders; 1923.

Coe JI. Postmortem chemistry update: emphasis on forensic applications. *Am J Forensic Med Pathol.* 1993;14:91–117.

Cone EJ, Buchwald WF, Darwin WD. Analytical controls in drug metabolism studies: 11. Artifact formation during chloroform extraction of drugs and metabolites with amine substitutes. *Drug Metab Dispos.* 1982;10:561–567.

Consensus Report. Drug concentrations and driving impairment. *JAMA.* 1985;254:2618–2621.

Coppola M, Mondola R. Synthetic cathinones: chemistry, pharmacology and toxicology of a new class of designer drugs f abuse marketed as "bath salts" or "plant food. *Toxicol Lett.* 2012;211(2):144–149.

Council on Scientific Affairs. Alcohol and the driver. *JAMA.* 1986;255:522–527.

Couper FJ, McIntyre IM, Drummer OH. Detection of antidepressant and antipsychotic drugs in postmortem human scalp hair. *J Forensic Sci.* 1995;40(1):87–90.

Cravey RH, Baselt RC. The science of forensic toxicology. In: Cravey RH, Baselt RC, eds. *Introduction to Forensic Toxicology.* Davis. CA: Biomedical Publications; 1981:3–6.

Dasgupta A. The effects of adulterants and selected ingested compounds on drugs-of-abuse testing in urine. *Am J Clin Pathol.* 2007;128(3):491–503.

Department of Health and Human Services, ADAMHA. Mandatory guidelines for federal workplace drug testing: final guidelines: notice. *Fed Reg.* 1988;53(69):11970–11989.

Dinis-Oliveira RJ, Carvalho F, Duarte JA, et al. Collection of biological samples in forensic toxicology. *Toxicol Mech Methods.* 2010;20(7):363–414.

Dowling GP, McDonough ET, Bost RO. "Eve" and "ecstasy": a report of five deaths associated with the use of MDEA and MDMA. *JAMA.* 1987;257:1615–1617.

Drummer O. Drugs in bone and bone marrow. In: Jenkins A, ed. *Drug Testing in Alternate Biological Specimens.* Humana Press. 2010:131–136:chap 8.

Edinboro LE, Nanco CR, Soghoian DM, Poklis A. Determination of ethylene glycol in serum utilizing direct injection on a wide-bore capillary column. *Ther Drug Monit*. 1993;15:220–223.

ElSohly MA, Jones AB. Morphine and codeine in biological fluids: approaches to source differentiation. *Forensic Sci Rev*. 1989;1:13–22.

ElSohly MA, Salamone SJ. Prevalence of drugs used in cases of alleged sexual assault. *J Anal Toxicol*. 1999;23(3):141–146.

Ernst MF, Poklis A, Gantner GE. Evaluation of medicolegal investigators' suspicious and positive toxicology findings in 100 drug deaths. *J Forensic Sci*. 1982;27:61–65.

Evans WED. *The Chemistry of Death*. Springfield, IL: Charles C Thomas; 1963.

Fehn J, Megges G. Detection of O6-monoacetylmorphine in urine samples by GC-MS as evidence for heroin use. *J Anal Toxicol*. 1985;9:134–138.

Ferrara DS, Tedeschi L, Frison G, Brusini G. Quality control in toxicological analysis. *J Chromatogr B Biomed Sci Appl*. 1998;713(1):227–243.

Ferslew KE, Nicolaides AN, Robert TA. Determination of chromate adulteration of human urine by automated colorimetric and capillary ion electrophoretic analyses. *J Anal Toxicol*. 2003;27(1):36–39.

Fisher RS, Hine CH, Stetler CJ (Committee on Medicolegal Problems). *Alcohol and the Impaired Driver: A Manual on the Medicolegal Aspects of Chemical Tests for Intoxication*. Chicago: American Medical Association; 1968.

Fitzgerald RL, Ramos JM, Bogema SC, Poklis A. Resolution of methamphetamine stereoisomers in urine drug testing: urinary excretion of R(-)-methamphetamine following use of nasal inhalers. *J Anal Toxicol*. 1988;12:255–259.

Flanagan RJ, Connally G, Evans JM. Analytical toxicology: guidelines for sample collection postmortem. *Toxicol Rev*. 2005;24(1):63–71.

Gagliano-Candela R, Aventaggiato L. The detection of toxic substances in entomological specimens. *Int J Legal Med*. 2011;114(405):19–203.

Gaillard Y, Pepin G. Screening and identification of drugs in human hair by high-performance liquid chromatography-photodiode-array UV detection and mass gas chromatography-mass spectrometry after solid phase extraction. A powerful tool in forensic medicine. *J Chromatogr*. 1997;762:251–267.

Gallagher CT, Assi S, Stair JL, et al. 5,6-Mehtylenedioxy-2-aminoindane: from laboratory curiosity to 'legal high'. *Hum Psychopharmacol*. 2012;27(2):106–112.

Gallardo E, Queiroz JA. The role of alternative specimens in toxicological analysis. *Biomed Chromatogr*. 2008;22(8):795–821.

Garside D. Drugs-of-abuse in nails. In: Jenkins A, ed. *Drug Testing in Alternate Biological Specimens*. Humana Press; 2010:43–63:chap 3.

Garriott JS, Simmons LM, Poklis A, Mackell MS. Five cases of fatal overdose from caffeine-containing "look-alike" drugs. *J Anal Toxicol*. 1985;9:141–143.

George S, Braithwaite RA. The effect of glutaraldehyde adulteration of urine specimens on syva EMIT II drugs-of-abuse assays. *J Anal Toxicol*. 1996;20(3):195–196.

Gettler AD. Poisoning and toxicology, forensic aspects: Part 1: historical aspects. *Inform*. 1977;9:3–7.

Goff ML, Brown WA, Omori AI, LaPointe DA. Preliminary observations of the effects of amitriptyline in decomposing tissue on the development of parasarcophagaruficornis (Diptera: Sarcophagidae) and implications of this effect to estimation of postmortem interval. *J Forensic Sci*. 1993;38:316–322.

Goldberger BA, Huestis MA, Wilkins DG. Commonly practiced quality control and quality assurance procedures for gas chromatography mass spectrometry analysis in forensic urine drug-testing laboratories. *Forensic Sci Rev*. 1997;9(2):59–80.

Granger RH, Condie LW, Borzelleca JF. Effect of vehicle on the relative up-take of haloalkanes administered by gavage. *Toxicologist*. 1987;40:1.

Gust SW, Walsh JM. *Drugs in the Workplace: Research and Evaluation Data*. NIDA Research Monograph 91. Washington, DC: US Government Printing Office; 1989.

Hambidge KM. Increase in hair copper concentration with increasing distance from the scalp. *Am J Clin Nutr*. 1973;26:1212–1215.

Harkey MR, Henderson GL. Hair analysis for drugs of abuse. *Adv Anal Toxicol*. 1989;2:298–329.

Hawks RL, Chiang CN. Examples of specific drug assays. In: Hawks RL, Chiang CN, eds. *Urine Testing for Drugs of Abuse*. NIDA Research Monograph 73. Rockville, MD: US Department Health and Human Services, PHS, ADAMHA; 1986:93.

Henderson GL. Designer drugs: past history and future prospects. *J Forensic Sci*. 1988;33:569–575.

Hime GW, Hearn WL, Rose S, Cofino J. Analysis of cocaine and cocaethylene in blood and tissues by GC-NPD and GC-Ion Trap mass spectrometry. *J Anal Toxicol*. 1991;15:241–245.

Inoue T, Seta S. Analysis of drugs in unconventional samples. *Forensic Sci Rev*. 1992;4:89–107.

Jacob P, Lewis ER, Elias-Baker BA, Jones RT. A pyrolysis product, anhydroecgonine methyl ester (methylecgonidine), is in the urine of cocaine smokers. *J Anal Toxicol*. 1990;14:353–357.

Jaffee WB, Trucco E, Levy S, Weiss RD. Is this urine really negative? A systematic review of tampering methods in urine drug screening and tresting. *J Subst Abuse Treat*. 2007;33(1):33–42.

Jones GR, Pounder DJ. Site-dependence of drug concentrations in postmortem blood—a case study. *J Anal Toxicol*. 1987;11:186–190.

Kaempe B. Interfering compounds and artifacts in the identification of drugs in autopsy material. In: Stolman A, ed. *Progress in Chemical Toxicology*. Vol 4. New York: Academic Press; 1969:1–57.

Kintz P. Drug testing in hair. In: Jenkins A, ed. *Drug Testing in Alternate Biological Specimens*. Humana Press; 2010:67–79:chap 4.

Kronstrand R, Druid H. Hair in postmortem toxicology. In: Kintz P, ed. *Analytical and Practical Aspects of Drug Testing in Hair [International Science and Forensic Investigation]*. CRC Press; 2006:223–240:chap 10.

Lanaro R, Costa JL, Fernandes LC, Resende RR, Tavares MF. Detection of paraquat in oral fluid, plasma, and urine by capillary electrophoresis for diagnosis of acute poisoning. *J Anal Toxicol*. 2011;35(5):274–279.

Larson SJ, Holler JM, Magluilo J Jr, Dunkley CS, Jacobs A. Papain adulteration in 11-nor-delta9-tetrahydrocannabinol-9-carboxylic acid-positive urine samples. *J Anal Toxicol*. 2008;32(6):438–443.

LeBeau M, Andollo W, Hearn WL, et al. Recommendations for toxicological investigation of drug-facilitated sexual assaults. *J Forensic Sci*. 1999;44:227–230.

LeBeau M, Montgomery MA, Brewer JD. The role of variations in growth rate and sample collection on interpreting results of segmental analyses of hair. *Forensic Sci Int*. 2011;210(1–3):110–116.

Lewis SA, Lewis LA, Tuinman A. Potassium nitrite reaction with 11-nor-delta-9-tetrahydrocannabinol-9-carboxylic acid in urine in relation to drug screening analysis. *J Forensic Sci*. 1999;44:951–955.

Marigo M, Tagliaro F, Poiesi C, Lafisca S, Neri C. Determination of morphine in the hair of heroin addicts by high performance liquid chromatography with fluorometric detection. *J Anal Toxicol*. 1986;10:158–161.

Martin BR, Lue LP, Boni JP. Pyrolysis and volatilization of cocaine. *J Anal Toxicol*. 1989;13:158–162.

Martz R. The identification of cocaine in hair by GC-MS and MS/MS. *Crime Lab Dig*. 1988;15:67–73.

Mason AP, McBay AJ. Ethanol, marijuana, and other drug use in 600 drivers killed in single-vehicle crashes in North Carolina. *J Forensic Sci*. 1984;29:987–1026.

McKenzie JM. Alteration of zinc and copper concentration of hair. *Am J Clin Nutr*. 1978;31:470–476.

Melethil S, Poklis A, Schwartz HS. Estimation of the amount of drug absorbed in acetaminophen poisoning: a case report. *Vet Hum Toxicol*. 1981;23:421–423.

Mills RA, Millis CD, Dannan GA, et al. Studies on the structure-activity relationships for the metabolism of polybrominated biphenyls by rat liver microsomes. *Toxicol Appl Pharmacol*. 1985;78:96–104.

Moenssens AA, Moses RE, Inbau FE. *Scientific Evidence in Criminal Cases*. Mineola, NY: Foundation Press; 1973.

Moore KA, Daniel J, Fierro M, et al. Detection of a metabolite of α-benzyl-N-methylphenylamine synthesis in a mixed drug fatality involving methamphetamine. *J Forensic Sci*. 1996a;41:524–526.

Moore KA, Ismaiel A, Poklis A. α-Benzyl-N-methylphenethylamine (BNMPA) an impurity of illicit methamphetamine synthesis: III. Detection of BNMPA and metabolites in urine from methamphetamine users. *J Anal Toxicol*. 1996b;20:89–92.

Muller C, Vogt S, Goerke R, Kordon A, Weinmann W. Identification of selectedpsychopharmaceuticals and their metabolites in hair by LC/ESI-CID/MS and LC/MS/MS. *Forensic Sci Int.* 2000;113(1–3): 415–421.

Murray JB. Munchausen syndrome/Munchausen syndrome by proxy. *J Psychol.* 1997;131:343–352.

National Highway Traffic Safety Administration, Office of Behavioral Safety Research, Prevalence of High BAC in Alcohol-Impaired-Driving Fatal Crashes, DOT HS 811 654, August 2012.

O'Neal CL, Poklis A. A sensitive HPLC assay for the simultaneous quantitation of lidocaine and its metabolites; monoethylglcinexylididie and glycinexylidide in serum. *Clin Chem.* 1996;42:330–331.

Oral R, Bayman L, Assad A, et al. Illicit drug exposure in patients evaluated for alleged child abuse and neglect. *Pediatr Emerg Care.* 2011;27(6):490–495.

Palmeri A, Pichini S, Pacifici R, Zuccaro P, Lopez A. Drugs in nails: physiology, pharmacokinetics and forensic toxicology. *Clin Pharmacokinet.* 2000;38(2):95–110.

Panel on Herbicides. Report on 2,4,5-T, In: *A Report of the Panel on Herbicides of the President's Science Advisory Committee.* Executive Office of the President, Office of Science and Technology. Washington, DC: US Government Printing Office; 1971.

Paul BD. Six spectroscopic methods for detection of oxidants in urine: implication in differentiation of normal and adulterated urine. *J Anal Toxicol.* 2004;28(7):599–608.

Peters FT, Drummer OH, Musshoff F. Validation of new methods. *Forensic Sci Int.* 2007;165(2-3):216–224.

Petersen F, Haines WS, Webster RW. *Legal Medicine and Toxicology.* Vol 2. 2nd ed. Philadelphia, PA: WB Saunders; 1923.

Pien K, Laloup M, Pipeleers-Marichal M, et al. Toxicological data and growth characteristics of single post-feeding larvae and puparia of Calliphoravicina (Diptera: Calliphoridae) obtained from a controlled nordiazepam study. *Int J Legal Med.* 2004;118(4): 190–193.

Poklis A. Pentazocine/tripelennamine (T's and blues) abuse: a five year survey of St. Louis, Missouri. *Drug Alcohol Depend.* 1982;10: 257–267.

Poklis A, Mackell MA, Tucker EF. Tissue distribution of lidocaine after fatal accidental injection. *J Forensic Sci.* 1984;29:1229–1236.

Poklis A, Moore KA. Response of EMIT amphetamine immunoassays to urinary desoxyephedrine following Vicks inhaler use. *Ther Drug Monit.* 1995;17:89–94.

Pounder DJ. Forensic entomo-toxicology. *J Forensic Sci Soc.* 1991;31: 469–472.

Pragst F, Balikova MA. State of the art in hair analysis for detection of drug and alcohol abuse. *Clin Chim Acta.* 2006;370(1–2):17–49.

Pragst F, Rothe M, Hunger J, Thor S. Structural and concentration effects on the deposition of tricyclic antidepressants in human hair. *Forensic Sci Int.* 1997;84(1–3):225–236.

Price LM, Poklis A, Johnson DE. Fatal acetaminophen poisoning with evidence of subendocardial necrosis of the heart. *J Forensic Sci.* 1991;36:930–935.

Prouty BS, Anderson WH. The forensic science implications of site and temporal influences on postmortem blood-drug concentrations. *J Forensic Sci.* 1990;35:243–270.

Prosser JM, Nelson LS. The toxicology of bath salts: a review of synthetic cathinones. *J Med Toxiol.* 2012;8(1):33–42.

Puschel K, Thomasch P, Arnold W. Opiate levels in hair. *Forensic Sci Int.* 1983;21:181–186.

Rollins DE, Wilkins DG, Gygi SP, Slawson MH, Nagasawa PR. Testing for drugs of abuse in hair—experimental observations and indications for future research. *Forensic Sci Rev.* 1997;9:23–25.

Rosenbaum CD, Carreiro SP, Babu KM. Here today, gone tomorrow... and back again? A review of herbal marijuana alternatives (K2, Spice), synthetic cathinones (bath salts), kratom, Salvia divinorum, methoxetamine, and piperazines. *J Med Toxiol.* 2012;8(10):15–32.

Ross EA, Reisfield GM, Watson MC, Chronister CW, Goldberger BA. Psychoactive "bath salts" intoxication with methylenedioxypyrovalerone. *Am J Med.* 2012;125:854–858.

Saady JJ, Narasimhachari N, Friedel RO. Unsuspected impurities in imipramine and desipramine standards and pharmaceutical formulations. *Clin Chem.* 1981;27:343–344.

San George RC, Hoberman RD. Reaction of acetaldehyde with hemoglobin. *J Biol Chem.* 1986;261:6811–6821.

Schroeder HA, Nason AP. Trace metals in human hair. *J Invest Dermatol.* 1989;53:71–78.

Scientific Working Group for Forensic Toxicology. www.swgtox.org.

Seely KA, Lapoint J, Moran JH, Fattore L. Spice drugs are more than harmless herbal blends: a review of the pharmacology and toxicology of synthetic cannabinoids. *Prog Neuropsychopharmacol Biol Psychiatry.* 2012;39(2):234–243.

Shapiro HA. Arsenic content of human hair and nails: its interpretation. *J Forensic Med.* 1967;14:65–71.

Shen M, Xiang P, Wu H, Shen B, Huang Z. Detection of antidepressant and antipsychotic drugs in human hair. *Forensic Sci Int.*2002;126(2):153–161.

Shiffman ML, Luketic VA, Sanyal AJ, et al. Hepatic lidocaine metabolism and liver histology in patients with chronic hepatitis and cirrhosis. *Hepatology.* 1994;31:933–940.

Skopp G. Preanalytic aspects in postmortem toxicology. *Forensic Sci Int.* 2004;142(2–3):75–100.

Smith H. The interpretation of the arsenic content of human hair. *J Forensic Sci Soc.* 1964;4:192–199.

Society of Forensic Toxicologists. www.soft-tox.org.

Spiehler V, Cooper G. Drugs-of-abuse testing in saliva and oral fluid. In: Jenkins A, ed. *Drug Testing in Alternate Biological Specimens.* Humana Press; 2010:83–95:chap 5.

Stockham TL, Blanke RV. Investigation of an acetaldehyde-hemoglobin adduct in alcoholics: alcoholism. *Clin Exp Res.* 1988;12:748–754.

Strang J, Marsh A, Desouza N. Hair analysis for drugs of abuse. *Lancet.* 1990;26:740.

Suzuki O, Hattori H, Asano M. Nails and hair as useful material for detection of methampetamine of amphetamine abuse. *Forensic Sci Int.* 1984;24:9–16.

Thorwald J. *The Century of the Detective.* New York: Harcourt; 1965.

Urey FM, Komaromy-Hiller G, Staley B, et al. Nitrite adulteration of workplace urine drug-testing specimens: Part 1: sources and associated concentrations of nitrite in urine and distinction between natural sources and adulteration. *J Anal Toxicol.* 1998;22:89–95.

Villain M, Concheiro M, Cirimele V, Kintz P. Screening method for benzodiazepines and hypnotics in hair at pg/mg level by liquid chromatography-mass spectrometry/mass spectrometry. *J Chromatogr B Analyt Technol Biomed Life Sci.* 2005;825(1):72–78.

Vorpahl TE, Coe JI. Correlation of antemortem and postmortem digoxin levels. *J Forensic Sci.* 1978;23:329–334.

Warren A. Interference of common household chemicals in immunoassay methods for drugs of abuse. *Clin Chem.* 1989;35:648–651.

White JM, Clardy MS, Groves MH, et al. Testing for sedative-hypnotic drugs in the impaired driver: a survey of 72,000 arrests. *Clin Toxicol.* 1981;18:945–957.

Yamaguichi S, Matsumoto H, Kaku S, Tateishi M, Shiramizu M. Factors affecting the amount of mercury in human scalp hair. *Am J Pub Health.* 1975;65:484–488.

Yang SH, Morgan AA, Nguyen HP, Moore H, Figard BJ, Schug KA. Quantitative determination of bisphenol A from human saliva using bulk derivatization and trap-and-elute liquid chromatography coupled to electrospray ionization mass spectrometry. *Environ Toxicol Chem.* 2011;30(6):1243–1251.

Yegles M, Mersch F, Wennig R. Detection of benzodiazepines and other psychotropic drugs in human hair in GC-MS. *Forensic Sci Int.* 1997;84(1–3):211–218.

Yin S. Malicious use of pharmaceuticals in children. *J Pediatr.* 2010; 157(5):832–836.

Clinical Toxicology

Louis R. Cantilena Jr.

HISTORY OF CLINICAL TOXICOLOGY

Historical Aspects of the Treatment of Poisoning

The history of poisons and poisoners dates back to ancient times. One of the earliest documented uses of poisons was for military use. The use of toxic smoke can be tracked to as early as 2000 BC in ancient India. Formulas for creating poisonous and noxious vapors have also been found from 1000 BC in Chinese writings. The incorporation of fire-generated arsenic containing smoke from the burning of wood covered with pitch and sulfur containing material was reportedly used by Sparta against Athens around 400 BC (Osius, 1957; Mayor, 2003). Documentation regarding the use of antidotes can be found in the Odyssey and Shastras from approximately 600 BC. What is believed to be the first documented use of a specific antidote may be found in Homer's Odyssey where it is suggested to Ulysses that he take moli to protect himself from poisoning. Moli may actually be *Galanthus* nivalis, a plant-derived cholinesterase inhibitor that might counteract the effects of the anticholinergic plant *Datura stramonium* (Plaitakis & Duvoisin, 1983).

Galen (129–200 AD) wrote three books called *De Antidotis I, De Antidotis II, and De Theriaca ad Pisonem* that described the development of a universal antidote known as a alexipharmic or theriac by King Mithridates VI of Pontus who lived from 132 to 63 BC (Wax, 1997). The antidote reportedly contained 36 or more ingredients and was ingested every day conferring protection against a broad spectrum of poisons such as venomous stings and bites from vipers, spiders, and scorpions (Jarcho, 1972).

The refinement of theriac (antidote) formulations is documented for nearly 2000 years. Andromachus (first century AD) was a physician to Nero and improved the Mithridates theriac by modifying the formula to include up to 73 ingredients (Wax, 1997). The use of these ancient antidotes included treatment of acute poisoning and prophylactic treatment to make one "poison proof." The Mithridates theriac with subsequent modifications remained in use until the early 20th century. William Heberden wrote *Antitheriaka: An Essay on Mithridatium and Theriaca* in 1745 in which he questioned the effectiveness of these products (Jarcho, 1972). Despite the skepticism concerning these antidote formulations, their use continued for two millenniums.

One of the earliest writings on the prevention of the gastrointestinal absorption of poisons was by Nicander (Major, 1934). In this ancient writing, the induction of emesis by ingestion of an emetic agent or mechanical stimulation of the hypopharynx was described as a method to prevent poison absorption. It would not be until the 1600s when the use of ipecacuanha for induction of emesis was recommended by William Piso (Reid, 1970).

The use of oral charcoal, now a mainstay in the treatment of many human poisonings, can be dated to early Greek and Roman civilization when wood charcoal was used for the treatment of maladies such as anthrax and epilepsy (Cooney, 1995). The antidotal properties of charcoal were demonstrated in the 1800s by the French with dramatic demonstrations of a reduction in lethality when charcoal was ingested with potentially lethal dosages of arsenic trioxide by Bertrand and strychnine by Touery (Holt & Holz, 1963). One of the earliest reported human studies examining the efficacy of charcoal in poisoning was in 1948 by the American physician Rand (Holt & Holz, 1963). As recently as the early 1960s, poison treatment center employees were known to start their work day by burning toast to create a supply of poison absorbent (charcoal) for the day's work. The use of superheated steam to treat the charcoal to enhance its absorption capacity was reported by Ostrejko, a Russian scientist in 1900 (Greensher *et al.*, 1987). By the 1960s, the use of activated charcoal was routinely recommended for the treatment of patients poisoned with substances thought to be absorbed by charcoal.

The Development of Effective Antidotes for Poisoning

The search for safe and effective antidotes has been challenging to say the least. From the time of the early, self-experimenting proponents of effective antidotes to as recently as the later part of the last century, discovery, refinement, and determination of conditions to permit optimal use of antidotes has been less than ideal. Much the same could be said for the state of drug development more broadly. It was not until the mid-20th century that a more informed scientific and systematic approach to drug development became possible and, in fact, became a requirement by newly created regulatory agencies in charge of controlling the sale and distribution of medicinal products. The therapeutic area of poison treatments and prophylaxis presents several additional hurdles compared to drug development for other, more prevalent disease categories. These challenges include the inability to perform controlled human studies to evaluate efficacy, in part due to the small numbers of poisoned patients available for enrollment in therapeutic trials and also due to the often sporadic occurrence of specific poisonings. These realities make it difficult to readily perform acceptable evaluations of poisoning antidotes. In addition, when trying to transition the nonclinical animal data for poison treatments to humans, there are sometimes significant interspecies differences encountered that make extrapolation of experimental efficacy or safety findings difficult.

INTRODUCTION OF THE POISON CONTROL CENTER

Advances in the field of clinical toxicology and improvements in the quality of care of the poisoned patient have paralleled the evolution of poison control centers. The introduction of the poison center and subsequent formation of associations involving healthcare professionals who work in these centers brought with it an opportunity to share information through publications and national conferences that ultimately resulted in systematic enhancements in the treatment of the poisoned patient. One of the earliest local efforts to systematically collect, analyze, and distribute to physicians, clinical information about poisoning was led by Jay Arena, MD, a Duke University pediatrician. In 1939, he published a case series detailing the clinical outcome of 50 cases of lye poisoning (Martin & Arena, 1939). Interest in clinical information regarding the treatment of poisoned patients and resultant patient outcomes was also growing in Europe during approximately the same time. During the 1940s, several European communities developed hospital-based treatment facilities for poisoning (Manoguerra & Temple, 1984). This local poison information effort continued for several years as further realization of the growing importance of the problem of poisoning occurred. A study by the American Academy of Pediatrics completed in 1952 reported that more than half of childhood accidents involved unintentional poisoning in the United States. Possibly in response to this study, Edward Press, MD, and Louis Gdalman, RPh, started the first United States poison control center in Chicago, Illinois. Mr Gdalman had collected toxicological information on more than 9000 commercial and noncommercial products throughout the 1940s and early 1950s. Their Chicago poison center provided telephone advice to healthcare professionals as well as collected poisoning data systematically during the telephone exchange. These centers grew to become valuable resources for information about product ingredients, potential toxicity, and recommendations for the treatment of poisoned patients. Poison control centers proliferated over the next two decades and peaked at

661 centers in 1978 (Scherz & Robertson, 1978). At the peak of this proliferation, each state in the US had at least one poison center; several states had more than 20 poison centers active at the same time; but there was little standardization throughout the specialty. Information resources gradually evolved from collected experiences of the individual poison center to a centralized collection of product contents, toxicities, and recommended treatments provided in a microfiche database to today's internet-based globally available database that is frequently updated and incorporates consensus recommendations for various treatment protocols for specific poisonings. Through regionalization, consolidation, and certification, the number of poison control centers have significantly decreased to 59 centers in 2011 (Bronstein et al., 2011).

Today, poison centers are generally staffed by a medical director (Medical Toxicologist), administrator or managing director, specialists in poison information, and educators for poison prevention programs. The medical toxicologist, managing director, and specialists in poison information are healthcare professionals who are credentialed by their respective Boards. The American Board of Medical Subspecialties offers a subspecialty certificate in Medical Toxicology to physicians who successfully complete the certifying examination. The American Board of Applied Toxicology (ABAT) offers a certification examination for nonphysicians and the American Association of Poison Control Centers (AAPCC) provides a certification of the specialists in poison information who are usually nurses, pharmacists, or other healthcare personnel. The managing director is usually either the same person as the medical director or a nonphysician certified by the ABAT.

Poison centers provide a significant service to the general public and to practicing medical caregivers. These services include direct information to patients with expert recommendations for needed treatment, critical diagnostic and treatment information for healthcare professionals, education for healthcare personnel, and poison prevention activities through public education. In addition, poison centers now receive partial funding from federal sources in part to serve as a potential early-warning system for potential chemical or biological terrorist attack. Central data collection via the National Poison Data System in near real time has demonstrated the capability of serving as an alert system. Recent food borne outbreaks resulted in clear early signals to alert public health authorities about a potential widespread medical issue (Bronstein et al., 2011).

In addition to this public health alert capability, ability to provide data that can lead to a recognition of improper use of medications, emergence of new illicit drug exposures or practice, prescription product diversion, and product tampering events, studies have shown that poison information centers are cost-effective. An often cited example of the economic benefit of a poison control center comes from a one-year forced closure of the Louisiana State Poison Center some years ago. Without a poison center to call, residents of the community were left with the expensive alternative of visiting a nearby hospital's emergency room or doctor's office visit for possible treatment of their exposure. It was estimated that the increased costs to the state for emergency medical services (EMS) were $1.4 million for that year (King and Palmisano, 1991). Studies have shown that for each dollar spent to operate a poison control center, a savings of approximately $3 to $6.50 can be realized for the healthcare system (Miller and Lestina, 1997).

Recently, the Institute of Medicine (IOM) affirmed the value and need for a poison center system by their commissioned in-depth study of poison prevention and control services in the United States. Their report (IOM, 2004) recommended further standardization of the regional poison centers, partial federal funding for the poison center system to stabilize core functions of each center and integration of poison control centers with public health agencies at the federal, state, and local level including integration with the Centers for Disease Control and Prevention for chemical and biological terrorism preparedness.

CLINICAL STRATEGY FOR THE TREATMENT OF THE POISONED PATIENT

The setting for the initial treatment of a seriously poisoned patient is usually in a hospital emergency room but can sometimes be in other, less ideal settings such as the battlefield, workplace, home, or street setting. In treatment environments that permit a complete assessment and initiation of treatments, most clinical toxicologists agree that a methodically executed, stepwise approach for the evaluation and treatment of the poisoned patient is recommended for optimal care (Goldfrank, 2006; Ellenhorn, 1997a,b). In this section, an overview of the general approach to the treatment of poisoned patients in the emergency department (ED) or acute intensive care setting of a hospital will be described. In that setting, the following general steps represent important elements of the initial clinical encounter for a poisoned patient:

1. Clinical stabilization of the patient
2. Clinical evaluation (history, physical, laboratory, radiology)
3. Prevention of further toxicant absorption
4. Enhancement of toxicant elimination
5. Administration of antidote (if available)
6. Supportive care, close monitoring, and clinical follow-up

Clinical Stabilization

The first priority in the treatment of poisoning is to stabilize the patient. Assessment of the patient's airway (ability to move air into and out of the lungs), breathing (the presence of spontaneous respirations), and circulation (adequate blood pressure and perfusion of vital organs) is the initial step of emergency treatment. Some poisoned patients, soon after even a potentially lethal exposure of the toxicant has occurred, will not show significant symptoms. Most poisoned patients, with a toxic exposure, will exhibit symptoms early in their presentation. For this reason, the initial triage of a poisoned patient can be difficult. On occasion, the patient is asymptomatic on presentation but by history has had a potentially serious toxic exposure. Clinicians and medical support staff, who may not be knowledgeable about the toxic exposure level of a specific drug or chemical, may mistakenly stratify the patient to a lower treatment priority, which can have disastrous results. The improper stratification sometimes can include a delay in calling for a clinical toxicology consultation from a regional poison control center or regional poison treatment center. Some drugs, such as a benzodiazepine, can cause significant sedation early after exposure but often have a comparatively mild clinical course, whereas other chemicals, such as camphor, show little clinical effects initially but can produce a fatal outcome. Some chemicals and drugs can cause seizures as part of their toxic-effect profile. Control of drug/toxicant-induced seizures can be an important component of the initial stabilization of the poisoned patient. A full discussion of the various methods available to treat abnormal conditions with a patient's airway, breathing, and circulation is beyond the scope of this chapter. The reader is referred to textbooks of *Emergency Medicine and Critical Care Medicine* for further information on this subject. After the initial stabilization of the patient, the remainder of the assessment and treatment steps

can proceed. On occasion, especially in critically ill patients, treatment interventions are initiated before a patient is completely stable.

Clinical History in the Poisoned Patient

The primary goal of obtaining the medical history in poisoned patients is to determine the substance the patient was exposed to and the extent and timing of exposure. Unfortunately, in contrast to most specialties of medicine, the clinical history from the initial clinical encounter with the poisoned patient is sometimes not available because either the patient is unresponsive and unable to provide the history or the history provided is unreliable. The history may be unreliable due to inability of the patient to recall pertinent facts relating to the ingestion or exposure or in the setting of an attempted suicide or patient who has taken illegal substances, the patient often is not willing to provide an accurate history. For these reasons, additional sources for the clinical history are often incorporated to aid the clinical team in determining the exposure history. Examples of additional resources sometimes employed to obtain an informative clinical history include interviewing family members, emergency medical technicians who were at the scene, a pharmacist who can sometimes provide a listing of prescriptions recently filled, or an employer who can provide a list of chemicals found in the work environment for an occupational exposure.

When estimating the extent of exposure to the poison, it is generally recommended that one maximize the estimate dose received. That is, one should assume that the entire contents of the prescription bottle were ingested, that the entire bottle of liquid was consumed, most of the body surface area was exposed to a topical chemical, or that the highest possible concentration of airborne contaminant was present for a patient poisoned by inhalation unless definite evidence exists to the contrary. Maximizing the potential dose or exposure level allows one to prepare adequately for the expected, likely toxic effects and reduces the probability of encountering an unexpected clinical outcome in a poisoned patient.

Once an appropriate estimate of the dose is made, the toxicologist can refer to various information resources to determine what the range of expected clinical effects might be from the estimated exposure. This is one of the most important early functions of the poison center. The estimation of expected toxicity greatly assists with the triage of poisoned patients. Poison information specialists working in Poison Information Centers routinely give telephone recommendations regarding the level of medical care required for a given ingestion based on the expected clinical effects from the reported ingestion. The vast majority of in-the-home accidental pediatric exposures are treated with at-home observation, home-administered activated charcoal, or less commonly the induction of emesis. In the hospital setting, ED staff use the estimation of expected clinical effects to effectively triage the poisoned patient. For example, a three-year-old patient who accidentally ingested 25 children's chewable multivitamins without iron would likely be triaged to a noncritical care area of the ED, whereas another similar patient who ingested a large amount of a potent anticholinergic chemical would be triaged to a high intensity of care section of the ED.

Estimating the timing of the exposure to the poison is frequently the most difficult aspect of the clinical history when treating the poisoned patient. Often the toxicologist must turn detective to determine the most likely window of time that the exposure occurred. For example, if a pediatric patient was being watched by a baby-sitter at all times except for a 20-minute period that preceded the onset of symptoms and the discovery of an open prescription bottle for digoxin is found, then it is straightforward to assume that the ingestion occurred in that 20-minute window. Other

Table 33-1

Clinical Features of Toxic Syndromes

	BLOOD PRESSURE	PULSE	TEMPERATURE	PUPILS	LUNGS	ABDOMEN	NEUROLOGICAL
Sympathomimetic	Incr.	Incr.	Slight Incr.	Mydriasis	NC	NC	Hyperalert, incr. Reflexes
Anticholinergic	Slight incr. or NC	Incr.	Incr.	Mydriasis	NC	Decr. Bowel sounds	Altered mental status
Cholinergic	Slight decr. or NC	Decr.	NC	Miosis	Incr. bronchial sounds	Incr. bowel sounds	Altered mental status
Opioid	Decr.	Decr.	Decr.	Miosis	NC or rales (late)	Decr. Bowel sounds	Decr. Level of consciousness

situations require estimation of a far broader window for exposure. For a person found down with several empty prescription bottles nearby who was not seen by anyone for the preceding 24 hours, one would not be able to accurately estimate the time of ingestion other than sometime in that 24-hour window. Therefore, in view of these often-encountered limitations, obtaining an accurate history in the poisoned patient can be very challenging and occasionally completely lacking. When the history is unobtainable or unreliable, the treating clinical toxicologist is left in the setting of empirical treatment of an "unknown ingestion" poisoning. This type of treatment will be discussed later in this chapter.

Physical Examination

One of the most important actions performed during the initial clinical encounter in the treatment of the poisoned patient is the physical examination. A thorough examination of the patient is required to assess the patient's condition, determine the patient's mental status and, if altered, determine possible nontoxicology explanations for the abnormal mental status such as trauma or central nervous system infection. In addition, findings from the physical examination allow one to categorize the patient's physical examination parameters into broad classes referred to as toxic syndromes. These toxic syndromes have been called toxidromes (Mofenson & Greensher, 1970). A toxidrome is a constellation of clinical signs and symptoms that, when taken together, are likely associated with exposure from certain toxicological classes of chemicals. The major toxic syndromes include narcotic, cholinergic, sympathomimetic, and anticholinergic. Table 33-1 lists the clinical features of these major toxic syndromes.

In certain treatment settings, the precise agent responsible for the poisoning is not known during the critically important phase of initial treatment of the poisoned patient. When the treating physicians are able to categorize the patient's presentation into a toxic syndrome, it permits initiation of rationale treatment based on the most likely category of toxin responsible without knowing the specific chemical causing the poisoning. For example, if a patient presents with altered mental status, mydriasis (dilated pupils), mild hypertension, tachycardia, warm skin, dry mucous membranes, and diminished bowel sounds in the abdomen, the clinical toxicologist can characterize the patient's presentation as consistent with the anticholinergic toxic syndrome. The treatment would then be directed at support of respiration and potentially administering a pharmacological antidote like physostigmine as well as additional situation-requiring supportive care.

Occasionally, a characteristic odor can be detected on the poisoned patient's breath or clothing, which may point toward exposure or poisoning by a specific agent. Table 33-2 lists some of the better recognized odors and the substance associated with the odor. Detection of one of these odors may provide an important historical clue as to the agent responsible for the poisoning.

Periodic re-examination of the patient is a very important aspect of clinical toxicology treatment procedures. Follow-up clinical examinations can help gauge the progression of the clinical course of poisoning as well as determine the effectiveness of treatment interventions and assess the need for additional treatment procedures.

Laboratory Evaluation

A common misconception concerning the initial treatment of poisoned patients is that a definitive diagnosis of the specific agent or poison responsible for the patient's clinical presentation is frequently made by the clinical laboratory during the initial patient evaluation. Unfortunately, the availability of an assay to identify the specific chemical on a rapid turn-around basis (STAT, eg, within one hour) is very limited. Table 33-3 lists drugs or other chemical tests that are typically available for STAT measurement in a medical center type hospital facility. As one can see, the number of chemicals for which quantitative detection is possible in the rapid turn-around timeline is extremely limited, compared to the number of possible chemicals that can poison patients. This further emphasizes the importance of recognizing clinical syndromes for poisoning and for the clinical toxicologist to be able to initiate general treatment and supportive care for the patient with poisoning from an unknown substance.

For the relatively few substances that can be measured on a rapid turn-around basis in an ED setting, the quantitative measurement

Table 33-2

Characteristic Odors Associated With Poisonings

ODOR	POTENTIAL POISON
Bitter almonds	Cyanide
Eggs	Hydrogen sulfide, mercaptans
Garlic	As, organophosphates, DMSO, thallium
Mothballs	Naphthalene, camphor
Vinyl	Ethchlorvynol
Wintergreen	Methylsalicylate

DMSO, dimethyl sulfoxide.

Table 33-3

List of Tests That are Commonly Measured in a Hospital Setting on a STAT Basis

Acetaminophen	Osmolality
Acetone	Phenobarbital
Carbamazepine	Phenytoin
Carboxyhemoglobin	Procainamide/NAPA
Digoxin	Quinidine
Ethanol	Salicylates
Gentamicin	Theophylline
Iron	Tobramycin
Lithium	Valproic Acid
Methemoglobin	

NAPA, N-acetylprocainamide.

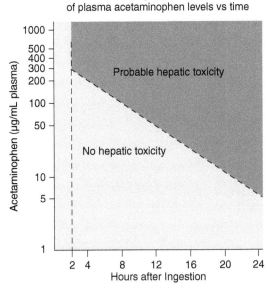

Figure 33-1. *Rumack-Mathew nomogram for acetaminophen poisoning.* SOURCE: From Rumack and Mathew, 1975, with permission. Copyright American Academy of Pediatrics, 1975.

can often provide both prognostic and therapeutic guidance. Several authors have suggested certain "action levels" for specific therapeutic drugs and chemicals, which when met or exceeded in the patient's plasma should trigger specific interventions or predict likely clinical outcomes. In some cases, measurement of an indicator of the biological effect of a poison provides sufficient information to render definitive treatment to the patient. Measurement of methemoglobin concentration in a patient poisoned by one of many chemicals that can cause this chemical transformation of the hemoglobin molecule is sufficient to initiate treatment for methemoglobinemia without identification of the specific toxicant that caused the condition. Similarly, most hospital laboratories have the capability for rapid measurement of carboxyhemoglobin concentrations, which permits treatment of carbon monoxide poisoning based on the laboratory test measuring a surrogate marker for carbon monoxide exposure.

For some commonly ingested drugs, a nomogram has been established to predict the severity of the poisoning and is important in some cases to guide therapeutic intervention based on the measured plasma concentration of the drug and the time elapsed from the expose. Proper use of such nomograms is necessary for the clinical management of poisoning cases.

The clinical usefulness of a drug plasma concentration measured by the clinical laboratory was suggested for salicylates approximately 50 years ago. In 1960, Done published a nomogram to predict the clinical outcome from poisoning with salicylates (Done, 1960).

In 1975, Rumack and Mathews published a nomogram for acetaminophen poisoning shown in Fig. 33-1 (Rumack & Mathew, 1975). This nomogram predicts clinical outcome and is also valuable to guide the clinician in the decision as to whether or not to administer *N*-acetylcysteine (NAC), an antidote for significant acetaminophen ingestion. Laboratory evaluation of a patient potentially poisoned with acetaminophen is crucial to assess what hepatic injury may have already occurred and to determine plasma concentrations of acetaminophen for prognostic purposes. Accurate estimation of acetaminophen in the plasma should be done on samples drawn at least four hours after ingestion, when or past the time that peak plasma levels can be expected. Once an accurate plasma concentration of acetaminophen has been obtained, it should be plotted on the Rumack–Matthew nomogram (Fig. 33-1) to determine whether NAC therapy is indicated. This nomogram is based on a series of patients with and without hepatotoxicity and their corresponding acetaminophen plasma concentrations at presentation.

In the appropriate patient, the decision to treat an acetaminophen-poisoned patient is based on the plasma concentration of parent acetaminophen plotted on the nomogram. Although some authors recommend that NAC treatment only be administered to a patient with an acetaminophen plasma concentration in the "definite toxic" range, most clinical toxicologist agree that NAC should be given at or above the "probably toxic" action level due to the often present uncertainty in the clinical history with respect to the exact time of the ingestion. It should be noted, however, that proper use of this nomogram is required, namely that certain conditions should be met to apply the nomogram to a specific clinical case. The nomogram was validated for a single acetaminophen ingestion, the time of ingestion is critically important to establish the X-axis coordinate for the data point and the plasma concentration should have been obtained at least four hours after ingestion to assure that the peak plasma concentration of parent acetaminophen has occurred.

Similar, though, perhaps less well established, predictive relationships of drug plasma concentration and clinical outcome and/or suggested concentrations that require therapeutic interventions are available for several other drugs including lithium, salicylates, digoxin, iron, phenobarbital, and theophylline. Some authors have identified "action levels" or toxic threshold values for the measured plasma concentrations of various drugs or chemicals (Ellenhorn, 1997a,b). Generally, these values represent mean concentrations of the respective substance that have been shown to produce a significant harmful effect during a retrospective analysis of clinical case series. The pharmaco- (or toxico-) dynamic variability for a given toxicant or for a combination of toxicant is significant, however. For example, a patient with a "normal" or "nontoxic" digoxin level may display significant toxic effects and conversely a patient with an elevated or "toxic" plasma concentration of digoxin may not show any sign of harmful effects. The clinical toxicologist is required to critically evaluate the measured drug concentration in context of the clinical presentation of the patient and not react to the measured value alone.

Because of the limited clinical availability of "diagnostic" laboratory tests for poisons, toxicologists can gain important insight into a suspected list of ingested drugs and other chemicals by performing simple calculations based on routine clinical laboratory data. Two examples of these calculated clinical parameters are the anion gap (AG) and the osmol gap calculations. An elevated AG or osmol

Table 33-4

Differential Diagnosis of Metabolic Acidosis With Elevated Anion Gap: "AT MUD PILES"

A	Alcohol (ethanol ketoacidosis)
T	Toluene
M	Methanol
U	Uremia
D	Diabetic ketoacidosis
P	Paraldehyde
I	Iron, isoniazid
L	Lactic acid
E	Ethylene glycol
S	Salicylate

Table 33-5

Differential Diagnosis of Elevated Osmol Gap

Methanol
Ethanol
Ethylene glycol
Isopropanol

gap suggests a differential diagnosis for significant exposures in a poisoned patient. Both calculations are used as diagnostic aids when the clinical history suggests poisoning and the patient's condition is consistent with exposure to chemicals known to cause elevations of these parameters (ie, metabolic acidosis, altered mental status, etc).

The AG is calculated as the difference between the serum Na ion concentration and the sum of the serum Cl and HCO_3 ion concentrations.

$$AG = [Na\ mEq/L - (Cl\ mEq/L + HCO_3\ mEq/L)]$$
$$Normal\ AG \leq 12$$

When there is laboratory evidence of metabolic acidosis (low blood pH and low serum HCO_3) in a poisoned patient, the finding of an elevated AG would suggest systemic toxicity from a relatively finite list of chemicals. A popular clinical pneumonic (AT MUD PILES) is commonly employed as a memory aid for this differential diagnosis. Table 33-4 lists the more common chemicals that have metabolic acidosis with an elevated AG as part of the clinical presentation that are included in this pneumonic.

The second calculated parameter from clinical chemistry values is the osmol gap. The osmol gap is calculated as the numerical difference between the measured serum osmolality and the serum osmolarity calculated from the clinical chemistry measurements of the serum sodium ion, glucose, and blood urea nitrogen (BUN) concentrations (Smithline & Gardner, 1976).

$$Osmol\ gap = measured\ serum\ osmolality\ (mOsm)$$
$$- calculated\ serum\ osmolarity\ (mOsm)$$

where calculated serum osmolarity = $2 \times Na\ mEq/L + glucose\ mg/dL\ /18 + BUN\ mg/dL\ /2.8$

Normal osmol gap < 10 mOsm

Note that the serum osmolality must be measured by freezing point depression and not boiling point elevation as the later method can fail to detect the osmolality contribution of volatile, low molecular weight substances due to vaporization of the substance during measurement.

An elevated osmol gap in the setting of a poisoned patient suggests the presence of an osmotically active substance in the plasma that is not accounted for by the Na, glucose, or BUN concentrations. Table 33-5 lists several substances that when ingested can be associated with an elevated osmol gap in humans.

Although calculation of both the AG and the osmol gap can provide very useful information from readily available clinical chemistry measurements, these determinations must be interpreted cautiously in certain clinical settings. For example, even though a patient may have ingested a large, significantly toxic amount of methanol, if measured late in the clinical course of the exposure, the osmol gap may not be significantly elevated as most of the osmotically active methanol has left the plasma and has been biotransformed or cleared but is still producing serious clinical effects.

Radiographic Examination

The utility of the radiographic examination to diagnose specific poisonings is relatively limited. This is due primarily to the lack of radiopacity of many oral forms of medication. Early radiographic surveys of the radiopacity of oral medications revealed that the vast majority of commercially available tablets and capsules surveyed were essentially undetectable by radiograph (Handy, 1971; O'Brien *et al.*, 1986). These and other studies have shown that relatively few formulations of drugs are radiopaque and would likely be detectable by plain X-ray of the abdomen. Generally, plain radiographs can detect a significant amount of ingested oral medication containing ferrous or potassium salts. However, a study of the in vitro and in vivo visualization of chewable oral formulations of iron supplements showed that once the chewable iron was ingested, it was no longer detectable by plain abdominal radiograph (Everson *et al.*, 1989). However, certain formulations that have an enteric coating or certain types of sustained release products are radiopaque and can be visualized (Savitt *et al.*, 1987; Nelson *et al.*, 1993).

The most useful radiographs ordered in an overdose or poisoned patient include the chest and abdominal radiographs and the computed head tomography study. The abdominal radiograph has been used to detect recent lead paint ingestion in children due to pica for many years. Although the presence of radiographic evidence of lead-based paint chips probably underrepresented the proportion of children with moderate-to-severe lead poisoning in one study, an abdominal radiograph showing pica was associated with significantly elevated blood lead concentrations (McElvaine *et al.*, 1992). Another situation in which an abdominal radiograph may be helpful is the setting of a halogenated hydrocarbon such as carbon tetrachloride or chloroform. If a sufficient amount of either liquid is ingested, it is likely that these organic solvents will be visualized as a radiopaque liquid in the gut lumen on the abdominal film relatively recently after ingestion (Dally *et al.*, 1987). Finally, abdominal plain radiographs have been helpful in the setting where foreign bodies are detected in the gastrointestinal tract. An example of this is in the situation where an international traveler coming to the United States becomes acutely ill with signs of severe sympathomimetic excess and numerous foreign bodies are visualized throughout the gastrointestinal tract. This type of patient is referred to as a body packer who smuggles illegal substances, such as cocaine or heroin, by swallowing latex or plastic storage vesicles filled with the substance (Beerman *et al.*, 1986; McCarron & Wood, 1983; Sporer & Firestone, 1997). Occasionally, these storage devices rupture and the drug is released into the gastrointestinal tract with serious and sometimes fatal results. Aside from these relatively uncommon situations, the overall clinical utility for detection and diagnosis of poisons by radiography is limited.

In contrast to the limited clinical utility of plain radiography for the identification of a specific poison or to diagnose poisoning, plain radiography and other types of diagnostic imaging in clinical toxicology can be extremely valuable for the diagnosis of toxicant-induced pathology and to aid the clinical toxicologist in the ongoing treatment and patient-management phases of the drug overdose. Detection of drug-induced noncardiac pulmonary edema is associated with serious intoxication with salicylates and opioid agonists (Stern *et al.*, 1968; Heffner *et al.*, 1990). Plain chest radiography can detect this abnormality, which would likely correlate with the findings observed during physical examination of the lungs. This radiographic finding would increase the severity stratification of the poisoning case and potentially alter the planned therapeutic strategy for the patient.

Another example of the use of radiological imaging in clinical toxicology is with computed tomography (CT) of the brain. Significant exposure to carbon monoxide (CO) has been associated with CT lesions of the brain consisting of low-density areas in the cerebral white matter and in the basal ganglia, especially the globus pallidus. Although not clinically employed for diagnostic purposes in the acute phases of a CO poisoning, these CT findings of the brain have been useful for estimating the prognosis for a patient who survives the initial phase of CO poisoning (Miura *et al.*, 1985; Jones *et al.*, 1994). Finally, concurrent intracranial pathology, such as trauma or hemorrhage can be detected by CT or MRI of the brain to aid in the diagnosis of additional injury or pathology previously not appreciated during the treatment of a poisoned patient.

The initial clinical evaluation of the poisoned patient is a critically important phase of the therapeutic process to treat poisoned individuals. The physical, laboratory, and radiological examination all contribute to the initial diagnostic steps for poison treatment. The physical and laboratory examinations are generally utilized more from a diagnostic and acute management standpoint, whereas the radiological examination tends to be more useful for detection and management of toxicant-induced pathology.

Prevention of Further Poison Absorption

During the early phases of treatment of a poisoned patient who has had a toxic exposure via the oral, inhalation, or the topical route, the opportunity to prevent further absorption of the poison to minimize the total amount of chemical that reaches the systemic circulation may be possible. For chemicals presented by the inhalation route, the main intervention to prevent further absorption is removal of the patient from the environment where the toxin is found and to provide adequate ventilation and oxygenation for the patient. For topical exposures, patient clothing containing the chemical must be removed and properly disposed in airtight wrappings or containers to ensure that the rescuers and healthcare providers are adequately protected from secondary exposure. Most topical exposures require gentle washing of the skin with water and mild soap taking care not to cause cutaneous abrasions of the skin that may enhance dermal absorption.

The optimal time to intervene to prevent continued absorption of an oral poison is as soon as possible after the ingestion. The four primary methods are currently available for this purpose: induction of emesis with syrup of ipecac, gastric lavage, oral administration of activated charcoal, and whole-bowel irrigation. Historically, induction of emesis was accomplished by a variety of concoctions such as tartar emetic, an antimony salt, mustard mixed in water, concentrated solutions of copper and zinc salts, and various botanical substances. In hospitals, apomorphine injection was given even in the 1980s to cause emesis in patients with a history of potentially toxic ingestion. At present, syrup of ipecac is the only agent available for induction of emesis in the treatment of a potentially toxic ingestion. Although a mainstay for poison center-directed induction of emesis for decades, this agent is rarely used today as efficacy and studies of clinical outcomes associated with use of syrup of ipecac have called into question the overall benefit of its use. Syrup of ipecac as a chemical for the prevention of toxicant absorption has largely been replaced by activated charcoal, which is discussed below. As stated, the efficacy to remove gastric contents, and therefore minimize subsequent absorption of the chemical declines with increase in the time interval between poison ingestion and syrup of ipecac administration (Neuvonen *et al.*, 1983). An important area of concern with the decline in use and eventually availability of syrup of ipecac is that, for chemicals not adsorbed by activated charcoal, there exists a potential void for effective therapy to prevent further absorption of orally ingested toxins. The American Academy of Clinical Toxicology and the European Association of Poisons Centres and Clinical Toxicologists issued a position paper regarding the use of syrup of ipecac in 2004, which stated that the syrup of ipecac should not be used routinely in the management of the poisoned patient and that there was insufficient data to either support or exclude ipecac administration soon after poison ingestion (Krenzelok *et al.*, 2004). Many clinical toxicologists believe that there remains a limited role for the clinical use of syrup of ipecac, mainly is rural areas where the length of time before a poisoned patient can reach medical care is significant, especially when the chemical ingested is poorly adsorbed to activated charcoal. The accepted contraindications for use of syrup of ipecac are (1) children less than six months of age; (2) in the ingestion of a caustic agent (acid or alkali); (3) in a patient with a depressed level of consciousness or gag reflex or when the toxicant ingested is expected to cause either condition within a short period of time; or (4) when there is a significant risk of aspiration of gastric contents such as for ingestion of a liquid hydrocarbon with high aspiration potential.

The use of gastric lavage, the technique of placing an orogastric tube into the stomach and aspirating fluid then cyclically instilling fluid and aspirating until the effluent is clear, has also diminished significantly in recent years. The reasons for the decline in use of this technique include a growing appreciation of the risk of aspiration during the lavage procedure and growing evidence that the effectiveness of gastric lavage may be more limited than originally thought. Like induction of emesis, where the efficacy of the procedure declines with increasing time interval between use of the procedure and the time of ingestion, gastric lavage too has this important limitation. Careful attention to the patient's gag reflex prior to initiation of this procedure is important. If the patient does not exhibit a gag reflex, then endotracheal intubation must be performed to adequately protect the airway and prevent aspiration. Most clinical toxicologists would agree that the current role of gastric lavage, if there is a role at all, would be in the initial treatment of the overdose patient who had a recent (within one hour) oral ingestion, especially in the cases where it is likely that activated charcoal will not be effective. It is essential that the orogastric tube be of sufficient size (40–44 French for an adult) to be useful. Even with a large bore orogastric tube some tablets or capsules may not be able to pass through the tube. In the pediatric patient, there are practical limitations to the use of large bore tubes. In this case, orogastric lavage may only be useful to attempt removal of liquid toxins or possibly dissolved tablets or capsules. Due to recent questioning of the effectiveness of the technique and the availability of data showing that other modalities for prevention of further toxin absorption (eg, oral activated charcoal) are possibly as or more effective, the use of gastric lavage has greatly diminished.

As described earlier, the medicinal use of charcoal dates back more than 150 years. The first reported medicinal use of oral charcoal to adsorb an ingested toxin is credited to the American physician, Hort, who, in 1834, used large amounts of powdered charcoal to successfully treat a patient poisoned with a chloride salt of mercury. A dramatic demonstration of the adsorptive effect of oral charcoal was that by Tourey, a French pharmacist who reportedly mixed a lethal dose of strychnine with charcoal and consumed the combination before his colleagues at the French Academy in 1930 (Andersen, 1946). Early in vitro investigations of the adsorptive properties of activated charcoal demonstrated the effect of charcoal on various chemical substances in aqueous solutions (Andersen, 1946), the effect of pH on charcoal adsorption properties (Andersen, 1947), and the effect of activated charcoal on the adsorption of strychnine from gastric contents (Andersen, 1948).

During the last 20 to 30 years there has been an increasing use of oral charcoal as a therapeutic intervention for oral poisoning. For many years, orally administered activated charcoal has been routinely incorporated into the initial treatment of a patient poisoned by the oral route. The term "activated" refers to the substantially increased adsorptive capacity that results from the processing of charcoal obtained from the burning of carbonaceous substances such as wood pulp, sugars, organic material, and industrial wastes. The processing involves extensive treatment with steam, carbon dioxide, oxygen, zinc chloride, sulfuric acid, or phosphoric acid at temperatures of 500°F to 900°F "activate" the residue oxidation, which leads to a significant increase in surface area through creation of small pores in the material. Many organic molecules are significantly bound to activated charcoal. Generally, low molecular weight and polar compounds such as ethanol tend to be less well bound to activated charcoal. Substances such as lithium, iron, and certain inorganic salts are also not appreciably bound. In acute oral overdose, activated charcoal is typically administered at a dosage of 1.0 to 1.5 g/kg. When the patient is unable to safely drink the charcoal it is placed into the stomach via orogastric or nasogastric tube.

The incorporation of the procedure of whole bowel irrigation for the treatment of the poisoned patient has gained acceptance in specific poisoning situations. Whole bowel irrigation is a procedure that cleanses the lumen of the gastrointestinal tract. The procedure is accomplished with a poorly absorbed, osmotically neutral polyethylene glycol electrolyte solution that is administered orally to expel the contents of the intestines via the rectal route. This procedure is the same as that used to prepare a patient for endoscopic medical procedures of the large intestine. The best evidence for efficacy of this procedure in the setting of poisoning is for removal of ingested packets of illegal drugs swallowed by people smuggling the material and hoping to avoid detection by concealing the agents in their intestines. Sometimes, these containers may leak and begin to cause symptoms that often lead the carrier to detection and treatment. Additional uses for this gastrointestinal decontamination technique are to prevent the ongoing absorption of sustained release formulations of drugs and for the early treatment of ingestions of substantial amounts of iron preparations (Tenebein et al., 2004).

Most clinical toxicologists agree that, for the prevention of further absorption following oral ingestion of most chemicals, the administration of oral activated charcoal provides the most consistent efficacy and best safety profile (Goldfrank, 2006). The other modalities described above have more limited roles (whole bowel irrigation, gastric lavage, syrup of ipecac) for use in the treatment of a poisoned patient. Most treatment centers favor the use of activated charcoal without gastric decontamination (lavage or ipecac)

for treatment of oral poisoning and drug overdose. Many poison control centers recommend home use of a premixed slurry of activated charcoal for immediate treatment of potentially significant poisonings. The use of ipecac syrup is largely limited to individual patients in whom it is likely to make a difference in outcome, who are in rural environments, hours away from more definitive medical treatment, in whom it appears to be the most effective method available in that particular set of circumstances, or in whom it is the only method available to attempt gastric emptying.

Enhancement of Poison Elimination

There are several methods available to enhance the elimination of specific poisons or drugs once they have been absorbed into the systemic circulation. The primary methods employed for this use today include alkalinization of the urine, hemodialysis, hemoperfusion, hemofiltration, plasma exchange or exchange transfusion, and the administration of oral activated charcoal serially during the treatment time course.

The use of urinary alkalinization results in the enhancement of the renal clearance of certain weak acids. The basic principle applied is to increase urinary filtrate pH to a level sufficient to ionize the weak acid and prevent renal tubule reabsorption of the molecule. This is also referred to as ion trapping. The ion-trapping phenomenon occurs when the pK_a of the chemical is such that after glomerular filtration into the renal tubules, alteration of the pH of the urinary filtrate can ionize and "trap" the agent in the urinary filtrate. Once the toxin is ionized, reabsorption from the renal tubules is greatly reduced and more of the drug remains in the urinary filtrate, and therefore is excreted in the urine. See Fig. 33-2 for a schematic representation of ion trapping for salicylate.

Clinical use of this alkalinization procedure requires adequate urine flow and close clinical monitoring including that of the pH of the urine. The procedure is accomplished by adding sterile sodium bicarbonate to sterile water with 5% dextrose for intravenous (IV) infusion and administering the mixture intravenously to titrate the urine pH to 7.5 to 8.5. The drugs for which this procedure has been shown clinically efficacious include salicylate compounds and phenobarbital that have pK_as of 3.2 and 7.4, respectively. The increase in total body clearance for salicylate for example, by increasing urinary pH from 5.0 to 8.0 can be substantial. The AAPCC and the European Association of Poisons Centres and Clinical Toxicologists 2004 Position Paper on Urinary Alkalinization recommends this procedure for moderately severe salicylate poisoning for patient not meeting criteria for hemodialysis (Proudfoot et al., 2004).

Theoretically, there are similar advantages to be gained from acidification of the urine regarding enhancement of clearance of drugs such as amphetamine and phencyclidine; however, there are significant adverse events associated with acidification such as acute renal failure and acid-base and electrolyte disturbances. For this reason, acidification of the urine is not recommended as a therapeutic intervention in the treatment of poisoning.

The dialysis techniques, either hemodialysis, continuous venous filtration, or peritoneal dialysis, relies on passage of the toxic chemical through a semipermeable dialysis membrane (or the peritoneal membrane for peritoneal dialysis) so that it can equilibrate with the dialysate and subsequently be removed. Hemodialysis incorporates a blood pump to pass blood next to a dialysis membrane to allow chemicals permeable to the membrane to pass through and reach equilibrium. In order for this method to be clinically beneficial, the chemical must have a relatively low volume of distribution, low protein binding, a relatively high degree of water solubility, and low molecular weight. Use of hemodialysis

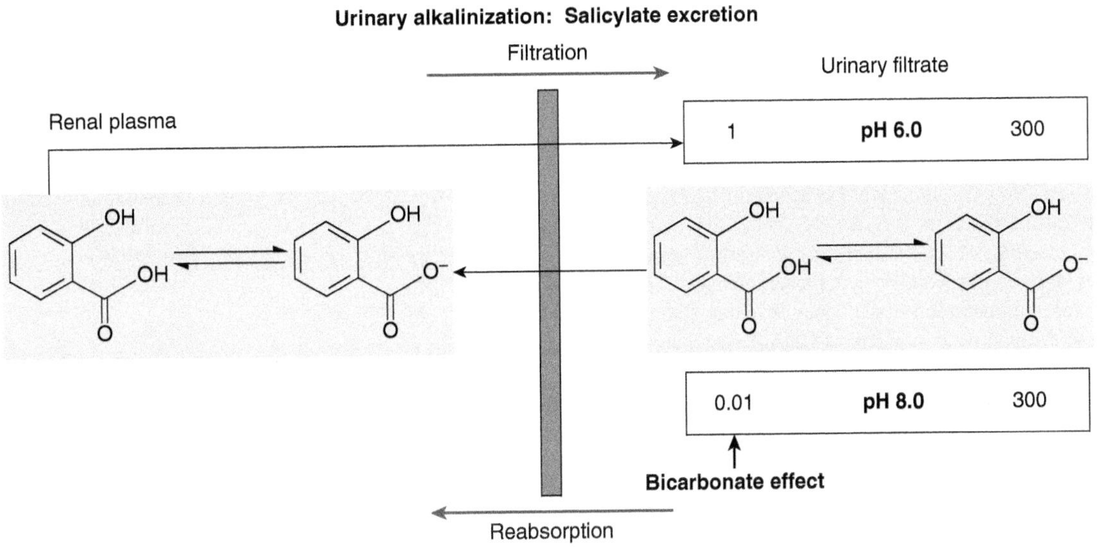

Urinary alkalinization: Salicylate excretion

Figure 33-2. *Ion trapping schematic for salicylate in the renal tubule.*

to attempt to remove a chemical with the later three characteristics but with a high volume of distribution such as digoxin would not be clinically beneficial, because the vast majority of the drug is not in the physiological compartment (blood) accessible to the dialysis membrane. Therefore, despite hemodialysis being able to effectively clear the digoxin in plasma during the dialysis run, most of the body burden of digoxin is located outside of the blood compartment and is not appreciably affected by the procedure. Similarly, if a drug is highly protein-bound, only a small percentage (the free fraction) would be available to pass through the dialysis membrane and be cleared from the body. Some drugs, such as phenobarbital, can readily cross these membranes and go from a high concentration in plasma to a lower concentration in the dialysate. Phenobarbital has a relatively low volume of distribution (0.5–0.7 L/kg) and protein binding (30%–50%), so there is a reasonable opportunity for enough drug to be removed from the total body burden to make the technique valuable in serious cases of overdose (Brown *et al.*, 1985; Cutler *et al.*, 1987). Drugs and chemicals for which hemodialysis has been shown to be clinically effective in the treatment of poisoning by these agents is shown in Table 33-6.

The technique of hemoperfusion is similar to hemodialysis except there is no dialysis membrane or dialysate involved in the procedure. The patient's blood is pumped through a perfusion cartridge where it is in direct contact with adsorptive material (usually activated charcoal) that has a coating of material such as cellulose or a heparin-containing gel to prevent the adsorptive material from

being carried back to the patient's circulation. The principle characteristics for a drug or other chemical to be successfully removed by this technique are low volume of distribution and adsorption by activated charcoal. This method can be used successfully with lipid soluble compounds and with higher molecular weight compounds than for hemodialysis. Protein binding does not significantly interfere with removal by hemoperfusion. Because of the more direct contact of the patient's blood with the adsorptive material, the medical risks of this procedure include thrombocytopenia, hypocalcemia, and leukopenia. This technique is primarily used for the treatment of serious theophylline overdose, and possibly amanita toxin exposure, as well as paraquat and meprobamate poisoning. The technique is seldom used currently and it is possible that access to the sterile hemoperfusion cartridge necessary for the procedure may be limited, even at major medical centers.

The use of the technique of hemofiltration for the treatment of poisoning has been suggested as an additional modality for enhancement of chemical elimination. During this procedure, the patient's blood is delivered through hollow fiber tubes and an ultrafiltrate of plasma is removed by hydrostatic pressure from the blood side of the membrane. Different membrane pore sizes are available for use so the size of the filtered molecules can be controlled during the procedure. The perfusion pressure for the technique is either generated by the patient's blood pressure (for arteriovenous hemofiltration) or by a blood pump (for venovenous hemofiltration). Needed fluid and electrolytes removed in the ultrafiltrate are replaced intravenously with sterile solutions. The procedure has the advantage of running continuously as opposed to the four- to six-hour limitation for a hemodialysis treatment cycle. One potential advantage of continuous filtration versus intermittent hemodialysis is that the rebound phenomenon (increase in plasma toxin concentration shortly after hemodialysis is terminated—due to redistribution of the toxicant from the nonvascular, tissue, compartment to the vascular space) is not seen with hemofiltration due to the continuous nature of the procedure. This rebound is commonly seen during hemodialysis for lithium overdose (Bosinski *et al.*, 1998). Whether or not hemofiltration becomes a more commonly employed technique in poisoning treatment is unclear at this time.

The use of either plasma exchange or exchange transfusions has been relatively limited in the field of clinical toxicology. Although the techniques afford the potential advantage of being able to remove high molecular weight and/or plasma protein-bound

Table 33-6

Chemicals for Which Hemodialysis Has Been Shown Effective as a Treatment Modality for Poisoning

Alcohols	Meprobamate
Antibiotics	Metformin
Boric acid	Paraldehyde
Bromide	Phenobarbital
Calcium	Potassium
Chloral hydrate	Salicylates
Fluorides	Strychnine
Iodides	Theophylline
Isoniazid	Thiocynates
Lithium	Valproic acid

toxicants, the clinical utility in poison treatment has been limited. Plasma exchange or plasma pheresis involves removal of plasma and replacement with frozen donor plasma, albumin, or both with IV fluid. The risks and complications of this technique include allergic-type reactions, infectious complications, and hypotension (Mokrzycki *et al.*, 1994). Exchange transfusion involves replacement of a patient's blood volume with donor blood. The use of this technique in poison treatment is relatively uncommon and mostly confined to the setting of inadvertent drug overdose in a neonate or premature infant in the setting of a neonatal intensive care unit.

Serial oral administration of activated charcoal, also referred to as multiple-dose activated charcoal (MDAC), has been shown to increase the systemic clearance of various drug substances. The mechanism for the observed increase in total body clearance associated with the use of repeated doses of oral charcoal is thought to be translumenal efflux of drug from blood to the charcoal passing through the gastrointestinal tract (Berg *et al.*, 1982). In addition, MDAC is thought to produce a further enhancement in clearance by interrupting the enteroenteric–enterohepatic circulation of drugs that undergo that pharmacological route of elimination and recirculation. After systemic absorption, a drug may reenter the gut lumen by passive diffusion if the intraluminal drug concentration is lower than that in blood. The rate of this passive diffusion depends on the concentration gradient and the intestinal surface area, permeability, and blood flow. The activated charcoal in the gut lumen serves as a "sink" for toxicants. A concentration gradient is maintained and the chemical passes continuously into the gut lumen, where it is adsorbed to charcoal. The characteristics of chemicals that favor enhanced elimination by MDAC include (1) significant enteroenteric–enterohepatic circulation, including the formation of active recirculating metabolites, (2) prolonged plasma half-life after an overdose, (3) small (<1.0 L/kg) volume of distribution, (4) limited (<60%) plasma protein binding, (5) a pK_a that maximizes transport of the drug across cell membranes, (6) sustained-release/resin-form tablets and/or capsules, and (7) onset of organ failure (eg, kidney) that results in reduced capacity of the major route of elimination of the toxicant (for renally excreted chemicals) so that MDAC may make a considerable contribution to total body clearance.

The technique involves continuing oral administration of activated charcoal beyond the initial dosage (described above) every two to four hours with approximately one-half the initial dose, or 0.5 g/kg. The charcoal is generally mixed as an aqueous slurry and a cathartic substance is not incorporated due to the potential for electrolyte abnormalities with repeated administration of cathartic agents. An alternative technique for MDAC is to give the activated charcoal via an orogastric tube or nasogastric tube a loading dose of 1.0 g/kg of an aqueous slurry of activated charcoal, followed by a continuous infusion intragastrically of 0.2 g/kg/h. The duration of gastric infusion depends on the clinical status of the patient and repeated monitoring of plasma drug concentrations where indicated (Ilkhanipour *et al.*, 1992; Ohning *et al.*, 1986; Chyka *et al.*, 1995; Goulbourne *et al.*, 1994; Mofenson *et al.*, 1985; Park *et al.*, 1983, 1986; Pollack *et al.*, 1981; Van de Graaff *et al.*, 1982; Weisman, 1998).

Studies in animals and human volunteers have shown that MDAC increases drug elimination significantly, but few prospective randomized controlled clinical studies in poisoned patients have been published demonstrating a significant reduction in patient morbidity or mortality when MDAC is employed. One recent study, however, does provide a striking example of clinical benefit from the use of MDAC (de Silva *et al.*, 2003). The study showed that patients who intentionally poisoned themselves with yellow oleander seeds (a cardiac poison) and were randomized to MDAC (after all patients received an adequate initial single dose of activated

Table 33-7	
Drugs for Which Multiple Dose Activated Charcoal Has Been Shown Effective as a Treatment Modality for Poisoning	
Carbamazepine	Nadolol
Dapsone	Phenobarbital
Digoxin	Salicylates
Digitoxin	Theophylline

charcoal) had a statistically improved outcome in both mortality and cardiac morbidity. The early use of MDAC is an attractive alternative to more complex methods of enhancing toxin elimination, such as hemodialysis and hemoperfusion, although only in a relatively small subset of patients. The decision to use MDAC depends on the clinical situation including the specific chemical involved, the presence of contraindications (eg, intestinal obstruction) to the use of MDAC, and the likely effectiveness of alternative methods of therapy. A list of agents for which MDAC has been shown as an effective means of enhanced body clearance is shown in Table 33-7.

Use of Antidotes in Poisoning

A relatively small number of specific antidotes are available for clinical use in the treatment of poisoning. There are several main reasons for the slow growth and little progress in drug development for antidotes for poisoning. These include the small projected market for antidotes making development cost recovery challenging and, as mentioned earlier, the practical difficulties in performing clinical trials in overdose patients, a prerequisite for a successful drug approval application. The typical standard for clinical proof of drug safety and efficacy is the prospective, randomized, double-blinded, placebo controlled clinical trial. Practical considerations make it very difficult to perform this type of clinical trial for rare conditions such as specific poisonings. Enrolling actual poisoned patients into a clinical trial is difficult as many, potentially important confounding factors will be encountered across the overdose patient population, the severity of poisoning, extent of toxicant exposure and interindividual variability in susceptibility to the chemicals effects, and the potentially beneficial effects of the antidote all contribute to a highly variable clinical course, which increases the difficulty to show a meaningful, statistically significant benefit from antidote usage. The United States Food and Drug Administration (FDA) placed incentives for sponsors to develop drugs for rare diseases or conditions through the Orphan Drug Act. Fomepizole (4-methylpyrazole), a chemical inhibitor of alcohol dehydrogenase, was approved as an antidote for ethylene glycol (and later methanol) poisoning via the Orphan Drug pathway in December 1997. Another Orphan Drug Act approval was hydroxocobalamin, a cyanide chelating agent. This was approved in the US in December 2006 after being approved in Europe many years earlier. Despite these early successes, there have not been a large number of antidote products approved to this point in time as a result of this regulatory incentive. Another potential stimulus for antidote drug development has been the "post 9/11" federal funding increase for antiterrorism efforts including research for prevention and treatment of chemical, biological, and radiological poisons. In addition, the FDA has made available the "animal rule" that will permit human-drug approval based on robust evidence of efficacy and safety from animal studies when human studies cannot be conducted. Hopefully, these important changes will facilitate the development and approval of new antidote agents.

The mechanism of action of various antidotes is quite different. For example, a chelating agent for heavy metal poisoning or Fab fragments specific to digoxin or crotalid venom work by physically binding the toxin, preventing the toxin from exerting a deleterious effect in vivo and, in some cases, facilitating body clearance of the toxin. In essence, the Fab fragments serve as biologically derived chelating agents to bind and render the specific toxin inactive. Other antidotes pharmacologically antagonize the effects of the toxicant. Atropine, an antimuscarinic, anticholinergic drug is used to pharmacologically antagonize at the receptor level, the effects of organophosphate insecticides or acetylcholinesterase-inhibiting nerve gases, which produce cholinergic, muscarinic effects, which if sufficient, can be lethal. Certain chemicals exert their antidote effects by chemically reacting with biological systems to increase detoxifying capacity for the toxicant. For example, sodium nitrite is given to patients poisoned with cyanide to cause formation of methemoglobin, which serves as an alternative binding site for the cyanide ion, thereby making it less toxic to the body. Other agents, such as L-carnitine, are approved to mitigate the biochemical toxicity of high exposures to valproic acid (an antiseizure medication) at the level of the mitochondria. Just as in other therapeutic areas of drug development, basic research into fundamental mechanisms can reveal viable drug targets that can be exploited to produce a point of intervention for a drug/antidote to lessen the effects of a toxic exposure.

The time course for antidote onset of action is highly variable across currently available antidotes. IV naloxone can have a dramatic effect on the level of consciousness of an opiate-poisoned patient within minutes of IV administration. Chelating agents such as desferoxamine may require multiple dosages over many days before a clinically detectable effect is seen.

The skillful therapeutic use of antidotes is essential to optimize the treatment of the poisoned patient. Many antidotes have a relatively narrow safety margin or low therapeutic index. Excessive dosing with an antidote can in some instances be more harmful than the expected effects of the toxicant itself. An example of this is when physostigmine (a cholinergic agent) is given at an excessive dose or dosing rate to a patient with mild-to-moderate anticholinergic poisoning, the antidote can cause a potentially fatal bradycardia that can progress to a fatal cardiac arrest. Some antidotes require an adjustment of their dosage based on a measured blood concentration of the chemical (eg, digoxin Fab fragments) or based on the clinical assessment of the patient such as with sodium bicarbonate usage in a tricyclic antidepressant overdose. A significant part of the clinical training in the field of medical toxicology is devoted to learning how to use antidotes skillfully.

An important area of research in clinical toxicology has been in the study of prognostic indicators of poisoning severity and predictors for the level of treatment required. For practical reasons much of this work has been retrospective in nature but has resulted in significant aids to guide the treatment rendered by clinical toxicologists. Several authors have proposed "action levels" that are a threshold for a certain level of clinical intervention based upon a measured plasma concentration of the chemical or a clinical manifestation of the poisoning. For example, a patient with a measured plasma valproic acid concentration of 900 mcg/mL after a single oral exposure would be expected to exhibit significant toxicity. If the patient's clinical condition correlated with the measured laboratory plasma concentration (ie, laboratory error was unlikely), the patient would likely require aggressive treatment measures such as hemodialysis instead of supportive care. Another way that prognostic information is studied is when a constellation of clinical signs and symptoms is proven to correlate with a clinical outcome following exposure to a specific poison. An example of this would be

a worker with a significant topical methanol exposure who demonstrates a metabolic acidosis with an elevated AG, an osmol gap, and visual symptoms. Based on clinical signs and symptoms, this patient would likely undergo hemodialysis even in the absence of a confirmatory measurement of the methanol concentration in serum. These relationships, the correlation of serious clinical effects with a valproic acid level above 900 mcg/mL or visual symptoms in a methanol-poisoned patient (Ellenhorn, 1997a,b) have been derived from many years of observational study of poisoning outcomes by investigators in the field of clinical toxicology. Early on in the field, the majority of publications were primarily case reports making it difficult to determine the relative effectiveness of various treatments being assessed. There were also significant discrepancies in the initial management of the patients confounding the ultimate outcomes of the cases. The case series or meta-analysis type of scientific analysis was an important step to advance the study of clinical outcomes and assess the quality of treatment provided to poisoned patients. An example of the case series study includes the publication that described the relationship of the QRS interval on the patient's 12-lead electrocardiogram (ECG) to the severity of poisoning by tricyclic antidepressant drugs (Boehnert et al., 1985). This important observational study helped to stratify patients poisoned with an overdose of first-generation tricyclic antidepressants into risk categories based on the lengthening of the QRS on the patient's ECG for development of seizures or cardiac arrhythmias. The highest level of evidence for establishing efficacy and safety for therapeutic interventions is the prospective, double blinded, controlled clinical trial. Whenever possible to successfully execute, these clinical investigations are most likely to result in objective data with the least confounding of results if properly conducted. These advantages better enable clinicians to validate (or dismiss) new therapeutic modalities and treatment strategies. Unfortunately, the ability to perform these trials in the evaluation of new treatments for poisoning is significantly limited due to ethical concerns when considering withholding effective treatment (placebo treatment), or the ability to effectively blind treatment groups in the poison treatment setting.

Supportive Care of the Poisoned Patient

Once the initial treatment phase in the clinical management of the poisoned patient has been completed, the care of the patient is generally shifted to an inpatient hospital setting for those patients who will require admission. This supportive care phase of poison treatment is very important. Poisoned patients who are unstable or at risk for significant clinical instability are generally admitted to a critical care unit for close monitoring. In addition, patients who are excessively sedated from their poisoning or those who require mechanical ventilation or invasive hemodynamic monitoring are also candidates for an intensive care stay. Not only are there certain poisonings that have delayed toxicity such as acetaminophen, paraquat, and diphenoxylate, but there are also toxicants that exhibit multiple phases of toxicity that include delayed effects (ie, ethylene glycol, salicylate, and buspirone).

Similar to other ill, hospitalized patients, patients admitted for continued treatment of poisoning are at risk for nosocomial infections, iatrogenic fluid, and electrolyte disturbances as well as potential harmful effects from the initial therapies that they received for treatment of their poisoning. For example, induction of emesis, gastric lavage, or orogastric infusion of activated charcoal can cause aspiration and lead to pneumonitis. Any drug that severely alters a patient's mental status causing obtundation can allow aspiration of gastric contents associated with a loss of the gag reflex. Organ system dysfunction due to profound hypotension caused by a poisoning can result in delayed complications such as acute renal failure, hepatic failure, and permanent brain damage. Close clinical monitoring can detect these later phase poisoning complications and allow for prompt medical intervention to minimize patient morbidity and mortality. These are but a few of the reasons that close vigilance is a very important component of the support phase of poison treatment.

Another important component of the supportive care phase of poison treatment is the psychiatric assessment. For intentional self-poisonings, a formal psychiatric evaluation of the patient should be performed prior to patient discharge. In many cases, it is not possible to perform a psychiatric interview of the patient during the early phases of treatment and evaluation. Once the patient has been stabilized and is able to effectively communicate, the psychiatric evaluation should be obtained prior to determining the patient's disposition. Generally, a patient who has attempted suicide should be constantly monitored until they have been evaluated by the psychiatric consultant and judged to be at low risk for being without constant surveillance.

CASE EXAMPLES OF SPECIFIC POISONINGS

Acetaminophen

A 16-year-old female patient arrives in the ED by ambulance after being found by a parent in what appeared to be an intoxicated state with empty pill bottles scattered about her room. The parent reports the patient was despondent recently after breaking up with her boyfriend. The patient is tearful and reports abdominal pain and admits to drinking alcohol and taking over-the-counter (OTC) pills in an apparent suicide attempt. The estimated time of ingestion is six hours prior to arrival in the ED. The patient does not use prescription, OTC medications, or dietary supplements and is not known to have a history of regular consumption of alcoholic beverages or use illicit drugs.

On physical examination the vital signs were blood pressure 118/80 mm Hg, pulse 88/min and regular, respiratory rate 18/min, and temperature 37.0°C. She was awake and oriented, responded to questions appropriately with slightly slurred speech. Other pertinent findings included normal bowel sounds with mild epigastric tenderness. The neurological examination was only significant for slightly slurred speech.

Routine clinical laboratory studies were ordered STAT (electrolytes, creatinine, BUN, glucose, complete blood count with differential, coagulation studies, urine analysis, and urine toxicology screen) and a plasma acetaminophen level. Chest and abdominal radiography were normal.

The patient was given 1.5 g/kg oral activated charcoal as a slurry in a sorbitol cathartic and placed in the intensive monitoring section of the ED while the laboratory tests were being performed. Forty minutes later, the laboratory results returned and showed a mildly increased white blood cell count, liver transaminase values were elevated at approximately three times the upper limit of normal, and an acetaminophen concentration was 308 ug/mL. She denied taking any other medications with the acetaminophen and alcohol. Based on the Rumack–Mathew nomogram (Fig. 33-1), a plasma acetaminophen concentration of 308 ug/mL at approximately six hours after ingestion is well within the "probable hepatic toxicity" range, and therefore treatment with NAC was required.

The patient received the first dose of IV NAC in the ED and was admitted to the medical ward to complete the treatment course of IV NAC. Transient increases of hepatic transaminases were measured over the ensuing two days of the hospitalization. The patient

was seen by the Psychiatry Consultation service, which determined she was not actively suicidal; she was discharged from the hospital two days after admission with scheduled psychiatric and medical follow-up appointments.

Acetaminophen has been used as an analgesic and antipyretic since the mid-1950s and has become more prominently recognized as a potential hepatotoxicant in the overdose situation since the original British reports in the late 1960s (Proudfoot & Wright, 1970). Work on the mechanisms of the liver toxicity of this drug has provided a scientific basis for therapy (Mitchell *et al.*, 1973).

The clinical presentation of patients poisoned with acetaminophen is sufficiently confusing in some cases; it is difficult to estimate the time of ingestion. Due to the paucity of clinical symptoms with acute overdose, waiting for the appearance of symptoms is an inadequate strategy for the clinical decision-making process regarding institution of treatment. Most clinicians will request an acetaminophen concentration be measured for any patient suspected of having a toxic exposure to any substance precisely for the reason highlighted above—that is the paucity of signs and symptoms associated with an acetaminophen overdose makes inadvertent missing of a potentially fatal overdose until the window for maximum antidote effectiveness has passed.

Acetaminophen in normal individuals is inactivated by sulfation (approximately 52%) and glucuronide conjugation (42%). About 2% of the drug is excreted unchanged. The remaining 4% is biotransformed by the cytochrome P-450 mixed-function oxidase system. The P-450 isozyme responsible for acetaminophen biotransformation is CYP2E1. Metabolism by CYP2E1 results in a potentially toxic metabolite that is normally detoxified by conjugation with glutathione and excreted as the mercapturate. Evidence extrapolated from animals estimates that when 70% of endogenous hepatic glutathione is consumed, the toxic metabolite becomes available for covalent binding to hepatic cellular components. However, patients who are concurrently using, or have recently used, agents that induce CYP2E1, such as in the case of chronic ethanol exposure or phenobarbital use, may produce more than 4% of the toxic metabolite. It is therefore important to determine, whenever possible, whether or not the patient's CYP2E1 system may be induced when assessing the risk of hepatic necrosis from acetaminophen overdose in any given individual. When there is evidence (medical history) of concurrent chemicals that induce CYP2E1, the treatment nomogram from acetaminophen should be modified to a lower threshold for treatment with NAC (Rumack *et al.*, 1981).

Follow-up liver biopsy studies of patients who have recovered three months to a year after hepatotoxicity have demonstrated no long-term sequelae or chronic toxicity (Clark *et al.*, 1973). A very small percentage (0.25%) of patients in the national multiclinic study conducted in Denver may progress to hepatic encephalopathy with subsequent death. The clinical nature of the overdose is one of a sharp peaks of serum glutamic-oxaloacetic transaminase (SGOT) by day three, with recovery to less than 100 IU/L by day seven or eight. Patients with SGOT levels as high as 20,000 IU/L have shown complete recovery and no sequelae one week after ingestion (Arena *et al.*, 1978).

Laboratory evaluation of a potentially poisoned patient is crucial in terms of both hepatic measures of toxicity and plasma levels of acetaminophen. Accurate estimation of acetaminophen in the plasma should be done on samples drawn at least four hours after ingestion, when peak plasma levels can be expected.

Once an accurate plasma level has been obtained, it should be plotted on the Rumack–Matthew nomogram to determine if NAC therapy is indicated (Fig. 33-1). This nomogram is based on a series of patients with and without hepatotoxicity and their corresponding measured plasma acetaminophen concentrations.

Treatment should be instituted in any patient with a plasma concentration in the potentially toxic range. Some clinical toxicologist recommend withholding NAC treatment unless the plasma concentration is at or above the "probably toxic" demarcation but most often, due to the inherent uncertainty in the history regarding the time of ingestion (the x-axis of the Rumack nomogram), the more conservative approach is recommended. Standard support with administration of activated charcoal or gastric lavage (a seldom used option for very recent acetaminophen ingestions) should be followed by administration of NAC. The protective effect of NAC in oral acetaminophen poisoning was demonstrated when contrasted with controls not receiving antidotal therapy (Rumack et al., 1981; Smilkstein et al., 1988). Because NAC is most effective if it is given within eight to 12 hours of acetaminophen ingestion, patients in whom blood levels cannot be obtained should have NAC treatment instituted and therapy terminated only if levels are nontoxic. The dosing regimen for oral NAC is a loading dose of 140 mg/kg orally, followed by 70 mg/kg orally for 17 additional doses (Peterson & Rumack, 1977). The dosage regimen for IV NAC is 150 mg/kg loading dose over 15 minutes, followed by 50 mg/kg over the next four hours then 100 mg/kg over 16 hours for a total dose of 300 mg/kg in 20 hours. Anaphylactoid reactions have been associated with the use of IV NAC; therefore, some authors do not recommend this route of administration for adults with asthma (Howland, 2006). Children can receive IV NAC but the volume required for the dilution can cause electrolyte abnormalities. The advantage from using the IV form is that the complete dosage regimen is completed in 20 hours in contrast to the 72-hour oral regimen. Children less than nine to 12 years of age have a lower incidence of hepatotoxicity after an overdose than do adults but are still treated with NAC according to the Rumack–Mathew nomogram. Patients with trivial or "nontoxic" acetaminophen ingestions should not be given NAC therapy because the antidote can produce clinical significant side effects.

Ethylene Glycol

A 37-year-old female was brought to the ED after being found unresponsive in her home. The patient was comatose and unresponsive to pain and without obvious signs of trauma. At the scene, emergency medical personnel administered oxygen and naloxone and performed a finger stick for glucose, (standard procedure for encountering a person with altered mental status and suspected toxic ingestion), which showed a normal value of 95 mg/dL. The patient's spouse reported that she had been depressed and despondent with the recent loss of her job. No empty pill bottles or liquid containers were found with her at home.

Upon arrival to the hospital, she remained comatose and had the following vital signs: blood pressure 105/65 mm Hg, pulse 78/min, respiratory rate elevated at 32/min, and her body temperature was normal. The remainder of the physical examination was significant for her pupils were 3 mm and sluggishly reactive to light; the lung and heart examinations were normal; the abdominal examination revealed diminished but present bowel sounds, no tenderness, organomegaly, or masses were detected. The rectal examination was normal; the stool was without detectable gross or occult blood. Neuro examination was nonfocal with a diminished gag reflex.

The patient was placed on a cardiac monitor, an IV line was started, clinical laboratory specimens were obtained, and she was placed on oxygen, given naloxone, thiamine, and dextrose (50%) intravenously. Similar to the EMS encounter, these treatments are standard for patients presenting with an altered mental status to an ED. Chest and abdominal radiography was without abnormality. A 12-lead ECG was also normal. Faced with the uncertainty of oral ingestion versus topical and inhalation exposure, a decision was made to proceed with gastric decontamination. Because no direct history from the patient was available, a mixed ingestion could not be ruled out as well. Because of a diminished gag reflex, the patient was endotracheally intubated to protect her airway before an orogastric tube was placed. Gastric lavage was performed and no blood was found. The fluid withdrawn from the stomach was bright yellow in appearance and slightly viscous. When a Wood's lamp illuminated this fluid in a darkened room, fluorescence was observed. This finding suggests the presence of automotive antifreeze that contains ethylene glycol. Activated charcoal (2.0 g/kg) was placed via the orogastric tube into the stomach with a cathartic even though the efficacy for binding ethylene glycol is limited; the use of activated charcoal here was for other, potentially unknown coingestants. Clinical laboratory results returned showing the following:

Serum Chemistries

Na = 140 mEq/L	K = 3.1 mEq/L
Cl = 94 mEq/L	HCO_3 = 8 mEq/L
BUN = 12 mg/dl	Glucose = 100 mg/dl

Arterial blood gas:

pH = 7.20; pCO_2 = 20 mm Hg; pO_2 = 98 mm Hg

The complete blood count was normal, the urine analysis was normal, measured serum osmolarity was 330 mOsm/kg, and acetaminophen and salicylate levels were below the limits of detection, and the urine toxicology screen was negative.

The laboratory results were interpreted as follows: a metabolic acidosis with elevated AG (AG = 38) and an elevated osmol gap (40 mOsm). These findings are consistent with either methanol or ethylene glycol poisoning (Tables 33-4 and 33-5). A blood sample for measurement of methanol and ethylene glycol was sent for analysis but based on the history and finding of fluorescent, yellow fluid in the stomach and the acid-base disorder detected, the working diagnosis of ethylene glycol poisoning was established. The patient was treated with IV fomepizole (4-methylperazole) and transfer to a nearby regional hospital that has hemodialysis capability was requested. Sodium bicarbonate was given intravenously for the profound metabolic acidosis and the patient was successfully transferred to the regional medical center where she underwent hemodialysis shortly after arrival. After four hours of hemodialysis, the acid-base and electrolyte abnormalities were corrected but the patient remained comatose. Approximately, nine hours after the blood specimen was sent, the laboratory reported a "toxic" serum ethylene glycol concentration of 366 mg/dL, most likely representing a fatal original plasma concentration. The patient underwent a second four-hour course of hemodialysis eight hours later to again correct a slight recurrence in her metabolic acidosis with the appearance of minor renal injury (serum creatinine increased to 1.8 mg/dL). She regained normal consciousness within 18 hours and her renal function recovered completely within three days. Subsequently, the patient admitted that she intentionally drank more than half a container of antifreeze with the intent of harming herself. She was evaluated by the psychiatry consultation service and transferred to their service for further care.

This case demonstrates the importance of utilizing the anion and osmol gap calculations in overdose patients as well as all available diagnostic tools (eg, the Wood lamp) in their initial evaluation. It also highlights the life-saving features of rapidly and competently applied therapeutic modalities in poisoning treatment. Without a readily available drug such as fomepizole (or sterile IV ethanol that also inhibits the alcohol dehydrogenase enzyme) and the ability to rapidly transfer to a facility with definitive care capability

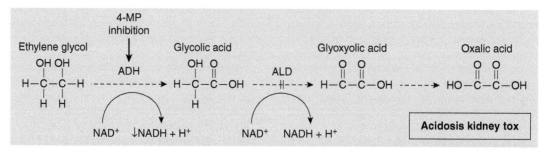

Figure 33-3. *Metabolic pathway for the metabolism of ethylene glycol.*

(hemodialysis), this patient would have likely succumbed to her poisoning. Initiation of antidote therapy and hemodialysis to increase removal of the poison prior to receipt of the confirmatory laboratory test (measured serum concentration of the specific poison—ethylene glycol) was also required in this case. Although not considered diagnostic (Walker *et al.*, 1986), the presence of both a metabolic acidosis with an AG and an osmol gap is highly suggestive of either methanol or ethylene glycol given the patient's presentation despite a scant history. It is commonplace for hospital clinical laboratories to have to "send out" blood specimens for ethylene glycol and methanol analysis as these are not routinely performed on-site. A turn-around time of six to 12 hours for this test result to be available is typical in most settings.

Ethylene glycol exerts is primary toxicity after undergoing biotransformation by alcohol dehydrogenase to glycolic acid and then to glycolic and oxalic acid by the action of aldehyde dehydrogenase. Fig. 33-3 contains a schematic representation of the metabolism of ethylene glycol to its toxic metabolites. The later two acid metabolites are thought to be responsible for both the renal and the acid-base toxicity observed during poisoning by ethylene glycol (Swartz *et al.*, 1981). If untreated or treated too late, ethylene glycol poisoning can result in fatal cerebral edema with seizures as well as irreversible renal damage. Hemodialysis can remove the unmetabolized ethylene glycol and toxic more polar metabolites, eliminating the substrate for production of the toxic metabolite and the damaging metabolites themselves. Administration of an inhibitor or competing substrate for alcohol dehydrogenase can be instituted while transporting the patient to a healthcare facility where hemodialysis is available. Fomepizole, (4-methylperazole) is a commercially available inhibitor of alcohol dehydrogenase that is FDA approved for the treatment of methanol and ethylene glycol poisoning. Ethanol (sterile, for IV administration) or oral, nonsterile ethanol (when the IV formulation is not readily available) can also be given to effectively inhibit the metabolism of methanol or ethylene glycol and prevent the potentially devastating effects of the poisoning. Finally, in the specific case of methanol poisoning, the administration of folic acid in animal models has been shown to enhance the in vivo clearance of formate, the toxic metabolite of methanol (McMartin *et al.*, 1977). Folate or folinic acid has been given to methanol-poisoned patients and is suggested to hasten formic acid metabolism, thereby accelerating its clearance. Many clinical toxicologists will include folic or folinic acid in their therapeutic regimen for methanol-poisoned patients.

Valproic Acid

A 33-year-old male is brought to the ED after being found unresponsive by his brother at home with two empty prescription pill bottles of extended release valproic acid at his side. He was last

seen eight hours prior to being found unresponsive and was then in normal health. No further history is available. The patient's pharmacy confirmed that three monthly prescriptions, each containing 30, 250 mg extended release valproic acid tablets had been dispensed within the preceding three months. A call to the office of the prescribing physician did not reach anyone who could verify the prescription or provide past medical history for the patient.

The patient was unresponsive to verbal or tactile stimulation with vital signs: blood pressure 85/55 mm Hg, pulse 94/min, respiratory rate 20/min, and temperature 33.2°C. IV access was obtained and IV fluids were administered as rapidly as possible. Naloxone was administered without effect. The patient was placed on a cardiac monitor that showed sinus rhythm. The remainder of the physical examination showed the patient to be without obvious signs of trauma; the skin was cool and without track marks. The pupils were 2 mm and poorly reactive to light. Other significant findings include the examination of the abdomen, which showed diminished bowel sounds. The rectal examination was negative for occult blood. The neurological examination revealed coma without focal motor abnormalities and an absent gag reflex.

Initial laboratories showed mild metabolic acidosis with elevated serum lactate, an increased anion, slightly increased serum ammonia, normal glucose, liver function tests, and renal function tests. The chest and abdominal radiographs were normal. The 12-lead ECG showed a prolonged QT interval without arrhythmia. The patient was endotracheally intubated to protect his airway prior to gastric lavage that yielded some pill fragments only. The patient was placed on a ventilator to support his respiration. Activated charcoal (1.5 g/kg) was administered via the orogastric tube immediately following the lavage procedure. The blood pressure continued to remain low despite IV fluid administration. A STAT valproic acid serum measurement showed the concentration was 572 mcg/mL.

Blood pressure responded to low-dose vasopressors (IV dopamine) with continued IV fluid administration. A repeat serum valproic acid concentration was 890 mcg/mL at two hours post-admission. Serial oral activated charcoal (every four hours) was initiated via the orogastric tube and hemodialysis was started three hours after admission. IV L-carnitine was given when a repeat serum ammonia concentration returned further elevated at 94 mg/dL. Subsequent measured plasma concentrations of vaproic acid gradually declined to <100 mcg/mL over the next 48 hours after one additional hemodialysis session was conducted. The patient regained consciousness 24 hours after admission and made a full recovery by hospital day four. He was evaluated by the Psychiatry consult service, which accepted the patient in transfer to their inpatient service after he was medically cleared by the Toxicology service.

This case illustrates the significance of increasing plasma concentrations of the toxic substance despite gastric decontamination procedures. In this case, the most likely cause for this observation is the ingestion of an extended release formulation, which is pharmaceutically designed to slowly dissolve in the gastrointestinal tract and provide for ongoing sustained release of the active drug product as opposed to immediate release of the agent. Other drug substances can demonstrate the "slow release" profile without having been formulated in a special sustained release dosage form. Examples of these drug "bezoars" include salicylates and barbiturates as well as formulations of iron supplements. The presence of a drug bezoar or concretion can be dangerous because, without serial drug concentration measurements, the treating team could erroneously stratify a patient based on the initial measured plasma concentration and be unprepared for severe toxicity or prolonged toxicity time course not expected from the initial concentration alone.

The use of L-carnitine is an example of the application of basic biochemical knowledge to apply and effective therapeutic intervention. In the case of valproic acid intoxication, the biochemical effects of valproate on fatty acid metabolism in liver mitochondria, specifically the depletion of L-carnitine, are thought to be causative for the hyperammonemia often observed in moderate and severe cases of valproic acid intoxication (Lheureux & Hantson, 2009; Bohan *et al.*, 2001). Based on these findings and other experimental date, the FDA has recently approved the use of IV L-carnitine for the treatment of valproic acid poisoning in the setting of hepatotoxicity, hyperammonemia, large overdoses of valproate by history, or measured serum concentrations of valproic acid exceeding 450 mcg/mL.

Finally, the benefit of employing multiple methods simultaneously to enhance the elimination of a toxicant is also demonstrated in this case example. The total body clearance of valproic acid is known to be enhanced when serial oral activated charcoal is administered (Table 33-7). Hemoperfusion, or the more available method of hemodialysis has been shown to increase the total body clearance of valproic acid in overdose (Guillaume *et al.*, 2004). This recommendation is based, in part, on the finding that the plasma protein binding of valproic acid is easily saturated and in large overdoses, the free fraction (unbound) drug increases from 10% to more than 30%, making more of the drug available for effective removal during hemodialysis. Both modalities were likely beneficially employed in this potentially fatal valproic acid ingestion.

SUMMARY

The practice of Clinical Toxicology encompasses the expertise of the specialties of Medical Toxicology, Applied Toxicology, and Clinical Poison Information Specialists. Basic and clinical science continues to provide new information that allows for more effective diagnosis and treatment of the poisoned patient. The evolution of the poison control (information) center and regional poisoning treatment centers has greatly aided advances in the field of Clinical Toxicology. The incorporation of evidence-based, outcome-driven practice recommendations has significantly improved and standardized the evaluation of treatment modalities for poisonings. Application of a stepwise approach to the poisoned patient as described above remains an essential approach to the effective evaluation and treatment of the poisoned patient. This methodically performed, clinical diagnostic and therapeutic approach, applied in a parallel fashion to the poisoned patient is essential especially when the medical history is absent or likely unreliable. Skillful use of antidotes is an important component of the practice of Medical Toxicology. Continued research will increase the repertoire of effective treatments for poisoning and ultimately improve patient outcomes.

REFERENCES

Andersen AH. Experimental studies on the pharmacology of activated charcoal; adsorption power of charcoal in aqueous solutions. *Acta Pharmacol Toxicol (Copenh)*. 1946;2:69–78.

Andersen AH. Experimental studies on the pharmacology of activated charcoal; the effect of pH on the adsorption by charcoal from aqueous solutions. *Acta Pharmacol (Copenh)*. 1947;3:199–218.

Andersen AH. Experimental studies on the pharmacology of activated charcoal. III. Adsorption from gastrointestinal contents. *Acta Pharmacol*. 1948;4:275–284.

Arena JM, Rourk MHJ, Sibrack CD. Acetaminophen: report of an unusual poisoning. *Pediatrics*. 1978;61:68–72.

Beerman R, Nunez D, Wetli C. Radiographic evaluation of the cocaine smuggler. *Gastrointest Radiol*. 1986;11:351–354.

Berg MJ, Berlinger WG, Goldberg MJ, et al. Acceleration of the body clearance of phenobarbital by oral activated charcoal. *N Eng J Med*. 1982;307:642–644.

Boehnert MT, Lovejoy FH. Value of the QRS duration versus the serum drug level in predicting seizures and ventricular arrhythmias after an acute overdose of tricyclic antidepressants. *N Eng J Med*. 1985;313: 474–479.

Bohan TP, Helton E, MacDonald I, et al. Effect of L-carnitine treatment for valproate-induced hepatotoxicity. *Neurology*. 2001;56:1405–1409.

Bosinski T, Bailie GR, Eisele G. Massive and extended rebound of serum lithium concentrations following hemodialysis in two chronic overdose cases. *Am J Emerg Med*. 1998;16:98–100.

Bronstein AC, Spyker DA, Cantilena LR, Green JL, Rumack BH, Dart RC. 2010 Annual Report of the American Association of Poison Control Centers' National Poison Data System (NPDS). *Clin Toxicol (Phila)*. 2011;49(10):910–941.

Brown TR, Evans JE, Szabo GK, et al. Studies with stable isotopes II: phenobarbital pharmacokinetics during monotherapy. *J Clin Pharm*. 1985;25:51–58.

Chyka PA. Mutiple-dose activated charcoal enhancement of systematic drug clearance: summary of studies in animals and human volunteers. *J Toxicol Clin Tox*. 1995;33:399–405.

Clark R, Borirakchanyavat V, Davidson AR, et al. Hepatic damage and death from overdose of paracetamal. *Lancet*. 1973;1:66.

Cooney DO. *Activated Charcoal in Medical Applications*. New York: Dekker; 1995.

Cutler RE, Forland SC, Hammond PG, Evans JR. Extracorporeal removal of drugs and poisons by hemodialysis and hemoperfusion. *Ann Rev Pharmacol Toxicol*. 1987;27:169–191.

Dally SL, Garneir R, Bismuth C. Diagnosis of chlorinated hydrocarbon poisoning by x-ray examination. *Br J Indus Med*. 1987;44:424–425.

de Silva HA, Foneska M, Pathmeswaran A, et al. Multiple dose activated charcoal for treatment of yellow oleander poisoning: a single-blind, randomized, placebo controlled trial. *Lancet*. 2003;361:1935–1938.

Done AK. Salicylate intoxication, significance of measurements of salicylate in blood in cases of acute intoxication. *Pediatrics*. 1960;26:800–807.

Ellenhorn MJ. Alcohols and glycols. In: Ellenhorn MJ, ed. *Ellenhorn's Medical Toxicology, Diagnosis and Treatment of Poisoning*, 2nd ed. Philadelphia, PA: Williams and Wilkins; 1997a.

Ellenhorn MJ. *Ellenhorn's Medical Toxicology, Diagnosis and Treatment of Poisoning*. 2nd ed. Philadelphia, PA: Williams and Wilkins; 1997b.

Everson GW, Oudjhane K, Young LW, et al. Effectiveness of abdominal radiographs in visualizing chewable iron supplements following overdose. *Am J Emerg Med*. 1989;7:459–463.

Goldfrank LR. In: Goldfrank NR, Flomenbaum NE, Lewin NA, et al., eds. *Goldfrank's Toxicologic Emergencies*. 8th ed. New York, NY: McGraw-Hill; 2006: chap 3.

Goulbourne KB, Cisek J, et al. Small-bowel obstruction secondary to activated charcoal and adhesions. *Ann Emerg Med*. 1994;24:108–109.

Greensher J, Mofenson HC, Caraccio TR. Ascendency of the black bottle (activated charcoal). *Pediatrics*. 1987;80:949–950.

Guillaume CP, Stolk L, Dejagere TF, et al. Successful use of hemodialysis in acute valproic acid intoxication. *J Toxicol Clin Toxicol*. 2004;42(3):335–336.

Handy CA. Radiopacity of oral non-liquid medications. *Radiology.* 1971;98:522–533.

Heffner JE, Harley RA, Schabel SI. Pulmonary reactions from illicit substance abuse. *Clin Chest Med.* 1990;11:151–162.

Holt LE, Holz PH. The black bottle: a consideration in the role of charcoal in the treatment on poisoning in children. *J Pediatr.* 1963;63:306–314.

Howland MA. Antidotes in depth: *N*-Acetylcysteine. In: Goldfrank LR, Flomenbaum NE, Lewin NA, et al., eds. *Goldfrank's Toxicologic Emergencies.* 8th ed. New York, NY: McGraw-Hill; 2006.

Ilkhanipour K, Yealy K, Krenzelok EP, et al. The comparative efficacy of various multiple-dose activated charcoal regimens. *Am J Emerg Med.* 1992;10:298–300.

Institute of Medicine. Forging a poison prevention and control system. Washington D.C.: National Academy Press; 2004.

Jarcho S. Medical Numismatic Notes. VII: Mithridates IV. *Bull NY Cad Med.* 1972;48:1059–1064.

Jones JS, Lagasse J, Zimmerman G. Computed tomographic findings after acute carbon monoxide poisoning. *Am J Emerg Med.* 1994;12:448–451.

King WD, Palmisano PA. Poison control centers: can their value be measured? *South Med J.* 1991;84:722–726.

Krenzelok EP, McGuigan M, Lheureuz P; and the American Academy of Clinical Toxicology and European Association of Poisions Centres and Clinical Toxicologists. Position Paper: Ipecac Syrup. *J Toxicol Clin Toxicol.* 2004;42(2):133–143.

Lheureux PE, Hantson P. Carnitine in the treatment of valproic acid-induced toxicity. *Clin Toxicol (Phila).* 2009;47(2):101–111.

Liebelt EL, Francis PD, Woolf AD. ECG lead aVR versus QRS in predicting seizures and arrhythmias in acute tricyclic antidepressant toxicity. *Ann Emerg Med.* 1995;26:195–201.

Major RH. History of the stomach tube. *Ann Med Hist.* 1934;6:500–509.

Martin JM, Arena JM. Lye poisoning and stricture of the esophagus: a report of 50 cases. *Southern Med J.* 1939;32:286–290.

Manoguerra AS, Temple AR. Observations on the current status of poison control centers in the United States. *Emerg Med Clin North Am.* 1984;2:185–197.

Mayor A. *Greek Fire, Poison Arrows, and Scorpion Bombs: Biological and Chemical Warfare in the Ancient World.* Woodstock, NY: Overlook Press; 2003.

McCarron MM, Wood JD. The cocaine "body packer" syndrome. *JAMA.* 1983;250:1417–1420.

McElvaine MD, DeUngria EG, Matte TD, et al. Prevalence of radiographic evidence of paint chip ingestion among children with moderate to severe lead poisoning. St. Louis, Missouri, 1989 through 1990. *Pediatrics.* 1992;89:740–742.

McMartin KE, Martin-Amat G, Makar AT, et al. Methanol poisoning V: role of formate metabolism in the monkey. *J Pharmacol Exp Ther.* 1977;201:564–572.

Miller TR, Lestina DC. Costs of poisoning in the united states and savings from poison control centers: a benefit-cost analysis. *Ann Emerg Med.* 1997;29(2):239–245.

Mitchell JR, Jollow DJ, Potter WZ, et al. Acetaminophen induced hepatic necrosis. *J Pharm Exp Ther.* 1973;187:185–194.

Miura T, Mitomo M, Kawai R, Harada K. CT of the brain in acute carbon monoxide intoxication: characteristic features and prognosis. *AJNR.* 1985;6:739–742.

Mofenson HC, Caraccio TR, Greensher J, et al. Gastrointestinal dialysis with activated charcoal and cathartic in the treatment of adolescent intoxications. *Clin Pediatr.* 1985;24:678–684.

Mofenson HC, Greensher J. The nontoxic ingestion. *Pediatr Clin North Am.* 1970;17(3):583–590.

Mokrzycki MH, Kaplan AA. Therapeutic plasma exhange: complications and management. *Am J Kidney Dis.* 1994;23:817–827.

Nelson JC, Liu D, Olson KR. Radiopacity of modified release medications. *Vet Hum Tox.* 1993;35:317.

Neuvonen P, Vartiainen M, Tokola O. Comparison of activated charcoal and ipecac syrup in prevention of drug absorption. *Eur J Clin Pharm.* 1983;24:557–562.

O'Brien RP, McGeehan PA, Helmeczi AW, et al. Detectability of drug tablets and capsules by plain radiography. *Am J Emerg Med.* 1986;4:302–312.

Ohning BL, Reed MD, Blumer Jl, et al. Continuous nasogastric administration of activated charcoal for the treatment of theophylline intoxication. *Ped Pharm.* 1986;5:241–245.

Osius TG. The historic art of poisoning. *Med Bull (Ann Arbor).* 1957;23:111–116.

Park GD, Radomski L, Goldberg MJ, et al. Effects of size and frequency of oral doses of charcoal on theophylline clearance. *Clin Pharm Ther.* 1983;34:663–666.

Park GD, Spector R, Goldberg MJ, Johnson GF. Expanded role of charcoal therapy in the poisoned and overdosed patient. *Arch Intern Med.* 1986;146(5):969–973.

Peterson RG, Rumack BH. Treatment of acute acetaminophen poisoning with acetylcysteine. *JAMA.* 1977;237:2406–2407.

Plaitakis A, Duvoisin RC. Homer's moly identified as Galanthus nivalis: physiologic antidote to stramonium poisoning. *Clin Neuropharm.* 1983;6:1–5.

Pollack MM, Dunbar BS, Holbrook PR, Fields AI, et al. Aspiration of activated charcoal and gastric contents. *Ann Emerg Med.* 1981;10:528–529.

Proudfoot AT, Krenzelok EP, Vale JA. Position paper on urine alkalinization. *J Toxicol Clin Toxicol.* 2004;42:1–26.

Proudfoot AT, Wright N. Acute paracetamol poisoning. *Br Med J.* 1970;2:557.

Reid DHS. Treatment of the poisoned child. *Arch Dis Child.* 1970;45:428–433.

Rumack BH, Matthew H. Acetaminophen poisoning and toxicity. *Pediatrics.* 1975;55:871.

Rumack BH, Peterson RC, Koch GG, et al. Acetaminophen overdose: 662 cases with evaluation of oral acetylcysteine treatment. *Arch Intern Med.* 1981;141:380–385.

Savitt DL, Hawkins HH, Roberts JR. The radiopacity of ingested medications. *Ann Emerg Med.* 1987;16:331–339.

Scherz RG, Robertson, WO. The history of poison control centers in the United States. *Clin Toxicol.* 1978;12(3):291–296.

Smilkstein MJ, Knapp GL, Kulig KW, et al. Efficacy of oral *N*-acetylcysteine in the treatment of acetaminophen overdose. *N Engl J Med.* 1988;319:1557–1562.

Smithline N, Gardner KD. Gaps: anionic and osmolal. *JAMA.* 1976;236:1594–1597.

Sporer KA, Firestone J. Clinical Course of crack cocaine body stuffers. *Ann Emerg Med.* 1997;29:596–601.

Stern WZ, Spear PW, Jacobson HG. The roentgen findings in acute heroin intoxication. *AJR.* 1968;103:522–532.

Swartz RD, Millman RP, Billi JE, et al. Epidemic methanol poisoing: clinical and biochemical analysis of a recent episode. *Medicine.* 1981;60:373–382.

Tenebein M. Lheureuz P; and the American Academy of Clinical Toxicology and European Association of Poisions Centres and Clinical Toxicologists. Position paper: whole bowel irrigation. *J Toxicol Clin Toxicol.* 2004;42(6):843–854.

Van de Graaff WB, Thompson WL, Sunshine I, et al. Adsorbent and cathartic inhibition of enteral drug absorption. *J Pharmacol Exp Ther.* 1982;221:656–663.

Walker JA, Schwartzbard A, Krauss EA, et al. The missing gap: a pitfall in the diagnosis of alcohol intoxication by osmometry. *Arch Intern Med.* 1986;146:1843–1844.

Wax PM. Analeptic use in clinical toxicology: a historical appraisal. *J. Toxicol Clin Toxicol.* 1997;35:203–209.

Weisman RS. Theophylline. In: Goldfrank, ed. *Goldfrank's Toxicologic Emergencies.* 6th ed. Stanford, CT: Appleton and Lange;1998.

Occupational Toxicology

Peter S. Thorne

INTRODUCTION

The work environment has played a significant role in the occurrence of adverse human health effects due to chemical and biological hazards for centuries. Early writings by Ulrich Ellenbog (1435–1499), Agricola (1494–1555), and Paracelsus (1492–1541) revealed the toxic nature of exposures in mining, smelting, and metallurgy. A systematic treatise by Ramazzini (1633–1714) described the hazards as they applied to miners, chemists, metal workers, tanners, pharmacists, grain sifters, stonecutters, sewage workers, and even corpse bearers. Legislation to protect worker health began in England with the Factory Act of 1883, which established a factory inspectorate and limited child laborers nine to 13 years old to a 48-hour workweek, and 14 to 18 years olds to a 68-hour workweek. Today we continue to be concerned with occupational health and safety in a wide variety of work environments. Although occupational settings in developed countries are safer now than in the past, the levels of risk deemed acceptable have decreased while the recognition of the causal link of exposures to chronic diseases or diseases with long latencies has increased. As new hazards arise with the emergence of new technologies, we must be prepared to assess the risks and protect the health of workers. With increased globalization, there exists a responsibility to extend health protection to workers in developing nations who too often bear the burden of high exposures to occupational toxicants.

Occupational toxicology is the application of the principles and methodology of toxicology to understanding and managing chemical and biological hazards encountered at work. The objective of the occupational toxicologist is to prevent adverse health effects in workers that arise from exposures in their work environment. Because nonoccupational exposures can act as confounders or can increase the susceptibility of individual workers, occupational toxicologists must evaluate the entire spectrum of exposures experienced by the work force under consideration. Occupational toxicology is a discipline that draws on industrial hygiene, epidemiology, occupational medicine, and regulatory toxicology. The occupational toxicologist must have an intimate knowledge of the work environment and be able to recognize and prioritize exposure hazards. Because the work environment can present exposures to complex mixtures, the occupational toxicologist must also recognize those that are particularly hazardous when occurring in combination.

It is often difficult to establish a causal link between a worker's illness and job. First, the clinical expressions of occupationally induced diseases are often indistinguishable from those arising from nonoccupational causes. Second, there may be a protracted but biologically predictable latent interval between exposure and the expression of disease. Third, diseases of occupational origin may be multifactorial with other environmental factors or personal (eg, genetic or epigenetic) risk factors, contributing to the disease process. Nevertheless, studies have repeatedly shown that the dose of toxicant is a strong predictor of the likelihood, severity, and type of health effect.

WORKPLACES, EXPOSURES, AND STANDARDS

The Nature of the Work Force

Approximately 40% of the global work force, some one billion people, work in agricultural production. Many of these workers are engaged in subsistence agriculture (International Labour Organization, 2011). In contrast, the demographics and distribution of the work force in industrialized nations have undergone a progressive shift over the past three decades, moving away from jobs in heavy industry and agriculture toward jobs in the service sector

US labor market sector

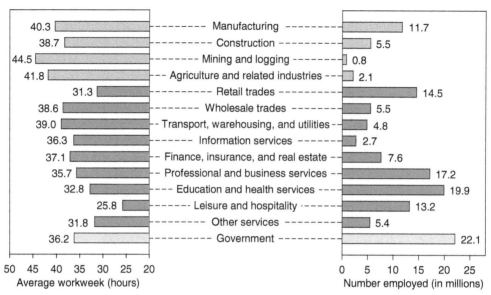

Figure 34-1. *Hours worked and number employed in the US civilian labor market.*

SOURCES: Current Employment Statistics Survey (Establishment Survey), US Bureau of Labor Statistics. Data as of June 2011. http://www.bls.gov/ces/#news accessed July 8, 2011.

National Compensation Survey: Occupational Wages in the United States, 2009. http://www.bls.gov/ncs/ncswage2009.htm#Wage_Tables accessed July 8, 2011.

Current Population Survey (Household Survey), US Bureau of Labor Statistics. Data for 2010. http://www.bls.gov/cps/tables.htm#annual accessed July 8, 2011.

and high-technology industries. In some instances, these manufacturing jobs have moved to less developed countries with less stringent worker health protection. There are currently 134 million people in the United States in the civilian, paid work force (seasonally adjusted data). The civilian labor force participation rate is 64.1% (United States Department of Labor [USDL], 2011b), a figure that has grown markedly over the past 50 years owing to the increased entry of women into the labor force. The 27 countries of the EU have an estimated 222.3 million workers (Employment in Europe, 2010), and Japan has about 62.6 million (Japan Monthly Statistics, 2011). Fig. 34-1 shows the breakdown of employment in the United States. This illustrates that there are about 20.1 million workers (15.0%) engaged in manufacturing, construction, mining and logging, and agriculture—occupations that have the potential for significant exposure to chemical and biological agents. Furthermore, there are occupations in the service sector, such as automobile repair; other repair and maintenance; work in gasoline stations, pipeline transportation, truck and rail transportation; waste management and remediation services; and employment in botanical gardens that can also include exposures to hazardous chemicals. Service-producing occupations (including government jobs) account for the majority (85%) of US jobs. On average, employees in the service sector work 6.7 fewer hours per week than in the goods-producing sector. Farm work employs an estimated 2.11 million workers, 16 years of age and older, and the US Bureau of Labor Statistics has documented an average of 41.8 hours worked per week. Work in agriculture is markedly different from most other occupations in four fundamental ways. First, 44% of those employed in agriculture are self-employed or unpaid family members. Second, the overwhelming majority of farm establishments (90%) have fewer than 20 employees, and these work sites represent 35% of the agricultural work force (USDL, 2011a). Third, although the annual national average hours worked per week is 41.8, many farmers, ranchers, and farm workers have periods (eg, harvest time) when they work as many as 20 hours per day, seven days per week. Fourth, according to the US Bureau of the Census,

there are in excess of 290,000 children who identify agricultural work as their major employment (GAO/HEHS, 1998). Department of Labor data indicate that, on average, 128,500 hired farm workers between the ages of 14 and 17 were working annually in crop production (GAO/HEHS, 1998). The presence of children in the work force has important ramifications for body burdens, disease latency, toxicokinetics, and biotransformation of toxicants.

Determinants of Dose

Dose is defined as the amount of toxicant that reaches the target tissue over a defined time span. In occupational environments, *exposure* is often used as a surrogate for *dose*. The response to a chemical is dependent on both host factors and dose. Fig. 34-2 illustrates the pathway from exposure to subclinical disease or to adverse health effect, and suggests that there are important modifying factors: contemporaneous exposures, genetic and epigenetic susceptibility, age, gender, nutritional status, and behavioral factors. These modifying factors can influence whether a worker remains healthy, develops subclinical disease that is repaired, or progresses to frank illness. Workplace health protection and surveillance programs (shown in blue) can reduce exposures, disrupt the exposure-dose pathway, or identify internalized dose and early effects before irreparable disease develops. These programs help to ensure a safe workplace and a healthier work force.

As illustrated in Fig. 34-2, dose is a function of exposure concentration, exposure duration, and exposure frequency. Individual and environmental characteristics can also affect dose. Exposure assessment is the process of quantifying the intensity, frequency, and duration of exposures and their determinants in order to better estimate dose. Table 34-1 indicates determinants of dose for exposure via the inhalation and dermal routes. For determining inhalation exposures, environmental conditions such as concentration, particle size distribution, and properties of the chemical are important. However, respiratory rate and breathing volume as well as other host factors contribute. Protection afforded by personal

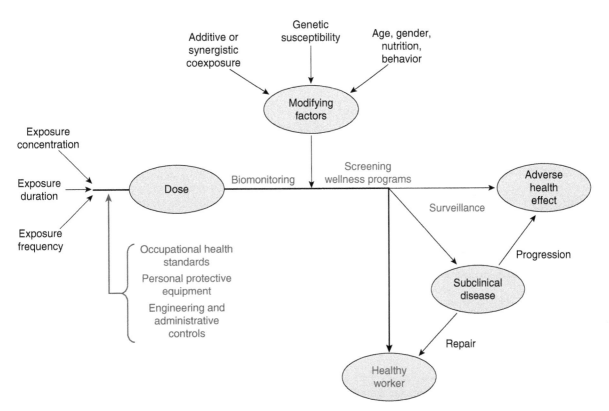

Figure 34-2. *Pathway from exposure to disease, showing modifying factors and opportunities for intervention.*

protective equipment (especially respirators) will reduce but not eliminate exposure. The degree of exposure reduction for a particular respirator (the workplace protection factor) varies with respirator design, fit, maintenance, manner of use, and environmental conditions from less than five to 10,000. A respirator with a workplace protection factor of 10, when used properly, will reduce particulate matter concentrations inside the mask to one-tenth that outside the mask. A commonly used two-strap fiber respirator for lowering

particulate matter exposure, the N95, should reduce exposures by 95% but may fail to meet this criterion for submicron aerosols (Balazy *et al.*, 2006).

Dermal exposures depend on toxicant concentration; work conditions, including the degree and duration of wetness; and the ambient conditions at the work site (Table 34-1). Some determinants of dermal dosing relate to the physicochemical properties of the chemical as they affect the percutaneous absorption rate. These include solubility, temperature, pH, molecular size, and chemical characteristics of the vehicle. Host factors also influence dermal absorption and distribution. Important factors include the surface area of the skin that is exposed, the integrity of the skin, blood flow, and biotransformation. Because the stratum corneum, the outer layer of the epidermis, is the principal barrier to dermal uptake, the thickness of this layer in the exposed area has great significance. As an example, the absorption of hydrocortisone through the plantar foot arch is 1/25 less than through the back and 1/300 less than through scrotal skin (Bason *et al.*, 1991). A classic human in vivo study by Maibach *et al.* (1971) using the pesticide parathion demonstrated a 12-fold range in percutaneous absorption between the anatomical site with the highest (scrotum) to that with the lowest (forearm) percent of dose absorbed. For malathion there was a 12-fold difference in absorbed dose between the jaw angle and the palm. The use of protective gloves and clothing or aprons and the application of barrier creams can greatly reduce exposure. For maximal protection, it is important that the glove be constructed of material tailored to the toxicant(s) of concern.

Table 34-1

Determinants of Toxicant Dose

Inhalation exposure
  Airborne concentration
  Particle size distribution
  Respiratory rate
  Tidal volume
  Other host factors
  Duration of exposure
  Chemical, physical, or biological properties of the
    hazardous agent
  Effectiveness of personal protective devices

Dermal exposure
  Concentration in air, droplets, or solutions
  Degree and duration of wetness
  Integrity of skin
  Percutaneous absorption rate
  Region of skin exposed
  Surface area exposed
  Preexisting skin disease
  Temperature in the workplace
  Vehicle for the toxicant
  Presence of other chemicals on skin

Occupational Exposure Limits

One of the roles of the occupational toxicologist is to contribute data to the process of establishing standards, or determining the appropriateness of those standards. Workplace exposure limits exist for chemical, biological, and physical agents, and are recommended as guidelines or promulgated as standards in order to promote worker health and safety. For chemical and biological agents, exposure limits are expressed as acceptable ambient concentration levels (occupational exposure limits [OELs]), or as concentrations of a toxicant, its metabolites, or a specific marker of its effects in biological systems (biological exposure indices).

OELs are established as standards by regulatory agencies or as guidelines by research groups or professional organizations. In the United States, the Occupational Safety and Health Administration (OSHA) under the Department of Labor promulgates legally enforceable standards known as permissible exposure limits (PELs). These standards are determined and supported by the best scientific evidence available and assure "to the extent feasible . . . that no employee will suffer material impairment of health or functional capacity" with regular exposure "for the period of his working life." OSHA has defined an eight-hour time-weighted average (TWA) PEL (US Federal Register, 1992) as the "employee's average airborne exposure in any eight-hour work shift of a 40-hour workweek which shall not be exceeded." The TWA PEL is established as the highest level of exposure to which an employee may be exposed without incurring the risk of adverse health effects (OSHA, 1995). Although approximately 500 PELs have been promulgated, there are not enough to regulate exposures to the vast number of compounds to which workers are exposed, and some of the existing PELs do not reflect current knowledge.

The National Institute for Occupational Safety and Health (NIOSH), under the Centers for Disease Control and Prevention, publishes recommended exposure limits (RELs) that are more frequently updated and are generally more stringent than PELs. NIOSH also performs research and disseminates information on workplace hazards and their prevention. Most developed countries have governmental inspectorate agencies, analogous to OSHA, that are responsible for establishing and enforcing OELs. In some countries, the insurance system also plays a significant role.

The European Commission has established legally enforceable binding occupational exposure limit values (BOELVs) and biological limit values (BLVs) for the protection of health and safety in the workplace. Socioeconomic and technical feasibility factors are also considered in setting these values. The OELs are established based on recommendations of the Scientific Committee on Occupational Exposure Limits (SCOEL), which evaluates published scientific data on hazardous compounds for regulation and provides assessment of exposure limits that "it believes will protect workers from chemical risks" (European Commission, 1995, 1998). Indicative Occupational Exposure Limit Values (IOELVs) are nonbinding, health-based OELs that do not consider technical or economic feasibility. A first list of IOELVs was established in 2000 followed by a second in 2006. EU member countries may not promulgate OELs less stringent than these values.

The American Conference of Governmental Industrial Hygienists (ACGIH) is a nonprofit scientific association that publishes OELs for chemicals and for physical agents. These take the form of threshold limit values (TLVs) and biological exposure indices (BEIs). They are frequently revisited and generally reflect current knowledge in occupational toxicology and industrial hygiene. They are developed as guidelines and are not enforceable standards; however, many industries adopt TLVs and BEIs as internal OELs. As stated by the ACGIH, "The TLVs and BEIs represent conditions under which ACGIH believes that nearly all workers may be repeatedly exposed without adverse health effects" (ACGIH, 2010). These guidelines are health based and do not include consideration of technical feasibility or economic effects of implementation.

Three types of TLVs are suggested, depending on the time scale of adverse effects inducible by the toxicants. The time-weighted average TLV (TLV-TWA) is an OEL for exposures, averaged over an eight-hour day, five-day workweek regimen. These are generally applied to toxicants that exert their effects over long periods. The short-term exposure limit (TLV-STEL) is an OEL for a 15-minute measurement period. The TLV-STEL should not be exceeded in any 15-minute sampling window, and there should be 60 minutes or more between exposures in this range. The ceiling limit (TLV-C) represents a concentration that should never be exceeded. These are usually applied to toxicants that cause acute effects (such as asphyxia or potent sensory irritation) and for which real-time monitoring devices are available. BEIs are guidelines for biological monitoring and represent levels "most likely to be observed in specimens collected from healthy workers who have been exposed to chemicals to the same extent, as workers with inhalation exposure at the Threshold Limit Value" (ACGIH, 2010). BEIs are recommended for analysis of urine, blood, and exhaled air. While hair, fingernails, adipose tissue biopsies, and other specimens are used in research and forensic toxicology, there are no BEIs for these.

It is important to recognize that OELs do not correspond to exposure conditions devoid of health risk. The concept of acceptable exposure level must be understood as the level of exposure, below which, the probability of impairing the health of the exposed workers is acceptable. The process of deciding what is an acceptable risk to occupational or environmental hazards blends the scientific disciplines of exposure assessment and toxicology with often vexing policy issues. Historically, acceptable risk in a society is related to the general health of the population and to a host of factors that influence how risks are perceived. To determine that the risks from an occupational hazard are acceptable, it is necessary to characterize the hazard, identify the potential diseases or adverse outcomes, and establish the relationship between exposure intensity or dose and the adverse health effects. If biological markers of exposure or early reversible effects are identified, this can aid in the risk-assessment process.

OCCUPATIONAL DISEASES

Routes of Exposure

Diseases arising in occupational environments involve exposure, primarily through inhalation, ingestion, or dermal absorption. In the vast majority of work environments, inhalation of toxicants is a primary concern. Inhalation exposures can occur with gases, vapors, liquid aerosols, particulate aerosols, fumes, and mixtures of these. Dermal exposures are also important and can arise from airborne materials as well as liquids splashed onto the skin, immersion exposures, or from material handling.

Additional exposure hazards exist for infectious agents. Exposures leading to occupational infections may arise through inhalation or ingestion of microorganisms, but can also arise from needlesticks in health care workers or through insect bites among farmers, natural resource workers, and others employed out of doors. Additionally, poisonings from toxic plants or venomous animals can occur through skin inoculation (eg, zookeepers, horticulturists, or commercial divers).

Agents Associated With Diseases

There are a myriad of agents responsible for occupational diseases. While some act on a particular organ such as the liver or kidney, others can affect multiple organ systems. Table 34-2 presents a list of the major occupational diseases and examples of agents that cause them. This is not intended to be all-inclusive. Rather it is meant to highlight what are historically the most prevalent and

Table 34-2

Examples of Occupational Diseases and the Toxicants That Cause Them

ORGAN SYSTEM OR DISEASE GROUP	DISEASE	CAUSATIVE AGENT
Lung and airways	Acute pulmonary edema, bronchiolitis obliterans	Nitrogen oxides, phosgene, diacetyl
	Allergic rhinitis	Pollens, fungal spores
	Asphyxiation	Carbon monoxide, hydrogen cyanide, inert gas dilution
	Asthma	Toluene diisocyanate, α-amylase, animal urine proteins
	Asthma-like syndrome	Swine barn environments, cotton dust, bioaerosols
	Bronchitis, pneumonitis	Arsenic, chlorine
	Chronic bronchitis	Cotton dust, grain dust, welding fumes
	Emphysema	Coal dust, cigarette smoke
	Fibrotic lung disease	Silica, asbestos
	Hypersensitivity pneumonitis	Thermophilic bacteria, avian proteins, pyrethrum, *Penicillium, Aspergillus*
	Metal fume fever	Zinc, copper, magnesium
	Mucous membrane irritation	Hydrogen chloride, swine barn environments
	Organic dust toxic syndrome	"Moldy" silage, endotoxin
	Upper respiratory tract inflammation	Endotoxin, peptidoglycan, glucans, viruses
Cancer	Acute myelogenous leukemia	Benzene, ethylene oxide
	Bladder cancer	Benzidine, 2-naphthylamine, 4-biphenylamine
	Gastrointestinal cancers	Asbestos
	Hepatic hemangiosarcoma	Vinyl chloride
	Hepatocellular carcinoma	Aflatoxin, hepatitis B virus
	Mesothelioma, lung carcinoma	Asbestos, arsenic, radon, bis-chloro methyl ether
	Skin cancer	Polycyclic aromatic hydrocarbons, ultraviolet irradiation
Skin	Allergic contact dermatitis	Natural rubber latex, isothiazolins, poison ivy, nickel
	Chemical burns	Sodium hydroxide, hydrogen fluoride
	Chloracne	TCDD*, polychlorinated biphenyls
	Irritant dermatitis	Sodium dodecyl sulfate
Nervous system	Cholinesterase inhibition	Organophosphate insecticides
	Neuronopathy	Methyl mercury
	Parkinsonism	Carbon monoxide, carbon disulfide
	Peripheral neuropathy	*N*-Hexane, trichloroethylene, acrylamide
Immune system	Autoimmune disease	Vinyl chloride, silica
	Hypersensitivity	See entries for allergic rhinitis, asthma, hypersensitivity pneumonitis, allergic contact dermatitis
	Immunosuppression	TCDD*, lead, mercury, pesticides
Renal disease	Indirect renal failure	Arsine, phosphine, trinitrophenol
	Nephropathy	Paraquat, 1,4-dichlorobenzene, mercuric chloride
Cardiovascular disease	Arrhythmias	Acetone, toluene, methylene chloride, trichloroethylene
	Atherosclerosis	Dinitrotoluene, carbon monoxide
	Coronary artery disease	Carbon disulfide
	Cor pulmonale	Beryllium
	Systemic hypotension	Nitroglycerine, ethylene glycol dinitrate
Liver disease	Fatty liver (steatosis)	Carbon tetrachloride, toluene
	Cirrhosis	Arsenic, trichloroethylene
	Hepatocellular death	dimethylformamide, TCDD*
Reproductive system	Male	Chlordecone (Kepone), dibromochloropropane, hexane
	Female	Aniline, styrene
	Both sexes	Carbon disulfide, lead, vinyl chloride
Infectious diseases†	Arboviral encephalitides	Alphavirus, Bunyavirus, Flavivirus
	Aspergillosis	*Aspergillus niger, A. fumigatus, A. flavus*
	Cryptosporidiosis	*Cryptosporidium parvum*

(continued)

Table 34-2		
(Continued)		
ORGAN SYSTEM OR DISEASE GROUP	**DISEASE**	**CAUSATIVE AGENT**
	Hepatitis B	Hepatitis B virus
	Histoplasmosis	*Histoplasma capsulatum*
	Legionellosis	*Legionella pneumophila*
	Lyme disease	*Borrelia burgdorferi*
	Psittacosis	*Chlamydia psittaci*
	Tuberculosis	*Mycobacterium tuberculosis hominis*

*TCDD, 2,3,7,8-tetrachlorodibenzo-para-dioxin.
†For more on occupational infectious diseases, see Douwes et al. (2003).

widely recognized occupational diseases, plus those that continue to be prevalent in the workplace. The toxicants listed are those for which there is a strong association with the disease or the most conclusive data to support causality. Examples are shown for cancer and for diseases of the lung and airways, heart, liver, kidney, skin, nervous system, immune system, and reproductive system. Several examples of occupational infectious diseases are also listed to highlight the fact that, in many work settings, infectious agents may constitute the major hazard and may coexist with chemical hazards. Most of the occupational diseases listed in Table 34-2 are associated with industrial chemicals. These are discussed in other chapters throughout this book.

Table 34-3 lists forty agents that are known by the International Agency for Research on Cancer (IARC) to be carcinogens in humans (Group 1) and for which there has been or is currently extensive occupational exposure. This list includes agents such as asbestos, arsenic, benzene, vinyl chloride, and coal tars. IARC Group 1 refers to agents or mixtures that are known to be carcinogenic to humans based on sufficient epidemiological evidence usually accompanied by limited or sufficient animal evidence.

Occupational Respiratory Diseases

Because inhalation generally represents the most significant route of exposure, many of the major occupational diseases affect the lung and airways. These diseases have been studied extensively and are largely responsible for the creation of the occupational regulatory framework. Deaths due to occupational lung diseases such as asbestosis, coal workers' pneumoconiosis, silicosis, byssinosis, and occupational asthma have been recognized for centuries and led to important legislation such as the 1970 US Occupational Safety and Health Act. These occupational lung diseases continue to have significant associations with morbidity. Table 34-4 lists the crude US death rate and annual deaths for 2005 (the most recent data available) and illustrates that while the death rates are fairly low, there are still about 2460 deaths per year attributable to asbestos, silica, coal dust, and other pneumoconiotic dusts; 2704 malignant mesothelioma deaths; and 67 deaths from hypersensitivity pneumonitis. However, fatalities are just the tip of the iceberg as some occupational lung diseases are rarely fatal, yet may still be debilitating. Every year in the United States, there are 20,000 hospital discharges related to cases of asbestosis, and 188,000 coal workers receive federal Black Lung Benefits (NIOSH, 2006). The US Mine Safety and Health Administration has compiled data on inspector- and mine operator-collected samples in coal mining operations and found that 29.3% of these

exceeded the PEL for respirable quartz and 7.5% were over the PEL for respirable coal dust.

Many of the diseases listed in Table 34-2 are known by other names that refer to a particular occupation or agent. One example is hypersensitivity pneumonitis, an allergic lung disease marked by interstitial lymphocytic pneumonitis and granulomatous lesions. Hypersensitivity pneumonitis is also known as extrinsic allergic alveolitis, farmer's lung disease, bagassosis (sugar cane), humidifier fever, Japanese summer house fever, pigeon breeder's lung, and maple bark stripper's lung, depending on the occupational setting in which it arises. Although we often think of these as the same disease, it is important to recognize that the exposures and physiological responses they induce are complex and may differ in the manifestation of the disease.

The US Bureau of Labor Statistics tracks data for nonfatal occupational injuries and illnesses, of which, there were 3.3 million in 2009. The vast majority of these were injuries, but there were still over 220,000 occupational illnesses reported in 2009 (USDL 2011c). There were 21,500 reported respiratory conditions arising from exposure to toxic agents and dust diseases of the lung. The former category includes pneumonitis, pharyngitis, rhinitis, and acute lung congestion. Table 34-5 shows data for rates and cases in 2009 by industry division. Poisonings were relatively rare, whereas skin diseases occurred at rates as high as 5.2 per 110,000 workers per year. The manufacturing sector accounted for approximately 29% of all occupational illnesses. Seven industry codes that had respiratory condition incidence rates that exceeded seven per 10,000 full-time workers were ambulance services, police and fire protection, urban transit systems, support activities for water transportation, adhesive manufacturing, grain and oil seed milling, and animal slaughtering. The relevant exposures for the first four of these are combustion products from fires and diesel engines. The rate for chemical manufacturing was much lower, 1.8 cases per 10,000 workers, down by 50% since a decade ago.

Toxic gas injuries are often characterized by leakage of both fluid and osmotically active proteins from the vascular tissue into the interstitium and airways. Important determinants of the severity and location of injury are the concentration and water solubility of the toxic gas or vapor. Anhydrous ammonia, with its extremely high solubility, primarily damages the eyes, sinuses, and upper airways. The vapors combine with water in the tissue and form ammonium hydroxide, quickly producing liquefaction necrosis. Chemicals with lower solubility, such as nitrogen dioxide, act more on the distal airways and alveoli and take longer to induce tissue damage.

Occupational asthma may be defined as a "disease characterized by variable airflow limitation, and/or airway hyperresponsiveness,

Table 34-3

Occupational Exposure Agents Classified by IARC as Group 1 Definite Human Carcinogens

AGENT	INDUSTRIES AND OCCUPATIONS WHERE SOME WORKERS MAY BE EXPOSED
Particulate matter	
Asbestos	Miners, abatement workers, construction workers, sheet metal workers, steam fitters, shipyard workers
Crystalline silica (quartz or cristobalite)	Stone and ceramics industry, foundries, construction, abrasives manufacturing
Erionite	Waste treatment workers, building materials manufacturing
Hematite	Underground mining
Talc containing asbestiform fibers	Ceramics industry
Wood dust	Wood and wood-products industries, pulp and paper industry, wood working trades
Metals	
Arsenic and arsenic compounds	Miners, nonferrous metal smelting, arsenical pesticide manufacturers and applicators
Beryllium	Specialty metallurgy workers, avionics, electronics, nuclear industry
Cadmium and cadmium compounds	Cadmium smelting, battery production, dyes and pigment making, electroplating
Gallium arsenide	Microelectronics manufacturing
Hexavalent chromium compounds	Chromate production plants, dye and pigment making, welders, tanners
Nickel compounds[*]	Nickel smelting, welding
Organic chemicals	
Aflatoxin	Animal feed industry, grain handling and processing
4-Aminobiphenyl	Chemical industry, dyes and pigment manufacturing
Benzene	Refineries, shoe industry, chemical, pharmaceutical and rubber industry, printing industry
Benzidine	Chemical industry, dyes and pigment manufacturing
Benzo(a)pyrene	Coke oven emissions, coal tar pitch volatiles, diesel exhaust, environmental tobacco smoke
Bis(chloromethyl) ether and Chloromethyl ether (technical grade)	Chemical industry, laboratory reagent, plastic manufacturing
1,3-Butadiene	Chemical industry, petrochemical plants, styrene–butadiene rubber manufacturing
Coal tars and pitches	Coke production, coal gasification, refineries, foundries, road paving, hot tar roofing
Ethylene oxide	Chemical industry, dry vegetable fumigation, hospital sterilizing
Formaldehyde	Textiles, composite wood industry, chemical industry, medical laboratories
4,4′-Methylenebis(2-chloroaniline)	Epoxy resin manufacturing, polyurethane product fabrication
Mineral oils, untreated and mildly treated	Metal machining and honing, roll steel production, printing
2-Naphthylamine	Chemical industry, dyestuffs, and pigment manufacturing
2,3,4,7,8-Pentachlorodibenzofuran	Hazardous waste processing, chlorophenoxy herbicide production and use, pulp and paper industry
3,4,5,3′,4′-Pentachlorobiphenyl	Hazardous waste processing, waterway dredging, transformer handling, pulp and paper industry
Shale oils or shale-derived lubricants	Mining and processing, cotton textile industry
Soots	Chimney sweeps, heating and ventilation contractors, firefighters, metallurgical workers
2,3,7,8-Tetrachlorobibenzo-para-dioxin (TCDD)	Hazardous waste processing, chlorophenoxy herbicide production and use, pulp and paper industry
Vinyl chloride	Plastics industry, production of polyvinyl chloride products and copolymers
Other agents with occupational exposure	
Environmental tobacco smoke	Restaurant, bar and entertainment industry; other smoke-exposed workers
Occupational exposures as a painter	Commercial painting
Leather dust	Garment industry, auto seat fabrication, saddle and tack manufacturing
Magenta dye (rosaniline, pararosaniline)	Dye manufacture, textile dying, commercial art and printing
Mustard gas	Production, soldiers, some research laboratories
Exposures in the rubber industry	Work in rubber manufacturing industries
Strong inorganic acid mists containing sulfuric acid	Steel industry, petrochemical industry, fertilizer industry, pickling industry
Physical Agents	
Ionizing radiation[†]	Radiology and nuclear medicine staff, nuclear workers, miners, hazardous waste workers
Solar radiation	Farmers, gardeners and landscapers, lifeguards, construction workers

[*]*Certain combinations of nickel oxides and sulfides.*
[†]*Includes x-rays, γ-rays, neutrons, radon gas, and α and β particle-emitting substances internally deposited.*
SOURCE: *IARC (2011), Siemiatycki et al. (2004).*

Table 34-4

US Deaths and Crude Death Rates Attributed to Selected Occupational Lung Diseases for 2005

DISEASE	NUMBER OF DEATHS	DEATH RATE PER MILLION WORKING AGE PEOPLE
Asbestosis	1423	6.04
Coal workers pneumoconiosis	653	2.77
Silicosis	161	0.68
Byssinosis	7	0.03
Other pneumoconioses*	216	0.92
Malignant mesothelioma	2704	11.47
Hypersensitivity pneumonitis	67	0.28

*This includes aluminosis, berylliosis, stannosis, siderosis, and fibrosis from bauxite, graphite fibers, wollastonite, cadmium, portland cement, emery, kaolin, antimony, and mica.
SOURCE: NIOSH Work-Related Lung Disease (WoRLD) Surveillance System 2005. Available from: http://www2a.cdc.gov/drds/World ReportData/. Accessed July 6, 2011.

and/or inflammation due to causes and conditions attributable to a particular occupational environment and not to stimuli encountered outside the workplace" (Bernstein *et al.*, 2006). Data from the NIOSH Work-Related Occupational Lung Disease Surveillance System has shown that 20% of occupational asthma cases represented aggravation of preexisting asthma by workplace exposures and 68% of cases represented new-onset asthma caused by occupational exposures. The remaining 12% could not be classified (NIOSH, 2011). The US National Health Interview Survey has provided data on the prevalence of asthma based upon usual industry and smoking status (Table 34-6). These data indicate that asthma prevalence is highest in health services; general merchandise stores; food, bakery, and dairy stores; and eating and drinking places. Also high are hospitals; transportation equipment; printing, publishing, and allied industries; utilities and sanitary; furniture, lumber, and wood products industries; and chemicals and allied products. Interestingly, in some industries, current smokers demonstrate the higher prevalence, while in other industries, the higher prevalence is seen among nonsmokers. This may reflect that many people diagnosed with these conditions quit smoking.

There are a variety of industries in which there is increased risk of developing work-related asthma. In chemical-based industries, plastic and rubber polymer precursors, diisocyanates, reactive dyes, and acid anhydrides are recognized low-molecular-weight sensitizing compounds. Biocides and fungicides used in metal fabrication and machining, custodial services, lawn and turf growing, and agriculture are also chemicals associated with occupational asthma. A number of metals can induce sensitization and asthma, including

Table 34-5

Rate of Nonfatal Occupational Illnesses 2009

INDUSTRY DIVISION	NUMBER TOTAL CASES	RATE			
		OVERALL	RESPIRATORY CONDITIONS*	POISONINGS	SKIN DISEASES OR DISORDERS†
Goods producing	57,300	29.1			
Manufacturing	47,900	39.0	1.4	0.2	4.0
Construction	6,800	11.6	1.2	0.3	3.4
Agriculture, fishing, forestry‡	2210	24.7	2.3	0.6	7.1
Mining	490	7.9	0.7	–	0.8
Service providing§	108,900	15.3			
Education and health services	45,400	32.0	3.6	0.2	5.2
Trade, transportation, public utilities	25,500	11.7	1.1	0.2	1.8
Leisure and hospitality	10,300	11.9	1.1	0.3	3.1
Finance, insurance, real estate	6,800	9.4	0.8	–	1.0
Professional and business services	12,500	9.2	0.7	0.3	2.2
Information	3,200	12.3	0.7	0.1	0.9
State and local government	58,300	39.1	4.6	0.8	–
Total number of reported cases	224,500		21,500	3,200	35,400

Rate per 10,000 full time workers.
*These conditions are pneumonitis; pharyngitis; rhinitis; acute congestions due to chemicals, dusts, gases, or fumes; and other dust diseases of the lung.
†These conditions are contact dermatitis, eczema, or rash caused by primary irritants and sensitizers or poisonous plants; oil acne; friction blisters; chrome ulcers; and inflammation.
‡Agricultural illnesses are grossly underreported because the data exclude farms with fewer than 11 employee.
§Includes auto repair, other repair, health care, hotel, personal, business, entertainment, educational, social, and engineering services.
SOURCE: Bureau of Labor Statistics, US Department of Labor (2011). Available from: http://www.bls.gov/iif/oshsum.htm. Accessed October 8, 2011.

Table 34-6

US Asthma Prevalence by Current Industry and Smoking Status for Selected Industry Codes* Age 18 and Over

INDUSTRY	ASTHMA PREVALENCE (%)		
	NONSMOKERS	FORMER SMOKERS	CURRENT SMOKERS
Health services except hospitals	9.8	12.1	12.9
General merchandise stores	8.0	12.7	11.8
Eating and drinking places	10.5	9.3	12.1
Food, bakery, and dairy stores	9.2	10.2	11.9
Hospitals	8.7	12.6	9.5
Transportation equipment	10.6	9.0	9.1
Printing, publishing, and allied industries	10.0	10.3	7.4
Utilities and sanitary	9.0	10.0	7.9
Furniture, lumber, and wood products	7.9	9.2	8.5
Chemicals and allied products	8.9	7.9	8.3
Fabricated metal industries	7.3	8.1	7.9
Trucking service and warehousing	7.6	6.8	8.5
Repair services	7.4	6.9	8.3
Construction	6.4	8.2	7.2
Agriculture	6.4	7.1	7.4
Mining	8.7	4.8	6.7
Textile mill and finished textile products	5.6	6.8	5.5
Primary metal industries	4.3	6.1	6.9

*The US adult self-reported lifetime asthma prevalence rate is 11.6% for males and 14.9% for females, and the prevalence rate for current asthma is 6.1% for males and 10.0% for females (BRFSS, 2004).

SOURCE: Data for 1997–2004. National Health Interview Survey, Work-Related Lung Diseases Surveillance System; 2011. Available from: http://www2. cdc.gov/drds/WorldReportData Accessed July 6, 2011.

chromium, cobalt, nickel, platinum, and zinc. Enzymes pose significant risks for occupational asthma (Heederik *et al.*, 2002). Examples include α-amylase among bakery workers and subtilisin, a protease used in laundry detergents. The enzyme production industry has had to adopt strict environmental and process controls to reduce the incidence of occupational asthma in their production facilities.

Those working with animals or animal products are at increased risk of developing allergy (Elliott *et al.*, 2005) and occupational asthma (Pacheco *et al.*, 2003). Animal handlers, processors, and laboratory technicians who work with animals can become immunologically sensitized to urine or salivary proteins in many vertebrates; proteins in bat guano and bird droppings; animal dander; serum proteins in blood products; dust from horns, antlers, and tusks; or the shells of crustaceans. Very high rates of sensitization can occur in shellfish processors (Glass *et al.*, 1998). Arthropods such as insect larvae, cockroaches, mites, or weevils are recognized inducers of work-related asthma. Plants and plant products (eg, soy flour, spices, and coffee beans) can also cause asthma among workers. In a variety of occupations, exposure to fungi, especially of the genera *Aspergillus*, *Penicillium*, *Rhizopus*, *Mucor*, and *Paecilomyces*, are associated with allergic rhinitis and asthma. These are especially present in sawmills, woodchip handling, and composting facilities (Duchaine *et al.*, 2000; Eduard *et al.*, 1992). Apart from the contaminating microorganisms, certain woods themselves produce chemical sensitizing agents. Examples include western red cedar, redwood, and some tropical hardwoods.

Asthma emerged in the 1980s as a major occupational health concern among health care workers. In order to reduce the risk of hepatitis B and other infectious diseases, health care workers adopted the use of natural rubber latex gloves for barrier protection. Proteins from the latex of the rubber tree, *Hevea brasiliensis*, led to immunological sensitization. Thirteen of these high-molecular-weight proteins have been characterized as allergens (Bernstein *et al.*, 2003). Many other plants of less commercial value produce a similar milky fluid when cut, and have similar sensitizing properties. A shift to powder-free and nonlatex examination gloves has reduced the incidence of latex allergy among health care workers and patients.

Studies of asthma prevalence in occupational settings with exposure to low-molecular-weight chemicals have suggested prevalence rates of 5% to 10% for toluene diisocyanate (Baur, 1996; Becklake *et al.*, 2006), 3.2% to 18% for anhydrides (Venables *et al.*, 1985; Wernfors *et al.*, 1986), 4% for plicatic acid from western red cedar (Chan-Yeung *et al.*, 1984), and 54% in a platinum refinery (Venables *et al.*, 1989). For high-molecular-weight allergens, prevalence among shellfish processors was estimated at 21% to 26% (Desjardins *et al.*, 1995; Glass *et al.*, 1998), 11% to 44% among lab animal workers (Cullinan *et al.*, 1994; Fuortes *et al.*, 1997; Hollander *et al.*, 1997), and 5% to 7% among bakers exposed to wheat and α-amylase (Heederik *et al.*, 2002).

Agricultural workers exposed to grain dust, cotton dust, or atmospheres in swine or poultry confinement barns are at risk for the development of an asthma-like syndrome. This syndrome is an acute nonallergic airway response characterized by self-limited inflammation with neutrophilic infiltrates and increased proinflammatory cytokines and chemokines (eg, TNFα, IL-6, and IL-8), but it does not include persistent airway hyperreactivity as in occupational asthma (Schenker *et al.*, 1998). Asthma-like syndrome includes cough, mild dyspnea, fever, malaise, and cross-shift declines in lung function. Endotoxin in combination with other inflammatory bioaerosols is the likely etiological agent (Douwes *et al.*, 2003; Schwartz *et al.*, 1994, 1995).

An emerging area of concern is adverse effects of respiratory exposures to manufactured nanomaterials. There are currently over one thousand consumer products that contain nanotechnology-based materials (Nanotechnology Consumer Products Inventory, 2011). Nanomaterials are engineered structures that have a primary size less than 100 nm in at least one dimension. Airborne nanoparticles generally form agglomerates in which groups of particles are held together by relatively weak forces (eg, van der Waals). They may also aggregate forming clusters that are fused, sintered, or chemically bonded to one another (Pettibone *et al.*, 2008). Manufactured nanomaterials find applications in electronics, construction materials including wall and floor coverings, cosmetics, drug delivery, medical imaging, food products, packaging materials, and textiles, to name a few. Occupational exposures occur in the manufacture of the nanomaterials and in their use in fabricating materials and consumer products. Exposures can also occur when nanomaterials are cut or shaped and when product waste is discarded. Engineered nanomaterials may be carbon-based, metal-based, or biological in nature (Adamcakova-Dodd *et al.*, 2010). Biological actions of nanoscaled materials may differ from the comparable bulk materials or micron-sized particles (Nel *et al.*, 2006; Grassian *et al.*, 2007). Inhaled nanomaterials may induce pulmonary toxicity or they can cause adverse effects in other tissues through adsorption and transport, generation of toxic substances by their dissolution or degradation, or by crossing key physiological barriers, or cell and nuclear membranes (Kim *et al.*, 2011). In early 2011, NIOSH issued a new guideline on TiO2 marking the first instance of two guidelines for the same compound based on particle size. In mid 2011, NIOSH has issued for peer review a draft *Current Intelligence Bulletin* on carbon nanotubes and nanofibers. Other research and regulatory bodies worldwide are studying nanomaterials and conducting human health risk assessments.

Other Occupational Diseases

Occupational diseases of the skin are common but less often fatal that those of the respiratory system. Irritant dermatitis and allergic contact dermatitis have the highest incidence of reported skin conditions. Table 34-5 shows data for rates of skin diseases or disorders in 2009 by industry division. These data indicate that agriculture, fishing, and forestry services; and manufacturing carry the highest risks. In the service sector, the education and health services division has the highest rate of skin diseases. This is due to the high rate of skin disorders in hospitals (7.2 per 10,000) and in nursing and residential care facilities (10.6 per 10,000). In 2009, 14% of reported occupational skin disorders were in manufacturing while 21% were in education and health services.

Occupational toxicants may induce diseases in a variety of body sites distant from the lung or skin. These include tumors arising in the liver, bladder, gastrointestinal tract, or hematopoietic system and are attributable to a variety of chemical classes. Further discussion of other occupational diseases and the toxicants listed in Table 34-2 can be found in the relevant chapters in Units IV and V of this text.

Nervous system damage can be central, peripheral, or both. It may be acute, as with some organophosphate exposures, or chronic, as with organomercury poisoning or acrylamide-induced neuropathy. Injury affecting the immune system may arise from the immunosuppressive effects of chemicals such as dioxins or toxic metals. Many occupational diseases of the immune system occur due to hypersensitivity leading to respiratory or dermal allergy or systemic hypersensitivity reactions. Autoimmune syndromes have been associated with occupational exposures to crystalline silica and vinyl chloride.

Occupational diseases of the cardiovascular system include atherosclerosis, a variety of arrhythmias, problems with coronary blood supply, systemic hypotension, and cor pulmonale (right ventricular hypertrophy usually due to pulmonary hypertension as with chronic obstructive pulmonary disease). Liver diseases such as carbon tetrachloride-induced fatty liver and hepatocellular death due to toxic concentrations of acetaminophen have classically been used to illustrate chemical mechanisms of cellular injury leading to organ failure. These are thoroughly discussed in Chap. 13. Occupational diseases of the reproductive system can be gender- and organ-specific; but several toxicants—including carbon disulfide, lead, and vinyl chloride—may affect both sexes.

Exposures to infectious agents are a part of a variety of occupations (Thorne and Duchaine, 2007). Veterinarians, health care workers, and biomedical researchers studying infectious agents have exposures that are largely known and infection control strategies can limit their risks. For others, such as farmers and foresters, specific risks may be less obvious. Zoonotic diseases such as Q-fever, rabies, leptospirosis, and brucellosis may affect abattoir workers, zookeepers, animal handlers, and veterinarians. Foresters, field biologists, and natural resource workers who spend time in wooded areas experience tick- and mosquito-borne illnesses at a higher frequency than that of the general population. These illnesses include the arboviral encephalitides, Rocky Mountain spotted fever, Lyme disease, and ehrlichiosis. Occupational infections may arise as a result of work settings, bringing people into close proximity with other people or animals, thus facilitating the transmission of microorganisms. Occupational infectious diseases attributable to the clustering of people affect workers in such facilities as day care centers, schools, health care settings, correctional facilities, dormitories, military barracks, or shelters for the homeless, among others. Industrial settings can place large numbers of workers in a shared space, leading to increased transmission of diseases. This is especially true for diseases with annual outbreaks, such as influenza and Norwalk-like viruses. Exposures to chemicals may increase the susceptibility of workers to infection through irritation of mucosa or the pulmonary epithelium or through immunosuppression leading to impaired host defense.

Both industrial and nonindustrial occupational environments may pose occupational hazards due to the presence of chemical or biological agents. Reports of work environments with ineffective ventilation or decreased ventilation rates and increased utilization of synthetic building materials have demonstrated a rise in complaints associated with occupancy in buildings. In some cases, service sector workers in a problem building develop specific clinical conditions with recognized etiology. This is defined as building-related illness. In other cases, symptoms are nonspecific and disappear when the worker leaves the problem building. When this occurs with sufficient prevalence, it is termed *sick building syndrome*. This can arise from volatile and semivolatile chemicals released from office materials, building materials, floor coverings, furniture, cleaning products, and microorganisms. Office buildings and residential settings comprise a complex ecology consisting of people, molds, mites, volatile organic compounds of microbial and nonmicrobial origin, and sometimes plants, pets, cockroaches, and other vermin (Thorne and Heederik, 1999b). Molds, house dust mites, and animal proteins are potent human allergens that can lead to allergy and asthma. Exposure to chemicals and biomolecules such as endotoxin may enhance this process (Douwes *et al.*, 2003). Workers in laboratory animal facilities exhibit a high prevalence of allergy to rodent urinary proteins. In some cases, the occupied space of a building may be clean and dry, but local amplification sites for molds may develop. These may arise in ventilation systems, utility closets, subfloors or basements that serve as return air plenums, or in local sites of water damage. Such sites can become sources of microorganisms and aeroallergens of sufficient volume to generate significant bioaerosol exposures throughout the environment. Airborne viruses, bacteria, and fungi are responsible for a variety of building-related illnesses arising from organisms that are pathogenic to humans. Nonpathogenic microorganisms may induce symptoms or diseases through inflammatory processes, by stimulating innate or adaptive immune response, or by releasing noxious odors, allergenic compounds, or bioactive macromolecules. These may combine with industrial chemicals released into the air to create complex exposure environments.

TOXICOLOGICAL EVALUATION OF OCCUPATIONAL AGENTS

Evaluation of Occupational Risks

In most instances of prolonged exposure to low levels of chemicals, there is a continuum between being healthy and being ill. The exposures may impart biochemical or functional changes that are without signs or symptoms, subclinical changes, or in cases of more significant toxicity, manifest as clinical disease. The health significance of the identified changes resulting from exposure to a particular agent must be assessed in order to determine which effects are adverse. Following this assessment, one must consider the interindividual variability or susceptibility factors that influence the risks. There is no single dose–effect relationship but a distribution of responses. Therefore, in order to recommend an acceptable exposure level to an industrial chemical, one must attempt to define the risk associated with adverse effects in the most sensitive populations exposed. It then remains to be determined what proportion of exposed subjects may still develop an adverse effect at the proposed acceptable exposure level. This acceptable risk level will vary according to a value judgment of the severity, permanence, and equality of the potential adverse effects, and the characteristics of the most susceptible population. Clearly, inhibition of an enzyme without functional consequences will be viewed as more acceptable than a more serious toxic effect, such as teratogenicity leading to a congenital malformation in the offspring of the exposed individual.

Establishing Causality In complex occupational environments, it may be difficult to establish a causal relationship between a toxic substance and a disease. For this reason, a number of systematic approaches have been devised to help define causation. In 1890, Robert Koch proposed postulates for "proving" that a specific organism caused a specific disease. TM Rivers extended this approach to viruses in 1937. Sir Austin Bradford Hill suggested epidemiological criteria for assessing causality in 1965 considering strength, specificity, consistency, temporality, exposure period, exposure gradients, and biological plausibility of the associations. These schema and modern weight-of-evidence determination criteria were later combined to suggest a set of postulates for the evaluation of evidence for disease agents in organic dust (Donham and Thorne, 1994). A matrix was developed and is extended here to evaluate the weight of evidence for a causal association between a toxicant and an occupational disease (Fig. 34-3). Evidence from well-conducted in vitro studies, animal studies, human challenge studies, case reports, and epidemiological investigations are evaluated with regard to data quality and clarity of evidence in support of the establishment of causality. This evaluation is guided by seven criteria (shown in blue). If a chemical were thoroughly studied in

	Assessment of exposure to specific agents	Consideration or control of confounders	Evidence of a dose – response relationship	Consistent results from different studies	Objective clinical data	Endpoints related to human pathology	Appropriate subjects or models
In vitro studies							
Animal studies							
Human challenge studies							
Case studies							
Epidemiology studies							

For each type of study listed in the first column weight the quality of data from existing studies based on the criteria listed in the column headings as follows:
- 0 No evidence or condition is not met
- 1 Equivocal evidence or condition is partially met
- 2 Some evidence or condition is mostly met
- 3 Clear evidence or condition is convincingly met

Figure 34-3. *Matrix for assessing the strength of an association between a toxicant and an occupational disease.*

animals, humans, and in vitro studies, and produced clear and convincing evidence of an exposure–response relationship in controlled studies that used appropriate models and relevant endpoints, that would constitute compelling evidence of a causal relationship between that chemical and that disease. Fig. 34-3 reminds us that a consortium of study types contributes data used for the evaluation of occupational hazards. These are discussed below.

To evaluate with some degree of confidence, the level of exposure at which the risk of health impairment is acceptable, a body of toxicological information is required. Five sources of data may be available to inform the occupational risk-assessment process.

- In vitro assays
- Animal toxicology studies
- Human challenge studies
- Case reports
- Epidemiology studies

In Vitro Assays A number of useful in vitro assays have been developed over the past several decades in order to provide screening data and, in some cases, mechanistic insight without the need or expense of exposing animal or human subjects. While at this time there are few validated methods to determine complex toxicological responses such as immune hypersensitivity or peripheral neuropathy, there are validated and very useful screening assays. Notable examples are the *Salmonella typhimurium* reverse mutation assay, or Ames test, the Corrositex assay for dermal corrosivity potential of chemicals (Interagency Coordinating Committee on the Validation of Alternative Methods [ICCVAM], 2003; NIH-99-4495, 1999), the in vitro ocular toxicity test for identifying severe irritants and corrosives (ICCVAM, 2006), and use of three in vitro test methods for assessment of eye irritation of antimicrobial cleaning products (ICCVAM, 2010). In addition, quantitative structure–activity relationships can help suggest potential toxicological effects for an unstudied compound if structurally similar compounds have been evaluated.

Animal Toxicology Studies Animal toxicology studies serve an important function in terms of identifying adverse effects, providing mechanistic data, establishing dose–response relationships, and aiding the process of establishing standards. Because animal studies can be conducted before there is any human exposure, these studies play an important role in hazard identification and prevention of human disease. There are numerous animal models for occupational injury and illness, which are described throughout this textbook in the context of the affected organ system and the classes of toxicants. Generation of animal toxicology data to predict health effects in workers is a central function of experimental toxicologists.

Toxicological investigations using animals often serve to establish a tentative acceptable exposure level. Other important information that may also be derived from these investigations concerns the relationships between the metabolic handling of the chemical and its interactions with target molecules (mechanism of action), identification of methods for biological monitoring of exposure and early health effects, and identification of preexisting pathological states that may increase susceptibility to the chemical. However, animal testing can provide only an estimate of the toxicity of a chemical for humans. Animals do not always respond to a chemical exposure in the same way as humans. For instance, there are very significant species and strain differences in responsiveness to aryl hydrocarbon receptor agonists, such as polychlorinated dibenzo-*p*-dioxins

(Abnet *et al.*, 1999; Boverhof *et al.*, 2006). In some instances, interspecies differences in metabolism or mechanism of action cause certain chemicals to induce cancer in rodents, but not in humans. One such example is kidney cancer, attributable to the accumulation of a rat-specific protein (α_{2u}-globulin) in proximal tubular cells, and produced in male rats chronically exposed to unleaded gasoline (Hard *et al.*, 1993). There are a few compounds for which predictive animal models have not been found. As discussed further, skin and internal cancers caused in humans by excessive oral exposure to inorganic arsenic were not reproduced during classic carcinogenicity studies in animals (Agency for Toxic Substances and Disease Registry [ATSDR], 2007).

Human Challenge Studies Human challenge studies, or clinical exposure studies, are a useful approach for verifying findings from animal toxicology studies in humans and for establishing whether biotransformation pathways in the animal models represent those in exposed humans. Human challenge studies with occupational toxicants are usually designed to answer very specific questions regarding rates of uptake, biotransformation pathways, the time course of metabolite excretion during and after exposure, evaluation of the threshold concentration for sensory responses (odor, irritation of the nasal mucosa, etc), and acute effects of toxicant exposure on perception, vigilance, and function. Human challenge studies help to establish biomarkers of exposure. For reversible conditions, they can be useful for testing therapeutic options. They may also be useful for investigating bronchial hyperresponsiveness to inhaled agents. Extreme caution must be exercised to ensure the safety of research subjects. Idiosyncratic responses can cause a subject to be exceptionally sensitive. For inhalation studies, equipment malfunction can result in overexposure, so real-time exposure monitoring is a necessity. In the past 25 years, there have been several serious injuries and fatalities associated with human challenge studies. These have been attributed to hypersensitivity reactions and generally used mock workplace simulations without rigorous control and monitoring of exposures, as is the current standard of practice. Thus, such studies should be undertaken only when the required data cannot be obtained through other means and under circumstances in which the risk for volunteers can reasonably be estimated as negligible.

Case Reports When new toxicants, new combinations of toxicants, or changes in process conditions occur in the workplace, a case or outbreak of cases can occur. These may be identified through workplace surveillance systems or through workers associating their disease with workplace exposures. In some cases, the problem is identified quickly and resolved, while others take years to resolve. These are often published as case reports and may give rise to animal or epidemiological studies. Hypersensitivity pneumonitis among machinists exposed to metalworking fluids contaminated with mycobacteria is one example (Thorne *et al.*, 2006; Weiss *et al.*, 2002). Another example is diacetyl-induced bronchiolitis obliterans that was first recognized in workers manufacturing artificially flavored microwave popcorn (Kreiss *et al.*, 2002). NIOSH has a Health Hazard Evaluation (HHE) program in place in which employees or their authorized representatives or employers at a job site can request an investigation to evaluate a potentially hazardous situation. This program issues HHE Reports to disseminate information regarding the hazard. NIOSH also publishes NIOSH Alerts, Criteria Documents, Special Hazard Reviews, Occupational Hazard Assessments, and Current Intelligence Bulletins. In addition, NIOSH publishes Joint Occupational Health Documents with similar entities in foreign governments. While useful for hazard identification and mitigation, case reports and HHE Reports generally do not establish incidence or prevalence of diseases associated with an occupational hazard.

Epidemiology Studies Epidemiology studies help to unravel the associations between occupational diseases, exposures, and personal risk factors. Exposure may be characterized using a surrogate measure such as job classification, or via questionnaire, or more directly through exposure monitoring or biomonitoring. Adverse effects may be expressed in terms of mortality, incidence or prevalence of clinical disease, irreversible or reversible functional changes, or critical biological changes.

Several types of epidemiological studies are used to gather data on the association of workplace exposures with human disease. Cross-sectional studies compare disease prevalence or health status between groups of workers classified according to job title, work site, or exposure status. Cohort studies compare exposed workers versus unexposed or less exposed workers either prospectively or retrospectively in order to associate the occurrence of disease with exposure. Because many occupational diseases have a long induction period or occur only rarely, prospective cohort studies may require a long time and need a large number of subjects to establish significant findings. Retrospective cohort studies can resolve the latency problem but require that relevant exposure data have been collected over time. In the absence of measured exposures, job titles, tasks routinely performed, and years of employment may allow exposure categorization (eg, low, medium, high). Exposure misclassification is frequently a problem in retrospective studies

that reduces the likelihood of associating a disease with a particular exposure.

Case–control studies are useful for investigating rare diseases or diseases with long induction periods. As the name suggests, case–control studies compare workers with disease to workers without disease with regard to their past exposure intensity, frequency, and duration, plus other postulated risk factors. In some instances, where the exposure–disease relationship is not understood, it may be difficult to identify an appropriate control group. Case–control studies are strongest when accompanied by a rich data set of measured exposures to the candidate causative agents spanning the relevant exposure period. If exposure history is assessed by questionnaire after workers have developed adverse health effects, there arises the potential for recall bias in which those with disease may recall past exposures differently than those who are free of disease. Error can also arise due to selection bias if those who agree to participate in the study are not representative of the population of interest.

Characteristics of observational epidemiology studies are listed in Table 34-7. Occupational epidemiology studies assess relationships between exposures and human health outcomes and, therefore, are particularly useful for risk assessment. Confounding may arise due to exposures of risk factors not associated with the work environment.

Because measures of effect may be subtle and may overlay a background level of incidence, results generally require sophisticated statistical comparisons between a group of exposed workers

---

Table 34-7

Comparison of Epidemiologic Studies and Experimental Exposure Studies

	OBSERVATIONAL EPIDEMIOLOGIC STUDIES	EXPERIMENTAL ANIMAL EXPOSURE STUDIES
Toxicant exposure Character	Reflects true exposure among population at risk	Controlled to represent major toxicant of interest
	Complex and variable in space and time	Usually one or two test compounds
	May include nonoccupational exposures to toxicant or related compounds	May not reflect complexity of human exposures
Frequency and duration	Work day, work week, and years in that job May be task specific	Acute, subacute, subchronic, chronic
Exposure route	Inhalation, ingestion, percutaneous, or a combination	Injection, inhalation, oral, or dermal. Rarely a combination by design
Appropriateness of dose	Reflect the actual range of exposure	Often doses studied are far higher than human exposures
Assessment	Environmental sampling, or measurement of biomarkers	Measurement of administered dose with or without measurement of biomarkers
	May be retrospective and based on employer records, group based approaches, or questionnaires	Sampling of exposure chamber air for inhalation studies
Species considerations	Humans—cohorts or cases and controls	Laboratory animals, usually inbred strains of mice or rats
	Must protect the safety and confidentiality of subjects	Must ensure proper care and use of animals
Representativeness	May exist a selection bias such that the study population may not represent the occupational work force	Experimental animal species may not represent humans
Relevance to human health	Directly relevant if appropriate outcomes are studied	Relevant if species differences are known
		Of limited relevance if species or strain effects on absorption, distribution, metabolism, and disease are unknown
Analytical challenges	Selection bias, misclassification, and confounding in characterization of outcomes	Control of genetics, feeding, and housing between exposed and control groups
	Within- and between-subject variance may be high	Low variance in outcomes

and a similar group of workers without the exposure of interest. Ideally, the group of unexposed workers should be matched on variables such as age, race, gender, socioeconomic status, and smoking habits. They should also undergo the same standardized clinical, biological, or physiological evaluation at the same time as the exposed group. Comparison with the general population is ill-advised because an employed population is a highly selected group and may have a higher degree of physical fitness. Because occupational epidemiological studies often last for several years, all methods of investigation—such as questionnaires, measurement instruments, and analytic techniques—must be validated and standardized before the start of the study. If results will be compared to prior or contemporaneous studies, the same questionnaires should be used. The number of subjects under study should be chosen based on a sample size calculation to be able to detect a difference between exposed and unexposed subjects (should there be a difference) and should take into account labor turnover and those declining participation in any aspects of the study. If exposures are high enough to induce an adverse effect, it is expected that these studies may permit establishment of the relationship between integrated exposure (intensity × time) and frequency of abnormal results and, consequently, a redefinition of the OEL.

In most cases, occupational epidemiological studies encompass the collection of samples from the subjects or data obtained through interaction with the subjects. Because this often includes identifiable private information, the confidentiality of the data must be protected. United States, European Union, and international laws require that subjects must always have the right to refuse participation and investigators must have written consent from a duly informed volunteer obtained without coercion.

Animal Toxicology Testing for Establishing Acceptable Levels of Exposure

It is evident that certainty as to the complete safety of a chemical can never be obtained, regardless of the extent of toxicological investigations performed on animals. Nevertheless, animal studies provide valuable data from which to estimate the level of exposure at which the risk of health impairment is acceptable. Table 34-7 compares the information gained from animal studies to epidemiology studies. To the extent possible, animal studies should employ species for which the metabolic pathways and disease processes reflect those of humans. Guidelines and protocols for assessing experimentally the toxicological hazards of chemicals have been formulated by various national and international agencies. These tests include local and systemic acute toxicity tests, tests of toxicity following repeated exposure, investigations of metabolism and mechanism of action, short-term tests for detecting potential mutagens and carcinogens, studies of effect on reproduction and of teratogenic activity, chronic studies to detect carcinogenesis and other long-term effects, interaction studies, tests for immunosuppression, and dermal and pulmonary hypersensitivity tests. The need for performing these testing protocols should be carefully evaluated for the inclusion of any occupational toxicant to which workers will be exposed. In selecting the studies most appropriate for safety evaluation, the toxicologist should be guided by an understanding of the following:

- physicochemical properties of the chemical
- potential for the generation of toxic derivatives when the chemical is submitted to heat, pH changes, and UV light
- conditions of use and route of exposure
- type of exposure (continuous, intermittent, or incidental)
- degree of exposure

Toxicological information already available on other chemicals with similar chemical structure and reactive chemical groups can suggest potential hazards and reactivity.

Conclusions drawn from any toxicological investigation are useful only if the composition and physical state of the tested preparation is known. This would include the nature and concentration of impurities or degradation products, speciation of inorganic compounds, characterization of physicochemical properties for inhaled materials, and characterization of the vehicle (the carrier, diluent or excipient of the toxicant). Sensitive and specific methods of analysis of the chemical in solution, air, and biological material should also be available. The assessment of the toxicity of malathion illustrates this point. Malathion is an organophosphate insecticide that normally has relatively low human toxicity. This pesticide was responsible for an episode of mass poisoning among malaria workers in Pakistan because the specific product contained impurities (mainly isomalathion) capable of inhibiting tissue and plasma carboxyesterases (Aldridge *et al.*, 1979) and inactivating acetylcholinesterase via formation of adducts (Doorn *et al.*, 2003). The toxicity evaluation for malathion had not anticipated isomalathion coexposure. A recent study evaluated the pulmonary toxicity of inhaled aluminum nanowhiskers (Adamcakova-Dodd *et al.*, 2012). The manufacturer of this material stated they were Al_2O_3 whiskers. Careful physicochemical analysis prior to toxicity evaluation using x-ray photoelectron spectroscopy and transmission electron microscopy revealed they were actually mixed phase aluminum hydroxy structures containing $Al(OH)_3$ and γ-AlOOH. Further, the whiskers were 100 to 400 nm in length, considerably shorter than the 2800 nm length claimed by the manufacturer.

The duration of tests necessary to establish an acceptable level for occupational exposure is primarily a function of the type of toxic action suspected. It is generally recognized that for systemically acting chemicals, subacute and short-term toxicity studies are usually insufficient for proposing OELs. Subacute and short-term toxicity tests are usually performed to find out whether the compound exhibits immunotoxic properties and cumulative characteristics. They also aid in selection of the doses for long-term-exposure studies and the kind of tests that may be most informative when applied during long-term exposures. A number of studies have drawn attention to the fact that the reproductive system may also be the target organ of industrial chemicals (eg, glycol ethers, styrene, lead, dibromochloropropane). Thus, studies designed to evaluate reproductive effects and teratogenicity should also be considered during routine toxicological testing of occupational toxicants.

Information derived from exposure routes similar to those experienced by workers is clearly the most relevant. For airborne pollutants, inhalation exposure studies provide the basic data on which provisional OELs are based. Experimental methodology is much more complicated for inhalation studies than for oral administration experiments and requires more specialized equipment and expertise (Thorne, 2000). For example, in the case of exposure to an aerosol, particle size distribution must be evaluated, and the degree of retention in the respiratory tract of the animal species under study should be established. Ideally, particle size should be selected according to the deposition pattern of dry or liquid aerosols in the particular animal species used in order to represent human lung deposition with occupational exposures. Particle deposition and retention curves have been published for human, monkey, dog, guinea pig, rat, and mouse (Asgharian *et al.*, 2003; Hsieh *et al.*, 1999; Schlesinger, 1985). Recent research coupling asymmetric multiple-path models of the bronchial tree and ventilation parameters can provide more accurate prediction of site-specific particle deposition (Asgharian and Price, 2006). It should also be kept in mind that the concentration of the material in the air and the duration of exposure do not give a direct estimate of the dose, because retained dose is also dependent on the minute volume and the proportion of inhaled particles retained. Measurement of pulmonary dust retention following exposure to a radiolabeled or fluorescently tagged test aerosol should be performed prior to conducting acute, subchronic, or chronic studies. This allows one to assess deposition and determine whether the selected levels of exposure may overwhelm pulmonary clearance mechanisms (ILSI, 2000; Oberdörster, 2002).

The choice of studies to perform and their routes of administration must be evaluated scientifically for each toxicant. Important considerations include its target sites and mechanism of action, metabolism, the nature of its adverse effects, and how workers are exposed to the toxicant. The morphological, physiological, and biological parameters that are usually evaluated, either at regular intervals in the course of the exposure period or at its termination, are described in Units IV and V of this text. Investigations that can make use of specific physiological or biochemical tests, based on knowledge of the principal target organ or function, produce highly valuable information and increase confidence in the OEL derived from them.

Worker Health Surveillance

The primary objective of worker health surveillance programs is to provide both periodic screening of general health and wellness plus health and exposure monitoring tailored to recognized hazards of the workplace. The monitoring of exposures to toxicants in the workplace may play an important role in detecting excessive exposures before the occurrence of significant biological disturbances and health impairment. A scheme for biological monitoring of exposure and of early biological effects is possible only when sufficient toxicological information has been gathered from in vitro, animal, or human studies on the mechanism of action and the metabolism of xenobiotics to which workers are exposed. When a new chemical is being used on a large scale, the careful clinical surveillance of workers and monitoring of workplaces should be instituted in order to address three aims: (1) to identify overexposure or adverse effects on the health of the workers and quickly intervene, (2) to evaluate the validity of an existing or proposed OEL, and (3) to test the validity of a proposed method for biological monitoring.

Evaluation of the validity of the proposed OEL derived from animal experiments through workplace surveillance is the major aim because studies and observations on humans are the final basis for deciding whether an OEL set originally on the basis of animal toxicity testing is truly acceptable as one that will not produce excess health risks. This means that sensitive clinical, biochemical, physiological, or behavioral tests for detecting an adverse effect of a toxicant should ideally be performed on the workers concurrent with exposure assessment. It is helpful if health surveillance programs can include the same biomarkers as used in prior animal or human exposure studies. Occupational toxicologists and occupational physicians cannot rely solely on the standard diagnostic tools used in clinical medicine, as they were established primarily to reveal advanced pathological states and not to detect early adverse effects at a stage when they are still reversible. For example, the measurement of serum creatinine is still a widely used clinical test for assessing renal integrity, yet it is known that the glomerular filtration rate of the kidney

must be reduced by more than 50% before serum creatinine rises significantly.

The main limitation of current OELs or BEIs is that some are based on limited experimental data or clinical studies in which only late effects have been investigated and correlated with past exposure. Furthermore, several BEIs are derived from the study of external–internal exposure relationships and not from relationships between internal dose and early adverse effects. The validity of an OEL is much stronger if it is based on the study of dose–response relationships in which the dose is expressed in terms of the cumulative target dose and the monitored effect reflects a critical biological event. However, for some chemicals and some adverse effects (eg, induction of hypersensitivity and possibly genotoxic effects), the frequency of peak exposure may be more important for health risk assessment than the integrated dose. For example, long-term low-level exposures to commercial enzymes rarely induce sensitization. However, a single exposure to a high concentration can produce hypersensitivity and occupational asthma.

In cases where a surveillance program was not instituted before the introduction of a new chemical, it is more difficult to establish the efficacy of the OEL. In this situation, evaluation depends on retrospective cohort studies or case–control studies on workers who have already sustained exposure. Evaluation of a "no observed adverse effect level" (NOAEL) is difficult because information on past exposures is often incomplete, and frank effects are generally the focus of retrospective or case–control studies. Provided that a satisfactory assessment of past exposure is possible, cross-sectional studies that rely on preclinical signs of toxicity may, to a certain extent, overcome these difficulties. Whether or not clinical investigations are planned from the introduction of a new chemical or process, it is essential to keep standardized records of occupational histories and exposure. The need may arise for mortality or case history studies in order to answer an urgent question on a suspected risk.

Careful investigation of overexposures resulting from specific incidents such as containment breaches, chemical spills, or vessel or pipe ruptures can provide useful information. Although, such observations are usually not helpful for determining the NOAEL in humans, they may indicate whether human symptomatology is consistent with medical signs found in animals and may suggest functional or biological tests that might prove useful for routine monitoring of exposed workers.

Linkage of Animal Studies and Epidemiological Studies

In the field of occupational toxicology, perhaps more than in other areas of toxicology, cooperation between those conducting animal studies and studies of workers is essential for examining risks associated with overexposure to chemicals and other toxicants. A few examples will serve to illustrate the complementarity of these disciplines.

Several occupational carcinogens have been identified clearly through combined epidemiological and experimental approaches. For example, the carcinogenicity of vinyl chloride was first demonstrated in rats (Viola et al., 1971), and a few years later, epidemiological studies confirmed the same carcinogenic risk for humans (Creech and Johnson, 1974; Monson et al., 1974). This observation stimulated several investigations on the metabolism of vinyl chloride in animals and on its mutagenic activity in in vitro systems. Identification of vinyl chloride metabolites led to the conclusion that there is microsomal oxidation leading to the formation of an epoxide derivative, which acts as a proximate carcinogen (ATSDR,

2006). This finding triggered further studies on the biotransformation of structurally related halogenated ethylenes, such as vinyl bromide, vinylidene chloride, 1,2-dichloroethene, trichloroethylene, and perchloroethylene. Comparison of their oncogenic activity in relation to their metabolism suggested that an interplay between the stability and reactivity in reaching the DNA target and reacting with it after being formed would determine their genotoxic risk. It is now recognized that vinyl chloride is metabolized to 2-chloroethylene oxide, which rearranges to 2-chloroacetaldehyde and produces promutagenic etheno-DNA adducts including etheno-guanine, etheno-cytosine, and lesser amounts of etheno-adenine (ATSDR 2006; Bolt, 2005; National Toxicology Program [NTP], 2011).

1,3-Butadiene is a known human carcinogen with more than 75% of its use in the manufacture of synthetic rubber products. Experimental studies in rats and mice demonstrated carcinogenicity, with mice being particularly sensitive. Subsequent to these findings, 1,3-butadiene was shown to follow the same metabolic pathway in humans as in rats and mice, forming mutagenic and carcinogenic epoxides. That led to cohort and case–control studies establishing 1,3-butadiene as a human carcinogen (NTP, 2011). Recent studies have considered the relative importance of the metabolic pathway leading to formation of the reactive metabolites, 3,4-epoxy-1-butene, 1,2:3,4-diepoxybutane, and 3,4-epoxy-1,2-diol, which react with DNA and with nuclear proteins. Under the assumption of a genotoxic mechanism and cross-species comparisons of DNA binding, these data facilitate a more informed cancer risk assessment. In vitro studies showed that human lymphocytes were less sensitive to 1,2:3,4-diepoxybutane-induced chromosomal abberations than mouse or rat cells (ATSDR, 2009). In vivo studies revealed a higher rate of formation of epoxides in mice than rats. Inhaled 1,3-butadiene produced N7-guanine DNA adducts in lung tissue due to 3,4-epoxy-1,2-diol (Koivisto and Peltonen, 2001) and 1,2:3,4-diepoxybutane (Goggin et al., 2009). These cross-links were more prevalent in mice than rats, and females than males, which agreed with the enhanced susceptibility to cancers of female mice. On this basis, rats were judged to be a more predictive species than mice for human risk assessment. This work illustrates that the measurement of DNA adducts is a sensitive method for monitoring 1,3-butadiene metabolism via the epoxide-forming pathway in workers.

In 1973, an outbreak of peripheral neuropathy occurred in workers exposed to the solvent methyl butyl ketone (2-hexanone, MBK) (McDonough, 1974; Allen et al., 1975). The same lesion was reproduced in animals (Mendell et al., 1974; Spencer et al., 1975). Bio-transformation studies were then undertaken in rats and guinea pigs, and some MBK metabolites (2,5-hexanedione, 5-hydroxy-2-hexanone) were also found to possess neurotoxic activity (Spencer and Schaumburg, 1975; DiVincenzo et al., 1976, 1977). Similar oxidation products are formed from n-hexane, the neurotoxicity of which is probably due to the same active metabolite as that produced from MBK. Because methyl ethyl ketone (MEK) cannot give rise to 2,5-hexanedione, it was suggested as a replacement solvent. Recent work has demonstrated the potentiation of neurotoxic effects of n-hexane upon coexposure with methyl ethyl ketone (Yu et al., 2002). Nevertheless, MEK remains a much less toxic solvent than MBK.

These examples demonstrate that studies of the metabolic handling of occupational toxicants in animals are instrumental in the characterization of reactive intermediates, and may suggest unsuspected risks or indicate new methods of biological monitoring. Conversely, clinical observations of workers may stimulate studies of the metabolism or the mechanism of toxicity of a toxicant in animals, thereby revealing the health significance of a biological disturbance.

Arsenic is one of the very few compounds for which there are limited data of predictive value from animal studies to human health effects. Arsenic has been used as a medicine since the time of Hippocrates. Initially used to treat ulcers, arsenicals achieved notoriety as medicinals for a wide variety of ailments, and then, in the first half of the 20th century, for the treatment of syphilis and parasites. Many foods and beverages contaminated with arsenic have been associated with accidental and intentional poisonings. Inorganic pentavalent arsenic (arsenate) is readily absorbed across tissues and converted to the trivalent form (arsenite). This is then methylated to form monomethyl arsenic acid and dimethyl arsenic acid (ATSDR, 2007). These are primarily transported in the blood bound to sulfhydryl groups in proteins. The half-life in humans for arsenic compounds is two to four days and the major excretion is via urine (Nriagu, 1994).

Inorganic arsenic was first noted as a human carcinogen by Hutchinson in 1887 (Hutchinson, 1887). Epidemiological studies led to classification of arsenic by the IARC as a skin and lung carcinogen in 1980 (IARC, 1980). Since then studies among occupationally exposed populations and populations with high arsenic in their drinking water have shown conclusively, that arsenic causes human cancers of the skin, lung, bladder, kidney, liver, nasal tissue, and prostate. There is also evidence for arsenic-associated cutaneous effects, cardiovascular and cerebrovascular disease, diabetes mellitus, and adverse reproductive outcomes (EPA, 2000; WHO, 2001).

A large number of carefully executed cancer bioassays in mice, rats, beagles, and monkeys have been performed using sodium arsenate, sodium arsenite, lead arsenite, arsenic trioxide, and dimethylarsinic acid. These studies have been uniformly negative for cancer. A number of subsequent studies that tested for tumor-promotion activity following dosing with recognized tumor initiators also yielded negative results. The ATSDR Toxicological Profile for arsenic states, "First and most importantly, no animal model exists for the health effect of greatest concern for human exposure: carcinogenicity in skin and other organs after oral exposure" (ATSDR, 2007). Recent studies using transgenic mice, high-dose in utero exposures, or administration of a cocarcinogen have yielded tumors in mice (Hughes, 2006). However, negative results in standard animal carcinogenicity screens have been problematic in the face of unquestionable oncogenic activity in humans.

The examples above demonstrate that the occupational toxicologist cannot rely solely on animal or epidemiological studies. A combined approach is necessary in order to identify, elucidate, and prioritize risks, and to develop interventions and techniques for worker health surveillance.

EXPOSURE MONITORING

Two important applications of occupational toxicological investigations are compared below: environmental monitoring and biological monitoring. As described above under "Occupational Health Standards," both are important in worker health surveillance, and are essential elements of toxicology studies with dosing via the inhalation or dermal routes.

Environmental Monitoring for Exposure Assessment

An important objective of experimental and clinical investigations in occupational toxicology is the proposal of safe levels of exposure. OELs must be reevaluated at regular intervals as new information on the toxicity of industrial chemicals develops. Adherence to OELs may not protect everyone and, therefore, cannot supplant close medical surveillance of workers. Various private and official institutions regularly review the toxicological information on chemicals in order to propose or update permissible levels of exposure. These include governmental organizations worldwide and professional organizations such as the ACGIH. A critical element of establishing OELs is the accurate and uniform assessment of exposure. Methodology for exposure assessment must be specifically tailored to the agent under study and the environment in which it appears. To assess airborne exposures for compliance purposes, personal samples taken in the breathing zone are generally used. In a few specific environments, area samples form the basis of an exposure standard (eg, the OSHA standard for exposure to raw cotton dust specifies use of the vertical elutriator or an equivalent method). Occupational environmental surveys may employ area sampling to determine areas with higher or lower toxicant concentrations. However, concentrations determined from personal samples typically exceed area concentrations depending on the work practices and environmental controls. For example, geometric mean concentrations of inhalable dust assessed from 159 personal samples in dairy barns were 1.78 mg/m³, compared with 0.74 mg/m³ for 252 area samples collected simultaneously in two locations in the same barns (Kullman *et al.*, 1998). Thus, in this environment, area sampling alone would underestimate personal exposures by a factor of 2.4.

Repeated random sampling is theoretically the best approach to developing unbiased measures of exposure. However, this is rarely the approach that is taken. Variability in exposure, especially variability over time, is often large; therefore, a considerable number of repeated measurements are needed to obtain an accurate proxy of the true exposure. When the number of repeats is insufficient, the slope of the exposure–response relationship will be biased, usually leading to considerable underestimation of the relationship (Heederik and Attfield, 2000). Recent studies have demonstrated that approaches assessing exposures to groups rather than to individuals are more efficient in terms of measurement effort for obtaining a desired level of accuracy (Vermeulen and Kromhout, 2005). In a group-based approach, workers are grouped by job title, task performed, or through exposure modeling studies to elucidate determinants of exposure, and the group mean is used as the average exposure for each worker (Kromhout *et al.*, 1996). Further statistical modeling of the exposure data can reduce problems of bias and large temporal and spatial variability (Preller *et al.*, 1995; Tielemans *et al.*, 1998). Whereas this approach is gaining acceptance among occupational epidemiologists for evaluating exposure–response data and assessing risks, it is not accepted for compliance monitoring.

Although, one cannot assess dose directly through exposure monitoring, it does have several distinct advantages over biomonitoring. Exposure monitoring allows one to quantify workplace exposure by route through selective air monitoring in the breathing zone of the worker and dermal dosimetry using absorptive material affixed to the workers' skin or clothing. Biomonitoring generally does not provide route-specific exposure data. Environmental monitoring techniques are generally less expensive and less invasive than techniques involving the collection and analysis of biological samples such as blood or urine. Thus, a larger population of workers can be studied for the same amount of money. New personal sampling devices incorporate global positioning system, accelerometers, and cellphone technology to provide enhanced data on location and activity. Workers are accustomed to wearing personal samplers for exposure assessment and are generally quite willing to do so. However, they are often unwilling to give a blood or urine sample, fearing that the sample will be surreptitiously used for drug testing, DNA testing, or experimentation. Another benefit of air sampling in the workplace is that

spatial, temporal, and work practice associations can be established, and can suggest better interventions and engineering controls to reduce exposures. Finally, analytic interferences and variabilities are generally lower with environmental samples than with biological samples.

A fully validated sampling and analysis method requires specification of the sampling methods; sample duration, handling, and storage procedures; the analytic method and measurement technique; the range, precision, accuracy, bias, and limits of detection; quality assurance issues; and known interferences. It is also important to document intralaboratory and interlaboratory variability. Once a standard method is established, it must be closely followed in every detail in order to assure consistency of results.

The development of accurate and precise analytic methods for environmental assessment is an ongoing effort. NIOSH publishes the extensive *NIOSH Manual of Analytical Methods* (NIOSH, NMAM, 2011) and these are widely used. ASTM International has also developed a rigorous system for the establishment of methods. It generally requires five or more years to establish a new ASTM method for exposure assessment. The International Organization for Standardization (ISO) is a global federation of national standards bodies with 162 member countries. The subcommittee on workplace atmospheres is administered by the American National Standards Institute (ANSI). ISO has completed harmonization on a number of air sampling methods—for example, the determination of the number concentration of airborne inorganic fibers by phase contrast optical microscopy. The American Industrial Hygiene Association (AIHA) and the ACGIH publish compilations with descriptions of analytic devices and methodology (Anna, 2010; Cohen and McCammon, 2001). Methods have also been developed for bioaerosol exposure assessment and these have been reviewed (Heederik *et al.*, 2003; Thorne and Heederik, 1999a).

Biological Monitoring for Exposure Assessment

Biomonitoring consists of the measurement of toxicants, their metabolites or molecular signatures of effect in specimens from humans or animals, including urine, blood, feces, exhaled breath, hair, finger or toenails, bronchial lavage, breast milk, and adipose tissue. These may serve as biomarkers of exposure, biological effect, or susceptibility. New technologies are emerging that will allow measurement and monitoring of chemicals in the body and transmission of the data from indwelling biosensors. Biomonitoring data provide a measurement of exposure based upon internalized dose and, thus, account for all exposures by all routes for the assessed analyte.

Depending on the chemical and the analyzed biological material, the term *internalized dose* may have different meanings. The measured biomarker may reflect the amount of chemical absorbed shortly before sample collection, as with the concentration of a solvent in exhaled air or in a blood sample obtained during the work shift. It may reflect exposure during the preceding day, as with the measurement of a metabolite in blood or urine collected after the end of exposure. For toxicants with a long biological half-life, the measured parameter may reflect exposure accumulated over a period of weeks or months, as with arsenic in toenails. *Internal dose* may refer to the amount of chemical stored in one or in several body compartments or in the whole body (*the body burden*).

When biological measurements are available to assess the internal dose, they offer important advantages over monitoring the air of the workplace or measuring deposition of chemicals onto dermal patches. The greatest advantage is that the biological measure of exposure is more directly related to the adverse health effects than environmental measurements, because it reflects the amount of toxicant absorbed. Therefore, it may offer a better estimate of the risk than can be determined from ambient monitoring. Biological monitoring accounts for uptake by all exposure routes. Many industrial chemicals can enter the organism by absorption through the skin or the gastrointestinal tract, as well as the lung. For example, some solvents (eg, dimethylformamide) and many pesticide formulations exhibit substantial exposure via the dermal route. In these situations, exposures determined through monitoring airborne concentrations alone underestimate true exposure. Monitoring of an early biomarker of effect is useful when the subjects are exposed to a complex mixture and the agents responsible for the effect are unknown or several agents are working in synergy.

Several factors can influence uptake. Personal hygiene habits vary from one person to another, and there is some degree of individual variation in the absorption rate of a chemical through the lungs, skin, or gastrointestinal tract. Use of size-selective air sampling to determine the inhalable or respirable fraction can strengthen the exposure estimate. However, biological factors such as ventilatory parameters can affect the strength of such a correlation because increased workload can markedly increase the respiratory uptake of an airborne toxicant. Because of its ability to encompass and evaluate the overall exposure (whatever the route of entry), biological monitoring can also be used to test the overall efficacy of personal protective equipment such as respirators, gloves, barrier creams, or aprons. Another consideration with biological monitoring is the fact that nonoccupational exposures (through hobbies, residential exposures, dietary habits, smoking, second jobs) may also be expressed in the biological sample. The organism integrates the total external (environmental and occupational) exposure into one internal load. Whereas this is beneficial for worker health and safety, it may be confounding in epidemiological studies or compliance monitoring. Thus, while biomonitoring is an important exposure measurement tool for health risk assessment, it generally does not allow one to relate sources and levels of exposure to adverse health effects (Albertini *et al.*, 2006).

The value of biological monitoring is heightened when the relationships between external exposure, internal dose, and adverse effects are established. Normally, biological monitoring of exposure cannot be used for assessing exposure to substances that exhibit their toxic effects at the sites of first contact and are poorly absorbed. Examples include dermally corrosive compounds and primary lung irritants. In this situation, the only useful relationship is that between external exposure and the intensity of the local effects.

Relationships between air monitoring and biological monitoring may be modified by genetic or external factors that influence the fate of an occupational toxicant in vivo. Metabolic interactions can occur when workers are exposed simultaneously to chemicals that are biotransformed through identical pathways. Exposure to chemicals that modify the activity of the biotransformation enzymes (eg, microsomal enzyme inducers or inhibitors) may also influence the fate of another compound. Furthermore, metabolic interferences may occur between occupational toxicants and alcohol, tobacco, food additives, prescription drugs, natural product remedies, or recreational drugs. Changes in any of several biological variables (weight, body mass, pregnancy, diseases, immune status, etc) may modify the metabolism of an occupational chemical. These factors have to be taken into consideration when the results of biomonitoring are interpreted. Whatever the parameter measured, whether it is the substance itself, its metabolite, or an early biomarker of effect, the test must be sufficiently sensitive and specific to provide meaningful data in the range of workplace exposures.

Some chemicals have a long biological half-life in various body compartments (eg, hydrophobic persistent organic pollutants), and the time of sampling may not be critical. For other chemicals, the time of sampling is critical because, following exposure, the compounds or their metabolites may be rapidly eliminated from the body. In these cases, the biological sample is usually collected during exposure, at the end of the exposure period, or sometimes just before the next work shift. When biological monitoring consists of sampling and analysis of urine, it is usually performed on "spot" urine specimens or on the first morning void. It is a standard practice for most organic compounds to adjust the results for urine output by expressing the results per gram of creatinine in the urine. Analyses performed on very dilute urine samples are not reliable. The WHO has specified acceptable limits for urine specimens of between 0.3 and 3.0 g/L creatinine or 1.010 and 1.030 specific gravity (ACGIH, 2010). When samples exhibit large interindividual variability or high "background" levels, the interpretation of a single measurement may be difficult. In such cases, it may be useful to analyze biological material collected before and after the exposure period and gauge exposure based upon the cross-shift change.

The majority of BEIs listed by the ACGIH refer to analysis of the parent compound or its phase I metabolite. Analytical advances over the past decade have yielded methods for detecting reactive intermediates of metabolism and macromolecular adducts that may induce mutations or cell cycle disruption. These methods are important for comparing human and animal toxicity data for risk assessment and may help to explain differential responses in animal models and susceptibility in human populations. These methods are also useful for occupational health surveillance programs.

Environmental monitoring plays an important role in the evaluation and prevention of excessive exposure to toxicants in the workplace. However, the prevention of acute toxic effects on the respiratory tract, skin, or eye mucosa can only be achieved by keeping the concentration of the irritant substance below a certain level or by eliminating the exposure. Local acute effects of chemicals do not lend themselves to a biological surveillance program. Likewise, biological monitoring is usually not indicated for detecting peak exposure to dangerous chemicals such as arsine (AsH_3), carbon monoxide, or prussic acid (HCN). Furthermore, identification of emission sources and the evaluation of the efficiency of engineering control measures are usually best performed by ambient air analysis. Table 34-8 lists the approaches most useful for controlling inhalation exposures in the workplace. These include process changes, engineering controls, and use of personal protective equipment. It should be emphasized that process changes and application of engineering controls are preferable to reliance on personal protective equipment.

In summary, environmental and biological monitoring should not be regarded as opposites but as complementary elements of an occupational health and safety program. They should be integrated

---

Table 34-8

Control Approaches for Occupational Inhalation Hazards

Change the process to use or produce less hazardous compounds.

Automate and enclose the process to isolate the compounds.

Incorporate administrative and work practice controls to reduce duration or intensity of exposure.

Install or upgrade local exhaust systems and dilution exhaust.

Institute a comprehensive program for personal protective equipment use where necessary.

as much as possible to ensure low levels of contaminants and optimal health for workers.

CONCLUSION

The working environment will always have the potential to overexpose workers to various toxicants. Recognition of these risks should not wait until epidemiological studies have uncovered hazardous levels. A combined experimental, clinical, and epidemiological approach is most effective for evaluating and managing the potential risks. One can then promulgate scientifically based occupational health standards, apply effective workplace controls to ensure adherence to those standards, and institute worker health surveillance programs to identify unexpected effects in susceptible individuals.

REFERENCES

Abnet CC, Tanguay RL, Heideman W, Peterson RE. Transactivation activity of human, zebrafish, and rainbow trout aryl hydrocarbon receptors expressed in COS-7 cells: greater insight into species differences in toxic potency of polychlorinated dibenzo-*p*-dioxin, dibenzofuran, and biphenyl congeners. *Toxicol Appl Pharmacol.* 1999;159(1):41–51.

Adamcakova-Dodd A, Stebounova LV, O'Shaughnessy PT, Kim JS, Grassian VH, Thorne PS. Thorne Murine pulmonary responses after subchronic exposure to aluminum oxide-based nanowhiskers. *Part Fibre Toxicol.* 2012;9:22.

Adamcakova-Dodd A, Thorne PS, Grassian VH. In vivo toxicity studies of metal nanoparticles. In: Casciano DA, Sahu SC, ed. *Handbook of Systems Toxicology.* Chichester, UK: John Wiley & Sons, Ltd; 2011:803–834.

Agency for Toxic Substances and Disease Registry. *Toxicological Profile for Vinyl Chloride.* Atlanta: Department of Health and Human Services; 2006. Available from: http://www.atsdr.cdc.gov/ToxProfiles/TP.asp?id=282&tid=51. Accessed October 20, 2011.

Agency for Toxic Substances and Disease Registry. *Toxicological Profile for Arsenic.* Atlanta: Department of Health and Human Services; 2007. Available from: http://www.atsdr.cdc.gov/ToxProfiles/TP.asp?id=22&tid=3. Accessed October 20, 2011.

Agency for Toxic Substances and Disease Registry. *Draft Toxicological Profile for 1,3-Butadiene.* Atlanta: Department of Health and Human Services; 2009. Available from: http://www.atsdr.cdc.gov/toxprofiles/TP.asp?id=459&tid=81. Accessed October 20, 2011.

Albertini R, Bird M, Doerrer N, et al. The use of biomonitoring data in exposure and human health risk assessments. *Environ Health Perspect.* 2006;114:1755–1762.

Aldridge WN, Miles JW, Mount DL, Verschoyle RD. The toxicological properties of impurities in malathion. *Arch Toxicol.* 1979;42:95–106.

Allen N, Mendell JR, Billmaier DJ, et al. Toxic polyneuropathy due to methyl n-butylketone. *Arch Neurol.* 1975;32:209–218.

American Conference of Governmental Industrial Hygienists. *2010 TLVs® and BEIs®: Threshold Limit Values for Chemical Substances and Physical Agents and Biological Exposure Indices.* Cincinnati, OH: American Conference of Governmental Industrial Hygienists; 2010.

Anna DH, ed. *The Occupational Environment—Its Evaluation and Control.* 3rd ed. Fairfax, VA: American Industrial Hygiene Association; 2010.

Asgharian B, Kelly JT, Tewksbury EW. Respiratory deposition and inhalability of monodisperse aerosols in Long-Evans rats. *Toxicol Sci.* 2003;71:104–111.

Asgharian B, Price OT. Airflow distribution in the human lung and its influence on particle deposition. *Inhal Toxicol.* 2006;18:795–801.

Balazy A, Toivola M, Adhikari A, et al. Do N95 respirators provide 95% protection level against airborne viruses, and how adequate are surgical masks? *Am J Infection Control.* 2006;34:51–57.

Bason M, Lammintausta K, Maibach HI. Irritant dermatitis (irritation). In: Marzulli FN, Maibach HI, eds. *Dermatotoxicology.* 4th ed. New York: Hemisphere; 1991;223–252.

Baur X. Occupational asthma due to isocyanates. *Lung.* 1996;174:23–30.

Becklake MR, Malo JL, Chan-Yeung M. Epidemiological approaches in occupational asthma. In: Bernstein IL, et al., eds. *Asthma in the Workplace.* 3rd ed. New York: Taylor & Francis Group; 2006:37–77.

Bernstein DA, Biagini RE, Karnani R, et al. In vivo sensitization to purified Hevea brasiliensis proteins in health care workers sensitized ti natural rubber latex. *J Allergy Clin Immunol.* 2003;111:610–616.

Bernstein IL, Bernstein DI, Chan-Yeung M, Malo JL. Definition and classification of asthma in the workplace. In: Bernstein IL et al., eds. *Asthma in the Workplace.* 3rd ed. New York: Taylor & Francis Group; 2006:1–4.

BRFSS. Adult Asthma Data Prevalence Tables and Maps. Atlanta: Department of Health and Human Services; 2004. Available at: http://www.cdc.gov/asthma/brfss/04/brfssdata.htm. Accessed October 10, 2012.

Bolt HM. Vinyl chloride—a classical industrial toxicant of new interest. *Crit Rev Toxicol.* 2005;35:301–323.

Boverhof DR, Burgoon LD, Tashiro C, et al. Comparative toxicogenomic analysis of the hepatotoxic effects of TCDD in Sprague Dawley rats and C57BL/6 mice. *Tox Sic.* 2006;94:398–416.

Chan-Yeung M, Vedal S, Kus J, et al. Symptoms, pulmonary function and bronchial hyperactivity in western red cedar workers compared with those in office workers. *Am Rev Respir Dis.* 1984;130:1038–1041.

Cohen BS, McCammon CS Jr, eds. *Air Sampling Instruments for Evaluation of Atmospheric Contaminants.* 9th ed. Cincinnati, OH: American Conference of Governmental Industrial Hygienists; 2001.

Creech JL, Johnson HM. Angiosarcoma of the liver in the manufacture of polyvinylchloride. *J Occup Med.* 1974;16:150–151.

Cullinan P, Lowson D, Nieuwenhuijsen MJ, et al. Work related symptoms, sensitisation, and estimated exposure in workers not previously exposed to laboratory rats. *Occup Environ Med.* 1994;51:589–592.

Desjardins A, Malo JL, L' Archevçque J, et al. Occupational IgE-mediated sensitization and asthma due to clam and shrimp. *J Allergy Clin Immunol.* 1995;96:608–617.

DiVincenzo GD, Hamilton ML, Kaplan CJ, Dedinas J. Metabolic fate and disposition of ^{14}C-labeled methyl *n*-butyl ketone in the rat. *Toxicol Appl Pharmacol.* 1977;41:547–560.

DiVincenzo GD, Kaplan CJ, Dedinas J. Characterization of the metabolites of methyl-*n*-butyl ketone, methyl iso-butyl ketone, and methyl ethyl ketone in guinea pig serum and their clearance. *Toxicol Appl Pharmacol.* 1976;36:511–522.

Donham KJ, Thorne PS. Agents in organic dusts. Criteria for a causal relationship. *Am J Ind Med.* 1994;25:33–39.

Doorn JA, Thompson CM, Christner RB, Richardson RJ. Stereoselective inactivation of *Torpedo californica* acetylcholinesterase by isomalathion: inhibitory reactions with (1*R*)- and (1*S*)-isomers proceed by different mechanisms. *Chem Res Toxicol.* 2003;16:958–965.

Douwes J, Thorne PS, Pearce N, Heederik D. Biological agents—recognition. In: Perkins JL, ed. *Modern Industrial Hygiene: Vol II. Biological Aspects.* Cincinnati, OH: American Conference of Governmental Industrial Hygienists; 2003:219–292.

Duchaine C, Meriaux A, Thorne PS, Cormier Y. Assessment of particulates and bioaerosols in Eastern Canadian sawmills. *Am Ind Hyg Assoc J.* 2000;61:727–732.

Eduard W, Sandven P, Levy F. Relationships between exposure to spores from *Rhizopus microsporus* and *Paecilomyces variotii* and serum IgG antibodies in wood trimmers. *Int Arch Allergy Immunol.* 1992;97:274–282.

Elliott L, Heederik D, Marshall S, Peden D, Loomis D. Incidence of allergy and allergy symptoms among workers exposed to laboratory animals. *Occup Environ Med.* 2005;62:766–771.

Employment in Europe 2010. European Commission Directorate-General for Employment, Social Affairs, and Equal Opportunities. October 2010. Available from: http://ec.europa.eu/social/main.jsp?catId=738&langId=en&pubId=593. Accessed July 14, 2011.

EPA. 40 CFR Parts 141 and 142, National primary drinking water regulations; arsenic and clarifications to compliance and new source contaminants monitoring; proposed rule. 2000; *Fed Reg.* 65(121):38888–38983.

European Commission. European Commission Directive 95/320/EC; 1995. Available from: http://eur-lex.europa.eu/LexUriServ/LexUriServ.do?uri=CELEX:31995D0320:EN:HTML. Accessed October 23, 2011.

European Commission. European Commission Directive 98/24/EC; 1998. Available from: http://osha.europa.eu/en/legislation/directives/exposure-to-chemical-agents-and-chemical-safety/osh-directives/75. Accessed October 22, 2011.

Fuortes LJ, Weih L, Pomrehn P, et al. Prospective epidemiologic evaluation of laboratory animal allergy among university employees. *Am J Ind Med.* 1997;32:665–669.

GAO/HEHS. Child *Labor in Agriculture—Changes Needed to Better Protect Health and Educational Opportunities.* GAO/HEHS-98-193. Washington, DC: US Government Accountability Office; 1998: 1–90.

Glass WI, Power P, Burt R, et al. Work-related respiratory symptoms and lung function in New Zealand mussel openers. *Am J Ind Med.* 1998;34:163–168.

Goggin M, Swenberg JA, Walker VE, et al. Molecular dosimetry of 1,2,3,4-diepoxybutaneinduced DNA–DNA cross-links in B6C3F1 mice and F344 rats exposed to 1,3-butadiene by inhalation. *Cancer Res.* 2009;69(6):2479–2486.

Grassian VH, O'Shaughnessy PT, Adamcakova-Dodd A, Pettibone JM, Thorne PS. Inhalation exposure study of titanium dioxide nanoparticles with a primary particle size of 2 to 5 nm. *Environ Health Perspect.* 2007;115(3):397–402.

Hard GC, Rodgers IS, Baetcke KP, et al. Hazard evaluation of chemicals that cause accumulation of α_{2u}-globulin, hyaline droplet nephropathy, and tubule neoplasia in the kidneys of male rats. *Environ Health Perspect.* 1993;99:313–349.

Heederik D, Attfield M. Characterization of dust exposure for the study of chronic occupational lung disease: a comparison of different exposure assessment strategies. *Am J Epidemiol.* 2000;151(10):982–990.

Heederik D, Thorne PS, Doekes G. Health-based occupational exposure limits for high molecular weight sensitizers: how long is the road we must travel? *Ann Occup Hyg.* 2002;46(5):439–446.

Heederik D, Thorne PS, Douwes J. Biological agents—monitoring and evaluation of bioaerosol exposure. In: Perkins JL, ed. *Modern Industrial Hygiene: Vol II. Biological Aspects.* Cincinnati, OH: American Conference of Governmental Industrial Hygienists; 2003:293–327.

Hollander A, Heederik D, Doekes G. Respiratory allergy to rats: exposur–response relationships in laboratory animal workers. *Am J Respir Crit Care Med.* 1997;155:562–567.

Hsieh TH, Yu CP, Oberdorster G. Deposition and clearance models of Ni compounds in the mouse lung and comparisons with the rat models. *Aerosol Sci Technol.* 1999;31:358–372.

Hughes MF. Biomarkers of exposure: a case study with inorganic arsenic. *Environ Health Perspect.* 2006;114:1790–1796.

Hutchinson J. Arsenic cancer. *Br Med J.* 1887;2:1280–1281.

ILSI Risk Science Institute Workshop Participants. The relevance of the rat lung response to particle overload for human health risk assessment: a workshop consensus report. *Inhal Toxicol.* 2000;12:1–17.

Interagency Coordinating Committee on the Validation of Alternative Methods. 2003. http://iccvam.niehs.nih.gov/methods/corrode.htm.

Interagency Coordinating Committee on the Validation of Alternative Methods. 2006. http://iccvam.niehs.nih.gov/methods/ocudocs/otmer102706.pdf.

Interagency Coordinating Committee on the Validation of Alternative Methods. 2010. http://iccvam.niehs.nih.gov/methods/ocutox/MildMod.htm.

International Agency for Research on Cancer. *Metals and Metallic Compounds. IARC Monographs on the Evaluation of Carcinogenic Risks to Humans*, Vol 23. Lyon, France: International Agency for Research on Cancer; 1980.

International Labour Organization. 2011. Available from: http://www.ilo.org/public/english/dialogue/sectors/agri/emp.htm. Accessed July 14, 2011.

Japan Monthly Statistics. 2006. Ministry of Internal Affairs and Communications, Statistics Bureau. 2011. Available from: http://www.stat.go.jp/english/data/getujidb/index.htm#g. Accessed July 22, 2011.

Kim JS, Adamcakova-Dodd A, O'Shaughnessy PT, Grassian VH, Thorne PS. Effects of copper nanoparticle exposure on host defense in a murine pulmonary infection model. *Part Fibre Toxicol.* 2011;8(1):29.

Koivisto P, Peltonen K. N7-Guanine adducts of the epoxy metabolites of 1,3-butadiene in mice lung. *Chem Biol Interact.* 2001;135–136: 363–372.

Kreiss K, Hubbs A, Kullman G. Correspondence. bronchiolitis in popcorn-factory workers. *N Engl J Med.* 2002;347:1981–1982.

Kromhout H, Tielemans E, Preller L, Heederik D. Estimates of individual dose from current measurements of exposure. *Occup Hyg.* 1996;3:23–39.

Kullman GJ, Thorne PS, Waldron PF, et al. Organic dust exposures from work in dairy barns. *Am Ind Hyg Assoc J.* 1998;59:403–413.

Maibach HI, Feldmann RJ, Milby TH, Serat WF. Regional variation in percutaneous penetration in man. Pesticides. *Arch Environ Health.* 1971;23:208–211.

McDonough JR. Possible neuropathy from methyl-*n*-butyl ketone. *N Engl J Med.* 1974;290:695.

Mendell JR, Saida K, Ganasia MF, et al. Toxic polyneuropathy produced by methyl-*n*-butyl ketone. *Science.* 1974;185:787–789.

Monson RR, Peters JM, Johnson MN. Proportional mortality among vinylchloride workers. *Lancet.* 1974;2(7877):397–398.

Nanotechnology Consumer Products Inventory. Available from: http://www.nanotechproject.org/inventories/consumer/. Accessed October 25, 2011.

National Institute for Occupational Safety and Health. *Work-Related Lung Disease (eWoRLD) Surveillance System*; 2006. Available from: http://www2a.cdc.gov/drds/WorldReportData/.

National Institute for Occupational Safety and Health. *Work-Related Lung Disease Surveillance Report.* Washington, DC: Department of Health and Human Services (NIOSH); 2011. Available from: http://www.cdc.gov/niosh/topics/surveillance/ords/nationalstatistics/WoRLDHighlights.html. Accessed on October 7, 2011.

National Institute for Occupational Safety and Health NMAM. 2011. Available from: http://www.cdc.gov/NIOSH/NMAM.

National Toxicology Program. *12th Report on Carcinogens.* Research Triangle Park, NC: National Toxicology Program. US Department of Health and Human Services, 2011. Available from: http://ntp.niehs.nih.gov/?objectid=03C9AF75-E1BF-FF40-DBA9EC0928DF8B15. Accessed on October 23, 2011.

Nel A, Xia T, Madler L, Li N. Toxic potential of materials at the nanolevel. *Science.* 2006;311(5761):622–627.

NIH-99-4495. *Corrositex: An in Vitro Test Method for Assessing Dermal Corrosivity Potential of Chemicals.* NIH-99-4495. Washington, DC: National Toxicology Program; 1999:1–236. Available from: http://iccvam.niehs.nih.gov/docs/reports/corprrep.pdf.

Nriagu JO. *Arsenic in the Environment: Part II: Human Health Effects and Ecosystem Effects.* New York: Wiley; 1994:1–91.

Oberdörster G. Toxicokinetics and effects of fibrous and nonfibrous particles. *Regul Toxicol Pharmacol.* 2002;27:123–135.

Occupational Safety and Health Administration. Standard Interpretations: 10/06/1995—8-hour total weight average (TWA) permissible exposure limit (PEL). 1995. Available from: http://www.osha.gov/pls/oshaweb/owadisp.show_document?p_table=INTERPRETATIONS&p_id=24470.

Pacheco KA, McCammon C, Liu AH, et al. Airborne endotoxin predicts symptoms in non-mouse-sensitized technicians and research scientists exposed to laboratory mice. *Am J Respir Crit Care Med.* 2003;167:983–990.

Pettibone JM, Adamcakova-Dodd A, Thorne PS, O'Shaughnessy PT, Weydert JA, Grassian VH. Inflammatory response of mice following inhalation exposure to iron and copper nanoparticles. *Nanotoxicology.* 2008;2(4):189–204.

Preller L, Kromhout H, Heederik D, Tielen MJM. Modeling long-term average exposure in occupational exposure-response analysis. *Scand J Work Environ Health.* 1995;21:504–512.

Schenker MB, Christiani D, Cormier Y, et al. Respiratory health hazards in agriculture. *Am J Respir Crit Care Med Suppl.* 1998;158(pt 2): S1–S76.

Schlesinger RB. Comparative deposition of inhaled aerosols in experimental animals and humans: a review. *J Toxicol Environ Health.* 1985;15:197–214.

Schwartz DA, Thorne PS, Jagielo PJ, et al. Endotoxin responsiveness and grain dust–induced inflammation in the lower respiratory tract. *Am J Physiol*. 1994;267:L609–L617.

Schwartz DA, Thorne PS, Yagla SJ, et al. The role of endotoxin in grain dust–induced lung disease. *Am J Respir Crit Care Med*. 1995;152: 603–608.

Siemiatycki J, Richardson L, Straif K, et al. Listing occupational carcinogens. *Environ Health Perspect*. 2004;112:1447–1459.

Spencer PS, Schaumburg HH. Experimental neuropathy produced by 2,5-hexanedione A major metabolite of the neurotoxic industrial solvent methyl-*n*-butyl ketone. *J Neurol Neurosurg Psychiatry*. 1975;38: 771–775.

Spencer PS, Schaumburg HH, Raleigh RL, Terhaar CJ. Nervous system degeneration produced by the industrial solvent methyl-*n*-butyl ketone. *Arch Neurol*. 1975;32:219–222.

Thorne PS. Inhalation toxicology models of endotoxin- and bioaerosol-induced inflammation. *Toxicology*. 2000;152:13–23.

Thorne PA, Adamcakova-Dodd A, Kelley KM, et al. Metalworking fluid with mycobacteria and endotoxin induces hypersensitivity pneumonitis in mice. *Am J Respir Crit Care Med*. 2006;173:759–768.

Thorne PS, Duchaine C. Airborne bacteria and endotoxin. In: Hurst CT, Crawford RL, Garland JL, Lipson DA, Mills AL, Stetzenbach LD, eds. *Manual of Environmental Microbiology*. 3rd ed. Washington, DC: ASM Press; 2007:989–1004.

Thorne PS, Heederik D. Assessment methods for bioaerosols. In: Salthammer T, ed. *Organic Indoor Air Pollutants—Occurrence, Measurement, Evaluation*. Weinheim, Germany: Wiley/VCH; 1999a:85–103.

Thorne PS, Heederik D. Indoor bioaerosols—sources and characteristics. In: Salthammer T, ed. *Organic Indoor Air Pollutants—Occurrence, Measurement, Evaluation*. Weinheim, Germany: Wiley/VCH; 1999b: 275–288.

Tielemans E, Kupper LL, Kromhout H, et al. Individual-based and group-based occupational exposure assessment: Some equations to evaluate different strategies. *Ann Occup Hyg*. 1998;42(2):115–119.

United States Department of Labor. *Career Guide to Industries: Agricultural Production*. 2011 ed. Washington, DC: US Department of Labor, Bureau of Labor Statistics; 2011a. Available from: http://www.bls.gov/oco/cg/cgs001.htm, 2011. Accessed October 23, 2011.

United States Department of Labor. *The Employment Situation June 2011*. Washington, DC: US Department of Labor, Bureau of Labor Statistics, USLD-11-1011; 2011b. Available from: http://www.bls.gov/news.release/archives/empsit_07082011.htm. Accessed July 8, 2011.

United States Department of Labor. *Workplace Injuries and Illnesses-2009*. Washington, DC: US Department of Labor, Bureau of Labor Statistics, USLD-10-1451; 2011c. Available from: http://www.bls.gov/iif/oshsum.htm. Accessed July 6, 2011.

US Federal Register. 1992;57(114):26539–26590.

Venables KM, Dally MB, Nunn AJ, et al. Smoking and occupational allergy in workers in a platinum refinery. *Br Med J*. 1989;299:939–942.

Venables KM, Topping MD, Howe W, et al. Interaction of smoking and atopy in producing specific IgE antibody against a hapten protein conjugate. *Br Med J*. 1985;290:201–204.

Vermeulen R, Kromhout H. Historical limitations of determinant based exposure groupings in the rubber manufacturing industry. *Occup Envir Med*. 2005;62:793–799.

Viola PL, Bigotti A, Caputo A. Oncogenic response of rat skin, lungs, and bones to vinyl chloride. *Cancer Res*. 1971;31:516–522.

Weiss LPC, Lewis R, Rossmoore H, et al. Respiratory illness in workers exposed to metal working fluid contaminated with nontuberculous mycobacteria–Ohio, 2001. *Morb Mortal Wkly Rep*. 2002;51:349–352.

Wernfors M, Nielsen J, Schültz A, Skerfving S. Phthalic anhydride-induced occupational asthma. *Int Arch Allergy Appl Immunol*. 1986;79:77–82.

WHO. *Arsenic and Arsenic Compounds*. 2nd ed. Environmental Health Criteria 224. Geneva: World Health Organization; 2001. Available from: http://whqlibdoc/ehc/WHO_EHC_224.pdf. Accessed October 23, 2011.

Yu RC, Hattis D, Landaw EM, Froines JR. Toxicokinetic interaction of 2,5-hexanedione and methyl ethyl ketone. *Arch Toxicol*. 2002; 75(11–12):643–652.

chapter 35

Regulatory Toxicology

Gary E. Marchant*

WHAT IS REGULATORY TOXICOLOGY?

Regulatory toxicology is a subfield of regulatory science, which addresses the intersection of science with regulation, namely how is science developed, evaluated, and applied in regulatory decision making. Toxicology is one of the most common fields of scientific knowledge utilized in regulatory science, as regulatory agencies often are required to identify and quantify the health risks of the products and activities they seek to regulate. Regulatory toxicology, which must straddle traditional scientific methodologies with the public policy world of regulation, strains to adhere to the standards of good toxicological science while also providing relevant inputs to decision making, which often asks questions that science cannot answer completely or with any certainty. It is the tension between these two different worlds of science and policy that raise many of the most important and challenging issues in regulatory toxicology, many of which will be addressed in this chapter.

Over the past 40 years, the field of regulatory toxicology has grown enormously as the intersection between regulation and toxicology has expanded dramatically. With the enactment of a series of

environmental, health, and safety statutes in the 1970s and 1980s, regulatory agencies increasingly rely on toxicological science to identify potential hazards, prioritize chemicals and other potentially toxic substances, and provide the data used for assessing risk. Regulators are not merely consumers of toxicological studies but also help shape toxicology science in important ways. Regulatory programs have provided a major impetus for improvements in toxicology methods, and they have stimulated a demand for toxicology studies that meet various regulatory requirements. Some programs, such as the programs of the Food and Drug Administration (FDA) for licensing drugs, devices, and food additives and that of the Environmental Protection Agency (EPA) for registering pesticides, explicitly demand toxicology studies as a condition for marketing products. Other statutory and regulatory requirements, such as the recent program requiring EPA to screen chemicals for their endocrine disruptor capability, or agencies to evaluate the safety of new nanotechnology applications are a major driver for the development of new types of toxicological assays.

Regulatory agencies have exercised important influence over the design and conduct of toxicology studies. For example, the EPA is empowered by the Toxic Substances Control Act (TSCA) to promulgate standards for different types of toxicology (and other scientific) investigations. Likewise, the FDA has long issued guidelines for laboratory studies submitted in support of food additives and drugs. Both agencies have adopted requirements governing laboratory operations and practice. Communication between

*The author acknowledges and appreciates the work of Professor Richard Merrill, a pioneer in the legal study of regulation, who authored previous versions of this chapter and upon whose work this chapter builds.

government officials and laboratory scientists flows in both directions. Government testing standards are influenced strongly by the prevailing consensus among toxicologists, many of whom work in regulatory agencies.

THE SCIENCE/POLICY INTERFACE IN REGULATORY TOXICOLOGY

There are critical differences between the objectives and methods of science and regulatory policy. Science seeks to understand natural phenomena through objective, empirical, and neutral methodologies, and is cautious, incremental, and evidence-based. In contrast, government regulation seeks to affect human behavior and resolve human disputes; it is episodic, peremptory, and normative, pursuing goals such as well-being, efficiency, and fairness.

Science is open-ended and can continue to study a problem indefinitely without coming to any final resolution. As the National Research Council noted, "the scientific process of seeking the truth, by design and to its credit, has no natural endpoint" (NRC, 2009). In contrast, regulation usually does not have the luxury of waiting until the science has matured, but rather must come to decisions based on legislative, political, and societal deadlines. This creates two problems. First, finality is essential for regulations, so that regulated entities and other stakeholders have certainty about the applicable regulatory requirements, which often involve significant resources and leadtime to achieve compliance. Consequently, regulations are adopted as final decisions, which can only be reconsidered at significant administrative burden. Science meanwhile continues to develop, resulting in regulations that often become increasingly out-dated in relationship to evolving scientific data and understanding.

The second problem created by the need to adopt regulations on a set timetable is often that the scientific inputs into that regulatory decision remain uncertain and underdeveloped. This leads to what Alvin Weinberg referred to as the "regulator's dilemma": "the regulator, by law, is expected to regulate even though science can hardly help him; this is the regulator's dilemma" (Weinberg, 1985). Regulatory agencies are therefore required to make numerous assumptions to fill the gaps in the available scientific data. This then has the inevitable effect of making agency determinations have a mixed science–policy nature, which can lead to confusion and obfuscation.

Scientists are also often frustrated by the political and administrative requirements (often referred to colloquially as "red tape") associated with regulatory utilization of toxicological data. A regulatory proposal incorporating scientific evidence has to pass through many layers within a regulatory office, including the agency scientists, economists, program officers, office of the general counsel, political appointees, various Centers, Programs and Offices within the agency that are affected by the proposed decision, external advisory committees, and finally the agency head, subject at every stage to a bevy of internal control requirements and processes. When the agency has finally made its proposed decision, the proposal is often then scrutinized by the Office of Information and Regulatory Affairs (OIRA) in the White House, courts conducting judicial review, Congressional oversight committees, and of course external stakeholders and the media. At every step along this pathway, the scientific findings of the agency are subject to challenge, prodding, and second-guessing.

This elaborate regulatory process has a number of implications. First, regulatory agencies tend to attempt to buttress their regulatory decisions with extensive analytical support. As a comparative study

of US and European regulation observed, "American regulators, being more politically exposed than their European counterparts, have a greater need to support their actions through formal analytical arguments. Their demand for expertise necessitates a continuing build-up of technical capabilities and the development of more sophisticated and detailed analytical methodologies. The structure of the American rule-making process subjects the analytical case for regulation to intense political scrutiny. Any weaknesses are quickly exploited, and the uncertainties and shortcomings of the relevant scientific base are readily exposed…." (Brickman *et al.*, 1985). In response to these pressures, regulatory agencies will often compile extensive scientific assessments of the toxicological and other data supporting their regulatory decisions, sometimes thousands of pages in length.

Another consequence of the highly politicized and adversarial nature of regulatory decision making is that regulatory agencies have an incentive to overstate the scientific basis of their decisions. Although scientific data are a critical input into sound-regulatory decision making, the actual decision of how much protection to provide and which requirements or limits to impose is inevitably a normative policy decision. Yet, agencies receive greater deference from Congress, the White House, reviewing courts, and even the media and public if they justify their decision on scientific rather than policy grounds. Accordingly, regulatory agencies are inclined to give disproportionate weight to scientific arguments and evidence in trying to justify their decisions, a tendency that has been labeled in the literature as the "science charade" (Wagner, 1995).

AN OVERVIEW OF REGULATORY APPROACHES

Different agencies and even different regulatory programs within the same agency use toxicological data in different ways. One important difference relates to the extent of premarket analysis or approval required before a new product may be commercialized. Some products require premarket approval from a regulatory agency (eg, drugs and medical devices by FDA and pesticides by EPA), other products require only premarket notification to the agency (eg, new chemical substances), whereas still other products require no premarket activity with a regulatory agency (eg, foods, cosmetics) before they can be sold commercially. There are also differences in who has the burden of proof to demonstrate safety or hazard. For example, the manufacturer of a new food additive has the burden to demonstrate to the FDA the lack of hazard before humans may be exposed, while laws such as the Occupational Safety and Health Act (1970) put the burden on regulators to show that a substance is hazardous before exposures can be restricted. The approach chosen by Congress for a particular type of product or activity greatly influences an agency's ability to require comprehensive toxicological investigation prior to commercialization.

In determining what level of a substance to allow, regulatory agencies generally use one of three different approaches: (i) acceptable risk, (ii) balancing, or (iii) feasibility. The determination of which of these three approaches is used for a particular hazard is generally determined by the applicable statutory framework.

Acceptable Risk

This approach determines the level of risk a substance presents, and then seeks to lower that risk (if necessary) to a level that is "acceptable." Because these risk-based programs only consider health evidence, toxicological data play a central role in these regulatory programs. In making the determination of acceptable risk, agencies have traditionally distinguished between carcinogens and noncarcinogens in their approach. For noncarcinogenic chemicals, regulators have generally embraced a standard safety assessment formula, built around the concept of acceptable daily intake (ADI) for the FDA or reference dose (RfD) or reference concentration (RfC) in the case of EPA. These levels are derived by applying a series of safety factors to the lowest "no observed adverse effect level" from animal experiments. Human exposures to a chemical that fall below the resulting ADI, RfD, or RfC are assumed to be "safe" or acceptable. This traditional approach to noncarcinogenic toxicants has not been considered appropriate for carcinogens. Regulators in the United States and many of their counterparts in other countries have operated on the premise that carcinogens as a class cannot be assumed to have "safe" or threshold doses. Furthermore, they have assumed that any chemical shown convincingly in animal studies to cause cancer should be considered a potential human carcinogen. Accordingly, for this group of compounds, regulators have generally assumed that no finite level of human exposure can be considered risk-free. As research has begun to illuminate the different mechanisms by which chemicals may cause cancer, however, regulatory agencies have cautiously accepted the possibility that "safe" thresholds may be established for some nongenotoxic carcinogens.

An example of an "acceptable" risk-regulatory program is the national ambient air quality program under the Clean Air Act (CAA). Under this program, EPA must set standards for criteria air pollutants such as particulate matter, ozone, and carbon monoxide that protect against "adverse effects" in the most susceptible subgroup with an adequate margin of safety. EPA may only consider risk data in setting these standards; no consideration of costs or feasibility is permitted (*Whitman v ATA*, 2001). A more stringent form of the acceptable risk approach is a "zero" or "negligible" risk requirement, epitomized by the famous Delaney clause, enacted in 1958 as part of the Food Additives Amendment. The amendment itself requires that any food additive be found "safe" before the FDA may approve its use [Food Additive Amendment, 1958]. The Delaney clause stipulated that this finding may not be made for a food additive that has been shown to induce cancer in humans or in experimental animals. In 1996, Congress amended the provisions of the Food, Drug, and Cosmetics Act applicable to pesticide residues in food, revoking the Delaney proviso as it applies to food additives (but not color additives), and adopting a standard that, though not expressed in these words, is understood to permit a tolerance for a carcinogenic pesticide if the estimated cancer risk is extremely small, on the order of one in one million (Food Quality Protection Act, 1996).

Balancing Approaches

Other regulatory programs require the agency to balance the health benefits of risk reduction against the costs of such reductions. These approaches known as cost-benefit or risk-benefit analysis generally require a quantified estimate of both the health risks and costs associated with various regulatory options, and the agency then chooses the regulatory option that offers the biggest estimated net benefit. Both toxicological and economic data play key roles in these statutory programs for calculating the benefits and costs of regulation, respectively. The TSCA (1976) is an example of a statute utilizing a balancing approach, requiring EPA to set standards for toxic substances based on a quantified cost-benefit analysis (*Corrosion Proof Fittings v EPA*, 1991).

Feasibility/Best Available Technology

The third major approach requires the agency to reduce exposures to the lowest feasible level, or to require companies to install the best available technology. This approach does not explicitly rely on any health data, and this skirting of the complexities and uncertainties of toxicological evidence is seen as a major advantage of this approach. The consequence of ignoring health impacts, though, is that the resulting standards may overprotect or underprotect health. An example of such a feasibility-based approach is the Clean Water Act's effluent standards, which requires dischargers of pollutants to install the best available technology determined to be feasible for that industrial category. A program using a hybrid feasibility/acceptable risk approach is the Occupational Safety and Health Act, which directs the Occupational Safety and Health Administration (OSHA) to set workplace standards for hazardous exposures to the level "which most adequately assures, *to the extent feasible* ... that no employee will suffer material impairment of health or functional capacity" (OSHA, 1970). This language has been interpreted by OSHA and the courts as requiring the agency to set occupational health standards at the lowest exposure level that is technologically and economically feasible, to the extent necessary to reduce a "significant" risk (*American Textile Manufacturers Institute v Donovan*, 1982).

SPECIFIC REGULATORY PROGRAMS UTILIZING TOXICOLOGICAL DATA

At the federal level, four agencies are chiefly responsible for regulating human exposure to toxic materials: the FDA, EPA, OSHA, and the Consumer Product Safety Commission (CPSC). Together they administer over two-dozen statutes whose primary goal is the protection of health. The statutes administered by these four agencies utilize different regulatory approaches and require divergent safety benchmarks. This diversity has several explanations. The statutes were enacted in different eras. They originated with different political constituencies and remain under their influence. Perhaps most significant, statutory standards often reflect differences in the technical capacity to control different types of exposures, and they embody different Congressional judgments about the economic implications of limiting exposures.

Food and Drug Administration

The oldest of the major health regulation laws, the FFD&C Act, was originally enacted in 1906 and, as amended over time, now covers food for humans and animals, human and veterinary drugs, medical devices, and cosmetics.

Food The initial Food and Drug Act enacted in 1906 prohibited "adulterated" foods that contain "any poisonous or deleterious substance, which may render it injurious to health." This provision, which remains in the statute to date [FFD&C Act § 402(a)], does not require premarket approval of foods and puts the burden of proof on FDA to demonstrate that a food meets the definition of "adulterated."

Congress has since amended the act several times to strengthen the FDA's ability to ensure the safety of foods (FFD&C, 1938). The most important of these amendments was the 1958 Food Additives Amendments that require the safety of food additives to be demonstrated prior to marketing (Food Additive Amendments, 1958). The manufacturer of a food additive must submit a petition demonstrating that the substance is "reasonably certain to be safe"; no inquiry into the benefits of an additive is undertaken or authorized (Cooper, 1978). Two categories of nonnaturally occurring food ingredients were exempted from this food additive requirement: (a) substances generally recognized as safe among experts qualified by scientific training and experience to evaluate safety; and (b) substances that either FDA or the US Department of Agriculture (USDA) had sanctioned for use in food prior to 1958 (so-called "prior sanction" substances).

Separate regulatory standards have been developed for several classes of indirect food constituents. For example, a food-contact substance requires approval as a food additive if, when used as intended, it "may reasonably be expected to become a component of food." In 1997 omnibus legislation that addressed most of FDA's regulatory programs, Congress created a new premarket notification system for food-contact materials that permits the agency to delay introduction if it questions a material's safety, but does not require affirmative agency approval (FDA Modernization Act, 1997).

Human Drugs Preclinical studies in animals play an important role in the FDA's evaluation of human drugs. The current law requires premarket approval, for both safety and efficacy, of all "new" drugs, a category that embraces virtually all prescription drug ingredients introduced since 1938 (Hutt *et al.*, 2007). Premarket approval of therapeutic agents for commercial use primarily relies on randomized controlled trials in human subjects to establish safety and efficacy. However, animal and in vitro studies are the primary source of information about a substance's biological effects before human trials are begun, and their results influence not only the decision whether to expose human subjects but also the design of clinical protocols. The FDA reviews the clinical evidence before authorizing human clinical trials through review of an Investigational New Drug (IND) application.

Medical Devices In 1976, Congress overhauled the FFD&C Act's requirements for medical devices, providing the FDA major new authority to regulate their testing, marketing, and use. The elaborate new scheme contemplates three tiers of control, the most restrictive of which (class III) is premarket approval similar to that required for new drugs. To obtain FDA premarket approval of a class III device, the sponsor must demonstrate safety and efficacy. The bulk of the data supporting such applications will be derived from clinical studies but also will include toxicology studies of any constituents likely to be absorbed by the patient.

Cosmetics The statutory provisions governing cosmetics do not require premarket approval of any ingredient, or demand that manufacturers test their products for safety, though many manufacturers routinely do so. The basic safety standard for cosmetics is similar to that for food ingredients: no product may be marketed if it contains "a poisonous or deleterious substance, which may render it injurious to health" [FFD&C Act § 601(a)]. The case law establishes that this language, too, bars distribution of a product that poses any significant risk of more than transitory harm when used as intended, but it places on the FDA the burden of proving a violation (Hutt *et al.*, 2007). The FDA has brought few cases under this standard, in part because acute toxic reactions to cosmetics are readily detected and immediately result in abandonment of the offending ingredient. The FDA also relies on the Cosmetic Ingredient Review (CIR), a private expert assessment body established in 1976 and operated by the Personal Care Products Council. The CIR appoints an expert panel that conducts safety assessments of cosmetics ingredients that are subject to public review and comment and then published as monographs.

Environmental Protection Agency

The EPA is responsible for administering most of the nation's environmental laws, which include protection of both human health and the environment. A comprehensive review of the EPA's numerous programs is not possible here; the following summary focuses on those EPA activities in which toxicology evidence plays a central role: the agency-wide Integrated Risk Information System (IRIS) program, pesticide regulation, regulation of industrial chemicals, regulation of drinking water supplies, hazardous waste control, and regulation of toxic pollutants of water and of air.

IRIS Program EPA's IRIS provides an agency-wide scientific assessment program to evaluate the carcinogenic and noncarcinogenic human health risks of various chemicals. EPA prepares a Toxicological Review for a chemical, which goes through a series of internal and external reviews before being finalized, that is then used to derive a RfD and/or inhalation RfC for noncarcinogenic effects, and a weight of evidence determination as well as oral and inhalation unit risks for carcinogenic effects. IRIS values are used to support a variety of agency regulatory programs, including many of those described below. As of 2011, the agency has established IRIS values for over 550 chemical substances. EPA is in the process of reforming its IRIS process in response to criticisms of recent reviews, including a critical National Research Council study of EPA's IRIS assessment of formaldehyde (NRC, 2011).

Pesticides Pesticides are subject to two types of regulation: (i) registration under the Federal Insecticide, Fungicide, and Rodenticide Act (FIFRA, 1972), which is required for a pesticide to be marketed in the United States; and (ii) tolerance (under the FFD&C Act), which sets the allowable level of pesticide residue in food for human consumption. Pesticide residues on raw agricultural commodities for years were initially regulated by the EPA under a 1954 amendment to the FFD&C Act, which allowed the agency to consider in setting tolerances both the potential adverse health effects of residues and the benefits of pesticide uses. If the concentration of a pesticide in a processed food exceeded the established tolerance, or the pesticide was a carcinogen, the Delaney clause prohibited its approval for that use (*Les v Reilly,* 1992). This framework was revised by Congress in 1996 by the Food Quality Protection Act (FQPA) to exempt pesticide residues from the operation of the Delaney clause but also restricted the consideration of pesticide benefits in setting tolerances.

The FQPA integrated the standard for registration and tolerance of a pesticide to require a pesticide to be shown to be safe, a standard defined as "reasonable assurance of no harm" (FQPA, 1996). The 1996 amendments also introduced some additional novel elements to the tolerance process. First, it required EPA to determine the safe level of a pesticide residue in a cumulative context, considering "all anticipated dietary exposures and all other exposures for which there is reliable information" [21 USC § 346a(b)(2)(A)(ii)]. This includes other nonoccupational sources of exposure, including food, drinking water, and residential exposures [21 USC § 346a(b)(2)(D)(vi)]. EPA must also base its safety determination on a consideration of exposures to other pesticides that share the same mechanism of toxicity [21 USC § 346a(b)(2)(C)(i)(III)].

Second, the 1996 FQPA required EPA to give special consideration to the health of infants and children, by ensuring "that there is a reasonable certainty that no harm will result to infants and children from aggregate exposure to the pesticide chemical residue...." [21 USC § 346a(b)(2)(C)(ii)(I)]. To implement this requirement, the statute directs EPA to "use an additional 10-fold margin of safety in assessing the risks to infants and children to take into account potential for pre- and postnatal toxicity and the completeness of the toxicology and exposure databases." EPA can deviate from the 10-fold margin of safety "only if, based on reliable data, the resulting margin would be safe for infants and children" [21 USC § 346a(b)(2)(C)(ii)(I)]. EPA's failure to provide a legally sufficient rationale for not applying the presumptive 10-fold extra safety factor for children has been found to be arbitrary and capricious by reviewing courts (*NRDC v EPA*, 2011; *Northwest Coalition for Alternatives to Pesticides v EPA*, 2008).

Third, EPA must develop a program to test for endocrine disrupting effects of pesticides. There has been a flurry of research over the past couple of decades addressing the identification and mechanisms of toxicity from endocrine-disrupting chemicals (Marty *et al.*, 2011). The FQPA required EPA to "develop a screening program, using appropriate validated test systems and other scientifically relevant information, to determine whether certain substances may have an effect in humans that is similar to an effect produced by a naturally occurring estrogen, or such other endocrine effect as the Administrator may designate" [21 USC § 346a(p)(1)]. Although EPA was required to establish this program by 1999, it did not meet this deadline.

EPA has been moving forward nevertheless and has created an Endocrine Disruptor Screening Program, which involves a two-tier screening and testing process: In Tier 1 testing, EPA seeks to identify chemicals that have the potential to interact with the endocrine system. Tier 1 consists of 11 different assays, which are being applied to 67 pesticide ingredients on EPA's initial list of chemicals to be tested, which was released in 2009. This initial round of testing was scheduled to be completed in February 2012. EPA proposed in 2010 a second list of 134 additional chemicals to be tested in Tier 1. In Tier 2, EPA will determine the endocrine-related effects caused by each chemical that indicated endocrine disruption activity in Tier 1, and obtain information about effects at various doses in order to enable risk assessment. The agency is in the process of developing and validating Tier 2 tests. One issue is whether in Tier 2 EPA should use traditional animal assays or in vitro and computational assays that are part of EPA's ToxCast program.

After the FQPA of 1996, the pesticide registration process now includes a broader review of the human health impacts of the pesticide from commercial use of the pesticides on applicators and other individuals, as well as effects on the environment. The manufacturer of a pesticide must produce a variety of data from tests done according to EPA guidelines. EPA's test guidelines, most recently revised in 2007, now encompass guidelines for 340 types of tests recommended for pesticides (40 CFR 158 and 161). These tests evaluate whether a pesticide has the potential to cause adverse effects on humans, wildlife, fish, and plants, as well as possible contamination of surface water or ground water from leaching, runoff, and spray drift. The potential human risks that are evaluated include both acute and chronic toxicity. The EPA then conditions the use of the pesticide on various protections to ensure that the pesticide is used safely, which are summarized on the pesticide label.

The EPA has been engaged in a comprehensive review of previously registered pesticides and "reregistration" of those that meet contemporary standards for marketing for approximately the past three decades. Under this program, many older pesticides have been subjected to comprehensive toxicology testing, including carcinogenicity testing, for the first time, and the results have required modification of the terms of approved use and, in some instances, cancellation for several agents. The FQPA required EPA to review the registration ("reregistration") and tolerance of

older pesticides. In addition, EPA initiated a new program in 2006 called "registration review" in which it intends to re-evaluate all pesticides every 15 years. Finally, EPA may initiate a "Pesticide Special Review" process whenever it discovers that the use of a registered pesticide may result in unreasonable adverse effects on people or the environment.

Industrial Chemicals The TSCA was promulgated in 1976 (TSCA, 1976) to regulate all chemical substances manufactured or processed in or imported into the United States, except for substances already regulated under other laws. *A chemical substance* is defined broadly as "any organic or inorganic substance of a particular molecular identity."

TSCA gives the EPA three main powers. First, the agency is empowered to restrict or even ban the manufacturing, processing, distribution, use, or disposal of a chemical substance when there is a reasonable basis to conclude any such activity poses an "unreasonable risk of injury to health or environment." In determining whether a chemical substance presents an unreasonable risk, the agency is instructed to balance the costs of restricting the substance against the health benefits of the proposed regulation [TSCA § 6]. This trade-off approach to regulation has proved a major challenge to the EPA. The agency has exercised its regulatory authority under section 6 against only a handful of substances, and it's most significant regulations, such as its attempted ban on asbestos products, have been struck down by the courts for failing to do an adequate cost-benefit analysis (*Corrosion Proof Fittings v EPA*, 1991).

Second, if the EPA suspects that a chemical *may* pose an unreasonable risk but lacks sufficient data to take action, TSCA empowers the agency to require testing to develop the necessary data. Similarly, it may order testing if the chemical will be produced in substantial quantities that may result in significant human exposure whose effects cannot be predicted on the basis of existing data. In either case, the EPA must consider the "relative costs of the various test protocols and methodologies" and the "reasonably foreseeable availability of the facilities and personnel" needed to perform the tests [TSCA § 4].

Finally, to enable the EPA to evaluate chemicals before humans are exposed, TSCA requires the manufacturer of a new chemical substance to notify the agency 90 days prior to production or distribution [TSCA § 5(a)(1)]. The manufacturer's or distributor's notice (called a pre-manufacturing notice or PMN) must include any health effects data it possesses. However, the EPA is not empowered to require that manufacturers routinely conduct testing of all new chemicals to permit an evaluation of their risks; Congress declined to confer the kind of premarket approval authority that the FDA exercises for drugs and food additives and the EPA exercises for pesticides.

In contrast, the European Union (EU) is implementing a much more aggressive regulatory program for chemical substances, known as the **R**egistration, **E**valuation, **A**uthorization, and Restriction of **Ch**emical substances (REACH) program. REACH puts the responsibility for ensuring the safety of chemicals on the companies that produce, import, and use chemicals. The program applies to both new and existing chemicals, and is phased-in over an 11-year period based primarily on the production volume of individual chemicals. REACH employs a tiered-testing approach, with the amount of initial testing determined by production volume. A technical dossier is required for all registered chemicals; however, only chemicals with a production volume of 10 or more tons per year require a chemical safety assessment documented in a chemical safety report. REACH allows the use of alternative testing strategies to evaluate specific endpoints in lieu of experimental testing; however, whole animal testing requirements exist for each level based on production volume.

In light of the limitations of TSCA and the more proactive approach of the EU REACH program, there are active proposals in Congress to modify and update TSCA. Although the details of TSCA reform remain undecided at the time of this writing, there is broad consensus that some type of reform is needed.

Hazardous Wastes The two primary statutes regulating hazardous wastes in the United States are the Resource Conservation and Recovery Act (RCRA, 1976) and the Comprehensive Environmental Response, Compensation, and Liability Act (CERCLA, 1980). With some exceptions, the primary purpose of CERCLA is the cleanup of contamination from pre-existing hazardous waste sites, whereas RCRA regulates the generation, transport, and disposal of new hazardous wastes. Both RCRA and CERCLA have their own extensive lists of substances and waste streams of toxic materials that are defined as hazardous wastes. In addition, under RCRA, wastes that meet any of four "characteristics" are also treated as hazardous wastes. The four characteristics are ignitability, corrosivity, reactivity, and toxicity, and EPA has identified standardized protocols for determining whether a particular waste stream meets one or more of these characteristics. Under RCRA, EPA has developed standards for generators, transporters, and those who treat, store, or dispose hazardous wastes that are required to "protect human health and the environment." The EPA's regulations applicable to generators and transporters establish a manifest system that is designed to create a paper trail for every shipment of waste, from generator to final destination, to ensure proper handling and accountability. The agency has the broadest authority over persons who own or operate hazardous waste treatment, storage, or disposal facilities. Pursuant to the RCRA, it has issued regulations prescribing methods for treating, storing, and disposing of wastes; governing the location, design, and construction of facilities; mandating contingency plans to minimize negative impacts from such facilities; setting qualifications for ownership, training, and financial responsibility; and requiring permits for all such facilities (RCRA, 1976).

CERCLA, often referred to as Superfund, authorizes the cleanup of hazardous waste sites and provides for liability of persons responsible for releases of hazardous waste at these sites. EPA can conduct cleanup of hazardous waste sites itself, and then seek recovery for the costs from potentially responsible parties (PRPs), or it can direct one or more PRPs to conduct cleanup, who may then seek contribution from other PRPs for their share of the cleanup. Under CERCLA, EPA has created the National Priorities List (NPL), which is a list of hazardous waste sites that are deemed the most hazardous sites and eligible for use of federal funds for long-term clean-up, and the National Contingency Plan (NCP), which provides the guidelines and procedures needed to respond to releases and threatened releases of hazardous substances, pollutants, or contaminants. For sites on the NPL, EPA conducts a Remedial Investigation and Feasibility Study to support the risk management process, which includes a site-specific human health and ecological risk assessment.

Toxic Water Pollutants The EPA has had responsibility for regulating toxic water pollutants since 1972. As originally enacted, Section 307 of the Federal Water Pollution Control Act required the EPA to adopt standards for toxic water pollutants that provided an "*ample margin of safety*"—a difficult criterion to meet for most toxic pollutants and arguably impossible for any known to be carcinogenic. Given EPA's difficulties in complying with this statutory directive, Congress amended the statute in 1977 to focus standards

on economic cost and technologic feasibility. In 1987, Congress amended the statute again to toughen standards for toxic pollutants. Under the prior law, the EPA had developed health-based "water quality criteria" for 126 compounds it had identified as toxic. These criteria essentially described *desirable* maximum contamination levels, which, because the EPA's discharge limits were technology-based, generally were substantially lower than the levels actually achieved. The 1987 amendments gave what had been advisory criteria real bite by requiring that states incorporate them in their own mandatory standards for water quality and impose additional effluent limits on operations discharging into below-standard waterways (Heineck, 1989).

Drinking Water The 1974 Safe Drinking Water Act (SDWA) was enacted to ensure that public water supply systems "meet minimum national standards for the protection of public health." Under the SDWA, the EPA is required to regulate any contaminants "which may have an adverse effect on human health." Over time and several Congressional amendments, this system has evolved into a two-tier system in which EPA adopts for each contaminant a maximum contaminant level goal (MCLG) that represents the optimal level to be achieved to ensure safety and the usually less stringent, feasibility-based maximum contaminant level (MCL). Only the MCL is legally enforceable. As part of the 1996 Safe Drinking Water Amendments, Congress directed EPA to use the "best available science" in setting MCLGs and MCLs.

Toxic Air Pollutants The original 1970 version of the CAA provision for regulation of hazardous air pollutants (section 112) required the agency to set emission standards for individual toxic pollutants that protect public health with "an ample margin of safety." The implication of this language—that standards were to provide absolute safety without regard to the costs of emissions control—generated intense debate from the beginning and contributed to the EPA's glacial pace of implementation. The EPA finally attempted to escape the strict language of section 112 when it issued a standard for vinyl chloride in 1986 in which the agency claimed it could consider costs and declined to adopt a standard dictated solely by safety. A court ruled that the EPA had improperly considered costs, but it did make clear that in determining what emissions level was safe, even for a carcinogen, the EPA was not obligated to eliminate exposure but rather was to "decide what risks are acceptable in the world in which we live" (*NRDC v EPA*, 1987).

Amendments to the CAA in 1990 responded to the difficulties presented by the strict health-based approach of old section 112. The statute now provides a list of 188 hazardous air pollutants, which EPA may modify by adding or deleting items. The EPA must establish national emissions standards for sources that emit any of the listed pollutants with a two-tier system of regulation. The EPA must first issue standards that are technology-based, designed to require the "maximum achievable control technology" (MACT) [CAA § 112(d)(2)]. If the MACT controls are insufficient to protect human health with an "ample margin of safety," the EPA must issue residual risk standards [CAA § 112(f)]. The 1990 Amendments essentially define "ample margin of safety" for carcinogens by requiring the EPA to establish added residual risk limits for any pollutant that poses a lifetime excess cancer risk of greater than one in one million. However, as subsequently clarified in a judicial decision, while EPA must promulgate residual risk standards if the MACT standards do not reduce risks to one in one million, the residual risk standards are not required to reduce the risks to one in one million, but rather to 100 in one million (*NRDC v EPA*, 2008).

Occupational Safety and Health Administration

The 1970 Occupational Safety and Health Act requires employers to provide employees with safe working conditions and empowers OSHA to prescribe mandatory occupational safety and health standards (OSHA, 1970). OSHA's most controversial actions involved its attempts to set occupational exposure limits for hazardous chemicals.

The Act specifies that in regulating hazardous occupational exposures, OSHA shall adopt the standard "which most adequately assures, to the extent feasible, on the basis of the best available evidence, that no employee will suffer material impairment of health or physical capacity" [OSHA § 6 (b)(5)]. Judicial challenges to OSHA standards have clarified OSHA's responsibilities. In a famous case, the US Supreme Court overturned OSHA's benzene standard because the agency had not shown that prevailing worker exposure levels posed a "significant" health risk (*Industrial Union Department, AFL-CIO, v American Petroleum Institute,* 1980). This prerequisite proved a major obstacle when OSHA attempted to establish standards for 428 air contaminants in a single proceeding in 1989. Although it found that OSHA's generic approach to regulation was permissible in theory, a court vacated the standards because OSHA failed to show that each individual contaminant posed a "significant risk" at current levels (*American Federation of Labor v OSHA,* 1992). However, the Supreme Court earlier upheld OSHA's cotton dust standard, rejecting arguments that the agency was obligated to balance the costs of individual standards against the benefits of reducing hazardous workplace exposures (*American Textile Manufacturers Institute v Donovan,* 1982).

Consumer Product Safety Commission

Of the four agencies discussed here, the CPSC has played the least important role in federal efforts to control toxic chemicals to date. The commission was created in 1972 by the Consumer Product Safety Act (CPSA, 1972) with authority to regulate products that pose an unreasonable risk of injury or illness to consumers. The commission is empowered to promulgate safety standards "to prevent or reduce an unreasonable risk of injury" associated with a consumer product. If no feasible standard "would adequately protect the public from the unreasonable risk of injury" posed by a consumer product, the commission may ban the product [CPSA § 8]. In assessing the need for a standard or ban, the agency must balance the likelihood that a product will cause harm, and the severity of harm it will likely cause, against the effects of reducing the risk on the product's utility, cost, and availability to consumers.

The CPSC also administers the older Federal Hazardous Substances Act (FHSA, 1976). The FHSA authorizes the CPSC to regulate, primarily through prescribed label warnings, products that are toxic, corrosive, combustible, or radioactive or that generate pressure. The FHSA is unusual among federal health laws because it contains detailed criteria for determining toxicity. It defines "highly toxic" in terms of a substance's acute effects in specified tests in rodents; substances capable of producing chronic effects thus fall within the "toxic" category. The FHSA contains another unique provision [FHSA § 2(h)(2)] specifically addressing the probative weight of animal and human data on acute toxicity: "If the [commission] finds that available data on human experience with any substance indicates results different from those obtained on animals in the above-named dosages or concentrations, the human data shall take precedence."

The CPSC has prescribed labeling for products containing numerous substances that are acutely toxic. It has also acted to ban from consumer products several substances that pose a cancer risk, including asbestos, vinyl chloride as a propellant, benzene, tris(hydroxymethyl)aminomethane, and formaldehyde (Merrill, 1981).

In 2008, Congress adopted the Consumer Product Safety Improvement Act (2008), which significantly strengthened the CPSC's enforcement authority, especially for children's products, in response to a number of high-profile recalls of children's toys. The Act imposes bans on products containing lead or phthalates that exceed stringent levels, and requires third-party testing of certain children's products.

INSTITUTIONAL OVERSIGHT AND CONTROLS

As the previous subsection describes, regulatory agencies are required to evaluate and apply toxicological and other scientific data in a variety of statutory contexts. In addition to the statutory language, a number of internal and external institutional control mechanisms and processes greatly influence the agencies' treatment of toxicological data.

Advisory Committees

Regulatory agencies frequently rely on scientific advisory committees composed of external scientific experts to help guide their scientific determinations, including toxicological evaluations. For example, the EPA has a Scientific Advisory Board (SAB), established by Congress in 1978, to advise the agency on the quality and relevance of the scientific and technical information being used in regulatory programs as well as to review the agency's research programs. The SAB's work is done by a relatively large number of subcommittees and panels that focus on special subjects. The EPA also has two other independent scientific advisory committees associated with specific regulatory programs—the Clean Air Science Advisory Committee for air pollution, and the Science Advisory Panel for pesticides. These committees consist of external scientists who are appointed to serve on the committees for specified terms. Similarly, the FDA has over 50 external advisory committees that provide advice on the agency's significant product approvals and other scientific issues.

Regulatory agencies are not required to automatically follow the advice of their external advisory committees, but frequently do. Failure to follow the independent advice of their own advisory committee tends to call into question the soundness of the agency's scientific findings, whereas advisory committee endorsement of the agency's position can provide important scientific credibility and political cover to the agency.

Peer Review

Beyond peer review by agency advisory committees, regulatory agencies frequently utilize external peer review of scientific reports and assessments. In December 2004, the Office of Management and Budget (OMB) formalized the requirement for peer review by issuing its Final Information Quality Bulletin for Peer Review (OMB, 2004). This Peer Review Bulletin requires federal regulatory agencies to ensure that all "influential scientific information" they disseminate is peer-reviewed. Influential scientific information is defined as "scientific information the agency reasonably can determine will have or does have a clear and substantial impact on important public policies or private sector decisions." The Bulletin specifically identifies "scientific assessments" as one type of information subject to the peer review requirement, which are defined as "an evaluation of a body of scientific or technical knowledge, which typically synthesizes multiple factual inputs, data, models, assumptions, and/or applies best professional judgment to bridge uncertainties in the available information." These assessments include, but are not limited to, state-of-science reports; technology assessments; weight-of-evidence analyses; meta-analyses; health, safety, or ecological risk assessments; toxicological characterizations of substances; integrated assessment models; hazard determinations; or exposure assessments.

The Peer Review Bulletin directs agencies to choose a peer review mechanism that is appropriate and commensurate with how the information will be used, giving due consideration to the novelty and complexity of the science involved, the relevance of the information to regulatory decision making, the extent of prior peer reviews, and the expected benefits and costs of additional review. The Peer Review Bulletin requires the most rigorous peer review requirements for highly influential scientific assessments.

Risk Assessment Guidance/Guidelines

Regulatory agencies often adopt guidelines to promote consistency and predictability in their treatment of toxicological data and the conduct of risk assessment. For example, EPA has adopted risk assessment guidelines for carcinogenicity, mutagenicity, developmental toxicity, chemical mixtures, exposure analysis, reproductive toxicity, neurotoxicity, and ecotoxicity. The genesis of EPA's risk assessment guidelines was a series of "cancer principles" prepared largely at the instigation of EPA lawyers in the mid-1970s (Albert, 1994). The agency lawyers were frustrated by the delays in regulating pesticides as a result of scientific disagreement about the mechanisms and causes of human cancer. In an attempt to circumvent such scientific disputes, the lawyers developed a series of 17 "cancer principles" with the assistance of EPA scientists during hearings on the pesticides heptachlor and chlordane. The 17 principles were intended to be nonrebuttable guidelines that would govern and simplify carcinogenicity determinations.

Shortly thereafter, EPA began to develop a more comprehensive set of guidelines for evaluating carcinogens. This led to EPA publishing its "interim" guidelines for carcinogenic risk assessment in 1976, which were subsequently updated and finalized in 1986 (EPA, 1986). The 1986 guidelines primarily consisted of a series of "default options" that were intended as presumptive principles that would apply in the absence of sufficient data to establish an alternative assumption. Some of the most important default options included in EPA's 1986 carcinogen guidelines included: (i) laboratory animals are assumed to be a valid surrogate for humans in assessing risk; thus, positive cancer results in animal bioassays are taken as evidence of human carcinogenicity; (ii) humans are assumed to be as sensitive as the most sensitive animal species, strain, or sex evaluated in an appropriately designed animal bioassay; (iii) benign tumors are assumed to be as significant as malignant tumors; (iv) the dose–response of humans to potential carcinogens is assumed to be linear all the way to the zero exposure levels with no threshold; and (v) a given intake of a substance is assumed to have the same effect regardless of the rate or route of intake (EPA, 1986). Most of the default options selected by EPA were deliberately chosen to be "conservative," in that they are intended to estimate the plausible upper-bound of actual risk (NRC, 1994).

EPA's risk assessment guidelines not only promoted consistency in risk assessment approach and procedure across the broad array of EPA regulatory programs, which use risk assessment, but also furthered the objective of efficiency, by sparing the agency the need to revisit the same controversial issues in each successive rule-making proceeding (Wiltse and Dellarco, 1996). The courts were generally supportive of the predictability and consistency provided by the agency's risk assessment guidelines, giving greater deference to EPA risk assessments that comported with the guidelines. As one court stated, "EPA's specific enunciation of its underlying analytical principles, derived from its experience in the area, yields meaningful notice and dialogue, enhances the administrative process, and furthers reasoned agency decision making" (*Environmental Defense Fund, Inc, v Environmental Protection Agency*, 1976).

Notwithstanding these benefits of risk assessment guidelines, EPA's implementation of its guidelines was criticized in a 1994 NRC report that found that EPA applied the default principles too rigidly and had failed to articulate clear criteria for departing from the defaults (NRC, 1994). EPA itself acknowledged that "[i]n practice, the agency's assessments routinely have employed defaults and, until recently, only occasionally departed from them. (EPA, 1996). EPA published draft revisions to its carcinogen guidelines in 1996 (EPA, 1996) that were finalized in 2005 (EPA, 2005) that take a more flexible, data-based approach to default options. As explained by EPA, the revised guidelines "are intended to be both explicit and more flexible than in the past concerning the basis for making departures from defaults, recognizing that expert judgment and peer review are essential elements of the process" (EPA, 1996). The revised guidelines incorporate "a weight-of-the-evidence approach that considers all relevant data in reaching conclusions about the potential human carcinogenicity of an agent" (EPA, 1996).

Judicial Review

Agency regulations are often subject to legal challenges by stakeholders who disagree with the agency's decision. Under the Administrative Procedure Act, such judicial review tends to be deferential to the agency's decision, overturning the decision only if it is "arbitrary and capricious" or lacking "substantial evidence." Nevertheless, a significant proportion of major agency regulations are overturned in whole or in part, or sent back to the agency for further explanation. Scientific determinations, such as toxicological findings, are generally given the highest level of deference under a decision by the US Supreme Court, which held that "[w]hen examining this kind of scientific determination, as opposed to simple findings of fact, a reviewing court must generally be at its most deferential (*Baltimore Gas & Elec v NRDC*, 1983).

Even with this deference to scientific determinations, there have been many important judicial decisions impacting the way regulatory agencies address toxicological information. One prominent example was a challenge to the EPA's decision to retain a MCLG of zero under the Safe Drinking Water Act for chloroform in the face of evidence, accepted by its own scientific advisory committee, that the mechanism by which chloroform produces tumors in rodents is threshold-limited. The reviewing court held that given its acceptance of the evidence of a threshold, the EPA was required by the SDWA's "best available" evidence provision to base its decision on that evidence (*Chlorine Chemistry Council v EPA*, 2000). This ruling marks the first time that a court has directed a federal regulatory agency to recognize a "safe" finite level of exposure for an animal carcinogen. Another example of proactive judicial oversight is two recent decisions where the court second-guessed EPA's determination that there was sufficient toxicological evidence to justify departing from the presumptive 10-fold extra safety factor to protect children in pesticide regulatory decisions (*NRDC v, EPA*, 2011; *Northwest Coalition for Alternatives to Pesticides v EPA*, 2008).

Congressional Oversight

Congress has ultimate oversight of regulatory agencies, both by delegating the authority to regulate in the form of statutes, and by controlling the purse strings for the agencies. Regulatory statutes determine many of the fundamental choices for regulatory programs by specifying what factors may be considered in adopting regulatory standards and the objectives of the standards in terms of the level of safety to be attained. Statutes differ greatly on these questions, with some mandating standards be based on technological feasibility, whereas others specifying health-based regulation. The statutes can provide additional guidance that can influence the agency's consideration of toxicological evidence, such as the 1996 amendments to the Safe Drinking Water Act, which direct EPA to use "the best available, peer-reviewed science and supporting studies conducted in accordance with sound and objective scientific practices"(SDWA, 1996).

Congress also controls regulatory programs through its budgetary authority. By directing how much money is directed to specific activities or programs, Congress can directly influence agency priorities and emphasis. If Congress is not pleased with an agency's actions, it can adopt appropriation riders prohibiting the agency from spending money on controversial topics. In the past, for example, Congress has prevented EPA from working on climate change or radiofrequency issues by imposing annual riders for a time period.

In addition to these primary legislative controls, Congress has a number of other ways it can influence agency decision making. Congress can pressure agencies toward a preferred policy outcome through oversight hearings, letters to agency officials, and press releases. Congress has also adopted some oversight statutes to further control agency rulemaking. The Congressional Review Act requires federal regulatory agencies to file final rules with Congress before the rules can become effective. If the regulation meets the definition of a major rule ($100-million impact on the economy), Congress has 60 days to introduce a resolution of disapproval that, if adopted by both the House and Senate and signed by the President, can nullify the agency's rule.

Congress also enacted section 515 of the Treasury and General Government Appropriations Act of 2001, known as the Information Quality Act (IQA), which required the OMB to promulgate guidance to agencies ensuring the quality, objectivity, utility, and integrity of information (including statistical information) disseminated by federal agencies (IQA, 2001). Federal agencies were also required by the IQA to publish their own agency-specific guidelines no later than one year after OMB's guidelines, and also provide a mechanism for stakeholders to file petitions challenging agency actions that allegedly fail to comply with the data quality objectives. Private parties have challenged a number of scientific determinations by federal agencies under this provision, but the courts have determined that the agency decisions on these petitions are not judicially reviewable (*Salt Institute v Leavitt*, 2006).

Executive Oversight

The Executive branch also exerts overview of regulatory decisions, particularly through the OIRA within the White House OMB. OIRA reviews all draft significant regulations proposed by regulatory agencies, and although its review most often focuses on the economic aspects of the proposed rule, it also reviews the agency's scientific assumptions and findings. Although OIRA cannot itself revise the proposed regulation, it can hold up its publication until it has reached agreement with the agency on acceptable revisions.

The Executive Branch has other mechanisms for oversight and influence of regulatory science determinations by agencies. The White House under various Presidents has put out a series of Executive Orders providing regulatory guidance that agencies must follow to the extent consistent with the governing regulatory statute. For example, Executive Order 13563 issued by President Obama in January 2011 requires that federal regulations "must be based on the best available science. It must allow for public participation and an open exchange of ideas. It must promote predictability and reduce uncertainty. It must identify and use the best, most innovative, and least burdensome tools for achieving regulatory ends. It must take into account benefits and costs, both quantitative and qualitative" (EO 13563, 2011).

The White House also issued a memorandum on Scientific Integrity in 2009 that required each regulatory agency to develop its own scientific integrity policy that implemented several principles of scientific integrity, including: "(a) The selection and retention of candidates for science and technology positions in the executive branch should be based on the candidate's knowledge, credentials, experience, and integrity; (b) Each agency should have appropriate rules and procedures to ensure the integrity of the scientific process within the agency; (c) When scientific or technological information is considered in policy decisions, the information should be subject to well-established scientific processes, including peer review where appropriate, and each agency should appropriately and accurately reflect that information in complying with and applying relevant statutory standards...." (White House, 2009).

REGULATORY INFLUENCES ON TOXICOLOGY

This chapter has focused thus far on how toxicological data are used in federal regulatory programs. Yet, the relationship between regulation and toxicology is reciprocal, in that regulatory programs have also shaped and influenced the practice of toxicology. Modern toxicology has developed, in substantial part, in response to the information needs of contemporary regulation. But government regulation impinges on the discipline of toxicology in more direct ways as well. Regulatory agencies often prescribe the specific objectives and design of studies that are conducted to satisfy regulatory requirements. In addition, pressure to protect animals used in research has produced laws and regulations that govern toxicologists themselves.

Testing Guidelines

An agency's influence over the conduct of toxicology studies depends on its regulatory responsibilities. An agency such as the FDA or the EPA, which must confirm the safety of new substances before marketing, can dictate the kinds of tests that manufacturers must conduct to gain approval. By contrast, an agency or program that has no premarket approval function has less leverage.

Agencies such as the FDA and EPA that have been authorized to require premarket approval for certain categories of products have generally specified the types of tests they require before they will consider the safety of a compound (eg, tests for acute toxicity, subchronic effects, and chronic effects). Within each of these categories, an agency might set out more detailed requirements, essentially enumerating its "base set" data demands. In addition, the agencies usually adopt guidelines that describe preferred or acceptable methods for executing particular tests, such as a bioassay for carcinogenesis (EPA, 2011a; FDA, 2000). In addition, the EPA has established guidelines for several of the tests that it may mandate by rule or consent agreement for individual chemicals under TSCA § 4 (EPA, 2011a). Multinational bodies such as the Organization for Economic Cooperation and Development have sought to secure multilateral adherence to standardized test guidelines and minimum testing requirements for new chemicals (Page, 1982).

Both the FDA and the EPA have adopted another set of requirements that specify laboratory procedures for conducting tests required or submitted for regulatory consideration. These good laboratory practice (GLP) regulations prescribe essential but often mundane features of sound laboratory science, such as animal husbandry standards and record-keeping practices (EPA, 2011b, 2011c; FDA, 20011a). All of these requirements are intended to contribute to sound-regulatory decision making by ensuring the quality and integrity of toxicology data submitted to support agency decisions.

Food and Drug Administration The FDA exercises premarketing approval authority over several classes of compounds, of which the most important, for present purposes, are new human drugs and direct additives to food.

Toxicology Testing Requirements for Human Drugs In 1962, Congress expressly authorized the FDA to exempt investigational drugs from the premarket approval requirement so that they could be shipped for use in clinical testing, subject to conditions the agency believed appropriate to protect human subjects [FFD&C Act § 505(i)]. One condition that the FDA established was that an investigational drug first must have been evaluated in preclinical studies, which are then submitted to FDA as an IND application. This requirement appears in current regulations that amplify, in the text and in referenced guidelines, the types of tests that are to be performed and the design they should follow (FDA, 2011b). A drug's sponsor is encouraged to consult agency personnel to get a precise understanding of what sorts of toxicology studies the agency expects prior to submitting the IND. Preclinical studies of substances that are candidates for use as human drugs must also meet the standards set by the FDA's GLP regulations (FDA, 2011a). These regulations apply to all laboratories—university, independent, and manufacturer-owned—in which such studies are conducted. The work of the International Conference on Harmonization of Technical Requirements for Registration of Pharmaceuticals for Human Use (ICH) highlights the trend toward international agreement on test methods. Since its founding in 1990, the ICH—comprising the pharmaceutical regulatory agencies and industries from the European Union, Japan, and the United States—has issued over 50 harmonized guidelines on various aspects of pharmaceutical regulatory approval, including numerous guidelines on toxicology testing methods for human drugs.

Testing Requirements for Food Additives The Food Additives Amendment and the Color Additive Amendments require premarket approval of new additives to human food. Both laws assume that laboratory studies in animals will provide the principal data for assessing safety. Thus, a petitioner must submit "full reports of investigations made with respect to the safety for use of such additives, including full information as to the methods and control used" [FFD&C Act § 409(c)]. The FDA has adopted regulations specifying the types of data that an applicant must submit (FDA, 2011c).

The FDA's regulations contain only general statements about the need for and features of toxicology studies. For many years, the agency maintained an advice-giving system in which it prescribed the type and design of tests to be performed. In 1982, the FDA

first codified this "common law" in *Toxicological Principles for the Safety Assessment of Direct Food Additives and Color Additives Used in Food,* known thereafter as the "Red Book." The Red Book, revised in 2000, describes the types of tests the FDA believes necessary to evaluate an additive's safety (FDA, 2000). The agency's requirements, which are in the form of guidelines rather than regulations, are calibrated to the purposes for which the additive will be used, to estimated levels of human exposure, and to the results of sequential studies. Tests of food color and additives must also comply with the FDA's GLP regulations (FDA, 2011a).

Environmental Protection Agency The EPA's premarket approval authority over pesticides places it, like the FDA, in a position to dictate the design and conduct of studies on such compounds. The 1976 TSCA gave the EPA authority to mandate testing of other chemicals in use or scheduled for introduction and to specify, by regulation, test standards.

Toxicology Requirements for Pesticides FIFRA requires the submission of toxicology studies, as well as other types of investigations, to support the EPA's evaluation of a pesticide [FIFRA § 136(b)]. The statute also requires the EPA to publish guidelines specifying the kinds of information that will be required to support the registration.

The agency has issued regulations outlining the procedures for submission of registration petitions and their basic content (40 CFR part 158 and 161). The Office of Chemical Safety and Pollution Prevention (formerly the Office of Prevention, Pesticides, and Toxic Substances) has issued Harmonized Test Guidelines for all toxicology testing done under both FIFRA (pesticides) and TSCA (chemicals) (EPA, 2011a). For example, the Health Effects Test Guidelines (Series 870) include guidelines for approximately 50 different specific assays for acute toxicity, subchronic toxicity, chronic toxicity, genetic toxicity, neurotoxicity, and other toxicity testing. EPA has attempted to harmonize these guidelines whenever possible with applicable Organization for Economic Cooperation and Development (OECD) guidelines. Animal studies of pesticides must also comply with EPA's own good laboratory practice regulations, which were inspired by the same investigations that led the FDA to promulgate its standards for testing laboratories and impose similar requirements.

Testing of Industrial Chemicals The primary means by which the EPA may mandate health effects testing of new or existing industrial chemicals is Section 4(a) of the TSCA. That provision states that the administrator "shall by rule require that testing be conducted to develop data with respect to the health and environmental effects for which there is an insufficiency of data and experience" to permit assessment of whether a substance presents an unreasonable risk. This obligation to order testing is triggered by an administrative finding that a chemical presents a potential risk (based on the suspicion of toxicity) or that humans or the environment will be exposed to substantial quantities. The statute creates an Interagency Testing Committee (ITC) with members from EPA, CPSC, FDA, Department of the Interior (DOI), OSHA, Council on Environmental Quality (CEQ), National Institute for Occupational Safety and Health (NIOSH), National Institute of Environmental Health Sciences (NIEHS), National Cancer Institute (NCI), National Science Foundation (NSF), Agency for Toxic Substances and Disease Registry (ATSDR), National Library of Medicine (NLM), USDA, and the Department of Commerce to recommend a list of chemicals that should be tested and in what order of priority. Once the ITC has recommended a chemical substance for testing, the EPA is required by statute to either initiate testing or publish its reasons for not doing so within 12 months, although given the administrative burdens of such action the agency has frequently failed to meet this deadline.

This last requirement to take action on ITC recommendations within 12 months, coupled with the statute's formal procedures for adopting test rules, led the EPA initially to rely on negotiations with chemical producers to secure voluntary agreements for the conduct of tests it thought appropriate for chemicals identified by the ITC (GAO, 1982). The practice was challenged by public interest organizations, which were excluded from the negotiations, and ultimately it was declared unlawful (*NRDC v EPA*, 1984). The agency amended its regulations to recognize two forms of mandates for testing: test rules and enforceable testing consent agreements.

TSCA test rules are subject to judicial challenge. Manufacturers challenged a 1988 test rule for cumene, arguing that the EPA had failed to support its finding that the substance enters the environment in substantial quantities with the potential for substantial human exposure. Although the court ultimately upheld the rule, it ordered the agency to articulate standards governing the definition of "substantial" (*Chemical Manufacturers Association v EPA*, 1990). Another court challenge to a test rule requiring neurotoxicity studies of 10 widely used and intensively marketed organic solvents resulted in a settlement with the EPA. The settlement required the EPA to enter into consent agreements with reduced testing requirements for seven chemicals, to eliminate testing requirements for two, and to postpone its decision on one. Both test rules and testing consent agreements specify what types of tests are to be done. Their design is governed by regulations promulgated at 40 CFR part 799, and can usually be satisfied by the EPA Harmonized Test Guidelines (EPA, 2011a). Compound-specific testing requirements are sometimes also written into individual TSCA test rules or consent agreements. All toxicology studies required by the EPA under the TSCA must also comply with its GLP regulations.

Validation of Alternative Test Methods

Regulatory agencies have also been instrumental in encouraging the development of new safety test methods. Federal agency validation of new toxicological test methods was formalized and harmonized by the Interagency Coordinating Committee on the Validation of Alternative Methods (ICCVAM) Authorization Act of 2000, which permanently established the ICCVAM. Some 15 federal agencies participate in ICCVAM. Congress directed that one of the purposes of ICCVAM was to "ensure that new and revised test methods are validated to meet the needs of Federal agencies" [Pub L 106-545, §3(b)(4)]. In that regard, ICCVAM is directed to review and evaluate new or revised or alternative test methods and to provide test recommendations to federal agencies. Each federal agency administering a program that "requires or recommends acute or chronic toxicological testing" is required to adopt an alternative test method recommended by ICCVAM unless the agency determines that the alternative test method would not be consistent with its statutory goals.

The ICCVAM statute also requires that each federal agency "that requires or recommends acute or chronic toxicological testing shall ensure that any new or revised acute or chronic toxicity test method, including animal test methods and alternatives, is determined to be valid for its proposed use prior to requiring, recommending, or encouraging the application of such test method" [Pub L 106-545, §4(c)]. ICCVAM has established detailed criteria for the validation and regulatory acceptance of toxicological test methods (NIEHS, 1997). ICCVAM defines validation as "the

process by which the reliability and relevance of a test method are evaluated for the purpose of supporting a specific use." The ICCVAM criteria stipulate that test methods that have been validated according to the ICCVAM criteria are not automatically acceptable for regulatory agencies. The ICCVAM criteria thus specify a second set of criteria for regulatory acceptance, which address the existence of standard operating procedures for the test method, its cost-effectiveness, its utility for agency risk assessment, its potential for harmonization with similar testing requirements by other entities, and its potential for reducing the use of animals. The ICCVAM statute preserves the individual agency's final authority to accept or reject a specific test method based on its statutory mandate and regulatory mission.

The ICCVAM process has now been used to validate a significant number of alternative test methods, including for acute oral toxicity, dermal irritation, ocular irritation, and allergic contact dermatitis. The ICCVAM Authorization Act also directs federal agencies to reduce, refine, and/or replace the use of animals in testing where feasible.

Computational Toxicology

Another area where regulatory demands and programs are pushing the development of new toxicology tests is the field of computational toxicology. Computational toxicology uses high-powered computers to discern patterns and findings from large data sets derived from quantitative structure–activity relationships, in vitro assays, and various 'omic technologies (eg, toxicogenomics, proteomics, metabolomics). The regulatory driver for computational toxicology is the need to evaluate much larger numbers of chemicals much quicker and at lower costs, and perhaps eventually even with more robust and relevant results, than traditional animal studies. The shift toward computational toxicology was boosted by a 2007 Natural Research Council report entitled *Toxicity Testing in the 21st Century: A Vision and a Strategy*, which endorsed greater reliance on computational methods (NRC, 2007). EPA has launched an ambitious program to implement computational methods into its regulatory programs, which is called the ToxCast program, and EPA and the National Institutes of Health (NIH) signed a memorandum of agreement in 2008 to work together to develop these new toxicological methods for regulatory applications (Collins *et al.*, 2008).

Animal Welfare Requirements

Researchers who conduct studies funded by federal agencies must comply with the Animal Welfare Act (AWA), and some are also subject to restrictions imposed by the Public Health Service (PHS). Recipients of grants from the Department of Education, the Department of Agriculture, or the EPA are subject only to the AWA. Those funded by the Department of Energy or by the PHS (which includes all research agencies within the Department of Health and Human Services, including the NIH) must also comply with PHS policies. Restrictions on animal use also appear in the GLP regulations adopted by the FDA and the EPA (Reagan, 1986).

Animal Welfare Act The AWA was initially adopted in 1966 and has been subsequently amended several times (1970, 1976, 1985, 1990, 2002, 2007, 2008). It is administered by the Animal and Plant Health Inspection Service (APHIS), a part of the USDA. The AWA, which protects only warm-blooded animals and excludes birds, rats, and mice bred for research, requires all covered research facilities to register with APHIS and agree to comply with applicable AWA standards for humane treatment of animals. Each facility must file an annual report signed by a responsible official that shows that "professionally acceptable standards governing the care, treatment, and use of animals" were followed for the year in question (AWA, 1998).

Pursuant to the AWA, APHIS has established specific requirements for the humane handling, care, and transportation of dogs and cats, guinea pigs and hamsters, rabbits, nonhuman primates, marine mammals, and other warm-blooded animals. The regulations governing facilities address living space, heating, lighting, ventilation, and drainage. The health and husbandry provisions address feeding, watering, sanitation, veterinary care, grouping of animals, and the number and qualifications of caretakers (APHIS, 2011).

The AWA requires each research facility to establish an Institutional Animal Care and Use Committee (IACUC), composed of three or more members, one of whom must be a veterinarian and one of whom must represent community interests and who may not be affiliated with the institution. In 1989, the APHIS expanded the responsibilities of the IACUC and increased the minimum size to five members, and must include a veterinarian, an animal research scientist, a nonscientist, and an individual not affiliated with the institution. At least one member of the IACUC must now review and approve the animal care and use components of all proposed research activities. Prerequisites to approval include the avoidance or minimization of discomfort, distress, and pain; the use of pain-relieving drugs where appropriate; the consideration of pain-free alternatives; and euthanization when an animal would otherwise experience severe or chronic pain or distress that cannot be relieved.

The IACUC is also responsible for conducting semiannual inspections of the facility itself and of the program for humane care and use of animals. Committee reports are filed with the APHIS and with any federal agency funding the research.

Public Health Service Policy The PHS Policy on Humane Care and Use of Laboratory Animals applies to research funded by the NIH and other federal agencies that uses any vertebrate animals, and thus has a broader reach than the AWA. The PHS policy requires each facility to submit an annual report, called an "Assurance," which is evaluated by the NIH Office of Laboratory Animal Welfare (OLAW) to determine the sufficiency of animal care.

The PHS policy imposes two primary obligations on researchers as a condition for receiving federal funding: each institution must adopt an Institutional Program for Animal Care and Use, and it must establish an IACUC. The IACUC must review all applications for research funding and review the institution's programs to ensure compliance with NIH standards. The Health Research Extension Act of 1985 requires that PHS-funded institutions provide training on methods to reduce animal suffering similar to that mandated by the AWA for its personnel. It also requires that researchers' grant applications justify any proposed use of animals (NRC, 1988).

Research facilities subject to either the AWA or PHS may wish to consult a National Academy of Sciences' report that details suggestions for developing institutional compliance programs (NRC, 1991). Scientists working with no federal funding who expect their research to be submitted to the FDA or the EPA are not subject to the AWA or PHS policies, but they must comply with the animal protection provisions of those agencies' GLP regulations. These regulations prescribe adequate living conditions, detail requirements for veterinary treatment, and impose specific record-keeping requirements (EPA, 2011b, 2011c; FDA, 2011a).

REFERENCES

CASES

American Federation of Labor v OSHA, 965 F2d 962 (11th Cir 1992).

American Textile Manufacturers Institute v Donovan, 452 US 490 (1982).

Baltimore Gas & Elec v NRDC, 462 US 87 (1983).

Chemical Manufacturers Association v EPA, 899 F2d 344 (5th Cir 1990).

Chlorine Chemistry Council v EPA, 206 F3d 1286 (DC Cir 2000).

Corrosion Proof Fittings v Environmental Protection Agency, 947 F2d 1201 (5th Cir 1991). *Environmental Defense Fund, Inc, v Environmental Protection Agency,* 548 F2d 998 (DC Cir 1976).

Industrial Union Department, AFL-CIO, v American Petroleum Institute, 448 US 607 (1980).

Les v Reilly, 968 F2d 985 (9th Cir 1992).

Natural Resources Defense Council, Inc., v United States Environmental Protection Agency, 595 F Supp 1255 (SD NY 1984).

Natural Resources Defense Council, Inc., v United States Environmental Protection Agency, 824 F2d 1146 (DC Cir 1987).

Natural Resources Defense Council, Inc., v United States Environmental Protection Agency, 529 F3d 1077 (DC Cir 2008).

Natural Resources Defense Council, Inc., v United States Environmental Protection Agency, 658 F3d 200 (2nd Cir 2011).

Northwest Coalition for Alternatives to Pesticides v EPA, 544 F3d 1043 (9th Cir 2008).

Salt Institute v Leavitt, 440 F3d 156 (4th Cir 2006).

Whitman v American Trucking Associations, Inc, 531 US 457 (2001).

SECONDARY SOURCES

Albert RE. Carcinogen risk assessment in the U.S. Environmental Protection Agency. *Crit Rev Toxicol.* 1994;24:75–85.

Brickman R, Jasanoff S, Ilgen T. *Controlling Chemicals: The Politics of Regulation in Europe and the United States.* Ithica, NY: Cornell U. Press; 1985.

Collins FS, Gray GM, Bucher JM. Transforming environmental health protection. *Science.* 2008;319:906–907.

Cooper R. The role of regulatory agencies in risk-benefit decision-making. *Food Drug Cosmet L J.* 1978;33:755–757.

GAO. *EPA Implementation of Selected Aspects of the Toxic Substances Control Act.* Washington, DC: U.S. General Accounting Office; 1982.

Heineck D. New clean water act toxics control initiatives. *Nat Resources Environ.* 1989;4(1):10–12, 49–50.

Hutt PB, Merrill R, Grossman LA. *Food and Drug Law: Cases and Materials.* 3rd ed. Mineola, NY: Foundation Press; 2007.

Marty MS, Carney EW, Rowlands JC. Endocrine disruption: historical perspectives and its impact on the future of toxicology testing. *Toxicol Sci.* 2011;120(S1):S93–S108.

Merrill R. CPSC regulation of cancer risks in consumer products: 1972–81. *Va L Rev.* 1981;67:1261.

National Research Council. *Use of Laboratory Animals in Biomedical and Behavioral Research.* Washington, DC: National Academy; 1988.

National Research Council. *A Guide for Developing Institutional Programs.* Washington, DC: National Academy; 1991.

National Research Council. *Science and Judgment in Risk Assessment.* Washington, DC: National Academy; 1994.

National Research Council. *Toxicity Testing in the 21st Century: A Vision and a Strategy.* Washington, DC: National Academy; 2007.

National Research Council. *Science and Decisions.* Washington, DC: National Academy; 2009.

National Research Council. *Review of the Environmental Protection Agency's Draft IRIS Assessment of Formaldehyde.* Washington, DC: National Academy; 2011.

Page NP. Testing for health and environmental effects: The OECD guidelines. *Toxic Substances J.* 1982;4:135.

Reagan K. Federal regulation of testing with laboratory animals: Future directions. *Pace Environ L Rev.* 1986;3:165.

Wagner W. The science charade in toxic risk regulation. *Columbia L Rev.* 1995;95:1613–1723.

Weinberg A. Science and its limits: the regulator's dilemma. *Issues Sci Tech.* 1985;Fall:59–72.

Wiltse J, Dellarco VL. U.S. Environmental Protection Agency guidelines for carcinogen risk assessment: past and future. *Mutation Res.* 1996;365:3–15.

Statutory and Regulatory Materials

Animal Welfare Act, 7 USC § 2131 et seq (1988).

APHIS, Animal Welfare, 9 *CFR* Parts 2 & 3 (2011).

Comprehensive Environmental Response, Compensation and Liability Act, 42 USC § 9601 et seq (1980).

Consumer Product Safety Act, 15 USC § 2051 et seq (1972).

Consumer Product Safety Improvement Act, 15 USC § 2051 et seq (2008).

EPA. Guidelines for Carcinogen Risk Assessment. *Fed. Reg.* 1986;51(185): 33992–34003.

EPA. Proposed Guidelines for Carcinogenic Risk Assessment, 61. *Fed Reg.* 1996;61(79):17960–18011.

EPA. Notice of Availability of the Document Entitled Guidelines for Carcinogen Risk Assessment. *Fed Reg.* 2005;70(66):17766–17817.

EPA. Harmonized Test Guidelines. Available at http://www.epa.gov/ocspp/pubs/frs/home/guidelin.htm (2011a).

EPA. Good Laboratory Practice Standards (FIFRA), 40 CFR Part 160 (2011b).

EPA. Good Laboratory Practice Standards (TSCA), 40 CFR Part 792 (2011c).

Executive Order 13563. Improving regulation and regulatory review, 76. *Fed Reg.* 2011;3821–3823.

FDA Modernization Act, Pub L No. 105–115 (1997).

FDA. *Toxicological Principles for the Safety Assessment of Food Ingredients: Redbook 2000.* Washington, DC: U.S. Food and Drug Administration; 2000 (periodically updated).

FDA. Good Laboratory Practice for Nonclinical Laboratory Studies, 21 CFR. Part 58 (2011a).

FDA. Investigational New Drug Application, 21 CFR Part 312 (2011b).

FDA. Food Additive Petitions, 21 CFR Part 171 (2011c).

Federal Food, Drug, and Cosmetic Act, 21 USC § 321 et seq (1938).

Federal Hazardous Substances Act, 15 USC § 1261 et seq (1976).

Federal Insecticide, Fungicide, and Rodenticide Act, 7 USC § 135 et seq (1972).

Federal Water Pollution Control Act Amendments of 1972, 33 USC § 307.

Food Additive Amendments to the Federal Food, Drug, and Cosmetic Act, 21 USC § 348 et seq (1958).

Food Quality Protection Act, Pub L No. 104–170 (1996).

ICCVAM Authorization Act of 2000, Pub L No. 106–545, 106th Congress.

Information Quality Act, Pub L No. 106–554, 31 USC § 3516 note (2001).

NIEHS. *Validation and Regulatory Acceptance of Toxicological Test Methods: A Report of the ad hoc Interagency Coordinating Committee on the Validation of Alternative Methods.* NIH Publication No. 97–3981. Research Triangle Park, NC: NIEHS, 1997.

Occupational Safety and Health Act, 29 USC § 651 et seq (1970).

OMB. *Memorandum for the Heads of Departments and Agencies*, M-05-03. Available at: http://www.whitehouse.gov/omb/memoranda/fy2005/m05-03.pdf (2004).

Resource Conservation and Recovery Act, 42 USCA § 6901 et seq (1976).

Safe Drinking Water Act, 42 USC §§ 300f to 300j-9 (1974, amended 1996).

Toxic Substances Control Act (1976), 15 USC § 2601 et seq.

White House. Memorandum for the Heads of Executive Departments and Agencies. Subject: Scientific Integrity (March 9, 2009).

Index

NOTE: Page numbers followed by a *t* refer to tables and page numbers followed by an *f* indicate figures.

INDEX